Professor, Department of Pediatrics, Case Western Reserve University School of Medicine;
Attending Physician, Rainbow Babies and Childrens Hospital, Cleveland, Ohio

Professor in Pediatrics, Temple University School of Medicine;
Attending Physician, St. Christopher's Hospital for Children;
Senior Medical Evaluation Officer, National Board of Medical Examiners,
Philadelphia, Pennsylvania

Professor of Pediatrics, Medical College of Pennsylvania and Temple University
School of Medicine;
Attending Pediatrician, St. Christopher's Hospital for Children,
Philadelphia, Pennsylvania

IGAKU-SHOIN/SAUNDERS INTERNATIONAL EDITION

NELSON

TEXTBOOK OF

PEDIATRICS

TWELFTH EDITION

RICHARD E. BEHRMAN, M.D.

VICTOR C. VAUGHAN, III, M.D.

SENIOR EDITOR
WALDO E. NELSON, M.D.

W.B.SAUNDERS COMPANY   1983

Philadelphia   London   Toronto   Mexico City   Rio de Janeiro   Sydney   Tokyo

IGAKU-SHOIN/SAUNDERS

W. B. Saunders Company: West Washington Square
Philadelphia, PA   19105

1 St. Anne's Road
Eastbourne, East Sussex BN21 3UN, England

1 Goldthorne Avenue
Toronto, Ontario M8Z 5T9, Canada

Apartado 26370—Cedro 512
Mexico 4, D.F., Mexico

Rua Coronel Cabrita, 8
Sao Cristovao Caixa Postal 21176
Rio de Janeiro, Brazil

9 Waltham Street
Artarmon, N.S.W. 2064, Australia

Ichibancho, Central Bldg., 22-1 Ichibancho
Chiyoda-Ku, Tokyo 102, Japan

Library of Congress Cataloging in Publication Data

Main entry under title:

Nelson textbook of pediatrics.

Rev. ed. of: Nelson textbook of pediatrics/Victor C. Vaughan,
III. 11th ed. 1979.

Includes bibliographies and index.

1. Pediatrics.   I. Behrman, Richard E., 1943– .   II.
Vaughan, Victor C., III, 1919– .   III. Nelson, Waldo
Emerson, 1898– .   Nelson textbook of pediatrics.   IV.
Title.   V. Title: Textbook of pediatrics.

RJ45.N42 1982   618.92   81–48409
ISBN 0-7216-1736-0   AACR2

Listed here is the latest translated edition of this book together
with the language of the translation and the publisher.

French—Vol. I (10th Edition)—Doin Editeurs, S.A.,
                   Paris, France

French—Vol. II (10 Edition)—Doin Editeurs, S.A.,
                   Paris, France

Nelson: Textbook of Pediatrics

ISBN 0-7216-1736-0 (US Edition)
ISBN 4-7557-0064-7 (Igaku-Shoin/Saunders International Edition)

Printed in Japan, 1983

Last digit is the print number: 9   8   7   6   5   4   3   2

CONTRIBUTORS

TARO AKABANE, M.D., Ph.D. Chairman and Professor of Pediatrics, Faculty of Medicine, Shinshu University, Japan

STEVEN C. ARANOFF, M.D. Assistant Professor of Pediatrics, Case Western Reserve University School of Medicine; Assistant Pediatrician, Division of Pediatric Infectious Diseases, Rainbow Babies and Childrens Hospital, Cleveland, Ohio

RUSSELL S. ASNES, M.D. Associate Professor of Clinical Pediatrics, College of Physicians and Surgeons, Columbia University; Attending Pediatrician, Babies Hospital, Columbia-Presbyterian Medical Center, New York, New York, and Englewood Hospital, Englewood, New Jersey

VICTOR H. AUERBACH, Ph.D. Research Professor of Pediatrics (Biochemistry), Temple University School of Medicine; Director, Department of Laboratories, St. Christopher's Hospital for Children, Philadelphia, Pennsylvania

HENRY W. BAIRD, M.D. Professor of Pediatrics, Temple University School of Medicine; Attending Pediatrician (Neurology), St. Christopher's Hospital for Children, Philadelphia, Pennsylvania

GIULIO J. BARBERO, M.D. Professor and Chairman, Department of Child Health, University of Missouri School of Medicine; Chief of Service, Child Health, University of Missouri Hospital, Columbia, Missouri

LEWIS A. BARNESS, M.D. Professor and Chairman, Department of Pediatrics, University of South Florida College of Medicine, Tampa, Florida

JOHN B. BARTRAM, M.D. Professor Emeritus of Pediatrics, Temple University School of Medicine; Honorary Attending Pediatrician, St. Christopher's Hospital for Children, Philadelphia, Pennsylvania

RICHARD E. BEHRMAN, M.D. Professor, Department of Pediatrics, Case Western Reserve University School of Medicine; Attending Physician, Rainbow Babies and Childrens Hospital, Cleveland, Ohio

CHARLES D. BLUESTONE, M.D. Professor of Otolaryngology, University of Pittsburgh School of Medicine; Director, Department of Otolaryngology, Children's Hospital of Pittsburgh; Senior Staff, Eye and Ear Hospital, Pittsburgh, Pennsylvania

THOMAS F. BOAT, M.D. Professor and Chairman, Department of Pediatrics, University of North Carolina, Chapel Hill, North Carolina

PHILIP A. BRUNELL, B.S., M.S., M.D. Professor and Head, Division of Pediatric Infectious Diseases, University of Texas Health Sciences Center; Attending Physician, Medical Center Hospital and Santa Rosa Children's Hospital, San Antonio, Texas

HUGO F. CARVAJAL, M.D. Professor of Pediatrics, University of Texas Medical Branch; Chief of Pediatrics, Shriners Burns Institute, Galveston, Texas

JAMES D. CHERRY, M.D. Professor of Pediatrics, Chief, Pediatric Infectious Diseases, UCLA School of Medicine; Attending Physician, UCLA Hospital and Clinics, Los Angeles, California

J. JULIAN CHISOLM, Jr., M.D. Associate Professor of Pediatrics, Johns Hopkins University School of Medicine; Senior Staff Pediatrician, Baltimore City Hospitals; Director, Childhood Lead Poisoning Prevention Program, John F. Kennedy Institute, Baltimore, Maryland

DAVID F. CLYDE, M.D., Ph.D., D.T.M.&H. Regional Malaria Adviser and Senior Public Health Adviser, World Health Organization, S-E Asia, New Delhi, India

MAIMON M. COHEN, Ph.D. Chief, Division of Human Genetics, Professor of Obstetrics/Gynecology and Pediatrics, University of Maryland; University of Maryland Hospital, Baltimore, Maryland

SANFORD N. COHEN, M.D. Professor of Pediatrics, Associate in Pharmacology, and Associate Dean, Wayne State University School of Medicine, Detroit, Michigan

WILLIAM A. DANIEL, Jr., M.D. Professor of Pediatrics, Chief, Division of Adolescent Medicine, University of Alabama School of Medicine; Staff, The Children's Hospital and University Hospital, Birmingham, Alabama

FRANKLIN L. DeBUSK, M.D. Professor of Pediatrics, University of Florida College of Medicine; Staff Physician and Director of Pediatric Clinic, University of Florida Teaching Hospital, Gainesville, Florida

FLOYD W. DENNY, M.D. Professor of Pediatrics, University of North Carolina School of Medicine; Attending Staff Member, North Carolina Memorial Hospital, Chapel Hill, North Carolina

ANGELO M. DiGEORGE, M.D. Professor of Pediatrics, Temple University School of Medicine; Chief, Endocrine and Metabolic Disease Section, St. Christopher's Hospital for Children, Philadelphia, Pennsylvania

CARL F. DOERSHUK, M.D. Professor of Pediatrics, Case Western Reserve University School of Medicine; Associate Pediatrician, University Hospitals and Rainbow Babies and Childrens Hospital, Cleveland, Ohio

ALBERT DORFMAN, M.D., Ph.D. Late Professor of Pediatrics and Biochemistry, University of Chicago; Late Director, Joseph P. Kennedy, Jr. Mental Retardation Research Center, Department of Pediatrics, University of Chicago, Chicago, Illinois

JOHN J. DOWNES, M.D. Professor of Anesthesia and Pediatrics, University of Pennsylvania; Anesthesiologist-in-Chief, and Director, Department of Anesthesia and Critical Care, The Children's Hospital of Philadelphia, Philadelphia, Pennsylvania

KEITH N. DRUMMOND, M.D., C.M., F.R.C.P.(C) Professor and Chairman, Department of Pediatrics, McGill University; Physician-in-Chief, The Montreal Children's Hospital, Montreal, Quebec, Canada

JOHN M. DUNN, M.D. Clinical Associate Professor in Psychiatry (Child), Temple University School of Medicine, Philadelphia; Staff Psychiatrist, Grandview Hospital, Sellersville, Pennsylvania

HEINZ F. EICHENWALD, M.D. William Buchanan Professor of Pediatrics, University of Texas Health Sciences Center at Dallas; Attending Physician, Children's Medical Center, Parkland Memorial Hospital; Consulting Pediatrician, St. Paul Hospital, Presbyterian Hospital, Baylor Medical Center, Dallas, Texas

ELLIOT F. ELLIS, M.D. Professor and Chairman, Department of Pediatrics, State University of New York at Buffalo School of Medicine; Pediatrician-in-Chief, Children's Hospital, Buffalo, New York

NANCY B. ESTERLY, M.D. Professor of Pediatrics and Dermatology, Northwestern University Medical School; Head, Division of Dermatology, The Children's Memorial Hospital, Chicago, Illinois

JAMES C. FALLIS, M.D., F.R.C.S.(C), F.A.C.S. Assistant Professor in Surgery and in Pediatrics, University of Toronto; Active Staff, Departments of Surgery and Pediatrics, and Director, Emergency Services, Hospital for Sick Children, Toronto, Ontario, Canada

AVROY A. FANAROFF, M.B., F.R.C.P. Professor of Pediatrics, Case Western Reserve University School of Medicine; Director of Nurseries, University Hospitals, Cleveland, Ohio

RALPH D. FEIGIN, M.D. J.S. Abercrombie Professor and Chairman, Department of Pediatrics, Baylor College of Medicine; Physician-in-Chief, Texas Children's Hospital; Physician-in-Chief, Pediatric Services, Ben Taub General Hospital and Jefferson Davis Hospital; Chief, Pediatric Service, The Methodist Hospital, Houston, Texas

HARRY A. FELDMAN, M.D. Professor and Chairman, Department of Preventive Medicine, State University of New York, Upstate Medical Center; Attending Physician, State University Hospital, Syracuse, New York

MARC A. FORMAN, M.D. Professor of Psychiatry, Professor in Pediatrics, Temple University School of Medicine; Child Psychiatry Center, St. Christopher's Hospital for Children, Philadelphia, Pennsylvania

GORDON FORSTNER, M.D., F.R.C.P.(C.) Professor, Department of Pediatrics, University of Toronto; Staff, Hospital for Sick Children, Toronto, Ontario, Canada

LAWRENCE A. FOX, D.D.S., M.P.H., M.Ed. Associate Professor, Community Dentistry and Behavioral Sciences, Case Western Reserve University School of Dentistry; Dental Staff Member, Lake County Memorial Hospitals; Associate in Dental Surgery, University Hospital of Cleveland, Ohio

EDWARD C. FRANKLIN, M.D. Late Professor of Medicine, Director, Irvington House Institute, and Chairman, Rheumatic Diseases Study Group, Department of Medicine, New York University Medical Center, New York, New York

WELTON M. GERSONY, M.D. Professor of Pediatrics, College of Physicians and Surgeons of Columbia University; Director, Division of Pediatric Cardiology,

Columbia-Presbyterian Medical Center, New York, New York

LOWELL A. GLASGOW, M.D. Late Professor and Chairman, Department of Pediatrics, University of Utah School of Medicine; Late Medical Director, Primary Children's Medical Center, Salt Lake City, Utah

ELI GOLD, M.D. Professor of Pediatrics, University of California at Davis; Professor of Pediatrics, University of California at Davis Medical Center, Sacramento, California

ARMOND S. GOLDMAN, M.D. Professor of Pediatrics, University of Texas Medical Branch, Galveston, Texas

I. BRUCE GORDON, M.D. Associate Professor of Pediatrics, Case Western Reserve University School of Medicine; Director, Department of Pediatrics, Cleveland Metropolitan General Hospital, Cleveland, Ohio

STEPHEN R. GUERTIN, M.D. Assistant Professor of Pediatrics, Michigan State University; Director, Pediatric Intensive Care Unit, Edward W. Sparrow Hospital, Lansing, Michigan

GABRIEL G. HADDAD, M.D. Assistant Professor of Pediatrics, College of Physicians and Surgeons, Columbia University; Assistant Attending Physician, Center for Women and Children, Presbyterian Hospital, New York, New York

SCOTT B. HALSTEAD, M.D. Professor and Chairman, Department of Tropical Medicine and Medical Microbiology, John A. Burns School of Medicine; Professor, School of Public Health, University of Hawaii at Manoa

J. RICHARD HAMILTON, M.D., F.R.C.P.(C.) Professor of Pediatrics, University of Toronto; Chief, Division of Gastroenterology, Hospital for Sick Children, Toronto, Ontario, Canada

JAMES BARRY HANSHAW, M.D. Professor and Chairman, Department of Pediatrics, University of Massachusetts Medical School; Lecturer, Department of Pediatrics, Harvard Medical School; Pediatrician-in-Chief, University of Massachusetts Medical Center; Consultant in Pediatrics, St. Vincent Hospital, Worcester City Hospital, and Memorial Hospital, Worcester, Massachusetts

HAROLD E. HARRISON, M.D. Professor Emeritus, Pediatrics, Johns Hopkins University School of Medicine; Pediatrician, Johns Hopkins Hospital and Bal-

timore City Hospital; Consultant in Pediatrics, Sinai Hospital of Baltimore, Maryland

ALFRED D. HEGGIE, M.D. Associate Professor of Pediatrics, Case Western Reserve University School of Medicine; Attending Pediatrician, Rainbow Babies and Childrens Hospital; Virologist-in-Charge, University Hospitals of Cleveland, Ohio

WERNER HENLE, M.D. Professor Emeritus of Virology, University of Pennsylvania; Director, Division of Research Virology, The Joseph Stokes Jr. Research Institute, The Children's Hospital of Philadelphia, Pennsylvania

JOHN J. HERBST, M.D. Professor of Pediatrics, University of Utah School of Medicine; Head, Division of Pediatric Gastroenterology, University of Utah Medical Center, Salt Lake City, Utah

WILLIAM H. HETZNECKER, M.D. Professor of Psychiatry, Professor in Pediatrics, Temple University School of Medicine; St. Christopher's Hospital for Children, Philadelphia, Pennsylvania

STEPHEN S. HIRSCHFELD, M.D. Associate Professor of Pediatrics and Director of Pediatric Cardiology, Tulane University School of Medicine, New Orleans, Louisiana

LEWIS B. HOLMES, M.D. Associate Professor of Pediatrics at the Massachusetts General Hospital, Harvard Medical School; Chief, Embryology-Teratology Unit, and Associate Pediatrician, Massachusetts General Hospital; Consultant in Pediatrics (Genetics), Brigham and Women's Hospital, Boston, Massachusetts

RICHARD HONG, M.D. Professor of Pediatrics and Medical Microbiology, University of Wisconsin Center for Health Sciences; Attending Physician, University of Wisconsin Hospitals and Madison General Hospital, Madison, Wisconsin

R. RODNEY HOWELL, M.D. David R. Park Professor and Chairman, Department of Pediatrics, University of Texas Health Science Center; Pediatrician-in-Chief, Hermann Hospital; Consultant in Pediatrics, Shriners Hospital for Crippled Children and M.D. Anderson Hospital and Tumor Institute, Houston, Texas

GEORGE HUG, M.D. Professor of Pediatrics, University of Cincinnati College of Medicine; Attending Pediatrician and Director, Divisions of Enzymology and the Clinical Research Center, Children's Hospital Medical Center, Cincinnati, Ohio

PETER R. HUTTENLOCHER, M.D. Professor of Pediatrics and Neurology, University of Chicago Medical School; Chief, Pediatric Neurology Section, Wyler Children's Hospital, Chicago, Illinois

RICHARD B. JOHNSTON, Jr., M.D. Chairman, Department of Pediatrics, National Jewish Hospital and Research Center; Professor of Pediatrics, University of Colorado School of Medicine, Denver, Colorado

KENNETH LYONS JONES, M.D. Associate Professor, Department of Pediatrics, University of California, San Diego, La Jolla, California; University Hospital, San Diego, California

BERNARD KAPLAN, M.B., B.Ch., F.C.P.(S.A.) Associate Professor of Pediatrics, McGill University; Director of Nephrology, The Montreal Children's Hospital, Montreal, Quebec, Canada

SHELDON L. KAPLAN, M.D. Assistant Professor of Pediatrics, Baylor College of Medicine; Attending Pediatrician, Texas Children's Hospital; Assistant Pediatrician, Ben Taub General Hospital; Chief, Infectious Diseases Service, Texas Children's Hospital, Houston, Texas

JAMES W. KAZURA, M.D. Assistant Professor of Medicine, Case Western Reserve University School of Medicine; Assistant Professor of Medicine, Department of Medicine, University Hospitals, Cleveland, Ohio

C. HENRY KEMPE, M.D. Professor of Pediatrics and Microbiology, University of Colorado School of Medicine, Denver, Colorado; Director Emeritus, National Center for the Prevention and Treatment of Child Abuse and Neglect

JOHN KIRKPATRICK, Jr., M.D. Professor of Radiology, Harvard Medical School; Radiologist-in-Chief, Children's Hospital Medical Center, Boston, Massachusetts

ROBERT M. KLIEGMAN, M.D. Assistant Professor of Pediatrics, Case Western Reserve University School of Medicine; Assistant Attending Physician, Rainbow Babies and Childrens Hospital, Cleveland, Ohio

R. LAWRENCE KROOVAND, M.D. Associate Professor of Urology, Wayne State University; Associate Chief, Department of Pediatric Urology, Children's Hospital of Michigan, Detroit, Michigan

MELVIN D. LEVINE, M.D. Associate Professor of Pediatrics, Harvard Medical School; Chief, Division of Ambulatory Pediatrics, The Children's Hospital Medical Center, Boston, Massachusetts

PAUL S. LIETMAN, M.D., Ph.D. Wellcome Professor of Clinical Pharmacology and Pediatrics, Johns Hopkins University; Director of Clinical Pharmacology, Johns Hopkins Hospital, Baltimore, Maryland

IRIS F. LITT, M.D. Associate Professor of Pediatrics, Stanford University School of Medicine; Director, Division of Adolescent Medicine, Stanford University School of Medicine, Stanford, California

BETSY LOZOFF, M.D. Assistant Professor of Pediatrics, Case Western Reserve University School of Medicine; Assistant Attending Physician, Rainbow Babies and Childrens Hospital, Cleveland, Ohio

C. CHARLTON MABRY, M.D. Professor of Pediatrics, University of Kentucky; Attending Pediatrician, University Hospital, Lexington, Kentucky

ADEL A. F. MAHMOUD, M.D., Ph.D. Professor of Medicine, Professor of Microbiology, Case Western Reserve University; Physician, University Hospitals of Cleveland, Ohio

MILTON MARKOWITZ, M.D. Professor and Head, Department of Pediatrics, University of Connecticut School of Medicine; Pediatrician-in-Chief, University John Dempsey Hospital, Farmington, Connecticut

LOIS J. MARTYN, M.D. Associate Professor of Ophthalmology, Associate Professor in Pediatrics, Temple University School of Medicine; Pediatric Ophthalmologist, St. Christopher's Hospital for Children; Honorary Staff, Wills Eye Hospital, Philadelphia, Pennsylvania

LeROY W. MATTHEWS, M.D. Professor of Pediatrics, Case Western Reserve University School of Medicine; Attending Physician, Rainbow Babies and Childrens Hospital, University Hospitals; Co-Director, Cystic Fibrosis and Pulmonary Disease Center, Cleveland, Ohio

ALVIN M. MAUER, M.D. Professor of Pediatrics, University of Tennessee Center for the Health Sciences; Director, St. Jude Children's Research Hospital, Memphis, Tennessee

KENNETH McINTOSH, M.D. Associate Professor of Pediatrics, Harvard Medical School; Clinical Chief, Division of Infectious Disease, Children's Hospital Medical Center, Boston, Massachusetts

R. JAMES McKAY, M.D. Professor and Chairman, Department of Pediatrics, University of Vermont College of Medicine; Chief of Pediatrics, Medical Center Hospital of Vermont, Burlington, Vermont

ROBERT B. MELLINS, M.D. Professor of Pediatrics, College of Physicians and Surgeons, Columbia University; Attending Physician, Center for Women and Children, Presbyterian Hospital, New York, New York

MICHAEL H. MERSON, M.D. Programme Manager, Diarrhoeal Diseases Control Programme, World Health Organization, Geneva, Switzerland

ALBERT MILLER, Ph.D. Associate Professor (retired) of Parasitology, Tulane University School of Public Health and Tropical Medicine, New Orleans, Louisiana

ROBERT W. MILLER, M.D. Chief, Clinical Epidemiology Branch, National Cancer Institute, National Institutes of Health, Bethesda, Maryland

GRANT MORROW III, M.D. Professor and Chairman, Department of Pediatrics, Ohio State University; Medical Director, Columbus Children's Hospital, Columbus, Ohio

E. A. MORTIMER, M.D. Professor and Chairman, Department of Epidemiology and Community Health, Professor of Pediatrics, Case Western Reserve University School of Medicine, Cleveland, Ohio

HENRY L. NADLER, M.D. Dean, Professor of Pediatrics, Wayne State University; Children's Hospital of Michigan, Detroit, Michigan

M. BERNADETTE NOGRADY, M.D. Associate Professor of Pediatrics, Associate Professor of Diagnostic Radiology, McGill University, Montreal, Quebec, Canada

MICHAEL E. NORMAN, M.D. Director of Pediatrics, Wilmington Medical Center, Wilmington, Delaware; Jefferson University Hospital, Philadelphia, Pennsylvania

JAMES C. OVERALL, Jr., M.D. Professor of Pediatrics and Pathology; Chief, Pediatric Infectious Diseases, Department of Pediatrics; Director, Diagnostic Virology Laboratory, Department of Pathology; Center for Infectious Diseases, Clinical Microbiology, and Immunology, University of Utah School of Medicine; Consultant in Infectious Diseases, Primary Children's Medical Center, Salt Lake City, Utah

DEMOSTHENES PAPPAGIANIS, M.D., Ph.D. Professor and Chairman, Department of Medical Microbiology and Immunology, School of Medicine, University of California, Davis, California

ROBERT H. PARROTT, M.D. Chairman and Professor of Child Health and Development, George Washington University; Director, Children's Hospital National Medical Center, Washington, D.C.

JEROME A. PAULSON, M.D. Assistant Professor of Pediatrics, Case Western Reserve University School of Medicine; Assistant Pediatrician, Rainbow Babies and Childrens Hospital; Assistant Visiting Pediatrician, Cleveland Metropolitan General Hospital, Cleveland, Ohio

HOWARD A. PEARSON, M.D. Professor and Chairman, Department of Pediatrics, Yale University School of Medicine; Chief of Pediatrics, Yale–New Haven Hospital, New Haven, Connecticut

ALAN D. PERLMUTTER, M.D. Professor of Urology, Wayne State University; Chief, Department of Pediatric Urology, Children's Hospital of Michigan, Detroit, Michigan

CAROL F. PHILLIPS, M.D. Professor of Pediatrics, University of Vermont College of Medicine; Attending, Medical Center Hospital of Vermont, Burlington, Vermont

STANLEY A. PLOTKIN, M.D. Professor of Pediatrics, University of Pennsylvania; Professor of Anatomy and Biology, Wistar Institute; Director, Infectious Diseases, Children's Hospital of Philadelphia, Pennsylvania

PAUL G. QUIE, M.D. Professor of Pediatrics, University of Minnesota Medical School, Minneapolis, Minnesota

RUSSELL C. RAPHAELY, M.D. Associate Professor of Anesthesia and Pediatrics, University of Pennsylvania; Director, Pediatric Intensive Care Unit, and Associate Director, Department of Anesthesia and Critical Care, The Children's Hospital of Philadelphia, Pennsylvania

THOMAS A. RIEMENSCHNEIDER, M.D. Professor of Pediatrics, Case Western Reserve University School of Medicine; Director of Pediatric Cardiology, Rainbow Babies and Childrens Hospital, Case Western Reserve University School of Medicine, Cleveland, Ohio

ALAN M. ROBSON, M.D., F.R.C.P. Professor of Pediatrics, Washington University School of Medicine; Director, Division of Pediatric Nephrology, St. Louis Children's Hospital, St. Louis, Missouri

IRA M. ROSENTHAL, M.D. Professor of Pediatrics, University of Illinois College of Medicine; Attending Pediatrician, University of Illinois Hospital and Cook County Hospital, Chicago, Illinois

JANE GREEN SCHALLER, M.D. Professor of Pediatrics, University of Washington School of Medicine; Head, Rheumatic Disease Division, Children's Orthopedic Hospital and Medical Center, Seattle, Washington

BARTON D. SCHMITT, M.D. Associate Professor of Pediatrics, University of Colorado School of Medicine; Attending Pediatrician for University Hospital, The Denver Children's Hospital, and Denver General Hospital; Pediatric Consultant, C. Henry Kempe National Center for the Prevention and Treatment of Child Abuse and Neglect

ROBERT SCHWARTZ, M.D. Professor of Pediatrics, Division of Biology and Medicine, Brown University; Director of Pediatric Metabolism and Nutrition, Rhode Island Hospital, Providence, Rhode Island

BARRY SHANDLING, M.B., Ch.B., F.R.C.S.(Eng.), F.R.C.S.(C), F.A.C.S. Associate Professor of Surgery, University of Toronto; Senior Staff Surgeon, Hospital for Sick Children; Consulting Surgeon, North York General Hospital and Sunnybrook Hospital; Staff Surgeon, Ontario Crippled Children's Centre, Toronto, Ontario, Canada

DAVID O. SILLENCE, M.D. (Melb.) F.R.A.C.P., F.R.C.P.A. Professor of Public Health Biology, Commonwealth Institute of Health, University of Sydney; Visiting Medical Geneticist, Royal Alexandra Hospital for Children, King George V Memorial Hospital and Westmead Centre, Sydney, Australia

WILLIAM T. SPECK, M.D. Gertrude Lee Chandler Tucker Professor of Pediatrics and Chairman, Department of Pediatrics, Case Western Reserve University School of Medicine; Director, Department of Pediatrics, Rainbow Babies and Childrens Hospital, Cleveland, Ohio

MARK A. SPERLING, M.D. Professor of Pediatrics, University of Cincinnati Medical School; Director, Division of Endocrinology, Children's Hospital Medical Center, Cincinnati, Ohio

ROBERT C. STERN, M.D. Associate Professor of Pediatrics, Case Western Reserve University School of Medicine; Associate Pediatrician, Rainbow Babies and Childrens Hospital, Cleveland, Ohio

MARSHALL L. STOLLER, M.D. Physician, University of California at San Francisco Affiliated Hospitals, San Francisco, California

LEON STREBEL, M.D. Ciba-Geigy Ltd., Basel, Switzerland

LAWRENCE T. TAFT, M.D. Professor and Chairman, Department of Pediatrics, University of Medicine and Dentistry of New Jersey—Rutgers Medical School; Attending, Middlesex General Hospital and St. Peters Medical Center, New Brunswick, New Jersey

M. MICHAEL THALER, M.D. Professor of Pediatrics, University of California, San Francisco; Chief, Division of Pediatric Gastroenterology and Nutrition, Department of Pediatrics, University of California Medical Center, San Francisco, California

NORBERT W. TIETZ, Ph.D. Professor, Department of Pathology, College of Medicine, University of Kentucky; Director of Clinical Chemistry, University of Kentucky Medical Center, Lexington, Kentucky

PHILIP TOLTZIS, M.D. Chief Resident, Department of Pediatrics, Rainbow Babies and Childrens Hospital, Case Western Reserve University School of Medicine, Cleveland, Ohio

CAROL C. TOWNE, Ph.D. Associate Professor in Pediatrics, Temple University School of Medicine; Director, Speech and Language Services, St. Christopher's Hospital for Children, Philadelphia, Pennsylvania

P. M. UDANI, M.D., D.C.H., F.A.M.S. (IND.), F.I.A.P., F.I.C.P., Hon.F.A.A.P.(U.S.A.) Director and Professor, Institute of Child Health, J. J. Group of Hospitals, and Department of Pediatrics, Grant Medical College; Director/Organizer, UNICEF/WHO Course for senior teachers in child health; Professor Emeritus, Pediatrics, Institute of Child Health, J. J. Group of Hospitals, and Grant Medical College, University of Bombay; Honorary Pediatrician, Bombay Hospital, Bombay, India

VICTOR C. VAUGHAN, III, M.D. Professor in Pediatrics, Temple University School of Medicine; Attending Physician, St. Christopher's Hospital for Children; Senior Medical Evaluation Officer, National Board of Medical Examiners, Philadelphia, Pennsylvania

HUGH G. WATTS, M.D.   Professor of Orthopedic Surgery, University of Pennsylvania; Chief of Orthopedic Surgery, Children's Hospital of Philadelphia, Pennsylvania

RALPH J. WEDGWOOD, M.D.   Professor, Department of Pediatrics, University of Washington School of Medicine; Attending Physician, Children's Or-

thopedic Hospital and Medical Center, Harborview Medical Center, and University Hospital, Seattle, Washington

DAVID WENGER, Ph.D.   Professor of Pediatrics and Biochemistry, Biophysics and Genetics, University of Colorado Health Sciences Center, Denver, Colorado

ROBERT E. WOOD, Ph.D., M.D.   Associate Professor of Pediatrics, Case Western Reserve University School of Medicine; Associate Pediatrician, Rainbow Babies and Children's Hospital, Cleveland, Ohio

PREFACE

With this twelfth edition of *Nelson Textbook of Pediatrics*, the contribution of Waldo E. Nelson to pediatric education and child care through this work approaches four and a half decades. His leadership, editorial talents, and standards continue to be invaluable to us as we strive to meet the needs of practitioners, medical students, and house staff in a comprehensive and concise one-volume edition.

New knowledge and concerns have resulted in substantial modifications and/or expansion of many sections and the addition of essentially new sections. We appreciate the cooperation of our contributors in the effort to achieve completeness, relevance, and conciseness. We have tried to produce an edition that will continue to be helpful to all those who care for children or want to know about them or their problems.

Since the last edition we have lost four contributors through death. Albert Dorfman, Edward Franklin, Lowell Glasgow, and David W. Smith are much missed.

In this edition we have had the invaluable assistance of the staffs of the Departments of Pediatrics at Case Western Reserve University and Temple University. We are particularly indebted to Constance McSweeney, who carried a major load as editorial assistant, and to Michiko Claflin and Margaret McCreary. Victor H. Auerbach, Ph.D., and Richard Hamilton, M.D., have served as associate editors for the sections on Inborn Errors of Metabolism and Gastroenterology, respectively.

The preparation of this twelfth edition has also required the help and cooperation of many other persons. To each of them we acknowledge our debt of gratitude and wish to indicate our heartfelt thanks.

Last, but certainly not least, this textbook would not have been possible without the understanding, forbearance, and active participation of Ann Behrman and Deborah Vaughan. In countless ways their contributions have been essential to the Twelfth Edition of *Nelson Textbook of Pediatrics*.

RICHARD E. BEHRMAN

VICTOR C. VAUGHAN, III

NOTICE

Extraordinary efforts have been made by the authors, the editors, and the publisher of this book to insure that dosage recommendations are precise and in agreement with standards officially accepted at the time of publication.

It does happen, however, that dosage schedules are changed from time to time in the light of accumulating clinical experience and continuing laboratory studies. This is most likely to occur in the case of recently introduced products.

It is urged, therefore, that you check the manufacturer's recommendations for dosage, *especially if the drug to be administered or prescribed is one that you use only infrequently or have not used for some time*.

THE PUBLISHER

CONTENTS

19. PEDIATRIC GYNECOLOGY AND ADOLESCENT ISSUES 1515

20. CONVULSIVE DISORDERS 1531

21. THE NERVOUS SYSTEM 1546

22. NEUROMUSCULAR DISEASES 1601

23. THE BONES AND JOINTS 1614

COLOR PLATES

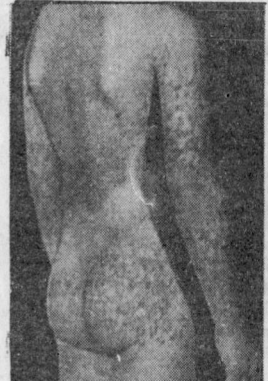
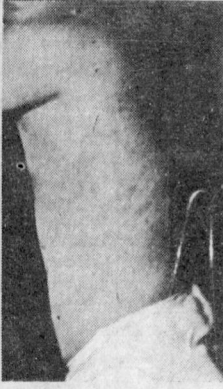

Figure 9–21   Henoch-Schönlein purpura (anaphylactoid purpura). (From Korting, GW: *Hautkrankheiten bei Kindern und Jugendlichen.* Stuttgart, FK Schattauer Verlag, 1969.)

Figure 9–15   Rash of rheumatoid arthritis.

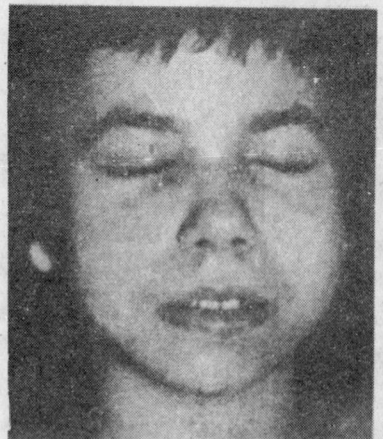
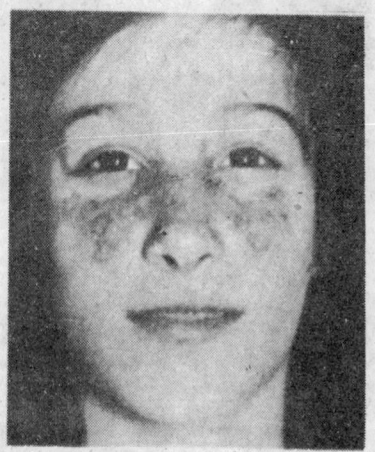

Figure 9–22   The facial rash of dermatomyositis. Note the faint erythema over the bridge of the nose and malar areas, and the heliotrope discoloration of the upper eyelids.

Figure 9–20   The butterfly rash of systemic lupus erythematosus.

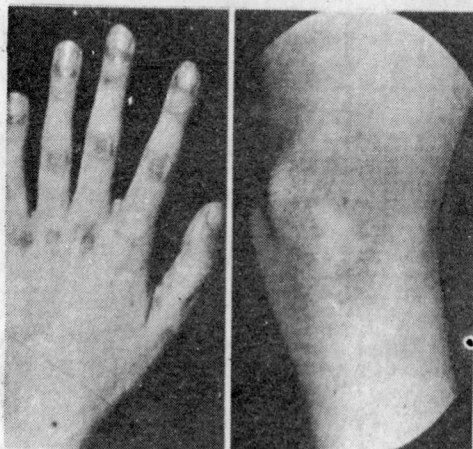
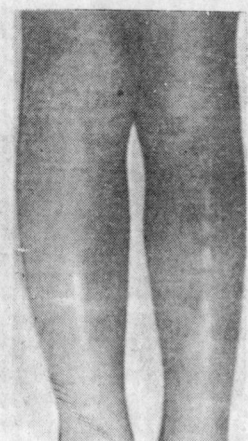

Figure 9–23   Rash of dermatomyositis. Skin changes over the knuckles (left) and over the knee (right).

Figure 9–26   Erythema nodosum.

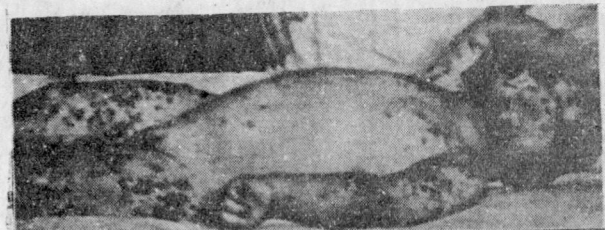

Figure 10–4   Fulminating meningococcemia in child 2½ yr of age. Onset 36 hr before admission, with vomiting and fever; 18 hr before admission, extensive purpuric eruption began, death 8 hr after admission. Blood culture positive. Meningococcus type II. Nasal and cerebrospinal fluid cultures negative. One sibling had meningitis; another was found to be a carrier.

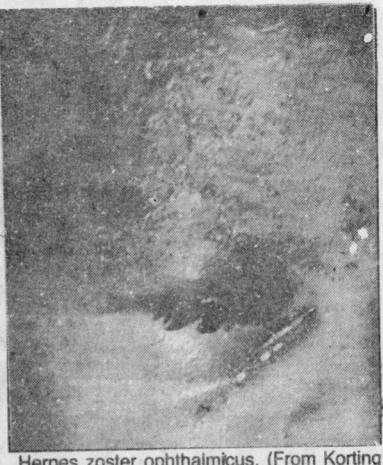

Figure 10–23   Herpes zoster ophthalmicus. (From Korting GW: Hautkrankheiten bei Kindern und Jugendlichen. Stuttgart, Germany, FK Schattauer Verlag, 1969.)

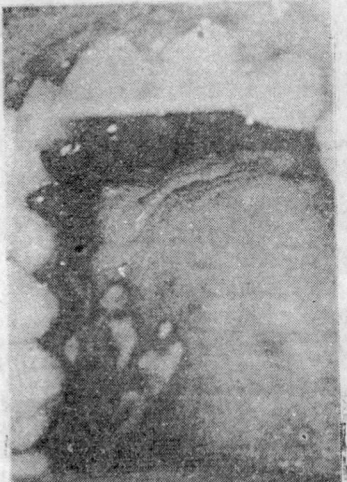

Figure 10–34   Herpangina. (From Korting GW: Hautkrankheiten bei Kindern und Jugendlichen. Stuttgart, Germany, FK Schattauer Verlag, 1969.)

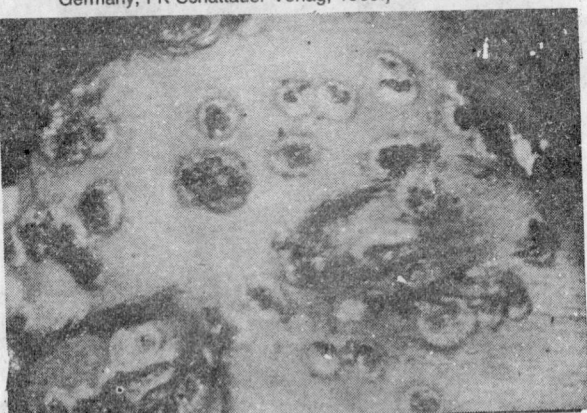

Figure 10–25   Eczema vaccinatum. (From Korting GW: Hautkrankheiten bei Kindern und Jugendlichen. Stuttgart, Germany, FK Schattauer Verlag, 1969.)

Figure 10–41   Creeping eruption of cutaneous larva migrans. (From Korting GW: Hautkrankheiten bei Kindern und Jugendlichen. Stuttgart, Germany, FK Schattauer Verlag, 1969.)

Figure 10–13 Maculopapular rash of measles. (From Korting GW: Hautkrankheiten bei Kindern und Jugendlichen. Stuttgart, Germany, FK Schattauer Verlag, 1969.)

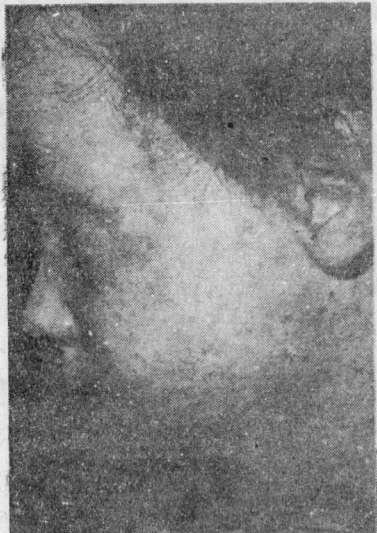

Figure 10–15 Rash of rubella (German measles). (From Korting GW: Hautkrankheiten bei Kindern und Jugendlichen, Stuttgart, Germany, FK Schattauer Verlag, 1969.)

Figure 10–16 Erythema infectiosum. (From Korting GW: Hautkrankheiten bei Kindern und Jugendlichen. Stuttgart, Germany, FK Schattauer Verlag, 1969.)

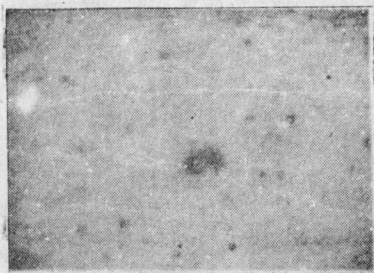

Figure 10–21 Skin lesions of chickenpox. Note the varying stages of development (macules, papules, and vesicles) present at the same time. (Courtesy of Dr. P. F. Lucchesi.)

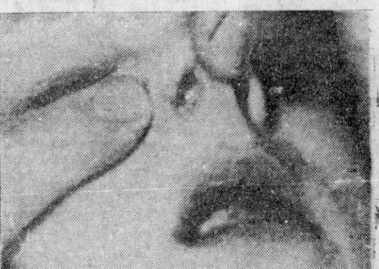

Figure 10–2 Nasal diphtheria. (Courtesy of Dr. Robert A. Lyon.)

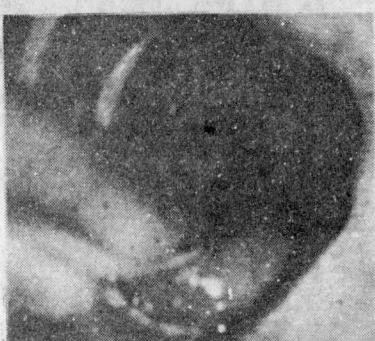

Figure 10–3 Pharyngotonsillar membrane of diphtheria. (Courtesy of Dr. Robert A. Lyon.)

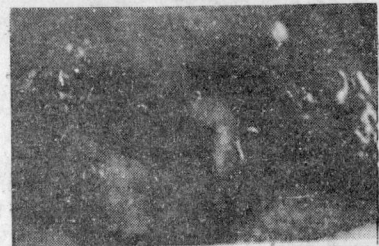

Figure 10–26 Tonsillitis with membrane formation in infectious mononucleosis. (Courtesy of Dr. Alex J. Steigman.)

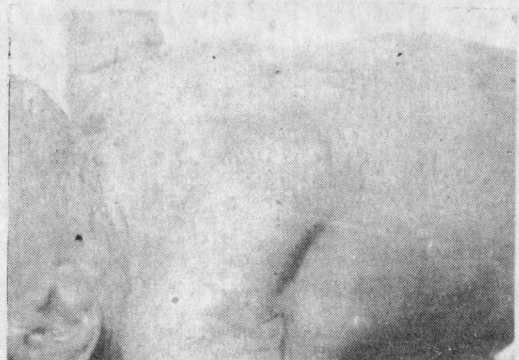

Figure 24–1 Widespread erythema toxicum on the trunk of a newborn infant.

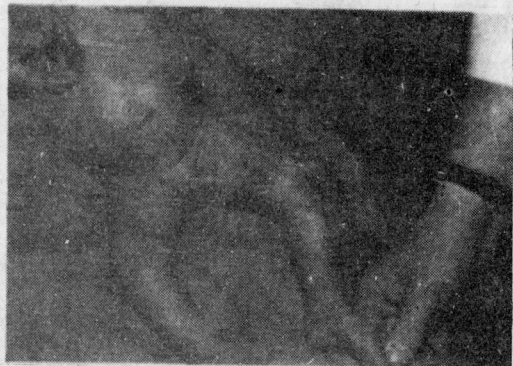

Figure 24–7 Marbled pattern of cutis marmorata telangiectatica congenita on the left leg.

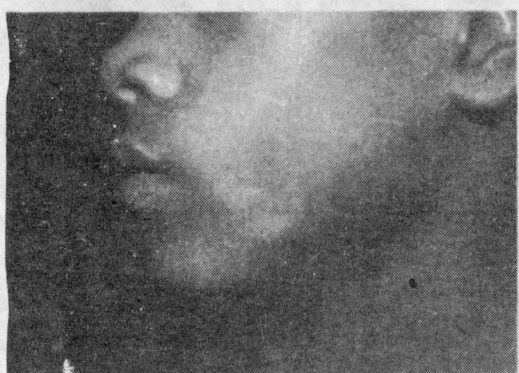

Figure 24–22 Patchy hypopigmented lesions with diffuse borders characteristic of pityriasis alba.

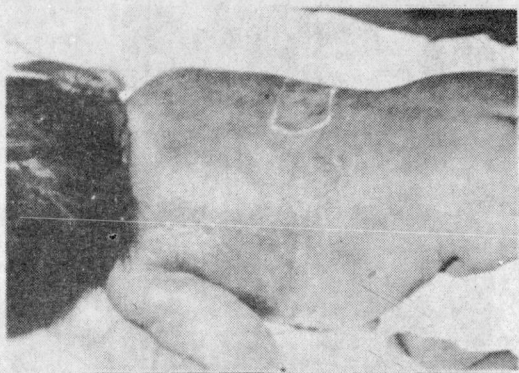

Figure 24–36 Red purple nodular infiltration of skin of back and upper arms due to subcutaneous fat necrosis.

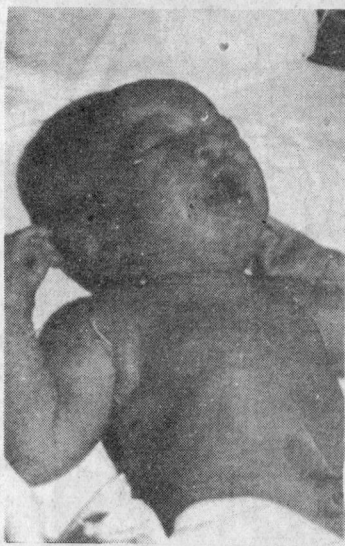

Figure 24–40 Infant with staphylococcal scalded skin syndrome.

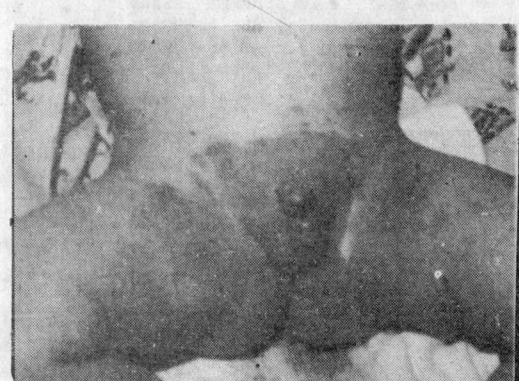

Figure 24–45 Erythematous confluent plaque with satellite pustules due to candidal infection.

NELSON
TEXTBOOK OF
PEDIATRICS

THE FIELD OF PEDIATRICS 1

Many specialties in the field of medicine deal primarily with problems in particular organ systems or with particular biologic processes or systems of care. Pediatrics, on the other hand, is concerned with disturbances of any system or function that might have impact upon the health or orderly growth and development of the child. The pediatrician's commitment, extending beyond purely physical matters, is to secure for all children the opportunity to achieve their full native potential. In the role of understanding guardians of children's physical, mental, and emotional progress from conception to maturity, pediatricians are in the vanguard of social concern for children and their families. The caring qualities of any society may best be measured by the concerns it manifests for its aged, its disadvantaged, and its young. The young and the disadvantaged are often the same.

History of Pediatrics

Pediatrics became differentiated as a medical specialty about a century ago in response to a growing appreciation that the problems of children are different in kind from those of adults and that the incidence of those problems and the child's reaction to them vary with age. The focus and scope of pediatrics have been continually revised.

The health and the health problems of children vary widely among the nations of the world in accordance with many factors which include (1) the prevalence and ecology of infectious agents and their hosts; (2) climate and geography; (3) agricultural resources and practices; (4) educational, economic, and sociocultural considerations; and (5), in many instances, the gene frequencies for some disorders. These factors are often interrelated.

Not only do problems differ in certain parts of the world, but priorities do also since they must reflect local concerns, resources, and needs. The assessment of the state of health of any community must begin with epidemiologic and other studies that describe the incidence of illness and must continue with studies that show the changes that occur with time and in response to programs of prevention, case finding, therapy, and adequate surveillance. As contemporary problems in any community have yielded to study and to improved management, new problems are recognized, or arise de novo, to attract the attention and efforts of pediatric clinicians and research workers. Accordingly, with time, there may be major changes in the relative importance of the various causes of childhood morbidity and mortality.

In the late 19th century in the United States, of every 1000 children born alive 200 might be expected to die before the age of 1 yr of such conditions as dysentery, pneumonia, measles, diphtheria, whooping cough, and the like. The early and continuing efforts of the young specialty of pediatrics, combined with those of immunologists and pioneers in public health, have led to such better understanding of the origin and management of many problems of infants that in the past half century the infant mortality in the United States has fallen from around 75/1000 live births in 1925 to about 13.0 in 1979. Fig 1–1 depicts this change and shows that both neonatal (1st mo) and postneonatal (1–11 mo) mortality have had major reductions. Fig 1–2 shows that, of all deaths of infants under 1 yr of age, 72% now occur within the 1st 28 days of life, 85% of these within the 1st 7 days; more than half of those within the 1st 7 days occur within the 1st day (40% of all deaths in the 1st yr of life). Table 1–1 extends similar observations to the remainder of childhood, showing that more than half of all deaths under 20 yr of age take place within the 1st yr.

Early in the 20th century the efforts of those who contributed to the control of infectious disease began to be complemented by those of nutritionists. New and continuing discoveries were translated into effective practice by those with an interest in public health who set up the earliest well child clinics. Acute infections and the chronic disturbances associated with deficits of calories, vitamins, minerals, or proteins were studied intensively, and the acute nutritional and metabolic disturbances such as the disorders of fluid and electrolyte balance that accompany acute diarrhea also received attention.

In the middle years of the 20th century, a profound revolution in child health was brought about by the introduction of antibacterial chemicals and antibiotic agents. With improved control of infectious disease through both prevention and treatment and with other concurrent scientific and technical advances, pediatric medicine turned its attention to the conditions affecting relatively small numbers of children. These included lethal conditions, such as diseases of the newborn infant, leukemia, and cystic fibrosis, and also temporarily or permanently handicapping conditions, such as congenital heart disease, mental retardation, genetic defects, rheumatic diseases, renal diseases, and metabolic and endocrine disorders.

More recently, increasing attention has been given behavioral and social aspects of child health, ranging from a re-examination of child-rearing practices to the creation of major programs aimed at prevention and management of abuse and neglect of infants and children. Developmental psychologists, child psychiatrists, sociologists, anthropologists, ethologists, and others have brought us new insights into human potential, including new views of the importance of the circum-

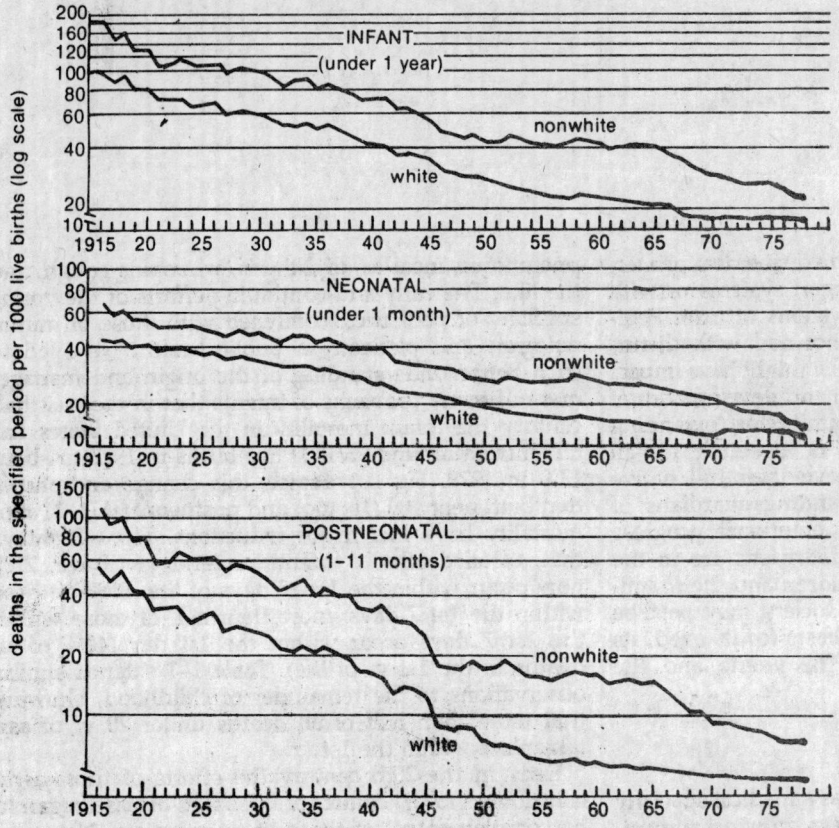

Figure 1-1 Mortality rate of white and of nonwhite infants by age, United States, 1915–1978 (birth registration area). (United States Department of Health and Human Services. Data from United States Public Health Service, National Center for Health Statistics.)

stances surrounding birth and the early hours together of infants and parents (Sec 2.3, 2.5, and 2.33).

Tables 1–2 and 1–3 show how problems of children have changed in the United States over a half century;

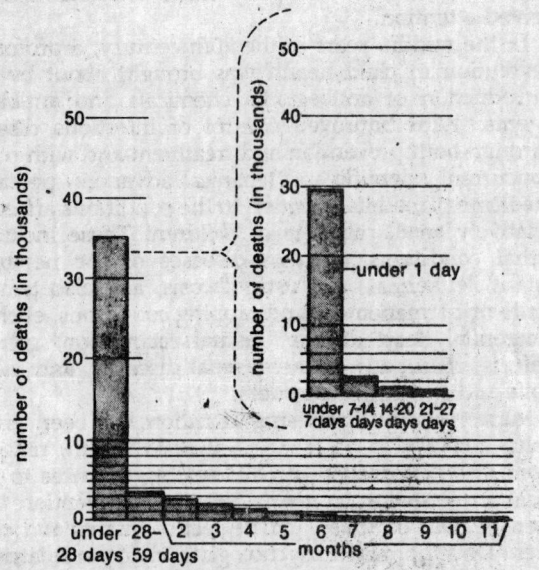

Figure 1-2 Infant mortality by age, United States, 1976. (United States Department of Health and Human Services; data from National Center for Health Statistics.)

the implications for priorities are evident. These tables list the 10 leading causes of death for children aged 1–4 yr and 5–14 yr of age for each 10th yr from 1920–1970. Table 1–4 gives data for the year 1978 and shows dramatically the impact of violent deaths upon the nation's statistics.

Figure 1–1 shows that the nonwhite children of the United States have not fully benefited from the changes in infant mortality in this century, because of a variety of socioeconomic and other disadvantages that have resisted the efforts of many who have struggled to reduce this disparity, including many pediatricians.

In 1981 a Select Panel for the Promotion of Child Health completed a comprehensive assessment of the health needs of children in the United States. General findings of the study were that existing programs for meeting child health problems are not available to all of those families in need, with gaps between eligibility for public support and ability to pay costs; that needed services are often nonexistent or fragmented among programs, agencies, or policies; that programs are poorly coordinated; that data collection is inadequate; and that the resources available for maternal and child health care services are generally inadequate. These findings reflect a need, not just in the United States but in many other parts of the world as well, for continuing re-examination and revision of the system of health care.

The above study reported that from 1970–1978 the percentage of mothers 25–30 yr old who were employed in the labor force had risen from 45% to 62% and that

Table 1-1 DEATHS AND DEATH RATES, BY AGE, COLOR, AND SEX: UNITED STATES, 1979
(Based on a 10% sample of deaths. Rates per 100,000 population in specified group. Due to rounding estimates of deaths, figures may not add to totals.)

AGE	TOTAL			WHITE			ALL OTHER		
	Both Sexes	Male	Female	Both Sexes	Male	Female	Both Sexes	Male	Female
Number									
All ages	1,906,000	1,042,960	863,350	1,670,310	908,040	762,270	236,000	134,920	101,080
Under 1 yr.	45,000	26,080	18,960	31,450	18,500	12,950	13,590	7,580	6,010
1-4 yrs.	7,750	4,290	3,460	5,800	3,160	2,640	1,950	1,130	820
5-14 yrs.	12,040	7,800	4,240	9,690	6,360	3,330	2,350	1,440	910
15-24 yrs.	48,920	37,490	11,450	40,410	31,200	9,210	8,530	6,290	2,240
Rate									
All ages*	866.2	974.7	763.4	879.3	980.0	783.4	783.2	940.5	640.3
Under 1 yr.	1,372.5	1,552.4	1,184.3	1,160.1	1,330.0	981.1	2,388.4	2,622.8	2,146.4
1-4 yrs.	62.7	67.8	57.2	57.2	60.8	53.4	87.3	100.1	74.3
5-14 yrs.	34.8	44.2	25.0	33.9	43.5	23.9	39.2	47.7	30.6
15-24 yrs.	118.2	179.9	55.7	115.4	176.1	53.2	134.2	201.5	69.2

*Figures for age not stated included in "All ages" but not distributed among age groups.
44Table adapted from Monthly Vital Statistics Report 28(13):22, 1980.

the children of working mothers had increased in numbers by 3.3 million between 1970–1977, 38% of them by 1977 under 6 yr old; these changes occurred even though the actual number of children under the age of 18 yr had fallen between the 1970 and 1980 censuses from about 70 million to 62 million. The study further reported that the number of children living in homes in which there was only 1 parent (usually the mother)

Table 1-2 MAIN CAUSES OF DEATH AMONG CHILDREN 1-4 YEARS OF AGE: UNITED STATES, 1970 AND SPECIFIED YEARS

CAUSE OF DEATH*	EIGHTH REVISION CATEGORY NUMBERS IN USE 1968 TO DATE	YEAR							SIXTH AND SEVENTH REVISION CATEGORY NUMBERS IN USE 1949–67	COMPARABILITY RATIO†
		1970	1965	1960	1950	1940	1930	1920		
		Rate per 100,000 children 1–4 years								
All causes	000–E999	84.5	92.9	108.8	139.4	289.6	563.6	987.2	001–E999	1.000
Main causes		64.4	72.3	83.5	98.0	198.4	409.7	794.4		
Accidents	E800–E949	31.5	31.8	31.5	36.8	48.7	61.2	80.2	E800–E962	0.957
Accidents, except motor vehicles	E800–E807, E825–E949	20.0	21.3	21.5	25.3	36.3	46.7	71.1	E800–E802, E840–E962	0.928
Motor vehicle accidents	E810–E823	11.5	10.5	10.0	11.5	12.4	14.5	—	E810–E835	0.992
Congenital anomalies	740–759	9.7	10.2	12.8	11.1	10.3	—	—	750–759	1.020
Influenza and pneumonia	470–474, 480–486	7.6	11.4	16.2	18.9	62.5	123.1	283.7	480–483, 490–493, 763	0.993
Malignant neoplasms, including neoplasms of lymphatic and hematopoietic tissues	140–209	7.5	8.6	10.8	11.7	—	—	—	140–205	1.002
Symptoms and ill defined conditions	780–796	2.1	2.4	2.8	—	—	—	—	780–795	0.994
Meningitis	320	1.9	2.6	2.8	2.8	—	—	—	340	0.959‡
Acute respiratory infections, including acute bronchitis (except influenza)	460–466	1.7	—	—	—	8.9	15.2	12.3	470–475, 500	————
Enteritis and other diarrheal diseases	008, 009	1.4	2.3§	3.2§	————	80.2	95.6	141.3	571, 764	1.185‡
Meningococcal infections	036	1.0	1.8	1.4	2.6	—	—	—	057	————
Gastritis, duodenitis, diverticula of intestine, chronic enteritis and ulcerative colitis	535, 562, 563	—	0.1	0.1	————	—	—	—	543, 572	————
Bronchitis	490, 491	—	1.1	2.1	2.5	—	—	—	501, 502	1.062
Measles	055	—	—	—	—	—	21.9	56.4	085	————
Tuberculosis, all forms	010–019	—	—	—	6.3	12.3	25.9	45.4	001–019	0.950‡
Whooping cough	033	—	—	—	—	9.7	23.4	57.7	056	————
Diphtheria	032	—	—	—	—	9.0	33.5	90.5	055	————
Appendicitis	540–543	—	—	—	—	6.8	—	—	550–553	————
Streptococcal sore throat and scarlet fever	034	—	—	—	—	—	9.9	23.2	050, 051	————
Dysentery	004, 006, 007	—	—	—	—	—	—	12.8	045–048	————
All other causes	Residual	20.1	20.6	25.3	41.4	91.2	153.9	192.8	Residual	————

*Causes of death listed each year are the 10 main causes in that year. For 1970, titles of the causes listed, and inclusions in each cause group, are those of the Eighth Revision, International Classification of Diseases; for 1960 and 1965, inclusions are those of the Seventh Revision; for 1950 and 1955, inclusions are those of the Sixth Revision; for 1940, inclusions are according to the Fifth Revision; for 1930, according to the Fourth Revision; and for 1920, according to the Second Revision. Rates are unadjusted for changes in the classification of causes of death in successive revisions of the lists. In 1950 and later years, "Diarrhea of the newborn" was included in Enteritis and other diarrheal diseases (ICDA Nos. 008, 009). Based on data from the National Center for Health Statistics, Public Health Service, Department of Health and Human Services.

Symbol: —Class or item not applicable.
————Class or item not available.

†Ratio of estimated total deaths assigned according to the Eighth Revision to total deaths assigned according to the Seventh Revision. Ratios by age are not available.

‡These ratios may be slightly underestimated because of the method of computation.

§These figures revised to correspond to the category numbers shown for the Sixth and Seventh Revisions.

Table 1–3   MAIN CAUSES OF DEATH AMONG CHILDREN 5–14 YEARS OF AGE: UNITED STATES, 1970 AND SPECIFIED YEARS

Cause of Death*	Eighth Revision Category Numbers in Use 1968 to Date	Year							Sixth and Seventh Revision Category Numbers in Use 1949–67	Comparability Ratio†
		1970	1965	1960	1950	1940	1930	1920		
		Rate per 100,000 children 5–14 years								
All causes	000–E999	41.3	42.2	46.6	59.8	103.7	171.7	263.9	001–E999	1.000
Main causes		33.2	32.8	35.9	44.7	67.6	111.8	196.3		
Accidents	E800–E949	20.1	18.7	19.2	22.6	28.6	36.1	44.3	E800–E962	0.957
Motor vehicle accidents	E810–E823	10.2	8.9	7.9	8.8	11.5	14.7	13.0	E810–E835	0.992
Accidents, except motor vehicle	E800–E807, E825–E949	9.9	9.8	11.3	13.8	17.1	21.4	31.3	E800–E802, E840–E962	0.925
Malignant neoplasms, including neoplasms of lymphatic and hematopoietic tissues	140–209	6.0	6.5	6.8	6.7	3.0	—	—	140–205	1.002
Congenital anomalies	740–759	2.2	2.8	3.6	2.4	2.1	—	—	750–759	1.020
Influenza and pneumonia	470–474, 480–486	1.6	2.1	2.6	3.2	9.0	18.8	45.1	480–483, 490–493, 763	0.993
Homicide	E960–E978	0.9	0.6	—	—	—	—	—	E964, E980–E985	0.897
Diseases of the heart	390–398, 402, 404, 410–429	0.8	0.4	1.3	3.9	10.6	15.1	21.8	400–402, 410–443	1.004
Cerebrovascular diseases	430–438	0.7	0.7	0.7	—	—	—	—	330–334	0.990
Symptoms and ill defined conditions	780–796	0.5	—	0.6	0.8	—	—	—	780–795	0.994‡
Benign neoplasms and neoplasms of unspecified nature	210–239	0.4	0.6	0.7	0.8	—	—	—	210–239	0.968‡
Anemias	280–285	—	0.4	0.5	—	—	—	—	290–293	0.944‡
Acute poliomyelitis	040–043	—	—	—	2.5	—	—	—	080	———
Appendicitis	540–543	—	—	—	—	0.8	13.1	—	550–553	———
Tuberculosis, all forms	010–019	—	—	—	1.8	5.5	11.9	22.4	001–019	0.950‡
Nephritis and nephrosis	580–584	—	—	—	—	1.7	—	3.5	590–594	0.886
Diphtheria	032	—	—	—	—	1.7	8.1	28.0	055	———
Typhoid fever	001	—	—	—	—	—	4.4	7.1	040	———
Meningococcal infections	036	—	—	—	—	—	4.3	—	057	———
Enteritis and other diarrheal diseases	008, 009	—	—	—	—	—	3.0	4.1	571, 764	1.185‡
Diabetes mellitus	250	—	—	—	—	—	—	3.5	260	0.997
All other causes	Residual	8.1	9.4	10.7	15.1	36.1	59.9	67.6	Residual	

*Causes of death listed each year are the 10 main causes in that year. For 1970, titles of the causes listed, and inclusions in each cause group, are those of the Eighth Revision of the International Classification of Diseases; for 1960 and 1965, inclusions are those of the Seventh Revision; for 1950 and 1955, inclusions are those of the Sixth Revision; for 1940, inclusions are according to the Fifth Revision; for 1930, according to the Fourth Revision; and for 1920, according to the Second Revision. Rates are unadjusted for changes in the classification of causes of death in successive revisions of the lists, but the category "Diseases of the heart" was adjusted to include rheumatic fever for each year specified. Based on data from the National Center for Health Statistics, Public Health Service, Department of Health and Human Services.

Symbol: —Class or item not applicable.
            ———Class or item not available.

†Ratio of estimated total deaths assigned according to the Eighth Revision to total deaths assigned according to the Seventh Revision. Ratios by age are not available.

‡These ratios may be slightly underestimated because of the method of computation.

has increased from 9% in 1960 to 19% in 1978. Many such 1-parent families live at poverty levels of income.

The above findings generated 3 sets of priority goals. The 1st set includes the following goals: that all families have access to adequate perinatal, preschool, and family-planning services; that governmental activities be effectively coordinated; that services be so organized that they reach populations at special risk; that there be no insurmountable or inequitable financial barriers to adequate care; that the health care of children have continuity from prenatal through adolescent age periods; and that ultimately every family have access to *all* needed services, including genetic, dental, and mental health services. A 2nd set of goals addressed factors influencing maternal and child health which lie beyond personal health services: accidents and environmental risks, nutritional needs, and health education aimed at fostering health-promoting life styles. A 3rd set of goals specified the need for research: in biomedical and behavioral science, in fundamentals of bioscience and human biology, and in the particular problems of mothers and children.

The unfinished business in the quest for physical, mental, and social health in the community is impres-

sively illustrated in Fig 1–3, 1–4, and 1–5, which show how unevenly deaths due to disease, to accidents, and to violence are distributed between white and nonwhite children. Fig 1–5 shows that homicide is a major cause of adolescent deaths. As a cause of death it has also increased steadily among the very young, in whom the increase may in part represent the more accurate identification of child abuse (Sec 2.67); among adolescents it may reflect unresolved social tensions and an unhealthy preoccupation in our society with violence. Some of the issues underlying these problems are discussed in Sec 2.30, 2.45, 2.54, 2.57, and 2.67.

Patterns of Health Care

The National Ambulatory Medical Care Survey of the NCHS estimates that in 1975 about 8.2% of all office visits for health care, representing about half the visits of children under the age of 15 yr, were made to the offices of pediatricians. Private offices or clinics or group practices either of pediatricians or other medical practitioners served 88.6% of children under 17 yr of age as their place of usual care, whereas 5.8% used the outpatient clinics of hospitals and 0.6% the emergency

Table 1-4 DEATHS AND DEATH RATES FOR THE 10 LEADING CAUSES OF DEATH, BY SPECIFIED AGE GROUPS: UNITED STATES, 1978
(Refers only to resident deaths occurring within the United States. Rates per 100,000 population)

RANK ORDER IN 1978	CAUSE OF DEATH AND AGE (EIGHTH REVISION INTERNATIONAL CLASSIFICATION OF DISEASES, ADAPTED, 1965)		1978 Number	Rate
	Under 1 yr—all causes		45,945	1,378.4
1	Congenital anomalies	740–759	8,404	252.1
2	Immaturity, unqualified	777	3,677	110.3
3	Respiratory distress syndrome	776.2	3,324	99.7
4	Asphyxia of newborn, unspecified	776.9	2,955	88.7
5	Hyaline membrane disease	776.1	2,667	80.0
6	Birth injury without mention of cause	772	1,851	55.5
7	Influenza and pneumonia	470–474, 480–486	1,533	46.0
8	Accidents	E800–E949	1,262	37.9
9	Septicemia	038	1,093	32.8
10	Conditions of placenta	770	768	23.0
—	All other causes	Residual	18,411	552.3
	1–4 yr—all causes		8,429	69.2
1	Accidents	E800–E949	3,504	28.8
—	Motor vehicle accidents	E810–E823	1,287	10.6
—	All other accidents	E800–E807, E825–E949	2,217	18.2
2	Congenital anomalies	740–759	1,027	8.4
3	Malignant neoplasms, including neoplasms of lymphatic and hematopoietic tissues	140–209	599	4.9
4	Influenza and pneumonia	470–474, 480–486	354	2.9
5	Homicide	E960–E978	313	2.6
6	Diseases of heart	390–398, 402, 404, 410–429	279	2.3
7	Meningitis	320	220	1.8
8	Meningococcal infections	036	112	0.9
9	Cerebrovascular diseases	430–438	100	0.8
10	Anemias	280–285	78	0.6
—	All other causes	Residual	1,843	15.1
	5–14 yr—all causes		12,030	33.9
1	Accidents	E800–E949	6,118	17.2
—	Motor vehicle accidents	E810–E823	3,130	8.8
—	All other accidents	E800–E807, E825–E949	2,988	8.4
2	Malignant neoplasms, including neoplasms of lymphatic and hematopoietic tissues	140–209	1,500	4.2
3	Congenital anomalies	740–759	650	1.8
4	Homicide	E960–E978	454	1.3
5	Diseases of heart	390–398, 402, 404, 410–429	357	1.0
6	Influenza and pneumonia	470–474, 480–486	304	0.9
7	Cerebrovascular diseases	430–438	199	0.6
8	Suicide	E950–E959	153	0.4
9	Anemias	280–285	87	0.2
10	Benign neoplasms and neoplasms of unspecified nature	210–239	83	0.2
—	All other causes	Residual	2,125	6.0
	15–24 yr—all causes		48,500	117.5
1	Accidents	E800–E949	26,622	64.5
—	Motor vehicle accidents	E810–E823	19,164	46.4
—	All other accidents	E800–E807, E825–E949	7,458	18.1
2	Homicide	E960–E978	5,443	13.2
3	Suicide	E950–E959	5,115	12.4
4	Malignant neoplasms, including neoplasms of lymphatic and hematopoietic tissues	140–209	2,588	6.3
5	Diseases of heart	390–398, 402, 404, 410–429	1,098	2.7
6	Congenital anomalies	740–759	648	1.6
7	Influenza and pneumonia	470–474, 480–486	553	1.3
8	Cerebrovascular diseases	430–438	473	1.1
9	Diabetes mellitus	250	140	0.3
10	Benign neoplasms and neoplasms of unspecified nature	210–239	136	0.3
—	All other causes	Residual	5,664	13.8

Table adapted from Monthly Vital Statistics Report 28(13):23, 25, 1980.

rooms of hospitals as the places of usual care. Nonwhite children under 17 yr old were about 4 times as likely as white children to use these hospital facilities for ambulatory care. About 25% of the visits made to pediatricians' offices in 1975 involved health assessment or health maintenance activities, the remainder made because of problems of acute or chronic illness, most often (about 35%) involving the respiratory tract or ears.

Hospitals, particularly in urban areas, are sources of both routine and intensive child care, with inpatient medical services which may cover the gamut of medical illnesses and with surgical services which may range from tonsillectomy and adenoidectomy to open heart surgery and renal transplantation. These latter procedures involving hyperintensive care are likely to be clustered in university-affiliated centers serving as regional resources. For many years the most common major surgical operation on children has been tonsillectomy and adenoidectomy. The incidence is falling, but it varies significantly with geographic region, the slow rate of fall giving impressive testimony to the tenacity with which a procedure of uncertain merit holds its place in the health care of children.

Planning a System of Care

Physicians caring for children have become more involved with the *quality of the child's life*. They find themselves increasingly called upon to advise in the management of disturbed behavior or of relationships between child and parent, child and school, or child and community and are increasingly concerned with problems of mental, social, and societal health. There is also an increasing concern with disparities in how the benefits of what we know about child health reach various groups of children. Just as in many developing countries, so in the United States the health of children lags far behind what it could be if the means and will to apply current knowledge could be brought to bear, the medical problems of the children being often intimately related to problems of mental and social health. The children most at risk are disproportionately represented among ethnic minority groups. Pediatricians have a responsibility to address themselves aggressively to problems such as these.

Linked to the broader notion of health implicit in these views of the scope of pediatric concern is the concept that health and health services are a right of the individual, to be maintained in aspects ranging from the molecular to the social by the commitments and efforts of the community or society to which the individual belongs. The failure of health services and health benefits to reach all who need them has led to re-examination of the design of the health care system in many countries; but there are in most systems unresolved problems such as the maldistribution of physicians, institutional unresponsiveness to the perceived needs of the individual, failure of medical services to be adapted to the need and convenience of the patient, and deficiencies in health education. Efforts to make the delivery of health care more efficient and effective have led imaginative pediatricians to the creation of new categories of health care providers who can magnify and multiply the effectiveness of the individual physician. We may expect allied professional persons to find increasingly productive roles in the health care of children which complement the work of the pediatrician.

New insights into the needs of children have pointed the way toward reshaping the child care system in other ways. Growing understanding of the need of the infant for certain qualities of stimulation and care has led to restudy and revision of the care of the newborn infant (Sec 2.3 and 2.33) and of procedures leading to adoption or to-foster care (Sec 2.41 and 2.42). Institutions for handicapped children have also been re-examined, and it seems likely that the massive centralized institutions of past years will be replaced by community-centered

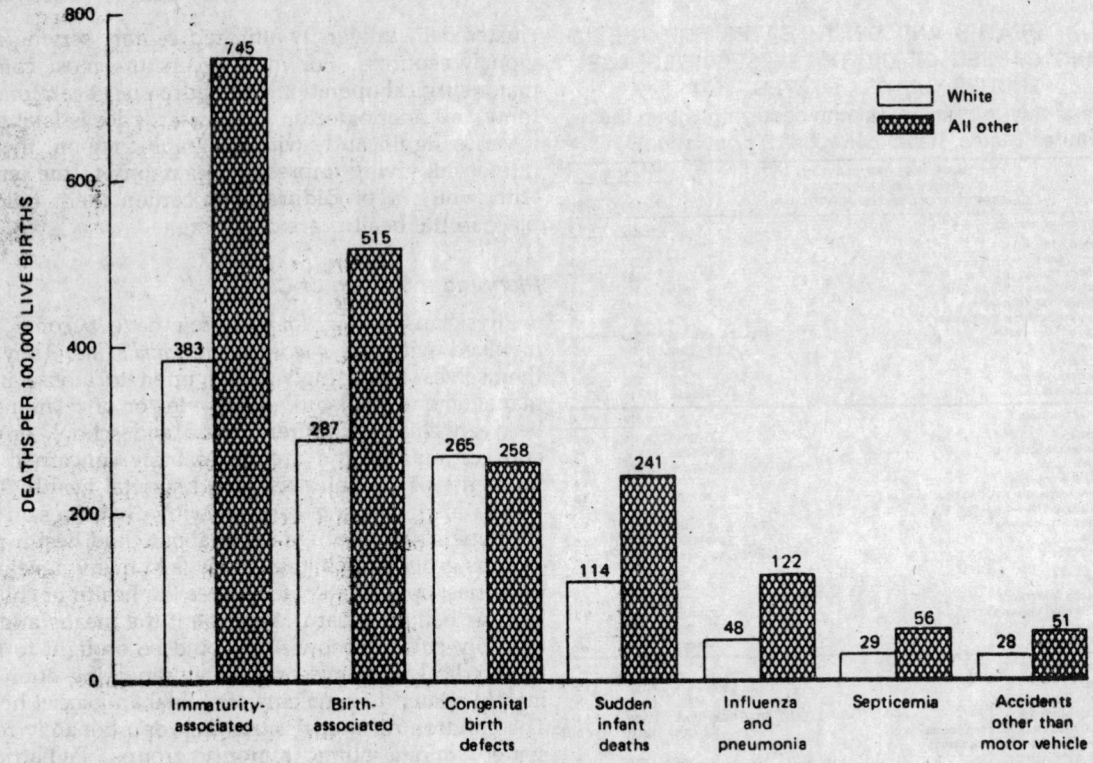

SOURCE: (Office of the Assistant Secretary for Health and the Surgeon General, 1979a)

Figure 1–3 Major causes of death among infants, according to color: United States, 1976. (Health, United States, 1980. Hyattsville, Md., Department of Health and Human Services, 1980.)

arrangements offering a better opportunity for these children to achieve their maximal potential. Pediatricians have been involved in shaping these institutions, and their insights and active contributions will continue to be needed.

Evaluation of Health Care

Akin to growing concern with the design of the health care system and its ability to distribute creative child care is a more intense preoccupation with the *quality of health care* and with the means for making care of the highest quality both efficient and effective. There is increasing public and political pressure for explicit, continuing evaluation of care in terms of what actually takes place rather than what modern medical knowledge has made possible. In this connection the problem-oriented system of keeping health care records (Sec 5.5) and, in the United States, the introduction of methods of assuring quality care through peer review on behalf of the community deserve mention.

Growth of Specialization

In the past quarter century the growth of specialization within pediatrics has taken a number of different forms: interests in problems of *age groups* of children have created neonatology and adolescent medicine;

interests in *organ systems* have created pediatric cardiology, allergy, hematology, nephrology, gastroenterology, pulmonology, endocrinology, and specialization in metabolism and genetics; interests in *the care system* have created pediatricians primarily devoted to ambulatory care on the one hand, and those specializing in intensive care on the other hand; and finally, multidisciplinary sub-specialties have grown up around the problems of *handicapped children*, to which pediatrics, neurology, psychiatry, psychology, nursing, physical and occupational therapy, special education, speech therapy, audiology, and nutrition all make essential contributions. This growth of specialization has been most conspicuous in university-affiliated departments of pediatrics and medical centers for children. The vast majority of pediatricians are generalists, though as many as 25% claim an "area of special interest." The development of such areas of special interest is particularly likely among pediatricians who practice in groups.

The amount of information relevant to child health care doubles about every 10 yr now, and no person can make herself or himself master of it all. Physicians are increasingly dependent upon one another for the highest quality of care for their patients; group practices in pediatrics are on the rise, each member developing some special knowledge and skills.

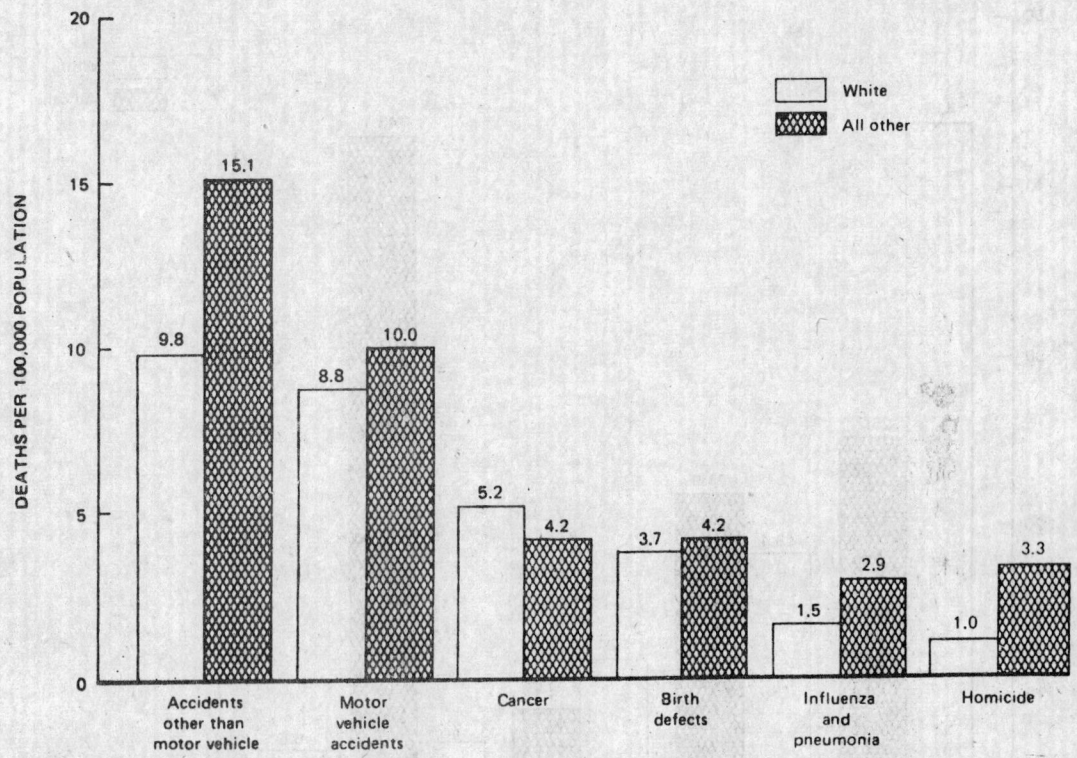

SOURCE: (Office of the Assistant Secretary for Health and the Surgeon General, 1979a)

Figure 1–4 Major causes of death among children 1–14 yr of age, according to color: United States, 1976. (Health, United States, 1980. Hyattsville, Md., Department of Health and Human Services, 1980.)

The Need for Continuing Self-Education

The explosion of information has also created a need for continuing education, which was much less keenly felt in earlier years, when the new information in any field of medicine was easily accessible through a relatively small number of journals, texts, or monographs. Now, relevant information is so widely scattered among the many journals published that elaborate electronic data systems have been implemented to facilitate its dissemination; new auditory and visual aids to learning abound as well as postgraduate courses through which the participating physician can be brought up to date on various aspects of child health care. The American Board of Pediatrics and the American Academy of Pediatrics have arranged for the close linkage of continuing education of the pediatrician to recertification in pediatrics.

There is no touchstone through which physicians can assure that the process of their own continuing education will keep them abreast of advancing knowledge in the field, but they must find a way if they are to discharge their responsibility to their patients. An essential element of this process may be that the physician take an *active* role in it. The passive role, reading or listening or watching, is far less effective than an active one in which the physician translates what is read, seen, or heard into some action of his or her own. Efforts in continuing self-education will be fostered, for example, if the physician can use them to teach, partic-

ularly if they are relevant to the problems actually encountered in practice. Each clinical problem can be made a stimulus for a review of standard literature, alone or in consultation with an appropriate colleague or consultant. This continuing review will do much to identify those inconsistencies or contradictions which will indicate, in the ultimate best interest of the patient, that things are not what they seem or have been said to be. Physicians still learn most from their patients but not if they fall into the easy habit of accepting their patients' problems casually or at face value because they appear to be simple.

The tools which the physician must use in dealing with the problems of children and their families fall into three main categories: *cognitive* (up-to-date factual information regarding diagnostic and therapeutic issues, available on recall or easily found in readily accessible sources); *interpersonal or manual* (the ability to carry out a productive interview, execute a reliable physical examination, perform a deft venipuncture, or manage cardiac arrest or the resuscitation of a depressed newborn infant, for example); and *attitudinal* (the physician's commitment to fullest possible implementation of knowledge and skills on behalf of children and their families in a climate of empathic sensitivity and concern).

The workaday needs of professional persons for knowledge and skills in care of children will vary widely. The primary care physician needs depth in

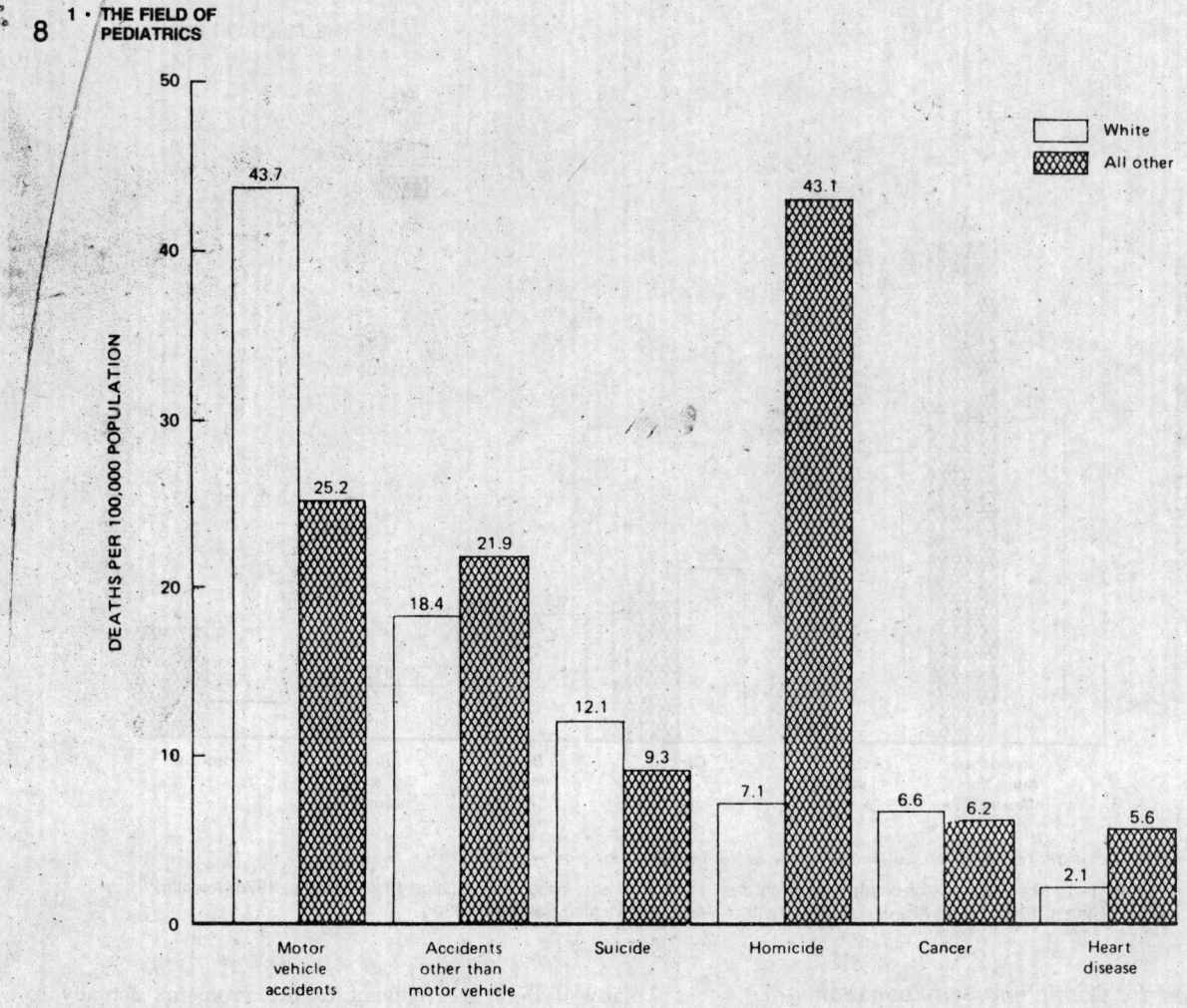

SOURCE: (Office of the Assistant Secretary for Health and the Surgeon General, 1979a)

Figure 1–5   Major causes of death among persons 15–24 yr of age, according to color: United States, 1976. (Health, United States, 1980. Hyattsville, Md., Department of Health and Human Services, 1980.)

developmental concepts and in the ability to organize an effective system for achieving quality and continuity in assessing and planning for health care during the entire period of growth. There may often be little or no need for immediate recall of esoterica. On the other hand, the consultant or subspecialist not only needs a comfortable grasp of esoterica within his or her field and perhaps within related fields, but also must be able to cope with controversial issues with the flexibility which will permit adaptation of a variety of points of view to the best interest of his or her unique patient.

At whatever level of care (primary, secondary, or tertiary), or in whatever role (as student, as pediatric nurse practitioner, as resident pediatrician, as a practitioner of pediatrics or of family medicine, or as a pediatric or other subspecialist), professional persons dealing with children must be able to identify their roles of the moment and their levels of engagement with a child's problem; each must determine whether his or her experience and other resources at hand are adequate to deal with this problem and must be ready to seek other help when they are not. Among the

resources to be kept at hand or called upon will be general textbooks, more detailed monographs in subspecialty areas, selected journals, audiovisual materials, and above all the human resources represented by colleagues with exceptional or complementary experience and expertise. The intercommunication of all these levels of interest in and engagement with medical and health problems of children offers the best hope that each generation may more closely approximate the goal of maximum achievement of the innate potential of every child.

VICTOR C. VAUGHAN, III*

Access to Ambulatory Health Care, United States, 1974. Advance Data, No 17, February 23, 1978.
Ambulatory Medical Care Rendered in Physicians' Offices. Advance Data, No 12, October 12, 1977.

*Acknowledgment.   We are indebted to the National Center for Health Statistics, Department of Health and Human Services for Tables 1–1, 1–2, 1–3, 1–4, and 1–5, and for the data from which Fig 1–1 and 1–2 were prepared.

Ambulatory Medical Care Rendered in Pediatricians' Offices. Advance Data, No 13, October 13, 1977.

Better Health for Our Children: A National Strategy. The Report of the Select Panel for the Promotion of Child Health (in 3 vols). DHHS (PHS) Publication No. 79-55071. Washington, D.C., U.S. Government Printing Office, 1981. (For sale by the Superintendent of Documents.)

Foundations for Evaluating the Competency of Pediatricians. Chicago, American Board of Pediatrics, Inc., 1974.

Healthy People: The Surgeon General's Report on Health Promotion and Disease Prevention. The Report and Background Papers. DHEW (PHS) Publications No. 79-55071 and 79-55071A. Washington, D.C., U.S. Government Printing Office, 1979. (For Sale by Superintendent of Documents.)

Health—United States, 1980: with Prevention Profile. DHHS Publication No. (PHS) 81-1232.

Morley D: Paediatric Priorities in the Developing World. London, Butterworths, 1973.

Program for Recertification in Pediatrics. Chapel Hill, N.C., American Board of Pediatrics, 1961.

Promoting Health/Preventing Disease: Objectives for the Nation. Department of Health and Human Services, Public Health Service, Office of the Assistant Secretary for Health and Surgeon General (JB Richmond, M.D.). Washington, D.C., U.S. Government Printing Office, 1980.

Inquiries regarding the publications of the National Center for Health Statistics (NCHS) can be made to National Center for Health Statistics, Center Building, Room 1-57, 3700 East-West Highway, Hyattsville, Md., 20782. Telephone: (301) 436-8500.

2 DEVELOPMENTAL PEDIATRICS

2.1 GROWTH AND DEVELOPMENT

The term *growth and development* in humans generally refers to the process by which the fertilized ovum attains adult status. *Growth* implies changes in size or in the values given certain measurements of maturity; *development* may encompass other aspects of differentiation of form or function, including those emotional or social changes pre-eminently shaped by interaction with the environment.

The degree to which an individual achieves biologic potential is the product of many interrelated factors. *Genetic* factors, which are sometimes thought of as establishing final limits to biologic potential, are intimately interwoven with the environment. *Trauma* affecting growth and development may be prenatal or postnatal; it may be chemical, residual from infection, physical, or immunologic. *Nutritional* factors affect growth and may be closely interwoven with *socioeconomic* factors. *Social and emotional* factors which may modify growth potential include the position of the child in the family, the quality of interaction between child and parent within the 1st hours, days, or weeks of life, the child rearing patterns, and the personal concerns and needs of the parents. *Cultural* considerations may limit children by establishing conventional expectations for their behavior throughout life and may conspicuously alter the schedule for acquisition of skills such as sitting or walking, which were once thought to be almost entirely determined by maturation alone. *Politics* and culture are closely related, the political life of any community providing the arena in which the community's priorities are set, including those that may have profound effects upon children.

Physical growth and development encompass changes in the size and function of the organism. Changes in function range from the molecular level, such as the activation of enzymes in the course of differentiation, to the complex interplay of metabolic and physical changes associated with puberty and adolescence.

In early infancy *intellectual growth and development* are difficult to differentiate from neurologic and behavioral maturation. In later infancy or early childhood, intellectual function is increasingly measured by communicative skills and the ability to handle abstract and symbolic material.

Emotional growth and development depend upon the infant's ability to establish supportive bonds of feeling, the capacity for love and affection, the ability to handle anxieties arising out of frustration, and the ability to control aggressive impulses. The relations established in infancy with parents are extended to other familial and to extrafamilial contacts.

Learning is an essential aspect of acculturation. Current learning theory suggests that the behavior of the infant is modified both by inner needs and tensions and by contingencies in the environment. Behavior is very responsive to the manner in which it is rewarded. If a pattern of behavior is reliably followed by pleasant circumstances such as reduction of need or by intrinsically satisfying stimuli, then that pattern of behavior will tend to occur with increasing probability; if by unpleasant circumstances, then with decreasing probability. This relationship exists both for desirable behavior and for undesirable behavior, whether viewed in personal, parental, or social perspective.

The *reinforcement* of behavior may be termed *positive* or *negative* in accordance with whether it consists of a pleasant, rewarding experience or the termination of some uncomfortable, unpleasant, or aversive situation. In contrast to negative reinforcement, *punishment* implies the creation of an unpleasant situation upon the exhibition of behavior. Behavior that produces neither positive nor negative reinforcement, nor punishment, tends not to recur, for an established or repetitive pattern of behavior, such disappearance is termed *extinction*.

There is a need to set limits to the behavior of children from time to time through restraint or other measures that might be construed as punishment, but there is evidence that positive reinforcement is a more effective way than punishment to elicit desirable behavior from children.

The techniques of *behavior modification* and *behavior shaping* have broad implications for socialization and discipline in childhood. Behavior shaping involves identifying the behavior ultimately desired and then rewarding actions that move toward or are partially successful in achieving that behavior or that show a willingness to move toward it. As behavior approaches in quality the desired goal, rewards are given only for behavior representative of goal conditions. Once the desired behavior has been achieved, it can be maintained through occasional further positive reinforcement (Sec 2.30).

A further consideration in the socialization and acculturation of children is the important role that *models* play; children even in the 1st months of life have a tendency to imitate the behavior of those around them. As they grow older, they are able to draw lessons and inferences not only from experiencing the consequences of their own behavior, but also from seeing that certain forms of behavior have predictable consequences for others. The importance of models to the child can scarcely be overemphasized. There is no doubt that what children see about them in reality or what they experience through mass media, such as television, newspapers, and literature, may profoundly affect their systems of values and their notions of what is expected of them. It is important that the value systems proposed for children by their parents and other significant persons be congruent with the actual behavior of these same individuals (Sec 2.30).

The broad picture of growth and development, then, is an intricate pattern of genetic, nutritional, traumatic, social, cultural, and political forces. The pattern is unique for each child and may be profoundly different for individual children within the broad limits that designate "normality." Indeed, patterns of growth and development have such variability that they can often be adequately expressed only in statistical terms.

VARIABILITY IN HUMAN GROWTH PATTERNS

Such measurements of growth as weight, height, and circumference of head will indicate the status of a child in relation to other children of the same age, but only sequential measurements will indicate the normal or abnormal dynamics of the process through which each child is achieving his or her growth potential. For example, a child below the 10th percentile point in weight for age may be suspected of being undernourished, but 10% of normal children will be below this level. If such children manifest regular sequential growth in height and weight within certain limits, they may be manifesting normal physical growth. On the other hand, other children whose height and weight approximate higher percentiles for their ages may be significantly below their own ideal levels when sequential measurements are evaluated.

Whenever one aspect of growth differs significantly from other aspects, possible reasons should be sought. For example, if height and bone age place a child at the 50th percentile for age, one would be concerned to find his or her weight at the 3rd or 97th percentile.

In the evaluation of physique, it is helpful to have standards that indicate the range of weights appropriate to the heights of children (see Tables 2–6, 2–7, and 2–8). Children whose weights are at less than the 5th percentile or over the 95th percentile for their actual heights should be evaluated. A physical assessment, along with a review of history of illness, of dietary habits, of family patterns of growth, and of the psychosocial circumstances of the child and family, will suggest whether more extensive studies are indicated.

It may be useful in evaluating a child's height to take into account familial patterns. Tanner and coworkers have developed for children between the ages of 2–9 yr standards for height appropriately adjusted for the parents' heights. Wingert and coworkers have also indicated how an appraisal of the preadolescent child's height can take parental height into account.

With allowance for normal influences that may put it at a given percentile at a particular time, the growth curve of each healthy child is sufficiently smooth that any substantial perturbations of the growth line are likely to reflect physical illness, nutritional disturbances, or psychosocial difficulties. In any case, the possibilities for early recognition of physical or emotional disturbances of growth and for useful intervention will depend on records of careful measurements made during infancy and early childhood; such records are an essential element of comprehensive and continuing care of children (Sec 2.11).

2.2 FETAL GROWTH AND DEVELOPMENT

Intrauterine life may be divided into 2 principal phases: *embryonic* and *fetal*. The embryonic period is usually considered to be the 1st 8 wk of growth, during which the fertilized ovum differentiates rapidly into an organism that has most of the gross anatomic features of the human form. Organogenesis continues beyond 8 wk in some systems, so that some prefer to designate the embryonic period as the 1st trimester of pregnancy, or the 1st 12 wk. The period after the 12th wk of gestation and through the 40th wk is distinguished by rapid growth and elaboration of function. Before the 24th–26th wk of gestation the fetus is generally considered *previable*; from 26–38 wk the infant is considered *viable*, with decreasing degrees of *prematurity*.

The mortality rate during the embryonic period is probably higher than at any other time of life. Causes include abnormalities of genes and chromosomes and alterations of maternal health, and these may at times be interrelated. Advanced maternal age, for example, seems to dispose to certain chromosomal abnormalities. Maternal infection during the 1st trimester of pregnancy may alter the differentiation of the fetus so as to produce congenital abnormalities. In general, intrauterine environmental factors responsible for defects in differentiation of the newborn infant exert their effects within the 1st trimester of pregnancy (Sec 7.6).

Morbidity during the fetal period may result from a variety of intrauterine factors. These include interference with *oxygenation* of the fetus through disturbances of the placenta or umbilical cord; *infections* such as syphilis, toxoplasmosis, cytomegalic inclusion disease, and other viral or bacterial conditions; *injury* by radiation, trauma, or noxious chemicals; *immunologic* disorders in which erythrocytes or other cells are altered by isoantibodies; or maternal *nutritional* disturbances.

Deficiencies in the maternal diet are more apt to affect the weight and general condition of the human infant than to produce such specific anatomic defects as occur in certain animals. Malnutrition in the pregnant woman leads to a high incidence of stillbirths or infants of low birth weight, and deficiency of calcium in the maternal diet may be related to osseous structure in the newborn infant. Life-long undernutrition of the mother, extended into pregnancy, may be more serious for the baby than an acute nutritional disturbance during pregnancy in the previously well-nourished mother. The long-term effects on the child are more severe and may be devastating when intrauterine malnutrition is followed by malnutrition in the 1st months of life.

The effects of intrauterine malnutrition upon cerebral structure or function in later life are not fully understood. The rate of increase in the number of neurons is high during gestation, and the number of the cells probably continues to increase at a decreasing rate in the human until about 18 mo of postnatal age. In this postnatal period there is also an increase in the number and complexity of dendritic connections, in the number of neuroglial cells, in the size of neurons and glial cells, and in myelinization. The effects on the central nervous system of malnutrition occurring after this time can be much more readily reversed than those that have occurred during the periods of increase in cell number.

FETAL DEVELOPMENT

The embryo is grossly inert during the 1st 7 wk of development except for the heart beat, which begins by about 4 wk. The 1st wk of embryologic life is germinal, consisting of active cell division. During the 2nd wk the tissues differentiate into 2 layers, entoderm and ectoderm, and during the 3rd wk the third layer, mesoderm, is added. During the 4th wk, the growing organism elaborates the somites and between the 4th–8th wk undergoes rapid differentiation into an essentially human form. At 8 wk of age the fetus weighs approximately 1 gm and is about 2.5 cm in length; at 12 wk it weighs about 14 gm and is about 7.5 cm long. By the end of the *1st trimester* the sex of the fetus can be distinguished by external features.

The *2nd trimester of pregnancy*, ending by about 28 wk, is characterized by rapid fetal growth, especially in linear dimensions, and by rapid acquisition of new functions. By the end of the 2nd trimester the fetus weighs approximately 1000 gm and is about 35 cm (14 in) in length. During the *3rd trimester* the further increase in size of the now viable fetus involves primarily subcutaneous tissue and muscle mass.

The *circulatory* system of the fetus attains its final form between the 8th–12th wk of gestation. Blood returning to the fetus from the placenta through the umbilical vein enters the inferior vena cava through the ductus venosus. As it enters the right atrium, this blood tends to be preferentially shunted through the patent foramen ovale into the left atrium. From the left ventricle it then enters the ascending aorta and is distributed to the head and the brain. Blood returning from the head by way of the superior vena cava tends to move across the right atrium into the right ventricle, and through the pulmonary artery and ductus arteriosus into the descending aorta, whence it is returned to the placenta by way of the umbilical arteries. In this way the head and brain receive proportionately more oxygenated blood than other parts of the body.

At birth, or shortly thereafter, there is closure of the ductus venosus, the ductus arteriosus, the foramen ovale, and the umbilical arteries and vein. Closure of the foramen ovale very likely becomes functionally effective within the 1st hr or so, owing to establishment of a lower pressure on the right side of the heart than on the left, after aeration of the lungs. Temporary reversal of flow through the foramen ovale may occur with crying and lead to mild cyanosis during the 1st few days of life. Closure of the ductus arteriosus probably occurs somewhat later, though usually within the 1st 10–15 hr of life. The stimulus for this closure is very likely the establishment of a high oxygen level in the arterial blood. Closure can be delayed or reversed by prostaglandin E₁, which probably maintains patency of the ductus in the fetus. Umbilical arteries undergo spasm with the cutting of the umbilical cord and are reduced ultimately to fibrous cords. The changes in blood flow at birth transform the circulatory system from one in which the 2 ventricles act in parallel, with shunts adjusting possible unequal outputs, to a system in which the 2 pumps act in series, which requires that their outputs be equal.

Although *respiratory* movements of the fetus may be seen as early as the 18th wk of gestation, the development of the alveolar structures of the lung will not generally be sufficient to permit survival until the 27th or 28th wk. The respiratory movements of the fetus result in a tidal flow of amniotic fluid into and out of the developing lung and may contribute to pulmonary arborization. Respiratory movements may be intensified by anoxia. Late in pregnancy, when amniotic fluid contains more cells and may contain meconium and other debris, aspiration may lead to deposition of these materials in the alveoli and to consequent respiratory embarrassment at delivery.

The hemoglobin of the fetus is predominantly fetal in type (hemoglobin F) and differs from that of adults (hemoglobin A) in its greater resistance to alkaline denaturation. Fetal hemoglobin carries more oxygen at a given oxygen tension than adult hemoglobin, which begins to be produced late in fetal life and represents about 30% of the hemoglobin of the mature newborn infant.

The fetus makes swallowing movements as early as the 14th wk of gestation; at 17 wk it may protrude the upper lip on stimulation in the oral area, and by the 20th wk it may protrude both lips on stimulation. At 22 wk the lips are pursed upon stimulation, and by 28–29 wk the fetus may actively suck in an attempt to gain nourishment.

Bile begins to be formed by about 12 wk of gestation, and digestive enzymes appear soon thereafter. Meconium, the distinctive intestinal content of the fetus, is present by 16 wk; it consists of desquamated intestinal cells and intestinal juices, and of squamous cells and lanugo hair swallowed by the fetus in amniotic fluid.

Neurologic activity in the fetus is first manifest by about 8 wk of gestation, when isolated local muscular reactions may be seen in response to stimulation. By 9 wk contralateral flexion may be followed by ipsilateral flexion, and some spontaneous movements may be seen. By 9 wk gestation the palms and soles have also become reflexogenic; by 13–14 wk graceful flowing movements may be produced by stimulation of all areas except the back, the back of the head, and the vertex. At this time the movement of the fetus may first begin to be perceptible to the mother. The grasp reflex is evident by 17 wk and is generally well developed by 27 wk. Respiration may occur in the fetus delivered at 18 wk; at 22 wk respiratory activity may be accompanied by weak phonation. By 25 wk the earliest signs of the Moro response can be elicited.

The amount of activity differs among fetuses, and there is evidence that fetal activity may be responsive to maternal emotions, possibly as a result of placental transfer of epinephrine or other substances. Virtually nothing is known about how the activity of newborn infants or the quality of the infant's demands during the 1st few wk of life may reflect aspects of gestation that are dependent upon maternal emotional states. The fetus is capable of habituation to certain sensory stimuli; e.g., changes in the fetal pulse rate in response to noise transmitted through the mother's abdomen are blunted by repetition of the noise. The comfort derived by some newborn infants from rhythmic motion or rhythmic sound may stem from similar sensations imparted in utero by maternal respiration or heart sounds.

The placenta is the principal avenue of metabolic interchange between mother and fetus. Its most urgent function is to provide for gas exchange between mother and fetus, which requires adequate perfusion on both sides. The placenta is a complex organ, elaborating hormones and enzymes that participate in the regulation of pregnancy, and effecting the selective transfer of nutrients and metabolites between mother and infant. Placental permeability is selective even for such closely related substances as antibodies against viruses and bacteria, the former being more readily transmitted (as IgG) than the latter (generally IgM). Much of the transfer of calcium, iron, and immunoglobulins to the infant occurs in the last trimester of pregnancy, with the result that the infant born prematurely may have unusual needs for calcium and iron and unusual susceptibility to infection.

2.3 THE NEWBORN INFANT

See also Chapter 7.

Physical Features. The body proportions of newborn infants differentiate them sharply from older infants, children, or adults (Fig 2-1). The head is relatively large, the face round, and the mandible relatively small. The chest tends to be rounded rather than flattened anteroposteriorly; the abdomen is relatively prominent, and the extremities are relatively short. The midpoint of the stature of the newborn infant is approximately at the level of the umbilicus, whereas in the adult it is at the symphysis pubis.

At birth there may be edema of the vertex or other presenting part, or an abnormal shape to the head molded by the forces of labor, with overriding of the bones of the cranial vault. The posture of the newborn infant tends to be one of partial flexion. It is often possible to establish what the predominant intrauterine position of the infant was by determining the most comfortable pattern into which the extremities can be fixed and adjusted to each other ("folded") to make the infant assume a more or less ovoid shape. Sometimes minor and occasionally major orthopedic abnormalities reflect the effect of intrauterine posture upon the growing fetus (Sec 23.2).

Localized anatomic variants which may be observed in the newborn infant include telangiectases of the eyelids and of the nape, Mongolian spot, milia, phimosis, and epithelial pearls of the oral mucous membrane. The external auditory canal of the newborn infant is short, and the drum is thicker and more opaque and is placed obliquely across the canal. The middle ear contains a mucoid substance which may be mistaken for an exudate of infection. The eustachian tube is short and broad. There is usually a single mastoid cell in the antrum; maxillary and ethmoid sinuses are small, and the frontal and sphenoidal ones undeveloped. The liver and spleen are commonly felt at or just below the costal margins, and the kidneys are often palpable.

An average newborn infant weighs approximately 3.4 Kg (7½ lb), boys being slightly heavier than girls. Approximately 95% of fullterm newborn infants weigh between 2.5-4.6 kg (5½-10 lb). The length averages about 50 cm (20 in), approximately 95% of infants being between 45-55 cm (18-22 in). The head circumference averages about 35 cm (14 in).

Physiology. The most critical need of the newborn infant is for the establishment of adequate respiratory activity with effective exchange of gases. The rate of established respirations varies from 35-50/min, with brief excursions outside this range relatively common.

The cardiac adjustments of the neonatal period are often associated with transient cardiac murmurs. The heart rate ranges from 120-160/min. The heart of the newborn infant often seems large with respect to the size of the chest when measured by adult standards.

The activity of newborn infants directed toward meeting their nutritional needs includes crying when hungry, a tendency when hungry to turn their heads toward and to "root" about for the nipple or other stimulus placed close to the oral area (rooting reflex), and sucking, gagging, and swallowing reflexes. The newborn infant is capable of manifesting nausea and of vomiting.

The infant initially expresses hunger at irregular intervals, but during the 1st wk will fall reasonably comfortably into patterns of feeding at intervals ranging from 2-5 hr. No schedule of feedings will meet the demands or needs of all infants; if infant and mother

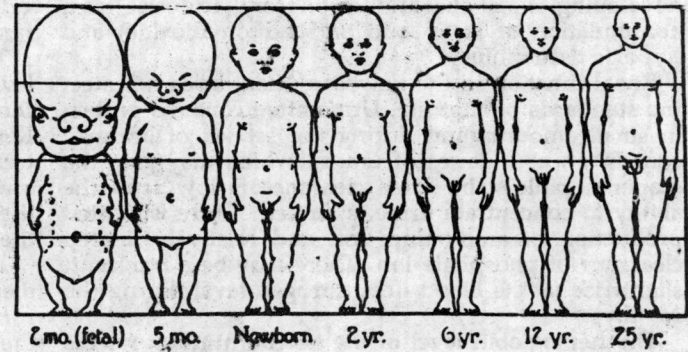

Figure 2-1 Changes in body proportions from 2nd fetal mo to adulthood. (From Robbins et al.: Growth. New Haven, Yale University Press. By permission of publisher.)

2 mo. (fetal)   5 mo.   Newborn   2 yr.   6 yr.   12 yr.   25 yr.

are close to each other during the immediate postnatal period, as in a rooming-in arrangement, the opportunities for comfortable meeting of the baby's needs are optimal.

The 1st stools will generally be passed within 24 hr and will consist of meconium. With the establishment of milk feedings, the meconium stools begin to be replaced on the 3rd–4th day by *transitional* stools, which are greenish brown and may contain milk curds. The typical milk stool of the older infant follows after an interval of 3–4 days. The frequency of stools in the newborn infant seems closely related to the frequency of feeding and the amount of food obtained, averaging 3–5 stools a day by the end of the 1st wk. On any given day during the 1st wk about 1 infant in 50 will have no stool at all; it is unusual for an infant to have as many as 6–7 stools after the 2nd day.

At delivery the body temperatures of mother and infant are likely to be virtually the same. After delivery the infant's temperature falls transiently, with restoration usual within 4–8 hr. The daily caloric need of the newborn infant to maintain body heat and basal activity is usually about 55 cal/kg/24 hr. By the end of the 1st wk the caloric needs will be approximately 110 cal/kg/24 hr, of which 50% supplies basal metabolic needs, 40% is invested in growth and in activity, 5% is for the specific dynamic action of protein, and 5% is lost in urine and feces.

The newborn infant is well supplied with body water, which in the extracellular compartment may constitute up to 35% of body weight. During the 1st few days of life there is a loss of excess fluid which, in the absence of unusual oral intake, generally averages about 6% of body weight and may occasionally exceed 10%. When this loss is excessive, there may be dehydration or inanition fever on the 3rd–4th day.

After the 1st wk of life the need for water will be in the range of 120–150 ml/kg/24 hr. Approximately half of this will be devoted to formation of urine and the rest to insensible loss by lungs and skin and to other losses. The insensible loss is in a relatively fixed relation to the calories metabolized by the infant (about 40 ml/100 cal). Losses in stool are variable; those in sweat, minimal.

The metabolism of newborn infants favors the anaerobic or glycolytic pathway, so that they are more tolerant of periods of deprivation of oxygen than older infants, children, or adults. This tolerance for anoxia is only relative, however. If oxygenation of the newborn infant is not quickly established, there may be a rapidly developing metabolic and respiratory acidosis (from accumulation of lactic acid and carbon dioxide) and hypoxic tissue injury.

Renal function in the newborn infant does not meet the standards of later life. Urine often contains protein in small amounts and during the 1st wk of life may contain an abundance of urates, which may give the diaper a pink stain. Urea clearance is low, and the ability to concentrate urine is limited. There is limited production of ammonium ion and relatively limited clearance of phosphate ion. There may be a transient, slight rise in the blood urea nitrogen level during the 1st days.

The hemoglobin level of the newborn infant ranges around 17–19 gm/dl, and mild reticulocytosis and normoblastemia may be observed for the 1st day or 2 of life. Leukocytes number about 10,000/mm³ at birth and generally increase in number for the 1st 24 hr, with a relative neutrophilia. Counts as high as 25,000–35,000 may be encountered. After the 1st wk the total white cell count is likely to be below 14,000 with the characteristic relative lymphocytosis of infancy and early childhood. Stressful situations in the newborn infant, including overwhelming infection, may be associated with little or no leukocytosis and even with leukopenia.

The transition from intrauterine to extrauterine life imposes upon the infant the need to activate a number of functions which have been dormant. Some of them, such as respiratory activity and the maintenance of body temperature, are usually quickly achieved. By contrast, there are delays in the development of certain enzymatic, hemostatic, and immunologic functions, so that infants may temporarily be subject to increased risk when exposed to infection or when given certain drugs which they are able to metabolize adequately only some weeks after birth (Sec 2.10).

There is little or no transfer of certain clotting factors from mother to infant. Establishment of normal hemostatic mechanisms depends upon establishment of normal intestinal flora and elaboration of vitamin K (Sec 14.59).

Placentally transmitted maternal hormones are responsible for temporary changes in the breasts (enlargement, and production of milk), uterus, and possibly other tissues; and the withdrawal of maternal hormones or other metabolites may contribute to temporary hypofunction of the fetal parathyroid. Blood levels of sugar and calcium are relatively low in the newborn infant, and further decreases (below about 20 mg/dl of sugar or about 7.5 mg/dl of calcium) may cause convulsions.

The gamma globulin level of the newborn infant (almost entirely IgG) is slightly higher than that of the mother, reflecting an active transport mechanism for gamma globulin. Protection is afforded against many viral and some bacterial diseases by antibodies of the IgG variety transferred from mother to infant. Antibodies against certain antigens of gram-negative enterobacteria, on the other hand, are, like isohemagglutinins, found in the IgM fraction of immune globulins, which do not cross the placenta in large amounts. IgM antibodies may be formed, however, by the fetus in response to intrauterine infection. IgA antibodies and IgE (reagins) do not generally cross the placenta. T lymphocyte functions are somewhat reduced in newborn infants.

The gamma globulin level of infants falls to a low level by about 3 mo of age, with a subsequent rise to those levels that characterize older children and adults. Responses to immunization are relatively sluggish in term newborn infants and markedly so in premature ones in comparison with older infants. Antibodies of the major blood group (ABO) system usually appear by the 2nd mo of life.

The digestive enzymes are usually adequate for the diet of the newborn infant, though fat is handled somewhat less well than protein or carbohydrate. At the cellular level, however, a number of deficiencies may have important clinical consequences. The red blood cells of newborn infants have relatively low levels of reduced glutathione, which may contribute to increased hemolysis of red blood cells under a variety of circumstances. A deficiency in capacity of the liver to conjugate bilirubin with glucuronic acid leads to hyperbilirubinemia, often with no evidence of abnormal hemolysis. When hyperbilirubinemia is severe, kernicterus becomes a threat. Evidences of metabolic immaturity generally do not persist beyond the 1st wk in fullterm infants; they may persist longer in the premature.

Behavior. The newborn infant has an unexpected capacity for interaction with the environment and a complex neurologic organization. Whereas traditional assessment of the newborn infant has been concerned with evidence of the level of maturity and with neurologic responses emphasizing reflexology, more attention is now given to more complex aspects of behavior.

Prechtl and others demonstrated that the behavior that can be elicited from the newborn infant is highly dependent upon the *behavioral state* or the level of arousal of the infant. Six levels of arousal have been defined: deep sleep; sleep with rapid eye movements (REM); a drowsy state; a quiet, alert state; an awake and active state; and a state in which the infant is crying intensely. It is in the quiet and alert state that newborn infants are capable of their most complex interactions with the environment. When the behavior of infants has not been modified by anesthetic or other agents given to their mothers and they have been examined under optimal conditions, in the quiet, alert state normal infants are from the moment of birth quite capable of visual fixation on objects and of following the movement of these objects; they will turn their eyes to the source of a sound; they are capable of visual scanning of simple geometric figures; and among somewhat similar and rather complex figures in the visual field they will give preferential attention to figures which more closely resemble the human face.

The mechanisms through which infants hold fixation of faces or of points of contrast, movement, or changing intensity of light within their visual fields are complicated. During the 1st wk of life they are able to maintain these fixations against passive movements of their bodies (doll's eye reflex), and responses originally partly vestibular become increasingly oculomotor alone.

Certain aspects of the behavior of infants in response to change in the environment have been called the *orienting response*. As a new stimulus is received in the auditory or visual fields or through some other sensory modality, the infant becomes more alert, with a suppression of spontaneous movement, with a likely turning of the head toward the stimulus, and with physiologic changes, including changes in heart rate. There is a tendency for the heart to decelerate when the baby orients to a more or less familiar stimulus, whereas cardiac acceleration occurs when a totally unfamiliar or noxious stimulus occurs. When a substantially unchanging new stimulus becomes repetitive the orienting response rapidly habituates; there is less startle reaction or cardiac acceleration, and as the stimulus becomes familiar, cardiac deceleration may supervene.

Brazelton has brought a number of observations together to form a behavior scale which may provide a more precise and predictive assessment of the newborn infant than a traditional neurologic examination or the Apgar rating. Brazelton's scale assesses the behavior of the infant in 4 dimensions: *interactive* processes with the environment (orientation; alertness; consolability; cuddliness); *motor* processes (muscular tone; motor maturity; defensive reactions; hand to mouth activity; general activity level; and reflex behavior); organizational processes involving *control of physiologic state* (habituation to a bright light, a rattle, a bell, and a pin prick; self-quieting behavior); and organizational processes in *response to stress* (tremulousness; lability of skin color; and startle reactions). This Neonatal Behavioral Assessment Scale has been used to identify deficits in neurobehavioral function, to describe the level and quality of normal behavior, to assess the impact on behavior of injury, drugs, and other interventions, and to attempt prediction of future development and function. As late as 1 wk after delivery use of this examination has detected changes in the infant's behavior due to drugs given to the mother (such as phenobarbital). The demonstration to parents of some of the items in the scale may foster healthy attachment as they reveal the infant's complexity and early evidence of the infant's personality and individuality.

The complexity of the behavior potential of the newborn is strikingly shown by the observation that the infant in the 1st minutes of life responds preferentially to figures that resemble a human face. Such behavior may be important in facilitating or eliciting those interactions leading to the formation of *social bonds*. For example, the steady gaze of the newborn infant into her eyes is often felt by the mother as a powerful stimulus to emotional attachment.

The auditory behavior of the infant is also complex. Newborn infants give attention preferentially to high pitched or female voices, and can be shown within the 1st wk of life to turn their heads more readily toward the sounds of their own mothers' voices than to voices not previously heard, and even to be able to distinguish a familiar sound in that maternal voice. Condon and Sander have shown that the motor behavior of infants is responsive to the cadences of speech of a person engaging them in a social relationship. This responsiveness to vocal stimulation may have importance for social bonding.

Other sensory modalities have been less well studied for their social implications. Prenatal and postnatal experiences involve kinesthetic, somesthetic, thermal, olfactory, and proprioceptive stimuli, such as those associated with the intrauterine position. The baby is exposed in utero to the regular rhythm and rate of maternal heart beat; and it has been shown that sounds having the quality, rhythm, and rate of a normal heart beat can sometimes comfort fretful infants. Infants are also capable within the 1st wk of life of differentiating breast pads containing the odor of the milk and breast of their own mothers.

Mother-Infant Bonding or Attachment (Sec 7.13). In the 1st hr or 2 after the normal delivery of a baby who has not been anesthetized or subjected to the effects of analgesic agents, the infant commonly spends a good deal of time in the quiet, alert state of arousal, during which the physiologic conditions fostering the earliest interactions with the environment seem at their best. Events at this time may have a profound influence upon the quality of the relationship established between mother and infant and, to a degree, between the infant and other persons who interact with the baby, even if only as onlookers. Within the next few days the amount of time spent by the baby in this state will constitute about 10% of the day, increasing with age. The sleep of the older fetus and newborn infant is predominantly REM; this predominance begins to change as early as the 2nd day, as new biologic rhythms become established, and changes in the state of the infant become signals for maternal intervention.

Whether there are *critical periods* generally for establishment of optimal mother-infant bonding in humans comparable to critical periods for imprinting in other vertebrate species is not fully resolved, but some losses of opportunities for making the most comfortable and harmonious conditions for interaction between infants and their families may be irretrievable within hours or days after the birth of the infant. These lost opportunities may be reflected in later life in emotional disorders, language or learning disabilities, child abuse and neglect, or failure to achieve potential levels of intellectual function.

Increasing attention to the circumstances surrounding childbirth, and growing concern with the care of mother and infant in the hospital and during the early weeks at home, should lead to substantial revision of some current practices. In particular, there is a need for greater involvement of both mothers and fathers in prenatal activities oriented to education for childbirth and for child rearing, for further encouragement of family-centered programs for pregnancy and childbirth, for greater restraint in the use of analgesic and anesthetic agents in labor, for further encouragement of breast feeding, and for rooming-in arrangements in the neonatal period that optimize the opportunities for newborn infants, their mothers, and their families to get to know each other within the 1st hours and days of life.

2.4 GROWTH AND DEVELOPMENT OF THE INFANT BORN PREMATURELY

See also Sec 7.16.

The fetus born prematurely begins to have substantial chance of survival by about 26–28 wk gestation, at a weight of about 800–1000 gm and length of about 33–35 cm. The premature infant faces difficulties from failure of adequate maturation of enzymatic, renal, metabolic, hematologic, and immunologic mechanisms (Chapter 7).

The behavioral characteristics of premature infants vary with their gestational age. The heads of infants whose birth weights are 1000–1500 gm tend to be rounded and large in relation to body size; the skin seems transparent. They tend to be predominantly atonic and to lie in a tonic neck attitude, often with little motion of the extremities. Vocalization is weak, as are the grasp and Moro responses. The sucking responses may also be weak, and these infants may show little evidence of hunger on deprivation of food. It is difficult to tell when they are awake and when asleep, though they can be stimulated to greater alertness.

Somewhat larger infants, those from 1500–2000 gm, have more subcutaneous tissue and relatively less enlargement of the head. These infants have good muscle tone when stimulated, more vigorous grasp, and complete Moro responses. A sleep pattern is easily discernible, and they are able visually to fixate some objects in their environment. The more vigorous of these babies are able to manage breast feeding.

Infants weighing between 2000–2500 gm at birth generally have the appearance of small fullterm infants, from which they cannot usually be differentiated by developmental examination. They have a good cry and sustained muscle tone.

The average premature infant is likely to gain 6–7 kg (13–15 lb) in the 1st yr, which is the average gain for the fullterm infant. Although a small premature infant, by the time he or she reaches the expected date of delivery, may seem more alert and active than a fullterm baby born on that day, the actual developmental level reached later in the 1st yr will generally be lower than that indicated by chronologic age. The deficit in level tends to correspond to the degree of prematurity. These differences will generally have disappeared by the end of the 2nd yr of life, so long as no complicating factors occur. Developmental defects are more common in premature infants than in fullterm infants and often include impairment of intellectual or motor function.

The premature infant is particularly vulnerable to the effects of sensory or social deprivation in the neonatal period, owing to the restrictions imposed by necessities of care and by the sometimes prolonged period of relative isolation. Recent studies emphasize the importance of involving the mothers of even the smallest babies in some aspects of their care as early as possible to enhance the opportunities for mutual emotional attachment (Sec 7.13).

2.5 GROWTH DURING THE FIRST YEAR

Most fullterm infants regain their birth weight by the age of 10 days. The fullterm infant will generally double the birth weight by 5 mo and triple it in 1 yr. The length of the normal infant increases during the 1st yr by 25–30 cm or 10–12 in. (The average length at birth is 50 cm, or 20 in.) There is a conspicuous increase of subcutaneous tissue in the early months of life, which reaches its peak by about 9 mo.

The anterior fontanel of the newborn infant may increase in size after birth, but generally diminishes after 6 mo and may become effectively closed at any time from 9–18 mo. The posterior fontanel is generally closed on palpation by 4 mo.

The circumference of the head, which is 34–35 cm at birth, increases to approximately 44 cm by 6 mo and to 47 cm by 1 yr (Table 2–1). The circumference of the head is somewhat larger than that of the chest at birth, but the two become approximately equal at 1 yr.

Table 2-1 MEDIAN HEAD CIRCUMFERENCES OF INFANTS AND CHILDREN

BOYS					GIRLS			
MEDIAN	PERCENTILES (5TH–95TH)	MEDIAN	PERCENTILES (5TH–95TH)	AGE	MEDIAN	PERCENTILES (5TH–95TH)	MEDIAN	PERCENTILES (5TH–95TH)
Centimeters		(Inches)			Centimeters		(Inches)	
34.8	32.6–37.2	(13.7)	(12.8–14.7)	Birth	34.3	32.1–35.9	(13.5)	(12.6–14.1)
37.2	34.9–39.6	(14.7)	(13.7–15.6)	1 mo	36.4	34.2–38.3	(14.3)	(13.5–15.1)
40.6	38.4–43.1	(16.0)	(15.1–17.0)	3 mo	39.5	37.3–41.7	(15.6)	(14.7–16.4)
43.8	41.5–46.2	(17.2)	(16.3–18.2)	6 mo	42.4	40.3–44.6	(16.7)	(15.9–17.6)
45.8	43.5–48.1	(18.0)	(17.1–18.9)	9 mo	44.3	42.3–46.4	(17.4)	(16.7–18.3)
47.0	44.8–49.3	(18.5)	(17.6–19.4)	1 yr	45.6	43.5–47.6	(18.0)	(17.1–18.7)
48.4	46.3–50.6	(19.1)	(18.2–19.9)	1.5 yr	47.1	45.0–49.1	(18.5)	(17.7–19.3)
49.2	47.3–51.4	(19.4)	(18.6–20.2)	2 yr	48.1	46.1–50.1	(18.9)	(18.2–19.7)
49.9	48.0–52.2	(19.7)	(18.9–20.6)	2.5 yr	48.8	47.0–50.8	(19.2)	(18.5–20.0)
50.5	48.6–52.8	(19.9)	(19.1–20.8)	3 yr	49.3	47.6–51.4	(19.4)	(18.8–20.2)

From Health Survey of National Center for Health Statistics, 1976 (see footnote to Table 2–6).

ESTIMATING FORMULA (FIRST YEAR ONLY):	BOYS AND GIRLS COMBINED	CENTIMETERS	(INCHES)
Normal range of head circumference (5th–95th percentile) = $\left[\dfrac{\text{Length (cm)}}{2} + 9.5 \right] \pm 2.5$	Median head circumference at 4 yr at 5 yr	50.4 50.8	(19.8) (20.0)
	From Studies of Harvard School of Public Health (see text).		

After Dine et al, 1981.

Deciduous teeth appear in most infants between 5–9 mo. The first to erupt are the lower central incisors, followed by the upper central and then the upper lateral incisors. The lower lateral incisors follow, the 1st deciduous molars, cuspids, and 2nd deciduous molars appearing in that order. By the age of 1 yr most children have 6–8 teeth. Occasionally an infant has as few as 2 teeth at 1 yr without other evidence of growth disturbance.

THE FIRST THREE MONTHS OF LIFE
(Table 2–6)

With the establishment of effective emotional and social bonds with their mothers, with comfortable reciprocal interaction, and with adequate nutrition, infants make rapid developmental progress in the first 3 mo of life. In the 1st days of life infants fixate best visually those objects that are placed close to or moved through their line of vision. Depending upon the quality of the stimulus, they may maintain fixation with movement of the eyes and head to nearly 90° to either side of the midline. By 2 mo of age a supine infant will be able to follow an object presented 90° from the midline through an arc of 180°. Infants very soon differentiate persons and objects in their environments, showing from as early as 2–6 wk of age that they are more comfortable with familiar persons than with strangers. A fully developed social smile becomes manifest usually between 3–5 wk of age. There is evidence that the smile of the very young infant may be elicited basically by the infant's discovery that he or she has control over some contingencies in the environment, such as securing care or attention from mother or another caretaker, or from being able to control the behavior of inanimate objects. The infant who does not have a social smile by the age of 8–12 wk should be regarded as severely deviant with respect either to developmental potential or to quality of antecedent experiences. The infant who at 4 wk was able to make small throaty noises will at 8 wk produce some vowel sounds, and will at 12 wk produce these sounds with evident pleasure on social contact.

A major part of the interaction between mother and infant in the 1st weeks of life is initiated by the infant, not simply as changes of state indicating distress or immediate need, but as part of a growing and complex system of signals between infant and mother (or other caretakers). Through these communicative exchanges emotional attachments are formed; the infant learns to sort out his or her own internal states for their meaning and to convey information regarding them; and the mother learns to read and to respond appropriately to the infant's signals, with activities which have the capacity to comfort, to reassure, or at times to make tolerable the appropriate or necessary frustration or postponement of gratification.

There is reason to feel that during this period the sense of security of the infant will be optimally fostered when care is given by mother or mother-figure in a prompt, loving, and confident manner. Both consistency and promptness seem important in the responses of the caretakers to the behavior of infant or child. In instances of defective mothering the infant's normal or appropriate behavior may not be consistently or reliably rewarded by reduction of tension, or an effective maternal response may come so late and after so much anxiety or tension that the infant cannot associate any specific action of his or her own with relief of tension. Such infants may come to feel that they have no way to affect their environment through their own actions. Long-term retreat, anxiety, or hostility may be the consequences.

The newborn infant placed prone upon a firm surface

is able to avoid suffocation by turning the face from side to side; by 4 wk of age the head is lifted above the surface. By then a rather symmetrical flexed posture has become more relaxed, and he or she is likely to lie, when supine, in a tonic neck posture (head turned to one side).

When the infant within the 1st 4–8 wk of life is pulled from a supine to a sitting position, the head lags, and with the infant in the upright position, head control is absent. By 12 wk of age there is some control of the head as the infant is drawn to a sitting position, but the head is tilted a little forward on the upright body; irregular head control results in a bobbing motion.

The grasp reflex persists until the age of about 8 wk, after which, with growing eye and hand coordination, active grasp becomes more evident. Reaching and grasping evolve out of early coordinate but incomplete motions of the arms and hands ("larval reach") in response to the sight of objects moving nearby; by 12 wk the infant attempts to make contact with an offered object and will hold it briefly if appropriate contact is made. The coordination of eye and hand implicit in this activity seems to be facilitated in some measure by the tonic neck attitude.

THREE TO SIX MONTHS
(Table 2–6)

By the age of 3 mo infants placed prone upon a firm surface are generally able to raise head and chest from the surface, with their arms extended before them. By 4 mo they are able in this position to raise the head to a vertical position and turn it easily from side to side. At 5–6 mo of age the infant begins purposefully to roll over, at first from the prone to the supine position and then in the reverse direction.

Between 3–4 mo of age the infant gradually abandons the tonic neck posture as the predominant posture, and the head becomes generally maintained in the midline, with the arms and legs in more or less symmetric positions, and the hands often brought together in the midline or at the mouth. In this position the 4–6 mo old infant often develops a bald spot over the occiput. By 4 mo the infant becomes more adept in making contact with objects brought within reach and will often bring these to the midline and to the mouth for oral exploration.

When the infant of 4 mo is pulled to a sitting position, the head is brought up without lag; in the upright position the head tilts a little forward, but is held steadily without bobbing. The head will be maintained erect and steady by 5 mo of age.

By 4–5 mo the infant will enjoy being supported in an upright posture and becomes increasingly attracted to objects presented on a plane surface. By 6 mo of age he or she is able to change the orientation of the entire body in order to extend a hand toward a desired object such as a rattle or ring.

At 4 mo of age the infant will be able to grasp an object of moderate size, but will have only limited interest in a small object, such as a pellet. By 7 mo the pellet is promptly seen and may be vigorously pursued by raking motions of the fingers, but the infant is not apt to be able to pick it up.

After 6 mo the functions of the hands are increasingly lodged in the structures on the radial side, the thumb being used in conjunction with the palm. By 6–6½ mo most infants can grasp a large object, such as a rattle, and transfer it from hand to hand.

At 6–6½ mo the infants are often able to sit alone, leaning forward upon their hands, or with slight support of the pelvis; they will not yet have developed a lumbar lordosis, and the spine will have a gentle kyphotic curve from sacrum to cervical region. At 5–6 mo they can often be pulled from a sitting to a standing position and will support their weight upon extended legs. At 6–6½ mo in this same position they will often flex the knees momentarily and return to a standing posture.

As infants become more intricately related to objects and persons in the environment, their smiles continue as catalysts of social exchange; and by 4 mo the infants are able to *laugh aloud* at pleasurable social contacts. They may also show displeasure by changes of expression, fussing, or crying. Between 4–7 mo of age infants become increasingly responsive to the emotional tone of social contacts, and by 7 mo will respond to changes in the facial expressions of those having close rapport with them. By the end of the 6th mo normal infants will have developed clear preferences for social contact with the persons giving the most care, and will, particularly when in mothers' arms, begin to show anxiety at the approach of strangers. In contrast, in a setting where they are alone with a stranger, new social contacts may be accepted without protest. Development of separation anxieties and fear of strangers may depend in some measure on the depth to which infants have developed comfortable patterns of communication and emotional exchange with primary caretakers.

SIX TO TWELVE MONTHS
(Table 2–6)

By 7 mo the infant in the prone position is able to *pivot* in pursuit of an object, but if it is not within reach, may be unable to attain it. By 9–10 mo most infants have learned to *creep* or to *crawl*.

Supine infants are able by 6 mo or so to lift their heads and become increasingly interested in their legs and feet. By 8–9 mo they are able to assume a sitting position without help and are soon able to maintain this with the back straight. They are often able at 8 mo to stand steadily for a short while so long as the hands are held, and by 9 mo may be able to take some steps with both hands held.

Between 6–9 mo the radial palmar grasp becomes clearly elaborated into movements involving thumb and forefinger. The index finger is used to poke at objects by 9 mo and at this time the thumb and forefinger can be brought into sufficiently accurate apposition to permit a pellet to be picked up with a pincer motion. This movement is apt to be made with the ulnar surface of the hand supported on the same surface upon which the pellet lies. By 12 mo the pincer movement will be executed without this ulnar support.

The infant is able to make repetitive vowel sounds at 6½ mo and by 8 mo is likely to execute repetitive consonant sounds, such as ba-ba, ma-ma, da-da, although not necessarily associating these sounds with objects. Children of 8–9 mo become attentive to the sounds of their own names. They may knowingly use a few words besides ma-ma or da-da by the age of 1 yr and may show by their behavior that they know the names of some objects.

The preference for their mothers which was manifested at 6 mo often evolves into separation anxiety between the ages of 6–8 mo. About this same time a mother may experience difficulty in putting a baby to sleep who always went willingly before. Sometimes a mother whose child is fretful when she leaves the room can comfort him or her by maintaining vocal contact. By 9–10 mo infants begin to be less dependent upon the physical presence of their mothers, partly because they are increasingly able to follow her around. Also at this time, if an object which has attracted attention and is covered with a cloth before the infant has an opportunity to grasp it, he or she will be able to uncover it and grasp it with the apparent sure knowledge that its being out of sight does not mean that it is not available. Peek-a-boo often becomes a pleasant game about this time, and gives the infant an opportunity to test and retest his or her ability to recreate the absent parent.

Between 6–12 mo one sees the earliest beginnings of imitative behavior. At 6 mo, if shown how to tap a table, the infant may crudely imitate this behavior. At 9 mo the infant will wave bye-bye or bring the hands together imitatively; at 12 mo a child may enter into very simple games with a toy such as a ball.

At 9 mo an infant may be able to release an object upon request, if the object is grasped as the request is made. By 1 yr most infants will extend the object and release it into an offered hand.

The demands on mother and infant during the 1st yr are for the development of comfortable interactions that will prepare for the infant's movement from a position of dependency to one of relatively independent activity. Failure of achievement of the developmental goals of the 1st yr may be the root of life-long emotional disorders.

2.6 GROWTH AND DEVELOPMENT DURING THE SECOND YEAR

During the 2nd yr of life there is a further deceleration in the rate of growth; the average child will gain about 2.5 kg (5–6 lb) and about 12 cm (5 in) (Tables 2–6 and 2–8). After 10 mo of age there is often a decrease in appetite extending well into the 2nd yr. The result is a loss during the 2nd yr of some of the subcutaneous tissue which reached its maximal development around 9 mo; the plump infant begins to change gradually to the lean and muscular child. The mild lordosis and protuberant abdomen appear that are characteristic of the 2nd and 3rd yr of life.

The growth of the brain decelerates during the 2nd yr; head circumference, which increased approximately 12 cm during the 1st yr, will increase only 2 cm during the 2nd yr. By the end of the 1st yr the brain has reached approximately two thirds, and at the end of the 2nd year four fifths, of its adult size.

A useful set of simple formulas for estimating the normal height and weight of children during the preschool and school years is given in Table 2–2.

During the 2nd yr 8 more teeth erupt, making a total of 14–16, including the first deciduous molars and the cuspids. The order of eruption may be irregular; the cuspids commonly appear after the 1st molars have erupted.

During the 2nd yr the infant moves from an awkward upright stance in which he or she could walk with support to a high degree of locomotor control. By 15 mo infants are generally able to walk alone, and by 18 mo may run stiffly.

At 18 mo the infant can climb stairs, with one hand held, going one step at a time; and by 20 mo he or she is able to go downstairs, one hand held, and may be able to climb stairs holding to the stair railing. By 24 mo the child is able to run well and has generally outgrown the tendency to fall. Between 18–24 mo children normally enter the "run about" age. They are able to move quickly from a safe environment into danger and will need constant surveillance.

With the 2nd yr infants enter a period when they will vigorously and imitatively exploit the objects in their environment. They can empty wastebaskets, drawers, and shelves and may try to examine everything within reach. Above all, household poisons, drugs, and chemicals must be kept in places inaccessible to them.

The child who at 12 mo was able to release a pellet into the hand of a person requesting it will at 15 mo generally be able to put the pellet into a small bottle. He or she may attempt to remove the pellet from the bottle by inserting a finger, and by 18 mo will be able to dump it from the bottle.

By 15 mo the child is able to put a 1-in cube on top of another in response to a demonstration; by 18 mo he or she is able to make a tower of 3 cubes and by 24

Table 2–2 FORMULAS FOR APPROXIMATE AVERAGE HEIGHT AND WEIGHT OF NORMAL INFANTS AND CHILDREN (AFTER WEECH)

WEIGHT	KILOGRAMS	(POUNDS)
(a) at birth	3.25	(7)
(b) 3–12 mo	$\dfrac{age(mo) + 9}{2}$	(age(mo) + 11)
(c) 1–6 yr	age(yr) × 2 + 8	(age(yr) × 5 + 17)
(d) 6–12 yr	$\dfrac{age(yr) \times 7 - 5}{2}$	(age(yr) × 7 + 5)

HEIGHT	CENTIMETERS	(INCHES)
(e) at birth	50	(20)
(f) at 1 yr	75	(30)
(g) 2–12 yr	age(yr) × 6 + 77	(age(yr) × 2½ + 30)

mo a tower of 6 cubes. Imitative behavior and conceptual behavior continue to evolve, with spontaneous scribbling and with imitation of vertical lines at 18 mo; by 24 mo the child imitates circular strokes and can make a horizontal line.

The normal infant commonly has a vocabulary of 10 words by 18 mo. There is wide variation in the times at which words begin to flow readily; it is not unusual for an entirely normal child to have few or no sounds conveying a definite meaning until 18 mo or later. Some children with delay in development of recognizable speech have a rich jargon before communicative sounds appear; this jargon often has many of the intonations and punctuations of human speech, but the sounds otherwise convey no meaning. In those normal children in whom speech is delayed to 18–20 mo, there is often rapid acquisition of words and meaning after this time, with the result that most normal children by their 2nd birthday are able to put 3 words together.

During the 2nd yr the child becomes highly imitative, and increasingly aware of and responsive to other persons, including siblings. Until the end of the 2nd yr, however, play is generally solitary and consists in active manipulation of available objects. During the 3rd yr of life children move increasingly into play activities in which other children are involved. By the end of the 4th yr the child is increasingly engaged in activity with other children in which the group begins to enact imaginative roles and activities. This tendency to role-playing will increase into the school years.

By 18–24 mo most children are able to verbalize their toilet needs and can be helped at this time to follow acceptable social patterns in meeting them. In settings in which the young child has adequate models to follow it seems increasingly evident that toilet training need not become the focus either of emotion-laden educational activity or of disciplinary concern on the part of parents.

The need for children to submit growing control of their bodies and of their environments to social and cultural pressures often produces frustration and anger. Temper tantrums, breath-holding spells, and less dramatic outbursts are common consequences. These episodes respond best to management by a firm and loving parent who is able to set the necessary limits for the child (Sec 2.30 and 2.55).

2.7 GROWTH AND DEVELOPMENT DURING THE PRESCHOOL YEARS

During the 3rd, 4th, and 5th yr of life gains in weight and height are relatively steady at approximately 2.0 kg (4.5 lb) and about 8–6 cm (3½–2½ in)/1 yr, respectively (Tables 2–6 and 2–7). Most children are lean relative to their earlier body configuration. The lordosis and protuberant abdomen of late infancy tend to disappear by the 4th yr along with the pads of fat that underlie the normal arches of the feet during the earlier years.

By 2½ yr the 20 deciduous teeth have usually erupted. During the rest of the preschool period the face tends to grow proportionately more than the cranial cavity and the jaw to widen preparatory to the eruption of permanent teeth.

The refinement of motor skills includes alternation of the feet in ascending stairs by 3 yr and alternation in descending stairs by 4 yr. By 3 yr most children can stand for a short period on 1 foot; by 5 yr they are generally able to hop on 1 foot and soon to skip.

By 3 yr a child may be able to imitiate crudely the drawing of a cross. By 4 yr the cross figure may be copied without previous demonstration, possibly as a 4-element figure. By 4–5 yr the child can make correctly proportionate copies of the figures and for the first time becomes able to handle figures with slanting lines, such as triangles. A diamond-shaped figure may not be accurately and proportionately reproduced until the 6th yr.

By 3 yr the child is able to count 3 objects correctly; a 4 yr old, 4; a 5 yr old, 10 or more.

By 3 yr most children can state their ages and whether they are boys or girls. With the increasing awareness that they are destined to become larger children and adults, children in the later preschool period begin to seek adequate models from whom to learn. The most accessible models are, of course, the parents and other members of the immediate family. The child's imperfect perception of the realities of the future often engenders conflicting pressures and anxieties. A child of 4, 5, or 6 yr assumes those habits of thought, feeling, and action that surround his or her growing perception or fantasy as to the future. Inside the home the child's fantasies about the future roles include playing the part of the parent of the same sex, and there may be increasing curiosity and concern as to what the realities of this role may be.

Outside the home, concerns and fantasies about future roles are likely to be expressed in dramatic play. The interest of children of this age in sex differences, which often appears as questions inside the home, may commonly appear in the form of sex play among children of each sex, which is entirely normal.

Changing patterns of parent-child interaction and of other relations in and out of the home often leave elements of hostility or aggression in the child's behavior, thoughts, and fantasies. Anxieties may be expressed as nightmares or as fears of separation, death, or bodily injury. Children with serious problems may display bedwetting or thumb-sucking, speech or learning difficulties, inability to enter into a comfortable sharing relation, temper tantrums, or other behavior appropriate to earlier developmental levels.

By the age of 6 the child begins to develop the ability to translate abstract conceptions into figures and structures (e.g., the sound of T into the letter T, the idea of two into the figure 2).

2.8 GROWTH AND DEVELOPMENT DURING THE EARLY SCHOOL YEARS

The early school years are a period of relatively steady growth ending in a preadolescent growth spurt by about the age of 10 in girls and about 12 in boys. The average gain in weight during these years is about 3–3.5 kg (7 lb)/1 yr, and in height approximately 6 cm (2½ in)/yr. Growth in head circumference is slowed, the circumference increasing from about 51 cm (20 in) to 53–54 cm (21 in) between the ages of 5–12 yr. At the end of this period the brain has reached virtually adult size.

The school years are a time of vigorous physical activity. The spine becomes straighter, but the child's body is supple, and postures may be assumed that are often disturbing to parents and to teachers. Mild degrees of knock-knee or flatfoot which may be apparent in the late preschool years tend to correct during the 1st yr or 2 of the school years. The motor activities of the earlier years, such as running and climbing, become increasingly directed to more specialized activities and games requiring particular motor and muscular skills.

The development of the facial bones continues actively during the school years, particularly with enlargement of the sinuses. The frontal sinus has usually made its appearance by the 7th yr.

The 1st permanent teeth, the 1st molars, most often erupt during the 7th yr of life. With these so-called 6-yr molars in place, the shedding of deciduous teeth begins, following approximately the same sequence as their acquisition. They are replaced at a rate of about 4 teeth/yr over the next 5 yr. The 2nd permanent molars commonly erupt by the 14th yr; the 3rd molars may not appear until the early 20's.

Lymphatic tissues are at the peak of their development during these years and generally exceed the amount of such tissue in the normal adult. The abundance of lymphoid tissue during this time of life bears some relation to the frequency with which tonsillectomy and adenoidectomy are incorrectly recommended. Respiratory infections are common during these years, and the response of the child to infection begins to be more like that of the adult than of the infant or young child. The usual number of respiratory infections during the school years is high; as many as 6–7 illnesses/yr is not uncommon.

With the removal of a large portion of the child's life from the home to the school environment, children begin increasingly to live independently and to look outside the home for goals and for standards of behavior. This shifting of interests is often anxiety-provoking for parents, and if earlier problems between parent and child have not been adequately resolved, adjustments to forces outside the home are apt to be difficult.

A large responsibility of the school years is the creation in the child of the senses of duty, of responsibility, and of realistic accomplishment. There is a possibility of great frustration for parents and children when the child's achievement does not measure up to parental hopes. The child unable to meet adequate standards may learn for the first time the sense of *failure* and may react with anxiety and hostility. Antisocial behavior may develop through which the child attempts to gain recognition which he or she cannot attain otherwise (Sec 2.72 and 2.76).

2.9 GROWTH AND DEVELOPMENT DURING ADOLESCENCE

Adolescence is the period during which sexual maturation occurs and the body takes final adult form (Sec 2.13). A trend toward increasing height and weight of adults has been evident for the past 100 yr and has probably existed for several centuries. It has been observed in the heights and weights of children as early as the 7th yr of life. This trend toward increasing height and weight may be reaching an asymptote in developed countries. Concurrently, there has been a tendency to earlier appearance of the menarche; in the United States the average age at menarche is now 1 yr earlier (just under 13 yr) than it was a half century ago.

The pace of general physical growth in adolescence can be most accurately assessed by examination of skeletal maturity (bone age); the pace of sexual maturation is closely related to bone age but can be more usefully assessed with sex maturity ratings (Sec 2.13). Physical and sexual changes go hand in hand with cognitive, emotional, social, and cultural changes and adaptations (Sec 2.13 and 2.40).

Medical problems of adolescence include overnutrition and undernutrition, sometimes related to dietary habits determined by social pressure rather than by absence of adequate diet at home. Fatigue is common in adolescence and may be related to protein or iron deficiency, the latter sometimes expressed not so much by anemia as by less than optimal function of enzyme systems using heme prosthetic groups. During adolescence there is heightened susceptibility to some illnesses and heightened reactivity to others. Myopia commonly has its onset during adolescence, as may some orthopedic conditions leading to kyphosis or scoliosis.

Acne, accompanied by a complex folklore and leading to some disfigurement, adds to the physical and emotional burden of adolescents. Adolescents are often reluctant to discuss their acne with the physician, who often must initiate its management (Sec 24.31).

The most significant health problem of adolescence is the frequency with which serious accidents and suicide occur. These are often directly related to the intense physical activity and emotional strivings of this age, particularly in boys. In the accident-prone child repeated accidents may be related to poorly solved problems of earlier life (Sec 2.22).

In adolescence the increasing emotional tension and pressure of biologic drives must meet and ultimately accommodate to increased demands and expectations from the environment. The process of attaining one's *ego identity* or "finding oneself" in adolescence and early adulthood has become prolonged in Western culture as the duration of formal education and dependency increases, and has become complicated by the breakdown of traditional patterns of family life and social class. The quest for one's own set of values involves gender identity, social class identity, and vocational and avocational identity, and takes place increasingly in the community outside the home.

A further stage in development involves an ability to relate to others besides one's parents and to avoid emotional isolation through facing the fear of rejection in shared physical activities such as sports, in close friendships, and in sexual experiences. An aspect of growing intimacy is the sharing of feelings, which is the essential quality of empathy.

The next stage in psychosocial development involves the commitments of persons to each other in love affairs, courtship, or marriage, or to other accepted responsibilities or tasks.

Erikson visualizes the final stage of growth as the ability "to accept one's individual life cycle and the people who have become significant to it as meaningful within the segment of history in which one lives. Integrity thus means a new and different love of one's parents, free of the wish that they should have been different, and an acceptance of the fact that one's life is one's own responsibility. It is a sense of comradeship with men and women of distant times and of different pursuits, who have created orders and objects and sayings conveying human dignity and love."

2.10 SPECIAL ASPECTS OF GROWTH

Many structural and functional details of growth and development are inconspicuous for the broad pattern outlined above, but take on significance as they become foci of clinical concern or contribute to the evaluation or management of a clinical problem. The physician who monitors the growth and development of the child will need to know or find the limits of normal variability in these details, not only quantitatively and qualitatively, but also with respect to their interrelations.

VARIABILITY IN BODY PROPORTIONS

Besides the profound changes in general body proportions between fetal life and adult life (Fig 2–1), there are also individual differences which express innate growth potential and environmental modifications. These variations in body forms of normal persons may be termed differences in *physique*. *Somatotype* connotes loosely the potentialities at the time of birth for the development of a particular physique: ectomorphic, mesomorphic, and endomorphic. The ectomorph is characterized by relative linearity, light bone structure, and small mass in respect to body length. The endomorph is characterized by relatively stocky build, with large amounts of soft tissue. The pattern of the mesomorph is between that of ectomorph and endomorph. Psychic and other functional attributes may be loosely related to somatotype.

Somatotype may be evident in early childhood or become clear only with the termination of the growth period. Somatotype does not seem to be closely related to the ultimate height or weight achieved, but the endomorph appears to mature earlier than the ectomorph. As a result of this early maturation the endomorphic child may have a tendency to be taller than

the ectomorphic one in late childhood, the differences being reduced as the ectomorph completes growth.

Other changes in bodily proportions depend not on somatotype but on different rates of growth of body parts: for example, head size relative to body length, and length of extremities relative to total body length. The size of the brain and cranial cavity approaches adult levels much more rapidly than the size of the face or the length of the legs. This relative preponderance of growth at the cephalad part of the body in fetal life, infancy, and early childhood, with corresponding early elaboration of function, followed by the growth of trunk and extremities, has been termed the cephalocaudad progression.

Alterations in proportionate sizes of trunk, extremities, and head are characteristic of certain disturbances of growth and may give insight into the underlying pathophysiologic process. The measurements which are usually most helpful are sitting and standing heights, span, body weight, and circumference of head. Normally, sitting height represents about 70% of body length in the newborn infant, 57% at 3 yr, and about 52% at the time of menarche in girls and at about 15 yr in boys. There is then a slight increase of 1–2 percentage points, as the trunk continues some growth after the extremities have finished growing.

Other variations in growth pattern, correlated with function, are distinctive for a number of body systems. Fig 2–2 illustrates the proportionate rates of growth for several body systems. Standards are available for the weights of organs at various ages, which indicate that organs follow characteristic patterns that may be des-

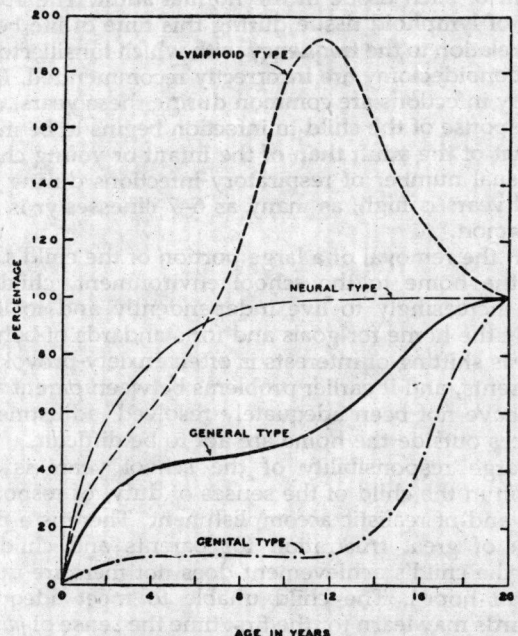

Figure 2–2 Main types of postnatal growth of the various parts and organs of the body. (After Scammon: The measurement of the body in childhood. *In* Harris et al.: The Measurement of Man. Minneapolis, University of Minnesota Press, 1930.)

ignated as lymphoid, neural, general, and genital. There are a number of deviations. For example, although the ovary and testes follow the designated genital pattern, the uterus and adrenals are relatively large at birth, and show involution in the early weeks of life. The spleen appears to follow the lymphoid pattern, and the liver the general growth pattern. Skeletal muscle follows the general pattern, but is slow to achieve its ultimate mass. Cardiac muscle is initially proportionately large to body size and thereafter follows the general growth curve.

The weight of the thymus is labile in childhood, decreasing rapidly during illness. It appears to follow the general pattern of growth during the 1st 5 yr of life, then maintains a relatively steady state, with involution at adolescence.

As indicated earlier, the proportionate mass of sub-

cutaneous tissue is greatest by about 9 mo; it then decreases steadily to about 6 yr, when the increase begins that presages the "fat spurt" in preadolescence, at which time sex differences become apparent (Fig 2–3).

EVALUATION OF OSSEOUS MATURATION

The ossification of the skeleton of the fetus begins by about the 5th mo and from that time makes considerable demands upon the maternal supply of bone-forming substances. Ossification occurs earliest in the clavicles and membranous bone of the skull, and follows rapidly in long bones and spine. The distal femoral and proximal tibial epiphyses are usually ossified in the normal fullterm infant. The fusion of the humeral capitellum with the shaft is said to mark the end of the period of most rapid growth in girls and to predict menarche within the next year.

There is no better index of general growth than bone age as determined from roentgenograms. This is based (1) on the number and size of epiphyseal centers at a given chronologic age, (2) on the size, shape, density, and sharpness of outline of the ends of bones, and (3) on the distance separating epiphyseal center and zone of provisional calcification or the degree of fusion between these 2 elements. The information gained from the various epiphyseal areas varies with chronologic age. The hand and wrist are useful at all ages of childhood; useful information can also be derived from the leg, especially in early infancy. Table 2–3 shows expected times of appearance and fusion of various ossification centers, with normal variabilities for each. Since girls are more advanced than boys in skeletal development at all ages, separate standards are necessary. No interpretation of skeletal age should fail to take into account that 1 normal child in 20 can be expected to have a skeletal age either advanced or retarded by 2 standard deviations from the mean for his or her chronologic age. In boys the standard deviation of bone age around chronologic age is about 2 mo in the 1st yr of life, and increases to 4 mo during the 2nd yr, to 6 mo during the 3rd yr, and to 10 mo by the 7th yr. Thereafter, for the rest of the growth period, the standard deviation is about 12–15 mo. The variability is less for girls than for boys, especially in later childhood.

EVALUATION OF DENTAL DEVELOPMENT

See also Chapter 11.

The calcification of teeth begins in fetal life about the 7th mo. This calcification involves principally deciduous teeth, but shortly before term, calcification begins in the permanent teeth which will be first to erupt.

Nutritional disorders and prolonged illness in infancy may interfere with calcification of deciduous and permanent teeth. Such nutritional disturbances, if temporary, may leave defects in the enamel ranging from a line of small pits across the tooth to a broader band of hypoplasia. It is possible at times to date a nutritional disturbance by these bands of hypoplasia.

The formation of healthy tooth structure is fostered

BREADTHS OF SOFT TISSUES IN CALF FROM A-P ROENTGENOGRAMS OF LEG

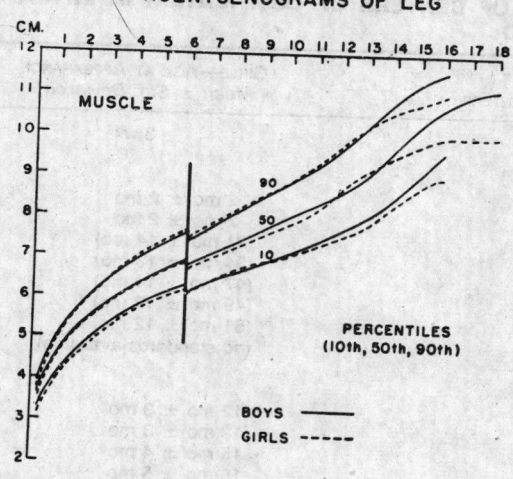

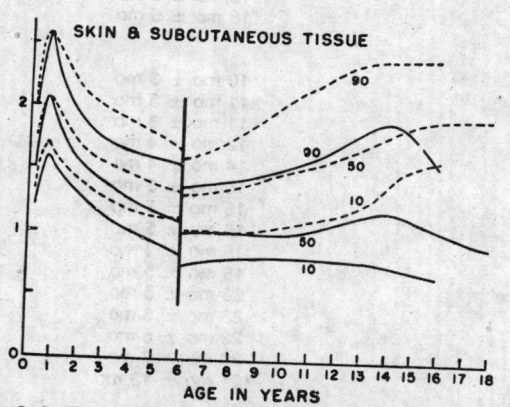

Figure 2–3 Breadths of muscle and of double layers of skin and subcutaneous tissue at greatest width of calf by age and sex from 3 mo to 18 yr of age. The graphs reveal the close similarity in pattern of the curves for muscle to those of general growth, but a unique pattern of increase and decrease and a sex difference in the skin and subcutaneous tissue. (For details, see Stuart and Sobel: J Pediatr 28:637, 1946, and Lombard: Child Dev, Vol 21, 1950. For distribution of subcutaneous fat in childhood and adolescence, see Reynolds: Monographs Soc Res Child Dev, Vol 15, 1950.)

by a diet adequate in protein, calcium, phosphate, and vitamins, especially C and D, and depends further upon an adequate supply of thyroid hormone. The resistance of teeth to dental caries is significantly increased when fluoride is available in optimal quantities.

Table 2–4 lists the times of eruption of the deciduous and permanent teeth. Delay in eruption of deciduous teeth occurs in hypothyroidism and in other nutritional and growth disturbances, but the normal variability in eruption prevents such delay from being useful as an index of a growth disorder. In some families the children have conspicuously early or late dentition without other signs of retardation or acceleration of growth.

The 1st permanent teeth to erupt are the 6-yr molars; they may be mistaken for deciduous teeth. The 1st permanent molars stabilize the dental arch and have a great deal to do with the ultimate shape of the jaw and the orderly arrangement of teeth. Caries or other defects

in them should receive prompt attention; extraction of these teeth should be avoided.

SPECIAL ASPECTS OF GROWTH IN THE RESPIRATORY TRACT AND THE CARDIOVASCULAR SYSTEM

Anatomically, the upper respiratory tract of the newborn infant is distinguished by the lack of well-developed accessory sinuses, by the close relation of the nasopharynx to the middle ear through a eustachian tube which is relatively short and broad, and by the absence of well-developed mastoid air cells. The sphenoidal sinuses appear by about the age of 3 yr, and the frontal sinuses between 3–7 yr of age.

Fig 2–4 and 2–5 show the pulse and respiratory rates for children of various ages and indicate the distinctive differences between boys and girls that become evident at adolescence. See Chapters 12 and 13 for other aspects of development of these systems.

Table 2–3A. TIME OF APPEARANCE IN ROENTGENOGRAMS OF CENTERS OF OSSIFICATION IN INFANCY AND CHILDHOOD

BOYS—AGE AT APPEARANCE Mean ± Std. Deviation*	BONES AND EPIPHYSEAL CENTERS	GIRLS—AGE AT APPEARANCE Mean ± Std. Deviation*
3 wk	*Humerus*, head	3 wk
	Carpal bones	
2 mo ± 2 mo	Capitate	2 mo ± 2 mo
3 mo ± 2 mo	Hamate	2 mo ± 2 mo
(30 mo ± 16 mo)	(Triangular)†	(21 mo ± 14 mo)
(42 mo ± 19 mo)	(Lunate)†	(34 mo ± 13 mo)
(67 mo ± 19 mo)	(Trapezium)†	(47 mo ± 14 mo)
(69 mo ± 15 mo)	(Trapezoid)†	(49 mo ± 12 mo)
(66 mo ± 15 mo)	(Scaphoid)†	(51 mo ± 12 mo)
(no standards available)	(Pisiform)†	(no standards available)
	Metacarpal bones	
18 mo ± 5 mo	II	12 mo ± 3 mo
20 mo ± 5 mo	III	13 mo ± 3 mo
23 mo ± 6 mo	IV	15 mo ± 4 mo
26 mo ± 7 mo	V	16 mo ± 5 mo
32 mo ± 9 mo	I	18 mo ± 5 mo
	Fingers (epiphyses)	
16 mo ± 4 mo	Proximal phalanx, 3rd finger	10 mo ± 3 mo
16 mo ± 4 mo	Proximal phalanx, 2nd finger	11 mo ± 3 mo
17 mo ± 5 mo	Proximal phalanx, 4th finger	11 mo ± 3 mo
19 mo ± 7 mo	Distal phalanx, 1st finger	12 mo ± 4 mo
21 mo ± 5 mo	Proximal phalanx, 5th finger	14 mo ± 4 mo
24 mo ± 6 mo	Middle phalanx, 3rd finger	15 mo ± 5 mo
24 mo ± 6 mo	Middle phalanx, 4th finger	15 mo ± 5 mo
26 mo ± 6 mo	Middle phalanx, 2nd finger	16 mo ± 5 mo
28 mo ± 6 mo	Distal phalanx, 3rd finger	18 mo ± 4 mo
28 mo ± 6 mo	Distal phalanx, 4th finger	18 mo ± 5 mo
32 mo ± 7 mo	Proximal phalanx, 1st finger	20 mo ± 5 mo
37 mo ± 9 mo	Distal phalanx, 5th finger	23 mo ± 6 mo
37 mo ± 8 mo	Distal phalanx, 2nd finger	23 mo ± 6 mo
39 mo ± 10 mo	Middle phalanx, 5th finger	22 mo ± 7 mo
152 mo ± 18 mo	Sesamoid (adductor pollicis)	121 mo ± 13 mo
	Hip and knee	
Usually present at birth	Femur, distal	Usually present at birth
Usually present at birth	Tibia, proximal	Usually present at birth
4 mo ± 2 mo	Femur, head	4 mo ± 2 mo
46 mo ± 11 mo	Patella	29 mo ± 7 mo
	Foot and ankle‡	

*To nearest month.
†Except for the capitate and hamate bones, the variability of carpal centers is too great to make them very useful clinically.
‡Standards for the foot are available, but normal variation is wide, including some familial variants, so that this area is of little clinical use.

Table 2-3B. MODAL AGE AT ONSET AND COMPLETION OF FUSION IN SKELETAL AREAS IN ADOLESCENCE

Boys—Modal Age Between	Area	Girls—Modal Age Between
	Elbow	
13.0–13.5 yr	Onset in humerus	11.0–11.5 yr
15.0–15.5	Complete in ulna	12.5–13.0
	Foot and ankle	
14.0–14.5	Onset in great toe	12.5–13.0
15.5–16	Complete in tibia, fibula	14.0–14.5
	Hand and wrist	
15.0–15.5	Onset in distal phalanges	13.0–13.5
17.5–18.0	Complete in radius	16.0–16.5
	Knee	
15.0–15.5	Onset in tibial tuberosity	13.5–14.0
17.5–18.0	Complete in fibula	16.0–16.5
	Hip and pelvis	
15.5–16.0	Onset in greater trochanter	14.0–14.5
after 18.0	Complete in symphysis	17.5–18.0
	Shoulder and clavicle	
15.5–16.0	Onset in greater tubercle of humerus	14.0–14.5
after 18.0	Complete in clavicle	17.5–18.0

The norms in Table 2-3 present a composite of published data from the Fels Research Institute, Yellow Springs, Ohio (Pyle SI, Sontag L. Am J Roentgenol Vol 49, 1943), and unpublished data from the Brush Foundation, Case Western Reserve University, Cleveland, Ohio, and the Harvard School of Public Health, Boston, Massachusetts. Compiled by Lieb, Buehl, and Pyle.

SPECIAL ASPECTS OF GROWTH IN NUTRITION AND METABOLISM

A child's nutritional requirements increase with growth in size, and many nutritional factors bear their most nearly constant relationship to body surface, which appears to be as closely related to the body's mass of metabolically active tissue as any other simple measurement. Owing, however, to fundamental differences in the metabolic activity of infants and children at various ages, adjustments may be necessary. This is particularly evident with respect to administration of drugs in the neonatal period (Sec 5.49).

Measurements of body surface which correspond to given heights and weights are available; reasonably accurate estimates of body surface can be obtained from nomograms (Chapter 29). Cruder estimates of body

Table 2-4 CHRONOLOGY OF HUMAN DENTITION
Primary or Deciduous Teeth

	CALCIFICATION		ERUPTION		SHEDDING	
	Begins at	Complete at	Maxillary	Mandibular	Maxillary	Mandibular
Central incisors	5th fetal mo	18–24 mo	6–8 mo	5–7 mo	7–8 yr	6–7 yr
Lateral incisors	5th fetal mo	18–24 mo	8–11 mo	7–10 mo	8–9 yr	7–8 yr
Cuspids (canines)	6th fetal mo	30–36 mo	16–20 mo	16–20 mo	11–12 yr	9–11 yr
First molars	5th fetal mo	24–30 mo	10–16 mo	10–16 mo	10–11 yr	10–12 yr
Second molars	6th fetal mo	36 mo	20–30 mo	20–30 mo	10–12 yr	11–13 yr

Secondary or Permanent Teeth

	CALCIFICATION		ERUPTION	
	Begins at	Complete at	Maxillary	Mandibular
Central incisors	3–4 mo	9–10 yr	7–8 yr	6–7 yr
Lateral incisors	Max., 10–12 mo Mand., 3–4 mo	10–11 yr	8–9 yr	7–8 yr
Cuspids (canines)	4–5 mo	12–15 yr	11–12 yr	9–11 yr
First premolars (bicuspids)	18–21 mo	12–13 yr	10–11 yr	10–12 yr
Second premolars (bicuspids)	24–30 mo	12–14 yr	10–12 yr	11–13 yr
First molars	Birth	9–10 yr	6–7 yr	6–7 yr
Second molars	30–36 mo	14–16 yr	12–13 yr	12–13 yr
Third molars	Max., 7–9 yr Mand., 8–10 yr	18–25 yr	17–22 yr	17–22 yr

Adapted from chart prepared by PK Losch, Harvard School of Dental Medicine, who provided the data for this chart.

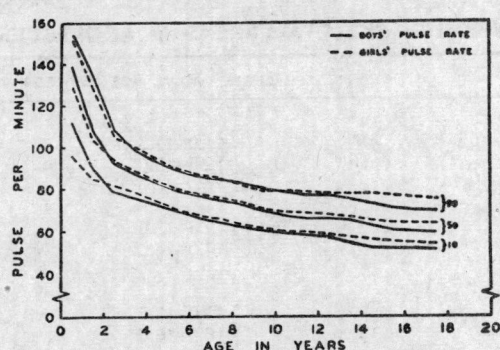

Figure 2–4 Pulse rates in infants and children.

**Table 2–5 APPROXIMATION OF SURFACE AREA (M²)
TO WEIGHT (KG)**

WEIGHT RANGE	APPROXIMATE SURFACE AREA
1 to 5 kg	$M^2 = (0.05 \times kg) + 0.05$
6 to 10 kg	$M^2 = (0.04 \times kg) + 0.10$
11 to 20 kg	$M^2 = (0.03 \times kg) + 0.20$
21 to 40 kg	$M^2 = (0.02 \times kg) + 0.40$

(The figures 5, 10, 20, and 40 are given in italics to indicate a simple mnemonic. The formula $M^2 = (0.02 \times kg) + 40$ is reasonably accurate from 21 to 70 kg.)

surface from weight only can be made for children whose physique is average; Lowe's formula is:

$$\text{surface area } (M^2) = \sqrt[3]{Wt^2} \text{ (kg)} \times 0.1$$

Other crude estimates for children of average physique are given by the simpler formulas in Table 2–5.

Basal caloric needs, when referred to body surface, appear to be somewhat lower in premature infants than in fullterm ones. They increase during the 1st yr of life from approximately 30 cal/M²/hr to about 50 by the 2nd yr, with a subsequent fall to adult levels of 35–40 cal/M²/hr. The rate of fall is slowed during prepubertal and adolescent years because of the need for additional energy for accelerated growth.

Needs for water and electrolytes remain roughly constant in their proportion to body surface through most of the growing period; the inevitable variations in intake are met by the capacity of homeostatic mechanisms to adjust to varying conditions of supply and demand.

DEVELOPMENTAL ASPECTS OF DRUG METABOLISM

Two developmental considerations modify the use of drugs in children. The first is the result of genetic variability, with the rate of metabolism or the pharmacologic effect of some substances being genetically determined through the activities of acetylation, methylation, demethylation, sulfation, and other processes. Specifically, for example, the rapidity of acetylation and

excretion of such drugs as isoniazid, hydralazine, and some sulfonamides is genetically set by autosomal recessive genes. Persons who are "fast acetylators" may need larger doses of drugs and respond poorly to them, whereas slow acetylators are at higher risk of toxic effects associated with elevated levels.

The second consideration is the rapidity with which the infant or child acquires a normal capacity to metabolize drugs for which the metabolic pathways are at birth incomplete or incompletely activated. Normal activities of glucuronidase, phenylalanine transaminase, and other enzymes may be achieved only after days, weeks, or months, sometimes with clinical consequences. Other developmental aspects of pharmacology not well understood include the paradoxic reactions of some children to some drugs; excitement as a response to phenobarbital and abatement of hyperkinesis with dextroamphetamine are examples. Moreover, children appear to have increased sensitivity to the effects of some drugs under other conditions; children with deficiencies of glucose-6-phosphate dehydrogenase (G-6-PD) have, for example, generally more severe reactions from ingestion of offending drugs than do susceptible adults.

2.11 ASSESSMENT OF PHYSICAL GROWTH AND DEVELOPMENT

Appraisal of growth and development in the infant and the child has its greatest usefulness only if it is accurate and continuous in each of the areas in which changes can be observed. In the infant the most useful physical measurements are head circumference, length, and weight (Fig 2–6 and 2–7 and Tables 2–6, 2–7, and 2–8). Note should also be made of the nutritional state, dentition, and the size or patency of fontanels.

In selected instances measurements of subcutaneous tissue (skinfold thickness) or of lengths of body segments (extremities, span, or sitting height) may be appropriate. Skinfold thickness will be useful in estimation of lean body mass and in study and management of obesity.

Charts depicting the course of normal growth, with indications of its variability, were developed a generation ago. Among them have been the Harvard and Iowa charts and the Wetzel grid, data for which were derived from Caucasian children of predominantly middle-class origin. Such charts may not reflect the characteristic

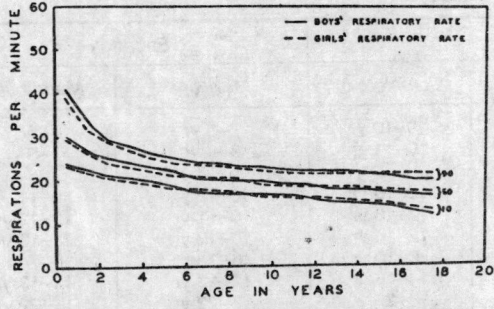

Figure 2–5 Respiratory rates in infants and children.

Text continued on page 33

Table 2–6 LENGTH, WEIGHT AND HEAD CIRCUMFERENCE BY AGE BOYS AND GIRLS: BIRTH TO 36 MONTHS

Age	BOYS: percentiles 5th	10th	25th	50th	75th	90th	95th	Measurement	GIRLS: percentiles 5th	10th	25th	50th	75th	90th	95th
	46.4 (18¼)	47.5 (18¾)	49.0 (19¼)	50.5 (20)	51.8 (20½)	53.5 (21)	54.4 (21½)	Length-cm (in)	45.4 (17¾)	46.5 (18¼)	48.2 (19)	49.9 (19¾)	51.0 (20)	52.0 (20½)	52.9 (20¾)
BIRTH	2.54 (5½)	2.78 (6¼)	3.00 (6½)	3.27 (7¼)	3.64 (8)	3.82 (8½)	4.15 (9¼)	Weight-kg (lb)	2.36 (5¼)	2.58 (5¾)	2.93 (6½)	3.23 (7)	3.52 (7¾)	3.64 (8)	3.81 (8½)
	32.6 (12¾)	33.0 (13)	33.9 (13¼)	34.8 (13¾)	35.6 (14)	36.6 (14½)	37.2 (14¾)	Head C-cm (in)	32.1 (12¾)	32.9 (13)	33.5 (13¼)	34.3 (13½)	34.8 (13¾)	35.5 (14)	35.9 (14¼)
	50.4 (19¾)	51.3 (20¼)	53.0 (20¾)	54.6 (21½)	56.2 (22¼)	57.7 (22¾)	58.6 (23)	Length-cm (in)	49.2 (19¼)	50.2 (19¾)	51.9 (20½)	53.5 (21)	54.9 (21½)	56.1 (22)	56.9 (22½)
1 month	3.16 (7)	3.43 (7½)	3.82 (8½)	4.29 (9½)	4.75 (10½)	5.14 (11¼)	5.38 (11¾)	Weight-kg (lb)	2.97 (6½)	3.22 (7)	3.59 (8)	3.98 (8¾)	4.36 (9½)	4.65 (10¼)	4.92 (10¾)
	34.9 (13¾)	35.4 (14)	36.2 (14¼)	37.2 (14¾)	38.1 (15)	39.0 (15¼)	39.6 (15½)	Head C-cm (in)	34.2 (13½)	34.8 (13¾)	35.6 (14)	36.4 (14¼)	37.1 (14½)	37.8 (15)	38.3 (15)
	56.7 (22¼)	57.7 (22¾)	59.4 (23½)	61.1 (24)	63.0 (24¾)	64.5 (25½)	65.4 (25¾)	Length-cm (in)	55.4 (21¾)	56.2 (22¼)	57.8 (22¾)	59.5 (23½)	61.2 (24)	62.7 (24¾)	63.4 (25)
3 months	4.43 (9¾)	4.78 (10½)	5.32 (11¾)	5.98 (13¼)	6.56 (14½)	7.14 (15¾)	7.37 (16¼)	Weight-kg (lb)	4.18 (9¼)	4.47 (9¾)	4.88 (10¾)	5.40 (12)	5.90 (13)	6.39 (14)	6.74 (14¾)
	38.4 (15)	38.9 (15¼)	39.7 (15¾)	40.6 (16)	41.7 (16½)	42.5 (16¾)	43.1 (17)	Head C-cm (in)	37.3 (14¾)	37.8 (15)	38.7 (15¼)	39.5 (15½)	40.4 (16)	41.2 (16¼)	41.7 (16½)
	63.4 (25)	64.4 (25¼)	66.1 (26)	67.8 (26¾)	69.7 (27½)	71.3 (28)	72.3 (28½)	Length-cm (in)	61.8 (24¼)	62.6 (24¾)	64.2 (25¼)	65.9 (26)	67.8 (26¾)	69.4 (27¼)	70.2 (27¾)
6 months	6.20 (13¾)	6.61 (14½)	7.20 (15¾)	7.85 (17¼)	8.49 (18¾)	9.10 (20)	9.46 (20¾)	Weight-kg (lb)	5.79 (12¾)	6.12 (13½)	6.60 (14½)	7.21 (16)	7.83 (17¼)	8.38 (18½)	8.73 (19¼)
	41.5 (16¼)	42.0 (16½)	42.8 (16¾)	43.8 (17¼)	44.7 (17½)	45.6 (18)	46.2 (18¼)	Head C-cm (in)	40.3 (15¾)	40.9 (16)	41.6 (16½)	42.4 (16¾)	43.3 (17)	44.1 (17¼)	44.6 (17½)
	68.0 (26¾)	69.1 (27¼)	70.6 (27¾)	72.3 (28½)	74.0 (29¼)	75.9 (30)	77.1 (30¼)	Length-cm (in)	66.1 (26)	67.0 (26½)	68.7 (27)	70.4 (27¾)	72.4 (28½)	74.0 (29¼)	75.0 (29½)
9 months	7.52 (16½)	7.95 (17½)	8.56 (18¾)	9.18 (20¼)	9.88 (21¾)	10.49 (23¼)	10.93 (24)	Weight-kg (lb)	7.00 (15½)	7.34 (16¼)	7.89 (17½)	8.56 (18¾)	9.24 (20¼)	9.83 (21¾)	10.17 (22½)
	43.5 (17¼)	44.0 (17¼)	44.8 (17¾)	45.8 (18)	46.6 (18¼)	47.5 (18¾)	48.1 (19)	Head C-cm (in)	42.3 (16¾)	42.8 (16¾)	43.5 (17¼)	44.3 (17½)	45.1 (17¾)	46.0 (18)	46.4 (18¼)
	71.7 (28¼)	72.8 (28¾)	74.3 (29¼)	76.1 (30)	77.7 (30½)	79.8 (31½)	81.2 (32)	Length-cm (in)	69.8 (27½)	70.8 (27¾)	72.4 (28½)	74.3 (29¼)	76.3 (30)	78.0 (30¾)	79.1 (31¼)
12 months	8.43 (18½)	8.84 (19½)	9.49 (21)	10.15 (22½)	10.91 (24)	11.54 (25½)	11.99 (26½)	Weight-kg (lb)	7.84 (17¼)	8.19 (18)	8.81 (19½)	9.53 (21)	10.23 (22½)	10.87 (24)	11.24 (24¾)
	44.8 (17¾)	45.3 (17¾)	46.1 (18¼)	47.0 (18½)	47.9 (18¾)	48.8 (19¼)	49.3 (19½)	Head C-cm (in)	43.5 (17¼)	44.1 (17¼)	44.8 (17¾)	45.6 (18)	46.4 (18¼)	47.2 (18½)	47.6 (18¾)
	77.5 (30½)	78.7 (31)	80.5 (31¾)	82.4 (32½)	84.3 (33¼)	86.6 (34)	88.1 (34¾)	Length-cm (in)	76.0 (30)	77.2 (30½)	78.8 (31)	80.9 (31¾)	83.0 (32¾)	85.0 (33½)	86.1 (34)
18 months	9.59 (21¼)	9.92 (21¾)	10.67 (23½)	11.47 (25¼)	12.31 (27¼)	13.05 (28¾)	13.44 (29½)	Weight-kg (lb)	8.92 (19¾)	9.30 (20½)	10.04 (22¼)	10.82 (23¾)	11.55 (25½)	12.30 (27)	12.76 (28¼)
	46.3 (18¼)	46.7 (18½)	47.4 (18¾)	48.4 (19)	49.3 (19½)	50.1 (19¾)	50.6 (20)	Head C-cm (in)	45.0 (17¾)	45.6 (18)	46.3 (18¼)	47.1 (18½)	47.9 (18¾)	48.6 (19¼)	49.1 (19¼)
	82.3 (32½)	83.5 (32¾)	85.6 (33¾)	87.6 (34½)	89.9 (35½)	92.2 (36¼)	93.8 (37)	Length-cm (in)	81.3 (32)	82.5 (32½)	84.2 (33¼)	86.5 (34)	88.7 (35)	90.8 (35¾)	92.0 (36¼)
24 months	10.54 (23¼)	10.85 (24)	11.65 (25¾)	12.59 (27¾)	13.44 (29¾)	14.29 (31½)	14.70 (32½)	Weight-kg (lb)	9.87 (21¾)	10.26 (22½)	11.10 (24½)	11.90 (26¼)	12.74 (28)	13.57 (30)	14.08 (31)
	47.3 (18½)	47.7 (18¾)	48.3 (19)	49.2 (19¼)	50.2 (19¾)	51.0 (20)	51.4 (20¼)	Head C-cm (in)	46.1 (18¼)	46.5 (18¼)	47.3 (18½)	48.1 (19)	48.8 (19¼)	49.6 (19½)	50.1 (19¾)
	87.0 (34¼)	88.2 (34¾)	90.1 (35½)	92.3 (36¼)	94.6 (37¼)	97.0 (38¼)	98.7 (38¾)	Length-cm (in)	86.0 (33¾)	87.0 (34¼)	88.9 (35)	91.3 (36)	93.7 (37)	95.6 (37¾)	96.9 (38¼)
30 months	11.44 (25¼)	11.80 (26)	12.63 (27¾)	13.67 (30¼)	14.51 (32)	15.47 (34)	15.97 (35¼)	Weight-kg (lb)	10.78 (23¾)	11.21 (24¾)	12.11 (26¾)	12.93 (28½)	13.93 (30¾)	14.81 (32¾)	15.35 (33¾)
	48.0 (19)	48.4 (19)	49.1 (19¼)	49.9 (19¾)	51.0 (20)	51.7 (20¼)	52.2 (20½)	Head C-cm (in)	47.0 (18½)	47.3 (18½)	48.0 (19)	48.8 (19¼)	49.4 (19½)	50.3 (19¾)	50.8 (20)
	91.2 (36)	92.4 (36½)	94.2 (37)	96.5 (38)	98.9 (39)	101.4 (40)	103.1 (40½)	Length-cm (in)	90.0 (35½)	91.0 (35¾)	93.1 (36¾)	95.6 (37¾)	98.1 (38½)	100.0 (39¼)	101.5 (40)
36 months	12.26 (27)	12.69 (28)	13.58 (30)	14.69 (32½)	15.59 (34½)	16.66 (36¾)	17.28 (38)	Weight-kg (lb)	11.60 (25½)	12.07 (26½)	12.99 (28¾)	13.93 (30¾)	15.03 (33¼)	15.97 (35¼)	16.54 (36½)
	48.6 (19¼)	49.0 (19¼)	49.7 (19½)	50.5 (20)	51.5 (20¼)	52.3 (20½)	52.8 (20¾)	Head C-cm (in)	47.6 (18¾)	47.9 (18¾)	48.5 (19)	49.3 (19½)	50.0 (19¾)	50.8 (20)	51.4 (20¼)

These data are those of the National Center for Health Statistics (NCHS), Health Resources Administration, DHEW. They were based on studies of The Fels Research Institute, Yellow Springs, Ohio. Metric data have been smoothed by a least-squares cubic spline technique. For details see Hamill PVV, et al: NCHS Growth Charts, 1976. Monthly Vital Statistics Report *25*(3):1, 1976, and page 33 of this volume. These data and those in Tables 2–7 and 2–8 were first made available to us with the help of William M. Moore, M.D., of Ross Laboratories, who supplied the conversion from metric measurements to approximate inches and pounds. This help is gratefully acknowledged.

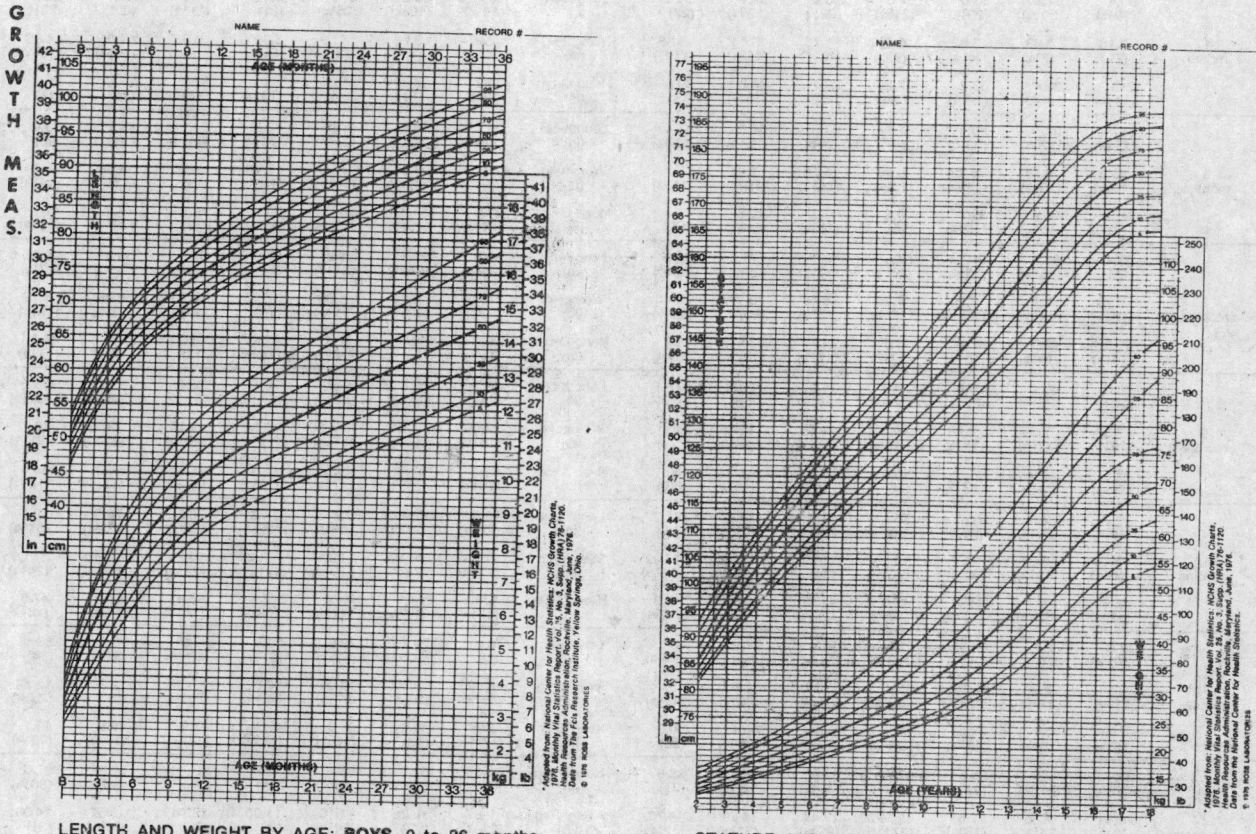

LENGTH AND WEIGHT BY AGE: **BOYS**, 0 to 36 months

STATURE AND WEIGHT BY AGE: **BOYS**, 2 to 18 years

Figure 2–6A

Figures 2–6A and 2–6B. (opposite). Charts for BOYS and GIRLS of *length [or stature] by age* (upper curves) and *weight by age* (lower curves), each curve corresponding to the indicated percentile level. These charts are based upon the data in Tables 2–6 and 2–7 and have been adapted from NCHS Growth Charts by Ross Laboratories. Permission to use them is gratefully acknowledged.

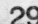

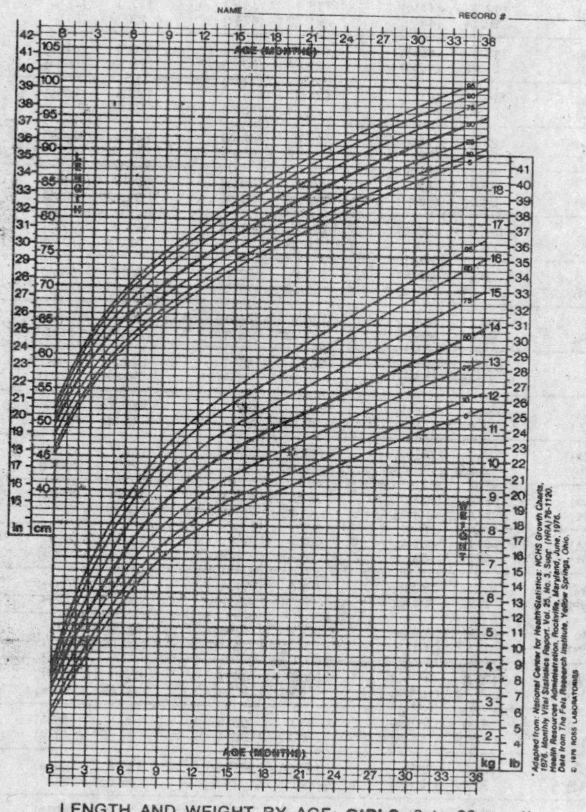

LENGTH AND WEIGHT BY AGE: **GIRLS**, 0 to 36 months

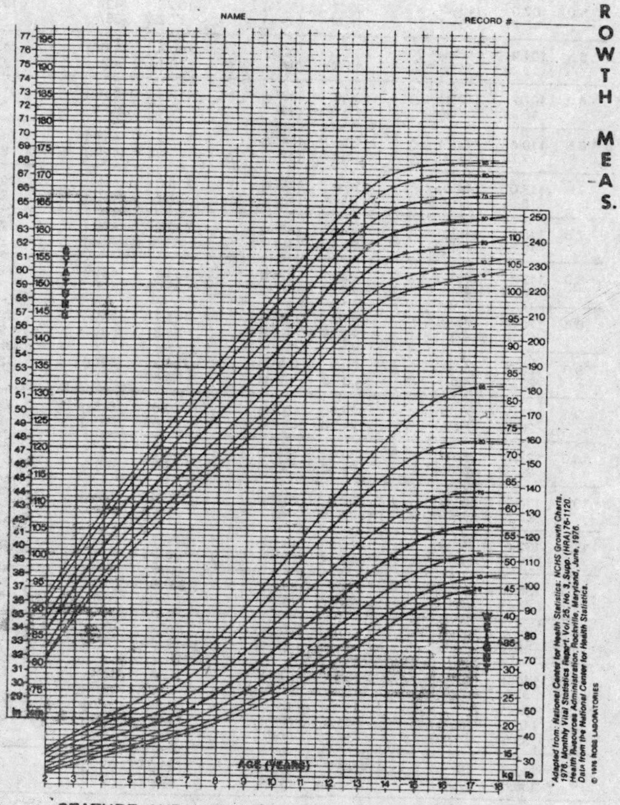

STATURE AND WEIGHT BY AGE: **GIRLS**, 2 to 18 years

Figure 2–6B (See Figure 2–6A, opposite.)

Table 2–7A STATURE AND WEIGHT BY AGE* BOYS: 2 TO 18 YEARS

{**STATURE:** centimeters and (inches)
{**WEIGHT:** kilograms and (pounds)

AGE years	BOYS: percentiles 5th	10th	25th	50th	75th	90th	95th
2.0†	82.5 (32½) 10.49 (23¼)	83.5 (32¾) 10.96 (24¼)	85.3 (33½) 11.55 (25½)	86.8 (34¼) 12.34 (27¼)	89.2 (35) 13.36 (29½)	92.0 (36¼) 14.38 (31¾)	94.4 (37¼) 15.50 (34¼)
2.5†	85.4 (33½) 11.27 (24¾)	86.5 (34) 11.77 (26)	88.5 (34¾) 12.55 (27¾)	90.4 (35½) 13.52 (29¾)	92.9 (36½) 14.61 (32¼)	95.6 (37¾) 15.71 (34¾)	97.8 (38½) 16.61 (36½)
3.0	89.0 (35) 12.05 (26½)	90.3 (35½) 12.58 (27¾)	92.6 (36½) 13.52 (29¾)	94.9 (37¼) 14.62 (32¼)	97.5 (38½) 15.78 (34¾)	100.1 (39½) 16.95 (37¼)	102.0 (40¼) 17.77 (39¼)
3.5	92.5 (36½) 12.84 (28¼)	93.9 (37) 13.41 (29½)	96.4 (38) 14.46 (32)	99.1 (39) 15.68 (34½)	101.7 (40) 16.90 (37¼)	104.3 (41¼) 18.15 (40)	106.1 (41¾) 18.98 (41¾)
4.0	95.8 (37¾) 13.64 (30)	97.3 (38¼) 14.24 (31½)	100.0 (39¼) 15.39 (34)	102.9 (40½) 16.69 (36¾)	105.7 (41½) 17.99 (39¾)	108.2 (42½) 19.32 (42½)	109.9 (43¼) 20.27 (44¾)
4.5	98.9 (39) 14.45 (31¾)	100.6 (39½) 15.10 (33¼)	103.4 (40¾) 16.30 (36)	106.6 (42) 17.69 (39)	109.4 (43) 19.06 (42)	111.9 (44) 20.50 (45¼)	113.5 (44¾) 21.63 (47¾)
5.0	102.0 (40¼) 15.27 (33¾)	103.7 (40¾) 15.96 (35¼)	106.5 (42) 17.22 (38)	109.9 (43¼) 18.67 (41¼)	112.8 (44½) 20.14 (44½)	115.4 (45½) 21.70 (47¾)	117.0 (46) 23.09 (51)
5.5	104.9 (41¼) 16.09 (35½)	106.7 (42) 16.83 (37)	109.6 (43¼) 18.14 (40)	113.1 (44½) 19.67 (43¼)	116.1 (45¾) 21.25 (46¾)	118.7 (46¾) 22.96 (50½)	120.3 (47¼) 24.66 (54¼)
6.0	107.7 (42½) 16.93 (37¼)	109.6 (43¼) 17.72 (39)	112.5 (44¼) 19.07 (42)	116.1 (45¾) 20.69 (45½)	119.2 (47) 22.40 (49½)	121.9 (48) 24.31 (53½)	123.5 (48½) 26.34 (58)
6.5	110.4 (43½) 17.78 (39¼)	112.3 (44¼) 18.62 (41)	115.3 (45½) 20.02 (44¼)	119.0 (46¾) 21.74 (48)	122.2 (48) 23.62 (52)	124.9 (49¼) 25.76 (56¾)	126.6 (49¾) 28.16 (62)
7.0	113.0 (44½) 18.64 (41)	115.0 (45¼) 19.53 (43)	118.0 (46½) 21.00 (46¼)	121.7 (48) 22.85 (50¼)	125.0 (49¼) 24.94 (55)	127.9 (50¼) 27.36 (60¼)	129.7 (51) 30.12 (66½)
7.5	115.6 (45½) 19.52 (43)	117.6 (46¼) 20.45 (45)	120.6 (47½) 22.02 (48½)	124.4 (49) 24.03 (53)	127.8 (50¼) 26.36 (58)	130.8 (51½) 29.11 (64¼)	132.7 (52¼) 32.73 (72¼)
8.0	118.1 (46½) 20.40 (45)	120.2 (47¼) 21.39 (47¼)	123.2 (48½) 23.09 (51)	127.0 (50) 25.30 (55¾)	130.5 (51½) 27.91 (61½)	133.6 (52½) 31.06 (68½)	135.7 (53½) 34.51 (76)
8.5	120.5 (47½) 21.31 (47)	122.7 (48¼) 22.34 (49¼)	125.7 (49½) 24.21 (53¼)	129.6 (51) 26.66 (58¾)	133.2 (52½) 29.61 (65¼)	136.5 (53¾) 33.22 (73¼)	138.8 (54¾) 36.96 (81½)
9.0	122.9 (48½) 22.25 (49)	125.2 (49¼) 23.33 (51½)	128.2 (50½) 25.40 (56)	132.2 (52) 28.13 (62)	136.0 (53½) 31.46 (69¼)	139.4 (55) 35.57 (78½)	141.8 (55¾) 39.58 (87¾)
9.5	125.3 (49¼) 23.25 (51¼)	127.6 (50¼) 24.38 (53¾)	130.8 (51½) 26.88 (58¾)	134.8 (53) 29.73 (65½)	138.8 (54¾) 33.46 (73¾)	142.4 (56) 38.11 (84)	144.9 (57) 42.35 (93¼)
10.0	127.7 (50¼) 24.33 (53¾)	130.1 (51¼) 25.52 (56¼)	133.4 (52½) 28.07 (62)	137.5 (54¼) 31.44 (69¼)	141.6 (55¾) 35.61 (78½)	145.5 (57¼) 40.80 (90)	148.1 (58¼) 45.27 (99¾)
10.5	130.1 (51¼) 25.51 (56¼)	132.6 (52¼) 26.78 (59)	136.0 (53½) 29.59 (65¼)	140.3 (55¼) 33.30 (73½)	144.6 (57) 37.92 (83½)	148.7 (58½) 43.63 (96¼)	151.5 (59¾) 48.31 (106½)
11.0	132.6 (52¼) 26.80 (59)	135.1 (53¼) 28.17 (62)	138.7 (54½) 31.25 (69)	143.33 (56½) 35.30 (77¾)	147.8 (58¼) 40.38 (89)	152.1 (60) 46.57 (102¾)	154.9 (61) 51.47 (113½)
11.5	135.0 (53¼) 28.24 (62¼)	137.7 (54½) 29.72 (65½)	141.5 (55¾) 33.08 (73)	146.4 (57¾) 37.46 (82½)	151.1 (59½) 43.00 (94¾)	155.6 (61¼) 49.61 (109¼)	158.5 (62½) 54.73 (120¾)
12.0	137.6 (54¼) 29.85 (65¾)	140.3 (55¼) 31.46 (69¼)	144.4 (56¾) 35.09 (77¼)	149.7 (59) 39.78 (87¾)	154.6 (60¾) 45.77 (101)	159.4 (62¾) 52.73 (116¼)	162.3 (64) 58.09 (128)
12.5	140.2 (55¼) 31.64 (69¾)	143.0 (56¼) 33.41 (73¾)	147.4 (58) 37.31 (82¼)	153.0 (60¼) 42.27 (93¼)	158.2 (62¼) 48.70 (107¼)	163.2 (64¼) 55.91 (123¼)	166.1 (65½) 61.52 (135¾)
13.0	142.9 (56¼) 33.64 (74¼)	145.8 (57½) 35.60 (78½)	150.5 (59¼) 39.74 (87½)	156.5 (61½) 44.95 (99)	161.8 (63¾) 51.79 (114¼)	167.0 (65¾) 59.12 (130¼)	169.8 (66¾) 65.02 (143¼)
13.5	145.7 (57¼) 35.85 (79)	148.7 (58½) 38.03 (83¾)	153.6 (60½) 42.40 (93½)	159.9 (63) 47.81 (105½)	165.3 (65) 55.02 (121¼)	170.5 (67¼) 62.35 (137½)	173.4 (68¼) 68.51 (151)
14.0	148.8 (58½) 38.22 (84¼)	151.8 (59¾) 40.64 (89½)	156.9 (61¾) 45.21 (99¾)	63.1 (64¼) 50.77 (112)	168.5 (66¼) 58.31 (128½)	173.8 (68½) 65.57 (144½)	176.7 (69½) 72.13 (159)
14.5	152.0 (59¾) 40.66 (89¾)	155.0 (61) 43.34 (95½)	160.1 (63) 48.08 (106)	166.2 (65½) 53.76 (118½)	171.5 (67½) 61.58 (135¾)	176.6 (69½) 68.76 (151½)	179.5 (70½) 75.66 (166¾)
15.0	155.2 (61) 43.11 (95)	158.2 (62¼) 46.06 (101½)	163.3 (64¼) 50.92 (112¼)	169.0 (66½) 56.71 (125)	174.1 (68½) 64.72 (142¾)	178.9 (70½) 71.91 (158½)	181.9 (71½) 79.12 (174½)
15.5	158.3 (62¼) 45.50 (100¼)	161.2 (63½) 48.69 (107¼)	166.2 (65½) 53.64 (118¼)	171.5 (67½) 59.51 (131¼)	176.3 (69½) 67.64 (149)	180.8 (71¼) 74.98 (165¼)	183.9 (72½) 82.45 (181¾)
16.0	161.1 (63½) 47.74 (105¼)	163.9 (64½) 51.16 (112¾)	168.7 (66½) 56.16 (123¾)	173.5 (68¼) 62.10 (137)	178.1 (70) 70.26 (155)	182.4 (71¾) 77.97 (172)	185.4 (73) 85.62 (188¾)
16.5	163.4 (64¼) 49.76 (109¾)	166.1 (65½) 53.39 (117¾)	170.6 (67¼) 58.38 (128¾)	175.2 (69) 64.39 (142)	179.5 (70¾) 72.46 (159¾)	183.6 (72¼) 80.84 (178¼)	186.6 (73½) 88.59 (195¼)
17.0	164.9 (65) 51.50 (113½)	167.7 (66) 55.28 (121¾)	171.9 (67¾) 60.22 (132¾)	176.2 (69¼) 66.31 (146¼)	180.5 (71) 74.17 (163½)	184.4 (72½) 83.58 (184¼)	187.3 (73¾) 91.31 (201¼)
17.5	165.6 (65¼) 52.89 (116½)	168.5 (66¼) 56.78 (125¼)	172.4 (67¾) 61.61 (135¾)	176.7 (69½) 67.78 (149½)	181.0 (71¼) 75.32 (166)	185.0 (72¾) 86.14 (190)	187.6 (73¾) 93.73 (206¾)
18.0	165.7 (65¼) 53.97 (119)	168.7 (66½) 57.89 (127½)	172.3 (67¾) 62.61 (138)	176.8 (69½) 68.88 (151¾)	181.2 (71¼) 76.04 (167¾)	185.3 (73) 88.41 (195)	187.6 (73¾) 95.76 (211)

*Data in Tables 2–7A and 2–7B are those of the National Center for Health Statistics, Health Resources Administration, DHEW, collected in its Health Examination Surveys. Metric data have been smoothed by the least-squares cubic spline technique. For details see footnote to Table 2–6 and text (page 33).

†Stature data for 2.0 to 3.0 years include some recumbent length measurements, which make values slightly higher than if all measurements had been of stature.

Table 2–7B STATURE AND WEIGHT BY AGE* GIRLS: 2 TO 18 YEARS
STATURE: centimeters and (inches)
WEIGHT: kilograms and (pounds)

GIRLS: percentiles							
5th	10th	25th	50th	75th	90th	95th	AGE *years*
81.6 (32¼) 9.95 (22)	82.1 (32¼) 10.32 (22¾)	84.0 (33) 10.96 (24¼)	86.8 (34¼) 11.80 (26)	89.3 (35¼) 12.73 (28)	92.0 (36¼) 13.58 (30)	93.6 (36¾) 14.15 (31¼)	2.0
84.6 (33¼) 10.80 (23¾)	85.3 (33½) 11.35 (25)	87.3 (34½) 12.11 (26¾)	90.0 (35½) 13.03 (28¾)	92.5 (36½) 14.23 (31¼)	95.0 (37½) 15.16 (33½)	96.6 (38) 15.76 (34¾)	2.5
88.3 (34¾) 11.61 (25½)	89.3 (35¼) 12.26 (27)	91.4 (36) 13.11 (29)	94.1 (37) 14.10 (31)	96.6 (38) 15.50 (34¼)	99.0 (39) 16.54 (36½)	100.6 (39½) 17.22 (38)	3.0
91.7 (36) 12.37 (27¼)	93.0 (36½) 13.08 (28¾)	95.2 (37½) 14.00 (30¾)	97.9 (38½) 15.07 (33¼)	100.5 (39½) 16.59 (36½)	102.8 (40½) 17.77 (39¼)	104.5 (41¼) 18.59 (41)	3.5
95.0 (37½) 13.11 (29)	96.4 (38) 13.84 (30½)	98.8 (39) 14.80 (32¾)	101.6 (40) 15.96 (35¼)	104.3 (41) 17.56 (38¾)	106.6 (42) 18.93 (41¾)	108.3 (42¾) 19.91 (44)	4.0
98.1 (38½) 13.83 (30½)	99.7 (39¼) 14.56 (32)	102.2 (40¼) 15.55 (34¼)	105.0 (41¼) 16.81 (37)	107.9 (42½) 18.48 (40¾)	110.2 (43½) 20.06 (44¼)	112.0 (44) 21.24 (46¾)	4.5
101.1 (39¾) 14.55 (32)	102.7 (40½) 15.26 (33¾)	105.4 (41½) 16.29 (36)	108.4 (42¾) 17.66 (39)	111.4 (43¾) 19.39 (42¾)	113.8 (44¾) 21.23 (46¾)	115.6 (45½) 22.62 (49¾)	5.0
103.9 (41) 15.29 (33¾)	105.6 (41½) 15.97 (35¼)	108.4 (42¾) 17.05 (37½)	111.6 (44) 18.56 (41)	114.8 (45¼) 20.36 (45)	117.4 (46¼) 22.48 (49½)	119.2 (47) 24.11 (53¼)	5.5
106.6 (42) 16.05 (35½)	108.4 (42¾) 16.72 (36¾)	111.3 (43¾) 17.86 (39¼)	114.6 (45) 19.52 (43)	118.1 (46½) 21.44 (47¼)	120.8 (47½) 23.89 (52¾)	122.7 (48¼) 25.75 (56¾)	6.0
109.2 (43) 16.85 (37¼)	111.0 (43¾) 17.51 (38½)	114.1 (45) 18.76 (41¼)	117.6 (46¼) 20.61 (45½)	121.3 (47¾) 22.68 (50)	124.2 (49) 25.50 (56¼)	126.1 (49¾) 27.59 (60¾)	6.5
111.8 (44) 17.71 (39)	113.6 (44¾) 18.39 (40½)	116.8 (46) 19.78 (43½)	120.6 (47½) 21.84 (48¼)	124.4 (49) 24.16 (53¼)	127.6 (50¼) 27.39 (60½)	129.5 (51) 29.68 (65½)	7.0
114.4 (45) 18.62 (41)	116.2 (45¾) 19.37 (42¾)	119.5 (47) 20.95 (46¼)	123.5 (48½) 23.26 (51¼)	127.5 (50¼) 25.90 (57)	130.9 (51½) 29.57 (65¼)	132.9 (52¼) 32.07 (70¾)	7.5
116.9 (46) 19.62 (43¼)	118.7 (46¾) 20.45 (45)	122.2 (48) 22.26 (49)	126.4 (49¾) 24.84 (54¾)	130.6 (51½) 27.88 (61½)	134.2 (52¾) 32.04 (70¾)	136.2 (53½) 34.71 (76½)	8.0
119.5 (47) 20.68 (45½)	121.3 (47¾) 21.64 (47¾)	124.9 (49¼) 23.70 (52¼)	129.3 (51) 26.58 (58½)	133.6 (52½) 30.08 (66¼)	137.4 (54) 34.73 (76½)	139.6 (55) 37.58 (82¾)	8.5
122.1 (48) 21.82 (48)	123.9 (48¾) 22.92 (50½)	127.7 (50¼) 25.27 (55¾)	132.2 (52) 28.46 (62¾)	136.7 (53¾) 32.44 (71½)	140.7 (55½) 37.60 (83)	142.9 (56¼) 40.64 (89½)	9.0
124.8 (49¼) 23.05 (50¾)	126.6 (49¾) 24.29 (53½)	130.6 (51½) 26.94 (59½)	135.2 (53¼) 30.45 (67¼)	139.8 (55) 34.94 (77)	143.9 (56¾) 40.61 (89½)	146.2 (57½) 43.85 (96¾)	9.5
127.5 (50¼) 24.36 (53¾)	129.5 (51) 25.76 (56¾)	133.6 (52½) 28.71 (63¼)	138.3 (54½) 32.55 (71¾)	142.9 (56¼) 37.53 (82¾)	147.2 (58) 43.70 (96¼)	149.5 (58¾) 47.17 (104)	10.0
130.4 (51¼) 25.75 (56¾)	132.5 (52¼) 27.32 (60¼)	136.7 (53¾) 30.57 (67½)	141.5 (55¾) 34.72 (76½)	146.1 (57½) 40.17 (88½)	150.4 (59¼) 46.84 (103¼)	152.8 (60¼) 50.57 (111½)	10.5
133.5 (52½) 27.24 (60)	135.6 (53½) 28.97 (63¾)	140.0 (55) 32.49 (71¾)	144.8 (57) 36.95 (81½)	149.3 (58¾) 42.84 (94½)	153.7 (60½) 49.96 (110¼)	56.2 (61½) 54.00 (119)	11.0
136.6 (53¾) 28.83 (63½)	139.0 (54¾) 30.71 (67¾)	143.5 (56½) 34.48 (76)	148.2 (58¼) 39.23 (86½)	152.6 (60) 45.48 (100¼	156.9 (61¾) 53.03 (117)	159.5 (62¾) 57.42 (126½)	11.5
139.8 (55) 30.52 (67¼)	142.3 (56) 32.53 (71¼)	147.0 (57¾) 36.52 (80½)	151.5 (59¾) 41.53 (91½)	155.8 (61¼) 48.07 (106)	160.0 (63) 55.99 (123½)	162.7 (64) 60.81 (134)	12.0
142.7 (56¼) 32.30 (71¾)	145.4 (57¼) 34.42 (76)	150.1 (59) 38.59 (85)	154.6 (60¾) 43.84 (96¾)	158.8 (62½) 50.56 (111½)	162.9 (64½) 58.81 (129¾)	165.6 (65¼) 64.12 (141¼)	12.5
145.2 (57¼) 34.14 (75¼)	148.0 (58¼) 36.35 (80¼)	152.8 (60¼) 40.55 (89½)	157.1 (61¾) 46.10 (101¾)	161.3 (63½) 52.91 (116¾)	165.3 (65) 61.45 (135½)	168.1 (66¼) 67.30 (148¼)	13.0
147.2 (58) 35.98 (79¼)	150.0 (59) 38.26 (84¼)	154.7 (61) 42.65 (94)	159.0 (62½) 48.26 (106½)	163.2 (64¼) 55.11 (121½)	167.3 (65¾) 63.87 (140¾)	170.0 (67) 70.30 (155)	13.5
148.7 (58½) 37.76 (83¼)	151.5 (59¾) 40.11 (88½)	155.9 (61½) 44.54 (98¼)	160.4 (63¼) 50.28 (110¾)	164.6 (64¾) 57.09 (125¾)	168.7 (66½) 66.04 (145½)	171.3 (67½) 73.08 (161)	14.0
149.7 (59) 39.45 (87)	152.5 (60) 41.83 (92¼)	158.8 (61¾) 46.28 (102)	161.2 (63½) 52.10 (114¾)	165.6 (65¼) 58.84 (129¾)	169.8 (66¾) 67.95 (149¾)	172.2 (67¾) 75.59 (166¾)	14.5
150.5 (59¼) 40.99 (90¼)	153.2 (60¼) 43.38 (95¾)	157.2 (62) 47.82 (105½)	161.8 (63¾) 53.68 (118¼)	166.3 (65¼) 60.32 (133)	170.5 (67¼) 69.54 (153¼)	172.8 (68) 77.78 (171½)	15.0
151.1 (59½) 42.32 (93¼)	153.6 (60½) 44.72 (98½)	157.5 (62) 49.10 (108¼)	162.1 (63¾) 54.96 (121¼)	166.7 (65¾) 61.48 (135½)	170.9 (67¼) 70.79 (156)	173.1 (68¼) 79.59 (176½)	15.5
151.6 (59¾) 43.41 (95¾)	154.1 (60¾) 45.78 (101)	157.8 (62¼) 50.09 (110½)	162.4 (64) 55.89 (123¼)	166.9 (65¾) 62.29 (137¼)	171.1 (67¼) 71.68 (158)	173.3 (68¼) 80.99 (178½)	16.0
152.2 (60) 44.20 (97½)	154.6 (60¾) 46.54 (102½)	158.2 (62¼) 50.75 (112)	162.7 (64) 56.44 (124½)	167.1 (65¾) 62.75 (138¼)	171.2 (67½) 72.18 (159¼)	173.4 (68¼) 81.93 (180½)	16.5
152.7 (60) 44.74 (98¾)	155.1 (61) 47.04 (103¾)	158.7 (62½) 51.14 (112¾)	163.1 (64¼) 56.69 (125)	167.3 (65¾) 62.91 (138¾)	171.2 (67½) 72.38 (159½)	173.5 (68¼) 82.46 (181¾)	17.0
153.2 (60¼) 45.08 (99½)	155.6 (61¼) 47.33 (104¼)	159.1 (62¾) 51.33 (113¼)	163.4 (64¼) 56.71 (125)	167.5 (66) 62.89 (138¾)	171.1 (67¼) 72.37 (159½)	173.5 (68¼) 82.62 (182¼)	17.5
153.6 (60½) 45.26 (99¾)	156.0 (61½) 47.47 (104¾)	159.6 (62¾) 51.39 (113¼)	163.7 (64½) 56.62 (124¾)	167.6 (66) 62.78 (138½)	171.0 (67¼) 72.25 (159¼)	173.6 (68¼) 82.47 (181¾)	18.0

*See footnotes to Table 2–7A.

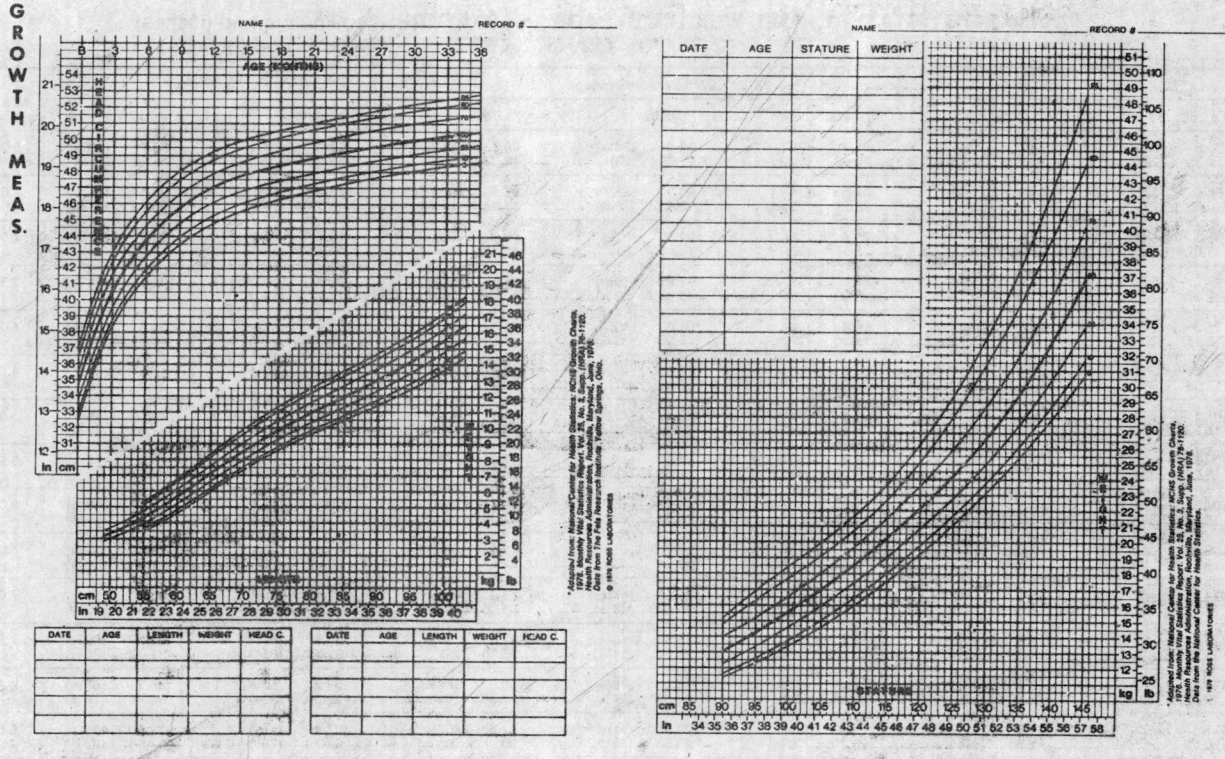

HEAD CIRCUMFERENCE AND WEIGHT BY LENGTH
GIRLS: BIRTH TO 36 MONTHS

WEIGHT BY STATURE
GIRLS: PREPUBESCENT

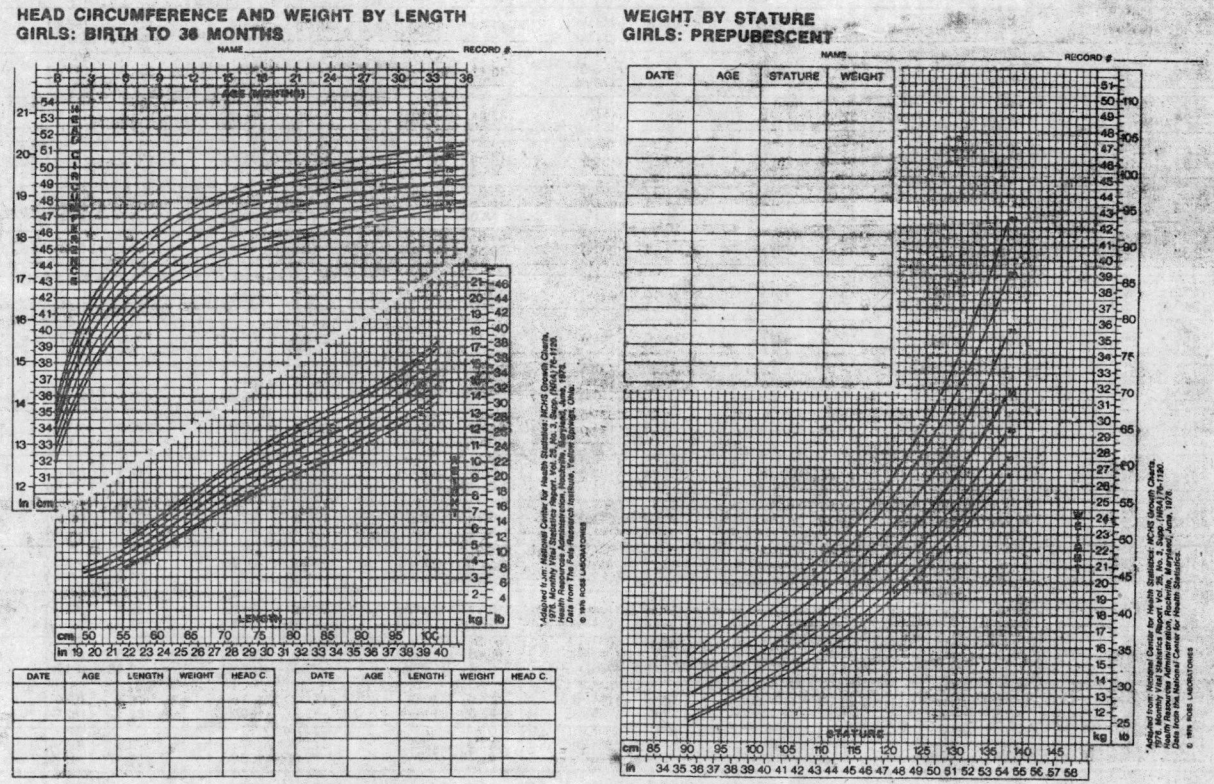

Figures 2—7A (above) and **B** (below). For legend, see bottom of opposite page.

growths of other ethnic, genetic, or socioeconomic groups. Although there is evidence that ethnic differences depend in largest measure upon differences in prevalence of malnutrition and infectious disease in various parts of the world, there can be no universal standard.

A recent large survey of characteristics of the growth of children in the United States has produced the data in Tables 2–6, 2–7, and 2–8 and in Fig 2–6 and 2–7. The children studied represented a cross-section of ethnic and economic groups; accordingly, some genetic, ethnic, and socioeconomic differences are imbedded in the final data. These data and the derived charts must be regarded, therefore, not as descriptive of any single racial, social, economic, or nutritional group, but simply as *reference standards*.

As reference standards, these data have certain justification and advantages: (1) they are more up to date than earlier standards; (2) they represent on the whole a well-nourished group of children whose general health has probably been as satisfactory as can now be achieved in an industrially developed country; and (3) they appear to indicate conditions close to asymptotic for the secular trend in increasing growth in height which has been evident for several centuries (Sec 2.9). In this last respect their utility as reference standards may be relatively long-lasting.

Tables 2–6 and 2–7 and Fig 2–6 present data of the NCHS survey regarding the distributions of length (or stature) and weight of infants and children at various ages. Table 2–8 and Fig 2–7A and 2–7B present data with respect to the distribution of weights of children of specified length (or stature). In the evaluation of the developmental or nutritional status of children these latter data may be particularly informative, in conjunction with the data relating height to age. For example, children with low heights for age who have normal weight for height may have experienced nutritional or growth failure in the past, whereas if both height for age and weight for height are strikingly low, then both past and current nutritional or growth failure may be suspected. By contrast, children with normal height for age who have conspicuously low weight for height are likely to have either relatively acute nutritional or growth problems or variant physiques (Sec 2.1 and 2.10).

TECHNIQUES OF MEASUREMENT

Accuracy of measurement is essential to the reliable interpretation of growth data; slight variations in technique may result in significantly large errors in the placement of children according to percentile rank.

Height. *Recumbent length* can be more accurately measured than standing height in children under the age of 5 yr, after which measurement of standing height is generally more convenient. Recumbent length is measured as the child lies on a firm table which has a measuring stick at least 125 cm or 50 in long fastened along one edge. The soles of the feet are held firmly against a fixed upright placed at the zero mark. A movable upright crosses the table above the head and is brought firmly against the vertex. If recumbent length is used after 5 yr of age, the value obtained may be reduced by 1 cm from that for standing height.

Standing height is measured as the child stands erect, with heels, buttocks, upper part of the back, and occiput against a vertical upright; the heels should be close together, and the arms should hang naturally at the sides. The external auditory meatus and the lower border of the orbit should be in a plane parallel with the floor. A wooden head piece having two faces at right angles may be placed firmly on the head against a 2-meter or 6-foot measuring scale attached to the vertical surface against which the child is positioned.

Head Circumference. This measurement is particularly valuable in infants; it need not be taken routinely after 3 yr of age. The tape is applied firmly over the glabella and supraorbital ridges anteriorly and that part of the occiput posteriorly that gives the maximal circumference. Difficulties with measurement of head circumference will sometimes arise when the head has an abnormal shape, as in hydrocephalus. Under these circumstances serial measurements of the changing size of the head may best be made by positioning the tape over whatever points on the forehead and occiput give the *maximal* circumference. If cloth tapes are used, they may stretch with aging and will need to be checked frequently against wooden or steel standards.

Chest Circumference. Measurement of chest circumference is made in midrespiration at the level of the xiphoid cartilage or substernal notch, in a plane at right angles to the vertebral column. Measurement is made recumbent up to the age of 5 yr, and standing thereafter.

Abdominal Circumference. This measurement is taken to 3 yr only and will be of value principally in recognizing and following the course of chronic intestinal disturbances. Measurement is made in the plane of the umbilicus when the infant is recumbent.

Other Measurements. Studies of nutritional status or of specific growth problems will often require other measurements, such as skinfold thickness or circumference of calf (in nutritional assessment), relationship of sitting height to length or span (in growth disturbances), pelvic breadth (in adolescence), and the like.

Text continued on page 38

Figures 2–7A and 2–7B on opposite page. Charts for BOYS (Fig. 2–7A, above), and for GIRLS (Fig. 2–7B, below) of *weight by length [or stature]*, for infants and young children (left) and for older [prepubertal] children (right). *Head circumference by age* is given for infants and young children (upper left). These charts are based upon the data in Tables 2–6 and 2–8, and have been adapted from NCHS Growth Charts by Ross Laboratories. Permission to use them is gratefully acknowledged.

Table 2–8A WEIGHT BY LENGTH*
BOYS AND GIRLS LESS THAN 4 YEARS

Recumbent Length	BOYS: weight percentiles, kg and (lb)							GIRLS: weight percentiles, kg and (lb)						
	5th	10th	25th	50th	75th	90th	95th	5th	10th	25th	50th	75th	90th	95th
48–50 cm (19–19¾ in)			2.86 (6¼)	3.15 (7)	3.50 (7¾)					3.02 (6¾)	3.29 (7¼)	3.59 (8)		
50–52 cm (19¾–20½ in)			3.16 (70)	3.48 (7¾)	3.86 (8½)					3.25 (7¼)	3.55 (7¾)	3.89 (8½)		
52–54 cm (20½–21¼ in)			3.52 (7¾)	3.88 (8½)	4.28 (9½)					3.56 (7¾)	3.89 (8½)	4.26 (9½)		
54–56 cm (21¼–22 in)	3.49 (7¾)	3.65 (8)	3.95 (8¾)	4.34 (9½)	4.76 (10½)	5.13 (11¼)	5.33 (11¾)	3.54 (7¾)	3.64 (8)	3.93 (8¾)	4.29 (9½)	4.70 (10¼)	5.02 (11)	5.21 (11½)
56–58 cm (22–22¾ in)	3.90 (8½)	4.09 (9)	4.43 (9¾)	4.84 (10¾)	5.29 (11¾)	5.69 (12½)	5.88 (13)	3.93 (8¾)	4.05 (9)	4.37 (9¾)	4.76 (10½)	5.20 (11½)	5.55 (12¼)	5.77 (12¾)
58–60 cm (22¾–23½ in)	4.37 (9¾)	4.58 (10)	4.94 (11)	5.38 (11¾)	5.84 (12¾)	6.28 (13¾)	6.47 (14¼)	4.38 (9¾)	4.50 (10)	4.85 (10¾)	5.27 (11½)	5.73 (12¾)	6.12 (13½)	6.36 (14)
60–62 cm (23½–24½ in)	4.88 (10¾)	5.10 (11¼)	5.49 (12)	5.94 (13)	6.42 (14¼)	6.88 (15¼)	7.08 (15½)	4.85 (10¾)	4.99 (11)	5.37 (11¾)	5.82 (12¾)	6.30 (14)	6.70 (14¾)	6.95 (15¼)
62–64 cm (24½–25¼ in)	5.43 (12)	5.65 (12½)	6.05 (13¼)	6.52 (14¼)	7.02 (15½)	7.50 (16½)	7.72 (17)	5.35 (11¾)	5.50 (12)	5.91 (13)	6.39 (14)	6.89 (15¼)	7.30 (16)	7.55 (16¾)
64–66 cm (25¼–26 in)	5.99 (13¼)	6.20 (13¾)	6.62 (14½)	7.11 (15¾)	7.63 (16¾)	8.13 (18)	8.36 (8½)	5.87 (13)	6.03 (13¼)	6.47 (14¼)	6.97 (15¼)	7.48 (16½)	7.90 (17½)	8.15 (18)
66–68 cm (26–26¾ in)	6.55 (14½)	6.76 (15)	7.19 (15¾)	7.70 (17)	8.23 (18¼)	8.75 (19¼)	8.99 (19¾)	6.38 (14)	6.56 (14½)	7.02 (15½)	7.55 (16¾)	8.07 (17¾)	8.50 (18¾)	8.75 (19¼)
68–70 cm (26¾–27½ in)	7.10 (15¾)	7.31 (16)	7.75 (17)	8.27 (18¼)	8.82 (19½)	9.35 (20½)	9.62 (21¼)	6.89 (15¼)	7.08 (15½)	7.56 (16¾)	8.11 (17¾)	8.64 (19)	9.08 (20)	9.33 (20½)
70–72 cm (27½–28¼ in)	7.63 (16¾)	7.84 (17¼)	8.26 (18¼)	8.82 (19½)	9.39 (20¾)	9.93 (22)	10.21 (22½)	7.37 (16¼)	7.58 (16¾)	8.08 (17¾)	8.64 (19)	9.18 (20¼)	9.63 (21¼)	9.88 (21¾)
72–74 cm (28¼–29¼ in)	8.13 (18)	8.33 (18¼)	8.78 (19¼)	9.33 (20½)	9.92 (21¾)	10.48 (23)	10.77 (23¾)	7.82 (17¼)	8.05 (17¾)	8.56 (18¾)	9.14 (20¼)	9.68 (21¼)	10.15 (22½)	10.41 (23)
74–76 cm (29¼–30 in)	8.58 (19)	8.78 (19¼)	9.24 (20¼)	9.81 (21¾)	10.43 (23)	10.99 (24¼)	11.29 (25)	8.24 (18¼)	8.49 (18¾)	9.00 (19¾)	9.59 (21¼)	10.14 (22¼)	10.63 (23½)	10.91 (24)
76–78 cm (30–30¾ in)	9.00 (19¾)	9.21 (20¼)	9.68 (21¼)	10.27 (22¾)	10.91 (24)	11.48 (25¼)	11.78 (26)	8.62 (19)	8.90 (19½)	9.42 (20¾)	10.02 (22)	10.57 (23¼)	11.08 (24½)	11.39 (25)
78–80 cm (30¾–31½ in)	9.40 (20¾)	9.62 (21¼)	10.09 (22¼)	10.70 (23½)	11.36 (25)	11.94 (26¼)	12.25 (27)	8.99 (19¾)	9.29 (20½)	9.81 (21¾)	10.41 (23)	10.97 (24¼)	11.51 (25¼)	11.85 (26)
80–82 cm (31½–32¼ in)	9.77 (21½)	10.01 (22)	10.49 (23¼)	11.12 (24½)	11.80 (26)	12.39 (27¼)	12.69 (28)	9.34 (20½)	9.67 (21¼)	10.19 (22½)	10.80 (23¾)	11.37 (25)	11.93 (26¼)	12.29 (27)
82–84 cm (32¼–33 in)	10.14 (22¼)	10.39 (23)	10.88 (24)	11.53 (25½)	12.23 (27)	12.83 (28¼)	13.13 (29)	9.68 (21¼)	10.04 (22¼)	10.57 (23¼)	11.18 (24¾)	11.75 (26)	12.35 (27¼)	12.72 (28)
84–86 cm (33–33¾ in)	10.49 (23¼)	10.76 (23¾)	11.27 (24¾)	11.93 (26¼)	12.65 (28)	13.26 (29¼)	13.56 (30)	10.03 (22)	10.41 (23)	10.94 (24)	11.56 (25½)	12.15 (26¾)	12.76 (28¼)	13.15 (29)
86–88 cm (33¾–34¾ in)	10.85 (24)	11.14 (24½)	11.67 (25¾)	12.34 (27¼)	13.07 (28¾)	13.69 (30¼)	14.00 (30¾)	10.39 (23)	10.78 (23¾)	11.33 (25)	11.95 (26¼)	12.55 (27¾)	13.19 (29)	13.57 (30)
88–90 cm (34¾–35½ in)	11.22 (24¾)	11.53 (25½)	12.08 (26¾)	12.76 (28¼)	13.50 (29¾)	14.13 (31¼)	14.44 (31¾)	10.76 (23¾)	11.17 (24½)	11.74 (26)	12.36 (27¼)	12.98 (28½)	13.63 (30)	14.01. (31)
90–92 cm (35½–36¼ in)	11.60 (25½)	11.94 (26¼)	12.52 (27½)	13.20 (29)	13.94 (30¾)	14.58 (32¼)	14.90 (32¾)	11.16 (24½)	11.58 (25½)	12.17 (26¾)	12.80 (28¼)	13.45 (29¾)	14.10 (31)	14.45 (31¾)
92–94 cm (36¼–37 in)	12.00 (26½)	12.37 (27¼)	12.97 (28½)	13.65 (30)	14.40 (31¾)	15.05 (33¼)	15.39 (34)	11.59 (25½)	12.02 (26½)	12.63 (27¾)	13.27 (29¼)	13.95 (30¾)	14.61 (32¼)	14.92 (33)
94–96 cm (37–37¾ in)	12.42 (27½)	12.81 (28¼)	13.45 (29¾)	14.14 (31¼)	14.88 (32¾)	15.54 (34¼)	15.90 (35)	12.05 (26½)	12.48 (27½)	13.12 (29)	13.77 (30¼)	14.48 (32)	15.14 (33½)	15.42 (34)
96–98 cm (37¾–38½ in)	12.88 (28½)	13.28 (29¼)	13.96 (30¾)	14.66 (32¼)	15.39 (34)	16.06 (35½)	16.43 (36¼)	12.55 (27¾)	12.98 (28½)	13.64 (30)	14.31 (31½)	15.04 (33¼)	15.71 (34¾)	15.99 (35¼)
98–100 cm (38½–39¼ in)	13.37 (29½)	13.78 (30½)	14.50 (32)	15.21 (33½)	15.94 (35¼)	16.62 (36¾)	17.00 (37½)	13.10 (29)	13.51 (29¾)	14.19 (31¼)	14.87 (32¾)	15.63 (34½)	16.32 (36)	16.64 (36¾)
100–102 cm (39¼–49¼ in)	13.90 (30¾)	14.30 (31½)	15.06 (33¼)	15.81 (34¾)	16.54 (36½)	17.22 (38)	17.60 (38¾)	13.68 (30¼)	14.08 (31)	14.77 (32½)	15.46 (34)	16.25 (35¾)	16.96 (37½)	17.39 (38¼)
102–104 cm (40¼–41 in)	14.48 (32)	14.85 (32¾)	15.65 (34½)	16.45 (36¼)	17.18 (37¾)	17.87 (39½)	18.24 (40¼)							

*Data in Tables 2–8A and 2–8B are those of the National Center for Health Statistics (NCHS), Health Resources Administration, DHEW. Data of Table 2–8A are based on studies of The Fels Research Institute, Yellow Springs, Ohio; those of Table 2–8B are based on the Health Examination Surveys of the NCHS. For details see footnote to Table 2–6 and text (p. 33).

Table 2–8B WEIGHT BY STATURE* BOYS AND GIRLS: PREPUBESCENT

Stature	BOYS: weight percentiles, kg and (lb)							GIRLS: weight percentiles, kg and (lb)						
	5th	19th	25th	50th	75th	90th	95th	5th	10th	25th	50th	75th	90th	95th
90–92 cm (35½–36¼ in)	11.70 (25¾)	11.97 (26½)	12.59 (27¾)	13.41 (29½)	14.35 (31¾)	15.25 (33½)	15.72 (34¾)	11.45 (25¼)	11.67 (25¾)	12.28 (27)	13.14 (29)	14.11 (31)	14.96 (33)	15.74 (34¾)
92–94 cm (36¼–37 in)	12.07 (26½)	12.36 (27¼)	13.03 (28¾)	13.89 (30½)	14.84 (32¾)	15.87 (35)	16.41 (36¼)	11.86 (26¼)	12.10 (26¾)	12.74 (28)	13.63 (30)	14.63 (32¼)	15.57 (34¼)	16.42 (36¼)
94–96 cm (37–37¾ in)	12.46 (27½)	12.77 (28¼)	13.49 (29¾)	14.38 (31¾)	15.34 (33¾)	16.45 (36¼)	17.06 (37½)	12.26 (27)	12.53 (27½)	13.21 (29)	14.12 (31¼)	15.14 (33½)	16.13 (35½)	17.05 (37½)
96–98 cm (37¾–38½ in)	12.87 (28¼)	13.21 (29)	13.98 (30¾)	14.89 (32¾)	15.87 (35)	17.01 (37½)	17.69 (39)	12.66 (28)	12.97 (28½)	13.70 (30¼)	14.62 (32¼)	15.66 (34½)	16.69 (36¾)	17.65 (39)
98–100 cm (38½–39¼ in)	13.31 (29¼)	13.67 (30¼)	14.48 (32)	15.43 (34)	16.41 (36¼)	17.56 (38¾)	18.29 (40¼)	13.06 (28¾)	13.42 (29½)	14.19 (31¼)	15.13 (33¼)	16.19 (35¾)	17.24 (38)	18.23 (40¼)
100–102 cm (39¼–40¼ in)	13.77 (30¼)	14.15 (31¼)	15.00 (33)	15.98 (35¼)	16.98 (37½)	18.11 (40)	18.89 (41¾)	13.48 (29¾)	13.88 (30½)	14.69 (32½)	15.65 (34½)	16.73 (37)	17.80 (39¼)	18.80 (41½)
102–104 cm (40¼–41 in)	14.25 (31½)	14.65 (32¼)	15.54 (34¼)	16.65 (36½)	17.57 (38¾)	18.67 (41¼)	19.50 (43)	13.91 (30¾)	14.36 (31¾)	15.21 (33½)	16.20 (35¾)	17.28 (38)	18.38 (40½)	19.36 (42¾)
104–106 cm (41–41¾ in)	14.76 (32½)	15.18 (33½)	16.10 (35½)	17.13 (37¾)	18.18 (40)	19.25 (42½)	20.12 (44¼)	14.36 (31¾)	14.85 (32¾)	15.75 (34¾)	16.75 (37)	17.86 (39¼)	18.98 (41¾)	19.98 (44)
106–108 cm (41¾–42½ in)	15.30 (33¾)	15.73 (34¾)	16.68 (36¾)	17.74 (39)	18.82 (41½)	19.86 (43¾)	20.76 (45¾)	14.84 (32¾)	15.37 (34)	16.30 (36)	17.33 (38¼)	18.46 (40¾)	19.62 (43¼)	20.61 (45½)
108–110 cm (42½–43¼ in)	15.85 (35)	16.31 (36)	17.28 (38)	18.37 (40½)	19.49 (43)	20.51 (45¼)	21.45 (47¼)	15.35 (33¾)	15.91 (35)	16.87 (37¼)	17.94 (39½)	19.09 (42)	20.30 (44¾)	21.29 (47)
110–112 cm (43¼–44 in)	16.43 (36¼)	16.91 (37¼)	17.90 (39½)	19.02 (42)	20.18 (44½)	21.22 (46¾)	22.18 (49)	15.90 (35)	16.48 (36¼)	17.47 (38½)	18.56 (41)	19.76 (43½)	21.03 (46¼)	22.03 (48½)
112–114 cm (44–45 in)	17.04 (37½)	17.53 (38¾)	18.54 (40¾)	19.70 (43½)	20.91 (46)	21.98 (48½)	22.98 (50¾)	16.48 (36¼)	17.09 (37¾)	18.08 (39¾)	19.22 (42¼)	20.47 (45¼)	21.81 (48)	22.84 (50¼)
114–116 cm (45–45¾ in)	17.66 (39)	18.18 (40)	19.20 (42¼)	20.39 (45)	21.66 (47¾)	22.82 (50¼)	23.85 (52½)	17.11 (37¾)	17.72 (39)	18.72 (41¼)	19.91 (44)	21.23 (46¾)	22.67 (50)	23.73 (52¼)
116–118 cm (45¾–46½ in)	18.32 (40½)	18.85 (41½)	19.89 (43¾)	21.11 (46½)	22.45 (49½)	23.73 (52¼)	24.80 (54¾)	17.77 (39¼)	18.40 (40½)	19.40 (42¾)	20.64 (45½)	22.04 (48½)	23.60 (52)	24.71 (54½)
118–120 cm (46½–47¼ in)	18.99 (41¾)	19.55 (43)	20.60 (45½)	21.85 (48¼)	23.28 (51¼)	24.73 (54½)	25.83 (57)	18.48 (40¾)	19.11 (42¼)	20.11 (44¼)	21.42 (47¼)	22.92 (50½)	24.62 (54¼)	25.81 (57)
120–122 cm (47¼–48 in)	19.70 (43½)	20.28 (44¾)	21.34 (47)	22.63 (50)	24.15 (53¼)	25.80 (57)	26.96 (59½)	19.22 (42¼)	19.85 (43¾)	20.87 (46)	22.25 (49)	23.88 (52¾)	25.73 (56¾)	27.03 (59½)
122–124 cm (48–48¾ in)	20.43 (45)	21.03 (46¼)	22.11 (48¾)	23.45 (51¾)	25.07 (55¼)	26.96 (59½)	28.18 (62¼)	19.99 (44)	20.64 (45½)	21.68 (47¾)	23.13 (51)	24.91 (55)	26.95 (59½)	28.37 (62½)
124–126 cm (48¾–49½ in)	21.20 (46¾)	21.82 (48)	22.92 (50½)	24.32 (53½)	26.05 (57½)	28.18 (62¼)	29.50 (65)	20.80 (45¾)	21.47 (47¼)	22.54 (49¾)	24.09 (53)	26.05 (57½)	28.27 (62¼)	29.87 (65¾)
126–128 cm (49½–50½ in)	21.99 (48½)	22.64 (50)	23.77 (52½)	25.24 (55¾)	27.10 (59¾)	29.48 (65)	30.92 (68¼)	21.65 (47¾)	22.34 (49¼)	23.47 (51¾)	25.11 (55¼)	27.28 (60¼)	29.71 (65½)	31.51 (69½)
128–130 cm (50½–51¾ in)	22.82 (50¼)	23.50 (51¾)	24.67 (54½)	26.22 (57¾)	28.21 (62¼)	30.86 (68)	32.44 (71½)	22.53 (49¾)	23.25 (51¼)	24.46 (54)	26.22 (57¾)	28.63 (63)	31.28 (69)	33.33 (73½)
130–132 cm (51¼–52 in)	23.69 (52¼)	24.59 (53¾)	25.62 (56½)	27.26 (60)	29.41 (64¾)	32.31 (71¼)	34.07 (75)	23.44 (51¾)	24.22 (53½)	25.52 (56¼)	27.40 (60½)	30.09 (66¼)	32.99 (72¾)	35.33 (78)
132–134 cm (52–52¾ in)	24.59 (54¼)	25.32 (55¾)	26.62 (58¾)	28.38 (62½)	30.68 (67¾)	33.82 (74½)	35.81 (79)	24.38 (53¾)	25.22 (55½)	26.66 (58¾)	28.68 (63¼)	31.68 (69¾)	34.84 (76¾)	37.53 (82¾)
134–136 cm (52¾–53½ in)	25.53 (56¼)	26.30 (58)	27.68 (61)	29.58 (65¼)	32.05 (70¾)	35.40 (78)	37.67 (83)	25.35 (56)	26.28 (58)	27.88 (61½)	30.06 (66¼)	33.41 (73¾)	36.84 (81¼)	39.93 (88)
136–138 cm (53½–54¼ in)	26.51 (58½)	27.32 (60¼)	28.80 (63½)	30.86 (68)	33.51 (74)	37.05 (81¾)	39.65 (87½)	26.34 (58)	27.39 (60½)	29.19 (64¼)	31.54 (69½)	35.29 (77¾)	39.01 (86)	42.54 (93¾)
138–140 cm (54½–55 in)	27.53 (60¾)	28.38 (62½)	29.99 (66)	32.23 (71)	35.08 (77¼)	38.77 (85½)	41.74 (92)							
140–142 cm (55–56 in)	28.59 (63)	29.48 (65)	31.25 (69)	33.70 (74¼)	36.75 (81)	40.55 (89½)	43.97 (97)							
142–144 cm (56–56¾ in)	29.70 (65½)	30.64 (67½)	32.58 (71¾)	35.27 (77¾)	38.54 (85)	42.39 (93½)	46.32 (102)							
144–146 cm (56¾–57½ in)	30.86 (68)	31.85 (70¼)	34.00 (75)	36.95 (81½)	40.45 (89¼)	44.29 (97¾)	48.80 (107½)							

*See footnote to Table 2–8A.

Table 2-9   EMERGING PATTERNS OF BEHAVIOR DURING THE FIRST YEAR OF LIFE*

NEONATAL PERIOD (FIRST 4 WEEKS)

Prone:	Lies in flexed attitude; turns head from side to side; head sags on ventral suspension
Supine:	Generally flexed and a little stiff
Visual:	May fixate face or light in line of vision; "doll's-eye" movement of eyes on turning of the body
Reflex:	Moro response active; stepping and placing reflexes; grasp reflex active
Social:	Visual preference for human face

AT 4 WEEKS

Prone:	Legs more extended; holds chin up; turns head; head lifted momentarily to plane of body on ventral suspension
Supine:	Tonic neck posture predominates; supple and relaxed; head lags on pull to sitting position
Visual:	Watches person; follows moving object
Social:	Body movements in cadence with voice of other in social contact; beginning to smile

AT 8 WEEKS

Prone:	Raises head slightly farther; head sustained in plane of body on ventral suspension
Supine:	Tonic neck posture predominates; head lags on pull to sitting position
Visual:	Follows moving object 180 degrees
Social:	Smiles on social contact; listens to voice and coos

AT 12 WEEKS

Prone:	Lifts head and chest, arms extended; head above plane of body on ventral suspension
Supine:	Tonic neck posture predominates; reaches toward and misses objects; waves at toy
Sitting:	Head lag partially compensated on pull to sitting position; early head control with bobbing motion; back rounded
Reflex:	Typical Moro response has not persisted; makes defense movements or selective withdrawal reactions
Social:	Sustained social contact; listens to music; says "aah, ngah"

AT 16 WEEKS

Prone:	Lifts head and chest, head in approximately vertical axis; legs extended
Supine:	Symmetrical posture predominates, hands in midline; reaches and grasps objects and brings them to mouth
Sitting:	No head lag on pull to sitting position; head steady, held forward; enjoys sitting with full truncal support
Standing:	When held erect, pushes with feet
Adaptive:	Sees pellet, but makes no move to it
Social:	Laughs out loud; may show displeasure if social contact is broken; excited at sight of food

AT 28 WEEKS

Prone:	Rolls over; may pivot
Supine:	Lifts head; rolls over; squirming movements
Sitting:	Sits briefly, with support of pelvis; leans forward on hands; back rounded
Standing:	May support most of weight; bounces actively
Adaptive:	Reaches out for and grasps large object; *transfers* objects from hand to hand; grasp uses radial palm; rakes at pellet
Language:	Polysyllabic vowel sounds formed
Social:	Prefers mother; babbles; enjoys mirror; responds to changes in emotional content of social contact

AT 40 WEEKS

Sitting:	Sits up alone and indefinitely without support, back straight
Standing:	Pulls to standing position
Motor:	Creeps or crawls
Adaptive:	Grasps objects with *thumb and forefinger*; pokes at things with forefinger; picks up pellet with assisted pincer movement; uncovers hidden toy; attempts to retrieve dropped object; releases object grasped by other person
Language:	Repetitive consonant sounds (mamma, dada)
Social:	Responds to sound of name; plays peek-a-boo or pat-a-cake; waves bye-bye

AT 52 WEEKS (1 YEAR)

Motor:	Walks with one hand held; "cruises" or walks holding on to furniture
Adaptive:	Picks up pellet with unassisted pincer movement of forefinger and thumb; releases object to other person on request or gesture
Language:	A few words besides mama, dada
Social:	Plays simple ball game; makes postural adjustment to dressing

*Data are derived from those of Gesell, Shirley, Provence, Wolf, Bailey, and others.

Table 2–10 EMERGING PATTERNS OF BEHAVIOR FROM 1 TO 5 YEARS OF AGE*

15 Months

Motor:	Walks alone; crawls up stairs
Adaptive:	Makes tower of 2 cubes; makes a line with crayon; inserts pellet in bottle
Language:	Jargon; follows simple commands; may name a familiar object (ball)
Social:	Indicates some desires or needs by pointing; hugs parents

18 Months

Motor:	Runs stiffly; sits on small chair; walks up stairs with one hand held; explores drawers and waste baskets
Adaptive:	Piles 3 cubes; imitates scribbling; imitates vertical stroke; dumps pellet from bottle
Language:	10 words (average); names pictures; identifies one or more parts of body
Social:	Feeds self; seeks help when in trouble; may complain when wet or soiled; kisses parent with pucker

24 Months

Motor:	Runs well; walks up and down stairs, one step at a time; opens doors; climbs on furniture
Adaptive:	Tower of 6 cubes; circular scribbling; imitates horizontal stroke; folds paper once imitatively
Language:	Puts 3 words together (subject, verb, object)
Social:	Handles spoon well; often tells immediate experiences; helps to undress; listens to stories with pictures

30 Months

Motor:	Jumps
Adaptive:	Tower of 8 cubes; makes vertical and horizontal strokes, but generally will not join them to make a cross; imitates circular stroke, forming closed figure
Language:	Refers to self by pronoun "I"; knows full name
Social:	Helps put things away; pretends in play

36 Months

Motor:	Goes up stairs alternating feet; rides tricycle; stands momentarily on one foot
Adaptive:	Tower of 9 cubes; imitates construction of "bridge" of 3 cubes; copies a circle; imitates a cross
Language:	Knows age and sex; counts 3 objects correctly; repeats 3 numbers or a sentence of 6 syllables
Social:	Plays simple games (in "parallel" with other children); helps in dressing (unbuttons clothing and puts on shoes); washes hands

48 Months

Motor:	Hops on one foot; throws ball overhand; uses scissors to cut out pictures; climbs well
Adaptive:	Copies bridge from model; imitates contruction of "gate" of 5 cubes; copies cross and square; draws a man with 2 to 4 parts besides head; names longer of 2 lines
Language:	Counts 4 pennies accurately; tells a story
Social:	Plays with several children with beginning of social interaction and role-playing; goes to toilet alone

60 Months

Motor:	Skips
Adaptive:	Draws triangle from copy; names heavier of 2 weights
Language:	Names 4 colors; repeats sentence of 10 syllables; counts 10 pennies correctly
Social:	Dresses and undresses; asks questions about meaning of words; domestic role-playing

*Data are derived from those of Gesell, Shirley, Provence, Wolf, Bailey, and others. After 5 years the Stanford-Binet, Wechsler-Bellevue, and other scales offer the most precise estimates of developmental level. In order to have their greatest value, they should be administered only by an experienced and qualified person.

2.12 ASSESSMENT OF NEUROLOGIC AND PSYCHOLOGIC DEVELOPMENT

See Sec 2.46 and Chapter 21.

The assessment of the functional status of the infant or child is an essential part of each examination but is all too often uncritical. Only with some knowledge of developmental standards can the physician be adequately sensitive to deviations that indicate slight or early impairment of development. Moreover, only if pediatricians can quickly and confidently compare their observations with the normal developmental pattern will they be able to handle the questions of parents or make appropriate suggestions for further study.

The observations made and the techniques used during the developmental examination must be appropriate to the age of the infant or child. The physician will often use readily available materials that have not been standardized but which will usually reveal whether a more comprehensive developmental evaluation is indicated, possibly by a psychologist. The casual examination should be interpreted with caution, particularly when an infant or child who is irritable, hungry, or ill fails to perform at his or her chronologic level. For such patients a future reassessment is in order. For the infant born prematurely an adjustment in chronologic age will need to be made.

In the young infant the examination may begin by observation of the child in the prone and supine positions, note being taken of spontaneous activity in each position, and then of the manner in which the infant adjusts to being pulled from a supine to a sitting position and being held in ventral suspension (*Landau response*). The reaction to moving persons or to objects brought within sight or grasp can be determined, both for relatively large objects such as a rattle or stethoscope and for such small objects as a pellet. Behavior when standing with support should also be observed.

After the 1st yr of life the child may be given blocks as well as a pencil and paper and the ability observed to mimic or copy the patterns of the physician. The standard blocks used in construction of various figures are 1-in red cubes. After 3–4 yr the child can be asked to "draw a man," to draw figures, and to count pennies.

Tables 2–9 and 2–10 list expected behavior of infants and children of various ages and circumstances.

A number of relatively simple tests permit the physician to make helpful assessments of the intellectual level of older children as part of normal office practice. Such tests include the Peabody Picture Vocabulary Test, the Quick Test, the Raven Matrices, the Thorpe Developmental Inventory, the Denver Developmental Screen-

ing Test, and the Revised Development Screening Inventory (Knobloch). Occasional or casual testing may be misleading. In using these or other tools for evaluation of performance the tester should become thoroughly familiar with the procedures, their rules for administration, and their limitations.

VICTOR C. VAUGHAN, III

Bayer LM, Bayley N: Growth Diagnosis. Chicago, University of Chicago Press, 1959.

Bower TGR: A Primer of Infant Development. San Francisco, WH Freeman, 1977.

Bower TGR: The Perceptual World of the Child. Cambridge, Harvard University Press, 1977.

Brazelton TB: Neonatal Behavior Assessment Scale. Clin Dev Med Ser No 50. London, William Heinemann, 1973.

Brazelton TB, Parker WB, Zuckerman B: Importance of assessment of the neonate. Curr Prob Pediatr 7:1, 1976.

Brazelton TB, Vaughan VC III (eds): The Family: Setting Priorities. New York, Science & Medicine Publishing Co, 1979.

Condon WS, Sander L: Neonatal movement is synchronized with adult speech: Interactional participation and language acquisition. Science 183:99, 1974.

Cravioto J: Mother-child interrelationships and malnutrition. In: Vaughan VC III, Brazelton TB (eds): The Family—Can It Be Saved? Chicago, Year Book Publishers, 1976.

Dine, MS, Gartside PS, Glueck CJ, et al: Relationship of head circumference to length in the first 400 days of life: A mnemonic. Pediatrics 67:506, 1981.

Erikson EH: Childhood and Society. Ed 2. New York, WW Norton, 1963.

Frankenburg WK, Goldstein AD, Camp BW: The Revised Denver Developmental Screening Test: Its accuracy as a screening instrument. J Pediatr 79:988, 1971.

Frankenburg WK, Thornton SM, Cohrs ME: Pediatric Developmental Diagnosis. New York, Thieme-Stratton Inc., 1981.

Greulich WW, Pyle SI: Radiographic Atlas of Skeletal Development of the Hand and Wrist. Stanford, Calif, Stanford University Press, 1950; 2nd ed, 1959.

Iliff A, Lee VA: Pulse rate, respiratory rate, and body temperature of children between two months and eighteen years of age. Child Develop 23:237, 1952.

Klaus MH, Kennell JH: Maternal-Infant Bonding. St. Louis, CV Mosby, 1976.

Knobloch H, Pasamanick B (eds): Gesell and Amatruda's Developmental Diagnosis. Ed 3. Hagerstown, Md, Harper & Row, 1974.

Knobloch H, Stevens F, Malone AF: Manual of Developmental Diagnosis. Hagerstown, Md., Harper & Row, 1980.

Lewis RC, Duval AM, Iliff A: Standards for the basal metabolism of children from 2 to 15 years of age, inclusive. J Pediatr 23:1, 1943.

McKay HE, McKay A, Sinisterra L: Behavioral intervention studies with malnourished children: A review of experiences. In: Kallen DJ: Nutrition, Development, and Social Behavior. Washington DC, DHEW Publication No 73–242.

Prechtl H, Beintema D: The Neurological Examination of the Full Term Newborn Infant. Clin Dev Med Ser No 12. Philadelphia, JB Lippincott, 1975. Repr of 1965 ed.

Pyle SI, Reed RB, Stuart HC: Patterns of skeletal development in the hand. Pediatrics 24:886, 1959.

Reynolds EL, Asakawa T: Skeletal development in infancy: Standards for clinical use. Am J Roentgenol Radium Ther 65:403, 1951.

Tanner JM, Goldstein H, Whitehouse RH: Standards for children's height at 2–9 years allowing for height of parents. Arch Dis Child 45:755, 1970.

Todd TW: Atlas of Skeletal Maturation (Hand). St. Louis, CV Mosby, 1937.

Vogt EC, Vickers VS: Osseous growth and development. Radiology 31:441, 1938.

Weech AA: Signposts on highway of growth. Am J Dis Child 88:452, 1954.

Wingert J, Solomon IL, Schoen, EJ: Parent-specific height standards for preadolescent children of three racial groups, with method for rapid determination. Pediatrics 52:555, 1973.

2.13   EVALUATION OF ADOLESCENTS

See also Chapter 19.

Adolescence is a time of major physical, cognitive, and psychosocial growth and change. It composes nearly half the growing period in man and is the only period of life after birth in which the velocity of growth

normally increases. It begins at about the age of 10 yr in girls and 12 in boys. The end of adolescence varies with physical, mental, emotional, social, or cultural criteria which characterize the adult. Puberty has been defined as that time when one becomes able to produce children: the menarche in girls, or a less clearly defined milestone found 1.5–2 yr later in boys. Pubescence, the time during which secondary sex changes occur, is not sharply demarcated in length, but is generally about 2–3 yr. Prepubescent changes precede the 1st secondary sex changes of adolescence.

At about 7 yr of age the earliest changes occur that will culminate in adolescence: a gradual increase in production of adrenal steroids occurs in both sexes, and somewhat later there is a gradual prepubertal increase in production of estrogen and a little later of androgen in each sex. At about the age of 9–11 yr in girls estrogen production increases greatly, attaining the levels for normal adults; a comparable increase in androgen production occurs in boys at a somewhat later age.

The complex mechanisms that regulate the onset of pubertal development are discussed in Sec 18.6 and 18.30.

SEX DIFFERENCES

Growth and development in adolescence must be considered separately for boys and girls. Boys are on the average larger than girls from birth to the prepubescent period, have slightly less subcutaneous fat during the middle years of childhood, and have a slightly higher basal metabolic rate in relation to body surface. Boys and girls have much the same degree of motor activity and coordination until 7–8 yr of age, but by 9 yr boys surpass girls in motor skills.

In both sexes the time of onset and the rate of acquisition of adolescent changes vary widely. Individual variability is often apparent during early childhood; for example, children who will be slow to mature at adolescence are usually smaller than their contemporaries as early as 2 yr of age. Girls who have menarche early have a greater velocity of growth but a shorter growth period, and have a higher ratio of weight to height in adult life than girls who mature more slowly.

The fat in subcutaneous tissue, which showed a steady decrease in amount proportionate to body weight from the ages of 1–6 yr in both sexes, begins to reaccumulate as early as 8 yr in girls and 10 yr in boys. Both boys and girls tend to become slightly chubby just before the onset of the increased velocity of growth that comes with puberty. The growth spurt begins about 1 yr after the increase in fat is first apparent; with it come signs of sexual maturation. During the pubescent period, fat is rearranged in girls, whereas most boys lose fat, which is not replaced until after the growth spurt.

Physical changes during adolescence almost always occur in the same sequence, but their time of onset, velocity, and age at completion vary greatly. The growth spurt in boys (Fig 2–8) begins between 13–15.5 yr of age; during this time the average increase in height is 20 cm (8 in), half of which occurs during the year of most rapid growth. In girls (Fig 2–9) the growth spurt begins about a year and a half before that of boys and is almost completed by 13.5 yr of age; during the year of peak change about 8 cm (3.25 in) is gained. Following these peaks, height growth decelerates, and by the age of 18 yr is nearly complete; for boys about 2.5 cm (1 in) of average height increase remains, slightly less for girls.

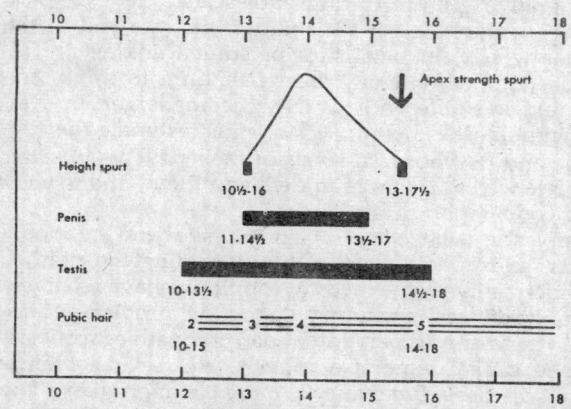

Figure 2–8 Sequence of growth in boys at adolescence. An average boy is represented. The age range for each event is given directly below its start and finish. (From Tanner JM: Growth at Adolescence. Ed 2. Oxford, England, Blackwell Scientific Publications, 1962.)

Widening of the pelvis occurs early in the pubescent period in girls. In both sexes the legs usually lengthen before the thighs, which then increase in breadth. Then shoulders widen and the trunk grows in length. Muscular strength normally increases in girls until menarche, whereas boys increase in strength until about 18 mo after the time of greatest height increase.

The changes in female breasts, in male genitalia, and in the pattern and quantity of pubic hair in both sexes form the basis of sex maturity ratings (see below).

MENTAL AND PSYCHOSOCIAL CHANGES

In middle childhood relatively uniform annual physical growth is associated with relatively comfortable feelings regarding the body. Adolescence disrupts this tranquility with tension among the physical, cognitive, and psychosocial aspects of growth.

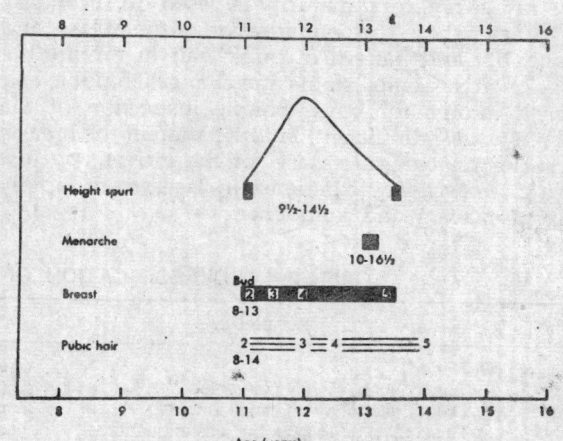

Figure 2–9 Sequence of growth in girls at adolescence. An average girl is represented. The age range within which some of the events may occur is given directly below them. (From Tanner JM: Growth at Adolescence. Ed 2. Oxford, England, Blackwell Scientific Publications, 1962.)

Cognitive growth during adolescence, like physical change, exhibits great variability in its rate and in the age at which characteristics of adult thinking are attained. Adults generally expect children to think, act, and respond differently as they become larger. In dealing with adolescents physicians must estimate the cognitive and psychosocial levels of their patients in order to relate well to them, to understand them, and to elicit their cooperation in health care.

Adolescents have age-specific physical and emotional needs, and various legal rights, including the right to confidentiality. Some medical conditions have relatively high incidences, including endocrine problems, anorexia nervosa, hyperventilation, idiopathic scoliosis, slipped capital femoral epiphysis, and sexually transmitted diseases. Pregnancy is more common than a few years ago. The responses of adolescent patients to disease may differ little from those of children or adults except in impact on physical or emotional growth; on the other hand, the emotional stage of development of the adolescent can markedly affect the course or outcome of illness.

2.14 SEX MATURITY RATINGS

The traditional estimates of the stage of biologic maturity have employed height, weight, skinfold thickness, dental changes, and the like, all of which, like age, are imprecise indicators of growth status. Skeletal age, as determined by roentgenography, is more closely related to the biologic changes of adolescence and gives more precise information about levels of physical maturity. Sex maturity ratings (SMR) have been useful in assessing growth and development during adolescence and correlate well with the level of skeletal maturity and with certain other biologic measurements. Sex maturity ratings can be easily made without need for special procedures, as part of any general physical examination.

ASSESSING SEXUAL MATURITY

The rating of sexual maturity is based on secondary sex characteristics. The configuration of the breasts and the quantity and pattern of pubic hair determine the ratings of girls. Genital status and changes in pubic hair establish ratings for boys. Simple inspection of the patient is usually sufficient, but palpation of the breasts or testicles may be necessary for the girl or boy just entering pubescence. Experience in assessment rapidly brings proficiency and confidence.

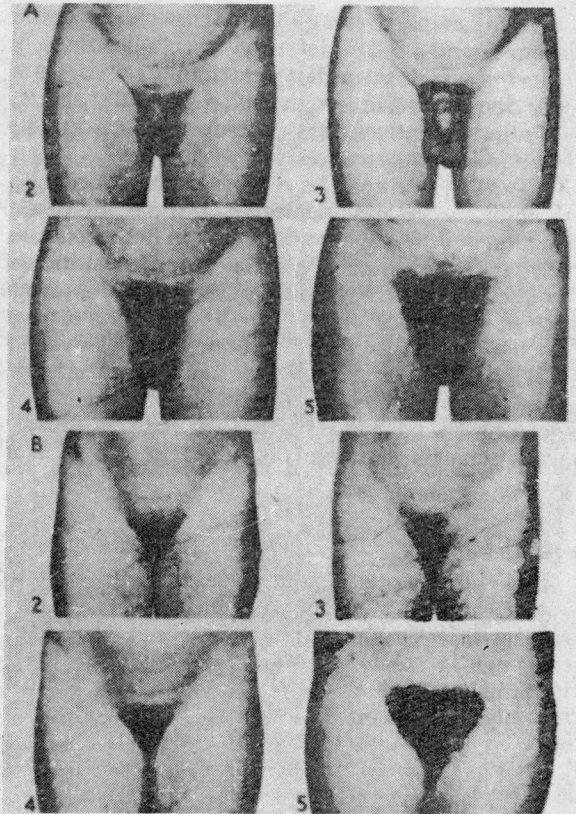

Figure 2–10   Sex maturity ratings of pubic hair changes in adolescent boys and girls. (Courtesy JM Tanner, M.D., Institute of Child Health, Department of Growth and Development, University of London, London, England.)

Sex maturity ratings range from 1–5; a score of 1 represents the prepubertal child and 5 corresponds to adult status. Sequential changes during adolescence are given in Table 2–11 for boys and in Table 2–12 for girls. In boys SMR 3 is characterized by the confluence of slightly curly hair across the pubic area, following medial extension from the sites of first appearance. SMR 4 in males is characterized by more nearly adult genitalia and by abundant pubic hair, usually curly, but less in quantity than expected in an adult male. The differentiation between SMR 3 and SMR 4 can be difficult at first. Similar difficulty may occur in assigning SMRs for girls, but experience will bring clarity and consistency. Changes in pubic hair for boys and girls

Table 2–11 CLASSIFICATION OF SEX MATURITY STAGES IN BOYS

Stage	Pubic Hair	Penis	Testes
1	None	Preadolescent	Preadolescent
2	Scanty, long, slightly pigmented	Slight enlargement	Enlarged scrotum, pink texture altered
3	Darker, starts to curl, small amount	Longer	Larger
4	Resembles adult type, but less in quantity; coarse, curly	Larger; glans and breadth increase in size	Larger, scrotum dark
5	Adult distribution, spread to medial surface of thighs	Adult size	Adult size

Adapted from Tanner JM: Growth at Adolescence. Ed 2. Oxford, Blackwell Scientific Publications, 1962.

Table 2-12 CLASSIFICATION OF SEX MATURITY STAGES IN GIRLS

STAGE	PUBIC HAIR	BREASTS
1	Preadolescent	Preadolescent
2	Sparse, lightly pigmented, straight, medial border of labia	Breast and papilla elevated as small mound; areolar diameter increased
3	Darker, beginning to curl, increased amount	Breast and areola enlarged, no contour separation
4	Coarse, curly, abundant but amount less than in adult	Areola and papilla form secondary mound
5	Adult feminine triangle, spread to medial surface of thighs	Mature; nipple projects, areola part of general breast contour

Adapted from Tanner JM: Growth at Adolescence. Ed 2. Oxford, Blackwell Scientific Publications, 1962.

are shown in Fig 2–10. Sequential changes in breast classification are shown in Fig 2–11.

Usually separate ratings are given to genitalia and pubic hair in boys and to breast development and pubic hair in girls. If the two ratings differ, they are averaged, and a single numerical indicator of the degree of maturity is obtained. Some changes correlate more closely with one rating than with another; for example, the peak height velocity in boys occurs at a pubic hair rating of 3 or at an averaged rating of 4.

CORRELATIONS OF SEX MATURITY RATINGS

The onset of puberty is evident in girls when a small breast bud is visible or palpable. In boys, the earliest sign is enlargement of the testicles, which is often difficult to assess; accordingly, a pubic hair SMR of 2 may be the first visible sign of puberty in a male. At this stage, pubic hair in a boy consists of small tufts of slightly pigmented hair at the sides of the base of the penis; the hair may be darker in boys of dark skin.

In girls, the most rapid increase in height is associated with a pubic hair rating of 2 (Fig 2–12). Menarche occurs most often at an average SMR of 4 (though many girls begin menstruation at SMR 3), and ejaculation occurs in boys as they approach SMR 3 but may not be consistent, nor does the semen contain sperm until between SMR 3 and 4.

During adolescence boys (Fig 2–13) become generally larger than girls. Many sex differences are attributed to testosterone, the production of which increases with SMR. It is presumed that testosterone stimulates erythropoiesis in bone marrow to bring about increases in the quantity of hemoglobin and higher hematocrit values. Fig 2–14 and 2–15 contrast the steady rise of

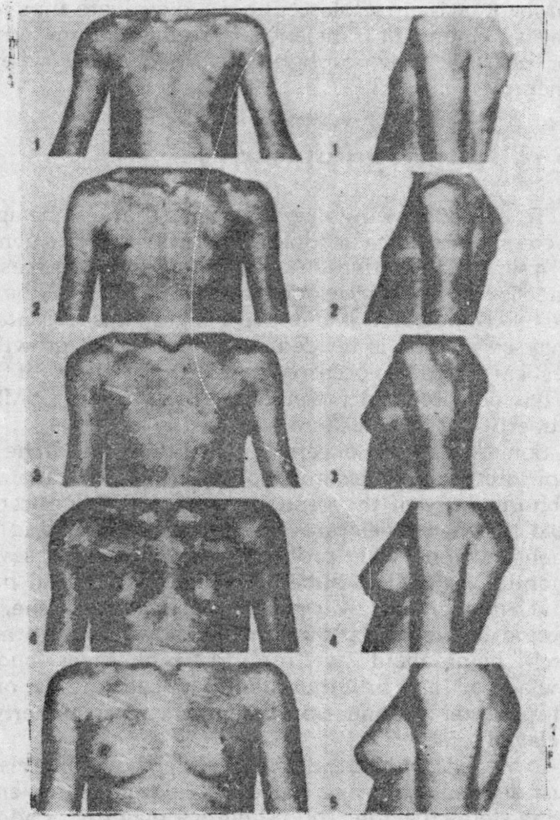

Figure 2–11 Sex maturity ratings of breast changes in adolescent girls. (Courtesy JM Tanner, M.D., Institute of Child Health, Department of Growth and Development, University of London, London, England.)

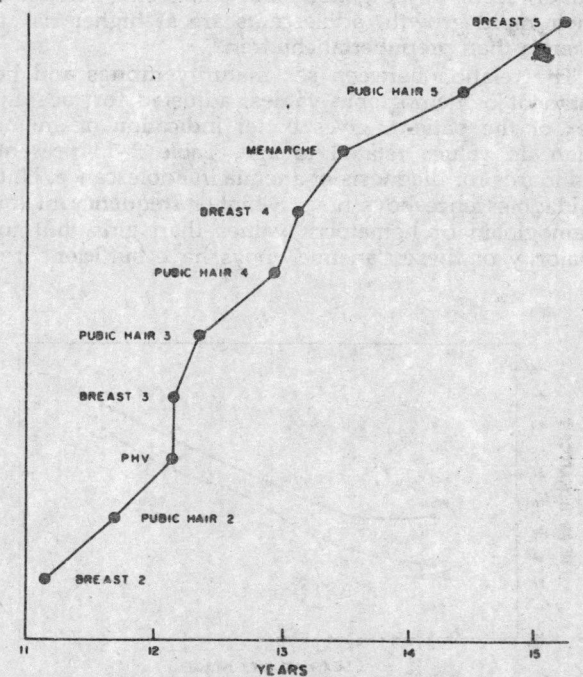

Figure 2–12 Sequential changes in sex maturity stages of breast and pubic hair in girls. PHV = peak height velocity. (Adapted from Root AW: J Pediatr 83:1–19, 187–200, 1973.)

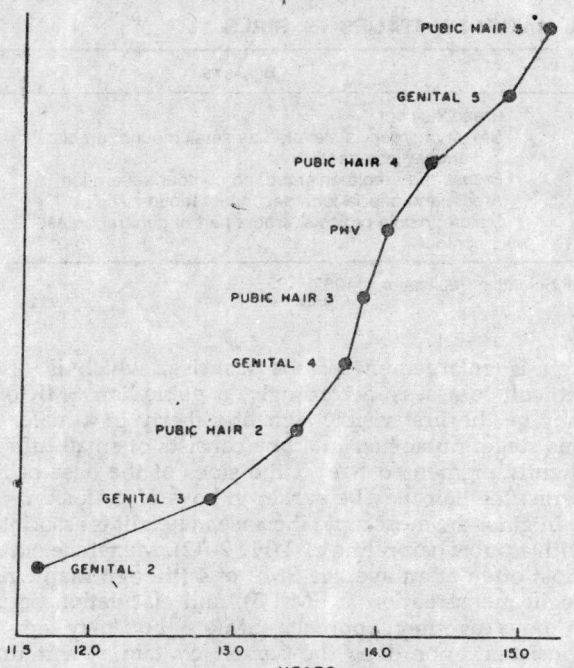

Figure 2–13 Sequential changes in sex maturity stages of pubic hair and genitalia in boys. PHV = peak height velocity. (Adapted from Root AW: J Pediatr 83:1–19, 187–200, 1973.)

hematocrit in boys with the relative stability in girls as both become more mature. Hemoglobin levels are lower for black adolescents than for white; this difference (1 gm/dl) seems to be genetic and persistent. Because of their rapid growth, adolescents are at higher risk of anemia than prepubertal children.

The relation between sex maturity ratings and hematocrit or hemoglobin values, adjusted for race and sex of the patient, gives better indication of anemia than do values related to age. Table 2–13 presents standards for diagnosis of anemia in adolescence. Until midadolescence boys have a higher frequency of low hemoglobin or hematocrit values than girls, but the majority of these "anemic" boys have sufficient iron

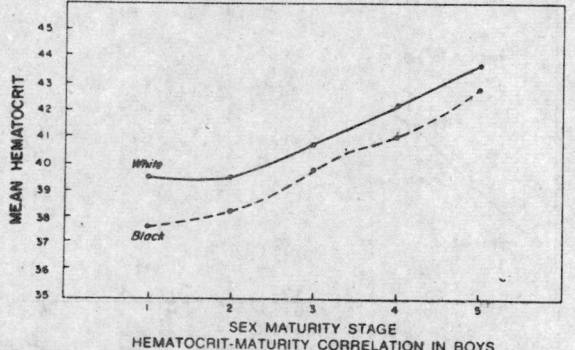

Figure 2–14 Hematocrit-sex maturity rating correlation in boys. (From Daniel WA Jr: Pediatrics 52:388–394, 1973.)

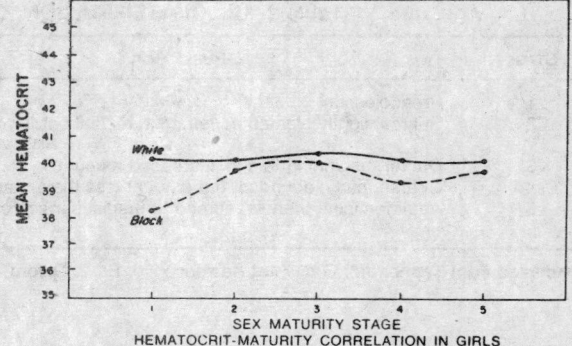

Figure 2–15 Hematocrit-sex maturity rating correlation in girls. (From Daniel WA Jr: Pediatrics 52:388–394, 1973.)

stores and normal iron-binding capacities, exhibit no clinical symptoms of anemia, and do not respond to supplemental dietary iron. Their low hematocrit levels may reflect increased plasma volume. Other factors may contribute; for example, a shift of the dissociation curve of oxyhemoglobin to the right may ensure that at lower levels of hemoglobin physiologic quantities of oxygen reach tissues. Whatever the reasons, many adolescent boys, particularly around the peak of the growth spurt, have hemoglobin or hematocrit levels indicating anemia, but are functionally healthy. It is probably wise in adolescent boys to evaluate anemia by measurements of transferrin saturation, serum ferritin, or red cell protoporphyrin before deciding whether therapy is needed.

2.15 DELAYED PUBERTY

To be not growing like other boys of the same age is a common concern of adolescent boys. If a boy's general physical examination discloses a pubescent increase in the size of the testicles or pubic hair at SMR 2, he can be told that sexual changes have begun; this reassurance may be all that is needed. If no pubescent growth in testicular size has occurred by 13.5 yr of age, or if SMR 3 has not occurred within 4 yr of the onset of SMR 2, puberty can be considered delayed.

Some girls feel concern because their menarche has not occurred. If examination indicates no anatomic abnormalities of the genitalia, a girl of SMR 3 can be told that her development is proceeding well and that menstruation will probably begin within several months. At SMR 2 pubertal change has begun, but a much longer time will pass before the menarche, the period between first budding of the breast and menarche being about 2 yr. If a girl has no breast bud by the age of 13 yr or if more than 5 yr separate the onset of pubertal change from menarche, her puberty is delayed.

If there is pubertal delay in either boys or girls, as just defined, it may be necessary to evaluate the endocrine status (Chapter 18). The great majority of adolescents with delayed onset of puberty, however, prove to be normal.

Table 2-13 RELATIONSHIP OF HEMATOCRIT TO SEX MATURITY RATING (SMR): STANDARDS USED FOR DETERMINING THE PRESENCE OF ANEMIA

SMR	1	2	3	4	5
Males					
White	35.6*	36.9	38.2	39.6	40.9
Black	34.9	36.0	37.1	38.2	39.3
Females					
White	35.8	36.6	37.0	36.7	35.9
Black	34.0	35.3	36.0	36.2	35.8

*Figures are the hematocrits (%) corresponding to the 15th percentile for the given sex and ethnicity.

2.16 SHORT STATURE

Adolescent boys worry more than girls about short stature. The boy with an SMR of 2-3 whose height is appropriate for skeletal age can be told that the endocrine system is active, and that he will grow taller, especially during the next year or year and a half, though his final height may not be all he desires. Short boys who have SMRs of 4 will be short when growth is completed. Such boys are often quite muscular and their participation in sports and other physical activities can give them status in their peer group and boost their self-esteem.

Short boys whose sexual development is lagging behind their ages and whose bone ages approximate their chronologic ages may need endocrinologic evaluation. The majority of boys who are short, however, are so presumably because of genetic factors; sexual maturation will occur at the appropriate time and in normal sequence.

2.17 GROWTH RETARDATION AND DISEASE

Growth retardation and delayed puberty can be associated with chronic illness; accordingly, investigation for associated disease is often indicated. In patients known to have illnesses that affect nutrition or growth, the progress of pubertal development can be followed with SMRs, which correlate with physical growth; when progress from one rating to another is unduly slow in a patient with chronic illness, attention should be given to conditions affecting growth.

2.18 NUTRITION AND ADOLESCENT GROWTH

Nutritional requirements are usually better correlated with sex maturity ratings than with chronologic age. Girls at SMR 2 and boys at SMR 3, for example, are at or close to their peak velocities of growth, and their intake of calories and specific nutrients should be assured adequate, without regard to their ages. Boys or girls at higher SMRs may need considerably fewer calories unless their expenditure of physical energy is great.

Participation in sports often increases during adolescence and nutritional requirements change accordingly. For participation in sports adolescents are usually assigned to groups according to chronologic age or weight, but some 13-14 yr old boys may be prepubertal in size and others almost as large as adults. To form groups in accordance with sex maturity ratings would help to lessen these physical differences, but unfortunately such arrangements are often impossible.

2.19 BIOCHEMICAL RELATIONSHIPS

Many biochemical measurements correlate better with sex maturity ratings than with chronologic age. Fig 2-16 relates activity of serum alkaline phosphatase to the SMRs for pubic hair. Similar correlations have been made for plasma folate, hematocrit, serum iron level, and many other constituents of the blood. These standards are preferred for adolescents to standards set by age.

2.20 COGNITIVE AND PSYCHOSOCIAL GROWTH

To know the status of an adolescent's maturation in cognitive and psychologic growth is useful in history

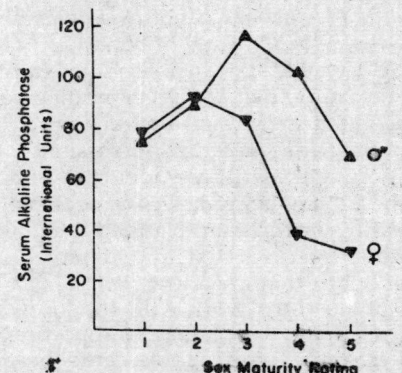

Figure 2-16 Relationship of serum alkaline phosphatase activity to sex maturity ratings in adolescents. (From Bennett DL, Ward MS, Daniel, WA Jr: J Pediatr 88:633-636, 1976.)

taking, in interviewing, and in providing health care. Estimations of the psychologic stage of development are less precise than those of physical growth or sexual maturation, but consideration of at least 3 variables provides much information: (1) an estimate of mental ability, (2) a tentative classification of early, middle, or late adolescence, and (3) the level of progress in the major psychosocial tasks of adolescence.

Usually mental ability is judged by school achievements, interests of the adolescent, and the scope of conversation and vocabulary used. Information obtained from formal tests may be available from schools. Mild mental retardation can remain undetected despite effects on psychosocial growth, and this possibility should be considered with each new patient. Young adolescents who are exceptionally bright may also have difficulties with interpersonal relationships. Their difference from their peers, which may be temporary, can produce a sense of isolation affecting psychosocial growth and misleading the physician in his evaluation of mental ability or emotional adjustment.

Chronologic age and sex maturity ratings will usually give satisfactory indication of early, middle, or late periods of adolescent change. Each of these arbitrary divisions has characteristics that are related to the tasks of adolescence. Normal psychologic growth during adolescence faces the individual with 4 major tasks that must be mastered before the fully mature adult emerges: (1) effecting emotional separation from the family, with acceptance of self-responsibility, (2) developing appropriate sexuality and a personal moral code, (3) dealing with the need for a future vocation and making the commitment to attain it, and (4) achieving the status of ego identity (Sec 2.9).

Early Adolescence. Early adolescents are fascinated with their changing bodies, wonder if they will be tall or short, fat or lean, attractive or ugly, and spend much time thinking about body parts and comparing themselves with age-mates or older members of the same sex. They have an ideal image of the body and often feel that their own bodies are out of control. Young adolescents are fascinated with secondary sex changes and are amazed, delighted, or frightened by erotic thoughts, dreams, and feelings. They observe and wonder about the actions of older adolescents or adults of the same sex and often attempt to imitate them. With increased curiosity about sexual matters and from discussions with friends, most young adolescents slowly evolve a personal moral code of conduct.

Increasing physical size, increased geographic mobility, and associations with a larger number of persons not only heighten the desire for freedom of action but also for money and material possessions. Teenagers often begin to get part-time jobs for which pay is received, the money being used for personal pleasures or clothes or in some instances added to family income. Work becomes an expected and accepted means of obtaining money, though few types of jobs are available. Most adolescents work with the knowledge that they must eventually become self-supporting.

There is a stage when adolescents become more aware of the past, of successes and failures, and whether they are accepted, admired, or rejected by others of the same age and sex. They come to a new recognition of parental status, and perhaps for the first time realize whether their parents are well educated, respected, rich or poor, or desirable models to imitate. At this time, the parents and their values may be rejected, temporarily or from time to time, other adults serving as confidants and advisors. In judging adults, adolescents begin to give consideration to the self, and to wonder what they will be like as adults. These thoughts are the beginning of a process of self-evaluation that should lead eventually to adolescents feeling comfortable with their bodies, knowing where they are going, and believing that they have inner resources adequate to permit them to live as effective adults.

Middle Adolescence. Middle adolescence is reached about a year and a half after the time of maximal growth, at approximately 13–15 yr of age for girls and 16 for boys. By this time there is again a feeling of being in control of the body, a realistic body image is held, and there is less concern about physical changes. With a greater sense of competence, demands emerge for more freedom of action and self-responsibility, and there is usually far more mobility than during earlier puberty. Sexual matters still receive much thought; desires become generally directed toward a particular member of the opposite sex, dating occurs, and much information and misinformation is obtained and shared about sexual matters. Association with a peer group has increased, and the group's influence may temporarily become greater than that of parents, though parental views are usually not completely rejected. More midadolescents work part-time and many become more interested in specific types of vocations. Cognitive growth has progressed, and there is greater ability to think in abstract terms, to form hypotheses, to evaluate plans of action, and to consider the future. Less uncertainty remains about who one is, what future role is desired, or what is expected of adulthood. On the other hand, few midadolescents have attained ego identity.

Late Adolescence. Though some ambivalence persists, during late adolescence the desire to leave home and family increases. The adolescent looks forward to higher education or to a job with separate living quarters, with some reluctance to leave the security of the home and parents and to separate from peers. More thinking is directed toward future education or a job. Uncertainty can be frightening for the youngster who feels inadequate to select a specific vocation, and this uneasiness often affects decisions regarding additional years of study or training. Most late adolescents have established a moral code and feel relatively comfortable with sexual relationships and decisions; some are still uncertain about themselves or their beliefs. Cognitive growth has usually continued, with thinking more logical and concerned with the future. Ego identity may not be achieved until a few more years have passed, but late adolescents are comfortable with their bodies, know what they wish to achieve, can commit their energies toward achieving a goal, and believe they are competent to function as adults.

For some boys or girls one or more of the major psychologic tasks of adolescence remain unsolved or not yet integrated into the personality, and the state that Erikson calls ego diffusion may continue until each task has been completed. Adults who never achieve ego identity remain inadequate, feel inferior, and have many failures in their lives.

ASSESSMENT OF COGNITIVE AND PSYCHOSOCIAL GROWTH IN ADOLESCENCE

Precise or detailed measurement of cognitive or psychologic growth during adolescence requires a skilled psychologist, and the results should be interpreted with caution. Physicians caring for teenagers can obtain useful estimates of the stages of psychosocial development as early, middle, or late through conversations with their patients and the correlation of information obtained with other findings, including the sex maturity ratings obtained on physical examination.

Cognition at the onset of puberty is generally based on experiential thinking; that is, on what has happened in the past or is happening concurrently. Most early adolescents' thoughts deal primarily with concrete dimensions and relationships, rather than abstractions. With further cognitive growth, more abstract thought develops, hypotheses can be produced, and plans can be made for the future which take account of many variables. This stage of cognitive growth, which Piaget calls formal operational thought, may not be reached until early adulthood. In assessing the cognitive growth of an adolescent, evidence is sought of progress from the concrete to the abstract, but clear, logical, conceptual thinking cannot be expected early. The clinical objective in assessment is generally to determine whether cognitive growth is occurring rather than the level of proficiency in ideation. If more specific information is required, psychologic testing will be appropriate.

DEVIATIONS FROM NORMAL

Psychosocial milestones are not always achieved at the expected age. Moreover, physical, cognitive, and psychosocial growth may frequently be at different or dissonant developmental stages.

As in the case of physical changes of puberty, the range between early and delayed cognitive or psychosocial growth is wide. Adolescents experiencing either greater or less physical, emotional, cognitive, or social development than others of their age may feel different, abnormal, or isolated. If, however, reassurance and emotional support can be given, the separation is usually temporary.

Many adolescents experience transitory or briefly traumatic emotional problems. Some may be serious, threatening the achievement of comfortable identity, but most can be dealt with in ways that can help the adolescent become more adult. The physician who can anticipate or recognize problems likely to be temporary at their onset can often offer useful and sometimes critical help in adjustment.

Society often adds external pressures to the personal problems of adolescence. For instance, the changing values assigned to sexual activity often involve adolescents before their ability to assess and assume responsibility for their personal activities is sufficiently developed. Further, an extended period of higher education may foster continued dependency and consequently widen the gap between physical maturity on the one hand and social maturity and autonomy on the other.

2.21 COMMUNICATING WITH ADOLESCENTS

Physicians who provide care for small children are accustomed to interviewing and discussing with parents the physical findings and plans of treatment. With adolescents the parents become more peripheral and the patient more central in the relationship with the physician. The physical examination of adolescent patients often takes place in the absence of parents, and history taking, a lengthy interview, or the discussion of therapy is conducted primarily with the adolescent, though the parent may be informed appropriately. The adolescent patient is being encouraged to accept responsibility for personal health care; it is, therefore, necessary that physician and patient understand each other, in a relationship in which the traditional confidentiality of communications between physician and patient needs to be respected, so long as personal safety and well being are not threatened for the patient or for others.

Adolescents differ greatly, in accordance with their levels of cognition or psychosocial development and in their abilities to provide or utilize information. In early or middle adolescence physical signs and body language are often more informative and significant than the words. Young teenagers are unsure how to express themselves verbally and often believe they will be misunderstood by adults, or that confidentiality will not be respected, and are reluctant to speak freely. Further, adolescents' words often have unexpected meanings. Their posture, behavior, and gestures, however, can often convey feelings and can indicate a need to discuss now or later certain aspects of life that are too painful or anxiety-laden to present initially in words.

Young adolescents often attribute almost miraculous powers to physicians and assume that their advice, procedures, or medications will provide almost instant cures. If this does not happen, the young patient may believe that the physician is uninterested or does not know the diagnosis or how to prescribe appropriate therapy. It is important that physicians be specific with adolescent patients about what is wrong, what is expected to follow, what will be done, what the probable outcome will be, and what the pace of change is likely to be.

With some illnesses the need of early and middle adolescents to take regular medication comes into conflict with aspects of psychologic and cognitive growth. Boys and girls oriented to the present, for whom the future is an unthinkable abstraction, frequently listen to the physician and indicate acquiescence without comprehending the significance or knowing the necessity for compliance. Reinforcement of the need for cooperation and expressions of the physician's interest in the patient at frequent follow-up visits can be effective. Adolescents more often comply because they wish to please the physician than because they fully understand the need and the possible dangers if plans of treatment are not followed.

Adolescents often come to the physician playing roles or stereotypes, or otherwise acting inappropriately. This is not only a type of communication but a means of getting to know or testing the physician. Such behavior may initially irritate or anger the physician, but such testing usually represents attempts to know the physician better, to decide whether he or she can be trusted, or to learn the limits set by the physician. Young adolescents are ambivalent, change rapidly in mood and actions, and present themselves differently from day to day, particularly if they are ill. Changes may occur in a relatively short time that radically alter clinical assessment. Adolescents, particularly those chronically ill or handicapped, must be allowed these inconsistencies, while they still receive emotional support and direction.

2.22 ADOLESCENCE AND CHRONIC HEALTH PROBLEMS

The impact of chronic illness or handicaps on physical, cognitive, or psychosocial growth depends on many factors: whether a condition is congenital or acquired, appears suddenly or over a long period of time, occurs before or after the onset of puberty, represents a single episode or the beginning of a chronic process, produces neurologic damage, alters body image, is apparent to others, or is disfiguring.

Just as physical care aims at specific diagnosis and therapy, so should psychologic consideration of disease. Assessment should be made of the impact of disease on cognitive and psychosocial growth. A chronic illness or handicap may affect the adolescent in all major tasks, but frequently centers on one developmental area. For example, a boy with cystic fibrosis

may have a distorted body image, be more dependent upon his parents than he wishes, worry about sexuality because of the probability of sterility, and be severely limited in future choice of vocation; but one problem may be of much greater concern to him than the others at a given moment and requires special consideration and emotional support. An obese girl may enter puberty already feeling that she is helpless to change her appearance, and the new feeling of loss of control of bodily changes during early adolescent growth may magnify her concern and increase her isolation. Adolescents who develop diabetes often resent their increased dependency on parents, doctors, and hospitals; alternatively, they may embrace this dependency and refuse to separate themselves or to assume responsibility for their own care. In every chronic problem affecting adolescents consideration of these effects on psychosocial growth must be part of the therapeutic plan.

WILLIAM A. DANIEL, JR.

Barnes HV: Physical growth and development during puberty. Med Clin North Am 59:1305, 1975.
Erikson EH: Childhood and Society. New York, WW Norton, 1950.
Frisch RE: Weight at menarche: Similarity for well-nourished and undernourished girls at differing ages, and evidence for historical constancy. Pediatrics 50:445, 1972.
Garn SM, Smith NJ, Clark DC: Lifelong differences in hemoglobin levels between blacks and whites. J Natl Med Assoc 67:91, 1975.
Greulich WW, Pyle SI: Radiographic Atlas of Skeletal Development of the Hand and Wrist. Stanford, Calif, Stanford University Press, 1950; 2nd ed, 1959.
Havighurst RJ: Developmental Tasks and Education. Ed 3. New York, Daniel McKay, 1972.
Marshall WA, Tanner JM: Variations in the pattern of pubertal changes in boys. Arch Dis Child 45:13, 1970.
Marshall WA, Tanner JM: Variations in pattern of pubertal changes in girls. Arch Dis Child 44:291, 1969.
Osofsky JH, Spitz D: Adolescent sexual behavior: Normative data and current trends. In: Gallagher JR, Heald FP, Garell D (eds): Medical Care of Adolescents. Ed 3. New York, Appleton-Century-Crofts, 1976.
Piaget J: Intellectual evolution from adolescence to adulthood. Hum Dev 15:1012, 1972.
Root AW: Endocrinology of puberty, parts I and II. J Pediatr 83:1, 187, 1973.
Tanner JM: Growth at Adolescence. Ed 2. Oxford, Blackwell Scientific Publications, 1962.
Tanner JM, Whitehouse RH: Clinical longitudinal standards for height, weight, weight velocity, and stages of puberty. Arch Dis Child 51:170, 1976.
Vaughan VC III (ed): Issues in Human Development. Washington DC, Government Printing Office, 1971.

2.23 PSYCHOSOCIAL DIMENSIONS OF PEDIATRICS

INTRODUCTION

The term *psychosocial* recognizes that the activities, functions, and behaviors of a child include a *psychic* or *internal* dimension, which consists of feelings, attitudes, thoughts, fantasies, memory, judgment, values, and self-image, as well as a *social*, *external*, or *interactional* dimension, encompassing relationships with the environment, people, and circumstances within which the child lives. The psychosocial orientation in no way neglects the biologic or organic aspects of development. Biologic (physiologic or pathologic) facts established as

significant to psychosocial development or disturbances will be cited.

The psychosocial viewpoint considers the child's emotional and social development and its deviations and disturbances in *interactional* terms between fetus, infant, or child and the environment. For example, to state that an infant's cry indicates hunger is to infer a physiologic or biologic state. The inference seems justified when the cry subsides after feeding. But the process of feeding has had, besides its nutritional significance, emotional and social aspects for both infant and mother. Holding, cuddling, crooning to, or talking to the infant expresses emotional and social states of the mother, and the infant perceives and feels ("ingests") these aspects of the feeding relationship and responds to them as surely as to the food substances.

Maturation involves those intrinsic processes that are genetically or otherwise organically programmed; but even maturational features of development are dependent for their healthy achievement upon environmental factors.

Development refers to the progressive differentiation, refinement, and specialization of the organism and its constituent parts. Development is interactional and depends upon both general and specific internal and environmental conditions. The major intrapsychic dimensions of psychosocial development include the *cognitive* and the *affective*. Cognitive processes are perceptual reasoning, judgment, and memory—generally, the intellectual features of intrapsychic function. Affective states include anxiety, depression, fear, anger, sadness, joy, elation, jealousy, calmness, and placidity (the dimensions of feeling or emotion).

Most activities of the child integrate both affective and cognitive processes. The risk for most clinicians is that attention to the affective may be neglected until it is blatant. The affective component in a child's temper tantrum is unmistakable; but a child's poor performance in school may be too easily construed as primarily a cognitive or perceptual difficulty, with little attention given to strong feelings of guilt, discouragement, fear of failure, displaced anger, and the like.

The formation of conscience and its exercise are psychic processes with important cognitive and affective features. Anxiety and the desire for approval are early affective precursors. Identification and remembering of approved and disapproved actions, and choosing among behavioral alternatives are cognitive aspects of the formation and function of conscience.

BASIC PRINCIPLES

1. All human experiences have psychosocial as well as biologic or organic contexts.

2. The biologic equipment with which the child is born is modifiable. Its function can be facilitated or impaired, sometimes reversibly, sometimes not, in both the physical and the psychosocial domains.

3. All behavior has meaning. This meaning can be known to both the actor and the observer; or this meaning may be obscure to both. Meanings may frequently be given one label by a child, and others by parents, teachers, physicians, or others.

4. Everyone has theories which explain his or her own behavior and the behaviors of others. The clinician will choose among various theories in attempting to comprehend the development and the behavior of children. Conceptual models such as those described below may give meaning to aspects of children's behavior by providing useful frameworks of assumptions, hypotheses, and empirical data.

FREQUENTLY OVERLOOKED ISSUES

1. Both acute and chronic illnesses frequently produce in children lassitude and affective dullness bordering on depression. Even common viral illnesses often leave residual depression and irritability for days or weeks after other signs and symptoms have disappeared. Emotional, social, and academic behavior may be slow to return to pre-illness levels of function. Patience is required of parents and teachers, and parents may need reassurance from the clinician.

2. Events such as a household move, father's travels, illness of a family member, a substitute classroom teacher, separation from a friend, or death of a pet always have some and may have major psychosocial effects on the child. Even when the child's overt reaction is minimal, it is important to inquire about these events. How a child handles separation and loss, whether temporary or permanent, provides important information about his or her psychosocial style and adaptability. The child having little or no reaction is not displaying optimal adaptability. Relationships should be important to children, and they should learn to invest emotions freely in them, and be able to show their feelings in some ways when significant relationships are interrupted or terminated. Children unable to make emotional investments or who have to protect themselves from open reactions to losses may have significant developmental disturbances.

3. The specific ways in which affection is given and received among family members are important determinants of the manner and comfort with which children will express positive regard for others. To label a mother "cold" or "aloof" is less useful than finding out whether and under what conditions she can or cannot express physical, verbal, or emotional affection. Such clinical data will help both in assessment and in planning appropriate intervention in support of family relationships.

2.24 SOME CONCEPTUAL MODELS OF CHILD DEVELOPMENT

No single psychosocial theory accounts adequately for all aspects of the development or behavior of children, whether normal or disturbed. On the other hand, the clinician needs to be familiar with the general outlines of the major theories, as a set of perspectives within which to understand children and with respect to which he or she can make clear and explicit his or her own theoretic stance. Common sense is not an adequate basis for intervention into either organic or psychosocial aspects of health or disease; unfortunately, many physicians well informed of the physiologic and pathologic aspects of physical illness have only primitive knowledge of the data and theories of psychosocial health and illness.

Children and their societies present complex interrelationships. *Systems theory* attempts to improve understanding of these relationships through descriptions of hierarchies of interrelated systems. Any conceptual model usually deals with only one or a few of the many systems within which the child lives. The following conceptual models for the development of children are generally listed from "inside out."

The first model is that generally (but narrowly) called

the *medical* or *physiologic* model. Consider this analogy: the liver has at different ages differing capacities for metabolism of drugs, and the child can be understood, for certain purposes, in terms of liver function and age; and in illness or in health this physiologic system has very direct communication with the intrapsychic system through nervous and hormonal subsystems. The impact upon the child of asthma, heart disease, central nervous system disorders, and a host of other conditions can sometimes be best understood or dealt with in such a physiologic perspective.

Sigmund Freud and Erikson, among others, have contributed to the development of the *psychoanalytic* or *psychosocial* models of development, in which the child is seen as motivated by basic sexual and aggressive drives and as passing through successive and critical stages of development, influenced at first primarily by parents and then by an enlarging group of social experiences. For instance, the oral stage (psychoanalytic) of the first half of the 1st yr of life is seen as a stage during which basic trust (psychosocial) is learned, so long as both the child's physical apparatus and the environment are intact and supportive. Anna Freud added a longitudinal concept to the same model in describing *developmental lines*. For instance, the only child of articulate parents might seem quite advanced in the language line over his or her peers, owing to the preponderance of time spent with adults. On the other hand, the emotional line with respect to tolerance for independence might be found lagging, creating a disparate psychosocial assessment along these two lines.

A more circumscribed conceptual model is the *cognitive*, to which Piaget has contributed through his studies of the step-by-step acquisition of knowledge. His observations help in understanding how a 5 yr old and a 15 yr old differ in their capacities to know or to think about concepts such as sex, the future, or death.

The *behavioral* model of child development is less concerned with what goes on in the mind or body than with predictable patterns in the child's overt response to external stimuli at different age levels. This model is based on learning theories, and emphasizes that most of the behavior of children is learned. Use of this model helps physicians to counsel parents how to *teach* children (for example, to go to bed without undue delay). The model helps parents to see how their own behavior determines the responses of their children. Some parents do not know that unwanted behaviors are just as learned as wanted ones. The child who finds that screaming is the only stimulus that gets a response from mother will use that behavior when the need for mother overrides the consideration that her attention may be aversive. The behavioral model can help plan strategies aimed at changing such specific behaviors as enuresis, avoidance due to phobias, and others (Sec 2.1).

The physician should be familiar with the *family system* as a conceptual model. The child develops within a complex set of interpersonal systems which include relationships with parents or parent-surrogates and other members of the family or household, as well as their relationships with each other. The standards of parents and others have a heavy impact upon the child's life. It is the parent who monitors the child's health and brings him or her to the physician; and a hyperkinetic child whose parents are opposed to drug therapy will not get the benefits of that treatment, no matter how important the physician may feel it to be. The parents and the family and their relationships and expectations acculturate the child. Their rules and ways of functioning are the basic standards which the child ultimately makes his or her own. Children often incorporate into their own repertoires of feeling and behavior the manners in which their parents become ill or respond to illness. An anxious parent, for example, can magnify a child's minor pain into a frightening experience for both.

The *social* or *cultural* model recognizes that children are at any age part of a larger community or society. The broader the scope of the notion of society or culture, however, the less certain we can be about what this means to a given child. At one level, a variety of socioeconomic and sociocultural considerations increase the chances of prematurity, lead poisoning, rat bites, malnutrition, child abuse, and sudden infant death; at another level, the child-rearing practices of any community have profound effects upon how children view themselves and their future.

One of the most influential social systems outside the family is the school, which is perhaps the most age-structured system the child will experience. School provides the setting and framework within which the child is measured and in turn measures himself or herself academically, emotionally, socially, and physically. Though parents may have adapted to a child's immature speech, he or she will face on entering school a need to re-evaluate and change modes of speech. A pediatrician who points out this potential problem early may be able to initiate changes that prevent a major confrontation when school begins. Such early intervention is more successful than that which is deferred to the time of imperative need.

The physician, too, is part of the child's social system, playing a part ascribed by the family and its subculture. Physicians may play this part comfortably or uncomfortably, depending upon their level of familiarity and comfort with that culture and upon their capacity for adjustment.

THE ROLE OF PARENTS IN CHILD DEVELOPMENT

2.25 FAMILY PLANNING

Unfortunately, the first encounters of pediatricians with the families of their patients generally occur after the birth of the first child. The timing of the birth of the first child has heavy influence upon parental relationships and sets the pattern for the spacing and number of future children. The pediatrician has an important role in examining with families questions and issues in family planning. Central to family planning is the notion of *choice*. The National Association for Social Work has made the following statement: "Potential parents should be free to decide for themselves without duress, and according to their personal beliefs and convictions, whether they want to become parents, how many children they are willing and able to nurture, and the opportune time for them to have children." Pediatricians should encourage parents to discuss family planning, but they must approach the sensitive areas of personal beliefs and values with caution and concern. Variations in the birth rate, the tendency of some prospective parents to wish to influence or control the sex of their unborn child, and the diagnostic role of amniocentesis in cases of genetic risk all reflect a growing personal and technologic sophistication in family planning.

Perhaps the most common question on family planning asked of pediatricians is: what is the optimal interval between the births of siblings? This is a matter ultimately for parents to decide. They may be guided, however, by the consideration that an interval of approximately 2.5 yr allows time for maternal replenishment from the first pregnancy, time for comfortable reciprocal attachment between parents and the first child, time for the older child to master locomotion, toilet training, and other self-care which will free the mother for care of the new infant, and opportunity for a reasonably close-in-age relationship between the siblings.

2.26 PARENTAL ATTITUDES AND EXPECTATIONS

All adults bring to parenthood certain attitudes toward the roles of mother and father and certain expectations of and attitudes about children. These ideas are strongly influenced by childhood experiences and by the notions, models, and beliefs that each culture holds about children. Our society has a variety of views about children, and these views are frequently incongruent. For example, the young infant is seen as both innocent and uncivilized, or as a tabula rasa and as almost totally genetically determined. These attitudes about childhood have deep historic, philosophic, religious, and, more recently, scientific roots. And when mother and father hold conflicting attitudes about children and child rearing, areas of compromise must be found so that they may develop an effective partnership as parents.

At the first encounter with each family the physician should elicit the parents' attitudes toward children and toward their own child by inquiring into *expectations*. Among the most common and abrasive sources of distress within and between human beings are the gaps between expectations and achievement, or between incompatible expectations. Even with regard to the infant in utero parents have attitudes and expectations. The content and quality depend on many factors, including the adequacy of the marriage, the couple's feelings about each other, the economic circumstances of the family, and the unmet emotional needs of the parents as individuals. The unborn child may be viewed as a "mistake" or as a "savior," or may represent an unconscious or deliberate attempt to hold a shaky marriage together or a compensatory substitute for an ungratifying partner. In more normal circumstances, parents tend to view children as extensions of themselves, and to see in children their genetic legacy and certain aspects of their own personalities. Such a perspective can become pathologic if children are expected to fulfill the unrealized dreams and ambitions of their parents, rather than to lead their own lives. The child who is planned as a replacement for one who has recently died is at particular risk, and may be treated as fragile, with overindulgence, and as though vulnerable to the same fate which befell the previous child. The first child to be born after one or more miscarriages may be viewed similarly. Anticipatory exploration of feelings by the physician, with guidance and counseling, can be of considerable benefit in these instances.

Parents of children who are chronically ill, emotionally disturbed, mentally retarded, or severely handicapped are at risk of development of unhealthy and destructive attitudes toward their children, society, or themselves. Such children may provide little gratification and represent serious disappointment. The pediatrician must help such parents recognize and express their feelings and must guard against conveying unprofessional negative or condemning attitudes toward them. Physicians need to be sure of their own systems of beliefs and values with regard to parental roles, child rearing, and children; but they must be careful lest they impose their own idiosyncratic values on the children and families they seek to help (Sec 2.82).

2.27 TEMPERAMENT IN PARENT-CHILD RELATIONSHIPS

The notion of *temperament* embraces the individual's particular pattern of physiologic organization, probably genetically determined, through which a uniquely personal way of thinking, feeling, and acting is predictably and more or less continually effected. Temperament is the core of the personality; personality may in turn be shaped by the environment, which can mellow or muffle temperament but never eradicate it. For example, the reaction times of newborn infants to certain stimuli and the adaptabilities of infants to change appear to be among the first signs of temperament, and may predict activity level of older children or adults. For the most part the temperaments of parents and the complex superstructures of their personalities will permit them to interact comfortably and effectively with the possibly differing temperaments of their children, but the interpersonal experiences of parents sometimes differ so much with different children that parents have a sense of awe at the degree to which their children are not alike. Policies of child management successful for one child may not at all suit another. In cases of uncomfortable interaction with a given child, parents may develop unrealistic guilt. If such guilt leads them to anxiety or withdrawal, the child may become irritable or withdraw in turn. Parents may turn to anger as a defense against frustration or guilt.

The physician is in a favorable position to evaluate the temperaments of infants and of mothers and fathers. The mother who says she has a "good" baby generally means that their temperaments are in a complementary and happy relationship. On the other hand, a hyporeactive ("good") infant and a placid, slow-moving mother may not engage each other sufficiently in growth-promoting interactions. The physician can encourage or train such mothers to provide more sensory stimulation or exchanges for such children. Such mother-infant pairs may need, for example, to have the times of picking up and rocking structured for them, rather than depending for interaction on their own low levels of exchange of cues. In the opposite case, an intrusive mother with a highly reactive child may need help in damping stimuli to the child, to prevent undue irritability. For the measurement of infant temperament, Carey has developed a 70-item questionnaire which yields ratings in 9 categories: activity, rhythmicity, adaptability, approach, sensory threshold, intensity, mood, distractibility, and persistence.

Mothers and fathers often differ in temperament, and either can sometimes provide relief to the other or to the child when one of the parent-child relationships is in trouble. A more active, expressive, or creative parent can, for example, give special attention to the child in activities contributing to adaptive learning, whereas a more placid and relaxed parent can take over child care when a period of quiet is needed to consolidate and assimilate new experiences. The physician can help both parents to coordinate their different temperaments and personalities in action for the child's benefit, in this way preventing parental blocking or stasis. Stasis occurs when each parent sees the other's temperament as being "bad" for the child. If the label can be changed from "bad" to "different and complementary," the parents can conceptualize their joint efforts as mutually effective and supportive rather than destructive. The same considerations apply to parent-surrogates, such as grandparents, and at times even to siblings. All family members can be encouraged to contribute something of their own to the child, so long as these contributions are orchestrated positively and comfortably by the primary caregiver, rather than being offered in a chaotic or oppositional way.

Both temperamental differences and the child's developmental stages become more or less effectively enmeshed with the temperaments and personalities of parents. A mother who has always found it exciting to deal with new challenges finds her child's adolescence a stimulating and positive experience. A nurturant, stable, hyporeactive father may, on the other hand, find that he is more effective with the preschool toddler than with the inquisitive 10 yr old.

Finally, parents, like children, go through developmental stages. The teenage mother has a host of problems of her own adolescence to integrate into her plans for a life with her child; and children born to parents in their late 30's will have to deal not only with their parents' temperaments and their own problems of childhood and adolescence, but with involvement in the possible midlife problems of their parents.

2.28 PARENTS AS TEACHERS

The parent is the child's first and most important teacher. Most parents do not view themselves as educators of their children, but they present in direct and indirect ways an essential and far-reaching curriculum. The parents "teach" the infant how to trust, rely on, and depend on people and circumstances—the basis for the child's future view of interpersonal relationships. Parents not only teach a son or daughter how to throw a ball, but also impart notions of sportsmanship and fair play. Parents who read to their children motivate reading. Parents who explain to and inform children foster language development, serve as models of a communicative style, and provide the ingredients for mastery of problem-solving techniques. Parents who display aggressive and temperamental outbursts in response to minor frustrations model a style of behavior which may find ready imitators. In all of these educative ventures, parents not only offer content, information, and advice, but also transmit the values of their families and of their cultures. Children as "students" may be willing, unwitting, or resistant.

Parents tend to be unaware of or to undervalue their educative role, deferring to school teachers as professionals who "know more" or can "teach better." In recent years, however, the community mental health movement and programs of compensatory education have re-emphasized the importance of the teaching skills of parents, both in their natural affective roles and in the cognitive domain. With appropriate training and support, parents have learned to use their talents as teachers of language development in infant stimulation programs, as therapists in behavior modification with children who have maladaptive behavior patterns, as classroom aides, and in a variety of other endeavors with their own and other children.

For these complex educative roles as well as for the nurturant and economic roles of parenthood, most prospective parents receive little or no preparation. Most persons "learn" how to be parents primarily from their relationships with their own parents and from caretaking responsibilities they may have had for younger siblings. But sociocultural changes and urbanization have increasingly limited these experiences for many children. Furthermore, maladaptive and conflictual patterns, as well as positive ones, learned from parents may be passed on to succeeding generations; children of child abusers, for example, tend to be child abusers. Courses on parenthood have been introduced into the curricula of some high schools, but it would be more useful if throughout the school years children had some types of organized experiences in relating to and in helping to take care of younger children.

2.29 DEPENDENCE VS. AUTONOMY

Psychologically, children become independent beings during the phase of development that Mahler has called *separation* and *individuation*, which extends between 6–30 mo of age. It does not evolve as a steady movement toward separation and individuation; rather, both psychologically and literally the child departs from and returns to the mother in a predictable pattern. The end of this process finds 3–4 yr old children in a stage of autonomy, wanting to do things themselves, but, within the parents' view of reality, still needing a great deal of support.

At adolescence the child goes through a second and more definitive emergence as a person separate from his or her parents, as he or she strives for an identity as an independent adult. The adolescent has many advantages over the 4 yr old, including the capacity for abstract reason, the physical equipment of a young adult, and a great deal more knowledge and experience; but periodic regressions again reflect the underlying tension between needs for dependence and for autonomy. The 19–22 yr old finally pulls up roots and establishes himself or herself apart. But the pendulum between dependence and autonomy never rests, even in successive stages of adult life. The more success parents have in helping children to be comfortable with both autonomy and dependence and with the relationships between, the more successfully will the children live as adults.

Infants appear totally dependent upon their mothers or caregivers, but their strivings for new sights, sounds, movements, and other growth-promoting experiences must be unhindered, within the bounds of safety, if learning is to occur. On the other hand, when 15 yr olds learn and test independent behavior by staying out at night and taking unreasonable chances, parents may need to show concern and provide limits which help the adolescent to consolidate gains before moving out again into new experiences.

All new learning represents a striving for autonomy, but it can only be successful and its effect positive if the child feels secure. Overly dependent children may feel that their nurturant base is threatened by illness in their mothers or fathers or by parental conflicts, so that they cling to home all the harder. Parents may themselves view the world as a dangerous and untrustworthy place and foster similar feelings in their children. Physical illness increases dependency; this dependency is counterproductive if, after physiologic systems are back to normal, parents do not expect the child to resume appropriate autonomy.

Some children are forced into premature independence by loss of a parent. A 12 yr old who, because of his or her mother's death or separation, has to take over the care of a household or of a younger sibling may be able to assume this responsibility and independence without regression. But sometimes the apparently successful child will have trouble in dealing later with the dependent needs of his or her own children or of others, basically feeling cheated and resentful.

There are periods when the striving of children for more independent behavior creates crises for their parents. The physician can be an important neutral consultant or arbitrator, who can help parents to decide whether it is more realistic to yield some independence or to hold their children to certain limits. This is a particularly difficult issue for handicapped children, who require more care and restrictions. Helping such children achieve an inner sense of independence calls for creativity from both parents and physicians.

Finally, children learn about independence by observing their parents and grandparents and older sib-lings. A mother who becomes overly involved in her own mother's waning years provides both a model and a dependency conflict for her 12 yr old daughter, who may both want and not want to be closer to her own mother.

2.30 SOCIALIZATION, DISCIPLINE, AND PUNISHMENT

Socialization is primarily an interactional process between the developing child and his or her parents and other significant adults. Socialization involves the knowledge, skills, and techniques that accomplish an adaptive fit between the child and the social environment. These are acquired both formally and informally, in conscious and unconscious ways, and by precept and example. Although successful socialization continues into adulthood, and is a lifelong process, generally, the time from birth to late adolescence is considered the period of establishment of primary adaptive social attitudes and behaviors.

Discipline has been defined as training in proper conduct and action. It has mental and moral aspects. As a verb, *discipline* means to educate, to train, and especially to bring under control. The term also carries notions of protection, prevention, and punishment. In the early life of the child discipline emerges from relationship with parents, involving conformity to their expectations and obedience to their commands; it becomes generalized as the child grows older, shaping responsiveness to persons in authority generally, and contributing to notions of personal autonomy, authority, and integrity that are later codified in rules, regulations, laws, morals, and religious and ethical principles.

The child begins at about 18 mo to experience discipline when he or she is faced with growing numbers of rules, regulations, and expectations within the family. As children mature physically, cognitively, emotionally, and socially, they progressively internalize these standards and develop those internal controls of behavior that are termed self-discipline. The purpose of discipline is to provide children with incentives, reasons, values, and the instrumental means to achieve self-discipline. Discipline is too often seen only in terms of punishment, whereas at its healthiest it is a complex set of attitudes, behaviors, formal and informal instruction, rewards, and punishments which serve not to inhibit, restrict, subjugate, or repress children but to help them internalize appropriate cognitive processes, ideals, and values. With these they will be able ultimately to exercise their own judgments and choose their own behaviors in ways best adapted to their situations.

Social and cultural factors strongly influence the kinds and effectiveness of discipline. In some relatively homogeneous communities, strong and commonly held traditions of national, ethnic, philosophic, or religious values give strong support to the socializing and disciplinary actions of parents toward their children. In such communities discipline may seem easier, both in the congruence of views among adults who support each other's parental behaviors and in the common experience of the children. However, kinship ties are often nonexistent or attenuated over long distances in many families who move from their communities of origin. Many parents, moreover, may have come together from competing or contradictory traditions and values, the basis for marriage transcending common religion, ethnic origin, or ties of community or class.

It is important that parents be secure and explicit in their attitudes and values regarding child rearing, especially as they concern discipline. Difficulties in control or in adaptive socialization in children often stem from the contradictions and conflicts between parents over the systems of expectations, rewards, and punishments which will be appropriate to the disciplining of children.

Certain principles can be stated with regard to parental approaches to discipline: (1) Parents must help children appreciate the value of learning from the results of their behaviors; parents who recognize and reward approved behavior and negatively sanction the disapproved help their children to recognize the consequences of their actions. (2) Parents need to settle clearly on the difference between hurting and retaliation, and between teaching through discipline and through punishment; they need to examine how to resist exerting either power or authority for its own sake, rather than as a tool for the edification and education of the child. (3) Parents need to recognize and resist the tendency of all people to demean or to humiliate those who oppose their will. (4) Parents need to review and understand their own childhood experiences with parental discipline and to recognize attitudes or behaviors of their own which are unreasonable residua; these can include overdemanding expectations, over-reliance on authoritarian and power-oriented discipline, a tendency to respond impulsively or angrily or cruelly, the use of discipline to humiliate or demean, or a tendency to be so vacillating or inappropriately oversympathetic with a child that discipline lacks firmness and consistency.

Chess and Thomas have described a group of basically normal but "difficult" children, whose temperamental characteristics include a high level of intensity, some degree of impulsivity, a low tolerance for frustration, negative mood, and a tendency to recoil from new experiences. Parents of many such children regard them as having disciplinary problems. On the other hand, the stubborn or difficult child may have qualities that the parents admire and want preserved or developed, such as that they have "a mind of their own," or are "not easily led." Such children may become rather independent and creative thinkers or leaders, but these qualities may emerge only in late adolescence or early adulthood; during childhood such children may be regarded as unpleasantly stubborn, defiant, and resistant.

Punishment. Punishment is an aspect of discipline; it includes a variety of techniques for fostering approved and discouraging disapproved behavior. Punishment is related to the general area of conscience formation, which depends upon attitudes, values, motivation, effects of adult models, and visibility of legal, social, and cultural expectations, rewards, and sanctions. Punishment, whether it be construed as physical or psychologic, may have a relatively limited role in the formation of a mature, autonomous conscience. Studies of animals and of preschool and early school-aged children have identified some of the variables determining the effectiveness of punishment. Some conclusions of these studies are as follows:

Timing. Most studies agree that the shorter the delay between an act of transgression and the punishment for it, the more effective the punishment will be in preventing repetition of the prohibited behavior. The implication for parents is that punishment should be effected as soon as possible after a transgression is observed or known, not "when your father comes home." Nor should a parent say to a child, "You just sit there until I get to you, and then I'm going to punish you." Warning or admonishing the child who appears about to perform a forbidden act is frequently effective in preventing transgressions.

Intensity. Studies of animals indicate that the higher the intensity of punishment, the more effective will be the prohibition. This relationship is not so clear for children since it is unacceptable to use a high intensity of physical punishment. It has been further shown that punishment of high intensity is likely to interfere with learning when the child must make relatively complex discriminations in order to comply with expectations. Two principal recommendations emerge: first, the intensity of punishment should be high enough so that a mild to moderate amount of anxiety is generated in the younger child, but not so high that the child is frightened, panicked, or terror-stricken (by physical punishment) or made so angry (by either physical or emotional punishment) that he or she cannot learn the lesson; second, for the preschool child the rules and the discriminations surrounding expected behaviors should be simple. The more complicated the discrimination needed, the less intense should be any punishment that follows transgression.

Emotional Context of Punishment. Both clinical and experimental studies indicate that punishment is most effective when it takes place in the context of a warm, affectionate, and generally accepting relationship between parent and child. In naturalistic studies of child rearing, relatively cold and aloof mothers who used spanking as a means of physical punishment found it less effective than other mothers who also used spanking frequently, but who were temperamentally warm and affectionate toward their children. Retrospective studies of delinquent boys indicate that often their fathers have been cruel, harsh, and punitive, with little love, respect, or affection. Parents should understand that being affectionate and kind toward their children and praising them is not in conflict with the need from time to time to punish them.

Another aspect of punishment, involving the relationship between child and parent, is termed the temporary withdrawal of nurturance or of love. The more children desire the approval of their parents and care about their parents' positive regard for them, the more sensitive they are to shame and to indications of their parents' diminished respect. This does not mean that for a parent to reject the child or to declare that he or she no longer loves the child is a good method of punishment. Rather, it indicates that a moderate amount of shaming or disapproval can help to promote prescribed behaviors in the context of a relationship in which the child values the parents' approval and affection. The flow of nurturance and warmth from fathers to sons is particularly important, and the development of these harmonious relationships is important in itself, as well as contributing to the increased effectiveness of paternal discipline. Parents who are particularly sensitive to threats to their own power or authority may be unduly punitive and harsh in the discipline of their children, and may be less likely to be warm and affectionate in their overall relationships with them. They may need particular help in finding comfortable ground in this area.

Association of Punishment with Cognitive Methods: Reasoning. Reasoning and physical punishment are more effective together than physical punishment alone in bringing about the incorporation of approved behaviors in children; moreover, combinations of reasoning with nonphysical forms of punishment, such as deprivation of privileges, or withdrawal of nurturance, are more effective than any one alone. On the other hand, reasoning alone is more effective than any punishment alone. And even when punishment is delayed after the transgression, its effectiveness is increased if the child is provided reasons for the punishment. Studies of effects of reasoning indicate the importance of explanation and of careful labeling of proscribed behaviors. Internalization of standards (the acquisition of self-discipline) requires a cognitively oriented training procedure. The cognitive elements include the careful *labeling* of the prohibited behaviors, a careful *description* and *reconstruction* with the child of the nature of any transgression, a parental *demonstration* of the deviant act before punishment, and an indication as to what *consequences* or *results* of the deviant action are to be avoided. The efficacy of reasoning increases, of course, as the growing child can better understand a cognitive approach.

The following recommendations may be used in guiding parents. For the child between 12–30 mo old techniques which are direct, clear, and immediate, and which produce a moderate amount of anxiety without unduly frightening or angering the child, seem to be the most effective in producing inhibition of transgressions. With increasing understanding of language, by 20–24 mo, clear and simple explanations of the reasons for punishment should be given, without elaboration. In older children techniques of punishment seem most effective which diminish anxiety and emphasize the verbal control of behavior through attention to general rules, appeals to reason and common sense, and other cognitively oriented techniques. For children of any age a moderate amount of disapproval or of shaming may be useful in promoting the child's self-control, so long as it is used in the context of a positive, supportive, and respectful relationship.

Consistency. Studies of delinquent children and of the child rearing practices of parents of normal children, as well as experimental studies, indicate that parental *consistency* is an important factor in promoting approved behavior in children. Erratic disciplinary procedures, alternating punitiveness and laxity, are highly correlated with increased delinquency. Consistency is a relative term; no individual, still less 2 parents, can be totally consistent in child rearing. It is important, however, that parents establish a general consistency of style in terms of what, when, how, and to what degree punishment is appropriate to each transgression. The pediatrician should encourage parents who are attempting to establish new disciplinary procedures or alter previously unsuccessful ones to be patient and persistent. Parents usually feel that a few trials at a changed pattern of discipline ought to produce immediate results in the child. This is quite unrealistic, both for themselves and for their children, since all of their patterns of behavior probably took months or years to develop. Moreover, studies indicate that inconsistent discipline builds resistance to changes in response to later, more consistent behavior. The physician must instruct and encourage parents in maintaining reasonable and appropriate disciplinary procedures, even if favorable results are not immediately forthcoming.

Undesirable Consequences of Punishment. A clearly undesirable consequence of punishment is the modeling of aggressive behavior, best illustrated by the father or mother who in correcting a child for a temper tantrum becomes angry and physically cruel. The angrier the parent, the more likely he or she is to lose control and to punish too severely. Such parents can look foolish to their children and feel so themselves, which may increase the parent's anger so that the child may be held accountable in such terms as "he's trying to make a fool of me." Such parents may feel involved in struggles with their children for control.

Loss of control tends to diminish the positive effects and increase the negative effects of punishment. It arouses anxiety and anger in children, which turn them against their parents and against their parents' desires. Severe and demeaning disapproval can make the child feel small, helpless, and inadequate. Feelings of resentment, fantasies of retaliation, or a sense of worthlessness may arise. Such feelings reduce the effectiveness of punishment as a positive learning experience.

As children get older, physical punishment becomes much less effective and its negative effects increase. At any age slapping or whipping a child can be cruel and abusive and lead to the results cited above, and to alienation of the child from the family. Even moderate degrees of spanking in 7, 8, 10, or 12 yr old children can make them feel humiliated and resentful. The intended lesson is lost. Some children may begin to use repetition of the specific transgressions for which they were punished as a means of retaliation against punitive, cruel, or humiliating parents. Others, when escape is impossible and retaliation too dangerous, react by passivity and withdrawal instead of becoming angry, developing passive-aggressive or passive-withdrawal personalities that may inhibit development.

Reinforcement of Approved Behavior. This method of discipline involves essentially the encouragement of positive behavior. The parent generally ignores or musters a mild reproof for undesirable behavior, while encouraging cooperation, helpfulness, and sympathetic, prosocial behavior. Encouragement by helpful and kind words has been shown to reduce aggressive behavior both in college students and in 8–12 yr old children. With this positive approach to discipline many of the unwanted side effects of punishment are avoided. This approach can often be incorporated as an element of discipline, and although it takes more time initially it may save time in the end.

Modeling. Studies by Bandura, Walters, and others of aggressive behavior in children indicate that adult models significantly influence children's learning. Bandura contends that modeling can produce learning on a single trial, in contrast to the learning with multiple trials that is posited by theories of classical and operant conditioning. Modeling is equivalent to the phrase "good example." Parents repeatedly demonstrate the power of deeds over words in their behavior toward each other, as well as in the behaviors they manifest toward their children. In displays of affection, of anger and its control, of respect, honesty, and openness of communication, parents model behavior with which children identify and which they *imitate*. Modeling also involves *identification*, the process by which one feels he or she is like another person. Both verbal and nonverbal aspects of behavior, such as tone of voice, facial expressions, gestures, and expressions of physical affection or aggression, are sources of imitation and identification that may be powerful influences on children.

2.31   CONSCIENCE FORMATION

Theories of conscience formation have sought to identify factors that cause children to learn approved behavior and to resist temptations to transgress against rules, first of parents and later of society. Psychoanalytic theory has postulated that the psychologic structure has 3 functional aspects: ego, superego, and id. The *superego* has the functions of conscience, with both conscious and unconscious aspects. The superego is primarily a negative governor (or inhibitor), incorporating the do's and don't's of parents and of society; the latter reach the child through parents, peers, teachers, laws. The concept of *ego ideal* represents positive aspects and goals of living toward which one strives. The strong affective component of the superego is *guilt*. Guilt serves as an internal punishment for transgression, and the avoidance of the pain of guilt is the major deterrent to contemplated aggression. The wish or desire to transgress can mobilize defense mechanisms aimed at avoidance of the awareness of guilt. Such mechanisms include repression, denial, anger, displacement, and projection. Psychoanalytic theory suggests that a healthy, stable, and mature superego requires appropriate resolution of the oedipal complex, which occurs around the 6th or 7th yr of life. In repressing both sexual feelings for the parent of the opposite sex and hostility toward the parent of the same sex, the young child "identifies with the aggressor," establishing a firm gender identity and internalizing the values, attitudes, beliefs, and standards of the parents, particularly the parent of the same sex.

Erikson has broadened psychoanalytic theory by giving attention to important social and cultural factors. To the concept of the oedipal complex he adds notions of the influence of social rules upon children at this critical stage. Socialization is for Erikson a matter of learning roles by observation, imitation, and rehearsal and has cognitive, affective, and behavioral components. In the young child much of thought is carried out as an internal monologue, often uttered aloud but intended for the child alone. Language is also a major tool for socialization. The voices of parents and others become internalized, often concretely as voices at first, then as statements, and rather later as thoughts. Children also internalize the behaviors and attitudes that they have seen, rehearsing and adapting them through imitation and fantasy in play. Children's consciences are built from the superegos and sociocultural traditions of their parents. Erikson holds that the superego can be construed as the child becoming "parent"—a carrier of tradition. Children internalize not just what their parents teach but what they are as persons. In Erikson's view the ego has an active role in formation of conscience, and the child's superego is as individual as his ego.

Other theories of the development of conscience can be called "cognitive developmental." Piaget, Kohlberg, and Aronfreed have studied both the reactions of children to temptation in various experimental situations and how children have attempted to explain their behaviors in reaction to moral dilemmas. Kohlberg's theory has outlined stages in development of conscience; they have no timetable, but the order is invariable. Some adults never reach the final, most mature stage, owing to constitutional, temperamental, or environmental factors, or to psychologic or social disturbances of the developing conscience. Kohlberg posits 3 major levels of conscience development with 2 stages within each level. In general, the stages move from a primary emphasis on the self or parents as referents for moral judgments and actions to more remote referents such as law or universal principles.

Level I: Preconventional. Moral reasoning is determined by the consequences of behavior: punishment, reward, exchange of favors, or the physical power of people in authority, particularly parents.

Stage 1: Behavior is determined primarily by efforts to avoid punishment or to seek pleasure of rewards. Obedience to the power embodied in adults is more or less automatic.

Stage 2: Behavior is based upon a desire to satisfy one's own needs and at times those of others. The child's view of reciprocity is concrete: "You scratch my back and I'll scratch yours." There is some consideration of feelings of others but only as a matter of secondary convenience. Notions of loyalty and justice are not strong at this stage.

Level II: Conventional. The child's moral reasoning at this level has the dual focus of the interests of others and of the desire to maintain the respect and support of others. There is also an aspect of reasoning that involves justifying the existing social order.

Stage 3: For the first time behavior is judged not only by its outcome but by its intention, which becomes important. Many moral decisions are now based upon a desire to please others, to help them, and in turn to receive their approval and aid.

Stage 4: The notion of duty now emerges. Right behavior is seen as doing one's duty or meeting one's obligations. A desire develops to ally one's self with the existing authority, rules, and social order, particularly as they are embodied in custom and law.

Level III: Postconventional. This level is not attained until adulthood, if at all. Here the individual begins to develop a set of moral principles and to use them in solving rather complicated problems of moral and ethical behavior. These principles become more or less universal in concept, extending beyond the immediate family, the community, or even the national mores as these last may be codified in rules, laws, or customs.

Stage 5: The notion of social contract which embodies personal rights and responsibilities within a society becomes important. An emphasis on the legal aspect of morality includes the possibility of changing laws or customs so that they may be more equitable or reasonable, or may deal more effectively with moral wrongs.

Stage 6: Morality is conceived now in universal terms or principles, such as justice, equality, reciprocity, and respect for the individual. These universal concepts are seen as applying to all humankind, regardless of status, nationality, class, race, sex, and the like.

Children of 2–3 yr of age do modulate behavior to avoid pain and to seek approval and reward. Available data indicate that Kohlberg's stages 1 and 2 are typically found in elementary school children. Stages 3 and 4 emerge in adolescence and early adulthood; stage 5 occurs in some adults; stage 6 may occur in only a few.

The value of Kohlberg's work lies in its assessment of the role of reasoning in the development of moral judgments. There is clearly no precise relationship between a person's capacity for reasoning and his or her actions; moreover, the individual may reason at one moral level in some situations and at higher or lower levels in others.

2.32 COMPETENCE AND MASTERY

Learning theory sees the infant, child, and adult as reactive primarily to external stimuli, whereas psychoanalytic and motivational theories hold that defense operations are involved in maintaining a steady or homeostatic state through reduction of drives. These theories tend to deny, neglect, or give cursory attention to the possibility that the infant may have intrinsic or inherent mechanisms for developing competence in affecting, manipulating, or mastering the environment. Notions of competence and mastery, emphasizing the proactive rather than the reactive aspect of the infant and child, first gained wide attention through the work of R. W. White, who gave the name *effectance* to such intrinsic motivation and pointed out that traditional theories neglected the importance of the feedback that the child obtains as a result of his or her actions.

Piaget's work on cognitive development has emphasized that infants and children play active roles in building "schemata," which are cognitive behavioral structures. The process involves "assimilation" of new experiences and "accommodation" of the prestimulus states to the features of the new experience that are not familiar. For example, during the sensorimotor period (birth to about 15–18 mo) the infant constructs schemata from various instrumental activities such as touching, crawling, reaching, grasping, and bringing closer for detailed examination by looking, tasting, smelling, and so on. Grasping a rattle establishes an additional sensory reality for the external object and conveys the ability to affect it by moving it, turning it for a new look, or putting it in the mouth. In such ways the infant gains power over the world of objects as growing cognitive structures help formulate the separateness of self and the external world. Piaget holds that the infant or child manipulates the environment to learn about it, developing concurrently the cognitive strengths that lead to further competence and mastery.

Stimulating interactions with impersonal as well as personal elements in the environment are also important for perceptual cognitive development. The interactions with persons and with inanimate objects support each other; for example, 1 yr old infants explore a controlled environment more actively in the presence of their mothers than with stangers. Infants appear to need and thrive on informational input as if it were analogous to a nutritional requirement. In an unchanging environment, lacking in a flow of new information, the infant may become apathetic, and ultimately retarded in cognitive and social development. A balanced and sensible approach is needed, however; too many mobiles or a constant barrage of music may overstimulate and some varieties of stimuli may be ineffective or irrelevant before 2–3 mo of age. Parents should be advised that the infant first needs adequate interpersonal stimulation, and that perceptual or sensory stimulation should be secondary and complementary. Parents should learn to judge what is interesting or pleasing for each child, how much becomes too exhausting, or what is too complex, beyond the child's capacity to exploit and enjoy.

SPECIFIC DEVELOPMENTAL ISSUES

2.33 ATTACHMENT BEHAVIOR

See Sec 2.3 and 7.13.

The continuing support of a nurturant family is vital for a child in all stages of his or her development, but when social and emotional deprivation occur within the 1st 2 yr of life, there may be psychologic and cognitive sequelae. Some deleterious effects may be reversible, but there is little doubt that children may experience lasting damage to social development, especially when deprivation occurs within the context of major familial conflict, psychotic illness in one or both parents, prolonged separation, or abandonment. "Failure to thrive" in an infant is commonly a subacute manifestation of maternal depression and reflects the inability of the mother to give her child adequate psychologic warmth and care. For treatment to be effective, the mother must be helped to emerge from her withdrawn or depressive state toward more active involvement with her child. Chronic social deprivation has been shown to contribute to intellectual retardation and to major emotional disturbances.

When mothers working outside the home have arranged for adequate day care for their children and see them daily, there appears to be little risk of serious harm to the children. Caldwell et al found that children in day care showed no significant differences in maternal attachment at the age of 30 mo, when compared with children reared at home. Day care–reared children, however, may be more aggressive and less cooperative when they later enter nursery school. Some children raised in depriving circumstances or by depressed mothers may benefit from the intellectual and social stimulation which good day care offers. Essentially nothing is known about the effects of "informal" day care, in which children are entrusted to untrained caretakers while their parents work. A national commitment to day care must provide a large pool of competent and dedicated personnel.

A mother who is to be separated from her child for a prolonged period of time should find a single consistent and stable surrogate, rather than a series of caretakers. Hospitalization of children under the age of 5–6 yr should, wherever possible, involve the rooming-in of the mother, in order to minimize the child's anxiety and to prevent subsequent maladaptive emotional responses (Sec 2.64). Normal children show separation anxiety at the age of 7–9 mo, the onset of this phenomenon reflecting an important step in the evolution of attachment behavior between mother and infant. The child becomes fretful when the mother leaves the room and fearful when persons outside the family attempt to remove him or her from the mother's arms. Parents can be reassured that such children have simply begun to recognize separateness from and dependence upon mother, and that after a few more months they will have a better understanding of her permanence, and separation anxiety will diminish.

Maternal care during the 1st 2 yr should be sufficiently reliable, predictable, and warm to give the child a sense of basic trust about the world, but not overindulgent. The infant's learning that he or she can survive and tolerate some frustrations, as well as inevitable or appropriate delays in the satisfaction of wishes, probably contributes positively to the quality of social development and to the strength and health of mother-child attachment.

Parents of infants handicapped by physical abnormalities may, owing to feelings of depression or shame, maintain an emotional distance from the children and create a situation of relative deprivation. Blind, deaf, and physically disabled infants and children require considerable interaction and stimulation to reach their full potential; a diminution of parental contact compounds their difficulties.

The role of the mother is vital in early infant-parent attachment. Less is known of the role of fathers, which may be quite variable; there is little doubt, however, that the participation of fathers and siblings in the care and stimulation of infants may be of paramount importance in their emotional development.

2.34   GENDER IDENTITY AND ROLE

The establishment of gender identity and appropriate gender role behavior is a complex process; it begins before the birth of the child on at least 2 levels. At the biologic level, the sex chromosomes predetermine the development of male or female gonads and sex organs, usually with congruence between genotype and phenotype. At another level, the gender of the unborn baby is involved in the wishes, hopes, anxieties, expectations, and projections of the parents, whose degrees of satisfaction in their own gender identities and roles and whose previous experiences as parents of boys or girls will establish certain expectations or wishes, both positive and negative.

The terms which refer to aspects of the development of sexual identity and role should be clearly understood. *Chromosomal sex* is the sex assignment determined by karyotype. *Somatotype* is the sex assigned at birth, in accord with the appearance of the external genitalia. Genitals and chromosomal sex are generally congruent. (Exceptions are discussed in Sec 18.44.) *Gender identity* is the *subjectively* felt conviction that one is male or female. *Gender role* or *sex role* consists of the personal and social expectations and behaviors through which the individual gives expression to being male or female.

Biologic Factors.   Neither gender identity nor gender role is determined finally by chromosomal sex. Individuals with ambiguous genitalia who have been assigned at birth to somatotypes inappropriate to their chromosomal sex have generally adopted gender identities, gender roles, and sex roles in accordance with the somatotype assigned. On the other hand, transsexuals, whose external genitalia and sex chromosomes are in accord, have a subjectively felt gender identity which is incongruent. Neither the true sex of the gonads, nor the influence of adrenal or other hormones, nor the form of the external genitalia determines finally what gender identity or role will be adopted. On the other hand, prenatal exposure to steroids of the progesterone type may influence certain stereotypic gender role behaviors; for example, masculine behavior has been found more evident in girls exposed prenatally to synthetic progestins, and study of boys and girls exposed prenatally to progestins found them higher than their siblings on scales of independence and self-sufficient behaviors.

Psychosocial Aspects.   It is the *social* determinants of gender identity and gender role that are critical in sexual typing. These arise from within the family and the large social environment. Money et al indicate that by 18 mo of age the child may have an irreversibly firm grip on his or her gender role. Others feel that the final identification of sexual self occurs between 2.5–3 yr. Two thirds of 3 yr olds and almost all 4 yr olds are able to identify their own gender correctly.

Among the factors determining gender identity and role behaviors are those standards, expectations, and behaviors of parents, other adults, and siblings, which have sexual implications for the child. If parents and other important persons in the environment of children label, raise, and treat them consistently as belonging to one sex, it is that gender identity they will internalize. The transsexual is a rare exception (Sec 2.61). Sexual standards, which are beliefs about the behaviors or attitudes appropriate to gender roles, serve as an internal guide to what is male and what is female. Standards arise from identification with important models of gender roles, parents especially, and out of growing expectations that certain behaviors or attitudes will be approved, and others not. By the age of 7 yr the child's notion of sex roles as dichotomous has been established. Physical attributes perceived by the child as identifying sex roles are fairly clear and direct. Young children's drawings distinguish gender on the basis of hair, clothing, jewelry, occasionally breasts, and only rarely by external genitalia.

Traditional Western cultural standards rate aggressive, assertive, and instrumental behavior as masculine, whereas dependent, socially compliant, more emotionally expressive behavior is regarded as typically feminine. These cultural stereotypes present boys as more dominant in interpersonal relationships, more interested in mechanical things, more interested and active in sports, developing greater skill in the use of large muscles, and more independent, whereas girls are typified as more expressive emotionally, more concerned and skilled in interpersonal relationships, and more nurturant, with athletic prowess limited to certain sports. These cultural stereotypes, however, are undergoing significant changes.

Preschool children choose their parents of the same sex as models for sex roles. Boys are usually required by cultural standards and expectations to make sex role preferences and a clear definition earlier, more consistently, and more stringently than girls. For example, parents will frequently be unnecessarily anxious if their 3–4 yr old boy is still interested in dolls or in "girls' activities and games," but girls seem to have more latitude in terms of "tomboy" behaviors. In traditional families, girls show a strong feminine preference in preschool years which seems to diminish as they get older, whereas the preference of boys for the male role increases steadily throughout the elementary years.

The most obvious behavioral differences between boys and girls in the preschool years lie in the greater assertiveness and aggressiveness of boys, which become manifest between 2–2.5 yr of age, along with their identification of their own sex. This may be the result of constitutional and temperamental differences between boys and girls that presumably exert their influence from birth or may reflect parental and cultural attitudes and expectations incorporated from the earliest weeks of life.

Gender identity, belief about one's own appropriate sexual traits, involves a very emotionally laden set of feelings. There is never perfect correspondence between sexual standards and sexual identity, but some congruity is necessary to the emotional health and successful adaptation of the child. Seeing one's self as similar to the parent of the same sex and different in certain critical ways from the other parent is important in achieving a secure gender identity. Children with weak or vague gender-related traits may have unusual difficulty in identifying themselves as female or male. Upon entry into school, the child's basis for comparison broadens in the world of peers; this may either strengthen or threaten the depth or nature of convictions about his or her own gender.

Academic achievement is not specifically sex typed, but our culture tends to stress academic success for boys, particularly in adolescence and in pursuit of vocational success. Girls in the elementary school years generally perform better than boys academically, except in mathematics, and are more fluent verbally, although boys may actually know more words. Learning disabilities are 3–6 times more frequent in boys than in girls. By adolescence, boys have generally caught up with and at times surpassed girls in many areas of academic achievement. Differential rates of maturation and development may influence these differences; other possibilities include the fact that striving for intellectual achievements may be viewed by girls or by their adult models as aggressive or assertive behavior in conflict with traditional female sex roles. An achievement-oriented girl will likely engage in behavior that puts her into competition with boys, and she may feel that the possibility of her being loved and cherished is threatened. Such attitudes reflect a cultural prescription designed to maintain psychologic and economic domination of women by men and to make the female attractive as a marital candidate. This attitude also supports the traditional notion that the female role is to be loved and provided for, and protected in her future role fulfillment in motherhood, and it assumes that her economic security will come from her husband's efforts to maintain her and her children.

In the late 1960's the women's liberation movement challenged the cultural stereotypes of gender roles both for adults and for children. Its supporters have questioned the child rearing techniques and sex role standards that may mold girls into passive, nonassertive, noncompetitive adults, emphasizing exclusively the nurturant or emotionally expressive sides of personality development. The movement challenges the cultural assumption that the principal task of little girls is to prepare for the role of wife-mother and contends that a cultural concern with the security of the male ego and with protection of the dominant socioeconomic position of men both wittingly and unwittingly supports traditional sex role standards and behaviors.

Pediatricians can expect some problems of child behavior and child rearing to reflect these new attitudes toward the behaviors, games, interests, and activities heretofore assigned to one gender or the other. Moreover, the way in which parents serve as sexual role models may undergo some marked shifts. All this may proceed smoothly and agreeably in any given family or be marked with conflict and strife. For a generation or more among some middle class couples gender roles have been blurred in respect to many household activities, but the persons primarily responsible for day to day care of children have continued to be mothers or their female helpers (grandmothers, baby sitters, and so on). There is now greater pressure on the husband and father to share more directly in child rearing responsibilities, and conflict may occur over whether and how this is done. Although studies are in progress, neither the immediate nor the long-term effect of these new life styles is as yet known.

The physician who is consulted regarding appropriate gender roles or who finds children caught in the struggle between such roles can help parents to see that they are engaged in a renegotiation of their family relationships (or social contract). The physician can promote an atmosphere for this negotiation in which each party states his or her terms and expectations and can then decide which conflicting areas or issues can be compromised or traded off. Physicians must help parents to avoid generating conflicting loyalties in the children and possibly confusing them about their own gender identities. Children are very vulnerable when caught in struggles between their parents for their loyalty and affection. A typical response of such children is to develop symptoms—physical, behavioral, or emotional.

Sex Activity. Boys may develop erections from the time of birth. Girls can produce lubrication of their vaginas also from birth. During the first year, all children explore their bodies and identify various areas or zones as particularly sensitive. Boys identify the penis as sensitive to both pleasurable and painful stimuli. One third of the mothers of 1 yr old infants have reported some sort of genital manipulation. Boys were noted mostly to simply pull at their penises, girls to do some sort of rubbing or other stimulation of the genital area. Between 2–5 yr approximately one half of boys and one third of girls are observed to be involved in some sort of genital handling. Girls engage in friction of the thighs together as well as in direct genital rubbing.

Very young children frequently touch their mothers' breasts, brothers' or fathers' penises, or buttocks of both parents, principally out of curiosity and interest. Preschool children often engage in thinly veiled sexual games such as playing "mother and father," "doctor and nurse," or other games that involve dressing and undressing. Such games allow for visual and at times manual exploration of each other's bodies, including the genitals of both sexes. Children at this age are curious about the sexual differences in their parents and will often intrude upon parents in the bathroom or when they are getting dressed.

These behaviors are to be viewed as a normal part of the curiosity that children have about themselves and the world they live in. Parents are well advised not to show shock, repugnance, anger, or shaming behavior toward children who engage in these various curiosity-seeking and harmless pleasure-seeking activities. Parents need not engage in exposure or nudity that they are not comfortable with, albeit some boys first urinate in a standing position only after their fathers model this behavior. Children should not share a bed with parents or sleep in the same room when this can be avoided. Nor should parents engage in erotic and explicit sexual behavior in the presence of their children, in hope of providing an enlightened household or encouraging their acceptance of sexuality as normal and good. Such affectionate displays as kissing, hugging, and a certain amount of sensual exchange between parents are healthy for children to see and be aware of. If a child accidentally or intentionally happens upon parents involved in sexual activities, the parents should be neither embarrassed nor ashamed, still less enraged. If the incident is handled calmly and casually, with the child requested to leave or return to his or her bedroom, it is likely that the incident will be treated quite naturally by the child. If the child asks, he or she should be provided with a simple, direct, and calm explanation of what he or she has seen, and the statement that this is one of the ways that parents show their love and affection for each other.

By 5–7 yr of age many children develop an increasing sense of modesty about their own dressing and undressing, toileting, and bathing behaviors, and this sense of privacy often increases toward puberty. It parallels the increasing privacy of the child's mind, which can become excessively valued and a preoccupation in adolescence.

Prepubertal children used to be thought to exhibit little sexual activity. This "latency period" of psychoanalytic theory is now known to contain considerable sexual activity and concern. One study found masturbation in 10% of 7 yr old boys and 80% of 13 yr olds. Heterosexual interests may include a boy's identifying a specific girlfriend, sharing activities with her and exchanges of affection, and at times experiences of erotic nature. A study has found that 5% of 5 yr olds, 33% of 8 yr olds, and two thirds of 13 yr olds can acknowledge heterosexual interests or curiosities, with the oldest age group claiming a fair amount of experience. Most 10–12 yr old girls or boys said that they had a boy- or girlfriend; two thirds of 10 yr olds and 85% of 12 yr olds stated that they had kissed their girl- or boyfriend. Sexual interests of girls and boys move from the notion of wanting to get married in a general way to wanting to marry a particular boy or girl, to actually having a boyfriend or girlfriend, and then to some social and heterosexual activities with the friend.

2.35 PHYSICAL ACTIVITY

Mobile exploration is a vital step in acquisition of knowledge and of a sense of initiative, but parental supervision is necessary to minimize the risk of accidents. Stairways must be barred, poisonous substances placed out of reach, electrical outlets plugged, and the handles of gas burners out of reach or removed. Physicians should see that parents receive careful instruction on safety measures; they also must encourage parents to allow the child considerable freedom to move about in safe places.

Data indicate that restraint of the child's mobility by surgical and medical procedures involving splints or casts, oxygen or mist tents, prolonged intravenous feedings, dressings for burns, and the like may contribute to the development of subsequent emotional or personality problems or to speech or learning difficulties. When restraint of the child's locomotion function is necessary, it should be with considerable emotional support, with rooming-in of parents and close contact with medical and other staff, and with diversions such as appropriate games, television, and so on.

Excessive motor activity in the toddler may be an early sign of the *hyperactivity syndrome* (Sec 2.56). Involved children may be reported to have many accidents, "to get into things," to wander away from home, "not to understand the meaning of the word *NO*," and to be "always on the go." However, except where there is evidence of constitutional hyperactivity, difficulties in managing the active toddler mostly reflect inconsistent discipline by the parents. This period can be a difficult one, the toddler "feeling his oats," exercising newly developed skills, and testing limits. Occasionally the setting is complicated by the birth of a new sibling. Effective discipline requires that parents know what they want, mean what they say, use a firm approach, and follow through in a consistent fashion (Sec 2.30). Usually parental reproach, sometimes repeated, and removal of the child from an undesired activity will suffice. Temper tantrums are common, with peak incidence around 2.5 yr of age. These excellent attention-getting devices should generally be accepted by parents as understandable expressions of the child's frustration with having no power to change the rules; when tantrums prove useless, the child tends to give up this unprofitable behavior (Sec 2.55).

2.36 TOILET TRAINING

The impact of conflicts around toilet training on the child's emotional development has been exaggerated. There is little to indicate that the experiences involved in the toilet training of most children are of major psychologic consequence. Only when toilet training becomes a field of battle between overdemanding parents and the child or is pursued unrealistically early or overzealously would one expect conflict over toilet training to have any effect on personality development.

Parents may wish to start toilet training when the child is old enough to verbalize needs for care after wetting or soiling, and when he or she can appreciate a simple reward system. The substitution of training pants for diapers is an important step in the toilet training process, though it is to be expected that accidents will occur. If resistance is significant, parents should not make toileting a battleground but merely postpone further efforts for several weeks or months. Though it may be disappointing, annoying, or irritating to parents, it is neither uncommon nor harmful for toilet training to be achieved even as late as the 3rd yr. Many children, by tuning in on the parents' implicit or gently expressed wishes, appear to train themselves; some are trained by the encouragement of siblings.

2.37 SIBLING RELATIONSHIPS

The impact of a new sibling upon a young child can be felt very early. As soon as she knows herself to be pregnant the mother may alter her attitudes toward her other children and sometimes begin to intensify her concern with activities such as feeding, toilet training, and so on, which she wants to have under a different level of control by the time the new baby is born. The physician should explore such areas of family dynamics, and may well caution mothers against letting the deadline of the date of expected delivery provoke conflict in these areas. With the birth of a new sibling, the older child may show responses ranging from denial of the sibling's birth through regressive behavior, such as wetting or soiling, to happy acceptance of the event.

The older child requires such preparation for the sibling's birth as will impart the reassurance that he or she remains loved and will have some caretaking responsibilities, even if minor, for the new sibling. Questions regarding babies, hospitals, and birth should be answered as factually and comfortably as possible.

The ordinal position of siblings has no proven effect on their development of personality. Firstborn children are not necessarily more neurotic or more gifted, and there is little evidence that they are reared essentially differently from subsequent children. Ordinal position may be used to rationalize other problems to which it bears no relationship.

Bickering and competition among siblings are normal and help to develop interpersonal skills. Rough and tumble play is probably beneficial to such growth. Severe problems in sibling relationship, however, frequently reflect marital difficulties or inadequacies in parental management. Sometimes one of several siblings may be unconsciously assigned a role by one or both parents which involves him or her in a conflict between them, and such a child may be implicitly encouraged by one parent to be an ally against the other. Similarly, a sibling may serve as a scapegoat for other family psychopathology, owing to the timing of birth, a birth defect, or his or her temperament, sex, or resemblance to or identification with a parent or grandparent. At times a child may unconsciously fall into or choose the role of scapegoat in order to maintain a level of homeostasis in family psychopathology such that more serious or threatening disintegration in family interaction is held off.

Parents frequently complain about sibling jealousies as one of the problems in raising more than one child, but older siblings are important in the education, socialization, and support of younger ones, and siblings may be the closest of friends.

2.38 NORMAL FEARS OF CHILDREN

Fears are normal and perhaps a necessary part of psychologic development. To be realistically afraid of real danger and to take steps to avoid it or to minimize its effects are necessary for adaptation and survival. Fear is the perception of an external threat, real or possible. Anxiety implies the feelings associated with fear in the absence of any immediate perception of external threat. It may be the result of fantasies reflecting internal conflicts. Though the object of fear or anxiety may be imaginary or fictitious, the sensation itself, of course, is not and has familiar physiologic components. The distinction between fear and phobia is essentially that between normal and pathologic, phobia being defined within a psychoanalytic framework as involving certain mechanisms of defense, such as repression, projection, or displacement.

The things children are likely to fear change with age, becoming more specific to their environment and experience as they grow older. The younger child's fears are centered on basic conditions or situations such as darkness, or being left alone or abandoned, or upon cultural stereotypes of fear-inducing objects, such as animals, monsters, ghosts, and goblins. Preverbal and even school-age children do not necessarily have fears that correspond to the concerns adults may have for them or may try to inculcate. They may not, for example, be concerned about fire, traffic, or the friendly stranger who may spirit them away. As they become older, their fears become more oriented toward specific culturally appropriate threats in the environment and toward specific past experiences of their own. They may generalize isolated experiences of their own that were threatening or fear-inducing, sometimes appropriately, sometimes not. The cosmologic threats adults feel, such as of destruction from nuclear weapons, war, flood, or hurricane, are not particularly fearful for the preadolescent child and may be of no major concern even to the adolescent.

Children's fears may readily reflect those of their parents, and these fears may be transmitted from parents to child explicitly, or more often implicitly. Among the common fears of preschool and young school-age children are those of thunder and lightning, punishment, pain, hospitals, and such people as physicians or dentists. Parents also may be feared. Even when parents are not punitive, cruel, or harsh, most children are afraid of them under some situations. The anger of a parent is particularly frightening for the child, even when the parent refrains from physical contact with the child.

Children manifest their fears in various ways, depending upon age and sophistication and upon ability to verbalize and willingness to do so. The preverbal child may cling, cry, scream and try to escape from situations that frighten, and it may be very difficult to identify the fear-provoking stimulus. The older child may be hesitant to discuss or even name what he or she is afraid of, because of fantasy and fear that talking about it will make it come true, the words being given magical powers.

The physician can help parents to be patient with children's fears. Even intense fears are not necessarily a sign of emotional disturbance, still less of cowardice. For the preverbal and young verbal child, the parents can be encouraged to give support through hugging, holding, and physical comforting, conveying reassurance through their availability and presence that the feared object or condition has no power actually to hurt. In such young children logical explanation is of little or no value and is incomprehensible to the anxious and excited child.

For the child of school age and older, verbal reassurance should supplement physical and emotional support, for the child can respond to it in terms both of its tone and of its realism. Simple, direct explanations often require repetition each time the feared situation or object is encountered; the child may gain strength and support even as the logical and reasonable explanation is repeated in the same way each time. After a while the child may internalize the formula and be heard saying it to himself or herself or to younger brothers and sisters when they show concern with the same object or situation. The child becomes able to distinguish the feeling of fear from the fact that the feared situation, object, or condition has no real power

to do harm. Parents should be advised neither to shame nor to demean fearful children, nor to try to force them into feared situations hoping that, in surviving them without support or in crying it out, they will overcome fear. This procedure may induce terror and complicate subsequent management of fears.

The unrealistically feared situation needs eventually to be faced by the child, and parents may need advice in devising appropriate ways to help children to master specific fears. Children afraid to be separated from their parents at night may be allowed to stay outside their bedroom sleeping on the hall floor, to be moved into their own bedrooms or into the bedrooms of siblings as they become more secure. It helps if they can be given some power over the situation, such as being able to turn on or keep a light on if they are afraid of the dark, to reach their parents by telephone when they have been left for an evening, or to have contact with a nonthreatening puppy or kitten if fears center on dogs or cats. Each time a child masters even in a slight way the fearful situation, he or she should be given praise and encouragement. Whatever is done, the parents' own capacities to be calm, reassuring, encouraging, and supportive are essential.

Parents whose own fears of the dark, of being alone, of thunder or lightning, or of dentist or doctor provide models to their children's fears have the responsibility to underplay those situations. If their children ask them if they are afraid, it is important that parents be able to acknowledge their own fears, since to deny them is to deny the child's accurate perception, and this denial could be confusing. Parents do not have to be fearless nor to appear so to the child. Parents should be able to say, "Yes, I have the same fear and I know it is not sensible, but I have learned to live with it." They may then be able to give their children some advice about how to handle fears and may encourage them to feel that they do not have to be burdened with the fears of their parents. With this approach children may learn to cope with fears with more success than their parents.

When fears last an inordinately long time, when one set of fears is replaced by another, or when fears become increasingly incapacitating to the child or to parental or family function, a more definitive psychologic and psychiatric evaluation will be needed.

2.39 PRESCHOOL AND SCHOOL

Preschool experiences can be of value to the young child, enhancing socialization, peer group interaction, and perhaps even cognitive learning. Four yr olds and, in selected instances, 3 yr olds who appear to be mature enough to spend a half day away from home should be enrolled in nursery school. Even at 18 mo of age some children may benefit from a half day or 2 or more each week in a supervised setting where they may interact with other children (Sec 2.33).

The refusal of a child to go to school (*school phobia*) is not uncommon in kindergarten or first or second grade children. The children involved are generally good students with obsessive traits, who often have had earlier problems in separating from parents or from home. Somatic complaints may accompany the refusal to attend school. The physician should first help parents to insist upon the young child's prompt return to school and continued attendance, and then try to determine and alleviate the cause. Otherwise, early and transient school refusal may evolve into an ingrained and chronic difficulty. In preadolescence and adolescence, though, an episode of school refusal may indicate rather serious psychopathology, and it is wise not to insist on a return to school until psychiatric assessment finds that appropriate.

Poor school performance in an intellectually able child may be the result of emotional problems, sensory deficits, other physical illness, or inadequate teaching. Boys may be less ready developmentally than girls to assume the passive role of student, and the normally exuberant activity of young grade school boys may present problems for teachers in the early school years. As a general principle, it may be wise not to have boys begin their first grade experience before the age of 6, or at times closer to 7 yr. Despite some dangers of inaccurate diagnoses and mislabeling, the early school years provide a good setting for identifying such health, psychologic or educational problems as mental retardation, reading disorders, hyperkinesis, sensory deficits, and emotional difficulties. Identification is of value, however, only if appropriate remedial programs are available. In recent years schools have been experimenting with new educational techniques, including "open classrooms," programmed learning, "family" groupings, and operant conditioning; these may be more useful for some children than others. For example, a withdrawn and inhibited child may function quite well in an open setting; an overactive child may require a more structured educational program. Most children, however, do well in school, and schools do well by most children. Wherever possible, it makes good sense for those interested in children to work closely with schools, both around individual children with problems and in collaborative efforts that will strengthen the ability of schools to foster children's emotional development.

2.40 PUBERTY AND ADOLESCENCE

See Sec 2.13 and Chapter 19.

Adolescence is a physical and psychosocial process of long duration, lasting in Western society from the age of 12–13 yr to the late teens or even the early 20's. Assignment of an end point to adolescence depends upon whether one is measuring it by relatively internalized psychologic processes or by more social benchmarks such as economic and social emancipation from the parental family.

Adolescent "Turmoil." Conventional psychoanalytic theory has held that adolescence is normally a period of "turmoil," marked by a desire for independence and a quest for sexual identity and maturity, and by a casting off of the old, parental images and values in order to solidify one's own personality structure. Turmoil was once regarded as inevitable, a necessary part of growth. This view holds, further, that if turmoil does

not occur in adolescence, the individual will pay the cost later in inhibition, constriction of personality, or dependency.

More recent studies of adolescents, comparisons of patients and controls, and examinations of large populations of boys and girls suggest less conflict. Rutter et al found in a review of normative studies that "most adolescents are not particularly critical of their parents, and very few reject them." Parents and adolescents may disagree and most adolescents would prefer their parents to be less restrictive; but the overwhelming majority of adolescents tend to admire their parents, get along quite well with them, and are generally satisfied and happy at home. Contrary to popular belief, they are more worried about parental disapproval than about the disapproval of friends. They are not particularly alienated unless they have psychologic disturbances, and there is no evidence that the increase in sexual activity, including intercourse, is correlated with psychiatric disturbances (see below). Normal adolescents experience anxiety and depression as inherent in growing up, but do not experience major turmoil, confusion, or withdrawal.

However, an adolescent who is clearly unhappy or whose recurrent crises suggest serious conflict requires careful evaluation. Among signs requiring attention are sudden declines in scholastic achievement, choices of new companions with whom parents are uncomfortable or of whom they disapprove, or evidence of a preference almost exclusively for activities outside the home, especially when there appears to be a breakdown in a communication within the home. The last-named conflict may occur not only between adolescent and parents but also between parents. When such signs appear, it is well for the family physician or pediatrician to suspect serious illness, such as may warrant psychiatric referral. A disturbed adolescent should not be regarded as a normal variant with a necessary and transient disturbance. An adolescent who is disturbed was likely disturbed as a child, and will be a disturbed adult unless intervention occurs.

Sexual Behavior. In recent years traditional standards of sexual conduct have been challenged, studies of the past 20 yr indicating that adolescents are becoming more experienced sexually. This change is real and marked. In 1971 Zelnik and Kantner found that 30% of unmarried female teenagers in the age group 15–19 residing in metropolitan areas had experienced sexual intercourse, with an increase to 43% by 1976 and to 50% in 1979. In 1976 more were using birth control, especially the pill, but more than a third were "unprotected" at the time of last intercourse. By 1979 contraceptive use had increased, but there had also been an increase in ineffective measures, such as withdrawal. Thirteen % of unmarried teenagers had been pregnant. Sorenson's 1973 study found that 59% of American adolescent boys and 45% of adolescent girls had had sexual intercourse. His studies of the attitudes and values of experienced adolescents indicated that they saw sexual activity as occurring in the context of a relationship, as a means of communication, as a part of self-realization, and as an aspect of love. About half of the boys and 62% of the girls 16–19 yr old had used contraception during their most recent intercourse. Many adolescents who did not use birth control relied on the possibility of abortion or of having and keeping a baby without getting married.

The physician who deals with adolescents, even those who may be sexually active, should not assume that their theoretical knowledge, particularly in the area of contraception, is measured by their experience. Many sexually active adolescents find it difficult to admit ignorance about sexual matters, bravado, airs of sophistication, and saving face being for them highly invested coping styles. Accordingly, the physician must often take the initiative in providing instruction and guidance.

The failure of some adolescents to use contraceptives involves motivational factors as well as ignorance. Obtaining and using contraceptives makes the intention to have intercourse explicit. By not being prepared, the adolescent attempts to avoid guilt through the fiction that intercourse resulted from overwhelming passion or a miscalculation. For some girls pregnancy fulfills conscious or unconscious needs; it can boost self-esteem, provide reassurance of femininity, become an act of defiance or of self-denigration, or be used as a weapon against family, boyfriend, or self. For some boys, impregnating their girlfriends serves as proof of virility.

Guidance. In guiding the adolescent, the physician must take into account the relationships between adolescents and parents, and those between adolescents and their peers. The young adolescent may vacillate between attempts at extreme independence and sudden reversions to overt or camouflaged dependence. The adolescent is testing new ideas and new relationships and trying to renegotiate the old relationship with parents to win somewhat new and different terms. Adolescence in Western society can be viewed as a time of rehearsal for a variety of adult roles, and it is natural that early attempts at adult performance may be clumsy, exaggerated, and not satisfactory either to the adolescent or to others. One of the most important roles of the physician is to point out to adolescent, and particularly to parents, that they are entering upon a new phase of relationship. Both parents and adolescents must get used to the idea that they are in a process of separating from each other, reaching the final stage of a process that began with birth. Anxiety and depression are to be expected at times, on the part either of the child or of the parent, as they modify their earlier closer bond. The parental attitudes most threatening to the adolescent may be either premature total emancipation on the one hand or a resort to inappropriate severe restrictions on the other. Parental indifference might be equally threatening. Adolescents also fear and do their best to avoid loss of face, the appearance of being fools to themselves or to their peers, siblings, or parents. The physician can be most helpful to parents if, as a semi-objective outsider, he or she can help them to avoid power struggles in which the loss of face by child or parent is a frequent outcome.

In treating drug-related problems, physicians must know such things as types of drugs; frequency of use; among which age groups the drugs are used; whether the use is distinctive by social class, by school, or by local community; and what parental, school, and other community resources are doing about drug problems. Only adequately informed physicians can help adolescents or their families who face problems of drug abuse (Sec 2.13 and 19.13).

The choice of career, whether it follows immediately upon high school or after college and postgraduate work, is an important preoccupation of adolescents. The physician can be helpful in knowing what resources are available for vocational training, with advice regarding choice of colleges, or regarding preparation needed for a career in which the adolescent is interested. Adolescents frequently need to discuss with experienced adults their concerns about their future.

Adolescents in the United States are today under great pressure to succeed both academically and vocationally. They are likely to expect too much of themselves, to become discouraged and give up, or to strive inordinately hard, paying a high price emotionally and socially, and sometimes with health. Suicide attempts are at peak incidence in the age group between 15–25 yr (Sec 2.54).

Piaget and other investigators have indicated that in the adolescent period the final stage is reached in development of abstract reasoning and facility with logic, along with increased sophistication in moral reasoning (Sec 2.31). The physician can help adolescents and their parents by providing developmental interpretations of behavior. Discussion and arguments around such issues as religion, philosophy, politics, social concerns, and ethical questions is one way in which some adolescents develop and test their new cognitive and logical skills.

The average adolescent is subject to anxiety and to episodes of depression. Fairly effective strategies for dealing with stress and avoiding too much self-preoccupation include development of goal-directed academic or extracurricular or social activities. Discussions with their peers support adolescents in coping with the stresses and strains of everyday life. Humor is a major coping strategy, the butts of which may be parents and adult-dominated institutions, but also themselves, and often each other.

SOCIAL ISSUES

2.41 ADOPTION

Most adopted children and their families handle the matter with considerable common sense and sensitivity, but some issues concerning adoption require comment.

Adoptions accomplished through approved agencies are preferred to independent adoptions, since they tend to have more adequate assessment of the psychosocial setting of the prospective adoptive family and perhaps better safeguards for the physical condition of the infant. Adoptive placement should be made as soon after birth as possible in order to foster a firm attachment and bonding between infant and adoptive mother (Sec 2.33). Adoptions of older children, or across religious and ethnic lines, or by single parents are, in appropriate instances, reasonable alternatives to having adoptable children languish in institutions or temporary foster homes, but adoptions of older children present some risks. For example, a family seeking to rescue a 4–5 yr old child with a history of severe emotional deprivation and multiple foster home placements may find that the child has been severely traumatized and will later display major psychologic disturbances, even in the best of adoptive homes.

The adopted child should be told of his or her adoption as soon as reasonably good verbal facility and comprehension have been achieved, by the age of 3 or at the latest 4 yr. The explanation can be repeated when circumstances are appropriate, such as during a family discussion about the birth of a neighbor's baby, but should not become ritual. Children's books on adoption can be read to young children; later they can read them themselves.

Controversy continues as to whether adopted children are at increased risk for development of emotional problems. If they are, it is likely to reflect problems of parental adjustment or management. Since the adopted child generally arrives in the context of marital infertility, he or she may be treated with considerable overindulgence as a "special child." Adoption need not be perceived by the child as a threat to self-esteem, but in the case of individual and family problems, the child's adoptive status may reinforce otherwise existing doubts about his or her competence and worth. Not infrequently a natural child is born following an adoption to previously "infertile" parents. For the adopted child the event may initiate a competitive struggle requiring both understanding and firmness on the part of the parents.

Occasionally, foster parents wish to adopt a child who has been in their care for a number of years, but who has not been legally relinquished by the natural parents. Traditionally, the courts have upheld the claim of biologic parents for the child, even in those instances in which the natural parents abandoned the child and the foster parents have been essentially the child's only long-standing, nurturant, and consistent (psychologic) parents. Such legal decisions reinforce the notion that children are to be treated as property, rather than having their own needs and rights. Several recent decisions to the contrary, however, show the courts' growing appreciation of the child's need for continuity of care.

In some states, adopted persons who have attained their majority are entitled to access to their adoption records and to information about their biologic parents. On the whole, this is a commendable development; this right-to-know must be weighed, however, against the rights of biologic parents to privacy, if they desire it.

2.42 FOSTER CARE

Placement in foster care is typically provided by local welfare authorities for abandoned, severely neglected, or abused children. For many children, foster care offers a life-saving environment which gives them the oppor-

tunity to be physically replenished, to grow, and to develop innate potential. For others, however, foster care represents yet another episode in a lifelong history of deprivation. Unfortunately, we have yet to develop in the United States a comprehensive and well-supervised system of foster care which provides integrated services for children already at risk. Undermanned and underbudgeted departments of public welfare are often unable adequately to prepare, supervise, and support foster parents who may have to deal with difficult, traumatized children. Children are transferred from one foster home to another, because foster parents move or because the child doesn't "adjust" or because unsupervised foster parents are deemed to be inadequate. Some children move in and out of placement according to the whims of natural parents who can neither care for them nor let them go permanently. For some children 5–12 foster care placements have disastrous effects on abilities to learn, trust, and relate to others. Such children, already made vulnerable by the circumstances which led to their placement, are placed at further risk by the vagaries of foster care. Serious retardation in reading, antisocial behavior, apathetic states, and defects in socialization have all been compellingly described by Eisenberg as the sequelae of such experiences. This distressing situation will not change until the needs of children receive high priority in social planning and legislation. Only recently have trends in state and federal legislation been aimed at "permanency planning," with the use of adoptive placement or permanent foster care, and with earlier relinquishment or termination of the rights of parents who are unwilling or unable to care for their own children.

2.43 EFFECTS OF A MOBILE SOCIETY

For the first 30 yr after World War II approximately 20% of the population of the United States changed residence each year, although there has been a slight decline in mobility in recent years.

The effects of this movement on children and families are frequently overlooked. For children the move is essentially involuntary; they move because a parent has obtained employment elsewhere, because the birth of a sibling has made a larger home desirable, or for other reasons. When such changes in family structure as divorce or death precipitate moves, children face the stresses created by both the precipitating events and moving itself. When parents are sad because of the circumstances surrounding the move, this unhappiness will be transmitted to their children. Children who move lose their old friends, lose the comfort of a familiar bedroom and house, and lose their ties to school and community. Not only must they sever old relationships, but they are faced with developing new ones in new neighborhoods and new schools. Because movement upward in social standing often accompanies a geographic move, children may enter neighborhoods with new and different customs and values. And since academic standards and curricula vary from community to community, children who have performed well in one school may find themselves struggling in a new one.

Frequent moves during the school years are likely to have adverse consequences on social and academic performance.

Parents should prepare children well in advance of any move, and allow them to express any unhappy feelings or misgivings. Parents should acknowledge their own mixed feeings and agree that they will miss their old home while looking forward to a new one. Visits to the new home in advance are often useful preludes to the actual move. Transient periods of regressive behavior may be noted in preschool children after moving, and these should be understood and accepted. Parents should assist the entry of their children into the new community, and exchanges of letters with old friends and visits, whenever possible, should be encouraged.

2.44 SEPARATION AND DEATH

The younger the child, the more likely he or she is to respond to the loss of a parent through separation or death in a manner characteristic of other young children. In older children the reactions are more individualized and reflect differential characteristics of their own experiences. Relatively brief separations and reunions usually produce rather transient effects, in response either to the separation or to the reunion. The potential impact of each event must be considered in the light of the age and stage of development of the child and the particular relationship with the absent person, as well as the nature of the separation. It is more frightening for children to be separated from a parent at a hospital than within the familiar surroundings of home (Sec 2.64).

In young children the initial reaction to separation may involve crying, either of a tantrum-like, protesting type or of a quieter, sadder type. After a few hours or a day or so of separation, the child may appear more subdued, withdrawn, quiet or irritable, fussy, moody, and resistant to authority. Children may repeatedly ask where the absent parent is and when he or she will return home; some children may not refer to parental absence at all. The child may go to the window or door or out into the neighborhood looking for the absent parent; a few may even leave home or their places of temporary placement to try to find where their parents are. This last rather unusual response needs to be considered when a child cannot be found for a while shortly after the separation or departure of a parent. Disturbance of appetite may occur, and there may be special difficulties at bedtime, such as reluctance in going to bed and problems in getting to sleep, with a resurgence of old fears, and in younger children perhaps such regressive behavior as bed wetting.

The child's response to reunion may surprise or alarm the parent who is not prepared. The parent who joyfully returns to the family may be met by wary or cautious children, who, after a brief interchange of affection, may move away from the parent and seem indifferent to his or her return and presence. The interpretation of this response will depend on the child and his or her style; it may indicate anger at being left and wariness

that the event will happen again, or since children tend to personalize, the child may have felt he or she caused the parent's departure. For instance, if the mother who frequently says, "Stop it, or you'll give me a headache," is hospitalized, the child may unrealistically feel at fault and guilty. As a result of these feelings children may seem to be more closely attached to the other parent than the absent one, or even to the grandparent or babysitter who cared for them during their parent's absence. Immediately after the reunion or after a few days, some children, particularly younger ones, may become more clinging and dependent than they were prior to separation, with continuation of any regressive behavior which had occurred during separation. Such behavior may engage the returned parent more closely and help to re-establish the bond that the child felt was broken. Usually such reactions are transient; within a week or two the child will have recovered usual behavior and equilibrium. Recurrent separations may tend to make the child more wary and guarded about re-establishing the relationship with the repeatedly absent parent, and these traits may affect other personal relationships. Parents should not try to ameliorate a child's behavior by threatening to leave.

Permanent or semipermanent loss such as divorce or placement in foster care can give rise to the same kinds of reactions listed above but more intense and possibly more lasting. School-age children may respond with evident depression, seem indifferent, or be markedly angry. Other children appear to deny or avoid the issue, behaviorally or verbally. Most children may cling to the hope or fantasy that the actual placement or separation is not real. Guilt may be generated by the child's feeling that this loss, separation, or placement represents rejection and perhaps punishment for misbehavior. The child may protect the parents at his or her own expense, believing and asserting that one's own badness caused the parent to depart or to place him or her with relatives or strangers, rather than that the parent has been bad or irresponsible. Besides having their own feelings of guilt, children cannot blame their parents because they sense it may be fairly risky. The parent who discovered that the child harbored resentment might punish further for these thoughts or feelings. Children may feel that it was their misbehavior that caused their parents to separate or become divorced. Such children have the fantasy that trivial or recurrent behavioral patterns of their own have caused their parents to become angry with each other. Some children develop behavioral or psychosomatic symptoms and unwittingly adopt a "sick" role as a strategy for reuniting the parents.

In response to separation and divorce of their parents older children and adolescents commonly show more intense anger. Almost all children cling to the magical belief that their parents will reunite. Wallerstein and Kelly found that 5 yr after the breakup more than 30% of the children were "consciously and intensely unhappy and dissatisfied with their life in the post-divorce family." Moderate to severe depression was common in this group. Good adjustments seemed related to ongoing involvement with two psychologically healthy parents and the support system offered by siblings.

As to the ultimate separation—death of a parent—most preadolescent children do not seem to go through a typical mourning process as psychoanalytically defined. The child's mourning may be masked by behavior not typically seen in adults. Among school-age to adolescent children who had lost a parent through death Wolfenstein found that immediately after the loss sad feelings were not markedly evident, nor was there much crying. Children continued in everyday activities, the major mechanism in dealing with catastrophe being denial, both overt and unconscious, and maintained by the magical wish and hope for reunion and reappearance. Any depressed moods which occurred were not connected with thoughts of the parent's death; this could be acknowledged intellectually as a fact but was isolated in the emotionally nurtured expectation of return. Some children seemed to maintain remarkably good moods; some were more active than usual. Wolfenstein saw these good moods as an effective accompaniment of denial: "If one does not feel bad, then nothing bad has happened." Some children show hostile and angry feelings toward the surviving parent and tend to identify with and idealize the lost parent, sometimes with reunion fantasies accompanying denial. Guilt may be present, which points up the child's tendency toward egocentricity. An orphan of the Hiroshima bomb said, "We did nothing bad—and still our parents died."

Children under the age of 5 yr view death as reversible, with possible belief in the dead coming back to life and in ghosts. In the 2nd stage, up to the age of 8–9 yr, death is personified, e.g., the "grim reaper" who punishes and avenges. Only after this age does the child realistically understand death as a universal and final biologic process.

The physician can help the child and surviving caretakers through a period of separation or adjustment to death of parent or sibling, first with recognition that the adults themselves are going through a period of grief and mourning. It is not unhealthy for children to see their surviving or remaining parent mourn the loss of a mate or grieve for a divorced or separated spouse. In the case of a dead parent the child needs the support and reassurance of having the remaining parent or other important caretakers available. Close physical contact and emotional exchange, with verbal explanations and reassurance for those children who can understand, are important aspects of support. Children should not be expected or forced to discuss all their feelings or to put into words their reactions to a parent's death. They should not be expected to interrupt usual social or recreational activities for weeks or months after death of a parent, either out of respect for that parent or in recognition of the remaining parent's sorrow or grief. Continuance of usual activities should not be interpreted by adults or older children as callousness or indifference. It should rather be recognized as the child's way of dealing at his or her stage of development with what is as much a catastrophe for him or her as it is for the adult. Further, the child should not be expected to serve as a primary support to the remaining parent or others in their grief.

In most cases it seems helpful for the child to participate in an appropriate way in the rituals which generally surround the death and burial of a parent. A young child can attend a funeral, viewing, or wake so long as there is no morbid preoccupation or demand that the child remain a long time or be involved in prolonged religious ceremonies. To keep the young child away from some participation in the burial rituals, whatever they are, will be a misguided effort to protect, and more confusing and isolating than helpful.

2.45 IMPACT OF TELEVISION

It is estimated that American children watch television for an average of 30–40 hr/wk. This is more time than they spend in school, and for many it is their major scheduled activity. Television places children in passive roles and offers them entertainment generally requiring little engagement or imagination. It entices them away from such important activities as reading, hobbies, physical exercise, and relationships with peers and with other family members.

Educational programs aimed at preschool children through television may enhance cognitive development in reading readiness and acquisition of vocabulary. At best, however, such programs can only supplement rather than substitute for the activities of parents in conveying knowledge, skills, and information, and in motivating learning (Sec 2.28). Television may inform older children of current events, politics, history, and science; it more commonly, however, displays scenes of violence which serve as models for aggressive behavior. Exposure to violence in films increases interpersonal aggressiveness among children. Optimists may hope that most children will be able to separate themselves from the steady diet of violence they witness on television; but children readily imitate all types of models, and the effects of television violence on children may be considerably more pervasive than we now know. It is certain that some children already emotionally disturbed may act out aggressively as the direct result of crime or horror programs, and that the action may follow the models presented.

All parents should know what their children are watching on television, should decide whether certain programs are appropriate, and should feel in no way reluctant to meet their own standards in imposing restrictions on the time and content of television viewing.

2.46 ASSESSMENT AND INTERVIEWING

THE CLINICAL INTERVIEW

The clinical interview is the most common procedure in medicine, but the nature of the process is often poorly defined. The interview is not simply history taking; still less is it a cross-examination of the patient that attempts to fulfill the requirements of a review of systems. It is basically a working alliance between the patient and the physician, aimed at the orderly exchange of any and all clinically relevant information between them. The patient is seeking reassurance or help, and the physician possesses knowledge, skills, and the social sanction to be helpful. *The most useful perspective for the clinical interview is to see it as a major means of engaging the patient in the active management of his or her own care.*

One well-practiced aspect of the clinical interview in most pediatric and general medical settings is the simple collection of those historical medical data that disclose and review the signs and symptoms of a presenting illness, the nature and course of past medical illnesses, the family history, and a review of systems. Other aspects of the patient's life, such as the psychosocial, often get less or scant attention in interviewing. Physicians need to find ways to use clinical interviews to assess the emotional states of their patients, their usual reactions to stress, their levels of self-concept, their systems of values, the natures of their personal relationships, something of their personalities, the quality of their coping abilities, and clues that might point to psychosocial distress or disturbance.

To become an effective interviewer requires motivation, skill, and continuous attentive practice. The skills required develop throughout the course of one's professional life. They are frequently overlooked in medical school, or poorly taught, or seen as related only to psychiatric patients, or taken for granted once medical school is completed. The development of effective interviewing skills is facilitated when the student has opportunity to practice with simulated patients, to make and hear recordings of his or her work with simulators or with actual patients, and to have these activities supervised by competent teachers or consultants.

Time. An interview that attempts comprehensively to explore both psychosocial and biomedical aspects of the condition of a stranger who has just become a new patient needs at least 30–40 min for significant exchange of the most basic relevant information. Physician and patient must have time to become comfortable with each other and to establish the rapport that facilitates the exploration of psychologic and social information. When patient and physician have had an adequate earlier initial interview, and the physician therefore knows some of the major aspects of the patient's psychosocial status, it is possible to focus on particular issues in periods as brief as 10 min, but an initial interview of 10 min is ineffective and it may communicate to the family a lack of respect for the sensitivity and importance of material given such casual attention.

Setting. Privacy is essential, but it is unfortunately often at a premium in children's hospitals or in busy outpatient clinics. The need for privacy is most likely to be overlooked with children, who are frequently managed with less respect and sensitivity than is given adults. It is difficult to carry on an interview in a relatively unsheltered cubicle in an outpatient department or at bedside, even with curtains drawn to shield the child or family from visual intrusion or distractions. If possible, it is often more productive to seat the hospitalized child in a chair next to the bed rather than to converse with the child while he or she lies in bed.

Adverse physical conditions negatively affect the quality and the effectiveness of the clinical interview. Though it may be difficult, it is worth considerable effort to find a private place; in hospitals this may be a treatment room, an empty conference room, or even an unoccupied office or patient's room. Privacy is more easily arranged in the office of the practicing physician, where closed doors and reasonable comfort are ordinarily routine.

Goals. The most common deficiency within an interview is the failure of the clinician to define clearly the goals of that particular encounter. No single interview can accomplish everything that needs to be done to complete a clinical assessment. The clinician must set, define, and state priorities. These will depend upon the nature of the patient's condition, whether the interview is an initial visit or a follow-up one, or whether the physician has to elicit sensitive material or to transmit unpleasant or unhappy diagnostic or prognostic information to patient or family. Physicians must become sufficiently familiar with their own styles and learn enough from past experiences to be able to judge accurately what can be accomplished in each interview. For example, if the work of the 1st interview is to establish a working alliance with a child and family and to identify the primary problems or concerns, then it may be a mistake to attempt a total developmental, family, or school survey on such an occasion.

Communication. The major purpose and process of the clinical interview is the exchange of information. When the patients are children, this exchange occurs between parents and physician, between child and parents, and between parents, as well as between child and physician. In any social interaction communication has two major features: one is the *content* or *message;* the other is the *process*, or the manner in which content is exchanged within the relationship.

The notion of content refers to the literal meaning of the words exchanged between communicating parties; content is the message or the *what* of communication. The notion of process refers to the relational or nonverbal aspects of communication. The tone of voice, the rate of speech, the inflection of words and phrases, facial expressions, head movements, hand gestures, body postures, and movement all communicate meaning, often more accurately than the words exchanged. The words usually capture the major conscious attention, but the process may frequently determine the success of the venture. The nonverbal features of communication are continually monitored by each sender and receiver, often preconsciously or subconsciously. The nonverbal conveys the cognitive, emotional, social, or rather global state of the sender with respect to what he or she is saying, and indicates to the receiver *how the content is to be interpreted.*

Children attend to and interpret nonverbal communication before they understand the meanings of words. Reciprocal communication of basic feelings and emotions between parent and infant takes place through sounds, gestures, and body contacts long before the infant or the toddler can identify feelings or know what words appropriately express them. Physicians should be aware of how their own facial expressions, tones of voice, or gestures influence children's reactions and determine how messages are interpreted; this knowledge contributes greatly to skill in interviewing. The complementary skill required of the physician is to recognize and correctly interpret the child's emotional state through careful observation of facial expression, tone and inflection of voice, body posture, gestures, and other responses. Children may be unresponsive to questions because they are upset by the loudness of the physician's voice, by the suddenness with which he or she initiates an examination, or even by the closeness of the physician's body. Some children have temperamental characteristics predisposing them to anxiety in new or unfamiliar situations and the physician has the responsibility for recognizing the signs and knowing how anxiety may be dealt with. Many children are frightened of unfamiliar office or hospital settings, of physical pain, of separation, of uncertainty, of persons or figures to whom they may attribute awesome authority and power, and of all else that goes with the word "doctor."

Children need continually to know what is happening and what is going to happen to them in the immediate future. Their anxiety will be significantly reduced when physicians take time to explain what they are doing and what they are going to do, and when they engage the child as an active participant as much as the clinical situation and good judgment will allow. Making life predictable, within the framework of a short or even a 50 min encounter in office or hospital can have a profound effect on the likelihood of obtaining the cooperation of children.

Some children as young as 3–4 yr and most children by the age of 8 can participate verbally as well as physically in their own health care. All too frequently, conversation involves only the clinician and the parent, with the interaction between clinician and child being limited to the physical examination and some pleasantries. Children can and will respond relevantly to seriously posed questions about themselves.

By the age of 13 yr the young person is to be considered the primary informant and dealt with directly in his or her own right as a patient. If parents are present, they may be interviewed with the adolescent or separately; but at this age all explanations of diagnostic and treatment procedures should be directed first to the young person rather than to the parents. This procedure does not imply that the patient has veto power over the recommendations of the physician. The patient is still dependent on his or her parents, and the parents are still the major decision makers. Physical examinations of adolescents should be conducted with their parents not present, unless the patient requests otherwise.

Script. The distinction between content and process as aspects of communication requires further discussion of the content or message aspect. The use of words to convey messages has an aspect called *script*.

Script is the specific set of words used to convey a message. The impact of nonverbal communication upon the meaning of messages has been stressed above. The notion of script recognizes that the specific word content of the message may also convey subtleties of meaning, quite apart from nonverbal cues. Certain words or phrases, in accordance with their connotation or their usual reception, will inhibit or impede communication, whereas other words or phrases conveying substantially the same message will facilitate or promote effective communication and elicit relevant responses.

An example may clarify this. A mother might ask her 6 yr old child, "Why did you do that?" Alternatively, she might have said, "What reason did you have in mind when you did that?" or "What made you decide to do that?" If the mother's purpose is really to know *why*, then the first question is semantically adequate; on the other hand, the pejorative context in which such a question is usually phrased renders it much less likely to be effective in opening and revealing communication than the alternatives, both of which ask the same question in words that invite a more creative or process-oriented dialogue.

The first form of the above question belongs to a rather large set of stock phrases which, we learned as children, have various meanings hidden behind the words. We use these same stock phrases or questions as adults in communicating with a new generation of children. These phrases may have one or more of several characteristics:

1. Some phrases are likely to put a respondent on the defensive, such as: Why? What on earth makes you think that?

2. Some phrases subtly or blatantly impugn the veracity of the respondent, such as: You really don't believe that! Everyone knows that. That's just an old wives' tale.

3. Some phrases can express moral reproach about feelings or opinions of the respondent, such as: A good boy doesn't feel that way about his mother (father, etc.). I can't imagine anyone feeling that way. That kind of behavior never bothers *me*.

4. Some such phrases state or imply that the speaker enjoys a position of particular wisdom or virtue which the respondent could adopt to his or her benefit if only he or she could come to think, feel, or act in the same way as the speaker. For example: If I were you . . . . Why don't you . . . ? It just takes patience (or understanding, or love, or firmness) to . . . .

5. Many such phrases convey the patronizing, formalistic, condescending flavor of the sloganeer: Stop worrying. Take it easy. Learn to relax.

On the whole, such stock phrases emphasize the power side of a relationship. The speaker is frequently in a role of traditional power—doctor, parent, or teacher, or an adult engaged with a child. These words and phrases are accompanied by congruent tones of voice, gestures, facial expressions, and body postures, and are intended to admonish or to convince the hearer to admit error or wrong-doing or stupidity, and to change his or her feelings, thoughts, or behaviors in directions indicated by the speaker. The effect is to inhibit, reduce, or close off communication, with the respondent feeling wounded, hurt, rejected, helpless, depressed, exhausted, irritated, angry, or (rarely) amused or entertained.

Physicians must identify and evaluate their own stock phrases and substitute others when they will facilitate communication. In a sense, a new script is substituted for a set of habitual questions and responses. The new script may have surprising and gratifying results.

1. I'd like to understand your reasons for that (idea, feeling, behavior). Can you explain them?

2. Disliking (hating) your daughter (mother, husband) must be a very unpleasant feeling. How does it affect you?

3. Not everyone looks at a stuffy nose in the same way. What do you think it means?

4. There are a lot of conflicting opinions about hyperactivity (toilet training, sex education) and it's often hard for parents to sort out which one is going to be the most useful. Here is an approach some people have found successful. You may not find it exactly right for you, but you can try it.

5. I strongly recommend that you . . . . (NOTE: there is nothing at all wrong with a physician taking a strong stand in making professional recommendations to parents regarding the health of their children, but the proper way is clearly and simply to state that position without contaminating it with demeaning or pejorative phrases or with such nonverbal communication as scowls, raised voices, bombast, finger pointing, or other inappropriate gestures.)

6. I know it's hard to take your mind off your child's leukemia. What have you found that sometimes helps?

7. Try to ignore his constant pestering. If you find you can't, then let's figure out some other strategies.

The alternatives to stock phrases are usually longer, and more tentative, allow the other person more autonomy and leeway in terms of possible choices, and promote an alliance rather than the dominance of one party over the other. Successful alternatives help the hearer feel that his or her position and integrity are respected, even when these alternatives convey the message that there is an area of disagreement.

Many physicians find that tape recordings of their interviews or even of their conversations at home with family members or friends will help them to identify the phrases, as well as the tones of voice and inflections that they may wish to change or modify. They should practice saying aloud the alternative phrases that they propose, to see how they sound to others as well as to themselves. The procedure and effort may seem awkward and artificial at first; the experience sometimes resembling learning to play a musical instrument correctly after using incorrect techniques for years; but the awkwardness gives way to a much improved performance.

Talking with Children. Professional conversations with children have certain rules:

1. Don't talk to children in a condescending way, but as a physician talks with any patient.

2. Don't convey to the child your thought that his or her feelings, concerns, or ideas are "childish."

3. Don't laugh at what a child says unless you are quite sure the child intends to be humorous.

4. Don't try always to be funny or amusing to children. Such efforts are best saved for few occasions only, and for children you know and who know you very well. Children know the difference between doctors and funny people.

5. Never tease a child unless you know him or her very well and the child knows he or she has permission to tease you in return.

6. Initial or casual encounters with young children are often made easier when introduced in a whisper which young children may find more personal, private, and reassuring than jollity; they commonly whisper in response.

7. When children are old enough, at 3–4 yr, form the habit of discussing with them their symptoms, diagnoses, and treatments in terms they can understand.

8. Never discuss in his or her presence the illness or treatment of a hospitalized child who has acquired receptive language functions unless you are discussing it with him or her as well.

9. When a child fails to cooperate in his or her care in office or hospital, the first assumption should be that negativism or struggling means that he or she is frightened and reacting to fear in a customary personal manner; such behavior is often erroneously perceived as immature and irritating, embarrassing, provocative, or frightening by parents and other adults.

In the last context it can be noted that one can always ultimately overpower a child, verbally or physically or both. Sometimes, though rarely, that may be necessary; but there is always a cost to the child, to the physician, and to the relationship. Physicians frequently delegate the task of enforcing control of children to parents, nurses, students, aides, or drugs. This may give the physician a sense of distance from the regrettable or unpleasant necessity, but he or she is ultimately responsible. Calling upon naked power, whether it be verbal or physical, has at least 3 undesirable results: it increases the patient's sense of helplessness and powerlessness; it models the technique for students, residents, and other health care staff; and it narrows and restricts the clinician's own rapport, sometimes dulling sensibility to the feelings of others as well as to his or her own.

Other Aspects of the Interview. Certain signs indicate that the progress of an interview or examination should be assessed or reassessed for the effectiveness of communication.

1. When parents do not appear readily reassured by the diagnostic and treatment procedures, look for hidden anxiety from unanswered questions which they may have difficulty recognizing or stating. Latent anger may have the same result. The physician should make it comfortable and easy for parents to ask "stupid" questions or to admit "shameful" thoughts or "ungrateful" or angry feelings.

2. When a child is giving evidence of feeling pain, it is a psychologic impossibility that nothing hurts. When parents scold a child with "That doesn't hurt," they must be helped to understand that pain is a purely subjective experience and needs to be respected. Their acceptance of this may help greatly to clear the air.

3. Parents will sometimes be heard denigrating or shaming a child by using such terms as "baby," which is almost as bad as being intentionally cruel or frightening. Such behavior should be dealt with by the physician promptly and its inappropriateness discussed, with as much empathy for the parents' position

as possible. "I can see that it's upsetting to you to have your child behaving this way, but I don't think that this approach is going to help us. Let's look at it from her (his) point of view . . ."

4. Exhortation and other emotional appeals to reason will be frequently heard used by parents and are among the weakest methods of attempting to alter behavior or attitudes. Again, " . . . Let's look at it from the child's point of view . . ."

5. When only one parent accompanies the child, it is almost always the mother. Physicians should feel increasingly uncomfortable as time passes and they have not yet met the fathers of children for whom they have assumed the responsibility of continuing care. The working hours of physicians and most men frequently coincide; on the other hand, many fathers will be found eager to see a physician who extends a specific invitation, has clearly stated expectations, and will accommodate his time and schedules.

6. The physician will often, if he or she adequately explores the matter, find that parents have not complied with recommendations made for the care of their children. Compliance is not simply a matter of hearing, understanding, and doing what the doctor says; nor is noncompliance to be explained simply as ignorance, neglect, or a personality clash. The parent who fails to comply with recommendations may do so for a number of reasons, and these must be accurately identified.

Did the parent really understand what was prescribed or recommended? Does noncompliance express the parent's reservations as to the appropriateness of the recommendations or were the recommendations beyond the capacity of these parents to execute them, for technical, emotional, or financial reasons? Had the parents enough opportunity to ask questions and to discuss the details and ramifications of the child's condition and treatment? Is a noncompliant parent being influenced or torn by information or advice contrary to that of the physician, which may come from the other parent, a grandmother, a friend, a newspaper or magazine article, or TV programs?

Does the parent or do the parents have personal or marital problems which so upset and distract them that they cannot be effective; or does the child's illness itself have them so emotionally upset that they cannot accept the initiative and responsibility that has been thrust upon them? Depressed mothers can be so psychologically depleted as to be unavailable to the child even though they may consciously want or intend to carry out recommendations. Is the parent expressing anger at the physician through noncompliance? Is the parent of an anxious and resistant child unable to execute a prescribed regimen that may be difficult or uncomfortable because he or she fears that the child may become hurt, resentful, or angry if the required firmness is exercised?

OTHER SOURCES FOR ASSESSMENT

Institutions or Agencies. Besides the clinical interview, psychosocial assessment can be greatly helped by other data. Birth records, for example, may help in questions of injury during pregnancy or at birth. Such records are often deficient, but they may provide the only objective view of events of the patient's birth and early days. Other health records, including those from other physicians or agencies who have cared for the patient, may provide essential information concerning acute or chronic illness, show a pattern of unusually frequent visits to the physician's office for relatively minor problems, or reveal an obsessive focus on certain areas of the body.

School reports are important to the psychosocial assessment, especially if they include both an academic assessment and a description of the child's relationships with schoolmates and teachers. Requests for school reports should be made only with the written permission of the child's parents or legal guardians.

Reports from child care agencies may also be helpful, especially in the case of adopted children or children in foster care. Such agencies often have extensive background material and may have reports of earlier psychologic examinations.

Psychologic Testing. Relatively simple screening tests such as the Peabody Picture Vocabulary Test, the Denver Developmental Screening Test (Sec 2.12), the Thorpe Developmental Inventory, and others may be administered by the trained pediatrician or by his or her assistant. They may indicate areas of possible or patent intellectual or perceptive dysfunction which need further study. The major danger of these tests is that they may be relied upon too heavily as giving definitive assessments, whereas they should be regarded purely as screening tests.

Some psychologic tests should be administered and interpreted only by or under the supervision of trained psychologists; others can be used by trained school personnel. They are generally of 4 types. The 1st type is concerned with *perceptual-motor* integrity. This type is felt to be especially sensitive to "organicity," or to reflect structural or physiologic abnormalities in the central nervous system. The Bender-Gestalt test is probably the best known in this category. The 2nd category is that of *intelligence* tests such as the Stanford-Binet or the Wechsler Intelligence Scale for Children (WISC). The WISC is a 10-category test that gives both verbal and performance IQ scores. The 3rd type of test includes the *achievement* tests that are usually administered in schools. Tests such as the Wide Range Achievement Test (WRAT) report the grade level of achievement in such subject areas as reading, spelling, and mathematics. The 4th type includes the *projective* tests such as the Rorschach test (ink blot) or the Thematic Apperception Test (TAT). These give some indication of the fantasy life of the child as well as the reality testing and personality characteristics. When tests have already been done by the school, the results should be examined before new tests that may prove redundant or unnecessary are requested.

The tests to be used should be chosen by the psychologist after physician and psychologist have discussed the nature of the problem and the reason for consultation. As much as possible, tests should be chosen to assess specific problems, rather than as an exhaustive battery some of which may have only vague relationships to any clearly defined problems or goals. When the physician is at all uncertain of the nature of the tests or the implications conveyed in their interpretation, a joint meeting should be arranged with the psychologist and parents for an interpretive review; otherwise, costly tests may be ordered, the results of which are never fully exploited.

Occasionally, genetic, endocrine, or neurologic studies will be required to determine whether organic problems may contribute to or be responsible for psychologic disorders.

Psychiatric Consultation. A psychiatric consultation may be a valuable part of the assessment of children in whom vague or unexplained physical symptoms may have substantial psychogenic determinants; it will often be most acceptable and useful when the child has been hospitalized for study. Other indications include the evaluation of depression in children with major acute or chronic illness, of chronic neurotic problems, of underachievement, and of serious aggressive difficulties. The physician should inform both parent and child of the reasons for the psychiatric consultation, obtain their consent, and prepare them for what to expect.

Correlation of Data. The physician must avoid early diagnostic closure even when the parents' initial description of their problem gives a reasonably clear idea of what is going on. So long as the physician remains a receptive and perceptive listener, new and important information will emerge, as parents and perhaps patient begin to feel more trusting, and as they are educated by the physician's questions. Furthermore, the weighing of data must be done in the context of the family's sociocultural pattern. It is important that the physician not use his or her personal value system or style of living as a yardstick against which to measure the family's behavior or their success or failure in coping with their life situation. Their own feelings of anger,

frustration, anxiety, failure, or depression are more valid indicators of where they need help.

It is important that the principal item of concern be accurately identified. Parents may present as the immediate prime concern, for example, a problem such as bedwetting which may have existed for many years. Why then have they come for help now? It is important to determine whether there may, in fact, be more important hidden issues not recognized, acknowledged, or able to be faced by the parents. By the same token it must be understood that the parents' assessment of the problem is critical for the child. Sometimes a physician, having collected and assessed appropriate data, can only conclude that a child presented by his or her parents as a problem is functioning within normal limits. In such a case it must be determined what personal, familial, social, or cultural considerations compel the parents to see the child's behavior as a major problem. It must then be determined what re-education they may need in order to feel reassured and not be left with the impression that their anxiety has been casually dismissed.

Referral. When problems have not been internalized by the child it may be sufficient simply to counsel the parents, school personnel, or both. If this has been done and a maladaptive child or situation continues to present problems, the child and family will probably require more intensive or extensive help and should be referred to a child psychiatrist or to a psychiatric clinic. It is important that physicians avoid the position that psychiatric referral is a last resort. The need for a psychiatric consultation or referral can perhaps best be expressed in terms of the joint need of the family and physician for help in areas where the psychiatrist has special expertise, with the understanding that the collaboration of physician and family in management of the other health needs of the child remains intact.

2.47 Psychosocial Problems

A psychosocial disorder in a child may become manifest as a disturbance in feelings (e.g., depression, anxiety), in bodily functions (psychosomatic disorders), in behavior (e.g., conduct disturbances, passive-aggressive behavior), or in performance (learning problems). Dysfunction may involve any or all of these areas. Psychosocial problems may be produced by a great variety of physical and emotional stresses, such as birth defect, physical injury, inconsistent and contradictory child rearing practices, marital conflict, child abuse and neglect, overindulgence, chronic illness, and so on. Particular agents, however, do not produce specific symptoms or disorders; rather, children's psychosocial problems are multifactorial in origin, their expression depending on many variables, including temperament, developmental level, the nature and duration of stress, past experiences, and the coping and adaptive abilities of the family. In general, chronic stresses, or a series of stressful events, are much more difficult for child and family to manage than a single acute stressful episode. Children may react immediately to traumatic events, or

may keep their feelings dormant until maladaptive reactions become apparent during later periods of vulnerability.

Anticipatory guidance during periods of stress may considerably help children and their families to achieve more positive outcomes. Parents should be encouraged to prepare their children in advance for potentially traumatic events that can be anticipated (e.g., elective surgery, separation, or divorce). Children should be allowed or encouraged to express their feelings of dismay, fear, or anger, rather than be told to be a "good girl" or "brave boy."

Infants and toddlers tend to react to stressful situations with impairment of physiologic functions, such as disturbances of feeding and sleep, with relatively global expressions of anger or fear, as in temper tantrums, or with withdrawal and avoidance behavior. School-age children demonstrate their difficulties through altered interpersonal relationships with peers and family members, through impairment of school performance, by the development of specific psychologic syndromes, such as phobias or psychosomatic disorders, or by "regressing" to earlier, more "childish" modes of functioning.

Parents are frequently concerned whether the particular behaviors of their children are "normal" or whether they represent problems which require intervention. Various "symptomatic" actions of children may be part of normal development. For example, a temper tantrum may express the normal negativism of a toddler; on the other hand, temper tantrums occurring at slight provocation in a 6 yr old may be a sign of psychosocial disturbance. Whether a particular behavior is judged to be a developmental variation or evidence of a more serious problem depends upon the age of the child, upon the frequency and intensity and number of symptoms, and especially upon the degree of functional impairment. The decision of parents to seek help is determined, in turn, by the characteristics of their children's behavior, by the amount of distress it causes the children, parents, teachers, and others, and by their past experiences in discussing psychosocial matters with their physicians.

2.48 PSYCHIATRIC CONSIDERATIONS OF CENTRAL NERVOUS SYSTEM INJURY

Psychiatric difficulties may follow infection, injury, or intoxication, or genetic, metabolic, or idiopathic illness involving the central nervous system. These are not to be confused with the manifestations of minimal cerebral dysfunction (also known as minimal brain dysfunction, dysfunctional child, learning disabilities, or, in behavioral terms, the hyperactive or hyperkinetic child. For the last condition see Sec 2.56).

There is no brain injury, intoxication, or disease in children that has typical psychiatric sequelae, nor are there any specific psychiatric symptoms, signs, or syndromes that point reliably to a particular injury, intoxication, or illness. The particular expression of a disturbance is more dependent on the child's developmental level, past history, temperament, and family relationships than on the nature of the insult. Psychosis is not a typical result of brain injury or illness in childhood. The autistic psychosis is probably the result primarily of genetic, physiologic, and organic factors, but these have not been specified (Sec 2.62). Chess has reported an autism-like syndrome in children who have had congenital rubella.

Psychiatric disorder accompanies or follows brain injury or illness or epilepsy in a significant percentage of children. The epidemiologic survey of the Isle of Wight found brain-injured or epileptic children 5–15 yr old to have 5 times the normal risk of psychiatric disorder. An uncontrolled study of children who had suffered major head injury found that about one third developed a psychiatric disorder, manifested chiefly by difficulties in controlling anger, and accompanied also by hyperactivity or restlessness.

Prenatal factors have long been suspected of causing brain damage and psychiatric or behavioral disorders. Prematurity and neonatal complications involving hypoxia have been seen as causing such conditions as hyperactivity, impulsivity, difficulties in socialization, and poor control of emotions, especially anger. On the other hand, Graham's study of 350 children with clearly documented neonatal asphyxia found no excess of behavioral or emotional disturbances at the age of 3.5 yr in comparison with a control group matched for social class and family factors.

Children under the age of 3 yr who survive encephalitis or meningitis seem to show more lasting personality and behavioral effects than those who have these illnesses later. The result seems to contradict the notion that the brain might in the earlier years have a greater potential for recovery without significant residual dysfunction.

Children with untreated phenylketonuria are reported to exhibit apathy, withdrawal, and autistic traits. Children with galactosemia are reported to display hostility in addition to withdrawal. These reports have not been well controlled, and some of the differences may be accounted for on temperamental grounds, family interaction, or other environmental factors. The most significant factor in the child's adjustments to a chronic handicapping organic condition is the capacity of his or her parents to adjust and cope.

Children with hydrocephalus and motor deficits have a 7 times greater than average incidence of psychiatric disorder. The additional findings of low IQ, language disorder, or bilaterality of the motor handicap increase the incidence of psychiatric disturbance significantly, but again there is no specificity in the type of disturbance encountered.

Children with idiopathic epilepsy have an increased risk of psychiatric disturbance. Their behavioral disorders include excess aggressive behavior, stubbornness, defiance, nonconformity, and passive-aggressive reactions. These disturbances correlate better with the psychosocial interactions of the child and family than with the type of abnormality in the electroencephalogram or with neurologic signs. Children in whom epilepsy is combined with high intelligence are reported to have increased risk of depression. Psychoses have been reported more common than usual in children with convulsions, embryopathies, toxoplasmosis, or congenital syphilis, but these reports generally have not been conclusive.

When children with brain damage or injury have problems with impulse or anger control, aggressivity, hyperactivity, or other emotional reactions, these do not differ in quality from those of children with intact nervous systems who have the same disturbances. Mentally retarded children have an increased risk of psychiatric disorder, particularly if they suffer brain injury or if brain injury is primary to the retardation.

How central nervous system illness or injury produces psychosocial effects is unclear. Two clinical features stand out: emotional reactivity seems increased, whether it be anxiety, anger, or depression; and social interactions become more conflict laden. Impaired integration of social perception and judgment may lead to vicious cycles: for example, a more irritable, impulsive, and demanding child may elicit reactive anger, criticism, and hostility from adults and peers, and the interaction becomes circular.

Among children with psychosocial disorders due to central nervous system disease or injury there is no predominant incidence of boys over girls. By contrast, with psychiatric disturbance in non-brain-injured children the ratio of boys to girls ranges from 2:1–4:1, depending on age, type of disturbance, and other factors.

Prognosis and Treatment. Hyperactivity has been reported to decrease in adolescence among the children who have evidence of possible central nervous system injury or disease, but deficits in attention, poor performance in school, and other behavioral and emotional problems persist. Antisocial behavior of varying degrees may appear, due in part to primary pathology, and in part to failures in academic or social adjustment. A pattern may develop, involving emotional lability, irritability, and a propensity to loss of control of anger.

In some affected children stimulant drugs improve the ability to perform in school, smooth out emotional reactivity, and facilitate social interactions with peers and adults. Such medication taken for extended periods may produce growth retardation, which must be weighed against possible beneficial effects. Tranquilizers may lessen anxiety and improve emotional control and behavior, but they tend also to produce obtundation and somnolence, which may interfere with learning.

Psychotherapy has not been rigorously proved effective in the children discussed here, any more than in most other disorders of childhood. Clinical experience, however, indicates that most such children benefit from understanding psychosocial support. A frequently beneficial approach is to help the child to identify his or her ineffective reaction patterns, along with more successful patterns. The approach combines "coaching" and education, with an opportunity to discuss depression, isolation, and anger and those feelings of being different, rejected, or exploited, that so much affect self-esteem. Parents and perhaps other family members must be involved in any treatment plan. The parents have their own needs and will need advice, counseling, and emotional support in dealing with their child's emotional and behavioral problems, both in family matters and in his or her life at school and with friends. Fair, firm discipline is always useful. Behavior modification techniques can be helpful to children in whom specific target behaviors can be identified; the technique may be used at home or at school. Both aberrant psychosocial behaviors and learning difficulties may respond (Sec 2.64).

2.49 PSYCHOSOMATIC DISORDERS

Psychologic conflict may lead to alterations in somatic function or so-called "psychosomatic disorders." Contrary to earlier views, particular types of feeling or conflict do not produce specific kinds of psychosomatic illness; rather, any kind of emotional distress may be associated with any type of psychosomatic disorder in a child. There appear to be both innate constitutional vulnerabilities and environmental factors, none well understood, which determine why one organ or system becomes dysfunctional rather than another. Psychosomatic illnesses are of two types: conversion ("hysterical") reactions, and psychophysiologic disorders.

Conversion reactions are sudden in onset, and can usually be traced to a precipitating environmental event. Voluntary musculature and organs of special sense are the most frequent target sites for the "hysterical" expressions of psychologic conflict. Such reactions may take many forms, including hysterical blindness, paralysis, diplopia, gait disturbances, and the like. Physical examination often fails to reveal objective abnormalities. Deep tendon reflexes can be elicited in a paralyzed leg, and pupillary responses to light are noted in hysterical blindness. Affected children and their families tend to be rather dramatic and hypochondriacal and often give a past history of previous conversion episodes.

Psychophysiologic disorders have a more insidious onset. Chronic anxiety produces functional abnormalities within the autonomic nervous system which lead to structural changes within organ systems. Eczema, bronchial asthma, ulcerative colitis, and peptic ulcer are considered to be psychophysiologic disorders or at least to have significant psychophysiologic components in some children. Children with psychophysiologic disorders tend to be obsessional, compulsive, perfectionistic, and somewhat constricted in social functioning. They are often superficially compliant, high achievers, and pseudomature.

There are several general principles which guide management of children with psychosomatic disorders. (1) The symptoms of affected children are not within their conscious control; they are not "acting" or malingering; their pain and their problems are real. (2) It is essential that a psychiatric assessment be arranged early in the management of these disorders; otherwise, after elaborate and expensive tests have been done, the child and family will often be convinced that he or she has a very serious illness for which a "real" cause exists that cannot be found. (3) An explanation of the role of the emotions in the genesis of these disorders must be accepted by the parents before truly effective intervention can be accomplished. (4) Psychotherapy for the child and counseling for the family are often indicated, combined with pediatric management; psychiatrist and pediatrician must be in close communication with each other in a therapeutic alliance; modest amounts of tranquilizing medication may be a useful adjunct. (5) Child and family should be encouraged and helped to live as normally as possible to avoid crippling psychologic invalidism with stress put on early return to school after acute illness, upon participation in recreational activities, and upon normal peer interactions. Parents should know that some children unconsciously use their symptoms to maintain dependency, and that firm, gentle insistence upon the fullest possible range of activities for the child is indicated. (6) The physician should be alert for indications of psychosomatic illness in parents, with which children may unconsciously identify; successful treatment of parental illness may be necessary for a favorable outcome in the child.

2.50 DISORDERS RELATED TO VEGETATIVE FUNCTIONS

Obesity. Sec 3.20.

Anorexia Nervosa. Anorexia nervosa is a serious psychosocial disorder characterized by voluntary starvation and severe weight loss. It is seen most often in girls in early adolescence; amenorrhea may accompany it. This disorder frequently begins with voluntary institution of a weight-reduction diet by the patient, who expresses concern about being "too fat," though her weight may be in the normal range. Refusal of food is extreme and weight loss continues far past normally desirable limits. Parental pleas, threats, and cajolery are ineffective. The patient may hide food and pretend that she has eaten it, may eat and then induce vomiting, or may use enemas and laxatives. Denial is prominent among defense mechanisms; the patient may insist that she feels and looks fine, though others who view her are shocked by her skeletal appearance. Curiously, physical activity generally remains at a fairly high level.

The premorbid personality of affected children is frequently marked by obsessive-compulsive traits and constriction of affect. They tend to be well behaved, good students, and to set somewhat perfectionistic standards for themselves and others. There may be a history of feeding problems or gastrointestinal disorders in one or both parents, or of early feeding difficulties in the child. Psychoanalytic theory suggests that this disorder may represent a defense against a threatening fantasy of pregnancy and a fear of sexual impulses. Patients with anorexia nervosa may display general immaturity and have difficulty in entering into appropriate adolescent peer group and social relations.

Management of the patient almost always requires an initial phase of hospitalization, though some milder cases may not. The possibilities of physical disorders, such as Simmonds cachexia, chronic infection, or malignancy should be excluded by appropriate studies. Separation of child from parents during a period of hospitalization may be beneficial. The patient should be instructed that she is expected to eat, and that when she has gained appropriate weight, she will leave the hospital. She should also be informed, but this should not be conveyed as a threat, that nasogastric feedings may be necessary if her survival is in danger. Beyond these measures, little attention should be paid to the patient's food intake; medical and other staff should be instructed to take a "matter of fact" attitude toward the patient's eating habits. Individual psychotherapy is often indicated, though these patients are often markedly resistant to psychotherapeutic intervention. Minuchin reports success with an approach using family therapy, initiated even during the period of hospitalization. Benefits have also been achieved through behavior therapy, the patient's inherent desire for activity being encouraged and used as a reward for weight gain. The prognosis for children with anorexia nervosa is variable, depending primarily on the magnitude and treatability of underlying personality problems. On the whole, the outlook for the acute episode is relatively good, and better than once thought.

Pica. Pica is a habit disorder involving repeated or chronic ingestion of inedible substances, which may include plaster, charcoal, clay, wool, ashes, paint, and earth. The tasting or mouthing of objects is normal in infants and toddlers, but pica after the 2nd yr of life is a symptom needing investigation. Pica is most often associated with family disorganization, poor supervision, and affectional neglect. It appears to be more prevalent in lower socioeconomic classes and may be related to poor nutrition. Pica may also be seen in severely retarded children, as part of their tendency to mouth objects indiscriminately. Children with pica are at risk for the development of lead poisoning (Sec 28.15) and parasitic infections.

Enuresis. Enuresis is one of the most common and perplexing problems brought to the attention of the pediatrician. It is defined as involuntary discharge of urine, occurring after the age by which bladder control should usually have been established. Because of wide variation in the age of achievement of bladder mastery, children are not generally labeled "enuretic" unless the symptom persists beyond the age of 5 yr. Nocturnal enuresis occurs once a month or more in 8% of school-age children. Persistent diurnal enuresis is much less common, usually represents a more serious problem, and, especially in girls, may be associated with infection.

Bedwetting occurs more frequently in boys than girls and becomes less common as the child approaches puberty. It will often have been present in one of the parents. Bedwetting may be divided into 2 types: the persistent type, in which the child has never been dry at night; and the regressive type, in which a previously continent child begins to wet the bed after a stressful episode. Persistent nocturnal enuresis is often the result of inadequate or inappropriate toilet training experiences. Parents who demand coercively that a child become toilet trained promptly may mobilize an angry response, the child unconsciously defying them by wetting the bed. On the other hand, parents who are not sufficiently close to the needs of the child to support toilet training may undermine his or her attempts at bladder mastery. Chronic psychologic stress unrelated to toilet training experiences but occurring during the toddler period can also impair the child's ability to learn effective bladder control.

The regressive type of bedwetting is related to precipitating stressful environmental events, such as a move to a new home, marital conflict, birth of a sibling, or death in the family. Bedwetting in these instances is often intermittent and transitory; prognosis is better and management less difficult than in those children who have never been continent.

In both types of bedwetting, organic pathology can be found in only a very small number of cases. Physical examination and urinalysis are indicated, but more strenuous procedures such as urograms and cystoscopies are usually not warranted, and should not be pursued unless there is definite suspicion of an organic lesion (Sec 16.52).

Treatment of the child with enuresis depends on an understanding of the possible specific causative factors suggested by an adequate psychosocial inventory and physical examination; for example, a child can be helped to deal with feelings about a new younger sibling, or the parents may be helped to establish proper attitudes and climate for a child's success in toilet training. Some general suggestions are: (1) It is important to enlist the cooperation of and to motivate the child to deal with the problem. Rewarding the child for being dry at night is a useful step. Child or parent can chart the dry nights, and with one or two dry nights a small token or reward can be given, with more substantial rewards with increasing success. (2) Older children should be expected to launder their own soiled bedclothes and pajamas. (3) Children should be given no liquids after dinner time. (4) The child should void before retiring. (5) Waking the child repeatedly to take him or her to the bathroom is useful in only a few children and may further mobilize or aggravate anger in child or parent. (6) Punishment or humiliation of the child by parents or others should be strongly discouraged.

The use of conditioning devices (such as a buzzer which rings when the child wets a special sheet) is usually not necessary, and should be reserved for persistent and refractory cases in which the child's self-esteem has been seriously eroded, and only with the consent of the child. Imipramine (Tofranil), in a dose of 25–50 mg at night, may effectively reduce frequency of voiding or wetting in a significant number of children. This medication has, however, a variety of side effects (hypotension, hypertension, tachycardia, restlessness, nightmares, dry mouth, rare blood dyscrasia) and its chronic use is not without risk (Table 29–1).

Encopresis. Encopresis is the involuntary passage of feces at an age by which bowel control should have been established. By the age of 4–5 yr it is viewed as a symptom, rather than a developmental variation. As in the case of enuresis, organic defects are rarely found. Encopresis is much less common than enuresis (though the two may coexist), and it indicates a more serious emotional disturbance. Chronic soiling may persist from infancy onward, or may appear as a regressive phenomenon. Encopresis is often associated with chronic constipation, fecal impaction, and overflow incontinence, and may progress to psychogenic megacolon. This symptom usually represents unconscious anger and defiance in the child, and the parents may respond with retaliatory, punitive measures. School performance and attendance may be affected, as the child becomes the target of scorn and derision from schoolmates because of the offensive odor. Chronic use of enemas and laxatives should be avoided; they are usually of no benefit, call further attention to the symptom, and make the child more defiant (Sec 11.17). Measures similar to those used in the supportive treatment of enuresis may be useful with encopretic children, but the fixed and disabling nature of the symptom frequently requires psychotherapeutic intervention with child and family.

Sleep Disorders. Sleep disorders are common in childhood, and may be temporary, intermittent, or chronic in nature. Infants who show difficulty in establishing regular night-time sleep patterns may also show general fussiness and irritability as a temperamental characteristic. Sleep disorders in infancy may also be a result of parental anxiety or strife. Older children may experience transient night-time fears of burglars, noises, thunder and lightning, being kidnapped, and so on, and this anxiety will interfere with their sleep. Children may express their fears overtly, or they may disguise them, often by invoking tactics designed to delay bedtime. The fearful child may also seek to sleep in the parents' bedroom or may attempt to come into their bedroom after they are asleep.

Separation anxiety is often a causative factor. Children may unconsciously and symbolically view sleep as a time when they are removed from parental love and concern. If there is conflict within the family, or if separation or divorce has occurred, such anxiety will be naturally exacerbated. Bedtime fears often relate to such normal separations as occur with the child's first attendance in nursery school or kindergarten. As growing children become more aware of death, they may be unwilling to go to sleep at night for fear that they may die. This fear will be heightened if a family member has recently died. Finally, anxiety related to any other areas of the child's life—family, peers, school performance—may be expressed as a sleep disorder.

Parental support, reassurance, and encouragement are vital for the alleviation of sleep disorders. Angry threats and punitive measures are to be avoided. Parents should adopt calm, understanding, but firm attitudes. Bedtime should be set for a regular and stated time, variations being kept to a minimum. The parents should discourage the child from sleeping in their room, but may temporarily allow a fearful child to sleep in a sibling's room. A night light and allowing the child to leave the door open are often reassuring. The interval before bedtime should be quiet and restful; stimulating television programs should be avoided. A warm bath, a light snack, and a quiet affectionate moment with parents are conducive to sleep. Some children may become drowsy if they are allowed to read a favorite book for a few minutes after they are settled in bed. Diphenhydramine (Benadryl) may serve as a mild sedative.

Nightmares in children are of 2 types: the more common anxiety dream or "bad" dream, and the rarer "night terror." The anxiety dream occurs during REM sleep; the child awakens, becomes lucid quickly, and usually remembers the content of the dream. He or she can be reassured and comforted by being held and by soothing words. *Night terrors* usually have their onset in the preschool years and occur with arousal from stage 4 (non-REM) sleep; the child is confused and disoriented, shows signs of intense autonomic activity (labored breathing, dilated pupils, sweating, tachypnea, tachycardia), may complain of peculiar visual phenomena, and appears to be very frightened. A period of somnambulism (sleep walking) may follow during which the child may be at risk of injury. Some minutes may pass before the child seems to be oriented. Usually he or she cannot recall dream content causing the night terror. Night terrors are often self-limited and may be related to a specific developmental conflict or to a precipitating traumatic event.

Persistent nightmares reflect chronic underlying anxiety and warrant a comprehensive evaluation of the child, including psychologic status. Diazepam (5–10 mg at bedtime) has been reported to be of benefit in the treatment of night terrors and somnambulism.

2.51 HABIT DISORDERS

Habit disorders include many tension-discharging phenomena, such as head banging, body rocking, thumb sucking, nail biting, hair pulling, and teeth grinding. Tics, which involve the involuntary movement of various muscle groups of the body, are included. Stuttering and masturbation will be discussed with the habit disorders, though the latter is not usually considered a disorder.

All children show at various developmental levels repetitive patterns of movement which can be described as habits. Whether they come to be considered disorders depends on the degree to which they interfere with the child's function—physically, emotionally, or socially. Some habit patterns may be learned by imitation of adults. Many begin as a purposeful movement which becomes for some reason repetitive, the habit losing its original significance and becoming a means of discharge of tension. For example, a child with an eye irritation or one attempting not to shed tears might try closing his or her eyelids several times in rapid succession. This activity might become repetitive, and incorporated into the child's behavior as an outlet for tension. Such symptoms are often reinforced by attention from parents or others. Other movements, such as rhythmic head banging and rocking in early life, can persist without parental reinforcement, occurring when the child is put to bed or is alone; they seem to provide a kind of sensory solace to the child feeling otherwise uncared for and understimulated by human touch or interaction. These movements represent in this sense a kind of internal stroking. Such patterns are often seen in the mentally retarded or in children suffering from maternal or emotional deprivation. Equivalent movements are evident in children who twist their hair or touch or play with parts of their bodies in repetitive ways. These rhythmic movements are often most prominent just before sleep or as the child passes from wakefulness into sleep, and they seem to help the child cope with anxieties. As involved children become older, they learn to inhibit some of their rhythmic habit patterns, particularly in social situations; but in the more seriously disturbed the rhythmic habit patterns may persist.

Teeth grinding (bruxism) seems to result from tension originating in unexpressed anger or resentment. It may create problems in dental occlusion. Helping the child to find other ways to express resentment may relieve the teeth grinding. Bedtime can be made more enjoyable and relaxed, with reading or talking with the child permitting re-experience and review of some of the fears or angers of the day. Praise and other emotional support for the child are useful at these times.

Thumb sucking is normal in early infancy. In the older child it has the unfortunate effects of making the child appear immature, and of interfering with the normal alignment of teeth. Like other rhythmic patterns it can be seen as a way in which the child secures extra self-nurturance. Providing the child with evidence of concern and with other forms of satisfaction is generally the best strategy for dealing with thumb sucking. Parents should ignore the symptom if possible, while they give attention to more positive aspects of the child's behavior. The child actively trying to restrain thumb sucking should be given praise and encouragement.

Tics involve repetitive movements of muscle groups, but have no apparent function. They may have been first intentional, sometimes becoming nonintentional very quickly. Parts of the body most frequently involved are muscles of the face, neck, shoulders, trunk, and hands. There may be lip smacking, grimacing, tongue thrusting, eye blinking, throat clearing, and so on. Tics appear to represent discharges of tension originating in emotional states which involve the muscular system. It is very difficult for the person with a tic to inhibit it. Tics can be distinguished from variants of minor seizures in that the child does not experience a transient loss of consciousness or amnesia. Tics occasionally accompany other psychiatric syndromes or follow encephalitis. Most cases seem to have had no physical antecedents and are transient. Undue parental attention can reinforce tics, whereas ignoring them may diminish their occurrence.

Gilles de la Tourette syndrome is a rare condition seen in children some of whom have severe psychopathology; it is characterized by tics, compulsive barking, or the shouting of obscene words. It can be helped to some extent by counseling the child and parents. Haloperidol (a potent dopaminergic inhibitor) has been found to lessen the frequency and intensity of the tics and to reduce anxiety.

Masturbation is manipulation of the genitals by the child for sexual pleasure. There may be movements or contractions of the musculature of the thighs, with copulatory movements. Younger children unaware of cultural taboos against masturbation may be observed by their parents in this activity, but most children sense parental disapproval, and the activity is carried out in privacy. Open masturbation by the older child suggests poor awareness of social reality or a lack of parental censorship. It is important for the parent to understand that masturbation may be normal at any age and is virtually universal among children and adolescents. It presents a self-gratification analogous to thumb sucking. In the older child or adolescent it serves the purpose of exploring and experimenting with newly developing sexual capacities. It also serves to discharge sexual tensions, and may aid in gaining control over sexual urges. Masturbation is most common at bedtime, when anxiety is increased owing to separation or to fear of loss of control over sexual or aggressive impulses. Children are most likely to masturbate when alone and feeling lonely, or when they are having sexual fantasies. Beyond normal release of sexual tension, masturbation can be done in a repetitious and compulsive way as a reassurance against fear of injury to the genitalia. Excessive masturbation suggests some problem or deficiency in the child's or adolescent's ability to relate to others.

It is appropriate for parents to discourage open masturbation and to be concerned about excessive masturbation. On the other hand, it is important that masturbation be accepted as a normal aspect of the child's sexual life, and that guilt or anxiety relative to it be avoided. By the time of puberty, children should be given explanations of its normality. This can be done in conjunction with explanations of ejaculation, orgasm, and menstruation, so that children can understand them, too, as normal bodily functions.

Stuttering is not generally regarded as a tension-releasing activity but it can become so in a secondary fashion. Most theories of stuttering agree that primary stuttering comes about as an atypical development during the learning of speech. As it becomes more fixed, secondary compulsive and repetitive movements of various muscle systems come into play as the child attempts to "force" out the words and release the buildup of tension. The physician can help parents accept the child's early patterns of dysfluent speech; the less emphasis paid to these early patterns, the better the outcome. The child can be made to feel successful and cared for in other areas. If the pattern persists, a speech therapist should be consulted. Approaches to treatment include breath control exercises or the use of a miniaturized metronome that "paces" the rhythm of speech (Sec 2.78).

EMOTIONAL DISORDERS

2.52 Neuroses

According to psychoanalytic theory, psychoneuroses arise from intrapsychic conflict between one's wishes for expression of sexual and aggressive drives and the prohibitions of the conscience against these expressions. This internalized conflict is outside conscious awareness, but the symptoms of anxiety become apparent. Anxiety can be expressed as irritability or whimpering, or as worry in older children. It can also appear as a phobia, such as fear of the dark or of going outside. Sometimes anxiety is converted into a somatic symptom, i.e., a conversion reaction, such as paralysis of a limb or inability to see clearly. The neurotic conflict may express itself also in obsessive-compulsive rituals.

Psychoneurotic conflict does not reach awareness owing to repression, a defense mechanism which may intermittently or generally keep the conflict from consciousness; when it fails, neurotic symptoms appear. Specific neuroses usually do not appear by themselves in children; rather, intermittently there may be multiple neuroses, or neurotic traits. Neurotic traits may be interwoven with underlying personality disorders. The essence of neurotic symptoms is that affected patients are aware of them, will admit to them, and find them unpleasant. The prognosis for most childhood neurosis is relatively good.

The overanxious child is upset beyond apparent reason. There may be excessive shyness, shaking, frequent crying, insomnia, tics, and so on. One form of overanxiety is seen in the so-called *school phobia* (Sec 2.39). Affected children have a problem of separation, rather than a true phobia. Besides showing anxiety in the morning, affected children become excessively anxious at night, when the gradual diminution of sensory input leaves them relatively more aware of their fearful fantasies. The physician should help the parents look for hidden sources of anxiety that can be dealt with openly by child and parents.

Children with *phobias* have organized their anxieties into focused and projected mental patterns. Instead of feeling generally anxious, they are anxious only under specific conditions: in the presence of a dog, in the dark, on high places, outside the home, at the sight of men with beards, and so on. The choice of object to be feared is in some unconscious way related to the origins of the anxiety; for example, aggressive or murderous thoughts unacceptable to the conscience are repressed, and projected into fears of the robber or of the monster lurking in the dark. Phobic neuroses may resolve spontaneously if they are not reinforced by new sources of anxiety. It appears also that children can be desensitized to their phobias by the techniques of behavioral modification, the phobias becoming attenuated and disappearing without their underlying sources necessarily having been revealed or dealt with. The extent, if any, to which these unresolved unconscious conflicts affect the future mental or emotional life of the individual is uncertain.

The parents of a phobic child should remain calm in the face of their child's anxiety or panic. If they become upset, the child will conclude that there is in fact something to fear. Calm acceptance provides a useful model for the child in dealing with the normal and unavoidable anxieties of growing up. The most powerful therapeutic tools physicians can use in these conditions are their listening, their understanding, and their own calmness.

The child with an *obsessive-compulsive* neurosis has further elaborated anxiety and conflict into a system of apparently pointless rituals. For example, a boy in conflict over sexual urges may become hyperalert to the genital area. He may next project the thought that others can see his penis, which may also represent a repressed exhibitionistic wish. He may begin looking down each time he enters a room to make sure that his pants are buttoned or zipped, or he may check his belt every few minutes to make sure that everything is in place. Obsessive-compulsive rituals are not always seen as pathologic. When they become so intense and persistent, however, as to interfere with comfortable function, they require psychiatric help. Obsessive-compulsive neuroses are generally harder to treat than phobias, and some theorists feel that there may be an inborn element to their formation. Affected children tend to be very serious children, "grown up," rigid, and finicky, and to find it hard to reach out to others with positive affect. On the other hand, within limits obsessive-compulsive traits may be healthy manifestations of self-discipline, may help children to stay organized, and may contribute to their success in various activities and their self-esteem. A good student striving for scholastic achievement, who puts off immediate gratification in order eventually to become a professional person, may have some obsessive-compulsive traits working to his or her advantage.

Children with *hysterical neuroses* are able to achieve massive repression of certain ego states without overt evidence of anxiety (equivalent to forgetting). In the *dissociated state* a child may at times feel that he or she is someone else. In a more organized rendition of this, the *fugue state*, the child may act out a complicated series of behaviors, return to his or her usual ego state, and have no memory of the period of fugue. This is not the same as sleepwalking (Sec 2.50), but more akin to the phenomenon of multiple personalities. Parents of many children report that their children have transient marked changes in personality, but these variant behaviors are almost always under the control of markedly divergent moods, rather than true fugues or dissociations. Temporal lobe epilepsy may produce strange behavioral sequences, but these rarely last more than a few minutes; they are unremembered, as in fugue states, but unlike the latter are followed by postictal sleepiness. Electroencephalography may be of help in differential diagnosis.

A more common hysterical neurosis is the *conversion neurosis*, which is a somatization of a repressed psychic conflict and often, if not always, follows a model in the child's experience (Sec 2.49). For example, a child with bronchitis may overcome the infection, but maintain or reintroduce later a chronic hysteric cough. The symptom appears to be an attempt to recreate an ego state which at the time of bronchitis served the purpose of conflict resolution, permitting the receipt of dependency gratifications without guilt. For another example, a young child with a crippled grandmother might get a twinge in the knee at times when he or she wishes to withdraw from stressful situations, these factors correlating with ego states in which the child pictures himself or herself at a certain level as an invalid, and acts out this internalized picture. Conversion symptoms often have a bizarre "unmedical" quality. They represent the notions of unsophisticated persons as to how it is to be paralyzed, blind, voiceless, in pain, and so on. Affected children are not pretending or malingering, and should not be so charged. They consciously believe in their condition, and their parents often join them in this belief. There is always less anxiety than one would expect, except when facing the physician. Referrals to psychiatric consultants can be difficult, since these challenge the integrity of the perceptions of the children, parents, or both. Referral is best accomplished by presenting the need for consultation as part of an adequate investigation (Sec 2.65). Probably most conversion symptoms will disappear with positive suggestion by the physician. The most important diagnostic and therapeutic considerations involve identifying the secondary gain being achieved by the symptom. If this can be reduced or eliminated, the symptom will often abate.

2.53 Depression

Anaclitic depression was first described by Spitz as the devastating effect of disruption of the mother-child relationship in early infancy. Spitz observed the condition in infants of mothers who were imprisoned and separated from them when they were a few months to a year old. The infants were then cared for in a babies' home which was clean, hygienic, and well-run. The staff, however, w s able to provide only minimal routine care, and not the same kind of close, affectionate, and stimulating relationships of the usual mother-child dyad. The infants showed profound disturbances in health and in motor, social, and language development. Some died.

There is a characteristic pattern to this type of separation-based depression of infancy. By 6 mo of age infants have formed a strong bond with a mothering figure. Separation for a significant period at this time leads to a profound reaction in many infants, especially in those who have had the warmest and most satisfying relationships. The initial reaction is protest: crying, searching, almost panic behavior, a good deal of motor activity in both arms and legs. Subsequently, when an adult who is not the usual mothering figure approaches, the infant will first search anxiously to see if the mother has returned, and then will turn away and reject the approaching figure. The final phase of reaction is a period of apathy, in which the infant is hypotonic and inactive, with a sad facial expression. Affected infants cry silently and stare into space. When picked up, they search again for the familiar face; they will cling to a stranger and cry, but are not consoled.

Estimates of the frequency of childhood depression vary widely, from as low as 2% to as high as 50%, depending upon the population studied.

In the school-age child it is convenient to distinguish between acute and chronic depressive reactions. *Acute depressive reactions* are almost invariably preceded by some precipitating event such as an illness requiring hospitalization, loss of a parent through separation, divorce, or death, loss of a significant relationship with a friend or a pet, or a move of the family from one residence or city to another. As children enter the preadolescent period, experiences that damage self-esteem can precipitate acute depressive responses. Included are such events as failures in school, social exclusion, the disruption of an intense friendship or early romantic relationship, or even the growing awareness that childhood is over and that significant responsibilities and concerns of adolescence are approaching.

Several different models, generally based on studies of adults, attempt to explain childhood depression. The biochemical model examines variations in the production, utilization, or degradation of monoamine neurotransmitters. Evidence that these substances are significant in the origin of childhood depression is as yet scanty, but promising enough that further studies are in progress. Other models include the genetic model, the learned helplessness model, the life stress model, the cognitive distortion model, and the behavioral reinforcement and sociologic models. Attempts are being made to examine each of these, with appropriate modification, in studies of children.

What the specific diagnostic criteria for childhood depressive disorders should be is still controversial and needs more research. Recently, the criteria set forth in the Diagnostic and Statistical Manual of the American Psychiatric Association (DSM-III) for adult depression have been applied to children and compared with other diagnostic instruments and inventories. Two clinical features are considered central: general dysphoria and a general loss or impairment of the pleasure previously derived from enjoyable experiences.

The obvious features of the depressed child include a sad or downcast face, easy tears, irritability, withdrawal from some usual activities and interests, and loss of pleasure in such things as friendships, sports, games, family outings, and so on. The depressed child may spend more time than usual alone, watching television. School performance may be impaired. Depending on his or her personality style, the child may become more clinging and dependent; more aloof, withdrawn, and seclusive; or more disruptive, aggressive, and defiant. Conflicts may often arise in relationships with family and friends; they may add to the child's negative feelings as well as provoke anger, criticism, and rejection from others. Depressed children may at times show some of the psychomotor retardation, slouched posture, and decreased activity characteristic of adult depression. When asked how they feel, they will frequently say that they are bored, or that they don't like anything, or that nothing is fun any more, rather than describing their state as depressed. Their capacity to look forward to pleasurable events is impaired or absent. They may express feelings of hopelessness or helplessness in terms appropriate to their age and verbal ability. They often communicate a sense of being unattractive and unloved, and complain that others in the family are favored or that everyone else is having a good time while they are not. Separation anxiety is frequently found in children who have depressive disorders; it may lead to school refusal (school phobia) in young children.

Sleep disturbances in acute depression occur more often than they are reported. Unless parents become aware of their children's inability to go to sleep or intermittent wakefulness, disorders of sleep may pass unnoticed. Disorders of appetite are hard to assess in many children, owing to fluctuating food preferences and normal variations in amounts eaten at meals or between meals. The marked decline in appetite, constipation, early morning awakening, and explicit expressions of depression, guilt, and hopelessness which mark severe depression in adults (endogenous or psychotic depression) are hardly ever seen in children. Depressions appear to cluster in some families.

Acute depressive responses may last only a few days or weeks and often resolve spontaneously. When physicians, parents, or teachers become aware of these changes in children, their solicitous concern, their recognition of feelings, their allowing the children to talk about it if they are able, and the emotional support given by verbal and physical expressions of affection can help depressed children to regain feelings of self-worth. When a clear-cut event has precipitated a depression, parents can discuss the matter with the depressed child, helping the child understand both the event and his or her feelings about it. Medication is rarely indicated.

Chronic depression is not so common as acute, and sometimes merges into a "depressive-reactive" style of personality. There is usually no clear-cut precipitating event. Affected children have often had frequent disruptions in important relationships, often from early infancy onward. There is usually, moreover, a history of depressive illness in one or both parents, and usually during the child's lifetime. Affected children often show a marginal emotional and social adjustment throughout their lives. Sometimes they present a picture of helpless, passive, clinging, dependent, and lonely children. At other times they relate to others in a more hardened, negativistic, aloof, or almost cynical manner. Having frequently experienced many disappointments in interpersonal relationships, they expect further disappointment from adults and others. They are reluctant to invest emotion or trust in relationships, and frequently develop rather manipulative or expedient approaches to human affairs.

Children with chronic depression may engage in potentially self-destructive behavior, risking physical danger, or exposing themselves to socially dangerous situations in which they can be harmed or exploited by adults. They are less likely than acutely depressed children to show episodes of crying, and they attempt to hide their depressive affect. They are often very wary and guarded in discussing anything that has to do with their personal feelings, thoughts, or attitudes.

Children with chronic depression usually require therapeutic help and are best referred to consultants or mental health facilities for diagnosis and management. Since effective treatment of the child is frequently possible only when one or both parents suffering from depressive symptoms can also be effectively treated, it is imperative that the family be involved in treatment, as well as the child. A long-term supportive and therapeutic relationship with the child or family is often necessary.

The efficacy in childhood depression of the psychopharmacologic agents used for adult depression is uncertain. The tricyclic antidepressant medications, which are not officially approved for children under 12 yr of age, may produce moderate to significant improvement in older children and adolescents. (See Table 2–14. It should be noted that these medications can have serious side effects.) In any case, the use of a psychopharmacologic agent in treatment of children's psychiatric disorders should only be one aspect of a program which should include psychologic therapy of the family as well, with attention to educational, social, and recreational lacks and needs. In certain unusually severe depressions or where the environment is unresponsive, intolerable, or very stressful, the depressed child may require a period of hospitalization.

The concept of *masked depression* is controversial, describing children with various behaviors who seem to be hiding an underlying depressed affect. For some the term identifies children who are aggressive and hyperactive, with poor school performance and psychosomatic and hypochondriacal complaints, and who may engage in delinquent behavior. The underlying depression has been inferred from projective tests, such as the TAT or Rorschach, or through diagnostic play or interpretations of drawings of figures. Affected children may occasionally reveal their depressive symptoms when their usual "masking" or camouflage behavior is not possible, or if they become comfortable enough in a relationship with an adult to allow the depressive symptoms to become conscious and manifest. Others feel increasing dissatisfaction with the concept of masked depression, which allows for diagnostic inferences of depression without substantial clinical criteria. A reassessment of 14 children originally thought to have masked depression (Cytryn and McKnew), using the DSM-III criteria, reclassified them as major recurrent depressive disorder (2), a typical depressive disorder (2), shyness disorder (1), introverted disorder of childhood (2), and unsocialized conduct disorder (7). Dysphoric or depressive affect can accompany conditions such as school failure, hyperactivity, or psychosomatic disorders without the depression being primary. The diagnosis of depression will depend on the presence of the primary clinical symptoms of depression, in the context of developmental and family history.

2.54 Suicidal Behavior

Myths of our culture deny that children before the age of adolescence are sexually interested and active, that they become depressed, or that they may at times have murderous wishes or behavior; we have also been slow to accept that young children have suicidal thoughts, and that with measurable frequency they act on suicidal thoughts and impulses.

Among children and adolescents predisposed to suicidal behavior there is no consistent clinical picture. Depression is quite common, but anger, jealousy, anxiety, feelings of rejection, and loneliness may all contribute to the suicidal thoughts and behaviors, which are generated by the pressure to reduce intense stress. An involved child may have tried many other means to reduce this stress. Suicidal threats or behavior may be directed both at the environment and at the self, a significant motive often being to cause people in the environment to react, either with a rescue attempt or with feelings of guilt, remorse, or sorrow. Although there is some skepticism as to whether young children with an inadequate concept of death can really intend suicide, in depth studies reveal that many of them have perceived death as a way of fulfilling their needs or even an experience of love.

Suicide has a low incidence in children under the age of 15 yr, but the rate has increased from 0.4/100,000 deaths in 1955 to 1.2/100,000 deaths in 1975 and studies of clinically distressed children indicate that both thoughts of and attempts at suicide are much more common than earlier believed. It has been reported that as many as one third of children referred for psychiatric hospitalization may have either threatened or attempted suicide. Among older adolescents and young adults (aged 15–24 yr) the rate of suicides in 1957 was 4/100,000 deaths; in 1977 this rate was 13.6/100,000 deaths. Suicide is second only to accidents as a cause of death in this age group (Sec 4.2).

The major methods selected for suicide include firearms, poisoning, and hanging. The likelihood that self-administration of a poison is a suicidal gesture or attempt increases with the age of the child. Any episode of self-poisoning that occurs after the age of 6 yr is less likely to be accidental and should be treated as if the behavior had suicidal potential or as a possible instance of child abuse or neglect. It is estimated that in the age group 5–14 yr there are 100,000, and in the age group 15–24 yr 150,000 self-poisoning events per year. About 46% of the self-poisoned children have symptoms, and about 24% are hospitalized. The fatality rate in the age group 5–14 yr is about 0.1 deaths/11,000 events, whereas in the 15–24 age group the mortality is about 6 fatalities/1000 self-poisonings. Self-poisoning is the most common method for suicidal gestures but accounts for only 25% of fatalities in the age group of 15–24 yr. In adolescents the ratio of suicidal gestures to completed suicide has been estimated to range from 16:1–200:1.

An international study found a marked increase in self-poisoning in girls at the age of 12 yr, with a decrease after the age of 16, whereas in boys the incidence of self-poisonings increased sharply at the age of 14 yr and continued through the age of 18. Girls accounted for approximately 2½ times more attempts than boys after the age of 12 yr, whereas boys were 1½ times more likely than girls to attempt suicide between the ages of 6–11 yr. This same study found about half of the children had evidence of a psychosocial disorder prior to the event; 10% were classified as having behavior disorders, 2% as psychotic. Personality disorders, school dropouts, and children with multiple problems accounted for nearly 20%. No significant problems were detected in the past histories of about 30% of the children. No information was available for 20%. Evidence of precipitating stress was more common in the age group 6–10 yr than in the age group 11–18 yr. In the younger children stresses related to aggression or hostility or fear of retribution, in older boys anxieties related to homosexual experiences, or other sexual matters, and in older adolescent girls to marriage experiences or pregnancy.

Studies both in the United States and in England have identified significant family and dynamic factors both in children who attempt and in those who succeed at suicide. Broken homes are prominent, whether through parental separation, divorce, or death. Other significant factors include acute or prolonged grief, loneliness, and despair over the loss of a loved person. Sometimes death is viewed as a means of reunion. Concern over failure at school may also be a prominent feature in some children. Guilty and self-deprecating children often used the attempt or threat of suicide as a cry for help directed outside the immediate family, which was seen as unresponsive or hostile. Abused children often internalize self-hate and have been found to be at high risk for self-harming behavior. In some adolescents who attempt suicide and in at least half of those who succeed, the notion of revenge or hostility is prominent, directed either outwardly or against self. Suicidal behavior may also be an attempt to obtain evidence of parental love. A small percentage of suicide attempts were felt to result from playing the "suicide game."

Many of the children studied have shown for a month or more some outward sign of distress, including signs of depression, as noted by teachers, family, or friends; others have had difficulties in adjustment for several months to a year or more. In those children under 12 yr, boys were more severely depressed than girls and were at continuing risk for suicidal behavior. At least half of the children who succeeded at suicide had personalities that were seen as irritable, easily hurt or aroused to anger, or impulsive. In over half of such cases suicidal mental illness had existed in another family member; and in at least a third of such cases actual suicide or suicidal attempts had been carried out by a parent, a sibling, or another first degree relative.

The above studies found that successful suicides had higher IQs, were more likely to be boys, and were more physically developed and taller than average. Two stereotypes of personality were generated: an isolated, solitary, aloof boy, depressed and withdrawn; an impetuous, aggressive child given to violent outbursts, hypersensitive, and frequently in trouble at school. Neither of these types is specific to suicide in any way.

Of possible importance is the familiarity that a child with problems may have with the idea or experience of suicide. Parents may have served as models of thinking about, talking about, or actually attempting suicide, sometimes with signs of clinical depression. Some children hear threats or discussion of suicide by peers, or in movies, television, or books; many know of the actual suicides of cultural idols in the entertainment world. These models and this familiarity make suicide seem a possible solution to intolerable stress, conflict, loss of self-esteem, or intense hostility, particularly in the early or middle adolescent years.

Recidivism in suicidal attempts is primarily related either to the adolescent's inability to change his or her life situation (which may involve depression, entrapment related to poverty, alcoholism in a parent, chronic illness, unwanted pregnancy, homosexual guilt, thought disorders, or acting out) or to inability to respond to changes that have occurred in the environment. Hospitalization or institutionalization has not been very helpful. Finding of a thought disorder bodes a poor prognosis. The most important risk factors for recurrence are severe depression, thought disorder, and deteriorating home environment.

Management of Suicidal Behavior in Children and Adolescents.   Threats of or attempts at suicide should be seen as acts communicating desperation, and all such threats or attempts should be taken seriously. Physicians, parents, and others must scrupulously avoid sarcasm or kidding, daring, or belittling them. If the physician labels such behavior "manipulative," power or control becomes the major issue influencing his or her response. Such a position reduces the psychologic flexibility required to deal effectively with child and family at a time of great stress.

The physician assessing suicidal behavior in a child or adolescent should carefully explore, with scrupulous attention to details, the child's life for the 48–72 hr prior to either the threat or the event of a suicide attempt. The physician must identify any precipitating events, as well as any possible hints or early warnings of a suicidal attempt that had been missed or ignored by family members, teachers, or friends. It is crucial to assess the degree of premeditation or impulsivity, whether the patient intended to be stopped or discovered by the timing of the action, and whether the behavior prior to or subsequent to the attempt would promote or impede the patient's being discovered in the attempt. The physician needs to judge the margin of error allowed by the patient in terms of the method used or proposed, the closeness or remoteness of available help, whether the patient actually called for help immediately after the attempt if it was not immediately discovered, and whether the patient calculated correctly whether the family would return in time to discover him or her or planned it so that he or she would not be discovered. *The factor most significant in assessing intended lethality is the possibility and probability of rescue as foreseen by the child or adolescent.*

When the patient is able or willing, the physician should investigate the child's frame of mind, the degree of hopelessness, helplessness, overwhelming shame or guilt, and the presence or absence of anger, and whether directed against others or self. The degree of depression should be carefully evaluated both in terms of the seriousness of the attempt and whether or not the patient presents a continued risk. It is also important to determine whether or not the child acted out of a psychotic delusion or paranoid ideation, or as the result of such hallucinatory experiences as might produce intolerable anxiety or panic—all of which are very high risk factors. Some psychotic and some young children have feelings of magical omnipotence that nothing can hurt or kill them; it is important to assess this possibility.

After the patient has recovered from the effects of attempted suicide, it is important to assess the frame of mind, to determine whether the intent to suicide persists or whether there is now a more optimistic sense of being able to solve or to seek help for problems in a manner other than through suicide. It is important to know whether the patient has some sense of what the immediate future may hold or feels that the future may not be totally hopeless or bleak.

When suicidal patients have been seen in the physician's office or in an emergency room, it is often best to admit them for a day or more to the hospital, so that a more adequate evaluation can be made of the patient's frame of mind and of the circumstances of the family or environment. Such admissions usually require only 2 or 3 days, unless medical needs require a longer stay or unless serious psychiatric disorders are found, such as severe depression or psychosis. If social services and psychiatric assessment are adequate and arrangements for appropriate follow-up care can be made, disposition can be fairly rapidly made. The physician must give careful attention to how family and friends have responded to the patient's act. A hostile and angry family, such as is frequently found, will indicate a different disposition or resolution than a family that is supportive, sympathetic, and understanding. Some families may deny completely the seriousness of the behavior; this can be quite discouraging or provocative to a patient whose desperate act has been an attempt to get another response. It is important that family members examine their roles in the interactions that preceded an attempted suicide, without being made overly guilty. Judgments about the supportiveness of the family are essential to deciding whether a patient can return home immediately or not.

In planning care of patients after suicidal threats or attempts, the physician must consider the following:

1. Has the patient been restored physiologically? For example, have the effects of drugs cleared? What is the state of consciousness, orientation, memory, attention, concentration, and so on? Many drugs produce an acute brain syndrome or delirium that persists after the coma or stupor has lifted.

2. Is the patient less depressed, or has the depression simply become submerged? This may be difficult to determine quickly, and may require a psychiatric consultant, particularly one who is familiar with children. The family may sometimes help determine whether or when the patient seems to be more like his or her usual self.

3. Does the patient appreciate the seriousness of what he or she tried to do, and did he or she want to die? Does the wish to die persist? Answers to these questions may indicate that the patient needs a psychiatric hospitalization or an immediate referral to a psychiatric facility before any final decision about a return to home and community can be made.

4. Are the precipitating events or other reasons that provoked the suicidal behavior still actively influential? The answer requires assessment of the family and of the environment by physician, social worker, nurse, or mental health professional.

5. Have the family, friends, teachers, or other persons significant to the patient responded in a relatively positive manner? It is important to determine whether parents or other significant adults have recovered from their anger or excessive guilt, since the child will need their functional support when he or she returns home. Have parents and child been able to identify for themselves some changes that they can make in order to improve relationships in the home, at school, or in the neighborhood?

6. Does the child show evidence of a future orientation? Has the child something to look forward to when he or she returns home? This may be as simple as going out with friends, attending a sports event, or an outing with the family.

7. Have the child's anger and disappointment, shame, guilt, depression, grief, and other strong feelings moderated or remitted to the point that he or she feels in better control and less at the mercy of impulses and feelings? It is particularly important to assess whether hopelessness and helplessness have declined and whether a sense of control over one's life or one's situation has reappeared.

Whenever possible, every suicidal attempt or threat should initiate a psychiatric or mental health consultation at the time of the event, or shortly thereafter. This may be in the emergency room or hospital, or on immediate referral to a local mental health practitioner or facility. Patients who have made suicide attempts should generally receive follow-up care. The motivation and willingness of the family may be crucial to the success of referral, since the child is frequently unable to accept this on his or her own. Usually it is best for the physician to make personal contact with the referral resource, in addition to encouraging and enabling the family to do so.

2.55 CONDUCT DISTURBANCES IN EARLY CHILDHOOD

Around the ages of 2–3 yr children begin to develop a need for some autonomy, a sense of wanting and being able to do things their own way. In many cases they do not have the motor or social skills to be successful at this. This can lead to frustration and to the expression of much anger. Common manifestations of anger are crying and screaming, breath-holding spells, temper tantrums, and physical aggression against objects or people.

Breath-holding is fairly common in the first 2 yr of life. Parents are best advised to leave the room when a child makes such attempts to control parental behavior; this leaves the child without reinforcement for the behavior, which soon disappears. A few children hold their breath until they lose consciousness for a few seconds. Such children have no increased risk of seizure disorders later on. In children with repeated episodes of breath-holding to the point of unconsciousness, small doses of mephobarbital will often reduce their frequency.

Defiance, oppositional behavior, and *temper tantrums* are all related to the child's learning how to express aggression. A child should learn that expression of anger in appropriate ways is an acceptable and important part of his or her life. Children can be frightened by the strength of their own angry feelings, or by the intensity of angry feelings that they arouse in their parents. It is not often apparent, though it is true, that children are as concerned as their parents about learning to control their own anger. When children successfully control themselves, they should be praised for this. And it is also of prime importance that parents provide those models in control of their own anger and aggressive feelings that they wish their children to follow. Many parents who are horrified at their children's loss of control of anger are unable to see that they have often lost control themselves; they are not, therefore, helping their children to internalize controls. Physicians must learn from the parents how they handle anger before making recommendations about how the child's problems are to be helped.

Defiant and oppositional behavior is to some extent normal in the older toddler, as an effort to achieve a sense of autonomy or individuality. To some extent this oppositional behavior should be accepted by parents so long as it does not go beyond the parents' own limits. The child at this age needs to know that his or her parents are going to be reassuring in a calm and firm way. A technique for dealing with children who have strong oppositional feelings is to provide them with choices, both or all choices being ones that the parents can accept. This gives the child a feeling that he or she has some options, with the knowledge also that the parents are still in the background, able to keep things from getting out of control. If a child becomes irrational and extremely angry, parents may have the child go to his or her room or leave the child and become busy in some other part of the house. Children sometimes substitute a younger brother or sister as the object for anger, when parents are too threatening to confront.

There is a distinction to be made between *temper outbursts* and full-blown *temper tantrums*. In the former the child is angry, but still has some control over feelings and can at times respond to a calm approach on the part of parents who accept the anger. When the stage of temper tantrum is reached, the child no longer has either control or an observing ego, except that he or she remains aware that the frustrating parent is still within scope. In this latter case, no form of verbalization will control the child's behavior. It is then important for the parent to separate physically from the child. Parents can sometimes divert their children to other activities before they reach the point of loss of control or help them to isolate themselves voluntarily until they feel better. It is important not to demean the child or make fun of his or her angry state. Such behavior tends to send confusing messages to children; they may develop the notion that their behavior is desired by parents who seem to be getting perverse pleasure from it. Children need to know that angry feelings are normal, but that the control of excessive anger is an important part of growing up and being mature.

Stealing can sometimes be an expression of anger or of revenge for real or imagined frustration by parents. It is also evidence that the child's internalization of controls has not reached a level where temptation can be resisted. Stealing is sometimes learned from parents. Parents, for instance, who boast of outwitting tax laws or of exceeding speed limits or getting away with other illegal practices are telling their children that these are acceptable forms of behavior. Another formulation that leads children to steal is their sense of the lack or loss of something, perhaps on an emotional level, such as a feeling of not being cared for. Stealing in these cases is a concrete effort to replace the loss. Finally, it appears that in many instances of children's stealing there is a strong element of the child's wanting to be caught, almost as if the theft were arranged so that a confrontation with the parents could serve the child's need for an "emotional reward." Children may find, in effect, that this is one way in which they can compel parents to show an intense feeling toward them, and this gives them a power over their parents that they cannot resist using.

Whatever the cause of stealing, it is important that parents help the child to undo the theft by returning the stolen articles, or by rendering their equivalent either in money that the child can earn or in services. When it is apparent that children are not able to control temptation, money and valuable objects should not be left in their paths to increase the chances of stealing. Almost all children steal something at some time during their childhood. It is important to respond to the event appropriately. It is also important that the act not be overemphasized, lest the behavior or the response to it become so exciting that it is reproduced in future periods of discontent.

Lying is another conduct disorder commonly brought to the attention of physicians by concerned parents. It is important first to determine whether a lying child is developmentally capable of understanding what he or she has said or whether the parents may be misinterpreting statements which sound untruthful to them but may not be so intended by the child. In one sense, lying is a form of fantasy for the child, who is describing things as they are wished rather than as they are. For instance, a child who has not done something that a parent wanted done may say that it has been done in order to avoid an unpleasant confrontation. The child's sense of time does not permit the realization that this only postpones an even angrier confrontation. Some children lie because they seem to enjoy masochistically the response of their upset parents. Most often, lying seems to represent children's not wanting to accept the pain of a relative loss of self-esteem. That is, most lying is an effort to cover up something that the child does not want to accept in his or her behavior. The lie is invented, therefore, to achieve temporary good feeling. Finally, lying, like stealing, can be the result of parental modeling, in which case the child's interpretations of reality are often conflicting, confusing, or unclear. For instance, when mothers and fathers accuse each other frequently of lying, the child may become hopelessly unsure of how the word is to be interpreted; moreover, a loyalty conflict is added to the already distorted process of reality testing.

For the child who presents a history of repeated accidents or of *accident-prone behavior*, a complete assessment of physical, psychologic, and developmental status should be made, together with a careful evaluation of family and especially parental interactions. The child's impulsivity and self-harm may be related to problems of marital discord, or the withdrawal or depression of a parent. The preoccupations of parents with their own needs and interests can markedly reduce their investment in activities as parents. Unresolved parental anger, resentment, or ambivalence toward the child can also result in neglect of normal considerations of safety. As children get older, their risky, careless behaviors may become intended or unconscious ways of getting parental attention, or such behavior may reflect the child's own perception of not being wanted. Children thus internalize negative views of themselves and behave as though they do not care about their safety.

When a physician judges that accident proneness does not primarily depend on a parental or marital disturbance, he can rely on careful instructions to the parents to protect the child and to decrease hazards and risk to health and safety. On the other hand, if accident proneness is judged to be a sign of emotional disturbance in the child or to reflect a parental or family disturbance, then the physician should refer the family to a family service or children's service agency or to a mental health clinic.

2.56 ATTENTION DEFICIT DISORDER
(Hyperactive Syndrome)

The term *attention deficit disorder* designates the central disturbances of children who heretofore had been labeled as suffering from hyperactivity, hyperkinesis, minimal brain damage, or minimal cerebral dysfunction. Subgroups of children with attention deficit disorder include those *with* hyperactivity, those *without*, and a residual type. Criteria for diagnosis of each of these types are detailed in the DSM-III Manual. The word hyperactivity as the primary designation for this syndrome has been misleading; objective measures of activity have failed to demonstrate consistent quantitative differences in physical activity between hyperactive and nonhyperactive children (see below). *Learning disability* has been used as synonymous, and many children with the hyperactivity syndrome have learning disabilities; on the other hand, many children with learning disabilities do not have hyperactivity (Sec 2.71 and 2.72). The syndrome probably represents a heterogeneous group of disorders.

Etiology. Opinions vary as to the origin, features, or even the reality of this disorder. Some believe that the disorder probably results from disturbances in the neurochemistry or neurophysiology of the central nervous system. The term "attention deficit disorder" refers to what many believe is the primary disturbance. The syndrome has been attributed to genetic, gestational, or noxious factors, to hazards of prematurity or immaturity, as well as to trauma, anoxia, or other complications of birth. Temperament has been studied as a possible predisposing factor, as have child-rearing practices and emotional difficulties in parental interactions. No causal factors have been conclusively shown.

Pathophysiology. There is no conclusive evidence of any pathophysiologic mechanism or biochemical disturbance. Hyperactive boys of ages 6–9 yr and of average IQ who have responded well to stimulant medication have shown a low level of arousal in the central nervous system before treatment, as measured by electroencephalography, auditory evoked potentials, and skin conductance. These boys had high scores for restlessness, distractibility, poor attention span, and impulsivity. With 3 wk of treatment, the laboratory measures became more nearly normal, and the ratings by teachers showed improved behaviors.

Incidence. Depending on its definition, an attention deficit disorder with hyperactivity is estimated to occur in 5–10% of school-age children. Specific learning disabilities overlap with hyperactivity. The incidence of hyperactivity in boys is 4–6 times that in girls.

Clinical Manifestations. Objective measures do not show that affected children are more physically active than normal controls, but their movements are less purposeful, and they are restless and fidgety. They have short attention spans, are distractible and impulsive, and tend to act without considering or reflecting upon the consequences. They have a low tolerance for frustration and are emotionally labile and excitable. Their moods tend to be neutral or oppositional; they are frequently gregarious, but socially clumsy. Some are hostile and negative, but these traits are often secondary to the psychosocial problems they experience (Sec 2.76). Some are excessively dependent; others are so independent as to be foolhardy.

Emotional and behavioral difficulties are common, and usually secondary to the negative social impact of the behavior. These children receive criticism and punishment from parents and teachers, and social ostracism from peers. They fail chronically at academic tasks, and many are not well enough coordinated or self-controlled to be successful at sports. They have a poor self-image and low self-esteem, and frequently suffer from depression. There is a high incidence of learning disabilities in reading, mathematics, spelling, and handwriting. Academic performances may lag by 1–2 yr and are less than would be expected from their measured intelligence.

Past and Developmental History. Probably the most important tools in evaluation are the developmental history and the teacher's report of academic problems and behavior in the classroom. The history is often diagnostic: typically, the mother remembers an alert, active, demanding baby who had intense emotional responses, with feeding and sleeping difficulties often in the early months, difficult to get quiet at bedtime, and slow to establish diurnal rhythms. Colic is rather commonly reported. Developmental milestones are usually normal; some children stand, walk, and run quite early. As toddlers, these children are "into everything," constantly intrusive and demanding, and their mothers learn that they need constant supervision to keep out of mischief, nuisance, or danger.

Diagnosis. It is difficult among 2–4 yr old children to identify those who will develop hyperactivity from those who are simply active, boisterous, and gregarious. The latter learn during the preschool period to master motor output, to maintain attention and concentration, and to modulate social behavior in preparation for school. The pediatrician should be alert to the possibility of nascent hyperactive syndrome in toddlers or preschool children as part of normal longitudinal assessment. Mothers who describe their children as hyperactive should not be told they "will outgrow it," nor should stimulant or other medication be given without adequate study (see below).

To assess accurately the term "hyperactive" the physician needs descriptions of behavior; these will clarify the expectations of parents and reveal their levels of tolerance for motor activity such as running, playing, shouting, and so on. Parents who value physical and emotional control may judge a normally active boy or girl as hyperactive or "bad." The physician must assess the psychosocial structure within which judgments of "normal," "hyperactive," "deviant," or "stubborn" are made.

The initial identification of children as "hyperactive" commonly occurs as they enter nursery or elementary school. Their teachers report that they are uncontrollable, can't sit still, intrude into the spaces and activities of other children, are boisterous and inattentive, won't concentrate, or won't follow instructions. They are often said to provoke others to anger, not to seem to hear instructions, not to learn from mistakes, and not to respond to the usual disciplinary actions. Parents may report many of the same traits, their prior management perhaps reflecting their range of tolerance or their experience with other children. Some children with attention deficit syndrome are clumsy, but others are well coordinated, meeting the physical requirements of sports or games but having difficulty with social requirements, with keeping to the rules, paying attention, and concentrating. They may be particularly disabled in activities requiring cooperation.

Affected children are frequently unable to sit still, even for television. They may quietly watch a television program they like but be disruptive and intrusive when they have little interest. The dinner table is an arena of frustration and conflict.

Clinical Evaluation.   Children with attention deficits not uncommonly maintain good control in the physician's examining room, sitting quietly, paying attention, and responding to directions. The physician should not be misled; these children may be suppressing characteristic behavior in this structured situation free of the distractions and demands of home or school.

Physical examination does not generally contribute to the diagnosis, although there is an increased frequency of minor congenital anomalies in children with behavioral difficulties, retardation, or neurologic disease. The reported anomalies include fine hair, malformed ears, epicanthal folds, high-arched palates, and single palmar creases.

Children with attention deficits are generally believed to show increased numbers of "soft" neurologic signs, such as mixed hand preference, impaired balance, astereognosis, dysdiadochokinesia, and problems in fine motor coordination. The most useful diagnostic tools are observation in the classroom and psychoeducational testing. Since the groups of learning-disabled and hyperactive children overlap, it is likely that the same lack of diagnostic specificity in neurologic signs exists for both. Standards for evaluation of "soft" neurologic signs are only gradually being set. In the absence of defined standards, it will be useful to establish for each child his or her baseline performance, particularly on tasks requiring sensory or motor integration, such as hopping, balancing, stereognosis, graphesthesia, alternating movements, heel to toe walking, throwing, and kicking (Sec 2.72).

Laboratory and Other Studies.   No laboratory studies establish the diagnosis of attention deficit disorder. Children with hyperactivity are reported to have increased amounts of slow waves in the electroencephalogram, without evidence of progressive neurologic disease or epilepsy, but this finding has doubtful significance. A computer-analyzed EEG may be helpful in evaluating some learning disabilities (Sec 2.72).

Psychologic and Psychoeducational Testing.   It is uncertain whether hyperactive children with attention deficit syndrome have significantly lower IQ scores than children who do not have this syndrome when appropriately matched for age, school grade level, socioeconomic status, and the like. Some hyperactive children have verbal scores more than 10 points higher than performance scores on the Wechsler Intelligence Scale for children (WISC) and lower scores on the attention/concentration subset. Psychoeducational tests which help identify concomitant learning disabilities in hyperactive children include the ITPA, Frostig, and Wepman tests; such tests also help delineate the strong and weak modes of learning in particular children (Sec 2.73).

Projective tests such as the TAT and Rorschach are not helpful in diagnosis of attention deficit disorder, though they may provide information on psychodynamics and on emotional strengths and weaknesses.

Differential Diagnosis.   Hyperactivity and learning disabilities often occur together; the child suspected of having one should be evaluated for the other. Children with problems in sustaining attention may also have problems in learning, but such problems are not called a "learning disability." The latter term refers to those problems which arise out of perceptual-motor difficulties, such as those described in Sec 2.72, which affect achievement in reading and/or mathematics. Seizure disorders, particularly petit mal, may produce apparent lack of concentration or attention, but children with petit mal do not have an attention deficit disorder unless these disorders coexist. Children whose activity, boisterousness, and assertiveness are at the upper extreme of normal usually respond to appropriate techniques of socialization and discipline, and rapidly learn to maintain the attention, concentration, and impulse control required in a structured environment. Children suffering from depressive episodes (Sec 2.53) may show increased activity and social disturbances, but they do not have the characteristic history of excessive activity and impulsivity in early life. Angry, aggressive, hostile children may resemble those with this syndrome, but they do not usually have the attentional or concentrating difficulties, nor the random and restless social intrusiveness of the latter. The aggressive child's antisocial behavior is usually more clearly intentional and directed at specific persons, the apparent motive being most often to retaliate against a real or imagined injury, or to initiate aggressive activity. Children with the attention deficit syndrome may develop similar negative and hostile characteristics when criticism, failure, and the absence of positive reinforcement have eroded self-esteem and made them unhappy and defensive.

Treatment.   Treatment of children with attention deficit disorders is directed at the social environment of the home and classroom and at the child's personal academic and psychosocial needs, with judicious use of medication. A clear explanation of the child's condition must be given both to the parents and to the child.

A program that will give "structure" to the child's environment will decrease the effects of the handicap and help in academic and social learning. The child should have a regular daily routine, with the child's prompt following of routine expected and rewarded with praise. Rules should be simple, clear, and as few as possible, and coupled with firm limits, enforced fairly and sympathetically through restrictions or deprivations for transgressions. Overstimulation and excessive fatigue should be avoided. The child will need time for relaxation after play, particularly after vigorous physical activity. The period before bedtime should be quiet, with avoidance of exciting television programs and rough and tumble games. It is probably best that young children with the attention deficit syndrome who are hyperactive not be taken on long trips by automobile or on extensive shopping trips. The confined space of the car and the excessive stimulation in large stores may intensify the child's symptoms. The home should be arranged so that all valuable, dangerous, or breakable objects are out of the reach of the young child. Parents should reward even partially successful efforts at control of behavior or academic responsibilities with recognition, affection, and regular praise. More formal operant conditioning techniques are often helpful, which reward the child with stars or tokens (exchangeable for toys and activities), contingent upon improved behavior.

Medication. (Sec 2.66 and 2.76 and Table 2–14). Pharmacotherapy is often used for children with attention deficit disorders. Dextroamphetamine and methylphenidate are most commonly used, the latter preferred because it has fewer side effects. Their action is probably to modify fundamental disturbances in attention span, concentration, and impulsivity. Since the response to medication cannot be predicted, a clinical trial is usually needed; 2–3 wk of daily medication may be required to determine whether a drug effect will occur. The drug is given after breakfast and lunch, in order to have minimal effect on appetite or sleep. To determine the effect, the physician should obtain reports both from family and from teachers every 5–7 days; standardized rating scales can be used for this purpose.

The therapeutic range of dose of stimulant medication may be rather narrow. Too small a dose has no effect; too large a dose will produce a jittery and agitated or socially withdrawn child. Some children develop with chronic medication a pale, sallow, drawn, glassy-eyed appearance; it is not thought to represent a significant disturbance, but can be distressing to child and parents. If these effects do not abate with decreases in dose, another medication may be tried.

Children who do not respond show little or no change in behavior with increasing doses. Parents or teachers may report that the child is worse. Before a child is judged to be unresponsive, a full therapeutic trial should be undertaken, so long as side effects are not serious.

Major short-term side effects include anorexia, upper abdominal pain, and difficulty in going to sleep. Upper abdominal pain is usually without nausea or vomiting and usually responds to a decrease in dose; suspension of medication is rarely required. Insomnia can be minimized by giving no stimulant medication after 3:00 P.M. and arranging that the period before bedtime be calm and nonstimulating. It is best to avoid the use of sedative drugs to treat the sleep disturbance.

With onset of treatment some children become tearful and sensitive to criticism, whereas they may have earlier seemed impervious to correction, criticism, or punishment. This change may indicate that the child will respond well to medication. The reaction should subside after 1–2 wk; if it persists, reduction of dosage or a change of medication should be considered. Other short-term side effects include drowsiness, headaches, tics, and nail biting.

Long-term side effects include increased heart rate and growth suppression. The implications of increased heart rate are not clear; there may be a chronic increase in the workload of the heart. After 3 yr treatment with more than 20 mg/24 hr of methylphenidate, a group of children were reported to have an average loss of 5 percentile units in expected height. Catch-up growth occurred on termination of medication. Growth suppression has not occurred when the level of medication was less than 20 mg/24 hr. Weight loss was also reported and found unrelated to anorexia.

There is no evidence that children treated with stimulant drugs are at increased risk of becoming abusers of such drugs in adolescence.

The benefits and disadvantages of medication must be weighed carefully by the physician, with full disclosure to parents, and to the child as well, within his or her limitations of understanding. Informed consent is a necessary condition for effective treatment, since adequate management of the hyperactive child with the attention deficit syndrome requires parents and child to sustain a regimen that may last for many years. The trust and confidence established in an initial working alliance between parents, child, and physician are of paramount importance. An important strategy is to engage the hyperactive child increasingly in responsibility for his or her own management to the degree permitted by age, understanding, and emotional stability. This assumption of responsibility involves not only medication but social and academic behaviors.

Although some children will have rebound effects, medication should be eliminated or reduced, if possible, on weekends, during summer vacations, or on school holidays. After 6–12 mo stimulant medication should be discontinued for a period of at least 2–3 wk to determine whether the child's own control has improved. If a positive adaptation is maintained, medication can be discontinued altogether.

The effective dose of methylphenidate varies with the age of the child. Body weight does not usually help determine the dose. Initially, 5 mg is given at breakfast and at lunch. If no response is noted, the dose can be increased by 2.5 mg at 3–5 day intervals. For children 8–9 yr of age the usual effective dose is 15–20 mg/24 hr. Older children may need up to 40 mg/24 hr (Table 2–14). The effect of methylphenidate lasts from 2–4 hr. As the effect wanes, some children have rebound hyperactivity, becoming weepy and irritable. This effect can last an hour or more. When this occurs, the dose can be increased to see if a favorable response can be prolonged, or a dose may be split. The FDA has not approved stimulant medication for children under 6 yr old.

Dextroamphetamine may be given in slowly released form, in initial doses of 10 mg with a duration of action of 8–18 hr, so that only 1 daily dose is needed at breakfast. The dose of dextroamphetamine is about one half that of methylphenidate, ranging from 10–20 mg/24 hr.

The effect of magnesium pemoline develops more slowly and lasts about 12 hr. Initial doses of 18.75 (half of the 37.5 mg tablet) have been suggested, to be increased by a half tablet/wk. Three–4 wk are required to determine its efficacy. About 1–2% of treated children may show changes in liver function; accordingly, pretreatment studies and the monitoring of liver function every 2 mo are required. Side effects of magnesium pemoline include increased nervousness and jitteriness.

Since pemoline is a relatively new drug, the physician should try the more thoroughly tested medications first.

Phenothiazine drugs, and particularly thioridazine, may decrease the child's motor behavior; they are less attractive than stimulant medication because of their side effects of somnolence, irritability, and dystonias. The more obtunded child will probably have no improvement in attention or concentration at school.

Some children unresponsive to stimulant medication may derive benefit from the mildly tranquilizing effects of diphenhydramine or hydroxyzine. Diphenhydramine has been used in children under 6 yr of age; fairly high doses are required. Phenytoin is not helpful.

Psychotherapy. When severe psychosocial difficulties have produced serious family distress and parents are ineffective in carrying out a prescribed regimen, referral to a mental health professional or an appropriate mental health clinic will be indicated. There is no conclusive evidence that psychotherapy is primarily beneficial in the attention deficit syndrome, but individual and family therapy will be indicated when it is complicated by depression, social withdrawal or negativism, eroded self-esteem, or chronic family conflict.

School. Management of the child at school follows the same principles as at home. The teacher's task may be more difficult, since he or she must deal as well with 20 or more other children. The physician should urge an extended trial in one or more regular classrooms before a decision is made to place the child in a special class, and when such a decision is made, it should be for educational reasons, not simply behavioral. The child with the attention deficit syndrome with hyperactivity often has a learning disability, and may need any of the special educational approaches prescribed for learning disabilities. Special classes frequently use contingency or operant conditioning for behavior modification; when carefully planned and carried out by teachers well grounded in theory and practice, such approaches can help these children. It is essential that physician and school personnel maintain close communication about the child's progress. Decisions about medication or about referral to a mental health facility may well depend foremost upon the information obtained from a cooperative and perceptive teacher.

Prognosis. The attention deficit syndrome may last through childhood and adolescence, and may also cause adult difficulties. The random motor movements and social intrusiveness may diminish, but learning disabilities and behavioral and psychosocial problems may become even more intense and handicapping in late childhood and adolescence. An optimistic prognosis can be made if the child can succeed sufficiently at learning to make progress through school approximately with his or her age group, and if the secondary psychosocial effects can be ameliorated by a supportive family.

2.57 AGGRESSIVE BEHAVIOR AND AGGRESSIVE DISORDERS

Aggression is a problem both of normal development and of psychosocial disturbance. There is no totally satisfactory theory of the nature and causes of human aggressive behavior, though various disciplines have contributed to partial understanding of its nature and control. Some believe that aggression is primarily innate or instinctual, studies of aggression in fish, birds and lower mammals, subhuman primates, and man revealing certain similarities. A common finding is that certain configurations of stimuli give rise to aggressive responses, especially those involving territory, mating, food, protection of the nest and young, and social hierarchy. A striking observation of many studies is that intraspecies aggression is rarely fatal, particularly in subhuman primates.

In the development of psychoanalytic theory Freud named aggression as 1 of the 2 basic drives, conceiving of it as a death instinct in contrast to a life instinct. Later theorists have paired an aggressive instinct with the sexual instinct as 2 basic drives. In accounting for the perpetuation of aggressive behaviors learning theories stress conditioning, and contingency theories stress positive reinforcement. Social theorists suggest that modern crowding, the breakdown in commonly shared values, the demise of traditional family patterns of child rearing in kinship systems, and social alienation both in individuals and in large groups are leading to increased aggression in children, adolescents, and adults.

There are individual constitutional differences within species. For example, boys are almost universally reported more aggressive than girls, possibly because of greater muscle mass. In many animals, giving male sex hormones to females produces more aggressive behavior. Larger children are often more aggressive than smaller ones. More active and intrusive children are perceived as more aggressive. Other dimensions of temperament also influence aggressive activity (Sec 2.27).

Descriptively, aggressive behavior that results in some kind of injury might be distinguished from initiative behavior which intrudes upon the environment for the sake of learning, mastering, or achieving. Many hyperactive, clumsy children are termed aggressive because of the accidental results of their behavior, their intentions being benign. Intentional aggression may be primarily *instrumental*, to achieve an end, or primarily *hostile*, part of the motivation of the latter being to inflict physical or psychologic pain. Clinically, it is important to attempt to differentiate among these motives. Other factors needing attention in assessment include the developmental level and circumstances of the child, the social acceptance accorded the child, the models the child may have for aggression, the possibility of emotional disturbances, and familial, social or subcultural patterns of behavior.

The child of 2–5 yr may show aggressive outbursts ranging from temper tantrums and screaming to hurting others or destroying toys and furniture. In these situations aggressive behavior frequently arises out of particular frustrations. Usually such aggressive behavior in 2–3 yr olds is directed toward the parents in response to demands for performance or compliance, or as a response to frustration of the wishes or intent of the child. By the age of 4–5 yr such behavior is more likely to be directed at siblings or peers, owing to the greater social interaction at these ages. Verbal aggression increases between the ages of 2–4 yr and after the age of 3 yr revenge and retaliation become more prominent as determinants of aggression.

Aggressive behavior in boys is relatively stable from the preschool period through adolescence; a boy with a high level of aggressive behavior in the period between 3–6 yr of age has a high probability of carrying this behavior into adolescence. On the other hand, girls under 6 yr old who were aggressive toward their peers did not continue to be aggressive at older ages, nor did this earlier aggression correlate with adult competitiveness. This is probably because aggressive girls suffer anxiety in the conflict between competitiveness and development of the traditional gender role.

Frustration is commonly viewed as the response to those conditions that bar an individual from achieving goals important to self-esteem or that create internal conflicts between incompatible responses. Frustration and aggression are closely associated: the frustrated individual responds with aggressive behavior to a degree depending on his or her personality. If a child learns that reacting aggressively against sources of frustration removes them, this experience reinforces the aggressive behavior, and may cause it to be perpetuated. But in making judgments about aggressive behavior one should take into account the age of the child, the stage of development, the nature of the environment, and whether what is termed aggression is a misplaced attempt to persevere in the face of obstacles or to engage in appropriate problem solving. It is important not to attribute malice to the child whose aggression is really self-assertion in response to anxieties or feelings of incompetence or low self-esteem.

Children exposed to aggressive models in play, whether these models be other children, adults, or cartoon figures, will display increased aggressive behavior when compared with children not exposed to these same models. Parents must understand that their anger and aggressive or harsh punishment will model behavior which children may imitate when they themselves have been physically or psychologically hurt.

Our culture provides universal support for violence and aggressive behavior through literature, films, and television, and the influence is significant. As nations attempt to solve problems by aggression, so adults attempt to satisfy their needs or to right wrongs through aggressive and violent behaviors ranging from personal assault, murder, and rape to terrorist activities against individuals or social institutions. Societies, in turn, respond with aggressive counterbehavior in dealing with suspected or actual perpetrators of crime. Reports of police brutality, of the violence of parents or teachers against children, and of riots and confrontations all create a climate in which, unfortunately, violence is seen as a legitimate and even valued means of solving human problems or of dealing with human conflict.

2.58 PASSIVE-AGGRESSIVE BEHAVIOR

The passive-aggressive child expresses hostility indirectly, as procrastination, "forgetting," dawdling, stubbornness, resistance, or "willful" behavior. Parents will often complain that such children don't hear them and that they fail to respond to repeated requests. Academic underachievement is common. Their early histories may reveal excessive negativism during the infancy and toddler periods, feeding disturbances, and problems in bladder and bowel training.

Children may unconsciously adopt passive-aggressive strategies for a variety of motives: to gain independence while maintaining dependency; to counter underlying low self-esteem; to maintain control and autonomy when threatened by anxiety; and to get revenge. Children using these strategies are essentially fearful of direct expression of aggression and hostility; consequently, anger is disguised through passive-aggressive maneuvers. The child-rearing styles of their parents are often intimidating, critical, and authoritarian, or on the other hand indulgent and permissive. Both children and parents may find it difficult to deal directly and overtly with anger, and neither may be able to acknowledge the anger which contributes to and is generated by the passive-aggressive behavior. Physicians should encourage parents to handle passive-aggressive behavior by setting firm limits and expectations for the child. The parents and the child should reach agreement upon what they will consider his or her most important tasks and responsibilities. Deficiencies in lesser or minor areas should be temporarily overlooked so that confrontations over unimportant issues are avoided. Age-appropriate assertiveness and independence should be promoted and rewarded. The more refractory cases require psychiatric intervention to reveal and modify the underlying psychodynamics.

2.59 DEPENDENCY

The *dependent child* is inhibited in self-expression, shy, and fearful in social situations, often described as "sensitive" and "easily hurt." Dependent children tend to cling to parents and to avoid taking initiatives, unconsciously wishing and arranging that others take care of them. Recreational activities and peer group interactions may be shunned because of fear of competition and injury. Dependent children have frequently been overprotected and overindulged by parents, and their development of normal independence and autonomy has been hindered. The child is often viewed by the parents as sickly and fragile, even when any physical illnesses have been minor.

Successful management depends on the parents' willingness to encourage the child to take the normal risks of growing up. The pediatrician should support and reassure parents, as they assist the child in meeting new situations in small, calibrated steps. Nursery school for the preschool child and organized recreational activities for the older child are helpful initial steps in aiding the child's psychologic separation from parents. Any small change toward more independent and autonomous function should be praised and rewarded. Expectations should not be raised too high too quickly. If supportive advice and direction are unavailing, psychiatric intervention should be considered.

2.60 THE SCHIZOID CHILD

The *schizoid child* is characterized not only by limited socialization skills but also by seeming not to desire any. Schizoid children are not out of touch with reality, delusional, or having hallucinations, but they resemble in some ways adults with simple schizophrenia. Their interests seem shallow, their energies limited. The schizoid child can often become obsessed with some limited activity and appear quite content. Since such children generate few demands on their parents or teachers, their illness can remain undetected. They are not mentally retarded but emotionally and socially immature. They may appear neither to have nor to want substantial friendships, whereas shy or withdrawn children want to be involved with others but are too fearful. The latter children may be quite animated and friendly in their family groups but not at school.

The schizoid child may have some inborn neurophysiologic disorder, but this is not proved. Schizoid children are at risk for more serious disorders in late adolescence and young adulthood unless they are well protected and their lives structured for them. Under stress they may become frankly psychotic or adopt antisocial behavior. As the child gets older, there may be deterioration in intellectual abilities; the child may come to resemble a person with organic brain damage.

Parents of schizoid children need long-term guidance and help in providing socialization experiences for their children. They will have to be firm in supporting and implementing activities that enhance ego growth, even though the child is reluctant. Medication is of little or no help. Diagnostic assessment should be made as early in the child's life as the above pattern can be recognized. Evaluation can be made through a child psychiatrist or a mental health clinic.

2.61 VARIATIONS IN SEXUAL ADAPTATIONS

Children are naturally curious—about the world around them, about other people, and about themselves. Their bodies are of particular interest, following the discovery of body parts in the 1st yr of life. The 2 yr old child can and ought to be told the proper names for the parts of his or her body, including the genital parts. It is to be hoped that the child's exploration, manipulation, and enjoyment of his or her own body, including the genitals, will be met with calm understanding on the part of the parents, rather than with anxiety or anger.

Young boys and girls commonly undress together and engage in looking and touching behavior involving the genitalia. In preschool children hugging, kissing, and perhaps lying on top of each other may be the extent of the physical contact, genital behavior being usually confined to mutual touching and stroking. Preschool children who engage in more explicit sexual behavior, such as oral contacts, attempts at simulated intercourse, or anal stimulation, have probably learned such behavior by watching or being involved in such activities by older children or adults. The majority of sexual abuses against young children are perpetrated by adolescents or adults well known to the child, often by family members, and sometimes with the tacit approval or in default of supervision on the part of other responsible adults (Sec 2.67 and 19.14).

Children can be advised that questions about sexual matters are natural and can be answered by their parents, by their doctor, or by books. There are many well designed, factual, and sensitive sex education materials, some distributed through such organizations as Planned Parenthood, religious groups, sex education societies, and other organizations, as well as through medical societies and public health organizations. Parents can be advised to explain to each child that his or her own body is private and personal, and that the same consideration applies to the bodies of other children.

Sexual interests and activities have had negative sanctions in western culture, and still evoke strong emotions in adults. All adults, and physicians above all, should be extremely cautious in inferring meaning for the current or future sexual development of children from any isolated act or even a series of sexual acts. This is especially true for preschool children, though gender identity and gender role development are well advanced in preschool children (Sec 2.34).

Transvestism may occur transiently as a part of normal development or it may be a chronic manifestation of a disturbance in gender identity or gender role. Preschool boys may frequently dress up in clothing of their mothers or sisters and strut around, sometimes to the delight and sometimes to the consternation of others. Parents rarely remark on "cross-dressing" in girls; in fact it is almost impossible to define the condition, since girls are permitted to wear "boys' clothing" from early childhood through adulthood. Both fathers and mothers should not become angry, accusatory, or anxious about transient cross-dressing in little boys; nor should they be entertained by or encourage it. Ignoring the behavior or firmly but calmly discouraging it is probably the best means of handling it. At the same time, physicians and parents should understand that the transient behavior may be a sign of a more fundamental anxiety or concern on the part of the young boy, having to do with his discomfort with what he believes to be the masculine role.

Parental concern is warranted when transient cross-dressing becomes chronic and recurrent, or furtive, and when the boy dresses in girls' or women's underwear, pays a great deal of attention to jewelry and cosmetics, and seems uncomfortable with the usual activities of boys of his age. When these behaviors recur regularly and persistently despite parental disapproval, the possibility of a disturbance in gender role or sex identity needs to be considered, especially if the child is more than 5–6 yr old.

The pediatrician should not label the child as a transvestite, but merely note that he is showing episodes of cross-dressing behavior. Neither should it be inferred immediately by parents or clinician that the child is becoming or will become a homosexual.

Transvestism usually appears after masculine identity has been established. The adult transvestite man does not question his being male, though he may be at times uncomfortable with his masculinity and manifest this discomfort by feminine behavior and cross-dressing. An essential characteristic of adult transvestite behavior is the man's knowledge that he has a penis. He may frequently become sexually aroused during periods of cross-dressing or develop fetishistic attachments to certain articles of women's clothing in order to obtain genital arousal and/or orgasm. The older pubertal child who persists in transvestite behavior may have the same experiences.

Transsexualism is the psychologic conviction in a person biologically (chromosomally, gonadally, hormonally, and genitally) belonging to one sex that he or she is a member of the other sex. This disorder is differentiated from homosexuality, transvestism, and effeminacy. In adults this has become a medically important condition, since hormonal and surgical treatment can accomplish a change of sex for both male and female transsexuals. The results of surgery, however, are controversial with respect to improvement in personal, social, or work adjustment. The true incidence of this disturbance among adults is unknown. In children the condition is rare; it has been reported, however, in male children ranging in age from 3 yr to puberty.

Transsexualism manifests itself in cross-dressing of an elaborate, persistent, and intransigent nature. It almost always arises from a psychologic conviction in the male child that he is or will become a woman. Studies of psychologic roots and early attitudes of transsexuals have found that evidence may have been apparent as early as within the 1st 18 mo of life. By all measures currently known there are no biologic determinants, nor does it seem due to genetically inherited behaviors or dispositions. Affected children adopt gestures, postures, gaits, voices, mannerisms, games, and interests that are feminine. They prefer to play almost exclusively with girls and willingly adopt female roles in various fantasy games.

Affected children are not psychotic; rather, they may be pleasant, creative, socially attractive to both peers and adults, intelligent, and articulate. Their behavior is not primarily characterized by overt erotic or sexual interaction with peers. Rather it is gender role behavior that belongs to the gender identity assumed, which may be encouraged and supported by the family dynamics. Stoller reports that the mothers of affected boys are uncertain about their own sexuality and not particularly active sexually, but not evidently homosexual. Their lives have frequently had a sense of emptiness, with no close interpersonal relationships. Their relationships with their own mothers seemed problematic and unrewarding. The fathers of these boys have been psychologically and physically absent, both to their children and to their wives. Stoller reports that the mothers of affected children lavish physical attention upon them, not only as infants but through the preschool years. They are held, cuddled, petted, and allowed to be close to mother in bed, during bathing, and in dressing, as if there were no psychologic or physical boundary or social distance between mother and child. Mothers of affected children characteristically gratify them completely, seeing their life's mission as giving these children pleasure and rewarding their every whim and wish.

Exploring and counseling with parents regarding questions of gender role dysfunction requires great sensitivity and tact. Clinicians must be aware of their own anxiety in dealing with problems in this area, which may be expressed as punitiveness, disgust, brusque referral, or denial and avoidance. A successful referral to a mental health practitioner or agency may be crucial to helping parents and child in understanding the possible sources and meaning of the behavior. Such a referral may also help the child adapt with less distress to the conflict between somatic sex assignment and psychosocial role behaviors.

HOMOSEXUAL BEHAVIOR

Developmental same-sex (homosexual) behavior. Sexual behavior between members of the same sex is not uncommon in children; its incidence in relation to age and sex is not known. The impression that it is more common between boys is biased by a cultural sensitivity and anxiety about male homosexual behavior, as well as by the cultural stereotype that boys are intrinsically more interested and active sexually than girls or women. In addition, adult male homosexuality has been more publicly recognized. The physician should not infer that sexual relations between boys or between girls is likely to be a sign either of a basic homosexual identity or of serious psychiatric disturbance. The important questions are similar to those addressed to any other behavior. What are the ranges of normal expectation as they relate to age, developmental level, the gender of the individual, and the circumstances under which the behavior occurred? Other judgments relate to whether or not the behavior is adaptive; its frequency and duration; whether it interferes with normal function; and whether it is an aspect of more generally disturbed psychosocial function. Sexual behavior is likely to be given the center of the emotional stage. The physician must be able to maintain his or her own perspective and help others to consider sexual behavior as only one aspect of the child's global development, interpersonal functioning, and personal adaptation.

If the physician judges that same-sex behavior reported by a parent in a child is normal developmental behavior or transient and circumstantial, he or she can adopt the following management: parents will need reassurance and some advice as to how to handle any recurrence of such behavior; the physician will need to help the parents control their anxiety, anger, disgust, guilt, or feelings that the child is destined to develop a deviant sexual orientation. Reassurance and guidance are crucial in helping the parents to achieve the attitudes and emotional control that will permit them to be helpful and supportive to their child.

The first task of physicians or parents is to help younger children feel safe and less guilty. Parents should avoid suspicious, scolding, threatening, shaming, or guilt-inducing attitudes or behaviors toward the child. The physician can serve as a model for the parent through his or her own calm, sensitive, careful and supportive exploration of feelings and behavior with the child. The physician should expect denials on the part of the child, and avoidance of and embarrassment with the subject, but discussion will help the child to understand that sexual behavior is comprehensible, and that sexual feelings and curiosity are normal. It is important to know whether the child's information and understanding of sexual matters are appropriate to his or her age. If the same-sex behavior involves another child in the family, he or she should be treated in the same manner. If an older child is the initiator or seducer, he or she should be told clearly and firmly that such behavior will not be tolerated and that he or she will be expected to act with responsibility and control. The older child should talk with a physician or mental health professional, and if there are concerns about emotional or social adjustment, referral for psychiatric evaluation is indicated.

The physician must not let his or her own negative feelings aggravate the disgust, anger, or punitive feelings that parents may have for an older child seen as perpetrator, especially if the older child is not a member of the younger child's family. The physician may need to help parents of exploited children refrain from ill-considered acts of revenge against offenders. If, on the other hand, there has been physical violence or psychologic coercion, both psychiatric and legal intervention are indicated.

Parents can be advised that it is appropriate to make a careful inventory of their children's activities and friends. Vigilance over the child may be increased, but it should not become punitive, suspicious, or guilt-inducing.

Circumstantial same-sex behavior occurs in situations where there are not opportunities for heterosocial or heterosexual behavior, especially among adolescents. Same-sex detention centers and prisons for youth, residential treatment centers, and group-living situations provide occasions for circumstantial homosexuality. In these settings, many involved in such behavior are not homosexual in psychologic orientation. Such circumstances may, however, bring latent homosexual orientations or desires to overt expression. Sexual exploitation and sadistic behavior, including rape, may occur in these situations. Most homosexual experimentation in adolescence is developmental or circumstantial and not premonitory of a later fixed homosexual orientation.

HOMOSEXUALITY

True homosexual orientation is a complex phenomenon, different from merely developmental or circumstantial same-sex behavior. It is essentially a psychologic orientation through which the individual has sexual desires toward or attraction to and gratification from sexual and sensuous contact with members of the same sex. The true homosexual orientation is not exclusively or even primarily genital, but rather a global psychosocial involvement. Only a minority of homosexual

persons demonstrate such discordant gender role behaviors as effeminacy in men or masculine behavior in women.

The cause of homosexual orientation is uncertain; there are probably various pathways to it. Theories have proposed genetic, biochemical, neurohumoral, and structural factors. There is no substantial indication of a biologic or physiologic causation. Homosexual orientation is probably not fixed until middle or late adolescence, or even later, if ever. Various forms of therapy (psychoanalytic, behavioral, group) have produced heterosexual orientations in some homosexual persons who have sought this goal.

Historically, acceptance of homosexuality has waxed and waned within given societies and over various time periods. The view is currently held by some that homosexuality is best regarded as an alternative life-style, and the American Psychiatric Association no longer lists homosexuality among mental disorders.

Homosexuality in Boys. Factors seen as influential in the development of homosexual orientation in boys have included lack of adequate male models and of support from parents, peers, and subculture for male behavior.

The potentially damaging father is psychologically distant, demeaning, or punitive, especially if such attitudes are aimed at his son's attempts at gender role behaviors. For example, a father who criticizes his son's interest in volleyball as "sissy" and is openly disappointed or angry at the boy's lack of interest in or skill at sports demanding physical contact may produce in the boy feelings of failure, inadequacy, and loss of self-esteem, with doubts about meeting the gender role expectations so vehemently valued within the family. Some fathers with intense, eroticized feelings toward their sons may inadvertently provoke anxiety-producing homosexual feelings.

The mother may, on the other hand, be overprotective and indulgent. She may also be intentionally or unintentionally seductive in her behavior, stimulating intense sensuous and sexual feelings which the boy finds intolerable, and which may reach consciousness only in the form of anxiety, placing the child in a situation of irreconcilable conflict. The boy who wants to be close to his mother and enjoy the rewards of her interest and affection is made very uncomfortable by the overt and covert erotic aspects of the relationship. This may compel him to avoid her or to develop an irritable, angry façade which keeps her at a distance and alleviates his own anxiety. The boy may then generalize this pattern of interaction to his relationship with girls. At adolescence this conflict may become so intensified that the boy orients himself to male company as a way of avoiding the anxiety generated by his neuroticized relationship with his mother.

Homosexual feelings in adolescents and young men may often also arise from excessive dependency, and other feelings of ineffectiveness or incompetency in male role behaviors; these feelings may produce an unconscious desire for a passive-dependent relationship with a strong man.

Some cautions are indicated. The intrafamilial dynamics just described, which correspond in a general way to the psychoanalytic theory of inadequate resolution of the oedipal conflict, do not necessarily lead to homosexual orientation in boys. It is important that physicians not accuse mothers or fathers of sexually seductive attitudes or behavior toward their children. Such accusations are extremely harmful. They impugn the intentions and integrity of parents, and even when only implied, make parents extremely guilty (or angry). Parents are then likely to reject further counsel from the physician and avoid further contact, reacting toward the child with increased psychologic distance owing to their anxiety, guilt, and self-disgust. The child suffers an attenuation of the relationship with parents and is in turn confused and guilty. The erotic aspects of parent-child relationships can usually be discussed only with professionals with special training and experience.

A physician who is concerned about the possibility of such an abnormal relationship between parents and child can approach the need for change by discussing the adverse effects of excessive dependency and the need to help the young boy become more grown up and autonomous. Suggestions about modesty in the home and about the privacy of adult sexual behavior can be given in the form of general counseling without the parents feeling accused of negligence or of seductive actions. It is important that both parents be involved in counseling around such issues, so that they can both understand what has been said and be supportive to each other, and so that the physician can assess the father's role in promotion or maintenance of the excessive closeness of mother and son, or assess the degree to which the father's relationship with his son is defective.

Some young boys who may be able to handle social contacts with girls become anxious or guilty or feel incompetent when the relationship begins to become sexualized. Such boys may also experience impotence in their early attempts at sexual activity with girls. The accompanying shame or feeling of failure may be augmented by the girl's reaction of disappointment or teasing. The boy may compare himself unfavorably with his peers' reports of sexual exploits. Such boys may turn to homosexual behavior as less anxiety-provoking than to risk further social or sexual failure with girls—a homosexual orientation by default.

Such boys and young men need professional help and referral to a mental health facility. Their parents need to be advised that such a referral is not a luxury, nor should they expect such boys simply to "outgrow" their shyness. Such referrals should at least promote opportunities for the adolescent to feel free to explore heterosexual orientation. He may otherwise be excluded from such options owing to paralyzing anxiety or to intermittent depression accompanying loss of self-esteem.

Boys of elementary school age who display effeminate traits (see below), who lack interest in boys as friends, or who have excessive attachment to their mothers and predominant interest in the activities of girls and women deserve an adequate psychiatric evaluation, and treatment if indicated.

Homosexuality in Girls. Knowledge of the development of homosexuality in girls and young women is more tenuous than for males. Women who as young adolescents become homosexually oriented often give a history of a very unsatisfying, non-nurturant relationship with their mothers, persistent from early childhood. Their mothers may have been aloof and distant, punitive and rejecting, or so involved elsewhere that the young girl felt a sense of rejection and abandonment. If mother or father shows an excessive interest in male siblings, the girl feels ashamed of or questions the value of her own sexual role. As she becomes older, she may become attracted to other girls for the opportunity they afford for nurturance, dependency, gratification, and attention.

Many girls go through a normal developmental stage marked by "crushes" on other girls. These positive emotional feelings can also involve inseparable social companionship and such physical contacts as hand holding. Such behavior is culturally more accepted in girls than in boys, girls being generally allowed much more latitude in physical interaction with other girls than boys with other boys. For some girls neither "crush" relationships nor such socially acceptable activities as dancing together or slumber parties provide any sexual or erotic stimulation. For others they may provide occasions for more deeply felt and strongly desired physical, erotic, or sexual contact with other girls. The eroticization of these relationships may both be exciting and fulfill needs for closeness and affection. A more firmly fixed homosexual orientation may evolve in a vulnerable girl.

Some homosexual girls may be extremely masculine in behavior, with hair cut short, and wearing such masculine clothes as leather jackets and heavy boots. They often quite explicitly reject all things feminine and female, but it is not necessarily correct to infer that they are homosexual in genital orientation. Some are asexual and have adopted the masculine façade as a way of avoiding any sexual or even social contact with boys owing to anxieties in this area. Such girls may have felt that male roles in their families were especially or excessively valued by parents, or may regard the male role in society as valued and prized over the female, and as perhaps essential to various social, academic, and economic rewards. They may also have underlying fears about passivity and dependency for which they compensate by adoption of the masculine gender role in behavior and dress, often in an exaggerated way. Some have had distant, unsatisfying relationships with their mothers and perhaps too close, affectionate, and eroticized relationships with their fathers. Anxiety arising from the sexual aspects of this relationship may have forced them to deny and abandon feminine sexuality as a way of denying incestuous wishes toward their fathers or competition with their mothers.

Management. There is probably a wide range of intrafamilial, interpersonal, and cultural dynamics besides the above that may give rise to homosexual orientation in girls or boys. It is important that the physician not conclude from apparent gender role or behavior that a masculinized girl or an effeminate boy has an underlying homosexual orientation. Children displaying these behaviors merit careful evaluation by a competent mental health professional. Their parents should be advised that punishment, castigation, shaming, or rejection will not support their children's attempts to struggle with whatever intrapsychic, interpersonal, or cultural conflicts they may have. Parents also need reassurance that they did not wish or intend for such behavior to develop. Homosexual orientations in their children are very threatening to parents, in terms both of their possible responsibility and of underlying uncertainties and fears about their own sexual identities. Some children act out the underlying unconscious or unfulfilled wishes of their parents, and this principle might extend to homosexual orientations; but such possibilities are not to be explored in the usual relationship between physician and the family. They require the evaluation and counsel of a fully trained and specifically qualified mental health professional.

EFFEMINACY IN BOYS

Effeminacy in boys may be noted by a physician or brought to his or her attention by an anxious parent. In either case, a full profile of the child's behavior should be reviewed before reassurance is given to the parent or a referral made to a psychiatrist. The attitudes and behaviors of parents are crucial to evaluation of the significance of this symptom. Newman distinguishes 2 categories of cross-sex behaviors: the 1st category includes cross-dressing, a verbal wish on a boy's part to be a girl, taking feminine roles in games and fantasies, and the imitation of the gestures of girls; the 2nd category includes dislike of rough or competitive games, disinterest in mechanical toys, preference for artistic activities, enjoyment of girls as playmates, gracefulness in body movements, and being teased as a sissy. Newman believes that the behaviors in the 2nd category do not themselves constitute serious effeminacy, but that the combination of any 1st category behavior with one or more 2nd category behaviors requires careful psychiatric evaluation and possible treatment. He found that for boys who wished to be girls the prognosis is good for reversal of the wish when therapy for child and parents is begun in early childhood, whereas after puberty, the prognosis for change is poor. Young boys exhibiting feminine behavior have a higher than normal incidence of serious problems of gender identity in adult life. The 2 parental factors that seem most commonly related to effeminacy in boys are a distant, disinterested father and a mother who covertly or overtly encourages the boy's identification with her, as revealed, for example, by her enjoying her son's dressing in feminine apparel.

INCESTUAL BEHAVIOR

Most *incestual behavior* involves sexual relations between a father and pubertal or teenage daughter. Incest is a form of child abuse and is required by law in many states to be reported by physicians to local child welfare authorities (Sec 2.67). Unfortunately, mothers are often reluctant to face consciously what they fear is taking place, and the daughter feels fearful and guilty. The fathers involved are manifesting arrested psychosexual development. The family needs not only to have the problem exposed and faced but to have the continuing support of the physician, since the revelation of incest can lead to the father's imprisonment, the mother's becoming dependent on public welfare, and the daughter's suffering great guilt and shame. Referral to a family counseling center is imperative, as incest is usually not a single event but a pattern of inappropriate sexual behavior between parent and child.

When younger children have been or are alleged to have been sexually molested by family members, the physician should try not to identify with the anger of a parent or both parents at the alleged molester; such parental anger may be a defensive reaction against feelings of guilt for not having prevented the event. The molested child may feel anger both at the molester and at the parents who failed to protect him or her. Fear and guilt are inevitable. The role of the physician is not simply to seek justice; that is left to public authorities. The physician can help alleviate unnecessary fear, conflict, and guilt by protecting the child from insistent or inappropriate questioning as well as preventing the child from developing an unhealthy attention-getting device. It is also helpful to point out to the parents that the child's understanding of the event is different from their own and that with adequate evaluation and counseling or other therapy, lasting adverse effects can generally be avoided.

EXHIBITIONISM

Exhibitionistic and voyeuristic activities (including undressing games, such as the "doctor" game) are common among preschool children. Exhibitionism diminishes through the early grade school years; intermittent episodes of voyeurism may occur as the child attempts to gain more knowledge about sexual activities, especially when parents have been unwilling or unable to impart sexual information.

Compulsive male exhibitionism may occur as a symptom of disturbance during adolescence. The adolescent exhibitionist is not only "seeking attention." He may be seeking reassurance as to his genital equipment and sexual identity, albeit in a perverse fashion; but the common underlying motive is frequently aggressive—the exhibitionist shocks and frightens his victims. The exhibitionist may also be reacting to covert seductive behavior or overly repressive sexual attitudes by parents. His unconscious guilt compels him into situations in which he will inevitably be caught and punished. Persistent exhibitionism generally indicates serious psychologic disturbance, and psychiatric intervention for both the adolescent and his family is essential. Overt sexual exhibitionism is seen less commonly in adolescent girls.

2.62 Psychoses in Childhood

Psychoses are rare but important disorders in children. They may be divided into those of early onset (infancy and preschool) and those of late onset (pre-adolescence and adolescence).

PSYCHOSES OF EARLY ONSET

Autism. Early infantile autism was first described by Kanner in 1943; it is characterized by profound impairment of the child's ability to relate to people, including his or her parents. Autism affects from 0.7–4.5/10,000 children. Typically, autistic children come to the attention of the physician because the emergence of speech is seriously delayed. Historical review may reveal that the autistic child did not appear to be "cuddly" as an infant, that social smiling was delayed or absent, and that the child did not assume anticipatory postures prior to being picked up.

The autistic child is withdrawn and may spend hours in solitary play, favorite toys and activities being preferred to human contact. Ritualistic behavior prevails and reflects the child's need to maintain a constant environment. The child has compulsive routines (e.g., the touching of objects in a prescribed sequence); disruption of routines may provoke tantrum-like rage reactions. Eye contact with others is minimal or absent, and the child is indifferent to the attempts of others to engage him or her in play. Head banging, teeth grinding, whirling, and rocking are noted. These activities may lead to self-mutilation of such degree that the child's life is in danger. Visual scanning of hand and finger movements, mouthing of objects, and rubbing of surfaces may indicate a heightened awareness and sensitivity to some stimuli, whereas diminished responses to pain and lack of startle responses to sudden loud noises reflect a lowered sensitivity to other stimuli. If speech is present, echolalia, pronominal reversal ("he" to refer to self, for example), nonsense rhyming, and other idiosyncratic language forms may predominate. IQ by conventional psychologic testing usually falls in the functionally retarded range, but deficits in language and socialization make it difficult to obtain an accurate estimate of the autistic child's intellectual potential. Some autistic children perform adequately in nonverbal tests, and those with developed speech may demonstrate adequate intellectual capacity. Occasionally, an autistic child may have an isolated, remarkable talent, analogous to that of the adult "idiot savant."

The cause of autism is speculative. Theories have centered on a variety of agents, including brain injury, constitutional vulnerability, developmental aphasia, and deficits in the reticular activating system. Recent evidence appears to indicate that autism is probably neurophysiologic in origin. Contrary to notions in vogue 20 yr ago, autism is not induced by parents.

Many different therapies have been attempted with autistic children, but success has been quite limited.

Some gains in acquisition of speech have been reported with approaches utilizing behavior therapy and operant conditioning. Behavior modification has also been useful in the control of destructive, self-mutilating, and nonfunctional perseverative behavior. Intensive psychotherapy has been of limited value. Tranquilizing medication is useful only in controlling aggressive outbursts. Treatment in a therapeutic residential setting may be indicated, especially when parents feel unable to manage the child at home.

The prognosis for autistic children is guarded. Some, especially those with speech, may grow up to live marginal, self-sufficient, albeit isolated, lives in the community; but for most, chronic placement in institutions is the ultimate outcome. Whether there is any relationship between autism and adult schizophrenia is not known.

Symbiotic Psychosis. Symbiotic psychosis is not so well defined a clinical syndrome as early infantile autism, and there is continuing controversy as to whether it exists as a separate entity. The disorder, as originally described by Mahler in 1952, has its onset between the ages of 2–5 yr. Early development is often described as normal, though traces of temperamental "oversensitivity" may have been noted in infancy. A precipitating event, such as the birth of a sibling, causes acute, sudden, panic-like anxiety, together with severe regression in social behavior and intellectual functioning. The symbiotic child clings intensely to his or her mother, but may also show marked dependent attachment to others in an indiscriminant manner. Speech, which may have been present prior to onset, becomes jargonistic and idiosyncratic, losing its communicative value. Regression may attain a state of "secondary autism," which is chronic and persistent, and resembles early infantile autism. Some of the same etiologic factors already described for autism have been imputed for the symbiotic psychosis, but the cause remains unknown. The prognosis is perhaps slightly more favorable than that of autism.

PSYCHOSES OF LATE ONSET

Psychotic reactions in older children tend more closely to resemble the psychotic reactions described in adults. Prominent signs and symptoms include disorders of thought, delusions, hallucinations, behavioral disorganization, withdrawal from interpersonal relations, and failure of reality testing. In contrast to the psychoses of early onset, psychoses occurring later in childhood occur in families with a higher than expected rate of schizophrenia. Prognosis is more favorable than in the types with early onset. Individual psychotherapy, family therapy, behavior modification, and tranquilizing medication are all useful therapeutic interventions. Hospitalization during periods of acute crises and prolonged residential treatment may also be indicated. The natural history includes periods of remission.

2.63   Prevention of Psychologic Disorders in the Sick Child

Whenever an illness alters children's functions or changes the way in which their parents or others feel about them, there may be psychologic disturbances. These effects can be minimized and psychogenic problems may be prevented through anticipatory guidance. The psychologic impact of illness may derive from discomfort, anxiety, and changes of sensorium (clouding of consciousness, hallucinations, delusions, and disorientation) and may be manifest as withdrawal, depression, irritability, and regression. Regression is normal for ill children and for ill adults as well. The caretaking process reinforces regression and can lead to prolongation of illness if excessive and inappropriate. The sick child withdraws interest from the outside world and invests it in self and his or her hurt. This is normal for a while, but parents should be advised to increase their expectations of the patient as clinical signs of illness subside.

2.64   PSYCHOSOMATIC INTERPLAY

Psychosocial factors modify responses to experiences, including illnesses. Every clinical phenomenon has reverberations at all organizational levels: molecular, anatomic, physiologic, intrapsychic, interpersonal, familial, and social. This leads to 3 important implications for the physician. (1) He or she must maintain an open attitude toward the cause of the patient's discomfort rather than a position that symptoms are *either* organic *or* psychologically determined. (2) The psychosocial aspects of illness should from the outset be examined along with the physiologic aspects. (3) The physician has the opportunity to act as a model for the parents and the child by showing an interest in the child's feelings and demonstrating that it is possible and appropriate to communicate discomfort in verbal, symbolic language, and not just in somatic language. A good opening question is "How are you feeling?" rather than "Where does it hurt?"

For the young child who is hospitalized potential challenges include coping with separation (Sec 2.44), adaptation to a new environment, adjustment to multiple caretakers, often association with very sick children, and sometimes experience in an intensive care unit, with submission to machines, to anesthesia, or to surgery. The most intense fears for the infant or the young child are created by separation from the parents, often felt as loss of love and/or abandonment. Bowlby has described the following sequence of reactions in hospitalized young children: angry protest with panic-like anxiety; depression and despair; eventual apathy and detachment. Older children may be more concerned with painful procedures, some of which carry the threat of bodily mutilation, and with the loss of control implicit in the use of anesthesia. Data indicate that repeated hospital admissions are significantly associated with disturbance in later childhood. All of these reactions may be reduced through preventive measures which ease adaptation to the hospital and lessen psychologic and behavioral consequences.

For the child under the age of 5–6 yr, the rooming-in of the parent is basic, if it is at all feasible. For the child whose future admission is arranged, an earlier visit to the hospital is very important: to see where he or she will be, to meet the people who will be caring for him or her, and to receive answers to questions as to what will happen. Creative and active recreational or socialization programs, with liberal or open visiting hours (including visits from siblings), and chances to act out feared procedures in play with dolls or mannequins are all helpful. The hospital staff should maintain sensitive, sympathetic, and accepting attitudes toward child and parent. Some nurses or physicians find themselves at times at odds with parents toward whom they take condescending or critical attitudes, overtly or unconsciously. Such nurses or physicians may feel, for example, that they are better able to meet the child's needs than parents who appear to be anxious or distraught or, alternatively, less concerned than circumstances seem to warrant. At these times, such nurses or physicians may convey to the parents an "I can be a better parent than you" feeling which may greatly impair the adjustment of the parents and child to hospitalization. Parents often already, albeit irrationally, feel guilty enough that their child became ill; they may react in a hostile manner to compensate for their feelings of guilt, or they may not be able to ask crucial questions for fear of "sounding stupid." The physician, nurse, and other professional persons all need to help to establish and to maintain effective communication and a climate of interest and affection for the child and family.

Ambulatory care presents particular problems in clinics in which patients receive discontinuous care from a series of physicians whose intercommunication is often negligible. Differences of language and culture may raise additional barriers to communication. Parents are often unable to verbalize their major concerns about their children. Recommendations for care may become inappropriate or irrelevant, and the compliance with which parents follow advice or directions becomes poor. At the end of any initial diagnostic or management activity, the physician should habitually inquire whether there are other things parents or children may wish to ask or talk about during this visit. In the busy emergency rooms of hospitals in urban centers, conflicting expectations exist between how professional staff expect the emergency room to be used (for trauma or for acute and serious illness of recent onset) and what the patients actually need (a local medical agency offering the services of a family-oriented physician). When these different expectations are critically examined, ways may be found to deal more effectively with the patterns of use of emergency services. The employment of ombudsmen in emergency rooms to whom patients and parents can turn for help has been shown often to clarify and resolve individual, social, and cultural differences and conflicts.

The *chronically or fatally ill child* presents special problems to the physician, some of which are discussed in Sec 2.81. Here we shall touch on certain preventive measures which can lessen the psychologic discomfort of child and parents during illness and prevent psychologic problems for surviving parents and siblings.

Every symptom experienced by children is vaguely or perhaps unconsciously perceived by them and by their parents as a threat to their physical integrity and, when carried to its extreme, as a threat to life and a reminder of their mortality. The more serious the clinical state, the greater the intensity of emotions aroused. The young child feels this primarily as discomfort, as an increase in manipulations, and perhaps as an anxiety that reflects parental anxiety. By the age of 9 yr, however, children begin to conceive of death as meaning more than just going away. By adolescence they can think of death in philosophic terms much like adults, albeit with limited experience.

In chronic illnesses that shorten life, such as cystic fibrosis, parents need the physician's early support in developing a relatively guilt-free understanding of the disease and how to help ameliorate it. They need guidance also in answering comfortably the child's questions about the disease. The young child will take most cues from the parent. With the older child, and especially the adolescent, parents must be prepared for the anger of the child at his or her fate. This anger will be less and easier to accept if the child has been given at each phase of illness such relatively consistent, accurate, and simple information as is needed and can be assimilated. The child needs both the parents' psychologic strengths and resources and the physician's availability and objectivity.

The role of the physician is difficult. He or she must stand for hope and for relief of discomfort, ready to help parents and child avoid emotionally crippling psychologic handicaps. For example, parents must be encouraged to meet their own needs, even when this requires temporary and perhaps recurrent separation from the child; at times this might help the child learn to tolerate frustration. Parents of chronically or fatally ill children may creatively support each other in groups meeting under the professional guidance of physician, psychologist, or social worker (Sec 2.81).

In more potentially fulminant lethal processes, such as leukemia, the intensity of parental anxiety, guilt, and despair may be greater than in more chronic illnesses. With most children over 9-10 yr of age it has been found most supportive to treat fatal illnesses such as leukemia factually with the child, so far as diagnosis and prognosis are concerned, but always offering realistic hope. Children do not usually ask the physician if or when they are going to die, though they may reveal their fears to others in the hospital. Young children primarily want to be reassured that their parents will not desert them and that they are loved. Both in and outside the hospital the team representing medical, nursing, psychologic, and social work disciplines, and perhaps others, should provide support. The primary physician also needs to stay involved and close to the child and to the clinical situation; he or she often knows the child and family best and can be most supportive. The hospital team needs frequent conferences for their own mutual support in the difficult situation of losing a patient. If objectivity is lost, physicians who feel they have failed may themselves become anxious or depressed and lose their supportive ability for patient and family.

After the death of a child the parents will need opportunities to talk out their feelings with the physician, one of whose goals should be to help them avoid psychologically encapsulating the lost child in an unmourned state (Sec 2.81). Many parents can be helped and comforted by being with and holding the dying infant or child or seeing and touching him or her after death.

Organ transplant in children has most often involved the kidney. Hemodialysis may precede renal transplant for varying lengths of time and begins in the hospital, but parents are often expected to learn to carry out this procedure at home. They may be ambivalent about being given control of a life-threatening process. The child receiving dialysis becomes psychologically dependent and often withdrawn. Bone marrow transplant also involves many psychologic considerations, such as donor relationships and the stress of isolation.

Family problems multiply with the question of who will donate an organ. If relatives are available as donors, there may be tension about who should "make the sacrifice." In some cases guilt may be relieved if the physician arbitrarily (but thoughtfully) makes this decision. A medical support team of carefully chosen staff is essential to decision making and continuing care. There is a high suicide rate among adults on hemodialysis, but it appears to be less traumatic to children, probably owing to the child's greater capacities for denial and acceptance of a support system. Adolescents are concerned with distortions of body image, which they cannot always express verbally. The physician needs the patience to listen (both to the stated and to the implied questions and misconceptions), to interpret, to set appropriate limits, and to help families and patients with technical details and with decision making.

2.65 Management of Established Psychologic Disorders

Planning Psychotherapy. When it has been determined that there is psychopathology in a child or family which requires intervention, the physician may develop and implement the therapeutic plan, or may refer to a more specialized level of care, if appropriate. Referral should not, however, end the role of the primary physician as the ongoing medical caretaker; there will be a need to assess the psychiatric intervention being offered and what the child or family appear to gain from it.

When referral for psychotherapy is considered, the resources in the community may include not only private practitioners in child psychiatry, social work, or psychology, but also child guidance agencies, child welfare and family service agencies, and children's psychiatric wards or hospitals. Some school districts have both psychologic evaluative and treatment services, as well as special classes. In justifying referral to child or parent, the simplest statement is the best, conveying the physician's confidence that it is necessary. The choice of treatment should be left to the consultant, with reassurance to the family and patient by the referring physician that close communication with the consultant will be maintained. The referring physician should ordinarily retain interest in and plan actively for the continuing medical care of the patient including their episodic illnesses. The child or parents should not be left with the feeling that "there is nothing more" the physician can do.

Treatment Methods Used by the Psychiatrist. In classic psychotherapy, the therapist works directly with the child in the task of resolving intrapsychic conflict. If intensive, it is called child psychoanalysis; if less intensive, it is termed child psychotherapy. Efforts may range from specific suggestions to the child for alteration of behavior to interpretive therapy aimed at giving the child an opportunity to change his or her intrapsychic structure and coping behavior. Some allegiance to the therapeutic effort is required on the part of the child. Parents may be involved in concurrent casework, may be seen occasionally, or sometimes not at all. The *psychodynamic* approach stresses the importance of having child and parents come to understand how past patterns of behavior have influenced current feelings and function. The *behavioral modification* approach stresses a complete analysis of the behavior of the child, in terms of the current behavior's immediate antecedents and consequences. Desirable behavioral changes are then brought about by changing the reward system.

A second approach involves working with the family as a group, in part or in whole, giving most attention to the relationships between family members, rather than to the inner emotional life of each individual. There is heavy stress on mending communication difficulties between family members and upon having each member learn what his or her healthy role is, accept it, gain acceptance for it, and function effectively within it.

A third approach involves group therapy for children, which is particularly useful for the child who has problems in development of social skills. Group therapy for preadolescent children tends to emphasize physical and other structured activities through which therapist and children alike can discover how they relate to each other and find ways to change.

Psychotherapy by the Nonpsychiatric Physician. Basic barriers to the involvement of the generalist or pediatrician in psychotherapeutic activities with children are a presumed lack of time and a lack of adequate conceptual background. The experience of successfully grappling with some of these problems will give many physicians the confidence that they *can* treat many of them.

The first therapeutic impact is conveyed by interest, in listening thoughtfully and in asking questions that evoke new thoughts in parents or children which help them to gain more objective views of their lives together as a family. This process is helped if parents can be given the opportunity from time to time to state at their level of understanding how *they* see a problem. When trusting and well-established relationships exist between physician and family, it may be appropriate to convey directly and simply some diagnostic impressions and suggestions for management. The physician may recommend that parents and children talk about their feelings about the problem and feel freer to express them.

Adolescents should usually be included in discussions which formulate the problem and suggest changes. Some supportive therapy of this kind can be viewed as representing a contract between physician, parents, and child, which indicates the actions to be taken by each party with respect to a focal point of concern. Progress toward solution of a problem is reviewed at successive visits with questions on how well or whether goals have been met and what new problems may have come up. If little or no improvement occurs, the primary physician may wish to seek the advice of a psychiatrist or refer the patient for more intensive study or therapy.

Psychotherapy by the nonpsychiatric physician emphasizes listening and interviewing, conceptualization of the problem (first to self and then to parents), exploration of problem-solving techniques with parents in one or more conferences, a willingness to stay involved as long as needed, and a readiness to accept limitations and to make referrals when these are appropriate.

Hospitalization. At times hospitalization of the disturbed or emotionally ill child in a general or pediatric hospital will be helpful or necessary, and may serve a number of functions. In the case of many psychosomatic disorders or of a suicidal or drugged adolescent, indications may be medical as well as psychiatric. If treatment of a child in a psychiatric hospital is thought to be necessary, consultation with a psychiatrist or a social agency is necessary in decision-making and planning. Admission to residential treatment reflects the family's decompensation as often as the child's.

2.66 PSYCHOPHARMACOLOGY

The use of drugs in modifying the behavior of children is controversial. The specific ways in which commonly used psychopharmaceutic agents act upon the central nervous system are generally unclear. Their effects on behavior are influenced by the maturity of the central nervous system, by intrapsychic and psychosocial factors, the personality or charisma of the physician prescribing them, and by the problem itself, the patient, the parents, the time of day given, and so on.

The psychopharmaceutic agents most commonly used outside of hospitals for the treatment of behavior disorders in ambulatory patients are listed in Table 2–

Table 2–14 PSYCHOPHARMACEUTIC AGENTS

MEDICATION	INDICATIONS	OUTPATIENT DOSAGE RANGE	SIDE EFFECTS AND TOXICITY
Major Tranquilizers			
Chlorpromazine (Thorazine) Thioridazine (Mellaril)	Severe anxiety, agitation, hyperactivity, agressivity, psychosis	Total daily dose: 30–150 mg, in divided doses	Sleepiness, irritability, dry mouth, tympanites, parkinsonism, dystonia, blood dyscrasias, hepatic abnormalities, cutaneous reactions, photosensitivity, alteration in pigment metabolism with high doses over prolonged time, cataracts, tardive dyskinesia
Haloperidol (Haldol)	Tics, psychotic conditions marked by agitation and aggressivity; not approved for children under 12 yr old	Total daily dose; 1–6 mg, in divided doses	
Stimulants			
Methylphenidate (Ritalin) Dextroamphetamine (Dexedrine)	Attention deficit (hyperactivity) syndrome; not approved for children under 6 yr old	Total daily dose: methylphenidate, 5–40 mg, in divided doses; dextroamphetamine, 2.5–20 mg, in divided doses	Anorexia, weight loss, irritability, abdominal pain, headache, insomnia, variable blood pressure response, tachycardia, increased hyperactivity; to date, addiction has not been reported; tolerance is rare
Antidepressants			
Imipramine (Tofranil)	Depressive states; not approved for children under 12 yr old; enuresis, age 6 yr and older (imipramine only)	For depression, 30–75 mg/day in divided doses; for enuresis, 25–50 mg at bedtime	Hypotension, hypertension, tachycardia, insomnia, restlessness, nightmares, ataxia, parkinsonism, dry mouth, blurred vision, blood dyscrasias
Amitryptyline (Elavil)		30 to 50 mg per day in divided doses	
Miscellaneous			
Diphenhydramine (Benadryl)	Hyperactivity, anxiety, sleep disorders	For hyperactivity, 25–150 mg/day, in divided doses; for sleep disorders, 25–50 mg at bedtime; can be given as elixir	Dry mucous membranes, skin rash

14, together with appropriate dosage schedules, indications, and contraindications. These medications are of 3 general types: stimulants, tranquilizers, and antidepressants.

Dextroamphetamine and methylphenidate for the child with an attention deficit syndrome are discussed in Sec 2.56 and 2.76.

Tranquilizers have been used in children, in doses proportional to those given to adults. Indications for their use, however, are not well established, especially in young children. In disturbed adolescents, these drugs may be used in much the same manner as they are in young adults. The use of tranquilizers should generally be reserved for children with serious disorders, characterized by *excessive* agitation, aggressiveness, anxiety, or psychosis.

Recent studies indicate that childhood depression is much more common than has been supposed in the past. With the exception of imipramine, which has been extensively used in the management of enuresis, there is little experience with antidepressant drugs in children (Sec 2.53).

During treatment with major tranquilizing and antidepressant drugs, baseline and periodic laboratory examinations should be obtained. These should include complete blood counts (including differential and platelet counts), studies of liver enzymes, and tests for urobilinogen in urine.

As some parents are adamantly opposed to the use of psychotropic drugs, the physician contemplating their use in children should make sure of the parental attitudes. If drugs are to be used, it should be for as short a period as possible. As in any clinical disorder, the physician should avoid using multiple medications and should not shift back and forth from one medication to another when no immediate response occurs. All psychotropic medications can have significant biochemical effects on the developing child, and it is important that the physician give an adequate and appropriate explanation to the parents and child about the rationale for medication. There is no "magic" pill that will immediately alter a child's behavior; medication is at best a sometimes useful adjunct to the child's overall therapeutic management. Drugs are certainly not a substitute for the human interaction and psychodynamic techniques that have been discussed above.

MARC A. FORMAN
WILLIAM H. HETZNECKER
JOHN M. DUNN

General

Chess S: An Introduction to Child Psychiatry. New York, Grune & Stratton, 1975.
Erikson EH: Childhood and Society. Ed 2. New York, WW Norton, 1963.
Flavell JH: The Developmental Psychology of Jean Piaget. Princeton, N.J., Von Nostrand, 1963.
Freud A: Normality and Pathology in Childhood. New York, International Universities Press, 1965.
Hetznecker W, Forman MA: On Behalf of Children. New York, Grune & Stratton, 1974.

Kessler JW: Psychopathology of Childhood. Englewood Cliffs, NJ, Prentice-Hall, 1965.

Rutter M: Helping Troubled Children, New York, Plenum Press, 1975.

Rutter M (ed): Scientific Foundations of Developmental Psychiatry. London, William Heinemann Medical Books Ltd, 1980.

Role of Parents in Enhancing the Development of the Well Child

Becker W: Parents Are Teachers. Urbana, Ill, Research Press, 1971.

Brazelton TB: Early parent-infant reciprocity. In: Vaughan VC III, Brazelton TB (eds): The Family—Can It Be Saved? Chicago, Year Book Medical Publishers, 1976.

Carey WB: A simplified method for measuring infant temperament. J Pediatr 77:188, 1970.

Deur JL, Parke RD: The effects of inconsistent punishment on aggression in children. Dev Psychobiol 2:403, 1970.

Dodson F: How to Parent. Los Angeles, Nash Publishing Corp, 1970.

Haselkorn F (ed): Family Planning: A Source Book and Case Material for Social Work Education. New York, Council on Social Work Education, 1971.

Kagan J, Moss HA: Birth to Maturity: A Study in Psychological Development. New York, John Wiley & Sons, 1962.

Kohlberg L: Stages of moral development as the basis for moral education. In: Beck C, Sullivan E, Crittendon D (eds): Moral Education. Toronto, University of Toronto Press, 1971.

Maccoby EE: The development of moral values and behavior in childhood. In: Clausen JA (ed): Socialization and Society. Boston, Little, Brown, 1968.

Nelson SH: Sex, family planning and population. In: Lieberman J (ed): Mental Health: The Public Health Challenge. Washington DC, American Public Health Association, 1975.

Parke RD: The role of punishment in the socialization process. In: Hoppe RA, Milton GA, Simmel EC (eds): Early Experience and the Process of Socialization. New York, Academic Press, 1970.

Siegel E: The biological effects of family planning—preventive pediatrics: The potential of family planning. J Med Educ 44:74, 1969.

Smith BM: Competence and socialization. In: Clausen JA (ed): Socialization and Society. Boston, Little, Brown, 1968.

Thomas A, Chess S, Birch HG: Temperament and Behavior Disorders in Children. New York, New York University Press, 1968.

White RW: Motivation reconsidered: The concept of competence. Psychol Rev 66:297, 1959.

Specific Developmental Issues

Aronfreed J: Conduct and Conscience: The Socialization of Internalized Control over Behavior. New York, Academic Press, 1968.

Bowlby J: Attachment. New York, Basic Books, 1969.

Bowlby J: Attachment and Loss. Vol II, Separation. New York, Basic Books, 1973.

Brown GW, Harris T: Social Origins of Depression. London, Tavistock Publications, 1978.

Caldwell BM, Wright CM, Honig AS, et al: Infant day care and attachment. Am J Orthopsychiatr 40:397, 1970.

Douvan E, Adelson Y: The Adolescent Experience. New York, John Wiley & Sons, 1966.

Ehrhardt AA, Money J: Progestin-induced hermaphroditism; IQ and psychosexual identity in a study of ten girls. J Sex Res 3:83, 1967.

Green R, Money J (eds): Transsexualism and Sex Reassignment. Baltimore, Johns Hopkins Press, 1969.

Green R: Sexual identity of 37 children raised by homosexual and transsexual parents. Am J Psychiatr 135:692, 1978.

Group for the Advancement of Psychiatry Committee on Adolescence: Normal Adolescence: Its Dynamics and Import. New York, GAP, 1968.

Hutt C: Biological bases of psychological sex differences. Am J Dis Child 132:170, 1978.

Kagan J: Acquisition and significance of sex typing and sex role identity. In: Hoffman ML, Hoffman LW (eds): Review of Child Development Research. Vol I. New York, Russell Sage Foundation, 1964.

Masterson JF: The psychiatric significance of adolescent turmoil. Am J Psychiatr 124:107, 1968.

Money J: Influence of hormones on sexual behavior. Ann Rev Med 16:67, 1965.

Money J: Psychosexual differentiation. In: Money J (ed): Sex Research; New Developments. New York, Holt, Rinehart and Winston, 1965.

Offer D: The Psychological World of the Teenager: A Study of Normal Adolescent Boys. New York, Basic Books, 1969.

Offer D, Offer JL: Profiles of normal adolescent girls. Arch Gen Psychiatr 19:513, 1968.

Ounstead C, Taylor DC (eds): Gender Differences: Their Ontogeny and Significance. Edinburgh, Churchill Livingstone, 1972.

Reinisch JM, Karow WG: Prenatal exposure to synthetic progestins and estrogens: Effects on human development. Arch Sex Behav 6:257, 1977.

Reiss IL: The Social Context of Premarital Sexual Permissiveness. New York, Holt, Rinehart and Winston, 1967.

Rutter M, Chadwick OFD, Yule W: Adolescent turmoil: Fact or fiction? J Child Psychol Psychiatr 17:35, 1976.

Rutter M: Normal psychosexual development. J Child Psychol Psychiatr 11:259, 1971.

Schofield M: The Sexual Behavior of Young People. Boston, Little, Brown, 1965.

Schooler C: Birth order effects: Not here, not now. Psychol Bull 78(3):161, 1972.

Schwartz J, Strickland RG, Krolick G: Infant day care: Behavioral effects at preschool age. Dev Psychol 10:502, 1974.

Sibinga MS, Friedman CJ: Restraint and speech. Pediatrics 48:116, 1971.

Sorensen RC: Adolescent Sexuality in Contemporary America. New York, World Publishing, 1972.

Thomas A, Chess S: Evolution of behavior disorders in adolescence. Am J Psychiatr 133:539, 1976.

Zelnik M, Kantner JF: Sexual activity, contraceptive use and pregnancy among metropolitan-area teenagers: 1971–1979. Family Planning Perspect 12:230, 1980.

Specific Environmental Issues

Anthony S: The Discovery of Death in Childhood and After. New York, Basic Books, 1971.

Eisenberg L: The sins of the fathers: Urban decay and social pathology. Am J Orthopsychiatr 32:5, 1962.

Eron LD, Heusmann LR, Lefkowitz MM, et al: How learning conditions in early childhood—including mass media—relate to aggression in late adolescence. Am J Orthopsychiatr 44:421, 1974.

Gardner RA: The Boys and Girls Book About Divorce. New York, Science House, 1970.

Kantor MB: Internal migration and mental illness. In: Plog SC, Edgerton RB (eds): Changing Perspectives in Mental Illness. New York, Holt, Rinehart and Winston, 1969.

Maluccio A, Fein E, Hamilton J, et al: Beyond permanency planning. Child Welfare 59:515, 1980.

Miller JBM: Children's reactions to the death of a parent: A review of the psychoanalytic literature. J Am Pyschoanal Assoc 19:697, 1971.

Nagy M: The child's meaning of death. In: Feifel H (ed): The Meaning of Death. New York, McGraw-Hill, 1959.

Wallerstein JS, Kelly JB: Surviving the Breakup: How Children Actually Cope with Divorce. New York, Basic Books, 1980.

Wolfenstein M: How is mourning possible? In The Psychoanalytic Study of the Child. New York, International Universities Press, 1966.

Assessment and Interviewing

Beiser HR: Psychiatric diagnostic interviews with children. Am Acad Child Psychiatr 1:656, 1962.

Rich J: Interviewing Children and Adolescents. London, Macmillan, 1968.

Schulman JL: Management of Emotional Disorders in Pediatric Practice. Chicago, Year Book Medical Publishers, 1967.

Simmons JE: Interviewing. In: Green M, Haggerty R (eds): Ambulatory Pediatrics. Philadelphia, WB Saunders, 1968.

Psychosocial Problems

Adams RM, Kocsis JJ, Estes RE: Soft neurological signs in learning-disabled children and controls. Am J Dis Child 128:614, 1974.

Amann MG, Werry JS: Methylphenidate in children: Effects upon cardiorespiratory function. Int J Ment Health 4:119, 1975.

American Psychiatric Association: Diagnostic and Statistical Manual of Mental Disorders. Ed 3. DSM-III, Washington, 1980.

Bandura A: Aggression: A Social Learning Analysis. Englewood Cliffs, NJ, Prentice-Hall, 1973.

Berg I: Day wetting in children. J Child Psychol Psychiatr 16:289, 1975.

Black P, Jeffries JJ, Blumer D, et al: The post-traumatic syndrome in children. In: Walker AE, Caueness WF, Critchley M (eds): The Late Effects of Head Injury. Springfield, Ill, Charles C Thomas, 1969.

Blinder BJ, Freeman DM, Stunkard AJ: Behavior therapy of anorexia nervosa: Effectiveness of activity as a reinforcer of weight gain. Am J Psychiatr 126:1093, 1970.

Camp BW, Blom GE, Herbert F, et al: "Think aloud": A program for developing self-control in young aggressive boys. J Abnorm Child Psychol 5:157, 1977.

Campbell SB: Mother-child interaction: A comparison of hyperactive, learning-disabled, and normal boys. Am J Orthopsychiatr 45:51, 1975.

Chess S: Autism in children with congenital rubella. J Autism Child Schizo 1:33, 1971.

Clements SD, Peters JE: Minimal brain dysfunction in the school age child. Arch Gen Psychiatr 6:185, 1962.

Conners CK: A teacher rating scale for use in drug studies with children. J Psychiatr 126:884, 1969.

Cytryn L, McKnew DH Jr, Bunney WE Jr: Diagnosis of depression in childhood: A reassessment. Am J Psychiatr 137:22, 1980.

Cytryn L, McKnew DH Jr, Logue M, et al: Biochemical correlates of affective disorders in children. Arch Gen Psychiatr 31:659, 1974.

Denson R, Nanson JL, McWatters MA: Hyperkinesis and maternal smoking. Can Psychiatr J 20:183, 1975.

Douglas VI: Stop, look, and listen: The problem of sustained attention and impulse control in hyperactive and control children. J Behav Science 4:259, 1972.

Dubey DR: Organic factors in hyperkinesis: A critical evaluation. Am J Orthopsychiatr 46:353, 1976.

Eron L, Walden L, Lefkowitz M: Learning of Aggression in Children. Boston, Little, Brown, 1971.

Fish B: The 'one child, one drug' myth of stimulants in hyperkinesis. Arch Gen Psychiatr 25:193, 1971.

Gittleman-Klein R, Klein DF: Controlled imipramine treatment of school phobia. Arch Gen Psychiatr 25:204, 1971.

Graham FK, Ernhardt CB, Thurston CB, et al: Development three years after perinatal anoxia and other potentially damaging newborn experiences. Psychol Monographs 76:1, 1962.

Graham PJ, Rutter M: Psychiatric disorders in the young adolescent—a follow-up study. Proc R Soc Med 66:1226, 1973.

Guilleminault C, Anders JF: Sleep disorders in children. In: Schulman I (ed): Advances in Pediatrics, Vol 22. Chicago, Year Book Medical Publishers, 1976.

Hackney IM, Hanley WB, Davidson W, et al: Phenylketonuria: Mental development, behavior and termination of low phenylalanine diet. J Pediatr 72:646, 1968.

Heston LL, Shields J: Homosexuality in twins. Arch Gen Psychiatr 18:149, 1968.

Hetznecker W, Forman MA: Developmental issues and psychosocial problems in children: I. Normal development and minor behavioral problems. II. More serious behavioral and performance disorders. In: Smith DW (ed): Introduction to Clinical Pediatrics. Ed 2. Philadelphia, WB Saunders, 1977.

Kashani JH, Husain A, Shekim WO, et al: Current perspectives on childhood depression: An overview. Am J Psychiatr 138:143, 1981.

Keith PR: Night terrors. J Am Acad Child Psychiatr 14:477, 1975.

Lapouse R, Monk MA: An epidemiologic study of behavioral characteristics in children. Am J Pub Health 48:1134, 1958.

Lebovitz P: Feminine behavior in boys: Aspects of outcome. Am J Psychiatr 128:10, 1972.

Levy D: Oppositional syndromes and oppositional behavior. In: Harrison SI, McDermott JJ: Childhood Psychopathology. New York, International Universities Press, 1972.

MacKeith R, Sandler J (eds): Psychosomatic Aspects of Paediatrics. London, Pergamon Press, 1961.

Malmquist C: Depression in childhood and adolescence. N Engl J Med 284:887, 1971.

Mattson A, Seese LR, Harkins JW: Suicidal behavior as a child psychiatric emergency. Arch Gen Psychiatr 20:100, 1969.

McIntire MS, Angle CR (eds): Suicide Attempts in Children and Youth. Hagerstown, Md, Harper & Row, 1980.

Meichenbaum DH, Goodman J: Training impulsive children to talk to themselves: A means of developing self-control. J Abnorm Child Psychol 77:115, 1971.

Minuchin S: Families and Family Therapy. Cambridge, Harvard University Press, 1974.

Newman LE: Treatment for the parents of feminine boys. Am J Psychiatr 133:683, 1976.

Pfeffer CR, Conte HR, Plutchik R, et al: Suicidal behavior in latency-age children: An empirical study. J Am Acad Child Psychiatr 18:679, 1979.

Poznanski E, Zrull JP: Childhood depression; clinical characteristics of overtly depressed children. Arch Gen Psychiatr 23:8, 1970.

Puig-Antich J, Blau S, Marx N, et al: Prepubertal major depressive disorder: A pilot study. J Am Acad Child Psychiatr 17:695, 1978.

Rutter M: Brain damage syndromes in childhood: Concepts and findings. J Child Psychol Psychiatr 18:1, 1977.

Safer D, et al: Depression of growth in children on stimulant drugs. N Engl J Med 287:217, 1972.

Safer DJ, Allen RP, Barr E: Growth rebound after termination of stimulant drugs. J Pediatr 86:113, 1975.

Satterfield JM, Cantwell DP, Satterfield BT: Pathophysiology of the hyperactive child syndrome. Arch Gen Psychiatr 31:839, 1974.

Schildkraut JJ, Kety SS: Biogenic amines and emotions. Science 156:21, 1967.

Schulterbrandt JG, Raskin A (eds): Depression in Childhood: Diagnosis, Treatment and Conceptual Models. New York, Raven Press, 1977.

Scott JP: Biology and human aggression. Am J Orthopsychiatr 40:568, 1970.

Shaffer D: Psychiatric aspects of brain injury in childhood: A review. Dev Med Child Neurol 15:211, 1973.

Shaffer D: Suicide in childhood and early adolescence. J Child Psychol Psychiatr 15:275, 1974.

Shaffer D, McNamara N, Pincus JH: Controlled observations on patterns of activity, attention, and impulsivity in brain-damaged and psychiatrically disturbed boys. Psychosom Med 4:4, 1974.

Spitz R: Anaclitic depression. In: Eissler RS (ed): Psychoanalytic Study of the Child. Vol II. New York, International Universities Press, 1946.

Spitz R: Hospitalism. In: Eissler RS (ed): Psychoanalytic Study of the Child. Vols I and II. New York, International Universities Press, 1945.

Teicher JD, Jacobs J: Adolescents who attempt suicide. Am J Psychiatr 122:1248, 1966.

Weinberg WA, Rutman J, Sullivan L, et al: Depression in children referred to an educational diagnostic center: Diagnosis and treatment. J Pediatr 83:1065, 1973.

Weiss G, Hechtman L: The hyperactive child syndrome. Science 205:1348, 1979.

Wender PH: Minimal Brain Dysfunction in Children. New York, Wiley Interscience, 1971.

Werry J: The use of psychotropic drugs in children. J Am Acad Child Psychiatr 16:446, 1977.

West DJ: Homosexuality. Ed 3. London, Duckworth, 1968.

Childhood Psychoses

Kanner L: Early infantile autism. Am J Orthopsychiatr 19:416, 1949.

Kolvin I: Psychoses in childhood. In: Rutter M (ed): Infantile Autism—Concepts, Characteristics, and Treatment. London, Churchill, 1971.

Mahler MS, Furer M, Settlage CF: Severe emotional disturbances in childhood psychoses. In: Arieti S (ed): American Handbook of Psychiatry. Vol 1. New York, Basic Books, 1959.

Ornitz EM, Ritvo ER: The syndrome of autism: A critical review. Am J Psychiatr 133:609, 1976.

Prevention of Psychologic Disorders of the Sick Child

Bergman T: Children in the Hospital. New York, International Universities Press, 1966.

Douglas JWB: Early hospital admissions and later disturbances of behavior and learning. Dev Med Child Neurol 17:456, 1975.

Lansky SB: Childhood leukemia. J Am Acad Child Psychiatr 13:499, 1974.

Prugh DG: Toward an understanding of psychosomatic concepts in relation to illness in children. In: Solnit AJ, Provence SA (eds): Modern Perspectives in Child Development; in Honor of Milton JE Senn. New York, International Universities Press, 1963.

Quinton D, Rutter M: Early hospital admissions and later disturbances of behavior: An attempted replication of Douglas' findings. Dev Med Child Neurol 18:447, 1976.

Robertson J: Young Children in Hospitals. New York, Basic Books, 1958.

Sampson TF: The child in renal failure: Emotional impact of treatment on the child and his family. J Am Acad Child Psychiatr 14:462, 1975.

Solnit AJ, Green M: Psychologic considerations in the management of deaths on pediatric hospital services. I. The doctor and the child's family. Pediatrics 24(1):106, 1959.

Tisza VB, Dorsett P, Morse J: Psychological implications of renal transplantation. J Am Acad Child Psychiatr 15:709, 1976.

Film: You See, I Had a Life. The Eccentric Circle Cinema Workshop, PO Box 1981, Evanston, Ill, 60204.

Management of Established Psychologic Disorders

Balint M: The Doctor, His Patient and the Illness. New York, International Universities Press, 1957.

Eisenberg L: Principles of drug therapy in child psychiatry with special reference to stimulant drugs. Am J Orthopsychiatr 41:371, 1971.

Wolberg LR: The technique of short-term psychotherapy. In: Wolberg LR (ed): Short-Term Psychotherapy. New York, Grune & Stratton, 1965.

2.67 ABUSE AND NEGLECT OF CHILDREN

Child abuse includes any maltreatment of children or adolescents by their parents, guardians, or other caretakers. Physicians must be able to recognize abused children and confirm the diagnosis; recognition is especially important in the first 6 mo of life because the risk of a fatal outcome is high if the diagnosis is missed at this age. Physicians have 3 main responsibilities toward abused children: detection, reporting, and prevention. In all 50 states the law requires that physicians report suspected cases of child abuse and neglect to a local child protective agency and protects physicians from liability if their suspicions should prove unfounded.

THE SPECTRUM OF CHILD ABUSE AND NEGLECT

The most common types of child abuse and neglect seen by physicians are approximately 80% physical abuse, 15% sexual abuse, and 5% failure to thrive due to underfeeding. Physical abuse or nonaccidental trauma inflicted by a caretaker may include bruises, burns, head injuries, fractures, and the like; their severity can range from minor bruises to fatal subdural hematomas. Corporal punishment that causes bruises or leads to an injury that requires medical treatment is outside the range of normal punishment; reckless and dangerous punishment (e.g., kicking a child in the abdomen) is also unacceptable, even if injuries do not occur. *Nutritional neglect* or deliberate underfeeding is the most common cause of underweight in infancy. Over half of the cases of failure to thrive may be due to this single cause. *Sexual abuse* is usually family-related (incest) and is probably the most unrecognized type of child abuse.

Intentional drugging or poisoning includes giving a child a prescription drug that is harmful and not intended for children, or sharing illegal drugs with them. *Neglect of medical care* recommended for a child with a treatable chronic disease may lead to serious deterioration in the condition and require court-enforced supervision or placement in foster care. Court orders to hospitalize and treat are also needed when an emergency exists for the child that parents will not acknowledge or will not permit to be treated. Accidents to children from *neglect of safety* constitute child neglect if there is gross lack of supervision, especially if the child involved is under 3 yr of age. Rare types of child abuse also include hypernatremic dehydration due to water deprivation, hypothermia due to cold water punishment, near drowning following forced immersion, intentional suffocation, deprivational dwarfism, and kwashiorkor due to cult diets.

Emotional abuse is the continual rejection or scapegoating of a child by caretakers; severe verbal abuse is usually part of this picture. Emotional abuse is difficult to prove. The diagnostic criteria include severe psychopathology in the child, as determined by a psychiatrist, with the persistent refusal by the parents of treatment for the child. Psychologic terrorism (e.g., locking a child in a dark cellar or threats of mutilation) may also occur.

2.68 PHYSICAL ABUSE

Epidemiology. During childhood 1–2% of children in the United States are abused, an incidence of approximately 700 new cases/1,000,000 population/yr. If physical neglect cases were included, these figures would be much higher. Approximately 10% of injuries seen in a hospital emergency room in children under 5 yr of age are due to abuse. The mortality is about 3% or 2000 deaths/yr. The victims of physical abuse are estimated to be one third under 1 yr of age, one third from 1–6 yr of age, and one third over 6 yr. Premature infants have a 3-fold greater risk of abuse.

Etiology. The abuser is a related caretaker in 90% of cases, a male friend of the mother in 5%, an unrelated babysitter in 4%, and a sibling in 1%. Parents who abuse their children come from all ethnic, geographic, religious, educational, occupational, and socioeconomic groups. Groups living in poverty may have an increased incidence of child abuse because of the increased number of crises in their lives (e.g., unemployment or overcrowding) and because they have limited access to economic or social resources. An increased incidence of physical abuse has been noted on military bases. The presence of spouse abuse doubles the frequency of child abuse. Women are more likely to be involved in abuse than are men, but this difference is not present in families in which the fathers are home, unemployed.

Over 90% of abusing parents have neither psychotic nor criminal personalities; they tend to be lonely, unhappy, angry adults under tremendous stress. They injure their children in anger after being provoked by some misbehavior and often themselves experienced physical abuse as children. They usually believe that all misbehavior is deliberate and that severe punishment is necessary in teaching children to respect authority. If the abuse profile is absent in the parents, suspicion should turn to babysitters and other parties.

The occurrence of physical abuse requires not only the particular parent but also a specific child and occasion. The child often has characteristics that make him or her provocative such as negativism or a difficult temperament; some of the more offensive misbehaviors are intractable crying, wetting, soiling, and spilling. The most common family crises include loss of a job, eviction, marital strife or upheavals, birth of a sibling, or physical exhaustion.

Clinical Manifestations. Many cases of physical abuse are first suspected because the injury is unexplained. Parents usually know to the moment where and when their children were hurt. More commonly an explanation is offered, but it is implausible. Inconsistencies between the history offered of a minor accident and the physical findings of a major injury, or between the history and the child's developmental level, are common. There is often delay in seeking medical help for abused children. Parents normally bring their injured children immediately for examination; Smith found that 40% of abused children were not brought to medical attention until the morning after the injury, another 40% 1–4 days later.

Bruises, welts, lacerations, and scars identify physical abuse. Bruises confined to the buttocks and lower back are almost always related to punishment. Finger and thumb prints may be found on the arms where a child has been forcefully grabbed. A slap mark leaves a bruise on the cheek with 2–3 parallel lines running through it. Attempts to silence a screaming child with impatient, forced attempts at feeding may lead to bruising of the upper lip and frenulum. Human bite marks are distinctive, paired, crescent-shaped bruises facing each other. When a blunt instrument is used in punishment, a bruise or welt will often resemble it in shape. Loop marks or scars on the skin are secondary to a doubled-over cord or rope. Lash marks are seen after beating with a belt, tree branch, or hard-edged ruler. Choke marks may be seen on the neck, or circumferential marks of ropes tied around the ankles or wrists. Traumatic alopecia may occur when the hair is yanked; the scalp has a normal appearance and the damaged hairs are broken off at varying lengths. A subgaleal hematoma may form under the site. Bruises and scars may be found at various stages of healing. The most common sites of accidental bruises are over the forehead, anterior tibia, and other bony prominences. Petechiae of the face and shoulders may follow intense retching, coughing, or crying. A mongolian spot may be mistaken for a bruise, but the color is blue-gray without any red hue.

Approximately 10% of cases of physical abuse involve burns. Hot solid burns are easiest to diagnose. These are usually 2nd-degree burns without blister formation and involve only one surface of the body. The shape of the burn is pathognomonic if the child is held against a heating grate or electric hot plate. Cigarette burns produce circular, punched-out lesions of uniform size. These are often found on the hands or feet and may be confused with bullous impetigo.

Hot water burns are the most common type of inflicted burn; blisters are usually present. A dunking burn occurs when a parent holds the thighs against the abdomen and places the buttocks and perineum in scalding water as punishment for enuresis or resistance to toilet training. This results in a circular type of burn restricted to the buttocks. With deeper, forced immersions, the scald extends to a clear-cut water level on the thighs and waist. The hands and feet are spared, which is incompatible with falling into a tub or turning on the hot water while in the bathtub. Forcible immersion of a hand or foot as punishment can be suspected when a burn goes well above the wrist or ankle. Toxic epidermal necrolysis can be confused with scalds.

Subdural hematoma is the most dangerous inflicted injury, often causing death or serious sequelae. Infants often present with coma, convulsions, and increased intracranial pressure. Subdural hematomas may be associated with skull fractures secondary to a direct blow to the head, but over one half of the cases have no skull fracture. They may also occur without bruises or swelling of the scalp. These cases are probably the result of violent, whiplash-type, shaking injuries; the rapid acceleration and deceleration of the head as it bobs about may lead to tearing of the bridging cerebral veins with bleeding into the subdural space, usually bilaterally. Retinal hemorrhages are nearly always present, and there may be grab mark bruises of the upper extremities, shoulders, or chest.

Intra-abdominal injuries are the second most common cause of death in battered children. Affected children may present with recurrent vomiting, abdominal distention, absent bowel sounds, localized tenderness, or shock. Because the abdominal wall is flexible, the force of the blow is usually absorbed by the internal organs and the overlying skin is free of bruises. The most common finding is a ruptured liver or spleen. Much rarer are tears or other injuries of the small intestine at sites of ligamental support such as the duodenum and proximal jejunum. Intramural hematomas at these sites can lead to temporary obstruction. Chylous ascites and pseudocyst of the pancreas have been reported.

Laboratory Data. Screening tests for a bleeding diathesis should be obtained if medically indicated or if the parents deny the possibility of inflicted injury or give a history of easy bruisability.

When physical abuse is suspected in a child under 5 yr of age, a roentgenologic bone survey consisting of films of skull, thorax, and long bones should be made; pelvis and spine films may be indicated if any of the preceding films are positive. These films are of great diagnostic value since the clinical findings of fracture often disappear in 6–7 days even without orthopedic care. For children over the age of 5 yr roentgenograms need be obtained only if there is bone tenderness or a limited range of motion on physical examination. If films of a tender site are initially negative, they should be repeated in 2 wk to detect any calcification of subperiosteal bleeding or nondisplaced epiphyseal separations that may have occurred. Bone trauma is found in 10–20% of physically abused children.

Most inflicted fractures are due to wrenching or pulling injuries that damage the metaphysis, and the classic early finding is a chip fracture where a corner of the metaphysis of a long bone is torn off, along with the epiphysis and periosteum. From 10–14 days later calcification of the subperiosteal bleeding becomes visible at the periphery. By 4–6 wk after the injury the subperiosteal calcification will be solid and start to smooth out and remodel. Inflicted fractures of the shaft are usually spiral rather than transverse, and spiral fractures of the femur prior to the age of walking are usually inflicted. Fractures of the ribs, scapula, or sternum are unusual and should arouse suspicion of nonaccidental trauma.

Diagnosis. A tentative diagnosis of physical abuse should be made if an injury is unexplained or inadequately explained. Often a child over the age of 3 yr will be able to tell a sensitive and skillful interviewer that a particular adult hurt him or her. Certain bruises, burns, and scars are pathognomonic, and subdural hematomas do not occur spontaneously. Roentgenographic findings of chip fractures or multiple bony injuries at different stages of healing, implying repeated assaults, are also diagnostic.

Rare bone diseases such as scurvy and syphilis may resemble nonaccidental bone trauma, but the bony changes are symmetrical. Children with osteogenesis imperfecta, severe osteomalacia, or sensory deficits (e.g., myelomeningocele or paraplegia) have an increased incidence of pathologic fractures, but not of the metaphysis.

Treatment. A child suspected of being abused or neglected should usually be hospitalized, regardless of the extent of injuries, in order to protect the child until evaluation of the family with respect to the safety of the home is complete. The reason given to the parents for hospitalization can be that the injuries need to be watched or that further studies are needed; incriminating questions should be kept to a minimum. If the parents refuse hospitalization, a police or court holding order should be obtained. Some cases of child abuse can be safely evaluated without hospitalization when the child can be placed in an emergency receiving home or the person inflicting the trauma no longer has access to the child. Children over age 6 with mild injuries may also be evaluated in the home under certain circumstances.

Once the child is in the hospital, the medical and surgical problems should receive appropriate care. The parents should be told by the physician that inflicted injury is suspected and of the legal obligation to report it before it is reported. It should be emphasized that this problem is treatable, that a child welfare agency will be involved (not usually the police), that the matter will be shared only with professional persons (not appear in the newspapers), and that everyone's goal is not to punish anyone but to help the parents find better ways of dealing with their child's needs. The protective service agency should then be contacted immediately by telephone; required written reports should be sent subsequently. Siblings should have a full examination within 12 hr of the reported child abuse in the family. Approximately 20% of them will also have signs of physical abuse.

Feeling angry with abusing parents is natural, but expressing the anger is very damaging to rapport and makes the cooperation of parents less likely. Repeated interrogations, confrontations, and accusations must be avoided. The parents should be encouraged to visit their children, and the hospital staff must do their best to be courteous and helpful. The primary physician should see the parents or telephone them daily. An evaluation by hospital social services should be obtained to determine the nature of the family and environmental problems and the safety of the home. A psychiatric evaluation may be appropriate in some instances.

Every hospital caring for children should designate a group of professional persons to respond to the needs of abused or neglected children and their families. The group should include a pediatric consultant, a hospital social worker, a pediatric nurse, a psychologist or psychiatrist, and an administrator. There should be clearly defined liaisons with public agencies and the courts, and legal consultants should be available. Within 1 wk of admission of any child for abuse or neglect, evaluations should be completed and the team should meet with the child's physician and nurse, the child protective service representative, and, as appropriate, the police or any other community agencies involved with the family, to decide on the best immediate and long-range plans for each problem.

The pediatrician is responsible for coordinating the health care of the abused child who needs more intensive surveillance and well-child care than the average child as well as care of any chronic disabilities resulting from physical abuse. Child welfare agencies are primarily responsible for home visits and coordination and evaluation of the therapy of the entire family. Because of the number of difficulties experienced by most abusive families, usually no single agency or discipline can provide all the needed services. Innovative types of therapy that have been successful when designed for individual families include Lay Therapists or Parent Aides, Homemakers, Parents Anonymous groups, telephone hotlines, environmental crisis therapy, child rearing counseling, and so on. Traditional psychotherapy is often not effective.

Prevention. A group of parents at high risk for being unable to adequately love and care for their offspring can be identified early if attention is given to such things as abuse of a previous child, drug addiction or serious psychiatric illness in a new mother, negative parental comments about the newborn infant, lack of evidence of maternal attachment, infrequent visits to a new baby whose discharge is delayed because of prematurity or illness, the spanking of a young infant, or the severe neglect of infant hygiene. Abuse and serious neglect may be prevented when such families receive an intensive form of well baby care, including prenatal classes, contact between mother and baby in the delivery room, rooming-in, increased parental contact with premature infants, extra help with the colicky infant, more frequent office visits, ongoing counseling regarding discipline, visits of public health nurses, nurseries to which infants and young children can be admitted for short-term respite care at the times of family crises, close follow-up of acute illnesses, telephone lifelines, arrangement for day care, and assistance in family planning.

Prognosis. With comprehensive, intensive treatment of the entire family, 80–90% of families involved in child abuse or neglect can be rehabilitated to provide adequate care for their child. Approximately 10–15% of such families can only be stabilized, and will require an indefinite continuation of supporting services until their children are old enough to leave home. Adoption or continued foster placement is required in 1–2% of cases.

If an abused child is returned to his or her parents without any intervention, 5% will be killed and 25% will be seriously injured. The child with repeated injuries to the central nervous system may develop mental retardation, an organic brain syndrome, seizures, hydrocephalus, or ataxia. Common emotional traits of abused children are fearfulness, aggression, and hyperactivity. Further, untreated families tend to produce children who become the juvenile delinquents and violent members of our society and the next generation of child abusers.

2.69 INCEST
(Family-Related Sexual Abuse)

See Sec 2.61.

Incest refers to any sexual activity between persons too closely related to marry; most legal codes include adopted and/or stepchildren in the definition. The most common type of sexual mistreatment of children is the family-related type. Sexual abuse by friends and acquaintances of the child or family is the second most common type. Least common is sexual abuse perpetrated by strangers. This section will not deal with extrafamilial child sexual abuse, although the steps in medical evaluation of both types are similar. Intrafamilial sexual abuse is more difficult to manage because the child must be protected from additional abuse at the same time that one tries to preserve the family unit.

Three types of incest are molestation, sexual intercourse, and family-related rape. Child molestation includes touching or fondling the genitals of the child or asking the child to fondle the adult's genitals; forced exposure to sexual acts or pornography is also part of this definition. Sexual intercourse includes vaginal, oral, or rectal penetration, or attempted penetration on a nonassaultive basis. Without detection and intervention molestation almost always progresses to full sexual intercourse. Less than 10% of incest is assaultive, forced intercourse (family-related rape).

Epidemiology. At least 0.2–0.3% of children have been involved in incestuous relationships for an average period of 5 yr. Brief sexual encounters occur more frequently. The victims are 90% female and 10% male. No age group is exempt. Approximately one third are less than 6 yr of age, one third 6–12, and one third 12–18. The process is often repeated with successive daughters. The offenders are 99% males. The problem occurs slightly more commonly with stepfathers than natural fathers. Incest cuts across all socioeconomic groups to a greater degree than physical abuse.

Etiology. Most incest involves fathers and daughters. Sexual relationships usually begin gradually and without any violence. The father brings to this relationship a need for sexual gratification, and the daughter brings a need for tender affection and nurturance. The father is usually rigid, patriarchal, and emotionally immature. He is unlikely to engage in any extramarital relationships, but he may have a drinking problem. Mothers are usually chronically depressed, unavailable to their husbands because of work or illness, and aware of the incest but able to overlook it on a conscious level; many of the mothers were sexually abused as children. The child victim tends to be pseudomature and has taken on many of the housekeeping tasks. The families are often closely knit and socially isolated. In the violent cases of family-related rape, the father is usually a sociopath and his sexual abuse extends outside the family circle.

Clinical Manifestations. Victims of family-related rape are usually brought to an emergency room in acute distress. The child may disclose the incestuous relationship to her mother and be brought to a physician at that time. If the mother does not believe the child, the child may later tell a girlfriend, friend's mother, or school counselor and be brought in. Some adolescents will disclose their secret to a physician in a private interview. At other times the physician must elicit the history of incest based on his suspicions, e.g., when the prepubertal child presents with vaginal bleeding or other unexplained genital symptoms. The main cause of venereal disease in the prepubertal child is sexual transmission from adults. A pregnant adolescent who is not dating and offers no information regarding the baby's father should be suspected as being an incest victim.

Incest cases require sensitive and thorough history taking because less than half of the victims have any physical or laboratory findings. A detailed explicit account of sexual experiences by a prepubertal child should be considered hard evidence in these cases. Physical findings are usually absent because of the long delay before the victim feels safe in telling someone about his or her plight. Interviewing should proceed gently and at the child's pace. Pictures or dolls should be used to clarify body parts; the child's vocabulary should be learned from the parent. If a social worker has performed the initial interview, the physician can review this material and need not repeat the interview.

Most female victims prefer a female physician to examine them, but this is not mandatory. An examination of the skin should be carried out for any signs of trauma, especially bite marks. The abdominal examination should assess the possibility of pregnancy. The mouth should be examined for signs of trauma such as redness, abrasions, or purpura. The rectum should be examined for signs of trauma or laxity. The external genitals should be visually examined for signs of trauma, laxity, or vaginal discharge. In prepubertal girls, a hymenal opening of 5 mm or greater is probably abnormal. A speculum examination of the vagina is indicated when the victim is postpubertal or when nonmenstrual vaginal bleeding or major trauma of the external genitals is present.

Laboratory Data. The amount of laboratory evidence sought depends on the history. Molestation victims usually receive a wet preparation for sperm. Sexual intercourse victims should have tests for sperm, acid phosphatase, and gonorrhea. In the vagina, sperm are motile for 6 hr and nonmotile for 72 hr or longer. Acid phosphatase is present for 24 hr. Sperm and semen may also be recovered from the mouth and rectum. While the presence of semen substantiates the victim's history, the absence of semen does not contradict the history of vaginal intercourse. Gonorrhea cultures should be taken from the mouth, vagina, and rectum; occasionally they are positive at sites initially denied by the child because of embarrassment. Less than 5% of the victims have positive cultures for gonorrhea. Additional tests that may help to identify the perpetrator include pubic hair, scalp hair, fingernail scrapings, blood samples, and sperm type. The specimens are usually transferred to the police laboratory in sealed, signed, and dated envelopes.

Diagnosis. The diagnosis of child molestation and most sexual intercourse rests on the graphic history offered by the victim. False accusations are rare except for psychotic patients or sexually active patients who are angry at their father or stepfather. If sexual intercourse has occurred within the previous 72 hr, laboratory evidence of acid phosphatase or sperm helps to confirm the diagnosis. The presence of a nonvirginal hymen suggests penetration, but the victim must clarify whether this was self-induced or inflicted. In family-related rape cases, the diagnosis is usually confirmed by evidence of recent trauma as well as positive laboratory findings.

Treatment. Evaluation and management of sexual abuse cases is similar to but more complex than physical abuse cases. All victims of sexual abuse require psychologic support. Often both parents deny the girl's accusation and turn on her for reporting the incident. Victims of a single nonviolent episode (e.g., some child molestation) may need only reassurance and a chance to ventilate about the event on one or two occasions. Usually they are less distressed by the incident than are their parents. In a single, violent episode of family-related rape the patient is usually in serious emotional distress and requires the services of a child psychiatrist and/or rape victim advocate. Most of these patients make a good adjustment after several sessions in age-appropriate psychotherapy. The victims of multiple episodes of sexual abuse almost always need long-term psychotherapy. The victim may be able to return home if the perpetrator is out of the home or has confessed and is in therapy. The child should be placed in foster care if this is his or her desire, the mother doesn't believe the child's story, family life is chaotic, or all evidence has not yet been collected. Medication to prevent pregnancy may be given to girls who are post-menarche, are in mid-cycle, and have experienced vaginal intercourse within the previous 72 hr. At a minimum all victims should revisit their physicians within 2 wk to assess their psychologic functioning and the services that have been implemented.

Most incest offenders are treatable. The offending parent requires a psychiatric evaluation, and the spouse should be evaluated by a social worker. Offenders are always investigated by the police, and criminal prosecution commonly occurs. Sentencing is usually deferred if the father becomes honestly involved in therapy. Both parents usually need psychotherapy and marital therapy. The offender in family-related rape cases is usually placed in jail, and criminal prosecution and sentencing do occur. The sociopaths are usually untreatable. Alcoholics may be helped by Alcoholics Anonymous groups.

Prognosis. With intervention most incest victims can lead a normal adult life; without intervention many of them run away from home and become adolescent prostitutes and drug addicts. Those who stay at home manifest depression, suicidal gestures, and conversion reactions. As adults most of them have difficulties with close relationships and need psychiatric help.

2.70 NONORGANIC FAILURE TO THRIVE

See Sec 5.36.

Failure to thrive (FTT) has several causes. Approximately 70% is nonorganic and 30% is organic. The nonorganic group is composed of 50% neglectful or psychologic FTT and 20% accidental, e.g., errors in formula preparation, errors in feeding techniques. This section focuses on neglectful failure to thrive, which rarely occurs after 2 yr of age because older children can obtain food for themselves. Under bizarre circumstances an older child can lose weight or gain poorly because he is confined to a room or deliberately starved. The main cause of FTT in infancy is that the baby is not fed enough. The mother may neglect feeding because she is busy with external problems (e.g., overwhelmed with work), preoccupied with inner problems, or doesn't like the baby. Emotional deprivation inevitably occurs concurrently with nutritional deprivation. Most of these mothers feel deprived and unloved themselves; many are also acutely or chronically depressed. The baby is usually unplanned and unwanted. Multiple and continuing crises, frequently compounded by the physical absence of the father, may overwhelm the mother who reacts with neglect of her infant.

Clinical Manifestations. The dietary history in infants with nutritional neglect usually is not helpful because the parent reports that the baby is receiving adequate calories. In some cases, the mother reports that the baby has vomiting and diarrhea which is not confirmed by the baby's hospital course. The parents have not usually sought medical care for their baby and immunizations are not up-to-date. By contrast, the details of the feeding history are extremely helpful in diagnosing accidental FTT because the parents are open about their feeding errors and misunderstandings.

The infant with FTT usually exhibits thin extremities, a narrow face, prominent ribs, and wasted buttocks. Hygiene neglect as evidenced by a rampant diaper rash,

unwashed skin, untreated impetigo, uncut fingernails, or filthy clothing is often present. A flattened occiput points to being left unattended for undue hours. Delays in social and speech development are common, but rarely seen before 4 mo of age. These findings include an avoidance of eye contact, an expressionless face, and the absence of a cuddling response. The amount of time the mother spends holding, playing with, and talking to her baby is usually reduced or inappropriate. A rejecting mother will often feed her baby with anger and unnecessary force.

Laboratory Data. Investigation of the etiology of failure to thrive is discussed in Sec 5.36. Extensive laboratory evaluation should usually be delayed until dietary management has been attempted for at least 1 wk and failed. A skeletal survey is indicated in those infants who have a rejecting parent or evidence for associated physical abuse.

Diagnosis. A feeding trial may establish the diagnosis. Most children should be hospitalized and given unlimited feedings for a minimum of 1 wk of a diet appropriate for age which approaches 150 cal/kg (ideal weight)/24 hr. The formula should be similar to the one allegedly given at home. Infants with neglectful FTT will gain over 2 oz/24 hr sustained for 1 wk (approximately 1 lb/wk) or have a gain that is strikingly greater than achieved during a similar time period at home. Most of these infants also display a ravenous appetite. If deprivational behaviors are also present, another diagnostic finding is their improvement or resolution in the hospital setting.

Treatment. All cases of FTT due to underfeeding from maternal neglect should be reported to a child protective agency. After appropriate hospital management approximately 75% of babies are discharged home with added services for the family, 20% go into temporary foster care while the parents receive therapy, and 5% enter long-term foster care with plans for relinquishment or termination of parental rights. This dispositional decision is based mainly on the potential responsiveness of the mother to treatment. Those babies who are discharged to their natural home require intensive intervention. The parents should be provided with clear, written dietary instructions at discharge and encouraged to hold the baby closely during feedings and offer unlimited stimulation. Many of these families require a homemaker, public health nurse, health visitor, and other types of services. Weekly medical follow-up is needed to monitor general progress and weight gain.

Prognosis. Without detection and intervention a small percentage of infants with nutritional neglect die from starvation. Approximately 5–10% of these infants sustain superimposed physical abuse. Weight loss and understature from malnutrition are reversible, but normal head circumference and brain growth may not be achieved if the infant has marasmus persisting beyond 6 mo of age. The most common sequelae are emotional and educational problems which occur in over half of these children.

BARTON D. SCHMITT
C. HENRY KEMPE

Physical Abuse

Bittner S, Newberger EH: Pediatric understanding of child abuse and neglect. Pediatr Rev 2:209, 1981.

Caffey J: The whiplash shaken-infant syndrome. Pediatrics 54:396, 1974.

Feldman KW, Schaller RT, Feldman JA, et al: Tap-water scald burns in children. Pediatrics 62:1, 1978.

Kempe CH, et al: The battered child syndrome, JAMA 181:17, 1962.

Kempe CH, Helfer RE (eds): The Battered Child. Ed 3. Chicago, University of Chicago Press, 1980.

Lenoski EF, Hunter KA: Specific patterns of inflicted burn injuries. J Trauma 17:842, 1977.

Schmitt BD, Beezley PJ: The long-term management of the child and family in child abuse and neglect. Pediatr Ann 5:164, 1976.

Wilson EF: Estimation of the age of cutaneous contusions in child abuse. Pediatrics 60:751, 1977.

Incest

Beezley-Mrazek P, Kempe CH (eds): Sexually Abused Children and Their Families. New York, Garland, 1981.

Ellerstein NS, Canavan JW: Sexual abuse of boys. Am J Dis Child 134:255, 1980.

Jones GJ: Sexual abuse of children. Am J Dis Child 136:142, 1982.

Orr DP, Prietto SV: Emergency management of sexually abused children. Am J Dis Child 133:628, 1979.

Rimsza ME, Niggeman EH: Medical evaluation of sexually abused children: A review of 311 cases. Pediatrics (in press), 1982.

Soules MR, Pollard AA, Brown KM, et al: The forensic laboratory evaluation of evidence of alleged rape. Am J Obstet Gynecol 130:142, 1978.

Woodling BA, Kossoris PD: Sexual misuse: Rape, molestation, and incest. Ped Clin North Am 28:481, 1981.

Failure to Thrive

Ayoub C, Pfeifer D, Leichtman L: Treatment of infants with non-organic failure to thrive. Child Abuse Neglect 3:937, 1980.

Jacobs RA, Kent JT: Psychosocial profiles of families of failure to thrive in infants—preliminary report. Child Abuse Neglect 1:469, 1977.

Rosenn DW, Loeb LS, Jura MB: Differentiation of organic from non-organic failure to thrive in infancy. Pediatrics 66:698, 1980.

2.71 DEVELOPMENTAL DYSFUNCTION IN THE SCHOOL-AGED CHILD

The disciplines of developmental and behavioral pediatrics are giving increased attention to handicaps of "low severity–high incidence" and to subtle impairments of development. Specific patterns of deficiency in such areas as attention, motor output, memory, perception, productivity, and language are being identified in a variety of clusters and degrees of severity. Estimates of the incidence or prevalence of developmental dysfunction in school-aged children range from 1–30%, depending upon definitions and diagnostic criteria. Developmental disabilities are expressed in a broad range of symptoms, and it is difficult to distinguish between statistical variability in normal behavioral or cognitive styles and true obstacles to learning and performance. These problems affect more boys than girls, the most commonly quoted ratio being approximately 4:1.

The role of the physician in the care of children with developmental dysfunction includes:

(1) The early detection of dysfunction (in infant, toddler, or preschool child) and prevention of its consequences.
(2) The developmental and neurologic evaluation of the dysfunctional child.
(3) Application of specific medical therapies.
(4) Participation in multidisciplinary assessment and management teams.
(5) Coordination of therapeutic, consultative, educational, and counseling services.
(6) Long-range continuity of monitoring and management.
(7) Integration of knowledge about the child's development, health, family function, and other factors.
(8) Advocacy for the child and family in the community.

Many labels have been proposed for children with constitutional handicaps. Such terms as hyperactivity, minimal cerebral dysfunction, learning disabilities, developmental dyslexia, the Gerstmann syndrome, and dozens of others have been suggested. Identifying stable clusters of such children may help to obtain appropriate services or guide research efforts, and refinements of nomenclature will continue; but there are hazards to classifications and to the identification of "syndromes." Some labels act as self-fulfilling prophecies, or lead to therapeutic inaction or to stigmatization.

The following discussion will focus not upon labels or upon descriptions of syndromes, but upon how specific deficits develop and are commonly encountered. Some techniques that may be used to assess competence within each area are also discussed, in the context of the learning tasks facing the school-aged child. The readiness of the child for the psychoeducational tasks of middle childhood requires adequate developmental function in a number of areas. These include visual-spatial organization; temporal-sequential organization; receptive and expressive language functions (joined by appropriate central processing); selective attention and activity; and increasingly higher orders of conceptualization. These functions are supported by the somewhat more general or pervasive functions of the apparatuses of memory (auditory, visual, sequential, short-term, and long-term) and of motor output (with elements of neuromaturation). All of these elements functioning serve the child in a psychosocial context shaped by past experiences and level of social development, by learned skills and coping styles, and by the child's emotional health and feelings of self-esteem.

This section concerns children with "low severity handicaps." The dysfunctions of youngsters with mental deficiency or multiple handicaps have similar elements. The retarded may often differ from the subtly handicapped only in the extent or multiplicity of their deficits.

2.72 THE ELEMENTS OF DEVELOPMENTAL FUNCTION

VISUAL-SPATIAL ORIENTATION

Normal Function. From birth, infants begin to comprehend spatial relations by moving their bodies and obtaining visual, kinesthetic, tactile, and proprioceptive feedback, integrating visual experience with somesthetic input. Piaget called the developmental period during which infants first and primarily employ sensory cues to construct a world of objects the stage of sensorimotor intelligence.

Perception is a process whereby the central nervous system organizes sensory data. Visual-perceptual function permits recognition or discrimination between patterns and relationships in space; it plays a central role in learning, particularly in the earliest grades. It entails the appreciation of details, relative position, size, contour, and orientation of stimulus patterns. Also involved are distinctions between background and foreground. The ability to differentiate visually among symbols and letters is critical for reading and ultimately for writing. Recognition is closely linked to the ability to perceive an overall pattern or gestalt, as opposed to a more fragmented or piecemeal appreciation of forms, patterns, or details.

Related to visual-motor integration, which may depend upon the adequacy of spatial perceptions and the constant monitoring of visual feedback for many tasks, a child must obtain and use visual data in order to plan and execute a motor movement (a process called *praxis*). Catching a ball, tying shoelaces, copying designs, and buttoning a shirt are examples of complex acts involving (among other things) visual-motor coordination.

Dysfunction. Children with delays in development of visual-perceptual or visual-motor function may be difficult to identify in infancy or in the early preschool years. Initial manifestations may include difficulty learning how to tie shoelaces, problems with discrimination between left and right, confusion and anxiety over recognition of letters, trouble in catching a ball or riding a bicycle, or delay in acquiring skills in drawing or copying. Ultimately, a child with visual-spatial disorientation may encounter problems in learning to read (Sec 2.73), to write, to arrange words and sentences on a page, and to deal with the written aspects of the arithmetic processes. Some children develop strong compensatory strategies, independently or with help, and may succeed despite significant visual processing handicaps.

Some children with visual-perceptual disorders are also delayed in motor function, but not all; nor do all children with motor dysfunction demonstrate visual-spatial disorganization.

Assessment. The diagnosis of deficits in visual perception can be difficult. Most commonly, children are asked to copy specific forms standardized for age (Table 2–15). Such tests, however, depend upon fine motor function, as well as upon visual-motor integration; moreover, a child who is reflective is likely to reproduce such forms more accurately than an impulsive youngster. The skill is also somewhat dependent on previous experience. For these reasons, one must interpret such assessments carefully. Delay in form-copying does not prove a visual-perceptual problem, but might be taken as evidence of such a deficit. Confirmatory evidence may come from some of the subtests on the Wechsler Intelligence Scale for Children (WISC) (in particular, object assembly, picture completion, and block design);

Table 2–15 EXAMPLES OF FORMS STANDARDIZED FOR AGE

FORMS TO COPY FOR THE SCREENING OF VISUAL-PERCEPTUAL-MOTOR FUNCTION

AGE (YEARS)	FORMS FOR DIRECT COPYING		COPY FROM MEMORY (10 SEC EXPOSURE)
5			
6			
7			
8			
9–10			
11–12+			

The above forms can be utilized by pediatricians as screening devices for visual-perceptual-motor deficits. Impaired performance on such a task might also be due to other problems, such as inattention, inexperience, fine motor difficulties, or problems with conceptualization. These forms should never be used as the ultimate diagnostic indicator; instead, they might indicate the need for further evaluation of a visual-perceptual-motor problem.

other standardized tests such as Frostig's Developmental Test of Visual Perception and Raven's Progressive Matrices are more direct measures of visual perception.

TEMPORAL-SEQUENTIAL ORGANIZATION

Normal Function. Just as children acquire schemata for vision and space, an appreciation of time and sequence emerges. This function is localized to a large extent in the left hemisphere of the brain. The appreciation of overall form and pattern is thought to be predominantly a function of the right hemisphere in most persons.

Much of a child's information gathering and daily activity depends upon sequence. Wristwatches, calendars, schedules, and routines testify to the importance attached to time and sequence in our society. Young children acquire an appreciation of sequence as they master the routine order of meals, days, months, and years, and comprehend concepts such as *before* and *after*, *today* and *tomorrow*, and *now* and *later*.

The retention of sequential information is essential for following instructions in school and at home. A sequential function organizes a variety of processes, visual, auditory, and motor. Sequential organization is closely related to memory.

Dysfunction. Children with deficits in sequential organization may show serious problems with short-term and immediate memory. Parents and teachers may complain that they seldom follow instructions, seem unable to retain what has just been said, or get "overloaded" or bewildered by a series of directions. They may have difficulty with story telling or reporting, may show confusion over temporal prepositions, and be delayed in learning to tell time. Such children may show maladaptive classroom behaviors, as protective strategies or as signs of frustration and anxiety.

Weak sequential organization can interfere with spelling and arithmetic, through an inability to grasp the concept of number or of a predictable order of letters within a word. Some children have sequencing difficulties primarily in the auditory channel, others more with visual or motor sequences; some have difficulties in all areas.

Deficits of temporal-sequential organization often have a fairly typical natural history. The earliest manifestations (such as problems with telling time or with multistep directions) are slowly mastered, but academic troubles arise, such as problems remembering the multiplication tables. Ultimately, these too improve, but in adolescence significant problems with organization and study habits arise, as does trouble with arranging ideas in appropriate sequences, and with scheduling and timing of long-range projects (sometimes for life).

Assessment. There are several methods of screening for temporal-sequential organization. The *digit span*, which tests immediate recall of a sequence of numbers, is sometimes interpreted as a test of auditory-sequential memory; but performance may be influenced by the strength of the child's number concept. Moreover, anxiety or inattention can interfere. In the *object span* assessment the child is asked to tap or point to a series of objects in an order demonstrated by the examiner. The *block tapping* exercise is done the same way, except that a series of squares is tapped instead of concrete objects, some perceptual clues being eliminated from the task. These tests of visual-sequential memory are also influenced by a child's attentional strength. *Serial commands* involve a sequence of oral instructions. *Motor sequencing* involves imitation of a sequence of motor activities, as demonstrated by the examiner. These tests for sequential organization are summarized in Table 2–16.

Standardized tests of visual-sequential and auditory-sequential memory form part of the Illinois Test of Psycholinguistic Abilities. The digit span and picture arrangement subtests of the WISC may also offer indications of sequencing problems.

MEMORY

Normal Function. Memory is fundamental to learning. Three basic stages of memory involve reception of information, data storage, and retrieval. To learn, children must select appropriate stimuli for retention, "file" these data for later use, and, when an appropriate occasion arises, retrieve what has been stored without undue effort or delay.

Some investigators have distinguished immediate recognition from recall; many have separated long-term from short-term memory and the latter from immediate recall (or parroting). Certain children demonstrate preferred learning modes. Some, for example, may be described as visual learners, others as auditory learners. Others learn best through active motor performance, demonstrating a kind of facilitated motor memory (learning by doing). The quality of memory within a particular modality depends upon the adequacy of information processing. A child's difficulties in appreciating patterns or form contours may, for example, be related to deficits in visual memory.

Dysfunction. Reductions of memory may be discrete deficits or parts of a broader picture of dysfunction. Affected children often have academic and behavioral difficulties. In particular, those with reduced short-term memory may have difficulty retaining instructions and lessons, and may be labeled poorly motivated or lazy. Deficits of visual memory may permit only vague impressions of the configuration of words and slow acquisition of an appropriate rate of reading based on an adequate sight vocabulary. Other problems can interfere with memory, and in some cases masquerade as primary deficits in the retention process. An inattentive child, for example, may lose information because he or she was distracted at the time the input was presented.

Table 2–16 TASKS FOR THE ASSESSMENT OF TEMPORAL-SEQUENTIAL ORGANIZATION

	TASK DESCRIPTION				
	Digit Span	Object Span	Block Tapping	Serial Commands	Motor Sequence
Age	Series of digits, given one per second, to be repeated by child	Series of objects tapped in order; child imitates in same order	Series of squares tapped in order; child then imitates in same order	Series of simple commands; child performs in correct order	Child performs act after examiner
5–6 yr	4 forward digits	4 objects	4 squares	3 steps	Simultaneously open and close both hands, arms extended
6–7 yr	4–5 forward digits	4 objects	4 squares	4 steps	Imitative finger tapping (both hands, 3–4 steps)
7–8 yr	5 forward digits	5 objects	5 squares	5 steps	Imitative mixed finger-foot tapping (4–5 steps)
9–10 yr	6 forward digits 4 reverse digits	5 objects	5 squares	5 steps	Alternate left and right open and close fists, arms extended
11–12 + yr	6 forward digits 5 reverse digits	6 objects	6 squares	6 steps	Imitate edge of hand on knee, then palm on knee, then clenched fist (4 cycles)

It may be difficult to separate problems of attention from those of retention. Memory can also be weakened by chronic anxiety or by low motivational power in the information presented.

Assessment.   Most measures of retentive ability assess immediate recall and short-term memory. Visual memory and auditory short-term memory may be tested as described above. To some extent, long-term memory is evaluated in gauging a child's store of general information and vocabulary; such evaluation is biased by cultural and other factors.

Many parents and teachers will give anecdotal clues to short-term memory deficits in reporting some children's inability to retain classroom instructions or to take telephone messages. Some children with short-term memory deficits who cannot follow simple instructions have a hypertrophied long-term memory. Their parents will comment on an uncanny ability to recall often irrelevant details from the distant past.

RECEPTIVE LANGUAGE AND CENTRAL AUDITORY PROCESSING

Normal Function.   The acquisition of the ability to decode words and sentences dramatically facilitates children's understanding and assimilation of their surroundings, their perception of themselves, their interactions with others, and their ultimate academic skills. Usable vocabulary helps them to establish associations such as those between words and objects, between their own bodies and the world around them, and between ideas and abstractions. In addition, children acquire the rules of syntax or grammar which give words meaning in context.

Language skills are presumed when the child enters school and become increasingly germane and complex with higher education, whereas visual-perceptual skills have their peak importance during the first 3 grades of elementary school.

Receptive language function involves interpretation of auditory stimuli and extraction of meaning from words and sentences. The first step involves selective attention to speech sounds. Auditory discrimination, which is a differentiation between or sorting of similar sounds, follows. Basic units of sound are then identified as words with meanings which can be examined in their syntactic relationships.

Dysfunction.   Auditory perceptual difficulties can involve both auditory discrimination and the decoding of complex syntactical structures, such as difficulty with recognition of discrete units of sound or with auditory figure-sound relationships, or difficulty in association of meanings with words or understanding the significance of grammatical structures. Affected children may be restless and inattentive in verbal environments.

Children with chronic lack of good language reception may have trouble analyzing words phonetically. Delays in reading, spelling, and written output can result from relatively subtle receptive weaknesses. Secondary inattention, emotional difficulties, and social maladjustment are common. Young children with these problems can become confused and anxious or panic-stricken, as they perceive the classroom experience as

Table 2–17 CLUES TO THE DIAGNOSIS OF RECEPTIVE AND EXPRESSIVE LANGUAGE DISORDERS IN SCHOOL-AGED CHILDREN*

History of delay in speaking full sentences
History of recurrent ear infections
Difficulty in understanding simple or complex sentences
Decreased receptive vocabulary (word recognition or comprehension)
Weak auditory memory
Difficulty in focusing attention
Difficulty in learning and applying phonetic word analysis skills, or phonetically inaccurate spelling errors
Significant disparity between visual-motor and language skills
Poor word-finding ability and poor expressive vocabulary
Poor narrative skills
Stuttering, stammering, or immature articulation
Maladaptive behaviors

*These findings are intended to suggest the need for further evaluation. A child with a language disability may have none of these findings. Conversely, any of them may reflect nonlanguage difficulties.

through a bad telephone connection or a poorly tuned radio.

Assessment.   Screening for speech and language disabilities begins with a careful history and informed, perceptive interaction with the child. No single speech and language screening test serves all ages. Such tests as the Preschool Language Scale (Zimmerman, Steiner, and Evatt) or the Screening Test for Preschool Children (Fluharty) are useful for children until the age of 5 yr (Sec 2.12). Table 2–17 lists some findings that might suggest the possibility of language disability. Clues such as these should be noted by the clinician and comprehensive evaluation arranged when indicated.

An expressive language disorder may be accompanied by difficulty with receptive processing. Children with difficulties in articulation, word finding, and narration may also have underlying auditory-perceptual deficits, weaknesses of auditory memory, or other language deficiencies. Physicians must be alert for receptive language problems, and not assume that conventional psychologic testing will reliably detect language disabilities interfering with school performance.

When a child is referred to a skilled consultant for evaluation of speech and language, testing can be pursued in greater depth. The Illinois Test of Psycholinguistic Ability is commonly used; its findings may have direct implications for teaching techniques. Other tests of receptive language include the Detroit Tests of Learning Ability and the Wiig-Semel Test, which explores the appreciation of syntax, tense, and other components giving sentences structure and meaning.

EXPRESSIVE LANGUAGE

See Sec 2.78.

Normal Function.   Useful language depends on the capacity to call up relevant words, arrangement of these words in phrases or sentences that conform to linguistic rules, development of ideas in a meaningful sequence or narrative, and planning and execution of the complex motor act of speech. During the school years, written and spoken language come to occupy the center stage in education, in self-monitoring, in controlling social interaction, in dealing with and understanding one's own feelings, and in demonstrating competence.

Dysfunction. Disorders of expressive language include:

(1) Deficits of resonance: abnormal oral-nasal sound balance, usually heard as hypernasality or hyponasality.
(2) Voice disorders: deviations in quality, pitch, or loudness of physiologic or psychologic origin.
(3) Fluency disorders: disruption in the natural flow of connected speech, most commonly as stuttering.
(4) Articulation disorders: a major group of problems in which the production of speech sounds is imprecise.
(5) Language disorders: problems in comprehension and manipulation of the symbol systems of language.

Disorders of resonance and voice are common and ordinarily require the assistance of a speech therapist (Sec 2.78). During the normal development of language, all children show some evidence of nonfluent speech between 1–4 yr of age. These may consist of pauses, repetitions of sounds, revisions of sentences, lapses in responding, or prolongation of sounds. Stuttering is felt by some to be due often to inappropriate response by a listener to this normal developmental dysfluency; the resulting feelings of inadequacy by the child aggravate the nonfluency. The majority of stuttering children are identified between the 3rd and 4th yr of life. Stuttering may appear later, with the first school experience or with the approach of adolescence. In all likelihood, stuttering is a symptom with multiple causes. Its association with wider neurologic dysfunction is unusual. It may occur in families, but it is not generally regarded as genetic or learned by imitation. The attitude of the family toward normal nonfluency and other expectations may explain its occurrence in siblings. The possibility that some children derive secondary gains from stuttering needs thoughtful assessment. Stuttering children need early, careful psychologic assessments and evaluations of speech and language. Most should be referred to a speech pathologist.

Disorders of articulation are the most commonly encountered speech problems in children, and involve 3 types of errors: *substitutions*, replacement of one sound with another (e.g., wight for light); *omissions*, failure to produce certain speech sounds (e.g., boo for book); and *distortions*, inappropriate sounds replacing the correct ones. Wide variability is observed in the number of consonants and vowels that are misarticulated. Errors may range from a few misarticulated sounds to speech that is sometimes unintelligible. Poor articulation may be caused by anatomic abnormalities within the oral cavity, including dental irregularities, or abnormal shape or structure of the hard palate. Paralysis or weakness of the tongue can affect speech production; occasionally, poor articulation is a symptom of hearing loss. Articulation deficits may be associated with developmental language disabilities. Environmental and psychologic factors may also predispose to poor speech sound production.

Evidence suggests that many children or adults with articulation disabilities have difficulty in using sensory information from the mouth (buccal somesthetic and kinesthetic feedback). Such an articulation disorder may be analogous to other perceptual-motor problems.

Disabilities of expressive language create a variety of problems for children. One is an inability to use syntax in a manner commensurate with developmental age. Affected youngsters are often shy; commonly, they rely on gestures and on communication through single words or phrases, appearing at times to speak in telegraphic style, deleting words. There may be a history of delay in the achievement of language milestones. Children with pronounced deficits in expressive language must be evaluated also for developmental delay, auditory sensory loss, emotional disturbance, autism, and elective (selective) mutism.

For some children who express themselves in appropriate syntax the process requires excessive time and effort; they have difficulty keeping pace in conversations and become reluctant to use narrative.

Word-finding disorders, as expressive language handicaps, are far more common than has been generally recognized. Parents of an affected child may report that "he can't say what he wants," or "it's as if it's just at the tip of her tongue." The child is momentarily unable to recall the name of an object or event for which previous knowledge exists, or may be slow to name pictures or objects. He or she may attempt to use gestures or pantomimes that conform closely to the object. Some children will speak in definitions or approximations rather than specific words; others will label things by association (e.g., rain for umbrella, or tobacco for pipe). Sometimes a word is substituted that sounds like the word sought (e.g., slow for low). Word-finding deficits often occur with other language handicaps, such as difficulties with syntax and auditory memory.

Disorders of narrative may take several forms, such as an inability to comment on content, or reduced storytelling skills. Affected youngsters may speak only in the most concrete way about events. Many cannot organize a narrative, but ramble and build incoherent structures.

Deficits of word-finding and of narrative organization may not be detected by parents or teachers. An affected child may, in fact, be verbose; but careful study will show that the content of expressive language is developmentally delayed, the words used being relatively simple and below the child's developmental level in other areas, and sentence structure relatively primitive.

Language impairments may disrupt seriously the development of social relationships within the family, or with peer groups. Secondary emotional problems can develop, and significant behavioral disorganization or regression may be observed. Many of the children with expressive language problems have difficulties in reading. Their difficulties mount when they are required to produce high volumes of written material (Sec 2.73). Early detection and intervention are particularly urgent.

Assessment. A history of recurrent otitis media, of delayed acquisition of intelligible speech, or of persistent articulation problems may point to dysfunction in this area. The evaluation of expressive language ability requires assessment of the child's ability to formulate sentences, to name, and to narrate. Picture-naming tasks can be used and the child can be asked to describe recent experiences, with attention given to the child's ability to organize narrative, to find words quickly, to use grammar appropriately, to produce at an adequate rate, and to articulate in a manner commensurate with age. Tests for articulation ability include the Hejna Test of Developmental Articulation. In addition to assessing the intelligibility of speech, one should judge the child's voice quality, pitch, and resonance. When there are doubts about any of these, a full-scale evaluation of speech and language should be undertaken (Sec 2.78).

VOLUNTARY MOTOR OUTPUT

Normal Function. Gross and fine motor control reflect the constant feedback of visual and somesthetic cue. which contribute to a sense of body position, to control over movement quality, to the maintenance of posture, and to decisions as to whether to continue, to modify, or to complete motor acts. Motor function involves also the facilitation and inhibition of muscle groups, the planning (praxis), execution, and monitoring of motor acts, and their integration with patterns established from previous experience. Fine motor function, such as dexterity with the hands, critical for writing skills, depends upon afferent stimuli involving visual, proprioceptive, and kinesthetic feedback and various aspects of memory. Effective gross motor control in school-aged children offers obvious dividends in the enhancement of self-image through recreation and sports. Though some professionals claim that motor therapy can improve learning, there is little evidence of a direct relationship between effective gross motor function and the early mastery of academic skills.

Dysfunction. Inefficiencies of fine motor performance may affect writing, copying, and drawing. Some children compensate by developing a maladaptive pencil grip, which may later impair their ability to produce a large volume of output. Such children may be overwhelmed by lengthy writing assignments or by tests taken under timed conditions. Problems in this area may emerge only in the later elementary school grades, when the demand for written output increases.

In some children poor fine motor performance actually reflects impulsivity or an attempt to perform the task too quickly. Sometimes illegible handwriting is the result not of poor fine motor function but of poor selective attention. In other cases writing difficulties stem from problems with visual memory, with poor retrieval of symbols.

Children with gross motor delays may develop profound feelings of inadequacy, avoiding interaction with their peers for fear of such humiliation as always being picked last for teams. Some degree of social ostracism may result from their visible awkwardness or clumsiness.

Difficulties with motor praxis or memory may disturb either gross or fine motor function. Children with *apraxia* have difficulties planning specific motor acts; they may know *how* to do something, but have difficulty integrating this know-how into a final motor pattern. Other youngsters show deficiencies of motor memory, unable to recall and apply readily motor patterns that were previously mastered; they need to relearn and overlearn patterns if they are to retrieve them efficiently.

Assessment. The examination of a child's gross and fine motor control involves presenting developmentally appropriate tasks. Table 2–18 lists examples of such activities as rough guidelines. Motor performance is poorly standardized for older children, however, owing to the effects of cultural differences and experience. The quality of performance may be more important than simply whether or not the child can perform a task.

In evaluating fine motor function, children of all ages should be observed using a pencil, with attention to the strength and effectiveness of the grasp and to

Table 2–18 TASKS FOR THE ASSESSMENT OF VOLUNTARY MOTOR FUNCTION

AGE	GROSS MOTOR	FINE MOTOR
5–6 years	Skip Walk on heels Tandem gait forward Hop in place	Six block tower (1 inch cubes, 15 sec) Six cube pyramid Button 2 buttons (20 sec)
6–7 years	Tandem gait backward Stand on one foot, eyes open (10 sec)	Tie shoelaces Alternate left-right index finger-to-nose from arms extended Sequential finger opposition forward
7–8 years	Crouch on tiptoes, eyes closed (10 sec) Hop twice in place on each foot in succession (3 cycles) Stand in tandem gait position (heel-toe), eyes closed (10 sec)	Sequential finger opposition (forward-backward, 5 seconds) Bead stringing on a shoelace
9–10 years	Tandem gait sideways Catch tennis ball in air, one hand Throw tennis ball at target	Draw horizontal lines parallel to lines on a page String beads
10–12 years	Balance on tiptoes, eyes closed (15 sec) Jump in air, clap heels together Jump in air, clap hands three times Catch ball in one hand	Place pennies in a box (one hand at a time) Draw 30 vertical lines connecting horizontal lines on notebook paper (15 sec with preferred hand)

control of the pencil's movement, as in the formation of the angles of figures. Some children with fine motor deficits have particular difficulties with the coding subtest of the WISC, or with such fine motor problems as using scissors, or manipulating eating utensils or buttons or zippers.

For gross movement, one should observe coordination, balance, visual-motor integration, and motor-sequential organization. For fine movements, it is particularly useful to note the way in which the hands and eyes work together, the smoothness of fine motor output, and the precision shown. The rate of fine motor output can have crucial bearing on ease of written expression.

For children with possible gross motor delays standardized examinations, such as the Lincoln-Oseretsky Test, can offer developmentally appropriate tests of motor function.

SELECTIVE ATTENTION AND ACTIVITY

See also Sec 2.56.

Normal Function. Attention is a continuing and self-reinforcing process of selection. At any instant, a host of internal and external stimuli compete for attention, including immediate auditory or visual sensations, data stored in long- or short-term memory, impulses originating in viscera, muscles, and joints, or fantasies, feelings, or associations. With the process of selection, one or a few of these inputs take priority, while the others are relegated to the background or to a level beneath conscious awareness.

The process of selective attention allows children to focus purposefully and for appropriate lengths of time on incoming data that will lead them toward productive activities or learning. When the process is operating optimally, the resistance to distraction and degrees of reflection and persistence are adequate for tasks involving comprehension and problem solving. Choice of activity also is dependent upon selectivity. Children with effective selectivity for activity may be exploratory, purposeful, efficient, and goal-directed much of the time, the level and quality of their activity adjusting to changing demands and expectations.

Dysfunction. Ineffective controls of activity and attention are not necessarily associated with learning handicaps, but chronic inattention and poorly controlled activity are frequent concomitants of academic and social failure in the school-aged child. Not all affected children are "hyperkinetic" or "overactive"; some children are extremely active but purposeful and effective, and should not be considered dysfunctional.

Four categories of disorders of activity and attention can be defined: Youngsters with *primary disorders of attention* demonstrate (possibly on a neurologic or biochemical basis) basic inefficiencies in selecting foci of attention and activity. They may not be appropriately aroused, alert, or organized in the function of selectivity. Other youngsters may be *secondarily inattentive*, owing to handicaps in one or more of the areas of information processing discussed above, or to emotional difficulties. For example, a child with an auditory sequential memory deficit may derive no reinforcement of efforts at attention in the classroom because what

should be attended to is so often missed or rapidly forgotten. Children who have emotional difficulties may be preoccupied by chronic anxiety, depression, or specific fears (sometimes of failure). Such preoccupations may "drain" attention. Children with *situational inattention* have no functional difficulty; rather, the problem lies in the classroom, at home, or elsewhere. Problems include inappropriate curriculum or materials, inadequate teaching, discrepancies between a child's cognitive style and expectations, cultural discordance between the child and the educational system, and inappropriate academic pressures at home. In such instances inattentive behaviors may be confined to specific situations and may be less global than in other attentional disorders. Finally, *mixed types* of attention deficits occur. A full discussion of the effects, assessment, and treatment of attention deficit (hyperactivity) is presented in Sec 2.56.

NEUROLOGIC MATURATION

Normal Function. With the maturation of structure and function within the central nervous system and the cumulative effects of experience, normal children achieve increasing efficiency and adaptability in behavior as they mature.

Dysfunction and Assessment. The observable indicators of the degree of organization and maturation of the central nervous system have often been referred to as "soft neurologic signs." They are nearly always found in young children, but rarely in older age groups. For this reason, these signs have been linked to central nervous system maturation. Many of them reappear during senescence. The persistence of neuromaturational signs beyond the ages at which they usually disappear has been associated with learning disorders, behavior problems, and other manifestations of developmental dysfunction. A single such sign in isolation may not have much meaning. Some very successful children may show one or more of these indicators, while others with significant developmental dysfunctions may have no such evidence of neuromaturational delay. Clusters of these signs may be more accurate discriminators than any one alone.

The most frequently examined neuromaturational indicators include:

(1) Synkinetic (mirror) movements: one side of the body mimics closely an activity conducted on the contralateral side (e.g., when a child is asked to oppose his thumb and forefinger repeatedly, the other hand mirrors the action). In older school children, such movements may be elicited by more complex unilateral acts. Persistence of true mirror movements in several different areas of the body beyond the age of 8 yr is unusual, except in children with learning and behavioral disorders.

(2) Other associated unnecessary or inefficient movements may also be interpreted as evidence of a neuromaturational lag in older children. For example, a child may consistently show rhythmic mouth movements, head bobbing, or foot tapping in conjunction with another activity concentrated in a distant anatomic region.

(3) Dysdiadochokinesis: difficulty in performing rapid alternating movements, most commonly tested by sequential and alternating pronation and supination of

the hands. Some children have difficulty suppressing activity in proximal muscle groups while performing this, exhibiting excess flailing of the limbs.

(4) Finger agnosia: the inability of the child to perceive and name the position of fingers in the absence of visual cues. The child, with eyes closed, may be asked how many of his or her digits an examiner is touching, or how many fingers are held between 2 of the examiner's fingers. Reduced finger awareness appears to have some validity in prediction of educational readiness.

(5) Stimulus extinction: a tendency for a young child to be unable to perceive a sensory stimulus when it is presented simultaneously with a second stimulus. In some cases, more proximal stimuli are dominant over distal, or two-point discrimination may be poor. For example, a child with eyes closed may be touched on a hand and then on the face and asked each time to locate the touch. When the hand and face are then stimulated simultaneously, the child may report only the touch on the face (sometimes called "rostral dominance"). This is not generally encountered after the age of 7 yr.

(6) Choreiform movements: involuntary rotatory and arrhythmic movements, most commonly seen in the outstretched fingers or the protruded tongue. They can be elicited by having a child close the eyes, extend both hands, spread the fingers, open the mouth, protrude the tongue, and sustain this posture for 30 sec. Studies have correlated such involuntary movements with school failure and behavior problems.

(7) Motor impersistence: inability to stand with hands outstretched, mouth open, eyes closed, and tongue protruding for 30 sec. The motor-impersistent youngster may show downward deviation of the arms, difficulty inhibiting the tongue from random movements such as darting in and out of the mouth, and an inability to keep the eyes closed. This tendency can be seen with attentional disorders and learning difficulties.

(8) Lateral dominance: the propensity to preferential use of one side of the body. With the development of each hemisphere of the brain for a particular set of functions, hand dominance is usually well established between 4–6 yr. Eye dominance is often established by the age of 2 yr. Ear and foot dominance can also be evaluated, but less is known about these. Children with delays in establishing clear dominance may have problems in other areas. Mixed dominance (e.g., a tendency to be left-eyed and right-handed) has been associated in some studies with an increased incidence of reading disabilities; these findings, however, are in doubt.

(9) Left-right discrimination: a sense of laterality, to be distinguished from the ability to name left and right. Children become progressively competent in these discriminations. Children may first be able to identify asymmetry about the sagittal plane. By the age of 6 yr, most can tell the left from the right on their own body coordinates. Before their 8th birthdays they are usually able, on request, to cross the midline (e.g., touch the right ear with the left hand). By 9–10 yr of age, they can identify right and left parts of another person's body. By early adolescence, they are often competent at rapidly distinguishing left and right, starting from new bases (e.g., turning to face left, then right, then left, and so on). Problems in left-right discrimination may involve problems of both maturation and basic processing. For example, many children with visual-spatial dysfunction have delays in the acquisition of left-right discrimination.

The above signs of neuromaturational delay are those used most commonly in evaluation of dysfunctional children. They do not have direct implications for intervention, but they may suggest the degree of constitutional or maturational deficit. In some cases, delays in neuromaturation are accompanied by other forms of maturational lag: in skeletal age, stature, dentition, emotional maturity, or social insight. Some affected children may have delayed onset of puberty.

"HIGHER-ORDER" PROCESSING AND INTEGRATION

Normal Function. Complex processes exist at the highest levels of cognitive function which the neurobehavioral sciences have only begun to elucidate. Higher cognitive processes include:

(1) Reasoning on an abstract or symbolic level.

(2) Developing and applying generalizations, classifications, or rules that facilitate further behavior and learning.

(3) Agility of movement back and forth from the concrete to the abstract-symbolic.

(4) Capacity to put concrete and/or abstract materials into new juxtapositions (i.e., creativity and imagination).

(5) Ability to identify textural discrepancies, as well as consistencies, within complex materials.

(6) Skill at inferential reasoning.

In young children, one can study the pace and the order of development of the above functions. Specific stages are dominated by the emergence of particular components of intelligence, which have implications both for learning and for behavior and moral development (Sec 2.30 and 2.31).

Dysfunction. Many children with difficulty in higher-order conceptualizations, abstractions, and so on, also have other developmental dysfunctions. The difficulties with higher-order processing may prevent them from developing strategies to deal with their other handicaps. On the other hand, some children with perceptual problems or other cognitive deficits may be able to compensate for them and develop effective learning and behavioral styles because they have relative strengths in such higher-order processes as reasoning, creativity, and generalization.

Assessment. The similarities and block design subtests of the WISC have been thought to measure conceptualization in verbal and nonverbal areas, respectively, and other assessments of higher order conceptual abilities have been based on the work of Piaget, but these kinds of assessments have not yet been proved useful in the evaluation of children with learning disorders. Through careful observation of children with learning problems at home and at school, parents and teachers can identify styles and strengths in cognitive function which may have implications for remediation.

The results of intelligence tests in children with developmental dysfunctions must be interpreted with care (Sec 2.71). Youngsters with attention deficits may show low test-retest reliability. Moreover, a child's calculated IQ may largely reflect a deficit in a single relatively narrow area of function. There are few tests which assess children's capacities to develop problem-solving strategies, to overcome adversity, to be creative, or to use imagination.

ATTITUDE AND MOTIVATION

All performance depends on motivation; on the other hand, the admonition "he can do it when he really wants to" may be very damaging, preventing a child from receiving needed services. It is critical that behavior and performance be assessed in relation to levels of motivation. A child with an attentional problem may show rapt concentration when observing a monster movie, but such a high level of motivation is not typical and may lack relevance to day-to-day performance capabilities.

Cultural and social values influence attitude and motivation toward learning. The drive for academic excellence may in some families tend to maximize a child's achievement. Alternatively, a poor performance may sometimes be due to excessive parental pressure.

A "poor attitude" may be a sign of a learning disorder rather than its cause. Labeling a child "poorly motivated" may lead to a failure to meet needs for special education and counseling.

2.73 AREAS OF PERFORMANCE

Systematic observation and analysis of a child's academic performance can identify various functional components, including degree of reflectivity, persistence, reactions to frustration, responses to positive reinforcement, preferred style or modalities of learning, and areas of processing deficit. Analysis of the components of a task and observation of the nature of a child's success or failure at it will permit the diagnosis or the description of developmental dysfunction. Many of the tests for language and learning disabilities lack standards for older children and adolescents. The direct observation of performance is especially important, therefore, in diagnostic evaluation of adolescents.

READING

During the early school years, a lag or deficit in one or more areas of development may lead to a serious impediment in reading which may sow the seeds of later inhibitions or negative attitudes toward learning. It is important, therefore, that reading difficulties receive prompt diagnosis and intervention.

Delays in learning to read may result from a variety of cognitive, psychologic, and social influences. In assessment of a child's reading performance, the following should be evaluated:

(1) Reading level or grade equivalent.
(2) Reading rate.
(3) Sight vocabulary (the ability to recognize words almost instantly).
(4) Word analysis skill (the capacity to sound out or analyze phonetically a word not remembered nor previously encountered).
(5) Tracking (the ability to keep one's place).
(6) Level of comprehension.

Deficits may include excessive use of finger pointing (a possible indication of a visual tracking problem); over-reliance on context; sequencing errors (incorrect juxtaposition of letters within a word or words within a sentence); deficits in visual discrimination (e.g., substituting b's for d's or misreading words for those of similar overall configuration); poorly established sound-symbol association; disregard of punctuation; word-by-word reading or monotony of tone; and word substitutions or omissions. Some professionals refer to children who misinterpret visual symbols during reading, but who have adequate peripheral sensory mechanisms, as dyslexic. By observing the types of errors and stylistic tendencies, a diagnostician or teacher may identify certain patterns consistent with specific neurodevelopmental deficits. Appropriate strategies for educational intervention may follow.

The health care team, but more likely the school, can easily administer such standardized tests as the Wide Range Achievement Test, the Stanford Reading Achievement Tests, and the Gray Oral Reading Paragraphs. When these are supplemented by developmental tests, specific themes of dysfunction may appear.

SPELLING

As with reading, careful analysis of the tasks and performances involved in spelling can yield valuable descriptive data about a child's learning style or handicaps. Difficulty with spelling (dysorthographia) may not in itself constitute a significant obstacle to success in life, but in combination with other areas of dysfunction, it may contribute to emotional anguish and to poor performance.

The manner in which a grade level for spelling achievement is measured is critical. Some youngsters who have great difficulty in spelling words from dictation will be highly accurate in selecting a correctly spelled word from a list of incorrect ones.

A careful analysis of a child's errors can be revealing. Some children produce spellings that are correct phonetically but inaccurate visually (e.g., lite for light). Others mistake similar configurations (e.g., laugh for light), or persistently commit errors of sequencing (e.g., lihgt for light). Still others show mixed errors. It may be useful to have a child read a list of words that are well ingrained in his or her sight vocabulary, and immediately thereafter try to spell them from dictation. Some youngsters have great difficulty with the revisualization of words, even those they have just seen.

Disorders of visual memory, sequencing, and receptive language are common in children with poor spelling, but in many cases problems with spelling appear to be isolated deficits without other developmental or psychologic correlates.

Spelling can be assessed using the Stanford or Wide Range Achievement Tests. The Boder Spelling Lists can be used to assess revisualization.

WRITING

In the middle and upper elementary school grades, earlier emphasis on relatively passive skills in recognition and discrimination gives way to increasing stress on written work. Most school-aged children respond to this transition effectively and welcome the opportunity to express themselves, but some children have difficulty with written compositions, one of the highest forms of language, and the last, therefore, to be learned. It is not unusual for children at the late elementary or early junior high school level to become discouraged with their writing; such children may or may not have had earlier reading problems.

A variety of dysfunctions may underlie disorders of writing. Some children have multiple deficits; others have isolated or discrete problems. The common disturbances are:

(1) Weakness of fine motor control: difficulty with eye-hand coordination, defective or inefficient pencil grasp, or problems executing the motor patterns needed to form letters, numbers, or words.

(2) Disorders of visual-motor integration: problems perceiving visual configurations and converting them into a blueprint from which written words or sentences can be drawn. Affected children may be able to spell, narrate, and read with fluency, but still encounter obstacles in writing.

(3) Problems with visual memory or revisualization: inability to retain visual images of letters, words, or shapes to permit their reproduction from memory (even in some children who can copy them well). Affected children would have difficulty writing or spelling from dictation.

(4) Dysnomia: slowness in finding words in either written or oral expression.

(5) Deficiencies in composition, organization, and syntax: inability to arrange thoughts in an organized way in writing and at times in speech.

(6) Spatial organization: difficulty arranging letters, words, or sentences in an orderly manner on a page.

(7) Diminished rate of processing: difficulty with accomplishing the task at an appropriate rate. Affected children become discouraged with the slow, laborious nature of writing effort, avoid writing when possible, and obtain less practice.

Three other factors need consideration in evaluating writing failure: (1) because poor writing can be a permanent exhibit of a child's inadequacies, some children may be embarrassed and reluctant to write, especially when perfection is demanded too soon; (2) children with little opportunity to write are unlikely to write well; and (3) writing is under strong cultural influence, there being low incentive for writing in families with little stress on the written word.

Children with developmental disorders of written language are frequently branded as unmotivated, lazy, disinterested, or depressed. They may become anxious or emotionally disturbed because of their limited productivity, further inhibiting written output.

In evaluating a child with writing difficulties, a writing sample may be sufficient. It is useful to have the child perform on at least 3 levels: first, copying some sentences or words; second, writing from dictation; and third, writing a paragraph on a particular subject. Observations can be made on grasp of pencil and on fine motor control, word finding, organizational skills, direct visualization and revisualization, and visual-motor integration. Data are needed also about the child's earlier development and experiences and about family dynamics.

MATHEMATICS

Dyscalculia, or disability in mathematics, subsumes a group of common but poorly understood disorders. Difficulties with mathematics may stem from dysfunctions described above. Visual processing problems may impair visual recognition of numbers; visual-spatial problems present obstacles to arranging numbers or columns of numbers systematically on a page, or difficulties with the geometric aspects of mathematics.

Some children with sequencing problems have particular difficulty learning the multiplication tables and integrating basic number concepts; some with language disabilities have difficulty relating the symbolism of arithmetic operations to everyday situations, and may meet insurmountable confusion in dealing with word problems. Attentional difficulties and excessive impulsivity may impair ability to organize details of written numerical problems. Some youngsters with fine motor problems have difficulty aligning numbers for addition, subtraction, or multiplication.

Higher-order conceptualizations are critical in arithmetic. Children with arithmetic disorders may have difficulties with the notion of conservation of quantity (e.g., 1 dime equals 2 nickels); with formulating and applying principles for problem solving; with associating auditory with visual symbols; with ideas of one-to-one correspondence (e.g., 4 people need 4 spoons to consume their soup); or with counting (as opposed to rote repetition of numbers in sequence).

In assessing arithmetic performance, it is useful to survey organizational skills, perceptual competencies, and basic concepts, as well as to look at the child's written arithmetic productions. Analysis of errors can be helpful. The Wide Range Achievement Test and the KayMath Test of Arithmetic Abilities cover a broad range of mathematical operations.

SOCIAL INTERACTION

Success in social interactions depends on appropriate experience, on emotional health, and on many other social and cultural factors. Some children may lack the capacity or sensitivity to read facial expressions of approval or disapproval, to perceive and respond to the needs of others, or to comprehend basic social skills such as sharing or offering support to another individual; or they may be persistently egocentric and insatiable.

Children with gross motor delays may have difficulty establishing gratifying social interactions in a milieu that accords a high value to athletic competence. Impulsive and inattentive children are often rejected by their peers and may experience isolation as early as the preschool years. Children with receptive or expressive language difficulties may have problems in building relationships, as may those with stuttering or other articulation problems. Failure often leads to a sense of inadequacy and a retreat from peers. Such youngsters may prefer the company of younger children or of the opposite sex. Some such young children may feel most comfortable in the company of adults. Others feel alienated from the adult world owing to their failure to meet its expectations.

For children with developmental dysfunction, a description of patterns of social interaction at home, in school, and in the neighborhood is important to understanding their needs. This can often be obtained from the child, supplemented by the insights of parents and teachers. The child's interactions with the physician may *not* offer a reliable sample of social performance.

2.74 ORIGINS AND OUTCOMES

Early History. In evaluating school-aged children with developmental dysfunction, the search for a specific etiology has rarely been fruitful. In pursuing an early medical and developmental history, one can often identify certain "risk factors" or predispositions, but one can rarely be certain that such associations are, in fact, causes of the child's current difficulties. Infants born prematurely, small for gestational age, or with traumatic deliveries have higher than expected likelihoods of developmental lags, but statistical associations between perinatal stresses and later development are weak and inconsistent. Although many children born of difficult pregnancies and deliveries, with stormy neonatal courses, function normally during the school years, it is important to record early life stresses, and to examine the possibility that they may have been elements of a process culminating in dysfunction. The support of family, early cognitive experiences, cultural values, and emotional factors may all modify developmental processes and compensate for mild physiologic impairments. Longitudinal studies of children with perinatal complications and of others with malnutrition in infancy have shown behavior and achievement to be influenced by socioeconomic class as well as the antecedent events; a poor outcome for the child is surer when biologic insult and lower socioeconomic class occur together.

A child's particular strengths and weaknesses may be mutually compensatory, allowing for resiliency. If dysfunctions are severe enough or sufficiently maladaptive, however, even strong environmental support may be inadequate to prevent failure. Finally, children with several areas of dysfunction may have greater difficulty bypassing a deficit than those with single deficits.

Some developmental dysfunctions are hereditary or genetic. Certain families have a high incidence of reading problems with no ready environmental explanation. Some children with attention deficits have parents whose behavior was similar during childhood; in such cases, it may be difficult to separate genetic effects from modeling. Some genetic syndromes have specific processing problems; girls with Turner syndrome, for example, have difficulties with visual-spatial organization.

Infections or other inflammations of the central nervous system may be followed by attentional weakness and deficits in cognitive processing, and encephalopathies such as lead poisoning may also produce developmental dysfunctions.

Increasing attention is being paid to the temperamental characteristics of infants as predictors of later developmental function, and neurologic examinations such as the Brazelton Neonatal Assessment Scale have revised the assessment of behavior and neurologic organization in the newborn. Insatiability, irritability, and unpredictability have been described as intrinsic traits of some infants who later develop behavioral disorganization and problems with learning. The predictive validity of observations of temperament or of the Brazelton Scale has yet to be established for children of school age. Developmental assessments in infancy are useful in the detection of severely handicapped children, but their ability to predict handicaps of low severity appears limited. In the preschool years, early detection may become increasingly feasible with use of educational readiness examinations which examine perceptual-motor, language, and memory functions more closely than do traditional developmental assessments.

Outcomes.   Resiliency in development may continue into adult life, but adult performance and life style may be influenced adversely by early life failure, and outcomes are sometimes tragic. Alcoholism, drug abuse, unemployment, serious automobile accidents, and crime have been linked to developmental dysfunctions. The comprehensive early evaluation and treatment of such dysfunctions may be essential to a future stable and productive adulthood.

2.75 THE DIAGNOSTIC PROCESS

Children with developmental dysfunction present complex and sometimes baffling diagnostic challenges. Their problems are not easily classified, each discipline tending to perceive problems in the context of its own subject matter.

The health care team can play a critical role in diagnostic evaluation and follow-up, in cooperation with educators, psychologists, and other specialists. Schools may seek medical help in identifying emotional and neurologic factors predisposing to failure. Parents may ask for assistance in obtaining evaluations free of distortions inherent in some school-based evaluations, in which personalities, budgets, and space may at times bias diagnosis and management.

The individual physician or nurse may collect the data leading to a plan for appropriate services, but in many cases a multi-professional team evaluation will be the most appropriate. An initial evaluation should include:

(1) A detailed review of early history, including a description of pregnancy and the perinatal period, early temperament, early development (motor, language, and social), health record, and family background, with particular attention to early life events that are frequently associated with developmental dysfunction. One should attempt to estimate the degree of stimulation or deprivation in the

child's life, as well as make a retrospective analysis of the interaction between parents and child. Most of the historical data can be captured economically through standardized questionnaires for parents and teachers, such as the ANSER System, a group of questionnaires designed for this purpose. Data so obtained can be elucidated further during an interview.

(2) A clear account of present function. Rating systems have been developed which measure a child's activity and attentional strength. These include the Conners Scales, the Werry Scales, and the ANSER System. Parents can fill these out prior to the child's visit. Behavioral inventories can record positive or maladaptive behaviors that may be associated with the child's dysfunction; other instruments elicit ratings by teachers of academic performance, attention, activity, and associated behaviors.

(3) A description of the child's present home and school settings. The structure, living arrangements, and style of the family should be noted so far as possible, with a sense of the child's activities, supports, and interactions at home, in the neighborhood, and in the classroom. There should be an analysis of the curriculum and of any extra help the child is receiving.

(4) A mental health assessment. Parents and child should be interviewed separately by the mental health member of the team. The child should be evaluated as to self-esteem, personality, affect, mood, relatedness, and evidence of organicity. A child's drawing of his or her family may be helpful.

(5) A complete physical examination. A careful evaluation of vision and hearing and a traditional neurologic examination are required, though few significant abnormalities can be expected from the latter. Note should be given to evidence of maturation delay, growth retardation, malnutrition, deprivation, and medical conditions that might interfere with attention and learning such as allergies, sinus infections, or chronic serous otitis.

(6) A neurodevelopmental screening assessment. This should screen for neuromaturational delay and for the specific deficits outlined earlier. The health care team can work with the psychoeducational specialist in direct observations of performance.

(7) Psychoeducational testing. This should include assessments of intelligence and achievement and, as indicated, of specific developmental areas, such as language, memory, or visual-spatial processing.

The diagnostic process should be able to describe a child on 5 levels: (1) *neurodevelopmental*, with an analysis of constitutional, maturational, and developmental factors interfering with function and underlying strengths; (2) *psychosocial*, elucidating factors in the environment, in the family, and in the past experience or present emotional climate of the child that interfere with performance; (3) *secondary psychologic*, with an account of the emotional effects of failure; (4) *supportive*, with a description of how the family, the school, and the community are attempting to cope with the child's dysfunction; and (5) *strategic*, with an analysis of the child's strategies for dealing with failure.

In the United States Public Law 94–142 mandates that children with developmental disabilities and other sources of learning difficulty have a right to a multidisciplinary assessment in school, which should lead to an Individualized Educational Plan (IEP) to meet their specific educational, developmental, and counseling needs. The roles of pediatricians or other health care providers in this planning vary from state to state. Physicians are commonly involved in "independent evaluations" when schools or parents seek an outside opinion. The health team and the school should collaborate in developing an educational plan, including specific recommendations for counseling of the parents and the child, and, when necessary, further study or consultation. A system for follow-up and accountability should be instituted. Children with developmental dysfunction need the same continuing care as children with chronic diseases.

2.76 INTERVENTION

EDUCATIONAL PLANS

Health care personnel are becoming increasingly involved with education in planning for children with developmental dysfunction, but the selection and utilization of curricular materials and classroom activities are functions primarily of educators. Educators must become more familiar with the medical and developmental aspects of school failure, and health professionals need to know more about educational systems and alternatives. Generic options for individualizing educational programs include:

The Alteration of Classroom Structure. Some children with chronic inattention or poor activity control may function far more effectively in smaller classrooms with higher teacher:pupil ratios and in highly structured or predictable programs. On the other hand, there is such great variation in the organization of classrooms that recommendations need to be based on knowledge of the specific settings available and objective information about their educational relevance.

Modification of Teacher-Student Interaction. Teachers aware of a child's developmental dysfunctions can apply specific educational strategies. Problems with sequencing require presentation of materials in small units and instructions one step at a time. The child may need to confirm receipt of multiple-step instructions by repeating them. Children with visual distractibility may benefit from a somewhat isolated carrel or a workspace; those with auditory distractibility, from sitting near the front of the room or having an opportunity to do some work in relatively quiet settings each day. Teachers need to discover whether a given child learns best through visual or auditory channels.

Children with output problems may require more time or reduced assignments. Youngsters chronically deprived of mastery will profit if their teachers can regularly assign tasks in which success is assured.

Additional Specialized Help. Many youngsters may require specialized assistance outside of regular classrooms. There is a growing trend in this country not to segregate children with educational problems into "special" classes. This trend is referred to as "mainstreaming." Children in need can leave the regular classroom for portions of the day for specialized help in special settings ("learning centers," "resource rooms"). There each child can receive individualized help from such specialists as learning disabilities teachers, speech and language pathologists, and reading specialists. Efforts of such specialists are aimed both at strengthening basic skills and at overcoming specific dysfunctions, with exercises directed at visual-perceptual motor function, sequencing, fine motor problems, or language disabilities.

Some children with attentional problems may learn best in a one-to-one relationship. Appropriate feedback and reinforcement, an emphasis on reflective behavior, and the elimination of distractions and peer pressure may dramatically facilitate performance and learning in such children.

For some children a multisensorial approach to learning is based on the assumption that a weak modality can be compensated for by input through several channels. For example, a youngster with a visual-perceptual problem might learn to recognize letters by an approach combining auditory, visual, tactile, and kinesthetic input, a child with difficulty in visual learning might be taught through the use of tape recordings, or a child with fine motor problems impairing writing might use a typewriter.

Remedial Help in Performance Areas. As children grow older, more emphasis is placed on direct tutorial help in subject areas, with less emphasis on readiness skills. Such intervention may be very beneficial to a child whose slow rate of processing creates difficulty with the tempo of a regular classroom.

Curriculum Modifications and Substitutions. The selection of curriculum and teaching methods should be directed by an understanding of the child's developmental status and learning style. There are differing, valid approaches to the learning of basic skills, and specific curricula may accommodate individual styles.

Modifications in course content may help dysfunctional children. For example, those with gross motor lags who are intimidated by physical education classes may flourish in other areas after being excused from regular gym classes or being enrolled in an adaptive physical education program.

Other curricular issues, such as the introduction of foreign languages, the special demands of the sciences, and the provision of specific vocational training, need to be considered as children with learning problems enter the upper grades. Whenever possible, highly motivating educational experiences need to be included.

Many educational interventions have not been adequately evaluated and are espoused on the basis of anecdotal reports and uncontrolled trials. Investigations need to allow for wide individual variations, for the inevitable effects of maturation, and for the tendency of all helping gestures to produce nonspecific gains.

COUNSELING PARENTS AND CHILDREN

Health care professionals can play major roles in the counseling of children with developmental dysfunction and of their parents, through a continuing relationship with the family. The interaction will focus upon the specific deficits and manifestations, upon the child's strengths, upon the social milieu, and upon associated issues, including coping with day-to-day situations. The physician or nurse can also interpret biomedical, developmental, and educational findings, helping to "demystify" the child's problem.

Health care professionals should avoid excessive reassurance. Such assertions as "she'll outgrow it," or "I was the same way when I was his age," are inappropriate. Reassurance can be beneficial, but its overuse can prevent a child from receiving appropriate services or impede further evaluation. The teacher's view of a child's performance is crucial.

Children should be included in discussions about their learning difficulties; they are likely otherwise to fantasize uncomfortably about secret conversations between professionals and their parents.

Provision should be made for counseling directly with children by a physician, nurse, guidance counselor, or other professional. Counseling should aim in part at elucidating for the children their specific problems and strengths in understandable language with encouragement to talk about such problems and to report how they are coping.

Professionals and parents can together seek to identify areas of strength in which children can achieve a sense of mastery or triumph. Parents should be encouraged to balance criticism with praise, and to be reasonable and consistent in their expectations.

Health care professionals, parents, and teachers should be careful not to moralize about a child's learning problem. Such terms as "bad," "lazy," and "poorly motivated" never motivate, probably intensify negative self-images, and may act as self-fulfilling prophecies.

Psychotherapy may be indicated in instances of family disorganization and conflict, or when significant psychopathology is evident in the child. When referral is necessary, the physician, child, and family may need to meet several times to plan the use of mental health services to increase the likelihood of a successful referral (Sec 2.65).

SPECIFIC MEDICAL INTERVENTIONS

The first responsibility of the health care team is to ensure that any medical problems interfering with function, such as sensory deficits, neurologic problems, seizures, or chronic medical problems, receive appropriate care. Children with allergies, for example, may have learning difficulties aggravated by serous otitis, chronic nasal congestion, or excessive fatigue. Antihistamines may produce chronic fatigue and inattention in the classroom. If teachers are aware of medication being taken, their observations may lead to helpful alterations of dosages or schedules.

Many children with developmental disorders have associated symptoms, such as abdominal pain, enuresis, encopresis, headaches, or other complaints. Alleviation of these can improve function in other areas.

PHARMACOTHERAPY

Drugs used for children with problems in learning and attention have included cerebral stimulants, tranquilizers, antidepressants, and anticonvulsants. Their efficacy has been a matter of controversy; ethical concerns have been expressed regarding "behavioral control" of children, though dramatic improvements in learning and life style occur in some children receiving such therapy (Sec 2.56 and 2.66).

In children with disorders of attention, activity, and organization, stimulant drugs have had the most widespread use and acceptance. However, placebo effects, heterogeneity in the groups investigated, confusion over measurements of effects, and variations in drug schedules have made it difficult to assess clinical trials. There is no clear evidence that specific disabilities in learning or motor function are significantly altered by these medications, but in many cases, restlessness, impulsivity, poorly modulated activity, and distractibility are diminished, and there may be enhancement of goal-directed behavior, organization, selectivity, attentional strength, and reflectivity.

The decision whether to use stimulants can be difficult. They should not be given without a comprehensive evaluation of psychopathology and specific learning deficits. The hasty offering of these drugs may delay other much needed help. Even among those children whose learning is particularly impaired by inattention and poorly controlled activity, who may be most likely to benefit from stimulant medication, some will not respond favorably.

The most commonly used stimulant drugs are dextroamphetamine (Dexedrine), methylphenidate (Ritalin), and pemoline (Cylert). Their use, side effects and contraindications are discussed in Sec 2.56.

THERAPEUTIC CAUTIONS

Other therapeutic offerings of varying degrees of quality and validity have included use of special diets, megavitamin therapy, allergic hyposensitization, optometric exercises, the use of thyroid medication and insulin, motor patterning exercises, and transcendental meditation.

It has been suggested that food additives may have a deleterious effect on the learning and behavior of certain children. The question is being studied, but data are still inconclusive. It is unlikely that an additive-free diet will benefit the usual child with learning problems. If a trial of diet is made, close supervision will be important.

Others have suggested that high levels of dietary carbohydrate impair learning and behavior in many young children. Use of a high protein, low carbohydrate diet has, however, meager data to support it. Dietary manipulation may produce nutritional deficiencies, elevate hopes unrealistically, or delay the child's receiving appropriate educational and counseling services. Advocates of special biochemical and orthomolecular approaches to learning disorders, or of optometric, motor, and other interventions, have yet to present adequately controlled studies. In some cases, schools themselves have endorsed questionably valid treatment programs.

As advocates for parents and children, pediatricians can help to minimize their susceptibility to irresponsible claims. Many parents seek help elsewhere when they feel abandoned by the health and educational systems.

Adequate continuing support and appropriate intervention with families will lessen their need to seek "miracle workers." The physician may also, as coordinating member of a team, help families to avoid the biases of single disciplines and to avoid rigid categorization or labeling.

PREVENTION

A variety of preventive programs have been proposed to minimize the effects of both blatant and subtle handicaps and to foster the nurturance of the developing child. Some have assumed responsibility for optimizing the early health, development, and education of children. Demonstration models, such as the Brookline Early Education Project, have "enrolled" children in public school programs before they were born. The ultimate gains of such programs and their cost:benefit ratios are under study.

During the first years of life the earliest screening for developmental dysfunction is a responsibility of the primary health care system, which has a critical role in uncovering historical and physical indicators of evolving handicaps.

COMMUNITY ACTION

Where resources for children with developmental dysfunction do not exist, physicians, nurses, and educators can lead the way to changes in public policy which will reallocate resources. Where school systems lack the personnel and facilities for special educational treatment and evaluation, the health care team can help document the need. Where multidisciplinary diagnostic programs do not exist, health providers can take the initiative in creating appropriate team efforts. Health care providers and other professionals can also educate the community about the nature of developmental dysfunctions, the predicament experienced by failing children and their families, and the ultimate high cost of neglecting failure in early life.

MELVIN D. LEVINE

Connors CK: Psychological assessment of children with minimal brain dysfunction. Ann NY Acad Sci 205:283, 1973.

Connors CK: Food Additives and Hyperactive Children. New York, Plenum Press, 1980.

Corballis MD, Beale IL: The Psychology of Left and Right. New York, John Wiley & Sons, 1976.

Dykman RA, Acherman PT, Clements SD, et al: Specific learning disabilities: An attentional deficit syndrome. In: Myklebust HR: Progress in Learning Disabilities. Vol 2. New York, Grune & Stratton, 1975.

Johnson DJ: The language continuum. In: Sapir SG, Mitzburg AC (eds): Children with Learning Problems. New York, Brunner Mazel, 1973.

Kirk SA, Kirk WD: Psycholinguistic Learning Disabilities. Chicago, University of Illinois Press, 1971.

Lerner JW: Children with Learning Disabilities. Boston, Houghton Mifflin, 1976.

Levine MD: The ANSER System: Questionnaires for Student Assessment. Cambridge, Educator's Publishing Service, 1980.

Levine MD, Brooks R, Shonkoff JP: A Pediatric Approach to Learning Disorders. New York, John Wiley & Sons, 1980.

Levine MD, Oberklaid F: Hyperactivity: Symptom complex or complex symptom. Am J Dis Child 134:409, 1980.

Levine MD, Oberklaid F, Meltzer L: Developmental output failure: A study of impaired productivity in school children. Pediatrics, 67:18, 1981.

Levine MD, Palfrey J, Lamb GL, et al: Infants in a public school system: The early indicators of health and development. Pediatrics 60(Suppl):579, 1977.
Palfrey J, Mervis R, Butler J: New directions in the evaluation and education of handicapped children. N Engl J Med 298:819, 1978.
Peters JE, Romine JS, Dykman RA: A special neurologic examination of children with learning disabilities. Dev Med Child Neurol 17:63, 1975.
Ross AO: Psychological Aspects of Learning Disabilities and Reading Disorders. New York, McGraw-Hill, 1976.
Sameroff AJ, Chandler MJ: Reproductive risk and the continuum of caretaking casualty. In: Horowitz FD (ed): Review of Child Developmental Research. Vol IV. Chicago, University of Chicago Press, 1975.

Stroufe LA: Drug treatment of children with behavior problems. In: Horowitz FD (ed): Review of Child Development Research. Vol IV. Chicago, University of Chicago Press, 1975.
Tarver SG, Hallahan DP: Attentional deficits in children with learning disabilities. J Learn Disab 7:560, 1974.
Touwen BCL, Prechtl HFR: The Neurologic Examination of the Child with Minor Nervous Dysfunction. Spastics International Medical Publications. Philadelphia, JB Lippincott, 1970.
Wender P: Minimal Cerebral Dysfunction. New York, John Wiley & Sons, 1971.
Wiig EH, Semel EM: Language Disabilities in Children and Adolescents. Columbus, Ohio, CE Merrill, 1976.

DISORDERS OF HEARING, SPEECH, AND LANGUAGE

2.77 HEARING DISORDERS

See also Sec 12.37.

Hearing is the primary sensory pathway by which children normally develop speech and language. Hearing disorders at any age, even of mild degree, can cause problems of speech, language, and learning. It is essential, therefore, that hearing loss in children be identified as early as possible and its management planned promptly. The skills of the audiologist are essential in identifying the existence, degree, and type of hearing loss.

TYPES OF HEARING LOSS

Conductive losses result from interference in the mechanical transmission of sound to the inner ear. Atresia, stenosis, and inflammation of the external auditory canal, cerumen or foreign bodies in the canal, perforations of the tympanic membrane, congenital or acquired anomalies of the ossicular chain, and otitis media are among the causes of conductive hearing loss. With conductive hearing losses up to 60 decibels (db) loss may be demonstrated for sounds conducted in air, whereas sounds transmitted to the inner ear by bone conduction will be heard at normal thresholds. Most conductive losses respond well to appropriate treatment. Early treatment is important, however, to avoid the possibility of sensorineural loss due to toxic materials passing into the inner ear and to reduce the risk to speech and language development.

Sensorineural losses result from destruction of or damage to the cochlea or the auditory nerve. Such loss is nearly always irreversible. Sensorineural losses may not be readily detected, since the external auditory canal and tympanic membrane will usually appear to be normal.

Mixed hearing losses result when conductive loss is superimposed on sensorineural loss. Typically, the conductive component of mixed losses is temporary. It must be treated promptly so that a bad situation not be made worse. Children who must wear hearing aids may find cerumen or ear infections extremely uncomfortable. They should be examined frequently to see that no problems exist in the external or middle ear.

Central auditory problems may be accompanied by normal audiograms, or may coexist with other types of hearing loss. They appear as difficulties with comprehension of auditory stimuli despite the ability of the hearing mechanism to transmit auditory signals. Audiologic methods for assessing this complex problem are still evolving (Sec 2.72).

ASSESSMENT

Hearing loss is commonly described as mild to profound, depending on the threshold level at which the child is able to detect sound. Table 2–19 illustrates the ranges of threshold for various hearing levels, with the corresponding effects of hearing loss on the child's communication and learning.

To define the needs of a child with hearing impairment, one must know the type of loss, the auditory thresholds, and whether the loss is unilateral or bilateral. It is also important to assess behavioral characteristics: the child's visual attentiveness, ability to relate to

Table 2–19 EFFECTS OF HEARING LOSS

THRESHOLD	DEGREE OF LOSS	EFFECTS
30 to 40 db	Mild (hard of hearing)	Difficulty hearing faint or distant speech; may require hearing aid; needs preferential seating in classroom
41 to 55 db	Moderate (hard of hearing)	Difficulty hearing distant speech; requires amplification, preferential seating, auditory training, and probably speech therapy
56 to 70 db	Moderate to severe	Difficulty with conversation unless loud; great difficulty in group/classroom discussion; requires hearing aid; may require special class for hard of hearing
71 to 90 db	Severe (deaf)	May hear loud voice close to ear; may hear some vowels, recognize some sounds in environment; needs special education for the deaf, with specific training in speech and language
Over 90 db	Profound (deaf)	May hear some loud sounds; does not rely on hearing for communication; requires special education for the deaf

others, communicative style and intent, vocal quality, distractibility, and relationship with parents.

Results of hearing tests are most commonly expressed as thresholds of sensitivity to pure tones presented by air and by bone conduction. The *audiogram* plots the responses to frequencies ranging from 125 or 250 Hz through 8000 Hz. "Degree of hearing loss" is often derived from the average levels of sensitivity of the better ear at the 3 frequencies considered to be most important for speech: 500, 1000, and 2000 Hz. This approach assumes that a hearing loss is functionally only as bad as the better ear. But unilateral deafness, though it usually allows for normal speech and language development, does create problems in localization of sound, in perception of sound in noisy or reverberant environments, and in reliable understanding of speech when the speaker's face is not visible.

Pure tone testing is usually accompanied by examination of the child's threshold for speech reception and discrimination. Such testing is usually possible only with children 3.5 yr of age and over, who have developed nearly adult language competence. The hearing acuity of younger children is apt to be expressed in terms of their *hearing awareness threshold* or *speech awareness threshold*. Before 7 mo of age these thresholds are identified through the infant's responses to calibrated noisemakers and to acoustically controlled speech presented through speakers in the free field of the testing room. From 7 to approximately 42 mo most children's thresholds can be identified through *visual response audiometry* (VRA) or *play audiometry*. In VRA the child is conditioned to anticipate some reinforcement from lighted or moving toys when he or she hears a pure tone. In play audiometry the child is conditioned to move toys from one place to another in response to pure tones presented through earphones or in a free field.

Impedance audiometry assesses objectively the integrity and function of the peripheral hearing mechanism and has become a routine and helpful aspect of the assessment of hearing function in young children. The evaluation consists of (1) *tympanometry*, measurement of the mobility (compliance) of the tympanic membrane; (2) measurement of *static compliance* (acoustic impedance) and assessment of the peripheral auditory system at rest; and (3) measurements of *acoustic reflex* thresholds, the sound levels at which the stapedial muscle contracts. These elements of impedance audiometry yield objective data as to aeration of the middle ear (patency of the eustachian tube), integrity of the tympanic membrane and ossicular chain, and loudness recruitment. The 3 tests are not nearly so informative individually as they are together; their combined results are especially helpful in evaluation of very young children and those difficult to test.

Brainstem evoked response (BSER) audiometry can help identify hearing losses in young children. This electrophysiologic method averages the electroencephalographic responses to auditory stimuli and can be used to verify suspected peripheral hearing loss.

The *central auditory processing (CAP) test battery* is held by some audiologists to be of significant help in identifying the type of auditory disorder in some children with learning disabilities. The CAP test battery consists of (1) a dichotic sentence listening task, (2) a monotic filtered word task, (3) a binaural fusion task, and (4) an alternating speech task. This battery requires that the child be able to respond verbally.

MANAGEMENT

Hearing Aids. Except in special habilitative situations, a child must be able to hear and comprehend speech to learn to speak. A hearing aid may provide hearing-impaired children with the auditory stimuli that their own deficits deny them. The audiologist can guide the selection of a hearing aid and determine the optimal age to begin its use. Working closely with the physician, the otologist, the hearing aid supplier, the parents, and the child, the audiologist can help to ensure the optimal use of amplification by young children. Decisions will involve (1) the type of hearing aid (body, ear-level, or in-the-ear; monaural or binaural); (2) training for parents in the care and use of the aid; (3) provision for new ear molds as the child grows; and (4) monitoring the use of the aid.

Habilitation. A paramount concern in the development of children with severe to profound hearing loss is their impaired ability to learn verbal communication and language. Deaf children do develop a language, and deaf children of deaf parents communicate with each other and their parents effectively. Deaf children of hearing parents, on the other hand, typically have difficulty learning to communicate with their parents, as well as with the rest of a hearing world. Efforts to teach deaf children oral communication have generally been frustrating, though successful in some cases. Until the late 1960's this was the most popular approach to education of the deaf. The method used amplification, speech-reading training, and specific speech production training for young deaf children, generally within residential schools for the deaf.

In the past decades there has been increasing use of Total Communication in the training of young deaf children. Total Communication uses sound amplification, sign language, and speech to help the child learn communication and language. Total Communication requires the full commitment and participation of parents and, in fact, of all family members; they, too, must learn to communicate by sign language as well as by speech. Advocates of Total Communication assert that this approach enables deaf children to develop more wholesome, normal relationships with their hearing families, and to develop language at a more nearly normal rate than is usually seen in deaf children trained exclusively in the oral method. Others express concern that deaf children trained in Total Communication will be able to communicate only with those who know sign language, and will, therefore, be limited for social relations to the deaf community. Available data now indicate that children (and their families) trained in Total Communication are, in fact, better able to communicate with each other and, further, that children so trained are more likely to use oral speech, to demonstrate higher levels of scholastic achievement, and to adjust more satisfactorily emotionally to both the hearing and the deaf communities than are deaf children trained exclusively in either the oral or the manual (sign language) method.

2.78 SPEECH AND LANGUAGE: DEVELOPMENT AND DISORDERS

Speech and language development is a significant indicator of later learning abilities. The normal child has learned within the 1st 4 yr of life most of the grammatical principles governing his or her native language. Amazingly, this occurs without specific or special strategies by the child's parents or other significant persons. Because speech and language appear to develop so naturally, parents who express anxiety at the lack of speech of their 18 mo to 2 yr old children may commonly be advised that the children will "outgrow" the speech problems. Typically, however, the child who talks early and well also performs well in later learning activities, and the child with late development of speech and language may show problems in school, especially when there are early and persistent problems in understanding and responding to verbal communication. The requirements for development of normal speech and language are few but pervasive: (1) The child must have intact hearing from the time of birth. Evidence now points, for example, to deleterious effects of early (before 2 yr of age) and recurring otitis media. Even in children who give little evidence of physical discomfort, the intermittent hearing loss that occurs with recurrent otitis media appears to inhibit the child's learning of the associations of speech sounds and their significance, which are important to the decoding of language. The effects of sensorineural hearing loss on speech, language, and learning have been discussed above. (2) The child must have an intact nervous system. Consideration of the effects of central nervous system disorders on the speech and language development of children is discussed in Sec 2.72. Impaired development of speech and language is a common early indicator of cerebral dysfunction or mild neurologic impairment which may later cause behavioral and learning difficulties (Sec 2.72). (3) The child must have the physical structures and physiologic control that permit the rapid, integrated, and complex motor acts required for intelligible speech. Early feeding and eating patterns can provide important clues to the child's later speech skills. (4) The child must live in an environment that encourages the development of verbal skills and verbal exchange.

Language may be defined as knowledge of the symbol system used for verbal communication; *speech* is the demonstration of that knowledge in audible behavior. Language can be considered the base on which speech is constructed, both developing in an orderly progression. Language is closely related to cognitive development, though many children with limited cognitive ability learn to produce speech clearly and intelligibly. Language ability can be demonstrated in a variety of ways: by the manner in which the child responds to verbal directions; by the gestures used by the child to communicate needs, desires, and knowledge of the environment; and by the child's creative, imaginative play.

SPEECH AND LANGUAGE DEVELOPMENT

The critical period for speech and language development has long been held to be the period between approximately 9–24 mo of age. Recent research indicates, however, that we can move the earlier age limit even lower. From earliest infancy the child's development of speech and language should be of concern to the pediatrician. Direct observation of communicative behavior during routine examinations can be supplemented by parental reports. Table 2–20 contains a checklist of behaviors indicating the young child's receptive language function, which normally involves increasing awareness of the visual as well as the auditory content of communication. The developing child can be seen to observe the speaker's face and gestures more and more closely until a point, as language skills develop, at which the visual cues may become less important, suggesting increased facility in decoding the auditory verbal signals alone.

Expressive language development follows an equally predictable pattern (Sec 2.72). Its content consistently lags behind that of receptive language. Table 2–20 lists behaviors helpful in assessing this aspect of language development.

As the child's expressive skills develop, evidence of increasing competence in language and speech becomes easier to observe. The period from 2–4 yr of age shows rapid increases in the quantity and complexity of speech development, as comprehension, expressive vocabulary and neuromotor controls all increase rapidly. Vocal inflection may be exaggerated; control of vocal intensity may be limited, as may articulatory control and control over the rhythm of speech. It is during this period that disturbances in the fluency of speech may become apparent, and parents may express concern over stuttering, especially if they are among those who eschew baby talk. The knowledge that nonfluency is part of the normal development of speech control will allay the anxiety of many parents. They may find the following suggestions helpful:

(1) Demonstrate (model) a more relaxed speech pattern for the child, rather than telling him or her to "slow down," "take a deep breath," and so on.
(2) Provide words for the child, in as conversational a manner as possible, when the child's own vocabulary falters in expressing ideas and experiences.
(3) Take the time to listen attentively to the child who has exciting news to report.
(4) Expect the child to have passed through the nonfluent stage within 3 mo. If not, re-evaluate.

Skill in the articulation of speech sounds also follows an orderly and predictable pattern. The easiest and most visible sounds are the first to appear; these are the lip sounds (represented by the letters *m*, *p*, *b*, and *w*). Next to be heard are the simple tongue-to-gum ridge (alveolar) sounds (*d*, *n*, *t*). As children begin to master tongue-to-velum contacts (*g*, *k*, and *ng*), it is often possible to hear them confuse *d* for *g* or *t* for *k*,

Table 2–20 DEVELOPMENT OF SPEECH AND LANGUAGE

AGE AT WHICH BEHAVIOR SHOULD BE ESTABLISHED (MONTHS)	RECEPTIVE LANGUAGE BEHAVIOR	EXPRESSIVE LANGUAGE BEHAVIOR
1	Random activity arrested by sound	Random vocalization; primarily vowel sounds
2	Appears to listen to speaker; may smile at speaker	Vocal signs of pleasure; social smile
3	Looks in direction of speaker	Cooing and gurgling; smile in response to speech
4	Responds differentially to angry vs. pleasant voice	Responds vocally to social stimuli
5	Responds to own name (see also 2.3)	Begins to mimic sounds
6	Recognizes words like "bye-bye," "Mamma," "Daddy"	Protests vocally; squeals with delight
7	Responds with gestures to words such as "up," "come," "bye-bye"	Begins to use wordlike sounds, some jargon
8	Stops activity when own name is called	Imitates sound sequences
9	Stops activity in response to "no"	Imitates intonation pattern of speech
10	Accurately imitates pitch variations	First words appear
11	Responds to simple questions ("where is the dog?") by looking or pointing	Jargon well established
12	Responds with gestures to a variety of verbal requests	Announces awareness of familiar objects by name
15	Recognizes names of various parts of body	True words heard embedded in jargon, often with gestures
18	Identifies pictures of familiar objects when they are named	Uses words more than gestures to express desires
21	Follows two consecutive, related directions ("pick up your hat and put it on the chair")	Begins combining words ("Daddy car," "Mamma up")
24	Understands more complex sentences ("after we get in the car we'll go to the store")	Refers to self by name

especially when both sounds appear in one word (e.g., for "dog" the child might say "dawd" or "gawg"). This kind of phonetic duplication is not uncommon in 2 yr olds, and may be heard in some 3 yr olds. As children learn to make these sound discriminations in their own speech, they are also learning the motor controls for more complex speech patterns and can be heard to articulate sounds represented by the letters *f, v, s,* and *z.* Because these sounds are similar, 3 yr old children may be heard to substitute *f* for *s* or *v* for *z.* By the time they are able to produce the difference between "shoe"

and "Sue," they have mastered the difference between "fine" and "sign." They have also learned to produce "thing" and "sing" as separate and distinct words, and are able to say "rabbit" rather than "wabbit."

Control of the various speech sounds is usually mastered first at the beginning of words. The 2 yr old may omit sounds at the end of words; the 3 yr old may slide over sounds in the middle of words. And 4 or even 5 yr olds may have difficulty with complex sounds such as *skw* (squirrel) or *tr* (tree). Occasional misarticulations should be considered within normal limits up to 7 yr of age so long as the child's conversational speech can be understood readily. The normal 4 yr old is a competent receiver of his or her native language. There may still be some misarticulations and some overgeneralization of grammatic rules (e.g., "goed" for *went* or "seed" for *saw*), but speech is normally intelligible to strangers and shows basic mastery of the rules of syntax, phonology, and semantics.

Table 2–21 lists signs that suggest an valuation of the child's developing speech may be required.

Table 2–21 SIGNS OF PROBLEMS IN LANGUAGE AND SPEECH DEVELOPMENT IN PRESCHOOL CHILDREN

1. At 6 mo of age does not turn eyes and head to sound coming from behind or to side
2. At 10 mo does not make some kind of response to his or her name
3. At 15 mo does not understand and respond to "no-no," "bye-bye," and "bottle"
4. At 18 mo is not saying up to 10 single words
5. At 21 mo does not respond to directions (e.g., "sit down," "come here," "stand up")
6. After 24 mo has excessive, inappropriate jargon or echoing
7. At 24 mo does not on request point to body parts (e.g., mouth, nose, eyes, ears)
8. At 24 mo has no 2-word phrases
9. At 30 mo has speech that is not intelligible to family members
10. At 36 mo uses no simple sentences
11. At 36 mo has not begun to ask simple questions
12. At 36 mo has speech that is not intelligible to strangers
13. At 3.5 yr of age consistently fails to produce the final consonant (e.g., "ca" for *cat*, "bo" for *bone*, etc.)
14. After 4 yr of age is noticeably dysfluent (stutters)
15. After 7 yr of age has any speech sound errors
16. At any age has noticeable hypernasality or hyponasality, or has a voice which is a monotone, of inappropriate pitch, unduly loud, inaudible, or consistently hoarse

DETERRENTS TO NORMAL DEVELOPMENT

Hearing loss should be the first possibility to exclude when speech and language fail to develop. Physicians should watch for signs of development of communicative intent even before true speech can be expected. Even severely to profoundly hearing-impaired children will use visual cues to relate to the environment. The absence of communicative behavior of any kind may suggest auditory perceptual problems with or without lesions of the receptive organs.

Mental retardation is probably the most common cause of delay in development of speech and language. With intense stimulation even severely retarded children have been able to acquire some speech skills. In the case of severe to profound retardation, however, language development can be expected to remain at a low level, generally commensurate with intellectual development.

Orofacial deviations may impede speech development. The physiologic effects of an unrepaired cleft palate or of a functionally inadequate velopharyngeal mechanism normally result in predictable patterns of misarticulation and deviant resonance. Early conductive hearing loss, common in children with cleft palate, compounds the problem of speech and language learning for them. Early and successful surgical repair of cleft palates improves the prospects for speech and language development; speech therapy is frequently required, however, to help the child with a repaired cleft make the best use of the mechanisms for intelligible speech.

Other orofacial deviations that have detrimental effects on speech development include severe malocclusions, maladaptive tongue habits (for example, tongue thrust), enlarged tonsils and adenoids, and tongue tie. Malocclusion and tongue thrust, sometimes causally related to each other, result in (and sometimes from) maladaptive tongue postures and movements that may impair articulation. Enlarged tonsils and adenoids may so restrict the airway as to produce changes in normal resonance of voice and may constrict tongue movements, resulting in faulty articulation. Habitual mouth breathing resulting from airway obstructions may result in low tongue postures that impede clear speech. Tongue tie is seldom a cause for faulty speech development. Rarely, however, the frenum binds the tongue tip so tightly to the floor of the mouth that the child cannot produce without some distortion those precise movements required for over 60% of the consonant sounds of speech.

Neurologic impairment may result in faulty integration of speech and language signals, and impaired neuromuscular control of the muscles involved in speech may produce certain predictable deviations in phonation, resonance, and articulation. Other symptoms of such involvement include persistent drooling, difficulties in chewing and swallowing, and weak or aberrant breathing patterns.

Bilingualism may result in mild delay in language development for the child who has normal potential. By the time they reach school age, however, normal children reared bilingually from birth are linguistically competent in both languages. For the normal child the mild delay associated with bilingual training may be a small price to pay for the mastery of 2 languages. On the other hand, for children who have any difficulty in learning language the need to decode and encode 2 languages may render them vulnerable to speech and language delay in both languages.

GETTING HELP FOR CHILDREN WITH SPEECH AND LANGUAGE PROBLEMS

Early detection of and intervention in speech and language problems can help both children and parents to avoid or minimize pain and suffering during the school years. Public Law 94–142 mandates public school systems in the United States to provide appropriate and free special education to all children with handicaps, including speech and language problems. In each community, therefore, the public school system's office for special education services can identify the services available and indicate how children may be enrolled. In addition, clinical services in speech/language and audiology are to be found in most teaching hospitals and children's hospitals. Academic programs in speech/language pathology and audiology at major universities also provide clinical services, both as part of their training programs and as a direct service to the community.

Carol C. Towne

Bar-Adon A, Leopold W (eds): Child Language: A Book of Readings. Englewood Cliffs, NJ, Prentice-Hall, 1971.
Bzoch K, League R: Assessing Language Skills in Infancy. Gainesville, Fla, Tree of Life Press, 1972.
Dale PS: Language Development: Structure and Function. Ed 2. New York, Holt, Reinhart and Winston, 1976.
Halliday M: Learning How to Mean. London, Arnold Press, 1975.
Jaffe BF (ed): Hearing Loss in Children. Baltimore, University Park Press, 1977.
Lewis M, Rosenblum L: Interaction, Conversation, and the Development of Language, New York, John Wiley & Sons, 1977.
Northern J, Downes M: Hearing in Children. Baltimore, Williams and Wilkins 1974.
Paradise JF: Otitis media in infants and children. Pediatrics 65:5, 1980.
Perkins W: Speech Pathology. St. Louis, CV Mosby, 1977.
Weiss C, Lillywhite H: Communicative Disorders. St. Louis, CV Mosby, 1976.

OTHER DEVELOPMENTAL ISSUES

2.79 MENTAL RETARDATION

Mental retardation is a symptom found in numerous disorders of known and unknown etiologies. It is often difficult to define or to grade as to its severity. The diagnosis should be made only when adequate evidence has made it certain; otherwise, the stigmatizing effect of the label itself can be seriously handicapping.

Mental retardation should be considered in any child who performs more than 2 standard deviations below the mean for his or her age on a standard psychometric examination measuring intelligence. The IQ, or intelligence quotient, is the ratio of mental age to chronologic age, multiplied by 100. It is important to recognize that almost 3% of any "normal" population falls 2 standard deviations below the mean on any "intelligence" test. Pitfalls of intelligence tests are discussed elsewhere (Sec 2.72). They generally measure several brain functions, including auditory memory, visual-spatial capability, and expressive and receptive language. The measured IQ is an average of these functions and does not indicate specific strengths and weaknesses. Binet, who designed the first IQ test, did not intend it as a measure of innate cognitive ability but simply as a tool to predict school performance, for which the IQ proves after the age of 3 yr to be a rather reliable, but far from perfect, predictor. The IQ may not reflect the optimal cerebral function or potential of the individual. It is in some respects insensitive to the adverse effects of cultural and environmental factors in preventing achievement of the fullest potential.

The limitations of the intelligence quotient as a criterion for diagnosis of mental retardation have led to development of scales which assess the ability to adapt successfully to environmental and societal demands. For example, adaptation may be measured in terms of a child's ability to care for personal needs such as dressing and feeding as compared to that of children of similar chronologic age. Social skills may be assessed as well as the ability to adapt to general educational demands in a normal school setting. Focus may center on the degree to which, as an adult, the individual can be expected to be personally independent, socially accepted, and vocationally competitive.

The need to adapt to changing environmental circumstances is a primary reason for the changes with age in reported incidence of mental retardation (Fig 2–17). The number of children recognized as "retarded" rises during the school years, for it is at this time that the social setting results in comparisons among large numbers of children of the same age. The incidence decreases in late adolescence when scholastic demands are no longer an obstacle to functional adequacy. Many young adults with mild mental retardation make satisfactory adaptations in the community, both vocationally and socially. They function independently and competitively notwithstanding that their intellectual handicap adds to their difficulties in reaching this goal. It is estimated

Table 2–22 LEVELS OF MENTAL RETARDATION AND ASSOCIATED FEATURES

Borderline (IQ 68–83) —	Children with IQ's above 69 are not retarded, strictly speaking, but are vulnerable to educational problems. They are usually able to function adequately in slow sections of regular classes. Most achieve independent social and vocational adjustment.
Mild (IQ 52–67) —	This group includes 90% of children formally classified as retarded. Most need special class placement, and some can achieve 4th–6th grade reading levels. Those who are well adjusted may be able to function independently as adults.
Moderate (IQ 36–51) —	Children in this group will usually function in classes for the trainable retarded, with emphasis on gaining maximal self-care and perhaps some academic skills. Those who are well adjusted may be able to function semi-independently in supervised living and sheltered workshop settings.
Severe (IQ 20–35) —	Children in this group can learn minimal self-care skills and simple conversational skills. They need much supervision and are often institutionalized.
Profound (IQ below 20) —	Children in this group need total supervision. Very minimal self-care skills are possible. Some may be toilet trained. Language development will be minimal.

that among persons with IQ's of 60–80, 30–75% make adequate adjustment as adults to community life without the assistance of health, social, or correction agencies.

None of the many adaptive scales proposed have been universally accepted as devices for classification. Accordingly, in spite of its limitations the intelligence quotient remains the principal diagnostic criterion used by the health professions and agencies that deal with the mentally handicapped. Table 2–22 gives the classification of mental retardation currently in general use. It is estimated that over 90% of retarded persons are in the mild or borderline range. Only 5% are severely or profoundly retarded.

Etiology.   Table 2–23 lists and classifies the principal causes of mental retardation. In the majority of patients whose mental retardation is in the mild to borderline range comprehensive medical evaluations have not found evidence of a defective brain. The majority of these mildly retarded individuals are in social classes 4 and 5 (the lower end of the socioeconomic scale [Hollingshead]); accordingly, one is led to the hypothesis that their poor adaptive function is likely to be secondary to adverse sociocultural influences, including the lack of a stimulating environment. This theory is in keeping with the observation that children of lower socioeconomic groups have gradual declines in IQ's with maturation. On the other hand, it is possible that

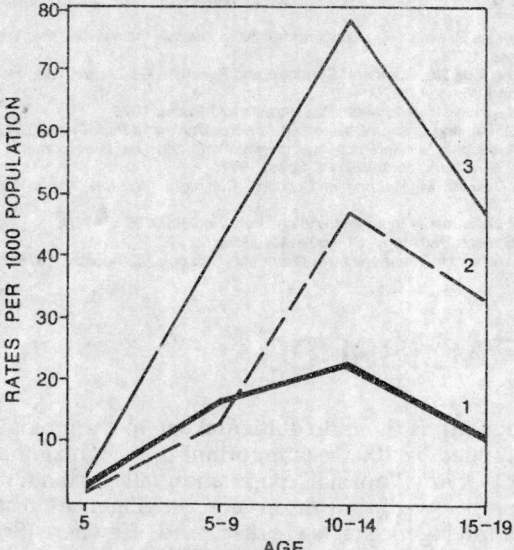

Figure 2–17. Incidence of mental retardation in different age groups as reported from three different surveys. 1. Report of the Mental Deficiency Commission. London, His Majesty's Stationery Office. 1929, Pts 1, 2, 3, and 4. 2. Lemkau P, et al.: Mental Hygiene Problems in an Urban District. 3. New York State Department of Mental Hygiene, Mental Health Research Unit: A Special Census of Suspected Referred Mental Retardation, Onondaga County, N.Y. Syracuse, N.Y., 1955, p 84.

Table 2–23 CAUSES OF MENTAL RETARDATION

Nonorganic — environmentally determined
  Sociocultural factors
  Emotional distrubances
Organic
  Static encephalopathies
    Prenatal origin
      Cerebral maldevelopment — 1st trimester
        Chromosomal aberrations
        Intrauterine infections (e.g., TORCH infections)
        Teratogens
        Placental dysfunction
        Unknown cause
      Cerebral maldevelopment — 2nd and 3rd trimesters
        Intrauterine infection (e.g., TORCH infections)
        Teratogens
        Maternal diabetes mellitus
        Maternal toxemia of pregnancy
        Placental dysfunction
        Maternal urinary tract infection (?)
        Maternal malnutrition
    Perinatal origin
      Complications of prematurity
      Asphyxia neonatorum
      Birth trauma
      Meningitis
    Postnatal origin
      Significant head and central nervous system trauma
      Cerebrovascular accident
      Neurotoxins (e.g., lead)
      Intracranial infections
      Anoxic episodes (e.g., near-drowning)
  Progressive encephalopathies
    Metabolic
      Aminoacidurias (e.g., PKU)
      Carbohydrate disorders (e.g., galactosemia)
      Polysaccharidoses (e.g., Hurler)
      Cerebral lipidoses (e.g., Tay-Sachs); with hepatomegaly
        (Gaucher)
      Leukodystrophies (e.g., metachromatic leukodystrophy)
      Uric acid disturbance (e.g., Lesch-Nyhan)
      Hormonal imbalance (e.g., hypothyroid,
        pseudohypoparathyroid)
      Nutritional deficiencies
      Neuroectodermal dysplasia (e.g., tuberous sclerosis)
      Other degenerative diseases (e.g., Alpers)
    Infectious
      Kuru
      Subacute sclerosing panencephalitis

Diagnosis and Clinical Manifestations. The assessment of a child who is functioning in the mentally retarded range must first answer the following questions: (1) Is the brain dysfunction on an organic basis? (2) If so, is the organic deficit due to a static or progressive lesion? (3) Is there a treatable condition present? (4) Is there an indication of a familial or hereditary disorder?

A comprehensive history can be the best aid to diagnosis. Certain high risk factors are associated (prenatally, perinatally, or postnatally) with the likelihood of brain damage (Table 2–24). The presence of one or more of these factors offers only circumstantial evidence that cerebral injury has resulted. It is not unusual to find in an infant at high risk who performs poorly on standard developmental testing that medical and neurologic examinations and comprehensive laboratory evaluations are normal. In such cases, to conclude that there is no relationship between the high risk factor and evidence of brain injury may be unjustifiable. Clinical judgment is required in assessing the relationship between high-risk events and later neurologic status.

During physical examination a variety of findings may give clues as to etiology or organicity. It is important to determine whether certain congenital stigmata are present (Table 2–25). Various patterns of stigmata indicate specific syndromes. Some are secondary to

Table 2–24 FACTORS INDICATING INFANTS OR CHILDREN AT RISK OF MENTAL RETARDATION

Prenatal
  Toxemia
  Placenta praevia
  Abruptio placentae
  Exposure to ionizing radiation during 1st trimester
  Syphilis
  TORCH infections
  Ingestion of teratogens
  Multiple pregnancy
  Previous miscarriage
  Family history of cerebral dysfunction, speech and language
    dysfunction, hearing impairment
  Maternal malnutrition
  Vaginal bleeding in the 2nd or 3rd trimesters
  Maternal age less than 16 yr or over 40 yr
  Consanguinity

Perinatal
  Prematurity
  Small birth weight for gestational age
  Birth anoxia or hypoxia
  Birth trauma
  Low 1 min and/or 5 min Apgar scores
  Neonatal seizures
  Abnormal neonatal neurobehavioral examination
  Early difficulty in sucking
  Hypoglycemia
Postnatal
  Disadvantaged socioeconomic environment
  Intracranial infection
  Significant head trauma
  Encephalitis
  Meningitis
  Ingestion or inhalation of neurotoxins (e.g., lead)
  Cerebral hypoxia secondary to near-drowning or carbon monoxide
    poisoning
  Cerebrovascular accident
  Severe malnutrition

the defective brain function may not be detected by present neuroinvestigative techniques or that polygenic determinants of intelligence may be playing a role. Moreover, there may be prevalent in the lower socioeconomic environment subtly detrimental "organic" effects that are not readily apparent. For example, blood lead levels are often higher in inner-city, economically deprived children than in suburban children from affluent families. Subclinical lead intoxication, acting over a prolonged period of time, can impair cognitive abilities. Cytomegalovirus infection is also more frequently noted among mothers of lower socioeconomic status, and their infants are more frequently found to excrete the virus than infants from more affluent families. The likelihood of nutritional deficiency also correlates with socioeconomic status (Sec 2.1). Malnutrition, smoking, and deficiencies in prenatal care are all more common among socioeconomically disadvantaged mothers and are known to have detrimental effects on fetal brain development.

Table 2–25 STIGMATA ASSOCIATED WITH MENTAL RETARDATION

Head
  Maximum occipitofrontal circumference at less than 3rd percentile or over 97th percentile
  Plagiocephaly
Hair
  Double whorl; sparse or absent hair
  Fine, friable, prematurely gray or white locks
Eyes
  Microphthalmia
  Hypertelorism
  Hypotelorism
  Upward-and-outward or down-and-outward slant
  Inner or outer epicanthal folds
  Colomboma of iris or retina
  Brushfield spots
  Eccentrically placed pupil
  Nystagmus
  Telangiectasia
Ears
  Low set ears
  Simple or abnormal helix formation
Nose
  Flattened bridge
  Small size
  Upturned nares
Face
  Increased length of philtrum
  Hypoplasia of maxilla and/or mandible
Mouth
  Inverted "V" shape of upper lip
  Wide or high-arched palate
Teeth
  Evidence of abnormal enamelogenesis
  Abnormal odontogenesis
Neck
  Short neck
  Lack of full mobility
  Webbing
Extremities
  Unusually short or long limbs
  Increased carrying angle at elbows
Hands
  Short stubby fingers
  Long, thin tapered fingers
  Broad thumbs
  Clinodactyly
  Abnormal dermatoglyphics (e.g., distal triradius)
  Simian line
  Abnormal nails (e.g., short 5th metacarpal)
Feet
  Overlap of toes
  Short stubby toes
  Long, thin tapering toes
  Broad, large big toes
  Deep crease leading from angle of 1st and 2nd toes
  Abnormal dermatoglyphics
Abdomen
  Protuberant abdomen
  Umbilical hernia
Genitalia
  Ambiguous genitalia
  Micropenis
  Abnormal placement of urethral meatus
  Undescended testicles
Chest
  Pectus excavatum or carinatum
  Supernumerary nipples
Skin
  Café-au-lait spots
  Depigmented nevi
  Adenoma sebaceum
  Malar flush
  Eczema

Table 2–26 SOFT NEUROLOGIC SIGNS

Poor fine and/or gross coordination
Strabismus
Verbal dyspraxia
Motor dyspraxia
Motor impersistence (positive Prechtl sign)
Immature overflow patterns
Microcephaly
Macrocephaly
Immature sequencing (motor, auditory, visual)
Graphomotor difficulties
Constructional dyspraxia
Choreiform movements
Mirror movements
Dysdiadochokinesia

chromosomal abnormalities or teratogenic effects; others may be of unknown cause. Identification of these syndromes has been made easier through compendia that index the stigmata to known syndromes. One is often unable to identify a syndrome even though the prevalence of stigmata clearly suggests that the central nervous system anomaly may have the same origin as the visible external abnormalities. On the other hand, each of these stigmata occurs in normal persons, albeit with much lower frequency than among the mentally retarded.

Head circumference may be of diagnostic significance if it is more than 2 standard deviations below or above the mean or if head circumference and height are significantly discrepant though both are within normal limits. Clues to progressive degenerative diseases of the brain or to metabolic diseases include choreoretinitis, optic atrophy, pigmentary degeneration of the retina, cataracts, uveitis, skin lesions (vitiligo, café-au-lait spots, port-wine stains, hemangiomas, incontinentia pigmenti, nevus unius lateris, and adenoma sebaceum), organomegaly, abnormal genitalia, excessively short or tall stature, abnormal body proportions, unusual smell to urine or skin, light hair color, and sparse or friable hair. A formal neurologic examination should evaluate the status of the entire neuraxis and peripheral nervous system, including assessment of cranial nerves; muscular strength, tone, and coordination; deep tendon and primitive reflexes; and cortical sensory function. Examination is also made for the presence of "soft" neurologic signs (Table 2–26 and Sec 2.72).

The laboratory investigations necessary to assess the patient with mental retardation should vary with the clinical findings. Table 2–27 lists laboratory tests that should be considered in the context of historical events and findings on physical and neurologic examination.

Treatment. The primary goal of management of the mentally retarded is that each affected person reach his or her optimal developmental potential and be able to cope as effectively as possible with the handicap. In helping to achieve this, the physician must assist the family as a whole in developing strategies that will allow each member to make a rapid and optimal adaptation to the stress of living with a handicapped person (Sec 2.80).

Treatment begins as soon as diagnosis is suspected. It is important that the physician be scrupulously honest

Table 2–27 DIAGNOSTIC STRATEGY FOR INFANT OR CHILD WITH MENTAL RETARDATION

Chromosomal karyotype indicated in children with
  Unusual number and/or character of physical stigmata
  History of maternal exposure to a teratogen
  Abnormal genitalia
Examination for *aminoaciduria* indicated in children with
  Unexplained seizures — neonatal period
  Unusual smell to urine or skin
  Unusually light-colored hair
  Microcephaly
  Family history
  Dermatitis
Examination of urine for *mucopolysaccharides* indicated in children with
  Coarse features
  Kyphosis
  Short extremities
  Short trunk
  Cloudy cornea
  Impaired hearing
  Dwarfism
  Stiff joints
Examination of urine for *reducing substances* indicated in children with
  Cataracts
  Hepatomegaly
  Seizures
Examination of *serum ammonia level* indicated in children with
  Episodic vomiting and metabolic acidosis
Examination of urine for *ketoacids* indicated in children with
  Seizures
  Short friable hair
Examination of *blood lead level* indicated in children with
  History of pica
  Anemia
  Unexplained mental retardation in inner-city child
Examination of *serum zinc level* indicated in children with
  Acrodermatitis
Examination of *skull roentgenograms* indicated in children with
  Microcephaly
  Macrocephaly
  Plagiocephaly
  Suspected intracerebral mass
Examination of *serum copper and ceruloplasmin levels* indicated in children with
  Involuntary movements
  Cirrhosis
  Kayser-Fleischer rings
Examination of *serum neuroenzyme activities* and/or *skin biopsy* indicated in children with
  Loss of milestones or functions in motor and/or cognitive areas
  Optic atrophy
  Retinal degeneration
  Recurrent cerebellar ataxia
  Myoclonus
  Hepatosplenomegaly
  Coarse loose skin
  Seizures
  Enlarged head beginning after 1 yr of age
Examination of *VMA levels* indicated in children with
  Episodic vomiting
  Poor suck
  Symptoms of autonomic dysfunction
Examination of *serum uric acid levels* indicated in children with
  Self-mutilation
  Rage attacks
  Gout
  Choreoathetosis
Computed axial tomography (CAT scan) of head indicated in children with
  Progressive enlargement of head
  Tuberous sclerosis
  Suspected gross malformation of brain
  Focal seizures
  Suspected intracranial mass

regarding the diagnosis and in estimating the potential of the child, and also be willing to share uncertainty or ignorance on certain points. This truthful approach must be tempered by compassion. Parents who are told for the 1st time that their child is mentally retarded will not infrequently deny that the problem exists. Denial may be accompanied by anger toward the physician and by a search for contrary medical opinions. These parental reactions are normal. A defensive or angry reponse on the part of the physician whose diagnosis and advice are thus rejected or disbelieved will only further alienate the parents and complicate future contacts. The physician will usually need to reassure parents that they are not themselves responsible for the child's handicap. Such reassurance is particularly important when the etiology is not known.

When a diagnosis conveying the probability or certainty of mental retardation is evident during the neonatal period, the physician should meet with both parents and explain his or her concern about the baby, avoiding a tendency to focus only upon abnormal findings or probable weaknesses. Attention of the parents should also be directed to normal features and positive attributes which the baby may have, such as vitality, muscular strength, nice appearance, or alertness. Such observations may help parents to accept the infant as a person and foster the healthy bonding important to the infant's later development. Parents who learn that they have a retarded child who is not the fantasied ideal extension of themselves may go into a period of mourning as though they had lost a family member (Sec 2.44).

Retarded infants should be referred early to infant stimulation programs. These programs may be based either in centers or in the home. They have 2 primary functions: (1) to help the infant develop optimally by helping the parents to understand their baby's developmental problem, strengths, and limitations; and (2) to offer a curriculum of multisensory stimulation aimed at facilitation of cognitive, physical, and emotional development. A 3rd function is to support parents and other family members through individual and/or group counseling. Infant stimulation programs vary in the strategies aimed toward sensorimotor development. Although their effectiveness has not been convincingly demonstrated, many clinicians believe that they have value in immediate supportive and educational counseling of parents, which may decrease their need to "shop" for other opinions and may shorten the time necessary for them to adapt to the experience of having and living with a handicapped offspring. The sapping of emotional energy and financial resources through searching for contrary opinions can adversely affect maternal-infant bonding and impair or frustrate the nurturance needed by the handicapped infant.

All retarded children in the United States, irrespective of the severity of their functional deficits, have the legal right to an education up to the age of 21 yr. Education does not necessarily mean learning academic subjects but can mean learning self-care activities and social skills. In school districts which have programs for 3–5 yr old children with developmental delays it is essential that children with mental retardation be referred for enrollment. Where the public school system does not have educational resources available for preschool children, voluntary agencies may have such programs. The Head Start program in the United States is required to enroll handicapped children.

For children of school age, federal legislation (PL 94–142) mandates that children with developmental disabilities receive education services in school settings, either in regular classes with the help of extra resources ("mainstreaming") or in special classes geared to the handicapped child's educational, social, and behavioral needs (Sec 2.80). Physicians should encourage parents to enroll their handicapped children in school programs, should, with the parents' permission, exchange information with the school about educationally relevant medical and physical findings, and should participate in the formulation of the child's educational needs. To be effective in securing an appropriate educational program for any child with a learning disability, the physician must become familiar enough with the operation of his or her own local school system to understand and cope with the administrative and political issues that may interfere with provision of the appropriate individualized educational program to which the child is entitled. The physician who accepts and meets the challenge of bringing about communication among various professional persons involved in services to children with disabilities and to their families can perform a unique service because of his or her understanding of human development.

Unfortunately, many retarded persons are not befriended by their normally functioning age-mates or classmates. Social and recreational activities must be planned for them. Organized activities for retarded persons are often available, and parents should become familiar with them. Attendance at summer camps for the retarded should be encouraged. Such programs help the retarded to acquire comfortable social interactions and to achieve more independent function.

Many communities have sheltered workshops for retarded adults capable of simple repetitive tasks who are unable to compete in the labor market. For severely retarded individuals who cannot function in sheltered workshops, community-based activity centers offer a chance for socialization and recreation.

The United States is moving toward "normalizing" as much as possible the lives of retarded individuals. Foster care or placement in small group homes is becoming available as an alternative to large residential institutions for children or adults who need to be cared for away from their own homes. Group homes are usually situated within the community where the retarded person's family lives, and in such homes "house parents" are responsible for care of a small number of compatible handicapped individuals; this care is coordinated with other resources of the community, such as public schools, recreational facilities, and sheltered workshops. Early residential placement of retarded children or adults outside the home should not be casually advised by the physician, but the possibility can be mentioned as an option when it becomes evident that a particular family is finding it difficult to cope with the situation and/or when the particular child's behavior is deteriorating. The physician should discuss all options

without passing moral judgments as to what the family should or should not do. When parents make decisions in accord with *their* needs and resources, all options considered, the physician should be supportive.

Every retarded child needs someone to take the responsibility for monitoring progress, for assisting with educational placement and obtaining social and recreational experiences, and for supporting and advising parents and siblings during periods of crisis. This individual should also inform the family about the programmatic and financial assistance to which they may be entitled. A concerned pediatrician can discharge this function particularly well; at routine health visits for preventive care more global issues can be explored with the family. Pediatricians who do not feel that they can provide these services should suggest that help be sought at a local chapter of the Association for Retarded Citizens or through the responsible governmental agency (generally, the Crippled Children's Program).

Parents of handicapped children are often excessively devoted to the care of their handicapped child, leaving no time for themselves. Many communities have respite centers in foster care or residential settings where parents can leave their children temporarily with responsible caretakers while they have relief for a weekend or longer from the continuing demands of the care of the handicapped child. The physician should suggest such arrangements to parents and help them not to feel guilty about their need for periodic relief or vacation.

The sexual drives of mild or moderately retarded persons do not differ from those of persons of normal intelligence. On the other hand, their levels of comprehension of socially acceptable sexual behavior may present a problem, depending on their particular levels of intellectual functioning. Many retarded persons will need family-planning services adjusted to their levels of understanding and function. In some instances, sterilization may warrant consideration as a form of contraception, though ethical and legal issues surround its use. Sterilization of retardates for eugenic purposes is not acceptable in the United States.

Prognosis. If a mildly retarded adult is to have a chance of functioning independently within the community, he or she must have socially acceptable behavior. This achievement is not easy given the environmental burden mentally handicapped children must cope with. They are frequently frustrated by their inability to attain either academic or social success and feel the effects of parental unhappiness or dissatisfaction at their slow progress. The result is loss of self-esteem and decreased motivation to achieve. Some retarded persons feel that they can achieve recognition only by aggressive or acting-out behavior, which further alienates them from peers and family. Retarded persons with cosmetic difficulties have additional experiences of rejection.

Mildly retarded persons usually require placement in special educational programs, though a few succeed in regular classes. Many can achieve a 5th grade level in reading or in mathematics. Usually, they can find employment only in unskilled jobs. Not infrequently, mildly retarded persons marry and raise children in a responsible fashion. Assuming responsibility for a family can be a risky venture, however, especially for retarded persons with poor judgment who must compete in an increasingly technologic society.

LAWRENCE T. TAFT

Alford CA: Prenatal infections and psychosocial development in children born into lower socioeconomic settings. In: Mittler P (ed): Research to Practice in Mental Retardation and Biomedical Aspects. Vol III. Baltimore, University Park Press, 1977.

Beatti AO, Moore MR, Goldberg A: Role of chronic low-level lead exposure in the aetiology of mental retardation. Lancet 1:589, 1975.

Birch HG: Functional effect of malnutrition. In: Chess S, Thomas A (eds): Annual Progress in Child Psychiatry and Child Development. New York, Brunner/Hazel, 1972.

Crowe G: The brain and mental retardation. Br Med J 1:897, 1960.

Cruickshank W: The relation of physical disability to fear and guilt feelings. Child Dev 22:291, 1951.

Denhoff E: Status of infant stimulation or enrichment programs for children with developmental disabilities. Pediatrics 67:32, 1981.

Diagnostic and Statistical Manual of Mental Disorder III. Washington DC, American Psychiatric Association, 1979.

Dobbing J, Hopewell JW, Lynch A: Vulnerability of developing brain. VII. Permanent deficits of neurons in cerebral and cerebellar cortex following early mild malnutrition. Exp Neur 32:439, 1971.

Green M: The management of children with chronic disease. In: Green AM, Haggerty RJ (eds): Ambulatory Pediatrics II. Philadelphia, WB Saunders, 1977.

Mattson A: Long-term physical illness in childhood: A challenge to psychosocial adaptation. Pediatrics 50:901, 1972.

Meier JH: Screening, assessment and intervention for young children at developmental risk. In: Tjossem TD (ed): Intervention Strategies for High Risk Infants and Young Children. Baltimore, University Park Press, 1976, p 251.

Richmond JB, Targan G, Mendelsohn RS (eds): Mental Retardation: A Handbook for the Primary Physician. Chicago, American Medical Association, 1976.

Rosen M, Clark GR, Kivitz MO (eds): The History of Mental Retardation. Baltimore, University Park Press, 1976.

Schneider AP, Hanshaw JB, Simeoussou RH, et al: The study of children with congenital cytomegalovirus infection. In: Mittler P (ed): Research to Practice in Mental Retardation and Biomedical Aspects. Vol III. Baltimore, University Park Press, 1977.

Solnit AJ, Stark MH: Mourning and the birth of a defective child. Psychoanal Study Child 16:523, 1961.

Sparrow S, Zigler E: Evaluation of a patterning treatment for retarded children. Pediatrics 63:137, 1978.

Turnbull AP, Turnbull HR III: Parents Speak Out, Views from the Other Side of the Two-Way Mirror. Columbus, Ohio, Charles E Merrill Publishing Co, 1978.

Zigler E: Dealing with retardation. (Review of The Mentally Retarded and Society, by MJ Begab and SA Richardson). Science 196:1192, 1977.

2.80 CARE OF THE CHILD WITH A PERMANENT HANDICAP

Permanent handicaps of children include a wide variety of disorders which limit the activity or developmental potential of children in various ways. The most salient features of the handicapping condition may include mental retardation; limitations of physical activity; sensory, learning, and communicative difficulties; conspicuous physical deformities; needs for special arrangements to achieve such normal functions as toileting, mobility, feeding, and the like; evidences of chronic illness or its treatment; and so on. Whatever the particulars, the handicapped child must live in a social world that is perceived as being somewhat apart. And, ultimately, the successful management of children who have chronic and perhaps permanent disabilities depends as often on the social, academic, and home adjustments that can be achieved as it does on purely technical and medical procedures. The parents and family have the major responsibility in caring for and

nurturing their children, including the child with the handicap; but the physician should play a direct and supportive role, with others, in helping the family to meet their responsibilities for identifying, finding, and providing those things needed for optimal development (Sec 2.79).

THE PHYSICIAN

Some physicians are not suited by temperament or training to manage the handicapped child and the family. The comprehensive care required is time-consuming, and many of the children as well as their parents appear at times uncooperative, unapprec tive, and even negative. Much time must be spent with parents whose emotional reactions frequently demand more attention than the condition of the child. The physician who extends his or her responsibility beyond the treatment of the "chief complaint," however, will find rewards in helping young handicapped patients and their families to live more comfortably and effectively.

Physicians may feel inadequate because the problems appear complex or insoluble or beyond the means at immediate command. Physicians must be aware of their own possible negative attitudes, prejudices, and limitations and must, above all, be able to utilize other professional persons or disciplines, to make appropriate referrals, and to use other resources in the community while they maintain the role of primary physician.

The physician may feel inadequate if a specific diagnosis cannot be made or if the evaluation cannot be completed at one visit. The physician to handicapped children and their families must be a patient, unthreatening listener, satisfied with small gains and able to understand the child's and the parents' positions sufficiently to offer intelligent support when cure or recovery is not possible. Such physicians should not cling to outmoded concepts or be unaware of either the possibilities or the limitations of habilitation. They must communicate and work effectively with others in the community in providing adequate general pediatric care for the child and support for an acceptable role for parents. Physicians who are uncomfortable in these roles should arrange for care of the child and family by others prepared and willing to assume these responsibilities. When such a transfer of care is arranged, it should not be implied that the reason for it is any shortcoming of the family.

MANAGEMENT OF THE CHILD

Management begins at the first meeting with the family, with a functional appraisal of the child and a simple explanation to the parents. Further management should include the same comprehensive health services given to all children. Through continuing contacts and interest in the child and family the physician can help in developing and periodically revising a realistic plan. The ultimate goal is that the child make use of his or her abilities as effectively as possible and become as socially acceptable and self-sufficient as limitations permit. Immediate goals should be sufficiently realistic that success is possible and likely since failure discourages further effort, whereas success and praise of effort encourage and motivate.

Children with single or multiple handicaps often have limited opportunities for the experiences upon which normal learning and development depend; accordingly, particular effort must be made to arrange appropriate experiences at each developmental level. Opportunities for learning, for social and group experiences, and for the achievement of self-discipline should be provided. A variety of sensory stimuli and of close, warm, and stimulating parent-child interactions are essential from birth for optimal child development. It is especially important that the parents of infants and children whose avenues to learning may be blocked be reminded to create adequate opportunities for early social and environmental stimulation and interaction. A balance between overprotection and overstimulation must be sought. Misguided protection or indulgence may deprive the child of normal experiences, such as being held to normal limits of acceptable behavior and discipline through self-control. Every effort should be made to minimize secondary handicaps in personality development which may otherwise become more serious than the primary defect.

The physician should above all else try to help the child lead a happy life. Every effort should be made to involve the child as well as the parents in understanding the problem, in planning, and in decision making. The wise and understanding physician takes time to explain to the child at the child's level of comprehension why he or she is different, what is planned, what is to be done, and why. The physician must interpret the child's condition and behavior to those who are in regular or occasional contact with him or her.

THE FAMILY'S PROBLEMS

The environment and emotional climate of the home of the handicapped child are often more crucial than medical care for the child's eventual adjustment; accordingly, the family must be helped to understand their own feelings and to fulfill their own needs. They must always be given something constructive to do. Parents' reactions to a child with a defect depend on the extent to which they feel that their competency, social standing, and anticipated way of life are threatened. Most parents attempt initially to deny the reality of the defect, particularly if it is not apparent physically. Denial is usually followed by frustration, disorganization, self-accusation, and questioning, and fears and anxieties about the future may become overwhelming. Simple explanation, support, and guidance for the family are particularly necessary at this time. As parents' defenses become organized further, denial, hostility, and attempts to assign responsibility develop. A physician who is not aware that the parents' feelings of guilt may be projected as anger with him or her will be unprepared to react with the necessary understanding and patience and may emerge with a bruised ego. If communication and counseling are not effective, the "no one ever told me" reaction sets in and "shopping around" ensues. Frequently, introduction of the family to group discussions with other parents will prove

helpful through providing opportunities for sharing of feelings or for education about the condition itself.

The physician's ability to communicate a genuine professional concern for the child and for the family's feelings often spells the difference between the family's active involvement and their rejection of help. Depending upon their maturity and emotional resources, the family can be helped to plan realistically and constructively for the long-term needs of the child. Parents and other family members should join in assessment and re-evaluation of the child's progress and have active parts in developing and carrying out recommendations. If the family cannot approve or accept recommendations, even ideal ones, or if recommended community services are not available, substitutes must be found. Group or individual counseling about problems of management may be appropriate. Physicians may overlook the support that the church can give to families in time of stress.

The problems are as varied as the people involved. Most parents, regardless of their backgrounds, have feelings of guilt which must be resolved lest attitudes of self-sacrifice, excessive overprotection, or rejection of the child develop. Most families have ambivalent feelings varying from overt hostility to gross overindulgence. The handicapped child may frequently be the precipitating factor in marital difficulties not basically related to him or her.

As the child grows older, the parents have to make adaptations, which would otherwise not be necessary, because of the child's prolonged dependency upon them. Problems of social isolation, schooling, sexual development, and sometimes unpleasant behavior become increasingly important.

In some circumstances the principles of behavior modification should be discussed with the family and help given in establishing and maintaining an appropriate program of conditioning for acceptable behavior. Parents should be given support and suitable materials for ongoing health and sex education for their children.

FAMILY THERAPY

Parents often complain in retrospect that the status of the child was not made clear to them, that the diagnosis was based on an incomplete examination or hasty judgment, that a poor prognosis was not justified, or that their part in helping the child was not explained. It must be remembered that many parents hear, retain, and comprehend only in part and that interpretations and suggestions must be given *and repeated* in an acceptable and understandable way to all those concerned. Reinforcement of information given the family may be made by other members of the physician's staff or by members of various other disciplines if consultation services are available.

The initial explanation of the facts about a child with a handicap should be made to the parents *together* as simply as possible. A statement as to what is wrong and what will be done about it is less confusing than a technical explanation. Emphasis should be placed on normalities and similarities to other children rather than on deficiencies and differences. Long-term prognosis and planning should be left for later interviews; attention should be focused on management of immediate problems and symptoms. If necessary, for example, simple techniques could be demonstrated: how to handle an infant who arches the back; how to help an infant in sucking, swallowing, or chewing or in the use of a spoon or cup; how to choose appropriate toys or activities to encourage language development.

Questions should be answered simply and reassurance given to minimize guilt feelings. The physician should also stress the need for patience because it will take time to clarify the child's developmental potential. Attention cannot be given too early to the need to avoid secondary emotional problems in the child and family. The practical problems of carrying out a reasonable program can be best appreciated by a visit to the home. Grandparents and other relatives who may be involved in family affairs should be brought into explanations and planning so that the parents' efforts with the child will be supported.

The parents need clear, simple, valid explanations and interpretations of what the referring physician and consultants have observed and recommended in the form of statements as to what has been found, along with copies of reports and consultations. Such reports should be factual, should contain relevant positive and negative observations about the child and his or her developmental progress, and should make appropriate recommendations. They should not become complex scientific treatises but efficient working papers.

Care should be taken to assure siblings an equal share of parents' time, attention, and interest. With inadvertent or intentional neglect their problems may become greater than those of the affected child. Their questions about the abnormal child should be answered simply and honestly. The experience of living with a seriously handicapped brother or sister may be used constructively to teach tolerance, patience, and understanding of others. If parents openly accept the child as an individual despite limitations, and if they accept failures as gracefully as they do more limited successes, a good example is set for others.

The question of the probable outcome of future pregnancies is frequently raised by parents. If the cause of the disability is clearly an accidental one, it is easy to be reassuring. If it is known to be genetically determined or to arise as a result of circumstances that might recur, the physician should explain the facts as simply and clearly as possible and help the parents to make their own decision based on available evidence and their own circumstances (Sec 2.82).

INSTITUTIONAL CARE

In the case of a seriously handicapped child who will always be completely or partially dependent on others for care, the question of suitability of institutional placement will arise. The physician should objectively discuss with the family the advantages and disadvantages of such care. Evidence suggests that infants and young children have a better developmental future if they live with a consistent mothering figure in an emotionally sound home environment. Moreover, parents generally feel more comfortable about later placement if they have gradually gained full understanding and acceptance of the child's limitations by fulfilling their normal roles as parents. Premature placement may lead to doubts and greater feelings of guilt. Before advising the use of supportive or education facilities away from home, as opposed to what may be available in the community, the physician should assess their appropriateness, their cost, and their availability. In any case, the decision is the family's and not the physician's, though he or she, if convinced that such a solution would be beneficial to all, may diplomatically initiate the discussion when the family appears reluctant to open the question.

Temporary care away from home is indicated when the child can profit by greater opportunities in a different environment, or for a short term when inevitable family emergencies arise, or when a vacation is needed by all.

USE OF COMMUNITY RESOURCES

The physician is in a unique position to interpret to others in the school, the church, and the community center the special problems presented by children with handicaps, and the physician should help to develop and make effective use of community resources. Needs may include medical facilities for early diagnosis, evaluation, and treatment; social case work; genetic counseling; psychologic evaluation and counseling; home care by nurses; "homemaker" services, babysitting, or temporary boarding home care; day care; special educational and recreational facilities; occupation and vocational placement; sheltered workshops; and smaller, local residential programs for respite care.

The physician should support current trends to centralize and coordinate diagnostic and treatment services for children with related handicaps in order to avoid discontinuity, waste of professional effort, frustration of parents, fragmentation of services for the child, and general administrative inefficiency. The "developmental disability" approach is an example of such an effort to bring together programs involving several categorical disorders.

Mainstreaming is an educational movement to channel children with major special needs into regular classes in the schools in the hope of providing a more normal environment and of avoiding the stigma associated with special programs which label such children as different. This has had limited success in comparison with classes offering special education of good quality, structured to meet pupils' individual learning needs. Mainstreaming may become more effective as teachers are better prepared, as more adequate resources and supports are provided in the classrooms, as teachers are able to communicate more effectively with parents and with other concerned professionals, and as the attitudes and expectations of all concerned become more tolerant and realistic. In the shift from placement of retarded or severely handicapped children in relatively large isolated institutions toward care in the home or in smaller, neighborhood facilities, many of the anticipated benefits have been delayed because of deficiencies of local services and in clarifying administrative responsibility. Still to be clarified also are the ideal size of the group, the best physical environment, and the kinds of disabilities and the ages at which affected children can best be served. The smaller units seem, however, to be providing a stimulus for more appropriate individualized programs and for better social behavior.

Parents' Organizations. Parents' organizations and groups of handicapped persons themselves have been outstandingly successful in affording those with common problems opportunities to share their anxieties, to gain strength and hope through identification with a group, and to bring about effective changes in legislation, in community health and educational programs, and in support of legal and civil rights of the handicapped. These and other efforts in behalf of community education, support of research, voluntary participation in a variety of services, and public recognition are psychologically important to the families of children with handicaps and are constructively helpful to the community.

JOHN B. BARTRAM

Gordon S: Facts about Sex for Exceptional Youth. New Jersey Association for Brain Injured Children, 61 Lincoln Street, East Orange, NJ 07017.

Kempton W, et al: Guide for Parents: Love, Sex and Birth Control for Mentally Retarded. Planned Parenthood Association of Southeastern Pennsylvania, 1402 Spruce Street, Philadelphia, Pa 19102.

Pattullo A: Puberty in the Girl Who Is Retarded. National Association for Retarded Citizens, 2709 Avenue E East, Arlington, Tex 76010.

White B: First Three Years of Life. Englewood Cliffs, NJ, Prentice-Hall, 1975.

2.81   CARE OF THE CHILD WITH A FATAL ILLNESS

From time to time every physician has the painful duty of caring for a child with a fatal illness. It is then his or her responsibility to help the family cope with their pain and grief in such ways that the experience may become growth-promoting rather than destructive of family integrity or of the emotional well-being of the family members. The acceptance by physicians of these goals as realistic and urgently in need of their professional skills will help to blunt their sense of frustration, grief, or professional inadequacy.

CARE OF PARENTS

When the physician is certain of a fatal outcome, there should ordinarily be no equivocation in conveying the diagnosis to the family in a direct and empathic way. If both parents are available, the fact that their child has an illness from which recovery is not expected should be conveyed to them when they are together. The words chosen and the manner of the physician should be gentle and honest, and he or she should be prepared to meet the parents' anguish or disbelief with answers to their questions and with information as to what measures will be taken to try to forestall what seems to be inevitable (Sec 2.64).

The place in which this conversation occurs should be carefully chosen. It should be apart from the other activities of the hospital or office and should be available for an adequate, uninterrupted time. Much of the conversation at this time will not be truly heard or registered by the parents of the sick child, and the physician should plan another session later in the day or on the next day when the information given can be reviewed and new or recurring questions answered.

Ordinarily the physician should avoid taking the position that nothing can be done in a situation which the parents sense as a disaster but should emphasize the positive steps which the physician and parents together can take to surmount the difficulties ahead. Physicians should generally avoid detailed predictions of the course of the illness, emphasizing that in such situations one generally lives from day to day and that it is usually possible to avoid undue suffering or pain. When the illness may endure for months or years, it may not be inappropriate to hold out the hope that medical research may provide methods of control which are not currently available.

Parents are often reluctant to ask whether some other physician or the resources of some other medical center may offer more hope, or even whether the diagnosis may be in doubt. They will need help in expressing these concerns and should be encouraged and helped to seek additional medical opinions if they wish. These matters should be discussed in such a way that the family should feel no embarrassment, and they should know that they are causing none. They can be helped to understand that medical communication is generally good enough to provide prompt dissemination of any real breakthrough in the management of the otherwise fatal illness of their child. It is also reasonable to advise them that they may do the ill child and the rest of the family a disservice if they dissipate the family's emotional and other resources in a frantic search for something that is not available.

It is natural and inevitable that parents will ask themselves whether the fatal illness of their child was not somehow avoidable. Some will seek causes in inadequate medical care, in incompetent physicians, or in other environmental circumstances; others will assume a burden of guilt at their own failure to recognize the symptoms of illness or to take action quickly enough so that a cure could have been effected. Each of these reactions may be irrational. When these feelings are implicit in questions or responses of parents, the physician should make them explicit, point out the inevitability of such feelings, and, when it can be honestly done, reassure the parents that there are no grounds for their shouldering blame for a situation which no one could say might have been averted. The feeling of guilt or of punishment may be particularly strong in genetic disorders. Here it may be helpful to encourage the family to regard genetic mutations as tragic accidents, almost always beyond the ability of man to avoid.

In the management of the affected child parents should be encouraged to handle the life situation of the child as normally as possible. This may be difficult for parents who may think that their usual disciplinary activities may make the child's pain or illness worse.

These feelings should be allayed, and the parents should be encouraged to maintain the child in the normal place in the family hierarchy. Special arrangements, such as the celebration of Christmas in the summertime or other public dramatizations of the child's illness, should be discouraged; they may be more anxiety-provoking for the child than fulfilling of some special need. As much as possible, the parents should be encouraged to participate in the care of the child in the hospital as long as their responsibilities to other children at home are adequately met. They may also need encouragement to take adequate respite from the care of the ill child.

As the physician follows the evolution of a fatal illness in a child, the manner in which the parents are coping with the situation should be observed. For example, the parents may increasingly turn their attention to other sick children in the hospital. This is a healthy sign if it is not premature; if it comes too early, it may represent the parents' unresolved burden of guilt or their pain in facing the ill child. This turning away to help other children is healthy as long as the parents still have adequate resources and strength for the needs of their own child.

At times the guilt of parents is intensified by a wish that the illness were all over or by an unexpected sense of relief or release at the terminal event itself. The considerate and skillful physician will be on the watch for signs of these reactions and find the right words of reassurance or encouragement that such feelings are normal and that the parents have given everything that could have been expected of them in a situation which they have found very trying and toward which they will forever have sensitive and tender feelings.

CARE OF THE CHILD

What to tell the child who has a fatal illness about the future will vary with the condition and circumstances. Most young children do not ask whether they are going to die. They can often be told that they have an illness which may last for some time and which has ups and downs and that it is important for them to get adequate rest and to be active when they feel up to it. Unrealistic reassurances that they look well and are doing fine will be less helpful than the frank recognition of the child's feeling that being ill is no fun and that having it going on so long is discouraging. If the child is in a stage of illness requiring temporary hospitalization, he or she needs assurance that school and normal activity will begin again as soon as possible. Meanwhile it is supportive, when appropriate, for the child to receive attention from schoolteachers and play therapists in the hospital, who will help blunt the sense of inevitability of worsening illness.

In the case of preadolescent or adolescent children with chronic and fatal illness, the plan for care may often include sharing the diagnosis with the child and examining with parents and child together the implications of diagnosis and prognosis, answering their questions, and laying out with them a program of action and support which will have as its goal keeping the patient as comfortable as possible and forestalling any

conclusion to the effort as long as possible. In this atmosphere of frankness, trust, and cooperation, free of secrets or evasions, many families and patients will find an unexpectedly healthy climate for the expression of tenderness and love toward each other, and the physician may find his or her own work easier. As a chronic illness becomes terminal, this climate makes it easier to meet the needs of the patient for a sense of not being abandoned, for assurances of the continuing love and affection of those around, and for reasonably prompt responses to needs for care. Needless to say, the decision as to when or how the diagnosis of a potentially fatal illness is to be shared with the child must have the full understanding, consent, and cooperation of parents, and the parents will need to have given some thought to how the news of the child's illness is to be handled with siblings, relatives, and neighbors.

OTHER RESOURCES

In dealing with the problems of patient and family around a fatal illness, the physician will often call upon other professional persons for help. The family minister or other spiritual advisor can be of immense comfort. When family problems are likely to be ameliorated by the use of community resources, the help of skilled social workers may be extremely important. When the family is not intact, owing to the death or previous separation of a parent, the likelihood of emotional difficulties complicating the management of the illness is sufficiently great that social service resources should probably be involved from the time the diagnosis is known.

The fatal chronic illnesses of children tend to be clustered around certain diseases such as leukemia or other malignancy, cystic fibrosis, and metabolic or degenerative disorders (such as Tay-Sachs disease). When numbers of families who share a common problem can be brought together to discuss aspects of the care of their children under the guidance of a knowledgeable and skillful professional person (physician, social worker, or nurse), they can often help one another in the management of the illness as well as in coping with the feelings that go with the inevitability of ultimate loss.

TERMINAL CARE

In the management of terminal illness physicians should not leave decisions about what is to be done for the child to parents but should give positive advice as to what they plan to do. The physician should be responsive, however, to the suggestions of parents when these represent helpful and realistic appraisals of their children's needs.

When death is imminent, the patient should be kept comfortable and the parents, as much as possible, should be close at hand. The physician should be available both to parents and to the patient. The physician's control of his or her own feelings is important; if the physician's personal distress is allowed to increase the distance from or decrease involvement with the patient, the anger of the child or parents with what may be perceived as abandonment of them may make terminal care much more difficult. The continued interest and concern of the physician are important in preventing the emotional situation from deteriorating at this time.

As the moment of death approaches, the child should be in a room where he or she can be alone with parents or loved ones at the bedside or nearby. The sensitive physician will see that the occasion is accorded appropriate dignity and not rendered more frustrating or agonizing by fruitless efforts to prolong vital functions in a climate of purposeless hyperactivity.

When death has occurred, the patient, bed, and room should be made neat, and the paraphernalia of illness removed. If the parents are not at hand, they should be asked to come to the hospital and be informed of the circumstances. Parents should be given the opportunity to be with the child a little while in the relatively peaceful and uncluttered setting which has been created. A brief and tender parting may help the parents in the adjustments which they must ultimately make.

When an infant or child has died, parent groups with similar experiences may be as important and as supportive after the death of the child as before, as long as professional guidance is adequate. Such groups can help with the process of mourning and can foster the reassurance that comes with sharing such common and otherwise frightening experiences as the guilt felt at the sense of relief that the illness is over or the fear of losing touch with reality that comes with having set a place at the table for the dead child or with finding one's self listening for his or her footstep or voice. Whether or not such parent programs exist, physicians should plan in the weeks after a child's death for a number of visits with the parents in order to review such matters with them, to answer their continuing questions, and to assess their status.

DEATH OF THE NEWBORN INFANT

Acute fatal illnesses have a major cluster in the neonatal period, and neonatal nurseries and intensive care units must be responsive to the needs of parents who have had no preparation for a catastrophic loss. Mother and infant are usually apart at the moment of death. The body of the newborn infant can often be taken to the mother or to both parents at her bedside or at some other point in the hospital where the chance to hold and examine the baby may be the mother's only opportunity to establish for herself the reality of the birth and death of her infant and to adjust toward reality her current or future fantasies as to what the baby might *really* have been like or what might *really* have happened. For the mother of the malformed infant this may be even more important than for the mother of the otherwise intact infant. The defects can be examined by her in reality rather than in fantasy and their implications gently discussed, with the observation perhaps that the baby was in every other way perfectly formed. Mothers whose infants have died are in critical need of help in mourning; they should be as involved

as they may wish or circumstances permit in decisions occasioned by the death.

Some neonatal intensive care units are finding it helpful to maintain small discussion groups for mothers who have lost infants, within which they can share their experiences with others during the 1st few wk of mourning. The quality of professional guidance of such groups is crucial to their success in meeting the needs of parents.

Physicians should make sure that parents understand that the mourning process for a dead infant or older child ought to be reasonably complete and a stable state reached before they decide to have another child. This generally requires 9 mo to a year or more. A new infant conceived too soon is likely to be too closely identified with the dead child and to be surrounded by inordinate anxiety or inappropriate expectations.

POST MORTEM EXAMINATION

A request for post mortem examination should be made by the responsible physician who knows the family best, often not the house officer but the attending or referring physician. The need for post mortem examination should be urged as strongly as conviction permits. Parents can be assured that such examinations are always helpful, that information is gathered and saved which may be useful in years to come in solving similar problems of other children or in providing definitive answers to questions of other children in the family or of their relatives or descendants concerning the patient's illness. Later the physician should describe the important and relevant findings of the gross post mortem examination for the parents in simple terms, and they should have a chance to discuss them as freely as they desire.

Bluebond-Langner M: The Private Worlds of Dying Children. Princeton NJ, Princeton University Press, 1978.
Davidson GW: Death of the wished-for child: A case study. Death Educ 1:265, 1977.
Howell DA: A child dies. J. Pediatr Surg 1:2, 1966.
Kübler-Ross E: On Death and Dying. New York, Macmillan, 1969. (Available also in paperback.)
Schulman JL, Kupst MJ: The child with cancer: Clinical approaches to psychosocial care—Research in Psychosocial Aspects. Springfield Ill, Charles C Thomas, 1980.

2.82   DIFFICULT DECISIONS IN PEDIATRICS

Among the more difficult decisions faced by the physician caring for children and their families are those which involve a variety of moral or ethical judgments with respect to which the community has no uniformity of feeling or of standards. Among these are informed consent for surgery or other procedures or for the enlistment of a child in an experimental procedure; decisions regarding organ transplantation; genetic counseling; amniocentesis; abortion or other interruption of pregnancy; euthanasia; and determination of the point at which the potential has been passed for vital processes to be restored and the patient who still has a beating heart is effectively dead.

Recent increases in attention given these decisions reflect increased public and professional concern that they be made only after adequate study of the issues involved and that they meet certain standards of objectivity and accountability.

Among the factors which may influence or ultimately determine the responses of physicians to such problems are such considerations as the educational level, culture, and religion of the involved families; the larger social issues of eugenics, overpopulation, or other interests of the community; and, in many instances, legal constraints. In some cases the rights of parents and the rights of their children may appear to be in conflict. There is a growing feeling in the United States that the child deserves his or her own advocacy before the law. The rights of adolescents to receive medical care without the consent or knowledge of their parents have been recognized in a number of states through legislation aimed particularly at helping the adolescent in difficulties with sexual problems or with drug abuse. Physicians who deal with adolescents need to be well informed as to local statutes governing the rights of minors to confidentiality in their relationship.

Physicians faced with difficult decisions involving moral or ethical judgment will generally assume positions which they regard as appropriate and rational, sometimes with the support of notions borrowed from the physiologic or psychologic disciplines of medicine. But they must accept that their own logical, scientific, and intellectual positions or attitudes may not at all be so construed by others. The investment of emotions in some issues may be great, with intense feelings of fear, guilt, anger, and anxiety.

In dealing with these matters, an overriding principle ought to be that the issues must be examined in the context of the value system of the *patient* and of the *patient's family*, not only that of the physician. The goal is to help the family to find a solution to their problem with which they can live most comfortably. With an assessment of the needs and resources of patients and their families, the physician serves as a catalyst through which the most satisfying or least damaging solutions of difficult problems may be found.

Some decisions, such as those which may have as their result the shortening or the termination of life or the prolongation of a life of limited potential, are of such nature that to require parents to choose between alternatives is to lay upon them a devastating burden. Sometimes, decisions of such difficulty must be made by the physician on behalf of the family, but he or she must be as sure as circumstances permit that the decision is one which the family can accept in terms of *their* system of values, not his or her own. When all the issues have been examined and when the physician has formed a reasonable judgment as to what decision will be most growth-promoting or least destructive, then the physician should move toward this decision in discussions with the family, subject to re-examination at any point. The aim will be to arrive jointly with the family at the best or least bad plan, which may sometimes be appropriately regarded as the lesser of two tragedies.

When decisions have been made which it can be anticipated will cause periods of continuing grief or requestioning, the physicians who have participated in these decisions must be available to the concerned families and ready to satisfy their continuing needs for information, understanding, and support.

If a physician becomes involved in moral or ethical issues concerning which the family cannot accept his or her judgment, then it should be made clear to the family that they should feel free to seek advice from another consultant.

It is tempting to provide guidelines and examples of how specific problems ought to be handled. But there are often no specific guidelines, and each occasion must be evaluated on its own merits. The skills most useful to the physician will be in the psychotherapeutic realm and will involve skillful listening, gentle and sensitive probing, and compassionate help in decision-making.

VICTOR C. VAUGHAN, III

3 NUTRITION AND NUTRITIONAL DISORDERS

NUTRITIONAL REQUIREMENTS

Nutritional requirements of individuals vary in respect to genetic and metabolic differences. For all infants and children, however, the basic goals include satisfactory growth and avoidance of deficiency states. Good nutrition contributes to the prevention of acute and chronic illness and to the development of physical and mental potential and should provide reserves for stress.

The Food and Nutrition Board (NAS–NRC, 1980) has identified appropriate dietary allowances for a number of substances that prevent deficiency states for most persons (Table 3–1). Because some essential substances are not identified, it appears prudent, except in early infancy, to provide these with a varied diet. Only human milk appears to supply all essentials for a prolonged time. While some essential foods should be included in the daily diet, others are stored by the body and may be supplied periodically.

Although the dietary intake for good nutrition has considerable variability, mild excesses of nutrients or calories may prove to be as undesirable as mild deficiencies. Inasmuch as the influence of diet upon the aging process, including atherosclerosis and longevity, is not adequately known, avoidance of excessive caloric and fat intake appears to be wise at all ages.

3.1 WATER

Water is second only to oxygen as an essential for existence; lack of it results in death in a matter of days. The water content of infants is relatively higher (70–75% of the body weight) than that of adults (60–65%). Assuming that water constitutes 70% of the body weight, 5% is blood plasma, 15% is interstitial fluid, and 50% is intracellular fluid. Although fluids provide the principal source of water, some is obtained from the oxidation of foods (mixed diets yield about 12 gm $H_2O/100$ Cal) and some from the oxidation of body tissues.

Requirements for water are related to caloric consumption, to insensible loss, and to the specific gravity of the urine. The infant must consume much larger amounts of water per unit of body weight than the adult, but when calculated per unit of caloric intake, the amounts required are nearly identical (Tables 3–2 and 3–3). The daily consumption of fluid by the healthy infant is equivalent to 10–15% of body weight, whereas it is only 2–4% in the adult. The natural food of infants and children is high in water content; most of the solid food in the child's diet contains 60–70% water, and many of the fruits and vegetables contain 90%.

Water is absorbed throughout the intestinal tract. The quantity of water in the interstitial compartment is readily changed to maintain homeostatic balance within the intracellular and vascular compartments. The interchange of water among these compartments is dependent on their respective protein and electrolyte concentrations. Depending upon the rate of growth, about 0.5–3% of the fluid intake will be retained. Fomon estimates that retention of water is in the range of 9–13 ml/24 hr for the "male reference infant" in the 1st yr of life.

Water balance depends on such variables as fluid intake, protein and mineral content of diet, solute load presented for renal excretion, metabolic and respiratory rates, and body temperature. Water requirements for low birth weight infants are estimated at 85–170 ml/kg/24 hr. Phototherapy for hyperbilirubinemia increases requirements approximately 20%. Fecal losses are small (3–10% of intake). Evaporation from lungs and skin accounts for 40–50% of intake (sometimes more) and renal excretion for 40–50% or more. The kidney preserves the fluid and electrolyte equilibrium of the body by varying the osmolar content and volume of urine. Urine usually has a greater osmotic pressure (300–1000 mosm/l) than the internal environment (293 mosm/l). Although nursing infants may be able to concentrate to 100 mosm/l, maximum normal urinary concentration is approximately 600–700 mosm/l.

3.2 CALORIES

The unit of heat in metabolism is the large calorie or kilocalorie (1 Cal = 1 kcal); it is used to refer to the energy content of food. A kilocalorie is defined as the amount of heat necessary to raise the temperature of 1 kg of water from 14.5° to 15.5° C. The production of heat varies in the oxidation of different foods, so that measuring the amount of oxygen consumed or measuring the end products of oxidation, carbon dioxide, and water approximates the values obtained by direct calorimetry.

There is great variation in the energy needs of children at different ages and under various conditions (Fig 3–1). The approximate average expenditures of energy by the child 6–12 yr of age are basal metabolism, 50%; growth, 12%; physical activity, 25%; and loss by way of feces, about 8%, mainly as unabsorbed fat.

Basal metabolism is measured at room temperature (20° C) 10–14 hr after a meal, with the patient physically and emotionally quiet. For each degree centigrade of fever, basal metabolism is increased approximately 10%. The basal requirement in infants is about 55 kcal/kg/24 hr; it decreases to 25–30 kcal/kg/24 hr at maturity. The term *specific dynamic action* (SDA) refers to the increase in metabolism over the basal rate by the

Table 3-1 FOOD AND NUTRITION BOARD, NATIONAL ACADEMY OF SCIENCES–NATIONAL RESEARCH COUNCIL
RECOMMENDED DAILY DIETARY ALLOWANCES,* Revised 1980

Designed for the maintenance of good nutrition of practically all healthy people in the U.S.A.

Age (Years)	Weight (kg)	Weight (lb)	Height (cm)	Height (in)	Protein (gm)	Vitamin A (μg RE)†	Vitamin D (μg)‡	Vitamin E (mg α-TE)§	Vitamin C (mg)	Thiamine (mg)	Riboflavin (mg)	Niacin (mg NE)¶	Vitamin B6 (mg)	Folacin** (μg)	Vitamin B12 (μg)	Calcium (mg)	Phosphorus (mg)	Magnesium (mg)	Iron (mg)	Zinc (mg)	Iodine (μg)	Energy Needs (kcal)
Infants																						
0.0–0.5	6	13	60	24	kg × 2.2	420	10	3	35	0.3	0.4	6	0.3	30	0.5††	360	240	50	10	3	40	kg × 115
0.5–1.0	9	20	71	28	kg × 2.0	400	10	4	35	0.5	0.6	8	0.6	45	1.5	540	360	70	15	5	50	kg × 105
Children																						
1–3	13	29	90	35	23	400	10	5	45	0.7	0.8	9	0.9	100	2.0	800	800	150	15	10	70	1300
4–6	20	44	112	44	30	500	10	6	45	0.9	1.0	11	1.3	200	2.5	800	800	200	10	10	90	1700
7–10	28	62	132	52	34	700	10	7	45	1.2	1.4	16	1.6	300	3.0	800	800	250	10	10	120	2400
Males																						
11–14	45	99	157	62	45	1000	10	8	50	1.4	1.6	18	1.8	400	3.0	1200	1200	350	18	15	150	2700
15–18	66	145	176	69	56	1000	10	10	60	1.4	1.7	18	2.0	400	3.0	1200	1200	400	18	15	150	2800
19–22	70	154	177	70	56	1000	7.5	10	60	1.5	1.7	19	2.2	400	3.0	800	800	350	10	15	150	2900
23–50	70	154	178	70	56	1000	5	10	60	1.4	1.6	18	2.2	400	3.0	800	800	350	10	15	150	2700
51+	70	154	178	70	56	1000	5	10	60	1.2	1.4	16	2.2	400	3.0	800	800	350	10	15	150	2400
Females																						
11–14	46	101	157	62	46	800	10	8	50	1.1	1.3	15	1.8	400	3.0	1200	1200	300	18	15	150	2200
15–18	55	120	163	64	46	800	10	8	60	1.1	1.3	14	2.0	400	3.0	1200	1200	300	18	15	150	2100
19–22	55	120	163	64	44	800	7.5	8	60	1.1	1.3	14	2.0	400	3.0	800	800	300	18	15	150	2100
23–50	55	120	163	64	44	800	5	8	60	1.0	1.2	13	2.0	400	3.0	800	800	300	18	15	150	2000
51+	55	120	163	64	44	800	5	8	60	1.0	1.2	13	2.0	400	3.0	800	800	300	10	15	150	1800
Pregnant					+30	+200	+5	+2	+20	+0.4	+0.3	+2	+0.6	+400	+1.0	+400	+400	+150	‡‡	+5	+25	+300
Lactating					+20	+400	+5	+3	+40	+0.5	+0.5	+5	+0.5	+100	+1.0	+400	+400	+150	‡‡	+10	+50	+500

*The allowances are intended to provide for individual variations among most normal persons as they live in the United States under usual environmental stresses. Diets should be based on a variety of common foods in order to provide other nutrients for which human requirements have been less well defined.

†Retinol equivalents. 1 retinol equivalent = 1 μg retinol or 6 μg β carotene = 3.3 IU vitamin A.

‡As cholecalciferol. 10 μg cholecalciferol = 400 IU of vitamin D.

§α-tocopherol equivalents. 1 mg d-α tocopherol = 1 α-TE.

¶1 NE (niacin equivalent) is equal to 1 mg of niacin or 60 mg of dietary tryptophan.

**The folacin allowances refer to dietary sources as determined by Lactobacillus casei assay after treatment with enzymes (conjugases) to make polyglutamyl forms of the vitamin available to the test organism.

††The recommended dietary allowance for vitamin B12 in infants is based on average concentration of the vitamin in human milk. The allowances after weaning are based on energy intake (as recommended by the American Academy of Pediatrics) and consideration of other factors, such as intestinal absorption; see text.

‡‡The increased requirement during pregnancy cannot be met by the iron content of habitual American diets or by the existing iron stores of many women; therefore the use of 30–60 mg of supplemental iron is recommended. Iron needs during lactation are not substantially different from those of nonpregnant women, but continued supplementation of the mother for 2–3 months after parturition is advisable in order to replenish stores depleted by pregnancy.

Table 3–2   WATER REQUIREMENTS

URINE SP.GR.	INFANT—3 KG 300 CALORIES* INTAKE WATER INTAKE			ADULT—70 KG 3000 CALORIES* INTAKE WATER INTAKE		
	ml	gm/100 cal	gm/ kg	ml	gm/100 cal	gm/ kg
1.005	650	217	220	6300	210	90
1.015	339	113	116	3180	106	45
1.020	300	100	100	2790	93	40
1.030	264	88	91	2430	81	35

*In this sense calorie = large calorie = 1 kcal = 1 Cal (see text).

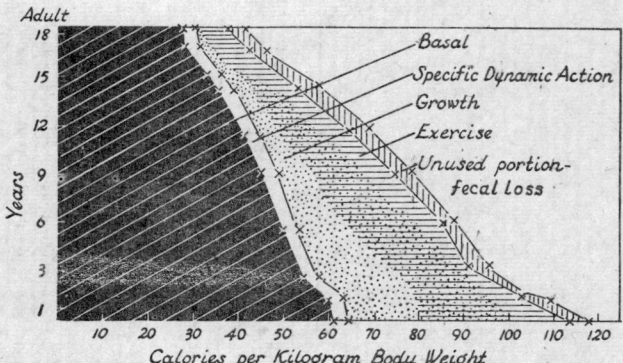

Figure 3–1 Total daily expenditure of calories with approximate distribution among individual factors in relation to age and weight (Calorie = large calorie = 1 kcal = 1 Cal).

ingestion and assimilation of food. Protein digestion may increase metabolism as much as 30% above the basal level, except when it is being deposited in tissues, whereas fat and carbohydrate, which have a "sparing" effect on the specific dynamic action of protein and upon each other, cause increases of only 4 and 6%, respectively. In infants, about 7–8% of the total caloric intake goes to specific dynamic action, whereas in older children on an ordinary mixed diet it is not likely to be more than about 5% of total intake. The energy necessary to build body tissue (*growth*) is estimated to be the difference between the calories ingested and those expended for other purposes. The average requirement for *physical activity* is 15–25 kcal/kg/24 hr, with peak utilizations being as high as 50–80 kcal/kg/24 hr for short periods of time. The amount of energy-producing food lost in the stools (*unused portion*), except when absorption is impaired, is not more than 10% of the intake.

Although caloric requirements can best be predicted from the surface area rather than from age or weight, the final criteria for evaluating the child's needs depend upon the growth pattern, the sense of well-being, and satiety. The daily requirement is approximately 100–120 kcal/kg for the 1st yr of life, with subsequent decreases of about 10 kcal/kg for each succeeding 3 yr period. Periods of rapid growth and development near puberty require increased caloric consumption. The distribution of calories in human milk, in most formulas, and in a well balanced diet is similar. Approximately 9–15% of

Table 3–3   RANGE OF AVERAGE WATER REQUIREMENTS OF CHILDREN AT DIFFERENT AGES UNDER ORDINARY CONDITIONS

AGE	AVERGE BODY WEIGHT IN KG	TOTAL WATER IN 24 HOURS, ML	WATER PER KG BODY WT IN 24 HOURS, ML
3 days	3.0	250–300	80–100
10 days	3.2	400–500	125–150
3 mo	5.4	750–850	140–160
6 mo	7.3	950–1100	130–155
9 mo	8.6	1100–1250	125–145
1 yr	9.5	1150–1300	120–135
2 yr	11.8	1350–1500	115–125
4 yr	16.2	1600–1800	100–110
6 yr	20.0	1800–2000	90–100
10 yr	28.7	2000–2500	70–85
14 yr	45.0	2200–2700	50–60
18 yr	54.0	2200–2700	40–50

the calories are derived from protein, 45–55% from carbohydrate, and 35–45% from fat.

Each gram of ingested protein or carbohydrate provides 4 kcal. One gram of short-chain fatty acids provides 5.3 kcal; medium-chain, 8.3 kcal; and long-chain, 9 kcal. A continued caloric intake greater or less than the body expenditure will result in an increase or decrease in body fat. In general, a consistent caloric imbalance of 500 kcal/24 hr results in a body weight change of about 450 gm (1 pound)/wk.

3.3   PROTEINS

Protein constitutes about 20% of the body weight of the adult. Its amino acids are essential nutrients in the formation of cell protoplasm. The kind, number, and arrangement of the amino acids in a protein molecule determine its characteristics. Twenty-four amino acids have been identified; 9 have been found to be essential for infants (threonine, valine, leucine, isoleucine, lysine, tryptophan, phenylalanine, methionine, and histidine). Arginine, cystine, and, perhaps, taurine are essential for low birth weight infants. Nonessential amino acids can be synthesized and need not be supplied in the diet. New tissue cannot be formed unless all of the essential amino acids are present in the diet simultaneously; hence the absence or deficiency of only 1 essential amino acid will result in a negative nitrogen balance.

Proteins are broken down in the digestive process to oligopeptides and α-amino acids. The hydrochloric acid of the stomach provides the optimal pH for peptide cleavage by pepsin. Rennin changes casein of milk to paracasein, which pepsin hydrolyzes along with other proteins. The various proteinases show preference for splitting specific peptide linkages; some cleave linkages in the interior of the peptide chain, and others act at more terminal junctures. In the alkaline medium of the intestine, trypsin, chymotrypsin, and carboxypeptidase from the pancreas hydrolyze these proteases and peptones to peptides and to some amino acids; other

Table 3–4 FUNCTIONS, EFFECTS OF DEFICIENCY AND EXCESS, REQUIREMENTS, AND SOURCES OF WATER, PROTEINS, CARBOHYDRATES, AND FATS

FOOD-STUFFS	FUNCTIONS	EFFECTS OF DEFICIENCY	EFFECTS OF EXCESS	REQUIREMENTS	SOURCES
Water	Structure of cells; solvent for cellular changes; medium for ions; transport of nutrients and waste products; regulation of body temperature	Thirst, dryness of tongue, dehydration, anhydremia, high sp. gr. of urine, loss of kidney function (acidosis, oliguria, uremia, death)	Abdominal discomfort, headache, cramps (water without salt), intoxication, convulsions, edema, and circulatory failure	See Tables 3–2 and 3–3 Related to calories consumed; greater in hot weather	Water as such All foods
Proteins	Supply amino acids for growth and repair of tissue cells; sols for osmotic equilibrium; ions in acid-base balance. With prosthetic groups to form hemoglobin, nucleoproteins, glycoprotein, and lipoproteins. Enzymes, hormones, cellular respiratory substance, antibodies. Protective structures (nails and hair). Source of energy	Lassitude, abdominal enlargement, edema; depletion of plasma proteins, negative nitrogen balance (no clinical syndrome due to lack of specific amino acid); kwashiorkor (protein malnutrition); marasmus (protein-calorie malnutrition)	Prolonged high protein intake probably not harmful. Important in certain anomalies involving amino acid and protein metabolism	See Table 3–1	Milk, eggs, meat, fish, poultry, cheese, soybeans, peas, beans, cereals, nuts, lentils
Carbo-hydrates	Readily available source of energy, antiketogenic, structure of cells, antibodies, source of stored calories (glycogen and fat), conversion to fat, resynthesis of amino acids, roughage	Ketosis if intake is less than 15% of calories or in starvation; underweight if total calories are low	Overweight if total calories are high. Various syndromes due to inborn errors of sugar metabolism	To supply 25–55% of calories	Milk, cereals, fruits, sucrose, syrups, starches, vegetables
Fats	Concentrated source of energy; physical protection for vessels, nerves, organs; insulation against changes in temperature; structure of body tissues, cell membranes, and nuclei; vehicle for absorption of vitamins (A, D, E, and K); appetite appeal; aids satiety (delays emptying time of stomach); avoids necessity of ingestion of large bulk of foods; spares protein, vitamin A, and thiamine; supplies linoleic acid	Lack of satiety (craving for fat); underweight; skin changes with intakes very low in linoleic acid	Overweight; abdominal symptoms in familial hyperlipidemia; high cholesterol intakes may be harmful to selected populations	Minimal not known; usually supplies 35% of calories; probably 1–2% of calories as linoleic acid	Milk, butter, egg yolk, lard, bacon, meat, fish, cheese, nuts, vegetable oils Breast milk usually supplies 4–5% of calories as linoleic acid; vegetable oils vary greatly, safflower, corn, soy, and others being especially rich

peptidases from the intestinal juices carry digestion to the amino acid stage.

Minute amounts of certain proteins may be absorbed unchanged, as evidenced by immunologic reactions, but it is the hydrolytic products, the amino acids and some peptides, that are normally absorbed through the intestinal mucosa. Large oligopeptides may be absorbed in the first few months of life or after episodes of gastroenteritis. The amino acids are carried to the liver by the portal circulation and from there distributed to other tissues. Amino acids are reconstituted to functional human proteins, e.g., albumin, hemoglobin, hormones. Excess amino acids undergo deamination, and the nitrogenous portions are converted to urea in the liver and excreted by the kidneys. The carbon from amino acids is oxidized much as that of carbohydrate or fat; some amino acids are glycogenic, others ketogenic. Proteins cannot be effectively stored. In protein depletion states, proteins from muscle may be broken down to supply amino acids for more essential sites such as brain and enzymes.

Aberrations in the metabolism of protein and the amino acids constitute a significant portion of the disease entities known as inborn errors of metabolism (Chapter 8).

Protein requirements at various ages are listed in Table 3–1. "Biologic value" of proteins indicates effectiveness of utilization; proteins of high biologic value have the quantity and distribution of essential amino acids appropriate for resynthesis of body tissues and provide little waste as determined by nitrogen balance studies. There is an abundant amount available for children in the United States, but the supply of protein in many countries is so limited that it is the greatest need of children throughout the world (Table 3–4).

3.4 CARBOHYDRATES

The greatest portion of the caloric needs of the body is supplied by carbohydrates, which also supply the necessary bulk of the diet. In the absence of sufficient carbohydrate, proteins and fats will be utilized for energy. Carbohydrates are stored chiefly as glycogen in the liver and muscles but probably make up no more than 1% of the body weight. The infant's liver is 10% the size of that of the adult; the muscle mass, 2%. Hence, the infant has only a small fraction (approximately 3.5%) of the glycogen reserve of the adult.

Carbohydrates are oxidized as glucose (dextrose) but are consumed in various forms: the monosaccharides (glucose, fructose, galactose), the disaccharides (lactose, sucrose, maltose, isomaltose), and the polysaccharides (starches, dextrins, glycogen, gums, cellulose). Pentoses are poorly absorbed.

Through a series of enzymatic and chemical reactions in the digestive tract, complex carbohydrates are split into simpler structures. Salivary and pancreatic amylases are principally involved in the breakdown of starch to oligosaccharides (dextrins) and disaccharides (primarily maltose). Intestinal amylase may be decreased during the 1st 4 mo of life. The disaccharides are absorbed intact into the intestinal brush border cells, where the various disaccharidases in the membrane fraction of the microvilli complete the hydrolysis to the monosaccharides: 1 molecule of maltose to 2 of glucose; sucrose to glucose and fructose; lactose to glucose and galactose. The monosaccharides are rapidly absorbed; glucose and galactose are actively taken up against concentration gradients, whereas fructose absorption is passive. During absorption, phosphoric acid "carrier" radicals combine with hexose sugars in the intestinal mucosa for transport across the cell membrane. Sodium must be present for absorption to continue when the intraintestinal sugar concentration is low. These hexose-phosphates separate again into their component parts, permitting the sugar to diffuse into the portal blood stream.

Some glucose may be oxidized directly, as in the brain and heart. Most of the absorbed sugar is converted to glycogen in the liver, though glycogenesis also occurs in other tissues of the body. Up to 15% of the weight of the liver and 3% of the muscle may be glycogen; small amounts are also found in the skin and in practically all other organs. Glycogenolysis in the liver yields glucose as the chief product, whereas glycogen breakdown in the muscle yields lactic acid. The overall oxidation of glucose has 2 phases, the anaerobic (glycolysis) and the aerobic (tricarboxylic acid cycle). In the former, glucose is broken down to pyruvic acid; in the aerobic cycle pyruvic acid is completely oxidized to carbon dioxide and water. Insulin and the pituitary and adrenal hormones are involved in these processes, and nicotinic acid, thiamine, riboflavin, and pantothenic acid take part in the enzymatic reactions. Carbohydrate which is not oxidized or stored as glycogen is converted to fat. High carbohydrate intake, particularly of refined sugars, may be associated with the development of atherosclerosis.

The principal carbohydrate metabolic disorders are diabetes mellitus, glycogen storage disease, galactosemia, fructose intolerance, and glucose intolerance; deficiencies of sugar-splitting enzymes in the intestines (lactase, invertase, maltase) are associated with diarrhea and malabsorption resulting from the osmotic effect of the unabsorbed sugar and from fermentation of the carbohydrate by intestinal bacteria.

3.5 FATS

Fats or their metabolic products form an integral part of cellular membranes and are efficient stores of energy. They impart palatability to food and serve as vehicles for fat-soluble vitamins A, D, E, and K. Approximately 98% of natural fats are triglycerides, 3 fatty acids combined with glycerol. The remaining 2% include free fatty acids, monoglycerides, diglycerides, cholesterol, and phospholipids (including lecithin, cephalin, sphingomyelin, and cerebrosides).

Naturally occurring fats contain straight-chain fatty acids, both saturated and unsaturated, varying in length from 4–24 carbon atoms. The degree of absorption generally varies with the melting point, the degree of unsaturation, and the positions of the fatty acids on the glycerol molecule.

Ingested triglycerides are partially hydrolyzed by lingual lipase and emulsified in the stomach. In the duodenum pancreatic lipase hydrolyzes the triglycerides to monoglycerides and fatty acids; intraluminal solubility is greatly enhanced by the presence of bile salts. The remaining unsplit diglycerides and triglycerides are insoluble even in the presence of bile salts. Low birth weight infants have decreased amounts of bile and hence decreased absorption of fat.

Long-chain fatty acids and monoglycerides (those with more than 10 carbon atoms) are presumably absorbed into the mucosal cell by diffusion. Transport across the cell involves re-esterification of these fatty acids and monoglycerides to triglycerides, which are then "coated" with lipoprotein to form the moiety known as the chylomicron, in which the fat is transported in the lymph system to the venous circulation via the thoracic duct. Transport proteins include very low density (VLDL), low density (LDL), and high density (HDL) lipoproteins synthesized in the liver.

Short- and medium-chain triglycerides are handled differently; they are readily hydrolyzed by pancreatic lipase to free fatty acids which are transported through the cell. Even when intraluminal hydrolysis is inadequate because of deficiency of pancreatic lipase or of bile salts, these fats will be absorbed and hydrolyzed to free fatty acids within the cell by mucosal lipase. With neither esterification to triglycerides nor subsequent chylomicron formation, these free fatty acids directly enter the intestinal veins and pass to the liver via the portal system. This alternate pathway for short- and medium-chain triglycerides is utilized in many nutritional formulations for children with severe absorptive problems.

Linoleic and Arachidonic Acids. Humans do not synthesize linoleic acid, an 18-carbon atom chain with 2 double bonds (dienoic acid); hence, it must be supplied in the diet. Linolenic (3 double bonds) and arachidonic (4 double bonds) acids also may be essential to infants. Unsaturated fatty acids are necessary for growth, skin and hair integrity, regulation of cholesterol metabolism, lipotropic activity, synthesis of the prostaglandins, decreased platelet adhesiveness, and reproduction. Diets containing less than 1–2% of the calories as linoleic acid require greater caloric consumption for comparable growth. In children with essential fatty acid deficiency, serum levels of trienoic acid increases relative to tetraenoic acids. Excess linoleic acids increase peroxidation and may cause membrane destruction. Rapidly growing young infants maintained on diets very low in linoleic acid undergo dryness, thickening, and desquamation of the skin, and intertrigo.

The relation of dietary fat intake to intimal fat streaking in the major arterial vessels in early life remains to be clarified. Reduction of total fat intake and an increase in the ratio of unsaturated to saturated fats are associated with reduction in serum cholesterol levels in adults with hyperlipidemia, particularly in those with the type II form. In the United States, polyunsaturated vegetable fats have been widely substituted for the more saturated butterfats in commercial milk formulas; it has not been established whether atheromatous changes are lessened by this substitution.

3.6 MINERALS

The physiologic roles and dietary sources of the principal minerals with nutritional significance are summarized in Table 3–5. Requirements are shown in Table 3–1, except for several of the trace elements.

The ash content of the fetus is about 3% of the body weight at birth. It increases continuously throughout childhood, both absolutely and relatively. In the adult the ash content is 4.35% of the body weight; 83% is in the skeleton and 10% in the muscle. It has been estimated that for each gram of protein retained, 0.3 gm of mineral matter is deposited. The principal cations are calcium, magnesium, potassium, and sodium; the comparable anions are phosphorus, sulfur, and chloride. Iron, iodine, and cobalt appear in important organic complexes. The trace elements fluorine, copper, zinc, chromium, and manganese have known metabolic roles; selenium, silicon, boron, nickel, aluminum, arsenic, bromine, molybdenum, and strontium are present in the diet and in the body, but their functions have not been clarified.

3.7 VITAMINS

The word "vitamin" refers to organic compounds that are required in minute amounts to catalyze cellular metabolism essential for maintenance or growth of the organism. Vitamin requirements for infants and children are listed in Table 3–1. For vitamin functions and disorders, see Table 3–6 and Sec 3.21–3.42.

MISCELLANEOUS FACTORS

Roughage. The quantity of indigestible vegetable fiber in acceptable diets may be as much as 170–300 mg/kg/24 hr. Most children who receive average, well balanced diets obtain sufficient amounts of roughage. Highly refined foods contain little fiber and may be associated with increased incidence of constipation, appendicitis, diverticulitis, and other intestinal disorders. High fiber intake may result in decreased absorption of zinc and other essential nutrients.

Digestibility. The relative amount of a given nutrient available for assimilation is high in most of the common food classes: carbohydrate is 97%; fat, 95%; protein, 92%. Cooking is a factor in digestibility. For example, the boiling of milk reduces the size of the curd and renders it more digestible; by contrast, heating destroys activity of vitamin C.

Satiety. The ingestion of a meal should provide a sense of well-being. Whole milk, cream, eggs, and fatty foods have high satiety values; sugar increases the flow of gastric juice and delays emptying of the stomach, thus increasing satiety. Bread and potatoes have relatively low satiety values, as do lean meat, fish, vegetables, and many fruits.

Availability. Poverty, ignorance, and lack of practical education in the buying and preparation of food are the main causes of malnutrition in children. Diets of families in the lower income brackets are likely to be deficient in milk, fruits, fresh vegetables, and meats. A suggested method for planning low cost meals is to divide the money available for food into fifths: one fifth each for vegetables and fruits; for milk and cheese; for meats, fish, and eggs; for bread and cereals; and for fats, sugar, and other food adjuncts.

Geographic location may influence the availability of foods, especially among low socioeconomic populations. The effects of geographic factors on deficiency diseases is evidenced by the high incidence of goiter because of a deficiency of iodine in certain areas and by the relation of dental caries to lack of fluoride in communal water supplies.

Bacterial Synthesis of Vitamins. Certain vitamins are synthesized in the human gastrointestinal tract; however, the extent to which they can meet the body needs is uncertain. Once the bacterial flora of the intestinal tract has been established, vitamin K is produced and is available to the body. Pantothenic acid and biotin, essential to human metabolism, can be supplied by bacterial synthesis alone. Thiamine, riboflavin, niacin, vitamin B_6, vitamin B_{12}, and folic acid are synthesized in some species, but synthesis is limited or does not exist in humans. The kind of food or the nature of intestinal flora may affect vitamin production or availability. For instance, 3% of the population in Kobe, Japan, were found to harbor intestinal bacteria which split thiamine; evidence of beriberi appeared in these persons.

Antimicrobial Factors. Administration of antimicrobial agents may influence nutritional status. Sometimes appetite is impaired or bacterial flora that produce vitamin K are altered sufficiently to precipitate borderline deficiency states. Several antibiotics are known to produce steatorrhea; penicillin and sulfonamides seem to provoke the syndrome only when used together. Neomycin may produce malabsorption in adults. Orally administered broad-spectrum antibiotics decrease nitrogen balance. Isoniazid combines with pyridoxal phosphate and may produce symptoms of vitamin B_6 defi-

Text continued on page 146

Table 3-5 PHYSIOLOGY AND SOURCES OF NUTRITIONALLY IMPORTANT MINERALS

MINERAL	FUNCTION AND METABOLISM	EFFECTS OF DEFICIENCY	EFFECTS OF EXCESS	SOURCES
Calcium	Structure of bone and teeth, muscle contraction, nerve irritability, coagulation of blood, cardiac action, production of milk Absorbed from upper small intestine: aided by vitamin D, ascorbic acid, lactose, acid reaction; hindered by excesses of dietary oxalic acid, phytic acid, fat, fiber, phosphate. Deposited in bone trabeculae and maintained in dynamic equilibrium with body tissues through action of parathyroid hormone and thyrocalcitonin About 70% excreted in feces, 10% in urine; 15–25% retained, depending on growth rate. Serum level 9–11 mg/dl, 60% ionized	Poor mineralization of bones and teeth; osteomalacia; osteoporosis; tetany; rickets; impairment of growth	Unknown	Milk, cheese, green leafy vegetables, canned salmon, clams, oysters
Chloride	Osmotic pressure; acid-base balance; HCl in gastric juice Readily absorbed; about 92% of intake is excreted, mainly in the urine, some in feces and sweat; comprises about 2/3 of the blood plasma anions; blood serum level, 99–106 mEq/l; in intracellular and extracellular fluids; parallels sodium intake and output	Hypochloremic alkalosis may occur with prolonged vomiting or excessive sweating, with parenteral administration of glucose without saline, with excessive ACTH therapy, and with congenital alkalosis	Unknown	Table salt, meat, milk, eggs
Chromium	Glycemia regulation and insulin metabolism	Diabetes in animals	None known	Yeast
Cobalt	Component of vitamin B_{12} (cobalamin) molecule and of erythropoietin Not utilized for synthesis of cobalamin by man; readily absorbed and excreted	None known	None (dietary); medicinally it may be goitrogenic or may produce cardiomyopathy	Widely distributed
Copper	Essential for production of red blood cells; catalyst in hemoglobin formation; absorption of iron. Associated with activities of tyrosinase, catalase, uricase, cytochrome C oxidase, delta-aminolevulinic acid dehydrase (porphyrin formation) Little known about effect on absorption; transported in plasma bound to plasma proteins and in ceruloplasmin; present in erythrocytes in a labile form and the more stable hemocuprein; highest concentration in liver and central nervous system (cerebrocuprein); excreted mainly via the intestinal wall and bile; deranged metabolism in Wilson disease (hepatolenticular degeneration)	May be cause of refractory anemia and osteoporosis	None (dietary)	Liver, oysters, meats, fish, whole grains, nuts, legumes
Fluorine	Tooth and bone structure Retained when intake is above 0.6 mg/day; excreted in urine and sweat; deposited in bones as fluorapatite (dynamic equilibrium)	Tendency to dental caries	Fluorosis: mottling of teeth with intake of more than 4–8 mg/24 hr	Water, sea foods, plant and animal foods (dependent upon content in soil and water)
Iodine	Constituent of thyroxine (T_4) and triiodothyronine (T_3) Readily absorbed from intestine; circulates as inorganic and organic iodide; selectively concentrated about 25:1 in the thyroid gland, quickly iodized and incorporated into a complex known as thyroglobulin; proteolytic enzymes release thyroxine and triiodothyronine into the blood. Excretion mainly in urine. Antithyroid compounds interfere with iodine metabolism: goitrins and brassicae; certain drugs	Simple goiter, endemic cretinism	Not harmful (less than 1 mg/24 hr); medicinally may cause goiter	Iodized salt, sea food, food grown in nongoitrous areas

Table continued on opposite page

Table 3–5 PHYSIOLOGY AND SOURCES OF NUTRITIONALLY IMPORTANT MINERALS (Continued)

MINERAL	FUNCTION AND METABOLISM	EFFECTS OF DEFICIENCY	EFFECTS OF EXCESS	SOURCES
Iron	Structure of hemoglobin and myoglobin for O_2 and CO_2 transport; oxidative enzymes: cytochrome C and catalase Absorbed in ferrous form according to body need, aided by gastric juice and ascorbic acid; hindered by fiber, phytic acid, steatorrhea Transported in plasma in ferric state bound to transferrin (a beta globulin); stored in liver, spleen, bone marrow, and kidney as ferritin and hemosiderin; carefully conserved and reused; minimal losses in urine and sweat; about 90% of intake excreted in the stool	Anemia: hypochromic, microcytic	Hemosiderosis in Bantu people of Africa due to low phosphorus and high iron contents of diet Poisoning by medicinal iron	Liver, meat, egg yolk, green vegetables, whole grains, legumes, nuts
Magnesium	Structure of bones and teeth; activation of enzymes in carbohydrate metabolism; muscle and nerve irritability. Important intracellular cation, essential to metabolic processes Principal cation of soft tissue; absorption from small intestine varies with intake; some urinary excretion, but excellent renal conservation; antagonist to calcium action	Not adequately understood; occurs in malabsorption and deficiency states; may be expressed clinically as tetany; associated frequently with hypocalcemia	None (dietary); toxicity from intravenous medication	Cereals, legumes, nuts, meat, milk
Manganese	Enzyme activation, especially in mitochondria; normal bone structure Poor absorption from intestine; transported in plasma; particularly high turnover rate in mitochondria; excretion mainly via the intestine in bile	Not known	None (dietary); toxicity from chronic inhalation (encephalopathy)	Legumes, nuts, whole grain cereals, green leafy vegetables
Molybdenum	Component of enzymes: xanthine oxidase for conversion to uric acid and mobilization of ferritin iron in liver, liver aldehyde oxidase Readily absorbed from intestine; excreted chiefly in urine, some in bile	Not observed in man	Not established	Legumes, grains, dark green leafy vegetables, animal organs
Phosphorus	Constituent of bones and teeth; structure of nucleus and cytoplasm of all cells; acid-base balance; key position in energy transformations and transmission of nerve impulses; metabolism of carbohydrate, protein, and fat About 70% of intake absorbed as free phosphates from intestine; vitamin D and parathormone implicated in intestinal absorption and kidney retention; excreted in urine and feces; occurs in blood as phospholipids, organic esters, and inorganic phosphates; inorganic phosphates in blood serum of infants and children, 4–7 mg/dl; ratio of inorganic-organic phosphates in whole blood is about 1:20	Not established; rickets may develop in rapidly growing, very low-birth-weight babies with low intakes of both P and Ca; muscle weakness	Possibility of tetany during recovery from rickets or in newborn on formula with low Ca: P (1:1) ratio	Milk, milk products, egg yolk, flesh foods, legumes, nuts, whole grains
Potassium	Muscle contraction; nerve impulse conduction; intracellular osmotic pressure and fluid balance; heart rhythm Primarily intracellular; absorption via intestine; excretion 80% in urine—some in sweat and feces; about 8% retained by growing child; blood serum level 4.0–5.6 mEq/l	In starvation or in such pathologic conditions as diarrhea, diabetic acidosis, ACTH excess: muscle weakness, anorexia, nausea, abdominal distention, nervous irritability, drowsiness, confusion, tachycardia; deficiency exaggerates effects of sodium	Heart block at serum levels of 10 mEq/l; important in Addison disease, renal failure, or administration of K-containing salts	All foods
Selenium	Cofactor for glutathione peroxidase in tissue respiration	Unknown in humans, muscle diseases in animals	Toxicity observed in animals	Vegetables, meats
Sodium	Osmostic pressure; acid-base balance; water balance; muscle and nerve irritability Readily absorbed from intestine; excreted chiefly in urine (98%); parallels chloride intake; renal excretion controlled by adrenal cortical hormone; extracellular cation, but small amount in muscle and cartilage; blood serum level, 135–145 mEq/l	Nausea; diarrhea, muscle cramps, dehydration	Edema if inadequate excretion or excessive parenteral fluids	Table salt, flesh foods, milk, eggs, sodium compounds as baking soda and powder, glutamate, seasonings, and preservatives

Table continued on following page

Table 3–5 PHYSIOLOGY AND SOURCES OF NUTRITIONALLY IMPORTANT MINERALS (Continued)

MINERAL	FUNCTION AND METABOLISM	EFFECTS OF DEFICIENCY	EFFECTS OF EXCESS	SOURCES
Sulfur	Constituent of all cellular protein; cocarboxylase; melanin; mucopolysaccharides of mucous secretions, vitreous humor, synovial fluid, connective tissues, cartilage, heparin; insulin; metabolism of nerve tissue; detoxification mechanisms; tissue metabolism as SH group in coenzyme A, cystathionine, and glutathione Only sources utilized are cystine and methionine; inorganic forms unavailable to body; excreted as inorganic sulfate or ethereal sulfate via urine and bile	Not known; growth failure from protein deficiency may be due in part to deficiency of S-containing amino acids	Not harmful; excreted in urine as sulfates	Protein foods contain about 1%
Zinc	Constituent of several enzymes: carbonic anhydrase (in erythrocytes) essential for CO_2 exchange; carboxypeptidase of intestine for hydrolysis of protein; dehydrogenase of liver Found in liver and organs, muscles, bones, red and white cells; higher tissue concentration in young subjects; excreted chiefly from intestine, competes with copper	Dwarfism, iron deficiency anemia, hepatosplenomegaly, hyperpigmentation and hypogonadism, acrodermatitis enteropathica	Gastrointestinal upsets (from galvanized iron cooking utensils)	Meat, grain, nuts, cheese

Table 3–6 PHYSICAL AND METABOLIC PROPERTIES AND FOOD SOURCES OF THE VITAMINS

NAME AND SYNONYMS	CHARACTERISTICS	METABOLISM	BIOCHEMICAL ACTION	EFFECTS OF DEFICIENCY	EFFECTS OF EXCESS	SOURCES
VITAMIN A: Retinol (vitamin A_1) is an alcohol of high molecular weight Provitamin A: The plant pigments, alpha-, beta-, and gamma-carotenes and cryptoxanthin	Fat-soluble; water-insoluble; heat-stable at usual cooking temperatures; destroyed by oxidation, drying, and very high temperatures	Bile is necessary for absorption of the provitamins. Conversion of provitamins takes place primarily in the walls of the intestine, to some extent in the liver. Vitamin A and provitamins stored in liver. Absorption of both facilitated by the presence of fat, impaired by intake of mineral oil or by defect in fat absorption. Vitamin E minimizes oxidation of both in the intestine	Vitamin A aldehyde combines with specific proteins to form the retinal pigments, rhodopsin and iodopsin, for vision in dim light; bone and tooth development; formation and maturation of epithelia of skin, eye, digestive, respiratory, urinary, and reproductive tracts	Nyctalopia, photophobia, xerophthalmia, conjunctivitis, keratomalacia leading to blindness; faulty epiphyseal bone formation; defective tooth enamel; keratinization of mucous membranes and skin; retarded growth	Dietary excess of vitamin A unlikely. Excessive carotene intake may produce carotenemia with xanthosis cutis. Individual variation in sensitivity to high intakes of vitamin A concentrates; 50,000 IU taken daily for prolonged periods may be toxic and cause anorexia, slow growth, drying and cracking of skin, enlargement of liver and spleen, swelling and pain of long bones, bone fragility, increased intracranial pressure	Liver, fish-liver oils, whole milk, milk fat products, egg yolk, fortified margarines. Carotenoids from plants—green vegetables, yellow fruits and vegetables
VITAMIN B COMPLEX: Thiamine: Vitamin B_1; antiberiberi vitamin; aneurin	Water- and alcohol-soluble; fat-insoluble; stable in slightly acid solution; labile to heat, alkali, sulfites	Readily absorbed from small and large intestines; combines with phosphate in all cells to form thiamine pyrophosphate (cocarboxylase); limited body stores; excess excreted in urine; destroyed in body by intake of raw fish or clams which contain thiaminases. Poor absorption in persistent GI disturbances	Component of carboxylases, which act in various oxidative decarboxylations, including that of pyruvic acid	Beriberi—early stages: fatigue, irritability, emotional instability, anorexia. Later: indigestion, constipation, headache, insomnia, tachycardia after exercise. Late stage: polyneuritis, cardiac failure, edema. Elevated pyruvic acid in the blood after exercise or after intake of standard amount of glucose and low urinary thiamine	None from oral intake	Liver, meat, especially pork, milk, whole grain or enriched cereals, wheat germ, legumes, nuts

Table continued on opposite page

Table 3-6 PHYSICAL AND METABOLIC PROPERTIES AND FOOD SOURCES OF THE VITAMINS (Continued)

Name and Synonyms	Character-istics	Metabolism	Biochemical Action	Effects of Deficiency	Effects of Excess	Sources
Riboflavin: Vitamin B₂	Sparingly soluble in water; sensitive to light and alkali; stable to heat, oxidation, acid	Absorbed from the intestines; limited storage in tissues; excess excreted in urine; careful economy when intake is low and rapid excretion when intake is high. Absorption poor with achlorhydria, diarrhea, vomiting. Utilization greater with increased metabolism	Constituent of 2 coenzymes which are components of a number of flavoprotein enzymes important in hydrogen transfer in a variety of reactions: amino acid, fatty acid, and carbohydrate metabolism and cellular respiration. Retinal pigment for light adaptation	Ariboflavinosis; early symptoms: photophobia, blurred vision, burning and itching of eyes, corneal vascularization, poor growth. One of the most common dietary inadequacies, often accompanying other B-vitamin deficiencies	Not harmful	Milk, cheese, liver and other organs, meat, eggs, fish, green leafy vegetables, whole or enriched grains
Niacin: Nicotinamide; nicotinic acid; antipellagra vitamin	Water- and alcohol-soluble; stable to acid, alkali, light, heat, oxidation	Readily absorbed from small intestine; limited storage; excess excreted in urine as several metabolites; synthesized in the body from tryptophan; vitamin B₆ is essential for conversion	Active constituent of coenzymes I and II, cofactors in a number of dehydrogenase systems	Pellagra: multiple B-vitamin deficiency syndrome. Early symptoms: fatigue, anorexia, weight loss, headache	Nicotinic acid (not the amide) is vasodilator; reactions include skin flushing and itching, circulatory disturbances, increased peristalsis	Meat, fish, poultry, liver, whole grain and enriched cereals, green vegetables, peanuts. Protein foods in general, from conversion of tryptophan (60 mg forms 1 mg of niacin)
Folacin: Group of related compounds containing pteridine ring, para-amino benzoic acid, and glutamic acid. Pteroylglutamic acid (PGA); folinic acid; citrovorum factor; leucovorin	Slightly soluble in water; labile to heat, light, acid	Excreted in urine and feces	Concerned with formation and metabolism of one-carbon units; hence participates in synthesis of purines, pyrimidines, nucleoproteins, and methyl groups	Megaloblastic anemia (infancy, pregnancy); usually is secondary to malabsorption disease	Unknown	Liver, green vegetables, nuts, cereals, cheese
Vitamin B₆: 3 active forms: pyridoxine, pyridoxal, pyridoxamine	Water-soluble; destroyed by ultraviolet light and by heat	Readily absorbed; phosphorylated in tissue to form coenzyme; intestinal synthesis important	Constituent of coenzymes for amino acid metabolism: decarboxylation, transamination, transsulfuration, conversion of tryptophan to niacin; fatty acid metabolism	Infants: irritability, convulsions, hypochromic anemia; peripheral neuritis in patients receiving isoniazid	Unknown	Meat, liver, kidney, whole grains, peanuts, soybeans
Cobalamin: Group of complex coordination compounds of cobalt—vitamin B₁₂; antipernicious anemia factor; Castle extrinsic factor; animal protein factor (APF)	Slightly soluble in water; stable to heat in neutral solution; labile in acid or alkaline ones; destroyed by light	Castle intrinsic factor of the stomach required for absorption	Transfer of one-carbon units in purine and labile-methyl group metabolism; essential for maturation of red blood cells in bone marrow; metabolism of nervous tissue	Juvenile pernicious anemia, due to defect in absorption rather than to dietary lack; also secondary to gastrectomy, celiac disease, inflammatory lesions of small bowel, long term drug therapy (PAS, neomycin)	Unknown	Muscle and organ meats, fish, eggs, milk, cheese
Biotin	Crystallized from yeast; soluble in water	Oxidation yields acetyl CoA	Coenzyme of acetyl coenzyme A carboxylase; involved in CO₂ transfer	Dermatitis, seborrhea; inactivated by avidin in raw egg white	None known	Yeast, animal products; synthesized in intestine
VITAMIN C: *Ascorbic acid:* Vitamin C; antiscorbutic vitamin	Water-soluble; easily oxidized; oxidation is accelerated by heat, light, alkali, oxidative enzymes, traces of copper or iron; fairly stable in acid solution at low temperature	Readily absorbed; blood plasma levels reflect daily intake, whereas concentration in leukocytes reflects tissue level; excess excreted in urine; little tissue storage, but high concentrations in glandular tissues; dehydroascorbic acid, first oxidation product, is biologically active	Integrity and maintenance of intercellular material in all tissues; facilitates absorption of iron and conversion of folic acid to folinic acid; probably coenzyme in the metabolism of tyrosine and phenylalanine. Contributes to activity of succinic dehydrogenase and serum phosphatase in infants, not in adults	Scurvy and poor wound healing	Not harmful	Citrus fruits, tomatoes, berries, cantaloupe, cabbage, green vegetables. Cooking has deleterious effect

Table continued on following page

Table 3–6 PHYSICAL AND METABOLIC PROPERTIES AND FOOD SOURCES OF THE VITAMINS (Continued)

NAME AND SYNONYMS	CHARACTERISTICS	METABOLISM	BIOCHEMICAL ACTION	EFFECTS OF DEFICIENCY	EFFECTS OF EXCESS	SOURCES
VITAMIN D: Group of sterols having similar physiologic activity. D_2-calciferol is activated ergosterol. D_3 is activated 7-dehydrocholesterol	Fat-soluble; stable to heat, acid, alkali, and oxidation	Absorbed from intestine with fat, bile salts being required. Provitamin D_3 is synthesized in the skin and is converted to the vitamin by ultraviolet irradiation and absorbed. Calciferol is converted to 25-HCC (25-hydroxycalciferol) in liver; 25-HCC is an intermediary of the most potent metabolite, 1,25-dihydroxycholecalciferol, which is secreted as a hormone by the kidney	Mechanism of action not known. Regulates absorption and deposition of calcium and phosphorus, presumably by affecting permeability of intestinal membrane. Regulation of level of serum alkaline phosphatase, which is believed to be concerned with calcium phosphate deposition in bones and teeth	Rickets (high serum phosphatase level appears before bone deformities); infantile tetany, poor growth, osteomalacia	Wide variation in tolerance; in general, 20,000–50,000 IU/24 hr toxic when continued for weeks; prolonged administration of 1800 IU/24 hr may be toxic (see Sec 3.30). Manifestations are nausea, diarrhea, weight loss, polyuria, nocturia, eventually calcification of soft tissues, including heart, renal tubules, blood vessels, bronchi, stomach	Vitamin D–fortified milk and margarine, fish-liver oils, exposure to sunlight or other ultraviolet sources
VITAMIN E: Group of related chemical compounds—tocopherols—with similar biologic activities	Fat-soluble; heat-stable in absence of oxygen; unstable to ultraviolet light, alkali; readily oxidized by oxygen, iron, lead, rancid fats. Antioxidant in foods and the body	Absorption may be affected by fat digestion. Some storage in fatty tissues, but not in liver	Mechanism of action unknown (cell maturation and differentiation). Minimizes oxidation of carotene, vitamin A, and linoleic acid in the intestine. Possibly related to muscle metabolism and to erythrocyte fragility	Antioxidant; important to cell membrane integrity, endoplasmic reticulum, and mitochondrial oxidative functions; requirements related to polyunsaturated fat intake; may be involved in red blood cell hemolysis in premature infants	Unknown	Germ oils of various seeds, green leafy vegetables, nuts, legumes
VITAMIN K: Group of naphthoquinones with similar biologic activities; K_1 is phytoquinone	Natural compounds are fat-soluble, but several water-soluble products have been developed (menadione). Stable to heat and reducing agents; labile to oxidizing agents, strong acids, alcoholic alkali, light	Bile salts necessary for intestinal absorption of fat-soluble forms. Limited storage in liver; synthesized by intestinal microorganisms	Mechanism of action unknown; necessary for prothrombin formation, hence normal blood clotting; coagulation factors II, VII, IX, X are K-dependent	Hemorrhagic manifestations are result of faulty intestinal synthesis of vitamin K (newborn, prolonged use of sulfonamides or antibiotics), faulty intestinal absorption, or inability to synthesize prothrombin (hepatic damage). Except in the last condition, menadione and bile salts effective. Dicumarol and salicylates act as vitamin K antimetabolites	Not established; medicinally may produce hyperbilirubinemia in premature infants	Green leafy vegetables, pork liver. Widely distributed

ciency. Antimicrobial compounds may be transmitted in breast milk or in foods from animals that have been fed these compounds.

Endocrine Factors. Antithyroid substances (goitrogens) have been found in turnips, rutabagas, cabbage, soybeans, cobalt-containing foods, food additives, and medications; they increase the requirement for iodine. Administration of ACTH or corticosteroids necessitates an increase in protein and calcium and a decrease in sodium intake. Transient hypoparathyroidism with tetany has been observed in the neonatal period after excessive intake of vitamin D or of phosphates.

Radioactivity. Apparently there is little danger from carbon-14 because of its low activity. Iodine-131 is removed from milk by aeration or storage. Cesium-137 may be found in meat and milk products and can be counteracted by a high potassium intake or by the use of Diamox. Only 10% of strontium-90 ingested by the cow is found in cow's milk.

Emotional Factors. Along with increased knowledge of the significance of various nutrients there has developed excessive parental and professional concern over the food intake of the individual infant or child. The mother may develop a sense of fear, even guilt, about her child's eating habits resulting in a battle of wits between mother and child which may have far-reaching effects. The physician must be well informed in the fundamentals of nutrition in order to recognize and manage emotional and behavioral problems arising from undesirable dietary practices.

3.8 EVALUATION OF DIET

The pediatrician should have a reasonable knowledge of the properties of various foods in order to take and evaluate a dietary history, to know which laboratory tests have value for diagnosis, and to interpret therapeutic responses. (See Tables 3–7, 3–8, and 29–9 and 29–10 of the Appendix.)

The recall-interview for determining food habits of children is satisfactory under usual circumstances, but for more accurate accounting the mother should be instructed to observe and record the actual food intake in terms of the standard measuring cup or tablespoon, weight, or size of pieces. The data may then be converted to "servings" appropriate to the age of the child (Table 3–7). It is important to include items that may not be consumed daily.

The dietary guide according to food groups provides flexibility for cultural, religious, and personal preferences and seasonal, regional, and economic availability. A food intake record is helpful in indicating possible nutritional imbalances. An excessive intake of foods of 1 group may result in a high caloric level producing an overweight child while at the same time leading to a dangerously low intake of some essential nutrients. A notable example is the overconsumption of milk and the underconsumption of meat and eggs, with the resultant danger of iron deficiency anemia. When certain key foods, such as milk, eggs, and citrus fruits, are eliminated for personal or medical reasons, the deficiencies imposed may be compensated by judicious substitutions. Following is a list of the principal nutrients in the food groups:

Milk: high-quality protein, calcium, and phosphorus; riboflavin; vitamin A; vitamin D (if fortified)

Meat and eggs: high-quality protein, iron, B vitamins; vitamin A from liver and eggs

Table 3–7 RECOMMENDED FOOD INTAKE FOR GOOD NUTRITION ACCORDING TO FOOD GROUPS AND THE AVERAGE SIZE OF SERVINGS AT DIFFERENT AGE LEVELS

Food Group	Servings per Day	Average Size of Servings					
		1 year	2–3 years	4–5 years	6–9 years	10–12 years	13–15 years
Milk and cheese (1.5 oz cheese = 1 C milk)	4	½ C*	½–¾ C	½–¾ C	½–1 C	½–1 C	½–1 C
Meat group (protein foods)	3 or more						
Egg		1	1	1	1	1	1 or more
Lean meat, fish, poultry (liver once a week)		2 Tbsp†	2 Tbsp	4 Tbsp	2–3 oz (4–6 Tbsp)	3–4 oz	4 oz or more
Peanut butter			1 Tbsp	2 Tbsp	2–3 Tbsp	3 Tbsp	3 Tbsp
Fruits and vegetables	At least 4, including: 1 or more (twice as much tomato as citrus)						
Vitamin C source (citrus fruits, berries, tomato, cabbage, cantaloupe)		⅓ C (citrus)	½ C	½ C	1 medium orange	1 medium orange	1 medium orange
Vitamin A source (green or yellow fruits and vegetables)	1 or more	2 Tbsp	3 Tbsp	4 Tbsp (¼ C)	¼ C	⅓ C	½ C
Other vegetables (potato and legumes, etc.) *or*	2	2 Tbsp	3 Tbsp	4 Tbsp (¼ C)	⅓ C	½ C	¾ C
Other fruits (apple, banana, etc.)		¼ C	⅓ C	½ C	1 medium	1 medium	1 medium
Cereals (whole-grain or enriched)	At least 4						
Bread		½ slice	1 slice	1½ slices	1–2 slices	2 slices	2 slices
Ready-to-eat cereals		½ oz	¾ oz	1 oz	1 oz	1 oz	1 oz
Cooked cereal (including macaroni, spaghetti, rice, etc.)		¼ C	⅓ C	½ C	½ C	¾ C	1 C or more
Fats and carbohydrates	To meet caloric needs						
Butter, margarine, mayonnaise, oils: 1 Tbsp = 100 calories (kcal)		1 Tbsp	1 Tbsp	1 Tbsp	2 Tbsp	2 Tbsp	2–4 Tbsp
Desserts and sweets: 100-calorie portions as follows: ⅓ C pudding or ice cream, 2 3" cookies, 1 oz cake, 1⅓ oz pie, 2 tbsp jelly, jam, honey, sugar		1 portion	1½ portions	1½ portions	3 portions	3 portions	3–6 portions

*C = 1 cup or 8 oz or 240 ml.

†Tbsp = Tablespoon (1 Tbsp = ca. 15 ml = ca. ½ oz).

Modified with Mildred J. Bennett, Ph.D., from "Four Food Groups of the Daily Food Guide," Institute of Home Economics, U.S.D.A., and Publication #30, Children's Bureau of the United States Department of Health, Education, and Welfare.

Table 3-8 COMPARISON OF NUTRIENT VALUES OF THE DIETS PRESENTED IN TABLE 3-7 WITH THE RECOMMENDED DIETARY ALLOWANCES [SHOWN IN ( )]

AGE AND WEIGHT (Boys and Girls 25–75th Percentiles)	CALORIES*	PROTEIN gm	CALCIUM gm	IRON mg	VITAMIN A IU	THIAMINE† mg	RIBOFLAVIN† mg	NIACIN† mg	ASCORBIC ACID mg	VITAMIN D IU
1 year (22 ± 2 lb)	1020 (1000)	42 (25)	0.6 (0.5)	5.4 (15.0)	2325 (1300)	0.47 (0.5)	1.0 (0.6)	3.4 (8.0)	40 (35)	300 (400)
2–3 years (30 ± 5 lb)	1320 (1300)	48 (25)	0.8 (0.8)	6.1 (15.0)	3225 (1300)	0.64 (0.7)	1.0 (0.8)	7.3 (9.0)	51 (45)	400 (400)
4–5 years (39 ± 6 lb)	1720 (1700)	67 (30)	1.0 (0.8)	8.4 (10.0)	4270 (1650)	0.85 (0.9)	1.5 (1.0)	11.7 (11.0)	60 (45)	500 (400)
6–9 years (56 ± 15 lb)	2130 (2400)	76 (35)	1.4 (0.8)	11.4 (10.0)	5140 (2300)	1.2 (1.2)	2.0 (1.4)	19.3 (16.0)	88 (45)	600 (400)
10–12 years (81 ± 20 lb)	2480 (2700)	93 (45)	1.4 (1.2)	13.0 (18.0)	4590 (3300)	1.4 (1.3)	2.5 (1.6)	23.0 (18.0)	102 (50)	600 (400)
13–15 years (108 ± 27 lb)	2580–3080 (2500–2800)	100 (45–60)	1.4 (1.2)	14.4 (18.0)	5540 (3900)	1.5 (1.5)	2.5 (1.7)	23.7 (18.0)	107 (60)	600 (400)

Recommended Dietary Allowances, Revised 1980, National Research Council, National Academy of Sciences.

*Selections from fats and carbohydrate group included for caloric values, but not for other nutrients. Calorie = large calorie = kcal = Cal. (See text.)

†Based on the following: thiamine, 0.4 mg/1000 calories riboflavin; 0.025 mg/gm of protein; niacin, 6.6 mg/1000 calories.

Fruits and vegetables: vitamin C; provitamin A from green and yellow ones; trace elements; fiber

Cereals: less expensive and supplementary amounts of protein, minerals, fiber, B vitamins

Suspected dietary insufficiencies may be corroborated by appropriate laboratory tests and clinical evaluation. When malnutrition, either as dietary deficiency or excess, or failure to thrive exists in spite of an apparently satisfactory food intake, the infant or child's family relationships must be evaluated, not only for organic causes but especially for psychosocial ones (Sec 2.70).

This section was originally prepared for this textbook by Arild E. Hansen and was subsequently revised by Mildred Bennett and William E. Laupus.

(References follow next section.)

3.9 FEEDING OF INFANTS

Successful infant feeding requires *cooperative* functioning between the mother and her baby, beginning with the initial feeding experience and continuing throughout the child's period of dependency. Prompt establishment of comfortable, satisfying feeding practices contributes greatly to the infant's and mother's emotional well-being (Sec 2.12). Feeding time should be pleasurable for both mother and child. Maternal feelings are readily transmitted to the baby and, in large measure, determine the emotional setting in which feeding takes place. Mothers who are tense, anxious, irritable, easily upset, or emotionally labile are more likely to experience difficulty in the feeding relationship, but frequently they become more comfortable and confident with appropriate guidance and support from an empathetic and experienced relative or friend.

As soon after birth as an infant can safely tolerate enteral nutrition, as judged by normal activity, alertness, suck, and cry, feedings should be initiated to maintain normal metabolism and growth during the transition from fetal to extrauterine life, promote maternal-infant bonding, and decrease the risks of hypoglycemia, hyperkalemia, hyperbilirubinemia, and azotemia. More mistakes are made by feeding the infant too much than too little. Inadequate fluid intake, particularly in hot weather, may result in "dehydration fever." Most infants may start feeding by 6 hr of life. When there is any question about the tolerance of feeding because of physical or neurologic status, it should be withheld and parenteral fluids substituted. The schedule of initial feeding in a hospital is less important than the principle of unhurried beginning and patient assistance and support for the mother. Mothers who wish to initiate breast feeding in the delivery room and continue on a demand basis thereafter should be supported. Alternatively, since some general feeding schedule is needed from the standpoint of the hospital when rooming-in is not available or desired and demand feeding is not practical, the following is suggested. The infant is taken to the mother for the 1st feeding at 10 A.M. or 6 P.M., whichever is nearer the end of a 6-hr postpartum rest. Subsequent formula or breast feedings are given every 3–4 hr/day and night by the mother, except for the 1st night, when the 2 A.M. feeding is given by the nursing staff. Artificially fed infants should receive sterile water for the 1st feeding, since regurgitation and aspiration of this liquid are less likely to cause significant irritation of the respiratory tract.

The feeding of infants requires practical interpretation

of specific nutritional needs and of the widely varying limits of the normal baby's appetite and behavior with regard to food. The emptying time of the infant's stomach may vary from 1–4 or more hr; thus, considerable difference in desire for food may be expected in the infant at different times of the day, and ideally the feeding schedule should be based on reasonable "self-regulation" by the infant. Variation in the time between feedings and in the amount taken per feeding is to be expected in the 1st few wk with such a plan of "self-regulation." By the end of the 1st mo more than 90% of infants will have established a suitable and reasonably regular schedule.

Most healthy bottle-fed infants will want 6–9 feedings/24 hr by the end of the 1st wk of life. Some will take enough at one feeding to satisfy them for approximately 4 hr; others who are smaller or whose gastric emptying time is more rapid will want milk about every 2–3 hr; breast-fed infants often prefer shorter intervals. Most term infants will rapidly increase their intake from 30 ml to 80–90 ml every 3–4 hr prior to discharge at 4–5 days of life. Feeding should be considered to have progressed satisfactorily if the infant is no longer losing weight by 5–7 days and is gaining weight by 12–14 days. Some infants will not awaken for a middle-of-the-night feeding after 3–6 wk of age; some may never want it. Many will not want a late evening feeding between 4 and 8 mo of age and will be satisfied with 3 meals a day by 9–12 mo.

In helping to fashion a schedule guided by the infant's needs and behavior, it is important to establish that babies cry for reasons other than hunger and *need not be fed every time they cry*; some infants are placid, some unusually active, some irritable. Sick infants are often uninterested in food. Babies who awaken and cry consistently at short intervals may not be receiving enough milk at each feeding or may have discomfort from some cause other than hunger, e.g., too much clothing; soiled, wet, or uncomfortable diapers and clothing; colic; swallowed air ("gas"); uncomfortably hot or cold environment; or illness. Some babies cry to gain sufficient or additional attention, whereas others deprived of adequate mothering become indifferent. Some infants simply need to be held. Those who stop crying when they are picked up or held do not usually need food, but those who continue to cry when held and when food is offered should be carefully evaluated for other causes of distress. The habit of offering frequent, small feedings or of holding and feeding to pacify all crying should not be cultivated.

The advantages in supplying the infant's needs as they are expressed are several: physiologic requirements are met promptly; the infant does not learn to associate prolonged crying and discomfort with feeding; and the infant is less likely to develop poor eating practices such as gulping the feedings or taking small amounts too frequently. Babies soon establish a regular schedule which permits the family to resume normal function. If this does not occur, individual feedings or the whole day's schedule can be moved ahead or delayed sufficiently to avoid conflicts with necessary family activities.

Some mothers will not understand the goals of "self-regulation" by the infant; some will misinterpret the physician's instructions, and others may not have the capacity to adjust themselves to the regimen of the infant. *The orderly, overanxious, and compulsive parent will do better with a more specific outline for the infant's activities.*

The postpartum period is often a time of great anxiety and insecurity for the 1st-time mother, who may be temporarily overwhelmed by the responsibilities of motherhood. It is important that the hospital setting and the attitude of the hospital personnel be comforting and supporting while the mother finds and develops confidence in her maternal abilities. *The questions of inexperienced or uncertain mothers will frequently go unanswered unless time is set aside to consider them at the hospital or in the home.* Simple procedures should be explained and potential problem areas discussed.

Fathers and other members of the household should not be neglected by physicians in these anticipatory guidance sessions. Knowledge of the personalities and expectations of both parents is invaluable in helping to avert physical and psychologic problems centered around feeding. Parental misconceptions and confusion concerning the dietary and satiety needs of infants and children are often the bases for abnormal parent-child relations which can be avoided by appropriate counseling.

3.10 BREAST FEEDING

Breast feeding continues to have practical and psychologic advantages that should be considered when the mother selects the method for feeding. Human milk is the most appropriate of all available milks for the human infant since it is uniquely adapted to his or her needs.

Advantages of Breast Feeding. *Breast milk is the natural food for full-term infants during the 1st months of life.* It is always readily available at the proper temperature and no time is required in preparation. The milk is fresh and free of contaminating bacteria so that the chances of gastrointestinal disturbances are lessened. Although there is little if any difference in mortality rates in formula-fed and breast-fed infants receiving good care, among the lower socioeconomic groups and where sanitary conditions are poor the breast-fed infant continues to have a much greater likelihood of survival.

Allergy and intolerance to cow's milk are responsible for significant disturbances and feeding difficulties not seen in breast-fed infants. The symptoms include diarrhea, intestinal bleeding, and occult melena. "Spitting up," colic, and atopic eczema are less common in infants receiving human milk. Heiner and others have correlated chronic pulmonary hemosiderosis with the presence of precipitins in milk proteins in the serum of infants and have described improvement when cow's milk is removed from the diet (Sec 11.45).

Human milk contains bacterial and viral antibodies, including relatively high concentrations of secretory IgA antibodies. Breast-fed infants of mothers with high antipoliomyelitis titers are relatively resistant to infection by the attenuated live poliomyelitis vaccine viruses. The effect may be pronounced in the neonatal period but does not seem to interfere with active immunization at 2, 4, and 6 mo of age. It has also been shown that growth of the mumps, influenza, vaccinia, and Japanese B encephalitis viruses can be inhibited by substances in human milk. These ingested antibodies from human colostrum and milk may afford local gastrointestinal immunity against organisms that enter the body via this route. Cunningham noted comparatively more respiratory and gastrointestinal diseases in formula-fed infants.

Macrophages are normally present in human colostrum and milk and may have the ability to synthesize complement, lysozyme, and lactoferrin. Breast milk is also a source of lactoferrin, the iron-binding whey protein. This is normally about one third saturated with iron and has an inhibitory effect on the growth of *E. coli* in the intestine. The stool of the breast-fed infant has a lower pH than that of the infant fed cow's milk, and its bacterial content is predominantly of the lactobacillus group in contrast to a preponderance of the coliform group in artificially fed infants. Human milk contains a "growth factor" which facilitates intestinal colonization by *Lactobacillus bifidus*. The intestinal flora of infants fed human milk may protect them against infections caused by some species of *E. coli.*

Milk from the mother whose diet is quantitatively adequate and properly balanced will supply the necessary nutrients, with the possible exception of vitamin D after several months (Sec 3.28 and 7.16) and fluoride. Iron stores are sufficient for the 1st 6–9 mo in term infants. The iron of human milk is well absorbed by the infant; breast-fed infants may not require supplemental iron during the 1st yr, but their diets should be supplemented after 6 mo of age by the addition of cereal and meat or by administration of one of the ferrous iron preparations. Even if the community water supply contains adequate amounts of fluoride, the breast-fed infant may receive little of it, and fluoride should be supplied during the 1st months of life. Human milk contains sufficient vitamin C for the infant's needs, provided the mother's intake is adequate.

The psychologic advantages of breast feeding for both mother and infant are well recognized, and successful breast feeding is a satisfying experience for both. The mother is personally involved in the nurturing of her baby, gaining both a feeling of being essential and a sense of accomplishment. The infant is afforded a close and comfortable physical relationship with the mother. Breast feeding offers increased opportunity for close sensual contact between mother and infant; studies suggest that early and intimate tactile and visual contact are important in determining the quality of attachment and mothering which is provided the infant (Sec 7.13).

The mother who is unable or does not wish to nurse her infant, however, need have no less sense of accomplishment or of affection for her baby. That the quality of attachment and mothering and the degree of security and affection provided can be very comparable deserves strong emphasis.

Contraindications to Breast Feeding. For the average, healthy, full-term infant there are no disadvantages to breast feeding, provided the mother's milk supply is ample and her diet contains sufficient amounts of protein and vitamins. Infrequently, allergens to which the infant is sensitized may be conveyed in the milk. In such instances an attempt should be made to find the specific allergen and to remove it from the mother's diet; its presence rarely is a valid reason for weaning the baby.

From the standpoint of the mother, there are few contraindications to breast feeding. Markedly inverted nipples may be troublesome. Fissuring or cracking of the nipples rarely necessitates cessation of nursing but does require special attention, such as exposure to air and application of pure lanolin. Mastitis was once considered cause for discontinuance of nursing, but many now recommend continued and frequent nursing on the affected breast to keep it from becoming engorged. Local heat applications and antibiotics are also helpful. Acute infection in the mother may contraindicate breast feeding if the infant does not have the same infection; otherwise there is no need to stop nursing unless the condition of either makes it mandatory. When the infant is not affected and the mother's condition permits, the breast may be emptied and the milk given to the infant. Septicemia, nephritis, eclampsia, profuse hemorrhage, active tuberculosis, typhoid fever, and malaria are permanent contraindications to nursing, as are chronic poor nutrition, debility, severe neuroses, and postpartum psychoses.

The resumption of menstruation should not be a deterrent to continued nursing, although temporary changes in the behavior of mother or baby may call for reassurance. Pregnancy does not necessitate immediate cessation of nursing, but the combined demands of supplying milk to the infant and nutrients to the fetus are formidable and require special attention to maternal nutrition.

Prematurely born infants weighing 2000 gm (4½ pounds) or more usually thrive on breast milk. Infants of lesser birth weights, however, may have such rapid rates of growth that human milk alone may not supply sufficient essential nutrients for normal growth. Low birth weight infants who are too weak to suck or those who tire before an adequate volume is ingested may be given human milk by gavage. Many such infants have thrived. Human breast milk has also been advocated in the management of necrotizing enterocolitis (Sec 11.39).

The low vitamin K content of human milk may contribute to hemorrhagic disease of the newborn. *Administration of 1 mg of vitamin K₁ parenterally at birth is recommended for all infants, especially for those who will be breast-fed.*

Unconjugated hyperbilirubinemia in breast-fed infants is discussed in Sec 7.44.

Hemolytic disease of the newborn (erythroblastosis fetalis) is not a contraindication to breast feeding if the infant's general condition warrants it since antibodies in the mother's milk are inactivated in the intestinal tract and do not contribute to further hemolysis of the infant's blood cells.

Preparation of the Prospective Mother. Most women are physically capable of breast feeding provided they receive sufficient encouragement and are protected from discouraging experiences and comments while the secretion of breast milk is becoming established. The physician interested in aiding the prospective mother to breast feed should discuss its advantages during the midtrimester of pregnancy or whenever the mother becomes naturally concerned with the planning for her baby. Many mothers who are ambivalent toward breast feeding will be able to nurse successfully if they are given reassurance and support. If the mother rejects the suggestion that she nurse her infant, it is probably wise to avoid overpersuasion, which may be detrimental to mother-infant relationships.

Physical factors conducive to breast feeding include establishing and maintaining a state of good health, proper balance of rest and exercise, freedom from worry, early and sufficient treatment of any intercurrent disease, and adequate nutrition. Nutritional deficiencies are contributory factors to inadequate lactation and to infant morbidity.

Retracted nipples are usually benefited by daily manual breast pump traction during the latter weeks of pregnancy; truly inverted nipples may be helped by the use of milk cups, starting as early as the 3rd mo of pregnancy.

The mother may be confidently told that she need not gain or lose weight if her diet is adequate. She should be reassured that breast tone will be preserved by the use of a properly fitted brassiere to support the breasts, especially before delivery and during the nursing period. During the latter part of pregnancy, the mother gains weight and stores fat which is utilized in lactation. Nutritional requirements for lactation are listed in Table 3–1.

ESTABLISHMENT AND MAINTENANCE OF MILK SUPPLY

The only known satisfactory stimulus to the secretion of human milk is regular and complete emptying of the breasts; milk production is reduced when the secreted milk is not drained. Once lactation is well established, mothers are capable of producing far more milk than their infants will need. There are many reasons for incomplete nursing, but the principal ones are unsupportive hospital practices, weakness of the infant, and failure to initiate the natural hunger cycle. Every effort should be directed toward the early establishment of normal, vigorous nursing by letting the infant empty the breast frequently during the time when only colostrum is being formed. The infant should be allowed to nurse when hungry whether or not there appears to be any milk.

Breast feeding should be begun as soon after delivery as the condition of the mother and of the baby permits, preferably within several hours. Infants who cannot be fed on demand should be brought to the mother for feeding about every 3 hr during the day and every 4 hr during the night. Many infants are hungry within 2 hr of a satisfying nursing episode, and about 75% of the breast's milk has been replenished by this time.

Appropriate care for tender or sore nipples should be instituted before severe pain from abrasions and cracking develops. Exposure of the nipples to air; application of pure lanolin; avoidance of soap, alcohol, and tincture of benzoin; and frequent changes of disposable nursing pads lining the brassiere cups are recommended. Nursing more frequently may be more helpful than nursing less often. When the tenderness causes apprehension in the mother, the *milk ejection reflex* may be delayed, leading to frustration in the baby and to increasingly vigorous nursing which further injures the nipple and areolar area. Manual expression of milk to start the flow will be helpful in re-establishing normal feeding relationships. Occasionally, nipple shields may be of help.

The 1st 2 wk of the neonatal period is the crucial time for the establishment of breast feeding. Lactogenic hormones are not effective in the stimulation of human breast secretion. Too much emphasis has been put on daily weight gains. When early supplemental milk feedings are given to achieve this false goal, attempts at breast feeding are compromised; usually the infant finds that it is easier to get milk from a bottle than from a breast. On the day the mother is discharged from the hospital lactation may not be well established, and the excitement of going home may not be conducive to an initially successful nursing experience there. A wise physician will anticipate this experience and discuss it with the mother. In some instances, providing the mother with enough isocaloric formula for 1 or 2 complementary feedings may prevent discouragement, which might prejudice further nursing.

Psychologic Factors. No factor is more important than a happy, relaxed state of mind. Worry and unhappiness are the most effective means for decreasing or abolishing breast secretions.

Mothers may worry that their babies are abnormal when they cry, are drowsy, sneeze, or regurgitate milk. Mothers are upset by any suggestion that their milk may be lacking in quantity or quality. They may be disturbed at the scanty supply of colostrum, at tenderness of the nipples, and at the fullness of the breast on the 4th or 5th day. Many mothers do not feel comfortable when trying to nurse in an open ward or with another person in the room. Mothers worry about what is going on at home while they are hospitalized and about what is going to happen when they arrive home. An alert physician is conscious of these worries, particularly if the baby is a 1st-born, and by tactful reassurance and explanation can help prevent or minimize worry, thus contributing to successful breast feeding.

Fatigue. Avoidance of fatigue is important, but the mother should have sufficient exercise to promote a sense of physical well-being.

Hygiene. Once a day the breasts should be washed. If soap is drying to the nipple and areolar area, it should be discontinued. The nipple area should be kept dry. *Boric acid must not be used.* Care should be taken to prevent irritation and infection of the nipples caused by prolonged initial nursing, maceration from wetness of the nipple, or rubbing of clothing.

Some mothers may be more comfortable if a properly fitted brassiere is worn day and night. Plastic liners should be removed. An absorbent pad (commercially available) or a clean cloth or handkerchief may be placed inside the brassiere to absorb any milk that leaks out.

Diet. The diet should contain enough calories to compensate for those secreted in the milk as well as those required for its production. A varied diet adequate to maintain weight and relatively high in fluid, vitamins, and minerals will suffice. Weight reduction diets should be avoided by the nursing mother. Milk is important but should not replace other essential foods. When the mother is allergic or has an aversion to milk, 1 gm of calcium may be added to her daily diet. The fluid intake should approximate 3 quarts daily; urinary output is a good measure of the adequacy of fluid in the daily diet.

There are mistaken ideas that such substances as milk, beer, oatmeal, and tea are galactogenic. Particular foods in the mother's diet seldom have a disturbing influence on the breast-fed infant. Occasionally, however, maternal ingestion of certain berries, tomatoes, onions, members of the cabbage family, chocolate, spices, and condiments may cause gastric distress or loose stools in the infant. No food need be withheld from the mother's diet unless it causes distress to the infant. Whenever possible, nursing mothers should not take drugs since the effects of many preparations on the neonate are harmful or have not been evaluated (Table 5–30). Antithyroid medications, lithium, anticancer agents, isoniazid, and phenindione are contraindicated. Temporary cessation of nursing is recommended if the mother requires diagnostic radiopharmaceuticals, chloramphenicol, metronidazole, sulfonamides, or anthroquinone-derivative laxatives. Lactating women should not eat sport fish from waters contaminated with polychlorinated biphenyls (PCB's). It is better to control maternal constipation by inclusion in her diet of raw and cooked fruits and vegetables, whole wheat bread, and an adequate amount of water than by use of laxatives. Smoking of cigarettes and drinking alcoholic beverages should be discouraged. Certain substances, such as the arsenicals, barbiturates, bromides, iodides, lead, mercurials, salicylates, opium, atropine, most antimicrobial agents, and cascara may be transmitted through the milk and exert an effect on the infant.

TECHNIQUE OF BREAST FEEDING

The technical aspects of breast feeding require careful consideration. It is not unusual for breast feeding to be deemed impossible simply because the attending physician fails to recognize that the difficulties are related to the manner of feeding.

The infant should be hungry at feeding time, dry, neither too cold nor too warm, and held in a comfortable, semisitting position for his or her enjoyment and for facilitation of eructation without vomiting. The mother, too, must be comfortable and completely at ease. When she is able to be out of bed, a moderately low chair with armrest is preferable, and a low stool is advantageous for resting her foot and raising her knee on the nursing side. The baby is supported comfortably with the face held close to the mother's breast by one arm and hand while the other hand supports the breast so that the nipple is easily accessible to the infant's mouth and yet does not obstruct the infant's nasal breathing. The baby's lips should be expected to engage considerable areola as well as nipple.

Success in infant feeding depends to a great extent upon the adjustments during the 1st few days of life. Difficulties are likely to result when attempts are made to adapt the infant to the nursing procedure rather than to try to satisfy the infant's natural desires. Rigid adherence to clock schedules and the "assembly line" manner in which babies are handled in many nurseries may make adjustment at home more difficult. Most problems can be avoided by conforming to the infant's spontaneous pattern. If the infant is put at the breast when there is normal hunger crying and the baby's appetite is satisfied, the fundamental requirements are met. Aldrich emphasized the natural initial responses to hunger; his account of one of them, the rooting reflex, is so well phrased that we have taken the liberty of reproducing it here.

At the time he is born, the normal infant is equipped with several reflexes, or behavior patterns, which are designed to make him a successful feeder from the breast. The most obvious of these reflexes are those concerned with the actual getting of food—rooting, sucking, swallowing, and satiety reflexes.

The *rooting reflex* is the first one of these to come into play. When a baby smells milk, he moves his head around and attempts to find its source. If one cheek is touched by a smooth object, he will turn his mouth toward that object and open it in anticipation of grasping the nipple. This obviously gives a clue as to how milk should be given to the baby. His cheek applied to his mother's breast will start him rooting with his mouth for the nipple.

The infant's rooting reflex brings the entire areolar area into the mouth; the contact of the nipple against the palate and posterior tongue elicits suckling or "milking," and the buccal fat pads help keep the nipple in place. This "sucking reflex" is a process of squeezing the sinuses of the areola rather than simply suction on the nipple. The infant's sucking results in afferent impulses to the mother's hypothalamus and then to both anterior and posterior pituitary. Prolactin from the anterior pituitary stimulates milk secretion in the cuboidal cells in the acini or alveoli of the breast. Finally, milk in the infant's mouth triggers the swallowing reflex.

Mothers should know that if the infant is not hungry, he or she will not search for the nipple or suck. Infants are usually sleepy for several days and most are not initially avid suckers. Particularly on the 3rd day, when there has been some weight loss, mothers are anxious about infants who do not seem particularly interested in nursing. It is reassuring for them to know that most healthy babies "wake up" and become good nursers on the 4th day. Kron and Brazelton have reported that infants whose mothers received obstetric sedation during labor sucked at lower rates and pressures and consumed less milk than comparable infants from mothers given no sedation.

Some infants will empty a breast in 5 min; others will be more leisurely and nurse well for 20 min. Most of the milk is obtained early in the feeding: 50% in the first 2 min and 80–90% in the first 4 min. The baby should be permitted to suck until satisfied unless the mother has sore nipples. Efforts to wake up a sleepy baby to nurse by snapping feet or pinching or shaking are rarely successful.

At the end of the nursing period the infant should be held erect over the mother's shoulder or on her lap to eructate swallowed air; often this "burping" procedure is necessary one or more times during the feeding as well as 5-10 min after the infant has been put into the crib. It is an essential procedure during the early months but should not be overdone. When nursing is completed, the infant should be placed in the crib on the abdomen or on the right side to facilitate emptying of the stomach into the intestines and to lessen the chances of regurgitation.

One or Both Breasts Per Feeding. The infant should empty at least one breast at each feeding; otherwise it will not be stimulated to refill. Both breasts should be used in the early weeks at each feeding to encourage maximal production of milk. After the milk supply has been established, the breasts may be alternated at successive feedings, and the baby will usually be satisfied with the amount obtained from one. If the secretion of milk becomes too great, both breasts may again be offered at each feeding and incompletely emptied with the intent of securing a partial decrease in lactation.

Determination of Adequacy of Milk Supply. If the infant is satisfied at the completion of the nursing periods, sleeps 2-4 hr, and gains weight adequately, it can be assumed that the milk supply is sufficient. Some babies are "light sleepers" and require a lot of body contact with the mother during the 1st months. Wakefulness and alertness in these babies should not be interpreted as poor milk supply. If the infant nurses avidly and is not satisfied after completely emptying both breasts, does not go to sleep, or sleeps fitfully and awakens after an hr or 2, and fails to gain weight satisfactorily, the milk supply is probably inadequate. The program of La Leche League,* which establishes close relationships between successful nursing mothers and mothers needing assistance, is often helpful in such circumstances.

The "let-down" or *milk-ejection reflex* is an important sign of successful nursing. Sucking or often psychologic stimuli associated with nursing lead to secretion of oxytocin by the posterior pituitary. As a result, the myoepithelial cells surrounding the alveoli deep in the breast contract, squeezing milk into the larger ducts, where it is more easily available to the sucking infant. When this reflex is functioning well, milk will flow from the opposite breast as the baby begins to nurse. It is frequently absent or erratic during periods of pain, fatigue, or emotional distress, and its malfunction is thought to be responsible for retention of milk in women who are unsuccessful in breast feeding.

Having the mother weigh her baby before and after nursing is generally neither a necessary nor a desirable way of judging the adequacy of milk supply. It wrongly focuses attention on how much the infant takes at a given time (normally there may be variations of 1 to several oz in the various feedings in a 24-hr period), and the results obtained are readily misinterpreted. Small gains may cause the mother additional worry,

*La Leche League International, 9616 Minneapolis Avenue, Franklin Park, Illinois 60131, has many local affiliates composed of successful nursing mothers who are willing to assist other mothers desiring to nurse.

and, in turn, her milk supply may diminish. She may think it necessary to give the baby a bottle to assure herself that the infant is getting enough and to see how many ounces can be taken. The result of the "test bottle" may so discourage her that subsequent breast feeding becomes impossible, even when she has an adequate supply of milk. Before it is assumed that the mother is unable to produce sufficient milk, 3 possibilities should be excluded: (1) errors in feeding technique responsible for the infant's inadequate progress; (2) remediable maternal factors related to diet, rest, or emotional distress; or (3) physical disturbances in the infant that interfere with eating or with gain in weight. Infrequently infants who seem to be nursing well may not thrive because of insufficiency of milk; increased frequency of feeding may be indicated. Nursing more frequently than every 2 hr may inhibit prolactin secretion of the anterior pituitary, with decreased production of milk, usually corrected by instruction to delay feedings to 2½-hr intervals. Other aids include stimulation of prolactin secretion by administration of small doses of chlorpromazine for a few days or by devices such as the Lact-aid which supplement the infant's intake.

Manual Expression of Breast Milk. This is achieved by 2 movements. First, the whole breast is compressed between the hands, starting at the base and continuing toward the areola. Firm pressure is maintained throughout the movement, which is repeated several times. The purpose is to impel milk to the lacteal sinuses. The 2nd movement empties the sinuses. The breast is supported with 1 hand while the tissue just behind the areola is repeatedly compressed between the thumb and 1st finger of the other hand. The direction of the force is backward toward the center of the breast rather than toward the nipple. The fingers are not moved from this initial position, nor is the skin rubbed over the breast tissue. The procedure should not be painful even if the nipples are sore and cracked.

Mechanical Expression of Breast Milk. Hand pumps are often ineffectual and may increase the irritation and pain in congested breast and nipple tissues. Many mothers prefer to use an electric breast pump.

Supplementary Feedings. An occasional replacement feeding, after the 1st 6 wk when nursing has been adequately established, has the advantage of permitting the mother greater freedom in her activities. For the otherwise normal and healthy baby who is getting insufficient breast milk, artificial feeding may be offered either immediately after or in place of one or more breast feedings. An attempt should first be made to increase the supply of breast milk. Any of the milk formulas described under Formula Feeding may be offered in amounts sufficient to satisfy the baby. If formula is to be given after the baby has completed a breast feeding, the bottle should be warmed and handy so that it can be offered immediately after the infant has been burped. The holes in the nipples should not be so large that the baby gets this portion of food without any effort or the baby will quickly abandon any efforts to suck adequately at the mother's breast.

Weaning. Most infants gradually reduce the volume and frequency of their demand for breast feedings at 6-12 mo of age as their mothers offer and they become accustomed to increasing amounts of solid foods and of liquids by bottle and cup. As the demand for breast milk decreases, the mother's supply will gradually diminish without causing the mother unnecessary discomfort from engorgement. Weaning should be initiated by substituting whole cow's milk by bottle or cup for part of a breast feeding, and subsequently for all of a breast feeding. Over several days, one of the breast feedings is replaced and then subsequently another, and so on, until the infant is weaned completely. Occasionally, the cup is taken as readily as the bottle, and the intermediate transfer from bottle to cup is avoided. It is important that these changes be made gradually and that they be a pleasant experience for mother and infant, not a cause for conflict. Praise, loving attention, and cuddling are vital to successful weaning.

When cessation of nursing is necessary at an earlier age because of maternal illness or prolonged illness or death of the infant, a tight breast binder may be used and ice bags applied for a day or so to decrease milk production. Restriction of the mother's fluid intake is also helpful. Hormones, such as small doses of estrogen for 1 or 2 days, also may help decrease milk production at the termination of nursing.

3.11 FORMULA FEEDING

Cow's milk in the whole state or in some modified form is the basis for most formulas, although other milks and milk substitutes are available for infants who cannot tolerate cow's milk. Marked reduction in the morbidity and mortality from gastrointestinal infections has resulted from sterilization and refrigeration of the formula. Milk processing (varying from simple boiling in the home to commercial pasteurization, homogenization, and evaporation) has so altered the casein that small and readily digestible curds are formed in the stomach, thereby eliminating the principal cause for indigestibility of cow's milk protein.

Though breast feeding is superior to formula feeding for normal infants, many infants in the United States receive formula from birth. Changing social and cultural patterns have contributed to this increased reliance on formulas. Many mothers are reluctant to nurse their infants because of employment outside the home or implied limitations on their activities; others refuse because of fear of failure or of worry that loss of physical attractiveness will ensue from gain of weight and loss of breast tone; some do not consider breast feeding socially acceptable. Whatever the mother's reasons, the present popularity of artificial feeding could not have been reached without prior improvements in the safety and quality of the substitute milks.

Objective studies of the state of nutrition in growing infants (rate of growth in weight and length, normality of various constituents in blood, performance in metabolic studies, body composition, etc.) show relatively small differences between infants fed human milk and those fed cow's milk. Such techniques* may not be sufficiently sensitive to record small but important variations. Nonetheless, these investigations attest to the ability of the normal infant to thrive by making satisfactory physiologic adjustments to relatively wide ranges of intake of protein, fat, carbohydrate, and minerals.

Conventional whole and evaporated cow's milk formulas provide approximately 3–4 gm of protein/kg/24 hr ("high protein" intake with a relatively large excess above basic need), whereas breast milk and many commercially prepared feedings simulating the composition of breast milk supply 1.5–2.5 gm/kg/24 hr ("low protein" intake supplying a smaller margin of excess).

Fomon has calculated the rate of increase in total body protein mass in the "male reference" term infant to average approximately 3.5 gm/24 hr in the 1st 4 mo of life. Assuming 0.5 gm/24 hr nitrogen loss from the skin, total protein need is estimated to be about 4.0 gm/24 hr during the 1st 4 mo and slightly less during the remainder of the 1st yr.

Commercial formulas are modified from a cow's milk base with protein and ash reduced to levels near those of human milk to decrease osmolality and renal excretory load. The saturated fat of cow's milk is replaced with some unsaturated vegetable fatty acids, and vitamins are added. The concentration of lactose is lower in cow's milk than in human milk. Some formulas include higher lactoproteins and lower casein as in breast milk. Low birth weight infants particularly may benefit from the increased cystine of lactoproteins. Until more information is available, it appears prudent to recommend breast feeding for all babies, but if this is not possible, then a formula as close in composition to breast milk as possible is desirable.

TECHNIQUE OF ARTIFICIAL FEEDING

The setting should be similar to that for breast feeding, with the mother and infant in a comfortable position, unhurried, and free from distractions. The infant should be hungry, fully awake, warm, and dry and be held as though being breast-fed. The bottle should be held so that milk, not air, is channeled through the nipple. Bottle propping, even with a "safe" holder, should be avoided as it not only deprives the infant of the physical contact, comfort, and security of being held but may also be dangerous to small infants, who may aspirate if unattended. Otitis media is more common in babies who are fed with the bottle propped.

The bottle of milk is customarily warmed to body temperature though no harmful effects have been demonstrated from feedings at room temperature or cooler, even when the bottle is taken directly from the refrigerator. The temperature may be tested by dropping

---

*For example, the commonly used gain in weight does not differentiate between accumulation in lean body mass and fat stores and includes increases in body water due to excess solute retention under certain circumstances, as has been demonstrated by the studies of Kagan et al. in the nutrition of premature infants.

milk on the wrist. The nipple holes should be of such size that milk will drop slowly.

Especially during the 1st 6–7 mo of life, the eructation of air swallowed during feeding is important for avoidance of regurgitation and abdominal discomfort. Holding the infant upright over the shoulder with or without gently rubbing or patting the back assists in expelling the air. A few babies relieve themselves best after being replaced in the crib. All babies will, at times, regurgitate or "spit up" a small amount of milk after feeding, a fact the mother should know. Spitting up occurs more often in the artificially fed than in the breast-fed infant. Aspiration of this milk is less likely if the infant lies on the right side or abdomen rather than on the back.

A feeding may require from 5–25 min, depending on the vigor and the age of the infant. Since the appetite varies from feeding to feeding, each bottle should contain more than the average amount taken per feeding. In no instance should the baby be urged to take more than desired, and excess milk should be discarded.

COMPARISON OF HUMAN MILK AND COW'S MILK

Average values for the various constituents of human milk and whole fresh cow's milk are listed in Table 3–9. Human milk and cow's milk differ during the various stages of lactation and among individuals, although the differences among women with adequate diets are insignificant. Milk late in pregnancy and early after birth contains more protein, calcium, and other minerals than later during nursing.

Colostrum. The secretion of the breasts during the latter part of pregnancy and for the 2–4 days after delivery is termed "colostrum." It has a deep lemon yellow color, its reaction is alkaline, and its specific gravity is 1.040–1.060, in contrast to the average specific gravity of 1.030 for mature breast milk. The total amount of colostrum secreted daily is 10–40 ml. Human or cow colostrum contains several times as much protein as mature breast milk and more minerals but less carbohydrate and fat. Human colostrum also contains some unique immunologic factors. After the first few days of lactation, colostrum is replaced by secretion of a transitional form of milk which gradually assumes the characteristics of mature breast milk by the 3rd or 4th wk.

Water. The relative amounts of water and solids in human and cow's milks are about the same, each having a water content of about 87–88%; the specific gravity of each is 1.030–1.032.

Calories. The energy value of each milk may vary slightly and is about 20 kcal/oz or 0.67 kcal/ml.

Protein. There are quantitative differences between the proteins of the 2 milks. Human milk contains only 1.0–1.5% (average 1.10) protein in contrast to about 3.3% in cow's milk. The increased protein of cow's milk is almost entirely accounted for by the 6-fold higher content of casein. In human milk the protein consists of approximately 60% whey proteins, largely lactalbu-

mins and lactoglobulins, and 40% casein; in cow's milk the ratio is reversed, to 18:82.

Carbohydrate. The sugars of the 2 milks differ only quantitatively; both contain lactose. Human milk contains 6.5–7.0% and cow's milk about 4.5%.

Table 3–9 APPROXIMATE COMPOSITION OF COLOSTRUM, HUMAN MILK, AND COW'S MILK*

CONSTITUENT gm/100 gm	HUMAN MILK	HUMAN COLOSTRUM	COW'S MILK
Water	88	87	88
Protein	0.9	2.7	3.3
Casein	0.4	1.2	2.7
Lactalbumin	0.4		0.4
Lactoglobulin	0.2	1.5	0.2
Fat	3.8	2.9	3.8
% polyunsaturated	8.0	7.0	2.0
Lactose	7.0	5.3	4.8
Ash	0.2	0.5	0.8
Calcium mg/100 gm	34	30	117
Phosphorus mg/100 gm	15	15	92
Sodium mEq/l	7	48	22
Potassium mEq/l	13	74	35
Chloride mEq/l	11	80	29
Magnesium mg/100 gm	4	4	12
Sulfur mg/100 gm	14	22	30
Chromium μg/l			10
Manganese μg/l	10	tr	30
Copper μg/l	400	600	300
Zinc mg/l	4	6	4
Iodine μg/l	30	120	47
Selenium μg/l	30		30
Iron mg/l	0.5	0.1	0.5
Amino acids (mg/100 ml)			
Histidine	22		95
Leucine	68		228
Isoleucine	100		350
Lysine	73		277
Methionine	25		88
Phenylalanine	48		172
Threonine	50		164
Tryptophan	18		49
Valine	70		245
Arginine	45		129
Alanine	35		75
Aspartic acid	116		166
Cystine	22		32
Glutamic acid	230		680
Glycine	0		11
Proline	80		250
Serine	69		160
Tyrosine	61		179
Vitamins (liter)			
Vitamin A (IU)	1898		1025
Thiamine (μg)	160		440
Riboflavin (μg)	360		1750
Niacin (μg)	1470		940
Pyridoxine (μg)	100		640
Pantothenate (mg)	2		3
Folacin (μg)	52		55
B_{12} (μg)	0.3		4
Vitamin C (mg)	43		11
Vitamin D (IU)	22		14
Vitamin E (mg)	2		0.4
Vitamin K (μg)	15		60

*Collated largely from Fomon SJ: Infant Nutrition. Ed 2. Philadelphia, WB Saunders Co, 1974, pp 360 ff, and Macy IG, Kelly HJ, Sloan RE: The Composition of Milks, NAS-NRC Publ. 254, 1953.

Fat. The fat content of milks is more variable than any other constituent, but the average content is about 3.5%. The amount in human milk varies somewhat with maternal diet; the fat content of milk obtained during a single nursing is higher in the latter portion of the feeding and may help satiate the infant at the conclusion of nursing. Fat and caloric contents are related and can be determined by the creamatocrit, a measure of the percentage of fat after centrifugation in a hematocrit tube.

The milks of different breeds of cattle vary in fat content. Most market milk in urban areas, however, is pooled, and the fat content is adjusted to a standard level, generally from 3.25–4%.

There are qualitative differences between the fats of human and cow's milks. The fats of each are composed principally of the triglycerides olein, palmitin, and stearin. Human milk, however, contains twice as much of the more readily absorbed olein. The volatile fatty acids (butyric, capric, caproic, and caprylic) account for only about 1.3% of the fat of human milk, in contrast to about 9% in cow's milk. The small amount of linoleic acid in most milks is sufficient to prevent deficiency. The premature or debilitated infant may have steatorrhea after ingesting cow's milk fat. For such infants it is wise to substitute a more readily assimilated vegetable fat or human milk.

Minerals. The total mineral content of human milk (0.15–0.25%) is considerably less than that of cow's milk (0.7–0.75%). With the exception of iron and copper, cow's milk contains much more of all the minerals. Cow's milk contains inadequate iron; breast milk iron, while low, may be sufficient for the infant because of better absorption. The deficiency is compensated for in the 1st 4 mo or so of life by iron stored during fetal life. Although the need for calcium and phosphorus is relatively great during periods of rapid growth, adequate balances are maintained on breast milk in spite of its comparatively low content of these minerals.

Vitamins. The vitamin content of each milk varies with the maternal intake. Each has relatively large amounts of vitamin A. Cow's milk is low in vitamins C and D. Breast milk usually contains adequate vitamin C if the mother consumes appropriate foods, as well as adequate vitamin D activity unless the mother receives insufficient exposure to sunlight or is darkly pigmented. Cow's milk contains more thiamine and riboflavin than human milk and about an equal quantity of niacin. It is assumed that each milk contains adequate amounts of vitamin A and the B-complex vitamins for the nutritional needs of infants in the 1st months of life.

Bacterial Content. Although human milk is essentially free from bacterial contamination, pathogenic organisms in significant numbers may gain access to the milk from mastitis. Both tubercle and typhoid bacilli and herpes, hepatitis B, rubella, mumps, and cytomegaloviruses may be found at times in the milk of women infected with these organisms. Cow's milk is regularly contaminated, but in most instances the bacteria are not harmful to man. Milk, however, is a good culture medium for pathogenic bacteria, and many infections are milk-borne, including streptococcal diseases, diphtheria, typhoid fever, salmonellosis, tuberculosis, and

brucellosis. Furthermore, certain bacteria which may not affect older children or adults may cause diarrhea in infants. For this reason, in most cities pasteurization of all marketed whole milk is required. In addition, boiling the milk immediately before mixing the infant's formula or terminal sterilization is advisable.

Digestibility. The emptying time of the stomach is more rapid for human than for whole cow's milk; however, there is no appreciable difference in gastrointestinal passage time during the 1st 45 days of life between human milk and processed milk formulas. The curd of cow's milk is reduced in size by boiling and is made considerably less tough and much smaller by the heating required in evaporation, by the addition of acid or alkali, and by homogenization. In contrast, the curd of breast milk is fine and flocculent and readily broken down in the stomach. The fat of cow's milk is less readily digested than that of breast milk.

MILK USED IN FORMULAS

Raw Milk. Raw milk is not advised for infant feeding; it forms large curds in the stomach, is slowly digested, and is easily contaminated with pathogenic organisms. Its sale is forbidden in most urban communities in the United States.

Pasteurized Milk. Pasteurization destroys pathogenic bacteria and modifies the casein so that smaller and less tough curds are produced in the stomach. It is accomplished by holding heated milk at a specified temperature for a specific length of time, e.g., at 145°F (63°C) for 30 min or, more commonly, at 161°F (72°C) for 15 sec followed by rapid cooling to 148°F (65°C) or lower (60°C). Standards for the bacterial content of pasteurized milk vary in different cities, tolerable counts ranging as high as 50,000 nonpathogenic bacteria/ml; average counts in many cities, however, are as low as 5000–10,000. Pasteurized milk should be boiled when used for infant feeding. If allowed to stand in the refrigerator for as long as 48 hr, a significant increase in bacterial count may occur.

Homogenized Milk. In the process of homogenization, the fat globules are broken into minute particles and remain dispersed, or, in other words, the cream does not separate. The principal advantage of homogenized milk lies in the smaller and less tough curd produced in the stomach.

Evaporated Milk. This milk has many advantages, including almost universal availability. The unopened can will keep for months without refrigeration. The casein curd produced in the stomach is softer and smaller than that of boiled whole milk; homogenization of the fat also contributes to smaller curd formation. The lactalbumin appears to be less allergenic than that of fresh milk. The sugar is unchanged. When necessary, evaporated milk can be fed in higher concentrations than whole milk formulas. The standard can contains 13 fluid oz* (384 ml). Each fluid oz is equal to about 44 kcal; in practice the value is generally considered to be

---

*One fluid oz is equivalent to approximately 29.57 ml.

40 kcal. Vitamin D is usually added in the processing so that each reconstituted quart contains 400 IU.

Prepared Milks. Numerous commercially prepared modified milks that require only the addition of water in a 1:1 proportion are widely used in infant feeding (Tables 3–10 and 3–11). Most are derived from cow's milk, and many are available in both liquid and powder forms. The majority have compositions that simulate breast milk in one or more ways: reduced protein contents; reduced mineral salts (sodium, potassium, chloride, calcium, phosphorus); fat modification by substitution of vegetable fat for butterfat; and addition of carbohydrate (lactose or dextrin-maltose). All are fortified with vitamin D; many contain other vitamins, and some have added iron.

These milks are nutritionally adequate for normal infants, simple to prepare, and convenient to use. Their cost is somewhat greater than evaporated milk–water formulas.

Other prepared milks that may have virtue for special circumstances are now available. Those with very low electrolyte content (mineral content similar to that in human milk) may be helpful for infants with congestive heart failure, nephrogenic diabetes insipidus, or marginal renal function. A low sodium milk, containing about 1 mEq of sodium per reconstituted quart, is commercially available for use in the management of infants with congestive heart failure but should be used with caution. Milks low in phenylalanine content are useful in the management of infants and children with phenylketonuria.

Condensed Milk. About 45% cane sugar has been added in sweetened condensed milk, making the carbohydrate content approximately 60% in the evaporated form before dilution. The usual dilutions (1:10–1:4) are disproportionately high in sugar and low in fat and protein. Although readily digestible, it has no use in infant feeding for more than short periods when a high caloric diet is desired.

Dried Whole Milk. The fat content of fluid milk is adjusted to 3.5%, and the milk is rapidly evaporated to powder form by spray-, freeze- or roller-drying. Reconstituted dried milk has most of the advantages of evaporated milk but does not keep well when exposed to air.

Dried Skim Milk. Available as either nonfat skim milk (fat content 0.5%) or half-skim milk (fat content 1.5%), these milks have limited usefulness (for infants with fat intolerance). Skim milk should not be used in the 1st yr of life for weight reduction. The high protein and mineral content in proportion to calories may cause severe dehydration. Many of these products do not contain added vitamin D.

Acid and Fermented Milk. So-called acid milks are prepared by addition of acid to previously boiled and cooled cow's milk formulas or are fermented by the addition of lactic acid–producing organisms. These milks require less hydrochloric acid for gastric digestion. The casein is altered so that smaller and less tough curds are formed in the stomach. Acidified milks are now rarely used in infant feedings as they are prone to cause acidosis.

Goat's Milk. In many countries goat's milk is used extensively for infant feeding; its use in the United States is limited to management of cow's milk allergies. Because of inconsistent antigenic cross-reaction between cow's and goat's milks, the latter is less popular than the soy "milks" or the formulas derived from lamb and beef and from casein hydrolysis.

Although goat's milk is similar in composition to cow's milk, it contains less sodium, more potassium and chloride, and more of the essential linoleic and arachidonic acids. Its fat may be more digestible and its curd tension lower than that found in cow's milk. It is low in vitamin D, iron, and folic acid; infants fed exclusively on goat's milk are prone to megaloblastic anemia due to folate deficiency. The goat is especially susceptible to brucellosis; the milk should be boiled before use. It is commercially available in evaporated and powdered forms.

Milk Protein. Powdered protein is used chiefly for increasing the protein content of some formulas fed to premature or debilitated infants or to infants with diarrhea. Because of the increased metabolic products and the easy conversion of a balanced to an unbalanced diet, such products should be used carefully and for short durations.

Milk Substitutes and Hypoallergenic Milks. There are a number of milks and milk substitutes for infants allergic to cow's milk. These include evaporated goat's milk, a preparation in which nutrient nitrogen is supplied as an amino acid mixture (casein hydrolysate), nonmilk foods in which the protein is derived from soybeans, and meat-base formulas (beef and lamb sources). All appear to be nutritionally satisfactory and have a place in the management of infants who cannot tolerate cow's milk; those which do not contain lactose are useful for infants with galactosemia. Powdered casein (Casec) and medium-chain triglycerides (MCT oil) are available for special purposes.

Milks, Filled and Imitation. Imitation milk products and nondairy "white" beverages in which vegetable fat is substituted for cow (butter) fat are being developed and tested for use in countries where milk and other high quality protein sources are in short supply. Many of these products lack the full nutritional benefits of fluid milk; they are not intended as formula for infants or as a substitute for breast milk. When they are used for older children, the physician should be aware of the composition and limitations of the product.

Elemental Dietary Substitutes for Milk. A number of specialty products have been developed to meet complicated dietary and nutritional problems in children and adults with malabsorption on the basis of primary disease or extensive surgical resection of small bowel. These include diets prepared with known quantities of purified chemical elements (free glucose, amino acids, and essential fatty acids). All are low residue, chemically defined, and nutritionally adequate, at least for short-term use. They have been most useful in treating severely ill infants with intractable diarrhea, in reducing stooling and/or "resting" the colon in inflammatory bowel disease, in making maximum use of short bowel segments after surgery, and in maintaining very

Table 3–10　NATURAL MILKS, PREPARED MILKS, AND MILK SUBSTITUTES USED IN INFANT FEEDING

	NORMAL DILUTION Kcal/oz*	APPROXIMATE PERCENTAGE COMPOSITION IN NORMAL DILUTION (GRAMS PER 100 ML)					APPROXIMATE ELECTROLYTE COMPOSITION IN NORMAL DILUTION (MILLIEQUIVALENTS PER LITER)			MILLIGRAMS PER LITER		
		Protein	Carbohydrate	Fat	PUFA	Minerals	Na	K	Cl	Ca	P	Fe
Human milk, mature, average	20	1.1	7.0	3.8	—	0.21	7	14	12	340	150	1.5
Cow's milk, market, average	20	3.3	4.8	3.7	—	0.72	25	35	29	1170	920	1.0
Cow's milk, evaporated	22	3.8	5.4	4.0	—	0.8	28	39	32	1300	1100	1.0
Prepared formulas, cow's milk based												
Alprem, Nestlé	20	1.9	7.5	3.2	0.28	0.28	6.9	17.0	7.5	522	295	0.8
Bebelac No. 1, Lijemph	—	1.8	8.6	3.0	—	0.4	—	—	—	950	540	0.4
Dumex Baby Food, Dumex	22	2.0	7.3	3.2	—	0.42	9.0	15	13	594	396	7.9
Dutch Baby Baby Food, Friesland	20	1.9	6.6	3.0	0.33	—	5.8	13.7	11.5	408	274	0.4
Enfamil, Mead Johnson	20	1.5	6.9	3.7	—	—	10	17	14	542	462	0.1
Frisolac, Friesland	20	1.4	7.4	3.4	0.60	—	5.5	12.8	10.3	455	274	0.4
Lactalac V, Friesland	20	3.5	4.9†	3.7	0.10	—	23.0	45.0	32.1	1340	1145	0.1
Lactogen, Nestlé	18	1.9	7.1	3.1	0.40	0.41	11.7	21.0	17.7	670	520	8.0
Lactogen FP, Nestlé	20	3.1	7.5	2.7	0.35	0.69	20.0	35.0	29.2	1110	860	12.0
Mamex, Dumex	22	1.6	7.3	3.5	—	0.26	6.0	14	10	500	333	7.7
Nan, Nestlé	20	1.7	7.4	3.4	0.43	0.30	7.8	18.7	14.1	450	300	8.0
Nativa 1, Nestlé	20	1.7	6.9	3.6	0.36	0.31	9.1	16	11	580	375	8.0
Pelargon, Nestlé	18	1.8	7.4	2.9	0.37	0.41	11.7	20.7	17.5	660	510	8.0
Similac, Ross (also 13, 24, 27 cal/oz)	21	1.5	7.3	3.6	0.86	—	13	28	14	510	390	1.5
Similac Advance, Ross	17	2.0	5.5	2.7	1.4	—	13	22	14	510	390	12
Similac PM 60/40, Ross	21	1.6	7.5	3.5	0.9	—	7	15	13	400	200	2.6
Similac with whey, Ross	20	1.6	7.2	3.6	—	6.34	10	19	12	400	300	12
SMA, Wyeth (also 13, 24, 27 cal/oz)	21	1.5	7.2	3.6	0.31	0.25	6.5	14	10	443	330	12.7
Hypoallergenic products, soy based												
Isomil (soy), Ross	21	2.0	6.8	3.6	1.0	—	13	18	15	700	500	12
Meat base (beef heart), Gerber	20	2.8	6.2	3.3	—	0.4	7.8	9.5	6	980	650	13.7
Nursoy (soy), Wyeth	20	2.1	6.9	3.6	0.53	0.3	8.7	18.9	10.4	634	443	12.7
Nutramigen (casein hydrolysate), Mead Johnson	20	2.2	8.7	2.6	—	—	14	17	13	630	465	12.7
Prosobee (soy), Mead Johnson	20	2.0	6.7	3.5	—	—	13	21	15	630	495	12.7
Soyalac (soy), Loma Linda	20	2.1	6.7	3.8	—	0.4	14.3	18.7	—	600	500	15.0
Specialty products												
Casec, Mead Johnson	20	16.0	—	0.3	—	—	12.0	4.7	21.5	2890	1430	—
Citrotein, Doyle, egg	20	2.3	7.0	0.5	0.1	—	17.3	10	15.1	600	600	21
Compleat B, Doyle, meat, vegetables	31	4.3	12.8	4.3	1.6	—	55.3	35	24.5	670	1340	12
Ensure Plus, Ross, casein, soy	50	5.5	20.0	5.3	3.0	—	46	48	45	630	630	1.4
Flexical, Mead Johnson, casein hydrolysate, AA‡	20	1.5	17.1	2.3	—	—	10.5	21.4	18.9	400	335	0.6
Isocal, Mead Johnson, casein, soy oil	20	2.1	8.4	2.8	—	—	14.6	21.4	18.9	400	335	0.6
Lactalac MCT,§ Friesland, carbohydrate hydrolysate	20	3.5	5.2	2.1	0.01	—	29	56.9	41.5	1675	1445	0.1
Lofenalac, Mead Johnson, casein hydrolysate	20	2.2	8.7	2.7	—	—	14	18	3.0	629	469	1.2
Lonalac, Mead Johnson, low sodium	20	3.5	5.0	3.7	—	—	1.1	31.0	0.1	1145	1045	0.1
MSUD Powder, Mead Johnson, AA	20	1.1	8.8	2.9	—	—	12	11	13	690	375	1.2
Phenyl-free, Mead Johnson, AA	20	3.4	11	1.1	—	—	18.2	30.0	23.6	1000	760	2.0
Portagen, Mead Johnson, casein	20	2.3	7.7	3.2	—	—	14	21	16	629	469	1.2
Precision, Doyle, egg	31	3.0	15.0	3.1	0.48	—	34.7	25.0	29.8	666	666	1.2
Precision LR, Doyle, egg	38	3.0	28.0	1.8	0.15	—	34.7	25.0	29.8	666	666	1.2
Pregestimil, Mead Johnson, casein hydrolysate, AA, MCT	20	1.9	9.0	2.7	—	—	14	19	16	629	415	12.7
Probana, Mead Johnson, casein hydrolysate, banana	20	4.0	7.5	2.1	—	—	27	31	21	1150	891	0.1
S-14, Wyeth	20	1.1	7.1	3.7	0.5	0.28	6.5	11.2	9.5	400	300	12
S-29, Wyeth, low solute	20	1.7	10.1	2.3	0.3	0.13	0.4	7.5	0.2	130	160	12
S-44, Wyeth, no vitamins	20	1.7	10.1	2.3	0.3	0.13	0.4	7.5	0.2	130	160	12
Vivonex, Norwich Eaton, elemental	32	2.1	24.6	0.15	—	—	37.4	29.9	51.8	555	555	10
Vivonex, HN, Norwich Eaton, elemental	32	4.2	22.6	0.10	—	—	33.5	17.9	52.4	333	333	6
3200 AB, Mead Johnson, casein hydrolysate	20	2.2	8.6	2.6	—	—	13.7	17.5	13.2	620	480	1.2
3200 K, Mead Johnson, soy	20	2.0	6.6	3.6	—	—	11.4	14.7	11.9	590	480	1.2
3232 A, Mead Johnson, casein hydrolysate	20	2.2	8.6	2.8	—	—	13.7	17.5	13.2	620	480	1.2
Formulas for low birth weight infants												
Enfamil LBW, Mead Johnson	24	2.4	8.8	4.1	—	—	13.8	23	19.4	950	470	0.19
Similac 24 LBW, Ross	24	2.2	8.5	4.5	6.0	—	16	31	25	730	560	3
Similac Special Care, Ross	24	2.2	8.4	4.4	1.0	—	15	26	18	1440	720	3
SMA Preemie, Wyeth	24	2.0	8.6	4.4	0.6	0.4	13.9	18.7	15	750	400	3

*Kcal = Kilocalories = Cal.
†Glucose-galactose.
‡AA = Amino acid.
§MCT = Medium-chain triglyceride.

Table 3–11 RECOMMENDED NUTRIENT LEVELS OF INFANT FORMULAS (PER 100 KCAL)—AMERICAN ACADEMY OF PEDIATRICS COMMITTEE ON NUTRITION, 1976 RECOMMENDATIONS WITH 1980 MODIFICATIONS

NUTRIENT	MINIMUM	MAXIMUM
Protein (gm)	1.8*	4.5
Fat (gm)	3.3 (30% of Cal)	6 (54% of Cal)
Including essential fatty acid (linoleate) (mg)	300 (2.7% of Cal)	
Vitamins		
A (IU)	250 (75 µg)†	750 (225 µg)†
D (IU)	40	100
K (µg)	4	—
E (IU)	0.7 (at least 0.7 IU/ gm linoleic acid)	—
C (ascorbic acid) (mg)	8	—
B₁ (thiamine) (µg)	40	—
B₂ (riboflavin) (µg)	60	—
B₆ (pyridoxine) (µg)	35 (at least 15 µg/gm of protein in formula)	—
B₁₂ (µg)	0.15	—
Niacin (µg)	250 (or 0.8 mg niacin equivalents)	—
Folic acid (µg)	4	—
Pantothenic acid (µg)	300	—
Biotin (µg)	1.5‡	—
Choline (mg)	7‡	—
Inositol (mg)	4‡	—
Minerals§		
Calcium (mg)	50¶	—
Phosphorus (mg)	25¶	—
Magnesium (mg)	6	—
Iron (mg)	0.15	2.5**
Iodine (µg)	5	—††
Zinc (mg)	0.5	—
Copper (µg)	60	—
Manganese (µg)	5	—
Sodium (mg)	20 (5.8 mEq)	60 (17.5 mEq)
Potassium (mg)	80 (13.7 mEq)	200 (34.3 mEq)
Chloride (mg)	55 (10.4 mEq)	150 (28.3 mEq)

*At least nutritionally equivalent to casein, quality recommended as outlined in statement: Commentary on Breast Feeding and Infant Formulas, Including Proposed Standards for Formulas. Pediatrics 57:278, 1976.

†Retinol equivalents.

‡Average amount in milk base formulas and should be included in this amount in other formulas.

§Formula should be made with water low in fluoride and should in any case contain less than 60 µg/100 kcal. (Pediatrics 63:150, 152, 1979.)

¶Calcium to phosphorus ratio should be no less than 1 nor more than 2.

**Prudence indicates an upper limit of iron. If formula is labeled "infant formula with iron," it must contain not less than 1 mg/100 kcal.

††Iodine is high in cow's milk based formulas and should be lowered by dairies.

ill patients in positive nitrogen balance while decreasing the bulk and bacterial content of the colon prior to and after major bowel surgery. (See Table 3–10.)

MILK FORMULAS

In its combination of milk, sugar, and water, the formula should contain about 20 kcal/oz and some

Table 3–12 AVERAGE NUMBER OF FEEDINGS PER 24 HOURS

AGE	AVERAGE NUMBER OF FEEDINGS IN 24 HOURS
Birth–1 wk	6–10
1 wk–1 mo	6–8
1–3 mo	5–6
3–7 mo	4–5
4–9 mo	3–4
8–12 mo	3

modification that results in a more desirable, smaller curd formation.

Caloric Requirements (Sec 3.2). The average caloric requirements of full-term infants are about 50–55 kcal/lb or 110–120 kcal/kg during the 1st few mo of life and about 45 kcal/lb or 100 kcal/kg by 1 yr of age; individual variations are significant, and for many infants intakes of this order are in excess of caloric need.

Fluid Requirements (Table 3–3). Fluid requirements are high during infancy. During the 1st 6 mo of life they range from 2–3 oz/lb/24 hr, or 130–190 ml/kg/24 hr. The requirements may be increased during hot weather. As a rule, the infant will regulate his or her own fluid intake provided adequate amounts are offered. Most of the fluid requirement is in the formula, but some is supplied in orange juice and other foods and by water between feedings.

Number of Feedings Daily. The number of feedings required per day decreases throughout the 1st yr so that by 1 yr of age most infants are satisfied with 3 meals a day (Table 3–12). The interval between feedings differs considerably among infants but, in general, ranges from 3–5 hr during the 1st yr of life, with an average of 4 hr for fullterm, healthy infants. Small and weak infants may prefer feedings at 2- to 3-hr intervals. For the 1st mo or 2, feedings are taken throughout the 24-hr period, but thereafter, as the quantity of milk consumed at each feeding increases and the infant adjusts his or her demand to the family pattern of daytime activity, the infant will usually sleep for longer periods of time at night. As the infant develops psychologically and the loving relationship between parent and infant evolves, there should be a gradual progression from demand feeding to a comfortable, regular, feeding regimen that takes into account the needs of both the infant and the parents.

Quantity of Formula. Although the quantity taken at a feeding will vary with different infants of the same age and with the same infant at different feedings, it is important to know the average amounts taken at various ages.

Table 3–13 AVERAGE QUANTITY OF FEEDINGS

AGE	AVERAGE QUANTITY TAKEN IN INDIVIDUAL FEEDINGS
1st and 2nd wk	2–3 oz (60–90 ml)
3 wk–2 mo	4–5 oz (120–150 ml)
2–3 mo	5–6 oz (150–180 ml)
3–4 mo	6–7 oz (180–210 ml)
5–12 mo	7–8 oz (210–240 ml)

Each infant must be given the primary responsibility in determining the quantity of intake (Table 3–13); therefore it is good practice to put more in each bottle than the infant is expected to take. Rarely will an infant want to take more than 7–8 oz of milk at one feeding if caloric and nutritional needs are adequately supplemented by other foods. The relative requirement for milk is somewhat less in the 1st 2 wk than in the succeeding 5–6 mo. After this time milk, though still of great value, has diminishing importance in meeting total nutritional requirements.

Rarely is it necessary to use more than 1 can (13 fluid oz) of evaporated milk or 1 quart of whole milk/day. By the time the infant is taking these quantities, other foods will be added to the diet in increasing amounts. There is no advantage in the ingestion of more milk, and there is the disadvantage that other essential foods may be displaced. Some of the milk may be incorporated in the cereal and in the preparation of such foods as custards, soups, and sauces.

During the 1st few mo the high quantity of protein and minerals in undiluted cow's milk makes such unmodified milk unsuitable for most infants. Free water is supplied by diluting the milk and increasing the caloric content with the addition of carbohydrate (Table 3–14).

While lactose is the milk sugar of most mammals, it is expensive and other carbohydrates are usually used in home-prepared formulas. Cane sugar, dextrin-maltose preparations, or other easily digestible sugars can be added.

Representative evaporated or whole milk formulas for the 1st 10 days of life are given in Table 3–15.

These formulas are satisfactory for an initial prescription. Subsequent adjustments of milk and water should be made in accordance with the infant's satiety and the growth curve.

Preparation of Formula. Several more bottles than the required number for feedings are needed for water and orange juice. Bottles should be made of heat-resistant glass, be smooth inside, and be marked in ounces. A wide-mouthed bottle is preferable because it is more easily cleaned, and those with adequate protection of the nipple are preferable if the baby is to be fed away from home. There should be several more nipples than the number required for feedings. Rubber caps or a plastic such as Pliofilm held in place by cardboard retainers may be used as bottle covers. Alternatively, disposable bottles are now widely used in some communities. The graduate should be made of heat-resistant glass

Table 3–14 HOUSEHOLD MEASURES OF SOME COMMONLY USED SUGARS*

	TABLESPOONFULS PER OUNCE
Lactose	3
Sucrose (cane)	2
Dextrin-maltose preparations:	
Mead's Dextri-Maltose	4
Karo	2
Certose	2
Dexin	6
Polycose fluid	2

*Caloric value of each is 120 calories per ounce, except Dexin, 115, and polycose, 60.

Table 3–15 REPRESENTATIVE FORMULAS

	1–3 DAYS	CALS	4–10 DAYS	CALS	10 DAYS	CALS
Evaporated milk	6 oz	240	7 oz	280	13 oz	520
Sugar	1 tbsp	60	1 tbsp	60	3 tbsp	180
Water	14 oz		14 oz		17 oz	
	20 oz	300	21 oz	340	30 oz	700
Cal/oz		14		16		22
Cal/100 ml		47		56		70
Whole milk	12 oz	240	14 oz	280	26 oz	520
Sugar	1 tbsp	60	1 tbsp	60	3 tbsp	180
Water	8 oz		7 oz		6 oz	
	20 oz	300	21 oz	340	32 oz	700

Total volume is divided into 6 bottles, and the total intake is regulated by the infant.

and marked in ounces. A saucepan for heating and mixing the formula, a container for nipples, a glass funnel if narrow-mouthed bottles are used, a large kettle or special bottle sterilizer, a measuring spoon, a can opener, a knife, a standard tablespoon, and a strainer complete the list of utensils.

All utensils required for the mixing and storing of the formula should be sterilized by boiling for 5–10 min. The rubber nipples and caps should not be boiled more than 5 min. After each feeding the bottle and nipple should be thoroughly flushed and the bottle filled with water until washed with water and a detergent.

The hands should be thoroughly scrubbed and the sterilized bottles and utensils arranged on a clean table. If whole milk is used, the bottle is shaken so that the contents are mixed, and the top is washed with hot water before the cap is removed. The water for the formula (it is necessary to allow for a slight loss in boiling) is brought to the boiling point in a saucepan; the amount of whole milk ordered is added; and the mixture is boiled for 5 min. Constant stirring is necessary. The sugar is added while the milk is still warm.

If evaporated milk is used, the top of the can is washed with soap and hot water and rinsed with hot water; 2 holes are punctured in it. The water for the formula is boiled for 5 min, and the evaporated milk and sugar are added to it. No further boiling is necessary.

The freshly prepared and sterile formula is poured in appropriate amounts into sterilized nursing bottles. The bottles are capped by aseptic technique and stored in the refrigerator until time for the feedings.

Terminal Heating. This method is most commonly used today; it has practical advantages and does not require presterilization of bottles or utensils. The formula is poured into clean nursing bottles, and the nipples are applied. The nipples are then loosely covered with glass, metal, or paper caps and the bottles placed in a rack in a container tall enough to prevent the bottles from touching the lid. The container is filled with water to about the midpoint of the bottles, covered, and placed over a moderate flame. The water is allowed to boil gently for 25 min. The bottles are then removed with tongs and placed in a container of cold water for 10 min. The caps are then tightened and the bottles stored in a refrigerator.

3.12 OTHER FOODS

Vitamins. Most marketed whole and artificial milks are fortified with 400 IU of vitamin D per reconstituted quart, and commercially prepared milks vary in the content of other vitamins. Therefore, it is essential to know the vitamin content of the milk before prescribing additional vitamins for the bottle-fed baby.

Orange and other citrus fruit juices are natural sources of *vitamin C*, but since many young infants do not seem to tolerate them in amounts large enough to supply an adequate vitamin intake, it is preferable to give 50 mg of ascorbic acid. When at least 2 oz of fresh, frozen, or canned orange juice (or equivalent amounts of other sources of vitamin C) is taken daily, the ascorbic acid may be discontinued.

Vitamin D should be started early in the neonatal period with a daily intake of approximately 400 IU only if the infant is taking a formula which does not contain vitamin D or is receiving an insufficient volume of milk to meet the daily requirement. Low birth weight infants require supplementation (Sec 7.16). Vitamin D supplement is not necessary during the 1st few mo of breast feeding of white infants but may be for black infants and those not exposed to adequate sunlight. Concentrates in water-miscible vehicles are desirable to avoid aspiration of oil.

Iron. Foods rich in iron tend to be limited in the diet of the least affluent groups in the population. The most effective way to prevent iron deficiency is to provide iron supplementation in the form of an iron-fortified milk formula or medicinal iron (2 mg/kg up to a total of 15 mg/24 hr) beginning at 6 wk of age. It is doubtful that iron-supplemented cereals can provide sufficient supplementation for infants with reduced iron stores.

"Solid" Foods. The caloric contents of the various prepared baby foods differ widely (Table 29–17). Egg yolk, cereals with added milk, meats, and puddings have greater caloric density than milk, whereas vegetables and fruits have a similar or lower energy value than milk. Without appropriate advice many mothers are not well enough informed to select foods for their infants. Among the potential errors is the tendency to select foods with high caloric values that result in obesity. There is little evidence that the addition to the diet of any solid foods before 4–6 mo of age contributes in any significant way to the well-being of the normal infant.

Any new food should be offered initially once a day in small amounts (1–2 teaspoonfuls). Any small spoon that easily fits the baby's mouth may be used. New foods are generally best accepted if fairly thin or dilute. Food is frequently pushed out rather than back by the tongue because the baby does not yet know how to swallow efficiently. This possibility should be mentioned to the mother, who might otherwise interpret the "spitting back" of new foods as dislike. It is usually wise to offer the same food daily until the baby becomes accustomed to it and not to introduce new foods more often than every wk or 2.

The feeding at which these foods are offered is not particularly important. They should be given when the baby's hunger is no longer satisfied by milk alone and when they logically fit into the daily schedule. There is no reason for persisting with or forcing a particular food that is definitely disliked. The family's dislikes and prejudices for particular foods are contagious and

should not be displayed before the infant. The physician should avoid prescribing a definite amount of a given food lest the mother interpret the suggestion too literally. *Many infants are overfed by overzealous parents who mistake acceptance of food for appetite.* The infant's appetite is the best index of the proper amount, and respect for the infant's wishes will avoid many problems.

Cereal. The various precooked cereals on the market provide in a convenient form a variety of grains excellent for infants. Most contain iron and factors of the vitamin B complex.

Fruits. Strained or puréed cooked fruits furnish minerals and some water-soluble vitamins and usually have a mildly laxative effect. Raw ripe banana is readily digested and enjoyed by most babies. It should be mashed with a fork. Many infants who are slow in accepting new foods seem to prefer fruits.

Vegetables. Vegetables are moderately good sources of iron and other minerals and of the vitamins of the B complex. They may be freshly cooked and strained, but many mothers prefer the commercially prepared vegetables because of their convenience. Vegetables are usually added to the infant's diet by about 7 mo of age.

Meats, Eggs, and Starchy Foods. Eggs and starchy foods are usually introduced during the 2nd 6 mo of life, although some physicians offer egg yolk at an earlier age. The yolk of the egg is used initially and is preferably hard-cooked. As with all new foods, a small amount is offered at first, with gradual increases up to a whole yolk 2–3 times a week. Egg white should be introduced with equal caution to minimize any possible allergic manifestations.

Potatoes, rice, spaghetti, bread, and similar starchy foods have principally a caloric value. As a rule, they are not included in the infant's diet until the more essential foods mentioned above are being taken regularly. Cooked potato, mashed with milk and butter, is a favorite. Zwieback, toast, or graham crackers may be offered to the infant when he or she shows an interest in "gumming" on coarser foods (usually 6–8 mo of age). It is with such foods that infants learn to chew and to feed themselves.

Meat is an excellent source of protein as well as of iron and vitamins. Ground fresh beef or liver or the strained canned meats may be used initially by about 6 mo of age. Meats may be more readily accepted when mixed with another food.

The commercial soups and meat and vegetable mixtures are relatively high in carbohydrate and are not considered optimal sources of iron or protein. Many home-prepared soups are bulky out of proportion to their food value, and much of the vitamin content is lost by overcooking.

Desserts. Puddings, junkets, and custards are good foods for older infants, particularly if they temporarily prefer milk in that form. If, however, such foods are given as a bribe or reward or only after other foods have been finished, poor eating habits are apt to be established. Sweet foods should be offered as casually as the rest of the meal and at any place in the meal that the child desires.

Salt Intake. To increase their palatability, particularly for the parent, excessive salt used to be added to baby foods. Recently this practice has been discontinued. The significance of large intakes of sodium, which are in the ranges seen in populations with a high incidence of hypertension, is not clear, but the possibility that they might contribute to the development of hypertension later in life cannot be ignored.

Food Additives. Naturally occurring chemicals and food additives, particularly the artificial flavors and colors, have been implicated in health problems. It has been estimated that more than 3000 flavors are currently being used, and few children are spared exposure to them in their daily diet. Artificial flavors and colors have been associated with respiratory allergic disorders, with urticaria and angioedema, with lesions of the tongue and buccal mucosa, with digestive disturbances, with arthralgia and hydrarthroses, and with headache and behavioral disturbances, including hyperkinesis in childhood.

3.13 FIRST-YEAR FEEDING PROBLEMS

Underfeeding. Underfeeding is suggested by restlessness and crying and by failure to gain weight adequately in spite of complete emptying of the breast or bottle. Underfeeding may also result from the infant's failure to take a sufficient quantity of food even when offered. In these instances the frequency of feedings, the mechanics of feeding, the size of the holes in the nipple, the adequacy of eructation of air, the possibility of abnormal mother-infant "bonding," and possible systemic disease in the baby should be investigated (Sec 5.36). The extent and duration of underfeeding determine the clinical manifestations. Constipation, failure to sleep, irritability, and excessive crying are to be expected. There may be poor gain in weight or an actual loss. In the latter instance the skin becomes dry and wrinkled, subcutaneous tissue disappears, and the infant assumes the appearance of an "old man." Deficiencies of vitamins A, B, C, and D and of iron and protein may be responsible for characteristic clinical manifestations.

Treatment consists of increasing the fluid and caloric intake, correcting deficiencies in vitamin and mineral intake, and instructing the mother in the art of infant feeding. If some underlying systemic disease or psychologic problem is responsible, specific management of these disorders will be necessary.

Overfeeding. Overfeeding may be quantitative or qualitative. Regurgitation and vomiting are frequent symptoms of overfeeding. As a rule, infants can be depended upon not to take excessive quantities, but occasionally an infant who has postprandial discomfort from eating too much may nonetheless gain weight excessively. Diets too high in fat delay gastric emptying, cause distention and abdominal discomfort, and may cause excessive gain in weight. Diets too high in carbohydrate are likely to cause undue fermentation in the intestine, resulting in distention and flatulence and in too rapid gain in weight. Such diets may be deficient in essential protein, vitamins, and minerals. Formulas too high in caloric content in the 1st wk or 2 of life are likely to result in loose or diarrheal stools. Obesity is undesirable at any time in life; all too frequently the excessively fed infant becomes the obese child and adult.

Regurgitation and Vomiting. The return of small amounts of swallowed food during or shortly after eating is termed "regurgitation" or "spitting up." More complete emptying of the stomach, especially when it occurs some time after feeding, is termed "vomiting." Within limits, regurgitation is a natural occurrence, especially during the 1st 6 mo or so of life. It can be reduced to a negligible amount, however, by adequate eructation of swallowed air during and after eating, by gentle handling, by avoidance of emotional conflicts, and by placing the infant on the right side or abdomen for a nap immediately after eating. One should also ensure that the head is not lower than the rest of the body during the rest period since gastroesophageal reflux is common during the 1st 4–6 mo.

Vomiting is one of the most common symptoms in infancy and may be associated with a wide variety of disturbances, both trivial and serious. It should be distinguished from rumination; its cause should always be investigated (Sec 11.17, 11.19, and 11.20).

Loose or Diarrheal Stools. Acute infectious diarrhea and chronic diarrheal conditions are discussed in Sec 10.12 and 11.36; only mild disturbances of dietary origin will be considered here.

The stool of the breast-fed infant is naturally softer than that of the infant fed cow's milk. From about the 4th to the 6th day of life the stools go through a transitional stage in which they are rather loose and greenish yellow and contain mucus; within a few days the typical "milk stool" appears. Subsequently, the use of laxatives or the ingestion of certain foods by the mother may be temporarily responsible for an infant's loose stools. Excessive intake of breast milk may also increase the frequency and the water content of the stool. Actual diarrhea in a breast-fed infant is unusual and should be considered infectious until proved otherwise.

Though the stools of artificially fed infants tend to be firmer than those of breast-fed infants, under certain circumstances loose stools may result from artificial feeding. In the 1st 2 wk or so of life, overfeeding is likely to cause loose, frequent stools. Later, formulas which are too concentrated or in which the sugar content is too high, especially in lactose, may be responsible for loose, frequent stools. Many of the temporary diarrheal disturbances in artificially fed infants are the result of contaminations of food that would not disturb an older child and are not serious enough to cause prolonged difficulty for the infant. The ease with which artificially fed infants acquire diarrheal disturbances and the potential seriousness of them are strong arguments for extreme care in providing a food supply free of pathogenic bacteria.

Mild diarrheal disturbances due to overfeeding respond quickly to temporary decrease or cessation of feeding. The withholding of all solid food and of one or several milk feedings, with the substitution of boiled water or 5% glucose in water or in a balanced electrolyte solution, is usually all that is required.

Constipation (Sec 11.17). Constipation is practically unknown in breast-fed infants who receive an adequate amount of milk and is rare in artificially fed infants receiving an adequate diet. The nature of the stool and not its frequency is the criterion of constipation. Although most infants have 1 or more stools daily, an occasional infant will have a stool of normal consistency only at intervals of 36–48 hr. Whenever constipation or obstipation is present from birth or shortly thereafter, a rectal examination should be performed. Tight or spastic anal sphincters may occasionally be responsible for obstipation, and correction usually follows finger dilatation. Anal fissures or cracks may also cause constipation. If irritation is alleviated, healing usually occurs quickly. Aganglionic megacolon may be manifest by constipation in early infancy; the absence of stool in the rectum on digital examination suggests this possibility.

Constipation in the artificially fed infant may be due to an insufficient amount of food or fluid. In other instances it may result from diets too high in fat or protein or deficient in bulk. Simply increasing the amount of fluid or sugar in the formula may be corrective in the 1st few mo of life. After this age better results are obtained by adding or increasing the amounts of cereal, vegetables, and fruits. Prune juice (½–1 oz) may be given as a temporary measure, but it is better to add foods with some bulk. Enemas and suppositories should never be more than temporary measures. Milk of magnesia may be given in doses of 1–2 teaspoonfuls but should be reserved for unresponsive or severe constipation.

Colic. The term "colic" describes a frequent symptom complex of paroxysmal abdominal pain, presumably of intestinal origin, and of severe crying. It usually occurs in infants under 3 mo of age.

The clinical pattern is characteristic: the attack usually begins suddenly; the cry is loud and more or less continuous; so-called paroxysms may persist for several hours; the face may be flushed, or there may be circumoral pallor; the abdomen is distended and tense; the legs are drawn up on the abdomen, though they may be momentarily extended; the feet are often cold; the hands are clenched. The attack may terminate only when the infant is completely exhausted, but often there is apparent relief with the passage of feces or flatus.

Certain infants seem to be peculiarly susceptible to colic. The cause of recurrent attacks is usually not apparent, though they may be associated with hunger and with swallowed air which has passed into the intestine. Overfeeding may also cause discomfort and distention. Certain foods, especially those of high carbohydrate content, may be responsible for excessive fermentation in the intestines, but only occasionally does a change in diet prevent further attacks of colic. Crying from intestinal discomfort is seen in infants with intestinal allergy, but colic is not limited to this group. Intestinal obstruction or peritoneal infection may mimic an attack of colic. Recurrent attacks commonly occur late in the afternoon or evening, suggesting that events in the household routine may serve as possible causes. Worry, fear, anger, or excitement may cause vomiting in an older child and may cause colic in an infant. Certainly, no single causative factor consistently accounts for colic, nor does any method of treatment consistently provide satisfactory relief. Careful physical examination is important to eliminate the possibility of intussusception, strangulated hernia, hair in eye, otitis, pyelonephritis, or other disorders.

Holding the baby upright or permitting the baby to lie prone across the lap or on a hot water bottle or heating pad is occasionally helpful. Passage of flatus or fecal material spontaneously or with expulsion of a suppository or enema sometimes affords relief. Carminatives before feedings are ineffective in preventing the attacks. Sedation is occasionally indicated for a prolonged attack and sometimes may be given to parent or child for a period of time if other measures fail. Temporary hospitalization of the infant, often without resorting to more than a change in the infant's feeding routine and providing a period of rest for the mother, may be helpful in extreme cases. The prevention of attacks should be sought through improved feeding techniques, including burping, the provision of a stable emotional environment, identification of possibly allergenic foods in the infant's or nursing mother's diet, and avoidance of underfeeding or overfeeding. The condition rarely persists after 3 mo of age. A supportive and sympathetic attitude in the physician is important to the successful resolution of this problem.

3.14 FEEDING DURING THE SECOND YEAR OF LIFE

Most infants naturally adapt themselves to a schedule of 3 meals a day by about the end of the 1st yr of life. Though considerable latitude in the diet of the individual infant must be permitted to allow for personal idiosyncrasies and family habits, the mother should be given an outline of the daily basic dietary needs (Table 3–16).

Reduced Caloric Intake. Toward the end of the 1st yr of life and during the 2nd yr, because of constantly decelerating rate of growth, there is a gradual reduction in the infant's caloric intake per unit of body weight. In addition, it is not unusual to have temporary periods of lack of interest in certain foods or even in food in general. Failure to recognize these features, especially the decreasing caloric needs, results in attempts to force feed. The natural reaction of the child is rebellion, and feeding problems ensue. Prevention is much more effective than are methods of correction, and the changing pattern of the infant's food habits during the 2nd yr of life should be explained to the mother before its appearance.

Self-Selection of Diet. Strong likes or dislikes of children for particular foods should be respected whenever possible and practicable. Spinach is an example of a nonessential food whose virtues have been overemphasized. When rejected foods consistently include such basic dietary staples as milk and eggs, the possibility of food allergy should be considered.

Children, including infants, tend to select diets which

Table 3–16 1100–1300 CALORIE DIET

Breakfast

1 orange, ½ grapefruit, or 1 cup of tomato juice
1 egg
1 slice of whole-wheat bread or 1 serving of cereal without sugar
1 teaspoonful of butter
6 oz of whole milk

Lunch

2 ounces of lean meat, 1 egg, or ½ cup of cottage cheese
1 serving of raw vegetable as salad—no dressing
1 slice of whole-wheat bread
1 teaspoonful of butter
1 serving of fresh or unsweetened fruit
6 oz of whole milk

Dinner

2 ounces of lean meat (liver once a week), poultry, or fish
2 servings of green, yellow, or red vegetables*
1 serving of fresh or unsweetened fruit
6 oz of whole milk
    (Part or all of bread and butter from one of the other meals
    may be included here)
    A 1000-calorie diet may be obtained by eliminating the butter or
cream from milk. In this case it becomes especially important to add
vitamin A to the daily diet.

---

*Does not include Irish or sweet potatoes, parsnips, dried peas or
beans, lima beans, or corn.

over a period of several days assume a balanced nature. Thus, the child may be permitted a rather wide choice of foods without concern so long as the eating performance is adequate over the longer period. Under normal circumstances the child should determine the quantity to be eaten with respect to both a given food and to the entire meal. At this age the development of eating habits may be strongly influenced by older children in the family, particularly in respect to food likes and dislikes. Eating patterns and habits developed in the 1st 2 yr of life are likely to persist for several years.

Self-feeding by Infants. Before 1 yr of age the infant should be permitted to participate in the act of feeding. By 6 mo or so the infant can hold a bottle; within another 2–3 mo, a cup. Zwieback, graham crackers, or other hand-held foods can be introduced by the age of 7–8 mo. A spoon may be used as soon as it can be held and directed to the mouth, possibly by 10–12 mo of age. Mothers often inhibit this learning process because of their objection to the messiness of learning adequate control.

Acquisition of the ability to feed one's self is an important step in the infant's development of self-reliance and of a sense of responsibility. By the end of the 2nd yr of life, the infant should be largely responsible for his or her own feeding.

The practice of permitting infants and children to go to sleep while holding and sucking intermittently from a bottle of formula, whole milk, sweetened fruit juice, or water should be discouraged. Pedodontists have called attention to the correlation of this habit with enamel erosion in deciduous teeth, terming it "the baby bottle syndrome." Bacterial action upon dissolved carbohydrate provides increased formation of lactic and other acids that are harmful to dental enamel, especially that of the young child.

Although the nutritional requirements per unit of body weight are constantly decreasing with increasing age (110 kcal/kg in infancy; 50 kcal/kg at 15 yr), at all times the need for calories as well as for protein, vitamins, and minerals is relatively greater than it is in the adult.

Daily Basic Diet. Parents should be given a daily basic diet for the child from which the family menu can be prepared. Daily selection from each of the food groups provides a balanced diet with sufficient macro- and micronutrients. The quantity of the intake after the basic requirements have been met can in most instances be determined by the healthy growing child. A history of the dietary habits of the child is essential for evaluation of the nutritive intake, but such histories are often unreliable unless an accurate dietary diary is kept for several days. From such information, corrections in the diet may be made more effectively. The recommended daily dietary intake is shown in Table 3–7.

The child should learn the content of a basic diet and its importance to proper growth and good health, but this information should never be presented as a threat to enforce rigid feeding practices.

Eating Habits. As stated previously, eating habits formed in the 1st yr or 2 of life have a distinct effect upon those of subsequent years. Feeding difficulties between the ages of 2–5 yr frequently result from excessive parental insistence on eating, with excessive anxiety when the child does not conform to some arbitrary standard. Negativistic reactions by the child are natural consequences of undue stress at mealtime, and correction requires improvement in parent-child relations. Other factors that disturb eating are too much confusion at mealtime, insufficient time for eating, either on the part of the adult or of the child, food dislikes of other members of the family, and poorly prepared and unattractively served food. A comfortable chair of proper height with a foot-rest is important for a child's ease at the table. Mealtimes should be happy and the conversation should be on subjects of interest to the entire family. The child's appetite should be respected; if his or her desire for food at times is below average, there should be no persuasion to eat more. Adults should realize that eating habits are taught better by example than by formal explanation.

Snacks Between Meals. During the 2nd yr and even for several years thereafter, orange juice or other fruit juice or fruit, together with a cracker, may be given in either or both of the between-meal periods. Snacks served in nursery schools and kindergartens should be nutritious. For older children, between-meal nourishment should be avoided if it reduces the appetite for the following meal. When a snack after school results in greater enthusiasm and energy for play and does not reduce the appetite for the evening meal, it should be encouraged. Fruits are especially recommended for such snacks.

VEGETARIAN DIET

All-vegetable diets supply all needed nutrients when vegetables are selected from different classes. Vegetables are high in fiber content, vitamins, and minerals. Vegetarians usually have faster gastrointestinal transit time, bulkier stools, and low serum cholesterol levels and are said to have less diverticulitis and appendicitis than meat eaters. Those who consume eggs are ovovegetarians. Those who consume milk are lactovegetarians. Those who consume neither are vegans. Vegans may develop vitamin B_{12} deficiency and, because of high fiber intake, may develop trace mineral deficiency. Nursing vegan mothers must be given added vitamin B_{12} to prevent methylmalonic acidemia in their infants. Vegetarian infants may not grow as rapidly as omnivores in the 1st 2 yr.

DIET FOR ATHLETIC ACTIVITIES

Adequate caloric intake is necessary for growth and activity. A varied diet supplies all necessary nutrients. Special food supplements are unnecessary and may be harmful. Water intake should be scheduled regularly before and during athletic events.

Aldrich CA: Ancient processes in scientific age: Feeding aspects. Am J Dis Child 64:714, 1942.
Bahna SL, Heiner DC: Cows' milk allergy. Adv Pediatr 25:1, 1978.
Burton BT: The Heinz Handbook of Nutrition. Ed 3. New York, Blakiston Division, McGraw-Hill, 1976.
Committee on Nutrition, AAP: Composition of milks. Pediatrics 26:1039, 1960.
Committee on Nutrition, AAP: Vitamin K supplementation for infants receiving milk substitute infant formulas and for those with fat malabsorption. Pediatrics 48:483, 1971.
Committee on Nutrition, AAP: Childhood diet and coronary heart disease. Pediatrics 49:305, 1972.
Committee on Nutrition, AAP: Filled milks, imitation milks, and coffee whiteners. Pediatrics 49:770, 1972.
Committee on Nutrition, AAP: Pediatric Nutrition Handbook. Chicago, 1979.
Committee on Nutrition, AAP: On the feeding of supplemental foods to infants. Pediatrics 65:1178, 1980.
Cunningham AS: Morbidity in breast-fed and artificially fed infants. J Pediatr 90:726, 1977.

Feingold BF: Food additives and child development. Hosp Pract (No 10) 8:11, 1973.
Fomon SJ: Body composition of the male reference infant. Pediatrics 40:863, 1967.
Fomon, SJ: Infant Nutrition. Ed 2. Philadelphia, WB Saunders, 1974.
Food and Nutrition Board: Recommended Dietary Allowances. Ed 9. National Academy of Sciences, 1980.
Friedman Z, Danon A, Stahlman MT, et al.: Rapid onset of essential fatty acid deficiency in the newborn. Pediatrics 58:640, 1976.
Garonger JD, Brown MS, Laster L: The columnar epithelial cell of the small intestine: Digestion and transport. N Engl J Med 283:1196, 1264, 1317, 1970.
Gartner LM, Arias IM: Studies of prolonged neonatal jaundice in the breast-fed infant. J Pediatr 68:54, 1966.
Goldfarb J, Tibbetts E: Breast-feeding Handbook. Hillside, NJ, Enslow Publ, 1980.
Gryboski J: Gastrointestinal Problems in the Infant. Philadelphia, WB Saunders, 1975.
Hambreus L: Proprietary milk versus human breast milk in infant feeding. Pediatr Clin North Am 24:17, 1977.
Hansen AE, Stewart RA, Hughes G, et al.: The relation of linoleic acid to infant feeding: A review. Acta Pediatr 51:Suppl, 1962.
Holt LE Jr, Snyderman SE: The amino acid requirements of infants. JAMA 175:100, 1961.
Howald H, Poortmans JR: Metabolic adaptation to prolonged physical exercise. Proc 2nd International Symposium on Biochemistry of Exercise, Magglingen, 1973. Basel, 1975.
Kagan BM, Stanincova V, Felix NS, et al.: Body composition of premature infants. Relation to nutrition. Am J Clin Nutr 25:1153, 1973.
Klaus MH, Jerauld R, Kreger NC, et al: Maternal attachment: Importance of the first postpartum days. N Engl J Med 286:460, 1972.
La Leche League International. The Womanly Art of Breast Feeding. Franklin Park, Ill, 1976.
Macy IG, Kelly HJ, Sloan RE: The composition of milks. A compilation of the comparative composition and properties of human, cow and goat milk, colostrum and transitional milk. Washington DC, Publication 254, National Academy of Science–National Research Council, 1953.
McMillan JA, Landaw SA, Oski FA: Iron insufficiency in breast-fed infants and the availability of iron from human milk. Pediatrics 58:686, 1976.
Pearson HA, Robinson JE: The role of iron in host resistance. Adv Pediatr 23:1, 1976.
Pitt J: Breast milk leukocytes. Pediatrics 48:769, 1976.
Powers GF: Infant feeding: Historical background and modern practice. JAMA 105:753, 1935.
Prasad AS (ed): Trace Elements in Human Health and Disease. Vol 1. Zinc and Copper. New York, Academic Press, 1976.
Raiha NCR, Heinonen K, Rassin DK, et al.: Milk protein quantity and quality in low birth weight infants. I. Metabolic responses and effects on growth. Pediatrics 57:659, 1976.
Reina D: Infant nutrition. Clin Perinatol 2:373, 1975.
Roy RN, Sinclair JC: Hydration of the low birth weight infant. Clin Perinatol 2:393, 1975.
Spock B: Baby and Child Care. New York, Pocket Books, 1962.
Watkins JB: Mechanisms of fat absorption and the development of gastrointestinal function. Pediatr Clin North Am 22:721, 1975.

NUTRITIONAL DISORDERS

3.15 MALNUTRITION

Malnutrition, from a worldwide perspective, is one of the leading causes of morbidity and mortality in childhood (Sec 4.4).

Malnutrition may be due to improper and/or inadequate food intake or may result from inadequate absorption of food. Deficient supply of food, poor dietary habits, food faddism, and emotional factors may limit intake. Certain metabolic abnormalities may also cause malnutrition. Requirements for essential nutrients may be increased during stress and disease and during the administration of antibiotics or of catabolic or anabolic drugs. Malnutrition may be acute or chronic, reversible or irreversible.

Precise evaluation of nutritional status is difficult. Severe disturbances are readily apparent, but mild disturbances may be overlooked, even after careful physical and laboratory examinations. The diagnosis of malnutrition rests on an accurate dietary history; upon evaluation of present deviations from average height, weight, head circumference, and past rates of growth; upon comparative measurements of midarm circumference and skinfold thickness; and upon chemical and other tests. Decreased skinfold thickness suggests protein-calorie malnutrition; excessive thickness indicates obesity. Muscle mass is calculated by subtracting skinfold measurements from arm circumference. For older children and adults midarm muscle circumference (cm) = arm circumference (cm) − (skinfold thickness [cm] × 3.14). Lean body mass can be estimated from 24 hr creatinine excretion. Deficiencies of some nutrients may be revealed by finding low blood levels of them or their metabolites, by observing biochemical or clinical effects of administration of the nutrients or their products, or by giving the patient substantial amounts of appropriate nutrients and noting the rate at which they are excreted. Protein reserves are assessed from serum albumin, transferrin, hemoglobin, prealbumin, or retinol-binding protein. Serum levels of essential amino acids may be lower than those of nonessential amino acids. Excretion of hydroxyproline is decreased and of 3-methylhistidine increased, and hair is easily pluckable in the severely malnourished child.

The most acute nutritional disturbances are those which involve water and electrolytes, especially sodium, potassium, chloride, and hydrogen ions (Chapter 5). Chronic malnutrition usually involves deficits of more than a single nutrient. Immunologic insufficiency is common in malnutrition and is demonstrated by total lymphocyte counts less than 1500/mm³ and anergy to skin test antigens, e.g., streptokinase-streptodornase, Candida, mumps, or tuberculin in exposed persons (Sec 9.20 and 9.26).

3.16 MARASMUS
(Infantile Atrophy, Inanition, Athrepsia)

Severe malnutrition in infants is common in areas with insufficient food, inadequate knowledge of feeding techniques, or poor hygiene. The synonyms listed above have been applied to patterns of clinical illness emphasizing one or more features of protein and calorie deficiency.

Etiology. The clinical picture of marasmus stems from an inadequate caloric intake due to insufficiency of the diet, to improper feeding habits such as those of disturbed parent-child relations, or to metabolic abnormalities or congenital malformations. Severe impairment of any body system may result in malnutrition.

Clinical Manifestations. Initially, there is failure to gain weight, followed by loss of weight until emaciation results, with loss of turgor in skin which becomes wrinkled and loose as subcutaneous fat disappears. Because fat is lost last from the sucking pads of the cheeks, the face may retain a relatively normal appearance for some time before becoming shrunken and wizened. The abdomen may be distended or flat, and the intestinal pattern may be readily visible. Atrophy of muscles occurs, with resultant hypotonia. Edema may be present.

The temperature is usually subnormal, the pulse may be slow, and the basal metabolic rate tends to be reduced At first the infant may be fretful but later becomes listless, and the appetite diminishes. The infant is usually constipated, but the so-called starvation type of diarrhea may appear, with frequent, small stools containing mucus.

3.17 PROTEIN MALNUTRITION
(PCM, Protein-Calorie Malnutrition, Kwashiorkor)

Children, because they are growing, must consume enough nitrogenous food to maintain a positive nitrogen balance, whereas adults need only maintain nitrogen equilibrium.

Etiology. Although deficiencies of calories and other nutrients complicate the clinical and chemical patterns, the principal symptoms of protein malnutri-

tion are due to deficient intake of protein of good biologic value. There may also be impaired absorption of protein, as in chronic diarrheal states, abnormal losses of protein in proteinuria (nephrosis), infection, hemorrhage or burns, and failure of protein synthesis, as in chronic liver disease.

Kwashiorkor is a clinical syndrome that results from a severe deficiency of protein and less than adequate caloric intake. It is the most serious and prevalent form of malnutrition in the world today and is especially so in industrially underdeveloped areas.

Kwashiorkor means "deposed child," i.e., the child who is no longer suckled; it may become evident from early infancy to about 5 yr of age, usually after weaning from the breast. Although gains in height and weight are accelerated with treatment, these measurements never equal those of consistently well-nourished children.

Clinical Manifestations (Fig 3–2 and 3–3). Early clinical evidence of protein malnutrition is vague and includes lethargy, apathy, or irritability. When well advanced, it results in inadequate growth, lack of stamina, loss of muscular tissue, increased susceptibility to infections, and edema. Secondary immunodeficiency is one of the most serious and constant manifestations. For example, measles, a relatively benign disease of the well nourished, can be devastating and fatal in malnourished children. The child may develop anorexia, flabbiness of subcutaneous tissues, and loss of muscle tone. Enlargement of the liver may occur early or late; fatty infiltration is common. Edema usually develops early; failure to gain weight may be masked by edema, which is often present in internal organs before it can be recognized in the face and limbs. Renal plasma flow, glomerular filtration rate, and renal tubular function are decreased. The heart may be small in the early stages of the disease but is usually enlarged later.

Dermatitis is common. Darkening of the skin appears in areas of irritation but not in those exposed to sunlight, in contrast to the situation in pellagra. Dyspigmentation may occur in these areas after desquamation or may be generalized. The hair is often sparse and thin and loses its elasticity. In dark-haired children, dyspigmentation may result in streaky red or gray color of the hair. Hair texture becomes coarse in chronic disease.

Infections and parasitic infestations are common, as are anorexia, vomiting, and continued diarrhea. The muscles are weak, thin, and atrophic, but there may, on occasion, be an excess of subcutaneous fat. Mental changes, especially irritability and apathy, are common. Stupor, coma, and death may follow.

Laboratory Data. Decrease in the concentration of serum albumin is the most characteristic change. Ketonuria is common in the early stage of inanition but frequently disappears in the later stages. Blood glucose values are low, but glucose tolerance curves may be diabetic in type. Urinary excretion of hydroxyproline relative to creatinine may be decreased. Plasma values of essential amino acids may be decreased relative to nonessential ones, and there may be increased aminoaciduria. Potassium and magnesium deficiencies are frequent. The serum cholesterol level is low, but it returns to normal after a few days of treatment. The

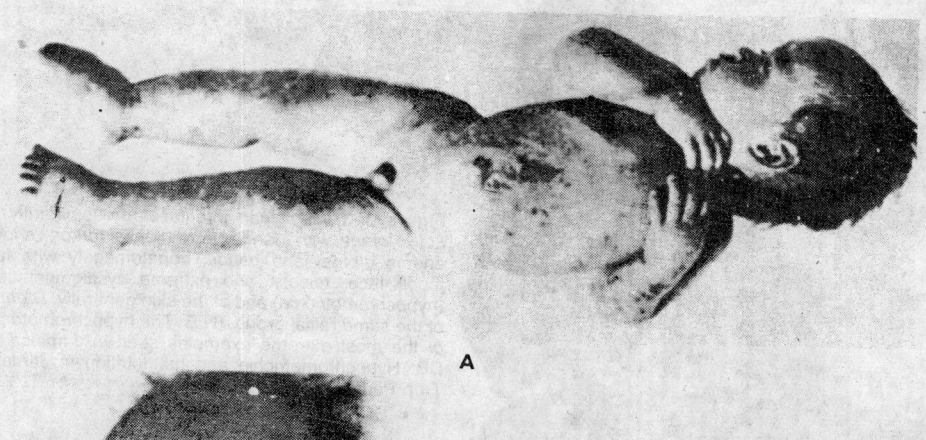

A

B

Figure 3–2 A, Kwashiorkor in a 2 yr old boy. Note the generalized edema, the typical skin lesions, and the state of prostration. B, Close-up of the same child showing the hair changes and psychic alterations (apathy and misery); the edema of the face and the skin lesions can be seen more clearly. (Photographs made available by the Institute of Nutrition of Central America and Panama [INCAP], Guatemala, C. A., through the courtesy of Dr. Moisés Béhar.)

serum values of amylase, esterase, cholinesterase, transaminase, lipase, and alkaline phosphatase are decreased. There is diminished activity of the pancreatic enzymes and of xanthine oxidase, but these values return to normal shortly after the onset of treatment. Anemia may be normocytic, microcytic, or macrocytic. Other nutritional deficiencies, as of vitamins and minerals, are usually evident. Bone growth is usually delayed. Growth hormone secretion may be increased.

Differential Diagnosis. Differential diagnosis of protein deprivation includes chronic infections, diseases in which there is an excessive loss of protein through urine or stools, and conditions with a metabolic inability to synthesize protein.

Prevention. This requires a diet containing an adequate quantity of protein of good biologic quality. Since kwashiorkor has not only a serious and often fatal course but often permanent and devastating aftereffects in recovered children and their offspring, adequate dietary instruction and food distribution are urgently needed in endemic areas.

Treatment. Immediate management of any acute problems such as those of severe diarrhea, renal failure, and shock (Sec 5.46) and, ultimately, the replacement of missing nutrients, is essential. Gradual increases in the dietary intake of calories and protein should be instituted only after nonprotein calorie rehabilitation is initiated. Skim milk, casein hydrolysates, or synthetic

amino acid mixtures may be used as supplements to the basic fluid and nutritional regimen. When high calorie and high protein diets are given too early and rapidly, the liver may become enlarged, the abdomen becomes markedly distended, and the child improves more slowly. Protein hydrolysates, when used alone, may result in hypoglycemia. Vegetable fat is better absorbed than cow's milk fat. Disaccharidase values in intestinal biopsies are low; lactose in particular should be limited in early treatment. Impaired glucose tolerance may be improved in some affected children by the daily administration of 250 mg of chromium chloride. Vitamins and minerals, especially vitamin A, potassium, and magnesium, are necessary from the outset of treatment. Iron and folic acid will usually correct the anemia.

Infections must be treated concomitantly with the dietary therapy, whereas treatment of parasitic infestations, if not severe, may be postponed until recovery is under way.

After treatment has been initiated, the patient may lose weight for a few weeks, due to loss of apparent or inapparent edema. Serum and intestinal enzymes return to normal, and intestinal absorption of fat and protein improves.

If impairment of growth and development has been extensive, mental and physical retardation may be permanent. Apparently, the younger the infant at the time

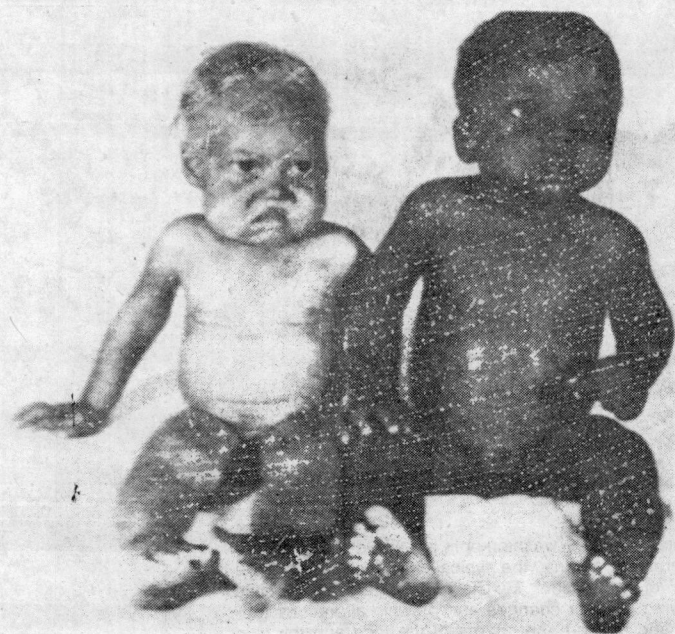

Figure 3–3 Jamaican infants of predominantly African stock. *Left,* Infant with "sugarbaby" kwashiorkor, showing stunting, edema of feet and hands, hepatomegaly with fatty infiltration, moon face, misery, and extreme dyspigmentation of the hair (hypochromotrichia) and of the skin generally. *Right,* Normal infant of the same racial group. (N.B. The hypochromotrichia here is one of the most extreme examples seen in Jamaica.) (From Jelliffe DB: Hypochromotrichia and malnutrition in Jamaican infants. J Trop Pediat, Vol 1.)

of deprivation, the more devastating are the long-term effects. Deficits in perceptual and abstract abilities are especially long-lasting.

3.18 MALNUTRITION IN CHILDREN BEYOND INFANCY

Etiology.   Malnutrition in children may be a continuation of an undernourished state begun in infancy, or it may stem from factors which become operative during childhood. In general, the causes are the same as those responsible for malnutrition in infants. The problem may be complex. Poor dietary habits may be associated with a generally poor hygienic situation, with chronic disease, with finicky eating habits of other members of the family, or with disturbed parent-child relations (Sec 5.36).

Poor eating habits in children under the age of 5 or 6 yr can often be traced directly to parental factors, of which overconcern about the quantity or quality of the diet is a common one. In children of all ages, insufficient sleep and too much emotional excitement, such as that associated with the movies and television, are important factors. School-age children often develop irregular or inappropriate eating habits, especially at breakfast and lunch, because sufficient time is not allotted or because the meals may be inadequate. During adolescence girls frequently restrict their dietary intake for esthetic reasons. Eating between meals, especially of such items as candy and snack foods, is likely to reduce the appetite at mealtime.

Clinical Manifestations.   Malnutrition does not invariably result in underweight. Fatigue, lassitude, restlessness, and irritability are frequent manifestations. Restlessness and overactivity are frequently misinterpreted by parents as evidences of lack of fatigue. An-

orexia, easily induced digestive disturbances, and constipation are common complaints, and even in older children the starvation type of mucoid diarrheal stool may be observed. Malnourished children often have a limited span of attention and do poorly in schoolwork. They have increased susceptibility to infections. Muscular development is inadequate, and the flabby muscles result in a posture of fatigue, with rounded shoulders, flat chest, and protuberant abdomen. Such children often look tired; the face is pale, the complexion is "muddy," and the eyes lack luster. Hypochromic anemia is common. In protracted cases there may be delayed epiphyseal development, irregularities in dentition, and delayed puberty.

Evaluation should always include a careful history of dietary habits, psychosocial maladjustments, physical hygiene, and illness; a thorough physical examination; and appropriate laboratory examinations.

Treatment.   There is a great need for individualization of treatment aimed at correction of the underlying psychologic and physical disturbances. An adequate diet (Sec 3.14) should be outlined; vitamin concentrates may be added and continued for a time after the dietary intake has become adequate. When anorexia is a problem, the essential items of the diet should be provided in as concentrated a form as possible, and the fat content should be low. Between-meal snacks need not be prohibited if they do not interfere with the appetite for the next meal; milk or candy should not be given at such times; fruit or fruit juices are appropriate. Re-education of the entire family in respect to eating habits may be necessary (Sec 5.36).

Cupoli JM, Hallock JA, Barness LA: Failure to thrive. Current Probl Pediatr 10, Nov 11, 1980.
Hegsted DM: Protein-calorie malnutrition. Am Scientist 66:61, 1978.

Katz M, Stiehm ER: Host defense in malnutrition. Pediatrics 59:490, 1977.

Robinson H, Picou D: A comparison of fasting plasma insulin and growth hormone concentrations in marasmic, kwashiorkor, marasmic-kwashiorkor and under-weight children. Pediatr Res 11:637, 1977.

Sleisenger MH, Kim YS: Protein digestion and absorption. N Engl J Med 300:659, 1979.

Zain BK, Haquani AH, Qureshi N, et al.: Studies on the significance of hair root protein and DNA in protein calorie malnutrition. Am J Clin Nutr 30:1094, 1977.

3.19 PROTEIN EXCESS

Excessive protein intake, especially in the absence of sufficient water, may lead to signs of dehydration—protein fever. Signs of protein excess are rare, but premature infants fed a high protein diet may have an increased morbidity. Marasmic infants fed high protein diets during the recovery phase may develop hyper-ammonemia; protein intoxication has also been noted in children with other liver disease. Some weight reducing diets with high protein content may be responsible for protein intoxication.

Barness LA, Omans WB, Rose CS, et al: Progress of premature infants fed a formula containing demineralized whey. Pediatrics 32:52, 1963.

3.20 OBESITY

There is no exact line of demarcation between good nutrition and overnutrition; practically, the diagnosis is made from the appearance of the child rather than from an arbitrary excess in weight. Children of the stocky type may have relatively large skeletal frames and more than the average amount of muscular tissue so that their weight and height as well as their appearance of bigness exceed those of the average child of their age, but they are not to be considered obese. Obesity or overnutrition is a generalized excessive accumulation of fat in subcutaneous and other tissues and can be quantitated by measuring skin fold thickness with calipers.

Etiology. Obesity is usually due to an excessive intake of food. Appetite may be influenced by a variety of factors that include psychologic disturbances; hypothalamic, pituitary, or other brain lesions; and hyperinsulinism. Genetic predisposition to obesity occurs in certain animals and may occur in man. In a study of adults, obesity was found to be 7 times more common in the lowest than in the highest socioeconomic class. Lack of activity may be responsible for obesity even though intake of food may not be unusual. Illnesses which keep a child in bed for prolonged periods of time may also result in obesity. Some inherited syndromes such as the Laurence-Moon-Biedl, Prader-Willi, and Cushing usually include obesity, on either an endocrine or inactivity basis.

Obesity may result from increases in numbers or in size of fat cells, adipocytes. Adipocytes appear to increase in number when caloric intake is increased, especially in the gestational months and during the 1st yr of life; this stimulus to increased numbers operates at a reduced intensity through puberty. During periods of weight reduction, the size but not the number of adipocytes decreases.

Resistance to insulin may occur in the obese and result in an increase in levels of circulating insulin. Insulin decreases lipolysis and increases fat synthesis and uptake. The obese have an increased insulin response to a carbohydrate meal and a decreased utilization of free fatty acids. During weight reduction regimens, the obese deliver less food to their cells than the lean, owing to decreased mobilization of free fatty acids. In starvation after obesity, fat is mobilized as serum insulin decreases. Protein conservation is facilitated as the brain utilizes ketones for energy. During starvation, serum alanine levels decrease and glycine levels rise.

Purified sugars as well as high protein diet may cause greater secretion of insulin than do complex carbohydrates.

The chronic and uncritical offering of a bottle as a means of dealing with a fretful or crying infant may lead to the development of a habit pattern so that for any frustration the infant may expect or seek food. If obesity is initiated early, it is likely to persist. Similarly, the uncritical early introduction of high caloric solid foods may lead to rapid weight gain and to obesity.

Clinical Manifestations. Obesity may become evident at any age, but makes its appearance most frequently in the 1st yr of life, at 5–6 yr of age, and during adolescence. The child whose obesity is due to excessively high caloric intake is usually not only heavier than his or her cohorts but also taller, and bone age is advanced. The facial features often appear disproportionately fine. The adiposity in the mammary regions of boys is often suggestive of breast development and therefore an embarrassing feature. The abdomen tends to be pendulous, and white or purple striae are often present. The external genitalia of boys appear disproportionately small but actually are most often of average size; the penis is often imbedded in the pubic fat. Puberty may occur early, with the result that the ultimate height of the obese may be less than that of their slower maturing peers. The development of the external genitalia is normal in the majority of girls, and menarche is usually not delayed. The obesity of the extremities is usually greater in the upper arm and thigh and is at times limited to them. The hands may be relatively small and the fingers tapering. Genu valgum is common.

Psychologic disturbances are common in obese children. Even in the apparently well adjusted child adequate psychologic evaluation often discloses significant underlying emotional problems. These may have initially contributed to the causes of obesity and usually are an additive factor in its maintenance.

Prevention and Treatment. Because obesity may be self-perpetuating for psychologic or physiologic reasons, children of obese parents or those with obese siblings should be encouraged to adhere to a systematic program of energetic exercise and a balanced low calorie diet. Idealized weight is desirable not only for esthetic reasons but also to prevent such complications of obesity as diabetes, shortness of breath, and early death. Untreated overweight infants almost always remain overweight as adults. Treatment of the obese child usually fails unless the child is motivated to lose weight. Modifying behavior to include increased activity is helpful.

In planning the diet, the basic nutritional needs must be met. All the essential dietary needs may be included in a 1100- to 1300-calorie diet for children 10–14 yr of age for several months (Table 3–16). Some children avoid excessive eating after they have been allowed to return to a free choice of diet. The diet should contain as much bulk as possible. At times greater cooperation is secured if small portions of the diet are permitted between meals, especially in the afternoon. If there is doubt that the daily vitamin intake is adequate, vitamin concentrates may be prescribed. Vitamin D should be included, as for all growing children. Rapid decreases in weight should not be attempted, and medical supervision should be maintained. During the growing years, maintenance of weight while the child increases in height is often a sufficient goal. There is at best a limited place for drug therapy. Psychologic support is often an essential element in management, and both dietary and psychologic treatment should involve the entire family.

The *pickwickian syndrome* is a rare complication of extreme exogenous obesity, in which there is severe cardiorespiratory distress. It is termed "pickwickian" for the fat boy, Joe, in Dickens' *Pickwick Papers.* The extreme obesity causes alveolar hypoventilation, with a decrease in pulmonary, tidal, and expiratory reserve volumes. The manifestations include polycythemia, hypoxemia, cyanosis, cardiac enlargement, congestive cardiac failure, and somnolence. High concentrations of oxygen may be dangerous in the treatment of the cyanosis since respiration may depend solely on the stimulatory effect of hypoxia. Reduction in weight is extremely important and should be accomplished as rapidly as feasible.

American Academy of Pediatrics Committee on Nutrition: Obesity in infancy and childhood. Pediatrics 68:880, 1981.
Bistrian BR, Blackburn GL, Stanbury JB: Metabolic aspects of a protein-sparing modified fast in the dietary management of Prader-Willi obesity. N Engl J Med 296:774, 1977.
Felig P, Wahren J: Fuel homeostasis in exercise. N Engl J Med 293:1078, 1975.
Striker EM: Hyperphagia. N Engl J Med 298:1010, 1978.

VITAMINS

Vitamins are essential nutrients which must be supplied exogenously. Functions of vitamins are summarized in Table 3–6, recommended daily allowances, in Table 3–1. Toxicity is more commonly seen with excesses of the fat-soluble vitamins A and D than with the water-soluble vitamins. The vitamin-dependent states are summarized in Table 3–17.

3.21   VITAMIN A DEFICIENCY

The term vitamin A is a generic label for all β-ionone derivatives other than provitamin A carotenoids. Retinol signifies vitamin A alcohol retinyl ester, vitamin A ester; retinal, vitamin A aldehyde; and retinoic acid, vitamin A acid.

"Provitamin A carotenoids" is the generic term for all carotenoids that have the biologic activity of β-carotene. They or their derivatives with vitamin A activity are required in the diets of infants and children.

Table 3–17   VITAMIN DEPENDENCY STATES

VITAMIN	DISEASE	UNTREATED STATE	DAILY DOSAGE
A	Darier	Hyperkeratosis follicularis	25,000 IU
B_1	Leigh—pyruvic-lactic acidosis	Ataxia, retardation	600 mg
	Thiamine-responsive anemia	Megaloblastic anemia	20 mg
	Maple syrup urine disease	Hypotonia, seizures	10 mg
Riboflavin	Pyruvate kinase deficiency	Hemolysis	10 mg
Niacin	Hartnup	Ataxia, eczema	200 mg
B_6	Cystathioninuria	No symptoms	200 mg
	Homocystinuria	Retardation	200 mg
	B_6-anemia	Hypochromic microcytic anemia	10 mg
	B_6-seizures	Seizures	25 mg
	Xanthurenic aciduria	Retardation	10 mg
	Gyrate atrophy of choroid	Blindness	100 mg
	Oxaluria	Oxalate crystals	100 mg
Folic acid	Formiminotransferase deficiency	Retardation	5 mg
	Folate reductase deficiency	Megaloblastic anemia	5 mg
	Homocystinuria	Retardation	10 mg
B_{12}	Methylmalonic acidemia	Retardation	1 mg
Biotin	Propionic acidemia	Retardation	10 mg
	β-Methylcrotonyl glycinuria	Coma	10 mg
C	Chédiak-Higashi	Infections	50 mg
D	Dependency	Rickets	4000 IU
	Familial hypophosphatemia	Rickets	100,000 IU

Beta-carotene is partly absorbed by the intestinal lymphatics and partly cleaved into 2 molecules of retinol. Dietary retinyl ester is hydrolyzed to retinol in the intestine. Retinol is esterified inside the mucosal cell with palmitic acid and is stored in the liver as retinylpalmitate; this in turn is hydrolyzed to free retinol for transport to its site of action. Zinc is required for this mobilization. Normal plasma values of retinol in infants are 20–50 µg/dl; in children and adults, 30–225 µg/dl.

Heavy ingestion of carotenoids may result in large amounts of carotene in the blood and in yellow discoloration of the skin but not of the sclera. This disorder, carotenemia, is especially apt to occur in children with liver disease, diabetes mellitus, or hypothyroidism and in those who have congenital absence of enzymes that convert provitamin A carotenoids.

Etiology. The liver at birth has a low vitamin A content which is rapidly augmented since colostrum and breast milk furnish large amounts of the vitamin. Breast milk and whole cow's milk are satisfactory sources of vitamin A. Other foods (vegetables, fruits, eggs, butter, liver) or vitamin supplements also provide vitamin A. Loss of it in cooking, canning, and freezing of foodstuffs is small; oxidizing agents, however, destroy it.

The danger of vitamin A deficiency is small in healthy children with balanced diets. Deficient diets commonly cause disease by 2–3 yr of age. Vitamin A deficiency also results from inadequate intestinal absorption, as, for example, with chronic intestinal disorders, celiac disease, hepatic and pancreatic diseases, iron deficiency anemia, chronic infectious diseases, or chronic ingestion of mineral oil. Low intake of dietary fat results in low vitamin A absorption. Vitamin A excretion is increased in cancer, urinary tract disease, and chronic infectious diseases. Low protein intake results in deficient carrier protein and in decreases in plasma concentration of vitamin A.

Pathology. The human retina contains 2 distinct photoreceptor systems: the rods are sensitive to light of low intensity, the cones to colors and to light of high intensity. Retinal is the prosthetic group of the photosensitive pigment in both rods and cones. The major difference between the visual pigments in rods (rhodopsin) and in cones (iodopsin) is the nature of the protein bound to retinal. All-*trans*-retinal isomerizes in the dark to 11-*cis* form. This combines with opsin to form rhodopsin. Energy from light quanta reconverts 11-*cis* retinal back to the all-*trans* form; this energy exchange, transmitted via the optic nerves to the brain, results in visual sensation. The energy factor can be measured by an electroretinograph to assess vitamin A status. Beta-carotene has been effective in ameliorating photosensitivity in patients with erythropoietic protoporphyria. It has also been suggested that retinitis pigmentosa may be related to a defect in retinol-binding protein.

Vitamin A is apparently necessary for membrane stability. Large doses of vitamin A lead to rupture of lysosomal membranes with release of hydrolases; deficiency may result in a similar phenomenon.

The vitamin plays a role in keratinization, cornification, bone metabolism, placental development, growth, spermatogenesis, and mucus formation. Characteristic changes in epithelium include proliferation of basal cells, hyperkeratosis, and the formation of stratified, cornified, squamous epithelium. Epithelial changes in the respiratory system may result in bronchiolar obstruction. Squamous metaplasia of the renal pelves, ureters, urinary bladder, enamel organs, and pancreatic and salivary ducts may lead to increase in infections in these areas. In experimental animals retinoids decrease the incidence of epithelial tumors.

Clinical Manifestations. Ocular lesions develop insidiously. Initially, the posterior segment of the eye is affected, with impairment of dark adaptation and night blindness. Later, drying of the conjunctiva (xerosis conjunctivae) and of the cornea (xerosis corneae) is followed by wrinkling and cloudiness of the cornea (keratomalacia) (Fig 3–4). Dry, silver-gray plaques may appear on the bulbar conjunctiva (Bitot spots), with follicular hyperkeratosis and photophobia.

Vitamin A deficiency may result in retardation of mental and physical growth and in apathy. Anemia with or without hepatosplenomegaly is usually present.

The skin is dry and scaly, and at times follicular hyperkeratosis may be found on the shoulders, buttocks, and extensor surfaces of the extremities. The vaginal epithelium may become cornified, and epithelial metaplasia of the urinary tract may contribute to pyuria and hematuria. Increased intracranial pressure with wide separation of cranial bones at the sutures may occur. Hydrocephalus, with or without paralyses of the cranial nerves, is an infrequent manifestation.

Diagnosis. Dark adaptation tests may be helpful. Xerosis conjunctivae can be detected by biomicroscopic examination of the conjunctiva. Examination of the scrapings from the eye and vagina is recommended as a diagnostic aid. The plasma carotene concentration falls quickly, but that of vitamin A decreases more slowly. A standard absorption test for vitamin A is

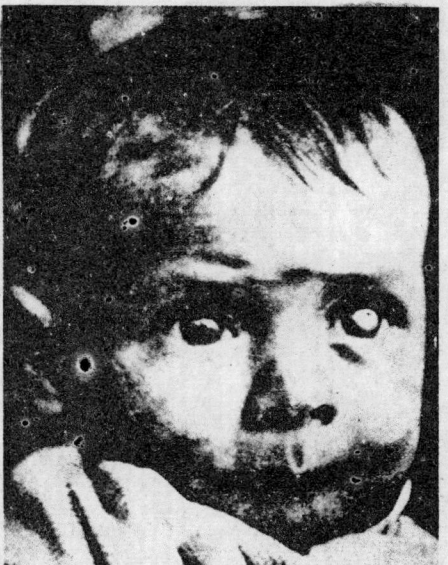

Figure 3–4 Recovery from xerophthalmia, showing permanent eye lesion. (Bloch: Am J Dis Child, Vol 27.)

available. Low absorption curves are obtained in children with cystic fibrosis, celiac disease, obliteration of the bile ducts, and cretinism (Sec 11.43).

Prevention. Infants should receive at least 500 µg* daily, older children and adults, 600–1500 µg of vitamin A or carotene. The average diets of infants and children in this country supply enough vitamin A to prevent symptoms of deficiency.

For therapeutic reasons low fat diets should be supplemented with vitamin A. In disorders with poor absorption of fat or increased excretion of vitamin A, water-miscible preparations of vitamin A should be administered in amounts several times the usual daily requirement. Premature infants, who absorb fats and vitamin A less efficiently than do full-term infants, should also receive water-miscible preparations. The World Health Organization recommends that, in areas of the world where vitamin A deficiency occurs, 100,000 IU of vitamin A be given orally in a water-miscible base 4 times yearly; the same dose should be given postpartum to mothers of breast-fed infants. -

Treatment. In cases of latent vitamin A deficiency, a daily supplement of 5000 IU of vitamin A is sufficient. For xerophthalmia, 5000 IU/kg/24 hr is given orally for 5 days and then continued with intramuscular injection of 25,000 IU of vitamin A in oil daily until recovery occurs.

---

*One international unit (IU) of vitamin A is equivalent to 0.3 µg of retinol (vitamin A alcohol).

Hypervitaminosis A. Acute hypervitaminosis A may occur in infants after the ingestion of 300,000 IU or more. The symptoms are nausea, vomiting, drowsiness, and bulging of the fontanel. Diplopia, papilledema, cranial nerve palsies, and other symptoms suggestive of brain tumor (*pseudotumor cerebri*) may also occur.

Chronic hypervitaminosis A appears after ingestion of excessive doses for several weeks or months. The child has anorexia, pruritus, and a lack of gain in weight. There is increasing irritability, limitation of motion, and tender swelling of the bones. Alopecia, seborrheic cutaneous lesions, fissuring of the corners of the mouth, increased intracranial pressure, and hepatomegaly may develop. Craniotabes and desquamation of the palms and soles are common. Roentgenograms reveal hyperostosis affecting several long bones; it is most notable at the middle of the shafts (Fig 3–5).

A history of excessive ingestion of vitamin A is helpful in the differentiation from cortical hyperostosis (Sec 23.17). The serum vitamin A level is also elevated. Hypercalcemia or liver cirrhosis occasionally occurs.

DeLuca HF: Retinoic acid metabolism. Fed Proc 38:2519, 1979.
Fisher KD, Carr CJ, Huff JE, et al: Dark adaptation and night vision. Fed Proc 29:1605, 1970.
Goodman DS: Vitamin A metabolism. Fed Proc 39:2716, 1980.
Gouras P, Chauder G: Retinitis pigmentosa and retinol-binding protein. Invest Ophthalmol 13:239, 1974.
Mahoney CP, Margolis T, Knauss TA, et al: Chronic vitamin A intoxication in infants fed chicken liver. Pediatrics 65:893, 1980.
Mathews-Roth MM, Pathak MA, Fitzpatrick TB, et al: Beta-carotene as an oral protective agent in erythropoietic protoporphyria. JAMA 228:1004, 1974.
McLaren DS, Shirajain E, Tchallian M, et al: Xerophthalmia in Jordan. Am J Clin Nutr 17:117, 1965.
Peck GL: Prolonged remissions of cystic and conglobate acne with 13-cis-retinoic acid. N Engl J Med 300:299, 1979.
Sporn MB, Newton DL: Chemoprevention of cancer with retinoids. Fed Proc 38:2528, 1979.

3.22 VITAMIN B COMPLEX DEFICIENCY

Vitamin B complex includes a number of factors that vary greatly in chemical composition and in function (Table 3–6). All are important constituents of enzyme systems. Since many of these enzymes are closely related functionally, lack of a single factor can interrupt an entire chain of normal chemical processes and produce diversified clinical manifestations.

Diets deficient in any 1 factor of the B complex are frequently poor sources of other B vitamins. It is, therefore, not unusual to find manifestations of several B deficiencies in 1 patient. It is usually advantageous to treat with the entire B complex.

Factors such as pantothenic acid, choline, biotin, and inositol are of importance for the normal function of the human organism, but at present no specific deficiency syndromes can be ascribed to lack of them in the diets of children.

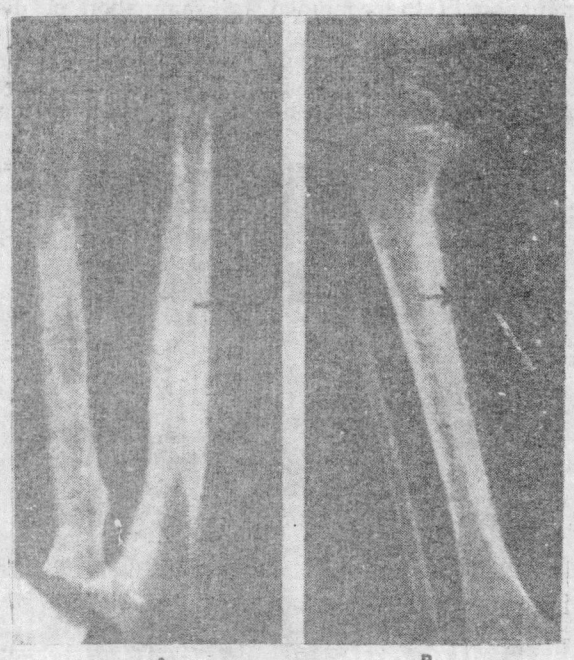

Figure 3–5 Hyperostosis of the ulna and the tibia in an infant 21 mo of age, resulting from vitamin A poisoning. *A,* Long, wavy cortical hyperostosis of ulna. *B,* Long, wavy cortical hyperostosis of right tibia; striking absence of metaphyseal changes. (From Caffey J: Pediatrics, Vol 5. Courtesy of Charles C Thomas, Publisher, Springfield, Ill.)

3.23 THIAMINE DEFICIENCY
(Beriberi)

Etiology. Vitamin B_1 (thiamine) is water-soluble and, as thiamine pyrophosphate or cocarboxylase, functions as a coenzyme in carbohydrate metabolism. Thiamine is required for the synthesis of acetylcholine, and deficiency results in impaired nerve conduction. It is the coenzyme in transketolation and in decarboxylation of α-keto acids. Transketolase participates in the hexose monophosphate shunt which generates NADPH and pentose.

Breast milk or cow's milk, vegetables, cereals, fruits, and eggs are sources of thiamine. Infants whose source of food is the milk of thiamine-deficient women may develop beriberi. Older children whose diet contains such good sources of thiamine as meats and legumes do not require supplements of thiamine.

Thiamine is easily destroyed by heat in neutral or alkaline media and is readily extracted from foodstuffs by cooking water. The presence of a destructive enzymatic factor in some fish explains why a diet low in thiamine induces beriberi rapidly when it contains such fish. Since the covering of grains of cereals contains most of the vitamin, polishing reduces its availability.

Thiamine absorption is decreased with gastrointestinal or liver disease. Requirements are increased with fever, surgery, or stress. Thiamine dependency has been described in a child with megaloblastic anemia and in an infant with otherwise typical maple syrup urine disease. In children with *Leigh encephalomyelopathy*, urine from them and their parents inhibits the formation of thiamine pyrophosphate. Large doses of thiamine improve some of the physical abnormalities associated with the disease.

Pathology. In fatal cases of beriberi, lesions are located principally in the heart, peripheral nerves, subcutaneous tissue, and serous cavities. The heart is dilated, and fatty degeneration of the myocardium is common. Generalized edema or edema of the legs, serous effusions, and venous engorgement may be present. The peripheral nerves undergo varying degrees of degeneration of myelin and axon cylinders, with wallerian degeneration, beginning in the distal locations. The nerves of the lower extremities are affected first. Lesions in the brain include vascular dilatation and hemorrhage.

Clinical Manifestations. Early manifestations of deficiency include fatigue, apathy, irritability, depression, drowsiness, poor mental concentration, anorexia, nausea, and abdominal discomfort. Progression, recognized as beriberi, includes peripheral neuritis with tingling, burning, and paresthesias of the toes and feet; decreased tendon reflexes; loss of vibration sense; tenderness and cramping of leg muscles; congestive heart failure; and psychic disturbances. There may be ptosis of the eyelids and atrophy of the optic nerve. Hoarseness due to paralysis of the laryngeal nerve is a characteristic sign. Muscle atrophy and tenderness of nerve trunks are followed by ataxia, loss of coordination, and loss of deep sensation. Paralytic symptoms are more common in adults than in children. Later, signs of increased intracranial pressure, meningismus, and coma occur.

In *dry* beriberi the child may appear plump but is pale, flabby, listless, and dyspneic; the heart rate is rapid and the liver enlarged. In *wet* beriberi the child is undernourished, pale, and edematous and has dysp-

nea, vomiting, and tachycardia. The skin appears waxy. The urine may contain albumin and casts.

The cardiac signs at first are slight cyanosis and dyspnea. Tachycardia, enlargement of the liver, loss of consciousness, and convulsions may develop rapidly. The heart is enlarged, especially to the right. The electrocardiogram shows increased Q-T interval, inversion of T waves, and low voltage, changes which rapidly revert to normal with treatment. Cardiac failure may lead to death in either chronic or acute beriberi.

Diagnosis. The early symptoms are encountered in many types of nutritional disturbances other than thiamine deficiency. Demonstrations of lowered red cell transketolase and of high blood or urinary glyoxylate values have been proposed as diagnostic tests. Excretion after an oral loading dose of thiamine or its metabolites, thiazole or pyrimidine, may help to identify the deficiency state. Clinical response to administration of thiamine remains the best test for thiamine deficiency.

Prevention. Thiamine deficiency in breast-fed infants is prevented by a maternal diet that contains sufficient amounts of this vitamin. The recommended daily dietary allowances of thiamine are 1.7 mg during pregnancy and lactation for the mother, 0.5 mg for infants, and 0.7–1.5 mg for older children. Thiamine requirements increase with a high carbohydrate content of the diet.

Treatment. If beriberi occurs in a breast-fed infant, both mother and child should be treated with thiamine. The daily dose for adults is 50 mg and for children 10 mg or more. Oral administration is effective unless gastrointestinal disturbances prevent absorption. Thiamine should be given intramuscularly or intravenously to children with cardiac failure. Such treatment is followed by dramatic improvement, though complete cure requires several weeks. The heart is not permanently damaged. There is often deficiency of other B vitamins in patients with beriberi; for this reason all other vitamins of the B complex should be administered in addition to large doses of thiamine chloride.

3.24 RIBOFLAVIN DEFICIENCY
(Ariboflavinosis)

Riboflavin deficiency is rarely encountered without deficiencies of other members of the B complex. Riboflavin is a water-soluble, yellow, fluorescent substance, stable to heat and acids but destroyed by light and alkalis. The coenzymes flavin mononucleotide (FMN) and flavin adenine dinucleotide (FAD) are synthesized from riboflavin and form the prosthetic groups of several enzymes important in electron transport. Riboflavin is essential for growth and tissue respiration; it may play a role in light adaptation and is required for conversion of pyridoxine to pyridoxal phosphate. Riboflavin occurs in large amounts in liver, kidney, brewer's yeast, milk, cheese, eggs, and leafy vegetables; cow's milk contains about 5 times as much riboflavin as human milk.

Riboflavin deficiency is usually due to inadequate intake. Faulty absorption may be a contributory factor in those with biliary atresia or hepatitis or in patients receiving probenecid, phenothiazine, or oral contraceptives. Phototherapy destroys riboflavin.

Clinical Manifestations. Evidences of riboflavin deficiency include cheilosis (perlèche), glossitis, keratitis, conjunctivitis, photophobia, lacrimation, marked corneal vascularization, and seborrheic dermatitis. Cheilosis begins with pallor at the angles of the mouth, followed by thinning and maceration of the epithelium. Superficial fissures often covered by yellow crusts develop in the angles of the mouth and extend radially into the skin for distances of 1–2 cm. Cheilosis occurs in epidemics in institutions and in families in which the diet is inadequate. With glossitis the tongue is smooth, and there is loss of papillary structure. A normocytic, normochromic anemia with bone marrow hypoplasia is common.

Diagnosis. Urinary excretion of riboflavin below 30 μg/24 hr is abnormally low. Levels of erythrocyte glutathionine reductase, a flavoprotein requiring FAD, may reflect the stores of riboflavin. A patient with hemolysis due to pyruvate kinase deficiency and reduced erythrocyte glutathionine reductase had both enzyme activities restored to normal on administration of riboflavin.

Prevention. Daily recommended amount of riboflavin for infants is 0.6 mg, for children and adults, 1–2 mg. Riboflavin deficiency is usually prevented by a diet that contains adequate amounts of milk, eggs, leafy vegetables, and lean meats.

Treatment. Treatment consists in the oral administration of 3–10 mg of riboflavin daily. If no response is obtained within a few days, intramuscular injections of 2 mg of riboflavin in saline solution may be made 3 times daily. The child should also be given a well balanced diet and, at least temporarily, more than the usual requirements of the B complex.

3.25 · NIACIN DEFICIENCY
(Pellagra)

Pellagra (*pellis*, skin; *agra*, rough) probably has existed under certain unfavorable conditions at all times in all parts of the world.

Etiology. Pellagra is a deficiency disease due mainly to a lack of niacin (nicotinic acid); it affects all the tissues of the body. Niacin forms part of 2 enzymes important in electron transfer and glycolysis: nicotinamide adenine dinucleotide (NAD) and nicotinamide adenine dinucleotide phosphate (NADP). Although 60 mg of dietary tryptophan can be utilized in place of 1 mg of niacin, other sources of niacin are necessary. Liver, lean pork, salmon, poultry, and red meat are good sources, but most cereals contain only small amounts of it. Pellagra occurs chiefly in countries where corn (maize), a poor source of tryptophan, is a basic foodstuff. Milk and eggs, which contain little niacin, are good pellagra-preventive foods because of their high content of tryptophan. Because niacin is a stable compound, there are only small losses in cooking.

Pathology. Histologically, there is edema and degeneration of the superficial collagen of the dermis. The papillary vessels are engorged, and there is perivascular lymphocytic infiltration in the dermis. The epidermis is hyperkeratotic and later becomes atrophic.

Changes comparable to those in the skin are present in the tongue, buccal mucous membranes, and vagina. These changes may be associated with secondary infection and ulceration. The walls of the colon are thickened and inflamed with patches of pseudomembrane; later the mucosa atrophies. Changes in the nervous system occur relatively late in the disease and consist of patchy areas of demyelinization and degeneration of ganglion cells; demyelinization in the spinal cord may involve the posterior and lateral columns.

Clinical Manifestations. The early symptoms of pellagra are vague. Anorexia, lassitude, weakness, burning sensations, numbness, and dizziness may be prodromal symptoms. After a long period of niacin deficiency the characteristic symptoms appear. The classic triad consists of dermatitis, diarrhea, and dementia. Manifestations in children who have parasites or chronic disorders may be especially severe.

The most characteristic manifestations are the cutaneous ones, which may develop suddenly or insidiously and may be elicited by irritants, particularly by intensive sunlight. They first appear as symmetric erythema of the exposed surfaces that may resemble sunburn and in mild cases may escape recognition. The lesions are usually sharply demarcated from the healthy skin

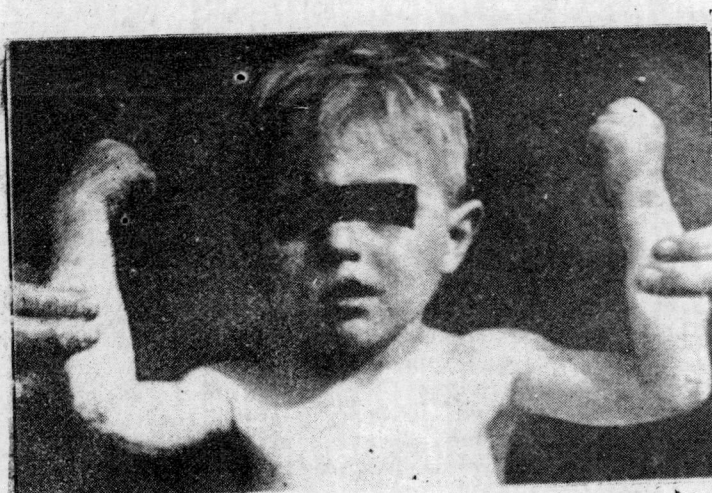

Figure 3–6 Pellagra in a boy 3 yr of age, showing lesions on the hands and elbows and an early lesion over the nose and malar eminences.

around them, and their distribution may change frequently. The lesions on the hands sometimes have the appearance of a glove (pellagrous glove) (Fig 3–6), and similar demarcations are occasionally seen on the foot and leg (pellagrous boot) or around the neck (Casal necklace). In some instances vesicles and bullae develop (wet type), or there may be suppuration beneath the scaly, crusted epidermis; in others the swelling disappears after a short time and desquamation begins. The healed parts of the skin may remain pigmented.

The cutaneous lesions are sometimes preceded by stomatitis, glossitis, vomiting, or diarrhea. Swelling and redness of the tip of the tongue and its lateral margins may be followed by intense redness of the entire tongue and of the papillae and even ulceration.

Nervous symptoms include depression, disorientation, insomnia, and delirium.

The classic symptoms of pellagra are usually not well developed in infants and children. Anorexia, irritability, anxiety, and apathy are common in "pellagra families." They may also have sore tongues and lips, and the skin is usually dry and scaly. Diarrhea and constipation may alternate and a moderate secondary anemia may occur. Children who have pellagra often have evidences of other nutritional deficiency diseases.

Diagnosis. Diagnosis is usually made from the physical signs of glossitis, gastrointestinal symptoms, and a symmetrical dermatitis. Rapid clinical response to niacin is an important confirming test. N-methyl-nicotinamide, a normal metabolite of niacin, is almost undetectable in urine during niacin deficiency.

Prevention. The recommended daily allowance of niacin is 8 mg for infants and 9–20 mg for older children. A well-balanced diet containing meat, vegetables, eggs, and milk meets this requirement so that supplements of niacin are necessary only in breast-fed infants whose mothers have pellagra or in children on restricted diets.

Treatment. Children respond rapidly to antipellagral therapy. A liberal and well-balanced diet should be supplemented with 50–300 mg of niacin daily; 100 mg may be given intravenously in severe cases or in cases of poor intestinal absorption. The administration of large doses of niacin is often followed within a half hour by a sensation of increased local heat and flushing and burning of the skin. These unpleasant effects are not produced by niacinamide, but in large doses it may cause cholestatic jaundice or hepatotoxicity.

The diet should be supplemented with other vitamins, especially with other members of the B complex. Sun exposure should be avoided during the active phase; the skin lesions may be covered with soothing applications. A blood transfusion may be helpful when there is severe anemia; less severe hypochromic anemia should be treated with iron. The diet of the cured pellagrin should be continuously supervised to prevent recurrence.

Thiamine Deficiency

Brin M: Erythrocyte as a biopsy tissue for functional evaluation of thiamin adequacy. JAMA 187:762, 1964.
McCandless DW, Schenker S: Neurologic disorders of thiamine deficiency. Nutr Rev 27:213, 1969.

Riboflavin Deficiency

Rillotson JA, Baker EM: An enzymatic measurement of the riboflavin status in man. Am J Clin Nutr 25:425, 1972.
Rivlin RS: Hormones, drugs and riboflavin. Nutr Rev 37:241, 1979.
Staal GEJ, Van Berkel TJC, Nijessen JG, et al: Normalization of red blood cell pyruvate kinase in pyruvate kinase deficiency by riboflavin treatment. Clin Chim Acta 60:323, 1975.

Niacin Deficiency

Darby WJ, McNutt KW, Todhunter EN: Niacin Nutr Rev 33:289, 1975.

3.26 PYRIDOXINE (VITAMIN B₆) DEFICIENCY

Vitamin B₆ includes pyridoxal, pyridoxine, and pyridoxamine. These are converted to pyridoxal-5-phosphate (or pyridoxamine-5-phosphate), which acts as a coenzyme in decarboxylation and transamination of amino acids, e.g., in the decarboxylation of 5-hydroxytryptophan in the formation of serotonin, and in the metabolism of glycogen and fatty acids. Vitamin B₆ is also essential for the breakdown of kynurenine. When this does not occur, xanthurenic acid appears in the urine. Adequate functioning of the nervous system is dependent on pyridoxine; its deficiency results in seizures and in peripheral neuropathy. Pyridoxal phosphate is the coenzyme for both glutamic decarboxylase and gamma-aminobutyric acid transaminase; each is necessary for normal brain metabolism. It participates in active transport of amino acids across cell membranes, chelates metals, and participates in the synthesis of arachidonic acid from linoleic acid. If it is lacking, glycine metabolism may lead to oxaluria. It is excreted largely as 4-pyridoxic acid.

Etiology. Pyridoxine is adequately available in human and cow's milk and in cereals, but prolonged heat processing of the latter two destroys it. Diseases with malabsorption, such as celiac syndrome, may contribute to vitamin B₆ deficiency.

There are several types of *vitamin B₆ dependency syndromes*, presumably the result of errors in enzyme structure or function, in which the patient responds to very large amounts of pyridoxine. These syndromes include B₆-dependent convulsions, a B₆-responsive anemia, xanthurenic aciduria, cystathioninuria, and homocystinuria.

Pyridoxine antagonists, such as isonicotinic acid hydrazide (isoniazid), which is used in the treatment of tuberculosis, increase the requirements for pyridoxine as do pregnancy and drugs such as penicillamine, hydralazine, and the oral progesterone-estrogen contraceptives.

Clinical Manifestations. Deficiency symptoms are not as common in children as in adults. Four clinical disturbances due to vitamin B₆ deficiency have been described in man: convulsions in infants, peripheral neuritis, dermatitis, and anemia.

Infants fed a formula deficient in vitamin B₆ for 1–6 mo exhibit irritability and generalized seizures. Gastrointestinal distress and an aggravated startle response are common.

Peripheral neuropathy may occur during treatment of tuberculosis with isonicotinic acid hydrazide. The neuropathy responds to administration of pyridoxine or to a decrease in the dose of the drug. Administration of isonicotinic acid also may be followed by manifestations of pellagra.

Skin lesions include cheilosis, glossitis, and seborrhea around the eyes, nose, and mouth. Microcytic anemia, oxaluria, oxalic acid bladder stones, hyperglycinemia, lymphopenia, decreased antibody formation, and infections occur.

Convulsions from B_6 *dependency* may occur several hours to as long as 6 mo after birth. Seizures are typically myoclonic with hypsarrhythmic patterns on the electrocardiogram. In several instances the mothers had received large doses of pyridoxine during pregnancy for control of emesis.

In B_6-*dependent anemia* the red cells are microcytic and hypochromic. There are increased serum iron concentrations, saturation of iron-binding protein, hemosiderin deposits in bone marrow and liver, and failure of iron utilization for hemoglobin synthesis.

Xanthurenic aciduria following tryptophan load tests is an apparently benign occurrence in some families. Xanthurenic acid excretion becomes normal following large doses of vitamin B_6. *Cystathioninuria* is similarly not accompanied by any clear clinical disturbance. Cystathioninase is vitamin B_6 dependent (Sec 8.4).

In some patients with *homocystinuria*, serum levels of homocysteine will fall following B_6 administration. Cystathionine synthetase is B_6-dependent (Sec 8.4).

Laboratory Data.   Anemia is not common in affected infants. After administration of 100 mg/kg of tryptophan, large amounts of xanthurenic acid will be found in the urine of patients with pryidoxine deficiency; in normal persons none is detected. The result of this test may be normal in patients with "pyridoxine dependency."

Diagnosis.   Infants with seizures should be suspected of having vitamin B_6 deficiency or dependency. If more common causes of infantile seizures, such as hypocalcemia, hypoglycemia, and infection, can be eliminated as causative factors, 100 mg of pyridoxine should be injected. If the seizure stops, B_6 deficiency should be suspected, and a tryptophan loading test is indicated. Similarly, in older children with seizure disorders, 100 mg of pyridoxine may be injected intramuscularly while the electroencephalogram is being recorded; a favorable response of the EEG suggests pyridoxine deficiency.

Erythrocyte glutamic pyruvic transaminase is reduced in pyridoxine deficiency; its concentration may be used as an indicator of vitamin B_6 status.

Prevention.   Balanced diets usually contain enough pyridoxine so that deficiency is rare. Children receiving high protein diets should have vitamin B_6 added. Infants whose mothers have received large doses of pyridoxine during pregnancy are at increased risk of seizures due to pyridoxine dependency. Any child receiving a pyridoxine antagonist such as isoniazid should be carefully observed for neurologic manifestations. If these develop, either pyridoxine should be administered or the dose of the antagonist decreased. Daily intake of 0.3–0.5 mg of pyridoxine in the infant, 0.5–1.5 mg in the child, or 1.5–2.0 mg in the adult prevents deficiency states.

Treatment.   For convulsions possibly due to pyridoxine deficiency, 100 mg of the vitamin should be given intramuscularly. One dose should suffice if the diet is adequate. For "pyridoxine-dependent" children, 2–10 mg intramuscularly or 10–100 mg orally may be necessary daily.

Aly HE, Donald EA, Simpson MHW: Oral contraceptives and vitamin B_6 metabolism. Am J Clin Nutr 22:97, 1971.
Cinnamon AD, Beaton JR: Biochemical assessment of vitamin B_6 status in man. Am J Clin Nutr 26:96, 1970.
Frimpter GW, Andelman RJ, George WF: Vitamin B_6-dependency syndromes. Am J Clin Nutr 22:794, 1959.
Hansson O, Hagberg B: Effect of pyridoxine treatment in children with epilepsy. Acta Soc Med Upsal 73:35, 1968.
Scriver CR: Vitamin B_6 deficiency and dependency in man. Am J Dis Child 113:109, 1967.

3.27   VITAMIN C (ASCORBIC ACID) DEFICIENCY
(Scurvy)

Ascorbic acid is essential for the normal formation of collagen; the defects in its structure that stem from deficiency of the vitamin are responsible for many of the metabolic deviations and clinical manifestations of scurvy. The alterations in collagen formation are, in part, represented by failure in the incorporation of hydroxyproline and proline.

Vitamin C is a potent reducing agent, easily oxidized and destroyed by heating. The adrenals and lenses have particularly high contents of vitamin C.

Ascorbic acid is operative in a number of enzymatic activities (Table 3–6 and Sec 8.3). Transient tyrosinemia in the neonatal period is relatively common among low birth weight infants and occasionally in fullterm ones who are fed high protein diets; it is corrected by administration of ascorbic acid (Sec 8.3).

Deficiency of ascorbic acid may also be a factor in some instances of megaloblastic anemia as a result of interference in the conversion of folic acid or other conjugates (Table 3–6 and Sec 14.10).

Etiology.   The infant is born with adequate stores of vitamin C if the mother's intake has been adequate; the vitamin C content of cord blood plasma is 2–4 times greater than that of maternal plasma. Under these circumstances breast milk contains about 4–7 mg/dl of ascorbic acid and is an adequate source of vitamin C. Deficiency of vitamin C in the mother's diet may result in scurvy in her breast-fed infant. Infants fed artificially must receive vitamin C supplements; such supplements will provide additional protection for the breast-fed infant.

The need for vitamin C is increased by febrile illnesses, particularly infectious and diarrheal diseases, and by iron deficiency, cold exposure, protein depletion, or smoking.

Pathology.   During vitamin C deficiency formation of collagen and of chondroitin sulfate is impaired. The tendencies to hemorrhage, defective tooth dentin, and loosening of the teeth are due to deficient collagen.

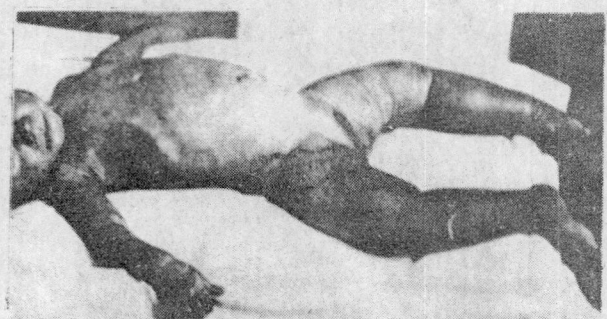

Figure 3–7 Scorbutic rosary, depression of sternum, and the so-called frog position.

Since osteoblasts no longer form their normal intercellular substance (osteoid), endochondral bone formation ceases. The bony trabeculae which have been formed become brittle and fracture easily. The periosteum be-

comes loosened, and subperiosteal hemorrhages occur, especially at the ends of the femur and tibia. In severe scurvy there may be degeneration in skeletal muscles, cardiac hypertrophy, bone marrow depression, and adrenal atrophy.

Clinical Manifestations. Scurvy may occur at any age but is extremely rare in the newborn infant. The majority of cases occur in infants 6–24 mo of age. Clinical manifestations require time for their development; after a variable period of vitamin C depletion, vague symptoms of irritability, tachypnea, digestive disturbances, and loss of appetite appear. The irritability becomes progressively greater, and there is evidence of general tenderness, especially noticeable in the legs when the infant is picked up or when the diaper is changed. The pain results in pseudoparalysis, and the legs assume the typical "frog position" (Fig 3–7), which consists of semiflexion of the hips and knees with the feet rotated outward. Edematous swelling along the shafts of the legs may be present, and in some cases a

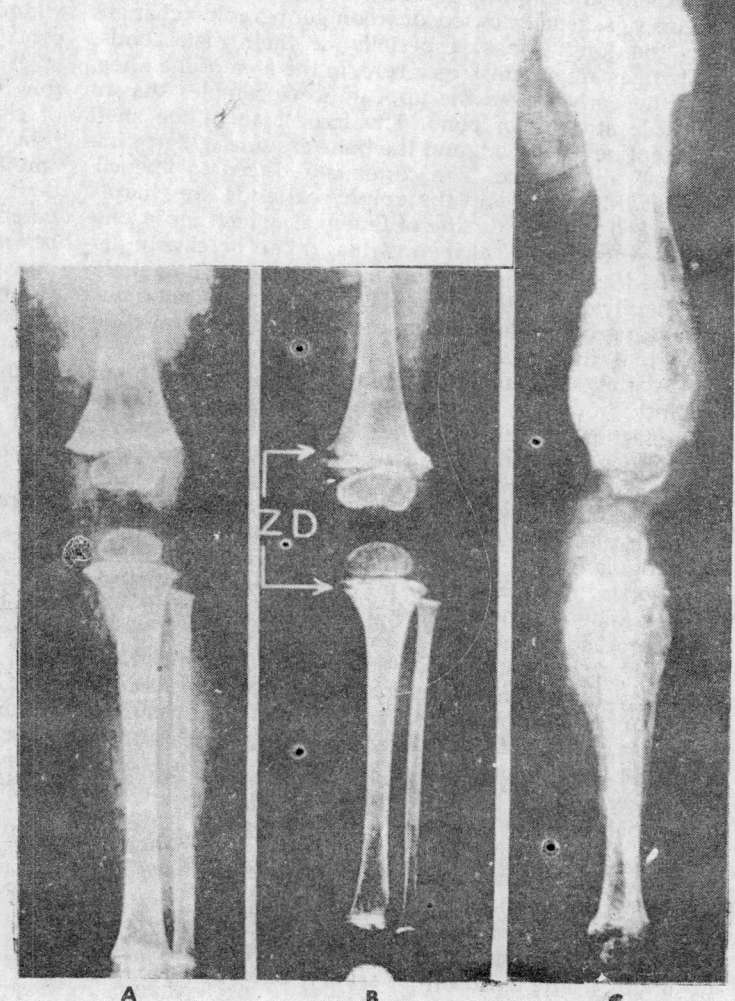

Figure 3–8 Roentgenograms of leg. *A*, Early scurvy: "white line" is visible on the ends of the shafts of the tibia and fibula; rings around epiphyses of femur and tibia. *B*, More advanced scorbutic changes; zones of destruction (ZD) in femur and tibia. *C*, Healing scurvy; calcification of subperiosteal hemorrhages.

subperiosteal hemorrhage can be palpated at the end of the femur. The facial expression is apprehensive. Changes in the gums, most noticeable when the teeth are erupted, are characterized by bluish purple, spongy swellings of the mucous membrane, usually over the upper incisors. There may be a "rosary" at the costochondral junctions and a depression of the sternum. The angulation of the "scorbutic beads" is usually sharper than that of the rachitic rosary since it is produced by a subluxation of the sternal plate at the costochondral junction (Fig 3–7) rather than by widening of the softened epiphyses as occurs in rickets (Sec 3.28).

Petechial hemorrhages may occur in the skin and mucous membranes. Hematuria, melena, orbital, or subdural hemorrhages may be found. Low-grade fever is usually present. Anemia may reflect inability to utilize iron or impaired folic acid metabolism (Sec 14.10). Wound healing is delayed, and apparently healed wounds may break down. Swollen joints and follicular hyperkeratosis may develop, as well as the "sicca" syndrome of Sjögren, which is usually associated with collagen disorders and includes xerostomia, keratoconjunctivitis sicca, and enlargement of the salivary glands.

Roentgenographic Manifestations. The diagnosis of scurvy is usually based on roentgenographic changes in the long bones, especially at their distal ends. Changes are greatest, as a rule, in the area of the knee. In the early stages the appearance resembles that of simple atrophy of bone. The trabeculae of the shaft cannot be discerned, and the bone assumes a "ground-glass" appearance. The cortex is reduced to "pencil-point thinness," and the epiphyseal ends are sharply outlined. The white line of Fraenkel, which represents the zone of well calcified cartilage, can be clearly discerned as an irregular but thickened white line at the metaphysis. The epiphyseal centers of ossification also have a ground-glass appearance and are surrounded by a white ring (Fig 3–8).

At this stage scurvy cannot be diagnosed with certainty from the roentgenogram unless the zone of rarefaction under the white line at the metaphysis becomes apparent. The zone of rarefaction is a linear break in the bone proximal and parallel to the white line. It often does not traverse the shaft in its entire width and may be seen only in its lateral parts as a triangular defect (Fig 3–8B). A spur, as a lateral prolongation of the white line, may be present. Epiphyseal separation may occur along the line of destruction, with linear displacement (Fig 3–9) or compression of the epiphysis against the shaft. Subperiosteal hemorrhages are not visible roentgenographically in active scurvy. During healing, however, the elevated periosteum becomes calcified, and the affected bone assumes a dumbbell or club shape (Fig 3–8C).

Diagnosis. Diagnosis is based mainly on the characteristic clinical picture, the roentgenographic appearance of the long bones, and history of poor intake of vitamin C. Occasionally, a mother may have been boiling the infant's fruit juices.

Laboratory tests for scurvy are unsatisfactory. A fasting vitamin C level of the blood plasma of over 0.6 mg/dl aids in the exclusion of scurvy, but a lower vitamin

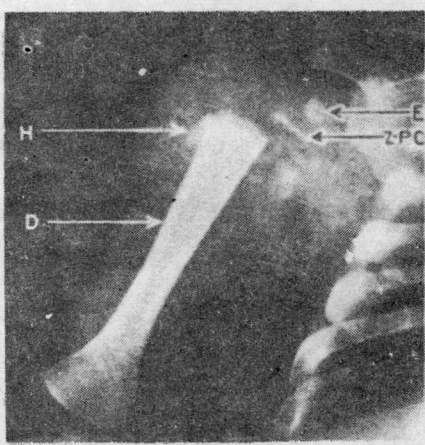

Figure 3–9 "Slipped diaphysis" in scurvy. The epiphysis (E) of the humerus and calcified cartilage of the zone of primary calcification (ZPC) remains in place and in contact with the glenoid fossa. The diaphysis (D) is displaced laterally and separated from the epiphysis. The shadow (H) at the proximal end of the diaphysis represents beginning calcification of a subperiosteal hemorrhage.

C level does not prove its presence. A better index of vitamin C deficiency is furnished by the ascorbic acid concentration in the white cell–platelet layer (buffy layer) of centrifuged oxalated blood. A level of zero in this layer indicates latent scurvy, even in the absence of clinical signs of deficiency. The saturation of the tissues with vitamin C can be estimated from the amount of urinary excretion of the vitamin after a test dose of ascorbic acid. During the 3–5 hr after the parenteral administration of the test dose, 80% of it can be found in the urine of normal children. A generalized, nonspecific aminoaciduria occurs in scurvy, while blood values of amino acids remain normal. After a tyrosine load the scorbutic infant excretes metabolites similar to those of the premature infant. Prothrombin time may be markedly increased.

Differential Diagnosis. The tenderness of the limbs and the pain elicited by movement have often led to a false diagnosis of arthritis or acrodynia. The patient's age aids in differentiating scurvy from rheumatic fever since rheumatic fever is rare in children under 2 yr of age. Suppurative arthritis and osteomyelitis should be considered in the differential diagnosis. The pseudoparalysis of syphilis usually occurs at an earlier age than does that of scurvy and is often accompanied by other signs of syphilis; a roentgenogram may aid in the diagnosis. Poliomyelitis causes a true flaccid paralysis, and, in infants, the exquisite tenderness present in the limbs in scurvy is absent. Henoch-Schönlein purpura, thrombocytopenic purpura, leukemia, meningococcemia, or nephritis may be suspected.

Prognosis. Recovery occurs rapidly in infants treated appropriately, except that the swelling of subperiosteal hemorrhage may require months to disappear. Body growth usually is quickly resumed.

Prevention. Scurvy is prevented by a diet adequate in vitamin C; citrus fruits and juices are excellent sources. Formula-fed infants should be supplied with 35 mg of ascorbic acid daily. Lactating mothers should have a daily intake of 100 mg; 45–60 mg daily is needed by children or adults.

Treatment. The administration of 3–4 ounces of orange juice or tomato juice daily will quickly produce healing, but ascorbic acid is preferable. The daily therapeutic dose is 100–200 mg or more, orally or parenterally.

Irwin MI, Hutchins BK: A conspectus of research on vitamin C requirements in man. J Nutr 106:823, 1976.

3.28 RICKETS OF VITAMIN D DEFICIENCY*

Rickets is the term employed to identify failure in mineralization of growing bone or osteoid tissue. As might be expected, the characteristic early changes are seen roentgenographically at the ends of long bones; there is also evidence of demineralization in the shafts. Subsequently, if healing is not initiated, clinically observable manifestations become apparent (see below). Failure in mineralization of mature bone is termed osteomalacia.

Etiology. Through the 1st third of this century, by far the predominant cause of rickets was nutritional deficiency of vitamin D due to inadequate direct exposure to the ultraviolet rays of sunlight (296–310 nm; these rays do not pass through ordinary window glass) or to inadequate intake of vitamin D or to both. Vitamin D deficiency rickets has been nearly eliminated among infants and children in the industrialized countries by prophylactic means but not in some of the countries of the third world, even though there are ample opportunities for adequate exposure to sunlight in many of them.

Currently in the United States and in other industrialized countries, conditions other than inadequate nutritional prophylaxis with vitamin D are collectively responsible for most of the observed rachitic lesions. These are listed in Sec 23.20, and some of them are described there; references are given for those described in other sections. The clinical varieties include those of genetic origin, such as familial hypophosphatemia (so-called vitamin D–refractory rickets), vitamin dependent rickets (hypocalcemic rickets would be a more appropriate designation), and hypophosphatasia; and those associated with clinical entities that interfere with the metabolic conversion and activation of vitamin D, such as hepatic and renal lesions, or that disrupt calcium and phosphorus homeostasis in other ways.

In spite of considerable elucidation of the metabolism, activation, and actions of vitamin D in man, much is still unknown. Two forms of vitamin D are of practical importance. Vitamin D_2 or calciferol is available as irradiated ergosterol; to a large extent it has replaced the fish liver oils (cod and percomorph) as a source of dietary and therapeutic vitamin D. Vitamin D_3, which is now also available synthetically, is naturally present in human skin in the provitamin stage as 7-dehydrocholesterol. It is activated photochemically to cholecalciferol and transferred to the liver. Each of these irradiated sterols is hydroxylated in the liver to 25-OH cholecalciferol and, subsequently, in the renal cortical cells to 1,25-dihydroxycholecalciferol. This end product is considered to be a hormone. Its antirachitic functions include facilitation of intestinal absorption of calcium and phosphorus and of reabsorption of phosphorus in the kidney and a direct effect on mineral metabolism of bone (deposition and reabsorption). In conjunction with parathormone and calcitonin, it plays a major role in homeostasis of calcium and phosphorus in the body's fluids and tissues.

The diet of infants may contain only small amounts of vitamin D; cow's milk contains only 5–40 IU/quart.* Cereals, vegetables, and fruits contain only negligible amounts. Egg yolk contains 140–390 IU/gm. Most marketed cow's milk is fortified with 400 IU of vitamin D per quart, and most commercially prepared milks for infant formulas are also fortified.

Besides lack of vitamin D in the diet or lack of access of skin to ultraviolet irradiation, several factors may predispose to vitamin D deficiency. Rickets or epiphyseal dysplasia is particularly apt to develop during rapid growth, such as occurs in low birth weight infants and in adolescents. Black children are singularly susceptible to rickets. Whether this is due to the pigmentation of their skin and inadequate penetration of sunlight has not been determined. Children with disorders of absorption, such as celiac disease, steatorrhea, pancreatitis, or cystic fibrosis, may acquire rickets because of deficient absorption of vitamin D and calcium or of both. Anticonvulsant therapy, as for example with the phenytoins or with phenobarbital, may interfere in the metabolism of vitamin D; rickets has been seen with some frequency in institutionalized children receiving such therapy who also have inadequate exposure to sunlight (Sec 23.20). Glucocorticoids appear to be antagonistic to vitamin D in calcium transport.

Pathology. New bone formation is initiated by the osteoblast, which is responsible for matrix deposition and its subsequent mineralization. Osteoblasts secrete collagen, and changes in polysaccharides, phospholipids, alkaline phosphatase, and pyrophosphatase follow until mineralization occurs in the presence of adequate calcium and phosphorus. Resorption of bone occurs when osteoclasts secrete enzymes on the bone surface, dissolving and removing matrix and mineral. Osteocytes covered by bone both resorb and redeposit bone. Factors affecting bone growth are poorly understood, but phosphorus, calcium, fluoride, and growth hormone all have some influence.

Defective growth of bone in rickets results from retardation or suppression of normal growth of epiphyseal cartilage and of normal calcification. These changes

---

*For a review of the rachitic lesions reference should be made to Table 3–5 and Sec 5.10 and 5.14 for calcium and phosphorus metabolism; Sec 3.29 and 5.34 for hypocalcemic tetany; Sec 18.17 for parathormone, vitamin D, and calcitonin activities, and Table 3–6 and Sec 23.20 for additional discussion of vitamin D metabolism and its activities.

---

*1 μg = 40 IU.

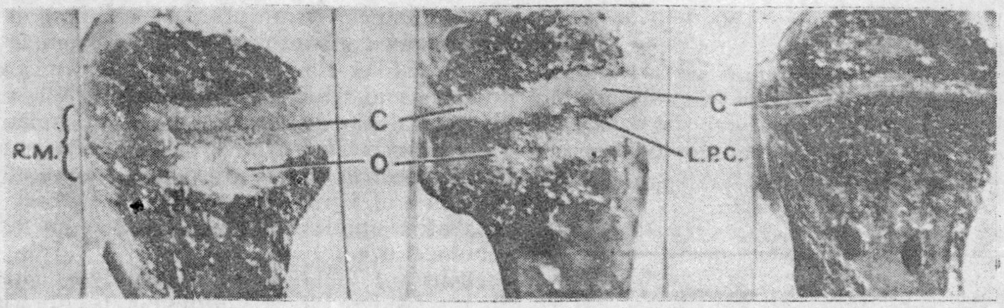

Figure 3–10 Line tests in rats (proximal end of tibia) (calcified tissue stained with silver appears black). *A,* Active rickets. The light broad zone between epiphysis and shaft represents the rachitic metaphysis (R.M.); C, cartilage; O, osteoid. *B,* Healing rickets. Line of preparatory calcification (L.P.C.) between zone of cartilage (C) and osteoid (O). *C,* Healed rickets. Cartilaginous disk (C) between epiphysis and normal shaft.

are dependent upon a deficiency in serum of calcium and phosphorus salts for mineralization. Cartilage cells fail to complete their normal cycle of proliferation and degeneration, and subsequent failure of capillary penetration occurs in a patchy manner. The result is a frayed, irregular epiphyseal line at the end of the shaft. Failure of mineralization of osseous and cartilaginous matrix in the zone of preparatory calcification followed by deposition of newly formed uncalcified osteoid results in a wide, irregular, frayed zone of nonrigid tissue (the rachitic metaphysis) (Fig 3–10). This zone is responsible for many of the skeletal deformities. It becomes compressed and bulges laterally, producing flaring of the ends of the bones and the rachitic rosary (Fig 3–11 and 3–14).

Mineralization is also lacking in subperiosteal bone; pre-existing cortical bone is resorbed in a normal manner but is replaced by osteoid tissues over the entire shaft, which fails to mineralize. If this process continues, the shaft loses its rigidity, and the resulting softened and rarefied cortical bone is readily distorted by stress; deformities and fractures result (Fig 3–14).

Healing Rickets. With healing, degeneration of cartilage cells occurs along the metaphyseal-diaphyseal border, capillary penetration of the resultant spaces is resumed, and calcification takes place in the zone of preparatory calcification. This calcification occurs approximately at the line at which normal calcification would have occurred had the rachitic process not supervened and produces a line clearly demonstrable in roentgenograms (Fig 3–15*A* and 3–15*B*). As healing progresses, the osteoid tissue between this line of preparatory calcification and the diaphysis also becomes mineralized (Fig 3–10). Osteoid tissue in the cortex and about the trabeculae in the shaft rapidly becomes mineralized. Months or years may be required to repair the deformities, and in extreme instances complete repair may be impossible.

Chemical Pathology. In healthy infants the inorganic serum phosphorus concentration is 4.5–6.5 mg/dl, whereas in rachitic infants it is usually reduced to 1.5–3.5 mg/dl. The serum calcium level is usually normal, but under certain conditions it too is reduced, and tetany may develop.

Vitamin D–deficient rickets can be understood if one assumes it to be an attempt of the body to maintain normal serum calcium levels, presumably because calcium is necessary for normal function of nerve, muscle, and endocrine glands and for intercellular bridging. In the absence of vitamin D, less calcium is absorbed from the intestine. With slightly lowered serum calcium, parathormone is secreted. This leads to mobilization of calcium and phosphorus from the bone. The serum calcium concentration is thus maintained, but secondary effects occur, which include the changes of rickets in bone, the lowered serum phosphorus concentration (because parathormone decreases phosphorus reabsorption in the kidney), and elevated serum phosphatase (due to increased osteoblastic activity).

The alkaline phosphatase of serum, which in normal children is less than 200 IU/dl, is elevated in mild rickets to more than 500 IU/dl. As rickets heals, the phosphatase value returns slowly to the normal range. Serum alkaline phosphatase may be normal in infants with rickets who are protein and/or zinc depleted.

Calcium and phosphorus homeostasis depends on the intestinal absorption of dietary calcium and phosphorus. Maximum calcium absorption occurs in man when the ratio of calcium to phosphorus in the diet is about 2:1; increase in phosphate decreases absorption of calcium. Acidity of intestinal contents increases absorption of calcium. An increase in calcium absorption also occurs when lactose is the dietary sugar. Chelating agents such as ethylenediaminetetraacetic acid (EDTA) or the phytates of cereals may decrease calcium absorption, and dietary iron may decrease absorption of phosphate. High dietary levels of stearic and palmitic acids, which are poorly absorbed, also decrease calcium absorption.

Calcium absorption is facilitated by 1,25-dihydroxycholecalciferol or similar hydroxylated forms of vitamin D. Calcium deficiency alone rarely leads to the failure of calcification as seen in rickets and osteomalacia; it results in a diminished amount of bone.

Vitamin D deficiency is also accompanied by generalized aminoaciduria, a decrease of citrate in bone and increased urinary excretion of it, decreased ability of the kidneys to make an acid urine, phosphaturia, and, occasionally, mellituria. The parathyroid glands hypertrophy in rickets, and urinary cyclic AMP is increased.

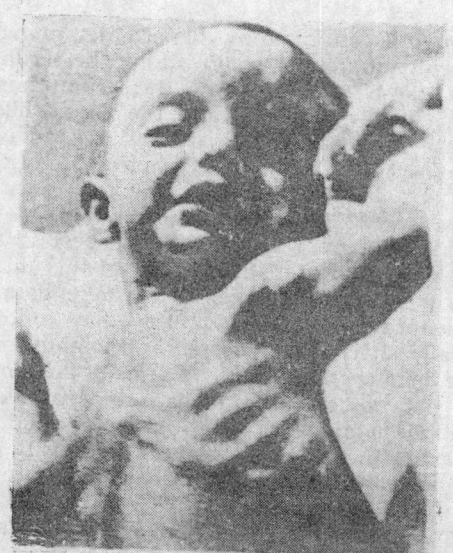

Figure 3–11 Rachitic rosary in a young infant. (Lyons and Wallinger: Pediatrics and Pediatric Nursing.)

Clinical Manifestations. Osseous changes of rickets can be recognized after several months of vitamin D deficiency. In breast-fed infants whose mothers have osteomalacia, rickets may develop within 2 mo. Florid rickets becomes apparent toward the end of the 1st and during the 2nd yr of life. In later childhood manifest vitamin D–deficient rickets is rare.

One of the early signs of rickets is craniotabes. It is due to thinning of the inner table of the skull and is detected by pressing firmly over the occiput or posterior parietal bones. A ping-pong ball sensation will be felt. Craniotabes near the suture lines is a normal variant. Low birth weight infants are particularly prone to early development of rickets and to craniotabes. Palpable enlargement of the costochondral junctions (the "rachitic rosary") (Fig 3–11) and thickening of the wrists and ankles (Fig 3–14) are other early evidences of osseous changes. Increased sweating, particularly around the head, may also be present.

Advanced Rickets. Signs of advanced rickets are easily recognized.

HEAD. Craniotabes may disappear before the end of the 1st yr, though the rachitic process continues. The softness of the skull may result in flattening and, at times, permanent asymmetry of the head. The anterior fontanel is larger than normal; its closure may be delayed until after the 2nd yr of life. The central parts of the parietal and frontal bones are often thickened, forming prominences or bosses, which give the head a boxlike appearance (caput quadratum). The head may be larger than normal and may remain so throughout life. Eruption of the temporary teeth may be delayed, and there may be defects of the enamel and extensive caries. The permanent teeth which are calcifying may be affected; usually, the permanent incisors, canines, and first molars show defects of the enamel.

THORAX. Enlargement of the costochondral junctions may become prominent; the beading of the ribs is not only palpable but also visible (Fig 3–11). The sides of the thorax become flattened, and the longitudinal grooves develop posterior to the rosary. The sternum with its adjacent cartilages appears to be projected forward, producing the so-called pigeon breast deformity. Along the lower border of the chest there develops a horizontal depression, Harrison groove (Fig 3–12), which corresponds to the costal insertions of the diaphragm. There may be a variety of other thoracic deformities, including those of the shoulder girdle.

SPINAL COLUMN. Slight to moderate degrees of lateral curvature (scoliosis) are common, and a kyphosis may appear in the dorsolumbar region of rachitic children who sit up (Fig 3–13). Lordosis of the lumbar region may be seen in the erect position.

PELVIS. In children with lordosis there is frequently a concomitant deformity of the pelvis, which is also retarded in growth. The pelvic entrance is narrowed by a forward projection of the promontory, the exit, by a forward displacement of the caudal part of the sacrum and the coccyx. In the female these changes, if they become permanent, add to the hazards of childbirth and may necessitate cesarean section.

EXTREMITIES. As the rachitic process continues, the epiphyseal enlargement at the wrists and ankles becomes more noticeable. The enlarged epiphyses can be seen (Fig 3–14) or palpated but are not distinct in roentgenograms since they consist of cartilage and uncalcified osteoid tissue. Bending of the softened shafts of the femur, tibia, and fibula results in bowlegs or knock knees; the femur and the tibia may also acquire an anterior convexity. Coxa vara is sometimes the result of rickets. Greenstick fractures occur in the long bones; often there are no clinical symptoms.

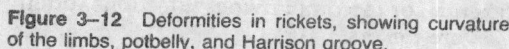

Figure 3–12 Deformities in rickets, showing curvature of the limbs, potbelly, and Harrison groove.

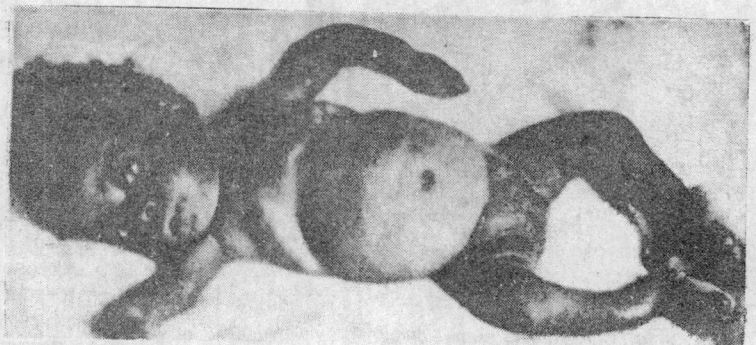

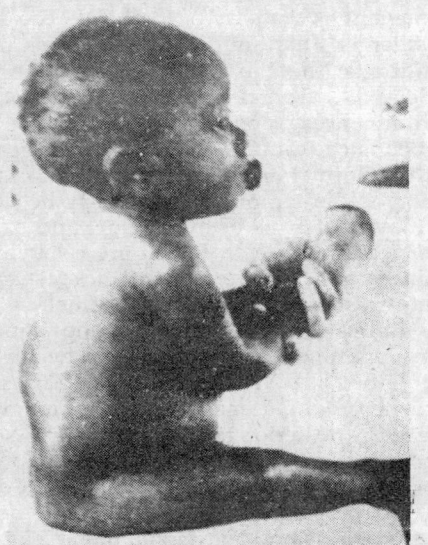

Figure 3–13 Rachitic spinal curvature, well marked when the child is sitting.

Deformities of the spine, pelvis, and legs result in reduction in stature, rachitic dwarfism.

LIGAMENTS. Relaxation of ligaments contributes to production of deformities and partly accounts for knock knees, overextension of the knee joints, weak ankles, kyphosis, and scoliosis.

MUSCLES. The muscles are poorly developed and lacking in tone. As a result, children with moderately severe rickets are late in standing and walking. The common condition of potbelly (Fig 3–12 and 3–14) depends to a large extent upon weakness of the abdominal muscles; weakness of the gastric and intestinal walls may be contributory.

Diagnosis. The diagnosis of rickets is based on a history of inadequate intake of vitamin D and on clinical

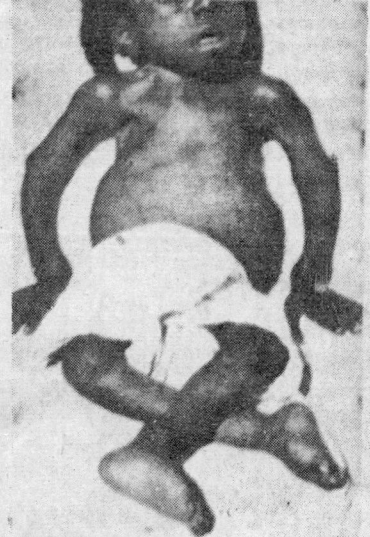

Figure 3–14 Curvature of arms, deformed "violin-shaped" chest, potbelly, enlarged epiphyses in a child 3 yr of age.

observation; it is confirmed by chemical determinations and by roentgenographic examination. The serum calcium level may be normal or low, the serum phosphorus level is below 4 mg/dl, and the serum alkaline phosphatase is elevated. Urinary cyclic AMP is elevated, and serum 1,25-dihydroxycholecalciferol is decreased.

Roentgenographic Changes (Fig 3–15). ACTIVE RICKETS. A roentgenogram of the wrist is best for early diagnosis since characteristic changes of the ulna and radius occur at an early stage. The distal ends appear widened, concave (cupping), and frayed, in contrast to the normally sharply demarcated and slightly convex ends. The distance from the distal ends of the ulna and radius to the metacarpal bones is increased since the large rachitic metaphysis, which is not calcified, does not appear on the roentgenogram. The density of the shafts is decreased, but the trabeculae are unusually prominent.

HEALING RICKETS (Fig 3–15). Initial healing is indicated by the appearance of the line of preparatory calcification. This line is separated from the distal end of the shaft by a zone of decreased calcification, the zone of the osteoid tissue. As healing progresses and the osteoid tissue becomes calcified, the shaft "grows" toward the line of preparatory calcification until it becomes united with it.

Differential Diagnosis. Nonrachitic craniotabes, at times present in the immediate postnatal period, tends to disappear before rachitic softening of the skull would become manifest (2nd–4th mo of life). Craniotabes also occurs in hydrocephalus and osteogenesis imperfecta, but it is not difficult to differentiate these conditions from rickets.

Enlargement of the costochondral junctions occurs in rickets, scurvy, and chondrodystrophy. The enlargements in rickets are rounded knobs, whereas in scurvy there is a ledgelike depression with the chondral or sternal portion displaced below the osseous ribs. In chondrodystrophy there may be irregular concave outlines of the distal ends of the bones, but there is no roentgenographic evidence of fraying. Other epiphyseal lesions that may require differentiation include congenital epiphyseal dysplasia, cytomegalic inclusion disease, syphilis, rubella, and copper deficiency. It is sometimes difficult to distinguish rachitic deformities of the chest from congenital ones. Bowlegs can be the result of rickets but may be a familial characteristic. Vitamin D–resistant rickets and other metabolic disturbances with osseous lesions resembling rickets must also be differentiated (Sec 23.20).

Complications. Respiratory infections such as bronchitis and bronchopneumonia are common in rachitic infants, and pulmonary atelectasis is frequently associated with severe deformities of the chest. Anemia due to iron deficiency or accompanying infections often develops in severe rickets.

Prognosis. If sufficient amounts of vitamin D are administered, healing begins within a few days and progresses slowly until the normal bony structure is restored. In many instances, the enlargement of the epiphyses of the long bones, including the ribs, and the deformities of the skull disappear only after months

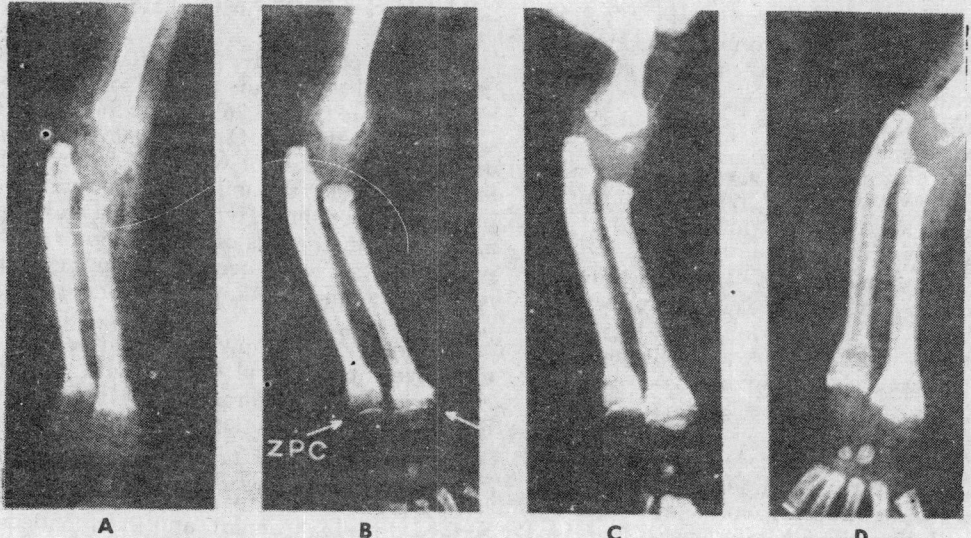

Figure 3–15 *A,* Active rickets; cupping and fraying of distal ends of radius and ulna; double contour along lateral outline of radius (periosteal osteoid). The 2 dense zones in the shaft of the ulna are calluses of greenstick fractures. *B,* Healing rickets after 12 days of treatment with vitamin D. Zones of preparatory calcification (ZPC); above them in the rachitic metaphyses there is beginning calcification. *C,* Healing rickets after 18 days of treatment. The zones of preparatory calcification are well defined, and the rachitic metaphyses appear well calcified. The epiphysis of the radius has become visible. *D,* Healing rickets after 29 days of treatment. Zones of preparatory calcification, rachitic metaphyses, and shafts have become united.

or years of treatment. Even rather severe bowing of the legs may disappear within several years without osteotomies. In advanced cases there may be permanent osseous alterations in the form of bowlegs, knock knees, curvature of the upper arms, deformities of the chest and spine, rachitic pelvis and coxa vara, and dwarfism.

Rickets in itself is not a fatal disease, but complications and intercurrent infections such as pneumonia, tuberculosis, and enteritis are more likely to cause death in rachitic than in normal children.

Prevention. Rickets can be prevented by exposure to ultraviolet light or by oral administration of vitamin D. Sunlight, as a prophylactic agent, can be considered effective in the temperate zones only during the summer months in haze-free areas.

The daily requirement of vitamin D is 10 μg or 400 IU/day. Much of the whole milk available in urban areas and evaporated milk are fortified by the addition of vitamin D concentrate so that 1 quart of fresh, whole milk or a can of evaporated milk contains this amount. Prematurely born infants or breast-fed infants whose mothers are not exposed to adequate sunlight should receive supplemental vitamin D daily.

Vitamin D should also be administered to pregnant and lactating mothers.

Treatment. Natural and artificial light are effective therapeutically, but oral administration of vitamin D is preferred. The daily administration of 50–150 μg or 0.5–2 μg of 1α- or 1,25-dihydroxycholecalciferol will produce healing demonstrable on roentgenograms within 2–4 wk except in the unusual cases of vitamin D–refractory rickets.

The administration of 1500 μg of vitamin D in a single dose, without further therapy for several months, may be advantageous. This is followed by more rapid healing, possibly earlier differential diagnosis from geneti-

cally vitamin D–resistant rickets, and less dependence on the parents for the daily administration of the vitamin. If no healing occurs, the rickets is probably resistant to vitamin D (Sec 23.20). After healing is complete, the dose of vitamin D should be lowered to 10 μg daily.

DeLuca HF: Some new concepts emanating from a study of the metabolism and function of vitamin D. Nutr Rev 38:169, 1980.
Harrison HE, Harrison HC: Rickets then and now. J Pediatr 87:1144, 1975.
Raisz LG: Physiologic and pharmacologic regulations of bone resorption. N Engl J Med 282:909, 1970.
Rasmussen H: Cell communication, calcium ion, and cyclic adenosine monophosphate. Science 170:404, 1970.
Root AW, Harrison HE: Recent advances in calcium metabolism. I. Mechanisms of calcium homeostasis. II. Disorders of calcium homeostasis. J Pediatr 88:1, 177, 1976.

3.29 TETANY OF VITAMIN D DEFICIENCY
(Infantile Tetany)

See also Sec 5.33.

Tetany due to deficiency of vitamin D is an occasional accompaniment of rickets. Formerly relatively common, it is now rare, due to the widespread prophylactic use of vitamin D. Occasionally, it is observed in association with celiac disease, probably as a result of deficient absorption of both vitamin D and calcium. Tetany of vitamin D deficiency occurs most frequently between the ages of 4 mo and 3 yr.

Chemical Pathology. When the serum calcium concentration falls below 7–7.5 mg/dl, there is muscular irritability, apparently due to the loss of the inhibitory control that ionized calcium of the serum exerts upon the neuromuscular junctions. Why serum calcium is occasionally decreased in association with rickets is not clear; failure of the parathyroids to compensate for the low serum calcium level may be a factor.

Clinical Manifestations. The symptoms are those of tetany, irrespective of the cause. Vitamin D–deficient tetany may exist in either a latent or a clinically manifest stage. In practically all instances there are concurrent manifestations of rickets.

Latent Tetany. Symptoms are not evident, but they can be elicited by means of the Chvostek, Trousseau, and Erb procedures. The serum calcium level is less than 7–7.5 mg/dl.

Manifest Tetany. Spontaneous clinical manifestations include carpopedal spasm, laryngospasm, and convulsions. The serum calcium level is often well under 7 mg/dl.

Diagnosis. The diagnosis is based on the combination of rickets, low serum calcium level, and the symptoms of tetany. The serum phosphorus level is usually low; the serum alkaline phosphatase level is increased. In the differential diagnosis causes of tetany such as hypoparathyroidism, hypomagnesemia, and ingestion of phenothiazine must be eliminated.

Prognosis. The prognosis is good unless treatment is delayed. Death rarely occurs in tetany, though it may result from laryngospasm and possibly from cardiac dilatation, as so-called cardiac tetany.

Prevention. Prophylactic treatment is identical to that for rickets (see above).

Treatment. Active treatment is designed to raise the serum calcium above the tetany level. This level may be attained by administration of calcium chloride in 1–2% solution in milk. For the 1st day or 2, 4–6 gm daily may be given in 1-gm doses, the initial dose being 2–3 gm; smaller doses of 1–3 gm a day should then be continued for 1 or 2 wk. Calcium chloride in more concentrated solution may cause severe gastric ulceration, and large doses may cause acidosis. Calcium lactate may be added to milk in doses of 10–12 gm a day for 10 days. When oral medication is impractical, calcium gluconate (5–10 ml of a 10% solution) can be administered intravenously but not subcutaneously or intramuscularly because of the dangers of local necrosis.

Oxygen inhalation is indicated during convulsive seizures. When intravenous administration of calcium gluconate does not quickly control the attacks, sodium phenobarbital may be given intramuscularly. Prolonged attacks of laryngospasm are usually controlled by sedation and the administration of calcium salts. Intubation is only occasionally necessary. After the acute manifestations have been controlled, administration of vitamin D in daily doses of 50–100 μg should be started and the oral administration of calcium continued (see above). When the rickets is healed, the dose of vitamin D should be decreased to the usual prophylactic one.

Fraser D, Kook SW, Scriver CR: Hyperparathyroidism as the cause of hyperaminoaciduria and phosphaturia in human vitamin D deficiency. Pediatr Res 1:425, 1967.

3.30 HYPERVITAMINOSIS D

Ingestion of excessive amounts of vitamin D results in signs and symptoms similar to those of idiopathic hypercalcemia (Sec 23.26), which may be due to hypersensitivity to vitamin D. Symptoms develop after 1–3 mo of large intakes of vitamin D; they include hypotonia, anorexia, irritability, constipation, polydipsia, polyuria, and pallor. Hypercalcemia and hypercalciuria are notable. Evidences of dehydration are usually present. Aortic valvular stenosis, vomiting, hypertension, retinopathy, and clouding of the cornea and conjunctiva may occur.

The urine may show proteinuria. With continued excessive intake, renal damage and metastatic calcification occur. Roentgenograms of the long bones reveal metastatic calcification and generalized osteoporosis.

Excessive intake of vitamin D may result from inadvertently substituting a concentrated form of vitamin D for a more dilute preparation, from increase of a prescribed dose by a parent, and from inadequate control of dosage in children receiving large amounts of vitamin D for chronic hyperphosphatemic states (Sec 23.21).

Differential Diagnosis. Metastatic calcification occurs in chronic nephritis, hyperparathyroidism, and idiopathic hypercalcemia. The latter two are accompanied by hypercalcemia.

Prevention. Prevention requires careful evaluation of vitamin D dosage.

Treatment. This includes discontinuance of vitamin D intake and a decrease in intake of calcium. For severely involved infants, aluminum hydroxide by mouth, cortisone, or sodium versenate may be used.

Forbes GB, Cafarelli C, Manning J: Vitamin D and infantile hypercalcemia. Pediatrics 42:203, 1968.

3.31 VITAMIN E DEFICIENCY

Vitamin E deficiency leads to varied effects in different animal species. It is a fat-soluble antioxidant and may be involved in nucleic acid metabolism. No precise biochemical action of vitamin E (α-tocopherol) has been found; it resembles in many of its actions ubiquinone (coenzyme Q) but is structurally unrelated. Vitamin E is present in many foods (Table 3–6).

Deficiency may occur in malabsorption states such as cystic fibrosis and acanthocytosis. Diets with a high unsaturated fatty acid content increase the vitamin E requirement in premature infants who absorb vitamin E poorly. Excess iron administration exaggerates signs of vitamin E deficiency.

Some patients deficient in vitamin E have creatinuria, ceroid deposition in smooth muscle, focal necrosis of striated muscle, and muscle weakness. Some improvement may occur after administration of vitamin E. Vitamin E deficiency has been suggested as a causative factor in the anemia of kwashiorkor. Premature infants may have low serum levels of tocopherol, with development of a hemolytic anemia at 6–10 wk of age which is corrected by administration of vitamin E.

Platelet adhesiveness is increased in deficiency states, and platelet levels in the blood are increased. Treatment of hemolysis in glucose-6-phosphate dehydrogenase deficiency, of sickle cell anemia, of leg cramps, or of coronary artery disease represents unsubstantiated use of vitamin E.

Diagnosis. If vitamin E has recently been administered, 3 days should elapse before determining blood levels, as oral vitamin E may circulate for 1–2 days. An in vitro test adds peroxide to the patient's erythrocytes, the susceptibility of the red cells to hemolysis reflecting the vitamin E status.

Prevention. Minimal daily requirements of vitamin E are not known; 0.7 mg/gm of unsaturated fat in the diet appears adequate. Intake should be increased in children with deficient fat absorption. Premature infants may be given 15–25 IU/24 hr.

Gross S: Hemolytic anemia in premature infants: Relationship to vitamin E, selenium, glutathione peroxidase, and erythrocyte lipids. Sem Hemat 13:187, 1976.

3.32 VITAMIN K DEFICIENCY

Vitamin K is a naphthoquinone that participates in oxidative phosphorylation. Absence of the vitamin or failure of its absorption from the intestinal tract results in hypoprothrombinemia and decreased hepatic synthesis of proconvertin. Prothrombin (factor II) and proconvertin (factor VII) are important to the 2nd stage of coagulation (Sec 14.59). The 2nd stage of coagulation is studied by the 1-stage prothrombin time (Quick). Administration of vitamin K to the newborn infant increases concentrations of prothrombin, proconvertin, plasma thromboplastin component (factor IX,PTC), and Stuart-Prower factor (factor X). Vitamin K–dependent calcium binding proteins promote phospholipid interactions in coagulation and in calcium metabolism.

Sources of Vitamin K. Naturally occurring vitamin K is fat soluble; it is found in high concentrations in hog's liver, soybeans, and alfalfa and in smaller amounts in some vegetables such as spinach, tomatoes, and kale. The natural vitamin (2-methyl-3-phytyl-1,4-naphthoquinone) has been labeled vitamin K_1 to distinguish it from synthetic naphthoquinones with vitamin K activity.

Many bacteria, including normal intestinal flora, are capable of synthesizing quinones with vitamin K activity. Suppression of intestinal bacteria by various antibiotics may be responsible for vitamin K deficiency, with resultant diminution of prothrombin. Irradiated

foods have produced vitamin K deficiency in animals. Cow's milk has more vitamin K than human milk.

Clinical Manifestations. Deficiency of vitamin K or hypoprothrombinemia should be considered in all patients with a hemorrhagic disturbance. The incidence of hemorrhagic disease of the newborn (Sec 7.46) has been sharply decreased by the prophylactic administration of vitamin K. Vitamin K deficiency in childhood is usually due to factors affecting absorption or utilization of fat or to factors limiting synthesis of vitamin K in the intestine, such as prolonged use of antibiotics. Diarrhea in infants, particularly breast-fed ones, may cause vitamin K deficiency. Diseases of the liver may lead to hypoprothrombinemia, which does not usually respond to administration of vitamin K.

Hypoprothrombinemia may also result from administration of certain drugs. Dicumarol, obtained from spoiled sweet clover, is used specifically for the production of hypoprothrombinemia in the prevention and treatment of venous thrombosis. Bishydroxycoumarin (dicumarol) is thought to prevent the liver from utilizing vitamin K without exerting an effect on prothrombin. Blood prothrombin is continually destroyed in the body; since dicumarol prevents its replacement, a fall in prothrombin occurs. If a dangerously low level results, massive doses of vitamin K_1 may be necessary to restore prothrombin, and whole blood transfusions may also be necessary.

Salicylic acid, a degradation product of dicumarol, produces hypoprothrombinemia by similar action. The fall in prothrombin resulting from the use of salicylates, however, is only mild in comparison with that of dicumarol. The hemorrhagic manifestations in acute rheumatic fever may be due in some instances to large doses of salicylates; vitamin K is effective in neutralizing this action. Its use in children receiving large doses of salicylates would appear to be justified.

Treatment. Mild prothrombin deficiency may be corrected by oral administration of vitamin K. One to 2 mg daily for an infant will usually suffice. If prothrombin deficiency is severe and hemorrhagic manifestations have appeared, 5 mg of vitamin K_1 daily should be given parenterally. Large doses of synthetic vitamin K analogues, but not of vitamin K_1, may result in hyperbilirubinemia and kernicterus in the glucose-6-phosphate dehydrogenase (G-6-PD)–deficient newborn and in the premature infant. When hypoprothrombinemia is due to liver damage, vitamin K_1 may be given, but whole blood is usually also necessary.

LEWIS A. BARNESS

Corrigan JJ: The vitamin K dependent proteins. Adv Pediatr 28:57, 1981.

4 PREVENTIVE PEDIATRICS AND EPIDEMIOLOGY

Preventive pediatrics comprises efforts to avert rather than to cure disease and disability. Traditionally, preventive medicine has been subdivided into primary, secondary, and tertiary prevention. Primary prevention, such as tetanus immunization or chlorination of water supplies, attempts to avoid disease before it begins. Secondary prevention involves the recognition and elimination of the precursors of disease and includes many screening programs such as those for elevated blood lead levels and the Pap smear; also included are efforts designed to identify and reverse disease in its early stages such as a screening program for scoliosis in adolescents. Tertiary prevention includes measures intended to ameliorate or arrest the disabilities arising from established disease, e.g., physiotherapy to prevent contractures in patients with chronic neurologic disorders.

The basic requirement for almost every successful primary preventive measure in pediatrics is understanding the cause, pathogenesis, and natural history of disease. In contrast, for secondary or tertiary prevention, knowledge of the natural history of the disease and of the means to recognize and treat it are necessary, but definition of the cause is not essential.

Remarkable changes have occurred in the emphases and priorities in child health in the United States during this century; many are a result of primary preventive medicine. Table 4-1 shows that the infant mortality rate was 162/1000 in 1900 compared to 14.9 in 1977; the provisional rate for 1980 was 12.5. In 1900, 53% of infant mortality was ascribed to infection; in 1977, under 10%. Because of the striking diminution of infant deaths due to controllable causes, certain other conditions loom proportionately larger in importance now than in the past. For example, congenital anomalies were respon-sible for 3% of infant deaths in 1900 and 18% in 1977. Similarly, there is no reason to believe that the sudden infant death syndrome has increased in frequency in recent years; it is now identified as causing between one sixth and one fourth of all infant deaths because of the declining mortality from other conditions. The death rate in the United States for children 1–4 yr of age decreased by more than 95% from 1900–1977 (Table 4-1). The major factor in the overall reduction in death rate has been the reduction of death due to infections. Neoplastic diseases, congenital anomalies, and violence, which caused less than 5% of all deaths in this age group in 1900, were the primary cause in 65% in 1977 and thus now are proportionately of much greater importance without an actual increase in incidence.

The reasons for these remarkable reductions in childhood mortality are multiple and include sanitary water supplies, hygienic food handling (especially of milk), nutrition, anti-infective drugs, active immunization, and social and economic improvements. Moreover, mortality from some diseases declined remarkably in the United States in the absence of any effective preventive or specific therapeutic measure. As an example, crude mortality rates from measles gradually declined 98% (from 13.3–0.3 per 100 000) from 1900–1955 before the advent of measles vaccine.

As a consequence of the decline in mortality, there have been remarkable changes in emphases in pediatric practices. With the major exception of accident prevention, there is little that pediatricians can do currently to reduce the residual mortality beyond tertiary care for malignant neoplasms, congenital anomalies, and neonatal problems, including prematurity. Thus increasing emphasis is placed on maintaining and enhancing the *quality* of life of children and on ensuring that each

Table 4-1 CERTAIN CAUSES OF DEATH OF U.S. CHILDREN LESS THAN 1 YEAR AND 1 TO 4 YEARS OF AGE, 1900 AND 1977

| ALL CAUSES (DEATHS/100,000) | 0–1 YEAR | | 1–4 YEARS | |
	1900	1977	1900	1977
	16,200	1486	1980	69
SPECIFIC CAUSES	%	%	%	%
Infections	53	9	84	12
Enteric infections	26	1	17	1
Tuberculosis	2	<1	5	<1
Neoplasms	<1	<1	<1	8
Congenital anomalies	3	18	<1	13
Perinatal	24	50	—	—
Violence	2	3	4	44
Homicide	<1	<1	<1	4
All other	21	18	12	24

Rates are deaths/100,000 children. Percentages are % of total deaths by age group. Data for 1900 are from Death Registration Areas only.

child reaches adult life as physically, intellectually, and emotionally intact and prepared as possible. Thus, such activities as anticipatory guidance, developmental counseling, assisting families with children's school-related problems, sexual counseling, secondary prevention by screening for incipient disease, and attempts to ameliorate the precursors of adult disease have become part of the pediatric practice.

4.1 PRIMARY PREVENTION

Primary prevention occurs both at the community level and in the pediatrician's office.

Community Primary Prevention. Several measures to prevent disease at the community level have had enormous effects on childhood morbidity and mortality in the United States: sewage disposal and sanitation of water, hygienic control of food including pasteurization of milk, iodination of salt, and control of arthropod vectors of disease (such as mosquito control by swamp drainage in malarial areas). In areas of the world where development of these measures is still incomplete, the spectrum of childhood mortality resembles that in the United States in 1900.

A number of other public health programs are of proven merit but have not been universally adopted.

Fluoridation of public water supplies is efficacious in reducing dental caries. Its safety and high benefit to cost ratio are well established. However, fluoridated water is currently available to only about half of all infants and children in the United States because about 20% of the population live in areas without communal water supplies and 30% or more reside in communities where fluoridation, although feasible, has not been instituted for social, political, or economic reasons. Community fluoridation programs should be supported. In unfluoridated areas school programs should be established to provide fluoride tablets or rinses as alternative approaches. Additional measures include fluoride supplements from birth as well as parent education.

Rat control is important in both rural and urban areas. Federally supported inner city rat control programs, initiated in 1969, resulted in eradication of rats by 1981 from neighborhoods in which approximately 7 million people resided. These programs, directed primarily at environmental cleanup and sanitation and secondarily at extermination by baiting, require local support for continuation after federal grants terminate. They should be continued and expanded. Unfortunately, rural rat control is more difficult to achieve.

Pasteurization of milk will prevent outbreaks of diarrheal disease caused by contaminating pathogenic bacteria. However, recent interest in "natural foods" among some segments of the population in the United States has led to increased consumption of ptw milk under the fallacious assumption that it is nutritionally superior to pasteurized milk. As a consequence, local outbreaks of diarrheal disease, including fatalities, have occurred due to strains of *Salmonella* and *Campylobacter* transmitted by milk. Pediatricians should educate par-

Table 4-2 DEATHS FROM EXTERNAL CAUSES, PERSONS 1-19 YEARS, U.S., 1977

| | AGE GROUPS | | | | |
	1-4	5-9	10-14	15-19	Total 1-19
All causes (no.)	8307	5834	6745	21,443	42,329
Accidents (%)	40	50	50	59	53
Suicide (%)	--	—	3	9	5
Homicide (%)	4	3	4	9	6
All violence (%)	44	53	57	77	64

Source: U.S. Vital Statistics.
Accidental poisoning included under accidents.

ents and local authorities concerning the risks of raw milk (certified or not).

Accidents (Sec 5.43) and *homicide* (Chapter 1) result in nearly two thirds of all deaths in children from 1-9 yr of age (Table 4-2). Nonfatal injuries, including poisoning, account for considerable acute childhood morbidity (Table 4-3), and many of these injuries result in permanent disability.

Prevention of accidents is difficult because of the diversity of childhood injuries. Three approaches to primary prevention of accidents in childhood have been explored in recent years. The 1st of these is public health education such as encouraging "childproofing" of the home or using car restraints for infants. Unfortunately, the few well-designed clinical trials that have been conducted have failed to show a salutary effect. A 2nd approach is a change in the environment of children, either mandated by law or voluntarily built in by manufacturers; such changes include flame-resistant fabrics, childproof containers, paint of minimum lead count, window guards for apartment buildings, safe spacing of crib rails, and others. These measures have been far more effective than public education.

A 3rd effective approach consists of one-on-one parent education by the child's physician, although this measure is utilized far too infrequently by pediatricians. To provide effective parental guidance, the physician should be aware of the household risk factors and the propensities of children at various ages for different types of accidents (Sec 5.43) and should urge parents to reduce these risks by such means as childproofing

Table 4-3 MORBIDITY IN CHILDREN FROM ACUTE INJURY,* INCLUDING POISONING, AND FROM ALL OTHER CONDITIONS, U.S., 1978

| | RATE/100 CHILDREN/YEAR | |
	0-5 Years	6-16 Years
Injuries	33.5 (8.6%)†	39.6 (14.5%)
Days of limited activity	50.3 (4.3%)	156.2 (17.5%)
Days of bed disability	17.6 (3.1%)	31.5 (7.0%)
School days lost		42.1 (8.8%)

*Acute injury is defined as any injury, including poisoning, requiring medical attention or resulting in 1 or more days of restricted activity.
†Percentage of all acute conditions, such as respiratory infections, etc.

Current estimates from the Health Interview Survey, United States, 1978, Series 10, Number 130, National Center for Health Statistics.

the house when there are toddlers about. Of particular importance are the medicine cabinet; areas where toxic household chemicals such as solvents, furniture polish, and the like are stored; the stove; matches; electrical wires and devices; and sharp objects such as glassware and knives. Outside the home the automobile and unprotected bodies of water endanger toddlers.

For older children and adolescents accident prevention requires a proper balance between excessive restriction and undue permissiveness. Most sports, whether competitive or not, are associated with some jeopardy, though usually minor. Some competitive sports, such as football and hockey, present greater risk; proper equipment, supervision, and instruction are required to minimize these risks. The risk of the trampoline is so great that it should not be available to children. Pediatricians should assume community responsibilities for certain aspects of accident prevention such as ensuring that playgrounds are reasonably safe and that sports programs are adequately supervised. Under some circumstances development and advocacy of mandatory regulations at the community or state level are indicated.

Poisoning has become a relatively more important child health problem as others have been ameliorated. In Greater Cleveland for the years 1971–1974, accidental poisoning was responsible for 3.1% of all hospital admissions and 2.2% of total hospital days for children 1–4 yr. In 1976 in the United States 115 children 1–4 yr died from accidental poisoning, accounting for 1.3% of deaths in this age group. Pediatricians should work for primary prevention of accidental poisoning not only in their offices but also in the community by supporting education of parents, childproof containers, proper storage and disposal of toxic substances, and the like. The poison control centers that have been developed since World War II represent preventive efforts at all levels: community education, emergency treatment before symptoms occur, and tertiary care for the symptomatic child. Poison control centers should provide immediacy of response and complete, up-to-date, accurate information and advice.

An alternative to the complete but self-contained, locally operated centers in smaller communities is the establishment of telephone linkage with highly sophisticated, round-the-clock services available in some large cities. Pediatricians should assume leadership in ensuring that poison control programs in their communities meet the above criteria.

Additionally, pediatricians should participate in developing approaches to 3 major community problems for which satisfactory solutions are not currently defined. These include homicide, adolescent pregnancy, and substance abuse.

The importance of *homicide* is shown in Table 4–2, which indicates that 6% of all deaths in individuals 1–19 yr of age resulted from murder in 1977, including 1 of every 11 deaths among those 15–19 yr of age. Mortality rates from homicide among persons 10–19 yr old increased 2½ times in the 25 yr from 1951–1976. In 1951 half of all murders of persons 10–19 yr old were committed with guns; in 1976 two thirds were so caused. The problem is particularly important among young Blacks, whose homicide rates at 10–19 yr are 4–5 times those of whites; males represent 80% of black homicides in this age group. The overall homicide rate among whites has increased 3-fold since 1951, compared to 2-fold in Blacks. How much permanent disability occurs in survivors of gunshot wounds can only be speculated. There is no easy, acceptable solution to this problem, though many believe that primary preventive measures such as licensing handguns or other forms of gun control and stringent penalties for misuse of firearms are necessary. Whatever the ultimate solutions, pediatricians should warn parents of the dangers associated with access to firearms and should participate in developing a public solution.

Adolescent Pregnancy. A problem that involves all aspects of prevention (primary, secondary, and tertiary) is that of sexuality and consequent pregnancy in adolescents. Teenage pregnancy causes major social, psychologic, educational, and financial burdens for the young parent(s). The infant of a teenage mother is at enhanced risk physically and developmentally, although, after adjustment for socioeconomic status and prenatal care, the only immediate consequences attributable to maternal youth are increases in preeclampsia and in low birth weight infants. In recent years rates of live births to teenage females have decreased slightly but absolute numbers of births to teenagers have not because of increases in the adolescent population. Fertility rates for girls under 15 yr, however, have changed very little since the mid-1970's, prior to which they rose rapidly. About 25,000 pregnancies occur annually in this age group in the United States; slightly more than half are terminated by abortion. About 1 female adolescent in 10 is pregnant before her 20th birthday.

The multiple and complex reasons for teenage pregnancies make control difficult to achieve. Moreover, not all are accidental. Though precise data are not available, teenage sexual activity and pregnancy affect all population groups, but pregnancy appears to occur more frequently in lower socioeconomic groups.

The optimal solution to the problem would be the reduction or avoidance of sexual activity during adolescence. Because this goal is unattainable, most efforts have been directed at encouraging and facilitating the use of contraceptives by teenagers (Sec 19.10). The key factors of the few programs that could be evaluated and did appear to be successful have been outreach, nonjudgmental counseling to reduce ambivalent feelings about pregnancy and contraceptives, and making contraceptives readily available. For pregnant teenagers counseling about options and encouraging regular prenatal care are important, as are helping to develop plans for care of the infant, continuing the mother's education, and preventing repeat pregnancies until maturity.

Substance abuse is discussed in Sec 19.13.

Primary Prevention in the Pediatrician's Office. The purposes of routine child health care are to foster the smooth, normal development of the child from infancy to adulthood and to help ensure that each child achieves adult life as physically, intellectually, and emotionally intact as possible. In infancy interaction between the pediatrician and the child is largely mediated through the parents; in later childhood and adolescence an increasingly direct relationship between the physician and the child develops. Regularly scheduled health maintenance encounters with children are evaluative and preventive. Evaluative activities include the usual interval history and inquiries for any perceived problem, assessment of growth and development by history and examination, and screening for various abnormalities or their precursors. Preventive management includes efforts to correct or ameliorate any abnormalities, specific preventive measures such as immunization, and anticipatory guidance. The following general recommendations derived from those of the American Academy of Pediatrics comprise general guidelines for the care of normal infants and children; the needs of individual children and their families may require deviation. For example, an experienced family with a 3rd child may require fewer visits than the anxious parents whose 1st pregnancy terminated in death due to prematurity.

Prenatal Period. It is desirable, particularly with 1st pregnancies, for the parents to talk with their pediatrician sometime during the 3rd trimester about any of their problems or concerns. At this time the pediatrician's role in the subsequent care of the child can be reviewed, including care in the newborn nursery, the proposed schedule of visits, planned immunizations, and the like. Financial arrangements may also be discussed. Other topics might include desirability of breast feeding, the pros and cons of circumcision, living arrangements for the baby, and what help may be available at home during the 1st wk or 2 after birth. The pediatrician may also help to instill confidence in the parents by pointing out there is no single correct method of caring for the baby and that for the most part their own instincts in dealing with the infant from day to day should be followed.

Newborn Care. A complete physical examination of the infant should be performed within 24 hr after birth; some pediatricians prefer to conduct the examination in the presence of the mother in her room. In high risk situations the pediatrician should examine the infant earlier or be present at the time of delivery. Every infant should receive prophylaxis for ophthalmia neonatorum and a single intramuscular dose of a vitamin K preparation (0.1–0.2 mg menadione sodium bisulfite or 0.5 mg vitamin K_1). A test for PKU should be done and T_4 measured. Ten to 15 ml of cord blood should be collected at birth and saved in the refrigerator for 7 days for typing, Coombs testing, and other tests if needed.

The results of the physical examination should be communicated immediately to the parents. Subsequently, it is important to visit the nursery and mother daily until discharge, although it is not necessary to examine the infant on each occasion unless problems occur. For infants without problems a brief discharge physical examination may be adequate before the mother and infant go home. Just prior to discharge it is important to sit down with the parents to review care at home, to reassure the parents that all is well, and, particularly, to encourage them to enjoy their baby. The parents also should be assured of the availability of the pediatrician by phone; a telephone conversation after the baby has been home 1–2 wk is desirable.

Follow-up. The optimal time for the 1st routine follow-up visit depends on the status of the infant and the experience of the parents. An office visit at 3–4 wk after birth ensures that feeding is going well, provides answers to questions that have arisen, identifies and solves minor problems, and reassures the parents. Table 4–4A and B suggests a schedule for evaluation and preventive measures at specific ages.

Routine Immunization. The schedule for immunization is that recommended for routine protection of children by the Committee on Infectious Diseases of the American Academy of Pediatrics and the Immunization Practices Advisory Committee, U.S. Public Health Service. Immunization with diphtheria and tetanus toxoids and pertussis vaccine, adsorbed (DTP), is ordinarily started at 6–8 wk of age; 2 additional doses are given at 1–2 mo intervals. A 4th dose is given at approximately 18 mo of age and a 5th dose at the time of school entry. DTP is not given after the 7th birthday. Instead, tetanus and diphtheria toxoids for adult use, combined (Td), containing a smaller amount of diphtheria toxoid are recommended at 10 yr intervals. DTP and Td should be given intramuscularly, preferably in the anterolateral thigh in young infants and either in the thigh or the deltoid in older children. Although the 1st of 3 doses of DTP may be given at 1 mo intervals if widespread pertussis is occurring, the 2 mo interval avoids unnecessary expense and inconvenience to parents.

There are 3 contraindications to administration of DTP: (1) an acute febrile illness, because confusion may result as to the causation of subsequent symptoms (a minor respiratory infection is not a contraindication); (2) an evolving neurologic illness (for the same reason); (3) a severe reaction to a prior dose of DTP.

Reactions that follow a DTP injection may be of 3 varieties. The 1st is minor, including local swelling and tenderness at the site of injection, slight fever, and irritability. A fever of greater than 105° F (40.5° C) is a contraindication to further doses of DTP. Second, reactions of unknown significance include excessive somnolence beyond that attributable to a visit to the physician and disruption of daily schedule, protracted inconsolable crying that may last 4 hr or more, and a peculiar shock-like syndrome that also may last for hours. The pathogenesis and sequelae, if any, of these reactions are unknown. The shock-like syndrome is a contraindication to further injections of DTP. The degrees of excessive somnolence or inconsolable crying sufficient to warrant discontinuation of DTP are matters of judgment. Third, neurologic reactions to DTP include occasional simple convulsions and, fortunately rarely, frank encephalopathy, sometimes with brain damage or death. These neurologic reactions are contraindications to further DTP. Because most of the reactivity of DTP is due to the pertussis component, the occurrence of 1 of these reactions does not contraindicate continuation of immunization against diphtheria and tetanus using diphtheria and tetanus toxoids for pediatric use (DT). Although local and febrile reactions to this preparation may occur, they are of less severity than those to DTP and, with the exception of extraordinarily rare anaphylactic reactions to tetanus toxoid, not dangerous.

Table 4–4A   EVALUATION AT SPECIFIC AGES

Note: Interval history, dietary and sleep patterns, height, and weight should be included in each routine visit and are not listed on the table. Items not previously performed, as with an older child who is a new patient, should be carried out at the initial visit.

Procedure	Months							Years									
	2	4	6	9	12	15	18	2	3	4	5	6	8	10	12	14	16
Interview																	
Family history	+											+					+
Pregnancy and delivery	+																
Neonatal course	+																
Other past history	+																
Immunizations		+															
Developmental evaluation																	
Motor	+	+	+	+	+	+	+	+	+	+							
Psychologic		+	+	+	+	+	+	+	+	+	+	+	+	+	+	+	+
Social									+	+	+	+	+	+	+	+	+
Educational status											+	+	+	+	+	+	+
Body systems																	
Hearing, vision	+	+	+	+	+		+										
GI (defecation, etc.)	+			+			+	+	+	+							
Urinary	+							+									
Dental care									+	+	+	+	+	+	+	+	+
Drugs, alcohol, tobacco															+	+	+
Pica					+	+	+	+	+	+							
Sexual behavior														+	+	+	+
Physical examination																	
Head circumference	+	+	+	+	+												
Blood pressure								+	+	+	+	+	+	+	+	+	+
Special items																	
Vision																	
Fixed eyes	+																
Red reflex	+																
Fundus			+					+									
Strabismus			+														
Snellen chart									+		+		+				
Hearing																	
Gross	+			+													
Audiometer										+	+	+	+				
Speech					+			+	+								
Hip dislocation	+	+	+														
Gait						+	+	+									
Scoliosis													+	+	+	+	+
Pubertal development														+	+	+	+
Laboratory																	
Hgb or Hct				+				+						+			+
Urinalysis				+				+									+
Urine culture (girls)					+				+					+		+	
Tuberculin					+			+					+	+	+	+	

Table 4-4B PREVENTIVE MEASURES AT SPECIFIC AGES

MEASURE	MONTHS							YEARS									
	2	4	6	9	12	15	18	2	3	4	5	6	8	10	12	14	16
Immunizations																	
DTP	+	+	+				+										
Td		+														+	
OPV	+	+	±	(optional)			+			+							
MMR						+											
Influenza (high risk only)				+				Annually hereafter									
Pneumococcal (high risk only)								+									
Counseling																	
Diet	+	+	+	+	+	+	+	+		+					+	+	+
Sleep	+	+	+		+	+	+	+	±			+		+	+	+	+
Toilet training						+	+	+									
Accidents																	
Falls (bassinet, etc.)		+															
Bathtub			+														
Infant car restraints			+														
Electrical cords				+	+												
Stove				+													
Poisoning (get ipecac)					+												
Open water, streets						+											
Parent-child interaction				+	+		+	+	+	+	+	+	+	+	+	+	+
Day care								+									
School problems										+	+	+	+	+	+	+	+
Puberty and sexuality														+	+	+	+
Adolescence															+	+	+
Substance abuse															+	+	+

Because there is no firm evidence that decreasing the dose of DTP reduces the reactivity of the pertussis component significantly, and because the administration of partial doses of DTP would have to be continued until the full 12 units of pertussis vaccine (1.5 ml) are given, such divided doses are not warranted.

Two types of polio vaccine are licensed in the United States: OPV, a live, attenuated trivalent polio vaccine (Sabin), and IVP, an inactivated (killed) trivalent polio vaccine (Salk). A full course of either vaccine protects the recipient against paralytic poliomyelitis almost without exception. Because rare cases of paralytic poliomyelitis occur in recipients of OPV or in their close contacts, some have advocated returning to IPV for routine immunization of children. Epidemiologic support for this recommendation comes from Sweden and other countries in which eradication of poliomyelitis has been achieved by IPV alone. However, immunization advisory groups in the United States have continued to recommend OPV for routine immunization of children because of the virtual eradication of poliomyelitis from the United States by OPV and because of the belief that, in view of less than optimal rates of immunization in the United States, circulation of wild virus in the community is controlled better by the greater intestinal immunity afforded by OPV.

The 1st dose of OPV should be given at approximately 2 mo of age and the 2nd 2 mo later. Ninety-five percent of recipients are protected against all 3 strains of poliomyelitis by this regimen. In communities close to areas of high endemicity of poliomyelitis, such as the southwestern United States, a 3rd dose at 6 mo of age is recommended. An additional dose is given to all children at approximately 18 mo of age and another prior to school entry. An interval of at least 2 mo between doses of OPV is required because intestinal carriage of vaccine virus may persist for up to 6 wk with consequent viral interference. The doses administered at 18 mo and prior to school entry are considered as "fillers" rather than boosters in case one of the original doses did not "take." The same schedule is recommended for IPV.

OPV should not be given to individuals proven or suspected to be immunocompromised, including those with congenital and acquired immunodeficiencies and those whose immune mechanisms are impaired by therapy. OPV also should not be given to household contacts of immunocompromised individuals or to subsequent siblings of a child who succumbed to congenital immunodeficiency until the present child is shown to be normal.

Unimmunized parents of infants scheduled for poliomyelitis immunization represent a special problem due to their risk, albeit remote, of acquiring paralytic poliomyelitis from the vaccinated infant. In this situation 2 courses of action are acceptable. The 1st is the administration of OPV to the infant regardless of the immune status of household contacts, the usual practice in the United States. The 2nd approach is to give 3 consecutive monthly doses of IPV to the adult household contacts, administering the initial dose of OPV to the infant at the time of the 3rd dose of IPV to the contacts. If the adult household contacts have been partially immunized with OPV or IPV, they should be given OPV or IPV, respectively, at the same time that the initial dose of OPV is administered to the infant. Adults and children traveling to areas where poliomyelitis is endemic should be fully immunized with polio vaccine.

For routine immunization of children, live attenuated

measles-mumps-rubella vaccine, combined (MMR), should be administered at 15 mo of age. Because of persistent maternal antibody, vaccine failures, particularly with the measles component, occur when MMR is administered prior to this time; the younger the infant, the more likely is failure. However, when outbreaks of measles occur, the vaccine should be given as early as 9 mo of age but repeated some time after 15 mo. Teenagers who escaped natural rubella and measles in childhood and who were unimmunized should be identified and immunized. Currently these two diseases are more frequent in children over 10 yr than in better immunized younger children. MMR ensures seroconversion to all 3 antigens in 90–95% of recipients. Most vaccine failures, particularly to measles, are attributable to improper refrigeration, exposure to light, administration at too early an age, or the simultaneous use of immune serum globulin. There is no justification for the routine use of monovalent measles, mumps, and rubella vaccines in children.

Contraindications to MMR are pregnancy, immunodeficiency or therapeutic immunosuppression, and an acute febrile illness. Although the accumulated experienced has not shown deleterious effects on the fetus when these vaccines were given in the 1st trimester, it is prudent to avoid giving MMR to pregnant women. Additionally, women of childbearing age given MMR should be cautioned to avoid pregnancy for the next 3 mo. As with any live virus vaccine, immunocompromised individuals should not be immunized. Immunization of individuals receiving immunosuppressive therapy should be delayed until at least 3 mo following discontinuation of therapy. The measles and mumps vaccines are grown in chick-embryo cell culture. Because allergic reactions to these vaccines have been reported in 3 children with prior anaphylaxis from egg ingestion, such children should not receive either vaccine. Other types of egg allergy are not contraindications. In contrast to OPV, transmission of measles, mumps, or rubella vaccine virus to susceptible contacts has not occurred. Therefore the presence of a pregnant or immunocompromised household contact does not contraindicate immunization with MMR.

Adverse reactions to MMR attributable to the measles component include transient rashes and fever up to 103° F (39.4° C) occurring in a few individuals at 6–11 days after immunization. Subacute sclerosing panencephalitis (SSPE) has been attributed on rare occasions to measles vaccine. If it occurs, it does so at a much lower rate than that following natural measles. Additionally, transient arthralgia, rarely arthritis, and paresthetic pains may occur in 1–2% of children and a higher percentage of adults, especially females, 2–8 wk following immunization as a consequence of the rubella component. These phenomena usually last only a few days; cases of rheumatoid arthritis occurring after rubella vaccine probably are coincidental. Recognizable reactions to the mumps component have not occurred.

Delayed Immunization. Infants more than 2 mo but less than 14 mo of age without any immunization should be started on the same sequence of immunizations and intervals between doses as those recommended for young infants. Infants and children who previously received 1 or more doses of any vaccine at intervals longer than those routinely recommended, no matter how long, do not require reinitiation of the series; completion of full immunization, counting the original doses, should be undertaken.

Children 14 mo–7 yr of age who have received no immunizations should receive DTP, OPV, and a tuberculin test at the 1st visit. To provide prompt protection against measles, MMR should be given 1 mo later, followed by DTP and OPV after an additional mo. Approximately 2 mo after the 2nd DTP and OPV (4 mo after the initial doses), the 3rd dose of DTP and, in poliomyelitis-endemic areas, the 3rd dose of OPV should be given. DTP and OPV should be repeated approximately 1 yr later. If the child is more than 4 yr of age at this time, further immunization prior to school entry is unnecessary; otherwise DTP and OPV should be given again between 5–7 yr of age. All children should receive a dose of Td in early adolescence.

When immunization is delayed, questions arise about the simultaneous administration of multiple antigens, such as giving DTP, OPV, and MMR at the initial visit. There is no interference between DTP and OPV (or IPV). Although 1 study suggested that DTP and MMR given at the same time resulted in reduced seroconversion rates to measles, others have shown no difference. MMR and the "filler" dose of OPV are effective when given simultaneously in the 2nd yr; whether giving MMR and the 1st dose of OPV at this time compromises immune response is not known. Likewise, it is not known whether giving initial doses of DTP and OPV with MMR to an unimmunized child 15 mo or older is fully effective. Nonetheless, when such an older unimmunized child is seen and when there is reason to doubt the adequacy of follow-up, it is reasonable to administer DTP, OPV, and MMR simultaneously. In all situations it should be borne in mind that an interval of at least 1 mo should be allowed between doses of the same or different vaccines (2 mo between doses of OPV) when they are not given simultaneously.

Special Vaccines. Annual immunization against influenza is inappropriate for normal children. It *should* be given to children at high risk from infections of the lower respiratory tract. Examples include children with susceptibility to pulmonary infections from congenital or acquired heart disease (such as left to right shunts); disorders that compromise pulmonary function, including cystic fibrosis, severe asthma, neuromuscular and orthopedic conditions that distort or weaken the thoracic cage, and pulmonary dysplasia as a consequence of the neonatal respiratory distress syndrome; chronic azotemic renal disease or the nephrotic syndrome; diabetes mellitus; and chronic severe anemia such as thalassemia or sicklemia. Immunodeficient and immunocompromised children may also benefit. Since the constituents of influenza vaccine must be changed yearly because of shifts in prevalent influenza viruses, annual recommendations of the U.S. Public Health Service, published in the *Morbidity and Mortality Weekly Report*, should be consulted for doses and schedules.

The 14-valent pneumococcal vaccine presently licensed in the United States is not recommended for routine use in children. As with other polysaccharide vaccines, its efficacy is minimal in children under 2 yr of age. Experience with children with sickle cell anemia indicates that the vaccine is useful in children older than 2 yr with functional or anatomic asplenia. The dose is 0.5 ml intramuscularly or subcutaneously; because antibodies persist and because reactivity is high, even as long as 4 yr after the initial dose, reimmunization with pneumococcal vaccine is currently contraindicated.

The indications for the occasional use of other vaccines, such as meningococcal polysaccharide vaccine and typhoid vaccine, are discussed under those disease sections. Mixed respiratory vaccines and autogenous respiratory vaccines, orally or by injection, are not effective. Smallpox vaccine is discussed in Sec 10.74.

A *tuberculin test* should be performed early in the 2nd yr of life. It may be given before or, for convenience, at the time of the administration of MMR. Subsequent tuberculin testing is advisable prior to school entry and in early adolescence, but the physician should deviate from this schedule when circumstances, such as the local prevalence of tuberculosis, dictate.

Prevention of Disease in Later Life. In 1979 there were nearly 2 million deaths at all ages in the United States. The leading cause, accounting for 41% of deaths, was degenerative vascular disease, including coronary heart disease, hypertension, stroke, and other arteriosclerotic diseases. Cancer, the 2nd most frequent cause, resulted in 21% of deaths. Because 4 major risk factors for these degenerative cardiovascular diseases (hypertension, hyperlipidemia, obesity, and smoking) may be amenable to amelioration and because it is estimated that up to 90% of cancer is environmentally caused, it has been hypothesized that these leading causes of death have some of their origins early in life—or at least that habit patterns conducive to these diseases may be established in childhood.

Guidelines for pediatric prevention of degenerative vascular disease in later life are not established. Children with strong family histories of arteriosclerotic disease who display such characteristics as obesity, elevated serum lipid values, and/or hypertension are probably at higher risk as adults. Children in families with excessive early cardiovascular disease, such as myocardial infarction, are more apt to exhibit hyperlipidemia and elevated blood pressure for age than other children. However, whether attempts should be undertaken to ameliorate these risk factors in children is uncertain for several reasons: (1) modification of dietary habits and compliance with anti-hypertension regimens are very difficult in children; (2) there continues to be controversy about the preventive efficacy and benefit of some of these measures (especially reduction of dietary lipids), even in adults; (3) there is a potentially untoward emotional impact on a child of being labeled "at risk." Nevertheless, the following recommendations seem appropriate. Every effort should be made to discourage smoking. Children from families with excessive coronary heart disease should be evaluated with respect to weight, blood pressure, and serum lipids (Sec 13.86). Children with elevated cholesterol or triglycerides should receive a modified diet, and attempts should be made to limit weight gain in those with

obesity. Efforts to create optimal dietary behavior from birth may be more important for *all* infants than trying to modify risk factors after they appear. This might include the encouragement of breast feeding, which tends to reduce obesity, delaying the addition of high caloric food such as meat, egg yolk, and puddings, and avoiding creating habits of excessive intake of food in infancy (it isn't necessary to drain the bottle). Additionally, salt should be limited inasmuch as taste for it is acquired.

Preventing cancer in later life is an even more difficult problem. Averting the initiation of smoking would produce enormous benefits because cigarettes are currently responsible for about a quarter of all cancer deaths in the United States. Other personal activities, including dietary habits, have shown variable associations epidemiologically with excessive rates of cancer at certain anatomic sites. For example, there appears to be a relationship between meat ingestion and bowel, breast, and prostate cancer (probably related to fat). Additionally, numerous other substances in our complex modern environment can be linked to various cancers (Sec 15.1). The responsibilities of physicians in the prevention of cancer fall into 2 categories. At the public level they should support efforts to minimize environmental pollution. With individual patients, in addition to advising against smoking, they should counsel that an excess of many substances (such as continuous or excessive use of spices) may be detrimental. They should also make sure that therapeutic drugs, especially hormones, are limited to situations with clear-cut indications.

4.2 SECONDARY AND TERTIARY PREVENTION

Many facets of primary, routine pediatric care (Table 4–4) represent secondary preventive efforts. Some evaluative elements of pediatric care, including the family history, monitoring of development, sensory evaluation, blood pressure, and the like, are designed to identify the susceptibilities to, or antecedents of, later disease and thus are secondary preventive measures. Similarly, screening for tuberculosis, urinary tract infections, albuminuria, scoliosis, early signs of congenital hip dysplasia, and other features of routine child health care are part of secondary prevention. Care for the common, acute childhood illnesses also largely represents secondary prevention in that treatment for such illnesses in many cases prevents sequelae that would occur in very few. For example, streptococcal pharyngitis is treated to prevent suppurative complications, such as peritonsillar abscess, and rheumatic fever. Further, acute bacterial otitis media will subside spontaneously in up to 95% of instances; the major benefit of antimicrobial therapy, which has little effect on the immediate course, is the prevention of mastoiditis and/or chronic perforation of the drum. These and other examples of secondary prevention are reviewed in specific sections.

Similarly, a great deal of care for chronic illness and

disability in childhood represents tertiary prevention. Examples include the many facets of care for children with cystic fibrosis, orthopedic measures for cerebral palsy and neural tube defects, anti-streptococcal prophylaxis for those who have had rheumatic fever, and physiotherapy for children with rheumatoid arthritis. Here the pediatrician has the additional responsibility of providing continuous support to the family while ameliorating as much as possible the social, psychologic, and financial effects of chronic illness on the child and other family members and at the same time ensuring that optimal care is received. Because such children often require the attention of subspecialists and various services such as physiotherapy, occupational therapy, nutritional counseling, and others, the pediatrician must function as "coordinator" of these activities while providing regular child health care and treatment of intercurrent illness. The pediatrician must ensure that care proffered or recommended by other providers, including subspecialists and nonmedical health care professionals, is considered in the light of the total child and the family. For example, whether an enuretic child requires invasive urologic investigation and whether a child with serous otitis media needs tympanostomy tubes are issues involving interventions that are traumatic to the child and family. They should be evaluated from the standpoint of the probabilities of diagnostic and therapeutic benefits versus the risks, untoward effects, and costs.

4.3   EPIDEMIOLOGY IN PEDIATRICS

Epidemiology is the study of disease and its control in populations. *Descriptive epidemiology* records the incidence and prevalence of death, disability, and disease of various types and causes. It provides information useful in determining priorities in health care (Table 4–1). In the United States, city, county, and state local health departments and other regional agencies tabulate current, local information about health and disease. The National Center for Health Statistics and the Centers for Disease Control publish detailed morbidity and mortality data for the entire United States, states, and, to a limited extent, counties and metropolitan areas. Available publications include *Vital Statistics of the United States*, which provides annual age-specific causes of death; the *Monthly Vital Statistics Report*, which includes more current, although provisional, mortality data; the *Vital and Health Statistics of the United States* (the so-called Rainbow Series), which periodically summarizes prevalence data about health, illness, and disability derived from interviews and examination of representative samples of the population; and the *Morbidity and Mortality Weekly Reports*, published by the Centers for Disease Control of the U.S. Public Health Service. Data derived from these sources should be readily available because of their value in indicating "what's going around" locally, comprehending what is the norm, and assisting in developing local health programs.

Analytic epidemiology is used to develop clues to the cause of disease and to assess the efficacy, safety, and costs of methods of intervention. This approach to disease causation has been applied to studies of legionellosis, the sudden infant death and toxic shock syndromes, Lyme arthritis, aspirin and Reye syndrome, and others. Analytic epidemiologic studies provide the scientific rationale for the many diagnostic, therapeutic, and preventive measures currently available and enable the physician to evaluate critically the vast amount of information with which he or she is bombarded from medical literature, colleagues, pharmaceutical representatives, and patients. Before accepting new therapeutic or preventive measures and employing them, the physician should be confident that there is no other explanation for the results than that offered by the authors ("internal validity"). There also must be assurance that the results are applicable to patient populations other than those studied by the authors ("external validity").

From the standpoint of internal validity, clinical trials of therapeutic and preventive measures may be looked at as simple comparisons, e.g., antibiotic A may be compared with antibiotic B in the treatment of otitis media, or the costs of care under fee-for-service health insurance plans may be compared with those under prepaid plans. For the results of such clinical trials to be valid, 3 important study criteria must be met: (1) the groups being compared must be similar to begin with; (2) except for the therapeutic or preventive modality under study, the groups must be managed identically; and (3) the groups, treated and control, must be observed with equal intensity for outcomes. An important corollary to these criteria is that any deviations from them must be judged for their potential effects on the results of the study. To assess such clinical comparison studies, the pediatrician must look at who the patients were, how they were selected, and how they were treated and evaluated and must apply basic knowledge of clinical pediatrics and common sense. For example, corticosteroid hormones, which appeared in the early 1950's, seemed initially to exhibit remarkable effects in the management of acute rheumatic fever; arthritis and fever responded promptly and dramatically. In order to determine whether similarly salutary effects were exerted on valvular heart disease, studies compared patients treated with these hormones in the 1950's with patients managed without steroids in the 1930's and 1940's. The results indicated amelioration of valvular damage by this new therapy. However, several factors other than steroids that might have explained these results were not considered adequately: (1) the treated and control groups may have been different to begin with because several studies showed that rheumatic fever was becoming a milder disease starting in the 1920's or earlier; because diagnostic criteria improved during World War II (the Jones criteria); and because the advent of this new, apparently dramatic measure plus more widespread health insurance may have resulted in admissions to hospitals of patients with milder illnesses who would otherwise have been managed at home; (2) there may have been intervening variables, such as penicillin and better drugs for the management of congestive heart failure; (3) improved diagnostic methods and the fact that the patients receiving cortisone were under closer scrutiny before, during, and after treatment suggest that the way in which outcomes were evaluated may have differed between the 2 groups. Most of the randomized clinical trials made more recently have failed to show a benefit of steroids on valvular heart disease.

More subtle problems with study design and analysis include self-selection of patients (those who volunteer are different from those who do not); physician selection of patients by eliminating patients from study whose problems are "too severe" to justify an experiment that may result in their being controls; and alteration of therapy or removing patients from the study when benefit is not immediately obvious. A major problem is that of unintentional bias in outcome evaluation, e.g., the relief of parents when the tonsillectomy and adenoidectomy have been accomplished without event and their belief in the magic of medicine and surgery can be expected to alter their reporting of subsequent illness.

For these reasons the randomized, double-blind clinical trial is the optimal means of ensuring that the characteristics of study and control patients are similar to begin with, that treatment is the same except for the variable under study, and that observational bias does not influence outcome assessment. Randomization ensures that each study subject has an equal opportunity to fall into the experimental or control group. When the experimenters are unaware of who is treated and who is not, there is little likelihood that unintentional modification of treatment will occur, and the fact that neither the experimenters nor the patients know who is receiving what treatment eliminates observer bias. The randomized double-blind clinical trial is of particular importance in evaluating therapy for diseases that exhibit a spectrum of outcomes and a majority of which subside without treatment, e.g., otitis media. Unfortunately, not all clinical trials are susceptible to being double-blinded; there is no way to perform a clinical trial of tonsillectomy and adenoidectomy without its being obvious who received surgery and who did not, a reason why the value of these procedures continues to be uncertain.

E. A. MORTIMER

General

Deisher RW, Derby AJ, Sturman MJ: Changing trends in pediatric practice. Pediatrics 25:711, 1960.
Mortimer EA Jr: Immunization against infectious disease. Science 200:902, 1978.

Fluoridation

Promoting the use of fluorides in communities: Past accomplishments and future perspectives. Presented at the annual session of the American Association for Dental Research, March 20, 1980, Los Angeles, California. J Pub Health Dent 40:211, 1980.

Rat Control

Centers for Disease Control: Morbidity and Mortality Weekly Report (Public Health Service) 30:205, 1981.

Raw Milk

Centers for Disease Control: Morbidity and Mortality Weekly Report (Public Health Service) 30:205, 1981.

Homicide

Rushforth NB, Ford AB, Hirsch CS, et al: Violent death in a metropolitan county: Changing patterns in homicide (1958–74). N Engl J Med 297:531, 1977.

Routine Child Health Maintenance

Standards of Child Health Care. Ed 3. American Academy of Pediatrics, Evanston, Ill, 1977.
Report of the Committee on Infectious Diseases. Ed 19. American Academy of Pediatrics, Evanston, Ill, 1981.

Handicapped Children

Breslau N, Weitzman M, Messenger K: Psychologic functioning of siblings of disabled children. Pediatrics 67:344, 1981.
Pless IB, Pinkerton P: Chronic Childhood Disorder: Promoting Patterns of Adjustment. Chicago, Year Book Medical Publishers, 1975.
Satterwhite BB: Impact of chronic illness on child and family: An overview based on five surveys with implication for management. Int J Rehab Research 1:7, 1978.

Prevention of Disease in Later Life

Glueck CJ: Detection of risk factors for coronary artery disease in children: Semmelweis revisited? Pediatrics 66:834, 1980.
Haggery RJ: Should pediatricians try to prevent coronary artery disease? Pediatrics 66:834, 1980.
Holtzman NA: Hyperlipidemia screening and Semmelweis re-revisited. Pediatrics 66:838, 1980.
Maclure KM, MacMahon B: An epidemiologic perspective of environmental carcinogenesis. Epidemiol Rev 2:19, 1980.
Report of the task force on blood pressure control in children. Pediatrics (Suppl) 59:797, 1977.

Epidemiology

Colton T: Statistics in Medicine. Boston, Little Brown and Co, 1974, p 315.
Friedman GD: Primer of Epidemiology. Ed 2. New York, McGraw-Hill Book Co, 1980.
Haynes RB: How to read clinical journals: II. To learn about a diagnostic test. Can Med Assoc J 124:703, 1981.
Hill AB: The clinical trial. N Engl J Med 247:113, 1952.
Sackett DL: How to read clinical journals: I. Why to read them and how to start reading them critically. Can Med Assoc J 124:555, 1981.
Sackett DL: How to read clinical journals: V. To distinguish useful from useless or even harmful therapy. Can Med Assoc J 124:1156, 1981.
Trout KS: How to read clinical journals: IV. To determine etiology or causation. Can Med Assoc J 124:985, 1981.
Tugwell PX: How to read clinical journals: III. To learn the clinical course and prognosis of disease. Can Med Assoc J 124:869, 1981.

4.4 DELIVERY OF HEALTH CARE TO CHILDREN IN DEVELOPING COUNTRIES

In spite of advances in medical technology and the enormous amount of money spent on health care, 80–85% of the underprivileged persons in the developing countries do not have access to health services. The underprivileged communities can be broadly classified into rural, urban and periurban, and nomadic and seminomadic groups (WHO/UNICEF).

Rural Population. In 1970 the rural population was approximately 1.91 billion or 75% of the total population in the underprivileged regions of the world. By the end of this century, despite family planning programs and uncontrolled urban migration, the rural population will increase to 3 billion. The cost of health service for these people will be beyond the resources of the world.

Urban and Periurban Population. The currently estimated 18–20% of the urban population who live in slums in developing countries are likely to increase to 30–35% in the next 2 decades with unchecked urban migration. In some countries of South America there has already been an increase in the urban slum population, now amounting to 40–50% of the total population. There is no possibility that the increased requirements for employment, energy, education, housing, sanitation, water supply, and distribution of food, health, and other services that would have a preventive impact will be met. Under the circumstances one can only envision a worsening of already subhuman living conditions. Urban migrants from the villages continue their rural way of life and, in addition, often acquire new problems, such as drinking, gambling, smoking of charas, and prostitution.

Nomadic and Seminomadic Population. The majority of this group of nearly 1 billion people live in the poorer countries of Africa and Asia. Their migratory patterns create health problems requiring separate recognition and attention.

Some of the features responsible for the prevalence of poor health and for inadequate delivery of health care within the underprivileged communities are discussed below.

Agricultural Deficits and Population Growth. The combination of these 2 factors contributes significantly to the problems of the underprivileged communities. Although food production has increased within the past 2–3 decades, the gains have been offset by an increase in population of 2.5–3.5%/yr in the developing countries (compared to 0–0.3% in the developed countries). Moreover, the principal benefits of increased food production are reaped by the urban and rural rich communities. The poor and underprivileged inhabitants, such as laborers, marginal landowners, small shopkeepers, and families with unemployed and underemployed persons, continue to have inadequate food, both in quantity and quality. Many families exist in a state of partial starvation; the mothers usually consume about 1600 calories/day, and children get only 500–1100 calories instead of the needed 1000–2200 calories/day. Ill health continues to be the way of life in such families.

Economy. Poverty and economic stagnation afflict large segments of these populations; 40–60% of them are below the poverty line; this rate is likely to increase to 70–75% by the end of the century. Lack of employment and underemployment are prevalent in both the industrial and agricultural sectors. Usually the daily per capita income is less than 40–50 cents (U.S.). This coupled with a galloping inflation rate has a tremendous impact on the health of people in developing countries.

Social Status. In many countries the lower social classes are not included in the mainstream of national life in spite of the efforts of voluntary agencies and governments. These people live in such isolation in their own sociocultural milieu that major socioeconomic, cultural, and educational improvements are difficult to achieve.

Inadequate Communication. The social and cultural characteristics of the rural populations and deficiencies in means of communication make physical contacts difficult and contribute to cultural gaps and illiteracy. There are often no or inadequate vehicular roads to connect the rural population with the urban areas. The only means of transportation may be the bullock cart or the donkey, and during the monsoon seasons villages may be completely cut off from the health stations.

Demographic Handicaps. Large families are the pattern in the underprivileged communities: 35–45% of the population is under 15 yr of age and about 20% is under 6 yr. Such large percentages of children, particularly in the vulnerable preschool years, contribute to the prevalence of protein-calorie malnutrition, communicable diseases, and high mortality rates.

Environmental Factors. Within the cities the poor people live in congested slums, and in the villages their dwellings are often dark huts with poor ventilation and sanitary facilities. The lack of adequately protected water supplies leads to gastrointestinal infections.

Nutritional Deficits (Chapter 3). Because of the poverty, ignorance, cultural fantasies about foods, and certain food taboos, the incidence of protein-calorie malnutrition, anemia, and vitamin deficiencies is exceedingly high. Seventy percent of preschool children are below the 80th percentile of the international standard referral weights (50th percentile of the Harvard Standards).

High Incidence of Infections. Poor nutrition, lack of sanitation, poor hygiene, and inadequate immunizations result in the high incidence of such communicable diseases as gastroenteritis, respiratory infections, tuberculosis, measles, whooping cough, diphtheria, and other bacterial, viral, and parasitic infections. Severe undernutrition contributes significantly to immune incompetence, leading to increased susceptibility to infection and inadequate handling of what otherwise are usually self-limiting diseases, such as pertussis and measles.

Sociopolitical Handicaps. The majority of the population suffers from apathy due to malnutrition, lack of education, and cultural isolation. There are inequitable land-tenure systems, and many of the communities have no tillable land or only a small area, insufficient to support the inhabitants. The rigid heirarchies and class structures are responsible for persistence of this oppressed state. The lowest social classes have inadequate or no representation or influence in making decisions at the national or even at the regional or local levels.

Educational Limitations. Seventy to 80% of the inhabitants in the underprivileged communities are illiterate because of the poor educational facilities. Some of these communities also have become hostile to academic educational programs because the educated members frequently leave their communities and become culturally alien.

Geographic and Climatic Factors. The underprivileged rural communities usually suffer more during droughts, floods, and famines than is the case in other areas.

4.5 Population and Health Statistics

A United Nations report has estimated that the total population of the developing regions may increase by 28% within the 1980's, with increases of 21 and 28% among preschool and school-age children, respectively. In 1965–1969 84% of the estimated 120 million births/yr in the entire world occurred in developing countries. In these regions the infant mortality rate was 120–140/1000 live births compared with 16–27/1000 live births in the developed countries; in some of the developing countries, the infant mortality rate was as high as 200/1000 live births, while that of one developed country was as low as 9.6. The preschool mortality rates (1–5 yr) were 30–40/1000 population in developing countries, while those of the developed countries were 0.5–1.5. The maternal mortality rates were 5–10/1000 births in developing countries, in contrast to rates of 0.06–0.2 in developed countries.

Malnutrition is prevalent in the total population of the developing countries and particularly in women of childbearing age. These women also frequently have nutritional anemia and infections. The incidence of tuberculosis among them may be as high as 5–7%, and recurrent and chronic gastrointestinal infections sap their vitality. The adverse effects of these and other environmental factors result in 20–25% incidence of infants with birth weights 2000 gm or less. These infants contribute disproportionately to the excessively high perinatal, infant, and preschool mortality rates of these countries. The rates of abortions and stillbirths are also excessively high.

Protein energy (calorie) malnutrition is the most widespread of the major health problems among children in developing regions of the world and contributes in large measure to their high morbidity and mortality rates. An analysis of 101 community surveys in 59 developing countries during the years 1961–1971 indicated that no fewer than 100 million children under 5 yr of age were affected by moderate to severe protein energy malnutrition.

The high incidence of intrauterine, neonatal, and postnatal malnutrition contributes not only to high mortality rates but also to poor physical growth, premature senility, and low life expectancy among those who survive beyond infancy. It has adverse effects on mental development that result in reduced mental and physical potential and impose a serious handicap on economic development in all fields, particularly in agriculture and industry. This cycle of events also cripples the social and cultural advancement of the communities.

4.6 Conventional Structure of Medical Education and Health Services

Until recently, medical education and health services of the developing countries were organized on the basis of the European model of the last century. Education in medicine ignored traditional health practices of the underprivileged communities. Instead of utilizing existing skills as a basis for additional training and improve-

ment, an effort was made to create groups of health professionals parallel to those in developed countries. This was associated with an emphasis on personal advancement rather than responsibility to the community. Medical services tended to be centered in the cities, based in hospitals, not sufficiently community-oriented, and, in particular, inaccessible to villages. The graduates of the training programs were not oriented to meet the existing health needs of the communities. Eighty percent of the medical manpower provided services to less than 20% of the population, most or all of whom lived in urban areas. In a large city there might be 1 doctor to 1000 or fewer of the population, whereas in rural areas there might not be 1 doctor for 50,000 persons. Moreover, a large cultural gap exists between hospital-trained city doctors and the people of rural communities, and health service emphasis has been placed mainly on curative approaches and the development of relatively sophisticated hospital services. Such services are beyond the financial resources of the average person in a developing country, and the government does not have the organizational or financial resources to provide adequate care for the rural and neglected communities.

4.7 Primary Health Care

A concentration on primary health care appears to be the best solution to providing health care to the poor, backward, and tribal rural population and to some extent to the slum population of cities in developing countries. The World Health Organization has estimated that a considerable improvement in the health of these populations can take place for as little as 0.2–2% of the yearly gross national product provided the money is wisely spent on primary health care.

Primary health care is defined as essential health care made universally available to individuals and families in the community by means acceptable to them through their full participation, and at a cost that the community and country can afford. It should be the nucleus of the developing country's health system. Primary health care should focus on the main health problems in the community and provide preventive, curative, and rehabilitative services. These problems and appropriate services will vary from country to country and community to community but, in general, will provide the following:

1. Limited prenatal, intranatal, and postnatal care and, in particular, recognition of high risk mothers.
2. Family planning services.
3. Careful supervision of children under 6 yr, with emphasis on identification of children at risk.
4. Nutritional education assessment and supplementation.
5. Immunizations.
6. Health education for the layman.
7. Diagnosis and treatment of minor illnesses and recognition of serious disease.
8. First aid.
9. Facilities for referral of patients who require special therapy.
10. Emergency treatment prior to referral of a patient to a suitable health station or a hospital.

11. Maintenance of standardized health records, including growth charts for children.
12. Simple laboratory services (collection of sputum when tuberculosis is suspected, blood samples from persons with suspected malaria, etc.)
13. Continuous protection of the water supply.
14. Sanitation—personal, home environment, community, school, etc.
15. Vector control.

Role of Community. In order to make primary health care universally acceptable, accessible, and successful in the community as quickly as possible, broad-based community participation and individualized self-

Table 4–5 MATERNAL AND CHILD HEALTH SERVICES—ROLE OF COMMUNITY HEALTH WORKER AS A MEMBER OF THE HEALTH TEAM

General
  Registration of children and pregnant women

Antenatal care
  Early diagnosis of pregnancy
  Routine prenatal care
  Early detection of women at risk and referral to a higher level of health care
  Immunization, especially with tetanus toxoid
  Preparation for domiciliary delivery

Postnatal care
  Special attention to breast feeding and neonatal care

Infant and child care
  Identification of infants at risk
  Early detection of abnormalities
  Charting of growth and milestones
  Immunizations
  Treatment of diarrhea; supply electrolyte tablets and teach mother oral rehydration
  Treatment of such emergencies as convulsions, high fever, trauma, and so forth, prior to referral
  Treatment of such ailments as fever, cough, pain, skin diseases, conjunctivitis, and common infectious diseases
  Supplying antituberculous, antileprosy, and antimalarial drugs for proved cases
  Organization of day care or seasonal care centers
  Nutritional education and assessment
  Education
    Promotion of breast feeding
    Introduction of mixed feeding when infant is 4–6 mo old or when there is flattening of weight curve
    Hygienic handling of food in the home
    Avoidance of feeding by a bottle; it is a dangerous source of infection and underfeeding in underprivileged communities and of obesity, bottle addiction, and anemia in privileged communities
  Nutritional assessment made on growth chart to identify risk cases, i.e., those below 65% of reference weight (50th percentile of Harvard Standard)
  Distribution of food supplements if there is such a program
  Follow-up and supervision of infants returned from a higher level medical station
  Encouragement of community support for those in need

Family planning
  Registration of eligible couples
  Motivation
  Distribution of conventional contraceptives
  Referral of acceptors for loop insertion or sterilization
  Follow-up and simple treatment of side effects
  Health education, including information concerning sexually transmitted diseases

reliance are essential. The community, including the lowest socioeconomic segments, should participate in planning, organization, and management. The participation of the community can be best mobilized through appropriate education which enables the population to understand the real health problems and deal with them in the most suitable manner. Primary health care also depends upon the community's supplying its own health workers or volunteers at a cost the community and the country can afford. The functions of such a local team are indicated in Table 4–5.

Relation to Other Levels of the Health Care System. The other levels of health care delivery have to be reorganized and strengthened to support community primary health care, e.g., to providing (1) technical knowledge, training, guidance, and supervision; (2) logistic support; (3) supplies; (4) information for financing; and (5) referral facilities. In the development of health manpower, the team of professionals and subprofessionals who reside in the community must be effectively integrated with the professionals involved at other levels of the health care system for purposes of consultation and continuing education.

Coordination with Other Nonhealth Sectors. Improved health in developing countries cannot be achieved by primary health care alone. Socioeconomic development, employment, proper food production and distribution, provision of uncontaminated water, improved sanitation and housing, environmental protection and education, and other antipoverty measures are critical components. It is important that there be proper coordination between the health and nonhealth sectors of the society in implementing such social programs.

4.8 Involvement of Medical Colleges in the Delivery of Health Care to the Masses

In many developing countries health services and medical education are now being integrated. Undergraduate students are being exposed to the underprivileged urban and rural communities from the beginning of the medical school curriculum. In the preclinical years the students learn the various social, cultural, economic, statistical, and environmental aspects that affect family health in rural areas. Later in the clinical years the students are stationed in the rural areas for a period to participate in comprehensive health care, gaining experience in smaller health centers and in the homes of patients. During internship the students, having already reached some degree of maturity in understanding the problem of the rural masses, participate in the health care delivery system. Medical students and interns should, when possible, also participate in research designed to evaluate and improve methods of delivery of medical services, including health maintenance. As a result of this integration the rural population should receive improved health care at a low cost from several levels of personnel; primary care from the health team of community health workers, medical assistants, and nurse midwives; when necessary, secondary health care from general medical practitioners; and tertiary care from specialists at district, regional, and teaching hospitals.

P. M. Udani

Chaudhuri SN: Community pediatrics. Pediatric care for the millions. Indian J Pediatr 42:10, 1975.

David JA, Bamford FN: The community pediatrician in an integrated child health service. Arch Dis Child 50:1, 1975.

Dogramaci I: Pediatric education in Turkey: Use of community health programs as a medium for training medical students. Am J Dis Child 126:757, 1973.

Knyvett AF: The health center hospital; the community hospital of the future. Med J Aust 2:569, 1974.

Morley D: Paediatric Priorities in the Developing World. London, Butterworth and Company, 1973.

Putnam SM, Wyse DH, Lawrence RS: A model for teaching primary care in a rural health center. J Med Educ 50:285, 1975.

Salus: Low-cost rural health care and health manpower training. Vol 6, 1980, Vol 7, 1981, Rosanna Bechtel (ed.). ILD.R.C., Ottawa, Canada.

Silver HK, Ott JE: The child health associate: A new health professional to provide comprehensive health care to children. Pediatrics 57:1, 1973.

Udani PM: Perspectives in Pediatrics (pertaining to developing countries). Perspectives in Pediatrics Series, New Delhi, Interprint, 1977.

Udani PM: Problems of children in developing countries. Bull Intl Pediatr Assoc 5:8, 1978.

Watson EJ: Meeting community health needs, the role of the medical assistant. WHO Chron 30:91, 1976.

WHO and UNICEF: Joint report of International Conference on Primary Health Care, Alma-Ata, 1978.

WHO: Health by the People, Newell KV (ed). Geneva, WHO, 1975.

5 GENERAL CONSIDERATIONS IN THE CARE OF SICK CHILDREN

5.1 CLINICAL EVALUATION OF INFANTS AND CHILDREN

Whether the immediate purpose is the diagnosis of illness or the maintenance of health, the evaluation of the infant, child, or adolescent should be comprehensive and continuing and should embrace psychologic and environmental as well as somatic factors. A careful and complete history and physical examination are generally more informative than are laboratory tests. The latter should be used (1) as screening procedures when direct observation is impossible or when specific and otherwise hidden conditions are being sought, (2) as confirmation or further definition of suspected conditions, (3) as a guide to complex therapy, or (4) as a means of gathering research data.

Certain qualities in the physician are appreciated by all patients and will enhance effective gathering of data, ensure greater therapeutic compliance, and increase mutual satisfaction in the doctor-patient relationship. Among them are:

Gentleness. The touch of the physician should be gentle, both literally and figuratively. Roughness, rudeness, or crudeness in manner, speech, or handling of the patient should be scrupulously avoided; they usually lead to resistance (conscious or unconscious).

Respect. Self-respect is essential to the healthy psyche and, therefore, to each healthy person. The child's self-evaluation depends partly on the perception of how others treat his or her parents. Children gain self-respect when they see their parents valued.

A basic form of respect is to care enough to learn and use a person's name. The name the child prefers should be asked at the 1st encounter and consistently remembered and used thereafter. It is an unfortunate practice of many physicians and other medical personnel to address adults whom they feel to be socially, educationally, or mentally inferior (including the aged) by their 1st names in the absence of previous 1st-name familiarity; this is a sign of condescension. The common practice of referring to boys as "males" and girls as "females" also tends to depersonalize the individual, whether child or parent, and to create or widen gaps in communication or feeling.

Understanding. Children and parents may be unpleasant, uncooperative, and hostile. No matter how distasteful this behavior, the physician must recognize that it may be dictated by forces beyond the control of the individuals concerned. Efforts to understand why parents are angry or depressed or withdrawn usually improve the doctor-patient relationship and the care of the child.

Sympathy. The warm expression of sympathy by

word or touch relieves the uncomfortable child or troubled parent of feeling alone with pain or worry. It is greatly appreciated and adds to the rapport between physician and parent. The empathetic physician can respond to negative attitudes and behavior with therapeutic rather than antagonistic or defensive behavior. Likewise, when the physician can share the feelings of his patients and their parents, he is better able to supply needed support and not likely to view an unhappy encounter as one that should be terminated as quickly as possible.

Kindness. The physician who willingly seeks small ways of making the patient feel more comfortable in mind or body increases the patient's trust and is rewarded by the patient's appreciation.

5.2 INITIAL CONTACT

At the initial contact the physician should identify himself or herself in a friendly manner to both parents and child, even if the latter is a small infant. In subsequent encounters a friendly greeting to both is always desirable. The establishment of a relaxed and friendly atmosphere facilitates taking a history and performing a physical examination. Expressions of concern for the comfort of both parent and child increase confidence in the physician as they reveal the degree of personal interest and sensitivity. The *infant* will usually remain in the parent's arms during an interview. The *small child*, if ill, may do the same but should otherwise be provided with a box of toys or other distraction to prevent boredom. If sensitive areas of the child's own behavior and management are going to be discussed, it may be better to arrange to talk with the parent or parents alone. Serious prognoses should also be discussed out of the child's presence until some decision is reached on how to handle probable questions.

The child of *school age* can usually be expected to remain quiet during an interview and should be included from time to time in the questioning. Interviews with parents alone may alarm excluded children of this age by the implication that something serious is being kept from them. Opinions differ about the degree to which the older child should be included in the discussion of serious illness and prognosis; it is probably best to make individual judgments in this regard (Sec 2.46). Speaking with parents alone is important when discussing behavior disorders; however, with parents' concurrence, the physician should frankly discuss with the child the subject, if not the content, of the earlier conversation with the parents.

The parents of *adolescents* often need opportunities to express their concerns about their children to the physician without the patient present, but the physician should always make it clear, both to them and to the adolescent, that the basic relationship exists between the physician and the adolescent. The interviewing procedures should be arranged accordingly.

5.3 HISTORY

The traditional initial medical history is made up of the following components:

Chief Complaint (C.C.), i.e., the chief reason for the visit.

Present Illness (P.I.), i.e., all details bearing directly on the chief complaint.

Past History (P.H.), including previous illnesses, a systems review, and data concerning prophylactic or screening measures, such as immunizations and the like.

Family History (F.H.), i.e., all medical conditions present in blood relatives which may by their presence or absence have a bearing on the health of the patient.

Social History (S.H.), i.e., environmental circumstances which may bear on the physical or emotional well-being of the patient.

The history obtained at subsequent contacts is usually limited to a C.C. and P.I.; new items of P.H., F.H., and S.H. are added as they come to light or become appropriate.

In eliciting the medical history of a child, the physician should initially ask the reason for the visit or hospitalization. With acutely ill patients the reason may be obvious and may be better regarded as implicit. In other situations, simple questions such as "Would you tell me what the problem is from your point of view?" are appropriate for opening communication. The physician should listen carefully and respectfully to what follows and should not interrupt with questions. At the end of the parent's or the child's free recital, the physician should recapitulate what was understood from the story to make certain that all are in agreement on what has been said and what it means. Often a number of problems other than the chief complaint are touched upon. They should be noted as they emerge for later investigation (the "problem-oriented" approach). During the recital the observant physician may gain important clues from parent-child and parent-parent interactions, also from near-tearfulness, blushing, nail-biting, changes in tone of voice, and neuromuscular tension during the telling or discussion of specific items of the history.

Particular care should be taken to allow the informant to answer each question fully before going on to another. Failure to do so implies impatience or disrespect and carries the impression to the parent or child that the interviewer is not really interested in or listening to what is

being related. It is important also to *avoid leading questions,* which may result in an inaccurate history. Sympathetic remarks (e.g., "All that activity must really tire you out at times") or oblique questions (e.g., "Does your husband's job often keep him away on weekends?") are frequently more effective than direct or blunt questions in eliciting data in sensitive areas. Material in such areas (family relations, sexual information, or behavior) may be withheld by parents until one or more visits have reassured them of the physician's interest, concern, empathy, and discretion.

At the conclusion of many interviews, it is well to formulate some question such as "I want to be sure that I have answered all your questions; can you tell me just what you expected or wanted to get from this visit?" Sometimes only in this way will the physician discover that the prime concern of the mother of a hypothyroid infant is constipation rather than the endocrine status; compliance in management of the latter may be obtained only after her concerns with the former are relieved.

5.4 PHYSICAL EXAMINATION

Setting. The room in which a child is examined contributes to the emotional climate. White is cold and buff impersonal to the small child; pastel walls achieve a cheerful and familiar effect, as do bright colors, comfortable furniture, and pictures. Glaring lights and unfamiliar equipment may be frightening. The latter should be introduced in familiar terms; the blood pressure cuff may be called a "special" or "funny" balloon, and the otoscope and ophthalmoscope "funny" or "special" flashlights. The warmth and texture of cotton flannel sheets instead of paper will make lying on the examining table more comfortable for the unclothed infant or child.

Approach. The approach to physical examination of the infant and child should be unhurried and not structured according to preconceived notions. The anxieties of even 6 or 8 wk old infants may be allayed and their cooperation obtained by getting them to smile in response to friendly voice sounds before beginning the examination. Such an approach is also reassuring to parents, whose anxiety at brusque manipulation may otherwise be transmitted to the infant by vocal or neuromuscular tension. Small children usually need to have a little time to get used to the examiner and to the place where they are to be examined. This is best accomplished by allowing the child freedom to explore while the history is being obtained. He or she should then be told ("I want you"), not asked ("Will you please?"), to remove all clothing, specifically excepting underpants since the latter seem to represent a last bastion of self-respect and protection against assault. At the end of the examination, when the child has confidence that the examiner does not intend to hurt him or her, the underpants can usually be lowered or removed without objection.

The physical examination may be performed on an examining table or on the mother's lap, whichever seems more opportune. Some children are very comfortable if examined standing. Small children are reassured if they are not required to be supine until the end of the examination when they have gained confidence in the examiner's gentleness and good intentions. The older child can be treated more like an adult; this implies no less gentleness, respect, and consideration for feelings of privacy or anxiety. The least threatening order of examination is usually inspection, palpation, percussion, auscultation, ophthalmoscopy (children 2½ yr or older will usually cooperate if not mentally retarded or emotionally disturbed), and otoscopy. Examination of the pharynx is left for last with small children since it is usually the most uncomfortable. On the other hand, many children of 3 yr and older are quite comfortable standing, with an examination "to look you over from tip to toe" that begins with "shining a light

in your ear" and moves easily to nose, mouth, teeth, pharynx, and so on to the soles.

Content. The content and order of recording of the physical examination should be reasonably standardized for ease of review and should differ little from those used in adult medicine except for (1) the inclusion of head circumference as a standard measurement for children under 2 yr; (2) the use of a growth chart (Fig 2–6, 2–7, and 2–8); (3) the inclusion of a developmental evaluation, especially for small children; and (4) an assessment of speech. The emphasis on developmental data is the major difference between the physical examinations of the child and of the adult and is essential to the interpretation of data in health and in disease since many physical signs (e.g., blood pressure, pulse, heart sounds, breath sounds, organ size, neurologic signs) are influenced by the developmental process.

5.5   THE PROBLEM-ORIENTED
MEDICAL RECORD

The problem-oriented medical record formalizes and gives structure to some time-honored principles of medical record-keeping in a way that discourages oversight, simplifies audit of performance in regard to management of individual conditions, reinforces logical thought, makes explicit the process followed, and facilitates computerization of medical data. Problem-oriented record-keeping is the cornerstone of problem-oriented medical practice, which consists of (1) establishment and use of a defined *data base*; (2) formulation and maintenance of a *problem list*; (3) a *plan for management* of each problem; (4) *education of the patient* in regard to items in the data base, problem list, plans, and their implementation; and (5) establishment and maintenance of some form of continuing audit.

Data Base. The data base in the medical record is the recorded information pertinent to the patient and the problem(s). It may be general and comprehensive or limited to the problem of immediate concern. The *basic components* of the pediatric data base are the medical history, physical examination, growth charts, developmental flow sheet, screening tests, and baseline laboratory data. The content of the data base will vary with the *age* of the patient, with the *population* from which the patient is drawn, and with the *reason* for any specific patient-physician encounter. Other factors affecting the content of the data base include the ability and willingness of the patient or others to pay for its development; the interests or concerns of individual physicians or health agencies initiating the collection of the data (these may reflect professional anxieties, confusions, or research interests); and changes in medical practice or knowledge.

Ideally, the standard or general data base should be completely defined and uniform; in practice it varies with the factors listed above. The additional data bases for individual patients, diseases, or circumstances (e.g., a defined data base for a specific complaint such as

diarrhea and vomiting) are added only as necessary. *Flow sheets* are a form of continuing data base which may be standard, as for health supervision (Fig 5–1) or diabetes, or tailored to the needs of an individual with a rare disease or complication. The self-discipline and potential anguish involved in the development of a defined data base are usually more than repaid by professional satisfaction that nothing important has been overlooked and by the long-term saving of professional time.

The initial defined data base is often best obtained through use of a questionnaire appropriate to the age and environment of the patient (see Margolis, 1977).

It is a convention of the problem-oriented record that all data are recorded under the headings of *"Subjective"* (related by the patient or other lay person) or *"Objective"* (observed directly by the physician or delegate or reported by another physician or a laboratory). Distinctions between "subjective" and "objective" sometimes become blurred under this convention, but it is generally useful, particularly in the recording of progress notes.

Once the initial data base has been recorded, a *problem list* is developed and further data are recorded in relation to the specifically named and numbered problems on the list. The *number* of the problem is entered in the left-hand margin of the page or is circled for easy reference, and the *name* of the problem is the 1st part of the entry. A more detailed data base is obtained and recorded for each problem if all relevant data are not contained already in the initial data base. In many instances it is convenient to develop defined data bases for specific illnesses or categories of illnesses. Fig 5–2 shows a check-off form for gastrointestinal illness that can save time and help ensure completeness.

Problem List. The problem list is developed from information contained in the data base. It should include any medical, social, developmental, psychologic,

HEALTH MAINTENANCE FLOW SHEET

SUBJECTIVE / EDUCATIONAL

ILLNESS	FOOD	MILK	SLEEP	ELIM	TEMPERAMENT & COMMENTS	MILESTONES			Date / Age	NUTRITION	HEALTH	SAFETY	PSYCHO-SOCIAL DEVELOPMENT
						Regards Face		Head Up	Wk.	Vits Fluoride Quan Milk Technique	URI Rash	Car Surface Bathing	Crying Colic Sibs Mother out
						Smiles	Babbles			Solids Schedule	Pain Fever ASA	Toys	Stimulation Sleeps Alone Father Mot. Child Rel
Shot Reaction?						Hands Together	Laughs	Rolls Over	2 mo.	WM Vits Schedule	Constipation Vomiting Diarrhea Bottle in bed	Peanuts Foreign Objects Ipecac Fire	Pacifier Sitter Spoiling
						Reaches		Head Steady	4 mo.	Quant Milk? Cup	Bottle in bed No Q-Tips	Head Injury E-R	Limits Toilet Trng High Chair
						Transfer Feeds Self Cracker	Mama-Dada	Sits - no Support *	6 mo.	✓Appetite Cup Jr. Foods	Shoes	Car Yard	Discipline Separation Strangers
						Pat-A-Cake	Mama Dada Specif	Gets to Sitting, Standing	9 mo.	Bottle? Feed Self	Dr. Kit	Mobility Sunburn Water	Crayons Peers Tantrums Exploration Mastery
						Indicates Wants	3 Words	Walks Well *	12 mo.	✓Fluoride Spoon	Teeth	Pets Matches	Sex Crib Negativism
						Scribbles	Combines 2 Words Body Part	Walks up Steps	18 mo.	Snacks Vitamins	Dentist	Poisons Strangers	Self-care Separation Toilet Trng
						Puts on Clothes Wash & Dry	School Readiness	Trike	2 yr.	Fluoride	Bedwetting Flossing	Getting Lost Matches Drowning	Nursery School Fantasies Responsible
						Dresses Separates	School Readiness Colors Knows Name		3 yr.		Exercise Flossing	Car Seats Ipecac	Money Sharing Independence
							School Readiness		4 yr.	Fluoride	Exercise Flossing TV	Seat Belt Fire Bike	Household Tasks Allowance Manners
									5 yr.	Fluoride	Exercise Sleep Hours	Seat Belt Fire Swimming	Home Work School on time
									6-7 yr.	Fluoride	Exercise Flossing	Seat Belt Fire Boating	Independence
									8-9 yr.	Fluoride	Exercise Menec Alcohol	Seat Belt Fire Gun	Limits
									10-11 yr.	Snacks	Exercise Flossing Smoking Breast	Seat Belt Fire	Dating
									12-13 yr.		Exercise Drugs Masturbating	Seat Belt Cars	Birth Control
									14-15 yr.	Snacks	Exercise VD	Seat Belt	Career Marriage Children
									16-17 yr.				

[INTERVAL QUESTIONNAIRE]

IMMUNIZATION RECORD

DPT DT TD						
OPV						
MEASLES						
MUMPS						
RUBELLA						

UNIVERSITY PEDIATRICS, BURLINGTON, VT.

Figure 5-1 Flow sheet for health supervision.

DATE _____

TEMP PROB

ONSET/DURATION

SUBJ	OBJ		LAB
VOMITING	TOXIC?	WT	URINE
NO. IN LAST 12 HRS.	TEMP	BP	SP GR
	RR	PULSE	SED
DIARRHEA	SKIN TURGOR		STOOL CULT
CONSIST/COLOR	MUCOUS MEMBRANES		HEMATEST
FREQ.. (NO. IN 6 HRS.)	EYES		HCT
BLOOD/PUS	FONTANELLE		WBC
PAIN	DTR'S		DIFF
LOCATION	ABD. TENDERNESS		X-RAY
QUALITY	GUARDING?		
FEVER	REBOUND?		
URINATING?	BOWEL SOUNDS		
FLUIDS?	RECTAL		ASST.
IRRITABLE?	NECK		ASST.
SLEEPLESS?	THROAT		
TREATMENT	EARS		
	CHEST		
	DEHYDRATION?		PLAN
	SIGNED		

Figure 5-2 Data base and record for acute gastrointestinal illness.

NAME: _Betty Doe_

DOB: _July 4, 1984_

PROBLEM LIST

Entry Date	#	ACTIVE PROBLEMS	Date Resolved	INACTIVE OR RESOLVED PROBLEMS
7/14/84	1	Health Supervision		
8/14/84	2	Vomiting — 8/28/84 → Pyloric stenosis	8/29/84	s/p Pyloromyotomy
1/15/85	3	Paternal grandfather has Huntington's chorea		
4/14/85	4	Both parents working outside the home		
11/12/87	5	Father lost job 9/30/87	6/15/88	
4/19/88	6	H. Flu meningitis	4/19/88	
	7			
	8			

TEMPORARY PROBLEM LIST

No.	Problem	Ons.	Res.	Ons.	Res.	Ons.	Res.	Ons.	Res.	Ons.
A	Vomiting	7/24/84	8/29/84	4/8/88	4/10/88					
B	Constipation	8/4/84	8/31/84							
C	Hyponatremia + hypokalemia	8/28/84	8/30/84							
D	"Otitis Media"	3/3/85	3/4/85	11/2/87	11/12/87					
E	Diarrhea	8/20/85	8/25/85	1/5/88	1/8/88					
F	Serous otitis	11/12/87	1/5/88							

Figure 5—3 Sample master problem list.

economic, or environmental problems that have been identified, and each should be assigned a number and a name. Each subsequent entry in the record, including those on the hospital order sheet, is identified with the number and name of the problem to which it refers. This form of record-keeping makes it easier to locate all entries relating to a single problem, simplifies an *audit* of the record, and is ideally adapted to computerization, with easy ultimate retrieval of the data, notes, and orders referable to specific problems.

The *name of a problem* is customarily entered as (1) a diagnosis, (2) a physiologic or behavioral manifestation, (3) a symptom or physical finding, (4) an abnormal laboratory finding, (5) the history of a disease in the patient or the family, or (6) a social, environmental, or demographic circumstance that bears significantly on the patient, the illness, or management.

Each problem should be expressed only at a level of understanding or confidence that can be substantiated by objective evidence, including the course of the illness. This consideration helps the formulator of the problem list keep an open mind about diagnostic possibilities and avoid jumping to potentially erroneous diagnostic conclusions. For example, the initial entry on the problem list of a child with suspected meningitis would be "Fever, vomiting, and stiff neck." If a spinal tap shows purulent fluid, an arrow is drawn and the problem updated to "meningitis." If the cerebrospinal fluid culture grows out *Hemophilus influenzae* 2 days later, the problem is again updated to the final diagnosis of "*H. influenzae* meningitis." Each time an arrow is drawn to update a problem, the date or time of the updating is indicated over the shaft of the arrow (Fig 5–3). The problem list thus encourages logical rather than intuitive thinking in the clinical appraisal of the patient.

Generally, a problem is entered into the problem list and given a number when it requires specific and separate attention or action. Several conventions may be employed to keep the problem list from becoming unwieldy. For children, *health supervision* may be entered routinely as Problem No. 1 and all items relating to the observation of normal development, anticipatory guidance, and immunization referred to it. If a developmental abnormality of major or continuing importance (such as enuresis or mental retardation) becomes apparent, it is then listed as a separate problem with a separate number. Minor or transient complaints without sequelae are often entered as "Temporary Problems." These are listed separately with space to indicate the dates of recurrences; if the latter are frequent, transfer to the main problem list may be justified. Certain problems may be critical at the time they occur but of little long-term significance. This is particularly likely with problems leading to hospitalization. Consider, for example, the case of a child whose appendicitis is complicated by wound infection and dehiscence, bacteremia, penicillin reaction, water intoxication with convulsions, hypokalemia, and a near-fatal accidental overdose of morphine. Each of these is a major problem at some time, but only appendicitis, appendectomy, and penicillin allergy would be appropriate for inclusion in the permanent problem list. This situation may be handled either (1) by entering the associated problems as subproblems of appendectomy, e.g., wound infection, or (2) by listing each complication as a separate problem on a "single-admission problem list" and transcribing only "appendicitis → status postappendectomy" and "penicillin allergy" onto the permanent problem list, which remains separate from the single-admission problem list.

Ideally, there should be only 1 problem list for a patient and it should be continuous from birth to death, but in practice this may become cumbersome. As a result, problem lists may have to be revised from time to time. Moreover, other health professionals who see patients may need their own problem lists to guide them. In any event, the *primary physician* should be responsible for keeping a "permanent" or "master" problem list which is shared with patient or parent and which can serve as a guide to maintaining perspective and to ensuring that individual problems are not forgotten.

Although disagreements may arise as to what should be entered as separate problems, all perceived problems should be specifically identified and management efforts directed accordingly. The list should help the physician to deliver comprehensive and auditable care.

Assessment. Ordinarily, regular assessments should be made of each problem, including in each instance a direct or implied statement of the goal of the *plan* which is to be followed. For instance, if the assessment is "Probable febrile convulsion, r/o (rule out) meningitis," the implied goal of the initial plan is the elimination of meningitis as a diagnostic possibility. Once that has been done, the fever may become a problem separate from the convulsion, each requiring its own assessment and plan (which may be merely that certain possibilities should be diagnostically eliminated). In each instance, the assessment should place in perspective a reasonable, explicit, or implicit goal and a logical plan of action that will achieve that goal; accordingly, the assessment might be not to work up a problem at all, or it might define the extent of therapeutic effort to be expended.

Plan. The plan should consist of 4 parts: (1) information related to diagnosis (Dx), (2) treatment (Rx), (3) patient or parent education (Ed), and (4) follow-up (FU). Each plan, whether initial or subsequent, should contain these components in a clearly stated manner, including "none" if no plan is being made under that heading.

Progress Notes. Progress notes should be identified by the number and name of the problem to which they refer. Each note should contain 4 sections: (1) *subjective* data, usually supplied by the patient or parent; (2) *objective*, for directly ascertained data such as a new physical or laboratory finding; (3) *assessment*, for a statement of the significance of the data, including an explicit or implied goal for the following plan; and (4) *a plan* which follows logically from the content of (1), (2), and (3). The mnemonic SOAP is often used to designate these 4 sections of the progress note.

Flow Sheets. Most good plans for continuing problems require flow sheets that list the appropriate variables to be followed, thus serving as both simplified progress notes and reminders that certain items should be or have been checked periodically. Fig 5–1, for example, is a flow sheet for health supervision. It serves both as a reminder and a checklist (the guidance items, for instance, may be checked off on the sheet as they are carried out, and thus the physician has a handy record of what has and has not been done in this regard). The use of flow sheets increases the efficiency of the physician; once they have been prepared, most of the data can be gathered by an assistant for review and decision-making by the physician.

Audit. Audit of the problem-oriented record consists of 2 phases: nonprofessional and professional. *Nonprofessional audit* can be done by other than a physician through use of a checklist. It chiefly focuses on aspects of thoroughness, such as:

Was a data base obtained?

Are all the components of the data base contained in the record?

Are the components completed as defined?

Is there a problem list?

Are all entries in the progress notes referred to specific problems?

Were plans carried out?

Was patient education done?

Was planned follow-up carried out?

Professional audit is for quality of care; it includes (1) review of the nonprofessional audit, if that has been done; (2) review of the data base to see if all problems have been identified and entered on the problem list; and (3) general review of the record for thoroughness, efficiency, analytic sense, reliability, and professional knowledge and competence.

Disadvantages. The relatively rigid and detailed structure of the problem-oriented record can result, when improperly and overcompulsively used, in a greatly increased expenditure of time and paper. The emphasis on identification and management of each problem as a separate entity may lead not only to fragmentation of the record but to a loss of perspective; the neophyte, for instance, may be so intent on handling his or her patient's fever, vomiting, convulsions, and stiff neck as separate problems that the diagnosis of meningitis may be elusive or delayed. The method is still undergoing modification. Some physicians fear that it will foster medical care by rote, and that it may lead to depersonalization of care or to an overemphasis on structure rather than substance. Problems encountered in its implementation and use are more easily handled if users recognize that arbitrary judgments must be made in the adaptation of any new system to local conditions and that the user must remain the master; the system, the tool.

R. JAMES McKay

Barness LA: Manual of Pediatric Physical Diagnosis. Ed 4. Chicago, Year Book Medical Publishers, 1972.
Korsch BM: The pediatrician's approach to his patient. Am J Dis Child 126:146, 1973.
Margolis CG: The Pediatric Problem-Oriented Record. A Manual for Implementation. Pleasantville, NY, Docent Corp, 1977.
Walker HK, Hurst JW, Woody MF (eds): Applying the Problem-Oriented System. New York, MEDCOM Press, 1973.

5.6   THE PATHOPHYSIOLOGY OF BODY FLUIDS

The physiology of body fluids should be considered from 3 perspectives: (1) *The total amounts of water and solutes in the body as a whole.* These are the result of carefully regulated balances between intake and output. Many of the controlling mechanisms, especially for substances of physiologic significance, are extremely complex. Those of special importance to the clinician will be discussed in some detail. (2) *The distribution of water and solutes in the various compartments of the body.* This is of critical importance. Because relatively few substances are kept in simple equilibrium free of energy-requiring processes, considerable energy is required to maintain steady states. (3) *The concentration of the solutes within each compartment.* This depends on the relative amounts of both solute and the solvent (water) in that compartment. Thus, concentration can be changed by altering the content of either solute or water or both.

Regulatory mechanisms appear designed to prevent large changes in concentrations of solutes, changes which can lead to profound alterations in function. In general, the rate and percentage of change in concentration of the various solutes are of greater physiologic and clinical significance than is absolute change. For example, an alteration of 3 mEq/l from normal in the extracellular fluid concentration of potassium represents a change of approximately 70% and may result in profound physiologic effects, whereas an alteration of 3 mEq/l in the extracellular fluid sodium concentration amounts to a change of only 2%, is well tolerated, and is of little clinical significance.

Changes in volume are relatively well tolerated. Here, too, percentage and rate of change are more critical than absolute change. Thus, the loss of 100 ml of blood in a few minutes would produce a negligible disturbance in an adolescent but would result in shock in a newborn infant; the same hemorrhage in the infant extended over several days could be fairly well compensated.

5.7   WATER

TOTAL BODY WATER

Water constitutes 78% of body weight at birth but declines to approximately 60% (the adult value) by 1 yr of age. Fig 5–4 illustrates a linear relationship between total body water (TBW) and body weight (wt). The equation describing this relationship is TBW (liters) = 0.611 wt (kg) + 0.251. Thus, approximate estimates of total body water can be obtained from body weight

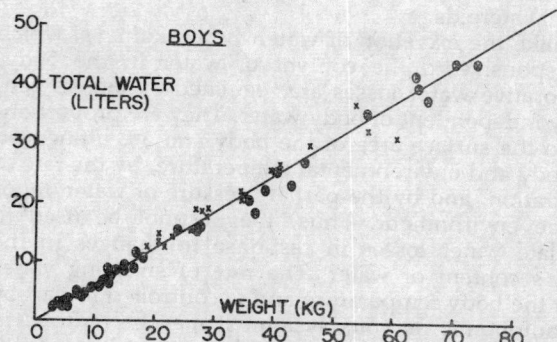

Figure 5–4 Total body water in boys plotted against body weight. The relevant equation is given in the text. The data of Cheek are indicated by X; those of Friis-Hansen, by ⊗. (From Cheek DB (ed.): Human Growth. Philadelphia, Lea & Febiger, 1968; and Friis-Hansen B: Changes in body water compartments during growth. Acta Paediatr 1957.)

alone. However, fat is low in water content, so TBW represents a smaller percentage of body weight in an obese than in a normal person, and a more exact estimate of TBW can be obtained from lean body mass (LBM) where the relationship is TBW (liters) = 0.72 LBM (kg).

Fluid Compartments. Body water is composed of intracellular and extracellular components (Fig 5–5). *Extracellular fluid* (ECF) volume is larger than the intracellular space in the fetus, but the ratio of extracellular water to intracellular water falls to the adult level by 9 mo of postnatal life. This relative loss of extracellular fluid is presumably the result of the increasing growth of cellular tissue and the decreasing rate of growth of collagen relative to muscle during the early months of life. Thereafter, extracellular fluid bears a fairly straight-line relation to weight (ECF = 0.239 wt (kg) + 0.325) and to total body water in normal infants and children. Under conditions of normal hydration in the older child (Fig 5–5) it constitutes 20–25% of body weight and is composed of plasma water (5% of body weight), interstitial water (15% of body weight), and transcellular water (1–3% of body weight).

The *transcellular water* compartment is composed primarily of gastrointestinal secretions plus cerebrospinal, intraocular, pleural, peritoneal, and synovial fluids. Transcellular fluid is usually considered a specialized fraction of extracellular fluid, although it is probably more accurate to consider fluid in the gastrointestinal tract as extracorporeal. The volume of the transcellular compartment varies greatly, depending on the absorptive and secretory activities of the intestine; during the fasting state it represents about 1–3% of body weight.

Intracellular fluid volume (ICF) is calculated as the difference between total body water and extracellular water. It approximates 30–40% of body weight. It is important to remember that, although frequently considered as a homogeneous phase, intracellular fluid represents the sum of fluids from cells in different locations with varying functions and differing intracellular compositions.

REGULATION OF BODY WATER

The plasma osmolality remains almost constant at 285–295 mOsm/kg H_2O regardless of day-to-day fluctuations in solute and water intake. This accomplishment is due in large part to precise control of the amount of water in the body through a finely regulated feedback system involving osmo- and volume receptors, the hypothalamus, the posterior pituitary, and the collecting ducts of the nephrons. To maintain a constant state, the amount of body water derived from intake and from oxidation of carbohydrate, fat, and protein of both exogenous and endogenous origin must equal losses from the kidneys, lungs, skin, and gastrointestinal tract. Water balance is controlled by regulating both intake and excretion, the latter being the more important regulatory mechanism.

Intake. Normally, intake of water is stimulated by a sensation of *thirst;* this mechanism represents a major defense against fluid depletion and hypertonicity. Thirst is regulated by a center in the midhypothalamus and occurs either when plasma osmolality increases by

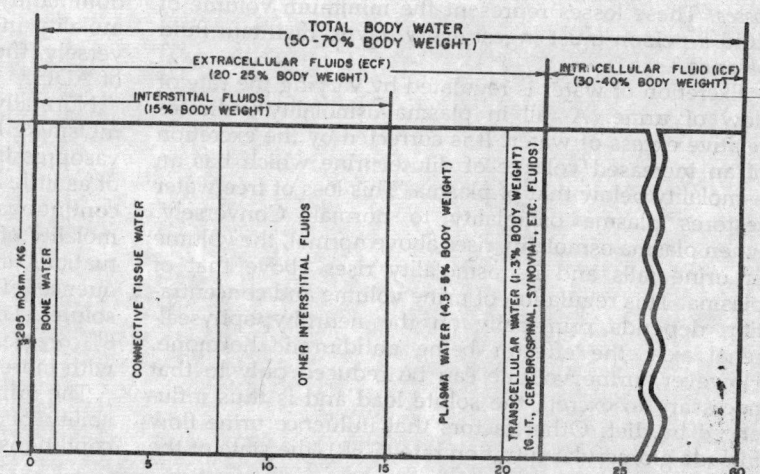

Figure 5–5 The distribution of water in the body of the older child. Percentages = % of body weight; G.I.T. = gastrointestinal tract.

as little as 1–2% or when there is a significant reduction in volume of body fluids, as occurs with hemorrhage or sodium depletion. The changes in osmolality are monitored by osmoreceptors (see below) located in the hypothalamus and possibly in the pancreas and hepatic portal vein. The mechanisms by which volume depletion induces thirst are less well understood, but it may be monitored by baroreceptors in the atria and elsewhere in the vascular bed. There is considerable circumstantial evidence to indicate that elevated plasma levels of angiotensin II stimulate drinking. They may be a mediator of thirst in hypovolemic and hypotensive states. The kidney may also be involved in regulating water intake, possibly through the renin-angiotensin system.

In clinical situations, when conflicting stimuli such as hypotonicity and decreased intravascular volume occur together, the volume signal is dominant and thirst causes increased water intake, restoring volume at the expense of tonicity.

The thirst mechanism and release of antidiuretic hormone (ADH) may be interrelated. However, at least some of the thirst centers are separated functionally and physically from those involved in release of ADH.

Disorders of the thirst mechanism may be seen in psychologic disorders associated with diseases of the central nervous system, in potassium deficiency, and in malnutrition. These may lead to increased drinking, even though the content of body water is greater than usual and osmolality is decreased.

Absorption.   Absorption of ingested water occurs in the gastrointestinal tract by passive diffusion in response to active transport of solute from intestinal lumen to interstitial fluid and plasma. The active transport of sodium is the chief process responsible for generating the osmotic gradient leading to movement of water. Any inhibition of sodium transport or failure of reabsorption of solute, as in disaccharidase deficiency, can lead to large volumes of unabsorbed intestinal water and result in diarrhea.

Excretion.   Losses of water occur from the lungs, skin, gastrointestinal tract, and kidneys. The losses from the lungs and skin are evaporative and, in conjunction with that part of the urine volume necessary to excrete its solute load, are referred to as *obligatory losses*. These losses represent the minimum volume of fluid a person must ingest every day to maintain fluid balance.

Excretion of water is regulated by varying the rate of flow of urine. A fall in plasma osmolality indicates relative excess of water. It is corrected by the excretion of an increased volume of dilute urine which has an osmolality below that of plasma. This loss of free water restores plasma osmolality to normal. Conversely, when plasma osmolality rises above normal, the volume of urine falls and its osmolality rises above that of plasma. This regulation of urine volume and concentration depends principally on the neurohypophyseal-renal axis, the effector being antidiuretic hormone. However, urine volume can be reduced only to that necessary to excrete the solute load and is thus influenced by diet. Other factors that influence urine flow include glomerular filtration rate (GFR), the state of the renal tubular epithelium, and plasma concentrations of adrenal steroids.

Unlike the excretion of water by the kidneys, which is responsive to the content of water in the body, evaporative water losses are regulated by factors generally independent of body water. They are proportionate to the surface area of the body and are influenced by body and environmental temperature, by the rate of respiration, and by the partial pressure of water vapor in the environment. Thus, they cannot be used to regulate water losses in response to changes in the body's content of water. The rate of sweating varies with the body temperature and is controlled in part by the autonomic nervous system. It may be reduced in heat stress, by *severe* deficits in volume of body fluids or by concentration of electrolytes, but still does not represent a major mechanism for regulation of body water.

Antidiuretic Hormone (ADH).   Human ADH (arginine vasopressin), a cyclic octapeptide, is synthesized in the supraoptic nuclei. This neurosecretory substance is transported down axons which descend through the infundibular stem to be stored in the terminal arborizations in the pars nervosa of the posterior pituitary. Release of ADH into the blood stream occurs by exocytosis in response to stimuli from the hypothalamus. Depletion of ADH in the posterior pituitary occurs in animals deprived of water; storage occurs when water loads are administered.

Secretion of ADH is regulated by the effective osmotic pressure of the extracellular fluid, i.e., that produced by solutes (primarily sodium and chloride) which do not readily penetrate cell membranes. This is monitored by vesicles in the supraoptic nuclei which act as osmoreceptors. They swell when the osmolality of extracellular fluid is less than that of the intracellular fluid and shrink when the osmolality of extracellular fluid is greater than that of the intracellular fluid. Thus, the administration of urea, which readily diffuses across cell membranes and increases the osmolality of both extracellular and intracellular fluids, produces little shift of water between cells and interstitial fluid and does not evoke consistent antidiuresis. On the other hand, the intravenous injection of hypertonic saline solution evokes intense antidiuresis; the sodium remains predominantly in the extracellular fluid, increasing its osmolality in relation to that of intracellular fluid. Conversely, the administration of water inhibits the release of ADH.

Normally, the threshold for release of ADH is 280 mOsm/kg H_2O. The initiation or inhibition of release of vasopressin occurs with changes in plasma osmolality of as little as 1–2%. Response is graded, permitting the continuous regulation of urine volume and of the osmolality of extracellular fluid, thus preventing the fluctuations in osmolality that would occur as a consequence of normal variations in intake of fluid and solutes. Levels of ADH also increase significantly after 8% or greater dehydration, the rise being exponential with more marked dehydration.

The primary action of ADH is to increase the permeability of the renal collecting ducts to water. Under conditions of antidiuresis, the interstitium of the renal medulla has an osmolality of up to 1200 mOsm/kg H₂O at the level of the papilla. This is accomplished by the actions of the countercurrent multiplier (loops of Henle) and exchange (medullary vasa recta blood vessels) systems. In the presence of ADH, luminal urine entering the collecting duct has an osmolality of about 285 mOsm/kg H₂O. It becomes progressively more concentrated along the course of the collecting duct as water diffuses out of the urine into the hypertonic medullary interstitium by passive osmotic diffusion. By the time the urine enters the calyces, it has achieved the same concentration as the fluid in the hypertonic medullary papillae. If ADH is absent, continued reabsorption of sodium in the distal tubule and collecting duct leads to further dilution of the urine. Since, in the absence of ADH, these segments of the nephron are impermeable to water, diffusion into the hypertonic medulla does not occur and dilute urine is formed.

Influence of Disease States. Interruption of the supraoptic hypophyseal system causes diabetes insipidus. A failure of the renal collecting ducts to respond to ADH results in nephrogenic diabetes insipidus. Both are accompanied by an inability to concentrate the urine. Release of ADH may be stimulated or inhibited by emotional factors. Stressful stimuli such as pain or the mass discharge of peripheral receptors resulting from trauma, burns, or surgery increase ADH output and are important considerations in fluid therapy. Nicotine, prostaglandins, and cholinergic and beta-adrenergic drugs are potent stimulators of ADH output. Demerol, morphine, and barbiturates are probably antidiuretic in this way although their reduction of GFR may contribute to their reduction of urine flow. Alcohol is a potent inhibitor of ADH release with a consistent dose-response relation. Diphenylhydantoin and possibly glucocorticoids also inhibit ADH release. Anesthesia reduces urinary flow, probably by altering renal hemodynamics. The presence of nonabsorbable, osmotically active solutes in the renal tubular lumen, e.g., glucose in diabetes mellitus, reduces the amount of water that can diffuse into the hypertonic medulla and thus limits the ability of ADH to conserve water.

MECHANISMS OF DISTRIBUTION OF FLUID IN THE BODY

The distribution of water between intracellular and extracellular spaces is determined by physical factors. *Intracellular volume* is maintained relatively constant by osmotic forces operating across cell membranes freely permeable to water. The maintenance of these forces is dependent upon active transport of potassium into and sodium out of cells by energy-requiring processes. There is no evidence for active transport or secretion of water per se. A rise in extracellular osmolality (e.g., with a sodium load) results in a fall in cell water. Conversely, water intoxication decreases extracellular osmolality and leads to an increase in cell volume. Disturbances in cellular function may also result in an increase in the fluid content of cells.

The volume of fluid in the *intravascular space* (plasma water) is maintained in a steady state by a balance between filtration and oncotic forces at the capillary level. Oncotic pressure (colloid osmotic pressure) represents only a small fraction of total osmotic pressure,* but its osmotic pressure is exerted by molecules, primarily albumin, which do not readily pass through the capillary pores. Thus, colloid osmotic pressure results in an effective osmotic gradient across capillary walls. At the arteriolar end of the capillaries the dominant effect of intracapillary hydrostatic pressure is a net loss of plasma ultrafiltrate. Normally, at the venous end of the capillary, oncotic pressure results in the net return of an equivalent amount of fluid and electrolytes.

Decreases in protein concentration (as in the nephrotic syndrome) lead to reductions in plasma volume with equivalent increases in *interstitial volume*. These changes may compromise the intravascular volume enough to reduce glomerular filtration rate and blood flow to other vital organs, but, since the volume of plasma is only one third that of interstitial fluid, reduction of plasma volume through shifts of water to the interstitial space may not be observed clinically as *edema*. An increase in permeability of capillaries to protein, as in angioneurotic edema, produces a rise in protein concentration of the interstitial fluid. This reduces net oncotic pressure and causes a net shift of fluid, which increases interstitial fluid volume. The increase may be localized, appearing as a wheal or urticaria, or may be generalized. Interstitial fluid volume may also be increased by an increase in the hydrostatic pressure at the venous end of the capillary, as occurs with increased venous pressure associated with heart failure or with retention of sodium and resultant hypervolemia in glomerulonephritis.

The *transcellular fluid* space normally represents 1–3% of body weight. It may increase markedly in inflammatory bowel disease, e.g., eosinophilic gastroenteropathy, in early severe diarrhea, or in ileus with multiple fluid levels.

OSMOLALITY OF BODY FLUIDS

The concentrations of individual solutes in the extracellular and intracellular fluids vary (Fig 5–6). However, the osmolality (concentration of solute particles) in each compartment is comparable (Fig 5–5); thus, the chemical activity of water (i.e., the tendency of molecules to escape to another compartment) is the same in each compartment. Nevertheless, the water content of the different body fluids does differ considerably, and variations in these values from normal can be of clinical significance. For example, when serum solids such as the proteins and lipids are elevated, as may occur in diabetic ketosis with hyperlipemia, the content of water

---

*The principal colloids in the plasma are the plasma proteins. They exert an osmotic pressure of approximately 28 mm Hg compared with the 5100 mm Hg exerted by the crystalloidal solutes of plasma. However, the capillary walls are very permeable to the crystalloidal solutes, which, therefore, exert no osmotic force across the capillary walls. Albumin, the most abundant plasma protein and the one with the lowest molecular weight, is the principal solute responsible for colloid osmotic pressure and for regulating net water movement across capillary walls.

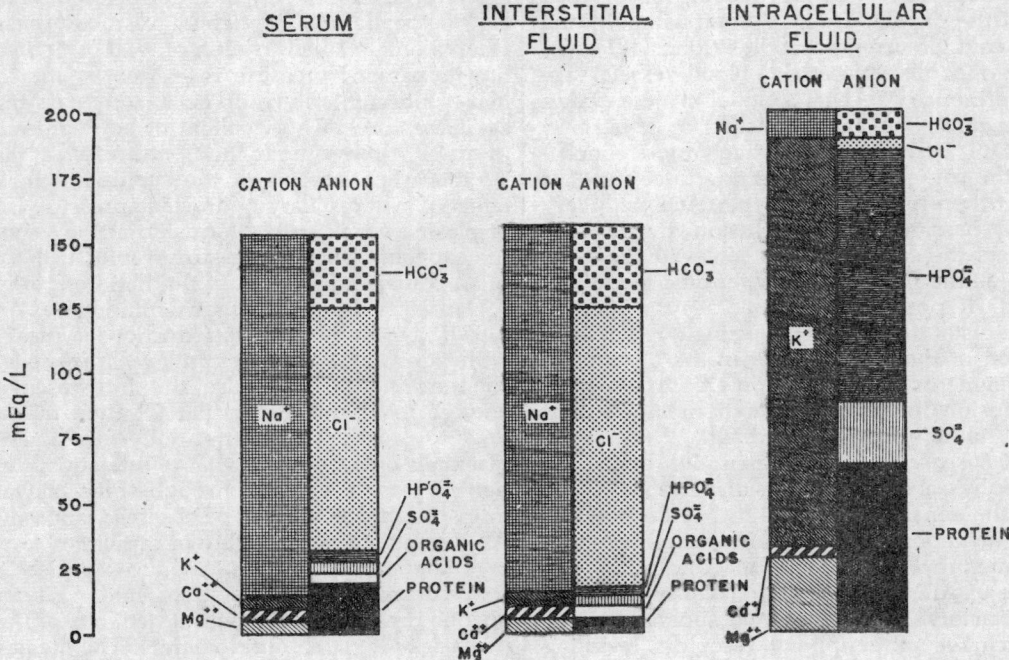

Figure 5–6 Differences in composition of intracellular and extracellular fluids.

in the serum is markedly decreased (when expressed per liter of serum) because of volume displacement of water by lipids. Since electrolytes are dissolved in the aqueous phase of serum, electrolyte concentrations determined and expressed in the usual way (as mEq per liter of serum) will appear decreased even though their concentration per liter of serum water will be normal. Spurious hyponatremia is most often noted in this circumstance. Treatment of such *pseudohyponatremia* is not necessary and may be detrimental to the patient. Its occurrence can be recognized by simultaneous measurement of osmolality by freezing point depression (osmometry). This determination measures solute content as related to the water fraction of serum only and provides a more accurate reflection of sodium concentration in the serum water. Alternatively, sodium concentration can be measured using ion-specific electrodes.

5.8 SODIUM

BODY CONTENT OF SODIUM

Sodium is the bulk cation of the extracellular fluid and is the principal osmotically active solute responsible for the maintenance of intravascular and interstitial volumes. The quantity of sodium in the body approximates 58 mEq/kg; more than 30% of this sodium is either nonexchangeable or only slowly exchangeable. The distribution of sodium in different body compartments is shown in Fig 5–7. Of total body sodium, 6.5 mEq/kg (11.2% of total) is present in the plasma sodium pool, 16.8 mEq/kg in the interstitial fluid, and 1.4 mEq/

kg in the intracellular fluid. About 25 mEq/kg (43.1% of total body sodium) is present in bone, but only one third of the sodium in bone is exchangeable.

The *sodium content of the fetus* is relatively higher than that of the adult; exchangeable sodium averages approximately 85 mEq/kg compared to the adult value of 40 mEq/kg because the fetus has relatively large

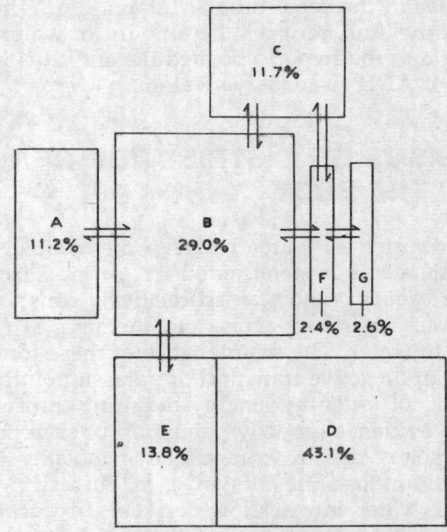

Figure 5–7 Distribution of sodium within the body of a normal young adult man. A, Plasma sodium; B, interstitial lymph sodium; C, dense connective tissue and cartilage sodium; D, total bone sodium (including E); E, exchangeable bone sodium; F, intracellular sodium; G, transcellular sodium. (From Edelman IS, Liebman J: Am J Med 27:256, 1959.)

amounts of cartilage, connective tissue, and extracellular fluid (all of which contain considerable amounts of sodium) and a relatively small mass of muscle cells (which have a low sodium content).

REGULATION OF SODIUM

Intake. The amount of sodium in the body is determined by the balance between intake and excretion. When compared to the thirst mechanism for water, the regulatory mechanism for sodium *intake* is poorly developed but may respond to gross changes, e.g., salt craving may occur in some patients with salt-wasting syndromes. However, under normal circumstances sodium intake depends on cultural customs. In the average adult in the United States it usually varies from 100–170 mEq per day, equivalent to 6–10 gm of salt. The sodium intake of children is less, in proportion to their smaller intake of food. However, infants generally have a relatively high sodium intake because of the high sodium content of cow milk.

Absorption. This occurs throughout the gastrointestinal tract, minimally in the stomach and maximally in the jejunum, probably by way of a sodium-potassium–activated ATPase (adenosine triphosphatase) system. This transport mechanism is augmented by aldosterone or desoxycorticosterone acetate (DCA).

Excretion. This occurs in the urine, sweat, and feces, with the kidney the principal organ for the facultative regulation of sodium output. Normally, the concentration of sodium in sweat usually ranges from 5–40 mEq/l. Higher values are seen in cystic fibrosis and Addison disease, lower values in sodium depletion and hyperaldosteronism, but there is little evidence that changes in the level of sodium in sweat are part of the excretory mechanism for regulating the sodium content of the body. In the absence of diarrhea, fecal concentrations of sodium are low.

Renal regulation of sodium excretion depends on a balance between glomerular and tubular functions. Under normal conditions the amount of sodium filtered daily by the kidneys is more than 100 times that ingested and more than 5 times the total amount of sodium in the body. However, less than 1% of the filtered sodium is excreted in the urine; the remaining 99% is reabsorbed along the length of the renal tubule.

Under normal conditions changes in glomerular filtration rate (GFR) do not affect sodium homeostasis; changes in the filtered load of sodium produced by alterations in GFR are compensated for by appropriate changes in tubular reabsorption of sodium. Moreover, sodium balance can be achieved even when sodium intake varies and GFR remains stable. However, the reduction in GFR that occurs with severe depletion of the volume of extracellular fluid and the increase that accompanies volume expansion may facilitate sodium regulation. Even then it has been shown that experimentally induced changes in GFR, over a wide range, are accompanied by proportional changes in sodium reabsorption in the proximal tubule. Such glomerular-tubular balance reduces changes in the delivery of sodium to more distal segments of the nephron, even

when the filtered load of sodium alters markedly, and presumably acts as a protective mechanism.

Approximately two thirds of the filtered sodium is reabsorbed by the *proximal convoluted tubule*. With contraction of extracellular fluid volume this fraction increases; with volume expansion, it decreases. The percentages of filtered sodium and water reabsorbed in the proximal tubule are proportional so that the fluid remaining at the end of the proximal convoluted tubule has a sodium concentration comparable to that in the blood. Sodium enters the tubular cell from the lumen across the brush border membrane. Traditionally, this process has been considered to be passive, but recent observations suggest that a more complex mechanism may be required to permit such a high net rate of sodium flux into the cell. The extrusion of sodium from the cell occurs at both the basilar and lateral surfaces and represents active transport against both electrical and concentration gradients. This sodium transport creates an osmotic gradient that results in the net movement of an equivalent volume of water out of the proximal tubule. The resulting hydrostatic force in the intercellular spaces and basilar infoldings stimulates the movement of salt and water toward the peritubular capillaries and entry into these vessels. This latter process occurs according to Starling forces and is also dependent on the oncotic pressure exerted by the plasma proteins of the blood in the peritubular capillary.

Glomerular-tubular balance may be maintained through changes in the concentration of protein in the peritubular capillaries. According to this theory, an increase in glomerular filtration rate without a change in renal plasma flow would result in an increased filtration fraction and a decreased blood volume in the glomerular efferent arterioles. Consequently, the concentration of protein in the efferent arterioles and the oncotic pressure in the peritubular capillaries would be increased and facilitate increased proximal tubular reabsorption of salt and water and maintenance of glomerulotubular balance.

The epithelium of the proximal convoluted tubule permits movement of sodium and water not only from the tubular lumen into the peritubular spaces but also in the opposite direction. This latter movement probably occurs principally through the intercellular spaces, with the net rate of sodium reabsorption representing the difference between these fluxes. Thus, the "tight junctions" present at the luminal end of the intercellular spaces may also regulate *net* movement of sodium out of the proximal tubules. Under certain conditions these structures appear patent and may provide a route for return of part of the sodium and water into the lumen since hydrostatic pressure in the intercellular spaces is higher than that in the lumen. Sodium reabsorption in the proximal tubule may also be regulated by a natriuretic hormone secreted from the midbrain or hypothalamic region. Although considerable indirect evidence supports this hypothesis, such a hormone has yet to be isolated.

Significant sodium reabsorption occurs in the *loop of Henle* and is central to the countercurrent multiplier system essential for water balance and the concentration of urine (see above). Water reabsorption occurs in the

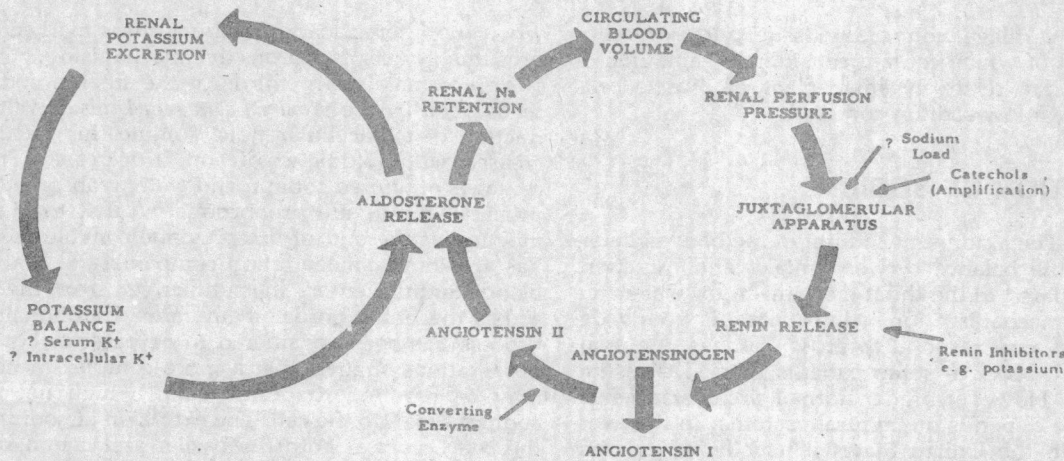

Figure 5–8 The interrelationship of the volume and potassium feedback loops with aldosterone secretion. Integration of signals from each loop determines the level of aldosterone secretion. (From Williams GH, Dluhy RG: Am J Med 53:595, 1972.)

descending limb of the loop of Henle, sodium reabsorption in the ascending limb. Sodium transport at this site may be secondary to the active transport of chloride rather than primary as it is at most other sites. Although the loop of Henle is clearly important in the overall control of sodium reabsorption, no precise mechanism for regulation has yet been delineated, nor has a maximal rate for sodium transport at this site been demonstrated. When the load of sodium delivered to the loop is increased, either by changes in glomerular filtration rate or in sodium reabsorption in the proximal tubule, most of the excess load is reabsorbed in the loop, providing a further protective mechanism and limiting the magnitude of changes of delivery of sodium to the distal convoluted tubule.

The fine regulation of sodium balance probably occurs throughout the distal nephron in both the *distal convoluted tubules* and the *collecting ducts*. Sodium reabsorption at these sites is stimulated by aldosterone; secretion of this hormone is governed by the renin-angiotensin system, by some aspect of potassium balance (Fig 5–8), and by a tropic hormone. The release of renin from the cells of the juxtaglomerular apparatus results in the conversion in the plasma of angiotensinogen into angiotensin I and in the production of angiotensin II. This latter compound stimulates aldosterone secretion from the adrenal. The stimulus for release of renin may be a decrease in renal perfusion pressure or a change in sodium concentration (or delivery) in the distal tubule at the level of the macula densa; either system provides a "servo-mechanism" to prevent excessive changes in sodium balance. Throughout the distal tubule and collecting duct, sodium is reabsorbed against a large concentration gradient from lumen to plasma; there appears to be no limit to the reduction in luminal sodium concentration that can be reached. However, in comparison with the proximal convoluted tubule and the loop of Henle, the total capacity for sodium reabsorption is more limited. Thus, if the load of sodium reaching the distal tubule increases significantly, reab-

sorption does not increase proportionately and the added load is excreted in the urine.

Additional mechanisms may be responsible for the renal regulation of sodium. It has been postulated that the cortical nephrons with their short loops of Henle may be sodium-losing nephrons and the juxtamedullary nephrons with long loops of Henle, sodium-retaining nephrons. Sodium balance could be accomplished by altering the proportion of renal blood flow directed to these 2 populations of nephrons. Such a regulatory mechanism could be intrarenal and respond to local release of renin.

In health, less than 1% of filtered sodium is normally excreted in the urine. However, to maintain sodium balance this figure may increase to 10% or higher with a high sodium intake and can decrease to very low levels in response to reduced dietary sodium. Thus, there is considerable flexibility in sodium intake which prevents a significant positive or negative sodium balance, accompanied respectively by edema or by volume contraction.

DISTRIBUTION OF BODY SODIUM

Although cell membranes are relatively permeable to it, sodium is predominantly extracellular in distribution. Intracellular concentrations are maintained at levels of approximately 10 mEq/l and extracellular ones at approximately 140 mEq/l. The low intracellular concentration is achieved by active extrusion of sodium from cells by the sodium-potassium and magnesium-activated ATPase systems. No other cation can replace sodium stimulation of ATPase, but potassium can be replaced by ammonium, rubidium, cesium, and lithium. Calcium inhibits ATPase, as do ouabain and related cardiac glycosides.

Although intracellular concentrations of sodium are low and represent a small part of total body sodium, they may be critical in modifying certain intracellular

Table 5–1 SODIUM, POTASSIUM, AND CHLORIDE CONCENTRATIONS IN TRANSCELLULAR FLUIDS

FLUID	SODIUM (mEq/L)	POTASSIUM (mEq/L)	CHLORIDE (mEq/L)
Saliva	33.1 ± 13.4	19.5 ± 3.4	33.9 ± 10.2
Gastric juice	60.4 (9–116)	9.2 (0.5–32.5)	84.0 (7.8–154.5)
Ileal fluid	129.4 (105.4–143.7)	11.2 (5.9–29.3)	116.2 (90–136.4)
Cecal fluid	52.5	7.9	42.5
Pancreatic juice	141.1 (113–153)	4.6 (2.6–7.4)	76.6 (54.1–95.2)
Bile	148.9 (131–164)	4.98 (2.6–12)	100.6 (89–117.6)
Cerebrospinal fluid	140.0 (130–150)	3.3 (2.7–3.9)	126.8 (115.5–132.4)
Aqueous humor (rabbits)	143.0 (141.7–145.0)	4.7	107.9 (106.2–109.5)
Sweat	See Table 5–6		

From Edelman IS, Liebman J: Am J Med 27:256, 1959.

enzyme activities. Thus, intracellular sodium content is usually relatively constant, and changes in total body sodium reflect mostly changes in extracellular sodium. However, redistribution of sodium between the intracellular and extracellular compartments may occur in the absence of significant changes in total body sodium. Such a change may be observed in the severely ill patient, where it usually is referred to as the "sick cell syndrome."

Because of the Donnan distribution of anionic proteins, the concentration of sodium in interstitial fluid is approximately 97% that of the serum sodium value; changes in concentration of sodium in the serum are reflected by proportional changes in the concentration of sodium in the interstitial fluid. Concentrations of sodium in transcellular fluids vary considerably because such fluids are not in simple diffusion equilibrium with plasma (Table 5–1). Unexpected changes in composition of these fluids may occur and may necessitate the changing of therapeutic regimens designed to replace their abnormal loss.

INFLUENCE OF DISEASE STATES

In many disease states the ability to maintain body sodium at normal levels is lost. Such abnormalities usually result in changes in volume rather than in changes in sodium concentration. Retention of sodium is typically accompanied by a compensatory retention of an equivalent amount of water so that edema develops. Sodium concentration remains in, or near, the normal range. Excessive losses of sodium may cause hyponatremia but are often paralleled by comparable losses of water so that they result in volume contraction with little change in sodium concentration.

Patients with *chronic renal disease* can usually modify the rate of excretion of sodium, but both the upper and lower limits of tolerance for sodium are characteristically limited. Some renal diseases, especially those affecting the tubules, are associated with a limited renal ability to conserve sodium. In such patients the unnecessary restriction of sodium will result in volume contraction and a further reduction in renal function. Conversely, exceeding the upper limit for sodium tolerance results in positive sodium balance and edema, a condition most often seen in patients with glomerular diseases. However, patients with chronic renal disease frequently do not develop positive sodium balance until their glomerular filtration rate (GFR) falls to levels below 5–10% of normal or unless they have a nephrotic syndrome. Positive sodium balance may be seen also in association with acute decreases in GFR in acute glomerulonephritis. It may also result from a decrease in the oncotic pressure of plasma (e.g., with the nephrotic syndrome), from a decrease in effective arterial volume (e.g., with congestive heart failure), or from the administration or increased secretion of steroids with mineralocorticoid effects.

In *diabetes mellitus* the high level of osmotically active solute in the tubular urine is due to the presence of glucose. This retards passive reabsorption of water and causes the limiting gradient for sodium transport to be attained inappropriately, thus reducing sodium transport. This osmotic effect, which is exerted principally beyond the proximal tubule, results in both natriuresis and diuresis and can cause negative sodium balance. Negative salt balance (with an inappropriate elevation of sodium in the urine) is also seen in Addison disease and in some patients with neurologic lesions. More commonly, it results from extrarenal losses of sodium, such as those that occur with severe or protracted diarrhea when urine sodium concentrations should be low.

Alterations in sodium concentration most often reflect an abnormality in the handling of water. *Hyponatremia* (serum sodium <135 mEq/l) indicates that there is relatively less sodium than water in the extracellular fluid (ECF) space. It can be due to ECF sodium depletion but often results from expansion of the ECF by water. This latter situation may arise from inappropriate reduction of water loss, e.g., with the inappropriate ADH syndrome, or from excessive water administration (Sec 5.32). Mild degrees of hyponatremia result in remarkably few symptoms. More severe decreases in sodium concentration typically result in confusion as the presenting symptom. When serum sodium concentrations fall to 120 mEq/l or less, they should be treated promptly since convulsions may occur as the osmotically induced movement of water into cerebral cells causes them to swell and produce seizures.

Hypernatremia (serum sodium >150 mEq/l) occurs when the amount of sodium in the ECF is increased in relation to the amount of water in this space. The content of sodium in the ECF may be increased but can be normal or even decreased if there have been major losses of water. Thus, as with hyponatremia, hypernatremia can result from derangements of sodium or water balance either alone or in combination. Examples include (1) sodium retention due to excess sodium administration either as saline or as salt tablets or with accidental substitution of salt for sugar in infant formulas and (2) negative water balance due to inadequate replacement of either excessive losses (e.g., patients with central or nephrogenic diabetes insipidus) or normal losses (e.g., a comatose patient). (See Sec 5.32.)

5.9 POTASSIUM

BODY CONTENT OF POTASSIUM

Potassium is the major intracellular cation. Its body content correlates well with lean body mass. Indeed, because potassium is predominantly intracellular, the change in body potassium content that occurs with growth is an excellent index of cellular mass at different ages. In the adult, potassium approximates 53 mEq/kg body weight, 95% being exchangeable. Intracellular potassium amounts to 48 mEq/kg (Fig 5–9); extracellular, only 5.5 mEq/kg, of which 4 mEq/kg is in bone.

Intracellular concentrations of potassium approximate 150 mEq/l of cell water. Most is unbound and osmotically active, but sequestration by active transport in subcellular particles, such as mitochondria, is likely. Extracellular concentrations of potassium are maintained normally at 4–5 mEq/l.

REGULATION OF POTASSIUM

Potassium is present in remarkably constant quantities in almost all animal and vegetable tissues. A daily intake of 1–2 mEq/kg body weight is recommended, but intakes vary widely. Absorption of potassium is reasonably complete in the upper gastrointestinal tract. More distally, body potassium is exchanged for sodium present in the lumen of the lower bowel.

Chronic potassium balance is primarily regulated by the kidneys, which can adjust the amount of potassium excreted over a wide range. Under normal conditions the rate of excretion of potassium in the urine approximates 10–15% of that filtered. With the administration of large amounts of potassium, urinary excretion may

be more than twice the amount filtered at the glomerulus. Conversely, urinary concentrations of potassium can be reduced to very low levels if potassium conservation is required. Thus, in the adult, rates of urinary potassium excretion may range from less than 5 mEq to 1000 mEq/day.

Potassium is freely filtered in the glomerulus. Its concentration along the length of the proximal convoluted tubule is similar to that of plasma. Thus, reabsorption of potassium in this segment of the nephron is proportionate to that of water with 60% or more of the filtered potassium being absorbed. Concentrations of potassium are increased in the loop of Henle. However, by the time tubular fluid reaches the early distal convoluted tubule, its potassium concentration is below that of plasma, with the amount of potassium delivered to more distal segments of the nephron being equal to less than 10% of the filtered load. Under states of maximal potassium conservation, continued reabsorption occurs in the distal tubule; when dietary intake is normal or when excretion is increased for other reasons, secretion of potassium takes place in the distal tubule and possibly the collecting duct. Indeed, most of the potassium in the final urine probably results from tubular secretion rather than glomerular filtration.

The mechanisms responsible for the control of net secretion of potassium in the distal nephron are extremely complex and not fully understood. Transfer of potassium across the luminal membrane is passive and depends on electrical and chemical gradients as well as on permeability of the membrane to potassium. The electrical gradient generated by reabsorption of sodium from the fluid in the distal tubule represents a major driving force for this potassium secretion. The rate of potassium secretion, however, is always less than that of sodium reabsorption. Moreover, that the ratio of the two rates is variable indicates that the processes are not tightly coupled. Furthermore, hydrogen ion is also excreted into the distal tubule in exchange for sodium. Indeed, renal production of ammonia, a regulatory system for acid-base balance, is also intimately related to potassium homeostasis. These observations may explain the interrelation between hydrogen ion excretion and potassium excretion and account for the effects of acid-base balance on urinary losses of potassium. For example, kaliuresis and hypokalemia frequently occur with systemic alkalosis.

The concentration gradient for potassium between the distal tubular fluid and distal tubular cells also modifies the addition of potassium to the fluid in the distal nephron. This may be regulated in large part by modulation of intracellular concentrations of potassium through the active transport of potassium at the contraluminal cell membrane. Such a scheme could account for the observation that potassium excretion frequently cannot be correlated with serum potassium levels but may be better correlated with intracellular concentrations of the cation. An increased rate of flow of distal tubule fluid increases the concentration gradient as well as the rate of loss of potassium in the urine.

There may also be active transport of potassium at the luminal membrane from tubular fluid back into the cells. It has been proposed that this could represent the

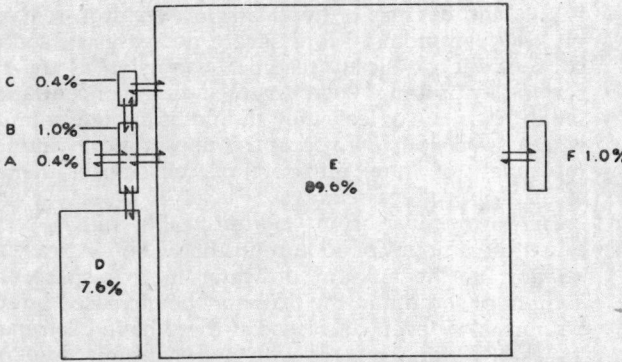

Figure 5–9 Distribution of potassium within the body of a normal young adult man. A, Plasma potassium; B, interstitial lymph potassium; C, dense connective tissue and cartilage potassium; D, bone potassium; E, intracellular potassium; F, transcellular potassium. (From Edelman IS, Liebman J: Am J Med 27:256, 1959.)

final regulating mechanism. In summary, factors affecting distal nephron potassium secretion include mineralocorticoid activity, dietary potassium, acid-base status, distal tubular flow rate, and sodium delivery to the distal tubule.

Aldosterone plays a major role in potassium regulation in the kidney as well as in other tissues. Injected intravenously into a patient with Addison disease, it reduces urinary excretion of sodium and increases that of potassium. It acts at the level of the distal tubule by altering permeability of the luminal membrane to sodium, thus allowing increased exchange between luminal sodium and intracellular potassium. Aldosterone secretion appears to be affected by both sodium and potassium balance (Fig 5–8).

Potassium is also lost in the feces and sweat. The exchange of plasma potassium for sodium present in the colonic contents contributes to sodium conservation and permits the colon to participate in potassium homeostasis. However, even under conditions of chronic potassium loading, fecal potassium constitutes only a small percentage of the total amount of potassium excreted. The human colon responds to mineralocorticoids by decreasing sodium and increasing the potassium content of the stool. Glucocorticoids have a similar effect.

The potassium content of sweat is normally 10–25 mEq/l. It is increased by mineralocorticoids and may be elevated in aldosteronism as well as in cystic fibrosis, but losses are not significant.

Acute potassium loads require well developed extrarenal mechanisms to prevent severe hyperkalemia and to avoid potassium toxicity. In the 1st 4–6 hr following a potassium load, only half of the potassium is excreted by the kidneys. Some is secreted into the intestinal tract. More than 40%, however, is translocated into cells, primarily in the liver and muscle. This process is an important protective mechanism. Both insulin and epinephrine play a major regulatory role in enhancing potassium uptake by liver and muscle. The catecholamine effect appears to be mediated through β-receptors. β-Agonists tend to increase rather than decrease plasma potassium concentration. Aldosterone also plays a key role in the extrarenal handling of potassium. Its primary site of action may be the gastrointestinal tract, although it also affects muscle transport of potassium. Glucocorticoids may also be important in extrarenal potassium homeostasis. Glucagon infusion causes a transient hyperkalemia, but its role in potassium regulation is not clear.

Acid-base balance also affects intracellular shifts of potassium. Systemic acidosis results in movement of potassium out of cells; alkalosis produces the opposite effect. For every 0.1 unit change in blood pH, the plasma potassium concentration changes 0.3–1.3 mEq/l in the opposite direction. The changes depend on numerous factors; for example, the increase in serum potassium accompanying respiratory acidosis is much less than that with metabolic acidosis.

Potassium Depletion. Abnormally low amounts of total body potassium have been demonstrated in a variety of disease states, such as muscular dystrophy, which are characterized by a decrease in muscle mass.

These disorders are not necessarily accompanied by *hypokalemia*. However, a low serum potassium may result from a prolonged decreased intake, from increased renal excretion, or from increased extrarenal losses. Renal losses may be increased by the use of diuretics including osmotic diuretics and carbonic anhydrase inhibitors; by tubular defects such as renal tubular acidosis; by acid-base disturbances; in endocrinopathies such as Cushing syndrome, primary aldosteronism, and thyrotoxicosis; in diabetic ketoacidosis; in Bartter syndrome; and in magnesium deficiency. Extrarenal losses may occur from the bowel, e.g., with diarrhea, chronic catharsis, frequent enemas, protracted vomiting, biliary drainage, or enterocutaneous fistulas, or from the skin if there is profuse sweating. Movement of potassium into cells during correction of a metabolic acidosis, for example, may also result in hypokalemia, as may familial hypokalemic periodic paralysis, a relatively rare disorder in which episodes of paralysis are usually accompanied by an abrupt and marked hypokalemia due to movement of potassium into an extravascular body compartment.

External losses of potassium result in a shift of potassium from the intracellular to the extracellular fluid. Intracellular potassium is replaced in part by sodium, hydrogen ions, and dibasic amino acids. If these changes become severe, intracellular acidosis in the renal tubular cells may result in excessive exchange of intracellular hydrogen for sodium in the distal tubular fluid. This results in aciduria with the increased urinary excretion of ammonia and in systemic alkalosis.

The relation of extracellular to intracellular potassium concentration is of vital importance to cell function. Membrane depolarization, the process responsible for initiating muscle contraction, requires the abrupt influx of sodium into cells and a comparable efflux of potassium out of them. The process is reversed with repolarization. With hypokalemia the ratio of intracellular to extracellular potassium concentrations is increased. The transmembrane electrical potential gradient increases so that there is a wider differential between the resting and excitation potentials, which interferes with impulse formation, propagation, and muscle contraction. Thus hypokalemia produces functional alterations in skeletal muscle, in smooth muscle, and in the heart. It is not possible to predict with accuracy the degree of loss of body potassium from measurements of serum potassium. In general, however, a 1 mEq/l decrease in serum potassium concentration secondary to potassium loss corresponds to a loss of approximately 5–10% of body potassium. Many patients will tolerate this degree of loss without symptoms. Rate of change in potassium levels as well as magnitude of losses probably affects severity of symptoms. Weakness is an early manifestation typically noted first in limb muscles before trunk and respiratory muscles. Areflexia, paralysis, and death from respiratory muscle failure can develop. Paralytic ileus and gastric dilation reflect smooth muscle dysfunction. Electrocardiographic abnormalities, especially a lowered T-wave voltage and the appearance of a U wave, are characteristic. In the kidney, potassium deficiency results in vacuolar changes in the tubular epithelium. If sustained for a long time, it leads to nephrosclerosis and interstitial fibrosis, pathologic lesions indistinguishable from those of chronic pyelonephritis. The kidney has a reduced ability to concentrate or dilute the urine, with polyuria and polydipsia developing. An increase in bicarbonate reabsorption and hydrogen ion secretion results in systemic alkalosis. When the source of potassium loss is not apparent, measurements of urinary potassium may be of help. A low urine concentration of 15 mEq/l, or less, indicates renal conservation of potassium and suggests that the loss occurred from a nonrenal source.

Increases in Body Potassium. Increases comparable in magnitude to the deficits already discussed have not been described and probably would be lethal. Indeed, *hyperkalemia* with serum potassium levels of 5.5 mEq/l or greater may result from surprisingly small increases in total body potassium. Because the kidney has such a large capacity to excrete excess potassium and to prevent hyperkalemia, this electrolyte abnormality is most often seen when renal excretory mechanisms are impaired. Thus it may occur in acute or chronic renal failure, in adrenal insufficiency, in hyporeninemic hypoaldosteronism, and with the use of potassium-sparing diuretics. Acute increases in potassium intake may also result in hyperkalemia, although it is typically transient in duration. Sources of such potassium include the use of potassium salts of penicillin (1.7 mEq/million units) and of salt substitutes by patients on a salt-restricted diet. Acute tissue breakdown, e.g., from trauma, major surgery, or burns, can also release sufficient potassium into the extracellular fluid to cause hyperkalemia. Finally, transcellular redistribution of potassium may cause an elevated serum potassium. This is seen typically in metabolic acidosis. It may occur also shortly before death or in severely ill patients. Certain drugs may increase the serum potassium by similar mechanisms. Succinylcholine inhibits membrane repolarization which requires cellular uptake of potassium. Severe digitalis overdose may cause severe hyperkalemia, presumably by inhibiting sodium-potassium exchange by cell membranes. Since intracellular levels of potassium are 30 times as high as those in the extracellular fluid, lysis of red cells during the collection or handling of a blood sample or release of potassium from platelets during clotting may result in pseudohyperkalemia, in which apparent elevations of serum potassium are recorded by the laboratory.

The major consequences of hyperkalemia are due to its neuromuscular effects. It reduces transmembrane potential toward threshold levels and therefore results in delayed depolarization, faster repolarization, and a slowing of conduction velocity. Paresthesias are followed by weakness and eventually by flaccid paralysis if treatment is not instituted. The heart is particularly vulnerable to hyperkalemia. The electrocardiogram typically shows peaking of the T waves. Lengthening of the P-R interval and widening of the QRS complex develop later and are particularly ominous as they often herald the development of ventricular fibrillation. Since the sequence of cardiotoxic events often progresses rapidly, hyperkalemia should be treated as a medical emergency.

5.10   CALCIUM

BODY CALCIUM

See Sec 3.6, 5.34, and 23.20.

This divalent cation is discussed here briefly because of its interrelations with other electrolytes. At all ages 99% of the body's calcium is in bone. The bones of infants are less densely mineralized than those of adults; the body contents of calcium in infants and adults approximate 400 and 950 mEq/kg of body weight, respectively.

In health the extracellular pool of calcium remains remarkably constant despite fairly free exchange with the enormous reservoir in bone. The concentration of calcium in serum is also maintained within narrow limits, averaging 2.5 mM/l (10 mg/dl). Approximately 40% is protein-bound, of which 80–90% is bound to albumin. The remaining 60% is ultrafilterable or diffusible; about 14% is complexed with anions such as phosphate and citrate, and the remaining 46% (1.2 mM/l or 4.8 mg/dl) is present as free ionic calcium. The ionized calcium is of greatest physiologic importance.

REGULATION

Body calcium content is regulated primarily through the gastrointestinal tract. The recommended daily dietary intake of calcium is 360 mg in the lst 6 mo of life, 540 mg in the 2nd 6 mo, 800 mg from ages 1–10 yr, and 1200 mg from ages 11–18. Dairy products constitute the most important single source. Dietary calcium is absorbed along the small intestine, primarily in the duodenum and early jejunum. This process is enhanced by 1,25-dihydroxy vitamin D_3. It is proposed that hypocalcemia stimulates release of parathyroid hormone (PTH) which, in turn, increases the renal conversion of 25-hydroxy vitamin D_3 to its 1,25 derivative.

The efficiency of intestinal absorption of dietary calcium is increased on a low calcium intake, in the growing child, in pregnancy, and during depletion of body calcium stores. The mechanisms responsible for this adaptation are not known. Administration of vitamin D and PTH also increases calcium absorption, the latter probably by its effect on vitamin D metabolism. Increases in absorption leading to hypercalcemia occur in sarcoidosis, carcinomatosis, and multiple myeloma. Decreased absorption of calcium results from the presence in the gastrointestinal tract of phytate, oxalate, and citrate (all of which complex the dietary calcium); from increased gastric motility; from reduction of bowel length; and from protein depletion, which may cause a deficiency of the calcium-binding protein in the intestinal mucosa. Although, in addition to the dietary calcium not absorbed, the feces contain small amounts of calcium secreted by the bowel, this process is not thought to represent a regulatory mechanism.

Excretion. Plasma non-protein-bound calcium (ultrafilterable calcium) is filtered at the glomerulus. Almost all (around 99%) of this filtered calcium is reabsorbed by the tubules, ionized calcium being transported more easily than the complexed form. Reabsorption occurs throughout the nephron. That which occurs in the proximal tubule (50–55%) and loop of Henle (20–30%) appears to parallel sodium reabsorption; factors influencing transport of one of these cations also affect the other. Calcium transport in the distal convoluted tubule (10–15%) and the collecting duct (2–8%) is independent of sodium transport; these sites probably represent the mechanisms that are specifically calciuric. Calcium reabsorption is stimulated specifically by 1,25-dihydroxy vitamin D_3 and inhibited by thyrocalcitonin. Parathyroid hormone increases reabsorption of calcium by the renal tubules, but this effect may be masked by the concomitant hypercalcemia and resultant increase in the glomerular filtered load of calcium seen in hyperparathyroidism. Urinary excretion of calcium is also increased by many nonspecific mechanisms. These include expansion of extracellular fluid volume; the administration of osmotic diuretics, furosemide, thiazides, growth hormone, thyroid hormone, or glucagon; metabolic acidosis; prolonged fasting; and an increase in serum phosphate.

There is a diurnal variation in the excretion of calcium, which peaks at the middle of the day. Alterations in dietary calcium result in only small changes in urinary excretion of calcium, probably reflecting adaptive changes in intestinal absorption of calcium. Physical inactivity is associated with increased urinary excretion of calcium and, if prolonged, may result in formation of renal stones.

Influence of Disease States. In the analysis of the significance of changes in plasma calcium concentration, it is the amount of ionized calcium that is of physiologic importance. Since some calcium is bound to protein, especially albumin, total calcium levels vary directly with the level of serum albumin. However, with hypoalbuminemia, a low total calcium level in the serum is rarely associated with symptoms or signs of hypocalcemia because the level of serum ionized calcium remains normal.

The balance between deposition and mobilization of calcium in bone determines to a large extent the concentration of ionized calcium in the blood. PTH and 1,25-dihydroxy vitamin D_3 promote increased calcium resorption from bone and elevate the serum calcium. Thyrocalcitonin has opposite effects. The amounts of calcium absorbed from the renal tubular fluid and from the bowel also affect concentrations of plasma-ionized calcium but to a lesser extent. Changes in hydrogen ion activity in the plasma modify the percentage of total calcium which is ionized; a pH change of 1.0 unit alters the concentration of ionized calcium by 10%. Acidosis increases and alkalosis decreases the proportion ionized so that symptomatic hypocalcemia may be seen during the rapid correction or overcorrection of acidosis. In addition, the serum concentrations of sodium and potassium may play some role in the balance between deposition and mobilization of bone calcium; thus, treatment of hypernatremia with fluids low in potassium content may result in hypocalcemia.

Symptomatic *hypocalcemia* due to a low concentration of ionized calcium results from vitamin D deficiency, which in turn is caused by nutritional deficiency, mal-

absorption, or abnormal metabolism of vitamin D. Hypocalcemia may also be due to hypoparathyroidism or pseudohypoparathyroidism, hyperphosphatemia, magnesium deficiency, and acute pancreatitis. The neonate is particularly susceptible to hypocalcemia in association with hypoparathyroidism, abnormal vitamin D metabolism, a low calcium intake, or a high phosphate intake.

Causes of *hypercalcemia* include primary or tertiary hyperparathyroidism, hyperthyroidism, vitamin D intoxication, immobilization, malignancies (especially those which metastasize to bone), use of thiazide diuretics, milk-alkali syndrome, and sarcoidosis. An idiopathic form may occur in infancy associated with typical "elfin" facies and supravalvular aortic stenosis; this syndrome may be due to hypersensitivity to vitamin D.

Calcium loading increases renal excretion of sodium and potassium and produces a profound reduction in ability to concentrate the urine, an effect that may explain the polyuria and polydipsia seen clinically in patients with hypercalcemia due to hypervitaminosis D. Concentrated calcium solutions should always be administered cautiously, using electrocardiographic monitoring whenever possible to minimize cardiac arrhythmias.

5.11 MAGNESIUM

Magnesium is the 4th most abundant cation in the body and plays a major role in cellular enzymatic activity, especially glycolysis.

Total body magnesium amounts to approximately 22 mEq/kg in the infant. It increases in the adult to 28 mEq/kg, approximately 2000 mEq in a 70 kg adult (the contents of calcium, sodium, and potassium in the same subject are approximately 60,000, 5500 and 3000 mEq, respectively). Sixty percent of body magnesium is in bone, of which about one third is freely exchangeable. Most of the remaining 40% is intracellular, playing an essential role in many enzymatic reactions, including the stimulation of the ATPases. Of the intracellular magnesium, more than 50% is in muscle and much of of the remainder in liver. Only 20–30% of the intracellular magnesium is exchangeable, the remainder being bound to proteins, RNA, and ATP.

Extracellular magnesium accounts for only 1% of body magnesium. Although freely exchangeable with the large exchangeable pools in bone and cells, extracellular concentrations of magnesium are maintained at low levels within a relatively narrow normal range. Serum magnesium normally ranges from 1.5–1.8 mEq/l, although wider normal ranges have been reported. Approximately 80% is ultrafilterable; this consists of 55% ionized and 25% complexed. The remaining 20% is protein bound.

The **intake** of magnesium in children ranges from 10–25 mEq per day depending on age; the highest intakes are required during periods of rapid growth. Green vegetables and many other foods contain high concentrations of magnesium; the intake of most subjects exceeds the minimum requirement of 3.6 mg/kg/day (12 mg magnesium is equivalent to 1 mEq or 0.5 mM). Absorption of dietary magnesium occurs primarily in the upper gastrointestinal tract by mechanisms which are not fully delineated. Vitamin D, parathyroid hormone (PTH), and increased sodium absorption enhance magnesium absorption; calcium, phosphorus, and increased intestinal motility decrease it. Absorption is far from complete; an amount of magnesium equal to about two thirds the intake is present in the feces. A small proportion of this magnesium is secreted by the bowel.

Maintenance of balance depends primarily on excretion in the urine. Normally, less than 5% of the filtered load of magnesium appears in the urine. Twenty to 30% is reabsorbed in the proximal tubule and most of the remainder in the loop of Henle, especially the thick ascending limb. Regulation of magnesium absorption is incompletely understood. Under a variety of conditions magnesium reabsorption parallels that of calcium and sodium. Indeed, there is competition between magnesium and calcium for transport. Urinary excretion of magnesium usually amounts to about one third of intake. It is increased by expansion of extracellular fluid volume; by osmotic, thiazide, mercurial, and loop diuretics; by glucagon; and by calcium loading. Conversely, volume contraction, magnesium deficiency, thyrocalcitonin, and PTH increase the renal reabsorption of magnesium.

The maintenance of magnesium balance and serum magnesium concentrations, however, requires a complex inter-reaction of both renal and nonrenal factors. For example, a low magnesium diet results in reduced urinary magnesium. This may be the consequence of modest reductions in the serum concentration of magnesium, which have been shown to increase the release of PTH. This, in turn, decreases urinary loss of magnesium. It also causes release of both magnesium and calcium into the extracellular fluid with increased concentrations of both cations. Tubular reabsorption of filtered magnesium can be almost complete. However, the gastrointestinal tract continues to secrete small amounts of magnesium, and depletion may result.

Influence of Disease States. In human *magnesium depletion*, particularly in severe nutritional insufficiency such as kwashiorkor, the content of magnesium in muscle is decreased. Since the concentration of magnesium in serum is dependent not only on intake and output but also on mobilization of magnesium from both bone and soft tissue, serum concentration of magnesium is not always a reliable indicator of magnesium balance. It may be normal during magnesium depletion. Conversely, reduced levels may be seen in the absence of appreciable losses.

Hypomagnesemia occurs in a variety of clinical states, including malabsorption syndromes, hypoparathyroidism, diuretic therapy, hypercalcemia, renal tubular acidosis, primary aldosteronism, alcoholism, and prolonged intravenous fluid therapy with magnesium-free fluids. At special risk are infants who undergo surgery and receive such fluids for protracted periods of time. Infants with either early or late neonatal tetany often also have hypomagnesemia. When associated with early neonatal tetany, it tends to be mild and transient and may not require treatment with magnesium. In late neonatal tetany, hypocalcemia may fail to respond to treatment until magnesium levels have been returned to normal.

The symptoms of hypomagnesemia are primarily those of increased neuromuscular irritability and include tetany, severe seizures, and tremors. Personality changes, nausea, anorexia, abnormal cardiac rhythms, and electrocardiographic changes may be seen also. Symptoms do not always correlate with serum magnesium levels, perhaps because serum levels do not always reflect the body content of magnesium, which is predominantly an intracellular cation. Alternatively, the symptoms of hypomagnesemia may be minor compared with the symptoms of the primary disease causing the magnesium depletion. A 3rd possibility is that symptoms may reflect whether hypomagnesemia is complicated by hypocalcemia. Severe hypomagnesemia interferes with release of PTH and induces skeletal resistance to the action of PTH. Thus, hypomagnesemia and hypocalcemia often coexist.

Hypermagnesemia or an increase in body magnesium rarely occurs in the absence of decreased renal function. Under most circumstances the kidney is effective in preventing elevations of serum magnesium to dangerous levels even when large magnesium loads are administered. However, hypermagnesemia with serum levels in excess of 5 mEq/l can occur. The usual sources of a magnesium load include magnesium-containing laxatives, enemas, and intravenous fluids. Severe hypermagnesemia may be seen in neonates born of mothers who received intramuscular injections of magnesium sulfate as treatment for the hypertension of preeclampsia. Neonates born prematurely with asphyxia and/or hypotonia are at special risk, although it remains to be determined whether the elevated magnesium is the cause or consequence of these abnormalities. Serum magnesium levels tend to return to normal spontaneously within 72 hr. There is also an increased incidence of hypermagnesemia in patients with Addison disease. Symptoms of hypermagnesemia occur when levels exceed 5 mg/dl. Hyporeflexia antedates respiratory depression, drowsiness, and coma. They are rapidly reversed by intravenous administration of calcium. Coma and death usually occur when the serum magnesium level increases above 15 mg/dl.

5.12   HYDROGEN ION
(Acid-Base Balance)

TERMINOLOGY

Acid-base balance has been complicated over the years by a confusion of terminologies, each with a reasonable but conflicting approach. Terminology used here was agreed upon under the auspices of the New York Academy of Sciences. Emphasis is placed on the hydrogen ion—or proton—which is a hydrogen atom with its neutralizing electron removed. *pH* is the negative logarithm of the concentration of free hydrogen ions. An *acid* is a proton (hydrogen ion) donor. Hydrochloric, sulfuric, phosphoric, and carbonic acids are conventional acids, each dissociating to liberate protons. A strong acid is one that is highly dissociated and, therefore, presents a high concentration of hydrogen ions; a weak acid is one that is poorly dissociated. A *base* is a hydrogen ion acceptor. Thus bases bind free hydrogen ions, reducing their concentration. Examples include hydroxyl ions, ammonia, and the anions of weak acids. A *buffer* is defined as a substance that reduces the change in free hydrogen ion concentration of a solution upon the addition of an acid or base. The presence of a buffer in a solution increases the amount of acid or alkali that must be added to cause unit change in pH. The addition of a strong acid to any of these buffer systems results in the production of a neutral salt and a weak acid. By generating a poorly dissociated acid, the buffer significantly reduces the increment in free hydrogen ion concentration when the reaction is compared to one that is not buffered. *Aprotes* are cations such as sodium, potassium, calcium, and magnesium that carry 1 or more positive charges, depending on valence, or anions such as chloride and sulfate that carry negative charges. Since aprotes are able neither to donate nor to accept protons, they are not acids, bases, or buffers.

REGULATING MECHANISMS

The daily turnover of hydrogen ions is large, amounting to more than 50% of the hydrogen ions usually present in the body buffers and 10% of the maximum storage capacity of the buffer (Table 5-2). Most diets result in net production of hydrogen ions; protein is the largest source, its metabolism accounting for approximately 65% of the total. Hydrogen ions derived from protein are generated primarily from the oxidation of sulfur-containing amino acids to yield sulfuric acid and from the oxidation and hydrolysis of phosphoproteins to yield phosphoric acid. The remainder of the hydrogen ions come from the incomplete catabolism of carbohydrates, fats, and organic acids such as pyruvic, lactic, acetoacetic, and citric acids. Complete oxidation of these compounds does not produce excess hydrogen ions since water and carbon dioxide are the final reaction products; incomplete metabolism results in the

Table 5-2 APPROXIMATE ORDER OF MAGNITUDE OF CERTAIN FACTORS IN HYDROGEN ION METABOLISM IN STANDARD MAN OF 1.73 M²

Total CO_2 turnover	24,000 mM/24 hr
Total hydrogen ion turnover	69 mEq/24 hr
Total buffer in body	2100 mEq
Total hydrogen ion in buffer (max. capacity)	700 mEq
Total hydrogen ion in buffer (normal amount)	105 mEq
Total free hydrogen ion in body fluids	0.0021 mEq

From Elkinton JR: Ann Intern Med 57:660, 1962.

formation of organic acids and adds hydrogen ions. Thus, milk and meat diets generate about 70 mEq of hydrogen ions/day in the adult and require the daily excretion by the kidney of an equal amount to maintain a normal blood pH of 7.35–7.45.

The number of potential hydrogen ions in the body is very large. Most are buffered and, therefore, are not in free form. Indeed, at the usual pH of 7.4 the concentration of free hydrogen ions in the blood is only 0.0000398 mEq/l or 3.98×10^{-8} Eq/l (often expressed as 40 nEq/l):

$$pH = -\log(H^+) = -\log(3.98 \times 10^{-8})$$
$$= -(0.60 - 8.0) = 7.4$$

Normally, the hydrogen ion concentrations of body fluids are maintained in relatively narrow ranges by the presence of buffers. Buffers represent the 1st line of defense against changes in pH; they cannot maintain acid-base balance. Indeed, in the presence of disease states or abrupt alteration of hydrogen ion production, buffer systems may not be able to maintain a normal pH for a prolonged period. The action of buffers needs to be supplemented by compensatory and corrective physiologic changes in the lungs and the kidneys.

Compensation of a primary acid-base disorder is a slower process than buffering, but it is more effective in returning pH to normal. In a primary metabolic disorder the respiratory system provides the compensating mechanism; the kidneys compensate in a primary respiratory disorder. Compensation reduces pH changes but must be followed by *correction* which returns all acid-base measurements to normal. This occurs when the primary disorder is cured and may be the responsibility of either the kidneys or the lungs. Although discussed separately, the buffering, pulmonary, and renal systems are interdependent and act in concert with one another.

Buffer Systems. The principal buffer in the extracellular fluid is the bicarbonate–carbonic acid system; intracellular buffers include various proteins and organic phosphates. In the urine, phosphate in its mono- and dihydrogen forms is the major buffer. Only the extracellular fluid buffer mechanisms will be considered in detail.

Hydrogen ions, when added to the plasma, are buffered in large part by bicarbonate with the generation of a neutral salt and carbonic acid.

$$HA + NaHCO_3 \rightarrow NaA + H_2CO_3$$

Carbonic acid is a weak acid with a relatively low solubility coefficient and is in equilibrium with dissolved carbon dioxide as follows:

$$[H^+] \cdot [HCO_3^-] \rightleftharpoons H_2CO_3 \rightleftharpoons CO_2 + H_2O$$

The addition of hydrogen ions drives this equation to the right, generating CO_2 and H_2O. Thus, despite the addition of hydrogen ions, the buffering mechanisms result in relatively little change in free hydrogen ion concentration and in pH. However, buffering is accomplished at the expense of a decrease in bicarbonate concentration (this has been referred to as representing *base deficit*) and an increase in carbon dioxide (pCO_2) levels. It is apparent from the Henderson-Hasselbalch equation that these changes must result in some change in pH:

$$pH = pK + \log \frac{Base}{Acid}$$

In the bicarbonate-carbonic acid system, pK (a constant derived from the dissociation of the acid-base pair) is 6.1. Thus:

$$pH = 6.1 + \log \frac{Bicarbonate}{Carbonic\ acid}$$

Since carbonic acid is in equilibrium with dissolved carbon dioxide, measurement of the partial pressure of carbon dioxide (pCO_2) can be used as a clinical estimate of carbonic acid concentration. It is apparent that by decreasing bicarbonate concentration and increasing pCO_2, the addition of hydrogen ion to the plasma will still result in some decrease in pH despite the presence of buffers. However, the changes are of lesser magnitude than would occur in the absence of the buffering mechanism.

Pulmonary Mechanisms. From the above equation it is apparent that pH is dependent not on absolute levels of bicarbonate and carbonic acid (pCO_2) but on the *ratio* of the 2 concentrations. A decrease or increase in concentration of bicarbonate will not modify pH if the pCO_2 is lowered or increased in proportion. Thus by altering the rate at which carbon dioxide is excreted, the lungs are able to regulate pCO_2 and modify pH. Although enormous quantities of carbon dioxide are produced from normal metabolic activity (Table 5–2), little change in pH results because of the unique properties of the bicarbonate–carbonic acid buffer system and a highly developed respiratory control mechanism. An increased respiratory rate, stimulated by increased levels of carbon dioxide, increases the excretion of carbon dioxide, decreases pCO_2, and thus increases pH. Conversely, a decreased respiratory rate will result in an increase in pCO_2 and a decrease in pH.

Even though the lungs can modify pH by changing pCO_2 and altering the ratio of carbonic acid to bicarbonate, this process cannot cause any loss (or gain) in hydrogen ions. The lungs are not capable of regenerating bicarbonate to replace that lost when hydrogen ion was buffered. The generation of new bicarbonate and, when required, the excretion of bicarbonate are the responsibilities of the kidneys.

Renal Mechanisms. The excretion of excess hydrogen ions with generation of new bicarbonate or the excretion of bicarbonate, occurs by regulation of 2 basic steps: (1) Reclamation of nearly all of the filtered bicarbonate occurs in the proximal tubule. No net hydrogen ion excretion results, but, in the adult, this process is responsible for the reclamation of up to 5000 mEq of bicarbonate which is filtered through the glomeruli each day. If this bicarbonate were not reclaimed, its loss would be equivalent to the retention of an equal amount of hydrogen ions and would result in severe systemic acidosis. (2) Generation of new bicarbonate occurs in more distal segments of the nephron and results in the

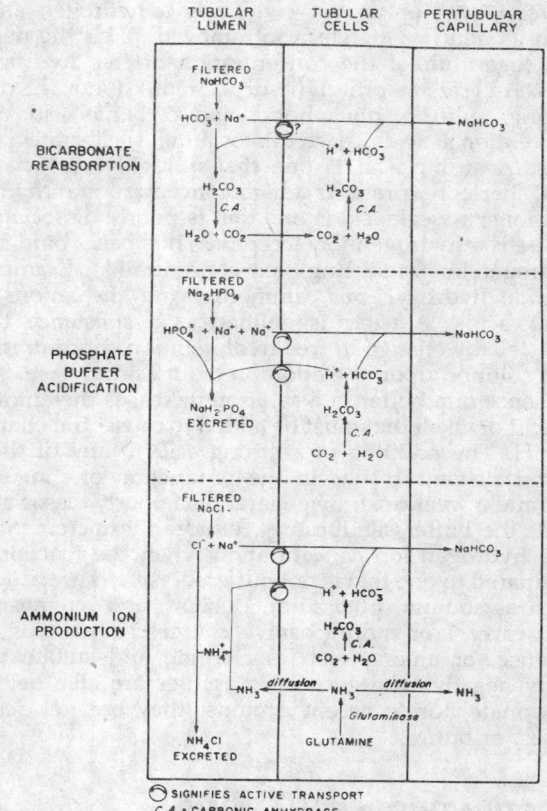

Figure 5–10 The renal mechanisms involved in acid-base homeostasis. Bicarbonate reabsorption normally occurs in the proximal tubule, where the presence of carbonic anhydrase on the luminal brush border facilitates the conversion of bicarbonate to carbon dioxide and water. This mechanism does not effect any net excretion of hydrogen ion from the body but results in the reclamation of bicarbonate in an amount equal to that lost from the plasma into the glomerular filtrate. Incomplete reabsorption of bicarbonate in the proximal tubule results in bicarbonate entering the distal nephron, where it decreases the amount of hydrogen ion available for the production of ammonium and the titration of phosphate to sodium dihydrogen phosphate and thus reduces net acid excretion. It is still uncertain whether the movement of sodium and hydrogen ions across the luminal border of the proximal tubular cell occurs by an active linked-transport mechanism.

net secretion of hydrogen ions needed to maintain hydrogen ion balance under most circumstances.

The mechanisms for both of these steps are highly developed, energy-requiring, active transport processes, in contrast to the pulmonary excretion of carbon dioxide, which results from simple, passive diffusion. Both steps require the generation of hydrogen ions by the same basic reaction. Fig 5–10 shows that the proximal renal tubular cells, under the influence of carbonic anhydrase, hydrolyze carbon dioxide to carbonic acid. This is then dissociated into hydrogen ion and bicarbonate. The hydrogen ions are transported into the proximal tubule and exchanged for filtered sodium, which is reabsorbed into the peritubular capillaries with the bicarbonate generated from the formation of hydrogen ion. In the lumen of the proximal tubule the hydrogen ion combines with filtered bicarbonate to form carbon dioxide and water. These mechanisms assure that virtually no bicarbonate passes to more distal segments of the nephron and that an amount of sodium bicarbonate equal to the amount filtered is returned to the peritubular capillaries.

Hydrogen ions are generated in the distal tubular cells by the same process as that described for the proximal tubular cells. They are also excreted into the lumen in exchange for sodium, probably by an active process. The transport of hydrogen ions at this site appears to be gradient-limited, with the distal tubule able to generate a gradient for free hydrogen ion from tubular lumen to tubular cell of up to 1000:1. Transport is thus facilitated by the presence in the tubular fluid of buffers that decrease the concentration of free hydrogen ion and permit increased movement of hydrogen ion from cells into the tubular fluid. The principal buffers at this site are phosphate and ammonia.

Under most conditions large amounts of *phosphate* are present in the distal tubular fluid. In the presence of a high concentration of free hydrogen ions, the phosphate is converted from a monohydrogen to a dihydrogen form (Fig 5–10), reducing the concentration of free hydrogen ion in the tubular fluid. The amount of hydrogen ion excreted in the urine in this form can be measured by determining the amount of alkali required to bring the urine to a neutral pH and is termed *titratable acidity.*

Ammonia, a hydrogen ion acceptor, is synthesized in tubular cells from the deamidation and deamination of glutamine in the presence of glutaminase; this reaction is stimulated by systemic acidosis. Ammonia diffuses through the lipid membrane of the cells into the tubular fluid, where it reacts with hydrogen ion to form ammonium ion, NH_4^+. This charged cation cannot readily diffuse back from luminal fluid.

These 2 processes, by reducing free hydrogen ion concentration in the tubular fluid, enable an increased rate of transport of hydrogen ions into the distal renal tubule fluid and allow the generation of new bicarbonate which can enter the plasma and replenish depleted levels of plasma bicarbonate (Fig 5–10).

The absolute net rate of excretion of hydrogen ions by the kidney is calculated as the sum of the excretion rates in the urine of titratable acid and ammonium ion minus urine bicarbonate. On an average mixed diet an adult in the United States must excrete about 70 mEq of hydrogen ions each day to maintain balance. Approximately one third is excreted as titratable acid, the remaining two thirds as ammonium.

A number of factors cause an increase in the rate of hydrogen ion secretion in the proximal tubules and lead to increased bicarbonate reabsorption with consequent elevation of serum bicarbonate. These include elevation of plasma pCO_2, hypokalemia, reduction in effective arterial blood volume (e.g., after vomiting or hemorrhage), and administration of mineralocorticoids. Conversely, hydrogen ion secretion, and thus bicarbonate reabsorption, is decreased by a decreased plasma pCO_2, by expansion of extracellular fluid volume, by inhibition of carbonic anhydrase (e.g., by drugs such as acetazolamide), and by mineralocorticoid deficiency. Reduction in plasma bicarbonate may occur in these situations. Similarly, disease states such as cystinosis or heavy metal poisoning associated with structural or functional damage to the proximal tubule may limit bicarbonate reabsorption at this site and result in systemic acidosis. The distal acidification mechanisms may be impaired by intrinsic defects in the tubule, which cause primary distal renal tubular acidosis, or by a variety of insults such as nephrocalcinosis, vitamin D intoxication, or amphotericin B administration which produce secondary forms of distal renal tubular acidosis.

DISTURBANCES OF ACID-BASE BALANCE

Systemic acidosis or alkalosis may result from either primary metabolic or respiratory abnormalities.

Metabolic Acidosis. Systemic acidosis may result from increased production or inadequate excretion of hydrogen ions or from excessive loss of bicarbonate in the urine or stools. Rapid expansion of the extracellular fluid space by a bicarbonate-free solution may also produce metabolic acidosis by diluting the bicarbonate in the extracellular fluid. The hydrogen ion load is buffered initially by bicarbonate in the extracellular fluid and by intracellular buffers such as hemoglobin and phosphate. Bone may be a further source of buffer. Serum bicarbonate and pH fall (but to a lesser extent than if no buffering mechanism were available) and pCO_2 rises. The resulting systemic acidosis and increased pCO_2 stimulate the respiratory center (and possibly peripheral chemoreceptors in the carotid artery and aorta) to increase the respiratory rate, thereby increasing the rate of excretion of carbon dioxide. Plasma pCO_2 and carbonic acid levels fall, partially or almost totally correcting the acidosis but at the expense of lowering both plasma bicarbonate and pCO_2. Thus blood pH is decreased but rarely as low as might be predicted from the low level of plasma bicarbonate.

The acidosis also stimulates the kidney to increase ammonia production and hydrogen ion excretion into the urine. As a result, there is an increased generation of new bicarbonate, returning plasma bicarbonate to normal if the primary disease process has been alleviated. In turn, the respiratory rate subsequently decreases, with the pCO_2 returning to normal. At this point the patient's acid-base status has returned to the normal state in existence before the hydrogen ion load was administered.

The clinical picture of metabolic acidosis is usually dominated by the underlying cause and by the deep, rapid respirations (*Kussmaul breathing*) needed for respiratory compensation. However, severe acidosis itself may cause a decrease in peripheral vascular resistance and cardiac ventricular function, resulting in hypotension, pulmonary edema, and tissue hypoxia. The laboratory findings are decreased serum pH, bicarbonate, and pCO_2. For every 1 mEq/l fall from normal in plasma bicarbonate there should be a 1.0–1.5 mm Hg decrease in arterial pCO_2. If this relationship does not occur, a mixed disturbance should be suspected (see below). When the acidosis is due to bicarbonate loss, the anion gap is normal and there is hyperchloremia. An increased anion gap usually signifies the increased production of hydrogen ion or its decreased excretion. A more detailed discussion of anion gap is presented in Sec 5.13.

Renal causes of metabolic acidosis are numerous. Diseases involving the proximal tubules may limit the ability of this segment of the nephron to secrete hydrogen ions and cause incomplete bicarbonate reabsorption. Increased amounts of bicarbonate are presented to the distal tubular fluid, resulting in the proximal form of *renal tubular acidosis*. In distal renal tubular acidosis the distal tubule is unable to maintain a normal hydrogen ion gradient so that urine pH remains relatively alkaline, rarely falling below 5.5. A reduction of titratable acid, decreased secretion of hydrogen ion, and systemic acidosis result. With *chronic renal insufficiency*, acidification mechanisms work normally or at supranormal rates. However, the reduced tubular mass limits the capacity of the kidney to generate sufficient ammonia and thus to excrete adequate amounts of hydrogen ions. A low glomerular filtration rate, as in the newborn, also limits the renal capacity to excrete hydrogen ion. In addition, the filtered load of phosphate is reduced, the bulk being reabsorbed in the proximal tubule; little is left for buffering of added hydrogen ion in the distal tubule. Hydrogen ion transport is thus reduced by rapid attainment of a maximal concentration gradient in the absence of buffer. Rarely, reduction in ammonia synthesis, as in the cerebro-oculo-renal syndrome of Lowe, limits the ability to excrete hydrogen ions.

Other Causes. Metabolic acidosis may also develop in *diabetic ketoacidosis*. Here it results from incomplete metabolism of body lipids and catabolism of body protein, with the production of large amounts of acetoacetic, β-hydroxybutyric, phosphoric, and sulfuric acids. In *salicylism*, metabolic acidosis results not only from hydrogen ion derived from salicylic acid but also from the uncoupling of oxidative phosphorylation by salicylate. In severe *diarrhea* the increased losses of bicarbonate in diarrheal fluid and, possibly, the formation of organic acids from incomplete breakdown of carbohydrate in the stools result in metabolic acidosis. *Hyperalimentation, lactic acidosis, starvation*, and *poisoning with either methyl alcohol or ethylene glycol* cause systemic acidosis by increased production of various strong acids. Metabolic acidosis is seen also in certain of the *inherited aminoacidurias* (e.g., methylmalonicaciduria), in hypoxemia, and in shock.

Metabolic Alkalosis. Metabolic alkalosis may result from any of 3 basic mechanisms: (1) excessive loss of hydrogen ion, as in prolonged gastric aspiration or persistent vomiting associated with pyloric stenosis; (2) increased addition of bicarbonate to the extracellular fluid—this may result from excessive administration by the parenteral route or by oral intake as in the milk-alkali syndrome, or from increased renal reabsorption of bicarbonate as in profound potassium depletion, primary hyperaldosteronism, Cushing syndrome, Bartter syndrome, or excessive intake of licorice; (3) contraction of the extracellular fluid volume, which increases bicarbonate concentration in this fluid space and increases bicarbonate reclamation in the renal tubule.

The buffer systems minimize pH change, but both plasma bicarbonate and pH are increased. Respiration may be depressed with some increase in plasma pCO_2, but this response is limited by increasing hypoxia so that respiratory compensation is always incomplete and never restores pH to normal. The renal threshold for bicarbonate is exceeded, and bicarbonate appears in the urine, which may have a pH as high as 8.5–9.0. However, factors such as volume depletion and hypokalemia often coexist and they, along with the increased pCO_2 itself, tend to increase renal reabsorption of bicarbonate, maintaining the metabolic alkalosis. Indeed, metabolic alkalosis is refractory to treatment in the presence of either hypokalemia or depletion of extracellular fluid volume and often can be corrected only after these deficiencies have been corrected.

The diagnosis of metabolic alkalosis should be considered in any patient with an appropriate history; there are no pathognomonic signs of this electrolyte disturbance. Patients may have cramps or feel weak and may have the signs of tetany if ionized calcium has been reduced by the alkalosis.

Characteristically, pH, plasma bicarbonate, and pCO_2 of arterial blood are elevated. Hypochloremia and hypokalemia are usually present, the latter principally due to increased urinary losses of potassium. Classically, the urine pH is alkaline, but in the presence of severe depletion of potassium, urinary potassium is low and there is paradoxic aciduria. Measurement of urinary chloride may help to identify those patients with volume depletion who will be responsive to sodium chloride. Their urine chloride concentrations should be less than 10 mEq/l. In contrast, patients who have metabolic alkalosis due to excessive mineralocorticoid activity or potassium depletion have a urine chloride in excess of 20 mEq/l and are resistant to treatment with sodium chloride.

Respiratory Acidosis. This disturbance results from inadequate pulmonary excretion of carbon dioxide in the presence of normal production of this gas. It may be seen acutely in neuromuscular disorders such as brain stem injury, Guillain-Barré syndrome, or sedative overdose; in airway obstruction such as that caused by a foreign body, severe bronchospasm, or laryngeal edema; in vascular diseases such as massive pulmonary embolism; and in other conditions such as pneumothorax, pulmonary edema, or severe pneumonia. Chronic respiratory acidosis may accompany the pickwickian syndrome, poliomyelitis, chronic obstructive airway disease, kyphoscoliosis, or chronic administration of sedatives.

In health, increased production of CO_2 stimulates its increased respiratory excretion so that a normal pCO_2 is maintained and acid-base status remains normal. In any of the disease states causing respiratory acidosis, the level of pCO_2 increases until it is elevated sufficiently to result in the pulmonary excretion of carbon dioxide that is once again equal to its production. Although a new steady state is reached, the increase in pCO_2 (hypercapnia) causes a systemic acidosis by increasing serum concentrations of carbonic acid and, therefore, of hydrogen ions.

Since pCO_2 is a major component of the principal buffer system of the extracellular fluid, the rise in pCO_2

must be buffered initially by the nonbicarbonate buffers, i.e., the proteins in the extracellular fluid and phosphate, hemoglobin, other proteins, and lactate in the cells. The acidosis and increased pCO_2 stimulate the kidney to increase hydrogen ion excretion as ammonium and titratable acid and to generate and reabsorb more bicarbonate; thus plasma bicarbonate levels may be increased somewhat above normal. At this stage the increase in plasma bicarbonate compensates for the primary increase in pCO_2 so that pH returns toward normal and the respiratory acidosis has been "compensated" by renal mechanisms. The only way to *correct* the abnormality is to reverse the primary disorder.

Causes of acute respiratory acidosis are often associated with hypoxemia, which usually dominates the clinical picture, along with the signs of respiratory distress. Hypercapnia results in vasodilatation, increases cerebral blood flow, and may be responsible for the headaches and raised intracranial pressure sometimes found in these patients. Severe hypercapnia may be a cerebral depressant; arterial pH is low, pCO_2 elevated, and plasma bicarbonate elevated moderately.

Respiratory Alkalosis. Excessive pulmonary losses of carbon dioxide in the presence of normal production results in a fall in pCO_2 and respiratory alkalosis. It may be observed with hyperventilation of psychogenic origin, with overventilation from mechanically assisted ventilation, and in the early stages of salicylate overdosage due to stimulation of the respiratory center by salicylate or to increased sensitivity of the respiratory center to pCO_2.

Plasma pCO_2 falls and pH rises. There is a rapid buffering of this change in pH, with hydrogen ions released from body buffers to decrease plasma bicarbonate. Approximately 99% of this hydrogen ion is released from intracellular buffers and the remaining 1% from extracellular buffers. The renal excretion of bicarbonate, slowly increasing by mechanisms that are incompletely understood, reduces plasma bicarbonate levels and compensates for the excessive loss of carbon dioxide, returning pH toward normal. However, correction cannot occur until the causative disorder is removed.

The clinical picture usually is that of the underlying disease process. However, acute hypercapnia may result in neuromuscular irritability and paresthesias in the extremities and periorally due to a decrease in the concentration of ionized calcium. Arterial pH is elevated, pCO_2 and plasma bicarbonate decreased. Despite systemic alkalosis the urine usually remains acid.

Mixed Disorders. It is apparent from the foregoing discussion that acid-base disturbances of respiratory etiology may have partial or almost complete compensation by renal mechanisms. Similarly, abnormalities induced by metabolic diseases may be partially compensated by respiratory changes modifying pCO_2. Under certain circumstances there may be mixed disturbances in which more than a single primary cause is responsible for the abnormal acid-base balance. For example, in respiratory distress syndrome metabolic and respiratory acidoses often coexist. The respiratory disease prevents the compensatory fall in pCO_2, and the metabolic component limits the ability to increase plasma bicarbonate, which would normally buffer a respiratory acidosis. In such a situation the decrease in pH is often profound, of greater magnitude than that seen when only a single disturbance exists.

Other types of mixed disturbances may be seen. Patients with congestive heart failure and chronic respiratory acidosis may develop a component of metabolic alkalosis if there is excessive use of diuretics. Plasma bicarbonate and pH will be higher than in a simple chronic respiratory acidosis. Indeed, pH may be normal or even slightly elevated. Patients with hepatic failure may have both a metabolic acidosis and a respiratory alkalosis. Plasma bicarbonate and pCO_2 may be lower than expected with a simple disorder, whereas pH may be little changed from normal. Respiratory and metabolic alkaloses may also coexist under some circumstances.

CLINICAL ASSESSMENT OF ACID-BASE DISORDERS

For clinical purposes acid-base status can be determined from serum pH, pCO_2, and bicarbonate levels. This approach has replaced the measurement of base excess or deficit and the estimation of buffer base as the sum of concentrations of the buffer anions of whole blood, i.e., bicarbonate, plasma proteins, and hemoglobin. Base excess was measured by titration of whole blood with a strong acid to pH 7.40 at a pCO_2 of 40 mm Hg at 37°C and base deficit, by titrating with base. Values were expressed as mEq/l.

Measurements. Blood pH can be measured accurately even with small samples of blood; normal values are from 7.35–7.45. The concentration of carbonic acid (H_2CO_3) in biologic fluids is quantitatively negligible compared with dissolved carbon dioxide. The latter is measured as the partial pressure of carbon dioxide (pCO_2) in a gas phase in equilibrium with the biologic fluid. The normal value approximates 40 mm Hg.

The concentration of bicarbonate ion in plasma can be measured directly, but the precision of this determination is not required for clinical purposes. It is customary to determine total carbon dioxide concentration of the serum as an estimate of bicarbonate level. This value is 1–2 mEq/l higher than that of true bicarbonate. It is obtained either by titration or by generation of carbon dioxide from serum with a strong acid. The carbon dioxide is derived principally from bicarbonate but also from dissolved carbon dioxide, carbonic acid, carbonate ion, and carbamino compounds. The normal value is 25–28 millimoles (mM)/l, except in the 1st yr of life when values are lower, often from 20–23 mM/l, probably because of the low renal threshold for bicarbonate.

If only 2 of these values are known, the 3rd can be derived from 1 of the nomograms developed for this purpose (Fig 5–11) or can be calculated by 1 of the several methods based on the Henderson-Hasselbalch

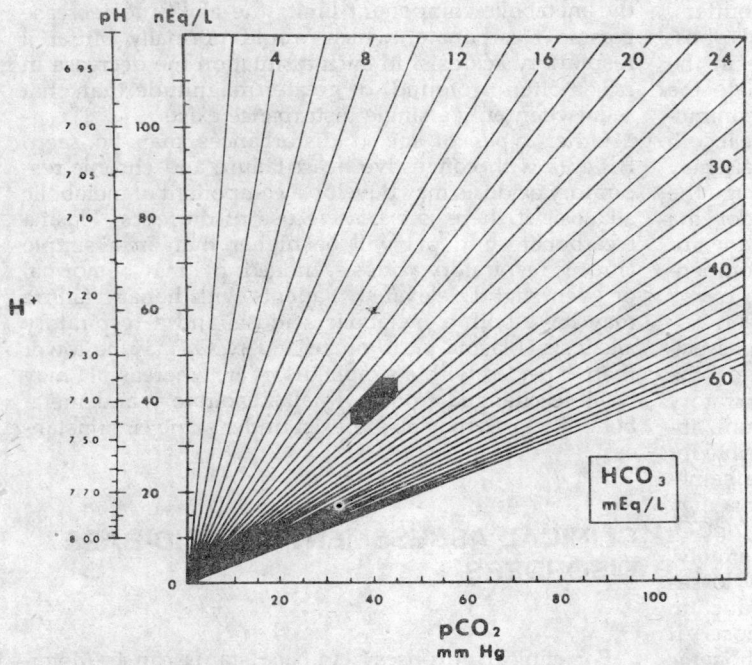

Figure 5–11 A nomogram permitting estimation of pH, pCO_2, or serum bicarbonate levels when only 2 of these measurements have been determined in the laboratory. The shaded area in the center of the plot represents the normal values. (From Cohen JJ: Ann Int Med **66**:159, 1967.)

equation.* If all 3 measurements have been determined in the laboratory, the same formulas can be used to check the validity of these values.

Interpretation. It is relatively easy to diagnose correctly a simple acid-base disorder, given blood pH, pCO_2, and bicarbonate levels and using an acid-base nomogram such as that shown in Fig 5–12 or the summary of laboratory findings shown in Fig 5–13. More difficulty may be experienced with a mixed disorder. In simple disorders pCO_2 and bicarbonate levels always change in the same direction. If any patient's values do not show this relationship, a mixed disorder should be considered. Similarly, results that plot outside any of the shaded areas shown in Fig 5–12 indicate a 95% chance of a mixed disorder. This can be diagnosed from the clinical setting, as discussed, and from the information presented in Fig 5–13.

INTRACELLULAR pH

Normal intracellular pH has been estimated to be 6.8; values as low as 6.0 have been obtained using micro-

---

*pCO_2 may be estimated from the equation

$$pCO_2 = \frac{[H^+] \times [total\ CO_2\ content]}{25}$$

$[H^+]$, expressed as nanoequivalents per liter (nEq/l), can easily be estimated from serum pH. At a pH of 7.40 $[H^+]$ is approximately 40 nEq/l (see Regulating Mechanisms). Each decrease in pH of 0.01 unit is associated with an increased $[H^+]$ of 1 nEq/l. Conversely, each increase in pH of 0.01 unit is associated with a decreased $[H^+]$ of 1 nEq/l. Thus, $[H^+]$ at a pH of 7.30 is 50 nEq/l and at 7.45 is 35 nEq/l. The maximum error in pCO_2 calculated by this simple formula is 7% for pH values from 7.10–7.50 and even less in the pH range of 7.28–7.45. (See N Engl J Med 272:1067, 1965.) Alternate methods are summarized by Kaehny (see References).

electrodes. Thus, intracellular pH appears to be maintained at a level lower than that of extracellular fluid. Mitochondrial pH may be even lower since intracellular pH is probably inhomogeneous.

Carbon dioxide diffuses readily across cell membranes so that intracellular and extracellular values for pCO_2 are similar. Thus, intracellular changes in hydrogen ion concentration may occur as a result of primary respiratory disorders and either hypocapnia or hypercapnia. With *hypo*capnia, intracellular alkalosis is proportional to the degree of extracellular alkalosis. With *hyper*capnia, however, because intracellular bicarbonate concentrations cannot be adjusted as rapidly as those in the extracellular fluid, intracellular acidosis may be proportionally greater than that seen in the extracellular fluid. In contrast to the situation in respiratory acidosis, intracellular pH may be maintained in the face of severe metabolic acidosis until extracellular pH drops below 7.0.

The effects of extracellular acidosis and alkalosis on cellular functions are not yet fully understood. A low pH produces a slight change in the Donnan distribution across the capillary membrane; therefore some decrease in oncotic pressure results in a reduced plasma volume. Low pH also seems to reduce myocardial contractility and impair catecholamine action, and it increases the likelihood of arrhythmia, particularly with hypoxia. Moreover, if hydrogen ion concentration rises rapidly, it may inhibit further transport of the ion in the kidney. Metabolic disturbances also lead to an alteration in exchange of sodium and potassium for hydrogen ion; deficiency of potassium may result in a decrease in the intracellular pH at the same time that extracellular pH is elevated.

Changes in intracellular pH probably affect the activities of many enzymes. Decrease in carbohydrate tol-

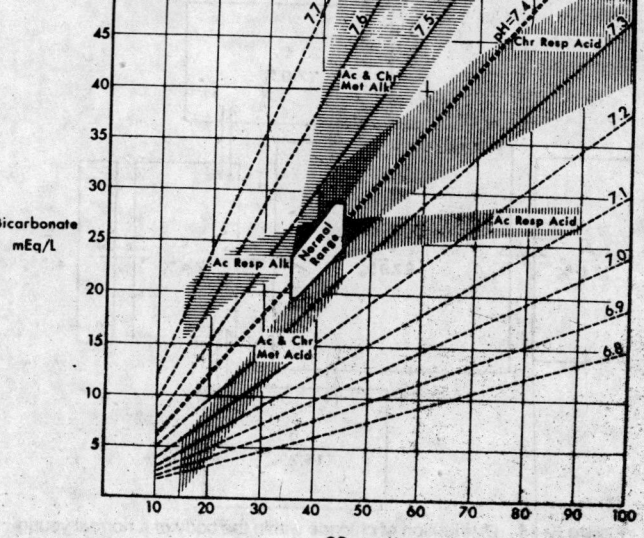

Figure 5–12 Determination of simple acid-base disorders from measurements of pH, pCO_2, and serum bicarbonate. Ac—acute, Acid—acidosis, Alk—alkalosis, Chr—chronic, Met—metabolic, Resp—respiratory. (From Arbus GS: Can Med Assoc J *109*:291, 1973.)

erance has been observed in acidosis, and increase in neuromuscular irritability (latent or manifest tetany) occurs in alkalosis. Hypocapnia leads to an increase in blood lactic acid with a decrease in bicarbonate concentration and production of acidosis of metabolic origin.

Cerebrospinal Fluid pH. Although difficulties with methodology have limited study of intracellular pH in systemic acidosis and alkalosis, pH changes in the cerebrospinal fluid have been evaluated in detail. Bicarbonate–carbonic acid represents virtually all the buffering capacity in this fluid. Carbon dioxide can diffuse freely between the blood and cerebrospinal fluid. Thus, increases or decreases in pCO_2 in the blood are reflected by similar changes in the cerebrospinal fluid, although this latter value is also modified by the rates of carbon dioxide production in the brain. In contrast, increases or decreases in concentration of bicarbonate in blood lead only slowly to small changes in bicarbonate in cerebrospinal fluid. In consequence, the concentration of hydrogen ion in the cerebrospinal fluid does not change instantaneously with changes in extracellular pH; the pHs of these fluids may differ significantly at

times, particularly if active respiratory compensation of a metabolic acidosis or alkalosis has occurred. Particular problems may be seen if a compensated metabolic acidosis is corrected too quickly. Correction results in an increase in both pCO_2 and bicarbonate levels in the extracellular fluid, but only the pCO_2 rises in the cerebrospinal fluid. The pH of the extracellular fluid returns to normal, but that of the cerebrospinal fluid falls even further. Thus, continuing neurologic symptoms and abnormalities in respiration may result.

5.13 CHLORIDE

Chloride is the major anion of extracellular fluid. Total body chloride amounts to 33 mEq/kg of body weight. Most of it is in the extracellular and transcellular fluid, with small quantities present in red blood cells and connective tissue (Fig 5–14). Exchangeable chloride also remains relatively constant per unit of body weight at different ages.

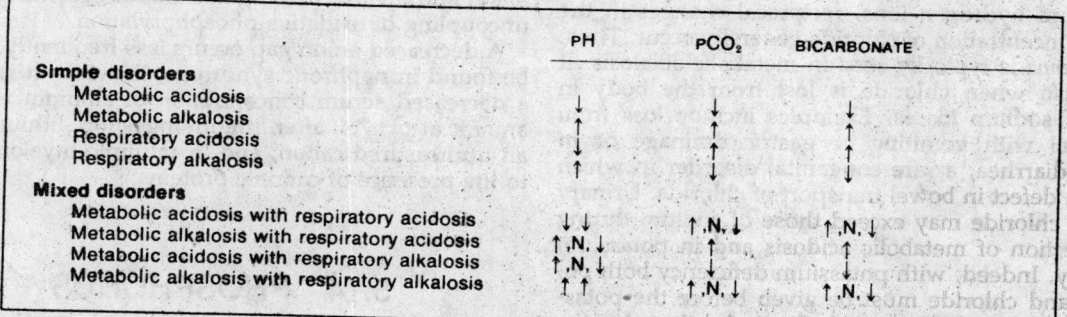

	PH	PCO₂	BICARBONATE
Simple disorders			
Metabolic acidosis	↓	↓	↓
Metabolic alkalosis	↑	↑	↑
Respiratory acidosis	↓	↑	↑
Respiratory alkalosis	↑	↓	↓
Mixed disorders			
Metabolic acidosis with respiratory acidosis	↓↓	↑,N,↓	↑,N,↓
Metabolic alkalosis with respiratory acidosis	↑,N,↓	↑,N,↓	↑,N,↓
Metabolic acidosis with respiratory alkalosis	↑,N,↓	↓	↑,N,↓
Metabolic alkalosis with respiratory alkalosis	↑↑	↑,N,↓	↑,N,↓

Figure 5–13 Typical serum findings in clinical disturbances of acid-base balance. In the simple disorders it has been assumed that the primary acid-base disturbance has been compensated (see text for details). ↑ = increased from normal, ↓ = decreased from normal, N = normal.

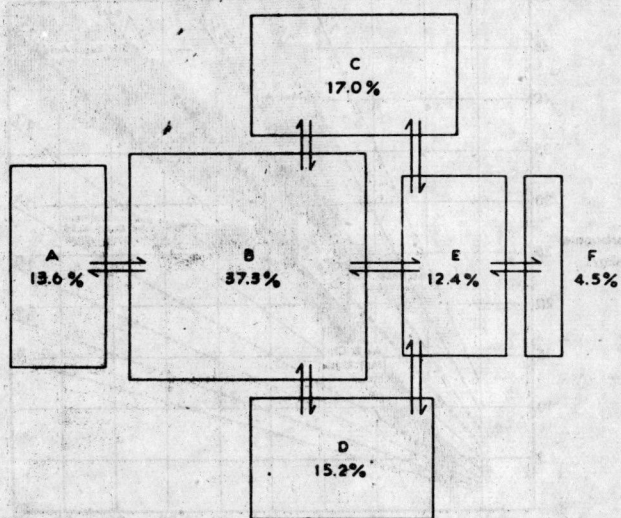

Figure 5-14 Distribution of chloride within the body of a normal young adult man. A, Plasma chloride; B, interstitial lymph chloride; C, dense connective tissue and cartilage chloride; D, bone chloride; E, intracellular chloride; F, transcellular chloride. (From Edelman IS, Liebman J: Am J Med 27:256, 1959.)

The intake and output of chloride parallel those of sodium. The transport of chloride is, to a large extent, passive and down an electrochemical gradient created in part by sodium transport. However, recent evidence indicates that chloride transport at several sites, including the thick ascending limb of the loop of Henle, may be active. That this mechanism is specifically inhibited by furosemide may account for the potency of this drug as a diuretic.

Under most clinical circumstances alterations in chloride concentration in the blood parallel those of sodium. Thus, hypo- and hyperchloremia are usually associated with comparable degrees of hypo- and hypernatremia, respectively, and are seen most often with dehydration secondary to diarrhea. On occasion, however, changes in chloride concentration are not accompanied by equivalent changes in sodium concentration.

Chloride is not directly involved in the regulation of the concentration of free hydrogen ion. Nevertheless, as metabolic adjustments within the kidney are made and plasma levels of bicarbonate change secondary to secretion of hydrogen ions, reciprocal changes in the plasma concentration of chloride generally occur. Thus, hypochloremia is typically seen in metabolic alkalosis. It occurs also when chloride is lost from the body in excess of sodium losses. Examples include loss from the bowel with vomiting or gastric drainage or in chloride diarrhea, a rare congenital disorder in which there is a defect in bowel transport of chloride. Urinary losses of chloride may exceed those of sodium during the correction of metabolic acidosis and in potassium deficiency. Indeed, with potassium deficiency both potassium and chloride must be given before the potassium deficits can be corrected. Similarly, the administration of chloride is necessary to correct most cases of metabolic alkalosis irrespective of whether or not it is

associated with potassium deficiency. In patients with metabolic alkalosis, the use of either potassium or sodium chloride, as appropriate, results in the prompt excretion of bicarbonate into the urine and correction of the alkalosis. Hypochloremia will also result from a protracted inadequate intake of chloride. For example, infants fed a chloride-deficient milk formula for several months developed chronic depletion of body chloride, severe hypochloremia (serum sodium levels usually remained normal), severe hypokalemic metabolic alkalosis, loss of appetite, failure to thrive, muscle weakness, and lethargy.

Hyperchloremia may result when chloride is conserved by the kidney in excess of sodium and potassium. This is observed with the formation of alkaline urine during the renal correction of alkalosis. An increased fractional reabsorption of chloride in the renal proximal tubule also results in hyperchloremia in distal renal tubular acidosis. Early amino acid solutions used in parenteral alimentation contained excessive amounts of chloride ion in the form of salts of the amino acids. Their administration resulted in hyperchloremic acidosis. Substitution of acetate has largely solved this problem.

Measurements of serum chloride are necessary to determine a patient's **anion gap.** The concentration of the most abundant serum cation (sodium) is greater than the sum of the 2 most abundant serum anions (chloride and bicarbonate). The difference, referred to as the anion gap, is normally about 12 mEq/l (range 8–16 mEq/l). This difference is due to the combined concentrations of the unmeasured anions such as phosphate, sulfate, proteins, and organic acids, which exceed those of the unmeasured cations, primarily potassium, calcium, and magnesium. The calculation of anion gap permits the detection of an abnormal concentration of an unmeasured anion or cation. An increased anion gap in renal failure is due to increased concentrations of phosphate and sulfate; in diabetic ketoacidosis, due to β-hydroxybutyrate and acetoacetate; in lactic acidosis, due to lactate; in hyperglycemic nonketotic coma, due to unidentified organic acids; and in disorders of amino acid metabolism, due to a variety of organic acids. Increased anion gap also follows the administration of large amounts of penicillin. After ethylene glycol ingestion, it is caused by glycolate production; with methanol ingestion, by formate production; and in salicylate poisoning, by the salicylate anion and a variety of organic anions secondary to the uncoupling of oxidative phosphorylation.

A decreased anion gap occurs less frequently. It may be found in nephrotic syndrome, in which it is due to a decreased serum concentration of albumin which is anionic at pH 7.4; after lithium ingestion, lithium being an unmeasured cation; and in multiple myeloma, due to the presence of cationic proteins.

5.14 PHOSPHORUS

Body Phosphorus.   Phosphate exists in the body in both inorganic and organic forms. Inorganic phosphate is the principal urinary buffer and plays a critical function in the regulation of free hydrogen ions (see above). It is present in massive quantities in bone and in high concentrations in cells. Intracellularly, it is essential for the synthesis of the important energy source, ATP, and is also present as creatine phosphate and various glucose-phosphate compounds, the largest quantities being present in muscle. Concentrations of inorganic phosphate are relatively low in extracellular fluids. Normal plasma levels vary from 1.0–3.0 mM/l depending on age (see below). In plasma at pH 7.4 and over the range of phosphate concentrations typically seen, approximately 90% of inorganic phosphate is ultrafilterable. Of this, slightly more than half is dissociated; 80% is present as the divalent anion (HPO_4^{--}) and 20% as the monovalent anion ($H_2PO_4^{-}$). The remaining ultrafilterable phosphate is composed of sodium, calcium, and magnesium salts. The nonultrafilterable inorganic phosphate is protein bound as is the plasma organic phosphate, which consists entirely of phospholipids.

The principal sources of *dietary phosphorus* are milk, milk products, and meat. The recommended daily intake is 800 mg/day for ages 1–10 yr and 1200 mg for older children. Up to two thirds of the dietary phosphate is absorbed from the bowel, primarily in the jejunum. This absorption is stimulated by vitamin D and its metabolites as well as by parathyroid hormone; it is decreased by thyrocalcitonin, by the presence in the bowel of binders such as aluminum hydroxide and carbonate, and, at least in animals, by a high dietary calcium intake.

Even though phosphate is actively transported across the bowel wall, it is the kidney which plays the major role in regulating body phosphate. Renal handling of phosphate consists of glomerular filtration with facultative reabsorption by the tubule. Ultrafilterable phosphate is freely filtered at the glomerulus with an average of 90% of this filtered load normally being reabsorbed. Sixty to 70% of the reabsorption occurs in the proximal tubule and the remainder in more distal segments. Under certain circumstances phosphate may also be secreted by the distal tubules. Although there is a maximal rate for tubular reabsorption of phosphate (Tm phosphate), this varies with filtration rate and is not approached under normal circumstances. Urinary excretion of phosphate shows a circadian rhythm—lowest in the morning and highest in early evening.

Tubular reabsorption of phosphate is regulated by *parathyroid hormone*, the effects of which are mediated by the adenylate cyclase system. This hormone reduces tubular reabsorption of phosphorus and is associated with phosphaturia. Conversely, large doses of vitamin D stimulate reabsorption of phosphate in the proximal tubule as does growth hormone. Under many circumstances renal tubular transport of phosphate appears to parallel that of sodium. Thus, expansion of extracellular fluid results in phosphaturia, as does the administration of diuretics, especially those that inhibit carbonic anhydrase. Phosphate transport also appears to be linked to that of glucose and to changes in pH; therefore hyperglycemia results in phosphaturia and reduced Tm

for phosphorus. Similarly, conditions that result in an alkaline urine also decrease reabsorption of phosphate.

Regulation of Plasma Phosphate. In addition to the factors already discussed, plasma phosphate concentration is affected by the continuous exchange of phosphate between the large stores in bone and those in the extracellular fluid. Net reabsorption of phosphate from bone is promoted by 1,25-dihydroxy–vitamin D_3 and PTH; it is opposed by thyrocalcitonin. Phosphate is also readily transported across all cell membranes. The administration of glucose or insulin decreases plasma phosphate concentration, probably because of an intracellular flux of phosphate secondary to the phosphorylation of glucose. Administration of epinephrine, hyperventilation, and alkalosis also decrease plasma phosphate concentration. Marked, acute increases in plasma phosphate concentration will result in hypocalcemia. Changes in calcium concentration, however, do not necessarily result in reciprocal alterations in plasma phosphate concentration.

Hyperphosphatemia is characteristic of hypoparathyroidism but rarely occurs in the absence of renal insufficiency. Although small changes in glomerular filtration rate (GFR) have little effect on phosphate excretion in health, *reduction in GFR* to below 25% leads to an elevation of serum inorganic phosphate and to reciprocal changes in serum calcium, resulting in secondary hyperparathyroidism. This process begins with small decreases in GFR but usually does not become clinically apparent until GFR has fallen to low levels. *In the young infant* GFR is low in relation to active cell mass and the dietary phosphorus intake is high; consequently, serum inorganic phosphorus is high. The premature infant has serum concentrations ranging from 2.5–3.0 mM/l (7.5–9.0 mg/dl), whereas in the adult the concentration is 1.0–1.3 mM/l (3–4 mg/dl). Hence, reduction in GFR or relative hypoparathyroidism in infants rapidly leads to very high serum values of phosphate, with depression of calcium concentration and latent or manifest tetany as consequences. The deficit of calcium results from its formation into bone salts. Hyperphosphatemia may also result from the excessive administration of phosphate by the oral or intravenous routes or as phosphate-containing enemas. Use of cytotoxic drugs to treat malignancies, especially lymphomas or leukemias, will result in cytolysis, with hyperphosphatemia due to release of phosphate into the circulation. The major clinical consequences of hyperphosphatemia are symptoms of the resulting hypocalcemia.

Hypophosphatemia may result from phosphate deficiency in association with, for example, starvation, protein-calorie malnutrition, and malabsorption syndromes. It may be the result of intracellular shifts of phosphate such as those which occur with respiratory or metabolic acidosis, during the treatment of diabetic ketoacidosis (typically during the 1st 24 hr), and following the administration of corticosteroids. Increased urinary losses of phosphate may be sufficiently severe to cause a reduction in plasma concentration; this reduction is observed in primary and tertiary hyperparathyroidism, in renal tubular defects, after ECF volume expansion, or after administration of diuretics. Often a combination of pathophysiologic mechanisms is responsible for the hypophosphatemia. Examples include vitamin D deficient and vitamin D resistant rickets (Sec 3.28). In most instances hypophosphatemia is mild or moderate in degree and is asymptomatic. Occasionally, plasma phosphate concentration may fall to very low levels (0.3 mM/l; 1.0 mg/dl or less). Such low levels have been observed with the prolonged use of intravenous alimentation without phosphate supplements and may result in a very severe, well-defined syndrome. Red cell concentrations of 2,3-diphosphoglycerate and ATP are decreased. The resulting decrease in release of oxygen by the red cells produces tissue anoxia. Increased hemolysis may also occur, as may leukocyte and platelet dysfunction. Some patients display the symptoms of a metabolic encephalopathy, including irritability, paresthesias, confusion, seizures, and coma, and there may be abnormalities in the electroencephalogram. Hypercalcemia, thought to be due to increased release of calcium from bone, rhabdomyolysis, cardiomyopathy, and possibly hepatocellular dysfunction, has also been reported. Renal tubular defects may occur, and the kidney's ability to excrete hydrogen ions is impaired. Prompt recognition and treatment of this syndrome, preferably by the oral administration of phosphate salts, is beneficial, but permanent defects may result. Thus, prevention of severe hypophosphatemia should always be the goal.

Ad Hoc Committee on Acid-Base Terminology: Report. Ann NY Acad Sci 133:25, 1966.

Bia MJ, DeFronzo RA: Extrarenal potassium homeostasis. Am J Physiol 9:F257, 1981.

Cooke RE (ed): The Biologic Basis of Pediatric Practice. New York, McGraw-Hill, 1968.

Earley LE, Daugharty TM: Sodium metabolism. N Engl J Med 281:72, 1969.

Emmett M, Narins RG: Clinical use of the anion gap. Medicine 56:38, 1977.

Grogono AW, Byles PH, Hawke W: An in-vivo representation of acid-base balance. Lancet 2:499, 1976.

Kaehny WD: Pathogenesis and management of respiratory and mixed acid-base disorders. In: Schrier RW (ed): Renal and Electrolyte Disorders. Ed. 2. Boston, Little, Brown, 1980.

Kassirer JP, Berkrnan PM, Lawrenz DR, et al: The critical roles of chloride in the correction of hypokalemic alkalosis in man. Am J Med 38:172, 1965.

Leaf A: The clinical and physiologic significance of the serum sodium concentration. N Engl J Med 267:24, 1962.

Omdahl JL, DeLuca HF: Regulation of vitamin D metabolism and function. Physiol Rev 53:327, 1973.

Plum, F, Price RW: Acid-base balance of cisternal and lumbar cerebrospinal fluid in hospital patients. N Engl J Med 289:1346, 1973.

Rocha AS, Kokko JP: Sodium chloride and water transport in the medullary thick ascending limb of Henle. Evidence for active chloride transport. J Clin Invest 52:612, 1973.

Roy S, Arant BS Jr: Hypokalemic metabolic alkalosis in normotensive infants with elevated plasma renin activity and hyperaldosteronism: Role of dietary chloride deficiency. Pediatrics 67:423, 1981.

Schrier RW (ed): Renal and Electrolyte Disorders. Ed 2. Boston, Little, Brown, 1980.

Schwartz, WB, Relman AS: A critique of the parameters used in the evaluation of acid-base disorders. N Engl J Med 268:1382, 1963.

Schwartz WB, Relman AS: Effects of electrolyte disorders on renal structure and function. N Engl J Med 276:383, 452, 1967.

Tannen RL (ed): Potassium homeostasis. Kidney Int 11:389, 1977.

Walser M: Magnesium Metabolism. Reviews of Physiology, Biochemistry and Experimental Pharmacology. Berlin, Springer-Verlag, 1967.

Winters RW (ed): The Body Fluids in Pediatrics. Boston, Little, Brown, 1973.

5.15 PARENTERAL FLUID THERAPY

Young children are especially susceptible to the consequences of illnesses that affect fluid balance. The usual daily turnover of water in the infant is equal to almost 25% of total body water. In contrast, the equivalent figure in the adult approximates only 6%. Thus the effects of diseases which reduce fluid intake (e.g., vomiting) or increase losses (e.g., diarrhea) appear much more rapidly in the infant than in the adult.

Calculation of Requirements. In most patients total fluid and electrolyte needs are calculated as the sum of deficit and maintenance requirements. *Deficit therapy* is designed to replace losses of fluids and electrolytes which resulted from an illness before the patient was brought for medical care and to return volume and composition to normal. *Maintenance therapy* is designed to replace ongoing losses, both normal and abnormal, of fluids and electrolytes, maintain patients in normal balance, and prevent deficits from developing. For example, after uncomplicated surgery a patient often requires only the replacement of fluids and electrolytes normally lost from the body through the lungs and as urine, sweat, and feces. A postoperative patient with gastric drainage, however, will require normal maintenance therapy plus replacement of the additional amounts of water and electrolytes lost in the gastric fluid. A dehydrated patient with severe diarrhea will require normal maintenance therapy, the replacement of continuing abnormal stool losses for as long as the

diarrhea persists, and replacement of the deficits which resulted from the diarrhea.

Patients with certain disease states may require specific fluids and electrolytes in addition to those for repair of deficits and maintenance. An example in which such *supplemental therapy* often is required is salicylate intoxication. Alkalinization and the induction of diuresis are frequently employed to increase salicylate excretion in the urine.

Each of these phases of fluid therapy will be considered separately. *As with potentially lethal drugs, amounts of fluids and electrolytes should preferably be calculated independently by at least 2 people and the results reconciled before administration is begun.*

Monitoring of Patient. Regardless of the accuracy of planning a therapeutic regimen, a patient's response is not always predictable. Consequently, frequent assessment is required so that appropriate modifications of therapy can be instituted promptly if needed. Typically, such monitoring consists of frequent physical examinations to determine clinical status, regular weighing to determine changes in body weight, and frequent review of intake and output charts. These clinical determinations may need to be supplemented by repeated laboratory determinations. Serial measurements of serum electrolytes, blood urea nitrogen, and serum creatinine may be essential; the interval between determinations depends on the patient's clinical status.

5.16 MAINTENANCE THERAPY

5.17 REPLACEMENT OF NORMAL LOSSES

Even in health, a person deprived of a normal oral intake will continue to lose basal amounts of fluids and electrolytes from the body as urine, sweat, and feces and will have additional losses of water from the lungs as evaporation in exhaled air. Water and electrolytes are required to replace these obligatory losses or deficits will result. Protein and calories are also required, but complete parenteral replacement is difficult and is not essential unless oral intake is restricted for a protracted period of time.

The amount and type of these losses may be modified by disease states. For example, pyrexia may be associated with increased sweating; renal disease may result in either oliguria or polyuria; both diarrhea and gastric suction will result in increased losses from the gastrointestinal tract. Less easily recognized but equally important losses are those that may result from sequestration of fluid in a body space, e.g., a patient with paralytic ileus may have pooling of fluid in the gastrointestinal tract. Under such circumstances, even though total body fluid and electrolyte content may not be changed, this pooled fluid may not be in equilibrium with the vascular compartment and may cause a functional deficit. Failure to replace any of these losses will result in the development of fluid and electrolyte deficits. The influence of disease states on maintenance requirements will be discussed after normal maintenance needs have been analyzed.

Calculation of Normal Maintenance Therapy. I: Basic Method. Fluid and electrolyte requirements for purposes of maintenance are directly related to metabolic rate. An increase in metabolic rate requires an increase in catabolism of metabolic fuels and has 3 effects: (1) it increases the rate of endogenous water production from the oxidation of carbohydrate, fats, and protein; (2) it increases urinary solute excretion which, in turn, increases obligatory urine flow rates and urinary water losses; and (3) it increases heat production, which increases water loss as sweat and water loss through respiration. Similarly, the turnover rates of electrolytes are related to water loss and to metabolic rate. In consequence, if a patient's caloric expenditure can be estimated, his maintenance requirements of fluids and electrolytes can be calculated because the amounts of water, sodium, and potassium required for every 100 kcal metabolized have been well established from numerous observations.

Calculation of Caloric Expenditure. Metabolic rate depends on age, body weight, degree of activity, and body temperature. *Basal metabolic rate* can be obtained from Table 5–3, which depicts the values for each sex at various ages and body weights. To calculate maintenance requirements from caloric expenditure, these basal values must be adjusted for the patient's activity, body temperature, and any pathologic state. *Adjustments for activity* are made from observation of the patient. No increments are needed for patients in coma

Table 5–3 STANDARD BASAL CALORIC OUTPUT

WEIGHT (KG)	KILOCALORIES/24 HOURS MALE AND FEMALE	
3	140	
5	270	
7	400	
9	500	
11	600	
13	650	
15	710	
17	780	
19	830	
21	880	
	Male	Female
25	1020	960
29	1120	1040
33	1210	1120
37	1300	1190
41	1350	1260
45	1410	1320
49	1470	1380
53	1530	1440
57	1590	1500
61	1640	1560

Modified from Talbot.
Increments or decrements:
1. Add or subtract 12% of above for each degree C (8% for each degree F) above or below rectal temperature of 37.8° C (100° F).
2. Add 0 to 30% increments for activity.

or under anesthesia. Usual activity in bed rarely increases basal expenditure by more than 30%. Caloric expenditure is increased by fever (12% per °C rise in body temperature) and by hypermetabolic states such as salicylism and hyperthyroidism (25–75%). It is decreased by hypothermia (12% per °C fall in body temperature) and by hypometabolic states such as hypothyroidism (10–25%).

These calculations permit a good estimate of caloric expenditure in all but the very young infant and the obese subject. In the neonate, activity during the 1st 3–5 days of life is low; total caloric expenditure does not usually exceed 50 kcal/kg of body weight per day, and this figure should be used to calculate maintenance requirements during this neonatal period. In obese infants and children, "ideal" weight (50th percentile for age and height) should be used to calculate basal metabolic rate.

Water and electrolyte requirements are calculated from these estimates of caloric expenditure. As shown in Table 5–4, the usual losses of water and electrolytes from lungs, skin, stool, and urine can be related to caloric expenditure. For every 100 kcal metabolized the patient requires approximately 125 ml of water, 3.2 mEq of sodium, and 2.4 mEq of potassium to replace normal losses. However, maintenance requirements for water have to be reduced by 10–15 ml/100 kcal metabolized to allow for the release of an equivalent volume of water during oxidation of endogenous and exogenous carbohydrate, fat, and protein. Thus water, sodium, and potassium requirements for normal maintenance therapy are estimated at 115 ml, 3 mEq, and 2.5 mEq respectively for every 100 kcal metabolized.

In health the kidney can adjust rates of urine flow and electrolyte excretion over wide ranges. The main-

Table 5–4 WATER AND ELECTROLYTE LOSSES PER 100 KILOCALORIES METABOLIZED UNDER NORMAL CONDITIONS AND IN DISEASE STATES

ROUTE OF LOSS	USUAL LOSS			RANGE OBSERVED IN DISEASE STATES		
	H_2O (ml)	Na (mEq)	K (mEq)	H_2O (ml)	Na (mEq)	K (mEq)
Evaporative						
Lungs	15	0	0	10–60	0	0
Skin	40	0.1	0.2	20–100	0.1–3.0	0.2–1.5
Stool	5	0.1	0.2	0–50	0.1–4.0	0.2–3.0
Urine	65	3.0	2.0	0–400	0–30.0	0–30.0
Total	125	3.2	2.4			

tenance requirements calculated above do not require maximal renal concentration or dilution of urine; they do not exceed the solute load which can be excreted by the kidney nor its ability to conserve electrolytes. The designated requirements thus provide some latitude in the amounts of fluids and electrolytes which can be administered safely. With renal damage, or in other disease states, this is frequently not the case, and maintenance requirements must be modified precisely, as outlined below.

The fluid requirement recommended above is less than that prescribed for bottle-fed infants, for whom 140 ml/100 kcal of food is suggested, because the infant's high protein diet, consisting principally of cow's milk, increases the solute load to be excreted by the kidney. This increases both obligatory water loss through the kidneys and fluid requirements.

Calculation of Normal Maintenance Therapy. II: Alternative Method. The calculation of maintenance therapy by the method outlined above is based on first principles and is accurate. However, difficulty may be experienced in calculating caloric expenditure if the appropriate reference tables are not available; therefore, several simpler methods have been devised. Most are derived from the principles already outlined but relate maintenance requirements to either body weight or body surface.

An alternative simple method is shown in Table 5–5. Caloric expenditure can be obtained from this easily remembered formula. The values are for the average hospitalized patient and allow for usual activity in bed. Although values for caloric expenditure are slightly higher than those used in the basic system, the derived values for maintenance requirements are identical since it is recommended that for every 100 kcal expended

Table 5–5 A SIMPLIFIED ALTERNATIVE METHOD TO CALCULATE CALORIC EXPENDITURE FROM BODY WEIGHT

BODY WEIGHT (KG)	CALORIC EXPENDITURE PER DAY
Up to 10	100 kcal/kg
11–20	1000 kcal + 50 kcal/kg for each kg above 10 kg
Above 20	1500 kcal + 20 kcal/kg for each kg above 20 kg

Modified from Holliday and Segar. Kcal = kilocalories = 1000 calories = 1000 Cal.

only 100 ml of fluid should be administered (compared to 115 ml with the basic system); this solution should contain 25 mEq of sodium and 20 mEq of potassium per liter, and 5% dextrose. Commercially prepared solutions with this composition are available (Table 29–8) and have the advantages of providing magnesium (3 mEq/l) and of giving some of the anion as phosphate (3 mEq/l) and either lactate or acetate (23 mEq/l). If such a solution is not readily available, an appropriate solution can easily be prepared from standard intravenous preparations.

Comparison of Methods. Maintenance requirements calculated by the newer alternative methods are virtually identical to those calculated by the basic method presented earlier. For example, to calculate daily maintenance requirements for an afebrile, previously healthy male child weighing 45 kg, basic caloric expenditure obtained from Table 5–3 would be 1410. Allowing a 20% increment for physical activity, the estimated caloric expenditure would be 1692 kcal. Based on this figure, daily water requirements would be $16.92 \times 115 = 1946$ ml; sodium requirements, $16.92 \times 3 = 51$ mEq (equivalent to 26 mEq/l of administered solution); and potassium requirements, $16.92 \times 2.5 = 42$ mEq (or 21 mEq/l of administered solution). The administered fluid should contain 5% dextrose. Using the alternative system presented in Table 5–5 caloric expenditure would be estimated as 2000 kcal, which would indicate the need to administer 2000 ml of the maintenance solution containing 5% dextrose, 25 mEq/l of sodium, and 20 mEq/l of potassium.

5.18 MODIFICATION OF MAINTENANCE REQUIREMENTS BY DISEASE STATES

Certain disease states may result in either markedly increased or decreased losses of water and/or electrolytes. This is illustrated in Table 5–4, which lists ranges of losses of water and electrolytes that have been observed in various disease states; maintenance therapy must be adjusted appropriately to maintain a patient's fluid and electrolyte balance.

Decreased Requirements. In *anuria* or extreme oliguria urine output may be negligible, often less than 10 ml/100 kcal, compared to a more normal 65 ml. Only stool and evaporative water losses occur, and the rate of fluid administration must be reduced accordingly. Rarely is more than 45 ml of exogenous water required for each 100 kcal. Indeed, it is preferable to underestimate rather than overestimate fluid requirements in such cases since it is easier to administer additional fluids later if needed than to attempt to remove excess fluid administered inappropriately. Administration of electrolytes should also be reduced in anuric patients. In the absence of complications such as diarrhea, sodium and potassium losses through the sweat and stools are usually negligible and no electrolytes may be required for maintenance in these subjects.

In some patients, particularly those with *meningitis*, excessive or inappropriate release of antidiuretic hormone may occur. The rate of flow of urine is markedly reduced, and fluid intake should be reduced to reflect

**Table 5-6 COMPOSITION OF
EXTERNAL ABNORMAL LOSSES**

FLUID	NA	K	CL	PROTEIN GM%
	——————mEq/L——————			
Gastric	20–80	5–20	100–150	—
Pancreatic	120–140	5–15	90–120	—
Small intestine	100–140	5–15	90–130	—
Bile	120–140	5–15	80–120	—
Ileostomy	45–135	3–15	20–115	—
Diarrheal	10–90	10–80	10–110	—
Sweat:*				
Normal	10–30	3–10	10–35	—
Cystic fibrosis	50–130	5–25	50–110	—
Burns	140	5	110	3–5

*Sweat sodium concentrations progressively increase with increasing sweat flow rates.

these decreased losses. *Patients in highly humidified atmospheres* (e.g., incubators or croup tents) also have reduced fluid requirements since the high humidity may reduce evaporative losses of water by 20–50%. In *congestive heart failure* restriction of sodium and water intake is indicated when planning parenteral as well as oral intake.

Increased Requirements. The principles underlying replacement of abnormally increased losses of fluids and electrolytes require little explanation. The amount and nature of the losses depend on the underlying disease process and the site of loss. Considerable variation exists in the composition of abnormal *gastrointestinal losses* from patient to patient and from time to time in the same patient. However, an estimate of the composition of the more common fluid losses can be made from the information in Table 5-6. These losses should be replaced as nearly as possible, volume for volume, as they occur to prevent physiologic readjustment that may further deplete the body of water and electrolytes. On occasion such estimates are too imprecise, and the electrolyte concentrations in the fluid being lost must be measured for an exact determination of replacement needs.

In general, losses in gastric or intestinal drainage can be replaced satisfactorily by isotonic or somewhat hypotonic solutions which contain more chloride than sodium for gastric replacement and more sodium than chloride for intestinal replacement. Although gastric fluid contains relatively little potassium, the alkalosis that develops from the loss of significant quantities of hydrogen ion in the gastric juice usually results in an increased urinary potassium loss; therefore, replacement fluid for a patient with gastric drainage should contain 10–20 mEq of potassium/l (provided renal function is well maintained).

Increased losses of sodium chloride in *sweat* usually are of little significance except in adrenal insufficiency and cystic fibrosis; heat stress should be avoided in such patients. In *hyperventilation* and *heat stress,* evaporative losses of water may increase as much as 90 and 120 ml/100 kcal, respectively.

When *renal* concentrating and diluting ability is lost, as in chronic renal disease, water requirements may rise to 150 ml/100 kcal and in diabetes insipidus of nephrogenic or hypothalamic origin, to as high as 400 ml/100 kcal. Precise replacement of such large quantities

of fluid may be difficult. In such instances, thirst, changes in body weight, and urinary output are usually more reliable indicators of the patient's needs than are the physician's estimates. As an additional precaution, oral feedings should be used whenever possible.

Under most circumstances fluid and sodium losses are replaced rapidly, patients with major losses often having to be re-evaluated every 8 hr or more frequently to see that balance is maintained. Typically, potassium losses are replaced over a more protracted period of time. Good reason for not replacing losses on a volume-for-volume and milliequivalent-for-milliequivalent basis may occur, e.g., in acute tubular necrosis. The increased urine output seen in the diuretic phase of this entity may eliminate fluid retained during the oliguric phase; these increased losses are not replaced since such therapy would only perpetuate the presence of edema.

ADMINISTRATION OF MAINTENANCE REQUIREMENTS

Maintenance therapy may be given by either oral or parenteral routes. When oral administration is not possible, the intravenous route is preferred. Use of subcutaneous injections of fluids is not recommended because of variable rates of absorption and other complications. However, if technical or other difficulties dictate that therapy be given by this route, glucose in water or in very dilute electrolyte solution should not be given because diffusion of sodium chloride into such an extravascular pool and the subsequent loss of fluid from the extracellular fluid may reduce plasma volume acutely and precipitate shock.

Caloric Intake

In a patient receiving maintenance fluids by the parenteral route it is difficult to match caloric expenditure with adequate caloric intake. Fortunately, this is not necessary if maintenance therapy is needed for only short periods of time. However, administration of maintenance electrolytes in a 5% dextrose solution is desirable as a routine measure. This provides approximately 20% of the calories metabolized and results in decreased catabolism of endogenous protein and a decreased solute load to be excreted by the kidney. Concentrations of dextrose above 5% are not recommended. When they are administered at infusion rates sufficient to meet water requirements, they frequently result in hyperglycemia and loss of dextrose in the urine. They may actually increase water requirements through an osmotic diuretic effect. At slower infusion rates, such as those used in the anuric patient or the neonate, higher concentrations may be effectively used, but they increase the risk of intravenous thrombosis and infection.

Intravenous Alimentation

Since the regimens for fluid and electrolyte replacement and maintenance already discussed are calorically

Table 5-7   COMPOSITION OF TYPICAL INFUSATE USED IN INTRAVENOUS ALIMENTATION

CONSTITUENT	CONCENTRATION (PER LITER)	APPROXIMATE INFUSION RATE (PER KG/DAY)
Amino acids*	25 gm	3.6 gm
Glucose	200 gm	27 gm
Sodium†	Up to 40 mEq	2-3 mEq
Potassium†	Up to 30 mEq	2-3 mEq
Chloride†	Up to 45 mEq	4-5 mEq
Acetate	15 mEq	2 mEq
Calcium	9.3 mEq	1-2 mEq
Magnesium	2.5 mEq	1 mEq
Phosphate	67 mEq	
Multivitamin	5.0 ml	
Folic acid	0.45 mg	

*Derived from an amino acid preparation Neoaminosol (Abbott Laboratories) or FreAmine (McGaw). Alternate sources of amino acids—5% beef fibrin hydrolysate (Aminosol:Abbott Laboratories) or casein hydrolysate (Amigen:Baxter Laboratories) — should be present in a higher concentration of 33 gm protein/l.

†Adjusted to meet individual patient's needs.

inadequate, they will not sustain growth. They are suitable, therefore, for short periods of time only. In some infants and children, especially newborns undergoing major surgery and children with protracted diarrhea, parenteral nutrition for prolonged periods is necessary. Regimens developed to meet this need may be effective in maintaining positive nitrogen balance and growth for periods of 60 days or longer. The infusate is prepared from an amino acid preparation; it contains 20% glucose plus sodium, potassium, calcium, magnesium, phosphorus, chloride, and vitamins (Table 5-7). Infused at a rate of 135 ml/kg/24 hr, it provides 122 cal/kg/24 hr. Essential fatty acids and trace metals are provided by the twice-weekly administration of plasma (10 ml/kg); vitamin K (5.0 mg) is given by intramuscular injection at weekly intervals; and a single intramuscular injection of vitamin B_{12} (500 μg) is also administered.

The solution is delivered by a constant-speed infusion pump into the superior vena cava through a long catheter. In an attempt to minimize the risk of infection, the catheter is tunneled subcutaneously for a considerable distance before entering the vein, and a Millipore filter is located in the circuit just before the tubing enters the patient.

Complications from this procedure are common and include sepsis, severe hyperglycemia, and marked electrolyte disturbances, including acidosis. The technique should be performed only in those centers experienced in the method with the facilities necessary for intensive monitoring.

5.19   DEFICIT THERAPY

Deficits in body water and electrolytes may result from reduced intake with continuing normal losses, from excessive losses occurring with or without usual intake, or from a combination of these mechanisms. The *absolute deficits* of water and electrolytes observed in dehydration produced by different disease states

Table 5-8   PROBABLE DEFICITS OF WATER AND ELECTROLYTES IN INFANTS WITH MODERATELY SEVERE DEHYDRATION

CONDITION	H_2O (ml)	Na (mEq)	K* (mEq)	Cl (mEq)
		PER KG OF BODY WEIGHT		
Fasting and thirsting	100-120	5-7	1-2	4-6
Diarrhea				
Isonatremic	100-120	8-10	8-10	8-10
Hypernatremic	100-120	2-4	0-4	-2--6†
Hyponatremic	100-120	10-12	8-10	10-12
Pyloric stenosis	100-120	8-10	10-12	10-12
Diabetic acidosis	100-120	8-10	5-7	6-8

*Converted for breakdown of tissue cells: – 1 gm N = 3 mEq of K.
†Negative balance of chloride indicates excess at beginning of therapy.

have been estimated by a variety of methods. Table 5-8 provides some representative values and illustrates the similarity in the magnitudes of deficits irrespective of the precipitating condition. This is not surprising, since deficits reflect not only the results of direct losses but also the physiologic readjustments by the patient. As a consequence, *patients with deficits resulting from many different causes can be treated successfully in a similar manner.* Thus, in most instances, management is dictated more by the severity and type of deficit than by its underlying cause. The *severity of the clinical disturbances* typically depends on the magnitude of the deficit in relation to body reserves and on the rate at which the deficit developed. The *type of deficit* depends on the relationship between the magnitude of loss of water and that of electrolytes, principally sodium.

SEVERITY OF DEFICIT

The magnitude or severity of a deficit can be gauged from change in body weight. Any loss of body weight in excess of 1%/day represents loss of body water. In young infants a weight loss of up to 5% is considered to indicate mild, 5-10% moderate, and 10-15% severe dehydration. The last of these is frequently associated with peripheral circulatory failure. Deficits in excess of 15% of body weight are rarely compatible with life.

In older children and adults total body water and extracellular fluid volume each represent a smaller percentage of body weight than in the infant. In these patients, any given percentage loss of body weight resulting from fluid and electrolyte deficits indicates more severe depletion than in infants. Thus comparable figures for severity of the deficit in older patients are 3% (mild), 6% (moderate), and 9% (severe).

The rapidity with which a deficit develops is also important. A 10% weight loss occurring over 24 hr in an infant is severe. The same weight loss developing over several days is better tolerated, and its effects typically are only moderately severe.

5.20   TYPES OF DEHYDRATION

The serum sodium in dehydrated patients may be normal, low, or high, depending on the relative losses of water and electrolytes. Dehydration is classified on this basis, being termed *isonatremic* when serum sodium levels are 130–150 mEq/l, *hyponatremic* when serum sodium levels are less than 130 mEq/l, and *hypernatremic* when serum sodium levels are above 150 mEq/l. Since plasma osmolality in large part reflects sodium concentrations, these forms of dehydration are usually *isotonic*, *hypotonic*, and *hypertonic*, respectively. Changes in tonicity do not always correspond to changes in sodium concentration, however, so the 2 sets of terms cannot be used interchangeably. For example, in diabetic ketoacidosis or in uremia, serum sodium concentration may be low, but the plasma is hypertonic as a result of elevated plasma levels of glucose or urea, respectively.

Classification of dehydration into these 3 types, based on sodium concentrations, is of practical importance. Each form is associated with different relative losses of fluid from intracellular (ICF) and extracellular (ECF) compartments. In *isonatremic* dehydration the fluid and electrolyte loss is from the extracellular fluid which remains isotonic. Since there is no osmotic gradient across cell walls, intracellular fluid volume remains virtually constant; thus, the majority of fluid loss is borne by the extracellular compartment. In *hyponatremic* dehydration the hypotonicity of the extracellular fluid results in an osmotically induced movement of fluid from the extracellular compartment into cells, resulting in even further depletion of extracellular fluid and some increases in intracellular fluid. Conversely, in *hypernatremic* dehydration the increase in osmolality of the extracellular fluid results in movement of fluid out of the cells so that the intracellular fluid volume is depleted; depletion of extracellular fluid is less than expected. This analysis assumes that the plasma does not contain pathologic concentrations of other molecules which are osmotically effective across cell walls. As a consequence of these differences, the 3 forms of dehydration are characterized by variations in clinical presentation and in physical findings. Each requires appropriate modification in therapeutic approach.

5.21 ESTIMATION OF MAGNITUDE AND TYPE OF DEFICIT

This assessment should consist of a detailed history and a thorough physical examination, often augmented by appropriate laboratory studies.

Table 5–9 HISTORICAL DATA REQUIRED IN ESTIMATING MAGNITUDE AND TYPES OF DEFICIT AND IN PLANNING DEFICIT THERAPY

Intake — during period of illness
  Quantity and how given
  Kind: water, electrolyte, protein, drugs
Output — during period of illness
  Quantity
  Kind: urine, vomiting, diarrhea, sweat, drainage
Balance
  Weight change
General medical
  Age
  Cardiovascular, respiratory, renal or central nervous system disease

History. Some important aspects are shown in Table 5–9. If a patient's preillness weight is known, the change from this value will provide an accurate estimate of the magnitude of fluid losses. Without such information, a detailed estimate of losses and the exact quantities and composition of the infant's feedings prior to being seen may permit a less exact assessment of the magnitude of the deficit. Such a history may also give an indication of the type of dehydration as well. Although deficits usually result from the loss of fluids that are hyponatremic in relation to serum (Table 5–6), it is important to remember that body composition of dehydrated patients is influenced not only by losses but also by *concomitant intake*. The severity and type of dehydration are the result of the sum of intake and losses of both water and electrolytes. For example, a patient with severe diarrhea, losing fluid with a sodium concentration as low as 40 mEq/l, may continue to drink tap water containing virtually no sodium. Water losses will be partially compensated for by the water intake but sodium losses will not be replaced. As a result, despite the primary loss of excessive quantities of a hyponatremic fluid (diarrhea), this patient may still present with hyponatremia. Conversely, the same patient treated with homemade electrolyte mixtures given by mouth may be hypernatremic, especially if the solution has been prepared with excessive amounts of salt or sodium bicarbonate, an all too common problem which has frequently been observed to result in severe hypernatremia.

The time and frequency of recent urinations, whether excessive or suppressed, may provide some appreciation of the severity of dehydration or give some indication of its cause. Urine output characteristically is decreased with dehydration, except in some low birth weight infants. Continued frequent and excessive urination with dehydration suggests diabetes mellitus, diabetes insipidus, or nephrogenic diabetes insipidus. Output of usual amounts of urine without increased intake of water, in association with physical signs of dehydration, indicates a loss in the capacity of the kidneys to conserve water and suggests the presence of renal disease.

Physical Examination. Table 5–10 details the physical findings associated with dehydration of different degrees of severity. Table 5–11 summarizes how different types of dehydration modify the physical signs.

Most infants and children appear ill when dehydrated. Frequently, the eyes appear sunken and the skin around them dark. Intraocular pressure, elicited by lightly pressing on the closed eyes, is low. The mucous membranes of the mouth are usually dry, but prolonged mouth breathing or the tachypnea of acidosis may cause dry mucous membranes in the absence of dehydration. Tissue turgor may be reduced. Normally, when the skin and subcutaneous tissue are pinched between the thumb and first finger and then released, they return to position immediately. Delay in return *(tenting)* indicates dehydration. Skin and subcutaneous tissue must be tested together or laxity of skin may be misinterpreted as dehydration. Skin over the abdominal and chest walls and of the thigh should be tested. Testing the abdomen alone may miss this sign since

Table 5–10   CLINICAL ASSESSMENT OF SEVERITY OF DEHYDRATION

SIGNS AND SYMPTOMS	MILD DEHYDRATION	MODERATE DEHYDRATION	SEVERE DEHYDRATION
General appearance and condition:			
Infants and young children	Thirsty; alert; restless	Thirsty; restless or lethargic but irritable to touch or drowsy	Drowsy; limp, cold, sweaty, cyanotic extremities; may be comatose
Older children and adults	Thirsty; alert; restless	Thirsty; alert; postural hypotension	Usually conscious; apprehensive; cold, sweaty, cyanotic extremities; wrinkled skin of fingers and toes; muscle cramps
Radial pulse	Normal rate and volume	Rapid and weak	Rapid, feeble, sometimes impalpable
Respiration	Normal	Deep, maybe rapid	Deep and rapid
Anterior fontanel	Normal	Sunken	Very sunken
Systolic blood pressure	Normal	Normal or low	Less than 90 mm; may be unrecordable
Skin elasticity	Pinch retracts immediately	Pinch retracts slowly	Pinch retracts very slowly (>2 sec)
Eyes	Normal	Sunken (detectable)	Grossly sunken
Tears	Present	Absent	Absent
Mucous membranes	Moist	Dry	Very dry
Urine flow	Normal	Reduced amount and dark	None passed for several hours; empty bladder
% body weight loss	4–5%	6–9%	10% or more
Estimated fluid deficit	40–50 ml/kg	60–90 ml/kg	100–110 ml/kg

Modified from World Health Organization guide.

abdominal distention may mask loss of turgor at this site. It should also be remembered that in the well-nourished infant or child, skin turgor may remain fairly normal in the presence of dehydration. Depression of the anterior fontanel in the infant is often an accurate indication of dehydration.

As suggested by Table 5–11, physical examination may also help to determine the type of dehydration. Patients with hyponatremic dehydration have increased losses of fluid from the extracellular compartment and are more likely to develop shock; conversely, evidence of depletion of intracellular fluid may be apparent in patients with hypernatremic dehydration and be reflected in a doughy or putty-like consistency of the skin and subcutaneous tissue on palpation.

Shock manifested by tachycardia, a thin and thready pulse, cyanosis, and low blood pressure may supervene with severe dehydration. Blood pressure is frequently hard to determine, but an estimate of systolic pressure only can often be obtained by palpation, and is useful. Alternatively, use of the Doppler technique may enable an accurate measurement of blood pressure. The state

Table 5–11   EFFECTS OF TYPE OF DEHYDRATION ON PHYSICAL SIGNS

	ISONATREMIC DEHYDRATION (PROPORTIONATE LOSS OF WATER AND SODIUM)	HYPONATREMIC DEHYDRATION (LOSS OF SODIUM IN EXCESS OF WATER)	HYPERNATREMIC DEHYDRATION (LOSS OF WATER IN EXCESS OF SODIUM)
ECF Volume*	Markedly decreased	Severely decreased	Decreased
ICF Volume*	Maintained	Increased	Decreased
Physical Signs			
Skin			
Color†	Gray	Gray	Gray
Temperature	Cold	Cold	Cold or hot
Turgor‡	Poor	Very poor	Fair
Feel	Dry	Clammy	Thickened, doughy
Mucous membrane	Dry	Slightly moist	Parched§
Eyeball	Sunken and soft	Sunken and soft	Sunken
Fontanel	Sunken	Sunken	Sunken
Psyche	Lethargic	Coma	Hyperirritable
Pulse†	Rapid	Rapid	Moderately rapid
Blood pressure†	Low	Very low	Moderately low

*ECF = extracellular fluid; ICF = intracellular fluid.
†Signs of shock rather than of dehydration itself.
‡Reflects magnitude of fluid loss from ECF.
§Tongue often has shriveled appearance due to loss of cellular fluid.

Table 5–12 PHYSICAL SIGNS OF VARIATIONS IN CONCENTRATION OF SPECIFIC IONS

Acidosis (metabolic)
  Respiration: increased depth and rate
Alkalosis (metabolic)
  Respiration: decreased depth and rate
  Latent or manifest tetany
Hypopotassemia
  Heart: fast or slow, poor quality to heart sounds
  Skeletal muscle: weakness or paralyses, diminished reflexes
  Smooth muscle: abdominal distention, ileus
Hyperpotassemia
  Heart: slow or fast, poor quality to heart sounds
  Skeletal muscle: fibrillation, paralyses
Hypocalcemia
  Latent tetany (Sec 5.33)
  Manifest tetany (Sec 5.33)
Hypercalcemia
  Gastrointestinal: fecal masses
  Hypotonia
Hypomagnesemia
  Latent or manifest tetany
  Muscular twitching
Hypermagnesemia
  Decreased deep tendon reflexes
  Central nervous system depression

of the peripheral circulation can be assessed by the warmth and color of the skin and by the rapidity of filling of the cutaneous capillary bed after pressure over the ear lobe, the nail bed, or the dorsum of the hand or the foot. However, peripheral circulation can be affected by local factors such as ambient temperature, and care must be taken when evaluating these signs.

Most physical findings in dehydration occur irrespective of the etiology of the volume depletion. Some disease states result in specific losses. For example, severe diarrhea is associated with marked losses of bicarbonate and results in systemic acidosis. In pyloric stenosis, major losses of hydrogen and chloride cause a hypochloremic alkalosis. Chronic diarrhea may result in hypomagnesemia from continuing losses of magnesium. The findings on physical examination that may indicate such deficits are summarized in Table 5–12. Such physical findings are not infallible or uniform. For example, the characteristic signs of metabolic acidosis (relatively slow, regular breathing with increased depth and a prolonged expiratory phase, sometimes referred to as *Kussmaul breathing*) may be less marked in the presence of severe circulatory insufficiency. The compensatory diminution in breathing associated with alkalosis, though usually absent in adults, may be seen in infants with pyloric stenosis. Deficiencies of potassium, calcium, or magnesium may exist without obvious physical findings. Hypokalemia may not always be present even when cells are depleted of potassium so that such deficits may have to be inferred from history alone.

In summary, mild dehydration may be indicated only by the presence of thirst. If 2 or more signs of moderate dehydration (Table 5–10) are present, the patient should be considered to have moderate dehydration even if all the signs are not present. A similar guide should be used for severe dehydration. In the absence of known changes in body weight, examination of the anterior

fontanel, skin elasticity, and the eyes, as well as a history of the recent pattern of urination, is most helpful in assessing the degree of dehydration in an infant.

Laboratory Data. Admission laboratory values are helpful in characterization of the type of deficit and in planning therapy. None is so essential, however, that adequate therapy cannot be initiated without it. Serial laboratory determinations are of greater importance. They permit the assessment of the results of treating deficits and guide subsequent maintenance therapy.

Hemoconcentration (increase in *hemoglobin, hematocrit,* and *plasma proteins*) may indicate the severity of dehydration. However, with pre-existing anemia, both hemoglobin and hematocrit may be normal even with severe dehydration. Similarly, the measurement of plasma proteins may have limited usefulness at the beginning of therapy, especially in a malnourished patient. Despite such limitations, these measurements, when correlated with physical findings, may be useful in planning therapy; serial determinations are of considerable help in assessing its effectiveness.

Dehydration may result in a decrease in glomerular filtration rate so that both *blood urea nitrogen* and *creatinine* levels will increase. Such elevations may also result from intrinsic renal disease. Measurement of urine concentration can help to separate these 2 entities; *urinalysis* showing a specific gravity of less than 1.020 with dehydration indicates a defect in urinary concentrating mechanisms and suggests intrinsic renal disease. With dehydration there may be mild to moderate proteinuria, and the urine may contain hyaline and granular casts, white blood cells, and, occasionally, red blood cells. Such findings do not necessarily indicate intrinsic renal disease, but urinalysis should be repeated after recovery from the dehydration. Serial measurements of urinary output and specific gravity are of value in evaluating the effectiveness of therapy and in guiding it.

Serum or *plasma electrolyte values* are especially useful. Serum sodium concentration reflects the relative losses of water to electrolytes. *Total body sodium is typically depleted in all patients with dehydration, even those with hypernatremia.* Serum potassium concentrations at the beginning of therapy are of limited value. They do not help to determine body content of this cation. Values may be elevated because of anoxia, diminished renal function, or acidosis, even when significant cellular deficits exist. Serial electrocardiograms may provide clues to disturbances of intracellular potassium as well as those of calcium. *Serum bicarbonate* concentrations help to define whether the patient has acidemia or alkalemia. Values may have to be supplemented by determination of blood pH and pCO_2. These determinations are particularly valuable as guides to the severity of metabolic disorders or in patients receiving assisted or artificial respiration. Measurement of *serum chloride* concentrations permits calculation of anion gap (Sec 5.13). Normally the difference between the sum of measured cations (sodium and potassium) and that of measured anions (chloride and bicarbonate) is 15 ± 5 mEq/l. This value is increased in renal disease, as a result of retention of phosphate and other unmeasured anions, as well as in ketosis and lactic acidosis. The difference may also be useful in indicating the possibility of laboratory error in electrolyte determinations.

5.22 PRINCIPLES OF THERAPY

In some dehydrated patients, e.g., those in shock, the administration of fluids must be treated as a medical emergency. A complete analysis of the patient can be undertaken after fluid therapy has begun and the patient's condition has been stabilized. However, most errors in fluid management occur in the initial stages of rehydration. When possible, it is preferable not to administer fluids until the patient's state of hydration has been assessed clinically and the type and amounts of fluids to be given for initial rehydration have been determined carefully. When planning this therapy for the dehydrated patient, the important considerations are the magnitude of deficits of sodium and water, the qualitative changes in body composition that have resulted from relative losses of electrolytes in relation to water (i.e., is the dehydration hypo-, iso-, or hypernatremic?), and the status of both potassium and hydrogen ion balances. *Similar basic therapeutic approaches with only minor modification may be utilized for patients with dehydration resulting from widely differing etiologies.*

Oral rehydration may be appropriate in patients with mild or moderate dehydration. It has been found that amounts of fluid and electrolytes adequate to correct the deficits often can be administered by mouth to such patients (Sec 5.24). Parenteral administration is required for patients with more severe dehydration or those who are nauseated or vomiting. As with maintenance therapy, the intravenous route is preferred for parenteral replacement of deficits although replacement fluids have been given intraperitoneally and subcutaneously.

It is convenient to consider parenteral rehydration therapy in 3 phases. The *initial phase* is designed to improve circulatory dynamics and renal function, which are of primary importance in the morbidity and mortality of dehydration. It consists of rapid re-expansion of extracellular fluid volume. *Subsequent therapy* is aimed at replacing the remaining intracellular and extracellular deficits of water and electrolytes but at a slower rate, with sodium replacement preceding potassium replacement. The *final phase* consists of the return of the patient's state of nutrition to normal and usually begins when the patient is able to return to oral feedings.

Initial Therapy. This phase is designed to treat shock or to prevent its occurrence by rapid expansion of the volume of extracellular fluid, especially the plasma. Ideally, the entire fluid used for the initial treatment of dehydration should remain in the vascular space. The administration of whole blood, however, is not the treatment of choice. Delays during the typing and cross-matching of the blood may occur and thrombosis accompanying the administration of blood in the dehydrated patient is a risk. Similarly, the risk of hepatitis makes the use of pooled plasma undesirable. Instead, an electrolyte solution with a sodium concentration similar to that of normal blood is recommended.

Glucose should be included in this fluid since the sick infant is susceptible to hypoglycemia. Suitable preparations which fulfill these criteria are commercially available (Table 29–8). Isotonic saline (0.9%; Na and Cl both 154 mEq/l) containing glucose, 5 g/dl, is one alternative especially useful in dehydrated patients with metabolic alkalosis (e.g., from pyloric stenosis). The use of this solution in a patient with acidosis is less optimal. It does not correct the acidosis unless renal perfusion is increased and permits increased excretion of hydrogen ions by the kidneys, and it might even aggravate the acidosis by further diluting the plasma bicarbonate. In an acidotic patient the use of a solution containing some bicarbonate or a bicarbonate precursor is preferred. A suitable solution containing bicarbonate is not commercially available but can easily be made by adding 28 ml of 7.5% sodium bicarbonate solution to 750 ml of 0.9% sodium chloride solution, increasing the final volume to 1 l with 5% dextrose in water. This solution contains 140 mEq of sodium, 115 mEq of chloride, and 25 mEq of bicarbonate/l. Similar commercial solutions containing lactate or acetate instead of bicarbonate are available but have the disadvantage that the bicarbonate precursor may not be readily metabolized to bicarbonate in severely dehydrated patients with impaired circulation; thus therapy with these solutions may aggravate the existing acidosis.

The solution chosen for the initial phase of therapy can be started immediately even though serum electrolyte values are not known. The volume given should equal 20–30 ml/kg of body weight and be administered as rapidly as possible if there are signs of shock, or within 1 hr in less severely ill patients. If clinical signs of shock persist, a 2nd and, rarely, a 3rd infusion of 20–30 ml/kg may be necessary to restore circulation. Ordinarily, however, normal circulation has been restored by the time 20 ml/kg has been administered, at which point the laboratory findings are available and one can proceed more slowly with logically planned subsequent therapy. If 3 infusions, each of 30 ml/kg, were to be given, the total of 90 ml/kg equals 9% of body weight and would be equivalent to the fluid deficit in moderate to severe dehydration. If such large volumes of fluid are administered, monitoring of central venous pressure is desirable to minimize the danger of volume overload.

This therapy is equally appropriate in hypo-, iso-, and hypernatremic dehydration; the administered fluid tends to return the serum sodium toward normal in most cases. In some patients with hypernatremic dehydration serum sodium may increase even further with the administration of isotonic saline solution. The mechanism for this is unclear. However, this increase in serum sodium is usually 5 mEq/l or less and does not appear to affect the clinical course adversely.

Potassium should not be administered at this stage of therapy unless the patient is known to be severely hypokalemic; it should be given only after it is established that the kidneys are functioning.

Occasionally, the therapy outlined above is inadequate to reverse shock; under such circumstances blood (10 ml/kg) or other plasma volume expander is required.

Subsequent Therapy. Once circulation has been restored, therapy during the remainder of the 1st 24 hr is aimed both at complete correction of the remaining deficits of sodium and water and at replacing ongoing abnormal and normal obligatory losses. Replacement of potassium losses may be started but is not essential. Frequently, it is not attempted until after the 1st 24 hr of treatment. The exception is the presence of proven hypokalemia or a situation known to be associated with severe losses of potassium. Examples include the hypochloremic alkalosis of pyloric stenosis, prolonged diarrhea, or diabetic acidosis, when potassium may be administered even when pretreatment serum levels are normal or only mildly reduced. Even in such patients, however, potassium should not be administered until urine flow has been established.

By the time this phase of therapy is reached, the patient's serum electrolytes should be known and therapy can be modified depending on the presenting serum sodium level.

Isonatremic Dehydration. In isonatremic dehydration there are not only external losses of sodium from the extracellular fluid but also movement of sodium from extracellular into intracellular fluid to compensate for intracellular potassium losses. Therefore, administration of sodium in an amount equal to the loss from the extracellular fluid would be excessive and would result in an increase in the patient's total body sodium; the increment of sodium in the intracellular fluid would later return to the extracellular fluid when potassium was administered, resulting in expansion of the latter compartment. To avoid this, therapy is planned so that only two thirds of the approximate losses of sodium and water from the extracellular fluid are replaced during the 1st 24 hr of treatment.

For example, in a patient with severe isonatremic dehydration and a 15% loss of body weight, the calculated fluid deficit would be 150 ml/kg (15% of body weight) and the sodium deficit 21 mEq/kg (assuming a serum sodium concentration of 140 mEq/l). In the 1st 24 hr of therapy only 100 ml/kg of water and 14 mEq/kg of sodium should be administered. Of this, 20–30 ml/kg of fluid and 3–4 mEq/kg of sodium (possibly more if the patient did not respond to this treatment) would be administered in the 1st 2–3 hr as initial therapy to expand the extracellular fluid. The remaining 70–80 ml/kg of water and 10–11 mEq/kg of sodium would then be given during the ensuing 21–22 hr. The fluid used for this phase of therapy should be similar to that used in the 1st 2–3 hr, i.e., 0.9% saline or its equivalent, and is aimed at replacing the bulk of the deficits of water and sodium.

In addition to replacing deficits, total fluid and electrolyte administration during this and subsequent phases of treatment must include replacement for both ongoing normal losses and any continuing abnormal losses such as those from diarrhea, intestinal suction, and so forth. Calculation of these additional requirements has been outlined in Sec 5.18; they are added to those needed to correct initial deficits, and thus an estimate of total requirements for the 1st 24 hr of treatment is obtained.

After the 1st 24 hr, the objective is to achieve complete replacement of sodium and water losses and to start replacing potassium losses. The sodium and water requirements at this point can be estimated by adding 25% to estimated normal maintenance requirements and by adding requirements for any ongoing abnormal losses. Potassium losses in dehydration may equal sodium losses, but potassium is lost almost exclusively from the intracellular fluid and has to be replaced by administration into the extracellular compartment. If potassium were replaced at a rate equal to that used to replace sodium, severe hyperkalemia would almost certainly result. Thus, potassium losses are usually replaced over a 3–4 day period. To minimize the risk of inducing severe hyperkalemia, potassium should not be administered if the serum potassium is elevated or until it is established that the kidneys are functioning. Moreover, it should be administered cautiously in the presence of severe acidosis. Except under unusual circumstances, the concentration of potassium in the administered fluid should not exceed 40 mEq/l, and the rate of potassium administration should not exceed 3 mEq/kg/24 hr.

Hyponatremic Dehydration. This condition results from relatively greater losses of sodium than of water. The extra sodium loss can be calculated from the formula:

$$\text{Extra sodium loss [mEq]} = (135 - S_{Na}) \times \text{total body water [in liters]}$$

where S_{Na} represents the serum sodium observed on admission (135 is a low normal value for serum sodium). Because the patient is dehydrated, total body water should be estimated as 50–55% of admission body weight rather than the usual value of 60%. Even though sodium is principally an extracellular cation, total body water is used for the calculation of sodium deficit. This allows for repletion of sodium lost from the extracellular fluid, for any expansion of the extracellular fluid that occurs with repletion, and for repletion of sodium lost from other pools of exchangeable sodium, such as that in bone.

Treatment of hyponatremic dehydration is similar to that of isonatremic dehydration, except that when calculating sodium administration, the extra losses of that ion should be taken into account. Administration of the extra amounts of sodium needed to replace the additional losses can be spread over several days so that gradual correction of the hyponatremia is accomplished as volume is expanded. No attempt is made to elevate sodium concentrations abruptly by the administration of hypertonic saline solutions unless symptoms of water intoxication, such as convulsions, are present. Such symptoms rarely occur unless serum sodium levels fall below 120 mEq/l. In such circumstances, symptoms are usually rapidly controlled by the administration of a 3% solution of sodium chloride given intravenously at a rate of 1 ml/min to a maximum of 12 ml/kg of body weight. *Hypotonic solutions should be avoided, especially in the initial phase of treatment, because of the risk of inducing symptomatic hyponatremia.*

Hypernatremic Dehydration. Severe hypernatremic

dehydration presents one of the more difficult problems in fluid therapy. Severe hyperosmolality may result in cerebral damage, with widespread cerebral hemorrhages and cerebral thromboses or subdural effusions. This cerebral injury may result in permanent neurologic deficit such as cerebral palsy. Even in the absence of such obvious pathologic lesions, seizures are common in patients with severe hypernatremia. The diagnosis of cerebral injury secondary to hypernatremia can be assisted by the finding of an elevated protein level in the cerebrospinal fluid.

Frequently, seizures occur when the serum sodium is returning to normal with treatment. They may result from an increase in the sodium content of cerebral cells during the period of dehydration. This results in an excessive movement of water into these cells during rehydration before excess sodium is eventually extruded. Although the mechanism by which this water movement may result in seizures is uncertain, the incidence of seizures may be reduced by correcting hypernatremia slowly over a period of days. Therefore, therapy is adjusted to return serum sodium levels toward normal by not more than 10 mEq/l/24 hr.

The sodium deficit in hypernatremic dehydration is relatively small and the extracellular fluid volume relatively well maintained so that the amounts of both sodium and water to be administered in this phase of therapy are reduced compared to those in hypo- or isonatremic dehydration. A suitable regimen is to administer 60–75 ml/kg/24 hr of a 5% dextrose solution containing 25 mEq/l of sodium as a combination of the bicarbonate and chloride.

Amounts of maintenance fluid and sodium should be reduced by about 25% during this phase of therapy because the hypernatremic patient has high levels of antidiuretic hormone (ADH), resulting in a low volume of urine. Replacement of ongoing abnormal losses does not require modification.

If seizures do occur, they may often be controlled by the intravenous administration of 3–5 ml/kg of a 3% sodium chloride solution or the administration of hypertonic mannitol.

Treatment of hypernatremic dehydration with large amounts of water, with or without salt, frequently results in expansion of the extracellular fluid volume before there is any notable excretion of chloride or correction of the acidosis. As a consequence, edema and cardiac failure may develop, necessitating digitalization. Hypocalcemia is also seen occasionally during treatment of hypernatremic dehydration; it may be prevented by administration of appropriate amounts of potassium during therapy. Once developed, it may require intravenous administration of calcium. Another complication is renal tubular injury with azotemia and loss of concentrating ability; this may necessitate modification of the therapeutic regimen.

Although hypernatremic dehydration can be successfully treated, management is difficult and seizures frequently occur even with the best-designed regimens. It is better to emphasize prevention since this particularly dangerous form of dehydration is frequently iatrogenic in etiology (Sec 5.24).

Correction of Nutritional Deficiencies. Although parenteral fluid therapy results in a caloric intake inadequate to meet the patient's needs, this is rarely a cause for concern because of the short periods of time usually involved. When the patient is able to return to a normal diet, any deficits in body fat and protein may soon be corrected.

Should parenteral fluid therapy be required for prolonged periods (e.g., when the patient is unable to eat or develops severe diarrhea whenever oral feeding is restarted), increased caloric and nutritional intake may be required to prevent the development of serious malnourishment. This is best accomplished by the technique of intravenous alimentation (Sec 5.18).

Assessment of Response. Many factors modify the amounts and types of fluids to be administered. Thus, it is of vital importance that the clinician monitor the response to therapy. This should include frequent clinical observation with special emphasis on the child's cry, degree of activity, skin turgor, and blood pressure. In addition, the careful charting of intake and output, with stool and urine volumes recorded separately, is of value in assessing response to therapy, as is frequent measurement of the body weight. Under certain circumstances, serial measurements of serum and urine electrolytes and osmolality and central venous pressure, as well as electrocardiographic monitoring, may be appropriate. In the severely ill child, the use of a carefully maintained flow sheet, on which these serial determinations are recorded as a guide to adjustment of therapy, may be lifesaving. Unpredicted responses to therapy are not uncommon; hence monitoring should be meticulous and, when indicated, appropriate modifications of the regimen should be instituted promptly.

SIMPLIFIED METHODS TO CALCULATE REQUIREMENTS

Alternative systems to estimate fluid and electrolyte requirements have been developed from the principles outlined. These newer methods usually estimate deficit and maintenance needs together. One method (Table 5–13) outlines suggested management of specific disease entities.

Another method in widespread use expresses fluid and electrolyte requirements per unit of body surface—the *meter-squared system*. Its basic principles are shown in Table 5–14. The ability of the kidneys to regulate and to alter markedly the excretion of water and electrolytes ensures that in health the administration of fluid and electrolytes can be tolerated over wide ranges. As shown in the table, various disease states may reduce the maximum (ceiling) or increase the minimum (floor) amounts of water or electrolytes that can be tolerated. However, the average dehydrated child with functioning kidneys still has relatively large ranges of tolerance. If water and electrolytes are provided in adequate quantities within the limits of tolerance, the patient will cure himself or herself, with renal function providing final regulation.

According to the meter-squared system, normal maintenance of water and electrolytes in older infants and children is provided by 1500 ml/M²/24 hr of a

Table 5–13 DEFICIT THERAPY OF INFANTS WITH MODERATELY SEVERE DEHYDRATION AND ELECTROLYTE DISTURBANCES

CLINICAL CONDITION	SOLUTION	ML/KG	TIME SCHEDULE IN HOURS FROM ONSET OF THERAPY	ROUTE
Fasting and thirsting	Ringer lactate	20	0–1	IV
	5% or 10% invert sugar or glucose in H_2O	60	1–8	IV
	Darrow K lactate*	20		
Diarrhea				
Isotonic dehydration	Ringer lactate	20	0–1	IV
	Blood or Plasmanate†	10	1–2	IV
	5% or 10% invert sugar or glucose in H_2O	40	2–8	IV
	Darrow K lactate*	60		
Hypotonic dehydration	Ringer lactate	20	0–1	IV
	Blood or Plasmanate†	10	1–2	
	5% invert sugar or glucose in Ringer lactate	40	2–8	IV
	Darrow K lactate*	60		
Dehydration in malnourished infants	5% invert sugar or glucose in Ringer lactate	40	0–1	IV
	Blood or Plasmanate†	10	1–2	IV
	5% invert sugar or glucose in Ringer lactate	40	2–8	IM
	Darrow K lactate*	60		
	$MgSO_4 \cdot 7H_2O \cdot 50\%$	0.1		
Hypertonic dehydration	Ringer lactate	20	0–1	IV
	Blood or Plasmanate†	10	1–2	IV
	5% or 10% invert sugar or glucose in H_2O	60	2–10	IV
	M/6 Na lactate	20		
	K acetate concentrate‡	0.5		
	Calcium gluconate§			
Pyloric stenosis	Isotonic NaCl	20	0–1	IV
	Blood or Plasmanate†	10	1–2	IV
	5% or 10% invert sugar or glucose in H_2O	40	2–8	IV
	Isotonic NaCl*	40		
	Isotonic KCl*	20		
Diabetic acidosis	Ringer lactate	20	0–1	IV
	Blood or Plasmanate†	10	1–2	IV
	5% or 10% invert sugar or glucose in H_2O	50	2–8	IV
	KPO_4 concentrate¶	0.5		IV
	Darrow K lactate*	50		

All of above to be followed by maintenance therapy.
*May be given separately subcutaneously.
†For shock not responding to Ringer lactate.
‡K acetate concentrate (Cutter) contains 4 mEq of K/ml.
§Total dose, 10 ml of 10% solution slowly IV.
¶Phosphate concentrate contains 2 mEq of K/ml.

solution containing 5% dextrose, 25 mEq/l of sodium, and 20 mEq/l of potassium. This basic rate of administration may be increased 2- or 3-fold in dehydration or reduced in overhydration. With experience the clinician can determine fluid and electrolyte requirements using these guidelines and does not necessarily go through the several stages of calculations presented earlier. The important exceptions to this generalization are patients with marked renal insufficiency, craniopharyngioma, adrenal insufficiency, or other defects in the homeostatic mechanisms responsible for regulation of water and sodium metabolism. In such patients severe impairment of renal or other regulatory mechanisms severely limits the ranges of tolerance and requires that each component of fluid and electrolyte therapy be carefully calculated for the individual on a daily or even more frequent basis.

5.23 THERAPY IN SPECIFIC DISEASE STATES

5.24 DIARRHEA

Acute. Despite improved infant care, diarrhea continues to be a serious problem in many areas of the world. As indicated in Table 5–8, it results in large losses of both water and electrolytes, especially sodium and potassium, and frequently is complicated by severe systemic acidosis.

In approximately 70% of patients, the losses of water and sodium are proportionate, with *isonatremic dehydration* developing. *Hyponatremic dehydration* is seen in approximately 10% of all patients with diarrhea; sodium losses are increased out of proportion to fluid losses. It

Table 5–14 PRINCIPLES OF METER-SQUARED SYSTEM FOR DETERMINING FLUID AND ELECTROLYTE THERAPY

SUBSTANCE	RANGE OF TOLERANCE (IN HEALTH)	CEILING LOWERED	FLOOR RAISED
Water	1–13 l/M²/24 hr (1–5 in first week of life)	General anesthesia Morphine and related drugs "Nephritis" Hypothalamic lesions Circulatory failure Neonatal period	Diabetes insipidus Nephrogenic diabetes insipidus Cellular K deficiency Na intoxication
Sodium	5–250 mEq/M²/24 hr	Zero potassium intake Hypoalbuminemia Cardiac failure Severe stress Corticosteroid therapy Cushing syndrome Renal disease	Hypoadrenocorticism Abnormal loss of GI fluids Extensive burns Renal tubular disease (diuretic therapy)
Potassium	10–250 mEq/M²/24 hr	Marked dehydration Circulatory failure Low Na intake Reduced GFR Hypoadrenocorticism Congenital adrenal hyperplasia	Diarrhea GI drainage High Na intake Corticosteroid therapy
Phosphorus	0–4000 mg/M²/24 hr (expressed as phosphorus)	Normal newborn Reduced GFR Hypoparathyroidism Pseudohypoparathyroidism Circulatory failure	Vitamin D intoxication Hyperparathyroidism
Chloride	0–250 mEq/M²/24 hr		
Bicarbonate	5–250 mEq/M²/24 hr		
Glucose	50–300 gm/M²/24 hr		

occurs when large amounts of electrolytes are lost in the stool. Thus, it is seen more frequently with bacillary dysentery or cholera. In these diseases, as opposed to diarrhea due to rotavirus, to other nonspecific (presumably virus) infections, and to many noninfectious causes, the concentration of sodium in the stool rises with increasing volume of stool. Hyponatremia may be accentuated or produced if, during the period of diarrhea, a considerable oral intake consisting of low electrolyte or electrolyte-free fluids is continued.

Disproportionately large net losses of water compared to electrolytes result in *hypernatremic dehydration*. It is seen in approximately 20% of patients with diarrhea and often is the result of the oral administration of homemade electrolyte solutions with too high concentrations of salt during the course of diarrhea. It may also occur in young infants with diarrhea if their renal ability to conserve water is limited, especially if the renal solute load is increased by feeding boiled skim milk. Such factors may be potentiated by fever, high environmental temperatures, or hyperventilation, each of which increases evaporative water loss significantly.

A significant development in recent years has been the demonstration that dehydration from diarrhea of any etiology can be treated effectively, in a wide range of age groups, using a simple glucose-electrolyte solution given by mouth. Such oral rehydration has been utilized in numerous countries around the world and has been found to reduce significantly the mortality rate from acute diarrhea and to lessen diarrhea-associated malnutrition. Patients in shock; those with severe dehydration or with uncontrollable vomiting; those unable to drink because of extreme fatigue, stupor, or coma; or those with other serious complications such as severe gastric distention require intravenous therapy. However, oral rehydration can be attempted in the remainder provided adequate supervision is available.

The composition of the oral rehydration solution (ORS) recommended by the Diarrhea Disease Control Program of the World Health Organization is shown in Table 5–15. It is made from sodium chloride, sodium bicarbonate, potassium chloride, and glucose. These chemicals are typically made available in powder form in preweighed packages using the formula shown in Table 5–15. The use of teaspoon or other household measures to "weigh" the amount of these solutes is

Table 5–15 COMPARISON OF COMPOSITION OF ORAL SOLUTIONS

	RECOMMENDED* BY WORLD HEALTH ORGANIZATION (mM/L)	TRADITIONAL SOLUTION
Sodium	90	30
Potassium	20	25
Chloride	80	25
Bicarbonate	30	30
Glucose	111	28

*Ingredients (gm/l water): NaCl, 3.5; NaHCO₃, 2.5; KCl, 1.5; Glucose, 20.0.

inaccurate and is not recommended. In the United States, a suitable preparation is available commercially (*Hydra-lyte*). Alternatively, an ORS with similar composition can be prepared from readily available solutions as follows: NaCl (0.95% saline solution) 450 ml; glucose (5% in water) 500 ml; KCl (2 mEq/ml) 10 ml; NaHCO$_3$ (1 mEq/ml) 30 ml. Glucose is the preferred sugar for use in ORS. Its high concentration facilitates the transport of sodium across the bowel wall. Sucrose can be substituted. It has a slightly lower success rate than glucose, possibly because it has to be hydrolyzed before being absorbed as glucose. When used, the concentration of sucrose in gm/l has been twice that of glucose in order to obtain the same osmolarity.

As a guideline for oral rehydration, 50 ml/kg body weight of the ORS should be given within 4 hr for patients with mild dehydration and 100 ml/kg over 6 hr for moderate dehydration. The amounts and rates should be increased if the patient continues to have diarrhea or if rehydration does not appear complete; they should be decreased if the patient appears fully hydrated earlier than expected or develops periorbital edema. Breast feeding should be allowed *ad libitum* after treatment has been started in infants who are breast fed; in other patients, plain water should be offered. Vomiting may occur during the 1st 2 hr of administration of ORS but does not prevent successful oral rehydration. To reduce vomiting, the ORS should be given slowly, in small amounts at short intervals. If sustained severe vomiting occurs, intravenous therapy should be used. Progress of the patient should be assessed frequently, with changes in body weight being monitored, if possible, to determine the degree of rehydration.

When rehydration is complete, maintenance therapy can be started. Patients with mild diarrhea can be treated at home. The use of 100 ml ORS/kg/24 hr until diarrhea stops is recommended. Breast feeds or supplemental water intake must be maintained. Those patients with more severe diarrhea require continued supervision. The volume of ORS ingested should equal the volume of stool losses. If stool volume cannot be measured, an intake of 10–15 ml ORS/kg/hr is appropriate.

This regimen has not been universally accepted. The sodium concentration of ORS (90 mM/l) is 3 times that of fluids (such as *Pedialyte* or *Lytren*; see Tables 5–15 and 29–8) which have traditionally been recommended for oral therapy in patients with diarrhea. These low-sodium solutions were advocated because ..., pernatremia was seen frequently when oral electrolyte solutions with sodium concentrations of 50 mEq/l or more were used to treat infantile diarrhea. The importance of low sodium concentrations in ingested fluids has also been recently redemonstrated—in the United Kingdom the use of low solute milk with a sodium concentration of less than 20 mEq/l has reduced the incidence of hypernatremia. Despite such concerns, extensive use of ORS in many developing countries has documented hypernatremia to be a rare complication, probably because ORS has been used primarily for rehydration (the major previous role for oral therapy was to prevent dehydration or for maintenance), because large amounts of water are ingested in addition to ORS, and because ORS has been administered under close supervision by trained personnel.

Occasionally, an infant receiving 2–3 liters of carbohydrate and electrolyte mixtures per day orally may have an apparently related increase in the volume of stools, but such instances are sufficiently rare that they do not contraindicate an initial trial. The use of intravenous fluids to treat dehydration from severe diarrhea is discussed in Sec 5.22. Persisting diarrhea may cause continuing large losses of fluid. These and the concomitant losses of electrolytes (Table 5–6) must be replaced.

It has been traditional to omit oral feedings initially when treating infants with more severe diarrhea. Recently, it has been reconfirmed that, even during acute diarrhea, the small intestine is able to absorb a variety of nutrients and may absorb up to 60% of the food eaten. Since better weight gain has been documented in infants given a liberal dietary intake during diarrhea when compared to others on a more restricted intake, since fasting has been shown to reduce further the ability of the small intestine to absorb nutrients, and since there is no physiologic basis for giving the bowel a "rest" during acute diarrhea, regimens for the treatment of acute diarrhea in developing countries have encouraged the continuing oral intake of nutrients. This approach may cause an increase in the volume of stool which can complicate the replacement of water and electrolytes and may extend the need for parenteral fluids for several days. However, several studies have shown that rehydration occurs as rapidly with oral as with parenteral therapy.

Typically, frequency and volume of stools will subside within 48 hr in fasted patients treated with intravenous therapy. When this occurs, provided gastric distention and vomiting are absent, oral feeding of one of the carbohydrate and electrolyte mixtures may be initiated. As soon as this is tolerated without exacerbation of the diarrhea, the caloric intake may be increased gradually by the substitution of mixtures that also contain fat and protein until the usual dietary intake is achieved. Usually this is accomplished within 7–8 days. Premature administration of large numbers of calories in the form of milk may exacerbate the diarrhea. In the young infant with a family history of allergy, the use of a hypoallergenic feeding mixture is recommended for the recovery phase since permeability of the gastrointestinal tract to whole protein may be increased during this time.

In addition to replacement of the deficits of water and electrolytes, efforts must be made to obtain an etiologic diagnosis so that specific antimicrobial therapy may be given if indicated. Antibiotics are required in cases in which the diarrhea is due to cholera, shigella, amebic dysentery, or acute giardiasis. Such treatment does not modify fluid therapy. Drugs such as opiates which inhibit peristaltic activity of the bowel or absorbents such as kaolin or pectin have relatively little or no effect on the course of infantile diarrhea and are not recommended.

Diarrhea in Chronically Malnourished Chil-

dren. Severe malnutrition complicated by diarrheal dehydration is a common problem in tropical and subtropical countries and an occasional one in the temperate zones. Therapy must be adapted to meet the specific disturbances in body composition characteristic of the dehydrated *and* malnourished infant, in whom there appears to be an overexpansion of the intracellular space, with extracellular and presumably intracellular hypo-osmolality. Serum sodium, potassium, and magnesium levels tend to be low, and tetany may occasionally result from magnesium deficiency. Serum proteins are frequently below 3.6 gm/dl. The sodium content of muscle is high; potassium and magnesium contents are low. The electrocardiogram frequently shows tachycardia, low amplitude, and flat or inverted T waves. Cardiac reserve seems lowered, and heart failure is a common complication.

Despite clinical signs of dehydration and reduced body water, urinary osmolality may be low in the chronically malnourished child. This defect in renal concentration may result from the relative absence of urea to contribute to a hypertonic fluid in the renal papillae, a defect associated with a low dietary protein intake and resulting in a failure of tubular conservation of water. However, the glomerular filtration rate is low, resulting in a smaller loss of water than would otherwise be expected, and renal concentrating ability returns after several days of high-protein feedings.

Survival of the malnourished infant with diarrhea is limited by caloric deficit to a greater extent than by water and electrolyte deficit. Reparative calories can be given by slow drip through an indwelling nasogastric tube while electrolytes and water are given parenterally. If appetite is poor and vomiting and gastric distention are absent, feeding is begun early at the level of 30–40 Cal/kg/24 hr, given by slow intragastric drip. Increases to 50–100 Cal/kg/24 hr and 1–2 gm of protein/kg/24 hr are made in a few days. Ad lib intake should be permitted in the succeeding weeks, up to 250–300 Cal/kg/24 hr and should include an adequate supply of iron and copper.

Initial parenteral therapy is designed to improve the circulation and to expand extracellular volume. The repair solutions recommended resemble those of hyponatremic dehydration. If edema is present, the quantity of fluid and rate of administration should be reduced from recommended levels to avoid pulmonary edema. Blood should be given if the patient is in shock, severely ill, or anemic. Potassium salts can be given early if urine output is good. Controlled trials suggest that survival can be improved by the intramuscular injection of 1.0–1.5 ml of a 50% solution of magnesium sulfate (4.0 mEq/ml) every 12 hr for 1–3 days. Clinical and electrocardiographic improvement may be more rapid with magnesium therapy, and seizures occurring during recovery from diarrhea complicating severe malnutrition may respond to magnesium.

Chronic Diarrhea. When diarrhea is severe and prolonged, intravenous administration of amino acids, divalent cations, vitamins, and additional calories is required in addition to the usual carbohydrate and electrolytes. Parenteral alimentation is effective in these patients.

Occasionally, parenteral fluid therapy must be supplemented by full oral feedings during chronic diarrhea, especially in severe malnutrition. Allergy to cow's milk protein or specific disaccharidase deficiencies should be suspected in infants with persistent diarrhea. Acquired disaccharidase deficiency (especially for lactose) may develop as a complication of many chronic disorders of the gastrointestinal or other systems. Hypoallergenic feeding mixtures containing monosaccharides as the sole carbohydrate should be administered until cessation of the diarrhea and improvement in nutrition have occurred. Specific tests of carbohydrate (disaccharide) splitting and absorption and of milk protein sensitivity can then be carried out but can be potentially dangerous, sometimes resulting in severe diarrhea with marked fluid and electrolyte losses.

Congenital Alkalosis of Gastrointestinal Origin. Rarely, chronic diarrhea may be the result of a congenital defect in the transport of chloride in both the small and large bowel. The watery stools of such patients have a high content of chloride, and alkalosis results from the ensuing volume depletion. Potassium is lost in the stools and in the urine, the latter losses being a consequence of the alkalosis. Treatment of fluid and electrolyte deficits is similar to that used in pyloric stenosis. Long term therapy must provide an adequate dietary intake of potassium and chloride. A rare acute chloride-losing diarrhea may also occur.

5.25 PYLORIC STENOSIS

This condition exemplifies the correction of deficits associated with alkalosis. The therapy differs little from that for diarrhea, except that potassium replacement should begin early, as soon as the child has urinated, and relatively more sodium and potassium should be given as the chloride salt than is usual in treating dehydration, partly because of the larger deficit of chloride seen in pyloric stenosis, and partly because this results in some correction of the alkalosis as volume is expanded. Correction of the hypochloremia by administration of ammonium chloride without correction of the deficit of potassium results in continued dysfunction of renal tubular cells and other cells and is not recommended.

Severe depletion of intracellular potassium will result in increased exchange of hydrogen ion for sodium in the distal tubules of the kidney. Thus, the paradoxic presence of an acid urine with systemic alkalosis should be interpreted as signifying a marked potassium deficit and a need to increase the amount of potassium used for repletion.

It is not uncommon for deficits to be replaced and serum levels of electrolytes returned to normal within 12 hr. However, except in the mildly ill infant without signs of dehydration, it is preferable to delay operation for at least 36–48 hr. This permits optimal readjustment of body functions. During this period of preparation, adequate fluid therapy prevents dehydration and the stomach may be decompressed by gentle suction (Sec 5.31 and 11.23).

5.26 FASTING AND THIRSTING

Parenteral fluid therapy is usually required in the initial treatment of the infant or child who has taken little or no water and food for 1–5 days. Such infants are deficient not only in water, which has evaporated from the lungs and skin, but also in electrolytes, particularly sodium and chloride, which have been excreted in the urine (Table 5–8). The administration of electrolyte-free solutions under such circumstances leads only to an increase in urine volume, with possible increased losses of electrolytes, and may actually increase the dehydration. If fasting and thirsting continue beyond 4–5 days, urinary output will fall to such a low level that there will be no significant continued loss of electrolytes. Further severe deficiency of water alone will occur because of evaporative losses and will result in hypernatremia.

Therapy is begun with an isonatremic solution to produce rapid and safe expansion of extracellular volume and improvement in renal function. A large part of the remaining deficiency of water and electrolytes may be made up by a solution containing carbohydrate, sodium chloride, some potassium and bicarbonate, and a bicarbonate precursor such as lactate or acetate. Because of relatively smaller extracellular reservoirs with increasing age, children and adults should be given approximately one fourth to one third less water and sodium/kg than infants for a given degree of clinical dehydration. Potassium deficits are relatively the same in infants, children, and adults since they have approximately the same quantity of potassium/kg. Water, carbohydrate, and electrolytes may be administered to the mildly ill patient by mouth. Infants, however, often vomit when they are dehydrated, and for this reason initial therapy is usually given parenterally.

5.27 DIABETIC ACIDOSIS

See also Sec 17.1.

The deficit therapy of diabetic acidosis approximates that of diarrheal dehydration. Initially, extracellular volume is expanded rapidly with Ringer lactate or an equivalent solution. The balance of the replacement therapy is carried out slowly over the remainder of the 1st 24 hr. The early administration of carbohydrate permits glycogenation of the liver after response to insulin and reduces the danger of hypoglycemia.

In the appraisal of deficits in patients with diabetic ketosis, laboratory studies may be misinterpreted. Hypo-osmolality may be assumed erroneously on the basis of measurement of the serum sodium concentration alone; if there is a high concentration of blood glucose, extracellular osmolality may be normal or high even with a low serum sodium concentration. Blood sugar levels of 1800 mg/dl increase plasma osmolality by 100 mOsm/l—equivalent to an additional 50 mEq/l of sodium with an attendant anion. Elevations of serum lipid and protein concentrations in diabetic acidosis may also reduce the water content of the serum so that sodium concentrations expressed per liter of serum are low, even though the sodium concentration of extracellular water is normal or high.

Early administration of potassium to these patients is essential. A rapid fall in extracellular potassium concentration occurs shortly after administration of insulin. Untreated, such changes may produce alterations in the function of the heart, liver, brain, and kidneys; contribute to gastric distention; and even lead to respiratory paralysis. A fall in concentration of serum inorganic phosphate during therapy parallels that of potassium. This fall is primarily due to cellular uptake of phosphorus as glycogen is formed. Though the clinical significance of such changes has not been established, it is probable that serum inorganic phosphorus should be sustained at low normal levels. For this reason some potassium should be administered as the phosphate salt.

Magnesium levels, like potassium levels, may be elevated at the beginning of therapy and fall rapidly to below normal; no clinical significance has been attributed to these changes.

No specific attempts are made initially to elevate the low carbon dioxide content and pH; rapid correction of the systemic acidosis with bicarbonate may paradoxically increase the degree of acidosis in cerebrospinal fluid. Rather, therapy is directed to expansion of the extracellular volume, using a fluid that resembles an ultrafiltrate of normal plasma, such as Ringer lactate; this frequently results in a significant reduction in acidosis with symptomatic improvement.

If extreme respiratory distress persists, the administration of sodium bicarbonate may be indicated. The dose required may be calculated from the formula given in Sec 5.32. There is, however, a large reservoir of potential bicarbonate in the form of ketone acids which are metabolized with improvement in carbohydrate utilization after administration of insulin. Therefore, bicarbonate concentration of the serum should not be elevated abruptly to more than 12–15 mEq/l.

The amount of insulin and glucose that can be safely administered is discussed in Sec 17.1.

Response to therapy should be closely monitored. Collection of urine at hourly intervals, preferably without resort to catheterization, is essential for modifying the dosage of insulin and carbohydrate as therapy progresses; only rarely in children will ketones be absent from the urine when the serum level is significantly elevated. Reduction of the blood sugar to a level that avoids excessive glycosuria prevents unusual loss of water in the urine, but reduction of the blood sugar to excessively low levels by administration of insulin without adequate carbohydrate leads rapidly not only to hypoglycemia but to a return or exacerbation of ketosis.

During the early stages of treatment of children with severe ketoacidosis, serum electrolytes, pH, and blood sugar may have to be monitored at regular 4 hr intervals. Blood gas determinations may also be of assistance in monitoring response. Dextrostix give a rapid estimate of blood sugar but are of more benefit in detecting hypoglycemia than in determining the precise value of an elevated blood sugar level.

5.28 BURNS

See also Sec 5.45.

Maintenance requirements for water are diminished when a large area of burned skin is covered by wet dressings which limit evaporative losses from this site; evaporation from the lungs is normal or increased. Urinary output of water is probably limited by some antidiuresis resulting from massive stimulation of nerve receptors. Thus, the fluid therapy of burns is concerned principally with the replacement of abnormal losses. Some of these losses are external, such as oozing of plasma from the burned surface, but the largest part of the abnormal loss is *internal* in the form of plasma and plasma ultrafiltrate sequestered around the burn site.

After 48 hr, fluid therapy should be sharply limited; the sequestered fluid may return at this time to the vascular compartment and produce acute pulmonary edema, particularly if there has been thermal injury to the lungs. Digitalis, diuretics (if there has been no renal injury), or even phlebotomy with removal of plasma and replacement of red blood cells may be helpful at this stage.

5.29 SALICYLATE POISONING

The treatment of salicylate intoxication provides a good example of the importance of supplemental therapy in some clinical circumstances; water and electrolytes are given above the usual needs even in the absence of specific deficits—the aim is to facilitate excretion of the drug.

The initial effect of a high concentration of salicylate is to sensitize the respiratory center to carbon dioxide. The resultant hyperventilation, with its characteristic marked prolongation of the expiratory phase of respiration, leads to increased evaporative losses of water and to respiratory alkalosis, for which the kidneys compensate by excreting large amounts of sodium and potassium bicarbonate. In addition, toxic levels of salicylate uncouple oxidative phosphorylation and may reduce hepatic glycogen, with ketonemia and ketonuria usually resulting. Hyperglycemia and glycosuria are common; hypoglycemia may be seen occasionally.

The loss of sodium and potassium in excess of chloride and the accumulation of acetoacetic and beta-hydroxybutyric acids eventually produce severe metabolic acidosis, which is aggravated by the release of 2 moles of free hydrogen ion from each mole of aspirin absorbed and hydrolyzed. Thus, a dose of salicylate of 200 mg/kg adds an acute hydrogen ion load of 2 mEq/kg. Transition from respiratory alkalosis to a mixed disturbance of acid-base balance with severe metabolic acidosis complicated by respiratory alkalosis may be relatively rapid; therefore therapy must be followed by periodic monitoring of the serum carbon dioxide content and the pH of the blood and urine.

Except in poisoning due to repeated therapeutic administration of salicylates, the significance of an isolated blood salicylate level depends in part on the interval between the time the drug was ingested and the time the blood sample was obtained; a level of 35

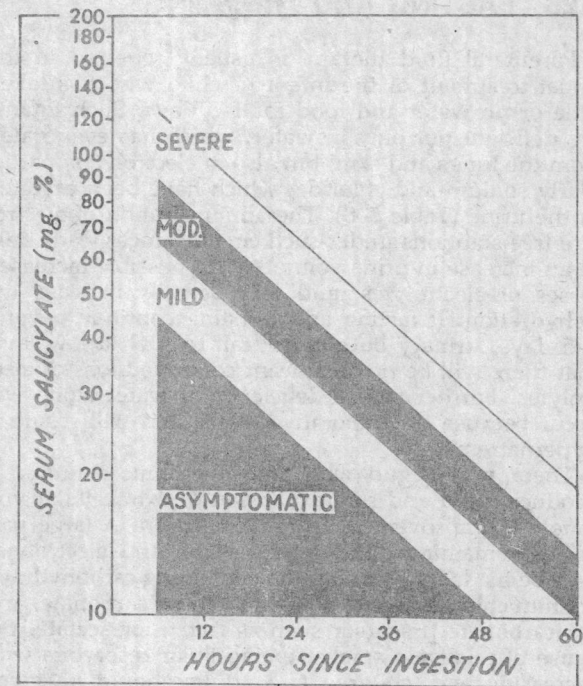

Figure 5–15 Nomogram relating serum salicylate concentration and expected severity of intoxication at varying intervals following the ingestion of a single dose of salicylate. (From Done AK: Pediatrics 26:800, 1960.)

mg/dl 36 hr after an acute ingestion or after the start of aspirin therapy may be more significant than a level of 60 mg/dl 2 hr after acute ingestion when peak levels may be expected. A nomogram (Fig 5–15) is available to help determine the severity of an overdose, given the serum salicylate level and the time since ingestion.

In chronic ingestion it should be remembered that even though a salicylate level of 35 mg/dl may be required to obtain therapeutic benefits in older children, fatal cases of salicylism have occurred in infants with lower blood levels; the need for active treatment depends only in part on blood levels of salicylate and on whether the overdose is acute or chronic. Coma, convulsions, marked hyperventilation, oliguria, respiratory depression, severe azotemia, or marked reduction in the plasma level of bicarbonate or pCO_2 are all indications for active therapeutic intervention.

Treatment is designed to prevent further absorption of salicylate, to correct deficits and replace ongoing losses of fluids and electrolytes (which are increased above normal), and to reduce tissue levels of salicylate by facilitating excretion of the drug.

The efficacy of attempting to empty the gastrointestinal tract of salicylate is in debate. However, in the absence of central nervous system depression, gastric emptying can be attempted for up to 10 hr following ingestion of the salicylate. Syrup of ipecac (dose in children over 1 yr of age: 1 tablespoon [15 ml] repeated after 20 min if vomiting does not occur) is probably still the most effective emetic, and a slurry of activated charcoal can be given later in an attempt to prevent further absorption of any remaining salicylate from the bowel. If the patient is in shock, an isonatremic solution will be required to expand plasma volume; otherwise a hyponatremic solution can be used to replace fluid and electrolyte deficits.

The amount of fluid required varies in individual patients from 2000–5500 ml/M²/24 hr. This fluid should contain sodium in a concentration of 40–50 mEq/l and, if there is adequate renal function, potassium in a concentration of up to 40 mEq/l. Oral potassium salts may be used to supplement the intravenous therapy. The administration of carbohydrate also appears to improve prognosis; intravenous fluids should contain at least 5% glucose.

Treatment is designed to replace maintenance losses of fluids and electrolytes, which may be twice normal due to increased evaporative losses, to replace deficits, and to maintain a diuresis to facilitate excretion of salicylate. A urine volume of at least 2000 ml/M²/24 hr with a specific gravity of less than 1.010 is a reasonable goal. The early administration of sodium bicarbonate to maintain an alkaline urine (pH higher than 7.5) facilitates excretion of salicylate by reducing its back-diffusion in ionized form from tubular urine through the lipid membranes of the renal tubular cells; the clearance of salicylate with a urine pH greater than 8.0 is 20 times that at a urine pH of 6.0. The dose of bicarbonate necessary to alkalinize the urine is approximately 2 mEq/kg, given over 1 hr. An additional 2 mEq/kg of sodium bicarbonate should be given if urine pH does not reach 7.0. The urinary pH should then be checked every 30 min. If the pH falls below 7.0, additional sodium bicarbonate should be given with appropriate amounts of potassium to avoid renal tubular potassium depletion and paradoxic aciduria.

Acetazolamide (5 mg/kg repeated 2–3 times in 24 hr) will also increase salicylate excretion; this therapy has not received general acceptance because of some reported complications, including seizures, and an increased mortality in experimental animals. Peritoneal dialysis or hemodialysis should be considered as a means to remove additional amounts of salicylate loosely bound to plasma proteins of severely ill patients, especially those with blood levels of salicylate above 100 mg/dl, those with an elevated pCO₂, those with severe acidosis, or those who have failed to respond adequately to alkalinization. The efficiency of dialysis in such patients is increased by the addition of albumin to the dialysis fluid. Exchange transfusion is a relatively inefficient means of removing salicylate in the critically ill patient. If done, heparinized blood should be used because of the often lethal exacerbation of acidosis if citrated blood is used.

Vitamin K₁ oxide (Konakion) should be given intramuscularly to offset possible prothrombin deficiency.

5.30 ELECTROLYTE DISTURBANCES ASSOCIATED WITH CENTRAL NERVOUS SYSTEM DISORDERS

Diseases of the central nervous system are not infrequently associated with disturbances in sodium concentration. Three types of changes have been described.

(1) Patients with diverse lesions, such as surgical or traumatic damage to the brain, encephalitis, bulbar poliomyelitis, cerebrovascular accidents, tumors of the 4th ventricle, and subdural hematomas, may lose large amounts of sodium in the urine. Dehydration, hypotension, and azotemia result unless large amounts of salt are administered and the intake of water is limited.

(2) Patients with tuberculous meningitis who are severely ill and comatose are frequently hyponatremic but exhibit no symptoms that can be attributed to hyponatremia. This situation may be analogous to the asymptomatic hyponatremia of severe malnutrition or pulmonary disease. Relatively large amounts of salt may be lost in the urine when attempts are made to correct the hyponatremia by salt loading. Careful clinical and laboratory observations are essential to ensure that salt depletion and water intoxication do not occur. Potassium should be administered in amounts at least 50% greater than with usual maintenance therapy.

(3) Patients with acute infections of the central nervous system occasionally have symptoms of acute water intoxication, with a rapid fall in serum sodium. These patients retain an excessive amount of water and have excessive thirst. Convulsions are severe and resistant to drug therapy but respond to the intravenous administration of hypertonic saline solution and subsequent restriction of fluid.

It is now being recognized that such changes may result from lesions involving the thirst center, osmoreceptors, or supraopticohypophyseal tract or from inappropriate secretion of antidiuretic hormone (ADH) or other lesions.

Convulsions or other symptoms from cerebral edema may respond to hypertonic mannitol solution, although care in its administration should be taken in patients with impaired renal function.

5.31 PREOPERATIVE, INTRAOPERATIVE, AND POSTOPERATIVE FLUIDS

Preoperative preparation of a patient who has no preexisting deficit or in whom the deficit has been repaired consists mainly in supplying carbohydrate to ensure adequate storage of glycogen in the liver. Usual maintenance requirements of water and electrolytes are appropriate. Small infants who are not vomiting should receive carbohydrate and sodium chloride mixtures by mouth until 3 hr before operation. Such fluids are readily absorbed from the gastrointestinal tract and will not produce aspiration pneumonitis if vomited and aspirated.

Preoperative preparation of the newborn involves certain unique hazards. Deficits of water and electrolytes from vomiting or from stasis owing to intestinal obstruction should be replaced before operation. If aspiration pneumonitis is suspected, it should be treated with antibiotics. Nasogastric suction may be inadequate. If so, gastrostomy should be performed to aid in decompression and in postoperative feeding. In intestinal obstruction conjugated bilirubin may be deglucuronidated by intestinal enzymes; an enterohepatic circulation of unconjugated bilirubin can then lead to high serum levels and kernicterus. Hypoprothrombinemia should be prevented by administration of 1.0 mg of vitamin K oxide.

Table 5–16 APPROXIMATE REQUIREMENTS OF WATER WITHOUT ELECTROLYTES DURING OPERATION

WEIGHT KG	BASAL KCAL/24 HOURS	EVAP. WATER, ML/HR (90 ML/100 KCAL/24 HOURS)*	URINE WATER, ML/HR (30 ML/100 KCAL/24 HOURS)†	TOTAL‡ ML/HOUR
3	150	6	2	8
5	270	10	3	13
7	410	15	5	20
10	550	21	7	28
20	850	32	10	42
30	1100	41	14	55
40	1300	49	16	65

From Harned HS Jr, Cooke RE: Surg Gynecol Obstet *104*:543, 1957. By permission.

*This value is assumed to be high because of possible sweating and hyperventilation.

†This value is assumed to be low because of probable antidiuresis.

‡Does not include abnormal losses of fluid (hemorrhage, wound edema, suction) which must be replaced by appropriate electrolyte-containing fluids.

The most common error in parenteral fluid administration during and after surgery is overadministration, particularly of dextrose in water. Table 5–16 lists water maintenance requirements during surgery. Additional amounts of blood, plasma, saline, or other volume expander must be given if blood loss or tissue trauma is significant. The magnitude of such losses is judged best by the experienced surgeon as he operates.

Under most circumstances it is preferable that no potassium be administered during this time since extensive tissue trauma or anoxia may result in the release of large amounts of intracellular potassium with the potential of causing hyperkalemia. Moreover, if shock occurs, it may be complicated by acute renal failure, making treatment of the hyperkalemia more difficult.

Postoperatively, intake should be limited for 24 hr. Thereafter, usual maintenance therapy is gradually resumed. The water intake should not exceed 85 ml/100 kcal metabolized because of antidiuresis resulting from trauma or circulatory readjustment unless renal capacity to concentrate the urine is limited (e.g., in sickle cell anemia). If the intake of water is not limited, whether given parenterally or by mouth, water intoxication may result. Sodium intake for maintenance should also be low because of the low caloric expenditure during anesthesia and postoperatively.

5.32 THERAPY OF ISOLATED DISTURBANCES IN CONCENTRATIONS OF ELECTROLYTES

Acidosis. *Respiratory acidosis*, in which the pH may be markedly lowered, primarily as a result of retention of carbon dioxide, may be seen with severe respiratory insufficiency, with respiratory distress syndrome in the newborn infant, and in patients receiving assisted ventilation for any reason. Mild metabolic acidosis may also exist because hypoxia leads to the accumulation of lactic and other organic acids in the extracellular fluid. Measurements of blood pH and blood gases facilitate correction of acidosis in such patients. The appropriate treatment of such disturbances is improvement of ventilation by assisted respiration rather than by administration of sodium bicarbonate, which may produce hyperosmolality and cardiac failure.

Metabolic acidosis, resulting, for example, from renal tubular acidosis or from accumulation of organic acids, may require the administration of alkali, especially if symptoms are evident. In lactic acidosis, in glycogen disorders, or in circulatory insufficiency and hypoxia, sodium lactate may not be adequately metabolized; in these situations sodium bicarbonate is the preferred agent. The usual initial dose is 1–2 mEq/kg. However, a more precise estimate of the dosage required is given by the following general formula:

$$[(C_d - C_a) \times f_d \times \text{body weight in kg} = \text{mEq required}]$$

where C_d and C_a represent, respectively, the serum bicarbonate concentration desired and the one actually present, expressed as mEq/l, and f_d represents that fraction of the total body weight in which the administered material is apparently (not actually) distributed (the value for f_d varies with the substance administered). The apparent distribution factor (f_d) for bicarbonate or potential bicarbonate approximates 0.5–0.6 of the body weight. Such calculations indicate that 0.5 ml/kg of a molar solution of sodium bicarbonate would raise the serum bicarbonate concentration approximately 1 mEq/l. There are, however, wide variations in response to administered bicarbonate since it may be sequestered in bone or muscle or lost in urine.

With glomerular insufficiency, caution must be exercised in correcting acidosis because the sodium administered with bicarbonate may result in further expansion of the extracellular fluid volume. It is rarely necessary to attempt to increase serum bicarbonate levels above 15 mEq/l unless the patient continues to be markedly symptomatic from the acidosis. In addition, overcorrection of acidosis may be complicated by the development of tetany. If hyperphosphatemia coexists with acidosis, it should be treated simultaneously with low phosphate diets and aluminum gels given orally.

The use of sodium bicarbonate in the treatment of metabolic acidosis should always be considered a temporizing measure; every attempt should be made to treat the underlying cause, e.g., using glucose and insulin in diabetic ketoacidosis, improving circulation in shock, or eliminating salicylates, methanol, or other toxins.

Alkalosis. Under normal circumstances the kidney has an enormous capacity to excrete bicarbonate, and increased amounts of bicarbonate which gain access to the blood are promptly excreted. However, under certain circumstances, *metabolic alkalosis* may develop and be maintained. Typically, it is caused by administration of excess amounts of alkali, by loss of hydrogen ion, or by volume contraction with disproportionate losses of chloride. Severe hypokalemia can result in alkalosis, too, or may perpetuate it.

Plasma bicarbonate is elevated and respiratory compensation results in hypoventilation and an increase in pCO_2. Rarely, respiration may be so depressed in infants with severe hypochloremic alkalosis that oxygenation of the blood is diminished. Severe alkalotic tetany may also occur. In such instances, the administration of ammonium chloride may effect symptomatic improvement; the dose may be calculated from the general formula presented above, with the probable f_d being 0.2–0.3. Such therapy is for relief of symptoms only and must not be used in place of correction of the contracted volume of body fluids or in place of administration of potassium chloride for repair of intracellular deficits.

Patients with metabolic alkalosis associated with volume contraction respond to measures designed to expand volume and replace the chloride and potassium deficits. They include those in whom the acid-base disorder is due to vomiting, gastric suction, congenital chloride diarrhea, dietary chloride deficiency, and administration of diuretics. Their urinary chloride concentration is low (10 mM/l or less). A minority of patients are "chloride-resistant." They have a higher urinary chloride concentration of 15 mM/l or greater. Causes include hyperadrenalism, Bartter syndrome, severe potassium depletion, and licorice ingestion. Potassium repletion and specific therapy directed to the underlying condition represent the appropriate therapeutic approach in these patients.

Respiratory alkalosis may be seen in salicylate intoxication; in various central nervous system diseases such as trauma, infection, or tumors; with anxiety or fever; and in congestive heart failure, hepatic insufficiency, and gram-negative septicemia. Treatment should be directed at removing the underlying cause, although measures designed to return pCO_2 to normal may be indicated. Use of an acidifying agent such as ammonium chloride is not an appropriate substitute.

Hyponatremia. Serum sodium is most commonly reduced as a result of either sodium depletion or water "intoxication" or a combination of these factors (Table 5–17). A low serum sodium, thought to be due to redistribution of total body sodium, may also be seen in association with severe illnesses or in the terminally ill patient. In addition, *apparent* hyponatremia may be observed as an artifact, e.g., in diabetic ketoacidosis when the water content of plasma is reduced by the presence of increased quantities of lipids.

Patients with a serum sodium below 120 mEq/l are usually symptomatic (i.e., convulsions, shock); those

Table 5–17 CLINICAL STATES COMPLICATED BY HYPONATREMIA

Expansion of extracellular space by water
Excessive intake
  Parenteral fluid therapy — glucose in water
  Oral (with diminished output)
  Tap water enemas
  Allergy to cow's milk (very rare)
Diminished output (usual intake)
  Renal
    Intrinsic: nephritis, nephrotic syndrome, tubular necrosis, prematurity
    Extrinsic
      Excess of antidiuretic hormone: acute and chronic central nervous system disease, vasopressin therapy, surgery, pulmonary disease
      Circulatory: heart failure, cardiovascular surgery, malnutrition
  Skin: premature infant in high humidity

Deficiency of extracellular sodium
Inadequate intake
  Low salt diet
  Parenteral therapy with glucose in water
Excessive losses
  Gastrointestinal: vomiting, salivary, gastric, biliary, pancreatic drainage, diarrhea, resin therapy, tap water enemas (especially in megacolon)
  Genitourinary
    Intrinsic renal disease: chronic nephritis, acute tubular necrosis (recovery phase), nephrotic syndrome (diuresis)
    Extrinsic influences: diuretics, acetazolamide, hypoadrenalism, central nervous system disease (rare), expanded volume (Pitressin, excessive water therapy)
  Skin
    Normal sweat
    Abnormal sweat: cystic fibrosis, adrenal insufficiency
    Burn therapy with silver nitrate (hypochloremia)
  Cerebrospinal fluid
    Draining myelomeningocele
    Arachnoureterostomy
    Continuous drainage of CSF, e.g., in lead encephalopathy
  Parenteral: thoracentesis, paracentesis, burns
Redistribution
  Severe malnutrition
  Potassium deficiency
  Trauma

with lesser degrees of hyponatremia are frequently asymptomatic. Treatment of *asymptomatic hyponatremia* depends on its cause. With water overload fluid restriction is the appropriate measure; serum sodium may return rapidly to normal in a patient with good renal function but may take several days or weeks with the inappropriate ADH syndrome. When sodium deficits are present, adding extra salt to the diet or increasing the sodium concentration of parenterally administered fluid will often be adequate to correct the deficit. Measuring urine sodium concentration will often help to determine the cause of hyponatremia. Typically with sodium depletion, urine sodium concentration is 10 mEq/l or less, although such low values are also found in nephrotic syndrome, congestive heart failure, or hepatic failure. Expansion of the extracellular fluid with water or renal tubular injury results in a higher urinary sodium concentration (often around 50 mEq/l). The wrong treatment will not correct the defect and may be detrimental. For example, the administration of sodium to a patient with hyponatremia due to water excess, such as that seen with the chronic edema of heart failure, nephrotic syndrome, or cirrhosis, may result only in further expansion of the extracellular fluid without correction of the serum sodium.

Treatment of *symptomatic hyponatremia* consists of the administration of a hypertonic saline solution. The dose may be calculated according to the formula in the preceding section on acidosis, except that C represents serum sodium rather than bicarbonate. Since there is osmotic equilibrium between cells and extracellular water, changes in osmolality are distributed over total body water so that the value for f_d should be 0.6–0.7. A dose of 12 ml/kg of body weight of 3% sodium chloride solution (6 mEq sodium/kg) usually raises the serum sodium approximately 10 mEq/l. Elevation of the sodium concentration should be effected in small increments (5–10 mEq/l) over 1–4 hr.

Hypernatremia. The treatment of hypernatremic dehydration has been discussed in Sec 5.23. It is seen with diarrhea and dehydration and may also result from faulty preparation of infant formulas: using condensed instead of evaporated milk or using heaped or packed instead of level measures of milk powder. These errors increase the solute load to be excreted by the kidney relative to the amount of water provided and may result in an osmotic diuresis and negative water balance. The accidental ingestion of excessive amounts of sodium chloride (*salt poisoning*) also may result in hypernatremia and lead to such serious residuals that special attention is warranted. The accidental substitution of salt for cane sugar in private homes as well as in institutions occurs with sufficient frequency to justify the routine use of liquid sugars in infant feeding. Hypernatremia resulting from the excessive intake of sodium, in contrast to hypernatremic dehydration resulting from diarrhea, is accompanied by increases in total body sodium and in the volume of extracellular water. Severe acidosis results from a shift of organic acids and free hydrogen ions to extracellular fluid. With shift of water from brain cells, distention of cerebral vessels occurs, leading to subdural, subarachnoid, and intracerebral hemorrhage. The complications and residuals of salt poisoning are similar to, but may be more severe than, those seen with hypernatremic dehydration.

Treatment is directed toward the rapid removal of excess sodium from the body. Intravenous fluids should consist of glucose in water, potassium acetate, and calcium as needed. *Intermittent peritoneal dialysis* with glucose solutions can remove large quantities of sodium, correcting the hyperosmolality without the danger of pulmonary edema and heart failure. Approximately 45 ml/kg of a dialysis solution containing 4.25% glucose can be injected intraperitoneally for severe hypernatremia (serum sodium concentration more than 200 mEq/l) and withdrawn 1 hr later. As the concentration of sodium in the serum falls, subsequent dialysis may be carried out using a solution with 1.5% glucose so as not to remove too much water and dehydrate the patient. Exchange transfusion is not a desirable substitute for dialysis because enormous quantities of blood would be required to effect a change in osmolality of total body water. Phenobarbital should be administered to prevent or control seizures. Digitalization may be necessary to counteract heart failure.

Hypokalemia. Disturbances in the concentration of potassium in the absence of disturbances of volume of body fluids have been described in primary hyperaldosteronism and in Bartter syndrome. Large amounts of potassium are lost in the urine, resulting in low serum potassium and high serum bicarbonate concentrations. In congenital alkalosis of gastrointestinal origin, large amounts of potassium and chloride are lost in the stools. The use of thiazide and loop diuretics (e.g., ethacrynic acid and furosemide) causes a kaliuresis as well as natriuresis; prolonged use may result in significant potassium loss and hypokalemia.

Severe hypokalemia may result in weakness of skeletal muscles, decreased peristalsis, ileus, and an inability of the kidney to concentrate urine. Prolonged hypokalemia results in characteristic pathologic changes in the kidney and a decrease in function which may persist even after potassium repletion.

Treatment consists of administration of large amounts of potassium (usually up to 3 mEq/kg/24 hr); in Bartter syndrome up to 10 mEq/kg may have to be given orally.

Hyperkalemia. Marked elevation of the serum potassium results in ventricular fibrillation and death. In consequence, levels above 6.5 mEq/l should be treated promptly. The possibility of oral or parenteral administration of excessive amounts of potassium should be considered and all potassium intake discontinued. The rapid intravenous administration of sodium bicarbonate (up to 2 mEq/kg of body weight over a 5–10 min period) or glucose and insulin (0.5 gm glucose/kg with 0.3 unit crystalline insulin/gm of glucose, given over a 2 hr period) will result in the intracellular movement of potassium and will lower serum potassium. Intravenous calcium gluconate (up to 0.5 ml of a 10% solution/kg given over 2–4 min) will counter the cardiac toxicity of potassium, but the EKG should be monitored while it is being administered. None of these measures removes significant quantities of potassium from the patient; they should be considered as temporizing measures until negative potassium balance is established by the use of ion exchange resins (Kayexalate, 1 gm/kg/24 hr, in divided oral doses twice daily or as a retention enema), by hemodialysis, or by peritoneal dialysis.

Hypocalcemia and **hypercalcemia** are discussed in Chapters 3, 7, 18, and 20.

Hypomagnesemia. The importance of magnesium in intravenous therapy is reviewed in Sec 5.11 and 5.24. The only definitive symptom complex associated with hypomagnesemia (serum magnesium less than 1.3 mEq/l) is that of latent or manifest tetany. Convulsions, muscular twitching, disorientation, athetoid movements, carpopedal spasm, and hyper-reactivity to mechanical and auditory stimulation have been observed. Lowered serum concentrations and whole body deficits of magnesium are found in chronic diarrhea or vomiting, sprue, celiac disease, prolonged parenteral fluid therapy, and hyperaldosteronism. Low serum magnesium levels have been observed in infantile tetany, presumably on the basis of transient hypoparathyroidism. The intramuscular injection of 0.1 ml of a 24% solution of $MgSO_4 \cdot 7H_2O$ (0.2 mEq/kg) repeated every 6 hr for 3–4 doses produces symptomatic and biochemical improvement. The addition of 3 mEq/l of magnesium to maintenance fluids for patients requiring long-term therapy may decrease the chance of serious deficiency. See Sec 7.54.

Hypermagnesemia. Levels of serum magnesium in excess of 10 mEq/l are accompanied by drowsiness and, occasionally, coma. Deep tendon reflexes may also be abolished, and respiratory depression may occur at higher concentrations. Disturbances in atrioventricular and intraventricular conduction may be detected at levels of 5 mEq/l. Acute renal failure and Addison disease are accompanied by significant elevations of serum magnesium. Iatrogenic poisoning can result from the use of magnesium in the treatment of hypertension or of toxemia of pregnancy; deaths have been reported from the use of magnesium sulfate enemas in megacolon and from oral administration for purging.

The intravenous administration of calcium gluconate, as in the treatment of tetany, rapidly reverses the depressant effects of hypermagnesemia as well as the associated cardiac abnormalities.

PARENTERAL SOLUTIONS

Table 29–8 lists some solutions commercially available for use in fluid therapy. The large number of carbohydrate and electrolyte mixtures available permits great flexibility and individualization of therapy.

ALAN M. ROBSON

Calagno PL, Rubin MI, Singh NSA: The influence of surgery on renal function in infancy: The effect of surgery on the postoperative renal excretion of water; the influence of dehydration. Pediatrics 16:619, 1955.

Colle E, Paulsen EP: The responses of the newborn to major surgery: Urinary electrolyte, water and nitrogen losses. Pediatrics 23:1063, 1959.

Cooke RE, Ottenheimer EJ: Clinical and experimental interrelations of sodium and the central nervous system. Adv Pediatr XI:81, 1960.

Darrow DC, Pratt EL: Fluid therapy: Relation to tissue composition and expenditure of water and electrolyte. JAMA 154:365, 1950.

Darrow DC, Pratt EL, Flett J Jr, et al: Disturbances in water and electrolyte in infantile diarrhea. Pediatrics 3:129, 1949.

Finberg L: Dehydration in infants and children. N Engl J Med 276:458, 1967.

Finberg L: The management of the critically ill child with dehydration secondary to diarrhea. Pediatrics 45:1029, 1970.

Finberg L: Hypernatremic (hypertonic) dehydration in infants. N Engl J Med 289:196, 1973.

Gordon P, Levitin H: Congenital alkalosis with diarrhea. A sequel to Darrow's original description. Ann Intern Med 78:876, 1973.

Harris F: Pediatric Fluid Therapy. Philadelphia, FA Davis, 1972.

Heird WC, Driscoll JM Jr, Schullinger JN, et al: Intravenous alimentation in pediatric patients. J Pediatr 80:351, 1972.

Hinton P, Allison SP, Littlejohn S, et al: Electrolyte changes after burn injury and effect of treatment. Lancet 2:218, 1973.

Hirschhorn N: The treatment of acute diarrhea in children. An historical and physiological perspective. Am J Clin Nutr 33:637, 1980.

Hogan GR, Dodge PR, Gill SR, et al: Pathogenesis of seizures occurring during restoration of plasma tonicity to normal in animals previously chronically hypernatremic. Pediatrics 43:54, 1969.

Miller NL, Finberg L: Peritoneal dialysis for salt poisoning. N Engl J Med 263:1347, 1960.

Nalin DR, et al: Oral rehydration and maintenance of children with rotavirus and bacterial diarrheas. Bull WHO 57:453, 1979.

Pierce AW Jr: Salicylate poisoning. Pediatrics 54:342, 1974.

Segar WE: Parenteral Fluid Therapy. Current Problems in Pediatrics. Chicago, Year Book Medical Publishers, 1972.

Weil WB: A unified guide to parenteral fluid therapy. J Pediatr 75:1, 1969.

WHO Treatment and prevention of dehydration in diarrheal diseases. Guide for use of primary health care personnel. Scientific Publication No. 336, 1977.

Winters RW (ed): The Body Fluids in Pediatrics. Boston, Little, Brown, 1973.

5.33 TETANY

Tetany is a state of hyperexcitability of the central and peripheral nervous sytems resulting from abnormal concentrations of ions in the fluid bathing nerve cells and peripheral nerves. Specifically, the abnormalities are decreases of H^+ (alkalosis), of Ca^{++}, or of Mg^{++}. The decrease in H^+ may precipitate tetany at concentrations of Ca^{++} or Mg^{++} which might otherwise be above the threshold for manifest tetany. A decrease of K^+ can prevent the development of tetany despite low Ca^{++} concentrations, whereas a rising K^+ can precipitate tetany in a patient with low Ca^{++}. Hypomagnesemic tetany on the other hand can occur despite reduction of K^+ concentration. There is thus a range of ionic concentrations at which tetany can be either latent or manifest.

The serum calcium, as usually measured, includes both Ca^{++} and undissociated calcium proteinate; albumin is the chief serum protein to form a complex with calcium. Ca^{++} can be measured, but this procedure is not available in most clinical laboratories. At normal concentrations of serum albumin about 40–50% of the total calcium is ionized, i.e., 4.0–5.2 mg/dl. When serum albumin is reduced, total serum calcium is decreased without a decrease in Ca^{++}; a rough rule of thumb states that each decrease of 1 gm/dl of albumin results in a decrease of 0.8 mg/dl of calcium. A nephrotic child with a serum albumin level of 1 gm/dl might, therefore,

be expected to have a total serum calcium concentration from 7.5–8.0 mg/dl without reduction of Ca^{++}.

At physiologic concentrations of H^+ and K^+, tetany may develop at Ca^{++} concentrations of less than 3.0 mg/dl and will almost always be manifest at Ca^{++} concentrations less than 2.5 mg/dl. At normal concentrations of serum albumin, these levels correspond to total serum calcium concentrations of approximately 7 mg/dl and 5 mg/dl, respectively.

The normal level of magnesium in serum ranges between 1.6 and 2.6 mg/dl, of which about 75% is Mg^{++}. A reduction of total serum magnesium to less than 1.0 mg/dl may be associated with hyperexcitability of the nervous system.

Manifest Tetany. The classic signs of peripheral hyperexcitability of motor nerves are spasms of the muscles of the wrists and ankles (carpopedal spasm) and of the vocal cords (laryngospasm). In *carpopedal spasm* the wrists are flexed, with extension of the fingers and adduction of the thumbs over the palms, the so-called obstetric position. The feet are extended and adducted. These muscular spasms can be quite painful. *Laryngospasm* causes inspiratory obstruction, with a high-pitched inspiratory crow; apnea may result. The sensory manifestations are paresthesias, particularly numbness and tingling of the hands and feet. Motor excitability of the central nervous system may be manifested by convulsions which are usually generalized but may be localized to 1 side of the body. They are often brief but recurrent. Between seizures the patient may be apparently conscious, but after a prolonged series of convulsions a postictal state may result. In young infants convulsions are frequently the only evidence of the hyperexcitability of the nervous system.

Latent Tetany. *Latent tetany* is defined as the condition in which ischemia or mechanical or electrical stimulation of motor nerves is required to produce the motor response characteristic of tetany. Carpopedal spasm may be induced in latent tetany through the production of ischemia of the motor nerves by cutting off the arterial supply with a tourniquet (*Trousseau sign*). The usual test employs a blood pressure cuff on the arm, inflated above the systolic blood pressure for 3 min. With a positive test the typical pattern of carpal spasm develops. Motor nerve impulses can be elicited by mechanical tapping, whereas this is not possible under normal physiologic conditions. The facial nerve can be stimulated by tapping anterior to the external auditory meatus. Contraction of the orbicularis oris occurs with a twitch of the upper lip or entire mouth (*Chvostek sign*). The peroneal nerve can be stimulated by tapping where it passes over the head of the fibula; a positive *peroneal sign* is dorsiflexion and abduction of the foot.

The motor nerves can also be stimulated electrically. *Erb sign* is a positive response of motor nerves to electrical stimulation with galvanic currents of amperage less than that required to stimulate them under normal physiologic conditions.

Another manifestation of reduced Ca^{++} concentrations is a prolonged Q-T interval on the electrocardiogram. This may be difficult to interpret unless the Q-T interval is carefully calibrated for variations in heart rate.

Alkalotic Tetany. This is very rare in infants and young children. Tetany can be induced through spontaneous overventilation, producing respiratory alkalosis; such hyperventilation is most often of psychogenic origin. In patients with low Ca^{++} concentrations tetany may be precipitated by overventilation or by a metabolic alkalosis following administration of sodium bicarbonate, but the metabolic alkalosis resulting from loss of gastric juice owing to pyloric obstruction is rarely associated with tetany. Alkalotic tetany has been seen in patients with renal disease who have been protected by concurrent metabolic acidosis from the consequences of low Ca^{++} concentration correction of the acidosis has caused tetany and convulsions. The treatment of alkalotic tetany due to hyperventilation is to rebreathe in a bag or balloon to increase pCO_2.

5.34 HYPOCALCEMIC TETANY

Disorders of Parathyroid Function. The most common disorder of parathyroid function is transient physiologic hypoparathyroidism of the newborn infant, sometimes referred to as *neonatal hypocalcemia*. Clinically, infants with transient hypoparathyroidism of the newborn can be separated into 2 groups, one with hypocalcemia during the first 36 hr of life, usually before the baby achieves a significant oral intake of milk, and a 2nd group with hypocalcemia due to high phosphate load, which develops only after the infant has been receiving cow's milk for a number of days. The onset of symptoms in the second group occurs most commonly from 5–10 days of life; clinical manifestations have occasionally appeared as late as 6 wk of age. Both forms are presumed to result from physiologically inactive parathyroid glands which fail to respond normally to low Ca^{++} concentrations.

Besides a relative lack of parathyroid hormone output, there may be in the newborn period a partial refractoriness of the target cells to parathyroid hormone. Moreover, excessive secretion of thyrocalcitonin may be a major contributing factor in persistent hypocalcemia of premature infants, particularly those stressed by anoxia. The low birth weight infant whose mother has had an inadequate intake of vitamin D and little exposure to sunshine also has a low plasma concentration of 25-hydroxy vitamin D_3, deficiency of which is associated with relative refractoriness to parathyroid hormone.

The relative hypoparathyroidism of the newborn has been attributed to the increased serum calcium of the fetus, which reflects a calcium gradient across the placenta. In addition, mild maternal hyperparathyroidism may augment inhibition of the fetal parathyroids by calcium ion. Physiologic hyperparathyroidism has been indicated by increased parathyroid hormone levels found during pregnancy and may be more intense in the diabetic woman. Occasional cases of transient hypoparathyroidism in infants have been associated with clinical hyperparathyroidism in the mother.

The infants at greatest risk for early hypocalcemia are low birth weight infants (prematurely born), infants born of diabetic mothers, and infants who have been subjected to prolonged, difficult deliveries.

The incidence of hypocalcemia in prematurely born infants is extremely high, particularly in those with respiratory distress. It is difficult to evaluate the role of hypocalcemia in the morbidity and mortality of such infants. Hypocalcemia should be suspected as one of the possible causes of convulsions. Diagnosis can be made only by determination of serum calcium concentrations. Treatment requires the intravenous injection of 10% calcium gluconate in a dosage of about 2 ml/kg (18 mg Ca/kg). This must be given slowly, with monitoring of the cardiac rate for bradycardia; excessive concentrations of calcium in blood reaching the right auricle may inhibit the rhythmic electrical activity of the sinus node causing cardiac arrest. Tissue necrosis and calcification may occur if this solution extravasates or is given intramuscularly. The intravenous dose of calcium gluconate can be repeated at 6–8 hr intervals until calcium homeostasis becomes stable, or the calcium gluconate can be added to a constant intravenous infusion. Administration in the 1st day of life of either 1,25-dihydroxy vitamin D_3 or 25-hydroxy vitamin D_3 to prematurely born infants at risk for hypocalcemia has been successful in preventing or reducing the severity and duration of hypocalcemia, but neither is recommended for routine prevention. Calcium gluconate or calcium lactate may be added to the feeding at the same time.

The hypocalcemia following feeding of high phosphate milks can occur in both fullterm and prematurely born infants and in infants whose clinical histories have been benign. The intake of a high phosphate food in relatively large volume leads to an elevated serum phosphate due to relatively high tubular reabsorption of phosphate and the physiologically low glomerular filtration rate of the newborn. The elevated serum phosphate depresses serum calcium through deposition of calcium in bone. The normal physiologic response would be an increased output of parathyroid hormone, which would increase both the solubilization of bone mineral and urine phosphate output by blocking tubular reabsorption of phosphate. This would restore serum levels of both calcium and phosphate to the normal range. If the infant's parathyroid glands are not yet able to respond with such an increase of parathyroid hormone, the level of serum calcium progressively falls and symptomatic hypocalcemia may result.

The most important manifestation of hypocalcemia in infants is convulsions; carpopedal spasm is not usually seen. Laryngospasm with cyanosis and apneic episodes may occur. In addition to the characteristic signs of increased excitability of the nervous system, there may be nonspecific symptoms such as poor feeding, vomiting, and lethargy rather than irritability. These clinical signs suggest sepsis; serum calcium determinations should be made in addition to other diagnostic studies in infants in whom sepsis is suspected. Rarely, bradycardia with heart block is noted. A prolonged Q-T interval on the electrocardiogram suggests hypocalcemia. A serum calcium concentration below 7 mg/dl establishes the diagnosis. The serum phosphate level is increased, sometimes to 10–12 mg/dl. The blood urea nitrogen is not elevated, distinguishing this condition from the hyperphosphatemia of severe renal dysfunction. Normal newborns being fed cow's milk have serum phosphate concentrations of 6–8 mg/dl, and concentrations in normal premature infants may be even higher.

For the convulsing infant the initial *treatment* is the intravenous injection of 10% calcium gluconate, 2 ml/kg, with the precautions given above. After this, specific treatment aims at reduction of the serum phosphate. Breast-fed infants rarely, if ever, develop hypocalcemia since human milk is low in phosphorus. Even "humanized" infant foods prepared from dialyzed whey of cow's milk are considerably higher in phosphate than human milk. The absorption of phosphate from the food can be suppressed, however, by adding to the formula a great excess of calcium, which precipitates as calcium phosphate in the lumen of the gut, e.g., adding calcium lactate or gluconate to the milk feeding to achieve a calcium to phosphorus ratio of 4:1 (see Table 5–18). Calcium lactate powder is preferred, and its addition to milk produces no important gastrointestinal disturbances. Since calcium lactate is 13% calcium, 770 mg of this salt provides 100 mg of calcium; calcium gluconate is 9% calcium, so that 1100 mg of this salt represents 100 mg of calcium. A soluble preparation of calcium gluconate is available (syrup of Neo-calglucon)

which contains 92 mg of calcium per teaspoonful, but this is a less desirable method of adding calcium and has caused diarrhea in the amounts necessary. Calcium chloride may cause gastric irritation and hyperchloremic acidosis.

Sample Calculation. An infant is taking a volume of prepared infant feeding estimated to contain 300 mg of P and 450 mg of Ca. To achieve a 4:1 ratio of Ca to P, 750 mg of calcium must be added to make a total calcium intake of 1200 mg. This requires addition of 6 gm of calcium lactate powder to the total feeding or 1 gm per feeding given every 4 hr. Since the salt must be dissolved in the milk, calcium lactate tablets should not be used as the compressed tablets are quite insoluble even if fragmented.

As the serum phosphorus level decreases with treatment, the serum calcium returns to normal and may even rise to somewhat hypercalcemic levels. At this point, the calcium supplement is reduced in steps, not stopped abruptly, since the serum phosphorus may rise precipitously and the calcium concentration fall again to tetanic levels. In most infants restoration of normal calcium homeostasis and presumably normal parathyroid responsiveness occurs in 1–2 wk.

Occasionally, a more prolonged period of calcium supplementation is needed. Therefore, the treatment must be individualized by serial measurements of calcium and phosphate concentrations. If there is poor response to treatment, the calculations should be checked to determine whether sufficient calcium is being added, and the feeding given the baby should be examined to see whether the calcium lactate or gluconate has been completely dissolved. If no errors are found and the therapeutic response is inadequate, the diagnosis of congenital hypoparathyroidism should be entertained, or, in older infants, vitamin D deficiency or an abnormality of absorption or metabolism of vitamin D.

Congenital absence of the parathyroids can occur either in association with aplasia of the thymus (*DiGeorge syndrome*), in combination with abnormalities of the great vessels of the heart, or as an isolated parathyroid aplasia. Such patients present the same symptoms as infants with transient physiologic hypoparathyroidism but respond incompletely to the simple treatment outlined above and have relapsing hypocalcemia which requires more definitive treatment. In total parathyroid deficiency, substitution for parathyroid hormone of pharmacologic amounts of vitamin D, vitamin D metabolites, or vitamin D analogues is required. We prefer to use dihydrotachysterol, which at pharmacologic doses is more potent than vitamin D in the correction of hypocalcemia; since it is also more rapidly inactivated in the body, it is not stored as is vitamin D and does not have so much cumulative toxicity. In the young infant 0.05–0.1 mg of dihydrotachysterol should be given daily and the dose adjusted by determination of serum calcium concentrations, which should be returned to levels of about 9–10 mg/dl. The highly active metabolite of vitamin D, 1,25-dihydroxy vitamin D_3, is now available and is effective in the treatment of hypoparathyroidism in doses of 0.25–0.5 µg/24 hr. As the child grows, the dosage of either steroid must be increased as indicated by serum calcium concentrations. The problem of hypoparathyroidism in older children is discussed in Sec 18.18.

Hypocalcemia and Tetany Due to Vitamin D Deficiency or Abnormalities of the Vitamin D Metabolism. The onset of vitamin D deficiency tetany occurs usually between 3–6 mo since this amount of time is necessary for the depletion of the infant's stores of vitamin D; on the other hand, an infant born of a vitamin D deficient mother may develop hypocalcemia due to vitamin D deficiency within the 1st wk of life. Nutritional vitamin D deficiency and tetany are now rare, but vitamin D deficiency will occasionally develop in a breast-fed infant whose mother is not aware that human milk is deficient in vitamin D and does not provide supplementary vitamin D.

Hypocalcemia may also be due to failure of normal metabolism of vitamin D. Vitamin D undergoes 2 hydroxylation steps, first in the liver and second in the kidney, before becoming the metabolically active 1,25-dihydroxy vitamin D_3. Infants with liver disease such as neonatal hepatitis, cytomegalic inclusion disease, or atresia of the bile ducts may show manifestations of vitamin D deficiency with hypocalcemia because of failure of liver metabolism of vitamin D. In atresia of the bile ducts, malabsorption of vitamin D may also contribute to the problem. In the genetic defect of vitamin D metabolism called vitamin D dependent (pseudodeficient) rickets, in which there is probably failure of the 1-hydroxylation step in the kidney, affected infants may also present with hypocalcemia. Vitamin D deficiency can also result from steatorrhea due to pancreatic lipase deficiency or to intrinsic intestinal mucosal disorders. In addition, rickets and osteomalacia are associated with the treatment of convulsive disorders by large doses of combined anticonvulsant drugs, principally phenobarbital, diphenylhydantoin, and primidone. These drugs alter the metabolism of vitamin D in the liver. Diphenylhydantoin also inhibits intestinal transport of calcium. The patients may present with hypocalcemia as well as skeletal changes.

Patients with tetany resulting from vitamin D deficiency or failure of normal metabolism of vitamin D can be given initial symptomatic relief by intravenous injection of 10 ml of 10% calcium gluconate, with the usual precaution of monitoring heart rate to prevent too rapid injection. The definitive treatment is vitamin D, and this should be given in amounts adequate to achieve a rapid physiologic effect, e.g., vitamin D, 600,000 units, in a single dose or divided into several doses over a 24 hr period. For this purpose a highly concentrated vitamin D preparation is needed. The common solution of vitamin D in propylene glycol (Drisdol), 10,000 units/gm, is not suitable for this type of therapy since the large volume of propylene glycol would be depressant. An alternative method of therapy is 10,000 units of vitamin D daily for 3 wk. These large doses of vitamin D given orally will be effective in true vitamin D deficiency. If there is impaired vitamin D absorption or a defect in the metabolism of vitamin D, larger doses may be required. The active metabolites of vitamin D, 25-hydroxy vitamin D_3 and 1,25-dihydroxy vitamin D_3, are now available for treatment. The hypocalcemia of hepatic disorders or of vitamin D dependent rickets will respond to large doses of vitamin D, but more precise treatment with 25-hydroxy vitamin D_3 or 1,25-dihydroxy vitamin D_3 is now possible. Treatment must be individualized and patients closely monitored to avoid vitamin D intoxication. (See also Sec 3.30.)

5.35 HYPOMAGNESEMIC TETANY

Hypomagnesemia has been reported as a cause of tetany in association with either low or normal serum calcium concentrations. In transient physiologic hypoparathyroidism of the newborn, low serum magnesium concentrations may accompany the hyperphosphatemia and hypocalcemia (Table 5–18). This hypomagnesemia usually responds to treatment directed at reducing the serum phosphate concentration. Occasionally, newborn infants with severe hypomagnesemia will require spe-

Table 5–18 EXAMPLES OF TREATMENT OF TRANSIENT PHYSIOLOGIC HYPOPARATHYROIDISM OF NEWBORN INFANTS WITH SUPPLEMENTARY CALCIUM

Age (Days)	Serum Levels (mg/dl)			Treatment	
	Ca	P	Mg	Diet	Ca:P Ratio
				I. Baby McC.	
10	6.9			Standard infant feeding*	
12	7.1	9.2	0.86	Calcium lactate supplement begun	4
14	9.2	8.3	0.91		
19	14.0	3.0	1.64	Supplement discontinued	1.5
22	6.9	8.8	0.77	Calcium lactate supplement restarted	3
32	10.7	6.2	1.80		
				II. Baby O.	
8	5.2			Standard infant feeding	1.5
9	5.0	10.5			
11	6.1			Calcium lactate supplement begun	4
14	9.4	5.7			
16	12.6	3.6			2.5
26	10.0	7.6		Standard infant feeding	1.5
38	10.5	7.4			

*Formula based on cow's milk.

cific magnesium therapy. This can be given by intramuscular injection of 0.2 ml/kg of a 50% solution of $MgSO_4 \cdot 7H_2O$ (25% solution of $MgSO_4$). This treatment will raise serum Mg concentrations into the normal range within an hour and should maintain adequate concentrations for several hours. Often, no further therapy is needed. The mechanism of this transient hypomagnesemia is not clear. Hypomagnesemic tetany and convulsions can be seen beyond the newborn period as the result of congenital disorders of magnesium transport, causing either failure of absorption of diet magnesium or failure of tubular reabsorption of magnesium with excessive urinary loss. Intestinal malabsorption of magnesium also is a consequence of acquired intestinal injury such as inflammatory bowel disease or resection of small intestine. Renal loss of magnesium may be secondary to nephropathy caused by aminoglycosides or cis-platinum. Magnesium depletion, whatever the pathogenesis, can be associated with hypocalcemia because of a need for magnesium for both secretion of parathyroid hormone and responsiveness of target tissues to the hormone. Treatment requires magnesium administration either intramuscularly as above or orally in the form of magnesium salts, such as the chloride or gluconate.

HAROLD E. HARRISON

Bakwin H: Tetany in newborn infants. Am J Dis Child 54:1211, 1937.

Booth BE, Johanson A: Hypomagnesemia due to renal tubular defect in reabsorption magnesium. J. Pediatr 84:350, 1974.

Colletti RP, Pan MW, Smith EWP, et al: Detection of hypocalcemia in susceptible neonates. The Q-oTc interval. N Engl J Med 290:931, 1974.

Gardner LI: Tetany and parathyroid hyperplasia in the newborn infant. Influence of dietary phosphate load. Pediatrics 9:534, 1962.

Harrison HE, Lifshitz F, Blizzard RM: Comparison between crystalline dihydrotachysterol and calciferol in patients requiring pharmacologic vitamin D therapy. N Engl J Med 276:894, 1967.

Harrison HE, Harrison HC: Disorders of Calcium and Phosphate Metabolism in Childhood and Adolescence. Philadelphia, WB Saunders, 1979.

Paunier L, Radde IC, Kooh SW, et al: Primary hypomagnesemia with secondary hypocalcemia in an infant. Pediatrics 41:385, 1968.

Richens A, Rowe DJF: Disturbance of calcium metabolism by anticonvulsant drugs. Br Med J 4:73, 1970.

Tsang RC, Light IJ, Sutherland JM, et al: Possible pathogenetic factors in neonatal hypocalcemia of prematurity. J Pediatr 82:423, 1973.

5.36 FAILURE TO THRIVE

The term failure to thrive is used for infants and children who, without superficially evident cause, fail to gain and often lose weight. This situation is observed more often in infants but also occurs later in childhood. It has occurred frequently among institutionalized children, especially those who are retarded.

Etiology. Most instances of failure to thrive result from psychosocial circumstances, not always apparent, which adversely affect the child's intake, absorption, or utilization of food. Emotional deprivation and physical neglect or abuse, including the withholding of food (Sec 2.67), are commonly associated. An increased incidence of failure to thrive, with malabsorption, has been reported among children with autism and adults with schizophrenia. Sometimes the physical or emotional deprivation of the child is related to a physical handicap, such as cerebral palsy or cleft palate, or to difficult behavior due to temperament or other causes. The syndrome may also result from obscure organic abnormalities as well as from easily discoverable diseases in which growth failure occurs. For many children who experience a period of failure to thrive with no ascertainable organic or environmental cause, retrospective analysis indicates the likelihood of psychosocial origin. Table 5-19 lists some of the psychosocial and organic conditions associated with failure to thrive.

Clinical Manifestations. Failure to gain weight or to grow at the expected rate may be the only signs. More characteristically, there are also signs of developmental retardation and of physical and emotional deprivation, such as apathy, poor hygiene, intense eye contact with people, withdrawing behavior, and disorders of oral intake which may be manifested as anorexia, voracious appetite, or pica. Vomiting, regurgitation, diarrhea, and general neuromuscular spasticity or hypotonia may be concurrent.

Table 5-19 SOME CAUSES OF FAILURE TO THRIVE AND SCREENING TESTS FOR THEM

CAUSE	SCREENING TESTS
Environmental	
Inadequate intake of food	History; observation in hospital
Emotional deprivation	History; observation in hospital
Environmental disruptions	History; observation in hospital
Rumination (Sec 11.20)	Observation in hospital
Organic	
Central nervous system abnormalities	Neurologic examination; developmental assessment; transillumination of skull; brain scan
Intestinal malabsorption	Observation in hospital; stool fat
Cystic fibrosis of the pancreas	Sweat test
Intestinal parasites (rarely a cause in temperate climates)	Stool for ova and parasites
Partial cleft palate	Physical examination; observation of feeding
Chronic heart failure	Physical examination; roentgenogram of chest
Endocrine disorders	Construction of growth chart; blood test for thyroid function; films for bone age
Idiopathic hypercalcemia	Serum calcium
Turner syndrome (girls)	Buccal smear
Other chromosomal disorders	Chromosomal analysis in patients with peculiar facies or multisystem defects
Renal insufficiency	Urinalysis; blood urea nitrogen
Renal tubular disorders	Urinalysis; urinary amino acid screen
Chronic infection (usually tuberculous or mycotic)	Tuberculin test; chest roentgenogram; temperature pattern in hospital
Chronic inflammation (e.g., rheumatoid arthritis)	Physical examination; sedimentation rate
Malignancies (especially of kidney, adrenal, brain)	Roentgenograms of abdomen, chest; intravenous urography; brain scan

Diagnosis and Differential Diagnosis. Hospitalization provides opportunity for quantitation of factors governing the net caloric intake (food intake, vomiting, stools) and for observation of interactions of the child, especially during feeding and play, with his mother, with health personnel, and with other children. It frequently leads to dramatic improvement in weight gain and in social responses and thus provides evidence that environmental factors are causative, rendering unnecessary any exhaustive and expensive search for underlying organic disease.

History-taking by different interviewers at different times is often helpful in turning up psychosocial problems which are inapparent or unexpressed at the initial interview. Information from friends, relatives, and neighbors may reveal unsuspected adverse factors in the child's family environment.

Construction and study of a growth chart and of a developmental flow sheet may identify the point in time when the child began to fail to thrive and may be useful in uncovering the environmental or physical factors responsible. On the other hand, if growth has been steady, though below the expected level (e.g., usually below the 3rd percentile), such diagnoses as constitutional short stature, hypopituitarism, or chromosomal abnormality must be considered.

If history and physical examination suggest disturbances in any particular organ systems, appropriate diagnostic study is warranted. This should begin with screening tests and proceed in detail only as these are positive. Routine blood counts and urinalyses serve as screening tests for the hematologic and renal systems. Extensive study to rule out most or all possible underlying organic lesions is justified only if the initial data base (Sec 5.5) has failed to provide clues pointing to a specific environmental or organic etiology; *in addition*, there should be demonstrated failure of a favorable response to hospitalization. Children chronically deprived of food may have stools consistent with malabsorption when an adequate dietary intake is initiated. They gain weight, however, and resume a normal stool pattern after some weeks or months.

Prevention. Environmental causes of failure to thrive may be prevented by such social measures as education for parenthood, encouragement of couples to have only as many children as they are economically and emotionally capable of supporting, reduction of social stresses that weaken the family relationship, and creation and maintenance of a social structure that will provide optimal nurturing of infants and children. The role of the physician and other health personnel in prevention of failure to thrive lies in early recognition of the syndrome and of the characteristics and circumstances of parents which may lead to it. These include general immaturity, drug addiction or abuse, irresponsible or antisocial behavior, dislike of children, low tolerance for stress, emotional instability, economic stress, marital discord, single parenthood, and sometimes severe temporary stresses such as family tragedies, which may lead to temporary failure to thrive in an otherwise healthy environment. Early counseling and adequate direct support in the care of the threatened child will often prevent the development of failure to thrive in these situations.

Treatment. A temporary change of environment, such as hospitalization for necessary evaluation, may be sufficient for transient relief of tension among family members. When this is coupled with advice, counseling, and support from a physician, social worker, and family service agency when appropriate, adjustments may be made that will ensure adequate care of the child when he or she returns home. However, temporary or permanent placement in a foster home may be necessary. Identified organic disease should be treated appropriately.

Prognosis. Most children with nonorganic failure to thrive eventually achieve physical development within the normal range. However, about half will later be identified as having neurotic or antisocial personality characteristics, two thirds will manifest a delay in learning to read, and one third will have lower verbal than performance scores on psychometric testing. A small but significant number will die later under suspicious circumstances. The relative roles of hereditary factors, of the period of failing to thrive, and of subsequent environmental factors in these sequelae have not been elucidated.

GIULIO J. BARBERO
R. JAMES McKAY

Barbero GJ, Shaheen E: Environmental failure to thrive: A clinical view. J Pediatr 71:5, 1967.
Hufton IW, Oakes RK: Nonorganic failure to thrive: A long-term follow-up. Pediatrics 59:73, 1977.
Smith CA, Berenberg W: The concept of failure to thrive. Pediatrics 46:661, 1970.

PREANESTHETIC AND POSTANESTHETIC CARE AND CARDIOPULMONARY RESUSCITATION

Pediatric anesthesiology encompasses not only administration of anesthesia to children, but also the closely related areas of intensive care, cardiopulmonary resuscitation, and associated uses of modern respiratory equipment for infants and children.

To provide safe and effective anesthesia for infants and children, a physician must thoroughly understand the basic principles of modern anesthetic practice and the pharmacology of the drugs used. The anesthesiologist must understand (1) the ways in which pediatric patients differ from adults in anatomy, physiology, and response to drugs; (2) the emotional reactions to anesthesia and surgery encountered in the various pediatric age groups; and (3) the physical status of the patient, the surgical lesion, and the operation to be performed.

With these factors in mind, the anesthesiologist can

make a preoperative evaluation, produce the desired degree of preanesthetic sedation, and select the least hazardous anesthetic agents, and techniques that will produce satisfactory operating conditions. The anesthesiologist also should determine the appropriate modes of monitoring various vital functions and provide for maintenance of an adequate circulating blood volume as well as fluid, electrolyte, and acid-base equilibrium.

5.37 PREANESTHETIC EVALUATION

A careful history will enable the anesthesiologist to plan the management of anesthesia and the postanesthetic period with greater effectiveness. It should include specific information about the following:

The child's previous anesthetic and surgical procedures
Family history of major anesthetic complications
Recent upper respiratory tract infection
Exposure to exanthems
Previous laryngotracheitis (croup)
History of allergies
Drug hypersensitivities
History of asthma or wheezing during respiratory infections
History of apnea or breathing irregularities
Abnormal weight loss
Exercise tolerance
Bleeding tendencies
Blood transfusion reactions
Current medications
Prior administration of corticosteroids
Emotional reactions of the child to the proposed operation
When and what the child last ate

A history of frequent croup will require special airway management during anesthesia; a familial history of abnormal response to muscle relaxants might indicate a genetically abnormal pseudocholinesterase which the anesthesiologist must consider when selecting a muscle relaxant; infants and children receiving cortisone, antiepileptic or sedative drugs, or certain antibiotics may have altered responses to anesthetic and adjuvant agents; a patient with a full stomach risks aspiration during induction of anesthesia.

The physical examination should emphasize the heart, lungs, and upper airways. The presence of heart murmurs, rales in the chest, or wheezing requires careful cardiac or pulmonary evaluation before the anesthesiologist proceeds. Small, narrow nares filled with secretions, loose teeth, tonsils and adenoids large enough to cause mouth-breathing, or a small, underdeveloped mandible with a protruding maxilla may contribute to upper airway obstruction after sedation or induction of anesthesia. Tracheal intubation may be difficult if the larynx lies anterior to its normal position.

Laboratory tests desirable before anesthesia include determination of hemoglobin or hematocrit, white cell count, and urinalysis. In patients with serious systemic disease or those about to undergo extensive surgery, a preoperative roentgenogram of the chest, and measurement of arterial pH, PaO_2 and $PaCO_2$, serum electrolytes, and blood glucose or urea nitrogen may be indicated.

5.38 PREANESTHETIC PREPARATION AND SEDATION

Children are frightened on leaving the security and familiarity of home, especially those 1–4 yr of age, who are unable to understand the purpose of hospitalization. Terrifying experiences during induction of anesthesia or in the immediate postoperative period can produce disabling psychologic changes such as night terrors, enuresis, and temper tantrums. Certain steps will minimize the psychologic trauma: (1) For the child over 3 yr of age, parents should explain the purpose of the proposed operation in simple terms, telling of the probable sequence of events and discomfort involved. (2) Parents must be encouraged to display confidence and cheerfulness; their tension and anxiety are readily transmitted to the child. (3) The anesthesiologist should visit the child prior to operation, in the presence of the parents if possible, so that the child will regard the anesthesiologist as a sympathetic, caring friend. (4) Preanesthetic sedation should permit the child to be transported to the operating room lightly asleep, allow induction of anesthesia without awakening, and provide some analgesia during postanesthetic recovery.

Improvements in pediatric anesthesia over the past 15 yr permit children with no organic disturbance or some mild to moderate abnormalities to be admitted to a surgical facility, undergo general anesthesia and superficial, noncomplex operative procedures, recover, and return home on the same day. The requirements for safe "day surgery" include a history and physical examination, basic laboratory studies, and a visit with the anesthesiologist within 30 days prior to operation; a brief preanesthetic review by the anesthesiologist on the day of operation; and an extended recovery period to ensure that the child can retain oral liquids, has voided, is not vomiting, and has adequate relief of pain.

Elective anesthesia and operation in the healthy infant less than 6 mo of age carries an increased risk of certain serious, even potentially lethal complications. Infants, in contrast to older children and adults, experience more rapid uptake from the lungs and require higher blood levels to achieve effective anesthesia with halothane, the most widely used volatile anesthetic agent. Severe systemic arterial hypotension at an effective anesthetic dose occurs more frequently in the infant, indicating a narrow margin of safety. Unexplained apneic episodes in apparently recovered infants may occur in the first 2 hr after anesthesia, resulting in severe brain damage and death if undetected. Hemoglobin concentration may be at its nadir and limit oxygen content reserves in the blood. Delayed or partial recovery from muscle relaxants may also occur during this period, especially if the infant's body temperature falls below 36° C. The retinal vasculature does not reach

Table 5–20   PREANESTHETIC MEDICATION

	AGE	DRUG
Intramuscular (IM)	0–6 mo	Atropine or glycopyrrolate
	6–12 mo	Atropine or glycopyrrolate + pentobarbital
	Over 12 mo	Atropine or glycopyrrolate + pentobarbital + morphine or meperidine
Oral (PO)	0–12 mo	None
	Over 12 mo	Atropine or glycopyrrolate + diazepam + meperidine

DRUG	ROUTE	Dosage DOSAGE
Atropine	IM, PO	0.02 mg/kg; minimum 0.15 mg, maximum 0.5 mg
Glycopyrrolate	IM, PO	0.01 mg/kg to maximum 0.35 mg
Pentobarbital	IM	3.0–4.0 mg/kg; maximum 120 kg
Morphine	IM	0.05–0.10 mg/kg; maximum 10 mg
Meperidine	IM, PO	1.0–2.0 mg/kg; maximum 100 mg
Diazepam	PO	0.2 mg/kg

maturity until 45–50 wk postconception so that hyperoxic retinal ischemia may still occur during anesthesia with a possible risk of retrolental fibroplasia. All of these complications are rare, yet are more likely to occur in the infant born preterm who is less than 40 wk postconception. Appropriate use of halothane, muscle relaxants, and oxygen provides safe, reliable anesthesia in infants; however, extended postanesthetic observation, use of the minimal inspired oxygen concentration required, and maintenance of body temperature will help ensure the safety of anesthesia in this age group.

A wide variety of drugs are used for preanesthetic sedation. Table 5–20 lists appropriate oral and intramuscular drugs and dosages for various age groups. Atropine provides more effective abolition of vagal reflexes than does scopolamine and, therefore, is preferred in infants under 1 yr of age, in whom vagal reflexes tend to be more active. Recent experience has verified the efficacy and safety in children over 1 yr of age of small volume oral preanesthetic sedation in a fruit-flavored syrup containing meperidine, diazepam, and atropine given 2 hr prior to anesthetic induction. A barbiturate in combination with an opiate and atropine given intramuscularly produces suitable preanesthetic sedation in most children requiring more profound sedation or those about to undergo painful and extensive operative procedures. (See Sec 5.31.)

Although the child's stomach should be free of solids prior to anesthesia, it is important not to interrupt fluid intake longer than necessary. No milk or solids should be given less than 12 hr prior to anesthesia. Clear fluids with glucose should be given up to 4 hr prior to induction of anesthesia in infants and up to 6–8 hr prior to induction in older children. Since this preoperative oral fluid regimen may not prevent mild dehydration, intravenous isotonic electrolyte solution with glucose is warranted for all but the shortest, minor procedures.

Before proceeding with an operation the anesthesiologist should correct dehydration, decrease excessive fever, compensate for acidosis, and restore a depleted blood volume.

The febrile, dehydrated child who requires emergency surgery, such as appendectomy, should receive at least partial rehydration rapidly, along with correction of any concomitant metabolic acidosis by intravenous sodium bicarbonate (2.0–3.0 mEq/kg). General endotracheal anesthesia with neuromuscular blockade and controlled ventilation followed by surface cooling with water mattresses on the anterior and posterior body surfaces can then be instituted. Cooling should be continued until the colonic or esophageal temperature is under 38° C (100.4° F). The anterior water mattress can be removed when the body temperature is below 39° C (102.2° F), and the operation safely started.

Newborn infants who require immediate surgery and who have made little or no recovery from birth asphyxia or who have a body temperature below 35° C (95° F) require oxygen, intravenous sodium bicarbonate (2–3 mEq/kg), and elevation of body temperature toward 37° C (98.6° F). Analysis of blood for pH, $PaCO_2$, PaO_2, electrolytes, glucose, osmolality, and hematocrit are essential to initial monitoring and evaluation of the patient's ventilation and metabolic status.

5.39   INTRAOPERATIVE MANAGEMENT

All the common inhalation agents have been used in children, but for the past 15 yr halothane (Fluothane) and nitrous oxide with neuromuscular blockade have replaced flammable agents such as cyclopropane and diethyl ether. For induction, most anesthesiologists prefer gravity flow of nitrous oxide and halothane over the face, with application of a face mask only after the child has lost consciousness. Intravenous induction, using a 25–27 ga scalp vein needle, may be achieved rapidly with intravenous thiopenthal (3–4 mg/kg); ketamine can also be used for intravenous induction in infants and young children, but is contraindicated in older children and adolescents because of the frequency of postanesthetic hallucinations in this age group. Newer inhalation agents such as enflurane (Ethrane) and isoflurane (Forane) also have been used for inhalation anesthesia induction in children and offer certain advantages over halothane in some patients. Regional anesthesia has limited application in infants and small children because of their fears.

Experience has shown that nondepolarizing muscle relaxants (metubine, *d*-tubocurarine, and pancuronium) can be used with effectiveness and safety even in the newborn infant. Tracheal intubation and controlled ventilation provide optimal gas exchange, and neostigmine preceded by atropine restores neuromuscular transmission at the conclusion of anesthesia.

Tracheal intubation is indicated in (1) operations about the head and neck, (2) intrathoracic and intraperitoneal procedures, (3) operations in the prone position, (4) most procedures in infants under 1 yr of age, and (5) virtually all emergency procedures because there is uncertainty about the contents of the stomach. Ventilation should be controlled manually or mechanically in all intrathoracic procedures and intraperitoneal operations and in patients in the prone position.

During anesthesia, monitoring of heart tones with a precordial stethoscope, a continuous electrocardiogram (lead 2), continuous measurement of rectal temperature with a thermistor probe, and assessment of arterial pressure by the Riva-Rocci or ultrasonic Doppler method are mandatory in all age groups. For children in poor physical condition or those undergoing extensive surgery, insertion of a plastic cannula into an artery for continuous direct measurement of arterial pressure as well as blood sampling usually is indicated.

Although the infant's heart and peripheral vasculature adapt remarkably to hypovolemia, decompensation may occur suddenly and cardiac arrest ensue. Awareness of the infant's approximate blood volume (80–90 ml/kg in the newborn, 75 ml/kg in the older infant) and immediate replacement of losses exceeding 10–15% of that volume can prevent hypovolemic shock. Blood for rapid infusion should be warmed to 37° C immediately before use because rapid infusion of cold blood may produce cardiac arrest. When the anticipated losses exceed one third of the patient's estimated blood volume, CPD (citrate-phosphate-dextrose) blood less than 10 days old should be used because older blood becomes extremely acidotic (pH 6.5–6.7) and depleted of clotting factors. Serial arterial pH, PCO_2, and electrolyte determinations will detect the acidosis, hypocalcemia, and hyperkalemia that may be associated with rapid, massive blood replacement. Selection of the appropriate blood products and balanced electrolyte solutions in many instances permits restoration of intravascular volume without the use of whole blood.

Continuous monitoring of body temperature is essential during general anesthesia. In modern air-conditioned operating rooms inadvertent hypothermia (colonic temperature under 35° C, 95° F) develops frequently in small infants undergoing laparotomy or thoracotomy and is associated with ventilatory depression, peripheral vasoconstriction, and a moderate metabolic acidosis in the immediate postanesthetic period. Overhead radiant heaters and circulating warm water mattresses, as well as heated humidification of inspired gases, can minimize this thermal stress. Malignant hyperpyrexia, the abrupt and unexplained rise in body temperature above 41° C (105.8° F) during or immediately following inhalation anesthesia, occurs in children over 1 yr of age and in young adults. The overall mortality rate exceeds 75%. Successful management demands immediate recognition of a rapid rise in temperature, cessation of anesthesia, and hyperventilation with oxygen. Treatment also includes packing the patient in ice, ice-water gastric lavage, rapid infusion of intravenous fluids at 5–10 times the maintenance rate until adequate urine output is established, intravenous administration of sodium bicarbonate (4–7 mEq/kg), and dantrolene (1 mg/kg to a total of 10 mg/kg). The patient at risk of malignant hyperthermia by prior personal or family history requires consultation with an anesthesiologist well in advance of the day of operation as well as special preanesthetic preparation.

5.40 POSTANESTHETIC RECOVERY

Recovery room facilities and nursing must be available to provide constant surveillance of airway patency, adequacy of ventilation, and circulatory stability. Infants less than 6 mo of age should be retained in the recovery room for a period of at least 2 hr to ensure full recovery of respiratory control, neuromuscular function, and upper airway reflexes. The common sequelae of general anesthesia in infants and children include postanesthetic excitement, vomiting, and pain. Postanesthetic excitement occurs most frequently in patients who have undergone painful procedures involving the head and neck and the abdomen; intravenous narcotics in an appropriate dose are most effective in managing this complication. Vomiting occurs commonly following myringotomy, tonsillectomy, procedures on the eyes, and intra-abdominal operations. The relief of vomiting can sometimes be achieved with intravenous diazepam or phenothiazines in small doses. For control of severe pain, such as that associated with extensive orthopedic procedures, morphine (0.05–0.10 mg/kg intramuscularly) should provide relief for at least 3 hr.

Following tracheal intubation, patients between 6 mo–6 yr of age may develop subglottic edema, especially if there is a history of croup or recent upper respiratory infection. This can often be relieved by inhalation of aerosolized racemic epinephrine (0.2%) in addition to supportive measures, including humidified oxygen and intravenous fluids. Intravenous corticosteroids appear to have no beneficial effect. Rarely, orotracheal intubation followed by nasotracheal intubation or tracheostomy may be required for 2–5 days to guarantee an adequate airway. Malignant hyperpyrexia may also occur in the immediate postanesthetic period; therefore careful monitoring of temperature remains important.

5.41 INTENSIVE CARE

The elements of intensive care are (1) physician, nursing, and paramedical personnel specially trained in the care of the critically ill; (2) monitoring and alarm systems for continuous assessment of vital functions; (3) respiratory therapy and resuscitation equipment and drugs; (4) immediately available physician specialists in anesthesiology, pediatrics, and surgery; and (5) 24 hr laboratory service for hematologic studies and rapid, precise determination of blood pH, gas tensions, and electrolytes on ultramicro samples. The objective is to provide maximal surveillance and care to patients with acute, temporary, life-threatening impairment of pulmonary, cardiovascular, renal, or nervous system functions.

Commercially available systems are adequate for continuous monitoring and have appropriate alarms for respiratory rate (impedance pneumograph), heart rate, arterial and central venous pressures, and body temperature (thermistor probes) in small infants and children. Cannulation of a peripheral artery permits continuous pressure monitoring and frequent blood sampling for pH and gas tensions in older infants and children. The recent development of special electrodes for continuous transcutaneous monitoring of O_2 and CO_2 tensions facilitates prolonged noninvasive monitoring. Continuous measurement of ambient oxygen concentrations with high and low alarm devices represents a major advance in oxygen therapy of the small infant.

Precise administration of intravenous fluids can be provided by mechanical syringe pumps. Total or partial caloric requirements may be infused parenterally in infants able to tolerate a hyperosmolar infusion into a major vein.

Patients with existing or impending **respiratory failure** require intensive respiratory therapy. Respiratory failure exists if the impairment of ventilation poses an immediate threat to life. An acute rise in $PaCO_2$ over 55 mm Hg or PaO_2 under 100 mm Hg at an inspired oxygen concentration over 50% (except in cyanotic heart disease) indicates life-threatening impairment of ventilatory function. Successful therapy usually requires an artificial airway (nasotracheal intubation or tracheostomy, Table 5–21), mechanical ventilation, continuous humidification of inspired gases, and sterile tracheobronchial toilet at 1–3 hr intervals. Infants and children with severe acute lung disease, especially those with an artificial tracheal airway, also require chest percussion, vibration, and postural drainage for removal of secretion and provision of airway patency.

Table 5–21   SPECIFICATIONS FOR PEDIATRIC OROTRACHEAL TUBES*†

AGE	INTERNAL DIAMETER (ID IN MM)	LENGTH‡ (CM)	15 MM MALE CONNECTOR SIZE (MM ID)
Newborn (<1.5 kg)	2.5	10	3
Newborn (≥1.5 kg)– 3 mo	3.0	11	3
3–7 mo	3.5	11	4
7–15 mo	4.0	12	4
15–30 mo	4.5	13	5
2.5–4 yr	5.0	14	5
5–6 yr	5.5	16	6
7–8 yr	6.0	18	6
9–10 yr	6.0 cuffed§	20	6
11–12 yr	6.5 cuffed	22	7
13–15 yr	7.0 cuffed	24	7

*The ID size for age is based on the average size of tracheal tube in that age patient during general anesthesia which permitted an audible tracheal air leak at 20 to 25 cm H_2O peak inspiratory airway pressure. (Lee KW, et al: Selection of tracheal tube size in infants and children. Submitted for publication, 1982.) For age over 2 yr, the size formula:

$$ID\ (mm) = \frac{16 + age\ (yr)}{4}$$

†Clear polyvinyl-chloride tracheal tubes which satisfy the USP tissue implant test for inertness and the American National Standards Institute specifications will be labeled "Z-79" and are recommended. Connectors should have an ID equal to or greater than that of the tube and should be of lightweight plastic material.

‡Nasotracheal tubes should be 2 to 4 cm longer.

§High volume, low pressure cuffs inflated to permit an audible leak at 20 cm H_2O peak pressure are recommended.

Interstitial pulmonary edema often can be the inevitable consequence of severe trauma, extensive cardiopulmonary surgery, septic shock, or severe pneumonitis. Decreased air-containing lung volume, increased work of breathing, and severe arterial hypoxemia result. The hypoxemia usually requires more aggressive therapy than mere increases in inspired oxygen concentration to achieve arterial gas tension compatible with intact recovery while avoiding toxic effects of oxygen on the lung. Fluid restriction and tubular diuretics reduce total body and intrapulmonary water; furosemide also may enhance pulmonary lymphatic flow in addition to its renal effects. Positive end-expiratory airway pressure (PEEP) increases alveolar gas volume and helps maintain peripheral small airway patency. This causes better matching of ventilation with perfusion resulting in improved arterial oxygen tensions at lower inspired oxygen concentrations. Because PEEP also decreases the work of breathing, most patients accomplish adequate alveolar ventilation by spontaneous efforts and need only infrequent ventilator breaths (intermittent mechanical ventilation, IMV). The frequency of mechanical ventilator breaths (tidal volume 12–20 ml/kg) can be adjusted to achieve a normal arterial pH and $PaCO_2$. The advantages of this technique over controlled mechanical ventilation with neuromuscular blockade or profound sedation include lower airway pressures with less risk of barotrauma; minimal interference with circulation; decreased need for sedation and neuromuscular blockade; and improved coordination of the patient with the ventilator, resulting in less work and better matching of alveolar gas with pulmonary blood flow.

Circulatory failure also can occur in patients with major trauma or sepsis and following complex cardiovascular operations (Sec 5.46). Pediatric patients can benefit from precise control of intravascular volume, vasomotor tone, and blood flow by assessment of directly measured systemic arterial and right atrial (central venous) pressures; cardiac output; and blood oxygen content, pH, and gas tensions. In more complex conditions, introduction of a quadralumen, flow-directed (Swan-Ganz) catheter into the pulmonary artery provides for evaluation of pulmonary arterial and pulmonary occluded (wedge) pressures which reflect right ventricular function as well as left atrial end-diastolic pressure. Treatment should be directed at the specific physiologic dysfunction by using the information obtained from extensive monitoring to precisely adjust *blood volume* with diuretics or fluid infusions and *tissue perfusion* with selected catecholamines and vasodilators to alter myocardial contractility, heart rate, and vasomotor tone (Sec 13.66).

Intracranial hypertension often occurs following severe head trauma and intracranial operations. Early recognition of increased intracranial pressure (ICP) and carefully monitored therapy can reduce the hyperemia and edema that impair cerebral perfusion, resulting in ischemia and permanent central nervous system damage. A hollow stainless steel threaded cannula (subdural bolt) inserted through a burr hole into the subarachnoid space provides a simple, safe, and usually reliable means of estimating ICP. The therapy for intracranial hypertension includes fluid restriction (one half to one third maintenance fluids), tubular diuretics to reduce cerebral edema, 30 degree head-up tilt with the head faced forward to enhance cerebral venous drainage and reduce intracranial blood volume, and dexamethasone (1.5 ml/kg initially, and 1.0 ml/kg/day for 5 days) for patients with cerebral swelling secondary to head trauma. Children whose ICP exceeds 15 mm Hg despite this therapy should undergo intubation, neuromuscular blockade, and mechanical hyperventilation to a $PaCO_2$ range of 22–28 mm Hg; if this fails to control ICP, barbiturate coma and total body hypothermia to depress cerebral metabolic rate and reduce pressure may be effective in preserving central nervous system function; these are, however, exceedingly complex forms of therapy requiring specialized medical and nursing skills and extensive monitoring of pulmonary, cardiovascular, and renal function.

5.42 CARDIOPULMONARY RESUSCITATION

Cessation of *effective* ventilation or circulation requires immediate treatment. The cardinal signs of respiratory arrest are apnea and cyanosis. Absence of heart tones and of carotid and femoral pulses denotes circulatory arrest. Primary respiratory arrest can be caused by airway obstruction, central nervous system depression, or neuromuscular paralysis. The 3 types of circulatory arrest that occur are asystole, ventricular fibrillation, and cardiovascular collapse associated with extreme arterial hypotension. If cardiopulmonary arrest is suspected, one should proceed with coordinated artificial ventilation and closed-chest cardiac massage even if in doubt.

Airway. A clear airway should be obtained immediately. Vomitus and secretions should be aspirated or removed with fingers and a handkerchief. Soft tissue obstruction can be overcome by extension of the occipitoatlantal joint and forward displacement of the mandible.

Ventilation. Inflation of the lungs with air or oxygen can be accomplished effectively by mouth-to-mouth or mouth-to-nose insufflation or by bag and mask devices. A good fit of the mask on the face with minimal or no leaks is essential. The hallmark of adequate lung inflation is synchronous thoracoabdominal motion. The lungs should be inflated rapidly, with a breath interposed between each 4–5 cardiac compressions.

Circulation. An effective cardiac output in the newborn or small infant can be produced by applying maximum pressure with the tips of 2 fingers over the middle third of the sternum while the vertebral column is firmly supported. In larger infants and children the pressure is applied by the heel of 1 hand over the sternum opposite the 4th interspace. In large children the heel of the left hand is placed over the right hand to provide the strength of both arms and shoulders. If the maximum compression is held for a fraction of a second, a larger stroke volume will be ejected. The usual rate in infants is approximately 100/min, and 60/min in older patients.

When ventilation and massage are effective, carotid and femoral pulses become palpable, pupils constrict, and the color of the mucous membranes improves.

Open thoracotomy and direct cardiac massage are rarely indicated outside the operating room or intensive care unit.

Drugs. As soon as artificial ventilation and cardiac massage are effectively established, sodium bicarbonate and epinephrine should be administered (Table 5–22). They may be given intravenously or directly into the

Table 5-22 DRUGS FOR RESUSCITATION

Drug	Concentration	Intravenous Drug	Intracardiac Dose	Frequency Dose
Sodium bicarbonate*	1 mEq/ml	2–4 mEq/kg, up to 200 mEq	1/2 intravenous	5–10 min
Epinephrine	1:10,000 (0.1 mg/ml)	0.01 mg/kg, up to 0.5 mg	Same as intravenous	5–10 min
	µg/ml numerically equal to wt in kg	0.2–2.0 µg/kg/min	—	Continuous infusion
Isoproterenol	1:10,000 (0.1 mg/ml)	0.01 mg/kg, up to 0.5 mg	—	Single dose
	µg/ml numerically equal to wt in kg	0.2–2.0 µg/kg/min	—	Continuous infusion
Dopamine	µg/ml numerically equal to wt in kg × 10	2.0–20.0 µg/kg/min	—	Continuous infusion
Dobutamine	µg/ml numerically equal to wt in kg × 10	2.0–20.0 µg/kg/min	—	Continuous infusion
Atropine sulfate	400 µg/ml	10–20 µg/kg	—	30 min
Calcium chloride	10% (100 mg/ml)	20 mg/kg	—	10 min
Calcium gluconate	10% (100 mg/ml)	60 mg/kg	—	10 min
Lidocaine	20 mg/ml	1 mg/kg		Single dose

Defibrillation: 2–5 watt-seconds/kg (external)

*Obtain arterial sample for pH, pCO_2, base excess, as soon as possible to guide alkali therapy.

Table 5–23 RECOMM_____ _ CONTENTS FOR A PEDIATRIC RESUSCITATION CART

Airway Equipment

1. Bag and masks (infant, child, adult) with nonrebreathing valve that has universal 15 mm female adapter for male 15 mm endotracheal tube connectors
2. Oropharyngeal airways (Guedel sizes 00, 0, 1, 2, 3, 4)
3. Orotracheal uncuffed tubes (complete sterile set of 2 of each size, 2.5 mm ID to 8.0 mm ID) with appropriate size straight 15 mm male connectors; cuffed tubes, 6.0 to 8.0 mm ID; all tubes cut to oral minimum length plus 2 cm (see Table 5–21)
4. Laryngoscope:
   Adult handle, pediatric handle
   Blades: Miller—premature
            Wis-Hipple 1 and 1½
            Flagg—child
            Macintosh—adult (no. 3, 4)
   2 extra batteries
   1 extra light
   1 extra light for each blade
5. Aspiration equipment
   Metal tonsil aspirator (Yankauer)
   Disposable sterile plastic suction catheters, sizes (French) 5, 8, 10, 14
6. Magill forceps
7. Stylets (Teflon coated for tubes sized 2.5–8.0 mm ID)
8. EKG paper

Drugs

Sodium bicarbonate (1 mEq/ml)	Dobutamine (0.2 µg/ml)
Epinephrine (1.0 mg/ml)	Dextrose (500 mg/ml)
Isoproterenol (0.2 mg/ml)	Diazepam (5 mg/ml)
Calcium chloride (100 mg/ml)	Mannitol (0.25 gm/ml
Calcium gluconate (100 mg/ml)	or 12.5 gm/50ml)
Atropine sulfate (400 µg/ml)	Lidocaine (20 mg/ml)
Dopamine (0.2 µg/ml)	Saline (for dilution)

Defibrillator

Direct current with range of 20–400 watt-seconds
   Saline-soaked 4 × 4 in gauze pads stored with external paddles
   Pediatric (5 cm diameter) and adult (10 cm diameter) external paddles

Miscellaneous

Intracardiac needles: 20 and 22 gauge, 6–8 cm length
Plastic intravenous cannulas (16, 18, 20, and 22 gauge) and scalp vein sets
Sterile cutdown tray with pediatric instruments

Tongue blades	Scissors
Alcohol swabs	Syringes (plastic disposable)
Sterile hemostat	Needles
Sterile 4 × 4 gauze sponges	Lubricant, water-soluble, disposable single-use packets

heart. Sodium bicarbonate compensates for the extreme metabolic acidosis which develops rapidly after cessation of circulation. Epinephrine, which increases myocardial contractile force without decreasing the systemic vascular resistance, should be given if artificial ventilation, cardiac massage; and sodium bicarbonate have not restored spontaneous, effective circulation within 3 min.

Defibrillation. An electrocardiogram should be obtained and run continuously as soon as possible after the diagnosis of circulatory arrest to detect ventricular fibrillation. External defibrillation can be achieved with an appropriate electric shock (2 watt-seconds/kg ini-

tially, 3–5 watt-seconds/kg up to total of 400 watt-seconds in subsequent shocks) applied through paddles of appropriate size to skin surfaces covered locally with a conductive electrode jelly or saline-soaked pads.

Postresuscitation Care. Subsequent care includes treatment of the cause of the collapse, plus monitoring and regulation of the electrocardiogram, arterial pressure, and arterial pH and gas tensions. Cerebral edema may occur, with increased intracranial pressure requiring insertion of a subdural transducer for pressure monitoring and therapy with corticosteroids, hyperventilation, furosemide, and moderate hypothermia (30–32° C).

Successful resuscitation cannot be achieved without careful preplanning, proper equipment (Table 5–23), and a coordinated team effort. One individual at a resuscitation should be designated the recorder, to note times and details of the entire resuscitation. A log of all resuscitations should be retained by a medical or nursing department of the hospital.

JOHN J. DOWNES
RUSSELL C. RAPHAELY

General

Downes JJ, Betts EK: Anesthesia for the critically ill infant. American Society of Anesthesiologist Refresher Courses (JB Lippincott, Philadelphia), 5:47, 1977.
Downes JJ, Raphaely RC: Pediatric anesthesia and intensive care. In: Ravitch MM (ed): Pediatric Surgery. Chicago, Year Book Publishers, 1978.
Gronert GA: Malignant hyperthermia. Anesthesiology 53:395, 1980.
Jordan WS, Graves CL, Elwyn RA: New therapy for post-intubation laryngeal edema and tracheitis in children. JAMA 212:585, 1970.
Salem MR, Bennett EJ, Schweiss JF, et al: Cardiac arrest related to anesthesia. Contributing factors in infants and children. JAMA 223:238, 1975.
Smith RM: Anesthesia for Infants and Children. Ed 4. St. Louis, CV Mosby, 1980.

Intensive Care

Downes JJ, Godinez RI: Upper airway obstruction in the child. American Society of Anesthesiology Refresher Courses (JB Lippincott), Philadelphia, 8:29, 1980.
Downes JJ, Raphaely RC: Pediatric intensive care. Anesthesiology 43:238, 1975.
Lyrene RK, Troug WE: Adult respiratory distress syndrome in a pediatric intensive care unit; predisposing conditions, clinical course, and outcome. Pediatrics 67:790, 1981.
Mager T, Walker ML, Johnson DG, Matlak ME: Causes of morbidity and mortality in severe pediatric trauma. JAMA 245:719, 1981.
Moylan F, O'Connell KC, Todres ID, Shannon DC: Edema of the pulmonary interstitium in infants and children. Pediatrics 55:783, 1975.
Raphaely RC, Swedlow DB, Kettrick RG, et al: Experience with pulmonary artery catheterizations in critically ill children. Crit Care Med 8:265, 1980.
Raphaely RC, Swedlow DB, Downes JJ, Bruce DB: Management of severe pediatric head trauma. Pediatr Clin North Am 27:715, 1980.
Shoemaker WC, Chang P, Czer LSC, et al: Cardiorespiratory monitoring in postoperative patients: I. Prediction of outcomes and severity of illness. Crit Care Med 7:237, 1979.
Shoemaker WC, Chang P, Bland R, et al: Cardiorespiratory monitoring in postoperative patients: II. Quantitative therapeutic indices as guides to therapy. Crit Care Med 7:243, 1979.

Resuscitation

Downes JJ, Goldberg AI: Airway management, mechanical ventilation, and cardiopulmonary resuscitation. In: Scarpelli E, Auld PAM (eds): Pulmonary Disease in the Fetus, Infant, and Child. Philadelphia, Lea and Febiger, 1978.
Ehrlich R, Emmett SM, Rodriguez-Torres R: Pediatric cardiac resuscitation team: A 6-year study. J Pediatr 84:152, 1974.
Standards for cardiopulmonary resuscitation (CPR) and emergency cardiac care (ECC). JAMA 244(Suppl):453, 1980.

5.43   ACCIDENTAL INJURIES

Accidents are a major cause of morbidity and mortality in children. For children 1–14 yr of age, accidents caused more deaths in the United States than the next 6 causes of death combined and about 4 times more deaths than cancer, the 2nd highest cause. For adolescents and young adults age 15–24 yr, accidents caused more deaths than all other causes combined and about 4 times more deaths than homicide, the 2nd highest cause in this age group.

SITES OF ACCIDENTAL INJURIES

Most accidental injuries and deaths in children occur in the road, the home, and the school.

The Road. Motor vehicle deaths are the leading cause of accidental deaths as well as the leading cause of all deaths for individuals 1–25 yr of age. Those under 20 account for 10% of drivers and 18% of fatal automobile accidents. Drivers' education programs have been instituted in many public school systems in an effort to reduce this morbidity and mortality, but no controlled prospective studies of the efficacy of drivers' education have been performed, and there is evidence that the fatal accident rate for 16–17 yr old drivers is about the same with or without drivers' education. Therefore, where drivers' education allows adolescents to obtain a license at a younger age than they would otherwise be able to, drivers' education may actually contribute to deaths.

Injuries can be reduced by improvements in motor vehicle design; the development of collapsible steering wheels, padded dashboards, and improved car window glass have all contributed to a decreased death rate. The improvement of roadside guardrails and signposts and the national speed limit of 55 mph have also lowered the highway death toll.

Another major effort in automotive safety has been to convince people to use individual restraint devices such as seat belts or seat restraints for young children, which keep people in place and distribute the forces of deceleration so that the body can tolerate them. The majority of adults do not wear their seat belts, and over 90% of children have been observed to ride unrestrained in automobiles. If seat belts were used by all adults, the morbidity and mortality from automobile accidents would be decreased. In Australia, a law requiring the use of seat belts resulted in a 21% decrease in automotive mortality in metropolitan areas and a 10% decrease in rural areas. Data from Washington state suggest that the appropriate use of seat belts or seat restraints could decrease infant deaths in automobile accidents by 91% and infant injury by 78%; corresponding decreases for older children would be 81% and 64%.

Children need to be restrained at all times when they travel in automobiles—even in utero. The largest single cause of fetal death in unrestrained automobile accident victims is the death of the mother; pregnant women wearing seat belts sustain fewer injuries and deaths.

Infants should be in a seat restraint on their 1st trip home from the hospital and during all other motor vehicle trips. Children in the 1st 3 yr of life have a higher death rate in motor vehicle accidents than do older children up to adolescence. Therefore, education on seat restraints should begin during the 1st encounter between the pediatrician and a new parent. Children are unsafe when carried in the arms of an adult. The body of an 8 kg, 6 mo old infant attains a force equivalent to almost 350 kg during a collision at 30 miles/hr. This is equivalent to a fall from a 3rd story window. For children over 1 yr of age who can sit up adequately, seat belts provide an acceptable alternative to infant seat restraints.

Various passive restraints, restraints which do not require the automobile driver or passenger to do anything in order for them to be effective, may be installed in motor vehicles. Passive shoulder harnesses and a knee bar are not protective for children who are less than 45 kg and 104 cm tall. Air bags offer some protection for children of all ages and all sizes; to be most effective, they should be used in conjunction with a lap type seat belt, which can also be used with various infant seat restraint systems.

Motorcycles, motorscooters, motorbikes, and mopeds, which in the past were used in the United States mainly for sport riding, have come into increased use as modes of transportation because of their low initial cost and relative fuel economy. Many of the riders of these vehicles are adolescents. Motorcycle accidents usually result in trauma to the musculoskeletal or central nervous systems; deaths are usually associated with trauma to the great vessels or to the central nervous system.

Motorcycles contribute to deaths out of proportion to their numbers in the United States. In 1971, there were 72 fatalities/100,000 registered motorcycles, about twice the rate for other registered motor vehicles. Also, while the death rate for all motor vehicles was 4.7 deaths/100,000,000 miles, there were 20 deaths/100,000,000 motorcycle miles. In 1974 motorcycles accounted for fewer than 4% of the registered motor vehicles but almost 7% of motor vehicle fatalities.

The use of helmets by riders of motorcycles and similar vehicles results in lower morbidity and mortality from accidents. In those states that have enacted laws requiring motorcycle riders to wear helmets, death rates have declined markedly; where the laws have been repealed, the death rate has increased. The use of bright-colored paints and clothing and of the headlight at all times will decrease accidents by making the rider and vehicle more visible.

Bicycle accidents result in relatively few deaths (approximately 1000/yr in the United States); however, they cause many injuries and lead the list of causes of product-related injuries compiled by the United States Consumer Product Safety Commission. In a study of all bicycle accidents reported to police over a 2 yr period, there was 1 death; about 10% of the cyclists required hospitalization; 40% had a minor injury requiring medical care; and 20% had no injury. In another study of 3–12 yr old children with injuries requiring medical treatment, about two thirds of the injuries were abrasions, contusions, and lacerations. In a study of patients admitted to the hospital, 67% had craniocerebral trauma, 18% had upper limb fractures, and 7% had lower limb fractures.

The majority of bicycle-related injuries to infants occur when they are carried as passengers. Their feet and legs may get caught in the wheel of the bicycle, where spokes can cause a laceration and where the extremity can become squeezed between the wheel and the frame of the bicycle and be subjected to crush and shearing injuries. Therefore, children should be carried on a bicycle only in a special seat equipped with leg guards. Parents also need to be aware that the addition of such an infant carrier may adversely affect the bicycle's handling capabilities.

The majority of fatal bicycle accidents involve a motor vehicle, and the injury leading to death is usually craniocerebral trauma. The type of bicycle–motor vehicle accident that causes the greatest proportion of deaths (24.6%) is the motor vehicle overtaking the bicyclist from the rear.

Children under 13 account for 10% of bicycle traffic but 28% of bicycle injuries. One study showed that in 38% of the accidents, motorists received traffic citations with failure to yield the right-of-way as the most common charge. Bicyclists were in violation of traffic laws in 70% of the accidents; most of them were guilty of wrong-way riding (riding facing traffic), failure to yield the right-of-way, and turning violations. It is likely that young children cannot process their perceptions of road situations quickly enough to ride safely in traffic.

One way to decrease bicycle accidents and thus bicycle-related injuries is to separate bicycle and motor vehicle traffic, e.g., by providing a separate bicycle path. Further, bicyclists, like motorcyclists, should make themselves and their bicycles as visible as possible by wearing light colors, such as yellow, and using adequate lights, especially at night. Bicyclists should also wear helmets.

Children are frequently involved in road accidents as pedestrians. These children are usually 3–7 yr old; as in most other types of accidents, boys outnumber girls. Usually the children are unsupervised by adults at the time of the accident and often dart out into the street. Frequently, prior to an accident, a child is hidden from the driver by parked cars, bushes, or other roadside objects. In addition, children of this age often do not see traffic signs or they misinterpret them.

In order for children to be safer as pedestrians, they should wear brightly colored reflective clothing so that they will be more easily seen. In addition, children should be separated from traffic by fences and closed streets, and under- or overpasses should be provided for crossing. Prohibiting parking and roadside obstructions near corners may allow drivers to see children sooner. Modification of motor vehicles to increase external padding, decrease external protuberances, and make bumper areas at better heights should decrease injuries.

The Home.   The home is frequently the site of both fatal and nonfatal accidents, and children in the 2–3 yr old age group are most commonly involved. The types of accidents which occur in the home are legion. See Sec 5.45 for discussion of burns and Sec 28.5 for discussion of poisoning.

Over half of the victims of drowning (Sec 5.44) are children, adolescents, and young adults (less than 25 yr old). The incidence of drowning varies with location: in Florida, it is the 3rd most common cause of death for all children under 14; and in Australia, drowning causes more deaths than motor vehicle accidents in children under 6. More males die from drowning than females and more Blacks than Whites in the United States. Between one third and two thirds of drownings occur in swimming pools. Various bodies of water such as creeks and rivers account for around half of the deaths, and the home bathtub is the site of drowning in almost 20% of the cases.

The majority of drownings that occur in swimming pools occur in home or apartment house pools. Pools have the highest accident and death rates for children 1–3 yr of age; and in about three fourths of the pool drownings, the children were in a pool that had no fence around it and were unsupervised. Bathtub drownings are also most likely to occur in children who are unsupervised at the time of the accident and usually happen in larger families to children who are 10–12 mo old, often to the youngest or next to the youngest child in the family.

The incidence of drownings and near-drownings could be decreased if all swimming pools were required to be enclosed on all 4 sides by a fence with a self-latching gate. In addition, parents need to be taught that young children should never swim or bathe unsupervised.

The School.   Between the ages of 5–18, children spend up to 20% of their waking hours in school. For children in the primary grades, physical education and unorganized activities have the highest accident rates. For older children, accidents most commonly occur in physical education, the school building in general, interscholastic sports, and shops and laboratories.

Playground equipment is number 8 in terms of frequency of product-related accidents. Approximately 118,000 children/yr have accidents related to playground equipment with injuries severe enough to require an emergency room visit. Most of these injuries relate to falls from the equipment, and approximately 50% of these falls result in injuries to the head and neck. Most of the problems relate to the surface over which the playground equipment is installed. Many times this surface is concrete or asphalt rather than an energy-absorbing material such as loose sand, wood chips, or foam mats. A fall from a height of 1 foot onto concrete or asphalt can create forces sufficient to cause death if the child lands directly on his or her head. A fall from 3 feet onto packed dirt can also lead to death. On the other hand, falls onto energy-absorbing material can be tolerated from a much greater height. All playground equipment should be installed over an energy-absorbing surface and should be adequately maintained, e.g., checked for weakness due to rust, for sharp edges and protrusions, and for loose nuts and bolts.

The older the children get, the more likely they are to be injured in physical education activities. Although these injuries are usually relatively minor, they are frequent, almost 4 injuries/100 participants/1 yr, and cause the loss of slightly more than 1 school day/injury.

The injury rate in interscholastic sports is higher in each succeeding level of school. It is highest for boys in high school football (2.3 accidents/100,000 student days) and highest for girls in high school basketball (0.23 accidents/100,000 student days). In one study, 92% of the injured athletes required the services of a physician; however, 73% of those injured were able to return to their sport in fewer than 5 days. Two thirds of the injuries occurred during practice rather than during competition.

INJURY REDUCTION

The cause of injuries is the uncontrolled transfer of energy (usually mechanical) to a susceptible body or, occasionally, as is the case in suffocation or drowning, the inhibition of normal transfer of energy. Moreover, the definition of the word "accident" as an unexpected, unavoidable, or unintentional event conveys the sense that nothing can be done to prevent accidents. It is useful to consider this problem in terms of injury reduction rather than accident prevention.

Measures directed toward injury reduction may attempt either to control the environment or to alter human behavior. Measures directed at changing the environment, "passive measures," usually require the cooperation of relatively few individuals on few occasions but influence the lives of many. On the other hand, measures directed at changing human behavior, "active measures," require the cooperation of many individuals on multiple occasions. There are 5 steps which must be taken to reduce injury: (1) define the frequency and severity of injuries that occur in a community and identify high risk groups and/or situations; (2) determine what caused the injuries and, when possible, predict situations that are likely to result in injuries in the future; (3) plan control measures; (4) implement the control measures; and (5) evaluate the control measures for effectiveness.

The active control measure of education is the most common approach to injury reduction, but it has been rigorously studied and demonstrated to be relatively ineffective, e.g., seat belts are unused and home hazards persist despite all efforts to educate the population. In contrast, passive interventions have frequently resulted in decreased injury rates, e.g., prevention of poisoning through the use of childproof bottlecaps, changes in dashboard design of automobiles, and breakaway highway lamp posts.

THE ACCIDENT-PRONE CHILD

This term has been used to describe a child with a personality characteristic that was thought to predispose the child to have accidents. Such a personality trait does not exist. The child with repeated injuries should alert physicians to families with psychosocial problems; to a child with motor, attention, or temperament problems; and to the possibility of child abuse (Sec 2.67).

JEROME A. PAULSON

General References

National Safety Council, Accident Facts, 1979 edition. Chicago, National Safety Council, 1980.

The Road Environment

Automobiles: Drivers and Passengers

Crosby W, Costiloe J: Safety of lap belt restraints for pregnant victims of automobile collisions. N Engl J Med 284:632, 1971.
Mohan D, Schneider LW: An evaluation of adult clasping strength for restraining lap held infants. Human Factors 21:635, 1979.
Robertson LS: Crash involvement of teenaged drivers when driver education is eliminated from high school. Am J Public Health 70:599, 1980.
Scherz R: Restraint systems for the prevention of injury to children in automobile accidents. Am J Public Health 66:451, 1976.

Motorcycles

Robertson LS: An instance of effective legal regulation: Motorcycle helmet and daytime head lamp laws. Law and Society Review 10:467, 1976.
Watson GS, Zador PL, Wilks A: A repeal of helmet use laws and increased motorcyclist mortality in the United States, 1975–1978. Am J Public Health 70:579, 1980.

Bicycles

Cross K, Fisher G: A study of bicycle/motor vehicle accidents: Identification of problem types and counter measure approaches, Vol I. Santa Barbara, Calif, Anacapa Sciences, Inc., 1977.
Kravitz HL: Preventing injuries from bicycle spokes. Pediatr Ann 6:713, 1977.

Pedestrians

Sandels S: Young children in traffic. Br J Educ Psychol 40:111, 1970.

The School Environment

Reichelderfer TE, Overbach A, Greensher J: Unsafe playground. Pediatrics 56:526, 1979.

Injury Reduction

Haddon W: Energy damage and the ten counter measure strategies. J Trauma 13:21, 1973.
Schaplowsky A: Community injury control—a management approach. Am J Public Health 53:252, 1973.
Schlesinger ER, Dickenson DG, Westag J, et al: Study of health education in accident prevention. Am J Dis Child 111:490, 1966.

The Accident-Prone Child—The Abused Child

Husband P: The accident prone child. Practitioner 211:335, 1973.

References for Parents

Action for Child Transportation Safety. PO Box 266, Bothwell Wash 98011.
Child Restraint Systems for Your Automobile. US Department of Transportation, National Highway Traffic Safety Administration. Washington DC 20590.
Don't Risk Your Child's Life! Physicians for Automotive Safety, 50 Union Avenue, Irvington NJ 07111.

5.44   DROWNING AND NEAR-DROWNING

The term *drowning* indicates death within 24 hr of submersion in water and *near-drowning*, survival for more than 24 hr. Death may occur from respiratory obstruction and asphyxia with or without the additional effects of aspiration of water while submerged. Near-drowning may also occur with or without aspiration of water. Death may be delayed after apparently successful resuscitation from near-drowning. Drowning causes over 7000 deaths per year in the United States; the highest incidence occurs in children 1–4 yr of age. Most drownings are accidental: inadequately attended toddlers and infants drown in swimming pools and bathtubs, respectively; accomplished swimmers overestimate their endurance; occupants of pleasure boats fall overboard without life jackets; small children fall into ponds, streams, and flooded excavations; and the incautious of all ages plunge through thin ice.

Pathophysiology. Hypoxemia is the most serious consequence of near-drowning either with or without aspiration and is accompanied by metabolic acidosis and transient hypercarbia. The severity depends on the duration of submersion, the occurrence of aspiration, and the amount of water aspirated.

Approximately 10% of victims of drowning do not aspirate, but die acutely of laryngospasm or breathholding. Similarly, 12% of near-drowned victims do not aspirate. Hypercarbia and hypoxia develop rapidly but are reversible. Near-drowning victims who apparently have not aspirated usually recover completely if they are given artificial ventilation before the occurrence of circulatory arrest and permanent hypoxic damage to the central nervous system.

The pathophysiology of near-drowning with aspiration is significantly different from that after submersion without aspiration. Aspiration by dogs of as little as 2.2 ml/kg of water produced a profound decrease in arterial oxygen tension and after aspiration of 11 ml/kg of fresh water or sea water, the PaO_2 consistently dropped to values of 30–40 torr and remained depressed for at least 72 hr in survivors.

Aspiration of sea water produces hypoxia by mechanisms that differ from those produced by the aspiration of fresh water. Because sea water is hypertonic, body fluid is initially drawn into the alveoli. Fresh water aspiration does not have this effect, but by altering the surface tension properties of pulmonary surfactant, it results in unstable alveoli which become atelectatic and thus produces intrapulmonary shunting and hypoxemia. After either fresh or sea water aspiration, pulmonary insufficiency with intrapulmonary shunting and ventilation/perfusion mismatching occurs. Lung compliance decreases, dead space to tidal volume ratio increases, and airway resistance increases. Near-drowned victims also may swallow large volumes of fluid, suffer gastric distention, and regurgitate and aspirate gastric contents, thus compounding the pulmonary injury.

In the recovery phase there may be hypoxia during breathing of room air which was not evident during oxygen breathing. This suggests the presence of some persistent areas of ventilation/perfusion mismatching. $PaCO_2$ initially increases with aspiration but rapidly returns to normal as experimental animals begin to hyperventilate. Measurements of $PaCO_2$ in human near-drowning victims are variable. They may be elevated by hypoventilation but rapidly return to normal with increased spontaneous or mechanical ventilation, indicating no barrier to the elimination of carbon dioxide.

Significant acidosis was found in approximately 80% of near-drowning victims when the pH of arterial blood was measured in the emergency room. The persistent metabolic acidosis is probably due primarily to tissue hypoxia, although a respiratory component may be present, especially if there has been aspiration.

Although much emphasis was previously placed on electrolyte imbalance as the cause of morbidity and mortality from drowning, most drowned victims die of other factors, presumably anoxia and acidosis. In general, higher serum sodium and chloride values are found in those who have been submerged in sea water than are found in fresh water victims. However, the survivor who arrives for treatment after an episode of near-drowning will likely manifest only transient electrolyte changes which will revert to normal without specific fluid and electrolyte therapy. Similarly, changes in blood volume are unpredictable and usually transient. After fresh water aspiration, there may be a rapid absorption from the lungs into the circulation with a transient increase in blood volume.

Hemoglobin and hematocrit are usually within normal ranges in victims of near-drowning in either fresh or sea water. Hemolysis does occur after aspiration of large quantities of fresh water, especially when combined with hypoxia, but seldom to a degree that necessitates specific therapy. Coagulopathies may occur in the severely asphyxiated.

Pathology. Post-mortem changes after drowning are nonspecific. Cutis anserina (goose flesh), water-wrinkling of the skin of the hands and feet, pale or sanguineous water foam from the nose and mouth, and vomitus and aquatic debris in the respiratory tract are common. The lungs may be hyperinflated and irregularly congested. Microscopic sections show varying degrees of alveolar distention, edematous protein precipitate, infiltrates, and focal intra-alveolar hemorrhage. The brain appears swollen and its microscopic appearance after near-drowning with delayed death varies with the degree and duration of anoxia. With early death, edema and anoxic perivascular hemorrhages may be the only changes. With prolonged and severe hypoxia, the changes may progress to cystic degeneration of the basal ganglia or midbrain. The liver, spleen, and kidneys appear congested, and the stomach may contain swallowed fluid.

Clinical Manifestations. Severe cardiovascular changes such as tachycardia, bradycardia, and cardiac standstill are rare after resuscitation and are usually related to the effects of hypoxia and acidosis on the myocardium. Pulmonary edema, decreased cardiac output, and hypotension also occasionally occur (Sec 5.46).

Submersion in cold water can result in hypothermia (body temperature $\leqq 30°$ C) which may decrease metabolic oxygen requirements by as much as 50%. Below 28° C arrhythmias, including ventricular fibrillation, are common. Preferential perfusion to the brain and heart, bradycardia, and decreased peripheral perfusion (the "diving reflex") may be protective during hypothermic submersion.

Central nervous system dysfunction may occur after near-drowning as the result of cerebral hypoxia, ischemia, or both. If cerebral edema develops, brain perfusion and cellular integrity may be further compromised.

Treatment. Immediate ventilation, oxygenation, and circulatory support are critical. If the victim is apneic when rescued, mouth-to-mouth ventilation should begin at once and be replaced as soon as possible with positive pressure ventilation. Closed chest cardiac massage should be added to ventilatory support if effective circulation is not present. Since occasional survival occurs without brain injury after prolonged submersion in cold water with resultant hypothermia, vigorous resuscitation is recommended for such patients even when vital signs are initially unobtainable. If a patient was diving into water, care must be taken to maintain the neck in a neutral position until cervical injury can be ruled out. All victims of near-drowning should be admitted to a hospital with cardiopulmonary resuscitation continued during transport. Patients with a history of significant submersion, even though asymptomatic, should be observed for at least 24 hr because of the risk of late development of pulmonary insufficiency. Intravenous administration of sodium bicarbonate may be indicated since severe metabolic acidosis commonly occurs in the near-drowned patient.

Subsequent intensive care should be suited to the condition of the patient. If the patient is *alert* with ventilation adequate to clear carbon dioxide, continuous positive airway pressure (CPAP) may be applied to the airway using a tight-fitting mask to increase functional residual capacity and prevent alveoli from collapsing to the completely airless state. A nasogastric tube should be inserted and the face observed for pressure points. The level of CPAP applied should be titrated to that level at which there is the least intrapulmonary shunt without deleterious effects on cardiovascular function. If hypovolemia is present, CPAP, particularly at high levels, may decrease cardiac output and increase the need for circulatory support. Just as CPAP is titrated to optimal levels, withdrawal from CPAP should be in decremental steps. Sudden discontinuation of CPAP or of routine suctioning may result in significant deterioration of oxygenation. If the patient cannot maintain a normal $PaCO_2$, respirations are labored, or PaO_2 does not significantly improve, the trachea should be intubated and intermittent mandatory ventilation (IMV) should be added at the rate determined by the arterial pH and pCO_2.

If the patient is *comatose*, intubation is necessary to protect the airway and to provide ventilatory support as indicated by the arterial blood gases. Maintaining a $PaCO_2$ of less than 30 torr and a PaO_2 of greater than 55 torr may diminish the development of cerebral edema. Inability of the patient to maintain an adequate arterial oxygen tension at inspired oxygen concentrations of less than 40% requires aggressive ventilatory therapy which may include mechanical ventilation with positive end-expiratory pressure (PEEP) and respiratory paralysis.

Nebulized isoproterenol, racemic epinephrine, or intravenous aminophylline may be useful if bronchospasm is present. Occasionally, diuretics may also be beneficial in mobilizing interstitial pulmonary edema, but they must be used cautiously in the hypovolemic patient. Inotropic agents may be necessary to maintain perfusion. Bronchoscopy is indicated only if food or solid material has been aspirated. Decompression of gastric dilatation with a nasogastric tube decreases the risk of regurgitation and aspiration and also may improve ventilation by decreasing intra-abdominal pressure. Prophylactic use of corticosteroids or of antibiotics is not recommended.

Only normal maintenance fluids are ordinarily required. However, with sea water aspiration, large amounts of protein may be lost through the lungs, and colloid replacement may be indicated. Pulmonary edema after aspiration of fresh or sea water may result in the loss of large volumes of fluid into the lung and require circulatory replacement. Pulmonary edema may also occur secondary to congestive heart failure and require fluid and pharmacologic management (Sec 13.66). Significant electrolyte imbalances, coagulopathy, or anemia should be appropriately diagnosed and corrected.

Near-drowning may precipitate multiorgan failure. Therefore, appropriate cardiopulmonary, renal, and central nervous system monitoring is required (Sec 5.41 and 5.46). It is important to remember that the initial chest roentgenogram may be relatively clear even in the face of extreme hypoxia, particularly after aspiration of fresh water. Atelectasis, shock lung, pneumothorax, and pneumomediastinum may occur. Associated injuries, such as those of the spinal cord and intracranial bleeding, also must be ruled out.

Intracranial pressure monitoring and treatment with hyperventilation, mannitol infusion, hypothermia, and barbiturates have been used to prevent subsequent anoxic and ischemic injury to the brain (Sec 21.6). The risks and benefits of the various treatment regimens advocated for the comatose near-drowned patient should be carefully and critically evaluated as no controlled studies of humans have documented the efficacy of the various treatment modalities.

Prognosis. The reported incidence of serious neurologic sequelae after near-drowning varies from 0–21%. There are no prospective studies, but retrospective studies suggest that those who are awake at the scene of rescue or unconscious at the scene and treated successfully with cardiopulmonary resuscitation so that they are fully awake on arrival at the emergency room did not suffer serious neurologic sequelae. The results seem similar in those patients with a blunted level of consciousness, e.g., lethargic, semi-comatose, agitated, confused, or combative, on arrival at the hospital. In these groups treatment consisted of cardiopulmonary support without aggressive cerebral resuscitation. In contrast, patients comatose on arrival at the hospital who received appropriate cardiopulmonary support have approximately 44% survival without brain damage whether treated only with mild hyperventilation and steroids or treated with aggressive hyperventilation, fluid restriction, hyperoxia, steroids, muscle paralysis, and barbiturate coma. Aggressive treatment may decrease morbidity and mortality in those with decerebrate or decorticate signs, but, in general, severe anoxic injury occurs in the flaccid comatose patient, in those submerged for more than 6 min, in patients requiring cardiopulmonary resuscitation in the emergency room, or in patients needing mechanical ventilation.

RICHARD E. BEHRMAN

Conn AW, Montes JE, Barker GA, et al: Cerebral salvage in near-drowning following neurological classification by triage. Can Anaesth Soc J 27:201, 1980.
Hoff BH: Multisystem failure: A review with special reference to drowning. Crit Care Med 7:210, 1979.
Modell JH: The Pathophysiology and Treatment of Drowning and Near-Drowning. Springfield, Ill, Charles C Thomas, 1971.
Modell JH, Graves SA, Kuck EJ: Near-drowning: Correlation of level of consciousness and survival. Can Anaesth Soc J 27:211, 1980.
Peterson B: Morbidity of childhood near-drowning. Pediatrics 59:364, 1977.

5.45   BURNS

Burns are due to the effects of thermal energy upon skin and other tissues. Tissue damage begins when the temperature reaches 44° C, and the rate of injury increases logarithmically as the tissue temperature rises. Burns are classified as 1st, 2nd, or 3rd degree according to the depth of tissue injured. *First degree burns*, such as sunburns, involve only the epithelium. *Second degree burns* destroy the epithelium and part of the corium but spare dermal appendages, from which re-epithelialization may occur. In *3rd degree burns* the entire thickness of the dermis is destroyed; re-epithelialization is consequently restricted to the periphery of the lesions. Burns covering less than 15% of the body surface may be of no major consequence unless they involve key areas such as the hands or face or flexural regions. Morbidity and mortality increase with increasing extent and degree of burn.

Incidence. Approximately 2,000,000 people receive medical attention, 100,000 are hospitalized, and 7800 die each year in the United States because of burn injuries. The death rate from fire in this country is the 2nd highest in the world and by far the highest among industrialized nations. Burns are the 2nd leading cause of nonvehicular accidental deaths; 30% of these deaths occur in children under 15 yr of age. Among children aged 1–4 yr, burns are the leading cause of accidental death in the home and 2nd only to vehicular injuries overall. Among children 5–14 yr old, burns are the 3rd leading cause of accidental deaths.

Etiology. The young, the elderly, and those in disadvantaged socioeconomic groups are particularly vulnerable to burns. Nearly all burns in children occur in the home during waking hours. The major vectors of heat energy are hot liquids and solids and materials such as flammable fabrics, volatile flammable liquids, and domestic dwellings. Combustible materials are most commonly ignited by matches, poorly guarded space heaters, kitchen ranges, or water heaters. Scalds are the leading cause of burn injuries in the 1st 3 yr of life and are usually limited to small areas. Chemical burns are rare and usually benign, with the exception of those involving the esophagus. Electrical burns are uncommon but may be devastating. Burns due to the ignition of combustible materials are most common after infancy, and the resultant injuries are usually large and life-threatening.

Prevention. Appropriate strategies to prevent burns by controlling the sources and expenditure of energy are outlined in Table 5–24. Prevention of burns requires (1) education of the public regarding potential risks and their avoidance, (2) regulation of product safety, and (3) technologic advances in attenuation of the vectors of heat energy and their ignitors. The physician has a major responsibility in educating parents and in encouraging appropriate legislative controls. For example, physicians strongly supported the federal regulation of flammability of children's sleepwear that reduced considerably the hazard of burn injury from flammable garments.

Pathophysiology. Hemodynamic, autonomic, cardiopulmonary, renal, and metabolic disturbances develop rapidly following severe burns. Within seconds of the injury, cardiac output falls, presumably because of exaggerated reflex responses and decreased venous return. Myocardial contractility does not seem to be

Table 5–24   PREVENTION OF TRAUMA, ADAPTED TO BURN INJURIES

GENERAL PRINCIPLES	EXAMPLES OF APPLICATION TO BURNS
Prevent marshaling of latent energy	Do not store gasoline in the home
Reduce the amount of marshaled energy	Reduce temperature of bath or shower water
Modify the rate at which energy can propagate	Use flame-retardant fabrics
Separate in time or space the energy from the susceptible structure	Locate water heaters away from flammable liquids
Separate by interposition of a barrier	Use safeguards for space heaters
Strengthen the structure that might be damaged by energy	Apply more stringent building and fireproofing codes
Detect the danger and counter its rapid continuation and extension	Use fire alarms, sprinkler systems, fire extinguishers

Table 5–25 PRIORITIES OF MEDICAL PROCEDURES IN THE EMERGENCY PHASE OF BURN INJURIES

PROCEDURE	INDICATION	COMMENT
Establish an adequate airway	Burns of the face Laryngeal edema Smoke inhalation Explosions	Avoid emergency tracheostomy
Examine for trauma to head, skeleton, or nervous system		Remove clothing; radiologic examination helpful
Begin intravenous infusion	To prevent intravascular dehydration	Use isotonic fluids
Empty stomach through a nasogastric tube	To prevent gastric dilatation, vomiting, or aspiration	Antacids may be helpful
Insert an indwelling urinary catheter	To monitor hourly urine output	Use a closed drainage system
Examine the burn wound	To estimate depth and extent	Use burn charts corrected for age
Clean, debride, and dress the burn area	To minimize microbial colonization	Use topical antimicrobial therapy
Medications	To treat infections; to prevent tetanus; for sedation	Use intravenous route for sedation
Begin fluid, electrolyte, and protein replacement	To correct antecedent deficits and concurrent losses	Use appropriate formula to estimate requirements

affected at this time. A plasma factor which depresses myocardial contractility has been isolated during the latter stages of shock from severely burned animals and humans, but its nature and role are poorly understood.

Soon after the injury the permeability of the entire vascular tree increases; as a result, water, electrolytes, and proteins are lost from the vascular compartment into interstitial tissues of injured and noninjured sites. These losses are maximal during the 1st 12 hr after injury and may amount to as much as one third of the blood volume. During the 1st 4 days as much as 2 plasma pools of albumin may be lost; thus, deficiencies of albumin and other plasma proteins are common.

Within minutes following a substantial burn, renal plasma flow and glomerular filtration rate are decreased. Severe oliguria may develop, and tubular function is at least transiently compromised. Increased secretion of antidiuretic hormone and aldosterone further contributes to reduction in urine formation; tubular reabsorption of sodium is stimulated, excretion of potassium is enhanced, and the urine is maximally concentrated. This antidiuresis is most prominent during the 1st 12–24 hr after the burn, but it may persist for several days.

Destruction of red blood cells in the period immediately after a burn seldom exceeds 10% of circulating erythrocytes. Additional losses may occur, however, in the ensuing days, as partly damaged cells are lysed and blood is lost from granulation tissues. For these and other reasons, anemia is likely to develop within 4–7 days of major burn injuries.

Emergency Management of Severe Burns. It is imperative that care be administered in an orderly fashion (Table 5–25). First, the adequacy of the airway must be established, especially in a child with facial burns or one who has inhaled smoke. Then, a rapid assessment is made, which includes (1) inspection of wounds, (2) evaluation of the cardiorespiratory status, and (3) determination of previously recognized injuries. An intravenous infusion is established through which isotonic fluids are given to expand the blood volume. Lactated Ringer solution, isotonic saline, or plasma may be infused at a rate of 20 ml/kg/hr until more accurate estimates of fluid requirements are made.

The stomach is emptied with a nasogastric tube to prevent gastric dilatation or vomiting. Before the tube is withdrawn, a small quantity of antacid is instilled to retard the development of stress ulcers. A urinary catheter is then inserted so that output can be monitored.

Since the quantities of fluids and medications to be administered depend upon the size of the patient and the extent of injury, the weight and length should be measured carefully, and the areas of the total body surface and the burned surface should be ascertained. Weight is measured before dressings, bedclothing, or restraints are applied, and afterward as well. The wounds are cleansed and debrided, their depth assessed, and the extent of 2nd and 3rd degree burns estimated by using body surface charts corrected for age (Fig 5–16). Then the wounds are covered with dressings saturated with an antimicrobial agent. In addition, circumferential 3rd degree burns must be recognized and escharotomies performed to prevent ischemia of extremities or respiratory embarrassment resulting from chest wall involvement.

Sedatives may be given if there are no injuries to the central nervous system, preferably via the intravenous route. Respiratory depressants should be avoided. Tetanus prophylaxis is given and penicillin administered parenterally to prevent β-hemolytic streptococcal infections.

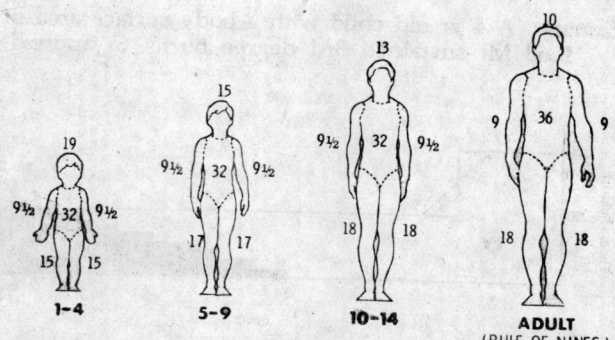

Figure 5–16 Burn assessment chart. (Body proportions modified from Lund and Brower.) Numbers under the figures indicate age; the others indicate % of body surface.

Fluid, Electrolyte, and Colloid Therapy. During the 1st 24 hr after a burn, the objectives of fluid therapy are (1) to correct hypovolemia; (2) to maintain the vascular volume; (3) to prevent abnormalities in plasma electrolytes, protein, or pH; and (4) to minimize edema. During this time errors in fluid therapy may have grave consequences. Underhydration can prolong the state of shock, worsen metabolic acidosis, and induce renal insufficiency; overhydration fosters edema formation and pulmonary congestion. At the same time, accurate prediction of fluid requirements is especially difficult since most formulas for fluid therapy of victims of burns were designed for adults (e.g., Evans, Brooke, and Parkland formulas) and their estimates of needed fluids are based solely on body weight and percentage of body surface burned. Consequently, they are not appropriate for burned children, particularly those with large burns and at the extremes of weight for age.

Repeated calculation of fluid needs in the 1st 24 hr is important. Compared with adults, children, particularly infants, have high rates of heat exchange relative to size and weight, high rates of water exchange in relation to total body water, and significant differences in muscle water and electrolyte composition. Children also require relatively larger volumes of urine for excretion of waste products, and insensible water losses, when expressed in terms of body weight, are significantly greater than in adults. Therefore, calculation of fluid and electrolyte requirements on the basis of body surface offers greater accuracy, consistency, and simplicity. The application of these concepts to the management of the burned child has led to the design of the formula for fluid replacement and maintenance that we currently recommend. The quantity of fluids to administer during the 1st 24 hr after the burn is estimated as follows:

$$2000 \text{ ml/M}^2 \text{ of body surface/24 hr}$$
plus
$$5000 \text{ ml/M}^2 \text{ of } burned \text{ body surface/24 hr}$$

Half this amount is administered during the 1st 8 hr and the other half during the subsequent 16 hr (Fig 5–17). No ceiling for size of the burn is used.

Fluids received prior to arrival at a center for definitive care must be reviewed and consideration given to adjusting the amounts of fluids administered subsequently.

Example. A 4 yr old child with a body surface area of 0.68 M^2 sustained 3rd degree burns to approximately 40% of his body surface. Despite having received 200 ml of lactated Ringer solution during the 1st hr, he appeared dehydrated on admission.

Comment. (1) Fluids received during the initial evaluation period (lactated Ringer, saline, or plasma) need not be included in the calculation of requirements for the 1st 24 hr. These fluids may be given at a rate of approximately 20 ml/kg/hr for 1–2 hr.

(2) Calculation of 1st 24 hr requirements:
$$2000 \text{ ml/M}^2 \text{ of body surface/24 hr}$$
Example.
$$2000 \times 0.68 = 1360 \text{ ml/24 hr}$$
plus
$$5000 \text{ ml/M}^2 \text{ of body surface burned/24 hr}$$
Example.
$$5000 \times 0.68 \times 0.4 = 1360 \text{ ml/24 hr}$$
Total requirement for 1st 24 hr (maintenance plus burn replacement) is 1360 ml + 1360 ml = 2720 ml.

(3) Half of the estimated amount is given during the 1st 8 hr and half during the subsequent 16 hr.
Example.
First 8 hr = 170 ml/hr
Second 8 hr = 85 ml/hr
Third 8 hr = 85 ml/hr

Although this surface area method offers definite advantages in children, it still provides only reasonable estimates of the quantities of fluid needed for the 1st 24 hr. Successful fluid resuscitation of the burned child requires not only use of an appropriate formula but also clear understanding of the fluid therapy program as a whole; this should include:

(a) Burn charts, properly corrected for age, to assess the extent of the injury (Fig 5–16).
(b) Careful measurement of height and weight to calculate surface area from standard nomograms (see Fig 29–1 and 29–2).
(c) Accurate prediction of fluid requirements using the surface area formula.
(d) Appropriate hydrating solutions.
(e) Well-defined guidelines to monitor the state of hydration.

Choice of Hydrating Solutions. The composition of fluids to be used is controversial; some recommend protein-free electrolyte solutions only. We recommend the use of isotonic solutions containing albumin, either lactate or bicarbonate, and adequate quantities of car-

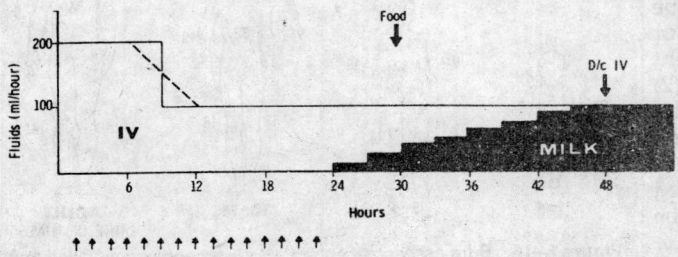

Figure 5–17 Graphic description of the fluid resuscitation program at the Shriners Burns Institute (Galveston Unit) to hydrate burned children. Half of the estimated fluid for the 1st day is given intravenously over the first 8 hr and the other half during the subsequent 16 hr. Oral fluids (milk) are begun during the 2nd day. After the first 8 hr, hourly fluid intake (intravenous and oral) remains constant. Only antacids are given orally during the first 24 hr. (IV, intravenous; D/c, discontinue.)

bohydrate (as 5% glucose) to provide a protein-sparing effect.

The addition of 12.5 gm of salt-poor albumin (50 ml of 25% solution) to 950 ml of lactated Ringer in 5% dextrose and water makes a suitable solution. Likewise, an electrolyte-protein mixture similar to the one proposed by Stone is appropriate; 1 l of this solution is prepared by mixing 920 ml of 5% glucose in 0.45% sodium chloride solution (77 mEq/l), 10 ml of hypertonic sodium chloride (3 mEq/ml), 20 ml of $NaHCO_3$ (1 mEq/ml), and 50 ml of 25% human serum albumin (salt-poor). The final composition of the mixture is as follows:

Na	127 mEq/l
Cl	107 mEq/l
HCO_3	20 mEq/l
Glucose	44 gm/l
Albumin	1.25 gm/dl

While this solution may be more effective in counteracting the metabolic acidosis of severely burned patients, a solution containing lactate instead of bicarbonate is quite adequate for burn injuries extending up to 70–75% of the body surface, and it is easier to prepare.

For burned children under 1 yr of age, the sodium concentration of any of the above solutions is greater than desirable; a more appropriate solution can be prepared by mixing 930 ml of 5% glucose in 0.3% sodium chloride solution, 20 ml of $NaHCO_3$ (1 mEq/ml), and 50 ml of 25% human serum albumin (salt-poor). The final composition of this mixture is as follows:

Na	79 mEq/l
Cl	52 mEq/l
HCO_3	20 mEq/l
Glucose	45 gm/l
Albumin	1.25 gm/dl

Potassium is not added during the 1st 24 hr since large amounts of this ion are released from injured cells into the extracellular fluids and acidosis and renal failure may result in dangerous hyperkalemia. After the 1st day, depending upon the blood urea nitrogen level, urine output, and condition of the patient, 20–30 mEq of potassium as the phosphate may be added to each liter of intravenous fluid.

The advantages of using composite burn solutions are (1) only 1 type of solution is required; (2) fluid, electrolyte, and protein are administered simultaneously; and (3) only the rate of the infusion may need adjustment. No oral fluids other than ice chips should be given for the 1st 24 hr; during this time, absorption of fluid and electrolytes from the gastrointestinal tract is unpredictable, and paralytic ileus and vomiting may develop. Antacids (Maalox, 20 ml/M^2 of body surface/hr) are administered orally to decrease the incidence of stress ulcers (Fig 5–17).

Monitoring Hydration Therapy. No one criterion suffices to guide adjustment of fluid therapy. Since renal function and antidiuretic hormone (ADH) secretion in burned patients are modified by factors other than blood volume, urine output may not adequately reflect the state of hydration. Extreme oliguria, how-

ever, usually does not occur unless there is renal damage or severe dehydration. The urine output usually varies considerably from hour to hour, but, ordinarily, 20–30 ml of urine/M^2 of body surface is produced hourly during the 1st 24 hr. Attempts to increase urine output beyond these limits usually cause increased peripheral edema and/or pulmonary edema. The state of hydration is better judged by frequent periodic assessment of the sensorium, pulse, blood pressure, venous capillary filling, body weight, hematocrit, BUN, and serum and urine electrolytes and osmolality rather than by urine output. Invasive techniques to measure other variables (e.g., cardiac output, central venous pressure) are usually unnecessary.

Calculation of Fluid Needs After the First 24 Hours. Fluid requirements for the 2nd and subsequent days usually average three fourths of the 1st day's allowance and may be estimated with the following formula:

$$1500 \text{ ml/M}^2 \text{ of body surface/24 hr}$$
$$plus$$
$$3750 \text{ ml/M}^2 \text{ of body surface } burned/24 \text{ hr}$$

From the 2nd day on, fluids are administered at a continuous rate. The hourly allowance should not be exceeded whether the oral and/or intravenous route is utilized. By the end of the 1st 24 hr, antacids are discontinued and homogenized milk is offered instead. Milk feedings are begun in small amounts and, if tolerated, they are progressively increased; intravenous fluids are reduced correspondingly (Fig 5–17). A soft diet is usually tolerated by the 2nd–3rd day.

During the next several weeks (subacute phase), the child is supported medically to facilitate the healing of 2nd degree burns and the autografting of 3rd degree burns. Management includes daily irrigation of wounds with antiseptic solutions, debridement of the wounds, topical antimicrobial therapy, splinting of affected parts, and other indicated surgical procedures. Body weight, serum electrolytes, plasma proteins, hematocrit, and hemoglobin should be monitored to detect any developing fluid or electrolyte disturbance, hypoalbuminemia, or anemia. Serum albumin levels should be maintained above 2 gm/dl and oncotic pressure above 15 mm Hg to prevent edema. This may be accomplished by infusing human serum albumin as a 5% solution over 12–24 hr. The usual quantity of human serum albumin needed to maintain the above serum level varies between 100–150 gm/M^2 of burned body surface per week, in 3 divided doses.

Blood lost as a direct result of the injury, or complications thereof, needs to be replaced during the 2nd–5th day after the burn, depending on its severity. Except in the patient with active bleeding or severe concomitant hypoproteinemia, transfusions of packed red blood cells are safer than whole blood and better tolerated. In most cases, packed cells in the amount of 10 ml/kg, given over a 3–4 hr period, are sufficient. Though transfusions may be needed at intervals of 3–4 days, quantities of blood in excess of 15 ml/kg should not be given within a 24 hr period unless the patient is actively bleeding. Giving packed cells in larger quantities frequently results in cardiopulmonary congestion and/or dangerous hypertension.

Caloric Requirements. Trauma usually increases basal energy expenditures. In burns this is accentuated by the calories spent in the evaporation of water from the wounds. Evaporative water losses may be estimated as 4000 ml/M^2 of burn area, and the caloric expenditure may be calculated by multiplying the evaporative water loss by 0.576, the number of kilocalories required to evaporate 1 ml of water. These increased caloric demands are usually met by oral feedings of milk and a well balanced diet, but nasogastric feedings may be necessary.

Example. A 4 yr old child has a surface area of 0.68 M^2 and 3rd degree burns over 40% of the body surface. The daily caloric requirements are estimated as follows: Surface area burned = 0.68 M^2 × 0.40 = 0.27 M^2

Evaporative water loss = 4 l/M^2 burn/24 hr = 4000 × 0.27 = 1080 ml/24 hr

Calories for evaporation = 0.576 kcal/ml × 1080 ml/24 hr = 622 kcal/24 hr

Daily caloric requirement for age = 1400 kcal
Calories required for evaporation = 622 kcal
Total daily caloric requirement = 2022 cal

Using the above calculations we have developed a simple formula to estimate caloric requirements in burned children:

$$2200 \text{ kcal/M}^2 \text{ burn/24 hr}$$
$$+$$
$$1800 \text{ kcal/M}^2 \text{ of body surface/24 hr}$$

Cardiovascular Complications. With appropriate fluid therapy, cardiac output usually returns to normal in 24–48 hr. The cause of persistent cardiac dysfunction in burns is unknown but may involve a circulating substance, presumably of pancreatic origin with a molecular weight of less than 1000, which has been reported in patients severely burned or with septic shock. This myocardial depressant factor (MDF) decreases myocardial contractility and reduces cardiac output. Burned children are prone to congestive failure and pulmonary edema during septic shock or renal failure. In addition to digitalis, diuretic agents (e.g., furosemide) may be required, and in extreme cases phlebotomy or peritoneal dialysis may be necessary. The development of overt congestive failure in burned children and septic patients can be prevented by cautious hydration; at present we maintain our patients slightly underhydrated.

Pulmonary Complications. Respiratory problems are common, particularly with smoke inhalation or facial burns. Phillips and Cope found that pulmonary lesions contributed to or were directly responsible for 80% of burn deaths (Sec 5.43). The most common respiratory problems are pulmonary edema, tracheobronchitis, bronchopneumonia, and the alveolar–capillary block syndrome. Moreover, poisoning by inhalation of toxic gases, such as carbon monoxide, may occur in burns. The management of these problems may require the participation of an expert respiratory therapist.

Renal Complications. Severe oliguria during the immediate postburn period is most likely the result of ADH secretion and a reduction in glomerular filtration rate, but the possibility of renal damage should not be discarded until normal renal function is evidenced. For example, in the presence of oliguria, the failure of the urine to become concentrated or to show conservation of sodium is indicative of renal dysfunction.

Renal failure in burns may be transient, in association with acute hypovolemia or shock, or persistent. With persistent azotemia the patient may or may not be oliguric. The prognosis for oliguric azotemia is extremely poor, but with adequate support recovery may occur. Recognition of nonoliguric renal failure is important since an adequate urine output may mask the fact that the urine volume is fixed; water and sodium are retained, and hypervolemia and congestive heart failure may develop. If, on the other hand, the condition is promptly recognized, appropriate restrictions of water, salt, and protein intake will usually sustain relatively normal fluid balance and allow for recovery of renal function. When renal failure, particularly of the oliguric type, complicates burns, peritoneal dialysis or hemodialysis is often required.

Infection. Sepsis is a leading cause of death in burned children. Besides the loss of the protective skin barrier, additional defects in host resistance such as deficiencies in thymic-dependent lymphocytes, in phagocytic function, in complement, and in macrophage activation may predispose the patient to infection for some weeks. Serum levels of immunoglobulins fall in the 1st wk because of loss of plasma into the interstitium, but antibody formation is spared. The infecting organisms vary with exposure, but the principal pathogens are *Staphylococcus aureus* and gram-negative bacteria such as *Psuedomonas aeruginosa*. The main portals of entry are the wound, the respiratory tract, the urinary tract, intravenous catheters, and possibly the gastrointestinal tract. Successful treatment of sepsis depends upon early diagnosis and prompt use of parenteral antibiotic therapy. No clinical signs are pathognomonic of sepsis. The diagnosis must be suspected when there is (1) wound infection, (2) hyper- or hypothermia, (3) tachypnea, (4) conspicuous leukocytosis or leukopenia, (5) thrombocytopenia, (6) sudden change in sensorium, (7) ileus, or (8) arterial hypotension.

With such findings, blood and other appropriate cultures are obtained and antibiotic therapy is begun. The bacteriologic history of the patient must be reviewed in order to choose the most appropriate antibiotic, but in most cases a combination of tobramycin and a penicillinase-resistant penicillin (oxacillin, dicloxacillin, methicillin) is adequate. Both drugs must be administered in maximal therapeutic doses and continued for a minimum of 2 wk. Whenever possible, therapy should be adjusted on the basis of in vitro antibiotic sensitivity tests, serum antibiotic levels, and assessment of the minimal inhibitory concentrations of the antibiotics in use.

The condition of burned children who are septic is unstable. It may change from one hour to another, and vascular collapse may lead to death within a few hours. Fluctuating body temperature, profuse sweating, anxiety, clouded sensorium, changes in vital signs, blood pressure, and urine output should be considered incipient signs of "septic shock." If no improvement occurs following institution of initial antibiotic therapy, carbenicillin and steroids (prednisolone) should be added. The usual amount of the latter is 40 mg/kg as a single intravenous dose.

It is important to recognize that the effects of endotoxemia are multiple and that both renal and cardiovascular functions are usually compromised. Therefore, fluid management should be conservative; a reasonable objective is to maintain the blood pressure just above shock levels and minimal urine output. Isotonic fluids containing albumin may be used initially, but subsequently, lower concentrations of sodium solutions should be administered. The cautious use of sympathomimetic amines (isoproterenol, dopamine) and digitalis is recommended to maintain blood pressure and avoid the administration of excessive quantities of fluids.

Rehabilitation. Since the physical and psychologic effects of burns are potentially crippling, a vigorous rehabilitation program to counter these effects should be instituted as soon as possible. Residual deformities or loss of function may greatly impair the child's body image and self-esteem, and prolonged hospitalization may lead to a dependency reaction which extends beyond the period of confinement. The child or parents may harbor guilt feelings about the injury. In the parents such feelings tend to interfere with their ability to cope with the illness of the child; the early facing of these issues with the child and family may, therefore, be essential. This may require the efforts of a mental health professional and social worker. To be effective, any program of emotional support should be closely coordinated with medical, nursing, and surgical procedures and other essential rehabilitative measures, including physical therapy, play therapy, and continuation of schoolwork.

Plans should be made to return the child to as normal a home life as possible. The parents and the child are instructed in home care procedures such as wound dressing, splints, pressure dressings, and physical therapy. These measures are particularly important in reducing hypertrophic scars. The child should return to school and other social activities as soon as possible. In most circumstances this is feasible within the 1st wk after the end of the hospitalization. The continuing rehabilitation of the child will involve the cooperative efforts of the family physician, physical therapist, mental health professional, and reconstructive surgeon. Their procedures should be planned so that they will interfere as little as possible with the child's schoolwork and other normal social activities.

HUGO F. CARVAJAL
ARMOND S. GOLDMAN

Artz CP: The Brooke formula. In: Contemporary Burn Management. Boston, Little, Brown, 1971.
Artz CP, Moncrief JA: The Treatment of Burns. Ed 2. Philadelphia, WB Saunders, 1969.
Baxter CR, Moncrief JA, Prager MH, et al: A circulating myocardial depressant factor in burn shock. In: Matter P, Barclay TL, Kowicfova S (eds): Research in Burns. Transactions of Third International Congress on Research in Burns, Prague. Bern, Hans Huber Publishers, 1971.
Berman W Jr, Goldman AS, Reichelderfer T, et al: Childhood burn injuries and deaths. Pediatrics 51:1069, 1973.
Brouhard BH, Carvajal HF, Linares HA: Burn edema and protein leakage in the rat. I. Relationship to time of injury. Microvasc Res 15:221, 1978.
Carvajal HF, Linares HA, Brouhard BH: Relationship of burn size to vascular permeability changes in rats. Surg Gynecol Obstet 149(2):193, 1979.
Carvajal HF: A physiologic approach to fluid therapy in severely burned children. Surg Gynecol Obstet 150:379, 1980.
Carvajal HF: Acute management of burns in children. South Med J 68:129, 1975.
Carvajal HF, Reinhart JA, Traber DL: Renal and cardiovascular functional response to thermal injury in dogs subjected to sympathetic blockade. Circ Shock 3:287, 1976.
Dubois J: Water and electrolyte content of human skeletal muscle—variations with age. Rev Europ Etudes Clin Biol 17:505, 1972.
Eagle JF: Parenteral fluid therapy of burns during the first 48 hours. NY J Med 66:1613, 1956.
Gump FE, Kinney JM: Energy balance and weight loss in burned patients. Arch Surg 103:442, 1971.
Haddon W Jr: On the escape of tigers: An ecologic note. Technology Review 72 (No 7), May, 1970.
Hutcher N, Haynes BW Jr: The Evans formula revisited. J Trauma 12:453, 1972.
Innes RL, Goldman AS, Schmitt R, et al: A study of the etiology and epidemiology of burn injuries in children. In: Matter P, Barclay TL, Kowicfova S (eds): Research in Burns. Transactions of the Third International Congress on Research in Burns, Prague. Bern, Hans Huber Publishers, 1971.
Metcoff J, et al: Losses and physiologic requirements for water and electrolytes after extensive burns in children. N Engl J Med 265:101, 1961.
Monafo WW: The treatment of burn shock by the intravenous and oral administration of hypertonic lactated saline solution. J Trauma 10:575, 1970.
Moncrief JA: Burns. N Engl J Med 288:444, 1973.
Phillips AW, Cope O: The revelation of respiratory tract damage as a principal killer of the burned patient. Ann Surg 155:1, 1962.
Shook CW, MacMillan BC, Altemeier WA: Pulmonary complications of the burned patient. Arch Surg 97:215, 1968.
Stoll AM, Chianta MA: Heat transfer through fabrics as related to thermal injury. Trans NY Acad Sci 33:649, 1971.
Stone HH: The composite burn solution. In: Polk HC Jr, Stone HH (eds): Contemporary Burn Management. Boston, Little, Brown, 1971.

5.46 SHOCK SYNDROMES

Shock is a syndrome of circulatory insufficiency which can be caused by a variety of illnesses and may present with prostration, hypotension, pallor, diaphoresis, cool skin, and oliguria. The inadequate blood flow can lead to hypoxia, acidosis, and death. The circulatory abnormalities are dynamic and evolve with time; careful, often invasive, physiologic monitoring is necessary to evaluate and treat the specific hemodynamic, respiratory, and metabolic abnormalities.

Etiology. Hypovolemia secondary to dehydration or hemorrhage is the most common cause of shock in pediatric patients. Cardiogenic shock, failure of the pumping action of the myocardium, has increased in frequency; it may follow open heart surgery or occur secondary to myocarditis, life-threatening arrhythmias, and advanced septic shock. Septic (endotoxic) shock often occurs in children requiring immunosuppression. Although gram-negative enteric bacilli and the meningococcus have been the chief pathogens in septic shock, the gram-positive cocci, such as the group B streptococcus, the pneumococcus, and *Staphylococcus aureus* have assumed increasing importance. Sudden vascular collapse occurs infrequently secondary to hypersensitivity reactions or anaphylaxis, central nervous system injuries, endocrine failure, such as adrenocortical insufficiency, and mechanical obstruction to the circulation by cardiac compression, pericardial tamponade, or pulmonary embolism.

Pathophysiology.   The basic defect in all shock states is inadequate blood supply to tissues; this may be produced by loss of blood or fluid or by myocardial depression with resultant pump failure and low cardiac output. Septic shock results from a complex interaction of endotoxin with the cardiovascular, hematologic, and metabolic systems.

Despite the different mechanisms producing circulatory insufficiency, certain common early cardiorespiratory adjustments occur in most patients in shock and begin immediately after the precipitating insult. There is an outpouring of catecholamines which increase heart rate, myocardial contractility, and myocardial oxygen consumption as well as cause vasoconstriction and enhanced alveolar ventilation. This early phase may be undetected because of minimal or absent hypotension. For example, in hypovolemic shock intense arteriolar and venular constriction will shift interstitial fluid into the circulatory volume; provided the volume loss is not overwhelming, hypotension and reduced cardiac output may be avoided. In cardiogenic shock, the myocardium cannot significantly improve its performance; thus the effect of sympathetic activity is usually intense vasoconstriction but little increase in cardiac output. The vasoconstriction may even be detrimental by increasing the workload of the myocardium. In early septic shock, when the myocardium is normal and fluid loss is absent, there is enhanced peripheral perfusion, often termed "hot shock" because of the increased cardiac output without perfusion failure.

The subsequent phase of shock is characterized by uneven organ and microcirculatory blood flow; flow is preferentially diverted to the brain and heart at the expense of the kidney, gastrointestinal tract, liver, and skin. If ischemia occurs, there may be hypoxia, acidosis, and cellular injury; lactic acid and other metabolic products from injured tissues accumulate. Late in this stage, the precapillary blood vessels no longer respond to vasoconstriction and their fluid is lost from the plasma into the interstitial space.

In endotoxic shock it is probable that the polysaccharide component of endotoxin (a lipid-polysaccharide-peptide macromolecule found in the outer layers of the bacterial cell wall) will activate the complement system, which leads to leukocyte and platelet aggregation and the release of vasoactive amines, including histamine, serotonin, and kinins. Blood pressure decreases secondary to diminished peripheral arterial resistance and an increased venous tone with a substantial portion of the total volume of fluid pooling in the venous capacitance vessels. Some capillary bed arteriovenous shunting is also promoted so that the capillary beds of many tissues are bypassed and the "effective circulating blood volume" is reduced.

During shock the pulmonary capillary is particularly sensitive to injury resulting in leakage of water, electrolytes, and protein into the interstitium and alveolar space. A ventilation-perfusion abnormality follows, which further complicates shock by accentuating hypoxia, reducing pulmonary compliance, and increasing the work of breathing. This syndrome has been termed "shock lung" or **adult respiratory distress syndrome** (ARDS). The capillary leakage may also result from the action of endotoxin on the pulmonary capillary or from a series of reactions involving the complement cascade, neutrophil aggregation, the coagulation system, and lung prostaglandins in acute endothelial injury. Intense systemic vasoconstriction may cause capillary leakage by forcing volume into the pulmonary circulation.

Diffuse intravascular coagulation (DIC) may also occur during shock and reduce nutrient blood flow to tissues (Sec 14.6).

The later stages of shock are a reflection of tissue ischemia and persistent anaerobic metabolism. Inadequate oxygenation eventually leads to irreversible damage of mitochondria and disruption of cell membranes. Cardiac function, generally adequate early in hypovolemic and septic shock, becomes compromised as the acidosis and hypotension persist. Coronary circulation receives two thirds of its blood flow during diastole; tachycardia and prolonged hypotension reduce this diastolic flow. Myocardial ischemia may be of such severity as to produce areas of endocardial infarction. Patients with cardiogenic shock generally tolerate little additional stress and may expire with moderate hypotension.

Central nervous system blood flow is normally about 15% of the cardiac output, and the brain tolerates any degree of hypoxia very poorly. Initially, the brain may reflexly preserve its blood flow in the face of moderate reduction in cardiac output, but with persistent hypotension and diminished cardiac output, cerebral anoxia and death ensue.

Clinical Manifestations.   Most patients with septic or cardiogenic shock have a history of significant antecedent illness or open heart surgery. In hypovolemic shock there is often a history of vomiting, diarrhea, gastrointestinal bleeding, or trauma.

There are signs of increased sympathetic activity such as cool, mottled, or moist skin, tachycardia, diaphoresis, and apprehension. Cold lower extremities suggest diminished perfusion. Blood pressure may be difficult to record because of intense vasoconstriction. In early shock hypotension may be absent or minimal, especially in patients who are bacteremic. Fever, petechiae, and ecchymoses generally suggest bacteremia. Profound hypothermia may occur as a late manifestation of any form of shock. Patients with septic shock often have edema of the extremities in contrast to hypovolemic patients, who may have loss of skin turgor and dry mucous membranes. There may be signs of intra-abdominal hemorrhage, pulmonary edema, myocardial dysfunction, or abnormalities of the central nervous system.

Monitoring and Laboratory Data.   The period from the onset of shock until death may be short, usually less than 48 hr. After a therapeutic decision has been made, it is essential to assess hemodynamic response

Table 5–26 DIRECT CIRCULATORY MEASUREMENTS

PARAMETER	NORMAL VALUES (MM HG)
Aortic pressure	100/60
Mean arterial pressure (MAP)	75
Pulmonary arterial pressure:	
Systolic	20
Diastolic	10
Mean (MPAP)	15
Wedge (PAWP)	6–10
Left ventricular pressure:	
Systolic	100
End diastolic	8–10
Right ventricular pressure:	
Systolic	25
End diastolic	3–5
Right atrial pressure	3–5
Central venous pressure (CVP)	3–5

immediately. The ability to do so has been facilitated by the introduction of thermodilution techniques which measure cardiac output and flow-directed intravascular catheters which measure central venous, right atrial, pulmonary arterial, systolic, mean, and wedge pressures and calculate pulmonary vascular resistance (Tables 5–26 and 5–27). Such monitoring is recommended for children with suspected septic and cardiogenic shock. For those with hemorrhagic shock, a central venous pressure line may be adequate.

The pulmonary artery wedge pressure is an excellent indication of left ventricular filling status and a useful guide to fluid and inotrope therapy; the pulmonary artery diastolic pressure is satisfactory provided pulmonary hypertension is not present. In contrast, the central venous or right atrial pressure may not reflect left ventricular (end diastolic) filling pressure in patients with myocardial dysfunction, which may occur in septic or cardiogenic shock or in patients with shock lung.

A cannula should be inserted in the radial artery to monitor blood pressure, to calculate systemic vascular resistance, and to sample arterial blood gases. Although measuring of arterial blood gases is routine in the management of acid-base disorders, the importance of evaluating mixed venous blood gases deserves emphasis. An elevated mixed venous pO_2 or percentage hemoglobin saturation with a narrowed or decreased arteriovenous oxygen difference is observed early in septic

Table 5–27 DERIVED HEMODYNAMIC VARIABLES

PARAMETER	FORMULA	NORMAL VALUE
Cardiac index (CI)	$\dfrac{\text{Cardiac output}}{\text{Body surface area}}$	3–5 liter/min/M²
Systemic vascular resistance	$\dfrac{\text{MAP} - \text{CVP}}{\text{Cardiac index}}$	15–25 resistance units
Pulmonary vascular resistance	$\dfrac{\text{MPAP} - \text{PAWP}}{\text{Cardiac index}}$	1–3 resistance units
Stroke index	$\dfrac{\text{CI}}{\text{Heart rate}}$	30–50 ml/beat/M²

CI = cardiac index; for other abbreviations, see Table 5–26.

shock and reflects increased cardiac output with arteriovenous shunting. A decreased mixed venous pO_2 or percentage saturation with an increased arteriovenous difference reflects the low cardiac output state that exists with cardiogenic and advanced septic shock.

Measurement of urine output is indicated and generally requires a urinary catheter. Urine production should be at least 1 ml/kg/hr and, if maintained at this level, indicates adequate renal perfusion and cardiac output. Red blood cells and casts in the urine indicate renal injury. The BUN may be elevated following gastrointestinal bleeding, but a urine/serum nitrogen ratio of less than 20:1 or a fractional excretion of sodium greater than 3% suggests acute renal failure.

The monitoring of heart rate, blood pressure, temperature, and respiratory rate may have little prognostic importance unless severe derangements are present as they will not differentiate the normal patient from one in a compensated shock state. However, the greater the difference between rectal temperature and skin temperature, the poorer the peripheral perfusion. In general, a poor prognosis will occur with depressed cardiac output, hypothermia, increased pulmonary vascular resistance, and increased systemic vascular resistance.

Laboratory evaluation may be helpful. The serum potassium may increase with cellular damage or renal insufficiency, while the serum sodium decreases when cell membranes lose their integrity. Serum albumin leaks through damaged capillaries and should be kept at normal levels to maintain intravascular oncotic pressure and retard further capillary losses. Serum calcium (ionized calcium in particular) is often depressed in patients with shock and should be normalized to prevent further loss of cardiac contractility. Serum enzymes such as SGOT, SGPT, LDH, and amylase may be elevated because of hepatic and pancreatic involvement. Stool blood may reflect primary intestinal lesions, and bleeding may occur secondary to intestinal ischemia. Serum glucose levels may be elevated early as a result of adrenergic activity but decrease as glycogen stores are depleted. An elevated arterial lactic acid level results from poor perfusion and anaerobic metabolism. Hemoglobin levels should be followed to ensure adequate oxygen carrying capacity. The patient with suspected septic shock should have a complete bacteriologic workup. The CBC, platelet count, and clotting factors, such as prothrombin time, partial thromboplastin time, and fibrinogen level, should be evaluated for evidence of intravascular coagulation. The electrocardiogram is commonly employed to monitor cardiac rhythm and electrical activity continuously. The chest roentgenogram with evidence of pulmonary edema should suggest the presence of the shock lung syndrome or congestive heart failure.

Treatment. The principles of therapy are (1) identification of the underlying disorders producing shock, (2) improvement of the cardiac output, and (3) relieving respiratory insufficiency. Therapy should be based on the monitored hemodynamic and blood gas parameters and titrated to attain optimal cardiorespiratory function.

Monitoring and treatment should be started as soon as the presence of early shock is suspected, but therapy beneficial in its earlier stages may subsequently lose effectiveness. The first priority is to control hemorrhage or fluid losses, restore the effective blood volume, and maintain adequate arterial pressures. A fluid push of 10 ml/kg should be given to patients with a central venous pressure less than 5–8 mm Hg and a pulmonary arterial wedge pressure less than 10 mm Hg. If no significant increase in pressure occurs, additional fluids should be administered until the central venous pressure is 10–12 mm Hg and the wedge pressure 16–18 mm Hg. Although these pressures are considered optimal ventricular filling conditions, each patient's response may vary depending on such factors as myocardial contractility, lung compliance, and level of respiratory support; serial cardiac output and blood pressure measurements performed during volume loading are necessary to determine the optimal cardiac filling pressures for each patient.

During early therapy, the administration of saline or Ringer lactate is acceptable to meet emergency volume needs. However, their effects are usually short-lived as fluid is quickly lost from the vascular into the interstitial space. This is especially true of patients with septic shock who have increased systemic and pulmonary capillary leakage and in whom aggressive therapy with excess crystalloids may produce serious pulmonary sequelae. Blood, plasma, or albumin should be employed for volume expansion when available. These colloids improve mean arterial pressure, cardiac output, oxygen consumption, and left ventricular stroke work to a far greater degree than crystalloids, and the benefits are prolonged. In advanced shock, however, even colloids may leak from the vascular space.

The response to fluids may unmask the presence of decreased myocardial contractility. An elevation in filling pressures without an increase in cardiac output indicates that the myocardium in depressed and inotropic support may be needed. Sympathomimetic amines are most commonly employed because of their rapid onset, ease of accurate dosage, and ultra-short half-lives (Table 5–28). *Isoproterenol* stimulates the beta-adrenergic receptors to produce a cardiac inotropic and chronotropic effect as well as dilatation of skeletal muscle vascular beds; it involves the risk of increasing myocardial oxygen consumption, reducing coronary blood flow, and predisposing to myocardial ischemia and arrhythmias. *Epinephrine* has the advantage of being strongly inotropic with a dose-dependent dual vascular effect: at lower dosage, its effect is to reduce systemic vascular resistance, while at higher dosage, increased resistance occurs. *Dopamine* is a precursor of norepinephrine and also activates the sympathetic receptors in a dose-dependent fashion. At very low dosage, its principal effect is renal and splanchnic vasodilatation with a reduction of systemic vascular resistance. At moderate doses, the inotropic effects occur, along with vasodilatation, while at larger doses, there is inotropy with vasoconstriction. *Dobutamine* is synthesized from isoproterenol. It has the unique action of being inotropic with little peripheral vascular effect and may be particularly helpful to patients with cardiogenic shock and an elevated peripheral vascular resistance. The high dose range of epinephrine and dopamine is recommended in the patient with septic shock and decreased systemic vascular resistance and hypotension. The use of digitalis to increase inotropy of patients in shock should be discouraged because of its slow onset of action and long half-life and the unstable electrolyte status and renal function of these patients.

Acidosis depresses myocardial function and interferes with the circulatory response to sympathomimetic amines. The pH should be maintained above 7.25 with sodium bicarbonate to ensure adequate response to these vasoactive amines. Persistent metabolic acidosis, despite therapy, indicates continued inadequate tissue perfusion and a poor prognosis. Calcium chloride should also be administered and may produce a positive inotropic response with increased blood pressure.

Myocardial failure coexists with elevated systemic vascular resistance in most patients with cardiogenic shock and many children in the later stages of septic shock. If the cardiac filling pressures are increased, with normal or elevated blood pressure and with depressed cardiac output, a vasodilator such as *sodium nitroprusside* should be employed for reduction of systemic vascular resistance. Adequate cardiac filling, supplemented by inotropic agents and/or afterload reduction, will improve cardiac performance unless irreversible myocardial damage has occurred.

Many patients with cardiogenic and septic shock require mechanical ventilation. It is indicated if the PaO_2 is less than 60–80 torr despite an enrichment of the inspired oxygen. Controlled ventilation will alleviate the patients' respiratory distress and reduce oxygen consumption. If extravasation of fluid has occurred into the alveolus or if shock lung is present, levels of positive end expiratory pressure (PEEP) of 10 cm H_2O or greater may be necessary. With very high PEEP levels (15 cm water or greater), the venous return may be impaired

Table 5–28 VASOACTIVE AGENTS

MEDICATION	DOSAGE (MICROGRAMS/KG/MIN)	ACTION
Isoproterenol	0.1–3	Tachycardia, increased contractility, vasodilatation
Epinephrine	0.1–1	Increased contractility, mild vasodilatation
	1–3	Increased contractility, vasoconstriction
Dopamine	0.5–2	Increased renal and splanchnic flow, mild vasodilatation
	2–10	Mildly increased contractility, mild vasoconstriction, and increased renal blood flow
	10–20	Moderately increased contractility, tachycardia, vasoconstriction
	>20	As above, but further vasoconstriction
Dobutamine	2–20	Increased contractility, decreased systemic vascular resistance

and cardiac output reduced. High levels require measurement of cardiac output and filling pressures to ensure adequate cardiac performance.

Corticosteroids have been reported to be useful when given in pharmacologic doses early in septic shock. The recommended dosage is 30 mg/kg for methylprednisolone and 1.5–3.0 mg/kg for dexamethasone.

STEPHEN S. HIRSCHFELD

Hodes HL: Endotoxin shock. In: Smith CA (ed): The Critically Ill Child. Philadelphia, WB Saunders Co, 1977.

Joly RH, Weil MH: Temperature of the great toe as an indication of the severity of shock. Circulation 39:131, 1969.
Rinaldo JE, Rogers RM: Adult respiratory-distress syndrome: Changing concepts of lung injury and repair. N Engl J Med 306:900, 1982.
Shoemaker WC: Pathophysiology, monitoring, and therapy of shock syndromes. In: Shoemaker SC, Thompson WL (eds): Critical Care. Fullerton Calif, Society of Critical Care Medicine, 1980.
Siegel JH, Greenspan M, Del Guercio LRM: Abnormal vascular tone, defective oxygen transport and myocardial failure in human septic shock. Ann Surg 165:504, 1967.
Stiem RE, Rich K: Recognition and management of shock in pediatric patients. Current Problems in Pediatrics, Year Book Medical Publishers, 1973.
The Organ in Shock. The proceedings of the second symposium on recent research developments and current clinical practice in shock. Thompson WL, Moderator. Kalamazoo, Mich, Upjohn Co, 1977.
Wiel MH: Current understanding of mechanisms and treatment of circulatory shock caused by bacterial infections. Ann Clin Res 9:181, 1977.

5.47 DRUG THERAPY*

Since 1962 extensive preclinical and clinical evaluations for safety and efficacy of drugs have been required in the United States, but these frequently have omitted evaluations of pharmacokinetic and pharmacodynamic properties in infants and children. Recent studies have led to a better understanding of the factors to be considered in planning therapeutic regimens, but the safe and effective use of drugs in infants and children continues to be a major problem.

Precise information on dosage and potential toxicity of drugs can be obtained only from extensive clinical studies. Frequently, the doses for adults have been applied to infants and children by use of various age-related formulas, but there is no predictable age-based relationship between a safe and effective dose in an adult and that in an infant or child. The rational basis for determining pediatric dosages is either clinical studies in infants and children or data gained from prolonged clinical use of available drugs. In either event, dosages should be calculated on the basis of weight or surface area (Fig 29–1) of the patient.

Legislation was passed in the United States in 1962 to protect immature individuals from inadequately tested new drugs. Ironically, this attempt to protect infants and children has led to the use of a "disclaimer" concerning pediatric indications and doses in the labeling of new drugs, resulting in the "unapproved" pediatric use drugs approved for adults. Studies in infants and children are now required to be under way prior to marketing of a new drug. This should eliminate the introduction of new drugs without data to guide those who care for infants and children in their use.

Pediatric pharmacology is concerned with pharmacokinetics and pharmacodynamics in the context of the developing individual. Pediatric pharmacotherapeutics combines basic and clinical pharmacology with knowledge of adverse effects of drugs and of the impact of disease upon pharmacokinetic and dynamic factors to develop dosage recommendations and other information essential to the safe medicinal treatment of infants and children.

*Consult Table 29–1A and B, for drugs and dosages.

5.48 PHARMACOKINETICS

The actions of a drug in human beings depend upon a number of factors which must be understood for rational therapeutic practice. The pharmacokinetic parameters (absorption, distribution, metabolism, and excretion), along with dosage, determine the concentration of a drug at its site of action and control the temporal course of the action. Each pharmacokinetic parameter may vary extensively with age. Pharmacodynamic factors, such as interaction with biologic receptors and mechanisms of action, are basic to the therapeutic or toxic effects produced.

During the early months of life some drugs may be absorbed more completely after oral administration than at any other time in life; the absorption of others may be impeded. This variation may be related to changes in gastric pH and emptying time which occur during development. The unpredictable eating habits and exercise patterns of children and adolescents may also modify absorption of drugs after oral administration. Thus, anatomic, physiologic, and behavioral factors can each lead at different ages to variation in absorption.

A number of factors determine the distribution of drugs in the body. The size of the drug molecule and its charge at physiologic pH influence the ease with which it passes through body membranes. Because of their specialized nature and structure, membranes vary in their permeability to individual drug molecules. Other factors include the relative size of the various water spaces, the ratio of lean body mass to total body weight, and the affinity of the drug for proteins in various body compartments.

Protein binding in the serum is especially important in influencing the distribution of drugs. A drug molecule bound to a serum protein, such as albumin, is not free to move across membranes and distribute into extravascular spaces. The apparent volume of distribution, V_d, of such a drug (see below) will depend upon the concentration of available protein binding sites in the vascular space. The dye Evans blue (T-1824), for example, is tightly and almost completely bound to serum albumin, and it has a volume of distribution equal to the volume of serum water since it diffuses out of the vascular space only very slowly, if at all. On the other hand, another compound may have high affinity for proteins in other spaces or for intracellular fat and have a very large V_d because of the rapidity with which it leaves the serum water to enter these other spaces. For example, thiopental has an affinity for lipids and therefore a very large V_d; the concentration of such a drug in serum water will be very low within minutes after administration because of rapid diffusion into fatty tissues.

The various penicillins and the aminoglycosides are sufficiently water soluble at physiologic pH to be excreted in the urine in an unchanged form. However, most drugs are highly lipid-soluble compounds which are filtered by the glomerulus but are reabsorbed so completely in the renal tubules that they would persist in the body in an active form for long periods of time if not modified chemically by enzymatic reactions. The 2 major categories of drug metabolizing reactions are nonsynthetic (oxidation, reduction, and hydrolysis) and synthetic (conjugation). For practical purposes, drug metabolism in vivo may be said to be carried out exclusively in the liver. The *nonsynthetic reactions* are catalyzed by mixed-function oxidases, which are fixed to the membranes of the endoplasmic reticulum. The resulting products may be less active, equally active, or even more active pharmacologically than the parent compound. *Synthetic reactions* generally result in the conversion of drugs or their (nonsynthetic) metabolic products into highly polar compounds that can be excreted in either the bile or the urine.

Drug metabolism is generally less efficient at early stages of development. However, the metabolic systems mature at different rates, and some drugs may be metabolized more rapidly during the postneonatal stages of infancy than they are in adults or older children. This may explain why infants require higher doses of phenytoin than do older children to achieve the same therapeutic serum concentrations. In most instances, however, it is still necessary to reduce doses during infancy and, perhaps, early childhood because

of inefficiency of metabolic processes and drug elimination in these age groups. Detailed studies of a given drug's metabolic developmental pattern are necessary before predictions can be made about its safe and effective use in pediatric patients.

Most drugs and drug metabolites are excreted in the urine; the rate of excretion varies as the rates of glomerular filtration and tubular secretion vary. Infants generally achieve an adult glomerular filtration rate by 1 yr of age, but some may do so by 3 mo. During the neonatal period, renal tubular secretion may be less than 5% that of adults but may reach mature levels at around 6 mo. Intrinsic renal disease and certain extrinsic factors, such as dehydration, may alter renal function significantly at any age or stage of development.

Because of the unpredictability of absorption, distribution, metabolism, and excretion at the various stages of human development, each drug requires clinical study to establish the dose and interval between doses appropriate to each developmental stage.

The Two-Compartment Pharmacokinetic Model

This model, which forms the basis for the application of general pharmacokinetic principles to the determination of drug doses, divides the body into a relatively small "central" compartment and a relatively large "peripheral" compartment. These are not defined anatomically, but the central compartment includes the serum and the extracellular fluid of highly perfused tissues (e.g., heart, lungs, liver, kidney), and the peripheral compartment the less well perfused tissues (e.g., muscles, body fat). This model assumes that the drugs are absorbed into and eliminated from the central compartment and that they distribute rapidly and to a uniform degree in the central compartment, while distribution in the peripheral compartment takes place more slowly.

A concept of major importance in understanding pharmacokinetic principles is that of apparent *volume of distribution* (V_d). V_d is the volume of water that would be required to dilute the administered dose of a drug to its concentration in the plasma, assuming no loss of drug from the body and uniform distribution of the drug in that volume of water. V_d is measured by extrapolating the straight line that results from a plot of the logarithm of the serum concentration (C) versus time, to t = 0 (Fig 5–18). The concentration at t = 0 (C_0) is then converted to volume by dividing C_0 into

the total dose (D) of drug administered: $V_d = \dfrac{D}{C_0}.$

The movement of drugs into and out of the 2 major theoretical compartments, their binding to proteins, their distribution and metabolism, and their rate of excretion are all assumed to be describable by a series of first-order rate constants. A first-order process is one whose rate is assumed to be directly related to concentration, i.e., absorption proceeds at the highest rate when the concentration of drug at the site of adminis-

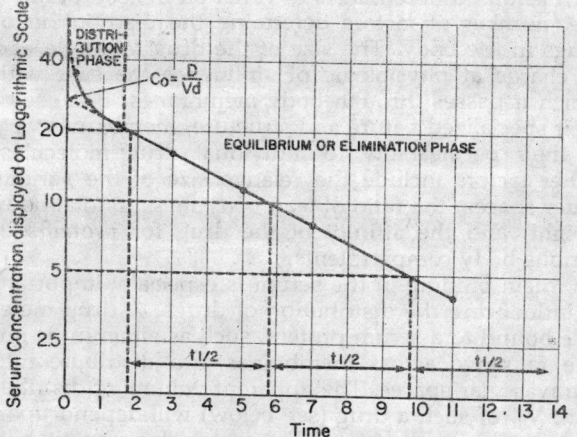

Figure 5–18 Time course of concentration of drug in the central compartment after administration of a single dose by the intravenous route. C_o and $T_{1/2}$ can be determined from such a graph and V_d and k_{el} can be calculated as noted in text.

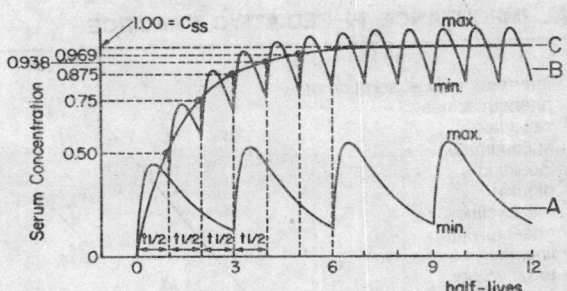

Figure 5–19 Repeated dosing at various constant dosing intervals. C represents the time course of serum concentration during constant intravenous infusion of a drug. After constant infusion for 5 half-lives the concentration reaches 96.9% of C_{ss}. In A, a fixed dose is administered (by the oral or intramuscular route) at a dosing interval of $3 \cdot T_{1/2}$. In B, the same dose and route are used but the dosing interval = $T_{1/2}$. Note that in a correct dosage regimen the same C_{ss} should be achieved by an appropriate dose irrespective of the route of administration, and the concentration maxima and minima should lie within the therapeutic range. The combination of an initial loading dose with subsequent doses sometimes offers the advantage of achieving an effective drug concentration rapidly and maintaining it safely.

tration is highest, and renal excretion proceeds at the highest rate when the plasma concentration is highest. Alternatively, processes proceed at a progressively slower rate as the concentration of drug is reduced. Since this results in the elimination of a fixed fraction, not a fixed amount, of the drug for each unit of time, the duration of each process is measured in half-lives (Fig 5–18). The half-life of a drug ($T_{1/2}$) is defined as the time it takes for the plasma concentration of the drug to be reduced to 50% of its value at the time of measurement, assuming equilibration and no further absorption of the drug.

K_{el} is the apparent first-order rate constant for elimination of a drug. K_{el} and $T_{1/2}$ bear the following relationship: $K_{el} = 0.693/T_{1/2}$. The total body clearance can be expressed as: Clear. $= V_d \cdot K_{el}$. Analogue computer studies and mathematical derivation have led to an equation that can be used to predict the steady-state blood level achieved in a specific individual during a multiple-dose regimen. The equation is $C_{ss} = \dfrac{F \cdot D}{V_d \cdot K_{el} \cdot t}$ where C_{ss} = concentration of the drug in serum in the steady state; F = fraction of dose absorbed (bioavailability); D = dose; t = the dosing interval; and K_{el} and V_d are experimentally determined in the individual (Fig 5–18) or assumed on the basis of age and disease-related standards. The dose required at the end of each dosing interval for a desired steady-state plasma concentration $= C_{ss} \cdot V_d \cdot K_{el} \cdot t$ when there is complete bioavailability or when the drug is administered intravenously (F = 1) (Fig 5–19).

5.49 INDIVIDUALIZATION OF DRUG DOSAGE

Individualization of drug dosage should be considered essential when a fixed dose or regimen yields an

unpredictable spectrum of effects in different individuals. There are 2 methods of accomplishing individualization. One aims at achieving a desired range of serum concentrations of drug, the other at maintaining an appropriate therapeutic effect regardless of serum level. The 1st is used when the therapeutic and toxic thresholds of the drug are known and the pharmacologic response is not readily quantifiable. The 2nd is important when the drug's effect is measurable but when there are several steps between the distribution of the drug to its site of action and the effect.

The optimal range of serum concentration of some drugs commonly used in pediatric pharmacotherapeutics is catalogued in Table 5–29. The anticonvulsant effects of *phenytoin* are difficult to quantitate because of the natural variability of epilepsy in children. It may produce severe toxic effects that can result in chronic

Table 5–29 THERAPEUTIC RANGE (SERUM CONCENTRATION) FOR SOME DRUGS USED IN PEDIATRIC PRACTICE

Antiarrhythmic/cardiotonic			
Digoxin			
Newborns and infants (birth–1 year)	0.0008–	0.0025	µg/ml
Children and adolescents	0.0008–	0.0016	µg/ml
Lidocaine	2	– 5	µg/ml
Procainamide	4	– 8	µg/ml
Propranolol	0.02	– 0.2	µg/ml
Quinidine	2	– 5	µg/ml
Anticonvulsants			
Carbamazepine	2	– 6	µg/ml
Clonazepam	0.02	– 0.07	µg/ml
Ethosuximide	40	–100	µg/ml
Phenobarbital	10	– 40	µg/ml
Phenytoin	10	– 20	µg/ml
Trimethadione (metabolized to dimethadione. This may attain levels of 500–1000 µg/ml on long-term use)	6	– 40	µg/ml
Valproic acid	80	–100	µg/ml
Antimicrobial agents			
Amikacin	15	– 25	µg/ml
Carbenicillin		around 100	µg/ml
Chloramphenicol	10	– 20	µg/ml
Gentamicin	6	– 8	µg/ml
Isoniazid	2.2	– 2.7	µg/ml
Antipyretic/analgesic/anti-inflammatory			
Acetylsalicylic acid (measured as salicylate)			
Antipyretic (short-term treatment)	50	–150	µg/ml
Antiarthritic (long-term use)	100	–300	µg/ml
Acetaminophen (short-term use)	50	–100	µg/ml
Meperidine	0.150	– 0.600	µg/ml
Phenylbutazone	40	– 80	µg/ml
Propoxyphene	0.05	– 0.2	µg/ml
Psychoactive drugs			
Amobarbital		around 5	µg/ml
Chloral hydrate	5	– 10	µg/ml
Chlordiazepoxide	1	– 3	µg/ml
Chlorpromazine	0.5	– 0.7	µg/ml
Diazepam	0.15	– 0.5	µg/ml
Imipramine	0.05	– 0.16	µg/ml
Pentobarbital		around 1	µg/ml
Miscellaneous			
Chlorothiazide	2	– 2.5	µg/ml
Theophylline	10	– 20	µg/ml

Table 5–30   DRUG INTERACTIONS OF POTENTIAL IMPORTANCE IN PEDIATRIC PRACTICE

1. Drugs interfering with gastrointestinal absorption of other drugs

Oral administration of:	Interferes with absorption of:
antacid	phenothiazines
	salicylate
	sulfonamides
antacid (aluminum-containing)	isoniazid
	digoxin
	tetracyclines
barbiturate	griseofulvin
kaolin-pectin	lincomycin
iron (ferrous)	tetracyclines
salicylate	fenoprofen
	indomethacin

2. Displacement of drug from protein binding site

Drug causing displacement	Drug displaced
phenylbutazone	phenytoin
phenytoin	thyroid hormone
salicylate	methotrexate
	naproxen
	phenytoin
sulfonamides	methotrexate
	phenytoin
quinidine	digoxin

3. Drugs with additive effect

Drugs increasing the action	Drugs in which action is increased (effect triggered)
digitalis glycosides	beta-adrenoceptor–blocking agents (bradycardia)
diazoxide	beta-adrenoceptor–blocking agents (bradycardia)
diuretics (potassium-losing)	corticosteroids (potassium depletion)
	curariform drugs (neuromuscular blockade)
ethanol (acute intoxication)	barbiturates (CNS depression)
	chloral hydrate (sedation)
	diazepam (CNS depression)
	meprobamate (CNS depression)
	salicylate (gastrointestinal bleeding)
phenothiazine	antihypertensives (hypotension)
	morphine (hypotension)
propranolol	phenothiazines (hypotension)
	phenytoin (cardiac depressant)
	quinidine (negative inotropic action)
	reserpine (sympathetic blockade)
	skeletal muscle relaxants (neuromuscular blockade)
quinidine	phenothiazines (cardiac depressant)
	skeletal muscle relaxants (neuromuscular blockade)
reserpine	beta-adrenoceptor–blocking agents (bradycardia)
tricyclic antidepressants	chlordiazepoxide (sedation)
	sympathomimetic amines (hypertensive crisis)

4. Drug-drug interaction by enhancement of the metabolism of one drug by another (induction of the drug-metabolizing enzyme system)

Drug causing induction	Drug of which metabolism is increased (pharmacologic effect diminished)
barbiturates (especially phenobarbital)	corticosteroids
	chloramphenicol
	clonazepam
	digoxin
	doxycycline
	estrogens
	phenothiazines
	phenytoin
	tricyclic antidepressants
	testosterone
carbamazepine	phenytoin
	valproic acid
phenytoin	corticosteroids
	diazepam
	thyroxine
	metapyrone
	primidone
salicylate	fenoprofen

(Drugs causing induction of their own metabolism: chlordiazepoxide, chlorpromazine, hexobarbital, meprobamate, pentobarbital, phenobarbital, phenylbutazone, phenytoin [weak effect], probenecid)

Table 5–30 DRUG INTERACTIONS OF POTENTIAL IMPORTANCE IN PEDIATRIC PRACTICE *(Continued)*

5. Drug-drug interaction by inhibition of metabolism of one drug by another
   Drug causing inhibition

	Drug of which metabolism is reduced (risk of toxicity increased)
allopurinol	azathioprine
	cyclophosphamide
	mercaptopurine
barbiturates (in large dose)	phenytoin
chloramphenicol	phenytoin
phenothiazines (especially chlorpromazine)	phenytoin
diazepam	phenytoin
erythromycin	theophylline
isoniazid	phenytoin
para-aminosalicylic acid	isoniazid
phenytoin	primidone
propoxyphene	carbamazepine
sulfonamides	phenytoin
valproic acid	phenobarbital
	phenytoin

6. Facilitation of a common adverse effect through combined use

aminoglycoside + second aminoglycoside or ethacrynic acid or furosemide	nephrotoxicity and ototoxicity
aminoglycoside + cephalosporin	nephrotoxicity, acute renal failure
aminoglycoside + polymyxin	nephrotoxicity
amphotericin B + digitalis glycoside	cardiac arrhythmia (hypokalemia)
cephaloridine + ethacrynic acid	nephrotoxicity
cephaloridine + furosemide	nephrotoxicity
corticosteroid + indomethacin	gastrointestinal ulceration
digitalis glycoside + sympathomimetic amine	cardiac arrhythmia
diuretic (K-losing) + digitalis glycoside	digitalis toxicity
isoniazid + rifampin	hepatotoxicity
phenytoin + isoniazid	neurotoxicity
tetracycline + diuretic	nephrotoxicity
tricyclic antidepressant + phenothiazine	cardiotoxicity
valproic acid + other anticonvulsants	neurotoxicity

impairment of central nervous system function if toxic plasma concentrations are maintained over long periods of time. It is common for phenytoin to fail to provide optimal effect or to cause intoxication if it is administered in a nonindividualized manner. Before it was possible to measure its serum concentration in small blood samples, phenytoin was administered according to a fixed regimen and the clinical course was followed. However, it is now known that there may be wide variation in the serum concentration achieved from the same weight-adjusted dose in different patients and that the potential therapeutic effectiveness can be evaluated only by maintaining serum concentrations above the known threshold for activity, regardless of the dose required to accomplish this. The variation in serum level is mainly from variation in the pharmacokinetic factors that govern the level following a given dose.

Antihypertensive agents, diuretics, analgesics, hypnotics, sedatives, and some antiarrhythmics and hormones can frequently be individualized by accurate quantitation of the intensity of their pharmacologic effect. Their concentration in the blood at the time of optimal therapeutic effect may vary widely because of differing modes of action. The pharmacokinetic factors that regulate serum concentration in such instances are far less important than the kinetic and dynamic factors that modify the intensity of the effects in the patient. These factors may involve diffusion or transport of the drug from the serum to the site of action, the number of receptors available at the site, the degree of respon-

siveness of the target tissue, and the effect of pathologic factors on the effector cells. The dose of such a drug prescribed for different patients may vary as much as 20-fold. There may even be wide variation from time to time in the dose required to achieve an effect in the same patient.

Appropriate practice in prescribing drugs varies with the drug to be administered and the state of knowledge about its pharmacokinetics and pharmacodynamics. Thus, for one drug it may be appropriate to aim at a fixed serum concentration; for another it may be necessary to achieve a state of measurable efficacy irrespective of the dose. Dosages for pediatric patients should be individualized whenever possible, and new drugs should be used according to the recommendations for determining appropriate dosages included in the labeling. Unfortunately, many drugs necessary for pediatric therapeutics must still be administered according to fixed dosage regimens because the data necessary to individualize are not yet available.

5.50 SPECIAL PROBLEMS OF DRUG TOXICITY

See also Sec 9.54.

Problems Linked to Growth and Development. The impact of a drug's action upon normal development must be considered in planning therapeutic regimens for pediatric patients. The increased incidence of kernicterus among jaundiced infants who were given drugs which displaced bilirubin from its intravascular binding sites is a widely appreciated example of such pediatric drug toxicity. Other adverse reactions specific to growing organisms that may make a drug approved for use in adults hazardous to infants and children include the damaging effects of tetracyclines upon permanent dentition when administered before completion of amelogenesis, and the possible adverse effect of treatment with steroid hormones, amphetamine, or methylphenidate on statural growth.

Drug-Drug Interactions.   When 2 or more drugs are administered to the same patient, the absorption, distribution, metabolism, excretion, and effect of each may be modified by interactions with the others. There are numerous examples which may be important in pediatric practice (Table 5–30). Not all of these interactions are bad, but most lead to suboptimal efficacy or to

Table 5–31   SOME SYNDROMES PRODUCED AS SIDE EFFECTS OF DRUG THERAPY*

1. Erythema multiforme and Stevens-Johnson syndrome†
   barbiturates
   codeine
   ethosuximide
   penicillins
   phenobarbital
   phenytoin
   salicylates
   sulfonamides
   tetracyclines
   thiazides

2. Erythema nodosum
   penicillins
   sulfonamides

3. Exfoliative dermatitis
   barbiturates
   penicillins
   phenytoin
   sulfonamides

4. Extrapyramidal symptomatology
   butyrophenones (haloperidol)
   diazoxide
   phenothiazines

5. Hemolytic anemia
   associated with G6PD deficiency:
   acetylsalicylic acid (in large doses)
   chloramphenicol
   dimercaprol
   nalidixic acid
   nitrofurantoin
   para-aminosalicylic acid
   primaquine
   probenecid
   quinidine
   sulfonamides (including salicylazosulfapyridine)
   water-soluble vitamin K analogues

   associated with positive Coombs test:
   cephalosporins
   chloramphenicol
   insulin
   isoniazid
   methicillin
   methyldopa
   para-aminosalicylic acid
   penicillins (in high doses)
   rifampin
   sulfonamides

6. Mental depression
   amphetamine withdrawal
   clonidine
   methyldopa
   phenothiazines
   prednisone (more commonly results in euphoria)
   propranolol
   reserpine
   tetrahydrocannabinol

7. Photosensitivity (phototoxic and photoallergic reactions can occur coincidentally or concomitantly)
   photoallergic (sensitization during first exposure, allergic reaction on continued exposure or re-exposure):
   antihistamines
   phenothiazines
   sulfonamides
   sunscreens (para-aminobenzoic acid)
   tetracyclines
   phototoxic (manifestations appearing 6 to 18 hr after exposure):
   antibacterial soaps (halogenated salicylanilides)
   coal tar and derivatives (perfumes, colognes, plants)
   griseofulvin
   nalidixic acid
   phenothiazines
   sulfonamides
   tetracyclines

8. Pseudomembranous colitis
   ampicillin
   chloramphenicol
   clindamycin
   lincomycin
   tetracyclines

9. Retrobulbar (optic) neuritis
   chloramphenicol
   clioquinol (iodochlorhydroxyquinoline)
   ethambutol
   isoniazid
   penicillamine
   phenothiazines

10. Serum sickness–like syndrome
    acetylsalicylic acid
    griseofulvin
    hydralazine
    penicillins
    sulfonamides
    thiouracil derivatives

11. Systemic lupus erythematosus
    hydralazine
    isoniazid
    penicillamine
    procainamide

12. Toxic epidermal necrolysis (Lyell syndrome, Ritter disease, scalded skin syndrome)
    acetylsalicylic acid
    allopurinol
    barbiturates
    methotrexate
    penicillins
    phenylbutazone
    phenytoin
    sulfonamides
    thiazides

*Hepatitis and nephritis syndromes, as well as fever and seizures, may be caused by a variety of agents and are not listed here. Consult a standard textbook of pharmacology for such relationships.
†Associated, but causality not established.

increased toxicity of 1 or more of the drugs in the combined regimen. The effect of each drug in such a regimen upon the others should be carefully considered.

Drug Toxicity. All drugs have the potential for producing adverse reactions. These usually represent an extension of the expected pharmacologic effects of the drug. Some adverse effects are referred to as *idiosyncratic* since their occurrence cannot be predicted from knowledge of the usual effects of the drugs that produce them. This type of adverse effect frequently takes the form of a complex of symptoms which may mimic naturally occurring syndromes (Table 5–31).

Pharmacogenetics. This branch of pharmacology concerns the genetically determined factors that affect drug responses, e.g., glucose-6-phosphate dehydrogenase and hemolysis (Table 5–31), or pseudocholinesterase isozymes and prolonged apnea after succinyl choline. Knowledge of the existence of a pharmacogenetic trait within a family is important in caring for members of that family. Whenever an unusual drug reaction is observed in a patient, the possibility that pharmacogenetic factors underlie such a reaction should be considered. In some instances the reaction will be a lack of response to a usual therapeutic dose and an increased threshold concentration of the drug in the serum. In others, it may be an increased sensitivity to the drug due to increased end-organ sensitivity or decreased K_{el}, leading to an increased effect of a standard dose or the early emergence of symptoms of a toxic reaction.

Drugs in Human Milk. Many drugs administered to lactating women are secreted into the milk and ingested along with feedings by the nursing infant. The effects of many of these drugs are unknown. Some drugs have been reported to affect the nursing infant adversely (Table 5–32); drug use should be kept to a minimum during lactation (Sec 7.12).

The concentration of a drug in breast milk is determined, among other factors, by its physicochemical characteristics, by its concentration in maternal serum, and by the pharmacokinetic behavior of it and its metabolites. Drugs such as cathartics in breast milk may affect the infant's gastrointestinal activity directly, but, in most instances, drugs taken in during nursing act only if they reach significant plasma and tissue concentrations in the infant. In most instances, the dose ingested and the total amount absorbed each day is small enough, and the infant's clearance of the drug is high enough, that there is no apparent pharmacologic effect.

5.51 PRESCRIBING PRACTICES

Factors such as taste, smell, color, consistency, and cost may affect compliance with the therapeutic drug regimen. The use of generic names in prescribing drugs may reduce the cost for an individual patient in some instances. However, the prescribing physician must ascertain that there is equal bioavailability, bioeffectiveness, and acceptability to the patient. In many instances information is available, but complete data are as yet not available on many drugs used in pediatrics.

Drugs familiar to the practitioner should be prescribed for the desired therapeutic effect. Newer preparations which are congeners of established agents and have no major therapeutic or cost advantage should be avoided; many of these are more expensive, and most have slightly different therapeutic actions or toxic potentials than the original drugs with which they were designed to compete on the market. These newer agents should be substituted for established drugs only after extensive clinical experience has demonstrated their added benefits.

Prescriptions should direct the dispensing of enough drug to treat the patient but not so much that a significant amount will be left over after the prescribed course of therapy. Parents should be instructed to discard residual doses to protect against accidental poisoning or improper self-medication at a later date. Simplified regimens should be employed whenever possible, and single ingredient preparations should be prescribed whenever appropriate. Complex regimens that require frequent dosing with one or another of several agents should be avoided since they frequently lead to over- or underadministration of the drugs by the parents or older child.

Compliance. Relatively little is known about the factors that determine the degree of compliance with a physician's instructions in an individual family. Compliance may be maximized in many instances by careful orientation of the family to the nature of the child's illness, to the action of the drugs prescribed, and to the importance of following the instructions precisely. If instructions are written down clearly and in detail for the family and if the regimen results in as little bother and interference as possible with the family living schedule, particularly the parental sleep habits, it probably will be followed with greater fidelity by more families.

SANFORD N. COHEN
LEON STREBEL

Table 5–32 SOME DRUGS EXCRETED IN BREAST MILK THAT PRODUCE ADVERSE EFFECTS ON NURSING INFANTS

Anthroquinones (laxatives)	Ethanol
Antithyroid agents	Iodides (expectorants)
Atropine	Narcotics (except morphine)
Bromides	Oral anticoagulants
Calciferol	Oral contraceptives
Diazepam	Primidone
Dihydrotachysterol	Propranolol
Ergot alkaloids	Reserpine
Estrogens	Tetracyclines

Avery GS (ed): Drug Treatment. Principles and Practice of Clinical Pharmacology and Therapeutics. Ed 2. New York, ADIS Press, 1980.

Melmon K, Morrelli HF (eds): Clinical Pharmacology. Basic Principles in Therapeutics. Ed 2. New York, Macmillan, 1978.

Morselli PL: Clinical pharmacokinetics in neonates. Clin Pharmacokinet 1:81, 1976.

Rane A, Wilson JT: Clinical pharmacokinetics in infants and children. Clin Pharmacokinet 1:2, 1976.

Shope JT: Medication compliance. Pediatr Clin North Am 28:5, 1981.

Yaffe SJ (ed): Pediatric Pharmacology: Therapeutic Principles in Practice. New York, Grune and Stratton, 1980.

6 PRENATAL DISTURBANCES

PRENATAL FACTORS IN DISEASES OF CHILDREN

Genetic Factors

Genetic abnormalities are a common cause of disease, handicaps, and death among infants and children. The primary diagnosis of 11–16% of patients admitted to the pediatric units of teaching hospitals is a genetic disease. One to 2% of newborn infants have a hereditary malformation and 0.5% have an inborn error of metabolism or an abnormality of the sex chromosomes which causes no physical abnormalities and can be detected only by specific laboratory tests.

The types of biochemical abnormalities that have been identified as the causes of genetic diseases include substitution of a single amino acid in a protein molecule; absence of a receptor site at the surface of a cell or within it; deficient activity of an enzyme located normally in the lysosomes, mitochondria, or extracellular space; or lack of production of a specific protein or protein-sugar complex (Table 6–1). Tissue culture techniques, such as hybridization of human and mouse cells, have made it possible to localize many of the human genes to their respective autosomes. New methods for staining human chromosomes and identifying subtle duplications and deficiencies of chromosomal material have also extended the understanding of human chromosomal abnormalities.

More complete understanding of the basic defect in many of the genetic diseases has altered current clinical classifications. For example, different types of hemophilia are now identified by the level of factor VIII antigen as well as by the clotting activity of factor VIII. Homocystinuria, once considered a single disease, has been shown to be the manifestation of several different metabolic abnormalities. Glucose-6-phosphate dehydrogenase deficiency has been found to be due not to a single genetic abnormality but possibly to over 100 separate genetic errors, mostly substitutions of 1 amino acid in this enzyme molecule.

Three categories of genetic defects have been identified in man: the single mutant gene, abnormalities of the chromosomes, and multifactorial inheritance. Other genetic abnormalities have been postulated but not proved, e.g., cytoplasmic inheritance, delayed mutation expressed in response to environmental factors, or a deletion in a chromosome which accentuates the effect of an adjacent gene or permits the expression of the effect of a mutant recessive gene on the homologous chromosome.

In the clinical appraisal and management of the child with an inherited disorder, 3 phases are critical: (1) recognition that the condition is inherited, (2) identification of the pattern of inheritance, and (3) clarification

Table 6–1 MOLECULAR BASIS FOR SOME GENETIC DISEASES

GENETIC DISEASE	PRIMARY DEFECT	REFERENCE
Familial hypercholesterolemia	Deficiency of a cell surface receptor for low density lipoprotein (LDL); this receptor normally regulates cholesterol metabolism by suppressing cholesterol synthesis and increasing LDL degradation	Brown MS, Goldstein JL: Science 185:61, 1974
Testicular feminization	Deficient cytoplasmic binding of androgen that leads to an inability to transport dihydrotestosterone to its acceptor site in the nucleus	Amrhein JA, et al: Proc Natl Acad Sci USA 73:891, 1976
Hemoglobin Constant Spring	A mutation of the terminating codon on an alpha-chain gene; the lack of the normal terminating codon allows the synthesis of an alpha-chain with 31 extra amino acid residues	Clegg JB, et al: Nature 234:337, 1971
Hereditary angioneurotic edema	Defective biosynthesis of the C1 esterase inhibitor	Rosen FS, et al: J Clin Invest 50:2143, 1971
Phenylketonuria due to deficiency of dihydropteridine reductase	An enzyme deficiency responsible for lack of the cofactor tetrahydrobiopterin, an essential for the metabolism of phenylalanine, tyrosine, and tryptophan; this is a rare form of PKU that does not respond to dietary management	Kaufman S, et al: N Engl J Med 293:785, 1975
Ehlers-Danlos syndrome, type VII	Deficiency of procollagen peptidase, required for conversion of procollagen to collagen	Lichtenstein JR, et al: Science 182:298, 1973
Macular corneal dystrophy	Failure to synthesize a mature keratan sulfate proteoglycan	Hassell JR, et al: Proc Natl Acad Sci USA 77:3705, 1980

of the clinical nature of the disorder, including understanding of the risk of occurrence of the disease in siblings or other members of the family. Recognition that a condition is hereditary may be difficult when the patient has no affected relatives. The physician should be familiar with the different types of genetic diseases and utilize appropriate references to identify their patterns of inheritance, such as *Mendelian Inheritance in Man* by McKusick, which catalogues conditions caused by single mutant genes. No catalogue is available for disorders attributed to multifactorial inheritance; recognition depends on the physician's awareness of these disorders. Only for chromosomal abnormalities is there a laboratory test to provide visible evidence of the underlying genetic disorder (Sec 6.8).

6.1 SINGLE MUTANT GENES

Each single mutant gene will exhibit 1 of the 4 patterns of mendelian inheritance: autosomal recessive, autosomal dominant, X-linked recessive, and X-linked dominant. This method of grouping genetic diseases is often helpful in understanding the clinical presentation of a disorder. Concepts like the basic structure of the DNA molecule and the transmission of genetic information, initially to messenger RNA and then to the formation of a specific polypeptide, become relevant in explaining the basis for such diseases as the many different disorders of hemoglobin structure, in which the primary abnormalities include amino acid substitutions and deletions, elongated globin chains, and fused or "hybrid" globin chains. Other mechanisms for the transmission of genetic information that are apparent in the study of microorganisms, such as the many different types of genetic mutation, repressor genes, and regulator genes, have not yet become applicable to the understanding of human genetic diseases.

A number of special terms are used in discussing single mutant genes. The 23 chromosomes in the sperm combine with the 23 chromosomes in the egg to form a *zygote* with 23 *pairs* of chromosomes. The *gene locus* is the particular location of a specific gene in a specific chromosome. Recent studies show that the coding portions of a gene, such as the beta globin gene, are interrupted by intervening sequences of DNA of variable lengths. These intervening sequences are not represented in the mature messenger RNA that corresponds to the gene. Each gene has an analogue with a similar location in the homologous (other of a pair) chromosome; the identical pair of loci are called *homologous loci*. The genes at the homologous loci are called *alleles*. Allelic genes are analogous (i.e., affect the nature of the same characteristic) but are often not identical; extensive variation may be observed in many of the products or characteristics they determine, such as different types of serum proteins among people of the same as well as different races. In view of the genetic variation that exists at many gene loci, it is arbitrary to consider some genes as mutant; usually the distinction is that the mutant gene has a major, harmful effect. When a person has a mutant gene at a locus in 1 chromosome but not at the homologous locus of the other of a pair of chromosomes, the person is *heterozygous* for that mutant gene. If the gene does not have an effect on the heterozygous individual, it is called a *recessive gene*. If the mutant gene has an effect in the heterozygous state, it is a *dominant gene*. A person who has the same mutant gene at both homologous loci is *homozygous* for that gene. Autosomal recessive genes manifest their clinical effect only in the *homozygote*. These distinctions between recessive and dominant genes become arbitrary when one can identify the heterozygote by means of biochemical testing or when the heterozygote has only a mild expression of the disorder.

Each mendelian pattern of inheritance has characteristics that may be useful in establishing a diagnosis or in planning family studies that may be important for a clear explanation to the parents of an affected child.

6.2 AUTOSOMAL RECESSIVE INHERITANCE

Some of the most common diseases transmitted in an autosomal recessive pattern are listed in Table 6–2. The pedigree illustrating this pattern of inheritance (Fig 6–1) shows the following characteristics: the child of 2 heterozygous parents has a 25% chance of being homozygous (that is, 1 chance in 2 of inheriting the mutant gene from each parent: $\frac{1}{2} \times \frac{1}{2} = \frac{1}{4}$); males and females are affected with equal frequency; the affected individuals are almost always born in only 1 generation of a family; the children of the affected (homozygous) person are all heterozygotes; the children of a homozygote can be affected only if the spouse is a heterozygote, a rare event because of the low incidence of most adverse recessive genes in the general population.

If the frequency of an autosomal recessive disease is known, the frequency of the heterozygote or carrier state can be calculated from the Hardy-Weinberg formula: $p^2 + 2pq + q^2 = 1$, in which p is the frequency of one of a pair of alleles and q is the frequency of the other. For example, if the frequency of cystic fibrosis among white Americans is 1 in 2500 (p^2), then the frequency of the heterozygote (2 pq) can be calculated: if $p^2 = 1/2500$, then p = 1/50 and q = 49/50; 2pq = 2 × 1/50 × 49/50 or approximately 1/25 (or 3.92%).

Every human probably has several rare, harmful, recessive genes. Since these mutant genes are frequently not identifiable by laboratory tests, the heterozygous adult usually learns about his or her harmful recessive genes after the birth of a homozygous (and therefore affected) child. Related parents are much more likely to be heterozygous for the same harmful recessive genes because they have a common ancestor. Consanguineous matings are rare in the United States and many other countries. Therefore, few genetic studies have been carried out to establish the overall risk for healthy but related parents. Based on the information available, the risk for parents who are first cousins of having a child with a birth defect is about double the 4% risk faced by healthy, unrelated parents.

6.3 AUTOSOMAL DOMINANT INHERITANCE

Some of the common diseases due to an autosomal dominant gene are shown in Table 6–2. The pedigree (Fig 6–2) shows that both males and females are affected, that transmission occurs from 1 parent to child, and that the responsible mutant gene can arise by spontaneous mutation. The risk is 50% that an offspring of the affected person will inherit the chromosome that contains the mutant gene.

Table 6–2 INCIDENCE OF DISEASES DUE TO SINGLE MUTANT GENES*

Genetic Disease	Frequency of Heterozygote	Number of Affected Individuals per Million Births
Autosomal recessive		
Adrenogenital syndrome		15
Albinism, tyrosinase negative		25
Albinism, tyrosinase positive		25
Alpha₁-antitrypsin deficiency, SZ Pi type		240 } Whites in Sweden†
ZZ		600
Cystic fibrosis	4% (U.S. Whites)	270 (Whites)
Galactosemia		25
Hemoglobin		
S-S (sickle cell anemia)	8% (U.S. Blacks)	1600 (U.S. Blacks)
S-C	(3% of U.S. Blacks have hemoglobin A-C)	1200 (U.S. Blacks)
		600 (U.S. Blacks)
S-β thalassemia	1% (U.S. Blacks)	100 (U.S. Blacks)
β thalassemia	Up to 16% of Italians	400 (U.S. citizens of Mediterranean origin)
Metachromatic leukodystrophy		25
Hurler syndrome α-iduronidase deficiency		25
Sanfilippo syndrome		20
Phenylketonuria		70 (Whites)
Tay-Sachs disease	3% (U.S. Jews)	400 (U.S. Ashkenazi Jews)
Autosomal dominant		
Achondroplasia		100
Acrocephalosyndactyly (Apert syndrome)		6
Aniridia		5–10
Dentinogenesis imperfecta		8000
Facioscapulohumeral muscular dystrophy		4
Huntington chorea		50
Hyperlipoproteinemia, type II (familial hypercholesterolemia)		10,000
Marfan syndrome		15
Neurofibromatosis		303
Polycystic kidneys (all types)		4000
Retinoblastoma		50
Thanatophoric dwarfism		15
Tuberous sclerosis		10
Waardenburg syndrome		250
X-linked recessive diseases	Frequency of female carriers	
Bruton agammaglobulinemia		10–15
Ocular albinism		10–15
Amelogenesis imperfecta		10
Fabry disease		2–5
Color blindness (deutan)		6% of males
(protan)		2% of males
Diabetes insipidus, nephrogenic		0.1
Glucose-6-phosphate dehydrogenase deficiency (African type or A-minus variant)	24% of American black females	10–14% of black Americans
Chronic granulomatous disease		1–5
Duchenne muscular dystrophy		200–220
Factor VIII deficiency (hemophilia A)		100–120
Factor IX deficiency (hemophilia B; Christmas disease)		20–30
Hunter syndrome		20
Ichthyosis		200
Retinitis pigmentosa		1–5

*Data from Benirschke K, Carpenter G, Epstein C et al: In Brent RL, and Harris MI (eds): Prevention of Embryonic, Fetal and Perinatal Disease. Washington, D.C., DHEW Pub. No. (NIH) 76–853, 1976, pp 219–261.
†Data from Sveger T: N Engl J Med 294:1316, 1976.

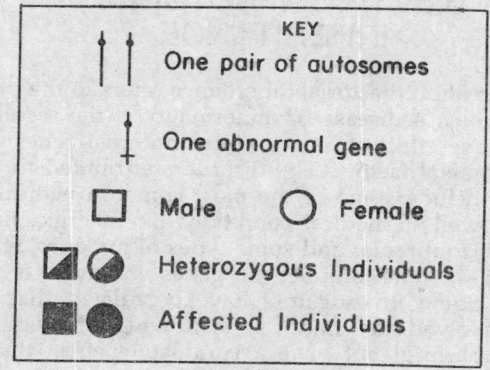

KEY

One pair of autosomes

One abnormal gene

Male ☐   Female ○

Heterozygous Individuals

Affected Individuals

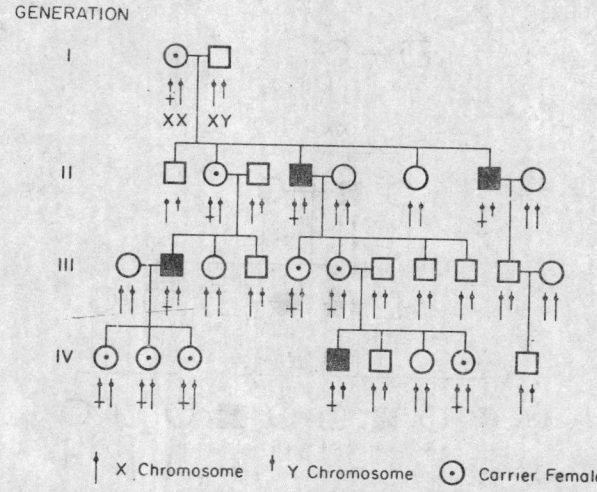

GENERATION

I

II

III

IV

↑ X Chromosome ↑ Y Chromosome ⊙ Carrier Female

Figure 6–3 X-linked recessive inheritance. (See Fig 6–1 for key.)

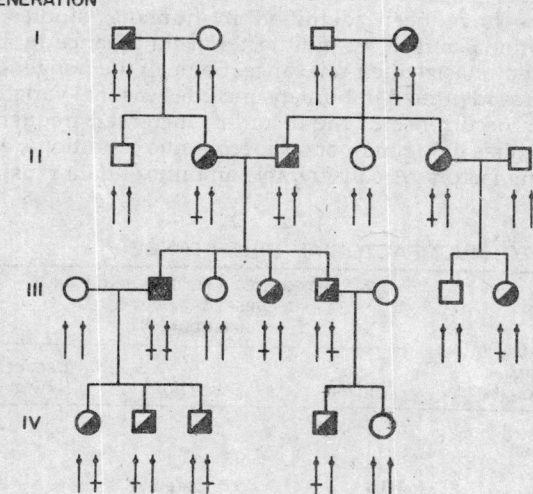

GENERATION

I

II

III

IV

Figure 6–1 Autosomal recessive inheritance.

6.4   X-LINKED RECESSIVE INHERITANCE

Common X-linked recessive diseases are listed in Table 6–2. The pedigree (Fig 6–3) shows that only males are clinically affected; that affected males are related through carrier females; that all daughters of affected males are carriers of the mutant gene; and that affected

males do not have affected sons but may have affected grandsons born to carrier females. The female carrier has a 50% chance of giving her chromosome that bears the mutant gene to each of her children. In other words, each daughter of a carrier has a 50% chance of being a carrier, and each son has a 50% chance of inheriting the mutant gene and having the disease that it causes. Therefore, in each pregnancy the female carrier has a 25% chance of having an affected son.

Initially, both X chromosomes of a female zygote are active. Random inactivation of one X in each cell occurs early in fetal development. The inactivated X, which replicates later than the active X, is the sex chromatin mass or Barr body, which may be observed in the nucleus of a cell near the nuclear membrane. This random inactivation, also called *lyonization* (the process was first proposed by Dr. Mary Lyon), protects the carrier female from the effect of the X-linked recessive mutant gene because there is as much chance that the X chromosome which carries the mutant gene will be inactivated as that the other X chromosome will. Therefore, the carrier expresses the effect of the mutant gene in an average of 50% of her cells. For this reason the female carrier of classic hemophilia will have a reduced level of factor VIII antigen and activity but a level not nearly as low as that in her affected son or brother.

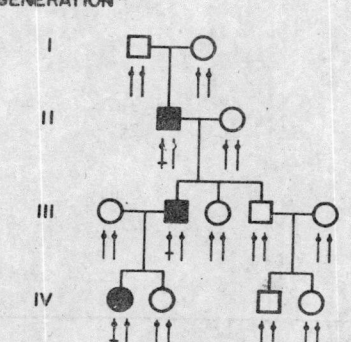

GENERATION

I

II

III

IV

Figure 6–2 Autosomal dominant inheritance. (See Fig 6–1 for key.)

6.5   X-LINKED DOMINANT INHERITANCE

Very few X-linked dominant genes have been identified in humans. Two examples are vitamin D–resistant rickets and the telecanthus-hypospadias (or BBB) syndrome of multiple malformations. The pedigree (Fig 6–4) shows the essential characteristics: both males and females are affected, but males are often more severely affected; the disorder is transmitted from generation to generation; all daughters of an affected father will be affected, but none of his sons.

GENERATION

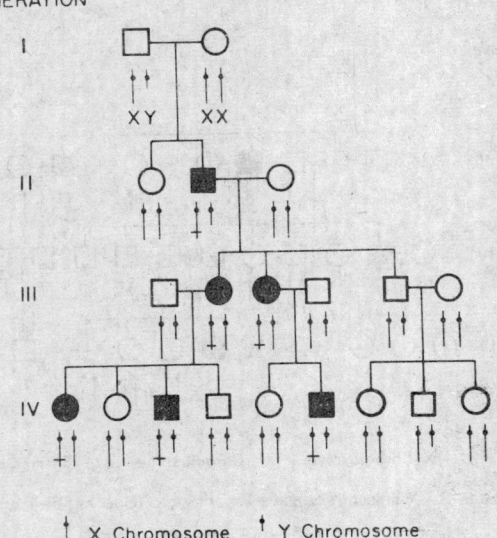

↑ X Chromosome   ↑ Y Chromosome

Figure 6–4 X-linked dominant inheritance. (See Fig 6–1 for key.)

6.6 MULTIFACTORIAL INHERITANCE

The term multifactorial inheritance refers to the process in which a disease or abnormality is the result of the additive effect of one or more abnormal genes and environmental factors. The disorders attributed to this process include some of the most common malformations as well as medical conditions like allergic disorders, schizophrenia, and some types of hyperlipidemia (Table 6–3). The number of genes involved is not known. Some investigators have postulated that the genes involved are "minor genes," which individually are not harmful but have a cumulative effect that is harmful; others postulate that genes that exert a major effect are also involved. Few of the environmental factors have been identified in humans; studies of conditions caused by multifactorial inheritance in animals emphasize their relevance. Some of the nongenetic features identified in humans include seasonal variation in the occurrence of the disorder, increased frequency in families living in poor socioeconomic conditions, and uterine factors. A considerable amount of data must be

Table 6–3 GENETIC DISORDERS ATTRIBUTED TO MULTIFACTORIAL INHERITANCE

Abnormality	Race	Prevalence in General Population (%)	Risk of Recurrence Among Family Members of an Affected Individual (%)		
			Siblings	Offspring	Identical Twin
Malformations					
Cardiac defects					
Ventricular septal defect		0.23	4.4	3.7	
Atrial septal defect		0.1 (1/1000)	3.3	3.5 (parents)	
Patent ductus arteriosus		0.05	1.4	2.8	
Tetralogy of Fallot		0.03	1.0	1.6	
Cleft lip and palate	Whites	0.13 (1/750)	3.9	3.5	31
	Blacks	0.04			
	Navajos	0.2			
	Japanese	0.16			
Cleft palate	Whites	0.05 (1/2000)	3.0	6.2	40
	Blacks	0.04			
	Navajos	0.03			
Club foot (talipes equinovarus)		0.01	2.9		33
Dislocation of hip, congenital		0.07 (1/1400)	4.3		35
Hirschsprung disease		0.02 (1.5000)	3.8* 12.5†		
Hypospadias	Whites	0.8 (1/120)	7.0	6.0 (fathers)	
	Blacks	0.2 (1/500)			
Legg-Perthes disease		0.07 (Canada)	3.7* 4.3†		
Meningomyelocele	Whites	0.3 (1/330) (London)	4.4	3.0	21
Anencephaly		0.14 (1/700) (Boston)	2		
Encephalocele	Jews	0.08			
	Blacks	0.07			
	Puerto Ricans	0.2			
Pyloric stenosis		0.2 (1/500) (London)	3.2* 6.5†	25.4‡ 4.2§	22
Other diseases					
Ankylosing spondylitis			7.0* 2.0†		
Atopic disease		2–3	5.8		24
Psoriasis		1–2	7.8		63
Schizophrenia		1–3	6–12		40

* = If brother affected.   ‡ = If mother affected.
† = If sister affected.   § = If father affected.

available on many affected persons and their families before the disease or malformation is attributed to multifactorial inheritance. This term should not be used whenever the cause of familial occurrence is poorly understood.

Some of the features of multifactorial inheritance are similar to mendelian inheritance of single mutant genes, e.g., the incidence of specific conditions varies according to racial background; this racial predisposition persists after migration to other countries.

Most of the features of multifactorial inheritance, however, are quite different from those observed in mendelian inheritance of a single mutant gene: (1) There is a similar rate of recurrence (usually 2–10%; Table 6–3) among all first-degree relatives (parents, siblings, and offspring of the affected infant). For example, if a couple has had 1 child with cleft lip and palate, the risk that the next one will be affected is about 4%; if 1 parent has cleft lip and palate, the chance that the 1st child will have the same malformation is also about 4%. (2) Some disorders have a sex predilection. For example, pyloric stenosis is much more common in males, whereas congenital dislocation of hips is much more common in females. (3) If there is an altered sex ratio, the affected person of the sex less likely to be affected is much more apt to have affected children. For example, a woman who had pyloric stenosis as an infant has a 25% chance of having a child similarly affected; the risk for the children of the father who had pyloric stenosis is only 4%. (4) The likelihood that both of identical twins will be affected with the same malformation is less than 100% but much greater than the chance that both nonidentical twins will be affected. The frequency of concordance for identical twins ranges from 21–63% for the disorders listed in Table 6–3. This distribution contrasts with that of mendelian inheritance, in which identical twins always share a disorder due to a single mutant gene. (5) The risk of recurrence in subsequent pregnancies depends on the outcome in previous pregnancies. For example, the risk of recurrence for cleft lip and palate is 4% for a couple with 1 affected child, but 9% after they have had 2 affected children. (6) The risk of abnormality in offspring is directly related to the severity of the malformation. For example, the infant who has congenital intestinal aganglionosis of a long segment of bowel has a greater chance of having an affected sibling than the infant who has aganglionosis of only a small segment.

6.7 GENERAL CLINICAL PRINCIPLES IN GENETIC DISORDERS

The Negative Family History. A child with a genetic disease or malformation is usually the only known affected member of his or her family. This reflects the fact that the rates of recurrence are very low for common abnormalities of the chromosomes and for conditions attributed to multifactorial inheritance. For example, the recurrence risk for Down syndrome associated with trisomy-21 is 1%; for conditions attributed to multifactorial inheritance it varies from 2–10% (Table 6–3). The recurrence risk for disorders with a mendelian pattern of inheritance is much higher (e.g., 25% for autosomal recessive disorders), but in small families it is more likely that an autosomal recessive disorder will affect only 1 of 3 or 4 children rather than 2. In the case of autosomal dominant disorders, the child may be affected by a spontaneous genetic mutation rather than by inheriting the mutant gene from an affected parent. Generally speaking, a negative family history may be misleading.

Environmental Factors. Since the family history is usually negative for the disorder under consideration, the parents often blame themselves and look for environmental factors which might have been the cause. The physician should anticipate their feelings of guilt and carefully discuss the events, including medications taken, to which congenital disorders may be attributed inappropriately by parents.

Genetic Heterogeneity. A single clinical manifestation may have more than 1 cause. An elevation in serum phenylalanine may be associated with classic phenylketonuria (either absence or deficiency of phenylalanine hydroxylase); absence or deficiency of the enzyme pteridin reductase (Table 6–1); or deficient biopterin synthesis. Arachnodactyly may be an isolated characteristic of a tall, thin person, or it may be a feature of a number of genetic disorders, including Marfan syndrome and contractural arachnodactyly.

Pleiotropism. Some genetic disorders have many different features, all of which are the pleiotropic effect of a single mutant gene. For example, in classic galactosemia, cataracts, hepatomegaly, malabsorption, neonatal sepsis, and mental deficiency are all related to deficiency of the transferase enzyme, which is the primary effect of the underlying autosomal recessive mutant gene. In neurofibromatosis, café-au-lait spots, subcutaneous nodules, solid tumors, scoliosis, and mental deficiency are caused by a single autosomal dominant gene.

Variable Expression. Reference books often illustrate the extreme manifestations of a clinical disorder and rarely describe its milder forms. The clinician must appreciate that 2 or 3 café-au-lait spots may be either innocent birth marks or the earliest signs of neurofibromatosis in which additional features may become manifest at an older age. This diagnostic dilemma can be resolved only by careful, long-term follow-up. In the case of hereditary disorders without progressive changes, such as the Treacher Collins syndrome (mandibulofacial dysostosis), the affected child may have microtia, severe hearing loss, colobomas of the lower eyelids, and marked maxillary hypoplasia, while the affected parent may have only mild hearing loss, a downward slant of the palpebral fissures, and a decreased number of lashes on the lower eyelid.

Not Everything Familial Is Genetic. Environmental factors, such as infection and teratogens, may simulate genetic conditions; on occasion, 2 or more children of healthy parents may be affected.

Establishing the Pattern of Inheritance Requires Extensive Data. There is a temptation to use data from a small number of families in establishing a pattern of inheritance. For example, when a presumed genetic disorder has occurred in a son and daughter of healthy parents, it is often concluded that each child is homozygous for an autosomal recessive mutant gene. However, it should be noted that a familial chromosomal abnormality and multifactorial inheritance could also cause the same pattern. Similarly, the pattern of occurrence in families with a disorder due to multifactorial inheritance may simulate mendelian inheritance; e.g., the parent and child with cleft lip and palate mimic autosomal dominant inheritance. With the rate of recurrence among parents and siblings only 4% for Caucasians, almost all children with cleft lip and palate are the only affected members of their families. Data on hundreds of families were needed to establish multifactorial inheritance as the basis for the disorder and to exclude the possibility of mendelian inheritance.

LEWIS B. HOLMES

Childs B, Der Kaloustian VM: Genetic heterogeneity. N Engl J Med 279:1205, 1267, 1968.
Day N, Holmes LB: The incidence of genetic disease in a university hospital population. Am J Hum Genet 25:237, 1973.
Forget BG: Molecular genetics of human hemoglobin synthesis. Ann Int Med 91:605, 1979.
Fraser FC: The multifactorial/threshold concept—uses and misuses. Teratology 14:267, 1976.
Harris H, Hopkinson DA, Robson EB: The incidence of rare alleles determining electrophoretic variants: Data on 43 enzyme loci in man. Ann Hum Genet (London) 37:237, 1974.
Scriver CR, Claw CL: Phenylketonuria: Epitome of human biochemical genetics. N Engl J Med 303:1336, 1394, 1980.

General

McKusick V: Mendelian Inheritance in Man: Catologs of Autosomal Dominant, Autosomal Recessive and X-linked Phenotypes. Ed 5. Baltimore, Johns Hopkins University Press, 1978.
Vogel F, Motulsky AG: Human Genetics: Problems and Approaches. New York, Springer-Verlag, 1979.

6.8   CHROMOSOMES AND THEIR ABNORMALITIES

The determination in 1956 that the correct somatic chromosome number of man is 46 and the discovery in 1959 that trisomy 21 is the basis for Down syndrome established cytogenetic abnormality as an important etiologic factor in human disease. During the ensuing 15 years, laboratory procedures were developed for the precise identification of the individual chromosomes (and segments thereof), enabling the interpretation of complex chromosomal rearrangements as well as minor morphologic variations. These techniques, including the differential staining methods (chromosome "banding"), the successful culture of amniotic fluid cells for prenatal diagnosis, studies of human meiosis, and the somatic cell hybridization procedures, have led to more accurate clinical diagnosis as well as to more precise genetic counseling.

These new developments have increased the demand for cytogenetic analyses. However, since chromosome studies are complicated and expensive, candidates for these procedures must be carefully identified. The most important clinical indications are congenital malformations, especially if more than 1 system is involved, and mental retardation of unknown origin. Some of the more common features of children with chromosome abnormalities are odd facies, abnormal ears, heart and kidney malformations, abnormal hands and feet, simian creases, a single crease on the 5th finger, and low birth weight. It has been estimated that 1 in 142 newborn infants has a chromosomal abnormality. Table 6–4 lists the incidence of various chromosomal abnormalities in liveborn infants.

In addition, the fact that 50–60% of the products of early spontaneous abortion have a chromosomal abnormality suggests that at least 7% of human conceptions have a karyotypic abnormality. At 16–18 wk of gestation, the incidence of chromosomal abnormalities is greater than in liveborn infants; one can thus assume the loss of additional cytogenetically unbalanced fetuses in mid- and late pregnancy. Approximately 90% of karyotypically abnormal conceptions, then, do not survive pregnancy. Of the chromosomal abnormalities observed in liveborn infants, about half involve the autosomes and half the sex chromosomes. The frequency of identifiable chromosomal abnormalities should increase as more accurate methods for detection of minor structural alterations become available.

METHODOLOGY

Cell Culture. The small lymphocyte, which is readily stimulated to divide with the plant mitogen phytohemagglutinin (PHA), is commonly used for chromosome investigation. The dividing cells are arrested in metaphase after about 72 hr in culture by exposure to demecoline (Colcemid), and the chromosomes are dispersed by exposure to hypotonic solution. Chromosome spreads are then prepared by air drying.

Cultures of fibroblasts, which are technically more demanding and time-consuming, may be necessary for studies of mosaicism and biochemical defects. For the diagnosis of blood dyscrasias, bone marrow prepara-

Table 6–4   INCIDENCE OF CHROMOSOMAL ABNORMALITIES AMONG LIVEBORN INFANTS

Down syndrome (21-trisomy)	1/800
18-trisomy syndrome	1/8000
13-trisomy syndrome	1/20,000
Turner syndrome (females)	1/10,000
Klinefelter syndrome (males)	1/1000
Poly-X anomalies (females)	1/1000
XYY karyotype (males)	1/1000
Balanced structural rearrangement	1/520
Unbalanced structural rearrangement	1/1700
Total	1/142

tions are best, but chromosomes of myelocytes can be prepared from peripheral blood leukocytes dividing after 24 hr in culture without mitogenic stimulation. The methodology for culture of amniotic fluid cells is similar to that for fibroblasts. Cytogenic analysis is complete in 2–3 wk. The conventional Giemsa or acetic orcein methods produce uniform staining along the entire length of the chromosome. These methods, however, have been largely supplanted by the development of techniques which yield a characteristic pattern of alternating light and dark (or bright and dull) bands for each chromosome. These bands appear to be associated with the composition of base pairs forming the DNA. Staining with quinacrine derivatives or similar compounds, followed by microscopic investigation using a UV light source, produces fluorescent bands called *Q bands*, while corresponding *G bands* are produced by a modified Giemsa staining procedure. Another method, using Giemsa or acridine orange, produces staining intensities opposite to Q and G bands which are called reverse or *R bands*. All qualified cytogenetic laboratories now use at least one of these banding methods to assure a reliable diagnosis. Other procedures available in more advanced laboratories include C-banding to stain constitutive heterochromatin found near the centromere of each chromosome; a *C-band* stain (G-11) specific for No. 9; NOR, using ammoniacal silver to stain the nucleolar organizing regions of satellited chromosomes; and SCE, a procedure that reveals exchanges between sister chromatids.

Karyotyping. Chromosomal DNA replicates during the S stage of interphase, but the double-structured nature of the chromosomes becomes clearly visible only at the beginning of mitosis. Thus, during mitosis, each chromosome consists of 2 identical long thin strands called sister chromatids, which coil progressively tighter, giving the appearance of short, thick arms held together by the centromere. At metaphase, when they are at their shortest length, the chromosomes are photographed and arranged in pairs. This systematized arrangement from a single cell is referred to as a karyotype. Presently, only "banded" karyotypes are acceptable for diagnoses, and most laboratories study 10–40 metaphase karyotypes per subject. If mosaicism is suspected, more cells, as well as cells of other tissues, should be analyzed.

6.9 THE NORMAL KARYOTYPE

The diploid number of human chromosomes is 46, consisting of 23 pairs. Thus, 23 is the haploid number found in the gametes. At metaphase each chromosome, consisting of 2 chromatids, has a characteristic morphology determined by the position of the centromere, or primary constriction, which delineates the long and short arms (Fig 6–5a). Examples of the three normal characteristic shapes are Nos. 1, 3, and 16 (*metacentric*), Nos. 4 and 5 (*submetacentric*), and Nos. 21 and 22 (*acrocentric*). The short arm of an acrocentric chromosome has a secondary constriction and satellite. The entire human complement of chromosomes was originally divided into 7 groups, designated A through G in order of descending size and according to morphologic similarities, with the exception of the sex chromosomes, which are placed last in the karyotype. Following the accurate identification of each chromosome, accomplished on the basis of size, morphology, and banding pattern, a numbering system was agreed upon (Fig 6–6), and the letters A to G lost their relevance except when referring in general terms to similarly shaped chromosomes.

A few morphologic variants have been observed in

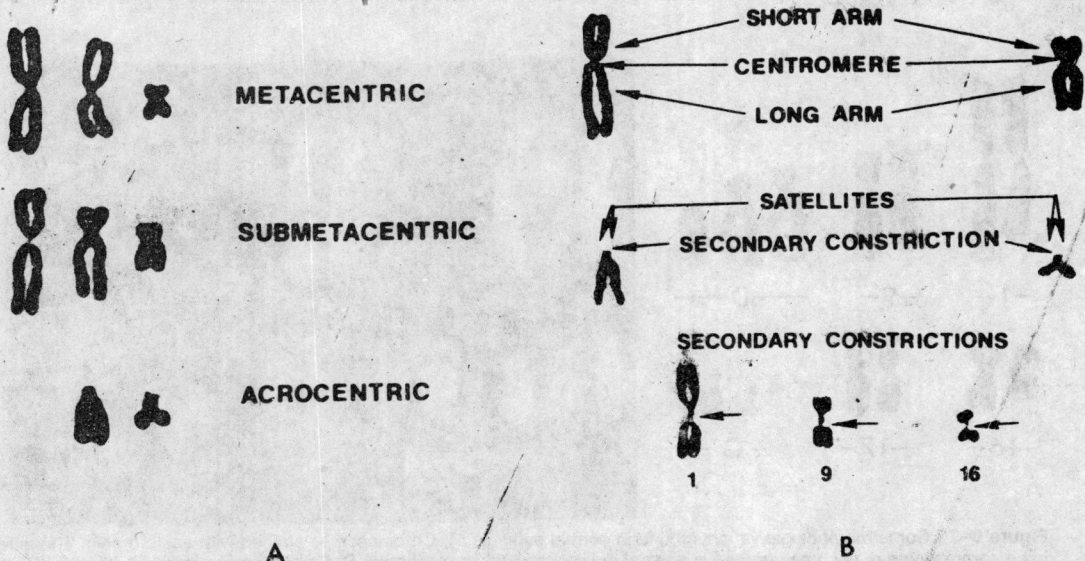

METACENTRIC

SUBMETACENTRIC

ACROCENTRIC

SHORT ARM
CENTROMERE
LONG ARM

SATELLITES
SECONDARY CONSTRICTION

SECONDARY CONSTRICTIONS

1   9   16

A   B

Figure 6–5 *a,* Centromere position determining the 3 types of chromosomes seen in the normal human karyotype—metacentric, submetacentric, and acrocentric. *b,* Morphologic landmarks useful in chromosome identification.

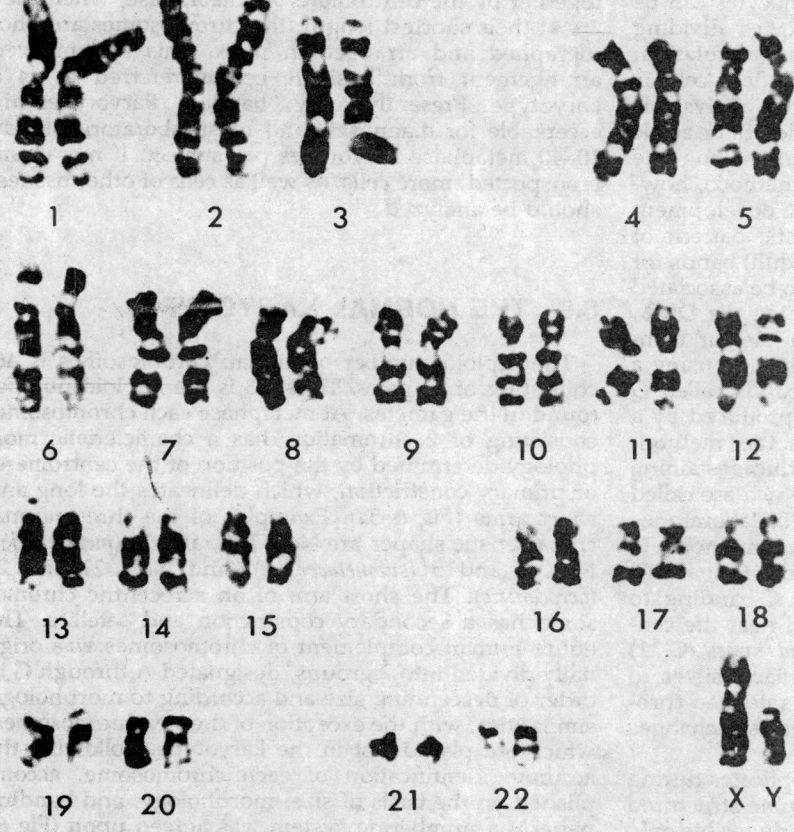

1 2 3   4 5

Figure 6–6 Karyotype of normal male. All chromosomes, pretreated with trypsin and stained with Giemsa, can be positively identified by characteristic banding patterns.

6 7 8 9 10 11 12

13 14 15   16 17 18

19 20   21 22   X Y

the normal karyotype with conventional stains. Best known are elongation of the paracentromeric region in the long arm of Nos. 1, 9, and 16 (Fig 6–5b), extended or deleted short arms or enlarged satellites of acrocentric chromosomes, and a secondary constriction on the short arm of No. 17 (Fig 6–7). The Y chromosome may

also vary in length and shape. Although the banding patterns are constant for each chromosome, normal variants have been revealed by fluorescent stains, e.g., variation in intensity of fluorescent bands near the centromeres of chromosomes 3 and 4 and satellites on the acrocentric chromosomes (Fig 6–7). The variation in

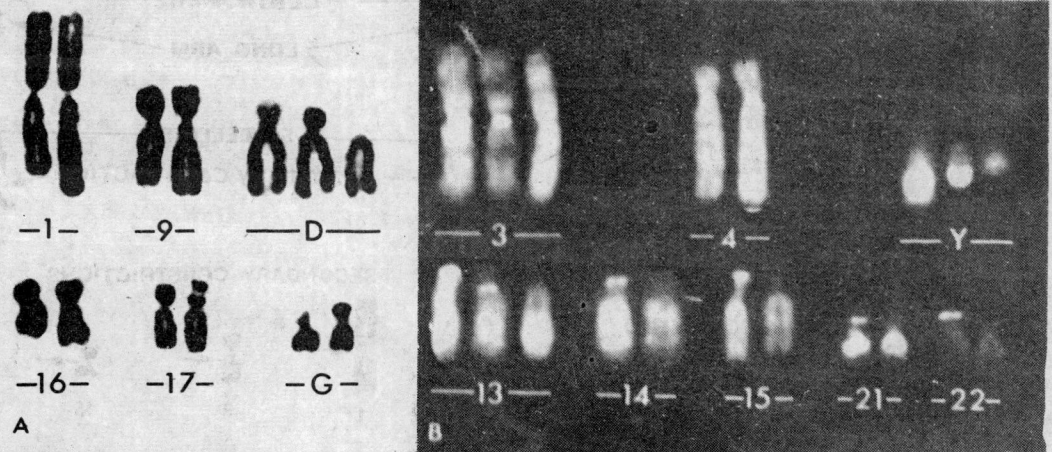

—1— —9— —D—   —3— —4— —Y—

—16— —17— —G—   —13— —14— —15— —21— —22—

A   B

Figure 6–7 Some morphologic variants found in normal subjects. *A*, Chromosomes stained with aceto-orcein. The left-hand chromosome of each pair or triad is a usual or "nonmarker" chromosome. *B*, Chromosomes stained with quinacrine dihydrochloride showing differences in intensity of fluorescent bands among homologues.

length of the Y chromosome is the result of extension or loss of the brilliant Q band, which appears to have no effect on the phenotype. Morphologic variants were first observed in abnormal subjects and thought to be associated with disease, but it soon became apparent that they were inherited in mendelian fashion, and some occur in sufficiently high frequencies to be considered polymorphisms ("normal variants"). Therefore, they are useful genetic markers and also help to localize genes to specific chromosomes. The possibility that such variants are etiologically related to normal chromosome behavior is under investigation.

Cell-to-cell variation in chromosome number has been found in older people. There is a tendency for loss of an X chromosome in women 55 and older and loss of a Y chromosome in men over 65.

6.10 ABNORMAL KARYOTYPES

Numerical Abnormalities. Chromosomal aberrations may be divided into numerical and structural types. A cell with the exact multiple of the haploid number, e.g., 46, 69, 92, etc., is referred to as *euploid*. Euploid cells with more than the normal *diploid* number of 46 chromosomes are termed *polyploid*. Cells deviating from one of the euploid numbers are termed *aneuploid*.

The most common type of aneuploidy is *trisomy*, i.e., 3 homologous chromosomes instead of the pair normally present. Lack of a chromosome is called *monosomy* (for the affected pair). Aneuploid individuals may be trisomic for more than 1 pair of chromosomes or may even combine trisomy and monosomy. During meiosis, synapsis occurs between each chromosome and its homologue; after separation each proceeds to an opposite pole of the dividing cell. Failure of synapsis or failure to separate (**nondisjunction**) interferes with orderly segregation and may result in aneuploidy (Fig 6–8). Monosomy may result from chromosome loss or *anaphase lag*, i.e., failure of a chromosome to reach either pole during anaphase. Nondisjunction occurring during mitotic division results in *mosaicism*, that is, the presence of more than 1 population of cells with differing chromosome numbers in the same individual. The older the mother, the greater the likelihood of nondisjunction and trisomy.

Pure polyploidy appears to be lethal in humans, but individuals with mosaicism have been known to survive. *Triploidy* (3 haploid sets, totaling 69 chromosomes) has been found most frequently among abortuses and stillbirths. It arises by fertilization of the ovum by 2 spermatozoa or by the union of a haploid with a diploid gamete. Tetraploid cells have been found in aborted material, in persons with malignant disease, and, rarely, in dysmorphic infants. *Tetraploidy* occurs occasionally in cultured cells, particularly amniotic fluid cells, and increases during culture.

Structural Aberrations. These abnormalities result from chromosome breaks. Terminal deletions may arise via a single break with the loss of the distal portion of the chromosome arm. *Deletion syndromes*, such as cri-du-chat (5p−), may result from a simple deletion or from the inheritance of a deleted translocation chromosome. Interstitial deletions result from the loss of a

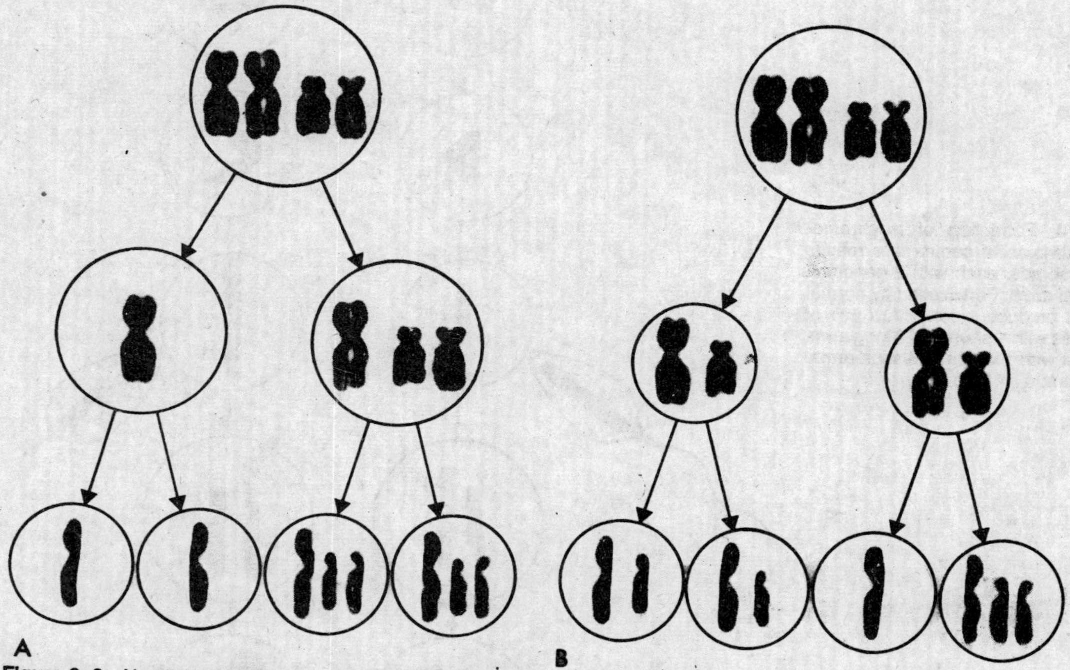

Figure 6–8 Nondisjunction during meiosis illustrated with 2 pairs of chromosomes. *A*, First division nondisjunction with failure of smaller homologues to separate gives rise to gametes with no small chromosome or with an extra one. *B*, Second division nondisjunction following division of centromere. Two newly formed chromosomes fail to separate in cell on the right.

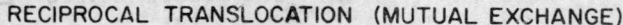

RECIPROCAL TRANSLOCATION (MUTUAL EXCHANGE)

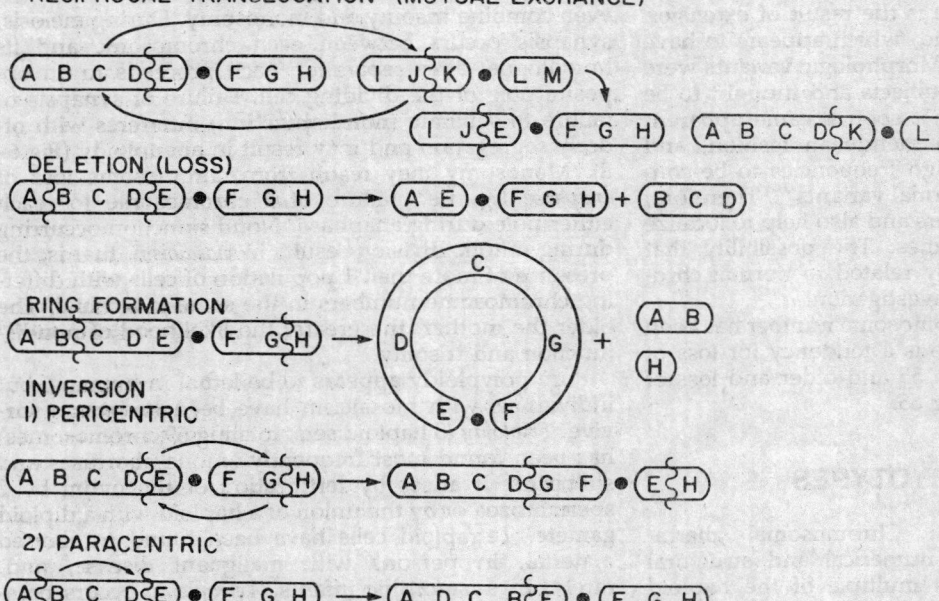

DELETION (LOSS)

RING FORMATION

INVERSION
1) PERICENTRIC

2) PARACENTRIC

Figure 6–9 Mechanisms leading to structural chromosome abnormalities. These aberrations are dependent upon the occurrence of at least 2 breaks (symbolized by a wavy line).

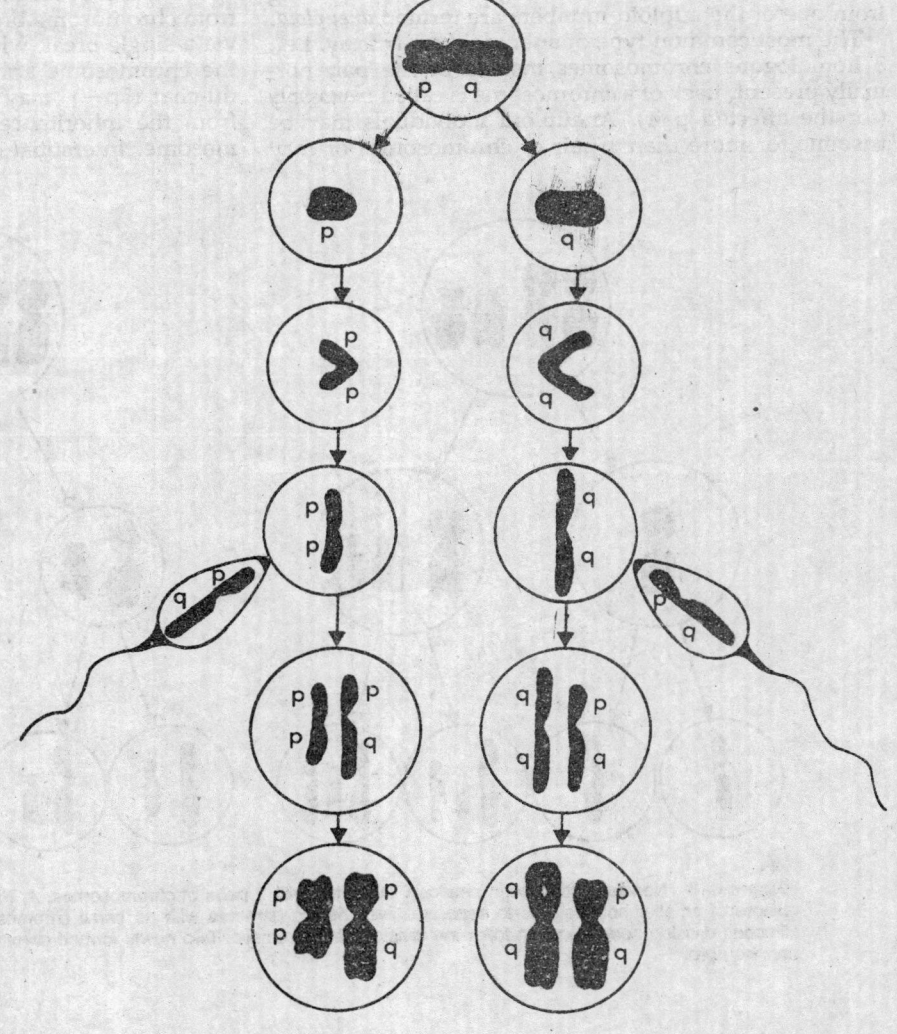

Figure 6–10 Formation of isochromosomes. Misdivision of centromere results in 2 chromosomes, each with 2 genotypically identical arms. Fertilization by normal gametes will produce 1 cell with a pair of chromosomes with 1 short and 3 long arms and the other with 1 long and 3 short arms. p = short arm, q = long arm.

segment within the chromosome arm (Fig 6–9). An *isochromosome* may also be formed by a single event, i.e., misdivision of the centromere; instead of longitudinal division producing 2 normal chromosomes, a transverse division through the centromere produces 2 chromosomes, each with duplication of 1 arm (Fig 6–10). Isochromosomes are formed most frequently from the X chromosome.

All structural defects require at least 2 chromosomal breaks followed by reunion of the broken ends. *Translocations*, which may be inherited or arise de novo, are most common. *Reciprocal translocations* result from the exchange of segments between 2 nonhomologous chromosomes (Fig 6–9). Carriers of reciprocal translocations are usually phenotypically normal since they have a full complement of genes. Children of such "translocation carriers" will be abnormal if they receive only 1 of the 2 translocation chromosomes and thus become affected by duplication-deficiency syndromes. Depending upon the amount of material duplicated or deficient, the aberration is referred to as *partial trisomy* or *partial monosomy*. A special type of translocation is the *centric fusion* or *Robertsonian translocation*, involving acrocentric chromosomes in which the breaks occur adjacent to the centromeres of "recipient" and "donor" chromosomes. The centromere of the donor chromosome and the short arms of both chromosomes are usually lost. Centric fusion commonly involves No. 13 and No. 21 and therefore may result in Down syndrome or 13-trisomy syndrome. Since the short arms of acrocentric chromosomes appear to be genetically inactive, loss of this material in such translocations has no apparent phenotypic effect on carriers.

Ring chromosomes are formed when both tips of a chromosome are broken and the ends of the centric fragment rejoin forming a chromosome with a deletion of both arms (Fig 6–9). This unstable closed structure leads to difficulties in mitosis. *Inversions* (Fig 6–9) of two types may result when the segment between 2 breaks in a single chromosome is inverted and the order of the genes reversed. Since an inversion may cause difficulty in synapsis, it may increase the risk of nondisjunction.

During meiosis, crossing over of genes between chromatids of homologous chromosomes is a normal phenomenon readily proved by the recombination or separation of genes originally linked on the same chromosome. Exchanges between chromatids may also occur during mitosis and may involve the chromatids of 2 homologous or nonhomologous chromosomes. Since at metaphase the sister chromatids have not yet separated, such exchanges result in *quadriradial* configurations that resemble crossroads. (See Fig 6–23 below.) It is somewhat more difficult to prove the existence of *sister chromatid exchanges* (SCE) in mitotic cells because replicated chromatids carry identical genes and no unusual configurations are formed. Proof involves treatment of cells with 5-bromodeoxyuridine (BrdU), following which the differential uptake of Hoechst stain by exchanged chromatid regions produces chromosomes with a harlequin effect. The various types of chromatid exchanges are found in breakage syndromes (see below) and in cells exposed to mutagenic agents.

Table 6–5 SOME REPRESENTATIVE KARYOTYPE NOTATIONS

46,XY	Normal male karyotype
47,XX, + 13	Female with 13-trisomy
47,XY, + 21	Male with 21-trisomy (Down syndrome)
46,XY, − 21, + t(21q21q)	Male with Down syndrome due to centric fusion-type translocation between 2 chromosomes 21, replacing 1 chromosome 21
45,XX, − 14, − 21, + t(14q21q)	Phenotypically normal female carrier of centric fusion-type translocation between chromosomes 14 and 21
46,XY,del(5p)	Male with cri du chat syndrome due to deletion of part of short arm of chromosome 5
46,XX,del(18q)	Female with deletion of all or a portion of the long arm of chromosome 18
46,XY,r(19)	Male with ring chromosome 19
45,X	Female with Turner syndrome due to monosomy X
47,XXY	Male with Klinefelter syndrome
46,X,i(Xq)	Female with Turner syndrome due to isochromosome for long arm of X chromosome
46,XY/47,XXY	Male with XY/XXY mosaic Klinefelter syndrome

NOMENCLATURE

The nomenclature for describing a karyotype has been standardized to avoid confusion. First, the total number of chromosomes is recorded, then the sex chromosome complement, followed by a description of any aberration (Table 6–5). The short arm is referred to as *p* (easily remembered by "petite") and the long arm as *q*. Any addition or loss of chromosomal material is denoted by a plus (+) or minus (−) sign placed before the chromosome number if a whole chromosome is involved and after a symbol denoting any increase or decrease in length. Chromosomes involved in a translocation are written in brackets preceded by a *t*; e.g., t(14q21q) denotes the translocation most frequently found in Down syndrome. (Most children with Down syndrome, however, have three No. 21 chromosomes, the extra denoted as + 21.)

The regions within the chromosomes are now also delineated by their characteristic bands. Each chromosome arm is divided and subdivided into regions (Fig 6–11) so that the breakpoints in chromosomal rearrangements can be identified and the aberration described with some accuracy. This nomenclature is complicated and necessitates constant referral to the diagram, but it allows for anticipated discovery of additional bands and for future adaptation to computer analysis. For the present, however, this system is more appropriate for the cytogeneticist than for the clinician.

DERMATOGLYPHICS

Before the advent of human cytogenetics, analysis of hand and footprints was used as one of the criteria for diagnosis of Down syndrome. The subsequent development of techniques for chromosomal analysis has decreased their relative importance in the clinical assessment of patients suspected of having a chromosomal abnormality.

Dermatoglyphics refers to those configurations

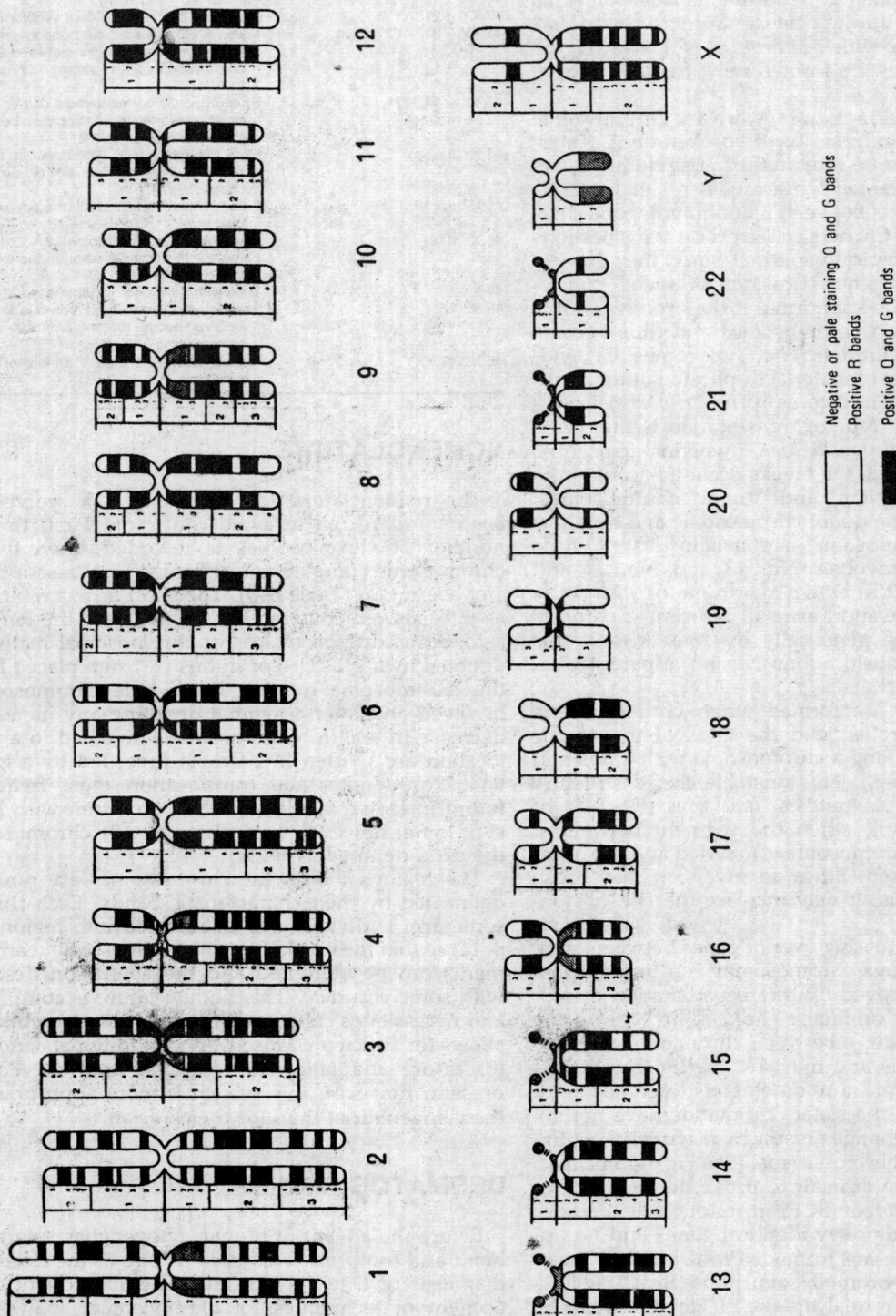

Figure 6–11 Diagrams of chromosome bands. (Paris Conference, 1971, © 1973 The National Foundation.)

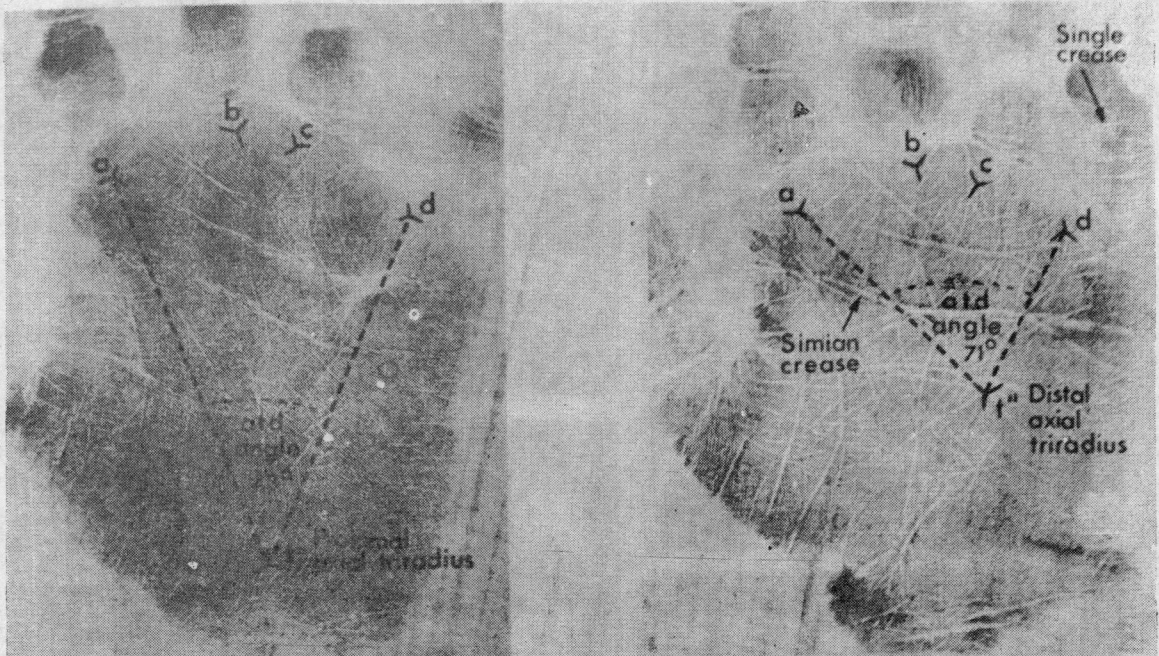

Figure 6–12 Normal palm print showing principal areas.

Figure 6–13 Palm print of child with Down syndrome showing typical dermatoglyphic features.

formed by the dermal ridges, not by the flexion creases. The most important landmarks are the patterns on the distal phalanges of the digits, the position of the triradius in the axis of the palm (Fig 6–12 and 6–13), and the pattern in the hallucal area of the soles.

The size of a pattern is determined by counting the number of dermal ridges between the center or core of the pattern and the triradius which determines its periphery. Whorls usually have the highest ridge counts while an arch has a count of 0 since it has no triradius. Digital pattern size is important in certain syndromes. In general, males have higher counts than females, but the reverse is true in the Klinefelter and Turner syndromes.

A strong correlation between dermatoglyphics and chromosomes was noted soon after the chromosomal basis for many congenital malformations was established. Characteristic dermal patterns are now well known diagnostic criteria for trisomies 13, 18, and 21 and in 18 and G deletion syndromes. They are described under the respective syndromes.

Dermatoglyphic indices have been developed to assist in the diagnosis of Down syndrome such as the Walker method and the *dermatogram* of Reed et al.

Clinical Abnormalities of the Autosomes

ANEUPLOIDY

6.11 21-TRISOMY SYNDROME
(Down Syndrome)

The presence of an extra chromosome No. 21 results in the best recognized and most frequent human chromosomal syndrome (Fig 6–14). The incidence in the general population is 1 in 600–800 live births. However, among all conceptuses, greater than twice this frequency occurs since more than half of the trisomy 21 fetuses are spontaneously aborted during early pregnancy. A high correlation exists between increasing maternal age and the nondisjunction resulting in the presence of an extra chromosome in the offspring. In New York State the frequency of 21-trisomic children rose from a low of 1 in 1925 births among mothers aged 20 yr to a high of more than 1% in women over 40 yr (Table 6–6). An even higher incidence of more than 5% has been found among fetuses of mothers over 40 yr of age who have been screened by genetic amniocentesis.

Heteromorphisms on fluorescent staining have furnished cytologic proof for the parental origin of nondisjunction in a number of instances (Fig 6–14B). Evidence is accumulating that abnormal segregation is paternal in origin in approximately one third of cases. This observation raises the question of whether paternal nondisjunction may be increasing and may account for the observed recent decline in mean maternal age for Down syndrome births from 34 to below 30 yr. There

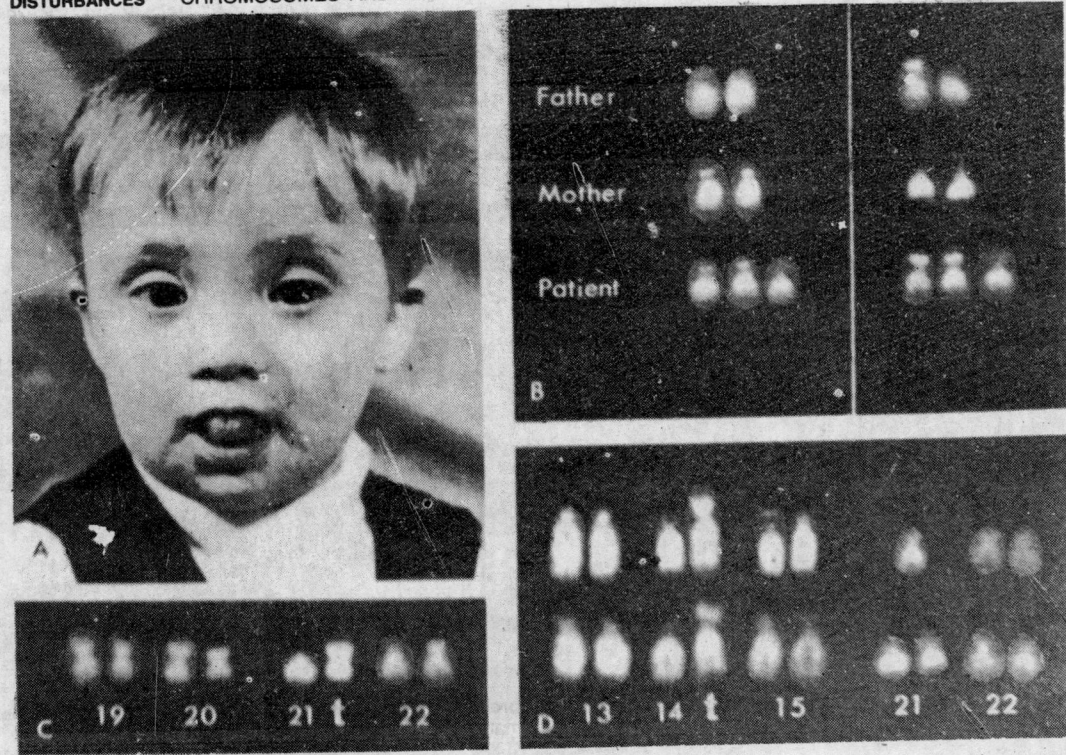

Figure 6–14 Partial karyotypes from patients with Down syndrome.
A, Patient with trisomy 21.
B, Chromosomes 21 from 2 patients and their parents. Left: 2 of a patient's chromosomes with brightly fluorescent satellites were transmitted by the mother. Right: 2 chromosomes with bright satellites resulted from paternal nondisjunction at second meiotic division.
C, 21q21q translocation.
D, 14q21q translocation in a mother (above) and her affected child (below).

are 2 distribution curves for maternal age: the age-independent curve, which includes cases due to translocation and probably paternal nondisjunction, and the age-dependent curve. In some cases it is possible to tell whether the nondisjunction occurred during the 1st or 2nd meiotic division; if all 3 No. 21 chromosomes have different markers, then misdivision occurred during 1st meiotic division, but if the aberration occurred during 2nd division, 2 No. 21s should be identical (Fig 6–14*B*).

The reason for the correlation between late maternal age and nondisjunction is still unknown. The incidences of both Down syndrome and maternal exposure to diagnostic roentgenograms of the abdomen correlate with maternal age. Virus-induced disturbance of chromosomal segregation has been suggested to account for the clustering of births of 21-trisomic infants following epidemics of infectious hepatitis. "Over-ripeness" of the ovum due to delayed fertilization because of decreased frequency of coitus with age has also been suggested. Significant increases in the frequency of thyroid autoantibodies have been observed in patients and mothers, but the mechanism responsible for this correlation is not known. Finally, a genetic predisposition to nondisjunction could account for the observed repetition not only of 21-trisomy but also of other aneuploidy, including that of the sex chromosomes within the same sibship.

The recurrence risk of trisomy to chromosomally normal parents is uncertain. Estimates range from increase in risk over the general population to a 50-fold increase in young mothers. Analysis of data using only chromosomally proven trisomy indicates that the risk

Table 6–6 ESTIMATED RATES OF DOWN SYNDROME (NEW YORK STATE STUDY)

MATERNAL AGE IN YEARS*	ESTIMATED RATE	MATERNAL AGE IN YEARS*	ESTIMATED RATE
20	1/1925	35	1/365
21	1/1695	36	1/285
22	1/1540	37	1/225
23	1/1410	38	1/175
24	1/1300	39	1/140
25	1/1205	40	1/110
26	1/1125	41	1/85
27	1/1050	42	1/67
28	1/990	43	1/53
29	1/935	44	1/41
30	1/885	45	1/32
31	1/825	46	1/25
32	1/725	47	1/20
33	1/590	48	1/16
34	1/465	49	1/12

*Age at last birthday at delivery.
(From Hook EB: Birth Defects *13*(3A):123,1977.)

Table 6–7 RISK OF RECURRENCE OF 21-TRISOMY ACCORDING TO MATERNAL AGE AT BIRTH OF PROBAND (MOSAICS AND TRANSLOCATIONS EXCLUDED)*

| MATERNAL AGE | TRISOMY BIRTH RATE (MANITOBA 1960–68) | CHILDREN BORN AFTER PROBAND | | RECURRENCE RISK |
		Total Sibs	21-Trisomy	
< 25	1/2000	181	2	1/90
25 – 34	1/1300	254	5	1/50
35 – 44	1/250	94	1	1/90
45 +	1/80	0	0	—
Totals	1/900	529	8	1/65

*Combined data from Manitoba study and Carter CO, Evans KA: Lancet 2:785, 1961.

of recurrence, regardless of maternal age, appears to be about the same as that for a mother who is over the age of 45 yr (Table 6–7). This increased risk may be due to undetected mosaicism in a parent or repeated exposure to the same environmental insult. In pregnancies subsequent to the birth of a 21-trisomic infant which were monitored prenatally, chromosomal aberrations were identified among 1% of fetuses of women under 35 yr of age, 4% of those of women 35 to 39 yr, and 15% of those of mothers 40 yr of age and over. These frequencies, based on study of very small samples, are for the 15th–16th wk of pregnancy and are considerably higher than for live births.

Translocation Down Syndrome. "Regular" trisomy comprises some 95% of cases of Down syndrome. Approximately 1% of cases are mosaic (this is doubtless a minimum since some mosaics probably remain undetected, particularly among phenotypically normal parents of trisomic offspring); the remainder are the result of translocation.

The majority of translocations giving rise to the Down syndrome consist of centric fusions between No. 21 and a D chromosome; approximately half of these are inherited. The vast majority are t(14q21q) (Fig 6–14D) and a few are t(15q21q). The rarity of t(13q21q) probably accounts for the absence of 13-trisomy syndrome, which would be expected to occur among the offspring of phenotypically normal carriers of the Dq21q translocation. Carrier mothers produce 3 types of viable offspring: normal phenotype and karyotype, phenotypically normal translocation carrier, and translocation trisomy-21 (Fig 6–15). Theoretically, these 3 types of offspring should occur with equal frequency, but only 10% have been abnormal, possibly because of an increased lethality to the unbalanced zygote or fetus. The expected frequency of one third affected has been observed, however, among fetuses studied early in gestation. Carrier fathers rarely have affected offspring, though they do produce both normals and carriers.

Only 5% of cases of translocation Down syndrome involving 2 G chromosomes are inherited from a carrier parent. The small metacentric translocation chromo-

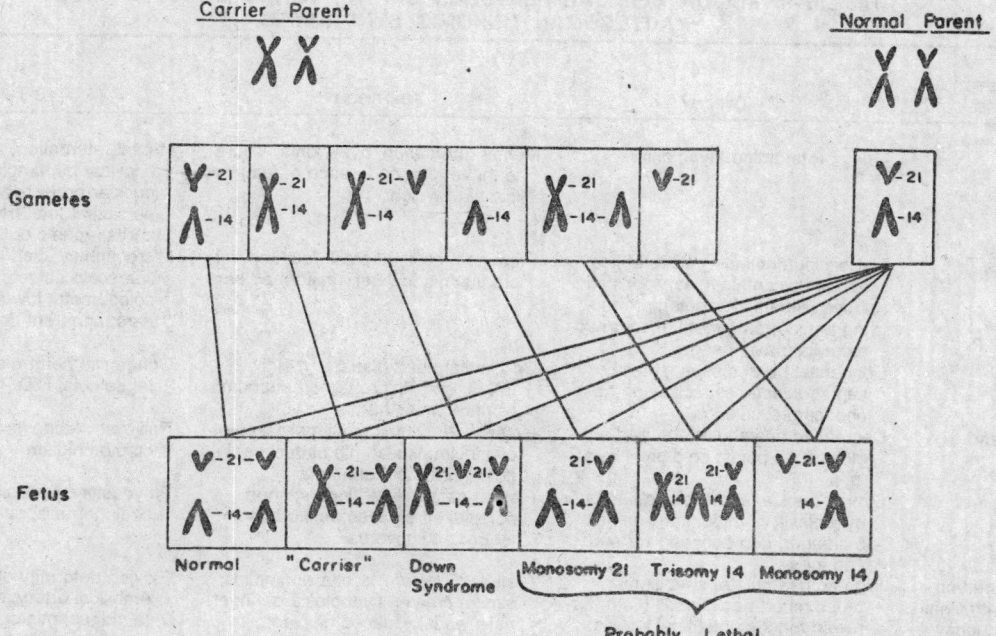

Figure 6–15 Possible outcomes of pregnancy in segregation products of a balanced carrier of a Robertsonian translocation.

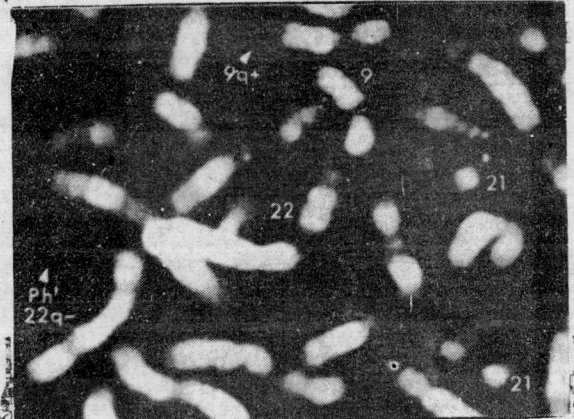

Figure 6-16 Partial spread showing small Ph¹ chromosome (No. 22) formed by translocation of distal portion of long arm of No. 22 to long arm of No. 9, seen as a band of pale fluorescence.

some may represent centric fusion of chromosomes Nos. 21 and 22 or of 2 No. 21 chromosomes (Fig 6-14C) or misdivision of the centromere to form an iso-21 chromosome (Fig 6-10). The low frequency of inherited cases suggests that most of these metacentric chromosomes are of the latter 2 types since a normal carrier of either could result only from the rare coincidence of translocation in 1 parent plus absence or loss of the 21 chromosome from the gamete of the other parent or from translocation occurring after the zygote stage. All viable offspring from a t(21q21q) carrier would have Down syndrome (with the possible exception of 21-monosomics). A t(21q22q) carrier, on the other hand, can produce carrier and normal as well as abnormal offspring.

Not all translocations producing the Down syndrome are of the centric fusion type. Some have been reported with increased length of the long arm of 1 chromosome No. 21. Other patients with Down syndrome and apparently normal karyotypes may have a hidden translocation, i.e., part of No. 21 attached to a larger chromosome, which can be demonstrated by banding techniques. However, most children with Down syndrome and apparently normal karyotypes are probably mosaics with low frequencies of trisomic cells.

The frequency of acute leukemia among individuals with Down syndrome is higher than in the general population. The majority of such cases are of the lymphoblastic type. When the Philadelphia (Ph¹) chromosome was first found in patients with chronic myeloid leukemia, it was thought to be a deleted No. 21; it has now been proved that the Ph¹ chromosome involves No. 22, in which the distal portion of the long arm has been translocated to the long arm of chromosome No. 9 or another autosome (Fig 6-16).

A number of biochemical alterations have been reported in patients with Down syndrome, but most have not been consistent enough to provide useful genetic information. Several gene loci have been assigned to chromosome 21. Studies of one of these, the gene for the soluble form of the *superoxide dismutase* (SOD_s), have revealed a dose relation proportional to the number of No. 21 chromosomes in a cell. The level of SOD_s in cells from patients with trisomy 21 has been shown to be approximately 1.5 times normal.

The important clinical features of Down syndrome are listed in Tables 6-8 and 6-9.

Table 6-8 MAJOR CLINICAL FEATURES OF THE THREE MOST COMMON AUTOSOMAL TRISOMIC SYNDROMES

CHARACTERISTIC FEATURES	21-TRISOMY	18-TRISOMY	13-TRISOMY
General	Mental retardation; hypotonia	Mental retardation; hypertonia; failure to thrive; preponderance of females; low birth weight	Mental retardation; failure to thrive; capillary hemangiomas; increased nuclear projections in neutrophils; persistent fetal hemoglobin; seizures; apneic episodes
Craniofacies	Flat occiput; oblique palpebral fissures; epicanthic folds; speckled irides (Brushfield spots); protruding tongue; prominent, malformed ears; flat nasal bridge	Prominent occiput; small features; micrognathia; low-set, malformed ears	Microcephaly; cleft lip ± palate; midline scalp defects; microphthalmia; colobomata; low-set malformed ears; apparent deafness
Thorax	Congenital heart disease, mainly septal defects, especially of the endocardial cushion	Congenital heart disease, mainly V.S.D. and P.D.A.;* short sternum; diaphragmatic hernia	Congenital heart disease, mainly septal defects, P.D.A.
Abdomen and pelvis	Decreased acetabular and iliac angles; small penis; cryptorchidism	Horseshoe kidney; small pelvis; cryptorchidism; limited hip abduction; inguinal or umbilical hernia	Polycystic kidneys; bicornuate uterus; cryptorchidism
Hands and feet	Simian crease; short, broad hands; hypoplasia of middle phalanx of 5th finger; gap between 1st and 2nd toes	Flexion deformity of fingers; short, dorsiflexed big toes; rockerbottom feet or equinovarus	Polydactyly; hyperconvex or hypoplastic fingernails; simian crease
Other features observed with significant frequency	High-arched palate; strabismus; broad, short neck; small teeth; furrowed tongue; intestinal atresia; imperforate anus	Cleft lip ± palate; ocular anomalies; simian crease; hypoplasia of fingernails; widely spaced nipples; webbed neck; single umbilical artery	Flexion deformity of fingers; single umbilical artery; shallow supraorbital ridges; micrognathia; retroflexible thumb; rockerbottom feet; omphalocele

*V.S.D. = ventricular septal defect; P.D.A. = patent ductus arteriosus.

**Table 6–9 IMPORTANT DERMATOGLYPHIC PATTERNS AND FLEXION CREASES
FOUND IN THE THREE COMMON AUTOSOMAL TRISOMIC SYNDROMES***

AREAS	21-TRISOMY	18-TRISOMY	13-TRISOMY
Digits	Ulnar loops on most fingers; radial loops on fingers 4 and 5	Arches on fingers and toes	—
Palms	Distal axial triradius or large *atd* angle	—	Distal axial triradius or large *atd* angle
Soles	Arch tibial or small loop distal in hallucal area	—	Arch fibular or arch fibular-S in hallucal area
Flexion creases	Simian crease; single crease on finger 5	Single crease on finger 5 or on all fingers	Simian crease

*See also Fig 6–12 and 6–13.

6.12 18-TRISOMY SYNDROME
(E-Trisomy Syndrome, Edwards Syndrome)

This is the second most common autosomal aberration (Fig 6–17), originally referred to as the E-trisomy syndrome until improved techniques permitted distinction between chromosomes 17 and 18.

Small, delicate facial features serve to distinguish children with 18-trisomy from other trisomics. The principal clinical characteristics are listed in Tables 6–8 and 6–9. Incidence is about 1 in 8000 births. Although infants are usually born after term, the birth weight is low. The sex ratio is 1 male to 4 females. Almost all have a cardiac malformation, a major factor in the characteristically early demise, most frequently within the first 3 mo of life. Exceptional long-lived cases have been reported, the oldest being 15 yr of age. As with 21-trisomy, advanced maternal age is etiologically important.

Translocations of Chromosome 18. These, though rare, have given rise to partial 18-trisomy syndromes, i.e., only part of 1 No. 18 chromosome is duplicated either by elongation of its long arm or by translocation to another chromosome. The diagnosis of partial tri-

somy has generally been based on the clinical picture since in the absence of a reciprocal translocation in 1 parent, it has not been possible to confirm cytologically the origin of the extra chromosomal material. As with translocation Down syndrome, offspring of 6 different chromosomal types can result from segregation of the chromosomes of a carrier parent, but probably only 3 are viable: normal karyotype, balanced translocation carrier, and partial 18-trisomy, theoretically in equal proportions. Mosaics and double trisomies have also been reported.

6.13 13-TRISOMY SYNDROME
(D-Trisomy Syndrome, Patau Syndrome)

Because the 3 chromosome pairs of the D group were indistinguishable from one another by conventional stains, patients with an extra D chromosome were called D_1 trisomics in anticipation of the future identification of trisomies involving the other 2 pairs. When autoradiographic techniques were developed, the 3 pairs could be distinguished by differential labeling. The most heavily labeled of the 3 was designated No. 13, and

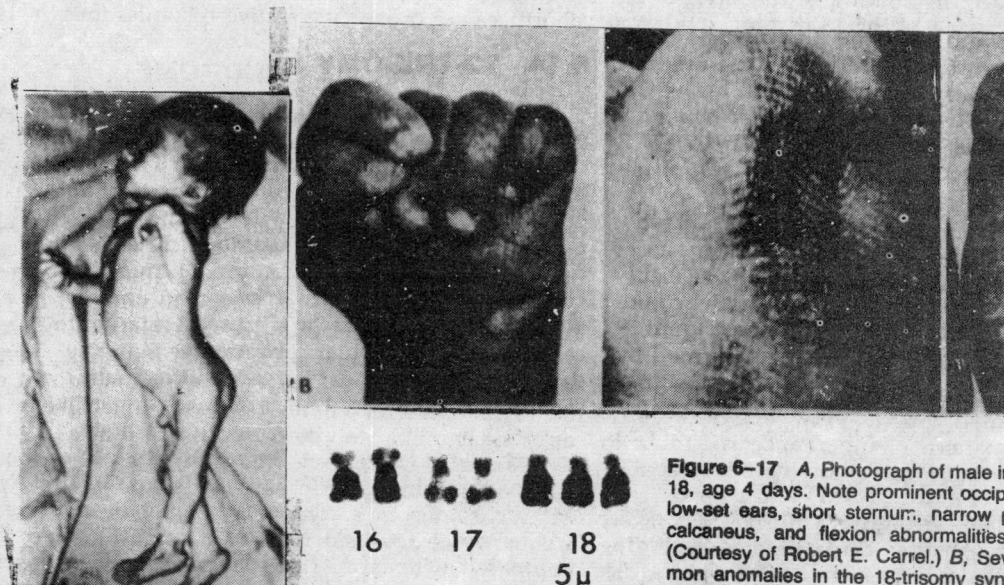

16   17   18
5μ

Figure 6–17 *A*, Photograph of male infant with trisomy 18, age 4 days. Note prominent occiput, micrognathia, low-set ears, short sternum, narrow pelvis, prominent calcaneus, and flexion abnormalities of the fingers. (Courtesy of Robert E. Carrel.) *B*, Several of the common anomalies in the 18-trisomy syndrome, including the unusual position of the fingers with hypoplasia of 5th fingernail; the simple arch pattern of the fingers; and the dorsiflexed hallux with hypoplasia of toenails. (From Smith DW: Am J Obstet Gynecol 90:1055, 1964.) *C*, Partial karyotype of trisomy 18 prepared with modified Giemsa stain.

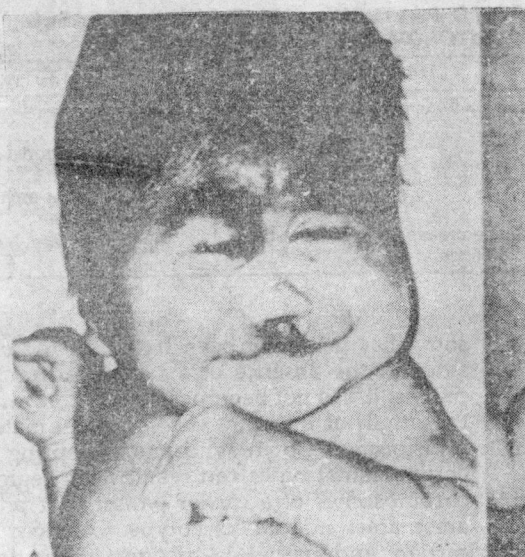
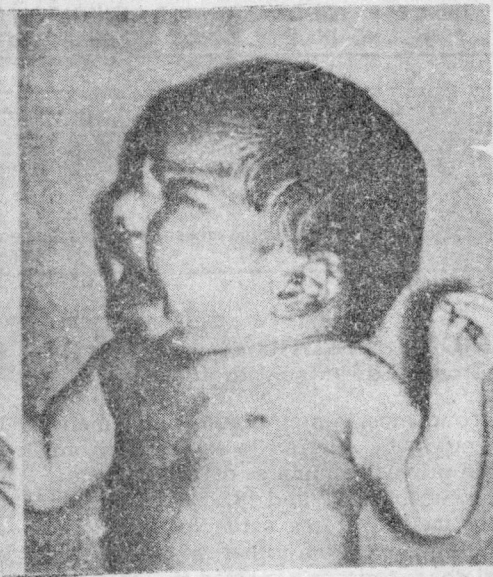
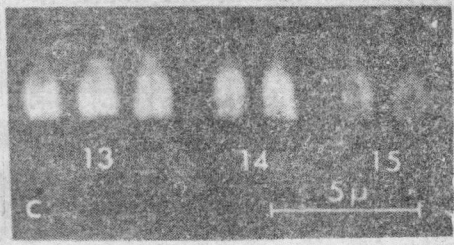

Figure 6–18 *A* and *B*, Female infants with 13-trisomy syndrome. Note midline cleft of the lip and palate, microcephaly, hypotelorism, microphthalmus, bulbous nose, polydactyly, and overlapping of fingers. Scalp defects (not shown) are also present. (Courtesy of Miriam G. Wilson.) *C*, Partial karyotype showing D-group chromosomes stained with quinacrine dihydrochloride.

this is the chromosome found in triplicate in this syndrome. Trisomies for the other 2 pairs have not been found and are probably lethal. All 3 pairs can now be identified by differences in banding patterns (Fig 6–18).

The phenotypic features of the 13-trisomy syndrome are listed in Tables 6–8 and 6–9. The prognosis is grave as in the 18-trisomy syndrome. Most infants affected die in the 1st year of life, but at least one is known to be alive at 10 yr of age. The incidence is approximately 1 in 20,000 live births; as with 18- and 21-trisomy, it increases with advancing maternal age. No sex predilection has been observed.

Translocations of D-Group Chromosomes. Translocations involving chromosome 13 have been more frequently reported than have those of No. 18, probably because of the greater tendency of acrocentric chromosomes to break and rearrange and the ease of identification due to chromosome length. Most are formed by centric fusion, but some consist of 2 D chromosomes attached in tandem to form a very long acrocentric chromosome. The pattern of inheritance is similar to that of the 21qGq translocation discussed under 21-trisomy.

There are many large pedigrees with phenotypically normal subjects who have 45 chromosomes, including a centric fusion t(DqDq), but such a carrier has a risk of less than 1% of producing trisomic offspring; larger chromosomes with symmetric arm lengths tend to segregate in an orderly fashion, giving rise to karyotypically normal individuals or balanced carriers. However, spontaneous abortion and infertility are encountered with increased frequency. Since the chromosomes forming these translocations are usually Nos. 13 and 14, the abortuses are probably effective trisomics for No. 14.

6.14 22-TRISOMY SYNDROME

Patients with an additional small acrocentric chromosome but without the clinical signs of Down syndrome were originally interpreted as having 22-trisomy, XYY, or partial trisomy resulting from deletions of larger chromosomes. However, with the aid of marker chromosomes and fluorescent banding, it has been possible to identify 22-trisomy in some of these patients. A clinical syndrome has now begun to emerge; its characteristics are mental and growth retardation; microcephaly; micrognathia; preauricular skin tags, appendages, and/or sinuses; low-set and/or malformed ears; cleft palate; congenital heart disease; finger-like or malapposed thumbs; and deformed lower limbs.

22-Trisomy is seen less frequently than 21-trisomy in spite of the similarity in size and shape of the 2 pairs of G chromosomes. The reason may be a decreased frequency of nondisjunction of chromosome No. 22 as compared with No. 21. G-trisomy has been observed with a relatively high frequency among abortuses; banding studies have shown 21- and 22-trisomics to occur with similar frequenices.

Table 6–10 MAJOR CLINICAL FEATURES OF THE TRISOMY-8 AND TRISOMY-9 SYNDROMES

Feature	Trisomy-8	Trisomy-9
General	Mental retardation, short stature, decreased weight, vertebral anomalies	Mental retardation
Craniofacies	Dysmorphic skull, prominent forehead, dysplastic ears, strabismus, plump nose with broad base, low-set ears, everted lower lip, high palate, cleft soft palate, micrognathia	Microcephaly, abnormal cranial sutures, prominent forehead, deep-set eyes, protuberant ears, prominent nose, fishmouth, micrognathia
Thorax	Congenital heart disease	
Abdomen and pelvis	Urinary tract anomaly, narrow pelvis	Congenital heart disease
Limbs	Patellar dysplasia, limited joint mobility, deep flexion creases on palms and soles	Urinary tract anomaly
		Congenital hip/knee dislocation, clinodactyly, digital hypoplasia, nail hypoplasia, syndactyly, simian palmar creases, absent B and C palmar digital triradii

6.15 TRISOMY INVOLVING OTHER AUTOSOMES

Accurate identification of chromosomes has led to the description of new autosomal trisomy syndromes involving primarily chromosomes of the C group. Syndromes due to trisomy-8 and trisomy-9 have been fairly well documented (Table 6–10). Full (i.e., not in mosaic association with a chromosomally normal cell line) trisomies for other chromosomes have also been reported, but documentation is lacking. Trisomy for virtually every autosome has been documented in the products of early spontaneous abortion; most full trisomies are probably lethal. Partial trisomy (duplication or duplication-deficiency state) for almost all the autosomes produced by segregation of a translocation or inversion has been described, as has partial trisomy for an unattached segment of an autosome.

6.16 AUTOSOMAL MONOSOMY

Several cases of monosomy involving a G-group chromosome have been reported, but few have been adequately documented as complete monosomy. Syndromes produced by deletion (partial monosomy) of part of the long arm of chromosome 21 or 22 have been well documented (Table 6–11).

STRUCTURAL ABERRATIONS

6.17 TRANSLOCATIONS

These are the most common structural aberrations. Exchange of segments between 2 nonhomologous chromosomes is known as a *reciprocal* or *balanced translocation*. Although early reports of translocations suggested the presence of *simple translocations*, i.e., a segment of 1 chromosome broken off and attached to the unbroken end of the recipient chromosome, no convincing evidence exists for the occurrence of simple translocations in humans.

In phenotypically normal individuals translocations are assumed to be *reciprocal* and *balanced* since loss or gain of chromatin material usually results in an abnormal phenotype. An exception is the balanced (Robertsonian) translocation discussed above. Unbalanced karyotypes associated with *duplication-deficiency syndromes* are found among the offspring of carriers of balanced translocations. Whether a syndrome is due to partial monosomy or partial trisomy will be determined by which interchange chromosome is transmitted.

Except for translocation resulting in well-known clinical syndromes, it is difficult and often impossible, even with the aid of banding patterns, to identify with certainty the origin of excess chromosomal material in the absence of a reciprocal translocation in a parent. Another exception is the translocation of a large segment of the X chromosome that can be positively identified by the X chromatin or thymidine-labeling pattern. When a parent is a translocation carrier, the origin of the extra (trisomic) chromosomal material can be accurately determined, and the delineation of new clinical syndromes becomes possible. Banding techniques can identify small duplications and deletions in karyotypes that were thought to be normal with conventional stains.

Syndromes have been described as the result of partial trisomy (duplication) for chromosomes 1q, 2p, 2q, 3p, 3q, 4p, 4q, 5p, 6q, 7q, 9p, 9q, 10q, 12p, 14q, 18q, and 22q. The best known and most frequently documented partial trisomy is the 9p-trisomy syndrome (Fig 6–19). Translocation of the short arm of chromosome 9 to a variety of autosomes has been reported, and many kindreds have been described in which reciprocal translocations are carried by many members and transmitted through several generations. Characteristic features include mental retardation, microcephaly, hypertelorism, oblique palpebral fissures, enophthalmos, bulbous nose, downward slanting mouth, low-set protruding ears, and single palmar crease.

Although all chromosomes are subject to breaks that result in structural aberrations, the chromosomes most frequently involved in translocations appear to be the acrocentrics of the D and G groups, probably because of their close association as nucleolar organizers, i.e., the stalks of the satellites have the capacity to organize diffuse nucleolar material into 1 or more compact bodies during interphase. Translocations and their modes of transmission have been discussed in the respective sections under *Aneupoloidy*.

Table 6–11   IMPORTANT CLINICAL FEATURES

FEATURE	4p–	5p–	9q–	13q–
General	LBW, severe MR, delayed ossification	LBW, MR, catlike cry	MR	LBW, severe MR, failure to thrive
Craniofacies	Microcephaly, hypertelorism, epicanthus, ptosis, colobomata, beaked nose, short broad philtrum, cleft palate, micrognathia, simple ears	Microcephaly, round face, hypertelorism, epicanthus, antimongoloid palpebral fissure, micrognathia, low-set malformed ears, preauricular tags	Trigonocephaly, upward slanting palpebral fissures, epicanthal folds, depressed nasal bridge, anteverted nares, long philtrum, low-set ears, high palate, micrognathia, short and webbed neck	Microcephaly; trigonocephaly; flat, wide nasal bridge; hypertelorism; ptosis, epicanthus, microphthalmia, colobomata; retinoblastoma; micrognathia
Thorax		CHD (occasional)	Widely spaced nipples, cardiac murmur	CHD
Pelvis and abdomen	Inguinal hernia, sacral dimples, hypospadias, cryptorchidism	Inguinal hernia, diastasis recti, small iliac wings		Hip dysplasia, cryptorchidism
Hands and feet		Short metacarpals or metatarsals, partial syndactyly, pes planus, simian crease	Long fingers, square nails	Hypoplastic or absent thumbs, clinodactyly of 5th fingers, syndactyly of toes

CHD = Congenital heart disease; LBW = low birth weight; MR = mental retardation; TRC = total ridge count.

6.18   DELETIONS

Chromosomal deletions were thought at first to be lethal in man, but several associated clinical syndromes have been documented. Some lead to a less severely affected phenotype than do trisomies. Clinical features of the more common deletions are listed in Table 6–11.

Chromosome Nos. 4 and 5 (4p– and 5p– Syndromes).   Clinical syndromes have been described as the result of deletion of part of the short arm of either of the B group chromosomes. Best known is the cri du chat syndrome (5p–) (Fig 6–20A), so named because

the cry of affected infants resembles that of a kitten and is characterized by high-pitched, tense phonation. The facilitation of diagnosis by this distinguishing trait probably accounts for the apparently greater frequency of 5p– compared to other deletions. However, the typical cry tends to disappear in late infancy, and a similar cry has been noted on occasion in other retarded infants. Most cases arise sporadically, but a few reports of reciprocal translocation in a parent have been made. Ring chromosomes with loss of material from both ends may produce the same syndrome.

Some patients with a deletion of a group B chromo-

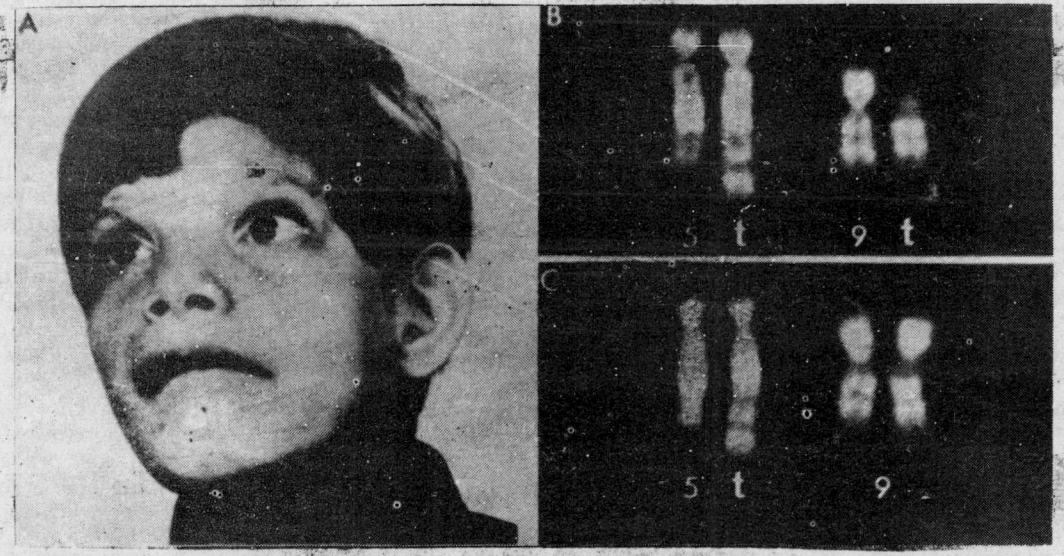

Figure 6–19   A, Patient with 9p-trisomy syndrome showing some of the characteristic features: hypertelorism, bulbous nose, downward slanting mouth, low-set protruding ears. B, Balanced t(5q/9p) translocation carried by mother. C, Unbalanced translocation resulting in 9p-trisomy syndrome in above patient. t = translocation chromosome.

OF THE DELETION SYNDROMES

18p−	18q−	21q−	22q−
LBW, variable MR, short stature, Turner syndrome–like stigmata	LBW, severe MR, seizures, hypotonia	MR, hypertonia, skeletal malformations, growth retardation	MR, hypotonia
Hypertelorism, epicanthus, flat nasal bridge, micrognathia, low-set, large floppy ears	Microcephaly, ophthalmologic defects, carp-shaped mouth, apparently protruding mandible, atretic ear canals	Microcephaly, downward-slanting palpebral fissures, high palate, large and/or low-set ears, prominent nasal bridge, micrognathia	Microcephaly, high palate, large and/or low-set ears, epicanthal folds, ptosis of eyelids, bifid uvula
	CHD (occasional), supernumerary ribs		
	Small penis, cryptorchidism, hypoplastic genitalia in females	Pyloric stenosis, inguinal hernia, hypospadias, cryptorchidism	
Stubby hands with high-set thumbs, partial webbing of toes, large digital patterns with high TRC	Long, tapering fingers; abnormal implantation of toes; large digital patterns with high TRC	Nail anomalies	Syndactyly of toes, clindodactyly

some are much more severely malformed and retarded and do not have the typical cry. The suspicion that these were deletions of chromosome No. 4 was confirmed with autoradiography and chromosome banding. The clinical signs are listed in Table 6–11 (Fig 6–20B).

Chromosome No. 9 (9p− Syndrome). A small number of infants have been described with deletion of the short arm of chromosome 9. The features of this deletion syndrome are enumerated in Table 6–11.

Chromosome No. 18 (18p− and 18q− Syndromes). Deletions of chromosome No. 18 take 3 forms: loss of

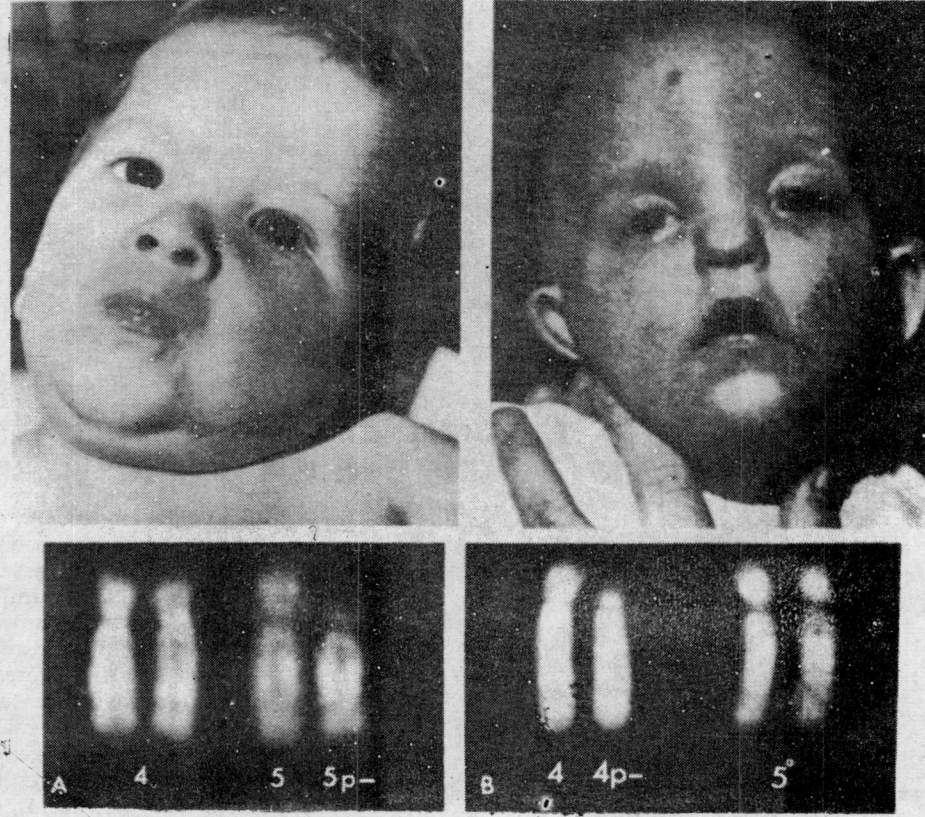

Figure 6–20 Patients with partial deletion of short arm of B group chromosomes. A, An 8 mo old boy with cri du chat syndrome and deletion of part of the short arm of 1 chromosome No. 5 (5p−). B, 1 yr old boy with partial deletion of the short arm of 1 chromosome No. 4. (Courtesy of W. R. Breg.)

the entire short arm, 18p−; loss of part of the long
arm, 18q−; and deletions of both ends to form a ring,
r(18). Patients with 18p− are phenotypically extremely
variable. A few are severely affected, with arrhinencephaly, cyclopia, or cleft lip and palate, but most have
only minor malformations and are only moderately
retarded (Table 6–11 and Fig 6–21). Turner syndrome
is often suspected. On the other hand, children with
18q− are severely retarded and have more characteristic
malformations (Fig 6–22). Children with a ring chromosome 18 have phenotypic features of both short and
long arm deletions since the ends of both arms of the
chromosome are lost during ring formation. The 18p−
syndrome is the only structural abnormality of the
chromosomes in which late maternal age appears to be
a factor.

A number of characteristics are common to the 3
types of deletion. Prognosis for survival seems to be
good. IgA deficiency has been noted in some patients.
Large dermal patterns are present on the digits, mainly
whorls, giving a very high total ridge count similar to
that seen in the Turner syndrome. This is in sharp
contrast to 18-trisomy syndrome, in which the presence
of arches results in a very low ridge count.

Chromosomes of the D Group. Loss of part of the
long arm of a D chromosome has been reported in a
few patients. It has not yet been definitely established
that the same chromosome is deficient, but a number
of cases have been shown by banding patterns to
involve chromosome 13 (Table 6–11).

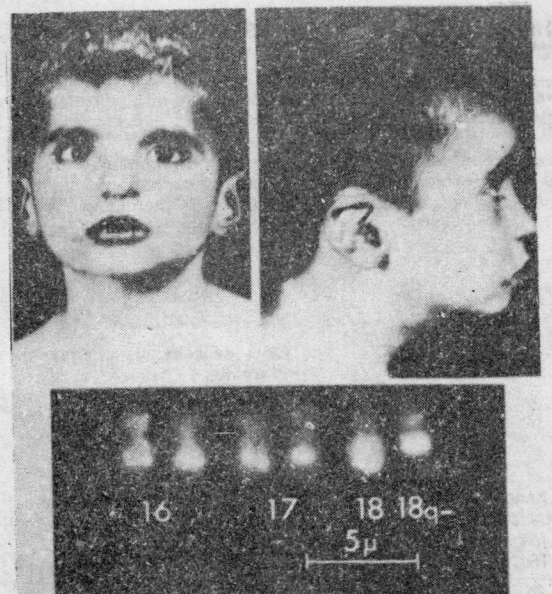

Figure 6–22 Patient with partial deletion of long arm of chromosome
No. 18. (Courtesy of P. S. Gerald and W. Wertelecki.) Partial karyotype
showing 18q−, stained with quinacrine dihydrochloride.

Chromosomes of the F and G Groups. Deficiencies
in these 2 groups have resulted mainly in formation of
ring chromosomes. Loss of material from the long arm
has occurred in some subjects, but deletions compatible
with life may often be too small to identify unless a
ring is formed. *F group aberrations* were first reported
only in studies of aborted material and patients with
blood dyscrasias. A few patients with severe mental
retardation and F group deletions have now been described; others with F deletions in only some of their
cells (mosaics) appear to be phenotypically normal.

Because many more cases have been described with
G deletions, 2 syndromes have emerged, one attributed
to 21q− and the other to 22q−. The phenotypic features of these syndromes, some of which are shared by
both, are enumerated in Table 6–11. Since some of the
clinical signs of 21 deletions are variations of those of
the Down syndrome, this syndrome has also been
referred to as "antimongolism."

6.19 BREAKAGE SYNDROMES

Chromosomal breakage, structural rearrangements,
and aneuploidy have been reported as inconsistent
findings during viral diseases such as measles, chickenpox, and infectious hepatitis. Similar aberrations have
been observed in both chronic and acute leukemia, but,
except for the Ph[1] chromosome, no consistent aberration
has been observed. There is, however, a group of
autosomal recessive diseases with high frequencies of
chromosome breaks and rearrangements, together with
an increased risk of leukemia and other malignancies:
Bloom syndrome (congenital telangiectatic erythema
with dwarfism, Sec 24.14), constitutional aplastic pan-

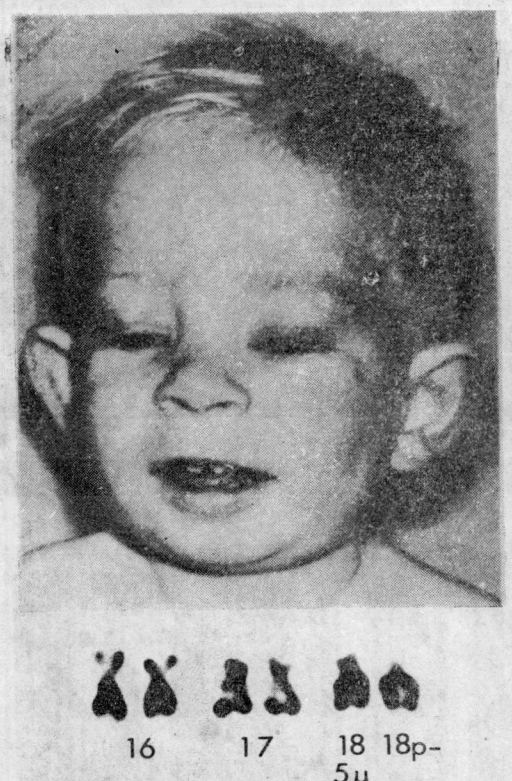

Figure 6–21 Patient with 18 short arm deletion, 18p−. Chromosomes
of E group showing Giemsa banding.

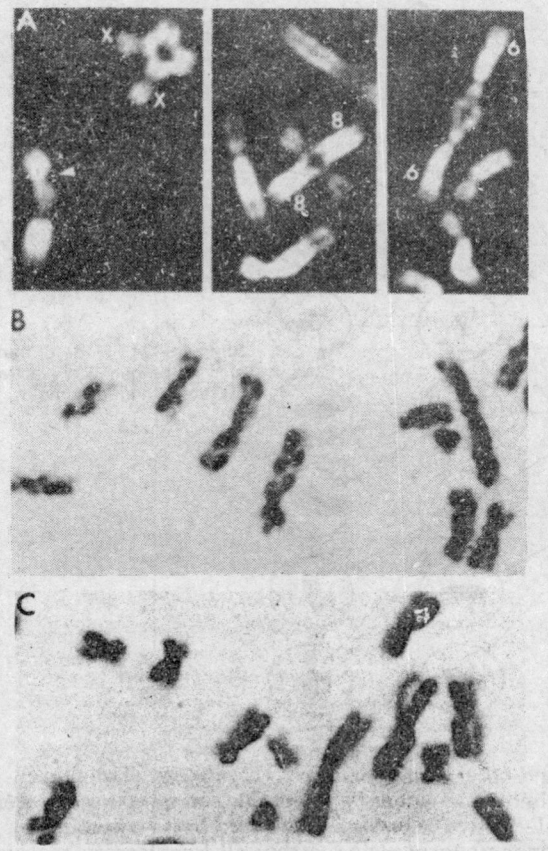

Figure 6–23 Partial spreads showing chromosome aberrations in cells from patient with Bloom syndrome, compared with a normal subject. *A,* Fluorescent-stained spreads with quadriradial figures formed by homologous chromosomes, typical of this syndrome. *B,* Harlequin effect resulting from high frequency of sister chromatid exchanges (SCE) in cells of patient with Bloom syndrome, treated with 5-bromodeoxyuridine (BrdU). *C,* Low rate of sister chromatid exchanges in cells of normal subject.

cytopenia (Sec 14.31), ataxia-telangiectasia (Louis-Bar syndrome, Sec 9.17 and 21.19), and xeroderma pigmentosum (Sec 24.14).

In addition to breaks and gaps, the characteristic chromosomal aberration of Bloom syndrome is the quadriradial, formed by the exchange of chromatid segments, usually between 2 chromosomes of the C and F groups. In almost all cases the breaks occur at corresponding sites in homologous chromosomes (Fig 6–23). The detection of sister chromatid exchanges (SCE) has led to the discovery that the number of such exchanges is much higher in cultured cells from affected children than in cells from homozygous normals *or* heterozygotes for the Bloom syndrome allele.

In the Fanconi pancytopenia syndrome endoreduplication and a variety of gaps, breaks, and rearrangements involving nonhomologues as well as homologues have been observed. The number of sister chromatid exchanges per cell is lower than that found in the cells of normal subjects. Chromosomal studies of the Louis-Bar syndrome have revealed an increase in gaps and breaks, an increase in rearrangements such as dicentrics and abnormal monocentrics, and the presence of distinct, stable cell subpopulations (clones) with translocations involving particularly chromosome 14.

Chromosomal gaps, breaks, and rearrangements have not been seen in xeroderma pigmentosum, but chromosomally abnormal clones have been observed in cultured skin fibroblasts from affected patients. An increased number of ultraviolet light-induced chromosome breaks and sister chromatid exchanges occur in cultured lymphocytes.

"Heritable fragile sites" form another category of chromosome breaks with clinical significance. These sites, reported to exist on several chromosomes, manifest themselves as spontaneous breaks inherited in a mendelian fashion whose appearance may be enhanced by the use of special tissue culture medium or specific pretreatments of the cells. The most important of such fragile sites occurs on the long arm of the X chromosome (band q27–28) and is associated with a syndrome of mental retardation, with or without macro-orchidism in males. It has been estimated that the "fragile-X syndrome" may account for up to 30% of X-linked mental retardation in males and perhaps 10% of all mild mental retardation in females (heterozygotes). The assessment of the mentally retarded male is incomplete without testicular measurement and chromosome study for this X chromosome marker.

6.20 The Sex Chromosomes

The normal sex chromosome complement in the female is XX and in the male XY. This section will deal with departures from that norm. In karyotype construction (Fig 6–6), the sex chromosomes are placed to the right of chromosome 22, at the lower right-hand corner of the karyotype. In the Q-banded karyotype, the Y is ordinarily the most brightly fluorescent chromosome. The brightly fluorescent segment of the long arm may be greatly extended or completely deleted (Fig 6–7*B*) without producing any discernible phenotypic effect. The only gene loci known to occupy the Y chromosome are those involving male sex determination; they are found in the pale-fluorescing region of the short arm.

Recent investigations have revealed the presence of an immunologically detectable product of a gene located on the short arm or the proximal long arm region of the Y chromosome. It is called the H-Y antigen and has been equated by some authors with the Y gene product which determines maleness. This hypothesis is supported by the fact that some phenotypic females who have an XY sex chromosome complement have no detectable H-Y antigen. This suggests a mutation in a gene locus which prevents the expression of the male-determining gene and also prevents the production of the H-Y antigen. On the other hand, XX males have been shown to be H-Y antigen-positive, which suggests

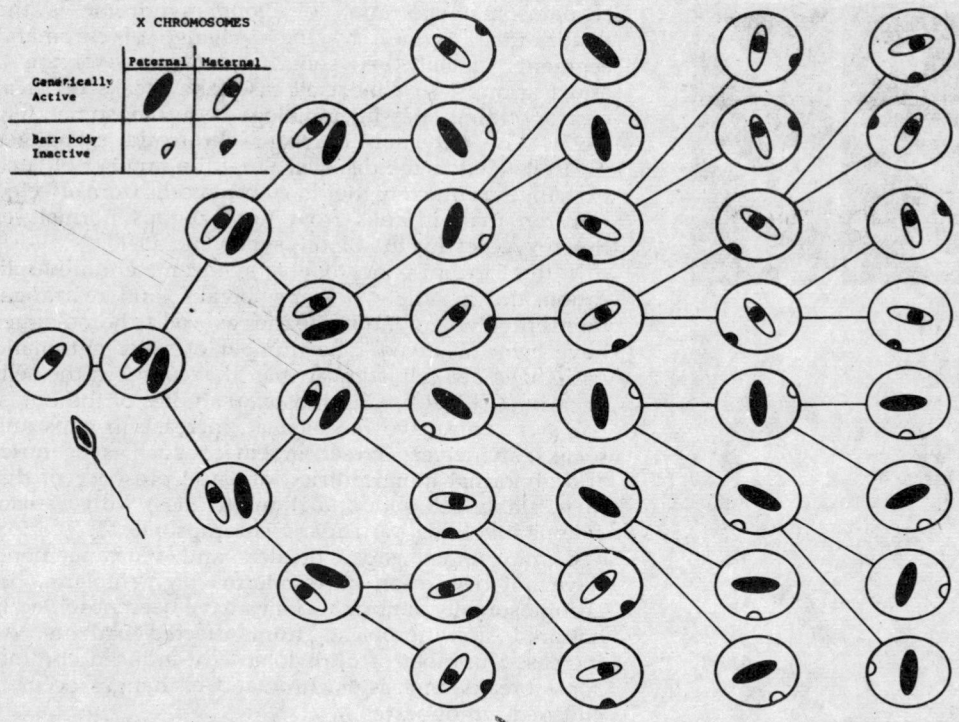

Figure 6–24 Mode of transmission of the genetically active and inactive X chromosomes.

that the male-determining segment of the Y chromosome is present but undetected.

6.21   SEX CHROMATIN

Tests for sex chromatin most often utilize cells scraped from the buccal mucosa, the *buccal smear*. Other tissues used include vaginal epithelial cells, hair root sheath cells, and cells from amniotic fluid. Because of limitations described below, X- and Y-chromatin determination should not be relied upon for the definitive diagnosis of an abnormal sex chromosome constitution. However, such determinations may be useful, along with chromosomal analysis by banding techniques, in genetic studies and in identification of structural rearrangements of the sex chromosomes.

X-CHROMATIN

Because females have 2 X chromosomes, they have 2 alleles for each X-linked gene; the male, with a single X, is therefore hemizygous for each X-linked allele. The lack of quantitative differences between the 2 sexes in the products of X-linked genes suggests *dosage compensation*. Lyon provided evidence that 1 of the 2 X chromosomes in the cells of females becomes genetically inactive at a point in early embryonic life. In each cell of a normal female the active X, whether paternally or maternally derived, is determined at random, but, once it is determined, all progeny of a particular cell will

have the same active X (Fig 6–24). Thus each cell, whether in a male or a female, contains only 1 genetically active X chromosome (the **Lyon hypothesis**). The genetic consequence is that all females are mosaic for any heterozygous alleles located in the X chromosome. The cytologic manifestation of the inactive X is the *X-chromatin mass* or "**Barr body**," found at the periphery of the resting or interphase nucleus (Fig 6–25A). All X chromosomes in a cell in excess of 1 are inactive and form X-chromatin masses. By counting the number of X-chromatin masses (in at least 100 cells), it is possible to obtain an index of the number of X chromosomes present in the cells of a subject, i.e., 1 more than the number of X-chromatin masses per cell. Because cell

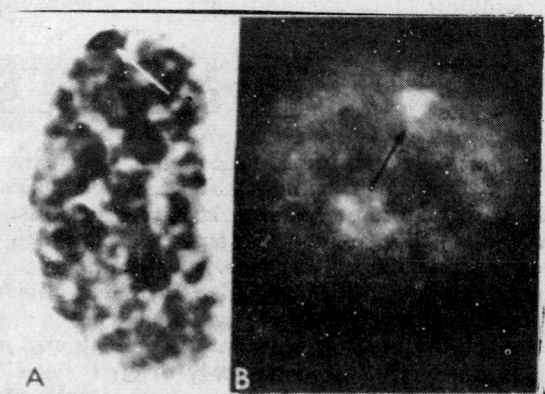

Figure 6–25 Sex chromatin bodies in interphase nuclei. *A*, X-chromatin mass (Barr body) seen at periphery of nucleus. *B*, Bright fluorescent Y-chromatin mass in nucleus of normal male.

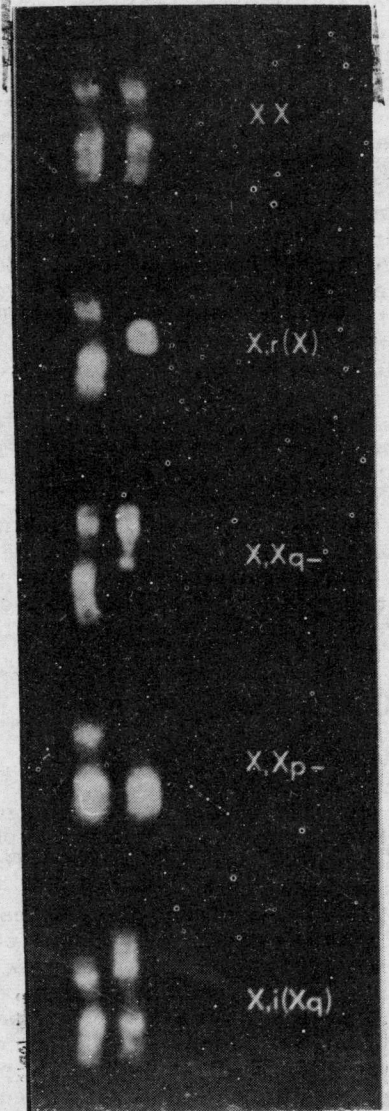

Figure 6–26 Structural aberrations of the X chromosome. Normal X chromosome on left of each pair. On right, from top to bottom: normal X, ring X, deletion of long arm, deletion of short arm, long arm isochromosome. All are X-chromatin positive.

survival requires the presence of 1 entire active X chromosome, any X with a deletion always forms the X-chromatin mass.

X-Chromatin in Turner Syndrome. X-chromatin determination is of value as a diagnostic and screening technique only if its limitations are kept in mind. Some patients with Turner syndrome have 2 X chromosomes, 1 of which is structurally altered (Fig 6–26), and are X-chromatin positive. If X-chromatin determination were the sole cytologic basis for the diagnosis of Turner syndrome, then the presence of an X-chromatin mass would erroneously exclude the diagnosis. In fact, almost 40% of patients with the Turner syndrome are X-chromatin-positive.

Y-CHROMATIN

Q-banding has led to a 2nd type of chromatin determination. In the interphase nucleus the Y chromosome remains tightly condensed and appears as a small, brilliantly fluorescent mass of chromatin (Fig 6–25B). The number of Y-chromatin masses in a nucleus bears a 1–1 relation to the number of Y chromosomes present. However, the Y-chromatin test also has limitations. Some acrocentric chromosomes bear fluorescent satellites which are large and brilliant enough to resemble a Y-chromatin body in an interphase nucleus. Moreover, if all or most of the brilliantly fluorescent segment of the Y chromosome has been deleted, a Y-chromatin mass will not be detected.

ABNORMALITIES OF THE SEX CHROMOSOMES

These make up about half of all chromosomal abnormalities encountered in newborn infants (Table 6–4). Their consequences may be varied, but almost all have some effect on gonadal function.

6.22 TURNER SYNDROME

See Sec 18.32 and 18.37 for clinical features.

This is defined as that spectrum of phenotypic features resulting from complete or partial monosomy of the *short arm* of the X chromosome. The most frequent abnormality, accounting for about 55% of cases, is complete monosomy-X, with a karyotype 45,X. Its frequency is approximately 1 in 10,000 live female births. However, this figure represents only a small proportion of conceptuses with a 45,X karyotype, at least 95% of which are estimated to be spontaneously aborted. The 45,X karyotype is one of the most common chromosomal aberrations found among the products of spontaneous abortion and is the only well documented chromosomal monosomy in humans. Turner syndrome may result from a number of abnormalities of the X chromosome other than 45,X (Table 6–12 and Fig 6–26). The most frequently encountered structural aberration is the isochromosome of the long arm produced by misdivision of the centromere and designated i(Xq). A metacentric X resembling the i(Xq) may be formed by a translocation following breaks in the paracentromeric regions of the short arms of 2 X chromosomes to form a dicentric. Simple deletion of the short arm of an X [del (Xp)] also produces Turner syndrome. However, patients with deletion of part or most of the long arm, while manifesting gonadal dysgenesis and its phenotypic results, do not have the other somatic features of Turner syndrome.

The characteristic features of Turner syndrome are listed in Table 6–13. Most important are short stature, gonadal dysgenesis with "streak" gonads, and primary amenorrhea. While mental retardation has not ordinar-

Table 6–12 ABNORMALITIES OF THE SEX CHROMOSOMES

	PER CENT OF CASES	POPULATION FREQUENCY
Turner syndrome		1/10,000 females
45,X	57	
Mosaics 45,X/46,XX;45,X/47,XXX, etc.	12	
Mosaics 45,X/46,XY	4	
46,X,i, (Xq) including mosaics	17	
46,X,del (Xq) including mosaics	1	
Other [del (Xp), r(X), mosaics]	9	
	100	
Klinefelter syndrome		1/1000 males
47,XXY	82	
48,XXXY	3	
49,XXXXY	<1	
Mosaics	8	
Other (XXYY, XXXYY)	6	
	100	
Poly-X females		1/1000 females
47,XXX	98+	
48,XXXX	Rare	
49,XXXXX	Rare	
Mosaics	Rare	
	100	
Y-polysomy		1/1000 males
47,XYY	98+	
Other (XXYY,XXXYY)	Rare	
	100	

ily been considered a feature of Turner syndrome, a recent review noted its presence in 18% of patients. In the absence of mental retardation, an abnormality in spatial perception has been reported in some cases. The characteristic dermatoglyphic feature is the large size of dermal patterns on the digits (high ridge count).

A mosaic karyotype is common in Turner syndrome; 45,X/46,XX is most frequent. In general, the presence of a 46,XX cell line in addition to the 45,X line mitigates

Table 6–13 CLINICAL FEATURES OF TURNER SYNDROME

	FEATURE	FREQUENCY (PER CENT)
General	Short stature	97
	Primary amenorrhea	96
	Sterility	>99
	Sexual infantilism	95
	Hypertension (primary)	27
	Mental deficiency	18
	Pigmented nevi	60
Craniofacies	Epicanthal folds	30
	High palate	45
	Defective vision	22
	Defective hearing	53
	Micrognathia	40
	Short neck	71
	Webbed neck	53
	Low nuchal hairline	73
Thorax	Pectus excavatum	38
	Shield chest	59
	Cardiac/vascular anomaly (e.g., coarctation of the aorta, aortic stenosis)	43
Abdomen	Urinary tract anomaly	43
Limbs	Peripheral lymphedema	41
	Cubitus valgus	58
	Short metacarpals or metatarsals	48
	Hypoplastic, hyperconvex nails	73

the effects of X-monosomy. Secondary sex development, menses, and even fertility have been reported in patients with 45,X/46,XX mosaicism. Fertility has also been described in a few cases of nonmosaic 45,X Turner syndrome. One form of mosaicism, 45,X/46,XY (mixed gonadal dysgenesis—Sec 18.37) presents a special and potentially serious problem. The presence of the 46,XY cell line predisposes the patient to gonadal neoplasia. Surgical removal of the gonads is mandatory in all patients with 45,X/46,XY Turner syndrome. A buccal smear for X-chromatin is misleading in 45,X/46,XY mosaicism since it does not reflect the presence of the XY cell line. Chromosomal analysis is needed in all patients suspected of Turner syndrome.

Unlike autosomal trisomy and 47,XXY Klinefelter syndrome, Turner syndrome is not associated with advanced maternal age. This suggests that the underlying mechanism can involve the loss of either a paternal or a maternal sex chromosome. In 75% of testable cases of 45,X Turner syndrome, the *paternal* X or Y is absent. The frequency of mosaic karyotypes implicates a postfertilization error in cell division as the cause of many cases. Once parents have had a child with Turner syndrome, their risk for producing a second affected infant is *not* increased.

6.23 KLINEFELTER SYNDROME

(See Sec 18.32 for clinical features.)

Klinefelter syndrome is defined as the spectrum of phenotypic features resulting from a sex chromosome complement that includes 2 or more X chromosomes and 1 or more Y chromosomes (Table 6–14). The 47,XXY Klinefelter syndrome occurs in approximately 1 per 1000 liveborn males but very rarely among spontaneous abortuses. The syndrome with karyotypes other than 47,XXY is rare. The somatic features are few and nonspecific. It is not often detected in the prepubertal male unless found in an X-chromatin screening program of a population, such as the males in an institution for the mentally retarded. However, retardation, if present, is usually mild and may not be much more frequent that in the general population. One helpful diagnostic feature is the presence of small patterns on the digits with

Table 6–14 PHENOTYPIC FEATURES OF KLINEFELTER SYNDROME WITH 47,XXY KARYOTYPE

FEATURE	FREQUENCY (PER CENT)
Histologic evidence of impaired spermiogenesis	100
Small testes	99
Azoospermia	93
Gynecomastia	55
Decreased facial hair	77
Decreased pubic hair	61
Decreased penile size	41
Decreased libido or potency	68
Decreased testosterone (plasma)	79
Increased gonadotropins (urine and plasma)	75
Mental retardation	5

Table 6–15 PHENOTYPIC FEATURES OF THE 49,XXXXY MALE

Feature	Frequency (Per Cent)
Skeletal abnormalities (radioulnar synostosis, coxa valga, rib anomalies, abnormal ossification centers in hands, fusion of vertebral arches, pseudoepiphyses in hands and feet, absent radial heads, short, bowed radius and ulna)	70
Genital anomalies	
Hypoplastic scrotum	70
Cryptorchidism	30
Small penis	85
Small testicles	80
Decreased or female distribution of pubic hair	40
Mental retardation	100
Facial features	
Upward slanting palpebral fissures	75
Epicanthal folds	80
Strabismus	57
Hypertelorism	87
Malformed ears	73
Broad nasal bridge	86
Depressed nasal bridge	68
Short neck	70
Increased frequency of digital arch patterns	

a low ridge count. Like autosomal trisomies, Klinefelter syndrome is associated with advanced maternal age.

Klinefelter syndrome is not a serious pediatric problem because, aside from infertility, most affected males lead normal lives; they are not identified until they are examined more closely because of the infertility and are found to have small testes and azoospermia.

Somatic abnormalities are more common in the Klinefelter syndrome caused by chromosomal abnormalities other than 47,XXY. A direct correlation is apparent between the increased occurrence and severity of mental retardation and increasing number of X chromosomes. A specific identifiable phenotype has been attributed to the 49,XXXXY karyotype (Table 6–15).

6.24 THE 47,XXX FEMALE

The 47,XXX female occurs with the same frequency among females as does 47,XXY among males (1/1000). There is no characteristic phenotype, and affected females are usually identified by chance, as in X-chromatin screening programs, newborn surveys, or amniocentesis ordered for other reasons; or they may be identified when an unrelated chromosomal abnormality is discovered in a child or other relative of a proband in a family study. They usually have normal gonadal function and are fertile, but they may have offspring with an abnormal sex chromosome complement. Recent studies suggest an increased frequency of delayed motor and speech development, mild intellectual deficit, and disturbed interpersonal relationships. More than 3 X chromosomes have been found in females, the largest number being 5 X. As in males, mental retardation appears to increase in females with increasing numbers of X chromosomes.

6.25 THE XYY MALE

A stigma has become attached to the 47,XYY sex chromosome complement because the original studies, carried out in a prison population, reported an association with aggressive antisocial behavior. The other feature claimed to be characteristic of XYY males is tall stature. A recent Danish-American study, while finding an elevated crime rate among XYY males, did not relate the criminal behavior to aggression. Difficult ethical problems are raised by such studies. Among children the XYY karyotype has occasionally been found in those referred for chromosomal analyses because of difficult personality problems in school. The frequency of XYY has been estimated from newborn surveys as 1 in 1000 live births.

See also Sec 18.32.

6.26 ATYPICAL SEX CHROMOSOME KARYOTYPES

46,XX in Phenotypic Males

A 46,XX karyotype has been reported in phenotypic males with characteristics resembling those of Klinefelter syndrome. Their internal and external genitalia are male. Most affected males are discovered at or after puberty because of sterility or failure of development of secondary sex characteristics (Sec. 18.32).

This occurrence of an XX sex chromosome constitution in a phenotypic male is contrary to the concept that a Y chromosome is necessary for male sex determination and differentiation. Possible explanations for the phenomenon include (1) undetected 46,XX/46,XY chimerism or 46,XX/47,XXY mosaicism, (2) translocation of the male sex-determining segment of the Y to the X chromosome or to an autosome, and (3) a mutant gene or genes. Evidence currently available suggests that the 1st explanation is most likely. The translocation of the male-determining segment of the Y to either the X or an autosome could produce an apparently XX male, although no cytologically documented Y to X translocation has been reported in an XX male; one possible Y-autosome interchange has been described. However, the translocation of a small, pale-fluorescing segment of the Y to another chromosome might go unnoticed. Increasing numbers of reports describing XX males who are positive for the Y-linked gene product, the H-Y antigen, support the idea of the presence of at least a portion of the Y. The occurrence in the same family of an XX male and an XX true hermaphrodite is consistent with the suggestion of a mutant gene that produces sex reversal in the 46,XX person.

46,XY in a Phenotypic Female

See also Sec 18.30 and 18.46.

The XY sex chromosome constitution exerts an effect on the early embryo to cause the gonads and the biopotential internal and external genitalia to differentiate into the definitive genital apparatus of the male. Without this influence the embryo will differentiate as a female. The influence of the XY chromosome constitution is not completely understood but is obviously mediated through induction of testicular differentiation. Testicular Leydig cells then secrete testosterone, which is converted peripherally to dihydrotestosterone. Target cells must have the capacity to respond to testosterone and dihydrotestosterone. If any of these steps fails, then masculinization of the embryo will not occur. Even though the infant's sex chromosome constitution is XY, that infant may have a female genital phenotype. A female phenotype may be seen in a 46,XY infant as the result of (1) complete insensitivity of target tissue to androgen, (2) testicular unresponsiveness to luteinizing hormone (LH) and human chorionic gonadotropin (hCG) (Leydig cell aplasia), (3) a severe defect in the biosynthesis of testosterone, and (4) the syndrome of XY pure gonadal dysgenesis (Swyer syndrome).

SPONTANEOUS ABORTIONS

Some 20% of all conceptuses are spontaneously aborted, at least half because of chromosomal aberrations, the most common being aneuploidy. Loss of a sex chromosome has been found most frequently. Chromosomal banding techniques have resulted in the identification of trisomies for all chromosomes except No. 1. Trisomy 16 is the most common, followed by trisomies of the small and large acrocentrics with the notable exception of No. 13. There is no evidence of an association of polyploidy or other types of aberrations with birth control pills.

6.27   GENETIC COUNSELING IN CHROMOSOMAL DISORDERS

With the many advances in cytogenetic procedures, counseling for chromosomal abnormalities is becoming more precise. The aberrant chromosome can usually be identified; small translocations, deletions, and inversions can often be distinguished. With further refinements and improvements, the outlook is optimistic. Fairly accurate risk figures can be given for inherited translocations. But the recurrence risks following aneuploidy or sporadic deletions and translocations are still based on empiric data.

Amniocentesis, with culture and karyotyping of cells obtained from amniotic fluid, has provided a practical tool to identify chromosomal defects in utero and, by selective abortion, to prevent the birth of chromosomally abnormal offspring. Because of the slight risks involved in this procedure, priority indications are situations in which a parent is known to be chromo-

somally abnormal, maternal age is over 35, or there has been a previous trisomic child. Pediatricians have a responsibility to ensure that mothers are aware of the availability of intrauterine diagnosis and the increased risk of chromosomal aberrations related to maternal age. Determination of fetal sex from amniotic fluid cells is also important in the prevention of X-linked recessive disorders.

Gene mapping of chromosomes is a field of investigation which eventually should produce valuable information for genetic counseling. If the locus of a gene is known to be on a specific chromosome, and this chromosome can be distinguished from its homologue by differences in structure or banding pattern, it should be possible to trace the transmission of an abnormal gene. At least 1 gene has been provisionally assigned to each of the 23 pairs of chromosomes. The autosome with the largest number of identified genes is No. 1. Genes located in the X chromosome have been known for some time, and the order in which they are linked together is rapidly becoming clear.

Acknowledgements. Acknowledgement is made to Mrs. Elizabeth Byrnes for preparing the fluorescence and trypsin-Giemsa karyotypes and to Paula R. Martens for the partial karyotypes prepared with modified Giemsa stain.

MAIMON M. COHEN
HENRY L. NADLER

Apgar V (ed.): Down's syndrome (mongolism). Ann NY Acad Sci 171:303, 1970.
Bergsma D (ed): Birth Defects—Atlas and Compendium. Baltimore, Williams & Wilkins, 1972.
Court-Brown WM: Human Population Cytogenetics. Vol 5, Frontiers of Biology. New York, John Wiley & Sons, 1967.
Hamerton JL: Human Cytogenetics. Vols I and II. New York, Academic Press, 1971.
Intrauterine Diagnosis. Birth Defects—Original Article Series. Vol VII. New York, The National Foundation—March of Dimes, 1971.
Levine H: Clinical cytogenetics. Boston, Little, Brown, 1971.
Opitz JM: Klinefelter syndrome. In: Bergsma D (ed): Birth Defects—Atlas and Compendium. Baltimore, Williams & Wilkins, 1973.
Paris Conference (1971): Standardization in Human Cytogenetics. Birth Defects—Original Article Series. Vol VIII. New York, The National Foundation—March of Dimes, 1971.
Paris Conference (1971) Suppl (1975): Standardization in Human Cytogenetics. Birth Defects—Original Article Series Vol XI. New York, The National Foundation—March of Dimes, Suppl 1975.
Reed TE, Borgaonkar DS, Conneally PM, et al: Dermatoglyphic nomogram for the diagnosis of Down's syndrome. J Pediatr 77:1024, 1970.
Simpson JL: Disorders of Sexual Differentiation: Etiology and Clinical Delineation. New York, Academic Press, 1977.
Summitt, RL: Disorders of sex differentiation. In: Givens JR (ed): Gynecologic Endocrinology. Chicago, Year Book Medical Publishers, 1977.
Summitt RL: Abnormalities of the Chromosomes. In: Jackson LG, Schimke RN (eds): Clinical Genetics. New York, John Wiley & Sons, 1979.
Wright SW, Crandall BF, Boyer L (eds): Perspectives in Cytogenetics. Springfield, Ill., Charles C Thomas, 1972.
Yunis JJ (ed): Human Chromosome Methodology. Ed 2. New York, Academic Press, 1974.
Yunis JJ (ed): New Chromosomal Syndromes. New York, Academic Press, 1977.

Patient Education

Apgar V, Beck, J: Is My Baby All Right? New York, Simon & Schuster, 1973.
Smith DW, Wilson AA: The Child with Down's Syndrome (Mongolism). Philadelphia, WB Saunders, 1973.

6.28 CONGENITAL MALFORMATIONS

About 2% of newborn infants have a major malformation. The incidence is as high as 5% if one includes malformations detected later in childhood, such as abnormalities of the heart, kidneys, lungs, and spine. Malformations are more common among spontaneous abortuses; many of these are severe and may be the cause of the abortion. About 9% of perinatal deaths are due to malformations. Treatment of malformations is one of the common reasons for the hospitalization of children.

A simple and arbitrary terminology has evolved for describing malformations. A *major malformation* has serious medical, surgical, or cosmetic consequences. A *minor anomaly* and a *normal variation* have no serious consequences and are differentiated on the arbitrary basis that a minor anomaly occurs in 4% or less of children of the same race, whereas a normal variation is more common. The incidence of features such as simian crease, clinodactyly of the 5th finger, extra nipples, Brushfield spots, and sacral dimple varies in each race (Table 6–16).

A *syndrome* refers to a recognized pattern of malformations considered to have a single and specific cause, such as the Holt-Oram syndrome, an autosomal dominant disorder with malformations of the heart and upper extremities. *Association* is used to indicate a pattern of malformations for which no specific etiology has been identified, such as the VATER association of *v*ertebral, *a*nal, *t*racheal, *e*sophageal, *r*adial upper limb and *r*enal anomalies. A *morphogenic complex* (which has also been called an *anomalad*) comprises a primary malformation and its derived structural changes but does not specify a cause.

Etiology. In a prospective study of 30,681 newborn infants Holmes found 810 major malformations (2.6%), 57% of which were attributed to genetic abnormalities. The 30,681 infants had 0.2% malformations attributed to chromosomal abnormalities, 0.1% to single mutant genes, 0.7% to multifactorial inheritance, and 0.5% to uncertain patterns of inheritance. The number of chromosomal abnormalities is less than the 0.6% incidence of all types of chromosomal abnormalities in newborn

infants because many of the common disorders, such as 47,XXY, 47,XYY, and 47,XXX, have no detectable physical characteristics in the newborn infant. Teratogens and other environmental factors were identified as a cause of malformations in 0.4% of the infants or 16.0% of all malformations, an incidence lower than many clinicians expect. Teratogens include drugs and maternal conditions such as diabetes mellitus; other environmental factors include amniotic constrictive bands and oligohydramnios. Twinning is associated with a higher incidence of malformations than that in singletons; the acardiac infant syndrome occurs only in monozygous twins.

The causes of 27% of the 810 major malformations were not detected. Malformations of unknown cause include many types of intestinal atresia, imperforate anus, megaloureter, Goldenhar syndrome, absence of the pectoralis major muscle, omphalocele, cloacal exstrophy, and diaphragmatic hernia through the foramen of Bochdalek.

Underlying Mechanisms. The understanding of malformations has been derived principally from the study of animals. Basic abnormalities identified include (1) abnormal cell shape; (2) abnormalities of the collagens or of the proteoglycans, major constituents of the extracellular matrix; (3) errors in circulation during fetal development; and (4) lack of appropriate death of cells during morphogenesis. An example of abnormal cell shape is the defect in the Bergmann glial cells which normally provide the latticework for migration of neuronal cells. When they are defective because of the autosomal recessive gene *weaver* in the mouse, hypoplasia of the cerebellum results. Several types of Ehlers-Danlos syndrome have been identified by clinical and genetic studies in humans; at least 3 have been shown to be due to different defects in collagen metabolism. For example, in type VI the collagen is deficient in hydroxylysine because of a deficiency of lysyl hydroxylase; in type VII there is an inability to convert procollagen to collagen; in type IV there is a lack of type III collagen.

The malformation *hemifacial microsomia* can be caused by a failure of the vascular supply to be transferred from the stapedial artery to the external carotid artery, a switchover that normally occurs during the 6th and 7th wk of gestation in humans. Lack of appropriate death of cells between the developing long bones in a limb can lead to synostosis of these bones. For the palatal shelves to meet in the midline and fuse, there must be death of cells in the epithelium preceding the fusion of the underlying palatal mesenchyme.

Clinical Evaluation. Any child with a major or with multiple minor malformation deserves diagnostic evaluation. This includes a history of defects in other family members and of any untoward events during the pregnancy as well as a thorough physical examination. In the examination it is helpful to use objective measurements when a physical feature seems too long, short, narrow, or wide. Many normal standards are included

Table 6–16 INCIDENCE OF MINOR ANOMALIES AND NORMAL VARIATIONS IN NEWBORN INFANTS*

PHYSICAL FEATURE	WHITE INFANTS (%) (N = 3989)	BLACK INFANTS (%) (N = 827)
Third sagittal fontanel	3.1	9.8
Epicanthal folds, bilateral	1.4	1.0
Brushfield spots, bilateral	7.2	0.2
Preauricular sinus, left or right	0.8	5.3
Extra nipple, left or right	0.5	4.6
Umbilical hernia	0.7	6.1
Sacral dimple	4.8	0.6
Clinodactyly of both 5th fingers	5.2	4.5
Simian crease, both hands	0.7	0.5
Syndactyly of toes 2 and 3, left or right	1.7	2.3

*From Holmes LB: The Malformed Newborn—Practical Perspectives. Boston, Developmental Disabilities Council, 1976.

in Smith's *Recognizable Patterns of Human Malformation.*
Chromosomal analysis by banding techniques should
be obtained when there are multiple malformations,
especially if the infant is mentally retarded, is stillborn,
or dies soon after birth. For such studies on a deceased
infant, cells obtained from biopsies of skin, gonad,
thymus, or spleen grown in tissue culture are preferable
to those obtained from a blood sample taken when the
infant is moribund. The likelihood of finding a chromosomal abnormality in infants in the above categories
is only 10 to 20%; hence the clinician must be prepared
to develop a differential diagnosis for other genetic and
nongenetic causes of the malformations.

The same clinical signs or malformations may be
caused by a variety of genetic accidents. For example,
the split-hand/split-foot syndrome, an unusual malformation in which there is a cleft in the middle of the
hand, foot, or both, may be due to lack of development
of the middle digits and metatarsals and metacarpals.
The same deformity occurs in focal dermal hypoplasia,
a multiple malformation syndrome, and in the autoso-

mal dominant disorder in which the deformities are
limited to the limbs.

Gorlin RJ, Pindborg JJ, Cohen MM Jr: Syndromes of the Head and Neck. Ed 2. New York, McGraw-Hill, 1976.
Holmes, LB: Inborn errors of morphogenesis. N Engl J Med 291:763, 1974.
Holmes LB, Moser HW, Halldorsson S, et al: Mental Retardation: An Atlas of Diseases with Associated Physical Abnormalities. New York, Macmillan, 1972.
Machin GA: Chromosome abnormality and perinatal death. Lancet 1:549, 1974.
Poswillo D: The pathogenesis of the first and second branchial arch syndrome. Oral Surg 35:302, 1973.
Pratt RM, Martin GR: Epithelial cell death and cyclic AMP increase during palate development. Proc Natl Acad Sci USA 72:874, 1975.
Smith DW: Recognizable Patterns of Human Malformation. Ed 3. Philadelphia, WB Saunders, 1982.
Spranger JW, Langer LO Jr, Wiedemann H-R: Bone Dysplasias: An Atlas of Constitutional Disorders of Skeletal Development. Philadelphia, WB Saunders, 1974.
Tharapel AT, Summitt RL: A cytogenetic survey of 200 unclassifiable mentally retarded children with congenital anomalies and 200 normal controls. Human Genetics 37:329, 1977.
Uitto J, Lichtenstein JR: Defects in the biochemistry of collagen in diseases of connective tissue. J Invest Dermatol 66:59, 1976.
Warkany J: Congenital Malformations. Chicago, Year Book Medical Publishers, 1971.

6.29   GENETIC COUNSELING

Genetic counseling is a process of communication
dealing with the human problems associated with the
occurrence or risk of occurrence of a genetic disorder
in a family. Those who should receive it can be divided
into a majority who are unaware of their risks and a
minority who request genetic information and counseling. The latter most commonly are couples whose 1st
child has just been born with a birth defect or medical
problem. Older parents also are frequently concerned
about genetic risks and wish to learn about prenatal
diagnosis. Others seek information prior to marriage or
before having children because of medical problems of
their relatives.

The challenge for the physician is to recognize which
birth defects and medical problems are hereditary and
to offer genetic information to all families, not just to
those who request it. Genetic counseling becomes more
complex when detection of carriers is possible or when
the relevance of prenatal diagnosis must be explained.

PRINCIPLES OF GENETIC COUNSELING

*The 1st step in genetic counseling is to make certain the
diagnosis is correct.* The physician must, for example,
distinguish isolated cleft lip and palate (multifactorial
inheritance) from cleft lip and palate with lip pits
(autosomal dominant); distinguish Duchenne muscular
dystrophy (X-linked recessive) from the Becker type of
muscular dystrophy (X-linked recessive), the latter
being much less severe; distinguish the perinatal type
of infantile polycystic kidney disease (autosomal recessive) from unilateral multicystic kidney (nonhereditary).

With diagnosis established, the steps in the counseling process follow:
1. Have both parents present for the discussion (a
teenage child should be offered the opportunity of a
separate discussion).
2. Discuss the medical consequences of the defect; if
relevant, the variability of associated features that might
develop in future years should be explained.
3. Review the family history of each parent and
identify any unrecognized genetic risks.
4. Review the interpretations the family has made or
which have been offered by others to explain the
condition under discussion.
5. Describe the genetic basis for the problem, using
visual aids (pictures demonstrating phenotypic or other
features of the problem, pictures of chromosomes, diagrams of patterns of inheritance) as much as possible.
6. Explain the genetic risks in terms the family can
understand.
7. Outline the options available, such as having no
children, having children and accepting the risks,
adopting a child if possible, artificial insemination (this
option is particularly pertinent in the case of all autosomal recessive disorders and serious paternal autosomal dominant disorders); note whether prenatal diagnosis is possible.
8. Provide the persons counseled with a summary of
the issues discussed and, if possible, meet with them
again to help them decide the option most appropriate
for them.
9. Stay in contact with families previously counseled
to provide new information that may become available,
such as new methods for carrier detection in a parent
or for prenatal diagnosis.

Often parents first become aware of their genetic

risks after the birth of a child with a birth defect. Coping with this knowledge usually includes periods of denial, anger, and depression before it is assimilated and accepted. Each family's situation is different and their reaction to counseling unique. A frequent problem for families is conceptualizing the genetic abnormality, such as a single mutant gene, an abnormal chromosome, or, in the case of multifactorial inheritance, the interaction of several genes and environmental factors. There is an obvious advantage in the case of chromosomal abnormalities in showing the abnormal karyotype in comparison with a normal one. Another problem is the fact that most infants and children with a genetic disorder are the 1st affected member of the family. Parents may assume a problem cannot be hereditary if no other relatives are affected. It is helpful for the counselor to bring up this issue and to discuss in detail how healthy parents with no affected relatives can have a child with a hereditary disorder.

GENETIC COUNSELING WHEN DETECTION OF CARRIERS IS POSSIBLE

Genetic counseling is simplified, more specific, and probably more effective when the carrier state for the genetic abnormality in question can be identified by laboratory tests. Those at risk can be identified, and their relatives who are tested and found not to be carriers can be reassured accordingly. The concept of genetic risk is more concrete when an individual has a venipuncture and can be shown the test results in comparison with the normal. Carrier detection is possible for biochemical disorders and certain abnormalities of the chromosomes.

Biochemical Disorders. Persons heterozygous for some autosomal recessive inborn errors of metabolism can be identified. These include abnormalities such as hemoglobins S and C, thalassemia, Tay-Sachs disease, and α_1-antitrypsin deficiency. If the assay is appropriate for the screening of large numbers of individuals, the testing of high-risk populations may be conducted. This type of testing has been used to screen Jews of Eastern European origin for Tay-Sachs disease, persons of Mediterranean ancestry for thalassemia, and Blacks for hemoglobins S and C. Screening for genetic diseases has been controversial for many reasons, such as the psychologic effects of focusing on a racial or ethnic group. Another limitation of screening for heterozygotes is lack of easy access to prenatal diagnosis for couples when both are heterozygous. This is particularly true of the hemoglobin abnormalities for which placental venipuncture, a technique available in only a few medical centers, is required.

Females can be identified as heterozygous for several X-linked recessive metabolic disorders, such as glucose-6-phosphate dehydrogenase deficiency, Fabry disease (α-galactosidase deficiency), and hypoxanthine–guanine phosphoribosyl transferase deficiency. Detection of female carriers is less precise in the 2 most common X-linked recessive disorders, Duchenne muscular dystrophy and hemophilia A. Testing for the carrier of Du-

chenne muscular dystrophy is indirect and still relies primarily on measuring the serum level of the muscle enzyme creatine phosphokinase (CPK). Only about 75% of known carriers can be identified by this method. Important factors in the testing are the establishment of a range of normal for the laboratory being used and testing women at risk at least 3 or 4 times, preferably in the resting state. Another variable is that the level of CPK in carriers is highest before age 30 and decreases thereafter. Some investigators use other serum enzymes, such as lactate dehydrogenase (LDH), to detect carriers. The diagnosis of Duchenne muscular dystrophy cannot be made with adequate consistency in the affected male fetus to make prenatal diagnosis available at this time. When proven female carriers are informed of their high risk of having affected sons, experience has shown that they often elect not to have more children.

The identification of women who carry the gene for hemophilia A has been improved in recent years by measuring both the activity of factor VIII and the amount of factor VIII antigen which is present. This test is available in only a few laboratories but effectively identifies about 80% of *known* carriers. Prenatal diagnosis in the 2nd trimester by means of immunoradiometric assays for factor VIII on fetal plasma obtained by fetoscopy is available. However, this option cannot be used by families in which hemophiliac males have circulating cross-reactive material.

Chromosomal Translocations. When a child is abnormal because of an excess or deficiency of chromosomal material, the parents should be studied to identify whether or not either is the carrier of a balanced translocation. A carrier parent can then be counseled as to his or her risk of having children with an unbalanced translocation, i.e., too much or too little chromosomal material, and other blood relatives may be tested to see if they, too, are carriers. Related chromosomal abnormalities of the fetus of the carrier of a balanced translocation may be identified through culture of fetal cells obtained by amniocentesis.

GENETIC COUNSELING WHEN PRENATAL DIAGNOSIS IS POSSIBLE

Many couples seek genetic counseling because they want to learn more about prenatal diagnosis. Discussing whether or not this would be helpful should be a routine part of genetic counseling. The most common indications for prenatal diagnosis are advanced maternal age (Table 6–6) and a previous child with either Down syndrome or anencephaly-meningomyelocele.

In general, prenatal diagnosis by amniocentesis is recommended for all women over 35, as their risk of having a child with any type of chromosomal abnormality is at least 1% (Table 6–6). There has been a steady decline over the last 20 yr in the percentage of infants born to women over 35. In the 1950's women 35 and older had half of the infants with Down syndrome, but by the 1970's the older mothers had only about 20% of these infants. Thus 80% of the infants with Down syndrome are now born to women under 35 yr of age, who are not routinely offered prenatal diagnosis as an option. The dilemma of whether or not to offer prenatal diagnosis to pregnant women under 35 has not been resolved. Another new finding pertinent to genetic counseling for the Down syndrome is the fact that in about 1 out of 4 instances, the extra No. 21 chromosome is derived from the father. Formerly it had been assumed that it was always derived from the mother.

Couples at risk for having children with metabolic diseases have a less common, but more complex, indication for prenatal diagnosis. Metabolic diseases that can be diagnosed in utero are listed in Table 8–2 (see footnote). Metabolic testing on amniotic cells should be done by those laboratories experienced in conducting such assays on amniotic cells.

Prenatal diagnosis is usually undertaken at 15–16 wk of gestation, when the uterus extends high enough out of the pelvis to allow amniocentesis. Ultrasound is used to locate the placenta and to determine whether there is more than 1 fetus, a realistic precaution since the incidence of twin pregnancy is about 1 in 80. Using aseptic technique and local anesthesia, a 22 gauge spinal needle with trocar in place is inserted through the abdomen at the most favorable site, as indicated by the ultrasonogram, and advanced into the amniotic cavity. The trocar is removed and the first 2 ml of fluid is discarded to minimize the risk of contamination of the sample with cells from the mother's skin; then 10–30 ml of amniotic fluid is withdrawn into a 2nd syringe, sealed in the syringe, and taken directly to the laboratory. The specimen is tested for the presence of fetal blood, and centrifuged to separate the fluid from the cells; the cells are then placed in tissue culture under sterile conditions in an incubator.

Fetal loss from amniocentesis is less than 0.5%. Three percent of women have transient cramps and leakage of amniotic fluid. In about 5–10% of instances the amniocentesis must be repeated, either because no amniotic fluid was obtained with the first amniocentesis or because there was insufficient growth of cells.

The objective is to provide the results within 14–21 days of the amniocentesis. If the results of the testing show that the fetus is abnormal and the parents elect to have the fetus aborted, most obstetricians prefer to terminate the pregnancy before 20 wk of gestation, although up to 24 wk is permissible by law. Fortunately, prenatal diagnosis usually shows that the fetus is unaffected.

Tissues and Technical Procedures Used in Prenatal Diagnosis

The Cells in the Amniotic Fluid. The cells obtained by amniocentesis can be used for chromosomal analysis or for biochemical assays. Two to 3 wk are needed for the cells to multiply and reach a number adequate for these tests; it is more difficult to obtain good metaphase preparations from the cells in amniotic fluid than from peripheral lymphocytes. Chromosomal abnormalities,

such as polyploidy and mosaicism with both normal and abnormal cell lines, are also more common in the cells of amniotic fluid obtained at 14–16 wk gestation than in those of infants at birth.

The Amniotic Fluid. *Alpha-Fetoprotein (AFP).* This is the constituent of amniotic fluid most frequently used in prenatal diagnosis. The level of this protein, which is synthesized by the fetal liver, gastrointestinal tract, and yolk sac, is increased whenever transudation across a thin membrane occurs, as in anencephaly, meningomyelocele, encephalocele, and omphalocele. The most common use of measuring AFP is to evaluate subsequent pregnancies of couples who have had a child with anencephaly, meningomyelocele, or encephalocele; omphalocele is not hereditary. AFP levels have also been used to identify the Meckel syndrome (an autosomal recessive disorder that includes encephalocele, polycystic kidneys, polydactyly, cleft lip and palate, and anomalies of the genitals and eyes) and congenital nephrosis (a rare autosomal recessive disorder).

The level of AFP is highest between 14–18 wk of gestation and falls steadily thereafter; it is important to confirm the clinical estimate of gestational age by ultrasound before amniocentesis. Since the concentration of AFP may be increased by the presence of fetal blood, each sample of amniotic fluid should be tested for fetal blood. The concentration is also increased by impending spontaneous abortion, fetal death, Rh sensitization, congenital nephrosis, and the presence of intestinal atresia. The measurement of acetylcholinesterase in amniotic fluid is helpful in confirming the presence of a neural tube defect and in eliminating false-positive elevations of AFP. The AFP level is often normal if a neural tube defect, such as meningocele or encephalocele, is covered by skin.

Measurement of AFP by radioimmunoassay in the pregnant woman's serum may become an effective means of identifying a larger percentage of affected newborns in the future. This is proposed as a screening test for all pregnant women at 16–18 wk of pregnancy. An elevated value would require a 2nd serum test. If the serum AFP is 2.5 times the median value on 2 occasions, the fetus would be examined by ultrasonography and amniocentesis. Essential to routine serum AFP screening is educating the parents about the issues involved. In addition to neural tube defects, serum AFP screening will also identify the presence of growth retardation and twinning.

Secretor Substance. Under certain conditions, either the presence or absence of the secretor substance in amniotic fluid can be used in some families to determine whether the fetus of an affected parent has myotonic dystrophy and the locus of the dominant gene responsible for the secretor substance.

The amniotic fluid can also be analyzed for steroid hormones and has been used to diagnose congenital adrenal hyperplasia due to a deficiency of 21-hydroxylase.

Ultrasound (Sec 7.4). Ultrasound is used primarily to determine gestational age, to localize the placenta, and to rule out multiple pregnancies. It has been used when the concentration of AFP is increased in the amniotic fluid in an attempt to identify anencephaly on the basis of the contour of the head, but the accuracy is low. Ultrasound is also effective in diagnosing chondrodystrophies, deficiencies of long bones, and kidney enlargement, as occurs in infantile polycystic kidney disease, but the accuracy of this method is unknown.

Amniography. When the AFP level is abnormally increased in the amniotic fluid, a water-soluble dye has been injected into the amniotic sac to look for the profile of the lumbar bulge caused by a meningomyelocele. Some large lumbar meningomyeloceles have *not* been identified by this technique.

Fetoscopy. Direct inspection of the fetus has been allowed only on an experimental basis at a few medical centers; the risk to the fetus is estimated to be about 5%. It has been used to obtain blood samples from placental vessels for identification of severe hemoglobin disorders, such as beta-thalassemia and sickle cell anemia, and of Duchenne muscular dystrophy. Fetoscopy has also been used to identify limb deformities. A difficulty with this technique is the small area that can be seen at one time.

Radiography. Roentgenograms of the fetus may be helpful when the fetus is at risk for a severe deficiency of the long bones, as in autosomal recessive thrombocytopenia with radial aplasia. However, this technique is being replaced by ultrasonography.

Genetic Counseling

Antley RM: Variables in the outcome of genetic counseling. Social Biology 23:108, 1976.

Fraser FC: Genetic counseling. Am J Human Genet 26:636, 1974.

Halloran KH, Hsia YE, Rosenberg LE: Genetic counseling for congenital heart disease. J Pediatr 88:1054, 1976.

Leonard CO, Chase GA, Childs B: Genetic counseling: A consumer's view. N Engl J Med 287:433, 1972.

Lippman-Hand A, Fraser FC: Genetic counseling, provision and reception of information. Am J Med Genet 3:113, 1979.

Carrier Detection

Klein HG, Aledort LM, Bourma BN, et al: Detection of the carrier state of classic hemophilia. N Engl J Med 296:959, 1977.

Hutton EM, Thompson MW: Carrier detection and genetic counselling in Duchenne muscular dystrophy: a follow-up study. CMA Journal 115:749, 1976.

Munsat TL, Baloh R, Pearson CM, et al: Serum enzyme alteration in neuromuscular disorders. JAMA 226:1536, 1973.

Prenatal Diagnosis

Bartley JA, Golbus MS, Filly RA, et al: Prenatal diagnosis of dysplastic kidney disease. Clin Genet 11:375, 1977.

Brock DJH, Barron L, Jelen P, et al: Maternal serum-alpha-fetoprotein measurements as an early indicator of low birth-weight. Lancet 2:267, 1977.

Firschein SI, Hoyer LW, Lazarchick J et al: Prenatal diagnosis of classic hemophilia. N Engl J Med 300:937, 1979.

Haddow J, Macri JN: Prenatal screening for neural tube defects. JAMA 242:515, 1979.

Lowry RB, Jones DC, Renwick DHG, et al: Down syndrome in British Columbia, 1952–1973: Incidence and mean maternal age. Teratology 14:29, 1976.

Magenis RW, Overton KM, Chamberlain J, et al: Parental origin of the extra chromosome in Down's syndrome. Hum Genet 37:7, 1977.

Marion KP, Kassam G, Fernhoff PM, et al: Acceptance of amniocentesis by low-income patients in an urban hospital. Am J Obstet Gynecol 138:11, 1980.

Midtrimester amniocentesis for prenatal diagnosis: Safety and accuracy. JAMA 236:1471, 1976.

Omenn GS: Prenatal diagnosis of genetic disorders. Science 200:952, 1978.

Schrott HG, Karp L, Omenn GS: Prenatal prediction in myotonic dystrophy: guidelines for genetic counseling. Clin Genet 4:38, 1973.

6.30 TERATOGENS

When an infant or child is malformed or mentally retarded, the parents often blame themselves and attribute the child's problems to events that occurred during pregnancy. Since infections occur and several drugs are taken during many pregnancies, the pediatrician must be able to evaluate the presumed viral infections and the drugs ingested to help parents understand their child's birth defect. The cause of about 40% of congenital malformations is unknown. While only a few teratogenic agents are recognized at this time (Table 6–17), it seems likely that additional environmental factors will continue to be recognized.

Several generalizations can be made about teratogens. None are harmful to every exposed fetus; some drugs (e.g., phenytoins) and maternal conditions, such as diabetes mellitus, may cause only a 2–3-fold increase in the overall incidence of malformations. Since the increase caused by a teratogen may be relatively small, harmful effects may be difficult to demonstrate. In general, exposure during the 1st trimester of pregnancy is probably the most harmful. The exact age of the fetus when a particular drug is most harmful has been established for only 1 drug, thalidomide (days 34–50). Even less information is available on the effects of exposure during the 2nd and 3rd trimesters.

If a child has multiple structural malformations, such as polydactyly, cleft palate, meningomyelocele, or absence of a long bone, it is inappropriate to consider intrauterine infections as a possible cause. It is true that rubella infection in utero causes cardiac anomalies, but its other effects, such as microcephaly, cataracts, and deafness, are the results of infection of the tissues concerned, not structural malformations. Likewise, congenital toxoplasmosis may cause hydrocephalus, and intrauterine infection with cytomegalovirus may cause cerebral cysts. However, none of these intrauterine infections cause multiple major and minor *structural* malformations, as can be caused by chromosomal abnormalities, single mutant genes, and teratogenic drugs.

The mechanism of action is known for only 2 teratogens: warfarin and drugs that cause hypothyroidism. Warfarin, an anticoagulant because it is a vitamin K antagonist, prevents carboxylation of gamma-carboxyglutamic acid (GLA). Inasmuch as this substance is a calcium-binding amino acid, normally part of the prothrombin molecule, deficiency of it interferes with normal clotting of blood. Gamma-carboxyglutamic acid is also present in human bones. Human fetuses exposed to warfarin in utero show abnormal cartilage, but the role of gamma-carboxyglutamic acid in chondrogenesis has not been determined. Hypothyroidism in the fetus may be caused by ingestion by the mother of an excessive amount of iodides or of propylthiouracil; each interferes with the conversion of inorganic to organic iodides.

Recognition of teratogens offers the opportunity for prevention of related birth defects. For example, if a pregnant woman who is a chronic alcoholic is informed of the potentially harmful effects of alcohol on her

Table 6–17   TERATOGENIC AGENTS IN HUMANS

TERATOGEN	PHENOTYPIC EFFECT	PERIOD OF GREATEST SENSITIVITY	LIKELIHOOD OF HARMFUL EFFECT
Drugs taken by pregnant mother			
Aminopterin or amethopterin (folic acid anatagonist)	Hydrocephalus, craniosynostosis, shortened limbs, absent digits, mental deficiency	?	?
Diethylstilbestrol	Carcinoma and adenosis of vagina in exposed females; genitourinary anomalies in exposed males	First 2 months	>50% of females 25% of males
Iodides and propylthiouracil	Goiter, fetal hypothyroidism	?	?
Phenytoin	Heart defects, nail hypoplasia, growth retardation	First trimester	10% (?)
Progestogens-estrogens			
Hormone pregnancy test	Anomalies of vertebrae, anus, heart, trachea, radius, and kidney	3–8 weeks	?
Therapeutic dosage	Heart defects	3–8 weeks	?
Older progestogens contaminated with testosterone	Masculinization of female fetus	Third trimester	?
Tetracyclines	Enamel dysplasia	Second and 3rd trimester	?
Thalidomide	Phocomelia, anomalies of ears, teeth, eyes, and intestine	Days 34–50 (menstrual age)	>90%
Warfarin (vitamin K antagonist)	Hypoplasia of nose, shortened digits, stippled epiphyses, mental deficiency in some	Weeks 6–8 (menstrual age)	?
Maternal conditions			
Chronic, severe alcoholism	Growth retardation, mental deficiency, microcephaly, heart defects, flexion contractures	?	30–50%
Diabetes mellitus	Heart defects; all types of birth defects; sacral agenesis; anencephaly	?	2-fold increase
Phenylketonuria	Microcephaly, mental deficiency, heart defects	?	
Trace metals			
Mercury	Microcephaly, spasticity, mental deficiency	?	?
Intrauterine infections			
Cytomegalovirus	Microcephaly, mental deficiency	First trimester	?
Rubella	Heart defects, microcephaly, cataracts, deafness, mental deficiency	First trimester	15–40%
Toxoplasmosis	Macrocephaly or microcephaly, microphthalmia, mental deficiency	First trimester	?
Varicella	Skin scars, hypoplasia of limbs, microphthalmus, cataracts, mental deficiency	?	?
Uterine factors			
Amniotic band deformity	Amputation or constriction bands on one or more extremities	?	?
Severe oligohydramnios	Lung hypoplasia, deformities caused by pressure from surrounding structures	Throughout	100%

unborn infant, experience has shown that she may be sufficiently motivated to control this problem during pregnancy.

Doctors are often asked about the risks of exposure in utero to drugs which have not been proved to be teratogenic. These include LSD (lysergic acid), marijuana, heroin, blighted potatoes, aspirin, and phenothiazine derivatives, such as Bendectin. The low incidence of abnormalities when they do occur and the possibility that some problems may not become apparent until later in life make it difficult to interpret negative reports about drug teratogenicity.

Genetic factors play a role in determining teratogenicity and may be 1 example of multifactorial inheritance in which the *inherited* factor is susceptibility to a teratogenic *environmental* factor. Variation in susceptibility to teratogens is apparent not only between different species of animals but also within species, e.g., different genetic strains of rats show different degrees of susceptibility to cortisone as a teratogenic agent which induces cleft palate in the rat fetus. The applicability of such observations to humans is likely but unproved.

Other conditions are also teratogenic, such as amniotic constriction bands, oligohydramnios, and uterine constraint. Bands of amniotic tissue cause either amputation or constriction of 1 or more extremities in about 1 in every 5000 pregnancies. Oligohydramnios may result from bilateral renal agenesis, severe polycystic kidney disease, chronic leakage of amniotic fluid, and extrauterine pregnancy. Its consequences are lung hypoplasia, club foot deformity, a flattened face, and amnion nodosum.

Clarren SK, Smith DW: The fetal alcohol syndrome. N Engl J Med 298:1063, 1978.
Dunn PM: Congenital postural deformities. Br Med Bull 32:71, 1976.
Hall JG, Pauli RM, Wilson KM: Maternal and fetal sequelae of anticoagulation during pregnancy. Am J Med 68:122, 1980.
Heinonen OP, Slone D, Shapiro S: Birth Defects and Drugs in Pregnancy. Littleton, Mass., Publishing Science Groups, 1976.
Lenke RR, Levy HL: Maternal phenylketonuria and hyperphenylalaninemia. N Engl J Med 303:1202, 1980.
Shepard TH: Catalog of Teratogenic Agents. Ed 3. Baltimore, The Johns Hopkins University Press, 1980.

6.31 RADIATION

Accidental exposure of the pregnant women to radiation is a common cause for anxiety among women, their families, and their physicians, usually about whether the fetus will have birth defects or genetic abnormalities. Fortunately, it is unlikely that exposure to either diagnostic or therapeutic radiation will cause gene mutations. Thus far, no increase in genetic abnormalities has been identified in the offspring exposed as unborn fetuses to the atomic bomb explosions in Japan in 1945.

A more realistic concern is whether the exposed human fetus will show birth defects or a higher incidence of malignancy. The recommended occupational limit of maternal exposure to radiation from all sources is 500 millirads for the entire 40 wk of a pregnancy. Estimates of the gonadal exposure for the mother and the whole body exposure of the fetus from several common roentgenographic examinations are shown in Table 6–18. The limited data on human fetuses show

Table 6–18 RADIATION EXPOSURE TO THE FETUS

	MILLIRADS*
Roentgenogram of:	
Chest	1
Thoracic spine	11
Abdomen	221
Pelvis	210
Hips	124
Roentgenographic contrast studies	
Upper G.I. series	171
Barium enema	903
Cholangiogram	78
Intravenous pyelogram	588

*Due to variation in techniques these estimates may be exceeded. (From U.S. DHEW: Gonad Doses and Genetically Significant Dose from Diagnostic Radiology; U.S., 1964 and 1970. Washington, D.C., U.S. Government Printing Office, 1976.)

that large doses of radiation (10,000–30,000 millirads) are harmful to the central nervous system. For that reason, therapeutic abortion is often recommended when exposure exceeds 10,000 millirads.

It is much more likely that a human fetus will be exposed to 1000–3000 millirads, an amount not shown to cause malformations. There is controversy as to whether this level of exposure is associated with an increased risk of developing cancer or leukemia. (See also Chapter 27.)

LEWIS B. HOLMES

Brent RL: Radiation teratogenesis. Teratology 21:281, 1980.
The Effects on Populations of Exposure to Low Levels of Ionizing Radiation (BEIR Report). Washington DC, National Academy of Sciences, National Research Council, November, 1972.
Griem ML, Meier P, Dobben GD: Analysis of the morbidity and mortality of children irradiated in fetal life. Radiology 88:347, 1967.
US Department of Health, Education, and Welfare: Gonad Doses and Genetically Significant Dose from Diagnostic Radiology; U.S., 1964 and 1970. Washington DC, US Government Printing Office, 1976.
Yamazaki NJ: A review of the literature on the radiation dosage required to cause manifest central nervous system disturbances from in utero and postnatal exposure. Pediatrics 37:877, 1966.

6.32 DYSMORPHOLOGY—THE APPROACH TO STRUCTURAL DEFECTS OF PRENATAL ONSET

The field of dysmorphology has expanded dramatically as the number of recognizable patterns of malformation has more than doubled over the last 10 yr; new insights have been gained into the pathogenesis of various structural defects, and the potential prenatal effect of various drugs, chemicals, and environmental agents has been better appreciated. Because of their vast number, a listing of all known recognizable patterns of malformation will not be presented. Rather, this section will set forth a method of approach to the child with the prenatal onset of structural defects. The approach is predicated upon the concept that the nature of the structural defects represents a clue to the time of onset, mechanism of injury, and potential etiology of the problem, all of which determine the necessary evaluation. This approach permits a systematic narrowing of the diagnostic possibilities so that other sections of this textbook or one of the basic compendiums on dysmorphology may be utilized to make a specific overall diagnosis.

Structural defects of prenatal onset can be separated into those which represent a single primary defect in development and those which represent a multiple malformation syndrome. In the majority of cases, the defect involves only a single structure, the child being otherwise completely normal. The 7 most common single primary defects in development are congenital hip dislocation (Sec 23.3), talipes equinovarus (Sec 6.6), cleft lip with or without cleft palate (Sec 11.10), cleft palate alone (Sec 11.11), cardiac septal defects (Sec 13.32), pyloric stenosis (Sec 11.23), and defects in neural tube closure (Sec 21.8). For most, the etiology is unknown, and counseling as to recurrence risk is difficult. However, most single primary defects are explained on the basis of multifactorial inheritance, which carries a recurrence risk of between 2–5% for the next child of unaffected parents with 1 affected child.

The extent to which multifactorial inheritance contributes to the etiology of some of the less common single defects in development is unclear. The fact that single primary defects are etiologically heterogeneous implies that some will have an environmental etiology whereas others will result from dominantly or recessively inherited single altered genes. Craniosynostosis (Sec 23.10) secondary to in utero constraint is an example of the former, whereas postaxial polydactyly (Sec 23.9) illustrates the latter. Before multifactorial risk figures are used for counseling when a single primary defect is recognized, references should be consulted to determine whether other risk figures are available.

In contrast to the concept of the single primary defect in development, the designation *multiple malformation syndrome* is used when several observed structural defects all have the same known or presumed etiology. The defects usually include a number of anatomically unrelated errors in morphogenesis. Multiple malformation syndromes are caused by chromosomal abnormalities, by teratogens, and by single gene defects inherited in mendelian patterns. Risks of recurrence range from 0 in cases which represent fresh gene mutations or are caused by teratogens to 100% in the case of a child with the Down syndrome in which the mother is a balanced 21/21 translocation carrier (Sec 6.11).

Single Primary Defects in Development. These defects are subcategorized according to the nature of the error in morphogenesis which has produced the observed structural defect: malformation, deformation, or disruption of developing structure. A *malformation* is a primary structural defect arising from a localized error in morphogenesis. A *deformation* is an alteration in shape and/or structure of a part which has differentiated normally. The term *disruption* is used for a structural defect resulting from destruction of a previously normally formed part. Of the deformations noted at birth, 90% will correct spontaneously; of those that do not, most can be corrected with early postural intervention. If correction of malformations or disruptions is at all possible, surgery is virtually always required.

Malformations. Most children with a localized malformation such as cardiac septal defect or pyloric stenosis are otherwise completely normal. Following surgical correction, prognosis is excellent. When neither dominant nor recessive inheritance has been established, multifactorial recurrence risk factors (2–5%) apply to unaffected parents.

Deformations. The vast majority of deformations involve the musculoskeletal system and are probably caused by intrauterine molding. The pressure to produce such molding may be intrinsic, due to neuromuscular imbalance within the fetus, or may be extrinsic, secondary to fetal crowding. In either case, the impaired ability of the fetus to kick results in decreased fetal movement, an important factor in development of the normal musculoskeletal system, particularly with respect to normal joint development. In addition, marked positional deformation of any body part can occur when the fetus is unable to change position and thus alter the direction along which potentially deforming extrinsic forces are being directed.

Intrinsically derived positional deformation of prenatal onset occurs in disorders involving muscle degeneration, such as the Steinert myotonic dystrophy syndrome, and disorders involving motor neurons, such as Werdnig-Hoffmann disease (Sec 22.2). Early defects in development of the central nervous system are more common causes of positional deformations and should be seriously considered whenever a structural defect is thought to be intrinsically derived.

Fetal crowding, the common cause of an extrinsically derived deformation of prenatal onset, is usually due to a decreased volume of amniotic fluid, a situation that occurs normally during the later weeks of gestation when the fetus is undergoing extremely rapid growth. However, it also occurs abnormally with diminished fetal urinary output and chronic leakage of amniotic fluid.

Other extrinsic factors associated with the development of deformations include breech presentation and the shape of the amniotic cavity. When a fetus is held in the breech position, the legs may be trapped between the body and the uterine wall. In that position, the fetus is unable to kick optimally. Dunn has reported that breech presentation is associated with a 10-fold increase in the incidence of deformations. The shape of the amniotic cavity, which has profound influence on the shape of the fetus that lies within it, is influenced by many factors, including uterine shape; volume of amniotic fluid; size and shape of the fetus; presence of more than one fetus; site of placental implantation; presence of uterine tumors; shape of the abdominal cavity, which is influenced by the pelvis, sacral promontory, and neighboring abdominal organs; and tightness of abdominal musculature.

The various forms of talipes and congenital hip dislocation are the most frequently observed congenital postural deformities. Most children with these deformations are otherwise completely normal, and their prognosis is excellent. Correction usually occurs spontaneously. However, recognition that a structural defect represents a deformation does not always imply "normal" fetal crowding and should lead to careful consideration of other etiologic possibilities that might have far greater significance to the child. For example, since decreased fetal movement can be secondary to serious neurologic abnormalities, multiple joint contractures should alert the physician to the possibility of a malformation in central nervous system development. Although the most common deformational single primary defects, congenital hip dislocations and talipes, have a 2–5% recurrence risk, the vast majority of deformations are the result of physiologic crowding and have a lower recurrence risk. Deformations which are due to pathologic crowding (e.g., uterine tumors or malformation) have a much higher recurrence risk unless the factors leading to crowding are altered prior to subsequent pregnancies. Deformations which are the result of an underlying malformation (e.g., renal agenesis) have a recurrence risk similar to that for the underlying malformation.

Disruption. These defects occur when there is destruction of a previously normally formed part. There are at least 2 basic mechanisms known to produce disruption. One involves entanglement followed by the tearing apart and/or amputation of a normally developed structure, usually a digit, arm, or leg, by strands of amnion floating within amniotic fluid, e.g., amniotic bands (Sec 24.5). The second involves the interruption of blood supply to a developing part leading to infarction, necrosis, and/or resorption of structures distal to the insult. If interruption of blood supply occurs early in gestation, the disruptive defect which is seen at term usually involves atresia or absence of a particular part. If the infarction occurs later, necrosis is more likely to be present. Examples of disruptive single primary defects for which infarctive mechanisms have been implicated include nonduodenal intestinal atresia, gastroschisis (Sec 11.75), and porencephaly (Sec 21.9). The extent to which disruption of a developing structure plays a role in dysmorphogenesis is unknown.

Genetic factors play a minor role in the pathogenesis of disruptions; most are sporadic events in otherwise normal families. The prognosis for a disruptive defect is determined entirely by the extent and location of the tissue loss. Thus a child with a limb amputation has an excellent prognosis for normal function, whereas a child with porencephaly does not.

Sequence. The pattern of multiple anomalies which occurs when a single primary defect in early morphogenesis produces multiple abnormalities through a cascading process of secondary and tertiary errors in morphogenesis is called a sequence. When evaluating a child with multiple anomalies, the physician must in counseling regarding risk of recurrence differentiate between multiple anomalies secondary to a single localized error in morphogenesis (a sequence) and a multiple malformation syndrome. In the former situation recurrence risk counseling for the multiple anomalies depends entirely upon the recurrence risk for the single localized malformation.

The words malformation, deformation, and disruption sequence are used to describe only the initiating error in morphogenesis of a sequence if it is known. For example, the Robin malformation sequence (Sec 11.3) is a pattern of multiple anomalies, all of which are produced by a single prenatal onset defect in development. The primary defect is mandibular hypoplasia, a malformation. Since the tongue is relatively small for the oral cavity, it drops back (glossoptosis), blocking closure of the posterior palatal shelves and causing a U-shaped cleft palate. Recognition that all of the ob-

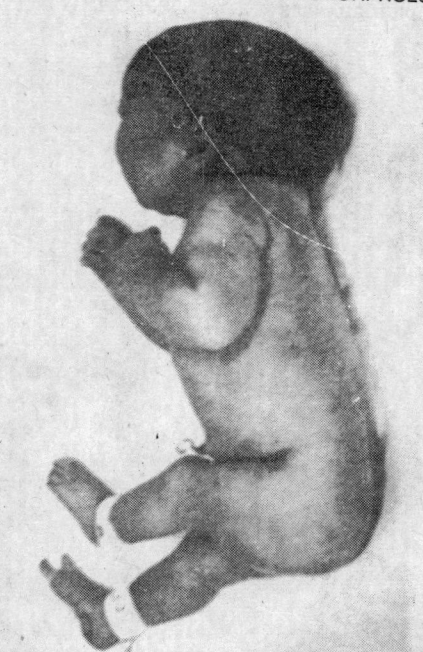

Figure 6–27   Breech deformation sequence.

served defects are due to a single localized error in morphogenesis (mandibular hypoplasia) permits recurrence risk counseling based upon the single defect.

The patient depicted in Fig 6–27 has bathrocephaly, torticollis, facial asymmetry, a dislocated hip, and valgus anomalies of both feet. All of the structural defects are the result of compression of developing fetal parts. This pattern of abnormalities is referred to as the breech deformation sequence. Intrauterine crowding here was due to large size of an infant delivered from a breech position to a small primigravida mother. Recurrence risk is therefore negligible. Recognition of the deformational nature of the abnormalities is helpful with respect to prognosis. All of the problems should resolve spontaneously or with postural therapy.

The patient depicted in Fig 6–28 has the amniotic band disruption sequence. All of the craniofacial and limb defects are secondary to constrictions caused by entanglement in multiple fibrous strands of amnion extending from the placental insertion of the umbilical cord to the surface of the amnion-denuded chorion or floating freely within the chorionic sac. These strands of amnion, which result from disruption of the normally formed membrane, cause secondary defects through any one or more of the following mechanisms. Malformations occur if a strand of amnion interferes with the normal sequence of embryologic development. For example, a strand of amnion may interrupt fusion of the facial processes so that a cleft lip results. Disruptions, on the other hand, are secondary to tearing apart of structures which have previously developed normally; an amniotic band might cleave areas in the developing craniofacies along lines not conforming to the normal planes of facial closure. Deformations due to fetal compression occur secondary to oligohydramnios and/

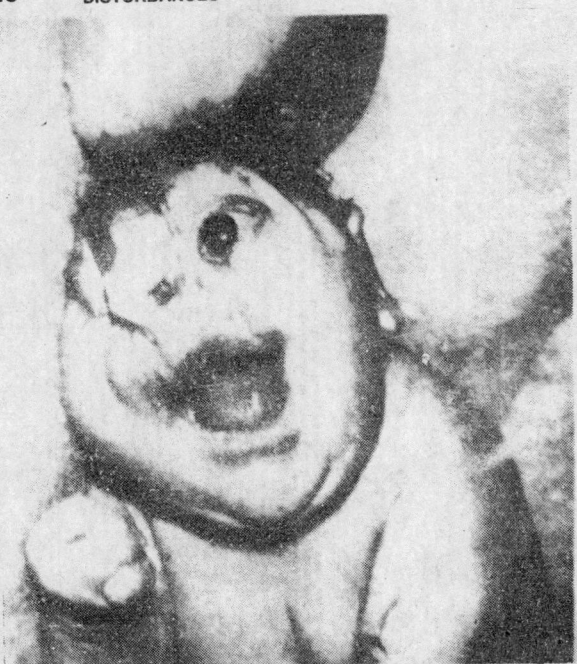

Figure 6—28 Amniotic band disruption sequence.

or tethering of a fetal part. The former situation may be the result of rupture of both amnion and chorion, leading to chronic leakage of amniotic fluid. Tethering occurs when the fetus or one of its parts becomes immobilized by the constraining effect of an amniotic band such that it is unable to change position and thus alter the direction along which potentially deforming forces are being directed. The recurrence risk is based upon the recurrence risk for the initiating event, amnion rupture. There has not yet been a family in which unaffected parents have given birth to more than 1 child affected with this disorder.

Finally, it is important to emphasize that a sequence like any other single defect in development can occur by itself in an otherwise normal individual or may be 1 feature in a multiple malformation syndrome. There are at least 7 multiple malformation syndromes in which the Robin malformation sequence represents 1 feature. In those disorders recurrence risk for the sequence depends on the primary diagnosis.

Multiple Malformation Syndromes. This category includes patients in whom 1 or more developmental anomalies of 2 or more systems have occurred, all of which are thought to be due to common etiology. Other than Down syndrome, which has an incidence of 1:660, and XXY syndromes (1:500 males), none of these disorders occurs more frequently than 1 in 3000 live births.

Multiple malformation syndromes may be caused by chromosomal and genetic abnormalities and by teratogens. The ability to perform chromosomal studies has led to the recognition of a number of multiple malformation syndromes (Sec 6.8).

Disorders known to be due to single mutant genes (dominant, or X-linked in males) or to pairs of mutant genes (autosomal recessive) cause a number of recog-

nizable multiple malformation syndromes of prenatal onset. Correct diagnosis in most of these disorders depends on clinical recognition since in the vast majority of cases there is no laboratory test to confirm the diagnosis. Family history indicating a similarly affected individual can be extremely helpful. However, in many patients with multiple malformation syndromes of genetic etiology, the occurrence is sporadic and thus represents fresh gene mutations. In such situations, all family members are normal, and diagnosis depends entirely on evaluation of the patient's phenotype.

Disorders caused by teratogens include multiple malformation syndromes due to the effect of specific infections or of pharmacologic and/or chemical agents with which the embryo and/or fetus has come into contact during gestation. They are the only groups of dysmorphologic conditions which may be prevented prior to conception, particularly in the case of drugs and chemicals if the mother is aware that the agent in question can affect her baby. It is difficult, on the other hand, for a pregnant woman to avoid contact with all infectious agents.

A careful history of drug intake (Sec 5.3) and chemical exposure (Sec 28.16) should be taken from the parents of all children with multiple malformation syndromes, especially when the etiology of the disorder is unknown. *A Catalog of Teratogenic Agents* by T. H. Shepard is an excellent reference for determining what agent the mother has been exposed to.

Specific and easily distinguishable phenotypes do not exist for each of the infectious diseases which are commonly associated with altered fetal development, but intrauterine infection can frequently be suspected if there is an overall pattern of malformation (Sec 7.69–7.73). Any patient should be suspected of having had an intrauterine infection if he or she is small for gestational age, otherwise developmentally delayed, and affected by microcephaly or hydrocephalus, ocular defects including microphthalmia, chorioretinitis, cataracts, and/or glaucoma, and hepatosplenomegaly and thrombocytopenia. It should be emphasized, however, that intrauterine infections have a wide spectrum of clinical manifestations from the severely affected newborn infant with multiple malformations to the child with no malformations who first manifests learning disabilities at school age.

There are also some well-recognized multiple malformation syndromes in which virtually all cases have been sporadic in otherwise normal families and the etiology is unknown. The Cornelia de Lange syndrome, the Williams syndrome, the Prader-Willi syndrome, and the Rubinstein-Taybi syndrome are 4 of the most common disorders included in this category. Each occurs with a frequency greater than 1 per 10,000. Despite the lack of knowledge of etiology, experience with many children with each of these disorders has provided a vast amount of information that can be extremely helpful to parents in understanding their child's behavior and to educators in planning an appropriate curriculum. For example, a specific behavioral phenotype has been delineated for the de Lange syndrome; awareness by parents that the child's aberrant behavior is "normal" for the de Lange syndrome rather than "their fault" can be extremely helpful in relieving anxiety and guilt. For the Williams syndrome, a characteristic psychologic profile that indicates delayed motor and perceptual development with relatively good verbal performance and sociability has been demonstrated. This knowledge of a child's particular strengths and weaknesses may allow educators to develop a curriculum that will give children with specific disorders a better chance to reach their potential.

Finally, there are certain nonrandom associations of malformations for which it has not yet been possible to determine whether the pattern is a sequence or a syndrome. These have been designated as associations. One important clinical example is the VATER association. This acronym designates some of the nonrandomly occurring complexes of anomalies which include *v*ertebral defects, *a*nal atresia, *t*racheo*e*sophageal fistula with atresia, *r*adial upper limb hypoplasia, and *r*enal defects. The spectrum also includes single umbilical artery and cardiac and genital anomalies. These defects are likely to occur together in almost any combination of 2 or more and usually represent a sporadic occurrence in an otherwise normal family.

It is important to emphasize that the ultimate goal in the evaluation of a child with structural defects is a specific overall diagnosis. When this is achieved, appropriate recurrence risk counseling for the parents, accurate prognostication about the child's future development, and an appropriate plan to help the child reach his potential usually are possible. When an overall diagnosis is lacking, the most that can be expected is a better understanding of the nature and onset of the problem which often may be helpful to parents and to others dealing with the child.

KENNETH LYONS JONES

Bennett FC, Vanderveer B, Sells CJ: The Williams elfin facies syndrome: A psychological profile. Clin Res 25:170a, 1970.

Dunn PM: Congenital postural deformities. Br Med Bull 32:71, 1976.

Gorlin RJ, Cohen MM Jr, Pinburg JJ: Syndromes of the Head and Neck. Ed 2. New York, McGraw-Hill, 1975.

Higginbottom MC, Jones KL, Hall BD, et al: The amniotic band disruption complex: Timing of amniotic rupture and variable spectra of consequent defects. J Pediatr 95:544, 1979.

Johnson HG, Ekman P, Frieseu W, et al: A behavioral phenotype in the deLange syndrome. Pediatr Res 10:843, 1976.

McKusick VA: Mendelian Inheritance in Man. Catalog of Autosomal Dominant, Autosomal Recessive and X-linked Phenotypes. Ed 5. Baltimore, The Johns Hopkins University Press, 1978.

Shepard TH: A Catalog of Teratogenic Agents. Ed 3. Baltimore, The Johns Hopkins University Press, 1980.

Smith DW: Recognizable Patterns of Human Malformation. Ed 2. Philadelphia, WB Saunders, 1976.

Warkany J: Congenital Malformations: Notes and Comments. Chicago, Year Book Medical Publishers, 1971.

7 THE FETUS AND THE NEONATAL INFANT

The neonatal period is defined as the 1st 4 wk of life. However, fetal and neonatal life is a continuum during which the growth and development of the human organism are affected by genetic and by intrauterine and extrauterine environmental factors, the latter being modified by social, economic, and cultural influences. For example, maternal toxemia may result in a decreased rate of fetal growth and an increased incidence of neonatal hypoglycemia. Low economic status is also a factor frequently associated with low birth weight (premature birth), which in turn is associated with high rates of morbidity and mortality, not only in the neonatal period but throughout infancy. Socioeconomic factors are reflected in the significantly higher neonatal and infant mortality rate in the United States of nonwhite infants than of white ones (Table 7–1). Although social influences such as the reluctance of physicians to live in areas of poverty affect the availability of medical care to those most in need of it, the failure of many mothers in these areas to make effective use of prenatal and other preventive medical care available also contributes to fetal and infant morbidity and mortality. This latter failure is also, in part, a result of inadequate public education about health. Social factors leading to illegitimate births and cultural practices such as the use of drugs also increase the incidence of fetal and neonatal death and disease.

Neonatal mortality has progressively decreased (Table 7–1); it is highest during the 1st 24 hr of life, when it accounts for about 40% of deaths under 1 yr of age. Further reduction in this mortality and related morbidity depends, in large part, upon prevention, prenatal diagnosis, and early treatment of diseases that result from factors acting during gestation and at delivery, as opposed to diseases arising from postnatal factors (Table 7–2). The term *perinatal mortality* designates fetal and neonatal deaths influenced by prenatal conditions and circumstances surrounding delivery. It is most often defined as deaths of fetuses and infants from the 20th wk of gestational life through the 28th day after birth. Some perinatal mortality statistics, however, may exclude infants weighing under 1000 gm, infants born before 28 wk of fetal life, or infants dying after 7 days of age.

Fetal and neonatal deaths contribute about equally to

Table 7–2 PRINCIPAL CAUSES OF NEONATAL MORTALITY

CAUSE	PERCENTAGE OF DEATHS
Congenital anomalies	15
Immaturity (unqualified)	13
Asphyxia of newborn (unspecified)	12
Respiratory distress syndrome or hyaline membrane disease	21
Respiratory infection	2
Nonrespiratory infection	4
Complications of pregnancy and labor	19
Other	14

From Seigel DG, Stanley F, *In:* Quilligan EJ, Kretchmer N (eds): Fetal and Maternal Medicine. New York, John Wiley and Sons, 1980.

perinatal mortality. The key position of the obstetrician in the reduction of perinatal mortality and morbidity is obvious. Further, in recent years intrapartum fetal deaths have declined more than antepartum fetal deaths. This may reflect an increasing utilization of fetal monitoring during labor and a more liberal use of cesarean section for fetal distress, breech delivery, and other obstetric complications. It also emphasizes the need to be able to predict the maturity and functional reserve of the fetus prior to the onset of labor.

Perinatal and infant mortality rates vary from country to country; they are lowest in the Scandinavian countries and The Netherlands and highest in the developing countries. Even though socioeconomic, cultural, and, perhaps, geographic factors may be the most important influences that determine perinatal mortality, autopsy findings on liveborn infants indicate that there are potentials for further reductions in perinatal mortality by prophylactic health measures.

The high incidence of disease and excessive mortality rate during the 1st few days of life emphasize the need to identify as early as possible those fetuses and infants who are at greatest risk. The obstetrician and pediatrician must maintain effective communication so that perinatal problems may be anticipated and preventive and therapeutic measures taken promptly.

Of equal importance with the need to lower perinatal mortality rates is the need to lower the incidence of

Table 7–1 INFANT AND NEONATAL MORTALITY RATES, UNITED STATES

	INFANT MORTALITY			NEONATAL MORTALITY		
YEAR	Total	White	All Other	Total	White	All Other
1974	16.7	14.8	24.9	12.3	11.1	17.2
1972	18.5	16.4	27.7	13.6	12.4	19.2
1962	25.3	22.3	41.4	18.3	16.9	26.1
1952	28.4	25.5	47.0	19.8	18.5	28.0

From Seigel DG, Stanley, F, *In:* Quilligan EJ, Kretchmer N (eds): Fetal and Maternal Medicine. New York, John Wiley and Sons, 1980.

handicapping conditions resulting from untoward perinatal factors. Since both mortality and permanent neurologic sequelae are in large measure caused by the same or similar disturbances, research and public health measures directed at reducing perinatal mortality should also reduce the incidence of handicapping conditions. For example, a reduction of the high incidence of mental retardation among infants who required vigorous and prolonged resuscitation at birth depends upon the early diagnosis of fetal asphyxia, appropriate obstetric management, and optimal resuscitation. However, some injury may be unavoidable; retinal and pulmonary damage may occur among those who had prolonged exposure to high concentrations of oxygen in the immediate postnatal period through attempts to reduce the risk of hypoxic brain damage.

The limitation of population growth makes it even more critical to combat diseases that may limit the biologic potential of the individual newborn infant.

Successful and timely provision of high quality care to perinatal patients requires not only excellence in the performance of health professionals but also a system that facilitates coordinated teams linking the prenatal care of expectant mothers with community hospital facilities, special programs for high-risk pregnancies and infants, and referral centers. Regional perinatal programs should provide continuing education and consultation in both the community and the referral center and transportation for pregnant women and newborn infants to appropriate hospitals; they should also include a regional center with facilities, equipment, and personnel for obstetric and neonatal intensive care.

National Commission for the Protection of Human Subjects of Biomedical and Behavioral Research: Report and Recommendations, Research on the Fetus. Washington, DC, Department of Health, Education, and Welfare Pub No (OS) 76:127, 1975.
Chamberlain G.: Background to perinatal health. Lancet 2:1061, 1980.
Lee, KS, Paneth N, Gartner L, et al: Neonatal mortality: An analysis of recent improvement in the United States. Am J Pub Health 70:15, 1980.
Shapiro S, McCormick M, Starfield B, et al: Relevance of correlates of infant deaths for significant morbidity at 1 year of age. Am J Obstet Gynecol 136:363, 1980.
Tudehope DI, Sinclair JC: Birth weight, gestational age, and neonatal risk. In: Behrman RE (ed): Neonatal-Perinatal Medicine. St Louis, CV Mosby, 1977.
Wigglesworth JS: Monitoring perinatal mortality. Lancet 2:684, 1980.

7.1 THE FETUS

Fetal life begins with the completion of organogenesis at about the 12th wk of gestation. Genetic and environmental influences that affect the fetus are at work even before conception. The genes from each parent play an important role not only in fetal development but also in fetal survival. Environmental factors may influence selection and expression of genes transmitted to the infant, as well as the mutations of parental genes.

The father's health may affect the motility of the spermatozoon and its ability to penetrate the ovum. The mother's health and state of nutrition may affect ovulation, the viability of the ovum and the zygote, and the availability of an adequate site for implantation; women who suffer from malnutrition or debilitating illness have diminished fertility and often diminished frequency of menstruation. Exposure of the zygote or embryo to drugs, chemicals, infectious disease, or other noxious influences may result in structural malformations or aberrant fetal growth; prenatal maternal exposure to methyl mercury may result in Minamata disease (Sec 28.14). The general health and nutrition of the mother, and possibly her emotional health during pregnancy, also affect the fetus; the infants of malnourished mothers may weigh less and be slightly shorter at birth than those of mothers with adequate nutrition. Illness of the mother may result in fetal death, abortion, or premature delivery.

The major emphases in fetal medicine are (1) fetal effects of maternal disease; (2) fetal effects of drugs administered to the mother; (3) identification of fetal defects and disease and untoward changes in fetal vital signs; and (4) treatment of fetal disease. Increasing knowledge of fetal physiology may pave the way for practical approaches to problems of adaptation of the newborn infant, particularly of the premature one, to extrauterine life. Some aspects of human fetal growth and development are summarized in Sec 2.2.

7.2 MATERNAL DISEASE AND THE FETUS

Infectious Diseases. Almost any maternal infection with severe systemic manifestations may result in abortion, stillbirth, or premature labor. Whether these results are due to infection of the fetus or are secondary to stress is not always clear. Maternal hyperthermia during infections may be associated with an increased incidence of congenital anomalies. Certain agents, however, do infect the fetus more or less regularly without relation to the severity of the maternal infection, infections frequently with a disastrous effect on life or development. Such fetuses are frequently of low weight for their gestational age. Some infections, such as rubella, may also produce congenital malformations if they occur during the period of organogenesis. Maternal infections that cause disease in the fetus or newborn infant include *Chagas disease, chickenpox* or *herpes zoster, Coxsackie B viruses, cytomegalovirus, hepatitis, herpes simplex, listeriosis, malaria* (abortion, premature delivery), *mumps* (fetal death and possibly endocardial fibroelastosis), *poliomyelitis* (abortion, congenital paralysis, or poliomyelitis), *rubella, rubeola* (abortion, prematurity, fetal measles, possibly congenital malformations), *smallpox* (fetal smallpox), *syphilis, toxoplasmosis, tuberculosis* (congenital tuberculosis), *vaccinia or vaccination* (fetal vaccinia), *vibrio fetus* (abortion, prematurity, meningitis), and *Western equine encephalitis* (encephalitis).

Table 7-3 MATERNAL NONINFECTIOUS DISEASE AFFECTING THE FETUS

MATERNAL DISORDER	FETAL OR NEONATAL EFFECTS
Cholestasis	Preterm delivery
Cyanotic congenital heart disease	Intrauterine growth retardation
Diabetes mellitus	Large for gestational age infants, hypoglycemia, hypocalcemia, immaturity
Endemic goiter	Neonatal hypothyroidism
Graves disease	Transient neonatal thyrotoxicosis
Hyperparathyroidism	Hypocalcemia
Hypertension	Intrauterine growth retardation, stillbirth
Hypoparathyroidism	Hypercalcemia
Idiopathic thrombocytopenia	Thrombocytopenia, bleeding diathesis
Malignant melanoma	Placental metastasis
Myasthenia gravis	Transient neonatal myasthenia
Myotonic dystrophy	Neonatal myotonic dystrophy
Preeclampsia-eclampsia (toxemia)	Intrauterine growth retardation, stillbirth
Phenylketonuria	Microcephaly, mental retardation
Renal disease	Intrauterine growth retardation, abortion
Rickets	Hypocalcemia, rickets
Sickle cell anemia	Intrauterine growth retardation
Systemic lupus erythematosus	Congenital heart block, transient rash, anemia, leukopenia, thrombocytopenia, pericardial effusion

Noninfectious Diseases (Table 7–3). *Maternal diabetes* may result in organomegaly, hypertrophy and hyperplasia of the beta cells of the fetal pancreas, and metabolic derangements in the neonate (Sec 7.56). There is a high incidence of intrauterine death after the 36th wk of gestation in unmonitored mothers. *Toxemia* of pregnancy results in small size of the fetus for gestational age, prematurity, and intrauterine death. These effects are probably due to diminished uteroplacental perfusion. Uncontrolled *hypothyroidism* or *hyperthyroidism* in the mother is responsible for relative infertility, a tendency to abortion, premature labor, and fetal death. Maternal *immunologic diseases*, such as systemic lupus, myasthenia gravis, and Graves disease, mediated by IgG autoantibodies which cross the placenta result frequently in a transient illness in the newborn. Untreated maternal *phenylketonuria* results in abortion, congenital malformations, and injury to the brain of the nonphenylketonuric fetus.

7.3 MATERNAL MEDICATION AND THE FETUS

The effects of drugs taken by the mother vary considerably, especially in relation to the time in pregnancy when they are taken. Abortion or congenital malformations result from maternal ingestion of teratogenic drugs during the period of organogenesis. Some drugs may be synergistic with others in their teratogenic effects. Maternal medications taken later, especially during the last few wk of gestation or during labor, tend to affect the function of specific organs or enzyme

systems and to exert their chief adverse function on the neonate rather than on the fetus (Tables 7–4 and 7–5). There also may be genetically determined differences in susceptibility to some drugs. In addition, the effects of drugs may be evident immediately in the delivery room or may be delayed, such as with the development of genital lesions in female offspring of women exposed to diethylstilbestrol during pregnancy. Exposure to drugs in pregnancy is frequent, with surveys indicating that 90% of pregnant patients have taken at least 1 drug. The average mother has taken 4 drugs other than vitamins or iron during pregnancy; 4% have taken 10 or more drugs.

In view of the limited current knowledge of fetal effects from maternal medication, no drugs should be prescribed during pregnancy without weighing the maternal need against the risk of fetal damage.

7.4 IDENTIFICATION OF FETAL DISEASE (INTRAUTERINE DIAGNOSIS)

Diagnostic procedures may be employed for the identification of disease in the fetus when interruption of the pregnancy is under consideration and when direct treatment of the fetus may be possible. In a broader context, the family history, reproductive history of the mother, and course of the pregnancy may lead to the nonspecific diagnoses of "high-risk pregnancy" and "high-risk infant" (Sec 7.6 and 7.14).

Amniocentesis, the transabdominal withdrawal of amniotic fluid during pregnancy for diagnostic purposes (Table 7–6), is frequently done to determine the need for fetal transfusion or the timing of the delivery of fetuses with erythroblastosis fetalis. It is also done for genetic indications, usually between the 16th–18th wk of gestation. The amniotic fluid may be directly analyzed for amino acids, enzymes, hormones, and abnormal metabolic products; uncultivated amniotic fluid cells may be subjected to sex chromatin analysis and Y chromosome fluorescence to detect male fetuses at risk for sex-linked disorders, such as hemophilia and progressive muscular dystrophy; and amniotic fluid cells may be cultivated to permit detailed cytogenic analysis for the prenatal detection of chromosomal abnormalities and enzymatic analysis for the detection of inborn metabolic errors. Analysis of amniotic fluid also may be helpful in identifying neural tube defects (elevation of α-fetoprotein), adrenogenital syndrome (elevation of 17-ketosteroids and pregnanetriol), and thyroid dysfunction. In addition, direct visualization of the fetus by transabdominal amnioscopy has been used to diagnose fetal anomalies and to facilitate sampling of fetal blood used to diagnose hemoglobinopathies and hemophilia.

The best available chemical indices of fetal maturity are provided by determinations of amniotic fluid creatinine and lecithin, which reflect the maturity of fetal kidney and lung, respectively. Lecithin (L) is produced in the lung by type II alveolar cells and eventually reaches the amniotic fluid via the effluent from the respiratory passages. Until the middle of the 3rd trimester, it is present in a concentration about equal to that

Table 7-4 MATERNAL MEDICATIONS THAT MAY ADVERSELY AFFECT THE FETUS

Drug	Effect on Fetus	Dependability of Evidence
Adrenal corticosteroids	Cleft palate	Suggestive
Alcohol	Congenital anomalies, IUGR*	Conclusive
Amphetamines	Congenital heart disease, transposition of the great vessels, IUGR	Suggestive
Aminopterin	Abortion, malformations	Conclusive
Azathioprine	Abortion	Suggestive
Busulfan (Myleran)	Stunted growth, corneal opacities, cleft palate, hypoplasia of ovaries, thyroid and parathyroids	Doubtful
Caffeine	Spontaneous abortion, stillbirth, anomalies, or premature birth	Doubtful
Chlorambucil	Renal agenesis	Suggestive
Chloroquine	Deafness	Doubtful
Chlorothiazide	Thrombocytopenia	Suggestive
Cigarette smoking	Low birth weight for gestational age	Suggestive
Cyclophosphamide	Multiple malformations	Suggesive
Dicumarol	Fetal bleeding and death, hypoplastic nasal structures	Conclusive
Dilantin	Congenital anomalies, IUGR	Conclusive
Lysergic acid diethylamide (LSD)	Skeletal defects	Doubtful
	Chromosome damage	Suggestive
Meclizine (Bonine)	Congenital malformations	Doubtful
Mepivacaine	Bradycardia, death	Conclusive
6-Mercaptopurine	Abortion	Suggestive
Methimazole	Goiter	Conclusive
Methyltestosterone	Masculinization of female fetus	Conclusive
17-Alpha-ethinyl-19-nortestosterone (Norlutin)	Masculinization of female fetus	Conclusive
Penicillamine	Cutis laxa syndrome	Suggestive
Progesterone	Masculinization of female fetus	Suggestive
17-Alpha-ethinyl testosterone (Progestoral)	Masculinization of female fetus	Conclusive
Propranolol	Hypoglycemia, bradycardia, respiratory depression, fixed heart rate in infants	Suggestive
Propylthiouracil	Goiter	Conclusive
Quinine	Abortion, thrombocytopenia	Conclusive
	Deafness	Doubtful
Radioactive iodine (^{131}I)	Destruction of fetal thyroid	Conclusive
Stilbestrol (diethylstilbestrol [DES])	Masculinization of female fetus	Suggestive
	Vaginal adenocarcinoma in adolescence	Conclusive
Streptomycin	Deafness	Suggestive
Tetracycline	Retarded skeletal growth	Suggestive
	Pigmentation of teeth, hypoplasia of enamel	Conclusive
	Cataract, limb malformations	Doubtful
Thalidomide	Phocomelia, other malformations	Conclusive
Trimethadione and paramethadione	Abortion, multiple malformations, mental retardation	Conclusive
Tolbutamide	Congenital malformations	Doubtful
Vitamin D	Supravalvular aortic stenosis, hypercalcemia	Doubtful

*IUGR = intrauterine growth retardation.

of sphingomyelin (S); thereafter, S remains constant in amniotic fluid while L increases. By 35 wk, on the average, the L/S ratio is about 2:1 and it continues to increase until term.

A more accelerated lung maturation may occur when there is severe nonfatal premature separation of the placenta, premature spontaneous rupture of the fetal membranes, narcotic addiction, or maternal hypertensive and renal vascular disease. A delay in pulmonary maturation may be associated with hydrops fetalis or maternal diabetes without vascular disease. The likelihood of hyaline membrane disease is greatly reduced with L/S ratios of 2 or more to 1, although hypoxia, acidosis, and hypothermia may increase the risk despite this "mature" L/S ratio. However, 20–25% of infants with L/S ratios less than 2:1 will not have hyaline membrane disease. Maternal and fetal blood have an L/S ratio of about 1:4; thus, contamination will not alter the significance of a ratio of 2:1 or more. Meconium contamination, storage, and centrifugation all may reduce the reliability of the L/S ratio. An alternative bubble stability or shake test is also used as an index of a "mature" level of pulmonary surfactant; after diluting amniotic fluid with isotonic saline and then shaking with 95% ethanol varying degrees of bubble formation develop. The greater the dilution (1:2, 1:3, 1:4) that results in a complete ring of bubbles, the lower the risk of hyaline membrane disease.

A determination of saturated phosphatidyl-choline (L) or phosphatidyl-glycerol (PG) concentrations in amniotic fluid may be more specific and sensitive predictors of hyaline membrane disease.

Although amniocentesis can be carried out with little discomfort to the mother, there is, even in experienced hands, a small risk of direct damage to the fetus, of placental puncture and bleeding with secondary damage to the fetus, of stimulating uterine contraction and premature labor, of amnionitis, and of maternal sensitization to fetal blood. The earlier in gestation amniotic puncture is done, the greater the risk to the fetus. The risks can be reduced by using ultrasound B scan for placental localization. The procedure should be limited

Table 7-5 MATERNAL MEDICATIONS THAT MAY ADVERSELY AFFECT THE NEWBORN INFANT

Anesthetic agents (volatile)—central nervous system depression
Adrenal corticosteroids—adrenocortical failure (rare)
Ammonium chloride—acidosis (clinically inapparent)
Aspirin—neonatal bleeding, prolonged gestation
Bromides—rash, CNS depression
Caudal anesthesia with mepivacaine (accidental introduction of anesthetic into scalp of baby)—bradypnea, apnea, badycardia, convulsions
CNS depressants (narcotics, barbiturates, tranquilizers) during labor—central nervous system depression
Cephalothin—positive direct Coombs test reaction
Coumarin derivatives—high perinatal mortality, anomalies
Hexamethonium bromide—paralytic ileus
Indomethacin—persistent fetal circulation
Intravenous fluids during labor, e.g., salt-free solutions—electrolyte disturbances, hyponatremia
Iodides—neonatal goiter
Isoxsuprine—ileus, hypocalcemia, hypoglycemia, hypotension
Magnesium sulfate—respiratory depression, meconium plug, hypotonia
Morphine and its derivatives (addiction)—withdrawal symptoms (poor feeding, vomiting, diarrhea, restlessness, yawning and stretching, dyspnea and cyanosis, fever and sweating, pallor, tremors, convulsions)
Naphthalene—hemolytic anemia (in glucose-6-phosphate dehydrogenase [G-6-PD]–deficient infants)
Nitrofurantoin—hemolytic anemia (in G-6-PD-deficient infants)
Oxytocin—hyperbilirubinemia
Phenolic disinfectant (nursery)—hyperbilirubinemia
Primaquine—hemolytic anemia (in G-6-PD–deficient infants)
Reserpine—drowsiness, nasal congestion, poor temperature stability
Sulfonamides (long-acting)—interfere with protein binding of bilirubin; kernicterus at low levels of serum bilirubin
Sulfonylurea—refractory hypoglycemia
Thiazides—neonatal thrombocytopenia (rare)
Vitamin K (excessive amounts)—hyperbilirubinemia

to those cases in which it is estimated that the value of the findings will outweigh the risk.

Ultrasonography, employing pulsed sound of short wavelength above the audible limit for man and of high resolution, is used to obtain serial, accurately measurable images of the fetus. Two-dimensional B-scan sonographic display techniques are used to determine the dimensions of the fetal head (cephalometry), thorax, and abdomen for purposes of estimating maturity and diagnosing intrauterine growth retardation or death; to localize the placenta prior to amniocentesis so that it can be avoided; to identify a placenta previa or a hydatidiform mole; to diagnose fetal position and number; to diagnose fetal hydrops; and to detect congenital abnormalities. The low energy levels employed in

Table 7-6 APPLICATIONS OF AMNIOCENTESIS DURING PREGNANCY

Biochemical and cytogenetic studies in early pregnancy
Diagnosis and prognosis of erythroblastosis fetalis
Diagnosis and treatment of polyhydramnios
Direct fetal visualization and blood sampling
Determination of amniotic fluid volume (indicator dilution)
Studies of amniotic fluid circulation
Determinations of fetal maturity
Induction of labor
Instillation of pharmacologic agents for inhibition of uterine contractions or treatment of the fetus

pulsed or continuous ultrasound have not been demonstrated to have a detectable effect on tissue culture, on chromosomes, or on the infants. Although more than 95% of fetuses whose biparietal diameters measure 9.5 cm or more by ultrasonography are of at least 37 wk gestational age, biparietal diameter data correlate poorly with the L/S ratio. Combining biparietal diameter and abdominal circumference estimates enhances the ability to detect intrauterine growth retardation before delivery. Sonography also has been used successfully to diagnose anencephaly, hydrocephaly, meningocele, polycystic kidneys, omphalocele, gastroschisis, diaphragmatic hernia, dextrocardia, gastrointestinal obstruction, and large fetal neoplasms.

Continuous fetal heart rate monitoring detects abnormal cardiac patterns by instruments that compute the beat-to-beat fetal heart rate from a fetal electrocardiogram signal. Signals are derived from an electrode attached to the fetal presenting part or the mother's abdomen; from an ultrasonic transducer placed on the maternal abdominal wall to detect continuous ultrasonic waves reflected from the contractions of the heart; or from a phonotransducer placed on the mother's abdomen. Uterine contractions are simultaneously recorded from an amniotic fluid catheter and pressure transducer or from a tocotransducer applied to the maternal abdominal wall overlying the uterus.

Fetal heart rate patterns show various characteristics, some of which suggest fetal distress. Baseline fetal heart rate is the average rate between uterine contractions, which gradually decreases from about 155 beats/min in early pregnancy to about 135 beats/min at term; the normal range at term is 120–160 beats/min. Tachycardia (over 160 beats/min) is associated with early fetal hypoxia, maternal fever, maternal hyperthyroidism, maternal β-sympathomimetic or atropine therapy, fetal anemia, and some fetal arrhythmias. The latter do not generally occur with congenital heart disease and tend to resolve spontaneously at birth. Fetal bradycardia (less than 120 beats/min) occurs with fetal hypoxia, the placental transfer of local anesthetic agents and beta adrenergic blocking agents, and, occasionally, cardiac arrhythmias associated with congenital heart disease.

Normally, the baseline fetal heart rate is variable with long-term changes of 3–5 cycles/min as well as short term beat-to-beat variation. This variability may be decreased or lost with fetal hypoxemia or the placental transfer of drugs such as atropine, scopolamine, diazepam, promethazine, magnesium sulfate, and most sedative and narcotic agents. Prematurity and fetal tachycardia may also diminish beat-to-beat variability.

Periodic accelerations or decelerations of fetal heart rate responses to uterine contractions may also be monitored (Fig 7–1). Early deceleration (type I dips) is a repetitive pattern of slowing synchronous with and proportional to the amplitude of the associated uterine contraction. Variable deceleration (associated with cord compression) is characterized by variable shape, onset and occurrence with consecutive contractions, and the return to baseline at or before the conclusion of the contraction. Late deceleration (type II dips) is associated with fetal hypoxemia, occurs repetitively after a uterine contraction is well established, is proportional to its

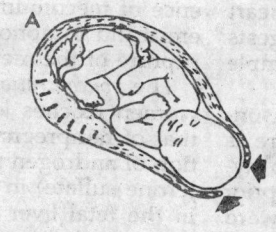

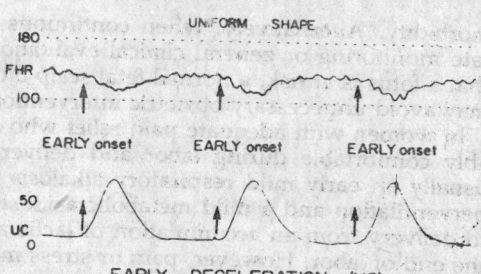

HEAD COMPRESSION

EARLY DECELERATION (HC)

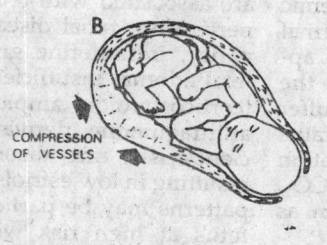

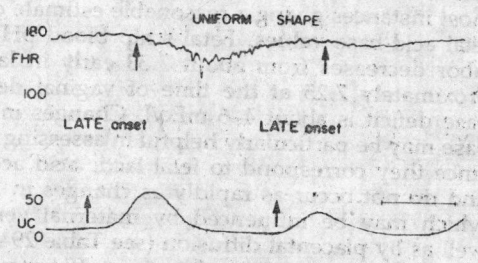

COMPRESSION OF VESSELS

UTEROPLACENTAL INSUFFICIENCY

LATE DECELERATION (UPI)

Figure 7–1 Patterns of periodic fetal heart rate decelerations. Tracing in *A* shows early deceleration which occurs during the peak of uterine contractions and is due to pressure on the fetal head; *B*, late deceleration due to uteroplacental insufficiency; *C*, variable deceleration due to umbilical cord compression. Arrows denote time relation between onset of FHR changes and uterine contractions. (From Hon EH: An Atlas of Fetal Heart Rate Patterns, New Haven, Conn., Harty Press, Inc., 1968.)

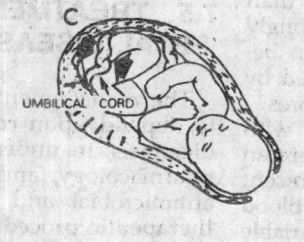

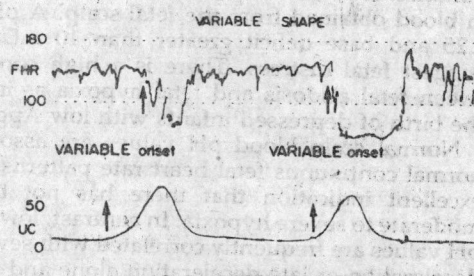

UMBILICAL CORD

UMBILICAL CORD COMPRESSION

VARIABLE DECELERATION (CC)

amplitude, and persists into the interval following contractions. The late deceleration pattern is usually associated with maternal hypotension or excessive uterine activity, but may be a response to any maternal, placental, umbilical cord, or fetal factor that limits effective oxygenation of the fetus. Early signs of fetal distress include mild late deceleration, loss of baseline variability, and increasing baseline rate.

Antenatal diagnosis of diminished uteroplacental perfusion also may be assessed using the *non-stress test* (NST) or the *oxytocin challenge test* (OCT). The NST relies upon the observation that a healthy fetus has an increased heart rate in association with fetal movements while the hypoxic or compromised fetus does not. During an OCT, oxytocin is infused at a rate sufficient to produce 3 uterine contractions within 10 min; if this results in 3 late (type II) decelerations, the fetus is judged to be at risk.

Roentgenographic examination is rarely the diagnostic procedure of choice to estimate fetal maturity or to establish a fetal diagnosis. The distal femoral epiphysis

may appear as early as 32 wk and is nearly always present by 40 wk, while the proximal tibial epiphysis may appear as early as 36 wk and is present in 50–75% of fetuses at 40 wk. Ultrasonography is substantially more accurate before 36 wk of gestation and avoids the remote risks of genetic or developmental injury from diagnostic radiation. Roentgenograms are necessary, however, to detect bony or calcific abnormalities such as achondroplasia, infantile cortical hyperostosis, osteogenesis imperfecta, or meconium peritonitis. The edema of fetal hydrops also can be detected roentgenographically. Lipid-soluble contrast medium injected into the amniotic fluid (amniography) can be used to outline the fetal soft tissues and diagnose congenital anomalies.

Fetal scalp blood sampling during labor through a slightly dilated cervix may aid in confirming fetal distress suspected on the basis of variations in fetal heart rate or the presence of meconium in the amniotic fluid. The proper use of this technique may result in the earlier delivery of depressed infants with a better chance of successful resuscitation, increased survival, and less morbidity. Alternatively, when continuous fetal heart rate monitoring or general clinical evaluation suggests that a fetus is at risk, a normal fetal scalp blood sample may avoid unnecessary obstetric intervention.

In women with adequate pain relief who are reasonably comfortable during labor and delivery, there is usually an early mild respiratory alkalosis due to hyperventilation and a mild metabolic acidosis just prior to delivery from an accumulation of lactic acid toward the end of labor. However, pain or stress may result in severe hyperventilation with marked reduction in maternal and subsequently fetal pCO_2 that may mask fetal acidosis. Fetal scalp blood pH and pCO_2 fall between values measured in the umbilical vein and artery, in most instances giving a reasonable estimate of systemic fetal acid-base values. Fetal scalp blood pH in normal labor decreases from about 7.33 early in labor to approximately 7.25 at the time of vaginal delivery; the base deficit is about 4–6 mEq/l. Changes in the buffer base may be particularly helpful in assessing fetal status since they correspond to fetal lactic acid accumulation and do not occur as rapidly as changes in fetal pCO_2, which may be influenced by maternal ventilation as well as by placental diffusion (see Table 29–2).

Fetal hypoxia and circulatory insufficiency result in a mixed placental respiratory and metabolic acidosis that often, but not invariably, can be detected by the determination of pH, base deficit, and carbon dioxide tension in blood obtained from the fetal scalp. A pH less than 7.25 and base deficit greater than 10 mEq/l strongly suggest fetal distress. There is a high correlation between fetal acidosis and fetal hypoxia as indicated by the birth of depressed infants with low Apgar scores.

Normal scalp blood pH values are associated with normal continuous fetal heart rate patterns and are an excellent indication that there has not been recent moderate to severe hypoxia. In contrast, low scalp blood pH values are frequently correlated with severe variable deceleration or late deceleration alone and with loss of beat-to-beat variability or baseline tachycardia associated with these deceleration patterns. However, a wide range of pH's is found with these patterns. Accordingly, heart rate–uterine contraction monitoring should be used as a screening technique, and acid-base analysis of fetal scalp blood and maternal blood should be obtained to properly evaluate many types of fetal heart rate abnormalities.

Complications of fetal scalp sampling and internal monitoring devices are relatively uncommon, but include bleeding (usually due to an underlying coagulation defect), puncture of the fontanel, and scalp abscesses with or without adjacent osteomyelitis. Abscesses may be due to *S. aureus* or gram-negative rods; more often they are sterile.

Fetal breathing movements also can be monitored antenatally and during labor with ultrasonic techniques. Changes in the incidence, duration, and patterns of normal human fetal respiratory movements are being evaluated to determine whether they will be useful adjuncts to other methods of identifying high-risk fetuses or detecting fetal distress during labor. Transcervical examination of the turbidity of amniotic fluid (*amnioscopy*) has also been employed to detect the presence of meconium in the amniotic fluid in severe toxemia and in abnormally prolonged gestations prior to rupture of the membranes or amniocentesis.

The *concentration of estriol* in the urine of pregnant women reaches levels of 100–1000 times greater than that of nonpregnant women as a result of the production of androgen precursors (mainly dihydroepiandrosterone sulfate) in the fetal adrenal, their hydroxylation in the fetal liver and conversion to estriol in the placenta, and the conjugation of estriol in the maternal liver. The 24 hr urine estriol excretion increases throughout pregnancy with a surge during the last 4–8 wk. Abnormally low serial urinary estriol determinations and depressed plasma unconjugated estriol levels are associated with fetal death, maternal diabetes, hypertension, renal disease or toxemia, prolonged pregnancy, intrauterine growth retardation, anencephaly, fetal adrenal insufficiency, and maternal drug therapy (corticosteroids, ampicillin, Mandelamine, dihydroxyanthraquinone derivatives). Placental sulfatase deficiency is a rare disorder affecting male infants and resulting in low estriols but no other abnormality. These patterns may be particularly helpful in identifying the fetus at high risk when combined with continuous monitoring of the fetal heart rate response to uterine contractions.

7.5 TREATMENT AND PREVENTION OF FETAL DISEASE

The management of diseases of the fetus continues to depend upon coordinated advances in accuracy of diagnosis; in understanding of fetal pathophysiology, pharmacology, and immunology; in the availability of antimicrobial and especially antiviral drugs; and in therapeutic procedures. Progress in providing specific treatments for accurately diagnosed diseases has been limited.

Fetal syphilis is nearly always present in untreated maternal disease and can be specifically and safely treated (Sec 10.55). Fetal mortality and prematurity associated with maternal bacterial urinary tract infections can be reduced with appropriate antibiotic treatment of the mother. Immunization has effectively reduced fetal mortality and morbidity from rubella (Sec 10.68).

The incidence of sensitization of Rh negative women by Rh positive fetuses has been reduced by the prophylactic administration of Rh(D) immune globulin to mothers early in pregnancy and after each delivery or abortion, thus reducing the frequency of hemolytic disease in their subsequent offspring. Fetal erythroblastosis (Sec 7.47) may now be accurately diagnosed by amniotic fluid analysis and treated with induced premature delivery, which may be combined with intrauterine intraperitoneal transfusions of packed Rh negative blood cells to maintain the fetus until mature enough to have a reasonable chance of survival.

Fetal asphyxia or distress may now be diagnosed with moderate success through monitoring the fetal heart rate and uterine pressure and through blood samples obtained by the scalp blood sampling technique. Treatment, however, remains limited to supplying the mother with high concentrations of oxygen, positioning the uterus to avoid vascular compression, and operative delivery before severe fetal injury occurs.

Pharmacologic approaches to fetal immaturity (e.g., administration of steroids to the mother to accelerate fetal lung maturation and decrease the incidence of hyaline membrane disease [Sec 7.34] in prematurely delivered infants) are promising. Inhibiting labor with β-sympathomimetic tocolytic agents is successful in some patients with premature labor. The treatment of definitively diagnosed genetic disease or congenital anomalies in a fetus consists of parental counseling and/or abortion; rarely, high dose vitamin therapy for a responsive inborn error of metabolism (e.g., biotin-dependent disorders) or fetal surgery to relieve obstructive hydrocephalus or genitourinary tract anomalies may be indicated. The nature of the defect and its consequences as well as ethical concerns of parents, society, and the physician must be taken into consideration.

Barden TP: Intrapartum fetal monitoring. In: Behrman RE (ed): Neonatal-Perinatal Medicine. St Louis, CV Mosby, 1977.
Clewell W, Johnson M, Meier P, et al: A surgical approach to the treatment of fetal hydrocephalus. N Engl J Med 306:1320, 1982.
Frantz T, Lindback T, Skjaeraasen J, et al: Phospholipids in amniotic fluid. II. Lecithin fatty acid patterns related to gestation, maternal disease and fetal outcome. Acta Obstet Gynecol Scand 54:33, 1975.
Freeman RK: The use of the oxytocin challenge test for antepartum clinical evaluation of uteroplacental respiratory function. Am J Obstet Gynecol 121:481, 1975.
Fuchs F: Prevention of premature birth. Clin Perinatol 7:3, 1980.
Gabert HA, Bryson MJ, Stenchever MA: The effect of cesarean section on respiratory distress in the presence of a mature lecithin-sphingomyelin ratio. Am J Obstet Gynecol 115:366, 1973.
Garite T, Freeman R: Antepartum stress test monitoring. Clin Obstet Gynecol 6:295, 1979.
Gluck L, Kuolvich MU, Borer RC Jr, et al: Interpretation and significance of the lecithin-sphingomyelin ratio in amniotic fluid. Am J Obstet Gynecol 120:142, 1974.
Golbus M, Harrison M, Filly R, et al: In utero treatment of urinary tract obstruction. Am J Obstet Gynecol 142:383, 1982.
Golbus M, Loughman W, Epstein C, et al: Prenatal genetic diagnosis in 3000 amniocenteses. N Engl J Med 300:157, 1979.
Hobbins J, Mahoney M: Fetoscopy in continuing pregnancies. Am J Obstet Gynecol 129:440, 1977.
Hobbins J, Grannum P, Berkowitz R, et al: Ultrasound in the diagnosis of congenital anomalies. Am J Obstet Gynecol 134:331, 1979.
Hon EH, Zannini D, Quilligan EJ: The neonatal value of fetal monitoring. Am Obstet Gynecol 122:508, 1975.
Liley AW: Liquor amnii analysis in management of pregnancy complicated by rhesus sensitization. Am J Obstet Gynecol 82:1359, 1961.
Low JA, Panchow SR, Worthington D, et al: The incidence of fetal asphyxia in six hundred high-risk monitored pregnancies. Am J Obstet Gynecol 121:456, 1975.
Olson EB, Jr, Hartline JV, Schneider JM, et al: The use of amniotic bubble stability, L/S ratio, and creatinine concentration in the assessment of fetal maturity. Am J Obstet Gynecol 122:755, 1975.
Parer JT: Fetal Monitoring. Semin Perinatol 2: Entire issue, 1978.
Pitkin RM: Estimation of fetal maturity. In: Behrman RE (ed): Neonatal-Perinatal Medicine. St Louis, CV Mosby, 1977.
Pleet H, Graham J, Smith D: Central nervous system and facial defects associated with maternal hyperthermia at 4–14 wk gestation. Pediatrics 67:785, 1981.
Porreco R, Young P, Cousins L, et al: Reproductive outcome following amniocentesis for genetic indications. Am J Obstet Gynecol 143:653, 1982.
Seeds AE: Fetal scalp acid-base monitoring. In: Behrman RE (ed): Neonatal-Perinatal Medicine. St Louis, CV Mosby, 1977.
Tejani N, Maran LI, Bhakthavathsalan A, et al: Correlation of fetal heart rate-uterine contraction patterns with fetal scalp blood pH. Obstet Gynecol 46:392, 1975.
Zuspan F, Quilligan E, Iams J, et al: NICHD Consensus Development Task Force Report: Predictors of intrapartum fetal distress – the role of electronic fetal monitoring. J Pediatr 95:1026, 1979.

7.6 HIGH-RISK PREGNANCIES

Pregnancies in which factors exist that increase the likelihood of abortion, fetal death, premature delivery, low birth weight, fetal or neonatal disease, congenital malformations, mental retardation, or other handicapping conditions are termed high-risk pregnancies (Table 7–7; also see Sec 7.14). Some factors, such as ingestion of a teratogenic drug in the 1st trimester, bear a causal relation to the risk; others, such as hydramnios, are associations that alert the physician to the existence of the risk or risks. Ten to 25% of pregnant patients can be identified as "high risk" on the basis of their medical history, and over half of all perinatal mortality and morbidity is associated with these pregnancies. Though antepartum risk assessment is important to reducing perinatal mortality and morbidity, a significant proportion of women become high risk only during labor and delivery; therefore, careful monitoring is critical throughout the intrapartum course.

The identification of high-risk pregnancies is important not only because it is the 1st step toward prevention, but also because in many instances therapeutic steps may be taken to reduce the risks to the fetus or to the neonate if the physician is alerted to the increased possibility of difficulty. A decreased incidence of low birth weight infants born to indigent women correlates with the provision and acceptance of good prenatal care. Identification and optimal management of high-risk pregnancies depend on careful attention to the family history, the reproductive history of the mother, and the course of the pregnancy and delivery, *together with close and continuing personal communication between the physician caring for mother and fetus and the physician who will care for the infant after birth.*

Genetic Factors. The occurrence of chromosomal abnormalities, congenital anomalies, inborn errors of metabolism, mental retardation, or, indeed, of any familial disease in blood relatives increases the risk of the same condition in the infant. Because many parents are not aware of the names or existence of these genetically determined diseases but only of 1 or more of their manifestations, specific inquiry should be made about any disease affecting more than 1 blood relative.

Maternal Factors. The lowest neonatal mortality rate occurs in infants of mothers 20–30 yr of age. Both teenage pregnancies and those among women over 35 yr of age, particularly primiparous women, carry an increased risk for intrauterine growth retardation, fetal distress, and intrauterine death.

Maternal illness (Table 7–9), multiple pregnancies, particularly those involving monochorionic twinning, and certain drugs (See 7.3) increase the risk for the fetus.

Table 7-7 FACTORS ASSOCIATED WITH HIGH-RISK PREGNANCY

Demographic factors
  Lower socioeconomic status
  Disadvantaged ethnic groups
  Marital status: unwed mothers
  Maternal age
    Gravida less than 16 yr of age
    Primigravida 35 yr of age or older
    Gravida 40 yr of age or older
  Maternal weight: nonpregnant weight less than 45 kg (100 lb) or
    more than 90 kg (200 lb)
  Stature: height less than 157 cm (62 in)
  Malnutrition
  Poor physical fitness
Past pregnancy history
  Grand multiparity: 6 previous pregnancies terminating beyond 20
    wk gestation
  Antepartum bleeding after 12 wk of gestation
  Premature rupture of membranes, premature onset of labor,
    premature delivery
  Previous cesarean section or mid- or high-forceps delivery
  Prolonged labor
  Previous infant with cerebral palsy, mental retardation, birth trauma,
    central nervous system disorder or congenital anomaly
  Reproductive failure: infertility, repetitive abortion, fetal loss,
    stillbirth, or neonatal death
  Delivery of preterm (less than 37 wk) or post-term (more than 42
    wk infant)
Past or present medical history
  Hypertension or renal disease or both
  Diabetes mellitus (overt or gestational)
  Cardiovascular disease (rheumatic, congenital, or peripheral
    vascular)
  Pulmonary disease producing hypoxemia and hypercapnia
  Thyroid, parathyroid, and endocrine disorders
  Idiopathic thrombocytopenic purpura
  Neoplastic disease
  Hereditary disorders
  Collagen diseases
  Epilepsy
Additional obstetric and medical conditions
  Toxemia
  Asymptomatic bacteriuria
  Anemia or hemoglobinopathy
  Rh sensitization
  Habitual smoking
  Drug addiction or habituation
  Chronic exposure to any pharmacologic or chemical agent
  Multiple pregnancy
  Rubella or other viral infection
  Intercurrent surgery and anesthesia
  Placental abnormalities and uterine bleeding
  Abnormal fetal lie or presentation, fetal anomalies, oligohydramnios,
    polyhydramnios
  Abnormalities of fetal or uterine growth or both
  Maternal trauma during pregnancy
  Maternal emotional crisis during pregnancy

Polyhydramnios and *oligohydramnios* are indications of a high-risk pregnancy. Although there is a rapid turnover rate, during normal pregnancy the amniotic fluid volume gradually increases at a rate of less than 10 ml/day until about the 34th wk of pregnancy, after which it slowly diminishes. The volumes vary widely in normal pregnancy; term volume may be 500–2000 ml. A volume estimated at greater than 2000 ml in the 3rd trimester constitutes polyhydramnios, and a volume estimated at less than 500 ml indicates oligohydramnios.

Acute polyhydramnios is rare, and is usually associated with premature labor and delivery before 28 wk. Chronic polyhydramnios is commonly diagnosed in the 3rd trimester, occasionally not until the patient has a dysfunctional labor or until an abnormally large amount of amniotic fluid is noted during delivery. Ultrasound is very helpful in establishing the diagnosis before labor. Polyhydramnios is associated with maternal diabetes (especially if severe), congenital malformations (Table 7–8), erythroblastosis fetalis, and multiple gestations (especially monochorionic twins); the association correlates with an increased perinatal mortality. Anencephaly and hydrocephaly are frequently associated congenital anomalies; about 50% of anencephalic pregnancies have polyhydramnios. The incidence of atresias of the upper intestinal tract, which presumably interfere with the reabsorption into the circulation of swallowed amniotic fluid, is also increased. When polyhydramnios occurs with erythroblastosis fetalis, hydrops fetalis is usually present.

Aplasia or hypoplasia of the fetal kidneys is often associated with oligohydramnios, presumably because fetal urine has not been formed. Oligohydramnios, from whatever cause, before the last few wk of pregnancy may result in mechanically induced abnormalities of the fetal limbs. It may also be associated with pulmonary hypoplasia, which can result in respiratory insufficiency and neonatal death.

Obstetric factors are of understandable importance when one considers that fetuses weighing more than 2500 gm make up a very high proportion of the total fetal deaths and that neonatal mortality is greatest during the 1st 24 hr after delivery. A pregnancy should be considered high risk when the uterus is inappropriately large or small. A uterus that is large for the estimated stage of gestation suggests multiple fetuses, hydramnios, or an excessively large infant; an inappropriately small one suggests retardation of intrauterine growth. Rupture of membranes earlier than 24 hr before delivery carries a risk of infection of the intrauterine contents and increased perinatal mortality. Prolonged and difficult labors increase the risks of mechanical and hypoxic damage. The risk of neonatal death in uncomplicated labors lasting 24 hr or less is approximately

Table 7-8 FETAL MALFORMATIONS FREQUENTLY ASSOCIATED WITH POLYHYDRAMNIOS OR OLIGOHYDRAMNIOS

POLYHYDRAMNIOS	OLIGOHYDRAMNIOS
Anencephaly (in approximately 20% of cases)	Renal agenesis
Meningocele and encephalocele	Ureteral dysplasia
Esophageal or duodenal atresia	Urethral atresia
Pyloric stenosis	Pulmonary hypoplasia
Klippel-Feil syndrome	Amnion nodosum
Cleft palate and harelip	
Achondroplasia	
Diaphragmatic defects	
Multiple anomalies (not central nervous system)	
Hydrocephaly	
Trisomy 18 or 21	
Nonobstructive hydronephrosis	

0.3%; it increases 6-fold in labors lasting over 24 hr and 20-fold (to 6%) in those over 30 hr. A tumultuous short labor, with a precipitate delivery, increases the risk of intracranial hemorrhage. Placental separation at any time prior to delivery and abnormal implantation or compression of the cord increase the possibility of brain damage from fetal anoxia; brown or muddy amniotic fluid at the time of rupture of the membranes or on prior endoscopic examination suggests that meconium has been passed during an episode of fetal anoxia.

Although the relative danger of any type of delivery depends upon the skill of the obstetrician, an increased hazard accompanies certain methods. Obviously this results not only from the method but also from the circumstances that dictated its use. Neonatal deaths following deliveries by mid and high forceps, breech extraction, and version are likely to be related to traumatic intracranial injury; those following vaginal delivery and cesarean section are more apt to be due to anoxia.

Infants born by cesarean section present problems that may be related to the unfavorable obstetric circumstance that necessitated the operation or to prolonged maternal anesthesia. In normal term pregnancies, when there is no indication of fetal distress, delivery through the abdomen carries a greater risk than delivery through the birth canal. However, there is controversy in regard to the safest type of delivery for the nondistressed viable immature fetus, especially in a breech presentation; cesarean section may involve less risk than the "stress" of labor and the potentially anoxic effects of uterine contractions during vaginal delivery. A small percentage of infants delivered by cesarean section have some degree of respiratory difficulty for a day or 2.

Although transient tachypnea is the most frequently associated problem, hyaline membrane disease may develop, particularly in infants born to diabetic mothers.

Anesthesia and analgesia affect the fetus as well as the mother; mild maternal hypoxemia or hypotension may result in severe fetal hypoxia and shock. Skilled use of medication avoids severe fetal narcosis while securing the benefits of gentle and unhurried delivery. Even skilled administration often results in a mildly depressed infant whose crying and breathing may be delayed 1–2 min and who may be somewhat inactive for several hr. When anesthesia and analgesia are carelessly used or when their milder effects are added to already unfavorable fetal circumstances such as prematurity, anoxia, or trauma, the result may be catastrophic.

Antonov AN: Children born during the siege of Leningrad in 1942. J Pediatr 30:250, 1947.
Barden TP: Management of premature labor. In: Behrman RE (ed): Neonatal-Perinatal Medicine. St. Louis, CV Mosby, 1977.
Berkowitz R: High Risk Pregnancy—1980. Clin Perinatol 7:Entire issue, 1980.
Bottoms S, Rosen M, Sokol R: The increase in the cesarean section rate. N Engl J Med 302:559, 1980.
Campbell S, Kurjak A: Comparison between urinary estrogen assay and serial ultrasonic cephalometry in assessment of fetal growth retardation. Br Med J 4:336, 1972.
Freeman RK: Diabetes in pregnancy. In: Behrman RE (ed): Neonatal-Perinatal Medicine. St Louis, CV Mosby, 1977.
Mann LI, Tejani NA, Weiss RR: Antenatal diagnosis and management of the small-for-gestational age fetus. Am J Obstet Gynecol 129:995, 1974.
Queenan J: Erythroblastosis fetalis and polyhydramnios. In Behrman RE (ed): Neonatal-Perinatal Medicine. St Louis, CV Mosby, 1977.
Zuspan FP: Pregnancy-induced hypertension. In Behrman RE (ed): Neonatal-Perinatal Medicine. St Louis, CV Mosby, 1977.

7.7   THE NEWBORN INFANT

See also Chapter 2.

The *newborn* period of life is a highly vulnerable time during which many of the physiologic adjustments required for extrauterine existence are completed. Its importance is attested to by the high morbidity and mortality rates; in the United States over two thirds of the deaths in the 1st yr of life occur in the neonatal period. Deaths during the 1st yr of life occur at an annual rate not equaled again until the 7th decade.

The transition from intrauterine to extrauterine life requires many biochemical and physiologic changes. Removal from dependence on the maternal circulation via the placenta requires activation of pulmonary function for purposes of exchange of oxygen and carbon dioxide, of gastrointestinal function for absorption of food, of renal function for excretion of wastes and maintenance of chemical homeostasis, of liver function for neutralization and excretion of toxic substances, and of function of the immunologic system for protection against infection. The cardiovascular and endocrine systems also undergo adaptations necessitated by removal from maternal and placental support. Many of the special problems of the newborn infant are related to interference with or failure of these biochemical and physiologic adjustments owing to premature birth, anatomic abnormalities, or adverse environmental influences, either intrauterine or arising at or after birth.

7.8   THE HISTORY IN NEONATAL PEDIATRICS

The medical history of the neonatal infant should (1) aim at early identification of diseases in which disability or mortality may be prevented by prompt treatment, (2) lead to anticipation of conditions that may be of later importance, and (3) uncover possible causative factors that may help to explain any pathologic condition regardless of its immediate or future significance. A detailed family history should be elicited and recorded for every newborn infant; the events of labor, delivery, anesthesia, and the immediate postpartum period are especially important.

7.9 PHYSICAL EXAMINATION OF THE NEWBORN INFANT

Many of the physical and behavioral characteristics of the normal newborn infant are described in Sec. 2.5, which should be consulted before reading this section.

The initial examination of the newborn infant should be performed as soon as possible after delivery to detect abnormalities and to establish a baseline for subsequent examinations. For high-risk deliveries this examination should occur in the delivery room and focus upon congenital anomalies and potential pathophysiologic problems that may interfere with a normal cardiopulmonary and metabolic adaptation to extrauterine life. Following a stable delivery room course, a 2nd, more detailed examination should be performed within 24 hr of birth. In well infants this examination should be done in the mother's presence. At this time even minor anatomic variations which seem insignificant should be explained because the mother may be disturbed if she or other relatives discover them or if the physician does not appear to give them adequate consideration. The explanation of any problem carries the possibility of unduly alarming otherwise unworried parents unless it is carefully and skillfully done. No infant should be discharged from the hospital without a final examination since certain abnormalities, particularly heart murmurs, frequently appear or disappear in the immediate neonatal period, or there may be evidence of acquired disease. Pulse and respiratory rates, weight, length, head circumference, and dimensions of any visible or palpable structural abnormality should be recorded.

The examination of the newborn infant requires patience, gentleness, and flexibility in routines of procedure. Thus, if the infant is quiet and relaxed when first approached, palpation of the abdomen or auscultation of the heart should be performed before other, more disturbing manipulations.

General Appearance. Physical activity may be absent in the relaxation of normal sleep or decreased by illness or drugs; the infant may be lying with motionless extremities because energy is being conserved for the effort of difficult breathing, or the infant may be vigorously crying with accompanying activity of arms and legs. Both active and passive tone and any unusual posture should be recorded. Coarse, tremulous movements with ankle or jaw clonus are more common and of less significance in newborn infants than at any other age. Such movements tend to occur when the infant is active, whereas convulsive twitching usually occurs in an otherwise quiet state. Nutritional status is evidenced by weight and length and by wrinkling or smoothness of the body surfaces. An appearance superficially suggesting good nutrition may be produced by edema. There may or may not be pitting after pressure, but the fingers and toes will lack the normal fine wrinkles over the knuckles when they are puffed out with fluid. Edema of the eyelids is a common result of irritation from silver nitrate administration. Generalized edema may occur with prematurity or with hypoproteinemia secondary to severe erythroblastosis fetalis (hydrops fetalis), congenital nephrosis, Hurler syndrome, or un-

known cause. Localized edema suggests a congenital malformation of the lymphatic system; when confined to 1 or more extremities of a female infant, it may be the presenting sign of Turner syndrome (Sec. 18.37).

Skin. Vasomotor instability and sluggishness of peripheral circulation are revealed by deep redness or purple lividity in the crying infant, whose color may darken profoundly with closure of the glottis preceding a vigorous cry, and by harmless cyanosis (acrocyanosis) of the hands and feet, especially when these are cool. Mottling is another example of general circulatory instability; it may be associated with serious illness or related to a transient fluctuation in skin temperature. An extraordinary division of the body from forehead to pubis into red and pale halves is called harlequin color change. This is transient and harmless. Significant *cyanosis* may be masked by pallor in circulatory failure; alternatively, the relatively high hemoglobin content of the 1st few days and the thin skin may combine to produce an appearance of cyanosis when the arterial oxygen saturation is adequate. Localized cyanosis is differentiated from ecchymosis by the momentary pallor which follows pressure. The same maneuver is also helpful in demonstrating *icterus*, which may be significant but pass unnoticed if the skin is suffused with blood. *Pallor* may represent asphyxia, anemia, shock, or edema. Early recognition of anemia may lead to a lifesaving diagnosis of erythroblastosis fetalis, rupture of the liver, subdural hemorrhage, or fetal-maternal or inter-twin transfusion. Postmature infants tend to have paler skin than do term or premature ones.

The vernix is described in Chapter 24, as are the common transitory capillary hemangiomas of the eyelids and neck. Slate blue, well demarcated areas of pigmentation are seen over the buttocks and back and sometimes other parts of the body in over 50% of black infants and occasionally in white ones. These have no known anthropologic significance in spite of their designation as mongolian spots; they tend to disappear within the 1st yr. The vernix, skin, and especially the cord may be stained a brownish yellow if the amniotic fluid has been colored by passage of meconium during or before birth, usually because of intrauterine anoxia. The skin of the premature infant is thin and delicate and tends to be deep red; in extreme degrees of prematurity the appearance is almost gelatinous. Fine, soft, immature hair—lanugo hair—frequently covers the scalp and brow in the premature infant; it may also cover the face. Lanugo hair has usually been lost or replaced by vellus hair in the term infant. Tufts of hair over the lumbosacral spines suggest an underlying abnormality such as an occult spina bifida, sinus tract, or tumor. The nails are rudimentary in very premature birth; conversely, they may protrude beyond the fingertips in infants born past term. Such post-term infants also tend to have a peeling, parchment-like skin (Fig 7-16), a severe degree of which suggests ichthyosis congenita (Sec 24.16).

Many neonates develop small, white, occasionally vesiculopustular papules on an erythematous base 1-3 days after birth. This benign rash, *erythema toxicum*, persists for as long as 1 wk and is usually distributed on the face, trunk, and extremities (Sec 24.3). *Pustular* melanosis, a benign lesion seen predominantly in black neonates, is present at birth as a vesiculopustular eruption around the chin, neck, back, extremities, and palms or soles; it lasts 2–3 days. Both lesions need to be distinguished from more dangerous vesicular eruptions such as herpes simplex (Sec 7.72) and staphylococcal disease of the skin (Sec 7.67).

The skull may be molded particularly if the infant is the firstborn and if the head has been engaged for a considerable time. The parietal bones tend to override the occipital and the frontal bones. The head of an infant born by cesarean section or from a breech presentation is identified by its characteristic roundness. The suture lines and the size and tension of the anterior and posterior fontanels should be determined digitally. There is great variation in the size of the fontanels at birth; if small, the anterior fontanel usually tends to enlarge during the 1st few mo of life. Persistence of excessively large anterior and posterior fontanels has been associated with several disorders (Table 7–9). Soft areas (craniotabes) are occasionally found in the parietal bones at the vertex near the sagittal suture; they are usually inconsequential, but, if they persist, the possibility of a pathologic cause should be investigated. Soft areas in the occipital region suggest the irregular calcification and wormian bone formation associated with osteogenesis imperfecta, cleidocranial dysostosis, cretinism, and, occasionally, Down syndrome. Transillumination of the abnormal skull in a dark room will rule out hydranencephaly or porencephaly (Sec 21.9).

The general appearance of the face should be noted with regard to dysmorphic features, such as epicanthal folds, widely spaced eyes, and low-set ears, which are often associated with congenital syndromes. The face may be asymmetric from a 7th nerve palsy, hypoplasia of the depressor muscle at the angle of the mouth, or an abnormal fetal posture (Sec 11.1); when the jaw has been held against a shoulder or an extremity during the intrauterine period, the mandible may deviate strikingly from the midline. The skull of the premature infant may suggest hydrocephalus because of the relatively larger brain growth as compared to that of other organs. The eyes often open spontaneously if the infant is held up and tipped gently forward and backward. This is a result of labyrinthine and neck reflexes. This maneuver is more successful than that of forcing the lids apart to inspect the eyes. Equality of pupils is normally established some weeks after birth. Conjunctival and retinal hemorrhages do not by themselves have serious significance. The pupillary reflexes are present after 28 wk gestation. The iris should be inspected for colobomata and hyperchromia. A cornea greater than 1 cm in diameter in a term infant suggests congenital glaucoma and requires prompt ophthalmologic consultation. The presence of bilateral red reflexes suggests the absence of cataracts or of intraocular pathology (Sec 25.11). Deformities of the pinnae of the ears are seen occasionally. Unilateral or bilateral preauricular skin tags occur fairly frequently; if pedunculated, they can be ligated tightly at the base, and dry gangrene and slough will result. The tympanic membrane is easily visualized otoscopically through the short, straight external auditory canal and is normally dull gray in appearance. There may be a slight obstruction of the nose from an accumulation of mucus in the narrow nostrils. The normal mouth rarely may show precocious dentition, with supernumerary teeth in the lower incisor position or aberrantly placed; these teeth are shed before the deciduous ones erupt. Alternatively, neonatal teeth occur in Ellis–van Creveld, Hallermann-Strieff, or other syndromes. Premature eruption of deciduous teeth is even more unusual.

The soft and hard palate should be inspected for a hidden cleft and the contour noted if excessively high arched. On the hard palate on either side of the raphe may be temporary accumulations of epithelial cells called Epstein pearls. Retention cysts of similar appearance may also be seen on the gums. Both disappear spontaneously, usually within a few wk of birth. Clusters of small white or yellow follicles or ulcers on an erythematous base may be found on the anterior tonsillar pillars, most frequently on the 2nd–3rd day of life. Their cause is unknown, and they clear without treatment in 2–4 days. There is no active salivation. The tongue appears relatively large; the frenulum may be short, but rarely, if ever, is this a reason for cutting it. Occasionally, the sublingual mucous membrane forms a prominent fold. The cheeks have a fullness on both the buccal and the external aspects due to the accumulation of fat which makes up the sucking pads. These pads, as well as the labial tubercle on the upper lip, disappear when suckling ceases.

The throat of the newborn infant is hard to see because of the arch of the palate; however, it should be clearly visualized because of the possibility of easily missed clefts of the posterior palate or uvula. The small tonsils give no clue to the size to be attained during later lymphoid tissue growth.

The neck appears relatively short. Abnormalities are not common; they include goiter, cystic hygroma, branchial cleft rests, and lesions of the sternocleidomastoid muscle, which are presumably traumatic (Sec 22.6). Redundant skin or webbing in a female infant suggests Turner syndrome (Sec 18.37). Both clavicles should be palpated for fractures.

As much can be learned about the lungs by observation of breathing as by auscultation and percussion. Variations in rate and rhythm are characteristic. The rate may vary from 20–100/min in normal infants, fluctuating according to physical activity, state of wakefulness, or presence of crying. Because fluctuations are rapid, counting of the respiratory rate should be done for a full minute with the infant in the resting state, preferably asleep. Under these circumstances the usual

Table 7–9 DISORDERS ASSOCIATED WITH A LARGE ANTERIOR FONTANEL

Achondroplasia	Osteogenesis imperfecta
Apert's syndrome	Prematurity
Athyrotic hypothyroidism	Pyknodysostosis
Cleidocranial dysostosis	Rubella syndrome
Hallerman-Streiff syndrome	Russell-Silver syndrome
Hydrocephaly	Trisomies 13, 18, 21
Hypophosphatasia	Vitamin D deficiency rickets
Intrauterine growth retardation	

rates for normal term infants are 30–40/min; for premature infants they are higher and fluctuate more widely. Rates that are consistently over 60/min during periods of regular breathing usually indicate cardiac or pulmonary insufficiency. The premature infant may normally breathe with a Cheyne-Stokes rhythm, known as periodic respiration, or with complete irregularity. Periodic respiration is rare in the 1st 24 hr of life. Irregular gasping, sometimes accompanied by spasmodic movements of the mouth and chin, strongly indicates serious impairment of respiratory centers.

The breathing of newborn infants is almost entirely diaphragmatic, with the result that the soft front of the thorax is commonly drawn inward during inspiration and the abdomen simultaneously protruded. If the baby is quiet, relaxed, and of good color, this "paradoxical movement" is not necessarily a sign of insufficient ventilation. On the other hand, labored respiration is important evidence of abnormal pulmonary ventilation, pneumonia, anomalies, or other mechanical disturbance of the lungs. The intercostal tissues are usually drawn in during respiration when the mechanical difficulty is either too much or too little air in the lungs, so that the differentiation between atelectasis and emphysema must be made from the size and shape of the chest, the percussion note, and a roentgenogram. A weak groaning or whining cry often accompanies expiration in severe disturbances of respiration. A method of "retraction scoring," which, along with the respiratory rate and the presence or absence of cyanosis, affords a convenient gauge of respiratory difficulty in newborn infants, is illustrated in Fig 7–2.

Normally, the breath sounds are bronchovesicular. Suspicion of diminished breath sounds should always be verified by inducing deeper breathing and, if a local area is suspicious, altering the position of the infant's head and body before final decision. This latter maneuver also applies to suspected percussion dullness. The fine, crackling rales of early pneumonia in the newborn may at times be heard only at the end of the deep inspirations induced by crying. Because of the many etiologies associated with respiratory distress a chest roentgenogram is indicated when clinical signs occur.

The size of the **heart** is difficult to estimate owing to normal variations in the size and shape of the chest.

The location of the heart should be determined to detect dextrocardia. There may be transitory murmurs; conversely, congenital malformations may not initially produce the murmur that will be present later. According to Richards, there is only a 1:12 chance that a murmur heard at birth represents congenital heart disease. Evaluation of the heart by roentgenogram, echocardiogram, and electrocardiogram is desirable when the possibility of significant lesions exists. The pulse may vary normally from 90/min in relaxed sleep to 180 during activity. The still higher rate of paroxysmal tachycardia may be counted better on an electrocardiogram than by ear. Premature infants, whose resting heart rate is usually 140–150, may have a sudden onset of **sinus bradycardia,** not infrequently associated with nodal escape.

Pulses should be palpated in the upper and lower extremity both on admission and on discharge from the nursery.

Blood pressure measurements may be a valuable diagnostic aid (Sec 13.1). The *auscultatory method* can often be used satisfactorily, provided the stethoscope head is small enough. The *Doppler method* utilizes a transducer in the cuff to transmit and receive ultrasound waves. It detects movements of the arterial wall to provide a more accurate measure of systolic and diastolic pressures. Other methods are the *palpatory method,* in which the systolic blood pressure is taken to be the point at which the pulse distal to the cuff becomes palpable in the course of deflation, and the *flush method,* in which compression of the extremity to render it relatively bloodless below the cuff is followed by deflation of the cuff, with the systolic pressure recorded at the point flushing appears in the arm and hand below the cuff. Each has the disadvantage that the pulse pressure is not obtained and that the reading lies between the systolic and diastolic pressures obtained by the auscultatory method. Continuous or intermittent direct measurement of blood pressure using an umbilical artery catheter may be indicated in special circumstances for infants under close observation in an intensive care unit (Fig 7–3).

In the **abdomen** the liver is usually palpable, sometimes as much as 2 cm below the rib margin. Less commonly, the spleen may be felt. The approximate size and location of each kidney can usually be deter-

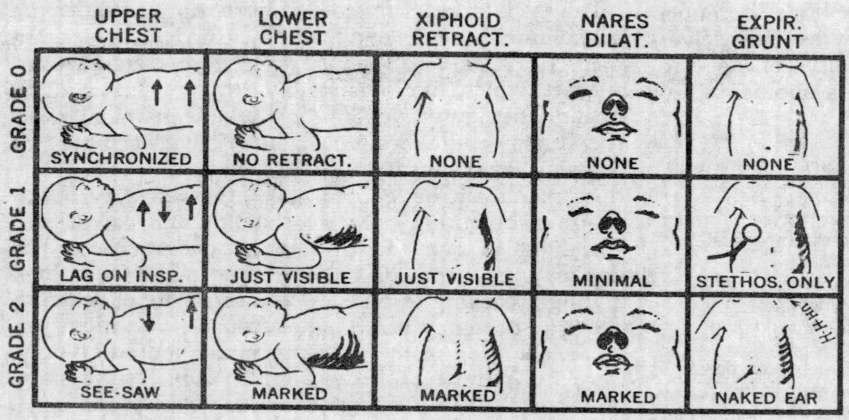

Figure 7–2 Criteria of respiratory distress. Grade 0 for each criterion indicates no respiratory distress; grade 2 for each criterion indicates severe respiratory distress. Abbreviations: DILAT., dilation; EXPIR., expiratory; INSP., inspiration; RETRACT., retraction; STETHOS., stethoscope. (Courtesy of Mead Johnson & Company, Evansville, Ind.: adapted from Silverman and Andersen: Pediatrics 17:1, 1956.)

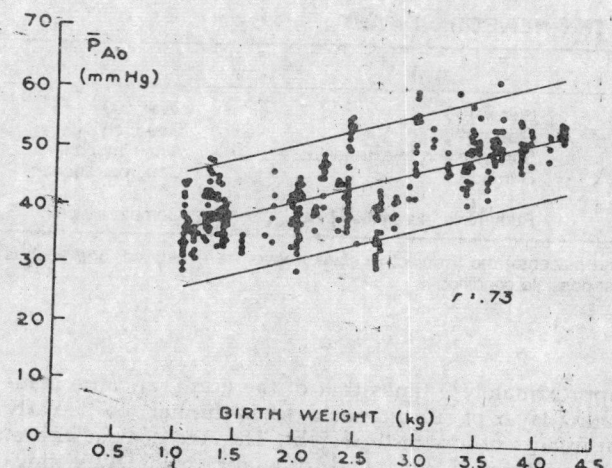

Figure 7–3 Linear regression and 95% confidence limits of mean aortic blood pressure in infants between 2–12 hr of age. (From Kitterman J, Philbs R, Todey W: Pediatrics 44:959, 1969.)

mined on deep palpation when this is indicated. Gallbladder distention may occur in septic neonates. Unusual masses should be investigated immediately by "flat plate" and cross-table lateral roentgenograms of the abdomen, followed by intravenous pyelography and exploratory laparotomy if their innocent nature cannot be established. Abdominal ultrasound may replace the intravenous pyelogram as a diagnostic aid in these infants. Urinary tract anomalies, renal embryoma, ovarian cysts, and intestinal duplications are the most common masses encountered. Abdominal distention at or shortly after birth suggests either obstruction or perforation of the gastrointestinal tract, which is often due to meconium ileus. Later it suggests lower bowel obstruction, sepsis, or peritonitis. A scaphoid abdomen in the newborn suggests diaphragmatic hernia. At no other period of life is the air content of the gastrointestinal tract so varied in amount, nor may it be so relatively great under normal circumstances. The abdominal wall is normally weak (especially in premature infants), and **diastasis recti** and umbilical hernias are common, particularly among black infants.

The **genitalia** and **mammary glands** normally respond to transplacentally obtained maternal hormones to produce enlargement and secretion of the breasts in both sexes and prominence of the female genitalia, often with considerable nonpurulent secretion. These are transitory manifestations requiring observation but no interference. The normal scrotum is relatively large; its size may be increased by the trauma of breech delivery or by a **transitory hydrocele,** which is distinguished from a hernia by palpation and transillumination. The testes may be in the scrotum or palpable in the canals or may not be felt until they descend spontaneously, perhaps not until later infancy. The male black infant usually has dark pigmentation of the scrotum before the rest of the skin assumes its permanent color.

The prepuce of the newborn infant is normally so tight and adherent that no information can be obtained as to later need for circumcision. Apparent hypospadias or epispadias should always arouse suspicion that the sex chromosomes are abnormal (Sec 18.30) or that the infant is actually a masculinized female with enlarged clitoris since this may be the 1st evidence of the adrenogenital syndrome (Sec 18.24). Erection of the penis is common and has no significance. Urine is usually passed during or immediately after birth; there may then normally follow a period without voiding. However, about 95% of preterm and term infants void within 24 hr.

Some passage of **meconium** usually occurs within the 1st 12 hr after birth; 99% of term infants and 95% of premature infants will pass meconium within 48 hr of birth. **Imperforate anus** is not always visible and may require evidence obtained by the gentle insertion of the examiner's little finger or a rectal tube. Roentgenographic study is required. The dimple or irregularity of skinfold often normally present in the sacrococcygeal midline may be mistaken for an actual or potential pilonidal sinus.

In examining the **extremities** the effects of fetal posture (Sec 23.2) should be noted if for no other reason than that their cause and usual transitory nature can be explained to the mother. This is particularly important after breech presentations. The suspicion of a fracture or nerve injury associated with delivery is more commonly aroused by observing the extremities in spontaneous or stimulated activity than by any other means. The head and feet should be examined for polydactyly, syndactyly, and abnormal dermatoglyphic patterns such as a simian crease.

All infants should have their hips examined to rule out a congenital dislocation (Sec 23.3).

Neurologic Examination.   See Sec 21.2.

7.10   ORDINARY CARE OF THE NEWBORN INFANT

The basic requirements of the newborn infant are immediate assistance at birth when needed, the *establishment of respiration,* and subsequent assistance in obtaining *adequate nutrition,* in maintaining a *normal body temperature,* and in *avoiding contact with infection.* These requirements should be met in an environment that not only provides constant nursing and medical alertness for any sign of specific illness but also keeps the time an infant is separated from his mother to a necessary minimum. The care of fullterm and premature infants differs only in the degree of emphasis on each of these requirements.

7.11   ROUTINE DELIVERY ROOM CARE

The low-risk infant should be suspended head downward immediately after delivery until the mouth, pharynx, and nose have been cleared of fluid, mucus, blood, and amniotic debris by gravity and gentle suction with a bulb syringe or soft rubber catheter. Wiping the palate

Table 7–10 EVALUATION OF THE NEWBORN INFANT

Sign	0	1	2
Heart rate	Absent	Below 100	Over 100
Respiratory effort	Absent	Slow, irregular	Good, crying
Muscle tone	Limp	Some flexion of extremities	Active motion
Response to catheter in nostril (tested after oropharynx is clear)	No response	Grimace	Cough or sneeze
Color	Blue, pale	Body pink, extremities blue	Completely pink

Sixty sec after the complete birth of the infant (disregarding the cord and placenta) the 5 objective signs above are evaluated, and each is given a score of 0, 1, or 2. A total score of 10 indicates an infant in the best possible condition.
Modified from Apgar V: Current Res Anesth Analg 32:260, 1953.

and pharynx with gauze may lead to abrasions and the development of thrush, pterygoid ulcers (Bednar aphthae), or, rarely, tooth bud infection with maxillary osteon yelitis and retrobulbar abscess formation. If infants appear to be in satisfactory condition, they should then be placed on their sides, head downward, in a bassinet tilted at an angle of about 30 degrees, to promote drainage from the respiratory tract for 4–8 hr. When there is a possibility of intracranial hemorrhage following difficult delivery, the reverse position may be indicated. As a guide to prognosis and the need for particularly close observation or care in the delivery room and nursery, the Apgar method of scoring is of practical value at 1 and 5 min (Table 7–10). *The score taken at 1 min is an index of asphyxia and of the need for assisted ventilation;* the 5-min score is a more accurate index of likelihood of death (Fig 7–4) or neurologic residual. Infants with prolapsed cord or delayed delivery and evidence of intrauterine asphyxia should receive prompt resuscitation and close observation subsequently (Sec 7.29). For reasons not clear, the stomachs of infants delivered by cesarean section may contain more fluid than those of infants delivered normally. Their stomachs should be emptied as soon as possible by gastric tube to prevent possible aspiration of gastric contents.

Maintenance of Body Heat. Relative to body weight, the body surface of the newborn infant is approximately 3 times that of the adult, and the insulating layer of subcutaneous fat is thinner, particularly in infants of low birth weight. The rate of heat loss in the newborn is estimated to be approximately 4 times that of an adult. Under the usual conditions in hospital delivery rooms (20–25° C), an infant's skin temperature falls approximately 0.3° C and the deep body temperature approximately 0.1° C/min during the period immediately after delivery, resulting usually in a cumulative loss of 2–3° C in deep body temperature (corresponding to a heat loss of approximately 200 cal/kg). The heat loss occurs by *convection* of heat energy to the cooler surrounding air, *conduction* of heat to colder materials on which the infant is resting, heat *radiation* from the infant to other nearby solid objects, and *evaporation* from moist skin and lungs (a function of alveolar ventilation).

Term infants exposed to cold after birth may develop metabolic acidosis, relative hypoxemia and hypoglycemia, and increased renal excretion of water and solutes owing to their efforts to compensate for heat loss. They augment heat production by increasing the metabolic rate and oxygen consumption and, indirectly, by releasing more norepinephrine, which results in nonshivering thermogenesis through oxidation of fat, particularly brown fat. In addition, muscular activity may increase. Hypoglycemic or hypoxic infants cannot increase their oxygen consumption when exposed to a

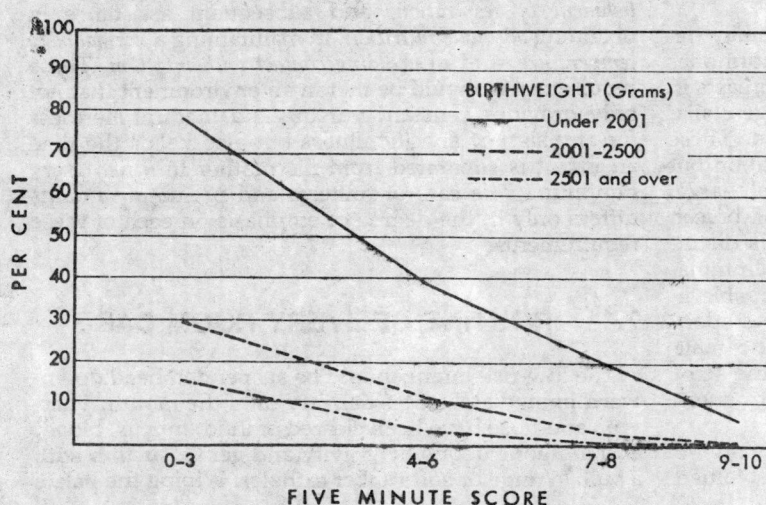

Figure 7–4 Mortality (percentage) during first 28 days of life of infants with various Apgar scores recorded at 5 min, arranged according to birth weight. (From Drage JS, Berendes J: Pediatr Clin North Am 13:635, 1966.)

cold environment and their central temperature decreases. After labor and vaginal delivery, many newborn infants have a mild to moderate metabolic acidosis, which may be compensated for by hyperventilation; this compensation is more difficult for depressed infants and infants exposed to cold stress in the delivery room. It is desirable, therefore, to make certain the infant is dried and wrapped in blankets; these procedures are frequently overlooked in the bustle of the delivery room, especially during resuscitation. Since it is difficult to carry out resuscitative measures on a covered infant or one in a closed incubator, a radiant heat source should be used for immediate reception of the baby.

Antiseptic Skin and Cord Care. To reduce the incidence of skin and periumbilical infections, the entire skin and cord should be cleansed in the delivery room or upon admission to the nursery with sterile cotton soaked in warm water and/or a mild soap solution. The infant may be rinsed with water at body temperature if care is taken to avoid chilling. The baby is then dried and wrapped in sterile blankets and taken to the nursery. To lessen the chance of carrying pathogenic organisms into the nursery, the outer blanket can be discarded at the nursery door. Daily bathing in the nursery or any other necessary washing should be done in a similar manner. Total body exposure to bathing with detergent solutions containing 3% hexachlorophene over prolonged periods may be neurotoxic, particularly in infants of less than 35 wk gestation or 1200 gm weight or with abraded skin, and is not recommended. A single bath with a 3% hexachlorophene solution at 2–4 hr of life, followed by an immediate, thorough rinse, significantly reduces the rate of colonization by *Staphylococcus aureus*. When a high risk of staphylococcal colonization exists in a nursery or when a baby has a minor skin infection, such baths may be used with discretion. Nursery personnel should continue to use hexachlorophene-containing detergents or similar effective agents for routine handwashing. Rigid enforcement of hand-to-elbow washing for 2 min in the initial wash and 15–30 sec in the 2nd wash is recommended for staff and visitors entering the nursery. Shorter, but equally thorough, washes between handling infants also should be required. Initial and daily painting of the umbilical cord stump with a bactericidal dye also may be used until hospital discharge in an attempt to reduce bacterial colonization.

Other Measures. The eyes of all infants must be protected against gonorrheal infection. The instillation of 1% *silver nitrate* drops is the best-proved and only generally lawful method. This may be delayed during the initial short alert period following birth to promote bonding, but once applied, drops should not be rinsed out. Also see Sec 7.64.

Though hemorrhage in the newborn may be due to factors other than *vitamin K deficiency*, an intramuscular injection of 1.0 mg of water-soluble vitamin K_1 is recommended for all infants immediately after birth to prevent any coagulation defect related to vitamin K deficiency. Larger amounts may predispose to the development of hyperbilirubinemia and kernicterus and should be avoided. Administration of vitamin K to the mother during labor is not recommended.

7.12 NURSERY CARE

Infants not in the "high-risk" category may be taken after examination in the delivery room to the "regular" newborn nursery or placed in the mother's room if the hospital has a rooming-in arrangement.

The bassinet should be easily and frequently cleaned and preferably be of clear plastic material to allow easy visibility. All professional care should be given in the bassinet; this includes physical examination, change of clothing, temperature-taking, skin cleansing, and other procedures which, if performed elsewhere, establish a common point of contact and may provide a channel for cross infection. The clothing and bedding should be the minimum needed for the infant's comfort; a constant temperature of approximately 24° C (75° F) in the nursery simplifies problems of clothing. The temperature of the infant may be taken by rectum or, if properly done, in the axilla. The interval depends on many circumstances, but need not be oftener than 4 hr during the 1st 2–3 days and 8 hr thereafter. Axillary temperatures of 36.0–37.0° C (96.5–98.5° F) are within normal limits. Little is gained by frequent weighing of the healthy infant. Weighing at birth and on alternate days thereafter is sufficient.

Vernix is spontaneously shed within 2–3 days; much of it will adhere to the clothing, which should be completely changed daily. The diaper should be checked before and after feeding and when the baby cries and changed when wet or soiled. Meconium or feces should be cleansed from the buttocks with sterile cotton moistened with sterile water. The foreskin of the male infant should not be retracted.

RICHARD E. BEHRMAN
ROBERT M. KLIEGMAN

Nurseries and Breast Feeding. See Sec 3.10 and 3.11 for full discussion of breast and formula feeding, respectively. Although breast feeding continues to be the optimal method of feeding infants, its incidence and duration are decreasing in many parts of the world (Sec 3.10). Its incidence in the United States, for example, declined to a low of 25% of mothers in 1970; only half of those women who currently start to nurse in the hospital continue for 3–4 mo, and many stop within the 1st few wk. The most common explanation of early weaning is a lack of milk supply, generally attributed to a failure on the mother's part; however, many hospital practices established during the decades of almost universal bottle feeding contribute to this failure. Hospital routines, such as enforcing 4-hr feeding schedules, limiting nursing time, using only 1 breast at a feeding, washing nipples with substances other than water, delaying the 1st feeding, and using heavy intrapartum sedation may lead to breast feeding problems by causing painful engorgement and sore nipples. If such problems occur, frequent nursing, even every 1–2 hr, is indicated. Since the infant should not be forced to feed, adequate milk drainage may sometimes require manual milk expression or mechanical pumping. Routine bottle supplementation is unnecessary and often disruptive because it may satiate the infant, thereby decreasing stimulation of the mother's nipples, and because the difference between breast and bottle nipples may confuse the baby. Breast feeding involves more effort, requiring the infant to squeeze out the milk from the areolar sinuses, while the bottle's free flow forces the baby to compress the nipple to avoid choking. The neonate may have difficulty in mastering 2 such different techniques and may treat the breast like the bottle, damaging the mother's nipples. Other hospital practices, such as weighing babies before and after nursing, should be avoided because they may undermine a mother's confidence in her ability to produce enough milk.

Sustained postnatal milk production depends upon adequate nipple stimulation and milk drainage. This, the major physiologic foundation of breast feeding, should provide the basis for maternity hospital practice. Hospital practices which encourage successful breast feeding include immediate postpartum mother-infant contact with suckling, rooming-in, true demand feeding day and night, inclusion of fathers in prenatal breast feeding education, and support from experienced women. The optimal duration of the initial nursing episode is not established, but at least 5 min at each breast is reasonable and allows the baby to obtain most of the available breast contents and to provide effective stimulation for increasing milk supply. Nursing episodes should then be extended according to the comfort and desire of mother and infant.

A confident and relaxed mother with adequate support is likely to nurse well despite hospital management detrimental to lactation. Even the inhibitory effects of anti-lactation medication may be overcome and breast feeding established by frequent feeding. However, appropriate physiologic management alone does not ensure success. The mother must be provided a supportive environment at home and in hospital.

BETSY LOZOFF

Committee on Nutrition, American Academy of Pediatrics: Breast feeding. Pediatrics 62:591, 1978.
Gussler JD, Briesemeister LH: The insufficient milk syndrome: A biocultural explanation. Medical Anthropology 4(2), 1980.
Lawrence RA (ed): Counseling the Mother on Breast-Feeding. Report of the Eleventh Ross Roundtable on Critical Approaches to Common Pediatric Problems. Columbus, Ohio, Ross Laboratories, 1980.
Lozoff B, Brittenham G, Trause MA, et al: The mother-newborn relationship: Limits of adaptability. J Pediatr 91:1, 1977.

7.13   MATERNAL-INFANT BONDING

See also Sec 2.3.

Normal infant development is dependent in part upon a constellation of reciprocal affectionate responses between a mother and her newborn infant which bind them together psychologically and physiologically. This bonding is facilitated and reinforced by the emotional support of a loving husband and family. The process of attachment may be an important factor in enabling some mothers to provide loving care during the neonatal period and subsequently during childhood. It is initiated before birth with the planning and confirmation of the pregnancy and with the growing acceptance of the fetus as an individual. After delivery and during the ensuing days, visual and physical contact between mother and baby triggers a variety of mutually rewarding and pleasurable interactions. The characteristic pattern of interlocking maternal and infant behaviors often includes the mother's touching the infant's extremities and face with her fingertips and encompassing and gently massaging the infant's trunk with her hands. Touching the infant's cheek elicits responsive turning toward the mother's face for eye to eye contact or toward the breast with nuzzling and licking of the nipple, which is a powerful stimulus for prolactin secretion. The initial quiet alert state of the infant facilitates the opportunity for eye to eye contact, which is particularly important to the loving and possessive feelings of many mothers for their babies. The infant's crying elicits the maternal response of touching the infant and speaking in a soft, soothing, higher-toned voice. It is desirable for the initial contact between mother and infant to take place in the delivery room and that there be an opportunity for extended intimate contact within the 1st hours after birth. Delayed or abnormal maternal-infant bonding may occur because of prematurity, infant or maternal illness, birth defects, or family stress with potentially untoward effects on infant development and maternal caretaking ability. Special efforts should be made to alter hospital routines to encourage parent-infant contact and to counsel the parents appropriately.

Klaus MH, Kennell JH: Maternal-Infant Bonding: The Impact of Early Separation or Loss on Family Development. St Louis, CV Mosby, 1976.
Klaus MH, Kennell JH: Care of the mother, father and infant. In: Behrman RE (ed): Neonatal-Perinatal Medicine. St Louis, CV Mosby, 1977.

7.14   The High-Risk Infant

See also Sec 7.6.

To decrease neonatal morbidity and mortality, it is useful to identify as early as possible those liveborn infants who are at particular risk during the neonatal period. The term high-risk infant designates infants who should be under close observation by experienced physicians and nurses. The duration of such observation is usually a few days but may range from a few hr to several wk. Some institutions may find it advantageous to provide a special or transitional care nursery for high-risk infants; it may be located within the labor and delivery suite. This facility should be equipped and staffed similarly to a neonatal intensive care area so that some well but high-risk term infants can be observed and cared for immediately after birth without transport away from their mothers.

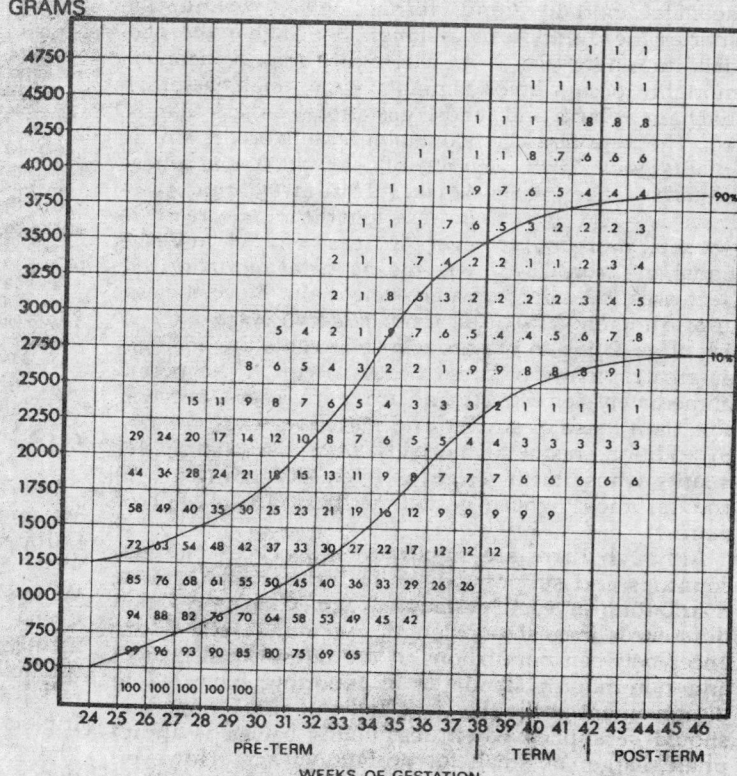

GRAMS

Figure 7–5 Curvilinear zones of mortality rates. Numbers indicate mortality rate per 100 newborn infants. Infants below the 10th percentile are small for gestational age (SGA) and those above the 90th percentile are large for gestational age (LGA). Those infants between the 10th and 90th percentiles have weights appropriate for gestational age (AGA). (From Lubchenco LO, Searls DT, Brazie JV: J Pediatr 81:814, 1972.)

Infants in the high-risk category include those (1) born before 37 or after 42 wk gestation; (2) weighing less than 2500 or more than 4000 gm; (3) deviating from expected size or development, e.g., low or very high weight for gestational age determined by the date of the mother's last menstrual period, by physical examination, or by intrauterine evaluation (Fig 7–5) (Sec 7.16); (4) with a history of serious neonatal illness or death of a sibling or of more than 2 fetal deaths of siblings; (5) in poor condition at delivery (Apgar 0–4 at 1 min) or requiring resuscitation in the delivery room or subsequently in the nursery; (6) born to mothers who have infections or a history of any illness during pregnancy (Table 7–3) or premature rupture of the membranes; a history of severe social problem such as teenage pregnancy, drug addiction, or absence of mate, of absent or long-delayed prenatal care, of minimal or no weight gain during pregnancy, of prolonged infertility, or of 4 or more previous pregnancies; who are 35 yr or more of age (especially if primiparous); or who have a history of taking any of the medications listed in Tables 7–4 and 7–5 during pregnancy; (7) of multiple pregnancy or of a gestation commencing within 3 mo of a previous pregnancy; (8) delivered operatively or with any unusual obstetric complication, including hydramnios, abruptio placentae, placenta previa or abnormal presentation; (9) having a single umbilical artery or any important malformation or suspicion of one; (10) being observed for anemia or blood group incompatibility; and (11) born to mothers who have had stressful events during gestation, such as severe emotional problems, hyperemesis gravidarum, serious accidents, or general anesthesia.

Examination of a fresh *placenta, cord,* and *membranes* may alert the physician to a newborn infant who is at high risk. Fetal blood loss may be indicated by placental pallor, **retroplacental hematoma,** and tears of a velamentous cord or of chorionic blood vessels supplying succenturiate lobes. **Placental edema** and subsequent deficiency of immunoglobulin G in the newborn may be associated with feto-fetal transfusion syndrome, hydrops fetalis, or congenital nephrosis or hepatic disease. **Amnion nodosum (granules on the amnion)** and **oligohydramnios** are associated with pulmonary hypoplasia, and small whitish **nodules** on the cord suggest a candida infection. **Short cords** occur with chromosome abnormalities and omphalocele. **Chorioangiomas** are associated with prematurity, abruptio, polyhydramnios and intrauterine growth retardation, and angiomas of the cord with increased mortality. **Meconium staining** suggests asphyxia, and opacity of the fetal placental surface suggests infection. **Single umbilical arteries** are associated with an increase in mortality and in the incidence of congenital abnormalities.

With or without the other conditions mentioned, many high-risk infants are born prematurely, have low weight for gestational age, have significant perinatal asphyxia, or are born with life-threatening congenital anomalies. Generally speaking, for any given duration of gestation, the lower the birth weight, the higher the neonatal mortality, and, for any given weight, the shorter the duration of gestation, the higher the neonatal mortality (Fig 7–5). The highest risk of neonatal mortality occurs among infants who weigh less than 1000 gm at birth and whose gestation was less than 30 wk. The lowest risk of neonatal mortality occurs among infants with birth weights of 3000–4000 gm whose gestational age was 38–42 wk. As birth weight increases from 500–3000 gm, there is a logarithmic decrease in neonatal mortality; for every increase of 2 wk in gestational age from 25–37 wk, the neonatal mortality rate decreases by approximately one half. Nevertheless, approximately 40% of all *perinatal deaths* occur after 37 wk of gestation in infants whose weights are 2500 gm or greater; many of these deaths occur in the period immediately before birth and are more readily preventable than those of smaller and more immature infants. In addition, neonatal mortality rates rise sharply for infants whose birth weight is over 4000 gm (Fig 7–6) and for those whose gestational period is 42 wk or more.

Although there are significant differences between countries and subpopulations in birth weight and its distribution at each gestational age, cross-population differences in gestation length are minor. The differences between populations in the rate of fetal growth and nonuniform standards in reporting have led to disagreement about the class limits of size-for-age that should be applied when designating babies as appropriate, large, or small for gestational age. However, since neonatal mortality is highly dependent on birth weight and gestational age, Fig 7–6 is useful for rapid identification of high-risk infants according to these variables. This analysis is based on total live births and therefore describes the mortality risk *at birth*. Since most neonatal mortality occurs within the 1st hours and days after birth, the outlook improves rapidly with increasing postnatal survival.

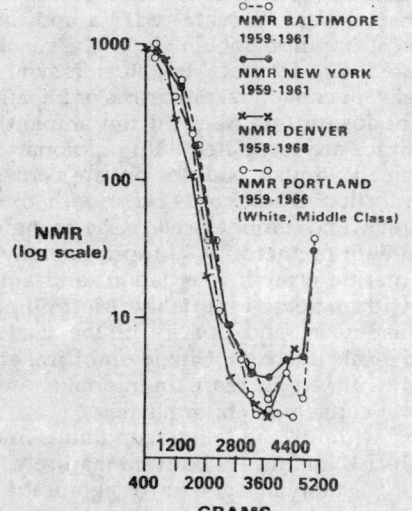

Figure 7–6 Neonatal mortality by birth weight. (From Tudehope D, Sinclair J, *In:* Behrman RE (ed): Neonatal-Perinatal Medicine. St. Louis, CV Mosby, 1977.)

Battaglia FC, Frazier TM, Hellegers AE: Birth weight, gestational age and pregnancy outcome with special reference to the high birth weight, low gestational age infant. Pediatrics 37:417, 1966.

Behrman RE, Babson GS, Lessel R: Fetal and neonatal mortality in white middle class infants. Am J Dis Child 121:486, 1971.

Benirschke K: Placental pathology. *In:* Behrman RE (ed): Neonatal-Perinatal Medicine. St. Louis, CV Mosby, 1977.

Bjerkedahl T, Bakketeig L, Lehmann EH: Percentiles of birth weights of single live births at different gestational periods. Acta Pediatr Scand 62:449, 1973.

Hobel C: Better perinatal health: U.S.A. Lancet 1:31, 1980.

Lubchenco LO, Searls DT, Brazie JV: Neonatal mortality rate; relationship to birth weight and gestational age. J Pediatr 81:814, 1972.

Tanner JM, Lejarraga H, Turner G: Within-family standards for birth weight. Lancet 2:193, 1972.

Whitby C, DeCates C, Robertson N: Infants weighing 1.8–2.5 kg: Should they be cared for in neonatal units or postnatal wards? Lancet 1:322, 1982.

Yerushalmy J: The classification of newborn infants by birth weight and gestational age. J Pediatr 71:163, 1967.

7.15 MULTIPLE PREGNANCIES

Incidence. The reported incidence of twins is highest among Blacks and East Indians, followed by North European Whites, and is lowest among the Mongolian races: Belgium, 1:56; American Blacks, 1:70; American Whites, 1:88; Italy, 1:86; Greece, 1:130; Japan, 1:150; China, 1:300. Differences in the incidence of twins mainly involve fraternal (polyovular) twins. Identical (monovular) twins constitute 25–33% of twins in all racial and ethnic groups. It is roughly estimated that triplets occur in 1 of 86^2 pregnancies and quadruplets in 1 of 86^3 pregnancies in the United States. The incidence of females increases with the number of fetal products of a multiple pregnancy, reaching approximately 53.5% for quadruplets as opposed to approximately 48.5% among single births.

Etiology. The occurrence of monovular twins appears to be independent of genetic or environmental influences. Polyovular pregnancies are more frequent beyond the 2nd pregnancy, in older women, and in families with a history of polyovular twins. They may result from simultaneous maturation of multiple ovarian follicles, but follicles containing 2 ova have been described as a genetic trait leading to twin pregnancies. Polyovular pregnancies occur in many women treated for infertility with human pituitary or menopausal urinary gonadotropins or other experimental drugs.

Conjoined twins (Siamese twins) are probably the result of relatively late monovular twinning, as is the presence of 2 separate embryos in 1 amniotic sac. The latter condition has a high fatality rate, owing to obstruction of the circulation secondary to intertwining of the umbilical cords. The prognosis for conjoined twins depends on the possibility of surgical separation.

Superfecundation, the fertilization of an ovum by an insemination that takes place after 1 ovum has already been fertilized, has occasionally been advanced as the cause of differences in size and appearance of twins. *Superfetation*, the fertilization and subsequent development of an ovum when a fetus is already present in the uterus, also has been proposed as a reason for differences in size of certain twins at birth, but evidence to support these theories is lacking.

Monozygotic versus Dizygotic Twins. The identification of twins as monozygotic or dizygotic (monovular or polyovular) is important because study of monozygotic twins is useful to determine the relative influence of heredity and environment on human development and disease. Twins who are not of the same sex are dizygotic. In twins of the same sex, zygosity should be determined and recorded at birth through careful examination of the placenta or later through comparison of physical characteristics, detailed blood typing, or tissue typing.

Examination of the Placenta. Inspection of the placenta is carried out with knowledge of the sex and birth of the twins and with identification of the cords as belonging to twin 1 or to twin 2. If the placentas are separate, they are always dichorionic, but the twins are not necessarily dizygotic since initiation of monovular twinning at the 1st cell division or during the morula state may result in 2 amnions, 2 chorions, and even 2 placentas. One third of monozygotic twins are dichorionic and diamniotic.

An apparently single placenta may be present with either monovular or polyovular twins. Yet inspection of the polyovular placenta usually reveals for each fetus a separate chorion that crosses the placenta between the attachments of the cords and 2 amnions. Separate or fused dichorionic placentas may be disproportionate in size. The fetus attached to the smaller placenta or portion of placenta is then usually smaller than its twin or is malformed. Monochorionic twins may be presumed to be monovular. They are usually diamnionic, and, almost invariably, the placenta is a single mass. Monoamnionic twins have a high rate of stillbirth of 1 or both twins because of interference with 1 or both fetal circulations due to extensive intertwining of the umbilical cords.

Placental vascular anastomoses occur with high frequency in monochorionic twins, and the resulting exchange of blood proteins and cells may have as much to do with later homograft tolerance between monovular twins as does their common genetic make-up.

Table 7–11 CHARACTERISTIC CHANGES IN MONOCHORIONIC TWINS WITH UNCOMPENSATED PLACENTAL ARTERIOVENOUS SHUNTS

TWIN ON	
ARTERIAL SIDE—DONOR	VENOUS SIDE—RECIPIENT
Oligohydramnios	Polyhydramnios
Small premature	Large premature
Malnourished	Well nourished
Pale	Plethoric
Anemic	Polycythemic
Hypovolemic	Hypervolemic
Shock	Cardiac failure
Microcardia	Cardiac hypertrophy
Glomeruli small or normal	Glomeruli large
Arterioles thin-walled	Arterioles thick-walled

Vascular anastomoses between dichorionic twins have not been described, although the possibility may be inferred from the reported existence of blood group chimeras in heterosexual twins.

In monochorionic placentas, the fetal vasculature is almost invariably joined, sometimes in a very complex manner. The vascular anastomoses in monochorionic placentas may be artery-to-artery, vein-to-vein, or artery-to-vein. Usually, they are well enough balanced so that neither twin suffers. Artery-to-artery communications cross over placental veins, and when anastomoses are present, blood can readily be stroked from 1 fetal vascular bed to the other. Vein-to-vein communications are similarly recognized and are less common. A combination of artery-to-artery and vein-to-vein anastomoses is associated with *acardiac fetus*. In rare cases 1 umbilical cord may arise from the other after leaving the placenta. In such instances the twin attached to the secondary cord is usually malformed or dies in utero. Table 7–11 lists the more frequent changes associated with a large uncompensated arteriovenous shunt from the placenta of 1 twin to that of the other (Fig 7–7);

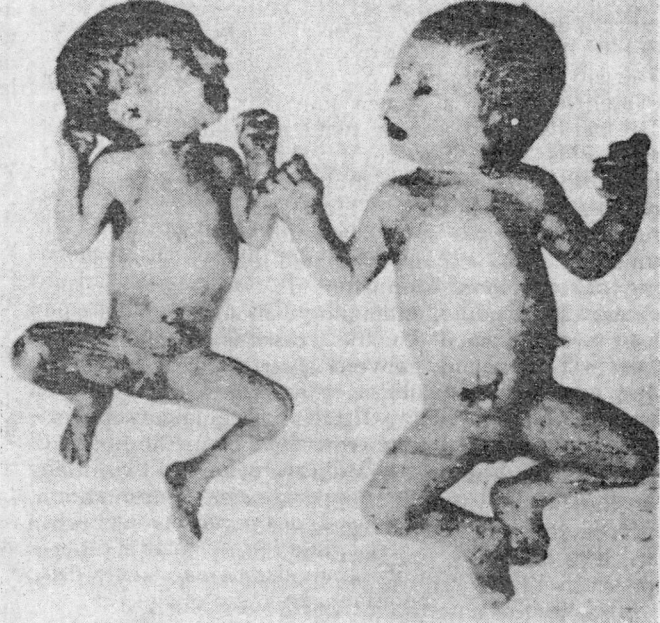

Figure 7–7 Slightly premature monochorionic "identical" twins at birth. Twin 1 at left weighed 3 lb 12 oz, and twin 2 at right weighed 5 lb 15 oz. (From Benirschke K: NY State J Med 61:1499, 1961.)

twins of widely discrepant size are usually monochorionic.

In the **fetal transfusion syndrome,** an artery from 1 twin delivers blood which is drained through the vein of the other. The latter becomes plethoric and large while anemia and small size characterize the other. Maternal hydramnios in a twin pregnancy should always lead to suspicion of the fetal transfusion syndrome. Anticipation of this possibility may lead to lifesaving readiness to give a transfusion to the donor twin or to bleed the recipient twin. Death of the donor twin in utero may result in generalized fibrin thrombi in the smaller arterioles of the recipient twin, possibly as the result of transfusion of thromboplastin-rich blood from the macerating donor fetus. The surviving twin may develop disseminated intravascular coagulation.

Postnatal Identification. Physical criteria for determining monovular twins are as follows: (1) both must be the same sex; (2) their features, including ears and teeth, must be obviously alike (but they need not resemble one another more than the lateral halves of 1 individual); (3) their hair must be identical in color, texture, natural curl, and distribution; (4) their eyes must be of the same color and shade; (5) their skin must be of the same texture and color (nevi may be differently apportioned and distributed); (6) their hands and feet must be of the same conformation and of similar size; and (7) their anthropometric values must show close agreement.

Although *detailed blood typing* can offer absolute proof only that twins are dizygotic, a reasonable presumption of monozygosity may be made if no blood group discrepancies can be demonstrated between twins. Tissue typing may provide even further support.

Prognosis. Most twins are born prematurely, and maternal complications of pregnancy are more common than with single pregnancies. Although Benirschke has shown that there is a significant increase in perinatal mortality among monochorionic twins, there is no significant difference between the neonatal mortality rates of twin and single births in comparable weight groups. Yet, since most twins are premature by weight, their overall mortality is higher than that of single births. The perinatal mortality of twins is about 4-fold that of singletons. The incidence of malformations incompatible with life is greater in multiple than in single pregnancies. There is also an increased incidence of ruptured vasa previa and velamentous insertion of the umbilical cord, with an associated higher risk of bleeding during labor. Monoamniotic twins have an increased likelihood of entangling their cords, which may lead to asphyxia. If 1 of the fetuses is macerated, the live twin is usually delivered first. Theoretically, the 2nd twin is more subject to anoxia than is the 1st because of the possibility that the placenta may separate after the birth of the 1st twin and before the birth of the 2nd. In addition, the delivery of the 2nd twin may be difficult as it may be in an abnormal presentation, uterine tone may be decreased, or the cervix may begin to close following the 1st twin's birth. Notable differences in size at birth of monovular twins usually disappear by the time the infants are 6 mo of age.

Treatment. Prenatal diagnosis enables the obstetrician and the pediatrician to anticipate the birth of infants who are at high risk because of twinning. Close observation is indicated during labor and in the immediate neonatal period so that prompt treatment of asphyxia or fetal transfusion syndrome can be initiated. The decision to perform an immediate blood transfusion in a severely anemic "donor twin" or to perform a partial exchange transfusion of a "recipient twin" must be based on clinical judgment.

Benirschke K, Chung KK: Multiple pregnancy. N Engl J Med 288:1276, 1329, 1973.
Rausen AR, Seki M, Strauss L: Twin transfusion syndrome. A review of 19 cases studied at our institution. J Pediatr 66:613, 1973.
Soma H, Yoshida K, Tada M, et al: Fetal abnormalities associated with twin placentation. Teratology 12:211, 1975.

7.16　PREMATURITY AND INTRAUTERINE GROWTH RETARDATION

Definitions. Liveborn* infants delivered before 37 wk from the 1st day of the last menstrual period are considered to have a shortened gestational period and are termed *premature* by the World Health Organization. The American Academy of Pediatrics uses 38 wk to delineate prematurity. Premature is also often used to denote immaturity. More recently, infants of extremely low birth weight, i.e., less than 750 gm, have been referred to as immature neonates. Historically, prematurity was defined by a birth weight of 2500 gm or less. However, today infants who weigh 2500 gm or less at birth, "low birth weight infants," are considered to have had either a shortened gestational period or a less than expected rate of intrauterine growth (referred to as intrauterine growth retardation), or both. Prematurity and low birth weight are associated with increased neonatal morbidity and mortality. Ideally, the definition of low birth weight should be set for individual populations which are genetically and environmentally as homogeneous as possible. Fig 7–5 shows observed variations in neonatal mortality based on birth weight with respect to gestational age.

Incidence. The incidence of preterm delivery (less than 37 wk) in the U.S. Collaborative Perinatal Study was 7.1% for Whites and 17.9% for nonwhites. Approximately one third to one half of the low birth weight infants have a gestational age of 37 wk or more. The incidence of infants weighing less than 2500 gm varied from 6–16%.

The Very Low Birth Weight (VLBW) Infant. This designation refers to those infants born weighing less than 1500 gm who constitute less than 1% of all births.

*Live birth is defined by the World Health Assembly (1950) as "the complete expulsion or extraction from its mother of a product of conception . . . which, after such separation, breathes or shows any other evidence of life such as beating of the heart, pulsation of the umbilical cord, or definite movement of the voluntary muscles, whether or not the umbilical cord has been cut or the placenta is attached." This definition is approved by the American Public Health Association.

Table 7–12 POSSIBLE ETIOLOGIES OF PREMATURE BIRTH

Abruptio placentae	Polyhydramnios
Amnionitis	Preeclampsia
Congenital malformations	Premature rupture of membranes
Erythroblastosis fetalis	Severe maternal illness
Iatrogenic	Twins, triplets, etc.
Incompetent cervix	Unknown
Placenta previa	Urinary tract infection

Their perinatal care and improved survival rate (see Table 7–14) has assumed great importance because of the latter's significant impact on overall premature mortality rates and the large commitment of resources required to achieve lower mortality in the VLBW infant. Concomitant with the decrease in mortality there has been a decrease in neurologic morbidity. However, VLBW infants have a higher incidence of rehospitalization during the 1st yr of life than larger infants for such causes as inguinal hernias, infections, treatment of chronic sequelae of prematurity, and caretaking disorders.

Factors Related to Premature Birth and Low Birth Weight. It is difficult to separate completely factors associated with prematurity from those associated with low birth weight. In about one third of low birth weight infants the birth weight is less than would be expected for gestational age calculated from the mother's last menstrual period. Thus, the small size is due primarily to a retarded rate of intrauterine growth; in the remainder the low weight is appropriate for the early date of delivery. In general the *premature birth* of infants whose low birth weight is appropriate for their preterm gestational age is associated with conditions in which there

Table 7–13 FACTORS IMPLICATED IN THE ETIOLOGY OF INTRAUTERINE FETAL GROWTH RETARDATION

Fetal factors
 Chromosomal disorders (e.g., autosomal trisomies)
 Chronic fetal infections (e.g., cytomegalic inclusion disease, congenital rubella, syphilis)
 Familial dysautonomia
 Radiation injury
 Multiple gestation
 Pancreatic aplasia
Placental factors
 Decreased placental weight or cellularity or both
 Decrease in surface area
 Villous placentitis (bacterial, viral, parasitic)
 Infarction
 Tumor (chorioangioma, hydatidiform mole)
 Placental separation
 Twin transfusion syndrome (parabiotic syndrome)
 Localized transfer lesion (?)
Maternal factors
 Toxemia
 Hypertensive or renal disease or both
 Hypoxemia (high altitude, cyanotic cardiac or pulmonary disease)
 Malnutrition or chronic illness
 Sickle cell anemia
 Drugs (narcotics, alcohol, cigarettes, antimetabolites)
Experimental factors
 Maternal uterine ischemia—rat
 Fetal placental ischemia—sheep and monkey
 Maternal protein deprivation—rat, guinea pig, and pig
 Maternal hyperinsulinemia—rat

is inability of the uterus to retain the fetus, interference with the course of the pregnancy, premature separation of the placenta, or a stimulus to effective uterine contractions prior to term (Table 7–12). *Intrauterine growth retardation* is associated with conditions that interfere with the circulation and efficiency of the placenta, with the development or growth of the fetus, or with the general health and nutrition of the mother (Table 7–13).

There is a positive correlation of both premature birth and low birth weight with low socioeconomic status. In such families there are relatively high incidences of maternal undernutrition, anemia, and illness; inadequate prenatal care; drug addiction; obstetric complications; and maternal histories of reproductive inefficiency (relative infertility, abortions, stillbirths, premature or low weight infants). Other less clearly associated factors such as illegitimacy, teenage pregnancies, close spacing of pregnancies, and mothers who have borne more than 4 previous children are also encountered more frequently. Although systematic differences in fetal growth have been described in association with maternal size, birth order, sibling weight, social class, maternal smoking habit, and other factors, how much of the variation in birth weight between various

EXTERNAL SIGN	SCORE				
	0	1	2	3	4
Edema	Obvious edema of hands and feet, pitting over tibia	No obvious edema of hands and feet, pitting over tibia	No edema		
Skin texture	Very thin, gelatinous	Thin and smooth	Smooth, medium thickness, rash or superficial peeling	Slight thickening, superficial cracking and peeling, especially on hands and feet	Thick and parchmentlike; superficial or deep cracking
Skin color (infant not crying)	Dark red	Uniformly pink	Pale pink; variable over body	Pale; only pink over ears, lips, palms, or soles	
Skin opacity (trunk)	Numerous veins and venules clearly seen, especially over abdomen	Veins and tributaries seen	A few large vessels clearly seen over abdomen	A few large vessels seen indistinctly over abdomen	No blood vessels seen
Lanugo (over back)	No lanugo	Abundant, long and thick over whole back	Hair thinning, especially over lower back	Small amount of lanugo and bald areas	At least half of back devoid of lanugo
Plantar creases	No skin creases	Faint red marks over anterior half of sole	Definite red marks over more than anterior half, indentations over less than anterior third	Indentations over more than anterior third	Definite deep indentations over more than anterior third
Nipple formation	Nipple barely visible, no areola	Nipple well defined, areola smooth and flat, diameter <0.75 cm	Areola stippled, edge not raised, diameter <0.75 cm	Areola stippled, edge raised, diameter >0.75 cm	
Breast size	No breast tissue palpable	Breast tissue on one or both sides <0.5 cm diameter	Breast tissue both sides, one or both 0.5 to 1.0 cm	Breast tissue both sides; one or both >1 cm	
Ear form	Pinna flat and shapeless, little or no incurving of edge	Incurving of part of edge of pinna	Partial incurving whole of upper pinna	Well-defined incurving whole of upper pinna	
Ear firmness	Pinna soft, easily folded, no recoil	Pinna soft, easily folded, slow recoil	Cartilage to edge of pinna, but soft in places, ready recoil	Pinna firm, cartilage to edge, instant recoil	
Genitalia Male	Neither testis in scrotum	At least one testis high in scrotum	At least one testis down in scrotum		
Female (with hips half abducted)	Labia majora widely separated; labia minora protruding	Labia majora almost cover labia minora	Labia majora completely cover labia minora		

Figure 7–8 External characteristics of the Dubowitz examination. Physical criteria are recorded and a final score is obtained following addition of each category's score. (From Dubowitz L, Dubowitz V: Gestational Age of the Newborn. Reading, Mass., Addison-Wesley Pub Co Inc, 1977.)

subgroups is due to environmental (extrafetal) rather than to genetic differences in growth potential is unknown.

Assessment of Gestational Age at Birth. The infant with retarded intrauterine growth is likely to be *shorter than expected for gestational age* and to appear to have a *disproportionately larger head relative to body size* than the premature infant of appropriate weight; infants of either group may lack subcutaneous fat. In most of these infants birth weight is usually severely affected and brain growth relatively spared; chronic fetal nonbacterial infections and certain chromosomal anomalies are exceptions in which head growth and body weight are reduced equally. In general, the functional development of the fetal nervous system continues to correlate with gestational age.

Physical signs may be useful in estimating gestational age at birth. After 34 wk, the anterior vascular capsule of the lens has usually completely atrophied. Until 36 wk of gestation there are only 1–2 transverse skin *creases on the anterior one third of the sole of the foot.* By 37–38 wk more creases have appeared, and by 40 wk there is a complex series of crisscrossed creases covering the entire sole. The *size of the breast nodule* correlates generally with gestational age. It is usually not palpable at 33–34 wk, is usually not over 3 mm in diameter at 36 wk, and is usually 4–10 mm in term infants. The *scalp hair* tends to be short and fuzzy up to 37 wk, but to consist mainly of more coarse individual strands by 40 wk. The *cartilaginous development of the ear lobe* which makes the folds of the helix and antihelix stand out occurs chiefly between 36–40 wk. At 36 wk the *testes* are usually not completely descended, and the *scrotal rugae* are few and limited to the anterior and inferior aspects of the scrotum; by 40 wk the testes are usually descended, and rugae cover the entire scrotal surface. Individually, these signs may result in considerable error in determining gestational age. Alternatively, the Dubowitz scoring system is commonly used and is accurate to ±2 wk (Fig 7–8, 7–9, and 7–10). An infant should be presumed to be at high risk of mortality or morbidity if there is a discrepancy between estimation of gestational

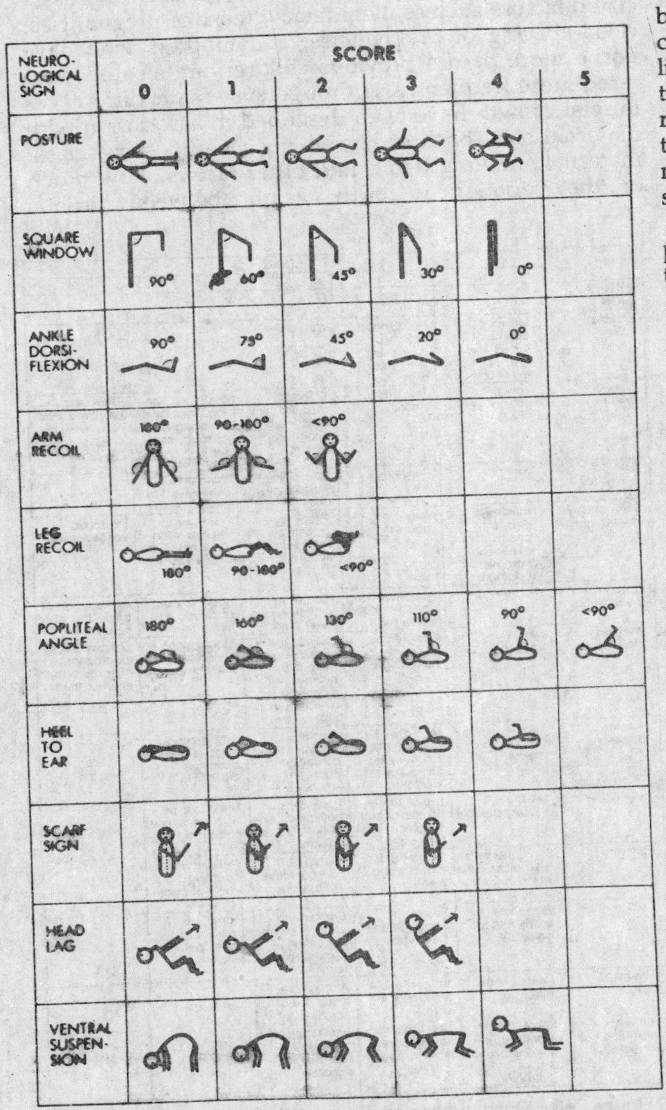

NEURO-LOGICAL SIGN	SCORE					
	0	1	2	3	4	5
POSTURE						
SQUARE WINDOW	90°	60°	45°	30°	0°	
ANKLE DORSI-FLEXION	90°	75°	45°	20°	0°	
ARM RECOIL	180°	90–180°	<90°			
LEG RECOIL	180°	90–180°	<90°			
POPLITEAL ANGLE	180°	160°	130°	110°	90°	<90°
HEEL TO EAR						
SCARF SIGN						
HEAD LAG						
VENTRAL SUSPEN-SION						

Figure 7–8 Neurologic characteristics of the Dubowitz examination. Neurologic criteria are recorded and added to a final score as performed for the physical assessment. (From Dubowitz L, Dubowitz V: Gestational Age of the Newborn. Reading, Mass., Addison-Wesley Pub Co Inc, 1977.)

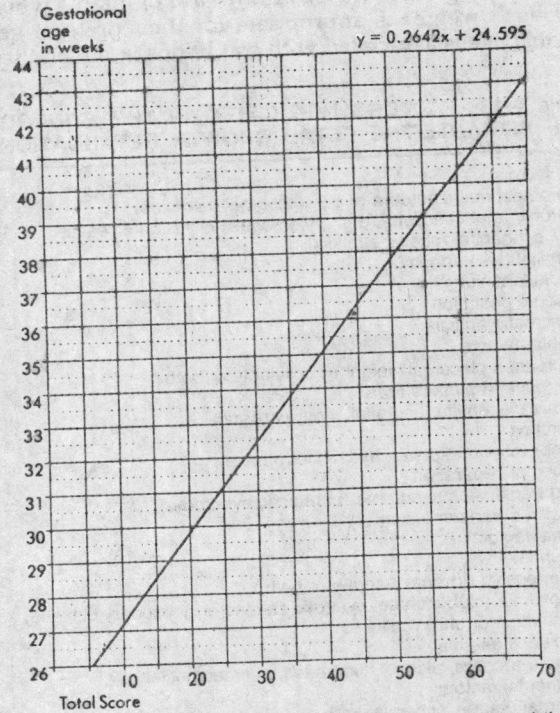

Figure 7–10 Both the external physical criteria score and that for the neurologic criteria are added together and gestational age (± 2 wk) may be read off this graph. (From Dubowitz L, Dubowitz V: Gestational Age of the Newborn. Reading, Mass., Addison-Wesley Pub Co Inc, 1977.)

age by physical examination, the mother's estimated date of last menstrual period, and amniotic fluid or fetal ultrasonic evaluation.

Pathology in Prematurity and Intrauterine Growth Retardation. The principal causes of death among premature, as well as term, infants are asphyxia, birth injuries (principally cerebral), malformations, hyaline membrane disease, septicemia, and intraventricular hemorrhage; prematurity itself should not be considered a cause of death in an infant born alive.

The incidence of certain neonatal risks varies with birth weight, gestational age, and birth weight for gestational age (Fig 7–11). Problems of major clinical significance associated with prematurity include respiratory distress (hyaline membrane disease, pulmonary hemorrhage, aspiration syndrome, congenital pneumonia, pneumothorax), recurrent apnea, hypoglycemia, hypocalcemia, hyperbilirubinemia, anemia, edema, neurologic signs related to cerebral anoxia, circulatory instability, hypothermia, bacterial sepsis, and disseminated intravascular coagulopathies. In addition, preterm infants frequently have poor feeding and prolonged failure to gain weight, apnea, anemia, bleeding, and late metabolic acidosis.

Small for gestational age infants are a very heterogeneous population even when those with congenital anomalies or congenital infections are not included. These infants tend to have neonatal problems related more to their gestational age than to their birth weight. In addition, preterm small for gestational age infants have a lower incidence of hyaline membrane disease

than expected for their low birth weight; this may be related to chronic intrauterine stress enhancing pulmonary maturity. Problems encountered in small for gestational age infants include perinatal asphyxia, hypoglycemia, hypothermia, pulmonary hemorrhage, meconium aspiration, necrotizing enterocolitis, polycythemia, and illnesses related to congenital anomalies, syndromes, or infections. The prognosis for these infants depends on the etiology of their growth retardation and on the acute management of these potentially lethal neonatal problems. Head circumference less than the 10th percentile at birth and abnormal neurologic examination in the newborn period are associated with poor growth, later microcephaly, and neurologic deficit in low birth weight infants.

Hemorrhage, whether associated with trauma, asphyxia, infection, or defect of clotting mechanism, is frequent and often severe in low birth weight infants. Subcutaneous ecchymoses and subependymal and intraventricular hemorrhage are frequent. Increased capillary fragility, vulnerable arterial and venous capillary networks in friable paraventricular germinal tissue, hypernatremia, and increased vascular pressures may be contributing causes. Sudden shock and collapse during the 1st few days of life are often due to massive **intraventricular hemorrhage,** which occurs predominantly in very small premature infants. It is uncommon in infants who weigh more than 2000 gm at birth or are of more than 34 wk gestational age. Less severe degrees of hemorrhage may be associated with lethargy, seizures, apnea, and an acute decline of the hematocrit.

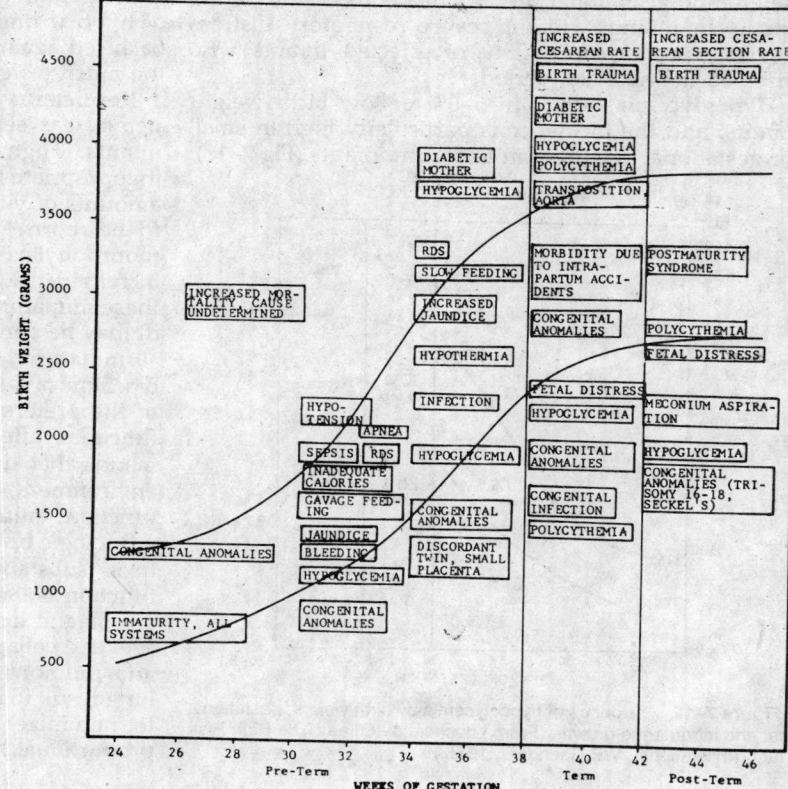

Figure 7–11 Neonatal problems according to birth weight, gestational age, and intrauterine growth. (From Lubchenco LO [ed.]: The High Risk Infant. Philadelphia, WB Saunders, 1976.)

Small intraventricular or subependymal hemorrhage may go undetected. Pulmonary hemorrhage has a similar pattern of increased incidence and high mortality in preterm low birth weight infants, especially those small for gestational age.

Hyaline membrane disease occurs most frequently, and mortality is highest, in infants of shortest gestation, and the incidence and mortality fall progressively with increasing gestational age. It is rare in large infants born at or near term, except in those delivered by cesarean section or born to diabetic mothers.

Congenital malformations occur with a greater frequency in infants of low birth weight than in all live births. There is a higher malformation rate both in preterm babies and in fullterm infants small for gestational age; those with the slowest intrauterine growth rates have the highest incidence of malformations (Fig 7–11). The incidence of ventricular septal defect is much higher in infants of birth weight less than 2500 gm and gestational age less than 34 wk than among larger or older infants. Infants with chromosome anomalies (e.g., trisomy 21, trisomy 18) and those with congenital rubella infection have a high incidence of congenital heart disease and tend to be small for gestational age. Babies with meconium ileus, intestinal obstruction, gastroschisis, and omphalocele are often born prematurely, especially if hydramnios is present.

Patent ductus arteriosus that persists beyond the 3rd day of life has an increased incidence in low birth weight infants, particularly in infants with hyaline membrane disease. Siassi found this condition in 21% of a group of low birth weight infants and noted the incidence was inversely related to increasing birth weight and gestational age. Spontaneous closure of the ductus in infants without severe respiratory distress syndrome occurred in 79% of affected infants who survived the neonatal period.

Hypoglycemia occurs in 5–6% of low birth weight infants, and the incidence is particularly high in small for gestational age preterm and term infants (Fig 7–12).

Hyperglycemia is a common problem in extremely premature infants receiving excessive intravenous glucose infusions but also occurs in other low birth weight infants.

Recurrent apnea, defined as cessation of breathing for more than 20 sec or long enough to produce cyanosis or bradycardia, has a very high incidence in infants under 1500 gm or under 32 wk gestational age (Table 7–15).

Necrotizing enterocolitis occurs most commonly in infants of the lowest birth weight. The highest incidence is among babies weighing less than 1500 gm, but it may also occur in term, normal weight infants (Sec 11.39).

Retrolental fibroplasia occurs in premature infants treated with oxygen at concentrations above ambient air levels. The increased arterial oxygen tensions that result may lead to severe arterial vasoconstriction with subsequent hypoxic damage to the immature retina (Sec 25.13). The eyes of premature infants exposed to oxygen should be examined after recovery from the illness requiring oxygen therapy, before discharge, and at 3 mo after discharge; retinal surgery has been proposed for severe detachment. The practice of administering oxygen only in such amounts and for such periods of time as are absolutely necessary for the relief of respiratory distress, apnea, hypoxemia, or cyanosis, along with the frequent monitoring of arterial oxygen tensions, has significantly reduced the incidence of this disease and the partial or complete blindness that may result from it. The exact level or duration of elevated arterial pO_2 that results in injury is unknown, but arterial oxygen tensions should be kept between 50–80 mm Hg. Immaturity is an important contributing factor and may, rarely, be the only identifiable cause. The risk of hypoxic brain injury from too little oxygen must be balanced against the risk of retrolental fibroplasia from too much oxygen.

Kernicterus (Sec 7.45) associated with hyperbilirubinemia was seen in 2–20% of autopsies of premature infants. High incidences are probably the result of inappropriate treatment, such as administration of large amounts of vitamin K analogues to mothers in labor or to newborn infants and use of sulfisoxazole as chemoprophylaxis. Very low birth weight infants are at increased risk, particularly if they have meningitis; in these immature infants bilirubin levels as low as 10 mg/dl may be dangerous.

Immaturity of anatomic structure or physiologic and biochemical functions is an index of the relative inability of the preterm infant to survive. Deficiencies in these functions affect the infant's ability to withstand demands that do not exist in the protective intrauterine environment, such as control of body heat, pulmonary function, nutrition, disposal of metabolic waste, immunologic function, and detoxification and excretion of toxic substances. The immature infant's respiratory function is limited by the underventilation of perfused alveoli and insufficient surface-active lipid surfactant to prevent collapse of alveoli. Underdeveloped airways and pulmonary tissue and persistence of fluid in the lung result in increased resistance to air flow. The ability to minimize heat loss in response to cold stress is proportional to body size. Decreased stores of hepatic

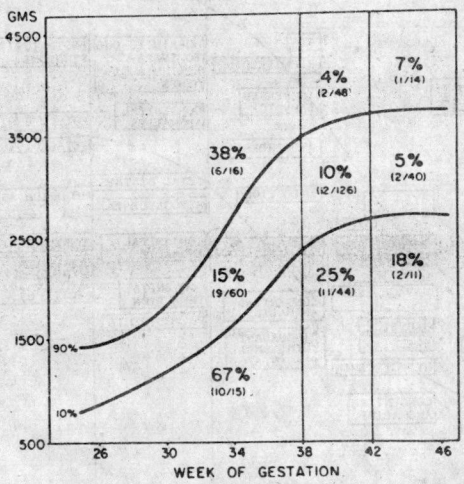

Figure 7–12 Incidence of hypoglycemia by birth weight, gestational age, and intrauterine growth. (From Lubchenco LO [ed]: The High Risk Infant. Philadelphia, WB Saunders, 1976.)

and myocardial glycogen compromise the immature infant's ability to withstand a moderate degree of asphyxia. Renal blood flow, glomerular filtration, and tubular functions are decreased. The cardiopulmonary circulation is transitional between that of a fetus and that of an adult; increased shunting through the ductus arteriosus and foramen ovale may occur in response to stress, hypoxia, or polycythemia and result in circulatory insufficiency or underperfusion of vital organs.

Care. At birth the same measures for clearing of airway, initiation of breathing, and care of the cord and eyes are required for immature infants as for those of normal weight and maturity. Special care is required to maintain a patent airway and avoid potential aspiration of gastric contents. Additional considerations are (1) need for incubator care and monitoring, (2) need for increased oxygen, and (3) need for special attention to the details of feeding. Safeguards against infection can never be relaxed. There must also be an awareness that routine procedures which disturb these infants may result in hypoxia. Finally, the need to have the parents regularly and actively participate in the infant's care in the nursery, the need of instructing the mother in the care of the infant at home, and the question of prognosis for later growth and development require special consideration. There can be significant untoward effects on the development of a normal mother-infant relationship as a consequence of separation during the neonatal period; these effects may contribute to subsequent behavioral and physical abnormalities, e.g., failure to thrive and deprivation syndromes, child neglect, and abuse (Sec 7.13).

Incubator Care. Modern incubators conserve body heat through provision of a warm atmospheric environment and standard conditions of humidity. They also may provide a regulated oxygen supply and reduced atmospheric contamination if they are scrupulously cleaned. The survival of low birth weight and sick infants is greater when they are cared for at or near their *neutral thermal environment.* This is a set of thermal conditions, including air and radiating surface temperatures, relative humidity, and air flow, at which heat production (measured as oxygen consumption) is minimal and the infant's core temperature is within the normal range. It is a function of the size and postnatal age of infants; larger, older infants require lower envi-

ronmental temperatures than smaller, younger infants. On the basis of current experience the optimal incubator temperature for minimum heat loss and oxygen consumption for the unclothed infant is that which will maintain the core temperature of the infant at 36.5–37.5° C. This depends on an infant's size and maturity (Fig 7–13). In many circumstances incubator care alone may be insufficient to keep a very small premature infant warm; these infants may require a plexiglass heat shield or head caps and body clothing.

Maintenance of a relative humidity of 40–60% aids in stabilizing body temperature by reducing heat loss at lower environmental temperatures, by preventing drying and irritation of the lining of respiratory passages, especially during the administration of oxygen and following or during endotracheal or nasotracheal intubation, and by thinning viscid secretions and reducing insensible water loss from the lungs.

The administration of oxygen to reduce the risk of injury from hypoxia and circulatory insufficiency must be balanced against the risks of hyperoxia to the eyes (retrolental fibroplasia) and oxygen injury to the lungs. When possible, oxygen should be administered by a head hood, CPAP apparatus, or endotracheal tube in order to maintain stable and safe inspired oxygen concentration. Although the presence of cyanosis, dyspnea, and apnea are definite clinical indications for treating with only as much oxygen as is needed to eliminate these signs, the potential harm from hypoxia or hyperoxia cannot be minimized without monitoring the oxygen tension (pO_2) of arterial blood and continuously readjusting the concentration of oxygen administered on the basis of this laboratory analysis. Lankowski has demonstrated that significant limitations of the ability and reliability of experienced observers to diagnose cyanosis clinically may result in errors of administering too little or too much oxygen unless both clinical and laboratory data are taken into consideration. The development of the transcutaneous oxygen electrode for routine clinical management of these infants has significantly improved the effectiveness of oxygen monitoring. Capillary blood gases are not adequate for the estimation of arterial oxygen levels.

If an incubator is not available, the general conditions of temperature and humidity control outlined above can be attained by the intelligent use of radiant warm-

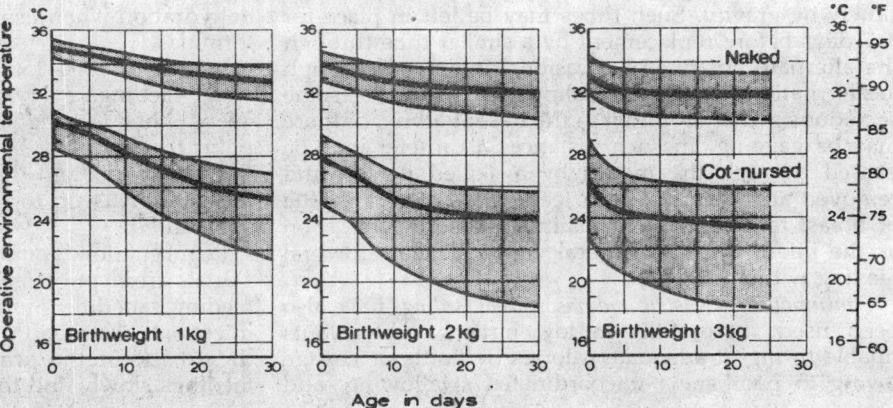

Figure 7–13 Air temperature required to provide warmth for newborn infants of varying birth weight and postnatal age in a crib (cot) or incubator. The dark line represents the mean while the shaded zone indicates the range to maintain a thermoneutral environment. Under these conditions rectal temperature should be normal while energy expenditure and heat loss are minimal. (From Oliver T, *In:* Behrman RE [ed]: Neonatal-Perinatal Medicine. St Louis, CV Mosby, 1977.)

Operative environmental temperature

Birthweight 1kg   Birthweight 2kg   Naked   Cot-nursed   Birthweight 3kg

Age in days

ers, blankets, heating lamps, heating pads, and warm water bottles, and by control of the temperature and humidity of the room. It may be necessary to administer oxygen temporarily by face mask or through an intubation tube.

The infant should be removed from the incubator only when the gradual change to the atmosphere of the nursery is not accompanied by a significant change of the infant's temperature, color, or activity, whether it be days or weeks after birth.

Feeding. The method or combination of methods optimal for the clinical problems of each infant should be used in feeding. It is important to avoid fatigue and the aspiration of food during feeding or by regurgitation. No method of feeding will avoid these risks unless the person using it has been well trained in the process. Oral feedings should not be initiated or should be discontinued in infants with respiratory distress, hypoxia, circulatory insufficiency, excessive secretions, gagging, sepsis, central nervous system depression, immaturity, or signs of serious illness. These infants will require parenteral therapy to supply calories, fluid, and electrolytes.

Large premature infants can often be fed by bottle or at the breast. Since the effort of sucking is usually the limiting factor, breast feeding is least likely to be successful. Bottle feeding of expressed breast milk may be a temporary alternative. In *bottle feeding*, effort may be reduced by use of special small, soft nipples with large holes. The process of oral alimentation requires, in addition to a strong suck, the coordination of swallowing, epiglottal and uvular closure of the larynx and nasal passages, and normal esophageal motility. This synchronized process is usually absent prior to 34 wk gestation.

Smaller or less vigorous infants should be fed by *gavage:* a soft plastic tube of No. 5 French external and approximately 0.05 cm internal diameters with a rounded atraumatic tip and 2 holes on alternate sides is preferable. The tube is passed through the nose until approximately 2.5 cm (1 in) of the lower end is in the stomach. The free end of the tube is then placed under water. If bubbles appear with each expiration, the catheter is in the trachea and must be reinserted into the proper position. The free end of the tube has an adapter into which the tip of a syringe is fitted, and the measured amount of feeding is allowed to flow in slowly by gravity. Such tubes may be left in place for 3–7 days before replacement by a similar tube through the alternate nostril. An occasional infant has enough local irritation from an indwelling tube that troublesome secretions gather around it in the nasopharynx, or there may be gagging. In such instances a catheter may be passed through the mouth by a skilled person and removed at the end of each feeding. Change to bottle or breast feeding may be instituted gradually as soon as the infant displays general vigor adequate for oral feeding without fatigue.

Continuous nasogastric and nasojejunal feedings have also been used successfully in low birth weight infants unable to ingest adequate calories by bottle or gavage owing to poor suck, uncoordinated swallowing, and delayed gastric emptying. However, intestinal perforation has occurred during nasojejunal feedings.

Gastrostomy feeding is contraindicated in premature infants because of an associated increase in mortality, except as an adjunct to the surgical management of specific gastrointestinal conditions. The routine use of partial or total *intravenous alimentation* for premature infants as a substitute for oral or gavage feedings is inappropriate; it should be used only when the latter are contraindicated by the infant's condition.

INITIATION OF FEEDING. The main principle in the feeding of premature infants is to proceed cautiously and gradually. Careful early feeding of glucose or formula tends to reduce the risk of hypoglycemia, dehydration, and hyperbilirubinemia without added risk of aspiration provided the presence of respiratory distress or other disorders is not considered an indication for withholding oral feedings and administering electrolytes, fluids, and calories intravenously.

If the infant is vigorous, making sucking movements, and in no distress, oral feeding may be attempted, though most infants under 1500 gm and many larger ones require initial tube feeding because they are unable to coordinate sucking and swallowing. A suggested schedule is to begin with 1 ml of a sterile solution of 5% glucose in water for infants under 1000 gm; 2–4 ml for infants between 1000–1500 gm; and 5–10 ml for infants over 1500 gm. If the beginning amount is 1 ml, feedings may be given hourly for the 1st 8 hr, increasing the amount by 1 ml at every other feeding. Feedings may then be given every 2 hr, with an increment of 2 ml at every other feeding until 12 ml is reached. Once dextrose water feedings have been tolerated, formula feeding may be substituted within 12–48 hr. Standard commercial formulas with caloric density of 20 kcal/oz are satisfactory for most premature infants. Amounts of formula may then be gradually increased so that the intake is approximately 150 ml/kg/24 hr. If the infant still seems hungry or fails to gain weight, the amounts should be further increased. The expected weight increments for infants of various birth weights can be projected from Fig 7–14. Certain infants with small gastric capacities fail to gain on tolerated amounts of formula containing 20 kcal/oz. In such instances more frequent feedings may be given to increase the total daily intake or the caloric content may be increased incrementally to as high as 30 kcal/oz. Care must be taken to avoid dehydration when using these hypercaloric high solute formulas.

Infants of 1000–1500 gm may be given glucose and water feedings every 2–3 hr, with 4-ml increments at every other feeding until 16 ml is reached, at which point formula may be substituted gradually. With infants over 1500 gm the interval may be 3–4 hr with 8-ml increments up to 32 ml when formula is gradually substituted.

Regurgitation, vomiting, abdominal distention, or residuals from prior feedings in the early stages of the feeding schedule should arouse suspicion of sepsis or intestinal obstruction; later, these are indications to drop back in the schedule and increase subsequent feedings slowly and to evaluate for more serious prob-

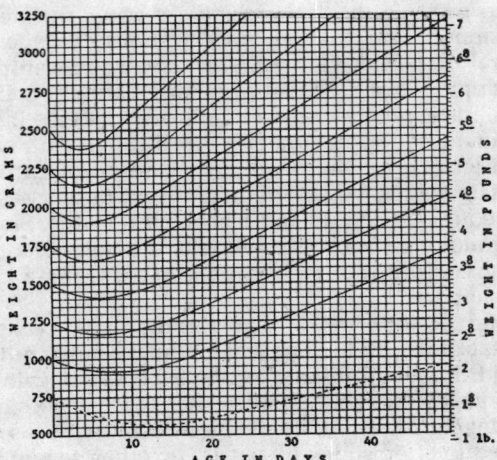

Figure 7–14 Grid for recording weights of premature infants. The average weight increments are indicated on the basis of weight at birth. (From Dancis J, et al: J Pediatr, Vol 33.)

lems such as sepsis or necrotizing enterocolitis. Gain in weight may not be achieved for 10–12 days, and a daily intake of 130–150 kcal/kg or higher may be necessary for some infants. Alternatively, in vigorous infants whose feeding schedule is advanced rapidly in calories or volume, there may be weight gain within a few days.

When tube feeding is used, the contents of the stomach should be aspirated before each feeding. If only air or small amounts of mucus are obtained, the feeding is given as planned. If greater than 10% of the previous feeding is obtained, it is advisable to reduce the amount of the feeding and to proceed more gradually with subsequent increases.

The digestive enzyme systems of infants greater than 28 wk gestation are mature enough to permit adequate digestion and absorption of protein and carbohydrate. Fat is less well absorbed due primarily to inadequate amounts of bile salt; unsaturated fats and the fat of human milk are absorbed better than those of cow's milk. Weight gain of infants weighing under 2100 gm at birth should be adequate when human milk or "humanized" milk (40% casein and 60% whey) with a protein intake of 2.25–2.75 gm/kg/24 hr is fed. This should provide all amino acids essential for premature infants, including tyrosine, cystine, and histidine. Higher protein intakes may be well tolerated and generally safe, especially for older, rapidly growing infants. However, protein intakes as high as 4.5 gm/kg/24 hr may be hazardous—although linear growth may be promoted, high protein formulas may cause abnormal plasma aminograms; elevations in blood urea nitrogen, ammonia, and sodium concentrations; metabolic acidosis (cow's milk formulas); and untoward effects on neurologic development. Further, the high protein and mineral contents of balanced cow's milk formulas of high caloric content constitute a large solute load for the kidney, a fact important in the maintenance of water balance, especially in the infant with diarrhea or fever.

Although formulas in amounts necessary for adequate growth probably contain sufficient amounts of all vitamins, the volume of milk sufficient to satisfy requirements may not be attained for several wk. Therefore, low birth weight infants should be given supplemental vitamins. Since exact requirements for these infants have not been established, the recommended daily allowances for term infants should be given (Chapter 3). Further, these infants may have a special need for certain vitamins. Intermediary metabolism of phenylalanine and tyrosine depends, in part, upon vitamin C. Decreased fat absorption with increased fecal fat loss may be associated with decreased absorption of *vitamin D*, other fat soluble vitamins, and calcium in premature infants. Very low birth weight infants are particularly prone to develop rickets. The total intake of vitamin D should not exceed 1500 IU/24 hr. *Folic acid* is essential for the formation of DNA and production of new cells; serum and erythrocyte levels decrease in preterm infants over the 1st few wk of life and remain low for 2–3 mo. Therefore, supplementation is recommended, though it does not result in improved growth or increased hemoglobin concentration. Deficiency of vitamin E is associated with increased hemolysis and, if severe, with anemia in premature infants. Vitamin E functions as an antioxidant to prevent peroxidation of polyunsaturated fatty acids in red blood cell membranes; the need for it may be increased because of the increased membrane content of these fatty acids. Vitamin K deficiency is discussed in Sec 3.32.

In the low birth weight infant, physiologic anemia due to postnatal suppression of erythropoiesis is exacerbated by smaller fetal iron stores and greater expansion of blood volume as a result of more rapid growth compared with the term weight infant; therefore, the anemia develops earlier and reaches a lower ultimate level. Fetal or neonatal blood loss accentuates this problem. Iron stores, even in the very low birth weight neonate, are usually adequate until the infant doubles his or her birth weight. In addition, iron supplementation during the period when these infants are at risk for vitamin E deficiency (less than 34 wk post-conception age) may enhance hemolysis and reduce vitamin E absorption. Therefore, vitamin E supplementation may be discontinued once the premature infant doubles his or her birth weight, at which time iron supplementation (2 mg/kg/24 hr) should be started.

The properly fed premature infant may have from 1–6 stools of semisolid consistency daily; sudden increase in number or a change to a watery consistency is reason for more concern than any arbitrarily stated frequency.

The premature infant should not vomit or regurgitate. He or she should be satisfied and relaxed after a feeding but may normally show the activity of hunger shortly before the next one.

Fluid Requirements. These vary according to gestational age, environmental conditions, and disease states. Assuming minimal water losses in stool in infants not receiving oral fluids, their water needs are equal to insensible water loss, renal solute excretion, and any unusual ongoing losses. Insensible water loss is indirectly related to gestational age; the very immature preterm infant (< 1000 gm) may require as much as 2 to 3 ml/kg/hr, partly because of thin skin, lack of subcutaneous tissue, and a large exposed surface area.

Insensible water loss is increased under radiant warmers, during phototherapy, and in the febrile infant. It is diminished when the infant is clothed, is covered by a plexiglass inner heat shield, breathes humidified air, or approaches term. Larger premature infants (2000–2500 gm) nursed in an incubator may have an insensible water loss of approximately 0.6–0.7 ml/kg/hr.

Fluids also need to be administered to permit excretion of the urinary solute load, e.g., urea, electrolytes, phosphate. The amount varies with dietary intake and the anabolic or catabolic state of nutrition. High solute load formulas, total intravenous alimentation, and catabolism increase the end products which require urinary excretion and thus increase the requirement for water. Renal solute loads may vary between 7.5–30 mOsm/kg. Newborn infants, especially those of very low birth weight, also have decreased ability to concentrate urine, thus increasing the fluid intake required to excrete solutes.

Water intake in term infants is usually begun at 60–70 ml/kg on day 1 and increased to 100–120 ml/kg by day 2–3. Smaller, more premature infants may need to be started with 100 cc/kg on day 1 and advanced to 150 cc/kg or more by day 3–4. Fluid volumes should be titrated individually. Daily weights, urine output and specific gravity, and serum urea nitrogen with electrolytes should be monitored carefully to detect abnormal states of hydration because clinical observations and physical examinations are poor indicators of the state of hydration of premature infants. Conditions which increase fluid losses, such as glycosuria, the polyuric phase of acute tubular necrosis, and diarrhea, may place additional strain on kidneys which are unable to conserve water and electrolytes adequately and result in severe dehydration. Alternatively, fluid overload may lead to edema, congestive heart failure, and a patent ductus arteriosus.

Total Parenteral Nutrition. When oral feeding is impossible for prolonged periods of time, total intravenous alimentation may provide sufficient fluid, calories, electrolytes, and vitamins to sustain growth of low birth weight infants. This technique has been lifesaving in infants who have had intractable diarrheal syndromes or extensive resection of bowel. Infusions may be administered through an indwelling central vein catheter or through a peripheral vein.

The goal of parenteral alimentation is to deliver enough nonprotein calories to allow the infant to use most of the protein for growth. The infusate should contain a protein equivalent (hydrolysates of beef fibrin and casein and synthetic amino acids are available) of 2.5 gm/dl and hypertonic glucose in the range of 10–25 gm/dl in addition to appropriate quantities of electrolytes, trace minerals, and vitamins. A crystalline amino acid mixture is recommended because it is less likely to produce acidosis. The initial daily infusion should deliver 10–15 gm/kg/24 hr of glucose and increase gradually to 25–30 gm/kg/24 hr when glucose alone is used to meet the full requirements of 100–120 nonprotein kcal/kg/24 hr. If a peripheral vein is used, it is advisable to keep the glucose concentration below 12.5 gm/dl. Intravenous fat emulsions such as Intralipid (11 kcal/gm) may be used to provide calories without an appreciable osmotic load, thereby decreasing the need for infusion of the higher concentrations of glucose by central or peripheral vein and usually preventing the development of essential fatty acid deficiency. Electrolytes, trace minerals, and vitamin additives are included in amounts approximating established intravenous maintenance requirements. The content of each day's infusate should be determined after careful assessment of the infant's clinical and biochemical status. Slow and continuous infusion is advisable. All solutions should be mixed by a well trained pharmacist using a laminar flow hood.

After a caloric intake of greater than 100 kcal/kg/24 hr is established by total parenteral intravenous nutrition, low birth weight infants can be expected to gain about 15 gm/kg/24 hr, with positive nitrogen balances of 150–200 mg/kg/24 hr, if there are not multiple operative procedures, episodes of sepsis, or other severe stress. This goal usually can be achieved and the catabolic tendency during the 1st wk of life reversed with subsequent weight gains by peripheral vein infusions of 2.5 gm/kg/24 hr of an amino acid mixture, 10 gm/dl of glucose, and 4 gm/kg/24 hr of Intralipid.

The complications of intravenous alimentation are related to both the catheter and the metabolism of the infusate. Sepsis is the most important known problem of central vein infusions and can be minimized only by meticulous catheter care and aseptic preparation of the infusate. *Staphylococcus aureus* and *Candida albicans* are the common infecting organisms. Once infection has occurred, the line must be removed and appropriate antibiotics given. Thrombosis, extravasation of fluid, and accidental dislodgment of catheters have also occurred. Sepsis is rarely attributable to peripheral vein infusions, but phlebitis, cutaneous sloughs, and superficial infection occasionally occur. The **metabolic complications** include hyperglycemia from the high glucose concentration of the infusate, which may lead to an osmotic diuresis; dehydration; azotemia; hypoglycemia from a sudden accidental cessation of the infusate; hyperlipidemia and possibly hypoxemia from intravenous lipid infusions; and hyperammonemia, which may be due to high levels of ammonia in beef fibrin hydrolysates or the lack of arginine in casein hydrolysates. Abnormal liver chemistries have also been noted. Hyperchloremic acidosis occurs in infants receiving synthetic amino acids unless there is an appropriate balance between cationic and anionic amino acids and salts. Abnormal elevations of blood amino acid levels are an additional potential hazard. If intravenous fat emulsions are not used, fatty acid deficiency also may occur. When the infusion is given through a peripheral vein, the osmolality of the solution may limit the duration of time an infusion site can be used while, at the same time, requiring greater volumes of fluid than can be tolerated. Continuous chemical and physiologic monitoring of infants receiving intravenous alimentation is indicated because of the frequency and seriousness of complications.

INTRAVENOUS SUPPLEMENTATION OF TOLERATED ORAL FEEDINGS. Glucose, amino acid mixtures, and lipid emulsions alone or in combination may be infused into peripheral veins when sufficient calories cannot be provided to low birth weight infants by oral feeding alone. Some infants weighing less than 1500 gm may regain their birth weight sooner and have fewer apneic episodes with a supplemental infusion containing nitrogen. Increases in weight, length, and head circumference approaching those expected in utero have been achieved with mixtures of protein hydrolysate, glucose, and Intralipid. Although the complications of both techniques may occur, the combination of nutrient delivery methods allows smaller volumes of enteral feedings, thus decreasing the risk of aspiration. Hyperglycemia, azotemia, hypermethioninemia, and hyperglycinemia have been reported.

Prevention of Infection. Premature infants have an increased susceptibility to infection which requires rigorous hand-to-elbow washing by personnel before and after handling the infant, measures to reduce contamination of food and the objects that come in contact with the infant, prevention of air contamination, avoiding overcrowding, and limiting direct and indirect contacts with nursery personnel (including other infants). No one with an infection should be permitted in the nursery. However, the risks of infection must be balanced against the disadvantages of limiting the infant's contacts with the family, which may be detrimental to the infant's ultimate development; early and frequent participation by parents in the nursery care of their infant does not increase the risk significantly when appropriate preventive precautions are maintained.

Prevention of transmission of infection from infant to infant is difficult because frequently neither term nor premature newborn infants manifest clear clinical evidence of an infection early in its course. If a unit admits infants born outside that hospital, it should be assumed that they are infected until 72 hr of observation in a special nursery or an incubator with an individual air supply proves otherwise. When epidemics occur within a nursery, cohort nursing and isolation rooms should be employed in addition to routine antiseptic care.

The most important factor in the successful care of premature infants is the skill, experience, and number of the nursing staff. It is the responsibility of the physician to insist upon an optimal amount of expert nursing.

General Considerations of Disease. Prematurity tends to increase the severity and to reduce the clinical manifestations of most neonatal diseases. Subcutaneous and intracranial hemorrhage, "primary" atelectasis, respiratory distress syndrome, pneumonia, bacteremia, hypoglycemia, and hyperbilirubinemia occur more frequently among premature than among term infants.

Retrolental fibroplasia is seen almost exclusively in premature infants.

DRUGS. Renal clearances for almost all substances excreted in the urine are diminished in newborn infants, but more so in premature ones. Dosing intervals may, therefore, need to be extended when administering drugs chiefly excreted by the kidney. For instance, highly satisfactory levels of penicillin, gentamicin, and kanamycin are maintained on doses given at 12-hr intervals. Drugs detoxified in the liver or requiring chemical conjugation before renal excretion should also be given with caution and in smaller than usual doses. Decision as to the choice, dose, and route of administration of antibacterial agents to possibly infected infants should be made on an individual rather than on a routine basis, owing to the dangers of (1) development of infections with organisms resistant to antibacterial agents, (2) destruction or inhibition of intestinal bacteria which manufacture significant amounts of essential vitamins (e.g., vitamin K and thiamine), and (3) possible deleterious interference in important metabolic processes (e.g., the role of sulfisoxazole in hyperbilirubinemia).

Since food and drug laws and regulations in the United States are based largely on toxicity studies on adult animals and human beings, apparently "safe" drugs may not be so for newborn infants, especially premature ones. Oxygen, vitamin K analogues, sulfisoxazole (Gantrisin), chloramphenicol, and novobiocin have proved toxic to premature infants in amounts not harmful to term infants. Thus, administration of any drug to newborn infants, particularly in large doses, should be done with care and with risk weighed against potential benefit.

The levels of some immunoglobulins of premature infants at birth are significantly lower than those of their mothers at the time of delivery or those of term infants, and they undergo further decrease during the 1st months of life. However, the routine or prophylactic administration of gamma globulin has not been proved to be of benefit.

Prognosis. There is now a 95% or greater chance of survival for infants born weighing between 1501–2500 gm, but those weighing less still have a significantly higher mortality (Fig 7–5 and Table 7–14). Intensive care has led to an extension of the period when a very low birth weight (VLBW) infant is likely to die from complications of perinatal disease, such as bronchopulmonary dysplasia, necrotizing enterocolitis, or secondary infection. The mortality rate of low birth weight

Table 7–14 SURVIVAL OF VERY LOW BIRTH WEIGHT INFANTS

BIRTH WEIGHT (GM)	CAMBRIDGE MATERNITY 1976–1978	RAINBOW BABIES AND CHILDRENS HOSPITAL				NEW YORK–CORNELL		
		1975	1976	1977	1978	1976	1977	1978
501–750	1/2(50%)	0/12(0%)	2/7(29%)	3/12(25%)	4/25(16%)	0/4(0%)	0/5(0%)	0/9(0%)
751–1000	15/23(65%)	15/35(43%)	19/36(53%)	23/39(59%)	25/44(57%)	1/4(25%)	3/6(50%)	10/18(56%)
1001–1250	33/51(65%)	18/33(55%)	38/50(76%)	30/42(71%)	34/47(72%)	8/10(80%)	13/14(93%)	19/24(79%)
1251–1500	40/45(89%)	44/58(56%)	53/60(88%)	37/43(86%)	54/62(87%)	15/18(83%)	20/23(87%)	14/14(100%)

From Clin Perinatol 7:135, 1980.

infants who survive to be discharged from the hospital is higher than that of term infants during the 1st 2 yr of life. Many of these deaths are attributable to infection and are, therefore, at least theoretically preventable. There is also an increased incidence of failure to thrive, the sudden infant death syndrome, child abuse, and inadequate maternal-infant bonding among premature infants. The possible roles of defects in the regulation of the cardiorespiratory system secondary to complications of underlying perinatal disease and immaturity and of high environmental risk factors secondary to low socioeconomic status in increasing the mortality rate have not been fully delineated.

Congenital anatomic anomalies are present in approximately 3–7% of low birth weight infants.

In the absence of congenital abnormalities, central nervous system injury, very low birth weight, or a marked reduction in birth weight for gestational age (intrauterine growth retardation), physical growth of low birth weight infants tends to approximate that of term weight infants during the 2nd yr; this occurs earlier in premature infants of larger size at birth. Very low birth weight infants may not catch up, especially if there has been severe chronic illness, insufficient nutritional intake, or an inadequate caretaking environment. Premature birth in itself may prejudice later development. In general, the greater the immaturity and the lower the birth weight, the greater the likelihood of intellectual and neurologic deficit (Fig 7–15). Small head circumference at birth may be similarly related to poor neurobehavioral prognosis. The incidence of neurologic and developmental handicap in VLBW infants ranges from 10–20%, including cerebral palsy (3–6%), moderate to severe hearing and visual defects (1–4%), and learning difficulties (20%). Mean global I.Q. is 90–97, and 76% have normal school performance.

Mothers of low socioeconomic status are more apt to have low birth weight babies who tend to develop less well than do those in better environments. Major neurologic defects were found to be uncommon in a prospective study of full-term small-for-dates infants, although there was an increased incidence of minimal cerebral dysfunction (hyperactivity, short attention span, learning difficulties), electroencephalographic abnormalities, and speech defects compared with appropriate-for-gestation term infants.

Behavior and personality problems may be more common in children born prematurely than in those born at term. The extent to which isolated care in early infancy, a defect in development of the normal maternal-infant relationship, and understandable parental anxiety and overprotectiveness may foster an abnormal emotional environment for the growing infant is unknown. However, avoiding unnecessarily prolonged hospitalization and encouraging parental visiting and participation in the nursery care of the infant might reasonably be expected to decrease such a possible untoward effect.

Discharge. Before discharge, a premature infant should be taking all nutrition by nipple, either bottle or breast. Growth should be at steady increments of approximately 10–30 gm/day. Temperature should be stabilized in an open crib. There should have been no recent apneas or bradycardias, and oxygen or parenteral drug administration should have been discontinued. Infants previously treated with oxygen should have an eye examination to determine the presence, stage, or absence of retrolental fibroplasia, and those who had indwelling umbilical arterial catheters should have their blood pressure measured to check for renal vascular hypertension. A hemoglobin level or hematocrit should be determined to evaluate possible anemia. If all major medical problems have resolved and the home setting is adequate, premature infants may then be discharged when their weight approaches 2000–2200 gm; close follow-up and easy access to health care providers are essential components of such early discharge protocols. Alternatively, if the medical or social environment is not ideal, high-risk neonates transported to neonatal intensive care units whose major illness has resolved may be returned to their hospital of birth for an additional period of hospitalization.

Home Care. While the infant is in the hospital the mother should be instructed about caring for the baby

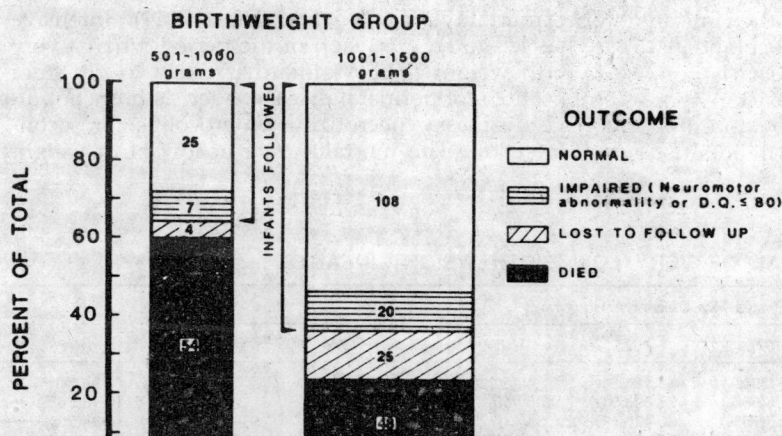

BIRTHWEIGHT GROUP

Figure 7–15 Prognosis of very low birth weight infants followed to a mean of 2 yr conceptual age at Rainbow Babies and Childrens Hospital, Cleveland, Ohio. (N Engl J Med 301:1162, 1979.)

after discharge. This program should include at least 1 visit to her home by a person capable of evaluating domestic arrangements and of advising about any needed improvements.

7.17 POST-TERM INFANTS

Post-term infants are those born after 42 wk of gestation, calculated from the mother's last menstrual period, irrespective of weight at birth. This designation is often used synonymously with the term "postmature" for infants whose gestation exceeds the normal 280 days by 7 days or more. Approximately 25% of all pregnancies end on or after the 287th day of gestation, 12% on or after the 294th day, and 5% on or after the 301st day. The cause of post-term birth or postmaturity is unknown. Large size of the infant correlates poorly with late delivery, but it does correlate with large size of either parent, multigravidity, or a prediabetic or diabetic state in the mother.

Clinical Manifestations. Post-term infants may be clinically indistinguishable from term infants, but some have received the designation postmature because of appearance and behavior suggesting those of an infant 1–3 wk of age. These post-term, postmature infants are characterized by the absence of lanugo, decreased or absent vernix caseosa, long nails, abundant scalp hair, white parchment-like or desquamating skin, and increased alertness. Occasionally, some of these clinical manifestations of postmaturity are observed in term and preterm infants.

Prognosis. When delivery is delayed 3 wk or more beyond term, there is a significant increase in mortality, which in some series has approximated 3 times that of a control group of infants born at term. Mortality has been lowered markedly through improved obstetric management. Primiparity and maternal age over 35 yr appear to increase the mortality rates.

Treatment. Careful obstetrical monitoring, including nonstress testing or oxytocin challenge tests, usually provides a rational basis for choosing a course of nonintervention, induction of labor, or cesarean section. Cesarean section may be indicated in older primigravidas who go more than a week or 2 beyond term, particularly if there is evidence of fetal distress.

7.18 PLACENTAL DYSFUNCTION SYNDROME

Incidence and Etiology. The incidence of some clinically recognizable form of placental dysfunction (abnormal fetal heart rate pattern, retarded intrauterine growth, low maternal levels of estriol, contamination of amniotic fluid by meconium) has been estimated to be as high as 12% of all births. The incidence of the clearly recognizable form of the syndrome, with yellow staining of the vernix and skin, is approximately 1.2% of all births. Although this syndrome is frequently confused with postmaturity, *only about 20% of infants with placental dysfunction syndrome are post-term.* The majority affected are term and preterm infants, particularly those of low birth weight for gestational age who

are infants of toxemic mothers, older primigravidas, and women with chronic hypertension or other serious illness. The placentas are often small or poorly attached. This syndrome has been postulated to be the result of degenerative changes in the placenta resulting in progressive reduction of oxygen and nourishment for the fetus.

Clinical Manifestations. Term or preterm infants who are born at weights lower than expected for gestational age have been discussed previously. Those who are born post-term in association with presumed placental dysfunction may have any of a variety of physical signs: desquamation, long nails, abundant hair, white skin, alert faces, and loose skin, especially around the thighs and buttocks, giving the appearance of recent loss of weight; meconium-stained amniotic fluid, skin, vernix, umbilical cord, and placental membranes, possibly a manifestation of fetal anoxia; bright yellow, meconium-stained nails and skin; and a yellow-green stained umbilical cord (Fig 7–16).

Prognosis. Prolonged gestation correlates with increased mortality, and up to one third of mildly affected infants show evidence of respiratory distress or central nervous system irritation. Infants with more prominent clinical signs are usually born after a moderate to severe intrauterine hypoxic episode close to the time of delivery; about two thirds of them have severe respiratory symptoms, and a smaller number show signs of anoxic cerebral damage. In some infants the clinical presenta-

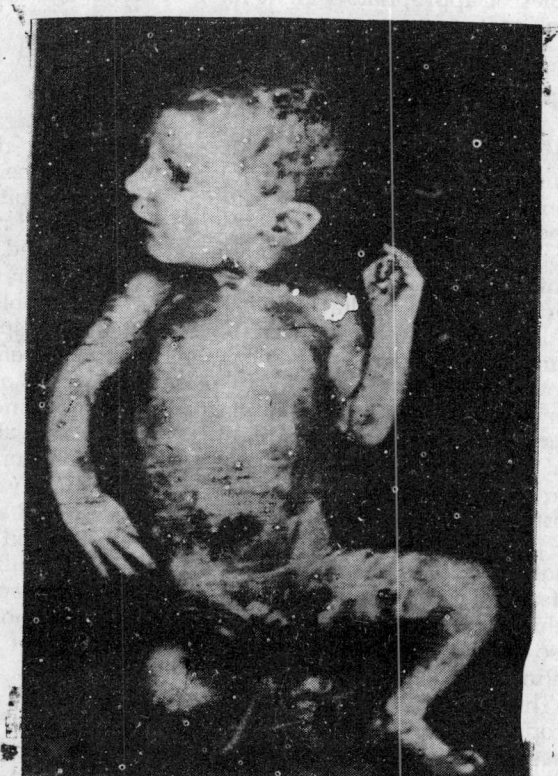

Figure 7–16 Placental dysfunction syndrome, stage III. Note long, thin infant with loose, peeling, parchment-like skin, alert expression, staining of skin and nails. (From Clifford: Advances in Pediatrics. Vol 9. Chicago, Year Book Medical Publishers, Inc.)

tion, e.g., long, yellow-stained nails, suggests that asphyxia took place at some time prior to labor and delivery.

Treatment. The treatment of placental dysfunction lies chiefly in preventing the conditions which predispose to it and in alleviating episodes of acute fetal distress that occur during labor. It therefore constitutes an obstetric and perhaps a genetic and social problem. Aspiration pneumonia and cerebral anoxia are treated symptomatically.

7.19   HIGH BIRTH WEIGHT

Perinatal and neonatal mortality rates decrease with increasing birth weight until approximately 4000 gm after which mortality increases (Fig 7–6). These oversized infants are usually born at term, but preterm infants with weights high for gestational age also have a significantly higher mortality than infants of the same size born at term. Infants who are very large, regardless of their gestational age, have a higher incidence of birth injuries, such as cervical and brachial plexus injuries, phrenic nerve damage with paralysis of the diaphragm, fractured clavicles, cephalhematomas, subdural hematomas, and ecchymoses of the head and face. The incidence of congenital anomalies is also higher than in term infants of normal weight. Intellectual and developmental retardation is also statistically more common in high birth weight term and preterm infants than in babies of appropriate weight for gestational age. (See also Sec 7.14.)

INFANT TRANSPORT

With the advent of regionalized care for high-risk neonates, increasing numbers of sick infants are being transported to neonatal intensive care units in hospitals other than where they were born. Ideally, high-risk mothers should be transported to and delivered at centers where these units are located. Neonatal transport includes consultation about the infant's problem and care before transport, ease of access to the transport team, and transport and stabilization by the team before moving the infant. Securing an airway, providing oxygen, assisted ventilation, antimicrobial therapy, and a warmed environment plus placing intravenous or arterial lines should all be initiated if indicated prior to transport. Infant and maternal records, laboratory reports, and a tube of clotted maternal blood should also be provided. Before departure, the mother should be spoken to briefly and allowed to see the stabilized infant, if practical; the father should follow the transport vehicle to the unit. The transport officer or nurse should also call ahead to inform the receiving unit about the nature of the patient's illness.

The transport vehicle should be equipped with appropriate medicines, fluids, oxygen tanks, catheters, chest tubes, endotracheal tubes, laryngoscopes, and an infant warming device. It should be well illuminated and have ample room for emergency procedures and monitoring equipment. With appropriate education of nursing and medical staff at the referring hospitals, combined with efficient transport, the mortality of "outborn" neonates should be no higher than that of those born within the tertiary care center.

American Academy of Pedriatrics: Hospital Care of Newborn Infants. Ed 5. Evanston, Ill., The Academy, 1971.
Anderson T, Muttart C, Bieber M, et al: A controlled trial of glucose versus glucose and amino acids in premature infants. J Pediatr 94:947, 1979.
Babson SG, Behrman RE, Lessel R: Fetal growth; liveborn birth weights for gestational age of white middle class infants. Pediatrics 45:937, 1970.
Bell E, Warburton D, Stonestreet B, et al: Effect of fluid administration on the development of symptomatic patent ductus arteriosus and congestive heart failure in premature infants. New Engl J Med 302:598, 1980.
Berg K, Celander O: Circulatory adaptation in thermoregulators of full term and premature newborn infants. Acta Pediatr Scand 60:278, 1971.
Bryan MH, Wei P, Hamilton JR, et al: Supplemental intravenous alimentation in low birth weight infants. J Pediatr 82:940, 1973.
Chen JS, Wong PWK: Intestinal complications of nasojejunal feeding in low birth weight infants. J Pediatr 85:109, 1974.
Chernick V, Raber MB: Electrical hazards in the newborn nursery. J Pediatr 77:143, 1970.
Cross KW, Hey EN, Kennard DL, et al: Lack of temperature control in infants with abnormalities of the CNS. Arch Dis Child 46:437, 1971.
Driscoll JM Jr, Behrman RE: Routine and special care; general. In: Behrman RE (ed): Neonatal-Perinatal Medicine. St Louis, CV Mosby, 1977.
Du JN, Oliver TK Jr: The baby in the delivery room; a suitable microenvironment. JAMA 207:636, 1967.
Duc G: Assessment of hypoxia in the newborn; suggestions for a practical approach. Pediatrics 48:469, 1971.
Eisenach KD, Reber RM, Eitzman DV, et al: Nosocomial infections due to kanamycin-resistant (R)-factor carrying enteric organisms in an intensive care nursery. Pediatrics 50:395, 1972.
Fanaroff AA, Wald M, Gruber HS, et al: Insensible water loss in low birth weight infants. Pediatrics 50:236, 1972.
Gaudy GM, Adamsons K, Cunningham N, et al: Thermal environment and acid base homeostasis in human infants during the first hours of life. J Clin Invest 43:751, 1964.
Gaull GE, Rassin DK, Raiha NCR, et al: Milk protein quantity and quality in low-birth-weight infants. III. Effects on sulfur amino acids in plasma and urine. J Pediatr 90:348, 1977.
Gordon HH, Levine SJ, McNamara H: Feeding of premature infants; a comparison of human and cow's milk. Am J Dis Child 73:442, 1947.
Gustafson A, Kjellmer I, Olegard R, et al: Nutrition in low birth weight infants. I. Intravenous infection of fat emulsion. Acta Pediatr Scand 61:149, 1972.
Heird WC, Anderson TL: Nutrition, body fluids, and acid-base homeostasis; I. Nutritional requirements of the low birth weight infant. In: Behrman RE (ed): Neonatal-Perinatal Medicine. St Louis, CV Mosby, 1977.
Heird WC, Anderson TL, Driscoll JM: Nutrition, body fluids and acid-base homeostasis; II. Methods of nutrient delivery for low birth weight infants. In: Behrman RE (ed): Neonatal-Perinatal Medicine. St Louis, CV Mosby, 1977.
Hittner HM, Hirsch NJ, Rudolph AJ: Assessment of gestational age by examination of the anterior vascular capsule of the lens. J Pediatr 91:455, 1977.
Hyman CJ, Pakravan P, Allen AC: Foot-abdomen skin temperature difference (FASTD) in the evaluation of neonatal fever. J Pediatr 83:149, 1973.
Kinsey VE, Arnold HJ, Kalina RE, et al: PaO₂ levels and retrolental fibroplasia: A report of the cooperative study. Pediatrics 60:655, 1977.
Kliegman R, King K: Intrauterine growth retardation: Determinants of aberrant fetal growth, In: Fanaroff AA, Martin RJ (eds.): Behrman's Neonatal Perinatal Medicine. St Louis, CV Mosby, 1983.
Levine SZ, Gorgon HH: Physiologic handicaps of the premature infant. I. Their pathogenesis; II. Clinical applications. Am J Dis Child 64:274, 1942.
Lewis R, Charles M, Patwary KM: Relationship between birth weight and selected social, environmental and medical care factors. Am J Publ Health 63:973, 1973.
Lubchenco LO, Hausman C, Boyd E: Intrauterine growth in length and head circumference as estimated from live births at gestational ages from 26 to 42 weeks. Pediatrics 37:403, 1966.
Lucy J: RLF resurgence haunts the nursery. News Bulletin Highlights issue. Am Acad Pediatr Spring Meeting 1982, Vol 18, No. 2.
Niswander KR, Gordon M: Collaborative Perinatal Study; The Women and Their Pregnancies. Philadelphia, WB Saunders, 1972.
Oliver TK: Routine and special care; thermal regulation. In: Behrman RE (ed): Neonatal/Perinatal Medicine. St Louis, CV Mosby, 1977.
Perlstein H, Edwards NK, Sutherland JM: Apnea in premature infants and incubator air temperature changes. N Engl J Med 282:461, 1970.
Raiha NCR, Heinonen K, Rassin D, et al: Milk protein quantity and quality in low birth weight infants. Pedriatrics 57:659, 1976.

Raiha NCR, Rassin D, Gaull G: Milk protein quality and quantity; biochemical and growth effects in low birth weight infants. Pediatr Res 9:679, 1975.

Rassin D, Gaull G, Neils CR, et al: Milk protein quantity and quality in low-birth-weight infants. IV. Effects on tyrosine and phenylalanine in plasma and urine. J Pediatr 90:356, 1977.

Roy R, Sinclair J: Hydration of the low birth weight infant. Clin Perinatol 2:393, 1975.

Silverman W: Retrolental Fibroplasia: A Modern Parable. New York, Grune and Stratton, 1980.

Speidel B: Adverse effects of routine procedures in preterm infants. Lancet 1:864, 1978.

Sterky G: Swedish standard curves for intrauterine growth. Pediatrics 46:7, 1970.

Tanner JM: Standards for birth weight or intrauterine growth. Pediatrics 46:1, 1970.

Tiffany FM, Dabiri CM, Hallock N, et al: Developmental effects of prolonged pregnancy and postmaturity syndrome. J Pediatr 90:836, 1977.

Van den Berg BJ, Yerushalmy J: The relationship of the rate of intrauterine growth of infants of low birth weight to mortality, morbidity and congenital anomalies. J Pediatr 69:531, 1966.

Diseases of the Newborn Infant: Premature and Fullterm

The child's physician should have an appreciation of the wide variety of disorders that may have their origin in utero, during birth, or in the immediate postnatal period, and of the need to distinguish them etiologically in respect to their time and place of origin.

Disorders that have their origin in utero may represent genetic mutations, chromosomal aberrations, or acquired diseases. Some of these disorders are described in this chapter in Sec 7.21, 7.30, 7.54, and 7.58; others are described in Chapters 3, 6, 8, 9, 10 and those discussing the various systems of the body.

7.20 CLINICAL MANIFESTATIONS OF DISEASE DURING THE NEONATAL PERIOD

Recognition of disease in the newborn infant is dependent upon knowledge and evaluation of a limited number of relatively nonspecific clinical signs and symptoms.

Cyanosis usually indicates respiratory insufficiency, which may be due to pulmonary conditions or may be secondary to intracranial hemorrhage or anoxic injury to the brain. If it is due to the former, respirations tend to be rapid and may be accompanied by retraction of the thoracic cage. If it is due to the latter, respirations tend to be irregular and weak and often slow. Cyanosis persisting for several days, unaccompanied by obvious signs of respiratory difficulty, is suggestive of cyanotic congenital heart disease or methemoglobinemia. Cyanosis from congenital heart disease may, however, on occasion be difficult to distinguish from cyanosis caused by respiratory disease in the 1st few days of life. Episodes of cyanosis also may be the presenting sign of hypoglycemia, bacteremia, meningitis, shock, or persistent fetal circulation.

In addition to anemia or hemorrhage, *pallor* should suggest hypoxia, hypoglycemia, sepsis, shock, or adrenal failure.

Convulsions (Chapter 20) usually point to a disorder of the central nervous system and suggest asphyxia, brain damage, intracranial hemorrhage, cerebral anomaly, • subdural effusion, meningitis, tetany, hypoglycemia, or, rarely, pyridoxine dependency, hyponatremia, hypernatremia, inborn errors of metabolism, drug withdrawal, or familial neonatal seizures. They may also be the 1st sign of bacteremia or other severe infection and may occur as a nonspecific sign in any severe illness, particularly if there is circulatory insufficiency. Seizures which begin in the delivery room or shortly thereafter may be due to unintended injection of maternal local anesthetic into the fetus. Convulsions may also result from the administration of large amounts of hypotonic fluids to the mother shortly before and during delivery, with subsequent hyponatremia and water intoxication in the infant.

Seizures should be distinguished from jitteriness which may be present in normal newborns, in infants of diabetic mothers, in those who experienced birth asphyxia or drug withdrawal, and in polycythemic neonates. Jitteriness which resembles simple tremors may be stopped by holding the infant's extremity, is often dependent on sensory stimuli, and is not associated with abnormal eye movements. Seizures in premature infants are often subtle and associated with abnormal eye or facial movements; the motor component is often that of tonic extension of the limbs, neck, and trunk. Term infants may have clonic or myoclonic movements but may also manifest more subtle seizure activity. *Apnea* may be the 1st manifestation of seizure activity, particularly in a premature infant.

Lethargy may be a manifestation of asphyxia or hypoglycemia, of sedation from maternal analgesia or anesthesia, of cerebral defect, of severe infection, and, indeed, of almost any severe disease including inborn errors of metabolism. Lethargy appearing after the 2nd day should, in particular, suggest infection.

Irritability may be a sign of discomfort accompanying intra-abdominal conditions, meningeal irritation, infections, or any condition producing pain. As in later infancy, the eardrums should always be examined as a possible source of pain.

Hyperactivity, especially of the premature infant, may be a sign of hypoxia, pneumothorax, emphysema, hypoglycemia, hypocalcemia, central nervous system damage, drug withdrawal, thyrotoxicosis, or a cold environment.

Failure to feed well is seen in most sick newborn infants and should always occasion a careful search for infection and other abnormal conditions.

Fever may be the result of too high an environmental temperature due to weather, overheated nurseries or incubators, or too many clothes or bedclothes. It is also seen in "dehydration fever" of newborn infants. If these causes of fever can be eliminated, then serious infection (pneumonia, bacteremia, viremia, meningitis) must be ruled out, although such infections often occur without

Table 7–15 POTENTIAL ETIOLOGY OF APNEA

Gastrointestinal: gastroesophageal reflux
Infections: sepsis, meningitis, necrotizing enterocolitis
Metabolic: ↓ glucose, ↓ calcium, ↓ pO₂, ↑ environmental temperature ↑ ammonia, ↑↓ sodium
Vascular: hypotension, hypertension, anemia, dehydration
CNS: drugs, hemorrhage, seizures, reflex, sleep state, immaturity
Respiratory: airway obstruction, alveolar collapse, chest wall instability, laryngeal reflex, intrapulmonary pathology
Idiopathic

provoking a febrile response in newborn infants. An unexplained *fall in body temperature* may accompany infection or other serious disturbances of the circulation or central nervous system.

Periods of *apnea*, particularly in the premature infant, may be associated with a variety of disturbances (Table 7–15). When apneas are recurrent and longer than 20 sec or associated with cyanosis or bradycardia, they warrant an immediate diagnostic evaluation.

Jaundice during the 1st 24 hr of life should be considered due to erythroblastosis fetalis until proved otherwise. Septicemia (especially in the low birth weight infant), cytomegalic inclusion disease, the congenital rubella syndrome, and toxoplasmosis should also be considered, especially if there is direct as well as indirect reacting bilirubin present.

Jaundice after the 1st 24 hr may also be due to septicemia, may be "physiologic," or may be due to hemolytic anemia, galactosemia, hepatitis, congenital atresia of the bile ducts, inspissated bile syndrome following erythroblastosis fetalis, syphilis, herpes simplex, or congenital infections.

Vomiting during the 1st day of life suggests obstruction in the upper digestive tract or increased intracranial pressure. Roentgenographic studies are indicated when obstruction is suspected. Vomiting also may be a nonspecific symptom of an illness such as septicemia. It is a common manifestation of overfeeding or inexperienced feeding technique, pyloric stenosis, milk allergy, duodenal ulcer, stress ulcer, or adrenal insufficiency. Infants placed in body casts for orthopedic treatment often vomit transiently. Vomitus containing dark blood is usually a sign of life-threatening illness. Bile-stained vomitus strongly suggests obstruction below the ampulla of Vater.

Diarrhea may be a symptom of overfeeding, acute gastroenteritis, malabsorption, or a nonspecific symptom of infection. It may be seen in conditions accompanied by compromised circulation of part of the intestinal or genital tract, such as mesenteric thrombosis, necrotizing enterocolitis, strangulated hernia, intussusception, and torsion of the ovary or testis.

Abdominal distention, usually a sign of intestinal obstruction or an intra-abdominal mass, may also be seen in infants with enteritis, ileus accompanying sepsis, respiratory distress, or hypokalemia.

Failure to move an extremity or part of it suggests fracture, dislocation, or nerve injury. It is also seen in osteomyelitis and other infections that cause pain on movement of the affected part.

7.21 CONGENITAL ANOMALIES

Congenital anomalies are important as a cause of stillbirths and neonatal deaths, but are perhaps even more important as causes of physical defects and metabolic disorders. (Anomalies are discussed in general in Chapter 6 and specifically in the chapters on the various systems of the body. For congenital mental defects, see Chapter 2; for congenital metabolic and chemical disorders, see Chapter 8; and for immunologic deficiency disorders, see Chapter 9.) Early recognition of anomalies is important for planning care; for some, such as tracheoesophageal fistula, diaphragmatic hernia, choanal atresia, or intestinal obstruction, immediate medical and surgical therapy is essential for survival. Parents are likely to be assailed by anxiety and guilt when they become aware of the existence of a congenital anomaly and will require sensitive counseling.

BIRTH INJURY

The term *birth injury* is used to denote avoidable and unavoidable mechanical and anoxic trauma incurred by the infant during labor and delivery. These injuries may result from inappropriate or deficient medical skill or attention, or they may occur despite skilled and competent obstetric care and independent of any acts or omissions of the parents. In order to avoid later misunderstandings, recriminations, or parental guilt, it is important to counsel parents who have a child with a residuum from birth trauma or anoxia about this broad use of the term birth injury. The definition does not include injury from amniocentesis, intrauterine transfusion, scalp vein sampling, or resuscitation procedures, which are discussed elsewhere.

The incidence of birth injuries has been estimated at 2–7/1000 live births. Predisposing factors include macrosomia, prematurity, cephalopelvic disproportion, dystocia, prolonged labor, and breech presentation. Although the incidence has decreased in recent years, in part owing to refinement in obstetric techniques and judgment, birth injuries still represent an important problem because even transient injuries are frequently readily apparent to the parents and result in anxiety and questions that require supportive and informative counseling. Some injuries may be latent initially, but later result in severe illness or sequelae.

7.22 CRANIAL INJURIES

Caput succedaneum is a diffuse sometimes ecchymotic, edematous swelling of the soft tissues of the scalp involving the portion presenting during vertex delivery. It may extend across the midline and across suture lines. The edema disappears within the 1st few days of life. Analogous swelling, discoloration, and distortion of the face are seen in face presentations. No specific treatment is needed, but if there are extensive ecchymoses, early phototherapy for hyperbilirubinemia may be indicated. *Molding* of the head and overriding of the parietal bones are frequently associated with caput succedaneum and become more evident after the caput has receded, but disappear during the 1st weeks of life. Rarely, a hemorrhagic caput may result in shock and require blood transfusion.

Erythema, abrasions, ecchymoses and *subcutaneous fat necrosis* of soft tissues may be seen after forceps deliveries. Their location depends upon the area of application of the forceps. Ecchymoses may be seen after manipulative deliveries and occasionally in premature infants for no discernible reason.

Subconjunctival hemorrhages are frequent, and *petechiae* of the skin of the head and neck are common. All are probably secondary to a sudden increase in intrathoracic pressure during passage of the chest through the birth canal. Parents should be assured that they are temporary and the result of *normal* hazards of delivery.

Cephalhematoma (Fig 7–17) is a subperiosteal hemorrhage, hence always limited to the surface of 1 cranial bone. There is no discoloration of the overlying scalp due to subcutaneous hemorrhage and swelling is usually not visible until several hr after birth, since subperiosteal bleeding is a slow process. An underlying skull fracture, usually linear and not depressed, is occasionally associated with cephalhematoma. Cranial meningocele may be differentiated from cephalhematoma by pulsation, increased pressure on crying, and the roentgenographic evidence of bony defect. Most cephalhematomas are resorbed within 2 wk–3 mo, depending upon their size. They may begin to calcify by the end of the 2nd wk. A sensation of central depression suggesting underlying fracture or bony defect is usually encountered on palpation of the organized rim of a cephalhematoma. A few remain as bony protuberances for years and are detectable roentgenographically as widening of the diploic space; cyst-like defects may persist for months or years. Despite these residuals, cephalhematomas require no treatment, although phototherapy may be necessary to ameliorate hyperbilirubinemia. Incision and drainage are contraindicated because of the risk of introducing infection in a benign condition. Rarely, a massive cephalhematoma may result in blood loss severe enough to require transfusion,

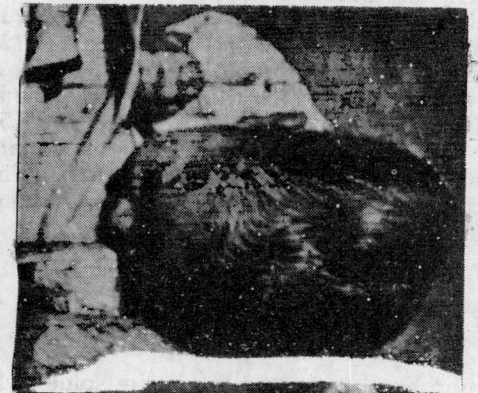

Figure 7–17 Cephalhematoma of the right parietal bone.

or there may be an associated skull fracture and intracranial hemorrhage.

Fractures of the skull may occur as a result of pressure from forceps or from the maternal symphysis pubis, sacral promontory, or ischial spines. Linear fractures are most common, cause no symptoms, and require no treatment. Depressed fractures are usually indentations of the calvarium similar to a dent in a ping-pong ball; usually they are a complication of forceps delivery. The infant may be asymptomatic unless there is associated intracranial injury; it is advisable to elevate such depressions to prevent cortical injury from sustained pressure. Fracture of the occipital bone with separation of the basal and squamous portions almost invariably causes fatal hemorrhage owing to disruption of the underlying sinuses. It may result during breech deliveries from traction on the hyperextended spine of the infant with the head fixed in the maternal pelvis.

7.23 INTRACRANIAL HEMORRHAGE

Intracranial hemorrhage may result from trauma or asphyxia and, rarely, from a primary hemorrhagic disturbance or congenital vascular anomaly. Traumatic hemorrhage is especially likely when the fetal head is large in proportion to the size of the mother's pelvic outlet; when for other reasons the labor is prolonged; when there are breech or precipitate deliveries; or when there is injudicious mechanical interference with delivery. The proper use of forceps may decrease the incidence of intracranial bleeding in prolonged hard labors. Intracranial hemorrhages may occur in infants, especially premature ones, delivered spontaneously without apparent trauma.

In premature infants subependymal, subarachnoid, intracerebral, and intraventricular hemorrhages are common. The highly vascularized periventricular subependymal germinal matrix is a particularly vulnerable region in the fetus and premature infant during the 1st wk of life. Anoxic injury, birth trauma, or neonatal circulatory disturbances such as hypervolemia and hypertension or shock may result in thrombosis, periventricular leukomalacia and/or bleeding, and intraventricular hemorrhage. Excessive use of sodium bicarbonate and elevated carbon dioxide tension have also been associated with intraventricular hemorrhage in premature infants. Massive subdural hemorrhages, often associated with tears in the tentorium cerebelli or less frequently in the falx cerebri, are rare but encountered more often in fullterm than in premature infants.

Primary hemorrhagic disturbances usually give rise to subarachnoid hemorrhage, and vascular anomalies to subarachnoid or intracerebral hemorrhage. Intracranial bleeding may be associated with disseminated intravascular coagulopathy or idiopathic thrombocytopenia.

Clinical Manifestations. Although intraventricular and subependymal hemorrhages may be present at birth in premature infants and occasionally are immediately symptomatic, clinical manifestations of intracranial hemorrhage usually appear at a variable time after delivery. The most common symptoms are a general failure to move normally, diminished or absent

Moro reflex, poor muscle tone, lethargy, and somnolence. Irregularity of respirations in the absence of other signs of respiratory distress is often a sign of severe hemorrhage. In premature infants with intraventricular hemorrhage there is often a precipitous deterioration on the 2nd or 3rd day of life. Periods of apnea, pallor, or cyanosis, failure to suck well, forceful vomiting, abnormal eye signs, anxiety and restlessness, a high-pitched, shrill cry, muscular twitchings, convulsions, decreased muscle tone, paralyses, and a deceased hematocrit or failure to increase it after transfusion may be the 1st indications. The fontanel *may* be tense and bulging, and an adder-like protrusion of the tongue may be seen. Retinal hemorrhage, ocular palsies, inequality in size and failure of the pupils to react to light, nystagmus, or hyperpyrexia may be observed. In a small percentage there may be no clinical manifestations.

Diagnosis. This is based chiefly on the history of delivery, the clinical manifestations, and the course. Since nonlocalizing signs of intracranial hemorrhage are identical with those caused by cerebral edema or anoxia, before carrying out any diagnostic procedure, the physician should weigh the chance of helping the patient against the risk of the procedure. In the absence of an obstetric history of intrapartum hemorrhage, of other signs of bleeding or of extensive bruising in the infant, or of iatrogenic removal of large quantities of blood, a significant fall in hematocrit should suggest the diagnosis of intracranial hemorrhage or that of subcapsular hemorrhage of the liver. Computed tomography (CT scan) of the head is a particularly sensitive method of diagnosing intracranial hemorrhage in the neonatal infant; ultrasonography may be similarly useful. Subdural taps, although occasionally valuable, are usually unrewarding, even in the presence of subdural hemorrhage, since it is likely that the blood will have clotted; they may, however, on occasion be lifesaving. Ventricular taps are rarely done because the possibility is remote that it will be either diagnostically or therapeutically efficacious. Lumbar puncture is indicated in the presence of signs of increased intracranial pressure or deteriorating clinical condition to identify gross subarachnoid hemorrhage or to rule out the possibility of bacterial meningitis; the cerebrospinal fluid usually has elevated protein levels with many red blood cells. Not infrequently there is hypoglycorrhachia and a mild lymphocytosis. Apnea, bradycardia, or circulatory insufficiency may occur as a consequence of the physical manipulation of performing a lumbar puncture in a premature infant.

Since a small amount of bleeding into the cerebrospinal fluid often occurs in the course of normal and even cesarean deliveries, small numbers of red blood cells or slight xanthochromia in subarachnoid fluid is not necessarily indicative of significant intracranial hemorrhage. Conversely, the subarachnoid fluid may be absolutely clear with severe subdural or intracerebral hemorrhage when there is no communication with the subarachnoid space.

Prognosis. Intrapartum death may occur in the more severe cases; postnatally, fatalities usually occur within the 1st wk and result from respiratory failure. If an infant survives, recovery may be complete, or there may be permanent residuals, mainly cerebral palsy and hydrocephalus. Some of the membrane-enclosed subdural effusions observed in later infancy may have their origin in subdural hemorrhage at birth. Prior to the availability of the CT scan, the diagnosis in the surviving or asymptomatic patient was rarely certain.

Because the majority of parents are aware of and fear the possibility of cerebral residuals following intracranial hemorrhage or cerebral anoxia, it is usually wisest to give them an opportunity to air their anxiety in a frank discussion of the problem, during which their questions should be invited rather than suppressed or evaded. As optimistic an attitude as possible, consistent with the physician's opinion of the prognosis of the individual case, should be maintained.

Prevention. Prophylactic measures include continuing improvements in obstetric and pediatric management; many instances of intracranial hemorrhage are avoidable. Wide swings of blood pressure and pCO_2 should be avoided. In addition, judicious use of sodium bicarbonate is indicated.

Treatment. The infant should be handled as little and as gently as possible and maintained in an incubator that allows good temperature control, continuous observation, and easy administration of oxygen for cyanosis. Phenobarbital or other anticonvulsant drugs in appropriate doses may be used to control convulsive movement. A small dose of vitamin K_1 oxide (Sec 7.49) and a transfusion of fresh frozen plasma are indicated in the presence of hemorrhagic disease of the newborn. The management of disseminated intravascular coagulopathy is discussed in Sec 14.69. There is lack of agreement about the advisability of serial spinal punctures for the relief of increased intracranial pressure and for removal of blood to reduce its irritant effect on the cerebral cortex or to prevent possible interference with the normal resorptive mechanisms for cerebrospinal fluid. Neurosurgical procedures are not indicated unless hydrocephalus is uncontrolled by other measures, such as repeated lumbar punctures.

Cerebral edema may result in any or all of the clinical signs produced by intracranial hemorrhage. Trauma and asphyxia are the most common causes. It is usually not possible to establish this diagnosis during life except by inference from the obstetric history. Anterior fontanel pressure may be monitored externally to detect changes in intracranial pressure, but the technique is not generally available or well established. Treatment includes avoidance or correction of dilutional hyponatremia. The indications for and benefits of reducing increased intracranial pressure from edema by removal of cerebrospinal fluid, by the parenteral administration of dexamethasone (10 mg/M^2 initially, then 5 mg/M^2 every 6 hr), or by intravenous infusions of mannitol in neonatal infants have not been established. They may be indicated if an infant's condition is deteriorating with rapidly progressing neurologic signs.

7.24 SPINE AND SPINAL CORD

Strong traction exerted when the spine is hyperextended or when the direction of pull is lateral, or forceful longitudinal traction on the trunk while the head is still firmly engaged in the pelvis, especially when combined with flexion and torsion of the vertical axis, may produce fracture and separation of the vertebrae. Such injuries are rarely diagnosed clinically. They are most likely to occur when difficulty is encountered in delivering the shoulders in cephalic presentations and the head in breech presentations. The injury is most commonly at the level of the 7th cervical and 1st thoracic vertebrae. Transection of the cord may occur, but hemorrhage and edema may produce neurologic signs indistinguishable from those of transection, except that they are not permanent. There is complete paralysis of voluntary motion below the level of injury, although the persistence of a withdrawal reflex mediated through spinal centers distal to the area of injury is frequently misinterpreted as representing voluntary motion. The infant may be in poor condition from birth with respiratory depression, shock, and hypothermia, and, if the injury is severe, may deteriorate rapidly to death within several hr, before neurologic signs are obvious. Alternatively, the course may be protracted with symptoms and signs appearing at birth or later in the 1st wk; immobility, flaccidity, and associated brachial plexus injuries may not be recognized for several days. Constipation may also be present. Some infants survive for prolonged periods with initial flaccidity, immobility, and areflexia being replaced after several wk or mo by rigid flexion of extremities, increased muscle tone, and spasms.

The differential diagnosis includes amyotonia congenita and myelodysplasia associated with spina bifida occulta. In the survivors treatment is supportive and there is often permanent injury. When there is compression from a fracture or dislocation, the prognosis is related to the time elapsing before the compression is removed.

7.25 PERIPHERAL NERVE INJURIES

Brachial Palsy. Injury to the brachial plexus may cause paralysis of the upper arm with or without paralysis of the forearm or hand or, more commonly, paralysis of the entire arm. These injuries occur when lateral traction is exerted on the head and neck during delivery of the shoulder in a vertex presentation, when the arms are extended over the head in a breech

presentation, or when there is excessive traction on the shoulders.

In **Erb-Duchenne paralysis** the injury is limited to the 5th and 6th cervical nerves. The infant loses the power to abduct the arm from the shoulder, to rotate the arm externally, and to supinate the forearm. The characteristic position consists of adduction and internal rotation of the arm with pronation of the forearm. The power of extension of the forearm is retained, but the biceps reflex is absent. The Moro reflex is absent on the affected side (Fig 7–18). There may be some sensory impairment on the outer aspect of the arm. The power in the forearm and the hand grasp are preserved unless the lower part of the plexus is also injured; the presence of the hand grasp is a favorable prognostic sign. When the injury includes the phrenic nerve, alteration of the diaphragmatic excursion may be observed fluoroscopically.

Klumpke paralysis is a rarer form of brachial palsy; injury to the 7th and 8th cervical nerves and the 1st thoracic nerve produces a paralyzed hand and ipsilateral ptosis and miosis if the sympathetic fibers of the 1st thoracic root are also injured.

The mild cases may not be detected immediately after birth. Differentiation must be made from cerebral injury; from fracture, dislocation, or epiphyseal separation of the humerus; and from fracture of the clavicle.

The *prognosis* depends upon whether the nerve was merely injured or was lacerated. If the paralysis was due to edema and hemorrhage about the nerve fibers, there should be a return of function within a few mo; if due to laceration, permanent damage may result. The involvement of the deltoid is usually the most serious problem and may result in a shoulder drop secondary to muscular atrophy. In general, paralysis of the upper arm has a better prognosis than paralysis of the lower arm.

Treatment consists of partial immobilization and appropriate positioning to prevent development of contractures. In upper arm paralysis, the arm should be abducted 90 degrees, with external rotation at the shoulder and with full supination of the forearm and slight extension at the wrist with the palm turned toward the face. This may be done with a brace or splint during the 1st 1–2 wk. Immobilization should be intermittent through the day while the infant is asleep and between feedings. In lower arm or hand paralysis, the wrist should be splinted in a neutral position and padding

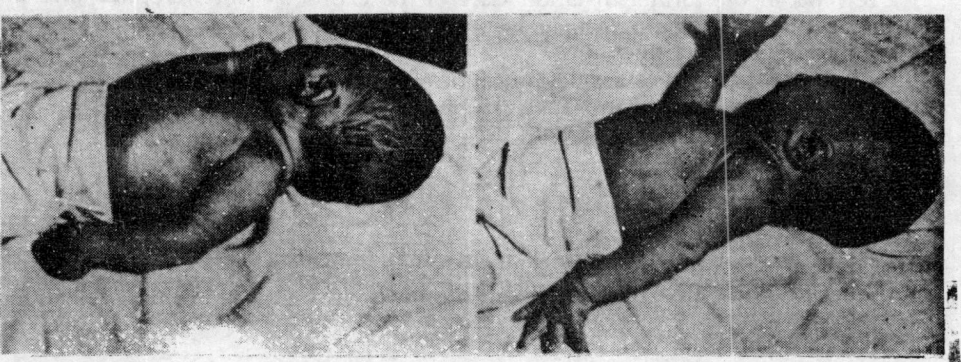

Figure 7–18 Brachial palsy of the left arm (asymmetric Moro reflex).

placed in the fist. When the entire arm is paralyzed, the same treatment principles should be followed. Gentle massage and range of motion exercises may be started by 7–10 days of age. Infants should be followed closely with active and passive corrective exercises. If the paralysis persists without improvement for 3–6 mo neuroplasty and tendon transfers offer hope for partial recovery but are usually not advisable before 3–4 yr of age when muscle development can be adequately assessed.

Phrenic Nerve Paralysis. Phrenic nerve injury with diaphragmatic paralysis must be considered when cyanosis and irregular and labored respirations develop. Such injuries are usually unilateral and associated with homolateral upper brachial palsy. Because breathing is thoracic in type, there is no bulging of the abdomen with inspiration. Breath sounds are diminished on the affected side. The thrust of the diaphragm, which often may be felt just under the costal margin on the normal side, is absent on the affected side. The *diagnosis* is established by fluoroscopic examination, which reveals the elevation of the diaphragm on the paralyzed side and seesaw movements of the 2 sides of the diaphragm during respiration.

There is no specific *treatment*; the infant should be placed on the involved side and given oxygen if necessary. Initially, intravenous feedings may be needed; later, progressive gavage or oral feedings may be started depending on the infant's condition. Pulmonary infections are a serious complication. Recovery usually occurs spontaneously by 1–3 mo; rarely, surgical plication of the diaphragm may be indicated.

Facial Nerve Palsy. Usually, facial palsy is a peripheral paralysis that results from pressure over the facial nerve in utero, during labor, or from forceps during delivery. Rarely it is nonobstetric, resulting from nuclear agenesis of the facial nerve. Peripheral paralysis is flaccid and, when complete, involves the entire side of the face, including the forehead. When the infant cries, there is movement on only the nonparalyzed side of the face, and the mouth is drawn to that side. On the affected side the forehead is smooth, the eye cannot be closed, the nasolabial fold is absent, and the corner of the mouth droops. The forehead will wrinkle on the affected side with central paralysis, since only the lower two thirds of the face is involved. Usually there are also other manifestations of intracranial injury, most commonly a 6th nerve palsy. The *prognosis* depends upon whether the nerve was injured by pressure or whether the nerve fibers were torn. Improvement occurs within a few wk in the former instance. Care of the exposed eye is essential. Neuroplasty may be indicated when the paralysis is persistent.

Other peripheral nerves are seldom injured at birth, except as they are involved in fractures or hemorrhages (Sec 12.56).

7.26   VISCERA

The liver is the only internal organ other than the brain injured with any frequency during birth. The damage usually occurs from pressure on the liver during delivery of the head in breech presentations. Large infant size, intrauterine asphyxia, coagulation disorders, and hepatomegaly are contributing factors. Incorrect cardiac massage is a less frequent cause. The liver is ruptured with formation of a subcapsular hematoma. The infant usually appears normal for the 1st 1–3 days. Nonspecific signs related to loss of blood into the hematoma may appear early and include poor feeding, listlessness, pallor, jaundice, tachypnea, and tachycardia. A mass may be palpable in the right upper quadrant. The hematoma may be large enough to cause anemia. Shock and death may occur if the hematoma breaks through the capsule into the peritoneal cavity reducing pressure and allowing fresh hemorrhage. Early suspicion and diagnosis, and prompt supportive therapy, can decrease the mortality of this disorder. Surgical repair of a laceration may be required.

Rupture of the spleen may occur in association with rupture of the liver. The causes, complications, treatment, and prevention are similar.

Although **adrenal hemorrhage** occurs with some frequency, especially after breech delivery, it is not known whether it is due to trauma, anoxia, or severe stress as in overwhelming infections. Calcified central hematomas of the adrenal have been identified roentgenographically or at autopsy in older infants and children suggesting that not all adrenal hemorrhages are fatal. In severe cases the diagnosis is usually made at post mortem examination. The symptoms are profound shock and cyanosis. There may be a mass in the flank with overlying skin discoloration; jaundice may also develop. If adrenal hemorrhage is suspected, abdominal ultrasonography may be helpful and treatment for acute adrenal failure may be indicated (Sec 18.22).

INJURY OF THE STERNOCLEIDOMASTOID

See Torticollis, Sec 23.7.

7.27   FRACTURES

Clavicle. This bone is fractured more frequently than any other bone during labor and delivery and is particularly vulnerable when there is difficulty in delivery of the shoulder in vertex presentations and of the extended arms in breech deliveries. The infant characteristically does not move the arm freely on the affected side; crepitus and bony irregularity may be palpated and occasionally discoloration is visible over the fracture site. The Moro reflex is absent on the affected side, and there is spasm of the sternocleidomastoid muscle with obliteration of the supraclavicular depression at the site of the fracture. In greenstick fractures there may be no limitation of movement and the Moro reflex may be present. Fracture of the humerus or brachial palsy may also be responsible for limitation of movement of an arm and the absence of a Moro reflex on the affected side. The *prognosis* is excellent. *Treatment*, if any, consists in immobilization of the arm and shoulder on the affected side. A remarkable degree of callus develops within a week at the site and may be the first evidence of the fracture.

Extremities. In fractures of the long bones spontaneous movement of the extremity is usually absent. The Moro reflex is also absent from the involved extremity. There may be associated nerve involvement. Satisfactory results for a fractured humerus are obtained with 2–4 wk of immobilization by strapping the arm to the chest, by applying a triangular splint and a Velpeau bandage, or by application of a cast. For fracture of the femur, good results are obtained with traction-suspension of both lower extremities, even if the fracture is unilateral; the legs, immobilized in a spica cast, are attached to an overhead frame. Splints are effective for treatment of fractures of the forearm or leg. Healing is usually accompanied by excess callus formation. The *prognosis* is excellent for fractures of the extremities.

Dislocations and **epiphyseal separations** rarely result from birth trauma. The upper femoral epiphysis may be separated by forcible manipulation of the infant's leg as, for example, in breech extraction or after version. There is swelling, slight shortening, limitation of active motion, painful passive motion, and external rotation of the leg. The diagnosis is established roentgenographically. The prognosis is good for the milder injuries, but coxa vara frequently results from extensive displacement.

Nose. The most prevalent injury of the nose is a dislocation of the cartilaginous portion of the septum from the vomerine groove and the columella. The infant may have difficulty in nursing with some impairment in nasal respiration. On physical examination the nares appear asymmetrical and the nose flattened. An oral airway should be provided immediately and surgical consultation obtained for definitive treatment.

7.28   ANOXIA

Anoxia is a term used to indicate the consequences of lack of oxygen from a number of primary causes. It is the leading immediate cause of perinatal death or of permanent damage to central nervous system cells, which is manifest later as cerebral palsy or mental deficiency. Its prevention and treatment are those of the basic conditions that cause it, though death and disability may sometimes be prevented through symptomatic treatment with oxygen or artificial respiration and the correction of associated metabolic acidosis with sodium bicarbonate.

Etiology. Fetal anoxia may result from (1) inadequate oxygenation of maternal blood as a result of hypoventilation during anesthesia, cardiac failure, or carbon monoxide poisoning; (2) low maternal blood pressure as a result of the hypotension that may complicate spinal anesthesia or that may result from compression of the vena cava and aorta by the gravid uterus; (3) inadequate relaxation of the uterus to permit placental filling as a result of uterine tetany caused by excessive administration of oxytocin; (4) premature separation of the placenta; (5) impedance to the circulation of blood through the umbilical cord as a result of compression or knotting of the cord; and (6) placental inadequacy from numerous causes, including toxemia and postmaturity (Sec 7.6).

After birth, anoxia may result from (1) anemia severe enough to lower the oxygen content of the blood to a critical level owing to severe hemorrhage or hemolytic disease; (2) shock severe enough to interfere with the transport of oxygen to vital cells from adrenal hemorrhage, intraventricular hemorrhage, overwhelming infection, or massive blood loss; (3) a deficit in arterial oxygen saturation from failure to breathe adequately postnatally, owing to narcosis or cerebral defect or injury; and (4) failure of oxygenation of an adequate amount of blood from severe forms of cyanotic congenital heart disease or deficient pulmonary ventilation.

Pathology. The pathologic changes of anoxia are principally those caused by congestion and increased capillary permeability. Congestion and petechiae are found in all organs but are especially noticeable in the pleura, pericardium, thymus, adrenals, brain, and meninges. Cerebral edema is common. Gross subarachnoid, intraventricular, or adrenal hemorrhage may be present without demonstrable tearing of blood vessels. Histologic study of the brain and liver, particularly the right lobe, may reveal cellular degenerative changes similar to those produced experimentally by anoxia. Fetal anoxia is characterized pathologically by the additional finding of large amounts of amniotic debris in the respiratory passages. Pathophysiologically, within minutes of the onset of total fetal anoxia there is bradycardia, hypotension, decreased cardiac output, and severe metabolic as well as respiratory acidosis. The initial circulatory response of the fetus to anoxia is with increased shunting through the ductus venosus, ductus arteriosus, and foramen ovale with transient maintenance of perfusion of the brain, heart, and adrenals in preference to the lungs (due to pulmonary vasoconstriction), liver, kidneys, and intestine.

Clinical Manifestations. The signs of anoxia in the *fetus* are usually noted a few min to a few days before delivery. The fetal heart rate slows, and the beat may become weak and irregular. Continuous heart rate recording may reveal a variable or late (type II dips) deceleration pattern, and scalp blood analysis may show a pH less than 7.20. The acidosis is made up of varying degrees of metabolic and/or respiratory components. Particularly in the infant near term, these signs should lead to the administration of high concentrations of oxygen to the mother and to immediate delivery to avoid fetal death or central nervous system damage.

At *delivery* the presence of yellow, meconium-stained amniotic fluid and vernix caseosa is evidence that there has been fetal distress, probably anoxic. At birth these infants are frequently depressed and fail to breathe spontaneously. During the ensuing hours they may remain hypotonic or change from hypotonia to extreme hypertonia, or their tone may appear normal. Pallor, cyanosis, apnea, slow heart rate, and unresponsiveness to stimulation also are signs of anoxia. Cerebral edema may develop during the next 24 hr and result in profound brainstem depression. During this time seizure activity may occur; it may be severe and refractory to the usual doses of anticonvulsants. Though most often a result of the hypoxic-ischemic encephalopathy, seizures in asphyxiated newborns may also be due to hypocalcemia and hypoglycemia.

In addition to central nervous system dysfunction, congestive heart failure and cardiogenic shock, persistent fetal circulation, respiratory distress syndrome, gastrointestinal perforation, hematuria, and acute tubular necrosis are also associated with perinatal asphyxia.

After delivery anoxia is due to respiratory failure and circulatory insufficiency (Sec 7.29 and 7.34).

Prognosis. Most of the deaths and cerebral damage that result from anoxia are probably due to late fetal or postnatal periods of anoxia. Early detection of signs of fetal distress by continuous monitoring of fetal heart rate and by serial determinations of acid-base balance in fetal scalp blood samples during labor may significantly decrease this morbidity and mortality by providing improved criteria for obstetric intervention in labor (Sec 7.4). Although the incidence of asphyxia is higher in the more premature infants, the increased risk of death from it is greater in more mature infants, e.g., increased over 100-fold for those greater than 36 wk gestation. Survival is directly related to gestational age, and postasphyxial seizures are associated with a poor prognosis.

7.29   PEDIATRIC EMERGENCIES IN THE DELIVERY ROOM

The most common and important emergency related to the newborn infant in the delivery room is the failure to initiate and maintain respirations. Less frequent, but of major importance, are shock, severe anemia, plethora, convulsions, and management of life-threatening congenital malformations.

Respiratory Distress and Failure. Disorders of respiration in the newborn infant can be categorized as either *central nervous system failure*, representing depression or failure of the respiratory center, or *peripheral respiratory difficulty*, indicating interference with the alveolar exchange of oxygen and carbon dioxide (Table 7–16). Cyanosis occurs in both groups. The respiratory problems encountered in the delivery room are most frequently those of airway obstruction and of depression of the central nervous system with the absence of adequate respiratory effort.

Respiratory distress in the presence of good respiratory effort should lead to an immediate consideration of peripheral causes; *it is an indication for a roentgenographic examination of the chest* if this is at all possible without undue risk for the infant.

If respiratory movements are made with the mouth closed but the infant fails to move air in and out of the lungs, bilateral choanal atresia (Sec 12.25) or other obstruction of the upper respiratory tract should be suspected. The mouth should be opened, and the mouth and posterior pharynx cleared of secretions by gentle suction. Nasal obstruction or hypoplasia of the

mandible, as in Pierre Robin syndrome, can be identified and relieved by pulling the tongue forward to allow air exchange. An oropharyngeal airway should be inserted and the source of the obstruction sought immediately. If effective respiratory flow is not produced by opening the infant's mouth and clearing the airway, laryngoscopy is indicated. With obstructive malformations of the epiglottis, larynx, or trachea, an endotracheal tube should be inserted; prolonged nasotracheal intubation or tracheostomy may be required. Respiratory failure from depression or injury of the central nervous system may require continuous artificial ventilation with a face mask and bag or through an endotracheal or nasotracheal tube.

Hypoplasia of the mandible (Sec 11.2) with posterior displacement of the tongue may result in symptoms similar to those of choanal atresia; they may be temporarily relieved by pulling the tongue forward. A scaphoid abdomen suggests a **diaphragmatic hernia** or **eventration**, as does asymmetry of contour or movement of the chest or shift of the apical impulse of the heart; these latter manifestations are also compatible with tension pneumothorax and cardiac abnormalities. Causes of peripheral respiratory difficulty are discussed in Sec 7.30.

Failure to Initiate or Sustain Respiration. This usually originates in the central nervous system; immaturity in itself is seldom a causative factor except in very low birth weight infants (< 800 gm). Intrapulmonary problems, such as the pulmonary hypoplasia associated with Potter syndrome and severe organized intrauterine pneumonia, may at times result in poorly sustained ventilation. The lungs in these infants are very noncompliant, and the initial efforts to begin respirations may be unable to start adequate ventilation.

Narcosis results from heavy doses of morphine, Demerol, barbiturates, reserpine, or tranquilizers administered to the mother shortly before delivery or from maternal anesthesia, especially if prolonged, during delivery. The infant is cyanotic at birth and slow to cry or breathe; when respiration is established, it is extremely slow.

Narcosis is rarely excusable and should be avoided by appropriate analgesic and anesthetic practices (Sec 5.50).

Treatment includes initial physical stimulation and securing a patent airway. If effective ventilation is not initiated, artificial breathing with a mask and bag must be instituted. At the same time, if depression is due to morphine or its derivatives, Narcan (naloxone hydrochloride), 0.01 mg/kg, should be given by either intravenous or intramuscular routes. Ventilation is essential prior to and during the administration of this antidote. If depression is due to other anesthetics or analgesics, artificial respiration should be continued until the infant is able to sustain his or her own ventilation. Central nervous system stimulant drugs should not be used as they are ineffective and may be harmful.

Prenatal or **perinatal anoxia**, whatever the cause, if sufficiently severe, will produce a central nervous system type of respiratory failure, secondary apnea, which does not respond to sensory stimulation. Death is due to apnea and may be prevented by resuscitation, pro-

Table 7-16 RESPIRATORY DISTRESS AND FAILURE IN NEWBORN INFANTS

TYPE	MANIFESTATIONS	CLINICAL ENTITY
Central nervous system failure	Apnea Slow, irregular, gasping respiratory efforts	Narcosis Prenatal or perinatal anoxia Intracranial hemorrhage or trauma CNS anomalies
Peripheral respiratory difficulty	Rapid respiratory rate Increasing respiratory rate Chest lag Intercostal retraction Subcostal retraction Xiphoid retraction Chin tug Expiratory grunt Frothing at lips	Primary atelectasis Congestive pulmonary failure Hyaline membrane disease Aspiration of amniotic fluid containing formed elements Pneumonia Diaphragmatic hernia Lung cysts Lobar emphysema Pneumothorax Aspiration of food or mucus

vided the basic cause of the anoxia can be eliminated within a reasonable time and while artificial respiration, if necessary, is being carried out. External cardiac massage, correction of acidosis, and circulatory support may be important adjuncts to ventilation. Hypothermia as a means of temporarily reducing metabolic needs for oxygen during the period of hypoxia or anoxia is contraindicated.

Intracranial hemorrhage and **trauma** are discussed in Sec 7.22 and 7.23. **Central nervous system anomalies** may be responsible for respiratory failure.

Resuscitation. Failure to breathe spontaneously within 1 min of birth is an indication for resuscitation. If the central mechanism can be revived, the infant will be more effective in ventilating the lungs safely than will any available artificial technique.

After the upper and central airway has been cleared as adequately as possible by removal of accumulated liquid contents, resuscitation should start with simple, gentle physical stimulation such as slapping the soles of the feet with a finger or repeatedly passing a nasal catheter. If this is unsuccessful, the upper respiratory passage should be suctioned again and a flow of oxygen directed at the infant's face. If the infant has an Apgar score of 4 or less, or if the pulse rate is less than 80 beats/min, artificial respiration or pulmonary inflation is indicated. Administration of oxygen at 16–20 cm of H_2O pressure for 1–2 sec, added to stimulus of chemoreceptors, initiates a gasp in about 85% of patients. If the Apgar score is 2 or less or if a gentle flow of oxygen at pressures up to 25 cm of H_2O administered either steadily or in puffs through a face mask does not produce improved color and tone followed by spontaneous respiratory movements, direct laryngoscopy and endotracheal intubation are indicated and should include suctioning of the lower respiratory passages and an attempt to inflate the lungs through the application of short bursts of oxygen at higher pressures.

Maintenance of the circulation through closed chest cardiac massage at a rate of 100 or more/min is an important adjunct to artificial respiration in infants in circulatory collapse with slow, weak heart beats. This must be synchronized with ventilation with 100% oxygen at a rate of 30–40 inflations/min. Laryngoscopy, intubation, and cardiac massage should be carried out by personnel skilled in the techniques, of whom there should be one in every delivery room. Negative intrathoracic pressures between 20–70 cm of H_2O have been recorded during the 1st few breaths; positive pressure much lower than 20 cm of H_2O is unlikely to introduce oxygen into the lungs. Pressures of greater than 25 cm may rupture the lung if only a small area is being expanded.

Mouth-to-mouth breathing has been successful in resuscitating some infants but may be harmful because of alveolar rupture from uncontrolled pressures or introduction of infection.

After the airway has been cleared and adequate ventilation provided, severely asphyxiated and acidotic infants often require the slow (1 ml/min) administration of sodium bicarbonate (2–3 mEq/kg) through an umbilical catheter to correct the associated metabolic acidosis; a solution containing 0.5 mEq of sodium bicarbonate/ml is used. It may also be necessary to administer epinephrine (0.1 ml/kg of a 1:10,000 solution) via catheter or intracardiac injection to combat hypotension, bradycardia, or poor cardiac output. The umbilical vein should be used if a catheter cannot be inserted in the artery as this procedure is easier during emergency conditions. Respiratory stimulants are contraindicated.

Shock. Circulatory insufficiency may present at birth as a result of internal hemorrhage; fetal bleeding during gestation, labor, or delivery (e.g., feto-fetal or feto-maternal transfusion syndrome); bleeding from the fetal circulation secondary to a placental tear; excessive bleeding from a severed or torn umbilical cord; or severe hemolytic anemia. Clinical manifestations include signs of respiratory distress; cyanosis; pallor; flaccidity; cold, mottled skin; tachypnea or bradycardia; hepatosplenomegaly; and, rarely, convulsions. **Edema** and hepatosplenomegaly also may present in erythroblastosis fetalis or congestive heart failure without shock.

Supportive treatment with type O, Rh negative blood, plasma, or electrolyte solutions is indicated for hypovolemia. Oxygen should be administered and metabolic acidosis corrected with sodium bicarbonate. β-Sympathomimetic agents such as dopamine may need to be employed. The diagnosis and treatment of erythroblastosis fetalis is discussed in Sec 7.47.

After supportive measures have stabilized the infant's

condition, a specific diagnosis should be established and appropriate continuing treatment instituted.

Adamsons K, Behrman R, Dawes GS, et al: The treatment of acidosis with alkali and glucose during asphyxia in fetal rhesus monkeys. J Physiol 169:679, 1963.

Apgar V, James LS: Further observations on the newborn scoring system. Am J Dis Child 104:419, 1962.

Behrman RE, James LS, Klaus MH, et al: Treatment of the asphyxiated newborn infant. J Pediatr 79:981, 1969.

Behrman RE, Mangurten HH: Birth injuries. In Behrman RE (ed): Neonatal-Perinatal Medicine. St Louis, CV Mosby, 1977.

Bejar R, Curbalo V, Coen R, et al: Diagnosis and follow-up of intraventricular and intracerebral hemorrhages by ultrasound studies of infant's brain through the fontanelles and sutures. Pediatrics 66:661, 1980.

Daniel SS, James LS: Abnormal renal function in the newborn infant. J Pediatr 88:856, 1976.

Dray JS, Kennedy C, Berendes H, et al: The Apgar score as an index of infant morbidity. A report from the collaborative study of cerebral palsy. Dev Med Child Neurol 8:141, 1966.

Gregory G: Resuscitation of the newborn. Anesthesiology 43:225, 1975.

Holden KR, Mellits ED, Freeman JM: Neonatal seizures. I. Correlation of prenatal and perinatal events with outcome. Pediatrics 70:165, 1982.

James LS: Acidosis of the newborn and its relation to birth asphyxia. Acta Pediatr (Upps) 49 (Suppl 122):17, 1960.

Lees MH: Cyanosis of the newborn infant. J Pediatr 77:484, 1970.

MacDonald H, Mulligan J, Allen A, et al: Neonatal asphyxia. I. Relationship of obstetric and neonatal complications to neonatal mortality in 38,405 consecutive deliveries. J Pediatr 96:898, 1980.

Mellits ED, Holden KR, Freeman JM: Neonatal seizures. II. A multivariate analysis of factors associated with outcome. Pediatrics 70:177, 1982.

Ment LR, Scott DT, Ehrenkranz RA, et al: Neonates of ≤1,250 grams birth weight: Prospective neurodevelopmental evaluation during the first year postterm. Pediatrics 70:292, 1982.

Mulligan J, Painter M, O'Donoghue P, et al: Neonatal asphyxia. II. Neonatal mortality and long term sequelae. J Pediatr 96:903, 1980.

Oliver TK Jr, Demis JA, Bates GD: Serial blood-gas tensions and acid-base balance during the first hour of life in human infants. Acta Pediatr 50:346, 1961.

Papile L, Burstein J, Burstein R, et al: Incidence and evolution of subependymal and intraventricular hemorrhage: A study of infants with birth weights less than 1500 grams. J Pediatr 92:529, 1978.

Schrager GO: Elevation of depressed skull fracture with a breast pump. J Pediatr 77:300, 1970.

Silverman SH, Liebow SG: Dislocation of the triangular cartilage of the nasal septum. J Pediatr 87:456, 1975.

Volpe J: Neonatal seizures. Clin Perinatol 4:43, 1977.

Volpe J, Pasternak JF: Parasagittal cerebral injury in neonatal hypoxic-ischemic encephalopathy: Clinical and neuroradiologic features. J Pediatr 92:472, 1977.

Zelson C, Lee SJ, Pearl M: The incidence of skull fractures underlying cephalhematomas in newborn infants. J Pediatr 85:371, 1974.

Disturbances of Organ Systems

7.30 DISTURBANCES OF THE RESPIRATORY TRACT

Disturbances of respiration in the immediate postnatal period may have had their origin in utero, in the delivery room, or in the nursery. A wide variety of pathologic lesions may be responsible for 1 or more of the signs of respiratory distress or failure (Table 7–16 and Fig 7–3); if respiratory embarrassment is severe, pallor or cyanosis may also be present. It is occasionally very difficult to distinguish cardiovascular from respiratory disturbances on the basis of clinical signs alone. Signs of respiratory distress in the newborn infant may suggest hyaline membrane disease (idiopathic respiratory distress syndrome), aspiration syndrome, pneumonia, congenital heart disease or congestive heart failure, choanal atresia, hypoplasia of the mandible with posterior displacement of the tongue, macroglossia, malformation of the epiglottis, malformation or injury of the larynx, cysts or neoplasms of the larynx or chest, pneumothorax, lobar emphysema, pulmonary agenesis or hypoplasia, congenital pulmonary lymphangiectasis, Wilson-Mikity syndrome, tracheoesophageal fistula, avulsion of the phrenic nerve, hernia or eventration of the diaphragm, intracranial lesions, neuromuscular disorders, and metabolic disturbances. *Any sign of postnatal respiratory distress is an indication for a roentgenogram of the chest.*

7.31 TRANSITION TO PULMONARY RESPIRATION

The establishment of adequate lung function at birth is related to gestational age or maturity. Fluid filling the fetal lung must be removed, functional residual capacity (FRC) established and maintained, and a ventilation-perfusion relationship developed that will provide optimal exchange of oxygen and carbon dioxide between alveoli and blood (Sec 12.3, 12.6, 12.8).

The First Breath. During vaginal delivery intermittent compression of the thorax facilitates removal of lung fluid. Some of the residual fluid enhances aeration of the gas-free lung by reducing surface tension and thereby lowering the pressure required to open alveoli. Nevertheless, the pressures required to inflate the airless lung are higher than those needed at any other period of life and range from 10–70 cm of H_2O for 0.5–1.0 sec intervals compared with about 4 cm for normal breathing in term infants and adults. The higher pressures are required to overcome the opposing forces of surface tension (particularly in small airways) and the viscosity of liquid remaining in the airways, as well as to introduce about 50 ml of air into the lungs, 20–30 ml of which remains after the 1st breath to establish the FRC. Most of the liquid in the lung is removed by the pulmonary circulation, which increases many fold at birth as all of the cardiac output perfuses the pulmonary vascular bed compared with only about 8% during fetal life. The remainder of the fluid is removed by the pulmonary lymphatics and expelled by the infant or aspirated from the oropharynx; this removal may be impaired following cesarean section or neonatal sedation.

The stimuli responsible for the 1st breath are multiple and their relative importance uncertain. They include a fall in pO_2 and pH and a rise in pCO_2 owing to the interruption of the placental circulation, a redistribution of cardiac output after the umbilical cord is clamped, a decrease in body temperature, and a variety of tactile stimuli.

The low birth weight infant with a very compliant chest wall may be at a disadvantage in accomplishing the 1st breath compared with the term infant. The FRC is least in the most immature infants, reflecting the presence of atelectasis. Abnormalities in the ventilation-perfusion ratio are greater and persist for longer periods of time, as does gas trapping. There may be a low PaO_2 (40–50 mm Hg) and elevated $PaCO_2$, reflecting atelectasis and intrapulmonary shunting. The smallest immature infants have the most profound disturbances, which may resemble hyaline membrane disease.

Breathing Patterns in Newborns. During sleep in the 1st months of life, normal fullterm infants may have infrequent episodes when regular breathing is interrupted 2 or more times within a 20 sec period. This **periodic breathing** pattern, shifting from a regular rhythmicity to intermittent apnea, is more common in the premature infant, who may have apneic pauses of 5–10 sec followed by a burst of rapid respirations at a rate of 50–60/min for 10–15 sec. There is rarely an associated change in color or heart rate, and it often stops without apparent reason. Periodic breathing persists intermittently usually until premature infants are about 36 wk of gestational age. An increase in inspired oxygen concentration or carbon dioxide concentration, lung volume, or external physical stimulation will often convert periodic to regular breathing. There is no prognostic significance to periodic breathing, which is a normal characteristic of neonatal respiration.

7.32   APNEA

Periodic breathing must be distinguished from prolonged apneic pauses because of the latter's association with serious illnesses (Table 7–15). Apnea of short duration may occur in normal term infants; the incidence and duration is greatest in the 1st wk of life and during active sleep. Apnea may also occur in premature infants in the absence of identifiable disease or as a complication of spontaneous or iatrogenic neck flexion; in preterm infants serious apnea is often defined as cessation of respiration for greater than 10–20 sec with or without bradycardia or cyanosis. Periodic breathing may precede a series of apneic spells; both patterns often occur in the same infant. Bradycardia, cyanosis, or both are almost invariably associated with significant apnea, and there is frequently marked hypoxemia with a lesser degree of carbon dioxide retention; these pauses occur most often from the 2nd–6th days of life but may occur earlier or later. The sudden onset of apnea in a previously well child beyond the 2nd wk of life is a critical event and warrants immediate investigation.

Physical stimulation of the infant is often adequate to get the infant breathing again. In severe cases, assisted ventilation with a bag and mask may be necessary to terminate an episode. An increase in ambient oxygen concentration usually decreases the frequency of apneic pauses, although it increases the risk of retrolental fibroplasia. Continuous positive airway pressure (CPAP) reduces the number of apneic periods, the need for higher ambient oxygen concentrations, and the duration of oxygen therapy required in infants with frequent apnea. Rocking incubators and water beds may also be helpful. In unresponsive patients, theophylline is indicated. Loading doses of 4–5 mg/kg followed by 1–2 mg/kg every 8–12 hr by oral or intravenous routes should be used with close monitoring of vital signs, the clinical course, and drug blood levels. Caffeine citrate may also be effective.

Aranda J, Turmen T: Methylxanthines in apnea of prematurity. Clin Perinatol 6:87, 1979.

Hoppenbrouwers T, Hodgman JE, Harper RM et al: Polygraphic studies of normal infants during the first six months of life: III. Incidence of apnea and periodic breathing. Pediatrics 60:418, 1977.

Kattwinkel J: Neonatal apnea: Pathogenesis and therapy. J Pediatr 90:342, 1977.

7.33   ATELECTASIS

Atelectasis is the incomplete expansion of a lung or a portion of a lung. The 1st few breaths taken by a vigorous newborn infant usually produce apparently complete expansion of most parts of the lung with air. However, lung function progressively improves during the 1st 72–96 hr, indicating that the expansion is not physiologically complete.

Failure of initial alveolar expansion is common at autopsy of premature infants dying without other apparent abnormality and is regarded as caused by the underdevelopment of the respiratory saccules, immaturity of the diaphragm and other respiratory muscles, hypermobility of the thoracic cage, other defects of the peripheral respiratory mechanism, or severe illness. It is also seen as a result of brain injury with damage to the respiratory center or of maternal oversedation prior to delivery. Incomplete initial expansion may also result from a relative inability to expand the thick-walled bronchioles, alveolar ducts lined with columnar epithelium, and thick-walled alveoli that are characteristic of the immature fetus.

Alveolar collapse after initial expansion by air may occur in any type of pulmonary disease in the newborn. Atelectasis also may be due to abnormal intrathoracic contents, such as an enlarged heart, intestines, liver, cysts, and tumors.

Clinical Manifestations. Persistent cyanosis and poor respiratory effort and air exchange are cardinal signs of atelectasis. Respiration may be irregular, with periods of apnea and intermittent cyanosis, especially when there is injury to or depression of the central nervous system. Auld has designated a group of small (800–1200 gm) premature infants with extensive atelectasis as having chronic pulmonary insufficiency. These infants are often well with minimal signs of respiratory distress until the 2nd or 3rd day, when they develop frequent episodes of prolonged apnea and cyanosis that may become progressively severe and terminate in death if not treated with mechanical ventilation or may gradually resolve over the ensuing 2–3 wk.

The signs of atelectasis usually merge with those of the underlying pulmonary problem. The infant with obstructive atelectasis may make vigorous efforts to breathe; there may be respiratory distress, cyanosis out of oxygen, rapid deep breathing with retractions, and grunting. A roentgenogram is indicated to diagnose the underlying pulmonary disease and to distinguish lobar or segmental from lobular or patchy atelectasis.

7.34 HYALINE MEMBRANE DISEASE
(Idiopathic Respiratory Distress Syndrome)

Incidence. This condition is a major cause of death in the newborn period; it is estimated that 50% of all neonatal deaths result from hyaline membrane disease or its complications and that it accounts for 10,000–40,000 deaths each yr.

The clinical incidence is difficult to determine because of differing diagnostic criteria. Hyaline membrane disease occurs primarily in premature infants; incidence is inversely proportional to the gestational age and weight. It occurs in about 60% of infants less than 28 wk of gestational age, in 15–20% of those between 32–36 wk, in about 5% beyond 37 wk, and rarely at term. An increased frequency is associated with infants of diabetic mothers delivered before 37 wk gestation, multiple pregnancy, cesarean section delivery, precipitous delivery after antepartum hemorrhage, asphyxia, and a history of prior affected infants.

Etiology and Pathophysiology. Small alveoli that are difficult to inflate and do not remain gas-filled between inspirations and a weak and compliant chest cage are closely interrelated developmental factors.

The failure to develop a functional residual capacity (FRC) and the tendency of affected lungs to become atelectatic correlate with high surface tensions and the absence of surfactant. The major constituents of surfactant are dipalmityl-phosphatidylcholine (lecithin), phosphatidylglycerol, two apoproteins, and cholesterol. With progressive maturation increasing amounts of phospholipids are synthesized and stored in type II alveolar cells. These active agents are released into the alveoli, reducing the surface tension and helping to maintain alveolar stability by preventing the collapse of small air spaces at end-expiration. However, the amounts produced or released may be insufficient to meet postnatal demands because of immaturity. Surfactant is present in high concentrations in fetal lung homogenates by 20 wk of gestation but does not reach the surface of the lung until later. It appears in the amniotic fluid between 28–38 wk.

Surfactant synthesis in the alveoli is also dependent, in part, on normal pH, temperature, and perfusion. Asphyxia, hypoxemia, and pulmonary ischemia, particularly in association with hypovolemia, hypotension, and cold stress, may suppress surfactant synthesis. The epithelial lining of the lung may also be injured by high oxygen concentrations, poor drainage of the upper airway, and the effects of respirator management, resulting in further reduction in surfactant.

Alveolar atelectasis, hyaline membrane formation, and interstitial edema make the lungs less compliant, requiring greater pressure to expand the small alveoli and airways. In these immature infants, the lower chest wall is pulled in as the diaphragm descends and the

intrathoracic pressure becomes negative, thus limiting the amount of intrathoracic pressure that can be produced, with a resulting tendency to atelectasis. The highly compliant chest wall of the preterm infant offers less resistance than that of the mature infant to the natural tendency of the lungs to collapse. Thus, at end-expiration, the volume of the thorax and lungs tends to approach the residual volume leading to atelectasis.

Deficient synthesis or release of surfactant, together with small respiratory units and compliant chest wall, results in atelectasis, rapid respiratory rate, small tidal volumes, decreased lung compliance, increased work of breathing, and, eventually, insufficient alveolar ventilation. The resultant hypercarbia, hypoxia, and acidosis produce pulmonary arterial vasoconstriction with increased right-to-left shunting through the foramen ovale and ductus arteriosus and within the lung itself. Pulmonary blood flow would thus be reduced, with ischemic injury to the cells producing lecithin and to the vascular bed, resulting in an effusion of proteinaceous material into the alveolar spaces (Fig 7–19).

Pathology. The lungs appear deep purplish red and are liver-like in consistency. Microscopically, there is extensive atelectasis with engorgement of the interalveolar capillaries and lymphatics. A number of the alveolar ducts, alveoli, and respiratory bronchioles are lined with acidophilic, homogeneous, or granular membranes. Amniotic debris, intra-alveolar hemorrhage, pneumonia, and interstitial emphysema are additional but inconstant findings; interstitial emphysema may be marked when an infant has been ventilated with a method that employs increased end-expiratory pressure. The characteristic hyaline membranes are rarely seen in infants dying earlier than 6–8 hr after birth.

Clinical Manifestations. Signs of hyaline membrane disease usually appear within minutes of birth, though they may not be recognized for several hr until rapid, shallow respirations have increased to 60 or more/min. The late onset of tachypnea should suggest other conditions. Some patients require resuscitation at birth because of intrapartum asphyxia or initial severe respiratory distress. Characteristically tachypnea, prominent (often audible) grunting, intercostal and subcostal retractions, nasal flaring, and duskiness are seen (Table 7–16). There is increasing cyanosis, often relatively unresponsive to oxygen administration. Breath sounds may be normal or diminished with a harsh tubular quality, and, on deep inspiration, fine rales may be heard, especially over the lung bases posteriorly. The natural course is characterized by progressive worsening of signs of air hunger and dyspnea (Fig 7–2). If inadequately treated, blood pressure and body temperature may fall; fatigue, cyanosis, and pallor increase and grunting decreases or disappears as the condition worsens. Apnea and irregular respirations occur as infants tire and are ominous signs requiring immediate intervention. There may also be edema, ileus, and oliguria. Signs of asphyxia secondary to apnea or partial respiratory failure occur when there is rapid progression of the disease. The condition may progress to death in severely affected infants, but in milder cases, the symptoms and signs may reach a peak within 3 days, after

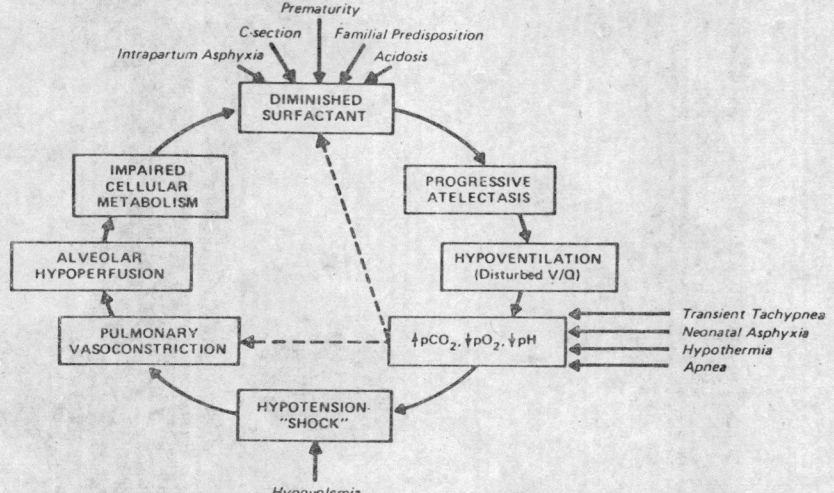

Figure 7–19 Contributing factors in the pathogenesis of hyaline membrane disease. Potential "vicious cycle" perpetuating hypoxia and pulmonary insufficiency. (From Farrell P, Zachman R, *In:* Quilligan EJ, Kretchmer N (eds): Fetal and Maternal Medicine. New York, John Wiley and Sons, 1980.)

which gradual improvement sets in. Death is rare after 3 days, except among infants whose fatal course has been forestalled by treatment.

The course may be dramatically altered by supportive therapy directed at maintaining adequate oxygenation, circulation, acid-base balance, and nutrition. Even in severe cases, clinical recovery may be complete within 10 days–2 wk. Alternatively, the natural course may be attenuated with persistence of mild to severe signs and superimposed complications associated with the treatment.

Diagnosis. The clinical course, roentgenogram of the chest, and blood gas and acid-base values help to establish the clinical diagnosis. Roentgenographically, the lungs may have a characteristic, but not pathognomonic, appearance which includes a fine reticular granularity of the parenchyma and an air bronchogram which is often more prominent early in the left lower lobe because of the superimposition of the cardiac shadow (Fig 7–20). Occasionally, the initial roentgenogram is normal, only to develop the typical pattern at 6–12 hr. There may be considerable variation among films, depending on the phase of respiration and the management (oxygen, CPAP, etc.), often resulting in poor correlation between the roentgenograms and clinical course. The laboratory findings are characterized by progressive hypoxemia, hypercarbia, and variable metabolic acidosis, depending on the presence of intrauterine asphyxia, neonatal circulatory insufficiency, and hypoxia.

In the *differential diagnosis*, group B streptococcal sepsis may be indistinguishable from hyaline membrane disease. In pneumonia presenting at birth, the chest roentgenogram may be identical to that for hyaline membrane disease; gram-positive cocci in the gastric aspirate and buffy coat smear and the presence of marked neutropenia may suggest this diagnosis. Cyanotic heart disease, persistent fetal circulation, aspiration syndromes, and congenital anomalies must also be considered. Transient tachypnea may be distinguished by its short and mild clinical course.

Prevention. Most important are the prevention of prematurity, including avoidance of unnecessary or poorly timed cesarean section, appropriate management of the high-risk pregnancy and labor, and the prediction and possible in utero treatment of pulmonary immaturity (Sec 7.4). In timing cesarean section or inducing labor, estimation of the fetal head circumference by ultrasound and determination of the lecithin concentration in the amniotic fluid by the lecithin to sphingomyelin (L/S) ratio or shake test decrease the likelihood of delivering a premature infant. Intrauterine antenatal and intrapartum monitoring may similarly decrease the risk of fetal asphyxia, which is associated with an increased incidence and severity of hyaline membrane disease.

Liggins and Howie reported that the administration of a synthetic corticosteroid to women who did not have toxemia, diabetes, or renal disease 48–72 hr before delivery of fetuses at 32 wk or less gestation significantly reduced the incidence and mortality from hyaline membrane disease. It may thus be appropriate to administer 1–2 doses of betamethasone intramuscularly to pregnant women whose lecithin in amniotic fluid indicates fetal lung immaturity and who are likely to deliver between 48–72 hr or whose labor can be delayed 48 hr or more.

Treatment. The basic defect that requires treatment is inadequate pulmonary exchange of oxygen and carbon dioxide; metabolic acidosis and circulatory insufficiency are secondary manifestations. Early supportive care of the low birth weight infant, especially the treatment of acidosis, hypoxia, hypotension, hypothermia, and atelectasis, appears to lessen the severity of hyaline membrane disease. Therapy requires careful and frequent monitoring of heart and respiratory rates, arterial pO_2, pCO_2, pH, bicarbonate, electrolytes, blood glucose, hematocrit, blood pressure, and temperature. Since most cases of hyaline membrane disease are self-limiting, the goal of treatment is to minimize abnormal physiologic variations and superimposed iatrogenic problems. The management of these infants is best

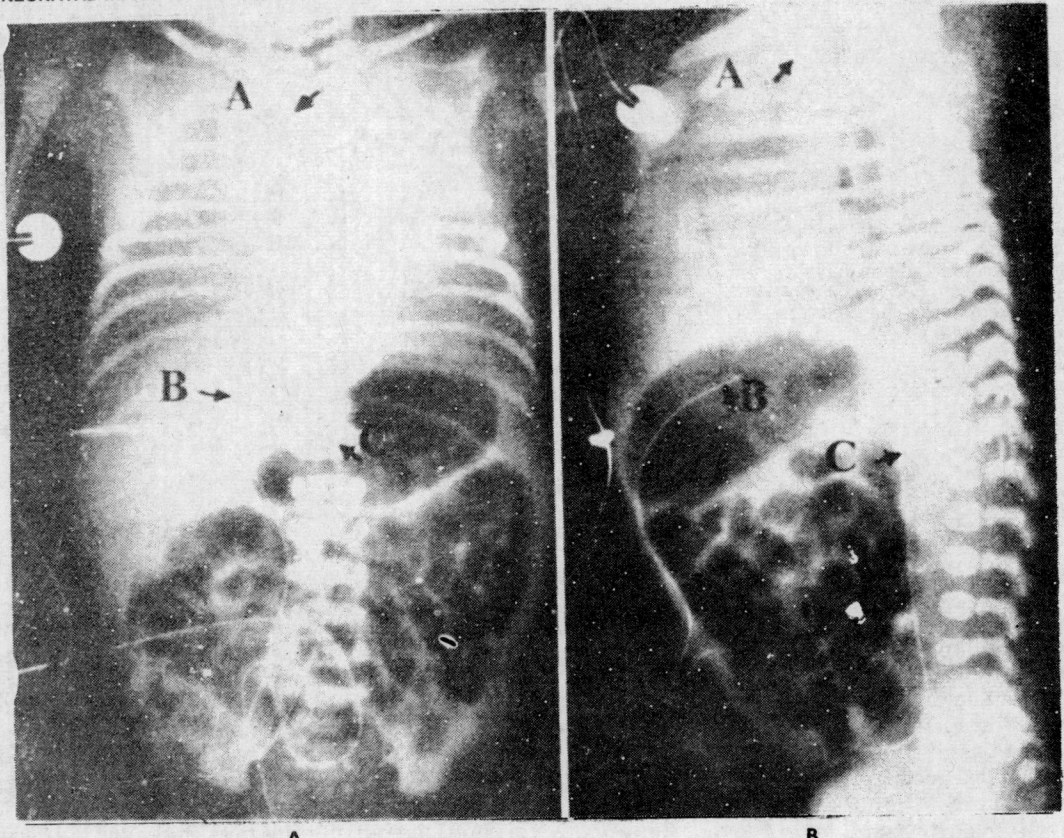

Figure 7–20   Infant with hyaline membrane disease. Note granular lungs, air bronchogram and air filled esophagus. Anteroposterior *(A)* and lateral *(B)* roentgenograms are needed to distinguish umbilical artery from vein catheter and to determine appropriate level of insertion. The lateral view clearly identifies that the catheter has been inserted into an umbilical vein and is lying in the portal system of the liver. A, endotracheal tube; B, umbilical venous catheter at the junction of the umbilical vein, ductus venosus and portal vein; C, umbilical artery catheter passed up the aorta to T-12. (Courtesy Walter E. Berdon, Babies Hospital.)

carried out in a specially staffed and equipped hospital unit, the neonatal intensive care nursery.

The general principles for supportive care of any low birth weight infant should be adhered to, including gentle handling and minimal disturbance consistent with management. To avoid chilling and minimize oxygen consumption, infants should be placed in an Isolette and core temperature maintained between 36.5–37°C (Sec 7.16). Calories and fluids should be provided intravenously. For the 1st 36–48 hr, 10% glucose and water should be infused through a peripheral vein at a rate of 65–100 ml/kg/24 hr. Subsequently, electrolytes should be added and fluid volumes increased gradually to 120–150 ml/kg/24 hr (Sec 5.22).

Warm humidified oxygen should be provided at a concentration sufficient initially to keep arterial levels between 60–80 mm Hg with stable vital signs to maintain normal tissue oxygenation while minimizing the risk of oxygen toxicity.

When the arterial oxygen tension cannot be maintained above 50 mm Hg at inspired oxygen concentrations of 70%, the application of *continuous positive airway pressure* (CPAP) at a pressure of 6–10 cm of H_2O by nasal prongs or head box or *continuous negative chest pressure* (CNCP) is indicated. This usually results in a sharp rise in arterial oxygen tension. Although the course may be protracted, the amount of pressure required usually decreases abruptly at about 72 hr of age and the infant can be weaned off CPAP shortly thereafter. If an infant on CPAP cannot maintain an arterial oxygen tension above 50 mm Hg while breathing 100% oxygen, assisted ventilation is required.

Infants with severe hyaline membrane disease or those who develop complications resulting in persistent apnea may require assisted ventilation. Reasonable indications for its use are (1) arterial blood pH <7.20; (2) arterial blood $pCO_2 \geq 60$ mm Hg; (3) arterial blood pO_2 ≤50 mm Hg at oxygen concentrations of 70–100%; or (4) persistent apnea.

The simplest method of assisted ventilation is the intermitent use of a **mask and bag resuscitator,** usually as an adjunct to nasal CPAP, for 5 min out of every 20 min or another time regimen adapted to the needs of the individual infant. A patient-cycled constant positive-pressure with variable volume or a constant volume with variable pressure **respirator** with a nasotracheal tube in place is widely used, but its use has been accompanied by serious upper airway complications, especially when nursery personnel are inexperienced. Negative-pressure respirators have the advantage of requiring neither a mask nor endotracheal tube and may be associated with a lower incidence of chronic lung disease. However, their construction makes them difficult to use on very low birth weight infants. In general, the extent to which the morbidity and mortality of severe hyaline membrane disease can be reduced with mechanical ventilation and the frequency with which complications secondary to the use of respirators can be minimized are directly related to constant maintenance of a high level of experience and skill by an intensive care team that regularly cares for critically ill newborn infants.

Although controlled studies have not shown a decrease in mortality as a result of **correcting the acidosis** associated with hyaline membrane disease, the severity of the disease seems to be lessened, and the risks of pulmonary vasoconstriction, ventilation-perfusion abnormalities, untoward shunting through the foramen ovale or ductus arteriosus, hypotension, and arrhythmias are probably diminished. These risks are increased when acidosis is coupled with hypoxia. There is a need to serially monitor pH, pCO_2, pO_2, bicarbonate, base deficit, and electrolytes and to correct significant abnormalities.

Respiratory acidosis may require short-term or prolonged assisted ventilation. In severe respiratory acidosis and hypoxia, treatment with sodium bicarbonate may exacerbate hypercarbia. A complicating intracranial hemorrhage with hypoventilation and hypercarbia may also occur.

Metabolic acidosis in hyaline membrane disease may be a result of perinatal asphyxia and hypotension and is often encountered when an infant has required resuscitation (Sec 7.29). The dosage of bicarbonate may be estimated as follows:

$$HCO_3^- \text{ needed (mEq)} = HCO_3^- \text{ deficit or}$$
$$\text{base excess (mEq/liter)} \times HCO_3^- \text{ space (liter)}$$

The values recommended for the HCO_3^- space range from 20–60% of the body weight, with 30% being the most frequently used. When 60% is used, it is advisable to give only one half of the calculated dose initially. The dose may be given diluted with 5–10% glucose (1:1) over a 10–15 min period through a peripheral vein with the acid-base determination repeated within 30 min, or it may be administered over several hr. More often, 2–3 mEq/kg of sodium bicarbonate, similarly diluted, is initially administered. In an emergency, an umbilical catheter may be used. Alkali therapy may result in skin sloughs from infiltration, increased serum osmolarity, hypernatremia, and liver injury when concentrated solutions are administered rapidly through an umbilical vein. The risk of complications is diminished when the circulation is adequately supported. More than 8 mEq/kg/24 hr of sodium bicarbonate should rarely be given unless serum sodium levels are normal and urine output adequate. In the presence of hypernatremia with edema, oliguria, or congestive heart failure, infusion of 0.3 M tris-hydroxymethyl aminomethane (THAM) at a rate of 1 ml/min, to provide 1.0 ml/kg for each pH unit below 7.4, may be preferred to bicarbonate.

Monitoring of *aortic blood pressure* through an umbilical arterial catheter or by Doppler technique may be useful in managing the shock-like state that may occur during the 1st hr or so after premature birth of an infant who has been asphyxiated or who has developed respiratory distress (Fig 7–3). Radiopaque catheters should always be used, and their position checked roentgenographically after insertion (Fig 7–20). The tip of an umbilical artery catheter should lie just above the bifurcation of the aorta or above the celiac axis. Placement and supervision should be done by skilled and experienced personnel. Catheters should be removed as soon as there is no indication for their continued use, i.e., when PaO_2 is stable and the FiO_2 is less than 40%.

Periodic monitoring of arterial oxygen and carbon dioxide tension and of pH is an important part of the management; if assisted ventilation is being used, it is essential. Blood should be obtained from the umbilical or radial artery. Tissue pO_2 and pCO_2 may also be estimated continuously from transcutaneous electrodes. Capillary blood samples are of limited value for the determination of pO_2 but may be useful to evaluate pCO_2 and pH.

Owing to the difficulty of distinguishing some group B streptococcal infections from hyaline membrane disease and the possible risk of infection complicating assisted ventilation and indwelling vascular catheters, the routine administration of antibacterial agents is advocated by some but rejected by those who are more fearful of increasing the numbers of resistant organisms. If used, penicillin or ampicillin with kanamycin or gentamicin is suggested, depending upon the recent pattern of bacterial sensitivities in the hospital where the infant is being treated (Sec 7.59 and 7.60).

Priscoline, glucocorticoids, acetylcholine, or adrenergic inhibitors are not effective in hyaline membrane disease and may cause serious untoward effects. Tracheal administration of a saline suspension of artificial surfactant within the 1st day has been reported to rapidly reduce the inspired oxygen requirement and roentgenographic abnormalities; this therapy requires further evaluation before it can be recommended.

Complications of Hyaline Membrane Disease and Intensive Care. The most serious complications of **tracheal intubation** are asphyxia from obstruction of the tube, cardiac arrest during intubation or suctioning, and the subsequent development of subglottic stenosis. Other complications include bleeding from trauma during intubation, difficult extubation requiring tracheostomy, ulceration of the nares due to pressure from the tube, permanent narrowing of the nostril from tissue damage and scarring from irritation or infection around the tube, avulsion of a vocal cord, laryngeal ulcer, papilloma of a vocal cord, and persistent hoarseness, stridor, or edema of the larynx.

Measures to reduce the incidence of these complications include skilled observation of the infant; use of polyvinyl endotracheal tubes that do not contain tin, which is toxic to cells; use of a tube of the smallest practicable size to reduce local ischemia and pressure necrosis; avoidance of frequent changes of the tube;

avoidance of motion of the tube in situ; avoidance of too frequent or vigorous suctioning; and avoidance of infection through meticulous cleanliness and frequent sterilization of all apparatus attached to or passed through the tube. The personnel inserting and caring for the endotracheal tube should be experienced and skilled.

The risks of **umbilical arterial catheterization** include vascular embolization, thrombosis, spasm, and perforation; ischemic and/or chemical necrosis of abdominal viscera; infection; accidental hemorrhage; and impaired circulation to a leg with subsequent gangrene. Although at necropsy the reported incidence of thrombotic complications varies from 1–23%, aortography has demonstrated that clots form in or about the tips of 95% of catheters placed in an umbilical artery. The risk of a serious clinical complication from umbilical catheterization is probably between 2–5%.

Transient blanching of the leg may occur during catheterization of the umbilical artery. It is usually due to reflex arterial spasm. The incidence is lessened by use of the smallest available catheters, particularly in very small infants. The catheter should be removed immediately; catheterization of the other artery may then be attempted. Persistent spasm after removal of

the catheter may be relieved by warming the opposite leg. Blood sampling from a radial artery may similarly result in spasm or thrombosis, and the same treatment is indicated. Intermittent severe spasm or unrelieved spasm may respond to the cautious local infusion of tolazoline (Priscoline), 1–2 mg injected intra-arterially over 5 min. Accidental lodgment of the catheter in a smaller artery so as to block it completely or cause unrecognized local vascular spasm may result in gangrene of the organ or area supplied by the vessel. To prevent this complication, the catheter should be removed promptly if blood cannot be obtained through it.

Serious hemorrhage on removal of the catheter is rare. Thrombi may form in the artery or in the catheter; their incidence is lowered by use of a smooth-tipped catheter with a hole only at its end, by rinsing the catheter with a small amount of saline solution containing 1.0 unit of heparin/ml or by continuously infusing a solution containing 1 unit/ml of heparin. The risks of thrombus formation with potential vascular occlusion can also be reduced by removing the catheter when there are early signs of thrombosis, such as narrowing of pulse pressure and disappearance of the dicrotic notch. Some prefer to use the umbilical artery for blood

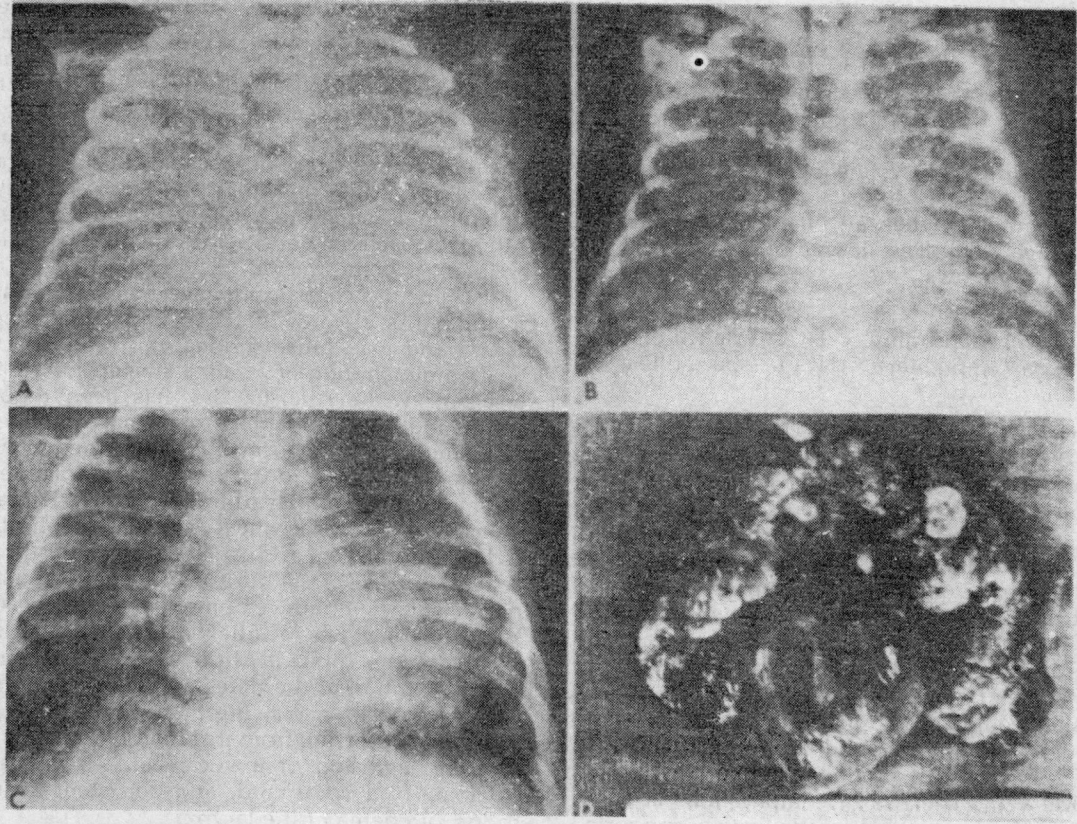

Figure 7–21 Pulmonary changes in infants who were treated in the immediate postnatal period for the clinical syndrome of hyaline membrane disease with prolonged, intermittent positive pressure breathing with air containing 80 to 100% oxygen. A, A 5 day old infant with nearly complete opacification of lungs. B, A 13 day old infant with "bubbly lungs" simulating the roentgenographic appearance of the Wilson-Mikity syndrome. C, A 7 mo old infant with irregular, dense strands in both lungs and cardiomegaly. D, Large right ventricle and cobbly, irregularly aerated lung of an infant who died at 11 mo of age; this infant also had a patent ductus arteriosus. (From Northway WH Jr, Rosan RC, Porter DY: N Engl J Med 276:357, 1967.)

sampling only, leaving the catheter filled with heparinized saline between samplings. Renovascular hypertension may occur days to weeks following umbilical arterial catheterization in a small number of neonates. Other long-term risks of catheterization of the umbilical artery or umbilical vein are as yet unknown.

The toxicity to the retina of elevated concentrations of oxygen administered for prolonged periods has been amply demonstrated (Sec 7.16).

Oxygen has been demonstrated to be toxic to the lung, particularly if administered by means of a positive pressure respirator, resulting in **bronchopulmonary dysplasia.** Instead of showing improvement on the 3rd–4th day, consistent with the natural course in survivors, some infants who have been on prolonged intermittent positive pressure breathing using increased concentrations of oxygen have roentgenographic evidence of worsening of their pulmonary condition (Fig 7–21A). Respiratory distress persists and is characterized by hypoxia, hypercarbia, and oxygen dependency, and they are prone to develop right heart failure. The chest roentgenogram is described as gradually changing from a picture of almost complete opacification with air bronchogram and interstitial emphysema to one of small, round, lucent areas alternating with areas of irregular density resembling a sponge (Fig 7–21B), similar to that seen in the "bubbly lung syndrome" of Wilson and Mikity. In the histologic picture at this stage (10–20 days after beginning oxygen therapy) there is less evidence of hyaline membrane formation, progressive alveolar coalescence with atelectasis of surrounding alveoli, interstitial edema, coarse focal thickening of the basement membrane, and widespread bronchial and bronchiolar mucosal metaplasia and hyperplasia. This corresponds with a severe maldistribution of ventilation. Most surviving neonates with persistent roentgenographic changes recover by 6–12 mo with about normal pulmonary function, but some require prolonged hospitalization with oxygen, diuretics, digitalization, and chest physiotherapy and may have respiratory symptoms persisting through infancy. Cor pulmonale, right heart failure, and infection are major causes of death. Pathology reveals cardiac enlargement and pulmonary changes consisting of focal areas of emphysematous alveoli with hypertrophy of the peribronchial smooth muscle of the tributary bronchioles, some perimucosal fibrosis and widespread metaplasia of the bronchiolar mucosa, thickening of basement membranes, and separation of the capillaries from the aveolar epithelial cells.

Extrapulmonary extravasation of air is another frequent complication of the management of hyaline membrane disease (Sec 7.38).

There may be clinically significant shunting through a **patent ductus arteriosus** in some neonates with hyaline membrane disease, the delayed closure being due to associated hypoxia, acidosis, increased pulmonary pressure secondary to vasoconstriction, systemic hypotension, immaturity of these infants, and local release of prostaglandins which dilate the ductus. The manifestations may include (1) persistent apnea for unexplained reasons in an infant recovering from hyaline membrane disease; (2) an active heaving precordium, bounding peripheral pulses, and a systolic or to-and-fro murmur; (3) carbon dioxide retention, occasionally with associated mixed acidosis; (4) increasing oxygen dependency; (5) roentgenographic evidence of cardiomegaly and increased pulmonary vascular markings; (6) enlarged left atrium demonstrated by echocardiography. Most infants respond to general supportive measures including digitalization and diuretics. In selected patients in whom spontaneous closure does not occur and there is progressive deterioration despite treatment, indomethacin, 1–3 doses of 0.1–0.3 mg/kg at 12–24 hr intervals for 48 hr, may induce pharmacologic closure by inhibition of prostaglandin synthesis. Indications for surgical closure are discussed in Sec 13.42.

Anemia secondary to frequent withdrawal of blood samples may also occur as a complication of intensive care. The cumulative amount of blood withdrawn should be carefully recorded. Replacement by transfusion may be indicated if more than 10–15% of estimated total blood volume is removed or if there is a significant decrease in the hematocrit. Oxygen-dependent infants should have their hematocrit maintained above 40%.

Prognosis. Early provision of intensive observation and care to high-risk newborn infants can significantly reduce morbidity and mortality due to hyaline membrane disease and other acute neonatal illnesses. However, good results depend on experienced and skilled personnel, specially designed and organized regional hospital units, equipment, and the lack of complications, such as severe fetal or birth asphyxia, intracranial hemorrhage, or irremediable congenital malformation.

Overall mortality for low birth weight infants referred to intensive care centers is steadily declining; about 50% of those under 1000 gm survive and the mortality progressively decreases at higher weights with over 95% of sick infants weighing more than 2500 gm surviving (Sec 7.16). Although 85–90% of all infants surviving hyaline membrane disease after requiring ventilatory support with respirators are normal, the outlook is much better for those above 1500 gm; about 80% of those under 1500 gm have no neurologic or mental sequelae. The long-term prognosis for normal pulmonary function in most infants surviving hyaline membrane disease is excellent.

Alden ER, Mandelkorn T, Wooddrum DE, et al: Morbidity and mortality of infants less than 1000 gms in intensive care nursery. Pediatrics 50:40, 1972.

Avery M, Fletcher B, Williams R: The Lung and Its Disorders in the Newborn Infant. Ed 4. Philadelphia WB Saunders, 1981.

Barr PA, Sumners J, Wirtshafter D, et al: Percutaneous peripheral arterial cannulation in the neonate. Pediatrics (Suppl) p 1058, 1977.

Behrman RE: The use of acid-base measurements in clinical evaluation and treatment of the sick neonate. J Pediatr 74:632, 1969.

Bryan MH, Hardie MJ, Reilly BJ, et al: Pulmonary function during the first year of life in infants recovering from the respiratory distress syndrome. Pediatrics 52:169, 1973.

Chernick V: Hyaline membrane disease—therapy with constant lung distending pressure. N Engl J Med 289:301, 1973.

Clements JA, Platzker ACG, Tierney DF, et al: Assessment of the risk of respiratory distress syndrome by a more rapid new test for surfactant in the amniotic fluid. N Engl J Med 286:1077, 1972.

Corbet AJ, Adams JM, Kenny JD, et al: Controlled trial of bicarbonate therapy in high-risk premature newborn infants. J Pediatr 91:771, 1977.

Edwards DK, Wayne DM, Northway WH Jr: Twelve years' experience with bronchopulmonary dysplasia. Pediatrics 59:839, 1977.

Farrell PM, Avery ME: Hyaline membrane disease. State of the art. Am Rev Resp Dis 111:657, 1975.

Fitzhardinge PM, Pope J, Arstikaitis M, et al: Mechanical ventilation of infants of less than 1500 grams' birth weight: health, growth, neurologic sequelae. J Pediatr 88:531, 1976.

Freedman WF, et al: Pharmacologic closure of patent ductus arteriosus in the premature infant. N Engl J Med 295:526, 1976.

Fujiwara T, Maeta H, Chida S, et al: Artificial surfactant therapy in hyaline membrane disease. Lancet 1:55, 1980.

Gluck L, Kulovich M: Lecithin-sphingomyelin ratios in amniotic fluid in normal and abnormal pregnancy. Am J Obstet Gynecol 115:539, 1973.

Gregory G, Kitterman J, Phibbs R, et al: Treatment of the idiopathic respiratory distress syndrome with continuous positive airway pressure. N Engl J Med 284:1333, 1971.

Ingram D, Pendergrass E, Bromberger P, et al: Group B streptococcal disease. Am J Dis Child 134:754, 1980.

Jacob J, Edwards D, Gluck L: Early onset sepsis and pneumonia observed as respiratory distress syndrome. Am J Dis Child 134:766, 1980.

Johnson JD, Malachowski NC, Grobstein R, et al: Prognosis of children surviving with the aid of mechanical ventilation in the newborn period. J Pediatr 84:272, 1974.

Kamper J: Long term prognosis of infants with severe idiopathic respiratory distress syndrome. Acta Paediatr Scand 67:71, 1978.

Krauss A: Assisted ventilation: A critical review. Clin Perinatol 7:61, 1980.

Kulovich M, Hallman M, Gluck L: The lung profile. Am J Obstet Gynecol 135:57, 1979.

LaMarre A, Lindao L, Reilly BV, et al: Residual pulmonary abnormalities in survivors of idiopathic respiratory distress syndrome. Am Rev Resp Dis 108:56, 1973.

Liggins BC, Howie RN: A controlled trial of antepartum glucocorticoid treatment for prevention of the respiratory distress syndrome in premature infants. Pediatrics 50:515, 1972.

Merrett TA, Farrell PM: Diminished pulmonary lecithin synthesis in acidosis: Experimental findings as related to the respiratory distress syndrome. Pediatrics 57:32, 1976.

Northway WH, Rosan RC, Porter DB: Pulmonary disease following respiratory therapy. N Engl J Med 276:357, 1967.

Outerbridge EW, Ramsay M, Stern L: Developmental follow up of survivors of neonatal respiratory failure. Crit Care Med 2:23, 1974.

Reynolds EOR, Taghizadeh A: Improved prognosis of infants mechanically ventilated for hyaline membrane disease. Arch Dis Child 49:505, 1974.

Robert MF, Neff RK, Hubbell JP, et al: Association between maternal diabetes and the respiratory distress syndrome in the newborn. N Engl J Med 294:357, 1976.

Shelly S, Kovacevic M, Paciga J, et al: Sequential changes of surfactant phosphatidylcholine in hyaline membrane disease of the newborn. N Engl J Med 300:112, 1979.

Stahlman M, Hedvall G, Dolanski E, et al: A six-year follow-up of clinical hyaline membrane disease. Pediatr Clin North Am 20:433, 1973.

Stewart AL, Reynolds EOR: Improved prognosis for infants of low birth weight. Pediatrics 54:724, 1974.

Stocker JT, Madewell JE: Persistent interstitial pulmonary emphysema: Another complication of the respiratory distress syndrome. Pediatrics 59:847, 1977.

Thibeault DW, Emmanouilides GC, Nelson RJ, et al: Patent ductus arteriosus complicating the respiratory distress syndrome in preterm infants. J Pediatr 86:120, 1975.

7.35   TRANSIENT TACHYPNEA OF THE NEWBORN

Transient tachypnea, occasionally termed **respiratory distress syndrome type II**, usually follows uneventful normal preterm or term vaginal delivery or cesarean delivery. It may be characterized only by the early onset of tachypnea, sometimes with retractions, or expiratory grunting and, occasionally, cyanosis that is relieved by minimal oxygen. Patients usually recover rapidly within 3–4 days, although they may rarely appear severely ill and have a more protracted course. The lungs are usually clear without rales or rhonchi, and the chest roentgenogram shows prominent pulmonary vascular markings, fluid lines in the fissures, overaeration, flat diaphragms, and, occasionally, pleural fluid. Hypoxemia, hypercapnia, and acidosis are uncommon. It may not be possible to distinguish the disease from hyaline

membrane disease except by the sudden recovery and the absence of a roentgenographic reticulogranular pattern. The syndrome is believed to be secondary to slow absorption of fetal lung fluid. It may be necessary to discontinue oral feeding to avoid the risk of aspiration and to treat with oxygen, but usually no other treatment is required.

Avery ME, Gatewood OB, Brumley G: Transient tachypnea of newborn. Possible delayed reabsorption of fluid at birth. Am J Dis Child 111:380, 1966.

Sundell H, Garrott J, Blankenship WJ, et al: Studies on infants with type II respiratory distress syndrome. J Pediatr 78:754, 1971.

7.36   ASPIRATION OF FOREIGN MATERIAL
(Fetal Aspiration Syndrome; Aspiration Pneumonia)

During prolonged labors and difficult deliveries, infants often initiate vigorous respiratory movements in utero, because of interference with the supply of oxygen via the placenta. Under such circumstances the infant may aspirate amniotic fluid containing vernix caseosa, epithelial cells, meconium, or material from the birth canal. This debris may block the smallest airways and

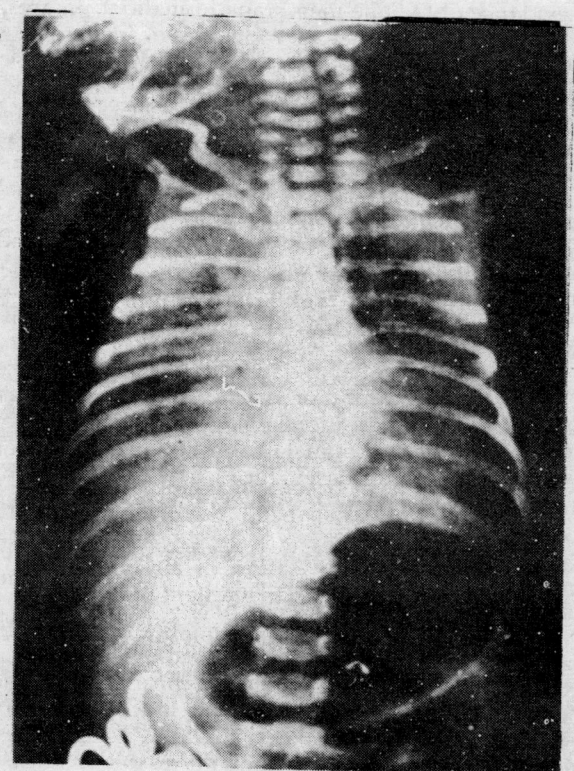

Figure 7–22   Fetal aspiration syndrome (aspiration pneumonia). Note the coarsely granular pattern with irregular aeration typical of fetal distress from aspiration of materials such as vernix caseosa, epithelial cells, and meconium contained in amniotic fluid.

interfere with alveolar exchange of oxygen and carbon dioxide. Pathogenic bacteria frequently accompany the aspirated material. When this is the case, pneumonia may ensue, but even in the noninfected cases respiratory distress and usually roentgenographic evidences of aspiration are seen (Fig 7–22).

Other situations in which pulmonary aspiration of foreign material may occur in the newborn infant include tracheoesophageal fistula, esophageal and duodenal obstructions, gastroesophageal reflux, improper feeding practices, the administration of medicines, and improper handling and placement of infants in their cribs.

The contents of the stomach should be aspirated through a soft rubber catheter just before operation or other procedures requiring anesthesia or significantly disturbing an infant. Once aspiration has occurred, treatment consists of general and respiratory support and treatment of pneumonia (Sec 7.60).

7.37 MECONIUM ASPIRATION

Meconium-stained amniotic fluid is seen in 5–15% of births, but this syndrome usually occurs in term or post-term infants who are often small for gestational age. Usually, there has been fetal distress and anoxia with passage of meconium into the amniotic fluid. These infants are frequently meconium-stained and depressed and require resuscitation at birth. Either in utero or more often with the 1st breath, thick meconium is aspirated into the lungs. The resulting small airway obstruction may produce respiratory distress within the 1st hours with tachypnea, retraction, grunting, and cyanosis in severely affected infants. Partial obstruction of some airways may lead to pneumothorax, pneumomediastinum, or both. Prompt treatment may delay the onset of respiratory distress, which may consist only of tachypnea without retractions. Overdistention of the chest may be prominent. Usually, there is improvement within 48 hr, but the course may be severe and the mortality high when assisted ventilation is required. Tachypnea may persist for many days or even several wk. The typical chest roentgenogram is characterized by patchy infiltrates, coarse streaking of both lung fields, increased anteroposterior diameter, and flattening of the diaphragm. Arterial pO_2 may be low, and if there has been anoxia, metabolic acidosis is usually present. Hypercapnia and respiratory alkalosis may be present late during recovery. The mortality of meconium-stained infants is considerably higher than that of nonstained infants, and meconium aspiration accounts for a significant proportion of neonatal deaths. Residual lung problems are rare, but the ultimate prognosis depends on the extent of central nervous system injury from anoxia and the occurrence of associated problems such as persistence of the fetal circulation.

Treatment of meconium aspiration should begin in the delivery room with atraumatic removal of oropharyngeal and tracheal meconium. Endotracheal tube insertion and suction are indicated when there is meconium staining. Supportive care for respiratory distress should be provided as indicated. The oxygenation benefit of positive end-expiratory pressure (or CPAP) must be weighed against its increasing the risk of air leaks. Hydrocortisone therapy is not of benefit.

Capitanio MA, Kirkpatrick JA: Roentgen examination in the evaluation of the newborn infant with respiratory distress. J Pediatr 75:896, 1969.
Gregory GA, Gooding CA, Phibbs RH, et al: Meconium aspiration infants; a prospective study. J Pediatr 85:848, 1974.
Marshall R, Tyrala E, McAlister W, et al: Meconium aspiration syndrome: Neonatal and follow-up study. Am J Obstet Gynecol 131:672, 1978.
Yeh TF, Srinivasan G, Harris V, et al: Hydrocortisone therapy in meconium aspiration syndrome: A controlled study. J Pediatr 90:140, 1977.

7.38 EXTRAPULMONARY EXTRAVASATION OF AIR
(Pneumothorax and Pneumomediastinum)

Asymptomatic pneumothorax, either unilateral or bilateral, is estimated to occur in 1–2% of all newborn infants; symptomatic pneumothorax and pneumomediastinum are less common. Pneumothorax is more common in males than in females and in term and post-term infants than in premature ones. The incidence is increased among infants with lung disease, such as meconium aspiration and hyaline membrane disease; in those who have had vigorous resuscitation or are receiving assisted ventilation, especially if high inspiratory pressure or a continuous elevation of end-expiratory pressure is used; and in infants with urinary tract anomalies.

Etiology and Pathophysiology. The most common cause of pneumothorax is overinflation and resulting alveolar rupture. It may be "spontaneous" or idiopathic or secondary to underlying pulmonary disease, such as lobar emphysema or rupture of a congenital or pneumonic cyst; to trauma; or to a "ball-valve" type of bronchial or bronchiolar obstruction resulting from aspiration. Air from a ruptured alveolus escapes into the interstitial spaces of the lung where it may cause interstitial emphysema and/or dissect along the peribronchial and perivascular connective tissue sheaths to the root of the lung. If the volume of escaped air is great enough, it may follow the vascular sheaths to cause mediastinal emphysema or a rupture with subsequent pneumomediastinum, pneumothorax, and subcutaneous emphysema. There may also be right-to-left shunting with persistent circulation through a collapsed area of lung. Rarely, increased mediastinal pressure may compress pulmonary veins at the hilum, interfering with venous return to the heart and cardiac output.

Tension pneumothorax occurs if an accumulation of air within the pleural space is sufficient to elevate intrapleural pressure above atmospheric pressure. Not only is ventilation impaired in the collapsed lung by a unilateral tension pneumothorax, but that in the normal lung also may be compromised by a mediastinal shift to the other side. Compression of the vena cava and torsion of the great vessels may interfere with venous return.

Clinical Manifestations. The physical findings of *asymptomatic pneumothorax* are hyperresonance and diminished breath sounds over the involved side of the chest.

Symptomatic pneumothorax is characterized by respiratory distress which varies from only an increased respiratory rate to severe dyspnea, tachypnea, and cyanosis. Irritability and restlessness or apnea may be the earliest signs. The onset may be sudden or gradual; an infant may rapidly become critically ill. The chest may appear asymmetric with increased anteroposterior diameter and bulging of the intercostal spaces on the affected side, and there are hyperresonance and diminished or absent breath sounds. The heart is displaced toward the unaffected side, and the diaphragm is displaced downward, as is the liver with right-sided pneumothorax. Since both sides are affected in approximately 10% of patients, symmetry of findings does not rule out pneumothorax. In tension pneumothorax there may be signs of shock and the apex of the heart is pushed away from the affected side. Rupture tends to occur early in meconium aspiration and later in hyaline membrane disease when the infant is beginning to make more vigorous efforts with improving lung compliance, or it may be a complication of assisted ventilation.

With **pneumomediastinum,** which occurs in at least 25% of patients with pneumothorax, the degree of respiratory distress is again dependent on the amount of trapped air. If it is great, there is bulging of the midthoracic area, the neck veins are distended, and the blood pressure is low. The last 2 findings are the result of blockage of the circulation by compression of the systemic and pulmonary veins. Although there may be few clinical signs, subcutaneous emphysema in the newborn infant is almost pathognomonic of pneumomediastinum.

Diagnosis. Pneumothorax and pneumomediastinum should be suspected in any newborn infant who shows signs of respiratory distress or who displays restlessness or irritability, or has a sudden change in condition. The diagnosis is established roentgenographically with the edge of the collapsed lung standing out in relief against the pneumothorax (Fig 12–18), and in pneumomediastinum with hyperlucency around the heart border and between the sternum and the heart border (Fig 7–23). Transillumination of the thorax is often helpful in the emergency diagnosis of pneumothorax; the affected side transmits excessive light.

Pneumopericardium may be asymptomatic requiring only general supportive treatment or may present as sudden shock with tachycardia, muffled heart sounds, and poor pulses suggesting tamponade which requires prompt evacuation of entrapped air. **Pneumoperitoneum** from air dissecting through the diaphragmatic apertures may also be confused with perforation of an abdominal organ.

Treatment. Without a continued air leak, asymptomatic and mildly symptomatic small pneumothoraces require only close observation. Frequent small feedings may prevent gastric dilatation and minimize crying, which can further compromise ventilation and worsen the pneumothorax. Breathing 100% oxygen accelerates the resorption of free pleural air into the blood by reducing the nitrogen tension in blood, with a resultant nitrogen pressure gradient from the trapped air into the blood, but the benefit must be weighed against the risks of oxygen toxicity. With severe respiratory or circulatory embarrassment, emergency needle aspiration is indicated. If this is unsuccessful in maintaining relief of distress or if there is adequate time, a chest tube should be inserted and attached to underwater-seal drainage. Severe localized interstitial emphysema may respond to selective bronchial intubation.

Chernick V, Avery ME: Spontaneous alveolar rupture at birth. Pediatrics 32:816, 1963.

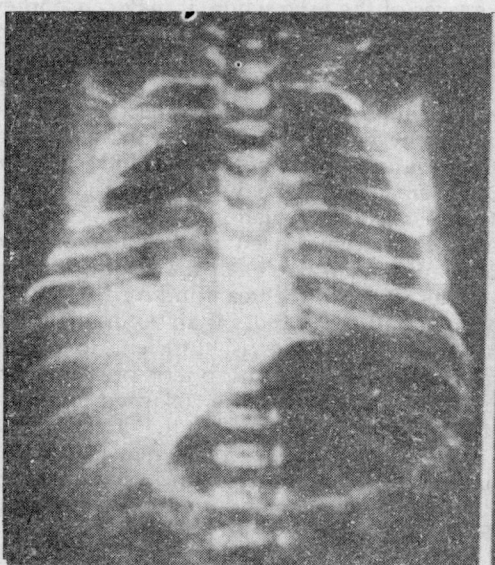 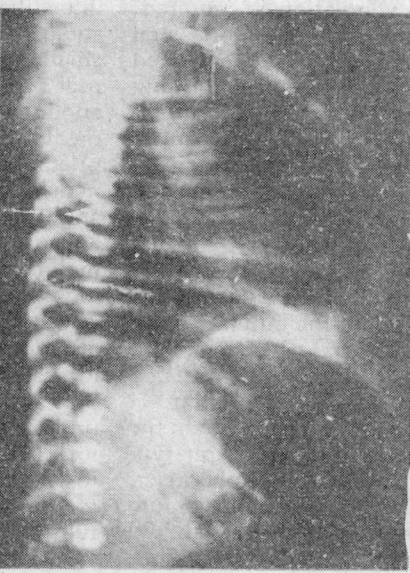

Figure 7–23 Pneumomediastinum in a newborn infant. Anteroposterior view demonstrates compression of lungs and the lateral view shows bulging of the sternum, each resulting from distention of the mediastinum by trapped air.

Hall RT, Rhodes PG: Pneumothorax and pneumomediastinum in infants with idiopathic respiratory distress syndrome receiving CPAP. Pediatrics 55:493, 1975.

Saldanha RL, Cepeda EE, Poland RL: The effect of vitamin E prophylaxis on the incidence and severity of bronchopulmonary dysplasia. Pediatr 101:89, 1982.
Wilson MG, Mikity VG: A new form of respiratory distress in premature infants. Am J Dis Child 99:489, 1960.

7.39 INTERSTITIAL PULMONARY FIBROSIS

(Wilson-Mikity Syndrome; Chronic Neonatal Pulmonary Disease; Pulmonary Dysmaturity; Bronchopulmonary Dysplasia)

See also Sec 7.34 for discussion of bronchopulmonary dysplasia.

Wilson and Mikity described a pulmonary syndrome of premature infants, usually of less than 32 wk gestation and birth weights below 1500 gm, characterized by insidious onset of dyspnea, tachypnea, retractions, and cyanosis during the 1st mo of life. Rarely, cases have been reported in fullterm infants, usually with a history of meconium aspiration or oxygen administration. Viral infections also have been implicated.

Several variations on the clinical presentation have been described with similar roentgenographic findings. Some infants have respiratory distress at birth which is occasionally severe, resembles hyaline membrane disease, and requires oxygen; these may be cases of bronchopulmonary dysplasia. Others have a more gradual development of dyspnea and cyanosis. Others have no early respiratory symptoms or history of exposure to oxygen, and the onset of symptoms is at several weeks of life.

Cough, wheezing, and rales may develop, but fever occurs only with concomitant infection. There may be collapse of a lobe or lung; other complications are right-sided heart failure, osteoporosis, and rib fractures. The symptoms usually increase over 2–6 wk with increasing oxygen dependency persisting for several mo, followed by gradual resolution or progressive respiratory and cardiac failure. Infants who recover from the severe form may have an increased number of lower respiratory tract infections in the 1st yr of life. The most characteristic features of this syndrome are roentgenographic. Early, they include bilateral coarse reticular streaky infiltrates and, often, overexpansion of the lungs with small areas of emphysema that develop into multicystic lesions. Subsequently, the cysts enlarge and coalesce to give a hyperlucent, bubbly appearance (Fig 7–21C). The roentgenograms tend to clear gradually over months to several yr. The roentgenographic changes in Wilson-Mikity syndrome may be indistinguishable from those of bronchopulmonary dysplasia (Sec 7.34).

The syndrome must be differentiated from pneumonia due to *Pneumocystis carinii* or chlamydia and cystic fibrosis. Treatment consists of supportive measures: oxygen for cyanosis, digitalization and diuretics for cardiac failure, acid-base correction, and assisted ventilation when indicated. Prophylaxis with vitamin E does not decrease the incidence or severity of bronchopulmonary dysplasia.

Krauss AN, Klain DB, Auld PAM: Chronic pulmonary insufficiency of prematurity (CPIP). Pediatrics 55:55, 1975.

PERSISTENT FETAL CIRCULATION (PFC)

See Sec 13.12.

LOBAR EMPHYSEMA

See Sec 12.48.

7.40 LUNG CYSTS

Most lung cysts observed during the neonatal period are acquired as the result of rupture of alveoli by overinflation or infection, often staphylococcal. Congenital cysts are rare; they may be solitary or multiple, air-containing or filled with fluid, and are believed to result as a developmental anomaly of the bronchial buds (Sec 12.50). Infants with congenital or acquired cysts may be asymptomatic or present with tachypnea and dyspnea at birth or any time thereafter or with recurrent or persistent pneumonia. Air-filled cysts on the surface of the lung, whatever their origin, sometimes rupture and cause pneumothorax. This is particularly true of multicystic disease. Since most cystic areas discovered only on roentgenographic examination will disappear spontaneously, treatment, which is surgical removal, should be reserved for those causing severe respiratory distress.

7.41 PULMONARY HEMORRHAGE

Massive pulmonary hemorrhage is present in 15% of neonates who come to autopsy in the 1st 2 wk of life. The reported incidence at autopsy varies from 1–4/1000 live births. About three fourths of the patients weigh less than 2500 gm at birth.

Most infants in whom pulmonary hemorrhage is demonstrated at autopsy have had symptoms of respiratory distress indistinguishable from those of hyaline membrane disease. The onset may occur at birth or be delayed several days. One fourth to one half of affected infants cough up or regurgitate material containing old or fresh blood from the nose, mouth, or endotracheal tube. Roentgenographic findings are varied and nonspecific, ranging from minor streaking or patchy infiltrates to massive consolidation.

The cause of massive pulmonary hemorrhage is unknown; the incidence is increased in association with acute pulmonary infection, severe anoxia, hyaline membrane disease, assisted ventilation, congenital heart disease, erythroblastosis fetalis, hemorrhagic disease of the newborn, kernicterus, inborn errors of ammonia metabolism, and cold injury. Although in the majority of instances bleeding into other organs is observed at autopsy, bleeding other than through the nostrils and mouth is relatively rare during life and should suggest the possibility of an additional bleeding diathesis such as disseminated intravascular coagulation (Sec 14.69). Bleeding is predominantly alveolar in about two thirds of cases and interstitial in the rest. In some infants the pulmonary hemorrhage represents hemorrhagic pulmonary edema due to severe left-sided heart failure from hypoxia.

There is little information about the prognosis of infants who bleed through the mouth or nostrils except that it is extremely poor. Death occurs in the 1st 48 hr of life in two thirds of the infants who come to autopsy. Treatment is supportive.

Cole VA, Norman ICS, Reynolds EOR, et al: Pathogenesis of hemorrhagic pulmonary edema and massive pulmonary hemorrhage in the newborn. Pediatrics 51:175, 1973.
Trompeter R, Yu VYH, Aynsley-Green A, et al: Massive pulmonary haemorrhage in the newborn. Arch Dis Child 51:123, 1975.

CONGENITAL PULMONARY LYMPHANGIECTASIA

See Sec 12.52.

CHYLOTHORAX

See Sec 12.101.

7.42 DISTURBANCES OF THE DIGESTIVE SYSTEM

Vomiting. Infants may vomit mucus, often blood-streaked, in the 1st few hr after birth. This vomiting infrequently persists after the 1st few feedings; it may be due to irritation of the gastric mucosa by material swallowed during delivery. If the vomiting is protracted, gastric lavage with physiologic saline solution may relieve it.

Vomiting is a relatively frequent symptom during the neonatal period. In the majority of instances it is simply regurgitation from overfeeding or from failure to permit the infant to eructate swallowed air. (See Sec 11.20 for discussion of gastric emptying and gastroesophageal reflux.) When vomiting occurs shortly after birth and is persistent, the possibilities of increased intracranial pressure and of intestinal obstruction must be considered. An accompanying history of maternal hydramnios suggests upper intestinal atresia.

Obstructive lesions of the digestive tract occur most frequently in the esophagus and intestines (Chapter 11). Vomiting from esophageal obstruction occurs with the 1st feeding. The diagnosis of **esophageal atresia** can be suspected if there is unusual drooling from the mouth and if resistance is encountered in the attempt to pass a catheter into the stomach. Diagnosis should be made before the infant chokes on oral feedings and risks aspiration pneumonia. Infantile **achalasia** (cardiospasm), a rare cause of vomiting in the newborn infant, is demonstrable roentgenographically by obstruction at the cardiac end of the esophagus, without organic stenosis. Regurgitation of feedings due to continuous relaxation of the esophageal-gastric sphincter, **chalasia,** is a cause of vomiting, which can be controlled by keeping the infant in a semi-upright position.

Vomiting from *obstruction of the small intestine* usually begins on the 1st day of life and is frequent, persistent, usually nonprojectile, copious, and, unless the obstruction is above the ampulla of Vater, bile-stained; it is associated with abdominal distention, visible deep peristaltic waves, and reduced or absent bowel movements. **Malrotation** with obstruction from midgut volvulus is an acute emergency that must be considered. Upright roentgenographic films of the abdomen will show the distribution of air in the intestine and often aid in locating the site of the obstruction; the use of contrast material is usually unnecessary. Normally, air can be demonstrated roentgenographically in the jejunum by 15–60 min, in the ileum by 2–3 hr, and in the colon by 3 hr after birth. Persistent vomiting may occur with congenital *hernia of the diaphragm* (Sec 11.75). The vomiting of **pyloric stenosis** may begin any time after birth but does not assume its characteristic pattern before the 2nd–3rd wk. Vomiting may occur with many other disturbances that do not obstruct the digestive tract, such as celiac disease, milk allergy, adrenal hyperplasia of the salt-losing variety, septicemia, meningitis, and other infections. It is common with urinary tract infections.

Thrush (Oral Moniliasis). Thrush of the mouth occurs in healthy infants; later, it is rare except in debilitated infants and children and in those receiving antibiotic or immunosuppressive therapy.

Transmission of the infection from maternal vaginal moniliasis to the infant's oral mucosa is the primary means of infection in healthy newborns. Secondary cases develop in the hospital nursery, presumably by contact with infected infants and contaminated supplies or caretakers.

Occasionally a heavy coating forms on the tongue which may be mistaken for thrush. It can be removed by 1–2 applications of a 1% aqueous solution of gentian violet.

Oral thrush in an otherwise healthy infant is usually a self-limited infection, but treatment is advised (Sec 11.13).

Diarrhea. See Sec 7.63, 10.29, and 11.36.

Constipation. More than 90% of newborn infants pass meconium within the 1st 24 hr, and most of the remainder do so within 36 hr; the possibility of intestinal obstruction should be considered in any infant who does not. Intestinal atresia or stenosis, congenital aganglionic megacolon, milk bolus obstruction, meconium ileus, or meconium plugs may present as constipation. Constipation not present from birth, but appearing during the 1st mo of life, suggests congenital aganglionic megacolon, cretinism, or anal stenosis. It must be kept in mind that infrequent bowel movements do not necessarily mean constipation. A breast-fed infant may rarely go 5–7 days without a bowel movement and without evidence of discomfort and then pass a large but otherwise normal stool.

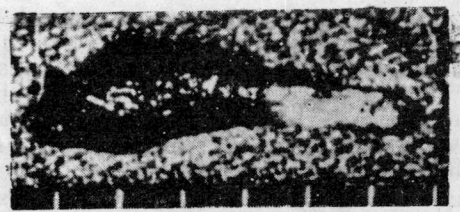

Figure 7-24 Anorectal plug, from child who had not passed meconium for 2 days after birth, is indistinguishable from normal plug. Pale end was adjacent to anus. (From Emery JL: Arch Dis Child, Vol 32.)

Meconium Plugs. Anorectal plugs (Fig 7-24) of lower water content than normal may cause intestinal obstruction. Rarely a firm mass of meconium may form elsewhere in the intestine and cause intrauterine intestinal obstruction and meconium peritonitis unrelated to cystic fibrosis. Anorectal plugs may also cause intestinal ulceration and perforation. The plug may be evacuated by irrigation with isotonic sodium chloride solution. Enemas with the iodinated contrast medium, *Gastrografin*, will usually cause passage of the plug, presumably because the high osmolarity (1900 mOsm/l) of the medium draws fluid rapidly into the intestinal lumen and loosens inspissated material. Since this rapid loss of fluid into the bowel may result in acute dehydration and shock, it is advisable to dilute the contrast material with an equal amount of water, to correct any existing dehydration, and to provide intravenous fluids during and for several hr after the procedure. *After removal of a meconium plug the infant should be observed closely for the possible presence of congenital aganglionic megacolon.*

Meconium Bodies. These light yellow particles are usually no more than 1 mm in diameter and are rarely large enough to cause distortion of the intestine. They are occasionally associated with intestinal atresia.

7.43 MECONIUM ILEUS IN CYSTIC FIBROSIS

In the newborn infant impaction of meconium is a relatively rare cause of intestinal obstruction associated with cystic fibrosis. The depletion or absence of pancreatic enzymes limits normal digestive activities in the intestine, and meconium is left in a viscid, mucilaginous state. It clings to the intestinal wall and is moved with difficulty, or not at all, by intestinal peristalsis. The inspissated and impacted meconium fills the intestinal canal but is most concentrated in the lower ileum.

Clinically, the pattern is that of congenital intestinal obstruction with or without intestinal perforation (see Meconium Peritonitis below). Abdominal distention is prominent, and persistent vomiting soon occurs. Infrequently 1 or more inspissated meconium stools may be passed shortly after birth.

The differential diagnosis involves other causes of intestinal obstruction; an exact diagnosis cannot be made except at laparotomy. A presumptive diagnosis can be made on the basis of a history of cystic fibrosis in a sibling, by palpation of doughy or cordlike masses of intestines through the abdominal wall, and by the

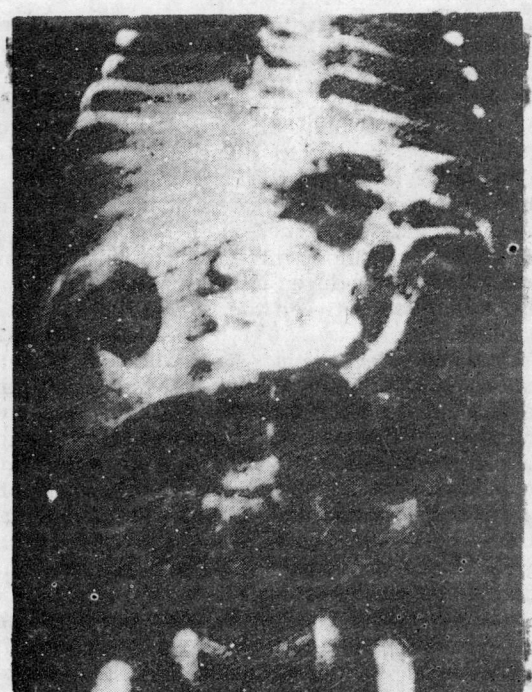

Figure 7-25 Meconium ileus. Impacted meconium with small amounts of air interspersed throughout it in loops of intestine on the right side of abdomen; intestinal loops above this impaction are greatly distended.

roentgenographic appearance. Roentgenographically, in contrast to the generally evenly distended intestinal loops above an atresia, the loops may vary in width and not be as evenly filled with gas. At points of heaviest meconium concentration the infiltrated gas may create a granular appearance (Fig 7-25 and 7-26). A negative sweat test in the neonatal period may not rule out cystic fibrosis.

The case fatality rate is high, but a number of infants

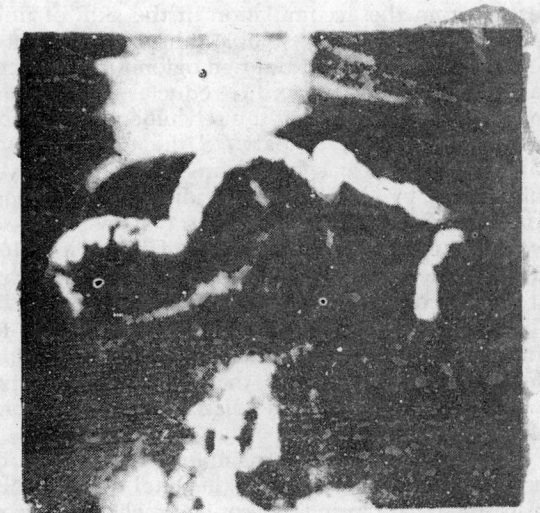

Figure 7-26 Meconium ileus. The colon, outlined by contrast material, is small because meconium has not reached it.

have survived the neonatal period; their subsequent prognosis is dependent upon the basic disturbance, cystic fibrosis (Sec 12.110).

Treatment is high Gastrografin enemas as described under meconium plugs above. If they are unsuccessful or if there is reason to suspect a perforation of the bowel wall, laparotomy is performed and the ileum opened at the point of greatest diameter of the impaction. The inspissated meconium is removed by gentle and patient irrigation with warm isotonic sodium chloride solution introduced through a fine catheter which may be passed between the impaction and the bowel wall.

Meconium Peritonitis. Perforation of the intestine may occur in utero or shortly after birth. The tear may be sealed by natural processes relatively quickly with only a small amount of meconium escaping or the meconial contents may largely be emptied into the peritoneal cavity. Such perforations occur most often as a complication of meconium ileus in infants with cystic fibrosis, but occasionally the perforation is due to a meconium plug, meconium bodies, or intestinal obstruction of another cause.

When the intestinal perforation is spontaneously sealed and only a small amount of meconium has escaped, the event may never be known, except as some of the meconial particles become calcified and are subsequently discovered fortuitously on roentgenograms of the abdomen. Alternatively, the clinical picture may be dominated by the signs of intestinal obstruction or peritonitis. Characteristically there is abdominal distention, vomiting, and absence of stools. The treatment is primarily elimination of the intestinal obstruction and drainage of the peritoneal cavity.

7.44 JAUNDICE AND HYPERBILIRUBINEMIA IN THE NEWBORN

Under usual nursery conditions jaundice is observed during the 1st wk of life in approximately 60% of term infants and 80% of preterm infants. The color usually results from the accumulation in the skin of unconjugated, nonpolar, lipid-soluble bilirubin pigment (indirect-reacting) formed from hemoglobin by the action of heme oxygenase, biliverdin reductase, and nonenzymatic reducing agents in the reticuloendothelial cells; it may also be due, in part, to the deposition of the pigment after it has been converted in the liver cell microsome by the enzyme uridine disphosphoglucuronic acid (UDPGA) glucuronyl transferase to the polar, water-soluble ester glucuronide of bilirubin (direct-reacting). The unconjugated form is neurotoxic for infants at certain concentrations and under various conditions.

Jaundice should be considered a sign of risk for the infant with the degree of danger that it may represent dependent upon factors that affect the production, metabolism, excretion, and distribution of bilirubin after birth.

Etiology. The newborn infant's metabolism of bilirubin is in transition from the fetal stage, when the placenta is the principal route of elimination of the lipid-soluble bilirubin, to the adult stage, when the water-soluble conjugated form is excreted from the hepatic cell into the biliary system and then into the gastrointestinal tract. Any factor that increases the load of bilirubin to be metabolized by the liver (hemolytic anemias, shortened red cell life owing to immaturity or to transfused cells, increased enterohepatic circulation, infection), any factor that may damage or reduce the activity of the enzyme (anoxia, infection, possibly hypothermia and thyroid deficiency), any factor that may compete for or block the enzyme (drugs and other substances requiring glucuronic acid conjugation for excretion), or any factor leading to absence of or decreased amounts of the enzyme or reduction of bilirubin uptake by the liver cell (genetic defect, prematurity) may be expected to cause or increase the degree of jaundice. The risk of toxic effects from elevated levels of bilirubin in the serum is increased by factors that reduce the retention of bilirubin in the circulation (hypoproteinemia, displacement of bilirubin from its binding sites on albumin by competitive binding of drugs such as sulfisoxazole, acidosis, hyperosmolality, increased free fatty acid concentration secondary to hypoglycemia, starvation, or hypothermia), or by factors that increase the permeability of the blood-brain barrier or nerve cell membranes to bilirubin or the susceptibility of brain cells to its toxicity. (See Table 7–17.) Early feeding decreases and dehydration increases the serum levels of bilirubin. Drugs such as oxytocin and chemicals employed in the nursery such as phenolic detergents may also produce hyperbilirubinemia.

Clinical Manifestations. Jaundice may be present at birth or may appear at any time during the neonatal period, depending on the condition responsible for it. *Its intensity bears no clinically dependable relation to the degree of hyperbilirubinemia*, particularly in infants receiving phototherapy (Sec 7.45). Therefore, bilirubin determinations should be done on all jaundiced infants. Jaundice resulting from deposition of indirect bilirubin in the skin tends to appear bright yellow or orange; jaundice of the obstructive type (direct bilirubin), a greenish or muddy yellow. This difference is usually apparent only in severe jaundice. The infant may be lethargic and feed poorly. Signs of kernicterus rarely appear on the 1st day of jaundice.

Differential Diagnosis. Jaundice present at birth or appearing within the 1st 24 hr of life may be due to erythroblastosis fetalis, sepsis, cytomegalic inclusion disease, rubella, or congenital toxoplasmosis. Jaundice in infants who have received intrauterine transfusions may be characterized by an unusually high proportion of direct-reacting bilirubin. Jaundice which first appears on the 2nd or 3rd day is usually "physiologic," but may represent a more severe form called hyperbilirubinemia of the newborn. Familial nonhemolytic icterus (Crigler-Najjar syndrome) also is seen initially on the 2nd or 3rd day. *Jaundice appearing after the 3rd day and within the 1st wk should suggest septicemia as a likely cause;* it may be due to other infections, notably syphilis, toxoplasmosis, and cytomegalic inclusion disease. Jaundice secondary to extensive ecchymosis or hematoma may occur during the 1st day or later, especially in premature infants. Polycythemia may lead to early jaundice.

Jaundice initially noted after the 1st wk of life sug-

Table 7–17 FACTORS INCREASING THE RISK OF KERNICTERUS

FACTORS	MECHANISM OF ACTION		
	Reduced Albumin Binding Capacity	Competition for Binding Sites	Increased Cell Susceptibility to Toxicity
Prematurity	+	–	?
Hemolysis	–	+	?
Asphyxia	+	–	+
Acidosis	+	–	?
Elevated nonesterified fatty acids	–	+	–
Hyperosmolality	+	–	?
Cold stress	–	+	–
Low levels of serum albumin	+	–	+
Hypoglycemia	–	+	?
Infection	+	–	?
Drugs	–	+	–
Male sex	–	–	?

Modified from Brown AK, In: Behrman RE (ed): Neonatology, St. Louis, CV Mosby, 1973; and Birth Defects Series, New York, The National Foundation, June 1972, Vol VI, No 2.

gests septicemia, congenital atresia of the bile ducts, homologous serum hepatitis, rubella, herpetic hepatitis, idiopathic dilatation of the common bile duct, galacto-semia, congenital hemolytic anemia (spherocytosis), or possibly the crises of other hemolytic anemias (such as pyruvate kinase and other glycolytic enzyme deficiencies, thalassemia, sickle cell disease, hereditary non-spherocytic anemia), or hemolytic anemia due to drugs (as in congenital deficiencies of the enzymes glucose-6-phosphate dehydrogenase, glutathione synthetase, reductase, or peroxidase) or to exposure to other substances.

Persistent jaundice during the 1st mo of life suggests the so-called inspissated bile syndrome (which may follow hemolytic disease of the newborn), hepatitis, cytomegalic inclusion disease, syphilis, toxoplasmosis, familial nonhemolytic icterus, congenital atresia of the bile ducts, idiopathic dilatation of the common bile ducts, or galactosemia. It also may be associated with total parenteral nutrition. Rarely, physiologic jaundice

may be prolonged for several wk, as in infants with hypothyroidism or pyloric stenosis.

Regardless of the gestational age or time of appearance of jaundice, significant hyperbilirubinemia requires a complete diagnostic evaluation, which should include the determination of the direct and indirect bilirubin fractions, hemoglobin, reticulocyte count, blood type, Coombs test, and an examination of the peripheral blood smear (Table 7–18). Indirect reacting bilirubinemia, reticulocytosis, and a smear demonstrating evidence of red cell destruction suggest hemolysis; in the absence of blood group incompatibility, nonimmunologically induced hemolysis should be considered. If there is direct-reacting hyperbilirubinemia, hepatitis, inborn errors of metabolism, cystic fibrosis, and sepsis are diagnostic possibilities. If the reticulocyte count, Coombs, and direct bilirubin are normal, physiologic or pathologic indirect hyperbilirubinemia may be present.

Physiologic Jaundice (Icterus Neonatorum). Under normal circumstances, the level of indirect-reacting bil-

Table 7–18 DIAGNOSTIC FEATURES OF THE VARIOUS TYPES OF NEONATAL JAUNDICE

DIAGNOSIS	NATURE OF VAN DEN BERGH REACTION	JAUNDICE		PEAK BILIRUBIN CONC.		BILIRUBIN RATE OF ACCUMULATION mg/dl/day	REMARKS
		Appears	Disappears	mg/dl	Age in Days		
1. "Physiologic jaundice":							1. Usually relates to degree of maturity
Full-term	Indirect	2–3 days	4–5 days	10–12	2–3	<5	
Premature	Indirect	3–4 days	7–9 days	15	6–8	<5	
2. Hyperbilirubinemia due to metabolic factors, etc.:							2. Metabolic factors: hypoxia, respiratory distress, lack of carbohydrate
Full-term	Indirect	2–3 days	Variable	>12	1st wk	<5	Hormonal influences: cretinism, hormones
Premature	Indirect	3–4 days	Variable	>15	1st wk	<5	Genetic factors: Crigler-Najjar syndrome, transient familial hyperbilirubinemia
							Drugs: vitamin K, novobiocin
3. Hemolytic states and hematoma	Indirect	May appear in 1st 24 hr	Variable	Unlimited	Variable	Usually >5	3. Erythroblastosis: Rh, ABO. Congenital hemolytic states: spherocytic, nonspherocytic. Infantile pyknocytosis Drugs: vitamin K. Enclosed hemorrhage—hematoma
4. Mixed hemolytic and hepatotoxic factors	Indirect and direct	May appear in 1st 24 hr	Variable	Unlimited	Variable	Usually >5	4. Infection: bacterial sepsis, pyelonephritis, hepatitis, toxoplasmosis, cytomegalic inclusion disease, rubella Drugs: vitamin K
5. Hepatocellular damage	Indirect and direct	Usually 2–3 days	Variable	Unlimited	Variable	Variable can be >5	5. Biliary atresia; galactosemia; hepatitis and infection as in (4)

From Brown AK: Pediatr Clin North Am 9(No. 3):589, 1962.

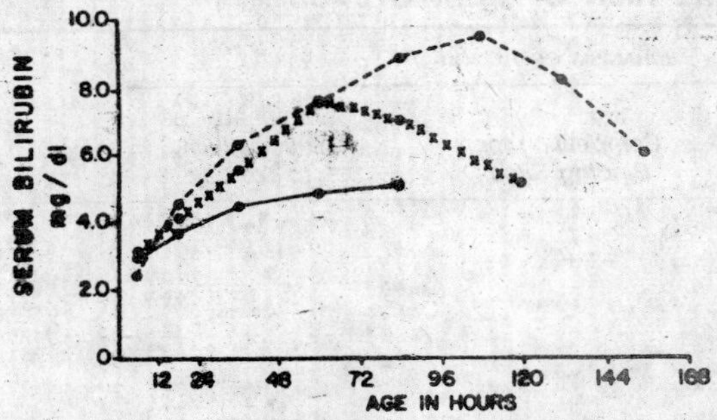

Figure 7–27 Mean serum bilirubin in relation to age in 3 groups of infants. AGA = appropriate for gestational age; SGA = small for gestational age. (From Behrman RE (ed): Neonatology. St. Louis, CV Mosby, 1973.)

irubin in umbilical cord serum is 1–3 mg/dl and rises at a rate of less than 5 mg/dl/24 hr; thus, jaundice becomes visible on the 2nd–3rd day, usually peaking between the 2nd–4th days at 5–6 mg/dl and decreasing to below 2 mg/dl between the 5th–7th days of life. Jaundice resulting from these changes is designated "physiologic" and is believed to be the result of breakdown of fetal red cells combined with transient limitation in the conjugation and excretion of bilirubin by the liver.

Among premature infants the rise in serum bilirubin tends to be the same or a little slower than in term infants but of longer duration, generally resulting in higher levels, the peak being reached between the 4th–7th days (Fig 7–27); the pattern depends upon the time required for the preterm infant to achieve mature mechanisms for the metabolism and excretion of bilirubin. Usually, peak levels of 8–12 mg/dl are not reached until the 5th–7th day and jaundice is infrequently observed after the 10th day.

The diagnosis of physiologic jaundice in term or preterm infants can be established only by excluding known causes of jaundice on the basis of history and clinical and laboratory findings (Table 7–18). In general, a search to determine the cause of jaundice should be made if (1) it appears in the 1st 24 hr of life; (2) serum bilirubin is rising at a rate greater than 5 mg/dl/24 hr; (3) serum bilirubin is greater than 12 mg/dl in fullterm or 14 mg/dl in preterm infants; (4) jaundice persists after the 1st wk of life; or (5) direct-reacting bilirubin is greater than 1 mg/dl at any time.

Genetic and *ethnic factors* may affect the severity of physiologic jaundice resulting in pathologic hyperbilirubinemia. Mean peak serum unconjugated bilirubin concentrations in Chinese, Japanese, Korean, and American Indian fullterm newborns are approximately double those of other populations. The incidence of kernicterus is increased in Oriental and in Greek infants from Lesbos and Rhodes independent of hemolysis from the increased incidence of glucose-6-phosphate dehydrogenase deficiency. Other factors that increase the risk of hyperbilirubinemia may result in severe jaundice in these infants.

Pathologic Hyperbilirubinemia. Jaundice and its underlying hyperbilirubinemia are considered patho-

logic if their time of appearance, duration, or pattern of serially determined serum bilirubin concentrations varies significantly from that of physiologic jaundice, or if the course is compatible with physiologic jaundice but there are other reasons to suspect that the infant is at special risk from the neurotoxicity of unconjugated bilirubin. It may not be possible to determine precisely the etiology for an abnormal elevation of unconjugated bilirubin, especially in premature infants; hence, the term **hyperbilirubinemia of the newborn** is used for those infants whose primary problem is probably a deficiency or inactivity of bilirubin glucuronyl transferase rather than an excessive load of bilirubin for excretion.

The *significance* of hyperbilirubinemia lies in the high incidence of kernicterus associated with serum bilirubin levels over 18–20 mg/dl in term infants. The correlation between serum bilirubin levels and kernicterus or milder forms of brain injury in infants with erythroblastosis fetalis probably holds for all newborn infants who develop bilirubin concentrations beyond the physiologic range for their weight and gestational age, independent of the etiology of the jaundice. Low birth weight infants develop kernicterus at lower levels (10–12 mg/dl) in association with asphyxia, respiratory distress syndrome, hypoglycemia, acidosis, sepsis, and meningitis. Sulfisoxazole also increases susceptibility to kernicterus at relatively low levels (12–15 mg/dl) of serum bilirubin.

Fewer than 3% of term infants without blood group incompatibility develop bilirubin levels greater than 15 mg/dl. Sixteen percent of white and 8% of black infants of low birth weight (presumably preterm) achieve these levels. Unconjugated hyperbilirubinemia has also been associated with the administration of vitamin K_3 or novobiocin, mongolism, and maternal diabetes.

Jaundice Associated with Breast Feeding. An estimated 1 of 200 breast-fed term infants develops significant elevations in unconjugated bilirubin between the 4th–7th days of life, reaching maximum concentrations as high as 10–27 mg/dl during the 3rd wk. If breast feeding is continued, the hyperbilirubinemia gradually decreases and then may persist for 3–10 wk at lower levels. If nursing is discontinued, the serum bilirubin level falls rapidly, usually reaching normal levels within a few days. Cessation of breast feeding for 2–4 days results in a rapid decline in serum bilirubin, after which nursing can be resumed without a return of the hyperbilirubinemia to its previously high levels. These infants have no other sign of illness, and kernicterus has not been reported. The milk of some of these mothers contains 5β-pregnane-3α,20β-diol and nonesterified long-chain fatty acids, which competitively inhibit glucuronyl transferase conjugating activity in approximately 70% of the infants nursed by them. In others, the milk contains a lipase which may be responsible for jaundice. This syndrome must be distinguished from a frequently claimed but inadequately documented relationship between accentuated unconjugated hyperbilirubinemia in the 1st wk of life and breast feeding.

Transient Familial Neonatal Hyperbilirubinemia. Severe unconjugated hyperbilirubinemia leading to kernicterus may occur rarely in the 1st 2 days of life because of a glucuronyl transferase-inhibiting factor present in the serum of mother and infant.

Neonatal Hepatitis. See Sec 11.89.
Congenital Atresia of the Bile Ducts. See Sec 11.91.
Inspissated Bile Syndrome. See Late Complications in Sec 7.47.

7.45 KERNICTERUS

Kernicterus is a neurologic syndrome resulting from the deposition of unconjugated bilirubin in brain cells. The risk in infants with erythroblastosis fetalis is directly related to serum bilirubin levels. It is probably similar for infants with hyperbilirubinemia of whatever cause.

The precise blood level above which indirect-reacting bilirubin or free bilirubin will be toxic for an individual infant is unpredictable, but kernicterus is rare in term infants with serum levels under 18–20 mg/dl. The duration of exposure necessary to produce toxic effects is also unknown. There is some evidence that motor disturbances in later childhood are more common among newborn infants whose total serum bilirubin rises above 15 mg/dl. *The less mature the infant, the greater the susceptibility to kernicterus.* Factors that potentiate the movement of bilirubin into brain cells and its adverse effects on them are listed in Table 7–17. In exceptional circumstances kernicterus in premature infants with serum bilirubin concentrations as low as 8–12 mg/dl has been associated with an apparently cumulative effect of a number of the factors listed in Table 7–17.

Clinical Manifestations. Signs and symptoms of kernicterus usually appear 2–5 days after birth in term infants and as late as the 7th day in premature ones, but hyperbilirubinemia may lead to the syndrome at any time during the neonatal period and, very rarely, later in childhood. The early signs may be subtle and indistinguishable from those of sepsis, asphyxia, hypoglycemia, intracranial hemorrhage, and other acute systemic illnesses in the neonatal infant. Lethargy, poor feeding, and loss of the Moro reflex are common initial signs. Subsequently, the infant may appear gravely ill and prostrated with diminished tendon reflexes and respiratory distress. Opisthotonos, with bulging fontanel, twitching of face or limbs, and a shrill high-pitched cry may follow. In advanced cases convulsions and spasm occur, with the infant stiffly extending his arms in inward rotation with fists clenched. Rigidity is rare at this late stage. Many infants who progress to these severe neurologic signs die; the survivors are usually seriously damaged, but may appear to recover and for 2–3 mo manifest few abnormalities. Later in the 1st yr of life opisthotonos, muscular rigidity, irregular movements, and convulsions tend to recur. In the 2nd yr opisthotonos and seizures abate but irregular, involuntary movements, muscular rigidity, or, in some infants, hypotonia increase steadily. By 3 yr of age the complete neurologic syndrome is often apparent, consisting of bilateral choreoathetosis with involuntary muscle spasm, extrapyramidal signs, seizures, mental deficiency, dysarthric speech, high-frequency hearing loss, squints, and defective upward movement of the eyes. Pyramidal signs, hypotonia, and ataxia occur in a few infants. In mildly affected infants the syndrome may be characterized only by mild to moderate neuromuscular incoordination, partial deafness, or "minimal brain dysfunction," occurring singly or in combination; these problems may be inapparent until the child enters school.

Pathology. The surface of the brain is usually pale yellow. On cutting, certain regions are characteristically stained yellow by unconjugated bilirubin, particularly the corpus subthalamicum, hippocampus and adjacent olfactory areas, striate bodies, thalamus, globus pallidus, putamen, inferior clivus, cerebellar nuclei, and cranial nerve nuclei. Nonpigmented areas may also be damaged. Loss of neurons, reactive gliosis, and atrophy of involved fiber systems are found in late disease. The pattern of injury has been related to the development of oxidative enzyme systems in various regions of the brain and overlaps with that found in anoxic brain damage. Evidence favors the hypothesis that bilirubin interferes with oxygen utilization by cerebral tissue, possibly by injuring the cell membrane; antecedent hypoxic injury increases the susceptibility of brain cells to injury. Gross bilirubin staining without hyperbilirubinemia or the specific microscopic changes of kernicterus may not be the same entity.

Incidence and Prognosis. Using pathologic criteria one third of infants with untreated hemolytic disease and bilirubin levels in excess of 20 mg/dl will develop kernicterus. The incidence at autopsy of hyperbilirubinemic premature infants is 2–16% and is related to presence of factors listed in Table 7–17. Reliable estimates of the frequency of the clinical syndrome are not available because of the wide spectrum of manifestations. Overt neurologic signs have a grave prognosis; 75% or more of such infants die, and 80% of affected survivors have bilateral choreoathetosis with involuntary muscle spasm. Mental retardation, deafness, and spastic quadriplegia are common. Infants who are at risk should have screening hearing tests.

Treatment of Hyperbilirubinemia. Irrespective of etiology, the goal of therapy is to prevent the concentration of indirect-reacting bilirubin in the blood from reaching levels at which neurotoxicity may occur; it is recommended that exchange transfusion and/or phototherapy be used to keep the maximum total serum bilirubin below the levels indicated in Table 7–19. The risk of injury to the central nervous system from bilirubin must be balanced against the risk inherent in the treatment for each infant. The criteria for initiating phototherapy are not generally agreed upon. Since phototherapy may require 12–24 hr to have a measurable effect, it must be started at bilirubin levels below those indicated in Table 7–19. When identified, the underlying cause of the icterus should be treated, e.g., antibiotics for septicemia. Physiologic factors that increase the risk of neurologic damage should also be treated, e.g., correction of acidosis.

Exchange Transfusion. This widely accepted treatment should be repeated as frequently as necessary to keep indirect bilirubin levels in the serum under 20 mg/dl in fullterm infants. (See Exchange Transfusion in Sec 7.47.) A variety of factors may alter this criterion in

Table 7-19   RECOMMENDED MAXIMAL TOTAL SERUM BILIRUBIN CONCENTRATIONS (MG/DL)*

BIRTH WEIGHT CATEGORY (GM)†	UNCOMPLICATED COURSE	COMPLICATED COURSE‡
Less than 1250	13	10
1250–1499	15	13
1500–1999	17	15
2000–2499	18	17
2500 and up	20	18

*Direct-reacting bilirubin concentrations are not subtracted unless they amount to more than 50% of the total serum bilirubin concentration. This table is applicable during the 1st 28 days of life.

†Equivalent gestational age categories may be used in lieu of birth weight for small for gestational age (SGA) infants.

‡Complications include perinatal asphyxia and acidosis, postnatal hypoxia and acidosis, significant and persistent hypothermia, hypoalbuminemia, meningitis and other significant infections, hemolysis, hypoglycemia, and signs of clinical or CNS deterioration.

From Gartner LM, *In:* Behrman RE (ed): Neonatal-Perinatal Medicine. St. Louis, CV Mosby, 1977.

either direction in an individual patient. Appearance of clinical signs suggesting kernicterus is indication for exchange transfusion at any level of serum bilirubin. A healthy fullterm infant may tolerate a concentration slightly higher than 20 mg/dl with no apparent ill effect, whereas a sick premature infant may develop kernicterus at a significantly lower level. A level approaching that considered critical for the individual infant may be an indication for exchange transfusion during the 1st day or 2 of life when a further rise is anticipated but not on the 4th day in term infants or on the 7th day in premature infants, when an imminent fall may be anticipated as the conjugating mechanism becomes more effective.

Phototherapy. Clinical jaundice and indirect hyperbilirubinemia are reduced on exposure to a high intensity of light in the visible spectrum. Bilirubin absorbs light maximally in the blue range (from 420–470 nm). Bilirubin in the skin absorbs light energy, which by photoisomerization converts the toxic unconjugated bilirubin into unconjugated isomers that are excreted in the bile and by autosensitization involving singlet oxygen may result in oxidation reactions producing breakdown products that are excreted by the liver and kidney without need for conjugation.

The use of phototherapy with fluorescent light bulbs has decreased the need for exchange transfusion in low birth weight infants without hemolytic disease and in infants with hemolysis as well as for repeated exchange transfusion of infants with hemolytic disease. However, when there are indications for exchange transfusion, phototherapy should not be used as a substitute.

Phototherapy is indicated only after establishment of the presence of pathologic hyperbilirubinemia. The basic cause(s) of the jaundice should be treated concomitantly. The effectiveness of phototherapy in lowering serum bilirubin levels varies inversely with the rate and degree of hemolysis, if present, and varies directly with the often unpredictable degree of activity of glucuronyl transferase.

Normal infants receiving phototherapy for 1–3 days have peak serum bilirubin concentrations about one half those of untreated infants. In premature infants without significant hemolysis serum bilirubin usually declines 1–3 mg/dl after 8–12 hr of exposure, and peak levels attained may be decreased by 3–6 mg/dl. The therapeutic effect depends upon the light energy emitted in the effective range of wavelengths, the distance between the lights and the infant, and the amount of skin exposed, as well as upon the rate of hemolysis and in vivo metabolism and excretion of bilirubin. It is not known whether phototherapy prevents kernicterus or milder forms of brain injury associated with bilirubin toxicity. Available commercial phototherapy units vary considerably in the spectral output and intensity of radiation emitted; therefore, the dose can be accurately measured only at the skin surface. Dark skin does not reduce the efficacy of phototherapy.

Phototherapy is applied continuously and the infant is turned frequently for maximal skin exposure. It should be discontinued as soon as the indirect bilirubin concentration has been reduced to levels considered safe in view of the infant's age and condition. Serum bilirubin levels and hematocrits should be monitored every 4–8 hr in infants with hemolytic disease or those with bilirubin levels near the range considered toxic for the individual infant. Others, particularly older infants, may be monitored at 12–24 hr intervals. Monitoring should continue for at least 24 hr after cessation of phototherapy since unexpected rises of serum bilirubin sometimes occur and require further treatment. Skin color cannot be relied upon for evaluating the effectiveness of phototherapy; the skin of babies exposed to light may appear almost without jaundice in the presence of marked hyperbilirubinemia. The infant's eyes should be closed and adequately covered to prevent exposure to light (excessive pressure from an eye bandage may injure the closed eyes or the corneas may be excoriated if the infant can open his or her eyes under the bandage). Body temperature should be monitored and the infant should be shielded from bulb breakage. If feasible, irradiance should be measured directly, and details of the exposure should be recorded (type and age of bulbs, duration of exposure, distance from light source to infant, etc.). *In the infant with hemolytic disease, care must be taken not to overlook developing anemia which may require transfusion.*

Complications of phototherapy include loose stools, skin rashes, overheating and dehydration from lights, chilling from exposure of the infant, and "bronze baby syndrome." Animal experiments suggest the possibility of eye injury from light, but it has not been observed in humans. Eye injury from the bandages is uncommon.

The term **bronze baby syndrome** refers to a dark grayish brown discoloration of the skin sometimes noted in infants undergoing phototherapy. Almost all infants observed with this syndrome have had a mixed type of hyperbilirubinemia with significant elevation of direct-reacting bilirubin and often with other evidence of obstructive liver disease. The discoloration may last for many months.

Wide clinical experience suggests that long-term adverse biologic effects of phototherapy are absent, no imal, or unrecognized. However, those employing phototherapy should remain alert to these possibilities and avoid its unnecessary use since in vitro untoward effects on DNA have been demonstrated.

Phenobarbital. Phenobarbital enhances the conjugation and excretion of bilirubin. Its administration will limit the development of physiologic jaundice in the newborn infant when administered to mothers in a dose of 90 mg/24 hr prior to delivery or to infants at birth in a dose of 5 mg/kg/24 hr. However, since its effect on bilirubin metabolism is usually not manifest until after several days of administration and since it is less effective than phototherapy in lowering serum bilirubin concentrations, may have an untoward sedative effect, and does not add to the response to phototherapy, it is not recommended for treating jaundice in the neonatal infant.

NECROTIZING ENTEROCOLITIS

See Sec 11.39.

Andres JM, Mathis RK, Walker WA: Liver disease in infants; Part I: Developmental hepatology and mechanisms of liver dysfunction. J Pediatr 90:686, 1977.

Broderson R: Bilirubin transport in the newborn infant, reviewed with relationship to kernicterus. J Pediatr 96:349, 1980.

Drew JH, Kitchen WH: The effect of maternally administered drugs on bilirubin concentration in the newborn infant. J Pediatr 89:657, 1976.

Gartner LM, Lee K: Jaundice and liver disease; I. Unconjugated hyperbilirubinemia. *In:* Behrman RE (ed): Neonatal-Perinatal Medicine. St. Louis, CV Mosby, 1977.

Mathis RK, Andres JM, Walker WA: Liver disease in infants; Part II: Hepatic disease states. J Pediatr 90:864, 1977.

Ritter DA, Kenny JD, Norton HJ, et al: A prospective study of free bilirubin and other risk factors in the development of kernicterus in premature infants. Pediatrics 69:260, 1982.

Scheidt PC, Mellito ED, Hardy JB, et al: Toxicity to bilirubin in neonates: Infant development during the first year in relation to maximum neonatal serum bilirubin concentration. J Pediatr 92:292, 1977.

Turkel S, Guttenberg M, Moynes D, et al: Lack of identifiable risk factors for kernicterus. Pediatrics 66:502, 1980.

Turkel S, Miller CA, Guttenberg M, et al: A clinical pathologic reappraisal of kernicterus. Pediatrics 69:267, 1982.

DISTURBANCES OF THE BLOOD

7.46 ANEMIA IN THE NEWBORN INFANT

Anemia at birth is manifest by pallor or shock. It is usually caused by hemolytic disease of the newborn but may also be the result of tearing or cutting of the umbilical cord during delivery, abnormal cord insertions, communicating placental vessels, placenta previa or abruptio, or hemorrhage from the fetal side of the placenta. The last may be caused by accidental incision of the placenta in the course of cesarean section or by so-called transplacental hemorrhage. Anemia at birth may also occur in 1 of twins with conjoined placental circulation, in which case the anemic twin "bleeds into" the other twin. Rarely, scalp blood sampling for fetal distress may result in anemia.

Transplacental hemorrhage, with bleeding from the fetal into the maternal circulation, is probably more common than is generally recognized and may occasionally be severe but is usually not sufficient to cause clinically apparent anemia at birth. The cause of transplacental hemorrhage is not clear, but its occurrence has been proved by demonstration of significant amounts of fetal hemoglobin and red cells in the maternal blood on the day of delivery.

Acute blood loss usually results in severe distress at birth, initially with normal hemoglobin level, no hepatosplenomegaly, and the early onset of shock. In contrast, chronic blood loss in utero produces marked pallor, less distress, low hemoglobin level with microcytic indices, and, if severe, congestive heart failure.

Anemia appearing in the 1st few days after birth is also most frequently the result of hemolytic disease of the newborn. Other causes are hemorrhagic disease of the newborn, bleeding from an improperly tied or clamped umbilical cord, large cephalhematomas or caput succedaneum, intracranial hemorrhage, or subcapsular bleeding from rupture of the liver, spleen, adrenals, or kidneys. Rapid decreases in hemoglobin or hematocrit values during the 1st few days of life may be the initial clue to these conditions.

Later in the neonatal period delayed anemia from hemolytic disease of the newborn, with or without exchange transfusion or phototherapy, may be seen. Vitamin K (as Synkayvite) in large doses may cause anemia in premature infants, characterized by inclusion bodies (Heinz bodies) in the erythrocytes. Congenital hemolytic anemia (spherocytosis) occasionally makes its appearance during the 1st mo of life, and hereditary nonspherocytic hemolytic anemia has been described during the neonatal period secondary to deficiency of such enzymes as glucose-6-phosphate dehydrogenase and pyruvate kinase. Bleeding from hemangiomas of the upper gastrointestinal tract or from ulcers caused by aberrant gastric mucosa in a Meckel diverticulum or duplication is a rare source of anemia in the newborn. Repeated blood sampling of infants requiring frequent monitoring of blood gases and chemistries may also produce anemia.

Since a further "physiologic" decrease in erythrocytes and in hemoglobin content is to be expected in all newborn infants (Table 14–3), treatment of any significant anemia (less than 8 gm of hemoglobin/dl) present at or shortly after birth consists not only in eliminating its cause, if it is still present, but also in transfusing small amounts of packed red blood cells (10–15 ml/kg; 2 ml/kg raises hemoglobin about 1 gm/dl).

7.47 HEMOLYTIC DISEASE OF THE NEWBORN
(Erythroblastosis Fetalis)

Erythroblastosis fetalis results from the transplacental passage of maternal antibody active against red cell antigens of the infant, leading to an increased rate of red cell destruction. It continues to be an important cause of anemia and jaundice in newborn infants despite the development of a method of prevention of maternal isoimmunization by Rh antigens. Although more than 60 different red cell antigens capable of eliciting an antibody response in a suitable recipient have been identified, significant disease is associated primarily with the D antigen of the Rh group and with incompatibility of ABO factors. Rarely, hemolytic disease may be caused by C or E antigens or by other red cell antigens, such as C", C", D", K(Kell), M, Duffy, S, and Kidd.

Hemolytic Disease of the Newborn Due to Rh Incompatibility

The Rh antigenic determinants are genetically transmitted from each parent either as a single gene or a group of closely linked genes that determine the Rh type and direct the production of a number of blood group factors (C, c, D, d, E, and e). Each factor can elicit a specific antibody response under suitable conditions.

Pathogenesis. Approximately 15% of Whites, 7% of Blacks, and 1% of Chinese do not have the D antigen and are designated Rh negative (d/d). As a consequence, isoimmune hemolytic disease from this antigen is approximately 3 times more frequent in Whites than in Blacks. When Rh positive blood is infused into an Rh negative woman through error or when small quantities (usually more than 1 ml) of Rh positive fetal blood containing D antigen inherited from an Rh positive father enter the maternal circulation during pregnancy, with spontaneous or induced abortion, or at delivery, antibody formation against D may be induced in the unsensitized Rh negative recipient mother. Once immunization has occurred, considerably smaller doses of antigen can stimulate an increase in antibody titer. Initially, there is a rise of antibody in the 19S gamma globulin fraction, which later is replaced by 7S (IgG) antibody; the latter readily crosses the placenta to agglutinate the infant's red blood cells, causing hemolytic manifestations.

Hemolytic disease rarely occurs during a 1st pregnancy since transfusions of Rh positive fetal blood into an Rh negative mother tend to occur near the time of delivery, too late for the mother to become sensitized in time to transmit antibody to the infant before delivery. The fact that 55% of Rh positive fathers are heterozygous (D/d) and may have Rh negative offspring reduces the chance of sensitization as does small family size, in which there are fewer opportunities for it to occur. Finally, the capacity of Rh negative women to form antibodies is variable, some producing low titers even after adequate antigenic challenge. Thus, the overall incidence of isoimmunization of Rh negative mothers at risk is low, with antibody to D detected in less than 10% of those studied, even after 5 or more pregnancies; only about 5% ever have babies with hemolytic disease.

Some Rh negative women sensitize easily, with the 1st pregnancy at risk; others have many Rh positive infants without producing antibodies. The woman whose husband is heterozygous will not be affected by an Rh negative fetus. When mother and fetus are incompatible with respect to groups A or B, the mother is protected to a degree against sensitization by the rapid removal of Rh positive cells from her circulation by her anti-A or anti-B which are IgM antibodies and do not cross the placenta. Once the mother is sensitized, the infant is likely to have hemolytic disease. There is a tendency in some families for the severity of the illness to worsen with successive pregnancies. The possibility that the 1st affected infant after sensitization may represent the end of the mother's child-bearing potential for Rh positive infants argues urgently for the prevention of sensitization when this is possible. Such prevention consists of injection into the mother of anti-D gamma globulin (RhoGam) immediately following the delivery of each Rh positive infant (see below).

Clinical Manifestations. A wide spectrum of hemolytic disease occurs in affected infants born to sensitized mothers, depending on the nature of the individual immune response. The severity of the disease may range from only laboratory evidence of mild hemolysis (15% of cases) to severe anemia with compensatory hyperplasia of erythropoietic tissue, leading to massive enlargement of the liver and spleen. When the compensatory capacity of the hematopoietic system is exceeded, profound anemia results in pallor, signs of cardiac decompensation (hepatosplenomegaly, respiratory distress), massive anasarca, and circulatory collapse. This clinical picture, termed **hydrops fetalis**, frequently results in death in utero or shortly after birth; it may also occur from other etiologies (Table 7–20). Failure to initiate spontaneous effective ventilation due to pulmonary edema results in birth asphyxia; following successful resuscitation, severe respiratory distress may ensue. Petechiae, purpura, and thrombocytopenia may also be present in severe cases and should suggest the presence of concurrent disseminated intravascular coagulation.

Jaundice is usually absent at birth because of placental clearance of lipid-soluble unconjugated bilirubin, but in severe cases bilirubin pigments stain the amniotic fluid, cord, and vernix caseosa yellow. Icterus is generally evident within the 1st day of life since the infant's bilirubin-conjugating and excretory systems are unable to cope with the load resulting from massive hemolysis. Indirect-reacting bilirubin therefore accumulates postnatally and may rapidly reach extremely high levels with a significant risk of bilirubin encephalopathy.

Table 7–20   ETIOLOGIES OF HYDROPS FETALIS

Hematologic: Rh incompatibility, rarer blood group incompatibility, α-thalassemia, twin-twin transfusion, feto-maternal hemorrhage
Infections: syphilis, cytomegalovirus, toxoplasmosis, Chagas disease, leptospirosis
Cardiovascular: paroxysmal atrial tachycardia, congestive heart failure, arteriovenous malformation, umbilical vein thrombosis
Tumors: congenital neuroblastoma, placental chorioangioma
Pulmonary: pulmonary lymphangiectasia, cystic adenomatoid malformation, hypoplasia
Hepatorenal: hepatitis, nephrosis, renal vein thrombosis, urethral atresia
Metabolic: maternal diabetes mellitus, Gaucher disease, achondroplasia
Idiopathic
Multiple severe congenital anomalies

There may be a greater risk of developing kernicterus from hemolytic disease than from comparable nonhemolytic hyperbilirubinemia, although the risk in an individual patient may only be a function of the severity of illness (anoxia, acidosis, etc.). Hypoglycemia occurs frequently in infants with severe isoimmune hemolytic disease and may be related to hyperinsulinism and hypertrophy of the pancreatic islet cells in these infants.

The availability of techniques for improved intrauterine diagnosis of the severity of disease in an affected fetus has led to the development of obstetric criteria for induced premature delivery. This has decreased the incidence of fetal death from the disease and increased the frequency of premature infants with clinical erythroblastosis, with the added risk of neurologic damage from the combination of immaturity and hyperbilirubinemia.

Infants born after intrauterine transfusion for prenatally diagnosed erythroblastosis are generally severely affected since the indications for the transfusion are evidences of already severe disease in utero. Such infants usually have very high (but this is extremely variable) cord levels of bilirubin, reflecting the severity of hemolysis and its effects upon hepatic function. Anemia from continuing hemolysis may be masked by the prior intrauterine transfusion, and the clinical manifestations of erythroblastosis may be superimposed upon various degrees of immaturity due to spontaneous or induced premature delivery.

Laboratory Data. Prior to treatment, the direct Coombs test* is usually positive. Anemia is usual. The cord blood hemoglobin varies, usually proportionally to the severity of the disease; with hydrops fetalis it may be as low as 3–4 gm/dl. Alternatively, despite hemolysis, it may be within the normal range owing to compensatory bone marrow activity. The blood smear usually shows polychromasia and a marked increase in nucleated red blood cells. The reticulocyte count is increased. The white blood cell count is usually normal but may be elevated, and there may be thrombocytopenia in severe cases. The cord bilirubin is usually between 3–5 mg/dl; only rarely is there a substantial elevation of direct-reacting (conjugated) bilirubin. The indirect-reacting bilirubin rises rapidly to high levels in the 1st 6 hr of life.

After intrauterine transfusions the cord blood may show a normal hemoglobin concentration, negative direct Coombs test, predominantly adult red cells, and a relatively normal smear. Marked elevation of both indirect- and direct-reacting bilirubin levels has been reported in these infants.

Diagnosis. The definitive diagnosis of erythroblastosis fetalis requires demonstration of blood group in-

compatibility and of corresponding antibody bound to the infant's red cells.

Antenatal Diagnosis. In Rh negative women a history of previous transfusions, abortion, or pregnancy should suggest the possibility of sensitization. Expectant parents' blood types should be tested for potential incompatibility and the maternal titer of albumin-active IgG antibodies to D should be assayed at 12–16, 28–32, and 36 wk. The presence of measurable antibody titer in albumin at the beginning of pregnancy, a rapid rise in titer, or a titer of 1:64 or greater suggests significant hemolytic disease, although the exact titer correlates poorly with the severity of disease. If a mother is found to have antibody against D at a titer of 1:16 or greater at any time during a subsequent pregnancy, the severity of fetal disease should be monitored by amniocentesis. Higher titers suggest a more severely affected fetus and the need for earlier amniocentesis. If there is a history of a previously affected infant and/or a stillbirth, an Rh positive infant is usually equally or more severely affected than the previous infant, and the severity of disease in the fetus should be followed by serial amniocenteses. Ultrasonography is indicated to determine if there is hydrops fetalis.

Amniocentesis. Spectrophotometric analysis of bile pigments in amniotic fluid obtained by direct transabdominal uterine aspiration after placental localization by ultrasound has proved to be a generally safe and reliable way of predicting the severity and progress of fetal hemolysis. In the affected fetus there is a positive deviation from the normal straight line curve of optical density of the amniotic fluid, measured at wavelengths from 350–700 nm and plotted on semilogarithmic paper. The peak of density deviation from the normal occurs at 450 nm (ΔOD450) and is used as an index of the risk of intrauterine death and severity of anemia when plotted against gestational age and compared with the outcome of a population of affected infants (Fig 7–28).

Postnatal Diagnosis. Immediately after the birth of any infant to an Rh negative woman, blood from the umbilical cord or from the infant should be examined for ABO blood group, Rh type, hematocrit *and* hemoglobin, and reaction of the direct Coombs test. If the Coombs test is positive, a serum bilirubin should be done as a baseline, and a commercially available red cell panel should be used to identify as many as possible of the specific red cell antibodies that are present in the mother's serum. This is done not only to identify antibody against the D antigen but against a broad group of other antigens as well and will help to ensure the selection of the most compatible blood for exchange transfusion, should it be necessary. The direct Coombs test is usually strongly positive in clinically affected infants and may remain so for a few days up to several mo.

Treatment. The main goals of therapy are (1) to prevent intrauterine or extrauterine death from severe anemia and its complications, and (2) to avoid neurotoxicity from hyperbilirubinemia.

Treatment of the Unborn Infant. The survival of moderately and severely affected fetuses has been markedly improved by inducing labor between 33–34

---

*The *Coombs test* detects the presence of antibody globulin attached to red blood cells. In the *direct* Coombs test antiserum against human gamma globulin (Coombs serum) causes agglutination of the red cells of an affected infant. The term *indirect* Coombs test refers to a technique that is used to detect antibody in plasma or serum. Normal red cells are exposed first to the suspected serum and then to Coombs serum, at which point agglutination occurs if antibody present in the suspected serum has attached itself to the red cells.

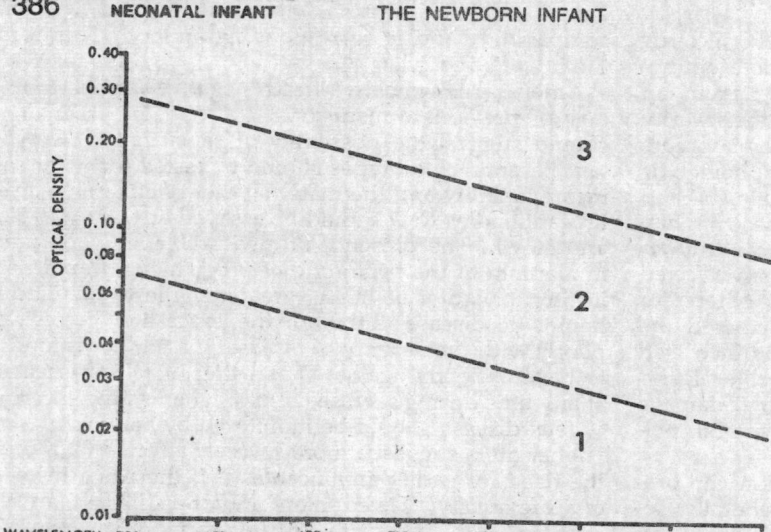

Figure 7–28 Plotting of the increase in optical density at 450 mµ according to gestational age, and zoning of the increase in optical density according to Liley's data. Zone 3, Severe disease; impending fetal death. Zone 2, Indeterminate disease. Zone 1, Rh negative infant or mildly affected Rh positive infant. Predictions should be based on the *trend* of readings from 2 or 3 amniotic fluid specimens serially obtained at 1- to 2-wk intervals beginning no later than about 10 wk before the gestational time at which the previous pregnancy ended. A high reading that remains flat or rises on serial determinations suggests the need for intrauterine transfusion and/or early delivery; a fall in serial readings suggests a good prognosis without interference. (From Bowman JM, Pollock JM: Pediatrics 35:815, 1965.)

wk when repeated amniocenteses show flat or rising ΔOD450's in high zone 2 or zone 3 (Fig 7–28). When the chance that a severely affected fetus will survive to a gestational age compatible with early delivery and neonatal survival is small, an intrauterine intraperitoneal transfusion of erythrocytes compatible with the mother's blood may be indicated. A judgment must be made whether at a particular gestational age the risk of dying from erythroblastosis or from premature delivery is greater than the risk of dying during or immediately following the procedure. At 33–34 wk or more of gestation, delivery should be induced since the risk of intrauterine transfusion is usually greater. Between 30–33 wk of gestation the decision should be based upon a comparison of the mortality rates of the transfusing team and of the premature intensive care unit where the newborn infant will be treated. Additional indications for intrauterine transfusion include several optical density readings in zone 3, especially if the trend is increasing and there is a family history of stillbirths, hydrops fetalis, or severely affected infants. Some use hydrops fetalis as an indication for intrauterine transfusion.

Treatment of the Liveborn Infant. The birth should be attended by the physician who will care for the affected infant afterward. Fresh, low titer, group O, Rh negative blood, crossmatched against the maternal serum using an indirect Coombs technique, should be immediately available. If clinical signs of severe hemolytic anemia (pallor, hepatosplenomegaly, edema, petechiae, or ascites) are evident at birth, immediate supportive therapy, temperature stabilization, and monitoring before proceeding with exchange transfusion may save some severely affected infants, though hydropic babies rarely survive. Such therapy should include correction of acidosis with 2–3 mEq/kg of sodium bicarbonate; a small transfusion of compatible packed red cells to correct anemia; volume expansion for hypotension, especially in those with hydrops; and provision of assisted ventilation, if needed.

Exchange Transfusion. When the clinical condition of the infant at birth does not require an immediate full or partial exchange transfusion, the decision to do it should be based on a judgment that there is a high risk of rapidly developing a dangerous degree of anemia or of hyperbilirubinemia. The criteria for this judgment include a cord blood hemoglobin of 10 mg/dl or less, verified by an equally low capillary blood hemoglobin (which tends to be higher than that of cord or venous blood), or a cord bilirubin of 5 mg/dl or greater. Some physicians consider previous kernicterus or severe erythroblastosis in a sibling, reticulocyte counts greater than 15%, and prematurity to be further factors supporting a decision for early exchange transfusion.

The hemoglobin, hematocrit, and serum bilirubin levels should be measured at 4–6 hr intervals at first, with extension to longer intervals if and as the rate of change diminishes. The decision to perform an exchange transfusion is based upon the likelihood that the trend of bilirubin levels plotted against hours of age indicates that the serum bilirubin will reach the level indicated in Table 7–19, above which there is an increased risk of kernicterus. Although most exchange transfusions are performed to prevent or reduce hyperbilirubinemia, one may rarely be indicated to deal with rapidly developing anemia. Ordinary transfusions of compatible Rh negative red cells may be necessary to correct anemia at any stage of the disease up to 6–8 wk of age when the infant's own blood-forming mechanism may be expected to take over. Weekly determinations of hemoglobin or hematocrit should be done until a spontaneous rise has been demonstrated.

Careful monitoring of the serum bilirubin level is essential until a falling trend has been demonstrated in the absence of phototherapy. Even then, an occasional infant, particularly if premature, may experience an unpredicted significant rise in serum bilirubin as late as the 7th day of life. Alternatively, predictions of the achievement of dangerously high levels of serum bilirubin based on observed levels exceeding 6 mg/dl in the 1st 6 hr or 10 mg/dl in the 2nd 6 hr of life, or on rates of rise exceeding 0.5–1.0 mg/dl/hr, are also uncertain. Indices of free bilirubin and bilirubin binding have not yet been shown to be routinely reliable aids in evaluating the risk associated with hyperbilirubinemia.

Blood for exchange transfusion should be as fresh as possible. Heparin, acid-citrate-dextrose (ACD), or citrate-phosphate-dextrose (CPD) may be used as anticoagulants. If the blood is obtained before delivery, it should be taken from a type O, Rh negative donor with a low titer of anti-A and anti-B, and be compatible with the mother's serum by indirect Coombs test. After delivery, blood should be obtained from an Rh negative donor whose cells are compatible with both the infant's and mother's serum; when possible, type O donor cells are usually employed, but cells of the infant's blood type may be used. A complete cross-match, including indirect Coombs test, should be performed prior to the 2nd and subsequent transfusions. Blood should be gradually warmed to and maintained at a temperature between 22–37°C throughout the exchange transfusion. It should be kept well mixed by gentle squeezing or agitation of the bag to avoid sedimentation; otherwise, the use of supernatant serum with a low red cell count at the end of the exchange will leave the infant anemic. Whole blood should be used rather than packed red cells. An elevated venous pressure may reflect severe peripheral and pulmonary vasoconstriction which will respond to the intravenous administration of 2–3 mEq/kg of sodium bicarbonate. Alternatively, it may suggest a failing heart from hypervolemia. The infant's stomach should be emptied prior to transfusion to prevent aspiration, body temperature should be maintained, and vital signs monitored. A competent assistant should be present to help monitor, tally the volume of blood exchanged, and perform emergency procedures.

The umbilical vein is cannulated, using strict aseptic technique, with a polyvinyl catheter to a distance no greater than 7 cm in a fullterm infant. When free flow of blood is obtained, the catheter is usually in a large hepatic vein or the inferior vena cava. Exchange should be carried out over a 45–60 min period, alternating aspirations of 20 ml of infant blood and infusions of 20 ml of donor blood. Smaller aliquots (10 ml) may be indicated for sick and premature infants. The goal should be an exchange of approximately 2 blood volumes of the infant (2×85 ml/kg). If heparinized blood is used, 0.45 ml (4.5 mg) of a 1% solution of protamine sulfate should be injected intravenously at the conclusion of the transfusion for each dl of blood exchanged.

The administration of albumin before an exchange transfusion is not recommended because of conflicting results concerning the increased efficiency of bilirubin removal that may result, the risk of redistribution of bilirubin from areas of innocuous deposition into the nervous system, the potential bilirubin-displacing effect of stabilizers added to injectable preparations of human serum albumin, the risk of resulting hypervolemia, and the increased difficulty in interpreting subsequent bilirubin levels that results from albumin-binding of bilirubin in the vascular space.

The venous pressure should be measured intermittently during an exchange transfusion; elevated umbilical venous pressure (higher than 10 cm of water) may occur among infants with severe hemolytic disease and hydrops fetalis or those born after intrauterine transfusions. This may represent hypervolemic congestive heart failure and indicate the need for the initial withdrawal of blood sufficient to reduce the venous pressure to normal levels (5–7 cm of water). The pressure may also be falsely elevated as the result of faulty catheter placement, pulmonary disease, or high intra-abdominal pressure from ascites. Direct or indirect measurement of blood pressure is important to detect hypovolemic hypotension or diagnose hypertension which may occasionally occur with exchange transfusion.

These infants and others with acidosis and hypoxia from respiratory distress, sepsis, hypothermia, or shock may be further compromised by the significant acute acid load contained in citrated (ACD) blood which usually has a pH between 6–7. The subsequent metabolism of citrate may result in a later metabolic alkalosis if ACD blood is used. Fresh heparinized blood avoids this problem. If sodium bicarbonate is administered either to correct or to prevent acidosis during the exchange, the blood pH must be serially monitored. Symptomatic hypoglycemia may occur before exchange transfusion in moderately to severely affected infants; it may also occur 1–3 hr after exchange. Prophylactic antibiotics are not indicated as a routine; sulfonamides and other drugs that may bind to albumin competitively with bilirubin are contraindicated.

After exchange transfusion the bilirubin level must be determined at frequent intervals (every 4–8 hr), and 2nd or repeated exchange transfusions should be carried out to keep the indirect fraction from exceeding the levels indicated in Table 7-19. Symptoms suggestive of kernicterus are mandatory indications for exchange transfusion at any time.

The risk of death from exchange transfusion carried out by skilled and experienced physicians is less than 1%. However, with the decreasing use of this procedure because of the use of phototherapy and the prevention of sensitization, the general level of competence is decreasing. Thus, it may be best to concentrate this mode of treatment in neonatal referral centers.

Late Complications. The infant with hemolytic disease and/or who has had an exchange or an intrauterine transfusion must be observed carefully for the development of anemia and hepatitis. Treatment with supplemental iron and/or blood transfusion may be indicated.

Inspissated bile syndrome refers to the rare occurrence of persistent icterus in association with significant elevations of direct as well as indirect bilirubin in infants with hemolytic disease. The cause is unclear but the jaundice clears spontaneously within a few wk or mo.

Portal vein thrombosis may occur among children who have been subjected to exchange transfusion as newborn infants. It is probably associated with prolonged, traumatic, or septic umbilical vein catheterization.

Prevention of Rh Sensitization. The risk of initial sensitization of Rh negative mothers has been reduced from between 10–20% to less than 1% by intramuscular injection of 300 µg of human anti-D globulin (1 ml of RhoGAM) within 72 hr of delivery or abortion. This quantity is sufficient to eliminate approximately 10 ml of potentially antigenic fetal cells from the maternal circulation. Large fetal-to-maternal transfer of blood may require proportionately more RhoGAM. The use of this technique, combined with improved methods of detecting maternal sensitization and quantitating the extent of the fetal to maternal transfusion, plus the use of fewer obstetric procedures that increase the risk of such fetal to maternal bleeding (versions, manual separation of the placenta, etc.) should eventually almost eliminate erythroblastosis fetalis.

Hemolytic Disease of the Newborn Due to A and B Incompatibility

Major blood group incompatibility between mother and fetus usually results in milder disease than does Rh incompatibility. Maternal antibody may be formed against B cells if the mother is type A or against A cells if the mother is type B. However, usually the mother is type O and the infant is A or B. Although ABO incompatibility occurs in 20–25% of pregnancies, hemolytic disease develops in only 1 in 10 of such offspring and usually the infants are of type A_1 which is more antigenic than A_2. Low antigenicity of the ABO factors in the fetus and newborn infant may account for the low incidence of severe ABO hemolytic disease relative to the incidence of incompatibility between the blood groups of mother and child. Although antibodies against A and B factors occur without prior immunization ("natural" antibodies), these are ordinarily present in the 19S (IgM) fraction of gamma globulin, which does not cross the placenta. However, univalent, incomplete (albumin active) antibodies to A antigen may be present in the 7S (IgG) fraction, which does cross the placenta, so that A–O isoimmune hemolytic disease may be seen in 1st-born infants; when high antibody levels are present, an infant may be severely affected. Those mothers who have become immunized against A or B factors from a previous incompatible pregnancy also exhibit antibody in the 7S gamma globulin fraction. These "immune" antibodies are the primary mediators in ABO isoimmune disease.

Clinical Manifestations. Most cases are mild, with jaundice as the only clinical manifestation. The infant is not generally affected at birth; pallor is not present and hydrops fetalis is extremely rare. Liver and spleen are not greatly enlarged, if at all. Jaundice usually appears during the 1st 24 hr. Rarely, it may become severe with symptoms and signs of kernicterus rapidly developing.

Diagnosis. A presumptive diagnosis is based on the presence of ABO incompatibility, a weakly to moderately positive direct Coombs test, and spherocytes in the blood smear which may at times suggest the presence of hereditary spherocytosis. Hyperbilirubinemia is often the only other laboratory abnormality. The hemoglobin level is usually normal, but may be as low as 10–12 gm/dl. Reticulocytes may be increased to 10–15%, with extensive spherocytosis, polychromasia, and increased numbers of nucleated red cells. In 10–20% of affected infants the unconjugated serum bilirubin level may reach 20 mg/dl or more unless phototherapy is employed.

Treatment. Phototherapy may be effective in lowering serum bilirubin levels. Otherwise, treatment is directed at correcting dangerous degrees of anemia or hyperbilirubinemia by exchange transfusions with blood of the same group and Rh type as that of the mother. The indications for this procedure are similar to those previously described for hemolytic disease due to Rh incompatibility.

Other Forms of Hemolytic Disease

Blood group incompatibilities other than Rh or ABO (c, E, Kell [K], etc.) account for less than 5% of hemolytic disease of the newborn. The direct Coombs test is invariably positive, and exchange transfusion may be indicated for hyperbilirubinemia and anemia. Congenital infections, such as cytomegalic inclusion disease, toxoplasmosis, rubella, and syphilis, may present with hemolytic anemia, jaundice, hepatosplenomegaly, and thrombocytopenia, but the direct Coombs test is negative, and there are usually other distinguishing clinical findings. Homozygous α-thalassemia may present with severe hemolytic anemia and a clinical picture resembling hydrops fetalis; it can be distinguished by a negative direct Coombs test and characteristic clinical and laboratory findings. Anemia and jaundice may occur in infancy from hereditary spherocytosis and, if untreated, can result in kernicterus. Hemolytic anemia producing jaundice in the 1st wk of life may also be secondary to congenital deficiencies in red cell enzymes, such as glucose-6-phosphate dehydrogenase (G-6-PD).

7.48 PLETHORA IN THE NEWBORN INFANT
(Polycythemia)

See also Sec 14.30.

Plethora or apparent cyanosis associated with abnormally high erythrocyte, hemoglobin, and hematocrit values has been reported with and without clinical findings suggestive of placental dysfunction syndrome. Polycythemia is defined as a central hematocrit value of 65% or more. Anorexia, lethargy, cyanosis, and convulsions may appear on the 2nd and 3rd days of life. Hyperbilirubinemia, congestive heart failure, necrotizing enterocolitis, respiratory distress, and persistent fetal circulation are associated problems. The pathophysiology of the condition is not clear but may, in part, be related to the increased viscosity of the blood. Plethora may also be due to a "placental transfusion" in the recipient twin of monozygotic twins with parabiotic placental circulations. Plethora as the result of transfusion from the maternal to the fetal circulation has also been described. It also may occur in large "cushingoid" infants of diabetic mothers, Down syndrome, adrenogenital syndrome, neonatal Graves syndrome, and Beckwith syndrome.

The *treatment* of symptomatic plethora of the newborn

is phlebotomy and replacement with plasma. A partial exchange transfusion is a technically simpler and therapeutically more effective approach.

7.49 HEMORRHAGE IN THE NEWBORN INFANT

Hemorrhagic Disease of the Newborn. A moderate decrease of factors II, VII, IX, and X normally occurs in all newborn infants by 48–72 hr after birth, with a gradual return to birth levels by 7–10 days of age. This transient deficiency of vitamin K–dependent factors probably is due to lack of free vitamin K in the mother, immaturity of the infant's liver, and absence of bacterial intestinal flora normally responsible for synthesis of vitamin K. Rarely among term infants and more frequently among premature infants there is an accentuation and prolongation of this deficiency between the 2nd–5th days of life, resulting in spontaneous and prolonged bleeding. Breast milk is a poor source of vitamin K, and hemorrhagic complications have appeared more commonly in breast-fed than cow's milk-fed infants. This form of hemorrhagic disease of the newborn, which is responsive to vitamin K therapy, must be distinguished from disseminated intravascular coagulopathy and from rarer congenital deficiencies of 1 or more of the other vitamin K–dependent factors or factor V which are unresponsive to vitamin K (Sec 14.59).

Hemorrhagic disease of the newborn resulting from severe transient deficiencies of vitamin K–dependent factors is characterized by bleeding which tends to be gastrointestinal, nasal, subgaleal, intracranial, or a result of circumcision. The prothrombin time, blood coagulation time, and plasma recalcification time are prolonged, and the levels of prothrombin (II) and factors VII, IX, and X are significantly decreased. Bleeding time, fibrinogen, factors V and VIII, platelets, capillary fragility, and clot retraction are normal for age and maturity. The administration of 1 mg of natural oil-soluble vitamin K, either intramuscularly or orally, at the time of birth prevents the fall in vitamin K–dependent factors in fullterm infants but is not uniformly effective in the prophylaxis of hemorrhagic disease of the newborn in premature infants. The disease may be effectively treated with an intravenous infusion of 5 mg of vitamin K_1, with improvement of coagulation defects and cessation of bleeding within a few hr. However, serious bleeding, particularly in premature infants or those with liver disease may require a transfusion of fresh frozen plasma or whole blood. The mortality rate is low among treated patients.

A particularly severe form of deficiency of vitamin K–dependent coagulation factors has been reported in infants born to mothers receiving anticonvulsive medications during pregnancy (phenobarbital and phenytoin). There may be severe bleeding with onset within the 1st 24 hr of life, usually corrected by vitamin K_1, although in some the response is poor or delayed. A prothrombin time (PT) should be obtained on cord blood and the infants given 1–2 mg of vitamin K intravenously. If the PT is greatly prolonged and fails to improve, then 10 ml/kg of fresh frozen plasma should be given.

Concentrated forms of vitamin K–dependent coagulation factors should be avoided in this group of infants because they may carry considerable risk of transmitting serum hepatitis.

Other forms of bleeding may be clinically indistinguishable from hemorrhagic disease of the newborn responsive to vitamin K but are neither prevented nor successfully treated with it. Treatment of the rare congenital deficiencies of prothrombin and factors V, VII, and X requires fresh whole blood or specific factor replacement.

Disseminated intravascular coagulopathy in newborn infants results in consumption of coagulation factors and bleeding. The infants are often premature; the clinical course is frequently characterized by hypoxia, acidosis, shock, or infection. Treatment is directed at correction of the primary clinical problem, such as infection, and at interruption of consumption and replacement of clotting factors. The prognosis is poor regardless of therapy (Sec 14.69).

A clinical pattern identical to that of hemorrhagic disease of the newborn may also result from any of the congenital defects in blood coagulation (Sec 14.54–14.62).

Infants with central nervous system or other bleeding constituting an *immediate threat to life* should receive a small transfusion of fresh, compatible whole blood or plasma, as well as vitamin K, as soon as possible after blood has been drawn for coagulation studies, including determination of the number of platelets.

The so-called swallowed blood syndrome, in which blood or bloody stools are passed, usually on the 2nd or 3rd day of life, may be confused with hemorrhage from the gastrointestinal tract. The blood may be swallowed during delivery or from a fissure in the mother's nipple. Differentiation from gastrointestinal hemorrhage is based on the fact that the infant's blood contains mostly fetal hemoglobin, which is alkali-resistant, whereas swallowed blood from a maternal source contains adult hemoglobin, which is promptly changed to alkaline hematin upon the addition of alkali. Apt devised the following test for this differentiation:

(1) Rinse a bloodstained diaper or some grossly bloody stool with a suitable amount of water to obtain a distinctly pink supernatant hemoglobin solution. (2) Centrifuge the mixture. Decant the supernatant solution. (3) To 5 parts of the supernatant fluid add 1 part of 0.25 normal (1%) sodium hydroxide. Within 1–2 min a color reaction takes place: a yellow-brown color indicates that the blood is maternal in origin; a persistent pink, that it is from the infant. A control test with known adult or infant blood, or both, is advisable.

Widespread subcutaneous ecchymoses in premature infants at or immediately after birth are apparently a result of fragile superficial blood vessels rather than of a coagulation defect. Vitamin K_1 administration to the mother during labor has no effect on their incidence. An occasional infant is born with petechiae or a generalized bluish suffusion limited to the face, head, and neck. These are probably the result of venous obstruction caused by sudden increases in intrathoracic pressure during delivery. It may take 2–3 wk for such suffusions to disappear.

Neonatal Thrombocytopenic Purpura. See Sec 14.65.

Bleyer WA, Hakami N, Shepard TH: The development of hemostasis in the human fetus and newborn infants. J Pediatr 79:838, 1971.

Desjardins L, Blaychman M, Chintu C, et al: The spectrum of ABO hemolytic disease of the newborn infant. J Pediatr 95:447, 1979.

Gross S, Stuart M: Hemostasis in the premature infant. Clin Perinatol 4:259, 1977.

Honig GR, Hruby MA: Disorders of the blood and hematopoietic system. In: Behrman RE (ed): Neonatal-Perinatal Medicine. St Louis, CV Mosby, 1977.

Liley AW: Liquor amnii analysis in management of pregnancy complicated by rhesus sensitization. Am J Obstet Gynecol 82:1359, 1961.

Mountain KR, Hirsch J, Gallus AS: Neonatal coagulation defect due to anticonvulsant drug treatment in pregnancy. Lancet 1:265, 1970.

Oski F, Naiman J: Anemia in the neonatal period. In: Hematological Problems in the Newborn. Philadelphia, WB Saunders, 1972.

Phibbs RH, Johnson P, Kitterman JA, et al: Cardio-respiratory status of erythroblastotic newborn infants; III. Intravascular pressures during the first hours of life. Pediatrics 58:484, 1976.

Queenan J: Erythroblastosis fetalis and polyhydramnios. In: Behrman RE (ed): Neonatal-Perinatal Medicine. St Louis, CV Mosby, 1977.

7.50 DISTURBANCES OF THE GENITOURINARY SYSTEM

See also Chapter 16.

One or both kidneys are often easily palpable in the newborn infant. When both are palpable and similar, there is usually no particular diagnostic problem, but when only 1 kidney can be felt, the impression that it is larger than normal or is displaced by an intrinsic or extrinsic mass is frequent. Fetal lobulation may contribute to this impression. Usually the problem resolves itself as the kidney becomes progressively less easily palpable during the early mo of life. Since palpable enlargement or displacement of the kidney in the newborn may be due to hydronephrosis, an embryoma, or a cystic malformation, an abdominal plain film, intravenous urogram, or ultrasound examination may be indicated. Because of the poor concentrating ability of the neonatal kidney, relatively large amounts of contrast material (10–20 ml of Diodrast) must often be injected to get satisfactory films. During the neonatal period moderate elevation of the blood urea nitrogen does not necessarily signify renal disease, and elevations may occur in association with polycystic disease and hydronephrosis without necessarily implying a poor prognosis. The urine may also contain casts and cellular elements simply as a manifestation of dehydration.

Thrombosis of the Renal Vein. See Sec 16.49.

7.51 DISTURBANCES OF THE CRANIUM

See Anencephaly, Microcephaly, Craniosynostosis, and Hydrocephalus in Chapter 21.

Craniotabes (Congenital Cranial Osteoporosis). Palpation of the skull of the newborn infant may reveal areas of softening along the suture lines, especially in the parietal area, which indent from pressure of the fingers as would a ping-pong ball. This phenomenon is more frequent in premature infants, but occurs in 10–35% of all newborn infants. Failure to observe it in breech presentations has led to an assumption that it may be the result of intrauterine pressure against the maternal pelvis. This condition is a harmless and physiologic result of incoordination between the rapid growth of the brain and the calcification processes in the vertex in the last mo of gestation and is associated with a generalized osteoporotic process in the newborn infant. Differentiation must be made from the craniotabes of rickets, from lacunar skull, in which honeycombed areas of porotic bone create a characteristic appearance in the roentgenogram of the skull, and from osteogenesis imperfecta.

7.52 DISORDERS OF THE SKIN

Skin disorders of the newborn are covered in Chapter 24.

Mastitis Neonatorum. Engorgement of the breasts is physiologic in newborn infants. Infection may be abetted by undue manipulation of the breasts and is manifest by redness, local heat, swelling, and pain. Fever and other general symptoms may also be present. The prognosis is favorable unless septicemia develops. Prophylaxis consists in avoidance of manipulation or other trauma of the engorged breasts. Treatment includes systemic antibiotic therapy and hot compresses applied locally. If an abscess develops, it should be incised and drained.

Scar formation after infection may distort the nipple and impair the secretory power of the mammary gland in a female later in life.

DISTURBANCES OF THE EYE

See Chapter 25.

7.53 THE UMBILICUS

Umbilical Cord. The cord contains the 2 umbilical arteries, the vein, the rudimentary allantois, the remnant of the omphalomesenteric duct, and a gelatinous substance called Wharton jelly. The sheath of the umbilical cord is derived from the amnion. The arteries have a strong contractile capacity; that of the vein is less so that it retains a fairly large lumen after birth. When the cord sloughs, portions of these structures remain in the base. The blood vessels are functionally closed but are patent anatomically for 20–25 days. The arteries become the lateral umbilical ligaments; the vein, the ligamentum teres; and the ductus venosus, the ligamentum venosum. During this interval the umbilical vessels are potential portals of entry for infection.

A **single umbilical artery** is present in about 5–10 of 1000 births; the frequency is about 35–70/1000 twin births. Approximately one third of infants with a single umbilical artery have congenital abnormalities, usually more than 1, and many such infants are stillborn or die shortly after birth. Trisomy 18 is 1 of the more frequent abnormalities. Since many abnormalities are not apparent on gross physical examination, it is important that at every delivery the cut cord and the maternal and fetal surfaces of the placenta be inspected. The number of arteries present should be recorded as an aid to the early suspicion and identification of abnormalities in such infants.

Patency of the omphalomesenteric duct may be responsible for an intestinal fistula, prolapse of the bowel, polyp, or a Meckel diverticulum (Sec 11.30).

A *persistent urachus* (urachal cyst) is due to failure of closure of the allantoic duct. Patency should be suspected if there is a clear, light yellow, urinelike discharge from the umbilicus.

Congenital Omphalocele. An omphalocele is a herniation or protrusion of abdominal contents into the base of the umbilical cord. In contrast to the more common umbilical hernia, the sac is covered with peritoneum without overlying skin. The size of the sac that lies outside the abdominal cavity depends upon its contents. There is herniation of intestines into the cord in about 1 of 5000 births and of liver and intestines in 1 of 10,000 births. The abdominal cavity is proportionately small because of deficient impetus to grow and develop. Immediate surgical repair, before infection has taken place and before the tissues have been damaged by drying or the sac has ruptured, is usually essential for survival. Silastic, Mersilene, or similar synthetic material may be used to cover the viscera if the sac has ruptured or if excessive mobilization of the skin would be necessary to cover the mass and its intact sac. Nonoperative treatment of giant omphaloceles may be successful through "tanning" the sac with a 2% aqueous solution of Merthiolate applied 2–3 times daily. Epithelialization as well as intra-abdominal containment of the viscera has been achieved by this method, which, under special circumstances, may also be applied to smaller lesions.

Tumors. Tumors of the umbilicus are rare; they include angioma, enteroteratoma, dermoid cyst, myxosarcoma, and cysts of urachal or omphalomesenteric duct remnants.

Hemorrhage. Hemorrhage from the umbilical cord may be due to trauma, to inadequate ligation of the cord, or to failure of normal thrombus formation. It may also be an indication of hemorrhagic disease of the newborn, septicemia, or local infection. The infant should be observed frequently during the 1st few days of life so that, if hemorrhage does occur, it will be detected promptly.

Granuloma. The umbilical cord usually dries and separates within 6–8 days after birth. The raw surface becomes covered by a thin layer of skin, scar tissue forms, and the wound is usually healed within 12–15 days. The presence of saprophytic organisms delays separation of the cord and increases the possibility of invasion by pathogenic organisms. Mild infection may result in a moist granulating area at the base of the cord with a slight mucoid or mucopurulent discharge. Good results are usually obtained by cleansing with alcohol several times daily.

The persistence of exuberant granulation tissue at the base of the umbilicus is common. The tissue is soft, vascular and granular, and dull red or pink, and it may have a seropurulent secretion. The *treatment* is cauterization with silver nitrate; it should be repeated at intervals of several days until the base is dry.

Umbilical granuloma must be differentiated from **umbilical polyp**, a rare anomaly resulting from persistence of all or part of the omphalomesenteric duct or the urachus. The tissue of the polyp is firm and resistant, bright red, and has a mucoid secretion. If there is a communication with the ileum or bladder, small amounts of fecal material or urine may be discharged intermittently. Histologically the polyp consists of intestinal or urinary tract mucosa. Treatment is surgical excision of the *entire* omphalomesenteric or urachal remnant.

Infections. Inflammation in the umbilical region, which may be caused by any of the pyogenic bacteria, is especially serious because of the danger of hematogenous spread or extension to the liver or peritoneum. Venous phlebitis may develop later, resulting in portal hypertension and cirrhosis. The general manifestations may be minimal even when septicemia or hepatitis has resulted. Daily baths or daily application of triple dye to the umbilical stump and surrounding skin may reduce the incidence of umbilical infection. *Treatment* includes prompt antibacterial therapy and, if there is abscess formation, surgical incision and drainage.

Umbilical Hernia. This is due to an imperfect closure or weakness of the umbilical ring and is often associated with diastasis recti. It is common, especially in low birth weight and black infants. It appears as a soft swelling covered by skin that protrudes during crying, coughing, or straining and can be reduced easily through the fibrous ring at the umbilicus. The hernia consists of omentum or portions of the small intestine. The size of the defect varies from less than 1 cm in diameter to as much as 5 cm, but large ones are rare.

Treatment. Few medical problems have given rise to more contradictory opinions and practices than has the management of umbilical hernia in infancy. Most umbilical hernias that appear before the age of 6 mo will disappear spontaneously by 1 yr of age. Even large hernias (5–6 cm in all dimensions) have been known to disappear spontaneously by 5–6 yr of age. Strangulation is extremely rare. There is considerable agreement that "strapping" is ineffective as usually practiced. At least 1 study indicates that any form of strapping has a deleterious rather than a beneficial effect. Another study suggests that careful strapping, in which the hernia is reduced by finger pressure and the defect closed by drawing each side of the adjacent abdominal wall toward the midline by means of interlocking straps of broad adhesive tape, increases the incidence of closure of hernias over 6 cm in diameter. Unfortunately neither strapping nor surgery can be accepted as efficacious because data of various studies are not comparable and, particularly, because a careful long term study of the natural history of umbilical hernias is not available. Surgery is not advised unless the hernia persists to the age of 3–5 yr, causes symptoms, becomes strangulated, or becomes progressively larger after the age of 1–2 yr.

7.54 METABOLIC DISTURBANCES

HYPERTHERMIA IN THE NEWBORN
(Transitory Fever of the Newborn;
Dehydration Fever)

Elevations of temperature (38–40° C or 100–104° F) are occasionally noted on the 2nd–3rd day of life in infants whose clinical course has been otherwise satisfactory. This disturbance is especially likely to occur in breast-fed infants whose intake of supplementary fluid has been particularly low or in infants exposed to high environmental temperatures, either in an incubator or in a bassinet near a radiator or in the sun.

The infant may be restless, and there may be a precipitous drop in weight. However, there may not be a consistent relation between the fever and the extent of weight loss or inadequacy of fluid intake. The urinary output and frequency of voiding diminish. The skin may lose some of its elasticity, and the fontanel may be depressed. The infant appears unhappy and takes fluids avidly. The apparent vigor of the infant contrasts with the usual appearance of "being sick" in the presence of infection. Rarely there may be marked tachypnea and tachycardia as the infant attempts to increase heat loss by way of the respiratory tract to compensate for a sudden increase in environmental temperature. The rise in temperature may be associated with an increase in serum protein and sodium and hematocrit. The possibility of local or systemic infection must be evaluated.

Oral or parenteral administration of fluids or lowering of the environmental temperature leads to prompt reduction of the fever and alleviation of symptoms.

A more severe form of neonatal hyperthermia occurs among both newborn and older infants when they are warmly dressed for an outside low temperature that does not exist in their immediate indoor environment. The diminished sweating capacity of the newborn infant is a contributing factor. Warmly dressed infants left near stoves or radiators, traveling in well heated automobiles, or left with bright sunlight shining directly on them through the windows of a closed room or automobile are likely victims. Overclothing in hot weather, especially when the infant is left in the sun, is a less common cause. Body temperature is often as high as 41–44° C (106–111° F). The skin is hot and dry, and initially the infant usually appears flushed and apathetic. This stage may be followed by stupor, grayish pallor, coma, and convulsions. Hypernatremia may contribute to the convulsions. The mortality and morbidity rates (brain damage) are high. The condition is prevented by clothing suitable for the temperature of the immediate environment. In the newborn infant exposure of the body to usual room temperature or immersion in tepid water usually suffices to bring the temperature back to normal levels. Older infants may require cooling for a longer time by repeated immersions or by use of a water-cooled mattress or other apparatus for induction of hypothermia. Attention to possible fluid and electrolyte disturbance is essential.

NEONATAL COLD INJURY

Neonatal cold injury usually occurs among infants in adequately heated homes during damp cold spells when the outside temperature is in the range of freezing. The presenting features are apathy, refusal of food, oliguria, and coldness to touch. The body temperature is usually between 29.5–35° C (85–95° F), and immobility, edema, and redness of the extremities, especially of the hands, feet, and face are observed. Bradycardia and apnea may also occur. The facial erythema frequently gives a false impression of health, delaying recognition that the infant is ill. Local hardening over areas of edema may lead to confusion with scleredema. Rhinitis is common, as are serious metabolic disturbances, particularly hypoglycemia and acidosis. Hemorrhagic manifestations are frequent; massive pulmonary hemorrhage is a common finding at autopsy. Treatment consists of gradual warming with scrupulous attention to recognition and correction of metabolic imbalances, particularly hypoglycemia. Prevention consists in provision of adequate environmental heat. The mortality rate is about 25%; about 10% of the survivors have evidence of brain damage.

EDEMA

Generalized edema occurs in association with hydrops fetalis (Table 7–20) and in the offspring of diabetic mothers. In the premature infant edema is often a consequence of a decreased ability to excrete water or sodium, although some have considerable edema without identifiable reason. Infants with hyaline membrane disease may become edematous even without congestive heart failure. Edema of the face and scalp may result from pressure from the umbilical cord around the neck, and transient localized swellings of the hands or feet may similarly be due to intrauterine pressures. Edema may be present with heart failure due to congenital cardiac lesions, even in the absence of a murmur; a lag in renal excretion of electrolytes and water may result in edema when there has been a sudden large increase in intake of electrolytes, particularly with feeding of concentrated cow's milk formulas. High protein formulas also may cause edema due to the excessive solute load, particularly in premature infants. It is difficult to show a relation between low serum protein or low hemoglobin and the occurrence of edema in older premature infants, but occasionally the therapeutic response to plasma or blood transfusion is prompt. Edema also occurs in association with anemia and vitamin E deficiency in premature infants. Rarely, idiopathic hypoproteinemia with edema lasting weeks or months is observed in term infants. The cause is unclear, and the disturbance is benign. Persistent edema of one or more extremities may represent congenital lymphedema (Milroy disease) or, in females, *Turner syndrome*. Generalized edema with hypoproteinemia may be seen in the neonatal period with congenital nephrosis and rarely with Hurler syndrome or after feeding hypoallergenic formulas to infants with cystic fibrosis of the pancreas. *Sclerema* is described in Sec 24.17.

HYPOCALCEMIA (TETANY)

Early neonatal hypocalcemia, the most common form of postnatal hypocalcemia, is being recognized with increasing frequency. About one third of preterm low birth weight infants, one half of infants born to insulin-dependent diabetic mothers, and 30% of infants with birth asphyxia develop hypocalcemia with total serum calcium levels of 7 mg/dl or less or signs of tetany within the 1st 48 hr of life. In each of these groups, the risk of developing hypocalcemia may be, in part, related to decreased calcium intake due to the infant's small size or illness; increased endogenous phosphate loading from glycogen or tissue breakdown; transient functional hypoparathyroidism with decreased excretion of phosphate; or correction of acidosis with alkali. Serum calcium values correlate directly with gestational age, and less mature infants also have a greater chance of developing hypoglycemia; small for gestational age infants who are not gestationally premature or asphyxiated are less likely to develop hypocalcemia. Decreased circulating vitamin D metabolites also increase the likelihood of hypocalcemia in premature infants, particularly if the mother is vitamin D deficient. The degree of hypocalcemia also varies with the severity of maternal diabetes, and the risk of its development in these infants is increased with concomitant prematurity and asphyxia. In early neonatal hypocalcemia there may be a gradual reversion to normal calcium levels after 1–3 days.

Late neonatal hypocalcemia occurs beyond the 1st 3–4 days of life but usually within the 1st few wk. It most commonly refers to *cow's milk–induced hypocalcemia* resulting from the high phosphate content of cow's milk and some modified cow's milk preparations. It may also be associated with feeding of cereals of high phosphate content. Other disorders that may present as hypocalcemia during this period are *intestinal malabsorption*, especially if the ileum, the site of calcium absorption, is involved (there may be associated malabsorption of magnesium or vitamin D); *acid-base disturbances* associated with alkali therapy for acidosis or hyperventilation; *transient congenital idiopathic hypoparathyroidism*, which may be an extension of early neonatal hypocalcemia and may on rare occasions persist despite dietary management; *true congenital hypoparathyroidism* as a sex-linked condition associated with ring chromosomes or as part of DiGeorge syndrome; *secondary hypoparathyroidism* in offspring of mothers with hyperparathyroidism; *dietary deficiency of vitamin D*; neonatal *liver disease*; and *vitamin D–deficiency rickets*.

Irritability, muscular twitchings, jitteriness, tremors, and convulsions are symptoms; laryngospasm and carpopedal spasm are less common. Since a positive Chvostek sign is common in newborn infants, it cannot be interpreted as a sign of tetany of the newborn. The serum calcium is below 7.5 mg/dl and the serum phosphate is elevated; an absolute diagnosis cannot be made in the absence of these chemical findings. Hypomagnesemia may also be present. The serum phosphatase is normal. A favorable response to administration of calcium is not sufficient in itself to make the diagnosis since calcium may act nonspecifically during seizures. Furthermore, symptoms such as irritability and tremors may subside spontaneously, and convulsions resulting from cerebral edema, anoxia, or injury may not be repeated during the neonatal period. The diverse etiologies of convulsions in the neonatal period call for establishment of a diagnosis by examination of spinal fluid (meningitis, intracranial hemorrhage) and blood chemistries.

The response to **calcium therapy** may be dramatic, convulsions and other symptoms being controlled by the administration of 2 ml/kg (18 mg of elemental calcium/kg) of 10% calcium gluconate into a peripheral vein over a 10 min period while monitoring the heart rate. The infusion should be discontinued if bradycardia occurs. Continued intravenous supplementation at the rate of 75 mg elemental calcium/kg/24 hr is sufficient to achieve normocalcemia. Intramuscular injection of calcium is contraindicated because local induration and necrosis may occur. Calcium should be given orally for approximately 1 wk, preferably as calcium chloride (1.0 gm/24 hr, divided in 3 or more doses) or calcium lactate (2–3/gm/24 hr, divided in 3 or more doses) in 10% solution. The hypocalcemia is usually self-limited as spontaneous improvement occurs in the physiologic functions regulating calcium homeostasis. In early neonatal hypocalcemia, the use of parathyroid extract or of dihydrotachysterol is not indicated. In hypocalcemia secondary to other disorders, therapy for the primary disease is important. If hypocalcemia is persistent, vitamin D or 1 of its metabolites may be helpful. Hypomagnesemia generally requires treatment before hypocalcemia can be successfully treated.

Asymptomatic hypocalcemia usually resolves spontaneously. However, whenever possible, oral calcium gluconate should be given as it will usually obviate the subsequent need for intravenous therapy with its attendant complications.

HYPOMAGNESEMIA

Rarely, hypomagnesemia of unknown etiology may occur in the newborn infant, usually in association with hypocalcemia. It may also be associated with insufficient stores of skeletal magnesium secondary to deficient placental transfer, decreased intestinal absorption, neonatal hypoparathyroidism, hyperphosphatemia, renal loss, a defect in magnesium and calcium homeostasis, or an iatrogenic deficiency due to loss during exchange transfusion or insufficient replacement during total intravenous alimentation. It has also been observed in uremic infants. Infants of diabetic mothers tend to have serum magnesium levels that are lower than the normal mean. The clinical manifestations of hypomagnesemia are indistinguishable from those of hypocalcemia and tetany and may, in fact, be secondary to the accompanying hypocalcemia.

Hypomagnesemia occurs when serum magnesium levels fall below 1.5 mg/dl, though clinical signs usually do not develop until serum magnesium levels fall below 1.2 mg/dl. During exchange transfusion with citrated blood, which is low in magnesium ion because of binding by citrate, the serum magnesium drops about 0.5 mEq/l; approximately 10 days are required for a return to normal. In noniatrogenic hypomagnesemia the serum magnesium may be less than 0.5 mEq/l. The serum calcium in either instance is usually at levels seen in hypocalcemic tetany, but the serum phosphorus value is normal or high. Since the hypocalcemia accompanying hypomagnesemia is inadequately corrected by administration of calcium, hypomagnesemia should also be suspected in any patient with tetany not responding to calcium therapy. Almost all the spontaneously occurring cases thus far reported have been in males.

Immediate *treatment* consists of the intramuscular injection of magnesium sulfate. For newborn infants 0.25 ml/kg of a 50% solution daily usually suffices. The accompanying hypocalcemia usually corrects itself as the hypomagnesemia is relieved. The same daily dose can be given for oral maintenance therapy. Four to 5 times higher doses may be required in malabsorptive states. In most cases the metabolic defect is transient and treatment can be discontinued after 2–3 wk. A few patients appear to have a permanent form of the disease that requires continuous oral supplementation with magnesium to prevent recurrence of hypomagnesemia.* No residual damage to the central nervous system is evident after prompt treatment.

HYPERMAGNESEMIA

Hypermagnesemia may occur in newborn infants of mothers treated with magnesium sulfate for eclampsia. At high serum levels there is depression of the central nervous system and total paralysis so that artificial respiration is required. Toxicity may also result from magnesium sulfate enemas. Lower levels may result in hypoventilation, hypotension, lethargy, flaccidity, and hyporeflexia. The upper limit of normal magnesium is 2.8 mg/dl. Rarely, hypermagnesemia may be associated with failure to pass meconium (meconium plug syndrome). Exchange transfusion has been used as a means of rapid removal of magnesium ion from the blood. Calcium salts and diuresis have also been used. Recovery appears to be complete.

*Four ml/kg/24 hr of the following solution:
Magnesium chloride (MgCl$_2$ · 6 H$_2$O) 4.0 gm (39.6 mEq)
Magnesium citrate (MgHC$_6$H$_5$O$_7$ · 5 H$_2$O) 6.0 gm (39.6 mEq)
Water to 100 ml
Solution provides approximately 0.8 mEq of magnesium/ml.

OTHER METABOLIC DISEASES

A number of inborn errors of metabolism may be manifest during the neonatal period; these include phenylketonuria, galactosemia, the urea cycle defects, methylmalonic acidemia, and maple syrup urine disease. Pyridoxine deficiency and dependency are considered in Sec 3.26.

NARCOTIC ADDICTION AND WITHDRAWALS

Physiologic addiction to narcotics exists in most infants born to actively addicted mothers since many opiates cross the placenta. It may be manifest even before birth by increased activity of the fetus at times when the mother feels the need for the drug or develops withdrawal symptoms. Morphine and methadone are the drugs most frequently involved, but withdrawal syndromes also occur with alcohol, phenobarbital, pentazocine, codeine, propoxyphene, and diazepam.

Pregnancy in an addict or alcoholic is, by definition, a high risk. Prenatal care is usually inadequate, and there is a higher incidence of venereal disease, toxemia, premature rupture of the membranes, breech presentations, prolapsed cords and limbs, preterm and small for gestational age infants, and prenatal morbidity and mortality.

Heroin addiction results in 50% incidence of low birth weight infants, half of whom are small for gestational age. Infections, maternal undernutrition, and a direct fetal growth inhibiting effect have been causally implicated. The rate of stillbirths is increased, but not the incidence of congenital anomalies. *Clinical manifestations* of withdrawal occur in 50–75% of infants, usually beginning within the 1st 48 hr, depending upon the daily maternal dose (<6 mg/24 hr is associated with no or mild symptoms); duration of addiction (>1 yr has a greater than 70% incidence of withdrawal); and time of last maternal dose (there is a higher incidence if within 24 hr of birth). However, symptoms may appear as late as 4–6 wk of age. The incidence of hyaline membrane disease and hyperbilirubinemia may be decreased in low birth weight infants of heroin addicts; hyperventilation leading to respiratory alkalosis or accelerated production of surfactant may explain the former, and enzyme induction of glucuronyl transferase, the latter.

Tremors and hyperirritability are the most prominent symptoms. The tremors may be fine or jittery and indistinguishable from those of hypoglycemia, but are more often coarse, "flapping," and bilateral; the limbs are often rigid, hyperreflexic, and resistant to flexion and extension. Irritability and hyperactivity are generally marked and may lead to skin abrasions. Other signs include tachypnea, diarrhea, vomiting, high-pitched cry, fist sucking, poor feeding, and fever. Sneezing, yawning, myoclonic jerks, convulsions, abnormal sleep cycles, nasal stuffiness, respiratory depression or apneic attacks, flushing alternating rapidly with pallor, and lacrimation are less common. The *diagnosis* is generally established by the history and clinical presentation.

Chromatographic examination of the urine for opiates may reveal only low levels during withdrawal, but quinine, which is often mixed with heroin, may be present in higher concentrations. Hypoglycemia and hypocalcemia should be excluded.

Methadone addiction is resulting in an increasing number of infants with withdrawal symptoms, the incidence varying from 20–90%. In general, mothers taking methadone have better prenatal care than those taking heroin; however, there is a high incidence of multiple drug abuse, including alcohol, barbiturates, and tranquilizers, and they are often heavy smokers. There is no increased incidence of congenital anomalies. The average birth weight of infants of mothers taking methadone is higher than that of infants of heroin-addicted mothers; the *clinical manifestations* are similar except that the former group has a higher incidence of seizures (10% to 20%) and of late onset (2–6 wk of age) of symptoms and signs.

Alcohol withdrawal is uncommon. The infants of women who have been drinking immediately before delivery may have alcohol on their breath for several hr as it rapidly crosses the placenta, and blood levels in the infant are similar to those in the mother. Infants who develop withdrawal symptoms often become agitated and hyperactive with marked tremors lasting for 72 hr, followed by about 48 hr of lethargy before return to normal activity. Seizures may develop. See Sec 28.17 for discussion of the **fetal alcohol syndrome.**

Phenobarbital withdrawal usually occurs in fullterm, appropriate for gestational age infants of addicted mothers. Symptoms begin at a median age of 7 days (range 2–14 days). There may be a brief acute stage consisting of irritability, constant crying, sleeplessness, hiccups, and mouthing movements, followed by a subacute stage that may last 2–4 mo consisting of voracious appetite, frequent regurgitation and gagging, episodic irritability, hyperacusis, sweating, and a disturbed sleep pattern.

Treatment of heroin, methadone, and alcohol withdrawals has been successful using various combinations of narcotics, sedatives, and hypnotics. Therapy is indicated for seizures, for diarrhea, or for such irritability that normal sleep and feeding patterns are disturbed and weight gain is poor. Methadone withdrawal may require larger amounts of medication for longer periods than heroin withdrawal to control clinical manifestations. Phenobarbital, 8–10 mg/kg/day in 4 divided doses, can effectively reduce irritability and prevent seizures. It is as effective as chlorpromazine, 2.2 mg/kg/24 hr, divided into 3–4 doses. It is usually not necessary to administer either drug for more than 5 days, but on occasion it may be necessary to treat for as long as 6 wk. Patients with severe autonomic symptoms may require gradually diminishing doses of methadone or paregoric for 2–10 wk. Paregoric at a beginning dose of 3–5 drops given every 3–6 hr, increased to 5–10 drops every 4 hr if necessary, depending on the size and response of the infant, will abolish most withdrawal symptoms, especially diarrhea. The dose and duration of therapy may be adjusted according to the clinical response. Parenteral administration of fluids may be necessary to prevent aspiration or dehydration until the symptoms are brought under control. Narcotic and phenobarbital withdrawal requires swaddling, frequent feedings, and protection from noxious external stimuli.

Current mortality is not over 10% and with early recognition and treatment may be negligible. *Prognosis* for normal development is affected by the adverse circumstances of high risk pregnancy and delivery and by the environment to which the infant is returned after recovery.

LATE METABOLIC ACIDOSIS

Between 5–40% of preterm low birth weight infants develop a metabolic acidosis during the 2nd or 3rd wk of life. Usually there is no history of asphyxia, respiratory distress, or other problems, and the infants are vigorous. However, they often have received cow's milk formulas of high protein and casein content shortly after birth and have had a delayed start of postnatal weight gain. Blood base excess values range from −10 to −16 mEq/l, and pCO_2 values are usually less than 40 mm Hg. The condition probably represents an abnormally high rate of endogenous acid formation.

Kildeberg P: Late metabolic acidosis of premature infants. *In* Winters RW (ed): The Body Fluids in Pediatrics. Boston, Little, Brown and Co., 1973.

Nervez CT, Shott RJ, Bergstrom WH, et al: Prophylaxis against hypocalcemia in low birth weight infants receiving bicarbonate infusion. J Pediatr 87:439, 1975.

Neuman L, Cohen S: The neonatal narcotic withdrawal syndrome. Clin Perinatol 2:99, 1975.

Scriver CR, Feingold M, Mamanes P, et al: Screening for congenital metabolic disorders in the newborn infant: Congenital deficiency of thyroid hormone and hyperphenylalaninemia. Pediatrics 3(Suppl):389, 1977.

Tsang R, Steichen J, Brown D: Perinatal calcium homeostasis: Neonatal hypocalcemia and bone demineralization. Clin Perinatol 4:385, 1977.

7.55   DISTURBANCES OF THE ENDOCRINE SYSTEM

The endocrinopathies are discussed in Chapter 18. The purpose of this section is to call attention to those endocrine disturbances that may be identified at birth or during the 1st mo of life.

Pituitary dwarfism is usually inapparent at birth, although panhypopituitary male infants may present with neonatal hypoglycemia and micropenis. Conversely, constitutional dwarfs usually demonstrate length and weight consistent with prematurity when born after a normal gestational period; otherwise their physical appearance is normal.

Thyroid deficiency may be apparent at birth in genetically determined **cretinism** or in infants of mothers treated with thiouracil or its derivatives during pregnancy. Constipation, prolonged jaundice, lethargy, or poor peripheral circulation as shown by persistently mottled skin or cold extremities should suggest *cretinism.* The early diagnosis and treatment of congenital deficiency of thyroid hormone may be greatly facilitated by screening all newborn infants for this deficiency.

Temporary hyperthyroidism may occur at birth in the

infants of mothers with hyperthyroidism or of those who have been receiving thyroid medication.

Transient *hypoparathyroidism* may be manifest as tetany of the newborn.

The *adrenal gland* is subject to numerous disturbances which may become apparent and require lifesaving treatment during the neonatal period. Acute adrenal *hemorrhage* and failure may be seen after breech or other traumatic deliveries or in association with overwhelming infection. *Adrenocortical hyperplasia* is suggested by vomiting, diarrhea, dehydration, convulsions, shock, or phallic or clitoral enlargement. Since the condition is genetically determined, newborn siblings of patients with the salt-losing variety of adrenocortical hyperplasia should be observed closely for manifestations of adrenal insufficiency. *Congenitally hypoplastic adrenal glands* may also give rise to adrenal insufficiency during the 1st few wk of life. Female infants with webbing of the neck, lymphangiectatic edema, hypoplasia of the nipples, cutis laxa, low hairline at the nape of the neck, low-set ears, high-arched palate, deformities of the nails, cubitus valgus, and other anomalies should be suspected of having *gonadal dysgenesis.*

Transient *diabetes mellitus* (Sec 17.1) is rare and only seen in the newborn. It usually presents as dehydration, loss of weight, or acidosis in small for gestational age infants.

7.56 INFANTS OF DIABETIC MOTHERS

The successful control of diabetes with insulin has led to the survival of increasing numbers of diabetic women who bear children. Their infants and the infants of women who later develop diabetes share certain distinctive morphologic characteristics, including large size and macrosomia and high morbidity risks. Diabetic mothers have a high incidence of polyhydramnios and over 10 times the fetal mortality rate of nondiabetic mothers, which is higher at all gestational ages, but especially after 32 wk. Fetal wastage throughout pregnancy is associated with poorly controlled maternal diabetes, especially ketoacidosis. Diabetic mothers produce an excess of high birth weight infants at all gestational ages and of low birth weight infants at 37–40 wk gestations. The neonatal mortality rate is over 5 times that of infants of nondiabetic mothers and is higher at all gestational ages and in every birth weight for gestational age category; the relative risk is highest in infants of normal and high birth weight.

Pathophysiology. No single physiologic or biochemical event explains the diverse clinical manifestations. The probable pathogenic sequence is that maternal hyperglycemia causes fetal hyperglycemia, and the fetal pancreatic response leads to fetal hyperinsulinemia; fetal hyperinsulinemia and hyperglycemia then cause increased hepatic glucose uptake and glycogen synthesis, accelerated lipogenesis, and augmented protein synthesis. Related pathologic findings are the hypertrophy and hyperplasia of the pancreatic islets with a disproportionate increase in the number of β cells; increased weights of the placenta and infant organs except for the brain; myocardial hypertrophy; increased amounts of cytoplasm in liver cells; and extramedullary hematopoiesis. The separation of the placenta suddenly interrupts glucose infusion into the neonate without a proportional effect on the hyperinsulinism, resulting in hypoglycemia and attenuated lipolysis during the 1st hours after birth.

Hyperinsulinemia has been documented in infants of gestational diabetic mothers and in those of insulin-dependent diabetic mothers without insulin antibodies. The former group also have significantly higher fasting plasma insulin levels than normal newborns despite similar glucose levels; they respond with a prompt elevation of plasma insulin and assimilate a glucose load more rapidly. Following arginine administration, they also have an enhanced insulin response and increased disappearance rates of glucose, compared with normal infants. In contrast, fasting glucose utilization rates are diminished. The lower free fatty acid levels in infants of insulin-dependent diabetic mothers are probably also a reflection of their hyperinsulinemia. With good prenatal diabetic control, the incidence of macrosomia has decreased.

Although hyperinsulinism is probably the main cause of hypoglycemia, the diminished epinephrine and glucagon responses that occur may be contributing factors. Cortisol and human growth hormone levels are normal.

Clinical Manifestations. The infants of diabetic and gestational diabetic mothers often bear a surprising resemblance to each other (Fig 7–29). They tend to be large and plump owing to increased body fat and

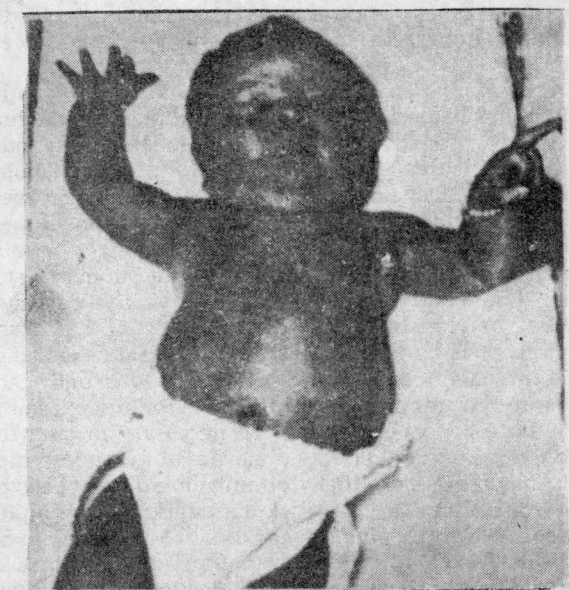

Figure 7–29 Large, plump, plethoric infant of a gestational diabetic mother. Baby was born at 38 wk of gestation but weighed 9 lb 11 oz (4408 gm). Mild respiratory distress was the only symptom other than appearance.

enlarged viscera, with puffy, plethoric facies resembling those of patients who have been receiving a corticosteroid. These infants may, however, also be of normal or low birth weight, particularly if delivered before term or if there is associated maternal vascular disease.

The infants tend to be "jumpy," tremulous, and hyperexcitable during the 1st 3 days of life, although hypotonia, lethargy, and poor sucking also may occur. They may have any of the diverse manifestations of hypoglycemia. Early appearance of these signs is more likely to be related to hypoglycemia and later appearance to hypocalcemia; these abnormalities also may occur together. Perinatal asphyxia or hyperbilirubinemia may produce similar signs. Rarely, hypomagnesemia may be associated with the hypocalcemia.

About 75% of infants of diabetic mothers and 25% of infants of mothers with gestational diabetes develop hypoglycemia (<30 mg/dl glucose), but only a small percentage of these infants become symptomatic. The probability of an infant developing hypoglycemia increases and the glucose levels are likely to be lower at higher cord or maternal fasting blood glucose levels. Usually, the nadir in the infant's blood glucose concentration is reached between 1–3 hr; spontaneous recovery may begin by 4–6 hr.

Many infants of diabetic mothers develop tachypnea during the 1st 5 days of life. This may be a transient manifestation of hypoglycemia, hypothermia, polycythemia, cardiac failure, or cerebral edema from birth trauma or asphyxia. There is a greater incidence of hyaline membrane disease in infants of diabetic mothers than in infants of normal mothers born at comparable gestational age, possibly related to an antagonistic effect between cortisol and insulin on surfactant synthesis. Cardiomegaly is common (30%) and heart failure occurs in 5–10% of infants of diabetic mothers. Asymmetrical septal hypertrophy may occur and become manifest as idiopathic hypertrophic subaortic stenosis. Neurologic development and ossification centers tend to be immature and correlate with the brain size (which is not increased) and gestational age rather than with total body weight. There is also an increased incidence of hyperbilirubinemia, polycythemia, and renal vein thrombosis; the latter should be suspected in the presence of a flank mass, hematuria, and thrombocytopenia. The incidence of congenital anomalies is increased 3-fold in infants of diabetic mothers; cardiac and skeletal are most common. These infants may also develop abdominal distention due to a transient delay in the development of the left side of the colon, the *small left colon syndrome*.

Prognosis. The subsequent incidence of diabetes mellitus in infants of diabetic mothers varies between 1–7%. Physical development is normal, but in oversized infants there may be a predilection to obesity in childhood that may extend into adult life. Disagreement persists about whether there is a slightly increased risk of impaired intellectual development unrelated to hypoglycemia; symptomatic hypoglycemia probably increases the risk.

Treatment. Management of these infants should be initiated before birth by frequent prenatal evaluation of all pregnant women with overt or gestational diabetes, by evaluation of fetal maturity, and by planning delivery of these infants in hospitals where expert obstetric and pediatric care is continuously available. All infants of diabetic mothers, regardless of size, should initially receive intensive observation and care. Asymptomatic infants should have a blood sugar determination within 1 hr of birth and then every hr for the next 6–8 hr; if clinically well and normoglycemic, oral or gavage feedings initially with sterile water or 5% glucose water, followed by milk formula, should be started at 2–3 hr of age and continued at 2-hr intervals. If there is any question about an infant's ability to tolerate oral feeding, it should be discontinued and glucose given by peripheral intravenous infusion at a rate of 4–8 mg/kg/min. Blood glucose values under 30 mg/dl should be treated, even in asymptomatic infants, with intravenous infusions of glucose sufficient to keep the blood levels well above this level. Bolus injections of hypertonic glucose should be avoided, except to stop hypoglycemic convulsions, as they may cause further hyperinsulinemia and potentially produce rebound hypoglycemia. A single intramuscular injection of glucagon (300 µg/kg) has been proposed, but its value is not established. The management of hypoglycemia in sick or symptomatic infants is discussed in the following section. For treatment of *hypocalcemia* and *hypomagnesemia*, see Sec 7.54; for *hyaline membrane disease* treatment, see Sec 7.34.

Infants with central nervous system symptoms should have spinal fluid examined to rule out meningitis or cerebral hemorrhage.

7.57 HYPOGLYCEMIA

Hypoglycemia is present when an infant's blood glucose concentration is significantly lower than the mean for a population of infants of similar age and weight. In term infants over 2500 gm, this is defined as plasma concentrations of less than 35 mg/dl in the 1st 72 hr and 45 mg/dl subsequently; in low birth weight infants, it is less than 25 mg/dl (Fig 7–12). Glucose is the major source of energy throughout fetal life, though amino acids and lactate constitute additional sources of nutrients during late gestation. The rate of glucose uptake by the fetus is related to the maternal blood glucose level, and the fetal blood level is approximately two thirds that of the mother. After their abrupt removal from the constant placental infusion of glucose, fullterm infants usually stabilize their blood levels between 50–60 mg/dl during the 1st 72 hr of life, and low birth weight infants at lower levels.

Four pathophysiologic groups of neonatal infants are at high risk of developing hypoglycemia: (1) Infants of mothers with diabetes mellitus or gestational diabetes and infants with severe erythroblastosis fetalis seem to suffer from hyperinsulinism. (2) Infants of low birth weight may have experienced intrauterine malnutrition resulting in reduced hepatic glycogen stores and total body fat; those who are small for their gestational age, the smaller of discordant twins (particularly if discordant by 25% or more in weight with a weight of less than 2.0 kg), polycythemic infants, infants of toxemic mothers, and infants with placental abnormalities are particularly vulnerable. (Other factors in the development of hypoglycemia in this group include abnormal insulin responsiveness, impaired gluconeogenesis, diminished free fatty acids, increased brain/liver weight ratio, low cortisol production rates, and possibly increased insulin levels and decreased output of epinephrine in response to hypoglycemia.) (3) Very immature or severely ill infants may develop hypoglycemia due to increased metabolic needs out of proportion to substrate stores and calories supplied; low birth weight infants with respiratory distress syndrome, perinatal asphyxia, polycythemia, hypothermia, and systemic infections, as well as infants in heart failure with cyanotic congenital heart disease, are at increased risk. The interruption of intravenous infusions, particularly those with high glucose concentrations, may also result in the precipitous onset of hypoglycemia. (4) Rare infants with genetic or primary metabolic defects, such as galactosemia, glycogen storage disease, fructose intolerance, propionic acidemia, methylmalonic acidemia, tyrosinemia, maple syrup urine disease, leucine sensitivity, insulinomas, β cell nesidioblastosis, functional β cell hyperplasia, panhypopituitarism, and Beckwith syndrome (see below), or infant giants are also susceptible.

The overall frequency of hypoglycemia is 2–3/1000 live births but appears to be significantly higher among infants of low birth weight for gestational age, especially those with a complicated prenatal history or severe illness. The incidence among infants of diabetic mothers may be as high as 75%. It is lower in infants of gestationally diabetic mothers and lower but still elevated among infants of low birth weight.

Clinical Manifestations. In contrast to the frequency of chemical hypoglycemia, the incidence of symptomatic hypoglycemia is highest in small for gestational age infants (Fig 7–12). These infants usually fall into (2) or (3) of the above pathophysiologic groupings and some are referred to as having *transient symptomatic idiopathic neonatal hypoglycemia*. Because many of the symptoms also occur together with other conditions such as infections, especially sepsis and meningitis; central nervous system anomalies, hemorrhage, or edema; hypocalcemia and hypomagnesemia; asphyxia; drug withdrawal; apnea of prematurity; congenital heart disease; or polycythemia, and because some may be seen in normoglycemic well infants, the exact incidence of symptomatic hypoglycemia has been difficult to establish. It probably varies between 1–3/1000 live births with about 5–15% of low birth weight infants being affected and with the higher incidence occurring in those who are below the 50th percentile for gestational age.

The onset of symptoms varies from a few hr to a wk after birth. In approximate order of frequency there are jitteriness or tremors, episodes of cyanosis, apathy, convulsions, intermittent apneic spells or tachypnea, weak or high-pitched cry, limpness or lethargy, difficulty in feeding, and eye-rolling. Episodes of sweating, sudden pallor, hypothermia, and cardiac arrest and failure also occur. There is frequently a clustering of episodic symptoms. Because these clinical manifestations may result from a variety of causes, it is critical to determine whether they disappear with the administration of sufficient glucose to raise the blood sugar to normal levels; if they do not, other diagnoses must be considered.

Treatment. When seizures are not present, an intravenous bolus of 200 mg/kg (2 ml/kg) of 10% glucose is effective in elevating the blood glucose concentration. In the presence of convulsions 10–25% glucose as a bolus injection resulting in a total loading dose of 1–2 gm/kg is indicated.

Following initial therapy a glucose infusion should be given at 4–8 mg/kg/min. If hypoglycemia recurs, the infusion rate should be increased until 15–20% glucose is employed. If intravenous infusions of 20% glucose are inadequate to eliminate symptoms and maintain constant normal blood glucose concentrations, hydrocortisone (2.5 mg/kg/12 hr) or prednisone (1 mg/kg/24 hr) should also be administered. Blood glucose should be measured every 2 hr after initiating therapy until several determinations are above 40 mg/dl. Subsequently levels should be obtained every 4–6 hr and the treatment gradually reduced and finally discontinued when the blood glucose has been in the normal range and the baby asymptomatic for 24–48 hr. Treatment is usually necessary for a few days to a wk, rarely for several wk. Diazoxide, epinephrine, and fructose are not of established benefit. Epinephrine and fructose may produce lactic acidosis. If neonatal hyperinsulinism is present, as in nesidioblastosis, and unresponsive to steroids and glucose given for a sufficient time, diazoxide and Sus-Phrine may be employed.

Surgery is the definitive treatment for nesidioblastosis and islet cell adenomas; glucagon plus somatostatin has been a helpful adjunct in some cases.

Infants who are at increased risk of developing hypoglycemia should have their blood glucose measured within 1 hr of birth and subsequently every 1–2 hr for the first 6–8 hr, then every 4–6 hr until 24 hr of life. Normoglycemic high risk infants should receive oral or gavage feedings with formula started at 2–3 hr of age and continued at 2-hr intervals for 24–48 hr. An intravenous infusion of glucose at 4 mg/kg/min should be provided if oral feedings are poorly tolerated or if *asymptomatic transient neonatal hypoglycemia* develops.

Prognosis. Prognosis for life is good in the absence of congenital anomalies severe enough in themselves to be lethal. There are recurrences of hypoglycemia in 10–15% of infants after adequate treatment. Some have been reported as late as the age of 8 mo. Recurrences are more common if intravenous fluids infiltrate or are too rapidly discontinued before oral feedings are well tolerated. Children who later develop ketotic hypoglycemia have an increased incidence of neonatal hypoglycemia. Prognosis for normal intellectual function must be guarded since prolonged and severe hypoglycemia may be associated with neurologic sequelae and death. Symptomatic infants with hypoglycemia, particularly low birth weight infants and large-sized infants of overtly diabetic mothers, have a worse prognosis for subsequent normal intellectual development than asymptomatic infants.

Hypoglycemia with Macroglossia
(Beckwith Syndrome)

Beckwith described a syndrome of intractable neonatal hypoglycemia occurring in infants with macroglossia, large size, visceromegaly, mild microcephaly, umbilical abnormalities, facial nevus flammeus, a characteristic earlobe crease, and renal medullary dysplasia. The visceromegaly involves chiefly the liver and the kidneys in which there is a noncystic hyperplasia. Some infants are also polycythemic. Hyperinsulinemia has been demonstrated. Treatment is that of hypoglycemia; in this syndrome hypoglycemia may be severe and persist for several mo. The prognosis is poor.

Severe hypoglycemia has also been demonstrated in extremely high birth weight infants who do not have the anomalies present in Beckwith syndrome. These *infant giants* weigh from 3.8 to 5.3 kg, and, in some, pancreatic hyperplasia has been described.

RICHARD E. BEHRMAN
ROBERT M. KLIECMAN

Adam P: Infant of a diabetic mother: Energy imbalance between adipose tissue and liver. Semin. Perinatol 2:329, 1978.
Cornblath M, Schwartz R: Carbohydrate Metabolism in the Neonate. Ed 2. Philadelphia, WB Saunders, 1976.
Haworth JC, Dilling LA: Relationship between maternal glucose tolerance and neonatal blood glucose. J. Pediatr 89:810, 1976.
Kalhan S, Savin S, Adam P: Attenuated glucose production rate in newborn infants of insulin dependent diabetic mothers. N Engl J Med 296:375, 1977.
Kolvisto M, Blanco-Sequiros M, Krause N: Neonatal symptomatic and asymptomatic hypoglycemia; a follow up study of 151 children. Dev Med Child Neurol 14:603, 1972.
Lilien L, Pildes R, Srinivasan G, et al: Treatment of neonatal hypoglycemia with minibolus and intravenous glucose infusion. J. Pediatr 97:295, 1980.
Pildes RS, et al: A prospective controlled study of neonatal hypoglycemia. Pediatrics 54:5, 1974.
Sosenko I, Kitzmiller J, Loo S, et al: The infant of the diabetic mother. Correlation of increased cord C-peptide levels with macrosomia and hypoglycemia. N Engl J Med 308:859, 1979.

7.58 INFECTIONS OF THE NEWBORN

GENERAL CONSIDERATIONS

Infections are a frequent and important cause of morbidity and mortality in the neonatal period (see Chapter 10). As many as 2% of fetuses are infected in utero, and up to 10% of infants are infected during delivery or the 1st mo of life. Inflammatory lesions are found in about 25% of newborn infant autopsies; these lesions are 2nd only to hyaline membrane disease in frequency.

Several general factors contribute to the frequency and severity of neonatal infections and emphasize the importance of early and accurate diagnosis and appropriate therapy. First, a variety of organisms, including bacteria, viruses, fungi, protozoa, chlamydia, and mycoplasma, are etiologic agents. Second, the presenting clinical features in the neonate with infection may be subtle and may mimic the features of other common diseases during this period. As a result, the diagnosis of infection is often missed or delayed until the process has become widespread. Third, some routine laboratory tests available to aid in the diagnosis of infection appear to be imprecise or do not provide the rapid results needed. Fourth, the host resistance mechanisms present in the newborn infant, particularly the sick premature infant, may be immature and easily overcome by invading microorganisms. Infections, therefore, may become fulminant and cause death within a few hr or days, despite appropriate and intensive antimicrobial therapy. Fifth, many bacterial infections are caused by organisms relatively resistant to antibiotics, particularly the gram-negative enteric bacilli. These infections are difficult to treat, and the dose of antibiotics that can safely be used is limited by toxic side effects. Finally, antiviral chemotherapy is now available for herpes infections of the neonate.

Frequency and Specific Predisposing Factors. Table 7-21 lists the frequency of the most common infections in the newborn infant and, when the fetus is infected in utero, the frequency of infection in the mother during pregnancy. A variety of maternal and neonatal factors are associated with increased frequency or severity of infections. Mothers susceptible to certain pathogens (e.g., rubella or cytomegalovirus) may acquire an acute primary infection and transmit the microorganism transplacentally to the fetus. On the other hand, mothers who are immune (e.g., to measles or a particular strain of group B streptococcus) have antibody in their serum that can pass transplacentally and provide passive protection for the neonate against infection after birth. During epidemic periods, the incidence of maternal and congenital disease may be several-fold higher. The use of vaccines against maternal infections, such as rubella, has reduced the frequency of congenital infections. Much higher rates of vaginal colonization

Table 7-21 APPROXIMATE FREQUENCY OF INFECTIONS IN THE MOTHER DURING PREGNANCY AND IN THE NEWBORN INFANT

INFECTION OR AGENT	APPROXIMATE FREQUENCY	
	Mother Per 1000 Pregnancies	Neonate Per 1000 Live Births
Bacterial infections		
Sepsis	—	1–5
Meningitis	—	0.2–0.5
Urinary tract infection	—	10–13
Viruses		
Cytomegalovirus		
During pregnancy	10–130	4–24
Perinatal	30–280	20–100
Rubella		
Epidemic	20–40	3–30
Nonepidemic	0.1–2.0	0.1–0.7
Hepatitis B	2–30	0–7
Herpes simplex	1–10	0.03–0.3
Protozoa		
Toxoplasma gondii	1–10	1–6

with group B streptococcus and genital infection with
herpes simplex virus occur in women with multiple
sexual partners; the rates of infection in neonates born
to such women are correspondingly higher.

An important variable in the increased risk of neonatal sepsis in infants born of mothers with prolonged
rupture of membranes is the development of ascending
infection of the amniotic fluid, which then leads to
congenital aspiration pneumonia (Sec 12.69) in the fetus
and subsequent neonatal sepsis. However, amniotic
and fetal infection can occur with rupture of membranes
for less than 24 hr, and membranes may be ruptured
for more than 24 hr without infection developing.
Maternal urinary tract infections are also associated with
an increased incidence of disease in the neonate. The
maternal genital tract may be colonized with a wide
variety of organisms that do not necessarily cause
disease in the mother, but may result in a heavy
inoculum for the neonate at the time of birth and cause
significant illness during the newborn period. These
organisms include group B streptococcus, *E. coli* (particularly the K1 capsular antigen-containing organisms),
gonococcus, *Listeria*, chlamydia, *Candida*, herpes simplex virus, and cytomegalovirus. Intrauterine asphyxia
may cause aspiration of infected amniotic fluid and
result in congenital pneumonia. Difficult or traumatic
delivery is associated with an increased frequency of
infections during the neonatal period.

The most important neonatal factor predisposing to
infection is prematurity; there is a 3–10-fold higher
incidence of sepsis, meningitis, or urinary tract infection
in premature infants than in fullterm newborns. Males
have an approximately 2-fold higher incidence of sepsis,
meningitis, and urinary tract infections than females,
suggesting the possibility of a sex-linked factor in host
susceptibility. Resuscitation at birth, particularly if it
involves endotracheal intubation, insertion of an umbilical vessel catheter, or both, is associated with increased risk of bacterial infection. The presence of
underlying diseases, such as hyaline membrane disease, or congenital defects, such as meningomyelocele,
predisposes to infection by acting as a portal of entry
for organisms or by compromising host resistance. The
majority of infants cared for in a neonatal intensive care
unit are exposed to a variety of diagnostic and therapeutic procedures that may also compromise host defenses and provide a portal of entry for organisms, e.g.,
umbilical vessel catheters, endotracheal tubes, EKG
monitor leads, fetal scalp electrodes, intravenous catheters, and so on. In addition, these infants may be
exposed to antibiotic-resistant organisms carried on the
hands of personnel or contaminated equipment.

Epidemiology and Pathogenesis. Infections in the
newborn infant may be acquired in utero (congenital),
at the time of birth (natal), or after birth and during the
neonatal period (postnatal). The transplacental route is
the most common means by which microorganisms
reach the fetus in utero (Fig 7–30). Some viruses,
Toxoplasma gondii, *Treponema pallidum*, and occasionally
bacteria are transmitted by this route. Infection acquired
in utero may result in resorption of the embryo, abortion, stillbirth, congenital malformation, intrauterine
growth retardation, premature birth, acute disease in
the immediate neonatal period, or an asymptomatic but
persistent infection that can cause neurologic sequelae
later in life (Table 7–22). Most infections acquired by
the newborn infant during birth are the result of aspiration of infected amniotic fluid or vaginal secretions,
which can result in colonization of the upper respiratory
tract or true infection of the lower respiratory tract. The
most common organisms causing infection at this time
are group B streptococcus, *E. coli*, *Neisseria gonorrhoeae*,
and herpes simplex virus, which often result in acute,
fulminant, systemic infections; *Candida albicans* and chlamydia, which usually cause less severe infection limited
to the mucous membranes; and cytomegalovirus, which
tends to result in asymptomatic infections. Symptoms
of infections acquired during birth are usually apparent
within a few days after birth. Those acquired after birth
are the result of environmental exposure in either the
hospital or the community. The respiratory or the
gastrointestinal tract is the primary route of infection in
the latter, while the umbilicus, a surgical wound, a
trachea with an endotracheal tube in place, or the site
of an intravascular catheter may be the portal of entry
in a hospitalized neonate.

Clinical Manifestations. Infection in the newborn
infant may simulate other common diseases, may be
subtle or nonspecific, and may involve a number of
organ systems (Table 7–23). In addition, infections with
different microorganisms may have overlapping patterns so that it is usually not possible to make a
definitive diagnosis of a specific etiologic agent from
clinical features alone. Finally, in the majority of congenital infections no symptoms are evident at birth.

Diagnosis. The maternal history may provide important clues to the diagnosis of infection in the newborn infant. Hepatitis B virus infection is much more
common in mothers with acute hepatitis than in asymptomatic chronic carriers. However, virtually all of the

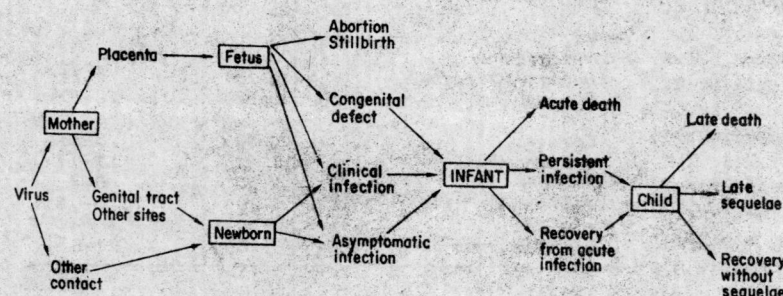

Figure 7–30 Pathogenesis of viral infections in
the fetus and newborn. (From Overall JC Jr, *In:*
Feigin RD, Cherry JD [eds]: Textbook of Pediatric
Infectious Diseases. Philadelphia, WB Saunders,
1981.)

Table 7-22 VIRAL, PARASITIC, AND SPIROCHETAL AGENTS ASSOCIATED WITH FETAL AND INFANT MORBIDITY AND MORTALITY

PATHOGEN	FETUS	NEONATAL DISEASE	CONGENITAL DEFECTS	LATE SEQUELAE
Rubella virus	Abortion	Low birth weight, hepatosplenomegaly, petechiae, osteitis	Heart defects, microcephaly, cataracts, microphthalmia	Deafness, mental retardation, thyroid disorders, diabetes, degenerative brain tissue, autism
Cytomegalovirus	—	Anemia, thrombocytopenia, hepatosplenomegaly, jaundice, encephalitis	Microcephaly, microphthalmia, retinopathy	Deafness, psychomotor retardation, cerebral calcification
Varicella-zoster virus	—	Low birth weight, chorioretinitis, congenital chickenpox or disseminated neonatal varicella, possibly zoster	Limb hypoplasia, cortical atrophy, cicatricial skin lesions	Fatal outcome due to secondary infection
Picornaviruses				
Coxsackie virus	Abortion	Mild febrile disease, exanthems, aseptic meningitis, disseminated disease, multiple organ involvement (CNS, liver, heart), gastroenteritis	Possible congenital heart disease, myocarditis	Neurologic deficits
Echo virus	—			
Poliovirus	Abortion	Congenital poliomyelitis		Paralysis
Herpes simplex virus	Abortion	Disseminated disease, multiple organ involvement (lung, liver, CNS), vesicular skin lesions, retinopathy	Possible microcephaly, retinopathy, intracranial calcifications	Neurologic deficits
Western equine virus	—	Congenital encephalitis	—	Neurologic deficits
Measles virus	Abortion	Congenital measles	—	
Vaccinia virus	Abortion	Congenital vaccinia	—	—
Variola virus	Abortion	Congenital variola	—	—
Hepatitis B virus	—	Asymptomatic HB Ag positive infection, low birth weight, rarely acute hepatitis	—	Chronic hepatitis, persistent HB Ag positive
Mumps virus	Abortion	Possible association with endocardial fibroelastosis		—
Influenza virus	Possible abortion	—	—	—
Toxoplasma gondii	Abortion	Low birth weight, hepatosplenomegaly, jaundice, anemia	Hydrocephalus, microcephaly	Chorioretinitis, mental retardation
Treponema pallidum	—	Skin lesions, rhinitis, hepatosplenomegaly, jaundice, osteitis	—	Interstitial keratitis, frontal bossing, saber shins, tooth changes
Malaria	—	Hepatosplenomegaly, jaundice, anemia, poor feeding, vomiting		—

primary infections due to cytomegalovirus and toxoplasma and half of those due to rubella are asymptomatic in the pregnant woman. A history of painful genital ulcers or of genital herpes in a sexual partner should suggest neonatal herpes, and the occurrence of prolonged rupture of the fetal membranes, maternal peripartum infection, or complications during labor or delivery should suggest the possibility of early onset bacterial sepsis.

The most direct means to diagnose a specific infection in the neonate is the recovery of an etiologic agent from body fluids or tissues, particularly from sites of infection. In the infant with suspected bacterial sepsis, samples of spinal fluid and urine, as well as blood, should be obtained for culture and other laboratory tests. Gram-stained smears of spinal fluid, urine, or material from sites of infection can provide an immediate diagnosis of bacterial infection and can assist in the choice of initial antibiotic therapy. In addition, within hours the antigens of group B streptococcus or K1 strains of E. coli can be identified in the spinal fluid

or urine by counterimmunoelectrophoresis (CIE). Since the prognosis and the duration of antibiotic therapy are quite different in the infant with sepsis alone as compared with the infant with sepsis complicated by meningitis and since neonates with urinary tract infection can present a picture resembling sepsis in the absence of bacteremia, the infant with suspected sepsis should have a complete evaluation.

The usual samples obtained for virus isolation are urine for cytomegalovirus; throat swab for rubella, herpes simplex, and enteroviruses; vesicle fluid for herpes simplex and varicella-zoster viruses; spinal fluid for herpes simplex, rubella, and enteroviruses; and stool for enteroviruses. Evidence of specific viral cytopathic effect in tissue culture may be evident within a few days with some viruses (herpes simplex, enteroviruses) but not for a wk or more with others (cytomegalovirus, rubella, varicella-zoster virus). Hepatitis B virus antigen is demonstrable in serum by a variety of techniques (Sec 7.71). Serologic tests are usually used in addition to virus isolation to diagnose viral infection in newborn

Table 7-23 CLINICAL MANIFESTATIONS OF INFECTION IN THE NEWBORN INFANT

GENERAL	CARDIOVASCULAR SYSTEM
Fever, hypothermia	Pallor, cyanosis, mottling,
"Not doing well"	cold, clammy skin
Poor feeding	Hypotension
Lethargy	
Scleredema	
GASTROINTESTINAL SYSTEM	CENTRAL NERVOUS SYSTEM
Abdominal distention	Irritability
Anorexia, vomiting	Tremors, seizures
Diarrhea	Hyporeflexia
Hepatomegaly	Abnormal Moro reflex
	Irregular respirations
	Full fontanel
RESPIRATORY SYSTEM	HEMATOLOGIC SYSTEM
Apnea, dyspnea	Jaundice
Tachypnea, retraction	Splenomegaly
Flaring, grunting	Pallor
Cyanosis	Petechiae, purpura
	Bleeding

infants. For this reason the TORCH (*Toxoplasmosis, Other, Rubella, Cytomegalovirus, Herpes simplex*) screen was developed. Serologic testing is the primary means used for diagnosis of *Toxoplasma gondii* (Sec 10.113). Since the antibodies measured in the TORCH screen are predominantly IgG, they are passed from mother to fetus and are found at approximately the same level in maternal sera and in cord blood or samples from the newborn infant. Serum levels obtained from the infant at the age of 4–5 mo will show a significant drop if the antibody was passively transferred from the mother but remain the same as in the neonatal period or even rise if active infection is present in the neonate. Although quantitative elevation of IgM in cord blood or early neonatal sera (IgM is not passed transplacentally under normal circumstances) has been used as a screening test to identify neonates with an intrauterine infection, there is a high rate of both false-positive and false-negative results. Furthermore, the test does not identify a specific etiologic agent. However, presence of IgM against specific antigens (cytomegalovirus, rubella, toxoplasma, herpes simplex, syphilis) can be used to make an etiologic diagnosis.

Routine laboratory tests may assist in the diagnosis of infection in the newborn infant. In neonatal sepsis elevation of the absolute band neutrophil count and thrombocytopenia often occur within the 1st 24 hr after onset of symptoms, and white blood cells may contain vacuoles and toxic granulation. Thrombocytopenia has also been observed in congenital cytomegalovirus, rubella, toxoplasma, and spirochetal infections. Erythrocyte sedimentation rate and C-reactive protein are elevated in most neonates with systemic bacterial infection. However, delays in the development of an abnormal test and the time required to perform the laboratory test have reduced their usefulness. Although inflammatory cells are present in sections of umbilical cord and increased numbers of neutrophils are seen in smears of gastric aspirates obtained within hours of birth in many infants with early onset sepsis, there is a

high incidence of false-positive results. Roentgenographic examination is a primary method of diagnosis in patients with suspected pneumonia, septic arthritis, or osteomyelitis.

Because of the rapidity with which bacterial infections can become fulminant and life-threatening in this age group and the lack of a definitive diagnostic test short of bacteriologic cultures, it is particularly important to maintain a high index of suspicion when the history indicates an increased risk of bacterial infection. If sepsis, pneumonia, or meningitis is suspected, treatment should be initiated after appropriate cultures have been obtained and diagnostic laboratory studies performed. The decision whether to continue antibiotics for a full course of therapy will depend on the results of cultures and other laboratory tests and the course of illness.

Nosocomial Nursery Infections. Outbreaks of infectious illness have occurred in nurseries and neonatal intensive care units due to a variety of bacterial and viral agents. Although the most common nosocomial infections in newborn intensive care units are surface infections (EKG lead abscesses, omphalitis, conjunctivitis, pyoderma), more serious infections such as pneumonia, bacteremia, surgical wound infection, urinary tract infection, and meningitis account for almost half of those occurring. *Staphylococcus aureus* has been a major cause of hospital-acquired infections and has resulted in outbreaks of pustules and cellulitis, pneumonia, septicemia, and the staphylococcal scalded skin syndrome (Sec 7.67). Group A beta hemolytic streptococcus has caused a low grade granulating omphalitis, cellulitis, pneumonia, septicemia, and meningitis, while enteropathogenic *E. coli* have caused outbreaks of diarrheal disease. A number of gram-negative enteric bacteria including *E. coli, Klebsiella pneumoniae, Pseudomonas aeruginosa, Proteus mirabilis, Serratia marcescens,* and *Flavobacterium meningosepticum* have resulted in epidemics of pneumonia, sepsis, and meningitis. Clusters of cases of fulminant viral infection consisting of hepatitis, encephalitis or aseptic meningitis, and myocarditis have been observed with Coxsackie and ECHO viruses. Adenovirus has caused cases of upper respiratory infection and gastrointestinal disease while respiratory syncytial virus, parainfluenza virus, and influenza viruses have resulted in predominantly lower respiratory tract disease (pneumonia and bronchiolitis).

The occurrence of a similar clinical illness due to the same organism in several infants from the same nursery unit over a short period of time should suggest the possibility of an outbreak. In fullterm infants whose nursery stay is usually only 2–3 days, the illness may not manifest itself for several days or maybe several wk after discharge; it is therefore difficult to recognize a nursery-acquired infection or a clustering of similar cases suggesting a nursery-associated outbreak. It may also be possible to demonstrate that 1 organism has caused the illness. This may require phage typing of *Staphylococcus aureus,* pyocin typing of *Pseudomonas aeruginosa,* serotyping for enteropathogenic *E. coli,* demonstration of a common antibiotic sensivity pattern in *Serratia marcescens,* or restriction endonuclease fingerprinting of the DNA from herpes simplex virus isolates.

An outbreak may need the following steps: (1) Cultures should be taken of infants and, depending on the pathogen, of nursery personnel to identify additional cases, those incubating the disease, or asymptomatic carriers. Even during an outbreak of staphylococcal disease in a nursery, most infant carriers are asymptomatic. (2) All symptomatic and asymptomatic infants colonized with the epidemic strain should be isolated, and a cohort system should be maintained until discharge of all infants from the unit. (3) Systemic antibiotic therapy is required for infants with significant disease, while topical antibiotics may be used for asymptomatic carriers of *S. aureus*, oral antibiotic therapy for infants colonized with enteropathogenic *E. coli*, and triple dye application to the umbilicus for a group A streptococcus outbreak. In some instances antibiotic treatment of nursery personnel may be required. (4) The extent of the epidemic should be defined. If the outbreak is confined to only a few infants in a single room in the nursery, limited infection control measures may suffice to curb the outbreak. However, more extensive steps may be required if a number of areas or numerous infants or personnel are involved. If the outbreak is extensive and serious disease results, closure of the nursery to new admissions may be required until the outbreak is brought under control. (5) Culturing of the environment for reservoirs of pathogens may be necessary in selected instances. Faucet aerators, sink traps and drains, eyewash solutions, resuscitation equipment, and humidification apparatus have been the source of outbreaks due to *P. aeruginosa*, *Serratia marcescens*, and *Flavobacterium meningosepticum*.

Alford CA Jr, Stagno S, Reynolds DW: Diagnosis of chronic perinatal infections. Am J Dis Child 129:455, 1975.

Baker CJ, Barrett FF, Clark DJ: Incidence of kanamycin resistance among *Escherichia coli* isolates from neonates. J Pediatr 84:126, 1974.

Harris H, Wirtschafter D, Cassady G: Endotracheal intubation and its relationship to bacterial colonization and systemic infection of newborn infants. Pediatrics 58:816, 1976.

Hemming VG, Overall JC Jr, Britt MR: Nosocomial infections in a newborn intensive care unit: Results of forty-one months of surveillance. N Engl J Med 294:1310, 1976.

Hill RR, Hunt CE, Matsen JM: Nosocomial colonization with Klebsiella type 26 in a neonatal intensive care unit associated with outbreak of sepsis, meningitis and necrotizing enterocolitis. J Pediatr 85:415, 1976.

Krugman S, Gershon RA (eds): Infections of the Fetus and Newborn Infant. New York, AR Liss Inc, 1975.

McCracken GH Jr: Managing neonatal infections. Hosp Pract 11:49, 1976.

Mims CA: Pathogenesis of viral infections of the fetus. Prog Med Virol 10:194, 1968.

Nahmias AJ: The TORCH complex. Hosp Pract 9:65, 1974.

Overall JC Jr, Glasgow LA: Virus infections of the fetus and newborn infant. J Pediatr 77:315, 1970.

Plotkin S, Starr S: Perinatal infections. Perinat Clin North Am 8:entire issue, 1981.

Sever JL, Larsen JW Jr, Grossman JH III: Handbook of Perinatal Infections. Boston, Little, Brown and Co, 1979.

Zipursky A, Palko J, Milrner R, et al: The hematology of bacterial infections in premature infants. Pediatrics 57:839, 1976.

7.59 SEPSIS AND MENINGITIS

Neonatal sepsis is a clinical syndrome characterized by symptomatic systemic illness and bacteria in the blood. Asymptomatic bacteremia may also occur in the neonate. Meningitis is present when the spinal fluid contains increased cells and protein, a low sugar, and bacteria or bacterial antigens. Sepsis and meningitis are considered together since the etiology, epidemiology, and pathogenesis have many common features and the clinical manifestations are similar. Suspected sepsis and/or meningitis is one of the most frequent diagnoses considered by the physician caring for sick newborn infants.

Etiology and Epidemiology. The most common organisms causing disease are *Escherichia coli* and group B streptococcus (which together account for 50–75% of cases at most medical centers), *Staphylococcus aureus*, enterococcus, *Klebsiella-Enterobacter* sp., *Pseudomonas aeruginosa*, *Proteus* sp., *Listeria monocytogenes*, and anaerobic organisms. Early-onset disease presents as a fulminant process involving multiple organs in the 1st wk of life, while late-onset disease is often manifested as meningitis after the 1st wk. In the former there are usually associated maternal factors, and the organisms are acquired from infected amniotic fluid or on passage through the birth canal, while in the latter the infant may acquire infection in the community or from a number of sources in the hospital. *E. coli* and group B streptococcus may be responsible for either early or late onset of infection, whereas *S. aureus*, *Klebsiella-Enterobacter* sp., *P. aeruginosa*, and *Serratia* sp. more commonly cause late-onset disease. Organisms that are the major cause of septicemia and meningitis in the older infant and child—*Hemophilus influenzae* type b, *Streptococcus pneumoniae*, and *Neisseria meningitidis*—are infrequent etiologic agents of disease in the neonatal period (Sec 10.13 and 10.21).

Clinical Manifestations. The usual manifestations of sepsis are abnormal temperature (either hyper- or hypothermia), jaundice, respiratory distress, hepatomegaly, abdominal distention, anorexia, vomiting, and lethargy. Similar findings occur with meningitis, along with convulsions and irritability; bulging fontanel and stiff neck are absent in 75% or more of the neonates with this disease. The initial signs of sepsis or meningitis may be subtle. Often the mother or nurse states that the infant "doesn't look well" or "feeds poorly." It is important, therefore, to maintain a high index of suspicion, particularly in a neonate with a history of 1 or more of the risk factors referred to in Sec 7.58.

Diagnosis. The diagnosis of sepsis or meningitis depends upon the isolation of the etiologic agent from the blood, CSF, urine, or other body fluids. Blood for culture should be obtained from a peripheral vein. Blood collected from an indwelling vascular catheter that has been used for exchange transfusions or present for some time will give a high incidence of false-positive results. Osteomyelitis and septic arthritis of the hip have been associated with femoral vein puncture, which is rarely indicated. Although 2 blood cultures will often aid in the interpretation of possible bacterial contaminants, a single sample will usually suffice since it is important to institute antibiotic therapy promptly; as little as 0.5–1.0 ml may suffice when smaller volumes of blood culture media are used. Culture of the urine is important in suspected sepsis as the kidney can be seeded with organisms during bacteremia and result in positive urine cultures. In addition, the neonate with an isolated urinary tract infection can present a clinical picture resembling sepsis.

Infants with meningitis will usually have cerebrospinal fluid (CSF) cell counts greater than 100/mm³ with a neutrophil predominance, although the cell count may be considerably less. The protein concentration in the CSF of normal neonates may be as high as 150 mg/dl, particularly in the premature, but in patients with meningitis, levels of several hundred to a few thousand are usually observed. Since hypoglycemia can occur in neonates, it is important to obtain a simultaneous blood sugar so that an isolated finding of hypoglycorrhachia can be interpreted. In meningitis the CSF glucose is usually lower than 40 mg/dl and less than 50% of a simultaneous blood level. Examining a Gram-stained smear of CSF allows an immediate diagnosis of meningitis along with a prediction as to the likely etiologic agent.

Cultures of other body sites should be performed whenever the clinical situation indicates that they may provide useful information: needle aspirate of cellulitis or an abscess; swab of purulent discharge from the eye, umbilicus, or surgical wound. Cultures of the external ear canal, axilla, gastric aspirate, or throat are usually not helpful as it is difficult to differentiate colonization from true infection.

Treatment. Once the diagnosis of sepsis or meningitis is suspected and after appropriate cultures have been obtained, antibiotic therapy should be instituted immediately. Initial treatment should consist of ampicillin and gentamicin or kanamycin by the intravenous or intramuscular route. Doses of the commonly used antibiotics are provided in Table 7–24. The choice of an aminoglycoside is influenced by (1) where the infection was acquired and (2) what the antibiotic susceptibility pattern of gram-negative enteric organisms is in a particular nursery or newborn intensive care unit. Gram-negative infections acquired from the mother or in the community are more likely to be susceptible to kanamycin, while gentamicin (or even tobramycin or ami-

kacin) may be required for infections acquired in the newborn intensive care unit. When the history or the presence of necrotic skin lesions suggests the possibility of *Pseudomonas* infection, initial therapy should be carbenicillin and gentamicin. When staphylococcal sepsis is suspected, treatment should be initiated with methicillin or nafcillin and gentamicin.

Once the pathogen has been identified and the antibiotic sensitivities determined, the most appropriate drug or drugs should be selected. With most of the gram-negative enteric bacteria and with enterococcus both a penicillin (ampicillin or carbenicillin) and an aminoglycoside (gentamicin, kanamycin, or 1 of the newer aminoglycosides) should be used since synergism has been demonstrated with this combination of antibiotics in a substantial proportion of the strains. Moxalactam is an alternative agent for gram-negative meningitis. Ampicillin alone is adequate for *Listeria*, while penicillin will suffice for group B streptococcus and most anaerobes. The combination of nafcillin and gentamicin is synergistic against staphylococcal infections.

Therapy in sepsis should be continued for a total of 10–14 days or for at least 5–7 days after clinical response, when there is no evidence of deep tissue involvement or abscess formation. Blood culture 24–48 hr after initiation of therapy should be negative. If the culture is positive, change in therapy may be indicated or the possibility of an occult abscess should be considered. Treatment for meningitis should be continued for at least 3 wk; longer treatment may be necessary if the clinical response is poor or if the spinal fluid cell count, protein, and sugar do not demonstrate a satisfactory response. Response to therapy in meningitis should be followed by repeat lumbar punctures until cultures are negative. It is not unusual for spinal fluid cultures to continue positive for 4–5 days with gram-negative enteric bacteria, while group B streptococcus and *Listeria* are usually negative in 1–2 days. Mortality and neurologic sequelae rates are no better with intrathecal gentamicin plus parenteral ampicillin and gentamicin than with parenteral therapy alone in treating gram-negative

Table 7–24 DOSAGES OF ANTIBIOTICS COMMONLY USED IN NEWBORNS

| DRUG | ROUTE | DAILY DOSAGE (NO. OF DOSES) | |
		Infants <1 Wk old	Infants 1 to 4 Wk old
Amikacin	IV, IM	15 mg/kg (2)	15–20 mg/kg (3)
Ampicillin	IV, IM	100 mg/kg (2)	200 mg/kg (2)
Carbenicillin	IV, IM	200 mg/kg (2)	300–400 mg/kg (3–4)
Chloramphenicol*	IV	25 mg/kg (1)	50 mg/kg (2)
Gentamicin	IV, IM†	5 mg/kg (2)	7.5 mg/kg (3)
Kanamycin	IV, IM	15–20 mg/kg (2)	15–30 mg/kg (2 or 3)
Methicillin	IV, IM	50 mg/kg (2)	100–150 mg/kg (3)
Nafcillin	IV	50 mg/kg (2)	100–150 mg/kg (3)
Penicillin G aqueous	IV, IM	100,000 units/kg (2)	150,000–250,000 units/kg (3 or 4)
Penicillin G procaine	IM	50,000 units/kg (1)	50,000 units/kg (1)
Tobramycin	IV, IM†	4 mg/kg (2)	6 mg/kg (3)

*Serum levels of chloramphenicol are highly variable. This drug should be given to newborns only if serum levels can be monitored.
†IM preferred. IV = intravenous; IM = intramuscular.
Adapted from McCracken, GH Jr, *In:* Remington JS, Klein JO (eds): Infectious Diseases of the Fetus and Newborn Infant. Philadelphia, WB Saunders, 1976.

enteric neonatal meningitis. Ventriculitis occurs in the majority of neonates with gram-negative meningitis, and poor response to therapy may be related to failure to sterilize the ventricular fluid. Although treatment of meningitis and ventriculitis due to gram-negative enteric bacilli with intraventricular aminoglycosides has not been proved to be beneficial in neonates, this form of therapy has been effective in adults. The decision to use intraventricular antimicrobial therapy in a neonate, therefore, should be individualized. The newborn infant with meningitis who is not doing well clinically and whose CSF cultures remain positive after 48–72 hr should be evaluated for possible ventriculitis. Infants who have adequate ventricular size by computed axial tomography and demonstrable ventriculitis may be considered for intraventricular therapy: 2–2.5 mg of gentamicin/24 hr until cultures are negative.

Supportive treatment, including management of fluid and electrolyte balance, ventilatory assistance, fresh whole blood transfusion, white cell transfusions, exchange transfusions, treatment for DIC, support of blood pressure with inotropic agents such as dopamine, dobutamine, or steroids, and other measures, is an important adjunct to antibiotic therapy. Appropriate management of complications, such as surgical drainage of a deep abscess, fluid restriction for inappropriate antidiuretic hormone secretion, and anticonvulsant therapy for seizures, should be instituted when they occur.

Prognosis. Current mortality rates in neonatal sepsis range from 10–40% and in meningitis from 15–50%. Rates vary depending on the time and manner of disease onset, the etiologic agent, the degree of prematurity of the infant, the presence and severity of associated disease, and the particular nursery or newborn intensive care unit. Significant neurologic sequelae, including hydrocephalus, mental retardation, blindness, hearing loss, motor disability, and abnormal speech patterns, occur in 30–50% of the survivors of neonatal meningitis. Milder forms of sequelae, such as perceptual difficulties, learning disability, and behavioral problems may also occur.

Prevention. Increased use of prenatal care facilities, the establishment of a high-risk pregnancy program for delivery of mothers at medical centers with newborn intensive care facilities, and the development of modern transport equipment may have a significant impact in reducing maternal and neonatal factors predisposing to infection in the newborn infant. Prophylactic antibiotics have been used to prevent infection in the neonate. However, appropriate controlled studies have not documented the efficacy of prophylactic antibiotics when there has been premature rupture of membranes, maternal peripartum infection, respiratory distress syndrome, exchange transfusion, surgical procedures in the neonate, or insertion of an umbilical catheter. Regular cleaning and decontamination of nursery equipment, emphasis on sound handwashing principles, regular surveillance for infection in nurseries and newborn intensive care units, and rapid identification and control of common source outbreaks are important in reducing the risk of infection. Vaccines against group B streptococcus and the K1 antigen-containing strains of

E. coli are being developed for use in the mother to provide passive protection for the neonate.

Baker CJ, Barrett FF, Gordon RC, et al: Suppurative meningitis due to streptococci of Lancefield group B: A study of 33 infants. J Pediatr 82:724, 1973.
Chow AW, Leake RD, Yamauchi T, et al: The significance of anaerobes in neonatal bacteremia: Analysis of 23 cases and review of the literature. Pediatrics 54:736, 1974.
Christenson R, Rothstein G, Anstoll M: Granulocyte transfusions in neonates with bacterial infection, neutropenia and depletion of mature marrow neutrophiles. Pediatrics 70:1, 1982.
Gotoff SP, Behrman RE: Neonatal septicemia. J Pediatr 76:142, 1970.
Lee EL, Robinson MJ, Thong ML, et al: Intraventricular chemotherapy in neonatal meningitis. J Pediatr 91:991, 1977.
McCracken GH Jr: The rate of bacteriologic response to antimicrobial therapy in neonatal meningitis. Am J Dis Child 123:547, 1972.
McCracken GH Jr: Neonatal septicemia and meningitis. Hosp Pract 11:89, 1976.
McCracken GH Jr, Mize SG: A controlled study of intrathecal antibiotic therapy in gram-negative enteric meningitis of infancy. J Pediatr 89:66, 1976.
McCracken GH Jr, Shinefield RR: Changes in the pattern of neonatal septicemia and meningitis. Am J Dis Child 112:33, 1966.
Overall JC Jr: Neonatal bacterial meningitis: Analysis of predisposing factors and outcome compared with matched control subjects. J Pediatr 76:499, 1970.
Sarff LD, Platt LH, McCracken GH Jr: Cerebrospinal fluid evaluation in neonates: Comparison of high risk infants with and without meningitis. J Pediatr 88:473, 1976.
Schaad U, McCracken G, Threlkeld N, et al: Clinical evaluation of a new broad spectrum oxabeta-lactam antibiotic, moxalactam, in neonates and infants. J Pediatr 98:129, 1981.
Siegel JD, McCracken GH Jr: Sepsis neonatorum. N Engl J Med 304:642, 1981.

7.60 PNEUMONIA

Pneumonia (Sec 12.66–12.68) is an important cause of morbidity and mortality in the newborn infant and is the most common inflammatory lesion found at autopsy in the neonatal period. Although pathologic evidence of inflammatory disease of the lung is evident in 15–20% of stillborns and 20–30% of neonatal deaths, not all of the inflammatory disease is due to infection, and its role as a cause of death is often unclear. Pneumonia due to infection may be acquired *transplacentally* as 1 component of a generalized intrauterine infection caused by cytomegalovirus, rubella virus, *Toxoplasma, Listeria,* and *T. pallidum* (Sec 7.68–7.70); *natally* by aspiration of infected amniotic fluid or birth canal secretions with onset of illness during the 1st several days of life (Sec 7.36), most commonly associated with group B streptococcus (Sec 7.66), gram-negative enteric bacilli (Sec 7.58), chlamydia (Sec 10.62), and herpes simplex virus (Sec 7.72); and *postnatally* with symptoms usually not evident until after several days of life, caused by *S. aureus, P. aeruginosa, Klebsiella* and *Serratia* sp., and respiratory viruses (Sec 12.66).

When pneumonia is acquired transplacentally or perinatally, it is often termed *congenital pneumonia* and frequently is associated with prolonged rupture of the membranes, chorioamnionitis, prolonged labor, premature labor, or fetal distress.

Pathology. Pneumonia in early infancy is usually bronchopneumonia in type, occasionally interstitial or lobar.

Clinical Manifestations. Infants with natal or postnatal pneumonia may initially exhibit nonspecific signs of illness such as poor feeding, lethargy, irritability, poor color, a rise or sudden fall in body temperature,

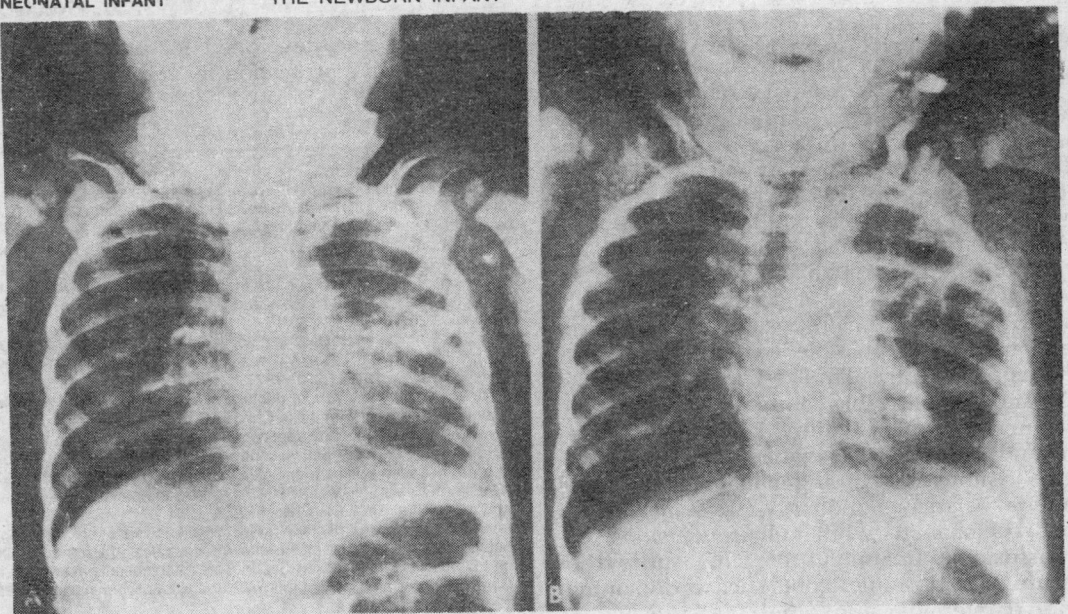

Figure 7–31 Staphylococcal pneumonia in an infant 7 mo of age. *A,* The diffuse inflammatory process involving the left lung and pleura is evident. *B,* Five days later, just before death, there are multiple air-containing cavities in the lung and pleura.

abdominal distention, sudden loss or gain in weight, and a general impression that the baby is doing less well than previously. Signs of respiratory distress, including tachypnea, flaring of the alae nasi, grunting, tachycardia, apnea, accentuation of periodic breathing, and retraction of the suprasternal, intercostal, and subcostal spaces, may rapidly ensue or be somewhat delayed.

Dullness to percussion is difficult to elicit, but, when present, suggests extensive consolidation or effusion. Auscultation may reveal fine, crackling rales in any portion of the lung or decreased breath sounds, but often these may not be present, even with extensive pneumonia. It is important to auscultate the chest with the baby crying as well as quiet since rales frequently are heard only at the end of the deep inspirations that come with crying in the newborn. Areas of hyperresonance may indicate compensatory emphysema. Roentgenograms of the chest are often helpful (Fig 7–31) and are essential to distinguish pneumonia from other causes of respiratory distress. Tracheal aspirate and blood cultures are helpful in making an etiologic diagnosis.

Treatment. Since the etiologic agents of bacterial pneumonia are the same as for sepsis and meningitis, similar antibiotic regimens are used except for chlamydial pneumonia, which is treated with erythromycin or trimethoprim/sulfamethoxazole.

An acute, often fulminant, form of group B streptococcal pneumonia associated with septicemia may present within the 1st day of life, or later, with respiratory distress, sometimes with shock, or with the sudden deterioration of an infant receiving assisted ventilation. The roentgenogram may be typical for bronchopneumonia or show a diffuse atelectasis resembling hyaline membrane disease.

Ablow RC, Driscoll SG, Effmann EL, et al: A comparison of early onset group B streptococcal neonatal infection and the respiratory distress syndrome of the newborn. N Engl J Med 294:65, 1976.
Beem MD, Saxon E, Tipple MA: Treatment of chlamydial pneumonia of infancy. Pediatrics 63:198, 1979.
Davis PA, Aherne W: Congenital pneumonia. Arch Dis Child 39:598, 1963.

7.61   OSTEOMYELITIS AND SEPTIC ARTHRITIS

See also Sec 10.14 and 10.15.

Because of the unique nature of the blood supply to the skeletal system in the neonate and young infant, these 2 infections often occur together. During the 1st several mo of life capillaries penetrate the epiphyseal plate and provide a direct communication between the metaphysis of the bone and the joint space. In addition, the capsules of the hip and shoulder joints attach distal to the metaphysis of the femur and humerus, respectively. Therefore, infections beginning in the metaphysis, the site of initial involvement in osteomyelitis, can readily spread to involve the joint space and vice versa. Although osteomyelitis and septic arthritis usually occur as a result of hematogenous seeding during the course of a bacteremia, extension from a subcutaneous infection (osteomyelitis of the calcaneus associated with multiple heel punctures for blood samples) or by direct inoculation during a procedure (septic arthritis of the hip associated with a femoral puncture) have been reported.

Etiology. *Staphylococcus aureus* is the causative agent in 85% of the cases of osteomyelitis. Other organisms causing osteomyelitis include group A and B streptococcus and pneumococcus; gram-negative bacteria are rarely encountered. In septic arthritis *S. aureus* is also the most common organism, but gram-negative enteric bacteria (*E. coli, P. aeruginosa, Proteus,* and *Klebsiella* sp.), *Candida,* and *N. gonorrhoeae,* agents which rarely cause osteomyelitis, also commonly cause septic arthritis.

Clinical Manifestations. The infant may demonstrate little or no sign of systemic illness, and there may only be diminished spontaneous movement, pain on passive motion of the affected limb, or localized swelling. In the more severe form systemic manifestations of sepsis predominate, and multiple sites of the skeletal system are often involved. The long bones and the major joints of the extremities are the most common areas involved.

Diagnosis. In osteomyelitis roentgenographic examination demonstrates soft tissue swelling followed by necrosis of bone, with rarefaction and periosteal elevation in the metaphyseal area. The radionuclide bone scan may be positive early in the course of osteomyelitis when roentgenograms show no or minimal change. Widening of the joint space may be observed in septic arthritis, and subluxation of the hip or shoulder joint is seen on occasion. Direct aspiration of the joint space or the subperiosteal area is indicated in all cases and may provide an immediate diagnosis. Orthopedic consultation should be obtained. Gram stain and culture of any purulent material aspirated should be performed and blood cultures obtained. The peripheral white count is often not helpful, but the sedimentation rate may be elevated in infants with osteomyelitis.

Treatment. The choice of initial antibiotic agents should be guided by the results of the Gram stain. If gram-positive cocci are seen, treatment should be initiated with methicillin or nafcillin, plus gentamicin; if gram-negative organisms are present, therapy should consist of ampicillin and gentamicin. Once the results of culture and antibiotic sensitivity are known, treatment should be continued with the appropriate drug or drugs. The antibiotics should be given by the intravenous or intramuscular route in the doses indicated in Table 7–24 for at least 3–4 wk after defervescence. Oral therapy is discussed in Sec 10.14. Direct instillation of antibiotic into the joint space or bone is not indicated as adequate levels are achieved with parenteral therapy. In general the infected bone or joint space should be drained by either aspiration or surgical incision. The hip and shoulder joints, in particular, require drainage since purulent material under pressure within the joint capsule can occlude the vascular supply and result in necrosis of the bone. The affected extremity should be immobilized until inflammation has subsided and roentgenographic evidence of healing is present.

Prognosis. Although death is infrequent, long-term morbidity may be significant. Chronic osteomyelitis, skeletal and joint deformities, or disturbed bone growth may occur in 25–50% of cases, particularly if the hip or knee is involved.

Klein JO, Marcy SM: Osteomyelitis and septic arthritis: In: Remington JS, Klein JO (eds): Infectious Diseases of the Fetus and Newborn Infant. Philadelphia, WB Saunders, 1976.
Nelson JD: Follow up: The bacterial etiology and antibiotic management of septic arthritis in infants and children. Pediatrics 50:437, 1972.

Ogden JJ, Lister G: The pathology of neonatal osteomyelitis. Pediatrics 55:474, 1975.
Weissberg ED, Smith AL, Smith DH: Clinical features of neonatal osteomyelitis. Pediatrics 53:505, 1974.

7.62 URINARY TRACT INFECTION

See also Sec 16.43.

Urinary tract infection occurs in about 1% of newborn infants. The incidence is much higher in low birth weight infants and is about 3 times more common in males than females. Over 75% of the infections are due to *E. coli;* the remainder are caused by other gram-negative enteric bacilli (*Klebsiella,* Enterobacter, and *Proteus* sp.) and gram-positive cocci (enterococci, *S. aureus,* and *S. epidermidis*). The major route of infection of the urinary tract in the neonate is hematogenous invasion. The incidence of anatomic obstructive lesions is around 5%.

Clinical Manifestations. The signs are varied and nonspecific. Infants may present a picture resembling sepsis, or there may be an insidious onset consisting of low grade fever, irritability, and failure to gain weight. Some infants may be completely asymptomatic while others may have localized signs such as balanitis, urethritis, a weak urinary stream, or a large flank mass.

Diagnosis. The diagnosis is confirmed by a positive urine culture. Since the collection of a satisfactory clean catch urine specimen is often difficult, obtaining an uncontaminated urine by suprapubic aspiration is advised. In infants who appear septic, blood and CSF cultures should also be obtained. Although pyuria is not a reliable indicator of infection in the neonate, the presence of white cells in the urine on a routine urinalysis should be evaluated for possible infection.

Treatment and Prognosis. If the infant with a urinary tract infection has signs of sepsis, the antibiotic regimens outlined in Sec 7.59 should be used. The urine culture should be negative in 36–48 hr in a successfully treated patient. If cultures continue positive, an obstructive lesion or an abscess should be suspected. Therapy is continued for 10–14 days in the uncomplicated patient. Recurrent infections may occur in 20–25% of cases, usually within the 1st few mo after the initial episode, and should be treated with a full course of antibiotics. Therefore, follow-up urine cultures should be obtained.

Every infant with a documented urinary tract infection should have roentgenologic evaluation of the urinary tract, but unless the infant fails to respond to antibiotic therapy, this should be deferred until recovery from the acute stages of the illness and attainment of a few wk of age. Vesicoureteral reflux can occur during the acute disease and clear with resolution of the infection, and excretion of the dye used in the intravenous pyelogram may be inadequate to provide proper visualization during the 1st 1–2 wk of life. Infants with obstructive lesions should be referred for urologic evaluation for potential corrective surgery.

Abbott GD: Neonatal bacteriuria: A prospective study in 1,460 infants. Br Med J 1:267, 1972.

Bergstrom T, Larson H, Lincoln K, et al: Studies of urinary tract infections in infancy and childhood: Eighty consecutive patients with neonatal infection. J Pediatr 80:858, 1972.

Edelmann CM Jr: The prevalence of bacteriuria in full term and premature newborn infants. J Pediatr 82:125, 1973.

Littlewood JM: Sixty-six infants with urinary tract infection in the first month of life. Arch Dis Child 47:218, 1972.

Nelson JD, Peters PC: Suprapubic aspiration of urine in premature and term infants. Pediatrics 36:132, 1965.

7.63 DIARRHEA

Although only a small percentage of neonates with diarrhea are infected with a recognized pathogen, the possibility of nursery outbreaks of infectious diarrhea, which can involve many infants with a potentially life-threatening illness, is a serious risk (Sec 10.12). Transmission occurs by the fecal-oral route, and the neonate is usually infected at the time of birth by organisms present in maternal stool or after birth by spread of organisms from other infected infants on the hands of personnel. Outbreaks of diarrheal disease in nurseries have occurred due to *E. coli*, salmonella, echovirus, rotavirus, and adenovirus.

Onset of the illness may be either slow and insidious or abrupt. Often, a period of listlessness and poor feeding is followed by vomiting and then diarrhea. Stools are initially yellow and loose, then become watery, green, and mucoid as they increase in frequency. The most serious aspect of disease is fluid loss with resultant dehydration and electrolyte disturbances; small premature infants may lose sufficient fluid into the bowel lumen to cause hypovolemic shock prior to the development of clinically significant diarrhea. Management of diarrhea occurring in a nursery includes maintenance of fluid and electrolyte balance, antibiotics when appropriate, and the prevention of spread of the disease to other infants (Sec 7.58) by an emphasis on good handwashing techniques, discharge of culture-positive infants from the hospital as soon as their condition allows, and follow-up stool cultures on patients who have received a course of therapy.

Blacklow NR, Cukor G: Viral gastroenteritis. N Engl J Med 304:397, 1981.

Boyer KM, Peterson NJ, Farzaneh I, et al: An outbreak of gastroenteritis due to E. coli 0124 in a neonatal nursery. J Pediatr 86:919, 1975.

Kapikian AZ, Kim KW, Wyatt RG, et al: Human reovirus-like agent as the major pathogen associated with winter gastroenteritis in hospitalized infants and children. N Engl J Med 294:965, 1976.

Kaslow RA, Taylor A Jr, Dweck HS, et al: Enteropathogenic Escherichia coli infection in a newborn nursery. Am J Dis Child 128:797, 1974.

Steinhoff MC: Rotavirus: The first five years. J Pediatr 96:611, 1980.

7.64 CONJUNCTIVITIS

See also Sec 25.9.

Conjunctivitis is encountered frequently in the newborn infant, secondary to inflammation caused by silver nitrate and to infection with *Neisseria gonorrhoeae*, *Chlamydia trachomatis*, and *Staphylococcus aureus*. Less common causes include infection with group A or B streptococcus, *P. aeruginosa*, other bacteria, or herpesvirus hominis type 2. *N. gonorrhoeae*, *C. trachomatis*, group B streptococcus, and herpesvirus hominis are acquired on passage through a colonized or infected birth canal; other bacteria are usually acquired after birth. Prematurity and prolonged rupture of membranes are associated with an increased incidence of conjunctivitis due to the organisms acquired at birth.

Clinical Manifestations. The onset of inflammation caused by silver nitrate drops is usually within 6–12 hr after birth, with clearing by 24–48 hr. The usual incubation period for conjunctivitis due to *N. gonorrhoeae* is 2–5 days and *C. trachomatis*, 5–14 days. The time of onset of disease with other bacteria is highly variable.

Gonococcal conjunctivitis begins with mild inflammation and a serosanguineous discharge. Within 24 hr the discharge becomes thick and purulent, and tense edema of the eyelids with marked chemosis is evident. If proper treatment is delayed, the infection may spread to involve deeper layers of the conjunctivae and the cornea. Complications include corneal ulceration and perforation, iridocyclitis, anterior synechiae, and rarely panophthalmitis. Conjunctivitis caused by *Chlamydia trachomatis* (inclusion blennorrhea) may vary from mild inflammation to severe swelling of the eyelids with copious purulent discharge. The process involves mainly the tarsal conjunctivae; the corneas are rarely affected. Conjunctivitis due to *S. aureus*, *P. aeruginosa*, or other organisms is similar to that produced by *C. trachomatis*.

Diagnosis. Conjunctivitis appearing after 48 hr should be evaluated for a possibly infectious cause. Gram stain of the purulent discharge should be performed and the material cultured. If a viral etiology is suspected, a swab should be submitted in tissue culture media for virus isolation. In chlamydial conjunctivitis the diagnosis is made by examining Giemsa-stained epithelial cells scraped from the tarsal conjunctivae for the characteristic intracytoplasmic inclusions or by isolating the organisms from a conjunctival swab using special tissue culture techniques.

Treatment. In the infant in whom gonococcal ophthalmia is suspected and the Gram stain shows characteristic organisms, treatment should be initiated immediately with aqueous penicillin G, given intravenously or intramuscularly in a dosage of 100,000–150,000 units/kg/24 hr in 2–3 divided doses for 5–7 days. In addition, saline eye irrigation should be done, every 10–30 min at first and gradually increasing to 2 hr intervals, until the purulent discharge has cleared. Some advocate the use of penicillin G or chloramphenicol as eye drops immediately after each saline irrigation. Inclusion blennorrhea is treated by local instillation of 10% sulfacetamide eye drops every 2 hr initially, gradually dropping to every 4 hr, then every 6 hr, for 2–3 wk. If topical therapy fails, treatment with oral erythromycin should be implemented. Staphylococcal and *Pseudomonas* conjunctivitis in the neonate are treated with systemic antibiotics plus local saline irrigation, with or without topical antibiotics.

Prognosis and Prevention. Prior to the institution of silver nitrate prophylaxis at birth, gonococcal ophthalmia was a common cause of blindness or permanent eye damage. If properly applied, this form of prophylaxis is highly effective. Drops of 1% silver nitrate are instilled directly into the open eyes at birth using wax or plastic single dose containers. Saline irrigation is not necessary but, if performed, should not be done until after the silver nitrate solution has been in contact with the eye for at least 15 sec.

Antigonococcal prophylaxis with silver nitrate has little effect on chlamydial ophthalmia. With prompt recognition and appropriate therapy, only a small percentage of such patients have demonstrable corneal scarring, rarely associated with any visual disturbance. Because of the increasing recognition of chlamydial infections, possible alternatives to silver nitrate prophylaxis of ophthalmia neonatorum include 1% tetracycline or 0.5% erythromycin ointment, which are active against *Chlamydia trachomatis* as well as *Neisseria gonorrhoeae*, or a single intramuscular injection of aqueous penicillin (50,000 μ in term or 20,000 μ in preterm infants).

American Academy of Pediatrics: Prophylaxis and treatment of neonatal gonococcal infections. Pediatrics 65:1047, 1980.

7.65 OTITIS MEDIA

Acute otitis media in the newborn period presents a special diagnostic problem since the signs and symptoms of disease are subtle and nonspecific and the tympanic membrane is difficult to examine. In examining the eardrum, it is important to determine its mobility since the tympanic membrane may appear dull and thickened in the normal infant. Nonspecific signs and symptoms include irritability and/or lethargy, decreased appetite or failure to thrive, mild respiratory symptoms, and low grade fever. Infants may be asymptomatic (Sec 12.41).

The incidence of otitis media in premature and term infants has not been well defined, although it occurs more frequently in preterm infants. In contrast with older children, the etiologic agents isolated from about one third of infants with otitis media during the 1st 6 wk of life include *E. coli*, *K. pneumoniae*, and *P. aeruginosa* as well as group B streptococci or *S. aureus*. *S. pneumoniae* and *H. influenzae*, the most common pathogens in older children, are found in approximately one third of the cases. In the remainder, nonpathogens are isolated or no organism is found.

When a diagnosis of otitis media is established, appropriate therapy should be instituted. In a neonate in whom sepsis is considered, the initial therapy should be similar to that of neonatal sepsis. In an older infant who appears otherwise well ampicillin or amoxicillin may be started, but the infant should be carefully reevaluated in 2–3 days to determine that the middle ear disease has responded. Alteration of the therapeutic regimen should optimally be based on tympanocentesis in order to identify the specific etiologic agent. Any infant with otitis media should be carefully followed to prevent the development of chronic middle ear disease.

Bland R: Otitis media in the first six weeks of life, diagnosis, bacteriology, and management. Pediatrics 49:187, 1972.
De Sa D: Infection and amniotic aspiration of middle ear in stillbirths and neonatal deaths. Arch Dis Child 48:872, 1973.
Shurin PA, Howe VM, Pelton SI, et al: Bacterial etiology of otitis media during first six weeks of life. J Pediatr 92:893, 1978.

7.66 GROUP B STREPTOCOCCUS

Since the early 1970's there has been a significant increase in serious infections caused by this organism; in some medical centers it is the leading cause of sepsis and meningitis in neonates. The reasons for this increase are not understood.

Epidemiology. The infant is commonly infected on passage through a birth canal colonized with group B streptococcus. Although maternal cervical and/or vaginal colonization rates vary from 5–30%, depending on the geography and the nature of the population sampled, group B streptococcus rarely results in clinically significant diseases in the mother. Colonization of the throat or umbilicus in newborn infants occurs at a rate of 1–35%, but only approximately 1 in 50–100 colonized infants gets systemic disease. The organism can also be transmitted to neonates after birth on the hands of personnel, and nosocomial outbreaks of infection in a nursery have been reported.

Clinical Manifestations. Two patterns of illness in the neonate have emerged: early-onset disease with fulminant pneumonia and sepsis and late-onset disease that is insidious and manifests primarily as meningitis. However, these patterns may vary considerably and may merge: infants have been seen early with meningitis and late with sepsis. The *early-onset disease* is associated with a high incidence of maternal obstetric complications, such as prolonged rupture of membranes, difficult traumatic delivery, or maternal peripartum fever. Characteristically, the infant's birth weight is low and respiratory distress begins within hours of birth and rapidly worsens. The clinical and roentgenographic features closely resemble those of hyaline membrane disease; infants with group B streptococcal infection often have prolonged rupture of membranes (>12 hr), gram-positive cocci in the gastric aspirate, and low white blood cell counts, especially in the 1st 12 hr. In most cases, a rapid downhill course brings death in 12–24 hr despite intensive support therapy and high intravenous doses of appropriate antibiotics. Mortality rates range from 60–90%, and the organisms usually can be cultured from multiple body fluids and orifices.

The *late-onset* disease usually presents more slowly the features characteristic of meningitis: fever, lethargy, vomiting, and a bulging fontanel. Other forms of late-onset disease may occur, such as septic arthritis, osteomyelitis, and cellulitis. Asymptomatic bacteremia has also been reported. Mortality rates in group B streptococcal meningitis range from 15–40%, with neurologic sequelae in approximately 30% of survivors.

Diagnosis. Group B streptococcus infection is established by isolation of the organism from blood, CSF, or urine. A rapid diagnosis can be made using counter-immunoelectrophoresis on these fluids. Although a number of infants with early-onset disease may have leukopenia, thrombocytopenia, or both, peripheral blood counts are not usually helpful. The most important aspect of diagnosis is maintaining a high index of suspicion. In the infant in whom the diagnosis is strongly considered, antibiotic therapy should begin promptly after appropriate cultures have been obtained.

Treatment. Virtually all strains of group B streptococcus are highly sensitive to penicillin G, but because some relapses of meningitis have occurred in patients infected with a relatively resistant strain, the current recommended treatment regimen is 200,000 units of aqueous penicillin G/kg/24 hr given intravenously in 2–3 divided doses depending on the age. Therapy should be continued for 10–14 days for sepsis uncomplicated by meningitis and for at least 3 wk in meningitis.

Because of the high mortality rates in these infections of neonates, particularly the early-onset disease, treatment of the colonized mother has been considered in an attempt to eradicate the organism from the vagina or cervix. This approach has not been successful. Prevention of early-onset group B streptococcal disease has been reported by the routine administration of 50,000 units of aqueous penicillin intramuscularly within minutes after delivery. Although conclusive random trials have not been completed, this approach could be considered in a situation in which group B streptococcal infections are a special problem. Several investigators have been able to demonstrate absence of protective antibody against the group B streptococcus in both the infected infant and the maternal sera. A vaccine to immunize mothers and provide passive protection for the neonate is being developed.

Anthony BF, Okada DM: The emergence of group B streptococci in infections of the newborn infant. Ann Rev Med 28:355, 1977.
Baker CJ, Barrett FF: Group B streptococcal infections in infants: The importance of the various serotypes. JAMA 230:1158, 1974.
Baker C: Summary of the workshop on perinatal infections due to group B streptococcus. J Infect Dis 136:137, 1977.
Hodes HL: Penicillin prophylaxis and neonatal streptococcal disease. Hosp Pract 15:115, 1980.
Howard JB, McCracken GH Jr: The spectrum of group B streptococcal infections in infancy. Am J Dis Child 128:815, 1974.

7.67 STAPHYLOCOCCUS

See also Sec 10.24 and 12.66.

During the 1st 5 days of life, 40–90% of infants are colonized by staphylococcal organisms. Periodic epidemics of neonatal staphylococcal infection are related in part to differences in the capacity of different strains to colonize and cause disease.

Despite the high colonization rates with *S. aureus* in neonates, the incidence of disease is probably no more than 1–3/1000 live births in the absence of epidemics. The most common source of infection for the newborn infant is medical personnel. Although those with clinically evident staphylococcal infections are more likely to disseminate the organism, asymptomatic carriers are extremely common and may be infectious on occasion. Medical personnel can carry staphylococci on their skin, in their anterior nares, axillae, or perineal areas.

Clinical Manifestations. *S. aureus* is associated with a wide spectrum of clinical disease. Skin lesions, the most frequent manifestation, are found mainly in the diaper area, axillae, groin, neck, and umbilicus and, in males, the site of circumcision. Staphylococcal **scalded skin syndrome** (toxic epidermal necrolysis or **Ritter disease**) is a generalized manifestation of a local staphylococcal infection (Sec 24.25). The initial focus of infection may be in the umbilicus, site of circumcision, conjunctiva, or oropharynx. A scarlatiniform rash may precede the development of superficial bullae, which readily rupture. Large areas of epidermis desquamate, leaving a raw, weeping, red, "scalded"-appearing surface (see Fig 24–40). Light rubbing of the skin results in wrinkling and separation of the outer layers of the epidermis (Nikolsky sign). The disease is usually caused by coagulase-positive, phage group II (3A, 3C, 55, 71) *S. aureus* which produces an exfoliative toxin. Intact, fluid-filled bullae are usually sterile and lack inflammatory cells. After rupture, staphylococci may often be isolated from the raw, denuded surface of the skin. The lesions heal without scarring over 7–10 days.

A number of host defense mechanisms in the sick neonate may be compromised, and organisms of relatively low virulence, such as *S. epidermidis*, may cause disease, particularly in the presence of a foreign body like a shunt for hydrocephalus or an umbilical catheter. If a neonate has clinical evidence of infection and *S. epidermidis* is a consistent or the only isolate from appropriate cultures, it should be considered the pathogen.

Prevention and Treatment. There is little evidence that caps, masks, and gowns contribute significantly to control of infection in a nursery unit except when isolating an infant with known infection. However, vigorous enforcement of handwashing techniques, hexachlorophene washes, and the application of antibiotic agents or triple dye to the umbilical cord decrease colonization rates.

Although milder forms of skin lesions may be treated with local cleansing, antibiotic therapy should be given to any infant who does not respond readily to local treatment or who develops signs of extensive disease or systemic illness. Penicillinase-resistant semisynthetic penicillins should be used except when staphylococci are resistant to these drugs. Under these circumstances systemic vancomycin therapy should be instituted.

Dunkle L, Nagvi S, McCollum R, et al: Eradication of epidemic methicillin-gentamicin resistant Staphylococcus aureus in an intensive care nursery. Am J Med 70:455, 1981.
Hurst V: The hospital nursery as a source of staphylococcal disease among families of newborn infants. N Engl J Med 262:951, 1960.
Hurst V: Transmission of hospital staphylococci among newborn infants. II. Colonization of the skin and mucous membranes of the infants. Pediatrics 25:204, 1960.
Kaslow RA, Dixon RE, Martin SM, et al: Staphylococcal disease related to hospital nursery bathing practices—a nationwide epidemiologic investigation. Pediatrics 51:418, 1973.
Melish ME, Glasgow LA: Staphylococcal scalded-skin syndrome: The expanded clinical syndrome. J Pediatr 78:958, 1971.

Melish ME, Glasgow LA: The staphylococcal scalded-skin syndrome. Development of an experimental model. N Engl J Med 282:1114, 1970.

Mortimer AE Jr, Lipsitz PJ, Wolinsky E, et al: Transmission of staphylococci between newborns. Importance of the hands of personnel. Am J Dis Child 104:289, 1962.

Shuman RM, Leech RW, Alvord EC Jr: Neurotoxicity of hexachlorophene in the human. I. A clinical-pathological study of 248 children. Pediatrics 54:90, 1974.

7.68 LISTERIA

See Sec 10.38.

7.69 CYTOMEGALOVIRUS (CMV)

Cytomegalovirus is a ubiquitous agent that usually results in subclinical infections in the normal adult or child but may cross the placenta in pregnancy to infect and damage the fetus (Sec 10.75). Although almost all infants with symptomatic congenital CMV disease are born to mothers who had a primary CMV infection during pregnancy, seropositive mothers may also transmit virus to subsequent offspring. The majority of these infants, however, have inapparent infections.

Although personal contact (including venereal) may be a source of infection, transmission from an infected baby to other infants or to other hospital personnel in a nursery does not represent a major risk under usual circumstances. It is advisable, however, to obtain antibody titers on nursery personnel, and seronegative pregnant personnel should not care for cytomegalovirus-infected infants. Isolation and strict handwashing techniques should be enforced in care of neonates with known or suspected cytomegalovirus disease.

Clinical Manifestations. Congenital cytomegalovirus infection or **cytomegalic inclusion disease** may be a systemic illness characterized by hepatosplenomegaly, jaundice, petechial rash, chorioretinitis, cerebral calcifications, and microcephaly (Fig 7–32). It is now evident, however, that this severe form of the disease represents less than 10% of congenitally infected neonates and that the majority of infections are asymptomatic in the neonatal period. A low birth weight for gestational age suggests intrauterine growth retardation. Hepatomegaly is usually associated with hyperbilirubinemia and with moderate elevations of the serum transaminase and alkaline phosphatase enzymes; direct involvement of the liver is indicated by isolation of virus and the presence of multinucleated giant cells and characteristic intranuclear inclusions. Extramedullary hematopoiesis may be the cause of organomegaly in the absence of hepatitis. Although the duration of hepatosplenomegaly may vary from several mo to several yr, cytomegalovirus probably does not cause persistent active hepatitis. A generalized, usually pinpoint, petechial rash is found in approximately 50% of severely involved infants. The virus appears to have a direct effect on the bone marrow, causing a thrombocytopenia that may clear in 48–72 hr or persist for weeks to months. Significant bleeding, however, rarely occurs. Infection of the central nervous system results in the most severe sequelae of the disease. Microcephaly is found with increasing frequency in severely involved

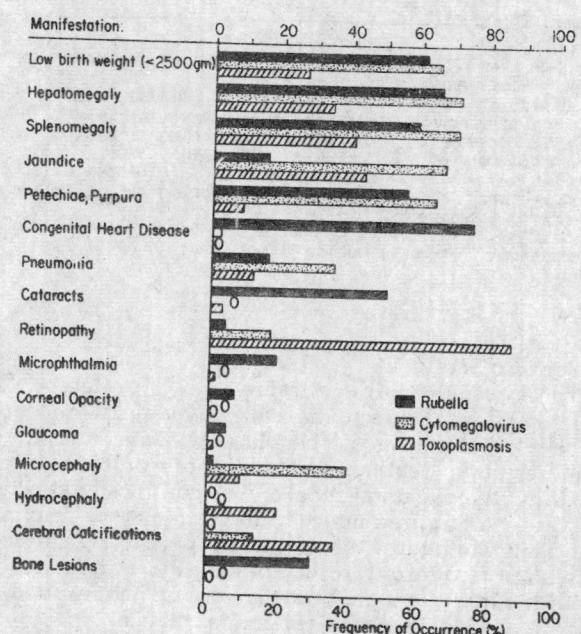

Figure 7–32 Manifestations of symptomatic congenital rubella, cytomegalovirus, and toxoplasma infections. (Overall JC Jr, In: Feigin RD, Cherry JD (eds): Textbook of Pediatric Infectious Diseases. Philadelphia, WB Saunders, 1981.)

infants and, when associated with cerebral calcifications, carries a high probability of psychomotor retardation. The cerebral calcifications are typically periventricular in distribution, in contrast to the more diffuse patterns observed in congenital *Toxoplasma* infection; these patterns, however, are not diagnostic. Microcephaly may not become apparent for several mo. The eye is less commonly involved in congenital cytomegalovirus infection than in rubella or toxoplasmosis. Chorioretinitis occurs in approximately 25% of the severely involved infants; strabismus and optic atrophy may occur. Microphthalmia and corneal opacities are rare. Cytomegalovirus can also directly infect the structure of the inner ear and result in deafness. Ear involvement may be unilateral or bilateral and can be progressive. The majority of infants with congenital CMV infection are asymptomatic during the neonatal period. However, these inapparent infections result in hearing loss and impaired intellectual functioning in at least one third of involved infants.

The respiratory tract may also be involved, although pneumonitis is not common during the typical course of congenital cytomegalovirus disease. On the other hand, a syndrome characterized by a septic appearance, hepatosplenomegaly, gray pallor, a deteriorating respiratory status, and atypical lymphocytosis has been associated with acquisition of cytomegalovirus during the neonatal period. The disease occurs in sick premature infants who are long-term residents of an intensive care unit, usually at 1–2 mo of age. Blood transfusions from seropositive donors have been associated with this syndrome. Whenever possible only cytomegalovirus seronegative donors should be used for blood transfusions in neonates.

Ballard RA, Drew WL, Hufnagle KG, et al: Acquired cytomegalovirus infection in preterm infants. Am J Dis Child 133:482, 1979.

Hanshaw JB: Cytomegalovirus. In: Remington JS, Klein JO (eds): Infectious Diseases of the Fetus and Newborn Infant. Philadelphia, WB Saunders, 1976.

Kumar ML, Nankervis GA, Gold E: Inapparent congenital cytomegalovirus infection; a followup study. N Engl J Med 288:1370, 1973.

Stagno S, Reynolds DW, Amos CS, et al: Auditory and visual defects resulting from symptomatic and subclinical congenital cytomegalovirus and Toxoplasma infections. Pediatrics 59:669, 1977.

Stagno S, Reynolds DW, Huang E, et al: Congenital cytomegalovirus infection: Occurrence in an immune population. N Engl J Med 296:1254, 1977.

7.70   RUBELLA

See also Sec 10.68.

The rubella syndrome represents a prototype for congenital viral infections. During maternal infection rubella virus can cross the placenta, infect the fetus, and result in death of the conceptus or birth of an infant with congenital rubella. The chronically infected infant who acquired infection in utero may be a source for maintaining the virus during periods when few cases are recognized in the community. Immunization with the live attenuated rubella vaccine has resulted in a decreased incidence of congenital rubella.

Pathogenesis and Pathology. Maternal infection is acquired through the respiratory tract. After an initial phase of replication at the local site of infection, target organs, including the placenta, may be seeded during the viremia. The placenta, in turn, may serve as a source of virus for the fetus. The gestational age of the conceptus at the time of infection is a critical factor in determining the outcome. Prior to the 8th wk of gestation, between 50–80% of fetuses exposed to maternal rubella become infected; by the 2nd trimester no more than 10–20% of infants become infected, and during the 3rd trimester infection of the fetus is relatively uncommon.

The possible courses of rubella virus infection are depicted in Fig 7–30. Early in pregnancy the clinical manifestations of infection in the fetus are more severe and multiple organ involvement is more frequent. Regardless of the degree of involvement, however, fetal infection is usually chronic and infants with congenital rubella may carry the virus in the nasopharynx, urine, cerebrospinal fluid, stool, eye, bone marrow, and peripheral leukocytes for extended periods of time.

Necrosis of vascular endothelium is common and may be accompanied by damage to organs secondary to vascular obstruction. Direct lysis of cells by rubella virus may occur in involved organs, particularly myocardial and skeletal muscle cells, and epithelial cells of the lens and inner ear. There is only a minimal infiltration of inflammatory cells, a characteristic which may be noted in a number of other viral infections of the fetus.

Clinical Manifestations. Congenital rubella may range from subclinical to severe disease involving multiple target organs and numerous anomalies. Infants of a mother with known or suspected rubella should be followed carefully throughout childhood since asymptomatic infants with chronic subclinical infection may subsequently develop defects or have specific organ involvement. The frequency of clinical manifestations identified in symptomatic infants during the neonatal period is illustrated in Fig 7–32. The incidence of thrombocytopenic purpura is relatively high as 1 group of patients was selected on the basis of the presence of purpura; the frequency of purpura in most series ranged from 15–50%. Thrombocytopenia usually resolves spontaneously during the 1st mo of life, but it is often found in severely affected infants with multiple organ involvement and congenital anomalies. Of 58 patients with purpura in 1 series, 35% died during the 1st yr of life, in contrast to an overall mortality rate of only 13% during the 1st 18 mo of life for the total series of 271 children with the rubella syndrome. Death is rarely due to hemorrhage, although the thrombocytopenia may be profound.

Congenital heart disease is observed frequently in the neonatal period. There also may be a viral interstitial pneumonia characterized by cough, tachypnea, and respiratory distress. In some infants the primary presenting syndrome may be respiratory; in 1 series, 6 of 7 patients with this syndrome died during the 1st yr of life as a result of their pulmonary disease. Low birth weight for gestational age is common and is believed to result from intrauterine growth retardation. Direct involvement of the liver by rubella virus may result in neonatal hepatitis, evidenced by hepatomegaly, a predominantly direct-reacting hyperbilirubinemia, and elevations of alkaline phosphatase and serum transaminase enzymes. Pathologic studies have usually demonstrated hepatocellular disease with necrosis, giant cell formation, bile stasis, and fibrosis, but extrahepatic biliary obstruction has also occurred.

Although cataracts are the most characteristic ocular lesion, they may not be recognized until after the neonatal period. The retina also may be involved and lesions may be widespread, mottled, or blotchy, with black pigmentary deposits that are variable in size and location—the "salt and pepper" retinitis. Retinal function is usually not adversely affected. Bone lesions are another typical finding but may exist in isolation; they consist of small linear areas of radiolucency and increased bone density in a longitudinal axis of the metaphyseal area in the long bones of the upper and lower extremities. The abnormality probably results from disturbances in the laying down and calcification of osteoid and usually resolves by 2–3 mo of age. The lesions may be differentiated from those observed in congenital syphilis by the absence of periosteal reaction.

Central nervous system involvement is frequent in symptomatic infants. Lethargy, irritability, disturbances of tone, and bulging fontanel are common. Seizures may occur but often are not observed until after the neonatal period. Elevation of protein in the cerebrospinal fluid is common, but elevation of cell counts is less frequent; rubella virus may often be isolated from the cerebrospinal fluid. The extent of impairment in infants at 18 mo of age is not predictable on the basis of clinical symptomatology or virus isolation in the 1st few wk of life. Severe involvement is more frequent, however, in infants with seizures and with high levels of protein in the cerebrospinal fluid during the neonatal period.

The majority of infected infants may be asymptomatic in the newborn period with as many as 70% subsequently developing evidence of congenital rubella. The most significant delayed manifestations include hearing loss (87% of 426 referred infants in whom hearing was tested), congenital heart disease (46%), mental retardation (39%), and cataract or glaucoma (34%). Children thought to have normal hearing when tested early in life have subsequently been found to have hearing loss when they reached school age. The hearing loss may be profound and a major contributor to speech impairment and learning disabilities. The lesions of the heart may not become significant until after the neonatal period; those most commonly associated with congenital rubella, in order of frequency, are patent ductus arteriosus, pulmonary artery stenosis, aortic arch anomalies, and ventricular septal defect. Children may have more than 1 cardiac defect. Mental retardation, when present, is frequently severe. Cerebral dysfunction and psychiatric disorders, including reactive behavior disorder and infantile autism, also have been recorded. Other late sequelae are increased frequency of diabetes or thyroid dysfunction and development of progressive rubella encephalitis.

Diagnosis. Although a history of an illness compatible with rubella in the mother during pregnancy may suggest the diagnosis, from one half to two thirds of the cases of maternal rubella are clinically inapparent. When congenital rubella is suspected, the diagnosis should be confirmed by virologic or serologic methods. Virus may be isolated from throat, urine, or CSF. If the eye is involved, a conjunctival swab may be a source for virus isolation. Maternal IgG antibodies against rubella cross the placenta, are present in the infant, and should decrease and disappear during the 1st yr of life in normal infants. In contrast, the congenitally infected infant usually maintains high levels of IgG antibody against rubella. A small number of infants, however, may have a gradually declining antibody titer to the rubella virus during the 1st several yr of life, apparently having lost their capacity to respond to the rubella virus antigen. The neonate with congenital rubella may have an elevated total IgM level, suggesting the possibility of intrauterine infection; however, a definitive diagnosis requires demonstration of IgM antibody specific for rubella.

Treatment. There is no specific chemotherapy for rubella virus. For discussion of immunization, see Sec 4.1 and 10.68.

Alford CA Jr: Rubella. In: Remington JS, Klein JO (eds): Infectious Diseases of the Fetus and Newborn Infant. Philadelphia, WB Saunders, 1976.

Cooper LZ: Congenital rubella in the United States. In: Krugman S, Gershon AA (eds): Infections of the Fetus and the Newborn Infant. New York, AR Liss Inc, 1975.

Desmond MM, Wilson GS, Melnick JL, et al: Congenital rubella encephalitis. J Pediatr 71:311, 1967.

Hardy JB, McCracken GH, Gilkeson MR, et al: Adverse fetal outcome following maternal rubella after the first trimester of pregnancy. JAMA 207:2414, 1969.

Korones SB, Ainger LE, Monif GRG: Congenital rubella syndrome; new clinical aspects with recovery of virus from affected infants. J Pediatr 67:166, 1965.

Phelan P, Campbell P: Pulmonary complications of rubella embryopathy. J Pediatr 75:202, 1969.

Rudolph AJ, Singleton EB, Rosenberg HS, et al: Osseous manifestations of the congenital rubella syndrome. Am J Dis Child 110:428, 1965.

Sever JL, Nelson KB, Gilkeson MR: Rubella epidemic, 1964; effect on 6000 pregnancies. Am J Dis Child 118:123, 1969.

Weller TH, Alford CA Jr, Neva FA: Changing epidemiologic concepts of rubella, with particular reference to unique characteristics of the congenital infection. Yale J Biol Med 37:455, 1965.

7.71 HEPATITIS

The etiologic agent responsible for neonatal hepatitis frequently cannot be identified. Hepatitis A appears to be transmitted across the placenta relatively rarely. Although non-A–non-B hepatitis may be transmitted from an infected mother to her offspring, infants exposed in utero are either uninfected or have only mild transient abnormalities of liver chemistries. Hepatitis B, on the other hand, is a common infection to which infants may be exposed during the perinatal period and which presents a problem in management. Other agents to consider in the etiology of neonatal hepatitis are cytomegalovirus, rubella, enteroviruses, syphilis, and toxoplasmosis.

The epidemiologic pattern of hepatitis B virus is complex and incompletely defined (Sec 10.83). An infant may be exposed through a number of different circumstances: (1) the mother may be asymptomatic but a chronic carrier of HB_sAg, (2) the mother may have active hepatitis B virus infection during pregnancy, or (3) the mother may have chronic active hepatitis. There appear to be 2 separate patterns of transmission of hepatitis B from chronic carrier mothers to their infants. In parts of Asia where the HB_sAg carrier state is common (5–20% of the population), direct transmission to the newborn is frequent. In 1 series 40% of infants born to mothers who were chronic carriers became HB_sAg-positive by 6 mo of age. In other countries, particularly in the United States and western Europe, a much lower rate (0–16%) of transmission from chronic carrier mothers to their infants has been observed. The rate of transplacental transmission appears to vary directly with the presence of the e antigen, Hb_eAg. Antibody also may develop against HB_eAg, and the presence of anti-HB_e in the serum of the mother is associated with the lack of transmission of the infection to her offspring.

The infant born to the mother who has acute hepatitis faces a different risk. When maternal hepatitis occurs during the 1st or 2nd trimester, only a small percentage of infants become infected. In contrast, 25–76% of infants become infected with the virus when maternal hepatitis occurs during the 3rd trimester or near the time of delivery. Although hepatitis B virus may cross the placenta causing infants to be born with antigenemia, most infants who acquire hepatitis B virus from mothers with acute hepatitis do not have Hb_sAg in their cord blood but rather develop antigenemia by 6–12 wk of age. This suggests that transmission occurs at delivery or shortly thereafter. Postpartum transmission of hepatitis B virus may infrequently occur by other routes since HB_sAg has been found in saliva, breast milk, urine, and stool.

Clinical Manifestations. Maternal hepatitis B has not been associated with congenital malformations, abortions or stillbirths, or intrauterine growth retardation. However, it has been correlated with prematurity, particularly during the last trimester of pregnancy.

Infants exposed to maternal hepatitis B (1) become HB₅Ag-positive and remain asymptomatic but develop persistent antigenemia with evidence of chronic liver involvement; (2) become Hb₅Ag-positive, remain asymptomatic, or develop mild hepatitis and then recover with clearance of their antigenemia; (3) become HB₅Ag-positive and develop severe fulminant hepatitis with liver necrosis and death; or (4) never acquire hepatitis B virus infection. Differences in the time of exposure, the route of inoculation, and the size of the viral inoculum may explain this wide variation in the time of antigenemia in the infected neonate. Some infants born to carrier mothers may have HB₅Ag in the cord blood but may not become infected, as evidenced by absence of HB₅Ag at 1–3 mo of life. The infant in whom an HB₅Ag-positive cord blood is obtained should have blood specimens assayed for HB₅Ag at follow-up visits. Apparent false positives may be due to contamination during the birth process and reflect the sensitivity of current laboratory assays in detecting the HB₅Ag.

The most common sequence of events in infants who acquire hepatitis B virus is to remain asymptomatic and become a chronic carrier, i.e., HB₅Ag-positive. In the series reported by Schweitzer, all such infants were antigen-positive for as long as they were followed (up to 5 yr). These children have persistently elevated transaminase levels but usually show no clinical evidence of liver disease. Biopsy specimens, however, indicate persistent hepatitis and evidence of ongoing liver disease. Long-term follow-up of these children is not yet available.

A small number of infants born either to mothers with acute hepatitis or to carrier mothers may become HB₅Ag-positive at any time during the 1st yr of life. These infants may have mild or no clinical signs of hepatitis, clear their antigenemia, and recover. Although most neonatal infections with hepatitis B virus are benign during infancy, a small number of infants have severe fulminant disease with massive liver necrosis and die; such cases may follow transfusions during the neonatal period or occur in infants of chronic carrier mothers. Several families have also been reported in which more than 1 infant born to the same carrier mother developed fulminant fatal neonatal hepatitis B. The reasons for these different patterns of illness are not understood.

Prevention and Treatment. Personnel should handle a known HB₅Ag-positive infant as a contagious patient, with emphasis on handwashing; use of gloves when handling, drawing blood, or processing excretions; and caution in handling needles. Anyone stuck by a needle used on an HB₅Ag-positive neonate should be tested for HB₅Ag or anti-HB₅Ag antibody. An individual negative for both should receive hepatitis B immune globulin, if available, or 8 ml of standard immune serum globulin. See Sec 10.83 for preventive use of hepatitis B immune globulin (HBIG).

There is no proven effective antiviral chemotherapeutic agent. However, HBIG may be effective when given early to the neonate and repeated during infancy.

HB₅Ag has been found in breast milk, and the virus could be ingested from cracked nipples while the infant is nursing. Although breast feeding did not alter the incidence of hepatitis B infection in Taiwan and transmission by this route has not been documented, the safest course may be to recommend that carrier mothers do not breast feed their infants.

Centers for Disease Control: Immune globulins for protection against viral hepatitis. Ann Int Med 96:193, 1982.
Crumpacker CS: Hepatitis. In: Remington JS, Klein JO (eds): Infectious Diseases of the Fetus and Newborn Infant. Philadelphia, WB Saunders, 1976.
Hieber JP, Dalton D, Shorey J, et al: Hepatitis and pregnancy. J Pediatr 91:545, 1977.
Krugman S: Viral hepatitis; recent developments and prospects for prevention. J Pediatr 87:1067, 1975.
Okada K, Kamiyama I, Inomata M, et al: e Antigen and anti-e in the serum of asymptomatic carrier mothers as indicators of positive and negative transmission of hepatitis B virus to their infants. N Engl J Med 294:746, 1976.
Schweitzer IL, Dunn AEG, Peters RL, et al: Viral hepatitis in neonates and infants. Am J Med 55:762, 1973.
Tong MJ, Thursby M, Rakela J, et al: Studies on the maternal-infant transmission of the viruses which cause acute hepatitis. Gastroenterology 80:999, 1981.

7.72 HERPES SIMPLEX VIRUS

Herpes simplex virus (Sec 10.71) may cause a severe generalized disease in the neonate with high mortality and devastating sequelae. The majority of cases are thought to be acquired during passage through the birth canal and are, therefore, type II virus. The specific source of infection may be difficult to elucidate since virus can be isolated from oral or genital sites in the absence of recognized clinical symptoms. Further, the majority (70%) of mothers of herpesvirus-infected neonates in 1 series had no clinical evidence of infection at the time of delivery. Thus, one should be extremely cautious in attributing neonatal infection to a family member or other contact with oral herpetic lesions. The virus can cross the placenta as indicated by several reports of infants with congenital malformations, typical vesicular lesions present at birth, and virus isolation from their placentas.

Clinical Manifestations. Neonatal herpes simplex infections may produce a spectrum of manifestations ranging from a local infection in the skin, eye, or mouth to a generalized disease involving multiple target organs. Virus is rarely found in the absence of signs or symptoms. Two thirds of the infants show the disseminated form, which involves the liver and adrenal glands and may produce a clinical picture resembling bacterial sepsis. In approximately 50% of infants the virus affects the central nervous system; death may occur before neurologic symptoms are apparent. Onset occurs usually within the 1st wk of life but is seen at birth or as late as 3 wk of age. The initial signs are usually nonspecific and include fever, lethargy, poor feeding, irritability, and vomiting; convulsions, jaundice, apneic spells, cyanosis, respiratory distress, and hepatosplenomegaly are frequently observed. Clinical evidence of central nervous system involvement includes irritability, bulging fontanel, local or generalized seizures, flaccid or spastic paralysis, opisthotonos, decerebrate rigidity, or coma. Involvement of the central nervous system in the absence of lesions in the skin, mouth, or eye is unusual but has been seen with subsequent development of the other manifestations.

Infants with disseminated infection in multiple organs or those with central nervous system involvement alone tend to have a poor prognosis with high mortality or major sequelae. Often the disease progresses rapidly to death following a deteriorating neurologic status.

The skin is the most common site of involvement with this virus; the majority of patients have a vesicular rash. Vesicles may be 1–2 isolated lesions or present in clusters. It is important to carefully evaluate infants with localized lesions of the skin only since some of these neonates have subsequently manifested psychomotor retardation. The vesicular eruption has also been distributed along a dermatome, simulating herpes zoster. A diagnosis of herpes zoster in the newborn should not be made without attempting to isolate and identify the specific etiologic agent. The eye may be involved alone or as one of several target organs in the disseminated form of the disease, with conjunctivitis, keratoconjunctivitis, keratitis, and, more rarely, chorioretinitis.

Prevention and Treatment. A cesarean section is indicated for mothers with a known genital infection at the time of delivery. This is most likely to decrease the risk when performed before, or less than 4 hr after, rupture of the membranes.

An infant born to a mother with genital herpes should be isolated and cultures of the infant obtained to determine whether infection has occurred.

Adenine arabinoside (ara-A) has been shown to be of benefit in adults with herpes encephalitis and to reduce mortality from 74% in the placebo control group to 38% in the treated infants. Therapy was most effective against localized disease, and the best prognosis occurred in neonates with superficial involvement of skin, eye, or mouth. The dose is 15 mg/kg/24 hr administered intravenously over 12 hr at a concentration of 0.7 mg/ml or less in a standard intravenous solution for 10 days. Higher doses may be more effective, but adequate data on benefits and toxicity are not available. Treatment should be started early, and the diagnosis should be confirmed by virus isolation.

Amstey MS: Management of pregnancy complicated by genital herpes virus infection. Obstet Gynecol 37:515, 1971.
Ch'ier. I, Whitley R, Nahmias A, et al: Antiviral chemotherapy and neonatal herpes simplex virus infection; a pilot study—experience with adenine arabinoside (ara-A). Pediatrics 55:678, 1975.
Echeverria P, Miller G, Campbell AGM, et al: Scalp vesicles within the first week of life: A clue to early diagnosis of herpes neonatorum. J Pediatr 83:1062, 1973.
Nahmias AJ, Visintine AM: Herpes simplex. In: Remington JS, Klein JO (eds): Infectious Diseases of the Fetus and Newborn Infant. Philadelphia, WB Saunders, 1976.
South MA, Tompkins WAF, Morris CR, et al: Congenital malformations of the central nervous system associated with genital (type 2) herpesvirus. J Pediatr 75:13, 1969.

7.73 ENTEROVIRUSES

The enteroviruses (Sec 10.84) are responsible for a wide spectrum of clinical manifestations in both mothers and neonates. Congenital infection is rare; it occurs by transplacental passage of the virus from mother to fetus. More commonly, infants are infected during the birth process or in the neonatal period. After delivery, infection is acquired in the same fashion as with older children and adults. Outbreaks have been reported in nurseries following introduction by an infected infant and spread from infant to infant through nursery personnel. When enterovirus disease is identified in a nursery setting, therefore, infected infants should be isolated and infection control techniques carefully followed.

Clinical Manifestations. There is no convincing evidence that Coxsackie virus and echovirus infections result in fetal loss. Congenital anomalies have not been reported with poliovirus or echovirus, but maternal Coxsackie virus infections may be associated with urogenital, digestive, and cardiovascular anomalies.

A wide variety of clinical manifestations may occur in neonates infected with the Coxsackie viruses and echoviruses. However, though infections with this group of agents are probably common, clinical symptoms are relatively infrequent. Severe forms of generalized enterovirus infection with multiple organ involvement and fatal outcome are particularly rare. Asymptomatic infections have been recognized with both Coxsackie virus and echovirus during surveys of nurseries and during epidemics in which other infants are symptomatic. The milder end of the clinical spectrum includes nonspecific febrile illness, gastroenteritis, or respiratory tract disease.

The occurrence of an exanthem in association with other signs of illness should suggest an enterovirus. Blotchy, erythematous, macular, papular, morbilliform, or petechial exanthems have all been associated with Coxsackie viruses and echoviruses (Sec 10.84). Distribution and duration of the rash is highly variable. In more severely ill infants in whom bacterial sepsis or meningitis is suspected, the absence of bacterial isolates from the blood or cerebrospinal fluid should suggest the possibility of an enterovirus infection. Clinical symptoms in the severe disease may be nonspecific, with lethargy, poor feeding, and irritability, or include evidence of specific target organ involvement such as cyanosis, apneic spells, seizures, jaundice, hepatosplenomegaly, or petechiae. Signs of cardiac involvement from myocarditis are often prominent.

Diagnosis. Certain characteristics associated with enterovirus infections may suggest the diagnosis. In temperate climates over 90% of infections due to these agents occur in summer and fall. When multiple cases occur in a nursery in the absence of any significant bacterial isolates, an enterovirus should be suspected. Other epidemiologic factors that should suggest infection are the presence of an outbreak in the community or the history of a nonspecific illness compatible with an enterovirus infection in the mother near the time of delivery. In addition, there is often a lack of the factors that commonly predispose an infant to bacterial infections: prematurity, low Apgar scores, prolonged rupture of membranes, or other complications of delivery. Finally, an exanthematous rash or aseptic meningitis should strongly suggest enterovirus infection, particularly if more than 1 case is observed in the nursery.

Enteroviruses can be isolated by most viral diagnostic laboratories (Sec 10.84).

Treatment.   There is no effective antiviral chemotherapy for these viruses. Gamma globulin is not effective in protecting an infant in those rare circumstances in which a maternal enterovirus infection is recognized at delivery.

Prognosis.   The prognosis depends upon the _____ity of the infection. Mortality in neonates with _____ illness is extremely low. In contrast, infants with multiple organ involvement, particularly myocarditis, hepatitis, and encephalitis, have a high mortality. It is probable that most infants recover without residual damage, but there are no data concerning the possible long-range sequelae of neonates with central nervous system disease.

Brightman VJ, Scott TFM, Westphal M, et al: An outbreak of Coxsackie B-5 virus in a newborn nursery. J Pediatr 69:179, 1966.

Kipps A, Naude WDT, Don P, et al: Coxsackie virus myocarditis of the newborn. Med Proc 4:401, 1958.

Lake AM, Lauer BA, Clark JC, et al: Enterovirus infections in neonates. J Pediatr 89:787, 1976.

Modlin JF: Fatal echovirus II disease in neonates. Pediatrics 66:775, 1980.

Modlin JF, Polk BF, Horton P, et al: Perinatal echovirus infection: Risk of transmission during a community outbreak. N Engl J Med 305:368, 1981.

7.74   VARICELLA-ZOSTER

The newborn may be exposed to varicella-zoster virus in utero or in the immediate postpartum period by the occurrence of either varicella or zoster in the mother or through contact with other neonates or medical personnel (Sec 10.72). Fetal wastage has not been associated with maternal varicella, though individual cases of abortion or stillbirth have been reported; there may be lesions in the placenta or in multiple fetal organs. Although a small number of infants delivered to women with a history of varicella during the 1st 15 wk of gestation have had a similar constellation of malformations at birth (low birth weight, hypoplastic limbs or digits, cicatricial skin lesions, cortical atrophy, growth retardation, delayed motor development, ocular abnormalities, enhanced susceptibility to infections), the failure to observe infants with the syndrome in prospective studies indicates that it is relatively uncommon.

Clinical Manifestations.   Varicella can be acquired congenitally when maternal chickenpox occurs within 21 days prior to delivery. Disease in the infant is seen in approximately 25% of the maternal infections. When the onset in the neonate is at 5–10 days of life, usually reflecting the occurrence of varicella in the mother within 5 days of delivery, the disease may follow a severe course, with a mortality of 25–30%. When clinical signs of varicella are present at delivery or begin within 4 days of life, the course usually is benign and fatalities rare. This amelioration may relate to the time of exposure of the fetus and the transfer of maternal antibody. Chickenpox may also be acquired by neonatal exposure, but spread within the nursery is rare and the disease is generally mild. The majority of infants exposed by nonmaternal sources probably have maternally acquired antibody and thus are protected against this virus. A diagnosis can usually be made by the characteristic distribution of vesicular lesions which closely resembles that in older children and a history of maternal or postnatal exposure. The differential diagnosis includes disseminated herpes simplex, impetigo, contact dermatitis, and the hand-foot-mouth syndrome.

On rare occasions zoster has been reported in infants, although varicella-zoster has not been isolated from any of these cases. The recovery of herpes simplex virus from at least 1 neonate with zoster indicated that the diagnosis should be made with caution and that cultures for virus isolation should be obtained.

Zoster immune globulin and pooled immune serum globulin can attenuate or prevent varicella when administered early during the incubation period. Infants born to mothers who have had varicella near the time of delivery should receive zoster immune globulin or, if that is not available, 0.6–1.2 ml/kg of normal immune serum globulin as soon as possible. With onset of maternal or neonatal varicella, the mother and infant should be isolated to prevent spread to susceptible individuals. Chemotherapy, including cytosine arabinoside (ara-C), adenine arabinoside (ara-A), and iododeoxyuridine, has not been established as effective or safe in the newborn infected with varicella-zoster virus. Therapy with ara-A may be considered in severe varicella-zoster virus infections when zoster immune globulin is not available or when it is too late to be used effectively; ara-A is efficacious in older immunosuppressed patients and has been used in neonatal herpes without apparent toxicity. Antiviral chemotherapy is not warranted in mild cases.

LOWELL A. GLASGOW*
JAMES C. OVERALL, JR.

Gershon AA, Steinberg S, Brunell PA: Zoster immune globulin. A further assessment. N Engl J Med 290:243, 1974.

Matscoane SL, Abler C: Occurrence of neonatal varicella in a hospital nursery. Am J Obstet Gynecol 92:575, 1965.

McKendry JBJ, Bailey JD: Congenital varicella associated with multiple defects. Can Med Assoc J 108:66, 1973.

Meyers JD: Congenital varicella in term infants: Risk reconsidered. J Infect Dis 129:215, 1974.

Music SI, Fine EM, Togo Y: Zoster-like disease in newborn due to herpes simplex virus. N Engl J Med 294:24, 1971.

Siegel M, Fuerst HT, Peress NS: Comparative fetal mortality in maternal virus diseases. A prospective study on rubella, measles, mumps, chickenpox and hepatitis. N Engl J Med 274:768, 1966.

Srabstein JC, Morris N, Larke RPB, et al: Is there a congenital varicella syndrome? J Pediatr 84:239, 1974.

*Deceased.

INBORN ERRORS OF METABOLISM 8

8.1 INTRODUCTION

Many disorders originate in mutational events that alter the genetic constitution of an individual and disrupt normal function. The number of human hereditary biochemical disorders, named "inborn errors of metabolism" by Garrod at the turn of the century, has grown into hundreds, and they are being discovered at an ever-increasing rate.

Modern biochemical genetics can now describe how genetic information is translated into the synthesis of proteins with specific metabolic or structural properties. Within the nucleus of each cell genetic information resides in the chromosomes, encoded in deoxyribonucleic acid (DNA) molecules. The code is made up of combinations of 2 purine and 2 pyrimidine bases arranged on the DNA helix. The genetic information contained in DNA is transcribed to messenger ribonucleic acid (mRNA), which is free to leave the nucleus. Proteins are synthesized from individual amino acids in the cytoplasm, where the information carried by the mRNA is translated into the linear array of amino acids comprising the polypeptide chain.

A mutation in DNA may alter the synthesis of a protein by introducing a structural error into the sequence of amino acids through substitution of 1 amino acid for another. If the integrity of the region of substitution is necessary for function, then, depending on the nature of the alteration, part or all of the normal function of this protein may be lost. Alternatively, an amino acid substitution may render the protein very labile, and it may be destroyed as rapidly as it is synthesized. Another mutation might affect another set of genes that control the rate of synthesis of a normally structured protein. Such a mutation can result either in lowered rate of synthesis of an enzyme or in its complete lack. In drug-induced hemolytic anemia, for example, a structurally altered form of erythrocyte glucose-6-phosphate dehydrogenase is synthesized which cannot carry out its normal function, whereas in analbuminemia plasma albumin is either not synthesized at all or is made in an altered and unstable form.

Much of what is known of human biochemical genetics has been garnered from studies of the hemoglobin molecule and the genetic factors that determine its chemical and physical properties. Information so obtained has been applied to the study of many other proteins and of the disease processes caused by their malfunction. Hemoglobin serves as a model substance because, unlike most enzymes, it is freely obtainable and can be easily separated from other protein contaminants. Certain changes in structure are revealed by alteration of electrophoretic mobility, and other analytic techniques can reveal the exact amino acid sequence of the polypeptide chain.

The predominant normal hemoglobin is hemoglobin A, which consists of 2 pairs of polypeptide chains (alpha and beta). Alpha and beta chains, as well as the common delta and gamma chains (Sec 14.2), differ slightly in the composition or sequential arrangement of their component amino acids. The composition of each polypeptide chain is under genetic control, and the sequential arrangement of the amino acids corresponds to the order of bases on the deoxyribonucleic acid molecule.

Studies of many varieties of hemoglobin, some of which are discussed elsewhere (Sec 14.18–14.22), indicate that approximately half the alpha chains and half the beta chains are synthesized under the control of a gene obtained from the father and the other half through a gene obtained from the mother. If a gene for an abnormal hemoglobin is obtained from only 1 parent, then only half the hemoglobin molecules will be affected (heterozygous). For all the hemoglobin to be affected (homozygous), the same gene must be obtained from each parent.

More than 1 defect can occur within the same polypeptide chain; there can be at least as many defects as there are positions for amino acids in the molecule. Within the same chain, different defects may occur at the same amino acid locus; in the beta chain of hemoglobin at a point normally occupied by glutamic acid, 1 mutation results in its replacement by valine (hemoglobin S), and another mutation results in replacement by lysine (hemoglobin C). Accordingly, if parents carry different abnormal genes at the same locus, e.g., 1 parent hemoglobin S, the other hemoglobin C, then all the hemoglobin in the offspring inheriting each parent's abnormal gene will be abnormal. Approximately half this child's hemoglobin will be hemoglobin S, and the other half, hemoglobin C (hemoglobin SC disease).

A genetic defect in hemoglobin structure may or may not have clinical significance, depending on how it affects the function of the hemoglobin molecule. As indicated, each mutation of a gene manifests itself as a chemically unique structure. Among persons with sickle cell hemoglobin (hemoglobin S), the heterozygote (hemoglobin A plus hemoglobin S) is identified clinically as having the sickle cell trait but may have little or no clinical disorder, whereas the homozygote (all hemoglobin S) has sickle cell disease and is seriously affected. In certain types of methemoglobinemia, on the other hand, the heterozygote (hemoglobin A plus hemoglobin M) has a significant clinical disorder. At the other extreme of the spectrum of hemoglobinopathies, alterations in hemoglobin structure are not reflected in functional disorders. For example, the homozygote for hemoglobin G is clinically normal.

Although the terms recessive and dominant, as well as incompletely recessive, incompletely dominant, penetrance, and expressivity, describe the patterns of inheritance (Chapter 6), it should be understood that alteration of a structural gene always leads to abnormal protein formation, even in the heterozygote without evidence of clinical disorder.

The mutations just described predominantly affect the amino acid composition of protein; other mutations alter the rate at which protein will be synthesized. For example, in the thalassemias (Sec 14.23) there may be decreased synthesis of either alpha or beta chains of hemoglobin A. In the latter instance, synthesis of fetal hemoglobin (2 alpha plus 2 gamma chains) and hemoglobin A_2 (2 alpha plus 2 delta chains) may continue; when synthesis of the alpha chain is not possible, hemoglobin molecules with only beta chains (4 beta, hemoglobin H) or only gamma chains (4 gamma, Bart hemoglobin) may appear.

For many enzymatic defects it is not known whether the enzyme is altered in such a way as to have no activity or is not synthesized in normal quantities. In any case, studies of the structure of purified enzymes of normal persons and persons with genetic defects indicate that what we have learned from the hemoglobinopathies applies without modification to the enzymopathies.

Other generalizations are germane to a discussion of hereditary defects. It should be appreciated that the absence of activity of a specific enzyme may have 1 or more of several effects.

1. The end-product is not made. If this is a substance essential to life, the result is lethal.

Table 8–1 SOME CLINICAL FINDINGS OFTEN ASSOCIATED WITH INBORN ERRORS OF METABOLISM

SYMPTOMS OR SIGNS	ASSOCIATED DISEASES
Neurologic abnormalities	Almost all categories
Metabolic acidosis with ketosis	See Table 8–3
Pernicious vomiting	Isovaleric acidemia, urea cycle or amino acid defects, methylmalonic acidemia, propionic acidemia, PKU, valinemia, α-methylacetoacetic acidemia, adrenal insufficiency, carnitine deficiency, multiple acyl-CoA dehydrogenase deficiency
Liver disease	Tyrosinemia, glycogen storage, galactosemia, Wilson disease, hereditary fructose intolerance, α_1-antitrypsin deficiency, cystic fibrosis, hemochromatosis, lipidoses

Miscellaneous
  Clinical: dislocated lenses, renal stones, thrombosis, deafness, microcephaly, cataracts, hematuria, self-mutilation, abnormal urine odor (see Table 8–4) or color, coarse facies, persistent eczema, abnormal hair
  Laboratory: osteoporosis, rickets, hypoglycemia, unexplained jaundice, bony x-ray change, increased anion gap, ketoacidosis, abnormal liver function

Table 8–2 INBORN ERRORS OF METABOLISM*

I. DEFECTS OF AMINO ACID METABOLISM
  A. Phenylalanine
    1. Phenylketonuria (PKU) (b — blood only)†
       (c — 80% detected)†
    2. Phenylalaninemia variants (b)
    3. Dihydropteridine reductase defect
    4. Dihydropteridine synthetase deficiency
    5. Methylmandelic aciduria (b)
    6. Parahydroxyphenylacetic aciduria (b)
  B. Tyrosine
    1. Tyrosinemia
       a. Transient neonatal (b)
       b. Acute (b)
       c. Subacute or chronic (b)
       d. Tyrosine transaminase deficiency (b)
       e. Richner-Hanhart syndrome (b)
    2. Albinism
       a. Oculocutaneous albinism (6 forms) (b)
       b. Other forms
    3. Alcaptonuria (b)
    4. Parkinsonism
  C. Methionine
    1. Methioninemia (b)
    2. Malabsorption of methionine (oasthouse disease) (b) (c)
    3. Homocystinemia
       a. Cystathionine synthase deficiency (type I)

       (1) Vitamin B_6 unresponsive (a) (b) (c)
       (2) Vitamin B_6 responsive (a) (b)
    b. ^5N-Methyltetrahydrofolate methyltransferase deficiency (type II)
       (1) Vitamin B_{12} unresponsive (a) (b)
       (2) Vitamin B_{12} responsive (a) (b)
    c. ^{5-10}N-Methylene-tetrahydrofolate reductase deficiency (type III)
       (1) Folic acid responsive (a) (b)
    4. Cystathioninemia
       a. Vitamin B_6 unresponsive (a) (b) (c)
       b. Vitamin B_6 responsive (a) (b) (c)
       c. Latent cystathioninuria (b)
  D. Cystine
    1. Cystinuria (a) (b) (c)
    2. Cystinosis (a) (b) (c)
    3. Sulfite oxidase deficiency (a) (b)
    4. β-Mercaptolactate-cysteine disulfiduria (b)
    5. Taurinuria (dominant) (b)
  E. Tryptophan
    1. Hartnup disease (a) (b)
    2. Tryptophanemia (b)
    3. Kynureninuria (b)
    4. Hydroxykynureninuria (b) (c)
    5. Pyridoxine-responsive xanthurenic aciduria (b)
    6. Indicanuria (b)
    7. Hydrindicuria (b)

*Unless otherwise indicated, an autosomal recessive form of inheritance is assumed. Many of the disorders listed are also discussed elsewhere in the text; consult the index.
  †(a) = Prenatal diagnosis is feasible or has been made.
  (b) = Early diagnosis is possible using easily accessible material such as blood, urine, tears, skin, etc.
  (c) = Heterozygous carrier state can be determined reliably.
  ‡See also VII. E. 13, this table.

Table 8-2 INBORN ERRORS OF METABOLISM* (Continued)

8. Indolylacroylglycinuria (b)
9. Glutaric acidemia (a) (b) (c)
10. α-Ketoadipic aciduria (a) (b)

F. Valine, leucine, isoleucine
  1. Maple syrup urine disease
    a. Classic form (a) (b) (c)
    b. Intermittent form (a) (b) (c)
    c. Mild form (a) (b)
    d. Vitamin B, responsive (a) (b)
  2. Valinemia (a) (b)
  3. α-Methylacetoacetic aciduria (a) (b) (c)
  4. Isoleucine-leucinemia (b)
  5. Isovaleric acidemia (a) (b)
  6. β-Methylcrotonyl glycinuria
    a. Biotin unresponsive (a) (b)
    b. Biotin responsive (a) (b)
  7. β-Methylglutaconic aciduria (b)
  8. β-Hydroxy-β-methylglutaric aciduria (a) (b) (c)
  9. Propionic acidemia
    a. Biotin unresponsive (a) (b)
    b. Biotin responsive (a) (b)
  10. Holocarboxylase synthetase deficiency (a) (b)
  11. Methylmalonic acidemia
    a. Vitamin B_{12} unresponsive (a) (b)
    b. Vitamin B_{12} responsive (a) (b)

G. Glycine
  1. Glycinemia (b)
  2. Sarcosinemia (b) (c)
  3. D-Glyceric acidemia (b)
  4. Trimethylaminuria (b)
  5. Glycinuria and glucoglycinuria (b)
  6. Primary oxaluria and oxalosis
    a. L-Glyceric aciduria (b) (c)
    b. Glycolic aciduria (b)

H. Serine
  1. Ethanolaminosis

I. Threonine
  1. Threoninemia

J. Proline and hydroxyproline
  1. Prolinemia (b)
  2. Hydroxyprolinemia (b)
  3. Familial iminoglycinuria (b)
  4. Prolidase deficiency

K. Glutamic acid
  1. Anemia due to γ-glutamylcysteine synthetase deficiency
  2. Anemia due to glutathione synthetase deficiency
  3. Pyroglutamic acidemia (a) (b) (c)
    a. Glutathione synthetase deficiency
    b. 5-Oxyprolinase deficiency
  4. Glutathionemia (a) (b)
  5. Vitamin B_6–responsive seizures
    (b — EEG response)
  6. Chinese restaurant syndrome

L. Urea cycle amino acids
  1. Ammonemia due to carbamyl phosphate synthetase deficiency (b)
  2. Ammonemia due to N-acetylglutamate synthesis deficiency
  3. Ammonemia due to ornithine transcarbamylase deficiency (X-linked dominant) (a) (b) (c)
  4. Citrullinemia (a) (b)
  5. Argininosuccinic acidemia (a) (b) (c)
  6. Argininemia (b) (c)
  7. Ornithinemia (a) (b)

M. Histidine
  1. Histidinemia (a) (b)
  2. Histidine and folic acid metabolism
    a. Formiminotransferase defect (b)
    b. Cyclohydrolase defect (b)
    c. Methyltransferase defect (a) (b) (see I, C, 3, b)
    d. Dihydrofolate reductase defect
  3. Histidinuria (b)
  4. Imidazole aciduria (b)

5. Serum carosinase deficiency (b)
6. Homocarnosinosis (b)

N. Beta-amino acids
  1. β-Alaninemia (b)
  2. β-Aminoisobutyric aciduria (b)

O. Lysine
  1. Lysinemia I (a) (b) (c)
  2. Lysinemia II (a) (b)
  3. α-Aminoadipic acidemia (b)
  4. α-Ketoadipic acidemia (a) (b)
  5. Glutaric acidemia (a) (b) (c)
  6. Congenital lysine intolerance (b)
  7. Pipecolatemia (b)
  8. Lysinuria (hyperdibasicaminoaciduria) (b) (c)
  9. Lysinuric protein intolerance (b)
  10. Hydroxylysinemia (b)
  11. Hydroxylysine-deficient collagen (a) (b) (c)

II. DEFECTS OF CARBOHYDRATE METABOLISM
A. Defects of carbohydrate absorption
  1. Sucrase-isomaltase deficiency
  2. Lactose intolerance
    a. Familial
    b. Congenital
    c. Late onset
  3. Glucose-galactose malabsorption
  4. Renal glycosuria (Chapters 16 and 23)

B. Defects of intermediary carbohydrate metabolism
  1. Defects without lactic acidosis or abnormal glycogen storage
    a. Deficiency of galactokinase (a) (b) (c)
    b. Deficiency of galactose-1-phosphate uridyl transferase (a) (b) (c)
    c. Deficiency of uridyl diphosphogalactose 4-epimerase (b) (c)
    d. Deficiency of fructokinase (b)
    e. Deficiency of 1-phosphofructaldolase (b)
    f. Deficient muscle phosphoglycerate mutase
    g. Deficiency of muscle type lactate dehydrogenase
  2. Defects in intermediary carbohydrate metabolism associated with lactic acidosis
    a. Deficiency of glucose-6-phosphatase
    b. Deficiency of fructose-1,6-diphosphatase
    c. Deficiency of pyruvate decarboxylase (b)
    d. Deficiency of dihydrolipoyl transacetylase (b)
    e. Deficiency of dihydrolipoyl dehydrogenase (b)
    f. Deficiency of pyruvate carboxylase
    g. Deficiency of pyruvate dehydrogenase phosphatase
    h. Congenital idiopathic lactic acidosis
    i. Leigh subacute necrotizing encephalopathy (SNE)
  3. Glycogen storage diseases
    a. Deficiency of glycogen synthetase (GSD 0)
    b. Deficiency of glucose-6-phosphatase (GSD I)
    c. GSD Ib (Pseudo-GSD I) (enzyme transport defect)
    d. Deficiency of lysosomal acid α-glucosidase (GSD II)
      GSD IIa (a) (b) (c)
      GSD IIb (b) (c)
    e. Deficiency of "debrancher" activity (GSD III) (a) (b)
    f. Deficiency of "brancher" activity (GSD IV) (a) (b)
    g. Deficiency of muscle phosphorylase (GSD V)
    h. Deficiency of liver phosphorylase (GSD VI)
    i. Deficiency of phosphofructokinase (GSD VII)
    j. Progressive brain disease and deactivated liver phosphorylase without demonstrated enzyme defect (GSD VIII)
    k. Deficiency of liver phosphorylase kinase (GSD IX)
      GSD IXa — autosomal recessive inheritance
      GSD IXb — X-linked recessive inheritance
    l. Deficiency of cyclic 3'5'-AMP-dependent kinase (GSD X)
    m. Hepatic glycogenosis with stunted growth (GSD XI)
  4. Miscellaneous

Table continued on following page

Table 8–2   INBORN ERRORS OF METABOLISM*   (Continued)

     a. Deficiency of gulonolactone pathway (scurvy)
     b. Deficiency of xyiulose dehydrogenase (essential benign pentosuria)
     c. Deficiency of acid α-mannosidase (mannosidosis) (a) (b)
     d. Deficiency of acid α-fucosidase (fucosidosis) (a) (b)
     e. Blood group substances

C. The mucopolysaccharidoses (Chapter 23)
   1. Mucopolysaccharidosis IH (Hurler) (α-L-iduronidase deficiency)
   2. Mucopolysaccharidosis IS (Scheie) (α-L-iduronidase deficiency)
   3. Mucopolysaccharidosis II (Hunter) (L-iduronosulfate sulfatase deficiency) (X-linked recessive)
   4. Mucopolysaccharidosis IIIA (Sanfilippo A) (Sulfamidase deficiency)
   5. Mucopolysaccharidosis IIIB (Sanfilippo B) (α-N-acetylglucosaminidase deficiency)
   6. Mucopolysaccharidosis IV (Morquio) (N-acetylgalactosamine 6-SO_4 sulfatase deficiency)
   7. Mucopolysaccharidosis VI (Maroteaux-Lamy) (arylsulfatase B deficiency)
   8. Mucopolysaccharidosis VII (β-glucuronidase deficiency)
   9. Mucopolysaccharidosis VIII (N-acetylglucosamine 6-SO_4 sulfatase deficiency)

III. DEFECTS OF PURINE AND PYRIMIDINE METABOLISM
   1. Hyperuricemia (gout)
     a. Hypoxanthine-guanine phosphoribosyl transferase (X-linked) (a) (c)
     b. Increased phosphoribosylpyrophosphate synthetase activity (X-linked)
     c. Increased adenine phosphoribosyl-transferase activity
     d. Increased glutathione reductase activity
     e. In Type I glycogenosis
   2. Lesch-Nyhan disease (hypoxanthine-guanine phosphoribosyl transferase)
     a. X-linked form (absent enzyme activity)
     b. Possible autosomal form
     c. Altered enzyme kinetics
   3. Xanthinuria (xanthine oxidase)
   4. Orotic aciduria
     a. Orotidylate phosphoribosyl transferase and orotidylate decarboxylase (a) (c)
     b. Orotidylate decarboxylase only
   5. Adenosine-deaminase deficiency (combined immunodeficiency syndrome)
   6. Nucleoside phosphorylase deficiency

IV. OTHER DEFECTS OF ENZYMES AND PROTEINS
A. Defects in plasma proteins
   1. Factors associated with clotting of blood (Chapter 14)
   2. Immunoproteins (Chapter 9)
   3. Other plasma proteins
     a. Analbuminemia
     b. Haptoglobin deficiency
     c. Abetalipoproteinemia
     d. Analphalipoproteinemia
     e. Absence of transferrin
     f. C1 esterase inhibitor deficiency
     g. $α_1$-Antitrypsin protein deficiency
     h. Transcobalamin II deficiency
     i. Defects of various complement components (Chapter 9)
B. Defects in plasma enzymes
   1. Pseudocholinesterase
   2. Lecithin-cholesterol acyltransferase deficiency
   3. Carnosinase deficiency
   4. Gamma-glutamyl transpeptidase deficiency
   5. Hypophosphatasia
C. Defects of proteins of other tissues
   1. Ceruloplasmin deficiency (Wilson disease, copper-thionein defect)
   2. Menkes kinky hair syndrome (X-linked)
   3. Molybdenum cofactor deficiency
   4. Myoglobin

     a. Variants
     b. Duchenne muscular dystrophy (X-linked)
     c. Carnitine palmityl transferase deficiency
   5. Xeroderma pigmentosum
   6. Macular corneal dystrophy
   7. Pancreatic enzyme deficiencies
     a. Lipase deficiency
     b. Trypsinogen deficiency
     c. Amylase deficiency
   8. Intestinal enterokinase deficiency
   9. Lysosomal acid phosphatase deficiency‡
   10. Procollagen peptidase deficiency
   11. Carnitine deficiency
   12. Succinyl-CoA, 3-keto-acid CoA transferase deficiency
   13. Acatalasia
   14. Aspartylglycosaminuria
   15. True cholinesterase deficiency
   16. Syndromes with impaired leukocyte function
D. Miscellaneous
   1. Defects of antibody formation
   2. Defects of receptor sites

V. DEFECTS IN ERYTHROCYTE METABOLISM (CHAPTER 14)
A. Hereditary methemoglobinemia
   1. Methemoglobin reductase
   2. Hemoglobin M diseases
B. Drug-induced hemolytic anemia
   1. Glucose-6-phosphate dehydrogenase
C. Hereditary hemolytic anemias
   1. Glucose-6-phosphate dehydrogenase (X-linked)
   2. 6-Phosphogluconate dehydrogenase
   3. Hexokinase
   4. Glucose phosphate isomerase
   5. Aldolase
   6. Triosephosphate isomerase
   7. Phosphoglyceric acid kinase
   8. 2,3-Diphosphoglyceric acid mutase
   9. Phosphofructose kinase
   10. Phosphoglycerate enolase
   11. Pyruvate kinase
   12. Lactate dehydrogenase
   13. PRPP synthetase
   14. Glutathione reductase
   15. Glutathione peroxidase
   16. Glutathione synthetase
   17. Adenylate kinase
   18. Adenosine triphosphatase
D. Other erythrocyte enzymes
   1. Catalase (acatalasia)
   2. True cholinesterase
   3. Elevated ATP production
   4. Carbonic anhydrase deficiency
   5. Nicotinamide adenine dinucleotide nucleosidase deficiency
   6. Glutathione reductase (increased activity — gout)

VI. DEFECTS IN OTHER FORMED ELEMENTS OF BLOOD (CHAPTER 14)
A. Platelet defects (several thrombocytopathies and thrombocytasthenias involving metabolic or membrane defects)
B. Granulocyte defects (defective oxidation following phagocytosis) (chronic granulomatous disease)

VII. DEFECTS OF LIPID METABOLISM
A. The hyperlipoproteinemias
   1. Type I
   2. Type IIa (autosomal dominant)
   3. Type IIb
   4. Type III
   5. Type IV
   6. Type V
B. Lecithin-cholesterol acyltransferase deficiency
C. The hypolipoproteinemias
   1. Abetalipoproteinemia (acanthocytosis)
   2. Analphalipoproteinemia (Tangier disease)
D. Steroid metabolism (Chapter 18)
   1. Congenital adrenal hyperplasia or hypofunction
     a. Defect of 20,22-desmolase
     b. Defect of 3-β-hydroxydehydrogenase

Table 8-2 INBORN ERRORS OF METABOLISM* (Continued)

    c. Defect of 21-hydroxylase
    d. Defect of 11-hydroxylase
    e. Defect of 17-hydroxylase
  2. Selective defects of aldosterone synthesis
    a. Defect of 18-hydroxylase
    b. Defect of 18-OH-corticosterone dehydrogenase
  3. Defects of androgen synthesis
    a. Defect of 20,22-desmolase
    b. Defect of 3-β-hydroxydehydrogenase
    c. Defect of 11-hydroxylase
    d. Defect of 17,20-desmolase
    e. Defect of 17β-hydroxyoxireductase
    f. Defect of 5α-reductase
  4. Steroid sulfatase defect
E. The lipidoses
  1. G_{M1} gangliosidoses (acid β-galactosidase deficiency)
    a. Type 1, generalized gangliosidosis (a) (b) (c)
    b. Type 2, late infantile G_{M1} gangliosidosis (a) (b) (c)
    c. Later onset forms with variable CNS and bone involvement (a) (b) (c)
  2. G_{M2} gangliosidoses (one or more β-hexosaminidases deficient)
    a. Type 1, Tay-Sachs disease (only hexosaminidase A deficient) (a) (b) (c)
    b. Type 2, Sandhoff disease (hexosaminidase A and B deficient) (a) (b) (c)
    c. Type 3, juvenile G_{M2} gangliosidosis (partial deficiency of hexosaminidase A) (a) (b) (c)
  3. Fucosidosis (α-fucosidase deficiency) (a) (b) (c)
  4. Fabry disease (X-linked, specific α-galactosidase isoenzyme deficiency) (a) (b) (c)
  5. Gaucher disease (glucosylceramide β-glucosidase deficiency)
    a. Type 1, adult or chronic type (a) (b) (c)
    b. Type 2, infantile or acute neuropathic type (a) (b) (c)
    c. Type 3, juvenile type (a) (b) (c)
  6. Niemann-Pick disease (sphingomyelinase deficiency in some types)
    a. Type A, classic CNS and visceral involvement (sphingomyelinase-deficient) (a) (b) (c)
    b. Type B, severe visceral involvement (sphingomyelinase-deficient) (a) (b) (c)
    c. Other types with sphingomyelin storage in juveniles or adults (sphingomyelinase normal or only partially deficient)
  7. Metachromatic leukodystrophies (cerebroside sulfate sulfatase deficiency)
    a. Late infantile form (a) (b) (c)
    b. Juvenile form (a) (b) (c)
    c. Adult form (a) (b) (c)
  8. Krabbe disease (galactosylceramide β-galactosidase deficiency) (a) (b) (c)
  9. Farber disease (acid ceramidase deficiency) (a) (b) (c)
  10. Wolman disease (acid lipase deficiency) (a) (b) (c)
  11. Cholesteryl ester storage disease (specific acid lipase deficiency) (a) (b) (c)
  12. Adrenoleukodystrophy (ALD) (X-linked)
  13. Acid phosphate deficiency (a) (b) (c)
  14. Refsum disease (phytanic acid α-hydroxylase deficiency) (a) (b) (c)
  15. Neuronal ceroid-lipofuscinosis
  16. Mucolipidoses
    a. Type I (lipomucopolysaccharidosis) (a) (b) (c)
    b. Type II (I-cell disease) (a)
    c. Type III (pseudo-Hurler)
    d. Type IV
  17. Sialidoses

VIII. DEFECTS OF PIGMENT METABOLISM
  A. Porphyrin metabolism
    1. Acute intermittent porphyria (autosomal dominant) (a) (b)
    2. Porphyria variegata (autosomal dominant) (b)
    3. Porphyria cutanea tarda (autosomal recessive)
    4. Hereditary coproporphyria (autosomal dominant) (b)
    5. Protoporphyria (autosomal dominant) (b)
    6. Congenital erythropoietic porphyria (autosomal recessive)
  B. Methemoglobinemias
    1. Methemoglobin reductase (autosomal recessive) (b)
    2. Hemoglobin M diseases (autosomal dominant)
  C. Primary hemochromatosis
  D. Glucuronide conjugation
    1. Crigler-Najjar disease
    2. Dubin-Johnson disease
    3. Gilbert disease
    4. Rotor syndrome
  E. Melanin metabolism
    1. Albinism
    2. Chédiak-Higashi syndrome
    3. Waardenburg syndrome
IX. DEFECTS OF VITAMIN METABOLISM
  A. Ascorbic acid
  B. Folic acid
    1. Formiminotransferase defect
    2. Cyclohydrolase defect
    3. ^5N-Methyltransferase defects
    4. Dihydrofolate reductase defect
  C. Niacin
    1. Hartnup disease
    2. Tryptophanemia
    3. 3-Hydroxykynureninuria
  D. Vitamin D
    1. Vitamin D dependent rickets (1-hydroxylase deficiency)
  E. Thiamine
    1. Thiamine pyrophosphate kinase defect (Leigh disease)
    2. Maple syrup urine disease
  F. Biopterin
    1. Dihydropteridine reductase defect (a variant form of PKU)
    2. Dihydropteridine synthetase deficiency
  G. Biotin
    1. β-Methylcrotonyl glycinuria
    2. Propionic acidemia
    3. Holocarboxylase synthetase deficiency
  H. Pyridoxine
    1. Xanthurenic aciduria
    2. Cystathionine synthetase deficiency
    3. Cystathioninemia
    4. Glutamic acid decarboxylase defect
X. PRIMARY DEFECTS OF RENAL TUBULAR TRANSPORT MECHANISM (CHAPTERS 16 AND 23)
  Many different disorders, e.g., nephrogenic diabetes insipidus, renal glycosuria, Fanconi syndrome
XI. GENETIC DEFECTS RESULTING IN INTESTINAL MALABSORPTION (CHAPTER 11)
  A. Carbohydrates
  B. Amino acids
  C. Lipids
  D. Proteins
    1. Cystic fibrosis
    2. Pancreatic enzyme defects
    3. Gluten-induced enteropathy
XII. DEFECTS INVOLVING MINERAL METABOLISM
  A. Copper
    1. Wilson disease (this chapter and Chapters 11 and 21)
    2. Menkes kinky hair disease (X-linked) (Chapter 21)

*Unless otherwise indicated, an autosomal recessive form of inheritance is assumed. Many of the disorders listed are also discussed elsewhere in the text; consult the index.
†(a) = Prenatal diagnosis is feasible or has been made.
  (b) = Early diagnosis is possible using easily accessible material such as blood, urine, tears, skin, etc.
  (c) = Heterozygous carrier state can be determined reliably.
‡See also VII. E. 13, this table.

Table continued on following page

Table 8–2 INBORN ERRORS OF METABOLISM* (Continued)

B. Iron (this chapter and Chapter 14)
 1. Hemochromatosis
 2. Absence of transferrin
C. Potassium (Chapter 22)
 1. Periodic paralysis
D. Phosphorus (Chapter 23)
 1. Hypophosphatemic resistant rickets (X-linked)
E. Iodine (Chapter 18)
 1. Defects of iodine transport
 2. Defects of thyroid hormone formation
F. Magnesium (Chapters 5 and 7)
 1. Hypomagnesemic tetany of infancy

G. Cobalt
 1. Transcobalamin II deficiency
 2. Vitamin B_{12} cofactor deficiency (homocystinuria and methylmalonic aciduria)
H. Zinc
 1. Hyperzincemia
 2. Hypozincemia (acrodermatitis enteropathica)
I. Molybdenum
 1. Sulfite oxidase and xanthine dehydrogenase deficiency
XIII. Defects About Which the Biochemical Aberration Is Unknown
 Many different disorders, e.g., achondroplasia, Marfan syndrome, Ehlers-Danlos disease and osteogenesis imperfecta

*Unless otherwise indicated, an autosomal recessive form of inheritance is assumed. Many of the disorders listed are also discussed elsewhere in the text; consult the index.

†(a) = Prenatal diagnosis is feasible or has been made.
 (b) = Early diagnosis is possible using easily accessible material such as blood, urine, tears, skin, etc.
 (c) = Heterozygous carrier state can be determined reliably.
‡See also VII. F 13, this table.

2. Precursor substances may accumulate. If they are toxic, specific dysfunction results.

3. Minor metabolic pathways may become manifest or more heavily utilized, and normal metabolites may accumulate or be excreted in unusual quantities.

Some enzyme functions may not be fully developed at birth but mature later, e.g., glucuronide transferase (Sec 2.10). These delays are not to be confused with true enzymopathies in which function will never develop, e.g., Crigler-Najjar disease (Sec 11.45).

Some disorders, such as the abnormal accumulation of glycogen in glycogen storage disease, once thought to result from absence of a single enzyme (glucose-6-phosphatase), are in fact a number of different entities, each associated with dysfunction of a different enzyme. All the involved enzymes, however, have roles in glycogen and glucose metabolism.

Even in those disorders in which only 1 enzyme is involved there is evidence that different mutations result in different degrees of enzyme activity, which, in turn, result in a spectrum of phenotypic effects. The possibility exists that for a given enzyme protein at least as many different abnormalities may exist as there are amino acids in the protein chain. The potential

Table 8–3 INBORN ERRORS OF METABOLISM THAT MAY HAVE METABOLIC ACIDOSIS AS A MAJOR COMPONENT

DISEASE	MAJOR METABOLITES (ACIDS)
AMINOACIDOPATHIES	
1. Maple syrup urine disease	α-Ketoisocaproic, α-keto-β-methylvaleric, α-ketoisovaleric, indoleacetic, ketones*
2. Isovaleric acidemia	Isovaleric, N-isovalerylglycine, β-hydroxyisovaleric, ketones*
3. β-Methylcrotonylglycinuria	β-Methylcrotonylglycine, β-hydroxyisovaleric, 2-oxoglutaric, ketones*
4. β-Hydroxy-β-methylglutaric aciduria	β-Hydroxyisovaleric, β-methylglutaric, β-methylglutaconic, β-hydroxy-β-methylglutaric
5. α-Methylacetoacetic aciduria	α-Methyl-β-hydroxybutyric, α-methylacetoacetic, ketones*
6. Propionic acidemia	Propionic, propionylglycine, β-hydroxypropionate, methylcitric, ketones*
7. Methylmalonic acidemia	Methylmalonic, propionic, ketones*
8. Pyroglutamic acidemia	Pyroglutamic (5-oxoproline)
9. α-Ketoadipic aciduria	α-Ketoadipic, α-hydroxyadipic, α-aminoadipic, 1,2-butenedicarboxylic
10. Glutaric acidemia	Glutaric, lactic, isobutyric, isovaleric, α-methylbutyric
11. Multiple carboxylase deficiency	α and β-Hydroxybutyric, β-hydroxyisovaleric, propionic, β-methylcrotonylglycine, lactic ketones*
12. Multiple acyl-CoA dehydrogenase deficiency (glutaric acidemia type II)	2-Ethylmalonic, adipic, glutaric hexanoylglycine, ketones*
DEFECTS IN CARBOHYDRATE METABOLISM	
13. Diabetes mellitus	Lactic, ketones*
14. Fructose-1,6-diphosphatase deficiency	Lactic, pyruvic, ketones*
15. Succinyl-CoA transferase deficiency	Ketones*
16. Glycogen storage disease, type I	Lactic, pyruvic, ketones*
17. Pyruvate carboxylase deficiency	Lactic, pyruvic

*Acetoacetic and β-hydroxybutyric.

Diagnosis of the diseases listed among the aminoacidopathies can be made through detection of the corresponding metabolite in urine by various techniques such as column or gas or high pressure liquid chromatography or by measuring enzyme activity in cultures of skin fibroblasts. Of the carbohydrate defects, only succinyl-CoA transferase deficiency can be detected in fibroblasts. Deficiency of fructose-1,6-diphosphatase can be demonstrated in white cells. Glycogen storage type I and pyruvate carboxylase defects must be detected in liver biopsies. In addition to the above, acidosis has been reported in a patient with acute tyrosinemia and in patients with oxalosis and renal tubular acidosis, in whom persistent acidosis is due primarily to a renal defect rather than being a direct effect of the metabolic error.

number may be large, but only mutations that affect enzyme activity sufficiently to produce clinical disease need be of concern.

A given biochemical block may result from a number of different genetic events. Usually the enzyme which carries out the blocked reaction is either absent or has lost all or most of its functional ability. Most of the defects discussed in this chapter are of this type. If the primary enzyme requires a cofactor (usually a derivative of a vitamin) or an activator, any distal block in the formation of the cofactor or activator will also result in diminished or absent activity of the primary enzyme. Such secondary blocks depend on the activities of other enzymes which are themselves under genetic control. Some enzymes such as many of those released into the gastrointestinal tract, as well as some found within cells, are produced in a precursor form which is larger (contains longer polypeptide chains) than the mature functioning enzyme. Nonspecific as well as specific proteinases are known which act upon the proenzyme yielding active enzyme. Some inborn errors of metabolism may prove to be due to genetically determined inactivity of these specific proteinases. In addition, other mechanisms, such as the phosphorylation of an already formed enzyme by a specific kinase, can be envisioned, aberrations of which will ultimately produce a given disorder.

Inborn errors of metabolism may have their important clinical effects in almost any body system and be manifest in most aspects of pediatric medicine (Table 8–1). A listing of the various inborn errors of metabolism appears in Table 8–2. Discussions of the following defects will be found in other chapters of this book in which the clinical considerations are germane to the system being discussed: the hemoglobinopathies (Chapter 14), disorders of clotting mechanisms (Chapter 14), the mucopolysaccharidoses (Chapter 23), defects of cellular transport (Chapter 16), defects of hormone synthesis (Chapter 18), and defects of immunoglobulin synthesis (Chapter 9). The disorders discussed in this chapter are those of clinical significance associated with metabolic defects involving amino acids, carbohydrates, lipids, purines and pyrimidines, or certain pigments, and some other disorders not easily categorized.

Neurologic abnormalities are well known complications of inborn errors of metabolism in children. Mental retardation is a major problem, and coma, seizures, spasticity, and progressive neurologic deterioration also occur. By the time neurologic effects become evident, irreversible damage may have taken place. In management of inborn errors of metabolism, therefore, the prime goal is to avert irreversible damage by instituting appropriate therapy. Specific therapy may involve limitations or exclusions of offending metabolites in the diet, as is the case in phenylketonuria or galactosemia, or the replacement of absent hormones as in hypothyroidism. A growing number of disorders of amino acid metabolism have been shown to be cofactor dependent. The addition to the diet of large amounts of a specific vitamin (thiamine, biotin, B_{12}, or pyridoxine) or of minerals (such as zinc) has proved most beneficial. Successful antenatal diagnosis of specific biotin-dependent disorders has been reported; the pregnant mothers

Table 8–4 INBORN ERRORS OF AMINO ACID METABOLISM ASSOCIATED WITH ABNORMAL ODOR OF URINE

INBORN ERROR OF METABOLISM	URINE ODOR
Glutaric acidemia (type II)	Sweaty feet
Phenylketonuria	Mousy or musty
Maple syrup urine disease	Maple syrup
Isovaleric acidemia	Sweaty feet
β-Methylcrotonylglycinuria	Tomcat urine
Methionine malabsorption	Cabbage
Trimethylaminuria	Rotting fish
Tyrosinemia	Rancid or fishy
Oasthouse disease	Hoplike

were treated with large doses of biotin, thus preventing the manifestation of the disorder at birth. Continuing treatment of the infant is then instituted. Early diagnosis is essential. Screening programs for phenylketonuria have been helpful in prevention of mental retardation, and screening programs for hypothyroidism are under development. Where screening programs do not yet exist, certain non-neurologic findings may suggest inborn errors of metabolism. Sensitivity of the clinician to these findings may permit an early diagnosis, whereas delay may impair the child's potential (see Table 8–1).

Vomiting is a common occurrence in infancy; when it is severe enough to produce or is associated with growth retardation, it should hint strongly at metabolic disease. Children with isovaleric acidemia, methylmalonic acidemia, propionic acidemia, and even phenylketonuria have been erroneously operated upon for pyloric stenosis when their vomiting was due to the metabolic error. Persistent acidosis in an infant or child, particularly if the CO_2 content of plasma is less than 10 or if there is a large anion gap, should suggest the possibility of an inborn error of metabolism (Table 8–3). Many of the errors of branched chain amino acid metabolism (see Fig 8–4) produce metabolic acidosis and are often associated with *ketosis*. Lethargy or coma associated with *liver disease* suggests an aminoacidopathy. An elevated prothrombin time is an early finding in acute tyrosinemia and may be present prior to overt signs of liver failure. Defects of the urea cycle often present with signs of hepatic insufficiency. As noted elsewhere, specific physical abnormalities may be frequently associated with defects of amino acid metabolism. Dislocated lenses are noted in errors of methionine metabolism. Renal stones are seen in various metabolic defects, with the most common being cystinuria. Deafness, rickets, and osteoporosis also have been noted in children with many of these disorders. Some disorders give rise to characteristic odors of urine or sweat which may aid in diagnosis (Table 8–4).

When an early diagnosis cannot prevent irreversible damage or make effective treatment possible, a proper diagnosis will still be essential for accurate genetic counseling of the parents and siblings of the affected patient.

VICTOR H. AUERBACH
GRANT MORROW III

DEFECTS IN METABOLISM OF AMINO ACIDS

8.2 PHENYLALANINE

Phenylketonuria (PKU). *Classic Form.* Phenylketonuria is the result of a genetic defect of phenylalanine metabolism. Mental retardation is the most serious manifestation. PKU occurs in approximately 1 in 14,000 births in the United States. The injury to the brain is caused by phenylalanine, which is present in all natural proteins and which accumulates in the blood at abnormal concentrations in the absence of activity of the hepatic enzyme phenylalanine hydroxylase.

Dietary phenylalanine not required for protein synthesis is normally degraded via the tyrosine pathway (Fig 8–1). In PKU, phenylalanine accumulates and is transaminated to phenylpyruvic acid or decarboxylated to phenylethylamine. These metabolites, along with excess phenylalanine, disrupt normal metabolism and may contribute to the clinical picture.

Genetics. PKU is transmitted by an autosomal recessive gene. Approximately 1 in 60 persons is an asymptomatic heterozygous carrier; about 80% of carriers can be identified through detection of an elevated ratio of fasting plasma phenylalanine to tyrosine.

Clinical Features. The untreated child with PKU may have clinical evidence of arrested brain development by 4 mo of age, and eventually the typical "classic" picture of a moderate to severely retarded child with schizoid behavior evolves. Such children are blonder than unaffected siblings; they have blue eyes, a musty odor, a tendency to seborrheic or eczematous skin lesions, and microcephaly. Many have abnormal electroencephalographic patterns, and approximately one third have seizures. There are no consistent abnormalities on the neurologic examination, though many of these children are hypertonic or hyperactive and have abnormal social behavior.

Diagnosis. Infants with PKU are clinically normal at birth, and tests of their urine for phenylpyruvic acid are negative in the 1st few days of life; accordingly, at this age the diagnosis *must* be made by measuring *blood* levels of phenylalanine. The bacterial inhibition assay method of Guthrie is widely used in the newborn period to screen for PKU. This test requires several drops of capillary blood; concentrations of phenylalanine may not be significantly elevated until the 3rd–6th day of life or until the infant has ingested dietary protein for 24–48 hr. When this test indicates an elevated level of phenylalanine, or when a test of urine for phenylpyruvic acid is positive at any age, before the diagnosis of PKU is made, the phenylalanine and tyrosine concentrations of the plasma should be measured. Classic PKU can be defined from these criteria: (1) a plasma phenylalanine level above 20 mg/dl; (2) a normal plasma tyrosine level; (3) increased urinary levels of metabolites of phenylalanine (phenylpyruvic and o-OH-phenylacetic acids); and (4) an inability to tolerate an oral challenge of phenylalanine. All newborn infants with positive Guthrie tests should have blood levels of phenylalanine measured within 2 wk after birth.

In most patients with PKU 10% ferric chloride added to their urine will produce an olive green color, which indicates a reaction with phenylpyruvic acid. Unfortunately, not all PKU patients have a positive test; moreover, color changes are also produced by ferric chloride in the urines of patients with other types of aminoaciduria and of those who have ingested medications, e.g., aspirin or certain phenothiazines. These considerations make urine testing unsuitable at any age for exclusion of PKU.

Treatment. The purpose of treatment in PKU is to prevent or minimize brain damage in susceptible children. A milk substitute has been prepared for use in infants that is an enzymatic hydrolysate of casein, containing a very small amount of phenylalanine but normal amounts of other amino acids, with added carbohydrate and fat.* Its use is continued for a variable time into childhood. Other natural foods for which the phenylalanine content is known are gradually added after an initial period of feeding limited to this milk substitute. Most natural food proteins contain approximately 5% phenylalanine, and their intake must be limited. The administration of the low phenylalanine diet demands close nutritional supervision of the child and frequent monitoring of the serum concentrations of phenylalanine. The optimal serum level to be maintained probably lies between 5–9 mg/dl. Since phenylalanine is not synthesized in the body, "overtreatment," particularly in rapidly growing infants, may lead to phenylalanine deficiency, which is manifested by lethargy, anorexia, anemia, rashes, and diarrhea; moreover, tyrosine becomes an essential amino acid and its adequate intake must be assured.

Restriction of phenylalanine in the diet is indicated for infants who have persistent serum phenylalanine concentrations over 20 mg/dl, with normal serum concentrations of tyrosine and with phenylketones in the urine. Dietary treatment should be begun as soon after birth as the diagnosis can be established. For infants receiving a normal diet who have serum phenylalanine concentrations in the range of 10–20 mg/dl, with normal tyrosine values and no PKU, a simple reduction of dietary protein intake may be sufficient to control serum concentrations of phenylalanine; if this is not effective, specific restriction of phenylalanine in the diet will be indicated. All infants for whom such specific dietary restriction is not undertaken should be systematically monitored with repeated urine and blood tests and with developmental evaluations to establish the safety of continuing partial treatment or nontreatment. Periodic challenges with natural protein may be helpful in determining the need for continued dietary restriction.

The dietary management of PKU is almost inevitably complicated by emotional problems resulting from the dietary restriction and the abnormal eating habits im-

---

*Dietary management with this milk substitute is described in Phenylketonuria—Low Phenylalanine Dietary Management with Lofenalac, a pamphlet available from Mead Johnson Laboratories, Evansville, Indiana 47721.

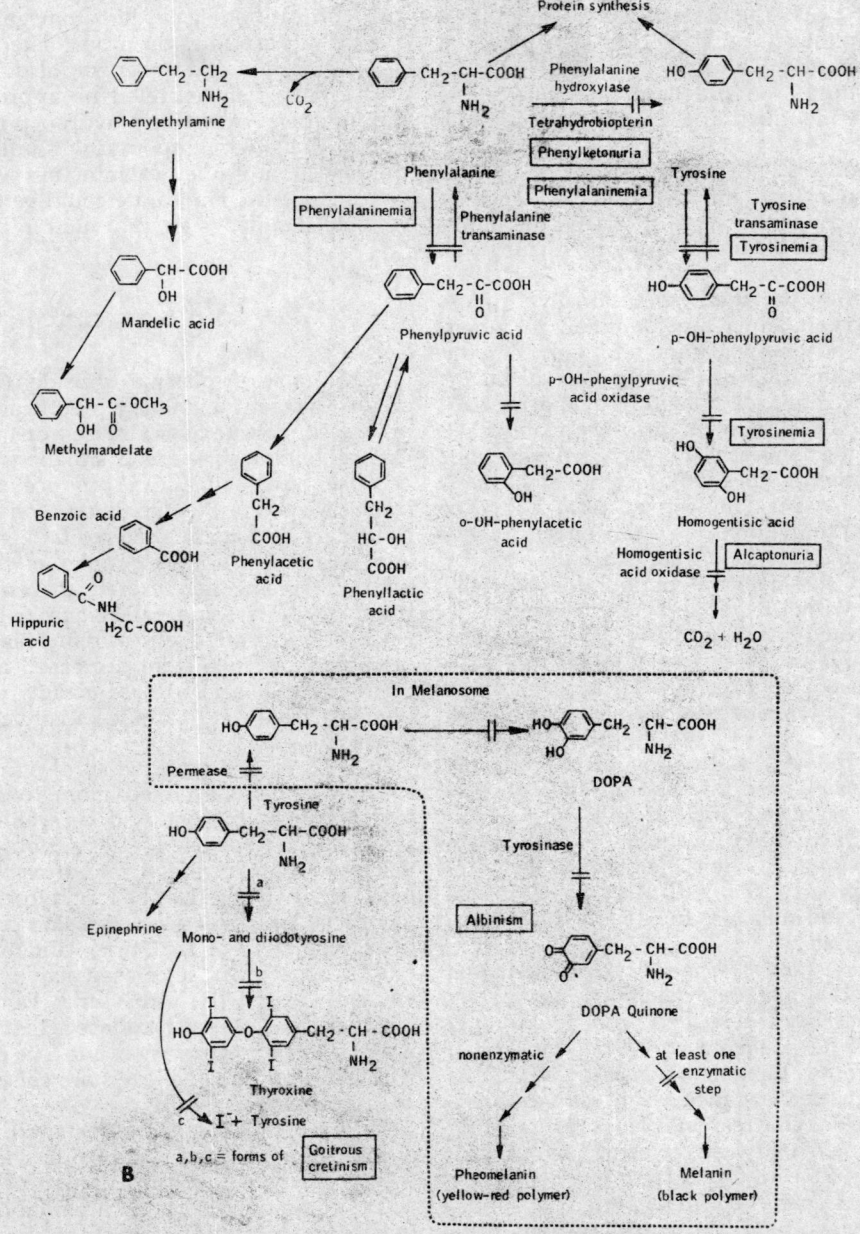

Figure 8–1 Pathways in the metabolism of phenylalanine and tyrosine. In this and subsequent figures the structural formulas and the names of various metabolites are shown. Inborn errors are depicted as bars crossing the reaction arrow or arrows, and the name of the associated defect or defects is given within the nearest box. In some figures the name of the enzyme is given in association with the reaction arrow. Some of the intermediates shown in some of the figures are metabolized via their coenzyme A (CoA) derivatives. For the sake of simplicity, this is not indicated.

posed upon child and family. The parents may have increasing difficulty in controlling the diets of children as they become ambulatory and an atmosphere of tension is created by the realization that ingestion of usual foods may provoke or increase mental retardation. The maintenance of adequate dietary control without psychologic problems is achieved with difficulty, and parents and children will need continuous skillful and empathetic support and guidance.

Preliminary results with feeding of the plant enzyme phenylalanine ammonia lyase (PAL) to PKU patients indicate that phenylalanine can be converted to cinnamic acid in the intestinal tract. The latter compound is nontoxic, and the conversion has been shown to reduce the blood level of phenylalanine while the patients were on an uncontrolled diet. A combination of dietary control and feeding of PAL may overcome some of the disadvantages of strict dietary control.

Mentally retarded children without PKU may be born to mothers with PKU; the occurrence suggests that cerebral damage in the fetus may be caused by placental transfer of excess phenylalanine from the maternal circulation. Therefore, the pregnant phenylketonuric woman should be identified and maintained on a low phenylalanine diet.

Offspring of mothers with either PKU or phenylalaninemia may also exhibit an increased incidence of microcephaly and congenital heart disease if the mother's blood level of phenylalanine during pregnancy was above 10–20 mg/dl.

Phenylalaninemia Variants. Occasionally infants with hyperphenylalaninemia are identified in whom the blood levels of phenylalanine are only slightly elevated, to levels insufficient (less than 15–20 mg/dl) to result in the excretion of phenylpyruvic acid. Like infants with classic PKU, these infants presumably have an abnormal phenylalanine hydroxylase enzyme, but one that has retained some of its activity; measured values of activity have usually ranged from 1–35% of normal, in contrast to the non-detectable enzyme activity found in classic PKU. Such infants are detected by screening tests in the neonatal period; they usually develop normally without special dietary treatment.

Moderately elevated levels of phenylalanine occur in transient tyrosinemia in the newborn infant (Sec 8.3). When the infant's ability to oxidize tyrosine matures, the elevated levels of tyrosine and phenylalanine return to normal.

Absence of or delayed maturation of the enzyme phenylalanine transaminase can also produce phenylalaninemia if the infant is being fed milk with a high protein content. Such infants cannot produce much phenylpyruvic acid even when their blood levels of phenylalanine approach 30 mg/dl; they have normal blood levels when fed milk products with the protein content of human milk.

Variants Unresponsive to Phenylalanine Restriction. Several children with initial phenylalanine levels greater than 20 mg/dl have been described who deteriorated neurologically despite adequate control of the serum level of phenylalanine. Enzyme analysis in fibroblasts and leukocytes revealed a deficiency in dihydropteridine reductase, the enzyme responsible for regenerating the phenylalanine hydroxylase cofactor, tetrahydrobiopterin (Fig 8–1). Since the reductase is essential for the biosynthesis of such neurotransmitters as dopamine, norepinephrine, and serotonin, restriction of phenylalanine will not permit normal development. Clinically similar variants have been described due to deficient dihydrobiopterin synthesis and delayed maturation of the involved enzyme system. This form of PKU is more similar to disorders responsive to vitamins than to other defects in amino acid metabolism.

Methylmandelic Aciduria. Two siblings with ataxia, convulsions, and mental retardation have been shown to excrete large amounts of methylmandelic acid. This compound results from the further oxidation of phenylethylamine, the decarboxylated product of phenylalanine. Symptoms could be produced by high protein feeding and abated by the restriction of protein to 0.5 gm/kg/24 hr.

Parahydroxyphenylacetic Aciduria. In a 14 wk old girl with cardiomegaly, hepatomegaly, hypotonia, and anemia, a defect has been postulated in the conversion of phenylacetic acid to benzoic acid, thence to hippuric acid. The patient excreted no appreciable amounts of hippurate but excessive p-hydroxyphenylacetate. Excretion of the latter compound was influenced directly by the ingestion of phenylalanine but was independent of tyrosine intake. Hippurate could be formed if benzoate was fed. Pathways are indicated in Fig 8–1.

8.3 TYROSINE

Elevations of plasma tyrosine (tyrosinemia) may either represent a primary inborn error of metabolism or be secondary to liver disease from a variety of causes. Differentiation of these 2 situations is often difficult because tyrosinemia can produce liver damage and some diseases of the liver have been shown to result in secondary tyrosinemia. Hereditary fructose intolerance and galactosemia are examples of the latter. Patients with tyrosinemia may excrete abnormal amounts of the products of tyrosine catabolism (p-hydroxyphenylpyruvic, -lactic, and -acetic acids). This situation, termed tyrosyluria, results from decreased hepatic p-hydroxyphenylpyruvic acid oxidase activity so that p-hydroxyphenylpyruvic acid cannot be converted to homogentisic acid.

In 1932, Medes reported studies in an asymptomatic adult male who excreted more than 1 gm/day of p-hydroxyphenylpyruvic acid, as well as other oxidative products of tyrosine. Medes proposed that the block resulted from decreased p-hydroxyphenylpyruvic oxidase activity (Fig 8–1). The term tyrosinosis was applied to this patient. However, tyrosine could not be measured accurately at that time, and other investigators have proposed that decreased activity of tyrosine transaminase caused the tyrosyluria. Doubt remains as to whether the depressed oxidase activity in these patients is a primary or secondary event. The clinical syndromes with elevated tyrosine levels are collectively referred to as "tyrosinemia."

Tyrosinemia (Transient Neonatal). Deficiency of p-hydroxyphenylpyruvic acid oxidase is most often transitory, due to delayed maturation of the enzyme, and occurs commonly in premature infants and occasionally in full-term infants. The levels of tyrosine in the plasma (normally less than 2 mg/dl) may be as high as 60 mg/dl. The defect is promptly corrected by the administration of vitamin C. Since vitamin C is necessary for optimal functioning of the oxidase, it is not surprising that tyrosyluria occurs in scurvy.

Tyrosinemia (Acute). Infants with this condition have a rapidly progressive, fulminating course that ends fatally unless appropriate therapy is initiated.

Clinical Manifestations. Onset usually occurs at 1–6 mo of age. Failure to thrive, irritability, fever, and hepatomegaly are the most frequent manifestations. Anorexia, vomiting, diarrhea, and abdominal distention are common. Bleeding manifestations, such as melena, hematemesis, hematuria, and ecchymoses occur early and may be severe. With hepatic failure, ascites, jaundice, lethargy, coma, and death follow.

Laboratory Data. Generalized aminoaciduria and tyrosyluria are constant findings and glycosuria may be present. Plasma amino acids are markedly elevated, particularly tyrosine and methionine, which may be 5–10 times normal. Tyrosine crystals have been found in bone marrow. Hypoproteinemia and hypoprothrombinemia are common; serum transaminase levels (SGOT and SGPT) may be only slightly increased. Hypoglycemia is common. The principal pathologic findings are dilation of the renal tubules and cirrhosis.

Treatment. Early restriction of dietary tyrosine and methionine has been very beneficial in some patients. Some who survive the acute hepatic decompensation are apparently cured and can be placed on an unrestricted diet. Others, despite adequate amino acid restriction, develop chronic cirrhosis.

Tyrosinemia (Subacute or Chronic). Most children with this variant do not manifest symptoms until after 1 yr of age. Failure to thrive, gastrointestinal symptoms, progressive cirrhosis, multiple renal defects, and rickets characterize the clinical picture. Amino acid elevations may involve only tyrosine early in the course of the disease, with later marked elevations of methionine. Death usually occurs by 10 yr of age. Hepatomas are often found at autopsy.

Most reported cases of tyrosinemia have hepatorenal damage and decreased p-hydroxyphenylpyruvic acid oxidase activity. In some, derangements of pyrrole metabolism have been noted, with increased excretion of δ-aminolevulinic acid in the urine, increased activity of δ-aminolevulinic acid synthetase activity in the liver or hepatoma tissue, and clinical symptoms of acute intermittent porphyria.

Nine mentally retarded patients have been described with persistent hypertyrosinemia but without hepatic or renal involvement. A deficiency of cytosol tyrosine transaminase with normal p-hydroxyphenylpyruvic acid oxidase was observed.

Tyrosinemia (Tyrosine Transaminase Deficiency). Blood levels of tyrosine as high as 70 mg/dl, with excretion of p-hydroxyphenylpyruvic acid, have been reported in a child with congenital malformations and mental retardation. In this instance the defect was shown to be absence of the soluble fraction of tyrosine transaminase. Mitochondrial tyrosine transaminase produces the p-hydroxyphenylpyruvic acid found in urine. Presumably, p-hydroxyphenylpyruvic acid oxidase is inhibited by the high levels of tyrosine.

Tyrosinemia (Richner-Hanhart Syndrome). This autosomal recessive genetic disorder results in mental retardation, palmar and plantar punctate hyperkeratosis, and herpetiform corneal ulcers. Patients with this syndrome have tyrosinemia and tyrosyluria, but there is apparently no liver damage. Treatment with a diet low in tyrosine has not only corrected the biochemical abnormalities but has also resulted in dramatic healing of the skin and eye lesions. Mental retardation may be prevented by early dietary restriction of tyrosine.

Albinism. *Oculocutaneous Albinism.* Generalized albinism (Sec 24.9) is a defect in the formation of the pigment melanin. There are at least 6 variants. In the most common form, the enzyme tyrosinase is not active. In the 2nd type, tyrosinase is present in the melanosome; thus, tyrosine can be converted to dopa and then to dopa quinone, but the permease for the transport of tyrosine into the melanosome is presumably absent (Fig 8–1). In both the tyrosinase negative and tyrosinase positive types of albinism neither melanin nor pheomelanin can be formed. Single hair roots incubated in tyrosine can be used to differentiate the tyrosinase negative and positive variants. In the former no melanin is synthesized in the hair bulb, whereas in the latter obvious darkening is noted. A 3rd type, found among the Amish, is due to a defect in an unidentified enzymatic step between dopa quinone and melanin. Affected patients can produce pheomelanin, a yellowish pigment, from dopa quinone; they develop normal skin color, but their ocular signs persist through life.

Three additional rare forms have been described. In the Chédiak-Higashi syndrome (Sec 14.49) the major features include incomplete oculocutaneous albinism, neutropenia, and susceptibility to pyogenic infections. The Hermansky-Pudlak syndrome is an autosomal recessive disorder characterized by oculocutaneous albinism and a hemorrhagic diathesis, in which there appears to be defective glutathione peroxidase activity. The Cross syndrome was first described in a consanguineous Amish family with 4 affected children. They presented with hypopigmentation, gingival fibromatosis, spasticity, athetoid movements, and microphthalmia.

Albinism occurs in all races, varying in incidence from 1 in 140 in the San Blas Indians of Panama to 1 in 100,000 in France. In the United States, the rate is approximately 1 in 20,000. It is transmitted as an autosomal recessive characteristic. Normal children have been born to parents both of whom had generalized albinism, but of different allelic forms.

In addition to extremely fair skin and fine silky hair, albinos have numerous ocular abnormalities. Traces of pigment may occur on the uveal borders, but it is absent from the iris, sclera, and fundus, and the iris appears gray or blue. Refractive errors, strabismus, nystagmus, and photophobia are common. Persistent loss of visual acuity and a red reflex are present in all tyrosinase-negative individuals. In tyrosinase-positive persons, the poor visual acuity may improve with age; the red reflex is found in white children and adults.

Other Forms. Partial albinism is characterized by localized areas of skin and hair devoid of pigment. In some instances a white forelock or a patch of depigmented hair elsewhere may be the sole manifestation. This form of albinism is inherited as a dominant trait.

In albinism limited to the eye, the depigmentation may be limited to the retina or may also involve the iris. Visual acuity is decreased, and there is nystagmus. Since this defect is sex-linked, this biochemical defect must be different from those occurring in generalized or oculocutaneous albinism. Waardenburg syndrome (Chapter 25) must be considered in the differential diagnosis of partial albinism.

Alcaptonuria. This disorder of tyrosine metabolism is characterized by accumulation in the body and excretion in the urine of homogentisic acid (Fig 8–1) and its oxidation products. It is transmitted by an autosomal recessive gene. Defective activity of the enzyme homogentisic acid oxidase arrests the catabolism of tyrosine, and large amounts of homogentisic acid are excreted in the urine.

Urine from affected patients becomes black on standing because of oxidation and polymerization of homogentisic acid. The darkness of the stain increases with continued exposure to air; a dried diaper has a pitch-black stain. The abnormality is usually noted in infancy, but in some instances the dark urine has not been observed until the 2nd or 3rd decade of life. The slow accumulation of the black polymer of homogentisic acid in cartilage and other mesenchymal tissues produces a black discoloration (alcaptonuric ochronosis) of the cheeks, nose, sclerae, and ears, which becomes evident by midadult life. Degeneration of pigmented cartilage leads to arthritis in about half of older patients with alcaptonuria. The connective tissue defects appear to be due to inhibition of the enzyme lysyl hydroxylase by homogentisic acid. The defect is otherwise asymptomatic.

The urine has reducing properties; it produces a positive reaction with Fehling or Benedict reagent. Homogentisic acid does not react with glucose oxidase. The dark urine of phenol poisoning and that associated with melanotic tumors do not have reducing properties.

There is no effective treatment for the disorder.

Parkinsonism. Another defect in tyrosine metabolism may occur in parkinsonism. The tyrosine hydroxylase of brain is distinct from the tyrosinase of melanocytes; both convert tyrosine to dopa. Patients with parkinsonism and some with schizophrenia excrete p-tyramine or decarboxylated tyrosine. Tyramine may accumulate in the brain in excessive amounts if the reaction from tyrosine to dopa is blocked.

8.4   METHIONINE

Methioninemia. Abnormal elevations of plasma methionine are observed in liver disease, tyrosinemia, and homocystinemia. Methioninemia has also been found in premature and newborn infants on high protein feedings, in whom it may represent delayed maturation of an enzyme. Lowering the protein intake usually resolves the situation. Two children (1 and 2½ yr) with prolonged methioninemia have been found to have a decrease in methionine adenosyltransferase activity (Fig 8–2). Both were asymptomatic, but abnormalities of hepatic morphology were found in the younger child.

Malabsorption of Methionine. A mentally retarded girl with diarrhea, convulsions, tachypnea, and a peculiar odor has been found to have a defect in the intestinal absorption of methionine and of other amino acids. Methionine is fermented by intestinal bacteria to α-hydroxybutyric, α-ketobutyric, and α-aminobutyric acids, which are absorbed and excreted in urine, producing the unusual odor. The finding of α-hydroxybutyric acid in urine and stools of both parents and of 3 siblings after methionine loading indicates autosomal recessive inheritance. Alpha-hydroxybutyric acid has also been found in the urine of a child with phenylketonuria; this latter association is referred to as oasthouse disease, referring to the urine odor.

Homocystinemia. Homocysteine, an intermediary in the production of cysteine, is produced when methionine is demethylated (Fig 8–2). Ordinarily, it is not found in plasma or urine. Many patients have been reported who excrete large amounts of homocystine (the dithiol of homocysteine) in the urine and have detectable amounts of both homocysteine and homocystine in the blood.

Defects at 3 enzymatic steps can produce homocystinemia. In the most common situation, type I, the biochemical defect has been shown to be a deficiency of the enzyme cystathionine synthase, which condenses homocysteine with serine to form cystathionine. Normal brain contains large amounts of cystathionine, whereas the brain of a patient who died with type I homocystinemia was shown to be devoid of this compound. Though many of the patients originally described were mentally retarded, about half of newly found affected persons are intellectually normal.

Type I homocystinemia is characterized clinically by ectopia lentis, an appearance resembling the Marfan syndrome, malar flush, osteoporosis, and an abnormality in intravascular clotting that leads to thromboembolic episodes. The methionine level is increased in blood. Homocystine can be readily detected in urine by the use of the cyanide-nitroprusside test. Some patients with defects of cystathionine synthase respond clinically to large doses of vitamin B_6. In some instances of the B_6-responsive form of the disorder, but not in others, it has been shown in vitro that pyridoxal phosphate can enhance the activity of the genetically altered cystathionine synthase. In those instances in which the defect is not at the coenzyme binding site, the administration of pharmacologic doses of B_6 may enhance alternate pathways that remove homocysteine.

In types II and III homocystinemia, blood methionine levels are normal or low; these patients do not have dislocated lenses, skeletal changes, or the thromboembolic episodes noted in type I. In forms II and III there is an inability to remethylate homocysteine to methionine.

Type II involves the enzyme $5N$-methyltetrahydrofolate methyltransferase, which requires methyl B_{12} for its activity. A genetic defect impairing the formation of active coenzyme B_{12} hampers methyltransferase activity as well as the conversion of methylmalonate to succinate (see Fig 8–4). Four children with this metabolic error have been described. The clinical spectrum varies widely; 2 died from their disease, at ages 7 wk and 7 yr. The latter patient suffered from progressive dementia and seizures, as well as megaloblastic anemia. The other 2 were mildly affected. Decreased methyltransferase activity can be detected in extracts of liver, kidney, brain, and cultured fibroblasts.

In type III, the defect is in the enzyme $5\text{-}10N$-methylene-tetrahydrofolate reductase, needed for production of the $5N$-methyltetrahydrofolate that provides the methyl group for forming methionine from homocysteine. Three patients with the reductase deficiency have been described. One 16 yr old boy had proximal muscle

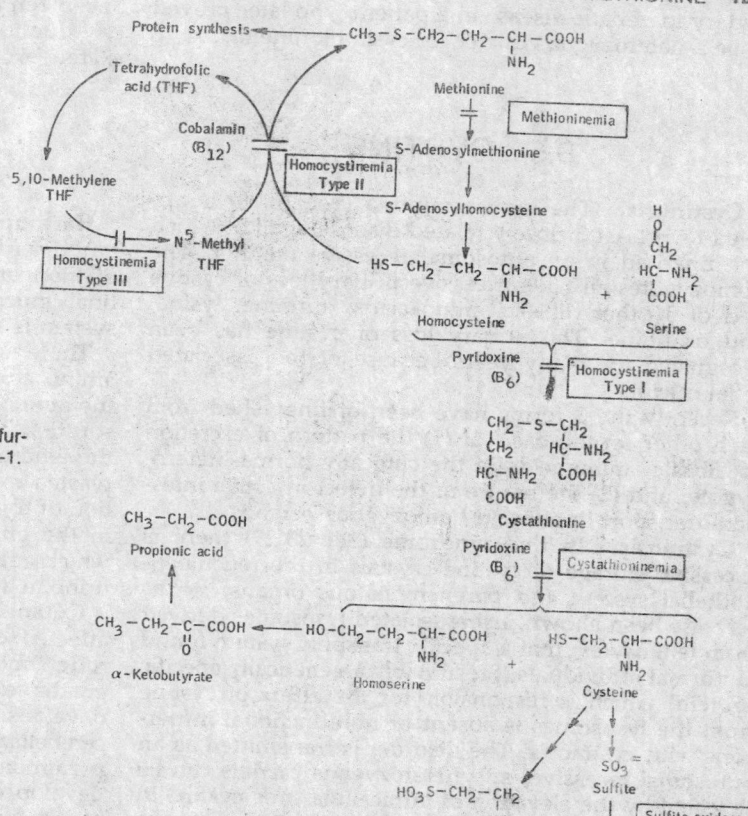

Figure 8–2 Pathways in the metabolism of the sulfur-containing amino acids. See also legend for Fig 8–1.

weakness and other neurologic signs. One of 2 sisters suffered from mild retardation; the other was considered to have schizophrenia. Folic acid therapy in the latter was accompanied by disappearance of her psychotic symptoms. Homocystinemia disappeared in all 3 patients with folic acid supplementation.

Proper therapy is predicated upon accurate differentiation of the 3 types of homocystinemia. Type I requires methionine restriction and may respond to vitamin B_6. In types II and III, methionine restriction would be harmful. Cofactor responsiveness differs also; vitamin B_{12} may benefit the type II patient, and folic acid the type III child.

Cystathioninemia. Cystathionine, an intermediate in the conversion of methionine to cysteine, is not normally found in plasma or urine. Cystathioninuria occurs in patients with neuroblastoma, other neural tumors, hepatoblastoma, or with other liver disease, and particularly when secondary to galactosemia. Cystathioninuria in association with cystathioninemia is inherited as an autosomal recessive trait; most affected persons have an aberrant form of the enzyme cystathioninase, which normally splits cystathionine to homoserine and cysteine (Fig 8–2). The binding site for its coenzyme, pyridoxal phosphate, is altered on the affected enzyme molecule. It has been shown both in vitro and in vivo that an increase in function of the enzyme occurs on addition of vitamin B_6 or of its coenzyme form. Two patients have been described with a different defect of the enzyme not responsive to vitamin B_6.

About 2 dozen patients with the disease have been studied; 1 also had phenylketonuria. Clinical manifestations have been variable and perhaps coincidental: 1 patient had convulsions; 2 sisters had mitral regurgitation; and 1 had thrombocytopenic purpura and renal calculi. Mental retardation has occurred in fewer than half of known cases. The association of retardation with this disorder may be the spurious result of selection due to increased use of screening programs among retarded patients. Therapy with vitamin B_6 of those with the predominant form of the defect has led to decreased urinary and blood levels of cystathionine, but its ultimate effects on mental development are unknown.

Cystathioninase is not present in normal fetal and newborn liver. As a result of this developmental lag, cysteine is most likely an essential amino acid during the newborn period, particularly in the low birth weight infant.

Latent cystathioninuria has been described in 2 mentally retarded brothers who excreted large amounts of cystathionine only when given excess methionine. Transient cystathioninuria has also been observed secondary to hepatic disease in a patient who later proved to be a heterozygous carrier for cystathioninemia.

8.5 CYSTINE

Cystinuria. The term cystinuria (Sec 16.28) is applied to at least 3 closely related disorders, all of which are inherited in an autosomal recessive manner. The homozygotes all have excessive urinary loss of cystine and of 3 other dibasic amino acids: arginine, lysine, and ornithine. The urinary loss of cystine has been recognized for many years because of the associated renal calculi.

Recently the 3 forms have been distinguished from each other on the basis of (1) the pattern of excretion of dibasic amino acids in the clinically normal heterozygote, and (2) the nature of the defect in active intestinal transport in affected homozygous persons.

Cystinosis. In this syndrome (Sec 23.29) there is excessive storage of cystine crystals in the reticuloendothelial system and parenchymatous organs. It has recently been shown, using isolated lysosomes derived from leukocytes, that a specific transport system found in normal individuals (presumably a genetically specific protein) which is responsible for the efflux of cystine from the lysosomes is absent or nonfunctional in persons with cystinosis. The disorder is transmitted as an autosomal recessive, and heterozygous carriers can be detected by the elevation of intracellular free cystine in peripheral leukocytes or in fibroblasts grown in tissue culture. When renal transplantation has been performed in patients with cystinosis, cystine has been found to accumulate even in the donor kidneys. However, it was later shown that the cystine was not deposited in the renal parenchymal cells (as is the case in the original kidneys) but was contained in macrophage which migrated from the host.

Sulfite Oxidase Deficiency. In the final step of cystine catabolism inorganic sulfate is formed and excreted in the urine. Absence of inorganic sulfate in the urine has been reported in a mentally retarded child with dislocated lenses who died at 3 yr of age; 3 of his 7 siblings died in infancy with neurologic abnormalities. The patient was shown to excrete large amounts of sulfite, thiosulfate, and S-sulfo-L-cysteine in his urine because of decreased sulfite oxidase (a molybdenum-containing enzyme) activity. A 2nd 3 yr old male with ataxia, seizures, hemiparesis, vomiting, and dislocated lenses has been shown to have decreased sulfite oxidase activity in his fibroblasts. The defect (Fig 8–2) is presumably inherited as an autosomal recessive.

β-Mercaptolactate-Cysteine Disulfiduria. β-Mercaptolactate-cysteine disulfide is a derivative of cystine in which 1 of the 2 amino groups is replaced by a hydroxyl group. This substance has been found in high concentration in the urine of a mentally retarded patient whose parents were siblings, in normal individuals, and in 1 with mild retardation and dislocated lenses. There were no other amino acid abnormalities.

Taurinuria. Taurine is normally excreted in the urine as an intermediate in the oxidation of cysteine.

Seventeen persons (in 4 families) who have camptodactyly due to a dominant gene have been shown also to excrete excess taurine (Fig 8–2).

8.6 TRYPTOPHAN

Hartnup Disease. Hartnup disease is a rare hereditary disorder in which there is a defect in the transport of monoamino-monocarboxylic amino acids by intestinal mucosa and renal tubules. A single transport system is affected.

There is massive generalized aminoaciduria. Plasma amino acid concentrations are not elevated; therefore the aminoaciduria must arise from faulty tubular reabsorption. The single exception to this generalization is the amino acid tryptophan; characteristically, levels in plasma are abnormally low. Impaired intestinal absorption of tryptophan results in its bacterial decomposition in the gut to various indole and indoxyl derivatives, which are absorbed, detoxified, and excreted in the urine in abnormally large amounts.

Cutaneous photosensitivity is seen early in most affected children. Unprotected areas of skin become rough and red after moderate exposure to the sun. With greater exposure, a rash identical to that of pellagra develops. Patients with Hartnup disease may also have cerebellar ataxia with evidence of involvement of the pyramidal tracts. During febrile illnesses, ataxia may develop without a rash. The clinical course is variable; severe cutaneous and nervous disturbances may alternate with periods of complete remission over many years. Mental deficiency was apparently an incidental finding in the original kindred and has not been observed in other cases. The disease is transmitted by an autosomal recessive gene. Hartnup disease must be considered in the differential diagnosis of pellagra.

The impaired intestinal absorption and urinary loss of tryptophan result in decreased synthesis of nicotinic acid. It is not surprising, therefore, that large doses of nicotinamide may cause sustained remission of the neurologic and cutaneous aspects of the disorder. Such remissions, however, may occur without therapy. The aminoaciduria and urinary excretion of indole compounds are not suppressed by such therapy, nor do they decrease during spontaneous remissions. It has been suggested that high protein diets compensate for the loss of amino acids.

Tryptophanemia. The catabolism of tryptophan (presumably in its conversion to kynurenine) is involved in this disorder (Fig 8–3). Two patients have been described with mental retardation, dwarfism, cerebellar ataxia, and a pellagra-like rash similar to that seen in Hartnup disease; they had tryptophanemia and tryptophanuria without generalized aminoaciduria or indicanuria. In 1 instance, parental consanguinity and the suspicion of a similar disorder in 2 cousins indicated autosomal recessive inheritance.

Kynureninuria. An abnormality of tryptophan metabolism consistent with a partial block of the enzyme kynurenine hydroxylase has been reported in 4 generations of a family. The propositus had scleroderma, but

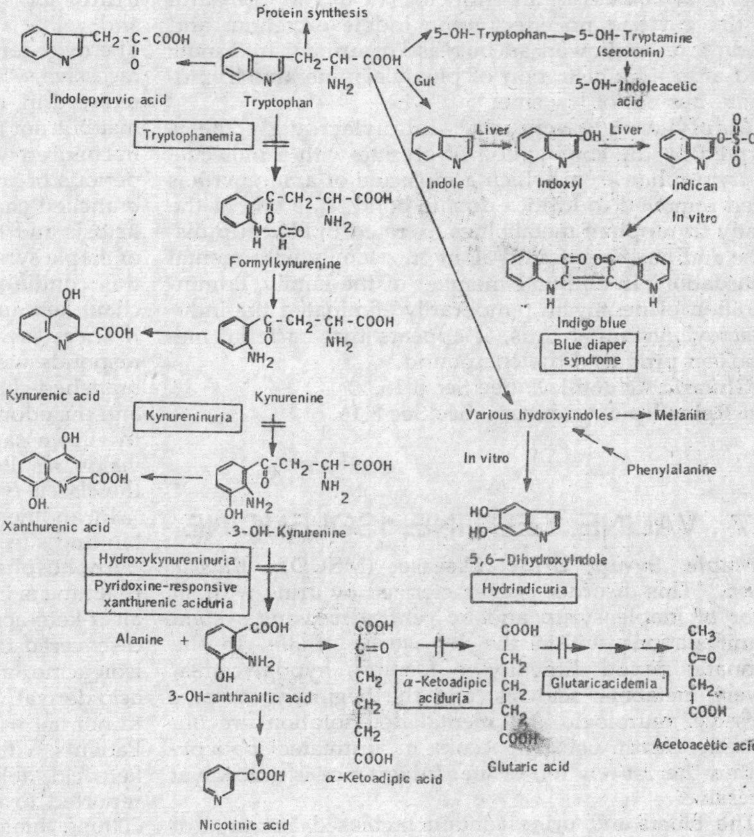

Figure 8-3 Pathways in the metabolism of tryptophan. See also legend for Fig 8-1.

the other members of the kindred were healthy. Abnormal amounts of kynurenine and other tryptophan metabolites proximal to hydroxykynurenine (Fig 8-3) are excreted in the urine both before and after administration of tryptophan. Pyridoxine did not affect the excretion pattern of tryptophan metabolites. The affected persons appear to be heterozygous for the condition.

Kynureninase Defects. *Hydroxykynureninuria.* A defect has been described in the tryptophan pathway consistent with lack of activity of the enzyme kynureninase. In this disorder large amounts of kynurenine, 3-hydroxy-kynurenine, and xanthurenic acid are excreted (Fig 8-3). Signs and symptoms of nicotinic acid deficiency develop in the absence of added dietary nicotinic acid since affected persons cannot synthesize it from tryptophan. A patient was mildly mentally retarded and had migraine-like headaches. Treatment with pyridoxine did not alter the excretion pattern of the tryptophan metabolites but did relieve the headaches.

Pyridoxine-Responsive Xanthurenic Aciduria. Children with pyridoxine deficiency may excrete several metabolites of tryptophan, mainly xanthurenic acid, since pyridoxal phosphate is the coenzyme for many enzymes involved in amino acid metabolism, including kynureninase. In pyridoxine-responsive xanthurenic aciduria, patients do not have anemia, convulsions, or pyridoxine deficiency. On the other hand, large doses of pyridoxine are required to normalize xanthurenic

acid excretion. In this disorder it has been shown in liver biopsies that there is a defect of the enzyme kynureninase so that it does not bind with the coenzyme form of the vitamin.

Excessive excretion of hydroxykynurenine, kynurenine, and xanthurenic acid, corrected by pyridoxine, has been observed in 5 unrelated patients with chronic granulomatous disease.

Indicanuria. Indicanuria arises when tryptophan is poorly absorbed from the gastrointestinal tract and is converted there by bacterial action to indole. Indole is absorbed, oxidized, sulfated, and excreted as an indican (Fig 8-3). Indicanuria is commonly observed whenever there is stasis in the bowels, such as with constipation or in the "blind loop syndrome"; it also occurs in Hartnup disease, in which tryptophan is poorly absorbed, and in phenylketonuria. The *blue diaper syndrome*, a familial disorder characterized by hypercalcemia, nephrocalcinosis, and indicanuria, derives its name from the fact that indican is oxidized to indican blue on exposure to air.

Hydrindicuria. Indole pigments related to both tryptophan and phenylalanine metabolism have been found in the urine of a mentally retarded child who had a persistent metabolic acidosis, presumably caused by carboxyindole derivatives. Laboratory manipulation of urine containing abnormal urinary indoles converts them to 5,6-dihydroxyindole (hydrindic acid); hence the name of the disorder (Fig 8-3). Prolonged administration of antibiotics in an effort to halt indole formation in the gut had no effect upon indole excretion, and loading tests showed an increase of urinary hydrindic acid after administration of phenylalanine and tryptophan, but not of tryosine.

Indolylacroylglycinuria. Indolylacroylglycine is formed by the conjugation of glycine with a molecule of tryptophan from which a molecule of ammonia has been removed to form a double bond. It is one of the many tryptophan metabolites excreted in Hartnup disease and has been found alone in a family with mental retardation. In all but 1 member of the family, administration of neomycin temporarily eliminated the indolylacroylglycinuria; thus, it appears that bacterial metabolism produced the compound.

Glutaric Acidemia.   See Sec 8.16.

α-Ketoadipic Aciduria.   See Sec 8.16.

8.7   VALINE, LEUCINE, ISOLEUCINE

Maple Syrup Urine Disease (MSUD). *Classic Form.* This disorder is characterized by urine with an odor of maple syrup and by central nervous system manifestations within the 1st weeks of life. In the neonatal period difficulty in feeding, hypoglycemia, severe metabolic acidosis, and the beginning of progressive neurologic and mental deterioration are observed. Death usually occurs in untreated patients within the 1st few mo of life. Inheritance is autosomal recessive.

The blood and urine contain increased amounts of the 3 branched-chain amino acids: valine, leucine, and isoleucine. The urine characteristically also contains increased amounts of the keto-acid derivatives of these amino acids. The defect is known to lie in oxidative decarboxylation of the keto-acids (Fig 8–4). There is some disagreement at present whether each keto-acid is decarboxylated by its specific decarboxylase. It appears, in any case, that the carboxylase has 2 binding sites for the substrate; the higher affinity site is nonfunctional in maple syrup urine disease. Alloisoleucine, a stereoisomer of isoleucine formed by way of the keto-acid and not normally found in blood, becomes readily detectable.

The enzymatic defect can be demonstrated in leukocytes in vitro; this method also serves to detect heterozygotes. Treatment with a diet low in the branched-chain amino acids has been successfully used to arrest the progressively downhill course of the disease. Variable degrees of central nervous system manifestations may persist, depending upon adequacy of dietary treatment and the amount of prior damage. During treatment it is necessary to monitor the blood levels of leucine and isoleucine carefully. When the ratio of leucine to isoleucine exceeds normal values, a condition resembling acrodermatitis enteropathica results. The rash abates when the isoleucine level of the diet is increased.

Variants of Maple Syrup Urine Disease. In the intermittent form, apparently healthy children suddenly become ill, develop the odor of maple syrup, exhibit neurologic symptoms, and excrete leucine, isoleucine, and valine and the corresponding keto-acids in urine. The disorder is genetically transmitted as an autosomal recessive. Activity of branched-chain decarboyxlase is reduced in leukocytes and fibroblasts to 8–16% of normal but not to the 0–2% level noted in the classic form. In children with ketotic hypoglycemia (Sec 17.10) during periods of acute illness, there is often a marked rise in branched-chain amino acids in urine, together with ketosis and hypoglycemia. There is, however, no odor of maple syrup to the urine, and one should not mistake this condition for the intermittent form of branched-chain ketonuria.

There is also a mild form of the disorder which responds well to a low protein diet. Elevations of the branched-chain amino and keto-acids persist in urine, and the odor of maple syrup may or may not be present. In vitro assay of branched-chain decarboxylase activity yields results that are intermediate between those of the classic type and the intermittent type.

In another variant, the defect is presumably at the binding site of the enzyme for the coenzyme thiamine pyrophosphate. The coenzyme form of the vitamin thiamine is involved in the oxidative decarboxylation of all α-keto-acids. A 13 mo old patient with ataxia was discovered to have elevation of blood levels of leucine, isoleucine, and valine, with no excretion of the keto-acid derivatives. The biochemical abnormalities reverted to normal with 10 mg/24 hr of thiamine hydrochloride. Patients with MSUD who have about 5% residual α-ketoacid dehydrogenase complex activity have been reported to improve biochemically when treated with 200 mg thiamine/24 hr for 4 wk.

Valinemia. A child with mental deficiency and growth failure has been observed who had elevated levels of valine in plasma and urine. The urine had neither keto-acids nor the odor of maple syrup. Impaired transamination of valine was demonstrated in leukocytes.

α-Methylacetoacetic Aciduria. In the normal pathway for isoleucine degradation, the compound α-methylacetoacetyl CoA is converted to acetyl CoA and propionyl CoA (Fig 8–4). Six children are known in whom the β-ketothiolase responsible for this conversion may be deficient inasmuch as they excreted large amounts of α-methylacetoacetate, α-methyl-β-hydroxybutyrate, and the glycine conjugate of tiglic acid. The children had intermittent acidosis, vomiting, lethargy, and coma, usually brought on by intercurrent infection. One child died during such an episode. The feeding of additional isoleucine aggravated the condition, whereas reduction of protein intake to 2 gm/kg/24 hr appeared to ameliorate the clinical course. There was no elevation of amino acid or propionate levels in blood or urine or any peculiar odor. A defect in isoleucine oxidation was demonstrated in cultured skin fibroblasts.

A defect of β-ketothiolase activity has been reported in an infant with ketotic glycinemia and hyperammonemia but no methylmalonic or propionic acidemia, though the clinical symptoms were those associated with the latter 2 findings (see below). Treatment with a low protein diet (1.5 gm/kg/24 hr) seemed advantageous.

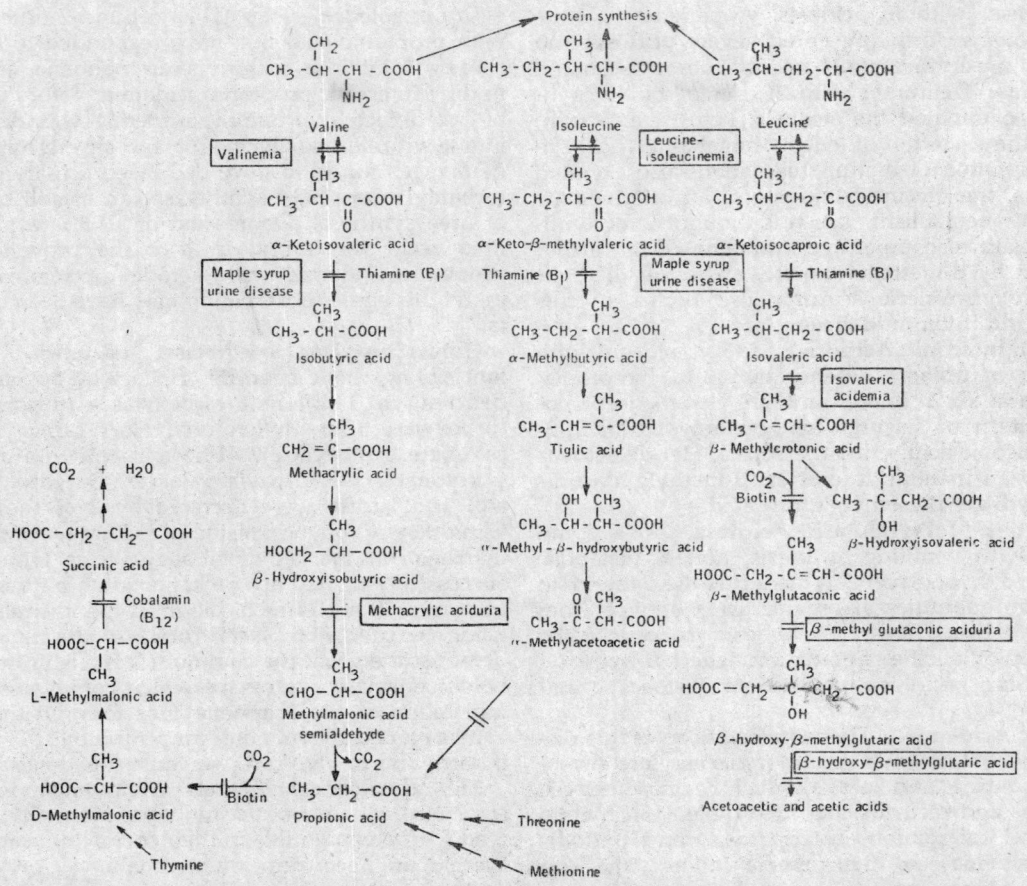

Figure 8–4 Pathways in the metabolism of the branched chain amino acids. (See also legend for Fig 8–1.) Lack of space prevents naming some of the defects depicted. In each case, the defect is called by the name of the substrate accumulating (e.g., Methylmalonic acidemia, Propionic acidemia, etc.).

For maple syrup urine disease genetic mutations can be postulated that correspond to variations in activities at each step in the entire catabolic pathway for leucine metabolism (Fig 8–4).

Isoleucine-Leucinemia.   Two siblings with severe neurologic symptoms, mental retardation, and failure to thrive have been reported to have type II prolinemia (see below) and mild (twice normal) to marked (8 times normal) elevations of blood valine, isoleucine, and leucine levels, with the latter 2 predominating. Assays of leukocytes revealed no abnormalities of branched-chain keto-acid decarboxylase activities or of valine transaminase but a 50% reduction of isoleucine and leucine transaminase.

Isovaleric Acidemia.   This condition was first described in 2 siblings with mild retardation, vomiting, severe acidosis, and coma. A more severe form of the disorder was reported in an infant who died in acidosis within a wk of birth. An odor described as the odor of sweaty feet, due to short-chain fatty acids, led to the biochemical elucidation of the defect. The defect is in the oxidation of isovaleryl CoA to β-methylcrotonyl CoA (see Fig 8–4) and has been demonstrated in leukocytes and in cultured fibroblasts.

Patients with isovaleric acidosis do not always have the odor of sweaty feet. One patient with periodic acidemia, lethargy, and coma had elevated plasma levels of glycine and excreted large amounts of isovalerylglycine and lesser amounts of isovalerate during her episodes of acidosis. Isovalerylglycine was demonstrated in thin-layer chromatography.

β-Methylcrotonyl Glycinuria.   Another condition involving leucine degradation gives rise to a peculiar odor resembling that of tomcat's urine. The enzyme β-methylcrotonyl CoA carboxylase fixes CO_2 and has biotin as a cofactor (Fig 8–4).

In this condition 2 errors of metabolism have been recognized which illustrate the fact that when specific cofactors of metabolic reactions are involved, genetic alterations may affect the protein either at the substrate binding site or at the cofactor binding site. If it is ability to bind cofactor that is reduced (but not abolished), then the in vitro or in vivo addition of massive amounts of cofactor can overcome the effects of the mutation.

In both forms of this disorder, β-methylcrotonyl CoA cannot be converted to β-methylglutaconyl CoA and large amounts of β-methylcrotonic acid are excreted, conjugated with glycine. A patient with the form of the disease unresponsive to biotin at 4.5 mo of age had neurologic symptoms similar to those of Werdnig-Hoffmann disease, without acidosis. A patient with the biotin-responsive form presented severe acidosis and ketosis and an erythematous rash of the buttocks and joint flexures. Treatment with 10 mg of biotin/24 hr completely eliminated the acidosis, ketosis, and rash, as well as the excretion of leucine metabolites. Prior to the administration of biotin, this patient also excreted tiglylglycine, the glycine conjugate of an intermediate of isoleucine metabolism, which is thought to accumulate as a result of competitive inhibition of its further degradation by β-methylcrotonate, an isomer of tiglic acid. Hydroxyisovaleric aciduria also occurs in this condition, and in biotin-deficient rats.

β-Methylglutaconic Aciduria. A 3 yr old girl with progressive neurologic deterioration and hypotonia, self-mutilation of 1 hand, and an electroencephalographic pattern of seizures had excessive urinary β-methylglutaconic acid without acidosis. Her defect was presumably an inability to convert β-methylglutaconic acid to β-hydroxy-β-methylglutaric acid.

β-Hydroxy-β-Methylglutaric Aciduria. In a 7 mo old infant with vomiting, cyanosis, apnea, metabolic acidosis, and hypoglycemia, the urine was found to contain large quantities of organic acids derived from leucine catabolism. The defect appears to occur at the terminal step of leucine degradation, where β-hydroxy-β-methylglutaric acid is converted to acetoacetic and acetic acids.

Propionic Acidemia. The manifestations of this disorder, formerly known as *ketotic glycinemia*, are severe acidosis, vomiting, and ketosis, which begin within the 1st few days and recur in later life (Table 8–3). Mental and physical retardation, osteoporosis, and periodic thrombocytopenia and neutropenia follow. The episodes of vomiting, ketosis, and acidosis appear to be related to the quantity of protein in the diet; reduction in dietary protein has led to decreased frequency and severity of the clinical attacks and to an increase in circulating neutrophils. Administration of methionine, threonine, valine, or isoleucine produces ketosis since all are converted to propionic acid and finally to succinic acid (Fig 8–4). In the absence of activity of the enzyme propionyl CoA carboxylase, propionic acid accumulates and ketones such as 2-butanone, presumably derived from isoleucine, appear in the urine during episodes of ketosis. Tiglic acid and tiglylglycine have also been found in the urine.

Treatment consists of careful reduction of the dietary intake of offending amino acids. The defect in propionate metabolism can be demonstrated in leukocytes and skin fibroblasts.

Since propionyl CoA carboxylase requires biotin, it is not surprising that a variant form of propionic acidemia has been observed. Treatment with biotin, 5 mg/24 hr, of a 2 yr old boy who had signs and symptoms of "ketotic glycinemia" has eliminated all the biochemical abnormalities.

The majority of patients with propionic acidemia have ketotic glycinemia; however, 2 patients with proven propionyl CoA carboxylase deficiency were exceptions. One 7 mo old male died without ever developing ketosis and a 10 mo old patient with mental retardation and seizures manifested ketoacidosis only when challenged

with an isoleucine load. This girl and 2 other patients with propionic acidemia have responded to an isoleucine or valine load with hyperammonemia, an unusual finding in classic propionic acidemia. Before the nature of the defect in propionic acidemia was defined, an infant with ketotic glycinemia and severe hyperammonemia was found to have decreased activity of hepatic carbamyl phosphate synthetase, an established defect of urea synthesis. Depression of all 5 enzymes of the urea cycle was found in 1 of the proven cases of propionic acidemia with ketotic glycinemia; accordingly, this earlier observation may have been coincidental.

Holocarboxylase Synthetase Deficiency. Three infant siblings have been described who appeared to be deficient in 3 different carboxylases (propionyl CoA carboxylase, β-methylcrotonyl CoA carboxylase, and pyruvate carboxylase). Abnormal amounts of β-methylcrotonate, β-hydroxyisovalerate, β-hydroxypropionate, and lactate were excreted by 2 of the children. Clinical symptoms consisted of lethargy, vomiting, and diarrhea with marked metabolic acidosis. One child was successfully treated after alkalinization by the administration of 10 mg/24 hr of biotin in the formula. Studies using cultured fibroblasts from 2 of the patients have demonstrated that the common defect is in the enzyme holocarboxylase synthetase which conjugates the vitamin biotin to the 3 apoenzymes forming the holoenzymes named above. High concentrations of biotin both in vitro and in vivo can overcome this deficiency.

Methylmalonic Acidemia. Methylmalonic acid is a structural isomer of succinic acid. Normally, both are readily interconvertible in their coenzyme A forms with the aid of the enzyme methylmalonyl CoA carbonylmutase, which requires the vitamin B_{12} coenzyme, adenosylcobalamin. With vitamin B_{12} deficiency, increased amounts of methylmalonic acid are excreted in urine. Methylmalonic acid is normally derived from propionic acid and therefore from the catabolism of isoleucine, methionine, threonine, and valine (Fig 8–2 and 8–4).

Methylmalonic acidemia and massive methylmalonic aciduria were first described in 2 unrelated children who failed to thrive and exhibited bouts of severe metabolic acidosis from birth (Table 8–3). One died at 2 yr of age in acute acidosis; the other, a 6 yr old girl, was treated with alkalinization and, despite episodes of vomiting and acidosis, had normal physical and mental development. A brother had died in infancy after vomiting and failure to thrive. Loading tests with protein, valine, or propionic acid led to hypoglycemia and ketosis as well as to slight increases in the excretion of methylmalonic acid. A number of additional patients with this disorder are now known; when glycinemia was sought, it was present in each (see below).

Multiple variants of methylmalonic acidemia are known. The most common varieties involve either the enzyme methylmalonyl CoA carbonylmutase, which converts L-methylmalonyl CoA to succinyl CoA, or the activation of vitamin B_{12} to its coenzyme forms. In vitro complementation studies distinguish 6 genetically distinct groups. Both vitamin B_{12}–responsive and B_{12}–unresponsive variants of the disorder have been identified. Four of the responsive forms are due to defects in the metabolism of vitamin B_{12} wherein cobalamin cannot be converted into either the adenosyl form or the 'methyl form. In the latter case, both homocysteine and methylmalonate metabolism are affected.

Prenatal diagnosis and successful prenatal treatment have been accomplished in 1 female infant with B_{12}–responsive methylmalonic acidemia. Maternal excretion of methylmalonate was monitored; since the mother did not excrete methylmalonate when she was not pregnant, the appearance of this compound in her urine could be used as a biochemical index of fetal status. During the last trimester, large doses of vitamin B_{12} produced a marked decrease in urinary methylmalonate. The infant was shown to have elevated vitamin B_{12} stores at birth as a result of the dose given the mother.

As more of the population is screened, asymptomatic persons are detected who have biochemical abnormalities corresponding to particular disease states. Two brothers have recently been found to excrete excessive methylmalonate and to have decreased white cell mutase activity. Neither one was vitamin B_{12}–deficient or –responsive. Further evidence of genetic heterogeneity in this disorder has been provided by several patients who did not respond in vivo to vitamin B_{12} but whose tissue samples responded to B_{12} coenzyme in vitro.

8.8 GLYCINE

Abnormal elevations of plasma glycine levels and episodes of ketosis are found in patients with a number of inborn errors of metabolism, such as methylmalonic acidemia or propionic acidemia, or some other defect of metabolism of leucine and isoleucine below the level of the block that occurs in maple syrup urine disease (Sec 8.7). The metabolic events producing high levels of glycine in these disorders are not known, but many of the metabolites that accumulate are excreted for the most part as glycine conjugates. Glycinemia may be an adaptive response to an increased need for detoxification of these acids normally present only in low concentration. Pathways are indicated in Fig 8–5.

Glycinemia. Besides the glycinemia that may occur secondary to the acidosis and ketosis in propionic or methylmalonic acidemia (see above), or, rarely, in propionic acidemia without acidosis or ketosis, there is *nonketotic glycinemia*, in which the primary defect is in glycine metabolism. Numerous patients with this entity have been studied and numerous hypotheses made about the nature of the biochemical defect(s).

The basic defect probably occurs in the cleavage of glycine to form CO_2, ammonia, and hydroxymethyltetrahydrofolate. Since the last compound normally reacts with another molecule of glycine to form serine, conversion of glycine to serine is also impaired. Some patients with nonketotic glycinemia have been reported to excrete less oxalic acid than normal; thus defects have been postulated in the pathway from glycine to glyoxylic acid and thence to oxalic acid. Except for 1 case with a possible defect in the conversion of glyoxalate to oxalate, these patients have been shown to have a defect of the cleavage enzyme. An additional

child with methylmalonic acidemia and glycinemia also was shown to have a block in hepatic glycine cleavage activity.

Patients with nonketotic glycinemia are mentally retarded and listless, fail to thrive, and have seizures, but they do not have episodes of acidosis or ketosis and do not exhibit neutropenia or thrombocytopenia. Symptoms often begin at birth and are quite severe. In children with nonketotic glycinemia, cerebrospinal fluid glycine concentrations are 15–30 times normal, though normal in patients with other forms of glycinemia. Glycine cleavage activity in brain was undetectable in the former group. The critical factor in producing mental retardation appears to be glycine concentration in the central nervous system rather than in plasma. Preliminary results suggest that strychnine may be useful in this disorder.

A patient with nonketotic glycinemia and a proven defect of the cleavage enzyme has been reported to have hyperammonemia. Normal values for carbamylphosphate synthetase, ornithine transcarbamylase, and argininosuccinic acid synthetase were found. Thus, in both propionic acidemia and nonketotic glycinemia, occasional patients have an as yet unexplained elevation of blood ammonia. For unknown reasons many children with nonketotic glycinemia develop profound coma after valine loads.

Sarcosinemia. Increased concentrations of sarcosine (N-methylglycine) have been observed in both blood and urine in 7 individuals; no consistent clinical picture can be attributed to this metabolic defect. Loading tests in family members suggest that this is a recessively inherited inborn error probably involving sarcosine dehydrogenase, the enzyme that converts sarcosine to glycine (Fig 8–5). In 1 of the original patients, who at 14 yr of age seemed to be a healthy girl with an IQ of 77, hepatic tissue obtained at biopsy contained no sarcosine dehydrogenase.

D-Glyceric Acidemia. Two retarded children have been described who excreted abnormal quantities of D-glyceric acid and normal amounts of oxalic acid. One child had nonketotic glycinemia without acidosis, whereas the other had normal plasma glycine but a persistent metabolic acidosis. There may be a block at D-glycerate kinase (Fig 8–5) so that glycerate cannot be converted to 2-phospho-D-glycerate.

Trimethylaminuria. Choline is an important dietary source of methyl groups. It is normally converted to betaine, thence to dimethylglycine, to sarcosine, and finally to glycine. Putrefaction, particularly in fish, yields trimethylamine. Several patients smelling of stale fish have been reported who excreted large amounts of trimethylamine. The 1st child described had pulmonary and hematologic problems, but these were probably fortuitous since the other patients were asymptomatic except for their foul smell. Because hepatic trimethylamine oxidase activity was decreased (Fig 8–5), noxious trimethylamine could not be oxidized to odorless trimethylamine-N-oxide.

Glycinuria and Glucoglycinuria. Glycinuria and glucoglycinuria have been identified as separate disorders of the renal tubules. Glycinuria is also observed in prolinemia and prolinuria since there exists a common

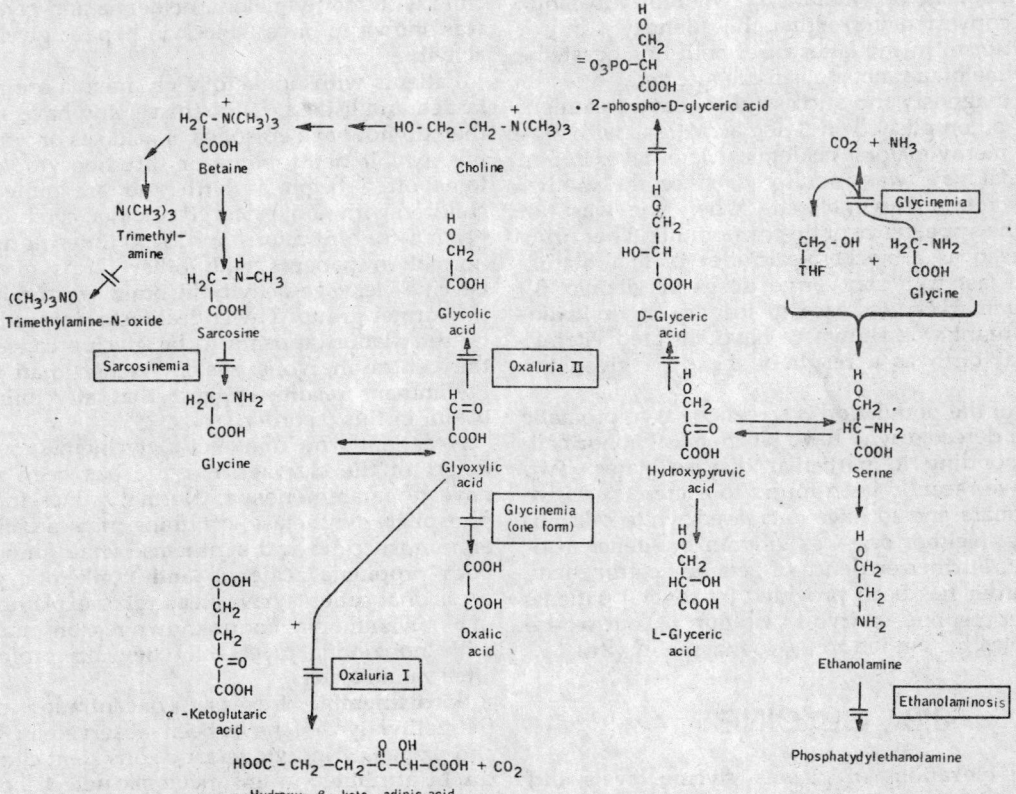

Figure 8-5 Pathways in the metabolism of glycine. See also legend for Fig 8-1.

transport system for proline, hydroxyproline, and glycine in addition to the specific renal transport system for glycine alone.

Primary Oxaluria and Oxalosis. Oxalic acid is a 2-carbon dicarboxylic acid derived mostly from the oxidation of the amino acid glycine via glyoxylic acid (Fig 8–5). Generalized *oxalosis* can occur after ingestion of ethylene glycol or use of the anesthetic agent methoxyflurane. A storage disease, oxalosis is characterized by the deposition of calcium oxalate crystals throughout body tissues and by excessive urinary excretion of oxalic acid, with renal and vesical lithiasis and nephrocalcinosis. Only occasionally have calcium oxalate crystals been found in the eye. Early in the course of the disease and in mild forms, only *oxaluria* may be present. Clinical manifestations appear in childhood, and death occurs in early adulthood. Primary oxaluria constitutes 2 distinct disorders, each caused by a different enzymatic deficit, both presumably with autosomal recessive inheritance.

In the 1st form, the more common and more severe, there is usually excess excretion of *glycolic acid* and glyoxylic acid as well as oxalic acid. The missing enzyme, α-,ketoglutarate-glyoxylate carboligase, normally removes glyoxylic acid to form α-hydroxy-β-ketoadipic acid. In the absence of this enzyme the glyoxylic acid floods the pathways leading to glycolic and oxalic acids.

In the 2nd type of hyperoxaluria, L-*glyceric acid* is also excreted in the urine in large amounts. This acid, which

is not produced by normal persons, arises from the reduction of hydroxypyruvic acid (the keto-acid of serine) by lactic dehydrogenase. Ordinarily, hydroxypyruvic acid is reduced to D-glyceric acid by the specific enzyme D-glyceric acid dehydrogenase. This enzyme is also capable of reducing glyoxylic acid to glycolic acid. In its absence hydroxypyruvic acid is converted to and excreted as L-glyceric acid, and glyoxylic acid is converted to and excreted as oxalic acid. Of about 30 fully studied cases with primary oxalosis, most have had glycolic aciduria and only 4, glyceric aciduria. Attempts at treatment, including renal transplantation, have not proved efficacious. In some patients, administration of large doses of pyridoxine has reduced the urinary excretion of oxalate, but values achieved remained well above normal limits.

8.9   SERINE

Ethanolaminosis. A brother and sister have been described with the clinical findings usually associated with GSD II (Sec 8.21) who had a new disorder. Both died before 2 yr of age and had cardiomegaly, hypotonia, and cerebral dysfunction. Many tissues contained material which stained with PAS and Best carmine. Glycogen content of the liver and heart was normal, as were all of the enzymes measured which are associated with the glycogenoses, the lipidoses, or the mucopolysaccharidoses. Ethanolamine was found to be present in excessive amounts in liver and urine and was undetected in serum. Measurements of activity of ethanolamine kinase (Fig 8–5) in liver revealed a 70% reduction of activity. Although it has been postulated that this disease represents a defect in the synthesis of phosphatidyl-ethanolamine, there currently exists no explanation of the nature of the stored material as free ethanolamine (although it reacts with PAS reagent, but not Best carmine) would be washed away during processing. Although listed among the aminoacidopathies, this disorder undoubtedly represents a new type of polymer storage disease.

8.10 THREONINE

Threoninemia. An infant with convulsions and growth retardation has been reported with threoninemia (13 mg/dl) and threoninuria. The parents were related.

8.11 PROLINE AND HYDROXYPROLINE

Proline and hydroxyproline, often referred to as imino acids because the nitrogen molecule is incorporated into the pyrrolidine ring, are found in high concentration in collagen. Neither of these imino acids is normally found in urine in the free form except in early infancy. Excretion of "bound" hydroxyproline (dipeptides and tripeptides containing hydroxyproline) reflects collagen turnover and is increased in disorders of accelerated collagen turnover, such as rickets or hyperparathyroidism.

Prolinemia. Two distinct types of prolinemia are known in which excessive amounts of proline are present in both blood and urine. Hydroxyproline and glycine are also excreted in abnormal amounts in urine because of inhibition of the common tubular reabsorption mechanism. In type I prolinemia the enzymatic defect involves proline oxidase (Fig 8–6). In type II the defect is presumed to be in the enzyme of the next step, a dehydrogenase, since pyrrolidine carboxylic acid, as well as proline, accumulates abnormally. Type I prolinemia has been associated with mild mental retardation, renal abnormalities, nerve deafness, and photogenic epilepsy. Type II prolinemia was originally observed in a young child who had only mild mental retardation.

Many asymptomatic individuals with both types of prolinemia have now been described. Since prolinemia is apparently a coincidental finding in these patients, diet therapy may not be indicated.

Hydroxyprolinemia. This disorder was first described in a severely retarded girl. Excessive hydroxyproline was found in serum and urine. In hydroxyprolinemia, in contrast to prolinemia, excessive urinary excretion of the other 2 amino acids (proline and glycine) that share the same transport mechanisms does not occur. The defect is in the enzyme hydroxyproline oxidase (Fig 8–6). This enzyme is distinct from the corresponding enzyme, which acts upon proline. The disorder is presumed to be inherited as an autosomal recessive. The association with mental retardation may be coincidental since in another family 2 adult siblings of an affected child were normal but had hydroxyprolinemia.

Familial Iminoglycinuria. A defect in renal tubular reabsorption of proline is inherited as an autosomal recessive. Since proline, hydroxyproline, and glycine are all transported by a common mechanism, patients with familial iminoglycinuria also excrete the other 2 amino acids in abnormal amounts. The concentrations of these amino acids in serum are normal. Many of the affected persons also have impaired intestinal transport

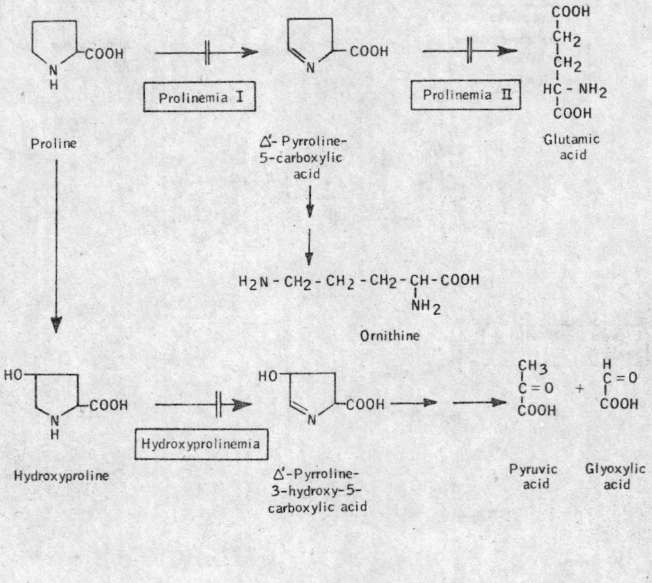

Figure 8–6 Pathways in the metabolism of the imino acids. See also legend for Fig 8–1.

of proline. An early impression of high coincidence of prolinuria and mental retardation may have arisen erroneously. In a screening program in Australia involving 200,000 infants, persistent iminoglycinuria was found in 15, none of whom had any clinical abnormalities.

Prolidase Deficiency Syndrome. During collagen degradation imidodipeptides are released and cleaved by the enzyme prolidase. Six patients with excessive imidodipeptides are described who have characteristic joints, dermatitis, skeletal and tendinous abnormalities, splenomegaly, frequent infection, and retardation. This presumed autosomal recessive disorder results from deficient prolidase activity.

8.12 GLUTAMIC ACID

There are a number of inborn errors related to the metabolism of glutamic acid. Glutathione (γ-glutamylcysteinylglycine) is involved in a nonspecific amino acid transport system, particularly in the renal tubule and intestinal villus; the cyclical synthesis and degradation of glutathione play a role in the formation of dipeptides with glutamic acid of the amino acids to be transported.

Anemia Due to γ-Glutamylcysteine Synthetase Deficiency. A 38 yr old man with intermittent jaundice, progressive spinocerebellar degeneration, speech impairment, and myoclonic spasms was found to have decreased γ-glutamylcysteine synthetase activity. His 36 yr old sister demonstrated mild neurologic symptoms and chronic hemolytic anemia. The anemias noted in disorders of the γ-glutamyl cycle presumably result from lowered intracellular glutathione concentration, as a result of which red cell membranes become more susceptible to lipid peroxidation.

Anemia Due to Glutathione Synthetase Deficiency. Seven patients in 4 families have been described with mild hemolytic anemia and intermittent jaundice but no neurologic findings. Glutathione synthetase activity and glutathione levels were markedly decreased in the patients' red cells. Pyroglutamic acid was not measured.

Pyroglutamic Acidemia (Glutathione Synthetase Deficiency). Twelve patients have been found to excrete massive amounts (6–20 gm/24 hr) of pyroglutamic acid (also known as 5-oxo-L-proline). This compound is an intermediate in the Meister γ-glutamyl cycle for the transport of amino acids (Fig 8–7).

Patients in the neonatal period may present severe metabolic acidosis and hemolysis. Progressive neurologic deterioration or apparently normal development may take place. Glutathione content and glutathione synthetase activity are quite low in red cells and fibroblasts. Overproduction rather than underutilization of pyroglutamic acid is the cause of the organic acidemia. This results from the release of feedback inhibition of the γ-glutamylcysteine synthetase by glutathione and the subsequent conversion of the overproduced γ-glutamylcysteine to pyroglutamic acid at a rate which exceeds the ability of 5-oxyprolinase to convert it back to glutamic acid. There is no explanation for the marked clinical contrast between pyroglutamic acidemia and the mild anemia of glutathione synthetase deficiency, though both lack activity of this enzyme. Patients with the latter condition may have only a red cell deficiency, whereas those with the former may have many tissues involved.

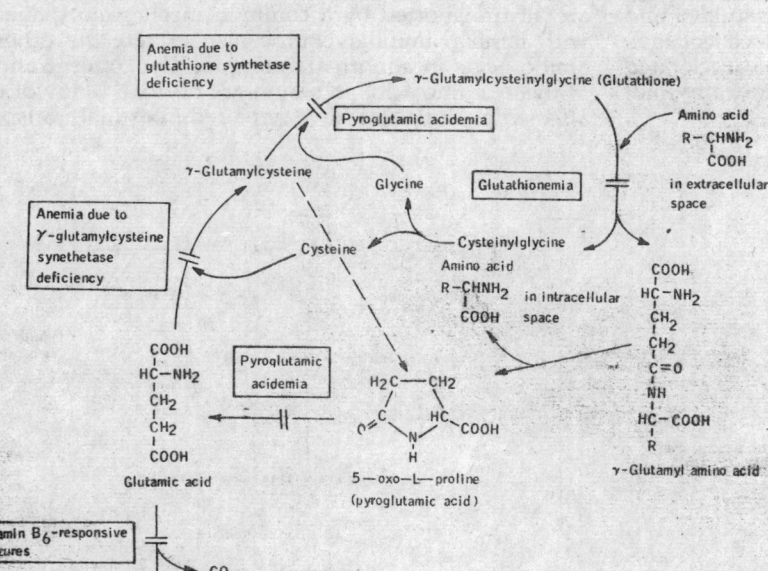

Figure 8–7 The γ-glutamyl cycle for nonspecific amino acid transport. Defects of glutathione synthesis and degradation are noted. See also legend for Fig 8–1.

Pyroglutamic Acidemia (5-Oxoprolinase Deficiency). In contrast to the disorder described above, this form of pyroglutamic acidemia is due directly to the inability to degrade the compound, as is most usually the case in other inborn errors of metabolism. Two teenage brothers have been described who have had recurrent episodes of vomiting, diarrhea, and abdominal pain since infancy. Urinary pyroglutamic acid excretion was up to 9 gm/24 hr. 5-Oxyprolinase was markedly reduced in the patients' fibroblasts and leukocytes, whereas the level in fibroblasts from their parents was intermediate between the patients and normal controls. Other enzymes of the γ-glutamyl cycle were normal as was the glutathione content of erythrocytes, and neither patient had neurologic symptoms or acidosis.

Glutathionemia. A routine screening program detected an adult male with mild retardation who excreted large amounts of glutathione and had elevated serum glutathione. Gamma-glutamyl transpeptidase activity in cultured fibroblasts was very low (Fig 8–7). Although this enzyme is necessary for nonspecific amino acid transport, his renal excretion of amino acids was normal.

Vitamin B₆–Responsive Seizures. Many children have been described in whom seizures in early life were poorly controlled with conventional anticonvulsant therapy but in whom parenteral administration of vitamin B_6 resulted in dramatic improvement of both seizure activity and EEG abnormalities. Analysis of tissues from several of these patients revealed a decrease in glutamic acid decarboxylase activity that was reversed with addition of the coenzyme pyridoxal phosphate. Since this defect cannot be detected in fibroblasts, the diagnosis is usually made on the basis of a clinical response to B_6.

Chinese Restaurant Syndrome. Monosodium glutamate (MSG), a widely used flavor enhancer, is one of the active components of soy sauce. It is responsible for the so-called Chinese restaurant syndrome. Certain individuals react to MSG by developing an acute syndrome that may last for 12 hr. Among other things, it consists of substernal pressure, headache, burning sensations, palpitations, and vomiting. Though there are no apparent sequelae in adults, animal experiments suggest possible central nervous system toxicity. Some investigators have postulated that this syndrome is a benign, undefined inborn error of glutamate metabolism.

8.13 UREA CYCLE

Catabolism of amino acids results in the production of free ammonia, which is highly toxic to the brain. Ammonia is catabolized to urea by a series of reactions known as the Krebs-Henseleit or urea cycle (Fig 8–8). Defects are now known for all of the enzymes of the urea cycle. In most instances the affected persons exhibit mental retardation, presumably the result of intoxication with ammonia. Pernicious vomiting is a common

and frequent finding in these children. Since most patients with defects of the urea cycle excrete normal amounts of urea, it is presumed either that the defect is not present in all tissues or that other pathways exist for synthesis of urea. Two genetically different forms of arginase have been found, only 1 of which is affected in argininemia. A pathway for urea synthesis involving guanidosuccinic acid has been postulated since this acid is found in the urine of patients with uremia. Although the results have been variable and usually discouraging, the accepted form of treatment consists of lowering dietary protein intake. Alpha-keto analogues of the essential amino acids may provide a more effective form of dietary therapy since diets containing these keto-acids reduce ammonia production. The anabolic requirements for amino acids are satisfied since there is adequate transamination of the α-keto analogues to their corresponding amino acids. Other attempts have been made to reduce ammonia levels in severely affected newborn infants. Arginine, ornithine, and citrulline have been administered in order to soak up ammonia or amino groups. Benzoate and phenylacetate have also been tried. Hemodialysis and plasmapheresis are effective in reducing ammonia levels.

Ammonemia Due to Carbamyl Phosphate Synthetase (CPS) Deficiency. At least 6 children have demonstrated a defect in the initial step of urea synthesis. The patient described in the original investigation of hyperammonemia of this type died at 5 mo of age after a stormy course that was aggravated by protein feeding. With restriction of dietary protein, the patient improved neurologically, blood ammonia levels became normal, but glycinemia and neutropenia were present and, terminally, acidosis. Vomiting, neurologic symptoms, and retarded development plague these patients. Ammonemia and decreased CPS activity have been associated with various organic acidemias. In primary CPS deficiency, urine orotic acid excretion is normal or low as opposed to the marked increase in orotic acid excretion noted in ornithine transcarbamylase deficiency.

Ammonemia Due to N-Acetylglutamate Synthetase Deficiency. Mitochondrial carbamyl phosphate synthetase activity (see above) requires the presence of N-acetylglutamate, which serves as an activator. A newborn boy with hyperammonemia but no orotic acidosis has been shown (using hepatic tissue obtained by biopsy) to have no demonstrable activity of the enzyme which forms N-acetylglutamate from acetyl CoA and glutamic acid. Carbamyl phosphate synthetase and ornithine transcarbamylase activities were normal. Two siblings had died shortly after birth; 1 was thought to have had hyperammonemia. Treatment with carbamylglutamate and arginine seems to be successful.

Ammonemia Due to Ornithine Transcarbamylase Deficiency. All of the patients described with this disorder of urea synthesis have had hyperammonemia. Many have died in the neonatal period. Most of the others experienced severe vomiting, coma, and either retardation or seizures. Some excreted increased amounts of orotic acid, presumably as a result of the accumulation of excess carbamyl phosphate and shunting of this compound into the pyrimidine biosynthesis pathway (Fig 8–8). In some instances the level of the

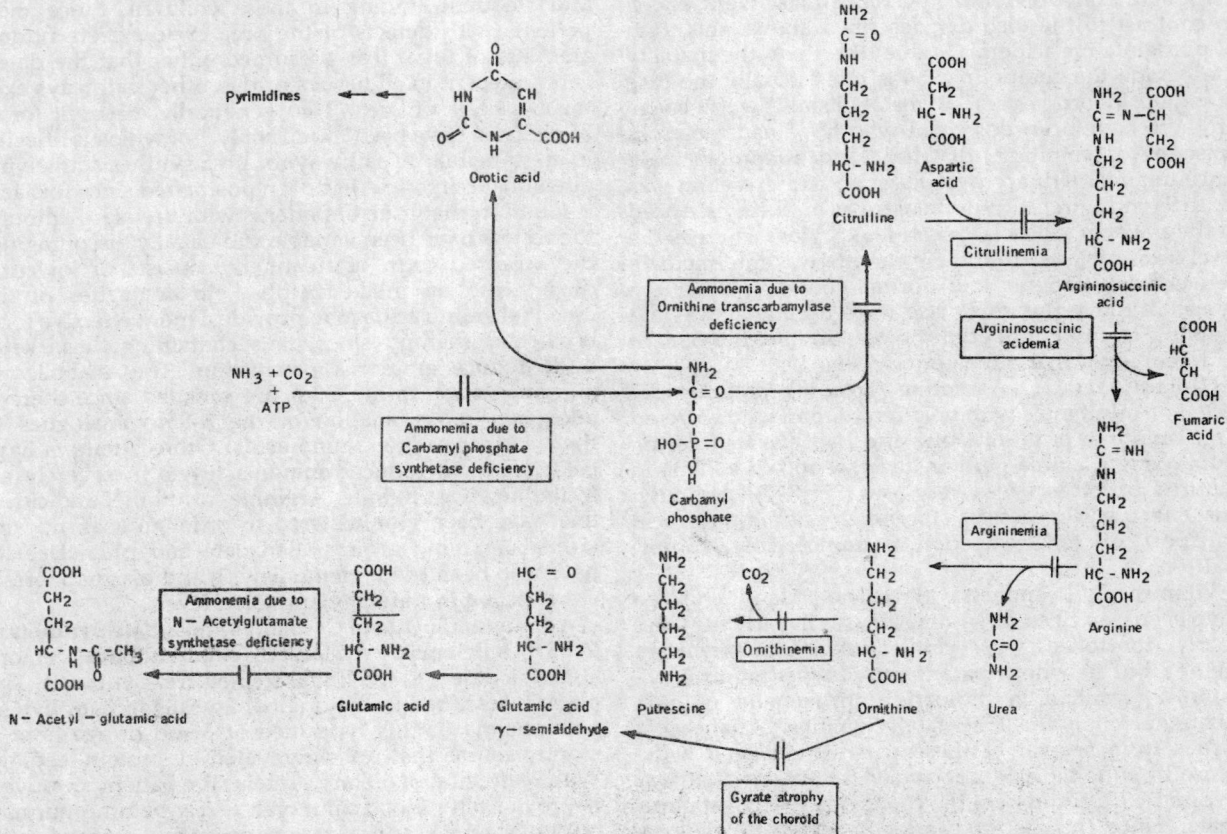

Figure 8—8 Pathways in the metabolism of ammonia and in the urea cycle. See also legend for Fig 8—1.

enzyme ornithine transcarbamylase was reduced to less than 10% of normal. In other cases the reduction in enzyme activity was much less severe. In 1 instance the total activity was not severely reduced, but it was shown that the K_m of the mutant enzyme for the substrate carbamyl phosphate was 4 times normal; accordingly, the affinity for this compound was much less than that of the normal enzyme. The affinity for the other substrate, ornithine, was normal. It is apparent, therefore, that ornithine transcarbamylase deficiencies are a heterogeneous genetic group. Despite the enzymatic heterogeneity, it would appear that this disorder follows X-linked inheritance and is lethal for males in the newborn period. Nearly all those surviving the neonatal period have been female. No father has transmitted the disorder, whereas some mothers of affected female patients have reduced enzyme activity and aversion to high protein foods. It has been shown, in accordance with the Lyon hypothesis, that carrier females have 2 populations of liver cells: some with normal and some with no ornithine transcarbamylase activity. Heterozygotes may be detected by finding abnormal urinary levels of orotic acid or increased blood ammonia after a protein challenge.

Citrullinemia (Argininosuccinic Acid Synthetase Deficiency). The reported cases of this disorder show considerable biochemical and genetic heterogeneity.

Mental retardation is a frequent feature. Some patients have hyperammonemia; others do not. The latter include an infant girl who died at 7 days of age and an adult male who is in apparently good health at 33 yr of age. In most of the patients there is a virtual absence of argininosuccinic acid synthetase activity; in others the affinity of a mutant enzyme toward citrulline is reduced 25-fold. It has been suggested that, in those cases without elevation of ammonia, citrulline is itself toxic to brain metabolism. Treatment with low protein diets or α-keto analogues may prove efficacious in this disorder, particularly in the mild variant.

Argininosuccinic Acidemia (Argininosuccinase Deficiency). About 4 dozen instances of this disorder have been reported, with hyperammonemia in some. Affected children have argininosuccinic acidemia and aciduria and have usually been mentally retarded; some have had abnormally friable hair (trichorrhexis nodosa). Not all patients with this type of hair abnormality, however, have argininosuccinic acidemia. The defect is in argininosuccinase, the enzyme that splits argininosuccinic acid to arginine and fumaric acid. The disorder is transmitted as an autosomal recessive. The defect can be demonstrated in erythrocytes; heterozygotes have lower than normal activity. Levels of argininosuccinic acid are higher in the cerebrospinal fluid than in the blood; concentrations of urea in the blood and urine are normal. The defect in the urea cycle in these patients may be limited to the brain. It has been postulated that there are at least 2 forms of the disorder: 1 with early onset, in which case failure to thrive and vomiting are noted in the 1st few mo of life; and a 2nd with late onset, in which developmental failure, seizures, and ataxia are observed after 1 yr of age. In 1 infant who died at 6 days of age, the enzyme was absent in liver, decreased in erythrocytes, and present in brain and kidney. In another *healthy* infant, who was found upon routine screening to have massive argininosuccinic aciduria, the enzyme was absent in erythrocytes. The clinical condition of this child at 1.5 yr of age suggests that the enzyme must be present in other tissues.

Argininemia (Arginase Deficiency). Three sisters with hyperammonemia, spastic diplegia, seizures, and severe mental retardation have been found to have deficient arginase activity in erythrocytes. Their parents had lower than normal activity and are probably heterozygous. The hyperammonemia and increased urinary excretion of other dibasic amino acids such as lysine and cystine disappeared on a low protein diet (1.5 gm/kg/24 hr). Argininemia, however, persisted.

Ornithinemia. Several mentally retarded patients are known with this finding. One had hyperammonemia and homocitrullinuria and responded well to a low protein diet. It has been postulated that in this patient the decarboxylase (Fig 8–8) is defective since its activity in fibroblasts is decreased. The other patients fall into a poorly defined group with no proven primary enzyme defect. *Gyrate atrophy* of the choroid, a chorioretinal degeneration, is found in patients with ornithinemia and deficient ornithine ketoacid transaminase activity.

Pyridoxal phosphate will produce beneficial responses both in vivo and in vitro in some of these patients.

8.14 HISTIDINE

Histidinemia. In histidinemia the activity of the enzyme histidase, which normally converts histidine to urocanic acid, is deficient in liver and skin. As a result, histidine is transaminated to imidazolepyruvic acid, which appears in the urine along with excessive amounts of histidine (Fig 8–9). Imidazolepyruvic acid, like phenylpyruvic acid, reacts with ferric chloride to produce a blue-green color. Many patients with histidinemia have been detected through screening tests for phenylketonuria, and some have been misdiagnosed as PKU. Demonstration of elevation in plasma levels of histidine is necessary for the correct diagnosis of this disorder, and a definitive diagnosis depends on measuring histidase activity of cornified epithelium or of liver.

Some affected persons have had impaired speech, a few were retarded in growth, and some were mentally retarded. The relation of these defects to histidinemia is unknown inasmuch as routine amino acid screening has uncovered a significant number of asymptomatic persons with histidinemia. The metabolic defect is transmitted as an autosomal recessive character; in some families the heterozygous state can be identified by demonstration of decreased histidase activity in skin.

Some evidence for genetic heterogeneity in histidinemia exists. In some but not in all affected children

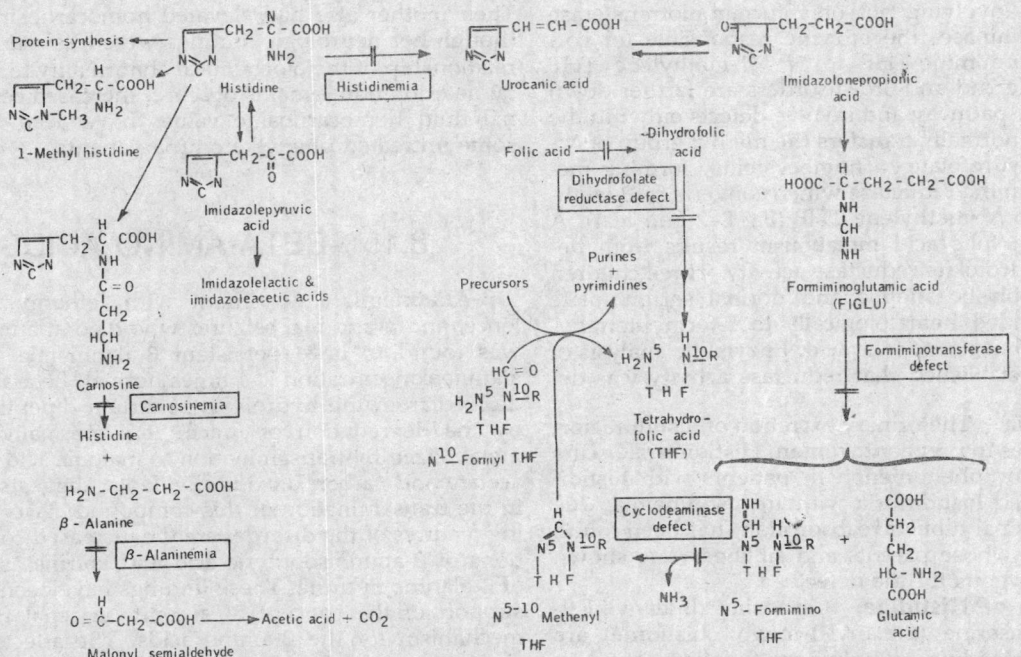

Figure 8–9 Pathways in the metabolism of histidine, beta amino acids, and folic acid. See also legend for Fig 8–1. (THF is an abbreviation for tetrahydrofolic acid.)

plasma levels of alanine as well as histidine were elevated. The reason for this association is unknown. In some families with histidinemia the level of histidase in skin is normal, and perhaps the defect in enzymatic activity is limited to the liver. Several children with Marfan syndrome also have histidinemia, but no relationship has been shown between these 2 genetic disorders.

Affected neonates do not excrete imidazole derivatives of histidine because there is a normal delay in the maturation of histidine transaminase.

Histidine and Folic Acid Metabolism. After histidine has been converted to urocanic acid, it is further metabolized to formiminoglutamic acid (FIGLU). The formimino group of this compound is normally transferred to folic acid, with the concomitant production of glutamic acid (Fig 8–9). Measurement of the urinary excretion of FIGLU after loading with histidine has been used as a method for the detection of folic acid deficiency states. Both FIGLU and urocanic acid are excreted by patients with megaloblastic anemia. Urocanic acid is found in the urine of children with kwashiorkor.

Four distinct defects in folic acid metabolism have been delineated, in each of which the blood values of folic acid are normal or elevated. In the 1st, formiminoglutamic acid is increased after administration of histidine; the enzyme formiminotransferase is deficient. A group of mentally retarded infants with defects in folic acid metabolism has been described in Japan. Microcephaly and electroencephalographic abnormalities were frequent findings. Other patients with normal folate levels and no hematologic abnormalities or retardation excreted massive amounts of FIGLU. These children responded to folate by decreasing FIGLU excretion, and they may represent a harmless variant of formiminotransferase deficiency. The more severely affected Japanese patients may represent a double enzyme defect involving not only formiminotransferase but cyclodeaminase, the enzyme responsible for correcting N^5-formimino-THF to N^5-N^{10}-methylene THF (Fig 8–9). The 2nd and 3rd disorders are farther down the metabolic pathway and involve defects either in the enzyme that normally transfers the methyl group of N^5-methyltetrahydrofolate to homocysteine, forming methionine, or in the reductase which converts 5,10-methylene THF to N^5-methylene THF (Fig 8–2 and text). A 4th defect in folic acid metabolism results from decreased dihydrofolate reductase activity. Three children with megaloblastic anemia and normal serum folate levels responded hematologically to 5-formyl-tetrahydrofolic acid but not to folic acid. Enzymatic analysis of liver tissue established that reductase activity was deficient.

Histidinuria. The urinary excretion of histidine normally increases in pregnant women. Histidinuria occurs as an overflow phenomenon in patients with histidinemia. Isolated histidinuria without histidinemia, due to defective renal tubular reabsorption, has been found in 3 children whose parents and siblings were shown to be heterozygous for the defect.

Dipeptides of Histidine. Carnosine (β-alanylhistidine) and anserine (β-alanyl-1-methyl histidine) are peptides of histidine of unknown function found in muscle. These peptides, as well as 1-methyl histidine derived from anserine, have been found in urine of normal persons, particularly after the ingestion of large amounts of turkey and chicken. Homocarnosine (γ-aminobutyryl-histidine) appears to be brain-specific since it is found only in the cerebrospinal fluid. In the disorders described below, the findings of the dipeptides of histidine in urine have been specific and independent of dietary intake.

Imidazole Aciduria. Excessive excretion of carnosine, anserine, and occasionally of homocarnosine (γ-aminobutyryl-histidine), as well as of histidine and 1-methyl histidine, has been reported in a number of patients with a form of cerebromacular degeneration resembling juvenile Tay-Sachs disease. The use of labeled histidine provided some evidence for increased synthesis of the dipeptides. The genetic basis of the disorder is not clear; in the 3 families studied the cerebromacular degeneration was inherited on a recessive basis, whereas the histidine peptiduria appeared to be transmitted on a dominant one. Isolated increased excretion of 1-methyl histidine without 1-methyl histidinemia has been reported in 3 male siblings with precocious puberty who had no other clinical abnormality.

Serum Carnosinase Deficiency. Seven patients are described with serum carnosinase deficiency. In all but one there was severe neurologic involvement. Persistent carnosinuria but not carnosinemia was noted. The defect is in the enzyme carnosinase, which normally hydrolyzes carnosine to histidine and β-alanine and can be assayed in plasma. The disorder appears to be recessively inherited.

Homocarnosinosis. Three siblings had cerebrospinal fluid homocarnosine concentrations that were 20 times normal. All suffered from progressive spastic paraplegia, mental deterioration, and retinal pigmentation. Their mother also had elevated homocarnosine levels, though her neurologic findings were less marked. The relationship of the biochemical abnormality to the mental deterioration remains obscure. Increased cerebrospinal fluid homocarnosine values have been found in some untreated phenylketonuria patients.

8.15 BETA-AMINO ACIDS

β-Alaninemia. An infant with lethargy, somnolence, and grand mal seizures who died at 5 mo of age was found to have persistent β-alaninemia, with β-alanine concentration 2–4 times normal. Beta-alanine is derived from the hydrolysis of certain dipeptides and by the degradation of uracil. It is normally further metabolized by transamination to malonic acid, then to acetate and carbon dioxide. Evidence suggests a block in the transamination of this compound. Two interesting features of the disorder are the increased concentrations of β-aminoisobutyric acid and taurine as well as of β-alanine in urine. These findings have been used in support of the concept of a common renal transport mechanism for the β-amino acids. The affected child also had increased concentration of γ-aminobutyric acid in cerebrospinal fluid, plasma, and urine. The neurologic symptoms have been attributed to the increase in β-alanine and the decrease in γ-aminobutyric acid within the brain. Abnormal urinary excretion of β-alanine and β-aminoisobutyrate has been reported in a 3 yr old girl with brittle hair. What appears to be an isolated transport defect for β-alanine has been reported in a 16 yr old girl with physical and mental retardation.

β-Aminoisobutyric Aciduria. Excessive excretion of β-aminoisobutyric acid (BAIB) is a genetic variant in metabolism in a small percentage of the normal population. In addition, β-aminoisobutyric aciduria occurs in a variety of illnesses in which there is tissue destruction and deoxyribonucleic acid is catabolized excessively. Beta-aminoisobutyric acid is a normal metabolite of both valine and thymine. Normal persons fed large amounts of β-aminoisobutyric acid can excrete it rapidly, which indicates that the renal tubular excretion of this compound is an adaptive process to an increased plasma level. In any case, increased excretion of β-aminoisobutyric acid is not evidence of a renal tubular defect since reabsorption in the tubules does not occur.

Affected persons with the congenital form are asymptomatic; they excrete 100–300 mg of β-aminoisobutyric acid daily, in contrast to 10–40 mg in normal persons. The condition is transmitted by a recessive gene.

8.16 LYSINE

Lysine is an essential amino acid that shares a common renal transport mechanism with other dibasic amino acids. Lysinuria has been observed in some children with malnutrition. There are at least 3 enzymopathies in which elevations of plasma lysine occur.

Lysinemia. Persistent lysinemia and lysinuria were originally described in a group of children with mental retardation and muscle weakness. As additional cases were detected and substantiated by appropriate enzyme analysis, many proved to be clinically normal children except for some with short stature.

Study of these patients has added to knowledge of the pathway of lysine degradation in man (Fig 8–10). One of the main routes of catabolism is the condensation of lysine with α-ketoglutaric acid to form the compound saccharopine. In patients with lysinemia, studies of cultured fibroblasts revealed marked reductions of activity of lysine ketoglutarate reductase, the enzyme which converts lysine to saccharopine. Minor pathways for lysine degradation have been shown; homocitrulline and homoarginine, pipecolic acid, and ε-N-acetyl-L-lysine and α-N-acetyl-L-lysine are formed and excreted. In those patients in whom the reductase was measured, all had reduced activity and the disease was attributed to the biochemical aberration at that step. More recently, in 8 patients with lysinemia studied in depth with analyses of fibroblasts and liver enzymes, all exhibited decreased saccharopine oxidoreductase (conversion of saccharopine to lysine) and saccharopine dehydrogenase activity (catabolism of lysine to saccharopine) in addition to the expected reduction of lysine-

ketoglutarate reductase activity. Lysinemia is an example of a single gene mutation producing multiple enzyme deficiencies in a patient. Analogous situations exist in maple syrup urine disease and orotic aciduria. In the former the oxidative-decarboxylation of the 3 branched-chain keto-acids is affected to the same extent despite evidence that the decarboxylases for the 3 ketoacids are distinct enzymes. In orotic aciduria (see Sec 14.13) 2 sequential steps are involved as the result of 1 defective gene.

The term saccharopinemia had previously been applied to a short, mentally retarded woman who had lysinuria, citrullinuria, homocitrullinemia, and saccharopinuria. Since it is now known that saccharopinuria is a common finding in lysinemia, the terminology for the complex of diseases has been changed to *lysinemia types I and II.* The former would apply to patients with major defects in both saccharopine dehydrogenase and lysine-ketoglutarate reductase activity, whereas the latter would designate those who retain significant lysine-ketoglutarate reductase activity.

α-Aminoadipic Acidemia. Two siblings were identified by screening who excreted large amounts of α-aminoadipic acid. There were multiple anomalies in the family, but no relationship could be made to the biochemical defect. One child had bony anomalies of the foot and a learning disability, but his sibling was normal. Since lysine loads increased the α-aminoadipic acid excretion, the block is presumed to be an inability to convert α-aminoadipic to α-ketoadipic acid.

α-Ketoadipic Acidemia. A 14 mo old with neonatal seizures, ichthyosis, and a mild metabolic acidosis was found to have elevated α-ketoadipic acid levels in her plasma and urine. She is now markedly retarded. Degradation studies in skin fibroblasts revealed a defect in the decarboxylation of α-ketoadipic to glutaric acid. Two additional siblings had similar metabolic findings. Though one was mentally retarded, the other was normal; there is thus doubt as to any relationship between the metabolic defect and the mental retardation.

Glutaric Acidemia. Glutaric acid is an intermediate in the degradation of lysine (Fig 8–10), hydroxylysine, and tryptophan (Fig 8–3). Two siblings with chronic metabolic acidosis and glutaric acidemia and aciduria were neurologically normal in infancy but later deteriorated with opisthotonos and posturing. Administration of lysine increased and lowering the protein intake reduced the excretion of glutaric acid. Leukocyte lysates were unable to metabolize glutaryl CoA, though oxidation of glutaric acid proceeded normally. Fibroblasts revealed a similar defect in glutaryl CoA oxidation. It is postulated that decreased glutaryl CoA dehydrogenase activity is responsible for the biochemical derangements in this disease. Other patients with a different form of glutaric acidemia have been described who also had hypoglycemia and metabolic acidosis and excreted many organic acids. This form, designated glutaric aciduria type II, represents multiple deficiencies of acyl-CoA dehydrogenase activity. Degradation of fatty acids as well as lysine is blocked.

Congenital Lysine Intolerance. This disorder was first observed in a 3 mo old infant who had episodes

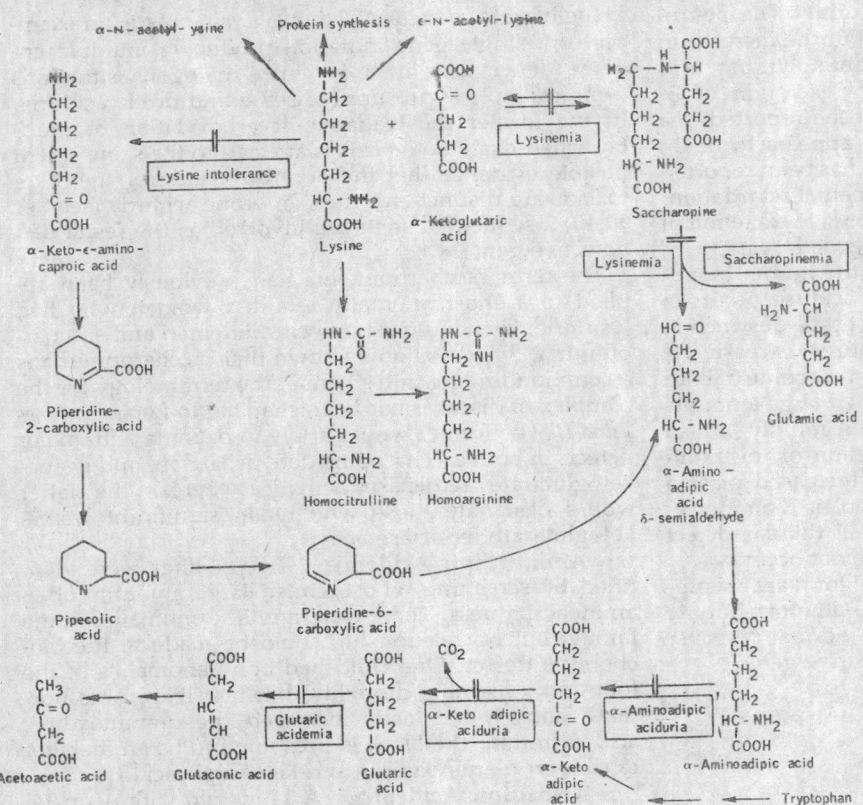

Figure 8-10 Pathways in the metabolism of lysine. See also legend for Fig 8-1.

of ammonia intoxication. With normal intake of protein, blood levels of lysine and arginine were normal, but when the protein intake was raised to 2.5–3 gm/kg/24 hr, plasma lysine, arginine, and ammonia levels increased to at least double their control values. The increases in arginine and ammonia were thought to be due to inhibition of arginase by lysine, with consequent inability to detoxify ammonia by the formation of urea. The administration of lysine orally depressed erythrocyte arginase activity and led to an increase of blood ammonia to 680 µg/dl and coma. There was a diminution in the activity of lysine dehydrogenase in liver; this enzyme converts lysine to α-keto-ε-aminocaproic acid (Fig 8–10).

A 2nd case, a 3 yr old child spastic at birth with frequent seizures, was found to have slight hyperammonemia and lysine intolerance. During a lysine load, blood arginine also rose dramatically.

Pipecolatemia. A single 18 mo old child with degenerative neurologic disease and hepatomegaly had marked elevations of pipecolic acid in his blood and cerebral tissue at autopsy. There was no defect in lysine metabolism and the site of the block remains obscure.

The experience with lysinemia, saccharopinemia, and lysine intolerance serves to point out how the study of inborn errors of metabolism contributes to knowledge of normal biochemical pathways. It was the studies of patients with these rare disorders that led to our present knowledge of the enzymatic steps involved in lysine metabolism.

Lysinuria (Hyperdibasicaminoaciduria). The dibasic amino acids (lysine, arginine, ornithine, and cystine) share a common transport mechanism in the intestine and kidney. Several genetic variants have been described that can affect the renal reabsorption of 1 or more of these dibasic amino acids. In cystinuria (Sec 8.5), all 4 amino acids are affected. Another group of patients who excrete lysine, arginine, and ornithine in excessive amounts have severe mental and physical retardation. Other mentally retarded individuals have been described with isolated defects of lysine transport or defects limited to lysine and arginine.

Lysinuric Protein Intolerance. This disorder, which has been studied in 20 Finnish patients, has much in common with 1 or more types of lysinuria described above. Earlier, this disorder was termed familial protein intolerance. The patients have an aversion to protein-rich foods, excrete large amounts of lysine and arginine, are physically retarded, and have low circulating levels of arginine, lysine, and ornithine. Some were mentally retarded. Hyperammonemia occurs particularly after high protein intake. Hepatomegaly, osteoporosis, and periods of diarrhea and vomiting have been noted in infancy. The hyperammonemia, which has been treated by the administration of arginine or ornithine, was not due to any demonstrable deficiency of enzymes of the urea cycle. The hyperammonemia stems from impairment of transport of arginine and ornithine from the gut into the hepatocyte, with diminished activity of the urea cycle because of inadequate substrate. Supplementation of the diet with citrulline has been quite beneficial by preventing hyperammonemia and improving the utilization of dietary proteins.

Hydroxylysinemia. At least 8 patients with a variety of symptoms (2 had trisomy 21) have been reported with hydroxylysinuria. As hydroxylysine is usually not detectable in plasma, the small amount found in the plasma of these patients indicates that the defect is not one of renal absorption. The nature of the defect, presumably in the degradation of free hydroxylysine, is not yet known.

Hydroxylysine-Deficient Collagen. Several patients with the clinical appearance of Ehlers-Danlos syndrome (q.v.) have been shown to have collagen with an abnormally low hydroxylysine content. Some patients exhibited severe scoliosis, joint laxity, hyperextensible skin, and thin scars, while another had, in addition, clubbed feet, retinal detachments, peptic ulcer, and hiatal hernia. The latter patient had a brother with the same clinical disorder. Measurements of the activity of the enzyme lysyl-protocollagen hydroxylase in cultured fibroblasts revealed approximately one eighth of the normal value. Another distinct form of Ehlers-Danlos

syndrome has the major complication of arterial rupture secondary to a type III collagen deficiency. At present there are at least 8 genetically separate variants of this syndrome. The biochemical defects have been delineated in 4 of them.

GRANT MORROW III
VICTOR H. AUERBACH

Bachmann C, Krähenbühl S, et al: N-Acetylglutamate synthetase deficiency: A disorder of ammonia detoxification. N Engl J Med 304:543, 1981.
Kaufman S: Differential diagnosis of variant forms of hyperphenylalaninemia. Pediatrics 65:840, 1980.
Larsson A, Mattsson B, et al: 5-Oxoprolinuria due to hereditary 5-oxoprolinase deficiency in two brothers—a new inborn error of the 8-glutamyl cycle. Acta Paediatr Scand 70:301, 1981.
Roth KS, Yang W, Forman JW, et al: Holocarboxylase synthetase deficiency. A biotin responsive organic acidemia. J Pediatr 96:845, 1980.
Smith I: The treatment of inborn errors of the urea cycle. Nature 291:378, 1981.
Wilcken B, Hammond JW, et al: Hawkinsinuria, a dominantly inherited defect of tyrosine metabolism with severe effects in infancy. N Engl J Med 305:865, 1981.

DEFECTS IN METABOLISM OF CARBOHYDRATES

8.17 INTESTINAL DEFECTS OF CARBOHYDRATE METABOLISM

Nutritional carbohydrates in man's diet include starch (the glucose polymers from plants) and glycogen (from animals), the disaccharides lactose and sucrose, and the monosaccharides glucose, galactose, and fructose.

There are 2 forms of starch: amylose and amylopectin. Amylose consists of α-1,4 linked glucose units that form straight chains. In amylopectin, the straight chains are branched by an α-1,6 linkage in about every 30th α-1,4 linked glucose unit. Glycogen averages 1 α-1,6 branch point per 10 α-1,4 linked glucose units.

Amylases in saliva and pancreatic juice hydrolyze starch and glycogen to maltose, maltotriose, and α-dextrin (isomaltose). Maltose consists of 2 glucose units joined in α-1,4 linkage. Maltotriose consists of 3 such units. Alpha-dextrin consists of several glucose units linked by an α-1,6 bond and a few α-1,4 linkages. In lactose, carbon 1 of galactose is attached to carbon 4 of glucose. The reducing end of the glucose unit, carbon 1, remains free. Thus lactose is a reducing sugar and gives a positive reaction with Clinitest but not with Testape. Strips of Testape, or of similar dipsticks such as Clinistix, contain glucose oxidase which acts on free glucose only. Clinitest tablets contain cupric sulfate that is converted to cuprous oxide by reducing substances.

The reducing sugars include glucose, maltose, maltotriose, and α-dextrin, but not sucrose. In sucrose, the reducing end of glucose is linked to that of fructose. Thus the reducing end of neither hexose is free to react, and sucrose is a nonreducing disaccharide.

The brush border of the intestinal villus cell exhibits the following hydrolytic activities (as demonstrated by hydrolysis of the substrates listed in parentheses): maltase (maltose, maltotriose), isomaltase (α-dextrin), lactase (lactose), and sucrase (sucrose). Glucose and galactose are actively transported across the intestinal epithelium. Hydrolysis or transport can be impaired either on a genetically determined (primary) basis or as the (secondary) consequence of another disease, such as infectious gastroenteritis or cystic fibrosis. In either case the clinical syndrome of malabsorption may develop. We are concerned here only with primary malabsorption (see also Sec 11.45).

A deficiency of maltase has not been reported. Deficiency states of the other 3 hydrolases and of the mechanism for glucose-galactose transport are here described briefly.

Sucrase-Isomaltase Deficiency

In patients with sucrase-isomaltase deficiency, chronic diarrhea and abdominal pain and discomfort occur when the diet contains sucrose (table sugar) or starch, i.e., with most solid foods. If this diet is replaced by one containing lactose, the symptoms disappear. Milk is tolerated well, as is glucose; but the usual "clear liquid diet" of water containing table sugar, fruit juices or carbonated beverages, and applesauce may aggravate the diarrhea. Oral administration of a test dose (1–2 gm/kg) of lactose, glucose, or galactose and of maltose produces a normal rise of blood sugar concentration. This is not observed after ingestion of sucrose, which may be followed by explosive diarrhea. Stool pH is low because lactic acid is formed by the bacterial fermentation of the unabsorbed carbohydrates. Lactic acid maintains diarrhea since it acts as an irritant and increases intraluminal intestinal osmolality.

Definite diagnosis depends on the demonstration of deficient activity of sucrase and isomaltase in a biopsy specimen of intestine. It is not known why both these enzymatic activities are defective together. Absence of steatorrhea and usually of villous atrophy serves to exclude celiac disease. Partial villous atrophy, if present, will revert to normal after a prolonged sucrose-free diet, as is provided by milk, meat, fish, fowl, eggs, animal fat, glucose, vegetables, and cheese.

Lactose Intolerance

This syndrome has been divided into 3 (at least) entities: familial lactose intolerance, congenital lactose intolerance, and late onset lactose intolerance.

Familial Lactose Intolerance. This is a rare and severe disorder, characterized by onset of vomiting after the initial feeding of milk or during the 1st few days of life. Intestinal lactase activity is normal. No enzymatic defect has been described.

Congenital Lactose Intolerance. Severe diarrhea, abdominal pain, and distention appear soon after birth when the diet begins to contain lactose. The symptoms disappear if milk is replaced by the usual "clear liquid diet." Steatorrhea is not an obligatory finding. Blood glucose concentrations increase normally after oral administration of glucose or galactose but not after lactose, which may induce explosive diarrhea, flatulence, and intestinal discomfort. Lactic acid produces an acid pH in stool and maintains the diarrhea.

Normal morphology is found in a biopsy specimen of the small intestine, with markedly deficient lactase activity. A lactose-free diet is effective as treatment.

Late Onset Lactose Intolerance. Clinical and pathologic observations are similar to those in congenital lactose intolerance except that the disorder may make its appearance gradually, beginning several yr after birth. People of northern European ancestry do not seem to be affected, whereas up to 90% of members of some other races may be affected. For example, 1 of 10 white and 7 of 10 black American adults develop moderate symptoms of lactase deficiency when challenged with oral lactose, either as milk or in a lactose tolerance test (the dose is not more than 50 gm of lactose, equivalent to 1 l of milk).

Children and adults may learn to adjust their diets so that the amount of dietary lactose is not greater than they can tolerate. It has been suggested that partial lactase deficiency accounts for the relative mildness of symptoms in many persons.

Glucose-Galactose Malabsorption

Inheritance of glucose-galactose malabsorption is autosomal recessive. The affected newborn develops se-vere diarrhea, abdominal distention, and discomfort after the 1st feeding of glucose water or milk. Symptoms are not relieved by formulas containing sucrose or maltose. Symptoms disappear if a carbohydrate-free (CHO-free) formula is fed that has been fortified with fructose. A normal rise in blood glucose concentration occurs after oral administration of fructose but not after lactose, glucose, or galactose.

The intestinal mucosa is normal morphologically, as is the activity of intestinal disaccharidases. The transport of glucose and galactose across the intestinal mucosa is thought to be defective.

Testing Procedures

Definitive diagnosis of intestinal hydrolase deficiency is made by measuring the specific enzymatic activity in the biopsy specimen. Techniques of peroral biopsy of intestinal mucosa and of hydrolase assay have become readily available. Their mastery requires some experience. There are, however, simple bedside tests for sugar intolerance that can be done on the liquid portion of a diarrheal stool. Immediately after collection, the liquid stool specimen is mixed with 2 volumes of water, and of this mixture, 15 drops are tested by Clinitest tablets for a presence of reducing sugars, and another drop is tested by Testape for the presence of glucose. A Clinitest reading of 0.5% or less is normal. Since sucrose is not a reducing sugar, it must be hydrolyzed prior to testing by boiling 1 part of liquid stool specimen in 2 parts of 0.1 N HCl for 2 min. After hydrolysis, the sucrose components, glucose and fructose, can be demonstrated by Clinitest.

In patients with sugar intolerance, the pH of the liquid stool specimen will likely be less than 6 and often less than 5.5 if there has been sufficient time for fermentation of the sugar by bacteria in the large bowel.

Peroral sugar tolerance tests are performed after several hr of fasting. The child drinks 50 gm/M^2 of body surface of the suspected sugar in a 10% solution. Normally the blood sugar concentration is expected to increase by 30 mg/dl or more within the following 2 hr; and, perhaps more reliably, liquid stool specimens should not indicate the (increased) presence of the administered sugar. In disaccharidase deficiency the unresponsive blood sugar curves observed following administration of the disaccharide may be found normal after an equivalent mixture of the respective monosaccharide moieties is ingested.

8.18   DEFECTS IN INTERMEDIARY CARBOHYDRATE METABOLISM

The intracellular conversion of glucose, fructose, and galactose proceeds as shown schematically in Fig 8–11, 8–13, and 8–14. Defects of the enzymes that are identified by name in the 3 figures have been associated with the disorders listed in Tables 8–5, 8–6, and 8–7.

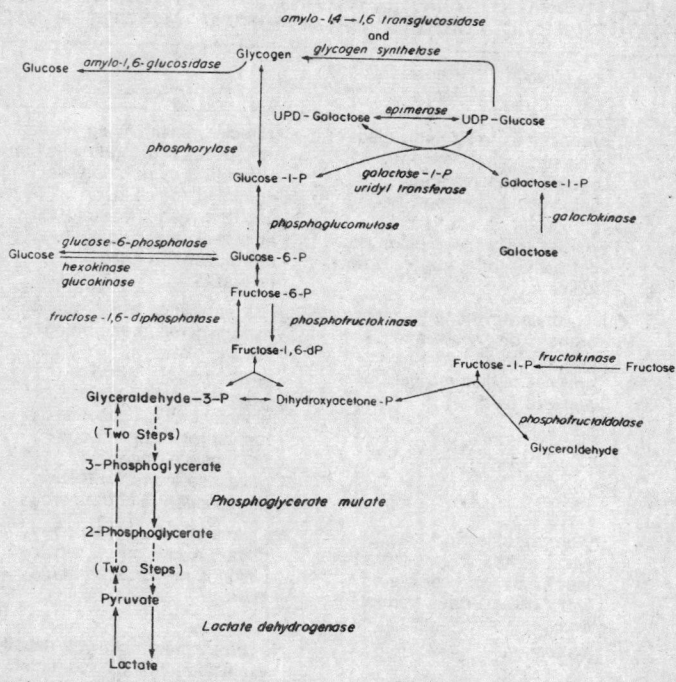

Figure 8–11 Pathway of cytoplasmic glycogen synthesis and degradation. Enzymes identified by name have been found deficient in diseases listed in Table 8–5.

An enzymatic defect affecting 1 tissue may not be demonstrable in another tissue for several reasons:

(1) The defective enzyme may normally be absent from muscle, as is glucose-6-phosphatase. Therefore, the deficiency of this enzyme in liver, kidney, and intestine of glycogen storage disease type I (GSD I) does not affect the skeletal muscle.

(2) An enzymatic activity may reflect several different enzyme proteins which are normal in muscle as is the case for glycogen synthetase, phosphorylase, or phosphorylase kinase. Thus the defective activities of these enzymes in the livers of GSD 0, GSD VI, or GSD IX do not affect their activity in skeletal muscle.

(3) There may not have been the opportunity to measure a defective activity in more than 1 tissue of the patient. Galactokinase deficiency of erythrocytes is likely to affect the liver. However, galactokinase has not been assayed in hepatic tissue of a patient with the defect of this enzyme in erythrocytes.

(4) An enzyme may not be effective in vivo although the usual assay indicates in vitro activity. This is the case in GSD Ib (pseudo-GSD I) that has the clinical and biochemical manifestations of GSD I except that in vitro activity of glucose-6-phosphatase in frozen liver specimens is normal.

(5) The enzymatic deficiency demonstrable in vitro may be the result of an artifact. For example, the activity of liver phosphorylase has been low or absent in autopsy tissue, even though it was normal in a premortem biopsy specimen.

Nonetheless, the demonstration of a defective enzyme activity must serve as the basis of diagnosis and therapy in inborn errors of metabolism.

8.19 DEFECTS WITHOUT LACTIC ACIDOSIS OR ABNORMAL GLYCOGEN STORAGE

DEFECTS IN METABOLISM OF GALACTOSE

See Table 8–5 and Fig 8–11.

Galactosemia: Deficiency of Galactokinase. This disorder is characterized by galactosemia, galactosuria, and cataracts without mental deficiency or aminoaciduria. Cataracts begin to form after birth when the diet contains galactose derived from the lactose in milk. By the time the diagnosis is made elimination of dietary galactose may come too late to reverse cataract formation, but possibly younger siblings of the patient may be helped; these should be tested at birth.

Galactokinase is responsible for the initial phosphorylation of galactose. In its absence, the ingestion of galactose leads to its increased concentration in blood and its excretion in urine as a reducing substance which is not glucose. Galactosuria can be identified by an enzymatic test specific for it. Urine specimens to be tested must be collected following the ingestion of a galactose-containing formula. If an affected infant were to receive glucose water for a substantial period prior to the urine collection, galactose would be absent from the urine and the diagnosis would be missed.

Postnatal institution of a galactose-free diet should prevent cataract formation. Since the children are otherwise normal, the prognosis can be good.

Definitive diagnosis is made when the erythrocytes are shown to be deficient in galactokinase activity. To date, other tissues have not been examined. The defect

Table 8–5 DEFECTS IN INTERMEDIARY CARBOHYDRATE METABOLISM WITHOUT LACTIC ACIDOSIS OR ABNORMAL GLYCOGEN STORAGE

ENZYME AFFECTED	TISSUE DISTRIBUTION OF DEFECT	SYMPTOMS AND SIGNS	COMMENTS
Galactokinase	Erythrocytes; presumably also liver (and other tissues) because administered galactose is not converted to glucose Feasibility of prenatal diagnosis not established; generally not indicated	Cataracts growing since infancy may become recognized when vision fails in an otherwise normal schoolchild; no hepatomegaly, hepatotoxicity, aminoaciduria, or mental retardation; prognosis favorable	Galactokinase has not yet been assayed in liver of patients; increased concentrations of galactose and galactitol (but not of galactose-1-phosphate); galactose or galactitol may produce cataracts
Galactose-1-phosphate uridyl transferase	Liver, erythrocytes, intestine; prenatal diagnosis is feasible and indicated, with enzyme analysis of cultured cells of amniotic fluid	Onset at birth or later; vomiting, hypoglycemia, hepatomegaly, hepatic cirrhosis, splenomegaly, jaundice, cataracts, aminoaciduria, galactosuria, glucosuria, mental retardation; poor prognosis if untreated; galactose tolerance test unnecessary and dangerous	Increased intracellular concentration of galactose-1-phosphate and galactitol; galactose-1-phosphate responsible for hepatotoxicity and mental retardation, and galactitol for cataracts
Uridyl diphosphate galactose 4-epimerase	Erythrocytes, leukocytes, lymphocytes; liver, cultured fibroblasts, and stimulated lymphoblasts have normal enzyme activity	No signs of disease; no need for dietary exclusion of galactose, which is metabolized in the liver	Condition discovered during neonatal screening, since erythrocytic galactose-1-phosphate concentration elevated
Fructokinase	Liver, kidney, intestine	No symptoms; fructosuria usually an incidental finding; affected individuals healthy	Also known as benign or essential fructosuria; Testape (= glucose oxidase) negative, Clinitest positive; urine must not be basis for incorrect diagnosis of diabetes mellitus
1-Phosphofructaldolase	Liver, kidney, intestine; prenatal diagnosis not established	Hepatomegaly and hepatic cirrhosis; vomiting and hypoglycemia after fructose ingestion; aminoaciduria; prognosis fair to good with dietary elimination of fructose; fructose tolerance test not necessary for diagnosis, and may produce irreversible coma, especially in infants and young children	Also called hereditary fructose intolerance; leukocytes and erythrocytes not involved (they normally lack 1-phosphofructaldolase); heterogeneity suggested by fact that some patients may die in infancy whereas others do well on similar management
Phosphoglycerate mutase (M unit)	Muscle	Myoglobinuria, muscle pain, exercise intolerance	Only muscle isozyme is deficient (Type MM); brain isozyme (Type BB) is present
Lactate dehydrogenase (M unit)	Muscle, RBC, WBC	Myoglobinuria, easily fatigued after exercise	M isozyme subunit absent, H isozyme present

may be presumed to involve the liver since the hepatocyte is the normal site of metabolism of galactose. Some of the excessive galactose overflows into the urine; some is converted into galactitol, which may be responsible for the cataract formation. The level of activity of erythrocyte galactokinase is below the limits of measurement in the patient; heterozygous parents and siblings have intermediate activity values. Inheritance is autosomal recessive. The incidence of the condition is about 1 in 40,000.

Galactosemia: Deficiency of Galactose-1-Phosphate Uridyl Transferase. "Classic" galactosemia is a serious disease with early onset of symptoms. The newborn infant normally receives up to 20% of caloric intake from the disaccharide lactose, which consists of glucose and galactose. Without the transferase the infant is unable to metabolize galactose-1-phosphate. The accumulation of the latter is injurious to the affected infant and is thought by some to be able to do damage in utero, as it may be elevated in the heterozygous mother's blood and may cross the placenta.

Uridyl transferase deficiency should be considered in newborn infants or older infants or children with any of the following symptoms: jaundice, hepatomegaly, vomiting, hypoglycemia, convulsions, lethargy, irritability, feeding difficulties, poor weight gain, aminoaciduria, cataracts, hepatic cirrhosis, ascites, splenomegaly, or mental retardation. When the diagnosis is not made at birth, damage to the liver (cirrhosis) and brain (mental retardation) becomes increasingly severe and irreversible. It is therefore important that galactosemia be considered for the newborn or young infant who is not thriving or who presents any of the above findings.

Since galactose is injurious for persons with galactosemia, diagnostic tests employing administration of galactose either by mouth or intravenously cannot be used. Though galactose tolerance tests are diagnostic, they result in high concentrations of intracellular galactose-1-phosphate, which can function as a competitive inhibitor of phosphoglucomutase. This inhibition impairs the conversion of glycogen to glucose transiently and produces hypoglycemia, which may be severe after administration of galactose as a test and which is observed in some patients on a diet containing normal amounts of lactose. Galactose-1-phosphate is responsible for hepatotoxicity and mental retardation but not for cataracts. Deficiency of either galactokinase or uridyl transferase produces elevations of galactitol.

Examination by light and electron microscopy of hepatic tissue reveals fatty infiltration, the formation of pseudoacini, and eventual macronodular cirrhosis. These changes are consistent with a metabolic disease; they do not indicate the precise enzymatic defect.

The preliminary diagnosis of galactosemia is made by the demonstration of a reducing substance in several urine specimens collected while the patient is receiving human or cow's milk or another formula containing lactose. The reducing substance found in urine by use of Clinitest or some similar procedure can be identified definitively by chromatography or by an enzymatic test specific for galactose. Examination of the patient's urine with Clinistix or Testape can show only that the reducing substance is not glucose since these test materials rely on the action of glucose oxidase, which is specific for glucose and nonreactive with galactose. The enzymatic defect is easily demonstrable in erythrocytes, which also exhibit increased concentrations of galactose-1-phosphate. Heterogeneity in the genetic defect is manifested by partial enzymatic defects, now being found with increasing frequency. In the complete absence of uridyl transferase activity, very small amounts of galactose may still be metabolized by alternate pathways. These pathways are of no clinical significance in most patients.

Prenatal diagnosis of defective galactose-1-phosphate uridyl transferase has been accomplished by examination of cultured amniotic fluid cells. Inheritance is autosomal recessive. The incidence of the disease is 1 in 50,000.

The term *galactosemia*, though adequate for the deficiencies of both galactokinase and uridyl transferase, generally designates the latter, for historical reasons.

An occasional infant with galactosemia may tolerate an unexpected amount of food containing lactose, but this is rare. As a rule, galactose must be excluded from the diet early in life to avoid severe cirrhosis of the liver, mental retardation, cataracts, and recurrent hypoglycemia. With good dietary control the prognosis is generally good.

Deficiency of Uridyl Diphosphogalactose 4-Epimerase. This defect is an incidental finding in an otherwise healthy individual. There are no known clinical abnormalities. The liver is not enlarged, nor are there cataracts or abnormal neurologic findings. Growth and development are normal on an unrestricted normal diet.

The initial patient was discovered during a newborn screening program that registered the increased concentration of galactose-1-phosphate in the child's erythrocytes. The activity of galactokinase and of uridyl transferase in erythrocytes was normal. There are at least 8 affected individuals known in 3 different families. Inheritance is autosomal recessive.

The epimerase deficiency affects leukocytes, lymphocytes, and erythrocytes. The normal epimerase activity in tissues other than blood cells of these patients, although less stable, may explain the normal tolerance tests for galactose and the absence of clinical symptoms.

No treatment is indicated, although the initial patient's diet contained galactose.

DEFECTS IN METABOLISM OF FRUCTOSE

See also Sec 8.20.

Deficiency of Fructokinase (Benign Fructosuria). This condition is not associated with any signs of disease. It is an incidental finding usually made because the asymptomatic patient's urine contains a reducing substance. No treatment is necessary. Inheritance is autosomal recessive. Incidence is 1 in 120,000.

Fructokinase deficiency is present in liver, intestine, and kidney. Ingested fructose is not metabolized. Its level is increased in the blood, and it is excreted in urine, there being practically no renal threshold for fructose. Positive Clinitest tests and negative Clinistix tests reveal the urinary reducing substance not to be glucose. It can be identified definitively by chromatography.

Deficiency of 1-Phosphofructaldolase (Hereditary Fructose Intolerance). This severe disease of infants makes its appearance with the ingestion of fructose-containing food. Either fructose or sucrose (table sugar), the disaccharide of glucose and fructose, may be added as a sweetener to baby foods or formulas. Symptoms may occur quite early in life, perhaps soon after birth if foods or formulas containing sucrose or fructose are then introduced into the diet. With early appearance the symptoms may resemble those of galactosemia and include jaundice, hepatomegaly, vomiting, lethargy, irritability, and convulsions. A reducing substance in urine which is not glucose can be identified as fructose by chromatography.

The deficiency of 1-phosphofructaldolase is practically complete in the liver. Fructose-1-phosphate accumulates in hepatocytes and can act as a competitive inhibitor for phosphorylase in concentrations similar to those of intracellular glucose-1-phosphate. The resulting transient inhibition of the conversion of glycogen to glucose leads to severe hypoglycemia. Some affected children show severe reduction in the hepatic conversion of fructose-1,6-diphosphate to the 2 appropriate trioses, in addition to the expected effects of deficiency of 1-phosphofructaldolase on the metabolism of fructose-1-phosphate. The latter effects may be eliminated by dietary elimination of fructose, but the cleavage of fructose-1,6-diphosphate is a major step in the pathway for glycogen degradation.

Perhaps it is a severe reduction in the activity of 1,6-diphosphofructaldolase that in some children results in progressive liver disease. This progression may occur despite a diet free of fructose in patients who appear

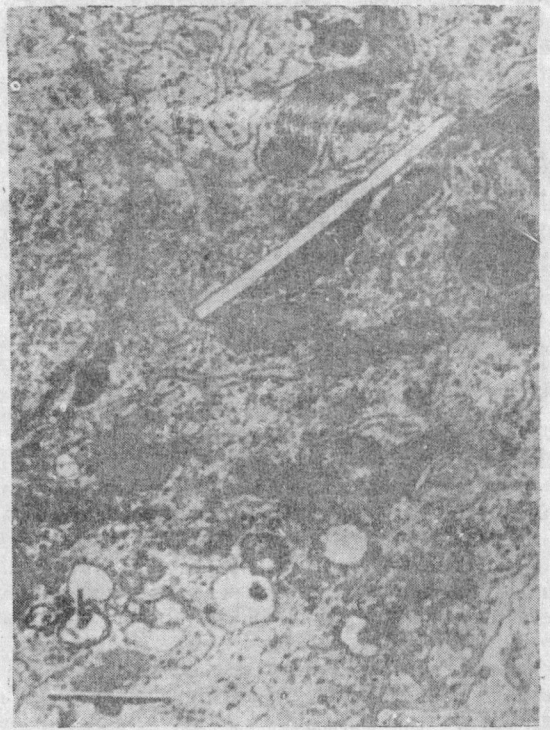

Figure 8–12   Liver biopsy specimen in phosphofructaldolase deficiency. Alpha-glycogen particles (g) are typical for liver tissue; they are scarce here. The circles surround individual α-particles. Lysosomes (L) are abundant. Unusual "crystals" (C) are seen regularly. M, mitochondria; N, nucleus. (Bar: 2 μm.)

clinically well except for hepatomegaly and elevated levels of serum transaminases. Successive biopsy specimens indicate increasing fatty infiltration and fibrosis, with focal cytoplasmic dissolution, an abnormal appearance of glycogen and mitochondria, and unusual plate-like and needle-like crystals in hepatocytes (Fig 8–12). The prognosis of fructose intolerance must be

guarded in some patients, even with good dietary control. Without such control, the disease can result in death during infancy or early childhood.

Fructose tolerance tests are contraindicated since they may be followed by hypoglycemia, shock, and death. Fructose must be eliminated completely from the diet. This may be difficult since fructose is a widely used additive, found even in some aspirin preparations. Some infants with hereditary fructose intolerance show fewer and relatively milder symptoms. Inheritance is autosomal recessive. Incidence (including a mild form in adults) is about 1 in 40,000.

Deficient Muscle Phosphoglycerate Mutase. This deficiency has been described in an adult who, although otherwise healthy, exhibited myoglobinuria and cramps after exercise. The patient was not able to increase lactic acid concentration after ischemic exercise, and examination of a muscle biopsy showed normal glycogen levels and normal levels for all the enzymes measured except for phosphoglycerate mutase. The small amount of activity of this enzyme was shown to be due to the presence of small normal amounts of the B (brain type) isozyme. The M (muscle type) isozyme was absent.

Deficient Muscle Type Lactate Dehydrogenase. A family has been described in which many members are unable to synthesize the M unit of lactate dehydrogenase (LDH). They still possess the ability to make the H unit of the enzyme. Thus in amounts of subtypes H4, H2M2, and M4, members of this family have only the H4 isozyme. The defect is inherited as an autosomal recessive and has been shown to reside on chromosome No. 11.

The propositus' main complaint was fatigue after strenuous exercise. He had myoglobinuria during such episodes and had slightly below normal activity of erythrocyte LDH with a disproportionately high ratio of creatine kinase to LDH activity. Ischemic work resulted in venous lactate levels below those of control subjects. However, his venous level of pyruvate was at least twice that of normal controls. Patients with deficient M type lactate dehydrogenase can convert muscle

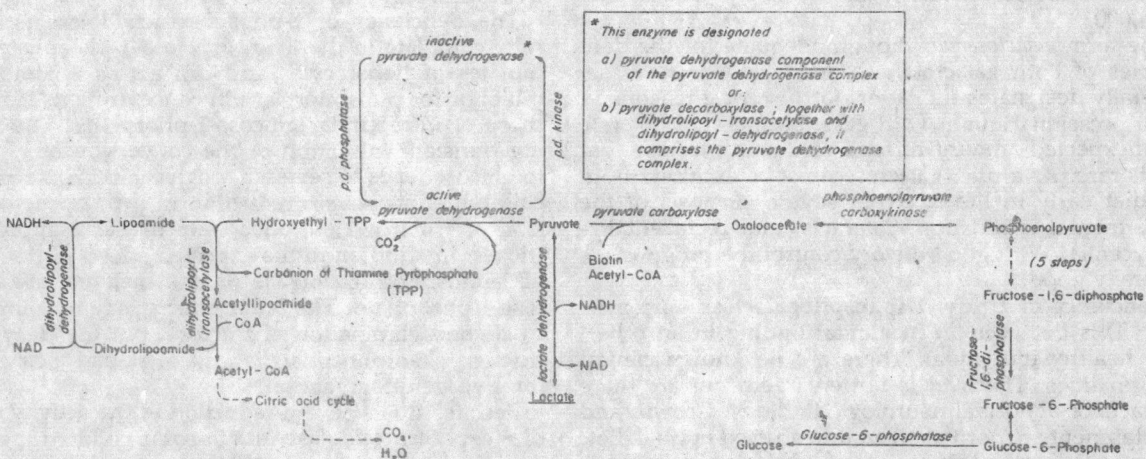

Figure 8–13   Enzymatic reactions of carbohydrate metabolism, deficiencies of which may give rise to lactic acidosis, pyruvate elevations, and/or hypoglycemia. Enzymes identified by name have been found deficient in diseases listed in Table 8–6.

glycogen to pyruvate, which is then released into the bloodstream rather than converted to lactate. Why this defect also results in damage to muscle tissue and easy fatigability remains to be elucidated.

8.20 DEFECTS IN INTERMEDIARY CARBOHYDRATE METABOLISM ASSOCIATED WITH LACTIC ACIDOSIS

The defects in carbohydrate metabolism associated with lactic acidosis are listed in Table 8–6; Fig 8–13 depicts the relevant metabolic pathways.

The normal concentration of lactic acid in blood is less than 18 mg/dl or 2 mM. Hyperlactic acidemia unrelated to an enzymatic defect occurs in hypoxemia. In this case the serum concentration of pyruvic acid may remain normal (<1.0 mg/dl), whereas it is usually increased when hyperlactic acidemia is the result of an enzymatic defect. It is useful, therefore, to measure lactic *and* pyruvic acid in the same blood specimen. These measurements should be made on multiple blood specimens obtained during a period of time when the patient is symptomatic since dramatic and ultimately fatal hyperlactic acidemia can be intermittent.

Hyperlactic acidemia occurs with those defects of carbohydrate metabolism that interfere with the conversion of pyruvate to glucose via the pathway of gluconeogenesis or to CO_2 and water via the mitochondrial enzymes of the citric acid cycle. Recognition of these defects depends on identification of hyperlactic acidemia. The concentration of blood lactic acid should be determined in infants and children with unexplained acidosis, especially if the anion gap in blood is greater than 16 mM. The anion gap is the difference between

Table 8–6 DEFECTS IN INTERMEDIARY CARBOHYDRATE METABOLISM ASSOCIATED WITH LACTIC ACIDOSIS

ENZYME AFFECTED	TISSUE DISTRIBUTION OF DEFECT	SYMPTOMS AND SIGNS	COMMENTS
Glucose-6-phosphatase	Liver, kidney, intestine	Lactic acidosis, hypoglycemia, tendency for hepatoma in later life (see Table 8–7)	Treatment (if necessary) by frequent small meals or by continuous night-time feeding, not by portacaval shunt and not by phenytoin or phenobarbital administration (see Table 8–7)
Fructose-1,6-diphosphatase	Liver	Infants with hypoglycemia, hyperventilation, convulsion, shock, elevated blood lactate, hepatomegaly; oral galactose converted to glucose; no conversion of fructose, alanine, or glycerol, which produce hyperlacticacidemia; may be fatal	Severe fatty infiltration of hepatocytes; hypoglycemia after oral fructose or glycerol (avoid such tolerance tests); hepatic glycogen concentration reduced to <1.4%; on diet free of fructose and sorbitol, mental and physical development will be normal
Pyruvate dehydrogenase component of the *pyruvate dehydrogenase complex;* or 1st enzyme (E_1) of the pyruvate dehydrogenase complex; or pyruvate decarboxylase	Liver, brain, white blood cells, cultured skin fibroblasts	Neurologic abnormalities from birth; increased blood concentration of pyruvate and lactate; death in infancy or Intermittent neurologic signs (ataxia, choreoathetosis); elevated blood lactate and pyruvate; normal psychomotor behavior and intelligence between attacks	In a patient with severe signs at birth who died at 6 mo, the enzymatic defect was complete; partial defect in an unrelated 9 yr old boy with intermittent symptoms, who was normal between attacks
Dihydrolipoyl-transacetylase; or 2nd enzyme (E_2) of the pyruvate dehydrogenase complex	Cultured skin fibroblasts (no other tissues analyzed)	Severe retardation; minimal blood pyruvate and lactate elevation; severe lactic acidosis on diet low in fat and high in carbohydrates	Data derived from cultures of skin fibroblasts in 1 patient suggest deficient activity of dihydrolipoyl transacetylase (not measured directly)
Dihydrolipoyl-dehydrogenase; or 3rd enzyme (E_3) of the pyruvate dehydrogenase complex	Liver, muscle, brain, kidney and "all tissues measured"; feasibility of prenatal diagnosis not established	In a male infant of consanguineous parents: at 2 mo of age, lethargy, hypertonia, optic atrophy, laryngeal stridor; twice normal blood pyruvate, lactate, and α-ketoglutarate concentration; not responsive to thiamine or dietary fat; death at 7 mo. In an unrelated 3 yr old girl of consanguineous marriage with severe neurologic disease, lactic acidosis, optic atrophy, and muscular hypotonia may have existed	Dihydrolipoyl-dehydrogenase can function in vitro as the 3rd component of the α-ketoglutarate dehydrogenase complex; simultaneously deficient activity of both dehydrogenase complexes may indicate that their 3rd components are similar, if not identical

Table continued on following page

Table 8-6   DEFECTS IN INTERMEDIARY CARBOHYDRATE METABOLISM ASSOCIATED WITH LACTIC ACIDOSIS (Continued)

ENZYME AFFECTED	TISSUE DISTRIBUTION OF DEFECT	SYMPTOMS AND SIGNS	COMMENTS
Pyruvate carboxylase	Liver	In an 11 mo old boy, anorexia, vomiting, lethargy, retardation, elevation of blood lactate and pyruvate	Complete loss of activity of enzyme in liver; enzyme was not found in *normal* control leukocytes or in skin fibroblasts
		In an unrelated newborn girl, hypoglycemia, psychomotor retardation, increased blood concentration of pyruvate, lactate, and alanine; symptoms aggravated by high carbohydrate diet, ACTH, or anorexia, but controlled by a diet low in carbohydrate and protein, or by thiamine or by both	Total liver enzyme activity in this patient reduced by less than 50%; the result of complete loss of 1 of 2 "isoenzymes"
Pyruvate dehydrogenase phosphatase	Liver, muscle, not brain	In a newborn male, lactic acidosis, blood elevation of pyruvate, free fatty acid, alanine, ketone bodies; lethargy, irritability, generalized seizures, death at 6 mo	Incubation of liver of patient with ATP deactivates pyruvate dehydrogenase in normal manner; enzyme not reactivated under conditions effective in controls
Congenital idiopathic lactic acidosis (no demonstrated enzyme defect)	Patients with this diagnosis usually have not had biochemical studies appropriate to all of the enzyme defects listed in this table	Convulsions, lethargy, hyperventilation, ataxia, vomiting, psychomotor retardation, muscular weakness, hypoglycemia, eye abnormalities, hepatomegaly; death in infancy or childhood, or intermittent attacks compatible with life	Diagnosis of "idiopathic lactic acidosis" requires demonstration that pyruvate dehydrogenase complex and gluconeogenic enzymes are normal; most patients so diagnosed have been incompletely studied
Leigh subacute necrotizing encephalopathy (SNE)	No enzyme defect consistently demonstrated as yet; total deficiency of liver pyruvate carboxylase in 1 patient (the 1st patient described in this table as having "pyruvate carboxylase deficiency")	Convulsions, lethargy, vomiting, psychomotor retardation, muscular weakness, blindness, etc.; fatal in infancy or longer lasting (some adults); symptoms do not distinguish SNE with certainty from several other entries in this table; an inhibitor in blood, CSF, and urine for thiamine pyrophosphate — adenosine triphosphate phosphoryl transferase (which catalyzes the reaction TPP + ATP ↔ TTP + ADP)	Comments on "congenital idiopathic lactic acidosis" apply; SNE and pyruvate carboxylase deficiency and "pyruvate dehydrogenase phosphatase deficiency showing cavitation and demyelination of basal ganglia" similar in autopsy findings in brain; the inhibitor is found in up to 10% of normal persons (significance uncertain)

the sum of the serum concentrations of cations (Na⁺, K⁺) and that of anions (Cl⁻, HCO₃⁻). An abnormally large anion gap may indicate abnormal levels of keto-acids, salicylates, lactate, or other organic acids.

Deficiency of Glucose-6-Phosphatase. Glycogen storage disease type I (GSD I) is the only 1 of the 12 types of glycogenosis that is associated with significant lactic acidosis. In most patients the resultant recurrent metabolic acidosis appears to be of minor clinical importance, but in some children with GSD I recurrent lactic acidosis is a life-threatening condition. GSD I is further discussed in Sec 8.21.

Deficiency of Fructose-1,6-Diphosphatase. Infants with this condition are free of symptoms as long as their diet is limited to human milk. If they receive formulas or food containing fructose or sucrose, they develop intermittent attacks of hypoglycemia, shock, coma, convulsions, and a metabolic acidosis due to

hyperlactic acidemia. In symptom-free intervals, physical examination may be normal except for hepatomegaly. If untreated, the disease can lead to psychomotor retardation or death. Inheritance is autosomal recessive.

Fructose-1,6-diphosphatase is 1 of the 4 key enzymes of gluconeogenesis. Its activity is markedly reduced or not detectable in hepatic biopsy specimens, which show fatty infiltration and have a reduced glycogen concentration. Other enzymes of fructose metabolism, gluconeogenesis, or glycogen degradation are normal. The normal increase in blood glucose concentration after glucagon administration is found after 6 hr of fasting but not after 18 hr. This may indicate rapid exhaustion of stores of liver glycogen. Galactose given by mouth or intravenously produces a normal increase in concentration of blood glucose, but fructose, glycerol, and alanine do not increase; the latter substances may produce acute hypoglycemia and lactic acidosis, and tolerance tests using them should be avoided. Fasting for 18–20 hr may cause hypoglycemia and lactic acidosis. The picture may resemble "ketotic hypoglycemia." Untreated fructose-1,6-diphosphatase deficiency is a serious disease with a poor prognosis. Growth and development are normal if the diet is kept free of fructose, sucrose, and sorbitol and reasonably restricted in fat and protein.

Deficiency of Pyruvate Decarboxylase. This enzyme has also been designated the pyruvate dehydrogenase component or the 1st enzyme (E_1) of the *pyruvate dehydrogenase complex*. No detectable activity of this enzyme was identified in a 1.3 kg newborn boy of 35 wk gestation who had rapid respirations and "several neurologic signs." Plasma concentrations of pyruvate and lactate were high. The patient died at 6 mo of age despite attempts at dietary control. In contrast, a 9 yr old boy had 20% of normal activity in cultured skin fibroblasts and white cells. He suffered intermittent episodes of cerebellar dysfunction and choreoathetoid movements, which began at 16 mo of age, occurred from 2–6 times a year, lasted a few hr to over 1 wk, and seemed to be triggered by febrile illnesses or other stresses. The episodes ranged in severity from generalized clumsiness to such severe incapacitation because of ataxia that locomotion was possible only by crawling. Serum concentrations of pyruvate, lactate, and alanine were moderately elevated during attacks, but normal between them, as was clinical appearance. Intelligence was normal. Dexamethasone relieved attacks but did not correct the blood chemical abnormalities.

Deficiency of Dihydrolipoyl Transacetylase. This enzyme is designated the 2nd enzyme (E_2) in the *pyruvate dehydrogenase complex*. The 1 reported patient who might have had this defect was a 9 yr old boy with profound motor and mental retardation. Blood concentrations of pyruvate and lactate were normal when the patient was fasting, but rose to twice the level of controls by 2 hr after a normal meal. A diet high in carbohydrates but not fat (65% and 15%, respectively) precipitated severe lactic acidosis. Dietary thiamine had no effect. Two sisters of the patient had died with severe lactic acidosis; their brains were severely deficient in myelin, but there were no signs of active demyelination. The boy's cultured skin fibroblasts had reduced activity of the pyruvate dehydrogenase complex; activity of pyruvate decarboxylase was normal. Since the α-keto glutarate dehydrogenase complex was not defective and since there is evidence that this complex includes an enzyme similar if not identical to E_3 of the pyruvate dehydrogenase complex, it can be assumed that E_2 of the complex, or dihydrolipoyl transacetylase, may have been defective in the boy's cultured fibroblasts and by inference in other tissues as well.

Deficiency of Dihydrolipoyl Dehydrogenase. This enzyme is designated also as the 3rd enzyme (E_3) of the *pyruvate dehydrogenase complex*. A deficiency was found in a 2 mo old boy of consanguineous parents; he had lethargy, hypertonia, irritability, optic atrophy, laryngeal stridor, irregular respirations, and metabolic acidosis, with episodes of hypoglycemia relieved by alanine. Blood concentrations of pyruvate, lactate, and α-keto glutarate were twice normal. Diets high in thiamine

or fat did not correct the hyperlactic acidemia. Death occurred at 7 mo of age.

Liver, muscle, brain, and kidney of the 1st patient showed only 10% of normal activity of the pyruvate dehydrogenase complex and of the α-keto glutarate dehydrogenase complex. The deficiency of activity in both complexes in the same patient suggested that the defect might reside in E_3, the activity of which is shared by both complexes. It was then demonstrated that the tissue of the boy had only 5% of normal activity of dihydrolipoyl dehydrogenase component (E_3). Pyruvate dehydrogenase component E_1 was normal. Examination of the brain at autopsy disclosed cavitation and lack of myelination in basal ganglia, thalamus, and brain stem, which resembled the findings of Leigh syndrome; the observation underscores the importance of precise enzymatic diagnosis.

An unrelated 3 yr old girl, also of consanguineous parents, had a similar severe illness, with signs including optic atrophy, muscular hypotonia, hyperactive reflexes, and spasticity of the lower extremities. There was a persistent lactic acidosis. High fat diet and thiamine supplementation were not helpful. Liver function tests were normal. Skin fibroblasts had deficient activity of pyruvate dehydrogenase complex, though not of E_1. A partial defect of the tricarboxylic cycle was also present. This might be consistent with the interpretation that defective E_3 impaired the activity of both the pyruvate dehydrogenase and the α-keto glutarate dehydrogenase complexes. This interpretation has not, however, been confirmed by the direct assay of E_3.

Deficiency of Pyruvate Carboxylase. This deficiency was 1st reported in a boy who was well until 4 mo of age. Three of 6 siblings had died with progressive psychomotor retardation. By 11 mo this patient showed vomiting, irritability, lethargy, and motor and mental retardation, with hypotonia, abnormal eye movements, and twice normal concentrations of lactate and pyruvate in serum.

An unrelated 2nd patient had no abnormal clinical signs during the 1st yr of life. An older brother had died of Leigh syndrome, as indicated by clinical findings and examination of the brain at autopsy. At 7 mo of age the level of protein in the patient's cerebrospinal fluid was elevated, and by 12 mo he had a persistently increased concentration of lactate in serum; during the 2nd yr of life he developed psychomotor retardation, hypotonia, hyporeflexia, abnormal eye movements, optic atrophy, and ataxia. Death occurred at 38 mo with autopsy findings typical of Leigh syndrome. Therapy with thiamine, biotin, and lipoic acid had no effect.

In a 3rd patient psychomotor retardation began at 3 mo of age; by 14 mo the patient had convulsions and hypertonia, had no head control, could not sit, and had no social interaction with her environment. Serum levels of lactate, pyruvate, and alanine were elevated. An extract of urine inhibited thiamine pyrophosphate–adenosine triphosphate phosphoryl transferase. On electron microscopy, glycogen appeared increased in liver and muscle of the 3rd patient. The size of the liver was normal, and there was a normal increase of blood glucose concentration following glucagon administration.

A 4th patient, an infant girl, had hypoglycemia; serum elevations of lactate, pyruvate, and alanine; and severe psychomotor retardation. Therapy with thiamine prevented episodes of acute metabolic acidosis for several yr, but psychomotor retardation remained.

The 1st 3 patients, all of whom had been thought to have Leigh syndrome, were shown to have pyruvate carboxylase deficiency. The 1st and 3rd children showed the defect in biopsy specimens of liver, whereas the 2nd patient had normal activity in a biopsy during life but not in a liver specimen examined at autopsy. The 4th patient was shown to have a deficiency of 1 of 2 different pyruvate carboxylases in liver, a deficiency of the one with a low K_m producing a partial defect of hepatic enzymatic activity. Activities of the 3 other key gluconeogenic enzymes were normal in tissue specimens of these 4 patients. Thiamine partially controlled the biochemical defect in the 3rd and 4th patients; in none of them did such therapy improve the clinical outcome.

Deficiency of Pyruvate Dehydrogenase Phosphatase. This deficiency has been found in a newborn boy who presented a metabolic acidosis with high serum concentrations of lactate (up to 7 times normal), of pyruvate (twice normal), and of free fatty acids (3 times normal). There was no hypoglycemia or hepatomegaly. The acidosis improved when the intake of glucose was increased and that of fat decreased. Periods of clinical stability and moderate hyperlactic acidemia were interrupted every few days by episodes of severe lactic acidosis. Neurologic damage was evident, with lethargy, convulsions, hypotonia, and irritability. The patient died at 6 mo of age.

The pyruvate dehydrogenase component F_1 of the pyruvate dehydrogenase complex exists in an active and in an inactive form. E_1 is inactivated when it is phosphorylated by pyruvate dehydrogenase kinase in the presence of ATP. E_1 is activated when it is dephosphorylated by pyruvate dehydrogenase phosphatase, which is stimulated by calcium. Pyruvate dehydrogenase phosphatase activity was reported deficient in liver and muscle but not brain of the described infant boy. The report was based on the observation that the addition of calcium to a homogenate of liver increased the activity of pyruvate decarboxylase in the patient by 4% and in a control by 50%. Deficiency of this activating phosphatase has been reported in another 7 mo old boy in whom brain autopsy findings were consistent with Leigh syndrome.

Carnitine Deficiency Syndrome (see also Sec. 8.28). This can present with recurrent attacks of severe metabolic acidosis (hyperlacticacidemia), hypoglycemia, and hepatomegaly. Carnitine concentration is reduced in serum, muscle, and liver. Cardiomegaly may be present. Untreated the patient may die during such a crisis, but correction of the acidosis and, in particular, the prompt intravenous administration of sufficient amounts of glucose will terminate the crisis, usually within 12–24 hr. Administration of DL-carnitine is without demonstrable benefit and may be harmful in acute episodes; it may be useful in chronic treatment.

Congenital Idiopathic Lactic Acidosis. This diagnosis may be considered when there is labored respiration in infancy associated with metabolic acidosis and hyperlactic acidemia. Liver and spleen may be enlarged. Convulsions, hypoglycemia, psychomotor retardation, and neurologic damage usually lead to death in infancy despite dietary administration of thiamine, biotin, steroids, lipoic acid, and other agents. Long-term survival in a few instances is possible.

There are increased serum concentrations of pyruvate, lactate, and alanine, as well as of other amino acids. Cerebral autopsy findings may show severe spongy degeneration and lack of myelination, or there may be only moderate or mild abnormalities.

A variety of deficiencies in enzymatic activities, including those reported above, may lead to lactic acidosis. In patients who have not been examined in a systematic way with exclusion of the defects described above, the diagnosis of congenital idiopathic lactic acidosis should probably not be used as though it described a discrete entity.

Leigh Subacute Necrotizing Encephalopathy (SNE). This condition is marked by seizures, psychomotor retardation, optic atrophy, hypotonia, vomiting, abnormal movements, lethargy, and lactic acidosis. It is difficult to distinguish this syndrome reliably from many of the enzymatic deficiencies that are associated with lactic acidosis. Gliosis, cavitation, and capillary proliferation in brain stem, basal ganglia, and thalamus are seen. These lesions may be visible on CT scan. Similar lesions viewed as characteristic have been encountered in patients shown to have pyruvate carboxylase deficiency, or, in 1 case, defective pyruvate decarboxylase activity in skin fibroblasts. Another boy with SNE by brain autopsy also had deficiency of pyruvate dehydrogenase phosphatase. The assessment of patients presenting symptoms and signs consistent with Leigh syndrome must include assays of those enzymatic activities, the deficiency of which results in lactic acidosis. These activities were normal in a 22 mo old boy who had the cerebral findings of Leigh syndrome associated with increased concentration of endorphin and norepinephrine in CSF and of enkephalins in cerebral cortex.

Thiamine is transiently effective in some patients with Leigh syndrome, but not in others. The use of thiamine was suggested by the report that extracts of blood, cerebrospinal fluid, and urine of patients with SNE inhibited thiamine pyrophosphate–adenosine triphosphate phosphoryl transferase. Thiamine in pharmacologic doses might have overridden this inhibitor, which is reported to be found in the urine of as many as 10% of clinically normal persons. For further discussion see Sec 21.17.

Attempts have been made to correct hyperlactic acidemia with dichloroacetate, which inhibits the inactivating kinase for pyruvate dehydrogenase (E_1; Fig 8–13), thereby maintaining dehydrogenase (E_1) activity. This treatment was not effective in 1 child with fatal lactic acidosis of unknown cause. This treatment was considered but not tried in lactic acidosis due to the deficiency of the activating phosphatase of dehydrogenase (E_1). Acute, life-threatening hyperlactic acidemia can be corrected by the intravenous infusion of trishydroxymethyl aminomethane (THAM). This avoids

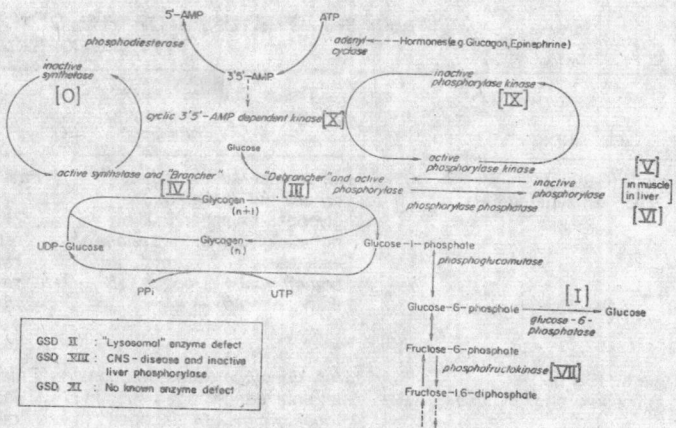

Figure 8–14 Pathway of phosphorylase activation and anaerobic glycolysis. Bracketed numbers refer to the type of glycogenosis in which the activity of the enzyme next to the number is defective. The various types are listed in Table 8–7.

the sodium overload of sodium bicarbonate administration. THAM treatment does not alter the poor prognosis for the majority of conditions that are associated with increased lactic and pyruvic acid.

8.21 THE GLYCOGEN STORAGE DISEASES

The glycogen storage diseases (GSD) are the result of metabolic errors that lead to abnormal concentrations or structure of glycogen. The GSD or glycogenoses can be divided into types in accord with the identified enzymatic defects, or sometimes on the basis of distinctive clinical features. The identification of a new type is useful only if the clinical or biochemical manifestations are sufficiently distinctive to permit their precise recognition in future patients.

A classification based on these considerations is listed in Table 8–7; Fig 8–14 depicts the relevant metabolic pathways. Table 8–8 indicates the concentrations of glycogen and the enzymatic activities found in liver and in skeletal muscle of normal individuals and of a patient representative of each type of glycogenosis that we have encountered.

Deficiency of Glycogen Synthetase (GSD 0). This disease has been identified in twins and in an unrelated 9 yr old girl. Early morning convulsions associated with hypoglycemia have been typical symptoms. There is an associated hyperketonemia. Serum concentrations of lactate are normal when the patient is fasting, but are increased after administration of glucose or after 12–24 hr of fasting. Hypoglycemia appears during such periods without food and is not responsive to glucagon (Fig 8–15). After administration of glucose the glucose level is elevated for longer than usual. It is important that the diagnosis be made expeditiously since hypoglycemic episodes and mental retardation can be avoided if the patient is given frequent meals rich in protein. The clinical picture is quite similar to that of "ketotic hypoglycemia"; some patients with the latter diagnosis should have an assay of hepatic glycogen synthetase.

Glycogen synthetase activity is deficient in liver, but normal in muscle and in white and red blood cells.

Concomitantly, glycogen concentration is low (less than 1%) but not absent in liver and normal in muscle. Differential involvement of tissues reflects the fact that different isozymes of glycogen synthetase exist for various tissues. The activation system for glycogen synthetase is normal.

A patient has been reported in whom analysis of the liver at autopsy found a deficiency of glycogen synthetase, phosphorylase, and glucose-6-phosphatase. These additional deficiencies may represent post mortem artifact, but it has been suggested that synthetase and phosphorylase may share certain peptide constituents. This possibility gains in attractiveness from the fact that the 9 yr old girl referred to above had 25% of normal phosphorylase activity in a biopsy specimen of liver.

Figure 8–15 Liver biopsy specimen during hypoglycemia. The total lack of glycogen is consistent with starvation (and/or shock) and requires glucose administration. Glucagon is ineffective. (Bar: 2 μm.)

Table 8-7 FEATURES OF THE GLYCOGEN STORAGE DISEASES, TYPES 0–XI (GSD 0–XI)

Type, Enzyme Affected	Tissue Distribution of Excessive Glycogen and Enzyme Deficiency	Clinical Symptoms and Signs*	Comments Alternate Names
Type 0 (GSD 0) Glycogen synthetase	Liver but not muscle (other tissues not analyzed); glycogen depletion in liver; hepatic glycogen synthetase less than 2% of normal, but some hepatic glycogen (1%) demonstrable	Fasting hypoglycemia; prolonged hyperglycemia after a meal or glucose administration; mental retardation follows hypoglycemic convulsions — when these are avoided by frequent protein-rich meals, psychomotor development can be normal	Aglycogenosis; defect convincingly demonstrated in 2 unrelated families; early diagnosis and dietary treatment important for prevention of retardation; some children with "ketotic hypoglycemia" may have GSD 0
Type I (GSD I) Glucose-6-phosphatase	Liver, kidney, intestine; frequent intranuclear glycogen seen in these organs not diagnostic; continuous nighttime feeding by tube and pump may alleviate clinical symptoms; portacaval shunt risky and clinically disappointing; treatment with phenytoin or phenobarbital ineffective	Enlarged liver and kidneys; "doll face," stunted growth, normal mental development; tendency to hypoglycemia, lactic acidosis, hyperlipidemia, hyperuricacidemia, gout, bleeding; IV galactose or fructose not converted to glucose (caution: these tests may precipitate acidosis); abortive or no rise in blood glucose after SC epinephrine or IV glucagon; normal urinary catecholamines; prognosis fair to good	Von Gierke disease, hepatorenal glycogenosis; no involvement of skeletal or cardiac muscle, or of leukocytes or cultured skin fibroblasts (glucose-6-phosphatase not normally present in these tissues)
Type Ib (GSD Ib; pseudo-GSD I) (in vitro activity of glucose-6-phosphatase is normal)	Despite normal glucose-6-phosphatase activity, liver glycogen concentration is increased	Symptoms are as those of GSD I	Transport defect for glucose-6-phosphate at microsomal membrane
Type IIa and IIb (GSD II) Lysosomal acid α-glucosidase (deficient activity of acid α-1,4- and of α-1,6-glucosidase; the latter could be considered "lysosomal glycogen debrancher")	In the fatal, infantile, classic form (GSD IIa), glycogen concentration excessive in all organs examined; acid α-glucosidase deficiency was generalized in 1 patient; in others normal renal acid α-glucosidase; amniotic fluid (in contrast to cultured amniotic fluid cells) contains acid α-glucosidase activity even if the fetus has the disease	Clinically normal at birth, though minimal cardiomegaly, abnormal ECG, increased tissue glycogen, abnormal lysosomes in liver and skin, and acid α-glucosidase deficiency demonstrable at birth. Within a few mo, marked hypotonia, severe cardiomegaly, moderate hepatomegaly; normal mental development; death usually in infancy (GSD IIa). Cases with involvement of muscle and liver but without cardiomegaly described in children and adults (GSD IIb). Normal blood glucose response to glucagon; normal urinary catecholamines	Pompe disease, generalized glycogenosis, cardiac glycogenosis; prenatal diagnosis within a few days after amniocentesis by the electron microscopic demonstration of abnormal lysosomes in uncultured amniotic fluid cells; for prenatal diagnosis by enzyme analysis, cultured amniotic fluid cells required, which also show the abnormal lysosomes GSD IIa: infantile fatal form GSD IIb: late juvenile-adult form
Type III (GSD III) Amylo-1,6-glucosidase, "debrancher enzyme"	Liver, muscle, heart, etc., in various combinations; designated types IIIA through D; cultured amniotic fluid cells have diagnostic biochemical abnormality	Moderate to marked hepatomegaly; none to moderate hypotonia; none to moderate cardiomegaly; ECG rarely abnormal; no acidosis, hypoglycemia, or hyperlipemia; glucagon produces a normal rise in blood glucose after a meal but not after fasting; normal mental development; failure of liver or heart rare; normal urinary catecholamines; prognosis fair to good	Limit dextrinosis, debrancher glycogenosis, Cori disease, Forbes disease; prenatal diagnosis by enzyme assay of cultured amniotic fluid cells feasible but perhaps unnecessary, owing to the usual benign course
Type IV (GSD IV) Amylo-1,4→1,6-transglucosidase, "brancher enzyme"	Generalized (?); low to normal levels of abnormally structured glycogen (amylopectin-like molecules with fewer branch points than normal in animal glycogen)	Hepatosplenomegaly, ascites, cirrhosis, liver failure; normal mental development; death in early childhood	Amylopectinosis, brancher glycogenosis, Andersen disease; prenatal diagnosis of this incurable disease may be feasible and indicated by enzyme analysis of cultured amniotic fluid cells

*IV, intravenous administration of; SC, subcutaneous administration of.

Table 8–7 FEATURES OF THE GLYCOGEN STORAGE DISEASES, TYPES 0–XI (GSD 0–XI) (Continued)

TYPE, ENZYME AFFECTED	TISSUE DISTRIBUTION OF EXCESSIVE GLYCOGEN AND ENZYME DEFICIENCY	CLINICAL SYMPTOMS AND SIGNS°	COMMENTS Alternate Names
Type V (GSD V) Muscle phosphorylase deficiency (congenital absence of skeletal muscle phosphorylase; phosphorylase-activating system intact)	Skeletal muscle; liver and myometrium normal	Temporary weakness and cramping of skeletal muscle after exercise; no rise in blood lactate during ischemic exercise; symptoms like those of type VII glycogenosis; normal mental development and urinary catecholamines; myoglobinuria in later life; fair to good prognosis	McArdle syndrome; liver and smooth muscle phosphorylase not affected; cardiac muscle phosphorylase not examined; prenatal diagnosis not feasible, does not seem indicated
Type VI (GSD VI) Liver phosphorylase deficiency (phosphorylase-activating system intact)	Liver; skeletal muscle normal; leukocytes unsatisfactory for diagnosis	Marked hepatomegaly, no splenomegaly; no hypoglycemia, acidosis, or hyperlipemia; no rise of blood glucose after SC epinephrine or IV glucagon; normal mental development; normal urinary catecholamines; good prognosis	Lack of glucagon-induced hyperglycemia distinguishes GSD VI from GSD IX; the latter shows a normal glucagon response; prenatal diagnosis not feasible, may not be indicated
Type VII (GSD VII) Phosphofructokinase	Skeletal muscle, erythrocytes (in initial report; other tissues not examined); not known whether cultured amniotic fluid cells are affected, but prenatal diagnosis not indicated	Temporary weakness and cramping of skeletal muscle after exercise; no rise in blood lactate during ischemic exercise; normal mental development; symptoms identical to those of type V glycogenosis; good prognosis	Reduction of phosphofructokinase activity severe in skeletal muscle, mild in erythrocytes, not established in other tissues; incapacity may be minimal
Type VIII (GSD VIII) No enzymatic deficiency yet demonstrated; total liver phosphorylase normal but most is in inactive form (liver phosphorylase activity reduced because control lost over extent of phosphorylase activation)	Liver, brain; skeletal muscle normal; cerebral glycogen increased; electron microscopy shows some cerebral glycogen in the form of α-particles within axon cylinders and synapses	Hepatomegaly; truncal ataxia, nystagmus, "dancing eyes" may be present; neurologic deterioration progressing to hypertonia, spasticity, decerebration and death; urinary epinephrine and norepinephrine are increased during acute phase of disease, not in stationary end phase	Predominant clinical problem of the 3 patients with this presumptive diagnosis was progressive degenerative disease of brain
Type IXa, IXb, and IXc (GSD IX) Liver phosphorylase kinase deficiency (total phosphorylase content normal but in inactive form, owing to the lack of phosphorylase kinase)	Liver; muscle tissue normal biochemically (in IXa and IXb) and microscopically; diagnosis not possible by using leukocytes; possible by using leukocytes; D-thyroxin induced liver phosphorylase kinase activity in 1 patient, but not in 2 others of a different family	Marked hepatomegaly, no splenomegaly; no hypoglycemia or acidosis; normal urinary catecholamines; normal rise in blood glucose after IV glucagon or SC epinephrine; prognosis good; treatment may not be necessary ("benign hepatomegaly" may disappear in early adulthood)	Liver phosphorylase can be activated in vitro by addition of exogenous kinase to the homogenate; not the human counterpart of muscle phosphorylase kinase deficiency in mice; normal glucagon response is a distinguishing feature vs GSD VI; GSD IXa, autosomal recessive; GSD IXb, X-linked recessive; prenatal diagnosis not demonstrated and is unnecessary
Type X (GSD X) Loss of activity of cyclic 3′5′-AMP–dependent kinase in muscle and presumably liver. (Total phosphorylase content of liver and skeletal muscle normal, but the enzyme completely deactivated in both organs; phosphorylase kinase activity 50% of normal, possibly owing to the loss of 3′5′-AMP–dependent kinase activity)	Liver and muscle (other organs not tested); identical biochemical findings were made in 2 muscle biopsy specimens taken 6 yr apart	Marked hepatomegaly; patient otherwise clinically healthy initially, but 6 yr after diagnosis mild recurrent muscle pain; no cardiomegaly or hypoglycemia; no rise in blood glucose after IV glucagon; the only individual known to have this condition not incapacitated at 12 yr of age	In vitro activation of the patient's phosphorylase occurs (1) under assay conditions not requiring 3′5′-AMP–dependent kinase, or (2) after the patient's muscle homogenate has been fortified with phosphorylase kinase–deficient mouse muscle that supplied 3′5′-AMP–dependent kinase; postulated defect restricted to the activity of the cyclic 3′5′-AMP–dependent kinase that phosphorylates phosphorylase kinase, other cyclic 3′5′-AMP–dependent phosphorylations being intact

Table continued on following page

Table 8–7 FEATURES OF THE GLYCOGEN STORAGE DISEASES, TYPES 0–XI (GSD 0–XI) (Continued)

Type, Enzyme Affected	Tissue Distribution of Excessive Glycogen and Enzyme Deficiency	Clinical Symptoms and Signs*	Comments. Alternate Names
Type XI (GSD XI) All enzymatic activities measured to date are normal (adenyl cyclase, 3'5'-AMP–dependent kinase, phosphorylase kinase, phosphorylase, debrancher, brancher, glucose-6-phosphatase)	Liver, or liver and kidney	Tendency for acidosis; markedly stunted growth; vitamin D–resistant rickets (that can be cured with high doses of vitamin D and oral supplementation of phosphate); hyperlipidemia, generalized aminoaciduria, galactosuria, glucosuria, phosphaturia; normal renal size; no rise in blood glucose after IV glucagon or SC epinephrine; urinary excretion of cyclic 3'5'-AMP increases markedly after administration of glucagon	Muscle usually not affected; GSD XI may include patients with glycogenoses with different enzymatic defects

*IV, intravenous administration of; SC, subcutaneous administration of.

This patient had an older brother who "outgrew" his clinical symptoms of hypoglycemia. These siblings might well have been labeled "ketotic hypoglycemia." Among patients so labeled, the persistent hyperglycemia and increase in serum lactate concentration after administration of glucose should reveal those with possible deficiencies of glycogen synthetase.

Deficiency of Glucose-6-Phosphatase (GSD I). In GSD I, glucose-6-phosphatase activity is defective in liver, kidney, and intestine. Concomitantly, glycogen concentration is increased in these tissues. Mild hypotonia is sometimes reported in GSD I, but the disease does not have a primary effect on muscle since muscle does not normally contain glucose-6-phosphatase.

In GSD I, the administration of galactose or fructose does not produce an elevation of blood glucose level; such tolerance tests should not be done since they can lead to severe acidosis. Administration of fructose, but not of galactose, is followed by increased concentrations of serum insulin. Intravenous administration of glucagon is not followed by a normal rise in blood glucose, regardless of how recently the patient may have eaten. The glucagon tolerance test can, therefore, differentiate between GSD I and GSD III; in the latter the concentration of blood glucose will increase if glucagon is given 2 hr after a meal. Subcutaneous administration of epinephrine has no advantage over the glucagon tolerance test and may produce unpleasant side effects.

Young children with GSD I have impressive hepatomegaly, but the involvement of the liver may be easily overlooked in the affected adult. In GSD I, the kidneys are moderately but consistently enlarged on roentgenographic examination. This finding helps to differentiate between GSD I and GSD III, in which renal size is normal. Marked hypoglycemia may be well tolerated; patients with blood glucose levels as low as 10 mg/dl have been known to display normal behavior. Hyperlipidemia and hyperuricacidemia are marked. In adults the latter produces gout, which must be appropriately treated. There is a secondary impairment of platelet function which may make bleeding a problem when biopsies are done.

Acute lactic acidosis may be a recurrent and life-threatening problem. Portacaval shunt has been advocated for its prevention or control, but we have not encountered any patients who have benefited from the operation, which has been complicated by closure of the anastomosis and by development of cirrhosis or encephalopathy. Patients difficult to control can be managed successfully with continuous night-time feedings by nasopharyngeal or gastrostomy tubes; children grow satisfactorily, hepatomegaly recedes, and hypoglycemia and lactic acidosis become manageable. How-

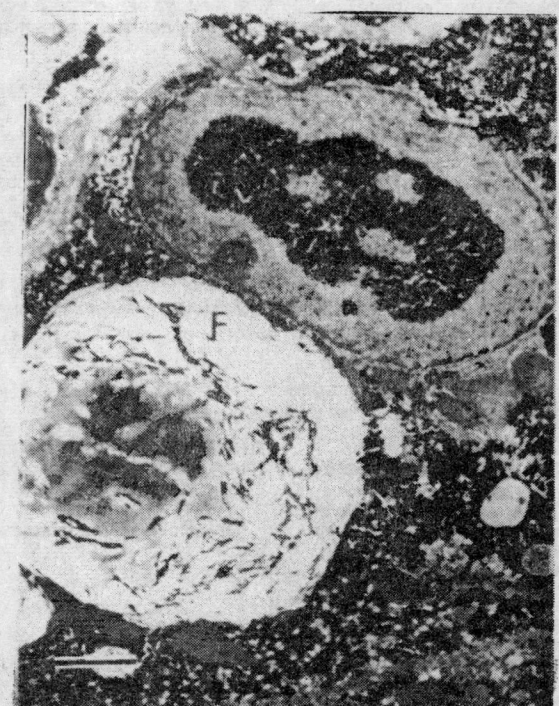

Figure 8–16 Liver biopsy specimen in GSD I. Visible are intranuclear glycogenosis, a medium-sized fat droplet (F), and abundant cytoplasmic glycogen. (Bar: 2 μm.)

Table 8-8 BIOCHEMICAL ANALYSIS OF TISSUES IN GLYCOGEN STORAGE DISEASES

Cases	Glycogen Concentration % Wt. of Wet Tissue	Phosphorylase Total μmoles Phosphate/gm/min	Active μmoles Phosphate/gm/min	Phosphorylase Kinase Active	Acid α-Glucosidase μmoles Glucose/gm/min	Amylo-1,6-Glucosidase*	Glucose-6-Phosphatase μmoles Phosphate/gm/Min
"Normal"							
Liver	2.5-6.0	44.3† ± 9.6	25.1 ± 6.5	100%	0.258 ± 0.093	3750 ± 490	4.7 ± 1.9
Muscle	0.1-1.5	78.0 ± 21.1	47.7 ± 13.2	100%	0.035 ± 0.011	7113 ± 553	
Type I							
Liver	8.9	42	23	Normal	0.242	Normal	0
Muscle	0.6	59	38		0.041		
Pseudo-Type I							
Liver	7.4	53	46	Normal	0.261	Normal	3.9
Muscle	1.1	77	28		0.037		
Type IIa							
Liver	8.8	47	26	Normal	0	Normal	3.2
Muscle	7.5	64	42		0		
Type IIb							
Liver	11.5	45	29	Normal	0.026	Normal	5.4
Muscle	1.6	80	31		0.0		
Type III							
Liver	9.3	40	19	Normal	0.210	45	2.9
Muscle	6.0	72	45		0.030	43	
Type V							
Liver	4.5	48	26	Normal	0.260	Normal	3.8
Muscle	3.8	0	0	Normal or increased	0.028		
Type VI							
Liver	7.6	2	1.8	Normal	0.176	Normal	3.4
Muscle	0.3	61	46		0.025		
Type VIII							
Liver	12.0	43	6	Normal	0.312	Normal	5.1
Muscle	0.4	58	35		0.040		
Type IXa							
Liver	9.9	46	2.3	<10%	0.155	Normal	3.7
Muscle	0.3	70	58	Normal	0.026		
Type IXb							
Liver	10.5	44	0.8	<10%	0.318	Normal	2.6
Muscle	1.4	100	72	Normal	0.029		
Type X							
Liver	10.5	39	0.1	Normal	0.292	Normal	6.8
Muscle	2.9	54	0	50% of normal‡	0.044		

*Glucose-^{14}C incorporated into -1,6-branch points expressed as cpm/mg glycogen/g tissue in 1 hr.

†Mean value ± 1 S.D.

‡Enzyme is demonstrable in GSD X only if I-strain mouse muscle and 3'5'-AMP have been added to homogenate of patient's muscle; in other types of GSD, the addition of mouse muscle is not needed.

ever, when the gastric tube feedings are discontinued, the pretreatment tolerance of hypoglycemia (well known in GSD I) may have been lost. Disease-related post-treatment hypoglycemia may thus result in convulsions. Frequent meals have similar effects to those of gastric tube feedings and may suffice for clinical control. As patients grow older, their metabolic problems become less severe and more easily manageable. Neither phenobarbital nor phenytoin corrects the biochemical or clinical abnormalities in patients with glycogenoses.

In GSD I, hepatocytes contain many lipid droplets ranging in size from smaller than mitochondria to several times that of the nucleus, and the nuclei themselves frequently contain glycogen (Fig 8-16). Nuclear glycogenosis can also occur in GSD III, in diabetes mellitus, and in Wilson disease. Heterogeneity of the defect is perhaps manifested by the development of

hepatoma in a few patients and by abnormalities of hepatic endoplasmic reticulum in some but not all children with GSD I. Prenatal diagnosis using amniotic fluid cells is not feasible since glucose-6-phosphatase is not normally present in cultured skin fibroblasts; neither can the enzyme be demonstrated in normal white cells.

GSD Ib (Pseudo-GSD I). Clinically GSD Ib is indistinguishable from GSD I. Hepatic glycogen concentration is increased. Glucose-6-phosphatase activity is normal in homogenates made of frozen liver tissue. The activity is decreased, however, in isotonic homogenates made from fresh liver tissue. This "latency" is interpreted as indicative of a defect in the transport of glucose-6-phosphate across microsomal membranes of GSD Ib hepatocytes. Further evidence that this variant of GSD I is due to a microsomal membrane defect is provided by the finding that when fresh liver homogenates from affected patients are treated with deoxycholate, the activity of glucose-6-phosphatase is normal. Deoxycholate is known to break up microsomal membranes.

Deficiency of Lysosomal Acid α-Glucosidase (GSD II). This disease occurs in at least 2 varieties, one affecting infants (GSD IIa), the other affecting older children and adults (GSD IIb). We know of no instance where both varieties have occurred in members of the same family. The study of fibroblasts indicated that in a case of GSD IIa, the lysosomal acid α-glucosidase was structurally altered, whereas in a case of GSD IIb the amount of the enzyme was reduced. The gene for acid α-glucosidase is localized on chromosome 17.

GSD IIa. This is the classic form of generalized glycogenosis, also known as *Pompe disease.* Abnormal lysosomes are the morphologic hallmark of the disease. GSD IIa is always fatal, usually within 2 yr after birth. Affected children appear clinically healthy at birth, but heart size and electrocardiogram are marginally abnormal. Muscle tone and liver size are normal at birth, but after a few wk or mo at home, the infant patient becomes completely flaccid. Sucking becomes weak, respirations shallow, and the cardiac silhouette huge. The liver is typically only moderately enlarged. The patients are alert and of normal intelligence. The mouth is kept open and the tongue thrust forward, perhaps

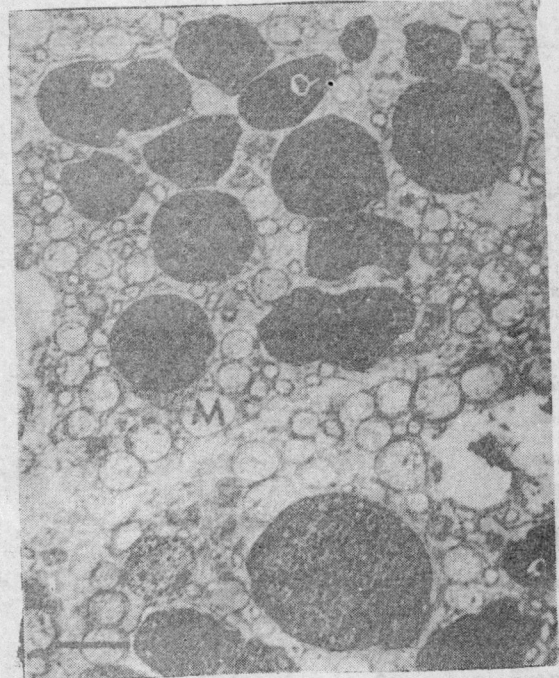

Figure 8–16   Liver autopsy specimen of GSD IIa. "Abnormal lysosomes" are ubiquitous but cytoplasmic glycogen is missing after starvation, and/or epinephrine treatment, or at autopsy. M, mitochondria. (Bar: 2 μm.)

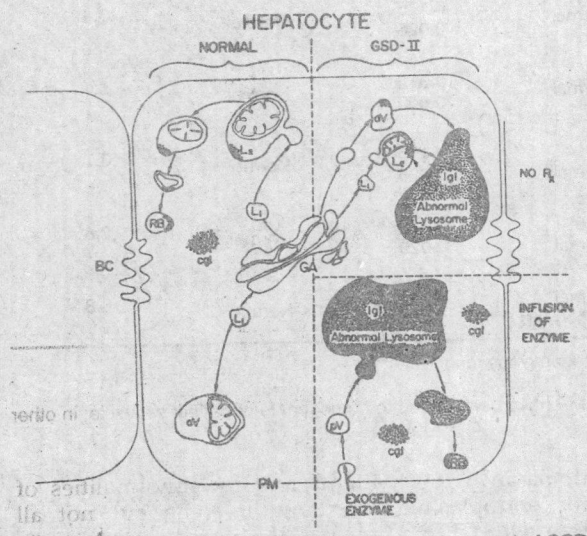

HEPATOCYTE

Figure 8–17   The lysosomal mechanism. During treatment of GSD IIa (right lower quarter), the exogenous enzyme is admitted to the cell in a pinocytotic vesicle (pV) and initiates the degradation of lysosomal glycogen (lgl) after the pinocytotic vesicle has fused with the abnormal lysosome. The cytoplasmic glycogen (cgl) is not degraded because it is shielded from the exogenous enzymes by the membrane of the pinocytotic vesicle that, presumably, derives from the plasma membrane (PM). Without treatment (right upper quarter), GSD IIa hepatocytes are characterized by the accumulation of membrane-surrounded glycogen (lgl) because the primary lysosome is deficient in lysosomal acid α-glucosidase.

aV, autophagic vacuoles that fuse with L₁, resulting in secondary lysosomes (L₂); BC, bile canaliculus; cgl, cytoplasmic glycogen; GA, Golgi apparatus; L₁, primary lysosomes containing acid hydrolases; L₂, secondary lysosomes; lgl, lysosomal glycogen; PM, plasma membrane; pV, pinocytotic vesicle; RB, residual bodies.

(From Hug G: Glycogen storage disease. Birth Defects 12:157, 1976.)

more because of air hunger than macroglossia; the resulting facial expression is characteristic. Aspiration pneumonia leads to chronic pulmonary infiltrates and atelectasis, and bronchial compression by the large heart to atelectasis. Death is due to failure of respiratory muscles. There is hardly any other condition in which such extreme cardiomegaly and muscular weakness occur in an infant who appears normal at birth. Blood glucose concentrations are normal, as are tolerance tests to glucagon and other carbohydrate test substances.

GSD II is the only lysosomal disease among the glycogenoses; the other types of GSD are associated with defects of enzymes located in the cytoplasm. The deficiency is of acid α-glucosidase, a glycogen-degrading enzyme associated with the lysosomal fraction of tissue homogenates. An isozyme present in kidney and leukocytes which has α-glucosidase activity at neutral pH can lead to misdiagnosis if synthetic substrates, rather than maltose, are used in the assay.

A schematic presentation of the normal lysosomal mechanism (Fig 8–17) indicates that fusion of a primary lysosome with an autophagic vacuole creates a secondary lysosome. If the primary lysosome is deficient in a lysosomal enzyme (such as α-glucosidase) then the secondary lysosome may become engorged with the material (such as glycogen) that should have been degraded by the defective enzyme. Besides deficiencies of enzymes there may be other errors in lysosomal mechanisms, such as membrane defects. In GSD IIa the deficiency of lysosomal acid α-glucosidase produces intracellular vesicles engorged with glycogen (Fig 8–18, 8–19, and 8–20). Such vesicles, the so-called "abnormal

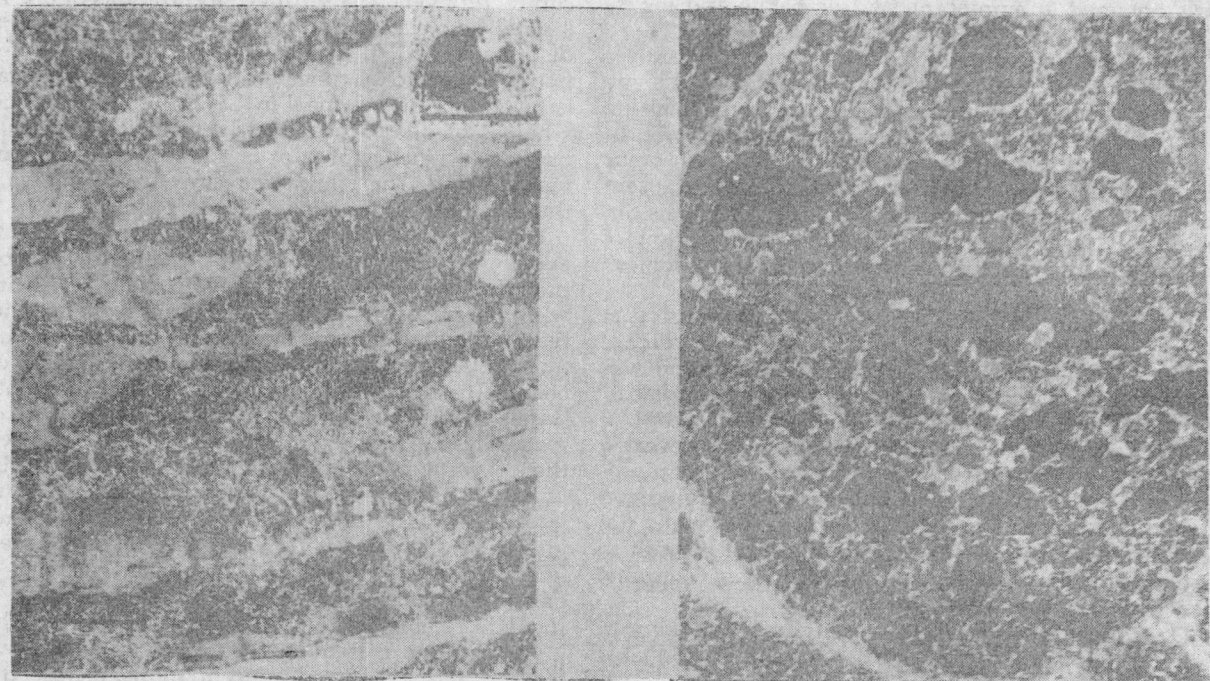

Figure 8–19 Muscle biopsy specimen in GSD IIa. Excessive glycogen (in the form of β-particles as is normal for muscle) is located in the sarcoplasm except for one glycogen-filled lysosome shown enlarged in the inset. (Bar of main figure: 2 μm; bar of inset: 1 μm.)

Figure 8–20 Liver biopsy specimen in GSD IIa. The presence of cytoplasmic glycogen indicates the specimen was *not* obtained after starvation or epinephrine treatment, or at autopsy. (Bar: 2 μm.)

lysosomes," are seen by light or electron microscopy in hepatic cells.

In tissues examined at autopsy in 5 untreated patients with GSD IIa we found increased glycogen concentrations in all of up to 17 tissues examined. In 1 patient, α-glucosidase deficiency was generalized; the kidneys had normal levels in the other 4 children. The deficiency of the lysosomal enzyme for glycogen degradation can explain the membrane-bound accumulations of glycogen in lysosomes, but the deficiency of a lysosomal enzyme does not explain the excessive accumulation of glycogen in the cytoplasm of heart and muscle cells. This cytoplasmic glycogen accumulates despite the fact that it is probably in contact with the normal glycolytic enzymes of cytoplasm, none of which are known to be defective in GSD II.

The excessive tissue glycogen as such is not a cause of death; we found the same 7-fold increase in glycogen in the muscle of a girl at birth when she was clinically healthy and 2 yr later in tissue obtained post mortem. Glucagon and epinephrine can mobilize cytoplasmic liver glycogen. When cytoplasmic glycogen is depleted, however, glucagon no longer produces a rise in blood glucose concentration. The lysosomal glycogen can be mobilized from hepatocytes by the administration of purified glycogen-degrading enzymes of fungal origin, and the abnormal lysosomes disappear. In 1 instance in which we have observed this, the normalization of the hepatic ultrastructure was of no clinical benefit.

The prenatal diagnosis of GSD IIa can be accomplished through electron microscopic examination of

Figure 8–21 Uncultured amniotic fluid cell obtained at 16 weeks of a pregnancy with a fetus having GSD IIa. Visible are parts of 3 disintegrating cells that each contain an "abnormal lysosome." Two of these are shown enlarged in the insets in which β-particles and lysosomal membrane are resolved. The diagonal alternating dark-light zones are artifacts of specimen preparation that do not interfere with interpretation. (Bar: 2 μm in main figure, 1 μm in inset.)

cells obtained at amniocentesis (see below and Fig 8–21).

GSD IIb. Patients with GSD IIb present weakness of skeletal muscle later in life than in GDS IIa. In some patients the disease is compatible with a normal life span, though it may demand a sedentary life style. In other patients death from respiratory failure can occur during the 3rd or 4th decade. Cardiomegaly is absent and the electrocardiogram is normal. The diagnosis can be made when electron microscopic examination of biopsy specimens of skin shows "abnormal lysosomes" packed with glycogen particles (Fig 8–22).

In a patient who died of unrelated hypertension at 24 yr of age we found a deficiency of acid α-glucosidase consistent with GSD IIa. Glycogen concentration was increased in all tissues except heart, though cardiac α-glucosidase activity was deficient. Light microscopy of heart muscle was normal; electron microscopy revealed occasional abnormal lysosomes but no excess of glycogen in cytoplasm. In skeletal muscle excessive glycogen accumulation seems to begin in the sarcoplasm and not in abnormal lysosomes. These findings are difficult to explain on the basis of the defective activity of lysosomal acid α-glucosidase.

Deficiency of "Debrancher" Activity (GSD III). In GSD III, hepatomegaly can be as impressive as in GSD I. If generalized, GSD III affects muscle and heart, though neither organ may be clinically involved. Electrocardiographic abnormalities and moderate cardiomegaly are usually found; the size of the kidneys is normal. Hypoglycemia is rare and does not present a

clinical problem. The serum concentrations of uric acid, lactate, ketones, and lipids are normal. These criteria distinguish GSD III from GSD I, as does this observation: blood glucose concentration increases if glucagon is given 2 hr after a meal in GSD III but not in GSD I, whereas blood glucose levels remain flat in both glycogenoses when glucagon is administered after overnight fasting. There may be recurrent pneumonia, but the long-term prognosis is usually good.

For "debranching" of the glycogen molecule, 2 enzymatic reactions need to occur in sequence after phosphorylase activity has reduced both the outer chains to within 4 glucose units of the 1,6-branch point. The 1st reaction is that of a transferase that transfers 3 glucose units of the branched outer chain onto the straight outer chain. The glucose molecule at the branch point becomes exposed and accessible to the action of α-1,6-glucosidase, which removes it. Both the transferase and the α-1,6-glucosidase activities are deficient in the livers of patients with GSD III. In some the activity of transferase in muscle may be low, whereas that of α-1,6-glucosidase remains normal. The overall effect in either liver or muscle is a loss of "debrancher" activity. Both enzymatic activities may be retained in muscle, with the defect being limited to the liver.

Perhaps more frequently GSD III is a generalized disease, with glycogen concentrations increased and "debranching" activity deficient in every (examined) tissue. In generalized GSD III, the concentration of glycogen in muscle may reach the same levels as in GSD II, though patients with the former are symptom-free and those with the latter are markedly hypotonic. In GSD III, starvation induces the degradation of glycogen to within 4 units of the branch point. Glycogen with such short outer chains is called a limit dextrin; hence *limit dextrinosis* is an alternative designation for GSD III. Light microscopic appearance of liver in GSD III is similar to that of GSD I except that GSD III exhibits formation of fibrous septa, more extensive nuclear glycogenosis, and a paucity of intracellular lipid droplets. Hepatic cirrhosis does not seem to be a progressive development in GSD III; the fibrous septa usually remain stable.

Deficiency of "Brancher" Activity (GSD IV). In GSD IV, hepatomegaly and splenomegaly are found. Progressive portal fibrosis leads to hepatic cirrhosis, ascites, and death in childhood from liver failure. Treatment with corticosteroids may induce temporary remission.

In this condition hepatic symptoms are associated with reduced rather than increased concentrations of tissue glycogen. The glycogen resembles amylopectin, since it has fewer than the normal number of branch points. This may be the consequence of deficiency of branching enzyme, though one would expect a defect of this enzyme to result in the synthesis of amylose, the glucose polymer with *no* branch points. The cirrhosis of the liver may be the result of the amylopectin-like glycogen since this glucose polymer is not normally even transiently present in the liver. The limit dextrin of GSD III may not have this effect since it is a transient form normally encountered during synthesis and degradation of glycogen.

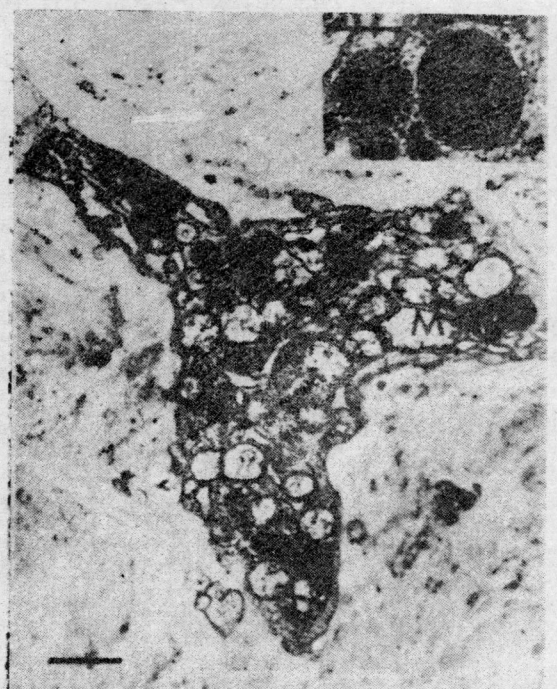

Figure 8–22 Skin biopsy specimen, *not* cultured, in GSD IIb. A fibrocyte contained several "abnormal lysosomes," one of which can be seen in the inset where β-particles and lysosomal membrane are resolved. M. mitochondria. (Bar of main figure, 2 μm; of inset, 0.5 μm.)

Deficiency of Muscle Phosphorylase (GSD V) (McArdle Syndrome). *McArdle syndrome* is characterized by muscular pains and cramps after exercise. GSD V is differentiated from more common causes of muscle cramps by the ischemic exercise test. The test requires inflation of a blood pressure cuff on the upper arm to above the arterial pressure. The patient is then asked to squeeze a rubber ball with the hand of the same arm about once every sec. The healthy person will easily squeeze 70–100 times, with some discomfort but without cramping of the muscle or residual symptoms after deflation of the blood pressure cuff. In the patient with GSD V, muscle cramps may limit the squeezes to 20–30 movements. When the cuff is released, the cramps persist, with the hand in a tetanic position (wrist bent, fingers extended) that cannot be corrected by the patient or by the examiner. After several min there is gradual release of the cramp. Pain may persist from 24–48 hr.

In the healthy person, blood samples taken from the antecubital vein of the ischemic arm during the above exercise will show a rise in serum lactate, such as in theory ought not to occur in GSD V because of the inability of muscle in GSD V to produce lactate from glycogen. The diagnosis of GSD V has been made using the noninvasive technique of nuclear magnetic resonance (NMR) by measurement of pH and ATP and phosphocreatine concentration following both aerobic and ischemic exercise. Lactic acid determinations are less helpful diagnostically than the dramatic muscle cramp elicited by ischemic exercise. The disease exhibits a wide clinical spectrum, varying from almost no symptoms to recurrent myoglobinuria and attacks of rhabdomyolysis. One patient experiencing unremitting muscle pain committed suicide.

In patients with GSD V, skeletal muscle is without demonstrable activity of phosphorylase. The activity in liver and smooth muscle is normal. The system of phosphorylase activation is intact; indeed, in 3 of 4 patients we found 3 times the normal activity of muscle phosphorylase kinase. Glycogen concentration is increased in muscle but usually not above 4%. Histologically, much of the excessive glycogen is deposited in the cytoplasm beneath the sarcolemma (Fig 8–23). In the patients with a deficiency in phosphorylase, the energy for muscle contraction can still be provided by glucose entering the myocyte. This might suffice for energy requirements at rest when there are no symptoms. Peak demands for energy, however, which can ordinarily be met by supplemental breakdown of muscle glycogen, cannot be met in GSD V because of the phosphorylase defect. The result is pain and cramping during and after exercise, with little or no production of lactic acid. The ischemic exercise worsens the situation by interrupting the normal supply of oxygen and glucose.

Deficiency of Liver Phosphorylase (GSD VI). In GSD VI, hepatomegaly may be massive. Otherwise, the affected children are without symptoms and lead normal lives, though there may be some elevation of serum lipids and transaminases. None of our patients has had hypoglycemia. The blood glucose concentration does not increase after glucagon administration; this finding can be used to separate GSD VI from GSD IX, in which

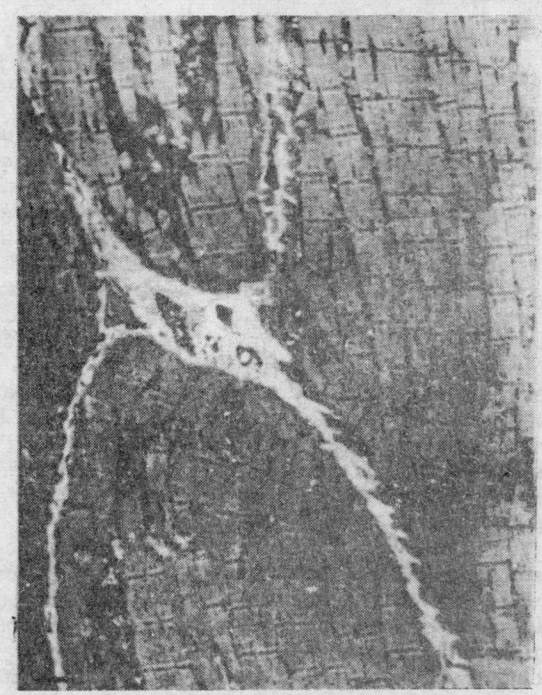

Figure 8–23 Muscle biopsy specimen of GSD V. Excessive glycogen (β-particles that are normal in muscle) appears between myofibrils close to the sarcolemma. (Bar: 2 μm.)

glucagon tolerance curves are normal. Separation from GSD I can be made on clinical evidence. GSD VI is probably an example of benign hepatomegaly that may recede as the children grow older.

The demonstration of low activity of the hepatic phosphorylase system is consistent with but not diagnostic of GSD VI since low activity may result from a number of defects within the phosphorylase activation system. The diagnosis of GSD VI rests on the biochemical demonstration of a deficiency in the liver phosphorylase enzyme itself. Leukocyte phosphorylase may also be affected; leukocyte assays cannot be relied on, however, since leukocyte phosphorylase may be inactivated to a varying and unpredictable degree during the isolation of the white cells. By light microscopy, liver specimens show slight formation of fibrous septa in portal areas. Whether this minimal change remains stationary or progresses to cirrhosis in adulthood is unknown. Phosphorylase activity in muscle is normal, as are glycogen concentration and histologic appearance.

Deficiency of Phosphofructokinase (GSD VII). The symptoms of GSD VII resemble those of GSD V. The muscle pain and cramping after exercise may be somewhat less severe in GSD VII, and the disease has been tolerated by a young man who plays tennis for pleasure.

Phosphofructokinase is deficient in skeletal muscle but apparently not in the liver; it is only partially defective in erythrocytes. Since this is a key glycolytic enzyme that affects the use of both glycogen and glucose in muscle, it is surprising that the deficiency may cause fewer symptoms than a deficiency in phosphorylase, which affects only the utilization of glycogen. The concentration of glycogen in muscle is moderately elevated, and its distribution is subsarcolemmal, like that observed in GSD V and GSD X.

Progressive Brain Disease and Deactivated Liver Phosphorylase without Demonstrated Enzyme Defect (GSD VIII). In GSD VIII, hepatomegaly is apparent soon after birth. On the other hand, the more impressive clinical features, unique for GSD VIII, are related to the central nervous system. Infants develop nystagmus and rolling of the eyes, ataxia, and truncal tremor. They become hypotonic and then spastic. They gradually lose rapport with their environment, become unresponsive and bedridden, develop swallowing difficulties, and may die of aspiration pneumonia. Urinary excretion of epinephrine and norepinephrine may be increased. The glucagon tolerance test is normal. Patients with GSD VIII are found among infants and toddlers with hepatomegaly and progressive degenerative disease of the brain.

Glycogen concentration is increased in biopsy specimens of liver and cerebral tissues; it has been normal in muscle and in the other tissues examined. Concomitantly, liver phosphorylase activity is low. Cerebral enzymes have not been assayed. The low activity of the hepatic phosphorylase system does not reflect a deficiency of phosphorylase enzyme or of any other specific enzyme in the hepatic system of phosphorylase activation. This is indicated by the fact that the glucagon tolerance curve is normal and by the fact that phosphorylase activity becomes normal within 2 min after the administration of glucagon or epinephrine to the patient. The low phosphorylase activity observed in vitro can be increased by the patient's own liver homogenate to normal values. Accordingly, the affected child appears to suffer from impaired control of phosphorylase activation. It is of interest that processes in the central nervous system of animals have been shown to affect rapid activation and deactivation of key enzymes involved in carbohydrate metabolism in the liver, including glycogen synthetase and phosphorylase.

On electron microscopy, specimens of cerebral tissue obtained at biopsy reveal increased amounts of glycogen, in the form of α-particles that average 10 times wider than the β-particles usually found in brain. Further pathophysiologic studies will depend on the recognition of additional patients among children with hepatomegaly and cerebral deterioration. Such children should have assays of liver phosphorylase in biopsy specimens.

Deficiency of Liver Phosphorylase Kinase (GSD IX). This defect occurs in 3 forms that differ in the pattern of inheritance and tissue distribution. GSD IXa follows autosomal recessive inheritance, GSD IXb, sex-linked recessive. Otherwise, these 2 forms are indistinguishable. Skeletal muscle is not affected and is normal biochemically as well as morphologically. In GSD IXc with autosomal recessive inheritance the phosphorylase kinase activity of liver and muscle is deficient. Hepatomegaly is massive in early life but recedes as the children grow older. The impressive protuberance of the abdomen may disappear completely in teenager or adult, though the liver can remain somewhat large.

Transaminases are minimally elevated. GSD IX can be classified as a benign hepatomegaly except in patients who also have defective debrancher activity. Glucagon produces a normal rise in blood glucose concentration in GSD IX; this serves to distinguish it from GSD VI, in which the glucagon tolerance curve remains flat. Affected children require no treatment, except perhaps in rare instances of combined deficiencies.

The concentration of glycogen in liver is increased (Fig 8–24) and phosphorylase activity low, as is the case in GSD VI. In GSD IX, however, the low activity of phosphorylase is the result of a deficiency in phosphorylase kinase. Other enzymes of the activating system, including phosphorylase, are normal, as is the enzymatic examination of muscle. Cultured skin fibroblasts and leukocytes have been reported to be affected; however, isolation of these cells may introduce unpredictable variations in kinase activity of these tissues, making them undependable for diagnosis.

Deficiency of Cyclic 3'5'-AMP-Dependent Kinase (GSD X). The 1 patient with this condition had marked hepatomegaly for which she was initially hospitalized at the age of 6 yr. The clinical picture was indistinguishable from GSD IX except that her blood sugar curve remained flat after intravenous administration of glucagon. She had no skeletal muscular symptoms at that examination. Six yr later she complained of muscular pain and cramping after exercise and of minimal degree of persistent muscular weakness. The ischemic exercise test was normal. Hepatomegaly has

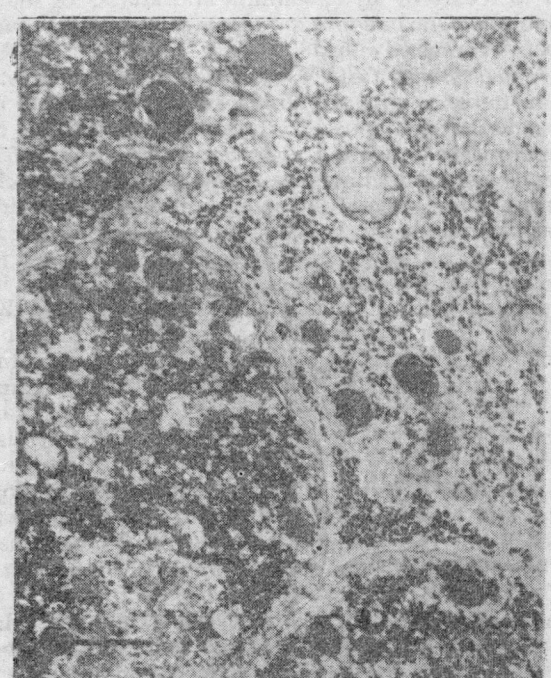

Figure 8–24 Liver biopsy specimen in GSD IX. Abundant glycogen is placed in intra- and intercellular space, but not next to plasma membrane, in such a way that the cellular circumference appears accentuated. This accentuation is visible on light microscopy and is also a feature of GSD VI, VIII, IX, and X, that is, in GSD with the symptom of low liver phosphorylase activity. (Bar: 2 μm.)

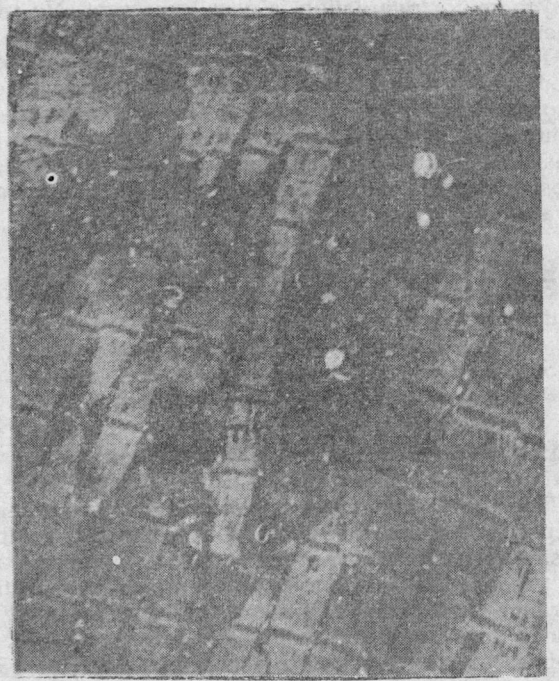

Figure 8–25 Muscle biopsy specimen in GSD X with abundant β-glycogen separating myofibrils (mf). (Bar: 2 μm.)

been persistent. The patient is otherwise doing well without specific therapy.

Concentration of glycogen in liver was high. Hepatic phosphorylase activity was low. Concentration of glycogen in muscle was increased to 2–4%. Light and electron microscopy showed increased glycogen deposition in cells of both liver and skeletal muscle (Fig 8–25). Phosphorylase in muscle was exclusively in the inactive form, whereas normal human muscle has 60–80% of its total phosphorylase in the active form. GSD X reflects a deficiency in activity of cyclic 3'5'-AMP-dependent kinase. It is of interest that the complete inactivation of muscle phosphorylase in GSD X is clinically well tolerated, whereas the complete lack of muscle phosphorylase in GSD V is characterized by cramps and pains. This difference may be explained by the ability of inactive phosphorylase *b* to degrade glycogen with the help of adenylic acid (5'-AMP) normally found in muscle tissue.

Hepatic Glycogenosis with Stunted Growth (GSD XI). GSD XI is a distinct clinical entity with greatly enlarged liver and stunted growth such that 12 yr olds may appear to be only 6 yr old. Affected children develop florid rickets in early life unless they receive oral phosphate supplementation and 50,000 units or more of vitamin D daily. Adequate growth is not attained through this regimen. Administration of arginine raises the level of growth hormone in serum. Intermittent aminoaciduria, galactosuria, and glucosuria are found.. Serum transaminase levels may be elevated, as are serum lipids. After puberty the growth rate may increase and hepatomegaly may recede.

Glycogen concentration is markedly increased in liver

and kidney but normal in muscle. All hepatic glycolytic enzyme activities that we have measured have been normal. The administration of glucagon did not increase the blood glucose concentration, but produced the increase of urinary excretion of cyclic AMP that is usually induced by glucagon administration.

Prenatal Diagnosis of GSD

The glycogenoses generally follow an autosomal recessive pattern of inheritance, except for GSD IXb, in which inheritance is sex-linked recessive. They should be detectable in the fetus through assay of cultured amniotic fluid cells when these cells normally produce the particular enzyme under study. This criterion is not fulfilled for GSD I since glucose-6-phosphate is not found in normal cultured amniotic fluid cells. GSD I, GSD III, GSD VI, GSD IX, and GSD X may not be candidates for prenatal diagnosis since most of the affected children with these conditions lead normal lives. In GSD IIa and GSD IV, on the other hand, antenatal diagnosis has been made through assay of cultured amniotic fluid cells. Uncultured cells are usually not adequate since only a small percentage of them are metabolically active and viable. Other restrictions may also be placed on the use of amniotic fluid; for example, we have found acid α-glucosidase activity in all amniotic fluid specimens tested, even in GSD IIa.

Amniocentesis is usually not carried out much before the 16th wk of gestation. Several wk may then be needed to culture the amniotic fluid cells. Reduction of this interval is sought. Short-term microcultures of cells have been used for microanalysis. Alternatively, prenatal diagnosis of GSD IIa is feasible within 1 day through electron microscopic examination of uncultured cells, which show abnormal intracellular lysosomes (Fig 8–21), whereas cells from healthy persons, presumably including those heterozygous for the disease, do not. GSD IIa is the only glycogen storage disease in which prenatal diagnosis by ultrastructural examination can currently be accomplished with the required reliability.

Concurrent Deficiencies of Enzymes in Patients with GSD

The delineation of defects in metabolism of glycogen has been complicated by technical problems involving activation of enzymes and the variability in distribution of the enzymes among body tissues and by the reasonably well established concurrence of double or multiple defects in the same person.

Deficiencies of 2 or more enzyme activities in the same patient are important. As a practical matter, the prognosis may be altered from that of an isolated deficiency. Liver sections in patients with deficiencies of debrancher or of phosphorylase generally exhibit a delicate fibrosis that remains essentially stationary. In a patient with both defects, however, the fibrosis may progress to frank clinical cirrhosis. Alternatively, an occasional combination of defects may mitigate or ameliorate the problem, though this might not be readily appreciated if the patient became well as a result. This situation is approximated if a defect is compensated for by the increased activity of a normal biochemical collateral pathway. For example, one would expect a deficiency of phosphohexoisomerase to result in arrested glycolysis and a clinical disaster. That this does not happen suggests that the defective interconversion of glucose-6-phosphate and fructose-6-phosphate can be bypassed by way of the pentose phosphate shunt.

DEFICIENCY OF GULONOLACTONE PATHWAY

Scurvy is discussed in Sec 3.27. The need for dietary L-ascorbic acid exists because man cannot synthesize its immediate precursor, 2-keto-L-gulonolactone, from L-gulonolactone. The latter is derived from D-glucose or myoinositol by way of D-glucuronate and L-gulonate. Hydroxylation of protocollagen is dependent on L-ascorbic acid as a reducing agent. In its absence the synthesized collagen does not form adequate fibers. The vascular fragility of scurvy is the result.

DEFICIENCY OF XYLULOSE DEHYDROGENASE
(Essential Benign Pentosuria)

This condition is typically discovered by the incidental finding of a reducing substance in the urine of an otherwise healthy individual. As in the case of benign fructosuria, one must not mistake the reducing substance for glucose or for evidence of diabetes mellitus. The pentose in the urine reacts with Clinitest but not with glucose oxidase test papers such as Testape or Clinistix dipsticks.

L-Xylulose dehydrogenase converts L-xylulose (which can arise from D-glucuronate) to xylitol. Xylitol is converted to D-xylulose, which becomes D-xylulose-5-phosphate and enters the pentose phosphate shunt. Deficiency of this enzyme leads to increased concentration of L-xylulose in blood and urine. The defect is rare and is most common in Jews. No therapy is required.

Pentosuria can be observed in normal individuals if the dietary pentose intake is increased, as with the excessive ingestion of fruit containing pentose. Under these circumstances there may be urinary excretion of xylose and arabinose up to 200 mg/24 hr in normal individuals.

DEFICIENCY OF ACID α-MANNOSIDASE
(Mannosidosis)

The appearance of the patient with mannosidosis is similar to that in Hurler syndrome. Liver and spleen are enlarged. The condition is a lysosomal disease; the lymphocytes contain vacuoles. Skeletal roentgenograms reveal structural abnormalities (dysostosis multiplex). Infections are frequent, especially of the middle ear and lungs. There may be corneal or lenticular opacities.

Psychomotor retardation is usually present. No treatment is available.

There is deficient activity of acid α-mannosidase in body fluids and tissues. Mannose-containing macromolecules are stored in "abnormal lysosomes" resembling those of the Hurler syndrome. They are observed easily in electron photomicrographs of liver. Mannosidosis exists in heterogeneous forms. No treatment is available.

DEFICIENCY OF ACID α-FUCOSIDASE
(Fucosidosis)

See Sec 8.31.

BLOOD GROUP SUBSTANCES

Blood group antigens are glycolipids or glycoproteins, depending upon whether they are cellular or soluble, respectively. In the synthesis of specific antigens, basic or fundamental macromolecules undergo modification through various transferases that are determined by genes designated H, A, B, Le, and so on. Gene H defines an enzyme that attaches fucose to the basic macromolecule in preparation for action by the other transferases. The attachment of this fucose molecule establishes the blood group O. Absence of the gene H results in a rare blood group (Bombay). The transferase dependent on gene A permits attachment of N acetyl galactosamine. Macromolecules so modified will become blood group A antigens. The transferase dependent on gene B attaches galactose, which will define group B antigens. To complete the synthesis of the respective antigen the attachment of several units of fucose (6-deoxy-L-galactose) is required. The exact sites and positions of these fucose units codetermine antigen specificity within the ABO and Lewis systems of blood group substances.

Incorporation of fucose is also decisive for whether an individual will secrete blood group substances into various body fluids, such as saliva. "Secretors" have the activity of a particular fucosyltransferase, whereas "nonsecretors" do not. The incidence of nonsecretors varies from 40% in black Americans to 25% in whites and to near zero in American Indians.

Patients with fucosidosis have the Lewis antigens in more than 5 times their usual concentration. Perhaps the accumulation of this macromolecule occurs because the deficiency of α-fucosidase in tissues of such patients impairs the disposal of fucose units that reside in the Lewis antigen.

8.22 DIAGNOSTIC PROCEDURES IN DEFECTS OF METABOLISM OF CARBOHYDRATES

Clinical awareness is essential to the recognition and diagnosis of the child who may have an inborn error of carbohydrate metabolism. A limited number of tests may provide a preliminary assessment: determinations of serum levels of lactate, pyruvate, transaminases, creatine phosphokinase, lipids, glucose, uric acid, and amino acids; measurement of urinary excretion of 3'5'-AMP and catecholamines; electrocardiography, roentgenographic examination of the sizes of the heart and kidney, determination of liver size by ultrasound; and carbohydrate tolerance tests with glucagon or glucose. The ultimate diagnosis depends on biochemical analysis of tissues. Biochemical diagnosis, moreover, provides the basis of treatment.

The tissue to be examined should be obtained preferentially from the organ or organs showing clinical signs of abnormality. Liver biopsy using the Menghini needle does not carry undue risks for the patient so long as adequate precautions are taken. However, needle biopsy provides only about 20 mg of tissue, which may not be enough for definitive studies. The interest of the patient may, therefore, be better served by open biopsy, which has the added advantage of providing easy access to specimens of skeletal muscle of the abdominal wall.

Analysis of white blood cells is valuable in selected instances, such as the determination of the carrier state of GSD IIa. Leukocytes have limitations, however, since low activity of leukocyte phosphorylase has been observed in persons without hepatomegaly. Our experience suggests that examination of blood cells is complementary to analysis of tissues of solid organs. Fibroblast cultures of biopsy specimens of superficial skin can be used for biochemical and electron microscopic examination but are of limited reliability.

Detailed advice on how to procure and handle specimens shipped to special laboratories should be obtained from the collaborating laboratory *before* the biopsy is made.

8.23 THERAPY OF DEFECTS IN METABOLISM OF CARBOHYDRATES

For many of the conditions discussed in this chapter, no treatment is effective; for others, none is necessary. The clinician's role may be limited to supportive care (see Sec 2.80 and 2.81) or to genetic counseling (Sec 6.7 and 6.29).

In a few conditions dietary regimens may offer some help; for some they are lifesaving (galactosemia, fructose intolerance, etc.). The therapies of the future depend upon research to find ways of replacing specific enzymes, adding pharmacologic doses of cofactors (vitamins, etc.) to the diet, or compensating for the enzymatic defect with hormones or drugs.

Enzyme replacement has been carried out with the transplantation of normal kidneys into patients with Fabry disease and of normal cultured fibroblasts into patients with Hunter or Hurler disease. In Fabry disease, characterized by α-galactosidase deficiency and the accumulation of ceramide trihexoside, angiokeratomatosis and attacks of pain and renal failure are seen. The transplantation of a normal kidney may provide the patient with a "filter" for circulating trihexoside with enough α-galactosidase to initiate its degradation. In 2 patients with Hurler disease, characterized by iduronidase deficiency, we repeatedly transplanted normal cultured fibroblasts under the skin of the back without apparent ultrastructural, biochemical, or clinical improvement.

The purified enzyme α-glucosidase of fungal origin was infused into a patient with GSD IIa. The infused enzyme normalized ultrastructure and glycogen concentration of hepatocytes; it did not gain entry into skeletal myocytes or cardiac cells, and death occurred in respiratory failure.

Vitamin therapy has recently been used successfully in patients with Chédiak-Higashi disease, which can be considered a lysosomal disease with no identified enzymatic defect as yet. Leukocytes are defective in bactericidal capacity, and this may lead to repeated severe and often fatal pyogenic infections. Patients' leukocytes have elevated concentrations of cyclic 3'5'-AMP. The administration of vitamin C corrected the defect in leukocytes and prevented pyogenic infections in patients with Chédiak-Higashi disease, although it was not equally effective in every patient. The abnormal cellular morphology was not corrected by vitamin C.

GEORGE HUG

Aynsley-Green A, Williamson DH, Gitzelmann R: Hepatic glycogen synthetase deficiency: Definition of the syndrome from metabolic and enzyme studies on a nine year-old girl. Arch Dis Child 131:573, 1977.

Bagnell P, Hug G, Walling L, et al: Biochemical and morphologic observations in severe infantile fructose intolerance. Pediatr Res 8:156, 1974.

Beratis NG, LaBadie GU, Hirschhorn K: Characterization of the molecular defect in infantile and adult acid α-glucosidase deficiency fibroblasts. J Clin Invest 62:1264, 1978.

Boxer LA, Watanabe AM, Rister M, et al: Correction of leukocyte function in Chédiak-Higashi syndrome by ascorbate. N Engl J Med 295:1041, 1976.

Brandt NJ, Terenius L, Jacobsen BB, et al: Hyper-endorphin syndrome in a child with necrotizing encephalomyelopathy. N Engl J Med 303:914, 1980.

Cederbaum SD, Blass JP, Minkoff N, et al: Sensitivity to carbohydrate in a patient with familial intermittent lactic acidosis and pyruvate dehydrogenase deficiency. Pediatr Res 10:713, 1976.

Dapergolas G, Gregoriadis G: Hypoglycaemic effect of liposome-entrapped insulin administered intragastrically into rats. Lancet 2:824, 1976.

DeVivo DC, Haymond MW, Obert KA, et al: Defective activation of the pyruvate dehydrogenase complex in subacute necrotizing encephalomyelopathy (Leigh disease). Ann Neurol 6:483, 1979.

Durand P, Borrone C, Gatti R: On genetic variants in fucosidosis. J Pediatr 89:688, 1976.

Farrell DF, Clark AF, Scott CR, et al: Absence of pyruvate decarboxylase activity in man: A cause of congenital lactic acidosis. Science 187:1082, 1975.

Gitzelmann R, Steinmann B, Mitchell B, et al: Uridine diphosphate galactose 4'-epimerase deficiency. IV. Report of eight cases in three families. Helv Paediatr Acta 31:441, 1976.

Greene HL, Slonim AE, O'Neill JA, et al: Continuous nocturnal intragastric feeding for management of type I glycogen storage disease. N Engl J Med 294:423, 1976.

Gregoriadis G: The carrier potential of liposomes in biology and medicine (part 1). N Engl J Med 295:707, 1976.

Gröbe H, von Bassewitz DB, Dominick HC, et al: Subacute necrotizing encephalomyelopathy: Clinical, ultrastructural, biochemical and therapeutic studies in an infant. Acta Paediatr Scand 64:755, 1975.

Hug G, Chuck G, Walling L, et al: Liver phosphorylase deficiency in glycogenosis type VI: Documentation by biochemical analysis of hepatic biopsy specimens. J Lab Clin Med 84:26, 1974.

Hug G, Garancis JC, Schubert WK, et al: Glycogen storage disease, types II, III, VIII, and IX. Am J Dis Child 111:457, 1966.

Hug G, Harris D, Grunt JA: Two types of glycogenosis (GSD) in the same girl: Combined deficiency of phosphorylase kinase in liver (GSD IX) and debrancher in liver and muscle (GSD III). Pediatr Res 10:366, 1976.

Hug G, Schubert WK, Chuck G: Phosphorylase kinase of the liver: Deficiency in a girl with increased hepatic glycogen. Science 153:1534, 1966.

Jolly RD, Thompson KG, Murphy CE, et al: Enzyme replacement therapy—an experiment of nature in a chimeric mannosidosis calf. Pediatr Res 10:219, 1976.

Kemp, CB, Knight MJ, Sharp DW, et al: Transplantation of isolated pancreatic islets into the portal vein of diabetic rats. Nature 244:447, 1973.

Lerner A, Iancu TC, Bashan N, et al: A new variant of glycogen storage disease type IXc. Am J Dis Child 136:407, 1982.

Lonsdale D, Hug G: D-Thyroxin induces phosphorylase kinase activity and normalizes glycogen concentration in the liver of a child with hepatic phosphorylase kinase deficient glycogenosis. J Cell Biol 70:157a, 1976.

Mehler M, DiMauro S: Late-onset acid maltase deficiency. Arch Neurol 33:692, 1976.

Ng WG, Donnel GN, Alfi O: Prenatal diagnosis of galactosaemia. Lancet 1:43, 1977.

Putschar W: Über angeborene Glykogenspeicherkrankheit des Herzens. Beitr Pathol Anat 90:222, 1932.

Robinson BH, Sherwood WG: Pyruvate dehydrogenase deficiency: A cause of congenital chronic lactic acidosis in infancy. Pediatr Res 9:935, 1975.

Robinson BH, Taylor J, Sherwood WG: Dihydrolipoyl dehydrogenase deficiency—a cause of congenital lactic acidosis. Pediatr Res 11:520, 1977.

Weil D, VanCong N, Gross M-S, et al: Localisation du gene de l'α-glucosidase acids (α-GLUa) sur le segment q21→qter du chromosome 17 par I-hybridation cellulaire interspecifique. Hum Genet 52:249, 1979.

DEFECTS IN METABOLISM OF PURINES AND PYRIMIDINES

Purines and pyrimidines are heterocyclic nitrogen-containing compounds. Combinations of purines and pyrimidines with ribose or deoxyribose and with phosphate create nucleotides. Combined with ribose and phosphate (hence, ribonucleotide), purines and pyrimidines form the elements of ribonucleic acid (RNA); combined with deoxyribose and phosphate (deoxyribonucleotides), they form deoxyribonucleic acid (DNA). The ability to synthesize the purine ring de novo is virtually universal among living organisms, including man. The final product of purine metabolism in man is uric acid.

Other than uric acid, the purines of clinical importance are adenine and guanine. The important pyrimidines are thymine, cytosine, and uracil. The importance of nucleotides as components of DNA rests on the genetic function of this material. RNA is of central importance in the regulation of protein synthesis and as a component of such important energy-producing compounds and nucleotide cofactors as ATP, UDPG, NAD and NADP, and others.

8.24 DISORDERS OF PURINE METABOLISM

Gout. The hallmark of gout is the elevation of serum uric acid concentration. This ancient disease primarily affects adults and rarely occurs in children. A notable exception is the child with type I glycogen storage disease (GSD I), in whom hyperuricemia routinely occurs and gouty arthritis and tophi appear in adolescence. As in this instance, when hyperuricemia and gout occur in childhood, they are almost always secondary to another disorder.

Elevations of concentrations of uric acid in serum can result from several general metabolic disturbances. Certain patients have an abnormally active production de novo of uric acid; others have reduction in the renal clearance of uric acid; and some represent combinations of these 2 major factors.

At least 95% of gouty arthritis is seen in postpubertal men. In a very small group of patients, the activity of the enzyme hypoxanthine guanine phosphoribosyl transferase (Fig 8–26) is reduced to only a few per cent of normal (a total deficiency leads to the Lesch-Nyhan syndrome). In another group of patients overproduc-

tion of uric acid and hyperuricemia could be clearly traced to an abnormally high activity of the enzyme phosphoribosylpyrophosphate synthetase or PRPP (Fig 8–27). In both of these situations, the increased availability of PRPP leads to an increase in the endogenous production of uric acid. Both enzymes are genetically transmitted as X-linked recessives. The increased availability of PRPP is the mechanism that also leads to hyperuricemia in type I glycogen storage disease; it is also probable that some of the reduction in uric acid clearance in GSD I is due to the hyperlactic acidemia, which reduces the renal clearance of uric acid.

Whether a patient with elevated levels of uric acid in serum develops gouty arthritis depends largely on the severity and duration of hyperuricemia.

Lesch-Nyhan Syndrome. Boys with this syndrome are usually normal at birth. The 1st abnormality consistently noted is a delay in motor development in the 1st few mo of life. Later, extrapyramidal choreoathetoid movements appear, and hyperreflexia, ankle clonus, and spasticity of the legs develop.

The most striking clinical abnormality is the dramatic compulsive self-destructive behavior usually observed. Older children begin to bite and chew their fingers, lips, and buccal mucosa. This behavior leads to mutilation. It is not the result of inability to feel pain but of a compulsive urge that appears so irresistible that it is necessary to restrain the patients.

In the Lesch-Nyhan syndrome, uric acid concentrations in serum are commonly in the range seen in the adult with gout (10–12 mg/dl), and there are marked increases in the production of uric acid and in its urinary excretion. There is an almost total absence of activity of the enzyme hypoxanthine guanine phosphoribosyltransferase, which can be demonstrated in many tissues, most easily and commonly in erythrocytes and fibroblasts. This enzyme is important to the "purine salvage" pathway, through which hypoxanthine and xanthine can be converted to nucleotides, to inosinic acid, and to guanylic acid (Fig 8–26). When this enzymatic pathway is not operative, PRPP synthetase activity increases and PRPP accumulates within the cell, giving rise to accelerated purine production de novo and to excesses of uric acid. The salvage pathway may be important in the synthesis of nucleotides within the brain; when this pathway is inactive, the brain may be unable to synthesize its own required nucleotides.

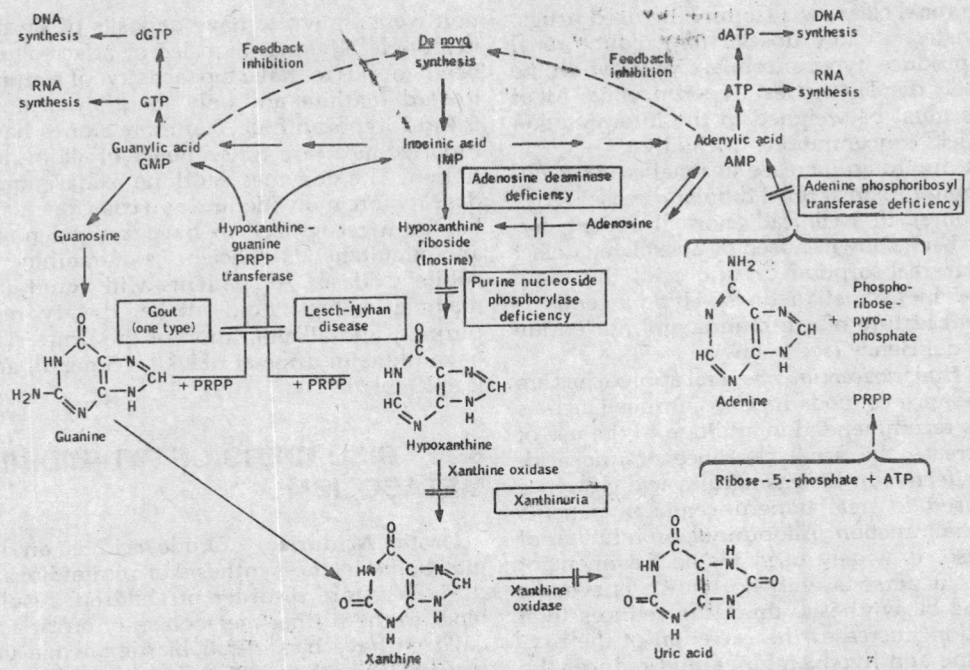

Figure 8-26 Pathways in purine metabolism and salvage. See also legend for Fig 8-1.

Gouty tophi and gouty arthritis are sometimes seen in older children with the Lesch-Nyhan syndrome. Tophi are the results of accumulation of sodium urate crystals in subcutaneous and other tissues; they traditionally occur over the extensor surfaces of the elbows, knees, fingers, and toes.

This syndrome is transmitted as an X-linked condition. Fibroblasts cultured from biopsies of skin of mothers of patients with Lesch-Nyhan syndrome can be shown by cloning techniques and by selective chemical treatment to represent 2 cell populations, 1 normal and 1 deficient in the crucial enzyme. Such studies lend support to the Lyon hypothesis concerning random inactivation of X chromosomes during development of females.

Other Abnormalities of Uric Acid Metabolism. Hyperuricemia is commonly encountered in situations of a marked increase in cell number and an increased turnover of these cells, as in myeloproliferative diseases. The excess of uric acid results from an increased intensity of degradation of nucleotides to purine end products (uric acid). In the treatment of acute leukemia or lymphoma masses, the sudden lysis of cells may provoke hyperuricemia and hyperuricosuria as serious clinical consequences (Sec 15.6–15.8).

Hyperuricemia may occur in any condition in which renal clearance is reduced. When the serum concentrations of β-hydroxybutyrate and acetoacetate are increased, as in starvation and diabetic ketoacidosis, there are elevations of serum uric acid concentrations-related

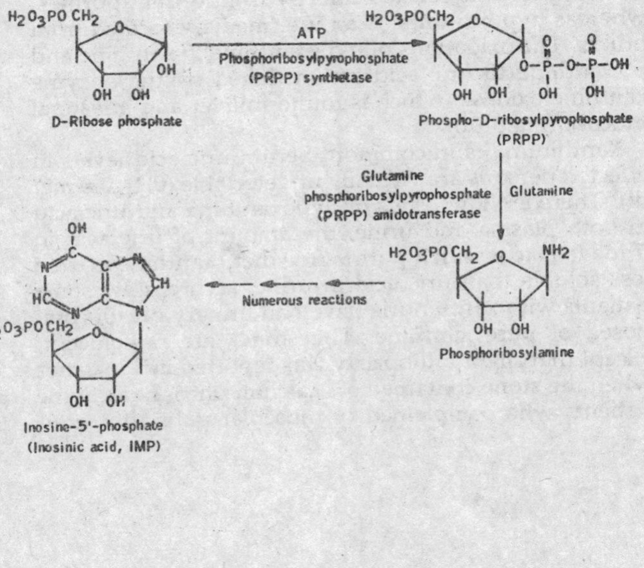

Figure 8-27 Early steps in the biosynthesis of the purine ring.

to reduction in renal clearance. Commonly used drugs, such as salicylates, in low doses, may reduce renal clearance and produce hyperuricemia. Down syndrome patients routinely display modest hyperuricemia. All of these variables must be weighed in the interpretation of serum uric acid concentrations in children.

Hypouricemia due to an increase in renal clearance of uric acid is seen in proximal renal tubular diseases (e.g., Fanconi syndrome). In 1 clinically normal patient, hypouricemia has been shown caused by an isolated defect of renal tubular reabsorption of uric acid; the same defect is found in Dalmatian dogs. Hypouricemia is also a prominent feature of xanthinuria and nucleoside phosphorylase deficiency (see below).

Treatment of Hyperuricemia. Several approaches are used. The avoidance of foods high in purines (such as sweetbreads) is recommended in addition to the use of drugs that increase the renal clearance of uric acid. Probenecid is effective in increasing uric acid clearance and may be used to treat hyperuricemia in patients with normal renal function. Allopurinol, an inhibitor of xanthine oxidase, is widely used in the treatment of hyperuricemia. In persons with no known enzymatic defect in purine biosynthesis, this drug reduces total purine production, increases the excretion of the oxypurines (xanthine and hypoxanthine), and reduces the excretion of uric acid. In Lesch-Nyhan syndrome, treatment with allopurinol reduces uric acid concentrations (and ameliorates gouty arthritis and tophi); there is no effect on the severe neurologic problems.

For any patient with hyperuricosuria, whether as a result of increased synthesis de novo or of drug therapy, it is essential that a high volume of urine be maintained and that its pH be maintained near neutrality (7.0). This can ordinarily be done effectively with a balanced mixture of salts, such as Polycitra, which is usually more effective than bicarbonate. The importance of adjusting the urine pH to 7.0 is illustrated by the fact that at pH 5.0 the solubility of uric acid is 15 mg/dl, whereas at pH 7.0 the solubility is 200 mg/dl.

The hyperuricemia associated with type I glycogen storage disease, like other significant hyperuricemias, should be treated; it does not respond to probenecid, but does respond appropriately to allopurinol.

Xanthinuria. Xanthine is the immediate precursor of uric acid. It is formed directly from certain purines, whereas hypoxanthine is an intermediary formed from others. The oxidations of hypoxanthine to xanthine and of xanthine to uric acid are mediated by the enzyme xanthine oxidase, which is found in liver and intestinal mucosa (Fig 8–26).

Xanthinuria is uncommon. Serum uric acid levels in affected persons are virtually undetectable (0.1–0.8 mg/dl). There are low levels of hypoxanthine and uric acid in both plasma and urine; the amount of uric acid in urine falls to 0 with a purine-free diet. Xanthine is even less soluble than uric acid in urine; accordingly, some patients with xanthinuria have had urinary calculi composed of pure xanthine. The stones are radiolucent, except that slight radiopacity was reported in 1 instance when the stone contained 5% calcium phosphate. Some patients who complained of muscular pain after exer-

tion were shown to have deposits of xanthine crystals in muscles. Jejunal biopsies of affected patients have been found to have no activity of xanthine oxidase toward xanthine and only about 5% of normal activity toward hypoxanthine. Xanthine stones have also been reported as a rare consequence of allopurinol administration. The enzymes xanthine oxidase and sulfite oxidase require molybdenum as a cofactor. A single patient has been recognized to have molybdenum deficiency and simultaneous deficiencies of xanthine oxidase and sulfite oxidase. All patients with xanthinuria should maintain a high fluid intake, dietary restrictions of purines, and alkalinization of the urine. The solubility of xanthine in urine at pH 5.0 is 5 mg/dl, and at pH 7.0 it is 13 mg/dl.

8.25   DISORDERS OF PYRIMIDINE METABOLISM

Orotic Aciduria. Orotic acid is an intermediate metabolite in the synthesis of pyrimidines. Orotic aciduria is a rare disorder of children, resulting from a block in the further metabolism of orotic acid. Affected children have had megaloblastic anemia unresponsive to therapy with vitamin C, folic acid, or vitamin B_{12}; they excreted up to 1.5 gm/24 hr of orotic acid and formed orotic acid crystals in urine. These patients were also retarded in their growth and development, but the hematologic manifestations were the more dramatic clinical features, probably because vigorous synthesis of RNA and DNA is so necessary for normal hematopoiesis. In 2 patients, therapy with corticosteroids has resulted in general improvement, but disappearance of abnormalities in the marrow or of the excretion of orotic acid was obtained only when pyrimidine compounds were administered, which are found beyond the metabolic block.

In most patients with orotic aciduria, orotidylic acid pyrophosphorylase and orotidylic acid decarboxylase are both deficient (Fig 8–28). A patient who lacks only the decarboxylase has been clinically indistinguishable from patients with the more usual genotype. The fact that 2 sequential enzymes are missing in most patients with orotic aciduria suggests that the 2 enzymes share some common subunit. These enzyme deficiencies have been demonstrated in liver, leukocytes, erythrocytes, and fibroblasts grown in culture. Heterozygotes have approximately half the normal levels of activities of both enzymes.

The administration of pyrimidine derivatives lowers the urinary excretion of orotic acid. This effect indicates that enzymes in the pathway leading to orotic acid synthesis are under feedback inhibition control. The hematologic response is directly due to the provision for DNA and RNA synthesis of essential material which cannot be made de novo.

Orotic acid excretion is increased in the urines of children who have primary genetic defects in the urea cycle. This is a result of the fact that additional carbamyl phosphate (which is usually utilized in urea synthesis) is shunted into de novo pyrimidine synthesis; this leads

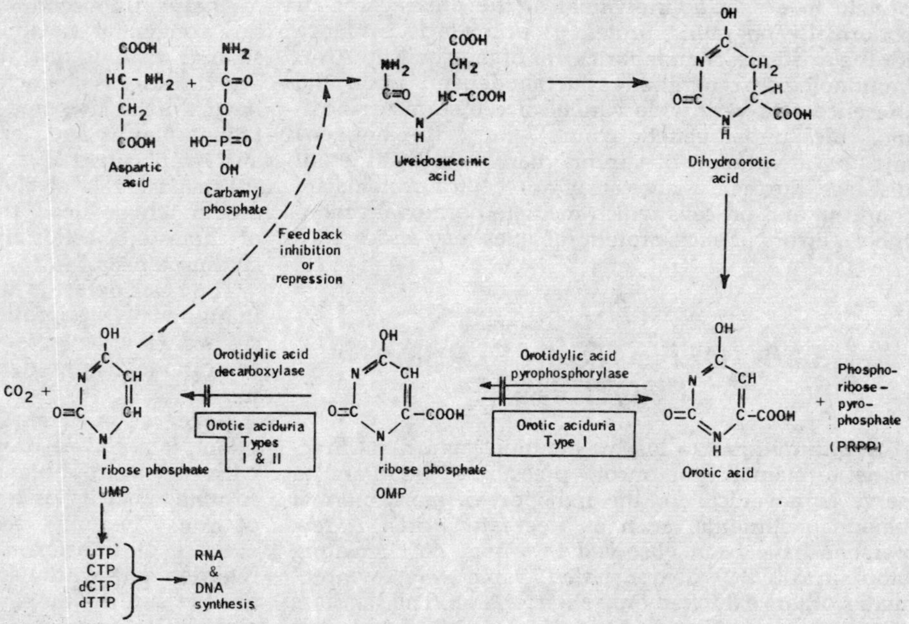

Figure 8–28 Pathways in pyrimidine biosynthesis. See also legend for Fig 8–1.

to an apparent overproduction of orotic acid. Orotic aciduria is also seen in nucleoside phosphorylase deficiency (see below).

Adenosine Deaminase Deficiency. Both cellular and humoral immunity are defective in children with severe combined immunodeficiency (SCID), a disorder of infancy with an invariably fatal outcome if untreated (Sec 9.14). In nearly half of patients with SCID inherited in an autosomal recessive fashion, a deficiency of adenosine deaminase activity has been demonstrated. Adenosine deaminase catalyzes the hydrolytic deamination of adenosine to produce inosine. The enzyme deficiency may be causally related to the immunodeficiency or, alternatively, be closely linked genetically.

Affected infants show lymphopenia, thymic aplasia (or hypoplasia), absence of delayed hypersensitivity, and defective synthesis of immunoglobulins and antibodies. Their lymphocytes do not respond to mitogens in vitro.

Currently the treatment of choice is histocompatible bone marrow transplantation; this, however, is severely limited by the availability of histocompatible donors. The infusion of frozen, irradiated erythrocytes has been beneficial in some but not all patients. These infusions have resulted in dramatic decrease of ATP in lymphocytes.

Nucleoside Phosphorylase Deficiency

Purine nucleoside phosphorylase effects the conversion of inosine and guanosine to their respective bases, hypoxanthine and guanine. This enzyme is present in most body tissues of man.

This enzyme is located on chromosome 14; genetic deficiencies of this enzyme, transmitted in an autosomal recessive fashion, are associated with marked deficiencies of cellular but normal humoral immunity. The clinical course is milder than that of adenosine deaminase deficiency.

These patients have profound hypouricemia and hypouricaciduria along with substantial orotic aciduria. There is increase in plasma guanosine and inosine.

No effective treatment has been shown; bone marrow graft is likely to be effective.

R. RODNEY HOWELL

Giblett ER, Polmar SH: Inherited immunodeficiency diseases: Relationship to lymphocyte metabolic dysfunction. In Steinberg AG, Bearn AG, Motulsky AG, Childs B (eds): Progress in Medical Genetics, Vol III. Philadelphia, WB Saunders, 1979, pp 177–219.

OTHER DEFECTS OF ENZYMES AND PROTEINS

We have thus far considered those inborn errors of metabolism that can be assigned naturally to certain biochemical systems, such as those involved in amino acid, carbohydrate, purine, or pyrimidine metabolism. Other defects involve the soluble proteins and formed elements of blood and certain proteins and enzymes of other organs or tissues.

At present a concerted effort is under way to map, via electrophoretic and chromatographic techniques, all of the proteins found in man. The absence of any given protein in a specific individual or the presence of an abnormally migrating protein is prima-facie evidence for the existence of an inborn error of metabolism. Also, immunologic recognition systems depend upon the presence of a very wide variety of cell surface macromolecules under genetic control, e.g., HLA antigens and the association of various markers with different diseases. Further, a large array of receptor proteins are found in and on cells which mediate hormonal action. Inborn errors of such protein moieties may also occur.

8.26 DEFECTS IN PLASMA PROTEINS

Analbuminemia. Plasma albumin has 2 main functions: to maintain the oncotic pressure of blood and to serve as a vehicle for the transport of many normal blood constituents, such as free fatty acids. A few persons have been observed in whom no circulating albumin could be demonstrated. Some were asymptomatic; others exhibited only slight edema. The 1st cases reported were siblings whose parents were double 2nd cousins, suggesting that the disorder is genetic in nature. Periodic administrations of albumin result in disappearance of edema, but usually no treatment is necessary.

It may be speculated that lack of symptoms in analbuminemia depends on lifelong compensations in fluid dynamics which patients with such disorders as nephrosis or protein-losing enteropathy are unable to make in the face of acutely lowered oncotic pressure.

Haptoglobin Deficiency. Haptoglobin is an α-2-globulin that binds free hemoglobin. There are numerous phenotypic variations (polymorphism) in the types of haptoglobins among normal persons. These are under genetic control. With severe hemolytic anemia, haptoglobin levels may be greatly decreased or absent. Healthy persons have been found who have no demonstrable circulating haptoglobin, on a genetic basis, without apparent ill effect.

Abetalipoproteinemia. Abetalipoproteinemia (Sec 11.49 and 21.17), a defect in synthesis of β-lipoprotein, is characterized by bizarrely shaped erythrocytes with thornlike projections (acanthocytes) and steatorrhea in infancy, followed by the development of ataxic neuropathy in childhood and retinitis pigmentosa in early adulthood. Characteristic pathologic changes have been observed in the intestinal mucosa; the columnar epithelium is filled with globules containing lipids. Plasma cholesterol, phospholipid, and triglyceride levels are sharply reduced. Beta-lipoprotein and chylomicra are absent. There appear to be at least 2 forms of abetalipoproteinemia, each associated with a deficiency of an antigenically different β-lipoprotein. In 1 form triglycerides are assimilated from jejunal epithelial cells; in the other the lipid cannot exit from the villous core. A patient with absent β-lipoprotein has been described who had chylomicra and normal postprandial triglyceride levels. The disorder is transmitted in an autosomal recessive manner.

Analphalipoproteinemia (Tangier Disease). This rare congenital metabolic defect was first described in siblings residing on Tangier Island in Chesapeake Bay. The disorder is characterized by enlarged tonsils which have a distinctive orange color. Other clinical manifestations may include enlargement of the liver, spleen, and lymph nodes.

Plasma levels of cholesterol and phospholipids are moderately reduced; there is storage of large amounts of cholesterol esters in reticuloendothelial tissues, including tonsils.

The basic defect is absence in serum of α-lipoprotein (high-density lipoprotein). Inheritance is autosomal recessive. Heterozygotes have about half the normal concentrations of high-density lipoprotein but are asymptomatic.

Absence of Transferrin. Transferrin, or siderophilin, is a plasma protein of molecular weight 90,000, with the electrophoretic mobility of a β-2-globulin. It is assumed that it has a prominent role in the transport of iron. The only recorded instance of a congenital absence of transferrin at birth involved a physically retarded girl with hepatomegaly, splenomegaly, and anemia sufficiently severe to require multiple transfusions. The anemia did not respond to any of the antianemic agents used. Iron was absorbed from the intestinal tract and transported to the tissues. Erythrocytes were hypochromic, and the marrow contained many immature erythroblasts. Liver biopsy revealed cirrhosis and siderosis. Immunochemical studies revealed complete absence of transferrin. Antibodies to transferrin developed after multiple transfusions. Sudden death at 7 yr of age was attributed to hemosiderosis. Both parents had lower than normal amounts of transferrin; this suggests autosomal recessive transmission.

C1 Esterase Inhibitor. Reduced levels of C1 esterase inhibitor, an α_2-neuraminoglycoprotein, are associated with hereditary angioneurotic edema (giant urticaria). The protein is an inhibitor of the esterase activity of the complement component designated C1. The esterase rises to high concentrations during an attack and is thought to be responsible for increased capillary permeability. The disorder can be caused by at least 2 different genetic defects: in one, concentration of C1 esterase inhibitor is low; in the other, an abnormally structured protein is produced. Transfusion of fresh frozen plasma may be of benefit if given during the acute phase of edema and/or abdominal pain.

Affected persons are apparently heterozygous for the condition and manifest their fluctuating levels of the inhibitor as episodic edema. No homozygous persons with the condition are known (Sec 9.23).

Complement Deficiencies. A number of patients have been described with a variety of complement deficiencies (Sec 9.21 through 9.28).

α_1-Antitrypsin Protein Deficiency. See Sec 11.65 and 12.78.

Transcobalamine II Deficiency. Two different serum proteins bind vitamin B_{12}. One of these, transcobalamine I (an α-globulin), has been reported deficient in 2 siblings; there were no discernible clinical or hematologic sequelae. The other protein, transcobalamine II (a β-globulin), has been reported deficient in several infants with severe megaloblastic anemia, some of whom have also had neurologic changes. No abnormalities were found in reactions involving the coenzyme forms of vitamin B_{12}, homocysteine methyltransferase, and methylmalonyl CoA mutase (Sec 8.7). Treatment consists of parenteral administration of large doses of vitamin B_{12}.

8.27 DEFECTS IN PLASMA ENZYMES

Pseudocholinesterase. Pseudocholinesterase is found in plasma, liver, and neural tissue; its physiologic function is poorly understood.

Numerous presumably allelic forms of the altered enzyme are known. Some with reduced enzyme activity are characterized by the extent of inhibition by dibucaine or fluoride, whereas a "silent" form has no activity. Homozygotes for each form and mixed heterozygotes are known. About 1 in 25 persons is heterozygous for one or another of these defects.

The 1 person in 3000 who is homozygous for one of these genes is ordinarily asymptomatic. The defect was discovered because the enzyme participates in the destruction of a commonly used muscle relaxant, succinylcholine. In the normal person this drug is rapidly destroyed by pseudocholinesterase and therefore has a transient effect. Persons homozygous for mutant pseudocholinesterase split the drug abnormally slowly or not at all and apnea results, lasting for hours. Artificial respiration is required, preferably through an endotracheal tube; the period of apnea can be shortened by transfusion with normal plasma.

Another genetic alteration of pseudocholinesterase has been described which leads to *increased* enzyme activity and hence to resistance to the pharmacologic effects of succinylcholine. These observations demonstrate how unusual sensitivity or resistance to the pharmacologic effects of drugs may be predetermined by the genetic constitution of the person. The study of such interactions is known as pharmacogenetics. Other well studied examples are primaquine sensitivity and genetic variation in response to isoniazid.

Lecithin-Cholesterol Acyltransferase Deficiency. Three sisters with corneal opacities, normochromic anemia, and proteinuria were shown to have decreased levels of alpha-lipoprotein and prebeta-lipoprotein, increased concentration of free cholesterol, almost absent esterified cholesterol, and, in 2 cases, hyperlipidemia. There were none of the changes of the tonsils seen in analpha-lipoproteinemia. The defect was demonstrated to be an almost complete absence of lecithin-cholesterol acyltransferase, a plasma enzyme that normally esterifies cholesterol; lecithin is the source of the fatty acid.

Carnosinase Deficiency. See Sec. 8.14.

γ-Glutamyl Transpeptidase Deficiency. A moderately retarded adult with increased levels of glutathione in blood and urine has been shown to have a deficiency in serum of γ-glutamyl transpeptidase, which catalyzes the 1st step in the degradation of glutathione. There was no other abnormality in amino acid excretion. These observations must be seen in the perspective of the involvement of this enzyme in amino acid transport (Fig 8–7). Apparently, the serum enzyme produced in the liver is under different genetic control from that synthesized in the renal tubule and intestine.

Hypophosphatasia. Several isoenzymes in plasma have alkaline phosphatase activity. The one presumably derived from bone is markedly low in homozygous individuals who excrete large amounts of phosphoethanolamine and have a defect of ossification leading to severe bone disease (Sec 23.25).

8.28 DEFECTS OF PROTEINS OF OTHER TISSUES

Mucopolysaccharidoses. The numerous defects of mucopolysaccharide metabolism are discussed in Chapter 23.

Ceruloplasmin Deficiency (Wilson Disease) (Sec 11.98). Ceruloplasmin, a blue-colored α_2-globulin containing 8 copper atoms per molecule, constitutes 0.5% of the total plasma proteins. The average normal serum concentration is 25 mg/dl (range, 16–33). Low levels are found in newborn infants and in patients with active nephrosis, who lose ceruloplasmin in urine. Wilson disease, or hepatolenticular degeneration, is a hereditary disorder transmitted by an autosomal recessive gene in which low serum levels of ceruloplasmin are characteristic; they average 5 mg/dl (range, 0–14). Several unequivocal cases, however, have been observed with normal levels of ceruloplasmin. Furthermore, the ceruloplasmin found in the blood of patients with Wilson disease has been shown to be of normal structure. An abnormal structure of the intracellular storage protein, *copperthionein*, results in a 4-fold increase in affinity for copper, and all the clinical and biochemical manifestations can be explained on this basis.

Menkes Kinky Hair Syndrome. This sex-linked disorder is characterized by abnormal hair, growth retardation, progressive neurologic degeneration, and death in the 1st few yr of life. Defective absorption of copper and decreased levels of ceruloplasmin and copper in plasma are seen. If copper is administered intravenously to these patients, the synthesis of ceruloplasmin occurs rapidly. Analysis of mitochondria from brain and muscle has revealed a diminished content of the copper-containing enzyme, cytochrome oxidase (cytochrome a + a₃). This finding may be secondary to the defect in copper absorption. Fibroblasts cultured from patients with this disease consistently have elevated copper concentrations compared to normal fibroblasts (Sec 21.17).

Molybdenum Cofactor Deficiency. A 3 yr old girl with the chemical findings of both sulfite oxidase deficiency (Sec 8.5) and xanthinuria (Sec 8.24) who also had ocular abnormalities (dislocated lenses, Brushfield spots, and nystagmus), neurologic abnormalities (tonic-clonic seizures), and mental retardation has been described. The defect appears to be an inability to form the molybdenum-pterin–containing cofactor whose presence is required for the activity of both enzymes. Treatment consisted of restriction of sulfur-containing amino acids and allopurinol administration. Two other patients with this combination are known.

Myoglobin. Myoglobin, a heme protein found in muscle, is responsible for the intracellular transport of oxygen. Two variants of myoglobin have been identified by starch gel electrophoresis. Changes in amino acid sequence producing myoglobinopathies are analogous to the changes responsible for the hemoglobinopathies. In each of 2 families observed, mother and son were heterozygous for the normal and for the aberrant molecules. Each family had a distinctive aberrant molecule. Neuromuscular diseases were not found in these families.

Spectrophotometric analyses of myoglobin from a number of patients with various neuromuscular diseases have revealed consistent changes in those with the sex-linked form of pseudohypertrophic muscular dystrophy (Duchenne) and the persistence of fetal myoglobin in 1 patient with facioscapulohumeral dystrophy. Fetal myoglobin has also been found in a patient with recurrent myoglobinuria. The myoglobin isolated from patients with progressive spinal muscular atrophy and the limb-girdle type of muscular atrophy appears to be normal spectrometrically. Myoglobinuria may also occur in a number of disorders of muscle metabolism such as deficient phosphorylase activity (Sec 8.21), deficient phosphofructokinase activity (Sec 8.21), deficient phosphoglycerate mutase activity (Sec 8.19), deficient lactate dehydrogenase activity (Sec 8.19), and absent carnitine palmityl transferase activity (see below), as well as in other disorders discussed in Chapters 16 and 22.

Carnitine Palmityl Transferase Deficiency. The enzyme carnitine palmityl transferase effects the transfer of long chain fatty acids across the mitochondrial membrane. This enzyme activity was markedly reduced in 2 brothers who, although otherwise normal, had repeated episodes of myoglobinuria; in 1 brother an acute episode of myoglobinuria resulted in renal failure.

Xeroderma Pigmentosum. Extreme dermal sensitivity to sunlight or ultraviolet light and the development of skin cancers that metastasize and lead to death are characteristic of this rare recessive disease (Sec 24.14). Skin fibroblasts grown in tissue culture have a defect of the enzymatic mechanism for repair of DNA. In normal persons the rupture of 1 strand of DNA in the double helical form by a mutagenic agent such as ultraviolet light is rapidly repaired by a set of specific enzymes that ensure integrity of the genetic material. Persons with xeroderma pigmentosum lack 1 of these enzymes and are therefore subject not only to skin damage by what would normally be small doses of radiation, but also to the immediate, potentially carcinogenic effects of other unrepaired breaks in DNA.

There seem to be at least 3 genetic forms of the disease, each with a different biochemical defect; in 1 patient with clinical xeroderma pigmentosum no defect in DNA repair could be demonstrated.

Macular Corneal Dystrophy. This is an autosomal recessive condition which results in progressive opacity of the cornea due to the deposition of an abnormal keratan sulfate in the stromal layers. Recent work has shown that the normal cornea contains a keratan sulfate proteoglycan which is chemically distinct and different from the keratan sulfate found in other tissues, such as cartilage. In macular corneal dystrophy the keratan sulfate proteoglycan found in the cornea contains an excess of oligosaccharides and appears to be a precursor for normal corneal keratan sulfate proteoglycan. Thus, it is presumed that this disorder, limited to the cornea, is due to an inborn error in which the enzyme which would normally "process" the keratan sulfate proteoglycan is absent or inactive. The presence of a precursor proteoglycan which has not been processed is thought to give rise to the opacity.

Pancreatic Enzyme Deficiencies. A number of patients have been described in whom malabsorption appears to result from a specific enzymopathy involving a pancreatic enzyme or proenzyme. They have none of the pulmonary or electrolyte abnormalities of cystic fibrosis.

A syndrome with inability to produce trypsin, lipase, and amylase in conjunction with hematologic evidence of bone marrow dysfunction has also been described, but in this case, as in cystic fibrosis, pancreatic dysfunction is presumed to be secondary to an underlying defect (Chapter 11).

Lipase Deficiency. Four children have been described with congenital inability to form active pancreatic lipase (2 formed none, and 2 synthesized small amounts). They had malabsorption of lipids and fatty (and sometimes malodorous) stools. Treatment with pancreatin was effective.

Trypsinogen Deficiency. A number of children with severe malnutrition, growth failure, and hypoproteinemic edema resembling kwashiorkor have been shown to lack the ability to synthesize pancreatic trypsinogen. As a result, chymotrypsin and carboxypeptidase activities are also low since these enzymes need to be formed from the corresponding proenzymes by trypsin activity. Treatment with a protein hydrolysate diet and exogenous pancreatic enzymes is recommended.

Amylase Deficiency. Less defined deficiencies of pancreatic amylase activity have been described in at least 2 children with malabsorption who were shown not to have cystic fibrosis. One of the children also had reduced trypsin activity.

Intestinal Enterokinase Deficiency. Enterokinase, an enzyme secreted by the small intestine, initiates the reactions for the conversion of the pancreatic proenzymes to their active forms. A number of children with a proven deficiency of enterokinase activity have been studied. The clinical findings and recommended treatment are identical with those described above for trypsinogen deficiency. Many if not all of the cases originally described as trypsinogen deficiency may be instances of enterokinase deficiency, with the lack of trypsin activity secondary to inability to form trypsin from trypsinogen.

Collagen Metabolism. A deficiency of the enzyme procollagen peptidase, which converts the protein procollagen to collagen, has been demonstrated in 3 patients with 1 of the variant forms of Ehlers-Danlos syndrome. Another form of this disorder has been shown to result from defective hydroxylation of lysine (Sec 8.16). In osteogenesis imperfecta it has been shown that 1 of the procollagen molecules (Type I) is produced with an excess of attached mannose. One of the enzymatic defects in this heterogeneous disorder may consist of a relative inability to remove this excessive amount of the sugar, resulting in abnormal transport and deposition of procollagen with attendant malformation of collagen.

Carnitine Deficiency (see also Sec. 8.20). The metabolism of long-chain fatty acids requires carnitine (γ-trimethylamino-β-hydroxybutyrate). A patient with longstanding muscle weakness was found to have muscle fibers filled with lipid vacuoles. Oxidation of long-chain fatty acids was depressed and the concentration of carnitine in muscle was shown to be one sixth of normal.

Succinyl-CoA, 3-Keto-Acid CoA-Transferase Deficiency. Acetoacetate and β-hydroxybutyrate cannot be further metabolized unless the acetoacetate is activated by the addition of a molecule of coenzyme A, which is donated by succinyl CoA via a specific transferase. A boy with severe ketoacidosis who died at 6 mo of age was shown to lack this transferase in all tissues studied. In another family, in which a 2 yr old boy died during his 3rd severe ketotic episode, the same enzymatic defect was found. Two siblings (1 male, 1 female) had died in infancy under similar circumstances. Consanguinity of the parents indicates the probability of autosomal recessive inheritance.

Acatalasia. Catalase is found in most tissues, including the erythrocytes. Persons with decrease of catalase activity in all tissues, to less than 1% of normal, can be detected through the demonstration that blood placed in contact with hydrogen peroxide turns brown and does not produce the oxygen bubbles usually seen. The disorder is heterogeneous; some instances appear to be mutations of the controller gene, whereas others are alterations of the structural gene. In all instances the mode of inheritance is autosomal recessive; the heterozygote can be detected by quantitative catalase assays. Of the 2 main types, the Japanese variants have oral gangrene (*Takahara disease*), whereas the Swiss variants are asymptomatic. A genetic strain of mice with acatalasia is known; catalase encapsulated in semipermeable membranes has been used successfully in their treatment.

Aspartylglycosaminuria. The compound 2-acetamido-1 (β-L-aspartamido)-1,2-dideoxyglucose (AADG) is a substituted hexose which forms 1 of the linkage points between the carbohydrate moiety and the amino acid groups of many glycoproteins. Large quantities of AADG (as well as other compounds containing AADG) have been found in the urine of 2 mentally retarded patients; 1 had petit mal seizures; the other, a manic-depressive psychosis. Other patients have had vacuolated lymphocytes, mental retardation, facial and osseous features similar to those of the mucopolysaccharidoses, hepatomegaly, and lenticular opacities. The defect of glycoprotein metabolism is in the lack of the enzyme, normally demonstrable in seminal fluid, which hydrolyzes AADG to glucosamine and aspartic acid. In this disorder the lysosomal enzyme is deficient in liver, brain, and spleen.

True Cholinesterase. True cholinesterase, an enzyme essential for neural and muscular function, is also found in erythrocytes, where its function is unknown. A brother and a sister have been observed whose erythrocyte cholinesterase activities were decreased to about one third of normal. They appeared to be homozygous for the condition, and their parents and 2 siblings to be heterozygous. There were no associated clinical manifestations. It has been suggested that a deficiency of true cholinesterase at the neuromuscular end-plate may account for the defect in myotonia congenita (Sec 22.6).

Syndromes with Impaired Leukocyte Function. The ability of leukocytes to phagocytose foreign particles such as bacteria and to destroy the ingested material depends on a number of factors, both extrinsic and intrinsic to the cell. The role of various opsonizing factors that act upon the particle undergoing phagocytosis and the effect of deficiencies of these factors are considered in Chapter 9. A tetrapeptide, L-threonyl-L-lysyl-L-prolyl-L-arginine, *tuftsin*, has been isolated from a leukophilic fraction of γ-globulin. Tuftsin is formed in the spleen, and splenectomized patients lack it. It has been shown to stimulate phagocytosis by acting directly upon leukocytes. A number of children with recurrent severe infections have been reported to have *tuftsin deficiency* (Sec 9.29).

Diminished bactericidal activity of leukocytes is observed in familial *chronic granulomatous disease*, in association with deficiency of the leukocytic enzyme, reduced nicotinamide-adenine dinucleotide phosphate (NADPH) oxidase. The failure to form the superoxide radical (O_2^-) is responsible for the diminished ability to kill phagocytosed bacteria (Sec 9.30).

Myeloperoxidase is an enzyme in leukocytes that, in the presence of hydrogen peroxide, oxidizes many compounds. Its activity seems to be important in the killing of phagocytosed microorganisms. A patient with disseminated candidiasis has been shown to have a *myeloperoxidase deficiency* in his polymorphonuclear leukocytes and monocytes. Phagocytosis was normal, but ingested *Candida albicans* were not killed, and the ability to kill other microorganisms was diminished. No other abnormalities of immune response were observed in this patient.

VICTOR H. AUERBACH

DEFECTS IN METABOLISM OF LIPIDS

The lipidoses or lipid storage diseases are a group of genetic diseases involving the accumulation of lipids in 1 or more of the body's organs usually due to a defect in their catabolism. Some of these disorders are associated with characteristic foamy histiocytes on examination of the bone marrow (Fig 8–29) (Niemann-Pick disease, Gaucher disease, G_{M1} gangliosidoses Type I, fucosidosis); others are not (Tay-Sachs disease, Krabbe disease, metachromatic leukodystrophy). Patients in the latter group show other characteristic cellular changes in organs of storage, such as nervous tissue. The signs and symptoms for each syndrome vary with the enzymatic defect and site of lipid accumulation. The amount of true storage depends on the organ involved and on the amount of catabolism required for maintenance of normal chemical composition.

In recent years research on the lipidoses has progressed rapidly and has even led to mass screening for the carrier status of 1 of these syndromes (Tay-Sachs disease). The enzymatic defect is recognized for many of these relatively rare syndromes; the complete elucidation of the disease processes is still under intense investigation. Clinical variants are being reported with increased frequency. Many variants do not fit the textbook descriptions of a given syndrome, though they are enzymatically closely related. In other cases a sign thought to be pathognomonic for a given disease has been found in patients with other syndromes. The diffuse angiokeratomatosis of Fabry disease, for example, has also been found in patients with fucosidosis and with glycoprotein sialidase deficiency.

When a symptom (or a group of symptoms) could indicate a genetic lipidosis, an enzymatic diagnosis should be requested from a laboratory that does these tests. No matter what preliminary studies may be done, the final diagnosis rests on the identification of an enzymatic defect. In most of the diseases to be described, the definitive diagnosis can be made on an easily obtained specimen, such as blood (serum and leukocytes) or a biopsy of skin which can be cultured and subsequently assayed. In most cases frozen serum or leukocytes can be shipped or heparinized blood can be sent at room temperature for preparation of leukocytes in the forewarned laboratory. Skin biopsies can also be sent by air mail for culturing, or a flask of cultured cells can be sent for subsequent subculturing and assaying.

When a diagnosis has been made in a child, other family members should be screened since studies on the parents, siblings, and other relatives can provide important genetic information. Carriers of most of the lipidoses can be reliably identified; and these studies can assist in genetic counseling and in alleviation of fear and guilt. Prenatal diagnosis may also be possible. In most cases, if a successful tap is obtained at 14–16 wk, enzymatic studies on cultured amniotic fluid cells can be completed before 20 wk gestation. The accuracy of prenatal studies should be confirmed by study of the aborted fetus or delivered infant. It should be noted that not many laboratories do these tests, and among those that do, conditions of enzyme assay vary, and activity levels reported for controls, patients, and carriers have not been standardized.

The sphingolipids have as their basic structure the long-chain amino diol sphingosine (sphingenine), in which the C-2 and C-3 carbon atoms have the D-configuration (Fig 8–30). The amino group of sphingosine usually has a long-chain fatty acid attached to it. This derivative is called ceramide. The C-1 hydroxyl group of ceramide can be substituted with a variety of different compounds to produce the different sphingolipids (Fig 8–30). For example, attachment of galactose in a beta-linkage to ceramide at C-1 creates galactosylceramide (commonly called galactocerebroside). Galactosylceramide with a sulfate group on C-3 of the galactose moiety is called sulfatide. Both these glycosphingolipids are found primarily in white matter.

Attachment of glucose in a beta-linkage to C-1 of ceramide produces glucosylceramide (glucocerebroside). Free glucosylceramide is found in small amounts

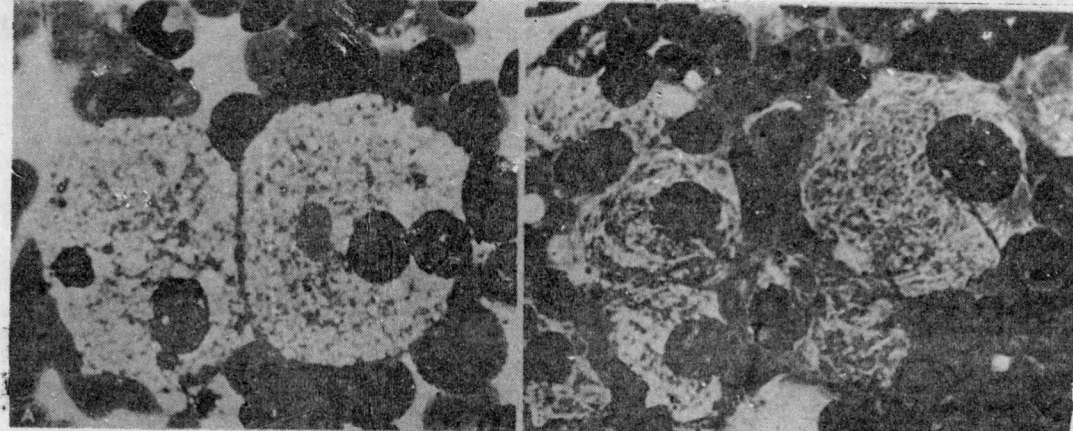

Figure 8–29 Smears from bone marrow aspirations (Giemsa stain) showing characteristic cells of Niemann-Pick disease (A) and Gaucher disease (B). Note the bubbly, vacuolated appearance of the Niemann-Pick foam cells, as contrasted with fibrillar texture of the Gaucher cell cytoplasm.

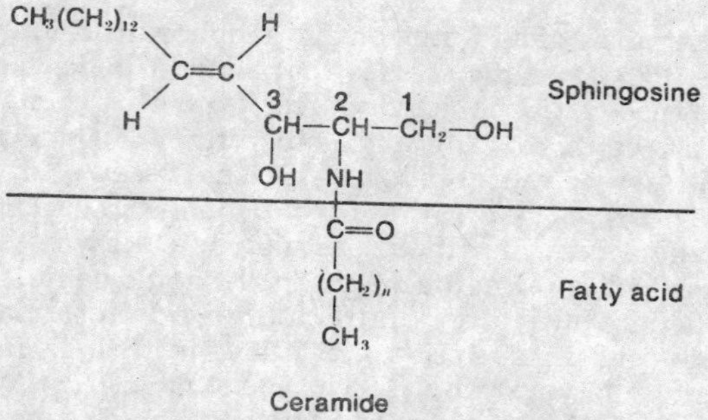

Figure 8–30 Basic structure of sphingolipids. All additions to ceramide are made through the hydroxyl group of carbon atom 1.

Glycosphingolipids= Ceramide plus one or more sugars attached to C-1
Gangliosides = Glycosphingolipids plus one or more sialic acid residues
Sphingomyelin = Ceramide plus phosphorylcholine attached to C-1

in normal tissues but is stored to great amounts in tissues of patients with Gaucher disease. Glucosylceramide is a portion of most larger glycosphingolipids and gangliosides. All degradation of these glycosphingolipids takes place sequentially from the nonreducing end of the molecule toward the lipid portion. Deficiency in enzyme activity results in the storage of the compound (or compounds) behind the block. In addition to the primary storage product other lipid compounds may be stored because of secondary factors.

8.29 G$_{M1}$ GANGLIOSIDOSES

G$_{M1}$ gangliosidoses are a group of lysosomal disorders with variable clinical findings. G$_{M1}$ ganglioside is a monosialoganglioside found in normal cerebral gray and white matter and in lesser quantities in the viscera. It is also formed during the normal catabolism of polysialogangliosides (Fig 8–31).

G$_{M1}$ gangliosidosis Type 1 (generalized gangliosidosis) is a severe cerebral degenerative disease with onset soon after birth. Edema and weakness and, in most cases, facial features not unlike those seen in Hurler syndrome and I-cell disease (mucolipidosis II) are observed. In many cases hepatosplenomegaly, hyperacusis, and cherry red spot of the macula occur. Roentgenographic changes of dysostosis multiplex are often found. Death usually occurs before 2 yr of age from respiratory infections.

Patients with G$_{M1}$ gangliosidosis Type 2 will usually have an onset of ataxia at 1–2 yr of age, with cessation of psychic and motor development. Within the next 6 mo deterioration leads to an unresponsive state. There will be little, if any, enlargement of the liver or other organs. Roentgenographic changes are minimal. Death usually occurs at 3–10 yr of age from bronchopneumonia.

Patients with significantly different phenotypes but with apparently the same enzymatic defect have been described. Two siblings, 19 and 25 yr, presented before 5 yr of age with clumsiness and mild roentgenographic bone changes but with normal intelligence. They developed dysarthria and mild CNS involvement as young adults. Other patients with β-galactosidase deficiency have severe bone involvement suggestive of Morquio

syndrome (mucopolysaccharidosis type IV). These children have normal intelligence. Other patients with moderate to severe mental retardation have survived until the 3rd or 4th decade. Another group of patients with myoclonus, cherry red spot in the macular region, and dementia has been recently demonstrated to have a glycoprotein sialidase deficiency which in some unknown way affects the activity of acid β-galactosidase. These patients will be discussed with the sialidoses.

All patients with G$_{M1}$ gangliosidosis have a profound deficiency of acid β-galactosidase activity in their leukocytes and cultured skin fibroblasts. In most suspected cases the use of a synthetic β-galactoside substrate to measure β-galactosidase activity can confirm the diagnosis. This enzyme is active with many β-galactoside–containing substrates in the body. The major compounds include the G$_{M1}$ ganglioside, glycoproteins (and oligosaccharides derived from them), and keratan sulfate–like mucopolysaccharides. Depending on the particular mutation in the enzyme, failure to hydrolyze some or all of these potential substrates will result in storage. Patients with G$_{M1}$ gangliosidosis Type 1 have little, if any, activity toward all potential substrates; hence severe involvement of brain, viscera, and bone occurs. Patients with connective tissue involvement paramount might be expected to have more residual β-galactosidase activity toward G$_{M1}$ ganglioside and less toward keratan sulfate–like mucopolysaccharides. Type 1 patients store G$_{M1}$ ganglioside in brain (10 times normal in gray matter) and viscera (20–50 times normal in liver), and keratan sulfate–like mucopolysaccharides and oligosaccharides in the viscera. The less severe forms have less storage of β-galactoside–terminal complex carbohydrates.

In Type 1 patients the neurons and the hepatic, glomerular, and renal tubular cells are vacuolated. Foamy histiocytes are found in all viscera. Storage in brain results in heavy damage to nerve cells, with demyelination and gliosis. Involved nerves show cytoplasmic membranous bodies, similar to those seen in Tay-Sachs disease. Secondary damage to white matter causes a decrease in the amount of cerebrosides and sulfatides found at autopsy. Similar, but milder, changes are found in juvenile forms of G$_{M1}$ gangliosidosis. Few mildly affected patients have been examined in detail.

The diagnosis of all forms of G_{M1} gangliosidosis must be made by enzymatic studies that show a deficiency of acid β-galactosidase activity. The Type 1 form may be initially confused clinically with certain mucopolysaccharidoses or mucolipidoses. In most cases of G_{M1} gangliosidosis, tests of urine for mucopolysaccharides will be negative. Enzymatic testing in leukocytes or fibroblasts will confirm the diagnosis. It should be noted that patients with Hurler and Hunter syndromes may have low acid β-galactosidase activities in their livers, due to secondary mucopolysaccharide storage. Tests on the parents (using leukocytes and/or cultured skin fibroblasts) will show about half normal β-galactosidase activity, indicating the autosomal recessive inheritance of these syndromes. Prenatal diagnosis using cultured amniotic fluid cells has been successful in the infantile and is possible in the milder forms also. There is no treatment currently available for these syndromes, though some orthopedic procedures may help older patients with problems related to bone. The prognosis of the older patients is unknown.

8.30 G_{M2} GANGLIOSIDOSES

See also Sec 21.17.

This group of genetic diseases includes those cases of cerebral degeneration in which the storage of G_{M2} ganglioside and related glycosphingolipids is due to deficiencies of specific hexosaminidases required for their catabolism (Fig 8–31 and 8–32). Tay-Sachs disease (or G_{M2} gangliosidosis Type 1) is the best known lipidosis because of the publicity given the role of the missing enzyme and its measurement to identify carriers in a high risk population.

Tay-Sachs disease or G_{M2} gangliosidosis Type 1 was known for many years as infantile amaurotic familial idiocy. Pathologic changes are mostly restricted to the central nervous system, though neurons throughout the body contain the characteristic membranous cytoplasmic bodies. With time, neurons are lost. There is proliferation of microglial cells, which are also swollen and filled with large granules. The spinal cord may have similar changes, with anterior horn cells more affected than those of the posterior and lateral horns. In the eye macular changes result in the cherry red spot seen in most patients. The liver and other organs show membranous cytoplasmic bodies with electron microscopy, though little actual storage may be measured. Foam cells are not usually found in the bone marrow. It is the failure of hexosaminidase A to degrade G_{M2} ganglioside that results in the 100-fold increase of this ganglioside found in the brains of children with Tay-Sachs disease. G_{M2} ganglioside is a minor component of normal brain, but it is in the degradative pathway for the major brain gangliosides.

The classic features of the onset of this disease include psychomotor retardation and deterioration after 4–6 mo of normal development and a startle response to sound. Hypotonia, loss of interest in surroundings, poor head control, and apathy also occur early. A cherry red spot in the macula may be found later. Seizures begin later, and in advanced stages of illness the child has little response to external stimuli. The head enlarges and in the final stage is obviously macrocephalic. No visceromegaly is found. Many cases are found in families of Eastern European Jewish heritage, but the diagnosis should not be excluded from consideration in non-Jewish or nonwhite children.

The diagnostic test for Tay-Sachs disease is measure-

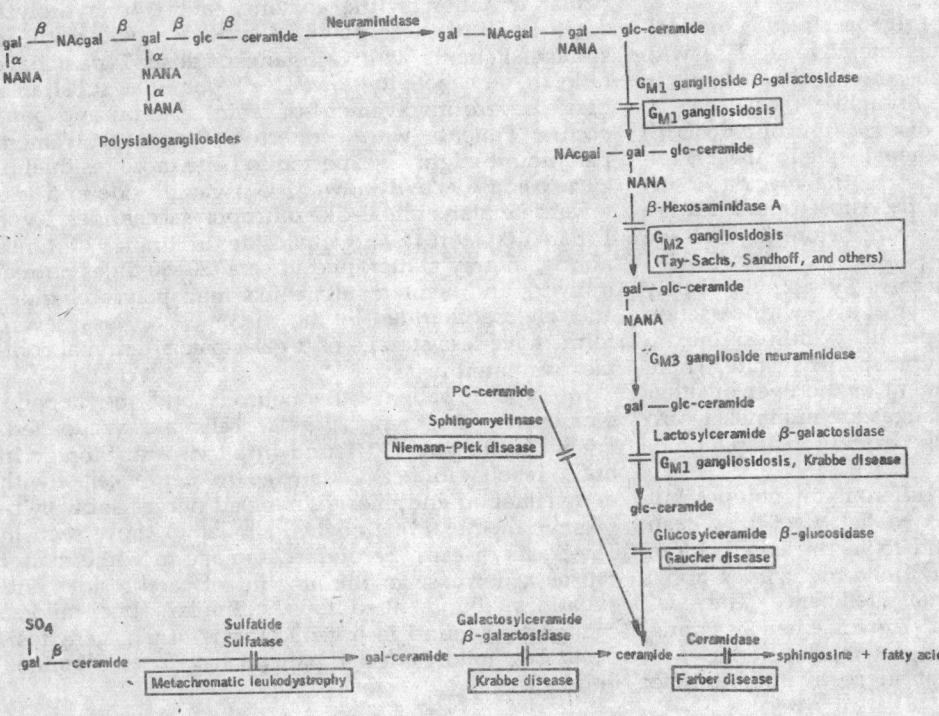

Figure 8–31 Pathways in the metabolism of sphingolipids found in nervous tissues. The name of the enzyme catalyzing each reaction is given along with the name of the substrate acted upon. Inborn errors are depicted as bars crossing the reaction arrows, and the name of the associated defect or defects is given within the nearest box. The gangliosides are named according to the nomenclature of Svennerholm. Anomeric configurations are given only on the largest starting compound.

gal, galactose; glc, glucose; NAcgal, N-acetyl-galactosamine; NANA, N-acetyl-neuraminic acid; PC, phosphorylcholine.

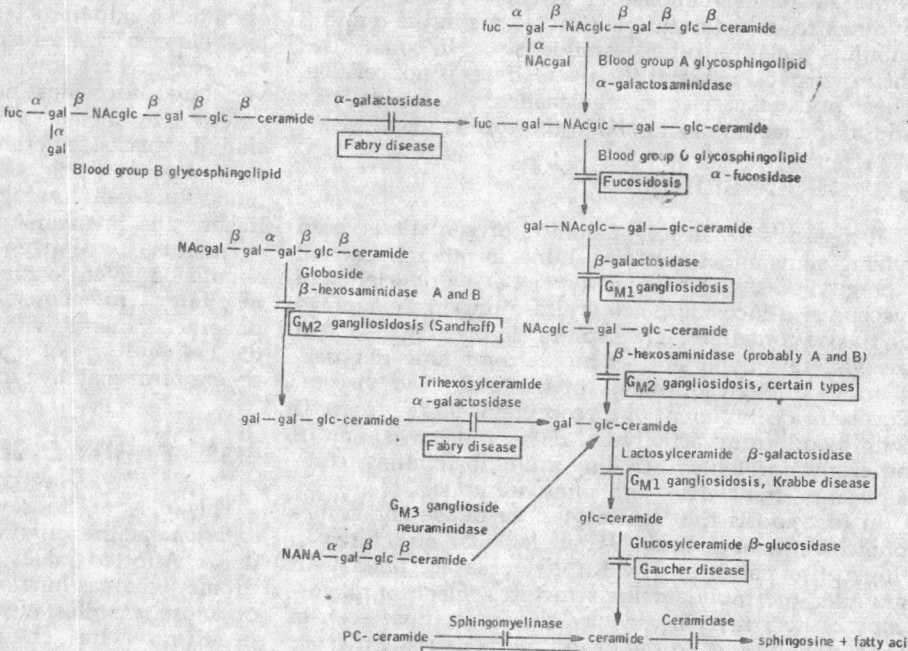

Figure 8–32 Pathways in the degradation of sphingolipids found in visceral organs and red or white blood cells. See also legend for Fig 8–31. Additional abbreviations: fuc, fucose; NAcglc, N-acetylglucosamine.

ment of the hexosaminidase A isoenzyme component of serum, leukocytes, tears, hair roots, or cultured skin fibroblasts. Total hexosaminidase activity may be normal in this disease, but an almost total deficiency of activity of the "A" component is diagnostic. Hexosaminidase A usually makes up over 50% of the total hexosaminidase activity. The use of heat inactivation to find the proportion of hexosaminidase A in the total hexosaminidase activity has led to the identification of carriers among people with no familial history of Tay-Sachs disease. Through this screening procedure couples at risk have been identified and counseled. Over 200,000 healthy people have been screened. Ashkenazi Jews have a carrier frequency of about 1 in 25. It is recommended that all Jewish couples of Eastern European ancestry be advised that tests for the carrier state are available and that prevention of this fatal disease is possible. Prenatal diagnosis is possible.

Little can be done for the affected child other than supportive care for recurrent infections in the late stages of the disease. Death usually occurs by 3–4 yr. Carriers have no symptoms.

Sandhoff disease, or G$_{M2}$ **gangliosidosis Type 2** (or 0 variant), is the result of total deficiency of hexosaminidase activity (both A and B isoenzymes of hexosaminidase are missing). This results in the storage not only of G$_{M2}$ ganglioside in the brain but also of other β-hexosaminide terminal glycolipids, glycoproteins, and oligosaccharides in brain and viscera. The clinical symptoms are similar to those seen in Tay-Sachs disease but with additional visceral involvement. The brain contains a 100–200-fold increase in G$_{M2}$ ganglioside and a 50–100-fold increase in G$_{A2}$, the asialo-derivative of G$_{M2}$. The liver, kidneys, and spleen have a great increase in the amount of globoside, the major glycosphingolipid

of red blood cells (Fig 8–32). The lack of hexosaminidase A and B activity prevents the degradation of all these glycosphingolipids (Fig 8–31 and 8–32). The diagnosis of Sandhoff disease can be made with serum, plasma, leukocytes, or cultured skin fibroblasts. Carriers can (with care) be identified using the same tissues, and prenatal diagnosis can be made. There is no increased incidence of Sandhoff disease in Eastern European Jewish families.

Juvenile G$_{M2}$ gangliosidosis or **Type 3** has a later onset than either Tay-Sachs or Sandhoff disease. Ataxia and progressive psychomotor retardation begin at 2–6 yr of age. Loss of speech, progressive spasticity, athetoid posturing of hands and extremities, and minor motor seizures become evident. Death occurs between 5–15 yr. Organomegaly, bony deformities, and foam cells are not found. Blindness occurs in the later stages of this disease. Neuronal lipidosis is prominent and G$_{M2}$ ganglioside is stored because of a partial deficiency of hexosaminidase A. Diagnosis, identification of carriers, and prenatal diagnosis are available through measurement of hexosaminidase A activity.

Other patients with unusual hexosaminidase patterns and ganglioside accumulation have been recently described. Some patients with typical symptoms of Tay-Sachs disease have been reported. These patients store G$_{M2}$ ganglioside, yet they have normal hexosaminidase activity; they are missing a noncatalytic effector protein required for the activity of hexosaminidase A in vivo. Other adult patients have been found to have low hexosaminidase A activity. Some of these patients have a variant form of spinocerebellar degeneration (ataxia, muscle atrophy, pes cavus, foot drop, spasticity, dysarthria, and normal intelligence), while others have psychotic behavior. Healthy adults have also been found with low hexosaminidase A activity. These unusual findings result from different mutations in the α and β subunits making up hexosaminidase A. In some cases the in vitro test using artificial substrates is not reliable. These unusual cases present a challenge to the clinician and to the laboratory to obtain the correct diagnosis.

8.31 FUCOSIDOSIS

Fucosidosis has at least 2 clinical presentations, both having signs and symptoms found in other lysosomal storage diseases. All clinical types have a deficiency of lysosomal α-fucosidase activity resulting in the storage of fucose-containing glycosphingolipids (Fig 8–32) in the visceral organs and of fucose-containing oligosaccharides and glycoproteins in the brain and viscera. Fucose is a component of glycoproteins and glycolipids with blood group activity (A, B, H, and Lewis) and of other glycoproteins, including immunoglobulins, ceruloplasmin, transferrin, and some hormones.

In fucosidosis the hepatocytes are dense and osmophilic, containing multilayered lamellar structures in fingerprint patterns. The Kupffer cells are filled with granular and multilamellar structures. Electron microscopy of liver reveals vacuoles similar to those seen in Hurler syndrome. In the central nervous system every nerve cell is enlarged, with a round to oval eccentric nucleus. The cells appear empty or filled with granular, weakly basophilic, and PAS-positive material. There is neuronal loss and the remaining neurons are vacuolated, as are the glial cells. Myelination is affected and the pathologic picture resembles that of sudanophilic leukodystrophy. Macrophages are numerous in liver and white matter. Cultured skin fibroblasts show clear vacuoles that sometimes show lamellar inclusions.

Most signs and symptoms are related to the abnormal accumulation of glycosphingolipids and glycoproteins in liver, heart, and brain. There is evidence also of lysosomal storage in vascular endothelium, eccrine sweat gland epithelium, and fibrocytes. The more severely affected patients have severe psychomotor retardation, neurologic signs including convulsions, and bony deformities evident before the end of the 1st yr of life (fucosidosis Type I). Myocarditis and cardiomegaly may occur. Short stature, macroglossia, frontal bossing, spastic ataxia, hepatomegaly, increased levels of sodium chloride in sweat, and delayed development are also reported. Skeletal changes include lumbar kyphosis, contractures of hips, knees, ankles, and elbows, and deformities of ribs. Patients with fucosidosis Type II may also have an onset in early childhood, but the course is slower. These patients initially have less severe psychomotor and neurologic signs, but severe mental retardation comes in the later stages. They also tend to have normal sweat electrolytes, less severe bone changes, and no hepatosplenomegaly. Skin lesions resembling the angiokeratoma corporis diffusum seen in Fabry disease usually appear at 5–7 yr of age.

The clinical picture of both types of fucosidosis could suggest a mucopolysaccharidosis or mucolipidosis. Urine does not contain mucopolysaccharides but rather fucose-containing oligosaccharides. Most patients have vacuolated lymphocytes that are characteristic. A suspected case can be confirmed when white blood cells or cultured skin fibroblasts are shown to have an almost total deficiency of α-fucosidase activity. Serum levels of this enzyme are low, but some normal people have very low α-fucosidase activity in serum. Carriers can be detected by means of white blood cells and cultured skin fibroblasts. Inheritance is autosomal recessive. Prenatal diagnosis has been reported using cultured amniotic fluid cells. A high incidence has been noted in Italians and Spanish-Americans.

Patients can be given only supportive care. Attention should be given to the hydration needs and repeated respiratory infections of the more severely affected patients. Patients with the more severe form usually die before 10 yr of age, whereas those with the less severe form may live into the 3rd decade.

8.32 FABRY DISEASE

This disease, formerly called *angiokeratoma corporis diffusum*, is the only well-characterized X-linked lipidosis. Affected males have the complete clinical syndrome, whereas heterozygous females may also have 1 or more manifestations which can present serious health problems. The purple punctate angiokeratomas in the "bathing suit" area were once pathognomonic for Fabry disease. Identical skin lesions have now been found in patients with certain types of fucosidosis and sialidosis. Recently, patients without skin lesions or corneal opacities have been determined to have Fabry disease.

Fabry disease is caused by the deficiency of α-galactosidase activity, which is responsible for the degradation of α-galactosyl terminal glycolipids. The main storage product is trihexosylceramide, which will be formed from the action of β-hexosaminidase on globoside, the major red blood cell glycosphingolipid (Fig 8–32). Further degradation of trihexosylceramide would require a specific α-galactosidase (called α-galactosidase A) which is missing in this syndrome. Another storage product is digalactosylceramide, which is found mainly in kidney tissue. In those patients having blood group B (Fig 8–32) an additional storage product may be found, not correlated with a more severe clinical picture. Storage of trihexosylceramide and digalactosylceramide takes place in visceral organs, especially in heart muscle and in renal tubules and glomeruli. Additional storage is evident in all vascular epithelia, the pituitary gland, autonomic neurons of the diencephalon and brain stem, the mesenteric and submucosal plexus of the gastrointestinal tract, and most skeletal muscles. Examination of the affected tissues reveals fine sudanophilic, PAS-positive granules and foamy storage cells. Bone marrow has shown granular material in histiocytes, with no evidence of anemia or other hematologic manifestations.

Storage of lipid material in the blood vessels leads to most of the symptoms. Fabry disease is not a disease of early childhood, but many patients are discovered before 10 yr of age because of complaints of pain in extremities, lack of sweating, unexplained proteinuria, attacks of fever, and the presence of a few purple skin lesions. As the disease progresses, there are complaints related to easy fatigability (due to storage in skeletal muscle), poor vision (corneal opacities, tortuosity of retinal and conjunctival vessels, and cataracts), and high blood pressure (due to continued vascular storage). This storage eventually leads to cardiac or renal failure in the 3rd or 4th decade of life. Psychologic disturbances have been reported and are probably due to decreased blood flow and thrombus formation in brain.

Increased levels of trihexosylceramide can be found in biopsy samples, urinary sediments, and cultured skin fibroblasts, but the best diagnostic method is measurement of α-galactosidase activity in one or more tissues. Using the synthetic substrate 4-methylumbelliferyl-α-D-galactoside, this disease can be easily diagnosed using plasma, urine, white blood cells, tears, and cultured skin cells. Cultured amniotic cells permit the prenatal diagnosis of this syndrome. Heterozygous females can be identified using serum, white blood cells, and cultured skin fibroblasts.

Though this disease can be quite benign until the 2nd or 3rd decade, it can lead to early death due to cardiovascular complications. Pain in the extremities, reported by almost all patients, has been treated with diphenylhydantoin (200 mg/24 hr) or carbamazepine (200 mg/24 hr) with variable success. Treatment of renal failure by dialysis and renal transplantation has had limited success. Attempts to supply the missing enzyme using whole plasma and purified α-galactosidase are still experimental.

Inheritance is X-linked. Many carrier females will have some symptoms. A family history of early male deaths with the above symptoms may suggest Fabry disease. There seems to be no ethnic group at increased risk.

8.33 GAUCHER DISEASE

Gaucher disease includes 2 or 3 clinically distinct genetic entities involving the storage of glucosylceramide (glucocerebroside) in the reticuloendothelial system. The initial report of Gaucher described the typical "adult" or "chronic" patient with splenomegaly and variable bone involvement. The eponym has been given to clinical variants that have the characteristic "Gaucher cell" in bone marrow aspirates and in visceral organs examined (Fig 8–29). The 3 clinical types of Gaucher disease are now called Type 1, adult, chronic, or nonneuropathic; Type 2, acute neuropathic or infantile; and Type 3, subacute neuropathic or juvenile. Unfortunately, these names do not always reflect the age of onset of symptoms or the severity of the disease. Some "adult" patients have obvious bone problems and splenomegaly leading to splenectomy before the end of the 1st decade, whereas others are not diagnosed until the 8th decade.

The finding of Gaucher cells is indicative of Gaucher disease, though similar cells are found in cases of myelogenous leukemia. There have been rare cases of confirmed Gaucher disease without the finding of this typical cell in bone marrow. These fusiform histiocytes are 15–85 μ in size and have 1 or more small dense nuclei eccentrically located. They have a blue staining cytoplasm with the appearance of wrinkled silk as opposed to the foamy cells found in other lipidoses. Gaucher cells are derived from reticular or sinusoidal endothelial cells and are found in bone marrow, spleen, liver, lungs, and lymph nodes. They may be found in the brain of patients who die of infantile Gaucher disease. These cells stain positive with PAS and stain strongly for acid phosphatase.

Splenomegaly is the initial finding in most patients, with spleens weighing over 3000 gm not unusual in adults. The liver is usually enlarged and in some cases liver failure occurs. Patients with infantile Gaucher disease have severe involvement of the central nervous system, as shown by decreased brain size, neuronal degeneration, and active neuronophagia. There is loss of neurons in the spinal cord. Skeletal complications are common, especially in the adult type, with fractures of the femoral neck and vertebral bodies and sometimes aseptic necrosis of the femoral head.

All the clinical problems in these patients appear to be caused by the storage of glucosylceramide due to deficiency of a specific β-glucosidase activity required for its degradation. Glucosylceramide is a portion of larger glycosphingolipids which is generated during the degradation of gangliosides, of red and white blood cell glycolipids, and of endogenous membrane glycosphingolipids (Fig 8–31 and 8–32). The reason for the great variation in clinical picture among patients is not clear as all patients are deficient in the same enzymatic activity. Within families, however, the clinical picture is relatively consistent; adult and infantile forms of Gaucher disease do not usually occur in the same family.

The onset of infantile Gaucher disease usually occurs within the 1st few mo of life with hepatosplenomegaly, slow development, strabismus, swallowing difficulties, laryngeal spasm, opisthotonos, and a picture of "pseudobulbar palsy." Recurrent aspiration and chronic bronchopneumonia lead to death usually at 6–18 mo. The juvenile form of Gaucher disease is less well defined; most cases have been reported in certain areas of Sweden. Dementia, often accompanied by behavior changes, seizures, and extrapyramidal and cerebellar signs, becomes evident in late childhood. Most patients have the chronic or adult type, but the clinical picture can vary greatly. Usually hypersplenism in early childhood causes anemia and thrombocytopenia. Bone pain and joint swelling are also evident in some patients. Pathologic fractures are a major problem in some patients, whereas others have few or no osseous difficulties. Roentgenograms will help identify osseous complications. Some adult patients have a yellow or patchy brown pigmentation in the exposed areas of the body. Pingueculae of the conjunctiva are also found in some adults. Liver necrosis and severe pulmonary involvement may rarely be found, with possibly a higher incidence in the black population.

Preliminary diagnosis of Gaucher disease is based on the clinical picture and the identification of Gaucher cells in bone marrow. Serum acid phosphatase levels are greatly elevated. A piece of spleen or liver can be extracted for lipids and the glycolipids separated by thin-layer chromatography. All patients with Gaucher disease show an elevation of glucosylceramide content in the organs checked. The best diagnostic method is measurement of glucosylceramide β-glucosidase activity in leukocytes and cultured skin fibroblasts. Inheritance is autosomal recessive. All patients have less than 20% of normal activity, whereas carriers have about 60% of normal activity. Prenatal diagnosis is available for all types of Gaucher disease, but care should be exercised when counseling families with the adult type. Type 1 (adult) Gaucher disease is most common in Ashkenazi Jewish people, but all ethnic groups are affected.

Splenectomy has been used to control the anemic and hemorrhagic symptoms of hypersplenism, and orthopedic supervision can help manage bone involvement. The periods of bone pain can be helped by rest, analgesics, and possibly the brief use of steroids. Problems in the hip joint may be serious and require surgery. No treatment is currently available for the infantile or juvenile forms; only supportive treatment for infections and feeding problems can be given. Attempts to treat Gaucher disease by transplantation of spleen or kidney have been made, with little success. Enzyme replacement therapy is experimental at this time.

8.34 NIEMANN-PICK DISEASE

Niemann-Pick disease is a group of genetic diseases in which sphingomyelin and, secondarily, cholesterol are stored in many organs. The classification of these patients is undergoing modification in light of recent clinical and biochemical findings. Basically, 4 subtypes are recognized: (1) classic Niemann-Pick disease (Type A according to Crocker), showing storage in viscera and severe CNS degeneration in infancy (with foam cells in bone marrow [Fig 8–29] and severe deficiency of sphingomyelinase activity); (2) Type B, showing severe visceral involvement in infancy (with foam cells in bone marrow and severe deficiency of sphingomyelinase activity); (3) juvenile types, showing moderate visceral involvement and variable CNS degeneration in early childhood (with foamy and/or sea blue histiocytes in bone marrow and partial sphingomyelinase deficiency in certain tissues); and (4) other patients with evidence of sphingomyelin storage who have normal sphingomyelinase activity and few, if any, neurologic abnormalities.

The disabilities of patients with classic infantile Niemann-Pick disease stem from extensive storage of sphingomyelin and cholesterol (and some glycosphingolipids, secondarily) in liver, spleen, and lungs, with less marked storage in brain. The brain, though, shows a marked increase in G_{M2} and G_{M3} gangliosides. Clinical onset typically comes after a period of normal development lasting several mo, with a slowing of motor and mental progress and hepatomegaly, followed by general deterioration of neurologic functions and health. Examination of bone marrow, blood, and organs reveals foamy cells loaded with lipid. Deterioration continues to a vegetative state, and death usually occurs before 4 yr of age. Cherry red spots in the macula are found in about 50% of the cases. Many cases of this type are found in Jews of Eastern European ancestry.

Patients with the less frequently occurring Type B form, who have visceral involvement only, show pronounced storage of sphingomyelin and cholesterol in visceral organs and foam cells in the marrow. Health problems related to this storage may be mild or severe. The lack of nervous system involvement in these patients is unexplained. Sphingomyelinase levels in visceral organs and cultivated skin fibroblasts are at the same low levels as in Type A patients.

The juvenile types present a variety of symptoms. Early jaundice may be followed by relatively normal development until 5–7 yr of age when unsteadiness of gait, ataxia, problems in vertical gaze, learning difficulties, emotional lability, and dementia become evident. The course is progressive at a variable rate, death occurring in the 1st, 2nd, or 3rd decade. Hepatosplenomegaly is not always evident, though some patients have evidence of excess sphingomyelin in biopsy or autopsy samples of liver. This group includes some with disease previously labeled Type C or D Niemann-Pick disease and with some forms of sea blue histiocyte syndrome. Sphingomyelinase levels are reported to be normal or partially deficient, with activities varying from tissue to tissue.

Some adult patients have been found to have storage of sphingomyelin in particular visceral organs, with no serious health problems or neurologic deterioration. These patients do not have the severe sphingomyelinase deficiency reported for Type B individuals. The prognosis for this group of patients cannot be stated; some have lived past the 5th decade.

Large lipid-laden foam cells are found in all groups of patients with sphingomyelin lipidosis. These cells differ from "Gaucher cells" and resemble the nondescript foam cells of G_{M1} gangliosidosis and other lipidoses. Sea blue and/or foamy histiocytes are found in increased numbers in a juvenile form of sphingomyelin lipidosis, as well as in other lipidoses and unrelated diseases. Hepatosplenomegaly is marked in most types, but especially so in the infantile forms. Lymph nodes, adrenal glands, and lungs frequently show evidence of storage. The brain is smaller than normal, with most regions atrophic. The neurons of the cortex and deep gray matter show marked distention of the cytoplasm and loss of Nissl bodies. A reduction in the number of Purkinje cells is found in the cerebellum, and a reduction of myelin and axonal fibers in cerebellar white matter. The juvenile and later-onset forms of Niemann-Pick disease show many of the same findings but to a lesser degree. The brain may reveal no significant pathologic changes. In some cases cirrhosis of the liver is found.

Any infant failing to thrive, with upper respiratory infections, hepatosplenomegaly, and impaired development, should be suspected of having infantile Niemann-Pick disease. In both Type A and Type B, enzymatic assays to confirm a deficiency of sphingomyelinase can be done with leukocytes or cultured skin fibroblasts. Because the level of sphingomyelinase activity is low in normal leukocytes, cultured skin fibroblasts are the preferred diagnostic tissue. Carriers can be identified in fibroblast cultures, and prenatal diagnosis can be done with cultured amniotic fluid cells. All forms of Niemann-Pick disease appear to be inherited in an autosomal recessive manner.

The juvenile forms are less well understood with respect to the relationship between specific sphingomyelinase deficiencies and sphingomyelin storage. Some patients have a partial deficiency of sphingomyelinase in cultured skin fibroblasts (15–50% of normal versus 0–2% of normal for Groups A and B). These patients have foam cells in their bone marrow and often bruise easily. Further studies of this latter group of patients are needed to correlate symptoms and signs, storage, and enzyme levels before accurate diagnosis, carrier identification, and prenatal diagnosis are available.

No treatment for this group of diseases has been effective.

8.35 METACHROMATIC LEUKODYSTROPHY

See also Sec 21.18.

Metachromatic leukodystrophy (MLD) has 3 clinical forms. Late infantile MLD usually has its clinical onset in the 2nd yr of life. The 1st signs are genu recurvatum and impairment of motor function. Patients with juvenile MLD present ataxia and intellectual deterioration at 5–20 yr of age. Patients with the adult type of MLD present ataxia, weakness, dementia, and psychosis after 20 yr of age. All forms of metachromatic leukodystrophy are caused by a deficiency of the sulfatase required for the degradation of sulfatide (Fig 8–31). Deposits of sulfatide are found in the peripheral and central nervous systems, as well as in kidney and gallbladder (where some is naturally found).

White matter from the brains of patients with MLD appears to have undergone demyelination with the deposition of many metachromatic bodies. The bodies stain strongly positive with PAS and alcian blue preparations. Oligodendroglial cells are markedly reduced in number. Neuronal inclusions are also reported in nerve cells in the midbrain, pons, medulla, retina, and spinal cord. Demyelination is noted in the peripheral nervous system. Biopsies of sural nerve stained with acid cresyl violet show many brown metachromatic deposits containing granules. These accumulate in the perinuclear cytoplasm of Schwann cells and in perivascular histiocytes. All involved areas show a loss of oligodendroglial elements.

The late infantile form of MLD is the most common. Initial signs consist of disturbances of gait and slowed development. Examination reveals reduced or absent tendon reflexes, weakness, and hypotonia. Within months or years the child with late infantile MLD will have gradual onset of nystagmus, cerebellar and Babinski signs, dementia, tonic seizures, optic atrophy, and quadriparesis. Juvenile patients will have many of the same symptoms seen in the late infantile form with a slower progression. "Adult" patients may initially present psychiatric problems, including emotional lability,

apathy, and change of character, followed by mental deficiency. Eventually, abnormal tendon reflexes, speech difficulties, muscular weakness, ataxia, tremor, and auditory and visual problems will be evident. There is progressive dementia and optic atrophy.

Diagnosis is based on the clinical picture and the findings of decreased nerve conduction velocities, increased cerebrospinal fluid protein, metachromatic deposits in biopsied segments of sural nerve, and metachromatic granules in urinary sediment. There are no hepatosplenomegaly, bone involvement, or foam cells in the bone marrow. Confirmation of the diagnosis can be made by enzymatic studies on serum, urine, leukocytes, and cultured skin fibroblasts, which will show the deficiency in activity of sulfatide sulfatase or arylsulfatase A (as measured with an artificial substrate). Enzymatic studies do not differentiate between the 3 clinical types of MLD. Enzymatic studies on family members confirm the autosomal recessive pattern of inheritance. Some carriers of MLD have arylsulfatase A levels near those found in affected children. This means that parents of affected children should be checked for their carrier status before prenatal testing is undertaken, in order to prevent abortion of a nonaffected but low activity carrier. Use of a different assay method in cultured cells can resolve this problem. Recently a patient with signs and symptoms of MLD was found to have normal arylsulfatase A activity. This patient may be deficient in a noncatalytic effector protein required for the action of the enzyme in vivo.

Prenatal diagnosis has been done for the late infantile and juvenile forms of this syndrome. There is no treatment for any form of MLD; only supportive care can be given. Patients with the late infantile form usually live 2–4 yr after the diagnosis; those with the juvenile form live 4–6 yr after diagnosis. Some with the adult form have lived to the 5th decade.

Another genetic disease with deficiency of arylsulfatase A (along with arylsulfatases B and C) has been reported, also inherited through an autosomal recessive gene. This is called multiple sulfatase deficiency. There is accumulation of sulfatides, glycosaminoglycan sulfates, steroid sulfates, and gangliosides in cerebral cortex. The neurologic picture is similar to late infantile MLD; the slight bony involvement, however, may lead to an examination of urine for mucopolysaccharides, which would be positive. A striking abnormality of granulation in the leukocytes may provide another clue to the diagnosis. Enzymatic studies will confirm the diagnosis.

8.36 KRABBE DISEASE

See also Sec 21.18.

Krabbe disease or globoid cell leukodystrophy is a progressive cerebral degenerative disease affecting primarily white matter. Descriptions of affected patients have been reported since early in this century, with a high incidence noted in persons of Scandinavian descent. Inheritance is autosomal recessive. The name globoid cell comes from the globular distended multinucleated bodies found in the basal ganglia, pontine nuclei, and cerebellar white matter. These globoid cells are found clustered around blood vessels; they may be derived from microglia by an accumulation of phagocytosed products from abnormal myelin. Globoid cells have a lacy, pink cytoplasm (with hematoxylin-eosin stain) and prominent staining of intracellular material with PAS. The pathologic abnormalities are almost entirely restricted to white matter of nervous tissue. There may, however, be some damage to cortical gray matter but without the intense intraneuronal deposition usually observed in other cerebral lipidoses. Visceral organs are usually not involved because of the paucity of galactosylceramide lipids.

There is severe demyelination throughout the brain, though the myelin that remains at autopsy appears to have a normal glycolipid composition. There is currently no universally accepted explanation for the severe lack of myelin. Some investigators feel that an abnormal myelin is made initially, which is subject to easier degradation. The patients with later onset forms of Krabbe disease may have had normal myelin that functioned adequately until some event (possibly a viral infection) started the degradative process. As the myelin is degraded by way of lysosomal enzymes, the lack of galactosylceramide β-galactosidase (galactocerebrosidase) activity results in the preservation of galactosylceramide; this results in globoid cell formation (Fig 8–31).

The clinical onset usually occurs before 6 mo of age, with irritability, hypertonicity, bouts of hypothermia, mental regression, and possibly optic atrophy and seizures. Within 9–12 mo there appear increased hypertonicity, opisthotonos, hyperpyrexia, blindness, and seizures. In the final stage the patient is blind, deaf, spastic, and decerebrate, death occurring usually before 2 yr of age. In forms of this disease with later onset, patients may reach late infantile developmental milestones before loss of vision and motor regression become evident. Other patients appear normal until 3–4 yr of age. Some have lived until 20 yr of age.

Most patients with Krabbe disease will have an elevated protein level in spinal fluid (values of 100–500 mg/dl are not unusual). As in MLD there is a decrease in velocity of nerve conduction. All patients have a severe deficiency of galactosylceramide β-galactosidase activity in leukocytes or cultured skin fibroblasts. Carriers have approximately half normal galactocerebrosidase activity in leukocytes and cultured skin fibroblasts. A few normal adults have been found to have low levels of galactosylceramide β-galactosidase activity; they appear to be carriers of the Krabbe defect, showing less than 15% of normal activity by the in vitro test.

Patients with onset before 6 mo rarely live longer than 2 yr. Feeding, seizures, and aspiration pneumonia increasingly become problems. There is no treatment. Genetic counseling is appropriate. Prenatal diagnosis is possible using cultured amniotic cells.

8.37 FARBER DISEASE

Farber disease (lipogranulomatosis) is an autosomal recessive disorder marked by widely disseminated granulomas containing foam cells. There are numerous subcutaneous nodules and plaques, and symptoms include arthropathy, hoarseness, irritability, and poor growth and development. Deformed and painful joints may simulate rheumatoid arthritis and are consistently found. Most patients die in the 2nd yr with respiratory infections and malnutrition; a few live into the 2nd decade with few, if any, neurologic problems.

The foam cells within the granulomas are found to contain PAS-positive material (possibly gangliosides); lymph nodes, liver, kidneys, and lung contain 10–60-fold excesses of free ceramide. Ballooning of neurons in the central and autonomic nervous systems is also reported. Visceral organs are not usually enlarged, though electron microscopic examination of liver cells reveals osmophilic deposits surrounding electron-lucent material in a dense granular matrix. Kupffer cells and liver macrophages contain dense bodies with an osmophilic matrix. Most patients have increased spinal fluid protein and excrete excess ceramide in the urine.

This disease is the result of a deficiency of acid ceramidase activity. Ceramide is the lipid component of all sphingolipids and is formed during the degradation of many glycosphingolipids and sphingomyelin (Fig 8–31 and 8–32). The deficiency of acid ceramidase in Farber patients has been demonstrated in kidney, cerebellum, and cultured skin fibroblasts. A partial deficiency in acid ceramidase activity has been found in some heterozygotic persons. Prenatal diagnoses have been made using cultured amniotic fluid cells. No effective treatment is available; some improvement of joint function has been reported with the use of chlorambucil.

8.38 WOLMAN DISEASE AND CHOLESTERYL ESTER STORAGE DISEASE

Wolman disease, or primary familial xanthomatosis with involvement and calcification of the adrenals, is an autosomal recessive disease marked by severe failure to thrive, diarrhea, vomiting, and abdominal distention with hepatosplenomegaly and calcification of the adrenals. Storage of lipid in histiocytic foam cells produces the hepatosplenomegaly. Onset occurs in the 1st few wk of life. Death usually occurs within 6 mo due to cachexia complicated by peripheral edema. Foam cells are found in bone marrow and other visceral organs, including intestinal villi. Hepatocytes stained with oil red O show vacuolation. There is evidence of storage of cholesterol and/or cholesteryl esters in liver cells, Kupffer cells, and histiocytes. Spleen and intestines also show evidence of storage. Neurons show changes like those in sudanophilic leukodystrophy. Storage in intestinal tissues can add to the nutritional problems. A large excess of cholesteryl esters and triglycerides in these organs has been reported.

Bone marrow examination reveals a large number of lipoid cells. Roentgenograms of the abdomen show enlargement and calcification of the adrenals. Enzymatic studies in leukocytes and cultured skin fibroblasts indicate acid esterase (acid lipase) deficiency. Patients with Wolman disease have no measurable activity with a variety of suitable substrates. Carriers of this disease can be identified by enzyme assays in leukocytes and cultured skin fibroblasts, and prenatal diagnosis has been accomplished by the use of cultured amniotic fluid cells. It is possible that roentgenograms of the pregnant mother might visualize the calcified adrenals in the affected fetus. No treatment is effective.

Cholesteryl ester storage disease is a relatively mild genetic disorder characterized by liver enlargement, short stature, chronic gastrointestinal loss of blood of uncertain etiology, and chronic anemia. Hyperlipidemia is found in most patients. Foam cells may be found in the bone marrow and lipids accumulate in the lamina propria of the intestine. Neurologic symptoms are minimal. Levels of cholesteryl esters are markedly elevated in liver, those of triglycerides only moderately elevated. A marked deficiency of cholesteryl ester hydrolase and triglyceride hydrolase has been found (as in Wolman disease). The hyperlipidemia seems to predispose the patient to atherosclerosis. A measurement of the acid lipase activity can confirm a diagnosis and presumably identify carriers of this autosomal recessive disease. Its relationship to Wolman disease is unclear at this time.

ADRENOLEUKODYSTROPHY

Adrenoleukodystrophy (ALD) is an X-linked disorder associated with progressive demyelination of cerebral white matter and adrenal insufficiency. The 1st symptoms, including change in behavior, loss of vision, gait disturbances, and dysarthria and dysphagia, are usually noted from 3–12 yr of age. The disease progresses rapidly with death in 1–4 yr from onset. Symptoms of Addison disease, including melanoderma, hypotension, and a failure of ACTH to induce a rise in plasma cortisol, are noted after the initial diagnosis. Later onset forms of this disorder are recognized in which adrenal insufficiency is associated with slowly progressive paresis and peripheral neuropathy. Patients with this slowly progressing form called adrenomyeloneuropathy (AMN) may survive to the 4th or 5th decade. In both ALD and AMN characteristic inclusions consisting of electron-dense leaflets enclosing an electron-lucent space are found in the cerebral white matter, peripheral nerves, and adrenal cortex. Examination of fatty acid content of the lipids in the involved tissues has demonstrated an accumulation of C_{24}–C_{30} fatty acids in both disorders.

Diagnoses have been made in suspected males by examination of biopsy samples from brain, adrenals, conjunctiva, and skin. Examination of the fatty acid composition from the total lipid extract of cultured skin fibroblasts reveals higher levels of C_{26} fatty acids in patients and mothers of patients when compared to controls or to other metabolic diseases involving lipid metabolism; the ratio of C_{26} to C_{22} is reported. This method identifies the cultures from patients with both ALD and AMN, confirming the close association of these 2 syndromes. The $C_{26}:C_{22}$ ratio in mothers of ALD patients was between that found in patients and controls. Using clones from these heterozygous females, 2 populations were identified, 1 with a normal ratio of $C_{26}:C_{22}$ and the other with a ratio similar to that found in affected males. This method should allow diagnosis of patients from only a skin biopsy and allow prenatal diagnosis by examination of the $C_{26}:C_{22}$ ratio in cultured amniotic fluid cells from at risk pregnancies. Since these long-chained fatty acids are found in many lipid classes, it is proposed that the primary defect involves an enzyme that degrades fatty acids with a chain length of 24 carbon atoms or more.

8.39 ACID PHOSPHATASE DEFICIENCY

Acid phosphatase deficiency is a rare lysosomal storage disease of early infancy. The few patients who have been described have had a clinical picture characterized by intermittent vomiting, hypotonia, lethargy, opisthotonos, terminal bleeding, and death within the 1st yr of life. Hepatomegaly is noted, and biopsy reveals widely scattered foci of necrosis of liver cells. Hepatocytes are enlarged with a prominent vacuolated cytoplasm. PAS-positive material, presumably lipid, is found in liver and kidneys. A "fatty" liver was found in 1 patient. The brain showed only focal neuronal degeneration. The initial patients reported by Nadler were deficient in lysosomal acid phosphatase activity in PHA-stimulated lymphocytes and cultured skin fibroblasts. Acid phosphatase levels were 20% of normal in the whole fibroblast homogenate and about 1% of normal in the lysosomal fraction. The deficiency was found using β-glycerophosphate, phenolphthalein phosphate, or p-nitrophenol phosphate as substrates. This genetic disease appears to be inherited as an autosomal recessive trait. Prenatal diagnosis has been accomplished by analysis of acid phosphatase levels in cultured amniotic fluid cells.

A 2nd syndrome involving low levels of acid phosphatase has been reported with opisthotonos and a bleeding tendency, death in this case occurring after 2 days of life. Physical examination was within normal limits, except for marked lethargy, a poor suck, and a poor Moro reflex. Fibroblasts grown from skin biopsy were found to have an almost total deficiency of acid phosphatase in the whole homogenate and lysosomal fraction.

In the 1st condition, the lysosomal acid phosphatase deficiency, prednisolone appears to stimulate acid phosphatase activity in the fibroblasts; it does not do so in total acid phosphatase deficiency.

8.40 REFSUM DISEASE

Patients with Refsum disease (phytanic acid storage disease or heredopathia atactica polyneuritiformis) have the onset before 20 yr of age of failing vision (night blindness), anosmia, ichthyosis, weakness in extremities, and unsteady gait. Examination of liver and kidneys reveals severe infiltration with neutral fat. Plasma contains a large amount of phytanic acid (a 20-carbon branched-chain acid), and this may constitute 5–30% of the total fatty acids. It may be the larger size of phytanic acid compared to other fatty acids that distorts cell membranes and results in nerve degeneration. Refsum disease is inherited as an autosomal recessive trait.

Most patients are identified before 20 yr of age, some after 50 yr. Almost all patients have retinitis pigmentosa, peripheral polyneuropathy, and cerebellar ataxia, and they may have dramatic exacerbations associated with ill-defined febrile illnesses, surgical procedures, or pregnancy. Lengthy periods of remission are not unusual. Diagnosis is indicated from clinical findings, increased spinal fluid protein (average 275 mg/dl), and the finding of elevated phytanic acid (up to 25 μg/ml) in the plasma. Studies on cultured skin fibroblasts indicate that in patients with Refsum disease phytanic acid is oxidized at 1–2% of the normal rate. Heterozygotes can be identified. There appears to be a high incidence among Norwegians.

Treatment of this disease is possible through elimination of precursors of phytanic acid in the diet. These include dairy products, ruminant fats, and other foods containing chlorophyll (to exclude phytol). With reduction of the content of phytanic acid in plasma and tissue there is some amelioration of the neuropathy in some patients. Supportive physiotherapy and orthopedic devices may help patients cope with neuropathy; extraction of cataracts may be indicated. Death due to cardiac and respiratory complications usually occurs before the 5th decade.

8.41 NEURONAL CEROID-LIPOFUSCINOSES

See also Sec 21.16 and 25.4.

The neuronal ceroid-lipofuscinoses encompass a group of genetic diseases including Batten disease, Spielmeyer-Vogt disease, Jansky-Bielschowsky syndrome, Kufs disease, and 3 types of amaurotic familial idiocy. All appear to be inherited as autosomal recessive diseases. Persons affected by this group of diseases have neuronal storage of lipopigments of the ceroid-lipofuscin type, with relatively normal ganglioside patterns. The age of onset varies: from 2–5 yr of age in the late infantile type; from 8–12 yr of age in the juvenile type; and over 20 yr in the adult type. In most of the younger patients (2–12 yr of age) clinical onset is marked by seizures, visual disturbances, intellectual retardation, and ataxia. Myoclonus and seizures can become refractory to all anticonvulsant medications. Blindness, with macular degeneration and retinitis pigmentosa, is common in the later stages of these syndromes. The course is variable, younger patients usually surviving 3–5 yr and juvenile patients 6–8 yr after initial signs. Adult patients present with ataxia and dementia or signs of involvement of basal ganglia and dementia.

In a suspected patient the diagnosis is usually made on the finding of abnormal neurons in a biopsy of rectum or brain. There is a severe loss of neuronal perikarya, which contain granules that stain with Sudan black B and PAS and give positive reactions with all stains for ceroid or lipofuscin. The cytoplasm of many neurons contains variable numbers of irregularly

shaped cytoplasmic inclusions called "curvilinear bodies." Other inclusions have the appearance of "fingerprint profiles." Studies of peripheral blood of patients with the late infantile form have revealed similar curvilinear bodies in lymphocytes. These may aid in the diagnosis without need for brain biopsy.

The clinical findings resemble those of other cerebral degenerative diseases, such as G_{M1} and G_{M2} gangliosidoses and the leukodystrophies, in which there are deficiencies of a specific lysosomal hydrolase. The exact enzymatic defect in the ceroid-lipofuscinoses has not yet been identified. Carriers cannot yet be accurately identified, and prenatal diagnosis has not been reported. The activity of leukocyte peroxidase has been reported to be low in some patients, but data from other laboratories have not confirmed this finding. The storage of these lipopigments, or "wear and tear pigments," in the neurons of these patients may be related to a defect in the oxidation of fatty acids.

Control of seizures should be attempted since uncontrolled seizures tend to hasten the course. No procedures have been successful in preventing death from aspiration pneumonia in the severely handicapped child.

8.42 MUCOLIPIDOSES

Patients with mucolipidoses exhibit clinical features of both lipidoses and mucopolysaccharidoses (Chapter 23). Despite their name, there is little evidence of true storage of lipids or mucopolysaccharides in the organs of affected patients. Technically, fucosidosis, G_{M1} gangliosidosis, and multiple sulfatase deficiency are mucolipidoses because there is evidence for storage both of lipids (as glycosphingolipids) and of glycosaminoglycans in various organs. All of the mucolipidoses are inherited as autosomal recessive traits.

Mucolipidosis (ML-I), lipomucopolysaccharidosis, or sialidosis Type 2 (infantile onset) produces symptoms in the 1st yr of life. There are Hurler-like features, with dysostosis multiplex, moderate mental retardation, visceromegaly, corneal clouding, cherry-red spot, seizures, vacuolated lymphocytes, and coarse fibroblast inclusions, but no mucopolysacchariduria. Sialic acid terminal oligosaccharides are excreted in large amounts in the urine. Kupffer cells and hepatocytes are vacuolated, and sural nerve biopsy reveals metachromatic myelin degeneration. These patients are deficient in glycoprotein sialidase activity, which can be measured using several water-soluble substrates. Ganglioside sialidase is normal. Carriers can be identified and prenatal diagnosis can be made using cultured amniotic cells.

ML-II or I-cell disease is manifest within the 1st few mo of life. The clinical pattern somewhat resembles Hurler syndrome and G_{M1} gangliosidosis (Type 1). Affected patients may have congenital dislocation of the hips, inguinal hernias, hypertrophy of the gums, restriction of motion in the shoulders, generalized hypotonia, thick and tight skin, and hepatomegaly. The coarse facial features become more conspicuous with age. Characteristic bone changes related to severe dysostosis multiplex occur, leading to a cloaking of the long tubular bones, to shortening of vertebral bodies, and to other significant changes in the pelvis, hands, ribs, and skull. Death from pneumonia or congestive heart failure usually occurs at 2–8 yr of age.

Urinary mucopolysaccharides are normal but sialyl-oligosaccharides are elevated. Fibroblast cultures viewed under phase contrast reveal the characteristic inclusions, which initially set this disease apart from the mucopolysaccharidoses. Enzyme studies reveal greatly increased lysosomal enzymes in serum, whereas values in leukocytes are near the normal range. Enzymes measured in most organs are normal except for a slight deficiency of β-galactosidase (which may be only a secondary effect). Diagnosis can also be made by examination of cultured skin fibroblasts for lysosomal enzyme activities. Activities of almost all lysosomal enzymes are deficient in the cells, whereas the culture medium has an excess of these enzymes when compared to that of control fibroblast lines. The primary defect in ML-II and ML-III is a deficiency of a specific N-acetylglucosaminyl phosphotransferase which phosphorylates newly formed lysosomal enzymes. This enzyme's activity can be measured in fibroblast cultures, and this will provide a specific diagnostic test for patient and carrier identification and for prenatal diagnosis.

ML-III or pseudo–Hurler polydystrophy appears to be a milder form of ML-II. After possibly delayed early psychomotor development, affected patients 3–4 yr of age may present progressive joint stiffness, short stature, mild dysostosis multiplex, mild gingival hyperplasia, and normal urinary mucopolysaccharide levels. Corneal clouding or nystagmus may be present. The IQ may range from normal to as low as 50. The prognosis is not known; some patients have attained the 3rd decade of life. Orthopedic treatment may be indicated in some cases. As in I-cell disease, serum lysosomal enzymes are elevated, and cultured skin fibroblasts reveal characteristic inclusions and decreased activities for many lysosomal enzymes. Prenatal diagnosis should be possible through examination of cultured amniotic fluid cells.

ML-IV is a recently described mucolipidosis. All cases reported so far have occurred in children of Ashkenazi Jewish descent. Affected children soon after birth present bilateral corneal opacities and strabismus. After 6 mo hypotonia and psychomotor retardation become more evident. There is no skeletal dysplasia or excess excretion of mucopolysaccharides in the urine. There are grossly abnormal storage bodies in the cells of liver, brain, conjunctiva, and fibroblasts. The prognosis is not yet certain. One patient has reached 24 yr of age. Treatment to correct the corneal opacities may improve the vision, but no other treatment is available.

Diagnosis is based on examination of fibroblast cultures for the characteristic lamellated multivesicular membrane bodies. The precise defect is unknown. A partial deficiency of G_{M3} ganglioside sialidase activity in cultured cells from a patient remains to be confirmed. Prenatal diagnosis has been accomplished by examination of the cultured amniotic fluid cells for characteristic storage bodies.

Sialidoses is the name given to a group of patients having a deficiency of sialidase (neuraminidase) activity when certain glycoprotein, oligosaccharide, or synthetic sialic acid–containing derivatives are used as substrates. Ganglioside sialidase activity is normal. The manifestations of disease in these patients vary greatly, from those presenting in the 1st yr of life (mucolipidosis I, sialidosis Type 2, infantile onset) to those having myoclonus, cherry-red spot, and vision loss but near normal intelligence (sialidosis Type 1) presenting in the 1st or 2nd decade and surviving until the 4th decade. One group of patients having a clinical picture between these 2 types (sialidosis Type 2, juvenile onset) has been mistaken for unusual forms of G_{M1} gangliosidosis because of low β-galactosidase activity also found in certain tissues. All types excrete sialyloligosaccharides in urine and store sialic acid–containing derivatives in cultured cells. The sialidoses can be enzymatically diagnosed in cultured fibroblasts and leukocytes, and prenatal diagnoses have been made. Carriers can be identified.

HYPERLIPIDEMIAS

See Sec 13.86 for discussion of hyperlipoproteinemias.

DAVID WENGER

Brady RO, Pentchev PG, Gal AE, et al: Replacement therapy for inherited enzyme deficiency. Use of purified glucocerebrosidase in Gaucher's disease. N Engl J Med 291:989, 1974.

Cortner JA, Coates PM, Swoboda E, et al: Genetic variations of lysosomal acid lipase. Pediatr Res 10:927, 1976.

Crocker AC, Farber S: Niemann-Pick disease. A review of 18 patients. Medicine 37:1, 1958.

Dulaney JT, Milunsky A, Sidbury JB, et al: Diagnosis of lipogranulomatosis (Farber disease) by use of cultured fibroblasts. J Pediatr 89:59, 1976.

Gilbert EF, Dawson G, ZuRhein GM, et al: I-cell disease, mucolipidosis II. Pathological, histochemical, ultra-structural and biochemical observations on four cases. Z Kinderheilk 114:259, 1973.

Hagberg B, Sourander P, Svennerholm L: Sulfatide lipidosis in childhood. Report of a case investigated during life and at autopsy. Am J Dis Child 104:94, 1962.

Kihara H, Ho C-K, Fluharty AL, et al: Prenatal diagnosis of metachromatic leukodystrophy in a family with pseudo arylsulfatase A deficiency by the cerebroside sulfate loading test. Pediatr Res 14:224, 1980.

Kousseff BG, Beratis NG, Strauss L, et al: Fucosidosis Type 2. Pediatrics 57:205, 1976.

Lowden JA, O'Brien JS: Sialidosis: A review of human sialidase deficiency. Am J Hum Genet 31:1, 1979.

Moser HW, Moser AB, Kawamura N, et al: Adrenoleukodystrophy: Elevated C26 fatty acid in cultured skin fibroblasts. Ann Neurol 7:542, 1980.

Nadler HL, Egan TJ: Deficiency of lysosomal acid phosphatase. A new familial metabolic disorder. N Engl J Med 282:302, 1970.

O'Brien JS: Molecular genetics of G_{M1} β-galactosidase. Clin Genet 8:303, 1975.

Okada S, O'Brien JS: Tay-Sachs disease: Generalized absence of a beta-D-N-acetylhexosaminidase component. Science 165:698, 1969.

Rapin I, Suzuki K, Suzuki K, et al: Adult (chronic) G_{M2} gangliosidosis. Atypical spinocerebellar degeneration in a Jewish sibship. Arch Neurol 33:120, 1976.

Wenger DA, Sattler M, Clark C, et al: An improved method for the identification of patients and carriers of Krabbe's disease. Clin Chim Acta 56:199, 1974.

Wenger DA, Sattler M, Mueller OT, et al: Adult G_{M1} gangliosidosis: Clinical and biochemical studies on two patients and comparison to other patients called variant or adult G_{M1} gangliosidosis. Clin Genet 17:323, 1980.

Wenger DA, Tarby TJ, Wharton C: Macular cherry-red spots and myoclonus with dementia: Coexistent neuraminidase and β-galactosidase deficiencies. Biochem Biophys Res Commun 82:589, 1978.

DEFECTS IN HEME PIGMENT METABOLISM

In this section, only the defects of iron and heme pigments are described. The defects involving melanin and bilirubin are discussed elsewhere (Sec 7.44, 8.3, and 11.80–11.82).

8.43 THE PORPHYRIAS

The porphyrias are a group of syndromes characterized biochemically by errors in pyrrole metabolism and clinically by photodermatitis and visceral and neuropsychiatric complaints. Incidence is estimated at 1:30,000 in the general population. Table 8–9 classifies them according to the organ system in which the error in pyrrole metabolism is localized: *erythropoietic* and *hepatic* forms are recognized. Most of the porphyrias have a dominant mode of inheritance. Family studies and close surveillance through adolescence are essential to identify cases in the latent stage; this is vital since most deaths occur during the late adolescent and early adult years and are attributable to delays in diagnosis that may lead to inappropriate and harmful therapy. Family studies entail determination of porphyrins in both urine and stool in all members; in cases of photosensitivity, measurements of erythrocyte protoporphyrin are also necessary. With early diagnosis, proper fluid and dietary therapy, and avoidance of contraindicated drugs, the prognosis for survival and symptomatic relief during acute visceral attacks is good. Enzyme diagnosis using blood, leukocytes, or skin is possible in most of the heritable forms of porphyria.

Relation of Abnormal Heme Biosynthesis to Disease States. Heme is the prosthetic group of hemoglobin, myoglobin, catalase, peroxidase, and the cytochromes (including P450). It is formed via the metabolic pathway shown in Fig 8–33. This pathway is common to all mammalian cells, each cell synthesizing its own heme for the formation of its own particular hemoproteins. The initial step, formation of δ-aminolevulinic acid (ALA),* is mediated by ALA synthetase (Fig 8–33). This mitochondrial enzyme is inductible, and its availability is rate-limiting for the entire process.

---

*See Table 8–10 for key to abbreviations used in this chapter.

Table 8–9 A CLASSIFICATION OF
THE PORPHYRIAS

HEPATIC PORPHYRIAS

Acute intermittent porphyria (AIP, Swedish genetic porphyria)
Porphyria variegata (PV, South African genetic porphyria)
Hereditary coproporphyria
The cutaneous porphyrias (PCT, porphyria cutanea tarda)
  Hereditary types
  Acquired (but possible genetic predisposition associated with
    alcoholism, etc.)
  Toxic (hexachlorobenzene-induced)

ERYTHROPOIETIC PORPHYRIAS

Protoporphyria (P)
Congenital erythropoietic porphyria

Four basic porphyrin isomers are known and are designated as types I, II, III and IV. Types I and III are the only naturally occurring isomers. Mammalian hemoproteins contain type III porphyrin isomers only. Protoporphyrin (PROTO) 9 is a type III isomer. Infinitesimal quantities of type I isomers are formed as byproducts of heme synthesis.

Increased activity of hepatic ALA synthetase is the enzymatic abnormality common to all dominantly inherited forms of hepatic porphyria. In *acute intermittent porphyria*, 1 of the 3 recognized types of heritable hepatic porphyria, the activity of URO I synthetase is reduced by about 50%. This apparently represents the primary defect and causes induction of ALA synthetase through negative feedback regulation by heme. This abnormality in regulation may well explain the precipitation of clinical attacks by drugs, chemicals, and steroids, which induce ALA synthetase and the formation of hepatic microsomal hemoproteins, particularly P450. This also accounts for the pattern of pyrrole excretion in acute intermittent porphyria (Table 8–10). Partial inhibition of coproporphyrinogen oxidase characterizes *hereditary coproporphyria*, while partial inhibition of protoporphyrinogen oxidase characterizes *porphyria variegata*. These enzymatic defects also account for the pyrrole excretion patterns seen in each disorder.

The fundamental metabolic defect in *congenital erythropoietic porphyria* resides in the inability of approximately half of the developing erythroblasts to convert PBG to uroporphyrinogen (UROGEN) III (Fig 8–33). Instead, URO I accumulates within the nuclei of these defective erythroblasts, diffuses into the circulation, is deposited in various tissues, including teeth and bone, and is excreted in the urine as a mixture of URO I and coproporphyrin (COPRO) I, with URO I predominant.

Protoporphyria is characterized by excessive amounts of free PROTO 9 in marrow reticulocytes and circulating erythrocytes, in which it has a short half-life and readily diffuses into plasma, skin, and liver. In iron deficiency and lead poisoning, which are not photosensitive disorders, the metalloporphyrin zinc protoporphyrin is found in erythrocytes rather than "free" PROTO 9. Activity of hemesynthase (ferrochelatase) is diminished in erythroid cells in the bone marrow and possibly in liver in *protoporphyria*. This results in substantial accumulation of PROTO 9 in circulating erythrocytes and liver. Excess PROTO 9 is excreted in feces but not in urine. There is a reciprocal relationship between caloric intake and PROTO excretion, similar to the "glucose effect" found in the hepatic porphyrias (see below).

Normally the urinary excretion of PBG and ALA does not exceed 3 mg/day. The qualitative Hoesch test for PBG (see below) is positive only with a pathologic excess of PBG. Porphyrins normally appear in the excreta in very small amounts: fecal COPRO and PROTO should not exceed 100 μg/gm of dry feces/day; COPRO appears in urine at a rate of 2.2 μg/kg (1 μg/lb) of body weight/day. Infections and accelerated erythropoiesis cause a 2–3-fold increase in urinary COPRO; hepatitis (infectious and toxic), a 10–40-fold increase in

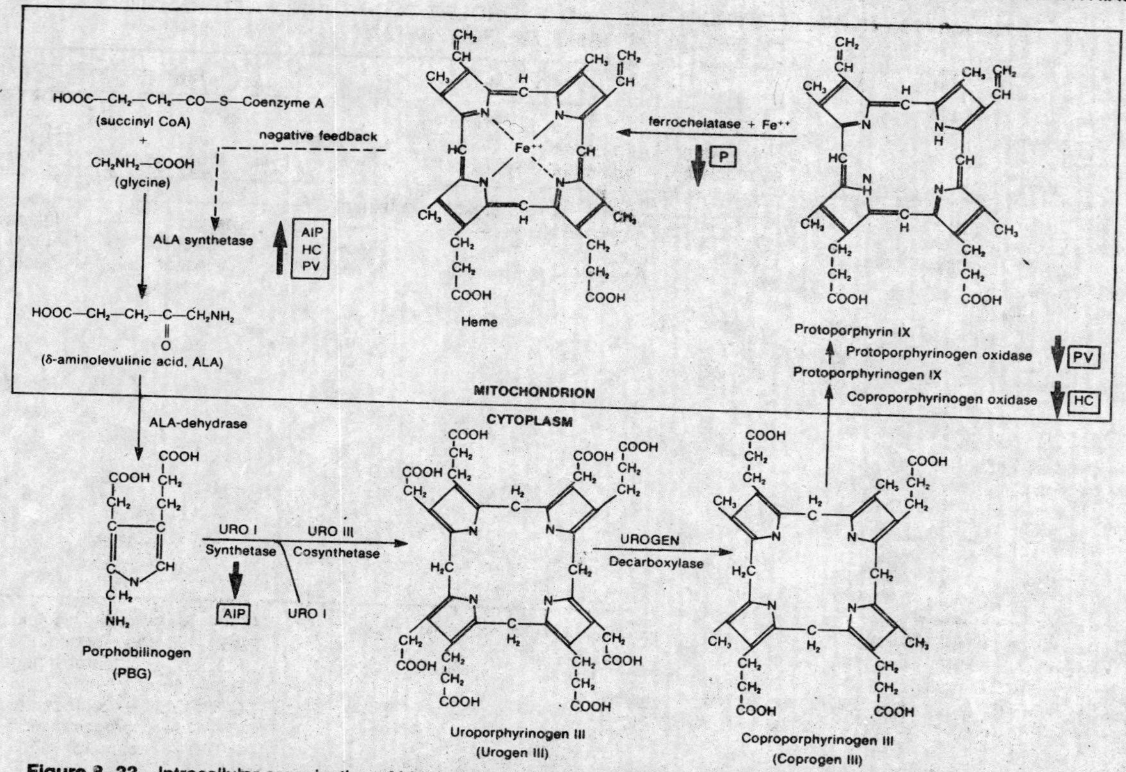

Figure 8–33 Intracellular organization of biosynthesis of heme. The initial and final steps in heme synthesis occur within the mitochondria. ALA is released in the cytoplasm. The metabolites formed in the cytoplasm are the ones found in the plasma and urine. ALA synthetase is the rate-limiting enzyme. Only the fully reduced porphyrin intermediates UROGEN III and coproporphyrinogen (COPROGEN) III are utilized for heme formation. These substances are colorless and unstable and do not exhibit fluorescence. Oxidation stabilizes porphyrin molecules and renders them fluorescent. Those portions of UROGEN and COPROGEN not utilized for heme synthesis are oxidized to UROs I and III and COPROs I and III, and it is in this form that these porphyrins are usually detected in the tissues and excreta. PBG and ALA are also colorless and do not fluoresce; they are measured by chemical methods. Lead (Pb) inhibits ALA dehydratase and heme synthetase (see Chapter 28).

urinary COPRO; and lead intoxication a 10–40-fold increase in both ALA and COPRO in urine. Porphyria may cause up to 1000-fold increases in pyrrole excretion. In acquired porphyria COPRO always exceeds URO in urine, but in the heritable forms the quantity of URO in urine always exceeds COPRO if both are present. Increased fecal porphyrins virtually always indicate a heritable form of porphyria.

Relation of Metabolic Errors to Clinical Manifestations. *Photosensitizing Effects of Porphyrins.* Some but not all the skin lesions of both erythropoietic and certain hepatic porphyrias are due to the photosensitizing effect of URO. Erythema, edema, and vesiculation of the exposed skin result when persons with increased uroporphyrinemia are irradiated with a combination of near ultraviolet (400 nm) and infrared (2600 nm) monochromatic lights. Protoporphyria is apparently unique among photosensitive dermatitides in that very brief exposure to sunlight can quickly cause intense pain and sensation of heat in the exposed skin. Repeated exposures to near ultraviolet light lead to urticarial and chronic eczematoid lesions. All the heme precursors (Fig 8–33) have at one time or another been injected into both healthy and porphyric human subjects without demonstrable adverse effect other than photosensitization.

Toxic and Experimental Hepatic Porphyria. The heritable hepatic porphyrias are characterized by induction and increased activity of hepatic ALA synthetase. In acute intermittent porphyria, reduced activity of URO I synthetase has been demonstrated in liver and blood in both symptomatic and asymptomatic patients and carriers. These abnormalities are not enough alone to explain the clinical phenomena. Attention is now focused on hepatic microsomal P450, an inductible hemoprotein with short biologic half-life and rapid turnover rate. The drugs and chemicals used experimentally to produce hepatic porphyria (Table 8–11) affect P450. Phenobarbital, for example, increases the requirement for P450; on the other hand, allylisopropylacetamide increases its destruction. Such findings suggest that patients with acute intermittent porphyria, because of impaired activity of URO I synthetase, may not be able to adjust the metabolism of P450 to the effects of the drugs, insecticides, other chemicals, and nutritional and hormonal factors. Though the sex steroid metabolites listed in Table 8–11 clearly modify the course of porphyria, their mechanism of action is not understood.

Table 8–10   CLINICAL SYNDROMES AND PYRROLE* EXCRETION PATTERNS IN HERITABLE FORMS OF PORPHYRIA

	HEPATIC PORPHYRIAS				ERYTHROPOIETIC PORPHYRIAS	
	Acute Intermittent Porphyria	Porphyria Variegata	"Porphyria Cutanea Tarda"	Hereditary Coproporphyria	Protoporphyria†	Congenital Erythropoietic Porphyria
Transmission	Autosomal dominant					Recessive
Onset of clinical manifestations	Puberty or later‡				Early childhood	Infancy
Acute visceral and neurologic attacks	Present	Present	Present	Present	Absent	Absent
Cutaneous lesions	Absent	Present	Present	?Absent	Present	Present
Pyrrole excretion§ during acute visceral and neurologic attacks *Urine* ALA, PBG¶	++++	++++	±	+ to ++		
URO, COPRO	± to +++	± to +++	±	+ to ++		
Feces COPRO	0	++++	++++	++++		
PROTO	0	++++	+++	±		
Pyrrole excretion§ during remission of visceral and neurologic symptoms *Urine* ALA, PBG	±	0	±	0	0	0
URO, COPRO	±	0	0	±	0	++++
Feces COPRO	0	++++	++++	++++	±	+++
PROTO	0	++++	++++	0	+++	±

*Strictly speaking, ALA is a heme precursor but not a pyrrole. PBG is a monopyrrole. URO, COPRO and PROTO are tetrapyrroles.
†Erythrocyte PROTO grossly increased in protoporphyria.
‡In each group rare cases have been observed before puberty.
§Increased URO in feces found in some cases of each group.

¶ALA — δ-aminolevulinic acid.
PBG — porphobilinogen.
UROGEN — uroporphyrinogen.
URO — uroporphyrin.
COPROGEN — coproporphyrinogen.
COPRO — coproporphyrin.
PROTO — protoporphyrin.

The experimental observation that glycuronide conjugates of these sex steroid metabolites do not induce porphyria suggests that maintenance of optimal liver function may be important in prevention of attacks. The roles of sex steroid metabolites as potent inducers of hepatic porphyria may explain why the onset of symptoms is so regularly delayed until after puberty.

Balance studies in patients with hepatic porphyria show that both severe caloric restriction and negative nitrogen balance are accompanied by a sharp increase in the excretion of pyrroles. This increase can be suppressed if adequate caloric intake is restored by the administration of carbohydrates. Return to positive nitrogen balance is also accompanied by diminution in pyrrole excretion. The maintenance of a diet high in carbohydrate and adequate in protein is of considerable clinical importance.

Diagnosis and Management of the Porphyrias. *Clinical Manifestations.* Though the porphyrias are generally genetically determined and the basic metabolic errors present from birth, clinical symptoms before puberty are rare in the hepatic forms. Three groups of clinical manifestations are recognized: cutaneous, visceral, and neuropsychiatric. Their onset is insidious, but once they occur, the complaints tend to run an undulating course throughout the remainder of the patient's life. The principal clinical syndromes and patterns of pyrrole excretion encountered in the porphyrias are summarized in Table 8–10.

Acute exacerbations of dermal lesions occur with exposure to sunlight. Visceral and neurologic complaints, which almost invariably occur together, may be precipitated by infection, menstruation, pregnancy, alcohol, barbiturates, and other agents listed in Table 8–11. Although the skin lesions are bothersome and may be disfiguring, it is the acute visceral and neurologic problems that threaten life. The relative frequency of various abnormal clinical findings encountered during an acute attack are shown in Fig 8–34 and 8–35; none are pathognomonic. Early diagnosis depends upon rec-

Table 8–11   AGENTS USED TO INDUCE CHEMICAL HEPATIC PORPHYRIA IN ANIMALS

Chemicals
Allylisopropylacetamide
Allylisopropylacetylurea (Sedormid)
Hexachlorobenzene
3,5-dicarbethoxy-1,4-dihydrocollidine

Drugs

Sulfonal	Griseofulvin
Barbiturates	Chloroquine
Sulfonamides	

Endogenous Sex Steroids

Potent porphyrin-inducing activity

C-19 Steroids	C-21 Steroids
Etiocholanolone	Pregnanediol
Etiocholandiol	Pregnanolone
Etiocholandione	11-Ketopregnanolone
Etiocholanolone-17	17-OH Pregnanolone

Weak porphyrin-inducing activity

Testosterone	Estrone
Progesterone	Estriol
Estradiol	

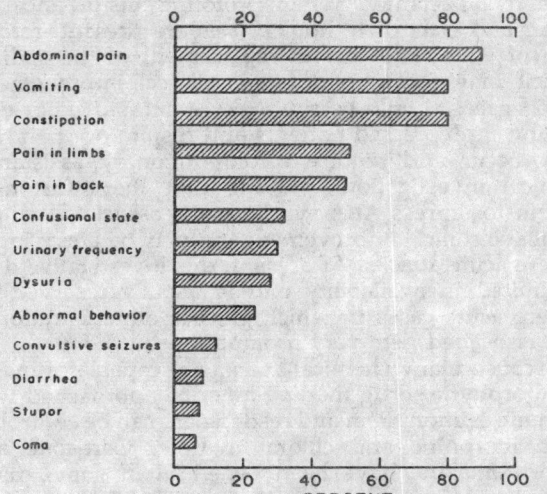

Figure 8–34 The acute attack of porphyria—relative frequency of symptoms. Based on an analysis of 107 acute attacks in 80 patients. (Adapted from Eales L: S Afr J Lab Clin Med 9:151, 1963.)

ognition of the sequence in which the clinical manifestations appear, intensify, and abate, and upon demonstration of excess pyrroles in the excreta. In vitro enzymatic assays can further substantiate the diagnosis. Colicky abdominal pain and varied neuropsychiatric symptoms are the usual presenting complaints.

Colicky abdominal pain is the initial symptom of an acute attack in most patients. The pain is most frequently in the epigastrium or right iliac fossa but may be located anywhere in the abdomen or pelvis. There is considerable variation in its intensity; the pain tends to worsen in an undulating manner over a period of days. Severe colic may persist for hours and often causes the patient to writhe about or assume bizarre positions in bed. Vomiting and constipation develop shortly in all but

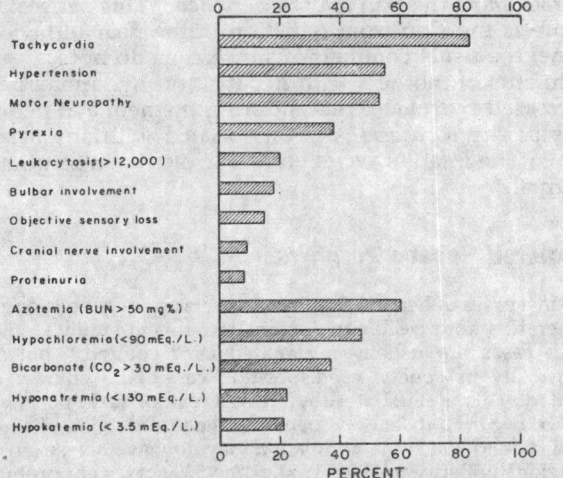

Figure 8–35 The acute attack of porphyria—relative frequency of signs and pertinent laboratory findings. Based on analysis of 107 acute attacks in 80 patients. (Adapted from Eales L: S Afr J Lab Clin Med 9:151, 1963.)

the mildest attacks. Examination of the abdomen and pelvis reveals minimal signs, which seem insignificant in comparison with the patient's pain. Diffuse tenderness of the abdomen is usually present, but does not localize; rigidity and muscle spasm are rare. Leukocytosis and fever are often present. The acute visceral pain of porphyria has been confused with virtually every acute surgical condition of the abdomen, various painful gynecologic disorders, and "hysteria." In the absence of other features and objective findings characteristic of these other conditions, the presence of tachycardia and hypertension makes porphyria a likely diagnosis.

Uncommonly, pain, weakness, and paresthesia in back and limb muscles occur as presenting complaints in the absence of abdominal pain. *Personality changes,* probably attributable to patchy cerebral demyelination, are observed in most patients suffering from visceral attacks, but they are rarely the predominating features. These patients are variously described as depressed, nervous, hysterical, lachrymose, or "peculiar." These traits wax and wane with the severity of the pain. In severe colic, mental confusion, hallucinations, and disorientation are often present.

After the patient with acute intermittent porphyria or porphyria variegata (Table 8–10) has had an exacerbation characterized by abdominal pain, vomiting, constipation, tachycardia, and, in more severe cases, hypertension, the end of the attack may often be heralded by the return of blood pressure, pulse, and weight to normal.

The urine is apt to be colorless at first, although PBG is always present in high concentration and is diagnostic. If the attack progresses, and especially if barbiturates are given, the urine usually becomes red, increasing motor restlessness is noted, and neurologic manifestations, rarely present initially, soon appear. These take the form of unpredictable, spotty weakness or paralysis, with diminished or absent tendon reflexes, and pain and tenderness in the involved muscle groups. These signs are attributable to patchy demyelination of peripheral nerves. Muscle paralysis is an ominous sign. Ill-advised abdominal or pelvic surgery may be quickly followed by catastrophic paralysis and coma. Weakness and paralysis may persist for months after the other features of an acute attack have subsided. Death, when it occurs, usually results from quadriparesis or respiratory failure.

There is a profound disturbance in water and electrolyte homeostasis in severe attacks of porphyria. The serum is hypotonic, with reduced concentrations of sodium and chloride (Fig 8–35). The urine is hypertonic, in part because of excessive loss of sodium, which is attributed to inappropriate secretion of antidiuretic hormone. The severity of neurologic injury may be related to the degree of hyponatremia. Hypocalcemia and hypomagnesemia may occur with and without tetany.

Burgundy red urine in the porphyric patient is due to the presence of URO. It is a constant finding in congenital erythropoietic porphyria and a frequent finding in patients with cutaneous manifestations of hepatic porphyria.

A variety of *dermal lesions* may be observed in porphyria. Exposure to sunlight produces vesicles, bullae, and edema on the exposed skin. These photosensitive lesions are prone to secondary infection and heal slowly, with chronic scars which become hyperpigmented. In some patients such lesions may also follow minor mechanical trauma and exposure to indoor sources of ultraviolet light. Macules, papules, eczematous plaques, and urticaria are also seen.

Nearly all patients with cutaneous forms of porphyria eventually have hypertrichosis and a violaceous hue to their skin. These changes develop insidiously over the years and are most prominent on the exposed parts of the body.

Differential Diagnosis. Examination of Fig 8–34 and 8–35 makes it clear that porphyria must be included in the differential diagnosis of essential hypertension, hyperthyroidism, painful gynecologic disorders, "hysteria," psychosis, and all surgical conditions of the abdomen. Whenever diagnosis of such surgical conditions as ulcer, gallbladder disease, or appendicitis cannot be made with confidence, a Hoesch test for PBG should be done prior to surgical exploration. A surprising number of porphyric patients are treated in error for hyperthyroidism. Serum protein-bound iodine may be elevated in hepatic porphyria without other laboratory evidence of hyperthyroidism. Cutaneous forms of porphyria should be included in the differential diagnosis of photosensitive dermatitides.

Laboratory Diagnosis. Accurate diagnosis of porphyria requires examination of both urine and feces, and, in the case of erythropoietic protoporphyria, of blood (Table 8–10). The excreta of patients and of their relatives must be examined to establish the type of pedigree and to identify latent cases. In the hepatic porphyrias, pyrrole excretion patterns may vary according to the presence or absence of visceral symptoms. Porphyrin excretion may be increased 1000-fold or more over the normal values. The red color imparted to urine by URO must be distinguished from that due to urates, bile, anthocyanin (from beets), melanin, eosin, hemoglobin, or myoglobin.

The Hoesch test for PBG is simple, specific, and virtually always positive in acute visceral attacks. It gives results comparable to those of the more complex Schwartz-Watson test. The Hoesch test can be performed at the bedside as follows:

To 1 ml of Hoesch reagent (2 g of *p*-dimethylaminobenzaldehyde in 100 ml of 6 N hydrochloric acid) add 1–2 drops of *freshly voided* urine. An instantaneous cherry red color at the top of the solution which spreads throughout the solution on brief agitation is specific for abnormally high amounts of porphobilinogen (PBG). False-positive results due to urobilinogen do not occur. Hoesch reagent is stable for 9 mo.

New simplified methods for measuring porphyrins in blood (primarily PROTO) should facilitate the clinical diagnosis of protoporphyria and possibly other porphyrias associated with photosensitive dermatitis. Enzymatic diagnosis can be helpful, especially in the detection of latent cases in family studies.

Treatment. Disturbances in water and electrolyte homeostasis are not usually seen in mild attacks; nevertheless, they should be anticipated and the patient treated expectantly. When profound disturbances in water and electrolyte homeostasis are present, restriction of water and careful replacement of the sodium deficit may result in dramatic clinical improvement. Blood gases should be routinely monitored. Poor ventilation in depressed patients and respiratory paralysis may occur and require cardiopulmonary assistance. Clinical investigations indicate that the infusion of hemin to repress ALA synthetase is associated with a dramatic clinical improvement and may be lifesaving in severe acute attacks. At present, this investigative drug is limited in availability and is usually reserved for severe acute cases in which glucose administration is not associated with very prompt improvement.

Because many chemical agents are capable of inducing porphyria, drug therapy must be approached with extreme caution. Pain and restlessness can be controlled with morphine and chloral hydrate. Cortisone and chlorpromazine have been beneficial in some cases, without obvious effect in others, and deleterious in a few. Adequate caloric and nitrogen intakes should be restored as rapidly as possible.

Successful long-term management requires careful control of infections and absolute avoidance of alcohol and of the drugs listed in Table 8–11. A calorically adequate diet high in carbohydrate content, adequate in protein, and low in fat is beneficial. Many patients are fearful of precipitating colicky episodes and indulge in food fads. In some women, attacks are clearly related to the menstrual cycle; some have been treated with ovulatory suppressants, androgens, and even oophorectomy, with apparent beneficial results. Oral contraceptives in the lowest effective dosage have been beneficial in some but not all cases of acute intermittent porphyria; they are contraindicated in pedigrees with dermal symptoms. Persons with latent or manifest hepatic porphyria should wear "Medic Alert" bracelets.

The cutaneous lesions are usually satisfactorily managed by avoidance of excessive exposure to sunlight. When this is inadequate, the application of *red veterinary petrolatum* to the skin may be beneficial. This petrolatum protects the skin from radiation in the near ultraviolet zone; the usual commercial sunscreens do not.

Infants of mothers with hepatic porphyria may have increased pyrrole excretion during the neonatal period; this *passive porphyria* is not associated with any symptoms. The infant's excretion of pyrroles soon returns to normal.

Acquired Hepatic Porphyria

Most cases of hepatic porphyria are clearly of genetic origin. When it is not possible to demonstrate this in family studies, such cases are usually designated as "acquired," but the possibility of genetic predisposition cannot be entirely excluded. This is illustrated by an outbreak of toxic porphyria which occurred in Turkey following the introduction of a new fungicide to which the population may not have been exposed previously. Between 1956–1960, some 5000 cases of porphyria in southeastern Turkey were traced to the eating of seed wheat which had been treated with a fungicide, hexachlorobenzene. The resultant syndrome, seen predominantly in children, was characterized by cachexia, hepatomegaly, bullous skin lesions, photosensitivity, hyperpigmentation, hypertrichosis, and increased porphyrin content of the excreta. "Rheumatoid" arthritic changes were noted ultimately in more than 50% of the patients. A chronic porphyric state with all the features just enumerated persisted in most patients for at least 2 yr after the cessation of hexachlorobenzene ingestion. Even 5 yr later most still had hepatomegaly, arthritis, hypertrichosis, and hyperpigmentation. Genetic factors were at first thought to be excluded, but later work by Dogramaci suggests that those affected may have been genetically predisposed.

The acquired forms of hepatic porphyria are clinically indistinguishable from the hereditary cutaneous syndromes (Table 8–10). Visceral manifestations are minimal or absent, and dermal features are usually less severe in the acquired disease, often being limited to hyperpigmentation and hypertrichosis. Acquired porphyria may occur as a rare complication of chronic alcoholism, cirrhosis, tumors involving the liver, and such systemic diseases as Hodgkin disease, disseminated lupus, and leukemia. Red urine due to the presence of URO is usually the clue that leads to the diagnosis.

Variants of Genetic Porphyria. *Congenital erythropoietic porphyria* is one of the rarest inborn errors of metabolism. Vastly increased amounts of URO I are found in bone marrow, circulating erythrocytes, plasma, urine, and feces. Lesser amounts of COPRO I are also found in the excreta. The excretion of other pyrroles is normal. The accumulation of URO I in the tissues (including the teeth) and the associated hemolytic anemia account for all the clinical manifestations of this disease. The photodermatitis of this disease is devastating, often causing severe permanent disfigurement. Splenomegaly results from the hemolytic anemia; splenectomy is beneficial in some cases. The excretion of urine which is burgundy red as passed, or becomes so upon exposure to light, begins at birth or shortly thereafter and continues for life.

Protoporphyria begins during childhood and continues through adult life. Pain, sensation of heat, and 2 types of skin lesions follow exposure to sunlight: (1) an urticarial response which resolves without chronic dermal changes, and (2) erythema and edema followed by an eczematous eruption on the exposed parts. This eczematous eruption is chronic rather than recurrent and leaves considerable scarring. These patients also have dull, opaque fingernails without lunulae. Increased amounts of PROTO 9 are always found in erythrocytes, and usually in feces.

Though the major symptoms are due to photosensitivity, recent reports suggest that a more important prognostic factor may be slowly progressive liver disease, culminating in cirrhosis and hepatic failure. Iron deficiency and other conditions stimulating erythropoiesis should be prevented, good nutrition maintained, hepatic function monitored, and hepatotoxic chemicals avoided. Rigorous avoidance of sunlight is indicated. Carefully monitored therapy with β-carotene has reduced sensitivity to sunlight in some patients.

Among the hepatic porphyrias the visceral, neurologic, and dermal manifestations and the pattern of pyrrole excretion are usually constant within a given pedigree. There is, however, considerable variation from one pedigree to another. The features of 4 typical variants are shown in Table 8–10. Of these, *acute intermittent porphyria* and *porphyria variegata* are perhaps the most common. In kindreds with acute intermittent ("Swedish") porphyria, visceral and neurologic attacks are both most frequent and most severe in females of childbearing age. In such kindreds, acute attacks often occur without obvious precipitating factors. The occurrence of visceral attacks before puberty is rare but has been reported. The disorder has an autosomal dominant mode of transmission. Preliminary studies suggest that both affected and latent cases can be identified either by an ALA loading test or with an in vitro assay for URO I synthetase in blood or in liver biopsy tissue.

In kindreds with porphyria variegata, "South African porphyria," symptoms are most common between puberty and the 5th decade of life. Skin lesions are relatively more common in males, whereas acute visceral attacks are more frequent in females. A striking feature is the great prominence of barbiturates in the precipitation of severe acute visceral attacks. There is an autosomal dominant mode of transmission; 50% of adult members of an affected family have a constant increase in excretion of porphyrins in the feces whether symptoms occur or not.

Porphyria cutanea tarda presents with visceral as well as dermal manifestations, but the visceral complaints tend to be mild in comparison with those seen in acute intermittent porphyria. The existence of a purely cutaneous, hereditary form of hepatic porphyria has been disputed; it can be argued that these patients have never encountered an environmental agent that would precipitate a visceral attack.

Hereditary coproporphyria appears to be transmitted as an autosomal dominant, and it is not a symptomless trait, as previously thought. Clinically it resembles acute intermittent porphyria, except that symptoms may begin during childhood. There may be chronic "nervousness" and other psychiatric complaints, with or without recurrent abdominal pain. The unique biochemical feature of this disease is increased excretion of COPRO III in the feces; urinary COPRO III may or may not be increased. In the majority of cases severe visceral attacks are provoked by barbiturates and possibly by other anticonvulsant and tranquilizing drugs; during such attacks urinary excretion of ALA, PBG, and COPRO III is increased as a consequence of reduced activity of coproporphyrinogen oxidase. Photosensitivity has been described in only 1 of 30 cases.

8.44 HEREDITARY METHEMOGLOBINEMIAS

Normally the iron of both oxygenated and deoxygenated hemoglobin is in the ferrous state; this is essential for its oxygen-transporting function. Oxidation of hemoglobin iron to the ferric state yields methemoglobin, which is nonfunctional and imparts a chocolate hue to the blood; in sufficient concentration it causes cyanosis. The blood of healthy persons contains methemoglobin, but the intraerythrocytic methemoglobin-reducing system maintains its concentration at less than 2% of the total hemoglobin. "Normal" methemoglobin has a characteristic spectral absorption band at 632 nm, which is abolished by treatment of the blood sample with cyanide. This test is specific for assaying methemoglobin produced by exposure to certain chemicals such as aniline dyes, but yields erroneous results when hemoglobin M type pigments are present. Among familial methemoglobinemias both recessive and dominant patterns of inheritance are recognized; each form has a distinct metabolic error.

Hereditary Methemoglobinemia Associated with Defective Methemoglobin-Reducing System. Reduction of methemoglobin in normal erythrocytes can be effected by 4 known systems: ascorbic acid, glutathione, triphosphopyridine nucleotide (NADPH) diaphorase, and diphosphopyridine nucleotide (NADH) diaphorase. Among these, NADH diaphorase (or NADH methemoglobin reductase) is by far the most active.

In hereditary methemoglobinemia with a recessive pattern of inheritance, there is complete absence of the NADH-dependent methemoglobin reductase. In these patients the methemoglobin formed has the spectral and chemical properties of "normal" methemoglobin. Methylene blue is therapeutically effective because it is reduced to leucomethylene blue by both glutathione and NADPH diaphorase; leucomethylene blue, in turn, can reduce "normal" methemoglobin to hemoglobin.

Clinically the disorder is characterized by cyanosis, the intensity of which varies with season and diet. The time at onset of the cyanosis also varies; in some patients it appears at birth, in others as late as adolescence. No associated abnormalities which might explain the cyanosis are found. Despite the fact that up to 50% of the total circulating hemoglobin may be in the form of nonfunctional methemoglobin, there is little or no cardiorespiratory distress except on exertion.

The daily oral administration of ascorbic acid (200–500 mg in divided doses) will gradually reduce the quantity of methemoglobin to about 10% of the total pigment and will alleviate the cyanosis as long as therapy is continued. Methylene blue given intravenously (1–2 mg/kg) promptly eliminates both methemoglobin and cyanosis, and this effect can be maintained by the daily oral administration of methylene blue (3–5 mg/kg). Mental deficiency has been associated in a few cases, but not in most, and there is insufficient evidence to indicate that it is causally related to the methemoglobinemia.

Hereditary Methemoglobinemia Associated with Abnormal Methemoglobins (Hemoglobin M Diseases). The dominantly transmitted forms of methemoglobinemia are collectively known as the hemoglobin M diseases. When all the hemoglobin pigment in a blood sample is first oxidized to methemoglobin by treatment with potassium ferricyanide, the abnormal methemoglobin M type pigments can be separated from normal methemoglobin by means of starch gel electrophoresis. Amino acid "fingerprinting" of several hemoglobin M pigments reveals the substitution of an abnormal amino acid residue in the globin chain. Dissimilar substitutions have been found in different pedigrees. This situation is analogous to that of other hemoglobinopathies (hemoglobin S, hemoglobin C, and others). Theoretic considerations strongly suggest that the abnormal amino acid residue in each of the hemoglobin M pigments lies in a portion of the globin chain in close proximity to the prosthetic heme group where it can alter the properties of the heme moiety. Thus, cyanosis is probably due to the unusual stability of the methemoglobin form of the M hemoglobins. Such a hypothesis would also explain the variable response of patients to ascorbic acid and methylene blue as well as the abnormal spectral properties and differing response to cyanide treatment of various hemoglobin M pigments. Among the several hemoglobin M pedigrees examined, 5 different hemoglobin M pigments have been identified. Some of their properties are summarized in Table 8–12. It is possible that the entity previously described as "congenital sulfhemoglobinemia" may fall within the hemoglobin M disease group.

Clinically methemoglobinemia of the hemoglobin M type should be suspected when family studies suggest an autosomal dominant pattern of inheritance and when the blood of the cyanotic patient does not show the absorption band at 632 nm which is characteristic of normal methemoglobin. The patient's methemoglobin may or may not react with cyanide to yield a normal cyanomethemoglobin absorption curve. This varies with the pedigree (Table 8–12). In the hemoglobin M diseases the quantity of methemoglobin does not exceed 25% of the total hemoglobin; the cyanosis, although persistent from early infancy, is not associated with any disability. There may be a compensatory polycythemia.

Table 8–12 SOME SPECTRAL AND CHEMICAL PROPERTIES OF THE HEMOGLOBINS M

Hb M Type*	Abnormal Hemoglobin Chain	Methemoglobin Spectral Absorption Maxima in Visible Range† (nm)	Cyanomethemoglobin Derivative Absorption Spectrum
Hb M Boston	α	495 and 602	Abnormal
Hb M Saskatoon	β	492 and 602	Normal
Hb M Milwaukee-1	β	500 and 622	Normal
Hb M Milwaukee-2	?β	490 and 588	Normal
Hb M Iwate	α	485 and 590	Abnormal
Normal Hb A	—	502 and 632	Normal

*Geographic designation refers to residence of first pedigree studied; types are often abbreviated as follows: Hb M_B, Hb M_S, Hb M_{M-1}, Hb M_{M-2}, Hb M_I.

†In M/15 sodium phosphate buffer, pH 6.5.

Adapted from Gerald PS: Pediatrics 31:780, 1963.

Affected members of some pedigrees do not respond to ascorbic acid or methylene blue (hemoglobin M_B and hemoglobin M_{M-1}). Fortunately, alleviation of cyanosis is not essential in the hemoglobin M diseases.

8.45 HEMOCHROMATOSIS

Hemochromatosis is 1 of several forms of iron storage disease. It is characterized by excessive deposition in many organs of hemosiderin, an iron hydroxide–protein complex which in liver, pancreas, heart, or gonad eventually causes impaired structure and function. The familial form of the disease is called *primary hemochromatosis* and is associated with increased gastrointestinal absorption of iron. The nature of the metabolic defect is unknown. It is not associated with any known cause of excessive iron absorption, such as increased erythroid activity or excessive dietary iron intake, which can cause *secondary hemochromatosis*. Untreated cases of primary hemochromatosis eventually exhibit the classic triad of hepatic cirrhosis, slate or bronze pigmentation of the skin, and diabetes mellitus. These symptoms and signs do not appear before adulthood. Serum iron levels are increased in both latent and symptomatic adult members of affected families, but not in the children. The pattern of inheritance has not been established. Depletion of iron stores is the aim of treatment and will improve both symptoms and the function of affected organs. This is most conveniently achieved by repeated phlebotomy; in anemic patients with secondary hemochromatosis or hemosiderosis, chelation therapy with deferoxamine is preferred.

J. JULIAN CHISOLM, JR.

Becker DM, Kramer S: The neurological manifestations of porphyria: A review. Medicine 56:411, 1977.

Bloomer JR, Phillips MJ, Davidson DL, et al: Hepatic disease in erythropoietic protoporphyria. Am J Med 58:869, 1975.

Brenner DA, Bloomer JR: The enzymatic defect in variegate porphyria: Studies with human cultured skin fibroblasts. N Engl J Med 302:765, 1980.

Brodie MJ, Thompson GG, Moore MR, et al: Hereditary coproporphyria. Demonstration of the abnormalities in haem biosynthesis in peripheral blood. Q J Med New Ser 46:229, 1977.

Dean G, Barnes HD: The inheritance of porphyria. Br Med J 2:89, 1955.

Debre R, et al: Genetics of haemochromatosis. Ann Human Genet 23:16, 1958.

Dogramaci I: In: Levine SZ (ed): Advances in Pediatrics, Vol 13. Chicago, Year Book Medical Publishers, 1964.

Editorial: Treatment of acute hepatic porphyria. Lancet 1:1024, 1978.

Goldberg A, Rimington C, Lochhead AC: Hereditary coproporphyria. Lancet 1:632, 1967.

Hellman ES, Tschudy DP, Bartter FC: Abnormal electrolyte and water metabolism in acute intermittent porphyria. Am J Med 32:734, 1962.

Lamon J, With TK, Redeker AG: The Hoesch test: Bedside screening for urinary porphobilinogen in patients with suspected porphyria. Clin Chem 20:1438, 1974.

Lamon JM, Frykholm BC, Hess RA, et al: Hematin therapy for acute porphyria. Medicine 58:252, 1979.

Matthews-Roth MM, Pathak MA, Fitzpatrick TB, et al: β-Carotene as an oral photoprotective agent in erythropoietic protoporphyria. JAMA 228:1004, 1974.

Meyer UA, Schmid R: The porphyrias. In: Stanbury JB, Wyngaarden JB, Frederickson DS (eds): The Metabolic Basis of Inherited Disease. Ed 4. New York, McGraw-Hill, 1978.

Meyer UA, Strand LJ, Doss M, et al: Intermittent acute porphyria—demonstration of a genetic defect in porphobilinogen metabolism. N Engl J Med 296:1277, 1972.

Pollycove M: Hemochromatosis. In: Stanbury JB, Wyngaarden JB, Fredrickson DS (eds): The Metabolic Basis of Inherited Disease. Ed 4. New York, McGraw-Hill, 1978.

Ridley A, Hierons R, Cavanagh JB: Tachycardia and the neuropathy of porphyria. Lancet 2:708, 1968.

Runge W, Watson CJ: Experimental production of skin lesions in human cutaneous porphyria. Proc Soc Exp Biol Med 109:809, 1962.

Sassa S, Solish G, Levere RD, et al: Studies in porphyria. IV. Expression of the gene defect of acute intermittent porphyria in cultured human skin fibroblasts and amniotic cells: Prenatal diagnosis of the porphyric trait. J Exp Med 142:722, 1975.

Schmid R, Schwartz S, Sundberg D: Erythropoietic (congenital) porphyria: A rare abnormality of the normoblasts. Blood 10:416, 1955.

Schwartz JM, Jaffe ER: Hereditary methemoglobinemia with deficiency of NADH dehydrogenase. In: Stanbury JB, Wyngaarden JB, Fredrickson DS (eds): The Metabolic Basis of Inherited Disease. Ed 4. New York, McGraw-Hill, 1978.

Stein JA, Tschudy DP: Acute intermittent porphyria; a clinical and biochemical study of 46 patients. Medicine 49:1, 1970.

Welland FH, et al: Factors affecting the excretion of porphyrin precursors by patients with acute intermittent porphyria. I. The effect of diet. II. The effect of ethinyl estradiol. Metabolism 13:232, 251, 1964.

Zimmerman TS, McMillin M, Watson CJ: Onset of manifestations of hepatic porphyria in relation to the influence of female sex hormones. Arch Intern Med 118:229, 1966.

EPILOGUE

The number of *recognized* inborn errors of metabolism is constantly increasing, partly because of the clinical identification of new syndromes and the description of the biochemical nature of the metabolic block responsible for the condition. In addition, as new biochemical techniques have become available, many disorders, such as phenylalaninemia and the glycogenoses, once thought to result from single enzymatic defects and presenting a broad spectrum of clinical manifestations, are now being subdivided into several distinct clinical entities, each with a different enzymatic error.

The detection of many inborn errors of metabolism can now be made early in life; large-scale detection programs utilizing screening tests for blood or urine are currently carried out. Analyses of enzymes in readily available cells such as erythrocytes, leukocytes, and cultured fibroblasts for confirmation of clinical diagnoses are becoming increasingly available. For many conditions, particularly those associated with mental retardation, the earlier detection takes place and effective therapy is instituted, the better is the prognosis. A vigorous effort at early detection and at subsequent treatment by dietary regulation has improved the mental development of children with phenylketonuria. Other inborn errors amenable to diet therapy include galactosemia, maple syrup urine disease, propionicacidemia, and homocystinemia. The administration of massive amounts of certain vitamins can effectively overcome an enzymatic error when the mutant enzyme can no longer effectively bind the cofactor derived from the vitamin. Specific examples are the beneficial effects of pyridoxine in 1 form of cystathioninemia and in hydroxykynureninuria (pyridoxine dependency) and the beneficial effects of cobamide in some patients with methylmalonic acidemia.

Replacement of a missing enzyme has always seemed a logical and desirable goal of therapy, but has not been possible except in a very limited way. In cystic fibrosis the extracellular enzyme required for proper digestion can be administered conveniently, though the underlying defect is not ameliorated. When one is dealing with an intracellular enzyme, the problem is more complex. Nevertheless, the experimental administration of hydrolytic enzymes such as α-glucosidase in the treatment of some forms of the glycogenoses is a step in this direction. It has been shown in tissue culture of cells derived from deficient patients that the direct addition of purified enzymes is efficacious in correcting the metabolic defect in some disorders, but this has not been the case in others. The feasibility of injection of microencapsulated purified enzymes, avoiding the immunologic difficulties encountered by the repeated introduction of foreign proteins, has been demonstrated in animal studies. One form of microencapsulation is the loading of intact red cell ghosts with purified enzymes; another is entrapment of enzymes in liposomes. A number of partially successful trials have been reported wherein a purified enzyme was injected directly into an individual lacking that enzyme.

Detection of some inborn errors of metabolism can now be made in utero through culture of cells obtained by amniocentesis. These techniques permit prenatal diagnosis with the possibility of interruption of pregnancy, or, where applicable, that therapeutic measures (such as the administration to the pregnant mother of large amounts of a specific vitamin) can be instituted in order to ameliorate the effects of the disorder.

There is now reason to anticipate that with increasing knowledge of genetic mechanisms it will be possible in the future to alter the genetic constitution of an individual and to overcome some of nature's more undesirable errors. For example, the Gunn rat, which lacks the hepatic enzyme bilirubin uridine diphosphate glucuronyltransferase, has been "cured" by the implantation into its liver of small pieces of normal rat liver. Whether this "cure," which spread throughout the recipient's liver, represented genetic alteration or was due to some other effect is not known. In any case, the results are promising, as are those involving the injection of protein-coated pseudovirus particles containing new genetic information. In both cases, however, we must remember that until it is possible to employ specific purified genes in this manner, other alterations may be produced that might prove even less tolerable than the disorder whose correction is attempted.

All of the defects described in this chapter have presumably been due to errors of the DNA found on the chromosomes in the nucleus of the cell. Recently it has been postulated that 1 form of familial mitochondrial myopathy may result from an alteration of the nonchromosomal DNA carried within the mitochondria. There is now substantial evidence that mitochondrial DNA is inherited in humans via the maternal line, and it behooves us to think of the possibility that some inborn errors of metabolism may indeed result from defects of nonchromosomal genetic material.

VICTOR H. AUERBACH
Associate Editor for Chapter 8

General

Anderson CM, Burke V (eds): Paediatric Gastroenterology. Oxford, Blackwell Scientific Publications, 1975.

Bergsma D (ed): Birth Defects; Atlas and Compendium. Baltimore, Williams and Wilkins, 1973.

Bondy PK, Rosenberg LE: Metabolic Control and Disease. Ed 9. Philadelphia, WB Saunders, 1980.

Callahan JW, Lowden JA (eds): Lysosomes and Lysosomal Storage Diseases. New York, Raven Press, 1981.

Giles RE, Blanc H, Cann HM, et al: Maternal inheritance of human mitochondrial DNA. Proc Natl Acad Sci USA 77:6715, 1980.

Hers HG, vanHoof F (eds): Lysosomes and Storage Diseases. New York, Academic Press, 1973.

McKusick VA: Mendelian Inheritance in Man. Ed 5. Baltimore, Johns Hopkins Univ Press, 1978.

Nyhan NWL (ed): Heritable Disorders of Amino Acid Metabolism: Patterns of Clinical Expression and Genetic Variation. New York, John Wiley & Sons, 1974.

Scriver CR, Rosenberg LE: Amino Acid Metabolism and Its Disorders. Philadelphia, WB Saunders, 1973.

Stanbury JB, Wyngaarden JB, Fredrickson DS (eds): The Metabolic Basis of Inherited Disease. Ed 5. New York, McGraw-Hill, 1982.

Stryer L: Biochemistry. San Francisco, WA Freeman, 1975.

IMMUNITY, ALLERGY, AND RELATED DISEASES 9

9.1   THE IMMUNOLOGIC SYSTEM

The immunologic system is that part of a host defense mechanism which includes the macrophages, the leukocytes, the lymphocytes, the complement system, and physical barriers such as an intact integument and motile cilia. Its primary function is to protect against invasion by infectious agents. The major costs of this protection are allergy, autoimmunity, and rejection of organ transplants.

PHYSIOLOGY

Source of Cells.   The cells destined to become lymphocytes arise as multipotential precursors from which derivatives of the hematopoietic and lymphoid systems will ultimately develop. In early intrauterine life the fetal liver serves as the repository for the cells. Subsequently, the bone marrow is populated and in extrauterine life serves as the major source of the precursor cells.

Differentiation.   The lymphoid stem cells differentiate into 2 major lines: the T cells and the B cells, which have different functions in their protective roles (Table 9–1). T cells are designated as such because of their intimate association with the thymus gland, which is their site of differentiation, and B cells because of their relationship to the bursa of Fabricius in chickens and the bone marrow in humans. Recent evidence suggests that the fetal liver assumes the bursal function in humans. The individual cell lines mature and acquire capabilities of subspecialization within the 2 major sites of differentiation. It is thought that most of the steps involved in the *early differentiation* of B cells are independent of antigenic stimulation and reflect an intrinsic capability of the cells to acquire a certain degree of maturation. At the end of early differentiation the cells are ready to react with antigen; appropriate interaction with antigens leads to a number of steps which are collectively denoted as *terminal differentiation* and lead to the immune state.

The steps of terminal differentiation are probably highly dependent upon divalent cations and cyclic nucleotides. The intracellular ratios of cyclic guanosine monophosphate (cGMP) to cyclic adenosine monophosphate (cAMP) are probably affected by antigen binding to surface receptors of the lymphocytes. Depending upon the degree of perturbation of its surface (e.g., by antigen), a lymphocyte may be triggered to further proliferation or, in some cases, placed in a resting or nonreactive state (e.g., to yield memory or tolerance). Similarly, receipt of antigen on the surface of lymphocytes can effect the influx of calcium ions. This induces the series of events that constitute terminal differentiation, which probably takes place in peripheral lymphoid organs such as the lymph node, spleen, and organized lymphoid tissues of the gastrointestinal tract.

A series of hormones produced by the thymus gland is important in the terminal differentiation of T cells. Studies of various extracts of the thymus gland have shown that these substances are probably of importance in promoting normal maturation and proliferation of thymus cells. In some cases many of the effects of thymectomy can be reversed by the injection of these hormonal substances. Material obtained from calf thymus, *thymosin*, has been used widely in clinical trials.

Traffic.   Since the events of the immune process, from differentiation to the receipt of antigen and elaboration of immune products, take place in different areas of the body, the lymphocytes must be quite motile. Although they circulate freely through the major lymphoid channels, the thoracic duct, and the vascular tree, the movement of cells into and from the lymphoid organs is highly controlled. For example, cells which leave the thymus gland apparently do not re-enter this site of primary differentiation. The traffic pattern appears to be controlled by various chemical groupings

---

Table 9–1   FUNCTIONS OF T AND B CELLS

Role of T cells
 T helper function
 T suppressor function
 T killer function
  Containment of acidfast bacteria
  Containment of certain viral infections after establishment (rubeola, varicella, herpes, cytomegalovirus, EBV, "slow" virus)
  Containment of fungal infections (especially *Candida*)
  Containment of protozoan infections
  Rejection of allografts (? tumors)
  Graft-versus-host disease (GVHD)
  Contact dermatitis

Role of B cells
 Synthesize and secrete major classes of immunoglobulin, which:
  Protect against staphylococcus, streptococcus, hemophilus, pneumococcus
  Neutralize viruses to prevent initial infection
  Act as barriers along gastrointestinal and respiratory passages
  Initiate killing of microorganisms by macrophages and null cells
  Cause the secretion of vasoactive amines from mast cells and basophils
  Actively lyse cells of autologous origin or engage in antigen-antibody complex disease
  Interfere with T killer cell activity by directly or indirectly blocking the reaction

From Horowitz SD, Hong R: The Pathogenesis and Treatment of Immunodeficiency. Basel, S. Karger, AG, 1977.

Table 9–2 LEVELS OF IMMUNOGLOBULINS

	IgG (MG/DL)	IgM (MG/DL)	IgA (MG/DL)	IgE (IU/ML)
Serum				
Newborn	1031 ± 200*	11 ± 5	2 ± 3	0–7.5
6 mo	427 ± 186	43 ± 17	28 ± 18	—
12 mo	661 ± 219	54 ± 23	37 ± 18	—
24 mo	762 ± 209	58 ± 23	50 ± 24	137 ± 147
8 yr	923 ± 256	65 ± 25	124 ± 45	251 ± 167
16 yr	946 ± 124	59 ± 20	148 ± 63	330 ± 212
Adult	1158 ± 305	99 ± 27	200 ± 61	200†
Secretions				
Colostrum	10	61	1234	—
Stimulated parotid saliva	0.036	0.043	3.9	—
Unstimulated whole saliva	4.86	0.55	30.4	—
Jejunal fluid	34	70	—	—
Seminal fluid	510	90	116	—
Cerebrospinal fluid				
Normal	3 ± 1	0	0.4 ± 0.5	—
Purulent infection	9	4	4	—
Viral infection	4	0.5	1	—

*Mean ± 1 standard deviation.
†Values up to 800 IU/ml are normal.
Adapted from Clin Immunobiol 3:13, 1976.

on the surface of the lymphocytes. Treatment of lymphocytes to remove surface carbohydrate or protein moieties alters the traffic pattern considerably.

Ontogeny. The newborn is immunologically quite competent. Fetal studies have shown various types of T cell function beginning as early as 7.5 wk of intrauterine life. By 8–9 wk lymphoid infiltration into the thymus begins; at 12 wk the thymus resembles the mature organ. The capacity to reject skin grafts is present even in premature babies.

Circulating B cells have been detected as early as 13 wk after conception; secretory capability is probably present for all major classes of immunoglobulins by 20 gestational wk. Extensive synthesis and secretion of antibody do not occur because of the relatively sheltered antigenic environment of the fetus. IgM antibodies are the 1st to develop; increased levels of IgM can, therefore, be taken as evidence of intrauterine infection. Postnatally, serum IgM usually rises to adult levels by 1 yr of age, IgG by about 4 yr, and IgA in adolescence (Table 9–2).

Cellular Events. The production of immune cell lines following exposure to antigens requires cellular interaction involving both the T and B cells as well as macrophages. Physical contact of at least 2 of the cell populations is probably necessary. Receptor molecules on the surfaces of the T and B cells have the capability to recognize antigens. The B cell receptor is classic antibody whereas the nature of that on the T cell remains elusive. The macrophages have the capability of adsorbing antibody molecules onto their surfaces. Simply put, antigen can be thought of as a ligand which binds 2 or more cells together. Following interaction initiated by this event, the cells are rendered immune and can then exert their protective capability upon subsequent exposure to the antigen. The actual mechanisms of developing immunity are much more complex and appear to require the activation of other groups, such as histocompatibility antigens and complement

receptor molecules which are also present on the cell surface.

Thus one can appreciate that the various cell lines involved in the immune response carry molecules on their surfaces which exert great control over their be-

Table 9–3 MONONUCLEAR CELL MARKERS

CELL LINEAGE	MARKER
B cell	
Stem cell	
Pre-B cell	Intracytoplasmic IgM
	(?) Mouse erythrocyte
B cell (mature)	Surface immunoglobulin (IgM, IgD)
	Mouse erythrocyte
	Epstein-Barr virus receptor
	Fc receptor for IgG, IgM, IgA
	Complement component (C3b, C3d)
	Ia-like
T cell	
Stem cell	
Pre-T cell	Terminal deoxynucleotidyl transferase (TdT)
	Peanut agglutinin
	OKT 6*
T cell (mature)	Sheep erythrocyte
	Fc receptors for IgG, IgM, IgA, IgE†
	TH 2 (suppressor)
	Histamine receptor (suppressor)
	OKT 3, Leu 1* (all T cells)
	OKT 4, Leu 3a (helper)
	OKT 8, Leu 2a (suppressor, killer)
Macrophage‡	IgG (Fc)
	Complement components

*OKT, Leu: designations of commercially available hybridoma antiserum.
†Cells showing receptors for Fc of IgM (T mu cells) and IgG (T gamma cells), formerly thought to be helper and suppressor cells, respectively. Recent studies do not confirm these earlier impressions.
‡Macrophages commonly adsorb Igs on their surface so the presence of certain markers does not necessarily reflect macrophage synthesis of that product.

havior. The ability to detect a number of these has provided a system of markers which serve to differentiate the T from B cells. The functional significance of some of the surface moieties is obvious, but the importance of others is unknown. The most commonly used marker for identification of T cells is the sheep erythrocyte rosette, while surface immunoglobulin M (IgM) marks the B cells, also known as surface immunoglobulin–bearing or SIg cells. The use of these markers has permitted enumeration of T and B cells in peripheral blood in a simple and convenient manner. Some other T and B cell markers are listed in Table 9–3. The recent availability of antibodies produced by tissue culture cell lines (hybridomas) will allow more precise characterization of T and B cell subpopulations.

The internal events triggered in T cells by surface reactions are poorly understood. However, the synthesis and secretion of immunoglobulins by B cells have been quite well studied; the events are schematically pictured in Fig 9–1. Basically, receipt of the appropriate signals on the surface of a B cell creates an internal signal that sets into motion the machinery which synthesizes immunoglobulins. After the assembly of the full immunoglobulin molecule, including the chains necessary for polymerization and carbohydrate groups that may be necessary to control traffic, the molecule is secreted into the lymph and thence enters the bloodstream so it may bathe the areas of need and combine with the appropriate antigen.

Amplification. This term describes the augmentation, by various collaborative processes, of the protective effect of antigen-binding by B and T lymphocytes. Amplification is necessary for complete elimination of infectious agents. Common modes of amplification include processes that lyse infectious agents or produce

Table 9–4   LYMPHOKINES

Chemotactic factor (for eosinophils, monocytes, neutrophils)
Clonal inhibitory factor
Interferon
Lymphotoxin
Lymph node permeability factor
Macrophage activation factor
Macrophage aggregation factor
Migration inhibition factor (MIF)
Mitogenic factor
Proliferation inhibitory factor
Skin-reactive factor
Transfer factor

From Horowitz SD, Hong R: The Pathogenesis and Treatment of Immunodeficiency. Basel, S Karger, AG, 1977.

a granulomatous response. Amplification of the protective function of B cells is accomplished chiefly by activation of the complement system, that of the T cells chiefly by lymphokines, though both B and T cells secrete lymphokines. It is doubtful that complement amplifies the protective function of T cells to any significant degree.

Lymphokines may have direct toxic effects (Table 9–4) or act indirectly as in the case of migration inhibitory factor (MIF), one of the best studied of the lymphokines. MIF attracts macrophages to an area where T cells have combined with an antigen; the macrophages then destroy the infectious agent through the release of lysosomal enzymes. They also release products that may lead to the formation of granulomas and may store or carry antibody. Primary quantitative or qualitative deficiencies of the macrophages, though poorly defined at present, could conceivably result in significant defects in host defenses.

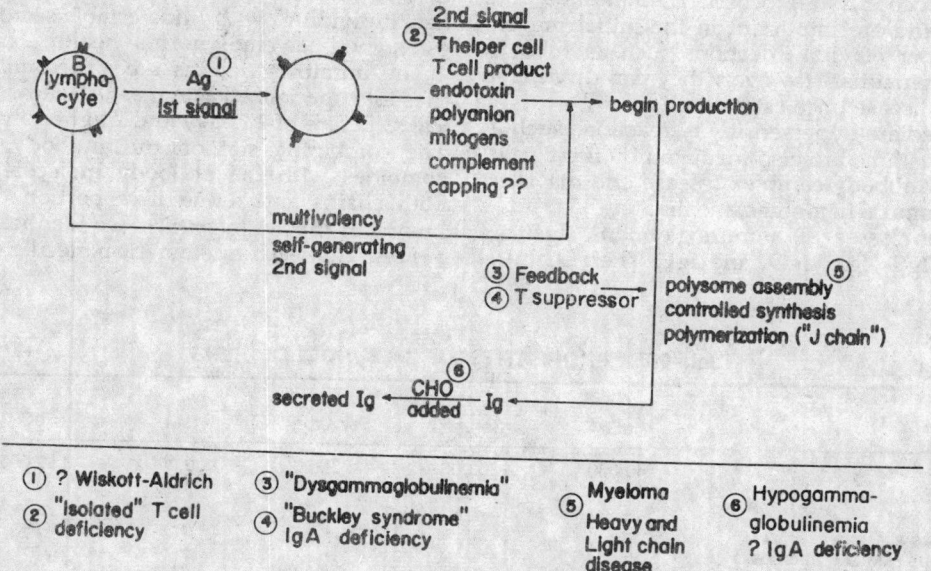

Figure 9–1   Mechanism of activation of synthesis and secretion of immunoglobulins. The numbers indicate points where a fault could result in clinical disease. Proposed disease correlates are shown at the bottom of the figure (see text). (From Horowitz SD, Hong R: The Pathogenesis and Treatment of Immunodeficiency, Monographs in Allergy, Vol 10. Basel, S Karger AG, 1977.)

COMPONENTS OF THE IMMUNOLOGIC SYSTEM

T Cell Subpopulations. The versatility of the immune system arises through the action of a number of subpopulations of the T and B cells. The major T cell subgroups currently defined are helper, suppressor, and killer populations. *Helper cells* are necessary in the initial antigen responses, especially to generate IgG and IgA responses; some IgM antibodies are formed in the absence of T helper cells. The immune response, because of its great potential for harm as well as good, must be modulated to prevent hyperimmune reactions. This process is thought to be accomplished by the T *suppressor cells*, which serve a homeostatic role in keeping the immune response within a tolerable level. T *killer cells* are the effector cells of the thymus-dependent system. They actually combine with the antigen to initiate the cytotoxic mechanisms which kill the invading organism.

T cells and their products are primarily concerned with acidfast bacteria, certain viral infections (e.g., rubeola, varicella, herpes, cytomegalovirus), and fungi. T cells are also the major immune factor involved in rejection of organ transplants and, in addition, are responsible for the disease known as the graft-versus-host reaction (Sec 9.19). Furthermore, the major immunopathologic mechanism in contact dermatitis is thought to be mediated by the T cell.

B Cell Subpopulations. Subspecialization of the B cells has not been as well defined as for the T cells. However, surface marker analysis (Sec 9.3) suggests that subpopulations also exist for the B cells. Also, B cell products, the immunoglobulins, can be divided into 5 major classes (isotypes), each of which is produced by a different cell line. Immunoglobulins are active against staphylococci, streptococci, *H. influenzae*, and pneumococci, and are important in the initial prevention of a number of viral infections such as rubeola, varicella, and hepatitis. However, they can do little to control a viral disease once established.

Typical immediate hypersensitivity reactions such as hay fever and asthma are also mediated by the B cells, as are antigen-antibody complex disease and disorders such as autoimmune hemolytic anemia.

The 5 major classes of immunoglobulins (Igs) are denoted IgM, IgG, IgA, IgD, and IgE. Their chemical characteristics and biologic functions are summarized in Table 9–5.

Of the immunoglobulins, IgM can be considered the 1st line of defense. It forms first in response to antigen, is mostly distributed in the vascular space, and has high efficiency in the ancillary functions that enhance immunity, such as complement fixation, agglutination, and opsonic activity. IgG has a long half-life and can cross the placenta, thus is ideally suited for passive immunization and recall immunity. IgA protects mainly the secretory surfaces (gastrointestinal tract and eyes) where there are nonvascular exposures to antigens and conditions that may interfere with usual antibody activity, such as acid secretion, presence of proteolytic enzyme, and intestinal motility. IgE effects the release of pharmacologically active agents from the mast cell and thus causes asthma, hay fever, and signs of anaphylaxis. IgD is primarily a lymphocyte receptor; the amounts detected in the serum probably represent effete receptors shed from young lymphocytes. IgD may be the strongest binding antibody and thus is important in directing antigen to B cell surfaces to accomplish initial immunization.

Recent studies indicate that secretory IgA and IgE play a greater role in the immune status of inhabitants of underdeveloped countries, where antibiotic therapy, nutrition, and general hygiene are less than optimal. Breast feeding is a major means of providing long-lasting protection in these countries, and weaning is followed by markedly increased death rates from infection. It is now known that (in addition to secretory IgA) macrophages and, perhaps, T cells are delivered to the infant in the breast milk. IgE is a major mechanism for the elimination of parasites. Macrophages armed with IgE antiparasite immune complexes are especially effective in eliminating parasitic infestation. Because these 2 defenses have become less necessary in modern societies, individuals with undetectable secretory IgA or IgE can sometimes enjoy normal health.

The immunoglobulins are structurally modified for these subspecialized activities. All show the same chemical structure of 2 heavy and 2 light polypeptide chains. The combining site on the antibody, when antigen combines with the antibody molecule, is formed by both chains and found in a portion of the molecule known as the *Fab fragment*. Two identical Fab fragments are found in each monomeric molecule of immunoglob-

Table 9–5 PROPERTIES OF IMMUNOGLOBULINS

	IgG	IgA Serum	IgA Secretory	IgM	IgD	IgE
Molecular weight	140,000	160,000	370,000	900,000	160,000	197,000
Complement fixation	+	−	?	+	−	−
Placental passage	+	−	−	−	−	−
Secreted by mucous surfaces	±*	±*	+	±†	?	±
Fixes to homologous skin and mast cells	−	−	−	−	−	+
"Blocking antibody"	+	?	+	?	?	?
Polymer formation	−	+	+	+	−	−

*In inflammatory conditions. + = positive; ± = weak or intermittent; − = negative.
†Frequently in selective IgA deficiency.
From Hong R: Immunobiol 1:29, 1972.

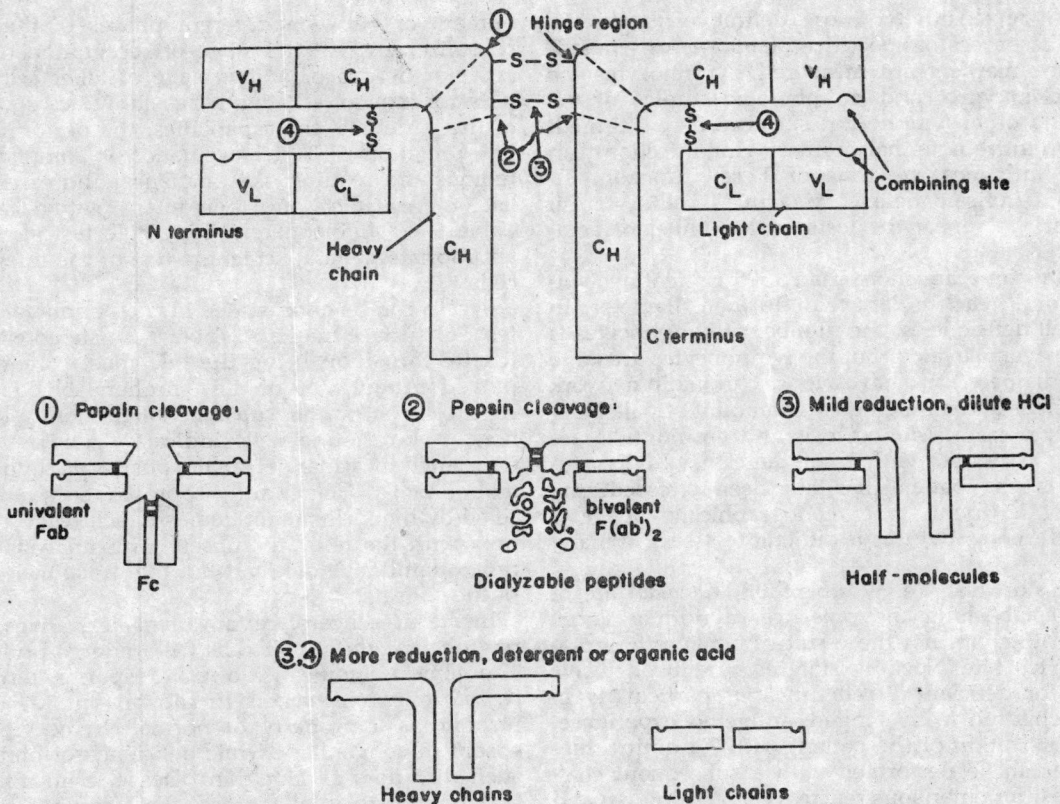

Figure 9–2 Basic structure of the immunoglobulins and the products obtained by chemical cleavage. The upper portion of the figure shows the monomeric subunit common to all immunoglobulins. The lower half shows the results of enzyme cleavage (1, 2) or disulfide bond cleavage (3, 4). C and V refer to constant and variable regions of the polypeptide chains. H and L refer to heavy and light chains. Fab, F(ab')₂, and Fc are fragments produced by cleavage. The N terminus contains the antigen-binding site; the C terminus attaches to cells or to other reactants. Heavy bars indicate disulfide bonds. (From Hong R, *In*: Ellis E, Middleton E, Reed C (eds): Allergy: Principles and Practice. St. Louis, CV Mosby, 1978.)

ulin. A 3rd fragment, composed of 2 portions of heavy chain, is known as Fc and contains the chemical structures that determine all the biologic characteristics of the immunoglobulin (complement fixation, placental passage, and so on) and the unique determinants that differentiate 1 immunoglobulin from another. For example, the Fab fragments of IgG and IgA are virtually identical, but the Fc portions are quite dissimilar (Fig 9–2).

Two immunoglobulins, IgM and secretory IgA, are polymers. The polymerization is probably initiated intracellularly by a short polypeptide chain known as the J *chain*. The IgA found in secretions (gastrointestinal, genitourinary, biliary, tears, saliva) has, in addition, a fragment known as *secretory component* (SC). IgA exists in 2 forms, monomeric in the serum and dimeric in the secretion.

Each isotype includes subgroups. Four are known for IgG (IgG₁, IgG₂, IgG₃, IgG₄) and 2 for IgA (IgA₁, IgA₂). Other isotypic subgroups are less well defined. Subgroups show unique biologic behavior; IgG₄ cannot fix complement. Different subgroups respond preferentially to various antigens (e.g., IgG₂ to polysaccharides, IgG₁ and IgG₃ to Rh antigens). Most secretory IgA is of the IgA₂ subgroup. This distribution suggested an enteric origin of the complexes found in IgA nephropathy which were shown to be essentially all of the IgA₂ subgroup. The subgroups thus provide a fine tuning of the immune response. Sometimes only some subgroups are absent, leading to clinical disease somewhat different from classical panhypogammaglobulinemic states.

Macrophages. Macrophages, once thought to be primarily scavenger cells without much specificity of function, have been found to play an important role in the acquisition of immunity and tolerance as well as to serve a key role in the effector mechanisms of T cell immunity. Disorders of macrophages and phagocytes are considered in Sec 9.30 to 9.41.

ASSESSMENT OF T AND B CELLS

9.2 T CELLS

A preliminary assessment of T cell function can be made from the peripheral blood lymphocyte count, lateral roentgenogram of the chest, and skin tests for delayed hypersensitivity. More definitive studies require the resources of specialized laboratories where T cell surface markers are measured, lymphocytes are stimulated in vitro, and morphologic studies of the thymus and other lymphoid tissues can be performed. It is important to note that ordinary viral infections can markedly influence the tests of T cell function. To confirm a significant deficiency of the T cell system it is necessary to repeat the tests on a number of occasions.

Normally there are more than 1500 circulating lymphocytes/mm³; each is less than 10 µ in diameter. In some T cell deficiencies, the number of lymphocytes is normal or even elevated, but the lymphocytes are large (>10 µ in diameter) and have a loose chromatin network in the nucleus and a much greater amount of pale blue-staining cytoplasm. Monocytosis and eosinophilia are commonly associated with T cell deficiency, as is neutropenia. If the patient has not been stressed, the absence of a thymus roentgenographically suggests thymic deficiency, but this is difficult to assess in many patients.

Positive skin tests (e.g., tuberculin, *Candida*) are of value in establishing the presence of normal T cell function if they are not the result of nonspecific irritation at the test site. Negative skin tests are inconclusive evidence for deficient T cell function, particularly in younger children with limited antigenic experience. Direct sensitization of the patient with 2,4-dinitrochlorobenzene can be performed with a subsequent challenge to test for cutaneous reactivity after a known and sufficient immunization. This procedure is moderately traumatic and should be supplanted by an in vitro test of T cell integrity. Phytohemagglutinin (PHA) has been utilized by some as a cutaneous stimulant in testing T cells but is not recommended. Application of skin grafts from nonrelated individuals tests T killer cell capability but can transmit hepatitis virus and could conceivably sensitize the recipient needlessly to donor antigens.

More specialized tests attempt to measure the capabilities of T cell subpopulations and can differentiate between deficiencies at various levels of T cell development or between different phases of the immune response, e.g., at the stage of recognition of antigen (affector defect) or at the stage of killer cell function (effector function). Patients may show lack of only some of the various T cell capabilities; the performance and interpretation of T cell evaluation is complicated and tedious and requires skill, patience, and experience. A list of T cell tests and their interpretation is given in Table 9–6. Unfortunately, no single test serves as an appropriate general screening test of the integrity of T cells.

T cells can be enumerated in the peripheral blood by tests of surface markers (Table 9–3), sheep erythrocyte rosette formation being the one most commonly employed. About 80% of the peripheral blood mononuclear cells show this capability. Persistently low numbers of E-rosetting cells indicate a degree of T cell deficiency in a manner analogous to panhypogammaglobulinemia. Helper and suppressor cells can be identified by monoclonal antibodies which react specifically only with the relevant subsets. This analysis provides only quantitative data but not the functional capability of the subsets.

In the presence of certain plant derivatives, such as phytohemagglutinin, T cells will undergo proliferation. The clinical significance of this response, termed *lymphocyte transformation*, is unknown, but the ability to respond is a property of normal thymocytes and is absent in congenital thymic deficiency or obtunded in such disorders as Hodgkin disease. Similarly, T cells will proliferate in the presence of concanavalin A or allogeneic cells (lymphocytes from an unrelated individual). The latter test, known as the mixed leukocyte culture (MLC), also tests histocompatibility, representing the phase of early recognition of foreignness in rejection of organ transplants. Some evidence indicates that nonreactivity of the proposed host in the MLC reaction is a good predictor of future organ acceptance. More relevant to immunodeficiency disorders is the fact that nonreactivity of *donor* cells in the MLC reaction is the best means of selecting prospective donors for attempts at reconstitution of bone marrow in the host. The proliferation of lymphocytes in response to soluble antigens is the in vitro correlate of the early recognition phase of skin tests showing delayed hypersensitivity. It is more sensitive than a cutaneous reaction and may be positive when the latter is negative.

The foregoing responses to mitogens, antigens, and allogeneic cells assess afferent responses, i.e., the ability to recognize and respond to a stimulator. The final phase of immunologic protection involves an effector phase in which cells lyse targets and generate inflammation. Only recently has assessment of this capability been performed in vitro. In assays for killer effect, the effector cell is "sensitized" by antigens of the potential target by a short in vitro incubation period. Subsequently, the target is presented to the "immunized" killer cell, whereupon the target is lysed (cell-mediated lympholysis [CML]). The target can be an allogeneic lymphocyte, a cell infected with a virus, or a tumor cell. The capacity of the lymphocyte to secrete lymphokines can be assessed by incubating the cells with the appropriate antigen and observing the ability of released substances to inhibit macrophage migration (MIF), stim-

Table 9–6   TESTS OF T CELLS

TEST	SIGNIFICANCE
Mitogenic stimulation	? Primitive recognition
	? Surface marker
	Proliferative capacity
Allogeneic stimulation	Ability to recognize foreign transplant
	Best matching test for bone marrow transplantation
Antigen stimulation	Specific recognition of antigen
Cell-mediated lympholysis	Effector function
Co-culture with B cells with pokeweed mitogen	Helper and suppressor functions of Ig synthesis and secretion
Co-culture with allogeneically stimulated cells (after concanavalin A)	Suppressor function
Lymphokine assays	Effector amplification
Thymopoietin, thymosin, facteur thymique serique	Hormonal activity

Modified from Hong R: J Allergy Clin Immunol 60:83, 1977.

ulate cell proliferation (blastogenic factor), etc. (Table 9–4).

The stimulation of lymphocytes by certain substances such as concanavalin A generates a large number of T cells capable of inhibiting other T cell responses. For example, supernatants of such stimulated cultures, or the stimulated cells themselves, will inhibit a mixed leukocyte culture reaction or the synthesis of immunoglobulin by B cells. Thus, concanavalin A–stimulated cells serve as a suppressor T cell assay.

Isolated T cells can be added to purified B cell preparations and T-dependent proliferative processes or the ability to synthesize immunoglobulin used as a T helper cell assay.

Morphology. The normal *thymus* has a characteristic structure consisting of lobules with a rich zone of thymocytes at the outer border and a less intense staining zone containing many epithelial elements in the center. These 2 areas are easily separated from each other at a well demarcated corticomedullary cleavage plane. Within the medulla are whorl-like bodies known as *Hassall corpuscles*. Absence of 1 or more of these features is found in various abnormalities of the T cell system. In the profound defects, there are virtually no normal elements; the gland consists only of reticular cells in a loose structure with broad fibrous bands. Hassall corpuscles and lymphoid elements (thymocytes) are conspicuously absent. The gland is very small, about 2–3% of normal size; often it does not descend into the mediastinum but remains high in the neck. In less severe deficiency, the thymus may appear to be involuted with a few remnants of normal structure. Some thymic abnormalities involve only mass (hypoplasia or aplasia), sometimes with a small gland of perfectly normal architecture.

The zone of lymphocytes just below the layer of follicles and germinal centers found in the periphery of *lymph nodes* is populated by T cells. This area is poorly developed and cell-depleted in isolated deficiency of the T cell system. In addition, although B cell follicles may sometimes be seen, formation of germinal centers does not occur. In the *spleen*, a collar of T lymphocytes surrounds the arterioles; absence of lymphocytes in this area is consistent with thymic deficiency.

9.3 B CELLS

B cells as well as T cells can be enumerated in peripheral blood. The most commonly employed markers are the IgM molecules present on the surface of B lymphocytes. Approximately 10% of mononuclear cells in the peripheral blood carry these markers, along with IgD. Other immunoglobulin classes are represented rarely, if at all. IgD molecules may have a greater affinity for antigen than those of the other immunoglobulins, and cells bearing this class of receptors may serve as the prime candidates for antigen binding to initiate immunization. Other markers of B cells are listed in Table 9–3, but their physiologic significance is as yet unknown.

The most commonly employed test of B cell function is quantitative measurement of serum immunoglobulin by single radial diffusion. A common error in this test is overinterpretation of slightly low values. Normal values for the immunoglobulins vary greatly (severalfold) and increase over a period of several yr from quite low values in infancy until adult levels are attained. Normal values also vary from laboratory to laboratory; it has been suggested that immunoglobulin levels be expressed in international units after comparing one's local values to an international reference standard.* This problem is less important in the diagnosis of immunodeficiency states if sufficiently stringent standards for the diagnosis of true deficiency are set and correlation with the clinical picture and physical examination is made.

Most states of true immunodeficiency in children show IgG values under 200 mg/dl, and IgA and IgM are undetectable. An unusual form of B cell deficiency is associated with higher than normal levels of IgM (dysgammaglobulinemia). These high values are in part due to the artifactually more rapid diffusion of the IgM because some of it is present as a low molecular weight monomer (rather than as the normal heavier polymer) whose rapid diffusion causes a large precipitin ring to develop, suggesting a higher than actual level of IgM.

Extremely high or at least normal values of 1 or more of the immunoglobulins are also seen in unusual forms of combined T and B cell deficiency. In these cases, the elevated immunoglobulins classically show an electrophoretic abnormality which causes the proteins to resemble the proteins of restricted mobility seen with myelomas. Usually the patients are immunologically inert and no specific antibodies can be detected either before or after antigenic stimulation. Finally, in cases of IgG subgroup deficiency, the total IgG levels are within normal limits, but specific subgroups are absent.

The pattern of levels of the various immunoglobulins in the serum is diagnostically uninformative, but some hints of the underlying or associated process can occasionally be found. Markedly elevated levels of IgA are often seen with thymic deficiency. Low levels of IgG and IgA in association with near-normal IgM values, as opposed to the immunoglobulin levels of typical hypogammaglobulinemia (e.g., IgG = 150 mg/dl, IgA = 0 mg/dl, IgM = 5 mg/dl), should alert one to the possibility of intestinal loss of protein. In such cases the levels of albumin and transferrin will also show marked diminution. Similar changes are also seen in the hypoproteinemic states of nephrosis and in cases of lymphangiectasia.

In selective deficiency of IgA, tests utilizing radial immunodiffusion present a special problem. Because of increased permeability of the gastrointestinal tract secondary to the deficiency of IgA, more dietary antigens are absorbed. As a result, higher levels of antibodies are formed to foodstuffs, especially to milk proteins. Precipitating antibodies to bovine proteins cross-react with many antisera (e.g., goat) used in anti-immunoglobulin reagents. As a result, in the diffusion analysis what is interpreted as goat antihuman IgA precipitating with serum IgA is actually human antibovine IgG pre-

---

*The standard is available from NCI Immunoglobulin Reference Center, 6715 Electronic Dr., Springfield, Va. 22151. The conversion units are as follows (μg/IU): IgG, 80.4; IgA, 14.2; IgM, 8.47.

cipitating because of cross-reaction with goat IgG. Either reaction would give a similar ring of precipitation; the interpretation would be that the patient has detectable levels of IgA when, in fact, he has none. The error can be avoided by the use of rabbit antisera to human IgA for quantitation or by testing the patient's serum in immunoelectrophoretic analysis in which no arc will be seen in the IgA region.

Ambiguous values of immunoglobulins require evaluation of immunoglobulin function for full interpretation. This is accomplished by measuring antibody response to specific antigens. One can use antigens to which the patient was exposed naturally (blood group substances, common bacteria) or as a result of immunization procedures (tetanus, diphtheria), or antigens purposefully injected to measure the response. Of the latter, bacteriophage φχ 174* is probably most informative; in cases of suspected B cell deficiency, the diagnosis can be made even at birth because normally even newborns will eliminate the phage by immune clearance. The transferred IgG levels of the mother offer no problem in interpretation, as they might if only quantitative levels were measured. Furthermore, there are different patterns of response which serve to define more precisely the nature of the B cell defect. *It is to be emphasized that live viruses other than φχ 174 should never be given to a patient suspected of immunodeficiency until the diagnosis of normality is confirmed, as severe disease or death may ensue.*

B lymphocytes stimulated with pokeweed mitogen and cultured in the presence of normal T cells will synthesize and secrete immunoglobulin. B cells which

---

*Available from Dr. R. J. Wedgwood, Department of Pediatrics, University of Washington School of Medicine, Seattle, Wash., 98195.

bear immunoglobulin on the surface (SIg cell) are in the early presecretory stage; the surface molecules are lost after the cell responds to the antigen and undergoes terminal differentiation enabling it to secrete the specific antibody. A study of the lymphocyte surface markers and the response to pokeweed mitogen can define the level at which the defect occurs in many cases. For example, SIg cells are usually absent in X-linked agammaglobulinemia but present in normal numbers in late-onset common variable immunodeficiency. In the latter, pokeweed mitogen will not induce further differentiation. Thus, X-linked agammaglobulinemia can be thought of as an early defect due to lack of B cells; common variable immunodeficiency represents a failure of the B cells to undergo terminal differentiation.

In some patients with common variable immunodeficiency, excessive T suppressor cell activity is found. Their T cells, incubated with normals, will completely prevent the synthesis and secretion of IgG, IgA, and IgM induced by pokeweed mitogen. In other patients deficiency of T helper cells is found. Thus, complete evaluation of B cells requires assessment of modulating influences as well as of the capability of the patient's lymphocytes to synthesize immunoglobulins.

Morphology. The thymus can be assumed to be normal in classic "pure" B cell deficiency disorders, of which congenital hypogammaglobulinemias of the X-linked or autosomal recessive types are prime examples. The thymus is abnormal in cases associated with paraprotein-like immunoglobulins. The lymph nodes show deficient or absent follicle formation, and germinal centers are absent in cases of deficient production of immunoglobulins. In selective deficiency of IgA there may be a compensatory increase of IgM-producing cells in the lamina propria of the intestine.

Diseases Due to Immunologic Deficiency

9.4 PRIMARY IMMUNODEFICIENCY

It is convenient to think of diseases as primarily involving the T cell or B cell systems, or both. In each case the clinical presentation and treatment are different. Generally, disorders of the T cell system are associated with a much graver prognosis than are those of the B cell system. Combined immunodeficiency involving both T and B cells carries the worst prognosis; if of the severe variety, death in the 1st 2 yr of life is the rule. Some patients with pure B cell disorders remain clinically well without any therapy.

A clinical diagnosis of whether the fault is a primary T or B cell deficiency cannot be made with certainty. However, certain clinical features are more suggestive of involvement of a particular system and are listed in Table 9–7.

Unusual response to usually benign infectious agents, or infection with unusual organisms, is a feature of immunodeficiency; this may occur either in isolated T or B cell diseases or in combined disorders. The major

organisms involved in immunodeficient patients are *Pneumocystis carinii*, cytomegalovirus, rubeola, and varicella; each often results in fatal pneumonia. Pneumonitis caused by any of these agents should raise the suspicion of immunodeficiency.

There is an increased incidence of malignancy in immunodeficiency. The explanations for this include increased susceptibility to infection by an oncogenic virus, the cancer representing another expression of the basic genetic fault, and a failure of immune surveillance. The last explanation is based on the theory that T cells eliminate newly formed populations of malignant cells as they arise, considering them foreign transplants. An alternative hypothesis, proposed by Melief and Schwartz, attributes the high incidence of lymphoid malignancy to failure of feedback control of antigen-induced lymphoproliferation. Since immunodeficient patients do not make antibody or other normal immune products following receipt of antigen, the stimulated aberrant lymphoid elements continue to respond by proliferation, with the repeated cell divisions increasing the random chance of malignant mutation.

Epstein-Barr virus (EBV) is particularly associated

Table 9–7 CLINICAL SYMPTOMS OF IMMUNODEFICIENCY

Suggestive of T cell defect
- Systemic illness following vaccination with any live virus or BCG; unusual life-threatening complication following infection with ordinarily benign viruses (e.g., giant cell pneumonia with rubeola; varicella pneumonia)
- Chronic oral candidiasis persisting after 6 mo of age and resisting adequate chemotherapy
- Chronic mucocutaneous candidiasis
- Features (fine, thin hair, short-limbed dwarfism with characteristic roentgenographic features) of cartilage-hair hypoplasia (CHH)
- Intrauterine graft-versus-host disease — most characteristic feature is scaling erythroderma and total alopecia (absence of eyebrows quite striking)
- Graft-versus-host disease after blood transfusion
- Hypocalcemia in newborn (DiGeorge syndrome, especially with characteristic facies, ears, and cardiac lesion)
- Small (less than 10µ diameter) lymphocyte, count persistently less than 1500/mm³; must rule out gastrointestinal loss or loss from lymphatics, however

Suggestive of B cell defect
- Recurrent proven bacterial pneumonia, sepsis, or meningitis
- Nodular lymphoid hyperplasia

Suggestive of B and T cell defect (combined immunodeficiency disease [CID])
- Features of all above except chronic mucocutaneous candidiasis and nodular lymphoid hyperplasia
- Features of Wiskott-Aldrich syndrome (draining ears, thrombocytopenia, and eczema)
- Features of ataxia-telangiectasia

Suggestive of immunodeficiency without clearly implicating T or B cell defect
- Pneumocystis carinii pneumonia
- Intractable eczema
- Ulcerative colitis in infants less than 1 yr of age
- Intractable diarrhea
- Unexplained hematologic deficiency (RBC, WBC, platelet)
- Severe generalized seborrheic dermatitis (Leiner disease) suggests C5 deficiency; seborrhea common in combined immunodeficiency disease
- Recurrent pyogenic infections seen in C3 deficiency

Suggestive of biochemical defect
- Features of combined immunodeficiency with characteristic bony lesions (adenosine deaminase deficiency)
- Features of Diamond-Blackfan aplastic anemia (nucleoside phosphorylase deficiency)

Suggestive of abnormality of polymorphonuclear leukocytes
- Primarily skin infections (if associated with asthma, eczema, and coarse facies, think of Buckley syndrome*)
- Chronic osteomyelitis with Klebsiella or Serratia species, draining lymph nodes (chronic granulomatous disease)

Suggestive that deficiency is secondary
- Concomitant or preceding viral infection
- Lymphoid malignancy (chronic lymphatic leukemia, Hodgkin disease, myeloma)

*Buckley RH, et al: Pediatrics 49:59, 1972.
From Hong R, In: Rose NR, Friedman H (eds): Manual of Clinical Immunology. Washington, D.C., American Society for Microbiology, 1976.

with oncogenesis in immunodeficient states. EBV has the capability to transform human B lymphocytes into cell lines capable of long-term survival under tissue culture conditions; possibly premalignant clones may be perpetuated in vivo as well. In the immunodeficient host, these clones are not eliminated because of the T killer cell deficiency. Genetic and other environmental factors may also play a role. In susceptible patients, the appearance of markedly enlarged nodes and persistent daily fever spikes is an ominous sign. Abnormal lymphocytes can be found in the bone marrow or peripheral smear. Central nervous system symptoms of a mass lesion are common as the brain is a site of frequent involvement. Lymph nodes show characteristic blood vessel proliferation, giving rise to the term angioimmunoblastic lymphadenopathy. Malignant transformation is frequent, resulting in immunoblastic sarcoma. Terminally, virtually every organ can be affected.

9.5 PRIMARY B CELL DISEASES

Clinically, the hypogammaglobulinemic syndromes can be divided into panhypogammaglobulinemia, selective deficiences of the immunoglobulins, and deficiencies of the immunoglobulin subgroups.

9.6 PANHYPOGAMMAGLOBULINEMIA
(Congenital Agammaglobulinemia; Bruton Disease)

Panhypogammaglobulinemia involving all 3 major classes of immunoglobulins is usually congenital in origin. X-linked (Bruton disease), autosomal recessive, sporadic, and "late-onset" forms are seen, but such differentiation is of little help in defining etiology, management, or prognosis. Since some patients with congenital deficiency remain amazingly asymptomatic until later in life, the term late-onset, implying an acquired or secondary disorder, is not justified.

Clinical Manifestations. Panhypogammaglobulinemia presents a history of repeated infections caused by pneumococcus, staphylococcus, and H. influenzae. Conjunctivitis secondary to H. influenzae is especially annoying. In older patients, chronic sinusitis is common, sometimes as the only complaint. Chronic pulmonary disease, with eventual bronchiectasis, pulmonary fibrosis, and cor pulmonale, characterizes adult disease. Fatal encephalitis and chronic viremia following echovirus, type 30, and other viral infections have been reported.

Autoimmunity is observed frequently. An increased frequency of malignancy also occurs (Sec 9.4).

Skin disorders are unusually frequent in immunodeficiency; intractable eczema and dermatomyositis have been reported. Eczema, recurrent skin abscesses, a history of allergy, and coarse facies have been observed in an unusual syndrome with extremely elevated serum IgE values and leukocyte dysfunction (Sec 9.32–9.40).

Approximately 25% of patients with hypogammaglobulinemic syndromes of the late-onset variety have significant malabsorption, most commonly involving vitamin B_{12}. Giardia lamblia infestation is especially common. Lactose intolerance, disaccharidase deficiency, villous abnormalities, and nodular lymphoid hyperplasia may be seen in association with B cell disorders. In nodular lymphoid hyperplasia, panhypogammaglobulinemia may occur, but selective deficiencies are more common.

Diagnosis. This is readily made by measuring serum immunoglobulins. Levels of IgG seldom exceed 200 mg/dl in childhood; IgA and IgM are barely, if at all, detectable. During the first 3 mo of life, the high levels of maternally derived IgG can make the diagnosis difficult, but normal levels of IgA and IgM will virtually rule out the presence of significant hypogammaglobulinemia. Inguinal lymph nodes are easily detected in normal infants, even at birth; the palpation of normal lymph nodes, along with visible tonsillar tissue, speaks strongly against the diagnosis of hypogammaglobulinemia. A rare syndrome of enlarged lymph nodes and histiocytosis-like skin lesions (Omenn disease) is discussed in Sec 9.15. Criteria as to what constitutes significant infections should be stringent. Upper respiratory infections are a common feature of the 1st few yr of life, and as many as 9–10/yr may occur normally. Unless there is a verified history of repeated bacterial pneumonias or other severe infections, frequent upper respiratory infections should not be used as an indication to investigate the patient exhaustively for immunodeficiency.

Treatment. This consists of the intramuscular injection of immune serum globulin (ISG) prepared by alcohol precipitation (Cohn Fraction II). A dose calculated to produce a serum level of 300 mg/dl is given (a loading dose of 1.4 ml/kg, followed by 0.7 ml/kg every 4 wk). For a larger person the large size of an individual dose may require shortening the interval to weekly and reducing the size of each dose proportionately. Local pain at the site of the injection can be partially controlled by mixing a small amount of local anesthetic with the immune serum globulin in the syringe.

The large dose of immune serum globulin required for the treatment of adults and older children may require intravenous administration. Rather than employ intravenous preparations of gamma globulin, which must be processed in a special manner to prevent anaphylaxis, we prefer to use plasma. In addition to IgG, this agent provides significant amounts of IgA and IgM which may offer therapeutic advantage not given by other preparations; e.g., chronic diarrhea may be diminished by plasma therapy. The main danger of repeated administration of plasma is transmission of serum hepatitis, the risk of which may be minimized by restricting the donors to 2–3 nonprofessionals or members of the patient's family. The plasma should be screened for hepatitis antigens by the most sensitive tests available. Continuous subcutaneous infusions may result in higher levels of all 3 major isotypes. Clinical trials are presently under way.

Chronic pulmonary disease is an ever-present danger in panhypogammaglobulinemia. Pulmonary function should be tested at least annually in all patients over 10 yr old, unless symptoms or roentgenograms suggest that earlier assessment should be performed. Unremitting pulmonary disease is probably a sign of failure of therapy with intramuscular gamma globulin and an indication for plasma therapy. However, there is no significant evidence that plasma is of benefit in cases of chronic pulmonary disease; this approach is entirely empiric. Daily prophylaxis with 10 mg/kg of trimethoprim and 50 mg/kg of sulfamethoxazole in 2 divided

doses may also be helpful in selected cases but is not established therapy.

SELECTIVE DEFICIENCIES

Selective deficiency of IgA or IgM has been adequately studied; that of IgE, whether or not associated with ataxia-telangiectasia, remains of unknown clinical significance. Selective total deficiency of IgG has not been described, but deficiency of subgroups is known.

9.7 Selective Deficiency of IgA

The major complications relate to the role of secretory IgA as the major immunoglobulin protecting the respiratory, gastrointestinal, and other secretory areas. As a result of the deficiency, recurrent respiratory infections and chronic diarrheal syndromes may occur. A striking association with autoimmune disorders, especially systemic lupus erythematosus and rheumatoid arthritis, is seen. The autoimmunity is believed to result from uncontrolled access to the lymphoid system of antigenic substances via the gastrointestinal tract, with the resultant undue stimulation causing generation of antigen-antibody complexes. Another reason for the association may be the profound dependency of the IgA system on intact thymic function. Thus, by inference, a deficiency in production of IgA implies a thymic abnormality. One such defect, lack or deficiency of T suppressor cells, could predispose to autoimmunity.

Some patients with selective deficiency of IgA show spontaneous recovery. Two reported patients with deficiency of serum IgA gradually acquired normal levels after periods of 3–5 yr without any specific therapy. Since all IgA-deficient patients studied to date possess normal numbers of nonsecreting lymphocytes bearing IgA molecules and since, in 1 study, these cells could be stimulated in vitro to become secreting cells, the potential for spontaneous recovery may exist in all patients. Selective deficiency of IgA may also be produced by external factors, e.g., by administration of phenytoin.

Patients with selective *total* deficiency of IgA have normal capacity for synthesizing IgG antibody, and their B cells can respond vigorously to most antigens. If such patients receive IgA from any source, formation of anti-IgA antibody is quite likely since their immune systems recognize IgA as a foreign protein. Immune serum globulin (ISG) is a common source, resulting from the frequent and, in our opinion, injudicious practice of empirically administering immune serum globulin as a prophylactic measure to children with frequent respiratory infections, which are usual in patients with total absence of IgA. Immune serum globulin contains trace amounts of IgA, which are adequate to sensitize the child with total deficiency of IgA but not to protect against agents that cause respiratory infections. If blood or blood products containing significant amounts of IgA are then administered to such IgA-sensitized patients, fatal anaphylaxis may result. Therefore, immune serum globulin should not be administered, particularly repeatedly, to children with frequent upper respiratory infections without justification. Likewise, patients with known total IgA deficiency should not receive blood or blood products without first ascertaining the absence of anti-IgA antibodies in their sera.

Selective IgA deficiency may be inherited either in an autosomal recessive or autosomal dominant manner. Often siblings of patients with panhypogammaglobulinemia show selective IgA deficiency. An interesting, but unexplained, association is that of chromosome 18 abnormality with selective IgA deficiency; the structural genes for immunoglobulins do not seem to be present on chromosome 18.

Although serum and secretory IgA appear to be under separate control, virtually all patients with serum IgA deficiency also have secretory IgA deficiency. Occasionally, a patient with deficiency of serum IgA will show IgA-staining plasma cells in the intestine. In these cases, full evaluation of the capability to produce secretory IgA in the gastrointestinal or respiratory tracts has not been carried out. Thus, it is unknown whether or not the number of IgA-producing cells was normal throughout the secretory system or whether their rate of synthesis of secretory IgA was adequate for protection. Therefore, although IgA function in the secretions is the most critical factor, as a practical matter in most situations measurement of serum IgA predicts the status of secretory IgA. Recently, 2 patients were described with deficiency of secretory IgA in the face of normal levels of serum IgA, in association with deficiency of secretory component (Sec 9.8). Thus, it now appears that, if symptoms warrant, specific determination of secretory IgA must be performed regardless of the level of IgA in the serum.

9.8 Selective Deficiency of Secretory Component (SC)

Secretory component is a protein produced by epithelial cells in many parts of the body. It is found on all molecules of IgA secreted into the lumen of the intestine; it may play an important role in the transport of IgA, and, perhaps, of IgM, from the site of synthesis in the plasma cells of the lamina propria. Recently, deficiency of secretory component has been observed in 2 different clinical situations. In the 1st, absence or deficiency of secretory component was reported in 5 of 8 children with sudden infant death syndrome (SIDS). In the 2nd, 2 children with deficiency of secretory component had chronic diarrhea. These patients also had a deficiency of secretory IgA but normal levels of serum IgA.

9.9 Selective Deficiency of IgM

This occurs as a primary deficiency state with a frequency of approximately 1:1000 in the general population. These patients tend to succumb from rapid hematogenous spread of bacterial infections; atopy and splenomegaly have also been noted. Whipple disease, regional enteritis, and lymphoid nodular hyperplasia have also been observed with increased frequency.

Patients should be treated aggressively with antibiotics at the 1st sign of infection. It has been recommended that their blood relatives also be treated empirically at the 1st sign of infection if the status of their serum IgM is unknown.

9.10 IgG Subgroup Deficiency

Generally speaking, in IgG subgroup deficiency the total levels of IgG are normal but the heterogeneity of its electrophoretic mobility may appear to be restricted. When tests of specific antibody formation are made, antibody formation to some antigens but not to others appears. Clinically, the patients show the same increased susceptibility to infection characteristic of panhypogammaglobulinemia, and some, but not all, will respond to gamma globulin therapy.

PRIMARY T CELL DISEASES

When the protection offered by the T cells is compromised but the B cells are operational, infections are primarily of a fungal or viral nature. Chronic interstitial pneumonia, nasal discharge, and neutropenia are also features associated with T cell deficiency. The major types of T cell defect in which the immunoglobulins are measurable (and usually functional) are the DiGeorge syndrome, Nezelof syndrome, cartilage-hair hypoplasia, some cases of adenosine deaminase deficiency, and nucleoside phosphorylase deficiency.

9.11 THE DiGEORGE SYNDROME

The thymus arises from the 3rd and 4th pharyngeal pouches in common with the parathyroid. An embryologic fault of these derivatives causes a combined deficiency of the thymus and parathyroids in association with congenital defects of the aortic arch and heart. Hypoplastic mandible, defective ears, and a short philtrum are other features of the disorder. A characteristic feature is the marked variability of expression of the syndrome, manifested by a range of clinical symptoms varying from minimal thymic deficiency with spontaneous acquisition of normal T cell function to involvement so severe that B cell deficiency is also present. Post mortem examination of thymuses from patients with DiGeorge syndrome reveals variable degrees of hypoplasia, but usually the architecture is preserved. To be included in the DiGeorge syndrome, the disorder must include both parathyroid deficiency (with lack of parathormone) and T cell dysfunction. The other features may or may not be present.

Hypocalcemia in the neonatal period is frequently the initial presentation. Should this occur, careful examination for associated facial and cardiac features should be made. Chest roentgenograms may be informative since sufficient stress to cause disappearance of the thymic shadow has usually not occurred. If hypocalcemia is mild, the diagnosis may first be made in the cardiac clinic. Recent reports suggest that the Zellweger syndrome may be confused with the DiGeorge syndrome. Lack of peroxisomes characterizes the former.

Thymic transplantation has been quite successful in treatment of DiGeorge syndrome, but it must be remembered that spontaneous cures do occur. Thymus implanted in a cell-impermeable Millipore chamber may also result in normalization of T cell tests, suggesting that humoral ("hormonal") factors play an important role in reconstitution.

9.12   NEZELOF SYNDROME

The absence of parathyroid or cardiac involvement in Nezelof syndrome differentiates it from DiGeorge syndrome. The most confusing point in delineation of Nezelof syndrome concerns the presence or absence of specific antibodies, which was not determined in Nezelof's original studies. Unfortunately, cases of T cell deficiency with detectable immunoglobulins are usually pooled together as Nezelof syndrome. Newer concepts of the role of the thymus in expression of the B cell system make this an important distinction. We prefer to classify patients with immunoglobulins of known specificity in the face of T cell deficiency as having Nezelof syndrome and believe them to be quite different from those whose immunoglobulins are measurable but are of nondefined specificity. The latter group of patients frequently does not produce all 3 major classes, and electrophoretic abnormalities are common. We believe that this group should be considered a variant of combined B and T cell deficiency.

9.13   CARTILAGE-HAIR HYPOPLASIA

In cartilage-hair hypoplasia (CHH) a unique form of bone dysplasia occurs, resulting in short-limbed dwarfism, sparse hair that lacks a central pigmented core, and neutropenia. The original patients were described in an Amish population, but cases have been observed in other ethnic groups. Only a small percentage of short-limbed dwarfs show the immune defect; furthermore, even though testing implies a virtual absence of T cell function, susceptibility to infection is limited and the major agents involved are vaccinia or varicella virus. Chronic candidiasis, for example, is not a feature of this T cell deficiency.

Little information is available on the response of cartilage-hair hypoplasia to therapy. Bone marrow transplantation has been performed in 1 case with apparent benefit.

COMBINED T AND B CELL DISEASE

In these disorders, both T and B cell functions are profoundly depressed. Originally, it was thought that combined T and B cell disease was best explained by a lesion of stem cells at the point in their development immediately preceding differentiation into T and B cells.

Recent evidence, however, suggests that B cell differentiation is highly thymus dependent. Consequently, at least some combined B and T cell disorders are probably caused by a primary thymic deficiency.

9.14   COMBINED IMMUNODEFICIENCY DISEASE (CID)

Originally, the term severe combined immunodeficiency was used to describe a syndrome beginning in infancy and usually resulting in death by 2 yr of age. Milder forms have now been described and early death is not inevitable. When the disorder involves both T and B cell systems, the disease is more severe than with either separate defect; the infectious processes that occur are of the varieties that characterize either deficiency state.

If combined immunodeficiency disease (CID) is defined as a disorder in which both T and B cell functions are diminished, *absence* of products of either system is not an absolute requirement for diagnosis. For example, patients with E-rosette cells but no other normal T cell functions and those with some or all classes of immunoglobulins but no detectable antibody activity ("cellular immunodeficiency with immunoglobulin") may also be included in the category of combined immunodeficiency disease. Certainly, the history of infection and susceptibility to disease seems to be as great in these children as in those without any detectable lymphocytes or immunoglobulins.

In addition to the symptoms already discussed for isolated deficiencies, a number of features are characteristic of combined immunodeficiency disease. Wasting, whether or not associated with chronic diarrhea, is common. If diarrhea is present, it is recalcitrant to therapy and hyperalimentation may be required. Unusual skin eruptions, total alopecia, excessive seborrhea, cutaneous laxity manifested by redundant skin folds, large umbilical hernias, and hyperelastic joints are also seen. One form of combined immunodeficiency disease is associated with short-limbed dwarfism, caused by metaphyseal or spondyloepiphyseal dysplasia.

Hematologic abnormalities, including thrombocytosis, neutropenia, anemia, monocytosis, and eosinophilia occur. Monocytosis and eosinophilia may occur in response to overwhelming infections such as pneumocystic pneumonia.

Combined immunodeficiency can be successfully treated with transplantation of bone marrow, with which there appears to be complete and long-lasting reconstitution of both B and T cell systems. The successful transplants have come from siblings who are matched at the major histocompatibility locus most important in determining the severity of graft-versus-host reaction, the HLA-D locus. Unfortunately, only about 25% of the siblings can be expected to match, and all attempts to modify the host or the donor to utilize non-D locus matches have been unsuccessful. In a few cases, it has been possible to utilize HLA-D matched, nonsibling, close relatives. In general, these transplants are not as successful as sibling transplants, and the graft-versus-host reaction may be more severe. A transplant from a completely unrelated HLA-D–matched individual has been successful, but several transplants were required, and administration of large doses of cyclophosphamide was finally necessary to prepare the patient for acceptance of the graft. However, the patient is substantially crippled by chronic graft-versus-host disease.

No significant benefit has resulted from treatment with transfer factor or thymic hormone. Transplants of fetal liver, fetal liver combined with fetal thymus, fetal thymus alone, or cultured thymic epithelium (CTE) have shown promise in some cases; it is probable that, for different varieties of combined immunodeficiency disease, different approaches will be necessary.

Pneumocystis infection is responsive to either pentamidine isethionate or trimethoprim-sulfamethoxazole; prophylaxis with the latter is advisable in a patient with combined immunodeficiency until curative transplantation of bone marrow is established. Treatment for cytomegalovirus, rubeola, and varicella infections is unsatisfactory. Zoster immune globulin is indicated to prevent infection upon exposure of a susceptible immunodeficient patient to varicella. In varicella pneumonia, therapy with adenosine arabinoside or interferon may be attempted.

9.15 COMBINED IMMUNODEFICIENCY DISEASE AND LETTERER-SIWE SYNDROME
(Omenn Disease)

In 1 variety of combined immunodeficiency disease, a chronic skin eruption, hepatosplenomegaly, eosinophilia, and histiocytic infiltration of the lymph nodes occur. The marked histiocytosis has led to an erroneous diagnosis of Letterer-Siwe syndrome, leading to reports of immunodeficiency and Letterer-Siwe syndrome occurring together. The skin eruptions of Letterer-Siwe syndrome, with its extreme seborrhea and characteristic histiocytic infiltration, are actually quite different from any form of combined immunodeficiency disease. Furthermore, in Letterer-Siwe syndrome there is no immunodeficiency unless cytotoxic drugs have been given. Combined immunodeficiency disease of this type is 1 of the few forms of severe immunodeficiency in which there is marked deficiency of both T and B cell systems but easily palpable lymph nodes. Usually, many of the tests of lymphocyte function are normal; thus, the diagnosis may require thymic biopsy for confirmation. A deficiency of the ectoenzyme 5'-nucleotidase may be characteristic of Omenn disease. *Pneumocystis* pneumonia is a common presenting symptom. Often the rash is really a manifestation of a chronic graft-versus-host disease.

9.16 WISKOTT-ALDRICH SYNDROME

This is an X-linked recessive disorder characterized by thrombocytopenia, draining ears, and eczema.

Serum IgA and IgE are markedly elevated, IgM is diminished, lymphopenia is common, and malignant reticuloendotheliosis is a frequent terminal event.

The reason for the susceptibility to infection in Wiskott-Aldrich syndrome is unknown. Although the most striking immunologic abnormality consistently found is an inability to form antibodies to carbohydrate antigens, poor responses to other antigens are found as the disease progresses. Detailed testing may show mild dysfunction of T cells but less than in the usual forms of T cell deficiency. The defects increase with time so that originally normal findings give way to abnormal responses; immunoglobulin levels change to a characteristic hyper-IgA, hypo-IgM pattern; and abnormalities of lymphoid tissues occur.

Three successful bone marrow transplants have been performed in Wiskott-Aldrich syndrome. In contrast to combined immunodeficiency disease, administration of near-lethal doses of cyclophosphamide or x-irradiation is necessary to prepare the patient for acceptance of the graft. This greatly increases the morbidity and mortality of the procedure. Transfer factor is said to be of some benefit in Wiskott-Aldrich syndrome, and a recent clinical trial with thymosin shows some encouraging results.

9.17 ATAXIA-TELANGIECTASIA

Ataxia-telangiectasia (AT) is characterized by ataxia, ocular and cutaneous telangiectasia, chronic sinopulmonary disease, endocrine abnormalities, and variable B and T cell deficiency. Deficiency of IgA and IgE, singly or together, constitutes the most common B cell abnormality. The disease may be due to a common embryologic fault resulting in failure of mesodermoentodermal interactions, leading to telangiectasia, neurologic disease, and lymphoid abnormalities. The finding of elevated alpha-fetoprotein in virtually all patients with ataxia-telangiectasia is consistent with an abnormal process of embryogenesis. Since only fetal-type cells synthesize this protein, continued postnatal production suggests an arrest at a fetal stage. In some as yet undefined way, similar arrests involving the many and varied organ systems in ataxia-telangiectasia could lead to the manifestations observed. Some workers have found evidence for autoimmune reactivity against various organ systems, including brain and thymocytes, implying autoaggression as a factor in the pathogenesis.

The disease is inherited as an autosomal trait, probably recessive. Cerebellar ataxia is usually the 1st neurologic sign; intellectual development is normal at first but seems to arrest at about the 10 yr level. A mask-like facies with excessive drooling gives a remarkable similarity of appearance to all affected patients. The telangiectases are most obvious in the sclerae, although involvement of the ear, lateral aspect of the nose, and antecubital and popliteal fossae is common.

Deficiency of both IgA and IgE is common and may be seen in 50–70% of cases; isolated IgE deficiency may occur in another 20–40%. Selective IgA deficiency is also found in high frequency. Variable degrees of T cell deficiency progressively worsen with time, and death by malignant lymphoma is a common terminal event.

9.18 CHRONIC MUCOCUTANEOUS CANDIDIASIS

This chronic, indolent candidiasis involves mucous membranes and spreads peripherally onto the skin. Satellite patches may occur on the trunk and extremities; onychomycosis may be present. Some patients have associated endocrine deficiencies, with hypoadrenalism, hypoparathyroidism; and hypothyroidism among the most common. Initially, these patients show increased susceptibility to infection with *Candida* only, with normal ability to resist other infectious agents. Gradually, however, their general immunity wanes and infection occurs from other opportunistic organisms.

The immunologic background for chronic mucocutaneous candidiasis is varied. There may be demonstrable defects of T cell immunity by the usual tests, deficiency of migration inhibitory factor (MIF), selective IgA deficiency, or biotin deficiency. In some patients no abnormalities are detectable with present methods.

Intravenous amphotericin (Sec 10.104) is extremely effective, but a return of symptoms frequently occurs upon cessation of therapy. In recalcitrant cases, clotrimazole, transfer factor, leukocyte infusions, and thymosin have all been used with variable degrees of success. It is important to remember that endocrinopathy, e.g., acute adrenal insufficiency, may occur at any time.

9.19 GRAFT-VERSUS-HOST DISEASE (GVHD)

A complication of T cell deficiency states occurs when a patient receives immunocompetent (T killer) cells with ordinary blood transfusions or bone marrow transplants. More rarely, it may occur in utero following transfusion for erythroblastosis fetalis or as a result of maternal cells which cross the placenta into the fetal circulation. In the intrauterine situation, whether the fetus must be T cell deficient or not has not been determined. The rarity of the event in the normal population and the frequency in immunodeficient individuals suggests that intrauterine graft-versus-host disease probably does not occur in normal fetuses.

Graft-versus-host disease may be acute or chronic. The *acute* variety is usually seen in recipients of blood or bone marrow from individuals who differ at HLA-D locus; the event most often occurs when a blood transfusion is unwittingly given to a T cell deficient patient. It may rarely occur after transplants of fetal tissue. Occasionally graft-versus-host disease is associated with blood product infusions in leukemic patients. It remains a rare event, however, and probably occurs only when a number of chance events happen simultaneously. *Chronic* graft-versus-host disease is seen with intrauterine transfusions, after transplantation from HLA-D matched bone marrow donors (especially in leukemia), and after transplants of fetal liver or fetal thymus.

The acute disease, which begins 7–14 days after grafting, is generally heralded by a skin eruption. This can be maculopapular in character or, in more explosive cases, can present as *"scalded skin syndrome."* Periportal necrosis of the liver, coagulation necrosis of the epidermis, and lesions of the crypts of the gastrointestinal tract are the characteristic histologic findings. When the source of killer T cells is from an HLA-D nonmatched donor, death can result. When the donor is HLA-D matched, the syndrome can vary from a fleeting skin rash and slight transient elevation of liver enzymes to a severe but usually nonfatal disease. The graft-versus-host reaction has an unusual capacity to activate latent virus infections. Thus, if the patient harbors cytomegalovirus, the infection may become widespread and overwhelm the patient before immunologic reconstitution occurs. *Pneumocystis* pneumonia often becomes manifest early in the post-transplant period, probably for the same reason.

The chronic disease is characterized by a scaling erythroderma, alopecia, and failure to thrive.

Treatment of established graft-versus-host disease is unsatisfactory. Some limited success with antithymocyte or antilymphocyte globulin has been reported in chronic graft-versus-host disease in leukemic patients who have received bone marrow transplants.

9.20 SECONDARY IMMUNODEFICIENCY DISEASES

In these disorders the primary cause is clearly outside the lymphoid system. The immune elements are involved either as part of a generalized process or as a result of some aspect of the primary disease which directly attacks or consumes the lymphoid products.

Adenosine Deaminase (ADA) and Nucleoside Phosphorylase (NP) Deficiency. These are the first biochemical defects described in association with immunodeficiency. Usually adenosine deaminase negative patients have combined immunodeficiency disease, but isolated defects of the thymus system are known. Nucleoside phosphorylase deficiency usually presents as an isolated T cell defect. However, with time, nucleoside phosphorylase deficiency eventually results in B cell deficiency as well. These biochemical defects cause immunodeficiency through a toxic effect on lymphocytes by products accumulated as a result of an inability to catabolize purines. Adenosine deaminase catalyzes the conversion of adenosine to inosine; in its absence, levels of lymphocyte ATP, cyclic AMP, and their deoxyanalogues increase. The reversible conversion of inosine to hypoxanthine, guanosine to guanine, and xanthosine to xanthine is catalyzed by nucleoside phosphorylase. A breakdown in normal catabolic processes results in the accumulation of inosine and guanosine. Whether these or other metabolites are the actual toxic factors is unknown as yet, but the principle of a slow toxic attrition of the lymphoid system appears to be valid.

Characteristically there is a period of normal lymphoid function followed by a gradual waning of immunity ("immunologic attrition").

The diagnosis is established by measurement of enzyme levels in erythrocytes. It can also be suspected from the clinical history suggesting an "acquired" defect of late onset and, in nucleoside phosphorylase deficiency, from finding a low serum uric acid. Characteristic splaying of the ends of the ribs and "squaring off" of the scapulae are seen in adenosine deaminase deficiency. In nucleoside phosphorylase deficiency, the metabolic defect may result in megaloblastic anemia, pure red cell aplasia, or spastic tetraparesis.

Repeated blood transfusions have been effective in managing some patients with adenosine deaminase deficiency. In nucleoside phosphorylase deficiency, experience with this form of treatment is not extensive but in a single reported case transfusions were without benefit. Another patient with nucleoside phosphorylase deficiency responded to thymosin injections but developed allergy to the hormone, necessitating cessation of the medication.

Transplantation of cultured thymus fragments offers additional help in management.

Loss of Immunologic Materials. Loss of protein, hence of immunoglobulins, may occur from the genitourinary and gastrointestinal tracts and from the lymphatic system. In *nephrotic syndromes* the glomerular sieve allows the escape of IgG and IgA but retains the larger molecules of IgM, which remain at near-normal levels. The ability to manufacture antibody is unimpaired, and susceptibility to infection is not increased (the susceptibility of nephrotic children to pneumococcal peritonitis appears to be related to ascites and lack of previous experience with pneumococcal infection rather than to an immunologic deficit). The situation with *protein-losing enteropathy* is analogous. Both are characterized by hypogammaglobulinemia associated with edema or hypoalbuminemia. Loss of immunologic materials from the *lymphatic system*, whether due to congenital malformations of the lymphatic vessels or to surgical accidents, includes loss of lymphocytes as well as of circulating immunoglobulins. The lymphocyte count may drop to one third of normal levels, and all 3 major classes of immunoglobulins may fall to one half of normal levels. Tests of T cell function show abnormal lymphocyte responses in vitro and retention of allogeneic skin grafts for up to 2 yr. Resistance to infections is surprisingly unimpaired, except in chylothorax; lymphangiectasia involving the thoracic cavity is associated with more infectious problems than that of other areas of the body.

Viral Infections. Intrauterine infections may cause altered development of lymphoid cells and organs, such as the thymus, in which primary differentiation takes place. B cell deficiency may occur following infection with Epstein-Barr virus. The disease (Duncan disease) appears to be X linked, and lymphoproliferative disease is commonly associated; the initial bout of Epstein-Barr virus infection is unusually severe and fulminant.

Nutritional Deficiency. In *protein-calorie malnutrition*, disseminated herpes infections and gram-negative sepsis are common. Death from measles may occur. Lymphopenia is marked, in vitro lymphocyte responses are defective, and tonsils and thymus are small. Usually B cell function is only slightly diminished; IgE may be markedly elevated.

Immune cellular functions are dependent upon divalent cations. For example, internal movement of calcium ions causes proliferation of lymphocytes, and immunodeficiency has been described in association with copper, zinc, iron, and calcium abnormalities. Acrodermatitis enteropathica is due to zinc malabsorption; chronic candidiasis may be associated with biotin deficiency.

Chemical or Physical Immunosuppression. The widespread use of immunosuppressive drugs in autoimmune disorders and transplantation has led to a number of immunologic deficiency states, as have cytotoxic agents employed in cancer chemotherapy. Preexisting immunity usually persists at pretreatment levels unless the dosage of medication is extremely high.

The addition of irradiation to chemotherapy adds significantly to the mortality of leukemic patients from infections. Deficiencies of both T and B cell systems are found. Immunologic recovery may require as long as 1 yr following cessation of such therapy.

When antilymphocyte serum or globulin is employed, marked depression of T cell functions is seen, with an associated increased incidence of fungal, protozoal, and viral infections.

RICHARD HONG

Ament ME, Ochs HD, Davis SD: Structure and function of the gastrointestinal tract in primary immunodeficiency syndromes. A study of 39 patients. Medicine 52:227, 1973.

Ammann AJ, Wara D, Salmon S: Transfer factor: Therapy with deficient cell-mediated immunity and deficient antibody-mediated immunity. Cell Immunol 12:94, 1974.

Bergsma D, Good RA, Finstad J, et al (eds): Immunodeficiency in Man and Animals. Birth Defects Original Article Series, Vol IV. White Plains, NY, The National Foundation, 1968.

Broder S, Waldmann T: The suppressor-cell network in cancer. N Engl J Med 229:1281, 1978.

Campbell AC, Hersey P, McLennan LC, et al: Immunosuppressive consequences in radiotherapy and chemotherapy in patients with acute lymphoblastic leukemia. Br Med J 2:385, 1973.

Cooper MD, Keightley RG, Wu LYF, et al: Developmental defects of T and B lines in humans. Transpl Rev 16:51, 1973.

Goldstein AL, Cohen GH, Rossio JL, et al: Use of thymosin in the treatment of primary immunodeficiency diseases and cancer. Med Clin North Am 60:591, 1976.

Good RA, Bach FH: Bone marrow and thymus transplants: Cellular engineering to correct primary immunodeficiency. In: Bach FH, Good RA (eds): Clinical Immunobiology. New York, Academic Press, 1974.

Hitzig WH, Grob PJ: Therapeutic uses of transfer factor. In: Schwartz RS (ed): Progress in Clinical Immunology. New York, Grune & Stratton, 1974.

Horowitz SD, Hong R: The Pathogenesis and Treatment of Immunodeficiency. Basel, S Karger, 1977.

Kersey JH, Spector BD, Good RA: Cancer in children with primary immunodeficiency diseases. J Pediatr 84:263, 1974.

Kirkpatrick CH, Smith TK: Chronic mucocutaneous candidiasis: Immunologic and antibiotic therapy. Ann Intern Med 80:310, 1974.

Pollara B, Pickering RJ, Meuwissen HG, et al: Inborn Errors of Specific Immunity. New York, Academic Press, 1979.

Polmar SH, Stern RC, Schwartz AL, et al: Enzyme replacement therapy for adenosine deaminase deficiency and severe combined immunodeficiency. N Engl J Med 295:1337, 1976.

Purtillo DT: Epstein-Barr virus–induced oncogenesis in immune-deficient individuals. Lancet 1:300, 1980.

Reinherz EL, Schlossman SF: Current concepts in immunology. Regulation of the immune response-inducer and suppressor T-lymphocyte subsets in human beings. N Engl J Med 303:370, 1980.

Seligmann M, Preud'homme JL, Brouet JC: B and T cell markers in human diseases. Transpl Rev 16:85, 1973.

Van Bekkum DW: Use and abuse of hematopoietic cell grafts in immune deficiency diseases. Transpl Rev 9:3, 1972.

Wilfert CM, Buckley RH, Mohanakumar T, et al: Persistent CNS ECHO virus infections and agammaglobulinemia. N Engl J Med 296:1485, 1977.

Complement and Associated Diseases

9.21   COMPLEMENT

It was noted in the late 19th century that certain bacteria could be killed in vitro by fresh serum from animals immunized against the organism. If the serum was heated to 56° C for 30 min or allowed to age for several days at room temperature, however, it lost its bactericidal capacity although its antibodies were retained. The addition of small amounts of fresh serum from unimmunized animals, itself incapable of effecting killing, restored the bactericidal ability of heated immune serum. Thus, bacteriolysis required antibody and a complementary, nonspecific, heat-labile principle, now termed *complement*. Within a few yr it was known that complement consisted of more than 1 factor; by the 1960's there were 9 known components, 1 of which had 3 subcomponents. By the early 1970's a 2nd major pathway of activation of complement, the *alternative* or *properdin pathway*, had been described. The latter system contains 3 unique factors. In addition, 6 regulators that control activity of either or both pathways have been identified. The original system of 11 interdependent factors is now referred to as the classical pathway of complement. The term *complement system* generally refers to both pathways, which interact to utilize together C3 through C9 and which depend upon each other for their full activity. All of the 20 components and regulators of both pathways are proteins. Together they make up about 10% of the globulin fraction of serum.

As knowledge of the components of complement and their biochemistry has grown, so has understanding of the biologic importance of the system. It acts as the principal mediator of the inflammatory response and plays an essential role in host defense against infection.

Nomenclature. The terminology applied to complement is cryptic but logical and consists of only a few rules: The components have been assigned a number in the order of their discovery and are preceded by the letter C. Unfortunately, the first 4 components do not interact in the sequence in which they were discovered, but rather in the order C1423. The remaining components react in the appropriate numerical order, C56789. C1 has 3 subcomponents, C1q, C1r, and C1s. Fragments of components resulting from cleavage by other components acting as enzymes are assigned small letters (a, b, c, d, or e); with the exception of C2 fragments, the smaller piece that is released into surrounding fluids is assigned the letter "a," and the major part of the molecule, bound to other components or to some part of the immune complex, is assigned "b," e.g., C3a and C3b. When a component is activated (becomes an active enzyme), a bar is placed above it, e.g., $\overline{C1}$.

Components of the alternative pathway have been assigned letters: B, D, and P (properdin). Factor B has an active form denoted $\overline{Bb}$. C3 (in particular, its major fragment, C3b) is a component of both the classical and alternative pathways.

General Concepts. Complement is a *system* of interacting proteins. The biologic functions of the system depend upon the interaction of individual components, which occurs in sequential fashion. This has been referred to as a "cascade," in analogy to the clotting system of blood; activation of each component (except the 1st) depends upon activation of the prior component or components in the sequence.

Interaction occurs along 2 pathways: the classical pathway, in the order antigen–antibody–C142356789; and the alternative pathway, in the order antibody–properdin system–C356789. Antibody accelerates the rate of activation of the alternative pathway, but some activation can occur in the absence of antibody. The classical and the alternative pathways interact with each other through the ability of both to activate C3.

The interaction of the early-acting components of complement (C1423) results in the generation of a series of active enzymes, $\overline{C1}$, $\overline{C42}$, and $\overline{C423}$. Thus, "activation" refers to transformation of the component into part of an active enzyme. In contrast, the interaction among C5b, C6, C7, C8, and C9 is nonenzymatic. In the case of C1, activation is a result of its interaction with antibody. Activation of C4, C2, C3, and C5, as well as factor B of the alternative pathway, is secondary to cleavage by a preceding component or components. Thus, activation of early components generates enzymes that fix to the antigen-antibody complex and catalyze a reaction on the next component, whereas later acting components (C6–C9) adsorb to the complex or the underlying cell by an interaction that depends on a change in their configuration.

These basic principles can be illustrated by a more detailed analysis of the activation sequence.

Sequence of Activation. The sequence in which the components of the classical pathway interact, the interdigitation between classical and alternative pathways, the chemical and functional by-products of these reactions, and the regulators of the system are summarized in Fig 9–3.

The sequence begins with fixation of C1, by way of C1q, to the Fc (Sec 9.1), nonantigen-binding part of the antibody molecule after antigen-antibody interaction. The C1 tricomplex changes configuration, and the C1s subcomponent becomes an active enzyme, "$\overline{C1}$ esterase."

C-reactive protein (CRP), which reacts with "C carbohydrate" from microorganisms and is elevated in certain inflammatory states, can substitute for antibody in the fixation of C1q and initiate reaction of the entire sequence. Thus, C-reactive protein functions like antibody though it can combine with only a few specific "antigens" and its size and structure are quite different. This reaction has the potential of initiating inflammation in the absence of antibody. Other agents can also activate C1 directly, without a requirement for antibody, including certain RNA viruses, uric acid crystals, the lipid A component of bacterial endotoxin, and the membranes of certain intracellular organelles.

In the next 2 steps of the classical pathway, polypeptide fragments are split from C4 and C2 during their

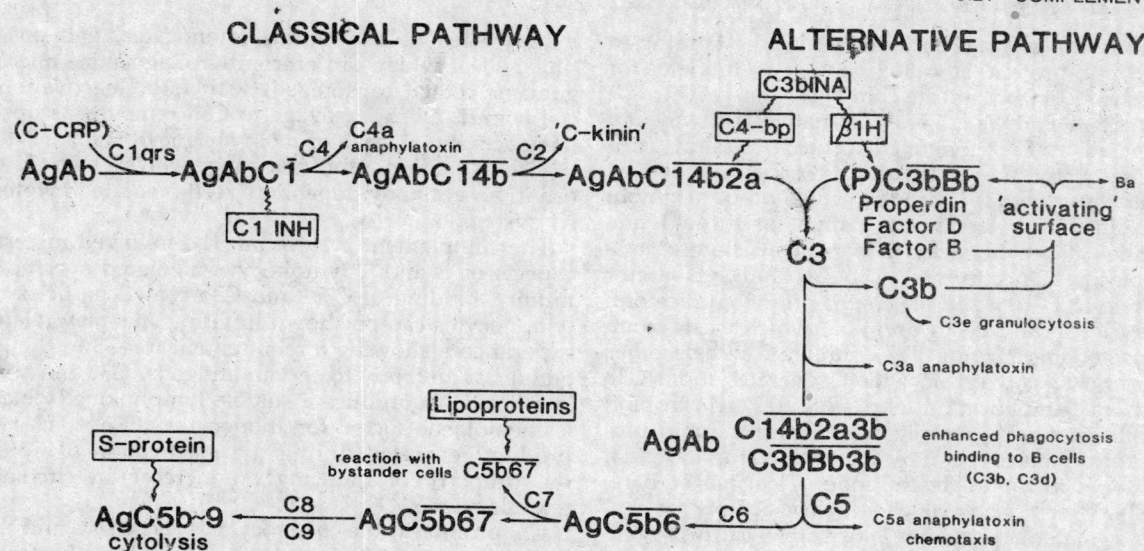

Figure 9-3 Sequence of activation of the components of the classical pathway of complement and interaction with the alternative pathway. Ag = antigen (bacterium, virus, tumor cell, or erythrocyte); Ab = antibody (IgG or IgM classes only); C-CRP = C carbohydrate–C-reactive protein; C1 INH = C1 inhibitor; C3b INA = C3b inactivator; C4-bp = C4-binding protein. Regulator proteins are each enclosed in a box. (Modified from Johnston RB Jr, Stroud RM: J Pediatr 90:169, 1977.)

activation and fixation by the enzymatic action of C$\overline{1}$. It appears that one of these, although not clearly characterized, is a kinin-like peptide that can induce vascular permeability, and thereby edema, through direct action on postcapillary venules. The peptide C4a has *anaphylatoxin* activity; it reacts with mast cells to release the chemical mediators of immediate hypersensitivity, including histamine. Fixation of the major part of the molecule C4b to the complex permits it to adhere to a variety of mammalian cells, including neutrophils, monocytes, and erythrocytes, a phenomenon termed *immune adherence*.

Cleavage of C3 and generation of C3b is the next step in the sequence and the most crucial in terms of biologic activity. Cleavage of C3 can be achieved through C$\overline{142}$, the "C3 convertase" of the classical pathway, or through the C3 convertase of the alternative pathway, C3bBb (see below). Once fixed to the complex, C3b permits adherence of the antigen-antibody complex to cells with C3b receptors, namely B lymphocytes, erythrocytes, and phagocytic cells (neutrophils, monocytes, and macrophages), leading, in the last case, to phagocytosis. In fact, without C3 bound to most microorganisms, phagocytosis in vitro, especially by neutrophils, is very inefficient. Judging from the severe pyogenic infections that occur commonly in C3-deficient patients, phagocytosis in vivo is also inefficient without C3. With time, the serum protein C3b inactivator cleaves C3b to C3c, which is released, and C3d, which stays bound. Binding to B lymphocytes can occur through bound C3d as well as C3b. Further cleavage of C3c creates C3e, which induces release of granulocytes from bone marrow.

The peptide C3a, generated when C3 is acted upon by either pathway, has anaphylatoxin activity. The action of C$\overline{423}$ or the alternative pathway "C5 conver-

tase" on C5 releases C5a, a 3rd anaphylatoxin. This same peptide serves as a potent chemical attractant for phagocytic cells.

The "membrane-attack" sequence leading to cytolysis begins with the attachment of C5b to C$\overline{423}$, the C5-activating enzyme (or to the alternative pathway enzyme). C6 is bound to C5b without being cleaved, stabilizing the activated C5b fragment. The C5b6 complex then dissociates from C$\overline{423}$ and reacts with C7. C5b67 complexes must attach to the cell membrane promptly or lose their activity and remain in the fluid phase. C8 and then C9 bind to C5b67. The assembled C5b6789 complex is inserted into the cell membrane, and lysis ensues.

Control mechanisms act at several points to prevent the system's consuming itself in activity that is unnecessary or deleterious to the host. An α-2 globulin, C1 inhibitor (C1 INH), inhibits C$\overline{1}$s enzymatic activity and, thus, the cleavage of C4 and C2. Activated C2 has a half-life of about 8 min at 37° C, and this relative instability limits the effective life of C$\overline{42}$ and C$\overline{423}$. The alternative pathway enzyme that activates C3, C3bBb, also has a short half-life, though it can be prolonged by the binding of properdin (P) to the enzyme complex. Serum contains the protein "anaphylatoxin inactivator," an enzyme that cleaves the carboxyterminal arginine from both C3a and C5a, thereby markedly reducing their anaphylatoxic activity and the chemotactic activity of C5a. C3b inactivator (C3b INA) cleaves C4b and C3b into inactive fragments, thus serving as an important means of controlling both pathways. β1H accelerates inactivation of C3b by C3b INA. An analogous factor, C4 binding protein (C4-bp), accelerates cleavage of C4b by C3b INA. Serum lipoproteins or circulating C8 can inhibit attachment of the C5b67 complex to cell membranes. Attachment of the C5b6789 complex to the cell can be inhibited by the binding to C5b6789 of S-protein, so called because it competes for membrane sites (S) with the complex.

Alternative Pathway. The alternative pathway can be activated by C3b generated through classical pathway activity, through leukocyte proteases released by degranulation, perhaps through activation of thrombin or plasmin during blood coagulation, or through the low-grade C3-cleaving activity that is consistently present in plasma. Once formed, C3b can bind to B. Factor B attached to C3b in the plasma or on the surface of a particle can be cleaved to Bb by D, which exists as an active proteolytic enzyme. The complex C3bBb becomes an efficient C3 convertase which generates more C3b through an "amplification loop" (Fig 9–3). P can bind to C3bBb, increasing stability of the enzyme and protecting it from inactivation by C3b inactivator and β1H, which serve to modulate the loop. Cleavage of B releases Ba, which has weak chemotactic activity.

Certain materials promote alternative pathway activation if C3b is fixed to their surface, e.g., teichoic acid from bacterial cell wall, endotoxic lipopolysaccharide, or immunoglobulin aggregates, especially of the IgA class. This activation depends on the ability of the C3bBb enzyme complex to escape the efficient control otherwise exercised by C3b inactivator and B1H. The surface of rabbit red blood cells also protects C3bBb from inactivation. This phenomenon serves as the basis for a diagnostic assay for serum alternative pathway activity. Endotoxin may act in vivo by altering normally "nonactivating" cell surfaces so that C3bBb is relatively protected from inactivation, which may partially explain the apparent activation of the alternative pathway in patients with gram-negative bacteremia.

Although C3bBb can activate C3 efficiently on only a limited variety of surfaces, significant activation of C3 can occur through this pathway, and the resultant biologic activities are qualitatively the same as those achieved through activation by C142, as illustrated in Fig 9–3.

Participation in Host Defense. Specific activities of the complement system in host defense against infection are summarized in Table 9–8. Neutralization of virus by antibody can be enhanced with C1 and C4. When antibody concentrations are low, the additional fixation of C3b to the viral antigen-antibody complex through the classical or alternative pathway is needed for improved neutralization; C5 and C6 add little to the effect. Therefore, complement may be particularly important in the early phases of a viral infection when antibody is limited. Antibody and complement can also eliminate infectivity of at least some viruses with the production of typical complement "holes" in the virus, as seen by electron microscopy. Animal RNA tumor viruses appear to interact directly with human C1q in the absence of antibody with resulting activation of the classical pathway and lysis of the virus. This may be a natural resistance mechanism that limits the infectivity of these viruses in man.

C4a, C3a, and C5a can bind to mast cells and thereby trigger release of histamine, leading to vasodilatation and to the swelling and redness of inflammation. C5a is the major chemical stimulus for the influx into inflam-

matory sites of neutrophils, monocytes, and eosinophils, all of which can efficiently phagocytize microorganisms coated (opsonized) with C3b. Inactivation of cell-bound C3b by cleavage to C3d removes its opsonizing activity, at least for most phagocytic cells. Fixation of C3b to a target cell can enhance its lysis by a "killer" cell in an antibody-dependent, cell-mediated cytotoxicity system.

The complement system may be involved in certain aspects of B and T lymphocyte–mediated specific immunity: binding of C3b- and C3d-coated particles to B lymphocytes can be shown in vitro. This may relate to experiments showing a requirement for C3 in the generation of antibody to certain antigens. C3b can stimulate B cells to produce a soluble lymphokine, which is a chemotactic factor for monocytes. C3e, a cleavage product generated during the inactivation of C3, has the property of inducing an increase in circulating granulocytes.

C5 promotes the phagocytosis of yeast and may further boost the phagocytosis of C3-coated bacteria to a slight extent. Neutralization of endotoxin in vitro and protection from its lethal effects in experimental animals require later-acting components of complement, at least through C6. Finally, activation of the entire complement sequence can result in lysis of virus-infected cells, tumor cells, and most types of microorganisms. Bactericidal activity of complement has not appeared to be important to host defense except for the occurrence of infections with *Neisseria* in patients lacking later-acting components of complement (Sec 9.24).

Fearon DT, Austen KF: The alternative pathway of complement—a system for host resistance to microbial infection. N Engl J Med 303:259, 1980.

Leddy JP, Simons RL, Douglas RG: Effect of selective complement deficiency on the rate of neutralization of enveloped viruses by human sera. J Immunol 118:28, 1977.

Mortenson RF, Osmand AP, Lint TF, et al: Interaction of C-reactive protein with

Table 9–8 ACTIVITIES OF COMPLEMENT IN HOST DEFENSE AGAINST INFECTION

COMPONENTS OR FRAGMENTS	FUNCTIONAL ACTIVITY
C14, C1423	Neutralization of viruses
C4a, C3a, C5a	"Anaphylatoxin" (capillary dilation)
C5a	Chemotaxis of neutrophils, monocytes, eosinophils
C3b	Opsonization
C3b	Enhancement of cell-mediated cytotoxicity
C3b	Stimulation of production of B cell lymphokines
C3b, C3d	Enhanced induction of antibody formation
C3e	Induction of granulocytosis
Bb	Macrophage adherence and spreading
C5	Opsonization of fungi
C1 ~ 6 (? additional components)	Inactivation of endotoxin
C1 ~ 9	Lysis of viruses, virus-infected cells, tumor cells, mycoplasma, protozoa, spirochetes, and bacteria

Adapted from Johnston RB Jr, Stroud RM: J Pediatr 90:169, 1977.

lymphocytes and monocytes: Complement-dependent adherence and phagocytosis. J Immunol 117:774, 1976.

Smith TF, Johnston RB Jr: The complement system: Implications for pediatrics. Pediatrics Update, 1981, p 305.

Spitzer RE: The complement system. Pediatr Clin North Am 24:341, 1977.

DISEASES OF THE COMPLEMENT SYSTEM

9.22 PRIMARY DEFICIENCIES OF COMPLEMENT

Congenital deficiencies of all 11 component proteins of the classical pathway and of C1 inhibitor and C3b inactivator have been described (Table 9–9).

9.23 Hereditary Angioedema

Hereditary angioedema occurs when an individual is born without the ability to synthesize normally functioning C1 inhibitor. In 85% of affected families the concentration of inhibitor is markedly reduced (5–30% of normal) in affected individuals; in the other 15% serum contains normal or elevated concentrations of an immunologically cross-reacting but nonfunctional protein. Both forms of the disease are transmitted as autosomal dominant traits.

In the absence of this α_2-globulin, activation of C1 leads to uncontrolled $\overline{C1s}$ activity with breakdown of C4 and C2 and release of a vasoactive peptide (kinin) from 1 or both of these substrates. Episodic, localized edema results from the vasodilatory effects of the kinin at the level of the postcapillary venule. The mechanism by which C1 is activated in these individuals is not known.

Swelling of the affected part accumulates rapidly, without associated urticaria, itching, discoloration, or redness, and often without any severe pain. Intense abdominal cramping can occur, however, from swelling of the intestinal wall. Concurrent subcutaneous edema is often absent, and patients have been subjected to abdominal surgery or psychiatric examination before the proper diagnosis was made. Laryngeal edema can be fatal. Attacks last 2–3 days, then gradually abate. They may occur at sites of trauma, after vigorous exercise, with menses, or with emotional stress. Attacks can begin in the 1st 2 yr of life but are usually not severe until late childhood or adolescence. The condition can be acquired in association with lymphoid cancer. Systemic lupus erythematosus (SLE) has been described in patients with the congenital disease. (Sec 9.27 and 9.28.)

9.24 Deficiencies of the Components of Complement

Complete deficiency of C1q has been detected in children with a syndrome of septicemia or meningitis, skin infections, and a florid maculopapular rash. Biop-

Table 9–9 CONGENITAL DEFICIENCIES OF THE COMPLEMENT SYSTEM

DEFICIENT COMPONENT	PROBABLE INHERITANCE†	ASSOCIATED CLINICAL FINDINGS‡
C1q	Not known	Recurrent infections, dermatitis, CGN
C1q dysfunction	AR(CD)	SLE syndrome
C1r	AR(CD)	CGN, SLE syndrome
C1s	Not known	SLE
C4	AR(CD)	SLE or SLE syndrome, discoid lupus erythematosus
C2	AR(CD)	SLE or SLE syndrome; MPGN; H-S purpura; dermatomyositis; septicemia, especially pneumococcal
C3	AR(CD)	Pyogenic infections, absence of expected neutrophilia, CGN
C5	AR(CD)	SLE; pyogenic infections; gonococcal, meningococcal infections
C5 dysfunction	AD	Pyoderma, septicemia, Leiner disease
C6	AR(CD)	Gonococcal, meningococcal infections; SLE syndrome
C7	AR(CD)	Sclerodactyly; chronic nephritis; gonococcal, meningococcal infections
C8	AR(CD)	Gonococcal, meningococcal infections; SLE syndrome
C8 dysfunction	Not known	Meningococcal infections
C9	AR(CD)	Meningococcal infections
C1 INH*	AD	Angioedema, SLE
C3b INA*	AR(CD)	Pyogenic infections

*INA = inactivator; INH = inhibitor.

†AD = autosomal dominant; AR = autosomal recessive; AR(CD) = autosomal recessive, co-dominant (heterozygotes have approximately half-normal serum levels); XLR = X-linked recessive. In some of the conditions the mode of inheritance is unproved.

‡CGN = chronic glomerulonephritis; H-S = Henoch-Schönlein; MPGN = membranoproliferative glomerulonephritis; SLE = systemic lupus erythematosus.

sies of the rash have shown deposition of immune complexes in the basal epidermis or walls of small blood vessels. C1q dysfunction was noted in 2 siblings who had complete deficiency of C1q activity but decreased amounts of an antigenically altered C1q molecule in their sera. The brother had a systemic lupus erythematosus–like syndrome; the sister was healthy.

Patients with C1q, C1r, C1s, C4, C2, C5, C6, C7, and C8 deficiency have had a strikingly high incidence of vasculitis syndromes (Table 9–9), especially systemic lupus erythematosus or a lupus-like syndrome in which antinuclear antibody may be undetectable. The reason for the concurrence of deficiencies of components of complement and these "autoimmune" diseases is not known; but, if these diseases originate as infections, the association might occur as a result of absence of 1 or more of the host defense properties described in

Table 9–8. Complement facilitates elimination of immune complexes, and inefficiency of this process is a possible alternative or additional explanation.

Several patients with C2 deficiency have had repeated life-threatening septicemic illnesses, especially those due to pneumococci. Most have not had problems with increased susceptibility to infection, presumably because of the protective function of the alternative pathway. A depression of factor B levels to about 50% of normal can occur in conjunction with C2 deficiency, however, and individuals with deficiency of both proteins might be at particular risk.

Since C3 can be activated by C142 or by the alternative pathway, a defect in the function of either pathway can be compensated, at least to some extent. Without C3, however, the chemotactic fragment from C5 is not generated, and opsonization of bacteria is inefficient. One would expect trouble from organisms that must be well opsonized in order to be cleared, and this has been the case; congenital absence of C3 has been associated with recurrent, severe pyogenic infections such as pneumococcal pneumonia and meningococcal meningitis. Some of the C3-deficient patients have had sluggish neutrophilic responses to infection, in agreement with reports that a cleavage factor of C3, C3e, elicits an increase in peripheral blood neutrophils.

The 1st patient found to have homozygous C5 deficiency was a girl who developed classic systemic lupus erythematosus in late childhood and had a life-long history of recurrent pyogenic infections, especially of the skin, presumably because of the absence of the critical chemotactic factor split from C5. Generation of chemotaxis by her serum in vitro was markedly depressed. Additional patients have had recurrent disseminated gonococcal infection or multiple episodes of meningococcal meningitis. Infants have been described with Leiner disease (generalized seborrheic dermatitis, severe diarrhea, and recurrent infections due to enteric bacteria and staphylococci) and dysfunction of C5 manifested by decreased opsonization of yeast by the patient's serum and by decreased generation of chemotactic activity. Sera from these infants had normal hemolytic complement activity, but purified C5 from 1 patient behaved abnormally in special studies of this component.

Over half of the approximately 20 individuals reported to have congenital C6 deficiency have had meningococcal meningitis or extragenital gonococcal infection. The combination of Sjögren syndrome, discoid lupus, and positive antinuclear antibody has occurred in a young man with C6 deficiency. Many of the individuals with deficiency of C7 or C8 also have had recurrent neisserial infections, and a boy with C8 dysfunction (absent function of C8 in spite of the presence of C8 protein) has had recurrent episodes of meningococcal meningitis or septicemia. It is not clear why patients with deficiency of 1 of the late-acting components suffer a particular predisposition to neisserial infections; one possibility would be that serum bacteriolysis is uniquely important in defense against this organism. Some individuals with such a deficiency have had no significant illness, however.

9.25 Deficiency of C3b Inactivator

Deficiency of C3b inactivator is a 2nd congenital abnormality of 1 of the regulatory proteins of complement that results in disease. This disorder was originally reported as a deficiency of C3 due to its hypercatabolism. The 1st patient described had suffered a series of severe pyogenic infections similar to those seen with agammaglobulinemia or congenital deficiency of C3. Further studies indicated that the primary deficiency was that of C3b inactivator, an essential regulator of the alternative pathway. This deficiency permits prolonged existence of C3b in the C3 convertase of the alternative pathway, C3bBb, resulting in constant activation of the alternative pathway and cleavage of more C3 to C3b, in circular fashion. Intravenous infusion of plasma or purified C3b inactivator induced a prompt rise in serum C3 concentration in the patient and a return to normal of C3-dependent in vitro functions such as opsonization.

9.26 SECONDARY DEFICIENCIES OF COMPLEMENT

Partial deficiency of C1q has occurred in patients with *severe combined immunodeficiency disease* or *hypogammaglobulinemia*, apparently secondary to the deficiency of IgG, which normally binds reversibly to C1q and prevents its rapid catabolism.

Serum from patients with *chronic membranoproliferative glomerulonephritis* contains a protein termed *nephritic factor* (NeF) that promotes activation of the alternative pathway. Nephritic factor appears to be an IgG antibody to the C3-cleaving enzyme of the alternative pathway that protects the enzyme from inactivation. The result is increased consumption of C3. Serum C3 concentrations vary widely from patient to patient, however. Pyogenic infections, including meningitis, may occur if serum C3 drops below about 10% of normal. This disorder has been diagnosed in children and adults with *partial lipodystrophy*. It is not known whether the lipodystrophy is a cause or a result of the NeF-C3 abnormality. An IgG nephritic factor that binds to and protects C42, the classical pathway C3 convertase, has been described in *acute postinfectious nephritis* and in *systemic lupus erythematosus*. The consumption of C3 that characterizes poststreptococcal nephritis and lupus could be due to this factor, to activation of complement by immune complexes, or to both.

Newborn infants are known to have mild to moderate deficiencies of most components of the classical pathway of complement and of factor B and properdin. Opsonization and generation of chemotactic activity in serum from full-term newborns can be markedly deficient through either the classical or the alternative pathway. Patients with *malnutrition, anorexia nervosa,* and severe *burns* also may have significant depletion of components and functional activity of complement. Although synthesis of components is depressed in these conditions, serum from some patients with malnutrition also appears to contain immune complexes which could accelerate depletion. On induction of therapy for *acute lymphoblastic leukemia*, supranormal levels of C3 and factor B fall to well below normal in about half of the cases, perhaps because of depressed synthesis. Severe chronic *cirrhosis of the liver* may also result in decreased synthesis of C3.

Individuals with *sickle cell disease* have normal activity of the classical pathway, but some have a defect in serum opsonization of pneumococci through the alternative pathway. Defects of alternative pathway activity in other test systems have also been reported, including bacteriolysis and opsonization of salmonellae and lysis of rabbit erythrocytes. Similar defects have been described in about 10% of individuals who have undergone *splenectomy* and in some patients with β-thalassemia major. The underlying mechanism for the defects in alternative pathway function in these disorders has not been fully defined. Children with *nephrotic syndrome* can have subnormal serum opsonizing activity in association with decreased serum levels of factor B.

Immune complexes, including those initiated by microorganisms or their byproducts, may induce consumption of components of complement. Activation occurs primarily through fixation of C1 to antibody and, thereby, initiation of the classical pathway. The immune complexes present in *systemic lupus erythematosus* activate the classical pathway, and C3 is deposited at sites of tissue damage, including kidneys and skin. Depressed synthesis of C3 is also seen in this disease. Formation of immune complexes and consumption of complement have been demonstrated in *lepromatous leprosy*, *subacute bacterial endocarditis*, *infected ventriculojugular shunts*, *malaria*, *infectious mononucleosis*, *dengue hemorrhagic fever*, and Australia antigen–positive *acute hepatitis*. Nephritis or arthritis may develop as a result of deposition of immune complexes and activation of complement in these infections. The syndrome of *recurrent urticaria, angioedema, eosinophilia, and hypocomplementemia* secondary to activation of the classical pathway may be due to circulating immune complexes, but this has not been proved. Circulating immune complexes and decreased C3 have been reported in some patients with *dermatitis herpetiformis, celiac disease*, and *Reye syndrome*.

In patients with *gram-negative shock*, endotoxin appears to initiate direct activation of the alternative pathway. *Intravenous injection of iodinated roentgenographic contrast medium* can induce a rapid and significant activation of the alternative pathway, which could explain at least some of the reactions that occur in 5–8% of individuals subjected to this procedure.

9.27 DIAGNOSIS OF DISORDERS OF THE COMPLEMENT SYSTEM

Testing for total hemolytic complement (CH_{50}) serves as a useful screening procedure for most of the diseases of the complement system. A normal result in this assay depends on the ability of all 9 classical pathway components to interact and lyse antibody-coated erythrocytes. The dilution of serum which lyses 50% of the cells determines the end point. In congenital deficiency of C1 through C8, the CH_{50} value will be about 0; in C9 deficiency, the value will be approximately half normal. Values in the acquired deficiencies will, of course, vary with the severity of the underlying disorder.

In hereditary angioedema, depression of C4 and C2 during an attack significantly reduces the CH_{50}. Serum concentrations of C4 and C3 can be determined by antibody precipitation in agar using commercially available radial immunodiffusion plates. In hereditary angioedema, C4 is characteristically low and C3 normal. Concentrations of C1 inhibitor can be determined with antibody, but a normal result can be anticipated in about 15% of cases (Sec 9.23). Since C1 acts as an esterase, the specific diagnosis can be made by showing increased capacity of patients' sera to hydrolyze synthetic esters.

Decreased serum concentrations of both C4 and C3 suggest activation of the classical pathway by immune complexes. In contrast, decreased C3 and normal C4 suggest activation of the alternative pathway. This difference is particularly useful in distinguishing nephritis secondary to complex deposition from that due to NeF (nephritic factor). In the latter condition and in deficiency of C3b inactivator, factor B is consumed, and its serum concentration is low as measured by radial immunodiffusion. Other assays of alternative pathway factors and functions currently are available only in specialized laboratories. A relatively simple and reproducible hemolytic assay depends on the capacity of rabbit erythrocytes to serve as both an "activating" (permissive) surface and a target of alternative pathway activity.

A defect of complement function should be suspected in any patient with collagen-vascular disease or with recurrent pyogenic infections, neisserial infections, or septicemia. The frequency with which complement disorders are being detected in such patients by an abnormality of the relatively simple hemolytic complement assay argues strongly that this procedure should be available as a screening test.

9.28 MANAGEMENT OF DISORDERS OF THE COMPLEMENT SYSTEM

Regular infusions of plasma have been an effective deterrent to infections in children with C5 dysfunction. Since these patients make C5 (though it is nonfunctional), they should not generate antibody that would nullify the effect of the infused C5 and perhaps induce anaphylaxis or a serum sickness reaction. The same argument might be invoked for the use of plasma infusions to treat the variant of the hereditary angioedema in which patients have nonfunctional C1 inhibitor. However, substrate for C1 (C4 and C2, the source of vasoactive kinin) would be infused along with normal C1 inhibitor and might precipitate or accentuate an attack. Specific therapy exists for adults with this disease in the form of danazol, a synthetic androgen with only weak virilizing and mild anabolic potential. The drug, given daily by mouth, increases the level of C1 inhibitor 3- to 4-fold and prevents attacks. It has not been recommended for use in children.

Only supportive management is available for other primary diseases of the complement system. Purified components are not obtainable for administration, and, if they were, the risk of inducing antibody to them probably would preclude their effective long-term use. It should be emphasized, however, that identification of a specific defect in the complement system could make an important difference to a patient's health. Certainly, concern for the associated complications (Table 9–9) would encourage more vigorous diagnostic efforts and earlier institution of therapy, including the obtaining of cultures and institution of antibiotic treatment with the onset of unexplained fever. Immunization of the patient and family members with bacterial capsular polysaccharides should also be considered. As defects are detected and carefully characterized, the likelihood of developing specific therapy of currently untreatable defects improves.

RICHARD B. JOHNSTON, JR.

Congenital Deficiencies

Altenburger KM, Johnston RB Jr: The complement system and its disorders in man. In: Chandra RK (ed): Immunodeficiency Disorders. Edinburgh, Churchill Livingstone, in press.
Berkel AI, Loos M, Sanal, Ö. et al: Clinical and immunologic studies in a case of selective complete C1q deficiency. Clin Exp Immunol 38:52, 1979.
Donaldson VH, Rosen FS: Hereditary angioneurotic edema: A clinical survey. Pediatrics 37:1017, 1966.

Hosea SW, Santaella ML, Brown EJ, et al: Long-term therapy of hereditary angioedema with danazol. Ann Intern Med 93:809, 1980.
Hyatt AC, Altenburger KM, Johnston RB Jr, et al: Increased susceptibility to severe pyogenic infections in patients with an inherited deficiency of the second component of complement. J Pediatr 98:417, 1981.
Lachmann PJ, Rosen FS: Genetic defects of complement in man. Semin Immunopathol 1:339, 1978.
Lee SL, Wallace SL, Barone R, et al: Familial deficiency of two subunits of the first component of complement: C1r and C1s associated with a lupus erythematosus–like disease. Arthritis Rheum 21:958, 1978.
Pussell BA, Bourke E, Nayef M, et al: Complement deficiency and nephritis: A report of a family. Lancet 1:675, 1980.
Thompson RA, Haeney M, Reid KBM, et al: A genetic defect of the C1q subcomponent of complement associated with childhood (immune complex) nephritis. N Engl J Med 303:22, 1980.

Secondary Deficiencies

Anderson DC, York TL, Rose G, et al: Assessment of serum factor B, serum opsonins, granulocyte chemotaxis, and infection in nephrotic syndrome of children. J Infect Dis 140:1, 1979.
Arroyave CM, Bhat KN, Crown R: Activation of the alternative pathway of the complement system by radiographic contrast media. J Immunol 117:1866, 1976.
Corry JM, Polhill RB Jr, Edmonds SR, et al: Activity of the alternative complement pathway after splenectomy: Comparison to activity in sickle cell disease and hypogammaglobulinemia. J Pediatr 95:964, 1979.
Day NK, Good RA. The complement system in human disease. In: Grieco MH (ed): Infections in the Abnormal Host. Yorke Medical Books USA, 1980, p 38.
Geha RS, Akl KF: Skin lesions, angioedema, eosinophilia, and hypocomplementemia. J Pediatr 89:724, 1976.
Halbwachs L, Leveillé M, Lesavre PH, et al: Nephritic factor of the classical pathway of complement: Immunoglobulin G autoantibody directed against the classical pathway C3 convertase enzyme. J Clin Invest 65:1249, 1980.
Johnston RB Jr, Alterburger KM, Atkinson AW Jr, et al: Complement in the newborn infant. Pediatrics 64:781, 1979.
Sissons JGP, West RJ, Fallows J, et al: The complement abnormalities of lipodystrophy. N Engl J Med 294:461, 1976.
Suskind R, Edelman R, Kulapongs P, et al: Complement activity in children with protein-calorie malnutrition. Am J Clin Nutr 29:1089, 1976.

The Phagocytic System and Associated Diseases

9.29 PHYSIOLOGY OF THE PHAGOCYTIC SYSTEM

The phagocyte system consists of sessile mononuclear cells and circulating polymorphonuclear and mononuclear leukocytes. Adequate numbers of properly functioning phagocytes are critically important for host defense against microbial disease.

Source and Storage of Phagocytes. Phagocytic leukocytes develop from pluripotent stem cells in the bone marrow. Leukocytes and erythrocytes are produced at nearly equal rates, but the shorter life of leukocytes (hours instead of months) results in the usual 2000:1 erythrocyte:leukocyte ratio in the peripheral circulation. Polymorphonuclear neutrophils are released into the circulation as highly differentiated mature phagocytes; monocytes are released as immature cells. Both cell types circulate in the bloodstream for a short time (4–10 hr) and migrate into tissues.

Mononuclear phagocytic cells develop into mature phagocytic cells (macrophages) in tissue with unique morphologic and metabolic characteristics depending on their resident organ system. Macrophages are found in the spleen, liver, lungs, lymph nodes, intestine, and central nervous system. Circulating mononuclear phagocytes also migrate into areas of inflammation, usually after infiltration by neutrophils, and are essential for "walling off" an infectious process and forming granulomas. Macrophages are the primary phagocytic cells in breast milk.

A large reserve of mature neutrophils is normally stored in the bone marrow and marginated in the circulation. Inflammation stimulates mobilization of these reserves and causes rapid multiplication of precursor cells and accelerated differentiation; enormous numbers of neutrophils are produced during acute infections. Circulating factors released from peripheral leukocytes appear to regulate production of phagocytic cells by the bone marrow.

Chemotaxis. Neutrophils and monocytes respond to inflammatory stimuli by adherence to capillary walls and by diapedesis into tissues. Once in tissue, phagocytic cells respond to inflammatory mediators and/or microbial factors by increased activity (chemokinesis) and unidirectional locomotion (chemotaxis). Chemotaxis involves perturbation of sequential segments of cell membrane with shifts in calcium concentration and change in surface charge; cytoplasmic contractile proteins, actin and myosin, polymerize into microfilaments, and the cells crawl toward the highest concentration of attractant. Once phagocytic cells reach a site of bacterial invasion, the invaders must be recognized as "non-self" and the complex process of phagocytosis begins.

Phagocytosis. Factors that prepare bacteria for phagocytosis are opsonins (primarily specific antibacterial antibodies and complement components) which neutralize antiphagocytic factors on bacterial surfaces and function as ligands binding bacteria to phagocytes. Phagocytic cells have membrane receptors for the Fc portion of antibodies and for activated fragments of complement; when recognition and attachment occur, contractile proteins are activated, and microbes or other particles are surrounded by pseudopods. When the phagocytic cell membrane completely surrounds the particle, a phagocytic vacuole is formed which migrates toward the nucleus; granular contents are contributed to the phagocytic vacuoles, and oxidative metabolism is stimulated.

Oxygen is consumed during phagocytosis and is univalently reduced to superoxide or divalently reduced to hydrogen peroxide. There is a shift of glucose metabolism to the hexose monophosphate pathway, and halides are oxidized. The rapid killing of most bacterial and fungal species requires the interaction of reactive oxygen molecules, myeloperoxidase (a constituent of cytoplasmic granules), and halides within phagocytic vacuoles. Critical factors required for this microbicidal activity are oxygen, reduced pyridine nucleotides, and oxidases. The presence of an intact oxidative response can be identified by either nitroblue tetrazolium reduction or chemiluminescence. Fig 9–4 represents the metabolic changes occurring in human polymorphonuclear neutrophils during phagocytosis.

DISEASES ASSOCIATED WITH DISORDERS OF THE PHAGOCYTES

9.30 Chronic Granulomatous Disease of Childhood

Chronic granulomatous disease (CGD) is a syndrome of recurrent bacterial or fungal infections associated with defective microbicidal capacity of the phagocytic cells and an abnormal oxidative metabolic response during phagocytosis. The morphology of the neutrophils and monocytes, as well as specific humoral and cell-mediated immunity, is normal.

Etiology. CGD occurs in both boys and girls; approximately 20% of reported patients are girls. There is clear evidence for X-linked inheritance in most boys with the disease, i.e., intermediate defects of neutrophil function are present in mothers and female relatives among whom 2 populations of neutrophils can be defined in peripheral blood after incubation with nitroblue tetrazolium (NBT). Although carrier females rarely suffer severe infections, several mothers of patients with CGD have had dermal infiltrates of lymphocytes similar to those seen in discoid lupus erythematosus.

The pattern of genetic transmission has not been identified in most female patients with CGD, although it has been suggested this might be an autosomal recessive disorder. Recent studies, however, using chemiluminescence as a measure of oxidative metabolism during phagocytosis suggest X-linked transmission in female as well as male patients with CGD. Markedly depressed neutrophil chemiluminescence (less than 2%

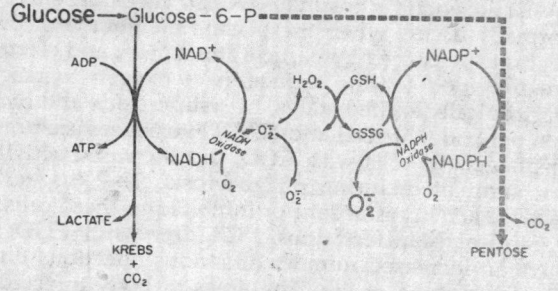

Microbicidal Metabolism of Phagocytes

Figure 9–4 Oxidative metabolic response during phagocytosis. Augmentation of hexose monophosphate shunt activity during phagocytosis is depicted by the heavy dashed line. Oxidase activity stimulated during phagocytosis results in oxygen uptake, and electrons from NADH and NADPH result in production of superoxide (O_2^-) and hydrogen peroxide (H_2O_2). These reactive oxygen radicals are associated with the microbicidal activity of phagocytic cells.

ADP = adenosine diphosphate, ATP = adenosine triphosphate, GSH = reduced glutathione, GSSG = oxidized glutathione, KREBS = Krebs cycle, NAD = oxidized nicotinamide adenine dinucleotide, NADH = reduced nicotinamide adenine dinucleotide, NADP = oxidized nicotinamide adenine dinucleotide phosphate, NADPH = reduced nicotinamide adenine dinucleotide phosphate.

of control) may be found in female patients, and their mothers and female relatives may have an intermediate chemiluminescence response during phagocytosis. Fathers and unaffected male siblings are always normal.

The Lyon hypothesis could explain X-linked transmission in females with CGD. Two distinct populations of neutrophils have been identified using the histochemical NBT dye reduction assay or autoradiographic technique for detection of bacterial iodination during phagocytosis in mothers of both male and female patients with CGD. Disproportionate inactivation of the normal X chromosome may result in a large population of defective phagocytic cells and clinical manifestations of CGD in females.

Certain patients with CGD lack Kell antigens on their erythrocytes (MacLeod phenotype), a condition making it exceedingly difficult to obtain compatible blood for transfusion; boys lack Kell antigen on their leukocytes, a deficiency suggesting that Kell antigens may be closely associated with membrane factors activating oxidative metabolism in phagocytic cells.

Pathogenesis. Attachment of bacteria and phagocytosis occurs normally in cells of patients with CGD, but the ingested microbes are not killed. Bacterial multiplication is inhibited, but intracellular bacteria survive and infections persist. Phagocytosis does not result in increased oxygen uptake, hexose monophosphate shunt activity, chemiluminescence, or generation of reactive oxygen radicals in neutrophils and monocytes of patients with the disease. When oxygen radicals are provided by ingested microbes that produce hydrogen peroxide (e.g., streptococci or pneumococci) or by particle-associated oxidases, the neutrophils kill bacteria at normal rates.

Defective oxidative metabolism and production of reactive oxygen radicals during phagocytosis are the essential defects in CGD. Stimulation of nicotinamide adenine dinucleotide (NADH) and nicotinamide adenine dinucleotide phosphate (NADPH) oxidase activity normally occurs when the plasma membrane of phagocytes is perturbed by particle attachment and electrons are provided for the reduction of oxygen to reactive electronically excited states, i.e., superoxide and hydrogen peroxide. NADH and NADPH oxidases are present in phagocytic cells with CGD, but increased activity is not stimulated during phagocytosis. The "trigger" of oxidase activity is absent or inhibited in these cells.

Clinical Manifestations. Children with CGD may have an increased number of serious infections during the 1st months of life. The areas of body infected are those constantly challenged with bacteria. Eczematoid lesions are frequently present around the nose and mouth, with development of purulent adenitis that requires surgical drainage. Hepatosplenomegaly is a nearly constant finding, staphylococcal abscesses of the liver occur with discouraging frequency, and osteomyelitis is common. The last of these may affect the small bones of the hands and feet as well as long bones. Gram-negative species such as *Serratia marcescens* are frequently found in bone lesions as well as in soft tissue abscesses; therefore, aggressive attempts to obtain material for culture are necessary to determine appropriate antibiotic treatment.

The infecting organisms include a variety of gram-positive and gram-negative bacteria. The predominant gram-positive organism is *Staphylococcus aureus; Serratia marcescens* and *Klebsiella* are frequent gram-negative organisms. Catalase-negative species, e.g., *S. pneumoniae*, *H. influenzae*, and streptococci, rarely cause serious infections in patients with CGD since these organisms produce hydrogen peroxide and are normally killed by the defective phagocytic cells.

Pneumonitis is frequent in patients with CGD. Lung infiltrates persist for several wk in spite of appropriate antibiotic therapy, and residual changes are visible on chest roentgenogram for many mo. Typical etiologic agents include *S. aureus* and gram-negative bacilli, but *Aspergillus fumigatus* has become an extremely serious problem in recent yr.

Granulomatous lesions or obstructive complications may involve any organ. Obstruction of the gastric antrum is frequent and must be considered if there is persistent vomiting in a patient with CGD. Biopsy material from the vicinity of abscesses or inflammatory lesions usually contains collections of macrophages with cytoplasmic lipoid material.

9.31 Chédiak-Higashi Syndrome

The Chédiak-Higashi syndrome (CHS) is an autosomal recessive disease characterized by recurrent infections, partial oculocutaneous albinism, photophobia, nystagmus, and neutrophils with giant cytoplasmic granules. The onset of symptoms usually occurs in early childhood, and death from infection or malignancy often results before the patient reaches 10 yr of age. The clinical course may be rapidly progressive in infancy, or it may be quiescent with recurrent minor infections until an "accelerated" phase later in childhood. Neurologic abnormalities include long tract and cerebellar involvement, peripheral neuropathies, and mental retardation.

Abnormal granules are found in the cytoplasm of all peripheral blood and bone marrow leukocytes, i.e., polymorphonuclear neutrophils, eosinophils, basophils, and monocytes. The abnormal granules contain both azurophilic and specific granular material such as lysosomal enzymes, peroxidase, and acid phosphates. Abnormal granules and inclusions are also observed in lymphocytes, erythrocytes, cultured skin fibroblasts, and platelets. As the disease progresses, anemia, thrombocytopenia, and absolute leukopenia frequently develop. At autopsy, widespread histiocytic infiltrations of almost all tissues of the body may be found. Histiocytes as well as neurons and renal tubular epithelium contain cytoplasmic inclusions. Neutrophils of patients with CHS are functionally abnormal, with defective chemotaxis, degranulation, and intracellular killing. The impaired chemotactic responsiveness has been demonstrated in vivo with Rebuck inflammatory skin window techniques and in vitro with the Boyden chamber assay.

The phagocytic rate of particle uptake and the ingestion capacity of leukocytes from patients with CHS are increased in relation to normal cells, and hexose monophosphate shunt activity (as measured by oxidation of $[1-^{14}C]$ glucose) is twice normal in both the resting and the phagocytizing state. Degranulation, however, is very abnormal since the giant lysosomes do not rupture into phagocytic vacuoles. Fifteen min after bacterial ingestion little peroxidase is found on the phagosomes. Unlike neutrophils from patients with CGD, cells from patients with CHS are significantly abnormal in intracellular killing of catalase-negative organisms (e.g., streptococci). Killing of *Escherichia coli* and *Candida albicans* by neutrophils from patients with CHS is abnormal during the 1st 20 min of incubation but returns to normal with longer incubation. The belief that degranulation and chemotaxis are dependent on intact microtubular function suggests that abnormal microtubular function may lead to defective function of the neutrophils. Microtubular function is regulated by the cyclic nucleotide guanosine 3':5'-cyclic phosphate (cyclic GMP), and cholinergic agents elevate intracellular cyclic GMP and enhance microtubule assembly in normal human neutrophils. These same agents improve the function of leukocytes from patients with CHS. Intraleukocytic concentrations of adenosine 3':5'-cyclic phosphate (cyclic AMP) may be markedly elevated in patients with CHS; an infant treated with ascorbic acid (200 mg/24 hr) had levels of cyclic AMP in the normal range and functionally normal neutrophils, but it is not known if such therapy will improve the long-term prognosis.

9.32 Myeloperoxidase Deficiency

The diagnosis of hereditary myeloperoxidase deficiency is based on the complete absence of peroxidase-positive granules on smears of neutrophils and monocytes stained histochemically for peroxidase. Eosinophil peroxidase is present in normal amounts. The metabolic response of myeloperoxidase-deficient neutrophils during phagocytosis is different from the response of neutrophils in individuals with CGD; there is normal or increased consumption of oxygen, oxidation of [1-^{14}C] glucose, production of superoxide anions, and reduction of NBT. All of these responses to phagocytosis are depressed in neutrophils from patients with CGD. The chemiluminescence response and killing of intracellular bacteria are initially depressed in myeloperoxidase deficient neutrophils during phagocytosis. Delayed bacterial killing does not appear to be a handicap to the defense of the host against bacterial infection, however, since patients with myeloperoxidase deficiency are not more susceptible to bacterial infections than are other individuals. In contrast, neutrophils from patients with congenital absence of myeloperoxidase cannot kill intracellular *C. albicans*; several patients with myeloperoxidase deficiency have had serious and prolonged candida infections.

9.33 Glucose-6-Phosphate Dehydrogenase (G-6PD) Deficiency

This deficiency is a relatively common, genetically determined error of metabolism that primarily affects erythrocyte function. Fortunately, profound deficiency (less than 5% of normal values) is quite rare, and only deficiency of this magnitude is associated with defective neutrophil function, phenotypically similar to that of CGD, such as recurrent infections and granulomatous lesions due to *S. aureus* or gram-negative bacteria. G-6PD activity is necessary for an increased hexose monophosphate shunt response during phagocytosis, which, in turn, is required for maintenance of adequate cellular levels of reduced pyridine nucleotide NADPH (the source of electrons for conversion of oxygen to superoxide) and for continued function of the glutathione system. Therefore, lack of substrate rather than lack of enzyme activity is the basis for defective respiratory metabolic response during phagocytosis in G-6PD deficient phagocytes.

9.34 Defective Glutathione System

This system plays an essential role in detoxifying the reactive oxygen metabolites that are formed in abundance during phagocytosis. Neutrophils from affected members of a family with neutrophil glutathione reductase deficiency had a normal initial burst of oxidative metabolism during phagocytosis, but after a few min there was an abrupt halt in metabolism and cell death. Further evidence for a protective role of glutathione was the observation that a patient with glutathione synthetase deficiency had neutropenia during infections; leukocytes accumulate large amounts of hydrogen peroxide, which damage the cells, and neutropenia is the result. Glutathione peroxidase deficiency has been described in several patients with CGD. Most patients with CGD, however, have normal glutathione peroxidase activity; therefore, patients with both CGD and

Table 9–10 DISORDERS OF BACTERICIDAL FUNCTION OF LEUKOCYTES

Chronic granulomatous disease	Bilobed nucleus and absent specific granules in neutrophils
Chédiak-Higashi syndrome	
Absent glucose-6-phosphate dehydrogenase	Myelogenous leukemia
	Down syndrome (tristomy 21)
Myeloperoxidase deficiency	Severe burn injury
Protein-calorie malnutrition	Overwhelming infection
Leukocyte alkaline phosphatase deficiency	Viral infection
	Cryoglobulinemia

glutathine peroxidase deficiency may have 2 separate metabolic abnormalities.

9.35 Transient Disorders of Leukocyte Bactericidal Function

These have been identified in patients with several clinical conditions (Table 9–10) such as overwhelming infection after severe burns or trauma. In these conditions there is a correlation between morphologic abnormalities of peripheral neutrophils and defective bactericidal function. Neutrophils which are vacuolated or contain toxic granules and Döhle bodies have defective bactericidal capacity. There is return to normal phagocytic function when patients recover clinically.

9.36 Defective Phagocytic Cell Chemotaxis

Abnormal locomotion of phagocytic cells has been identified in many patients with recurrent serious infections. Dysfunction may result from cellular defects, from inhibitors of chemotaxis in circulation, or from deficiency of chemotactic factors (Table 9–11). Abnormal locomotion of neutrophils may be the basis of neutropenia in certain patients. Patients with the so-called "lazy leukocyte syndrome" have normal neutrophils in the bone marrow, but they display abnormal random migration and chemotaxis. The defect appears to be in

Table 9–11 DISORDERS OF CHEMOTAXIS

Cellular defects	
Chédiak-Higashi syndrome	Kartagener syndrome
Panhypogammaglobulinemia	Anchor disease
Neutropenia	Shwachman syndrome
Hyperimmunoglobulin E	Microtubule abnormality
Hyperimmunoglobulin A	Ichthyosis
Chronic renal failure	Down syndrome (trisomy 21)
Acrodermatitis enteropathica	Measles
Mannosidosis	Severe eczema with
Leukemia	infections
Circulating inhibitors	
Wiskott-Aldrich syndrome	Periodontitis
Rheumatoid arthritis	Bone marrow transplant
Hodgkin disease	Cirrhosis
IgA myeloma	Felty syndrome
Chronic mucocutaneous candidiasis	
Deficient production of chemotactic factor	
Absent C5	Abnormal activation of C3
Hageman factor abnormality	Immunoglobulin deficiency
Systemic lupus erythematosus	

the capacity for locomotion from the bone marrow into the circulation. Clinical manifestations include stomatitis and skin and upper respiratory infections.

HYPERIMMUNOGLOBULIN E RECURRENT INFECTION (JOB) SYNDROME

A clinical syndrome characterized by unusual susceptibility to serious staphylococcal disease, chronic skin lesions similar to eczema, and "cold" abscesses was reported in 1966 as "Job syndrome." Several years later 2 boys with chronic dermatitis and recurrent severe lung, skin, and joint abscesses primarily due to staphylococci were found to have extremely elevated levels of IgE, suggesting a possible association between dermatitis, extremely elevated levels of IgE, and susceptibility to severe staphylococcal infection. Many, but not all, patients with very elevated levels of immunoglobulin E and recurrent infection have depressed chemotaxis of neutrophils and monocytes. Typically these patients have recurrent severe staphylococcal infections, cellulitis, subcutaneous abscesses, and deep muscle abscesses.

Patients with hyperimmunoglobulin E syndrome frequently have red hair, but the clinical association of recurrent severe staphylococcal infections, defective phagocytic cell chemotaxis, and hyperimmunoglobulin E occurs in males and females, adults and children, and persons of all hair colors. While there appears to be little association between defective chemotaxis and eczema or atopic dermatitis per se, this abnormality of phagocyte function is associated with hyperimmunoglobulin E and recurrent severe infections. Abnormal neutrophil and monocyte chemotaxis is highly variable in patients with hyperimmunoglobulin E syndrome; neutrophil chemotactic responsiveness may be low, slightly depressed, or normal. Material from lesions in patients with the hyperimmunoglobulin E recurrent infection syndrome does contain neutrophils; however, delay in accumulation of phagocytic cells may be related to pathogenesis of lesions. Patients generally develop severe bacterial infections during the 1st months of life, and pulmonary lesions are especially serious since pneumatoceles develop. Surgical removal of affected lung tissue has been a frequent necessity. A genetic basis for this disease is suggested since recurrent infections and extremely elevated levels of IgE have been identified in several family members.

Patients with hyperimmunoglobulin E recurrent infection syndrome have antibodies to *Staphylococcus aureus* of the IgE class in their sera; indeed, IgE antibodies to bacterial antigens were first demonstrated in these patients. Microbial species other than *Staphylococcus aureus* may be associated with serious infections. That cryptococcal meningitis and *Pneumocystis carinii* pneumonia have been diagnosed in patients with extremely elevated levels of IgE suggests an underlying defect in cell-mediated immunity.

9.37 OTHER DISORDERS OF LEUKOCYTE LOCOMOTION

Patients with Kartagener syndrome (Sec 13.28) have abnormal ciliary function of the respiratory tract, are highly susceptible to recurrent sinusitis and lower respiratory infections, and often demonstrate abnormal neutrophil chemotaxis. Abnormal respiratory tract ciliary function and chemotaxis may also be found in patients without Kartagener syndrome, but abnormal cilia suggest that neutrophil locomotion and ciliary activity have a common physiologic basis. Abnormal neutrophil chemotaxis and phagocytosis have been described in infants with delayed separation of the umbilical cord and recurrent serious bacterial infections and in a patient with defective neutrophil adherence (Anchor disease) (Table 9–11).

Patients with Shwachman syndrome (Sec 11.78) have pancreatic insufficiency and metaphyseal chondroplasia and are susceptible to recurrent infections and depressed neutrophil chemotaxis. Parents as well as patients have abnormal chemotaxis; therefore, neutrophil dysfunction, like other features of Shwachman syndrome, may be inherited as a recessive characteristic.

9.38 TRANSIENT DISORDERS OF NEUTROPHIL LOCOMOTION

Transient disorders of neutrophil chemotactic responsiveness have been reported in several clinical conditions (Table 9–11). For example, depressed neutrophil locomotion was found in children with measles, but it returned to normal with resolution of the rash and clinical improvement. Chemotaxis may be abnormal in bone marrow transplant recipients during graft-versus-host reactions, and transient chemotactic disorders are present in patients with overwhelming bacterial infections. Children with severe protein-calorie malnutrition have depressed neutrophil chemotaxis and increased susceptibility to bacterial, fungal, and viral infections. Since these children have decreased antibody production, decreased cell-mediated immunity, low levels of complement components, and defective intraleukocyte killing of bacteria and fungi, they have several reasons for increased susceptibility to infections.

9.39   Inhibitors of Chemotaxis

The clinical presentation in patients with cellular defects of neutrophilic chemotaxis and in patients with circulating inhibitors of chemotaxis is similar, i.e., recurrent severe infections of the skin and lower respiratory tract. Polymeric IgA may be a chemotactic inhibitor since a circulating inhibitor of chemotaxis has been identified in several patients with increased levels of IgA. This immunoglobulin is cytophilic for neutrophils. Other plasma factors also inhibit chemotaxis and have been identified in diverse clinical conditions (Table 9–11). For example, patients with Wiskott-Aldrich syndrome have high circulating levels of lymphocyte-derived chemotactic factors which inhibit chemotactic responsiveness of neutrophils and monocytes. Physiologic inhibitors of chemotaxis are present in normal plasma, and the levels of these normally occurring plasma proteins may be elevated in certain conditions such as Hodgkin disease. Increased levels of circulating chemotactic factor inhibitors may also contribute to the lack of delayed-type hypersensitivity in certain conditions such as cirrhosis or sarcoidosis. Monocytes may be prevented from migrating to the site of skin test antigen as a result of circulating inhibitors, thereby preventing a delayed-type hypersensitivity response in spite of normal recognition of antigen.

9.40 Deficiency of Chemotactic Factors

The absence of potential chemotactic factors can result in abnormal chemotaxis. Since most of the well-characterized chemotactic factors are components of the complement system, it is not surprising that patients with deficient or abnormal function of complement have chemotactic abnormalities. These include absence of C3 and C5 and hypercatabolism of C3. There are frequent serious infections of multiple organ systems with encapsulated gram-positive and gram-negative bacteria in patients with abnormalities of complement. Depressed immunoglobulin as well as deficient complement results in abnormal chemotaxis since the generation of biologically active factors from complement requires the participation of immunoglobulin.

Chemotactically active C3 and C5 fragments of complement are produced via the alternative complement pathway as well as the classical pathway. Therefore, patients with deficient early components of complement (C1, C4, C2) do not have unusually severe or recurrent microbial infections. Patients with C5 deficiency, however, have serious chronic infections which respond poorly to antimicrobial therapy. Plasma from patients with C5 deficiency has normal opsonic function (since C3 is the primary source of complement-related opsonic activity) but nearly absent chemotactic activity (Sec 9.21).

9.41 Treatment of Diseases Associated with Disorders of the Phagocytes

The identification of defective intracellular bacterial killing in phagocytic cells from patients with CGD has resulted in improved therapy of patients with disorders of the phagocytic system. Patients are highly susceptible to recurrent serious lesions of soft tissues and bones caused by staphylococci, gram-negative aerobes, and fungi. The diversity of microbial agents that cause severe disease in these patients makes prevention difficult, and every effort must be made to identify infectious microorganisms. Early, aggressive, and prolonged antimicrobial therapy is necessary for treatment. Surgical intervention is often required for abscesses developing in patients with phagocyte dysfunction. The presence of "saprophytic" or "poorly virulent" organisms in lesions is as serious as that of highly pathogenic species in these patients.

Patients with defective chemotaxis associated with underlying systemic illnesses often demonstrate improved resistance to infection when the underlying disorder is corrected. For example, when eczematoid skin lesions are improved, there is less danger of deep abscesses. Recovery of phagocytic cell function often coincides with clinical recovery in patients with severe eczema, trauma, or overwhelming infection.

Transfusion of leukocytes from normal donors may be used as adjunct therapy when life-threatening infections do not respond to antibiotic therapy in patients with CGD and other disorders of the phagocytic cells. The successful replacement of myelocytic precursor cells with bone marrow from HLA- and mixed lymphocyte-identical normal donors has the theoretic capacity to cure patients with disorders of phagocytic cells.

Chronic anemia is common in CGD, but blood transfusions may be hazardous because these patients possess a very rare red cell genotype of the Kell system called K_0. Transfusion almost inevitably leads to isoimmunization.

PAUL G. QUIE

Chemotaxis

Gallin JI, Quie PG (eds): Leukocyte Chemotaxis: Methods, Physiology, and Clinical Implications. New York, Raven Press, 1978.

Gallin JI, Wright DG, Malech HL, et al: Disorders of chemotaxis. Ann Intern Med 92:520, 1980.

Hill HR, Quie PG: Raised serum IgE levels and defective neutrophil chemotaxis in three children with eczema and recurrent bacterial infections. Lancet 1:183, 1974.

Schopfer K, Boeriocher K, Price P, et al: Staphylococcal IgE antibodies, hyperimmunoglobulin E and staphylococcus infection. N Engl J Med 300:835, 1979.

Snyderman R, Pike MC: Disorders of leukocyte chemotaxis. Pediatr Clin North Am 24:377, 1977.

Phagocytic Cell Function

Babior BM: Oxygen-dependent microbial killing by phagocytes. N Engl J Med 298:659, 1978.

Cohn ZA, Morse SI: Functional and metabolic properties of polymorphonuclear leukocytes. I. Observations on the requirements and consequences of particle ingestion. J Exp Med 111:667, 1960.

Klebanoff SJ, Clark RA (eds): The Neutrophil: Function and Clinical Disorders. North Holland, 1978.

Stossel TP: Phagocytosis. N Engl J Med 290:774, 1974.

Chronic Granulomatous Disease

Johnston RB Jr, Baehner RL: Chronic granulomatous disease: Correlation between pathogenesis and clinical findings. Pediatrics 48:730, 1971.

Mills EL, Rholl KS, Quie PG: X-linked inheritance in females with chronic granulomatous disease. J Clin Invest 66:332, 1980.

Quie PG, White JG, Holmes B, et al: In vitro bactericidal capacity of human polymorphonuclear leukocytes: Diminished activity in chronic granulomatous disease of childhood. J Clin Invest 46:668, 1967.

Quie PG, Davis AT: Disorders of the polymorphonuclear phagocytic system. In: Stiehm ER, Fulginiti V (eds): Immunologic Disorders in Infants and Children. Ed 2. Philadelphia, WB Saunders, 1980, p 349.

Chédiak-Higashi Syndrome

Blume RS, Wolff SM: The Chédiak-Higashi syndrome. Studies in four patients and a review of the literature. Medicine 51:247, 1972.

Boxer LA, Watanabe AM, Rister M, et al: Correction of leukocyte function in Chédiak-Higashi syndrome by ascorbate. N Engl J Med 295:1041, 1976.

Other Disorders

Eliasson R, Mossberg B, Camner P, et al: The immobile cilia syndrome: A congenital ciliary abnormality as an etiologic factor in chronic airway infections and male sterility. N Engl J Med 297:1, 1977.

Hayward AR, Leonard J, Wood CBS, et al: Delayed separation of the umbilical cord, widespread infections, and defective neutrophil mobility. Lancet 1:1099, 1979.

ALLERGIC DISORDERS

Allergic disorders are adverse physiologic reactions resulting from the interaction of antigen with humoral antibody and/or lymphoid cells. This definition precludes the use of the term allergy for disorders in which immunologic mechanisms have not been demonstrated. For example, adverse reactions following food or drug ingestion in some individuals may resemble typical allergic reactions, but there is frequently no evidence of an immunologic basis. In some instances a biochemical basis for the reaction can be identified, as in diarrhea following milk ingestion in individuals with disaccharidase deficiency. When there is no reason to suspect that allergy is responsible for signs or symptoms, the use of immunologic methods in diagnosis or treatment has no rational basis.

Use of the term allergy to designate only those reactions involving humoral antibody or cellular immune responses and occurring in a host sensitized by prior exposure to the antigen perhaps imposes an unintended restriction on the term. Von Pirquet coined the word to refer to a "state of changed reactivity" in a host occurring as a result of contact with a foreign substance. This altered reactivity could be either beneficial to the host, as in the case of immunity, or detrimental, as in anaphylaxis. In modern usage allergy refers only to the adverse consequences.

The terms antigen and allergen are often used interchangeably, but not all antigens are good allergens or vice versa. For example, tetanus and diphtheria toxoids are excellent antigens but are only rarely responsible for adverse reactions. On the other hand, ragweed pollen protein, one of the most potent allergens, is not a particularly potent antigen by immunologic criteria. Most naturally occurring allergens share several common characteristics. They are protein in part, are acidic with isoelectric points between 2–5.5, and have molecular weights of 10,000–70,000 daltons. Molecules smaller than 10,000 daltons would be unable to bridge adjacent IgE antibody molecules, a requirement necessary for mediator release. Molecules larger than 70,000 daltons would encounter difficulties in traversing mucosal surfaces and reaching IgE-forming plasma cells.

"Atopy" and "atopic" refer to certain allergic diseases. Atopy may be viewed as an abnormality with the following characteristics: (1) a *hereditary factor* expressed in a high incidence of hay fever, asthma, and *atopic* eczema in the families of affected individuals; (2) *eosinophilia* of the blood and tissue secretions; (3) a predisposition to *selective synthesis of IgE antibody* on exposure to environmental substances; (4) a *hyperreactivity of the airways in asthmatics* upon exposure to various environmental factors (cold air, irritant odors) and to certain endogenous body chemicals (acetylcholine, histamine), and/or *hyperreactivity of the skin in eczema* to certain physical and chemical factors (stroking, acetylcholine); and (5) evidence of beta-adrenergic hyporesponsiveness and cholinergic hyperreactivity. The former is manifested as diminished response to the cardiovascular effects of infused isoproterenol and the latter as increased response to cholinergic stimulation

of the pupillary sphincter muscle or the eccrine sweat apparatus.

The tendency to form IgE antibodies is revealed in atopic persons by "wheal and flare" reactions upon skin testing with allergenic extracts. However, the capacity to form IgE antibody is not limited to atopic individuals as IgE is found in the serum and on mast cells of virtually all normal individuals. Under intense allergen exposure, as in certain occupations, or in response to particular allergens, such as ascaris, nonatopic individuals may form large quantities of allergen-specific IgE antibodies. Atopic persons, however, form IgE antibodies on exposure to such common environmental substances as pollens and house dust, and this distinguishes them from the nonatopic. The cause of increased production of reaginic IgE has not been identified; atopic individuals may have a diminished capacity to dampen selectively the IgE antibody responses, although some evidence suggests that atopic and normal persons differ in the disposition of antigens coming in contact with mucosal surfaces.

The above characteristics of atopy vary in degree among individuals with asthma, hay fever, or eczema; they are rarely fully expressed by persons not afflicted with atopic disorders.

9.42 IMMUNOLOGIC BASIS OF ATOPIC DISEASE

The lymphoid system has a primary role in immunity to infections and in the elimination of malignant cells. Paradoxically, the same system is responsible for a broad spectrum of diseases and much chronic illness, ranging from relatively mild conditions like ragweed hay fever to such serious disorders as disseminated lupus erythematosus. Attempts to modulate the deleterious effects resulting from antigen-antibody or antigen-lymphocyte interaction by immunosuppression of the lymphoid system may result in serious infections or in the development of malignancy.

Allergic reactions in man result from a complex concatenation of factors. Tissue injury may be completely reversible or produce permanent pathologic change. The extent of tissue damage depends upon both the character of the antigen and the target organs involved, but perhaps most important may be the nature and degree of involvement of various components of the immune system, which include circulating antibodies, lymphoid and other hematopoietic cells, the complement system of proteins, and a wide variety of physiologically active molecules generated or released as a result of interactions of antigen with antibodies or lymphoid cells.

It is useful to attempt to characterize immunologic reactions in terms of the reactants involved in order to appreciate the mechanism by which injury occurs (Gell and Coombs classification). Immunologically mediated tissue injury may occur as a result of the interaction of humoral antibody with antigen or of the interaction of antigen with lymphocytes (cell-mediated or delayed hypersensitivity). Humoral antibody-antigen reactions are recognized in 3 forms, 2 of which occur on the surface of cells and the 3rd in the extracellular fluids. Of the 2 reactions occurring on the surface of the cells, the type mediated by IgE (immediate or anaphylactic) is of greatest interest to the allergist. In this circumstance, circulating basophils and tissue mast cells, the latter strategically located around blood vessels, become "sensitized" through the binding of IgE antibodies to surface receptors. Although this scheme is reasonable to describe the initial triggering event in production of immune tissue injury, a broad spectrum of secondary events involving various types of lymphoid cells, inflammatory cells, mediator-producing cells, and the soluble products derived not only from all of these cells but from other tissues (platelets, endothelial cells) at the site of the reaction as well influences the ultimate outcome of the reaction. For example, histamine, a major mediator of IgE-dependent reactions in addition to its many important effects on smooth muscle and endothelial cells, also affects other inflammatory cells (chemotaxis), lymphocytes (inhibition of T cell responses), the generation of prostaglandins, and cyclic nucleotide metabolism. Basophils and mast cells, principal reactants in IgE-mediated disorders, also play a role in the various forms of delayed-type hypersensitivity responses such as cutaneous basophil hypersensitivity (Jones-Mote reaction). To complete the circle, a subpopulation of T lymphocytes produces a lymphokine that modulates basophil and mast cell activities.

The terms reaginic IgE, IgE reagins, and homocytotropic antibodies refer to molecules with activities against specific allergens, such as ragweed pollen, whereas "nonspecific" IgE molecules are found in the serum and tissues of all normal individuals. The "normal" role of IgE antibody appears to be defending the host against tissue-invasive parasites. In man the ability to induce antigen-specific release of mediators from mast cells and basophils is principally confined to antibodies of the IgE class.

IgE antibodies, like IgA antibodies, are synthesized by plasma cells located predominantly under mucosal surfaces and particularly in the respiratory and gastrointestinal tracts. IgE-forming plasma cells arise following antigen-stimulated differentiation of B cells or their precursors. Antigen also reacts with several subpopulations of T cells to generate (1) suppressor cells which inhibit IgE synthesis by antigen-stimulated B cells and (2) helper cells which augment IgE production by B cells. IgE production is also modulated by antigen-nonspecific suppressor T cells and by serum-suppressive molecules which have yet to be fully characterized.

Various chemical modifications of antigens used in immunotherapy of allergic diseases have been documented to suppress IgE responses (Sec 9.47). While the control of IgE antibody production has been largely worked out in experimental animals, there is good reason to believe that similar mechanisms occur in the human. The association of IgE responses with HLA-linked Ir genes has been shown with several allergens (ragweed antigen Ra3 and HLA-A2, ragweed antigen Ra5 and HLA-B7, rye grass antigen I and HLA-B8). Once formed, IgE antibody has the unique property of

becoming reversibly bound or "fixed" to surface receptors of mast cells and basophils, which in the human number from 40,000–100,000 and are of very high binding affinity. The binding of IgE to its receptor involves the C_H4 and C_H3 domains of the Fc portion of the immunoglobulin molecule. In nonatopic individuals, only 20–50% of the receptors are occupied by IgE molecules. Atopic individuals with high serum IgE concentrations have a larger percentage, up to almost 100%, of their basophil and mast cell receptors occupied by IgE. Once binding of IgE occurs, the basophils and mast cells may be considered "sensitized," and upon subsequent contact with antigen specific for the bound IgE, a sequence of biochemical reactions occurs resulting in release of pharmacologically active substances (such as histamine), which are known as chemical mediators. The released mediators act on tissue receptors to cause symptoms in the patient. The reaction is largely reversible; the mast cells and basophils participating in the reaction are not lysed, and the effects of mediators are only temporary. Though aggregated IgE can fix late components of the complement system through an alternative pathway, participation of the complement system in IgE-mediated hypersensitivity disorders has not been shown.

The usual tests for inhalant or food sensitivity make use of the reaction that occurs on the surface of mast cells between antigen and IgE antibody. Small amounts of extracts of pollens, molds, danders, and foods are introduced into the patient's skin by scratch, puncture, or intradermal techniques. If IgE antibody specific for the test antigen is bound to the subject's mast cells, the interaction of injected antigen with cell-bound IgE will release histamine, a potent vasoactive material that causes increased capillary permeability and dilatation and axon reflex stimulation, leading to the familiar wheal and flare reaction. The prototypic anaphylactic or IgE-mediated disease is ragweed hay fever.

In the 2nd type of interaction between antigen and antibody at cell surfaces, IgG or IgM immunoglobulins react with antigenic determinants* that either are an integral part of the cell membrane or have become adsorbed to or incorporated in the membrane. In contrast to the IgE or anaphylactic type of reaction, this 2nd kind activates the complement system in most instances, and the involved cell is destroyed. An example of this type of immunologic injury occurs when incompatible red blood cells are transfused. The recipient's isohemagglutinins (antibodies directed against determinants on the surface of the red cells) react with the incompatible cells, the complement system is activated, and sequential action of complement proteins leads to lysis of the cell. Analogous immune injury may involve platelets or leukocytes and is sometimes induced by drugs.

The 3rd immunopathologic mechanism of tissue injury

---

*An antigenic determinant is a restricted portion of an antigen molecule that determines the specificity of an antigen-antibody reaction. Antigenic determinants may consist of only 4 or 5 amino acid residues. In complex antigens found in nature, such as pollens, there may be several hundred determinants on the surface of an antigen molecule, each capable of initiating immune responses and reacting with specific antibody.

involving humoral antibody and antigen does not occur on the surface of cells but in the extracellular spaces. At certain ratios of antigen to antibody, antigen-antibody complexes are formed which are "toxic" to tissues in which they are deposited. For example, complexes may lodge in the filtering organs of the body such as the kidney and lung or infiltrate the walls of small blood vessels, activating the complement cascade. There is release of biologically active substances, including factors that are chemotactic for polymorphonuclear (PMN) leukocytes, which are attracted to the site. With phagocytosis of the complexes, the polymorphonuclear leukocytes are lysed, and basic proteins and proteolytic enzymes are released which damage tissue. Immune complex disease is responsible for up to 90% of immunologic glomerulonephritis in man.

Toxic complex injury involves cooperation between different antibodies in the production of tissue injury. The deposition of immune complexes containing IgG_1, IgG_2, IgG_3, and IgM in small blood vessels in the kidney in experimental serum sickness in animals depends on an increase in the permeability of these vessels. This is brought about by histamine liberated in the course of a simultaneous interaction of IgE antibody and antigen which leads to "leakiness" of the capillaries and prepares them to receive the toxic complexes. Such deposition can be largely prevented by pretreatment with antihistamine drugs in the animal model.

In *cell-mediated or delayed hypersensitivity* pathologic changes occur following interaction of antigen with T lymphocytes of at least 2 of the 5 presently identified functional subclasses (helper cells, suppressor cells, amplifier cells, cytotoxic cells, and lymphokine-producing cells). While the basis for the tissue injury in classic cell-mediated immune reactions is not completely understood, it is clear that macrophages and cytotoxic cells play a major role. Both basophils and eosinophils are involved in the evolution of delayed-type hypersensitivity reactions, and they and the inflammatory cells that they attract may also contribute to the tissue injury observed. Contact allergy (poison ivy, chemical-induced contact dermatitis) is the prototypic delayed-type hypersensitivity-mediated allergic disease. Contact reactions in the human are typically infiltrated with basophils and hence represent a subtype of cutaneous basophil hypersensitivity. Drug reactions with involvement of liver, lung, and kidney may be further examples of T cell–mediated disease. Cell-mediated immunity is also involved in certain of the infiltrative hypersensitivity lung diseases in which granuloma formation is a pathologic feature.

9.43 CHEMICAL MEDIATORS OF ALLERGIC REACTIONS AND MECHANISMS OF RELEASE

The critical triggering event in mast cell degranulation and release of chemical mediators of allergic injury is the cross-linking of receptor-bound IgE antibodies (which may be viewed as an extension of the receptor) by multivalent specific antigen. Although antigen is usually the principal factor in causing the approximation of IgE receptors, this can be accomplished in the absence of antigen or even of IgE antibody, e.g., by purified antibody to the IgE receptor itself. Other stimuli can also cause mast cell activation without involvement of antigen and cell-bound IgE. These include products of activation of the complement system (C3a, C5a), kinins, neutrophil-derived lysosomal basic proteins, and a lymphokine. Whatever the nature of the mast cell surface signal that acts as the degranulation stimulus, a series of biochemical reactions takes place that results in granule discharge. Activation of a serine esterase, utilization of intracellular energy stores, calcium influx or remobilization of intracellular calcium, changes in the mast cell cytoskeleton such as polymerization of microtubules, and activation of actinomycin fibrils have all been observed during mediator release. Recent studies have shown that changes in membrane phospholipid metabolism occur, including methylation and activation of phospholipases and generation of phospholipid byproducts, which participate in the fusion of the mast cell granules with the cell membrane, leading to extrusion of the granules. Once discharged from the mast cell, the granules, which are relatively water insoluble, remain intact for hours. The preformed mediators, such as histamine, ECF-A, and other chemotactic factors, are rapidly eluted from the granule matrix and act immediately on local tissues—smooth muscles and endothelial cells in blood vessels. Another set of mediators which are preformed but granule associated, e.g., heparin, arylsulfatase, enzymes such as trypsin and chymotrypsin, and inflammatory factors, is thought to be responsible for the late phase reaction; these mediators express their activity either while part of the intact granule or only after the granule begins to dissolve. A further set of mediators which are generated by the action of the primary mediators upon target tissue, e.g., histamine stimulation of H_1 receptor sites to initiate prostaglandin synthesis, also has important biologic activities. The properties of the various mediators are listed in Table 9–12.

The relationship of changes in cyclic nucleotides (cAMP and cGMP) to the process of mast cell activation-secretion is basic to understanding the mechanism of drug action in IgE-mediated disorders. In vitro studies based upon intervention with pharmacologic agents (catecholamines, theophylline, etc.) suggest that mast cell mediator release is dependent upon a fall in intracellular cAMP, a rise in cGMP, or both. Other studies suggest that there are separate pools of cAMP which may be increased by pharmacologic agents independently but only one of which impedes the coupled activation-secretion process.

Non-Mast-Cell–Derived Factors Which Participate in Immediate-Type Hypersensitivity Diseases

Kinins are a system of proteins activated in inflammatory processes which have amplifier and effector properties. Their activities include chemotaxis, in-

Table 9–12 MAST CELL PRODUCTS

MEDIATOR	STRUCTURAL CHARACTERISTICS	FUNCTION/ACTIVITIES
I. Predominant smooth muscle contracting and vasoactive activities		
Histamine (preformed)	5-β-Imidazolylethylamine MW 111	H₁: Increased venular permeability Contraction of smooth muscle Increase in cyclic GMP levels Generation of prostaglandins Positive chemokinetic effect on neutrophils and eosinophils* Positive chemotactic effect on neutrophils and eosinophils Bronchial irritant receptor stimulation Pruritus H₂: Positive chemokinetic effect on neutrophils and eosinophils* Negative chemotactic effect on neutrophils and eosinophils Inhibition of T-cell responses Inhibition of basophil (not mast cell) mediator release Augmentation of gastric acid secretion Stimulation of mucus secretion Increase in cyclic AMP Increase in chronotropic and inotropic effects on heart
SRS-A† (newly formed)	Leukotrienes (LTC₄, LTD₄, LTE₄) (lipoxygenase-dependent derivatives of arachidonic acid) MW 400	Bronchoconstriction, particularly of peripheral airways Vasoconstriction (LTC₄) Vasoconstriction (LTD₄)
PAF's (newly formed)	AGEPC‡ MW 551 (hexadecyl) MW 523 (octadecyl)	Aggregation of platelets and secretion of amines Neutrophil aggregation and enzyme release Production of prostaglandins and thromboxanes by platelets Increase in vascular permeability Mimics physiologic and intravascular sequelae of IgE-mediated human systemic anaphylaxis
PGI₂ (prostacyclin)† (newly formed)		Stimulates adenylate cyclase Vasodilatation Platelet anti-aggregation Pulmonary vasodilator
PGD₂ (newly formed)		Stimulates adenylate cyclase Bronchoconstriction Peripheral vasodilatation ? Central vasoconstriction Stimulates granulocyte chemokinesis Bronchoconstriction
PGF₂α† (newly formed) PGE₂† (newly formed)	Products of oxidative metabolism of arachidonic acid via cyclo-oxygenase pathway	Stimulates adenylate cyclase Bronchodilatation Inhibits macrophage spreading and adherence
TₓA₂ (thromboxane A₂) (newly formed)		Bronchoconstriction Vasoconstriction Platelet aggregation
II. Predominant chemotactic activities		
ECF-A-tetrapeptides (preformed)	Val/Ala-Gly-Ser-Glu MW 360–390	Chemotactic attraction and deactivation of eosinophils and neutrophils
ECF-oligopeptides (preformed)	Peptides MW 1500–3000	Chemotactic attraction and deactivation of eosinophils and neutrophils
HMW-NCF (preformed)	Neutral protein MW >750,000	Chemotactic attraction and deactivation of neutrophils
Lipid-derived factors (newly generated via lipoxygenase pathway of arachidonic acid metabolism)	Hydroxy-eicosa-tetraenoic acids (HETE's) Hydroxy-hepta-decatrienoic acid (HHT) MW 300–400 LTB₄	Chemotactic attraction and deactivation of eosinophils and neutrophils Chemokinesis

Table continued on following page

Table 9–12   MAST CELL PRODUCTS Continued

MEDIATOR	STRUCTURAL CHARACTERISTICS	FUNCTION/ACTIVITIES
III. Enzymes§		
Chymase (preformed)	Protein MW 25,000	Proteolysis of chymotrypsin substrates
Arylsulfatases (preformed)	Protein A MW 100,000 B MW 60,000	Inactivates SRS-A
N-Acetyl-β-D-glucosaminidase (preformed)	Protein MW 150,000	Cleavage of glycosaminoglycans
β-Glucuronidase (preformed)	Protein MW 300,000	Cleavage of glucuronide Residues
β-D-Galactosidase (preformed)	Protein	Cleavage of galactoside Residues
Basophil lung kallikrein of anaphylaxis (preformed)	Protein MW ~400,000	Proteolysis with tryptic activity Cleavage of Hageman factor Cleavage of kinin from kininogen
IV. Structural components		
Heparin (preformed)	Acidic proteoglycan MW 60,000 (human)	Anticoagulation (anti-thrombin III binding activity) Anti-complementary activity (at several sites) Augmentation of inactivation of histamine

*Chemotactic migration requires a concentration gradient from the stimulus side. Movement in the absence of a gradient of the stimulus is termed "positive chemokinesis."

†Although strictly speaking these arachidonic acid products are not mast cell products in the same sense as histamine, they are generated during allergic inflammatory reactions by various tissues (PMN's, endothelial cells, platelets).

‡AGEPC = 0-1-hectadecyl/octadecyl-2-acetyl-sn-glyceryl-3-phosphorylcholine.

§Not all of these enzymes have been identified in the human; however, known analogues exist.

creased vascular permeability, and smooth muscle contraction. Bradykinin, a nonapeptide (molecular weight 106), is the most important product of the kinin system. The kinin, complement, and clotting systems are interrelated. Activation of the Hageman factor (Factor XII) is the initial step in kinin generation and amplification, and positive feedback loops occur which resemble those in the complement pathway. The Hageman factor is activated by a tissue injury and a number of agents, including IgG aggregates or immune complexes. Hageman factor and complexes of high molecular weight kininogen and prekallikrein and high molecular weight kininogen and factor XI are bound. Hageman factor appears to autoactivate to form activated Hageman factor (HF_a) which converts prekallikrein to kallikrein. Kallikrein digests high molecular weight kininogen to liberate the vasoactive peptide bradykinin. Bradykinin has potent contractile effects on smooth muscle, causes increased vascular permeability, and dilates peripheral arterioles. It also stimulates pain receptors. At least 2 other plasma kinins have biologic activities similar to those of bradykinin. The role of bradykinin in allergic disease is uncertain. Several patients with cold urticaria have had increased concentrations of bradykinin in plasma.

Serotonin (5-hydroxytryptamine) is a vasoactive amine which, in experimental animals, induces contraction of smooth muscle and increases vascular permeability. Ninety per cent of the body's stores of serotonin are found in the gastrointestinal tract, with the remainder divided between central nervous system and platelets. In rodents, serotonin is also found in mast cells of the skin and connective tissue. Serotonin is lacking from human mast cells. Human smooth muscle is much less sensitive than rat smooth muscle to serotonin in vitro. On the other hand, serotonin has been reported to induce bronchoconstriction in asthmatics but not in normal humans. Serotonin has no significant role in immediate hypersensitivity in humans. Its distinctive role in disease is its association with diarrhea in the carcinoid syndrome.

While not mediators in the same sense as products released from mast cells or basophils, certain components of the complement system have activities that may contribute to allergic reactions. (1) Though antigen-IgE interaction does not activate the classical complement pathway, aggregated IgE can initiate complement system activity in vitro through the alternative pathway; this probably does not occur in vivo because of the large quantities of IgE required. (2) Certain so-called "split" or "cleavage" products of the complement cascade, C3a and C5a, can induce mediator (histamine) release from basophils and from mast cells in the skin, producing wheal and flare reactions. C3a and C5a have been termed *anaphylatoxins* because they release histamine and resemble components of serum recognized years ago as capable of causing guinea pig anaphylaxis. C5a and to a much lesser extent C3a are chemotactic for various leukocytes. Neutrophils attracted to the site of complement activation by C5a may degranulate, releasing basic lysosomal proteins which trigger mediator liberation from mast cells. The result in the skin is urticaria mimicking an antigen-IgE mechanism. Small N-formylated peptides, derived from bacterial products, also possess potent granulocyte chemotactic activity and may operate in a manner similar to that of C5a to cause urticaria. (3) A kinin-like peptide derived from C2 as a result of reduced functional activity of the inhibitor of

C1-esterase (C1s̄) is thought to mediate the angioedema observed in hereditary angioedema (HAE).

From the above considerations it is evident that the signs and symptoms of typical, immediate-type allergic reactions, such as anaphylaxis, though most often involving the IgE mechanism, may result from non-IgE immunologic mechanisms or from nonimmunologic mechanisms as well.

9.44 GENERAL AND SPECIFIC METHODS OF DIAGNOSIS

Allergic History. A careful history is the most important method of arriving at a correct diagnosis in allergic diseases. After the general medical history has been obtained, information of particular interest to the allergist is sought, such as whether the patient's symptoms are perennial or seasonal. Seasonal symptoms suggest an etiologic role for seasonal allergens, such as pollens, whereas perennial symptoms suggest exposure either to multiple seasonal allergens or to factors not influenced by season. Questions concerning the home environment should focus on the heating system, composition of the furniture, the rugs, the furnishings in the child's bedroom (pillows, mattress, rugs, drapes, etc.), and the presence of domestic animals. Are the symptoms continuous or intermittent? Are they subject to diurnal variation? Has a change of location had any effect? These questions help to identify particular etiologic agents. In assessing the role of foods as etiologic agents, it is important to distinguish between what the parents have actually observed following ingestion of a food and what they may have been told by a physician, possibly on the basis of skin tests to foods, which are commonly subject to misinterpretation (Sec 9.57). One must be particularly critical in interpreting cause and effect relationships when foods are concerned as it is very easy for parents to arrive at erroneous conclusions based on inconsistent relationships between ingestion of a particular food and the appearance of symptoms. The value of properly conducted double-blind food challenges cannot be overemphasized. Significant improvement in symptoms following the use of antiallergic drugs such as antihistamines, sympathomimetics, xanthines, or corticosteroids supports the notion that an allergic reaction is the basis of symptoms; unfortunately, symptoms occurring on a nonimmunologic basis may also respond to such therapy.

In Vitro Tests. A white blood cell count and a differential count are useful in establishing the presence or absence of *eosinophilia*. A total eosinophil count gives a more accurate determination. Eosinophils are subject to a diurnal rhythm with numbers being highest in the early hours of the morning. Because eosinophilia may be intermittent, 2–3 normal results should be obtained before it is concluded that eosinophilia is not present. Eosinophilia in excess of 5% on peripheral smear or of 250 cells/mm³ is considered elevated. Eosinophilia of respiratory tract secretions in a patient with rhinorrhea or cough is a useful diagnostic sign. A smear of nasal secretions or bronchial mucus is easily prepared and stained on a microscope slide, preferably with an eosin–methylene blue stain (Hansel stain). A finding of more than 5–10% eosinophils supports the diagnosis of allergic rhinitis. Eosinophils in bronchial mucus are highly suggestive of asthma. Blood eosinophilia in allergic conditions does not generally exceed 15–20%, but may occasionally be as high as 35% in allergic children in the absence of other disorders known to cause eosinophilia. Other than atopic disorders, eosinophilia is associated most commonly with metazoan parasitoses, drug reactions, and a number of infiltrative pulmonary disorders. Corticosteroids cause eosinopenia for up to 6 hr following a dose; the timing of a blood specimen collection should be appropriately adjusted.

A number of in vitro immunologic tests are of value in allergy diagnosis. These include measuring the total and specific IgE content of serum and determining the sensitivity of the patient's leukocytes for antigen-induced histamine release. Quantification of total IgE can be accomplished by the paper radioimmunosorbent test (PRIST) or by a double antibody radioimmunoassay procedure. Table 9–13 shows the serum concentrations of IgE in normal subjects of different ages. Mean concentrations of IgE in individuals with such allergic

Table 9–13   LEVELS OF SERUM IgE IMMUNOGLOBULIN OF NORMAL SUBJECT AT DIFFERENT AGES*

AGE	NUMBER OF SUBJECTS	RANGE (IU/ml)	GEOMETRIC MEAN (IU/ml)	GEOMETRIC MEAN − 2 SD (IU/ml)	GEOMETRIC MEAN + 2 SD (IU/ml)
0 days	24	<0.1–1.5	0.22	0.04	1.28
6 wk	17	<0.1–2.8	0.69	0.08	6.12
3 mo	15	0.3–3.1	0.82	0.18	3.76
6 mo	15	0.9–28.0	2.68	0.44	16.26
9 mo	16	0.7–8.1	2.36	0.76	7.31
1 yr	12	1.1–10.2	3.49	0.80	15.22
2 yr	18	1.1–49.0	3.03	0.31	29.48
3 yr	6	0.5–7.7	1.80	0.19	16.86
4 yr	7	2.4–34.8	8.58	1.07	68.86
7 yr	18	1.6–60.0	12.89	1.03	161.32
10 yr	17	0.3–215	23.66	0.98	570.61
14 yr	19	1.9–159	20.07	2.06	195.18
18–83 yr	96	1–178	21.20	(Modal values 10–20 IU/ml)†	

*Ages 0–14 years from Kjellman, N-IM, Johansson SGO, Roth A: Clin Allergy 6:51, 1976; ages 18–83 years from Nye L, Merrett TG, Landon J, White RJ: Clin Allergy 1:13, 1975. The method used was a double antibody assay.

†Modal values — the most common values observed.

Table 9–14 DISORDERS ASSOCIATED WITH INCREASED CONCENTRATIONS OF SERUM IgE

Allergic (extrinsic) asthma (40–60% of patients)
Bronchopulmonary aspergillosis
Pulmonary hemosiderosis
Hyperimmunoglobulin E syndrome (increased IgE, dermatitis, susceptibility to infection)
Wiskott-Aldrich syndrome
Some T cell immunodeficiency states
Hodgkin disease
IgE myeloma
Atopic dermatitis associated with allergic rhinitis and/or asthma
Bullous pemphigoid
Chronic acral dermatitis
Parasitic infestations (Ascaris, Toxocara, Necator, Echinococcus, and Capillaria)

disorders as hay fever, asthma, and atopic dermatitis are higher than normal, though a significant number of allergic individuals have normal or low IgE concentrations. In cases of atypical forms of atopic dermatitis, however, the finding of grossly elevated IgE levels, which are very common in active atopic dermatitis, will support the diagnosis. The finding of an increased total IgE during infancy provides useful predictive information regarding the likelihood of the subsequent development of atopic diseases. Table 9–14 shows disorders associated with increased concentrations of serum IgE.

Determination of IgE levels against specific antigens is available for ragweed, grass, house dust or other inhalants, and various foods through the radioallergosorbent test (RAST). The principles of the RAST are shown in Fig 9–5. A comparison of RAST and skin testing in the diagnosis of IgE-mediated disorders is seen in Table 9–15.

There is good correlation among RAST results, other in vitro tests that measure specific antibody such as the leukocyte histamine release test, mucous membrane provocation tests, and the likelihood of symptoms upon exposure to the allergen under study. Allergy skin tests, on the other hand, are subject to errors due to use of inactive or too concentrated extracts, to poor technique (particularly with the intracutaneous method), and to overinterpretation of skin reactions.

In the *leukocyte histamine release test*, the patient's leukocytes are tested for their sensitivity to antigen-induced histamine release. For example, when leukocytes (actually, basophils) from persons with ragweed hay fever are exposed to various concentrations of ragweed antigen E (the major allergen of ragweed pollen), they will, under appropriate in vitro conditions, release histamine into the suspending medium. The leukocytes of individuals with high degrees of cell sensitivity release histamine on exposure to very small amounts of specific antigen, whereas leukocytes with lesser degrees of cell sensitivity require higher concentrations of antigen for release of comparable amounts of histamine. In the ragweed system, there is reasonably good correlation between sensitivity of leukocytes to histamine release on exposure to an antigen, the amount of specific IgE antibody measured by RAST, the titer of passive transfer (P-K) activity, mucous membrane provocation testing, and clinical sensitivity to the antigen on environmental exposure.

In Vivo Tests. Determination of allergic reactivity through direct *skin testing* of the patient is an important tool in the diagnosis of IgE-mediated sensitivity. A small quantity of allergenic extracts is introduced into the skin by scratch, prick/puncture, or intracutaneous technique. If the patient's mast cells have IgE antibodies specific for the allergen on their surfaces, an allergen-IgE interaction will trigger a sequence of biochemical events which culminate in release of histamine and other mediators from the mast cell. The histamine acts upon histamine receptors in capillaries, causing increased permeability and dilatation and axon reflex stimulation, which are observed clinically as the wheal and flare reaction. A biphasic late-phase reaction has also been described in these patients; this reaction begins with an influx of neutrophils over a 2–8 hr period and is followed by a mononuclear infiltrate at 24–48 hr. The late phase reaction is due to slowly eluted inflammatory factors of anaphylaxis from mast cell granules which attract neutrophils and mononuclear cells to the site of the reaction. The immediate wheal and flare reaction indicates that specific IgE antibody is present also on the mast cells in the tissue of the clinically affected organ. *It does not indicate that the patient will necessarily have clinical symptoms on exposure to the allergen.* A significant number of atopic persons have no symptoms following natural exposure to allergens which give positive wheal and flare reactions on skin testing. A general rule for the interpretation of the immediate wheal and flare skin test is: the larger the size of the wheal and flare reaction, the more clinically relevant is the test antigen. But one must be cautious about overinterpreting allergy skin tests.

Positive skin tests obtained by the puncture technique have a higher correlation than intracutaneous tests with measurements of specific IgE antibody and with appearance of clinical symptoms upon exposure to the allergen under test. With the intracutaneous technique, only those positive tests obtained with high dilutions (weak concentrations) of extract have as high correlations. If concentrated solutions of allergenic extract (e.g., 1 to 100 or 1 to 10 weight/volume) must be used

Radio Allergo Sorbent Test

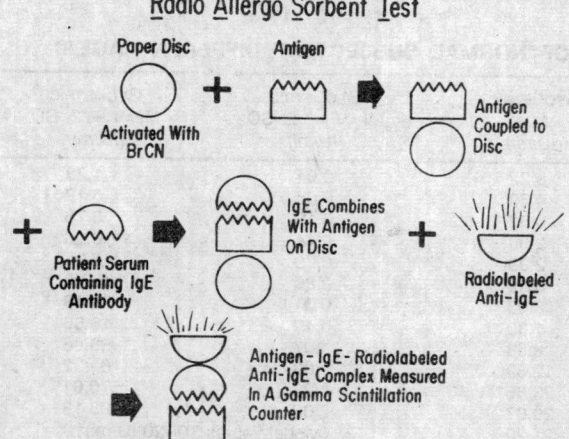

Figure 9–5 The principle of the radioallergosorbent test (RAST). The test is available in kit form, and with care and experience reliable results can be obtained. See text.

Table 9–15 RAST VERSUS SKIN TESTING IN DIAGNOSIS OF IgE-MEDIATED ALLERGY

Radioallergosorbent Test (RAST)	Skin Test
Advantages	
Safe	Immediate results
Convenient	Broad selection of allergens
Semi-quantitative	Relatively inexpensive
Not influenced by drugs	High degree of sensitivity
Useful in testing infants and patients with widespread dermatitis or dermographism	
Allergens on disk stable	
Good correlation with clinical symptoms, skin testing by end-point dilution, bronchial challenge, and in vitro leukocyte-histamine release	
Disadvantages	
Limited selection of allergens	Allergens labile in dilute solution
Expensive	Influenced by drugs
	Risk of systemic reaction
	Liable to misinterpretation

Modified from Yunginger JW, Gleich GJ: Pediatr Clin North Am 22:3, 1975.

to elicit a positive intracutaneous test, the result will more often than not be of little clinical significance. Overinterpretation of such reactions is responsible for considerable overuse of allergenic extracts in the United States.

Various drugs, extracts that contain irritant materials, and improper techniques can induce histamine release from tissue mast cells on a nonimmunologic or "toxic" basis. The resulting wheal and flare reaction cannot be differentiated from that which occurs as a result of IgE-allergen interaction; thus, IgE sensitivity may be mistakenly identified. Other drugs may inhibit full expression of clinically relevant positive skin tests. Among these are certain adrenergic drugs such as epinephrine and ephedrine and the antihistamines, particularly such potent ones as hydroxyzine. These drugs should be withheld prior to skin testing (ephedrine for at least 12 hr and antihistamines for at least 24 hr). To make sure that the skin is capable of reacting to endogenously released histamine, a positive histamine control (histamine phosphate (1%) should always be used. Corticosteroids to the equivalence of 60 mg of prednisone/24 hr have no appreciable inhibitory effects on IgE-mediated wheal and flare reactions and need not be withheld prior to skin testing.

In the *passive transfer test* (Prausnitz-Küstner [P-K] test) serum from an allergic individual is injected intracutaneously into a nonallergic recipient. The specific IgE antibodies in the donor serum passively sensitize the recipient's mast cells at the injected sites. The passively sensitized sites are challenged 24–48 hr later with various allergens, and the effects of histamine release are read in the same way as with direct skin tests. Passive transfer testing is time consuming and less sensitive than direct skin testing; it may also transmit hepatitis B.

Because the appearance of symptoms on natural exposure may be poorly correlated with results of skin testing, *provocation testing* by direct exposure of the mucous membrane of the affected organ to the suspected allergen (usually in the form of an extract of the material) has received considerable attention, particularly in Scandinavian countries. Provocation testing using mucous membranes has been applied mostly to asthma, to a lesser extent to allergic rhinitis. As commonly performed, the test requires that increasing concentrations of extracts of various allergens be inhaled by the patient after nebulization with a suitable device. A positive response will be manifested by an increase in airway obstruction as monitored carefully with an instrument that measures expiratory flow rate. The patient's degree of sensitivity should be determined by skin tests prior to provocation testing to permit appropriate initial concentrations of allergic extract to be used. With reasonable precautions the method is safe, and the results of provocation testing correlate well with clinical data. It is time consuming, however, and not suitable for general use in office or clinic. Bronchial challenge testing may have its greatest utility in patients who have many positive skin tests, and it will allow the rational selection of those allergens that may be most clinically significant for inclusion in a hyposensitization mixture. Selection in this way permits a greater concentration of the more clinically significant allergens in the mixture than would be possible if all the allergens possibly implicated by ordinary skin testing were to be included. Recent studies have shown excellent correlations between the results of provocative bronchial challenge testing, RAST, and quantitative intradermal skin tests (end-point dilution method); accordingly, the use of bronchial challenge is not likely to increase. On the other hand, bronchial provocative testing with methacholine and histamine is valuable when the degree of airway reactivity in asthma must be determined and when the diagnosis of asthma is uncertain.

Provocation testing with foods has used both subcutaneous injection and sublingual administration of food extracts, but reports are controversial. Symptoms referable to various organ systems are said to be provoked by positive tests and then "neutralized" by the injection of weaker concentrations of extract of the same foods that provoked the reactions, a response difficult to understand on immunologic or other grounds. In individuals who have IgE-mediated sensitivity to a food, there is little doubt that symptoms can be provoked when that food is ingested or injected; neutralization of such a reaction has not been convincingly shown. The relationship of this reaction to provocative food testing is unclear, however, and the above technique has not yet been validated by adequately critical studies.

The Rebuck skin window test has been used primarily as an investigational tool. The test involves abrading the skin with a sharp edge to the point of producing pinpoint areas of bleeding, applying the allergen to the abraded area under a coverslip, and then examining the stained coverslip at various time intervals. Eosinophils predominate in the positive response.

9.45   PRINCIPLES OF TREATMENT OF ALLERGIC DISORDERS

Successful treatment of allergic disorders is based upon 4 principles in management: avoidance of allergens, pharmacologic therapy, immunotherapy (hyposensitization or desensitization), and prophylaxis.

When allergens are identified by history and judicious use of allergy skin tests, their elimination or *avoidance* will be all the treatment needed in many cases of IgE-mediated disease. For example, if history and skin testing indicate reactivity to such household inhalants as house dust or molds, or dog or cat dander is contributing to the patient's symptoms, these allergens should be eliminated. The recommendation that a family pet be removed from a home is frequently difficult to implement, and occasionally one encounters families in which pets seem to be as deeply embedded in the social fabric of the family as the child or children. However, when the allergic disorder is a serious one, such as asthma, and when the child has a positive skin test to the dander of the pet, parents can generally be persuaded to remove the animal. When skin tests to danders are negative, the problem may be more difficult; most allergists feel that elimination of potentially sensitizing pets from the household of the allergic child is desirable on prophylactic grounds.

Instructions for preparation of an "allergen-free" indoor environment, emphasizing the bedroom, are found in standard allergy texts and are distributed by manufacturers of allergenic extracts. In significant numbers of patients, a great deal can be accomplished by the proper application of environmental control measures and the appropriate use of pharmacologic agents in the management of allergic disorders without resort to hyposensitization.

Pharmacologic therapy is a major element in management of allergic diseases (Sec 9.46). Drugs used for treatment have specific roles in the interruption of pathways leading to tissue damage as a consequence of antigen-antibody interaction. Certain drugs, for example, modulate the antigen-induced release of mediators (histamine, SRS-A); others affect tension of smooth muscle; and others prevent the migration to the site of an allergic reaction of inflammatory cells having the potential for producing tissue injury. In some patients with "allergic" disorders, such as asthma, there is no evidence that immunologic factors are involved. In such instances avoidance of allergens or attempts to increase the tolerance to allergens (hyposensitization or immunotherapy) have no value. Drug therapy, on the other hand, will be effective whether or not an allergic mechanism is involved. Individuals with nonimmunologic or nonallergic asthma may respond as well to drug treatment as those in whom allergy plays a major role.

Immunotherapy or *hyposensitization* is used for allergic disorders mediated by IgE antibody-antigen interaction which involves allergens that can either not be or only partially be avoided (Sec 9.47).

If a predisposition to form IgE antibodies to substances of "high" allergic potential is an important characteristic of the atopic state, then *prophylaxis* through the prevention of exposure of infants and children at risk has a rational basis. Thus, it is appropriate to recommend breast feeding in the case of infants born into families with strong histories of hay fever, asthma, or atopic dermatitis and to delay until at least 6 mo of age the introduction of solid foods into the diet of such infants, with special attention to foods of high allergic potential, such as eggs, wheat, and fish. It is not definitively established whether postponing cow's milk feeding in an atopic infant can prevent the development of cow milk allergy, of allergic diseases in general, or of atopic dermatitis in particular, though there is evidence of such effects. Nor are there convincing prospective studies indicating that avoidance of environmental exposure of atopic infants and children to inhalant allergens (e.g., dog and cat dander) will lessen the likelihood of their sensitization, though the result seems intuitively reasonable.

9.46   PHARMACOLOGIC THERAPY

Much relief can be provided children suffering from allergic diseases through the appropriate use of pharmacologic agents. The most useful drugs are of 5 distinctive types: adrenergics, theophylline, antihistamines, cromolyn sodium, and corticosteroids.

Adrenergics.   These drugs exert their activity by combining with specialized receptor areas on cell surfaces. Adrenergic receptors exist in a dynamic state and are subject to regulation in terms of numbers and properties by a variety of hormonal and other influences. There are two general types of adrenergic receptors, termed α and β. In general, with several exceptions, drugs that affect α receptors cause physiologic responses that are excitatory, whereas drugs that influence β receptors produce inhibitory responses. In a given tissue the response to a drug depends not only upon the relative proportion of α and β receptors but also upon the intrinsic properties of the drug, i.e., whether it stimulates predominantly α receptors, β receptors, or both. The identification of adrenergic receptors has been made possible largely through the development of drugs that specifically block various classes of these receptors. The adrenergic blocking agents have in turn become important in therapy of diseases in which it is advisable to block the physiologic responses resulting from stimulation of a given receptor.

Variations in sensitivity of β receptors in different organs to β agonists (stimulants) and differences in response to β blocking drugs of diverse chemical structure have led to separation of β receptors into 2 sub-

Table 9–16 EFFECTS OF ADRENERGIC DRUGS ON STIMULATION OF ADRENERGIC RECEPTORS IN SMOOTH MUSCLE AND THE HEART

α	$β_1$	$β_2$
Peripheral vasoconstriction	Cardiac chronotropy (rate) and inotropy (force)	Bronchodilatation (smooth muscle relaxation)

CNS effects not well studied
Epinephrine stimulates α, $β_1$, and $β_2$ receptors
Isoproterenol stimulates $β_1$ and $β_2$ receptors
New adrenergic agents stimulate $β_2$ receptors more selectively

classes, $β_1$ and $β_2$; $β_1$ and $β_2$ receptors are operationally defined in terms of their affinities for epinephrine and norepinephrine. $β_1$ receptors have approximately equal affinity for epinephrine and norepinephrine, whereas $β_2$ receptors have an approximately 10-fold higher affinity for epinephrine than norepinephrine. Agents with more $β_2$-selective activity can provide effective bronchodilation in asthma without the significant increase in heart rate that may occur with isoproterenol or epinephrine since the latter drugs stimulate both bronchial $β_2$ receptors and cardiac $β_1$ receptors, producing cardioacceleration. However, it is important to appreciate that $β_2$ selectivity is a relative phenomenon, and some patients will develop typical $β_1$ responses, e.g., cardioacceleration, after administration of a putative $β_2$-selective agent. Selective $β_2$ drugs have essentially no α-adrenergic activity and thus no pressor effect; accordingly, the patient does not develop the pallor that may occur with epinephrine administration (Table 9–16). At least 2 subtypes of α receptors exist, including $α_1$ and $α_2$; the significance of the α-adrenergic receptor subtypes is not yet apparent.

While in vitro experiments with human tissues have shown that adrenergic drugs can inhibit allergen-induced mediator release from mast cells and basophils, these drugs are used in allergic disorders principally because their effects on smooth muscle in blood vessels and in the bronchial airways can reverse physiologic responses resulting from IgE-mediated injury. Stimulation of α-adrenergic receptors reduces edema of nasal mucous membranes through vasoconstriction and decreases capillary permeability, for example, whereas β-adrenergic stimulation causes smooth muscle relaxation, which relieves at least 1 component of obstruction of the airway in asthma.

Adrenergic drugs include catecholamines (epinephrine, isoetharine, and isoproterenol) and noncatecholamines (ephedrine, albuterol, metaproterenol, and terbutaline). The former group should not be administered orally since they are rapidly inactivated by enzymes found in the gastrointestinal tract and liver. Accordingly, the use of epinephrine and isoproterenol is limited largely to injection, inhalation, and topical application to mucous membranes. Ephedrine, the oldest and most widely used of the noncatecholamine sympathomimetics, has relatively weak β-stimulant activity and a significant incidence of adverse side effects, principally involving the central nervous system. Newer noncatecholamine adrenergic agents (metaproterenol, terbutaline, and albuterol), which may also be given orally, have a somewhat longer duration of action (up to 6 hr) than ephedrine (4 hr), and have relatively selective activity on the $β_2$ receptors in the airways with less of the cardiovascular effects of isoproterenol and epinephrine. Since several-fold lower doses of adrenergic drugs are effective when the agents are given by the aerosol rather than the oral route, aerosol administration is preferred wherever possible, in order to minimize adverse drug effects.

Methylxanthines (Theophylline). Theophylline is the only methylxanthine used in the treatment of asthma. Theophylline's effect appears to result in part through inhibition of the activity of phosphodiesterase, the enzyme that hydrolyzes cyclic AMP. Theophylline's activity may also be due to an influence on calcium flux across cell membranes.

Theophylline is now recognized as a major therapeutic agent for treatment of both acute and chronic asthma. In order to use theophylline effectively and safely, the physician needs to be aware of the following: (1) The amount of anhydrous theophylline differs in various formulations of the drug. Because it is relatively insoluble in aqueous solution, theophylline has been combined with various salts and bases to improve solubility. The amount of theophylline base, the major determinant of plasma concentration, varies from 1 combination to another. There are many formulations of anhydrous theophylline with good bioavailability. Recently, reliable products which release the drug at a relatively constant rate during the dosing interval have become available. These formulations are particularly valuable in children whose rapid elimination of theophylline from the body makes it difficult to maintain therapeutic serum concentrations with quickly absorbed formulations even if administered every 6 hr. (2) Theophylline is eliminated from the body principally through biotransformation in the liver. Normal individuals may differ substantially in their rates of elimination of theophylline. Some diseases, particularly those that affect the liver, and other conditions affecting liver function have important effects on kinetics of theophylline. For example, liver disease, congestive heart failure, and cigarette smoking all influence the rate of theophylline clearance from the body, as do diet (low carbohydrate, high protein, dietary methylxanthines such as caffeine and theobromine), other drugs taken concurrently, particularly the macrolide antibiotics (troleandomycin and erythromycin salts), cimetidine, and acute viral illnesses (Table 9–17). Such considerations require the individualization of therapy in terms of dose and dose interval. (3) Both the therapeutic efficacy and the toxicity of theophylline are related to serum concentrations. The

Table 9–17 FACTORS INFLUENCING THEOPHYLLINE CLEARANCE

FACTORS	DECREASED	INCREASED
Age	Prematures Neonates ? Age >50 years	Age 1–16 years
Weight	Obesity (in relation to total body water)	
Diet	Dietary methylxanthines High carbohydrate	Low carbohydrate High protein Charcoal-broiled meats
Habits		Cigarette smoking (tobacco or marijuana)
Drugs	Troleandomycin Erythromycin Cimetidine Propranolol ?Influenza vaccine Oral contraceptives	? Phenobarbital
Disease	Cirrhosis Congestive heart failure Chronic obstructive pulmonary disease Acute pulmonary edema Acute viral illnesses	

monitoring of such concentrations is indicated, particularly in patients who do not derive therapeutic benefit or in those who develop signs or symptoms of toxicity on the usual regimens. (4) Analytic methods for measuring theophylline in biologic fluids are readily available, e.g., EMIT (enzyme-multiplied immunoassay), high-performance liquid chromatography (HPLC), and a new substrate-labeled fluorescence immunoassay procedure.

Adverse Side Effects. Though adverse reactions to theophylline are common, they are usually not serious. Most cases of significant toxicity in children have occurred because of excessive serum concentration due to overdosage, either iatrogenic or accidental. Signs and symptoms of toxicity most often involve the gastrointestinal tract (nausea and vomiting) and the central nervous system (restlessness, agitation, and seizures). Less often, the cardiovascular system is involved, disturbances of rhythm being most commonly reported. Theophylline may produce a hemorrhagic gastritis with hematemesis regardless of the route of administration. Hematemesis is a sign of serious intoxication.

Antihistamines. These are drugs of diverse chemical structure that compete with histamine for combination with receptors in various tissues. Two histamine receptors are now recognized, H_1 and H_2. Until recently, only H_1-receptor blockers were used in treatment of allergic disorders. It now appears that a combination of H_1 and H_2 antagonists may be beneficial in some patients with chronic urticaria and in treatment of anaphylactoid reactions typified by those due to intravenous pyelogram contrast agents. Cimetidine, an H_2 antagonist, inhibits delayed-type hypersensitivity skin responses, suggesting a role for H_2-receptor blocking agents in the modulation of cell-mediated immune injury. The H_1-type antihistamines, as a group, are nitrogenous bases with aliphatic side chains that resemble histamine. The side chains are attached to cyclic or heterocyclic rings of various configurations. The antihistamines may be classified clinically into the following types:

Type I — ethylenediamines (tripelennamine [Pyribenzamine]), (methapyrilene [Histadyl, Copyronil]).

Type II — ethanolamines (diphenhydramine [Benadryl]), (carbinoxamine [Clistin, Rondec]).

Type III — alkylamines (chlorpheniramine [Chlor-Trimeton, Teldrin, Novahistine, Demazin]), (brompheniramine [Dimetane]), (triprolidine [Actidil, Actifed]).

Type IV — piperazines (cyclizine [Marazine]), (meclizine [Bonine]).

Type V — piperidines (cyproheptadine [Periactin]).

Type VI — phenothiazines (promethazine [Phenergan]).

Hydroxyzine (Atarax, Vistaril), which has potent antihistaminic activity, does not belong to any of the 6 types listed. *The antihistamines may be found alone or in combination* in the above commercial preparations.

In general, the H_1 antagonists are rapidly absorbed after oral administration, with onset of action within 30 min, peak plasma concentration within 1 hr, and complete absorption within 4 hr. Antihistamines are eliminated from the body by biotransformation in the liver; little nonmetabolized drug is found in urine. Some antihistamines (diphenhydramine and chlorcyclizine) stimulate liver microsomal drug-metabolizing enzymes in animals and may accelerate their own metabolism and that of other drugs. There have been relatively few pharmacologic studies of the antihistamines, and most of our prescribing patterns are empirically based upon clinical experience. Diphenhydramine (Benadryl) has a relatively short serum half-life of 3–4 hr. Yet the drug is effective in suppression of wheal and flare response to allergy skin testing for over 24 hr. Thus, with this antihistamine there appears to be little correlation between serum concentration and therapeutic effect in the tissue. A recent study of chlorpheniramine in children showed a mean serum half-life of 13.7 hr (range 6–34 hr). Significant suppression of clinical symptoms of allergic rhinitis was observed for as long as 30 hr after injection of a single dose at which time chlorpheniramine was not detectable in the serum. The scant data available indicate that perhaps the customary 3 or 4 doses of antihistamines/day may not be necessary and that 2 or even 1 dose/day may suffice. In addition to histamine antagonism, the antihistamines have pharmacologic effects on exocrine secretions, the central nervous system, and the cardiovascular system.

Since antihistamines act as competitive antagonists, they are more effective in preventing than in reversing the action of histamine. To be effective, they must be administered in such dosage and at such intervals as will keep tissue histamine receptor sites saturated. Histamine is released explosively at the site of an IgE-mediated reaction; accordingly, antihistamines are less potent in antagonizing the effects of endogenous than of exogenous histamine. Their relative inefficacy in asthma is related both to this and to the fact that mediators of bronchoconstriction other than histamine are involved in allergic reactions in the lung. Many antihistamines possess anticholinergic activity, which is valuable in allergic rhinitis for controlling rhinorrhea. Anticholinergic activity may account for the occasional asthmatic patient who seems to have a favorable response to antihistamines. There is little support for an old notion that antihistamines are contraindicated in asthma because of their drying effect on mucous secretions. A well designed study has shown that in children with asthma, in the usual doses given for hay fever, antihistamines had neither favorable nor deleterious effects on the course of asthma.

There is little reason to choose 1 antihistamine over another. The ethanolamines (e.g., diphenhydramine) and the phenothiazines seem to have greater sedative effects than the alkylamines (e.g., chlorpheniramine); accordingly, if excessive sedation is noted, substitution of a drug from another group may be tried. The physician should learn to use 1–2 of these drugs effectively rather than occasionally use each of a large number of different drugs.

In general, antihistamines are extraordinarily safe and are sold without prescription. They have adverse effects, however, particularly in high dosages. Sedation is the most common side effect, to which some tolerance develops. Combinations of antihistamines with other central nervous depressants (e.g., alcohol) should be avoided. In high doses or in certain sensitive patients, the anticholinergic properties of antihistamines cause undesirable adverse reactions. These include excitation, nervousness, tachycardia, palpitations, dryness of the mouth, urinary retention, and constipation. Seizures are common in antihistamine poisoning. Skin eruptions, blood dyscrasias, fever, and neuropathy are rarely observed.

H_2-receptor antagonists, e.g., cimetidine, have no clearly defined indication in allergic disease at present.

Cromolyn Sodium (Sodium Cromoglycate). Cromolyn sodium is the disodium salt of 1,3,-bis (2-carboxychromone-5-yloxy)-2-hydroxypropane. It is a chemical analogue of the drug khellin, which has smooth muscle–relaxing properties. The drug is administered as a powder (Intal) with a special turboinhaler, the Spinhaler. A solution form designed for use in young children has just been marketed. It is principally used in asthma, but it has some value in allergic rhinitis and conjunctivitis and in vernal conjunctivitis. It has been used with varying results in aphthous ulcers, food allergy, systemic mastocytosis, ulcerative colitis, and chronic proctitis. The drug has no bronchodilator properties; it is not, therefore, used in treatment of acute attacks but is given prophylactically, 2–4 times/day. Cromolyn has no antimediator or anti-inflammatory properties. It is soluble in water, but insoluble in lipids; only 1% is absorbed from the gastrointestinal tract. Cromolyn prevents both antibody-mediated and non-antibody-mediated mast cell degranulation and mediator release. This effect may be due to the ability of cromolyn to block antigen-stimulated calcium transport across the mast cell membrane. Cromolyn inhibition of histamine release may also occur by regulation of a phosphorylation of a mast cell protein. The drug also has weak phosphodiesterase inhibitor activity. Cromolyn also inhibits bronchoconstriction that occurs in response to stimuli such as frigid air, exercise, and sulfur dioxide. Since these stimuli do not cause release of mast cell–derived mediators, cromolyn may have a unique effect on neural control of the airway.

Cromolyn is of greatest value in allergic or extrinsic asthma, but patients with nonallergic or intrinsic asthma may also respond. About 70% of asthmatic patients receive some degree of benefit from inhalation of the drug. The incidence of toxic reactions to cromolyn is extremely low; dry throat and transient bronchoconstriction have been the most frequently reported side effects. The latter is most likely due to inhalation of the dry powder into irritable airways and is not an intrinsic effect of the drug itself. Rare reports have associated urticaria, angioedema, and pulmonary eosinophilia with the use of cromolyn. There are no known contraindications to its use except that in some patients, during an acute attack of asthma, the powder may act as an airway irritant.

Corticosteroids. Corticosteroids are the most potent drugs available for treatment of allergic disorders. Although absorption problems exist with some products, following administration of a well absorbed tablet, peak plasma concentration is attained at 1–2 hr. There is then extensive 1st-pass conversion of prednisone to its active metabolite, prednisolone. The systemic availability of the active drug is over 80% of the oral dose. Regardless of the route of administration, there is interconversion of prednisone and prednisolone with prednisolone concentrations present at 4–10 times the prednisone concentration. There appears to be little effect of liver disease or renal insufficiency on the conversion of prednisone to prednisolone or on prednisolone disposition. The increase in volume of distribution, metabolic clearance, and renal clearance of prednisone that is observed with increasing dose is due to the partially saturable binding of prednisolone to transcortin in plasma which provides more unbound drug at higher plasma concentrations of this steroid.

While some effects of prednisolone are evident within 2 hr after oral or intravenous administration (fall in peripheral eosinophils and lymphocytes), other responses may be delayed to 8 hr or longer, e.g., hyperglycemia and improvement in pulmonary function in asthmatics. The delayed responses are due to the indirect mechanism of action of glucocorticoids. Steroid activity depends upon simple diffusion through the cell membrane, binding to cytosol glucocorticoid receptors (found in most mammalian cells), translocation of the steroid-receptor complex to the nucleus, binding of the complex to chromatin which affects nuclear gene expression, and subsequent synthesis of messenger RNA and proteins with enzyme activity. It is the newly synthesized enzymes that mediate the effects of glucocorticoids. The biologic half-life of the steroid is determined by the turnover time of the newly synthesized enzymes. Thus, steroid plasma concentrations do not directly determine the duration of corticosteroid response. Plasma half-lives of commonly used steroids vary from 1.5–5 hr, while biologic half-lives vary from 8–54 hr.

Pharmacokinetic studies of prednisolone have shown no differences in distribution, protein binding, plasma clearance, or disposition of unbound drug between males and females and adults and children. Steroid-dependent asthmatics do not differ from normal individuals in prednisolone binding, distribution, or clearance. Clinically significant drug interactions occur with phenobarbital and phenytoin, both of which increase steroid clearance. The anti-inflammatory actions of glucocorticoids result from their effect on (1) alteration in leukocyte number and activity (redistribution, suppression of migration to sites of inflammation, decreased response to mitogens, decreased cytotoxicity, and suppression of delayed hypersensitivity responses in the skin); (2) suppression of mediator release (decreased histamine synthesis and release, decreased synthesis of prostaglandins and other products of arachidonic acid metabolism); (3) enhanced response to agents which increase cAMP (PGE_2 and histamine via the H_2 receptor); and (4) enhanced response to catecholamines (increased synthesis of β-adrenergic receptors, increased availability of epinephrine due to decreased extraneuronal uptake of catecholamines). Humoral antibody synthesis is little affected by glucocorticoids in the dosage usually given for treatment of allergic disorders. Chronic corticosteroid administration may lower total immunoglobulin concentrations.

The short-term use of corticosteroids in self-limited allergic conditions, such as contact dermatitis due to poison ivy, rhinoconjunctivitis due to IgE-mediated allergy to tree pollens, or only occasional episodes of severe asthma, is not associated with significant adverse effects. Long-term use, on the other hand, may have substantial and undesirable side effects. In children the most common is suppression of linear growth. Posterior subcapsular cataracts develop occasionally in children on long-term steroid therapy.

Before any decision is made to initiate long-term corticosteroid therapy, all other modalities of management should be tried. Despite these measures, a small proportion of allergic children, most having asthma, will have severe and continuing symptoms which interfere with normal school attendance, play activities, and the like. The judicious use of glucocorticoids, particularly in alternate-day regimens, can produce substantial improvement in such children with little adverse effect.

A few considerations in the systemic use of corticosteroids bear emphasis. (1) When given in equivalent anti-inflammatory doses, available drugs do not differ qualitatively in anti-inflammatory effects. Prednisone or prednisolone is the preferred drug for oral administration and methylprednisolone or hydrocortisone for intravenous use. Other steroids with longer duration of biologic activity have greater propensities for adverse effects, are not suitable for alternate-day therapy, and are more expensive. (2) When corticosteroid therapy is initiated, a sufficient amount should be given in divided doses to bring the disease under control. As soon as this is accomplished, an attempt should be made to adjust the dose and the dosing interval to suppress activity of the disease without adverse effects. Whenever possible, alternate-day regimens using prednisone or prednisolone should be tried. In the alternate-day regimen, the drug is given as a single dose every 48 hr between 6:00–8:00 A.M. If daily steroid medication is required, a single dose is given, again between 6:00–8:00 A.M.; this regimen mimics endogenous cortisol secretion and causes less suppression of the hypothalamic-pituitary-adrenal axis or other adverse side effects than the same daily dose of drug given in divided doses. When exacerbations of the disease process occur during low dose maintenance therapy, then high dose suppressive therapy in divided dosage is indicated for a few days with prompt return to low dose alternate-day treatment as soon as the acute process is brought under control.

A new generation of highly surface-active corticosteroids is available for aerosol administration to corticosteroid-dependent asthmatics. Their high surface activity enables them to be given in minute doses which have little systemic effect in the usual therapeutic regimens. The relative merits of low-dose alternate-day steroids vs aerosol corticosteroids are unknown.

9.47 IMMUNOTHERAPY

Historical Aspects. Immunotherapy (hyposensitization) was introduced in 1912 as a treatment for hay fever induced by grass pollen upon the mistaken notion that the symptoms observed in patients were from a toxin in the pollen and that favorable results obtained with pollen extract injections were due to antitoxin. The original technique has been modified remarkably little.

Immunologic Changes. In the early weeks following the institution of regular injections of ragweed pollen extract, IgE antibody against ragweed pollen antigen increases; as regular treatment is continued, however, the titer of specific IgE ragweed antibody decreases. In untreated patients with ragweed hay fever, a rise and a fall of specific ragweed IgE occur during the year; the rise is temporally related to seasonal exposure to ragweed. Injection therapy appears to blunt this anamnestic rise in ragweed IgE. With continuing treatment ragweed antibodies of the IgG class ("blocking" or "antigen-binding") appear in the serum; the ultimate titer achieved is related to the quantity of ragweed extract injected but does not necessarily correlate with clinical changes, if any occur.

A further change with therapy involves the capacity of leukocytes (the basophils) from ragweed-sensitive individuals to release histamine on challenge in vitro with ragweed antigen E. Leukocytes from treated individuals require exposure to increased amounts of antigen E in order to release the same amount of histamine as prior to therapy. Leukocyte preparations from some treated patients behave as if they have been completely desensitized and do not release histamine upon challenge at any concentration of ragweed antigen E. The fundamental nature of this change in cell sensitivity is unknown; it does not appear to be related to titers of either ragweed IgE or IgG. There is thought to be some intrinsic change in receptors for IgE or in the biochemical pathways leading to histamine release. Experimentally, in animals it is possible both specifically to suppress IgE antibody production and to induce tolerance to certain chemically modified or conjugated antigens.

Studies of Efficacy. Critical review of studies of treatment of ragweed hay fever with ragweed extract injections leads to the conclusion that *some* individuals receive *some* degree of benefit. Data supporting the efficacy of grass and tree pollen extract immunotherapy in rhinitis induced by these allergens are less substantial, but the results appear similar to those with ragweed. Substantial proof of efficacy of hyposensitization therapy in asthma, despite its widespread use, is lacking, although there is some evidence that it may be beneficial in asthma induced by house dust or grass pollen. Before immunotherapy can be adequately assessed as a treatment for allergen-precipitated asthma or recommended for widespread use, additional carefully controlled, well designed studies must be done. Immunotherapy with bee venom in patients with anaphylactic sensitivity to bee venom antigen has been shown to protect against anaphylaxis upon subsequent sting in a convincing double-blind study.

The cost of therapy, its inconvenience, the possibility of making the disease worse, and other factors must be considered. There is no acceptable evidence for efficacy of injection therapy with allergens other than those noted above. Specifically, the injection of danders (cat, dog, horse), molds, bacterial vaccines, and food has not been shown to influence favorably the course of rhinitis or asthma.

Indications, Materials, and Procedure. Immunotherapy is indicated in individuals suffering from allergic rhinitis, IgE-mediated asthma, or allergy to stinging insects. Atopic dermatitis and food allergy are not improved by immunotherapy with allergenic extracts. A patient is a candidate for a trial of immunotherapy when there is a good correlation between symptoms and exposure to an inhalant allergen which cannot be adequately avoided, when the patient has evidence of IgE-mediated allergy by either in vivo (skin testing) or in vitro (RAST) criteria, and when disabling symptoms are not easily controlled with medication. There should also be a reasonable likelihood of good patient compliance since the treatment involves the administration of injections of allergenic extracts at regular intervals for several yr.

Aqueous extracts are used most commonly. Alum-precipitated pollen extracts and alum-precipitated pyridine-extracted extracts (Allpyral) do not appear to offer any substantial advantages over aqueous extract therapy. Furthermore, the immunogenicity of certain Allpyral extracts (ragweed in particular) has been questioned by several groups of investigators. Allergenic extracts are considered drugs by the FDA, but standards of potency do not exist. Extracts have been sold in the United States for diagnosis and therapy that were totally lacking in allergenic activity when tested by the RAST inhibition methods. Some of the antigens in allergenic extracts (e.g., ragweed antigen E) are quite labile. Methods of extraction, antigen concentration, and storage temperature are all critical factors in the activity and shelf life of an allergenic extract. Pollen extracts are being modified in attempts to reduce their allergenicity without reducing their immunogenicity. Allergens polymerized with gluteraldehyde retain their immunogenicity but are much less allergenic. Thus, the initial dose of extract may be substantially increased, the maintenance dose can be reached in about 2 mo compared to 5–6 mo with conventional therapy, and there is a greatly reduced incidence of local and systemic reactions.

In practice, immunotherapy with aqueous extracts involves the repeated injection of increasing amounts of allergenic extract until the patient reaches an "optimal" maintenance dose. The dose considered optimal is often arbitrary; the clinical trials involving ragweed referred to above reported better results with "high dose" than with "low dose" treatment. High dose therapy is possible only when a limited number of allergens are included in the extract treatment set. No more than 4–5 allergens should be included in a single injection. Children tolerate the same doses as adults.

The injections are given 1–3 times/wk until the patient reaches the maintenance dose, usually after 5–6 mo. In the "rush" method of immunotherapy used in Scandinavia, the initial injection period is compressed into a few days with apparently satisfactory results. The interval between injections is then extended to 2, 3, and then 4 wk. If more than 4 wk elapse between injections, the subsequent dose is reduced to avoid the possibility of a systemic reaction. There is little reason to continue weekly injections for prolonged periods of time as this greatly increases the cost of the treatment. During the course of the initial injections, the patient is observed carefully for evidence of excessive local reactions. Large local reactions are thought to predict systemic reactions, but this is uncertain. If an extensive local reaction or a systemic reaction occurs, the subsequent dose is reduced and then cautiously increased according to the patient's tolerance. Failure to see a local reaction at any time indicates either that the patient is not allergic to the constituents of the extract or that the extract is inactive.

Perennial treatment, in which injections are given throughout the yr, is preferred to preseasonal treatment, in which the treatment regimen is renewed each yr, beginning several mo prior to the pollen season. During the pollen season the maintenance dose of extract is unchanged except for the patient who develops systemic reactions, presumably due to the combined exposure to seasonal and injected allergen. For these patients, the dose may need to be reduced.

The optimal duration of treatment is not known and probably differs from patient to patient. Many allergists believe that if the patient is significantly improved after 3 yr of therapy, it is reasonable to discontinue the injections and observe for recurrence of symptoms. Some children have received "allergy shots" for many yr with no evidence that they have been beneficial. Immunotherapy should not be continued if there is no substantial improvement in the condition for which the patient is being treated. Since skin test reactivity changes little during the early yr of immunotherapy, it is unnecessary to retest the child yearly.

Precautions and Adverse Reactions. Allergenic extracts should *always* be administered in a physician's office where treatment of a systemic reaction or of anaphylactic shock is readily available. The patient should always remain under observation for at least 20 min after each injection since life-threatening reactions are most likely to occur within this time. Occasionally children will have delayed symptoms; for example, an exacerbation of asthma may occur in the evening of the day on which an injection of extract was given. Rarely, because of distance from a physician's office, it may be necessary to administer allergenic extracts in another setting. Under such circumstances, however, the non-physician who administers an injection must be prepared to treat a systemic reaction. Except for the possibility of constitutional reactions, no short- or long-term adverse effects of administration of allergenic extracts to children are known.

RESPIRATORY ALLERGY

The respiratory tract is the organ system most frequently affected by allergic disorders during childhood.

9.48 ALLERGIC RHINITIS

Seasonal allergic rhinitis, seasonal pollinosis, and hay fever all describe a symptom complex seen in children who have become sensitized to windborne pollens of trees, grasses, and weeds. Estimates indicate that 5–9% of children in unselected samples meet diagnostic criteria. The prevalence is age related; ragweed hay fever is rarely observed before 4–5 yr of age. There is little evidence that allergic rhinitis predisposes to the development of asthma, which follows allergic rhinitis in only an estimated 3–10% of cases.

In *perennial allergic rhinitis* the patient is symptomatic the yr round. The causative agents, when they can be identified, are generally found to be allergens to which the patient is exposed more or less continually, though exposure may vary during the yr. Indoor inhalant allergens are implicated most often, such as house dust, feathers, and danders of household pets; in certain climates, particularly where the humidity is high, mold spores are frequent offenders. In an occasional patient foods appear to cause symptoms of allergic rhinitis, but their role must be critically evaluated. Some patients are said to be able to ingest certain foods with impunity except during a pollen season, when ingestion causes an aggravation of nasal symptoms.

Diagnosis. The symptoms of allergic rhinitis include sneezing, which is frequently paroxysmal; rhinorrhea, which is often watery and profuse; nasal obstruction; and itching of the nose, palate, pharynx, and ears. Itching, redness, and tearing of the eyes may also occur, causing severe discomfort.

The typical case of allergic rhinitis presents bilateral nasal obstruction resulting from edema of the mucous membranes. Frequently, redundant mucosa is piled up on the floor of the nose. The mucous membranes are bluish in hue and rather pale, and a clear mucoid nasal discharge is seen. The child often has mannerisms involving the nose, which stem from itching or from attempts to increase the airway. The child wrinkles the nose (rabbit nose), and may rub it in characteristic ways (allergic salute). Rubbing in an upward direction may lead to a horizontal crease on the dorsum of the nose near the tip. The dark circles under the eyes which may be seen in some patients have been attributed to venous stasis resulting from interference with blood flow through the edematous nasal mucous membranes. Mouth breathing is common. The diagnosis of allergic rhinitis is substantiated by the finding of a predominance of eosinophils in a smear made of the nasal secretions. A nasal smear is best prepared by having the child blow the nose into wax paper. The mucus sample is then transferred to a glass slide and stained selectively for eosinophils.

Differential Diagnosis. *Vasomotor rhinitis* designates a poorly understood disorder in which symptoms similar to those of allergic rhinitis occur but in which an allergic etiology cannot be identified. Nasal obstruction is the predominant symptom, with minimal itching, sneezing, and rhinorrhea. The obstruction appears to be aggravated by environmental changes, such as in temperature or humidity, and by exposure to such irritants as tobacco smoke and other nonimmunologic inhalants. The patients characteristically do not have eosinophils in their nasal secretions. The underlying nature of the disorder is not clear; the peculiar hyper-reactivity of the vessels in the nasal mucous membranes seems most likely due to disturbance of autonomic neural control.

Other causes of nasal obstruction include *unilateral choanal atresia* in infants who characteristically have a unilateral nasal discharge; *deviated septum; hypertrophy of the adenoids; encephalocele;* and *nasal polyposis.* Nasal polyposis occurs in as many as 20% of children with cystic fibrosis. Fewer than 0.5% of patients in a typical allergy practice will have nasal polyps on a simple allergic basis. In addition to cystic fibrosis, nasal polyposis occurs in *Kartagener syndrome* and in *immunologic deficiencies.* The syndrome of nasal polyps, asthma, and aspirin intolerance is known as *triad asthma.* A foul-smelling, unilateral purulent or blood-tinged purulent nasal discharge in a child suggests a *foreign body.* A persistent bloody discharge always suggests *malignancy;* nasal obstruction with epistaxis in a male in late childhood or early adolescence suggests *benign nasopharyngeal fibroma,* also known as *angiofibroma.* Nasal obstruction occurs in *hypothyroidism.* Adolescents may suffer from *rhinitis of pregnancy.* A profuse, clear nasal discharge should suggest *cerebrospinal fluid rhinorrhea,* which can be confirmed by measuring the level of glucose in the fluid. Excessive use of vasoconstrictor nose drops or sprays can lead to *rhinitis medicamentosa,* in which nasal obstruction can be severe. Reserpine can produce marked nasal congestion.

Swelling of the mucous membranes of the sinuses frequently occurs with allergic rhinitis in childhood and may be seen in roentgenograms of the involved sinuses, occasionally with fluid levels. The sinuses appear abnormal so often on roentgenography, not only in children with allergic rhinitis but also in those with viral upper respiratory infections and in entirely asymptomatic children, that such examination is of little value. Sinus infection may complicate allergic rhinitis; the symptoms generally are fullness, discomfort, and persistent mucopurulent nasal and pharyngeal discharge.

Treatment. Treatment of either seasonal or perennial allergic rhinitis includes avoidance of exposure to suspected allergens, immunotherapy for those that cannot be avoided or can only partially be avoided, and drug therapy.

Avoidance. It is difficult or impractical to avoid exposure to seasonal pollens, but a great deal can be done to eliminate exposure to such indoor inhalant factors as house dust, danders, and molds. Control of house dust, with special attention to the child's bedroom, often ameliorates symptoms in the dust-allergic child. Elimination of exposure to danders and feathers is mandatory for a child with perennial allergic rhinitis when these factors appear to contribute to the symptoms. For the child sensitive to indoor molds, avoidance of damp basements and the application of measures designed to discourage mold growth in the house frequently lead to good results. These measures include dehumidifiers, air conditioners with efficient filters, and air cleaning devices, either the electronic precipitator type or one containing an HEPA filter. A 1:750 solution of Zephiran chloride is an effective agent in controlling mold growth. In areas that can be closed off, such as damp cellars, volatilization of paraformaldehyde (25–50 gm, depending upon the size of the area to be treated) from several open jars is also frequently effective in inhibiting growth of mold. For infants with persistent rhinorrhea and nasal obstruction, an elimination diet has been recommended, with particular avoidance of cow's milk. Such diets are only rarely effective, but a brief period of dietary manipulation is innocuous and should be given a trial.

Immunotherapy is discussed in Sec 9.47.

Drug Therapy. Relief can usually be obtained in allergic rhinitis by the appropriate use of drugs. *Antihistamines* are extremely useful, especially in the treatment of the seasonal variety of allergic rhinitis (Sec 9.46). To achieve the desired effects, it is frequently necessary to increase the dosage beyond that routinely recommended. Nasal itching, sneezing, and rhinorrhea are usually well controlled by antihistamine therapy, whereas nasal obstruction is relieved to a lesser degree. The major adverse side effect of antihistamine therapy is somnolence, which usually lessens with continued therapy. Sometimes it requires a change to another class of antihistamine.

If nasal obstruction is particularly troublesome, *sympathomimetics* such as pseudoephedrine or phenylpropanolamine may be tried alone or in combination with an antihistamine. Nose drops or sprays containing sympathomimetic drugs should be avoided except for short-term use; continued use may lead to progressively severe nasal obstruction due to rebound vasodilatation. Treatment of this latter complication requires complete cessation of use of medicated nose drops and the substitution of nose drops of physiologic saline solution.

Cromolyn sodium nasal solution has been effective to some degree in patients with perennial rhinitis. The nasal solution has also been used with moderately good results in hay fever but is not yet available in the United States.

By far the most effective drug for treatment of allergic rhinitis is the new generation of *topical corticosteroids.* Beclomethasone (Vancenase or Becomade) or flunisolide (Nasalide) should be used in children whose nasal symptoms are resistant to antihistamine-decongestant therapy. A dose of 2 inhalations in each nostril 3–4 times a day is given initially. After 3–4 days, as symptoms improve, the dose and frequency of use are reduced until a minimal effective dosage, on the order of 1–2 inhalations once or twice a day, is reached and continued as maintenance therapy. Occasionally, temporary use of corticosteroid eye drops is necessary in a child with hay fever and particularly severe eye symptoms. Treatment of vasomotor rhinitis, while often unsatisfactory, may be approached with the same drugs as for allergic rhinitis.

9.49 ASTHMA

Asthma is a leading cause of chronic illness in childhood, responsible for a significant proportion of school days lost because of chronic illness. It is estimated that 5–10% of children will at some time during childhood have signs and symptoms compatible with asthma. Prior to puberty about twice as many boys as girls are affected; thereafter, the sex incidence is equal. Asthma can lead to severe psychosocial disturbances in the family. With proper treatment, however, much relief can be provided. There is no universally accepted definition of asthma; it may be regarded as a diffuse, obstructive lung disease with (1) hyperreactivity of the airways to a variety of stimuli and (2) a high degree of reversibility of the obstructive process, which may occur either spontaneously or as a result of treatment.

Both large (>2 mm) and small (<2 mm) airways may be involved to varying degrees. Irritability or hyperreactivity of the airways is manifest as bronchoconstriction following exercise; natural exposures to strong odors or irritant fumes, such as sulfur dioxide (SO_2), tobacco smoke, or cold air; and intentional exposures in the laboratory to inhalations of parasympathomimetic agents, such as methacholine (Mecholyl) or histamine. Hyperreactivity of the airways, while not limited to asthmatics, is present in virtually all of them. It is the most sensitive objective indicator of asthma and is present to some degree when patients are asymptomatic, are free of physical findings, and have normal spirometry. Airway hyperreactivity, which relates to the overall severity of the disease, may vary from patient to patient but generally is stable over time in the same patient except for temporary fluctuations as follows: Increased responsiveness occurs during viral respiratory infections, following exposure to air pollutants and to allergens or occupational chemicals in sensitized individuals, and following administration of β-receptor antagonists. An acute decrease in airway responsiveness is observed following administration of β-receptor agonists, theophylline, and anticholinergics and after chronic administration of cromolyn and beclomethasone.

Data regarding the inheritance of asthma are most compatible with polygenic or multifactorial determinants. Lability of bronchoconstriction with exercise has been found concordant in identical twins but not in dizygotic twins. Bronchial lability in response to exercise testing also has been demonstrated in healthy relatives of asthmatic children.

Epidemiology. Asthma may have its onset at any

age; about 80–90% of asthmatic children have their first symptoms before 4–5 yr of age. The course and severity of asthma are difficult to predict. The majority of affected children have only occasional attacks of slight to moderate severity, managed with relative ease. A minority will develop severe, intractable asthma, usually perennial rather than seasonal, which is incapacitating and significantly interferes with school attendance, play activity, and day-to-day functioning. Although the relationship of age of onset to prognosis is uncertain, studies of Williams and McNichol in Australia indicate that most severely affected children have onset of wheezing during the 1st yr of life and a family history of asthma and other allergic diseases (particularly atopic dermatitis). These children may have growth retardation unrelated to corticosteroid administration, chest deformity secondary to chronic hyperinflation, and persistent abnormalities on pulmonary function testing.

The prognosis for young asthmatic children is generally good. Most will have an ultimate remission dependent in significant part upon growth in the cross-sectional diameter of the airways. Longitudinal studies indicate that about half of all asthmatic children will be virtually free of symptoms by the time they reach adulthood. Whether the hyperirritability of their airways ever disappears is unknown; continuing abnormal responsiveness to methacholine inhalation in former asthmatics has been reported as long as 20 yr after symptoms have abated.

Pathophysiology. The 3 elements that contribute to airway obstruction in asthma are spasm of smooth muscle; edema and inflammation of the mucous membranes lining the airways; and intraluminal exudation of mucus, inflammatory cells, and cellular debris. The obstruction produces increased airway resistance, which lowers forced expiratory volumes and flow rates, premature closure of the airways, hyperinflation of the lungs, increased work of breathing, and changes in the elastic properties and frequency-dependent behavior of the lung. Although the airway obstruction is diffuse, it typically is nonuniform from 1 part of the lung to another. This results in perfusion of inadequately ventilated portions of the lung and leads to abnormalities in blood gases, particularly decreased pO_2. Early in the course of an acute asthmatic attack, arterial pCO_2 is commonly decreased because of hyperventilation. As the obstructive process worsens, net alveolar hypo-

ventilation supervenes, pCO_2 rises, and when buffer mechanisms are exhausted, blood pH falls. Pulmonary hypertension, right ventricular strain, and impaired left ventricular filling may be observed.

Etiology. Asthma is a complex disorder involving biochemical, autonomic, immunologic, infectious, endocrine, and psychologic factors in varying degrees in different individuals. The control of the diameter of the airways may be considered a balance of neural and humoral forces (Fig 9–6). Neural bronchoconstrictor activity is mediated through the cholinergic portion of the autonomic nervous system. Vagal sensory endings in airway epithelium — termed cough or irritant receptors, depending upon their location — initiate the afferent limb of a reflex arc which at the efferent end stimulates bronchial smooth muscle contraction. On the neural bronchodilator side a nonadrenergic inhibitory system (purinergic) is found like that in the ganglion cells of the myenteric plexus. Humoral factors favoring bronchodilation include the endogenous catecholamines which act on β-adrenergic receptors to produce relaxation in bronchial smooth muscle. When humoral substances such as histamine and slow-reacting substance of anaphylaxis are released through immunologically mediated reactions, they produce bronchoconstriction, either by direct action on smooth muscle or by stimulation of the vagal sensory receptors described above.

One theory (Szentivanyi) considers asthma to be due essentially to abnormal β-adrenergic receptor–adenylate cyclase function, with decreased adrenergic responsiveness. The recent reports of decreased numbers of β-adrenergic receptors on leukocytes of nonadrenergic, drug-treated asthmatics may provide the morphologic basis for the observed hyporesponsiveness to β-agonists. Alternatively, increased cholinergic activity in the airway has been proposed as a fundamental defect in asthma, perhaps due to some intrinsic or acquired abnormality in irritant receptors, which seem in asthmatics to have lower than normal thresholds for response to stimulation. Neither theory reconciles all the data. In individual patients a number of factors generally contribute in varying degrees to the activity of the asthmatic process.

Immunologic Factors. In some patients with so-called extrinsic or allergic asthma, attacks follow exposure to environmental factors such as dust, pollens,

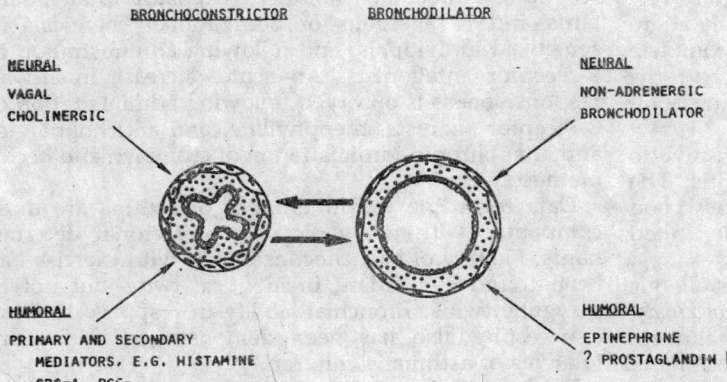

BRONCHOCONSTRICTOR   BRONCHODILATOR

NEURAL   NEURAL
VAGAL   NON-ADRENERGIC
CHOLINERGIC   BRONCHODILATOR

HUMORAL   HUMORAL
PRIMARY AND SECONDARY   EPINEPHRINE
MEDIATORS. E.G. HISTAMINE   ? PROSTAGLANDIN E_1
SRS-A, PGF_2

Figure 9–6 Airway diameter is regulated by both neural and humoral factors. See text for discussion.

danders, and foods. Often but not always, these patients have increased concentrations both of total IgE and of specific IgE against the allergen implicated. In other asthmatics with clinically similar asthma, no evidence of IgE involvement can be found; skin tests are negative and IgE concentrations low. This form of asthma, which is seen most often in the 1st 2 yr of life and in older adults ("late onset" asthma), has been called intrinsic or nonimmunologic, though no differences in general immunologic reactivity have been found between the intrinsic and extrinsic groups. In view of the scant evidence that the fundamental abnormality is immunologic, the interests of many asthmatics, particularly children, have not been well served by excessive emphasis on the role of allergy in their disease and by the overutilization of immunotherapy.

Viral agents are the most important infectious provocateurs of asthma. Early in life respiratory syncytial virus (RSV) and parainfluenza virus (PV) are most often involved; in older children rhinoviruses have also been implicated. Influenza virus infection assumes importance with increasing age. Viral agents may act to initiate asthma through stimulation of afferent vagal receptors of the cholinergic system in the airways. A recent study has shown an IgE response to RSV in infants and children with RSV-associated wheezing but not in those with non-wheezing-associated RSV respiratory disease.

Endocrine Factors. Exacerbations of asthma may occur in relation to menses, particularly premenstrually, or asthma may have its onset in women around the menopause. It improves in some children at puberty. Little else is known about the role of endocrine factors in the etiology and pathogenesis of asthma. Thyrotoxicosis increases the severity of asthma; the mechanism is unknown.

Psychologic Factors. Asthma is influenced to a great extent by emotional factors. However, "deviant" emotional or behavioral characteristics are not significantly more common among asthmatic children than among children in general. Nevertheless, emotional incidents are important precipitants of symptoms in many children and adults. The effects of severe chronic illness such as asthma on children's views of themselves, their parents' views of them, or their lives in general can be devastating. Emotional or behavioral disturbances are related more closely to poor control of asthma than to the severity of the attack itself; accordingly, skillful medical intervention can have important impact.

Clinical Manifestations. The onset of an attack of asthma may be acute or insidious. Acute episodes are most often brought on by exposure to irritants such as cold air and noxious fumes (tobacco smoke, wet paint) or exposure to allergens. When airway obstruction develops rapidly in a few min, it is most likely due to smooth muscle spasm in large airways. Attacks precipitated by viral respiratory infections are slower in onset, with gradual increases in frequency and severity of cough and wheezing over a few days. The signs and symptoms of asthma include cough, which sounds tight and is nonproductive early in the course of an attack; wheezing, tachypnea, and dyspnea with prolonged expiration and use of accessory muscles of respiration; cyanosis; hyperinflation of the chest; tachycardia; and abdominal pain, which may be present to varying degrees depending upon the stage and severity of the attack.

When the patient is in extreme expiratory distress, the cardinal sign of asthma, wheezing, may be strikingly absent; in such patients, only after bronchodilator treatment gives partial relief of the airway obstruction can enough movement of air occur to evoke wheezing. Shortness of breath may be so severe that the child has difficulty walking or even talking. The patient may assume a hunched-over, tripod-like sitting position which makes it easier to breathe. Expiration is typically more difficult because of premature expiratory closure of the airway, but many children complain of inspiratory difficulty as well. Abdominal pain is common, particularly in younger children, and is due presumably to the use of abdominal muscles and the diaphragm during expiration. The liver and spleen may be palpable because of hyperinflation of the lungs. Vomiting is not uncommon and may be followed by temporary relief of symptoms.

During a severe attack respiratory effort may be great, and the child may sweat profusely; a low grade fever may develop simply from the enormous work of breathing; fatigue may become severe. Between attacks the child may be entirely free of symptoms and have no evidence of pulmonary disease on physical examination. A barrel chest deformity is a sign of the chronic, unremitting airway obstruction of severe asthma. Clubbing of the fingers is rarely observed in uncomplicated asthma, even in severe cases. Clubbing suggests other causes of chronic respiratory illness, particularly cystic fibrosis.

Diagnosis. Recurrent episodes of coughing and wheezing, particularly accentuated by exercise, are so characteristic of asthma that the diagnosis is easily made in the majority of cases. There are, however, a significant number of young children with asthma who have a persistent chronic nonproductive cough, particularly at night after going to bed, who cough and become short of breath on exercise, but in whom wheezing has not been documented. A diagnosis of "allergic cough," "allergic bronchitis," "wheezy bronchitis," or chronic bronchitis is often erroneously made. Williams and McNichol in their long-term etiologic studies of asthmatic children were unable to separate those diagnosed as having "wheezy bronchitis" from those considered to have asthma. Both groups had similar family histories of atopic disease, an increased incidence of hay fever, eosinophilia, and positive allergy skin tests as compared to controls. Pulmonary function testing, sometimes in conjunction with exercise challenge if the child is old enough to cooperate (usually around 6 yr of age), is useful in arriving at the correct diagnosis. Furthermore, when treated by measures that are specific for asthma, they show remarkable improvement, strongly suggesting that the cough is a sign of asthma.

Laboratory Evaluation. Eosinophilia of the blood and sputum occurs with asthma. Blood eosinophilia above 250–400 cells/mm³ is usual. A total eosinophil count is preferable to the usual estimation from differential white counts. Asthmatic sputum is grossly tenacious, rubbery, and whitish. With an eosin-methylene blue stain, numerous eosinophils and the granules from disrupted cells may be seen. Few diseases in children other than asthma are likely to present eosinophilia in sputum. Sputum cultures are generally not useful in asthmatic children since bacterial superinfection is rare and they are frequently contaminated with oropharyngeal organisms. Serum protein and immunoglobulin concentrations are generally normal in asthma except that IgE levels may be increased.

Allergy skin testing is useful in identifying potentially important environmental allergens (Sec 9.44).

Inhalation bronchial challenge testing is occasionally done to explore the clinical significance of allergens implicated by skin testing, but since there is excellent correlation between RAST results and bronchial challenge testing, the latter procedure is only rarely indicated. Where the diagnosis of asthma is uncertain, testing for the asthmatic's heightened sensitivity to inhalation of Mecholyl and histamine may be helpful in children who are old enough to be monitored by pulmonary function testing.

The response of the asthmatic to *exercise testing* is quite characteristic (Sec 12.19).

Every child suspected of asthma should have a *roentgenogram of the chest* with posteroanterior and lateral exposures. Lung markings are commonly increased in asthma. Hyperinflation occurs during acute attacks and may become chronic when airway obstruction is persistent. Atelectasis is very common during acute exacerbations and is particularly likely to involve the right middle lobe, where it may persist for months.

Pulmonary function testing (Sec 12.19) is valuable in the evaluation of children in whom asthma is suspected. In those known to have asthma, such tests are useful in assessing the degree of airway obstruction and the disturbance in gas exchange, in measuring response of the airways to inhaled allergens and chemicals (bronchial provocation testing), in assessing the response to therapeutic agents, and in evaluating the long-term course of the disease. Assessments of pulmonary function in asthma are most valuable when made before and after administration of an aerosol bronchodilator; with this procedure the degree of reversibility of the airway obstruction at the time of the testing can be determined (Sec 12.8 and 12.19).

In mild cases of asthma in remission, no abnormalities may be detected. In others a variety of abnormalities may be found. Total lung capacity (TLC), functional residual capacity (FRC), and residual volume (RV) are increased. Vital capacity (VC) is usually decreased. Dynamic tests of air flow, forced vital capacity (FVC), forced expiratory volume in 1 sec (FEV$_1$), and maximum expiratory flow between 25–75% of the vital capacity (MEF$_{25-75}$) may also show reduced values which tend to normalize following administration of aerosolized bronchodilators. With the availability of small, relatively inexpensive instruments that measure peak expiratory flow rate (Mini-Wright Peak Flow Meter), it is feasible to monitor expiratory flow rate at home on a 2–3 times a day basis year round. This gives the physician an objective measurement of the degree of airway obstruction between office visits. Fall in peak expiratory flow predicts the onset of an exacerbation and encourages early intervention with additional drug therapy.

Determination of arterial blood gases and pH is essential in evaluation of the patient with asthma. During remission pO$_2$, pCO$_2$, and pH may be normal. During symptomatic periods, low pO$_2$ is regularly found and may persist days to wk after an acute episode is over. pCO$_2$ is generally low during the early stages of an asthmatic attack. As the obstruction worsens, pCO$_2$ rises; this is an ominous sign. Blood pH remains normal until the buffering capacity of the blood is exhausted, and then acidosis develops.

Differential Diagnosis. Most children subject to recurrent episodes of coughing and wheezing will be shown to have asthma. Other causes of airway obstruction include congenital malformations (of the respiratory, cardiovascular, or gastrointestinal systems), foreign bodies in the airway or esophagus, infectious bronchiolitis, cystic fibrosis of the pancreas, immunologic deficiency disease, hypersensitivity pneumonitis, allergic bronchopulmonary aspergillosis, and a variety of rarer conditions that compromise the airway, including endobronchial tuberculosis, fungal diseases, and bronchial adenoma. Very rarely in the United States, tropical eosinophilia and other parasitic infections may involve the lung and mimic asthma.

Asthma in Early Life. Wheezing in the infant merits special mention because it is common and presents substantial diagnostic and therapeutic problems. A significant number of children subsequently shown to have asthma have had symptoms of obstructive airway disease early in life (39% under 1 yr of age and 57% under 2 yr of age in 1 series).

A number of anatomic and physiologic peculiarities of early life predispose to obstructive airway disease: (1) Decreased amount of smooth muscle in the peripheral airways compared to adults, which results in less support. (2) Mucous gland hyperplasia in the major bronchi compared to adults, a factor that favors increased intraluminal mucus production. (3) Disproportionately narrow peripheral airways that last up to 5 yr of age. This results in decreased conductance relative to adults and renders the infant and young child vulnerable to disease affecting the small airways. (4) Decreased static elastic recoil of the young lung, predisposing to early airway closure during tidal breathing and resulting in mismatching of ventilation and perfusion and hypoxemia. (5) Highly compliant rib cage and mechanically disadvantageous angle of insertion of diaphragm to rib cage (horizontal vs oblique in the adult). Diaphragmatic work of breathing is thus increased. (6) Decreased number of fatigue-resistant skeletal muscle fibers in the diaphragm. The diaphragm is thus poorly equipped to maintain high work output. (7) Deficient collateral ventilation. The pores of Cohn are deficient in numbers and size, as are Lambert's canals. The infant and young child are therefore predisposed to the development of atelectasis distal to obstructed airways. The combination of the above factors with the normal susceptibility of infants and children to viral respiratory infections renders this age group particularly vulnerable to lower respiratory tract obstructive disease.

The clinical, roentgenographic, and blood gas findings in asthma and bronchiolitis are quite similar. It is helpful to remember that the incidence of bronchiolitis due to respiratory syncytial virus peaks during the 1st 6 mo of life, principally during the cold weather months, and that 2nd and 3rd attacks are uncommon. Some clinicians have proposed using the response to epinephrine to help decide whether an episode is asthma or bronchiolitis, with a favorable response favoring asthma. The validity of this test has not been established; the degree of response may be related more to the severity of the obstructive process than to its underlying nature. Trials of epinephrine or other bronchodilators are worthwhile, however, as will be discussed below.

The onset of symptoms is rather typical; many parents come to recognize and dread the sequence of events that leads to severe respiratory distress. In typical cases, previously well infants or young children will develop what seems to be a cold with rhinorrhea, rapidly followed by irritability, a tight cough, tachypnea, and wheezing. The symptoms may progress with frightening rapidity and often require hospitalization.

During the early years, respiratory tract infections with viruses or chlamydia may cause symptoms of airway obstruction that can be confused with asthma. Bacterial infections of the lower airway are rare, and the concept that allergic reactions to bacteria cause asthma is unproved. A child with recurrent episodes of coughing and wheezing associated with bacterial infections should be investigated for cystic fibrosis or immunologic deficiency. Chronic aspiration due to swallowing mechanism dysfunction (usually in developmentally delayed children) or cardioesophageal reflux also may cause recurrent cough and wheezing in early life. In these infants the symptoms of respiratory distress often occur in relationship to feeding or shortly thereafter, and a chest roentgenogram is commonly abnormal. Other rarer causes of obstructive airway disease in early life include obliterative bronchiolitis (usually a sequela of a severe viral insult, most often adenovirus, to the lungs), bronchopulmonary dysplasia, and homozygous α_1-antitrypsin deficiency.

The role of food allergy as a major cause of obstructive airway symptoms during early life is controversial. Positive skin tests for IgE-mediated sensitivity to foods are unusual in early life, and elimination diets and provocative food tests rarely give consistent results. The temporary elimination of milk, wheat, eggs, and chocolate from the diet of the asthmatic patient is recommended by some practitioners.

For an infant who has had several episodes of obstructive airway disease, a history of asthma, hay fever, or atopic dermatitis in mother, father, or siblings is an important predictor of subsequent obstructive airway problems. Eczema is also frequently associated with the subsequent appearance of asthma. Eosinophilia greater than 400 cells/mm³ (and especially greater than 700 cells/mm³) and high serum IgE concentrations predict continuing respiratory tract problems.

Treatment. The principles of avoidance of allergens outlined under treatment of allergic rhinitis also serve the child with asthma. The hyperreactivity of the asthmatic airway is an additional factor and is dealt with by minimizing exposure to nonspecific irritants such as tobacco smoke and strong odors such as wet paint and disinfectants, and by avoiding ice cold drinks and rapid changes in temperature and humidity. Proper maintenance of humidified air is important in dry, cold climates in the winter. If the clinical history suggests IgE-mediated sensitivity to inhalant factors that cannot be avoided or can be only partially avoided, hyposensitization therapy should be considered. The indications for hyposensitization and evidence for its efficacy in asthma are discussed in Sec 9.47.

Pharmacologic therapy is the mainstay of treatment of asthma. Oxygen administered by mask or nasal prongs at 2–3 l/min is indicated in most children during an acute attack of asthma. Not only is the pO_2 almost always reduced during an acute episode, but drugs used in therapy (isoproterenol or intravenous aminophylline) may cause a further fall in pO_2 secondary to worsening of ventilation-perfusion mismatching, which results from the action of these agents in causing pulmonary vasodilatation and/or increased cardiac output. Injection of epinephrine has been the treatment of choice for acute asthma for many yr, but bronchodilator aerosols are being increasingly used.

When epinephrine is used, a dose of 0.01 ml/kg of the 1:1000 concentrations of the aqueous preparation may be given. It may be necessary to repeat the same dose once in 20 min to obtain optimal relief. In infants and small children a dose of 0.05 ml is often effective. The unpleasant side effects of epinephrine (pallor, tremor, and headache) can frequently be minimized if doses of no more than 0.2–0.3 ml are given at any age. Terbutaline, one of the new selective β_2 agonists (Sec 9.46), is available in an injectable form and is an alternative to epinephrine. The usual dose of 0.25 cc (0.25 mg) does not cause peripheral vasoconstriction and produces less cardioacceleration than epinephrine. An additional advantage of terbutaline is its longer duration of activity, up to 4 hr. The more prolonged action of the drug has diminished the need for repository forms of epinephrine such as Sus-Phrine or Asmolin.

In children old enough to use them effectively, inhalation of bronchodilator aerosols is rapidly effective in relieving the signs and symptoms of asthma. Aerosols have the advantage that substantially less drug is given than would be required by the subcutaneous route; the unpleasant side effects of injected drugs such as epinephrine are avoided. Isoproterenol (Isuprel) 1:200, in a dose of 5 drops in 2 ml of water or saline, is aerosolized from a plastic nebulizer with a source of compressed air (or preferably oxygen). Alternatively, isoetharine (Bronkosol) 1:100 may be used in a dose of 10 drops in 2 ml of saline. A solution form of metaproterenol (Alupent), another of the β_2 selective agonists, also may be used as an alternative to isoproterenol or isoetharine in a dose of 5 drops diluted as above. All 3 drugs are also available for inhalation from hand-held Freon-propelled units, which deliver from 0.05–0.125 mg of isoproterenol, 0.34 mg of isoetharine, or 0.65 mg of metaproterenol/dose.

If the response to epinephrine and to isoproterenol is not satisfactory, some form of theophylline should be administered. Aminophylline (85% theophylline and 15% ethylenediamine) may be given intravenously in a dose of 4 mg/kg over 5–15 min at a rate no greater than 25 mg/min. This dose is safe in the patient who has had no theophylline in the past 4–6 hr. Studies have shown that theophylline serum concentrations obtained at the time of arrival in the emergency room are almost always low enough to permit the administration of the dose recommended above. However, if there is reason to believe that the patient may already have a significant serum theophylline concentration, the intravenous dose may be reduced by half to avoid the possibility of theophylline toxicity.

Most acute exacerbations of asthma respond to the treatment regimen described above. Unless the patient either is corticosteroid dependent or has had corticosteroids in the recent past, administration of steroids as part of the emergency room treatment program is unnecessary. However, in certain cases the prescription of prednisone in decreasing doses over a few days may be useful in hastening resolution of the exacerbation and causes no harm. The patient should be discharged from the emergency room with sufficient oral medication to continue therapy at home and appropriate arrangements made for follow-up. Good ambulatory management will almost always reduce the need for emergency room visits for acute attacks.

Status Asthmaticus

If a patient continues to have significant respiratory distress despite administration of sympathomimetic drugs and theophylline, the diagnosis of status asthmaticus should be considered. Status asthmaticus is a clinical diagnosis defined by increasingly severe asthma not responsive to drugs that are normally effective. A patient in whom the diagnosis is made should be admitted to a hospital, preferably to an intensive care unit, where the condition can be carefully monitored. A respiratory score should be determined initially and monitored at regular intervals according to a scheme originally proposed by Downes (Table 9–18). An indwelling arterial line may be indicated. Baseline complete blood counts and serum electrolytes should be measured. Since hypoxemia and acid-base disturbances predispose to cardiac arrhythmias and potentially cardiotoxic drugs (theophylline, adrenergics) will be used, cardiac monitoring is almost always indicated. Analysis of arterial blood for determination of pO_2, pCO_2, and pH is indicated. For these determinations well arterialized capillary blood is adequate but less desirable than arterial blood, particularly if the patient has received epinephrine, which constricts the peripheral vascular bed.

Patients in status asthmaticus are invariably hypoxemic. Oxygen in carefully controlled concentrations is therefore always indicated to maintain tissue oxygenation. In the face of hypercapnia, particular care should be taken to administer oxygen continuously and not intermittently. It may be administered very effectively by nasal prongs or mask at a flow rate of 2–3 l/min. A concentration of oxygen sufficient to maintain a PaO_2

Table 9–18   RESPIRATORY SCORING SYSTEM

	0	1	2
PaO_2 (torr)	70–100	≤70 in room air	≤70 in 40% O_2
Cyanosis	None	In room air	In 40% O_2
$PaCO_2$ (torr)	<40	40–65	>65
Pulsus paradoxus (torr)	<10	10–40	>40
Use of accessory muscles of respiration	None	Moderate	Marked
Air exchange	Good	Fair	Poor
Mental status	Normal	Depressed or agitated	Coma

Interpretation of respiratory scoring system:

0–4	No immediate danger
5–6	Impending respiratory failure
7 or greater	Respiratory failure

At the 5–6 range, all those caring for patients in respiratory failure should be notified that there is a patient who may require assisted ventilation.

of 70–90 torr is optimal. A mist tent should not be used; the water does not reach the lower airway to any significant extent, and mists have an irritant effect on the airways of many asthmatics, leading to coughing and worsening of the wheezing. Furthermore, it is not possible to observe adequately a patient who is enveloped in a dense fog.

Dehydration due to inadequate fluid intake, greatly increased insensible water loss due to tachypnea, and the diuretic effect of theophylline may be present. Care should be taken not to overhydrate the patient since increased secretion of antidiuretic hormone occurs during status asthmaticus promoting fluid retention, and the large negative-peak inspiratory pleural pressures that occur in children favor accumulation of fluid in the interstitial spaces around the small airways. Thus, no more than 1–1.5× maintenance fluids should be given. Sodium bicarbonate, 1–3 mEq/kg, should be administered every 4–6 hr or more often if signs of metabolic acidosis appear.

Bronchodilator therapy initiated in the emergency room should be continued. Aminophylline, 4–5 mg/kg, should be given intravenously over 20 min every 6 hr. Alternatively, a 6 mg/kg loading dose followed by a constant infusion in a dose of 0.75–1.25 mg/kg/hr may be administered. If the patient has received intravenous aminophylline in the emergency room, the loading dose should be omitted. It is essential to adjust aminophylline dosing by monitoring serum theophylline concentrations, since there are many physiologic derangements that occur during the course of status asthmaticus that may affect the disposition of theophylline. If the every-6-hr regimen is used, a serum sample should be obtained 1 hr after the intravenous injection and just before the next dose. During constant infusion theophylline concentration should be monitored at least at 1, 12, and 24 hr intervals as a basis for dose adjustments. A steady state serum concentration of approximately 12–15 µg/ml should be sought. Adrenergic drugs are best administered by aerosol using either isoproterenol or isoetharine as previously described. Bronchodilator treatments may be repeated every 2–3 hr or more often if necessary. Since the response to bronchodilators in status asthmaticus is by definition inadequate and short lived, we have repeated aerosol treatments as often as every 30 min in the very distressed patient who, by blood gas and other criteria, is not yet a candidate for intubation and assisted ventilation. In such a patient isoproterenol is often administered intravenously with gratifying results. Cardiac monitoring in this circumstance is essential. The drug is administered with a constant infusion pump in a dose of 0.1 µg/kg/min for 10–15 min; if the patient does not improve clinically, the dose is increased by 0.1 µg/kg/min for another 10–15 min. The dose may be increased by a similar increment until clinical or blood gas improvement occurs or the heart rate exceeds 200 beats/min. Blood gases should be measured before each incremental increase. This form of therapy has been used most effectively when the $PaCO_2$ is less than 40 torr and the patient is resistant to all other drugs and very distressed.

Corticosteroids in the form of methylprednisolone (Solu-Medrol) or hydrocortisone (Solu-Cortef) should be administered in large doses (2 mg/kg of prednisone, or its equivalent, every 4–6 hr). Because of its lesser effect on mineral metabolism when given in high doses over several days and lower cost for equivalent anti-inflammatory dose, methylprednisolone is preferred over hydrocortisone.

Treatment is guided by serial measurement of blood gases and pH every few hr or more often if indicated. If gas and pH analysis both indicate that respiratory failure is impending, an anesthesiologist should be alerted and facilities and equipment for nasotracheal intubation and respiratory support with a volume-cycled respirator should be available.

Sedation of patients with status asthmaticus is hazardous unless careful monitoring of blood gases is done. If sedation is necessary, chloral hydrate is the safest drug to use. The best sedative for the anxious patient' is the presence of a competent, compassionate physician and nurse at the bedside. Chest roentgenograms should be obtained in all cases and repeated as indicated to detect complications such as mediastinal emphysema or pneumothorax. Routine administration of antibiotics has not been shown to alter the course of status asthmaticus in children or the incidence of infectious complications.

Day-to-Day Management of the Asthmatic Child

On the basis of history, physical examination, laboratory data, pulmonary function testing, and need for medication, patients may be classified as having mild, moderate, or severe asthma. The day-to-day management of these different degrees of illness will vary.

Mild Asthma. Children with mild asthma have attacks of varying frequency, up to once a wk, which are not severe and which respond to bronchodilator treatment within 24–48 hr. Generally, medication is not required between attacks when the child is essentially free of symptoms of airway obstruction. Children with mild asthma have good school attendance, good exercise tolerance, and little or no interruption of sleep by asthma. They have no hyperinflation of the chest; their chest roentgenograms are essentially normal. Pulmonary function testing may show mild and reversible airway obstruction, with none to minimal degrees of increased lung volume.

Moderate Asthma. Children with moderate asthma have symptoms more frequently than those with mild asthma and often have cough and mild wheezing between exacerbations. School attendance may be impaired, exercise tolerance will be diminished because of coughing and wheezing, and the child may lose sleep at night, particularly during exacerbations. Such children will generally require continuous rather than intermittent bronchodilator therapy to achieve satisfactory control of symptoms. Corticosteroids are not required on a continuing basis in this group. Hyperinflation may be evident clinically and roentgenographically. Signs of airway obstruction on physiologic testing are more marked than in the mild group; lung volumes will be increased.

Severe Asthma. Children with severe asthma have virtually daily wheezing and more frequent and more severe exacerbations; they require recurrent hospitalization, which is rarely required for mild or moderate asthma. Severely affected children may miss significant amounts of school, have their sleep interrupted often by asthma, and have poor exercise tolerance. They have chest deformities due to chronic hyperinflation and abnormal roentgenograms. Bronchodilator medication will be required continuously, and regimens may include the regular systemic or aerosol administration of corticosteroids. Physiologic testing will show more severe airway obstruction than in mild or moderate asthma, less reversibility in response to aerosol bronchodilators, and more severe disturbances of lung volumes.

Children with mild asthma should receive bronchodilator medication only when symptomatic, and most exacerbations may be satisfactorily treated with adrenergic agents, by aerosol (isoproterenol, isoetharine, or albuterol), by injection (aqueous epinephrine), or by oral administration (metaproterenol or terbutaline). Theophylline may be added to an oral regimen when indicated. Drug therapy usually can be discontinued after a few days.

For children with moderate asthma who require round-the-clock therapy, theophylline is the drug of choice. Dose and dosing regimen should be individualized and, if required, monitored by measurement of plasma theophylline concentrations. Some experienced allergists reserve monitoring for those patients who fail to have a favorable bronchodilator response or who have symptoms of toxicity (gastrointestinal or central nervous system) on an average dosing regimen. When sustained-release formulations of theophylline are used, the peak plasma concentration occurs 3–4 hr after the dose, at which time a blood sample for monitoring should be obtained. Blood sampling should be delayed until after a few days of therapy with sustained-release drugs to assure that a steady state situation prevails. Significant peaks and troughs of serum concentration are not generally observed with sustained-release theophylline formulations when given at 8-hr dosing intervals. However, in children with unusually rapid theophylline elimination, an additional blood sample at the end of the dosing interval may be needed to see whether a trough of excessive magnitude exists.

While younger children (ages 1–9) generally eliminate theophylline more rapidly than older children and adolescents and hence require more theophylline on a mg/kg basis over 24 hr, it is safest to begin all children on a dose of 16 mg/kg/24 hr in 3 divided doses. If this dose is well tolerated, one may increase by 25% increments at 3–4 day intervals to a maximum of 24 mg/kg/24 hr at 1–9 yr of age, to 20 mg/kg/24 hr from 9–12 yr, and 18 mg/kg/24 hr from 12–16 yr. If adequate control of symptoms is not achieved at the maximum doses or adverse effects become evident, adjustment in the dosing regimen must be guided by determination of serum theophylline concentration. Rapidly absorbed liquids and uncoated tablets, while suitable for children with mild asthma who require a few days of therapy for an exacerbation, have no place in the therapeutic regimen of children who require round-the-clock theophylline therapy because wide fluctuations in serum theophylline concentrations are observed when rapidly absorbed products are used. The decision to use 1 of the sustained-release products will depend upon the dosage form, tablet vs capsule, and the amount of drug in the dosage form (Table 9–19). Capsule formulations that can be opened are virtually tasteless (unless chewed), may be mixed with food, and are particularly suitable for young children. Crushing a sustained-release tablet destroys its constant release properties. Exacerbations of asthma in patients receiving round-the-clock theophylline medication should be treated with adrenergic drugs, as described above for children with mild asthma. When theophylline and an adrenergic bronchodilator must be used together, they should be prescribed separately rather than in a fixed-combination formulation; this will permit the dose of each drug to be adjusted independently.

Cromolyn sodium is discussed in Sec 9.46.

In certain children with mild or moderate degrees of asthma, significant flareups occur from time to time which may require the use of corticosteroids for a few days. Early use of steroids in the child who is known to become severely ill may reduce the need for hospitalization. Steroids should be given in adequate doses (1–2 mg/kg/24 hr of prednisone in 2–3 doses) and should be discontinued as quickly as possible; a long "weaning" period following an acute attack of asthma is unnecessary. In patients who only rarely require steroid administration, return of normal hypothalamic-pituitary-adrenal function is hastened by the *prompt* discontinuation of the drug when the acute episode is over.

In a few children who have severe asthma despite the best available allergic management, unacceptable degrees of coughing and wheezing persist, which severely limit the child's play activities and school attendance. In such children the judicious administration of corticosteroids on an alternate-day basis frequently results in significant amelioration of symptoms and allows the child to lead a normal life without suffering the adverse effects of corticosteroids. If alternate-day therapy is indicated because of either chronic disability or the severity or frequency of attacks of status asthmaticus, the patient is given 5–7 days of intensive daily therapy and then switched to an alternate-day regimen with a short-acting steroid (prednisone, prednisolone, or methylprednisolone). A 12 yr old child might be given 60 mg, 40 mg, 30 mg, 20 mg, and 10 mg of prednisone/24 hr over a 5 day period for an exacerbation of asthma, to be followed by alternate-day therapy at a dose of 20 mg/24 hr given as a single dose at 7–8 A.M. every 48 hr. If the patient responds well to this regimen, the prednisone may be reduced by 5 mg per dose at 10–14 day intervals until the lowest dose compatible with acceptable control of symptoms is reached, usually 5–10 mg on alternate days. Concurrent therapy with theophylline and/or cromolyn should be continued since this reduces the dose of steroid required. Low-dose alternate-day therapy is associated with minimal adverse effects and, thus, may be justified in a disease that can be life-threatening and capable of causing chronic invalidism. However, steroid therapy should not substitute for or delay comprehensive management of the disease.

Inhalational corticosteroids, such as beclomethasone diproprionate (Vanceril, Beclovent), may provide an alternative to the use of every-other-day oral corticosteroid. While beclomethasone is well absorbed from mucosal surfaces, it is rapidly inactivated in the liver into metabolites devoid of glucocorticoid activity. Thus, systemic effects in children given less than 420 μg/24 hr (usual dose is 2 inhalations or 84 μg 4 times a day) are minimal. Oropharyngeal candidiasis occasionally may occur. Its frequency is diminished by rinsing the mouth after inhaling the aerosol. Effective use of the inhaled steroid requires a degree of compliance in the patient not often found in children under 6–7 yr of age. Although studies following up to 18 mo of inhaled steroid treatment showed no evidence of epithelial atrophy or thinning of underlying connective tissue, the possible long-term adverse effects of the drug on the pharynx and airways are unknown.

Emotional tensions surrounding asthma are best handled by unhurried discussion of the child's difficulty with the parents, by avoidance of overdramatization of the child's illness, and by careful examinations with the parents of those areas in which parent and child seem

Table 9–19 SELECTED SUSTAINED-RELEASE THEOPHYLLINE PREPARATIONS

DOSAGE FORM	BRAND NAME	MANUFACTURER	ANHYDROUS THEOPHYLLINE CONTENT
Tablet	Theo-Dur	Key	300 mg scored 200 mg " 150 mg "
Tablet	Theolair-SR	Riker	500 mg 250 mg
Capsule*	Slo-Phyllin Gyrocaps	Dooner	60 mg 125 mg 250 mg
Capsule*	Sprinkle Theo-Dur	Key	50 mg 125 mg 200 mg
Capsule*	Theovent	Schering	125 mg 250 mg
Capsule*	Somophyllin-CRT	Fisons	50 mg 100 mg 250 mg

*The capsules may be opened and mixed with food and are particularly useful in young children.

to be in conflict. The use of tranquilizers or sedatives as a substitute for more direct attempts to solve emotional problems should be avoided. As the asthma is brought under control, the emotional climate is often improved.

9.50 ATOPIC DERMATITIS
(Infantile or Atopic Eczema)

Atopic dermatitis is an inflammatory skin disorder characterized by erythema, edema, intense pruritus, exudation, crusting, and scaling. In the acute stages intraepidermal vesiculation (spongiosis) is present. There appears to be a genetically determined predilection. Infants with atopic dermatitis tend subsequently to develop allergic rhinitis and asthma.

About 80% of patients with atopic dermatitis have serum IgE concentrations increased 5–10-fold over normal. There is conflicting evidence about whether the level of IgE is related to either the severity or the extent of the dermatitis. The concentration of IgE, however, does fluctuate with the stage of the disease, serial studies indicating that the level returns to normal when the disease has been quiescent for several yr. The high levels of IgE have not been satisfactorily explained. It is by no means established that atopic dermatitis is primarily an IgE-mediated allergy; in fact, it is often difficult to demonstrate any role for allergens, whether foods or inhalants, in the pathogenesis of eczema. Moreover, the relationship of atopic dermatitis to allergy or immunology is made more uncertain by reports that IgE does not seem to be increased in affected patients who have neither family history nor clinical evidence of rhinitis or asthma.

The typical dermal manifestation of the interaction of IgE antibody with antigen is the hive (wheal and flare) rather than the erythematous papule of atopic dermatitis; and, while patients with atopic dermatitis frequently possess IgE antibody specific for inhalants or food allergens, it is not generally possible to induce skin lesions of atopic dermatitis by intradermal injection of the suspected allergen. Typical lesions of atopic dermatitis may occur in individuals with X-linked agammaglobulinemia, who are virtually without IgE.

Increased concentrations of IgE in atopic dermatitis may be related to defective T cell function, specifically to a deficiency of IgE "suppressor" T cells. Impairment of cell-mediated immunity in some patients with atopic dermatitis is indicated by (1) absence of the reactions of delayed hypersensitivity upon intradermal skin testing with certain antigens; (2) inability to be sensitized with potent contact sensitizers (e.g., dinitrochlorobenzene [DNCB]); (3) diminished proliferative response of lymphocytes to mitogens such as phytohemagglutinin (PHA); and (4) decreased numbers of T lymphocytes in peripheral blood as measured by sheep red cell rosette formation.

The hyperreactive skin of atopic dermatitis differs from normal skin in its response to a variety of physical and pharmacologic stimuli. For example, a light mechanical stroke results within 1 min in a white line with a surrounding blanched area. This phenomenon ("white dermographism") is not seen in normal skin. Involved skin has abnormal rates of cooling and warming in response to temperature changes, particularly in flexural areas. Paradoxical responses occur to injections of various pharmacologic agents, such as histamine, acetylcholine ("delayed blanch phenomenon"), and nicotinic acid ester. The observation that adrenergic responses are decreased in lymphocytes and granulocytes from patients with atopic dermatitis suggests that imbalance of autonomic homeostasis is a basis for the abnormalities in the skin. The abnormal reactivity of the skin has a counterpart in the airway hyperreactivity of asthma; in both disorders such hyperreactivity seems to be an intrinsic part of the disease and is independent of immunologic factors.

Clinical Manifestations. Atopic dermatitis typically occurs in 3 stages with fairly distinctive features. The disease most often *begins in infancy*, usually during the 1st 2–3 mo of life. The onset is sometimes delayed until the 2nd or 3rd yr. The earliest lesions of infantile atopic dermatitis are erythematous weepy patches on the cheeks, with subsequent extension to the remainder of the face, neck, wrists, hands, and extensor aspects of the extremities. Typical involvement of flexural areas characteristically appears later but may occur as popliteal and antecubital dermatitis in early life.

The disease is markedly pruritic; the affected infant makes incessant efforts to scratch the skin by rubbing the face on bedclothes and against the sides of the crib. This trauma to the skin rapidly leads to weeping and crusting; secondary infection is common and may be extensive.

The onset of dermatitis frequently coincides with the introduction of certain foods into the infant's diet, particularly cow's milk, wheat, or eggs. In most infants, however, a prime role of reaginic sensitivity in the pathogenesis of skin eruption is hard to prove, and there is disagreement concerning the importance of food allergy in initiating or maintaining atopic dermatitis. In certain infants, on the other hand, there is unequivocal evidence of reaginic sensitivity as manifested in the appearance of urticaria, colic, and a diffuse erythematous flush following ingestion of the offending food. The erythematous flush appears to be accompanied by intense itching, which results in scratching and then in the appearance of the skin lesions characteristic of eczema. The major role of scratching in the production of skin lesions has been demonstrated when 1 extremity has been encased in surgical dressings and the other left uncovered; the lesions of atopic dermatitis occur only in the uncovered extremity.

Atopic dermatitis shows a tendency to *remission at 3–5 yr of age*. In most cases the disease will become quiescent by the age of 5 yr; in some, a mild to moderate eczema may persist in the antecubital and popliteal fossae, on the wrists, behind the ears, and on the face and neck. During childhood, antecubital and popliteal involvement becomes common; extensor surfaces of the extremities may still be actively affected. With increasing age there is a tendency toward *drying and thickening of the skin* in the involved areas, particularly in the antecubital and popliteal fossae, and on the neck, forehead, eyelids, wrists, and the dorsa of the hands and feet. The face takes on a whitish hue (due to increased capillary permeability and dilatation resulting in edema and blanching of surrounding tissues), sometimes called the "mask of atopic dermatitis." Hyperpigmentation of the skin, scaling, and lichenification (a particular kind of papular thickening of the skin, with accentuation of the normal surface lines) become prominent. There is a marked tendency toward healing of the disease in the 4th and 5th decades of life.

Diagnosis. When pruritus is intense and the lesions characteristic, the diagnosis of atopic dermatitis may be easy. A family history of asthma, hay fever, or atopic dermatitis, the finding of elevated serum IgE concentrations and of reaginic antibodies to a variety of foods and inhalants, the presence of eosinophilia, and the demonstration of white dermographism support the diagnosis. Some patients have accentuated lines or grooves below the margin of the lower eyelids called the atopic pleat, Dennie line, or Morgan fold and an increased number of creases of the skin of the palm. The skin has a tendency to lichenify in response to chronic irritation or rubbing, a phenomenon that is not seen in normal persons. Generalized dryness of the skin, even in uninvolved areas, and sparsity of the hair of the lateral portion of the eyebrows, thought to be secondary to chronic rubbing, are also characteristic.

Differential Diagnosis. The eczematoid skin reaction characterized by erythema, edema, exudation, crusting, and scaling is not specific for atopic dermatitis. In infants and children the differential diagnosis includes seborrheic dermatitis, scabies, primary irritant dermatitis, allergic contact dermatitis, infectious eczematoid dermatitis, ichthyosis, phenylketonuria, acrodermatitis enteropathica, histiocytosis X, and 2 primary immunologic deficiency disorders: the Wiskott-Aldrich syndrome and X-linked agammaglobulinemia.

Seborrheic dermatitis typically begins on the scalp, often as "cradle cap," and involves the ear and contiguous skin, the sides of the nose, and eyebrows and eyelids with greasy, brownish scales that are usually distinguished easily from the erythematous, weeping, crusted lesions of infantile atopic dermatitis. On the other hand, it is sometimes difficult during the 1st few mo of life to distinguish clearly between seborrhea and atopic dermatitis, particularly when the face is primarily involved. The course of seborrhea in infancy is shorter than that of atopic eczema, and it responds much more rapidly to treatment. The difficulty in differentiating the 2 conditions is recognized in the use of the term seborrheic eczema by some dermatologists. In infancy, *scabies* may be confused with atopic dermatitis. The location of the lesions helps differentiate the 2 entities. Atopic dermatitis most often begins on the cheeks and does not involve the palms and soles, where scabies commonly starts with large papules on the upper back and with vesicles on the palms and soles. The mite of scabies or its ova can be seen in scrapings from the vesicles. The response of scabies to gamma benzene hexachloride will establish its diagnosis.

Primary irritant dermatitis is a nonallergic reaction due to various irritants and most common in infancy in the diaper area. The location and rapid response of lesions to therapy indicate the correct diagnosis.

The skin lesions of *allergic contact dermatitis* (the prototype is poison ivy) are usually limited to the sites of exposure to the offending allergen and do not typically involve the flexural areas. Occasionally, contact dermatitis is superimposed upon atopic dermatitis when sensitization occurs to chemicals used in treating the latter, such as neomycin, the parabens (used as preservatives in many ointments), or iodochlorohydroxyquin (Vioform).

Infectious eczematoid dermatitis is most often seen as a result of discharge of purulent material from a draining ear or other site of infection. The typical location of the lesions and rapid response to therapy support the diagnosis.

In *ichthyosis vulgaris*, dryness of the skin may lead to confusion with atopic dermatitis, but the scales in ichthyosis are usually larger than those in atopic dermatitis, and the pruritus of ichthyosis, if any, is generally mild. The two disorders may be associated. Infants and children with *untreated phenylketonuria* develop an eczematous dermatitis often confused with atopic eczema. The rash of phenylketonuria is responsive to a diet low in phenylalanine.

Histiocytosis X (Letterer-Siwe disease) and *acrodermatitis enteropathica* are serious systemic diseases occurring early in life in which failure to thrive is prominent. Hemorrhagic manifestations in the skin are common in histiocytosis X, in addition to eczematous eruption. The skin around the oral, nasal, genitourinary, and rectal orifices is typically involved in acrodermatitis (Sec 24.12).

Patients with Wiskott-Aldrich syndrome and X-linked agammaglobulinemia may have an eczema that is indistinguishable from atopic dermatitis.

Complications. During early infancy and childhood, secondary infection of the lesions of atopic dermatitis with bacterial or viral agents is common. Staphylococci and β-hemolytic streptococci are the bacterial agents most often recovered from infected lesions. Herpes simplex (Kaposi varicelliform eruption) is also of particular concern. Infants and children with eczema should not be exposed to adults with herpes simplex infection ("cold sores"). Vaccinia may be a major problem if routine smallpox vaccination is utilized. Keratoconus is occasionally seen in children with atopic dermatitis and is thought to occur as a consequence of chronic rubbing of the eyelids. Cataracts occur in 5–10% of adults with severe atopic dermatitis but are rarely seen during childhood.

Treatment. Effective treatment of atopic dermatitis requires control of the environmental precipitants of the itch-scratch-itch cycle that perpetuates the disease, beginning with avoidance of ingestant, injectant, contactant, and atmospheric factors that are known or can be shown to trigger itching or scratching. Extremes of temperature and relative humidity should be avoided. A warm climate of moderate humidity appears to be optimal for the majority of patients. Sweating leads to itching and to aggravation of the disease. Exposure to sunlight and salt water has a beneficial effect on the skin of many patients.

Garments should be made of a smooth-textured cotton; wool should be avoided. Infants should not be allowed to crawl on wool carpeting.

For the dry skin of atopic dermatitis, use of soaps and detergents that defat the skin should be avoided as much as possible. Bathing should be kept to a minimum. The purpose of the bath oil or other creams applied to the skin is to seal the water into the skin; used correctly, bath oil is added to the tub after the patient has soaked for 20 min. Thus, the bath oil seals the moisture in the hydrated skin instead of excluding it as would occur if the oil were added before the patient enters the bath. The same principle applies to application of creams and lotions to the skin. They should be applied to the damp skin following a bath. Should bathing appear to make the patient worse, a nondrying cleansing agent such as Cetaphil, a commercially available nonlipid lotion, can be applied to the skin.

If it appears that a food or other ingestant makes itching worse, then that food must be excluded from the diet. On the other hand, the arbitrary exclusion of numerous foods from the diets of infants with atopic dermatitis without clear-cut evidence that they are involved in the disease is irrational and can lead to malnutrition. The possibility that inhalant factors are related to the activity of the disease must be evaluated with the same critical concern.

Local therapy is the mainstay of management of atopic dermatitis. During acute flare-ups of the disease, wet dressings (e.g., Burow solution, 1:20) have an antipruritic and anti-inflammatory effect. Topical corticosteroid lotions or creams may be applied between changes of wet dressings. The continuous application of wet dressings also has the advantage of immobilizing and protecting the affected parts and preventing scratching. Unless scratching can be controlled, it will be almost impossible to manage the disease successfully, particularly during infancy and early childhood. Fingernails must be kept cut as short as possible; restraints for the elbows to keep the hands from the face are sometimes necessary to control scratching at night. Itching is difficult to control with drugs. Drugs with both sedative and antihistaminic activity, such as diphenhydramine (Benadryl), hydroxyzine (Atarax, Vistaril), or promethazine (Phenergan), appear to be of greatest value. In some patients aspirin has a marked antipruritic effect.

When infection is present, antibiotics should be given systemically. Antibiotics incorporated in topical medicaments not only are of little therapeutic value but can lead to sensitization to the agents applied, particularly in the case of neomycin. The possibility that contact sensitization is superimposed upon atopic dermatitis must be considered when there is a sudden exacerbation of eczema to which a topical medicament has been applied. Parabens, mercurial compounds, and lanolin can all cause contact sensitization.

After the acute phase has subsided, topical application of corticosteroid creams and ointments is of great value in management of the disease. Their cost may be a serious problem. Cost can be reduced by purchasing relatively concentrated creams in bulk, which the pharmacist can dilute to half strength with Aquaphor or Eucerin, rather than purchasing equivalent material in 15 or 30 gm amounts. Small amounts of steroid rubbed in well at frequent intervals give better results than large amounts applied only infrequently. Percutaneous absorption of corticosteroid occurs but is not generally clinically significant. Long-term topical use of steroids leads to an increase in growth of hair in some patients and to atrophy of the skin. The more potent topical steroids should not be applied to the face.

Systemic administration of corticosteroids should be avoided in treatment of atopic dermatitis in infancy and childhood. Such treatment is effective in clearing the skin, but its termination is almost always followed by severe exacerbation of the disease. The possible role of alternate-day steroid treatment in management of atopic dermatitis has not been adequately investigated.

Topical treatment with corticosteroids has largely superseded the use of coal tar preparations. Tars stain clothes and skin, and compliance of the patient in their use is often poor. However, newer preparations, Estargel (Westwood) and Psorigel (Owen), are effective and more acceptable cosmetically. Tars are considerably less expensive for long-term topical use than corticosteroids. Coal tar is photosensitizing, and occasionally its use results in a sterile, pustular folliculitis.

Prognosis. With adequate control of factors known to trigger itching, appropriate local treatment, and understanding support for the parents of a child for whom no immediate cure is to be expected, reasonable control of the disease can generally be accomplished.

9.51 URTICARIA
(Hives)

Clinical Manifestations. Urticaria, or hives, is a common skin disorder characterized by the appearance of usually well circumscribed but sometimes coalescent, localized, or generalized erythematous raised skin lesions (wheals or welts) of various sizes. The lesions may be intensely pruritic or itch little, if at all. The individual hive usually resolves within 48 hr, but new ones may continue to appear singly or in crops. When urticaria persists for longer than 6–8 wk, the condition is arbitrarily called chronic urticaria. Physiologically, urticaria has been attributed to edema of the upper corium due to dilatation and increased permeability of the capillaries.

In angioedema (angioneurotic edema or giant urticaria) the deeper skin layers or submucosa and subcutaneous or other tissues are involved; the upper respiratory tract and the gastrointestinal tract are common target organs. The distinction between urticaria and angioedema is frequently not clear; the lesions appear to differ only in the depth of tissue involvement.

Incidence. As many as 20% of persons experience hives at some time during life. Urticaria is somewhat more frequent in females than in males.

Pathogenesis. The principal noncytotoxic mechanism by which urticaria and angioedema are produced involves the interaction of antigen with mast cell- or basophil-bound IgE antibodies. The release of histamine from these cells causes vasodilatation and increased vascular permeability and stimulates an axon reflex, which produces a typical wheal and flare reaction. Slow-reacting substance of anaphylaxis (SRS-A) may contribute to the edema of the IgE-mediated reaction. A 2nd mediator pathway for urticaria involves the complement system. Two complement component split products, C3a and C5a, act as anaphylatoxins and trigger histamine release from mast cells and basophils by direct action on the cell surfaces, independent of antibodies. C3a and C5a can be generated through both the classical and the alternative complement pathways. A 3rd mediator pathway involves the plasma kinin–forming system of the coagulation scheme. Bradykinin is at least as potent as histamine in increasing vascular permeability. Both non-IgE immunologic reactions and nonimmunologic events can produce urticaria and angioedema when they activate the complement and kinin-forming systems.

Etiology. A clinical classification of urticaria is given in Table 9–20.

Differential Diagnosis. With a few exceptions no laboratory tests establish or exclude the diagnosis of urticaria and angioedema. Allergy skin testing is generally not helpful. In the absence of any clue suggesting an ingestant etiology, elimination diets are not generally useful. The diagnosis is clinical and requires that the physician be aware of the various forms of urticaria. A carefully taken history will usually allow the type to be identified. Except when there are obvious associations with IgE-mediated reactions, naming the "cause" of acute urticaria may be difficult; in chronic urticaria this is accomplished in less than 20% of cases.

Some forms of urticaria need special mention. *Papular urticaria* is usually seen in small children, generally on the extremities and other exposed parts at the site of insect bites. *Cholinergic urticaria* appears as wheals 1–2 mm in diameter surrounded by large areas of erythema (flares) and frequently involves the skin in the neck area. It is brought on by exercise, by hot showers, and in some instances by anxiety. Affected individuals seem to have an increased sensitivity to cholinergic mediators, which can be demonstrated when an intradermal injection of 0.01 mg of methacholine (Mecholyl) in 0.1 ml of saline produces a localized hive surrounded by smaller, satellite lesions. Urticaria is probably due more often to *viral infection* than is commonly appreciated. It is particularly associated with hepatitis, especially during the prodromal stages, and with infectious mononucleosis. Viral infections can also produce *erythema multiforme*, a form of the urticaria-angioedema symptom complex in which typical iris or target lesions are seen and mucosal involvement is common. In some patients typical hives appear to change spontaneously into lesions of erythema multiforme (Sec 5.50). These can be a sign of drug allergy.

Urticaria pigmentosa typically occurs during the 1st few yr of childhood and has a distinctive presentation. *Systemic mastocytosis* is a serious form of urticaria pig-

Table 9–20 TYPES OF URTICARIA

Due to ingestants (IgE mechanism in some cases)
 Foods, particularly fish, shellfish, nuts, and peanuts; food additives
 Drugs
Due to contactants (IgE mechanism in some cases)
 Plant substances (e.g., stinging nettle)
 Drugs applied to the skin
 Animal saliva
Due to injectants (IgE mechanism in some cases)
 Drugs (particularly penicillin), transfused blood, therapeutic antisera, insect stings and bites, allergenic extracts
Due to inhalants (IgE mechanism)
 Pollens, danders, and ? molds
Due to infectious agents (mechanism unknown)
 Parasites
 Viruses (e.g., hepatitis, infectious mononucleosis)
 ? Bacteria
 ? Fungi
Due to physical factors (mechanism mostly unknown)
 Cold urticaria
 Pressure urticaria
 Solar urticaria
 Aquagenic urticaria
 Dermographism
 Vibratory angioedema
Cholinergic urticaria (a distinctive entity)
Associated with systemic diseases (mechanism mostly unknown)
 Collagen-vascular
  Cutaneous vasculitis
  Serum sickness–like disease
 Malignancy
 Hyperthyroidism
 Urticaria pigmentosa (systemic mastocytosis)
Associated with genetic disorders (various mechanisms)
 Familial cold urticaria
 Hereditary angioedema
 Amyloidosis with deafness and urticaria
 C3b inactivator deficiency
Chronic urticaria and angioedema (mechanism unknown)
Psychogenic urticaria (existence as an entity uncertain)

mentosa in which mast cells infiltrate skeleton, liver, spleen, and lymph nodes. In adults, and to a lesser extent in children, urticaria may be associated with *malignancy* or *collagen-vascular disorders*.

Cold urticaria is the most common form due to physical factors. Urticarial lesions which may be either pruritic or described as painful or burning appear upon exposure to cold and are confined to the exposed parts of the body. The lesions develop not only on exposure to cold weather but also with local application of cold (e.g., a cold glass causing lesions on the hands, an iced drink causing swelling of the lips). The cooling of skin associated with evaporation upon emerging from water can produce urticaria. Swimming in cold water is hazardous; death may occur in patients so exposed. There are 2 forms: a primary acquired form and a familial form. Cold urticaria may be seen in adults with such systemic diseases as cryofibrinogenemia, cryoglobulinemia, cold-agglutinin disease, and secondary syphilis. In some cases of primary acquired urticaria, the phenomenon has been passively transferred using purified IgE and IgM fractions of serum from affected patients. Primary acquired cold urticaria appears and disappears spontaneously; in some cases, its onset occurs with a viral illness.

Hereditary angioedema (HAE), a potentially life-threatening form of angioedema (Sec 9.23 and 9.27), is the most important familial form of angioedema.

Treatment. In most instances urticaria is a self-limited illness requiring little treatment other than that aimed at relieving the associated pruritus. Antihistamines are the drugs of 1st choice. Diphenhydramine (Benadryl), 1.25 mg/kg, or hydroxyzine, 0.5 mg/kg, may be given every 4–6 hr as required.

In particularly acute situations epinephrine, 0.1–0.2 ml, gives rapid relief of itching. Hydroxyzine (0.5 mg/kg every 4–6 hr) is the drug of choice for cholinergic and chronic urticaria. The combined use of H_1- and H_2-type antihistamines has been reported to be beneficial in chronic urticaria. Cyproheptadine (Periactin) (2–4 mg every 8–12 hr) is especially useful as a prophylactic agent in cold urticaria. Cyproheptadine produces appetite stimulation and weight gain and perhaps other central nervous system–endocrine effects in some patients. Sun screens are the only effective treatment for solar urticaria. Corticosteroids have varying results in chronic urticaria; the doses required to control the urticaria are often so large that they cause serious side effects. Chronic urticaria does not often respond favorably to dietary manipulation, but a diet that includes only foods of low allergenic potential and eliminates all food colors (tartrazine, FD&C yellow #5, in particular) and additives is worth a 1–2 wk trial. For treatment of hereditary angioedema, see Sec 9.23 and 9.27.

9.52 ANAPHYLAXIS

Definition. The term anaphylaxis describes sudden life-threatening reactions which are most often, but not necessarily, immunologic. Many anaphylactic reactions are the result of IgE-mediated sensitivity to foreign substances, most commonly drugs. Anaphylaxis is uncommon in children. It is most commonly observed as a consequence of penicillin administration and Hymenoptera sting. The frequency may be higher in atopic persons. Fatal anaphylactic reactions follow about 1 in 7.5 million injections of penicillin and 1 in 8.6 million urograms.

Etiology. Virtually any foreign substance is capable of producing anaphylaxis under appropriate circumstances. Drugs, sera, pollen extracts, venom of stinging insects, foods, injectable agents for roentgenographic contrast studies, and hormone preparations have all produced anaphylactic reactions.

Pathogenesis. In the individual who has developed IgE-mediated anaphylactic sensitivity to a given antigen, subsequent administration of even minute amounts of the antigen may result in an explosive antigen-antibody reaction with massive release of chemical mediators such as histamine and slow-reacting substance of anaphylaxis (SRS-A). The action of the mediators on various tissue receptors throughout the body is responsible for the symptoms observed. Though histamine plays a central role in the pathogenesis of human anaphylaxis, other vasoactive substances (kinins, SRS-A, arachidonic acid metabolites) should also be considered. Decreased levels of factor V and factor VIII have been reported, suggesting consumption of coagulation factors due to intravascular coagulation.

Levels of high molecular weight kininogen, C3, and C4 have been depressed in several patients studied during severe episodes of systemic anaphylaxis. When an immunologic mechanism cannot be identified (anaphylactoid reactions), it is presumed that mediator release occurs as a direct effect of the causative agent on basophils and mast cells or perhaps by activation of the alternative complement pathway, with generation of anaphylatoxins (see above).

Clinical Manifestations. Anaphylactic reactions are characteristically explosive, particularly when the antigen is injected. Surviving patients describe a "feeling of impending doom." The more rapidly symptoms appear after administration of the foreign material, the more serious is the reaction. Often the 1st symptom noted is a tingling sensation around the mouth or face, followed by a feeling of warmth, difficulty in swallowing, and tightness in the throat or chest. The patient becomes flushed; urticaria and angioedema then appear, along with varying degrees of hoarseness, inspiratory stridor, dysphagia, nasal congestion, itching of the eyes, sneezing, and wheezing. Abdominal cramps, diarrhea, and contractions of the uterus and other organs of smooth muscle may also occur. The patient may lose consciousness and, on examination, be found hypotensive, with feeble heart sounds, bradycardia, and sometimes an arrhythmia. Cardiorespiratory arrest and death may ensue. In fatal cases death has most often resulted from acute upper airway obstruction, though profound circulatory collapse may occur without upper airway obstruction.

Treatment. Treatment of anaphylaxis depends on anticipation that the event may occur and being prepared for it. In particular, physicians who administer allergen extracts must be ready to treat this life-threatening complication of hyposensitization. If, for example, a generalized reaction follows an injection of pollen extract into an upper extremity, aqueous epinephrine 1:1000, 0.2–0.3 ml, should be administered immediately subcutaneously into the other arm and a tourniquet placed above the site of injection of extract. If the allergenic material has been given subcutaneously, an additional injection of epinephrine may be administered subcutaneously at the site of injection to retard absorption; but if the extract has been given intramuscularly, aqueous epinephrine should *not* be injected into the site since epinephrine has a vasodilatory effect on the blood vessels of skeletal muscle but a vasoconstrictive effect on subcutaneous blood vessels. An intravenous infusion must be started immediately to administer aminophylline should wheezing occur and to facilitate administration of drugs (principally epinephrine) and volume expanders for hypotension. Measurement of central venous pressure is a valuable guide to plasma volume expansion therapy. Oxygen should be administered by mask, and if there is upper airway obstruction (stridor, hoarseness), the patient may need prompt intubation or a tracheostomy. Diphenhydramine (25–50 mg) should be given intravenously. Corticosteroids are not useful as emergency drugs, but may be useful in preventing the recurrences of symptoms during the 12–24 hr following the acute reaction. While serious anaphylactoid reactions to intravenous radio-contrast media are rare in children compared to adults (1–2% of all procedures), they occasionally occur. A preventive regimen has been developed for patients known to be at risk by virtue of previous reactions. They are pretreated with prednisone, 50 mg orally every 6 hr for 3 doses, ending 1 hr before the procedure. Diphenhydramine, 50 mg, is given 1 hr before the procedure. This regimen is effective in preventing adverse reactions of any degree in over 90% of the high-risk patients.

The incidence of drug-induced anaphylaxis would drop substantially if drugs were given only when indicated and only by the oral route unless some compelling reason for injection exists. Not only is anaphylactic sensitivity more easily induced by injection of drugs than by oral administration, but in the sensitized individual anaphylaxis occurs more commonly following parenteral than oral administration. The incidence of anaphylaxis following Hymenoptera stings can be reduced significantly by the appropriate use of immunotherapy (Sec 9.47 and 9.55).

9.53   SERUM SICKNESS

The serum sickness syndrome is a characteristic systemic immunologic disorder which follows the administration of foreign antigenic material.

Etiology.   The disorder was first described in 1905 by von Pirquet and Schick as a consequence of antitoxin therapy for such diseases as diphtheria and tetanus. The illness was shown to be due to an adverse reaction to the serum proteins of the animal in which the antitoxin was prepared. Therapeutic antisera of animal origin, especially equine, are still occasionally used, but today the major cause of the serum sickness syndrome is drug allergy, particularly that due to penicillin. Cases have also followed use of other therapeutic agents, including human gamma globulin, and they also result from Hymenoptera stings. Preparations of immune globulin of human origin are presently available for treatment of diphtheria and tetanus in humans, but antitoxins for treatment of rabies, crotalid envenomation, and clostridial intoxication (botulism, gas gangrene) and the antilymphocyte serum used for immunosuppression in transplantation procedures are still prepared in the horse. Fractionation of these antitoxins to eliminate the nonantibody equine plasma proteins has reduced the incidence of serum sickness to far below that which followed the administration of whole serum.

Pathogenesis.   Serum sickness is the classic example of "immune complex" disease in the experimental animal. After a single large dose of isotopically labeled antigen is injected into the rabbit, the symptoms of serum sickness occur coincidentally with the appearance of antibody formed against the injected antigen, at a time when the latter is still present in the circulation. Antigen-antibody complexes formed under conditions of moderate antigen excess lodge in small vessels and in filtering organs throughout the body (deposition being aided in the rabbit by the actions of IgE antibody, basophils, and platelet-activating factor

and by the release of vasoactive amines that increase the permeability of blood vessels); these complexes activate the complement sequence. Complement components bound at the site of complex deposition encourage accumulation of neurotrophils through at least 2 general processes: adherence of neutrophils to the site of bound complement and chemotactic activity of the C567 complex and C3a and C5a fragments. Tissue injury results from the liberation of toxic molecules from the neutrophils. In this animal model, healing of the lesions occurs following elimination of the complexes from the circulation.

There are certain similarities between the rabbit model and serum disease in man but also outstanding differences. For example, glomerulonephritis is a major lesion of serum sickness in the rabbit but generally develops in humans only with severe serum sickness.

Serum sickness demonstrates how the differing biologic activities of the several species of antibodies formed against a complex antigen may be responsible for diverse parts of the clinical picture; the urticaria of serum sickness is thought to be due to IgE antibody molecules reacting with horse serum proteins, whereas the joint symptoms are thought to occur as a result of deposition of antigen-antibody complexes of the IgG and IgM classes. In both rabbits and humans it is suspected that histamine release from basophils and mast cells, mediated by IgE antibodies, facilitates the deposition of immune complexes through increases in vascular permeability.

Clinical Manifestations.   Typically the symptoms of serum sickness begin 7–12 days following injection of the foreign material. Urticaria, usually generalized, is the most common finding; edema, particularly around the face and neck, fever, myalgia, lymphadenopathy, arthralgia, and/or arthritis involving multiple joints also occur. Intense pruritus accompanying the urticaria is the most distressing symptom in many patients. The site of injection of the foreign material generally becomes red and swollen, commonly 1–3 days before systemic symptoms appear. If there has been earlier exposure or previous allergic reaction to the same foreign antigen, symptoms may appear in accelerated fashion, within 1–3 days following injection, or as anaphylaxis. The disease generally runs a self-limited course, and the patient recovers in 7–10 days. Carditis and glomerulonephritis rarely occur; the most serious complications of serum sickness are Guillain-Barré syndrome and peripheral neuritis, especially involving the brachial plexus (C5–C6).

Laboratory Findings.   The peripheral leukocyte and eosinophil counts are variable. Mild proteinuria and microscopic hematuria may be seen. Plasma cells in the peripheral circulation have been reported. The erythrocyte sedimentation rate is often increased. A sheep cell agglutinin titer of the Forssman type is usually elevated. Serum complement levels are generally normal to only slightly reduced except in patients with severe disease, who may have depressed concentrations of both early and late components. In serum sickness due to horse serum proteins, antibodies of the IgG, IgA, IgM, and IgE classes may be found directed against various horse serum proteins.

Treatment. Patients generally respond well to aspirin and antihistamines. During a diphtheria epidemic in San Antonio, Texas, the incidence of serum sickness due to equine antitoxin was significantly reduced by prophylactic administration of antihistamines. When the symptoms are particularly severe, corticosteroids have been used with great efficacy. High doses are given and rapidly reduced as the patient improves.

Prevention. The use of horse serum or other animal serum in therapy should be limited to cases for which no alternative is available. The availability of tetanus antitoxin of human origin makes the use of equine tetanus antitoxin unwarranted. When only equine antitoxin is available, skin tests should be employed prior to administration of serum, beginning with a puncture test using a 1:10 dilution. If the reaction is negative, one may then begin the intradermal testing with 0.02 ml of a 1:10,000 dilution. If there is no reaction, a subsequent skin test should be performed with a 1:1000 dilution. If a negative result again is obtained, a final test with a 1:100 dilution of horse serum is done. A negative reaction to the strongest intradermal solution indicates that anaphylactic sensitivity to horse serum is very unlikely; skin tests do not predict the likelihood of development of serum sickness.

Occasionally, a patient will require horse serum therapy who has evidence of anaphylactic sensitivity to horse serum by virtue of either a previous reaction or a positive immediate wheal and flare skin test. In such a case the antitoxin can be successfully administered by a process of rapid desensitization. Some allergists prefer to medicate the patient with epinephrine and antihistamines prior to beginning the desensitization procedure. Others prefer not to mask possible evidence of a reaction at an early stage when it still might be of a minor degree and serve as a warning to proceed more slowly with the desensitization. The desensitization process is begun with 0.1 ml amounts of antitoxin, diluted to 1:100,000–1:10,000, depending upon an estimate of the degree of the patient's sensitivity, and injected intravenously at 20 min intervals. If the patient tolerates the previous injection without adverse reactions, the amount administered may be doubled every 20 min. Generally, the entire amount of antitoxin can be administered safely over a 4–6 hr period. The desensitization, unfortunately, is of a transient nature and the patient will often regain his or her previous anaphylactic sensitivity within a few mo.

9.54 ADVERSE REACTIONS TO DRUGS

See also Sec 5.50.

Definition. An adverse reaction to a drug may be defined as any unwanted consequence of administration of the agent during or following a course of therapy. Adverse reactions fall into 2 broad categories: those dependent upon pharmacologic mechanisms and those dependent upon immunologic mechanisms. The majority of adverse drug reactions are pharmacologic; the Boston collaborative drug surveillance program found only 6% to have an allergic basis. In a study of hospitalized children who suffered adverse drug reactions, no more than 15% were thought to be of an allergic nature.

Certain generalities apply to adverse drug reactions: (1) Virtually any organ system may be involved. (2) After the neonatal period, children are less often affected than adults. (3) The incidence of reactions increases almost exponentially with the number of drugs given simultaneously. (4) Certain diseases predispose to adverse drug reactions, particularly those in which multiple drug therapy is common (in cardiovascular and infectious diseases and in psychiatric illnesses). Diseases that affect organs responsible for absorption (gastrointestinal tract), metabolism (liver), or excretion of drugs (kidney) also increase the likelihood of adverse reaction. (5) The pharmacokinetic properties of a drug (for example, the extent of protein-binding) also affect the incidence of adverse reactions.

Classification. Adverse drug reactions can be classified in terms of their underlying mechanisms. *Toxicity* may result from a high concentration of drug in the body due to excessive intake—accidental or intentional—or to abnormalities in absorption, metabolism, or excretion of the drug. Various diseases, genetic factors, or drug interactions may permit accumulation of a drug. Some patients for unknown reasons have excessive pharmacologic responses (*intolerance*) to average drug doses. The signs and symptoms are generally intensifications of the expected pharmacologic effects of the agent.

Side effects are undesirable but essentially unavoidable effects of drugs and largely reflect the fact that a given drug rarely affects only 1 tissue. When theophylline is given as a bronchodilator agent in asthma, for example, central nervous system stimulation is considered a side effect, though this 2nd well known effect of theophylline warrants its use in neonatal apnea. *Secondary effects* of drugs are those not related to their primary pharmacologic actions. An example is disturbance of the bacterial flora of the intestine as a consequence of antibiotic therapy. In drug *idiosyncrasy* the signs and symptoms of the reaction are unrelated to the known pharmacologic properties of the agent, sometimes because of metabolic abnormalities. An example is the hemolytic anemia that follows ingestion of primaquine in patients with glucose-6-phosphate dehydrogenase (G-6-PD) deficiency (Sec 5.47).

Drug interactions are discussed in Sec 5.50 (Table 5–30).

Allergic drug reactions occur on the basis of recognized models of immune injury. These include (1) IgE-mediated reactions; (2) cytotoxic reactions resulting from hapten binding to cell membranes and subsequent reaction with anti-hapten antibodies; (3) immune complex reactions in which drug-antibody immune complexes with affinity for cell membranes activate the complement system, resulting in cell membrane damage; (4) reactions due to autoantibody formation; and (5) reactions due to cell-mediated mechanisms. Most drugs are simple chemicals with molecular weights under 1000 and are rarely immunogenic. Substances with low molecular weights may act as haptens and become immunogenic after covalent chemical bonding with tissue proteins to form drug-protein conjugates. Hapten-protein complex formation is necessary for the macrophage–T cell–B cell interaction that leads to formation of hapten-specific humoral antibodies and cellular immunity. In general, only drugs (or their degradative or metabolic products) with sufficient chemical reactivity to bind irreversibly with proteins are capable of inducing hypersensitivity reactions. The major impediment to both study and diagnosis of drug allergy is that the chemically reactive substance is often not the native drug itself but a metabolic or degradative product. Since little is known about the metabolic fate of many drugs in common use, it is often not possible to identify the chemically reactive intermediates necessary for investigative or diagnostic use.

The complexities of understanding allergic reactions to drugs are illustrated by considering the penicillin model. Benzyl penicillin (penicillin G) has produced a wide variety of allergic reactions, including systemic responses such as anaphylaxis, serum sickness, and vasculitis; hematologic disorders, including hemolytic anemia, thrombocytopenia, and granulocytopenia; a broad spectrum of dermatologic entities; pulmonary disease; and renal disease. Under physiologic conditions, both in vivo and in vitro, a number of highly protein-reactive compounds are formed from penicillin. These metabolic products become immunogenic following conjugation with tissue proteins as described above. The penicilloyl group, formed by the combination of benzyl penicillenic acid with amino groups of proteins, is the antigenic determinant formed in largest amounts. Ninety-five per cent of all benzyl penicillin that conjugates with tissue proteins in vivo forms benzylpenicilloyl haptenic groups (BPO), and thus benzyl penicillin has been designated the "major" haptenic determinant of penicillin hypersensitivity. A large percentage of individuals who have been treated with penicillin can be shown to possess antibodies to the benzylpenicilloyl determinant, but most will not develop symptoms of penicillin allergy. BPO-specific IgE antibodies can be detected through a benzylpenicilloyl-polylysine skin test reagent in which BPO haptenic groups are attached to a "backbone" of lysine. Benzylpenicilloyl polylysine is available as a skin test reagent and for coupling to cyanogen bromide–activated disks in the RAST.

Unfortunately, the most feared consequence of penicillin allergy, anaphylaxis, is not due to IgE sensitization to the major BPO haptenic group but to less well defined, so-called minor haptenic determinants. These include penicilloate, penilloate, and penicillenate and its oxidation products. Though only 5% or less of the benzyl penicillin that reacts with proteins forms minor haptenic determinants, these have major clinical significance; unfortunately, antigens with minor determinant specificity are not available for testing either in vivo or in vitro.

Allergy to benzyl penicillin is further complicated by the development of related semisynthetic penicillins and cephalosporins which share a degree of immunologic cross-reactivity. Among the penicillins, the specificity of the antibody formed by the patient, e.g., whether directed toward the 6-amino-penicillin acid core common to all penicillins or directed toward a unique determinant on a distinctive side chain, determines the degree of cross-allergenicity. Thus, some individuals allergic to benzyl penicillin can tolerate the semisynthetic penicillins and vice versa. While substantially different structurally, penicillin and cephalosporins share the highly protein-reactive beta-lactam ring structure. Although uncommon, cases of anaphylaxis following administration of cephalosporins to individuals with penicillin allergy have been reported. Adverse reactions to ampicillin which occur in upwards of 10% of patients who receive the drug merit special consideration. The ampicillin rash is nonurticarial and appears in a high percentage of patients with infectious mononucleosis (about 90%) and also in patients with hyperuricemia. That the rash causes no other ill effects and typically disappears with continuing therapy casts doubt upon its immunologic nature; the pathogenesis of ampicillin rash remains an enigma.

Clinical Manifestations. Rashes are the most common manifestation of adverse drug reactions in children. Urticarial, exanthematous, and eczematoid eruptions predominate, but almost any morphology can be seen: exfoliative dermatitis (penicillin, sulfonamides, phenothiazines, anticonvulsants), bullous dermatoses (including epidermal necrolysis), erythema multiforme, Stevens-Johnson syndrome (sulfonamides, penicillin, barbiturates, anticonvulsants, phenytoin in particular), petechial eruptions, Lyell syndrome (penicillin, barbiturates, anticonvulsants, isoniazid), acneiform eruptions (iodides in postpubertal patients), lichenoid eruptions, photodermatitis (demethylchlortetracycline and phenothiazines), and fixed drug eruptions.

Renal or pulmonary disease following drug therapy rarely occurs during childhood. There have been occasional reports of interstitial nephritis associated with phenytoin with in vitro evidence of a cellular immune reaction. Fever, cough, and pulmonary infiltration occurring in a child being treated with nitrofurantoin strongly suggest an adverse drug reaction.

Drug fever, often suspected, rarely proved, does not generally occur as the sole manifestation of an adverse drug reaction. Often there is a concomitant skin rash. However, when a child who has received prolonged antimicrobial therapy has persistent fever without other cause, drug fever should be considered. The diagnosis is easily made when the drug is discontinued and defervescence occurs within 24–48 hr.

In contrast to those in adults, immunologically mediated drug-induced reactions in children are extremely rare. The same is true for drug-induced disorders of granulocytes and platelets; the overwhelming majority of these are based on toxicity.

Diagnosis. Diagnosis of an allergic drug reaction rests most often on a carefully taken history. Urticaria or angioedema following use of a drug is more relevant than nondescript rashes, for the former are the expression of IgE-mediated reactions. Even under the best of circumstances, however, a definitive diagnosis of an allergic drug reaction is frequently difficult to establish.

Only in the case of penicillin is there any indication that in vivo skin tests detect anaphylactic sensitivity. Skin testing with benzylpenicilloyl-polylysine (BPL; Pre-Pen) (Kremers-Urban Co., Milwaukee), penicillin G, and sodium benzyl penicilloate (Kremers-Urban Co.) will identify the overwhelming majority of children who are at risk of anaphylactic reactions following penicillin administration. The BPL is tested in a concentration of 6.0×10^{-5} M (as supplied by the manufacturer), first by prick or puncture test and, if negative, then by intradermal test according to the manufacturer's instructions. Benzyl penicillin (penicillin G) supplied as potassium penicillin G for injection, USP 1,000,000 U/ vial, is freshly diluted with saline to a concentration of 10,000 U/ml. Penicillin G is first tested by prick or puncture and then by intradermal technique up to a final concentration of 10,000 U/ml. Sodium benzyl penicilloate, 1×10^{-2} M, as supplied by the manufacturer, is also tested by the prick or puncture technique and then by the intradermal test as above. If the skin tests (interpreted in the same way as skin tests with pollen or other allergenic extracts) are negative, anaphylaxis is highly unlikely, and, if there is a compelling reason to do so, treatment may be initiated with a small test dose, usually one tenth of the usual dose, given either intravenously or orally. It is, however, impossible to exclude anaphylactic sensitivity due to other haptenic determinants formed in vivo from penicillin for which no skin test reagents are available. Furthermore, penicillin skin tests are predictive only of anaphylaxis and not of serum sickness or other reactions associated with use of the drug.

Patch testing to determine delayed hypersensitivity to a drug is helpful but should be carried out by someone familiar with the technique to avoid both false-positive and false-negative reactions due to improper procedure.

In vitro testing for drug allergy is principally carried out with the use of the RAST for detection of BPO-specific IgE antibodies. RAST for the other haptenic determinants of penicillin allergy is not available. As is the case with RAST for other allergens, the properly performed skin test is preferred on the basis of speed, sensitivity, and cost. Search for serum antibodies to formed elements of the blood in patients with what appear to be drug-induced blood disorders is rarely productive. Assays of cellular immunity have been used in the investigation of drug allergy. Their validity in this context has not been established.

Treatment of Drug Reactions. Treatment of a drug reaction depends upon its mechanism and the clinical manifestations produced. Discontinuation of the drug is indicated in most cases. Under certain conditions, and especially in infants and small children who develop rashes while receiving antibiotics, the circumstances may support a decision to continue administration of the drug until the etiology of the rash becomes clear. If, for example, an infant or small child with a febrile illness develops an exanthematous and nonurticarial rash on 1st exposure to penicillin, ampicillin, or another antibiotic, the rash is much more likely that of a viral illness than a cutaneous manifestation of allergy to the drug. Rather than labeling the child allergic to the drug on tenuous grounds and compromising its future use, it may be reasonable to continue therapy for a further period while the course of the rash is observed. If the history suggests that an adverse reaction has a pharmacologic basis, the drug may be introduced again at a later date, at a lower dosage or a longer interval between doses, while the serum concentration of the drug is measured, if possible. Ampicillin presents a special problem. There is little to suggest an allergic basis to the rash. However, many physicians will discontinue the ampicillin. If there are special circumstances that dictate the need for the drug, therapy may be continued with the expectation that the rash will disappear and no other problems develop. On the other hand, *if an allergic etiology is likely, the drug should not be reintroduced into the patient*, and an alternative drug should be sought. An exception to this principle arises with penicillin in special circumstances. Desensitization to penicillin of anaphylactically sensitive individuals has been carried out successfully without harm in instances in which penicillin therapy was mandatory (in SBE, for example). The procedure essentially is the same as that previously described for horse serum.

Treatment of systemic anaphylaxis is discussed in Sec 9.52.

As noted, drug allergy in children most commonly manifests itself in the skin. The eruptions are generally self-limited and disappear when the drugs are discontinued. Treatment is therefore symptomatic. Antihistamines are most useful for urticarial rashes. Diphenhydramine (Benadryl) and hydroxyzine (Atarax, Vistaril) possess antihistaminic and sedative properties, which may be useful. It may be necessary to give from 1.5–2 times the ordinarily recommended dose to achieve satisfactory control of symptoms. Epinephrine 1:1000 in doses of 0.1–0.3 ml provides short-term relief. For a more sustained effect, a suspension of epinephrine (Sus-Phrine) in doses of 0.1–0.2 ml subcutaneously every 6 hr may be prescribed. Corticosteroids are reserved for those severe cases in which relief is not obtained from the foregoing measures. The dose and dose interval are determined by the severity of the reaction.

Prevention. To minimize adverse drug reactions, physicians should use drugs only when indicated, be wary of new drugs, and know the relationships between drugs. Concurrent use of 2 or more drugs should be avoided unless genuinely indicated. Oral administration is less sensitizing than parenteral and preferred whenever possible. Topical application should be avoided when possible because of increased risk of sensitization by this route. Drug interactions should be anticipated, and patients should be warned against self-medication.

9.55 INSECT ALLERGY

Allergic reactions to insects are commonly seen in 3 clinical forms: (1) respiratory allergy secondary to inhalation of particulate matter of insect origin, (2) local cutaneous reactions to insect bites, and (3) anaphylactic reactions to stinging insects.

Etiology. Sensitization to antigenic material found in the debris and disintegrated bodies of dead insects may produce conjunctivitis, rhinitis, or asthma. Inhalation of scales from the wings of insects such as the mayfly, caddis fly, and moths is a particularly common cause of respiratory symptoms in the Great Lakes area, where large numbers of these insects appear each summer. Local cutaneous reactions are commonly observed following bites by mosquitoes, flies, and various bugs. Anaphylactic reactions of both immediate and delayed type due to insect allergy are almost entirely caused by the Hymenoptera order of the class Insecta, including the bee family, the wasp, hornet, and yellow jacket family, and the ant family. About 0.4% of persons give histories of systemic reactions to stinging insects, which produce about 40 deaths/yr in the United States.

Pathogenesis.   Inhalant allergy to insects is in many cases due to IgE-mediated sensitivity to antigenic materials found in the insects' bodies. The antigenic components responsible for the inhalant symptoms have not been thoroughly studied, but the allergenic material appears to reside usually in the cuticle or integument of the insect's body.

In the case of biting insects, the local reaction is frequently a wheal and flare lesion; it appears to be due to vasoactive or irritant materials deposited in the skin while the insect is feeding but may, particularly with recurrent bites, be mediated by IgE. The mechanism of late or persisting cutaneous reactions is unknown.

The biochemical and immunologic properties of stinging insect venoms have been well studied. They have at least 8–9 identified components, including vasoactive materials such as histamine, acetylcholine, and kinins, a number of enzymes (phospholipase A, hyaluronidase), apamine, melittin, and formic acid. Phospholipase A is the major allergen of honeybee venom. Hymenoptera venom and whole-body extracts have some antigens that are common to the Hymenoptera order and others that are family-specific. There is substantial cross-reactivity among vespid venoms. Other antigens are specific for venom sac material. The majority of patients who experience systemic reactions following Hymenoptera stings have IgE-mediated sensitivity to antigenic material in the venom. There are, however, a number of patients with convincing histories of sting anaphylaxis who have both negative skin tests and RAST to venoms.

Clinical Manifestations.   The clinical findings in inhalant allergy due to insects are quite similar to those seen with the usual inhalant allergens such as pollens. Rhinitis, conjunctivitis, and asthma have all been described.

The cutaneous reactions to biting insects are most often urticarial but may be papular, vesicular, and erythematous, particularly as the lesion progresses. Lesions that resemble typical delayed hypersensitivity reactions are also seen.

Clinical reactions to stinging insects range in severity from minimal pain and local erythema to life-threatening anaphylactic episodes. Local reactions vary from a papule or wheal at the site of the sting to edema of an entire extremity. The clinical manifestations of anaphylaxis due to sensitivity to stinging insects are identical to those observed in anaphylactic reactions from other causes. The patient may develop generalized urticaria, symptoms particularly of upper and to a lesser extent of lower airway obstruction, and circulatory collapse. Death may occur within a few min if appropriate measures are not taken. Typical serum sickness, nephrotic syndrome, vasculitis, neuritis, or encephalopathy may be seen as late sequelae of the reaction to stinging insects.

Diagnosis.   The diagnosis is usually easily made on the basis of history and, in the case of biting insects, by examination of skin lesions. Papular urticaria, which is common in children, occurs almost always as a result of insect bites, particularly of fleas and bedbugs.

Whole-body extracts should not be used for the diagnosis and treatment of Hymenoptera sensitivity. They vary widely in potency depending upon the amount of venom antigen they contain. Venom-specific antigens to which the patient may be allergic are not present in sacless whole bodies but vary with the content of venom sac material in the whole body preparation. Venoms of all 5 Hymenoptera (honeybee, vespids [yellow jacket, yellow hornet, white-faced hornet], polistes [wasp]) are available for skin testing and treatment. The skin tests should be done in accordance with the manufacturer's recommendations. While there is a general consensus that appropriately performed skin testing with potent materials is useful in identifying those individuals at risk of systemic anaphylaxis, there are reports of venom skin test–negative subjects who developed anaphylaxis when stung. Furthermore, in some investigators' experience, as many as 40% of skin test-positive, nonimmunized subjects may *not* experience anaphylaxis upon sting challenge. Unfortunately, in vitro testing with RAST has not substantially improved the ability to predict anaphylaxis as compared to skin testing. There is a 20% incidence of both false-positive and false-negative results with venom RAST.

Treatment.   Hyposensitization is occasionally undertaken when it can be established that inhalant allergy is due to a specific insect such as the mayfly or caddis fly. Beneficial results from hyposensitization treatment have not been thoroughly documented, and avoidance of the insect appears to be the preferred management.

For cutaneous reactions due to biting insects, treatment with topical medicaments to relieve itching and local discomfort and occasionally the systemic use of an antihistamine are all that is generally required.

In case of an anaphylactic reaction following a Hymenoptera sting, the acute treatment is essentially that of anaphylaxis. Epinephrine 1:1000 in a dose of 0.2–0.3 ml subcutaneously will be effective in combating both upper (glottis) and lower airway obstruction and symptoms of peripheral vascular collapse. Blood volume expanders must be given for persistent hypotension. An antihistamine (e.g., Benadryl 25–50 mg) may be given, although its efficacy has not been established. Corticosteroids are of little use in treatment of the acute systemic reaction but may be useful for treatment of sequelae.

Kits are available commercially for emergency use in case of anaphylaxis following insect sting. Each contains a syringe filled with epinephrine and an antihistamine tablet; one should be in the possession at all times of persons who have had previous severe or anaphylactic reactions. Patients at risk of anaphylaxis from an insect sting should also wear an identification bracelet (Medic-Alert) indicating their allergy.

Individuals at risk from insect sting should avoid using perfumes or cosmetics and wearing bright or pastel-colored clothing when outdoors. They should always wear gloves when gardening and long pants or slacks and shoes when walking in the grass or through fields.

Present recommendations for venom immunotherapy are marked by uncertainties because the natural history of the disease is not adequately understood. IgE-mediated reactivity to insect venoms as measured by skin test or RAST may decline spontaneously in untreated individuals, particularly children. During the 1st months of venom therapy, venom-specific IgE antibodies increase by as much as 3-fold but usually fall to pretreatment levels at the end of 1 yr of therapy. Whether the patient's clinical sensitivity is actually increased during the early course of immunotherapy is unknown. In children, who very frequently lose their venom-specific IgE antibodies without treatment, it is possible that immunotherapy may perpetuate their anaphylactic sensitivity. Venom-specific IgG antibody, which appears to be the most important protection against anaphylaxis in the majority of patients (there are exceptions), peaks at 2–4 mo following initiation of immunotherapy and declines according to the half-life of the immunoglobulin; therefore monthly injections of aqueous extracts are indicated. IgE antibodies may remain detectable for many yr in the serum of treated patients. How long treatment needs to be continued is unknown. There is a consensus that those who experience severe systemic reactions (airway involvement or hypotension) and have a positive skin test should receive immunotherapy. In over 300 patients treated at Johns Hopkins, there was a better than 95% success rate in treated patients who were intentionally challenged with a sting. For patients who, following stings, have urticarial or erythematous reactions which are not considered to be serious, especially in children, immunotherapy is not mandatory. These patients should practice avoidance procedures and carry an anaphylaxis kit. Immunotherapy is not indicated in patients with a history of sting anaphylaxis and negative skin test and RAST; one would not know which venom to use. Patients with large local reactions, even with positive skin tests or RAST, may not need to be treated with immunotherapy, but considerable judgment is needed in this group. The incidence of side effects during the course of treatment is significant with 50% of treated adults experiencing large local reactions and about 15% a systemic reaction. The incidence of both local and systemic reactions is much lower in children. A major problem, particularly for indigent patients, is the high cost (related to the difficulty in obtaining vespid and polistes venom) of venom immunotherapy. A conservative estimate of the cost of treatment for 1 yr of a patient with multiple venom sensitivities is in excess of $600.

9.56 OCULAR ALLERGIES

Allergic reactions involving the eye occur much less commonly in children than in adults. The eye may be involved as part of a generalized allergic reaction, in urticaria and angioedema, for example, or the eye alone may be affected. Allergic reactions in the eye are known to occur on the basis of IgE-mediated allergy, as conjunctivitis in a child with ragweed hay fever, for example, or on the basis of a cell-mediated (delayed hypersensitivity) immune reaction as is seen in contact dermatitis of the eyelids.

Eyelids. Eyelids are particularly prone to swelling because of their loose areolar connective tissue. Swelling may result from contact dermatitis to a variety of environmental substances. The lids are particularly involved because of the frequency with which offending contact sensitizers are carried to the eyelids with the hands. Occasionally, contact dermatitis appears as a result of sensitization to medication applied to the eyes. Cosmetics and topical ophthalmic medications head the list of sensitizing agents. Sulfonamides, neomycin, scopolamine and atropine, pilocarpine, and topical anesthetics have all been reported to cause contact sensitization. The lids become inflamed and indurated, and a scaly eczematoid reaction is evident. The conjunctiva becomes red, and a follicular conjunctivitis may develop.

Blepharitis is an inflammatory eczematous reaction of the eyelid margins, which may be caused by infection, allergy, or both. A chronic staphylococcal infection has been implicated as the major cause of chronic eczema of the eyelid margins. The lid margins, particularly of the lower lids, are affected with an itchy, scaly, erythematous eruption and the presence of exudate at the base of the lashes. The eyelids may be crusted together in the morning. The diagnosis is confirmed by slit lamp examination.

Allergic Conjunctivitis. Allergic conjunctivitis is a frequent concomitant of allergic rhinitis in individuals with hay fever, particularly when it is due to pollens. In affected children, both eyes itch, the conjunctivae are reddened and edematous, and there may be profuse tearing. Rubbing of the eyes aggravates the condition. On occasion, in a very sensitive child, edema of the conjunctiva will occur to such an extent that the conjunctiva will prolapse over the lower lid in a gelatinous-appearing mass that causes great concern to parents. The eye secretions are frequently watery but, if persistent, may become purulent in appearance. On examination, however, even the discharges that appear purulent consist predominantly of eosinophils; these permit differentiation from infectious conjunctivitis, in which the discharge is composed of polymorphonuclear leukocytes and bacteria.

Vernal Conjunctivitis. Vernal conjunctivitis is more common in children, with a 3:1 male:female predominance, than in adults and appears most often during the spring and summer. The disease affects both eyes and occurs in palpebral and limbal forms. In the palpebral form, which is most common, the tarsal plate of the upper lid presents a characteristic "cobblestone" appearance as a result of hyperplasia and thickening of the conjunctiva. A thick, ropy, whitish discharge may be present over the hypertrophied papillae responsible for the "cobblestone" appearance. In the limbal form of the disease, there is involvement at the junction of the cornea and sclera with thickening and opacity of the tissue in the area. Whitish Trantas dots, which represent accumulations of eosinophils, are pathognomonic of the disease. Progression of the limbal form may scar the cornea ultimately and lead to blindness in the most severe cases. Symptoms of vernal conjunctivitis include lacrimation, extreme itching, burning, and a particularly distressing photophobia. The seasonal occurrence, the finding of eosinophils, and the frequent coexistence with other atopic diseases such as asthma, hay fever, and eczema suggest that IgE-mediated sensitivity is responsible for the condition; but a detailed study of patients with the condition usually fails to prove any specific etiologic agent, and immunotherapy is of little if any value. The etiology of vernal conjunctivitis is unknown.

Treatment. Contact dermatitis of the lids is best managed by identification of suspected sensitizers and their elimination. Topical corticosteroids are of value in managing the acute reaction.

Blepharitis is best treated by good lid hygiene, using cotton-tipped applicators and half-strength baby shampoo mixed with water to remove scales and exudate, followed by the use of antistaphylococcal ointments. If an excessive reaction to the treatment results, steroids are applied topically for a few days. Since the disease tends to recur, regular lid care is in order.

Allergic conjunctivitis in the patient with hay fever generally responds well to topical application of sympathomimetics (naphazoline or phenylephrine) in the form of eye drops or, failing that, to eye drops or ointments containing corticosteroids. Immunotherapy for allergic conjunctivitis in the absence of allergic rhinitis gives poor results.

Vernal conjunctivitis may be treated with sparing use of corticosteroid eye drops or ointments. Medrysone (HMS), a topically active, poorly absorbed corticosteroid, in a dose of 1–2 drops 4 times/day, is particularly indicated in allergic conjunctivitis when there is involvement of only the superficial layers of the eye. The drug is less likely to cause increased intraocular pressure than the more readily absorbed preparations such as dexamethasone or methylprednisolone. Whenever topical steroids are used in the eye for more than a few days, intraocular pressure should be monitored. Ophthalmic preparations of disodium cromoglycate in 1–2% solution, 1–2 drops 4 times a day, provide modest relief of the symptoms of vernal conjunctivitis.

9.57 ADVERSE REACTIONS TO FOODS

The incidence of adverse reactions to foods is not known and unquestionably varies in different parts of the world. The average United States diet contains many food antigens, chemical food additives, antibiotics, and other substances; accordingly, a significant frequency of adverse reactions to foods should not be surprising. Food reactions caused by allergic mechanisms are estimated to occur in from 0.3–0.7% of persons, but the prevalence of food allergy is a subject of substantial disagreement. In the overwhelming majority of cases in which individuals react adversely to the ingestion of various foods, these reactions cannot be shown to have an immunologic basis. In these cases the use of immunologic methods of diagnosis (skin testing or provocative testing [injection or sublingual administration of food antigen]) is inappropriate. Treatment based upon immunologic principles is similarly unwarranted.

Etiology. Possible mechanisms for adverse reactions to foods are summarized in Table 9–21. There is little doubt that intact macromolecules may pass through the epithelium of the gastrointestinal tract and gain access to the systemic circulation. Studies in animals have shown that the intestinal absorption of intact proteins occurs more readily in animals that lack antibody to the proteins. In humans, individuals with IgA deficiency have higher levels of antibodies to milk proteins and of immune complexes containing milk than do normal controls. Secretory IgA limits the intestinal absorption of intact macromolecules. IgE-mediated reactions are characteristically rapid in onset and may present as angioedema of the lips, mouth, uvula, or glottis; as generalized urticaria; as asthma; or occasionally as shock. In such cases the patient usually recognizes that the symptoms have followed ingestion of a certain food. Individuals with such IgE-mediated food allergy are at constant risk of exposure to the offending food hidden in a food mixture. For example, a nut-sensitive individual may have a serious reaction to ingestion of a cookie coated with almond extract.

Individuals with IgE-mediated food reactions consistently show positive skin tests to the suspected food. In fact, skin testing itself, particularly if done by the intracutaneous technique, can precipitate the clinical reaction in individuals with anaphylactic allergy to a food. Foods that have the highest potential to cause IgE-mediated sensitivity are fish, shellfish, peanuts (a legume), various nuts and seeds, eggs, cow's milk, and wheat.

More difficult to diagnose are reactions that begin a few to 24 hr after ingestion of the offending food. Such reactions have been attributed without much convinc-

Table 9–21 MECHANISMS OF ADVERSE REACTIONS TO FOODS

Immunologic
  IgE mediated
  ? Toxic complex (α-gliadin)
  ? Cell (lymphocyte) mediated injury
Biochemical
  Enzyme deficiency (e.g., disaccharidase)
  "Hot dog" headache — nitrite sensitivity
  Tyramine headache
  "Toxic" effect — α-gliadin
Unknown
  Reactions to food additives (F.D. & C. colors and flavorings)

ing evidence to allergy to a digestive product of the food such as a proteose or polypeptide. The role of antigen-antibody complexes and cell-mediated immunity (delayed hypersensitivity) in the pathogenesis of these late-occurring reactions is unknown.

A variety of reactions have been reported to follow ingestion of *cow's milk* by infants and children. In some cases an IgE mechanism has been established. In others, however, even with antibodies to milk proteins (particularly α-lactalbumin, β-lactoglobulin, and casein) present in sufficient quantities to be demonstrable by gel diffusion methods, no immunologic mechanism has been established. During the 1st yr of life, vomiting and watery, blood-streaked, mucoid diarrhea may follow milk ingestion. An enteropathy with loss of both protein and blood has been found in other young infants fed large volumes of whole pasteurized milk (but not heat-processed formula). In older infants ingestion of milk has been associated with occult fecal blood loss, recurrent roentgenographic pulmonary infiltrates, and multiple precipitating antibodies to cow's milk proteins (Sec 12.81). Some cases of pulmonary hemosiderosis are said to be responsive to withdrawal of milk from the diet.

Adverse reactions to milk due to *disaccharidase* deficiencies are discussed in Sec 11.62.

A number of *enteropathies* with varying combinations of malabsorption, steatorrhea, hypoalbuminemia, and fecal blood loss have been reported due to cow's milk or wheat intolerance. Despite close associations between symptoms or signs and the feeding of these foods, a precise mechanism of immunologic injury has not been identified. It is not known whether wheat-sensitive individuals who have adverse symptoms from the gluten fraction of wheat are reacting to α-gliadin as a toxin or as an antigen in an immune complex type of injury.

Other nonimmunologic adverse reactions to foods principally in adults include headaches after ingestion of wine and cheese (tyramine), cured meats or "hot dog" headache (sodium nitrite), or the Chinese restaurant syndrome (monosodium glutamate). Affected persons apparently have idiosyncratic, but no allergic, reactions to these simple chemicals. In other cases nonimmunologic adverse reactions may be due to food additives, particularly the dyes used in foods and drugs. The best example is tartrazine (F.D. & C. Yellow No. 5), which will precipitate asthma in *some* aspirin-intolerant asthmatics. A report of the National Advisory Committee on Hyperkinesis and Food Additives concluded that there was no direct causal connection between artificial food colors and flavors and hyperactivity in children.

Diagnosis. An etiologic diagnosis in a child suspected of an adverse food reaction requires careful objective study. Elimination from the diet for a period of 7–10 days of a food causing difficulty should generally result in improvement in the patient's symptoms. Reintroduction of the food, preferably in large amounts for several meals, should result in the return of symptoms in a reasonable period of time, within 7 days at most. An equally critical diagnostic approach should be undertaken in children felt possibly to have "allergic tension-fatigue."

The critical testing of foods by the elimination and provocation method is difficult if either patient or parent anticipates an unfavorable reaction because of the emotional bias incident to the ingestion of the suspected food. Food challenges are best done in a blind manner, the food being given in a disguised form, for example, in opaque capsules or mixed with another food. When the patient's symptoms are present on a more or less continuous basis, the results of elimination of a given food are readily appreciated. On the other hand, when symptoms such as headache are only intermittent, results of elimination and provocation testing are frequently equivocal.

Skin testing utilizing properly prepared food antigens will reveal the presence of any IgE antibody to the test antigen. A positive skin test does not necessarily indicate, however, that the particular food causes symptoms. In anaphylactic food allergy, skin tests almost invariably show a positive reaction to the offending food, but in this instance the history alone usually establishes the diagnosis and skin testing is superfluous. Occasionally, a positive skin test to a food not previously suspected of causing trouble will be clinically corroborated when the history is re-examined in light of the positive test. All too often, undue attention paid to clinically irrelevant skin reactions to food extracts has led to very restricted diets with no attempt made to confirm the clinical importance of suspected foods through elimination and provocative testing. Overdiagnosis of food allergy has sometimes produced malnutrition in infants and children as well as anxiety and depression in mothers who have found it impossible to adhere to severely restrictive diets.

The RAST assay has been used to identify the presence of IgE antibodies to foods. The correlation between clinical history, puncture skin test, and RAST is excellent for codfish, egg white, nuts, peanuts, and peas. Positive RAST and skin tests to cereals correlate poorly with the results of cereal challenge. RAST for soybeans and white beans is unreliable, apparently because of nonspecific binding of IgE to the RAST disk. RAST does not appear to offer any substantial advantage over skin testing with potent food extracts.

In the provocative/neutralizing method of diagnosis of food allergy, dilutions of food extracts are injected intracutaneously in an attempt to reproduce the patient's symptoms, which are then said to be relieved by successive intracutaneous injections of other dilutions of the same extract. The techniques vary among users of the method. For example, some users both "provoke" and "neutralize" by *sublingual* administration of the antigen solutions. The validity of all of these methods has not been established, and their use in diagnosis and therapy is unwarranted.

Treatment. The treatment of an adverse food reaction is directed at the clinical manifestations, which may be anaphylaxis, urticaria, diarrhea, rhinitis, asthma, and so on. Offending foods should be removed from the diet. If elimination diets are prescribed, care must be taken to ensure that they are nutritionally adequate.

For reasons that are unclear, some children shown to be highly reactive to foods will become "tolerant" as they grow older; this is particularly likely in infants and small children. With the passage of time, therefore, cautious reintroduction of offending foods into the diet may be tried, particularly in the case of those common foods that are difficult to avoid in the average diet. A few studies report that cromolyn sodium, 60–200 mg, given orally 30 min before a food challenge, has blocked the appearance of symptoms in food-sensitive individuals. Cromolyn sodium may be tried, therefore, in those rare instances when an offending food cannot be avoided. The cost of such therapy is prohibitive because of the large amounts of drug required. Hyposensitization by injection or sublingual or oral administration of extracts of offending foods is not efficacious.

RELATIONSHIP BETWEEN THE PEDIATRICIAN AND ALLERGIST

Most of the common conditions discussed above can be effectively managed by pediatricians comfortable with the principles of allergy diagnosis and treatment. Consultation with an allergist is indicated if the pediatrician is not prepared to undertake measures such as skin or pulmonary function testing or if the case is difficult. The referral should be made for the evaluation of the role that IgE-mediated allergy may be playing in the disease and not just for "skin tests and shots" since, not uncommonly, no evidence of IgE-mediated allergy will be found and anticipated "shots" will not be indicated. The best results are obtained for the patient when pediatrician and allergist are in frequent communication and work together harmoniously.

ELLIOT F. ELLIS

General

Bierman CW, Pearlman DS (eds): Allergic Diseases of Infancy, Childhood and Adolescence. Philadelphia WB Saunders, 1980.
Ellis EF (ed): Symposium on Pediatric Allergy. Pediatric Clinics of North America. Philadelphia, WB Saunders, 1975.
Middleton E Jr, Reed CE, Ellis EF (eds): Allergy: Principles and Practice. St. Louis, CV Mosby, 1978.
Parker CW (ed): Clinical Immunology. Philadelphia, WB Saunders, 1960.
Patterson R (ed): Allergic Diseases: Diagnosis and Management. Philadelphia, JB Lippincott, 1980.

Immunologic Basis of Allergic Disease

Askenase PW: Basophil arrival and function in tissue hypersensitivity reactions. J Allergy Clin Immunol 64:79, 1979.
Cantor H, Gershon RK: Immunological circuits: Cellular composition. Fed Proc 38:2058, 1979.
Editorial: Is a mast cell a mast cell a mast cell? J Allergy Clin Immunol 66:1, 1980.
Katz DH: Control of IgE antibody production by suppressor substances. J Allergy Clin Immunol 62:44, 1978.
Marsh DG, Hsu SH, Hussain R, et al: Genetics of immune response to allergens. J Allergy Clin Immunol 65:322, 1980.
Metzger H, Bach MK: The receptor for IgE on mast cells and basophils: Studies on IgE binding and on the structure of the receptor. In: Bach MR (ed): Immediate Hypersensitivity—Modern Concepts and Developments. New York, Marcel Dekker, 1978, p 561.
Sehon AH, Lee WY: Suppression of immunoglobulin E antibodies with modified allergens. J Allergy Clin Immunol 64:242, 1979.
Solley GO, Gleich GJ, Jordan EK, et al: The late phase of the immediate wheal and flare skin reaction. Its dependence upon IgE antibodies. J Clin Invest 58:408, 1976.

Sullivan TJ, Kulczycki A Jr: Immediate hypersensitivity responses. In: Parker CW (ed): Clinical Immunology. Philadelphia, WB Saunders, 1980, p 115.

Principles of Treatment

Altounyan REC: Review of clinical activity and mode of action of sodium cromoglycate. Clin Allergy 10(Suppl):481, 1980.
Editorial: Histamine H₁ and H₂ antihistamines, and immediate hypersensitivity reactions. J Allergy Clin Immunol 63:371, 1979.
Fauci AS, Dale DC, Balow JE: Glucocorticosteroid therapy: Mechanism of action and clinical considerations. Ann Intern Med 84:304, 1976.
Fraser CM, Venter JC: The synthesis of beta-adrenergic receptors in cultured human cells: Induction by glucocorticoids. Biochem Biophys Res Comm 94:390, 1980.
Hendeles L, Weinberger M, Johnson G: Monitoring serum theophylline levels. Clin Pharmacokinet 3:294, 1978.
Jack D, Harris DM, Middleton E Jr: Adrenergic agents. In: Middleton E Jr, Reed CE, Ellis EF (eds): Allergy: Principles and Practice. St. Louis, CV Mosby, 1978, p 404.
Morris HG: Factors that influence clinical responses to administered cortiosteroids. J Allergy Clin Immunol 66:343, 1980.
Norman PS: An overview of immunotherapy: Implications for the future. J Allergy Clin Immunol 65:87, 1980.
Ogilvie RI: Clinical pharmacokinetics of theophylline. Clin Pharmacokinet 3:267, 1978.

Allergic Rhinitis

Broder I, Higgins MW, Matthews KP, et al: Epidemiology of asthma in allergic rhinitis in a total community, Tecumseh, Michigan. IV. Natural history. J Allergy Clin Immunol 54:100, 1974.
Mygind N: Nasal Allergy. Oxford, Blackwell, 1978.

Asthma

Blair H: Natural history of childhood asthma. Arch Dis Child 52:613, 1977.
Boushey HA, Holtzman MJ, Shelan JR, et al: State of the art. Bronchial hyperreactivity. Am Rev Respir Dis 121:389, 1980.
Clark TJH, Godfrey S: Asthma. Philadelphia, WB Saunders, 1977.
Ellis EF: Role of infection in asthma. Adv Asthma Allergy Pulm Dis 4(3):28, 1977.
Hogg JC, Williams J, Richardson JB et al: Age as a factor in the distribution of lower-airway conductance and in a pathologic anatomy of obstructive lung disease. N Engl J Med 282:1283, 1970.
McNichol KN, Williams HE: Spectrum of asthma in children. I. Clinical and physiological components. II. Allergic components. III. Psychological and social components. Br Med J 4:7, 1973.
Norrish M, Tooley M, Godfrey S: Clinical, physiological and psychological study of asthmatic children attending a hospital clinic. Arch Dis Child 52:913, 1977.
Souhrada JF, Buckley JM: Pulmonary function testing in asthmatic children. Pediatr Clin North Am 23:249, 1976.
Svedmyr N, Simonson BG: Drugs in the treatment of asthma. In: Widdecombe JG (ed): International Encyclopedia of Pharmacology and Therapeutics. Respiratory Pharmacology. Section 104. Oxford, Pergamon Press, 1981.
Weinberger M, Hendeles L, Ahrens R: Clinical pharmacology of drugs used for asthma. Pediatr Clin North Am 28:47, 1981.

Adverse Reactions to Drugs

Amos HE: Allergic Drug Reactions. Current Topics in Immunology Series, No 5. London, Edward Arnold Publishers, 1976.
Davies DM (ed): Textbook of Adverse Drug Reactions. New York, Oxford, 1977.
Gilmore NJ, Yang WH, Del Carpio J: Penicillin allergy: A simple, rapid intravenous method of desensitization" (Abstr). J Allergy Clin Immunol 63:185, 1979.
Green JR, Rosenblum AH, Sweet LC: Evaluation of penicillin hypersensitivity; value of clinical history and skin testing with penicilloyl-polylysine and penicillin G. J Allergy Clin Immunol 60:339, 1977.
Kerns DL, Shira JE, Go S, et al: Ampicillin rash in children: Relationship to penicillin allergy and infectious mononucleosis. Am J Dis Child 125:187, 1973.
Szefler SJ, Ellis EF: Adverse reactions to drugs. In: Brenneman-Kelly, Practice of Pediatrics, in press.
Whyte J, Greenan E: Drug usage and adverse drug reactions in pediatric patients. Acta Paediatr Scand 66:767, 1977.

Atopic Dermatitis

Ellis EF, Goltz RW: Atopic dermatitis. In: Tice's Practice of Medicine, Vol 1. Hagerstown, Md, Harper and Row, 1978.
Hanifin JM, Lobitz WC: Newer concepts of atopic dermatitis. Arch Dermatol 113:663, 1977.
Jacobs AH: Local management of atopic dermatitis in infants and children. Clin Pediatr 8:201, 1969.
Norins AL: Atopic dermatitis. Pediatr Clin North Am 18:801, 1971.

Rajka G (ed): Atopic Dermatitis. Major Problems in Dermatology Series No 3. London, WB Saunders, 1975.

Urticaria and Angioedema

Matthews K: Management of urticaria and angioedema. J Allergy Clin Immunol 66:347, 1980.
Soter NA, Wasserman SI: Physical urticaria/angioedema: An experimental model of mast cell activation in humans. J Allergy Clin Immunol 66:358, 1980.
Wanderer AA, St. Pierre J-P, Ellis EF: Primary acquired cold urticaria: Double-blind study of treatment with cyproheptadine, chlorpheniramine, and placebo. Arch Dermatol 113:1375, 1977.
Warin RP, Champion RH: Urticaria. London, WB Saunders, 1974.

Anaphylaxis

Delage C, Irey NS: Anaphylactic deaths: A clinicopathologic study of 43 cases. J Forensic Sci 17:525, 1972.
Greenberger PA, Patterson R, Simon R, et al: Pretreatment of high-risk patients requiring radio-contrast media studies. J Allergy Clin Immunol 67:185, 1981.
James LP, Austen KF: Fatal systemic anaphylaxis in man. N Engl J Med 270:597, 1964.
Smith PL, Kagey-Sobotka A, Bleechner ER, et al: Physiologic manifestations of human anaphylaxis. J Clin Invest 66:1072, 1980.

Serum Sickness

Cochrane CG, Dixon FJ: Antigen-antibody complex induced disease. In: Miescher PA, Müller-Eberhard HJ (eds): Textbook of Immunopathology. Ed 2. New York, Grune & Stratton, 1976.
Edgington T, Tonietti G: Mechanisms of deposition of immune complexes in tissues. Prog Immunol 5:333, 1974.
Knicker WJ, Guerra FA, Richards SEM: Prevention of immune complex disease (serum sickness) by antagonists of vasoactive amines. Pediatr Res 5:381, 1977.

von Pirquet C, Schick B: Die Serumkrankheit. Baltimore, Williams & Wilkins, 1951.

Insect Allergy

Hunt KJ, Valentine MD, Sobotka AK, et al: A controlled trial of immunotherapy in insect hypersensitivity. N Engl J Med 299:157, 1978.
James FK, Pence HL, Driggers DP, et al: Imported fire ant venom: Studies of human reactions to fire ant venom. J Allergy Clin Immunol 58:110, 1976.
Lichtenstein LM, Valentine MD, Sobotka AK: Insect allergy: The state of the art. J Allergy Clin Immunol 64:5, 1979

Ocular Allergy

Allansmith MR: Ocular allergy—diagnosis and management. In: Golden B (ed): Ocular Inflammatory Disease. Springfield, Ill, Charles C Thomas, 1974.
Theodore FH: Allergy in relation to ophthalmology. In Locatcher-Khorozoi D, Seegal B (eds): Microbiology of the Eye. St. Louis, CV Mosby, 1972.

Adverse Reactions to Foods

Bock SA: Food sensitivity. Am J Dis Child 134:973, 1980.
Bock SA, Buckley J, Holst A, et al: Proper use of skin tests with food extracts in diagnosis of hypersensitivity to food in children. Clin Allergy 7:375, 1977.
Goldstein GB, Heiner DC: Clinical immunological perspectives in food sensitivity. J Allergy 46:270, 1970.
Henderson WR, Raskin NH: "Hot-dog" headache: Individual susceptibility to nitrite. Lancet 2:1162, 1972.
May CD: Food hypersensitivity. In: Gupta S, Good RD (eds): Cellular, Molecular and Clinical Aspects of Allergic Disorders. New York, Plenum Press, 1979, p 321.
May CD, Bock SA: A modern clinical approach to food hypersensitivity. Allergy 33:166, 1978.
Walker WA, Isselbacher KJ: Uptake and transport of macromolecules by the intestine: Possible role in clinical disorders. Gastroenterology 67:531,1974.

RHEUMATIC DISEASES OF CHILDHOOD
(Inflammatory Diseases of Connective Tissue, Collagen Diseases)

The disorders described in this section are grouped because of similarities in symptomatology and pathology; in general, they are associated with inflammatory changes in various connective tissues throughout the body. Included are:

I. Rheumatic fever (Sec 9.81)
II. Juvenile rheumatoid arthritis (JRA)
III. Ankylosing spondylitis and other spondyloarthropathies
IV. Systemic lupus erythematosus (SLE)
   A. Lupus phenomena in the newborn period (Sec 9.63)
V. The vasculitis syndromes
   A. Schönlein-Henoch vasculitis
   B. Polyarteritis nodosa
      1. Infantile polyarteritis
      2. Kawasaki disease (Sec 9.68)
      3. Wegener granulomatosis
   C. Takayasu arteritis
VI. Dermatomyositis
VII. Scleroderma
   A. Morphea
   B. Progressive systemic sclerosis
VIII. Miscellaneous
   A. Mixed connective tissue disease

   B. Erythema multiforme exudativum (Stevens-Johnson syndrome)
   C. Erythema nodosum
   D. Goodpasture syndrome
   E. Relapsing nodular nonsuppurative panniculitis
   F. "Rheumatoid" nodules without rheumatic disease
   G. Fasciitis
   H. Lyme disease

Certain diseases discussed elsewhere have points of similarity to these disorders, i.e., serum sickness, glomerulonephritis, the idiopathic nephrotic syndrome, ulcerative colitis, regional enteritis, and thrombotic thrombocytopenic purpura.

The causes and pathogenesis of these disorders are unknown, and precise diagnostic criteria are lacking. They usually appear as clinically distinct entities, each generally presenting a characteristic picture. For example, rheumatoid arthritis is associated with chronic arthritis, dermatomyositis with inflammation of muscle, scleroderma with induration of skin, and the like. However, each of these diseases can affect many organs, and overlapping symptoms and signs sometimes make precise diagnosis difficult.

9.58 LABORATORY STUDIES IN THE RHEUMATIC DISEASES

Although laboratory studies are often helpful, few, if any, are diagnostic or specific for rheumatic diseases. Currently available laboratory studies include tests for acute phase phenomena, rheumatoid factors, antinuclear antibodies, serum complement and its components, immune complexes, serum proteins and immunoglobulins, and histocompatibility antigens. Other tests that are also useful at times in evaluating patients include blood counts, urinalyses, joint fluid analyses, studies of renal and liver function, and roentgenograms. Biopsies are frequently performed in rheumatic diseases; although tissue histology may provide confirmatory evidence of tissue involvement or aid in classification of disease, it is rarely diagnostic of any specific disease.

THE ACUTE PHASE PHENOMENA

The acute phase phenomena or acute phase reactants are plasma constituents which appear or increase during the inflammatory state. They include the sedimentation rate, C-reactive protein, serum mucoproteins, various alpha globulins, gamma globulins, some complement components, and certain proteins such as transferrin. Because patients with rheumatic diseases have an active inflammatory process, acute phase phenomena are usually present during periods of active disease. Such tests are not invariably positive during inflammation, however, and their absence does not exclude the possibility of an active disease process. These tests are of little diagnostic usefulness since they may be positive in a wide variety of conditions associated with inflammation (such as malignancy, infection, tissue trauma, and tissue necrosis). At times, acute phase phenomena are helpful in following the course of disease in individual patients. Of these tests, the sedimentation rate is the simplest and most readily available; rapid sedimentation rates result from increased plasma levels of serum fibrinogen, gamma globulins, or other proteins. Specific biologic roles for acute phase reactants have not been identified.

RHEUMATOID FACTORS

Rheumatoid factors are a group of antibodies which react with IgG immunoglobulins. These antibodies are not specific for host immunoglobulin but may react with immunoglobulin from other individuals or from other species. Rheumatoid factors detected by standard agglutination techniques such as the latex agglutination test or the sheep cell agglutination test are 19S IgM immunoglobulins; anti-immunoglobulin antibodies of the IgG and IgA classes can also be identified by methods other than agglutination tests. The occurrence of rheumatoid factors in disease states such as chronic infections or in experimental situations such as hyper-

immunization of animals suggests that protracted immune stimulation or chronic infection or inflammation may underlie their production.

Rheumatoid factors, particularly IgM rheumatoid factors detected by classic agglutination techniques, are strongly associated with classic adult rheumatoid arthritis; in such patients they are present in high titer and on consecutive tests throughout the course of disease. A small subgroup of juvenile rheumatoid arthritis resembling classic adult rheumatoid arthritis also is characterized by the presence of rheumatoid factors. However, rheumatoid factors are neither specific for nor diagnostic of rheumatoid arthritis. They occur also in other rheumatic diseases (lupus erythematosus, scleroderma), chronic active hepatitis, chronic infections (such as bacterial endocarditis, parasitic infections), leukemia and lymphoid malignancies, and certain viral infections; in addition, they can be found following immunizations, open heart surgery, or organ transplantation as well as in normal aging human beings. Many children with transiently positive low titer rheumatoid factor tests have probably had antecedent viral illnesses. Rheumatoid factors do not in themselves cause disease, nor are they necessary for the occurrence of chronic synovitis; they may play a role in perpetuation of synovial inflammation in rheumatoid arthritis by forming immune complexes with immunoglobulin.

ANTINUCLEAR ANTIBODIES
(Antinuclear Factors)

The antinuclear antibodies are a group of antibodies which react with various nuclear constituents, including deoxyribonucleoprotein (DNP), deoxyribonucleic acid (DNA), ribonucleoprotein (RNP), ribonucleic acid (RNA), SM antigen (a soluble nuclear protein antigen), and many others. Stimuli for production of these antibodies remain unkown. Antinuclear antibodies do not seem specific for organs, individuals, or species of cell origin. They are generally detected by immunofluorescent staining techniques utilizing frozen tissue sections.

Antinuclear antibodies are neither entirely diagnostic of nor specific for any disease. They are demonstrable in virtually 100% of patients with systemic lupus erythematosus (SLE) but are also found in patients with rheumatoid arthritis and scleroderma. The syndrome called mixed connective tissue disease is defined by the presence of antibody to RNP. Nonrheumatic conditions associated with antinuclear antibodies include drug ingestion (e.g., anticonvulsants, procainamide, birth control pills), certain infections (notably EB virus infection), certain malignancies, and the normal aging process. High titers of antinuclear antibodies are most common in SLE and mixed connective tissue disease. Antibodies reactive with DNA are usually found only in patients with active SLE.

The LE cell is the result of an antinuclear antibody reaction with DNP. The antibody reacts in vitro with nuclei of peripheral blood cells, rendering them susceptible to phagocytosis; the LE cell is a polymorphonuclear leukocyte which has ingested such a nucleus. The LE test is not a very sensitive method of seeking antinuclear antibodies; although of historical significance, it is no longer a necessary laboratory test when the more sensitive antinuclear antibody test is available.

COMPLEMENT

Complement consists of a group of serum proteins which react in sequence after activation; these proteins mediate certain aspects of inflammation and cell injury (Sec 9.21). Serum complement levels can be useful in indicating the activity of SLE and other diseases associated with formation of immune complexes; in such situations low serum complement levels reflect complement consumption by immune complexes and are thus associated with active disease. Measurement of the total serum hemolytic complement is probably the most meaningful test. Measurement of individual complement components C3 or C4 determines only the amount of protein without regard to its biologic activity. Complement studies are not diagnostic of any disease except the rare hereditary deficiencies of serum complement components.

IMMUNE COMPLEX DETERMINATIONS

Immune complexes of antigen and antibody are responsible for tissue damage in some rheumatic diseases, notably SLE, and also in a wide variety of other conditions (such as infectious diseases). However, these tests are of limited clinical usefulness in evaluation of patients. Most commonly available methods are C1q binding and the Raji cell assay. The ultimate role for such determinations in clinical medicine remains to be determined.

SERUM PROTEINS AND IMMUNOGLOBULINS

Elevated levels of gamma globulins and alpha$_2$ globulins are frequently found in patients with active inflammation; there is nothing specific about these tests. Most notable elevations are generally found in SLE. Elevations of 1 or more specific immunoglobulins may also be found in rheumatic disease patients; however, there are no diagnostic patterns. Serum albumin levels may be low in patients with chronic inflammation of various causes. Rarely, patients with immunodeficiency (especially IgA) or hypogammaglobulinemia appear with rheumatic disease states.

THE HISTOCOMPATIBILITY (HLA) SYSTEM

Associations of histocompatibility antigens (HLA antigens) with certain diseases provide insights into genetically determined susceptibility to disease. Histocompatibility antigens are located on the surfaces of most human cells. They determine the acceptance or rejection of tissue grafts. Loci determining HLA antigens are located on the 6th chromosome; A, B, C, D, and DR types are now recognized. The HLA system is complex, with multiple alleles for each locus (20 alleles now recognized for the A locus, 42 for the B locus, 8 for the C locus, 12 for the D locus, and 10 for DR). The prevalences of various HLA alleles vary in different racial groups. Each individual carries 2 alleles for each HLA locus, 1 from the mother and 1 from the father. HLA typing requires antisera of known specificity to type A, B, C, and DR loci and cells of known specificity to type the D locus; because obtaining and standardizing such typing sera and cells are difficult, HLA typing is not yet a readily available laboratory procedure.

The biologic roles of HLA antigens, other than those determining tissue compatibility, are not yet wholly known. The HLA system is located on the 6th chromosome in close proximity (linkage) to several genes known to be important in the immune system, including loci determining synthesis or deficiency of various components of complement and perhaps loci determining immune responsiveness. Since the HLA antigens are genetically determined traits which can be accurately identified, they can be used to provide information concerning both disease associations (the occurrence of particular diseases in association with particular HLA antigens) and disease linkages (the passage of a trait along with HLA antigens from generation to generation within the same family, implying the proximity of genes responsible for the trait to those of the HLA system on the 6th chromosome).

The most significant association of a human disease with the HLA system is that of HLA B27 with ankylosing spondylitis; 95% of patients with ankylosing spondylitis have HLA B27, as compared with only 6% of a control white North American population. An individual carrying HLA B27 has 90 times greater relative risk of developing ankylosing spondylitis than an individual who does not carry HLA B27. An estimated 3–20% of individuals with HLA B27 actually have ankylosing spondylitis or a related disease. Reiter syndrome, the spondylitis of inflammatory bowel disease and psoriasis, acute iridocyclitis, pauciarticular arthritis of teenage and adult patients, and the "reactive" arthritis following infections with salmonella, shigella, or *Yersinia enterocolitica* are also associated with HLA B27. It is not known whether susceptibility to these diseases is conferred by HLA B27 itself or by a linked genetic trait, perhaps of immune nature. The associations of these "spondyloarthropathy" diseases with HLA B27 hold true in various racial populations. No corresponding HLA D associations have been made for these diseases.

HLA B27 is associated with only 1 subgroup of childhood arthritis—that of older-onset pauciarticular patients (type II) who may well have early ankylosing spondylitis or 1 of the other spondyloarthropathies. DR5, DR6, and DR8 may be associated with pauciarticular juvenile rheumatoid arthritis (type I) and chronic iridocyclitis, and DR4 with rheumatoid factor–positive polyarthritis.

A different group of diseases is associated with HLA B8 and HLA DW3/DR3 in North American and European populations. These include chronic active hepatitis, celiac sprue, dermatitis herpetiformis with malabsorption, insulin-dependent diabetes mellitus, thyroiditis, Graves disease, Addison disease, myasthenia gravis, Sjögren syndrome, childhood dermatomyositis, and perhaps systemic lupus erythematosus. All of these diseases share the common property of chronic inflammation, often associated with formation of antibodies reactive with human tissues ("autoantibodies") and often resulting in inflammation of endocrine organs. Risks for any of these diseases are relatively low for individuals carrying B8–DW3/DR3, and the D associations are stronger than the B associations. Histocompatibility studies have revealed heterogeneous subgroups in several of these diseases: for example, diabetes mellitus (only insulin-dependent diabetes is associated with B8–DW3/DR3) and dermatitis herpetiformis (only dermatitis herpetiformis with malabsorption is associated with B8–DW3/DR3). The specific HLA antigens associated with these diseases may vary among racial groups.

Other human diseases, notably multiple sclerosis and psoriasis, have yet other HLA B and D associations. Few diseases have been associated primarily with antigens in the A locus; 1 such disease is hemachromatosis. Adult-onset rheumatoid arthritis is the 1 known human disease with only an HLA-D association (DW4/DR4) but no demonstrable A, B, or C associations.

Human conditions which have been *linked* to the HLA system, or transmitted along with antigens of the histocompatibility system from generation to generation, include deficiencies of the 2nd and 4th components of complement, congenital adrenal hyperplasia, and, possibly, predisposition to ragweed hay fever.

HLA typing is not currently diagnostic of any disease and has little practical use in clinical medicine other than the matching of tissue donors to recipients. There is a potential use in prenatal diagnosis of linked diseases such as deficiency of the 4th component of complement. Histocompatibility studies remain of great interest both in classifying diseases and in seeking possible genetic factors that predispose human beings to disease. Explanations for the associations of histocompatibility antigens with human diseases remain to be found.

9.59 JUVENILE RHEUMATOID ARTHRITIS

Juvenile rheumatoid arthritis (JRA) is a disease or group of diseases characterized by chronic synovitis and associated with a number of extra-articular manifestations. The terminology is difficult since more than 1 distinct disease is probably represented. Other names which have been used include Still disease, juvenile chronic polyarthritis, and chronic childhood arthritis; the term juvenile rheumatoid arthritis (JRA) will be used synonymously here with these terms. This disease differs from rheumatoid arthritis of adult onset in both articular and extra-articular manifestations.

JRA is an extremely variable disease which encompases several broad clinical subgroups (Table 9–22). Rheumatoid factor–positive polyarticular disease most closely resembles adult-onset rheumatoid arthritis; rheumatoid factor–negative polyarthritis is also well recognized in adults. Pauciarticular disease type II resembles those diseases described in adults as "spondyloarthropathies" (including early ankylosing spondylitis, Reiter syndrome, and the arthritis of inflammatory bowel disease). Systemic-onset disease occurs rarely in adults, and pauciarticular disease type I with chronic iridocyclitis has not been described in adults. Recognition of these patterns is useful in diagnosis, follow-up, and appropriate care of children with chronic arthritis.

Etiology and Epidemiology.   The etiology of rheumatoid arthritis and the mechanisms for perpetuation of chronic synovial inflammation in the disease are unknown. Two frequently mentioned hypotheses are that the disease results from an infection with as yet unidentified microorganisms or that it represents a hypersensitivity or "autoimmune" reaction to unknown stimuli. Various microorganisms have been isolated from rheumatoid synovium but none consistently. Organisms such as mycoplasma can cause chronic synovitis resembling rheumatoid arthritis in experimental animals. The possible roles of virus infections remain under investigation. Evidence that immune mechanisms are involved in pathogenesis is supplied by the association of rheumatoid factors (antibodies reactive with IgG) with adult-onset rheumatoid arthritis. Although these antibodies do not cause the disease, immune complexes of rheumatoid factor and immunoglobulin may perpetuate synovial inflammation and are responsible for the rheumatoid vasculitis seen in seropositive rheumatoid arthritis. Low levels of complement in the synovial fluid of some rheumatoid patients and low serum complement levels in patients with rheumatoid vasculitis are consistent with such a mechanism. However, this mechanism fails to explain all rheumatoid inflammation since chronic synovitis can occur in the absence of rheumatoid factors and with normal levels of complement in joint fluid. The occurrence of chronic arthritis in patients with IgA deficiency and hypogammaglobulinemia suggests that immunodeficiency may somehow predispose to rheumatoid arthritis; however, no blatant immunodeficiency has been identified in rheumatoid patients. Clinical onset may follow an acute systemic infection or physical trauma to a joint, but no direct relation to such events has been shown. Exacerbations may follow intercurrent illness or psychic stress.

There is no evidence that polyarticular, pauciarticular type I, or systemic-onset JRA is hereditary; they rarely occur in siblings or in multiple family members. Pauciarticular disease type II, however, is frequently found in association with a positive family history for ankylosing spondylitis, Reiter syndrome, acute iridocyclitis, or pauciarticular arthritis.

JRA is not a rare disease; it is estimated that there are a quarter million affected children in the United States. About 5% of all cases of rheumatoid arthritis begin in childhood. The disease may start at any age, though not usually before the 2nd birthday.

Pathology.   Rheumatoid arthritis is characterized by chronic nonsuppurative inflammation of synovium. Microscopically, affected synovial tissues are edematous, hyperemic, and infiltrated with lymphocytes and plasma cells. Secretion of increased amounts of joint

Table 9–22 SUBGROUPS OF JUVENILE RHEUMATOID ARTHRITIS

	POLYARTICULAR RHEUMATOID FACTOR–NEGATIVE	POLYARTICULAR RHEUMATOID FACTOR–POSITIVE	PAUCIARTICULAR TYPE I	PAUCIARTICULAR TYPE II	SYSTEMIC-ONSET
Per cent of JRA patients	25	10	30	15	20
Sex	90% girls	80% girls	60% girls	90% boys	60% boys
Age at onset	Throughout childhood	Late childhood	Early childhood	Late childhood	Through childhood
Joints	Any multiple (×2)	Any multiple (×2)	Few (×2) large joints: knee, ankle, elbow	Few (×2) large joints: hip girdle	Any
Sacroiliitis	No	Rare	No	Common	No
Iridocyclitis	Rare	No	50% chronic iridocyclitis	10–20% acute iridocyclitis	No
Rheumatoid factor	Negative	100%	Negative	Negative	Negative
Antinuclear antibodies	25%	75%	60%	Negative	Negative
HLA studies	?	HLA DR4	HLA DR5, DR8	HLA B27	?
Ultimate morbidity	Severe arthritis, 10%–15%	Severe arthritis, >50%	Ocular damage, 10%	Subsequent spondylo-arthropathy, ?%	Severe arthritis, 25%

fluid results in joint effusions. Projections of thickened synovial membrane form villi which protrude into joint spaces; hyperplastic rheumatoid synovium may spread over and become adherent to articular cartilage (pannus formation). With continuing synovitis, articular cartilage may become eroded and progressively destroyed. The mechanism of destruction of articular cartilage and other joint structures by chronic proliferating synovium remains unknown. The period of time before synovitis causes permanent joint damage varies from patient to patient; in general, lasting damage to articular cartilage occurs later in the course of JRA than in adult-onset disease, and many children with JRA never incur permanent joint damage despite prolonged synovitis. Joint destruction occurs more often in children with rheumatoid factor–positive disease or systemic-onset disease. Once joint destruction has commenced, erosions of subchondral bone, narrowing of the "joint space" (loss of articular cartilage), destruction or fusion of bones, and deformity, subluxation, or ankylosis of joints may result. Tenosynovitis and myositis may be present. Osteoporosis, periostitis, accelerated epiphyseal growth, and premature epiphyseal closure can occur adjacent to affected joints.

Rheumatoid nodules, less frequent in children than in adults and occurring primarily in rheumatoid factor–positive children, are characterized by fibrinoid material surrounded by chronic inflammatory cells. Pleura, pericardium, and peritoneum may show nonspecific fibrinous serositis; chronic constrictive pericarditis occurs rarely if ever. The rheumatoid rash appears histologically as a mild vasculitis, with a few inflammatory cells surrounding small vessels in subepithelial tissues.

Clinical Manifestations. *Polyarticular Disease.* This is characterized by involvement of multiple joints, typically including the small joints of the hands (Fig

9–7 and 9–8). Polyarticular disease unassociated with prominent systemic manifestations occurs in 35% of children with JRA. Two subgroups are included: *rheumatoid-factor–negative polyarthritis* (25% of total JRA patients) and *rheumatoid-factor–positive polyarthritis* (10% of total JRA patients). Rheumatoid-factor–positive patients have disease onset in late childhood, more severe arthritis, frequent rheumatoid nodules, and occasional rheumatoid vasculitis. Rheumatoid-factor–negative disease may begin at any time during childhood, is frequently mild, and is rarely associated with rheumatoid nodules. More girls than boys are affected in both types of disease. Both the polyarticular pattern and the nature

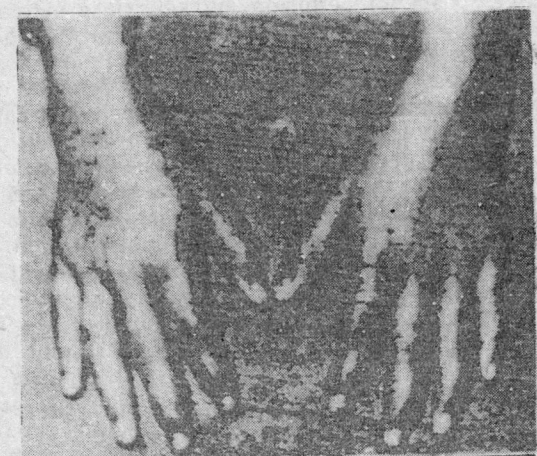

Figure 9–7 Hands and wrists of a girl with rheumatoid factor–negative polyarticular juvenile rheumatoid arthritis. Note symmetric involvement of the metacarpophalangeal joints, proximal interphalangeal joints, and distal interphalangeal joints. Both wrists are also affected.

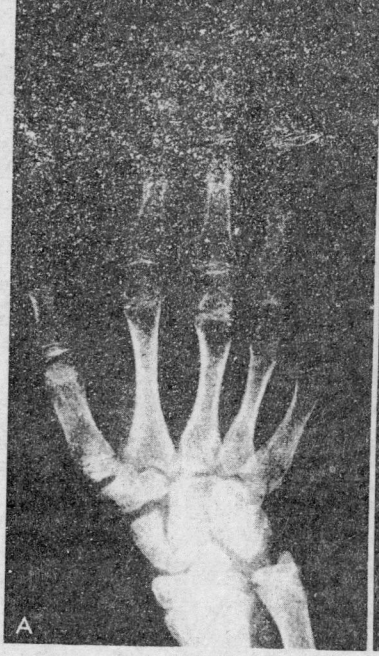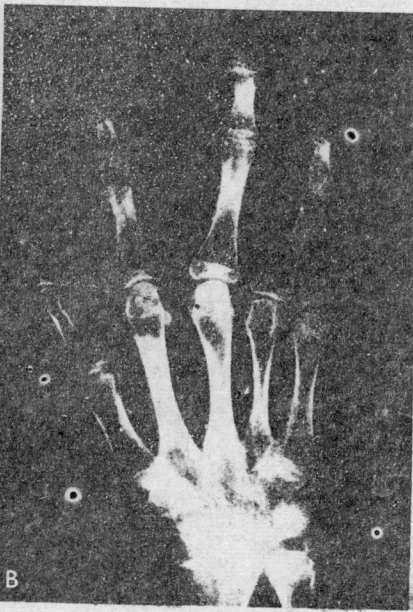

Figure 9–8 Progression of joint destruction in a girl with rheumatoid factor–positive juvenile rheumatoid arthritis despite doses of corticosteroids sufficient to suppress symptoms in the interval between *A* and *B*. *A*, Roentgenogram of hand at onset; *B*, roentgenogram 4 yr later, showing loss of articular cartilage and destructive changes in the distal and proximal interphalangeal and metacarpophalangeal joints and destruction and fusion of wrist bones.

of the rheumatoid factor tests are generally established early in the course of disease.

Onset of arthritis may be insidious, with gradual development of joint stiffness, swelling, and loss of motion, or fulminant, with sudden appearance of symptomatic arthritis. Affected joints are swollen and warm but rarely red. Swelling results from periarticular edema, joint effusion, and synovial thickening. Some children have joint stiffness and discomfort before objective changes appear. Affected joints may be tender to touch and painful on motion; however, severe tenderness and pain are unusual, and many children do not complain of any pain in obviously inflamed joints. Early in the disease limited joint motion is related to muscle spasm, joint effusion, and synovial proliferation; later, limited motion may result from joint destruction and ankylosis or from contractures of soft tissues. Pronounced synovial proliferation may produce cystic swellings about affected joints; occasionally herniations of synovium and extravasation of synovial fluid occur into neighboring structures, particularly in the popliteal area (popliteal cyst). Morning stiffness and "gelling" following inactivity are characteristic of rheumatoid arthritis in children, as in adults. Young children, particularly those with multiple joint involvement, are often irritable and assume a typical posture of anxious guarding of their joints against movement (Fig 9–9).

Arthritis, which may affect any synovial joint, often begins in large joints such as knees, ankles, wrists, and elbows. The involvement is often symmetrical. Inflammation of proximal interphalangeal joints produces spindling or fusiform changes of the fingers; metacarpophalangeal joint involvement is equally common, and distal interphalangeal joints may also be affected (Fig 9–7 and 9–8). Arthritis of the cervical spine, characterized by neck stiffness and pain, occurs in about half

the patients. Temporomandibular involvement with limited ability to open the mouth is common; the pain may be referred to as earache by young children. Hip involvement occurs in at least half the children with polyarthritis, usually beginning later in the disease process. Destruction of the femoral heads may ensue; severe hip disease is a major cause of disability in late JRA (Fig 9–10). Roentgenographic changes in the sacroiliac joints occur in some patients, usually in association

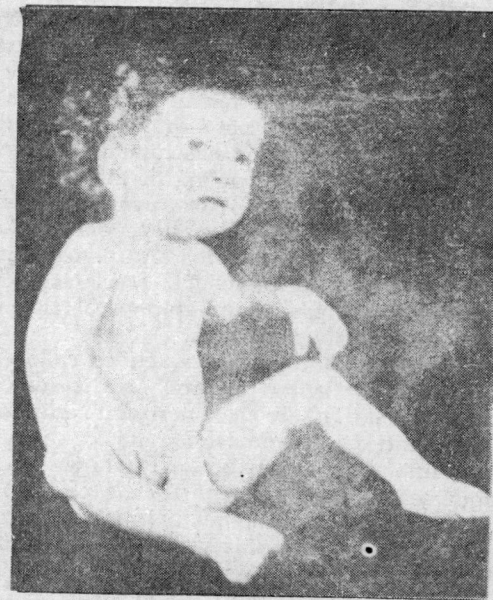

Figure 9–9 Characteristic posture of a child with juvenile rheumatoid arthritis, showing the anxious appearance and guarding of joints.

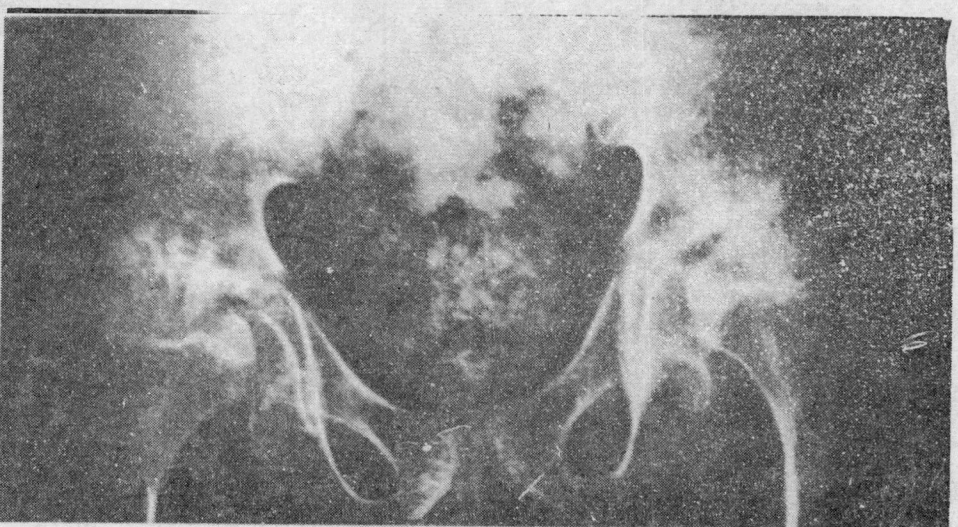

Figure 9–10 Severe hip disease in a 13 yr old boy with long-active, systemic-onset juvenile rheumatoid arthritis, showing destruction of femoral heads and acetabula, joint space narrowing, and subluxation of the left hip. The patient had received corticosteroids systemically for 9 yr.

with hip disease; these changes differ from those of ankylosing spondylitis and are not associated with involvement of the lumbodorsal spine. Rarely, cricoarytenoid arthritis causes hoarseness and laryngeal stridor. Involvement of sternoclavicular joints and costochondral junctions may cause chest pain.

Growth disturbances adjacent to inflamed joints may result in either overgrowth or undergrowth of the affected part. For example, increased leg length may follow chronic arthritis of the knee, and micrognathia after temporomandibular arthritis is 1 of the late hallmarks of JRA. Small, deformed feet may result from foot involvement in early childhood, as may shortened fingers from early hand involvement.

Extra-articular manifestations are not so dramatic as in systemic rheumatoid arthritis. However, the majority of patients with active polyarticular disease have malaise, anorexia, irritability, and mild anemia. Low-grade fever, slight hepatosplenomegaly, and lymphadenopathy may be present. Pericarditis is infrequent and iridocyclitis rare. Rheumatoid nodules may occur over pressure points, usually in patients with positive agglutination tests for rheumatoid factor. Rheumatoid vasculitis occurs at times in rheumatoid factor–positive patients, as does Sjögren syndrome. Growth may be retarded during periods of active disease; growth spurts often occur with remission.

Pauciarticular Disease. This illness is characterized by arthritis that remains limited to only a few joints (Fig 9–11). Large joints are primarily affected, and the distribution of arthritis is often asymmetrical or spotty. Two distinct subgroups are included: 1 includes primarily girls who are young at onset and are at risk for chronic iridocyclitis (pauciarticular disease type I); the other includes primarily boys who are older at onset and who are at risk for subsequent spondyloarthropathies (pauciarticular disease type II).

Pauciarticular disease type I affects about 30% of patients with JRA. Girls are predominantly affected, and the disease generally begins before age 4. Tests for rheumatoid factors are negative, but 60% of patients

have positive tests for antinuclear antibodies. HLA B27 is not associated. The most commonly affected joints are the knees, ankles, and elbows; occasionally, there is spotty involvement of other joints such as the temporomandibular joints, single toes or fingers, wrists, or neck. The hips and hip girdle are spared, and sacroiliitis is not associated. The clinical appearance and the synovial histology of affected joints are indistinguishable from those of polyarticular JRA. If arthritis remains limited to a few joints for the initial 6 mo, the disease generally remains pauciarticular throughout its course; additional large joints may be affected over the years, but widespread polyarticular disease does not usually occur. Although the arthritis may be chronic or recurrent, serious disability or joint destruction is uncommon. However, patients with pauciarticular disease type I are at high risk for eye complications; chronic iridocyclitis occurs in about 50% of such children at some time during the course of disease.

The *chronic iridocyclitis* of JRA is characteristically not associated with early symptoms or signs, activity of arthritis, or elevated sedimentation rate. Occasionally, children note redness, pain, photophobia, or decreased visual acuity early in the course of iridocyclitis. One or both eyes may be affected. If initial involvement is unilateral, the other eye usually remains uninvolved. Iridocyclitis is sometimes the presenting manifestation of JRA but generally begins at or up to 10 yr after onset of joint complaints. Patients with iridocyclitis frequently have positive tests for antinuclear antibodies. The earliest signs of inflammation of the iris and ciliary body are increased numbers of cells and amounts of protein in the anterior chamber of the eye, changes detectable only by slit lamp examination. The ocular inflammation often remains active for years. Sequelae (Fig 9–12) include posterior synechiae, complicated cataracts, secondary glaucoma, and phthisis bulbi (degeneration of the globe). Loss of vision may result; in severe cases permanent blindness occurs. Early detection and therapy before scarring occurs are important for preservation of vision. For this reason all children with pauciar-

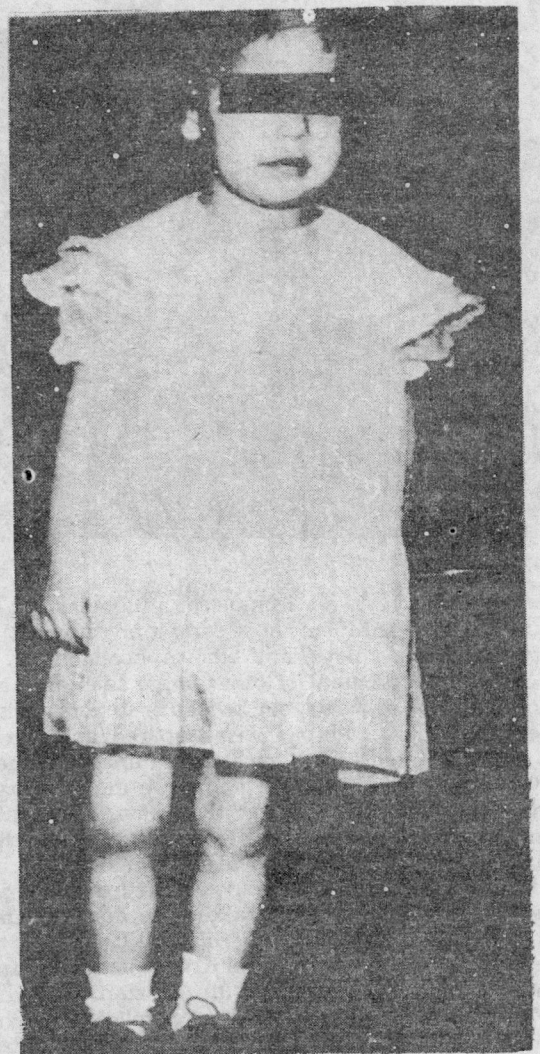

Figure 9–11   Characteristic appearance of a child with pauciarticular arthritis with onset in early childhood; note swelling of right knee.

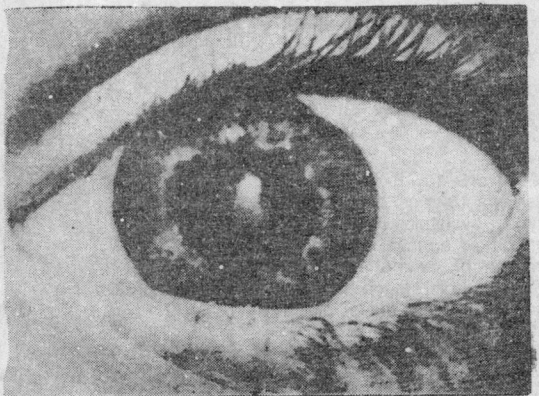

Figure 9–12   Chronic iridocyclitis of juvenile rheumatoid arthritis; extensive posterior synechiae have resulted in a small irregular pupil. There is a well developed cataract, and early band keratopathy can be seen at 3 and 9 o'clock positions in the cornea.

ticular disease should have slit lamp examinations 3–4 times yearly for the 1st 5 or more yr of disease regardless of the activity of the joint disease.

Other extra-articular manifestations are usually mild in pauciarticular JRA; low-grade fever, malaise, modest hepatosplenomegaly and lymphadenopathy, and mild anemia may occur in association with active joint disease.

Pauciarticular disease type II affects about 15% of patients with JRA. Boys are predominantly affected, and the onset is usually after the age of 8 yr. Family histories are often positive for pauciarticular arthritis, ankylosing spondylitis, Reiter disease, or acute iridocyclitis. Tests for both rheumatoid factors and antinuclear antibodies are negative; 75% of patients have HLA B27. Large joints, particularly those of the lower extremities, are affected; foot joints, temporomandibular joints, and joints of the upper extremities are also involved at times. Heel pain or Achilles tendinitis is

common, and there may be inflammation at the sites of tendon insertion into bone (enthesopathy). Hip girdle involvement is frequent early in the disease, and sacroiliitis can often be demonstrated on roentgenography. The peripheral arthritis is generally benign and often quite transient. Hip and foot pain may be severe at times, though, and may be incapacitating; such changes are often reversible with therapy.

As patients with pauciarticular disease type II are followed for years, some develop changes typical of ankylosing spondylitis with involvement of the lumbodorsal spine, changes consistent with Reiter syndrome (hematuria, urethritis, acute iridocyclitis, or mucocutaneous manifestations), or even inflammatory bowel disease. The ultimate morbidity for these children lies in the possible occurrence of any of these chronic spondyloarthropathies; the exact percentage of such occurrences is not known. Following children with pauciarticular disease type II requires recording of measurements of back flexion and chest expansion because extra-articular manifestations are associated with it. Though chronic iridocyclitis is not associated, 10–20% of patients have self-limited attacks of acute iridocyclitis, which is associated with prominent early symptoms and signs of eye inflammation but few scarring residua.

Systemic-Onset JRA.   Systemic JRA is characterized by prominent extra-articular manifestations (Table 9–23), particularly high fevers and rheumatoid rash. This type of disease occurs in 20% of patients. In contrast to most other types of JRA, as many boys as girls are affected. Systemic symptoms are generally the presenting manifestations of disease.

The fever is intermittent, with daily or twice-daily elevations to 39.5° C (103° F) or higher and rapid return to normal or subnormal levels (Fig 9–13). Temperature elevations usually occur in the evening but sometimes in the morning as well. Shaking chills are frequently associated. Patients may seem alarmingly ill during the period of fever and surprisingly well during its remission. Rheumatoid rash (Fig 9–14 and 9–15 [p. xxxi]) is characterized by its appearance and by its evanescent,

Table 9–23 MANIFESTATIONS OF SYSTEMIC JUVENILE RHEUMATOID ARTHRITIS

	%
High intermittent fever	100
Rheumatoid rash	95
Hepatosplenomegaly and/or lymphadenopathy	85
Pleuritis and/or pericarditis	60
Abdominal pain	20
Marked leukocytosis	85
Severe anemia	40
Rheumatoid factors	0
Antinuclear antibodies	0
Arthritis/arthralgia/myalgia during febrile periods	100
Chronic arthritis	90
Iridocyclitis	0

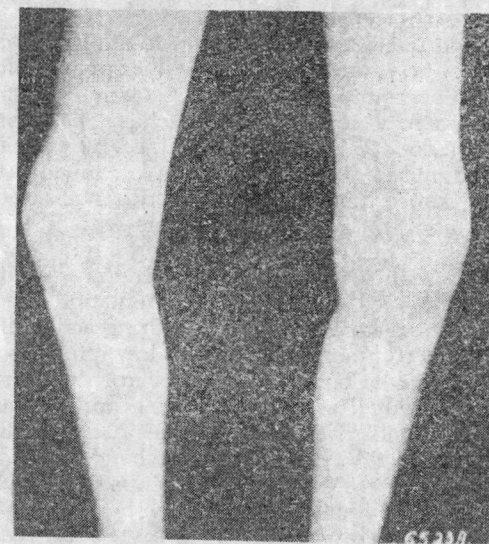

Figure 9–14 The rash of systemic-onset juvenile rheumatoid arthritis. (From Schaller JG, *In* Instructional Course Lectures, American Academy of Orthopedic Surgery, Vol XXIII. St. Louis, CV Mosby, 1974.)

recurrent nature. Individual lesions are small (several mm), pale, red-pink macules, often with central pallor; extensive lesions may coalesce. The rash is most frequently found on the trunk and proximal extremities but may occur anywhere on the body including the palms and soles. It usually appears during febrile periods but may also be induced by skin trauma (isomorphic response), heat, and embarrassment. Hepatosplenomegaly and generalized lymphadenopathy occur in most children with active systemic disease. The degree of organomegaly may be great. Mild hepatic dysfunction may be present, and lymph node histology may simulate lymphoma. About one third of affected children have detectable pleuritis or pericarditis, often subclinical. Chest roentgenograms may show pleural thickening or small pleural effusions; pericardial effusion may be large and electrocardiographic changes present. The pericarditis of JRA is generally benign. Rarely, severe chest pain, dyspnea, or cardiac failure, with or without evidence of myocarditis, demands vigorous therapy. Occasionally, interstitial lung infiltrates occur during periods of active systemic disease, but chronic rheumatoid lung disease rarely if ever occurs in children. A few children have episodes of severe abdominal pain during active disease. Leukocytosis and even leukemoid reactions are common. Anemia is also common during active disease and may occasionally be profound. Disseminated intravascular coagulation and acute liver failure have been reported; whether these are manifestations of disease or drug therapies (aspirin, gold) remains to be determined.

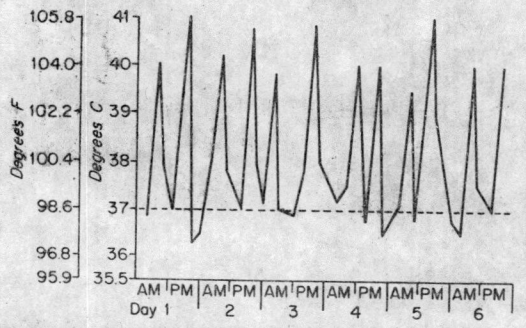

Figure 9–13 Characteristic fever of systemic juvenile rheumatoid arthritis; there are 1 or 2 daily temperature elevations to 39° C or greater, with rapid return of temperature to normal or subnormal levels.

Most children with systemic JRA have joint manifestations at or within a few mo of onset, although arthritis may initially be overlooked because of the overwhelming systemic symptoms. Some patients initially have only severe myalgia, arthralgia, or transient arthritis. A few patients do not develop arthritis until months or years later. The pattern of joint involvement is ultimately polyarticular and resembles that described in polyarticular disease. The systemic manifestations generally run a self-limited course for several mo but may recur. The real morbidity of systemic (polyarticular) JRA lies in arthritis that becomes chronic in some patients and persists after systemic symptoms have remitted. Systemic manifestations rarely recur after patients reach adulthood, even though chronic arthritis may persist.

Course and Prognosis. The major cause of morbidity in polyarticular and systemic JRA is chronic joint disease; in pauciarticular disease, the major morbidity is chronic iridocyclitis in type I patients and subsequent spondyloarthropathy in type II patients. The outcome is unpredictable in any individual patient. Even with severe systemic involvement, the disease is rarely life-threatening. There may be exacerbations and remissions, or symptoms may continue for years with mild arthritis causing little disability or, less commonly, with severe arthritis which progresses to joint destruction and permanent deformity. The disease does not always remit at puberty; some patients continue to have active arthritis into adulthood, and some have exacerbations after many yr of apparently complete remission. Exacerbations may be associated with intercurrent illness; hepatitis and other forms of liver disease may be followed by transient remission of arthritis.

Patients with rheumatoid factor–positive polyarthritis and systemic-onset disease have the poorest prognosis for joint function. The overall prognosis is good, however. At least 75% of JRA patients eventually enter long remissions without significant residual deformity or loss of function. A few patients are left with crippling joint deformities. Severe hip disease is particularly debilitating, as is loss of vision from iridocyclitis. Secondary amyloidosis (Sec 26.2), generally heralded by proteinuria and diagnosed by demonstration of amyloid in tissues, may cause morbidity; in England and Europe amyloidosis affects about 5% of patients with JRA; in the United States this complication is very rare.

' **Laboratory Manifestations.** There are no specific laboratory or diagnostic tests. The sedimentation rate is usually, but not invariably, elevated during active disease. Anemia is common, usually with low reticulocyte counts and negative Coombs test results; iron deficiency may also be present. The white blood cell count is often elevated; leukemoid reactions sometimes occur, particularly in systemic JRA, in which counts of 10,000–30,000/mm³ are the rule, and counts may sometimes be as high as 75,000/mm³. Urinalyses are normal; during salicylate therapy a few erythrocytes and renal tubular cells may be seen. Serum proteins may be altered, with increase in the alpha-2 and gamma globulin fractions and decrease in albumin. Any or all of the serum immunoglobulins may be elevated. *Antinuclear antibodies* are found in children with rheumatoid factor–negative (25%), rheumatoid factor–positive (75%), and pauciarticular type I (60%) disease but are rarely if ever present in systemic or pauciarticular type II disease. There is a strong correlation of antinuclear antibodies with chronic iridocyclitis but not with severity of arthritis. Lupus erythematosus (LE) cells can at times be demonstrated.

Rheumatoid factors are found in about 5% of children with JRA and correlate with older age at onset. Tests do not convert from negative to positive despite long-active JRA. Positive tests are most commonly associated with polyarticular disease, late childhood onset, severe destructive arthritis, and rheumatoid nodules; rheumatoid vasculitis and Sjögren syndrome are also associated at times.

Histocompatibility studies are described above.

Synovial fluid in JRA is cloudy, may clot spontaneously, and usually contains increased amounts of protein. The cell count varies from 5000–80,000 cells/mm³; the cells are predominantly neutrophils. Levels of glucose may be low in the joint fluid; levels of complement may be normal or decreased.

Early *roentgenographic changes* consist of soft tissue swelling, osteoporosis, and periostitis about affected joints (Fig 9–16). Regional epiphyseal closure may be accelerated and local bone growth increased or decreased. In long-active joint disease subchondral erosions and narrowing of cartilage spaces may occur, as may varying degrees of bony destruction and fusion. Late roentgenographic changes, i.e., in the wrist and hand (Fig. 9–8), are characteristic. Characteristic changes may occur in the neck, with narrowing and eventual fusion of neural arch joints (most frequently seen at C2 and C3, Fig 9–17), erosions of the odontoid process, atlantoaxial subluxation, and underdevelopment of vertebral bodies. Roentgenographic sacroiliitis resembling ankylosing spondylitis is often seen in pauciarticular disease type II.

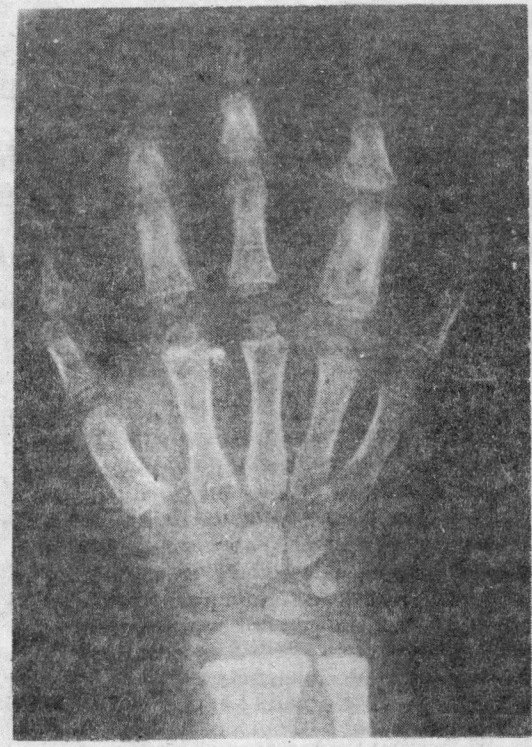

Figure 9–16 Early (6 mo duration) radiographic changes of JRA; soft tissue swelling and periosteal new bone formation appear adjacent to the 2nd and 4th proximal interphalangeal joints.

Diagnosis and Differential Diagnosis. The diagnosis is clinical and depends on the presence of persistent arthritis or typical systemic manifestations for 3 or more consecutive mo as well as on the exclusion of other diseases.

Early in the disease *pyogenic* or *tuberculous joint infection, osteomyelitis, sepsis,* or *arthritis associated with other*

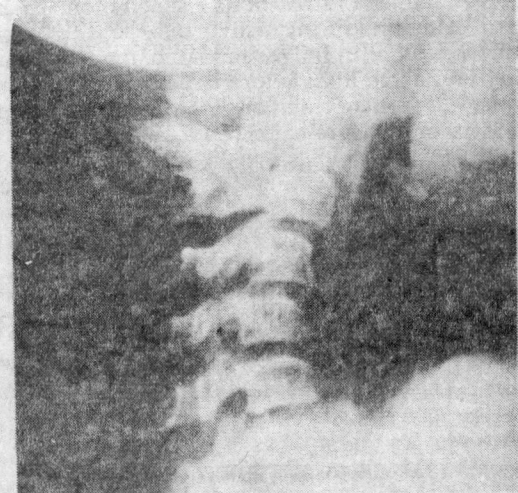

Figure 9–17 Cervical spine in long-active juvenile rheumatoid arthritis, showing fusion of neural arch between joints C2–C3, narrowing and erosions of the remaining neural arch joints, and resulting abnormal curvature.

acute infectious illnesses may be considered. Culture of joint fluid, tuberculin test, and roentgenograms of affected joints are helpful. Arthritis of limited duration may occur in association with a number of viral infections and after rubella immunization. Gonococcal infection may also result in arthritis. *Acute leukemia* and other malignancies occasionally present with pain and swelling of 1 or more joints and should be considered when onset is recent, particularly if severe anemia, thrombocytopenia, or abnormalities of peripheral white blood cells are present.

In *acute rheumatic fever* the transient, migratory nature of the arthritis and the presence of valvular carditis help in differentiation. *Systemic lupus erythematosus* (SLE) and *mixed connective tissue disease* can cause arthritis indistinguishable from rheumatoid arthritis, but the joint changes are usually milder, and other clinical manifestations of lupus are usually present; it should be noted that antinuclear antibodies and occasionally LE cells occur in JRA as well as in systemic lupus erythematosus. *Ankylosing spondylitis* may present with arthritis of a few peripheral joints which is indistinguishable from JRA (particularly pauciarticular disease, type II) before characteristic involvement of the spine becomes manifest; the presence of early roentgenographic sacroiliac joint changes associated with pain in the low back and hip girdle is suggestive. *Reiter syndrome* (arthritis, urethritis, conjunctivitis) is uncommon in children but should be considered in those with pauciarticular disease type II. The *vasculitis syndromes, dermatomyositis, ulcerative colitis, regional enteritis, psoriasis,* and *sarcoidosis* may be associated with arthritis similar to that of JRA but are generally distinguishable on clinical grounds. *Immunodeficiency diseases* may rarely be associated with chronic arthritis resembling JRA.

Various conditions such as *joint trauma, Legg-Perthes disease, Osgood-Schlatter disease,* and *slipped capital femoral epiphysis* may initially mimic JRA. *Acute toxic synovitis* of the hip is a self-limited condition of uncertain origin; JRA rarely begins in or affects solely the hip. Pigmented villonodular synovitis, an uncommon synovial overgrowth, usually affects only 1 joint.

Synovial biopsy may be useful, especially to exclude infection in monarticular disease; however, synovial histology does not distinguish the various subgroups of JRA, various other rheumatic disorders, or even so-called postinfectious states.

Treatment. In planning therapy physicians must realize that although JRA may be of long duration and has no specific cure, the ultimate prognosis is good for most patients and life is rarely threatened. Management of these children and their families tests the physician's ability to treat the whole child with sympathy, patience, and understanding. Unpredictable exacerbations are discouraging and make evaluation of therapy difficult. There is an understandable tendency for parents to shop for medical help and adopt fad or quack cures. The chronic nature of the disease, on the other hand, may cause the family to give up, allowing unnecessary crippling to occur.

The aims of immediate and long-term treatment are 2-fold: (1) to preserve joint function and to provide adequate care of extra-articular manifestations without

therapeutic harm; and (2) to support the family and child in achieving an optimal psychosocial adjustment. Such care ideally requires the devoted attention of a primary physician in consultation with specialists including a physiatrist or physical therapist, or orthopedist, an ophthalmologist, and sometimes a rheumatologist, an orthodontist, and a psychiatrist or social worker.

A number of drugs are effective in suppressing the inflammatory process. Acetylsalicylic acid (aspirin) is the safest and most satisfactory; in doses sufficient to maintain blood levels of 20–30 mg/dl it usually alleviates both arthritis and systemic manifestations. Such blood levels can be reached by using doses of about 100 mg of aspirin/kg daily for children of 25 kg or less and total daily doses of 40–60 grains (2.4–3.6 gm total) for older, heavier children. There is considerable individual variation in required doses, and patients must be watched carefully for toxicity. Full therapeutic response may require weeks to months. When dosage and response are determined and stabilized, the medication can be continued for years. Chronic therapeutic salicylate administration is relatively safe even in small children if physicians, patients, and parents are aware of the potential toxic effects. Intoxication from overdosage can be avoided if the dose is calculated with care and parents watch for the rapid or heavy breathing and drowsiness or other central nervous system changes that are often the earliest signs of salicylism in children. Tinnitus, a common complaint of adults with salicylism, is rarely noted by children. Salicylates should be given with food because of the possibility of gastric irritation. If patients complain of stomach ache, antacids can be added or buffered salicylate preparations or choline salicylate substituted for ordinary aspirin. Children with persistent gastrointestinal complaints should be investigated for peptic ulcer. Hemorrhagic phenomena and hypersensitivity reactions are extremely uncommon with therapeutic doses of aspirin. Elevated levels of hepatic enzymes have been described in the sera of patients with rheumatic diseases who were receiving large doses of salicylates; association of clinically significant liver disease is rare. Recent epidemiologic studies suggest that aspirin injection may be associated with Reye syndrome in children with either chickenpox or influenza; until this matter is clarified the physician may wish to withdraw aspirin temporarily from children exposed to these infections.

A number of drugs described under the heading of nonsteroidal anti-inflammatory agents are available for the therapy of arthritis in adults. These drugs are roughly as potent as aspirin in relieving pain and inflammation; some may provide particular relief for patients with spondyloarthropathies. These drugs include phenylbutazone, indomethacin, tolmetin, ibuprofen, naproxen, and fenoprofen. Of these drugs, only tolmetin is currently approved for use in children in the United States; this agent may provide a useful alternative to aspirin in some patients. The side effects are few.

There are few indications for systemic corticosteroids in JRA. Although they dramatically suppress symptoms, they do not induce permanent remission or prevent the occurrence of joint damage (Fig 9–8). It is suspected that destruction of cartilage and aseptic necrosis of bone, particularly in the femoral heads, may be related to long-term steroid therapy (Fig 9–10). Therapeutic doses of corticosteroids cause adrenal suppression, may suppress growth, and may produce a host of other potentially dangerous side effects. The dose required for suppression of symptoms is unpredictable and may actually increase with prolonged therapy.

Indications for use of corticosteroids in JRA include severe systemic disease unresponsive to an adequate trial of salicylates and iridocyclitis uncontrolled by topical steroids. In the former, or in rare instances of cardiac decompensation from pericarditis or myocarditis, prednisone in initial doses of 1–2 mg/kg/24 hr is indicated. As soon as symptoms are suppressed, the dose should be decreased and the drug gradually discontinued under a cover of salicylates. With decreasing doses there is often transient rebound of symptoms, which should be waited out. Since the systemic manifestations of JRA generally run a self-limited course, prednisone can usully be successfully discontinued within weeks or months. In iridocyclitis unresponsive to topical steroid therapy, systemic administration in doses sufficient to suppress ocular inflammation, as monitored by the slit lamp, are indicated; single doses given daily or on alternate days may be sufficient. Therapy should be managed jointly with an ophthalmologist.

Corticosteroids should rarely be used for relief of joint manifestations alone since they do not cure arthritis or prevent joint damage and since their chronic side effects may be even less tolerable than the joint disease. Other reasonable therapeutic possibilities should always be exhausted first. If corticosteroids are used, every effort should be made to employ the lowest effective dose, to use alternate day or single daily dosage, and to minimize the period of treatment.

Gold salts have not been widely used in JRA but appear to be no more toxic in children and as effective as in adults. They are useful if arthritis does not respond to an adequate trial of salicylates. Gold therapy requires weekly injections, *each* preceded by careful weekly follow-up for any signs of toxicity (rash, mucosal ulcers, leukopenia, thrombocytopenia, anemia, and proteinuria). Initially 2.5–5.0 mg of gold sodium thiomalate (Myochrysine) should be given intramuscularly and repeated 1 wk later, followed by a maintenance dose of 1 mg/kg/wk intramuscularly; a total weekly dose of 25 mg is appropriate for children weighing 25–60 kg; 50 mg can be given to larger teenagers. Several mo are required for therapeutic response, but if none has been noted after 20–24 weekly injections, the drug should be discontinued. If response occurs, injections should be gradually spaced out to 3–4 wk intervals and continued indefinitely. *Continuous surveillance for side effects must be maintained throughout the period of therapy; their appearance is almost always an indication for discontinuing the drug.*

Chloroquine and hydroxychloroquine may benefit some children with JRA but must be used with extreme care because of possible retinal toxicity; ophthalmologic examinations should be made every 3 mo. D-Penicillamine is currently being evaluated in the therapy of childhood arthritis but is a potentially toxic agent and still experimental. Although agents such as azathioprine and cyclophosphamide have been advocated as therapeutic agents in rheumatoid arthritis, their use in children for symptomatic relief of a disease which rarely threatens life does not seem warranted until more is known of their long-term side effects. Preliminary studies suggest that chlorambucil and azathioprine may be effective in treating potentially fatal amyloidosis associated with JRA.

Physical and occupational therapy are important to improve motion and muscular strength about affected joints and to restore and maintain the function of the whole individual. Patients and parents should be instructed in an appropriate exercise program to be carried out at home on a regular daily basis. Activities such as tricycle riding and swimming are beneficial and should be encouraged. Night splints for knees and wrists may aid in preventing and correcting deformity. Cylindrical casts or prolonged immobilization of joints should be avoided. Bed rest has little role in treatment. Children can usually determine their own activity; in general, they should avoid only those activities that cause overtiring and joint pain. Orthopedic surgery is sometimes required to correct joint deformities. Synovectomy of selected joints is occasionally helpful but does not appear to be curative. Total replacement of destroyed joints, particularly hips and knees, is now possible when full growth has been attained. Injection of corticosteroids into selected joints may be helpful at times, but repeated injections should not be used. Children with micrognathia may require orthodontic management or subsequent oral surgery.

Iridocyclitis requires prompt diagnosis and therapy to preserve vision. The eyes should be examined at each medical visit. Ophthalmologic slit lamp examinations should be made at least once a yr in children with systemic and polyarticular disease and 4 times yearly in children with pauciarticular disease. Parents should be cautioned to report any eye symptoms or decreased visual acuity at once. Therapy of iridocyclitis should be supervised by an ophthalmologist. Initially, it consists of topical steroids and dilating agents. Systemic steroids or subconjunctival injections should be used if prompt resolution of ocular inflammation is not achieved with topical agents. Frequent and long-term follow-up of eyes is essential. Ophthalmologic surgery may be required for chronic sequelae.

Children with JRA should be encouraged to lead as normal lives as possible. They and their parents need to know what to expect and to be treated optimistically. Affected children should not be led to believe that they are invalids but should be taught to be as self-sufficient as possible. With encouragement most can lead active lives, attend school, and participate in usual activities except strenuous sports. Long hospitalizations should be avoided. Children with residual handicaps need help in vocational planning.

9.60 ANKYLOSING SPONDYLITIS

Ankylosing spondylitis is characterized by stiffness and pain in the back, with involvement of sacroiliac joints and variable progression to joints and periarticular tissues of the lumbodorsal and cervical spine. About half of patients also have arthritis of peripheral joints. It is usually a disease of young and middle-aged adults but may begin in childhood, usually in males over 8 yr of age. There is striking association of ankylosing spondylitis with HLA antigen B27. The pathology of synovial tissue from affected joints is similar to that seen in rheumatoid arthritis.

Clinically, ankylosing spondylitis differs from rheumatoid arthritis in several respects: (1) characteristic involvement of sacroiliac joints and lumbodorsal spine, (2) predilection for males, (3) rarity of rheumatoid factor in affected adults, (4) extreme rarity of rheumatoid nodules, (5) high frequency of acute iridocyclitis, (6) occurrence of aortitis with resulting aortic insufficiency, and (7) significant familial incidence.

Clinical Manifestations. Peripheral arthritis may be the 1st manifestation and is often transient. Large joints, particularly those of the lower extremities, are affected most frequently. Heel pain is common. Shoulders, feet, and temporomandibular joints are also involved in a significant number of patients. Affected joints may be warm, swollen, and painful.

Characteristic involvement of sacroiliac joints and lumbodorsal spine may be present at the onset of disease or appear months to years later. Pain in the low back, hip girdles, and thighs is characteristic. The pain is often transient, more severe at night, and relieved by moving about. Stiffness in the low back with loss of normal spinal mobility follows (Fig 9–18). Spinal involvement characteristically begins in the sacroiliac joints and proceeds in an ascending fashion, involving the lumbar, the dorsal, and, finally, the cervical spine. In contrast, in JRA the neck is involved but the lumbodorsal spine spared. Decreased expansion of the chest, related to involvement of costovertebral joints, may occur early in disease. Low-grade fever, anemia, anorexia, fatigability, and growth retardation may occur. The family history is frequently positive for individuals with similar arthritis or acute iridocyclitis.

Ankylosing spondylitis may arrest at any stage, or the entire spine may become involved over a number of yr, with loss of virtually all vertebral mobility. Prognosis for functional outcome is usually good if good posture is maintained. Deformity of peripheral joints is uncommon, although some patients develop destructive hip disease. Acute iridocyclitis occurs in about 25% of patients at some time; aortitis has not been described in children but occurs in a significant number of adults with ankylosing spondylitis.

Laboratory Manifestations. There are no specific laboratory tests. Although HLA B27 is present in 95% of patients, it is not diagnostic. Sedimentation rates may be elevated. Anemia similar to that of rheumatoid arthritis occurs. However, rheumatoid factors are rarely found. Involvement of the sacroiliac joints is demonstrable roentgenographically (Fig 9–19), usually within the 1st 3–4 yr; destruction is progressive, with eventual obliteration of the joints. Characteristic roentgenographic changes in the lumbodorsal spine occur some yr later in the disease.

Differential Diagnosis. Ankylosing spondylitis should be suspected in any child with persistent pain in hips, thighs, or low back, with or without peripheral arthritis. Such children are often considered to have pauciarticular JRA. Roentgenographic changes in the sacroiliac joints are necessary for diagnosis, but several yr may elapse before they appear. In addition to ankylosing spondylitis, *spinal cord tumors, anatomic defects or infections of vertebrae or intervertebral discs,* and *Scheuermann* disease must be considered in any child with persistent back pain. *Legg-Perthes* disease and *slipped capital femoral epiphysis* may cause persistent hip and thigh pain. *Ulcerative colitis, regional enteritis, psoriasis,* and *Reiter syndrome* may have an associated spondylitis resembling ankylosing spondylitis.

Treatment. The aims of therapy are to relieve pain and to maintain good posture and function. For relief of pain, salicylates may suffice. Indomethacin and phenylbutazone may be helpful but must be used with caution in children and are considered experimental

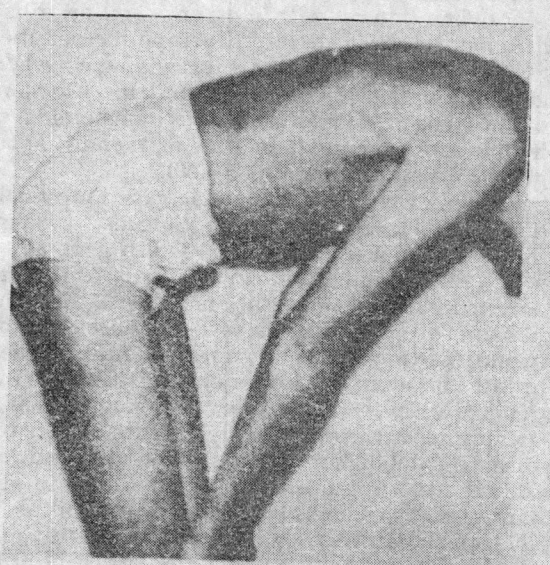

Figure 9–18 Loss of lumbodorsal spine mobility in a boy with ankylosing spondylitis: the lower spine remains straight when the patient bends forward.

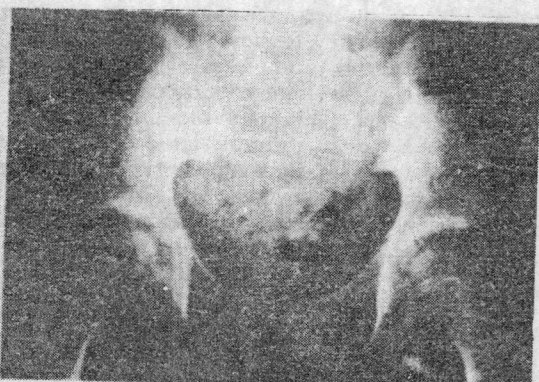

Figure 9–19 Well developed sacroiliitis in a boy with ankylosing spondylitis; both sacroiliac joints show extensive sclerosis, erosions of joint margins, and apparent widening of the joint space.

agents. Other newer nonsteroidal agents may also prove useful; only tolmetin is now approved for use in children. Gold is not thought to be effective, and corticosteroid therapy is rarely, if ever, indicated. Radiation therapy is contraindicated because of possible induction of leukemia. Maintenance of good posture is essential for preservation of good function; exercises designed to promote good posture and strengthen paraspinal muscles may be employed. A firm mattress or bed board should be used for sleeping, and thick pillows should be avoided.

9.61 OTHER SPONDYLOARTHROPATHIES IN CHILDREN

The spondyloarthropathies described in adults include those seronegative types of arthritis associated with sacroiliitis and spinal arthritis: ankylosing spondylitis, Reiter disease, psoriatic arthritis, the arthritis of inflammatory bowel disease, and the "reactive arthritis" of yersiniosis and other gastrointestinal infections. Although these types of arthritis are rarer in children than in adults, some of them, notably ankylosing spondylitis and Reiter disease, may sometimes be mislabeled as JRA during the childhood years. All of the spondyloarthropathies are associated with HLA B27 in some degree, although not generally as strongly as is ankylosing spondylitis; all share the property of being unassociated with either rheumatoid factors or antinuclear antibodies. The pathology of affected synovial tissues is not distinct from that of rheumatoid arthritis. Some of the spondyloarthropathies, notably Reiter disease and reactive arthritis, have been shown to occur after identifiable environmental events such as infections with Shigella or Yersinia. Various spondyloarthropathies may cluster in some families, with several family members having 1 or the other of these types of arthritis; acute iridocyclitis may also be similarly associated. Except for psoriatic arthritis, the spondyloarthropathies affect boys and girls equally or have a male preponderance. Diagnoses of the various spondyloarthropathies rest on clinical grounds.

The pauciarticular disease type II subgroup of JRA probably represents early ankylosing spondylitis or 1 of the other spondyloarthropathies. Although 3 of the other JRA subgroups are also seronegative (seronegative polyarthritis, systemic onset JRA, and pauciarticular disease type I), none is associated with sacroiliitis, HLA B27, or subsequent spondyloarthropathy.

Reiter Disease. In its full-blown form Reiter disease consists of a combination of sterile urethritis, arthritis, and ocular inflammation; other manifestations may include gastroenteritis and various skin rashes. Males are predominantly affected. In younger children Reiter disease has been reported following infections with Shigella, Yersinia enterocolitica, and Chlamydia; in older children, as in adults, Reiter disease has been reported following sexual exposure. Reiter disease is strongly associated with HLA B27, and the arthritis is generally pauciarticular, predominantly affecting large joints. Achilles tendinitis and heel pain are common. Some cases of pauciarticular disease type II may represent

"partial" Reiter disease, but this concept remains to be tested. The long-term prognosis of childhood-onset Reiter disease is unknown. The majority of reported children have recovered within a few mo. However, some individuals can be expected to have subsequent ankylosing spondylitis, some will continue with recurrent or chronic arthritis, and some will have recurrent attacks of ocular or urethral inflammation. Diagnosis is clinical. Infectious urethritis and gonococcal disease must be excluded. Salicylates or 1 of the other nonsteroidal anti-inflammatory agents, as in pauciarticular JRA or ankylosing spondylitis, are used for treatment. Physical therapy also plays an important role in therapy. Evidence of sacroiliitis should be sought and patients followed for possible subsequent ankylosing spondylitis.

Arthritis of Inflammatory Bowel Disease. Both ulcerative colitis (Sec 11.37) and regional enteritis (Sec 11.38) can be associated with arthritis during the childhood years; about 10% of children with inflammatory bowel disease will at some time have joint manifestations. Affected children are generally older than age 8, and the arthritis generally affects a few large peripheral joints in a pauciarticular pattern. Periods of arthritis usually coincide with periods of active bowel disease or follow the appearance of identifiable bowel disease by months or years; however, in a few patients arthritis may be the 1st disease manifestation. The arthritis of inflammatory bowel disease in children follows 2 patterns, as it does in adulthood. The majority of affected children have only peripheral arthritis, which waxes and wanes with activity of the bowel disease and causes neither joint destruction nor permanent joint deformity. However, a few children have early ankylosing spondylitis which may progress to disability regardless of control of the underlying bowel disease. For this reason it is important to follow children with inflammatory bowel disease for evidence of sacroiliitis or spinal arthritis. HLA B27 is associated with the ankylosing spondylitis but not with the peripheral arthritis of inflammatory bowel disease. Therapy for peripheral arthritis includes control of the underlying bowel disease, generally with corticosteroids, and the occasional additional use of salicylates or other nonsteroidal agents. If ankylosing spondylitis occurs, therapy should be given for that condition (Sec 9.60).

Reactive Arthritis. Following gastrointestinal infection with Yersinia enterocolitica, Shigella, or Salmonella there may be a sterile arthritis which generally affects a few peripheral joints in a pauciarticular fashion. Affected patients frequently have HLA B27. The relationship of such arthritis to Reiter disease and other spondyloarthropathies remains to be determined. The arthritis is generally transient and the ultimate outcome good. However, some affected patients may subsequently have chronic spondyloarthropathy. Any child with a combination of gastroenteritis and arthritis should have appropriate stool cultures and serologic studies made for possible offending organisms.

Psoriatic Arthritis. Although psoriasis is a relatively common skin condition of children, psoriatic arthritis is uncommon during the childhood years. Girls are predominantly affected in a 2.5:1 ratio. Psoriatic arthritis in childhood is similar to that in adulthood. Arthritis begins in 1 or several joints, often in an asymmetric fashion. More than half of patients have involvement of distal interphalangeal joints; tendinitis is also a frequent finding. In about half of patients, psoriasis precedes arthritis by months or years; in others the arthritis is the initial event, with psoriasis occurring in later years. Nail pitting is commonly associated. The prognosis of psoriatic arthritis in children appears to be quite good, though there are as yet few long-term follow-up studies. A few patients with psoriatic arthritis are found to have sacroiliitis and subsequent ankylosing spondylitis which is associated with HLA B27. Therapy of psoriatic arthritis is similar to that in adults; salicylates and other nonsteroidal anti-inflammatory agents are generally used. There is little experience with agents such as methotrexate in childhood psoriatic arthritis, and they should be avoided. As in JRA, physical and occupational therapy play important roles in maintenance of good function.

9.62 SYSTEMIC LUPUS ERYTHEMATOSUS

Systemic lupus erythematosus (SLE) is a systemic disease characteristically affecting many organ systems. Its natural history is unpredictable; it is often progressive, terminating in death if untreated, but may remit spontaneously or smolder for many yr. Lupus in children is generally more acute and severe than in adults.

Etiology and Epidemiology. The cause is unknown. Many observations are consistent with the hypothesis that SLE is a disease of altered immune reactivity, perhaps genetically determined. Viruses may also play a role in pathogenesis. A variety of immune phenomena occur. Serum levels of immunoglobulins are increased. Antibodies are found which react with various nuclear constituents (the **antinuclear antibodies**), ribonucleic acid, gamma globulin (rheumatoid factors), red blood cells (positive Coombs test), platelets, white blood cells, antigens used in serologic tests for syphilis (false-positive serology), and coagulation factors. There is also an association between inflammation and circulating immune complexes, particularly complexes of deoxyribonucleic acid (DNA) and antibodies reactive with DNA. Such immune complexes are deposited in tissues, fix complement, and initiate an inflammatory response that results in tissue injury. In SLE nephritis, for example, immunoglobulins and complement can be demonstrated in renal tissues by immunofluorescent techniques and DNA and anti-DNA antibodies eluted from affected glomeruli; active LE with nephritis is associated with decreased levels of serum complement and with circulating antibodies reactive with DNA.

The onset or exacerbations of disease may appear related to intercurrent infections; it is suspected that there is increased susceptibility to infections, perhaps on the basis of faulty immune mechanisms. Available evidence, including studies showing alterations in T and B lymphocyte function in patients with SLE, suggests that an immunodeficiency state may underlie the disease. It is sometimes familial and has occurred in identical twins; hypergammaglobulinemia, antinuclear antibodies, and other immune abnormalities have been found in relatives of patients with lupus.

Lupus-like disease occurs following exposure to a number of drugs, notably hydralazine, sulfonamides, procainamide, and anticonvulsants. Drug-induced disease is generally mild and reversible when the inciting drug is withdrawn. Cutaneous manifestations and sometimes systemic manifestations may be exacerbated by sunlight.

The incidence is not known, but the disease is not rare. SLE begins in childhood in 20% of cases, usually in children over 8 yr of age. Females are predominantly affected (8:1) in all age groups, except perhaps in prepubertal patients in whom the sex incidence seems nearly equal between girls and boys. All races may be affected; indeed, the prevalence of lupus may be higher in certain dark-skinned peoples including Blacks, Latin Americans, and certain native American tribes.

Pathology. Changes occur at multiple sites and involve many organ systems. Masses of amorphous, purple-staining extracellular material in hematoxylin-stained affected tissues are characteristic. These *hematoxylin bodies* probably represent degenerated cell nuclei similar to the inclusions of LE cells. Fibrinoid, an acellular, deeply eosinophilic material, is found in loose connective tissue or in walls of blood vessels of affected tissues. This substance, of uncertain composition, is not specific for SLE and is usually accompanied by inflammation, predominantly a mononuclear cell reaction. In the spleen perivascular fibrosis around affected vessels results in characteristic "onion ring" lesions. Granulomas are sometimes found in affected tissues. (See Sec 16.20 for renal pathology.)

Clinical Manifestations. The disease may begin insidiously or acutely. Sometimes symptoms antedate the diagnosis of SLE by years. The most frequent early symptoms in children are fever, malaise, arthritis or arthralgia, and rash. Fever occurs at some time in most affected children; it may be intermittent or sustained. Malaise, anorexia, weight loss, and debility are common.

Cutaneous manifestations occur in most affected children at some time. The "butterfly" rash (Fig 9–20 [p. xxxi]), an erythematous blush or scaly erythematous patches, involves the malar areas and usually extends over the bridge of the nose. The rash may be photosensitive, may spread to the face, scalp, neck, chest, and extremities, and may become bullous and secondarily infected. *Discoid lupus* (cutaneous manifestations only) is unusual in children. There are also other skin eruptions. Erythematous macules and punctate lesions on the palms, soles, and fingertips are distinctive; such lesions are secondary to vascular changes, and local infarction of tissue may occur. Raynaud' phenomenon may be present. Vascular changes are seen at times in the nail beds. Macular and ulcerative lesions also occur on the palate and mucous membranes of the mouth and nose. Purpura, sometimes associated with thrombocytopenia, may appear on dependent or traumatized areas. Erythema nodosum or erythema multiforme are occasionally associated. Alopecia, from inflammation about hair follicles, may be patchy or generalized, and the hair coarse, dry, and brittle.

Arthralgia and joint stiffness are common and often occur without objective changes. Sometimes affected joints are warm and swollen, but persistent deforming arthritis is rare. Aseptic necrosis of bone, particularly in the femoral heads, has been described, presumably secondary to vasculitis. Tenosynovitis and myositis may occur.

Polyserositis with pleurisy, pericarditis, and peritonitis is characteristic. Hepatosplenomegaly and generalized lymphadenopathy are common. Cardiac involvement may be manifested by variable murmurs, friction rubs, cardiomegaly, electrocardiographic changes, or congestive heart failure, with myocarditis, pericarditis, or verrucous endocarditis (Libman-Sacks endocarditis) found at postmortem examination. Myocardial infarctions may be a cause of death in relatively young lupus patients, including children. Parenchymal lung infiltrates may occur; infection must be excluded, however, before pneumonia can be ascribed to SLE. Acute pneumonia, pulmonary hemorrhage, or chronic pulmonary fibrosis may occur. Involvement of the nervous system may cause personality changes, seizures, cerebral vascular accidents, and peripheral neuritis. Gastrointestinal manifestations include abdominal pain, vomiting, diarrhea, melena, and even bowel infarction secondary to vasculitis. Ocular changes may include episcleritis, iritis, or retinal vascular changes with hemorrhages or exudates (cytoid bodies). Most children have clinical renal involvement (Sec 16.20).

Laboratory Manifestations.   Antinuclear antibodies should be demonstrable in all patients with active SLE and provide the best screening test for the disease; recent claims for "ANA-negative lupus" remain to be clarified. Antibodies to DNA are relatively specific and are associated with active disease, particularly nephritis; DNA antibodies thus provide a useful index of severity and activity. Serum hemolytic complement and some of its components (C3 is most frequently measured) are decreased in patients with severe active SLE, particularly in those with nephritis; measurement of serum complement therefore provides another useful guide to the activity and severity of disease. Other antibodies may be demonstrated by biologic false-positive tests for syphilis or positive Coombs tests. Serum gamma globulin levels are usually elevated; alpha-2 globulin levels may be increased and albumin decreased. One or more of the individual immunoglobulins may be elevated. An increased prevalence of HLA B8 and DW3/DR3 has been reported in some series of lupus patients.

Anemia related to chronic inflammatory disease or hemolysis is common. Difficulties in typing and cross-matching blood may arise from the presence of erythrocyte antibodies. Thrombocytopenia and leukopenia occur frequently. Platelet antibodies may be demonstrable; idiopathic thrombocytopenic purpura may be the 1st manifestation of SLE. The urine may contain red cells, white cells, protein, and casts. Renal insufficiency is manifested by elevation of the blood urea nitrogen or creatinine and abnormal renal function studies.

Diagnosis and Differential Diagnosis.   SLE may mimic any rheumatic disease and many other diseases as well. Diagnosis is clinical and is confirmed by laboratory tests. Antinuclear antibodies are always present even though they are not diagnostic; their absence makes the diagnosis unlikely. Antibodies to DNA are virtually diagnostic but are present only in severe or widespread disease. LE cells are not always demonstrable. Hypergammaglobulinemia, positive Coombs test, false-positive test for syphilis, anemia, leukopenia or thrombocytopenia, and signs of nephritis may also be diagnostically helpful. Serum hemolytic complement and some of its components are lowered in some patients with active disease. Renal biopsy may confirm the diagnosis, but histologic changes are not entirely specific. Thrombocytopenic purpura and hemolytic anemia may be presenting features; the differential diagnosis of these manifestations should include SLE.

Treatment.   Therapy should be based on the extent and severity of disease in the individual patient. Patients must be thoroughly evaluated, particularly for renal involvement. The type and severity of the renal lesion should be determined by renal biopsy on patients with clinical evidence of nephritis. There is no specific therapy; drugs used to treat the disease suppress inflammation and perhaps suppress the formation of immune complexes and the activities of immunologically active effector cells (although the latter mechanism remains unproved). In general, patients should be treated to maintain clinical well-being and normal serum complement levels.

In patients with mild disease without nephritis, salicylates or other nonsteroidal agents should be used to provide symptomatic relief of arthritis and other discomforts. Careful follow-up for possible development of nephritis is important. Chloroquine and hydroxychloroquine have long been used in discoid and systemic lupus, but extreme care must be taken because of retinal toxicity. Topical steroid preparations may suppress the facial rash. Corticosteroids in doses sufficient to suppress symptoms may be required. In patients with SLE and mild renal disease (viz., lupus glomerulitis), therapy is also symptomatic, with careful follow-up. Doses of corticosteroid sufficient to suppress symptoms should be given initially (1–2 mg/kg/24 hr may be required) and then tapered to the lowest suppressive dose. Antimalarials may be useful adjunctive drugs. In patients with SLE and severe nephritis (lupus glomerulonephritis or membranous glomerulonephritis with the nephrotic syndrome) therapy must be geared to maintain not only the clinical well-being of the patient but also suppression of the renal disease, as reflected by return of serum complement levels to normal and reduction of circulating antibodies to DNA. Large doses of corticosteroids for prolonged periods may be required; initial doses of prednisone of 1–2 mg/kg/24 hr are usual. All the undesirable side effects of steroid therapy may be expected if large doses are required for any significant period of time. Other schedules of steroid administration including intravenous pulses with large doses or alternate day dose schedules are used at times. Agents such as azathioprine, cyclophosphamide, or chlorambucil may be effective in suppressing severe SLE; however, such therapy remains experimental and must be used with extreme care. Little is known of the long-term effects of such drugs, particularly in children; side effects include increased susceptibility to severe viral and other infections, gonadal suppression, and possible induction of malignancies. Such agents should never be used in mild SLE or in patients whose disease can be satisfactorily controlled with corticosteroids alone.

Seizures and other central nervous system manifestations should be treated with large doses of prednisone; they are generally associated with severe active disease. Central nervous system disease occurs episodically in SLE and may never recur if the patient is helped over the acute episode and the disease can be subsequently controlled.

Because of the possibility of drug-induced disease, inquiry should be made about possible offending agents; drugs known to be associated with SLE should not be used in patients with the disease.

Meticulous follow-up is of paramount importance in the treatment of all patients with SLE; this requires monitoring of clinical, renal, and serologic status. Any signs of worsening disease should be promptly recognized and appropriately managed. Since there is no cure, the disease is potentially lifelong, and patients must be followed for years.

Prognosis. SLE has generally been considered a potentially or even uniformly fatal disease, particularly in children. Now, however, some children with milder disease are being recognized, and it is apparent that not all children with the disease have severe nephritis. Although spontaneous exacerbations and remissions occur, prolonged spontaneous remission is unusual in children. Therapy with antibiotics, corticosteroids, and, possibly, anticancer drugs has prolonged survival and brightened the short-term prognosis for many patients with lupus. The 5 yr survival for children with lupus has greatly improved, now approaching 90%. However, a significant number of patients still die later from the disease. Major causes of death in SLE patients today include nephritis, central nervous system complications, infections, pulmonary lupus, and, perhaps, myocardial infarctions. Whether the ultimate prognosis of severe lupus can be modified by vigorous therapy remains to be determined.

9.63 LUPUS PHENOMENA IN THE NEWBORN PERIOD

Infants of mothers with SLE may have transient manifestations of lupus in the newborn period, presumably mediated by transplacental factors. Transiently positive antinuclear antibody tests or LE cells are the most frequent abnormalities; there are generally no associated clinical manifestations, and the serologic abnormalities regress after several wk. The most frequent clinical abnormality of infants born to mothers with SLE is a rash clinically and histologically typical of discoid lupus, which fades over a period of several mo. Tran-

sient thrombocytopenia related to transplacental platelet antibodies has been noted, as have transient hemolytic anemia and leukopenia. Maternal SLE or other rheumatic disease is associated with a majority of infants with congenital heart block, although the mechanism for this is unknown. Endocardial fibroelastosis has also been reported in infants of mothers with SLE. Few, if any, cases of true SLE in infants have been reported.

9.64 VASCULITIS SYNDROMES

In these syndromes of inflammation of blood vessels the various patterns of disease depend on the size and location of affected vessels. When small nonmuscular vessels are involved, the disease takes the form of Schönlein-Henoch vasculitis (anaphylactoid purpura). With involvement of larger muscular arteries the disease is called polyarteritis nodosa; many variants have been described, including infantile polyarteritis, Wegener granulomatosis, and, probably, Kawasaki disease (Sec 9.68). Some overlap of these syndromes occurs; it is reasonable to expect that vessels of various sizes may sometimes be involved in the same patients. In Takayasu arteritis the aorta and other great vessels are sites of inflammation.

Inflammation of blood vessels also occurs in other rheumatic disease in children, notably lupus erythematosus, dermatomyositis, and scleroderma; in hypertension; and in vessels exposed to local infection, trauma, or thromboemboli.

The causes of these disorders are unknown. Both Schönlein-Henoch vasculitis and polyarteritis may follow exposure to drugs or allergens. In serum sickness, a usually self-limited type of vasculitis occurring after exposure to foreign substances, vasculitis is caused by deposition of immune complexes. Several cases of polyarteritis nodosa have been associated with Australia antigen, vascular damage presumably being caused by immune complexes of Australia antigen and its antibody. In contrast to most other rheumatic diseases, Schönlein-Henoch vasculitis and polyarteritis nodosa predominantly affect males. In childhood Schönlein-Henoch vasculitis is the most commonly encountered type; polyarteritis and its variants are extremely rare in children.

9.65 SCHÖNLEIN-HENOCH VASCULITIS
(Anaphylactoid Purpura)

This distinctive syndrome was described by Heberden before 1800; Schönlein in the 1830's described the typical rash in association with joint manifestations, and Henoch in the 1870's recognized the association of gastrointestinal and renal manifestations. Osler pointed out the similarity between this disease and the hypersensitivity reactions, erythema multiforme, and serum sickness. The skin lesion, which is not always purpuric, is the most obvious sign; the visceral lesions are less easily recognized but are far more serious. The primary manifestations are due to vasculitis of small blood vessels.

The cause is unknown. Allergy or drug sensitivity seems to play a role in some cases. The disease may follow an upper respiratory tract infection, sometimes streptococcal, but this sequence (or phenomenon) is of uncertain significance. The syndrome is not rare and may occur at any age; it is more common in children than in adults, most cases occurring in the age range from 2–8 yr. Boys are affected twice as often as girls.

Pathology. In the skin small vessels of the corium are surrounded with an acute inflammatory exudate of polymorphonuclear and round cells; eosinophils and varying numbers of red blood cells may be present. Capillaries are most frequently involved, but small arterioles and venules may be affected. Scattered nuclear debris, edema, and swelling of collagen fibrils are found adjacent to affected vessels. Inflammation or hemorrhage may occur at other sites, notably in synovium, the gastrointestinal tract, and the central nervous system. For the pathology of the renal lesion, see Sec 16.21.

Clinical Manifestations. Onset may be acute, with simultaneous appearance of several manifestations, or gradual, with sequential appearance of different manifestations over a period of weeks. Various combinations of symptoms and signs may occur. Malaise and low-grade fever are present in half the patients.

Skin lesions are present in all identified patients; it is not known whether visceral manifestations occur in the absence of rash. The lesions usually appear on the lower extremities but may involve buttocks, upper extremities, trunk, and face as well (Fig 9–21 [p. xxxi]). Dermatologic manifestations are extremely variable. The classic lesion begins as a small wheal or an erythematous maculopapule. Lesions initially blanch on pressure but later lose this ability and generally become petechial or purpuric. Purpuric areas progress in the usual manner of ecchymoses, changing from red to purple, becoming rusty, and eventually fading. Skin lesions appear in crops, and at any time a variety may be present. In addition to these characteristic lesions, the various patterns of erythema multiforme and erythema nodosum may occur. Such rashes are rarely pruritic. Angioedema involving the scalp, eyelids, lips, dorsa of the hands and feet, back, and perineum is common and may be striking, especially in young children. Rarely an entire limb segment, such as the forearm, may be transiently swollen and tender.

Arthritis occurs in two thirds of affected children. Large joints, particularly knees and ankles, are most commonly involved. Affected joints may be swollen, tender, and painful on motion. Effusions may be present; joint fluid is serous, with leukocytosis, not hemorrhagic. Joint symptoms usually resolve after a few days without residual deformity or articular damage but may recur during the period of active disease.

Gastrointestinal symptoms appear in two thirds of affected children. The most common complaint is colicky abdominal pain, which may be severe and is often associated with vomiting. Stools show gross or occult blood in over half of patients, and hematemesis may occur. Failure to recognize this syndrome in children with sudden onset of acute abdominal pain may lead to unnecessary laparotomy. In such cases peritoneal exudate and enlarged mesenteric lymph nodes are usually found; segmental edema and hemorrhage into bowel wall may be present. Gastrointestinal roentgenograms may show decreased motility and segmental narrowing, presumably related to submucosal edema and hemorrhage. Rarely intussusception, obstruction, or infarction and perforation of bowel may occur.

Renal involvement is potentially the most serious manifestation since it can result in chronic renal disease. It occurs in 25–50% of children during the acute phase, the frequency depending in part on the adequacy of examination. It is usually manifest during the 1st few wk of illness but sometimes appears after other manifestations have become quiescent. Moderate azotemia and hypertension, and even oliguria and hypertensive encephalopathy, can occur. Most children with renal involvement recover, although some continue to have abnormal urinary sediment, with or without abnormal renal function; a few suffer chronic renal disease within a few yr of the acute phase. See also Sec 16.21.

A rare but potentially serious manifestation is central nervous system involvement, with seizures, pareses, and coma. Hepatosplenomegaly and lymphadenopathy may occur during acute phases of the disease. Rarely, intramuscular hemorrhage, rheumatoid-like nodules, cardiac involvement, eye involvement, or testicular swelling and hemorrhage have been reported.

Prognosis is excellent in the absence of significant renal disease. The course is variable. Often the disease is mild, lasting a few days and manifested only by transient arthritis and a few purpuric spots. In more seriously affected children the average duration is 4–6 wk, but subsequent exacerbations and remissions may occur. Sometimes the illness may smolder for 1 or more yr.

Laboratory Manifestations. Laboratory tests are not diagnostic. The sedimentation rate may be elevated. The white blood cell count is often increased, and eosinophilia may be present. Coagulation studies are normal. With renal involvement red cells, white cells, casts, and albumin are present in the urine. There may be gross or occult blood in the stools. Lupus erythematosus cells, rheumatoid factor, and antinuclear antibodies are not associated. Serum complement titers are normal or elevated. Serum levels of IgA may be elevated.

Diagnosis and Differential Diagnosis. The full-blown picture of Schönlein-Henoch vasculitis with rash, arthritis, and gastrointestinal and renal manifestations is characteristic. However, diagnostic confusion may result when 1 symptom predominates or multiple system involvement is not recognized. The rash may suggest a *hemorrhagic diathesis* or *septicemia*; platelet counts, blood clotting tests, and cultures will exclude these possibilities. In addition, the patient with septicemia usually appears more acutely ill. When gastrointestinal manifestations predominate, the syndrome may suggest a number of *intra-abdominal emergencies*. The possibility of Schönlein-Henoch vasculitis should be considered in any child with acute abdominal pain and inquiry made for associated rash, nephritis, or arthritis. With prominent renal findings, *acute glomerulonephritis* may be suggested; the presence of other manifestations of

Schönlein-Henoch vasculitis should allow differentiation. In children with chronic renal disease a history of acute Schönlein-Henoch vasculitis in the past should be sought. Differentiation from other rheumatic diseases is rarely difficult. In polyarteritis nodosa, peripheral neurologic changes and cardiac manifestations are more common, but clinical distinction from Schönlein-Henoch vasculitis may occasionally be difficult.

Treatment. There is no specific therapy. In the rare instance in which a specific allergen can be proved, the patient should be kept from contact with it. When the disease seems to follow a bacterial infection, particularly streptococcal, the organism should be eliminated and, if the disease recurs, prophylaxis considered. Symptomatic treatment only is indicated for arthritis, rash, edema, fever, and malaise. Salicylates will often alleviate these self-limited discomforts.

Intestinal hemorrhage, obstruction, or perforation may be life-threatening in the acute phase; these complications may perhaps be prevented by the early use of corticosteroids. Therapy with prednisone in dosage of 1–2 mg/kg/24 hr is often associated with dramatic improvement. Corticosteroid therapy is also indicated in the rare instances of central nervous system manifestations. Steroids do not, however, affect renal involvement in the acute phase or prevent chronic renal disease. Acute renal failure should be managed in the same way as acute glomerulonephritis. Therapy of severe nephritis with drugs such as azathioprine and cyclophosphamide remains experimental (Sec 16.21).

Prognosis. Rarely, death may occur during the acute phase from gastrointestinal complications (hemorrhage, intussusception, bowel infarction), acute renal failure, or central nervous system involvement. Chronic renal disease may cause later morbidity in a few patients. About 25% of children with initial renal involvement have persistence of abnormal urine sediment for years; the eventual outcome for these patients is not known.

9.66 POLYARTERITIS NODOSA

Medium-sized and small arteries are the sites of inflammation in polyarteritis nodosa. The disease can affect all age groups but is rare in childhood. Males are affected more frequently than females. As with Schönlein-Henoch vasculitis, the cause is not known, but the disease has been reported to follow drug exposures. Hepatitis B antigen has been associated with a few cases as have streptococcal infections and serous otitis media. Inflammation with polymorphonuclear leukocytes, eosinophils, and round cells may involve the entire vessel walls. Necrosis, thrombosis, or aneurysm formation may occur in affected vessels and result in infarction. Healed vessels become scarred or recanalized.

Clinical manifestations are diverse and depend on sites of vascular involvement. Signs of systemic illness, such as fever, anorexia, lethargy, weakness, and loss of weight, are usually present. Arthralgia and arthritis are frequent; myalgia and myositis may be present. Various cutaneous manifestations are common and include erythematous rashes, nodular lesions, petechiae

and purpuric spots, cutaneous ulcers, and edema. Rarely, gangrene of extremities occurs. Peripheral neuropathy with pain, numbness, paresthesias, and muscle weakness results from involvement of peripheral nerves adjacent to affected vessels. Abdominal pain, bleeding, ulcerations, and infarction can follow involvement of gastrointestinal vessels. Renal involvement is a potentially serious manifestation which may result in kidney failure and death. Involvement of large renal vessels results in flank pain and gross hematuria; that of small vessels and glomeruli causes microscopic hematuria, proteinuria, and cylindruria. Associated hypertension is usual. Inflammation of pulmonary vessels may cause cough, wheezing, pulmonary infiltrates, and pleuritis. Central nervous system manifestations include seizures, encephalitic symptoms, and stroke. Cranial nerve palsies and iridocyclitis may occur. Involvement of coronary vessels may produce tachycardia, congestive heart failure, and myocardial infarction; pericarditis may also be present. Orchitis and epididymitis are common. Iridocyclitis may occur.

There are no specific laboratory tests. The sedimentation rate may be elevated and acute phase reactants be present. Anemia is common; eosinophilia is sometimes found. There may be gross or microscopic hematuria, and renal function studies may be deranged.

Polyarteritis nodosa is readily confused with many other diseases. Differentiation from other rheumatic diseases may be particularly difficult. The diagnosis is based primarily on clinical suspicion and on histologic changes in involved tissues on biopsy. Muscle biopsies may fail to identify vasculitis. Testicular biopsies are said to be helpful but are seldom done. Arteriograms of liver or kidney may be diagnostically helpful. The diagnosis in children is probably most frequently made at autopsy.

The prognosis is poor; death can occur from renal failure, heart failure, or severe gastrointestinal or central nervous system disease. Corticosteroids may suppress acute manifestations of the disease and effectively lengthen survival. Various anticancer drugs have been employed sporadically with variable success.

9.67 INFANTILE POLYARTERITIS

Polyarteritis in infants under 1 yr of age, though rare, presents a characteristic clinical pattern. Both sexes are affected. The cause is not known, but, as in other forms of vasculitis, this disease has been reported in association with drug exposure (sulfonamides, penicillin). There is also a suggestive relation to immunization and to viral and bacterial illnesses. Pathologic changes are similar to those of polyarteritis in older patients; fibrinoid necrosis of vessels is said to be less prominent. On the basis of similar pathologic changes, a relationship between infantile polyarteritis and mucocutaneous lymph node syndrome has been proposed.

The disease usually begins with a combination of fever, rhinitis, conjunctivitis, and macular erythematous rash, suggesting an acute viral infection, but the illness persists. Involvement of the coronary arteries has been the predominant manifestation in most reported cases, resulting in tachycardia, cardiomegaly, congestive heart failure, or pericarditis. The electrocardiogram may show right, left, or combined ventricular hypertrophy, as well as evidence of myocardial ischemia or infarction. At autopsy, aneurysms of coronary arteries are frequently found as well as myocardial infarcts and pericarditis. Aneurysms may perforate causing hemopericardium.

Other manifestations include renal involvement (abnormal urinary sediment), hypertension, decreased blood pressure in or ischemia of an extremity, central nervous system manifestations (nuchal rigidity, pareses, cranial nerve palsies, seizures), hepatosplenomegaly, lymphadenopathy, gastrointestinal symptoms, and cough. Involvement of vessels in skeletal muscle is uncommon, and muscle biopsy is of little diagnostic usefulness. At autopsy widespread arteritis involving many organs has been found.

There are no specific laboratory tests. The white blood cell count is often elevated, with eosinophilia; sedimentation rates may be high. Diagnosis is usually made at autopsy, although awareness of this syndrome should permit presumptive clinical diagnosis.

The prognosis is very poor, all reported cases having terminated in death within an average of 1 mo after onset. Death is usually sudden or related to progressive cardiac decompensation.

No satisfactory treatment has been found, but corticosteroid therapy appears worthy of trial.

9.68 KAWASAKI DISEASE
(Mucocutaneous Lymph Node Syndrome)

This syndrome, previously well known in Japan, is now increasingly recognized in the United States, sometimes occurring in epidemic form. Japanese children seem predisposed to this syndrome, although it has been reported now in many racial groups. The disease is characterized by prolonged high fever, conjunctivitis, stomatitis, palmar and solar erythema with subsequent desquamation of the digits, lymphadenopathy, and erythema multiforme–like rashes. Myocarditis, pericarditis, arthralgia or arthritis, pyuria or proteinuria, aseptic meningitis, and mild hepatitis may also occur. One to 2% of affected children die because of coronary vasculitis which is inseparable pathologically from that of infantile polyarteritis nodosa. Studies in Japanese children with this disease suggest that as many as 40% of affected patients may actually have coronary vasculitis, with most recovering. The cause of this association is unknown.

The diagnosis of Kawasaki disease rests on clinical grounds with demonstration of a combination of the features noted above. The diagnosis of associated coronary artery vasculitis is difficult to make in the living patient; echocardiography or coronary arteriography may be diagnostic. Electrocardiograms and chest roentgenograms should be obtained but may be normal even in the face of advanced coronary vascular disease. There are no specific laboratory tests. Sedimentation rates are generally elevated; leukocytosis and mild anemia may be present. Tests for rheumatoid factors and antinuclear

antibodies are negative, and serum complement values are normal or elevated. Studies for environmental or infectious agents have been unrewarding. The differential diagnosis includes various infectious diseases, poststreptococcal disease, and the Stevens-Johnson syndrome. Corticosteroids are not thought to be helpful and may be contraindicated. Salicylate therapy may be useful in suppressing fever and discomfort. The natural course of the disease runs from 1 to several wk. Recovery is usually complete in individuals who do not succumb to coronary vasculitis, though some instances of residual heart disease or aneurysms of large vessels are known.

9.69 WEGENER GRANULOMATOSIS
(Lethal Midline Granuloma)

Wegener granulomatosis is a rare syndrome in which destructive granulomatous lesions of the upper respiratory tract and lungs are associated with a systemic necrotizing vasculitis, most prominent in lungs and kidneys. The upper respiratory and pulmonary granulomas may predominate in some cases, antedating recognition of systemic vasculitis by years. Limited forms of this syndrome, with only upper respiratory or pulmonary involvement, may occur. Males are predominantly affected (2:1). The cause is not known; as in other vasculitis syndromes, an association with drug sensitivity and allergy has been noted.

Respiratory symptoms are prominent. Persistent nasal stuffiness and/or discharge may be an early symptom, with crusted or pustular lesions in the nares. Lesions are progressively destructive and may result in perforation of the nasal septum, obliteration of nasal sinuses, and ulcerations of the palate, pharynx, larynx, and trachea. Pulmonary symptoms of cough or hemoptysis occur, and fever and prostration are common. Associated in most instances are other manifestations such as arthritis, neuropathy, rash, splenomegaly, and severe progressive glomerulitis often terminating in renal failure. In cases with clinically inapparent systemic involvement, diffuse vasculitis may yet be found on post mortem examination. Limited forms of the disease with only upper respiratory or pulmonary lesions have been reported.

There are no specific laboratory findings; eosinophilia may be present. Roentgenograms may reveal bone destruction in the nose and sinuses and pulmonary infiltrates suggestive of tuberculosis or neoplasm. Urinalyses usually show evidence of nephritis, and renal function studies may be abnormal.

Diagnosis is based on the clinical picture and confirmed by demonstration of granulomatous lesions of the respiratory tract and systemic vasculitis, particularly nephritis. Without therapy, the prognosis is poor. Patients with more limited forms of the disease may survive for long periods of time, but the destructive lesions of the upper respiratory tract may be extremely disfiguring.

Corticosteroids may suppress systemic vasculitis and prevent progression of destructive lesions in the upper respiratory tract. Therapy with drugs such as azathioprine and cyclophosphamide may arrest the disease in some patients.

9.70 TAKAYASU ARTERITIS
("Pulseless Disease")

This uncommon condition, an inflammatory process involving the aorta and its major branches, occurs primarily in young women. Some cases have been reported in late childhood, a few in infants. Most reported cases have been from Asia or Africa. The cause is unknown; associated congenital defects of great vessels have been recorded.

The underlying pathology is a segmental panarteritis of the aorta and its major branches. Smaller vessels are spared. Aneurysmal dilatation and rupture may occur. Involvement of the great vessels can cause weak or absent pulses in the upper extremities, hence, "pulseless disease." Blood pressure in the legs may exceed that in the arms, the opposite of coarctation of the aorta. Renal arterial involvement may cause renal ischemia, resulting in hypertension. Decreased brain blood flow can result in neurologic disturbances. Visual disturbances are common in older patients.

Various rheumatic complaints, including arthritis, myalgia, pleuritis, pericarditis, fever, and rashes, have been associated, sometimes antedating the symptomatic aortitis by years. There are no specific laboratory data. Sedimentation rates and gamma globulin levels may be elevated; LE preparations may be positive. Angiography may demonstrate changes in affected vessels.

The condition should be considered in any child with obscure hypertension, particularly when fever and an elevated sedimentation rate are associated. The prognosis is variable. Some adults have survived; most children have died. No specific therapy is known. Corticosteroids have been used. Endarterectomy or nephrectomy may be warranted.

9.71 DERMATOMYOSITIS

Dermatomyositis is a multisystem disease characterized principally by nonsuppurative inflammation of striated muscle. Affected children usually have characteristic associated cutaneous lesions.

Etiology and Epidemiology. The cause of dermatomyositis is unknown. Available evidence suggests that cellular immune mechanisms play a basic role in pathogenesis. Lymphocytes from patients with dermatomyositis release lymphotoxins and kill muscle cells in tissue culture. Immunoglobulin and complement deposition have also been described in vessels in affected muscle. In adults, but not children, there is a frequent (20% of cases) association with malignancies, chiefly carcinomas. Preliminary studies suggest an association of childhood dermatomyositis with HLA B8/DR3.

Dermatomyositis is less common than rheumatoid arthritis, SLE, or Schönlein-Henoch vasculitis. It rarely begins before the 2nd yr of life. Girls are affected more frequently than boys (3:2). There is no familial or racial predilection.

Pathology. Lesions in skin, subcutaneous tissues, and muscles are irregularly distributed; care must be taken to choose an involved site for biopsy. The most prominent lesion in children is a vasculitis involving arterioles, venules, and capillaries in connective tissues of skin, subcutaneous tissue, and muscle. In muscle there is patchy degeneration, atrophy, and regeneration of muscle fibers, interstitial edema, and proliferation of connective tissue. In affected skin there is thinning of the epidermis and edema and vasculitis in the dermis. In the gastrointestinal tract vasculitis may result in mucosal ulcerations and tissue infarction. Mild renal glomerular changes have been described.

Clinical Manifestations. Onset is usually insidious, with slowly developing muscle weakness, generally first apparent in proximal muscles of the extremities and trunk. The child may develop an awkward gait and slowly lose capacity for functions such as climbing stairs, riding a bicycle, and dressing. Affected muscles tend to be stiff and sore and sometimes brawny, indurated, and tender. Nonpitting edema and thickening of the skin and subcutaneous tissues may be present. Although myositis is generally most pronounced in proximal muscles, any muscles can be affected, with varying sites and degrees of atrophy. Severe involvement of palatorespiratory muscles may lead to respiratory difficulty, aspiration, and death. Arthralgia and arthritis sometimes occur.

The skin lesions are characteristic and often have a distinctive violaceous hue. The upper eyelids assume a pathognomonic violaceous discoloration (heliotrope eyelids) (Fig 9–22, [p. xxxi]). Periorbital and facial edema may be associated. A butterfly rash similar to that of SLE may be present. Lesions of palatal and nasal mucous membranes may occur in association with the malar rash. The skin over extensor surfaces of joints, particularly the knuckles, knees, and elbows, becomes erythematous, atrophic, and scaly (Fig 9–23 [p. xxxi]). These areas later develop pigmentary changes resulting in hyperpigmentation or vitiligo. A dusky erythema may cover the upper trunk and proximal extremities. Other nonspecific skin changes may also occur. The skin over involved extremities may appear tight and glossy; in longstanding disease there may be cutaneous atrophy with binding of skin to underlying structures. Calcium may be deposited in affected subcutaneous tissues, muscles, and fascia; these deposits sometimes break down and are extruded in semisolid or solid form.

Low-grade fever is often present, and other evidence of systemic involvement such as lymphadenopathy, hepatosplenomegaly, and gastrointestinal manifestations may occur.

In untreated cases mortality is about 40%. Most deaths are related to palatorespiratory involvement or such gastrointestinal complications as hemorrhage and perforation and occur within 2 yr of onset. Otherwise, the disease slowly becomes inactive over several yr and subsequent exacerbations are unusual. Infrequently, the disease may smolder for years. Most surviving patients are able to lead active lives, although they may have residual abnormalities. A few have severe contractures and crippling deformities. The course of dermatomyositis can be favorably modified by early, vigorous treatment with corticosteroids, and the prognosis in adequately treated children is good.

Laboratory Manifestations. Muscle inflammation is responsible for elevated serum levels of such enzymes as transaminases, creatine kinase, and aldolase. The electromyogram of affected muscles is abnormal. The sedimentation rate may be elevated or normal. Tests for rheumatoid factors and antinuclear antibodies are generally negative or show them to be present in low titer. Urinalyses are usually normal. In patients with gastrointestinal involvement there may be gross or occult blood in the stool. Roentgenograms may reveal calcium deposits in soft tissues.

Diagnosis and Differential Diagnosis. In its typical form dermatomyositis should present little diagnostic difficulty. The combination of muscle weakness and characteristic rash, elevated serum levels of enzymes, and abnormal electromyogram is diagnostic; muscle biopsy is not usually necessary. In the differential diagnosis various neuromuscular disorders such as poliomyelitis, Guillain-Barré syndrome, muscular dystrophy, and myasthenia gravis should be considered, as should illnesses having predominantly muscular lesions, such as trichinosis. Transient myositis has been reported in association with influenza and may occur with other viral infections as well. SLE, mixed connective tissue disease, juvenile rheumatoid arthritis, and scleroderma are distinguishable clinically and by laboratory tests. In the chronic phase, features of dermatomyositis and generalized scleroderma may overlap and thus make precise categorization difficult. When the onset is insidious, a period of observation may be needed to establish the diagnosis.

Treatment. During the acute phase, evaluation of palatorespiratory function may be lifesaving. If swallowing mechanisms are impaired, soft or liquid diets should be provided under close observation. The patient should be closely watched for possible deterioration in respiratory function. Constant nursing care is mandatory for any child with palatorespiratory involvement, and equipment for nasopharyngeal suction, endotracheal intubation, and tracheostomy should be available. A respirator may be required. The possibility of serious gastrointestinal manifestations during the acute phase of disease must also be considered.

Functional recovery depends on preservation of adequate muscle strength and prevention of crippling contractures. Corticosteroids effectively suppress the inflammatory process in most patients. Serial serum levels of transaminase, creatine kinase, or aldolase provide a helpful gauge of activity and therapeutic response. Prednisone in initial dosage of 1–2 mg/kg/24 hr (or 60 mg/M² of body surface area/24 hr) usually reduces enzyme levels toward normal values within 1–2 wk; clinical improvement with decreased pain and swelling in muscles and increasing muscle strength usually follows. When enzyme levels have declined to normal, the steroid dosage should be slowly decreased, with continued monitoring of the clinical course and serum enzyme levels. If the dose of steroids is reduced too rapidly, rebound in enzyme levels may occur; such

rebounds are followed by deterioration in the clinical condition within a few wk unless corticosteroid dosage is promptly increased. A low dose of steroids sufficient to suppress clinical symptoms and serum enzyme levels should be found and maintained for months. Steroid therapy can generally be discontinued in 1–2 yr. Steroid preparations such as triamcinolone and dexamethasone, which are associated with "steroid myopathy," should be avoided. Salicylates may occasionally be helpful as adjunctive drugs in relieving symptoms. Agents such as methotrexate and cyclophosphamide are rarely warranted in childhood dermatomyositis.

Physical therapy is essential to avoid contractures and to rebuild muscle strength. During the acute phase when muscle weakness is pronounced, passive exercises can be used to maintain range of motion. With clinical improvement active exercises to strengthen muscles should be added. Appropriate splints to maintain good position of the limbs may be needed. Bed rest is not necessary, and immobilization without exercise is to be avoided at all times. Skin hygiene, especially around the neck, skin creases, and axillae, is important.

9.72 SCLERODERMA

Scleroderma ("hard skin") is a chronic inflammatory disturbance of connective tissue which classically involves skin but may also affect the gastrointestinal tract, heart, lung, kidney, and synovium. Cutaneous involvement, the hallmark of the disease, may occur in focal patches (*morphea*), in a linear distribution (linear scleroderma), or in a generalized, symmetric distribution. The last is usually associated with systemic involvement (*progressive systemic sclerosis*) and is the usual form seen in adults. Scleroderma in children usually has a patchy, focal distribution (morphea); systemic involvement is uncommon.

The disease is rare and of obscure origin. It affects girls more frequently than boys and may begin at any time during childhood. There is no familial predisposition.

Histology of affected cutaneous tissues shows increased thickness and density of dermal collagen with perivascular infiltrates of mononuclear cells.

Clinical Manifestations. *Morphea and Linear Scleroderma.* The 1st signs are patchy lesions of skin and subcutaneous tissues. These often have a linear pattern similar to the distribution of peripheral nerves and may occur primarily on 1 side of the body. During the early phases involved areas are slightly erythematous and edematous or have an atrophic, shiny appearance. The child may complain of pain or a prickly sensation. As the disease progresses, the skin lesions become indurated with violaceous, sometimes elevated borders and pale, waxy-appearing centers. Lesions enlarge peripherally and may coalesce to involve an entire extremity or a large portion of the body. Extensive scarring and fibrosis of the involved area can occur with firm binding of cutaneous tissues to underlying structures ("hidebinding"). This may be severe enough to limit growth

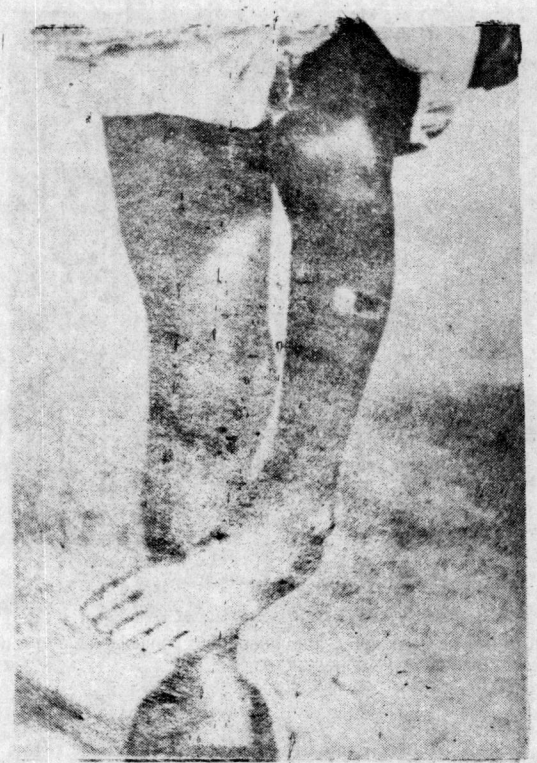

Figure 9–24 Extensive morphea involving the entire left leg, causing scarring, shortening, and flexion contractures. Note the shiny appearance and patches of hyperpigmentation and vitiligo of affected skin.

of the affected part and produce crippling contractures (Fig 9–24). Chronically involved areas may be hyperpigmented or depigmented. Active disease may arrest over a period of months to years or may smolder for years. Prognosis for life is good in the absence of systemic involvement.

Progressive Systemic Sclerosis. Cutaneous involvement is symmetrical. It includes hands, feet, and distal extremities and sometimes the trunk and face as well. Induration, pigmentary changes, and hide-binding of involved cutaneous tissues occur as with focal forms of the disease. Raynaud phenomenon may be associated and cutaneous ulcers occur. Synovitis, particularly about small hand joints, may mimic rheumatoid arthritis; tenosynovitis and nodules about tendon sheaths may be associated. The disease may involve the gastrointestinal tract, heart, lungs, and kidneys. Systemic manifestations, particularly renal, cardiac, and pulmonary, may be fatal. Esophageal dysfunction may result in chronic aspiration pneumonia. Severe hypertension may occur.

Laboratory Manifestations. There are no specific laboratory tests. The sedimentation rate is frequently normal. Rheumatoid factors and antinuclear antibodies may be found in both focal and disseminated forms of the disease. Roentgenograms may show dysfunction of esophageal and small bowel motility. Pulmonary function studies, electrocardiograms, and chest roentgeno-

grams may disclose cardiopulmonary involvement. Urinalyses and renal function studies are abnormal in the presence of renal involvement.

Diagnosis. The clinical picture is characteristic in both morphea and progressive systemic sclerosis. The disease may bear some superficial resemblance to *dermatomyositis*, but absence of myositis and the characteristic rash of dermatomyositis should allow differentiation. *Subcutaneous fat necrosis* and *Weber-Christian nonsuppurative panniculitis* may be suggested in morphea, but the course and histology are distinctive. *Scleredema adultorum*, a self-limited benign induration of subcutaneous tissues, occurs acutely, sometimes following streptococcal infection; subcutaneous tissues of the neck, upper trunk, and arms become indurated, but skin is spared.

Treatment. No specific therapy is known. Many therapeutic agents, including corticosteroids, salicylates, chelating agents, chloroquine, radiation, dimethyl sulfoxide, para-aminobenzoic acid, penicillamine, and anticancer drugs have been tried without clear-cut benefit. Surgical excision of local patches of morphea does not arrest the process. Systemic therapy with corticosteroids, penicillamine, or anticancer drugs may be tried for severe systemic disease. Topical corticosteroids have been used for morphea. Vigorous physical therapy is important early in the course of morphea to prevent or minimize crippling contractures.

MISCELLANEOUS DISORDERS

9.73 MIXED CONNECTIVE TISSUE DISEASE

Mixed connective tissue disease is a recently defined rheumatic disease syndrome combining features of SLE, rheumatoid arthritis, dermatomyositis, and scleroderma. It is characterized by the invariable presence of high serum titers of antibody to ribonucleoprotein (so-called "ENA") and high titers of speckled antinuclear antibody. Clinical features include polyarthritis, sclerodermal skin changes, Raynaud phenomenon, fever, cardiac involvement (particularly pericarditis), rashes suggestive of either SLE or dermatomyositis, myositis, esophageal abnormalities, lymphadenopathy and organomegaly, pulmonary disease, and thrombocytopenia. Renal disease occurs in some patients, and neurologic abnormalities and parotitis have also been described. Diagnosis of mixed connective tissue disease is made on clinical grounds by recognition of the overlapping clinical symptoms and requires the demonstration of serum antibodies to ribonucleoprotein and high titers of speckled antinuclear antibodies.

When this syndrome was first described, it was thought to have a better prognosis than SLE and to be readily amenable to corticosteroid therapy. Although corticosteroid therapy does produce symptomatic improvement in many patients, and although life-threatening disease manifestations are perhaps not so common as in SLE, mixed connective tissue disease is at times more severe than had been originally suggested. The ultimate prognosis is unknown. Also remaining in doubt are relationships of this syndrome to other rheumatic diseases. Appropriate therapy consists of symptomatic treatment with corticosteroids, alertness to possible serious complications such as nephritis, and physical therapy and careful attention to function of the musculoskeletal system.

9.74 ERYTHEMA MULTIFORME EXUDATIVUM
(Stevens-Johnson Syndrome)

Erythema multiforme exudativum (bullosum), characterized by lesions of skin and mucous membranes with fever and systemic prostration, was described by Hebra and Bazin over 100 yr ago.

The disease occurs in children and young adults and affects males more frequently than females. Onset often follows an upper respiratory tract infection. Evidence for a viral etiology agent, especially herpes virus, has been inconclusive. The association of Stevens-Johnson syndrome with patchy pneumonia, increased titers of cold agglutinins, and the isolation of *Mycoplasma pneumoniae* has suggested a relation to mycoplasma infection. Association of the syndrome with ingestion of drugs, including sulfonamides, anticonvulsants, penicillin, and barbiturates, has also been observed. The LE phenomenon has been demonstrated in a few patients.

The hallmark of the syndrome is an erythematous papular skin lesion that enlarges by peripheral expansion and usually develops a central vesicle. This eruption may involve most cutaneous surfaces, including the palms and soles, but spares the scalp. Lesions may be scattered or confluent. New lesions appear for 1–2 wk after onset. Vesiculobullous lesions also occur on mucous membranes of the conjunctivae, nares, mouth, anorectal junction, vulvovaginal region, and urethral meatus. Lesions have been described in the larynx, trachea, bronchi, bladder, and gastrointestinal tract.

The rash is often preceded by fever and general malaise. Severe prostration may occur at the height of the syndrome. About one third of the affected patients have pulmonary involvement, with a harsh, hacking cough and patchy changes on the chest roentgenogram. Periarticular swelling has been described. Involvement of cardiovascular and renal systems does not usually occur. As the disease process reaches its peak, the patient presents a striking picture (Fig 9–25). Stomatitis is particularly distressing; lesions erode, ulcerate, bleed, and crust. Meatal involvement may make urination painful. Conjunctivitis results in photophobia, and purulent conjunctival discharge may be profuse. Corneal ulcerations can occur with resulting scarring and even blindness.

The mortality may be as high as 10% during the acute phase, particularly in patients with pulmonary involvement. Subsequently, the disease is self-limiting: skin lesions gradually subside without scarring in 1–4 wk; mucous membrane lesions may persist for months. In

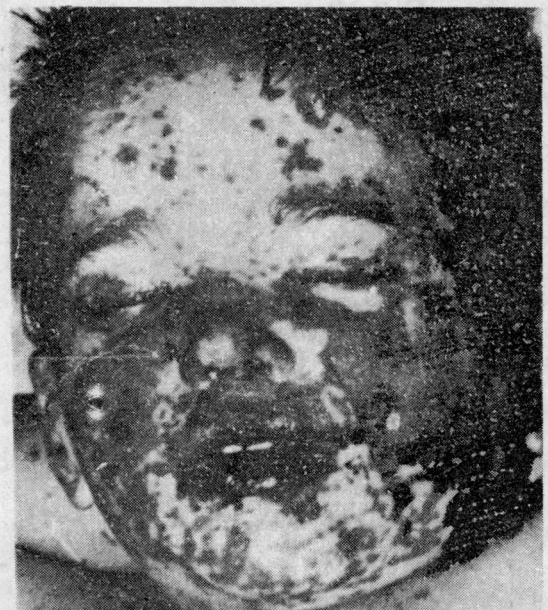

Figure 9–25 Cutaneous, oral, nasal, and conjunctival involvement in severe Stevens-Johnson syndrome.

about 20% of patients the disease recurs, often in association with re-exposure to an offending drug.

During the acute phase symptomatic treatment is of great importance. Fluid requirements are high, and intravenous administration is often required. Cutaneous hygiene should be maintained to prevent secondary infection. Ophthalmologic consultation should be sought if serious conjunctivitis is present. Prednisone, 1–2 mg/kg/24 hr, is often used in children with serious disease. The efficacy of such therapy is not proved; it should be carefully supervised and is contraindicated whenever there is a possibility of herpetic infection of the eye. Appropriate antibiotic therapy is indicated if there is reasonable suspicion of infection with *Mycoplasma pneumoniae*.

9.75 ERYTHEMA NODOSUM

Erythema nodosum is characterized by the development of painful, indurated, shiny, red, hot, elevated, ovoid nodules 1–3 cm in diameter. They are most frequently distributed symmetrically over the shins (Fig 9–26 [p. xxxi]) but may also occur on the calves, thighs, buttocks, and upper extremities. Fever, malaise, and arthralgia may precede or accompany the rash, and hilar adenopathy may be present on chest roentgenograms. The skin lesions have a characteristic progression: over a period of several days they become protuberant and present a brilliant display of violaceous colors; after 1–2 wk, as induration decreases, a dull purple discoloration predominates and then fades in the manner of a large bruise, leaving a brown residuum. The lesions come in crops, usually over a period of 3–

6 wk. The disease then becomes quiescent and rarely recurs. Erythema nodosum is uncommon in children under the age of 6 yr, becoming progressively more frequent up to the 3rd decade of life. Females are affected more frequently than males.

These skin lesions represent a reaction to a variety of stimuli. The eruption has been induced experimentally in patients with the disease by local injection of a single specific bacterial antigen. Epidemiologically, the disease was previously linked closely to tuberculosis, especially in Europe. In both the United States and Europe streptococcal infections are now more frequently implicated as stimuli. The eruption may also appear as a concomitant of sarcoidosis, histoplasmosis, coccidioidomycosis, and Yersinia infections or in association with the administration of some drugs, including birth control pills. It may also occur with diseases such as SLE, vasculitis, regional enteritis, and ulcerative colitis.

Search for a precipitating infection, drug, or underlying disease should be instituted. The sedimentation rate is usually elevated, and other nonspecific evidences of inflammatory disease, such as acute phase reactants, are found. Suggestive etiologic evidence may include the demonstration of beta-hemolytic streptococci in throat cultures or a rising antistreptolysin O titer; conversion of a previously negative tuberculin, histoplasmin, or coccidioidin skin reaction; roentgenographic evidence of pulmonary tuberculosis or fungus disease; or evidence of an underlying disease such as SLE, inflammatory bowel disease, or sarcoidosis.

Salicylates are usually adequate for symptomatic relief of erythema nodosum. The skin lesions and their constitutional manifestations may respond to corticosteroids, but such therapy is usually not warranted in a self-limited disease and may be contraindicated because of the presence of underlying active infection.

9.76 GOODPASTURE SYNDROME

The combination of pulmonary alveolar hemorrhage and glomerulonephritis, called Goodpasture syndrome, appears to be a distinctive clinical entity, although there is some overlap with polyarteritis nodosa and with idiopathic pulmonary hemosiderosis. Young adult males are predominantly affected, but the disease also occurs in children. The cause is unknown. The disease often begins after an acute illness and has been associated with influenza. It has also occurred after exposure to certain drugs, including penicillamine. Antibodies reactive with glomerular and alveolar basement membranes are involved in pathogenesis.

The syndrome is characterized clinically by hemoptysis, anemia, and nephritis. Dyspnea, cough, malaise, and fever are often present; and rales and rhonchi may be heard on auscultation of the chest. Chest roentgenograms characteristically show bilateral flocculent infiltrates spreading from hilus to periphery of the lung fields. Hemosiderin-laden macrophages can be demonstrated in the sputum. Anemia, presumably related to pulmonary hemorrhage, is prominent. Urinalyses reveal varying degrees of proteinuria, hematuria, pyu-

ria, and cylindruria. Azotemia is frequent; progressive renal failure often ensues. Histologically, focal glomerulitis or widespread glomerulonephritis may be demonstrated. Intra-alveolar hemorrhages, hemosiderinladen macrophages, and thickening of alveolar septa are present in the lungs. Generalized vasculitis is not found; patients with concomitant vasculitis are usually considered to have polyarteritis nodosa.

The disease is usually rapidly fatal. Corticosteroid therapy has been considered helpful in a few cases; alkylating agents and antimetabolites have been used on an experimental basis.

9.77 RELAPSING NODULAR NONSUPPURATIVE PANNICULITIS
(Weber-Christian Syndrome)

Recurrent nodular nonsuppurative panniculitis is a rare disorder of unknown cause; infection, drug reaction (especially to bromides and iodides), abnormal fat metabolism, and hypersensitivity have all been suggested. It is probable that panniculitis does not represent a single disease. It occurs in association with several rheumatic tissue diseases and with corticosteroid withdrawal. Adults are predominantly affected, although the syndrome has been reported in all age groups. Females are affected more frequently than males.

Histologically, there are foci of degeneration and inflammation in subcutaneous fat. Mesenteric, perivisceral, and periarticular adipose tissues may be affected; fatty metamorphosis of the liver and reticuloendothelial hyperplasia have been recorded. Laboratory findings are not specific. Leukopenia and elevated sedimentation rates may be present; rheumatoid factor, LE cells, and cryoglobulins have been observed.

Clinically, the disease is characterized by the appearance of crops of subcutaneous nodules on any part of the body; thighs, abdomen, breasts, and arms are most frequently involved. Nodules vary in size from mm to several cm and may be painful, with redness and warmth of the overlying skin. Nodules regress in days to weeks, usually leaving a pigmented depression. Fever is common, and a variety of rheumatic complaints may occur, including arthritis, arthralgia, and myalgia. Hepatosplenomegaly, abdominal pain, and episcleritis have been reported. Crops of nodules and systemic symptoms generally recur over long periods of time.

Diagnosis of Weber-Christian syndrome is made by the clinical picture and histologic changes. Differential diagnosis includes erythema induratum, sarcoidosis, and postinjection subcutaneous fat necrosis. Fat necrosis with subcutaneous nodules, arthritis, and visceral involvement can occur as a manifestation of pancreatic disease, presumably from enzymatic action on fat cells.

No specific therapy is known. Symptomatic relief may occur after therapy with corticosteroids, chloroquine, and phenylbutazone. Patients with underlying pancreatic involvement are benefited by therapy of the pancreatic disease.

9.78 "RHEUMATOID" NODULES WITHOUT RHEUMATIC DISEASE
(Benign Rheumatoid Nodules)

Rheumatoid nodule–like lesions unassociated with rheumatic disease occur occasionally in children. Single or multiple lesions may be present. Nodules occur over various sites, including the pretibial areas, dorsa of the feet, scalp, hands, and elbows, and may appear over pressure points or after trauma, as do true rheumatoid nodules. Clinically, the nodules are subcutaneous or fixed to deeper tissues and resemble rheumatoid nodules. Histologically, these lesions show central areas of fibrinoid necrosis with surrounding histiocytes and mononuclear cells; they may resemble adult-type rheumatoid nodules or the intracutaneous lesions of granuloma annulare and may occur in association with typical granuloma annulare.

The etiology of these nodules is unknown. Affected children are well; there are no associated rheumatic complaints. Laboratory tests are normal; tests for rheumatoid factor and antinuclear antibodies are negative. The nodular lesions wax, wane, and may recur, but recurrences generally cease after months or years. This is a benign condition; affected children are not at risk for rheumatic disease, and no therapy other than reassurance is required.

Nodules which occur in association with rheumatic disease (rheumatoid arthritis, acute rheumatic fever, scleroderma, SLE) rarely if ever occur as sole manifestations but rather appear in association with other signs of active rheumatic disease. Rheumatoid nodules in rheumatoid arthritis are generally associated with positive tests for rheumatoid factor.

9.79 FASCIITIS
(Diffuse Fasciitis, Eosinophilic Fasciitis)

Fasciitis is an unusual disorder characterized by diffuse inflammation of fascial tissues. It was first described in 1975, and there are as yet no long-term studies to define the extent and natural history of the disease. It may be a variant of scleroderma. Reported patients have been mostly adults, but the disorder has been noted in children. Inflammation of fascial tissues occurs in the limbs and trunk; hands, feet, and face are generally spared. The onset usually follows periods of heavy physical exertion. Affected tissues are swollen and tender; however, since the overlying skin is not affected, these areas appear puckered. Loss of musculoskeletal function and contractures may result. Involvement of internal organs and Raynaud phenomenon have not been associated. There are no diagnostic laboratory tests; tests for rheumatoid factors and antinuclear antibodies are generally negative. Some patients have striking eosinophilia (as high as 50%), and increased numbers of eosinophils may be found in affected tissues. Diagnosis is clinical and supported by biopsy evidence of fascial inflammation. Therapy with corticosteroids may be helpful, although long-term follow-up studies are not available.

9.80. LYME DISEASE
(Lyme Arthritis)

This condition may be caused by the tick-transmitted agent *Treponema borrelia* along the coast of southern New England and eastern Long Island and in Wisconsin, and by *Ixodes pacificus* in California and Oregon. These vectors are also associated with erythema chronicum migrans in Scandinavia and northern Europe.

Lyme disease usually begins with skin lesions with or without systemic complaints; joint, cardiac, and neurologic abnormalities follow weeks to months later. Onset of arthritis is often sudden and may be either persistent or migratory. The distinctive skin lesion, erythema chronicum migrans, begins as an erythematous papule which expands, often with central clearing, to reach diameters as large as 50 cm; these lesions are generally nonpainful. Large joints are usually then affected, especially the knees. Attacks of arthritis may last for weeks or months; recurrent attacks are common, and a few patients have chronic arthritis. Neither morning stiffness nor iridocyclitis is associated. Tests for antinuclear antibodies and rheumatoid factors are negative. Extra-articular manifestations include fever, malaise, fatigue, headache, aseptic meningitis, cranial nerve palsies, and myocardial conduction defects.

Erythema chronicum migrans and arthritis may respond to a 7–10 day course of penicillin (250,000 U orally 4 times a day) or tetracycline (250 mg orally 4 times a day), begun as soon as the diagnosis is made.

JANE GREEN SCHALLER
RALPH J. WEDGWOOD

Patient Education

Arthritis in children. Arthritis Foundation, 3400 Peachtree Road NE, Atlanta, Ga. 30326 (obtainable from the Arthritis Foundation or from its local chapter offices).

General

McCarty DJ Jr, Hollander JL: Arthritis and Allied Conditions. Ed 9. Philadelphia, Lea & Febiger, 1978.
Mikkelsen WM, et al: Twenty-fourth Rheumatism Review. Arth Rheum 24(2), 1981.
Proceedings of the First American Rheumatism Association Conference of the Rheumatic Diseases of Childhood. Chaired by Schaller JG, Hanson V. Arthritis Rheum (Suppl 2) 20:145, 1977.
Rodnan GP (ed): Primer on the rheumatic diseases. Ed 8. JAMA 224:552, 1973. (Also available in bound form from the Arthritis Foundation.) Ed 9 in press, 1981.)
Schaller JG, Hansen JA: Histocompatibility and human disease. Hospital Pract 16:41, 1981.

Juvenile Rheumatoid Arthritis

Ansell BM, Bywaters EGL: Prognosis in Still's disease. Bull Rheum Dis 9:189, 1959.
Ansell BM, Bywaters EGL: Diagnosis of "probable" Still's disease and its outcome. Ann Rheum Dis 21:253, 1967.
Bianco NE, Panush RS, Stillman JS, et al: Immunologic studies of juvenile rheumatoid arthritis. Arthritis Rheum 14:685, 1971.
Bywaters EGL: Heberden Oration, 1966. Categorization in medicine: A survey of Still's disease. Ann Rheum Dis 26:185, 1967.
Calabro JJ, Katz RM, Maltz BA: A critical appraisal of juvenile rheumatoid arthritis. Clin Orthop 74.101, 1971.

Calabro JJ, Marchesano JM: The early natural history of juvenile rheumatoid arthritis. Med Clin North Am 52:567, 1968.

Hanson V, Drexler E, Kornreich H: The relationship of rheumatoid factor to age of onset in juvenile rheumatoid arthritis. Arthritis Rheum 12:82, 1969.

Isdale IC, Bywaters EGL: The rash of rheumatoid arthritis and Still's disease. Quart J Med 25:377, 1956.

Laaksonen AL: A prognostic study of juvenile rheumatoid arthritis. Analysis of 544 cases. Acta Paediatr Scand (Suppl) 166:1, 1966.

McMinn FJ, Bywaters EGL: Differences betwe--, the fever of Still's disease and that of rheumatic fever. Ann Rheum Dis 18:293, 1959.

Schaller JG: The diversity of JRA: A 1976 look at the subgroups of chronic arthritis. Arthritis Rheum 20:S52, 1977.

Schaller JG, Johnson GD, Holborow EJ, et al: The association of antinuclear antibodies with the chronic iridocyclitis of juvenile arthritis (Still's disease). Arthritis Rheum 17:409, 1974.

Schaller J, Kupfer C, Wedgwood RJ: Iridocyclitis in juvenile rheumatoid arthritis. Pediatrics 44:92, 1969.

Schaller, JG, Ochs HD, Thomas ED, et al: Histocompatibility antigens in childhood-onset arthritis. J Pediatr 88:926, 1976.

Schaller J, Wedgwood RJ: Is juvenile rheumatoid arthritis a single disease? A review. Pediatrics 50:940, 1972.

Still GF: On a form of chronic joint disease in children. Med Chir 80:47, 1937. (Reprinted in Arch Dis Child 16:156, 1941.)

Ankylosing Spondylitis

Brewerton DA, Caffrey M, Hart FD, et al: Ankylosing spondylitis and HL-A 27. Lancet 1:904, 1973.

Ladd JR, Cassidy JT, Martel W: Juvenile ankylosing spondylitis. Arthritis Rheum 14:579, 1971.

Schaller J, Bitnun S, Wedgwood RJ: Ankylosing spondylitis with childhood onset. J Pediatr 74:505, 1969.

Schlosstein L, Terasaki PI, Bluestone R, et al: High association of an HL-A antigen, W27, with ankylosing spondylitis. N Engl J Med 288:704, 1973.

Wilkinson M, Bywaters EGL: Clinical features and course of ankylosing spondylitis; as seen in a follow-up of 222 hospital referred cases. Ann Rheum Dis 17:209, 1958.

Reiter Disease

Arnett FC, McClusky EO, Schacter BZ, et al: Incomplete Reiter's syndrome: Discriminating features and HL-A W27 in diagnosis. Ann Intern Med 84:8, 1976.

Russell AS: Reiter's syndrome in children following infection with Yersinia enterocolitica and Shigella. Arthritis Rheum (Suppl) 20:471, 1977.

Singsen BH, Bernstein BH, Koster-King KG, et al: Reiter's syndrome in childhood. Arthritis Rheum (Suppl) 20:402, 1977.

Arthritis of Inflammatory Bowel Disease

Lindsley CB, Schaller JB: Arthritis associated with inflammatory bowel disease in children. J Pediatr 84:16, 1974.

Reactive Arthritis

Aho K, Ahvonen P, Lassus A, et al: HL-A 27 in reactive arthritis. A study of Yersinia arthritis and Reiter's disease. Arthritis Rheum 17:521, 1974.

Psoriatic Arthritis

Lambert JR, Ansell BM, Stephenson E, et al: Psoriatic arthritis in childhood. Clin Rheum Dis 2:339, 1976.

Systemic Lupus Erythematosus

Baldwin DS, Lowenstein J, Rothfield NF, et al: The clinical course of proliferative and membranous forms of lupus nephritis. Ann Intern Med 73:929, 1970.

Cook CD, Wedgwood RJ, Craig JM, et al: Systemic lupus erythematosus. Description of 37 cases in children and a discussion of endocrine therapy in 32 of the cases. Pediatrics 26:570, 1960.

DuBois EL: Systemic Lupus Erythematosus. Ed 2. Los Angeles, University of Southern California Press, 1974.

Estes D, Christian CL: The natural history of systemic lupus erythematosus by prospective analysis. Medicine 50:85, 1971.

Fish AJ, Blau EB, Westberg NG, et al: Systemic lupus erythematosus within the fist two decades of life. Am J Med 62:99, 1977.

Hayslett JP, Kashgarian M, Cook CD, et al: The effect of azathioprine on lupus nephritis. Medicine 51:393, 1972.

Jacobs JC: Systemic lupus erythematosus in childhood: Report of 35 cases, with discussion of seven apparently induced by anticonvulsant medication, and of prognosis and treatment. Pediatrics 32:257, 1963.

King KK, Kornreich HK, Bernstein BH, et al: The clinical spectrum of systemic lupus erythematosus in childhood. Arthritis Rheum (Suppl) 20:287, 1977.

Koffler D, Agnello V, Thoburn R, et al: Systemic lupus erythematosus: Prototype of immune complex nephritis in man. J Exp Med 134:169s, 1971.

Kukla LG, Reddy C, Silkalns G, et al: Systemic lupus erythematosus presenting as chorea. Arch Dis Child 53:345, 1978.

Lehman TJA, Hanson V, Singsen BH, et al: Serum complement abnormalities in ANA positive relatives of children with SLE. Arthritis Rheum 22:954, 1979.

Meislin AG, Rothfield N: Systemic lupus erythematosus in childhood. Pediatrics 42:37, 1968.

Peterson RD, Vernier RL, Good RA: Lupus erythematosus. Pediatr Clin North Am 10:941, 1963.

Pollak VE, Pirani CL, Schwartz FD: The natural history of the renal manifestations of systemic lupus erythematosus. J Lab Clin Med 63:537, 1964.

Ropes MW: Observations on the natural course of disseminated lupus erythematosus. Medicine 43:387, 1964.

Schur PH, Sandson J: Immunologic factors and clinical activity in systemic lupus erythematosus. N Engl J Med 278:533, 1968.

Singsen BH, Bernstein BH, King KK, et al: Correlations between changes in disease activity and the serum complement levels. J Pediatr 89:358, 1976.

Singsen BH, Fishman L, Hanson V: Antinuclear antibodies and lupus-like syndromes in children receiving anticonvulsants. Pediatrics 57:529, 1976.

Wallace C, Schaller JG, Emery H, et al: Prospective study of childhood systemic lupus erythematosus. Arthritis Rheum 21:599, 1978.

Wallace C, Striker G, Schaller JG, et al: Renal histology and subsequent course in childhood systemic lupus erythematosus. Arthritis Rheum 22:669, 1979.

Walravens PA, Chase HP: The prognosis of childhood systemic lupus erythematosus. Am J Dis Child 130:929, 1976.

Lupus Phenomena in the Newborn Period

Beck JS, Rowell NR: Transplacental passage of antinuclear antibody. Lancet 1:134, 1963.

Chameides L, Truex RC, Vetter V, et al: Association of maternal systemic lupus erythematosus with congenital complete heart block. N Engl J Med 297:1204, 1977.

Esscher E, Scott JS: Congenital heart block and maternal systemic lupus erythematosus. Br Med J 1:1235, 1979.

Jackson R: Discoid lupus in a newborn infant of a mother with lupus erythematosus. Pediatrics 33:425, 1964.

McCue CM, Mantakas ME, Tingelstad JB, et al: Congenital heart block in newborns of mothers with connective tissue disease. Circulation 56:82, 1977.

Schönlein-Henoch Vasculitis

Ackroyd JF: Allergic purpura, including purpura due to foods, drugs and infections. Am J Med 14:605, 1953.

Allen DM, Diamond LK, Howell DA: Anaphylactoid purpura in children (Schönlein-Henoch syndrome): Review with a follow-up of the renal complications. Am J Dis Child 99:833, 1960.

Ayoub EM, Hoyer J: Anaphylactoid purpura: Streptococcal antibody titers and B 1C globulin levels. J Pediatr 75:193, 1970.

Bywaters EGL, Isdale I, Kempton JJ: Schönlein-Henoch purpura: Evidence for a group A β-haemolytic streptococcal aetiology. Quart J Med 26:161, 1957.

Emery H, Schaller JG, Larter W: Henoch-Schönlein vasculitis: Long-term follow-up study. Proceedings of the First Conference on Childhood Rheumatic Diseases. Arthritis Rheum 20:385, 1977.

Hurley RM, Drummond KN: Anaphylactoid purpura nephritis: Clinicopathological correlations. J Pediatr 81:904, 1972.

Osler W: The visceral lesions of purpura and allied conditions. Br Med J 1:517, 1914.

Vernier RL, Worthen HG, Peterson RD, et al: Anaphylactoid purpura. Pathology of the skin and kidney and frequency of streptococcal infection. Pediatrics 27:181, 1961.

Wedgwood RJ, Klaus MH: Anaphylactoid purpura (Schönlein-Henoch syndrome): Long-term follow-up study with special reference to renal involvement. Pediatrics 16:196, 1955.

Polyarteritis Nodosa

Fager DB, Bigler JA, Simonds JP: Polyarteritis nodosa in infancy and childhood. J Pediatr 39:65, 1951.

Frohnert PP, Sheps SG: Long-term follow-up study of periarteritis nodosa. Am J Med 43:8, 1967.

Gocke DJ, Hsu K, Morgan C, et al: Vasculitis in association with Australia antigen. J Exp Med 134:330s, 1971.

Owano LR, Sueper RH: Polyarteritis nodosa—a syndrome. Am J Clin Pathol 40:527, 1963.

Rose GA, Spencer H: Polyarteritis nodosa. Quart J Med 26:43, 1957.

Infantile Polyarteritis Nodosa

Munro-Faure H: Necrotizing arteritis of the coronary vessels in infancy. Case report and review of the literature. Pediatrics 23:914, 1959.

Roberts FB, Fetterman GH: Polyarteritis nodosa in infancy. J Pediatr 63:519, 1963.

Kawasaki Disease

Kato H, Koike S, Yamamoto M, et al: Coronary aneurysms in infants and young children with acute febrile mucocutaneous lymph node syndrome. J Pediatr 86:892, 1975.

Kawasaki T, Kosaki F, Okawa S, et al: A new infantile acute febrile mucocutaneous lymph node syndrome (MLNS) prevailing in Japan. Pediatrics 54:271, 1974.

Landing CH, Larson EJ: Are infantile periarteritis nodosa with coronary artery involvement and fatal mucocutaneous lymph node syndrome the same? Comparison of 20 patients from North America with patients from Hawaii and Japan. Pediatrics 59:651, 1977.

Melish ME: Kawasaki syndrome: A new infectious disease? J Infect Dis 143 (3):317, 1981.

Melish ME, Hicks RM, Larson EJ: Mucocutaneous lymph node syndrome in the United States. Am J Dis Child 130:599, 1976.

Wegener Granulomatosis

Blatt IM, Seltzer HS, Rubin P: Fatal granulomatosis of the respiratory tract (lethal midline granuloma—Wegener granulomatosis). Arch Otolaryngol 79:707, 1959.

Carrington CB, Liebow AA: Limited forms of angiitis and granulomatosis of Wegener's type. Am J Med 41:497, 1966.

Fauci AS, Wolff SM: Wegener's granulomatosis: Studies in 18 patients and a review of the literature. Medicine 52:535, 1973.

Novack SN, Pearson CM: Cyclophosphamide therapy in Wegener's granulomatosis. N Engl J Med 284:938, 1971.

Orlowski JP, Clough JD, Dyment PG: Wegener's granulomatosis in the pediatric age group. Pediatrics 61:83, 1978.

Takayasu Arteritis

Danaraj TJ, Wong HO, Thomas MA: Primary arteritis of the aorta causing renal artery stenosis and hypertension. Br Heart J 25:153, 1963.

Lee T, Sohn S, Hong C, et al: Primary arteritis (pulseless disease) in Korean children. Acta Pediatr Scand 56:526, 1967.

Nakao K, Ikeda M, Kimata Si, et al: Takayasu's arteritis. Clinical report of 84 cases and immunological studies of 7 cases. Circulation 35:1141, 1967.

Strachan RW, Wigzell FW, Anderson JR: Locomotor manifestations and serum studies in Takayasu's arteriopathy. Am J Med 40:560, 1966.

Dermatomyositis

Banker BQ, Victor M: Dermatomyositis (systemic angiopathy of childhood). Medicine 45:261, 1966.

Middleton PJ, Alexander RM, Szymanski MT: Severe myositis during recovery from influenza. Lancet 2:533, 1970.

Pachman LM, Cooke W: Juvenile dermatomyositis; a clinical and immunologic study. J Pediatr 96:226, 1980.

Pearson CM: Patterns of polymyositis and their response to treatment. Ann Intern Med 59:827, 1963.

Proceedings of the First American Rheumatism Association Conference of the Rheumatic Diseases of Childhood, chaired by Schaller JG, Hanson V: Arthritis Rheum (Suppl 2) 20:145, March, 1977.

Sullivan DB, Cassidy JT, Petty RE, et al: Prognosis in childhood dermatomyositis. J Pediatr 90:555, 1972.

Wedgwood RJ, Cook CD, Cohen J: Dermatomyositis: Report of 26 cases in children with a discussion of endocrine therapy in 13. Pediatrics 12:447, 1953.

Ziff M, Johnson RL: Polymyositis and cell-mediated immunity. N Engl J Med 288:465, 1973.

Scleroderma: Morphea and Progressive Systemic Sclerosis

Bradford WO, Cook CD, Vawter GF, et al: Scleroderma of childhood. J Pediatr 68:391, 1966.

Cassidy JT, Sullivan DB, Dabich L, et al: Scleroderma in children. Arthritis Rheum 20:351, 1977.

Chazen EM, Cook CD, Cohen J: Focal scleroderma. J Pediatr 60:385, 1962.

Christianson HB, Dorssy CS, O'Leary PA, et al: Localized scleroderma: Clinical study of 235 cases. Arch Dermatol 74:629, 1956.

Jaffe MO, Winkelmann RK: Generalized scleroderma in children. Arch Dermatol 83:402, 1961.

Kass H, Hanson V, Patrick J: Scleroderma in childhood. J Pediatr 68:243, 1966.

Proceedings of the First American Rheumatism Association Conference of the Rheumatic Diseases of Childhood, chaired by Schaller JG, Hanson V: Arthritis Rheum (Suppl 2) 20:145, 1977.

Winkelmann RK: Symposium on scleroderma. Mayo Clin Proc 46:77, 1971.

Mixed Connective Tissue Disease

Bennett RM, Spargo BH: Immune complex nephropathy in mixed connective tissue disease. Am J Med 63:534, 1977.

Sharp GC, Irvin WS, Tan EM, et al: Mixed connective tissue disease: An apparently distinct rheumatic disease syndrome associated with a specific antibody to an extractable nuclear antigen (ENA). Am J Med 52:148, 1972.

Singsen BH, Bernstein BH, Komreich HK, et al: Mixed connective tissue disease in childhood. J Pediatr 90:893, 1977.

Erythema Multiforme Exudativum (Stevens-Johnson Syndrome)

Ashby DW, Lazar T: Erythema multiforme exudativum major. Lancet 1:1091, 1951.

Bukantz SC: The Stevens-Johnson syndrome. Disease-A-Month, p 1. Chicago, Year Book Medical Publishers, Oct, 1968.

Foy HM, Kenney GE, Koler J: Mycoplasma pneumoniae in Stevens-Johnson syndrome. Lancet 2:550, 1966.

Stevens AM, Johnson FC: A new eruptive fever associated with stomatitis and ophthalmia. Am J Dis Child 24:526, 1922.

Erythema Nodosum

A Group of Pediatricians: Aetiology of erythema nodosum in children. Lancet 2:14, 1961.

Blomgren SE: Erythema nodosum. Semin Arth Rheum 4:1, 1974.

Doxiadis SA: Erythema nodosum in children. Medicine 30:283, 1951.

Kirby JF, Kraft GH: Oral contraceptives and erythema nodosum. Obstet Gynecol 40:409, 1972.

Weinstein L: Erythema nodosum. Disease-A-Month, p 1. Chicago, Year Book Medical Publishers, June, 1969.

The Goodpasture Syndrome

Benoit FL, Rulon DB, Theil GB, et al: Goodpasture's syndrome. Am J Med 37:424, 1964.

McCombs RP: Diseases due to immunologic reactions in the lungs. N Engl J Med 286:1186, 1972.

Relapsing Nodular Nonsuppurative Panniculitis

Hallahan JD, Klein T: Relapsing febrile nodular nonsuppurative panniculitis. Review of the literature and report of a case. Ann Intern Med 34:1179, 1951.

Perry HO, Winkelmann RK: Subacute nodular migratory panniculitis. Arch Dermatol 89:170, 1964.

Sanford HN, Eubank DF, Stenn F: Chronic panniculitis with leukopenia (Weber-Christian syndrome). Am J Dis Child 83:156, 1952.

"Rheumatoid" Nodules Without Rheumatic Disease

Altman RS, Caffrey PR: Isolated subcutaneous rheumatic nodules. Pediatrics 34:869, 1964.

Burrington JD: "Pseudorheumatoid" nodules in children. Report of 10 cases. Pediatrics 45:473, 1970.

Messara BW, Brody GL, Oberman HA: "Pseudorheumatoid" subcutaneous nodules. Am J Clin Pathol 45:684, 1966.

Simons FER, Schaller JG: Benign rheumatoid nodules. Pediatrics 56:29, 1975.

Fasciitis

Shulman, L: Diffuse fasciitis with eosinophilia: A new syndrome. Arthritis Rheum 20:S205, 1977.

Lyme Disease

Steere AC, Hardin JA, Malawista SE: Lyme arthritis: A new clinical entity. Hospital Pract 13:143, 1978.

Steere AC, Malawista SE, Hardin JA, et al: Erythema chronicum migrans and Lyme arthritis. The enlarging clinical spectrum. Ann Intern Med 86:685, 1977.

9.81 RHEUMATIC FEVER

Rheumatic fever is an inflammatory disease involving mainly the joints and the heart and less frequently the central nervous system, skin, and subcutaneous tissues. It has a marked tendency to recur, and both initial and recurrent attacks are nonsuppurative complications of group A streptococcal upper respiratory infections. Although the incidence of rheumatic fever in developed countries has fallen sharply in recent years, the disease has not been eradicated and is always potentially serious because it may lead to permanent cardiac damage.

History.   Rheumatic fever emerged as a separate entity in the 17th century under the name of "acute articular rheumatism." Although deformities of heart valves were noted frequently in the autopsies of patients with histories of acute articular rheumatism, it was not until 1836 that the 1st clinical description of heart disease in patients with rheumatic fever was published. Fifty yr later Cheadle described the major manifestations of the rheumatic fever syndrome much as we know it today. In 1931 the streptococcal etiology was proved by bacteriologic and epidemiologic studies; in 1939 Coburn and Moore showed that recurrences of rheumatic fever could be prevented by continual antistreptococcal prophylaxis; and a decade later Massell and Wannamaker demonstrated that adequate treatment of streptococcal pharyngitis with penicillin could prevent 1st rheumatic attacks.

Etiology and Epidemiology. Group A streptococcal infections of the upper respiratory tract are a prerequisite for the development of initial and recurrent attacks of rheumatic fever. Skin infections lead to acute glomerulonephritis but rarely, if ever, to acute rheumatic fever; such infections are caused by group A serotypes that do not generally cause clinical pharyngitis. Also, the ASO response is often feeble following skin infections, presumably because skin lipids inhibit streptolysin O. However, it is not clear whether the site of infection is critical because of these differences or whether anatomic or other factors play a role.

Not all rheumatic fever patients have a history of a preceding upper respiratory infection, and streptococci are not always found on throat culture at the time of acute rheumatic fever since the organisms often disappear from the pharynx during the 2–5 wk *latent* period between the upper respiratory infection and the onset of rheumatic fever. However, an elevated streptococcal antibody titer can be found in virtually all patients.

The rheumatic fever attack rate varies from 0.3% or less following sporadic streptococcal infections in the general population to approximately 3% documented during epidemics of untreated severe exudative pharyngitis. This suggests a relationship between the severity of the pharyngeal infection and the attack rate, although subclinical infections also may be followed by this complication.

Rheumatic fever occurs at all ages except infancy, but incidence peaks between 5–15 yr, an age period when streptococcal infections are most frequent. In the United States rheumatic fever is seen in late winter and early spring, when streptococcal respiratory infections are most common. The disease also has a high incidence in tropical and subtropical climates. The disease occurs with about equal frequency in both sexes, and there are no significant racial differences. There may be a genetic factor involved since the illness runs in families and monozygotic twins have a higher concordance rate for rheumatic fever than dizygotic twins. However, efforts to find a genetic marker that correlates with susceptibility have thus far failed.

Environmental factors could account for the familial incidence. Rheumatic fever has been called a "social disease" because its incidence is strikingly higher among the poor; overcrowding may be one of the most critical factors in this association. The importance of environmental factors is illustrated by the decline in the incidence of rheumatic fever prior to the introduction

of antibiotics (Fig 9–27). The annual incidence in Denmark fell from 200/100,000 population in 1862 to about 70/100,000 in 1940 chiefly because of better socioeconomic conditions. By 1962, the incidence had fallen to 10/100,000, a figure that approximates the annual incidence in the United States at present. The acceleration in the rate of decline since 1945 is due to earlier case detection, prevention of recurrences, and antibiotic treatment of upper respiratory infections.

In contrast to economically advanced countries, many developing countries show rheumatic fever as the etiology in 30–40% of all heart disease and a major cause of morbidity and mortality. Increased incidence in these countries in recent years is probably due to increasing industrialization and the migration from rural areas to crowded urban slums.

Pathogenesis. Although the streptococcal etiology of rheumatic fever is established, how these organisms in the pharynx cause the varied, multisystem manifestations of rheumatic fever is unknown. Streptococci cannot be found anywhere other than in the upper respiratory tract. These organisms exude a large number of toxins and enzymes (extracellular products) which diffuse out from the site of infection, and some, such as streptolysin, are cardiotoxic in animals. However, none of these has been shown to have a direct toxic action in humans. Since many of the extracellular substances are antigenic and provoke an antibody response, 1 objection to the toxin theory is that the potential deleterious effect of these substances would be neutralized by circulating antibodies. However, it has been hypothesized that 1 of the extracellular products, streptolysin O, may exist as an antigen-antibody complex that subsequently dissociates, allowing streptolysin O to exert its toxic effect.

A more widely held theory is that rheumatic fever is an autoimmune disease. Several streptococcal antigens cross-react with human tissue antigens, and cross-reactive ("anti-heart") antibodies have been found in rheumatic fever patients. According to this hypothesis, streptococcal antigens immunologically similar to human tissue antigens may elicit antibodies capable of reacting not only with microbial products but also with the host's antigens. However, anti-heart antibodies have been found in individuals who do not develop rheumatic fever. Furthermore, immunologic cross-reactions between bacterial components and human tissues are a common biologic phenomenon, and whether they are the cause or the effect of tissue injury remains uncertain.

Pathology. During the acute stage of rheumatic fever, there is an exudative inflammatory reaction in the connective tissues of the heart, joints, and skin characterized by edema of the ground substance and a cellular infiltration of lymphocytes and plasma cells. The inflammatory process may involve all segments of the heart. Within the myocardium there is cellular infiltrate in the interstitial tissues and damage to muscle cells. The valve leaflets are edematous and infiltrated mainly with lymphocytes. The serous surface of the pericardium is covered with a fibrinous exudate. On gross inspection the heart is dilated. There is swelling of the articular and periarticular structures with infiltra-

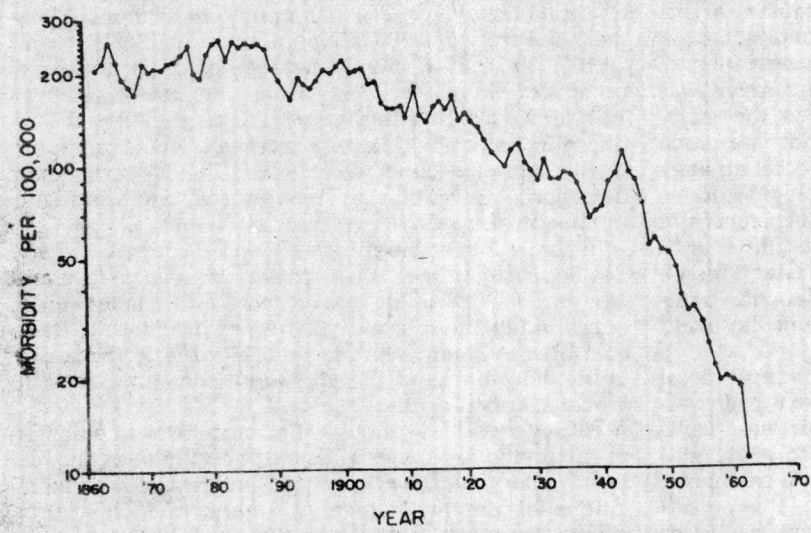

Figure 9–27 Reported rheumatic fever incidence in Denmark, 1862–1962. (From Stollerman GH: Rheumatic Fever and Streptococcal Infection. New York, Grune and Stratton, 1975.)

SOURCE : PUBLIC HEALTH BOARD OF DENMARK , COPENHAGEN , DENMARK.

tion of the synovial membrane and serous effusion into the joint space. However, there is never erosion of joint surfaces or pannus formation.

The changes seen during the acute stage are not diagnostic for rheumatic fever. This stage lasts for 2–3 wk and is followed by a proliferative phase that is essentially limited to the myocardium and endocardium. During this phase there is a perivascular aggregation of large, multinucleated cells arranged around an avascular core of fibrinoid material. This lesion is the myocardial *Aschoff body*, the pathognomonic lesion of rheumatic fever. Subsequently, fibrotic scarring occurs in the vicinity of Aschoff nodules. During the proliferative phase rheumatic vegetations made up of masses of eosinophilic material appear along the edge of the valves. These verrucous lesions, becoming progressively fibrotic, result in scarred, thickened valve cusps.

The histologic findings in the central nervous system are not characteristic of rheumatic fever, nor can they be correlated with the clinical findings. There is cellular degeneration and hyalinization of small blood vessels scattered throughout the cortex, cerebellum, and basal ganglia. No site is consistently involved, and Aschoff bodies have never been found in the brain. Subcutaneous nodules contain a central area of fibrinoid necrotic material surrounded by fibroblasts and occasional lymphocytes. Their structure resembles the Aschoff body.

Clinical Manifestations. The clinical findings vary greatly and are determined by the site of involvement, the severity of the attack, and the stage at which the patient is first examined. The onset is usually acute when arthritis is the presenting manifestation and more gradual when carditis or chorea is the initial clinical feature.

Joint symptoms are the most common presenting complaint, occurring in about 75% of patients during the acute stage of rheumatic fever. The severity ranges from pain in a joint without objective findings, to arthralgia, to frank *arthritis* with swelling, redness, and heat. In rheumatic fever more than in any other joint disease, the pain is often disproportionate to the objective findings. Knees, ankles, elbows, and wrists are commonly affected, less often the hips, and rarely the small joints of hands and feet. Successive rather than concurrent involvement of joints results in the characteristic picture of *migratory* polyarthralgia or polyarthritis. If left untreated, each joint is inflamed for only a few days, and all joint symptoms usually disappear spontaneously in 3–4 wk, leaving no permanent deformities.

Carditis is the most serious manifestation of rheumatic fever because it can be fatal during the acute stage or cause permanent valvular damage. Carditis occurs in 40–50% of initial attacks. The highest incidence occurs in young children, but overall carditis is less frequent and less severe in the United States than in the past.

The clinical picture is variable. Usually, rheumatic fever is heralded by fever and joint symptoms, and cardiac involvement is found on initial examination. At times, the cardiac findings are normal or equivocal at onset and become apparent after several days, or at most, within a wk or 2. Rarely is there a long delay in the appearance of carditis in acute onset rheumatic fever. Carditis may also present as an organic heart murmur in patients who initially appear with choreiform movements.

When carditis is the sole clinical manifestation, it can be difficult to determine when the attack began. Children have no symptoms referable to the heart unless pericarditis or heart failure is present. The history is vague. There is loss of appetite; the child appears pale and chronically ill and tires easily. The signs of cardiac involvement may be unequivocal, and often there is evidence of early heart failure. Carditis also can be entirely asymptomatic, so-called "silent carditis." This is a retrospective diagnosis when valvular heart disease is discovered years later and other causes of acquired heart disease have been excluded.

Carditis should be suspected if there is tachycardia disproportionate to the degree of fever. However, the most distinctive sign of rheumatic carditis is a new significant murmur. An apical high-pitched, blowing, holosystolic murmur of at least grade II intensity indicative of mitral valvulitis is the most common heart bruit. It may be accompanied by a low-pitched mid-diastolic (Carey-Coombs) murmur. A decrescendo diastolic murmur along the left sternal border indicating aortic regurgitation is much less frequent. Enlargement of the heart, a pericardial friction rub or effusion, and congestive failure may be present at the onset or occur during the course of the acute attack.

The duration of rheumatic carditis varies from 6 wk–6 mo. However, in patients with severe carditis the active rheumatic process may continue beyond 6 mo, so-called "chronic" rheumatic fever. Nowadays this occurs in a very small proportion of patients following an initial attack of rheumatic fever.

Chorea occurs in 10–15% of patients. It may be the only sign of rheumatic fever, or it may be associated with other manifestations such as carditis. Chorea is often heralded by emotional liability, deterioration in school performance, and poor coordination. Within a wk or 2 thereafter, involuntary, purposeless movements appear. These are random, nonrhythmic, rapid movements affecting any group of muscles but most often the face and upper extremities. The affected muscles are weak; at times the weakness is severe enough to resemble paralysis. The deep reflexes are variable, and there are no other neurologic findings.

Chorea is a self-limited condition with a variable course. Mild cases subside within a few wk, but a 3 mo course is average; occasionally, choreiform movements continue for 6 mo–1 yr.

Subcutaneous nodules are round, hard, freely movable painless swellings, usually overlying bone prominences. They occur in 5–10% of rheumatic patients, usually when severe carditis is present, and they often do not appear until several wk after onset of the attack. *Erythema marginatum* is the characteristic skin rash of rheumatic fever. It occurs in fewer than 5% of patients. The lesions begin as slightly red, barely raised, nonpruritic macules that extend outward to form wavy lines or rings with sharp margins; they occur mainly over the trunk and inner surfaces of arms and legs. These lesions are evanescent and may come and go for several mo.

Fever is usually present at the onset of an acute attack. It ranges from 38.3–40° C (101–104° F) without characteristic pattern. In children with an insidious onset the fever is low grade; it is completely absent in patients with pure chorea. *Abdominal pain* may precede other manifestations. The pain is not localized but can be severe enough to suggest a surgical condition. Spontaneous *epistaxis*, once frequent, is now rarely seen.

Laboratory Manifestations. Evidence of a recent streptococcal infection should be sought in every patient suspected of rheumatic fever. The throat culture may not be helpful for this purpose because by the time rheumatic fever develops, the culture is often negative. Tests for streptococcal antibodies are much more useful because they are specific for infections caused by the

bacteria and antibodies usually reach their peak at about the time of onset of rheumatic fever. Approximately 80% have an elevated anti-streptolysin O (ASO) titer. Titers ranging from 200–300 units are common in healthy school-age children so that only levels of over 300 units are considered abnormal. Patients suspected of rheumatic fever who do not show an abnormal ASO titer should be tested for other streptococcal antibodies, e.g., anti–DNase B and anti-DPNase. If these tests are not available, there is a commercial multiple antibody test (Streptozyme); it is considered positive at dilutions over 1:200. The Streptozyme test should not be used in lieu of the ASO titer, which is the best standardized and most reproducible test available.

Because streptococcal antibody levels may begin to decline after 2 mo, titers in patients with insidious rheumatic carditis discovered several mo after onset may have returned to normal levels. This is also true in patients with "pure" chorea since this manifestation may not appear until several mo after streptococcal infection. There is no correlation between the height and duration of the antibody titer and the severity or persistence of rheumatic activity. Thus, once it has been established that the patient has an elevated titer, there is no reason to repeat antibody studies.

The tests generally used to measure the presence and degree of inflammatory process are the erythrocyte sedimentation rate (ESR) and C-reactive protein (CRP). Neither is specific for rheumatic fever, but they are useful for determining when the acute process has terminated. The CRP is somewhat better because the sedimentation rate can be influenced by extraneous factors such as anemia. Mild to moderate anemia is common in active rheumatic fever; it is normocytic and normochromic.

Prolongation of the P-R interval occurs in about one third of the patients with acute rheumatic fever. While heart block can be a diagnostic aid, it is not of itself a sign of carditis and it has no prognostic significance. Other electrocardiographic changes include flattened or inverted T waves due to myocarditis as well as elevation of the S-T segment produced by pericarditis.

Roentgenograms of the chest are useful to detect cardiac enlargement and pericardial effusion. Patients with rheumatic polyarthritis do not require roentgenograms of the joints.

Diagnosis. Rheumatic fever may affect a number of organs and tissues, singly or in combination. No single clinical manifestation or laboratory test is characteristic enough to be diagnostic. The need to bring uniformity to the diagnosis led T. D. Jones to formulate diagnostic criteria based on combinations of clinical manifestations and laboratory findings. Clinical signs that are most useful are designated *major manifestations* and include carditis, arthritis, chorea, subcutaneous nodules, and erythema marginatum. The term "major" relates to diagnostic importance and not to frequency, severity, or prognostic significance of the particular manifestation. Other signs and symptoms, while less characteristic, may still be helpful. These *minor manifestations* include fever, arthralgia, past history of rheumatic fever or rheumatic heart disease, prolongation of the P-R interval, and positive acute phase reactants. Two major

Table 9–24 JONES CRITERIA (REVISED) FOR GUIDANCE IN THE DIAGNOSIS OF RHEUMATIC FEVER

MAJOR MANIFESTATIONS	MINOR MANIFESTATIONS
Carditis	*Clinical*
Polyarthritis	Fever
Chorea	Arthralgia
Erythema marginatum	Previous rheumatic fever or
Subcutaneous nodules	rheumatic heart disease
	Laboratory
	Acute phase reaction
	ESR, leukocytosis
	C-reactive protein
	Prolonged P-R interval

Plus supporting evidence of preceding streptococcal infection: increased ASO or other streptococcal antibodies; positive throat culture for group A streptococcus; recent scarlet fever.

From Circulation 32:664, 1965.

or 1 major and 2 minor manifestations indicate a high probability of rheumatic fever. The Jones criteria were revised in 1965 to include supporting evidence of a recent streptococcal infection (Table 9–24).

Clinical criteria can neither encompass the full spectrum of a disease nor totally exclude overlapping conditions. Thus, not all bona fide rheumatic fever patients fit the criteria, especially if the attack is mild or patients are seen early in the course of the illness. There are also clinical conditions which fulfill the criteria but are not due to rheumatic fever. Nevertheless, the criteria are useful, especially for avoiding overdiagnosis. Many errors in diagnosis occur because the history, physical, or laboratory findings have been misinterpreted.

Differential Diagnosis. The frequent occurrence of combinations of rheumatic manifestations makes the diagnosis fairly straightforward in many cases. When the patient presents with a single clinical feature, the differential diagnosis varies according to the presenting manifestation.

Joint pains without objective findings, arthralgia, can be difficult to distinguish from *nonspecific limb pain,* a common complaint in children. Pains behind the knees and in calf muscles that awaken children at night (so-called growing pains) are not due to rheumatic fever. Abnormalities of the feet, patellar chondromalacia, osteochondroses, and other orthopedic conditions can simulate rheumatic arthralgia. Limb pains may also be an expression of a functional disorder. The sedimentation rate is a helpful screening test to distinguish many of these conditions from true rheumatic arthralgia.

Acute onset polyarticular *rheumatoid arthritis* can mimic rheumatic fever early in the course of the illness. Polyarthritis in children under 3 yr of age is almost always due to rheumatoid disease. It is less migratory, less responsive to salicylates, and often accompanied by a high intermittent fever, splenomegaly, lymphadenopathy, and an evanescent macular rash, none of which occur in rheumatic fever. Arthralgia and arthritis can occur during infections with *Yersinia enterocolitica, salmonella, shigella, rubella,* and *viral hepatitis. Hypersensitivity reactions, sickle cell disease,* and *leukemia* can also cause periarticular pain and swelling and mimic rheumatic fever.

The most common diagnostic error related to the heart is misinterpretation of *innocent murmurs,* especially in children with ill-defined extremity pain and low grade fever. Innocent murmurs are common in children and are of 2 types: the ejection pulmonic systolic murmur and the musical parasternal systolic murmur. Since these murmurs are often loud, it is the quality, duration, and location rather than the intensity which distinguish them from the blowing pansystolic apical murmur of mitral regurgitation.

Viral myocarditis can usually be distinguished from rheumatic myocarditis since the latter is almost always accompanied by valvular disease and a significant murmur. An exception is the fulminant form of rheumatic myocarditis in very young children. Rheumatic pericarditis is also accompanied by other signs of carditis; when pericarditis is an isolated finding, a viral etiology should be suspected. Acute rheumatic carditis is rarely mistaken for congenital heart disease, although chronic rheumatic valvular disease can be confused with congenital abnormalities of the heart.

Abnormal movements due to other causes can be mistaken for Sydenham chorea when there is no other evidence of rheumatic fever. The repetitive stereotyped movements of *multiple tics* are fairly easy to distinguish from the random, jerky, choreiform movements. The *tic of Gilles de la Tourette* may resemble chorea at the onset, but its chronicity and other distinctive features soon distinguish it. *Huntington chorea* may start in childhood, but the movements tend to be choreoathetoid and there is a positive family history.

The significance of an elevated ASO has been a source of misdiagnosis. *An elevated ASO titer, no matter how abnormal, does not by itself confirm the diagnosis.* There must also be well documented clinical evidence of rheumatic fever. Questionable rheumatic manifestations plus an elevated ASO titer are insufficient for a diagnosis, but they may require careful observation of the patient.

Treatment. All patients with acute rheumatic fever should be placed at bed rest, if at all possible in a hospital. They should be examined daily to detect carditis, which almost always appears within 2 wk of onset. Thereafter, the duration and degree of bed rest should vary with the nature and severity of the attack. A guide for bed rest and ambulation is outlined in Table 9–25. In general, restrictions are continued until the rheumatic process has become quiescent. It is considered active when any of the following is present: joint

Table 9–25 GUIDE FOR BED REST AND AMBULATION IN PATIENTS WITH ACUTE RHEUMATIC FEVER

CARDIAC STATUS	MANAGEMENT
No carditis	Bed rest for 2 wk and gradual ambulation for 2 wk even if on salicylates
Carditis, no enlargement	Bed rest for 4 wk and gradual ambulation for 4 wk
Carditis, with enlargement	Bed rest for 6 wk and gradual ambulation for 6 wk
Carditis, with heart failure	Strict bed rest for as long as heart failure is present and gradual ambulation for 3 mo

symptoms, new organic murmurs, enlarging heart size, a sleeping pulse of greater than 100, or subcutaneous nodules. Heart failure in the absence of longstanding valvular disease is also a sign of activity. Persistence of an elevated ESR for more than 6 mo should not be considered a sign of rheumatic activity if no clinical signs are present.

Anti-inflammatory drugs are very effective for suppressing the acute manifestations of rheumatic fever. However, in patients with arthralgia only or with mild arthritis, anti-inflammatory agents should be withheld and other analgesics used if needed. This is particularly wise when the diagnosis is uncertain since analgesics will not interfere with the development of migratory polyarthritis.

Patients with definite arthritis, or with carditis but no cardiomegaly, should be treated with salicylates: 100 mg/kg/24 hr in divided doses for the 1st 2 wk and 75 mg/kg/24 hr for the following 4–6 wk. Occasionally, 150 mg/kg/24 hr may be necessary to control arthritis.

Patients with carditis and cardiomegaly should be treated with prednisone, starting with a dose of 2 mg/kg/24 hr in divided doses. After about 2 wk, prednisone may be withdrawn, decreasing the daily dose at the rate of 5 mg every 2–3 days. When tapering is started, salicylates, 75 mg/kg/24 hr, should be added and continued for 1 mo after prednisone is stopped. Overlapping therapy reduces the incidence of post-therapeutic rebounds which may occur within a wk or 2 after anti-inflammatory drugs are discontinued. Laboratory rebounds and all but the most severe clinical rebounds are best left untreated.

The recommendations outlined above and in Table 9–26 limit the use of steroids to patients with moderate to severe carditis because of the clinical impression that such patients respond more rapidly, tolerate steroids better than salicylates, and may be at less risk of death during the acute attack. However, most well controlled studies have failed to prove that treatment with steroids decreases the incidence of residual heart disease.

Mild heart failure can often be controlled by complete bed rest, oxygen, fluid restriction, and steroids. If severe failure is present, diuretics and digitalis are indicated. However, digitalis should be used with caution because some patients with acute myocarditis have an unusual sensitivity to digitalis.

Patients with chorea may benefit from barbiturates or chlorpromazine. More recently, haloperidol has been used, but no drug has proved uniformly effective. Steroids are not recommended unless there are also signs of an active rheumatic inflammatory process.

Prognosis. The sequelae of rheumatic fever are essentially limited to the heart and depend on the presence and severity of carditis. When there is no clinical evidence of carditis during the acute attack, complete recovery is the rule. The prognosis is also excellent if the findings are limited to prolongation of the P-R interval. When there is cardiac involvement, the incidence of residual heart disease mirrors the severity of the carditis. Three quarters of the patients with congestive heart failure during the initial attack will have chronic valvular disease after 10 yr. On the other hand, when the cardiac findings are limited to a systolic murmur, only about 25% of the patients are left with residual heart disease. Thus, in patients with mild carditis, the number of patients who heal completely is remarkably high *if they remain free of recurrent attacks.*

Recurrences of rheumatic fever markedly influence the prognosis, and the availability of antistreptococcal prophylaxis is the main reason for improved outcome in recent yr. Recurrences are more likely when the initial attack occurs early in life and when the attack includes carditis. They are more apt to occur in the years immediately after an attack, in patients with residual heart disease, and in those with previous recurrences.

Death during the acute attack has become exceedingly rare. The mortality from chronic rheumatic heart disease has also dropped markedly. The 10 yr mortality rate in a recent series was 4%, which contrasts with the 20–30% 10 yr mortality rate that prevailed prior to 1950.

Prevention. The attack rate after streptococcal infections in patients who have had rheumatic fever is much higher than in the general population. Therefore, once the diagnosis of rheumatic fever has been established, *continual antimicrobial prophylaxis* should be started to prevent streptococcal infections and recurrences of rheumatic fever. Intramuscular benzathine penicillin G, 1.2 million units every 4 wk, is the most effective prophylactic medication. It is the treatment of choice for *all* patients and especially for high risk patients, i.e., those with heart disease, those with a history of multiple attacks, or those unlikely to take oral medication regularly. There may be persistent pain for 1–2 days at the site of injection, but rarely does benzathine penicillin have to be discontinued for this reason. Allergic reactions in children are infrequent and generally mild.

Sulfadiazine is the drug of choice for the exceptional patient who cannot tolerate injections or who is allergic to penicillin. The dose is 0.5 gm once daily in children less than 30 kg and 1.0 gm in the others. Although reactions are rare, a blood count is advised after the 1st several wk, and patients should be advised to report immediately the appearance of any rash.

Oral penicillin is also effective in a dose of 200,000 units twice daily. Patients on oral penicillin can be monitored for compliance by a simple urine test for penicillin. Oral penicillin, however, causes the emergence of resistant alpha streptococci in the mouth, whereas benzathine penicillin and sulfadiazine do not. Resistant alpha streptococci in the oral cavity are a potential hazard for patients with rheumatic heart disease since they are at risk for bacterial endocarditis.

Prophylaxis should be maintained at least throughout childhood and adolescence. Young adults with children

Table 9–26 RECOMMENDED ANTI-INFLAMMATORY AGENTS FOR ACUTE RHEUMATIC FEVER

CLINICAL MANIFESTIONS	TREATMENT
Arthralgia	Analgesics only
Arthritis only, and/or carditis without cardiomegaly	Salicylates 100 mg/kg/24 hr for 2 wk and 75 mg/kg/24 hr for 4–6 wk
Carditis with cardiomegaly or failure	Prednisone 2 mg/kg/24 hr for 2 wk and taper over 2 wk; salicylates 75 mg/kg/24 hr at 2 wk and continue for 6 wk

in the home should also be urged to continue prophylaxis. The risk to individuals over 40 yr of age is very small, but lifetime prophylaxis is recommended if the patient has rheumatic valvular disease.

Initial attacks of rheumatic fever can be prevented by treatment of the preceding streptococcal pharyngitis. It is essential to eradicate the organisms, and 10 days of antimicrobial treatment are required to achieve maximum cure rates. A single injection of benzathine penicillin is the most reliable treatment. A 10 day course of oral penicillin is effective, but it is less reliable because it depends on compliance. Patients who are allergic to penicillin should receive erythromycin for 10 days. Sulfonamides should not be prescribed since they fail to eradicate streptococci. The tetracyclines are also contraindicated because many strains of group A streptococci have become resistant to this antibiotic.

The prevention of 1st attacks of rheumatic fever is hampered by failure to recognize streptococcal pharyngitis, by the subclinical nature of many of these infections, and by the lack of easy access to medical care. Some of these difficulties have been overcome in recent yr by the widespread use of throat cultures and greater availability of medical care through Medicaid and other programs. A study in 1 city demonstrated a significant reduction in the incidence of 1st attacks of rheumatic fever after comprehensive care clinics were established in deprived areas and a concerted effort was made to identify and treat streptococcal infections. An antistreptococcal vaccine is under development.

MILTON MARKOWITZ

DiSciascio G, Taranta A: Rheumatic fever in children: A review. Am Heart J 99:635, 1980.

Gordis L: Effectiveness of comprehensive care programs in preventing rheumatic fever. N Engl J Med 289:331, 1973.

Inter-Society Commission for Heart Disease Resources: Prevention of rheumatic fever and rheumatic heart disease. Circulation 61:A–1, 1970.

Jones criteria (revised) for guidance in the diagnosis of rheumatic fever. Circulation 32:664, 1965.

Jones TD: The diagnosis of rheumatic fever. JAMA 126:481, 1944.

Markowitz M, Gordis L: Rheumatic Fever. Ed 2. Philadelphia, WB Saunders, 1972.

Stollerman GH: Rheumatic Fever and Streptococcal Infection. New York, Grune and Stratton, 1975.

United Kingdom and United States Joint Report: The natural history of rheumatic fever and rheumatic heart disease: Ten year report of a cooperative clinical trial of ACTH, cortisone and aspirin. Circulation 32:457, 1965.

Wannamaker LW: Medical Progress: Differences between streptococcal infections of the throat and of the skin. N Engl J Med 282:23, 78, 1970.

Wannamaker LW, Matsen JM: Streptococci and Streptococcal Diseases. New York, Academic Press, 1972.

INFECTIOUS DISEASES 10

CLINICAL USE OF THE MICROBIOLOGY LABORATORY

The responsibility for attaining satisfactory laboratory diagnosis of infectious diseases rests with the clinician. He or she, not the laboratory worker, decides what specimens to collect, when to collect them, how to obtain them, and which laboratory procedures to request. The clinician must also see that the specimens are delivered promptly to the laboratory in a properly preserved state and should be competent to make the correct interpretation of the results.

The choice of specimens to be examined often makes the difference between diagnostic success and failure. The clinician will, in many instances, be guided by the patient's signs and symptoms as to the type of causative agent to be suspected. Sometimes, however, the signs and symptoms may be so nonspecific that the laboratory must help in ruling out a variety of agents. Material from the system of the body chiefly involved should be collected, e.g., cerebrospinal fluid from a patient with meningeal symptoms or joint fluid from a patient with arthritis. Consideration should also be given to possible portals of entry, such as the upper respiratory tract in patients with meningeal involvement.

The clinician must decide whether an attempt should be made to isolate the causative agent or to demonstrate an antibody response, or both. More than 1 culture is advisable when seeking a pathogen.

10.1 LABORATORY DIAGNOSIS OF BACTERIAL INFECTIONS

For bacterial infections the preferred diagnostic method is the demonstration of the responsible organism by smear and culture.

Culture of Feces. Rectal swabs or stool specimens are cultured for 2 reasons: to identify common bacterial pathogens such as *Salmonella* and *Shigella* or to determine the predominant flora of the intestine in a patient with weakened host defenses whose endogenous flora may become pathogenic. It should be remembered that feces contain mostly anaerobic bacteria and that routine cultures identify only the predominant aerobic organisms among the billions of bacteria contained in each gram. Fortunately, enteric pathogens usually replace the normal aerobic flora when they cause acute infection, thus rendering their isolation easier. Even so, selective media are needed to suppress growth of other organisms.

A number of organisms recently have been added to the list of bacterial pathogens to be searched for in feces, including *Campylobacter fetus*, *Yersinia enterocoli-*

tica, and *Clostridium difficile* (see Table 10–1 for selective media). In certain epidemiologic situations vibrios (*Vibrio cholerae, V. parahaemolyticus*) may need to be sought by culture on TCBS agar.

Nasopharyngeal, Throat, and Skin Swabs. A dry cotton or alginate swab is most efficient for the collection of specimens from the skin and mucous membranes. Since drying is rapidly destructive to some pathogenic bacteria, swab specimens should be placed promptly in a transport medium. Packaged swabs are available containing transport medium in a breakable ampule which is crushed after the specimen is taken.

Interpretation of results of cultures from skin and mucous membranes is difficult because microbial flora are normally recovered from these areas. Some organisms will be considered pathogenic whenever found, such as *Corynebacterium diphtheriae*, *Bordetella pertussis*, and *Neisseria gonorrhoeae*; others, such as *Streptococcus pyogenes*, *Neisseria meningitidis*, *Hemophilus influenzae*, or staphylococci, may be pathogenic or nonpathogenic, or there may be evidence of a carrier state, depending on circumstances. Still others, such as *Branhamella catarrhalis*, are rarely considered pathogenic. It cannot be emphasized too strongly that there is poor correlation between flora of the upper airway and that of the lower airway in lower respiratory tract disease; because spu-

Table 10–1 SELECTIVE PATHOGENS REQUIRING SPECIAL MEDIA FOR CULTIVATION

SUSPECTED ORGANISM	APPROPRIATE SPECIAL MEDIUM
Anaerobic organisms	Prereduced media, incubated under inert gas
Bordetella pertussis	Bordet-Gengou medium; charcoal agar with cephalexin and horse blood
Brucella sp.	Biphasic blood culture medium in 5–10% CO_2
Campylobacter fetus	Brucella blood agar with antibiotics (Campy-BAP)
Clostridium difficile	Cycloserine cefoxitin fructose agar
Corynebacterium diphtheriae	Loeffler and cystine-tellurite media
Francisella tularensis	Blood-dextrose-cystine agar
Free-living amebae	Non-nutrient agar seeded with *E. coli*
L-forms of bacteria	PPLO agar with horse serum and 20% sucrose
Legionella	Charcoal yeast extract agar
Leptospira sp.	Semisolid medium with rabbit serum
Mycobacterium sp.	Löwenstein-Jensen or Middlebrook media
Mycoplasma pneumoniae	E agar with horse serum
Neisseria gonorrhoeae	Thayer-Martin and chocolate agar
Yersinia enterocolitica	Saline enrichment at 4°C

595

tum cultures are seldom reliable, tracheal aspirates and lung punctures are often necessary for accurate diagnosis.

Blood Culture. Culture of the blood is one of the most fruitful procedures in the diagnosis of bacterial disease. It should be done carefully *before* administration of antibiotics, using iodine-alcohol for skin disinfection. After the venipuncture a fresh needle should be attached to the syringe and used for inoculating the blood into at least 2 bottles of medium prewarmed to room temperature. If only 1 sampling of blood is possible before antibiotic therapy begins, a generous sample should be obtained; e.g., 10 ml from a term newborn, 60 ml from an adult, and proportional amounts between these ages. Not more than 5 ml should be inoculated into each 50 ml flask; some bacteriologists add penicillinase to help destroy the antibiotic, whereas others consider this step unnecessary. Sodium polyanethanol sulfonate is included in modern blood culture media to prevent coagulation and to inactivate leukocytes. Some blood culture bottles also contain an oxygen-free CO_2-enriched atmosphere that allows for the recovery of anaerobes. If an isolate is reported, blood cultures should be repeated to determine (1) whether treatment has been successful when the patient is already on antibiotics, (2) whether the isolate is a contaminant when the organism reported is usually nonpathogenic, or (3) whether the organism is still present if the patient has not been given antibiotics in the interim. The question of whether an organism isolated from blood is a pathogen or a contaminant should be carefully considered since nonpathogens may cause disease in hosts with compromised immune mechanisms.

Examination of Cerebrospinal Fluid. Fluid obtained by lumbar puncture or ventricular tap should be collected in sterile capped containers and transported quickly to the laboratory, where centrifugation is done to concentrate organisms. Gram stains of CSF sediment are helpful; the presence of organisms distinguishes bacterial from viral disease, but impressions gained from smears should not be relied on to limit treatment to that for 1 kind of bacterial organism. Errors are possible, even by experienced clinicians; it is better to use broad-spectrum initial therapy in life-threatening disease and to wait for the culture report before ordering specific treatment. The coagulation of fluids containing blood or plasma may make the detection of organisms difficult and accurate cell counts impossible. When such fluids are encountered, a portion of each specimen should be collected in an oxalate tube for smear and cell count. If there are enough organisms in the CSF, a quellung reaction can be performed with antisera to *Hemophilus influenzae* type b or to various types of meningococci and pneumococci. Counterimmunoelectrophoresis and agglutination of antibody-coated latex beads are additional rapid, accurate methods for diagnosis. Specific antisera can be used to detect antigens such as those of *H. influenzae* type b, *N. meningitidis*, *S. pneumoniae*, group B streptococci, and *E. coli* K1. When the etiology of meningitis is unclear, acid-fast smear, culture for *M. tuberculosis*, India ink preparation, test for cryptococcal antigen, and fungal culture may be indicated.

Urine Culture. Urine for culture and colony count can be obtained in midstream (clean catch), by catheterization, or by suprapubic puncture. The last method is the most reliable; urine so obtained should normally be sterile. Urine collected by catheter is likely to reflect infection if there are 10^4 organisms/ml or more. Clean catch urine, if obtained after adequate cleansing, can be considered abnormal if more than 10^5 organisms/ml are present, and possibly abnormal if between 10^4 and 10^5 organisms are counted/ml. These limits apply only in uncomplicated urinary tract infection due to enteric gram-negative rods; different criteria may have to be used for gram-positive organisms, for yeasts, for patients in diuresis or with chronic pyelonephritis, or for patients on antibiotics. Although patients with low counts are statistically less likely to be infected than those with high counts, serial cultures and clinical assessment are sometimes necessary in order to make a decision regarding treatment. In practice it often happens that urine specimens from girls are obtained by the clean catch technique after inadequate washing and allowed to sit at room temperature for some time before being transported to the laboratories. This accounts for the high frequency in girls of putatively positive urine cultures which are not confirmed when repeated. Urine cultures should be done carefully since false positives may condemn a patient to long courses of antibiotics.

Exudates and Transudates. Abscesses, pleural fluids, joint fluids, urethral exudates, and other miscellaneous exudates and transudates can be cultured directly on agar. Prompt delivery of these specimens to the laboratory is essential. In addition to cultures and stains, sugar and cell count determinations should be done on all transudates for the same reasons they are done on CSF.

Gram Stain. The examination of a Gram stain should be carried out on all cultured fluids, including centrifuged urine. In addition to giving rapid results, the Gram stain may be useful in interpreting the subsequent cultural data.

Special Cultures. Most medically important bacteria can be cultivated on blood agar, chocolate agar, and eosinmethylene blue or MacConkey agar. The frequency of recovery of anaerobic organisms has increased in recent years as media with low redox potentials have gained wide use. Thioglycollate broth, while an excellent general culture medium, will not foster growth of strict anaerobes. For collection of anaerobic cultures material should be transported to the laboratory in a capped syringe, or special swabs supplied in oxygen-free tubes should be used. In some cases clinical circumstances may call for the use of additional media, such as those listed in Table 10–1. When an organism on this list is suspected, the microbiology laboratory should be informed in advance of sending the specimen. If the hospital's laboratory is not proficient in a particular culture technique, prior arrangements should be made with a reference laboratory that can do the necessary culture.

Fluorescent Techniques. Fluorescent antibody (FA) technique has widened the diagnostic scope of direct microscopy. Specific antisera are now available commercially for several common pathogens. In these sera the antibody molecules have been conjugated with a fluorescein dye. The specific dye-labeled serum is added to the smear containing the suspected organism and the slide examined microscopically under ultraviolet light. If the organism is present, the antibody molecules are concentrated about it and the observer sees a bright fluorescence. The presence of even a small number of organisms in the smear can be detected in this manner. This *direct method* can be used if specific fluorescein-labeled antisera are readily available. In the absence of such sera, the *indirect method* is useful, though more complex. The indirect method requires 2 steps: (1) the smear is covered with the unlabeled specific antiserum, time is allowed for antibodies to fix, and then the excess of unfixed antibody is washed off; and (2) the slide is then overlaid with a fluorescein-labeled gamma globulin containing antibodies against gamma globulin of the animal species in which the antiserum was made. The anti-gamma globulin antibodies are concentrated and fluoresce at the sites of specific microorganism-antibody complexes. FA is used principally for identifying *Mycobacterium tuberculosis*, *Bordetella pertussis*, *Corynebacterium diphtheriae*, *Legionella pneumophila*, *Neisseria gonorrhoeae*, and group A streptococci. The case of *M. tuberculosis* is special in that no antibody is used; rather, the smears are stained with the auramine-rhodamine, which is taken up by the organisms and fluoresces under UV light. This fluorescent stain is more sensitive but less specific than the acid-fast stain.

Skin Tests. The Schick test and the Dick test (for susceptibility to diphtheria and to scarlet fever, respectively) are no longer in general use. The principal indication for skin testing is suspicion of mycobacterial infection. Purified protein derivatives of *M. tuberculosis* (PPD-S) and other mycobacteria (PPD-B, PPD-Y, etc.) are not sensitizing in themselves, but dermal hypersensitivity to them often provides the quickest means of diagnosis. If skin tests are negative but clinical suspicion of tuberculosis remains high, skin testing for anergy should be conducted with a panel of antigens such as *Candida* and *Trichophyton*. Skin tests are available for some pathogenic fungi but should be used for epidemiologic surveys rather than individual diagnosis.

Serologic Tests. Bacteria are often typed through agglutination by specific sera (sometimes attached to latex particles), but titration of serum antibodies is useful in only a few bacterial infections, among which are those caused by streptococci, salmonella, brucella, Legionnaires bacillus, and leptospira. In the case of streptococci, antibodies against exotoxins are assayed to determine whether there has been recent significant invasion. Slide tests such as Streptozyme (Wampole) detect antibodies to multiple exotoxins in a rapid, accurate manner. Salmonella antibodies (Widal test) must be measured for each group (A, B, C, D, etc.) and for both flagellar and somatic antigens. Unless positive and negative control sera are also tested, the results may be misleading. In any case, because of cross-reactions and the presence of antibodies from previous exposure, only a 4-fold or greater rise is significant, and undue diagnostic weight should not be placed on the presence of salmonella antibodies.

Antibiotic Sensitivity Tests. Most laboratories routinely test bacterial isolates for sensitivity to various antibiotics. Clinicians have come to depend on this information for selection of therapy but are not always aware of how to obtain the best information from the laboratory and how to interpret it. The most prevalent technique of antibiotic testing is the Kirby-Bauer method, in which a standardized inoculum of the organism is seeded onto a plate. Filter paper discs, each impregnated with an antibiotic, are placed on the plate, and the zone of inhibition of bacterial growth around each disc is measured. The concentration of antibiotic in the disc presumably reflects an achievable blood level, and the zone diameter is directly related to the sensitivity of the organism. Standard zone diameters indicating sensitivity or resistance have been designated, according to previous tests correlating zone sizes and sensitivity by dilutions made in tubes of broth inoculated with bacteria. However, there are many pitfalls in the disc diffusion method of testing the sensitivity of bacteria to antibiotics. The geometry of the test is such that the difference in area between a zone of 13-mm diameter and one of 12-mm diameter is 17%, presumably equivalent to a 17% difference in antibiotic activity. Small differences, therefore, have large implications, and the control of inoculum size, the rate of diffusion of antibiotics, and the accurate measurement of zones are critical.

For more accurate measurement of antibiotic sensitivity, dilutions made in tubes or in wells on microtiter plates are coming into wide use. Antibiotic dilutions in growth medium are prepared in steps through the range of attainable blood levels; then each tube or well is inoculated with the test organism (about 10^5 bacteria), but varying with the particular organism and the volume of medium. After 24 hr the tubes or wells are examined for turbidity; the 1st clear tube or well gives the bacteriostatic concentration of the particular antibiotic for the organism (minimal inhibitory concentration, or MIC). The tubes or wells are then subcultured to agar plates; the concentrations of antibiotic in tubes or wells that yield a 99.9% decrease in organisms on subculture are bactericidal (minimal bactericidal concentration, or MBC).

Apart from the technical artifacts in antibiotic testing, clinicians may misapply valid results. Antibiotic sensitivities cannot be interpreted correctly except in the pharmacologic context. Certain clinical situations, such as endocarditis or osteomyelitis, call for the use of bactericidal rather than bacteriostatic drugs. Although a staphylococcus might be sensitive to both semisynthetic penicillins and erythromycin, the former would be a better choice than the latter in a bloodstream infection. Toxicity of drugs must also be taken into account: the use of less toxic agents is preferable when possible. Finally, attainable blood and tissue levels are the true measure of clinical efficacy: polymyxin B gives good zones of inhibition in vitro, but the highest blood levels that can be tolerated are often insufficient to achieve sterilization; on the other hand, carbenicillin may appear ineffective in vitro, but the high blood levels that are possible with this drug and its synergism with certain other antibiotics, such as gentamicin, may make it useful even when in vitro results do not appear promising.

The bacteriostatic and bactericidal activity in the serum or other body fluids of a patient receiving antibiotics can be measured by inoculation of the organism originally isolated from the patient into dilutions of serum obtained at specified times after infection or infusion of antibiotics. The actual concentrations of certain antibiotics in the blood can be measured by chemical assays or by microbiologic assays using susceptible stock strains of bacteria. These measurements are mandatory when patients with renal disease are treated with aminoglycosides.

The usefulness of the above procedures is illustrated in the management of streptococcal endocarditis. First, the organism is tested by tube dilution against penicillin G. If it is sensitive, the bacteriostatic and bactericidal activities of serum are measured 0.5 hr and 6 hr after infusion of penicillin. Killing at 0.5 hr and at 6 hr should occur at dilutions at least as high as 1:8 and 1:2, respectively.

OFFICE BACTERIOLOGY

Bacteriology done in hospital or private laboratories tends to be inconvenient and expensive for outpatients. Fortunately, in recent years commercial manufacturers have developed disposable materials which lend themselves to rapid, inexpensive bacterial diagnosis in the physician's office. Kits for the detection of streptococci, gonococci, and urinary tract infection are those most widely used. The only additional purchase required is a small incubator.

Every pediatrician should be able to do throat cultures for group A streptococci in the office to distinguish patients with pharyngitis who need antibiotic treatment from those who do not. A unit for this purpose with a built-in incubator is commercially available (Clinicult, SmithKline). An alternative is the use of a separately purchased incubator and blood agar plates, which can be purchased cheaply. A bacitracin disk (e.g., Taxo-A) must be placed on the plate after streaking; group A streptococci will usually be sensitive.

In prepubertal vaginitis and in circumstances suggesting sexual abuse, cultures for gonococci should be obtained. Thayer-Martin medium under CO_2 is the basic medium and is available in convenient form as Neigon (Flow Labs) or Clinicult Transgrow (SmithKline). Thayer-Martin medium is selective by means of inhibitors to which some strains of gonococci may be sensitive. Blood or joint fluid from which gonococci may be expected to be present in pure culture should be cultivated on chocolate agar.

Culture of urine has now become quite simple through the development of inexpensive disposable units. In fact, in the usual outpatient circumstances in which clean-catch urines may be delayed in reaching the laboratory, the commercial units are more accurate than full-scale cultures. Three examples are Bactercult (Wampole), Uricult (Medical Technology Corporation), and Clinicult-Bacteriuria (SmithKline). Some of the units are based on an agar-coated dipstick placed in the freshly voided urine. In all cases the numbers of colonies can be quantitated by inspection and subcultures made for identification and for testing for antibiotic sensitivity.

Although urine cultures are preferable to less specific techniques, a rapid method for presumptive detection of infected patients is the nitrite strip test. Nitrate is reduced to nitrite by many bacteria, and a chemical strip is available to register nitrite by color change (Uristix, Ames).

10.2   LABORATORY DIAGNOSIS OF SPIROCHETES

Serologic procedures are heavily relied on for the diagnosis of treponemal infection: complement fixation, precipitin, and fluorescent antibody methods. Darkfield examination of lesions of skin and mucous membranes may strongly suggest the diagnosis, but serologic confirmation is necessary. Leptospira can be cultivated directly in special media, but serologic tests are more generally available. Other spirochetes can be visualized directly.

10.3   LABORATORY DIAGNOSIS OF MYCOPLASMA AND L-FORMS

These organisms are discussed together because they both lack cell walls. *Mycoplasma pneumoniae* is an important cause of pneumonia and can be isolated on agar medium. Serologic tests on paired sera (by complement fixation, for example) are more often positive than cultures. If cold agglutinins are found in the blood, a presumptive diagnosis of mycoplasmal infection can be made, but both false negatives and false positives are common. L-forms of bacteria must be grown on hypertonic medium.

10.4   LABORATORY DIAGNOSIS OF FUNGI

The diagnosis of fungal disease is often difficult; all possible procedures should be employed. Direct visualization of fungal elements in pus or exudates, using various stains, is particularly helpful in candidiasis, cryptococcosis, and actinomycosis. Culture on Sabouraud dextrose agar is desirable for all fungi except *Candida* and other yeasts which grow well on ordinary bacterial media. Urine culture helps to identify candidal pyelonephritis. Blood and bone marrow cultures are frequently positive in disseminated histoplasmosis.

Fungal serology has come into wide use, including precipitin, hemagglutinating, complement-fixing, and agglutinating antibody systems. Currently, serologic tests are most valuable in candidiasis, coccidioidomycosis, histoplasmosis, and blastomycosis. In addition, cryptococcal antigen can be sought in serum or cerebrospinal fluid by latex slide-agglutination.

Reliance on skin tests for the diagnosis of acute fungal

infection is to be condemned; many patients do not manifest hypersensitivity, and many normal people have been sensitized by previous exposure. Skin test antigens also may produce confusing rises in serum antibody.

10.5 LABORATORY DIAGNOSIS OF RICKETTSIAE

Ordinarily no attempt is made to culture rickettsiae. Instead, diagnosis relies on nonspecific and specific serologic tests. The latter are accomplished with complement-fixing antigens prepared from yolk sacs infected with each species of rickettsia. The nonspecific test is the familiar Weil-Felix reaction, which depends on a heterologous antibody response to Proteus OX organisms. All serologic tests can be negative early in rickettsial infection.

10.6 LABORATORY DIAGNOSIS OF CHLAMYDIAE

Chlamydiae have come into prominence as a cause of pneumonia in the infant, in addition to the previously described inclusion conjunctivitis and psittacosis. The cytoplasmic inclusion bodies characteristic of chlamydiae may be demonstrated directly by Giemsa stain or by FA staining. More sensitive is the isolation of the organism in tissue culture of HeLa type cells that have been treated to prevent cell division.

10.7 LABORATORY DIAGNOSIS OF PROTOZOA

Protozoan infection is identified mainly by direct visualization, for example, of amebae in feces, of *Pneumocystic carinii* in lung aspirates, or of sporozoans in blood. Serologic tests, however, are extremely valuable in the diagnosis of malaria, invasive amebiasis, and toxoplasmosis. The absence of malarial antibodies indicates that malaria has not occurred in the past, but in attacks of short duration treated early, serum antibodies may be evanescent. Screening for toxoplasma antibodies is widely used to identify newborns with possible congenital infection.

10.8 LABORATORY DIAGNOSIS OF HELMINTHS

Traditionally, direct examination of stool or of other materials has been the method of diagnosis of helminthic infection. When tissue invasion occurs, as in trichinosis, echinococcosis, and toxocariasis, serologic procedures become crucial in efforts to identify the parasite before biopsy. These tests are done at the Center for Disease Control, Atlanta, Georgia, United States.

10.9 LABORATORY DIAGNOSIS OF VIRUSES

If viral disease is a diagnostic possibility when the patient is first seen, immediate steps should be taken to confirm the diagnosis since delay usually nullifies attempts at isolation and makes serologic results more difficult to interpret.

Microscopic Observation. Electron microscopy and fluorescent-antibody techniques provide opportunities for quick identification of viruses. Vesicle fluid can be examined by electron microscopy to distinguish smallpox (a poxvirus) from varicella (a herpesvirus). Smears of mucosal cells or urinary sediment can be stained by fluorescent antibody to identify the antigens of any virus for which there is a good animal antiserum, e.g., influenza and respiratory syncytial viruses. Hepatitis A and the rotavirus agents which are a cause of infantile gastroenteritis can be ascertained by immune electron microscopy, but these agents and others can be more conveniently detected by enzyme-linked immune serum assay (ELISA) or radioimmunoassay (RIA) using specific antisera.

Cytologic examination is an aid in diagnosis when inclusion bodies or syncytia are found, as in the urine of patients infected with cytomegalovirus, for example, and in the noses of patients with measles; but such demonstration should be buttressed with actual isolation of the virus.

Isolation. Viruses and rickettsiae require living cells for propagation; the cells used may be in the form of intact laboratory animals, embryonated hens' eggs, or tissue cultures of human or animal cells. Some viruses are difficult to isolate, and since many different tissue culture systems must be employed to isolate a wide range of viruses, the unspecified request from the clinician for "virus isolation" is impractical. Virus laboratories can screen for the most common agents and are materially assisted if the clinician can name the virus suspected or at least can state the type of illness.

Prompt delivery of specimens to the laboratory is essential. In some cases bedside inoculation of cultures may increase the chance of virus recovery. Routinely, throat and stool or rectal swab specimens should be submitted. Throat specimens are best taken by means of vigorous throat swabbing, which results in removing some superficial cells. For certain viruses, e.g., rubella, swabs should be taken from the nasal turbinates. The swab should be rinsed thoroughly in a fluid medium (nutrient broth or 0.5% gelatin in Hanks solution) containing antibiotics to inhibit bacterial growth, squeezed against the glass, and discarded. If the laboratory is reasonably close, specimens may be stored at 4° C for a few hr. If mailed, the specimen should be frozen and packed in dry ice.

Rectal swabs should not be heavily covered with feces as the antibiotics present in viral transport media may be insufficient to kill a large inoculum of bacteria. Rectal swabs should be collected even in respiratory and central nervous system syndromes since many viruses replicate in the intestine as well as in target organs.

Cerebrospinal fluid is often positive during the acute stages of central nervous system inflammation. A small extra amount of spinal fluid for viral diagnostic studies should be obtained at the initial lumbar puncture. This can always be discarded if a positive diagnosis of bacterial meningitis is made.

Urine culture for viruses is most useful for the isolation of cytomegalovirus, but urine is also a good source of mumps and adenoviruses. Urine should not be frozen but rather transported in ordinary ice.

Vesicular fluid can be cultured to distinguish among vaccinia, variola, varicella, herpes, and enteroviruses.

Blood is not routinely cultured for viruses, though viremia is part of many viral infections. The diagnosis of hepatitis B is made by demonstration of the viral antigen which is present in high titer in serum.

The principal difficulties with virus isolation are the fragility of some viruses such as the respiratory syncytial virus on removal from the patient, the need for living cell cultures or organisms as substrates for virus growth, the long time required for some agents to grow, and the uncertainty with which pathogenicity can be attributed to some isolates from the respiratory or gastrointestinal tracts.

Serologic Tests. Serologic tests are likely to be positive even when virus isolation fails. Correct diagnosis requires at least 2 blood specimens: the 1st should be obtained during the early acute phase of the disease ("acute serum"), the 2nd ("convalescent"), 14–21 days later. If the 2nd is taken earlier than 14 days, it is advisable to take a 3rd blood specimen 4–6 wk after the onset since the rise of antibodies may be delayed, especially in infants. Great care must be taken to avoid contamination and hemolysis. If it is not possible to

Table 10–2 MICROBIOLOGIC APPROACHES TO THE DIFFERENTIAL DIAGNOSIS OF FOUR SYNDROMES*†

SYNDROME	TESTS TO BE DONE	SYNDROME	TESTS TO BE DONE
Exanthem of uncertain origin (See also specific conditions mentioned)	Blood culture for bacteria (e.g., meningococci, *Salmonella typhosa*) Throat culture for streptococcus Serologic test for antibodies to streptococcal toxins Serologic test for syphilis Serologic test for toxoplasmosis Serologic test for rickettsiae (Proteus OX and specific CF antibodies) Nose and throat swabs for viruses (measles, rubella, enteroviruses) Rectal swab for viruses (e.g., enteroviruses) Serologic tests for heterophile antibodies and EB virus antibodies (infectious mononucleosis) Serologic tests for viruses (e.g., measles, rubella)	**Pulmonary infiltrates of uncertain nature** (Continued)	Fluorescent stain of sputum or gastric washings for mycobacteria Fluorescent stain of sputum for *Legionella* Sputum or gastric washings for mycobacterial culture PPD–S skin test for mycobacterial hypersensitivity Sputum stain and culture for fungi Serologic tests for fungal antibodies Lung biopsy (preferred) or aspiration for *Pneumocystis carinii* (patient on immunosuppressive therapy) Throat culture for *Mycoplasma pneumoniae* Serologic test for cold agglutinins (*Mycoplasma pneumoniae*) Serologic test for antibodies to *M. pneumoniae* Cultures for *Chlamydia* Serologic test for psittacosis Serologic test for Q fever antibodies Nasopharyngeal and rectal swabs for viruses Urine culture for cytomegalovirus Serologic tests for viral antibodies (e.g., adenoviruses, respiratory syncytial viruses)
Meningitis, suspected (See also specific conditions mentioned)	CSF stain and culture for bacteria Blood culture for bacteria CSF fluorochrome stain for mycobacteria CSF culture for mycobacteria PPD–S skin test for mycobacterial hypersensitivity CSF culture for leptospira Serologic test for leptospirosis CSF culture for fungi India ink preparation for cryptococci CSF and serum for cryptococcal antigen Serologic tests for fungal antibiotics CSF culture for free-living amebae on HeLa cells or on special agar plates CSF culture for viruses Nasopharyngeal and rectal swabs for viruses (e.g., mumps, enteroviruses) Serologic tests for viruses (e.g., mumps, arboviruses)	**Neonatal infection, suspected** (See also Neonatal Septicemia, Sec 7.59, and specific conditions)	Blood culture for bacteria Throat cultures for bacteria Rectal cultures for bacteria Urine cultures for bacteria Gastric aspirate for bacterial stain and culture Serologic test for syphilis Serologic test for toxoplasma antibodies Nasal swab for rubella virus Throat swab for viruses (e.g., herpes, Coxsackie B) Rectal swab for viruses (e.g., Coxsackie B, echo) Urine culture for viruses (cytomegalovirus, herpes) Serologic tests for cytomegalovirus, rubella, western equine encephalitis Serologic test for hepatitis B antigen
Pulmonary infiltrates of uncertain nature (See also Chapter 12, and specific conditions)	Blood culture for bacteria Tracheal aspirate or sputum culture for bacteria Gram stain of tracheal aspirate or sputum Fluorescent stain of nasopharyngeal swabs for pertussis		

*Not all tests will necessarily need to be done in any given situation, but when the diagnosis is obscure many of these will be indicated.
†Where serologic tests are suggested, paired sera are required.

send blood to the laboratory promptly, serum may be removed for preservation by freezing. Whole blood should never be frozen. To establish the etiologic diagnosis, it is necessary to demonstrate a 4-fold rise in titer of specific antibody in the convalescent as opposed to the acute phase serum. A battery of antigens is tested, including the viruses most likely to be the cause of the clinical syndrome.

Although finding a substantial titer against a suspected agent in a single late acute or convalescent specimen of serum will not differentiate between a recent and a past infection, under the following circumstances the study of a single serum specimen can strongly support a clinical diagnosis: (1) a high antibody level in comparison with that of the population in general; (2) particularly in neonates and in patients in the acute stage of hepatitis A, antibody in the IgM fraction; (3) antibody in the young infant not present in the mother; (4) antibody in both infant and mother which persists at the neonatal level in the infant; (5) in suspected mumps, the presence of antibody to the soluble ("S") fraction of the mumps virus in the acute serum (this antibody may be found as early as the 2nd or 3rd day of the disease, when that to the viral ("V") antigen may be absent or very low); and (6) in infectious mononucleosis, the presence of antibody to the early antigen found in cells infected by EB virus under specific conditions of preparation.

Methods of Detecting Antibody. Antibody can be detected by a variety of specific serologic methods, some being more appropriate than others for specific viruses. Complement-fixation (CF) antigens are available for a great range of viruses, and CF antibodies have the advantage of being generally correlated with recent infection. In poliomyelitis, for example, CF antibodies appear during acute infection and often disappear within a yr. Neutralizing antibodies, on the other hand, remain for life; unless one has obtained serum early in the disease, a rise may be difficult to show. Furthermore, neutralization tests have the technical disadvantage of needing to be done in tissue cultures or in whole animals. Hemagglutination-inhibition (HI) antibodies correlate fairly well with neutralizing antibodies. Fortunately, many viruses such as the myxoviruses, rubella, and some enteroviruses have the capacity to agglutinate erythrocytes. The presence of antibodies can be detected by the extent to which a particular serum specifically inhibits hemagglutination. Many of the viruses that agglutinate red cells will also cause adsorption of red cells to the membranes of infected cell monolayers. Inhibition of adsorption is a particularly useful test for parainfluenza virus antibodies. Fluorescent antibodies (FA) can be detected by the technique of indirect fluorescence (see above). For their demonstration FA require slides bearing cells infected with the specific virus against which antibodies are being sought. Indirect hemagglutination tests are now in greater use in virology; these depend on the attachment of viral antigens to glutaraldehyde or tannic acid treated sheep erythrocytes. Radioimmunoassays and enzyme-linked immunoassays are also being used more widely.

APPLICATION OF MICROBIOLOGY TO DIAGNOSTIC PROBLEMS

When the diagnosis is uncertain but infection is a possibility, a systematic approach involving multiple cultures and serologic procedures is necessary. Diagnostic strategies will, of course, depend on the severity of the illness, the epidemiology, and the clinical likelihood of certain infections. Table 10–2 presents examples of complete microbiologic approaches to certain diagnostic problems, indicating the tests that *might* be considered for patients presenting (1) an exanthem, (2) the possibility of meningitis, (3) pulmonary infiltrates of uncertain nature, or (4) possible infection in the neonatal period.

STANLEY A. PLOTKIN

Drew WL (ed): Viral Infections: A Clinical Approach. Philadelphia, FA Davis, 1976.
Lennette EH, Balows A, Hausler WJ, et al: Manual of Clinical Microbiology. Washington DC, American Society for Microbiology, 1980.
Lennette EH, Schmidt NJ: Diagnostic Procedures for Viral, Rickettsial and Chlamydial Infections. Washington DC, American Public Health Association Inc, 1979.
Shackelford PG, Campbell J, Feigin RD: Countercurrent immunoelectrophoresis in the evaluation of childhood infections. J Pediatr 85:478, 1974.

SOME CLINICAL SYNDROMES USUALLY OF INFECTIOUS ORIGIN

The purpose of this section is to provide a rational approach to the management of children with certain recognizable clinical syndromes, signs, or symptoms which may or may not be of infectious origin. Other syndromes, signs, and symptoms (e.g., vomiting, pneumonia, upper respiratory infection, urinary tract infection, failure to thrive) are discussed elsewhere (see Index).

10.10 FEVER OF UNKNOWN ORIGIN

Many physicians use the diagnosis of fever of unknown origin (FUO) for any febrile child admitted to the hospital without an apparent diagnosis. The term should be reserved for children with (1) documented fever of more than 1 wk duration, (2) fever also documented in hospital, and (3) no apparent diagnosis after an investigation of 1 wk in hospital.

A number of generalizations about this diagnosis can be substantiated: (1) Most fevers of unknown origin result from common diseases that may be atypical in their presentations. In some cases the presentation of a fever of unknown origin is typical of the disease (juvenile rheumatoid arthritis), but a definitive diagnosis can be established only after a prolonged period of observation because there are no associated findings on physical examination and all laboratory results are negative or normal. (2) The principal causes of fever of unknown origin in children are infections and collagen-vascular diseases. Neoplastic disorders are a serious consideration, but most children with malignancies do not have fever alone. (3) In the United States the infectious diseases implicated most consistently in children with fever of unknown origin have been salmonellosis, tularemia, tuberculosis, rickettsial diseases, brucellosis, syphilis, leptospirosis, rat-bite fever, infectious mononucleosis, cytomegalic inclusion disease, and hepatitis. (4) Juvenile rheumatoid arthritis and systemic lupus erythematosus are the collagen diseases associated most frequently with fever of unknown origin. (5) Fever should be documented in hospital by an individual who remains in attendance through the period of time in which the temperature is taken to rule out factitious fever. (6) Prolonged and continuous observation of the patient is imperative. Repetitive evaluation including history, physical examination, and roentgenographic studies may be required. (7) If the patient is receiving drugs, the possibility of drug fever should be considered. It is not usually associated with other symptoms, and temperature remains elevated at a relatively constant level. Withdrawal of the drug is associated with resolution of the fever, generally within 72 hr (when drugs, such as iodides, are excreted over a prolonged period of time, fever may persist for up to 1 mo after drug withdrawal).

Table 10–3 lists diseases that have presented as fever of unknown origin in children with sufficient frequency to merit serious consideration. Specific signs and symptoms of each of these diseases and methods of diagnosis are detailed elsewhere.

Table 10–3 SOME CAUSES OF FEVER OF UNKNOWN ORIGIN IN CHILDREN

Bacterial diseases
  Abscesses: dental, liver, pelvic, perinephric, subdiaphragmatic
  Bacterial endocarditis
  Brucellosis
  Leptospirosis
  Mastoiditis (chronic)
  Osteomyelitis
  Pyelonephritis
  Salmonellosis
  Sinusitis
  Tuberculosis
  Tularemia
Viral diseases
  Cytomegalic inclusion disease
  Hepatitis (chronic active)
  Infectious mononucleosis
Chlamydial diseases
  Lymphogranuloma venereum
  Psittacosis
Rickettsial diseases
  Q fever
  Rocky Mountain spotted fever
Fungal diseases
  Blastomycosis (nonpulmonary)
  Histoplasmosis (disseminated)
Parasitic diseases
  Malaria
  Toxoplasmosis
  Visceral larva migrans
Unclassified
  Sarcoidosis
Collagen vascular diseases
  Juvenile rheumatoid arthritis
  Polyarteritis nodosa
  Systemic lupus erythematosus
Malignancies
  Hodgkin disease
  Lymphoma
  Neuroblastoma
Miscellaneous disorders
  Anhidrotic ectodermal dysplasia
  Diabetes insipidus (non-nephrogenic and nephrogenic)
  Drug fever
  Factitious fever
  Familial dysautonomia
  Granulomatous colitis
  Infantile cortical hyperostosis
  Pancreatitis
  Periodic fever
  Serum sickness
  Thyrotoxicosis
  Ulcerative colitis

Diagnostic Approach to the Child with Fever of Unknown Origin

History. (1) A history of *exposure to wild or domestic animals* must be solicited. The incidence of zoonotic infections in the United States has been increasing yearly. They frequently are acquired from pets who are not overtly ill. For example, immunization of dogs against specific disorders such as leptospirosis may prevent canine disease but does not always prevent the animal from carrying and shedding leptospires which may be transmitted to household contacts. A history of ingestion of rabbit or squirrel meat may provide a clue to the diagnosis of oropharyngeal, glandular, or typhoidal tularemia. (2) A history of *pica* should be sought. Ingestion of dirt is a particularly important clue to infection with *Toxocara* (visceral larva migrans) or *Toxoplasma gondii* (toxoplasmosis). (3) A history of *travel* reaching back to the birth of the child should be sought. There may be re-emergence of malaria, histoplasmosis, and coccidioidomycosis years after visiting or living in an endemic area. It is important to ask about prophylactic immunizations and precautions taken by the individual against the ingestion of contaminated water or food during foreign travel. Rocks, dirt, and artifacts from geographically distant regions which have been collected and brought into the home as souvenirs may serve as vectors of disease. (4) A *medication* history should be pursued rigorously. This must include over-the-counter preparations and topical agents, including eye drops (atropine-induced fever). (5) The *genetic background* of the patient also is important. Descendants of the Ulster Scots may have fever of unknown origin because they are afflicted with nephrogenic diabetes insipidus. Familial dysautonomia (Riley-Day syndrome, a disorder in which hyperthermia is recurrent) is more frequent among Jews than other population groups.

Physical Examination. (1) Sweating in a febrile child should be noted. The continuing absence of sweat in the presence of an elevated or changing body temperature suggests dehydration from vomiting, diarrhea, or central or nephrogenic diabetes insipidus. Absence of sweat in the presence of fever also suggests anhidrotic ectodermal dysplasia, familial dysautonomia, or exposure to atropine. (2) Red, weeping eyes may be a sign of collagen-vascular disease, particularly polyarteritis nodosa. (3) Palpebral conjunctivitis in the febrile patient may be a clue to measles, coxsackieviral infection, tuberculosis, infectious mononucleosis, lymphogranuloma venereum, or cat-scratch or Newcastle disease virus infection. In contrast, bulbar conjunctivitis in a child with fever of unknown origin suggests leptospirosis. (4) Fever of unknown origin sometimes is due to hypothalamic dysfunction. A clue to this disorder is failure of pupillary constriction due to absence of the sphincter constrictor muscle of the eye. This muscle is derived from ectoderm rather than mesoderm and develops embryologically when hypothalamic structure and function also are undergoing differentiation.

(5) Lack of tears or an absent corneal reflex may suggest fever from familial dysautonomia. (6) Tenderness to tapping over the sinuses and teeth should be sought, and the sinuses should be transilluminated. (7) A smooth tongue may reflect absence of fungiform papillae and suggest a diagnosis of familial dysautonomia. Oral candidiasis may be a clue to various disorders of the immune system. (8) Fever blisters are common findings in patients with pneumococcal, streptococcal, malarial, and rickettsial infection. They also are common in children with meningococcal meningitis (which usually does not present as fever of unknown origin) but rarely are seen in children with meningococcemia. Fever blisters rarely are seen with salmonellal or staphylococcal infections. (9) Repetitive chills and temperature spikes are common in children with septicemia (regardless of etiology), particularly when associated with renal disease, liver or biliary disease, endocarditis, malaria, brucellosis, rat-bite fever, or loculated collections of pus. (10) Hyperemia of the pharynx, with or without exudate, may suggest infectious mononucleosis, cytomegalic inclusion disease, toxoplasmosis, salmonellosis, tularemia, or leptospirosis. (11) The muscles and bones should be palpated carefully. Point tenderness over a bone may suggest occult osteomyelitis or bone marrow invasion from neoplastic disease. Tenderness over the trapezius muscle may be a clue to a subdiaphragmatic abscess. Generalized muscle tenderness suggests dermatomyositis, trichinosis, polyarteritis, or mycoplasmal or arboviral infection.

(12) Rectal examination may reveal pararectal adenopathy or tenderness and suggest a deep pelvic abscess, iliac adenitis, or pelvic osteomyelitis. A guaiac test should be obtained on any stool found on the examining finger; occult blood loss may suggest granulomatous colitis or ulcerative colitis as the cause of fever of unknown origin. (13) The general activity of the patient and the presence or absence of rashes must be noted.

(14) Hyperactive deep tendon reflexes may suggest thyrotoxicosis as the cause of fever of unknown origin.

Laboratory Studies. These should be directed toward the diagnostic tests most likely to provide a definitive diagnosis promptly; the general tendency to order a large number of tests in every child with fever of unknown origin according to a predetermined sequence wastes time and money. The tempo of diagnostic evolution should be adjusted to the tempo of the illness; haste may be imperative in a critically ill patient, but if the illness is more chronic, the evaluation can proceed more slowly and deliberately.

Routine *white blood cell counts* and *urinalyses* generally have been of minimal diagnostic value in children who fulfill a rigorous definition of fever of unknown origin. An absolute neutrophil count below 5000, however, is strong evidence against nonoverwhelming bacterial infection other than typhoid. Conversely, patients with more than 10,000 polymorphonuclear leukocytes or 500 nonsegmented polymorphonuclear leukocytes/mm^3 have an 80% chance of having a severe bacterial infection.

An elevated *erythrocyte sedimentation rate* (>30 mm/hr, Westergren method) indicates inflammation and the need for further evaluation. A *nitroblue tetrazolium dye (NBT) test* may suggest the presence of bacterial infection.

Blood cultures should be obtained aerobically and anaerobically. The isolation of leptospires, *Francisella*, or *Yersinia* may require selective media or specific conditions not routinely employed.

Tuberculin *skin testing* should be performed carefully with polysorbate 80 (Tween) stabilized purified protein derivative (PPD) which has been kept appropriately refrigerated.

Urine culture should be obtained routinely. Roentgenographic study of the urinary tract may be indicated.

Roentgenographic examination of the chest, sinuses, mastoids, or gastrointestinal tract may be suggested by specific historic or physical findings. Roentgenographic evaluation of the gastrointestinal tract for granulomatous colitis may be helpful in the evaluation of selected children with fever of unknown origin and no other localizing signs or symptoms.

Examination of the *bone marrow* may reveal leukemia; metastatic neoplasm; mycobacterial, fungal, or parasitic diseases; and histiocytosis or other-storage diseases. If a bone marrow aspirate is performed, cultures for bacteria, *Mycobacterium*, and fungi should be obtained routinely.

Serologic tests may permit the diagnosis of infectious mononucleosis, cytomegaloviral disease, toxoplasmosis, salmonellosis, tularemia, brucellosis, leptospirosis, and, on some occasions, juvenile rheumatoid arthritis. For histoplasmosis, yeast and mycelial phase complement fixation tests may suggest the diagnosis. *Lymph node biopsies* and *exploratory laparotomies* seem helpful in children only when physical examination suggests they may be indicated.

Radioactive scans may be helpful in detecting osteomyelitis and abdominal abscesses. *Echocardiograms* may suggest the presence of vegetations on the leaflets of heart valves as in subacute bacterial endocarditis. Total body scanning permits the detection of neoplasms and collections of purulent material without the use of surgical exploration or radioisotopes.

Treatment. Fever and infection in children are not synonymous; antibiotics should not be used as antipyretics; empiric trials of medication should generally be avoided. An exception may be the use of antituberculous treatment in critically ill children with possible disseminated tuberculosis. Empiric trials of other antibiotics may be dangerous and can obscure the diagnosis of endocarditis, meningitis, parameningeal infection, or osteomyelitis. Hospitalization may be required for laboratory or roentgenographic studies which are unavailable or impractical in an ambulatory setting, for more careful observation, or for temporary relief of parental anxiety.

Prognosis. The child with fever of unknown origin has a better prognosis than that reported in adult studies, which suggest a mortality rate of 25–40%. In many cases no diagnosis can be established, but fever abates spontaneously. In as many as 25% of cases in which fever persists, the cause of fever will remain unclear even after thorough evaluation.

Felgin RD, Shearer WT: Fever of unknown origin in children. Curr Probl Pediatr 6:1, 1976.
Naiman JL, Bergman GE: Hematologic clues to systemic disease in childhood. Semin Hematol 12:287, 1975.

10.11 RASH

Rashes accompany many infectious diseases. They may be so characteristic of a particular disease that a specific diagnosis can be made without difficulty, but frequently the skin manifestations produced are common to many infections. Skin lesions may be the result of direct inoculation of the skin (e.g., anthrax or tularemia); hematogenous dissemination of microorganisms (e.g., septicemia due to meningococci or other bacteria); or contiguous spread from adjacent foci of infection (e.g., impetigo, herpetic lesions). The skin also may reflect the effect of toxins (e.g., scarlet fever), antigen-antibody reactions (e.g., rheumatic fever), or delayed hypersensitivity to the infecting agent (e.g., erythema nodosum).

Accurate diagnosis of patients with rashes presumed to be of infectious origin depends upon a careful history and an accurate, careful description of the skin lesions. Of specific interest are the nature and duration of any prodromal symptoms and an accurate description of the initial appearance and the evolution of the skin signs and symptoms. Pathognomonic signs (e.g., Koplik spots of measles) simplify diagnosis. In many cases the best the clinician can do is classify the disorder tentatively as viral, bacterial, or rickettsial or develop a list of a variety of infections that might be identified by appropriate cultural or serologic tests.

Rashes can be classified as macular eruptions, erythematous maculopapular eruptions, papulovesicular or bullous eruptions, petechial or hemorrhagic eruptions, ulcerative eruptions, and nodular eruptions; Tables 10–4 through 10–12 are arranged accordingly. Since some infections produce lesions that fall into more than 1 of these categories, the differential diagnostic lists in the tables are not always mutually exclusive.

Some infectious diseases and their agents are associated with erythema multiforme eruptions or with erythema nodosum (Tables 10–11 and 10–12). In some patients, meningitis and pneumonia are associated with exanthems; agents that have been associated with exanthems and meningitis or pneumonia are shown in Tables 10–13 and 10–14, respectively.

After an appropriate list of potential diagnoses has been assembled on the basis of the appearance of the skin lesions, further attempts to modify the list can be made through pertinent historic data. In most cases the specific diagnosis can be made, sometimes only retrospectively, if appropriate cultures and serologic data are obtained. Antibiotic therapy for possible bacterial infections should be initiated promptly but only after cultures of blood and skin lesions have been obtained. It is important to use media capable of supporting the growth of the organisms suspected of causing the infection. Skin biopsy may aid in the diagnosis of some of these disorders (e.g., rickettsial diseases or noninfectious papulovesicular eruptions). Vesicular or pustular skin lesions suspected to be due to viruses also should be cultured appropriately if the diagnosis cannot be established clinically. In some cases viruses may be recovered directly from the fluid of unruptured vesicles (e.g., varicella-zoster, herpes).

RALPH D. FEIGIN

Duncan WC: Cutaneous manifestations of infectious disease. In: Hoeprich PD (ed): Infectious Diseases. Ed 2. Hagerstown Md., Harper and Row, 1977.
Krugman S, Ward R, Katz SL: Infectious Diseases of Children. Ed 6. St. Louis, CV Mosby, 1977, p 472.

Table 10–4 INFECTIOUS AGENTS ASSOCIATED WITH ILLNESSES IN WHICH A MACULAR EXANTHEM HAS BEEN OBSERVED

INFECTIOUS AGENT	ILLNESS
Epstein-Barr virus	Infectious mononucleosis
Coxsackieviruses B1, B2, B5	—
Echoviruses 2, 4, 5, 14, 17, 18, 19, 30	—
Enterovirus 71	—
Dengue virus	Dengue fever
Lassa virus	Lassa fever
Marburg virus	Marburg fever
Chlamydia psittaci	Psittacosis
Rickettsia typhi	Murine typhus
Rickettsia prowazekii	Epidemic typhus
Rickettsia quintana	Trench fever
Mycoplasma pneumoniae	
Staphylococcus aureus	Septicemia
Streptococcus pyogenes	Scarlatina, septicemia
Bacillus anthracis	Anthrax
Salmonella typhi	Typhoid fever
Salmonella sp.	Septicemic salmonellosis
Spirillum minus	Rat bite fever
Yersinia pestis	Plague
*	Erythema infectiosum

From Cherry JD, In: Feigin RD, Cherry JD (eds): Textbook of Pediatric Infectious Diseases. Philadelphia, WB Saunders, 1981.
*Presumed to be of infectious etiology.

Text continued on page 610

Table 10–5 AGENTS OR DISEASES ASSOCIATED WITH MACULOPAPULAR RASHES

AGENT OR DISEASE	COMMENT
Viral	
Alphavirus: chikungunya, Sindbis, O'nyong-nyong fever, Ross fever	Discrete or confluent lesions
Arbovirus	May produce scarlatiniform maculopapules
Colorado tick fever virus	Discrete lesions
Coxsackieviruses	Types A5, A10, A16 and A9 also may produce vesicular or pustular lesions, as in hand, foot, and mouth disease
Cytomegalovirus	
EB virus (infectious mononucleosis)	Ampicillin increases incidence of rash
Echovirus	Particularly types 4, 6, 9, 11, 16, 18
Enterovirus 71	Lesions may be discrete or confluent
Flavivirus: dengue, kunjin	
Hepatitis B virus	Discrete lesions
Influenza viruses A, B	Discrete lesions
Marburg virus	Discrete or confluent lesions
Measles	Koplik spots pathognomonic
Mumps virus	Discrete lesions
Parainfluenza viruses 1-4	Discrete lesions
Reovirus 2, 3	Discrete or confluent lesions
Respiratory syncytial viruses	Discrete lesions
Rhinoviruses (many types)	Discrete lesions
Rubella virus	
Varicella-zoster (chickenpox, herpes zoster)	Maculopapular lesions early in course progress to vesiculopustular lesions; lesions of various types present on body at same time that new crops appear
Smallpox (variola), vaccinia	Lesions progress to vesicles and pustules and tend to be in same stage at same time
Presumed viral	
Roseola infantum	Rash appears when fever abates, preceded by 4–6 days of fever of 40–41° C (104–106° F) without localizing signs
Erythema infectiosum (fifth disease)	Slapped-face appearance; lesions on trunk may be evanescent and reticulated
Chlamydial	
Psittacosis	Faint macules may be evanescent
Rickettsial	
Endemic typhus, epidemic typhus, trench fever, tsutsugamushi fever	Rash appears on trunk and extends to extremities
Rocky Mountain spotted fever	Rash appears on extremities and moves to trunk; petechial or purpuric lesions may develop
Rickettsialpox	Rash varies from maculopapular to vesicular; initial lesion may be a vesicle
Bacterial	
Erysipelothrix	Red macules; may become purplish in color and extend slowly on hands and fingers
Leptospirosis (leptospires)	Rash may involve entire body, palms, soles, and may desquamate
Listeria monocytogenes	Macules may develop central necrosis with pustule formation
Mycobacterium leprae (leprosy)	Lesions may become depigmented or remain permanently pigmented
Salmonella	Evanescent rash (rose spots) on trunk
Streptococcus pyogenes (scarlet fever)	Rash due to toxin; gooseflesh or sandpaper texture; most marked in body creases; circumoral pallor; desquamation develops with time
Streptococcus pyogenes (rheumatic fever)	Erythema marginatum: macules coalesce, with annular patterns on trunk and extremities
Streptobacillus moniliformis (Haverhill fever)	Generalized maculopapular rash, including palms and soles
Spirillum minus (rat-bite fever)	Red-purple macules on trunk, extremities, palms, and soles
Staphylococcus aureus (scalded skin syndrome)	Due to exfoliative toxin; lesions ultimately desquamate
Treponema pallidum (syphilis)	Lesions can be localized or generalized; mucosal ulcerations may be noted
Treponema carateum (pinta)	Erythematous macules become depigmented with time
Fungal	
Tinea versicolor	Brownish-white maculopapules, particularly on trunk
Tinea (*Trichophyton, Epidermophyton*)	Erythematous macules become papular, confluent, or vesiculated; hair loss may be noted
Coccidioides immitis (coccidioidomycosis)	Produces discrete or confluent lesions

Table continued on following page

Table 10–5 AGENTS OR DISEASES ASSOCIATED WITH MACULOPAPULAR RASHES *Continued*

AGENT OR DISEASE	COMMENT
Protozoan	
Malaria	Erythematous, maculopapular, urticarial rash observed in chronic cases
Toxoplasma gondii (toxoplasmosis)	Rash evanescent; palms and soles generally spared
Other parasites	
Ancylostoma duodenale, Necator americanus (hookworm disease)	Pruritic papules may become vesicular
Ancylostoma braziliensis (creeping eruption or cutaneous larva migrans)	Lesions may become linear and pruritic
Wuchereria (filariasis)	Edema develops over involved lymphatics
Onchocerca volvulus (onchocerciasis)	Erysipeloid lesions may be pruritic
Schistosomiasis	Swimmer's itch; erythematous macules become pruritic and then vesiculate
Trichinella spiralis (trichinosis)	May develop erythema multiforme; lesions may be urticarial
Scabies	Lesions pruritic, most marked in skin folds
Pediculosis (lice)	Pruritic macules
Flea bites	Pruritic, grouped macules
Collagen diseases	
Juvenile rheumatoid arthritis	Small, pale, red-pink macules, often with central pallor; tend to appear during febrile periods
Systemic lupus erythematosus	Erythematous blush or scaly, erythematous patches over malar areas; vasculitic changes may occur, chiefly on extremities
Dermatomyositis	Violaceous, scaly erythema, especially over extensor surface of joints
Anaphylactoid purpura	Vasculitic rash, becoming purpuric, then rusty as it fades; predilection for buttocks and upper legs
Unclassified	
Erythema multiforme	Erythematous macules and papules; may be vesicular on mucous membranes or, rarely, on skin; follows infection by various bacteria, viruses, fungi, and noninfectious diseases (e.g., granulomatous colitis, hypersensitivity to drugs)
Mucocutaneous lymph node syndrome	Vasculitis of unknown etiology; rash desquamates

Table 10–6 AGENTS OR DISEASES ASSOCIATED WITH VESICULAR OR BULLOUS ERUPTIONS

AGENT OR DISEASE	COMMENT
Viral	
Alphaviruses: chikungunya, O'nyong-nyong fever, Ross River, Sindbis	
Coxsackievirus A4, A5, A8, A10, A15, A16	Hand, foot, and mouth syndrome; mucous membranes involved
Coxsackievirus B1, B2, B3	
Herpes simplex	Vesicles on skin, lips, mouth, pharynx, genitalia
Kunjin	
Measles virus	
Monkeypox virus	As atypical measles
Mumps	
Orf virus	
Reovirus 2	Produces ecthyma contagiosum
Smallpox	
Tanapox virus	Maculopapules → vesicles → scabs
Vaccinia	
Varicella-zoster (chickenpox)	Maculopapules → vesicles → scabs
Bacterial	Maculopapules → vesicles → scabs
Bacillus anthracis	
Mycobacterium tuberculosis	In selected cases of anthrax
Pseudomonas aeruginosa	
Streptococcus pyogenes and Staphylococcus aureus	Erythema → weeping vesicles → crusting; Organisms can be recovered from lesions
Rickettsial	
Rickettsia tsutsugamushi	Tsutsugamushi fever
Rickettsialpox	Seen in urban dwellers due to rodent mite bite; self-limited disease
Fungal	Vesicles that do not contain fungi develop in various fungal diseases (id reaction)
Parasitic	
Leishmania braziliensis	
Necator americanus	Hookworm disease
Others (noninfectious)	Hookworm disease
Insect bites	See index
Drug eruptions	See index
Dermatitis herpetiformis	See index
Incontinentia pigmenti	See index
Epidermolysis bullosa (various forms)	See index
Pemphigus	See index
Pemphigoid	See index

Table 10–7 AGENTS OR DISEASES ASSOCIATED WITH PETECHIAL OR PURPURIC LESIONS

AGENT OR DISEASE	COMMENT
Bacterial	
Anthrax	Hemorrhagic necrosis develops in center of original papular lesions
Neisseria meningitidis and many other bacteria, fungi, and rickettsiae	Petechial and purpuric lesions may be few in number or disseminated widely; lesions may contain the organism
Pseudomonas or Aeromonas	Ecthyma gangrenosum (red erythematous) lesions that become purplish and nodular; may develop central hemorrhagic necrosis
Rickettsial	
Endemic typhus; epidemic typhus; Rocky Mountain spotted fever	Basic pathophysiology is endothelial damage; petechial or purpuric lesions may reflect that damage or be due to thrombocytopenia or, rarely, disseminated intravascular coagulation
Viral	
Alphaviruses: chikungunya, O'nyong-nyong fever, Ross River, Sindbis	
Arbovirus (dengue, hemorrhagic fevers)	Diffuse petechial and purpuric lesions; history of residence in or travel to endemic areas helpful
Colorado tick fever virus	
Coxsackieviruses A4, A9	
Coxsackieviruses B2, B3, B4	
Echoviruses 4, 7, 9	
Infectious mononucleosis; cytomegaloviral disease; hepatitis	Petechial lesions may be seen as evidence of vasculitis
Lassa virus	Lassa fever
Marburg virus	
Measles virus	Hemorrhagic (black measles)
Respiratory syncytial virus	
Rubella virus	Congenital rubella
Varicella-zoster	Hemorrhagic chickenpox
Variola virus	Hemorrhagic smallpox
Mycoplasma	
Mycoplasma pneumoniae	
Parasitic	
Toxoplasma gondii	Congenital toxoplasmosis
Trichinella spiralis	Trichinosis
Others	
Spider bite	Painful, purpuric-necrotic lesions may be noted

Table 10–8 AGENTS OR DISEASES ASSOCIATED WITH ULCERATIVE LESIONS

AGENT OR DISEASE	COMMENT
Candida albicans	Superficial ulcerations of skin and mucous membrane on erythematous base
Chancroid	Painful, shallow, purulent ulcer
Diphtheria (cutaneous)	A shallow ulcer with a firm body may be noted
Leishmaniasis	Maculopapular lesions; may ulcerate
Lymphogranuloma venereum	Ulcerations of external genitalia or genital mucous membranes
Sporotrichosis	Nodule at site of inoculation; may ulcerate
Syphilis	Ulcers with indurated borders at site of primary inoculation
Tuberculosis and atypical mycobacteria	Papules or nodules of skin, may ulcerate
Tularemia	Ulcers at site of initial entry of organism
Yaws	Ulcerating granulomatous lesions of skin

Table 10–9 DISEASES ASSOCIATED WITH NODULAR SKIN LESIONS

DISEASE	COMMENT
Erythema nodosum (see also Table 10–12)	Erythematous nodules of extensor surfaces of body presumably reflect hypersensitivity reaction; reported in patients with infections due to streptococci, meningococci, mycobacteria, F. tularensis, Coccidioides immitis, Histoplasma capsulatum, Blastomyces, leishmania, EB virus, cat-scratch disease; also may be seen in patients without infectious diseases, including collagen-vascular diseases, drug sensitivity, granulomatous colitis, ulcerative colitis
Leishmaniasis, Oriental sore, Leishmania tropica	Purple papules or nodules may ulcerate and become crusted
Leprosy	Nodules may develop on face, ears, elbows, knees, and buttocks
Tuberculosis (lupus vulgaris)	Papules enlarge and become nodular and finally pustular

Table 10–10 INFECTIOUS AGENTS ASSOCIATED WITH ILLNESSES IN WHICH URTICARIAL EXANTHEMS OCCUR

INFECTIOUS AGENT	ILLNESS
Epstein-Barr virus	Infectious mononucleosis
Coxsackieviruses A9, A16, B4, B5	
Echovirus 11	
Mumps virus	Mumps
Hepatitis B virus	
Mycoplasma pneumoniae	
Neisseria meningitidis	Meningococcemia
Plasmodium sp.	Malaria
Giardia lamblia	Giardiasis
Entamoeba histolytica	Amebiasis
Trichomonas vaginalis	Vulvovaginitis
Enterobius vermicularis	Pinworm infestation
Necator americanus	Hookworm disease
Trichinella spiralis	Trichinosis
Schistosoma sp.	Schistosomiasis
Trichobilharzia sp.	Swimmer's itch; collector's itch
Wuchereria bancrofti	Filariasis
Echinococcus sp.	Echinococcosis
Sarcoptes scabiei	Sabies
Trombicula irritans	Chigger bites
Other mites	Mite bites
Pediculus humanus	Pediculosis
Bedbugs, kissing bugs, ants, fleas, flies and mosquitoes	Bites and stings

From Cherry D, In: Feigin RD, Cherry JD (eds): Textbook of Pediatric Infectious Diseases. Philadelphia, WB Saunders, 1981.

Table 10–11 INFECTIOUS AGENTS ASSOCIATED WITH ERYTHEMA MULTIFORME

AGENT	ILLNESS
Adenovirus 7	Respiratory infection
Herpes simplex virus 1	Perioral or respiratory infection
Epstein-Barr virus	Infectious mononucleosis
Coxsackieviruses A10, A16, B5	Enterovirus syndrome
Echovirus 6	Enterovirus syndrome
Poliomyelitis virus	Poliomyelitis
Vaccinia virus	Smallpox vaccination
Variola virus	Smallpox
Orf virus	Ecthyma contagiosum
Paravaccinia virus	Milker's nodules
Influenza A virus	Influenza
Mumps	Mumps
Hepatitis B virus	Serum hepatitis
Chlamydia psittaci	Psittacosis
Chlamydia trachomatis group	Lymphogranuloma venereum
Mycoplasma pneumoniae	Respiratory symptoms
Staphylococcus aureus	Septicemia
Streptococcus pyogenes	Respiratory symptoms
Neisseria gonorrhoeae	Gonorrhea
Corynebacterium diphtheriae	Diphtheria
Pseudomonas aeruginosa	Septicemia
Salmonella sp.	Gastroenteritis
Francisella tularensis	Tularemia
Yersinia sp.	Gastrointestinal symptoms
Vibrio parahemolyticus	Gastroenteritis
Treponema pallidum	Syphilis
Mycobacterium tuberculosis	Tuberculosis
Mycobacterium leprae	Leprosy
Coccidioides immitis	Coccidioidomycosis
Histoplasma capsulatum	Histoplasmosis
Trichomonas vaginalis	Vulvovaginitis
Presumed infectious etiology	Cat scratch fever

From Cherry JD, In: Feigin RD, Cherry JD (eds): Textbook of Pediatric Infectious Diseases. Philadelphia, WB Saunders, 1981.

Table 10–12 INFECTIOUS AGENTS ASSOCIATED WITH ERYTHEMA NODOSUM

AGENT	ILLNESS
Herpes simplex virus	Perioral or respiratory infection
Chlamydia psittaci	Psittacosis
Chlamydia trachomatis group	Lymphogranuloma venereum
Streptococcus pyogenes	Respiratory infection
Neisseria meningitidis	Meningococcemia
Corynebacterium diphtheriae	Diphtheria
Hemophilus ducreyi	Chancroid
Yersinia sp.	Gastrointestinal symptoms
Treponema pallidum	Syphilis
Mycobacterium tuberculosis	Tuberculosis
Mycobacterium leprae	Leprosy
Histoplasma capsulatum	Histoplasmosis
Cryptococcus neoformans	Cryptococcosis
Coccidioides immitis	Coccidioidomycosis
Blastomyces dermatitidis	Blastomycosis
Ascaris lumbricoides	Roundworm infestation
Wuchereria bancrofti	Filariasis

From Cherry JD, In: Feigin RD, Cherry JD (eds): Textbook of Pediatric Infectious Diseases. Philadelphia, WB Saunders, 1981.

Table 10–13 INFECTIOUS AGENTS ASSOCIATED WITH EXANTHEM AND MENINGITIS

AGENT	ILLNESS
Herpes simplex virus 2	Recurrent genital herpes
Coxsackieviruses A2, A9, B1, B2, B4, B5	Enterovirus syndrome
Echoviruses 4, 6, 9, 11, 14, 17, 25, 33	Enterovirus syndrome
Colorado tick fever virus	Colorado tick fever
Reovirus 2	Respiratory infection
Neisseria mehingitidis	Meningococcemia
Listeria monocytogenes	Listeriosis
Toxoplasma gondii	Toxoplasmosis

From Cherry JD, In: Feigin RD, Cherry JD (eds): Textbook of Pediatric Infectious Diseases. Philadelphia, WB Saunders, 1981.

Table 10–14 INFECTIOUS AGENTS ASSOCIATED WITH EXANTHEM AND PULMONARY INVOLVEMENT

AGENT	ILLNESS
Adenoviruses 7, 7a	Respiratory infection
Herpes simplex virus 1	Respiratory infection
Varicella-zoster virus	Chickenpox pneumonia
Epstein-Barr virus	Infectious mononucleosis
Coxsackievirus A9	Enterovirus syndrome
Echovirus 11	Enterovirus syndrome
Reovirus 3	Respiratory infection
Measles virus	Measles pneumonia and atypical measles
Chlamydia psittaci	Psittacosis
Mycoplasma pneumoniae	M. pneumoniae pneumonia
Neisseria meningitidis	Meningococcal pneumonia
Mycobacterium tuberculosis	Tuberculosis
Histoplasma capsulatum	Histoplasmosis
Cryptococcus neoformans	Cryptococcosis
Coccidioides immitis	Coccidioidomycosis

From Cherry JD, In: Feigin RD, Cherry JD (eds): Textbook of Pediatric Infectious Diseases. Philadelphia, WB Saunders, 1981.

10.12 DIARRHEA

See also Sec 7.63, 10.29, and 11.36. Diarrhea is 1 of the most frequent problems encountered by physicians who provide care for children. It is defined as an increase in frequency, fluidity, and volume of feces, and it is estimated that during the 1st 3 yr of life a child will experience 1–3 acute, severe episodes of diarrhea. Although most acute episodes of acute diarrhea subside within 72 hr with fluid administration and change in diet, 1–4% of these episodes, worldwide, will be fatal.

Diarrhea may follow invasion of the intestinal mucosa (e.g., *Staphylococcus aureus*, enteroinvasive *E. coli*, *Shigella*, *Yersinia enterocolitica*, *Entamoeba histolytica*) or may be induced by exposure of the bowel to a microbial toxin (e.g., *Vibrio cholerae*, enterotoxigenic *E. coli*, *Shigella dysenteriae* type 1, *Clostridium perfringens*, *Salmonella*). It also may be induced by adherence of bacteria to the mucosa of the gastrointestinal tract (*E. coli*) or infestation by *Giardia lamblia*.

Viruses are the major cause of wintertime diarrhea in infants. Rotavirus is the etiologic agent in over 50% of cases of acute diarrhea in children. Other viruses documented to cause diarrhea include parvovirus-like agents (Norwalk, Hawaii, and Montgomery), coxsackie-, echo-, and adenoviruses. More than two thirds of patients with rotavirus-associated diarrhea have a history of preceding or concurrent respiratory illness with rhinorrhea, cough, erythematous throat, or otitis media; most of these individuals are under 2 yr of age. Food intake does not appear to be a vector in transmission of this infection.

Differential Diagnosis. An approach to the etiologic diagnosis of diarrhea is presented in Fig 10–1. Common infections extrinsic to the gastrointestinal tract (pneumonia, otitis media) may be accompanied by diarrhea. Diarrhea also may accompany a variety of anatomic defects, endocrinopathies, neoplasms, disorders accompanied by malabsorption, and inherited diseases (Fig 10–1 and Table 10–15).

History and Physical Examination. A chief complaint of diarrhea should first be verified for accuracy (increase in number, volume, or fluidity of stools). The usual clinical features of infectious diarrheas are presented in Table 10–16. A history of recent travel to Mexico may suggest diarrhea related to enterotoxigenic *E. coli*, and travel to the Rocky Mountains or Soviet Union may suggest giardiasis. A history of blood or mucus in the stool, abdominal pain, tenesmus, fever, abdominal mass, weight loss, or consumption of dairy products or contaminated meats or water should also be sought. The degree of dehydration and state of consciousness should be described specifically (Sec 5.24). The presence or absence of arthralgia, arthritis, skin rashes, and bradycardia also may suggest an appropriate etiologic diagnosis. These findings coupled with a history of fluid intake, the frequency of urination, and an assessment of concurrent stool losses permit determination of whether hospitalization is required.

Laboratory Diagnosis. The routine total and differential white blood cell count may be normal, increased, or decreased, but over 50% of the patients have 10–40% band forms in the differential forms.

The stool should be examined for volume, color, and consistency, and for the presence of mucus, blood, and leukocytes. Leukocytes may be noted by mixing a small amount of stool with 1–2 drops of methylene blue; generally, they are not seen when diarrhea is related to disease of the small bowel, but are observed in patients with salmonellosis, enteroinvasive *E. coli*, shigellosis, staphylococcal enterocolitis, *Entamoeba histolytica*, granulomatous colitis (regional enteritis), ulcerative colitis, and pseudomembranous enterocolitis. Stool should be cultured in patients with fecal leukocytes, hospitalized children, patients with persistent or chronic diarrhea, and individuals who have been exposed to other persons who have diarrhea related to a previously documented bacterial pathogen. Examination of the stool for ova and parasites should be carried out on an individual basis when the history, physical examination, course of the patient, or negative laboratory data suggest that a parasitic disease is a possibility. A diagnosis of *Giardia lamblia* can be made by examination of the stool but may require examination of a duodenal aspirate or a duodenal biopsy. Stool may be sent for immune fluorescent microscopy to confirm diagnosis of infection by rotavirus.

In some patients examination of stool pH, stool glucose content, and stool chloride concentration may be helpful. If the stool glucose content is low or stool pH is less than 5.5, various noninfectious causes of diarrhea should be considered. However, low stool pH may also be found in children with acquired lactase deficiency that has followed a persistent infectious diarrheal illness. Significant stool chloride losses occur in cholera;

Table 10–15 NONINFECTIOUS CAUSES OF DIARRHEA

Feeding difficulty
Anatomic defects
    Malrotation
    Intestinal duplications
    Hirschsprung disease
    Fecal impaction
    Short bowel
Malabsorption
    Disaccharidase deficiencies
    Glucose-galactose monosaccaride malabsorption
    Cystic fibrosis
    Hereditary fructose intolerance
    Pancreatic insufficiency
    Abetalipoproteinemia
Endocrinopathies
    Thyrotoxicosis
    Addison disease
    Adrenogenital syndrome
    Hypoparathyroidism
Neoplasms
    Neuroblastomas
    Ganglioneuromas
    Pheochromocytomas
    Carcinoid
Miscellaneous
    Familial dysautonomia
    Immune deficiency diseases
    Protein-losing enteropathy
    Granulomatous colitis
    Ulcerative colitis
    Acrodermatitis enteropathica
    Niacin deficiency
    Methionine malabsorption syndrome
    Hartnup disease

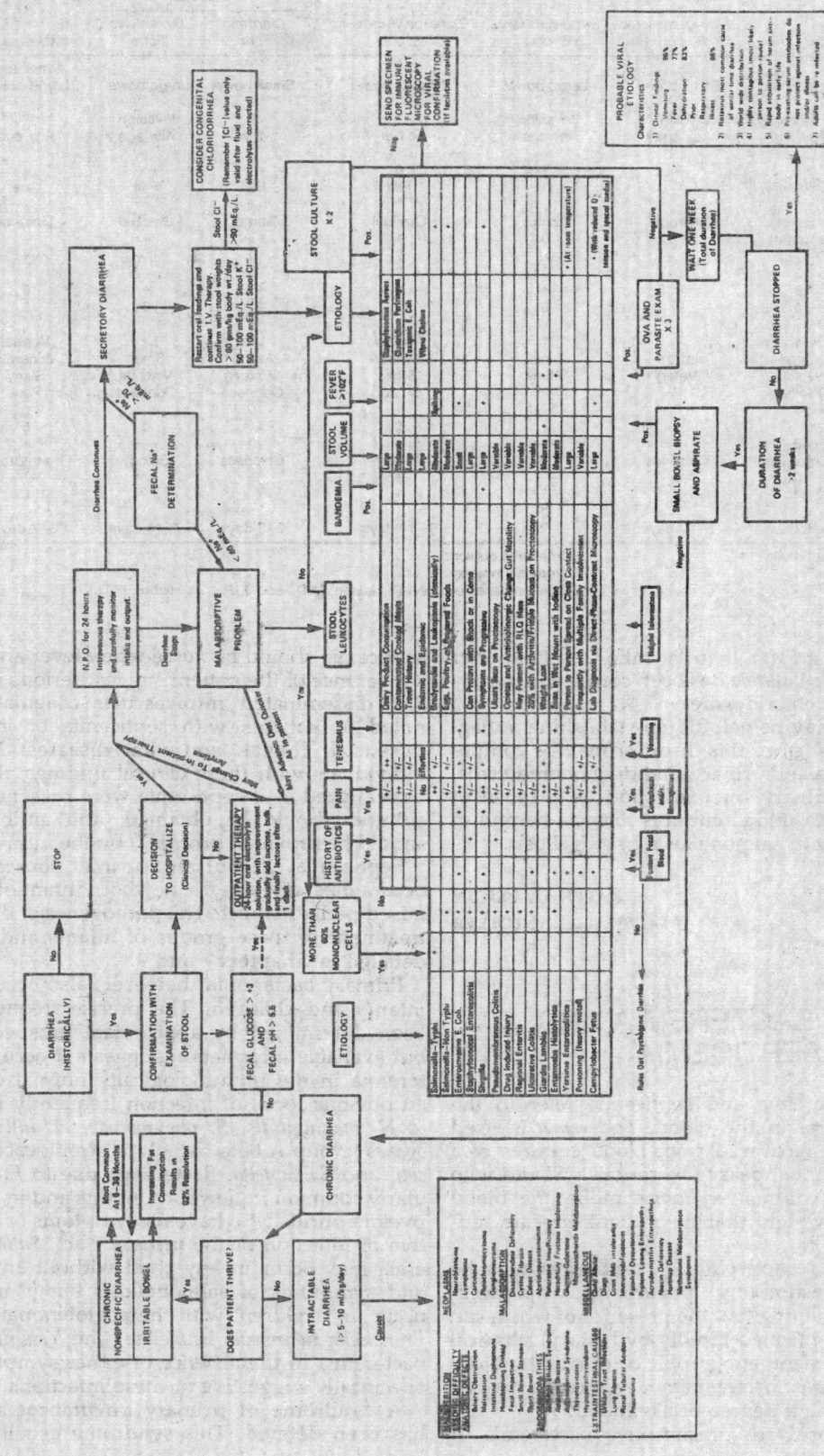

Figure 10-1 Algorithm for the approach to diarrhea.

Table 10-16   USUAL CLINICAL FEATURES OF INFECTIOUS DIARRHEAS

	CHOLERA	ENTEROTOXIGENIC E. COLI*	ENTEROINVASIVE E. COLI*	"ENTEROPATHOGENIC" E. COLI	SHIGELLA Diarrheic Form	SHIGELLA Dysenteric Form	SALMONELLA	ROTA (REO-LIKE) VIRUS
Site of action	Small bowel	Small bowel	Large bowel	? Small bowel	Small bowel	Large bowel	Small and Large bowel	Small bowel
Mechanism of action	Toxin	Toxin	Invasion	?	?	Invasion	?	?
Age	Any age	Any age?	Any age?	<1 yr	>2 yrs	Any age	Any age	<7 yrs
Diarrhea in household	++	?	?	0	++	++	+	+
Season	Epidemic	?	?	Fall	Fall	Fall	Any	Winter
Character of onset	Abrupt	Abrupt	Abrupt	Gradual	Abrupt	Gradual	Gradual	Abrupt
Vomiting	+ (Late)	++	0	+	++	+	+	++
Cramps	++	++	++	?	0	++	+	?
Tenesmus	0	0	?	?	0	++	+	?
Fever 39° C (102° F)	0	0	++	0	++	+	0	0
Convulsions	0	0	0	0	++	0	0	0
Anal sphincter tone	Normal	?	?	Normal	Lax	Lax	Normal	Normal
Stool: Volume	Large	Large	Small	Moderate	Large	Small	Moderate	Large
Consistency	Watery	Watery	Slimy	Slimy	Watery	Viscous	Slimy	Watery
Odor	Odorless	?	?	Musty	Odorless	Odorless	Foul	Odorless
Blood	0	0	++	+	0	++	0	0
Mucus shreds	++	++	+	0	++	0	0	0
Pus	0	0	++	+	0	++	+	0
Color	Colorless	Colorless	?	Green	Colorless	Bloody	Green/Brown	Colorless
Leukocytes	0	0	++	+	+	++	++	0
Bandemia	?	?	?	+	++	++	0	0
Duration (untreated)	3-6 days	5-10 days	?	7-14 days	2-3 days	7-14 days	3-7 days	5-7 days

*Based on observations in adults.
?Insufficient data available.
0Usually absent.
\+ Sometimes present.
\+ + Commonly present.
(Table prepared by John D. Nelson, M.D., and J. Patrick Hieber, M.D.)

chloride losses of greater than 90 mEq/l of stool after fluid and electrolyte balance has been corrected strongly suggest congenital chloridorrhea.

Urine cultures may be helpful in establishing a diagnosis of shigellosis, since this disorder may be complicated by bacteremia and urinary shedding of organisms, or in excluding urinary tract infection as a cause of nonspecific diarrhea. Blood cultures may be helpful in selected patients with salmonellosis or shigellosis.

RALPH D. FEIGIN
MARSHALL L. STOLLER

10.13   BACTEREMIA AND SEPTICEMIA

The terms bacteremia and septicemia refer to the presence of bacteria in the blood. *Bacteremia* is used when bacteria are recovered from blood cultures of a patient who does not appear to be seriously ill and who may be afebrile. In contrast, *septicemia* implies that blood cultures are positive and that the patient appears seriously or critically ill.

In some patients bacteremia or septicemia may be related to focal infection (e.g., pneumonia, osteomyelitis, endocarditis, meningitis), the presence of which can be suspected or confirmed rapidly by history, physical examination, and roentgenographic or other laboratory studies. In such cases, bacteremia or septicemia may be suspected with a high degree of likelihood.

A clinical diagnosis of presumptive bacteremia or septicemia should be made when fever and the general appearance of the patient suggest serious illness. Shock and disseminated intravascular coagulation may be noted in patients with septicemia or in those with rickettsial, fungal, and viral diseases. Nevertheless, individuals with these clinical findings always should be managed as if septicemia were present; appropriate cultures should be obtained, and antibiotic therapy should be provided promptly by the intravenous route.

Septicemia without an apparent source of infection occurs most often in the newborn infant or the compromised pediatric host. The pathogenesis, diagnosis, and treatment of these groups of infants and children are detailed in Chapters 7 and 9.

Primary bacteremia, however, also occurs in normal infants and children. The precise frequency has not been determined by appropriate prospective studies, but available information suggests it occurs often. Bacteremia in the immunologically normal child without an obvious focus of infection frequently has been due to *N. meningitidis, S. pneumoniae, H. influenzae, S. pyogenes* (group A beta-hemolytic streptococci), *Escherichia coli,* and *Salmonella.* Bacteremia due to *E. coli* is particularly common in newborn infants and in children with pyelonephritis who have no symptoms or signs suggestive of infection of the urinary tract. *Salmonella* bacteremia may occur in any child without any other signs and symptoms of salmonellosis but is most likely to occur in children with hemoglobinopathies. Rarely, *Francisella tularensis,* brucellae, and *Yersinia pestis* cause bacteremia in the absence of either symptoms or signs specifically suggestive of these infections.

A syndrome of **primary pneumococcal bacteremia** has been defined. This syndrome usually is noted in normal children 6–24 mo of age who do not appear to be seriously ill. Signs of an upper respiratory infection may be minimal or absent. In most patients rectal temperature exceeds 38.9° C and the white blood cell count is more than 20,000/mm³. Blood culture should be obtained from children who fulfill these criteria. Many of these patients will improve without therapy, but the incidence of subsequent otitis media, pneumonia, and meningitis is greater in untreated children with this presentation than in children whose clinical illnesses do not fulfill these criteria. Therefore, children with pneumococcal bacteremia who have not been treated should be recalled by the physician after receipt of the blood culture results. If they are now afebrile and well upon re-examination, they may be managed at home if the physician is confident that contact with the family can be maintained. Otherwise, another blood culture and treatment with oral penicillin in a dose of 50,000 units/kg/24 hr in 4 divided doses are appropriate. If the 2nd blood culture is negative and the child remains well, treatment may be discontinued after 5 days; if it is positive, treatment should be continued for 10 days.

In a child with untreated pneumococcal bacteremia who reveals a focus of infection upon re-examination, a 2nd blood culture should be obtained and the patient treated with penicillin provided in a dose, route, and duration appropriate to the disease process. If a child with pneumococcal bacteremia is re-examined and remains febrile but no focus of infection is yet apparent, the child should be hospitalized. In the hospital, blood cultures should be repeated and a lumbar puncture performed. The patient should be treated with aqueous penicillin intravenously and treatment modified subsequently according to the clinical course, blood culture, and lumbar puncture results.

Recent studies documented that the majority of children with fever of 39.7° C or greater (103.5° F) who were over 3 mo of age did not have bacteremia. A white blood cell count greater than 15,000/mm³ occurred more frequently in children with bacteremia than in those whose blood cultures were negative. The majority of children, however, with white blood cell counts greater than 15,000 cells/mm³ and with fever greater than 39.7° C had negative blood cultures; viruses were proved to be the causes of infection in a number of these children. These studies also suggest that a skilled clinician can differentiate as effectively as simple laboratory tests between children who may have bacteremia and those who do not. However, the economic and health costs of the failure to identify the few febrile children with bacteremia are greater than the costs of obtaining blood cultures on all of these children.

When a clinical diagnosis of septicemia is made in any patient beyond the neonatal period and no focus of infection is apparent, the patient should be hospitalized and blood cultures obtained. A clean voided specimen of urine should be examined carefully and sent for culture. In the absence of physical findings a chest roentgenogram is recommended in children under 1 yr of age, for it may disclose the focus of infection. If the urinalysis is normal, treatment may be initiated with ampicillin and a semisynthetic penicillinase-resistant penicillin (methicillin, oxacillin, nafcillin) intravenously. These antibiotics provide effective coverage for *S. aureus, S. pyogenes, S. pneumoniae,* most strains of *H. influenzae, N. meningitidis,* and *N. gonorrhoeae.*

In the compromised pediatric host or in the child with possible urinary tract infection and associated septicemia, the use of a semisynthetic penicillinase-resistant penicillin and gentamicin is favored.

McCarthy P, Jekel J, Dolan T: Temperature greater than or equal to 40° C in children less than 24 months of age: A prospective study. J Pediatr 59:663, 1976.
Teele D, Marshall R, Klein J: Unsuspected bacteremia in young children. Pediatr Clin N Amer 26:773, 1980.
Wright PF, Thompson J, McKee KT Jr: Patterns of illness in the highly febrile young child: Epidemiologic, clinical and laboratory correlates. Pediatrics 67:694, 1981.

OSTEOMYELITIS AND SEPTIC ARTHRITIS

The term *osteomyelitis* refers to bacterial infection of bone; *septic arthritis* refers to bacterial joint disease. These disorders must be differentiated not only from each other but also from cellulitis; viral, rickettsial, fungal, and parasitic disease of bones and joints; collagen-vascular diseases; rheumatic fever; metabolic disorders; and malignancies.

Early diagnosis of osteomyelitis or septic arthritis in childhood depends upon a high index of suspicion; in many patients the initial signs and symptoms may not suggest an infectious etiology. Experience indicates that about 30% of children with osteomyelitis are afebrile and have normal white blood cell counts when initially seen. Since chronic infection or other permanent debilitating sequelae may develop if diagnosis and treatment are delayed, appropriate antibiotics should be given to children suspected of osteomyelitis or septic arthritis as soon as relevant cultures have been obtained, but prior to definitive diagnosis.

Limp is a frequent presenting complaint, but the diagnosis of osteomyelitis or septic arthritis is often overlooked because of the absence of accompanying fever at the time of initial encounter. In 1 prospective study a diagnosis of osteomyelitis or septic arthritis was established in 25% of all children who presented to an emergency room with the chief complaint of unexplained limp. Unless some other reasonable explanation for limp can be established, a diagnosis of bone or joint infection must be considered seriously. Close observation, in the hospital if necessary, is essential until the diagnosis is clarified.

10.14 OSTEOMYELITIS

Acute osteomyelitis may occur at any age but occurs most often between 3–12 yr. It occurs twice as frequently in boys as in girls and requires early diagnosis and intensive therapy to achieve optimal results.

Etiology.   Osteomyelitis continues to be caused primarily by coagulase-positive staphylococci, although the proportion of infections caused by other organisms, particularly *H. influenzae* type b, the group B beta-hemolytic streptococcus, anaerobic microorganisms, and gram-negative enteric bacteria, may be increasing. Factors that predispose to the development of osteomyelitis include impetigo, furunculosis, infected lesions of varicella, infected burns, prolonged intravenous or central parenteral alimentation, drug addiction, and direct trauma to an area adjacent to the site of osteomyelitis.

Pathogenesis and Pathology.   Osteomyelitis generally begins as a hematogenous abscess in the metaphysis. Subsequently, if untreated, this abscess ruptures subperiosteally and spreads along the shaft of the bone or may penetrate to the marrow cavity. The periosteum may separate and form a shell of new bone about the infected portion of the shaft. Pieces of dead bone are known as *sequestra*, and the new bone formed by the periosteum is known as an *involucrum*. In some cases the infectious process in the metaphysis ruptures into the joint cavity and a secondary suppurative arthritis develops.

Osteomyelitis is most commonly hematogenous in origin but may be secondary to direct inoculation of organisms due to trauma or to contiguous spread of infection from cellulitis in adjacent or overlying soft tissues. In infants osteomyelitis frequently is associated with septic arthritis because infantile bone has vessels that perforate the growth plate, thereby delivering infection to the epiphysis and potentially causing both joint disease and permanent epiphyseal damage.

Clinical Manifestations.   These vary with the age of the child affected and depend upon the differing nature of the vascular pattern of bone in infants up to 1 yr of age, in children between 1 and puberty, and in adults following cessation of bone growth. In the infant, membranous bones are affected as well as long bones.

Osteomyelitis in the *infant* may be an acute illness with fever. More commonly, there is little evidence of systemic toxicity. Local signs generally are absent except for pseudoparalysis or failure to move the affected limb. *Staphylococcus aureus* is the predominant organism; group B streptococci and gram-negative bacteria are other organisms that deserve serious consideration. Distinctive features of infantile osteomyelitis are the tendency to produce permanent arrest in bone growth and involvement of multiple sites within the same bone or of multiple bones.

Hematogenous osteomyelitis in *children* beyond the neonatal period may occur as an abrupt illness with fever and systemic signs of toxicity or as a subacute illness in which local complaints at the involved bone dominate the clinical picture. Osteomyelitis localizes most often in the long bones. However, osteomyelitis of the pelvis and small bones of the hands and feet occurs with sufficient frequency to warrant consideration of this diagnosis in any child with pain in the pelvic region, hands, or feet. Osteomyelitis may be associated with swelling, erythema, tenderness, and decreased movement of the involved part. When these findings are coupled with an elevated white blood cell count, elevated erythrocyte sedimentation rate, and roentgenographic evidence of bone disease, the diagnosis is established readily. Recently, an increasing proportion of patients has presented with less striking clinical findings, possibly reflecting suppression of disease by antibiotics administered for another reason. In both acute and subacute osteomyelitis roentgenographic evidence of disease may not be apparent for 10–14 days after the appearance of signs and symptoms.

In *adolescents and adults* hematogenous osteomyelitis may involve the vertebrae in addition to other sites. Clinically, vertebral osteomyelitis is notable for its insidious onset, vague symptomatology, and lack of fever or systemic toxicity. Patients may complain of back pain for several wk with no other findings. *Staphylococcus aureus* is the usual cause, but streptococci, gram-negative enteric organisms, and *Mycobacterium tuberculosis* may also cause the disease. An increased frequency of vertebral osteomyelitis due to *Pseudomonas* has been reported among heroin addicts.

Diagnosis.   Careful examination may reveal marked tenderness over the involved bone; the tender areas may be small and sharply defined. The total white blood cell count may be elevated but is normal so frequently that it is of no help in diagnosis. The erythrocyte sedimentation rate, although a nonspecific finding, frequently is elevated. It is of help in monitoring the progress of the patient as well as in supporting the diagnosis of osteomyelitis.

Blood cultures and an aspirate of the soft tissue, bone, or both should be obtained for culture prior to institution of antibiotic therapy. A tuberculin test should be administered. A chest roentgenogram may be obtained in some cases for evidence of granulomatous disease, particularly in children who have subacute or chronic osteomyelitis. Roentgenograms of the affected areas should be obtained but generally are normal during the acute stages of the disease process. The radionuclide bone scan, particularly with ^{99m}technetium, is valuable in establishing a diagnosis of osteomyelitis in the face of negative roentgenographic studies and a normal white blood cell count. However, radionuclide imaging has several limitations. In some patients areas of increased uptake are detected roentgenologically at an early stage of septicemia due to *S. aureus*, but progression to osteomyelitis does not occur. Osteomyelitis has sometimes been documented bacteriologically and histologically when bone scans were initially negative. Radionuclide imaging does not consistently permit the differentiation of cellulitis from osteomyelitis. Bone scanning with 99m Tc–polyphosphate performed following a fracture or bone surgery does not distinguish between bone repair and infection. Scanning with gallium citrate-67 may allow detection of osteomyelitis early and may be positive even when a 99m Tc–polyphosphate scan is negative since it accumulates in inflammatory exudates. Scans may remain positive for extended periods of time despite effective therapy; thus the extent of healing cannot be ascertained by scanning.

Differential Diagnosis.   Other disorders may mimic acute osteomyelitis: neoplastic diseases; histiocytosis; pancreatitis with lytic lesions of bone; scurvy; deep cellulitis; viral, rickettsial, fungal, and parasitic diseases of bones and joints; collagen-vascular diseases; rheumatic fever; metabolic disorders; and malignancies.

Treatment. Management of suppurative bone infection may include symptomatic therapy, immobilization in some cases, adequate drainage of purulent material, and antibiotic therapy. Standard therapy consists of parenteral administration of antibiotics for a minimum of 3 and preferably 4 wk. In some cases parenteral antibiotic therapy has been advised for 6 wk or longer. When administered systemically, the penicillins and cephalosporins penetrate infected bones adequately. The tissue concentrations of antibiotic obtained are independent of binding by serum protein and uniformly are several-fold greater than the minimal bactericidal concentrations for the commonly encountered pathogens.

Treatment should be started as soon as the appropriate diagnostic studies have been concluded. The choice of antibiotic is based on the results of Gram stain of bone aspirate or biopsy and on other clinical considerations. Initial coverage should always be provided for penicillinase-producing staphylococci. In selected cases consideration may be given to treatment effective against the group B streptococcus and *H. influenzae*. In patients with sickle cell disease, coverage for *Salmonella* must be considered. Gram-negative enteric organisms should be covered where soil-contaminated contiguous wounds are present. *Pseudomonas aeruginosa* should be considered in drug addicts and *Candida*, *Aspergillus*, and *Rhizopus* in patients having compromised host defenses or receiving long-term parenteral hyperalimentation.

Recommended treatment for *Staphylococcus aureus* usually consists of methicillin in a dose of 200 mg/kg/24 hr in 6 divided doses *intravenously* for 4 wk; when such therapy has been provided, a treatment failure rate of 4% or less generally is found. In children who receive 3 wk of intravenous methicillin therapy, a 19% failure rate or progression to chronic osteomyelitis or recurrent disease has been reported. After the 4-wk recommended period of treatment, decision to discontinue therapy should be based upon review of the course of the patient, roentgenographic evidence of healing, and a sedimentation rate that has returned to normal. Oral therapy may be provided after 4 wk of intravenous therapy for certain patients who are doing well but who have a persistently elevated erythrocyte sedimentation rate. In these patients dicloxacillin at a dose of 75 mg/kg/24 hr or oxacillin in a dose of 100–150 mg/kg/24 hr will provide good serum levels and therefore should provide adequate bone levels.

Theoretically, it is possible to obtain serum levels of antistaphylococcal antibiotics 10–20 times the minimal inhibitory concentration for the organism with high oral doses of certain antibiotics. This has the advantage of shortening hospitalization significantly, but tolerance of the oral dose, compliance, and adequate follow-up if the patient is discharged from the hospital pose major problems. A number of recent studies have demonstrated that after an initial period of 1–7 days of intravenous antibiotic therapy, patients may be treated adequately by the oral route. Clindamycin in a dose of 30 mg/kg/24 hr, dicloxacillin 50–75 mg/kg/24 hr, cephalexin 100 mg/kg/24 hr, penicillin V 100 mg/kg/24 hr, and

ampicillin 100 mg/kg/24 hr all have been demonstrated to provide adequate oral treatment of osteomyelitis.

Because inadequate antibiotic therapy of osteomyelitis is very likely to lead to chronic disease and permanent orthopedic deformity, it is recommended that the following conditions be assured if antibiotics are to be administered orally to infants and children with acute osteomyelitis: (1) patients should be hospitalized for the entire period of antibiotic therapy; (2) antibiotics should be provided parenterally for an initial period of 5–7 days; (3) satisfactory activity of the orally administered drug in vitro against *Staphylococcus aureus* or the organism isolated from the individual patient must be demonstrated. Absorption of whatever oral drug is provided should be assessed by measurement of *serum bactericidal activity* against the pathogen isolated from the patient. Dosage must be tailored to achieve a peak bactericidal titer of at least 1:8–1:16. The total duration of therapy must be based upon the clinical response of the patient, roentgenographic findings, and return of the sedimentation rate to 20 mm/hr or less. After antibiotics have been discontinued, patients may be discharged from the hospital but should be followed closely in the physician's office for the possibility of recurrence of disease.

It is emphasized that oral treatment of osteomyelitis has been assessed adequately only for patients with documented *Staphylococcus aureus* infections and should not be attempted at present in individuals with osteomyelitis caused by other organisms. Optimal treatment for subacute or chronic osteomyelitis has not been established. Since antibiotics frequently must be provided for months or years for patients with this form of disease, oral therapy at home may be the only practical mode of treatment.

Prognosis. The prognosis of acute osteomyelitis has improved significantly in recent yr. The number of patients who progress to subacute or chronic disease has decreased with growing awareness of the subtlety of signs and symptoms of this disorder and consequent prompt diagnosis and adequate therapy. Mortality is rare, but sequelae still occur. The course and prognosis depend upon the age of the child, the rapidity with which diagnosis is established, the early institution of appropriate therapy, and treatment for an adequate period of time.

10.15 SEPTIC ARTHRITIS

Septic arthritis occurs most commonly during the 1st yr of life. It frequently follows infection of the skin or upper respiratory tract.

Etiology. Staphylococci are frequent etiologic agents of septic arthritis in all age groups. In the newborn, *Staphylococcus aureus* is the most common causative organism, but group B beta-hemolytic streptococci and gram-negative enteric bacteria also are involved. In the child from 2 mo–4 yr of age, *Hemophilus influenzae* type b now is the most frequent etiologic agent, followed by staphylococci, streptococci, pneumococci, and meningococci. Beyond 2 yr of age *S. aureus* predominates, though a great variety of other organisms may be involved. Sexually active adolescents may develop gonococcal arthritis or, occasionally, sterile inflammatory arthritis associated with gonococcal disease.

Pathogenesis. Septic arthritis may occur with or without osteomyelitis. In children under 2 yr of age, the metaphyseal plexus of veins traverses the epiphyseal plate; thus metaphyseal osteomyelitis is more frequently complicated by concurrent septic arthritis in patients of this age. Septic arthritis may be the result of hematogenous dissemination of bacteria, direct inoculation of organisms into the joint space, or contiguous spread of infection from surrounding soft tissues.

Clinical Manifestations. The onset may be sudden, with systemic symptoms and fever. Local swelling may appear rapidly with pain and muscular rigidity. Erythema, tenderness, warmth, pain on motion, and decreased mobility of the involved joint may be noted. Generally, fever, an elevated white blood cell count, and an elevated erythrocyte sedimentation rate are present. Children may be brought to a physician because they have developed a limp. The most frequent error in diagnosis of septic arthritis is to exclude it from further consideration because of the absence of fever at the time of initial encounter. Unless some other reasonable explanation for limp can be established on the basis of history, physical examination, and roentgenographic and laboratory studies, a diagnosis of bone or joint infection must always be entertained.

Diagnosis. Rapid diagnosis of suppurative arthritis is best done by arthrocentesis if the presence of fluid is suspected or observed clinically or roentgenographically. It is important, if possible, to avoid traversing an overlying area of cellulitis during the performance of the joint tap since the underlying joint may be uninvolved and a deep cellulitis may be converted into septic arthritis by carrying organisms into the joint.

The joint fluid should be examined morphologically, examined by Gram and Kenyoun stain (for mycobacteria), and cultured aerobically and anaerobically. Protein and glucose determinations should be obtained. Blood cultures and a blood glucose concentration should be obtained concomitantly. Joint fluid also may be sent to a laboratory for antinuclear antibody studies and for determination of hepatitis-associated antigen.

When septic arthritis is present, the joint fluid is usually purulent, the white blood cell count markedly elevated (more than 50,000 cells/mm^3), the glucose concentration depressed, and the Gram stain positive. Cultures of joint fluid that has the chemical and morphologic characteristics described may be negative in up to 30% of patients who have never received antibiotic therapy since the fluid itself may exert a bacteriostatic effect upon microorganisms. Blood cultures always should be obtained to aid in establishing a definitive diagnosis. In selected cases of subacute or chronic septic arthritis, synovial biopsy may be helpful in distinguishing between a septic and a noninfectious process.

If a diagnosis of septic arthritis cannot be established by joint aspiration but is still suspected, antibiotic therapy should be provided until cultures of both joint fluid and blood prove to be negative. Concomitantly, a diagnostic evaluation aimed at elucidating other possible causes of joint effusion should be initiated. Since septic arthritis may precede osteomyelitis or osteomyelitis may be present but not demonstrable roentgenographically at the time that the diagnosis of septic arthritis is established, roentgenograms of the adjacent bone are usually indicated 10–14 days after therapy is initiated.

The hip joint presents special problems in diagnosis. In the neonate or young infant the clinical signs of hip involvement may be minimal. Warmth, erythema, and swelling may not be appreciated because of the considerable amount of soft tissue surrounding the joint. Pain on movement and refusal to move the limb may be the only signs.

Differential Diagnosis. Suppurative arthritis must be differentiated from deep cellulitis; viral, mycoplasmal, mycobacterial, and fungal arthritis; acute rheumatic fever; rheumatoid arthritis or other collagen disease; toxic synovitis; Lyme arthritis; ulcerative colitis; granulomatous colitis; serum sickness; leukemia; Henoch-Schönlein (anaphylactoid) purpura; metabolic diseases affecting joints (e.g., ochronosis, Farber disease); and traumatic arthritis. As many as 10% of children with involvement of multiple joints have septic arthritis. In such patients rheumatic fever, rheumatoid arthritis, serum sickness, and anaphylactoid purpura must also be seriously considered.

Treatment. When a diagnosis of septic arthritis has been established, the choice of antibiotics should be based upon the results of microscopic examination of a Gram-stained smear of the joint fluid and a consideration of the agents likely to produce disease in a child of that particular age. Irrigation of the joint spaces with antibiotics is unnecessary except in cases of fungal arthritis. Surgical drainage should be performed immediately in hip joint involvement and seriously considered when the shoulder joint is involved. There are special characteristics of the hip joint which mandate drainage: (1) the joint capsule limits the amount of expansion possible, and therefore blood supply to the head of the femur may be compromised; (2) osteomyelitis from spread of infection to adjacent bone is a possibility because the articular cartilage covers only the articular surface of the head of the femur; the periosteum of the neck of the femur is therefore exposed and in contact with the infected fluid.

Surgical drainage of other joints may be required occasionally when rapid reaccumulation of fluid occurs after the initial diagnostic drainage is performed by arthrocentesis.

The minimum duration of antibiotic therapy for septic arthritis has not been determined. It is prudent to provide intravenous therapy for 14–21 days in most cases, but septic arthritis of the hip should be treated for 4 wk.

Methicillin in a dose of 200 mg/kg/24 hr intravenously in 6 divided doses is recommended for patients with suppurative arthritis due to *Staphylococcus aureus*. Disease due to *H. influenzae* should be treated with chloramphenicol in a dose of 100 mg/kg/24 hr in 4 divided intravenous doses and ampicillin in a dose of 200 mg/kg/24 hr in 6 divided doses until the organism has been shown to be sensitive to ampicillin, at which time chloramphenicol may be discontinued. If the *H. influ-*

enzae is resistant to ampicillin, ampicillin is discontinued and chloramphenicol therapy continued.

The specific antibiotic provided for other forms of septic arthritis must be related to the nature of the organism producing disease and the in vitro sensitivities of that organism. Therapy with oral antibiotics also has been suggested for septic arthritis, and various modes of therapy (clindamycin, dicloxacillin, cephalexin, ampicillin, and penicillin) have been tried. The precautions described in Sec 10.14 should be followed if oral therapy is used.

If there is no evidence of clinical improvement within 48 hr, surgical drainage of the infected joint should be undertaken immediately. If an area of osteomyelitis adjacent to the infected joint is discovered by roentgenograms obtained 10–14 days after the initiation of antibiotic therapy, the antibiotic must be continued since the recommended duration of treatment for osteomyelitis to prevent possible chronic or recurrent disease is longer than that required for the treatment of septic arthritis.

Dich VQ, Nelson JD, Haltalin KC: Osteomyelitis in infants and children. Am J Dis Child 129:1273, 1975.

Lisbona R, Rosenthall L: Observations on the sequential use of ^{99m}Tc–phosphate complex and ^{67}Ga imaging in osteomyelitis, cellulitis, and septic arthritis. Radiology 123:123, 1977.

Nelson JD: Follow-up. The bacterial etiology and antibiotic management of septic arthritis in infants and children. Pediatrics 50:437, 1972.

Nelson JD, Howard JB, Shelton S: Oral antibiotic therapy in skeletal infections of children. 1. Antibiotic concentrations in suppurative synovial fluid. J Pediatr 92:131, 1978.

Nelson JD, Koontz WC: Septic arthritis in infants and children: A review of 117 cases. Pediatrics 38:966, 1966.

Tetzlaff TR, Howard JB, McCracken GH, et al: Antibiotic concentrations in pus and bone of children with osteomyelitis. J Pediatr 92:135, 1978.

Tetzlaff TR, McCracken GH Jr, Nelson JD: Oral antibiotic therapy for skeletal infections in children. II. Therapy of osteomyelitis and suppurative arthritis. J Pediatr 92:485, 1978.

Waldvogel FA, Medoff G, Swartz MN: Osteomyelitis: A review of clinical features, therapeutic considerations and unusual aspects. N Engl J Med 282:198, 260, 1970.

Waldvogel FA, Vasey H: Ostmyelitis: The past decade. N Engl J Med 303:360, 1980.

10.16 CENTRAL NERVOUS SYSTEM SYNDROME WITH FEVER

Fever may be associated with a variety of diseases that affect the central nervous system (Table 10–17). In children, acute infection of the central nervous system is the most common cause of fever associated with signs and symptoms of central nervous system involvement.

Regardless of etiology, most patients with acute central nervous system infection present similar signs and symptoms, including fever, headache, nausea, vomiting, anorexia, restlessness, and irritability. Photophobia, back pain, nuchal rigidity, obtundation, stupor, coma, seizures, and focal neurologic signs also may be noted.

The neurologic expression of various parameningeal infections depends to some extent on the site of the lesion or lesions, and this in turn is determined by the manner in which the intracranial or intraspinal infection

Table 10–17 DISEASES OF THE CENTRAL NERVOUS SYSTEM WITH WHICH FEVER MAY BE ASSOCIATED

Acute bacterial meningitis
Viral meningitis: echo, coxsackievirus, poliovirus, mumps, herpes simplex, etc.
Mycoplasma
Leptospirosis
Syphilis
Tuberculosis
Sarcoidosis
Fungal meningitis: aspergillosis, North American blastomycosis, candida, cladosporiosis, coccidioidomycosis, cryptococcosis, histoplasmosis, paracoccidioidomycosis, phycomycosis (mucor), allescheriosis, alternariasis, cephalosporiosis, paecilomycosis, penicillosis, rhinosporidiosis, sporotrichosis, torulopsosis, ustilagomycosis
Parasitic meningitis: cysticercosis, amebiasis, trichinosis, toxoplasmosis
Infectious encephalitis (usually viral, including herpes simplex, varicella, rubeola, rubella, infectious mononucleosis, arboviruses)
Acute hemorrhagic encephalitis
Subdural empyema
Ventricular empyema
Brain abscess
Intracranial or spinal epidural abscess
Thrombophlebitis (often associated with subdural empyema)
Encephalopathies: Reye syndrome, poisons (e.g., arsenic), metabolic disorders (thyrotoxicosis), uremia
Subdural hematoma
Intrathecal injections (chemical meningitis)
Serum sickness
Collagen-vascular diseases
Acute multiple sclerosis
Hemolytic-uremic syndrome

was established. If an ear infection is present, the clinician might anticipate epidural, subdural, or parenchymatous lesions of the adjacent temporal lobe or of the cerebellum. Infection of the frontal sinuses and, less often, of the maxillary sinuses may be followed by cerebral abscess, corticothrombophlebitis, or subdural empyema. Metastatic cerebral lesions may be solitary or multiple but usually occur in the distribution of the middle cerebral artery. Bacterial endocarditis leads most often to embolic occlusion of medium-sized vessels with subsequent infarction of the brain. This may result in secondary abscess formation or in the development of a mycotic aneurysm that may declare itself by a subarachnoid hemorrhage.

The diagnosis of acute bacterial meningitis and its differentiation from other central nervous system disorders associated with fever depend in large part upon careful examination of cerebrospinal fluid obtained by lumbar puncture. Cerebrospinal fluid findings characteristic of various central nervous system disorders associated with fever are shown in Table 10–18.

Unfortunately, in some cases a definitive diagnosis cannot be made on the basis of either clinical or cerebrospinal fluid findings, and a thorough search for foci of infection adjacent to or remote from the meninges must be performed. The extent of dysfunction of the nervous system must be defined by repeated neurologic examinations and appropriate laboratory studies. The presence of focal neurologic findings; a lymphocytic reaction within cerebrospinal fluid in which the glucose concentration is normal; associated infection of the ears, sinuses, or lung; or the presence of bronchiectasis or

Table 10–18 CEREBROSPINAL FLUID FINDINGS IN VARIOUS CENTRAL NERVOUS SYSTEM DISORDERS ASSOCIATED WITH FEVER

CONDITION	PRESSURE (MM H₂0)	LEUKOCYTES/MM³	PROTEIN (MG/DL)	GLUCOSE	COMMENTS
Acute bacterial meningitis	Usually elevated	100–60,000 +; usually a few thousand; PMN* predominate	Usually 100–500	Depressed compared to blood glucose; usually <40 mg/dl	Organism may be seen on Gram stain and recovered by culture
Partially treated bacterial meningitis	Normal or elevated	1–10,000; PMN* usual but mononuclear cells may predominate if pretreated for extended period of time	100 +	Depressed or normal	Organisms may or may not be seen; in disease due to *H. influenzae*, organism may grow despite pretreatment; pretreatment may render sterile CSF of patients with pneumococcal and meningococcal disease
Tuberculous meningitis	Usually elevated; may be low due to block in advanced stages	10–500; PMN* early but lymphocytes predominate through most of course	100–500; may be higher in presence of block	<50 mg/dl usual in most cases; decreases with time if treatment is not provided	Acid-fast organisms may be seen on smear; organism can be recovered in culture
Fungal meningitis	Usually elevated	25–500; mononuclear cells predominate except PMN* early	25–500	50 mg/dl, decreases with time if treatment is not provided	Budding yeast may be seen; organism may be recovered in culture; India ink preparation may be positive in cryptococcal disease
Syphilis (acute) and leptospirosis	Usually elevated	200–500, usually lymphocytes	50–200	Generally normal	Positive CSF serology; spirochetes not demonstrable by usual techniques of smear or culture; darkfield exam may be positive
Viral meningitis or meningoencephalitis	Normal or slightly elevated	PMN* early; rarely more than 1000 cells except in Eastern equine encephalomyelitis where counts of up to 20,000 have been recorded; mononuclear cells predominate during most of course	50–200	Generally normal; may be depressed to <40 mg/dl in various viral diseases, particularly mumps (15–20% of cases)	Enteroviruses may be recovered from CSF by appropriate viral cultures
Sarcoidosis	Normal or elevated slightly	0–100; mononuclear	40–100	Normal	No specific findings
Amebiasis	Elevated	500–20,000 +; PMN* predominate	50–100	Normal or slightly depressed	Amebae may be seen rarely in CSF
Chemical (drugs, dermoids, cysts, myelography dye)	Usually elevated	100–1000 +; PMN* predominate	50–100	20–40 mg/dl	Epithelial cells may be seen within CSF in some children with dermoids by use of polarized light
Subacute bacterial endocarditis with embolism	Normal or slightly elevated	0–100; mixed PMN* and mononuclear cells	50–100	Normal	No organisms on smear or culture
Subdural empyema	Usually elevated	<100–5000; PMN* predominate	100–500	Normal	No organisms on smear or culture of CSF unless meningitis also present; organism found on tap of subdural fluid
Brain abscess	Usually elevated	10–200; fluid rarely acellular; lymphocytes predominate; if abscess ruptures into ventricle, PMN* predominate and cell count may reach >100,000	75–500	Normal unless abscess ruptures into ventricular system	No organisms on smear or culture unless abscess ruptures into ventricular system
Cerebral epidural abscess	Normal to slightly elevated	0–500; lymphocytes predominate	50–200	Normal	No organisms on smear or culture
Spinal epidural abscess	Usually low, with spinal block	10–100; lymphocytes predominate	50–400	Normal	No organisms on smear or culture
Thrombophlebitis (sometimes with subdural empyema)	Normal or elevated	0–500; PMN* and lymphocytes	50–200	Normal	No organisms on smear or culture
Acute hemorrhagic encephalitis	Usually elevated	0–1000; PMN* predominate	100–500	Normal	No organisms on smear or culture
Collagen-vascular disease	Slightly elevated	0–500; PMN* may predominate; lymphocytes may be present	100	Normal or slightly depressed	No organisms on smear or culture; LE preparation may be positive
Tumor, leukemia	Slightly elevated to very high	0–100 +; mononuclear or blast cells	50–1000	May be depressed to 20–40 mg/dl	Cytology may be positive

*PMN = polymorphonuclear leukocytes.

cyanotic heart disease should heighten suspicion of brain abscess, epidural or subdural infection, venous thrombophlebitis, or venous sinus thrombosis.

Additional Diagnostic Studies. *Blood cultures* should be obtained in every patient with fever and signs of central nervous systemic infection. If petechial lesions are present, they can be punctured by a small lancet; a Gram-stained smear of the material obtained may reveal microorganisms. This procedure has been helpful in some patients with meningococcal, pneumococcal, and staphylococcal disease. When the concentration of bacteria within the bloodstream is very high, a smear and Gram stain of the buffy coat obtained from a sample of blood may be helpful.

Transillumination of the head should be performed routinely. Use of this technique, coupled with serial measurements of head circumference, may suggest the presence of subdural effusion, subdural empyema, or subdural hematomas. *Roentgenograms* of the skull, sinuses, and mastoids can provide evidence of infection in these sites.

Radionuclide scanning also may be helpful. Suppurative lesions are characterized by increased uptake of ^{99m}technetium. Increased uptake of isotope may also be seen in patients with vascular malformations and tumors. A suprasellar and parasellar accumulation of isotope may be particularly prominent in tuberculous meningitis. Subdural effusions may be recognized by a crescentic accumulation of isotope over the convexities of the cerebral hemisphere.

Computed tomography (CT scan) provides an image of intracranial structures and has been of inestimable value in permitting diagnosis of a variety of central nervous system disorders quickly and noninvasively.

Angiography is performed less frequently with the advent of CT scans but remains useful in some cases in defining the location and extent of a brain abscess. It is also of value in the diagnosis of subdural empyema and, in the venous phase of study, in the diagnosis of thrombosis of the venous sinuses.

Pneumoencephalography and ventriculography have diminished in frequency of use since CT scans have been available. The introduction of air into the ventricles may be helpful in localizing a brain abscess; the process is slightly superior to angiography in localizing masses in the posterior fossa. In rare cases *brain biopsy* may be useful; it may be particularly helpful in establishing diagnoses of herpes simplex encephalitis or collagen-vascular disease. A definitive diagnosis is important in these cases because herpes can be treated with adenine arabinoside, and symptoms of collagen-vascular disease of the central nervous system can be controlled with steroids.

10.17 ACUTE BACTERIAL MENINGITIS BEYOND THE NEONATAL PERIOD

Bacterial meningitis in children is still encountered frequently despite the availability of chemotherapeutic agents that, in vitro, are capable of killing the microorganisms that cause most of these infections. Although the number of reported fatalities from many infectious diseases has decreased by 10- to 20-fold since 1935, the reported deaths from bacterial meningitis have decreased by only one half. The incidence of bacterial meningitis in general and that due to *Hemophilus influenzae* type b and *Streptococcus agalactiae* (group B, beta-hemolytic streptococci) in particular has increased in recent yr. Bacterial meningitis in the neonatal period is discussed in Sec 7.59.

Etiology. This is related to the age of the patient and a number of factors that may predispose the host to bacterial infection or alter host response to an invading microorganism. It is important to remember, however, that any microorganism can produce disease in an occasional patient of any age.

During the 1st 2 mo of life, the organisms that cause meningitis most frequently are those that reflect the maternal flora or the environment in which the infant has been placed, e.g., gram-negative enteric bacilli and the group B streptococcus. An increasing number of cases caused by *Listeria monocytogenes* and *Hemophilus influenzae* type b in the neonatal period is also being reported.

Most bacterial meningitis in children 2 mo–12 yr of age is due to *H. influenzae* type b, *Streptococcus pneumoniae*, or *Neisseria meningitidis*. Disease due to *H. influenzae* may be noted at any age, but its frequency decreases beyond 5 yr of age.

In children over 12, meningitis usually is due to *S. pneumoniae* or *N. meningitidis*. When host response has been compromised or anatomic defects are present, infection with other microorganisms, including *Pseudomonas*, staphylococci, salmonellae, or *Serratia*, may occur.

Epidemiology. In general, bacterial meningitis occurs more frequently in males than in females. This sex distribution is most prominent in infancy. Conditions that lead to an increased incidence of respiratory infection appear to enhance the incidence of bacterial meningitis.

H. influenzae Type b (see also Sec 10.27). Nonencapsulated strains of *H. influenzae* may be found in the throat or nasopharynx of up to 80% of children or adults; a smaller percentage carry *H. influenzae* type b. Carriage of type b occurs predominantly in children of the age at which frequency of disease due to this organism is greatest, but data are insufficient to implicate prolonged carriage with subsequent development of septicemia and meningitis. The risk of such disease occurring in a child exposed within the household to another with the disease is discussed in Sec 10.27. Otitis media caused by *H. influenzae* type b, particularly if inadequately treated, appears to predispose to development of meningitis due to this organism.

Streptococcus pneumoniae. The risk of developing septicemia and meningitis with the pneumococcus depends to some extent upon the pneumococcal serotype with which the child is infected. Experience indicates that meningitis most commonly is caused by serotypes 1, 3, 6, 7, 14, 18, 19, and 23. The risk is 5.5-fold greater in Blacks than in Whites, independent of income or population density. Fraser and associates suggested that 1 in every 24 children with sickle cell disease may develop pneumococcal meningitis by 4 yr of age. This incidence is 36-fold greater than that of pneumococcal meningitis in a black population without sickle cell disease and 314-fold greater than in white children.

Meningococcal Meningitis.   See Sec 10.25.

Pathology.   A meningeal exudate of varying thickness may be distributed widely but may accumulate around veins and venous sinuses, over the convexity of the brain, in the depths of the sulci, in the sylvian fissures, within the basal cisterns, and around the cerebellum. The spinal cord may be encased in pus. Ventriculitis (purulent material within the ventricles) has been observed repeatedly in children who have died of their disease. Invasion of the ventricular wall with perivascular collections of purulent material, loss of ependymal lining, and subependymal gliosis may be noted. Subdural empyema (to be differentiated from subdural effusion) occurs rarely.

Meningeal signs during the acute illness probably relate to inflammation of the pain-sensitive spinal nerves and roots. Residual sensory or motor paralysis following recovery is explained best on the basis of pressure on the peripheral nerves during the early phases of the illness.

Hydrocephalus is an uncommon complication of meningitis beyond the neonatal period. Most often it is communicating and is the result of adhesive thickening of the arachnoid about the cisterns at the base of the brain. Less frequently, the aqueduct of Sylvius or the foramina of Magendie and Luschka are obstructed by fibrosis and reactive gliosis. Ventricular dilatation which ensues may be associated with necrosis of cerebral tissue due to the inflammatory process itself or to occlusion of cerebral veins or arteries.

Vascular and parenchymatous cerebral changes have been demonstrated at necropsy. Polymorphonuclear infiltrates extending to the subintimal region of small arteries and veins have been associated with the exudative meningeal process. Thrombosis of small cortical veins, occlusion of 1 of the major venous sinuses, subarachnoid hemorrhages secondary to a necrotizing arteritis, and, rarely, necrosis of the cerebral cortex in the absence of identifiable thrombosis of small vessels may be observed. Reactive microglia and astrocytes may be identified in the cerebral cortex. Since no bacteria are found in the cerebral cortex, these lesions should be viewed as a noninfectious encephalopathy.

Damage to the cerebral cortex reflecting the effects of vascular occlusion, hypoxia, bacterial invasion or toxic encephalopathy, or some combination of these factors provides an adequate explanation for impaired consciousness, deficits in motor and sensory function, seizures, and retardation which may be observed.

Pathogenesis.   Bacterial meningitis most commonly is the result of hematogenous dissemination of microorganisms from a distant site of infection; bacteremia frequently precedes it or occurs concomitantly. Meningitis also may follow bacterial invasion from a contiguous focus of infection, i.e., paranasal sinuses or mastoids. Bacterial meningitis in children with otitis media generally follows bacteremia, though direct invasion of

the meninges may occur. Infection may spread to the meninges hematogenously in children with infective endocarditis, pneumonia, or thrombophlebitis.

Head trauma may precede bacterial meningitis, which in such cases is usually due to the 3 organisms most commonly causing meningitis in general. Recurrent meningitis due to *S. pneumoniae* and *H. influenzae* has been noted following a fracture through the paranasal sinuses. Direct invasion of the central nervous system also may be noted in individuals with dermoid sinus tracts or meningomyeloceles where a direct communication between the skin and meninges is present; the infection is most commonly caused by organisms found on the skin. Meningitis also may follow neurosurgical procedures, particularly those designed for diversion of cerebrospinal fluid, or may follow osteomyelitis of the skull or vertebral column.

Infection of the central nervous system may be the result of environmental contamination or manipulation. The child with cystic fibrosis or with severe burns may develop meningitis due to *Staphylococcus aureus* or *Pseudomonas aeruginosa*. Children placed in a humidified atmosphere may develop septicemia and meningitis from organisms that proliferate in a moist atmosphere. Indwelling catheters used for parenteral alimentation, blood transfusion, or repeated venipunctures with contaminated equipment (as in narcotic addicts) predispose to infection by bacterial (and fungal) organisms, which generally are of low virulence for the normal host.

Congenital or acquired deficiencies in host response to infection may predispose to bacterial meningitis. In part, meningitis in children between 1 mo–1 yr of age reflects qualitative or quantitative differences between the inflammatory and immunologic responses seen in infants as compared with older children.

Congenital deficiency of the 3 major immunoglobulin classes may predispose to severe bacterial infection. Congenital defects of T lymphocyte function or combined T and B cell defects each are detrimental to host defense. An increased incidence of meningitis has been reported following splenectomy, but the likelihood of such infection is related to the age of the child at the time of splenectomy, the number of years elapsed since splenectomy, and the indications for splenectomy. Congenital asplenia or splenosis also has been associated with an increased incidence of septicemia and meningitis due to *S. pneumoniae*.

Children with sickle cell anemia and other hemoglobinopathies experience meningitis due to *S. pneumoniae* and salmonellae more frequently than do normal children. Children with malignancies, particularly those involving the reticuloendothelial system, are prone to develop meningitis with organisms of low virulence.

Central nervous system infection also has been noted with increased frequency in children with malnutrition, diabetes mellitus, and renal insufficiency.

Susceptibility to meningitis with *H. influenzae* type b is not due to a deficiency of bactericidal antibody to this organism. Children with *H. influenzae* meningitis have high titers of bactericidal antibody at the time of admission to hospital, and the titers do not increase during convalescence. However, the quantity of capsular polyribosephosphate (PRP) of *H. influenzae* type b to which the child has been exposed and the duration of exposure correlate directly with the frequency of complications or sequelae of *H. influenzae* meningitis.

Antibody against polyribosephosphate can be detected by radioimmunoassay and appears to protect against *H. influenzae* infection. In general, such antibody has not been found at the time of admission of children with *H. influenzae* meningitis. Conversely, development of this antibody correlates with protection from the disease. Few children under 1 yr of age develop this antibody.

The pathogenesis of subdural effusions in children with bacterial meningitis is discussed in Sec 21.23.

Clinical Manifestations. Symptoms and signs of bacterial meningitis may be preceded by several days of upper respiratory or gastrointestinal symptoms. In some children, particularly young infants, signs of meningeal inflammation may be minimal; only irritability, restlessness, and poor feeding may be noted. Fever generally is present; its absence in a child with signs of meningeal inflammation, however, is common.

Inflammation of the meninges generally is associated with nausea, vomiting, anorexia, photophobia, and nuchal rigidity. The older child may appear confused and may complain of back pain. Frequently, Kernig and Brudzinski signs will be noted. Increased intracranial pressure is the rule and may be reflected by complaints of headache in older children and by a bulging fontanel and diastasis of sutures in the infant. Papilledema is an uncommon finding in acute meningitis; when it is observed, occlusions of the venous sinuses, subdural empyema, or brain abscess should be suspected.

Often, meningitis is associated with inappropriate secretion of antidiuretic hormone. If the patient is then given excessive amounts of water, a further increase in intracranial pressure will be observed. Signs of excessive brain swelling also may develop in patients with meningococcal disease, possibly reflecting a response to endotoxin.

Seizures occur in about 30% of children with bacterial meningitis. Seizures noted prior to or during the 1st several days of hospitalization are of no prognostic significance. Seizures which are difficult to control or which persist beyond the 4th hospital day, as well as those which develop for the 1st time late in the hospital course, have been associated with permanent neurologic sequelae.

Stupor, coma, and focal neurologic signs may be seen in children with bacterial meningitis. When these findings are present at the time of hospital admission, a relatively poor prognosis can be anticipated.

Transient or permanent paralysis of cranial nerves may be noted. Deafness or disturbances in vestibular function are relatively common. Involvement of the optic nerve, with blindness, is rare. Paralysis of the 6th cranial nerve, usually transient, is noted frequently early in the course.

Collections of fluid in the subdural space (Sec 21.23) have been demonstrated in up to 50% of infants during the acute illness. When appropriate corrections are made to normalize differences in age, the incidence of subdural effusion has been shown to be independent of the bacterial type causing the meningitis. The effu-

sions appear to be more frequent in the very young, more readily detectable in infants, or both.

Subdural effusions may cause enlargement in head circumference or result in abnormal transillumination of the skull. Occasionally, vomiting, seizures, focal neurologic signs, or persistent fever may be noted. These signs and symptoms occur in children with bacterial meningitis without subdural effusions so frequently that one can rarely attribute their occurrence confidently to the subdural effusion per se.

Arthralgia and myalgia are noted in many children with bacterial meningitis. Transient arthritis may occur and is most common with meningococcal disease.

Petechial or purpuric lesions may be seen in 50% of children with meningococcal meningitis but also may accompany any infectious or noninfectious disease process in which vasculitis is noted.

Shock may be associated with any bacteremic illness. Profound hypotension has been noted in 9% of children with meningococcal and 5% of children with *H. influenzae* meningitis. Signs of disseminated intravascular coagulation may accompany hypotension in these patients.

Differential Diagnosis. Many of the signs and symptoms described above suggest meningeal or intracranial pathology, but none are pathognomonic of acute bacterial infection. Tuberculous meningitis, fungal meningitis, aseptic meningitis, brain abscess, intracranial or spinal epidural abscesses, bacterial endocarditis with embolism, subdural empyema with or without thrombophlebitis, and brain tumors may present with similar signs and symptoms. Differentiation of these disorders depends upon careful examination of cerebrospinal fluid obtained by lumbar puncture and additional immunologic, roentgenographic, and isotope studies delineated below.

Diagnosis. Lumbar puncture should always be performed when bacterial meningitis is suspected. Measurement of pressure is an important component of each cerebrospinal fluid examination. When the pressure is very high, just enough fluid should be removed to permit a careful examination. Compression of the jugular vein should be avoided unless compression of the spinal cord is suspected.

Cerebrospinal fluid should be examined immediately. The total number of white blood cells should be enumerated in a counting chamber, and, following centrifugation, a differential cell count should be performed on a Wright-stained smear of the sediment. Separate smears should be made and then should be Gram-stained for bacteria and Kenyoun-stained for mycobacteria.

If the lumbar puncture has been traumatic, a total cell count should be performed. The red blood cells then can be lysed with acetic acid and the count repeated. If the total number of white blood cells compared to the number of red cells is in excess of that in whole blood, one can assume the presence of cerebrospinal fluid pleocytosis.

Cerebrospinal fluid protein should be measured (it is usually elevated in bacterial meningitis). Cerebrospinal fluid glucose should be compared with blood glucose concentration obtained concomitantly. In bacterial meningitis depression of CSF glucose and of the CSF:blood glucose ratio (normally about 66%) is the rule.

Treatment of bacterial meningitis with antibiotics prior to initial lumbar puncture usually does not alter markedly the morphologic or chemical results obtained. Generally, in patients with *H. influenzae* meningitis, cultures of cerebrospinal fluid will not be sterilized by prior oral antibiotic therapy. There is a tendency for pretreatment to render sterile the cerebrospinal fluid of children with pneumococcal or meningococcal disease.

Quellung and agglutination reactions can provide immediate identification of various organisms if they are visible on smear and if appropriate type-specific antisera are available. Countercurrent immunoelectrophoresis (CIE) has proved a useful technique for the rapid (within 1 hr) diagnosis of bacterial meningitis due to *H. influenzae* type b, *S. pneumoniae*, and *N. meningitidis* groups A, C, and D. This technique can detect nonviable bacteria. It is imperative to use antisera with the greatest possible sensitivity and specificity in this technique. Cerebrospinal fluid, serum, and urine should be screened concomitantly; results are enhanced if urine is concentrated prior to screening. A negative CIE result does not exclude the diagnosis of bacterial meningitis. Latex agglutination also may be used for rapid etiologic diagnosis of *H. influenzae* meningitis. This technique, somewhat more sensitive than CIE, yields false-positive results more frequently than CIE. An indirect enzyme-linked immunosorbent assay for the quantitation of type-specific antigen of *Hemophilus influenzae* type b also has been described and is more sensitive than CIE or latex agglutination; no false-positive reactions were noted. This test is more difficult to perform than CIE or latex agglutination and more time consuming (4 hr).

The cerebrospinal fluid should be cultured on a blood agar plate, on a chocolate agar plate, on Fildes or Leventhal medium, and in broth. When meningitis is suspected, the cerebrospinal fluid should be cultured and a Gram-stained smear made even if it is crystal clear and acellular since bacteria may be present before pleocytosis or chemical changes become apparent.

In some cases a definitive diagnosis cannot be made from either the initial clinical or cerebrospinal fluid findings. When available, the limulus lysate assay may permit the identification of endotoxin within cerebrospinal fluid; when performed appropriately, a positive test indicates meningitis with gram-negative organisms.

Blood cultures should be obtained in every patient. A thorough search for foci of infection adjacent to or remote from the meninges should be performed. Cultures of the throat and nasopharynx have not been particularly helpful in identifying the pathogen.

When the concentration of bacteria within the blood is high, a Gram-stained smear of a buffy coat obtained from the blood may reveal the presence of microorganisms. If petechial lesions are present, a smear of the lesions following puncture with a small lancet may reveal microorganisms on Gram stain.

Roentgenograms of the chest, sinuses, skull, or spine should not be routine but may be helpful in disclosing a focus of infection in selected patients. Radioisotope scanning may also be helpful in selected patients; the pattern of distribution of radioactivity recorded by the gamma camera coincides with the accumulation of purulent material. Localized concentration of radionuclide may be seen in children with meningitis, most likely as a result of cerebral vasculitis or infarction.

Computed tomography (CT scan) detects ventricular dilatation, subdural effusion, decrease in brain mass, and the presence of vascular lesions or of brain infarcts. Ventricular dilatation has been noted acutely by CT scan in many children who do not develop hydrocephalus following recovery from their disease.

Prevention. *H. influenzae Meningitis.* Immunization of adults and children with purified *H. influenzae* type b capsular polysaccharide has been followed by a long-lasting serum antibody response in individuals over 18 mo of age. Unfortunately, the response is relatively poor in infants under 18 mo, the very population at greatest risk for this disease. Prophylaxis is indicated for children under 4 yr of age who are family contacts or nursery school and day-care center contacts of individuals with *H. influenzae* disease. Rifampin appears to be the prophylactic agent of choice; the dosage is 20 mg/kg/24 hr once a day for 4 days (maximum dose, 600 mg/24 hr). The use of ampicillin is inherently unsound, because at the time that prophylaxis is instituted the sensitivity of the *H. influenzae* isolate may be unknown and the rate of eradication of nasopharyngeal carriage of *H. influenzae* when these organisms are sensitive to ampicillin is only 70%.

Meningococcal Infection. The use of chemoprophylaxis is reasonable in all household and day-care nursery contacts of a case of meningococcal infection. Schoolroom and hospital contacts usually are not given prophylaxis. Infections caused by sulfonamide-sensitive meningococci may be prevented by giving sulfadiazine orally in a dose of 0.5–1.0 gm twice daily for 3–5 days.

Minocycline and rifampin have proved to be 80–90% effective in eradicating carriage of meningococci. However, frequent and significant vestibular reactions to even a single 100 mg dose of minocycline limit its prophylactic use. The prophylactic dose of rifampin is 600 mg twice daily in 4 doses in adults and 10 mg/kg/dose for 4 doses in children 1 mo–12 yr of age. A dose of 5 mg/kg every 12 hr for 4 doses can be used in children who are less than 1 mo of age. The emergence of rifampin-resistant strains in treated meninogococcal carriers occurs with a frequency of 0–27%.

Penicillin in dosage regimens practical for ambulatory patients has not proved to be effective prophylaxis for meningococcal disease.

Serogroup A and C meningococcal polysaccharide vaccines have been developed and are licensed in the United States. A single dose of serogroup C vaccine is about 70% effective for a period of 6–9 mo in preventing meningococcal disease in children who are over 2 yr of age. Single 50 μg injections in children under 2 yr old are not followed by adequate antibody responses. A serogroup A polysaccharide vaccine field-tested by the World Health Organization is effective in persons over 3 mo of age. An effective meningococcal serogroup B vaccine has not been prepared. Meningococcal serogroup C vaccine is recommended in addition to rifampin prophylaxis for children 2 yr of age and above who are exposed within the household or day-care nursery to a confirmed case of serogroup C meningococcal disease. Meningococcal serogroup A vaccine is recommended, in addition to rifampin prophylaxis, for children 3 mo of age and above who are exposed within the household or day-care nursery to a confirmed case of serogroup A meningococcal disease.

Treatment. *Prompt treatment* of bacterial meningitis with an appropriate antibiotic is essential. Grossly cloudy (not bloody) cerebrospinal fluid at the time of initial lumbar puncture, rarely seen with viral meningitides other than that due to mumps, is ordinarily an indication for the immediate administration of an initial intravenous dose of 50–100 mg/kg of ampicillin and 25–50 mg/kg of chloramphenicol pending results of smear and culture. This affords adequate initial treatment for meningococcus, pneumococcus, and most strains of *H. influenzae* and will prevent a significant number of deaths from the rapid progression of a potentially overwhelming infection.

The appearance of strains of *H. influenzae* type b resistant to ampicillin has required a change in the subsequent therapy given to children with bacterial meningitis. The recent identification of strains of *H. influenzae* resistant to chloramphenicol may require further changes in recommended therapy.

Generally, treatment should be initiated with ampicillin and chloramphenicol. Ampicillin is provided intravenously in a dose of 300 mg/kg/24 hr in 6 divided doses. Chloramphenicol is administered separately in a dose of 100 mg/kg/24 hr in 4 divided intravenous doses. If *N. meningitidis*, *S. pneumoniae*, or *H. influenzae* sensitive to ampicillin is identified, chloramphenicol is discontinued. If an ampicillin-resistant strain of *H. influenzae* is identified, ampicillin is discontinued. Strains of *H. influenzae* type b that are resistant to ampicillin by a standardized disc susceptibility test should be reassessed by the tube-dilution method. Colorimetric assays permit the identification of β-lactamase production (suggesting resistance to ampicillin) within 15 min. *The appropriate antibiotic should be continued intravenously until the patient is afebrile for at least 3 days, but total duration of treatment should be at least 10 days for every patient.*

If clinical improvement is noted within 24 hr, a second examination of cerebrospinal fluid is not necessary during the course of treatment. If clinical improvement is slower than anticipated or does not occur, a re-examination of cerebrospinal fluid is indicated at any time. In some medical centers re-examination is routinely made 48 hr after treatment is discontinued in an attempt to detect relapse as soon as possible following treatment of *H. influenzae* meningitis with ampicillin and document bacteriologic sterility at the conclusion of treatment. At this time the total number of cells generally is less than 50/mm³ (most are mononuclear). Cerebrospinal fluid protein concentration and the CSF:blood glucose ratio may not have returned to normal at the conclusion of treatment, but Gram stain should show no organisms, and cultures of cerebrospinal fluid should be sterile. Retreatment is mandatory if they are not, and may be necessary if more than 10% of the cells are polymorphonuclear leukocytes and if the CSF glucose or the CSF:blood glucose ratios are less than 30 mg/dl and 30%, respectively.

Strains of *H. influenzae* resistant to both ampicillin and chloramphenicol have been reported. A new antibiotic, moxalactam, is now approved for use in children and has been utilized for the treatment of *H. influenzae* meningitis. To date, all isolates of *H. influenzae* (including ampicillin and chloramphenicol-resistant strains) have been sensitive to this antibiotic at 0.25 μg/ml or less. Pharmacokinetic studies indicate that concentrations of moxalactam within CSF can be achieved at doses of 150 mg/kg/24 hr that are at least 4–8 fold greater than those required to kill all *H. influenzae* isolates. This antibiotic is an effective alternative for the treatment of *H. influenzae* meningitis when the organism is resistant to both ampicillin and chloramphenicol. Newer 3rd generation cephalosporins (e.g., cefotaxime, ceftriaxone, cefuroxime) are being tested and also may prove to be effective therapy for *H. influenzae* resistant to ampicillin and chloramphenicol.

When meningitis is due to *Streptococcus pyogenes* or *agalactiae*, ampicillin, as above, provides effective therapy. If meningitis is due to *Staphylococcus aureus* or *epidermidis* resistant to penicillin, use of oxacillin, methicillin, or nafcillin is indicated; 200 mg/kg/24 hr in 6 divided doses should be administered. The treatment of meningococcal meningitis is described in Sec 10.25.

Supportive Care. This is vital and is directed toward the anticipation and prevention of complications of the disease. Pulse rate, blood pressure, and respiratory rate must be monitored frequently. A screening neurologic examination should be performed at the time of admission and daily thereafter.

Initially, the patient should receive nothing by mouth since vomiting may occur and the risk of aspiration is thus reduced. In addition, delivery of all fluid intravenously during the early days of treatment ensures greater accuracy in the measurement of intake and output. Every child with meningitis should be evaluated carefully for identification of inappropriate secretion of antidiuretic hormone (ADH), recognition of seizure activity, and the development of subdural effusions. Body weight, serum electrolytes, serum and urine osmolalities, and urine volume and specific gravity should be monitored.

If retention of fluid in excess of solute is suspected or documented, fluid administration should be restricted to 800–1000 ml/M²/24 hr. Fluid restriction is continued until it can be established that inappropriate ADH secretion is not a factor or has dissipated. The best indicators of retention of fluid in excess of solute are the body weight and serum sodium concentration. As serum sodium increases toward normal (140 mEq/l), fluid administration may be liberalized progressively to normal maintenance levels of 1500–1700 ml/M²/24 hr.

Head circumference should be measured, and the head should be transilluminated at the time of admission and daily thereafter. These simple techniques detect possible development of subdural effusions, though an enlarging head may be due to other causes.

Treatment of subdural effusions should consist of subdural paracentesis only to curtail specific symptoms of increased intracranial pressure or to determine whether the effusions may be responsible for seizure activity or the presence of focal neurologic signs. Usually, no subdural taps are required.

When seizures are noted, a patent airway must be

maintained and appropriate anticonvulsants administered. Sodium phenobarbital (7 mg/kg as an initial dose) may be administered parenterally. Seizure control may be sustained with diphenylhydantoin (5 mg/kg/24 hr) provided in 2 divided doses intravenously. Diphenylhydantoin generally does not depress the respiratory center to the same extent as phenobarbital; it also may benefit the patient by inhibiting the secretion of ADH. Diphenylhydantoin should not be administered in solutions containing glucose, in which this drug will precipitate. If necessary to terminate an episode of seizure activity, diazepam (Valium), 1 mg/yr of age to a maximum of 10 mg, may be provided intravenously as a bolus.

Heparin therapy should be considered for patients with the syndrome of disseminated intravascular coagulation (Sec 14.69). The efficacy of this form of therapy has not been unequivocally established by controlled studies.

Corticosteroids have been suggested as a therapeutic adjunct that may reduce cerebral edema and inflammation. In 2 controlled studies, however, steroids had no significant effect on the course or outcome of bacterial meningitis. An acute increase in intracranial pressure may necessitate the use of mannitol.

Despite appropriate antibiotic therapy and recovery of the patient, colonization of the nasopharynx by *H. influenzae* type b may persist. The American Academy of Pediatrics recommends that prior to or at the time of discharge, rifampin should be provided in a dose of 20 mg/kg/24 hr for 4 days (maximum dose, 600 mg/kg/24 hr) to prevent introduction or reintroduction of the organism into the household or day-care nursery.

Prognosis. Appropriate antibiotic therapy reduces the mortality rate for bacterial meningitis in children who are beyond the neonatal period to between 1–5%, but as many as 50% of the survivors have some sequelae of their disease. Prognosis depends upon many factors: (1) age, (2) duration of illness prior to effective antibiotic therapy, (3) the specific microorganism causing disease, (4) number of organisms or quantity of capsular polysaccharide material present in the meninges and cerebrospinal fluid at the time of diagnosis, and (5) presence of disorders that may compromise host response to infection. Generally, the younger the patient, the longer effective treatment is delayed, the greater the number of organisms present in the CSF at the initial lumbar puncture, and the larger the amount of capsular polysaccharide in the CSF at that time, the worse the prognosis.

Specific sequelae or complications of bacterial meningitis include cranial nerve involvement, including deafness and blindness; hemi- or quadriparesis; muscular hypertonia; ataxia; permanent seizure disorders; and the development of obstructive hydrocephalus, mental retardation, or learning disabilities. *Hearing impairment* can be detected in 25% of children following bacterial meningitis; 12% have a hearing impairment that may interfere with normal speech. In 1 large prospective study no correlation was noted between the loss of hearing and either the age of the patient at the onset of meningitis or the duration of illness prior to admission. Loss of hearing may occur early during

the evolution of disease in many children and may not be prevented by early diagnosis and treatment. Tympanometry and hearing evaluation are recommended for all children following recovery from bacterial meningitis. *Subdural effusions* (as noted above) are so frequent in young children that most can be considered a part of the general disease process rather than as a persistent or troublesome complication. *Brain abscess* following bacterial meningitis is rare; when it is found, the possibility that it preceded the development of meningitis must be entertained and a careful search for other sites of infection, e.g., endocarditis, should be initiated.

Bacteriologic relapse may follow treatment of meningitis, particularly that due to *H. influenzae* treated with ampicillin. Relapse of *H. influenzae* meningitis after chloramphenicol treatment also has been reported, but in almost all such cases failure occurred in patients who received a portion of treatment intramuscularly, a route now known to be unreliable.

A large prospective study of bacterial meningitis in children revealed that approximately 40% have abnormalities detectable on neurologic examination at the time of discharge, but that by 2 yr after discharge specific deficits were noted in only about 10% of the total group. In many patients even major neurologic defects such as hemi- or quadriparesis cleared with time. This important observation suggests the need to maintain cautious optimism in discussing long-term complications of meningitis with parents.

RALPH D. FEIGIN

Barken RM, Greer CC, Schumacher CJ, et al: *Hemophilus influenzae* meningitis. Am J Dis Child 130:1318, 1976.

Deal WB. Sanders E: Efficacy of rifampin in treatment of meningococcal carriers. N. Engl J Med 281:641, 1969.

DeLemos RA, Haggerty RJ: Corticosteroids as an adjunct to treatment in bacterial meningitis. A controlled clinical trial. Pediatrics 44:30, 1969.

Dodge PR, Swartz MN: Bacterial meningitis. A review of selected aspects. II. Special neurologic problems, postmeningitic complications and clinicopathological correlations. N Engl J Med 272:1003, 1965.

Feigin RD, Dodge PR: Bacterial meningitis: Newer concepts of pathophysiology and neurologic sequelae. Pediatr Clin North Am 23:541, 1976.

Feigin RD, Stechenberg BW, Chang MJ, et al: Prospective evaluation of treatment of *Hemophilus influenzae* meningitis. J Pediatr 88:542, 1976.

Feldman WE: Concentrations of bacteria in cerebrospinal fluid of patients with bacterial meningitis. J Pediatr 88:549, 1976.

Gessert C, Granoff DM, Gilsdorf J: Comparison of rifampin and ampicillin in day care center contacts of *Haemophilus influenzae* type b disease. Pediatrics 66:1, 1980.

Gilday DL: Various radionuclide patterns of cerebral inflammation in infants and children. Am J Roentgenol 120:247, 1974.

McCracken GH Jr, Ginsburg CM, Zweighaft TC, et al: Pharmacokinetics of rifampin in infants and children: Relevance to prophylaxis against *Haemophilus influenzae* type b disease. Pediatrics 66:17, 1980.

Munford RS, deVasconcelos ZJS, Phillips·CJ, et al: Eradication of carriage of *Neisseria meningitidis* in families: A study in Brazil. J Infect Dis 129:644, 1974.

Norden CW, Michaels RH, Melish M: Serologic responses of children with meningitis due to *Haemophilus influenzae*, type b. J Infect Dis 134:495, 1976.

Peltola H, Kayhty H, Sivonen A, et al: *Haemophilus influenzae* type b capsular polysaccharide vaccine in children: A double-blind field study of 100,000 vaccines 3 months to 5 years of age in Finland. Pediatrics 60:730, 1977.

Pepple J, Moxon ER, Yolken RH: Indirect enzyme-linked immunosorbent assay for the quantitation of the type-specific antigen of *Haemophilus influenzae* b: A preliminary report. J Pediatr 97:233, 1980.

Robbins JB, Parke JC Jr, Schneerson R, et al: Quantitative measurement of "natural" and immunization induced *Haemophilus influenzae*, type b capsular polysaccharide antibodies. Pediatr Res 7:103, 1973.

Sell SHW, Merrill RE, Doyne EO, et al: Long-term sequelae of *Hemophilus influenzae* meningitis. Pediatrics 49:206, 1972.

Sell SHW, Webb WW, Pate JE, et al: Psychological sequelae to bacterial meningitis. Two controlled studies. Pediatrics 49:212, 1972.

Shackelford PG, Campbell J, Feigin RD: Countercurrent immunoelectrophoresis in the evaluation of childhood infections. J Pediatr 85:478, 1974.

Shapiro ED, Wald ER: Efficacy of rifampin in eliminating pharyngeal carriage of Haemophilus influenzae type b. Pediatrics 66:5, 1980.

Stovring J, Snyder RD: Computed tomography in childhood bacterial meningitis. J Pediatr 96:820, 1980.

Ward JI, Fraser DW, Baraff LJ, et al: Haemophilus influenzae meningitis: A national study of secondary spread in household contacts. N Engl J Med 301:122, 1979.

10.18 ACUTE ASEPTIC MENINGITIS

Acute aseptic meningitis, an inflammatory process of the meninges, is a relatively common illness caused by a large number of different etiologic factors. The cerebrospinal fluid is characterized by pleocytosis and the absence of microorganisms on Gram stain and on routine culture. In most instances the illnesses are self-limited; with some etiologies, however, the resulting diseases are severe and progressive and lead to disability and death.

Etiology. Etiologic agents and factors in aseptic meningitis are listed in Tables 10–19 and 10–20. At present the etiologic agent is not identified in about 90% of all cases of aseptic meningitis. However, epidemiologic study and intensive investigations at some centers indicate that the vast majority of cases result from viral infections. Enteroviruses account for approximately 80% of all cases of aseptic meningitis; the most common specific types are coxsackievirus B5 and echoviruses 4, 6, 9, and 30. Other types are listed in Table 10–21. Arboviruses account for about 5% of cases of aseptic meningitis, St. Louis encephalitis and California encephalitis being the most common. In the prevaccine era mumps was the agent responsible for the greatest occurrence of aseptic meningitis; today in the United States use of vaccine has made mumps meningitis uncommon.

Table 10–19 ETIOLOGIC VIRUSES IN ACUTE ASEPTIC MENINGITIS PRESENTED BY FREQUENCY OF OCCURRENCE IN NORTH AMERICA

VIRUSES	FREQUENCY
Enteroviruses (coxsackieviruses, echoviruses, and polioviruses)	80%
Arboviruses* (Eastern equine encephalitis, Western equine encephalitis, Venezuelan equine encephalitis, St. Louis encephalitis, Powassan encephalitis, California encephalitis, Colorado tick fever)	5%
Mumps†	5%
Herpes simplex type 2	1%
Adenoviruses	<1%
Varicella-zoster	<1%
Epstein-Barr	<1%
Lymphocytic choriomeningitis	<1%
Encephalomyelitis	<1%
Cytomegalovirus	<1%
Rhinoviruses	<1%
Measles	<1%
Rubella	<1%
Influenza viruses	<1%
Parainfluenza viruses	<1%
Live virus vaccines (measles, vaccinia, polio)	<1%

*In other areas of world many other arboviruses are important.

†In areas where mumps vaccine is not routinely used, this agent is a common cause of aseptic meningitis.

Table 10–20 CLINICAL CONDITIONS AND INFECTIOUS AGENTS OTHER THAN VIRUSES ASSOCIATED WITH ASEPTIC MENINGITIS

Bacteria; meningitis
  M. tuberculosis
  Pyogenic—partially treated
  Leptospira sp. (leptospirosis)
  T. pallidum (syphilis)
  Borrelia sp. (relapsing fever)
  Nocardia sp. (nocardiosis)
Bacteria; parameningeal focus
  Sinusitis
  Mastoiditis
  Brain abscess
Rickettsia
  R. rickettsii (Rocky Mountain spotted fever)
Mycoplasma
  M. pneumoniae
  M. hominis
Fungi
  C. immitis (coccidioidomycosis)
  B. dermatitidis (blastomycosis)
  C. neoformans (cryptococcosis)
  H. capsulatum (histoplasmosis)
  C. albicans (moniliasis)
Protozoa
  T. gondii (toxoplasmosis)
Other parasites
  Angiostrongylus cantonensis (eosinophilic meningitis)
  Trichinella spiralis (trichinosis)
Presumed infections
  Cat scratch fever
  Erythema infectiosum
  Kawasaki disease
Malignancy
  Leukemia
  CNS tumor
Postvaccination
  Rabies
  Influenza
  Pertussis
Miscellaneous
  Heavy metal poisoning
  Intrathecal injections (contrast media, serum, antibiotics, etc.)
  Foreign bodies (shunt, reservoir)

The most common cause of nonviral aseptic meningitis is partially treated bacterial disease (Table 10–20). *M. pneumoniae* is also a frequent cause of aseptic meningitis. Of the other etiologies listed in Table 10–20, the following are those most frequently seen: tuberculosis, leptospirosis, parameningeal bacterial infection, toxoplasmosis, Kawasaki disease, and malignancy.

Epidemiology. Since approximately 80% of cases of aseptic meningitis are due to enteroviral infections, the basic epidemiologic pattern reflects these agents. In temperate climates most cases occur in the summer and fall; infection with enteroviruses is spread directly from person to person, and the incubation period is usually 4–6 days. Epidemiologic considerations in aseptic meningitis due to agents other than enteroviruses depend markedly upon season, geography, climatic conditions, animal exposures, and many other factors related to the specific pathogens.

Clinical Manifestations. The clinical manifestations of enteroviral aseptic meningitis are presented in Sec 10.84. The onset of illness is generally acute, although it may be insidious over a wk or so or may be preceded by a nonspecific acute febrile illness of a few days' duration. The presenting manifestations in older children are headache and hyperesthesia, in infants, irritability and resentment at being handled. Fever, nausea, and vomiting are frequent, but convulsions are rare. Preceding or accompanying exanthems may occur, especially with the echoviruses and coxsackieviruses.

Examination reveals nuchal-spinal rigidity (Sec 10.90) without significant localizing neurologic changes.

Laboratory Manifestations. The cerebrospinal fluid contains from 20–several thousand cells/mm^3; early in the disease the cells are often polymorphonuclear; later they are chiefly mononuclear. No organisms are seen on direct smears (bacteria, mycobacteria, protozoans, yeasts), and there are normal or slightly elevated levels of protein. The glucose level is usually normal. A decrease in glucose level can occur with medulloblastoma, leukemic infiltration, *M. pneumoniae* infection, and tuberculosis and, rarely, with certain viral infections. The spinal fluid should be cultured for bacteria, fungi, and mycobacteria, and in some instances special examinations are indicated for protozoa, mycoplasma, and other pathogens. Careful examination of the spinal fluid is most important, especially to assure that stains used for smears do not introduce artifacts and that the tests used for glucose levels are accurate. A simultaneous blood glucose level is taken at the time of spinal puncture. For special laboratory procedures used in the identification of viruses and other agents, refer to the sections on various agents.

Differential Diagnosis. Careful analysis of the history and epidemiologic circumstances may point toward 1 of the specific causes listed in Tables 10–19 and 10–20. During the summer and autumn the presence of pleurodynia, herpangina, or unexplained febrile eruptions in the community suggests the possibility of coxsackievirus or echovirus infections; the coexistence of acute paralytic disorders in other patients suggests poliomyelitis; encephalitic infections in horses point to the possibility of an arbovirus infection; a history of swimming in waters contaminated by dead animals may suggest leptospiral infection. Knowledge of clear-cut exposure to or concurrent evidence of mumps or of one of the common exanthems is helpful in the differential diagnosis.

The association of pneumonia or other respiratory illness preceding aseptic meningitis strongly suggests the possibility of *M. pneumoniae* as the etiologic agent.

Most difficult from the diagnostic, therapeutic, and prognostic points of view are instances of incipient or partially treated bacterial (especially when due to *H. influenzae*) or mycobacterial meningitis. The clinical findings, the dosage of antibiotic previously used, and the spinal fluid smear, culture, and glucose level may be helpful in bacterial meningitis. When tuberculous meningitis is suspected, a careful evaluation of contacts, a careful examination of an appropriately stained smear from the pellicle of the cerebrospinal fluid that was allowed to settle, and a positive tuberculin reaction may confirm that diagnosis as correct. Since combined bacterial and viral infection has occurred, examinations of CSF should be repeated if there is the slightest doubt. The possibility that the observed meningeal reaction is of neither viral nor bacterial origin must be considered. Finally, medulloblastoma must be considered in the differential diagnosis, particularly if there are hypoglycorrhachia and prominent signs of increased intracranial pressure.

Treatment. Symptomatic measures, including aspirin, and a cool room for relief of headache, hyperesthesia, and fever are useful. The withdrawal of spinal fluid for diagnosis often relieves headache. Codeine, morphine, and the phenothiazine derivatives should be avoided since they may induce misleading signs and symptoms. Assurance that recovery is likely may be considered part of therapy.

Several wk after apparent recovery, careful neuromuscular assessment should be conducted to assure that muscular weakness is not a sequel. Bilateral audiometry is recommended, especially when mumps virus was involved.

Center for Disease Control: Aseptic Meningitis Surveillance, Annual Summary 1976. Issued January 1979.

Cherry JD: Nonpolio enteroviruses: Coxsackieviruses, echoviruses, and enteroviruses. *In*: Feigin RD, Cherry JD (eds): Textbook of Pediatric Infectious Disease. Philadelphia, WB Saunders, 1981, p 1316.

Middlekamp JN: Aseptic meningitis and viral meningitis. *In*: Feigin RD, Cherry JD (eds): Textbook of Pediatric Infectious Diseases. Philadelphia, WB Saunders, 1981, p 319.

10.19   ENCEPHALITIS

Encephalitis is an inflammation of the brain, and the diagnosis can be established with absolute certainty only by the microscopic examination of brain tissue. In clinical practice the diagnosis is frequently made on the basis of neurologic manifestations and epidemiologic findings without the aid of histologic material. When neurologic manifestations suggest encephalitis but inflammation of the brain has not occurred (such as in Reye syndrome), the condition is called an *encephalopathy*.

Usually when encephalitis occurs, other areas of the nervous system are also involved and diagnostic terms reflect this involvement: *meningoencephalitis*, *meningoencephalomyeloradiculitis*, *Guillain-Barré syndrome*, and *acute cerebellar ataxia*.

Etiology. A classification of encephalitis by etiology and source is presented in Table 10–21. Many of the agents listed in Table 10–21 produce other illnesses and are discussed more fully elsewhere (see Index). Table 10–22 provides an analysis of 1536 cases reported to the Center for Disease Control in 1977. Although only about 30% of the cases of encephalitis reported to the Center for Disease Control had established etiologies, the seasonal pattern of disease in the United States indicates that the etiologic agents in the vast majority of unknown cases are enteroviruses (Sec 10.84) or arboviruses (Sec 10.87–10.90).

Epidemiology. Since there are many different causes of encephalitis, there is not a unified epidemiologic pattern. However, the vast majority of cases occur in the summer and fall reflecting arboviral and enteroviral etiologies. Encephalitis due to arboviruses occurs in localized outbreaks and epidemics with boundaries

Table 10-21 CLASSIFICATION OF ENCEPHALITIS BY ETIOLOGY AND SOURCE

I. Infections—viral
  A. Spread man to man only
    1. Mumps: frequent; often mild
    2. Measles: may have serious sequelae
    3. Enterovirus group: frequent all ages; more serious in new-borns
    4. Rubella: uncommon; sequelae rare except in congenital rubella
    5. Herpesvirus group
      a. Herpes simplex (types 1 and 2: relatively common; sequelae frequent; devastating in newborns
      b. Varicella-zoster virus: uncommon; serious sequelae not rare
      c. Cytomegaloviruses—congenital or acquired: may have delayed sequelae in congenital CMV
      d. EB virus (infectious mononucleosis): not common
    6. Pox group
      a. Vaccinia and variola: uncommon, but serious CNS damage occurs
  B. Arthropod-borne agents
    Arboviruses: spread to man by mosquitoes or ticks: seasonal epidemics depend upon ecology of the insect vector; the following occur in the U.S.A.:

Eastern equine	St. Louis
Western equine	California
Venezuelan equine	Powassan

  C. Spread by warm-blooded mammals:
    Rabies: saliva of many domestic and wild mammalian species
    Herpesvirus simiae ("B" virus): monkeys' saliva
    Lymphocytic choriomeningitis: rodents' excreta
II. Infections—nonviral
  A. Rickettsial: encephalitic component from cerebral vasculitis
  B. *Mycoplasma pneumoniae:* interval of some days between respiratory and CNS symptoms
  C. Bacterial: tuberculous and other bacterial meningitis; often has encephalitic component
  D. Spirochetal: syphilis, congenital or acquired; leptospirosis
  E. Fungal: immunologically compromised patients at special risk; cryptococcosis; histoplasmosis; aspergillosis; mucormycosis; moniliasis; coccidioidomycosis
  F. Protozoal: *Plasmodium sp.; Trypanosoma sp.; Naegleria sp.; Acanthamoeba; Toxoplasma gondii*
  G. Metazoal: trichinosis; echinococcosis; cysticercosis; schistosomiasis

III. Parainfectious—postinfectious, allergic
  Patients in whom an infectious agent or one of its components plays a contributory role in etiology, but the intact infectious agent is not isolated in vitro from the nervous system. It is postulated that in this group the influence of cell-mediated antigen-antibody complexes plus complement is especially important in producing the observed tissue damage
  A. Associated with specific diseases (These agents may also cause direct CNS damage—see I and II above)

Measles	Rickettsial infections
Rubella	Pertussis
Mumps	Influenza
Varicella-zoster	Hepatitis
Mycoplasma pneumoniae	

  B. Associated with vaccines:

Rabies	Pertussis
Measles	Yellow fever
Influenza	Typhoid
Vaccinia	

IV. Human slow-virus diseases.
  Accumulating evidence that viruses acquired earlier in life, not necessarily with detectable acute illness, participate somehow in later chronic neurologic disease (similar events also known to occur in animals) (see Chapter 21)
  A. Subacute sclerosing panencephalitis (SSPE); measles; rubella?
  B. Jakob-Creutzfeldt disease (spongiform encephalopathy)
  C. Progressive multifocal leukoencephalopathy
  D. Kuru (Fore tribe in New Guinea only)
V. Unknown—complex group
  This group constitutes more than two-thirds of the cases of encephalitis reported to the Center for Disease Control, Atlanta, Georgia (see Table 10-22).

  There is also a miscellaneous group with eponyms which are based on clinical criteria: Reye syndrome is one current example. Others include the extinct von Economo encephalitis (epidemic from 1918 to 1928); myoclonic encephalopathy of infancy; retinomeningoencephalitis with papilledema and retinal hemorrhage; recurrent encephalomyelitis (? allergic or autoimmune); pseudotumor cerebri; and epidemic neuromyasthenia—Iceland disease.

  An encephalitic clinical picture may be presented by a patient who has ingested unknown toxic substances, as well as in recognized instances of lead or methyl mercury ingestion, with excessive percutaneous absorption of hexachlorophene, with gamma benzene hexachloride as a scabeticide, and with other toxic medications.

---

determined by the range of particular mosquito vectors and the prevalence of natural reservoir animals. Although enteroviral disease including aseptic meningitis occurs in epidemics, severe encephalitis due to these agents is usually a sporadic event.

Sporadic cases of encephalitis occur in any season; epidemiologic considerations which must be reviewed in a search for the causative agent include geographic area; climatic conditions; animal, water, food, soil, and personal exposures; and host factors.

Arboviruses are zoonoses in which man is infected accidentally by an arthropod vector, man not being essential in the life cycle of arboviruses. Most commonly mosquitoes or other insects are infected through biting birds, which often have prolonged viremia without illness. The insect vectors, though preferring birds, bite other vertebrates, including man and horses. Encephalitis in horses and mules ("blind staggers") may be the 1st indication of incipient trouble in an area; veterinarians are often the 1st to detect an impending epidemic. Rural exposure is not a sine qua non; urban and suburban outbreaks are frequent.

Eastern equine encephalitis has a predilection for young infants; it is devastating, with high mortality and severe sequelae.

St. Louis virus encephalitis produces inapparent infection (demonstrated only by seroconversion) as well as disease and has a lower incidence in young children than in adolescents and adults.

Western equine encephalitis is usually mild or clinically inapparent, demonstrated only by seroconversion. Mortality is much lower than with Eastern equine encephalitis, but sequelae may be severe in young children and adolescents.

California virus encephalitis outbreaks occur mostly in the midwestern United States. Some cases are mild, but a significant number are severe with important sequelae.

Powassan virus encephalitis is transmitted by the bite of infected wood ticks. More cases occur in Canada than in the United States; few cases have been found in children.

Venezuelan equine encephalitis also occurs in the United States. Thus far the incidence of human disease has

Table 10–22 CASES OF ENCEPHALITIS AND DEATHS, BY ETIOLOGY, IN THE UNITED STATES IN 1977

CATEGORY	CASES		DEATHS	
	Number	% of Total	Number	% of Total
Arboviral	239	15.6	10	5.8
Western equine	41		0	
Eastern equine	1		1	
St. Louis	132		9	
California	65		0	
Enteroviral	17	1.1	1	0.6
Associated with childhood infections	119	7.7	9	5.3
Measles	32		5	
Mumps	43		3	
Chickenpox	43		1	
Rubella	1		0	
Associated with respiratory illness	5	0.3	0	0
Parainfluenza	1			
Adenovirus	1			
M. pneumoniae	1			
Respiratory syncytial virus	1			
Influenza A	1			
Associated with other known etiologies	80	5.2	33	19.3
Herpes simplex	63		25	
Herpes zoster	14		7	
Infectious mononucleosis	3		1	
Unknown or inconclusive etiology	1076	70.1	118	69.0
Total	1536		171	

From the Center for Disease Control: Encephalitis Surveillance Annual Summary 1977. Issued December 1979.

been low and the illness mild, though devastating outbreaks have occurred.

The **Human Herpesvirus Group** consists of 4 DNA viruses of which man is the sole source: (1) herpes simplex types 1 and 2, (2) varicella-zoster virus, (3) cytomegalovirus, and (4) the Epstein-Barr virus (EBV) associated with infectious mononucleosis and other conditions. In addition to the more usual clinical syndromes caused by these agents, acute encephalitis may occur. These viruses may become latent and induce late neurologic damage as a result of a variety of circumstances which compromise host resistance, especially conditions associated with depressed cellular immunocompetence (e.g., malignancy, immunodepressant drugs, organ transplants).

Herpes simplex types 1 and 2 are relatively frequent causes of sporadic acute encephalitis which may occur during primary contact with the virus or in persons who had an earlier primary infection, either subclinical or long forgotten. Herpesvirus encephalitis in newborn infants (Sec 7.72) is part of a generalized viremia; the infection may be due to either type 1 ("oral") or type 2 ("genital") herpesvirus. In older patients herpes simplex virus may produce diffuse encephalitis or simulate brain abscess or fatal bulbospinal poliomyelitis, even when the patient's serologic status indicates a nonprimary infection. Characteristically, fluid obtained by nontraumatic spinal tap may contain erythrocytes. Progressive focal neurologic signs and evidence of localization on arteriography, electroencephalography, and radionuclide or CT brain scan are frequent and are indications for prompt brain biopsy and early therapy with adenine arabinoside (Sec 10.71).

Varicella-zoster virus (VZV) may cause acute encephalitis in close temporal relationship to chickenpox. The VZV is also capable of secluding itself in spinal and cranial nerve roots and ganglia as a latent or suppressed infection, to express itself later as herpes zoster.

Cytomegalovirus (CMV) may produce intrauterine infection with involvement of the central nervous system (Sec 7.69). Severe cases may be recognized at birth, but more often subtle evidence of brain damage is not apparent for months or several yr after birth. CMV may remain latent in various tissues and in leukocytes. Therefore, blood transfusions may be responsible for transmission of disease. Under situations compromising host immunity, recrudescence may occur.

Epstein-Barr virus (EBV) encephalitis may occur during infectious mononucleosis but has also been verified in patients without hematologic changes. There is no evidence at present for its becoming latent in any portion of the nervous system.

Enteroviruses (Sec 10.84) are small RNA-containing viruses; 68 specific serotypes have been identified. The serotypes of poliovirus have become less important as agents of disease among well-vaccinated populations. Not all the coxsackievirus and echovirus serotypes have been definitely associated with neurologic disease. The severity of disease ranges from mild meningoencephalitis (aseptic meningitis) to severe encephalitis with death or significant sequelae. Epidemics, some devastating, have been observed in newborn nurseries in many parts of the world.

Pathogenesis. The sequence of events varies with the agent of disease and with the host. In general, the viruses of encephalitis get into the lymphatic system, whether from ingestion of an enterovirus or from a mosquito or other insect bite. There multiplication begins, and seeding of the bloodstream leads to infection of several organs. At this stage (the extraneural phase) a nonpleural, systemic, febrile illness is present, but if further viral multiplication takes place in the seeded organs, a secondary propagation of large amounts of virus may occur. Invasion of the central nervous system is followed by clinical evidence of neurologic disease.

It is likely that neurologic damage is caused (1) by a direct invasion and destruction of neural tissues by actively multiplying viruses, or (2) by a reaction of the patient's nervous tissue to antigens of the virus. Neuronal destruction is probably due directly to viral invasion, while the host's vigorous tissue response probably results in demyelinization and vascular and perivascular destruction. Vascular damage leads to impaired circulation and to corresponding signs and symptoms. The determination of how much of the damage to the central nervous system is inflicted directly by virus and how much represents immunologically mediated injury has therapeutic implications; agents to limit viral multiplication would be indicated for the former and agents to suppress the host's cellular immune response for the latter.

The etiology and pathogenesis of cases of inflammatory encephalitis in which there is no evidence of the direct or indirect involvement of any infectious agent are poorly understood.

Pathology. It is difficult to determine the etiology of encephalitis at autopsy, although morphologic identification of falciparum malaria, trypanosomiasis, and fungal encephalitis is possible. In viral encephalitides, the histopathologist may recognize rabies (Negri bodies) or an agent of the herpesvirus group (intranuclear inclusion bodies), but special viral studies are usually needed. Viral isolation and identification require that tissues be collected *without fixation in preservatives*; immunofluorescent and electron microscopic studies may provide critical diagnostic information.

Tissue sections of the brain generally reveal meningeal congestion and mononuclear infiltration, perivascular cuffs of lymphocytes and plasma cells, some perivascular tissue necrosis with myelin breakdown, neuronal disruption in various stages including ultimately neuronophagia, and endothelial proliferation or necrosis. A marked degree of demyelination with preservation of neurons and their axons is considered predominantly "postinfectious" or "allergic" encephalitis. The severity and the extent of observed lesions vary with the viral agent as well as with the degree of reaction of the host. The cerebral cortex, especially the temporal lobe, is often severely affected by herpes simplex virus; the arboviruses tend to affect the entire brain; rabies has a predilection for the basal structures. Involvement of the spinal cord, nerve roots, and peripheral nerves is quite variable.

Extraneural pathology varies with the etiology, the duration of the illness, and the complications of intensive treatment. Pneumonia may occur with or without tracheostomy; congestive heart failure, urinary tract infection with catheterization, thrombophlebitis at the sites of infusions, hemolytic-uremic syndrome, and the syndrome of disseminated intravascular coagulation are seen.

Clinical Manifestations. The clinical findings in encephalitis are determined by (1) the severity of involvement and anatomic localization of the affected portions of the nervous system, (2) the inherent pathogenicity of the offending agent, and (3) the immune and other reactive mechanisms of the patient ("host factors"). There is, accordingly, a wide range of severity of clinical manifestations even with the same etiologic agent. Some children may appear to be mildly affected initially only to lapse into coma and sudden death. Others may have their illness ushered in by high fever, violent convulsions interspersed with bizarre movements, and hallucinations alternating with brief periods of clarity and then emerge with relatively few sequelae.

Most commonly the initial manifestations resemble an undifferentiated acute systemic illness with fever; with headache or, in infants, with screaming spells; and with abdominal distress, nausea, and vomiting. Signs of an associated mild nasopharyngitis may suggest a respiratory infection. As the temperature rises, new findings direct attention to the nervous system: mental dullness eventuating in stupor; bizarre movements; convulsions; nuchal rigidity, often not as pronounced as in purely meningitic illness; and focal neurologic signs which may be stationary, progress, or fluctuate. Loss of bowel and bladder control and unprovoked emotional bursts may occur.

Specific forms of encephalitis or complicating manifestations of encephalitis include Guillain-Barré syndrome, acute transverse myelitis, acute hemiplegia, and acute cerebellar ataxia. **Acute cerebellar ataxia** is characterized by an abrupt onset of truncal ataxia resulting in varying degrees of gait disturbance. Children with this illness will have tremulousness of the head and trunk when in the upright position and of the extremities when attempting to move them against gravity. The duration of illness varies from 3–4 days to several wk, but complete recovery usually occurs.

Diagnosis and Differential Diagnosis. A meticulous history is essential and must evaluate exposure in the past 2–3 wk to illness in contacts; exposure to mosquitoes, ticks, and animals during recent vacations, picnics, etc.; awareness of illness in animals, especially horses and other equidae, in the patient's environment; recent travel from the home area; recent injections of any kind; and the possibility of accidental exposure to heavy metals, pesticides, or other questionable substances.

The cerebrospinal fluid must be carefully examined to exclude other disorders which will respond to specific therapy. Smears for bacteria and cultures of the cerebrospinal fluid are mandatory; the history and clinical findings may indicate the need for acid-fast stain and culture of the sediment for mycobacteria. Other circumstances may indicate the need for excluding fungal or protozoal infection; atypical cells may require cytopathologic study to exclude neural neoplasms which may present acutely.

In viral encephalitis the cerebrospinal fluid is generally clear; the leukocyte count ranges from none to several thousand, often with a significant percentage of polymorphonuclear cells initially, moderate or no elevation of protein, and an initially normal level of glucose relative to the simultaneously determined blood glucose level. Expert advice should be sought early for any patient suspected of having an encephalitic illness. In any patient suspected of having viral meningoencephalitis, spinal fluid, blood, feces, and throat swabs should be collected and sent to a laboratory offering viral diagnostic services. An additional serum specimen should be collected 10–14 days later. Though these studies may not provide an immediate diagnosis, they may give early warning of a specific epidemic; the cautious experimental use of specific antiviral chemotherapy may be indicated by the preliminary results. If there is evidence for a specific virus, the patient can generally be assured of subsequent lasting immunity to that virus.

A patient with concurrent or recent mumps, measles, etc. (see Table 10–21, I, A) is a likely candidate for encephalitis, but neurologic involvement at times precedes the classic disease. Mumps meningoencephalitis commonly occurs without parotitis. When mumps parotitis occurs without clinical evidence of involvement of the central nervous system, cerebrospinal fluid pleocytosis often indicates that such involvement is present. In measles, moreover, some 40% of patients without clinical evidence of encephalitis have electroencephalograms suggestive of neurologic disturbance. The relation of acute non-neural diseases in early life to debilitating neural syndromes appearing in later life ("slow virus effects") is important (Table 10–21).

Inquiry regarding recent illness, recent injections, and especially recent exposures away from the home environment are sometimes helpful. The incubation periods of some arboviruses are such that mosquito bites acquired 1 wk or more earlier or insect bites now healed may give a clue. Occasionally patients who have traveled in Africa or Asia in recent wk will present encephalitis due to viruses, trypanosomiasis, or falciparum malaria with bizarre systemic and central nervous system signs and symptoms.

Immunologically compromised children (e.g., by lymphoma, cytotoxic drugs, immunogenetic defects) are at increased risk, especially with respect to infections in which protective cell-mediated immunity is important (e.g., chickenpox, cytomegalovirus, fungal infections). Children with leukemia who have had prophylactic radiation to the central nervous system and intrathecal drugs may develop an acute meningoencephalitis *after* cessation of such prophylaxis and despite bone marrow remission.

Prevention. The introduction of effective attenuated viral vaccines for measles, mumps, and rubella has sharply reduced central nervous system complications in these diseases. The control of encephalitis due to arboviruses has been less successful as specific vaccines for humans are not available. Control of insect vectors by suitable spraying methods and eradication of insect breeding sites is useful.

Treatment. With the exception of the use of adenine arabinoside for herpes simplex encephalitis (Sec 10.71), treatment is nonspecific and empirical, aimed at maintaining life and supporting each involved organ system. The effectiveness of various recommended regimens has not been objectively evaluated.

Until a bacterial etiology and, in particular, a brain abscess are substantially excluded, parenteral antibiotic therapy should be administered.

It is crucial to anticipate and be prepared for *convulsions, cerebral edema, hyperpyrexia, inadequate respiratory exchange, disturbed fluid and electrolyte balance, aspiration and asphyxia, abrupt cardiac and respiratory arrest of central origin,* and *cardiac decompensation.* The syndrome of *disseminated intravascular coagulation* may be an additional complication. For these reasons all patients with severe encephalitis should be cared for in intensive care units. Cardiac monitoring should be maintained. In patients with evidence of increased intracranial pressure, placement of a pressure transducer in the epidural space is often indicated for monitoring intracranial pressure as a guide to therapy aimed at reducing cerebral edema. All fluids, electrolytes, and medications are initially given parenterally. In prolonged states of coma, parenteral hyperalimentation is indicated. The syndrome of *inappropriate secretion of antidiuretic hormone* is fairly common in acute central nervous system disorders; its possible occurrence adds to the importance of frequent clinical and laboratory evaluation of the fluid and electrolyte equilibrium. Normal blood levels of glucose, magnesium, and calcium must be maintained in order to minimize the threat of convulsions.

Phenobarbital, 5–8 mg/kg/24 hr, is given in an effort to prevent convulsions. Its use may make clinical assessment of progress difficult, but the importance of preventing convulsions is paramount. If frequent or sustained convulsions appear, intravenous diazepam (0.1–0.2 mg/kg) in a 3-min infusion may be necessary.*

A number of methods are proposed to minimize cerebral edema and to diminish the consequences of cerebral anoxia; these measures are difficult to evaluate and are generally reserved for patients with very severe illness whose condition appears desperate:

1. *Dexamethasone,* 0.5 mg/kg/24 hr, is given intramuscularly. This large dose should be reduced gradually after a few days if recovery or improvement is evident. Dexamethasone probably should not be used in acute viral diseases because steroids may potentiate the viral infection.

2. Substances employed in an effort to reduce elevated intracranial pressure include: (a) *Mannitol,* given intravenously, as a 20% solution in a dose of 1.5–2.0 gm/kg over a 30–60 min period. This may be repeated every 8–12 hr.† (b) *Glycerol,* by nasogastric tube, using 0.5–1.0 ml/kg diluted with twice that volume of orange juice. This is nontoxic and may be repeated every 6 hr for an extended period of time.

Equipment and personnel for handling emergencies such as cardiac and respiratory arrest must be constantly at hand. Early consultation with an anesthesiologist is useful in anticipation of the need for artificially assisted respiration (Sec 5.42). For the management of associated cardiac arrhythmias and congestive failure, see Sec 13.67 and 13.77.

---

*Manufacturer's precaution: Efficacy and safety of parenteral diazepam in the neonate has not been established.

†Manufacturer's precaution: The use of mannitol in pediatric patients has not been studied comprehensively.

Supportive and **rehabilitative** efforts are very important after the patient recovers. Motor incoordination, convulsive disorders, squint, total or partial deafness, or behavioral disturbances may appear only after an interval of time. Visual disturbances due to chorioretinopathy and perceptual amblyopia may also make a delayed appearance. Special facilities and, at times, institutional placement may become necessary.

Prognosis. Prognosis is guarded with respect to both immediate outcome and sequelae. Sequelae involving the central nervous system may be intellectual, motor, psychiatric, epileptic, visual, or auditory. Cardiovascular, intraocular, pulmonary, hepatic, and other systems are sometimes permanently affected. The short-term and long-term prognoses depend to some extent on etiology and age. Young infants usually have severe disease and sequelae. In general, herpes simplex viruses carry a worse prognosis for survival and residual disability than do the enteroviruses. Fetal rubella encephalitis is very ominous, as is acute generalized cytomegaloviral infection accompanied by encephalitis.

The latter may be insidious, with evidence of disability deferred for some months.

JAMES D. CHERRY

Table 10–23 PERIODS OF INFECTIVITY OF SELECTED INFECTIONS

DISEASE	INFECTIVE	RECOMMENDED ISOLATION
Diphtheria	Two–4 wk; 1–2 days after start of therapy	Until 2–3 consecutive cultures are negative
Scarlet fever (scarlatina)	Variable; 1–2 days after start of therapy	One day after start of therapy
Measles (rubeola)	From 5th day of incubation through several days of rash	From onset of catarrhal stage through 3rd day of rash
Rubella (German measles)	Seven days before rash to 5 days after; up to 10–12 mo for congenital	None, except that women in the 1st trimester of pregnancy should not be exposed, nor should sexually active, nonimmune women in child-bearing years not using contraceptive measures
Smallpox (variola)	Onset of rash until all crusts are shed	Until all crusts are shed
Chickenpox (varicella)	One–2 days before rash until 5–6 days after onset, when all lesions crusted; longer in patients with immune deficiency; may be longer in actively or passively immunized patients	Until all lesions crusted; usually 5–6 days
Pertussis	From catarrhal stage through 4th wk	Four weeks or until cough has ceased; protect infants from exposure
Poliomyelitis (enterovirus)	Shortly before and after onset; virus in throat for 1 wk after onset, in feces intermittently for 3–4 wk	Enteric precautions
Mumps	Up to 7 days before and 9 days after onset of parotitis or other manifestation	Until swelling subsides
Infectious hepatitis	Variable; in feces up to 3 wk before and after jaundice; may be most communicable 1 wk before and 1 wk after onset of jaundice	Enteric precautions

Adapted from Report of the Committee on Infectious Diseases (Red Book, Ed. 18). American Academy of Pediatrics, 1977.

after thorough bathing with soap and warm water, including a shampoo. They should not return to the contaminated area.

Other materials, as well as the floor and furniture of the room, should be thoroughly washed with a disinfectant and water and the room aired for at least 24 hr before again being occupied.

Material in the unit area that cannot be burned is cleansed as follows: all clothing and linen as already described; mattresses and pillows aired for 6–8 hr, preferably on 2 successive days; all glass, rubber, china, enamelware, and any instruments which permit it boiled for 5–10 min, autoclaved, or wiped down with an antiseptic solution.

When a patient is taken to an operating or radiology room or is transferred to another unit area, the accompanying attendant must wear a clean gown and the patient should be wrapped in a clean sheet. Equipment in the operating or radiology room that has been contaminated should be cleaned in the manner described for the unit area.

R. JAMES McKAY

BACTERIAL INFECTIONS

10.21 STREPTOCOCCAL INFECTIONS

Streptococci are 1 of the most common causes of bacterial infection in infancy and childhood. Group A streptococci, the most common bacterial cause of acute pharyngitis, also produce a large variety of other infections. In addition to the acute illness, nonsuppurative sequelae are a risk to patients. Infection during the 1st 3 mo of life with group B β-hemolytic streptococci has increased markedly during the past 5–10 yr.

Etiology. Streptococci are gram-positive spherical cocci, members of the order Eubacteriales and the family Lactobacillaceae. Streptococci are classified on the basis of their ability to hemolyze red blood cells: those with hemolysins producing complete hemolysis (beta-hemolytic), those producing partial hemolysis (alpha-hemolytic), and those producing no hemolysis (gamma-hemolytic).

Lancefield further separated the streptococci into groups by precipitin tests on the basis of differences in carbohydrate components (C-carbohydrate) within the cell wall; streptococcal groups A through H and K through T have thus been identified. The cell wall is composed of 3 distinct layers. The outer portion contains several antigenic proteins; the most important is M protein. Group A β-hemolytic streptococci can be divided into more than 55 immunologically distinct types that are based on differences in the M protein. M antigen is antiphagocytic and relates directly to virulence of the streptococcus.

Two other cell-wall proteins have been identified: T and R. More than 26 types have been recognized on the basis of T agglutination. Two immunogenically distinct R proteins also have been identified. The T and R antigens are unrelated to virulence.

Streptococci elaborate toxins, enzymes, and hemolysins. More than 20 extracellular antigens released by group A hemolytic streptococci growing in human tissues have been identified. The extracellular products of greatest clinical significance are erythrogenic toxins (A, B, and C), streptolysin O, streptolysin S, diphospho-

Table 10–24 RELATIONSHIP OF STREPTOCOCCI IDENTIFIED BY LANCEFIELD GROUPING AND HEMOLYTIC REACTIONS TO SITES OF HUMAN COLONIZATION AND TO DISEASE

LANCEFIELD GROUP	SPECIES	USUAL REACTION ON SHEEP BLOOD AGAR	USUAL HUMAN HABITAT	MOST COMMON HUMAN DISEASE
A	S. pyogenes	β	Pharynx, skin, rectum	Pharyngitis, erysipelas, impetigo, septicemia, wound infections, rheumatic fever, acute glomerulonephritis, necrotizing fasciitis, cellulitis, otitis media, meningitis, pneumonia, conjunctivitis, acute endocarditis
B	S. agalactiae	β	Pharynx, vagina	Puerperal sepsis, endocarditis, neonatal sepsis, meningitis, otitis media, osteomyelitis, pneumonia
C	S. equi equisimilis dysgalactiae zooepidemicus	β	Pharynx, vagina, skin	Wound infections, puerperal sepsis. cellulitis, endocarditis
D	S. faecalis* faecium* bovis* equinus	γ	Colon contents	Endocarditis, urinary tract infections, biliary tract infections, intestinal infection, peritonitis
E F	S. infrequens	?	?	?
	S. minutus anginosus	β	Mouth, pharynx	Sinusitis, meningitis, brain abscess, pneumonia
G	S. cariis	β	Pharynx, vagina, skin	Puerperal infection, skin or wound infection, endocarditis
H	S. sanguis†	α	Mouth	Endocarditis, brain abscess
K	S. salivarius†	α	Mouth	Endocarditis, sinusitis, meningitis, brain abscess
L	—	β or α	Mouth	Endocarditis, abscess, parotitis, neonatal sepsis
M	—	β or α	Mouth, pharynx, vagina	Endocarditis, septicemia
N	S. lactis cremoris	α or γ	Pharynx	?Meningitis, ?septicemia
O	—	α or β	Pharynx, conjunctiva, vagina	Pneumonia endocarditis, septicemia
Nontypable	S. viridans	α	Pharynx	Endocarditis
Nontypable	S. mutans	α	Pharynx	Endocarditis

*"Enterococcus."

†These organisms are frequently isolated from the bloodstream as α-hemolytic streptococci. Along with many nongroupable α streptococci, they are often called S. viridans, a term that incorrectly implies a specific species. Nevertheless, as a group, they cause the majority of episodes or endocarditis and are usually, but not invariably, exquisitely sensitive to penicillin. (Reproduced from Keusch GT, Weinstein L: Streptococcal Disease, Upjohn Company Publ.)

pyridine nucleotidase, streptokinases (A and B), deoxyribonucleases (A, B, C, and D), hyaluronidase, proteinase, amylase, and esterase. Erythrogenic toxins are responsible for the rash of scarlet fever. Generally, the elaboration of erythrogenic toxin depends upon bacteriophage infection (lysogeny) of the streptococcus. Streptolysin S is largely cell bound; recent evidence suggests that it exerts a leukotoxic action. Exposure to streptolysin O is followed by the development of antibodies that aid in the diagnosis of streptococcal infection. Elaboration of streptolysins S and O produces the clear zone of hemolysis permitting classification of the organisms as β-hemolytic strains. Streptokinases are immunogenic and induce antistreptokinase antibodies; their detection also may aid in the diagnosis of streptococcal disease. Hyaluronidase may play a role in permitting the spread of streptococci in human tissues.

Separation by type of hemolysis and Lancefield typing as methods of classifying streptococci are not mutually exclusive; therefore classification is difficult. See Table 10–24 for classifications by both methods as well as for the relationship of streptococci to human colonization and disease.

Group A Streptococci

Sequelae of group A β-hemolytic streptococcal disease (rheumatic fever, glomerulonephritis) are discussed in Sec 9.81 and 16.16.

Epidemiology. Group A streptococci are normal inhabitants of the nasopharynx; reported prevalence rates vary from 15–20% throughout the year. The incidence of disease depends upon the age of the child, the season of the year, the climate in a specific geographic location, and the degree of contact between individuals.

Generally, incidence is lowest in the infant, who may be protected by transplacental acquisition of type-specific antibodies. Subsequently, the incidence increases and peaks from 10–18 yr of age. Streptococcal infection of the skin is most common in children under 6 yr; streptococcal pharyngitis is most common between 6–12 yr. The incidence of streptococcal pharyngitis is higher in temperate climates, and incidence and severity appear to increase in cold weather. Streptococcal skin disease is more prevalent in tropical climates or in warmer weather in the temperate climates.

Group A β-hemolytic streptococci are spread from

person to person or occasionally from animals to people. Infection may be spread by droplets; nasal and pharyngeal carriers of the organism are effective disseminators. Infection also may be spread by contact with skin lesions or transmitted by food, milk, and water contaminated with streptococci. Dried streptococci found in dust are probably noninfectious.

Since infection is spread most commonly by droplets or by direct contact, acquisition of streptococci generally is associated with crowding in the home, school, military installation, or other institution. Immunity, which is type-specific, may be induced either by carriage of the organism or by overt infection. The incidence of streptococcal disease diminishes during adult life as immunity develops to the more prevalent serotypes.

Pathology. Streptococcal infection is associated with an acute inflammatory response. Local lesions are characterized by edema, hyperemia, and infiltration by polymorphonuclear leukocytes. Pathologic changes seen in patients with scarlet fever are related to the organisms and to toxin elaboration. Toxin elaboration is accompanied by a skin rash due to hyperemia, edema, and polymorphonuclear cell infiltrates in the corium of the skin.

Pathogenesis. Approximately 20 million group A β-hemolytic streptococci must be deposited on the pharyngeal mucosa to cause infection. Streptococci proliferate rapidly following inhalation. Leukocytes are attracted to the mucosal surface but may or may not be successful in phagocytosis. The hyaluronic acid capsule and the M protein of streptococci exert antiphagocytic activity; if the organism is phagocytized, it may be killed promptly. Sometimes engulfment does not result in death because the polysaccharide-glycopeptide cell wall complex is resistant to enzymatic degradation. In addition, the organisms may elaborate leukotoxic DPNase and streptolysin S. Nonphagocytized streptococci may elaborate streptolysin O. The enzyme also has a leukotoxic effect. Lysis of leukocytes, erythrocytes, and host cells produces an inflammatory focus. Streptokinase may activate plasminogen in the inflammatory exudate. In turn, activated plasminogen may act on fibrin to provide nutrients for further bacterial growth. Production of hyaluronidase may aid in the spread of infection. If erythrogenic toxin is elaborated in an individual who does not possess immunity to the toxin, scarlet fever will result.

Clinical Manifestations. The most common infections caused by group A β-hemolytic streptococci involve the respiratory tract, skin, soft tissues, and blood.

Respiratory Tract Infection. The incubation period of streptococcal respiratory disease is 1–3 days. The clinical expression of upper respiratory infection depends upon the age of the host. In children under 6 mo of age, illness is characterized by a thin, clear, nasal discharge which may be associated with anorexia, irritability, and other nonspecific symptoms. Temperature may be slightly elevated or normal. The acute symptoms may last 1 wk and may be indistinguishable from the common cold. In some cases symptoms and signs persist for 4–6 wk. This syndrome and that caused by streptococci in children between 6 mo–3 yr of age have been termed streptococcosis.

Streptococcosis in children between 6 mo–3 yr of age is characterized by low-grade fever, nasopharyngitis, and anterior cervical lymphadenopathy. The nasal discharge may be purulent. Otitis media and sinusitis may be complications. Symptoms may persist for 1–2 mo and weight loss may occur.

In older children disease is characterized by acute tonsillitis or pharyngitis. Fever and vomiting may be prominent. Listlessness, anorexia, headache, dysphagia, and abdominal pain may occur. The tonsils and pharynx are extremely hyperemic and covered by a purulent patchy or confluent yellow exudate. Palatal erythema, petechiae, and edema may be present. Respiratory obstruction may develop secondary to extensive edema and inflammation of the soft tissues. Streptococcal pharyngitis also may be associated with contiguous spread of infection, producing sinusitis or otitis media. Rarely, purulent material coalesces, and streptococcal parapharyngeal or retropharyngeal abscess results. Streptococci also may disseminate hematogenously and produce septicemia, pneumonia, and meningitis. Cervical lymphadenopathy is usual. Pain associated with pharyngitis and lymphadenopathy may cause meningismus. In some cases, signs and symptoms may be minimal.

Scarlet Fever. Scarlet fever is the result of infection by streptococci that elaborate an erythrogenic toxin against which the host has no antibodies. The incubation period ranges from 1–7 days with an average of 3 days. The onset is acute, characterized by fever, vomiting, headache, pharyngitis, and chills. Within 12–48 hr the typical rash appears. Abdominal pain may be present; when this is associated with vomiting prior to the appearance of the rash, an abdominal surgical condition may be suggested.

Generally, temperature increases abruptly and may peak at 39.6–40° C (103–104° F) on the 2nd day of illness. A gradual return to normal is noted over the next 5–7 days in the untreated patient; temperature usually drops to normal within 12–24 hr after the initiation of penicillin therapy. An exanthem will be noted. The tonsils are hyperemic and edematous and may be covered with exudate. The pharynx is inflamed and covered by a membrane in severe cases. The tongue may be edematous and reddened. During the early days of illness the dorsum of the tongue has a white coat through which the red and edematous papillae project (*white strawberry tongue*). After several days the white coat desquamates; the red tongue studded with prominent papillae persists (*red strawberry tongue*). The palate and uvula may be edematous, reddened, and covered with petechiae.

The exanthem is red, punctate, or finely papular. In some individuals it may be palpated more readily than it is seen, having the texture of gooseflesh or coarse sandpaper. The rash appears initially in the axillae, groin, and neck but within 24 hr becomes generalized. Punctate lesions generally are not present on the face. The forehead and cheeks appear flushed, and the area around the mouth is pale (*circumoral pallor*). The rash is most intense in the axillae and groin and at pressure sites. Areas of hyperpigmentation which do not blanch with pressure may appear in the deep creases, particularly in the antecubital fossae (*Pastia lines*). In patients with severe disease, small vesicular lesions (*miliary sudamina*) may be noted over the abdomen, hands, and feet.

The skin begins to desquamate on the face in fine flakes toward the end of the 1st wk, and desquamation proceeds over the trunk and finally to the hands and feet. The duration and extent of desquamation vary with the intensity of the rash; desquamation may continue for as long as 6 wk.

Scarlet fever may follow infection of wounds (surgical scarlet fever), burns, or streptococcal skin infection. Clinical manifestations are similar to those described above, but the tonsils and pharynx generally are not involved. A similar picture may be observed with occasional strains of staphylococci-which produce an erythrogenic toxin.

Pneumonia. Streptococcal pneumonia frequently begins as an interstitial bronchopneumonia. Subsequently, the inflammation may become confluent; lobar consolidation results. The disease may be rapidly progressive, and severe, diffuse, necrotizing pneumonia may be observed. Pleuritis and empyema are common.

Fever, chills, cough, and chest pain are noted. Older children may produce purulent sputum; hemoptysis may be observed.

Severe, necrotizing, streptococcal pneumonia is more common in newborn infants and in individuals whose response to infection has been compromised. Streptococcal pneumonia is also more frequent in children with chronic lung disease or with respiratory viral infections.

Skin Infections. The most common form of skin infection due to group A β-hemolytic streptococci is superficial pyoderma (impetigo). Disease develops frequently with an outbreak of vesicular lesions on the arms and legs or about the mouth, nose, and scalp. The lesions generally become pustular and subsequently are covered by a thick crust. The patient may complain of itching, but pain and systemic symptoms are unusual. Lymphangitis and regional lymphadenitis may be noted. Bacteremia is rare. Bullous lesions suggest concurrent infection with staphylococci.

Deeper soft tissue infections may occur secondary to impetigo. Streptococcal cellulitis is a painful, erythematous, indurated infection of the skin and subcutaneous tissues. Lymphangitis and regional lymphadenitis are common. Fever and other systemic manifestations of disease may be noted.

Erysipelas is a cellulitis and acute lymphangitis of the skin which spreads marginally. The skin is erythematous and indurated; the margins of the lesions have a raised firm border. The skin lesion usually is associated with fever, vomiting, and irritability. These symptoms subside when progression of the rash ceases. In some cases streptococci break through the lymphatic barrier, and cellulitis, subcutaneous abscesses, bacteremia, and metastatic foci of infection are observed.

Bacteremia and death have been associated with streptococcal cellulitis in the newborn infant. Progression of this disease may be so rapid that there is no response to treatment with penicillin.

Bacteremia. Streptococcal bacteremia may follow localized streptococcal disease of the skin or respiratory tract. Malaise, vomiting, chills, fever, prostration, and delirium may be observed. Group A streptococcal bacteremia also has been noted in children without an obvious focus of infection. This form of disease is most common in young children and is more frequent in children with cancer, diabetes, and other debilitating diseases. Rarely, disseminated intravascular coagulation and peripheral gangrene are noted. An unusual disseminated nodular papulosquamous eruption has been reported in a 15 mo old child with streptococcal bacteremia. The skin lesions were presumed to represent a hypersensitivity response to the group A β-hemolytic streptococcus.

Hematogenous infection of various organs may result in *meningitis, osteomyelitis, arthritis,* or *pyelonephritis.* Rarely, *acute* or *subacute bacterial endocarditis* has been due to group A β-hemolytic streptococci.

Vaginitis. The β-hemolytic streptococcus is a common cause of vaginitis in prepubertal girls. There is usually a serous discharge and marked erythema and irritation of the vulvar area, accompanied by discomfort in walking and urination. *Proctitis* is rare but may be seen in either sex.

Diagnosis. The diagnosis of streptococcal infection is suggested by characteristic clinical findings but established with certainty only by isolation of the organism. Identification of group A β-hemolytic streptococci is relatively easy. The organisms can be grown on a 5% sheep blood agar plate. If colonies are β-hemolytic, a clear zone of hemolysis will be apparent. Single colonies are then picked and streaked heavily onto a new plate. A 0.02 unit bacitracin disc is placed in the center; group A colonies will not grow around the disc (bacitracin-sensitive). Colonies also can be identified as group A by fluorescent antibody staining or Lancefield precipitin grouping.

Throat culture is the most useful laboratory aid in patients with acute tonsillitis or pharyngitis. A positive throat culture may indicate streptococcal pharyngitis, but hemolytic streptococci are common inhabitants of the nasopharynx in well children. Moreover, some children with a viral upper respiratory infection have positive throat cultures for β-hemolytic streptococci. Thus, isolation of a group A streptococcus from the pharynx of a child with pharyngeal infection does not necessarily indicate that the disease is caused by this organism. When streptococci are isolated from children with moderate or severe exudative pharyngitis who have petechiae on the palate and cervical adenitis, the diagnosis is more secure.

The immunologic response of the host following exposure to streptococcal antigen can be assessed. Antistreptolysin O (ASO) titers are commonly measured. An increase in ASO titer to greater than 166 Todd units has been reported in more than 80% of untreated children with streptococcal pharyngitis within the 1st 3 wk following infection. This response may be modified or abolished by early and effective antibiotic therapy. ASO titers may be very high in patients with rheumatic fever; in contrast, they are weakly positive or not elevated at all in patients with streptococcal pyoderma; responses in patients with glomerulonephritis are variable.

Individuals with impetigo may react strongly to stimulation by other streptococcal extracellular products. Anti-DNase (deoxyribonuclease) B appears to be the best serologic test for streptococcal pyoderma. Most patients with streptococcal pharyngitis also develop elevated titers to this enzyme.

Patients with pyoderma and pharyngitis also may develop antibody responses to hyaluronidase. Antihyaluronidase (AH) titers are elevated with less regularity than are ASO titers. For this reason, this test may supplement but should not replace the ASO test.

A response to DPNase (NADase, nicotinamide adenine dinucleotidase) may indicate present or past infection and also may provide information with regard to the infecting serotype. This enzyme is made in particularly large quantities by serotypes 4, 12, and 49.

Antistreptokinase titers are of limited value.

A 2 min inexpensive slide test (Streptozyme), designed to detect antibodies involved in all of the tests mentioned above, has been developed. Several studies have demonstrated that this test detects more patients with increased antibody titers than any other single test presently available. Nonspecific (false positive) reactions have been limited in number, and the performed test is capable of detecting antibody responses early in the course of disease. However, the strength of the Streptozyme reagent varies from lot to lot. Further, evaluation of the group specificity of the Streptozyme test suggested that it may not be specific for antibodies to extracellular products of group A streptococci since a response to this test was observed in individuals with only non-group A strains isolated from their upper respiratory tracts. In patients with group A streptococci in their respiratory tract cultures, the antibody response as measured by Streptozyme was comparable to but no greater than the ASO or anti-DNase B tests. Thus, although these factors suggest that the Streptozyme test is a valuable adjunct to the diagnosis of streptococcal disease, further standardization is needed.

Immunity to erythrogenic toxin can be measured by the Dick test. This is performed by inoculating 0.1 ml of a standardized dilution of erythrogenic toxin intracutaneously. The reaction is read at 24 hr and is positive if local erythema measures 10 mm or more in diameter. A negative reaction indicates neutralization of toxin (immunity); a positive reaction implies absence of antitoxin.

The white blood cell count may or may not be elevated. Leukocytosis may be noted in many bacterial and viral childhood diseases; hence, this finding is nonspecific. Similar elevations in erythrocyte sedimentation rate and C-reactive protein do not help to establish a specific diagnosis.

Differential Diagnosis. Acute pharyngitis indistinguishable clinically from that caused by group A β-hemolytic streptococci may be caused by many viruses, including EB virus (infectious mononucleosis) and cytomegalovirus. A viral etiology may be suggested by failure to isolate streptococci and may be identified specifically (if desired) by viral culture and serologic studies. Infectious mononucleosis may be suggested by clinical manifestations, the presence of atypical lymphocytes in the peripheral blood, and a rise in heterophile and EB viral antibody titers. Acute pharyngitis similar to that caused by β-hemolytic streptococci may be noted in patients with diphtheria, tularemia, and toxoplasmosis, and, rarely, in individuals with tonsillar tuberculosis, salmonellosis, and brucellosis. These diseases can be differentiated by appropriate cultures and serologic tests. An ulcerative pharyngitis may be noted in children with agranulocytosis, regardless of etiology.

Scarlet fever must be distinguished from other exanthematous diseases, including measles (characterized by its distinct prodrome of conjunctivitis, photophobia, dry cough, Koplik spots), rubella (disease is mild, postauricular lymphadenopathy usually is present, and throat culture is negative), and other viral exanthems. With infectious mononucleosis there is generally pharyngitis, rash, lymphadenopathy, and splenomegaly as well as atypical lymphocytes. The exanthems produced by several enteroviruses can be confused with scarlet fever. Generally, differentiation can be established readily by the course of the disease, the associated symptoms, and the results of culture. Fifth disease (Sec 10.70) is distinguished by its reticulated rash, lack of pharyngeal exudate, and negative bacterial cultures; roseola is characterized by the cessation of fever with the onset of rash and the transient nature of the exanthem. Severe sunburn can be confused with scarlet fever.

Reversion of the reaction to the Dick test from positive to negative during scarlet fever may confirm the diagnosis.

Streptococcal pyoderma must be differentiated from staphylococcal skin disease. Often these bacterial species coexist. The lesions produced are clinically indistinguishable; distinction is made only by culture.

Streptococcal septicemia, meningitis, septic arthritis, and pneumonia present signs and symptoms similar to those produced by other bacterial organisms. The offending pathogen can be established only by culture.

Complications. Complications generally reflect extension of streptococcal infection from the nasopharynx. This may result in sinusitis, otitis media, mastoiditis, cervical adenitis, retropharyngeal or parapharyngeal abscess, or bronchopneumonia. Hematogenous dissemination of streptococci may cause meningitis, osteomyelitis, or septic arthritis. Nonsuppurative late complications include rheumatic fever and glomerulonephritis.

Prevention. Administration of penicillin will prevent most cases of streptococcal disease if the drug is provided prior to the onset of symptoms. Indications for prophylaxis are not clear. Generally, we have obtained throat cultures from children who are close family contacts of patients with streptococcal disease. These include individuals living or eating with the family. If these cultures are positive, oral penicillin G or V, (400,000 units/dose) is provided 4 times each day for 20 days. Alternatively, 600,000 units of benzathine penicillin in combination with 600,000 units of aqueous procaine penicillin may be given as a single intramuscular injection. A similar approach may be used for institutional epidemics. Children exposed to an individual case at school may be observed carefully.

Management of carriers of group A β-hemolytic streptococci is controversial. Some authorities have suggested that treatment of the carrier precludes the development of type-specific immunity, thereby leaving the individual susceptible to reinfection and deferring illness until late in life.

No streptococcal vaccines are available for clinical use at this time.

Treatment. Penicillin is the drug of choice for the treatment of streptococcal infections. All strains of group A β-hemolytic streptococci isolated to date have been sensitive to concentrations of penicillin achievable in vivo. Optimal treatment eradicates streptococci, prevents septic complications, and diminishes the likelihood of rheumatic fever.

The goal of therapy is to maintain for at least 10 days blood and tissue levels of penicillin sufficient to kill streptococci. The dose utilized and the route chosen for delivery of medication depend upon a number of factors including clinical manifestations of infection, patient compliance, and cost, which also affects compliance.

Studies have documented that streptococcal pharyngitis and simple pyoderma can be eradicated by 800,000 units of penicillin G taken orally in 4 divided doses for 10 days, but children are customarily treated with 1.2–1.6 million units of penicillin daily in 4 divided doses. Penicillin G or penicillin V may be employed; the latter is preferable because satisfactory blood levels are achieved even when the stomach is not empty. Amoxicillin given orally in a dose of 125 mg 3 times each day regardless of the weight of the child may be as effective as penicillin but is associated with a greater frequency of adverse reactions and with higher cost.

Erythromycin (40 mg/kg/24 hr), lincomycin (40 mg/kg/24 hr), or clindamycin (30 mg/kg/24 hr) may be used for treatment of streptococcal pharyngitis in patients allergic to penicillin. Generally, relapse rates are greater with regimens other than penicillin. Tetracyclines and sulfonamides should not be used for treatment of streptococcal disease; sulfonamides may be used for prophylaxis of rheumatic fever.

A single dose of 1,200,000 units of benzathine penicillin intramuscularly provides adequate therapy for streptococcal pharyngitis. This circumvents the problem of patient compliance in use of an oral antibiotic. In addition, relapse rates are lower, presumably because compliance is superior. Some have suggested that the clinical manifestations of streptococcal pharyngitis are of shorter duration if a combination of 600,000 units of procaine penicillin and 600,000 units of benzathine penicillin is given.

Patients with scarlet fever, streptococcal bacteremia, pneumonia, meningitis, deep soft tissue infections, erysipelas, or complications of streptococcal pharyngitis should be treated parenterally with penicillin, preferably intravenously. The dose and duration of therapy must be tailored to the nature of the disease process with daily doses as high as 400,000 units/kg/24 hr required in the most severe infections.

Prognosis. The prognosis for adequately treated streptococcal infections is excellent, and most suppurative complications are prevented or readily treated. When therapy is provided promptly, nonsuppurative complications are prevented and complete recovery is the rule. In rare instances, particularly in the newborn infant or in children whose response to infection is compromised, fulminant pneumonia, septicemia, and death may occur despite usually adequate therapy.

Infections Due to Other Streptococci

In many centers the group B streptococcus has become the leading cause of neonatal septicemia and meningitis (Sec 7.59). Disease due to group B hemolytic streptococci has also become increasingly prevalent in infants 1–6 mo of age, in whom the organism has been associated with septicemia, meningitis, otitis media, osteomyelitis, and septic arthritis. Parenteral treatment with aqueous penicillin G is effective; the dose and duration depend upon the nature of the disease process.

Human infection with streptococci of groups C to H and K to O, as well as with nontypable strains, has been reported in normal infants and children. The classification of these organisms and the infections with which they have been associated are shown in Table 10–24. Penicillin G provides effective therapy for nongroup A streptococci, except for those belonging to group D (enterococci) and selected α-hemolytic strains; these organisms generally are susceptible to ampicillin. When endocarditis is caused by enterococci, therapy with ampicillin plus an aminoglycoside is recommended.

Bacterial endocarditis in children is commonly due to infection with *Streptococcus viridans*. A variant of this organism which requires vitamin B6 or thiol compounds for optimal growth has caused endocarditis in adults and children. It is important to recognize these organisms as a possible cause of endocarditis because supplemented media are needed for their isolation and sensitivity testing; spuriously low MIC's may be reported when nonsupplemented media are used. Some of these organisms are relatively tolerant to penicillin; therapy with penicillin and an aminoglycoside is recommended until results of sensitivity studies are available.

Breese BB: Beta-hemolytic streptococcal infections in children. Pediatr Clin North Am 7:843, 1960.

Breese BB, Disney FA, Tapley W, et al: Streptococcal infections in children. Comparison of the therapeutic effectiveness of erythromycin administered twice daily with erythromycin, penicillin phenoxymethyl, and clindamycin administered three times daily. Am J Dis Child 128:457, 1974.

Burech DL, Koranyi KI, Haynes RE: Serious group A streptococcal diseases in childhood. J Pediatr 88:972, 1976.

Feder HM Jr, Olsen N, McLaughlin JC, et al: Bacterial endocarditis caused by vitamin B6–dependent viridans group streptococcus. Pediatrics 66:309, 1980.

Kaplan EL, Howe BB: The sensitivity and specificity of an agglutination test for antibodies to streptococcal extracellular antigens: A quantitative analysis and comparison of the Streptozyme test with anti-streptolysin O and anti-deoxyribonuclease B tests. J Pediatr 96:367, 1980.

Silverman BK, Bierman RH, Atkin D, et al: Comparative serological changes following treated group A streptococcal pharyngitis. Am J Dis Child 127:498, 1974.

Stillerman M, Isenberg HD, Facklam RR: Treatment of pharyngitis associated with group A streptococcus: Comparison of amoxicillin and potassium phenoxymethyl penicillin. J Infect Dis 129:S169, 1974.

Wannamaker LW: Differences between streptococcal infections of the throat and of the skin. N Engl J Med 282:23, 78, 1970.

Wannamaker LW, Denny FW, Perry WD, et al: The effect of penicillin prophylaxis on streptococcal disease rates and the carrier state. N Engl J Med 249:1, 1953.

10.22 PNEUMOCOCCAL INFECTIONS

The pneumococcus, a normal inhabitant of the upper respiratory tract, can be an invasive pathogen. The name *Diplococcus pneumoniae*, which was adopted by American toxonomists in 1920, has been changed to *Streptococcus pneumoniae*.

Etiology. *Streptococcus pneumoniae* is a gram-positive, lancet-shaped, encapsulated diplococcus. In body fluids and tissues the organisms may be found as individual cocci or in chains. More than 80 serotypes have been identified on the basis of their type-specific capsular polysaccharide. Antisera to some pneumococcal capsular polysaccharides cross-react with other pneumococcal types or with other bacterial species. Only smooth, encapsulated strains are pathogenic for humans. Virulence is related, in part, to the size of the capsule, but pneumococcal types with capsules of the same size may vary widely in virulence. Fully encapsulated strains (e.g., type 3) are extraordinarily virulent. Capsular material impedes phagocytosis; the mechanism is unclear.

Somatic antigens also have been isolated. C substance is a cell-wall antigen which is related to species rather than to specific pneumococcal serotypes. R antigen is a species-specific protein on or near the cell surface. A *type*-specific protein (M antigen) also has been detected, but it does not confer any significant antiphagocytic properties upon the pneumococcus. Antibodies to the C, R, or M antigens produce only a negligible degree of immunity. In contrast, antibodies to the capsular polysaccharide are protective. The pneumococcus produces a hemolytic toxin called pneumolysin and a toxic neuraminidase. During autolysis pneumococci release a purpura-producing principle that causes both dermal and internal hemorrhages when injected into rabbits. The role of these substances, if any, in the pathogenesis of human disease is unknown.

On solid media, the pneumococcus forms unpigmented, umbilicated colonies surrounded by a zone of incomplete (α) hemolysis. Pneumococcal capsules can be seen and the organisms typed by exposing them to homologous type-specific antisera, which combine with their respective capsular polysaccharides and thus render the capsules refractile (quellung reaction).

Epidemiology. Many healthy individuals carry *S. pneumoniae* in their upper respiratory tracts. Serotypes 6, 19, and 23 constitute almost 50% of all isolates in children. These, plus types 3, 9, 11, 14, 15, and 18 account for 80% of all pneumococcal isolates. Frequently, the same serotype is carried continuously for extended periods (45 days–6 mo). However, carriage of a particular serotype does not induce local or systemic immunity sufficient to prevent later reacquisition of the same serotype. Most surveys have demonstrated that multiple serotypes may coexist in the same nasopharynx. Children in close contact with one another over long periods of time do not necessarily show the same pneumococcal serotype. Pneumococcal isolation rates peak during the 1st 2 yr of life and decline gradually thereafter; carriage rates are highest between December and April and lowest in July, August, and September.

Pneumococcal disease in adults is caused predominantly by low-numbered serotypes (1–8). In 305 hospitalized children with pneumococcal bacteremia, 90% of the organisms isolated were serotypes 1, 3, 4, 6, 7, 8, 9, 14, 18, 19, and 23. Reasons for these differences are not apparent. The greatest incidence of pneumococcal disease occurs in children between 6 mo–4 yr of age and in adults over 50. It is most prevalent in children who lack type-specific serum antibody.

Pneumococcal disease generally occurs sporadically. Its frequency and severity are increased in patients with sickle cell disease, asplenia, splenosis, deficiencies in humoral (B cell) immunity, and complement deficiencies.

Pathogenesis and Pathology. Pneumococci must invade to produce disease. Nonspecific local host defense mechanisms, including the presence of other bacteria in the nasopharynx, generally limit the multiplication of pneumococci. Aspiration of secretions containing pneumococci is prevented by the epiglottic reflex and by the cilia of the respiratory epithelium, which continuously move infected mucus upward toward the pharynx. Whether or not disease develops when pneumococci reach the alveoli depends upon the outcome of the interaction of the organism and the alveolar macrophage.

Pneumococcal infection frequently follows a viral respiratory tract infection which may produce mucosal damage, diminish the epithelial ciliary activity, and depress the function of alveolar macrophages. Phagocytosis may be impeded by respiratory secretions. In the tissues pneumococci multiply and spread via the lymphatics or bloodstream (bacteremia) or by direct extension from a local site of infection.

The severity of disease is related to the virulence of the organism, the number of organisms causing bacteremia, and the integrity of specific host defense mechanisms. Generally, a poor prognosis is associated with very large numbers of pneumococci in blood or with significant concentrations of capsular polysaccharide in the circulation; despite effective antibiotic therapy, many patients with antigenemia have a severe and protracted illness.

Additional factors important in the pathogenesis of pneumococcal infection have become apparent from recent studies of the compromised host. Homozygous C3 deficiency or hypercatabolism of C3 has been associated with severe and recurrent pneumonia and meningitis due to *S. pneumoniae*. Disease in such patients presumably reflects deficient opsonization and phagocytosis of the pneumococcus. The increased propensity for pneumococcal disease in patients who have been splenectomized or who are born asplenic presumably is related to deficient opsonization of the pneumococcus as well as to absence of the filtering function of the spleen on circulating bacteria. Pneumococcal disease also is more prevalent in patients with sickle cell disease and other hemoglobinopathies. Such patients become unable to activate C3 via the alternative pathway and to fix this opsonin to the pneumococcal cell wall. The efficacy of phagocytosis also is diminished in patients with B and T cell immunodeficiency syndrome because of a lack of opsonic anticapsular antibody and a failure to produce lysis and agglutination of bacteria. These observations suggest (1) that opsonization of the pneumococcus depends upon both the classical and the properdin (or alternative) complement pathways and (2) that recovery from pneumococcal disease depends upon the development of anticapsular antibodies which act as opsonins, thereby enhancing phagocytosis and ultimately killing the pneumococcus.

Recently, low levels of factor B of the properdin pathway (and defective opsonization) have been noted in normal individuals during acute pneumococcal disease. This finding suggests that pneumococcal infection may develop in some individuals because of a transient pre-existing depression of factor B; alternatively, acute pneumococcal infection may be accompanied by consumption of this component of complement.

In the lung and other body tissues the spread of infection is enhanced by the antiphagocytic properties of capsular-specific soluble substance; an edema-promoting factor also plays a role. In the lung, once infection is established, the alveoli are filled with acellular serous fluid. Soon thereafter polymorphonuclear leukocytes accumulate in the infected alveoli (consolidation), and phagocytosis of pneumococci may be noted. Macrophages subsequently replace the leukocytes in the exudate, and the lesion resolves. This sequence of events evolves over a period of 7–10 days but may be modified by appropriate antibiotic therapy or by administration of type-specific serum. The pathologic sequence in pneumococcal pneumonia is detailed in Sec 12.66.

Clinical Manifestations. These are related to the site of infection. Upper and lower respiratory tract infections are most common and frequently follow or occur concomitantly with a viral respiratory illness. Pneumonia, otitis media, or sinusitis may be noted. *S. pneumoniae* remains the most common bacterial cause of acute otitis media in children over 1 mo of age. Local spread of infection may occur, causing empyema, pericarditis, mastoiditis, epidural abscess, or, rarely, meningitis. Bacteremia may be followed by meningitis, septic arthritis, osteomyelitis, endocarditis, and brain abscess. Pneumococcal osteomyelitis, septic arthritis, and meningitis are more frequent in children with asplenia or sickle cell disease and after splenectomy.

Recent reports highlight the occurrence of pneumococcal bacteremia in young children with unexplained fever but no localizing signs or symptoms. The index of suspicion for this condition should be highest for children 6–24 mo of age with a body temperature of 38.9° C or higher and a white blood cell count greater than 20,000/mm³. Many of these patients appear minimally ill, and in some the bacteremia is a transient event, recovery ensuing without treatment. In others, however, bacteremia persists, and otitis media, pneumonia, and/or meningitis develops.

In recent years pneumococcal bacteremia, meningitis, endocarditis, and endophthalmitis have been documented in an increasing number of infants under 1 mo of age.

Primary peritonitis is frequently pneumococcal in origin. The route of entry of organisms is unknown, but bacteremia, ascending spread of organisms from the genital tract, transdiaphragmatic lymphatic spread, and bacterial migration from the intestine all have been suggested. Sudden onset of fever, abdominal pain, nausea, and vomiting occur. In some cases a history of preceding upper respiratory infection or diarrhea can be elicited. Generalized tenderness and guarding of the abdomen occur. Children with nephrotic syndrome are particularly prone to develop pneumococcal peritonitis.

Renal glomerular-capillary and cortical arteriolar thromboses have been associated with pneumococcal bacteremia. Localized gingival lesions, gangrenous areas of skin on the face or extremities, and disseminated intravascular coagulation have also been reported as manifestations of pneumococcal disease.

Diagnosis. This can be established definitively by recovery of pneumococci from the site of infection or the blood. Pneumococci found in the nose or throat of patients with otitis media, pneumonia, septicemia, or meningitis may not be related causally to their disease.

Blood cultures should be obtained in all children with pneumonia, meningitis, arthritis, osteomyelitis, peritonitis, pericarditis, or gangrenous skin lesions. It is also advisable to obtain blood cultures in children 6–24 mo of age with high fever and leukocytosis who have no localized signs of infection.

Pneumococci can be identified in body fluids as gram-positive, lancet-shaped diplococci. A direct quellung test utilizing pneumococcal omniserum (containing high titers of antibody to 82 pneumococcal types) may help to establish a definitive diagnosis rapidly. Early in the course of pneumococcal meningitis, many bacteria may be noted in a relatively acellular cerebrospinal fluid. Countercurrent immunoelectrophoresis of serum, cerebrospinal fluid, and urine, utilizing pneumococcal omniserum, may be helpful in establishing the diagnosis of pneumococcal meningitis or bacteremia. Pneumococcal antigen also may be detected in blood or urine of patients with localized pneumococcal disease (i.e., pneumonia, otitis media). Type-specific antisera enhance the sensitivity of this technique significantly; the diagnostic value of this technique is not affected significantly by previous antibiotic therapy. Countercurrent immunoelectrophoresis of sputum can be helpful in distinguishing between persons with pneumococcal pneumonia and those in whom colonization with the pneumococcus has occurred. This test generally is positive in the former and negative in the latter.

Leukocytosis generally is pronounced, with total white blood cell counts of 30,000/mm³ a common occurrence. The sedimentation rate may be elevated.

Differential Diagnosis. Unexplained fever in a child with leukocytosis may be noted in many bacterial, viral, and rickettsial diseases (Sec 10.10). Differentiation depends upon identification of the offending pathogen by culture (usually of blood). A chest roentgenogram is recommended, particularly in young children, even if physical examination reveals no signs of pneumonia.

Pneumococcal pneumonia characteristically assumes a lobar pattern in adults and older children. Lobar consolidation is less characteristic in young children. Chest roentgenograms of children with pneumonia due to viruses, mycoplasma, other bacteria, and fungi may be indistinguishable from those obtained in children with pneumococcal disease. Differentiation can be made by culture of material obtained by needle aspiration of the lung, by blood culture, and by appropriate serologic tests.

The signs and symptoms of pneumococcal meningitis are those of any acute bacterial meningitis. Specific diagnosis is established by culture of cerebrospinal fluid and blood. Upper lobe pneumonia may cause *meningismus* (resistance to anterior flexion of the neck) in patients without meningitis. Neither this finding nor abdominal pain in patients with lower lobe pneumonia is specific for pneumococcal disease.

Complications. Pneumococcal otitis media may be complicated by mastoiditis. Bronchiectasis may follow pneumococcal pneumonia. The complications of pneumococcal meningitis are those which may follow any bacterial meningitis (Sec 10.17), but deafness and hydrocephalus seem particularly prominent.

Postpneumococcal glomerulonephritis also has been observed. Recent studies suggest that pneumococcal polysaccharide can activate the alternative complement pathway and that it and C3 are bound to the glomerulus. A mesangial proliferative glomerulitis develops; this appears to be reversible.

Prevention. In adults polyvalent pneumococcal vaccines have been tested. They have proved to be highly immunogenic and associated with a low level of untoward reactions. Responsiveness to pneumococcal polysaccharide has been unpredictable in young children. An octavalent pneumococcal vaccine utilized in high risk children older than 2 yr of age has proved to be immunogenic and apparently protective against some fatal bacteremic pneumococcal infections. Pneumovax presently is recommended for children older than 2 yr of age with (1) asplenia regardless of etiology, (2) nephrotic syndrome, (3) sickle cell disease, and (4) related hemoglobinopathies. A single dose (0.5 ml) containing 50 µg of each polysaccharide type given subcutaneously or intramuscularly is recommended; optimal revaccination requirements are unknown. Immunization in accord with these recommendations will not prevent pneumococcal disease related to serotypes not found in the vaccine; it will not invariably prevent morbidity and mortality from pneumococcal bacteremia even when the bacteremia is related to a pneumococcal strain that is serotypically identical to 1 of the vaccine strains. Vaccination with the recently licensed tetradecavalent vaccine appears to have greater efficacy in children 10 yr of age or older than it does in younger children. Administration of gamma globulin to children with hypogammaglobulinemia (IgG less than 200 mg/dl) will diminish the frequency of pneumococcal bacteremia and meningitis but not of pneumococcal respiratory infections. Penicillin G or V, 25,000–50,000 units/kg/24 hr in 4 divided oral doses, may be given to patients who are asplenic or functionally asplenic or whose spleens have been removed. Controlled studies to document that this form of prophylaxis diminishes significantly the incidence of pneumococcal bacteremia in these patients are not yet available.

Treatment. Penicillin is the antibiotic of choice for pneumococcal disease. The dose and duration of treatment must be varied with the site of infection. Patients with uncomplicated pneumonia or otitis media can be treated with 50,000 units/kg/24 hr in 4 divided oral doses for 7–10 days. Patients with meningitis, osteomyelitis, or endocarditis should be given aqueous penicillin G intravenously in a dose of 400,000 units/kg/24 hr. Patients with uncomplicated meningitis may be treated until afebrile for 5 days but with a minimum course of at least 10 days. Patients with endocarditis or osteomyelitis may require 4–6 wk of therapy.

The child with unexplained fever who has pneumococcal bacteremia but who has been untreated must be re-examined as soon as the culture results have been received. If a focus of infection is now apparent, penicillin should be given in a dose and course appropriate for the disease. If no focus of infection is apparent but fever persists, hospitalization is recommended. Blood culture should be repeated and CSF examined, and treatment initiated with penicillin parenterally. The previously untreated child who is afebrile and well at the time initial culture results are available may be managed at home if the physician is confident that contact with the family can be maintained and that medication will be administered appropriately. A 2nd blood culture is obtained and penicillin V, 50,000 units/kg/24 hr, is prescribed in 4 divided oral doses. If the 2nd blood culture is negative and the child remains well, treatment is discontinued after 5 days.

Pneumococci with a decreased susceptibility to penicillin (MICs of 0.2–0.4 µg/ml) have been isolated. The existence of these strains emphasizes the need to use high-dose penicillin therapy for patients with meningitis. Ideally, pneumococci isolated from the cerebrospinal fluid of patients with meningitis should be tested by tube dilution as a guide to appropriate therapy. More recently, strains of pneumococci resistant to many antibiotics and to sulfonamides have been reported. Several of these multiply resistant pneumococci have been recovered from children with bacteremia or meningitis who were hospitalized in the United States. Since no reliable predictions of future distribution or prevalence of these strains are possible, routine sensitivity tests should be performed on all pneumococcal isolates from blood and cerebrospinal fluid. In those areas where such strains are encountered, intravenous treatment with vancomycin may be required.

Erythromycin, cephalosporins, clindamycin, and chloramphenicol provide effective alternatives for patients who are allergic to penicillin. Clindamycin and cephalosporins should not be used in patients with pneumococcal meningitis or endocarditis. Sulfadiazine and sulfisoxazole also are effective in pneumococcal pneumonia. Tetracycline should not be used since many strains of pneumococci resistant to it have been reported.

Prognosis. This depends upon the integrity of host defenses, the virulence of the infecting organism, the age of the host, and the site of infection. Mortality is greatest in patients with pneumococcal meningitis (about 5–10%). Estimates of mortality following pneumococcal bacteremia or pneumonia in previously healthy children are not available. Morbidity and mortality rates are greatest in patients with leukopenia or thrombocytopenia, in very young infants, and in the compromised host (sickle cell disease, asplenia, splenectomy, immunosuppression, T and B cell deficiency disease, complement deficiency disease, malignancy).

Ammann AJ, Addiego J, Ward DW, et al: Polyvalent pneumococcal polysaccharide immunization of patients with sickle cell anemia and patients with splenectomy. N Engl J Med 297:897, 1977.

Coonrod JD, Drennan DP: Pneumococcal pneumonia: Capsular polysaccharide antigenemia and antibody responses. Ann Intern Med 84:254, 1976.

Cowan MJ, Ammann AJ, Ward DW, et al: Pneumococcal polysaccharide immunization in infants and children. Pediatrics 62:721, 1978.

Feigin RD, Shearer WT: Opportunistic infection in children. II. In the compromised host. J Pediatr 87:677, 1975.

Finland M, Garner C, Wilcox C, et al: Susceptibility of pneumococci and Haemophilus influenzae to antibacterial agents. Antimicrob Agents Chemother 9:274, 1976.

Jacobs NM, Lerdkachornsuk S, Metzger WI: Pneumococcal bacteremia in infants and children: A ten year experience at the Cook County Hospital with special reference to the pneumococcal serotypes isolated. Pediatrics 69:296, 1979.

Klein JO: Pneumococcal bacteremia in the young child. Am J Dis Child 129:1266, 1975.

Loda FA, Collier AM, Clezen WP, et al: Occurrence of Diplococcus pneumoniae in the upper respiratory tract of children. J Pediatr 87:1087, 1975.

Michaels RH, Poziviak CS: Countercurrent immunoelectrophoresis for the diagnosis of pneumococcal pneumonia in children. J Pediatr 88:72, 1976.

Myers MG, Wright PF, Smith AL, et al: Complications of occult pneumococcal bacteremia in children. J Pediatr 84:656, 1974.

Paredes A, Taber LH, Yow MD, et al: Prolonged pneumococcal meningitis due to an organism with increased resistance to penicillin. Pediatrics 58:378, 1976.

Reed WP, Davidson MS, Williams RC Jr: Complement system in pneumococcal infections. Infect Immun 13:1120, 1972.

Winkelstein JA, Lambert GH, with the technical assistance of Swift, A: Pneumococcal serum opsonizing activity in splenectomized children. J Pediatr 87:430, 1975.

10.23 DIPHTHERIA

Diphtheria is an acute infectious disease caused by *Corynebacterium diphtheriae*. Generalized or localized symptoms follow production and elaboration of a toxin that is an extracellular protein metabolite of toxigenic strains of *C. diphtheriae*.

Records suggesting the existence of diphtheria date back to the 4th century B.C. In 1883 the causative agent was identified by Klebs in stained smears from diphtheritic membranes, and a year later Loeffler grew the organism on artificial media and produced in guinea pigs a fatal infection which closely resembled the human disease.

Etiology. *Corynebacterium diphtheriae* (Klebs-Loeffler bacillus) is an irregularly staining gram-positive, nonmotile, nonsporulating, pleomorphic bacillus. The club-shaped appearance of the bacillus is not a true morphologic feature but rather results from attempts to grow it under nutritionally inadequate circumstances (Loeffler medium). The organism can be recovered most readily on media containing selective inhibitors that retard the growth of other microorganisms (tellurite).

Colonies of *C. diphtheriae* appear grayish white on Loeffler medium. On tellurite media, 3 colony types can be distinguished: mitis colonies are smooth, black, and convex; gravis colonies are gray and semirough; intermedius colonies are small and smooth and have a black center. These 3 types also display differences in fermentation and hemolytic reactions.

Both smooth and rough strains may be either nontoxigenic or toxigenic; no differences have been detected in the exotoxins elaborated by the 3 strains of *C. diphtheriae*. Infection of *C. diphtheriae* with a bacteriophage carrying the gene for toxin production is required to render most strains toxigenic, but multiplication of phage is not a necessary prerequisite for toxin production. The capacity to synthesize toxin depends upon both genetic and nutritional factors. Toxin-producing cells apparently are those in which spontaneous induction of prophage to the phage occurs. The amount of toxin produced increases with longer periods of multiplication of the intrabacterial virus (phage). Growth of *C. diphtheriae* in iron-deficient media prolongs the duration of induction lysis and is associated with a high yield of toxin.

The ability of a strain of *C. diphtheriae* to elaborate toxin can be demonstrated by either of 2 tests: necrosis of tissue in guinea pigs or agar gel diffusion. The latter test is dependent upon demonstration of a precipitin band between toxin and antitoxin. Diphtheria toxin is lethal for man in an amount of about 130 µg/kg.

Epidemiology. Diphtheria is distributed worldwide, but its incidence declined markedly following the extensive use of diphtheria toxoid after World War II. The mortality, however, has remained relatively constant at about 10% of cases.

The incidence of diphtheria peaks during the autumn and winter months. Eighty per cent of cases still occur in (primarily unimmunized) individuals under 15 yr of age. In any given epidemic, however, the age incidence depends upon the immune status of the population. Recent outbreaks of diphtheria support the concept that disease occurs among the poor who reside in crowded conditions and who have limited access to health care facilities. Most fatalities occur among unimmunized individuals.

Diphtheria is acquired by contact with either a carrier or a person with the disease. The bacteria may be transmitted by droplets spread by coughing, sneezing, or talking. Some reports suggest that diphtheritic infections of the skin predispose to respiratory colonization. Fomites and dust may serve as vehicles of transmission but are comparatively unimportant.

Pathogenesis and Pathology. Diphtheria is initiated by entry of *C. diphtheriae* into the nose or mouth where the bacilli remain localized on the mucosal surfaces of the upper respiratory tract. Occasionally, the skin or the ocular or genital mucous membranes serve as the site of localization. Following a 2–4 day period of incubation, strains infected with bacteriophage may elaborate toxin, which is initially adsorbed to the cell membrane, then penetrates that membrane and interferes with protein synthesis within the bacterial cell. The toxin produces an enzymatic cleavage of nicotinamide adenine dinucleotide (NAD) with subsequent formation of an inactive transferase–adenosine diphosphoribose. Protein synthesis ceases because this enzyme is required for the transfer of amino acids from RNA to the elongating polypeptide.

Tissue necrosis is most marked in the vicinity of colonization. A local inflammatory response follows, and this, coupled with the necrotic tissue, produces a patchy exudate which initially can be removed. As toxin production increases, the area of infection widens and deepens, and a fibrinous exudate develops. A tough adherent membrane is formed that varies from gray to black depending on the amount of blood it contains. In addition to fibrin, the membrane contains inflammatory cells, red blood cells, and superficial epithelial cells. Since the latter are an integral part of the membrane, attempts to remove it are followed by bleeding. The membrane sloughs spontaneously during the recovery period.

Edema of the soft tissues beneath the membrane may be marked. Occasionally, secondary bacterial infection (classically streptococcal) develops. The membrane and edematous tissue may encroach upon the airway to cause respiratory embarrassment or suffocation with extension to the larynx or tracheobronchial tree.

Toxin produced at the site of infection is distributed via the bloodstream throughout the body; it reaches the bloodstream most readily when the pharynx and tonsils are covered by a diphtheritic membrane. The toxin can damage any organ or tissue, but lesions of the heart, nervous system, and kidneys are particularly prominent. Although diphtheria antitoxin can neutralize circulating toxin or toxin adsorbed to cells, it is ineffective once cell penetration has occurred. After toxin has become fixed to tissues, a variable latent period occurs before clinical manifestations caused by it appear. Myocarditis generally is observed 10–14 days after the onset of illness. Nervous system manifestations, particularly peripheral neuritis, generally do not appear until 3–7 wk after the onset of disease.

The most prominent pathologic findings are toxic necrosis and hyaline degeneration of various organs and tissues. In the heart one may observe edema, congestion, and mononuclear cell infiltration of muscle fibers and the conducting system. If the patient survives, muscle regeneration and interstitial fibrosis can be seen. A toxic neuritis with fatty degeneration of myelin sheaths may be noted. Liver necrosis may occur, possibly associated with hypoglycemia. Adrenal hemorrhage and acute tubular necrosis of the kidney are also noted in some cases.

Clinical Manifestations. The signs and symptoms of diphtheria will depend upon the site of infection and the immunization status of the host and upon whether or not toxin has escaped into the systemic circulation.

The incubation period may range from 1–6 days. Diphtheria is classified clinically on the basis of the anatomic location of the initial infection and of the diphtheritic membrane (nasal, tonsillar, pharyngeal, laryngeal or laryngotracheal, conjunctival, skin, and genital). More than 1 anatomic site may be involved.

Nasal diphtheria initially resembles a common cold and is characterized by mild rhinorrhea and a paucity of systemic symptoms. Gradually, the nasal discharge becomes serosanguineous and then mucopurulent and excoriates the nares and upper lip. A foul odor may be noticed, and careful inspection will reveal a white membrane on the nasal septum (Fig 10–2 [p. xxxiii]). Slow absorption of toxin coupled with the lack of systemic symptoms frequently delays an accurate diagnosis. This form of the disease occurs most often in infants.

Tonsillar and pharyngeal diphtherias begin as an insidi-

ous but more severe form of the disease. Anorexia, malaise, low-grade fever, and pharyngitis are noted initially. Within 1–2 days a membrane appears that may vary in extent according to the immune status of the host; in partially immune individuals a membrane may not develop. The membrane initially is thin and gray, resembling a spider web which gradually extends from the tonsil to the contiguous soft or hard palate; when present, this characteristic distinguishes diphtheria from other forms of membranous tonsillitis. The adherent membrane may spread to cover the tonsils and pharyngeal walls (Fig 10–3 [p. xxxiii]) or progress down into the larynx and trachea. Attempts to remove it are followed by bleeding. Cervical lymphadenitis is variable. In some cases it is associated with edema of the soft tissues of the neck and may be so severe as to give the appearance of a "bull neck." The edema may be characterized by obliteration (erasure) of the sternocleidomastoid muscle border, the mandible, and the median border of the clavicle. "Erasure" edema is brawny, pitting, warm to the touch, and tender to palpation; occurs most commonly in children over 6 yr of age; and is generally associated with infection due to the gravis or intermedius strains of *C. diphtheriae*.

The course of pharyngeal diphtheria depends upon the extent of the membrane and the amount of toxin produced. In severe cases respiratory and circulatory collapse may occur. The pulse rate is increased disproportionately to the body temperature, which generally remains normal or slightly elevated. Palatal paralysis may occur. If it is unilateral, the palate deviates away from the paralyzed side; if bilateral, paralysis may cause a nasal voice, nasal regurgitation, and difficulty in swallowing food. Stupor, coma, and death may follow within 7–10 days. In less severe cases, recovery may be slow or may be complicated by the development of myocarditis or neuritis. In mild cases the membrane sloughs off in 7–10 days, and recovery is uneventful.

Laryngeal diphtheria generally reflects downward extension of the membrane from the pharynx. Occasionally, only laryngeal involvement is present, and in these patients toxicity is less prominent. The clinical findings of noisy breathing, progressive stridor, hoarseness, and a dry cough are indistinguishable from those of other types of infectious croup. Suprasternal, subcostal, and supraclavicular retractions reflect severe laryngeal obstruction, which may be fatal unless alleviated. Occasionally, even in a mild case, acute and fatal obstruction may occur when a partially detached piece of membrane occludes the airway. In severe cases of laryngeal diphtheria the membrane may extend downward and invade the entire tracheobronchial tree. Signs of toxemia generally are few in children with primary laryngeal diphtheria, but both obstruction and toxemia are seen in the frequent association of laryngeal with pharyngeal disease.

Cutaneous, vulvovaginal, conjunctival, and aural diphtheria also occur. *Cutaneous diphtheria* usually appears as an ulcer with a sharply defined border and a membranous base. It is more common in warmer climates and may serve as an important source of person-to-person transmission of diphtheria. *Conjunctival lesions* usually are limited to the palpebral conjunctiva, which appears red, edematous, and membranous. *Aural diphtheria* is characterized by otitis externa with a persistent purulent and frequently foul smelling discharge.

Diagnosis. This should be made on the basis of clinical findings because any delay in therapy poses a serious risk to the patient. Definitive diagnosis depends upon isolation of *C. diphtheriae*. Microscopic examination of material from diphtheritic lesions is unreliable; the fluorescent antibody technique may be used but is reliable only when done by highly experienced personnel.

Material from beneath the membrane or a portion of the membrane itself should be obtained for culture. *C. diphtheriae* is relatively resistant to drying; use of nonnutritive, moisture-reducing transport medium helps to prevent the overgrowth of other microorganisms. The laboratory should be notified about the suspicion of diphtheria so that appropriate Loeffler, tellurite, and blood agar media are inoculated. Diphtheria bacilli that are recovered should be tested for toxigenicity by inoculating 2 guinea pigs intracutaneously with a broth suspension of the microorganism. One of the animals is given diphtheria antitoxin prior to intracutaneous challenge. An inflammatory lesion will appear at the site of inoculation in 24 hr and will become necrotic in 72 hr in the control animal. No skin reaction should occur in the animal given antitoxin.

Other laboratory studies are of little diagnostic value. The white blood cell count may be normal or elevated. Rarely, anemia may develop as a result of rapid hemolysis. In diphtheritic neuritis the cerebrospinal fluid may show a minimal elevation of protein and, rarely, mild pleocytosis. Hypoglycemia, glycosuria, or both may reflect hepatic toxicity. An elevation in blood urea nitrogen may develop in patients with acute tubular necrosis. Electrocardiography may reveal arrhythmias or S-T segment and T-wave changes indicative of myocarditis.

Schick Test. This skin test has been used to determine the immune status of the patient. It is not helpful in early diagnosis since it cannot be read for several days, but it is useful in determining the susceptibility of contacts and in the diagnosis and management of immunodeficiency.

Method: 0.1 ml (1/50 of a minimum lethal dose for a guinea pig) of a standard solution of diphtheria toxin is injected intracutaneously. In the absence of circulating antitoxin, a local inflammatory response characterized by erythema, swelling, and tenderness occurs and peaks at about 5 days after injection. If sufficient antitoxin is present, no reaction should occur. Many individuals become hypersensitive to the toxin itself or to other antigens in the toxin preparation. Therefore, a control injection of toxoid (0.005 Lf [limit flocculation unit]) is administered intradermally in the opposite arm. The individual who is immune but sensitive to the toxin preparation will react to both toxin and toxoid. These skin reactions generally are maximal at 48–72 hr and then fade in contrast to a positive Schick test, which persists for many days. If the individual has no antitoxin in his or her serum but is allergic to the toxoid, a reaction will be noted on both arms, but the reaction at the site of toxin injection will peak on day 5 and persist, whereas the reaction to toxoid will subside by 5–7 days. A positive Schick test consists of more than 10 mm of induration and indicates susceptibility to diphtheria.

Differential Diagnosis. Mild forms of nasal diphtheria in the partially immunized host may resemble the common cold. When a more serosanguineous or purulent nasal discharge is present, nasal diphtheria must be distinguished from foreign body in the nose, sinusitis, adenoiditis, or the *"snuffles"* of congenital syphilis. Careful examination of the nose with a nasal speculum, sinus roentgenograms, and appropriate serologic tests for syphilis are helpful in excluding these disorders.

Tonsillar or pharyngeal diphtheria must be differentiated from streptococcal pharyngitis which generally is associated with more severe pain on swallowing, higher temperature, and a relatively nonadherent membrane limited to the tonsils. In some patients pharyngeal diphtheria and streptococcal pharyngitis coexist.

Tonsillar and pharyngeal diphtheria also must be differentiated from infectious mononucleosis, which is usually accompanied by lymphadenopathy and splenomegaly, atypical lymphocytes, and heterophile antibodies. Nonbacterial membranous tonsillitis is usually characterized by a low white blood cell count, normal throat flora, and a course unaffected by antibiotics; primary herpetic tonsillitis, by gingivitis, stomatitis, and discrete lesions of the tongue and palate; and thrush, by lesions on the buccal mucosa and tongue and by absence of constitutional symptoms. Tonsillar and pharyngeal diphtheria also must be differentiated from blood dyscrasias, such as agranulocytosis and leukemia; from post-tonsillectomy faucial membranes, in which the membranes are stationary and do not spread; and from oropharyngeal involvement by *Toxoplasma*, cytomegalovirus, *F. tularensis*, and salmonellae. Vincent angina may be indistinguishable.

Laryngeal diphtheria must be differentiated from spasmodic or nonspasmodic croup, acute epiglottitis, laryngotracheobronchitis, aspirated foreign bodies, peripharyngeal and retropharyngeal abscesses, and laryngeal papillomas, hemangiomas, or lymphangiomas. A careful history followed by visualization in hospital under controlled conditions is helpful in arriving at a correct diagnosis.

Complications. Penicillin utilized for eradication of *C. diphtheriae* has reduced significantly the frequency of secondary bacterial complications of diphtheria, especially streptococcal disease. Nevertheless, respiratory obstruction and death may occur suddenly in young children with laryngeal or tracheal diphtheria as a result of occlusion of the airway by the diphtheritic membrane; edema of the neck may compromise the airway. Myocarditis (Sec 13.74) may follow both severe and mild cases of diphtheria and is most common in patients with extensive local lesions who have experienced a delay in the administration of antitoxin. It generally occurs in the 2nd wk of the disease but may appear as early as the 1st wk or as late as the 6th wk of illness and is manifested by tachycardia, a muffled 1st heart sound, murmurs, and arrhythmias; cardiac failure may also occur.

Neurologic complications generally appear after a variable latent period, are predominantly bilateral and motor rather than sensory, and usually resolve completely. Paralysis of the soft palate is most common, generally appearing in the 3rd wk. Ocular paralysis is most common during the 5th wk but may appear as early as the 1st wk of illness. It may cause blurring of vision, difficulty with accommodation, and internal strabismus. Neuritis of the phrenic nerve may cause paralysis of the diaphragm, usually between the 5th and 7th wk. Paralysis of the limbs with loss of deep tendon reflexes and an elevated cerebrospinal fluid protein may be noted and is clinically indistinguishable from Guillain-Barré syndrome.

Rarely, 2–3 wk after onset of diphtheria the vasomotor centers may be affected and hypotension and cardiac failure ensue. Gastritis, hepatitis, and nephritis may develop.

Prevention. *Immunization.* The most effective preventive measure against diphtheria is active immunization. The preferred agent for children under 6 is diphtheria toxoid given in combination with tetanus toxoid and pertussis antigen (DTP). Primary immunization is conveniently and effectively carried out by giving DTP as indicated in Sec 4.1.

Primary immunization of children more than 6 yr of age may be carried out using adult-type diphtheria and tetanus toxoids, adsorbed (Td). This preparation contains no more than 2 limit flocculation units (Lf) of diphtheria toxoid per dose, compared with the 7–25 Lf in the pediatric DTP-adsorbed preparations used for younger children. Two doses are given intramuscularly or subcutaneously at least 4 wk apart with a booster dose 1 yr later. Administration of Td is not followed by the high incidence of reactions associated with the use of pediatric DTP or DT. For this reason Td may be administered safely without prior skin testing. Subsequent booster doses of Td given at 10 yr intervals will maintain protective levels of antibody in most people.

Although a few individuals fully immunized against diphtheria may develop the carrier state or mild disease, the most important problem of diphtheria today is inadequate immunization of the population. Immunization rates are unsatisfactory for infants and children in many areas, but immunity of adults is even lower because of failure to maintain it through appropriate booster immunization.

Contacts. Prevention of diphtheria also depends upon isolation of the patient to minimize spread of disease and upon management of contacts of known cases. The patient is infectious until diphtheria bacilli can no longer be cultured from the site of infection; 3 consecutive negative cultures are required before the patient is released from isolation.

Intimate contacts are likely to contract the disease if they are not immune. Cultures of the nose and throat should be done. Previously immunized carriers should be given a booster injection of diphtheria toxoid *and* should be treated with aqueous procaine penicillin, 600,000 units daily for 4 days, benzathine penicillin, 600,000 units intramuscularly as a single dose, or erythromycin, 40 mg/kg/24 hr for 7–10 days. Nonimmunized asymptomatic carriers should receive diphtheria toxoid and penicillin and be examined daily by a physician. If daily surveillance is not possible, 10,000 units of diphtheria antitoxin should be administered intramuscularly. If a contact already is experiencing symptoms,

treatment as a case of diphtheria is indicated. Prophylactic therapy with toxoid, penicillin, and, if indicated, antitoxin, should be carried out in nonimmunized contacts prior to receipt of culture results.

Treatment. Treatment of diphtheria is predicated upon neutralization of free toxin and eradication of C. *diphtheriae* by the use of antibiotics. The only specific treatment is antitoxin of equine origin. Antitoxin should be administered on the basis of the site of the membrane, the degree of toxicity, and the duration of illness.

Antitoxin must be administered as early as possible by the intravenous route and in a dosage sufficient to neutralize all free toxin. A single dose is used to avoid the risk of sensitization from repeated doses of horse serum. Tests for sensitivity to horse serum must be performed prior to administration of antitoxin. For this purpose, 0.1 ml of a 1:1000 dilution of antitoxin in saline can be given intracutaneously or placed in the conjunctival sac. A positive reaction (>10 mm of erythema at site of infection within 20 min or the development of conjunctivitis and tearing) necessitates desensitization. If a patient shows sensitivity to horse serum, it should be provided in slowly increasing dosage given at 20 min intervals. Several procedures have been recommended. One commonly employed regimen is:

```
0.05 ml of a 1:20 dilution subcutaneously
0.1  ml of a 1:20 dilution subcutaneously
0.1  ml of a 1:10 dilution subcutaneously
0.1  ml undiluted subcutaneously
0.3  ml undiluted intramuscularly
0.5  ml undiluted intramuscularly
0.1  ml undiluted intravenously
```

If no reaction has occurred, the remaining material is given by slow intravenous infusion. Reactions should be treated with aqueous epinephrine (1:1000) intravenously. Antitoxin dosage is empiric. Mild nasal or pharyngeal diphtheria can be treated with 40,000 units of antitoxin; 80,000 units should be used for moderately severe pharyngeal diphtheria. Severe pharyngeal or laryngeal diphtheria should be treated with 120,000 units. The latter dose also should be given to patients with mixed clinical symptoms as well as to those with brawny edema or disease of longer duration than 48 hr.

·Antibiotics are not a substitute for treatment with antitoxin but are needed to stop the production of diphtheria toxin. Penicillin and erythromycin are effective against most strains of C. *diphtheriae*. Penicillin may be given as aqueous procaine penicillin G, 600,000 units intramuscularly once daily for 7 days. Patients sensitive to penicillin should be given erythromycin in a daily dosage of 40 mg/kg/24 hr in 4 divided doses for 7–10 days. The end point of therapy is 3 consecutive negative cultures. Each of these antibiotics is also effective in eradicating group A β-hemolytic streptococci, which may complicate up to 30% of cases of diphtheria. Amoxicillin, rifampin, and clindamycin provided in appropriate dosage also may be effective. Lincomycin and tetracycline have proved to be less effective; cephalexin, oxacillin, and colistin have been evaluated as ineffective. The carrier state has been treated effectively with benzathine penicillin G or oral erythromycin.

Supportive Treatment. Because of the frequency of myocarditis, bed rest is extremely important and should be required for 2–3 wk. Serial electrocardiograms should be obtained 2–3 times each wk for 4–6 wk to detect myocarditis as early as possible.

Hydration should be maintained and a high calorie liquid or soft diet provided. Secretions should be suctioned. The gag reflex and the quality of the voice should be checked regularly.

Laryngeal diphtheria may require relief of obstruction with a tracheostomy. This procedure should be carried out before the child has become exhausted.

Absolute bed rest must be enforced if myocarditis is detected. Sudden death has been precipitated by excessive activity. The patient with myocarditis may be digitalized if congestive heart failure develops. Digitalization for arrhythmias due to diphtheria may be contraindicated. In severe cases, prednisone, 1–1.5 mg/kg/24 hr for 2 wk has been shown to lessen the incidence of myocarditis.

Palatal and pharyngeal paralysis may be complicated by aspiration. Gavage via a polyethylene tube is indicated in these patients.

Immunization is necessary following recovery of the patient. At least half of the patients who recover from diphtheria do not develop adequate immunity and remain subject to reinfection.

Prognosis. Prior to the use of antitoxin and the availability of antibiotics, the mortality from diphtheria was 30–50%. Death was most common in children under 4 yr of age and was the result of suffocation due to the diphtheritic membrane. At present, the mortality is less than 5%, is most frequently associated with myocarditis, and is not associated with age.

The prognosis in the individual patient remains guarded until the child has recovered. Laryngeal obstruction may develop suddenly or unexpectedly. Myocarditis may be associated with congestive heart failure that responds poorly to digitalization. Occasionally, diphtheritic myocarditis is followed by permanent damage to the heart. Phrenic nerve paralysis may occur late and produce respiratory paralysis.

Generally, the prognosis in diphtheria depends upon the virulence of the organism, the location and extent of the diphtheritic membrane, the immunization status of the host, the rapidity with which medical care was sought and an accurate diagnosis suggested, the timeliness of treatment, and the adequacy of general nursing care.

Diphtheria caused by the *gravis* strain usually carries a poor prognosis. The more extensive the diphtheritic membrane, the more severe the disease. Laryngeal diphtheria is more likely to be fatal in infants or in patients whose respiratory status is not monitored closely. The development of amegakaryocytic thrombocytopenia or of myocarditis with atrioventricular dissociation heralds a poorer prognosis. If specific treatment is provided on the 1st day of disease, mortality may be reduced to less than 1%; delay in treatment until the 4th day may be associated with a 20-fold increase in mortality.

Nasopharyngeal persistence of *C. diphtheriae* may be noted in 5–10% of convalescing patients. Recovery is followed by immunity that is demonstrable for at least 1 yr after illness in 50% of patients. Second attacks are rare. Nevertheless, immunization should be carried out following recovery.

Belsey MA, Sinclair M, Roder MR, et al: *Corynebacterium diphtheriae* skin infections in Alabama and Louisiana. N Engl J Med 280:139, 1969.

Brooks GF: Recent trends in diphtheria in the United States. J Infect Dis 120:500, 1969.

Burch GE, Sun SC, Sohal RS, et al: Diphtheritic myocarditis. Am J Cardiol 21:261, 1968.

McCloskey RV, Eller JJ, Green M, et al: The 1970 epidemic of diphtheria in San Antonio. Ann Intern Med 75:495, 1971.

Miller LW, Older JJ, Drake J, et al: Diphtheria immunization. Effect upon carriers and the control of outbreaks. Am J Dis Child 123:197, 1972.

Pappenheimer AM Jr: Diphtheria toxin. *In:* Ajl SJ, Kadis S, Montie TC (eds): Microbial Toxins, Vol 2B. New York, Academic Press, 1973.

Report of the Committee on Infectious Disease. Evanston Ill., American Academy of Pediatrics, 1977, p 61.

Tasman A, Minkenhof JE, Vink HH, et al: Importance of intravenous injection of diphtheria antiserum. Lancet 1:1299, 1958.

Zamiri I: Diphtheria today: Some experiences in Iran. Lancet 1:1222, 1970.

10.24 STAPHYLOCOCCAL INFECTIONS

For staphylococcal infections of the newborn, see Sec 7.67.

Staphylococci are a common cause of pyogenic infections in infants and children. These organisms belong to the family Micrococcaceae, which grow in clusters. Staphylococci may grow aerobically or as facultative anaerobes. Strains are classified as *S. aureus* if they are coagulase-positive and as *S. epidermidis* if they are coagulase-negative, irrespective of their pigment production on solid media. Generally, strains of *S. aureus* produce a yellow pigment and those of *S. epidermidis*, a white pigment. Strains of *S. aureus* generally are mannitol-deoxyribonuclease– and acid phosphatase–positive and produce β hemolysis on blood agar. Strains of *S. epidermidis* generally are mannitol- and acid phosphatase–negative; production of β hemolysis on blood agar is variable.

Infections Due to Staphylococcus aureus

Staphylococcus aureus is a common cause of infection in children. The most common cause of pyogenic infection of the skin, it also may cause furuncles, carbuncles, osteomyelitis, septic arthritis, wound infection, abscesses, pneumonia, empyema, endocarditis, pericarditis, meningitis, and food poisoning.

Etiology. Disease due to *Staphylococcus aureus* may be the result of tissue invasion or reflect a reaction to a variety of toxins and enzymes elaborated by these organisms. Strains of *S. aureus* can be identified and classified by means of bacteriophage typing. Generally, typing is performed with 5 sets of pooled phages: Group I (phage numbers 29, 52, 52A, 79, and 80); Group II (phage numbers 3A, 3C, 55, and 71); Group III (phage numbers 6, 7, 42E, 47, 53, 54, 75, 77, 83A, 84, and 85);

Group IV (phage number 42D); and miscellaneous (phage numbers 81 and 187). The organism is then classified as a member of 1 of these groups. If more precise identification is required, a large panel of individual phages is required.

When grown in artificial media, many strains of S. aureus release a number of different exotoxins. Four immunologically distinct hemolysins (alpha, beta, gamma, delta) have been identified. Alpha toxin is lethal when injected parenterally into mice and rabbits. It also may cause tissue necrosis, injure human leukocytes, and produce aggregation of platelets and spasm of smooth muscle. The beta hemolysin appears to be responsible for hemolysis of red blood cells incubated at 39° C and then exposed to cold. The delta hemolysin is toxic to leukocytes. Little is known about gamma hemolysin other than that it also appears to act on cell membrane.

Leukocidin is produced by most strains of S. aureus. It combines with the phospholipid of the cell membrane, producing increased permeability of the membrane, leakage of protein, and eventual death of the cell. It has the capacity to destroy leukocytes in vitro.

Exfoliative toxin, associated with phage group II staphylococci, is the cause of "scalded skin syndrome" (Lyell disease, toxic epidermal necrolysis), generalized exfoliative disease of infants (Ritter disease), bullous impetigo, and staphylococcal scarlatiniform eruption (Sec 24.24).

Staphylococcal enterotoxins (types A, B, C, D, E) are elaborated by most strains of S. aureus. Ingestion of preformed enterotoxin A or B is associated with vomiting and diarrhea and in some cases with the development of profound hypotension.

A variety of enzymes also may be released by staphylococci. Production of coagulase (causing plasma to coagulate) differentiates S. aureus from S. epidermidis. Other enzymes elaborated by staphylococci include staphylokinase (activator of plasma plasminogen), penicillinase or β-lactamase (inactivator of penicillin at the molecular level), hyaluronidase (spreading factor), lipase, and DNase.

Most strains of S. aureus possess an agglutinogen (protein A). This material can react with the Fc fragments of IgG molecules and is known to cause hypersensitivity reactions in rabbits and guinea pigs. This protein also generates complement-derived chemotactic factors and has antiphagocytic properties. Several other capsular antigens have been identified which serve to block the agglutinating and opsonizing action of anticapsular antibodies.

Epidemiology. Twenty–30% of normal individuals carry S. aureus in the anterior nares at all times. The minimum inoculum for carriage for 5 days or more appears to be 10^4 organisms. In some individuals nasal carriage of a given strain persists for months, whereas others reject the strain almost immediately.

The organisms may be transmitted from the nose to the skin, where colonization seems to be more transient. Repeated recovery of S. aureus from the skin suggests repeated transfer of the organism from nose to skin rather than persistent skin colonization. Persistent umbilical or perianal carriage has been described.

Transmission of S. aureus generally occurs by direct contact or by spread of heavy particles over a distance of 6 ft or less. Spread by fomites is very rare. Acquisition of staphylococci is dependent upon the efficiency of the disseminator and the susceptibility of the host. Heavily colonized individuals and perianal carriers are particularly effective disseminators. Newborn infants are extremely susceptible to staphylococci; 10^2 organisms or fewer may be sufficient to effect colonization. The nasopharynx, skin, and umbilical stump are the most common sites of colonization. Colonized infants contaminate the hands of nursery personnel. If handwashing between patients is not performed meticulously, spread of staphylococci from patient to patient will result. Older children and adults are more resistant than the newborn infant to colonization. Generally, colonization through close household contact for 2 or more days is required to spread staphylococci.

Infection may follow colonization. Antibiotic therapy with a drug to which S. aureus is resistant favors both colonization and the development of infection. Other factors that increase the likelihood of infection include wounds, skin disease, ventriculoatrial shunts, intravenous or intrathecal catheterization, corticosteroid treatment, diabetes mellitus, starvation, acidosis, and azotemia. Viral infections of the upper and lower respiratory tract also may predispose to secondary bacterial infection with staphylococci.

Pathology. Suppuration is the hallmark of staphylococcal disease. Local multiplication of staphylococci within tissues produces necrosis and formation of abscesses. Elaboration of hyaluronidase may promote spread of the infection. Granulocytes appear in large numbers at the site of infection. Thrombosis of blood vessels and formation of fibrin clots may be noted. The well-developed local lesion has a necrotic center filled with dead leukocytes surrounded by a fibroblastic wall. Viable bacteria and leukocytes are within the abscess cavity. Rupture of the abscess results in bacteremia and disseminated disease.

Pathogenesis. The intact skin and mucous membranes serve as barriers to invasion by staphylococci; when they are breached or by-passed, phagocytosis and intracellular killing of these organisms by polymorphonuclear leukocytes are essential to prevent or limit the spread of infection.

The development of staphylococcal disease is related to resistance of the host to infection and to virulence of the organism. Studies with human volunteers have documented that it requires large numbers of S. aureus to induce infection even when the organism is injected under human skin. A foreign body at the site of inoculation markedly diminishes resistance to infection. Resistance to staphylococcal infection is also decreased by dietary deficiencies, injections of bacterial endotoxin, diabetes mellitus, the use of indwelling catheters, and implantation of prosthetic valves.

The pathogenesis of infection also is related to factors of bacterial virulence. A factor that appears to be a cell wall mucopeptide can be extracted only from virulent strains of S. aureus. This material inhibits chemotaxis and accumulation of fluid at the site of infection. The ability of virulent staphylococci to establish infection may be related directly to their capacity to inhibit chemotaxis.

Protein A, present in most strains of *S. aureus* but not in *S. epidermidis*, reacts specifically with IgG1, IgG2, and IgG4. It is located on the outermost coat of the organism and can absorb immunoglobulin found in serum, preventing antibacterial antibodies from acting as opsonins and thus inhibiting phagocytosis. Leukocidin, causing degranulation of leukocytes, and staphylococcal hemolysis toxic to erythrocytes and leukocytes also contribute to the virulence of *S. aureus*.

Proliferation of staphylococci in the gastrointestinal tract is controlled by the prevalence of other bacterial species. If this balance is upset during antibiotic therapy, resistant staphylococci may proliferate and invade the bowel wall. Elaboration of enterotoxin by staphylococci within the gastrointestinal tract or ingestion of preformed enterotoxins may produce disease in the absence of tissue invasion.

The infant may acquire type-specific humoral immunity to staphylococci transplacentally. Older children and adults develop antibodies to staphylococci as a result of intermittent minor infections of the skin and soft tissues; the antistaphylococcal titer of serum generally increases after overt staphylococcal disease. The presence of antibody, however, for reasons given above, does not always protect the individual from staphylococcal disease.

Formation of antibody and delayed hypersensitivity reactions can be induced by the cell wall, by a protein, and by ribotol teichoic acid components of the organism. The specific protection afforded by antibodies to any of these components remains unclear.

Following staphylococcal infection in rabbits, macrophages exhibit increased capability to kill staphylococci. It is unknown whether the same phenomenon is associated with infection in man.

Individuals with congenital or acquired defects in the complement system (required for chemotaxis), defective phagocytosis, and defective humoral immunity (antibodies required for opsonization) as well as those with an impaired intracellular bactericidal capacity are at increased risk of infection with staphylococci. Patients with chronic granulomatous disease, in which phagocytosis proceeds normally but killing of ingested bacteria is severely impaired, are particularly susceptible to staphylococcal disease. Impaired mobilization of polymorphonuclear leukocytes has been documented in children with diabetes mellitus and in healthy individuals following ingestion of alcohol.

Clinical Manifestations. Clinical manifestations and the incubation period of staphylococcal infection vary with the site of involvement.

Skin. Pyogenic skin infections are 1 of the most frequent forms of staphylococcal disease. They may be primary or secondary to wounds or superinfection of a primary noninfectious skin disease. They include impetigo, folliculitis, furunculosis, carbuncles, cellulitis, bullous impetigo (pemphigus neonatorum, Ritter disease), and toxic epidermal necrolysis (Lyell disease). All are discussed in Sec 24.24.

Staphylococcal scarlet fever is characterized by fever and a rash resembling that seen in streptococcal scarlet fever. Pharyngitis is not present. Only staphylococci can be recovered from the primary skin lesions. Presumably, those staphylococci elaborate an erythrogenic toxin. An identical clinical picture may be seen in patients with wounds, especially burns, secondarily infected with staphylococci.

Muscle. The development of localized staphylococcal muscle abscesses associated with elevation in muscle enzymes but without septicemia has been called tropical pyomyositis. Although this disorder has been reported most frequently from tropical areas, it also has been reported in the United States in otherwise healthy children. Multiple abscesses occur in 30–40% of cases. Prodromal symptoms include coryza, pharyngitis, diarrhea, and prior trauma to the site of the abscess. Surgical drainage is the most important aspect of therapy; appropriate antibiotics also should be utilized.

Adamski and associates have recently documented generalized staphylococcal myositis with rhabdomyolysis but without suppuration in a previously healthy adolescent with staphylococcal septicemia. Diffuse muscular inflammation without suppuration or localization and with marked elevation of serum levels of muscle enzymes was noted. Appropriate antistaphylococcal antibiotics given intravenously were curative, but residual muscle wasting, weakness, and stiffness occurred.

Respiratory Tract. See Sec 12.66. Infections of the upper respiratory tract due to *S. aureus* are rare considering the frequency with which this area is colonized. Otitis media and sinusitis due to *S. aureus* may occur. Staphylococcal sinusitis is more common in children with cystic fibrosis or defects in white blood cell function. Suppurative parotitis is a rare infection, but when it occurs, *S. aureus* is one of the most common causes. Staphylococcal tonsillopharyngitis is rare except in children whose response to infection has been compromised.

Pneumonia due to *S. aureus* may be primary or secondary to a viral infection. In children under 1 yr of age the onset may be heralded by expiratory wheeze briefly simulating bronchiolitis. More common are high fever, abdominal pain, tachypnea, dyspnea, and localized or diffuse bronchopneumonia or lobar disease. Staphylococci cause a necrotizing pneumonitis; hence empyema, pneumatoceles, pyopneumothorax, and bronchopleural fistulas develop frequently. Occasionally, staphylococcal pneumonia produces a diffuse interstitial disease characterized by extreme dyspnea, tachypnea, and cyanosis. Cough may be nonproductive. Oxygen therapy may not significantly improve the oxygen saturation of the blood.

Sepsis. Staphylococcal bacteremia may be associated with any localized staphylococcal infection. The onset may be acute and marked by nausea, vomiting, myalgia, fever, and chills. Organisms may localize subsequently in the lung, heart, joints, bones, kidneys, or brain.

In some cases disseminated staphylococcal disease occurs, characterized by fever, bone or joint pain, and urticarial, petechial, maculopapular, or pustular skin rashes. Less frequently, hematuria, jaundice, seizures, nuchal rigidity, and cardiac murmurs are noted. Leukopenia or leukocytosis, proteinuria, and red and white blood cells in the urinary sediment may be noted.

Heart. Acute bacterial endocarditis may follow staphylococcal bacteremia and occur in the absence of valvular heart disease. Perforation of heart valves, myocardial abscesses, acute hemopericardium, purulent pericarditis, and sudden death may ensue.

Central Nervous System. Meningitis due to S. aureus may follow bacteremia or occasionally result from direct extension of infection in patients with otitis media or osteomyelitis of the skull or vertebrae. Trauma or infection of meningomyeloceles also may predispose to S. aureus meningitis. Staphylococcal infection following neurosurgical procedures most commonly is due to S. epidermidis. S. aureus can be recovered from about 25% of brain abscesses. A staphylococcal etiology should be suspected more strongly in abscesses occurring in patients with known or possible staphylococcal bacteremia from whatever primary lesion.

Bones and Joints. S. aureus is the most common cause of osteomyelitis and septic arthritis in children. Generally, disease is acquired hematogenously rather than by direct extension of infection from an adjacent skin or soft tissue lesion.

Kidney. S. aureus is a common cause of renal and perinephric abscess. Urinary tract infection due to S. aureus is unusual.

Intestinal Tract. Staphylococcal enterocolitis follows the overgrowth of normal bowel flora by staphylococci. This most commonly follows use of oral broad-spectrum antibiotic therapy. Diarrhea associated with blood and mucus may be noted.

Food poisoning (Sec 28.1) may be caused by ingestion of enterotoxins preformed by staphylococci contaminating foods (particularly mayonnaise or mayonnaise-containing foods such as deviled eggs, salads, or sandwiches) left out at room temperature or above. Two–7 hr after ingestion of the toxin, sudden, severe vomiting begins. Watery diarrhea may develop, but fever is absent or low grade. Symptoms rarely persist longer than 12–24 hr. Rarely, shock and death may occur.

Diagnosis. The diagnosis of staphylococcal infection depends upon isolation of the organisms from skin lesions, abscess cavities, blood, cerebrospinal fluid, or other sites of infection. The organisms can be grown readily in liquid and on solid media. Following isolation, identification is made on the basis of Gram stain and coagulase and mannitol reactivity. Patterns of sensitivity to antibiotics can be assessed and the organism phage-typed if necessary for epidemiologic reasons.

Diagnosis of staphylococcal food poisoning generally is made on the basis of epidemiologic and clinical findings. Food suspected of contamination should be examined by Gram stain, cultured, and tested for enterotoxin. This last test can be done by the Center for Disease Control. Serologic assays for enterotoxin including gel-diffusion, passive hemagglutination-inhibition, and fluorescent antibody techniques have been developed but are not available in most hospitals. Teichoic acid antibodies in patients with S. aureus bacteremia can be measured by double diffusion in agar.

This test may be of value in the diagnosis of patients with staphylococcal endocarditis.

Differential Diagnosis. Skin lesions due to S. aureus and those due to group A β-hemolytic streptococci may be indistinguishable. Staphylococcal pneumonia can be suspected on the basis of chest roentgenograms that may reveal pneumatoceles, pyopneumothorax, or lung abscess. These changes suggesting a necrotizing pneumonitis are not pathognomonic for staphylococcal infection and may be seen in patients with pneumonia due to other bacteria, including Klebsiella and many anaerobes. Fluctuant skin and soft tissue lesions also can be caused by many organisms, including Mycobacterium, F. tularensis, and various fungi and may be seen in patients with cat-scratch disease (Sec 10.91).

Complications. Rarely, staphylococcal pneumonia is followed by fibrothorax or by congestive heart failure. Staphylococcal osteomyelitis may be complicated by the development of chronic osteomyelitis (particularly if treatment is delayed), by secondary septic arthritis, and by subperiosteal and subcutaneous abscesses. Scalded skin syndrome may be complicated by dehydration, anemia, and shock.

Prevention. Staphylococcal infection is transmitted primarily by direct contact. Strict attention to handwashing techniques is the most effective measure for preventing the spread of staphylococci from 1 individual to another. Use of a detergent containing an iodophor or hexachlorophene is recommended, but even placing hands under running water and drying them with a towel decreases markedly the likelihood of transmitting staphylococci. In hospitals or other institutional settings, all persons with acute staphylococcal infections should be excluded until they have been treated adequately. Nosocomial staphylococcal infections within hospitals should be sought actively by the infection control committee and infection surveillance coordinator. The use of bacterial interference has been helpful in some instances in arresting both nursery and family epidemics.

Food poisoning may be prevented by excluding individuals with staphylococcal infections of the skin from the preparation and handling of food. Prepared foods should be eaten immediately or refrigerated appropriately to prevent multiplication of staphylococci with which the food may have been contaminated.

Treatment. Antibiotic therapy alone is rarely effective in individuals with undrained abscesses or with infected foreign bodies. Loculated collections of purulent material should be incised and drained. Foreign bodies that have served as a nidus of infection should be removed, if possible. Therapy always should be initiated with a penicillinase-resistant antibiotic; in some areas, more than 90% of all staphylococci isolated, regardless of source, are resistant to penicillin.

For serious infections parenteral treatment is indicated; methicillin, oxacillin, and nafcillin are equally effective. Generally, a dose of 200 mg/kg/24 hr should be employed intravenously in 6 divided doses. Daily doses as high as 400 mg/kg/24 hr have been used without toxicity in selected patients.

The antibiotic employed as well as the dose, route,

and duration of treatment is dependent upon the site of infection, the response of the patient to treatment, and the sensitivity of the organisms recovered from blood or from local sites of infection. In patients with staphylococcal pneumonia, intravenous treatment is recommended until the patient has been afebrile for 72 hr and other signs of infection have disappeared. Oral therapy is continued for a total of 3 wk, longer in selected cases. For osteomyelitis 3–4 wk of intravenous therapy is the preferred treatment. Oral treatment of staphylococcal osteomyelitis may be effective when therapy is carefully monitored (Sec 10.14). In patients with meningitis intravenous treatment is continued until the patient has been afebrile for at least 5 days, but the minimum course of treatment is 10 days. Staphylococcal endocarditis should be treated for 4–6 wk intravenously. In all of these infections, oral treatment should be provided when parenteral therapy has been discontinued; dicloxacillin is penicillinase resistant, absorbed well orally, and quite effective. This drug is administered in a dose of 50–75 mg/kg/24 hr in 4 divided oral doses. Duration of oral therapy depends also upon the response of the patient as determined by the clinical, roentgenographic, and laboratory findings and by culture results. In selected patients with osteomyelitis, oral therapy may be required for 12 wk or longer, depending on the time it takes the erythrocyte sedimentation rate to return to normal.

Skin and soft tissue infection and minor upper respiratory infection may be managed by oral therapy alone or by an initial brief course of antibiotics provided parenterally, followed by oral medication. Dicloxacillin (25–50 mg/kg/24 hr), oxacillin (100 mg/kg/24 hr), or nafcillin (100 mg/kg/24 hr), each in 4 divided oral doses, provides excellent blood and tissue concentrations of these antibiotics. In very mild, localized skin infection, repeated cleansing with a mild antiseptic and use of topical antibiotics (bacitracin) may be effective. Penicillin should not be applied topically.

Penicillin G can be used to treat infections due to *S. aureus* if the organism proves sensitive to this antibiotic in vitro. The dose, route, and duration of treatment depend upon the severity of the disease process.

Individuals sensitive to penicillin and its derivatives must be treated with other antibiotics or desensitized to the penicillin derivative to be employed. About 5% of penicillin-sensitive children are also sensitive to cephalosporins. Clindamycin and lincomycin have proved effective for the treatment of skin, soft tissue, bone, and joint infections due to *S. aureus*. Clindamycin may be provided in 3–4 divided doses parenterally or orally (total daily dose 30–40 mg/kg/24 hr). Clindamycin and lincomycin should *not* be used to treat endocarditis, brain abscess, or meningitis due to *S. aureus*. Erythromycin, chloramphenicol, kanamycin, and gentamicin can be used but are inferior to the penicillins. Vancomycin can be used to treat penicillin-sensitive individuals with endocarditis, but serum levels of this antibiotic should be monitored when it is used. Peak serum concentrations should be 25–40 μg/ml. It can be administered in a dose of 10–15 mg/kg/dose given every 6 hr intravenously.

Staphylococcal infection of the central nervous system

can be treated by intravenous chloramphenicol or by a combination of chloramphenicol and erythromycin.

Prognosis. Untreated staphylococcal septicemia is associated with a mortality rate of 80% or greater. Mortality rates have been reduced to 20% by appropriate antibiotic treatment. Staphylococcal pneumonia can be fatal at any age but is more likely to be associated with high morbidity and mortality in young infants or in patients whose therapy has been delayed.

A total white blood cell count below 5000 or a polymorphonuclear leukocyte response of less than 50% is a grave prognostic sign. Prognosis also may be influenced by numerous host factors, including nutrition, immunologic competence, and the presence or absence of other debilitating diseases.

RALPH D. FEIGIN

Adamski GB, Garin EH, Ballinger WE, et al: Generalized nonsuppurative myositis with staphylococcal septicemia. J Pediatr 96:694, 1980.

Boris M, Shinefield HR, Ribble JC: Bacterial interference: Its effect on nursery-acquired infection with Staphylococcus aureus. IV. Louisiana epidemic. Am J Dis Child 105:674, 1963.

Cohen JO (ed): The Staphylococci. New York, Wiley-Interscience, 1972.

Davis JP, Jones RE Jr: Morbidity and Mortality Weekly Report 29:297, 1980.

Fine RN, Onslow JM, Erwin ML, et al: Bacterial interference in the treatment of recurrent staphylococcal infections in a family. J Pediatr 70:548, 1967.

Hieber JP, Nelson JD, McCracken GH Jr: Acute disseminated staphylococcal disease in childhood. Am J Dis Child 131:181, 1977.

Jessen O, Rosendal K, Bulow P, et al: Changing staphylococci and staphylococcal infections. A ten-year study of bacteria and cases of bacteremia. N Engl J Med 281:627, 1969.

Larinkari UM, Valtonen MV, Sarvas M, et al: Teichoic acid antibiotic test. Arch Intern Med 137:1522, 1977.

Melish ME, Glasgow LA: Staphylococcal scalded-skin syndrome: The expanded clinical syndrome. J Pediatr 78:958, 1971.

Melish ME, Glasgow LA, Turner MD: The staphylococcal scalded-skin syndrome: Isolation and partial characterization of the exfoliative toxin. J Infect Dis 125:129, 1972.

Schoenbaum SC, Gardner P, Shillito J: Infections of cerebrospinal fluid shunts: Epidemiology, clinical manifestations, therapy. J Infect Dis 131:543, 1975.

Toxic Shock Syndrome

Toxic shock syndrome (TSS) is a severe illness characterized by the acute onset of high fever, hypotension, an erythematous rash, vomiting, abdominal pain, diarrhea, myalgias, and nonfocal neurologic abnormalities.

Etiology and Epidemiology. TSS was originally described in 1978 in 7 children presenting with high fever, mental confusion, a scarlatiniform rash, vomiting, and diarrhea which progressed to oliguria, disseminated intravascular coagulation, and hypotension. A toxin-producing strain of *Staphylococcus aureus* phage group I was isolated from 5 of these children. Subsequent cases have been identified worldwide, and over 1000 confirmed patients have been reported in 48 of the United States. The syndrome typically occurs in young, healthy, menstruating women who use tampons, particularly highly absorbent brands. However, a substantial number of cases in men and nonmenstruating women have been reported. Recurrences occur in 30% and the mortality approaches 8%. Epidemiologic studies have established a significant association between continuous tampon use throughout the menstrual period and TSS as well as a relationship between this syndrome and *Staphylococcus aureus* colonization of the cervix and/or vagina. A pyogenic exotoxin or enterotoxin (F) has been identified in many of these staphylococcal isolates; however, a relationship between toxin production and TSS remains unproven.

Clinical Manifestations. TSS begins with an abrupt onset of high fever, vomiting, and diarrhea and is often accompanied by sore throat, headache, and diffuse myalgias. A diffuse erythematous macular rash appears within 24 hr and may be associated with hyperemia of pharyngeal, conjunctival, and vaginal mucous membranes. Symptoms often include alterations in the level of consciousness, oliguria, and hypotension, which in severe cases may progress to shock and disseminated intravascular coagulation. Recovery occurs within 7–10 days and is associated with desquamation, particularly of palms and soles; hair and nail loss has also been reported following recovery.

A number of nonspecific laboratory abnormalities are present reflecting involvement of multiple organ systems including the hepatic, renal, muscular, gastrointestinal, cardiopulmonary, and central nervous system. Vaginal cultures performed prior to administration of antibiotics usually yield *Staphylococcus aureus*.

Differential Diagnosis. Kawasaki disease (mucocutaneous lymph node syndrome) closely resembles TSS. Both illnesses are associated with fever unresponsive to antibiotics, hyperemia of mucous membranes, and an erythematous rash with subsequent desquamation. However, many of the clinical features of TSS are absent or rare in Kawasaki disease including diffuse myalgia, vomiting, abdominal pain, diarrhea, azotemia, hypotension, adult respiratory distress syndrome, and shock. Kawasaki disease typically occurs in children under 5 yr of age, and many of the reported cases of "adult Kawasaki disease" may actually be cases of TSS. Scarlet fever, Rocky Mountain spotted fever, leptospirosis, toxic epidermal necrolysis, and measles must also be considered in the differential diagnosis.

Prevention and Treatment. The low risk of TSS (6.2 cases/100,000 menstruating women) can be eliminated by not using tampons or reduced by using them intermittently during each menstrual period.

Management of women suspected of having TSS includes the careful removal of any retained tampons at the time of initial cervical and vaginal cultures. In addition to aggressive fluid replacement to prevent or treat cardiovascular collapse, parenteral administration of a beta-lactamase resistant antistaphylococcal antibiotic (e.g., nafcillin, oxacillin, methicillin) is recommended after appropriate cultures have been obtained. Antibiotic treatment is discontinued if cultures are negative for *Staphylococcus aureus*; however, positive cultures for this organism require prolonged treatment (parenteral followed by oral) until the organism has been eradicated from the vagina.

WILLIAM T. SPECK

Anonymous: Toxic shock syndrome—United States. Morbid Mortal Weekly Report 29:229, 1980
Anonymous: Follow up on toxic shock syndrome. Morbid Mortal Weekly Report 29:441, 1980
Anonymous: Toxic shock syndrome—United States, 1970–1980. Morbid Mortal Weekly Report 30:25, 1980.
Wannamaker, LW: Toxic shock: Problems in definition and diagnosis of a new syndrome. Ann Intern Med 96:775, 1982.

Infections Due to *Staphylococcus epidermidis*

S. epidermidis is a normal inhabitant of the skin, throat, mouth, conjunctiva, vagina, and urethra. Rarely, it has been identified as a cause of meningitis, septicemia, osteomyelitis, or septic arthritis in normal, previously healthy children. More commonly, *S. epidermidis* has been identified as a cause of urinary tract infection; in 1 study this organism was responsible for 40% of such infections in children 11–16 yr of age.

Otitis media may be attributed to this organism if (1) the organism is grown on solid media following needle tympanocentesis, (2) a swab of the external auditory canal obtained concomitantly fails to grow this organism, and (3) smears of exudate from the middle ear reveal this organism within polymorphonuclear leukocytes.

S. epidermidis is a common cause of infection in children with shunts inserted for diversion of cerebrospinal fluid and in individuals in whom other foreign bodies have been implanted. It also is a cause of subacute bacterial endocarditis after cardiac surgery.

Most infections with *S. epidermidis* are indolent and difficult to treat. Therapy must be guided by testing for sensitivity to various antibiotics; many isolates are resistant to penicillin. Selected isolates may be resistant to semisynthetic penicillins but unlike *S. aureus* may remain sensitive to cephalosporins. Sensitivity of *S. epidermidis* to various antibiotics should be assessed using tube dilution sensitivity tests.

Hermanson G, Boligren I, Bergstrom T, et al: Coagulase-negative staphylococci as a cause of symptomatic urinary infections in children. J Pediatr 84:807, 1974.

INFECTIONS DUE TO NEISSERIAE

Neisseriae are gram-negative, nonsporulating, spherical or oval cocci. In smears prepared from clinical specimens or from cultures, they are commonly arranged in pairs (diplococci) and appear biscuit- or pear-shaped. Neisseriae are aerobic and can be recovered on blood agar. They are extremely sensitive to various physical and chemical agents and to drying; recovery is enhanced by use of appropriate media.

Neisseriae normally are found in the nasal and oral cavities, pharynx, vagina, and lower intestinal tract. Human disease most commonly is due to infection with *N. meningitidis* and *N. gonorrhoeae*. Neisseriae of low virulence, including *N. catarrhalis*, *N. subflava*, *N. flavescens*, *N. sicca*, *N. mucosa*, *N. lactamica*, and *N. flava*, have been reported as causative agents of septicemia, meningitis, ophthalmitis, or endocarditis in normal children. In several cases petechial hemorrhages have been noted. In at least 1 case disseminated intravascular coagulation was associated with septicemia and meningitis due to N. catarrhalis.

Meningitis due to N. catarrhalis occurs more frequently in children than in adults; meningitis caused by chromogenic neisseriae (N. subflava, N. perflava, N. flavescens, and N. flava) has no predilection for children. The signs and symptoms of sepsis and meningitis caused by these organisms of low virulence are similar to those of recognized pathogens. Penicillin or ampicillin provides effective treatment for disease due to "nonpathogenic Neisseria."

10.25 MENINGOCOCCAL INFECTIONS

Etiology. Neisseria meningitidis (meningococcus, N. intracellularis) may be recovered from the nasopharynx of healthy individuals. Disease occurs when organisms invade the bloodstream (meningococcemia) and then disseminate to other organ systems. These bacteria are seen frequently within polymorphonuclear leukocytes in smears prepared from clinical specimens. Various serogroups of N. meningitidis have been identified (types A, B, C, D, X, Y, Z, 29E, 135) and differentiated on the basis of specific capsular polysaccharides. The cell walls of meningococci contain lipopolysaccharide, which appears to be responsible for the endotoxin-like effect associated with meningococcemia.

Epidemiology. N. meningitidis may be found in the nasopharynx of normal individuals. Carriage rates vary from 2–5% of healthy children to as high as 90% in groups of military personnel during epidemics. Children under 3 mo of age rarely develop meningococcal disease.

Meningococcal meningitis generally is a disease of children who acquire N. meningitidis from an adult carrier, usually in the same family. Sometimes acquisition follows exposure to individuals with disease or to adults or children carrying the organism in a day care center. The estimated likelihood of severe meningococcal disease in family contacts, usually occurring simultaneously with the first case, is 1%. This rate is 1000-fold greater than the risk in the community. The risk of meningitis in day care center contacts of children with meningococcal disease is 1/1000. Age-specific attack rates per 100,000 population are greatest for infants under 1 yr. Eighty per cent of cases of meningococcal disease occur in children under 10 years. In recent years in the United States, serogroup B has been associated most commonly with human disease (45% of isolates). Thirty-two per cent of isolates were of group C, 18% of group Y, 2% of group A, and 3% of other serogroups.

Pathology. Disease due to N. meningitidis is associated with an acute inflammatory response. Endotoxemia may be associated with diffuse vasculitis and disseminated intravascular coagulation. Small blood vessels may be filled with leukocyte-rich fibrin clots. Hemorrhage and necrosis may be noted in any organ system; bleeding into the adrenals in patients with septicemia and shock (Waterhouse-Friderichsen syndrome) may be observed.

Pathogenesis. Initially, meningococci colonize the nasopharynx. In certain individuals the organism penetrates the mucosa and is transported by leukocytes to the bloodstream and, in turn, to other organs, including ears, eyes, lungs, joints, meninges, heart, and adrenal glands. Circulating serum antibodies and specific secretory IgA seem to be important in protecting the human host. Children and adults develop group-specific antimeningococcal antibody following prolonged carriage of meningococci. Nasopharyngeal carriage of nontypable meningococci, of those belonging to serogroups X, Y, and Z, or of lactose-fermenting meningococci evokes the production of bactericidal antibodies against groups A, B, and C. Bactericidal antibodies which cross-react with meningococci also may be induced by contact with unrelated gram-positive and gram-negative organisms. Presumably, meningococcemia is prevented in many individuals by these antibodies. Children may receive antibodies transplacentally; these persist up to the 3rd mo of life after which they are generally undetectable until approximately 8 mo of age. Subsequently there is a gradual rise in the prevalence of antibodies; in 1 study 97% of children over 5 yr of age had antibody levels of 0.479 mg/ml or more. Group-specific hemagglutinating antibody has been detected in nasal washings of patients following recovery from meningococcal disease. Development of group-specific antimeningococcal secretory IgA antibody is associated with enhancement of the pharyngeal defense mechanism.

Clinical Manifestations. Upper respiratory infections resembling the common cold are observed most frequently during epidemics of meningococcal infection. The patient may improve within a few days without specific therapy, but blood cultures may grow N. meningitidis, apparently reflecting a transient self-limited bacteremia. Maculopapular skin eruptions may be observed in some of these patients. Acute meningococcemia may occur as an influenza-like illness with fever, malaise, myalgia, and arthralgia. Headache and gastrointestinal symptoms also may be noted. Within hours to days of onset, morbilliform, petechial, or purpuric lesions may be observed. Hypotension, oliguria, and renal failure may develop. The presence of coma, purpura, hypotension, thrombocytopenia, leukopenia, or high serum antigen concentrations usually presages a fatal outcome.

Meningitis follows hematogenous dissemination of meningococci. In addition to the preceding signs and symptoms, lethargy, vomiting, photophobia, seizures, and other signs of meningeal irritation may be observed. Chronic meningococcemia is rare in children. When it occurs it is characterized by anorexia, weight loss, chills, fever, arthralgia or arthritis, and maculopapular lesions. Purulent arthritis, while more common with chronic meningococcemia, may complicate any meningococcal infection accompanied by bacteremia. Acute nonsuppurative polyarthritis has been observed in some patients with meningococcal bacteremia. Erythema nodosum may be observed. Subacute meningococcal endocarditis usually is associated with chronic meningococcemia. *Acute endocarditis, myocarditis,* and *pericarditis* tend to be associated with acute meningococcemia. *Primary meningococcal pneumonia* also has been reported. *Endophthalmitis* is extremely rare. Symptoms develop 1–3 days after the onset of septicemia or meningitis. The patient complains of photophobia and ocular pain. Ciliary injection, exudate in the anterior chamber, and a swollen, muddy iris may be noted. *Vulvovaginitis* rarely is due to *N. meningitidis.* Clinical manifestations are similar to those of any bacterial infection of the vagina. A white vaginal discharge, itching, and excoriation of the vulva are noted. Meningococcal infections frequently reactivate latent infection with *herpesvirus,* usually manifest as "cold sores."

Diagnosis. The diagnosis of meningococcal disease is established by culture of blood, cerebrospinal fluid, skin lesions, or other sites of infection. The nasopharynx also should be cultured, but isolation of meningococci from this site provides only presumptive evidence of infection. Petechial or papular lesions can be lanced and smeared, to look for gram-negative diplococci. When meningitis is present, the morphologic and clinical characteristics of cerebrospinal fluid are those of an acute bacterial meningitis. Cerebrospinal fluid culture may be negative if the lumbar puncture has been performed early in the course of disease or if the patient has received previous antibiotic treatment.

Blood, cerebrospinal fluid, and urine also can be evaluated by countercurrent immunoelectrophoresis (CIE). This technique can detect capsular antigen whether or not the organism is viable. Commercially available antisera for *N. meningitidis,* types A, C, and D, are effective. Commercial antisera for group B meningococci are unreliable. No antisera are available for detection of groups X, Y, and Z meningococci at present. Cerebrospinal fluid also can be evaluated by the limulus lysate assay; a positive assay indicates the presence of endotoxin and suggests infection by a gram-negative organism. It does not, however, identify the etiologic agent.

Ancillary laboratory data may reveal polymorphonuclear leukocytosis, thrombocytopenia, proteinuria, and hematuria. In patients with disseminated intravascular coagulation, decreased serum concentrations of prothrombin, factors V and VIII, and fibrinogen may be observed.

Differential Diagnosis. The petechial or purpuric rash of meningococcemia (Fig 10–4 [p. xxxii]) is similar to that noted in any patient with a disease characterized by generalized vasculitis. These include septicemia due to many gram-negative organisms; overwhelming septicemia with gram-positive organisms; bacterial endocarditis; Rocky Mountain spotted fever; infection with echoviruses, particularly types 6, 9, and 16; and coxsackieviruses, predominantly types A-2, A-4, A-9, and A-16. The morbilliform rash occasionally observed may be confused with any macular or maculopapular viral exanthem.

Complications. Meningococcal meningitis may be complicated by deafness, blindness, paresis of cranial nerves 3, 4, 6, and 7, hemi- or quadriparesis, seizures,

obstructive hydrocephalus, and, rarely, brain abscess. Endophthalmitis, which can develop during the course of meningococcemia, is found more commonly in patients with meningococcal meningitis. Panophthalmitis and suppurative iridochoroiditis also may be observed.

Meningococcemia may be complicated by adrenal hemorrhage, encephalitis, arthritis, myocarditis, pericarditis, pneumonia, lung abscess, peritonitis, and disseminated intravascular coagulation. In patients with hypotension and purpura, serum cortisol levels generally are increased considerably above the normal range. A lack of responsiveness to further stimulation by ACTH has been noted by some investigators, and this could not be ascribed entirely to the higher basal cortisol levels in these patients. These findings suggest that patients with meningococcal disease with purpura may have a "relatively" decreased adrenal response to ACTH. Death may follow overwhelming meningococcemia, meningococcal meningitis, pericarditis, or myocarditis.

Prevention. See Sec 10.17.

Treatment. Aqueous penicillin G (penicillin V has only 10–25% the efficacy of penicillin G against meningococci and gonococci), 400,000 units/kg/24 hr, should be given intravenously in 6 divided doses. When the etiology is in doubt, ampicillin may be used (300 mg/kg/24 hr in 6 divided doses intravenously). Chloramphenicol sodium succinate, 100 mg/kg/24 hr intravenously in 4 divided doses, provides effective treatment for patients allergic to penicillin. Therapy for meningococcemia should be continued for at least 7 days *and* until the patient has been afebrile for 72 hr. If pericarditis, pneumonia, or other complications develop, more prolonged treatment may be necessary. Meningitis should be treated for at least 10 days *and* until the patient has been afebrile for at least 5 days.

Patients with acute meningococcal infections should be monitored carefully. Hourly or half-hourly blood pressure determinations are indicated during the 1st hours of treatment until the infection appears to be under control. White blood cell counts of 7000/mm^3 or less or total blood eosinophil counts of over 25 cells/mm^3 suggest overwhelming infection and impending shock, especially if purpuric lesions are present or beginning to appear. In this situation intravenous administration of hydrocortisone 10 mg/kg immediately, followed by 10 mg/kg/24 hr given in 4–6 divided doses for 24–48 hr may be beneficial but remains controversial.

If shock or disseminated intravascular coagulation develops, appropriate support of blood pressure with osmotically active fluids may be required. Fresh whole blood, heparinization, or both may be helpful in hypotensive patients with disseminated intravascular coagulation (Sec 14.69). For additional information concerning supportive care, see Sec 10.17.

Prognosis. Mortality from acute meningococcemia may be as high as 15–20%. Mortality of patients with meningococcal meningitis is less than 3% in most major medical centers. Thus, survival of the untreated patient for the period of time required to develop meningitis is a good prognostic sign. Poor prognostic signs include the development of hypotension, disseminated intravascular coagulation, leukopenia, thrombocytopenia, high serum antigen concentrations, and a low sedimentation rate. Survival for 48 hr following initiation of therapy is a good prognostic sign. Later sloughing of skin over purpuric areas may occur but usually heals uneventfully.

Abildgaard CF, Corrigan JJ, Seeler RA, et al: Meningococcemia associated with intravascular coagulation. Pediatrics 40:78, 1967.

Altmann G, Egoz N, Bogokovsky B: Observations on asymptomatic infections with Neisseria meningitidis. Am J Epidemiol 98:446, 1973.

Burian V, Gotschlich E, Kuzemenska P, et al: Naturally occurring antibodies to Neisseria meningitidis. Bull WHO 55:653, 1977.

Center for Disease Control, The Meningococcal Disease Surveillance Group: Analysis of endemic meningococcal disease by serogroup and evaluation of chemoprophylaxis. J Infect Dis 134:201, 1976.

Gotschlich EC: Development of polysaccharide vaccines for the prevention of meningococcal diseases. Monogr Allergy 9:245, 1975.

Jensen AD, Naidoff MA: Bilateral meningococcal endophthalmitis. Arch Ophthal 90:396, 1973.

Lewis LB: Prognostic factors in acute meningococcemia. Arch Dis Child 54:44, 1979.

Munford RS, de Vasconcelos ZJS, Phillips CJ, et al: Eradication of carriage of Neisseria meningitidis in families: a study in Brazil. J Infect Dis 129:644, 1974.

Wajchenberg B, Leme CE, Tambascin M: The adrenal response to exogenous adrenocorticotrophin in patients with infection due to Neisseria meningitidis. J Infect Dis 139:267, 1978.

10.26 GONOCOCCAL INFECTIONS

Gonorrhea, an acute infectious disease caused by *Neisseria gonorrhoeae*, afflicts children of all ages. The dramatic increase in the number of reported cases, more than 428/100,000 population, coupled with increasing or absolute resistance of the causative organism to penicillin, makes this a disease of increasing importance to those who provide care for children.

Etiology. *N. gonorrhoeae* are aerobic gram-negative diplococci, difficult to cultivate in vitro because of their fastidious growth requirements. They grow best on chocolate agar to which vancomycin, colistimethate sodium, and nystatin (Thayer-Martin media) have been added. This selective medium inhibits the growth of organisms other than gonococci or meningococci. Gonococci grow best in an atmosphere of 2–10% carbon dioxide at pH 7.2–7.6 and at a temperature of 35–37° C. In clinical specimens the organism may be found within polymorphonuclear leukocytes.

N. gonorrhoeae can be subdivided on the basis of colony variation into 4 types. Pili can be visualized by electron microscopy on colony types 1 and 2 only; these are the types that produce human disease. Autotyping has permitted discrimination of approximately 20 types based upon growth characteristics on 11 chemically defined media. Sixteen serotypes of gonococci have been identified according to the antigenic specificity of the protein antigen that is contained in the outer membrane of the gonococcus.

Epidemiology. Gonorrhea is the most commonly reported infectious disease in the United States, where at least 2 million cases occur each yr, one quarter in persons 10–19 yr of age.

In the newborn period gonorrhea generally is ac-

quired during delivery or by contact with fomites. Young children may acquire disease through contact with infected parents or other caretakers. Most cases in adolescents follow venereal contact.

Pathology. An inflammatory response is initiated beneath the epithelium at the point of entry of the gonococcus. This response, apparently caused by release of endotoxin, is characterized by a yellow-white discharge containing polymorphonuclear leukocytes, serum, and desquamated epithelium. The discharge may block the ducts of paraurethral or vaginal glands and thus cause cysts or abscesses. In the untreated patient the inflammatory exudate is replaced by fibroblasts; fibrous tissue produced may lead to stricture of the urethra.

Gonococci which invade the lymphatics and blood vessels lead to inguinal lymphadenopathy; perineal, perianal, ischiorectal, or periprostatic abscesses; or disseminated gonococcal disease.

Pathogenesis. The gonococcus has the capacity to invade columnar epithelium and, occasionally, immature stratified squamous epithelium. Fully mature stratified squamous epithelium is resistant to invasion. When gonococci are introduced onto a mucosal surface (urogenital, conjunctival, pharyngeal, or rectal), they adhere by means of hairlike protein structures (pili) which extend from the cell wall. The pili may protect the gonococcus from the action of antibody and complement and also may be responsible for antiphagocytic properties of the organism. Recently, a capsule has been demonstrated for *N. gonorrhoeae*. The presence of multiple capsular types may help to explain why multiple attacks of gonorrhea may occur. Local factors, such as the thickness of the vaginal wall and the pH of vaginal mucus, may influence the development of disease. The vaginal epithelium of prepubertal females is thin, and the pH of vaginal mucin is alkaline; these factors predispose to vaginitis. The peroxidase-mediated bactericidal capacity of cervical secretions also is pH dependent and is least active during menses. Thus, extension of gonococcal disease from the cervix, as well as dissemination, is more likely to occur during menses. Disseminated infection more frequently follows pharyngeal or anorectal inoculation.

Gonococcal infection is followed by a measurable immunologic response in many but not all individuals. Antigonococcal secretory IgA antibody, sensitized lymphocytes, and serum antibodies have been detected; immunologic responses have been most prominent in those with repeated infections and in asymptomatic female carriers.

Apparently, the presence of secretory antibodies, serum antigonococcal antibodies, and sensitized lymphocytes does not provide solid immunity to gonococcal disease; reinfection is common. *N. gonorrhoeae* isolates from patients with disseminated gonococcal disease differ from other gonococcal isolates. They have unique nutritional requirements and are susceptible to lower concentrations of antibiotic agents. Moreover, sera from patients with uncomplicated gonorrhea are bactericidal for more strains of *N. gonorrhoeae* than sera from patients with disseminated gonococcal disease. This observation suggests that disseminated disease may result from selective failure of the immune system to respond to gonococci or from infection by strains of *N. gonorrhoeae* that lack immunogenicity. Attention has been called to deficiencies of C8 or other factors at the end of the complement cascade in some patients particularly susceptible to dissemination of gonorrhea.

Clinical Manifestations. The clinical manifestations of gonococcal infection depend upon (1) the site of infection, (2) differences between strains of *N. gonorrhoeae*, and (3) the host response.

Asymptomatic Gonorrhea. The incidence of this form of gonorrhea in children has not been ascertained. In 1 study of females 12–19 yr of age admitted to a school for delinquents, the incidence of gonorrhea was 12%; most were asymptomatic. It is recognized that as many as 80% of adult women and 40% of adult men with gonorrhea are asymptomatic. Asymptomatic rectal carriage of *N. gonorrhoeae* has been documented in 40–60% of females with genital infection and in 33–90% of such males (generally homosexuals). Asymptomatic pharyngeal infection also has been documented principally but not exclusively in patients who practice fellatio. Individuals with asymptomatic gonorrhea serve as an important reservoir of infection and may develop disseminated disease.

Uncomplicated Gonorrhea. Genital gonorrhea has an incubation period of 2–6 days. Primary infection develops in the urethra of the male, the vulva and vagina of the prepubertal female, and the cervix of the postpubertal female. Neonatal ophthalmitis occurs in both sexes.

Gonococcal urethritis is characterized by a purulent urethral discharge and by burning on urination. Gram stain of the discharge shows gram-negative intracellular diplococci.

The prepubertal female develops a vaginal discharge, and the vulva may be swollen, erythematous, and excoriated. Dysuria may be noted.

Symptomatic gonococcal cervicitis is characterized by a purulent discharge, dysuria, and dyspareunia. The cervix may be inflamed and tender. Pain is not enhanced by moving the cervix, and the adnexae are not tender to palpation.

Gonococcal ophthalmitis may be unilateral or bilateral. The eyes are red and swollen with a purulent discharge. Corneal ulceration, opacification, and rupture may follow if the disease is not treated.

Disseminated Gonococcal Disease. Disseminated disease results from hematogenous spread from the initial site of infection and follows asymptomatic more commonly than symptomatic gonorrhea. The most common manifestations of disseminated infection are arthritis, tenosynovitis, dermatitis, carditis, and meningitis.

Two forms of gonococcal arthritis have been described. The 1st is associated with fever, chills, skin lesions, and involvement of multiple large and small joints. Blood cultures frequently are positive, and, less commonly, *N. gonorrhoeae* may be recovered from the joint effusion. The 2nd is associated with minimal systemic symptoms and signs, and monoarticular arthritis is more common; blood cultures tend to be

negative, but the organism is commonly recovered from the joint effusion.

Dermatologic lesions may be macular, maculopapular, vesicular, pustular, or purpuric. The mucous membranes and scalp generally are spared. Lesions may be noted on the palms and soles. Rarely, gonococci can be recovered from the lesions themselves.

Endocarditis is a rare and often fatal manifestation of disseminated gonococcal disease. Arthritis or arthralgia may precede findings of endocarditis. Both left- and right-sided endocarditis have been noted; aortic valve involvement is most frequent.

Meningitis with *N. gonorrhoeae* has been documented. Signs and symptoms are similar to those of any acute bacterial meningitis.

Diagnosis and Differential Diagnosis. A definite diagnosis of gonococcal disease depends upon isolation of *N. gonorrhoeae*. In the male with urethritis, a presumptive diagnosis can be made by identification of gram-negative intracellular diplococci in the urethral discharge. A similar finding in females is not sufficient since *Mima polymorpha* and *Moraxella* (normal vaginal flora) have a similar appearance. In some culture-positive cases the Gram stain may be negative. Fluorescent staining has been employed but is inaccurate; the antibody utilized cross-reacts with other species of *Neisseria* and with other organisms.

Cultures should be obtained with noncotton swabs and should be placed immediately in a transport medium (Transgrow) or plated directly on Thayer-Martin medium. Colonies of *N. gonorrhoeae* are oxidase-positive. Further differentiation of *N. gonorrhoeae* from oxidase-positive *Mima polymorpha* and *Neisseria lactamicus* (both found in normal vaginal and oral secretions) can be made by fluorescent antibody and sugar fermentation techniques; gonococci ferment only glucose.

Gonococcal urethritis and vulvovaginitis must be distinguished from other infections that produce a purulent discharge, including β-hemolytic streptococci, *Mycoplasma*, *Trichomonas vaginalis*, and *Candida*. Rarely, infection with herpesvirus type 2 may produce symptoms similar to gonorrhea. Gonococcal arthritis must be distinguished from other forms of septic arthritis as well as from rheumatic fever, rheumatoid arthritis, and arthritis secondary to rubella or rubella immunization.

Complications. Complications of gonorrhea result from the spread of gonococci from a local site of invasion. The time interval between primary infection and development of a complication varies from days to years. Endometrial invasion by gonococci (endometritis) occurs more frequently during menses. This may be followed by acute, subacute, or chronic salpingitis, pyosalpinx, hydrosalpinx, tubo-ovarian abscess, and eventual sterility. Gonococci may gain access to the peritoneum and accumulate over the capsule of the liver. Perihepatitis may develop (Fitz-Hugh–Curtis syndrome), characterized by right upper quadrant pain associated with signs of acute or subacute salpingitis.

The most frequent complication of gonococcal urethritis in the male is local extension to the prostate. Prostatitis, epididymitis, and urethral strictures may develop. Gonococcal infection of joints may be associated with destruction of cartilage and ankylosis.

Gonococcal ophthalmitis may be associated with corneal ulceration, opacification, and blindness. Enucleation may be necessary.

Prevention. Prevention of gonorrhea can be achieved by educational efforts and by initiation of bactericidal measures immediately following exposure. Prevention by immunization is not possible at present.

The use of a condom during intercourse helps to prevent acquisition of gonorrhea by the male; it also may prevent transmission of disease from the infected male to his female partner. Vaginal foam, jelly, and cream contraceptives also may be effective in destroying gonococci.

Gonococcal ophthalmitis in the newborn infant can be prevented by instillation into the conjunctival sac of a 1% solution of silver nitrate shortly after birth. Ophthalmic ointments containing erythromycin, tetracycline, or neomycin are also probably effective.

Treatment. Progressive resistance of *N. gonorrhoeae* to penicillin has been observed since the early 1950's. By 1975, 20–35% of isolates were relatively insensitive to penicillin (minimal inhibitory concentrations to penicillin were 0.5 $\mu g/ml$ or higher). In 1976, cases of gonorrhea due to β-lactamase–producing gonococci (completely resistant to penicillin and ampicillin) were reported within the United States. Nevertheless, penicillin remains the drug of choice for initial therapy.

Uncomplicated urethritis or vulvovaginitis can be treated with aqueous procaine penicillin G, 100,000 units/kg intramuscularly, and probenecid, 25 mg/kg orally. Alternatively, amoxicillin, 50 mg/kg orally, with probenecid, 25 mg/kg (maximum 1.0 gm), can be provided. For adults or children who weigh more than 45 kg (100 lb) the United States Public Health Service currently recommends injection of a single dose of 4.8 million units of aqueous procaine penicillin accompanied by 1.0 gm of probenecid orally. Alternatively, ampicillin 3.5 gm or amoxicillin 3.0 gm (orally) with 1.0 gm of probenecid (orally) can be used. Tetracycline can be provided for individuals over 8 yr of age in a dose of 40 mg/kg/24 hr orally in 4 divided doses for 5 days (total dosage 10 gm). Single dose treatment with penicillin, ampicillin, or amoxicillin is recommended for patients who are unlikely to complete the multiple dose tetracycline regimen. Uncomplicated gonococcal disease in the penicillin-allergic child who is under 8 yr of age also can be treated with erythromycin, 40 mg/kg/24 hr in 4 divided oral doses, for 7 days. Patients with disseminated gonococcal disease should be hospitalized and treated with aqueous penicillin G intravenously, 100,000–200,000 units/kg/24 hr in 6 divided doses for 7–10 days.

Orogastric, rectal, and blood cultures should be taken from infants who are born to mothers with known gonococcal infection. Aqueous penicillin G should be administered if cultures or Gram-stained smears reveal gonococci. Dosage and duration of therapy are determined by the clinical disease that develops. Patients with neonatal gonococcal ophthalmitis must be hospitalized. Aqueous penicillin G, 50,000–75,000 units/kg/24 hr in 3 divided doses, is provided intravenously for 7–10 days. Saline irrigations of the eyes and instillation of penicillin, tetracycline, or chloramphenicol eyedrops may be utilized concomitantly.

Patients who are allergic to penicillin and who have gonococcal cervicitis, urethritis, epididymitis, or prostatitis may be treated with spectinomycin in a dose of 2 gm for men and 4 gm for women administered once intramuscularly. Patients with disseminated gonococcal disease who are over 8 yr of age can be treated with tetracycline. An initial dose, 25 mg/kg, should be administered orally, followed by 40–60 mg/kg/24 hr in 4 divided doses for 7 days. When intravenous therapy is necessary, 15–20 mg/kg/24 hr of tetracycline should be given in 4 divided doses for 7 days. For children under 8 yr of age, complicated disease can be treated with cephalothin, 60–80 mg/kg/day in 4 divided doses, intravenously for 7 days. Cephalothin should not be used in children with a previous history of anaphylaxis, urticaria, or exfoliative dermatitis associated with penicillin administration.

Some studies suggest that trimethoprim-sulfamethoxazole may be effective for the treatment of gonococcal disease. This drug is not approved for treatment of gonorrhea in children at this time. The increasing number of gonococci resistant to both penicillin and tetracycline may necessitate the use of reasonably effective alternative modes of therapy in the future.

All patients with gonorrhea should have a serologic test for syphilis performed at the time of diagnosis and 3 mo later. Patients who also have syphilis should be given additional treatment appropriate to the stage of syphilis (Sec 10.55).

Prognosis. Prompt diagnosis and adequate therapy virtually assure complete recovery from uncomplicated gonococcal disease. Complications and permanent sequelae may be associated with delayed treatment.

RALPH D. FEIGIN

Brooks GF, Israel KS, Peterson PH: Bactericidal and opsonic activity against *Neisseria gonorrhoeae* in sera from patients with disseminated gonococcal infection. J Infect Dis 134:450, 1976.

Center for Disease Control: Gonorrhea: Recommended treatment schedules: 1979; Morbidity and Mortality Weekly Reports, Vol 28 (Jan 19), 1979.

Gutman L, Wilfert C: Venereal disease. In: Feigin RD, Cherry JD (eds): Textbook of Pediatric Infectious Diseases. Philadelphia, WB Saunders, 1981.

Kaufman RE, Johnson RE, Jaffe HW, et al: Neonatal gonorrhea, monitoring study. Treatment results. N Engl J Med 294:1, 1976.

Litt IF, Edberg SC, Finberg L: Gonorrhea in children and adolescents: A current review. J Pediatr 85:595, 1974.

Thompson TR, Swanson RE, Weisner PJ: Gonococcal ophthalmia neonatorum. Relationship of time of infection to relevant control measures. JAMA 228:186, 1974.

10.27 INFECTIONS DUE TO *HEMOPHILUS INFLUENZAE*

See also Sec 10.78. *Hemophilus influenzae*, first described in 1892 by Richard Pfeiffer, was mistakenly considered to be the etiologic agent in influenza.

Epidemiology and Pathogenesis. *Hemophilus influenzae* is a fastidious, gram-negative, pleomorphic coccobacillus which requires factors X (hematin, heat stable) and V (phosphopyridine nucleotide, heat labile) for growth. Encapsulated strains are classified by the polysaccharides of the soluble capsular substance and designated as types a through f. Types a, b, c, and f contain phosphate, while d and e contain neither phosphorus nor sulfur. Almost all the serious, invasive infections in children are due to type b. Nonencapsulated strains (nontypable) have been considered etiologic factors in chronic lung disease and in otitis media. Hemophilus can be further classified by biochemical characteristics into 6 biotypes. Biotype I is the most common biotype isolated from blood and cerebrospinal fluid. Hemophilus influenzae type b can be further classified using derivatives of outer membrane proteins which fall into 6 major molecular weight categories.

Hemophilus influenzae is usually an endemic organism but may be responsible for outbreaks of disease, particularly in day care centers or chronic care facilities. Ward et al have documented that in the 30 days after onset of meningitis due to Hemophilus influenzae, the risk of H. influenzae type b infection in household contacts is 585 times greater than the age-adjusted risk in the general population. The greatest risk of a secondary case is 6% and occurs in contacts under 1 yr of age; the risk in children under 4 yr of age is 2.1%. Thus, the risk of secondary cases of H. influenzae infection in household contacts under age 6 is very similar to the risk of secondary meningococcal disease in household contacts. Hemophilus influenzae type b meningitis occurs more commonly in black than in white children, and Hispanics have rates of infection 1.6 times that of Whites. The highest incidence of systemic disease occurs among Alaskan Eskimos, 491 cases/100,000 children below 5 yr of age. Individuals with sickle cell anemia appear to be at greater risk for infections due to H. influenzae; children with asplenia or those who have undergone surgical splenectomy are at increased risk for overwhelming infection due to H. influenzae type b.

Antibodies directed against the capsular polysaccharide of H. influenzae type b play an important role in host defense against this organism. Anti-polyribophosphate (PRP) antibody is related in part to the opsonic activity of serum for H. influenzae type b; other antibodies directed against non-PRP antigens also play a role in the opsonization of this organism. In addition, both the classical and alternative complement pathways may be important in the opsonization of H. influenzae type b.

Children 2 yr or less of age demonstrate a poor or absent immunologic response to PRP following either natural infection or immunization; H. influenzae type b capsular polysaccharide vaccine is not protective when children under 18 mo of age are vaccinated. Anti-PRP response to both natural infection and immunization appears in part to be under genetic control. When immunized with type b polyribosephosphate vaccine, children with allotype Km(1) fail to respond with antibody production to the extent noted in children without this allotype. The converse is true for meningococcus C polysaccharide vaccine. The frequency of HL-A-W17

antigen is increased in children with either epiglottitis or meningitis compared to control populations.

INFECTIONS DUE TO *HEMOPHILUS INFLUENZAE*

Hemophilus influenzae type b accounts for approximately 95% of serious infections due to *H. influenzae*. Other typeable and nontypeable *H. influenzae* strains infrequently account for serious systemic diseases but are isolated commonly from the middle ear of children with otitis media. The rapid diagnosis of *H. influenzae* type b can be accomplished by several laboratory techniques including countercurrent immunoelectrophoresis (CIE), latex particle agglutination, and enzyme-linked immunosorbent assays (ELISA).

Meningitis. See also Sec 10.17. *Hemophilus influenzae* type b is the leading cause of bacterial meningitis in the United States in children between ages 1 mo–3 yr, occurring almost exclusively before school age. It is accompanied regularly by bacteremia. The annual incidence in the United States is about 40/100,000 children under 4 yr of age, similar to that of poliomyelitis in the preimmunization era. The peak incidence occurs in infants 6–9 mo of age, with one half of the cases occurring during the 1st yr of life. The highest attack and mortality rates occur in November, December, and January, but cases occur throughout the year. Clinically, meningitis due to *H. influenzae* cannot be distinguished from that due to *N. meningitidis* or *S. pneumoniae*. The case fatality rates vary from 2–18%, depending upon the facilities for rapid diagnosis, treatment, and supportive care. Bacterial meningitis due to *H. influenzae* type b may be complicated by other infections due to this organism including pneumonia, arthritis, osteomyelitis, pericarditis, and endophthalmitis. Approximately 20% of the survivors have long-term neurologic sequelae ranging from severe and obvious (retardation, paralysis, and seizure disorders) to more subtle difficulties (decreased intelligence quotient relative to siblings, hyperactivity, language and learning problems); approximately 5–10% will have a significant hearing loss. Anemia due to accelerated red blood cell destruction is more common with *H. influenzae* type b meningitis than with meningitis due to other bacteria.

Acute Epiglottitis. See also Sec 12.54. This dramatic, potentially lethal condition usually occurs in children from 2–7 yr old. It is characterized by a fulminating course of fever, sore throat, dyspnea, rapidly progressive respiratory obstruction, and prostration. Within a matter of hours, epiglottitis may progress to complete obstruction of the airway and death unless adequate treatment is administered. On physical examination the child may have only mild hoarseness and a large, shiny, cherry-red epiglottis brought into view when the posterior portion of the tongue is properly depressed. Direct visualization of the epiglottis may result in trauma to the already inflamed region and initiate an acute airway obstruction requiring immediate intubation. Establishment of an airway by either nasotracheal intubation or tracheostomy is indicated in the face of clear evidence of epiglottitis even though the degree of apparent respiratory distress may not seem severe when the patient is initially evaluated. Bacteremia is present in a majority of patients; therefore, parenteral antibiotic therapy including ampicillin and chloramphenicol should be instituted promptly. Concomitant infection is unusual, but meningitis, pneumonia, cervical adenitis, and otitis media may occur.

Patients with acute epiglottitis have cellular antigens that are genetically different from those of siblings who contract meningitis. After epiglottitis, subjects develop high serum antibody titers against type b, whereas postmeningitic children do not. This may be a function of their older age, but recent evidence indicates that erythrocyte and genetic marker lymphocyte antigens differ significantly in the 2 groups of patients.

Pneumonia. The true incidence of *H. influenzae* pneumonia in children is unknown, but it appears to be more common in children 4 yr of age or less. The signs and symptoms of pneumonia due to *H. influenzae* cannot be distinguished from those due to other microorganisms, and associated infections such as otitis media, meningitis, and epiglottitis are common. There is no characteristic chest roentgenogram. The diagnosis may be established by a positive blood or pleural culture or by CIE or latex agglutination of serum, pleural fluid, or urine. If pneumonia due to *H. influenzae* type b is suspected in a community where ampicillin-resistant strains of *H. influenzae* type b are prevalent, chloramphenicol should be included in the initial antibiotic therapy of the patient.

Septic Arthritis. See also Sec 10.15. *Hemophilus influenzae* type b is the most common organism responsible for septic arthritis in children 2 yr of age or less. Large joints, such as knee, hip, ankle, and elbow, are affected most commonly. Associated infections such as meningitis may occur. The signs and symptoms of septic arthritis due to *H. influenzae* type b are not distinguishable from those due to other organisms. Blood and/or joint cultures are positive in up to 85% of patients; Gram stain and/or CIE of joint fluid may establish the diagnosis. Antibiotic therapy for at least 2 wk with chloramphenicol and/or ampicillin, depending upon the sensitivities of *H. influenzae* type b in the community, should be instituted in any child with a diagnosis of septic arthritis at the time of admission to the hospital. The indications for aspirations and surgical incision and drainage of joints are discussed in Sec 10.15. There are usually no long-term sequelae of septic arthritis due to *H. influenzae* in children.

Cellulitis. *Hemophilus influenzae* type b is responsible for 5–14% of the cases of cellulitis in young children; over 85% of children with *H. influenzae* type b cellulitis are 2 yr of age or less. Frequently, these children have a nonspecific upper respiratory infection which is followed by the acute onset of cellulitis. There is usually no prior history of trauma to the area of cellulitis. The head and the neck, particularly the cheek and the periorbital region, are the most common sites of infection. The lesion has generally indistinct margins and is tender and indurated. A violaceous or bluish purple color may be present but does not specifically indicate *H. influenzae* type b. Conversely, a lack of a violaceous color does not exclude infection due to *H. influenzae*

type b. In buccal cellulitis an ipsilateral otitis media may occur and may be the initial focus of infection, which spreads to the buccal region by way of lymphatic vessels. Other infections such as meningitis and septic arthritis may complicate cellulitis. Blood cultures are positive in approximately 80% of the patients. *H. influenzae* type b may be recovered directly from an aspirate of the cellulitis or from an aspirate following injection of 0.1 ml of a nonbacteriostatic sterile solution into the cellulitis. Cellulitis due to *H. influenzae* type b should be treated with parenteral antibiotics until the patient is afebrile and the cellulitis has resolved; antibiotics should be continued until approximately 1 wk after all signs and symptoms have resolved.

Osteomyelitis. See also Sec 10.14. *Hemophilus influenzae* type b is a relatively uncommon cause of osteomyelitis in children, accounting for about 3% of cases. Most patients are 2 yr of age or less; large bones such as the humerus, femur, and tibia are usually involved. The etiologic diagnosis can be established by culture of a bone marrow aspirate, by Gram stain, or by CIE. Treatment is discussed in Sec 10.14.

Pericarditis. See also Sec 13.79. *Hemophilus influenzae* type b is the etiologic agent of bacterial pericarditis in up to 15% of children with this infection. The children are generally older (most commonly 2–4 yr of age). An antecedent upper respiratory infection is very common. Fever, respiratory distress, and tachycardia are constant findings. Associated infections also are very common and occur in up to 80% of these children. The etiologic diagnosis may be established by blood culture or by culture, Gram stain, or CIE of pericardial fluid. Ampicillin and/or chloramphenicol should be provided intravenously. A pericardiectomy may be important to drain the purulent material effectively and prevent pericardial tamponade and constrictive pericarditis.

Bacteremia Without an Associated Focus. See Sec 10.10. Bacteremia due to *H. influenzae* type b may occur without any apparent focus of infection other than signs of an upper respiratory infection or pharyngitis. Although these children may appear only mildly ill at the initial visit, they are at substantial risk for the development of a serious focal infection such as pneumonia or bacterial meningitis.

Neonatal Disease. In the neonate nontypeable *H. influenzae* is more common than type b. Septicemia, pneumonia and respiratory distress syndrome, conjunctivitis, meningitis, mastoiditis, septic arthritis, and a congenital vesicular eruption have been reported.

Miscellaneous Infections. Urinary tract infection, epididymo-orchitis, cervical adenitis, acute glossitis, and infected thyroglossal duct cysts have been associated with *H. influenzae.*

Otitis Media. See also Sec 12.41. *Hemophilus influenzae* has been identified in cultures of middle ear fluid removed by tympanocentesis from 20–35% of children with acute otitis media. Eighty-five–90% of the strains isolated from the middle ear are nonencapsulated. Of the typeable strains of *H. influenzae*, type b is the most common; a significant proportion of patients also have had systemic infection with the same organism.

Treatment. Since 1974 resistance to ampicillin, recognized in type b as well as in nontypeable strains of

H. influenzae, has been related primarily to the production of a plasmid mediated β-lactamase enzyme. The prevalence of ampicillin-resistant strains varies throughout the country and must be monitored in each region. If one is in an area where any ampicillin-resistant *H. influenzae* have been isolated, invasive infections presumed to be due to *H. influenzae* should be treated initially with chloramphenicol in addition to ampicillin. Invasive illnesses include meningitis, pneumonia, cellulitis, septic arthritis, and pericarditis but not otitis media. Once an isolate has proved sensitive to ampicillin, chloramphenicol can be discontinued. β-lactamase activity can be rapidly determined by a pH indicator system. If β-lactamase production is present, the isolate is considered to be resistant to ampicillin. If the β-lactamase test is negative, one should not discontinue chloramphenicol until disc or tube sensitivity tests prove that the isolate is sensitive to ampicillin since a small percentage of β-lactamase negative strains may be resistant to ampicillin because of other mechanisms. In some patients a β-lactamase negative isolate can be recovered from 1 site and a β-lactamase positive isolate from another site of infection; specific sensitivities of both isolates must be determined prior to discontinuing chloramphenicol. Strains of *H. influenzae* have also been reported to be resistant to chloramphenicol because of the production of a plasmid mediated acetyl-transferase. Moxalactam as well as 3rd generation cephalosporins hold significant promise for the treatment of such resistant *H. influenzae* infections since they are effective in vitro against both ampicillin and chloramphenicol-resistant strains of *H. influenzae*.

Prevention. No available vaccine adequately protects infants and young children from disease due to *H. influenzae* type b. Current vaccines are being modified to improve immunogenicity in young children.

Since the risk for secondary infection due to *H. influenzae* type b is equivalent to that of *N. meningitidis*, antibiotic prophylaxis has been suggested as 1 method of preventing secondary cases. One study has shown rifampin to be useful in preventing a secondary infection due to *H. influenzae* type b. Rifampin is recommended for children under 4 yr who are family or day-care center contacts of individuals with *H. influenzae* disease. Parents of children with invasive *H. influenzae* type b disease should be told that there is an increased risk of secondary infection due to this organism in other young children in the same household and should be alerted to any signs or symptoms that might be related to such an infection.

INFECTIONS DUE TO *HEMOPHILUS APHROPHILUS*

This tiny, gram-negative, nonmotile, pleomorphic coccobacillus may be confused with *H. influenzae* on stained smears. It must be distinguished also from other microaerophilic or fastidious gram-negative bacilli. The natural habitat of the organism and the source of the infrequent infections related to it have not been established conclusively; *Hemophilus aphrophilus* has been isolated from gingival scrapings, interdental material,

and tonsils. It has been associated with pet contact, particularly dogs, and has been isolated from dog bite wounds. However, a history of canine contact is absent in many cases of *H. aphrophilus* infection.

A serious underlying illness is generally present in the patients with *H. aphrophilus* infection. The symptoms are those of the illness caused by the localization of the organism. Endocarditis occurs most frequently; less commonly, brain abscess, sinusitis, miscellaneous abscesses and wounds, pneumonia and/or empyema, septicemia, otitis media, septic arthritis, osteomyelitis, or meningitis may be noted. Children with cyanotic congenital heart disease are at increased risk for brain abscess due to this organism.

Standard disc susceptibility tests are not reliable for determining the in vitro antibiotic sensitivity of *H. aphrophilus*. Therefore, broth dilution tests are indicated for determining treatment of serious infections. In general, most *H. aphrophilus* strains are susceptible to chloramphenicol, tetracycline, and streptomycin. Sensitivity to penicillin, ampicillin, erythromycin, and cephalosporins is variable.

SHELDON L. KAPLAN
RALPH D. FEIGIN

Anderson P, Smith DH, Ingram DL, et al: Antibody to polyribophosphate of *Haemophilus influenzae* type b in infants and children: Effect of immunization with polyribophosphate. J Infect Dis 136:357, 1977.

Bieger RC, Brewer NS, Washington JA: *Haemophilus aphrophilus*: A microbiologic and clinical review and report of 42 cases. Medicine 57:345, 1978.

Dajani AS, Asmur BI, Thirumoorthi MC: Systemic *Haemophilus influenzae* disease: An overview. J Pediatr 94:355, 1979.

Echeverria P, Smith EWP, Ingram D, et al: *Hemophilus influenzae* b pericarditis in children. Pediatrics 56:808, 1975.

Elwell LP, DeGraaff J, Seibert D, et al: Plasmid-linked ampicillin resistance in *Haemophilus influenzae* type b. Infect Immun 12:404, 1975.

Fraser DW, Darby CP, Koehler RE, et al: Risk factors in bacterial meningitis: Charleston County, South Carolina. J Infect Dis 127:271, 1973.

Ginsburg CM, Howard JB, Nelson JD: Report of 65 cases of *Haemophilus influenzae* b pneumonia. Pediatrics 64:283, 1979.

Goldenberg DL, Cohen AL: Acute infectious arthritis. Am J Med 60:369, 1976.

Kaplan SL, Feigin RD: Rapid identification of the invading microorganism. Pediatr Clin North Am 27:783, 1980.

Lilian LD, Yeh TF, Novak GM, et al: Early onset *Haemophilus influenzae* sepsis in newborn infants: Clinical, roentgenographic and pathologic features. Pediatrics 62:299, 1978.

Marshall R, Teele DW, Klein JD: Unsuspected bacteremia due to *Haemophilus influenzae*: Outcome in children not initially admitted to hospital. J Pediatr 95:690, 1979.

Peltola H, Kayhty H, Sivomen A, et al: *Haemophilus influenzae* type b capsular polysaccharide vaccine in children: A double-blind field study of 100,000 vaccines 3 months to 5 years of age in Finland. Pediatrics 60:730, 1977.

Todd JK, Bruhn FW: Severe *Haemophilus influenzae* infections. Spectrum of disease. Am J Dis Child 129:607, 1975.

Ward JI, Fraser DW, Baraff LJ, et al: *Haemophilus influenzae* meningitis. A national study of secondary spread of household contacts. N Engl J Med 301:122, 1979.

Ward JI, Siber GR, Scheifele DW, et al: Rapid diagnosis of *Hemophilus influenzae* type b infections by latex particle agglutination and counterimmunoelectrophoresis. J Pediatr 93:37, 1978.

Whisnant JK, Rogentine GN, Gelnick MA, et al: Host factors and antibody response in *Haemophilus influenzae* type b meningitis and epiglottitis. J Infec Dis 133:448, 1976.

10.28 PERTUSSIS (Whooping Cough)

Pertussis is an acute respiratory infection which can affect any susceptible host but is most common and serious in young children. Pertussis means intensive cough. The 1st written description of this epidemic disease appeared in 1578, but the etiologic agent was not isolated until 1906 by Bordet and Gengou.

Etiology. Pertussis usually is caused by *Bordetella pertussis* (*Hemophilus pertussis*). A similar illness has been associated with infection by *B. parapertussis*, *B. bronchiseptica*, and adenovirus types 1, 2, 3, and 5. *B. pertussis*, and to a lesser extent *B. parapertussis*, are the etiologic agents which can be implicated in most unimmunized children with pertussis.

B. pertussis is a small, nonmotile, gram-negative rod with extremely fastidious requirements for growth. It is recovered most readily on glycerin–potato–blood agar media (Bordet-Gengou) to which penicillin has been added to inhibit growth of other organisms. Freshly recovered organisms generally belong to an antigenic type designated phase I. Passage in culture may result in induction of variant forms (phase II, III, or IV organisms). Phase I strains are required for transmission of disease and production of an effective vaccine. *B. parapertussis* and *B. bronchiseptica*, similar morphologically to *B. pertussis*, have similar requirements for growth but can be differentiated by specific agglutination reactions.

Epidemiology. Pertussis is one of the most contagious diseases. Attack rates of 97–100% have been recorded in susceptible populations. Risk of disease is highest in children under 5 yr. Mortality is greatest in young infants (between 1960–1967, 72% of all reported deaths due to pertussis in the United States occurred in children under 1 yr).

Pertussis exhibits little seasonal variation. Females are affected more frequently than males, in contrast with trends noted for most other infectious illnesses. *B. pertussis* rarely has been isolated from asymptomatic individuals; transmission of disease generally requires contact with a patient.

The incidence of pertussis remains high in developing countries. In the United States the incidence has decreased dramatically since the use of pertussis vaccine, but the disease still affects several thousand persons each yr. Immunization reduces the incidence and mortality of pertussis, but immunity is neither complete nor permanent. Pertussis has been reported with increasing frequency in recent yr in adolescents and medical personnel immunized appropriately during the 1st 6 yr of life. Formerly, most young infants acquired their illness from siblings or other children; more recently, the waning immunity of adults in the household has made mildly affected adults the most common source of infection in infants too young to be immunized.

Pathology. Inflammation of the mucosal lining of the respiratory tract is noted. The organisms multiply only in association with ciliated epithelium. There is congestion and infiltration of the mucosa with lymphocytes and polymorphonuclear leukocytes, and inflammatory debris accumulates in the lumen of the bronchi. Peribronchial lymphoid hyperplasia occurs early, followed by a necrotizing process that affects the midzonal and basilar layers of the bronchial epithelium. A bronchopneumonia develops with necrosis and desquamation of the superficial epithelium of small bronchi. Bronchiolar obstruction and atelectasis result from accumulation of mucus secretions. Bronchiectasis may develop and persist.

Pathologic changes have also been described in brain and liver. Microscopic or gross cerebral hemorrhages may be noted, and cortical atrophy has been observed, possibly as the result of anoxia. Fatty infiltration of the liver has been noted in patients with pertussis encephalopathy.

Pathogenesis. Infection follows inhalation of phase I organisms. An antigen is associated with the capsule of *B. pertussis*, but it does not appear to be associated with immunologic protection. Pili project from the outer layer of the cell wall. Other identifiable antigenic components on the surface of these organisms include lipopolysaccharide with endotoxin-like activity, protective antigen, agglutinogens, histamine-sensitizing factor, lymphocytosis-promoting factor, and adjuvant. A heat labile toxin is a cytoplasmic component of *B. pertussis*.

Understanding the pathogenesis of pertussis in man depends upon knowledge of the host response to these capsular, cell-wall, or cytoplasmic antigens. The endotoxin of *B. pertussis* is not important in the pathogenesis of the disease. The role of histamine-stimulating factor in human infection is unclear.

Lymphocytosis-promoting factor presumably plays a role in human infection by mobilizing lymphocytes from lymphatic organs; both T and B lymphocyte populations are affected in a similar manner. The role played by cell-mediated immunity in the human host is unclear. The association of lymphocytosis-promoting factor with the lymphocytosis in patients with pertussis must be viewed cautiously; although this factor is not present in *B. parapertussis*, lymphocytosis is prominent in children infected with this organism.

Exposure of humans to *B. pertussis* is followed by the development of agglutinins and of hemagglutination-inhibiting, bactericidal, complement-fixing, and immunofluorescent antibodies, but resistance to infection does not correlate with their presence. The existence of protective antigen in the cell wall of *B. pertussis* suggests that antibody directed against this antigen may offer protection from disease. An immunologically active material which correlates directly with immunity has not been identified in human sera.

The pili or surface appendages of *B. pertussis* apparently are responsible for its attachment to epithelial cells. In cell cultures protective antibody to *B. pertussis* inhibits attachment. Secretions of individuals immune to pertussis contain IgG and IgA with antipertussis activity. Secretory IgA can inhibit bacterial adherence specifically, and prolonged resistance to infection may be mediated by serum IgG. These observations suggest that local and systemic humoral immunity plays an important role in human protection against pertussis.

Clinical Manifestations. The incubation period for pertussis has a mean of 7 and a range of 6–20 days. Symptomatic illness is generally divided into 3 stages: catarrhal, paroxysmal, and convalescent. Illness generally lasts 6–8 wk. The clinical manifestations depend to some extent on the specific etiology of the syndrome as well as on the age and immunization status of the host. Illness due to *B. parapertussis* or *B. bronchiseptica* is less severe and of shorter duration than that described below.

Catarrhal Stage (1–2 wk). Symptoms of an upper respiratory infection predominate. Rhinorrhea, conjunctival injection, lacrimation, mild cough, and low grade fever are noted; a diagnosis of pertussis usually is not considered during this stage. Infants tend to have a profuse, viscid, mucoid, nasal discharge which may cause upper respiratory obstruction.

Paroxysmal Stage (2–4 wk or longer). Episodes of coughing increase in severity and number. Characteristically, repetitive series of 5–10 forceful coughs during a single expiration are followed by a sudden massive inspiratory effort which produces the whoop as air is inhaled forcefully against a narrowed glottis. Facial redness or cyanosis, bulging eyes, protrusion of the tongue, lacrimation, salivation, and distention of neck veins are noted during the attack. Episodes of severe paroxysmal coughing may occur sequentially until the child succeeds in dislodging the mucous plug obstructing the airway. Vomiting in association with the paroxysms is characteristic enough that the child who vomits with a cough should always be suspected of having pertussis, even in the absence of a whoop. The episodes are exhausting; it is not unusual for the patient to appear dazed and apathetic and to lose weight. Attacks may be triggered by yawning, sneezing, eating, drinking, and physical exertion or even by suggestion. Between attacks the patient may appear to be minimally ill and is usually comfortable. Not all patients with pertussis have a whoop.

Convalescent Stage (1–2 wk). Paroxysmal episodes of coughing, whooping, and vomiting gradually decrease in frequency and severity. Cough may persist for several mo. Recurrent paroxysmal cough is noted in some patients for months or years in association with subsequent upper respiratory infections.

Physical examination is generally uninformative. In the paroxysmal stage petechial or conjunctival hemorrhages may be noted over the head and neck. In some patients diffuse rhonchi and rales are noted.

Diagnosis and Differential Diagnosis. Pertussis can be recognized readily during the paroxysmal stage of disease if the diagnosis is considered. A history of contact with a known case is helpful but generally will be negative in a highly immunized population.

The white blood cell count may be helpful in establishing the diagnosis. Leukocytosis (counts of 20,000–50,000 cells/mm³ of blood) with an absolute lymphocytosis is characteristic at the end of the catarrhal and during the paroxysmal stage of disease. The white cell count may not be helpful in infants since they respond with lymphocytosis to any infection. Chest roentgenograms may show perihilar infiltrates, atelectasis, or emphysema.

Specific diagnosis depends upon recovery of the organism, best accomplished during the early phases of illness by nasopharyngeal swabs which are cultured on Bordet-Gengou media at the bedside. Cough plates are no longer recommended. Fluorescent antibody staining of pharyngeal specimens may provide a specific diagnosis rapidly.

Spasmodic attacks of coughing may be observed in infants with bronchiolitis, bacterial pneumonia, cystic fibrosis, tuberculosis, and any lymphadenopathy causing extrinsic compression of trachea and bronchi. A foreign body may produce paroxysms of coughing but can be distinguished by the sudden onset of symptoms as well as by roentgenographic and endoscopic findings.

Infections with *B. parapertussis*, *B. bronchiseptica*, and adenoviruses may produce clinical syndromes indistinguishable from that caused by *B. pertussis*. Differentiation may be made by isolation of these agents and, in the case of adenovirus, by demonstrating a rise in antibody titer to this agent.

Complications. The most frequent complication of pertussis is pneumonia. It is responsible for more than 90% of deaths in children under 3 yr of age. Pneumonia may be related to *B. pertussis* itself but more commonly is caused by secondary bacterial invaders. Atelectasis may develop secondary to viscid mucous plugs. The forcefulness of the paroxysm can cause rupture of alveoli, producing interstitial or subcutaneous emphysema. Bronchiectasis may develop and persist.

Otitis media is common and frequently is due to *Streptococcus pneumoniae*. Pertussis also has been associated with activation of latent tuberculosis. Convulsions and coma may be observed. These findings probably are a reflection of cerebral hypoxia related to asphyxia. Rarely, subarachnoid and intraventricular hemorrhage may be observed. Tetanic seizures may be associated with alkalosis from loss of gastric contents due to persistent vomiting. Other complications include ulcer of the frenulum of the tongue, epistaxis, melena, subconjunctival hemorrhages, spinal epidural hematoma, rupture of the diaphragm, umbilical hernia, inguinal hernia, rectal prolapse, dehydration, and nutritional disturbances.

Prevention. Immunity to pertussis is not acquired transplacentally. Although detectable concentrations of agglutinins to pertussis are found in the serum of one third of newborn infants, there is no evidence that these antibodies prevent disease. Active immunity can be induced by a total dose of 12 protective units of pertussis vaccine in 3 equal doses given 8 wk apart. Ideally, immunization is accomplished by providing pertussis in combination with diphtheria and tetanus toxoids (DTP adsorbed); primary immunization is initiated at 2 mo of age. If pertussis is prevalent in the community, immunization can be started at 1 mo of age. Subsequently, DTP should be given 1 yr after completion of the primary series and upon entry into kindergarten or elementary school.

If anaphylaxis, convulsions, focal neurologic signs, collapse, or encephalopathy follows a DTP immunization, no further injections of pertussis vaccine should be given. Other adverse reactions include screaming episodes, excessive somnolence, fever, malaise, and local induration and tenderness. There is no firm statistical evidence that children with brain damage or seizure activity antedating immunization are in greater danger from pertussis vaccine than the general population. Reported efficacy of the vaccine varies from 70-90%.

The risk of serious neurologic complications following pertussis immunization in the United States has been estimated at about 1 in 180,000. Objections to the use of pertussis vaccine began to appear in the British literature in 1974, and an increased number of cases were noted subsequent to decreased use of the vaccine. The British Joint Committee on Vaccination and Immunization conducted a survey to determine the frequency of complications due to pertussis immunization and agreed unanimously that vaccine use should be continued. Kaplan et al predicted a 71-fold increase in cases and a 4-fold increase in deaths from pertussis without immunization. With a vaccination program, 0.1 case of encephalitis associated with pertussis and 5 cases of post-vaccination encephalitis were predicted; without a program, there would be 2.3 cases of encephalitis associated with pertussis. Community vaccination would reduce the cost related to pertussis by 61%. Careful surveillance of the risk and effectiveness of pertussis vaccine should be maintained as there may be differences in populations and vaccines. Pertussis immune serum globulin (human), 1.5 ml intramuscularly, repeated in 3-5 days, has been given to unimmunized infants under 2 yr of age who have been intimately exposed to pertussis. Controlled studies fail to document the efficacy of this approach. Erythromycin was effective in preventing pertussis in newborn infants exposed to pertussis in a newborn nursery.

Close contacts less than 7 yr of age who have been immunized previously against pertussis should receive a booster dose of DTP unless a booster dose has been given within the preceding 6 mo. They also should be given erythromycin, 50 mg/kg/24 hr in 4 divided oral doses for 10 days. Children who are more than 7 yr of age and who have been immunized also should receive prophylactic erythromycin. Individuals in contact with a case of pertussis who have not been immunized previously should receive erythromycin for 10 days after contact has been eliminated. If the contact cannot be broken, erythromycin should be given until cough in the index case has stopped or until the index case has received erythromycin for 7 days. Although erythromycin eliminates carriage of pertussis, its effectiveness in preventing the development of disease is not completely established.

Treatment. Antibiotic therapy does not shorten the duration of the paroxysmal stage of the disease. Erythromycin (50 mg/kg/24 hr) or ampicillin (100 mg/kg/24 hr) may eliminate pertussis organisms from the nasopharynx within 3-4 days, thereby shortening the period of communicability. Erythromycin may abort or eliminate pertussis when given to patients in the catarrhal stage of the disease. Pertussis immune globulin has been used in children under 2 yr of age (1.25 ml daily for 3-5 doses). Controlled studies have not documented the efficacy of this form of treatment.

Supportive care includes avoidance of factors that provoke attacks of coughing and maintenance of hydration and nutrition. Oxygen and gentle suction to remove profuse, viscid secretions may be required, particularly in infants with pneumonia and significant respiratory distress.

Prognosis. Mortality rates have fallen to fewer than 10/1000 cases in the United States; they may reach 40% in infants under 5 mo. Most deaths are due to pneumonia or other pulmonary complications. The risk of chronic disease, including bronchiectasis, is unknown.

RALPH D. FEIGIN

Altemeier WA III, Ayoub EM: Erythromycin prophylaxis for pertussis. Pediatrics 59:623, 1977.

Bass JW, Klenk EL, Kotheimer JB, et al: Antimicrobial treatment of pertussis. J Pediatr 75:768, 1969.

Kaplan JP, Schoenbaum SC, Weinstein MC, et al: Pertussis vaccine—an analysis of benefits, risks, and costs. N Engl J Med 301:906, 1979.

Linnemann CC Jr, Bass JW, Smith MHD: The carrier state in pertussis. Am J Epidemiol 88:422, 1968.

Nelson KE, Gavitt F, Batt MD, et al: The role of adenoviruses in the pertussis syndrome. J Pediatr 86:335, 1975.

Shaw EB: Commentary on immunization. Am J Dis Child 134:130, 1980.

10.29 INFECTIONS DUE TO DIARRHEOGENIC *ESCHERICHIA COLI*

Escherichia coli may cause acute diarrheal disease in children. These organisms are classified as (1) enteropathogenic, (2) enterotoxigenic, (3) enteroinvasive, and (4) adherent. Enteropathogenic strains of *E. coli* (EPEC) are certain serotypes that historically have been associated with infantile diarrhea. Enterotoxigenic strains elaborate an enterotoxin that may induce diarrhea. Enteroinvasive *E. coli* are capable of invading and destroying intestinal epithelial cells, thereby causing a dysentery-like illness similar to shigellosis.

Etiology. *E. coli* are gram-negative, aerobic (facultatively anaerobic) rods that generally are motile. *E. coli* can be serotyped; immune sera are directed to the O or somatic antigens that are heat-stable, to the K-antigens that also are somatic antigens but heat-labile, and to the H (flagellar) antigens that also are inactivated by heat. According to this system, *E. coli* can be classified into more than 150 O, 93 K, and 52 H antigen groups, all of which occur independently.

Epidemiology. During the 1940's and 1950's certain serotypes of *E. coli* were associated with outbreaks of diarrhea in hospital nurseries; such serotypes came to be known as enteropathogenic *E. coli* (EPEC). When fed to volunteers, these strains caused diarrhea. However, later studies revealed that EPEC serotypes could be isolated from individuals without diarrhea, and outbreaks of diarrhea did not necessarily occur in nurseries when EPEC serotypes were isolated.

Enterotoxigenic *E. coli* (ETEC) which produce heat-labile enterotoxin are the major cause of diarrhea in adults from the United States traveling in Mexico, and they cause about 4% of diarrheal disease in children in the United States. Higher percentages have been noted in Mexico City, Brazil, and the Philippines. Since a large inoculum of ETEC, 10^6–10^9 organisms, is required to cause disease, water or food sources of ETEC must be highly contaminated. ETEC have been implicated in outbreaks of diarrhea in newborn nurseries. E. coli that possess certain O and H antigens are likely to be strains that produce an enterotoxin; almost all O78:H11, O78:H12, and O6:H16 strains are enterotoxigenic. O78 strains without H11 or 12 antigens generally are non-enterotoxigenic. ·

Enteroinvasive E. coli are not important causes of diarrhea in children in the United States, nor is person-to-person spread an important mode of transmission of enteroinvasive E. coli; outbreaks related to contaminated food have been reported.

Pathogenesis. The mechanism by which EPEC cause diarrhea is not completely understood. Levine et al have shown that EPEC that do not produce heat-labile or stable enterotoxins and are not invasive definitely produce diarrhea in human volunteers; large doses such as 10^{10} organisms were necessary to induce disease. However, highly concentrated supernatants of E. coli E51–71 cultures decreased absorption significantly in canine acute jejunal-loop tests, suggesting the presence of an enterotoxin.

E. coli may produce heat-stable, heat-labile, or both types of enterotoxin. Genetic control for the production of either type of enterotoxin resides on transferable plasmids. Heat-labile (LT) enterotoxin is related closely to the enterotoxin produced by cholera. It binds to G_{MI} ganglioside of epithelial cells as its receptor and activates cellular adenyl cyclase. The result is increased intracellular concentrations of cyclic AMP, which promote the net secretion of water and chloride. Heat-stable (ST) enterotoxin activates guanylate cyclase, which also increases the secretory activity of the gastrointestinal tract. The genetic information that codes for antibiotic resistance may be carried on the same plasmid as that responsible for coding enterotoxin production. Thus, the widespread use of antibiotics may promote the distribution of both antibiotic-resistant and enterotoxigenic E. coli.

Enteroinvasive E. coli are capable of invading and multiplying within the gastrointestinal epithelial cells much like Shigella. Local inflammation with hyperemia, edema, ulceration, and intraluminal exudate may result. The diarrheal stools may contain blood and mucus, and fecal leukocytes can be identified. Invasive E. coli usually are limited to serotypes O28, O32, O112, O115, O214, O36, O143, O144, O147, O152, and O164.

A 4th possible pathogenic mechanism for E. coli diarrhea involves adherence of bacteria to gastrointestinal epithelium with brush border damage and reduction in brush border enzymes as described by Ulshen and Rollo.

Clinical Manifestations. The diarrhea induced by EPEC is not pathognomonic. In general, patients have watery diarrhea with low grade fever and no other systemic symptoms. Stools may contain mucus but usually not blood. The patient may have up to 10 stools/day, and the gastroenteritis usually resolves spontaneously in 3–7 days. In young infants vomiting, dehydration, and electrolyte disturbances with acidosis may result.

The clinical picture of "traveler's diarrhea" due to ETEC is fairly typical. Within 1–2 wk of arrival, the traveler may have the abrupt onset of acute watery diarrhea that may be explosive in nature. As many as 10–20 diarrheal stools/day may be noted. The diarrhea is frequently associated with severe abdominal pain or cramps, nausea, and vomiting; malaise and fever are variable. Disease due to the labile toxin may be less severe with little or no complaint of abdominal pain or nausea and only low grade fever.

Patients with enteroinvasive E. coli diarrhea develop symptoms after an incubation period of approximately 18–24 hr. There is an abrupt onset of fever with severe diarrhea, urgency, and tenesmus. Bloody stools containing mucus may be present. Nausea, abdominal pain, myalgias, chills, and headache also may occur. E. coli which adhere to intestinal brush borders may be found more commonly in patients with protracted and chronic diarrhea.

Diagnosis. EPEC gastroenteritis may be suspected in outbreaks of diarrhea, particularly those occurring in nurseries. When the same serotype is isolated from the stools of many infected infants, a presumptive diagnosis of EPEC diarrhea may be made. In addition to the stool, nasopharynx, throat, and upper intestinal contents also may be colonized with the same EPEC serotype. Routine serotyping of E. coli for EPEC spectrum probably is not warranted except during outbreaks of diarrhea in nurseries or other enclosed populations. Detection of enterotoxigenic or enteroinvasive strains of E. coli requires special laboratory procedures that, at present, can be performed only in certain research laboratories.

In adults with severe ETEC diarrhea, stool losses of sodium are very high; in 1 study the mean ±1 SE stool sodium concentration was 108 ± 4 mEq/l. Mean stool sodium concentrations in children were 44–67 mEq/l, depending on the duration of diarrhea. The high stool sodium and bicarbonate losses are consistent with the pathogenesis of ETEC diarrhea, which is secretory in nature. High stool concentrations of sodium are consistent with but not diagnostic of ETEC diarrhea. The adherent form of E. coli diarrhea can be diagnosed definitively only by intestinal biopsy.

Prevention. During institutional outbreaks of EPEC diarrhea, enteric precautions must be maintained. In nurseries a cohort system of admission should be instituted.

In 1 study doxycycline, 100 mg/day, was an effective prophylactic agent for traveler's diarrhea in adults visiting Kenya. Such prophylactic therapy should be avoided in children under 8 yr of age. Trimethoprim-sulfamethoxazole administered twice daily prevented diarrhea in students traveling to Mexico. The prophylactic administration of lactobacilli preparations does not reduce the incidence or duration of traveler's diarrhea. The ingestion of 60 ml of Pepto-Bismol 4 times each day decreased the incidence of diarrheal illness significantly in student travelers compared to students who received a placebo. Similar studies are not available for children, but this quantity of Pepto-Bismol is contraindicated in young children because of the amount of bismuth subsalicylate contained in this volume.

Treatment. In infants and children correction of fluid and electrolyte disturbances is the major therapeutic concern. Severe diarrhea and vomiting may result in significant dehydration that may require hospitalization and intravenous fluid therapy. Oral glucose-electrolyte solutions have been recommended by the World Health Organization for the oral treatment of diarrheal dehydration of infants and children in developing regions (Sec 4.4).

Over-the-counter antidiarrheal preparations such as kaolin and pectins do not influence the frequency or the water content of stools in children with acute diarrhea. Diphenoxylate-atropine (Lomotil) also has no role in the treatment of diarrhea due to *E. coli*.

Neomycin, 10 mg/kg/day, given in 3–6 divided doses orally for 3–5 days is effective in the treatment of diarrhea due to EPEC, particularly among infants. Stool cultures become negative within 24 hr of therapy in approximately 75% of the children. A clinical response is generally noted when EPEC are eliminated from the stool. Relapse rates of 20% have been reported after therapy has been discontinued. Antibiotic therapy of diarrhea due to ETEC has not been evaluated adequately. In 1 study in Bangladesh, a slightly earlier termination of diarrheal illness was noted in adult patients, compared to placebo-treated controls, who harbored LT-ST ETEC strains and were treated with tetracycline. Tetracycline had no effect on duration of illness in patients infected with ST-producing ETEC strains. The duration of positive stool cultures for ETEC was decreased in the tetracycline-treated patients compared to the placebo patients. Tetracycline had no significant effect on the stool volume or intravenous fluid requirements. Since ETEC diarrheal illness can be treated with oral rehydration therapy alone, the use of tetracycline may not be indicated except in patients who are severely ill.

Treatment of diarrhea due to enteroinvasive *E. coli* also has not been evaluated critically. In general, patients do not require hospitalization and are asymptomatic within 1 wk of onset of illness without antibiotic therapy. However, like *Shigella*, diarrhea due to enteroinvasive *E. coli* may respond to ampicillin when therapy is indicated.

SHELDON L. KAPLAN
RALPH D. FEIGIN

DuPont HI, Evans DG, Rios N, et al: Prevention of travelers' diarrhea with trimethoprim-sulfamethoxazole. Rev Infect Dis 4:533, 1982.

DuPont HI, Formal SB, Hornick RB, et al: Pathogenesis of *Escherichia coli* diarrhea. N Engl J Med 285:1, 1971.

DuPont HI, Sullivan P, Pickering LK, et al: Symptomatic treatment of diarrhea with bismuth subsalicylate among students attending a Mexican university. Gastroenterology 73:715, 1977.

Echeverria P, Murphy JR: Enterotoxigenic *Escherichia coli* carrying plasmids coding for antibiotic resistance and enterotoxin production. J Infect Dis 142:273, 1980.

Klipstein FA, Rowe B, Engert RF, et al: Enterotoxigenicity of enteropathogenic serotypes of *Escherichia coli* isolated from infants with epidemic diarrhea. Infect Immunol 21:171, 1978.

Levine MM, Nalin DR, Hornick RB, et al: *Escherichia coli* strains that cause diarrhea but do not produce heat-labile or heat-stable enterotoxin and are noninvasive. Lancet 1:1119, 1978.

Merson MH, Morris GK, Sack DA, et al: Traveler's diarrhea in Mexico: A prospective study. N Engl J Med 294:1299, 1976.

Merson MH, Sack RB, Islam S, et al: Disease due to enterotoxigenic *Escherichia*

coli in Bangladesh adults: Clinical aspects and a controlled trial of tetracycline. J Infect Dis 141:702, 1980.

Molla AM, Rahman M, Sarker SA, et al: Stool electrolyte content and purging rates in diarrhea caused by rotavirus, enterotoxigenic *E. coli* and *V. cholerae* in children. J Pediatr 98:835, 1981.

Ryder RW, Wachsmuth IK, Buxton AE, et al: Infantile diarrhea produced by heat stable enterotoxigenic *Escherichia coli*. N Engl J Med 295:849, 1976.

Sack DA, Kapinsky DC, Sack B, et al: Prophylactic doxycycline for traveler's diarrhea. N Engl J Med 298:758, 1978.

Sack RB: Enterotoxigenic *Escherichia coli*: Identification and characterization. J Infect Dis 142, 279, 1980.

Ulshen MH, Rollo JL: Pathogenesis of *Escherichia coli* gastroenteritis in man: Another mechanism. N Engl J Med 302:99, 1980.

10.30 INFECTIONS DUE TO SALMONELLAE

Salmonella organisms are important pathogens for animals and man. Generally, human infections are caused by the ingestion of contaminated water or food. Currently, gastroenteritis due to *Salmonella* is one of the most common infectious diseases in the United States. Although systemic infection with *Salmonella typhosa* (typhoid fever) is infrequent in the United States, it remains endemic and epidemic in many parts of the world.

The causative organism of typhoid fever was found in mesenteric lymph nodes by Eberth in 1880. This group of organisms is called *Salmonella* after Dr. D. E. Salmon, who isolated *S. choleraesuis* in 1885.

Etiology. Salmonellae are motile, gram-negative, nonencapsulated, nonsporulating bacilli that do not ferment lactose or sucrose but utilize glucose, maltose, and mannitol. The principal antigens of salmonellae are the flagellae (H) antigens, the cell wall (O) antigens, and the envelope (Vi) heat-labile antigens that block the O antigen-antibody agglutination. An elaborate typing scheme utilizing O and H antigens (Kaufman-White) has permitted the differentiation of over 1400 *Salmonella* serotypes. A system of nomenclature has been suggested in which all salmonellae are classified into 3 groups (*S. enteritidis*, *S. typhi*, and *S. choleraesuis*). The 1st group contains all salmonellae except the latter 2. Each species, then, is classified as a bioserotype such as *S. enteritidis* bio *typhimurium*. In the United States selected *Salmonella* strains have been present consistently; about 95% of all salmonellae can be typed by utilizing a set of 51 absorbed and 32 unabsorbed O and H antisera. Phage typing permits further separation of strains of the same serotype which are otherwise indistinguishable by biochemical or serologic methods and allows identification of strains according to the phage type of Vi antigen. There are 33 types identified and categorized by letter and/or subtype; in the United States type E is most common.

Salmonellae are resistant to many physical agents. They can be killed by heating to 130° F (54.4° C) for 1 hr or 140° F (60° C) for 15 min. They remain viable at ambient or reduced temperature for many days; contaminated organisms may survive for days to weeks in sewage, dried foodstuffs, pharmaceutical agents, and fecal material.

The properties of salmonellae responsible for their pathogenicity remain incompletely defined. The O antigen (an endotoxin) enhances resistance of the organism to phagocytosis, and strains deficient in it are avirulent. The effects of endotoxin in the host may be responsible for selected clinical manifestations of the systemic disease, but no evidence suggests that they are important in gastroenteritis. Selected serotypes of salmonellae have marked host preferences and produce characteristic patterns of disease. *Salmonella typhosa* infects only man. Salmonellae of groups A and C are generally isolated from human sources, whereas *S. abortus equi* infects only horses. Despite the apparent propensity of selected strains to seek a specific host, 7 of the 10 types of *Salmonella* most commonly recovered from animal sources in the United States each year are among the 10 types most commonly isolated from humans.

NONTYPHOIDAL SALMONELLOSIS

Epidemiology. The opportunity to acquire an infection with 1 of the serotypes of *Salmonella* appears to be increasing; there are close to 30,000 culture-proven cases of salmonellosis reported in the United States annually. The actual number of cases may be more than 100-fold greater than those that have been reported. More than two thirds of the individuals with reported salmonellosis are under 20 yr of age; the attack rates within this age group are higher for those under 9 yr, particularly for infants and for males.

Man ingests *Salmonella* primarily through food and occasionally contaminated water. Meat and poultry products are the most common sources of salmonellae. Modern day methods of feeding, holding, and transporting farm animals lead to contamination. Animals may acquire *Salmonella* in the 1st few days of life from their environment, from contaminated milk, from suckling animals, or from animal byproducts which frequently contain salmonellae. On some farms the use of antibiotic-containing feed, especially for poultry, can lead to increased numbers of salmonellae and a higher incidence of *Salmonella*-carrying chickens. These animals continue to shed salmonellae, perpetuating the infection on the farm and contaminating other animals during transport. In the holding pens or during the butchering process, personnel may also be infected. Large poultry processing plants must be particularly careful that a few infected birds do not contaminate conveyor belts, water baths, and other equipment with the subsequent unsuspected contamination of large numbers of chickens or turkeys.

Salmonella can infect many species of animals, but those of particular hazard to human health are meat-producing animals, poultry, and reptiles (particularly pet turtles). Most of the animal infections are asymptomatic. The prevalence of salmonellosis in chickens creates a high risk for the contamination of eggs. Salmonellae can contaminate the shell surface, penetrate the egg, or be transmitted from an ovarian infection directly to the egg yolk. Pooling large numbers of eggs prior to freezing, drying, or use in the preparation of food materials increases the risk of human infection. All eggs utilized in processed foods should be pasteurized as a means of eliminating *Salmonella*. Up to 50% of poultry, 5% of beef, 16% of pork, and 40% of frozen egg products purchased in retail stores contain salmonellae. These foods pass inspection because contamination is not appreciated. In turn, *Salmonella* introduced into kitchens on these contaminated foods may be transferred to other materials including utensils, table surfaces, and personnel. *Salmonella* can resist boiling within an egg for even 2–3 min. Contamination of equipment and processing plants has been responsible for outbreaks associated with baker's yeast, dried milk, dried coconut, cotton seed protein, and various dyes. Carmine red dye derived from female scale insects and larvae, sometimes used in hospitals for determination of intestinal transit time, has caused hospital outbreaks of salmonellosis. This dye is also used as an artificial coloring in drugs, foods, and cosmetics.

Humans are important carriers of *Salmonella* species and can cause localized epidemics of food poisoning by contaminating food at large gatherings such as picnics. Outbreaks in hospitals and nursing homes which are traced to a carrier are of considerable concern because of the increased morbidity and mortality observed in infants, young children, and the compromised host. Cross-contamination also can occur within institutions by means of contaminated fingers, clothes of the staff, or aerosols. A more recently recognized and unlikely source of *Salmonella* is breast milk; *S. kottbus* was recovered from the stools of the donor of the milk as well as from the milk itself. Improper refrigeration led to multiplication of *S. kottbus* within the milk. Contaminated marijuana has also been reported.

During the acute stages of infection, 10^6–10^9 salmonellae are excreted/gm of stool; 70–90% of infected individuals will have a positive stool culture 2 wk following infection, about 50% at 4 wk, and 10–25% at 10 wk. The duration of *Salmonella* excretion is similar whether the infection has been asymptomatic or symptomatic but appears to be longer in individuals under 1 yr than it is for older children. Excretion is prolonged by antibiotic therapy regardless of the agent used for treatment of the infection.

Pathogenesis and Pathology. There is limited information concerning the number of salmonellae required to cause disease in man. Studies in volunteers document that 1 billion cells of *Salmonella typhosa* will produce disease in 95% of human volunteers; 100,000 virulent typhoid bacilli will induce disease in about 30% of healthy men. Similar numbers of *Salmonella typhimurium* have been required to cause diarrhea in human volunteers. Infants and children may be infected by smaller numbers of organisms, but the specific dose presumably varies widely depending upon the host and type or even subtype of *Salmonella* with which the host is infected.

Diarrhea initiated by *Salmonella* may be produced by several mechanisms. Many patients present with a nonspecific watery diarrhea clinically identical to that caused by enterotoxigenic *E. coli*; several toxins have been identified, and 1 of these has physiologic properties similar to the heat-labile enterotoxins of *E. coli*. Whether this or other toxins are responsible for the excess intestinal fluid production in humans remains to be proved. It also has been suggested that *Salmonella* can initiate diarrhea by indirect stimulation of the energy system within epithelial cells which allows these cells to secrete water and electrolytes. Strains of *Salmonella* associated with diarrhea evoke a neutrophil cellular response when they reach the lamina propria. Prostaglandins released from the inflammatory exudate may stimulate the adenylate cyclase–cyclic AMP system that would enable the epithelial cells to secrete fluid and electrolytes actively.

For *Salmonella* species to cause diarrhea, they must gain access to the mucosal lining of the small and large intestine. A stomach pH of 2 will kill swallowed salmonellae, but higher values of pH of gastric juice have a varying effect; there is no killing effect at pH 5 and above. Persons with gastrectomies or gastroenterostomies are especially prone to *Salmonella* infection. The absence of the gastric acid barrier plus the associated disturbed emptying time permits a larger inoculum of *Salmonella* to reach the intestine and produce disease. There are also numerous nonspecific defense mechanisms within the intestinal tract that may affect *Salmonella* survival adversely, e.g., rapid transit, lysozymes, and enzymes, but their role in preventing human disease is unknown.

Salmonellae can penetrate the superficial layers of the mucosal lining without destroying epithelial cells. A phagosome is created around the salmonellae in the epithelial cell, but no damage to the bacteria occurs as they travel through or between cells into the lamina propria. Serotypes that usually cause diarrhea evoke a polymorphonuclear leukocyte response in the lamina propria area. The infection extends no farther, and the patient develops only diarrhea. There may be low grade fever associated with diarrhea. The frequency of bacteremia is not known, but it is usually transient, and no metastatic phase of infection occurs in healthy individuals. Bacteremia is more frequent in infants, and this propensity may reflect a relatively incompetent bacterial localizing immune system.

Systemic invasion by *Salmonella* is much more common in individuals at the extremes of age as well as in those with diseases that impair reticuloendothelial or cellular immune function. A high percentage of patients with *Salmonella* septicemia have leukemia, lymphoma, Hodgkin disease, cirrhosis of the liver, collagen vascular disease, or disorders associated with hemolysis (malaria, bartonellosis) and hemoglobinopathies. Children with sickle cell disease are prone to develop *Salmonella* septicemia and osteomyelitis. The numerous infarcted areas of the gastrointestinal tract, bones, and reticuloendothelial system may initially permit organisms greater access to the circulation from the intestine and then furnish an optimal environment for localization. The decreased phagocytic and opsonizing capacity of patients with SS hemoglobin disease also contributes to the enhanced infection rate. Defects in the intracellular killing by phagocytes have led to unusual forms of chronic *Salmonella* infection. Individuals with chronic granulomatous disease of childhood or other white blood cell disorders have an increased propensity for infection with this microorganism. Possibly related defects in phagocytosis also are responsible for the associated chronic *Salmonella* bacteremia and bacilluria noted in individuals suffering from chronic schistosomiasis (Sec 10.128).

Clinical Manifestations. Gastroenteritis due to *Salmonella* has its peak incidence in the late summer and early fall, correlating with the increased number of foodborne outbreaks. Large epidemics occur during these periods, but sporadic cases involving small family units occur throughout the year.

The incubation period ranges from 8–48 hr. Onset often occurs the morning following an evening meal at which contaminated food was ingested. It is usually abrupt and is characterized by nausea, vomiting, and crampy abdominal pain followed by loose, watery diarrhea, which occasionally contains mucus and blood. Vomiting is usually not severe and, when it does occur, is clearly not protracted. Fever of 101–102° F is seen in as many as 70% of patients; however, chills are present in only 33%. Symptoms subside within 2–5 days in healthy individuals; in patients who are debilitated by the extremes of age, malignancy, or other illnesses or who are recipients of antibiotic therapy or steroids, the illness may persist. Fatalities are rare (about 1%), although higher rates are recorded in individuals at special risk. Some patients remain afebrile and have only mild intestinal symptoms. Others develop severe disease with higher fevers, headache, drowsiness, confusion, meningismus, and seizures. Moderate abdominal distention and severe and even localized pain with associated rebound tenderness have been reported.

Septicemic spread of salmonellae is accompanied by chills and high fever. Symptoms of enteric fever are those described subsequently for typhoid fever but generally are shorter in duration and associated with a lower mortality rate. Salmonellae can localize in any organ or tissue, causing pneumonia, empyema, abscesses, osteomyelitis, septic arthritis, pyelonephritis, or meningitis.

Complications. Complications of nontyphoidal salmonellosis are unusual and generally are limited to the extraintestinal manifestations of disease. Recently, however, several children have developed *Salmonella*-reactive arthritis about 2 wk after the initial diarrheal episode. The arthritis tends to be polyarticular, with knees and ankles affected most frequently. Swelling and tenderness are more prominent features than joint erythema. The arthritis is frequently migratory with rapid recurrence and regression of symptoms. Exacerbations may be accompanied by fever and malaise. Sedimentation rates may be high, but white blood cell counts are minimally elevated. When joint effusions are tapped, they are sterile. Roentgenograms of the involved joints reveal only soft tissue swelling. There is a highly significant association between the presence of histocompatibility antigen HLA B27 and the postsalmonella reactive arthritis syndrome.

Diagnosis. The stool of many individuals with *Salmonella* gastroenteritis contains polymorphonuclear leukocytes; these can be demonstrated by staining a freshly passed specimen with methylene blue. Mucus and red blood cells also may be present. Culture of the stool is positive more frequently than are specimens collected via rectal swabs. Bacteriologic results are enhanced by the incubation of the specimen in an enrichment medium (e.g., tetrathionate broth) prior to plating on selective medium. Promising results have also been obtained with a rapid direct fluorescent antibody technique with specimens incubated in enrichment broth prior to examination. Although 3 consecutive negative stool cultures are suggested as evidence that infection has ceased, excretion may be intermittent. Salmonellae can be recovered from blood, urine, cerebrospinal fluid, or other tissues that are infected.

Serologic tests are helpful in the diagnosis of typhoid fever and other forms of *Salmonella* infection, although as many as one third of patients may show insignificant increases in titer or no rise in titer at all; a 4-fold or greater rise in serum titer is diagnostic. A titer change can be noted as early as 1 wk after the onset of disease. Not all patients will have an increase in antibodies, and some will have significant increases of O or H antibodies but not of both. A single titer of 1:320 or greater for O antibody, particularly in a child, should alert the physician to consider salmonellosis as the cause of infection. Patients with acute and chronic liver disease may have high O and H agglutinin titers, but these represent cross-reacting antibodies and may not signify salmonellosis.

Differential Diagnosis. *Salmonella* gastroenteritis must be distinguished from other viral and bacterial causes of diarrhea, including those relating to rotavirus, *E. coli, Shigella, Yersinia enterocolitica,* and *Campylobacter fetus.* Rarely the clinical course and roentgenographic findings suggest ulcerative colitis, which should be excluded.

Treatment. Correction of dehydration and electrolyte disturbances as well as the symptomatic management of the patient are the most important aspects of the therapy of *Salmonella* gastroenteritis. Antibiotics do not eliminate susceptible salmonellae from the gastrointestinal tract and rarely, if ever, alter the clinical course. Antibiotics are indicated in gastroenteritis only for individuals at high risk for spread of disease (infants under 3 mo of age, children with immunologic deficiency, or those who are suffering a severe and protracted course). The clinical course of the gastroenteritis syndrome is no more severe or prolonged in children with cancer than that seen in otherwise normal children.

Children with septicemia, enteric fever, or metastatic sites of infection should be treated with systemically administered ampicillin (200–300 mg/kg/24 hr), amoxicillin (100 mg/kg/24 hr), or chloramphenicol (50–100 mg/kg/24 hr for older children or 25 mg/kg/24 hr for newborn infants). Each of these drugs should be given in 4 divided doses at 6 hourly intervals. In vitro susceptibility of the organism should dictate which agent should be utilized in each case. Resistance to chloramphenicol is unusual among *Salmonella* isolated in the United States, but it is not uncommon among those recovered in other areas of the world. Twenty per cent of *Salmonella* isolated from humans in this country are resistant to ampicillin.

Many antibiotics that have excellent bactericidal in vitro activity have no in vivo effect. Thus, the aminoglycosides, polymyxins, and tetracyclines should not be used for systemic *Salmonella* infections despite their in vitro activity. There is limited evidence that large intravenous doses of cephalosporins have therapeutic value; these drugs, however, generally should not be utilized.

Prognosis. The prognosis for patients with *Salmonella* gastroenteritis is excellent except in very young infants or debilitated children with underlying disease. The prognosis for individuals with *Salmonella* meningitis or endocarditis is poor unless effective therapy is provided early.

10.31   TYPHOID FEVER

Epidemiology. Between 300–500 new cases of *Salmonella typhosa* infection are reported each yr in the United States. The incidence of this disease has declined steadily since 1900. The majority of individuals with typhoid fever are under 20 yr of age. Several thousand chronic carriers of *Salmonella typhosa* are known to health departments throughout the country.

The typhoid bacillus infects only humans, and infected patients excrete *Salmonella typhosa* in respiratory secretions, urine, and feces for variable periods of time. Chronic carriers are responsible for most of the disease in the United States. Characteristically, the implicated carrier is an adult who may have had an enteric illness and who has had contact, often as a preparer of food, with the index case. Long survival of *S. typhosa* in food facilitates transmission. Water transmission generally involves inadequate plumbing or sanitation and is responsible for individual cases in the United States and for endemic disease in developing countries. Oysters and other shellfish cultivated in waters polluted by sewage and consumed without cooking to sterilizing temperature may also serve as sources of an outbreak of typhoid fever.

Pathogenesis. Studies in adult volunteers infected with various strains of *Salmonella typhosa* indicate that 10^7 organisms can produce disease in 50% of individuals. That typhoid fever can be induced by as few as 1000 organisms, however, suggests that differences exist in the resistance of individual hosts as well as in the pathogenicity of individual strains, particularly in those found in nature as opposed to those that have been utilized for controlled laboratory experiments.

A neutrophil leukocyte response that would release prostaglandins is evoked by typhoid bacilli because they lack enterotoxin activity on intestinal epithelial cells that would activate the adenylate cyclase system. Thus, there are significant differences in clinical and histologic findings between infection with *Salmonella typhosa* and infection with other serotypes. Reasons for different behavior of the typhoid bacilli are unclear. Virulent typhoid bacilli inhibit the postphagocytic oxidative metabolism of a neutrophil in contrast to nonvirulent typhoid strains and other bacteria. This inhibitory activity allows these organisms to resist destruction in the white cells. Monocytes are unable to destroy typhoid bacilli early in the disease process and also serve to carry these organisms into the mesenteric lymph nodes and other portions of the reticuloendothelial system, where multiplication occurs. Carriers are unique in that a large number of virulent typhoid bacilli pass into the gut daily without entering the epithelium of the host, move through the bowel, and are excreted in the stool.

The outside portion of the cell wall of salmonellae is a complex lipopolysaccharide structure (endotoxin). It has many properties, paramount among them its pyrogenicity, a property that makes endotoxin attractive as an explanation for the pathogenesis of the signs and symptoms of systemic forms of *Salmonella* infection. Collections of typhoid bacilli and the local release of endotoxin also may be partially responsible for the histologic changes in the gut, liver, skin, and elsewhere seen in patients with typhoid fever. Monocytic infiltrate of lamina propria, enlarged Peyer patches and mesenteric nodes, typhoid nodules in the liver consisting of monocytes and neutrophils, and hepatitis and myocarditis with the same cellular picture probably are initiated by small concentrations of endotoxin. Rose spots are characteristic skin lesions that also have a monocytic pattern. This same cellular response has been induced in volunteers with repeated local injections of minute quantities of endotoxin. Circulating endotoxin, however, is not usually demonstrable during typhoid fever. The bacteremia of typhoid fever is quantitatively different from that noted in other gram-negative rod infections (generally fewer than 50 organisms/mm^3); this may explain the lack of detectable circulating endotoxin.

A coagulopathy also has been demonstrated in many individuals with typhoid fever. This may be related to the local concentrations of endotoxin that indirectly stimulate the release of procoagulants from leukocytes by causing internal vascular damage and perhaps also by causing release of clotting factor proteases.

Infection with *S. typhosa* always results in clinical disease. Organisms rapidly invade the bloodstream from sites of minimal inflammation; the upper small bowel is the predominant site of invasion. Septicemia is cleared by organs of the reticuloendothelial system, where the bacteria multiply primarily within cells. Local inflammation is thereby produced in lymph nodes, liver, and spleen. The bacteria then re-enter the bloodstream from these sites. Secondary septicemia is usually prolonged, and many organs may be seeded. The gallbladder is particularly susceptible and is infected from the liver via the biliary system or the blood. Local multiplication of microorganisms in the wall of the gallbladder produces large numbers of *Salmonella* which are discharged into the large intestine.

Pathology. Morphologic changes of *Salmonella* infection are less striking in younger children than in older children and adults. The mesenteric lymph nodes, liver, and spleen are hyperemic and generally reveal areas of focal necrosis. Hyperplasia of reticuloendothelial tissue with proliferation of mononuclear cells is the predominant finding. Hepatic cells may reveal cloudy swelling. The mucosa and lymphatic tissue of the intestinal tract show marked inflammation and necrosis. Ulceration that heals without scarring is common. Hemorrhages may occur. The inflammatory lesion occasionally may penetrate the muscularis and serosa of the intestine producing an intestinal perforation. A mononuclear response also may be seen in the bone marrow associated with areas of focal necrosis. Inflammation of the gallbladder is focal, inconstant, and modest in propor-

tion to the extent of local bacterial multiplication. Bronchitis is common. Inflammation also may be observed in the form of localized abscesses, pneumonia, septic arthritis, osteomyelitis, pyelonephritis, endophthalmitis, and meningitis. Bacteria may be observed in all organ systems.

Clinical Manifestations. The clinical picture of typhoid fever in infants is that of a mild gastroenteritis or of a severe septicemia. Vomiting, abdominal distention, and diarrhea are common. The temperature may be variable but can reach as high as 106° F. Seizures may be observed. Hepatomegaly, jaundice, anorexia, and weight loss can be marked.

In older children the incubation period ranges from 5–40 days with an average of 10–20 days. It is followed by an irregular course characterized by fever, malaise, lethargy, myalgia, headache, and abdominal pain and tenderness. Diarrhea occurs in only half of the infected children at this stage of the disease; constipation occurs less frequently. Epistaxis may occur, and cough is common. Within 1 wk the fever rises and becomes less variable. Fatigue, anorexia, weight loss, cough, abdominal pain, and diarrhea increase in severity. The patient may become severely obtunded. Mental depression, delirium, and stupor all have been observed. The child now appears acutely ill, disoriented, and lethargic. At this stage of disease the spleen generally is enlarged, and abdominal tenderness is present. Abdominal distention may be appreciated, and rhonchi and scattered rales may be heard upon auscultation of the chest. A maculopapular rash may be observed in as many as 80% of patients. It occurs in the skin of the lower chest and abdomen, appearing in successive crops of 10–30 lesions that are 1–6 mm in diameter and last 2–3 days. The paradoxical relationship of a high temperature and low pulse rate is observed less commonly in children than in adults. If no complications occur, the symptoms and physical findings resolve within 2–4 wk, but malaise and lethargy may persist for an additional 1–2 mo.

Complications. Intestinal perforation has been observed in 0.5–3% and severe hemorrhage in 1–10% of children with typhoid fever. Most complications occur during the 2nd stage of disease and generally are preceded by a fall in temperature and blood pressure and an increase in pulse rate. Perforation rarely occurs without preceding hemorrhage, and the site is usually in the lower ileum. Perforation is accompanied by a marked increase in abdominal pain, tenderness, vomiting, and signs of peritonitis. A toxic encephalopathy or cerebral thrombosis may also occur. Neurologic sequelae of typhoid fever, however, are rare. Peripheral and optic neuritis as well as chorea have been reported. Acute cholecystitis has been observed, often presenting as a toxic dilatation of the gallbladder. Thrombosis and phlebitis occur rarely. Pneumonia is common during the 2nd stage of illness but often is caused by a superinfection related to organisms other than *Salmonella*. Pyelonephritis, endocarditis, and meningitis as well as osteomyelitis and septic arthritis occur rarely in the normal host. Septic arthritis and osteomyelitis occur more frequently in individuals with hemoglobinopathies.

Laboratory Manifestations. A normochromic normocytic anemia may be noted in individuals with typhoid fever who have suffered from intestinal blood loss or toxic suppression of the bone marrow. Leukopenia is observed rarely; peripheral leukocyte counts generally are low in relation to the patient's fever and toxicity but seldom decline to fewer than 3000 cells/mm³. When a pyogenic abscess due to *Salmonella typhosa* develops, leukocytosis as high as 20,000–25,000 per mm³ will be observed. Thrombocytopenia may be striking and persist for several days to 1 wk. Melena and proteinuria related to fever are common.

Diagnosis.   Examination of the stool microscopically generally reveals a large number of leukocytes, more than 90% of which are mononuclear. Bacteriologic cultures are diagnostic, but the identification of *Salmonella typhosa* requires 3–5 days in most laboratories. Specimens grown on selective media and examined with fluorescein-labeled antibody to the Vi antigen may provide specific and rapid identification. Blood cultures are usually positive early in the disease, whereas urine and stool cultures become positive following the secondary septicemia. Cultures are positive in as many as 40% of children during the initial stage of typhoid fever. Cultures of the bone marrow and involved lymph nodes or other phagocytic tissues often remain positive after the blood has been sterilized. Aspirates of the rash may be culture positive in up to 50% of the cases. Stool and urine of chronic carriers should be cultured as bone marrow and blood cultures are not likely to be positive. Enteric carriers generally excrete 10^6–10^9 *Salmonella typhosa*/gm of stool. In suspected cases with negative stool cultures, a culture of aspirated duodenal fluid to evaluate possible biliary infection may be helpful.

O and H antigens of *Salmonella typhosa* are not unique to that serotype or even to salmonellae. Treatment with chloramphenicol may depress an antibody response; conversely, high titers of H agglutinins may result from prior typhoid immunization. Moreover, nonspecific agglutinins often are observed in the serum of individuals with underlying disease accompanied by macroglobulinemia. With these reservations in mind, a 4-fold rise in agglutinin titer of a nonimmunized individual usually is diagnostic when performed in the same laboratory. An increase in O agglutinins in an individual immunized more than 6 mo earlier also is suggestive of infection.

In the nonimmunized child who has lived in a nonendemic area, O agglutinin titers of greater than 1:160 are suggestive evidence of infection during the 1st wk of symptoms. Titers of Vi agglutinins of 1:5 or greater generally identify a chronic carrier in nonendemic populations.

Differential Diagnosis.   During the initial stages of typhoid fever the individual may be diagnosed as having bronchitis, bronchopneumonia, gastroenteritis, or influenza. Subsequently the disease can be confused with other infections due to intracellular microorganisms, including tuberculosis, systemic fungal infections, brucellosis, tularemia, and rickettsial diseases as well as shigellosis and, where applicable epidemiologically, malaria. Septicemia of unknown etiology, leukemia, lymphoma, and Hodgkin disease also may be

suggested. Concern about acute surgical disease of the abdomen may lead to operative intervention.

Prognosis and Treatment.   The prognosis in typhoid fever is dependent upon the patient's age and previous state of health and the type of complications that may occur. Individuals who are not treated with antibiotics may die (10% of infants and a small percentage of older children succumb). Therapy with chloramphenicol has reduced the mortality rate to less than 1% in most areas. The presence of an underlying debilitating disease, perforation of the gastrointestinal tract, or severe hemorrhage increases the chances of death. Morbidity and mortality may also be related to the development of meningitis or endocarditis. Several studies suggest that *Salmonella* meningitis is particularly severe, but in our institution during the last 10 yr morbidity or mortality from *Salmonella* meningitis has not been greater than in those age-matched individuals with other forms of gram-negative meningitis.

Relapse occurs in up to 10% of those who are not treated with antibiotics. Clinical manifestations of relapse generally become apparent about 2 wk after cessation of antibiotic therapy and resemble the acute illness. The relapse, however, is generally milder and more abbreviated. Multiple relapses in the same individual may occur.

Individuals who excrete *S. typhosa* 3 mo or more after infection are usually excreters at 1 yr and often for life. The risk of becoming a chronic carrier is low in children but increases with age. Up to 5% of acutely infected adults become chronic carriers; generally they have chronic gallbladder infections and excrete the organisms in their stool. Chronic urinary carriage also may occur but is rare except in individuals with schistosomiasis.

The maintenance of appropriate fluid and electrolyte balance is important in children with typhoid fever. If shock accompanies intestinal perforation or severe hemorrhage, intravascular volume expansion is required.

Chloramphenicol is the antibiotic preferred by most infectious disease experts for the therapy of typhoid fever. It can be provided orally, but intravenous administration is indicated when the patient is acutely ill. Chloramphenicol should not be administered by the intramuscular route. Doses of 50–100 mg/kg/24 hr are given to children and 25 mg/kg/24 hr to infants under 2 wk of age, divided into 4 doses and given at 6 hr intervals. Most children become afebrile within 7 days of the initiation of therapy, but treatment of uncomplicated cases should be continued for at least 10–14 days or for 5–7 days following defervescence. In children who have underlying significant malnutrition and a high rate of complications, optimal results have been achieved by using therapy for a period of 21 days. Complications including intestinal hemorrhage and perforation have been observed during therapy. Treatment with chloramphenicol may increase the chance of relapse and does not prevent development of the chronic carrier state.

Ampicillin therapy results in a slower clinical response and more treatment failures than does treatment with chloramphenicol. Patients who have a favorable response to ampicillin, however, are less likely to experience relapses or become chronic carriers. Ampicillin should be used in a dose of 100–200 mg/kg/24 hr divided at 6 hr intervals. Systemic administration is preferred. Amoxicillin (100 mg/kg/24 hr given in equal divided doses at 6 hr intervals) provides results that are superior to those for ampicillin and equal to those obtained with chloramphenicol. A combination of sulfamethoxazole and trimethoprim is effective against typhoid fever (185 mg/M²/day TMT plus 925 mg/M²/day SMZ orally in 3 equally divided doses). However, some patients treated with this drug respond less predictably than with chloramphenicol or ampicillin. In 1972 a large epidemic of typhoid fever caused by chloramphenicol-resistant strains occurred in Mexico and lasted for 2 yr. The origin of this resistant strain is unknown, but its disappearance coincided with a reduction in the widespread use of chloramphenicol. Similar episodes of chloramphenicol-resistant strain–induced illness also were reported from Southeast Asia and the Middle East. Most chloramphenicol-resistant strains are susceptible to ampicillin, amoxicillin, and trimethoprim-sulfamethoxazole, and therapy of such infections with these drugs is successful. Ampicillin-resistant strains have been noted, but these strains are sensitive to chloramphenicol or to trimethoprim-sulfamethoxazole.

Corticosteroid therapy has been suggested for individuals with severe toxemia or prolonged symptoms. Corticosteroids do not increase the incidence of complications if antibiotic therapy is adequate. Thrombocytopenia can be sufficiently severe to play a causative role in intestinal hemorrhage. Platelet transfusions have been suggested for these individuals if surgery is contemplated. Up to 80% of carriers with chronic gallbladder infection can be cured by cholecystectomy even without antibiotic therapy. High dose ampicillin therapy provided for 4–6 wk has cured many carriers including some with cholecystitis.

Prevention. Immunity to typhoid fever is a relative phenomenon. Reinfection occurs in 20–25% of adults exposed naturally or experimentally. Typhoid fever stimulates host resistance by inducing a temporary nonspecific increase in phagocytic activity within the reticuloendothelial system as well as a more lasting enhancement of specific bactericidal activity in the form of type-specific antibodies. Antibodies enhance the immunity of the host by slowing extracellular bacterial multiplication and by promoting opsonization, but susceptibility to initial or subsequent attacks of typhoid fever does not correlate with the titers of antibodies to O, H, or Vi antigens. Preliminary studies with an attenuated oral typhoid vaccine suggest that local antibody activity may be important in the host response to salmonellae.

Parenteral vaccine presently is not indicated for routine use in children. Although available vaccines will prevent disease in most individuals exposed to small numbers of typhoid bacilli such as could occur with water-borne disease, exposure to a larger inoculum can overcome whatever immunity is induced by the vaccine. The indications for use of typhoid vaccine in the United States are as follows: (1) intimate exposure to a known household carrier, (2) an outbreak of typhoid fever in the community or an institution, and (3) travel to an endemic area in an attempt to prevent disease acquired via contaminated water. It is not indicated to administer killing vaccines to children attending summer camps or traveling to endemic areas. For children residing in endemic areas, the vaccine may provide some protection against water-borne disease, but a booster dose is not indicated as field tests failed to show any benefit in terms of increased protection when more than 1 dose was given. Immunity appeared to last at least 10 yr.

A dose of 0.5 ml administered subcutaneously is recommended for both primary and booster immunizations of individuals 10 yr or more of age; 0.25 ml is recommended for younger children. Local reactions, including fever, are common, and prophylactic administration of antipyretics in young children may be indicated. An intradermal dose of 0.1 ml may have immunogenicity and produce fewer side reactions than the larger subcutaneous dose; it may be used as a booster injection. Unacceptable reactions occur with the intradermal administration of acetone-extracted vaccine.

Control of *Salmonella* Infections. Attention to personal hygiene, hand washing, and sanitary practices is essential for personnel involved in the preparation of food and in patient care in order to minimize person-to-person and person-to-food transmission. Urine and feces of hospitalized patients should be handled with special precautions until 3 consecutive stool cultures are negative.

Every effort should be made to eradicate *Salmonella typhosa* from individuals excreting this organism. When these efforts are unsuccessful, the individuals must be kept under careful surveillance by health departments and prevented from working in food and water processing plants, in kitchens, and in occupations related to patient care. Such individuals should be made aware of their potential contagiousness and the importance of hand washing and personal hygiene. Antibiotic therapy of exposed individuals is contraindicated; prophylactic ingestion of nonspecific antimicrobial agents (oxyquinolines) does not prevent infection.

Attention to the preparation of foodstuffs, the use of proper temperature for cooking, and the avoidance of holding potentially infected foods at warm temperatures are important control measures. The requirement that pets be certified as *Salmonella* free before sale would eliminate, to some extent, an unnecessary problem.

The control of typhoid fever in endemic areas can be accomplished only by improved sanitation and housing and by the availability of pure water. Large scale immunization programs may reduce but will not eliminate this disease.

RALPH D. FEIGIN

Aserkoff B, Bennett JV: Effect of therapy in acute salmonellosis on salmonellae in feces. N Engl J Med 281:636, 1969.

Cherry WB, Thomason BM: Fluorescent antibody techniques for salmonella and other enteric pathogens. Pub Health Rep 84:887, 1969.

France GL, Mormer DJ, Steele RW: Breast-feeding and salmonella infection. Am J Dis Child 134:147, 1980.

Gianella RA: Importance of the intestinal inflammatory reaction on salmonella mediated intestinal secretion. Infect Immun 23:140, 1979.

Gianella RA, Formal SB, Dammin GJ, et al: Pathogenesis of salmonellosis. J Clin Invest 52:441, 1973.

Hornick RB: Salmonella infections. In: Feigin RD, Cherry JD (eds): Textbook of Pediatric Infectious Diseases. Philadelphia, WB Saunders, 1981.

Overturf G, Marton KI, Mathies AW: Antibiotic resistance in typhoid fever. N Engl J Med 289: 463, 1973.

Robertson RP, Wahab MFA, Raasch FO: Evaluation of chloramphenicol and ampicillin in salmonella enteric fever. N Engl J Med 278:171, 1968.

Rosenstein BJ: Salmonellosis in infants and children. Epidemiologic and therapeutic considerations. J Pediatr 70:1, 1967.

Ryder RW, Crosby-Ritchie A, McDonough B, et al: Human milk contaminated with Salmonella kottbus. JAMA 238:1533, 1977.

10.32 SHIGELLOSIS
(Bacillary Dysentery)

Shigellosis is an acute inflammatory disease of the gastrointestinal tract produced by bacteria of the genus *Shigella*. This illness may be characterized by fever, crampy abdominal pain, and loose stools which may contain mucus, pus, and blood or may be a nonspecific diarrhea.

Etiology. *Shigella* species are nonmotile, short, gram-negative rods which are characterized biochemically by very slow or absent fermentation of lactose. *Shigella* must be distinguished by other biochemical properties from those *Escherichia coli* which do not ferment lactose or form gas. The genus *Shigella* is subdivided into 4 groups (A, B, C, and D) in accordance with biochemical reactions and antigenic composition. Group A contains 10 serologic types of which *Shigella dysenteriae* is the most important. However, *Shigella dysenteriae* is rarely encountered in the United States except when it is imported. *Shigella* Group B contains 6 serologic groups of which *Shigella flexneri* is commonly isolated in the United States; Group C strains include *S. boydii*, which is not common in the United States; *S. sonnei* is the single serotype in Group D and the most common *Shigella* serotype isolated in the United States.

Epidemiology. Shigellae are found worldwide. In 1979, 20,135 cases of *Shigella* were reported to the Center for Disease Control. The highest incidence occurred in children 1–4 yr of age. *Shigella* is more common during the late summer, but its seasonality is not as marked as that of *Salmonella*. American Indians have a higher incidence of *Shigella flexneri* infection.

Man is the major reservoir for *Shigella* since there are no natural animal hosts. This organism is transmitted primarily by direct fecal-oral route. There have been outbreaks of water-borne or food-borne illnesses. Spread of infection via inanimate objects, such as toys, also may occur. Flies may be vectors for this organism. Personal hygiene is of the utmost importance in prevention of this illness. Persons in close contact in unsanitary conditions are at high risk for outbreaks of shigellosis. Thus, individuals in mental institutions, prisons, military installations, and Indian reservations frequently have outbreaks of *Shigella* gastroenteritis. *Shigella* may persist in institutionalized children because of a low level of personal hygiene, the existence of asymptomatic *Shigella* carriers, and the minute inocula of *Shigella* which are capable of causing illness. Children may acquire *Shigella* at a day care center and transmit it to the rest of the family.

Pathogenesis. The ingestion of as few as 200 *Shigella* bacilli may result in infection, and *Shigella* can survive the acidity of gastric secretions for as long as 4 hr. *Shigella* must penetrate epithelial cells in order to induce infection. Noninvasive strains of *Shigella* are not associated with clinical illness. Once inside the epithelial cell, the organisms multiply in the submucosa and lamina propria. Local inflammation, edema, hyperemia, and epithelial cell dysfunction occur. Microabscesses form behind obstructed crypts. Superficial ulcers may lead to bleeding. A fibrinous exudate containing polymorphonuclear leukocytes covers the mucosal lining of the colon. Because of the superficial nature of the *Shigella* infection, intestinal perforation does not occur and bacteremia is unusual. These gastrointestinal changes resolve spontaneously within 4–7 days.

Shigella dysenteriae produces an enterotoxin, but its role in the pathogenesis of disease is unknown. Toxigenic strains that are noninvasive do not result in disease. In contrast, invasive nontoxigenic strains result in shigellosis in experimental animals and man.

Clinical Manifestations. During the incubation period, usually 36–72 hr following ingestion, shigellae reach the colon. Initially, the patient may complain of fever and crampy abdominal pain. Fever may be greater than 40.0° C, and the patient may appear very toxic. After 48 hr of illness, diarrhea usually appears; the child may have up to 20 stools/day containing blood and mucus. Later in the illness, bloody diarrhea may occur without the presence of fever or abdominal cramps. On physical examination the child may have some lower abdominal tenderness to palpation without evidence of localization.

In 1 study seizures occurred in 12% of patients with *Shigella* gastroenteritis. Seizures are more likely to occur in children whose body temperatures exceed 40.0° C than in those whose temperatures remain below 39° C. Convulsions are much more likely to occur in children under 7 yr of age, particularly in those under 3 yr. Other central nervous system symptoms may include headache, delirium, nuchal rigidity, fainting, and lethargy. Fluid and electrolyte losses may result in significant dehydration, acidosis, and electrolyte disturbances. Children may complain of urgency and tenesmus. In severe cases, particularly in patients with malnutrition, rectal prolapse may occur.

Shigellae have been associated with infections in areas other than the gastrointestinal tract. Conjunctivitis may result from local inoculation by contaminated fingers or objects. A blood-tinged purulent vaginitis which is unresponsive to conventional outpatient medication may result from *Shigella* infection. Vaginal discharge may be present for months before diagnosis, and prior *Shigella* gastroenteritis may be associated with the development of vaginitis. *Shigella* may occur in neonates with a wide variety of clinical manifestations including an asymptomatic carrier state, explosive bloody diarrhea, and/or meningitis and sepsis. In Central America and Bangladesh, *Shigella dysenteriae* type 1 has been associated with anemia, thrombocytopenia, and acute renal failure (*hemolytic-uremic syndrome*). In such patients, circulating endotoxin and immune complexes are important in the pathogenesis of the hemolytic anemia, coagulopathy, and renal microangiopathy.

Diagnosis. *Shigella* should be considered a possible etiologic agent in any patient presenting with diarrhea, particularly those with accompanying fever. When examined under a microscope with methylene blue, stool samples reveal fecal leukocytes and red blood cells. The presence of fecal leukocytes indicates colitis but does not establish a diagnosis of *shigellosis* since patients with *Salmonella* and enterotoxigenic *E. coli* and those without an established pathogen associated with their diarrhea may have fecal leukocytes. The absence of fecal leukocytes does not exclude *Shigella* as the etiologic agent. The blood count may reveal a marked leukocytosis with a shift to immature polymorphonuclear leukocytes.

The diagnosis of shigellosis is established by isolating this organism from stool or rectal cultures. Selected media such as xylose-lysine deoxycholate (XLD) and SS agar should be inoculated promptly with a fresh stool sample. If these media are not available, the stool should be placed in a buffered glycerol-saline solution for preservation prior to transport to laboratory. Shigellosis must be distinguished from other causes of dysentery such as enterotoxigenic *E. coli*, amebic dysentery, and *Campylobacter fetus* as well as *Salmonella*, rotavirus gastroenteritis, intussusception, acute appendicitis, and iliac adenitis. Shigellosis may mimic central nervous system infection such as meningitis and encephalitis, particularly when high fever is present with associated seizures.

Treatment. Antibiotic treatment of gastroenteritis due to *Shigella* decreases the duration of excretion of the organism as well as the duration of symptomatic diarrhea. The choice of antibiotic is dependent upon the current sensitivities of this organism in the community. Resistance transfer factors are responsible for mediating multiple resistance to ampicillin, cephalosporins, chloramphenicol, aminoglycosides, sulfonamides, and tetracyclines. Susceptibility patterns may vary between serotypes of *Shigella*. When *Shigella* strains are sensitive to ampicillin, ampicillin is effective at doses between 50–100 mg/kg/day in 4 divided doses. Parenteral administration of ampicillin may be required initially if the patient is extremely ill and unable to tolerate oral medication. Amoxicillin, although better absorbed than ampicillin, is less effective than ampicillin in the treatment of *Shigella* gastroenteritis. When ampicillin-resistant strains are suspected or proved, trimethoprim-sulfamethoxazole is the drug of choice for treatment of shigellosis (trimethoprim at 10 mg/kg/day and sulfamethoxazole at 50 mg/kg/day in 2 divided doses for 5–7 days). In adults a single dose of tetracycline has been shown to be effective in the treatment of *Shigella* gastroenteritis. This form of therapy should be avoided in children under 8 yr of age.

Antibiotic therapy usually eliminates *Shigella* from the gastrointestinal tract. Rarely a long-term *Shigella* carrier state may develop. In such instances lactulose, a synthetic derivative of lactose, will transiently decrease the excretion of *Shigella*. The metabolism of lactulose by normal gut flora results in an increased production of short chain fatty acids and a decrease in stool pH, both of which are thought to inhibit the growth of *Shigella*. Lactulose is not effective for acute shigellosis. Drugs which decrease peristalsis are contraindicated in the treatment of shigellosis. Diphenoxylate hydrochloride with atropine (Lomotil) prolongs fever and the excretion of organisms in shigellosis. Fluid and electrolyte therapy is dependent upon the state of hydration of the patient.

Prognosis and Prevention. In most healthy children shigellosis is a self-limited illness which usually resolves spontaneously. Organisms occasionally can be cultured up to 3 mo following an acute episode of shigellosis. Increased morbidity and mortality may be seen in enclosed populations, such as those of mental institutions, or in underdeveloped countries, where malnutrition is common. Arthritis with sterile joint fluid is uncommon with shigellosis in children. Reiter syndrome has been associated with *Shigella dysenteriae* in individuals who are HLA B27 positive.

Proper hygiene and environmental standards are the most important factors in preventing disease due to *Shigella*. Rigid handwashing is mandatory for individuals caring for children with shigellosis. In the hospital enteric precautions must be initiated promptly. No efficacious and reliable vaccine is available. Patients with shigellosis should be reported to public health officials.

SHELDON L. KAPLAN
RALPH D. FEIGIN

Barrett-Connor E, Connor JD: Extraintestinal manifestations of shigellosis. Am J Gastroenterol 53:234, 1970.
Grady GF, Keusch GT: Pathogenesis of bacterial diarrheas. N Engl J Med 285:831, 1971.
Murphy TU, Nelson JD: *Shigella* vaginitis: Report of 38 patients and review of the literature. Pediatrics 63:511, 1979.
Reller LB, Gangarosa EF, Brachman PS: Shigellosis in the United States: 5 year review of nationwide surveillance, 1964–1968. Am J Epidemiol 91:161, 1970.
Weissman JB, Schmerler A, Weiler P, et al: The role of preschool children and day care centers in the spread of shigellosis in urban communities. J Pediatr 84:797, 1974.

10.33   CHOLERA

Cholera is an acute intestinal disease caused by an enterotoxin elaborated by *Vibrio cholerae*, serotype O1. Its severity ranges from asymptomatic infection to the most severe form, *cholera gravis*, in which sudden, profuse, watery diarrhea results in hypovolemic shock, metabolic acidosis, and, if untreated, death.

Etiology. *V. cholerae* is a short, slightly curved, motile, gram-negative rod with a single polar flagellum. Many serotypes of *V. cholerae* exist and may cause acute diarrhea. *V. cholerae* grows readily on various nonselective laboratory media (e.g., nutrient agar), on MacConkey agar, and on some selective media, including bile salt agar, glycerin-tellurite-taurocholate agar, and thiosulfate–citrate–bile salt–sucrose (TCBS) agar. *V. cholerae* O1 can be readily identified by its distinct opaque, yellow, colonial appearance on TCBS agar. There are 2 recognized biotypes of *V. cholerae* O1: classic and El Tor. Each biotype is separable into 2 main serotypes: Ogawa and Inaba. Reversion of serotypes has occurred in the intestine of patients with cholera.

Epidemiology. Cholera has been endemic in the Ganges Delta throughout history, with annual epidemics in West Bengal and Bangladesh. From 1817–1926 the disease spread worldwide in 6 pandemics. A 7th pandemic, caused by the El Tor biotype, began in 1961 in Indonesia and by 1977 had spread to most of Southeast and South Asia, the Middle East, Africa, Southern Europe, and the Western Pacific regions.

In the United States only a few laboratory-acquired cases were identified from 1911–1973, when a single case was reported in Texas. In 1978 2 more infections were found in Louisiana, and in 1981 19 more cases were identified in Texas, 17 of which occurred in 1 outbreak in employees on an oil rig. The strains from all these cases have been essentially identical. No other indigenous cases have been identified during the present pandemic in other countries in the Western Hemisphere.

Endemic and epidemic cholera often have a seasonal pattern. Contaminated water and food, especially shellfish, play a major role in transmission. Person-to-person transmission is uncommon because of the large infectious dose required to cause disease and the formidable gastric acid barrier in the stomach, which kills most ingested vibrios. Secondary cases are rare in medical personnel who have close contact with patients.

Persons with asymptomatic or mild infection play an important role in dissemination of cholera. The ratio of asymptomatic or mild infections to severe disease is generally 5–7:1 in classic cholera and as high as 50–100:1 in El Tor cholera. A prolonged carrier state with the gallbladder as the reservoir has been documented in adults convalescing from El Tor cholera but has not been observed in children. Family contacts of hospitalized patients are frequently infected.

In endemic areas cholera is predominantly a disease of children; in rural Bangladesh attack rates are 5–10 times greater for childen aged 2–9 than for adults. Serologic studies demonstrate increasingly high titers of vibriocidal antibody with age, suggesting that the lower attack rate for adults is due to immunity induced by recurrent exposure to *V. cholerae* O1 and that sub-

clinical or symptomatic reinfection probably occurs frequently. In contrast, when cholera spreads to a previously uninfected area, attack rates are usually equal for all age groups exposed. For unknown reasons cholera has been rarely reported in children under 1 yr of age; breast feeding may offer some protection.

Both human and nonhuman reservoirs of *V. cholerae* O1 may exist in endemic areas. The organism may be transmitted as a subclinical infection during interepidemic periods by persons who are asymptomatic or have mild disease, or the organism may survive for prolonged periods in an aquatic environment. Animals appear to have no role in the human disease cycle.

Pathology and Pathophysiology. The site of infection is the small intestine, primarily the jejunum. After being ingested, the vibrios multiply in the lumen and adhere to the surface of epithelial cells within the mucous layer, where they elaborate an enterotoxic protein. The binding subunit of this enterotoxin attaches to a receptor (GM_1 ganglioside) on the surface membrane of epithelial cells. The active subunit of the toxin then enters the cells and activates the intracellular enzyme adenylate cyclase to produce increased amounts of cyclic adenosine monophosphate (CAMP). This leads to a decrease in active absorption of sodium and chloride in villus cells and an increase in active secretion of chloride by crypt cells, resulting in a net loss of water and electrolyte in the bowel.

Biopsy specimens from the small intestine of patients with cholera reveal an intact epithelium with minimal cellular response. Histologic studies demonstrate clearing of goblet cells indicating an increase in mucus secretion by these cells. Slight edema of the lamina propria and moderate dilatation of capillaries and lymphatics in tips of villi are also seen.

The diarrheal fluid lost is isotonic with plasma and has relatively high concentrations of bicarbonate and potassium. Stools from children with cholera contain more potassium and less sodium, chloride, and bicarbonate than stools from adults (Table 10–25). This fluid loss usually results in an isotonic deficit of sodium and water, acidosis due to deficit of base, and potassium depletion. Bicarbonate loss continues even when systemic acidosis develops. Although some impairment of activity of jejunal disaccharidases, including lactase, often occurs, glucose absorption is usually preserved.

Clinical Manifestations. Typically, after an incubation period of 6 hr–5 days, there is sudden onset of profuse watery diarrhea. In the most severe cases stools

Table 10–25 ELECTROLYTE CONTENT OF CHOLERA STOOL AND OF SOLUTIONS RECOMMENDED FOR INTRAVENOUS AND ORAL TREATMENT OF CHILDREN

	Na	APPROXIMATE ELECTROLYTE CONCENTRATION (MM/L)			
	Na	K	Cl	HCO_3	Glucose
Cholera stool, adult	140	13	104	44	—
Cholera stool, child	101	27	92	32	—
Ringer lactate solution*	130	4	109	28	—
Diarrhea treatment solution†	117	13	82	48	55
Oral glucose-electrolyte solution*‡	90	20	80	30	111

*Solutions recommended by World Health Organization.
†Prepared in gm/l: NaCl, 4; Na acetate, 6.5 (or Na lactate, 5.4); KCl, 1; glucose, 10.
‡Prepared in gm/l: NaCl, 3.5; NaHCO$_3$, 2.5; KCl, 1.5; glucose, 20. This solution is referred to as ORS = Oral Rehydration Salts.

are passed frequently and effortlessly, become rice watery in appearance (i.e., clear fluid with only flecks of mucus visible), and have a slight fishlike odor. In less severe cases the stool is more yellow in appearance. Abdominal cramps in the umbilical area occur in about 50% of cases; tenesmus is absent. Vomiting is common in severe cases, usually occurring after onset of diarrhea. In about 25% of children, the rectal temperature is slightly elevated (38–39° C) on admission or in the 1st 24 hr of hospitalization.

Massive diarrhea can result in loss of 10% or more of body weight, causing profound dehydration and circulatory collapse. In these severe cases, cholera gravis, the blood pressure falls and is often unobtainable, the radial pulse becomes imperceptible, respirations are rapid and deepened, and urine flow ceases. The eyes and fontanel are deeply sunken; the skin is cold and clammy, with poor turgor and the skin of the fingers becomes shriveled. Cyanosis and painful muscle cramps in the extremities, especially in the calves, occur. The patient is restless and extremely thirsty. Lethargy, thick speech, and a somnolent state are common. Stool losses may continue for up to 7 days. Subsequent manifestations depend on the adequacy of replacement therapy. An early sign of recovery is usually the reappearance of bile pigment in the stool. Cessation of diarrhea is usually rapid.

Mild cases of cholera are considerably more common than the cases of cholera gravis described above. They usually present as simple diarrhea with little or no dehydration and are more commonly observed in children than in adults.

Diagnosis. Definitive diagnosis of cholera depends on isolation of *V. cholerae* O1 from stool. Light microscopic examination usually reveals fewer than 5 polymorphonuclear cells/high power field. Retrospective diagnosis is possible by determination of vibriocidal, agglutinating, and toxin-neutralizing antibodies; peak titers of all 3 antibodies usually occur 7–14 days after onset of illness. Vibriocidal and agglutinating antibody titers return to baseline levels 8–12 wk after onset; antitoxin titers remain elevated for up to 12–18 mo. A 4-fold or greater rise during acute disease or a fall in titer during convalescence is usually considered diagnostic. A 4-fold rise in vibriocidal antibody occurs in response to infection with other organisms, such as *Yersinia* and *Brucella*, making it imperative to interpret antibody titers in light of clinical and epidemiologic findings. Illness with *V. cholerae* O1 is more likely to occur in persons with lower vibriocidal titers, although those with high titers can have severe disease. Asymptomatic infection often results in 4-fold rises in vibriocidal titer.

A diagnosis of cholera should be considered in a person with a severely dehydrating diarrhea, especially when the patient has been in a cholera-infected area within 5 days of onset of illness. Severe cholera is indistinguishable from severe diarrhea produced by enterotoxigenic *Escherichia coli* or non-O1 *V. cholerae*. Milder disease may be similar to that caused by other bacterial pathogens (e.g. *Salmonella*), or certain viruses (e.g. rotavirus).

Complications. These are more frequent and more severe in children than in adults. Before the importance of rapid and sufficient fluid replacement in treatment of cholera was known, acute renal failure from tubular necrosis was common; with adequate therapy this complication is avoidable. Inadequate potassium replacement can result in hypokalemic nephropathy and cardiac arrhythmias and, in children, may cause paralytic ileus. Rarely, pulmonary edema has occurred in persons treated with excessive and rapid fluid replacement without correction of severe acidosis. Transient tetany during correction of acidosis has been reported infrequently. Prolonged drowsiness, coma, or convulsions may occur before or during treatment in as many as 10% of small children. In some cases these are caused by marked hypoglycemia, but the etiology is more often unknown. Hypoglycemia is preventable by inclusion of dextrose in replacement solutions. An increase in fetal death during the 3rd trimester of pregnancy has been observed primarily in severely dehydrated patients who delay seeking hospital care.

Prevention. Avoidance of contaminated food and water is the best preventive measure against cholera. Commercially available cholera vaccine containing phenol-inactivated suspensions of classic Inaba and Ogawa strains of *V. cholerae* O1 is of low efficacy and provides only limited protection of short duration. High-potency vaccines have demonstrated 50–80% protection for up to 6 mo in endemic areas; no data are available on the efficacy of vaccine in newly infected areas, but it is likely that it is less in these areas where naturally acquired immunity is not present. Vaccine does not reduce the rate of inapparent infections and thus does not prevent transmission of cholera within families or in communities. Vaccination is not required for entry into the United States from a cholera-infected area. It is recommended primarily to facilitate travel in countries where vaccination is required. A number of oral vaccines are being developed in the hope of attaining greater production of local immunity in the intestinal tract.

Chemoprophylaxis for 3 days with tetracycline, given in 500 mg doses every 6 hr in persons 10 yr of age and older and 250 mg in persons under 10 yr of age, reduces injection rates in household contacts. However, for ease of administration a single dose of doxycycline (300 mg in adults; 6 mg/kg in children) is the preferred tetracycline compound. The efficacy of mass chemoprophylaxis in a large community is doubtful.

Treatment. Successful management primarily requires prompt replacement of gastrointestinal losses of fluid and electrolytes (Sec 5.19). Antibiotic therapy is adjunctive. Cholera patients do not require strict isolation but can be more easily managed when hospitalized if they are placed in 1 location. Enteric precautions, including careful handwashing and proper disposition of stool and vomitus, should be followed. When possible, patients should be weighed on admission and subsequent stool output measured. A "cholera cot," made of canvas or burlap on a wooden frame with a plastic or rubber sheet extending through a 4–6 inch opening where the patient places his or her buttocks facilitates accurate measurement of stool volume. Urine output should be followed for at least 24 hr. Measurement of plasma specific gravity and serum electrolytes, especially bicarbonate, is helpful and complementary to clinical evaluation in planning fluid replacement.

When a cholera patient is first seen, the extent of dehydration should be quickly determined (Sec 5.21). By the time physical findings of dehydration appear, a child has already lost a significant amount of body fluid and electrolyte; the danger in treatment usually lies in underestimation of losses.

Patients presenting with severe dehydration and hypovolemic shock should be given intravenous replacement immediately. Younger children should receive about 30 ml/kg during the 1st hr, 40 ml/kg within the next 2 hr, and then about 40 ml/kg over the next 3 hr; older children and adults can usually be given the total amount in 3–4 hr. The exact rate and amounts of fluid replacement and maintenance should be adjusted according to the results of frequent monitoring of the patient's state of hydration and continuing stool losses. A good intravenous line is essential; sometimes 2 are required. If no peripheral vein is available, the external jugular or femoral veins may be used; time should not be wasted in infusing fluid subcutaneously or intraperitoneally or in performing a cutdown. Careful monitoring of vital signs, of the neck veins for distention, of the lungs for rales of pulmonary edema, and of the eyelids for edema should prevent overhydration. The intravenous fluid chosen should replace isotonic fluid and electrolyte loss of the choleric stool (Table 10–25); the World Health Organization (WHO) suggests Ringer lactate as the best commercial solution. Potassium chloride should be added to the bottle (10 mEq/l) or given orally if renal function is adequate. Specially prepared intravenous solutions that approximate the "ideal" composition (Table 10–25) are also recommended as they do not require additional electrolyte supplementation and contain glucose. Isotonic saline can be used to correct hypovolemia if base, potassium, and glucose supplementation are given. Electrolyte-free isotonic dextrose solution should not be used.

Patients presenting with moderate to mild dehydration (e.g., with diminished skin turgor, neck vein distention, and pulse volume but without shock, or with thirst alone) may be given initial replacement fluid orally (Table 10–25 and Sec 5.17), thus avoiding the need for sterilized intravenous fluid, special equipment, or skilled attendants. The solution may be made using ordinary clean drinking water, but it should be prepared daily to minimize bacterial contamination. Patients with moderate dehydration should be given 100 ml/kg of *oral rehydration salt solution* (ORS) over 4 hr; and 50 ml/kg over the same period is given for mild dehydration. When a patient is tired, a nasogastric tube can be used to give fluid. Vomiting is not a contraindication to oral use of fluids; when it occurs, smaller amounts should be administered more frequently. In fewer than 1% of patients there is malabsorption of glucose from the oral fluid and diarrhea worsens; in this situation the intravenous route must be used.

After replacement fluid has been given, maintenance therapy must be started to match insensible water loss (500–1000 ml/M² of body surface//24 hr in hot climates) and continuing diarrhea losses. During the 1st few hr of treatment stool output is often minimal, but once shock is corrected, it generally increases, reaching levels as high as 200–350 ml/kg/24 hr. In older children, hourly losses may be over 800 ml. Except for patients with very high rates of stooling and those with glucose malabsorption, continuing losses can usually be replaced with oral glucose-electrolyte fluid. Patients with severe diarrhea should have continued supervision and receive 10–15 ml/kg/hr of ORS until diarrhea becomes mild. If signs of dehydration reappear and losses cannot be adequately replaced, intravenous therapy should be instituted. For patients with mild diarrhea oral solution can be given at home at a rate of 100 ml/kg/day until diarrhea stops. Breast-fed infants should be encouraged to breast feed *ad libitum* during maintenance therapy; other infants can be offered water or milk feeds diluted with an equal volume of water if desired.

Since cholera is endemic in many areas where malnutrition is common and there is evidence that most nutrients are absorbed during illness, a normal diet for age should be started during maintenance therapy as soon as the patient can eat. This will help prevent further deterioration of nutritional status. Foods that are energy rich and contain potassium should be given. In infants 4–6 mo of age or older who have not previously been given semi-solid foods, this is a good time to start feeding such foods.

As soon as the patient is alert (within 2–6 hr), oral tetracycline should be given (50 mg/kg/24 hr every 6 hr for 3 days). Tetracycline shortens the duration and volume of diarrhea by 50–70% and the duration of carriage of vibrio organisms. Isolation of strains of *V. cholerae* O1 resistant to tetracycline is rare. Single dose doxycycline (4 mg/kg), furazolidone (5 mg/kg/24 hr given every 6 hr for 3 days), and erythromycin (30 mg/kg/24 hr given every 8 hr for 3 days) are as effective as tetracycline in decreasing duration and volume of diarrhea but are not as effective in shortening the period of excretion of vibrios. Both chloramphenicol (75 mg/kg/24 hr given every 6 hr for 3 days) and trimethoprim-sulfamethoxazole (as 8–10 mg/kg/24 hr of trimethoprim, given every 6 hr for 5 days) are beneficial but less so than tetracycline; most sulfonamides are ineffective. Parenteral antibiotic therapy is unnecessary. Antidiarrheal medications such as opiates, paregoric, other antimotility drugs, and steroids should not be used. Blood and plasma are not required.

Prognosis. The outcome of pediatric cholera should be as favorable as that of the adult disease, which has an overall mortality of less than 1%. The high mortality (20–70%) reported in earlier studies has not occurred since the pathophysiology of cholera has been better understood and fluid management adjusted accordingly

MICHAEL H. MERSON

Carpenter CCJ Jr, Hirschhorn N: Pediatric cholera: Current concepts of therapy. J Pediatr 80:874, 1972.

Cholera and other Vibrio Associated Diarrhoeas. WHO Scientific Working Group Report. Bull. WHO 58:373, 1980.

Holmgren J: Actions of cholera toxin and the prevention and treatment of cholera. Nature 292:413, 1981.

Lindenbaum J, Akbar R, Gordon RS, et al: Cholera in children. Lancet 1:1066, 1966.

Mahalanabis D, Watten RH, Wallace CK: Clinical aspects and management of pediatric cholera. *In:* Barua D, Burrows W (eds): Cholera. Philadelphia, WB Saunders, 1974.

Manual for the Treatment of Acute Diarrhoea. Geneva, World Health Organization, 1980.

Ouchterlony O, Holmgren J (eds): Cholera and Related Diarrheas. Molecular Aspects of a Global Health Problem. 43rd Nobel Symposium. Basel, S. Karger, 1980.

10.34 INFECTIONS DUE TO *PSEUDOMONAS*

Pseudomonads are gram-negative bacilli which live in soil and water and are rarely pathogenic for man. However, they may produce disease, particularly in newborn infants and children with impaired host defenses, such as those with cystic fibrosis, immunodeficiency disease, malignancies, other chronic diseases, burns, or malnutrition and those receiving immunosuppressive therapy. The most important species of the opportunistic pseudomonads is *P. aeruginosa.*

Etiology. *Pseudomonas* species are strict aerobes. Since they can utilize any source of carbon, pseudomonads can multiply in almost any moist environment containing minimal amounts of organic compounds.

P. aeruginosa is a gram-negative rod. Most strains are motile, and most possess a single polar flagellum and fine projections (pili or fimbriae). *P. aeruginosa* grows readily on standard laboratory media at temperatures up to 42° C. Strains from clinical specimens may produce beta-hemolysis on blood agar. More than 90% of strains produce a bluish-green phenazine pigment (blue pus) as well as fluorescein, which is yellow-green and fluoresces. These pigments diffuse into and color the medium surrounding the colonies. Strains of *Pseudomonas* can be differentiated from one another for epidemiologic purposes by serologic, phage, and pyocin typing.

Epidemiology. From 5–30% of normal individuals have *Pseudomonas* in their gastrointestinal tracts, but the organism rarely predominates. *Pseudomonas* frequently enters the hospital environment on the clothes, skin, or shoes of patients or hospital personnel. Colonization of any moist environment ensues. Thus, these organisms may be found growing in distilled water, hospital kitchens and laundries, antiseptic solutions, and equipment used for respiratory care or inhalation therapy.

Pathogenesis. The requirement of oxygen for growth may account for the lack of invasiveness of *Pseudomonas* after it has colonized or even infected the skin. It produces endotoxin which is extremely weak compared to that produced by other gram-negative organisms but which may produce a diarrheal syndrome. *Pseudomonas* also elaborates a number of extracellular products including lecithinase, collagenase, lipase, and hemolysins which may be responsible for localized necrosis of skin. One of the hemolytic factors is a heat-resistant glycolipid which may dissolve and destroy lecithin (surfactant), and this may cause the

atelectasis seen in pulmonary infections caused by *Pseudomonas.* The pathogenicity of *P. aeruginosa* also depends upon its ability to resist phagocytosis, which, in turn, seems to depend primarily upon the production of protein toxins by the organism. The host responds to infection by *Pseudomonas aeruginosa* with the production of antibodies to *Pseudomonas* exotoxin (exotoxin A) and lipopolysaccharide.

Clinical Manifestations. In healthy normal children *P. aeruginosa* may be introduced into a minor wound and be followed by cellulitis and a localized abscess which exudes green or blue pus. The skin lesions of *Pseudomonas,* whether due to direct inoculation or secondary to septicemia, may begin as pink macules which progress to small cutaneous hemorrhagic nodules and eventually to areas of necrosis with eschar formation, surrounded by an intense red areola *(ecthyma gangrenosum).* Multiplication of bacteria occurs locally; occasionally (in normal children), septicemia, meningitis, orbital cellulitis, mastoiditis, folliculitis, pneumonia, or urinary tract infections may ensue. Rarely, *Pseudomonas* may be associated with gastroenteritis. Pseudomonads other than *P. aeruginosa* rarely cause disease in healthy children, but pneumonia and abscesses due to *P. cepacia,* otitis media due to *P. putrefaciens,* abscesses due to *P. fluorescens,* otitis media due to *P. stutzeri,* and cellulitis and septicemia due to *P. maltophilia* have been reported.

Pseudomonas septicemia occurs with increased frequency in children with indwelling intravenous or urinary catheters; pneumonia and septicemia occur with increased frequency in children receiving artificial respiratory support or inhalation therapy. *Pseudomonas* may cause abscesses or meningitis in children with dermal sinus tracts or dermoids extending down to or communicating with the meninges or neural tissue and in children with meningomyeloceles. It may produce acute or subacute endocarditis in children with congenital heart lesions prior to or following cardiac surgery. Septicemia may occur in children with congenital or acquired neutropenia or in individuals with a functional deficit in polymorphonuclear leukocyte function.

Burns and Wound Infection. The surfaces of wounds or burns are frequently populated by *Pseudomonas* and other gram-negative organisms; this does not necessarily imply infection but is a necessary prerequisite to invasive disease. Septicemia with *P. aeruginosa* is a major problem in the burned patient. It may be related to multiplication of organisms in devitalized tissues, followed by invasion, or associated with prolonged use of intravenous or urinary catheters. Administration of antibiotics may diminish the susceptible microbiologic flora but permit selected strains of *Pseudomonas* to flourish. In burned patients, impaired killing of *Pseudomonas* by neutrophils has been described preceding the onset of septicemia. Burn injury also is associated with abnormal responses to antigens, delayed rejection of homografts, abnormal vascular responses, impaired delayed hypersensitivity responses, and diminished uptake of particles by the reticuloendothelial system.

Cystic Fibrosis (Sec 12.110). *P. aeruginosa* can be recovered from the sputa of most children with cystic fibrosis. This does not necessarily imply infection and destructive pneumonitis related to this organism but rather may reflect the use of mist tents and continuous broad-spectrum antibiotic therapy. Recent observations, however, suggest that the relationship between *Pseudomonas* and the patient with cystic fibrosis may be more specific; children with cystic fibrosis almost always harbor mucoid *P. aeruginosa* which produce an excessive amount of capsular slime. Usually, the tracheobronchial trees of these patients are chronically colonized, and the organism is eradicated infrequently either spontaneously or by antibiotic therapy. In contrast, mucoid isolates of *P. aeruginosa* are recovered infrequently from patients without cystic fibrosis. There is also a clustering of serotypes among isolates obtained from patients with cystic fibrosis, and there may be a specific local defect in pulmonary resistance to *Pseudomonas* in these patients. A progressive specific lymphocyte unresponsiveness to *Pseudomonas* may play an important role in the destructiveness of chronic pulmonary *Pseudomonas* infection in cystic fibrosis. Also a higher frequency of immune complex activity has been noted in the sputum of patients with cystic fibrosis who were chronically infected with *P. aeruginosa* than has been found in the sputum of those not infected.

Pseudomonas infection in cystic fibrosis is chronic and limited almost entirely to the lung; septicemia is very rare.

Malignancy. Children with leukemia, particularly those who are receiving immunosuppressive therapy and who are neutropenic, are extremely susceptible to septicemia from invasion of the bloodstream by *Pseudomonas* with which the patient is already colonized (i.e., from the gastrointestinal tract). Anorexia, malaise, nausea, vomiting, diarrhea, and fever may be noted. A generalized vasculitis develops, and hemorrhagic necrotic lesions may be found in all organs, including skin, where they appear as purple nodules or ecchymotic areas which become gangrenous. A hemorrhagic or gangrenous perirectal cellulitis or abscess may be noted. Ileus and profound hypotension may occur.

Titers of heat stable opsonins, specific for *P. aeruginosa*, may fall precipitously in children with acute leukemia who are receiving intensive combined chemotherapy; fatal infections with *Pseudomonas* may, in part, be related to deficiency of this specific opsonin.

Diagnosis and Differential Diagnosis. Diagnosis of *Pseudomonas* infection depends upon recovery of the organism from the blood, cerebrospinal fluid, urine, or purulent material obtained by aspiration of subcutaneous abscesses or areas of cellulitis. A diagnosis of *Pseudomonas* pneumonia can be made by needle aspirate of the lung and, less conclusively, by recovery of the organism from sputum obtained by postural drainage of a child with cystic fibrosis who has failed to respond to appropriate antistaphylococcal therapy. Recovery of the organism from the surface of the skin or from the throat, tracheal aspirate, or bronchial secretions reflects colonization but is not necessarily diagnostic of infection.

Bluish, nodular skin lesions and ulcers with ecchymotic and gangrenous centers and bright areolae (ecthyma gangrenosum) have been considered to be virtually pathognomonic of *Pseudomonas* infection of the skin. Rarely, skin lesions clinically indistinguishable from those caused by *P. aeruginosa* may follow septicemia due to *Aeromonas hydrophila*.

Prevention. In part, this depends upon continuous surveillance of the hospital environment to identify and subsequently eradicate sources of the organism as quickly as possible. *Pseudomonas* may grow to a concentration of 10^6 organisms/ml in distilled water which appears perfectly clear; growth of *Pseudomonas* in distilled water, disinfectants, and medications is the factor cited most commonly in single source outbreaks of *Pseudomonas* infection in hospitals. In newborn nurseries infection generally has been transmitted to the infants by the hands of personnel, from washbasin surfaces, and from solutions used to rinse suction catheters. Strict attention to hand washing, particularly with an iodophor-containing liquid, before and between contacts with newborn infants may prevent or interdict epidemic disease. Growth of *Pseudomonas* on suction catheters can be prevented by rinsing catheters in a 3% solution of acetic acid.

Meticulous care in the preparation of solutions for total parenteral alimentation and in the insertion and care of catheters as well as daily replacement of all apparatus used for intravenous administration greatly reduces the hazard of extrinsic contamination by *Pseudomonas* and other gram-negative organisms.

Recent studies have demonstrated the efficacy of active immunization of the burn patient with specific strains of *Pseudomonas* and of the administration of specific hyperimmune globulin in the prevention of septicemia. A polyvalent *Pseudomonas* vaccine has been tested in controlled clinical trials in children and adults with more than 15% full skin thickness burns; none of the vaccinated patients developed positive blood cultures with *P. aeruginosa*. Vaccinees developed protective antibodies, and increased phagocytic activity against *P. aeruginosa* could be demonstrated. The mortality in children with burns was 20.8% in the unvaccinated group but only 4.8% in the vaccinated group. Infection in the burn patient also may be minimized by careful protective isolation and by the topical application of silver nitrate (0.5%) solution or 10% mafenide acetate cream. Debridement of devitalized tissue also is of great importance.

Pseudomonas infection of dermal abnormalities communicating with the cerebrospinal axis is prevented by early discovery and surgical repair. *Pseudomonas* infection of the urinary tract may be minimized or prevented by early identification and corrective surgery of obstructive lesions.

Treatment. Systemic infections with *Pseudomonas* should be treated promptly with an antibiotic to which the organism is sensitive in vitro. Response to treatment may be impaired and prolonged treatment necessary for systemic infection in the compromised host.

Septicemia usually should be treated with gentamicin in a dose of 5–7.5 mg/kg/24 hr in 3 divided doses. The higher dose may be used after the 1st wk of life. This drug may be given intramuscularly or intravenously (if it is infused slowly over a period of 1 hr). Carbenicillin (200–400 mg/kg/24 hr in 6 divided doses) or ticarcillin

(200 mg/kg/24 hr in 6 divided doses intravenously) should be used concomitantly for a possible synergistic effect. Carbenicillin or ticarcillin alone is not recommended because strains of the organism rapidly become resistant to these agents. Tobramycin (3–5 mg/kg/24 hr) or amikacin (15–25 mg/kg/24 hr) in 3 divided doses intramuscularly or intravenously (over 1 hr) may be used to replace gentamicin in the therapeutic regimen. Polymyxin B and colistin (polymyxin E), previously widely used but now largely superseded by the preceding regimens, may still be useful in patients infected with strains of *Pseudomonas* resistant to other agents.

Meningitis should be treated with gentamicin and carbenicillin given intravenously as above. Concomitant intraventricular or intrathecal treatment with gentamicin (1–2 mg once daily, independent of body weight, until the cerebrospinal fluid is sterile) may be required.

Abscesses should be incised and drained. Failure to do so may be associated with a poor response despite prolonged systemic antibiotic treatment.

Prognosis. This depends in large part upon the nature of the underlying disease; e.g., the leading cause of death in childhood leukemia is septicemia, and half of these cases are due to *Pseudomonas*. Likewise, *Pseudomonas* is recovered from the lungs of most children who die of cystic fibrosis and may be responsible for the deaths of many of them. The prognosis for normal development is poor in the few infants who survive *Pseudomonas* meningitis.

Disease Due to Other Pseudomonads

Glanders

Glanders is a severe infectious disease of horses due to *P. mallei*, occasionally transmitted to man. It occurs more commonly in Asia, Africa, and the Middle East than in the United States, where it is very rare. An acute or chronic pneumonitis and hemorrhagic necrotic lesions of the skin, nasal mucous membranes, and lymph nodes may be noted.

Melioidosis

This rare disease of Southeast Asia has been seen with increasing frequency in the United States in Vietnamese children and in Americans returned from Vietnam. The causative agent is *P. pseudomallei*, an inhabitant of soil and water in the tropics. Infection follows inhalation of dust or direct contamination of abrasions or wounds. Pulmonary infection may be subacute and mimic tuberculosis. Occasionally, septicemia occurs and multiple abscesses are noted in every organ of the body except the gastrointestinal tract. Melioidosis may present as an encephalitic illness with fever and seizures; generally, antibiotic therapy results in recovery. This disease may remain latent and appear when host resistance is reduced, sometimes years after initial exposure. Both glanders and melioidosis are treated with tetracycline or chloramphenicol, supplemented with a sulfonamide, over a period of many mo. Aminoglycosides and the penicillins are ineffective.

Bobo RA, Newton EJ, Jones LF, et al: Nursery outbreak of *Pseudomonas aeruginosa*: Epidemiologic conclusions from five different typing methods. Appl Microbiol 25:414, 1973.
Feigin RD, Shearer WT: Opportunistic infection in children. Parts I, II and III. J Pediatr 87:507, 677, 852, 1975.
Jones RJ, Roe EA, Gupta JL: Controlled trials of a polyvalent *Pseudomonas* vaccine in burns. Lancet 2:977, 1979.
Liu PV: Biology of *Pseudomonas aeruginosa*. Hosp Pract Jan 1976, p 139.
Pennington JE, Reynolds HY, Wood RE, et al: Use of *Pseudomonas aeruginosa* vaccine in patients with acute leukemia and cystic fibrosis. Am J Med 58:629, 1975.
Reed RK, Larter WE, Sieber OF Jr, et al: Peripheral nodular lesions in *Pseudomonas* sepsis: The importance of incision and drainage. J Pediatr 88:977, 1976.
Reynolds HY, Di Sant'Agnese PA, Zierdt CH: Mucoid *Pseudomonas aeruginosa*. JAMA 236:2190, 1976.
Schiotz PO, Nielsen H, Hoiby N, et al: Immune complexes in the sputum of patients with cystic fibrosis suffering from chronic *Pseudomonas aeruginosa* lung infection. Acta Path Microbol Sect C 86:37, 1978.
Sorensen RU, Stern RC, Polmar SH: Lymphocyte responsiveness to *Pseudomonas aeruginosa* in cystic fibrosis: Relationship to status of pulmonary disease in sibling pairs. J Pediatr 93:201, 1978.

10.35 BRUCELLOSIS
(Undulant Fever, Mediterranean Fever, Goat's Milk Fever)

Brucellosis is an acute or chronic infectious disease of animals transmissible to man. Human infection is usually caused by the 4 main species of *Brucella* that may be transmitted from the cow, goat, hog, or dog. *Brucella* organisms also have been recovered from wild rats, field mice, wild guinea pigs, jack rabbits, ground squirrels, rams, camels, gazelles, water buffalo, chamois, deer, elk, bison, and fowl.

Etiology. Six *Brucella* species are known to be transmissible to man: *abortus* (cows), *melitensis* (goats), *suis* (hogs), *canis* (dogs), *ovis* (sheep and hares), and *neotomae* (desert wood rats). The organisms are small, gramnegative, nonmotile, nonspore-forming, nonencapsulated, and aerobic.

Epidemiology. Most cases of brucellosis in man result from direct contact with sick animals. Individuals working in food processing plants, dairy farmers, and other individuals with an opportunity for frequent contact with domestic animals are most commonly infected. The milk of infected animals serves to transfer brucellae to man following ingestion. The organisms also may invade the eye, nasopharynx, and genital tract, but unbroken skin is resistant to invasion. Brucellae may remain viable for up to 3 wk in a refrigerated carcass and can survive the curing of ham. The organisms are killed by pasteurization and cooking.

Most epidemics of brucellosis are due to ingestion of unpasteurized milk, cream, butter, cheese, or ice cream that contains *B. abortus* or *B. melitensis*.

As a result of compulsory pasteurization of milk and control measures in cattle, the reported incidence declined to 0.1/100,000 persons in the 1970's. The disease is infrequent in children. In a seroepidemiologic investigation of *Brucella canis* antibodies, 67.8% of individuals tested were positive. Eleven of 193 newborn infants (5.7%) had antibodies to *B. canis* as a result of transplacental transfer from seropositive mothers. The prevalence of *B. canis* antibodies in humans who are exposed to dogs is high, and it should be considered as a cause of febrile illness in children who have intimate contact with dogs. Although *Brucella* sp. have been recovered from the urine of patients with brucellosis, human to human transmission has not been documented. Congenital infections have not been reported.

Pathogenesis and Pathology. Brucellae are primarily intracellular parasites. The organisms are phagocytized by leukocytes and monocytes following entry into the body and are distributed throughout the reticuloendothelial system. Intracellular growth may occur in many cell types, including red blood cells.

Delayed or tuberculin-type hypersensitivity to brucella antigen characteristically develops. This reaction depends upon multiplication of living organisms; dead organisms, or fractions thereof, rarely produce sensitization.

The host responds to brucellosis by elaborating a variety of antibodies, including agglutinins, opsonins, bactericidins, precipitins, and complement-fixing antibodies. Multiplication of organisms within the host appears to be essential for induction of immunity. Infection is followed by early development of specific serum IgM antibodies and then shortly thereafter by the appearance of IgG antibodies, which ultimately predominate.

Serum or plasma from normal individuals and from patients with acute brucellosis may, in the presence of complement, have significant nonspecific bactericidal activity against brucellae. In chronic infections, however, a specific inhibitor appears and prevents the lethal activity of the serum-complement system. The specific antibody which is produced acts as an opsonin and promotes phagocytosis by polymorphonuclear leukocytes and fixed phagocytes. Thus, brucellae are cleared rapidly from the blood of individuals with demonstrable antibodies. They are not, however, killed; once sequestered within cells, they are protected from further bactericidal action of the blood. Smooth strains of *Brucella*, which are more virulent than rough strains, multiply within cells, including those obtained from immune individuals.

Smooth and intermediate strains of *Brucella* contain endotoxin, which does not appear to be important in the virulence of the organism but may play a role in human disease after infection has been established.

All species of *Brucella* produce granulomas that may be noted histologically in the liver, spleen, lymph nodes, and bone marrow. In addition to granuloma formation, centrilobular necrosis and cirrhosis of the liver have been described. Granulomatous inflammation of the gallbladder, interstitial orchitis with scattered areas of fibroid atrophy, endocarditis with vegetations of the aortic and mitral valves, granulomatous lesions of the myocardium, and involvement of the brain, kidney, and skin also have been described.

Clinical Manifestations. The incubation period of brucellosis varies from a few days to several mo. The onset may be sudden but most commonly is insidious. Prodromal symptoms include weakness, fatigue, anorexia, headache, myalgia, and constipation. As the disease progresses, evening elevations in temperature are observed and become increasingly prominent, with temperatures as high as 41–42.5° C (106–108° F). Chills, diaphoresis, epistaxis, abdominal pain, and cough may be observed. Weight loss may be prominent.

Physical findings generally are limited to hepatomegaly, splenomegaly, and cervical and axillary lymphadenopathy. Rales may be heard; in such instances, pulmonary lesions may be demonstrable by chest roentgenogram.

Chronic brucellosis may be difficult to diagnose and is a cause of "fever of unknown origin." Patients may complain of fatigue, myalgia, arthralgia, sweating, nervousness, and anorexia; depressive or psychotic episodes have been reported. A maculopapular or, rarely, morbilliform rash may be observed. The organisms may localize in various organs; uveitis, endocarditis, hepatitis, cholecystitis, epididymitis, prostatitis, osteomyelitis, encephalitis, and myelitis due to *Brucella* have all been reported.

The white blood cell count may be normal, elevated, or reduced. Relative lymphocytosis is common, as in anemia.

Diagnosis. The most useful method for diagnosis is the brucella agglutination test, which will reveal titers greater than 1:160 in almost all acute cases. Generally, the titer correlates with the activity of the infection, but brucella antigen in skin tests or food may produce an anamnestic response. Prozones of inhibition by blocking antibodies may obscure serum agglutination, but this can be avoided by use of the Coombs antiglobulin method. Cross-reactions occur with agglutinins against *F. tularensis;* thus tests against both should be performed. Later in the course of disease, the complement-fixation titer rises and usually is considered to be diagnostic if it is 1:16 or higher.

Skin tests, when negative, exclude infection but should not be performed if serologic studies are available because the skin test antigen may stimulate production of antibody and thereby confuse subsequent serologic results.

Isolation of *Brucella* by culture provides a definitive diagnosis. Blood cultures are most helpful in acute disease; cultures of infected tissues or abscesses also may be valuable. Cultures should be incubated under 10% carbon dioxide. Primary cultures should be incubated for at least 4 wk before they are discarded as negative.

Differential Diagnosis. Acute brucellosis can mimic many diseases, including tularemia, typhoid fever, rickettsial diseases, influenza, tuberculosis, histoplasmosis, coccidioidomycosis, and infectious mononucleosis. Chronic brucellosis may resemble lymphoma or other neoplastic diseases. Appropriate historic, roentgenographic, and serologic studies and culture results help to differentiate these disorders. Biopsy of appropriate tissues may also be required.

Complications. Complications are the result of localization of brucellae in various organs and tissues. Osteomyelitis is the most frequent complication in man, particularly suppurative spondylitis involving an intervertebral disc and the adjacent vertebrae. Acute suppurative arthritis may be seen, but destructive joint disease is rare. Neurologic complications may occur early or late and assume the form of an acute or subacute meningitis or encephalitis. Adhesive arachnoiditis has been described.

Myocarditis and endocarditis are serious complications which may lead to death. A Herxheimer reaction may develop at the time that therapy is initiated.

Prevention. This depends upon avoidance of exposure to the organism. Infection of domestic animals with which man has close contact can be prevented by immunization. In addition to immunization of animals and pasteurization of milk, periodic agglutination tests performed on milk and blood should be used to identify infected animals. Positive reactors should be slaughtered. Ingestion of unpasteurized milk or other dairy products derived from unpasteurized milk or cream must be avoided.

Treatment. Brucellosis can be treated with tetracycline in a dose of 30–40 mg/kg/24 hr in 4 divided oral doses. Treatment is continued for 3–4 wk. If relapse occurs (and it may in as many as 50% of cases), the dose may be increased and streptomycin added in amounts of 15–30 mg/kg/24 hr in 2 equally divided doses administered every 12 hr for 14 days; the initial dose may be halved during the 2nd wk. Trimethoprim-sulfamethoxazole has been used to treat some patients with good results.

Localized abscesses should be drained. Steroids may be of value in reducing the risk of a Herxheimer reaction at the onset of therapy.

Patients with brucellosis should be encouraged to rest, and adequate dietary intake should be encouraged.

Prognosis. The mortality of untreated brucellosis is about 3%. Most untreated patients survive, but recovery may require 6 mo. Prognosis following specific antibiotic therapy is excellent; a prolonged course of disease in patients with brucellosis who are receiving antibiotics usually is the result of a delay in diagnosis.

Boycott JA: Diagnosing brucellosis. Lancet 1:255, 1969.
Bradstreet CMP, Tannahil AJ, Pollock TM, et al: Intradermal test and serological tests in suspected brucella infection in man. Lancet 2:653, 1970.
Busch LA, Parker RL: Brucellosis in the United States. J Infect Dis 125:289, 1972.
Coghlan JD, Weir DM: Antibodies in human brucellosis. Br Med J 2:269, 1967.
Hall WH, Khan MY: Brucellosis. In: Hoeprich PD (ed): Infectious Disease. Ed 2. Hagerstown, Md., Harper & Row, 1977.
Street L Jr, Grant WW, Alva JD: Brucellosis in childhood. Pediatrics 55:416, 1975.

10.36 YERSINIAL INFECTIONS

Three organisms of the *Yersinia* sp. are responsible for human disease: *Yersinia pestis* (formerly *Pasteurella pestis*), *Yersinia enterocolitica,* and *Yersinia pseudotuberculosis.* Disease caused by *Y. pestis* (plague) has played a prominent role in world history.

Plague

A reservoir of plague infection exists in the rodent community throughout most of the western United States, extending into Canada and Mexico. This vast endemic area of infection is equivalent to any of the older plague foci of Europe and Asia and is a constant reminder that the threat of plague must be continually reviewed. Although reports of plague in the United States are infrequent, an epidemic in the Americas is a distinct possibility, considering the probable susceptibility of the population.

Etiology. *Yersinia pestis* is a nonmotile, nonsporulating, pleomorphic, gram-negative bacillus. The characteristic "safety-pin" or bipolar appearance is demonstrated best in smears of infected secretions or tissue stained by the Giemsa method.

Epidemiology. Plague of domestic and wild animals occurs in 2 forms: enzootic and epizootic. *Enzootic plague* implies a stable rodent-flea cycle of infection which is found in a relatively resistant host population. Enzootic foci are inconspicuous and serve effectively as reservoirs of infection, as in the United States at the present time. *Epizootic plague* occurs when the disease is introduced into a highly susceptible mammalian population, causing a high mortality rate among infected animals.

Plague is transmitted to man by the bite of fleas, which have sucked blood from infected animals. Transmission from animals to man usually causes bubonic plague and is referred to as *zootic plague.* Person-to-person transmission can occur and is called *demic plague* (pneumonic plague is the most serious form of demic plague).

In the United States reported cases of plague have been increasing since 1966; two thirds have occurred in individuals under 25 yr of age. Infection is more common in males than in females (2:1).

Pathology and Pathogenesis. Plague bacilli ingested by the flea proliferate and eventually block the lumen of the proventriculus. These are regurgitated into dermal lymphatics of the human host by the flea and are then transmitted to regional lymph nodes, which become tender and enlarged (buboes). In severe bubonic plague the lymph nodes fail to filter out all multiplying bacilli which gain entrance to the efferent lymphatics and disseminate to the vascular system. Once entry into the bloodstream has occurred, any organ of the body may be involved. Septicemia, meningitis, disseminated intravascular coagulation, and pneumonia (secondary) may develop.

Primary pulmonic plague may result from human-to-human transmission or from a laboratory accident. Droplets containing large numbers of virulent bacilli may be inhaled, causing severe pneumonia, septicemia, and, frequently, death within 24 hr.

When plague bacilli are introduced into man, they are susceptible to phagocytosis; those which survive are resistant to phagocytosis. The virulence of pneumonic plague may relate, in part, to the inhalation of organisms which have survived infection within another human host.

The pathogenic response of human tissues to *Y. pestis*

generally is pyogenic. Necrotic foci may develop within lymph nodes, spleen, and liver. Hemorrhagic lesions may be found in many organs and tissues, particularly if disseminated intravascular coagulation develops.

Clinical Manifestations. The incubation period of bubonic plague is 2–6 days. The incubation period of pneumonic plague varies from 1–72 hr.

The onset of bubonic plague may be acute or subacute. In the subacute forms, the initial findings are a tender lymphadenitis and associated lymphadenopathy. Patients are febrile but not particularly toxic in appearance. If treatment is delayed, septicemia may occur, associated with prostration, shock, and hemorrhagic pneumonitis.

Bubonic plague may present more acutely, with high fever, tachycardia, and myalgia. The disease progresses to delirium, shock, and death within 3–5 days.

The course of primary pneumonic plague is even more virulent. Pulmonary signs and symptoms may be lacking until within 24 hr of death. Symptoms of plague have included nausea, vomiting, abdominal pain, bloody diarrhea, and petechial and purpuric rashes. During epidemics a mild form of the disease may occur in which lymphadenopathy and vesicular or pustular skin lesions develop, serious symptoms are absent, and recovery can occur without therapy.

Diagnosis. The diagnosis of plague depends upon a careful history and physical examination and a high index of suspicion. Sputum, blood, purulent exudates, and aspirates of lymph nodes should be examined by smears stained with Giemsa or Wayson stain and by culture. Cultures may be made in blood broth or blood agar, and organisms that are recovered may be identified by biochemical methods, by the fluorescent antibody technique, or by lysis with specific bacteriophage. Serologic tests may be helpful in selected patients; passive hemagglutination antibody titers to Fraction I antigen of *Yersinia pestis* may be detectable by day 5 of illness; titers peak at 14 days.

Differential Diagnosis. Plague may be confused with other disorders causing localized lymphadenitis and lymphadenopathy, including infection due to *S. aureus*, *S. pyogenes*, and *F. tularensis*. Septicemic plague may be indistinguishable clinically from any other form of overwhelming bacterial septicemia or from rickettsial diseases.

Prevention. A heat-killed vaccine prepared from *Y. pestis* may produce immunity following administration of a primary series of 3 injections at 2 wk intervals. Biannual boosters are required for maintenance of immunity. Routine vaccination is not recommended, even for individuals living in plague enzootic areas of the United States. Immunization may be useful for those whose occupation regularly brings them into contact with infected rodents or with the organism itself in the laboratory.

The primary method for preventing plague in urban areas consists of environmental sanitation directed toward reducing rodent populations and their fleas. Patients with plague should be isolated until treated. Purulent exudates should be handled with rubber gloves. Face masks and goggles should be worn by personnel caring for individuals with pneumonic pla-

gue. *Y. pestis* may be found in the feces; accordingly, disinfection of the stools of patients with plague infection should be performed routinely before disposal.

Treatment. Streptomycin is bactericidal and can be used in a dose of 30 mg/kg/24 hr in 2–3 equally divided doses given intramuscularly for 5–10 days. Herxheimer reactions are not uncommon when streptomycin is given; thus this drug is usually reserved for pneumonic or septicemic forms of the disease. Tetracycline may be added after 2–3 days of streptomycin therapy in a dose of 30 mg/kg/24 hr in 4 divided oral doses continued for 10 days. Chloramphenicol, 50 mg/kg/24 hr in 4 divided doses, can be substituted for tetracycline.

Bubonic plague can be treated with tetracycline (40 mg/kg/24 hr in 4 divided oral doses) for 10 days, or chloramphenicol (50 mg/kg/24 hr in 4 divided oral doses).

Contacts of patients with pulmonic plague should be quarantined and may be given tetracycline (20 mg/kg/24 hr) in 4 divided oral doses prophylactically for 10 days.

Prognosis. The mortality of untreated bubonic plague is 60–90%. Pneumonic plague is virtually 100% fatal if untreated.

When bubonic plague is treated early, the mortality rate is less than 10%. Prognosis in primary pneumonic plague is poor if the diagnosis is not made and specific treatment provided within 18 hr of the onset of symptoms.

Yersinia enterocolitica and Yersinia pseudotuberculosis

Formerly considered rare, disease from these organisms has been recognized with increasing frequency in recent years.

Yersinia may be confused with coliform organisms. *Yersinia enterocolitica* and *Y. pseudotuberculosis* are oxidase-negative, gram-negative rods which are motile at 22° C but not at 37° C. It is this 3rd characteristic that aids in differentiating them from *Y. pestis* and Enterobacteriaceae. *Yersinia enterocolitica* and *Y. pseudotuberculosis* can be distinguished from each other by biochemical tests, by agglutination with specific antisera, and by the susceptibility of *Y. pseudotuberculosis* to specific bacteriophages. Serotypes 3, 8, and 9 of *Y. enterocolitica* and 1 of *Y. pseudotuberculosis* are found most frequently as causes of disease in humans.

Yersinia enterocolitica has been recovered from many wild and domestic animal species, raw milk, oysters, and water supplies. Recently, human infection following exposure to infected household dogs and human-to-human spread has been documented. Young infants and children are infected most commonly. In 1 prospective study *Y. enterocolitica* was recovered from the stools of 181 of 6364 children with gastroenteritis seen over a 15 mo period.

Y. enterocolitica has been associated with diarrhea, acute mesenteric adenitis, pharyngitis, abscesses, arthritis, osteomyelitis, hepatitis, carditis, meningitis, ophthalmitis, hemolytic anemia, Reiter syndrome, septicemia, and some rashes, including erythema nodosum. The most serious manifestation of *Yersinia* infection (septicemia) is associated with a case-fatality ratio of almost 50% despite antibiotic treatment. In patients with gastrointestinal disease, abdominal pain may be severe and suggest a diagnosis of appendicitis. Diarrhea is common and persistent, lasting 1–2 wk. The stool may be watery, mucoid, or bilious but generally is guaiac-negative. Ulceration of the small bowel has been described. The stool of patients with diarrhea due to *Y. enterocolitica* may contain polymorphonuclear leukocytes. Children with severe diarrhea due to *Y. enterocolitica* may develop hypoalbuminemia and hypokalemia; these findings suggest extensive disruption of the small bowel mucosa. The duration of illness generally is 2–3 wk, but occasionally diarrhea may persist for several mo.

Diagnosis of infection due to *Y. enterocolitica* may be established by identification of the organism in stool of infected patients. Passive hemagglutination tests may help to confirm the diagnosis. Antibodies are detectable 8–10 days after the onset of illness and may persist for several mo. Children under 1 yr of age are less likely to have a serologic response than are older children.

Diarrhea due to *Y. enterocolitica* usually resolves in time without therapy.

Most strains of *Yersinia* are sensitive to streptomycin, tetracycline, chloramphenicol, and sulfonamides.

Yersinia pseudotuberculosis has been associated with mesenteric adenitis and terminal ileitis. Abdominal pain may be severe and suggest acute appendicitis. Septicemia is unusual but may occur. Postdiarrheal hemolytic-uremic syndrome associated with *Y. pseudotuberculosis* septicemia has been reported. *Y. pseudotuberculosis* is generally sensitive to ampicillin, kanamycin, tetracycline, and chloramphenicol.

Kohl S: *Yersinia enterocolitica* infections in children. Pediat Clin North Am 26:433, 1979.

Marks MI, Pai CH, Lafleur L: *Yersinia enterocolitica* gastroenteritis: A prospective study of clinical, bacteriologic and epidemiologic features. J Pediatr 96:26, 1980.

Martin AR, Hurtado FP, Plessala RA, et al: Plague meningitis. A report of three cases in children and review of the problem. Pediatrics 40:610, 1967.

Poland JD: Plague. *In:* Hoeprich PD (ed): Infectious Diseases. Ed 2. Hagerstown Md., Harper & Row, 1977.

Weber J, Finlayson NB, Mark JBD: Mesenteric lymphadenitis and terminal ileitis due to *Yersinia pseudotuberculosis*. N Engl J Med 283:172, 1970.

10.37 TULAREMIA

Tularemia is an infectious disease caused by *Francisella tularensis (Pasteurella tularensis)*. Its clinical manifestations depend upon the virulence of the infecting organism and the route of infection, which may be subclinical but more frequently is characterized by the occurrence of specific syndromes. Ulceroglandular forms account for about 80% of cases, glandular, 10%, oculoglandular, 1%, and typhoidal, 6%. The precise frequency in children of exudative pharyngitis or pneumonia due to *F. tularensis* is unknown, but oropharyngeal tularemia is not uncommon.

Etiology. The organism is a short, nonspore-form-
ing, nonmotile, unencapsulated, gram-negative bacillus which may be markedly pleomorphic in culture. The use of special containment facilities is recommended when cultures are handled to avoid accidental acquisition of disease.

Strains of *F. tularensis* are antigenically homogeneous, but virulence is variable. One strain (Jellison type A), found only in North America, is highly virulent for humans. A 2nd strain (Jellison type B), found in North America, Europe, and Asia, is avirulent for rabbits and causes only mild disease in man.

Epidemiology. Tularemia is not an uncommon disease in the United States. No age group is immune and there is no sex or racial predilection. Most of the reported cases have been from the West–South Central States, but a large outbreak was reported in Vermont in 1969.

F. tularensis has been recovered from over 100 types of mammals and arthropods. Type A bacteria generally are acquired from cottontail rabbits or ticks. Type B strains are more commonly acquired from rats, mice, squirrels, muskrats, beavers, moles, birds, and ticks. Tularemia may also be acquired from horseflies, deerflies, fleas, and lice.

Disease follows direct contact of the skin or mucous membranes with tissues or body fluids of infected animals, the bite of infected arthropod vectors, and even inhalation and direct penetration of the pharyngeal mucosa by ingested organisms. The gastrointestinal tract is relatively resistant to penetration by *F. tularensis*, but infection by this route may occur. In humans, more than 10 million *F. tularensis* bacilli must be ingested to cause disease, whereas fewer than 50 Jellison type A bacilli may cause disease following inhalation or intradermal inoculation.

Tularemia has been considered to be a disease of hunters, cooks, trappers, muskrat farmers, and others with occupational exposure to the organism. It may occur in children who have ingested food (rabbit or squirrel meat) or water contaminated with *F. tularensis* or who have been bitten by infected ticks, flies, or other vectors. In 1 outbreak that occurred in Baltimore, Maryland, tularemia pneumonia resulted from an aerosol established by the affected children who beat a rabbit carcass with a stick.

Pathology and Pathogenesis. The host may be infected by inoculation through broken or intact skin, ingestion, or inhalation. Within 48–72 hr after the organisms enter the skin, an erythematous maculopapular lesion may be noted, followed shortly by ulceration and regional lymphadenopathy. The organisms multiply and produce granulomas within lymph nodes. Subsequently, bacteremia may occur. Although any organ of the body may be involved, infection of the reticuloendothelial system is most prominent and common.

Bronchopneumonia and, rarely, lobar pneumonia may follow inhalation of *F. tularensis*. An inflammatory reaction develops about the site of bacterial deposition, and necrosis of alveolar walls may be observed. In some cases inhalation of *F. tularensis* is followed by bronchitis rather than by pneumonitis. The organisms that reach the lung are ingested by alveolar macrophages, enter the hilar lymphatics, and then enter the blood. A typhoidal form of tularemia results when the mastication of contaminated food releases *F. tularensis*, which is then inhaled.

Direct invasion of the mucosa of the nasopharynx or conjunctival sac may occur.

Factors responsible for the virulence of *F. tularensis* remain poorly defined. No exotoxin has been identified, nor have virulent strains been identified to have anti-phagocytic properties.

F. tularensis is an intracellular parasite capable of surviving for extended periods of time within mono-cytes and other body cells. Although the immune re-sponse is usually persistent, chronic or relapsing dis-ease may occur, related probably to the prolonged intracellular survival of the organism. Cell-mediated immunity may be of greater import than are circulating antibodies in determining complete recovery.

Clinical Manifestations. The incubation period of tularemia varies from a few hr to 1 wk. The onset of illness is acute and characterized by myalgia, arthralgia, chills, fever of 40–41° C (104–106° F), nausea, vomiting, and diaphoresis. Headache is prominent but may not be reported by young children. Photophobia may be present. A generalized maculopapular rash may accom-pany any of the forms. A mild anemia may be present. The white blood cell count may be normal, depressed, or increased, and the sedimentation rate can be normal. Transient proteinuria has been observed.

In the *ulceroglandular* form of the disease, the primary maculopapular lesion is noted within 72 hr and ulcer-ates within 4–5 days. The ulceration is painful and requires an average of 4 wk to heal. Regional lymph-adenopathy occurs, usually without discernible inter-vening lymphangitis. The lymph nodes are tender and become fluctuant in about 25% of untreated cases. Generalized lymphadenopathy, splenomegaly, or both may develop.

Oropharyngeal tularemia is characterized by purulent tonsillitis and pharyngitis and occasionally by ulcerative stomatitis. Systemic manifestations of disease are simi-lar to those described above.

Glandular tularemia is similar to ulceroglandular dis-ease, but no local lesion is apparent on the skin or mucous membranes.

Oculoglandular disease is similar to the ulceroglandu-lar type except that the primary lesion is a severe conjunctivitis accompanied by regional lymphadenitis.

As the name implies, *typhoidal* tularemia resembles typhoid fever. Fever is protracted, and cutaneous or mucous membrane lesions may not be apparent. A dry cough, severe retrosternal chest pain, and hemoptysis may be noted. Clinical evidence of bronchitis, pneu-monitis, and pleuritis may be found in 20% of cases; roentgenographic evidence of pleural or pulmonary involvement, including nodular enlargement of the hilus of the lung, has been observed in 90% of cases in some series. Splenomegaly is common, and hepatic enlargement may be noted.

Meningitis, encephalitis, pericarditis, endocarditis, neuralgias, thrombophlebitis, and osteomyelitis due to *F. tularensis* have all been reported.

Diagnosis. The history and clinical manifestations should suggest the disease, particularly a history of ingestion of rabbit or squirrel meat, contact with rabbits, or bites by ticks, flies, or other vectors. A negative history, however, does not exclude the diagnosis.

Smear and Gram stains of sputum are usually unre-warding. Examination of pleural fluid may occasionally reveal *F. tularensis*. The cellular response within pleural fluid generally is mononuclear.

The *serum agglutination test* is a reliable method for the diagnosis of tularemia, but it usually is not positive until after the 1st wk of illness, and fatal cases have been reported in the absence of agglutinins. Agglutinins are first detectable between the 10th–14th days. The titer then rises abruptly to 1:640 or greater within 1 wk and may be in excess of 1:1280 by the 4th–8th wk of illness. A titer of 1:80 or greater may be considered positive, but serially rising titers are of greater signifi-cance in establishing a diagnosis. Low titers due to cross-reactions with brucella, heterophile, and OX-19 agglutinins have been reported. Prior immunization with cholera vaccine may also produce cross-agglutin-ation.

A preparation of phenolized organisms may be used for *skin-testing*. Positive reactions may be observed by the 4th–7th day of infection. Skin test material may be obtained from the Rocky Mountain Laboratory of the National Institute of Allergy and Infectious Disease.

Direct *culture* of organisms is possible but requires appropriate media and is hazardous to inexperienced laboratory personnel. The organism may be isolated from blood, gastric washings, and drainage from wounds by culture or by inoculating guinea pigs intra-peritoneally with these body fluids. Infected animals are even more hazardous to laboratory personnel than are cultures.

Differential Diagnosis. Ulceroglandular tularemia may resemble cat-scratch disease, infectious mononu-cleosis, sporotrichosis, plague, anthrax, melioidosis, glanders, rat-bite fever, or lymphadenitis due to *Strep-tococcus pyogenes* or *Staphylococcus aureus*. Oropharyngeal tularemia must be differentiated from the same diseases but also from acquired cytomegaloviral disease, ac-quired toxoplasmosis, and infection due to adenovi-ruses and herpes simplex.

Tularemic pneumonitis must be differentiated from other bacterial and nonbacterial pneumonias, particu-larly those due to mycoplasma, chlamydia, mycobac-teria, fungi, and rickettsia. These distinctions can be made on the basis of isolation of the organisms, sero-logic studies, skin tests, and response to various forms of therapy.

Typhoidal tularemia must be differentiated from ty-phoid fever, brucellosis, and other severe septicemic illnesses.

Prevention. Tularemia can be prevented by avoid-ance of exposure to mammals and arthropod vectors which may be infected. Rabbits that appear to be ill should be destroyed without direct handling. Rubber gloves should be worn to handle the flesh of wild animals. In areas infested with ticks, tight wristbands and boots are recommended. A careful search for ticks should be made as frequently as practical if one remains within a wooded area for an extended period of time and promptly after departure. Ticks should be removed by an instrument or the gloved hand and should not be squeezed during the removal process. The area of attachment should be cleansed with 70% ethanol.

Tularemia can be prevented by intradermal immunization with a live attenuated strain of *F. tularensis*, developed in Russia but tested in the United States. The vaccine is safe; the duration of immunity is at least 3–5 yr. Vaccine can be obtained for use in persons requiring special protection against tularemia, but it has not been evaluated for use in children.

Treatment.   Streptomycin, 30–40 mg/kg/24 hr in 2 divided doses intramuscularly for at least 7 days, is the treatment of choice. Tularemia also responds to treatment with tetracycline; chloramphenicol is also effective, but relapses are common with both. Retreatment with tetracycline has been followed by clinical recovery. The efficacy of kanamycin and gentamicin in treatment of tularemia has not been adequately evaluated.

Prognosis.   Untreated ulceroglandular tularemia has a fatality rate of about 5%. Untreated patients who survive experience symptoms for 2–4 wk and a subsequent period of disability of 8–12 wk. Mortality in untreated patients may reach 30% if pneumonia develops, irrespective of whether it is primary or secondary to ulceroglandular disease. Recovery from tularemia is associated with lifelong immunity. Second attacks may occur but are mild. Prognosis following infection with Jellison type B strains may be considerably better than that reported above. If treatment is provided promptly, recovery generally is rapid and fatality exceedingly rare.

Bloom ME, Shearer WT, Barton LL: Oculoglandular tularemia in an inner city child. Pediatrics 57:564, 1973.

Halsted CC, Kulasinghe HP: Tularemia pneumonia in urban children. Pediatrics 61:660, 1978.

Hughes WT: Tularemia in children. J Pediatr 62:495, 1963.

Miller RP, Bates JH: Pleuropulmonary tularemia. A review of 29 patients. Am Rev Resp Dis 99:31, 1969.

Tyson HK: Tularemia: An unappreciated cause of exudative pharyngitis. Pediatrics 58:864, 1976.

Young LS, Bicknell DS, Archer BG, et al: Tularemia epidemic: Vermont, 1968. Forty-seven cases linked to contact with muskrats. N Engl J Med 280:1253, 1969.

10.38   LISTERIOSIS

During the last 50 yr, listeriosis has emerged as a septicemic or meningitic illness which most frequently affects the newborn infant and the compromised pediatric host. Human infections with *Listeria monocytogenes*, unlike those in animals, generally are characterized by a polymorphonuclear response in blood, cerebrospinal fluid, and other body tissues.

Etiology.   *L. monocytogenes* is a small, gram-positive, nonspore-forming rod. It displays tumbling motility at room temperature but not at 37° C. Generally, it produces beta-hemolysis on blood agar, but alpha-hemolysis has been observed.

Listeria can be divided into 4 serologic types on the basis of somatic (O) and flagellar (H) antigens. Groups I, III, and IV can be differentiated on the basis of the (O) antigens and Group II on the basis of a distinctive (H) antigen. Major groups can be subdivided further as follows: Group I (Ia Ib); Group II; Group III (IIIa, IIIb); and Group IV (IVa, IVb, IVc, IVab, IVd, and IVe). Most human disease is due to organisms belonging to Groups I and IV.

On routine culture media *Listeria* frequently is mistaken for a diphtheroid and discarded as a nonpathogen or a contaminant. On Gram stains from clinical specimens, coccoid forms appear that may be mistaken for streptococci. In poorly stained smears the cells may appear gram-negative and resemble *Hemophilus influenzae*.

Epidemiology.   *Listeria* has been reported as a cause of disease in 42 domestic and feral mammalian and 22 avian species. It has been isolated from soil, where survival for more than 295 days has been reported, and from streams, sewage, silage, dust, and slaughterhouse waste. It also has been recovered from the intestinal tract, vagina, cervix, nose, ears, and, rarely, blood or urine of apparently healthy humans. The minimum number of fecal excreters of *Listeria* has been estimated at 1% of the population. The true frequency may be higher since recovery of *Listeria* from feces is difficult and a higher frequency of excreters has been documented in selected population groups. The role played by healthy carriers in the perpetuation and transmission of *Listeria* remains ill defined.

Listeria infection in the newborn infant has been attributed to acquisition of the organism transplacentally or by aspiration or ingestion at the time of delivery. Older children may acquire infection by inhalation or ingestion or, less commonly, by direct contact or venereal transmission. In some cases carriers may develop overt disease when their immune responses are altered by underlying disease (e.g., leukemia, lymphomas, Hodgkin disease) or by administration of immunosuppressive agents. Transmission to humans by ingestion of unpasteurized milk has been strongly suggested. Transmission by insect vectors has not been documented.

Risk of infection is greatest in newborn infants and in children with malignancies. Older studies suggest that the incidence of human infection is lowest in the spring; a more recent study performed in Sweden between 1958–1974 reveals no seasonal variation.

Pathology.   *L. monocytogenes* produces disease in many organs, including liver, lung, adrenals, kidneys, and brain. The abscesses do not differ from those found in other pyogenic infections. Necrotizing changes may be noted in the kidneys and the lung, particularly in the bronchioles and alveolar walls.

Listeria produces a pyogenic meningitis and also may cause suppurative ependymitis, encephalitis, choroiditis, and gliosis.

Pathogenesis.   *Listeria* is a facultative intracellular parasite. Cellular mechanisms are involved in the immune response to infection by these organisms. Any inherited or acquired disorder in which T cell function is impaired may predispose the host to infection by *Listeria*.

Listeriosis may develop at birth or be noted subsequently in the newborn infant or older child. Early-onset disease may be acquired transplacentally from a mother with subclinical or clinical infection. Infection acquired early in pregnancy may lead to abortion and, more commonly, if acquired later, to stillbirth or premature delivery.

Listeria may be recovered with great frequency from mothers of infants who develop *Listeria* infection during the 1st 5 days of life. The development of late-onset neonatal disease is not usually associated with maternal illness or carriage of the organism; epidemic neonatal disease has been described, presumably reflecting patient-to-patient transmission. Early-onset neonatal disease has been associated with maternal fever or other signs of maternal infection and with recovery of serotypes Ia and Ib. Late-onset disease is primarily associated with recovery of serotype IVb and is predominantly a meningitis rather than septicemic illness.

At any age all organs of the body may be involved after bloodstream invasion.

Clinical Manifestations. *Listeria* may cause septicemia or meningitis in infants and children. Listeriosis also may present as pneumonia, an influenza-like septicemic illness of pregnant women, infectious mononucleosis–like illness, endocarditis, localized abscesses, papular or pustular cutaneous lesions, conjunctivitis, and urethritis. It has also been blamed for habitual spontaneous abortion, but evidence for this association is not conclusive.

In the newborn infant (Sec 7.68), a spectrum of disease is apparent. Clinical presentation depends upon the time and route of infection. If *Listeria* infection occurs late in pregnancy, abortion, stillbirth, or an acutely ill infant who expires within a few hr of birth may be noted.

In the liveborn infant whose disease becomes apparent within the 1st wk of life (early-onset disease), whitish granulomas may be found on the mucous membranes and disseminated papules on the skin. Anorexia, lethargy, vomiting, jaundice, respiratory distress, pulmonary infiltrates, cyanosis, petechial rashes, evidence of myocarditis, and hepatomegaly all have been noted. These babies frequently are premature, and the mortality rate is high.

Late-onset neonatal disease also may occur. The infant appears well at birth, but septicemia or meningitis develops during the 1st mo of life. Signs and symptoms are similar to those noted in any form of pyogenic meningitis.

In older children meningitis or meningoencephalitis may be noted. Generally, there are no characteristics that distinguish meningitis due to *Listeria* from that due to other causes. In some cases, however, the onset is subacute and characterized by headache, low grade fever, and malaise of several days' duration prior to the time that symptoms and signs referable to the central nervous system are first noted.

Meningitis may occur in association with conjunctivitis, otitis media, sinusitis, pneumonia, endocarditis, and pericarditis. An oculoglandular syndrome due to *Listeria*, characterized by keratoconjunctivitis, corneal ulceration, and regional lymphadenitis, also has been described. Primary skin infection due to *L. monocytogenes* is rare but does occur.

An infectious mononucleosis–like syndrome was the 1st disorder of humans with which *L. monocytogenes* was associated. The Paul-Bunnell heterophile antibody test is negative in these patients. The organism may be a secondary invader in the sense that the disease may be due to EB virus, but *L. monocytogenes* in some manner interferes with heterophil antibody production.

Diagnosis. A history of animal contact should be noted. However, listeriosis occurs as frequently in individuals without history of exposure to domestic or wild animals as in those with it. *Listeria* infection should be suspected in every newborn child with signs and symptoms of septicemia, pneumonia, or meningitis and in children with malignancies who are receiving therapy with immunosuppressive agents. Appropriate materials for culture vary with the clinical diagnosis. If neonatal listeriosis is sought, cultures of the blood, cerebrospinal fluid, meconium, urine, and exudate expressed from an incised skin papule should be cultured. Cultures should also be obtained from the vagina and cervix of the mother and, if possible, from the placenta and lochia. Cerebrospinal fluid findings in cases of *Listeria* meningitis, similar to those observed in patients with other forms of bacterial meningitis, show a preponderance of polymorphonuclear leukocytes or elevated protein concentration and depressed glucose.

· The microbiology laboratory should be alerted when the possibility of listeriosis is considered so that confusion with diphtheroids can be minimized. Most strains of *Listeria* can be primarily isolated on conventional media within 1–2 days. Although a rise in agglutinins may occur 2–4 wk after the onset of infection, most investigators feel that serodiagnosis is unreliable because agglutinins to *Listeria* may be found in up to 90% of animals and man.

Differential Diagnosis. Listeriosis must be differentiated by appropriate cultures from all other forms of bacterial septicemia and meningitis. In the rare cases in which atypical lymphocytes are noted, toxoplasmosis and infection due to EB virus, cytomegalovirus, and hepatitis viruses must be excluded by appropriate cultures and serologic tests.

Prevention. Listeriosis of the newborn infant might be preventable by prompt recognition and vigorous treatment of maternal listeriosis. Since *Listeria* infection in pregnancy is generally mild and symptoms and signs nonspecific; prevention may be difficult. The ingestion of unpasteurized milk or contaminated water should be avoided.

Treatment. The sensitivity of strains of *L. monocytogenes* varies considerably. Most strains are sensitive by tube dilution in vitro to concentrations of erythromycin, tetracycline, penicillin G, and ampicillin that can be achieved in vivo. Many strains also are sensitive to chloramphenicol.

Generally, therapy should be initiated with ampicillin in a dose and route appropriate for the type of infection and the age of the patient. The sensitivity of each isolate should be tested and changes in therapy made if necessary. Tetracycline should not be used in pregnant women or in children under 8 yr of age because this drug may stain the deciduous or permanent teeth.

Prognosis. If listeriosis is acquired transplacentally,

the fetus is almost always aborted. The death rate of infants affected at or near term is greater than 50%. The mortality of listerial pneumonia noted within the 1st 12 hr of birth approaches 100%. Mortality varies from 20–50% if disease develops between the 5th–30th days of life. Early treatment of listerial septicemia and meningitis in older infants and children who are not immunologically compromised is associated with recovery in as many as 95% of cases. Mental retardation, paralysis, and hydrocephalus have been noted in survivors of *Listeria* meningitis.

Albritton WL: Neonatal listeriosis: Distribution of serotypes in relation to age at onset of disease. J Pediatr 88:481, 1976.

Dykes A, Baraff LJ, Herzog P: Listeria brain abscess in an immunosuppressed child. J Pediatr 94:72, 1979.

Gordon RC, Barrett FF, Yow MD: Ampicillin treatment of listeriosis. J Pediatr 77:1067, 1970.

Halliday HL, Hirata T: Perinatal listeriosis—a review of twelve patients. Am J Obstet Gynecol 133:405, 1979.

Larsson S: Epidemiology of listeriosis in Sweden 1958–1974. Scand J Infect Dis 11:47, 1979.

10.39 ANTHRAX

Anthrax is a well-known infection of animals which is transmissible to humans. The name is derived from the Greek word for *coal* and refers to the black eschar characteristic of cutaneous forms of the disease.

Etiology. *Bacillus anthracis* is a nonmotile, encapsulated, spore-forming, gram-positive bacillus. Spores are formed under aerobic conditions and are relatively resistant, surviving for years in soil and various animal products.

Epidemiology. Anthrax has decreased progressively in incidence in the United States since 1910. Worldwide, 10,000–100,000 cases occur each yr. In the United States 80% are the result of contact with goat hair, wool, or other animal products imported from Asia, Africa, and the Middle East. Skin infections have followed contact with commercially available products, including imported wool and shaving brushes.

Pathogenesis and Pathology. *Cutaneous anthrax* is the result of subepidermal inoculation of anthrax spores. The spores multiply and produce toxin with resultant tissue necrosis and formation of a black eschar.

Pulmonary anthrax is the result of inhalation of anthrax spores into the alveolar spaces. After phagocytosis the spores are transported to regional lymph nodes where replication and production of toxin may ensue. Septicemia and, occasionally, meningitis and death may follow. Mediastinal nodes may become edematous and hemorrhagic. As they enlarge, compression of the bronchi may occur. Direct depression of the central nervous system due to toxin may occur. Primary pneumonitis following inhalation is unusual, but respiratory failure and death may follow thrombosis of pulmonary capillaries.

When spores of *B. anthracis* are ingested, *gastrointestinal anthrax* may develop. The spores multiply and elaborate toxin, producing a necrotic lesion of the terminal ileum or cecum. Hemorrhage may follow.

Clinical Manifestations. The incubation period of cutaneous anthrax is usually 2–5 days. A small macule develops and rapidly becomes vesicular. As the initial lesion enlarges, the center becomes hemorrhagic and necrotic. A black eschar forms and enlarges. The eschar may be surrounded by vesicles and by firm nonpitting edema. Systemic symptoms include low-grade fever, malaise, and, occasionally, regional lymphadenopathy. Sometimes, atypical skin lesions may be the only cutaneous manifestation of disease; these may be small pinpoint black macules that never become vesicular. More than 90% of all cases of anthrax are cutaneous in form. Lesions on the arms are more common than those on the fingers; anthrax lesions on the legs rarely occur.

The incubation period of pulmonary anthrax is 1–5 days. Malaise, myalgia, and low-grade fever are noted initially. A nonproductive cough may develop and rhonchi may be heard. After a period of 2–4 days severe respiratory distress may develop. Pulse, respiratory rate, and temperature increase; dyspnea and cyanosis may be severe. Moist rales, pleural effusion, and subcutaneous edema of the chest and neck may be noted. Death within 24 hr generally follows the development of severe respiratory distress.

Gastrointestinal anthrax is the result of ingestion of contaminated meat. After an incubation period of 2–5 days, anorexia, nausea, vomiting, and fever may be observed. Hematemesis and bloody diarrhea may be noted. Shock and death may occur.

Meningitis follows untreated cutaneous anthrax in 5% of cases. The skin has been implicated as the primary site of infection in more than 50% of cases, but the skin lesion may no longer be apparent at the time signs and symptoms of meningeal infection are noted. Cerebrospinal fluid of most patients with anthrax meningitis is hemorrhagic but may be purulent. Cultures of cerebrospinal fluid generally are positive for *B. anthracis*. Encephalomyelitis and cortical hemorrhages may be noted.

Diagnosis. This should be considered when there are typical skin lesions and a history of exposure to the organism. Recovery of *B. anthracis* from the exudate or the eschar confirms the diagnosis. Pulmonary anthrax may be identified by recovery of the organism from pleural fluid or, rarely, from sputum. A history of the ingestion of contaminated meat should suggest gastrointestinal anthrax.

Differential Diagnosis. Cutaneous anthrax must be differentiated from skin lesions due to *S. aureus*, *F. tularensis*, *Y. pestis*, *P. aeruginosa*, *A. hydrophila*, and vaccinia.

Prevention. This depends upon avoidance of contacts with infected animals or animal products. A cell-free vaccine is available for individuals who are at high risk from occupational exposure.

Treatment. The drug of choice is penicillin. Mild disease can be treated with penicillin V in a dose of 50,000 units/kg/24 hr in 4 divided oral doses, continued for 7–10 days. Moderate or severe cutaneous disease can be treated with procaine penicillin, 30,000–40,000 units/kg/24 hr, administered intramuscularly in 3 divided doses for 7 days. Tetracycline, 15 mg/kg/24 hr in 4 divided doses orally for 7 days, can be used for the treatment of those sensitive to penicillin. The cutaneous lesion should be cleansed and covered; excision is not recommended and may lead to intensification of symptoms.

Pulmonary and meningeal anthrax are treated with aqueous penicillin G intravenously in a dose of 400,000 units/kg/24 hr in 6 divided doses continued for at least 10 days. Specific antitoxin has been used in some cases; its use has been associated with a decrease in mortality from 28% to 6% in patients without meningeal or pulmonary anthrax. Supportive care must also be provided.

Prognosis. Despite antibiotic treatment the mortality rate in anthrax meningitis approaches 100%; that of pulmonary anthrax exceeds 90%. The mortality rate in untreated cutaneous anthrax is 10–20% but is less than 1% with penicillin treatment. The mortality rate of gastrointestinal anthrax is 25–50%.

Brachman PS: Anthrax. In: Hoeprich PD (ed): Infectious Diseases. Ed 2. Hagerstown, Md., Harper & Row, 1977.
Manios S, Kavaliotis I: Anthrax in children: A long forgotten potentially fatal infection. Scand J Infect Dis 11:203, 1979.
Plotkin SA, Brachman PS, Utell M, et al: An epidemic of inhalation anthrax, the first in the twentieth century. Am J Med 29:992, 1960.

10.40   TETANUS

Tetanus is an acute toxemic illness caused by a soluble exotoxin (tetanospasmin) of the bacterium *Clostridium tetani*. The toxin is ordinarily produced by the vegetative forms of the organism at a site of injury and is subsequently transported to and fixed within the central nervous system.

Etiology. *Clostridium tetani*, an obligate anaerobe, is a gram-positive, nonencapsulated, slender, motile rod. The organism forms terminal spores which resemble drumsticks. The spores are resistant to many injurious agents, including boiling, but can be destroyed by autoclaving. They can survive in soil for years if not exposed to sunlight. They may be found in house dust, soil, salt and fresh water, and the feces of many animal species. Both spores and vegetative organisms may be found in the intestinal contents of humans. The vegetative forms of *C. tetani* are susceptible to heat and many disinfectants.

Tetanus bacilli are not invasive. Two toxins are produced, tetanospasmin and tetanolysin. The tetanospasmins produced by several types of antigenically different tetanus bacilli are immunologically identical. Tetanospasmin is a neurotoxin and is responsible for the clinical symptoms and signs of disease. With the exception of botulinum toxin, this diffusible protein is the most potent poison known; as little as 130 μg may be lethal for human adults.

Epidemiology. Tetanus occurs throughout the world; in developing countries it is an important cause of neonatal death. Morbidity and mortality rates in the United States generally have been decreasing since 1950, but case fatality rates have remained unchanged at 50–65% for the past 2 decades. Most of the reported cases have occurred between May and October with the highest incidence in the southern states. Factors contributing to the geographic distribution may include climate, the prevalence of spores of *C. tetani* in the soil, and immunization levels in selected population groups. Attack rates for the United States are approximately 1 case/million/yr.

In the United States the incidence of tetanus has been higher in newborn infants than in older children; in 1975, however, the number of reported cases was greatest in children 1–5 yr of age. Males are affected more frequently than females in a ratio of 3:2. Mortality rates for females also have been lower than those for males of the corresponding age group. Newborn males and females are affected with equal frequency, and there is no seasonal variation in the distribution of cases. Most newborn infants with tetanus have been delivered outside a hospital to unimmunized mothers under unsterile conditions.

Pathology. Infections with *C. tetani* remain localized and elicit minimal tissue reaction. Pathologic changes which may occur are secondary events. Pneumonia due to other microorganisms may be related to difficulty in clearing secretions. Degeneration of striated muscles, including the diaphragm, intercostal, psoas, rectus abdominis, and other muscles, may be noted. The principal pathologic changes include loss of stripes, lysis and disappearance of myrofibrils, and bleeding and rupture of muscle bundles. Degenerative changes in the intercostal muscles and diaphragm may contribute, in part, to the ventilatory failure of the patient and also explain the myasthenia which may be observed during convalescence. Vertebral fractures also may occur as a result of tetanic contractions.

Pathogenesis. *C. tetani* is usually introduced into an area of injury as spores. Disease develops only after spores are converted to vegetative organisms, which produce tetanospasmin only under conditions of reduced oxygen potential. Contamination of the umbilical cord is the most common source of infection in the newborn infant. In older children the organisms may be acquired at the time of a traumatic injury. The risk of tetanus is greatest following a deep puncture wound or an injury associated with tissue necrosis, conditions which favor toxin elaboration. However, tetanus has followed minor injuries, and occasionally no portal of entry is found. Under these circumstances it has been presumed that spores previously introduced persisted in normal tissue for months or years and germinated when conditions were favorable. Alternatively, the site of infection may have been the gastrointestinal tract or the tonsillar crypts. Tetanus has followed introduction of *C. tetani* in contaminated sera, vaccines, or suture material.

Tetanospasmin may reach the central nervous system (1) by absorption at myoneural junctions, followed by migration through perineural tissue spaces of nerve trunks, or (2) by transfer by the lymphocytes to blood and then to the central nervous system.

Tetanospasmin acts on the motor end plates in skeletal muscles, the spinal cord, the brain, and the sympathetic nervous system. The toxin interferes with neuromuscular transmission by inhibiting release of acetylcholine from nerve terminals in muscle. Its effects on the spinal cord lead to dysfunction of polysynaptic reflexes. Within the central nervous system tetanospasmin is bound to gangliosides and suppresses inhibitory influences on the motor neurons and interneurons without directly enhancing excitatory synaptic action. The antidromic inhibition of evoked cortical activity is reduced. These actions are similar to those of strychnine and explain the hypertonicity, spasms, and seizures which may be noted. The toxin also produces a fluctuating overactivity of the sympathetic nervous system: tachycardia, labile hypertension, cardiac arrhythmias, peripheral vasoconstriction, profuse sweating, hypercarbia, and increased urinary excretion of catecholamines can be observed.

Once bound to tissue, toxin is neither dissociated nor neutralized by tetanus antitoxin. Antitoxin may prevent binding in the central nervous system if binding has occurred only in the periphery. Antitoxin has no effect upon the germination of the spores of C. *tetani* or multiplication of its vegetative organisms in tissues.

Clinical Manifestations. The incubation period is 3–14 days after injury but may be as short as 1 day or as long as several mo.

There are 3 clinical forms: localized, generalized, and cephalic. *Localized tetanus* produces pain and continuous rigidity and spasm of muscles in proximity to the site of injury. These symptoms may persist for weeks and disappear without sequelae. Occasionally, this form of the disease precedes the development of the generalized disorder. Localized as well as a mild form of generalized tetanus has been seen occasionally in children with chronic otitis media; C. *tetani* may be recovered from the middle ear fluid. The fatality rate of localized tetanus is about 1%.

Generalized tetanus is the most common form of the disease. The onset may be insidious, but trismus is the presenting symptom in over 50% of cases. Spasm of the masseter muscle may be associated with stiffness of the neck muscles and difficulty in swallowing. Restlessness, irritability, and headache are also early findings. Spasm of the facial muscles produces a fixed sardonic grin (risus sardonicus). Shortly, tonic contractions of the somatic musculature become widespread. The lumbar and abdominal muscles may become rigid, and persistent spasm of the back muscles may result in opisthotonos. Tetanic seizures develop, characterized by sudden bursts of tonic contractions of various muscle groups, producing flexion and adduction of the arms, clenching of the fists, and extension of the lower extremities. Initially the spasms are mild, lasting for seconds to several minutes, and are separated by periods of relaxation; with time, they become severe, powerful, and exhausting. Spasms may be precipitated by almost any visual, auditory, or tactile stimulus. The patient is completely conscious during the course of the disease and experiences intense pain. Apprehension is prominent. Spasm of the laryngeal and respiratory muscles may produce respiratory obstruction; cyanosis and asphyxia may ensue. Dysuria or urinary retention may develop secondary to spasms of the bladder sphincter. Alternatively, involuntary defecation and urination may be noted. The forcefulness of the contractions may produce compression fractures of the spine and hemorrhage into muscle. Weakness and sensory loss compatible with a peripheral neuropathy may be noted. The pattern of involvement is usually asymmetrical; the nerves involved most commonly are the ulnar, median, and lateral popliteal. Electrophysiologic studies may reveal no conduction initially with variable rates of recovery over a period of weeks to months.

Elevation of the body temperature generally is mild, but temperatures of 40° C have been noted and are due to the intense output of energy which accompanies tetanic seizures. Hyperhidrosis, tachycardia, hypertension, and cardiac arrhythmias may be observed.

Signs and symptoms increase over a period of 3–7 days, plateau during the course of the 2nd wk, and then abate gradually. Complete recovery takes place in 2–6 wk.

Cephalic tetanus is an unusual form of the disease. It has an incubation period of 1–2 days and follows otitis media or injuries to the head and face, including foreign bodies placed in the nose by the patient. Dysfunction of cranial nerves III, IV, VII, IX, X, and XI is the most prominent feature of the disease. The 7th cranial nerve is affected most frequently. Cephalic disease may be followed by generalized tetanus.

Tetanus neonatorum usually begins when the newborn infant is 3–10 days of age and is generalized in type. Progressive difficulty with sucking and excessive crying are noted. Difficulty in swallowing is soon apparent; shortly thereafter the body becomes stiff, and spasms develop. Opisthotonos may be extreme or absent.

Diagnosis and Differential Diagnosis. The diagnosis of tetanus is made on clinical grounds. Most cases occur in individuals who are unimmunized or in infants of unimmunized mothers. The majority of patients have a history of trauma during the preceding 14 days. When this history is obtained from a patient who develops trismus, generalized muscular stiffness or rigidity, and spasms, and whose sensorium is clear, the diagnosis of tetanus is suggested.

The usual laboratory studies are of little value. The white blood cell count may be normal, or mild polymorphonuclear leukocytosis may be noted. Examination of the cerebrospinal fluid reveals no abnormalities, but the pressure may be elevated by the muscular contractions. The electroencephalogram is normal; electromyography is nonspecific. Wound cultures of patients are positive for C. *tetani* in about one third of patients with clinical evidence of disease. Gram stains of material from the wound may or may not show characteristic organisms. Identification of the organism by Gram stain and isolation in anaerobic cultures are presumptive evidence of tetanus in a patient with appropriate historic and clinical findings; isolation of C. *tetani* from contaminated wounds does not mean that the patient has, or will develop, tetanus.

Tetanus must be differentiated from other local and systemic diseases. Trismus may be associated with alveolar, parapharyngeal, or retropharyngeal abscesses. These conditions can be differentiated from tetanus by careful history, physical examination, and appropriate roentgenographic studies.

Poliomyelitis may be accompanied by stiffness and

spasm early in the course of the illness. In this disease, however, trismus is absent, flaccid paralysis develops, and the cerebrospinal fluid usually shows an elevated protein concentration and pleocytosis. Poliovirus can be isolated from the stool, and the diagnosis can be confirmed by demonstration of a rise in neutralizing antibody.

Other forms of acute or postinfectious encephalitides rarely are associated with trismus, generally have abnormal cerebrospinal fluid findings, and display a clouded sensorium. Bacterial meningitis also is unaccompanied by trismus; examination of cerebrospinal fluid can establish or strongly suggest this diagnosis.

Both *rabies* and tetanus may follow animal bites, and trismus has been noted in some patients with the former. Rabid spasms tend to be intermittent, and clonic rather than tonic. Cerebrospinal fluid pleocytosis may be noted. *C. tetani* is not a common inhabitant of the mouth of the dog. Tetanus toxoid may be given following dogbite to prevent tetanus, which may result from contamination of the wound (a relatively anaerobic environment) by *C. tetani* that may have been present on the skin of the patient at the time of the bite or that may be subsequently introduced into the wound.

A history of ingestion of poisons containing *strychnine* is most helpful in distinguishing this intoxication from tetanus. Trismus is rare and, when it occurs, develops after the onset of generalized tonic activity. Usually, there is complete relaxation between convulsions. Trismus has also been noted in children with phenothiazine poisoning.

Tetany may be characterized by carpopedal spasm and laryngospasm, but trismus is rare. The diagnosis is confirmed by a low serum calcium concentration.

Intestinal obstruction and perforation with development of peritonitis are associated with abdominal rigidity. Generalized muscular spasms and trismus are absent.

Complications. Complications of tetanus can be minimized by strict attention to supportive care and by appropriate therapy. Interference with pulmonary ventilation by respiratory muscle spasm and laryngospasm or by the accumulation of secretions may lead to aspiration pneumonia, atelectasis, mediastinal emphysema, or pneumothorax. The latter 2 findings may complicate tracheostomy. Lacerations of the tongue or buccal mucosa, intramuscular hematomas, and vertebral fractures may follow severe tetanic seizures. If the course is prolonged, malnutrition and dehydration may develop unless strict attention is paid to fluid balance and caloric intake.

Prevention. This is best achieved by active immunization, accomplished usually by a series of 3 intramuscular injections of tetanus toxoid, diphtheria toxoid, and pertussis vaccine. The injections ideally should begin at 2 mo of age and be separated by 8 wk intervals. A 4th dose should be given approximately 1 yr later. A booster is also provided at the time of entrance into kindergarten or elementary school; thereafter a dose of adult-type tetanus and diphtheria toxoid (Td) is recommended once every 10 yr. This approach can be altered to meet local situations. Immunization of previously nonimmune pregnant mothers will provide the

newborn infant with protection immediately following delivery. This is advocated in areas where the incidence of neonatal tetanus is high. Preferably, tetanus immunization should be carried out prior to pregnancy.

Children who have not been immunized by 6 yr should receive a series of 3 doses of adult-type Td intramuscularly. The 2nd dose should be given 4–6 wk after the 1st, and the 3rd 6–12 mo after the 2nd. Thereafter, a Td booster should be given every 10 yr.

Alum-precipitated or aluminum hydroxide–adsorbed tetanus toxoid is preferable for basic immunization. When these toxoids are used and when at least 4 doses have been given, protective levels of tetanus antitoxin (0.01 IU/ml by the toxin neutralization assay) are maintained for at least 10 yr. The actual duration of protection is unknown. For this reason, and because they may be associated with an increased incidence and severity of reactions, routine yearly boosters are not indicated.

Following injury, the preventive measures employed must be dictated by the immunization status of the injured patient and by the characteristics of the injury itself. Immediate and thorough surgical treatment of wounds is mandatory. The wound should be cleansed, necrotic tissue and foreign bodies removed, and, if necessary, more extensive debridement performed. Persons who have not been immunized actively or who have been immunized inadequately should be protected with human tetanus immune globulin (TIG). TIG is given intramuscularly in a dose of 250–500 units. Skin testing for sensitivity prior to injection is not necessary because TIG does not produce serum sickness. If TIG is not available, tetanus antitoxin (TAT) of bovine or equine origin can be given in a dose of 3000–5000 units intramuscularly. Careful screening and testing of the patient for sensitivity to TAT prior to its administration are mandatory; serum sickness may follow use of this material. Tetanus toxoid should be given to initiate active immunity. It may be given at the same time as TIG or TAT if it is administered in another site and in a separate syringe. Neither TIG nor TAT is indicated for prophylaxis following injury in fully immunized children.

If a child who has had at least 4 DTP immunizations is injured and 5 or more yr have elapsed since the last injection, a tetanus toxoid booster is indicated. Fluid toxoid is preferred under these circumstances since it produces a more rapid secondary immune response than precipitated or adsorbed tetanus toxoids. If tetanus immunization is incomplete at the time of the wound, the remainder of the recommended series should be given.

Treatment and Supportive Care. The principal objectives of therapy are to remove the source of tetanospasmin, to neutralize circulating toxin, and to provide supportive care until tetanospasmin which is fixed to neural tissue can be metabolized. Supportive care must be intensive and performed meticulously.

Tetanus immune globulin of human origin, 3000–6000 units, should be given intramuscularly as soon as possible; it should not be given intravenously. Administration of TIG is not followed by allergy or anaphylaxis; higher and more persistent titers of antitoxin are produced than with antitoxin from nonhuman sources. Protective levels are obtained rapidly and decline slowly (half-life, 24 days). Repeated doses are not required. TIG has no effect on toxin that is already fixed to neural tissue and does not penetrate the blood–cerebrospinal fluid barrier, but it can neutralize circulating or uncombined tetanospasmin.

If TIG is not available and skin testing shows no hypersensitivity, TAT can be given in a single dose of 50,000–100,000 units. This antitoxin is divided equally; half the dose is given intramuscularly and half intravenously, with careful observation of the precautions detailed in the package insert. If sensitivity to TAT is demonstrated, desensitization should be carried out as described in the package insert.

Wounds should be cleansed and debrided if necessary. Foreign bodies must be removed and the wound left open. Surgical efforts should be delayed until the patient has been sedated and antitoxin has been administered.

Antibiotic therapy may eradicate vegetative C. tetani organisms, which grow in areas of devitalized tissue where blood supply is poor or absent. For this reason large doses of penicillin G are favored in an effort to promote diffusion into the devitalized area. Penicillin G (200,000 units/kg/24 hr) may be used intravenously in 6 divided doses for 10 days. In patients who are sensitive to penicillin, tetracycline (30–40 mg/kg/24 hr, but not more than 2 gm) in 4 divided oral doses is effective.

Meticulous nursing care is imperative. The patient should be placed in a quiet environment and every effort made to control or eliminate auditory and visual stimuli. A respirator, oxygen, suction, and equipment for tracheostomy should be available. Although tracheostomy need not be considered a routine procedure, it should be performed prior to the development of severe involvement of respiratory muscles or laryngospasm.

Muscle relaxants should be given to all patients with tetanus. Diazepam has proved to be quite effective in controlling hypertonicity and spasms. It may be used in a dose of 0.1–0.2 mg/kg every 3–6 hr intravenously or intramuscularly as needed. Chlorpromazine and mephenesin also have been utilized but seem to be less effective. Two–6 wk of therapy may be required; the dose may be tapered as tetanic activity decreases.

Neuromuscular blocking agents such as D-tubocurarine and, more recently, pancuronium bromide (0.05 mg/kg/dose given every 2–3 hr intravenously as needed) have been used either to control seizures while sparing respiration or to produce complete respiratory paralysis which is then managed by artificial ventilation. The latter technique has produced the best survival rates but can be utilized only in centers where continuous intensive care and highly trained respiratory care teams are available.

Patients receiving sedation and muscle relaxants must be monitored continually and suctioned frequently. Adequate ventilation must be ensured. Respiratory depression should be avoided and treated promptly if it occurs.

The patient should be weighed daily. Intake and output of fluids should be monitored carefully. An adequate intake of fluid, electrolytes, and calories should be maintained. The oral route may be used in some patients; generally, intravenous infusion and/or nasogastric intubation are required. In selected patients gastrostomy may be necessary. Attention must be paid to care of the mouth, skin, bladder, and bowel.

The newborn infant has special problems relating to ventilation, hydration, and sedation. If possible, therapy should be aggressive and utilize endotracheal intubation, neuromuscular blocking agents, and assisted ventilation. Where facilities are not available, sedatives and muscle relaxants may be given orally. Syrup of chlorpromazine (3 mg every 6 hr), elixir of phenobarbital (10–20 mg every 6 hr), or elixir of mephenesin (130–160 mg every 6 hr) may be used. Diazepam may be given intravenously in a dose of 0.3 mg/kg and repeated as needed to control severe spasms. Excision of the umbilicus is no longer recommended.

Prognosis. The average mortality of tetanus is 45–55%; rates for neonatal tetanus are at 60% or greater.

Prognosis is affected by a number of factors. The highest mortality is found at the extremes of life; the lowest occurs in patients 10–19 yr of age (less than 20%). Extensive muscle involvement, high fever, and a short interval between injury and appearance of clinical manifestations or between the 1st evidence of trismus and the 1st generalized convulsion correlate with low survival rates. Patients who have localized disease or whose disease begins after a longer incubation period as well as those who remain afebrile have a better chance of recovery. Fatalities in severe cases usually occur during the 1st wk of disease. Prognosis also depends to a large extent upon the quality of supportive care provided for the patient.

Recovery from tetanus does not confer immunity; therefore, active immunization of the patient following recovery is imperative.

Adams JM, Kenny JD, Rudolph AJ: Modern management of tetanus neonatorum. Pediatrics 64:472, 1979.
Armitage P, Clifford R: Prognosis in tetanus: Use of data from therapeutic trials. J Infect Dis 138:1, 1978.
Blake PA, Feldman RA, Buchanan TM, et al: Serologic therapy of tetanus in the United States, 1965–1971. JAMA 235:42, 1976.
Corbett JL, Kerr JH, Prys-Roberts C, et al: Cardiovascular disturbances in severe tetanus due to overactivity of the sympathetic nervous system. Anesthesia 24:198, 1969.
LaForce FM, Young LS, Bennett JV: Tetanus in the United States (1965–1966): Epidemiologic and clinical features. N Engl J Med 280:569, 1969.
Peebles TC, Levine L, Eldred MC, et al: Tetanus-toxoid emergency boosters; a reappraisal. N Engl J Med 280:575, 1969.
Shahani M, Dastur FD, Dastoor DH, et al: Neuropathy in tetanus. J Neurol Sci 43:173, 1979.
Stanfield JP, Gall D, Bracken PM: Single-dose antenatal tetanus immunization. Lancet 1:215, 1973.
Weinstein L: Tetanus. N Engl J Med 289:1293, 1973.

OTHER CLOSTRIDIAL INFECTIONS

Clostridia other than C. tetani have been associated with a variety of disorders, including gas gangrene, food poisoning, necrotizing enteritis, and botulism.

Some of these disorders are the result of elaboration of toxin by vegetative organisms.

10.41   Gas Gangrene

Gas gangrene is an invasive anaerobic infection of soft tissues, including muscle, characterized by extensive tissue necrosis, variable degrees of gas production, and profound toxemia.

Etiology.   Six species of *Clostridium* are capable of producing gas gangrene: *C. perfringens* (formerly *C. welchii*), *C. novyi*, *C. septicum*, *C. histolyticum*, *C. bifermentans*, and *C. fallax*. These organisms are gram-positive rods which rarely produce spores in tissue or in culture media. All are obligate anaerobes measuring 0.5 × 1–5 μm. In the vegetative form they can be destroyed by many chemical and physical agents. Vegetative forms also produce a variety of toxins; the most significant are lecithinase (α-toxin), collagenase, hyaluronidase, leukocidin, deoxyribonuclease, protease, and lipase.

Epidemiology.   Gas gangrene is uncommon in the United States. The incidence in postoperative wounds or in civilian trauma has been estimated at less than 0.1%. Spores of clostridia associated with gas gangrene may enter tissues from the soil or may gain entry from the gastrointestinal or female genital tracts, their sites of carriage in normal individuals.

Pathogenesis and Pathology.   Development of gas gangrene depends on (1) contamination of a traumatized area with clostridia, and (2) the presence of devitalized tissue with decreased oxidation-reduction potential. Trauma, ischemia, the presence of a foreign body, or the presence of infection due to other bacteria may induce an anaerobic environment. The toxins elaborated by the multiplying clostridia are responsible for the gas gangrene syndrome. Lecithinases, particularly those elaborated by *C. perfringens*, destroy cell membranes and alter capillary permeability. A toxin produced by *C. histolyticum* also can digest tissues rapidly. Necrosis in tissues surrounding a local lesion and thrombosis of regional blood vessels develop. As bacterial multiplication proceeds, gas (hydrogen and carbon dioxide) is liberated and may be palpated in the tissues. Edema and swelling intensify, and overwhelming septicemia, shock, and death finally ensue. The precise nature of the toxemia and the ultimate cause of death remain poorly defined.

Clinical Manifestations.   The syndrome of *simple clostridial contamination* results from multiplication of clostridia in a wound, with little pain and no systemic reaction. Typical lesions appear deep and ragged, and a foul-smelling, brownish-black, seropurulent exudate may be noted. Healing proceeds slowly. Generally, anaerobic streptococci are recovered from these wounds in addition to the various species of clostridia.

Anaerobic cellulitis may appear de novo or may complicate simple contamination in about 5% of cases. The incubation period of anaerobic cellulitis is 3–4 days. Anaerobic cellulitis (gas abscess, localized gas gangrene, brown form of gas gangrene) is a clostridial infection of necrotic tissue already devitalized by ischemia or trauma. Healthy muscle remains uninvolved. Constitutional reactions are minimal. The wound appears dirty, has a foul odor, and may be locally crepitant. A moderate or profuse brownish, seropurulent discharge is present. Pain is minimal, and discoloration and edema of areas of skin surrounding the lesion are rare.

Anaerobic myonecrosis is the most serious form of gas gangrene. The incubation period may be as short as hours or as long as 1–2 mo; generally, it is less than 3 days. The onset of disease is acute, beginning with pain in the region of the wound. Localized edema and swelling are noted. The patients appear extremely ill and become pale and sweaty. Hypotension, delirium, or agitation can be noted. Jaundice may be a late manifestation. A profuse serosanguineous discharge with a sweet odor is noted at the site of the local lesion. Gas is minimal or absent. The discharge contains numerous organisms but no polymorphonuclear leukocytes. Muscle at the site of infection may be edematous and pale; as the infection progresses, its color changes to brick red, contractility is lost, and bleeding from the muscle surface ceases. Invasion of the bloodstream is a rare and unusual complication of myonecrosis; the systemic clinical findings are a reflection of elaboration of toxin. Bloodstream invasion may follow anaerobic endometritis (as in septic abortion or after prolonged rupture of membranes) or necrotizing infection of the gastrointestinal tract. The presence of clostridia in the bloodstream is not always apparent clinically. Conversely, clostridial bacteremia can lead to massive hemolysis of red blood cells, acute tubular necrosis, and death.

Infection caused by toxigenic clostridia also may involve the eye, brain, pleural cavity, lung, or liver. Gas gangrene may follow penetrating wounds of the chest wall which have been contaminated by soil.

Diagnosis and Differential Diagnosis.   The diagnosis of clostridial infection must be made early and be based on clinical findings. The appearance of the site of infection usually suggests the diagnosis; the specific clinical syndrome should be defined since this dictates the choice of therapy. Large gram-positive rods may be found in smears of the discharge. *C. perfringens* does not sporulate in tissues, but other clostridia may do so. Toxigenic clostridia may be recovered if anaerobic cultures are obtained; their isolation from a site of injury does not necessarily indicate that they are causing the disease. Roentgenograms may help to document the presence and location of gas in tissues.

Two disorders must be differentiated from gas gangrene. *Postoperative synergistic gangrene* usually begins the 2nd wk after surgery or injury. An enlarging ulcer with a gray purulent center surrounded by a red area of cellulitis is noted. The lesion evolves slowly. Fever and anemia develop, and death may ensue. This disorder is due to the synergistic multiplication of *Staphylococcus aureus* and microaerophilic *Streptococcus* series.

Necrotizing fasciitis is an infection of subcutaneous tissues following surgery or trauma. This disease also is associated with *Streptococcus* sp. or with *S. aureus*. Fever and hypovolemia occur, and death may follow within 3 days. In contrast to clostridial myositis, necrotizing fasciitis is characterized by hypesthesia or anesthesia of skin over the involved fascia, and the skin can be elevated readily from the necrotic fascia. No gas is found and no delirium is noted.

Prevention. The cornerstone of prevention is recognition of wounds prone to develop gas gangrene. Early, careful, and adequate debridement is imperative. All foreign bodies should be removed. Primary wound closure is best avoided. Penicillin G may be administered parenterally, but there is no evidence to suggest that its use will prevent gas gangrene in the absence of adequate surgery. There is no effective active immunization against gas gangrene. The effectiveness of antitoxin given prophylactically to patients with wounds contaminated by clostridia has not been established.

Treatment. Surgical excision of infected tissue is the accepted method of management. Penicillin G (250,000 units/kg/24 hr) in 6 divided doses intravenously should be provided to eradicate organisms not removed surgically. Chloramphenicol, erythromycin, and cephalosporins may be effective alternatives in patients allergic to penicillin.

Hyperbaric oxygen therapy may be helpful if suitable facilities are available. The value of polyvalent antitoxin in therapy of gas gangrene is unproved. Since this serum is of equine origin, its administration may be followed by serum sickness. In addition, commercially available antisera neutralize only a few of the many toxins elaborated by clostridia.

Altemeier WA, Fullen WD: Prevention and treatment of gas gangrene. JAMA 217:806, 1971.
Darke SG, King AM, Slack WK: Gas gangrene and related infection: Classification, clinical features, and aetiology, management and mortality: A report of 88 cases. Br J Surg 64:104, 1977.
Weinstein L, Barza MA: Gas gangrene. N Engl J Med 289:1129, 1973.

10.42 Food Poisoning, Necrotizing Enteritis, and Antibiotic-Associated Pseudomembranous Colitis Due to Clostridia

Etiology. C. perfringens is a common cause of food poisoning. Disease follows ingestion of C. perfringens type A. Necrotizing enteritis is extremely rare and is associated with ingestion of C. perfringens type F. Pigbel, an epidemic disease seen during periods of pig-feasting among New Guinea highlanders, has been related to ingestion of C. perfringens type C. Antibiotic-associated pseudomembranous colitis is related to elaboration of a toxin by C. difficile.

Epidemiology. Disease is acquired by ingestion of strains of C. perfringens capable of forming spores. These organisms can be found in the feces of normal individuals or animals and in raw meat. When food contaminated with C. perfringens is cooled to temperatures that permit spores to survive and then is permitted to stand, growth of vegetative organisms and elaboration of toxin may occur. The symptoms produced after ingestion appear to be the result of both tissue invasion and toxin production.

Antibiotic-associated pseudomembranous colitis is the result of administration of an antibiotic that alters the flora of the gastrointestinal tract permitting an overgrowth of C. difficile with elaboration of toxin which has cytopathic effects on the mucosa. This condition has been associated most commonly with clindamycin therapy, but it also may follow administration of other antibiotics (penicillin, ampicillin, cephalosporins, amoxicillin, tetracycline).

Clinical Manifestations. Within 12–24 hr following ingestion of food contaminated with C. perfringens type A, abdominal pain and diarrhea develop. Nausea and vomiting are rare. Fever is absent or low grade, and other constitutional symptoms are minimal. Duration of illness generally is 24–48 hr.

Necrotizing enteritis is an illness with an acute onset characterized by severe abdominal pain, vomiting, diarrhea, and shock. Necrosis of gastrointestinal mucosa, associated with submucosal gas cysts, hemorrhage, and thrombosis of submucosal vessels, may occur and explain the severity of the clinical picture. Fatalities are common.

Antibiotic-associated pseudomembranous colitis is characterized by the development of abdominal pain, diarrhea with mucus and blood, and occasional intestinal perforation. Symptoms usually abate when the antibiotic that has played a causative role in the illness is discontinued.

Diagnosis. C. perfringens may be isolated by appropriate anaerobic cultures of contaminated food. The same bacteria also may be recovered from the stools of infected patients. Studies may be performed to document toxin elaboration, and antibodies against C. perfringens enterotoxin can be measured in the serum of the patient following recovery.

The diagnosis of antibiotic-associated pseudomembranous colitis can be made by recovery of C. difficile from the stools and documentation in vitro that the organism recovered produces a cytopathic toxin.

Prevention. Disease can be prevented by cooking food thoroughly. If it is necessary for food to stand prior to ingestion, it should be stored at temperatures below 5° C or above 50° C.

Treatment. Gastroenteritis due to C. perfringens type A is usually self-limited. Adequate hydration should be maintained. Necrotizing enteritis and antibiotic-associated pseudomembranous colitis must be treated in hospital with appropriate fluids and electrolytes and by surgery designed to remove gangrenous portions of the bowel. The offending antibiotic must be discontinued when pseudomembranous colitis follows antibiotic administration. Antibiotics designed to prevent septicemia by organisms normally found in the gastrointestinal tract may be administered. Vancomycin, 2000 mg/1.73M²/24 hr in 4 divided doses, has been well tolerated and effective in eliminating C. difficile and its toxin from the stools of children with antibiotic-induced colitis.

Bartlett JG, Chang TW, Gurwith M, et al: Antibiotic-associated pseudomembranous colitis due to toxin producing clostridia. N Engl J Med 298:531, 1978.
Johnson WD, Hook EW: Gastroenterocolitis syndromes. In: Hoeprich PD (ed): Infectious Disease. Ed 2. Hagerstown Md., Harper & Row, 1977.
Killingbac MJ, Williams LK: Necrotizing colitis. Br J Surg 48:175, 1961.

10.43 Botulism

Three forms of botulism have been described: (1) food-borne botulism (an intoxication that results from improperly preserved food that contains preformed botulinum toxin); (2) wound botulism (the result of wound infection by toxin-producing *C botulinum* organisms); and (3) infant botulism (caused by germination of spores of *C. botulinum* in the gastrointestinal tract with toxin production in vivo).

Etiology. *C. botulinum* is a motile, anaerobic, gram-positive bacterium which produces heat-resistant spores. If the spores survive food-processing, they may germinate and elaborate toxins. Six antigenically distinct toxins have been identified (A, B, C, D, E, F), but only types A, B, E, and F have been associated with human disease.

Epidemiology. Between 1899–1969, 659 outbreaks of botulism affecting 1696 individuals were reported in the United States, resulting in 959 fatalities. Home-preserved foods were the most frequent cause of intoxication. In North America botulism is most frequently associated with type A toxin. In Scandinavian countries, Japan, and Canada, 50% of outbreaks are caused by type E toxin. In Europe type B toxin has produced most outbreaks.

Rarely, botulism may follow contamination of a wound by *C. botulinum* with subsequent toxin production in vivo. Recently, botulism has been reported in infants. Ingestion of honey appears to be an important risk factor in producing the disease as exposure has been documented in about 35% of cases. A California study also suggests an increased risk of infantile botulism in bottle-fed babies compared to breast-fed babies and in both bottle- and breast-fed infants who are supplemented with iron. Spores also have been found in a sample of vacuum cleaner dust collected at the home of 1 afflicted infant and in 3 soil samples from the yards of several affected infants.

Pathology and Pathogenesis. Following ingestion, toxins are absorbed from the gastrointestinal tract and are transported by lymphocytes or blood to the motor nerve terminals. Affinity of the toxins for nervous tissue varies. Type A is bound with great affinity; type E binds more slowly than type A but more quickly than type B. Type B botulinum toxin has been demonstrated in serum as long as 3 wk after ingestion of contaminated food.

The toxin inhibits release of acetylcholine at the prejunction region of terminal nerve fibers. A suppressive effect on motor neurons in the spinal cord has been demonstrated. In general, the effect of toxin on the brain is negligible, but cranial nerve terminals are affected early, and patients may aspirate or develop asphyxia and cardiac arrhythmias.

Clinical Manifestations. Signs and symptoms are similar for all types of botulinal intoxication. The usual incubation period is 12–36 hr with a range of several hr to 8 days.

Nausea, vomiting, diplopia, dysphagia, dysarthria, and dry mouth are common manifestations. Weakness, postural hypotension, urinary retention, and constipation may develop. The patient remains alert at the outset but, with time, may become somnolent.

Physical examination generally reveals an afebrile patient with normal pulse rate. Ptosis, meiosis, nystagmus, and paresis of extraocular muscles may be perceived. Mucous membranes of the mouth, tongue, and pharynx are dry, and lacrimation may cease. Respiratory efforts may be impaired. Sensory examination is normal.

In the *newborn infant* signs and symptoms are similar. When poor sucking or swallowing, weakness, poor head control, hypotonia, ptosis, mydriasis, and ophthalmoplegia are observed in an afebrile infant with a normal cerebrospinal fluid examination, botulism must be considered.

C. botulinum organisms were isolated from the stools of 10 California infants who died suddenly and unexpectedly; 9 deaths were ascribed to sudden infant death syndrome (SIDS). *C. botulinum* also has been recovered from the stools of several infants with SIDS from Utah and Washington. These findings coupled with the concordant age distribution of infantile botulism (1–6 mo of age) and SIDS suggest that infantile botulism may be a cause of SIDS in some cases.

Diagnosis and Differential Diagnosis. The diagnosis is confirmed by demonstrating botulinal toxin in food the patient has ingested or in the patient's serum or stool. The diagnosis of infantile botulism is established only by identification of *C. botulinum* organisms in the feces since they are not part of the normal bowel flora of infants. Inoculation of mice with serum from the affected patient identifies toxin by neutralization with specific known antitoxins.

Botulism must be differentiated from myasthenia gravis, poliomyelitis, Guillain-Barré syndrome, other forms of chemical or food poisoning, trichinosis, diphtheria, and various forms of electrolyte or mineral imbalance. A characteristic electromyographic pattern known as brief, small, abundant motor-unit action potentials (BSAP) frequently has been found. Its absence, however, does not exclude the diagnosis of botulism. An EMG pattern of post-tetanic facilitation also has been observed in infantile botulism.

Myasthenia gravis is differentiated by the fatigability of muscle noted in this disease and by response to edrophonium chloride (Tensilon) or neostigmine.

Guillain-Barré syndrome is associated with myalgia, paresthesias, occasional sensory deficits, and an elevated concentration of cerebrospinal fluid protein.

Cranial nerve involvement is usually absent in other forms of food poisoning, and diarrhea is more prominent.

Other infectious diseases, including poliomyelitis and encephalitis, are generally accompanied by fever, and cranial nerve involvement is less prominent than that noted in patients with botulism.

Prevention. Boiling for 10 min will destroy the toxin. A pressure cooker (115.5° C or 240° F) is required to kill spores of *C. botulinum*; pressure requirements vary with the food being processed.

Treatment. All individuals known to have ingested toxin should be hospitalized. Vomiting should be induced and gastric lavage initiated. Magnesium sulfate or other cathartics may be placed in the stomach at the conclusion of lavage. A high enema should be given to facilitate elimination of unabsorbed toxin.

Cardiac and respiratory function must be monitored carefully. Tracheostomy should be performed before respiratory impairment becomes severe.

Antitoxin has been efficacious. Three preparations of equine origin are available and can be obtained in the United States on a 24 hr basis from the Center for Disease Control, Atlanta, Georgia. The polyvalent preparation is preferred until the toxin type has been identified. Skin sensitivity testing is mandatory prior to administration of the antitoxin.

Penicillin G is recommended to kill *C. botulinum*, which may continue to produce toxin. Aqueous penicillin G should be given parenterally in a dose of 50,000 units/kg/24 hr in 4–6 divided doses. Penicillin G may also be given orally in a dose of 1,600,000 units/24 hr in 4 divided doses after lavage has been concluded.

Hypotension should be treated with appropriate intravenous fluids; fluid and electrolyte balance must be maintained.

Newborn infants with this disease seem to be less severely affected. Most have responded to supportive treatment and recovered without antitoxin. Penicillin therapy has been provided for infants with botulism, but neither oral nor parenteral penicillin administration has succeeded in producing discernible clinical benefit in some patients. Moreover, it does not eradicate either *C. botulinum* organisms or botulinal toxin from the intestine. In some cases parenteral aminoglycoside antibiotics may act synergistically with botulinal toxin at the neuromuscular junction and exacerbate the paralysis.

Prognosis. Severity of illness is directly proportional to the quantity of toxin ingested. A short incubation period is associated with more severe disease. The earlier specific treatment is given, the better the prognosis. Recovery will be complete with appropriate supportive care. Prognosis is excellent in infantile botulism; recovery generally occurs over a period of weeks. Long after recovery, fecal excretion of *C. botulinum* organisms may persist. Excretion of type A organisms and type A botulinum toxin persists longer than does excretion of type B organisms or type B botulinum toxin.

Arnon SS: Infant botulism. Ann Rev Med 31:541, 1980.

Gangarosa EJ: Botulism. *In:* Hoeprich PD (ed): Infectious Diseases. Ed 2. Hagerstown Md., Harper & Row, 1977.

Gangarosa EJ, Donadio JA, Armstrong RW, et al: Botulism in the United States, 1899–1969. Am J Epidemiol 93:93, 1971.

Merson MH, Dowell VR Jr: Epidemiologic, clinical and laboratory aspects of wound botulism. N Engl J Med 289:1105, 1973.

Pickett J, Berg B, Chaplin E, et al: Syndrome of botulism in infancy; clinical and electrophysiologic study. N Engl J Med 295:770, 1976.

Wilke BW Jr, Midura TF, Arnon SS: Quantitative evidence of intestinal colonization by *Clostridium botulinum* in four cases of infant botulism. J Infect Dis 141:419, 1980.

10.44 ANAEROBIC INFECTIONS OTHER THAN CLOSTRIDIAL

Anaerobic bacteria have been recognized as a cause of human disease since 1896. As recently as 1968, Sanders and Stevenson revie·d the literature and could identify only 36 children with anaerobic infections. Recent advances in techniques for recovering anaerobic bacteria, coupled with an increasing awareness of the possible role they play in producing clinical disease, have permitted a more reliable assessment of the prevalence and significance of anaerobic microorganisms as a cause of infection in infants and children.

Etiology. Anaerobic bacteria are present in soil and constitute a part of the normal human flora; they are found on all mucous membranes, particularly in the mouth and gastrointestinal tract. In the mouth and vagina and on the skin anaerobic bacteria outnumber aerobic bacteria by 10 to 1. In the colon anaerobic bacteria outnumber facultative bacteria by 100 to 1.

Anaerobic bacteria are microorganisms to which oxygen is toxic, but strains vary considerably in their ability to tolerate oxygen. Some strains survive in the presence of oxygen but grow better when the oxygen in their environment is reduced *(facultative anaerobes)*. *Obligate anaerobes* do not grow on the surface of blood agar plates incubated aerobically or even in an environment enriched with CO_2. Obligate anaerobes predominate in the normal human flora. A classification of anaerobic microorganisms is given in Table 10–26.

Epidemiology. Blood, intra-abdominal sources, and soft tissues are the principal sites from which anaerobes are recovered during infection in infancy and childhood. Except in blood cultures, several anaerobes or both anaerobes and aerobes are recovered concomitantly from sites of infection.

Symptomatic anaerobic infection occurs infrequently in a general pediatric population. In a large prospective study in which anaerobes were sought routinely, only 0.3% of blood cultures during a 1 yr period contained anaerobic organisms that were involved in the pathogenesis of the patients' diseases. In contrast, pathogenic aerobic microorganisms were recovered from 9% of the cultures. Anaerobes accounted for 5.8% of all bacter-

Table 10–26 CLASSIFICATION OF REPRESENTATIVE ANAEROBES

Nonspore-forming gram-negative bacilli
  Bacteroides: B. fragilis, B. oralis, B. melaninogenicus, B. corrodens
  Fusobacterium: F. nucleatum, F. varium, F. necrophorum, F. mortiferum
Spore-forming gram-positive bacilli
  Clostridia: C. perfringens (welchii), C. tetani, C. botulinum, C. novyi, C. septicum, C. ramosum
Nonspore-forming gram-positive bacilli: *Actinomyces, Arachnia, Bifidobacterium, Eubacterium, Propionibacterium, Lactobacillus*
Gram-positive cocci: *Peptococcus, Peptostreptococcus,* microaerophilic cocci
Gram-negative cocci: *Veillonella, Acidaminococcus, Megasphaera*

emic episodes (8.7% in the newborn period and 4.8% in children over 1 yr of age); 10.1% of newborn infants whose clinical disease was associated with bacteremia had anaerobic sepsis (aerobes were not recovered concomitantly).

The major clinical settings in which anaerobic infection of children might be anticipated are (1) birth following prolonged rupture of the membranes, amnionitis, or obstetrical difficulty; (2) peritonitis or septicemia associated with intestinal obstruction and perforation or with appendicitis; and (3) congenital or acquired disorders that impair the response of the host to infection.

Pathogenesis.   Normally, anaerobes are of low virulence for humans. Multiplication and invasion are favored by any process which creates a more favorable environment by removing oxygen or by adding reducing substances which lower the oxidation-reduction potential. In some cases removal of aerobes facilitates anaerobic invasion. More frequently, however, aerobes destroy healthy tissue, thereby facilitating the establishment of anaerobic infection in previously well-oxygenated sites.

Anaerobic *pleuropulmonic disease* may be initiated by aspiration (general anesthesia, esophageal dysfunction, tonsillectomy, tooth extraction); preceding extrapulmonic anaerobic infection (otitis media, pharyngitis, bacterial endocarditis, peritonitis); penetrating chest wounds or open heart surgery; and systemic disease that impairs host response to infection. Anaerobic *brain abscesses* may follow chronic otitis media, mastoiditis, sinusitis, lung abscess, congenital heart disease with right to left shunt, bacterial endocarditis, infections of the face or scalp, head trauma, or intracranial surgery.

Anaerobic *bacteremia* or *peritonitis* may be preceded by perforation of the large or small bowel, appendicitis, gastroenteritis, or cholecystitis.

Neonatal anaerobic infection most commonly follows prolonged rupture of the fetal membranes or is associated with necrotizing enterocolitis.

Pathology.   Abscess formation and widespread tissue destruction with necrosis are associated with anaerobic infection. The specific pathology observed varies with the site.

Clinical Manifestations.   Infections produced by anaerobic microorganisms occur in any part of the body.

Anaerobic infections of the *upper respiratory tract* are not unusual. Periodontal infection (trench mouth) may develop if an anaerobic environment is created by poor dental hygiene or by malocclusion. A foul odor is noted. The gingival tissues are inflamed and edematous, and a foul-smelling discharge may be elicited by pressing along the gums. Periapical abscesses or anaerobic osteomyelitis of the mandible or maxilla may develop.

Anaerobic microorganisms also may be recovered from patients with chronic sinusitis, otitis media, mastoiditis, peritonsillar or retropharyngeal abscesses, parotitis, and cervical lymphadenitis. Since potentially pathogenic aerobic organisms are generally recovered concomitantly, it is difficult to establish the precise role of anaerobes in these disease processes.

Fusobacteria appear to be important in the development of **Vincent angina.** This tonsillar infection is characterized by the presence of ulcers covered by a brown or gray foul-smelling exudate. Extensive tissue destruction can develop quickly and lead to perforation of the carotid artery.

Ludwig angina is an acute cellulitis of the sublingual and submandibular spaces. The infection spreads rapidly without lymph node involvement or abscess formation. Respiratory obstruction may be noted and require tracheostomy.

Anaerobic infection of the *lower respiratory tract* generally takes the form of necrotizing pneumonia, putrid empyema, or lung abscess. A history of aspiration can usually be elicited. Ordinarily, pneumonia develops first, and abscess formation is the result of liquefaction of lung tissue. Any sputum produced is foul-smelling.

Anaerobic infection of the *central nervous system* may occur as brain abscess, subdural empyema, or septic thrombophlebitis of cortical veins and venous sinuses. The initial predisposing lesion may be contiguous with the brain, or infection may follow hematogenous spread from a distant site (lungs or heart). Signs or symptoms of brain abscess may include headache, drowsiness, confusion, stupor, seizures, and focal motor, sensory, or speech deficits. Fever may be low grade or absent. Papilledema is rare in children. Purulent meningitis is rarely caused by anaerobes; recovery of anaerobes from the cerebrospinal fluid of a child with meningitis suggests brain abscess or subdural empyema.

Since the concentrations of anaerobes are highest in the lower gastrointestinal tract, it is not surprising that the spillage of gastrointestinal contents is associated with a high incidence of anaerobic intra-abdominal infection. Generally many aerobes and anaerobes are recovered from peritoneal contents concomitantly. The clinical manifestations produced depend upon the nature of the primary lesion as well as upon subsequent localization of the disease process but are independent of the number and type of bacterial species present.

Anaerobic bacteremia is clinically indistinguishable from aerobic bacteremia. Fever, leukocytosis, jaundice, hemolytic anemia, and shock may occur. Anaerobic bacteremia is frequently associated with disease of the gastrointestinal (e.g., necrotizing enteritis) and genitourinary (e.g., calculi) systems.

Anaerobic microorganisms also may cause osteomyelitis, septic arthritis, urinary tract infections, liver and subphrenic abscesses, lymphadenitis, and skin and soft tissue infections.

Diagnosis.   The diagnosis of anaerobic infection depends upon (1) awareness of those infections with which anaerobes are associated, (2) appropriate selection and collection of specimens for culture, and (3) use of media and techniques that will facilitate recovery of anaerobic microorganisms.

Clinical clues to the diagnosis of anaerobic infection include the presence of a foul-smelling exudate or discharge, evidence of necrotic tissue or gangrene, infection located in proximity to a mucosal surface, gas in tissue or discharges, infection following an animal or human bite, infection associated with tissue destruction (trauma or malignancy), or infection that persists or follows prolonged use of aminoglycosides. Additional clues may include endocarditis with negative routine blood cultures, septic thrombophlebitis, or bacteremia associated with unexplained jaundice.

Anaerobic infection can be acceptably documented only by cultures from the infected site. The principal consideration is to avoid contamination of cultures with normal anaerobic flora. Clinical specimens which should be cultured for anaerobes routinely include blood; bile; pericardial, peritoneal, pleural, or cerebrospinal fluid; abscesses; deep aspirates of wounds; transtracheal aspirates; and surgical specimens obtained from normally sterile sites (tissue, appendix, gallbladder, lymph nodes).

The following sites or specimens should not be cultured anaerobically except in rare cases: nose, mouth, throat, sputum, tracheostomy sites, bronchoscopic washings, gastric washings, feces, ileostomy or colostomy material, urine, vaginal swabs, or fistulas. Anaerobic microorganisms are normally found in these specimens and it is generally impossible to implicate them in a causative relationship with any disease process.

Bacteriologic clues that suggest infection with anaerobes include no growth on routine cultures (sterile pus); failure to grow aerobically but presence confirmed by Gram stain of the original exudate; growth in thioglycolate broth or on media containing 100 μg/ml of kanamycin, neomycin, or paromomycin; production of gas and foul odor in culture; and development of characteristic colonies on agar plates incubated anaerobically.

Rapid diagnosis of Bacteroides infection has been made utilizing an indirect immunofluorescence assay with specific antisera against the capsular polysaccharide of B. fragilis and pooled antisera against a number of serotypes of Bacteroides sp. The assay is sensitive, false-negative results unusual, and false-positive results within an acceptable range (9.7%). Rapid diagnosis of anaerobic infections also has been achieved using gas-liquid chromatography of purulent material.

Treatment. Identification of anaerobes is frequently delayed because they grow slowly. In addition, in vitro sensitivity patterns of anaerobes do not reliably predict response in vivo. Fortunately, the type of anaerobes causing infection can usually be predicted from knowledge of the site of infection, and since the vast majority have predictable susceptibility to antibiotic agents, the clinician can usually select an appropriate drug before the results of culture and tests for sensitivity to antibiotics are available.

Penicillin G is effective against virtually all gram-positive and most gram-negative anaerobic microorganisms. An important exception is B. fragilis, which is resistant to penicillin, ampicillin, and cephalosporins in most cases. Most anaerobes are susceptible to chloramphenicol, clindamycin, and carbenicillin. Erythromycin is effective against anaerobic cocci. Previously, tetracycline provided effective therapy for many anaerobes, but the prevalence of resistance to this antibiotic has increased in recent yr; in our opinion, it should not be used. Aminoglycosides (kanamycin, gentamicin) are not effective against anaerobes. Cefoxitin has been used successfully in some patients, but experience with this agent in children is limited. Cefoxitin is active against 80% of B. fragilis but is relatively inactive against species of Clostridium other than C. perfringens. Metronidazole has been used successfully in the treatment of anaerobic infection; oral administration has been effective even in a child with a brain abscess.

A combination of penicillin and chloramphenicol should be used to treat suspected anaerobic bacteremia or anaerobic infection in sites other than the respiratory tract, where penicillin alone will suffice. Clindamycin is an effective alternative to chloramphenicol in most situations but should never replace chloramphenicol for treatment of brain abscess since it does not penetrate the blood-brain barrier. For mixed aerobic and anaerobic infections, particularly those involving the gastrointestinal tract, peritoneal cavity, genitourinary system, or retroperitoneal space, a combination of chloramphenicol or clindamycin with gentamicin or kanamycin may be appropriate.

The dosages of all antibiotics utilized to treat anaerobic infections are similar to those employed to treat aerobic infections with the same drugs. Duration of therapy varies with the nature of the disease process.

Prognosis. This depends upon the age of the host, the nature of the disease process, and the rapidity with which the correct diagnosis is suspected and appropriate therapy provided. In the neonatal period anaerobic bacteremia has been reported to have mortality rates varying from 4-37.5%. These differences may reflect, in part, differences in patient population and the anatomic sites chosen for obtaining blood cultures. The highest rates of positive anaerobic blood cultures and lowest mortality rates have been reported when blood has been obtained from the umbilical cord. These positive cultures more likely reflect transient neonatal bacteremia occurring at the time of delivery than active infection. Lowest recovery and higher mortality rates have been reported from centers which obtain anaerobic blood culture only from peripheral veins.

Mortality associated with anaerobic infection is increased in patients with extensive tissue necrosis with inadequate debridement and in those with necrotizing enterocolitis.

Chow AW, Leake RD, Yamauchi T, et al: The significance of anaerobes in neonatal bacteremia: Analysis of 23 cases and review of the literature. Pediatrics 54:736, 1974.

Dunkle LM, Brotherton TJ, Feigin RD: Anaerobic infections in children: A prospective study. Pediatrics 57:311, 1976.

Finegold SM: Clinical experience with clindamycin in anaerobic bacterial infections. I. Therapy for infections due to anaerobic bacteria: An overview. J Infect Dis 135:S25, 1977.

Gorbach SL, Bartlett JG: Anaerobic infections. Parts 1, 2, and 3. N Engl J Med 290:1177, 1237, 1289, 1974.

Klastersky J, Coppens L, Mombelli G: Anaerobic infection in cancer patients: Comparative evaluation of clindamycin and cefoxitin. Antimicrob Agents Chemother 16:366, 1979.

Ladas S, Arapakis G, Malamou-Ladas H, et al: Rapid diagnosis of anaerobic infections by gas-liquid chromatography. J Clin Pathol 32:1163, 1979.

Law BJ, Marks MI: Excellent outcome of Bacteroides meningitis in a newborn treated with metronidazole. Pediatrics 66:463, 1980.

10.45 OPPORTUNISTIC INFECTIONS

Opportunistic infections are due to ordinarily nonpathogenic bacterial or fungal organisms either com-

Table 10–27 OPPPORTUNISTIC INFECTION IN THE HOST COMPROMISED BY CHANGES IN THE SKIN OR MUCOUS MEMBRANE BARRIERS TO INFECTION OR BY ANATOMIC DEFECTS

PREDISPOSING CAUSES: DEFECTS IN ANATOMIC BARRIERS	OPPORTUNISTIC ORGANISMS ISOLATED MOST FREQUENTLY	SUGGESTED MECHANISMS
Cerebrospinal fluid shunts	Staphylococcus epidermidis, Staphylococcus aureus, Bacillus sp., diphtheroids	By-pass skin as barrier to infection; act as nidus for infection
Intravenous catheters	Staphylococcus epidermidis, Bacteroides, Mimeae, Pseudomonas, Candida, Cryptococcus	By-pass skin as barrier to infection; may serve as nidus for infection
Urinary catheters	Pseudomonas sp., Serratia, Herellea, Staphylococcus epidermidis, Candida	Serve as nidus for infection and new portal of entry for microorganisms
Inhalation therapy equipment	Pseudomonas, Serratia	Serve as new portal of entry; equipment and medication frequently contaminated with opportunistic organisms
Burns	Pseudomonas, Serratia, Staphylococcus, Candida, Mucor	Change ecology of skin flora and physicochemical properties of skin; neutrophil dysfunction, abnormal responses to antigenic stimulation, impairment of delayed hypersensitivity
General surgery	Staphylococcus epidermidis, Pseudomonas, Alcaligenes fecalis, Candida	Prophylactic use of antibiotics alter normal flora
Cardiac surgery	Staphylococcus epidermidis, diphtheroids, Mimeae, Pseudomonas, Candida, Aspergillus	Prophylactic use of antibiotics may alter normal flora; foreign bodies inserted may serve as nidus of infection
Dermal sinus tracts	Staphylococcus epidermidis, diphtheroids	Skin by-passed as barrier to infection
Congenital and acquired cardiac defects	Streptococcus viridans, Corynebacterium, Pseudomonas, nonpathogenic Neisseria	Damaged tissue serves as nidus for infection

From Feigin RD, Shearer WT: J Pediatr 87:507, 1975.

monly found in the environment or indigenous to the host. They usually result from an identifiable congenital, acquired, or environmentally induced increase in susceptibility of the host. Unusual clinical infections with common pathogens may likewise be opportunistic in nature. Opportunistic infection must be anticipated as a possibility in every child with a derangement in host defense.

Changes in the Skin or Mucous Membranes. The skin and mucous membranes are important barriers to infection. The intact skin can destroy most bacteria with which it may be contaminated, and few microorganisms are able to penetrate it. Table 10–27 shows situations in which the barriers to infection provided by the skin and mucous membranes have been bypassed or compromised, thereby predisposing the host to opportunistic infection; it shows also the organisms incriminated most frequently and suggested mechanisms of infection.

Shunts. Schoenbaum et al noted that infection occurred in 24% of 289 children in whom cerebrospinal fluid was shunted to another site for absorption. Most of the infections were acquired in the perioperative period. Staphylococcus epidermidis was isolated from 65% of infected ventriculoatrial shunts and from most of the infected ventriculoperitoneal shunts; it rarely was associated with infection of ventriculoureteral shunts. Gram-negative enteric organisms were implicated in only 6% of ventriculoatrial and ventriculoperitoneal shunts but were responsible for 35% of infections of ventriculoureteral shunts. Underlying disease did not significantly affect the rate of shunt infection. Lumbar puncture, ventricular taps, ventriculograms, and ventricular drainage unrelated to shunt surgery did not increase significantly the risk of development of infection. Shunts for renal dialysis and other purposes are also prone to infection.

Fever is an almost constant manifestation of shunt infection; erythema of the skin overlying the tubing used for diversion of cerebrospinal fluid is virtually diagnostic. Children with infection of ventriculoatrial shunts generally have bacteremia, whereas blood cultures are rarely positive and cerebrospinal fluid cultures may be negative in patients with infected ventriculoperitoneal shunts. When fever is observed in a child with a ventricular shunt, multiple blood cultures should be obtained. Direct aspiration of the shunt reservoir is a helpful diagnostic procedure in patients who are not receiving antibiotics.

Hypocomplementemic glomerulonephritis is a well recognized complication of shunt infection. Most commonly, S. epidermidis has been implicated as the organism associated with this syndrome.

Children with infected shunts should be treated with antibiotics specific for the offending organism. Prior to the isolation and identification of the etiologic agent, treatment should include coverage for S. epidermidis, diphtheroids, and Bacillus species. Generally, this can be effected by the use of penicillin and chloramphenicol. In recent years many strains of S. epidermidis have become resistant to both penicillin and semi-synthetic penicillin derivatives (methicillin, oxacillin, etc.) but have remained sensitive to cephalosporins. In institutions where this is known to be a problem, initial therapy should include a cephalosporin (cefazolin or cefamandole) and chloramphenicol. Usually, removal of the infected shunt is required.

The temporal association of surgery with infection of shunts, particularly with staphylococci, has suggested the use of antibiotics prophylactically in the perioperative period, but controlled studies to evaluate their efficacy are not available.

Intravenous Catheters. Bacteremia or fungemia with organisms commonly found on the skin have been reported in 2–5% of patients with intravenous catheters. A higher rate of septicemia has been associated with prolonged intravenous catheterization as used for total parenteral nutrition.

The hazard of extrinsic contamination can be decreased significantly by inspecting all bottles containing fluid for intravenous administration for cracks and turbidity immediately prior to use and by replacing daily all apparatus used for intravenous administration of fluids. Whenever possible, small needles rather than plastic catheters should be employed.

Bacteremia related to intravenous therapy may occur in the absence of local signs of inflammation. More frequently, however, signs of inflammation or thrombosis are noted at the site of catheterization. In such instances the catheter tip should be cultured when withdrawn and blood cultures should be obtained.

When clinical signs suggest infection or when positive cultures are obtained, administration of fluid should be discontinued; bacteremia may resolve spontaneously without specific antibiotic therapy. If clinical signs or positive cultures persist, appropriate antibiotics should be administered.

Urethral Catheters. Urethral catheterization, particularly with indwelling catheters, bypasses the mucosal barrier and frequently results in infection of the urinary tract (Sec 16.62). *E. coli* are the bacteria most frequently involved. The elimination of "routine" indications for catheterization is an important preventive measure.

Inhalation Therapy Equipment. Opportunistic infection, particularly during the neonatal period, has been associated with increasing use of respiratory life support systems. Reservoir nebulizers represent the greatest hazard. *Pseudomonas aeruginosa* and *Serratia marcescens* have been implicated most frequently. Risk of infection may be decreased by effective programs for surveillance and maintenance of respirators, nebulizers, and tubing used for inhalation therapy.

Burns. Opportunistic infection in children with burns may relate to interruption of the skin and mucous membrane barriers to infection, to long-term administration of antibiotics, or to prolonged intravenous or urinary catheterization. Septicemia with *Pseudomonas aeruginosa*, *S. aureus*, and *S. epidermidis* is frequent.

Burn injury has been associated with the development of neutrophil dysfunction, abnormal responses to specific antigens, and delayed rejection of homografts. Thus, the host response of the burned patient may be blunted. Although altered, primary and secondary immune responses remain intact and permit the successful application of active immunization of the burned patient with specific strains of *P. aeruginosa.*

Surgery. Cardiac surgery is associated with a significant risk of postoperative infection due to opportunistic microorganisms. The greater frequency of systemic opportunistic infection may be related to extensive use of intravenous and intra-arterial catheters as well as of blood and blood products. Opportunistic microorganisms also may be responsible for contamination of wounds. Wilson and Stuart noted that 4.4% of all episodes of wound infection associated with septicemia were due to *S. epidermidis.*

When fever develops postoperatively, opportunistic infection must be considered. The organisms that may produce disease postoperatively are so varied that a single specific antibiotic regimen appropriate for all patients cannot be given. Certainly, coverage for staphylococci should be included.

Dermal Sinus Tracts. Children with dermal sinus tracts which communicate with the subarachnoid space or neural tissue may develop meningitis due to *S. epidermidis* or other microflora of the skin.

Cardiac Defects. Both congenital cardiac defects and those acquired through rheumatic fever or surgery, especially intracardiac shunts and prostheses, provide a nidus for opportunistic infection.

Inherited or Acquired Disorders Affecting Host Defense Systems (see also Chapter 9). These disorders, the organisms recovered most frequently, and the mechanisms that may be responsible for the infections are shown in Table 10–28.

Disorders of White Blood Cell Function or Number. The leukocytes of patients with *chronic granulomatous disease* do not respond to phagocytosis with increased oxygen consumption or with a significant increase in hexose monophosphate shunt activity, and hydrogen peroxide production is impaired (Sec 9.30). Infection in these individuals most often is due to catalase-positive organisms, such as *S. aureus*, many strains of *Pseudomonas, Proteus, Enterobacter, Salmonella,* paracolon bacillus, *Alcaligenes,* and some strains of *Herellea.*

Specific treatment must be dictated by the sensitivity patterns of the organisms producing the infection. When sepsis is suspected, parenteral treatment with a semisynthetic penicillinase-resistant penicillin and with gentamicin is recommended until results of culture are available. Drainage of abscesses is imperative. Continuous prophylactic antibiotic therapy with nafcillin or sulfonamide has been advocated by several groups.

Chédiak-Higashi syndrome has been associated with recurrent pyogenic infection related to defective bactericidal activity and abnormal chemotaxis (Sec. 9.31).

Opportunistic bacterial infection has been seen repeatedly in children with all forms of *congenital* and *acquired neutropenia.* Treatment requires use of antibiotics (preferably bactericidal). Transfusions of white blood cells may be helpful temporarily in selected patients who are critically ill.

Congenital and Acquired Immunodeficiency Syndromes (Sec 9.4). Disorders associated with defective humoral or cellular immunity have been associated with recurrent infection, frequently due to opportunistic microorganisms. Treatment depends upon identification of the offending agent. An approach to prevention and treatment of opportunistic infections in B- and T-cell deficiency syndrome is presented in Table 10–29.

Malignancy, Immunosuppression, and Transplantation. Infection is a major problem and may be the terminal event in children with *cancer.* Therapeutic maneuvers associated with a minimal risk of infection in the normal host (e.g., intravenous infusions, indwelling catheters, transfusions, use of respirators, broad-spectrum antibiotic therapy) become significant hazards to children with cancer.

The single most important factor that predisposes the child with cancer to infection is neutropenia (granulocyte count less than 1000/mm³). Granulocytopenia may

Table 10–28 OPPORTUNISTIC INFECTION IN INHERITED AND ACQUIRED DISORDERS THAT DIMINISH HOST RESISTANCE

Predisposing Causes: Inherited and Aquired Disorders of Inflammation or Immunity	Opportunistic Organisms Isolated Most Frequently	Suggested Mechanisms
Chronic granulomatous disease	Staphylococcus, gram-negative enteric organisms, Serratia, Nocardia	Impaired production of H_2O_2 with defective bactericidal function
Job syndrome	Staphylococcus aureus	Unknown
Myeloperoxidase deficiency	Candida	Failure to kill Candida
Glucose-6-phosphate dehydrogenase deficiency	Staphylococcus, Serratia	Deficient cellular NADH and NADPH; deficient HMPS activity; decreased H_2O_2 production; defect in bacterial killing
Chédiak-Higashi syndrome	Usual pyogens	Defective bactericidal activity, impaired chemotaxis, neutropenia
Congenital neutropenia	Herellea, Serratia, Pseudomonas, Staphylococcus epidermidis	Insufficient number of neutrophils
Complement deficiencies (C3, C3 inactivator)	Pathogens, i.e., Streptococcus pneumoniae, Streptococcus pyogenes, Neisseria meningitidis	Defective chemotaxis; impaired opsonization
Splenic insufficiency	Streptococcus pneumoniae, Salmonella	Defective opsonization; defective clearing of organisms
Sickle cell disease and other hemoglobinopathies	Streptococcus pneumoniae, Salmonella, Edwardsiella	Reticuloendothelial blockade; defective opsonization
Humoral immunodeficiency syndromes (predominantly B cell defects)	Bacterial pathogens, Pseudomonas	Reduced phagocytic efficiency; failure of lysis and agglutination of bacteria; inadequate neutralization of bacterial toxins
Cellular immunodeficiency syndromes (predominantly T cell defects)	Mycobacterium, Listeria, Nocardia, cytomegalovirus, varicella, Cryptococcus, Candida, Pneumocystis, Strongyloides stercoralis	Absence or impaired delayed hypersensitivity response; absent T cell cooperation for B cell synthesis of antibodies to T cell specific antigens
Severe combined immunodeficiency syndrome	Many bacteria, fungi, viruses, and Pneumocystis	Absence of T and B cell response
Cancer	Pseudomonas, Klebsiella, Escherichia coli, Listeria, Cryptococcus, varicella-zoster, herpes simplex, Pneumocystis, Mycobacterium; incidence of infection with gram-negative organism increases in presence of neutropenia	Granulocytopenia; decreased neutrophil chemotaxis; decreased bacterial activity of neutrophils; lymphopenia, defective cell-mediated immunity; impaired antigenic response to challenge
Immunosuppression	Pseudomonas, Klebsiella, Escherichia coli, Herellea, Serratia, herpes simplex, varicella-zoster, cytomegalovirus, EB virus, papovavirus, hepatitis virus, Candida, Aspergillus, Mucor, Cryptococcus	Dependent upon agent utilized
Transplantation	Staphylococcus, Pseudomonas, Klebsiella, Candida, Aspergillus, Nocardia, Pneumocystis, cytomegalovirus, hepatitis virus, herpes simplex, varicella-zoster	Probably related to use of immunosuppressive agents
Malnutrition	Measles, herpes simplex, varicella-zoster, Mycobacterium	Impaired T cell function; reduction in complement activity; impaired migration of phagocytes; reduced bactericidal activity
Cystic fibrosis	Staphylococcus, Pseudomonas	Presence of ciliary dyskinesia factor; impaired phagocytosis of Pseudomonas
Diabetes mellitus	Staphylococcus, Escherichia coli, Proteus, Clostridium, Actinomyces, Candida, Mucor, Torulopsis	Impaired phagocytic activity; decreased serum opsonizing capacity; decreased chemotaxis of neutrophils
Polyendocrinopathy	Candida	Unknown
Nephrotic syndrome	Streptococcus pneumoniae, enteric bacteria	Unknown
Uremia	Bacteroides, Serratia, Enterobacter, Staphylococcus, Candida, Mucor, herpesvirus, varicella-zoster	Defects in early phases of inflammatory response; lymphopenia; impaired T cell function
Exudative enteropathy	Streptococcus pneumoniae, enteric bacteria, Giardia lamblia	Low levels of IgG; depressed T cell function in intestinal lymphangiectasia
Inflammatory bowel disease	Candida, Mucor, herpesvirus, varicella-zoster	Probably not related to basic disease but to use of corticosteroids
Collagen diseases	Candida, Mucor, Aspergillus, Pneumocystis, diphtheroids, Listeria, Pseudomonas, Serratia, Staphylococcus, Nocardia, cytomegalovirus, herpesvirus, varicella-zoster	Probably related to use of immunosuppressive agents; may relate to involvement of reticuloendothelial system

From Feigin RD, Shearer WT: J Pediatr 87:677, 1975.

Table 10–29 INFECTIONS IN THE HOST COMPROMISED BY B- AND T-CELL IMMUNODEFICIENCY SYNDROMES

IMMUNODEFICIENCY SYNDROME	APPROACH TO TREATMENT OF INFECTIONS	PREVENTION OF INFECTIONS
Humoral immunodeficiency syndromes (predominantly B-cell defects)	1. Gamma globulin 1.4 ml/kg 2. Vigorous attempt to obtain cultures prior to antimicrobial therapy 3. Incision and drainage if abscess present 4. Antibiotic selection based upon sensitivity reports	1. Maintenance gamma globulin (0.7 ml/kg/mo) administration 2. In chronic recurrent respiratory disease vigorous attention to postural drainage 3. In selected cases (recurrent or chronic pulmonary; middle ear) prophylactic administration of ampicillin or penicillin
Cellular immunodeficiency syndromes (predominantly T-cell defects)	1. Vigorous attempt to obtain cultures prior to antimicrobial therapy 2. Incision and drainage if abscess present 3. Attempt to use antimicrobial agent with the most narrow spectrum 4. Topical and non-absorbable antimicrobial agents frequently useful	1. Prophylactic administration of trimethoprim-sulfamethoxazole for the prevention of *Pneumocystis carinii* pneumonia 2. Protective environments for some patients 3. Oral nonabsorbable antimicrobial agents to lower concentration of gut flora 4. No live virus vaccines or BCG 5. Careful tuberculosis screening
Combined immunodeficiency syndromes	1. Gamma globulin 1.4 ml/kg 2. Same as T-cell defects above	1. Gamma globulin maintenance 2. Same as T-cell defects above

Modified from Cherry JD, and Feigin RD, *In:* Stiehm ER, Fulginiti VA (eds): Immunologic Disorders in Infants and Children. Philadelphia, WB Saunders, 1980, p. 726.

be related to the primary disease or be the result of therapy provided. In some cases neutrophil function may be impaired in children with leukemia both in relapse and remission even though the number of circulating neutrophils is normal.

Although any agent may produce disease in children with malignancy, certain patterns emerge. Fever due to septicemia in patients with acute lymphocytic leukemia commonly involves gram-negative organisms, although in recent years the frequency of septicemia due to gram-positive organisms has increased. Protracted fever in patients with leukemia in relapse usually is the result of infection with fungal organisms. The majority of infections in patients with chronic lymphocytic leukemia and multiple myeloma are due to gram-positive organisms. When neutropenia develops in these patients, however, the incidence of gram-negative infection increases. Infections with intracellular organisms (*Listeria, Salmonella, Brucella,* mycobacteria, *Cryptococcus, Pneumocystis carinii*) are most prevalent in patients with Hodgkin disease. The lowest incidence of infection has been reported in children with solid tumors.

Infections also are responsible for significant morbidity and mortality in patients receiving *immunosuppressive therapy* for the management of malignancy, collagen vascular diseases, or transplantation. The microorganisms involved and the location of the infectious process depend, to some extent, upon the underlying disease process. In the immunosuppressed host, infection occurs more commonly with aerobic gram-negative than with aerobic or anaerobic gram-positive microorganisms.

Immunosuppressive therapy is an integral part of the process of *transplantation;* predictably, infections following transplantation are similar to those associated with immunosuppression. Recent evidence, however, suggests that transplantation and the rejection process per se predispose the host to infection. Hill and associates noted that opportunistic microorganisms, including *Pseudomonas, Klebsiella, E. coli,* and staphylococci, were responsible for 75% of infections in a series of 123

patients who had received organ transplants (primarily renal). Infection with cytomegalovirus in recipients of transplanted organs is even more frequent; clinical or subclinical infection with this virus may be seen in 90% of patients at some time following transplantation.

An approach to the treatment and prevention of infection in the host compromised by malignancy, immunosuppression, or transplantation is shown in Table 10–30.

Cystic Fibrosis of the Pancreas (Sec 12.110). Children with cystic fibrosis have recurrent or persistent pulmonary infection due to *S. aureus, P. aeruginosa,* coliform bacteria, and *Hemophilus* sp. Little evidence supports the concept that continuous aerosolized and oral antibiotic prophylaxis diminishes pulmonary infection; continuous administration of antibiotics may predispose the patient to colonization and infection with saprophytic strains of bacteria which are resistant to multiple antibiotics.

Diabetes Mellitus. Children with diabetes mellitus have a decreased resistance to bacterial and fungal infections (Sec 17.1). Pyelonephritis and perinephric abscesses due to *S. aureus, S. epidermidis, E. coli,* proteus and clostridia, mucor, *Torulopsis glabrata,* and *Candida* have been reported frequently. Decreased chemotactic activity of polymorphonuclear leukocytes, ineffective phagocytosis, and decreased opsonizing capacity of serum have been noted.

Exudative Enteropathy. This may accompany gastrointestinal infection, Menetrier syndrome (protein loss with giant hypertrophy of gastric mucosa), gluten-induced enteropathy, intestinal lymphangiectasia, kwashiorkor, Hirschsprung disease, gastrointestinal neoplasms, allergic gastroenteritis, regional enteritis, ulcerative colitis, jejunal malformations, gastrocolic fistula, angioneurotic edema, postgastrectomy syndrome, congestive heart failure, constrictive pericarditis, and aminopterin administration. Infection with *Streptococcus pneumoniae,* enteric bacteria, and *Giardia lamblia* occurs with increased frequency in these patients. Increased susceptibility to infection may relate, in part, to the

Table 10-30 INFECTION IN THE HOST COMPROMISED BY MALIGNANCY, IMMUNOSUPPRESSION, OR TRANSPLANTATION

Category	Approach to Treatment of Infections	Prevention of Infections
Malignancy	1. Appropriate Gram-stained smears and cultures (blood, urine, CSF, IV sites, wounds) even of minor lesions prior to the onset of therapy 2. When possible choose specific antibiotics for specific etiologic agents (employ bactericidal rather than bacteriostatic antibiotics) 3. When the etiology is not apparent initial therapy should be aimed at *Pseudomonas* and other gram-negative bacilli and *Staphylococcus aureus;* cefazolin and gentamicin (or another aminoglycoside antibiotic to which *Pseudomonas* is sensitive) is a good initial choice 4. Once therapy has been started allow ample time for effect; therapy should rarely be less than 7 days 5. Fresh frozen plasma, whole blood, and leukocyte transfusions are frequently helpful	1. Prophylactic administration of trimethoprim-sulfamethoxazole to prevent *Pneumocystis carinii* pneumonia 2. Avoidance of unnecessary hospitalization 3. Avoidance of antibiotics and catheters unless specifically indicated 4. Protective isolation in the hospital 5. Routine surveillance cultures (throat, stool, and axilla) at regular intervals 6. Use of zoster, vaccinia, and measles immune globulins if exposed
Immunosuppression	Same as Malignancy, above	1. Avoidance of unnecessary hospitalization 2. Avoidance of antibiotics and catheters unless specifically indicated 3. Protective isolation in the hospital 4. Use of zoster, vaccinia, and measles immune globulins if exposed
Transplantation	Same as Malignancy, above	Same as Malignancy, above, plus: 1. Reduction of total bowel flora of microorganisms with nonabsorbable antibiotics 2. Removal of diet items that contain microbial contamination 3. Possible use of special environmental units (laminar air flow rooms) for protective isolation

Modified from Cherry JD, Feigin RD, *In:* Stiehm ER, Fulginiti VA (eds): Immunologic Disorders in Infants and Children. Philadelphia, WB Saunders, 1980, p. 728.

Table 10-31 OPPORTUNISTIC INFECTION IN NORMAL CHILDREN

Organism	Frequent Types of Infection	Suggested Treatment
Actinomyces israelii	Cellulitis, pneumonia, osteomyelitis	Penicillin; alternate: tetracycline
Aeromonas hydrophila	Abscesses, cellulitis, diarrhea, peritonitis, pneumonia, septicemia, urinary tract infection	Chloramphenicol, gentamicin, kanamycin
Alcaligenes faecalis	Abscesses, cellulitis, otitis media, septicemia	Chloramphenicol, gentamicin, kanamycin
Bacteroides	Abscesses, peritonitis, septicemia	Chloramphenicol; alternate: clindamycin
Fusobacterium gonidia formans	Peritonsilitis, subdural empyema	Penicillin; alternates: tetracycline, erythromycin
Bacillus subtilis	Abscess, cellulitis, conjunctivitis, septicemia	Penicillin; alternate: chloramphenicol
Chromobacterium	Abscess	Carbenicillin; sensitivity varies and should be checked
Diphtheroids	Endocarditis, meningitis	Penicillin; alternate: erythromycin
Gaffkya tetragena	Meningitis	Penicillin
Hemophilus parainfluenzae	Endocarditis, meningitis, otitis media, septicemia	Ampicillin; alternate: chloramphenicol
HB group	Brain abscess, cellulitis, meningitis, otitis media, pneumonia	Chloramphenicol, tetracycline; alternate: ampicillin; sensitivity variable
Lactobacillus	Lung abscess	Check sensitivities
Mimae, Moraxella, Herellea	Cellulitis, conjunctivitis, endocarditis, meningitis, pneumonia, septicemia, septic arthritis, stomatitis	Gentamicin; alternate: kanamycin; oxidase-positive strains may be sensitive to penicillin
Nonpathogenic *Neisseria*	Meningitis, septicemia, otitis media	Penicillin, ampicillin
Nocardia	Osteomyelitis, pneumonia, septicemia	Sulfonamides or sulfonamides plus penicillin
Nonpathogenic *Pasteurella*	Brain abscess, meningitis	Penicillin, chloramphenicol
Pseudomonads	Abscesses, otitis media, pneumonia, septicemia	According to sensitivity studies
Serratia	Diarrhea, pneumonia, otitis media, osteomyelitis	Gentamicin; alternate: kanamycin or chloramphenicol according to sensitivity studies
Nonpathogenic *Spirillum*	Septicemia	Penicillin; alternate: tetracycline or chloramphenicol
Staphylococcus epidermidis	Meningitis, otitis media, osteomyelitis, septic arthritis, septicemia, urinary tract infection	Penicillin, or semisynthetic penicillin derivative if strain resistant to penicillin
Nonhemolytic streptococci	Abscess, cellulitis, endocarditis, gingivitis, pneumonia	Penicillin; alternate: erythromycin, ampicillin, or penicillin plus streptomycin
Vibrio	Abscess, pneumonia, septic arthritis	Chloramphenicol
Aspergillus	Abscess, endocarditis, pneumonia, osteomyelitis	Amphotericin B
Cryptococcaceae	Thrush, pneumonia, meningitis	Amphotericin B

From Feigin RD, Shearer WT: J Pediatr 87:852, 1975.

hypogammaglobulinemia which may be found. In patients with intestinal lymphangiectasia, lymphopenia and impaired homograft rejection also may be noted.

Opportunistic Infection in the Normal Host. Infection by saprophytic microorganisms has been reported in normal, healthy children with increasing frequency in recent years. The normal individual is at greatest risk of infection by organisms that constitute the indigenous flora of the host or by organisms commonly found in the environment during the neonatal period (Sec 7.58).

Saprophytic microorganisms that have produced infection in normal children, the types of infection encountered most frequently, and the antibiotic therapy most likely to be effective (to be modified on the basis of specific sensitivity testing) are shown in Table 10–31.

Evaluation and Treatment. The principles are the same as those applied when infection is caused by organisms normally considered to be pathogenic. The physician should suspect and alert the laboratory to the possibility of opportunistic infection in certain clinical situations. In turn, the microbiologist must not regard the isolation of a saprophytic microorganism as a contaminant, particularly if it is recovered repeatedly from the same patient.

Once appropriate cultures and serologic tests designed to establish an etiologic diagnosis have been obtained, therapy should be initiated immediately. Prior to identification of a specific infectious agent, initial treatment should be guided by the disease process with which the patient is afflicted and the types of organisms most often responsible for infection in these individuals.

Prevention. Prevention is best accomplished by a program that permits the systematic identification of infection in hospitalized patients. Sources of infection and the microorganisms involved must be identified early to permit corrective measures. The principles of infection control should be taught to all individuals with responsibility for patient care. Unrestricted or routine use of antibiotics, particularly for prophylaxis, should be discouraged except in selected circumstances.

Cherry JD, Feigin RD: Infection in the compromised host. *In:* Stiehm ER, Fulginiti VA (eds): Immunologic Disorders of Infancy and Childhood. Philadelphia, WB Saunders, 1980, p 715.
DeClerck Y, DeClerck D, Rivard GE, et al: Septicemia in children with leukemia. Can Med J 118:1523, 1978.
Donaldson SS, Glatstein E, Vosti KL: Bacterial infections in pediatric Hodgkin's disease: Relationship to radiotherapy, chemotherapy and splenectomy. Cancer 41:1949, 1978.
Feigin RD, Shearer WT: Opportunistic infection in children. J Pediatr 87:507, 677, 852, 1975.
Hill RB Jr, Dahrling BE II, Starzl TE, et al: Death after transplantation; an analysis of sixty cases. Am J Med 42:327, 1967.
Neiman PE, Reeves W, Ray G, et al: A prospective analysis of interstitial pneumonia and opportunistic viral infection among recipients of allogeneic bone marrow grafts. J Infect Dis 136:754, 1977.

ACQUIRED IMMUNE DEFICIENCY SYNDROME (AIDS)

Acquired immune deficiency syndrome (AIDS) is a newly described disease. It may be characterized by (1) opportunistic infections which include pneumonia, meningitis, or encephalitis, due to *Pneumocystis carinii*, aspergillosis, candidiasis, cryptococcosis, cytomegalovirus, nocardiosis, strongyloidosis, toxoplasmosis, zygomycosis, or atypical mycobacteriosis (*Mycobacterium avium–intracellulare*); esophagitis due to candidiasis, cytomegalovirus, or herpes simplex virus; progressive multifocal leukoencephalopathy; chronic enterocolitis (more than 4 wk) due to cryptosporidiosis; or unusually extensive mucocutaneous herpes simplex of more than 5 wk duration; (2) unusual malignant neoplasms such as Burkitt lymphoma, diffuse undifferentiated non-Hodgkin lymphoma, or Kaposi sarcoma; (3) autoimmune phenomena including thrombocytopenia; and (4) defective cell-mediated immunity characterized by alterations in T lymphocyte responses and T lymphocyte subpopulations.

Alternatively, AIDS may present without symptoms despite laboratory evidence of immune deficiency or with nonspecific symptoms (e.g., fever, weight loss, generalized, persistent lymphadenopathy). The pathogenesis of this life-threatening illness (mortality exceeds 40%), which is being reported with increasing frequency in homosexual males, intravenous drug abusers, Haitian immigrants, hemophiliacs, and nontransfused infants born to either Haitians or intravenous drug abusers, remains unknown; however, epidemiologic evidence suggests a blood-borne transmissible agent. Hospital personnel caring for AIDS patients should use isolation procedures similar to those recommended for patients with hepatitis B virus infections.

Acquired immune deficiency syndrome (AIDS): Precautions for clinical and laboratory staff. Mortal Morbid Wkly Rep 31:507, 1982.
Siegal FP, Lopez C, Hammer GS, et al: Severe acquired immunodeficiency in male homosexuals manifested by chronic perianal ulcerative herpes simplex lesions. N Engl J Med 305:1439, 1981.
Update on acquired immune deficiency syndrome (AIDS)—United States. Mortal Morbid Wkly Rep 31:365, 1982.

10.46 *CAMPYLOBACTER FETUS* INFECTIONS

Campylobacter fetus, subspecies *intestinalis*, and *Campylobacter fetus*, subspecies *jejuni*, were formerly classified as *Vibrio fetus* and "related vibrios," respectively. These organisms were a well known cause of abortion in domestic animals prior to 1947 but until recently were considered to be a rare cause of human disease. With the development of special isolation techniques permitting the recovery of *Campylobacter fetus*, this organism has now been established as a frequent cause of gastroenteritis in children.

Etiology. There are 3 species within the genus *Campylobacter*; 3 subspecies of *Campylobacter fetus* (ss. *fetus*, ss. *intestinalis*, and ss. *jejuni*) are of particular importance as a cause of human and animal disease. *Campylobacter* are spirally curved, thin, gram-negative rods. Short, S-shaped, and longer, multispiraled, filamentous organisms may occur. In older cultures coccal forms may appear. The organisms are motile with a single flagellum at 1 or both poles of the bacterium. *Campylobacter* will grow on blood agar, albimi-*Brucella* agar, Mueller-Hinton agar, and thio-blood agar when incubated under appropriate conditions. Human strains can be divided into 2 groups on the basis of serologic cross-reactions. These 2 groups are presumed to represent ss. *intestinalis* and ss. *jejuni* isolates.

Diagnostic human serology is useful primarily when the serum of the patient can be tested against his own isolate. The majority of patients have elevated antibody titers (greater than 1:40 by hemagglutination or bacterial agglutination), and paired acute and convalescent sera may show 4-fold titer increases.

Epidemiology. The epidemiology of human infections is only partially understood. Venereal transmission has been suggested as a cause of perinatal infections. *Campylobacter fetus* has been found as a part of the mouth flora, and it has been suggested that periodontal disease might predispose to bacteremia. Contaminated formula has been proposed as the source of several neonatal cases of *Campylobacter* infection. *Campylobacter* enteritis involves person-to-person spread, particularly among children and within families. Contaminated food or water may be a source of these infections. Contact with infected dogs and chickens has also been implicated as a source of human disease.

Pathogenesis and Pathology. The pathogenesis of systemic *Campylobacter* infections is unclear. Fewer than one third of patients have had documented environmental or occupational exposure. The occurrence of profuse watery stools suggests a small bowel secretory process perhaps mediated by an enterotoxin. Guerrant et al, however, have published evidence that *Campylobacter fetus* ss. *intestinalis* does not produce enterotoxins that are detectable by classic in vivo or cytotoxic tests of the type used for the detection of *Escherichia coli* or cholera enterotoxins. The same investigators could not document invasive properties of *Campylobacter fetus* ss. *intestinalis*. In vitro or in vivo evidence for invasiveness or cytotoxicity for ss. *jejuni* is also lacking at present. Extensive hemorrhagic ulcerations of the bowel wall and edema extending from the jejunum through the proximal ileum have been noted at autopsy.

Clinical Manifestations. The most common manifestation of systemic *Campylobacter* infection is **bacteremia** without localized infection. The majority of blood-stream isolates are *Campylobacter fetus* ss. *intestinalis*. Bacteremic illness generally begins with fever, headache, and malaise. The fever follows a relapsing or intermittent course. Night sweats and chills are prominent, and weight loss may occur when illness is prolonged. Central nervous system manifestations including lethargy and confusion are common, but specific neurologic signs are unusual in the absence of cerebrovascular disease or meningitis. Abdominal pain is described by the majority of patients with *Campylobacter* bacteremia, but diarrhea is noted in only 35% of these individuals. Cough may occur, but pulmonary parenchymal involvement is unusual. Physical examination is generally unimpressive except for the appearance of toxicity. Hepatomegaly and icterus have been noted but are unusual. Laboratory findings are usually nonspecific. A mild to moderate leukocytosis may occur.

Transient asymptomatic bacteremia that clears without antibiotic therapy has been noted. Fulminant and fatal septicemia may also occur. Prolonged bacteremia of 8–13 wk duration has been reported with symptoms that wax and wane as spontaneous relapses and remissions occur.

Bacterial endocarditis has been caused by *Campylobacter*. The majority of patients were male, and all were adults. Five had pre-existing heart disease and several had dental extractions performed prior to the onset of their illness. Four of the patients died, but none succumbed who had received adequate or appropriate antibiotic therapy.

Meningitis related to *Campylobacter* infection has been reported in both adults and children. *Campylobacter* meningeal involvement in childhood is generally confined to the neonatal period. Most patients who developed *Campylobacter* meningitis beyond the neonatal period have survived. Antibiotic therapy has been successful; a variety of antibiotics have been employed including chloramphenicol, tetracycline, gentamicin, and kanamycin.

Perinatal disease is suggested by the recovery of *Campylobacter* from the placenta and fetus of women who have had a febrile illness during pregnancy and an association with abortion and prematurity. *Campylobacter* neonatal meningitis is heralded by signs and symptoms similar to those engendered by other organisms that cause neonatal sepsis and meningitis. Apnea, cyanosis, shock, hemolysis, jaundice, poor feeding, lethargy, seizures, and fever may be noted. Perinatal infection with bacteremia and meningitis has been reported with the recovery of both *Campylobacter fetus* ss. *jejuni* and *Campylobacter fetus* ss. *intestinalis*. The onset occurs in the 1st 3 wk of life. These infants are often premature, and mortality is high.

Diarrhea associated with *Campylobacter fetus* bacteremia was reported in several children prior to 1972. In 1977 Skirrow reported recovery of *Campylobacter fetus* ss. *jejuni* from the stool of 7.1% of 803 patients with diarrhea and from none of 194 patients without diarrhea. Spread of infections from child to child or to parents was noted. Live or dressed chickens or dogs with diarrhea were also implicated as possible sources of infection. Outbreaks in day-care centers have been described. The incidence is similar to that caused by *Salmonella* or *Yersinia enterocolitica*, and ages of patients range from 2 wk–15 yr. Fever, diarrhea, and bloody stools occur in 90% of the patients. Blood appears in the stools characteristically 2–4 days after the onset of symptoms. Over 90% of older children complain of abdominal pain. Vomiting occurs in 30% of patients. The organism may persist in stools for up to 7 wk in untreated patients but cannot be recovered after 48 hr of therapy with erythromycin. Significant serologic responses are detected on a serum bactericidal assay. The incubation period of *Campylobacter* enteritis is estimated to be 2–11 days. The diarrhea is generally watery, profuse, and foul-smelling. Abdominal pain is periumbilical, and cramping may antedate other symptoms or may persist after the return of stools to normal. The disease has simulated appendicitis or intussusception.

Mesenteric adenitis has been reported in several patients subjected to laparotomy because of abdominal pain of unknown etiology. *Campylobacter* has been recovered from the stomach, jejunum, ileum, and stool of such individuals.

Thrombophlebitis has been reported in a number of instances in which *Campylobacter fetus* has been recovered from the bloodstream. A nonspecific febrile illness with prominent findings of thrombophlebitis should suggest the possibility of *Campylobacter fetus* as the etiologic agent. *Campylobacter* also has been reported to produce pericarditis, peritonitis, salpingitis, septic arthritis, lung abscess, and chest wall abscess.

Diagnosis. The diagnosis of *Campylobacter* enteritis is suggested by the occurrence of watery diarrhea followed by blood-streaked stools and preceded by or accompanied by severe abdominal pain. The organism may be recovered on blood agar or Colombia agar with added antimicrobials designed to suppress the majority of the fecal flora. The cultures are incubated under reduced oxygen tension. Visible growth in blood culture often is not evident until 5–14 days after initial inoculation of the media. Direct phase microscopy of feces is a specific and sensitive rapid diagnostic test.

Treatment. No controlled studies of the treatment of *Campylobacter* diarrhea exist. Most isolates are sensitive in vitro to gentamicin, kanamycin, chloramphenicol, and tetracycline; variable resistance has been reported to colistin, carbenicillin, and cephalothin. Gentamicin may be the antibiotic of choice for the treatment of *Campylobacter* septicemia and nonenteric *Campylobacter* disease when the antibiotic sensitivity pattern is not known. Chloramphenicol should be considered for use in patients with meningitis. *Campylobacter* enteritis may be treated successfully with oral tetracycline (50 mg/kg/24 hr), erythromycin (40 mg/kg/24 hr), furazolidone (5 mg/kg/24 hr), and oral neomycin (50 mg/kg/24 hr). Treatment of diarrheal disease should be provided for at least 1 wk. Treatment of systemic infections for 4 wk is recommended.

Prognosis. *Campylobacter* septicemia in the immunocompromised host or in the newborn is associated with a high mortality rate. The rarity of cases precludes providing a precise estimate of mortality, particularly when early or effective antimicrobial therapy is provided.

Prognosis of *Campylobacter* enteritis is good; antibiotics apparently shorten the duration of clinical symptoms.

Cadranel S, Rodesch P, Butzler JP, et al: Enteritis due to a "related vibrio" in children. Am J Dis Child 126:152, 1973.
Eden AN: *Vibrio fetus* meningitis in a newborn infant. J Pediatr 61:33, 1962.
Karmali MA, Fleming PC: *Campylobacter* enteritis in children. J Pediatr 94:527, 1979.
Pai CH, Sorger S, Lackman L, et al: *Campylobacter* gastroenteritis in children. J Pediatr 94:589, 1979.
Rettig PJ: *Campylobacter* infections in human beings. J Pediatr 94:855, 1979.
Skirrow MB: *Campylobacter* enteritis: A "new" disease. Br Med J 2:9, 1977.
Torphy DE, Bond WW: *Campylobacter fetus* infections in children. Pediatrics 64:898, 1979.

10.47 LEGIONNAIRES DISEASE
(Legionellosis; Pontiac Fever)

Legionnaires disease is an acute infection caused by a fastidious gram-negative bacillus called *Legionella pneumophila*. It occurs in at least 2 epidemiologic and clinical forms: a long incubation period pneumonic form (Legionnaires disease) and a short incubation period form (Pontiac fever). The long incubation form is frequently mistaken for a viral pneumonia, whereas the short incubation period form of the disease resembles influenza without pneumonia.

Legionnaires disease is a term initially used to describe an outbreak of pneumonia that primarily involved persons attending an annual convention of the American Legion in Philadelphia in 1976; 221 of those attending were affected and 34 died. Early in 1977, McDade reported the recovery of a gram-negative rod, *Legionella pneumophila*, from lung tissue of patients who had died of the disease and demonstrated that other patients had a specific antibody response to this organism during convalescence. Subsequently, it was demonstrated that the same organism, or one antigenically similar, had caused outbreaks in Washington, D.C., in 1965, in Pontiac, Michigan, in 1968, and in Memphis and Atlanta in 1978.

Epidemiology. The incidence of pneumonia due to *L. pneumophila* is estimated at 7–20 cases/100,000/yr in the United States. Nosocomial cases apparently occur more commonly among immunosuppressed patients than do community-acquired cases, and the case fatality rate in immunosuppressed patients is high.

Numerous common-source outbreaks of Legionnaires disease have been recognized; 0.5–5.0% of those exposed have been affected. This incidence contrasts sharply with outbreaks of Pontiac fever in which the attack rate has been 95–100%. Many of the outbreaks of Legionnaires disease have been associated with buildings or institutions including hotels and hospitals. Few children have been proved to have Legionnaires disease, but sporadic cases have been noted in children as young as 16 mo of age.

Increasingly, Legionnaires disease is being recognized as a major cause of hospital-acquired pneumonia, of both sporadic cases and outbreaks. The risk of nosocomial Legionnaires disease is increased 2–3-fold in patients with cancer or other disorders with immunosuppression. Therapy with corticosteroids is a significant risk factor for the disease, and several outbreaks have been noted among renal homograft recipients. Diabetes mellitus and the use of diuretic agents have also been associated with increased risks of sporadic community-acquired Legionnaires disease.

Only airborne spread of *L. pneumophila* has been documented. *L. pneumophila* has been recovered from air conditioning systems as well as from stream water and mud. Person-to-person spread of Legionnaires disease has not been proved. However, hospital staff members who had direct or indirect contact with persons with Legionnaires disease had a higher prevalence (9.3%) of serum antibody titers (128 or higher as measured by hemagglutination) than did staff members without known exposure (3.7%). These observations and the presence of L. pneumophila in respiratory secretions imply that person-to-person spread may occur under certain circumstances.

Etiology. L. pneumophila is a typical gram-negative bacillus with a double envelope of unit membrane and no evident cell wall. Cell suspensions induce gelation of Limulus amebocyte lysate and are pyrogenic to rabbits. The organism survives for several mo in distilled water and over 1 yr in tap water held at room temperature. On agar the organism grows most rapidly at 35° C. Four serogroups of Legionella have been defined by direct immunofluorescence staining with group specific antigens. Other strains do not stain with currently available antisera.

Pathogenesis. Legionnaires disease presumably begins with inhalation of L. pneumophila, which induces pneumonia after an incubation period of 2–10 days. The pulmonary infiltrate consists primarily of macrophages and polymorphonuclear leukocytes in alveolar spaces, fibrin, and proliferating alveolar lining cells. Terminal and respiratory bronchioles may be involved, but the bronchi and proximal bronchioles are generally spared. The cellular infiltrate commonly is necrotic, but the underlying pulmonary structure usually remains intact. The resolution of Legionnaires disease pneumonia may not be complete; a residual defect in diffusing capacity may be caused by the deposition of fibrin.

Bacteremia has been demonstrated in Legionnaires disease, but involvement of other organ systems either directly or indirectly through toxin elaboration has not been noted.

The pathogenesis of Pontiac fever syndrome is not understood. This disorder usually occurs within 24–48 hr after L. pneumophila is inhaled. The disease is not fatal, and no pathologic material has been examined. It is also not known whether bacterial proliferation is required to produce the syndrome and, if so, where the proliferation occurs.

Mechanisms of immunity to L. pneumophila are not well defined. Hotel staff members in the Philadelphia outbreak who had a high prevalence of elevated antibody titers to L. pneumophila Serogroup 1 were apparently protected against disease; this suggests that humoral immunity may be effective. The role of cellular immunity in L. pneumophila infection is unknown.

Clinical Manifestations. Legionnaires disease is a multisystem illness characterized by pneumonia, headache, high fever, chills, cough, myalgia, chest pain, diarrhea, and confusion, with laboratory evidence of mild hepatic involvement and mild renal disease. Renal failure may necessitate dialysis in 3% of patients. The white blood cell count is usually normal or slightly elevated with an increased proportion of segmented polymorphonuclear leukocytes. The erythrocyte sedimentation rate typically is elevated.

The pneumonia progresses over the 1st wk of illness with daily temperatures of 39–40° C; with treatment subsequent resolution is gradual. Chest roentgenograms obtained soon after onset of illness reveal patchy infiltrates that become nodular areas of consolidation which coalesce in severe cases. Pleural effusion is usu-

ally small except in patients with impaired immunity. In immunosuppressed patients pneumonia with cavitation may occur. In the absence of specific therapy, mortality averages 15–20% with death usually resulting from progressive pneumonia with concomitant hypoxemia or from shock. Weakness and shortness of breath may persist for months in a minority of patients, and roentgenographic clearing of the pneumonia is slow.

Pontiac fever is characterized by high fever, myalgia, headache, and extreme debilitation persisting for 2–7 days. Cough, diarrhea, confusion, and chest pain have been observed but are not prominent features. All of the patients known to have had this form of the disease have recovered completely.

Diagnosis and Differential Diagnosis. Legionella pneumonia must be distinguished from common bacterial pneumonias and from infections caused by Mycoplasma pneumoniae, Coxiella burnetii, Chlamydia psittaci, influenza viruses, or any other respiratory viruses. Legionellosis is diagnosed by isolating L. pneumophila in cultures from blood, pleural fluid, respiratory secretions, or lung tissue; by demonstrating the presence of L. pneumophila in respiratory secretions, lung tissue, pleural fluid, or urine by direct immunofluorescence or enzyme-linked, immunosorbent assay; or by demonstrating at least a 4-fold rise in antibody titer in paired serum specimens assayed by indirect immunofluorescence or other methods to titer of more than 128. This commonly occurs by the 21st day of the illness, although seroconversions may not occur in some cases until the 6th wk. Similar rises in titer have been observed in some patients with plague and tularemia, and elevated titer to L. pneumophila has also been observed in patients with rising titers to M. pneumoniae, Rickettsia rickettsii, and Leptospira interrogans.

Treatment. The therapy of Legionnaires disease is both specific and supportive. The disease responds to both erythromycin and tetracycline. In epidemics mortality has been markedly reduced in those treated with erythromycin. Erythromycin should be administered in a dose of 40 mg/kg/24 hr in 4 divided doses intravenously for 14 days (other than for neonates). Oral treatment with 40 mg/kg/24 hr of erythromycin in 4 divided doses also may be utilized. Relapse has been reported in several patients in whom treatment was stopped after 14 days; if relapse is noted, erythromycin therapy should be resumed.

It is presently recommended that rifampin, 15 mg/kg/24 hr, be reserved for combined therapy with erythromycin for those patients with confirmed Legionnaires disease who are not responding to high dose intravenous erythromycin therapy alone.

Specific therapy is not required for Pontiac fever.

Supportive therapy including supplemental oxygen and assisted ventilation may be required. Renal failure requires management of fluid and electrolyte balance and even dialysis on a temporary basis. Vasoactive drugs may be of assistance in the management of shock.

Prevention and Control. No method for preventing epidemics or sporadic cases of Legionnaires disease is effective, but in some instances outbreaks can be stopped. When an epidemic is traced to a cooling tower or an evaporative condenser, these implicated sources should be removed. Individuals at high risk for the disease should not be exposed to other individuals who have Legionnaires disease. Respiratory isolation of patients with Legionnaires disease is recommended, although person-to-person spread has not been proved.

Cohen ML, Broome CV, Paris A, et al: Fatal nosocomial Legionnaires' disease: Clinical and epidemiologic characteristics. Ann Intern Med 90:611, 1979.
Fraser DW, Tsai TF, Orenstein W, et al: Legionnaires' disease: Description of an epidemic of pneumonia. N Engl J Med 297:1189, 1977.
Glick TH, Gregg MD, Berman B, et al: Pontiac fever: An epidemic of unknown etiology in a health department. I. Clinical and epidemiologic aspects. Am J Epidemiol 107:149, 1978.
Lattimer GL, Rhodes LV III, Salventi JS, et al: The Philadelphia epidemic of Legionnaires' disease: Clinical, pulmonary, and serologic findings two years later. Ann Intern Med 90:522, 1979.

10.48 PITTSBURGH PNEUMONIA AGENT

Etiology.   In 1979 Pasculle et al reported the isolation of unique gram-negative, weakly acid-fast bacteria from the lung tissue of 2 renal transplant recipients who had pneumonia. This agent was designated tentatively as the Pittsburgh pneumonia agent (PPA) and is distinct from *Legionella pneumophila* as determined by bacteriologic, ultrastructural, tinctorial, and serologic analyses. Subsequently, pneumonia due to the PPA was documented in 8 immunosuppressed patients.

Pathology.   Touch-imprint smears of biopsied lung may reveal numerous polymorphonuclear leukocytes and many faintly staining gram-negative bacilli. Many of the organisms are intracellular. They are also weakly acid-fast. A fibrinopurulent intra-alveolar infiltrate may be noted. Alveolar septa are congested, but the basic lung architecture usually is preserved. Bronchopneumonia or pneumonia with lobar consolidation may be observed.

Clinical Manifestations.   The patients described to date have been adults in whom pneumonia developed during hospitalization or within several days of discharge. However, it is not unreasonable to suspect that this agent may cause pneumonia in children with malignancy who are immunosuppressed or in children who are immunosuppressed following renal transplantation procedures.

The initial clinical manifestations are mild. If fever is not present at the onset, it usually develops subsequently. There may be pleuritic pain, cough, and sputum production. Disease has progressed in all patients despite treatment with broad-spectrum antibiotics and in several instances with anti-tuberculous therapy as well. The hospital course of surviving patients was one of gradual, slow clinical improvement and even slower resolution of roentgenographic findings, which included patchy bronchial pneumonic alveolar infiltrates, nodular and well circumscribed infiltrates, and pleural effusions.

Diagnosis.   This depends upon an awareness that this new agent has been described and a high index of suspicion of the possibility of this disease in patients who are immunosuppressed. Lung biopsies that reveal gram-indifferent or gram-negative bacilli that are also weakly acid-fast can be cultured in embryonated eggs or guinea pigs. Serum antibody to the PPA can be detected by an indirect fluorescent antibody (IFA) technique.

Treatment.   Erythromycin, rifampin, and the combination of trimethoprim-sulfamethoxazole appear to be efficacious in vitro. When the diagnosis of pneumonia due to PPA is established, treatment with one of these agents is indicated.

Prognosis.   The prognosis is poor, a fact that may, however, be related to the nature of the underlying disease process and the abnormal state of the host rather than to the virulence of the organism.

Myerowitz RL, Pasculle AW, Dowling JN, et al: Opportunistic lung infection due to "Pittsburgh Pneumonia Agent." N Engl J Med 301:953, 1979.
Pasculle AW, Myerowitz RL, Rinaldo CR Jr: New bacterial agent of pneumonia isolated from renal-transplant recipients. Lancet 2:58, 1979.

10.49 INFECTIONS RELATED TO BITES

Human, dog, or cat bites or those of other animals may be followed by a variety of immediate and/or long-term infectious complications. Bite wounds can be presumed to be contaminated with bacteria. Wounds following human bites are usually infected with anaerobic bacteria found in the oropharynx of humans or with *Staphylococcus aureus*. *Pasteurella multocida* is a pathogen commonly associated with cat bites and, less frequently, with the bites of dogs and other animals. *Pasteurella pneumotropica* has also been implicated as a cause of infection from dog and cat bites. The development of tetanus is always a serious additional risk.

The possibility of rabies following animal bites must be considered on an individual basis (Sec 10.85). The risk is dependent upon the species of the biting animal; skunks, coyotes, foxes, wolves, raccoons, cats, and dogs are most likely to harbor this virus. Farm animals, squirrels, opossums, weasels, muskrats, and mongooses also may be infectious. The bite of a bat must always be considered potentially contaminated with rabies virus. The circumstances relating to the bite itself are another important consideration. An unprovoked animal attack suggests rabies as contrasted with the more usual provoked attack that occurs when children intentionally or unintentionally bother an animal. The vaccination status of the biting animal (when known) is also helpful in assessing the risk of rabies. Similarly, the presence of rabies in the region as determined by adequate surveillance enters into the decision with regard to the most appropriate method for treatment of the patient who has been bitten. Finally, the extent and location of the bite, e.g., multiple wounds, deeply penetrating wounds, bites on the head, neck, or hands, may dictate the form of treatment that one desires to provide. It should be emphasized, however, that any open wound or abrasion can be contaminated by the saliva of an animal that is rabid if the animal simply licks the lesion.

Diagnosis. A history of bite, the time of the bite referable to the time the physician sees the patient, and the appearance of the lesion(s) are the most important factors in evaluating infection. If the local wound already reveals erythema, swelling, and a purulent discharge, a diagnosis of infection is indicated. A Gram stain of any exudate from the wound will provide information permitting a rational selection of an antibiotic before culture and sensitivity reports are available. If the purulent material has no foul odor and if gram-positive cocci in clumps are seen, staphylococcal infection may be suspected. If the purulent discharge has no foul odor but gram-negative rods are present, infection with enteric or soil organisms or with *Pasteurella multocida* or *Pasteurella pneumotropica* should be suspected. Gram-negative anaerobes may be present in purulent material even in the absence of a foul-smelling discharge. If there is a foul odor and/or crepitation in the wound, anaerobic infection should always be considered. Gram-negative rods may suggest *Bacteroides* infection, whereas gram-positive rods with spores suggest *Clostridium sp.* Gram-positive cocci in chains may suggest infection with anaerobic streptococci.

Treatment. The care of the bite wound generally is similar to that for any comparable trauma from a contaminated source. The wound should be cleaned thoroughly and nonviable tissue removed by debridement. Quarternary ammonia compounds, such as 1:100 benzalkonium chloride (Zephiran), may be used when exposure to rabies is considered a possibility.

Primary closure of dirty wounds favors infection, particularly in the case of human, dog, or cat bite. Deep puncture wounds or crush injuries which cannot be cleaned adequately and debrided should be left unsutured. Many surgeons suggest that all bites inflicted by humans be left unsutured because of the high probability of local infection. If the wound is potentially disabling or disfiguring, the patient should be referred to a plastic surgeon, hand surgeon, or other qualified individual for an appropriate decision with regard to suturing to promote cosmetic healing.

Tetanus prophylaxis should be given for bites (Sec 10.40). Prophylactic immunization for rabies is instituted immediately if the biting animal is suspected of being rabid or known to be (Sec 10.85).

Because bite wounds can be presumed contaminated with bacteria, prophylactic antibiotic therapy is justified after culture if there is more than a superficial tissue injury. Generally, individuals who have been bitten by dogs or cats should be given penicillin G in doses of 125–150 mg orally 4 times a day for a period of 7–10 days. Human bites are more commonly infected with *Staphylococcus aureus* than animal bites; thus, a penicillinase-resistant drug such as dicloxacillin (50 mg/kg/24 hr in 4 divided doses) may be more effective prophylactically than penicillin. Individuals who are allergic to penicillin can be treated with a cephalosporin (provided that allergy to penicillin has not included anaphylaxis,

exfoliative dermatitis, or an urticarial reaction to penicillin) or alternatively with clindamycin, tetracyclines, or erythromycin.

If purulent drainage already is present and gram-negative rods are seen, ampicillin or amoxicillin plus an aminoglycoside such as gentamicin should be prescribed. A foul-smelling discharge suggesting anaerobic infection should be treated with high doses of penicillin (75,000 units/kg/24 hr) or with clindamycin (if *Bacteroides fragilis* is a consideration). Clindamycin can be given in a dose of 30 mg/kg/24 hr in 3 divided doses. *Pasteurella multocida* and *Pasteurella pneumotropica* both respond to penicillin treatment; tetracyclines are suitable alternative drugs.

Patients who have high fever and other complications of bites such as septic arthritis, osteomyelitis, septicemia, visceral abscesses, or endocarditis should be hospitalized, and appropriate blood cultures should be obtained. The individual should be treated with parenteral antibiotic therapy.

In rare cases certain gram-negative rods have been recovered from the mouth of dogs and have been implicated as a cause of infection in dog bite. These organisms have been designated II$_j$ and EF-4. These organisms are sensitive to ampicillin, tetracycline, and chloramphenicol. Most of the strains of II$_j$ are sensitive to penicillin, but isolates of EF-4 are penicillin-resistant.

RALPH D. FEIGIN

10.50   ACTINOMYCOSIS

Actinomycosis is a chronic suppurative disease of man and animals characterized by abscess formation, multiple draining sinuses, and subcutaneous spread. Infection is caused by an anaerobic actinomycete of the genus *Actinomyces* and may involve the cervicofacial region, the thorax, the abdomen, or the pelvis.

Etiology. *Actinomyces* are gram-positive filamentous bacilli with branching hyphae. Laboratory isolation is infrequent because of the strict anaerobic requirements of these slow-growing microorganisms. Human disease is primarily due to *A. israelii;* however, other species including *A. naeslundii, A. viscosus,* and *A. odontolyticus* have been incriminated.

Epidemiology. Actinomycosis has a worldwide distribution but is decreasing in incidence in the United States. It is uncommon in children and more common in males than females by a ratio of 4:1. *Actinomyces,* not found free in nature, are normal inhabitants of the nasopharynx and gastrointestinal tract. Infection occurs when these bacteria enter damaged tissue following infection, trauma, or surgical instrumentation. There is almost always concurrent infection with other anaerobic microorganisms.

Pathology. Actinomycosis is characterized by areas of suppuration surrounded by extensive fibrosis. Sinus tract formation is common and may extend to the skin surface or deep into internal organs. "Sulfur granules" are scattered throughout the suppurative areas and appear in tissue secretions as rounded basophilic masses representing clumps of myceliae cemented together with calcium phosphate. These hard, yellow-white granules with an average diameter of 2 mm are more common in infections with *A. israelii;* however, they have been reported in infections with other actinomyces, fungi, nocardia, and staphylococci.

Clinical Manifestations. *Cervicofacial actinomycosis* is the most common form of infection in children. The microorganisms gain access to the subcutaneous tissue of the neck from an infected tooth or after surgery or other traumatic injury of the dental structures and oral mucous membranes. Following inoculation, an enlarging area of painless swelling is noted along the margin of the mandible; the fluctuance gradually extends into the neck. The overlying skin becomes tense and develops a red or purple hue, and the mass is characteristically "woody" or indurated. With time, draining cutaneous fistulas appear, and the mass may temporarily decrease in size. Involvement of lymph nodes, the thyroid gland, and underlying bone is uncommon. Pain is minimal, and the infected child has no evidence of systemic disease. Roentgenographic examination of the involved area is typically normal; however, with long-standing disease periosteal reaction and bone destruction become apparent.

Thoracic actinomycosis is uncommon in children and occurs following aspiration of infected oral secretions or, less commonly, after extension of esophageal disease into the mediastinum. The clinical pattern is one of chronic pulmonary infection with fever, night sweats, weight loss, chest pain, productive cough, and hemoptysis. Extension of the pulmonary disease may lead to pleural involvement; however, massive empyema and the classic findings of a draining chest-wall sinus discharging granules are rarely seen. Involvement of the heart and other mediastinal structures is uncommon. Roentgenographic examination is not specific but may demonstrate an extensive pulmonary lesion involving the chest wall and associated with destruction of ribs, sternum, and shoulder girdle.

Abdominal actinomycosis most commonly follows surgical treatment of an acute appendicitis or a perforated abdominal viscus and presents as abdominal pain with fever, weight loss, and a palpable mass in the ileocecal region. Intra-abdominal extension occurs and may involve the entire abdomen. Diagnosis is often delayed. A small percentage of cases of actinomycosis involve the female pelvic organs; these characteristically occur in women using an intrauterine contraceptive device.

Diagnosis. The diagnosis of actinomycosis is established when histologic examination of biopsy material reveals sulfur granules and gram-positive filamentous bacilli with branching hyphae in an area of suppuration. The diagnosis is confirmed by isolating the infecting microorganisms anaerobically.

Treatment. Prolonged antibiotic therapy, surgical drainage of abscesses, and excision of infected tissue are indicated. Massive doses of penicillin (400,000 units/kg/24 hr) given intravenously for 6–8 wk followed by oral penicillin (phenoxymethyl penicillin 2–4 gm/24

hr) for an additional 6–12 mo are used to treat deep-seated infections. In vitro studies suggest that actinomycetes are susceptible to a number of additional antimicrobial agents including chloramphenicol, erythromycin, tetracyclines, and clindamycin. Therapeutic success has been obtained with each of these agents alone or in combination in patients allergic to penicillin.

Drake DD, Holt RJ: Childhood actinomycosis—report of 3 recent cases. Arch Dis Child 51:979, 1976.
Lerner PI: Susceptibility of pathogenic actinomycetes to antimicrobial compounds. Antimicrob Agents Chemother 5:302, 1974.

10.51 NOCARDIOSIS

Nocardiosis is a subacute or chronic suppurative disease of man and animals which occurs following inoculation of the skin, gastrointestinal tract, or lungs with a soil-borne actinomycete of the genus *Nocardia.* Infection in man usually presents as 1 of 3 distinct clinical syndromes: pulmonary (systemic nocardiosis), actinomycete mycetoma, or a localized lymphocutaneous infection resembling sporotrichosis.

Etiology. *Nocardia* species are aerobic, gram-positive, weakly acid-fast bacilli with delicate branching hyphae which appear microscopically as fragmented coccobacillary elements. These microorganisms are nonfastidious and grow over a wide temperature range (25–37° C) on a number of antibiotic-free culture media. *N. asteroides* is the predominant human pathogen in the United States and Europe and most often responsible for pulmonary or systemic nocardiosis. Other human pathogens include *N. brasiliensis* and *N. caviae*, which are typically associated with localized infection of the skin and adjacent soft tissue. Animal pathogens (*N. farcinica*) have recently been incriminated in human disease.

Epidemiology. Nocardiosis is being diagnosed with increasing frequency in the United States; recent studies estimate that 500–1000 culture-proven cases occur annually. Nocardiosis occurs at any age but is more frequent in adults; it demonstrates no particular geographic distribution; males are affected twice as often as females; and it occurs almost exclusively as an opportunistic infection in patients with a serious underlying disease or an alteration in their immunologic status. The respiratory tract is the initial site of involvement in 70% of cases.

Pathology. Nocardiosis produces a suppurative lesion characterized by tissue necrosis and abscess formation which microscopically resembles that seen with the common pyogenic bacteria. Branching filaments of *Nocardia* are often scattered throughout the area of suppuration, and there is no granule formation. There is little localization other than an occasional wall of loose granulation tissue, and local spread with the formation of daughter abscesses is common. Hematogenous dissemination from a pulmonary focus occurs in approximately one third of patients. Though the heart, liver, and spleen are occasionally affected, the secondary infection most often involves the central nervous system, where nocardiosis characteristically presents as a poorly encapsulated multilocular brain abscess.

Clinical Manifestations. In the United States nocardiosis typically presents as a subacute or chronic pulmonary infection in an immune-compromised patient with debilitating underlying disease. Pulmonary involvement begins as a confluent bronchopneumonia which progresses to consolidation, cavitation, pleural effusion, and empyema formation. The clinical findings are nonspecific and include fever, night sweats, a productive cough, anorexia, weight loss, dyspnea, and chest pain. Untreated pulmonary nocardiosis runs a chronic course and may be confused with tuberculosis except that lower lobe involvement is more common. Clinical manifestations may also include tracheitis, bronchitis, pericarditis, and mediastinitis with obstruction of the superior vena cava. Extension through the chest wall and subcutaneous abscess formation are extremely rare. Patients whose disease is complicated by hematogenous dissemination present a miliary picture with multiple subcutaneous abscesses and diffuse organ involvement. Brain abscesses may dominate the clinical picture; extension into the subarachnoid space may lead to a purulent meningitis.

Diagnosis. The signs and symptoms of nocardiosis are not diagnostic; however, a subacute or chronic suppurative pneumonitis with cavity formation and hematogenous dissemination to soft tissue and the central nervous system in an immunosuppressed patient suggests a diagnosis of nocardiosis. Sputum, bronchoscopic washings, pleural fluid, or material obtained by lung aspiration should be Gram stained and cultured for Nocardia. Branching gram-positive filamentous bacilli suggest the diagnosis of nocardiosis or actinomycosis. Nocardia are distinguished by the absence of granule formation and their acid-fast staining characteristics. Diagnosis by culture is difficult, especially in the case of heavily contaminated specimens.

Treatment and Prognosis. Sulfonamides (150 mg/kg/24 hr) in combination with appropriate surgical drainage of abscesses are the treatment of choice for nocardiosis. Antimicrobial susceptibility testing is helpful in selecting alternative therapeutic regimens when sulfonamides cannot be administered because of allergy or intolerance. Alternative drugs (minocycline, erythromycin, ampicillin, cycloserine, tobramycin, and amikacin) may be used in combination with sulfonamides in patients with serious, life-threatening infections. However, the efficacy of combination treatment for nocardiosis is not established. Therapy should be continued for a minimum of 6 wk, but sulfonamide administration is often continued for many mo after apparent cure because of the tendency of nocardiosis to relapse. Since the introduction of sulfonamide therapy, the mortality rate for all forms of this disease has fallen from 75 to 40%; however, only 35% of patients with disseminated disease survive.

WILLIAM T. SPECK

Beaman BL, Burnside J, Edwards B, et al: Nocardial infections in the United States, 1972–1974. J Infect Dis 134:286, 1976.
Curry WA: Human nocardiosis—a clinical review with selected case reports. Arch Intern Med 140:818, 1980.
Lerner PI, Baum GL: Antimicrobial susceptibility of nocardia species. Antimicrob Agents Chemother 4:85, 1973.

10.52   TUBERCULOSIS

Tuberculosis remains among the 10 leading causes of death in the world. Considerable progress in controlling the disease has been achieved in most industrial societies; its mortality rate in the United States, for example, has fallen steadily since the beginning of the 19th century to its present level of about 1.4/100,000 population. Over 30,000 cases of tuberculosis continue to occur annually in the United States, with severe disease found primarily among young children and adolescents. Thus, tuberculosis, in its many forms, remains an important clinical problem in both developing and developed countries.

Etiology. The tubercle bacillus belongs to the genus Mycobacterium, a member of the family of Mycobacteriaceae of the order Actinomycetales. Mycobacterium tuberculosis is responsible for cases of serious disease in humans and is also the most common cause of infection. However, other pathogenic mycobacteria exist, including Mycobacterium bovis, M. leprae, M. paratuberculosis, and a variety of others such as M. ulcerans, M. kansasii, and M. balnei (marinum), variously referred to as nontuberculous, atypical, unclassified, or "anonymous" mycobacteria.

Tubercle bacilli within tissue occur as rod-shaped microorganisms, varying in length from 1–4 microns and in diameter from 0.3–0.6 micron. Their shape is often slightly curved, and the bacteria may appear beaded or segmented. When grown in vitro, the organism may assume a coccoid or filamentous appearance.

Mycobacteria are difficult to stain with basic dyes and resist decoloration with 3–5% HCl and 95% ethanol (Ziehl-Neelsen stain), a property referred to as acid-fastness. Staining with auramine or rhodamine makes tubercle bacilli fluoresce brightly upon exposure to ultraviolet light, a phenomenon which has been employed as a diagnostic method when examining fluids thought to contain small numbers of organisms.

In vivo and in vitro, these microbes grow relatively slowly. They are obligate aerobes and require carbon dioxide for growth. Culture media capable of supporting multiplication of relatively fastidious bacteria are not appropriate for the isolation of most strains of mycobacteria; special substrates are required. More recently developed culture systems incorporate oleic acid and albumin and permit considerably more rapid growth. Differentiation of various mycobacteria is made on the basis of colony appearance, pigment production, growth rate, and a number of biochemical tests. The inoculation of animals, especially guinea pigs, is employed as a means of primary isolation, as a test for pathogenicity, and as a way to differentiate tuberculous from nontuberculous mycobacteria. Tubercle bacilli can survive for several wk in dried sputum and other excreta and possess unusual resistance to ordinary antiseptics. They are, however, rapidly inactivated by sunlight, ultraviolet rays, or temperatures above 60° C.

Of the 3 major strains of organisms causing tuberculosis, *Mycobacterium tuberculosis* is the principal agent of disease. Bovine tuberculosis is now almost unknown in the United States, although it continues to occur in other parts of the world. Avian tuberculosis is exceedingly rare in humans and appears to be caused by organisms considerably less pathogenic than either the bovine or human variants.

Epidemiology. Infants and children are most frequently infected by an adult member of the household, usually a close relative. Casual exposure outside the home is much less likely to produce infection, although on occasion individual cases or small outbreaks have been reported following exposure to an infected teacher, school bus driver, or medical personnel. The usual mode of infection consists of inhalation of droplets of sputum an infectious individual expels on coughing, sneezing, or even speaking. Rarely is the organism spread by dried sputum or by such events as kissing or mouth-to-mouth resuscitation. While the urine of patients with renal tuberculosis may contain numerous organisms, it is not a frequent source of disease. Likewise, discharges from open sinuses are rarely responsible for dissemination. Dogs can acquire the infection from humans and perhaps act as reservoirs. Congenital tuberculosis is acquired when the placenta becomes seeded with microorganisms during maternal bacteremia.

Bovine tuberculosis is acquired via the oral rather than the respiratory route by the ingestion of raw milk from infected cows. Pasteurization destroys infectivity of contaminated fluids.

Immunity and Resistance. Immunity to tuberculosis is exceedingly complex and differs from that found with most other bacterial diseases. While the appearance of agglutinating, precipitating, and complement-fixing antibodies occurs following infection as well as after the injection of dead bacteria or chemical fractions derived from organisms, these antibodies seem to play no detectable role in the development of immunity. Their transfer to other humans and experimental animals has not been shown to enhance resistance to infection. Nevertheless, while initial infection with mycobacteria is followed by their rapid multiplication, the rate sharply diminishes with time. It is possible that this relative state of immunity is mediated through phagocytes and mononuclear cells rather than through antibodies.

In a specific patient, the course of disease is determined by a number of factors, including the virulence of the strain of mycobacteria; the size of inoculum; the hypersensitivity of the individual's tissues; age, nutritional, or social status; presence of intercurrent diseases, infectious and noninfectious; and genetic background. All forms of malnutrition facilitate progressive disease; an improved food intake seems to exert a favorable effect. Similarly, there is little doubt that certain ethnic groups such as Jews are less susceptible to disease than,

for example, American Indians. Twin studies have demonstrated that when 1 homozygous twin has clinical disease, the other is more likely to be affected than is the case in heterozygous pairs. Age has long been recognized as the most important factor in susceptibility. In general, the younger the subject, the greater the likelihood of activity and dissemination. Increased risk also occurs around puberty. Female adolescents have more serious disease than their male counterparts. It is likely that these differences in age- and sex-related susceptibility rates are determined by metabolic activities of the host and not by any specific immunologic defects.

Of the intercurrent infections favoring progression, rubeola and pertussis are most significant. Rapid progression during or after measles remains a common phenomenon in developing countries; with whooping cough this effect is less striking. Other infections can produce similar, if less serious, deleterious effects.

The severity of tuberculosis is enhanced by diabetes mellitus, sickle cell disease, lymphoma, and other malignancies. The administration of glucocorticoid drugs or ACTH enhances tuberculous activity and favors dissemination, perhaps by suppression of local inflammatory response.

Allergy and Immunity. Tubercle bacilli synthesize various proteins responsible for the production of a delayed type of allergy, mediated by a cellular rather than a humoral mechanism and passively transferable by leukocytes. The presence of this allergy is detectable by a "tuberculin test." Whether a relationship exists between this type of allergy and resistance to tuberculosis has not been established; it is likely that these phenomena operate independently. It is known that dissemination is enhanced when drugs are administered that suppress hypersensitivity, but immunity to tuberculosis may persist in the absence of allergy.

Pathology and Pathogenesis. Since pulmonary tuberculosis represents by far the most frequent form of the disease, this process will be described in some detail. When the infection is acquired by routes other than through the respiratory tract, the pathogenesis and pathology are generally similar.

Almost immediately following the inhalation of viable tubercle bacilli into the lungs, histiocytes begin to carry organisms to the regional lymph nodes. Thus, the so-called primary complex is formed. It consists of the initial focus at the site of invasion and tuberculous lymphangitis leading from the focus to the regional nodes. The lymphadenitis may be marked by extensive inflammation and by a tendency toward caseation necrosis in the regional nodes.

The initial primary invasive focus, on the other hand, is often small, measuring only a few mm in diameter. When allergy develops to the products of the organism about 3–8 wk after initial infection, local histology changes and the initial focus becomes surrounded by a perifocal reaction. Mononuclear cells change to epithelioid cells, which cluster to form tubercles. Giant cells appear and the whole area is surrounded by lymphocytes. The regional lymph nodes enlarge. This primary focus may then dissolve and disappear, or central caseation may develop, which consists of incomplete cell autolysis. This lesion, too, may resolve spontaneously, or it may "soften" or liquefy or, if the multiplication of tubercle bacilli is inhibited by developing immunity or therapy, become encapsulated by fibroblasts and collagen fibers. The final process consists of hyalinization and calcification.

When the lesion progresses, the area of caseation will slowly enlarge and often perforate into a bronchus, which results in emptying of the semiliquid material, creating a pulmonary cavity. Aspiration of the contents of the cavity into other parts of the lung may follow, producing multiple foci in 1 or both lungs.

Calcification, a late stage of healing, occurs more rapidly in children than in adults. Viable mycobacteria may persist for many yr in calcified areas. Calcification may be permanent or may begin to resorb within 3–5 yr and eventually disappear completely.

Bacteremia, either directly from a primary focus or from the lymph nodes, seems to take place in every patient, beginning during the incubation period and persisting continuously or intermittently for several days or weeks. It is probably the quantity of tubercle bacilli released into the bloodstream and the host's susceptibility which determine whether this process remains permanently asymptomatic or is initially silent but is then followed by the appearance of metastatic lesions months or years later. More severe forms of bacteremia also occur, such as protracted hematogenous tuberculosis which is accompanied by fever, leukocytosis, and evidence of the formation of multiple metastases. The most dangerous form of disease, acute miliary tuberculosis, represents the extreme end of the spectrum of severity.

Since bacillemia occurs in every patient with primary tuberculosis, and since most complications of the disease in children are due to hematogenous spread from a primary focus, it is evident that even asymptomatic initial infection must never be considered a benign or normal process.

Diagnosis. In general, diagnosis utilizes a number of approaches, either separately or simultaneously: (1) epidemiologic history, (2) clinical history, (3) physical examination, (4) roentgenographic examination, (5) tuberculin testing, and (6) isolation and identification of tubercle bacilli.

Epidemiologic History. Most children with tuberculosis have a history of exposure to a known or suspected tuberculous adult. Any child with a history of contact with an infected adult, especially within the household, must be suspected of having tuberculosis; this possibility can be eliminated only by careful investigation utilizing the approaches discussed below.

Clinical History. As a rule, the initial onset of tuberculosis is symptomless; even children with progressive illness may have only minimal symptoms, usually far less than might be expected from the associated disease process. Hence, clinical history is of relatively little importance.

On occasion, the so-called typical symptom complex may be found: failure to thrive, or even loss of weight, chronic cough, fatigue, anorexia, and night sweats.

Persistent fever of 1–2 wk duration may accompany the development of primary tuberculosis, and erythema nodosum may occur when hypersensitivity to tuberculin develops. When the major disease process is found in organs other than the lung, such as in the central nervous system, bone, lymph node, or kidney, involvement of these organs is readily demonstrable.

Roentgenographic Examination of the Chest. This should always be done and should include lateral and oblique, as well as posteroanterior views, since enlarged nodes may be demonstrable by the former films but be missed in the latter.

The findings most characteristic of tuberculosis are enlarged lymph nodes; hilar, pulmonary, cervical, or abdominal calcifications; lesions of the vertebral bodies; and enlargement of the spleen. If associated with a positive Mantoux test, the presence of any 2 of the above findings is considered diagnostic of active tuberculosis. Individuals with positive tuberculin tests may have no detectable pulmonary lesion on roentgenographic examination. However, one must assume that the infection is present but that the lesions are too small for identification or have completely healed.

Tuberculin Skin Tests. These are by far the most important diagnostic tool. Two antigens are available for diagnostic use: purified protein derivative (PPD) and the Old Tuberculin (OT) of Koch. Applications are intracutaneous (Mantoux) and multiple puncture (e.g., Tine and Heaf).

Both of the available antigens are satisfactory, although PPD possesses certain advantages, especially that of consistent potency. It is produced by precipitation of the proteins of tubercle bacilli after growth in synthetic media. The precipitate is further refined into PPD-S, which was adopted in 1952 by the World Health Organization as the international standard tuberculin. Somewhat similar products are produced by a number of institutions, e.g., Weybridge Laboratories in England and the Statens Seruminstitut, Copenhagen; these differ slightly from PPD-S, but are equally satisfactory. The Danish product is widely used outside the United States; 1 unit corresponds to approximately 3 units of the PPD-S.

While concentrated solutions of both OT and PPD are stable, more dilute solutions are unreliable since they are inactivated by heat and by sunlight. Furthermore, tuberculin is adsorbed onto glass surfaces. The currently available diagnostic PPD solutions, when kept refrigerated in filled glass containers protected from light, may retain their potency for about 6 mo. PPD-S is also available as a tablet to be dissolved in an appropriate amount of buffered diluent prior to use. The concentrated solution of OT is regarded as containing 1000 mg/ml; it must be diluted prior to use with the proper buffered solution.

Potency of tuberculin is expressed in tuberculin units (TU). One TU is approximately equal to 0.01 mg of OT and 0.00002 mg of PPD.

To assure reproducibility, the tuberculin test should be performed in a standardized manner. Since antigen is adsorbed firmly to glass, a syringe used for tuberculin should not be employed for any other purpose or for injection of less concentrated tuberculin materials. An appropriate syringe is fitted with a 26 or 27 gauge needle with the bevel directed upward and then used to introduce 0.1 ml of either OT or PPD into the most superficial layer of the epidermis of the forearm, producing an immediate wheal. The needle should not be withdrawn for a few sec, to minimize leakage. The usual dose for both diagnostic and survey work is 5 TU (equivalent to 0.0001 mg PPD). If the patient is suspected of possessing marked hypersensitivity, smaller amounts such as 1 TU may be employed for the initial dose.

Mantoux tests with larger amounts of tuberculin (such as 100 TU) were often performed in the past, but should be done now only under special circumstances, as in malnourished children in whom marked suppression of dermal hypersensitivity is common.

The reaction should be read at 48 and 72 hr. Induration (not erythema) is measured in millimeters with a caliper or a ruler at right angles to the long axis of the arm.

It is crucial that the results of the Mantoux test be properly interpreted. A reaction less than 5 mm in diameter is considered negative. Induration measuring from 5–9 mm in diameter is doubtful and should be repeated, while a lesion 10 mm or more in diameter indicates a positive test. When the reaction is severe, considerable local swelling and redness may occur, occasionally with ulceration, local lymphangitis, and lymphadenopathy. Rarely, constitutional signs develop, such as fever and malaise.

The reasons why doubtfully positive tuberculin reactions occur are probably many. Studies in various parts of the world have shown great variation in the frequency of reactions measuring less than 10 mm. It is thought that other cross-reacting antigens, such as atypical mycobacteria, may be responsible.

Because organisms other than Mycobacterium tuberculosis may produce positive tuberculin tests, and because other events such as drug therapy or intercurrent infection, may inhibit the production or size of the skin reaction, individualized interpretation is required despite the general definition of positive, intermediate, and negative. For example, a child should be considered to have tuberculosis even with a "doubtful" skin test if there is a positive history of contact and compatible clinical findings or if the child is less than 2 yr of age.

Other factors may suppress the skin test. Live measles vaccine produces temporary anergy lasting 2–3 wk, similar to that from natural measles. Chickenpox less commonly produces a similar effect, of relatively short duration. It is possible that other viral vaccines suppress local dermal hypersensitivity on occasion, but do so apparently more rarely than rubeola vaccine.

Adrenocortical hormones may reduce allergy to OT and PPD, with peak inhibition found 4–6 wk after steroid therapy has begun. This effect is not completely predictable; generally, the skin test is completely suppressed in fewer than one third of patients. Children with clinical malnutrition syndromes may have diminished or negative tests. On occasion, individuals receiving isoniazid therapy lose their positive skin test at some time during the late stages of treatment or following its completion. Infants less than 6 mo of age, but more commonly less than 3 mo, may be unable to produce sufficient local inflammation for a positive skin test despite infection with tubercle bacilli.

Repeated testing does not confer tuberculin allergy on the individual, nor is there evidence that the injection of 5 TU can produce an exacerbation of an active or quiescent tuberculous process. As many as 30 injections a year have not resulted in the acquisition of positive tests by individuals previously negative. On the other hand, a "booster" phenomenon has been described in patients in whom skin test reactivity has waned with the passage of time; the intradermal injection of tuberculin may then result in an anamnestic response so that a 2nd skin test performed after a relatively short interval may result in a considerably enhanced reaction. This series of events can readily be confused with conversion due to recent infection.

Although the Mantoux procedure is considered the standard by which other tests must be judged, 3 other methods are in use in public health screening programs and in physicians' offices because of their relative ease of application.

The Heaf test is convenient for mass screenings but requires a special apparatus. The Heaf gun makes 6 simultaneous skin punctures 1 mm deep through a layer of concentrated PPD. The test is read from 3–7 days later and the presence of 4 or more papules constitutes a positive reaction. In general, this procedure is not as reliable as the Mantoux; it is so sensitive that a number of false positive reactions occur. Therefore, all positive tests should be corroborated with a Mantoux reaction.

The Tine test, a disposable unit with 4 small blades predipped in an Old Tuberculin concentrate, is commonly employed in physicians' offices. A positive reaction is considered to consist of 1 or more papules, each measuring at least 2 mm in diameter. The test is read in 48–72 hr. Perhaps because of technical factors, false-negative reactions do occur and all doubtful or positive reactions need to be compared with a standard Mantoux test.

The Mono-Vacc test utilizes a plastic scarifier mounted on the outer side of a ring. A plastic tube containing Old Tuberculin is sealed around the points. The tube is removed just prior to application and the tuberculin solution squeezed onto the points. The material is applied by pressing the points into the skin of the forearm. A doubtful reaction measures 2 mm, while positive reactions are larger with frequent vesiculation. Less information is available about the reliability of this test than about the Heaf and Tine procedures.

Bacteriologic Examination. The definitive method of diagnosis of tuberculosis is the isolation and identification of M. tuberculosis from appropriate fluids or tissues. Generally, guinea pig inoculation is no more sensitive than in vitro culture; thus, most institutions prefer to rely solely on the latter method. For definitive diagnosis, direct microscopic examination of appropriate materials is not as reliable as culture, since sputum, gastric contents, and urine may contain acid-fast bacteria other than M. tuberculosis; false-positive results may occur.

Since most tuberculosis affects pulmonary tissue,

examination of sputum is an important diagnostic procedure. Unfortunately, infants and children frequently do not cough, or, if they do, produce little expectoration, which is usually promptly swallowed. Thus, examination of gastric contents generally replaces sputum examination in these age groups, although, on occasion, material from the lungs can be obtained after appropriate stimulation by ventilatory therapy or by direct bronchoscopy.

Gastric aspiration should be carried out early in the morning on a fasting patient, preferably upon awakening. Gastric contents are aspirated into a glass syringe attached to a suitable catheter and placed in a sterile container. Following this, the stomach is washed with 30–50 ml of sterile water and the content again aspirated; this is added to the initial material. The procedure should be repeated at least twice on separate days.

Tubercle bacilli may also be grown from materials such as biopsy specimens; pleural, pericardial, or peritoneal effusions; spinal fluid; or drainage from abscesses or sinuses. In hematogenous tuberculosis, the organisms may occasionally be recovered from bone marrow aspirates or from biopsy specimens of the liver. Urine culture is useful in the diagnosis of renal tuberculosis.

Biopsy specimens should also be examined histologically. Often the classic tissue changes combined with the microscopic demonstration of the presence of acid-fast bacteria in lesions suffice for diagnosis.

Other Laboratory Investigation.   There are no characteristic hematologic changes. On occasion, with severe hematogenous disease, a leukemoid reaction may occur and some of the more severely affected children may develop thrombocytopenia and a declining hematocrit. Some children with primary tuberculosis demonstrate a rising gamma globulin level, while children with progressive disease, tuberculous meningitis, or miliary tuberculosis may show low serum levels of these proteins. The alpha$_2$-globulins increase progressively with activity and extent of disease and this measurement has been used, though not reliably, as a measure of progression and healing. The sedimentation rate is too erratic to be employed as a measure of activity.

Prevention.   Three approaches are in use: protection against exposure, immunization, and chemoprophylaxis.

Children acquire their disease from adults, and thus they must be protected by systematic surveillance of individuals whose occupation brings them into intimate contact with children and adolescents, such as school personnel, babysitters, food handlers, and so on. Furthermore, children should not be exposed to known tuberculous adults, even those on appropriate therapy. The rate of tuberculosis can be reduced only by a program of active case finding and protection of children. Other methods of control, such as vaccination and chemoprophylaxis, are far less effective and, even when widely used, do not result in the same sharp decline of disease incidence.

Vaccination with BCG (*bacille Calmette-Guérin*, an attenuated strain of *M. bovis*) still must be considered controversial despite wide use. The basic premise behind the method was that infection with this organism would result in immunity similar to that resulting from primary infection. However, for many yr following its introduction in France, no suitably controlled studies were carried out; thus the procedure is still regarded with some suspicion by many physicians. Part of the problem in evaluating BCG was due to technical factors, many of which are not relevant to the freeze-dried preparations presently employed. There are no simple laboratory tests to measure the efficacy of 1 batch versus another. Perhaps the only useful method of evaluating potency is to determine tuberculin conversion rates in susceptible human beings.

The degree of protection from BCG, if any, varies among different population groups but is never absolute, or even nearly so. In general, those individuals most susceptible to progressive and hematogenously disseminated disease by virtue of age and race benefit more than children whose resistance is greater. The duration of protection conferred by the vaccine is a matter of dispute; experience obtained in several large studies suggests that it lasts for 7–12 yr, but even 50 yr after the development of the vaccine it is not known whether booster doses are indicated or advisable.

In general, BCG vaccine should be administered as early in life as possible; in many countries it is given immediately after birth. At other ages, it should be employed only in tuberculin-negative individuals. Criteria for its application to population groups differ; 1 approach is to advise routine use in newborns if the tuberculin reactor rate at puberty is in excess of 10–15%. The vaccine is also recommended for children traveling to areas of the world where tuberculosis is prevalent or who are otherwise likely to be exposed to adults with active or recently arrested disease.

The dose is usually 0.05 ml for newborns and 0.1 ml for older individuals, injected superficially into the skin. A small papule forms and gradually enlarges, crusts, and then disappears in 8–12 wk. On occasion, local abscesses form, more commonly following deep injections. If abscesses occur or if there is evidence of spread, antituberculous drugs such as isoniazid and rifampin should be administered. Since these agents inhibit the multiplication of the vaccine organisms, it is likely that their use may reduce the efficacy of immunization.

The major drawback to BCG is the fact that it causes conversion of the tuberculin test. Thus, the physician can no longer employ the Mantoux test for diagnosis, and it becomes useless as a survey tool among populations in which BCG is frequently administered. In countries such as the United States, where tuberculosis among children is relatively uncommon, the value of the Mantoux test far outweighs the potential benefits of widespread administration of BCG.

Chemoprophylaxis is sometimes used when an individual must live in a highly contaminated environment for variable periods of time, e.g., an infant sent to a household with an active or recently arrested case of tuberculosis. There are adequate data derived from animal experiments to suggest that the regular administration of isoniazid protects effectively against infection. However, as with all long-term prophylactic regimens, compliance of patients tends to be poor.

PULMONARY TUBERCULOSIS

While tuberculosis may affect any organ, disease occurs most commonly in the lung. Two classifications of pulmonary tuberculosis are currently employed: initial disease (primary disease) and reactivation tuberculosis (adult or chronic pulmonary tuberculosis).

Initial Tuberculosis
(Primary Tuberculosis)

A majority of children and adults do not demonstrate any symptoms with initial infection, but some may be mildly ill and a few go on to more diffuse, progressive or miliary disease. In most children, the only evidence of tuberculous infection may be the conversion of a previously negative skin test. Lack of symptoms does not indicate benign infection; on occasion, patients with extensive disease involving lung or other organs may be asymptomatic.

Symptoms of initial pulmonary infection, when they do occur, are usually nonspecific and may consist of fever (rarely above 39° C, or 102° F) lasting only a few days but occasionally persisting for 2–3 wk. There may also be anorexia, weight loss, irritability, malaise, and easy fatigability. These findings are observed more frequently in young children. In older individuals they are often erroneously attributed to overwork, worry, school problems, etc.

Frequently, temperature elevation is too mild to be readily detectable unless regular determinations are made. An occasional young child may demonstrate signs and symptoms of an upper respiratory tract infection. This may be related to an intercurrent disease or a manifestation of tuberculosis.

Only rarely is the classic pulmonary infiltrate with hilar adenopathy detectable roentgenographically. More commonly, there are no roentgenographic changes; occasionally, modest mediastinal lymphadenopathy may be noted. Once a pulmonary infiltrate does appear roentgenographically, it may persist for many mo despite adequate therapy. Calcifications may or may not occur during healing. They persist for many yr, eventually disappearing in a few patients. Occasionally, erythema nodosum and phlyctenular conjunctivitis may occur during the initial infection, more commonly in some racial groups. Currently, however, erythema nodosum is rarely caused by tuberculosis.

Pneumonic tuberculosis represents a less common mode of onset. This process generally begins abruptly and may mimic lobar bacterial pneumonia with high fever, cough, and respiratory distress; physical findings include dullness on percussion, increased breath sounds, and moist rales. Even when the patient remains untreated, these signs and symptoms persist for only a few days, occasionally for up to 2 wk. While major roentgenographic findings may disappear at a similarly rapid rate, a small infiltrate will generally remain. Despite its apparent greater immediate severity, the ultimate prognosis of pneumonic tuberculosis is no different from that of asymptomatic or minimally symptomatic disease.

Because of the small numbers and the location of organisms involved, and despite the presence or absence of cough, patients with initial tuberculosis are virtually noninfectious and need not be isolated.

The mediastinal lymph nodes are regularly involved in initial infection but rarely cause symptoms. If problems do occur, they are related to partial or complete obstruction of a bronchus by enlargement of the peritracheal or peribronchial nodes. Partial obstruction results in asthmatic or stridorous breathing, usually associated with a loud and brassy cough, and there may be local hyperresonance related to overexpansion of the affected pulmonary segment. Complete obstruction leads to atelectasis of the distal segment, with dullness to percussion, decreased breath sounds, and, if the process is extensive, tachypnea. Compression of pulmonary parenchyma and bronchi may rarely result in secondary bacterial pneumonia. Extensive bronchiectasis and pulmonary fibrosis in the area distal to the obstruction may occur, but generally do not cause symptoms.

More rarely, a lymph node erodes through the wall of a bronchus and slowly discharges its content into the lumen; endobronchial spread of disease results. Widespread bronchitis and pneumonitis occur, with accompanying cough, respiratory distress, and cyanosis. The severity of illness is inversely related to the age of the patient and directly to the extent of disease. Physical findings may consist of rhonchi and rales; roentgenograms demonstrate varying degrees of bilateral alveolar consolidation.

Tuberculous pleurisy is a late complication but usually appears within the 1st yr after initial infection. The patient complains of cough, pleuritic pain, and usually shortness of breath and demonstrates objective evidence of fluid in the chest, with dullness on percussion and decreased breath sounds. The degree of pulmonary involvement is not related to the occurrence of pleurisy. Roentgenograms readily demonstrate the effusion. On thoracentesis the fluid is straw-colored, with a high protein content, and contains several hundred or, rarely, several thousand lymphocytes/mm^3. Occasionally, organisms can be seen on smear; more commonly, they are isolated only on culture. Even if untreated, spontaneous resolution of pleurisy usually occurs within 3–4 wk. However, because of the fact that patients are uncomfortable and may experience severe dyspnea, prompt treatment is indicated.

Reactivation Tuberculosis
("Adult" Tuberculosis, "Chronic" Tuberculosis)

Once the initial infection has healed, no further problems occur in most individuals. In a few patients, however, areas of the lung seeded during the initial hematogenous dissemination may become sites of active bacterial multiplication. The apices of the lung are most commonly involved, but the same process may occur anywhere in the pulmonary parenchyma. The early lesion consists of a small infiltrate which enlarges, rapidly becomes encapsulated, then caseates and liquefies. The liquid material eventually empties into a bronchus, forming a cavity and resulting in spread of bacteria to other areas of the lung. Coughing aerosolizes this infected liquid and thus spreads infection to other individuals.

Severity of symptoms is related to the extent of the process and its rate of progression. The most common early symptom is dry cough; as the lesions progress, the patient begins to produce sputum which is initially mucoid but then changes to mucopurulent and frequently becomes blood streaked. Rarely, erosion of a blood vessel produces a pulmonary hemorrhage. A variety of nonspecific symptoms are initially quite mild and readily overlooked: low-grade fever, malaise, anorexia, weight loss, and night sweats all increase in severity and intensity with time. Objective pulmonary signs are generally not observed until disease is extensive; even then they may remain quite subtle.

The earliest roentgenographic change usually is a well-circumscribed, homogeneous shadow, most commonly in the apex of a lung. As the lesion enlarges, it may resemble a patchy infiltrate or a globular or lobar consolidation. As liquefaction necrosis occurs, the classic cavitary lesion becomes visible.

Untreated reactivation tuberculosis may heal spontaneously or develop into progressive pulmonary disease. Serious complications may ensue, such as bronchial and tracheal ulceration, spontaneous pneumothorax, pleurisy and empyema, widespread bronchiectasis, tuberculous laryngitis, intestinal tuberculosis, or miliary dissemination with involvement of many organs.

Differential Diagnosis. Histoplasmosis and coccidioidomycosis (Sec 10.106 and 10.105) may be confused with tuberculosis. Diagnosis depends on an appropriate geographic setting, isolation of the offending microorganism, the application of suitable skin tests, and, if possible, confirmation by serologic diagnosis. More rarely, pulmonary abscesses or chronically progressive pneumonias produced by measles, adenovirus, cytomegalovirus, pneumocystis, and other agents may be confused with tuberculosis, especially in the immunosuppressed patient. Differential diagnosis can often be accomplished by means of the tuberculin test (although this may be nonreactive in the presence of some malignancies or medications) or appropriate cultures of sputum and gastric contents. On occasion, lung puncture or pulmonary biopsy may be necessary for differentiation, especially in patients with malignant disease in whom enlargement of the hilar or mediastinal lymph nodes, commonly found in tuberculosis, may be produced by the tumor. The absence of a positive tuberculin test in sarcoidosis helps differentiate that disease. Occasionally, children with pertussis or other forms of laryngotracheobronchitis mimic the clinical presentation of tuberculous endobronchitis. In these patients, a positive tuberculin test and the presence of enlarged hilar nodes should permit appropriate identification.

EXTRAPULMONARY TUBERCULOSIS

Tuberculosis in organs other than the lung usually results from hematogenous spread, which occurs soon after the initial pulmonary focus is established. Bacter-emia ceases with the development of cellular immunity and delayed hypersensitivity.

Most hematogenously spread disease occurs within 1 yr after the initial pulmonary focus was established and prior to puberty, except for genitourinary tuberculosis, which is found from early puberty through adulthood and affects females more frequently than males. Some forms produce early symptoms (superficial lymph nodes, central nervous system, and skeleton) while others become apparent only after a longer period of time (genitourinary).

Tuberculosis of the Upper Respiratory Tract

The various structures of the upper respiratory tract may become infected either by direct inoculation following ingestion of contaminated milk or sputum or by hematogenous spread. Tonsils, adenoids, buccal mucosa, larynx, middle ear, and mastoids may be involved separately or in combination. Tonsillar and adenoidal disease is usually asymptomatic but, on occasion, may be associated with recurrent fever of varying degree and a persistent sore throat. The appearance of granulomas or tuberculous ulcerations in the mucosa of the mouth is rare in children. Involvement of the larynx is usually manifested by pain on swallowing, hoarseness, and a croupy cough. Middle ear disease usually remains asymptomatic until perforation of the tympanic membrane and drainage of pus into the external canal occur. Mastoid disease may be associated with middle ear disease and represents a specific form of tuberculous osteomyelitis.

Occasionally, retropharyngeal nodes are involved, either secondarily from infection of the cervical vertebrae or by spread from other affected nodes.

Retropharyngeal abscesses caused by tuberculosis do not differ in their symptomatology from those produced by pyogenic organisms. Symptoms consist primarily of difficulty in swallowing or breathing, with local pain and discomfort. Lateral roentgenograms of the neck will show typical widening of the retropharyngeal space. Since the response to antituberculous therapy is good, incision of the abscess need be carried out only in those patients with respiratory distress.

Miliary Tuberculosis

This disease is most common in infants and young children and occurs within the 1st 3–6 mo after initial pulmonary infection. Its pathogenesis consists of invasion of a blood vessel by a caseous focus, followed by discharge of infectious microorganisms into the circulation. To some extent the clinical presentation depends on the number of organisms in the bloodstream and the rate at which they are entering. In acute miliary disease, large numbers of mycobacteria circulate and seed many organs within a short period of time. Numerous tubercles develop in various tissues, ranging in size from that of millet seed to 1 cm or more.

Fever of 39–40° C (102–104° F) is usually the 1st sign. At the same time, the child may develop fatigue, malaise, anorexia, and weight loss, all of which may be erroneously attributed to an initial pulmonary lesion. Seven–14 days later, the classic roentgenographic changes begin to appear; often the 1st finding is a mottling of the lungs. As these lesions progress, the patient may develop dyspnea, cyanosis, and widespread fine rales over both lung fields. Liver, spleen, and superficial lymph nodes enlarge in about half of the cases.

The laboratory is of little help in diagnosis. The tuberculin test is positive in about 90% of patients at the time of the appearance of symptoms. The sedimentation rate is markedly elevated, and the white blood cell count may be as high as 15,000–40,000/mm³, with a moderate shift to the left.

With time, other lesions may become apparent. Rare findings are cutaneous metastases and tubercles visible in the choroid on ophthalmologic examination. Meningitis was common in the preantibiotic era, but is now a far less frequent consequence of miliary tuberculosis. However, even in the absence of clinical meningitis, the spinal fluid may show a modest increase in cells and protein.

The untreated patient develops increasing respiratory distress, weight loss, and irritability, and death usually occurs within 3 mo of onset. Despite the severity of disease, appropriate chemotherapy results in rapid and often dramatic clinical improvement, except that the fever may not respond for 7–10 days. Roentgenographic changes in the lungs do not regress for 1 mo or more.

A somewhat different clinical picture is produced if organisms are discharged intermittently into the bloodstream in small amounts over an extended period of time. While this form of miliary tuberculosis is frequently seen in developing countries, it is rare in the Western world. Tubercles form in many organs and vary in size from tiny to several cm in diameter. The most common clinical presentation consists of "fever of unknown origin," with a continuous or remitting pattern of elevation to 39–40° C. Liver and spleen are usually enlarged and firm but not tender. Superficial lymph nodes are generally greatly enlarged but rarely caseate and drain. Large mediastinal and abdominal lymph nodes may compress or obstruct neighboring organs and produce a variety of confusing clinical signs and symptoms such as obstruction of biliary drainage, abdominal pain, compression of a ureter, bronchial obstruction, or atelectasis. Involvement of bones occurs commonly; and perifocal disease such as joint effusion also is seen. The white blood cell count may rise to as high as 40,000/mm³ or greater. The majority of patients have positive tuberculin tests, but anergy may occur. Roentgenographic findings in the lung demonstrate many lesions of varying or similar size throughout the pulmonary parenchyma.

As with the acute disease, response to appropriate chemotherapy is excellent, although these patients do not improve as rapidly.

Differential Diagnosis. The roentgenographic appearance of miliary tuberculosis is often not diagnostic, and the tuberculin test may be negative. A similar clinical picture may result from mycotic infections, such as coccidioidomycosis and histoplasmosis (Sec 10.105

and 10.106), which occur only in specific geographic areas and can generally be recognized by appropriate skin or serologic tests. Similar pulmonary findings may also be produced by sarcoidosis, reticuloendotheliosis, eosinophilic pneumonia, lymphosarcoma, and leukemia. On occasion, pulmonary or other organ biopsy may be necessary for precise differentiation.

Tuberculosis of Superficial Lymph Nodes

Involvement of superficial lymph nodes is a common manifestation of tuberculous infection. Rarely this may result from drainage from an adjacent initial lesion (such as inguinal adenopathy following skin tuberculosis of the leg or auricular node involvement from tuberculous conjunctivitis). Much more commonly, superficial lymph node involvement occurs from seeding of the node by hematogenous dissemination. The process therefore generally develops within 6 mo after the initial infection. The disease is usually bilateral, involves multiple groups of nodes, and occurs most commonly in the cervical chain. Whatever the site, the nodes slowly enlarge, unaccompanied by any specific or nonspecific systemic symptoms, and are initially firm, nontender, and easily demarcated. Gradually the masses become less distinct, appear to be matted together, adhere to the skin, and eventually may become fluctuant and drain through a sinus tract.

Tuberculous adenopathy is readily confused with other conditions; most commonly the process resembles that produced by nontuberculous mycobacteria and may, in fact, be virtually indistinguishable except through appropriate laboratory investigation. Moreover, it may also resemble pyogenic infection, fungal involvement of lymph glands, cat-scratch disease, brucellosis, lymphoreticular malignancy, or, occasionally, infectious mononucleosis.

Because of the close resemblance to nontuberculous mycobacterial disease, accurate diagnosis can often be accomplished only by biopsy and culture of the tissue removed at surgery. Surgical intervention also has therapeutic benefit; a caseous node which would heal only very slowly on chemotherapy may be excised entirely in order to shorten the duration of antimicrobial therapy. This is often recommended when a diagnosis of tuberculosis is strongly suspected. Needle aspiration of the affected node may prove satisfactory for diagnosis but does not permit removal of the major part of the lesion.

Lymph node tuberculosis generally responds to appropriate antimicrobial therapy. Affected smaller nodes may disappear completely; larger nodes fibrose and may continue to be palpable as irregular, firm-to-hard masses after the infection has been cured.

Tuberculous Infection of the Central Nervous System

Meningitis occurs most frequently within 6 mo after the onset of initial infection and represents the major cause of death from childhood tuberculosis.

Prior to the advent of effective therapy, meningitis

was always fatal, resulting in death usually less than 20 days after appearance of the 1st symptoms. While antimicrobial agents have considerably reduced the mortality, survival and reduction of the incidence of neurologic residua depend on early diagnosis.

The condition is most commonly found in young children (age 6-24 mo) but may occur in all age groups. Meningitis results from the seeding of tubercle bacilli in the cerebral cortex, meninges, and choroid plexus during the time of initial hematogenous spread. Within a short time, organisms established at these sites produce caseous foci. Depending on their size and location, these foci then can produce 3 separate types of central nervous system disease: meningitis, tuberculoma, and serous meningitis.

Tuberculous Meningitis

The onset is usually insidious but may be fulminant if a caseous lesion discharges directly into subarachnoid space. Clinical manifestations may be conveniently grouped into 3 stages: stage 1 (general, nonspecific symptomatology), stage 2 (appearance of definite neurologic signs), and stage 3 (coma).

It is difficult to suspect the correct diagnosis during stage 1 because of the nonspecific nature of the symptomatology. The child seems uninterested in playing, has periods of idly staring into space, and may be febrile. The older child may show rather abrupt mood changes, declining school performance, lethargy, and apathy. Because these early manifestations may occur intermittently, they may be disregarded or blamed on other problems.

With time, irritability becomes worse and may alternate with apathy. Approximately half the children will experience episodes of vomiting, a symptom which is, however, not prominent. Some patients may complain of headache. Children under 2 may have seizures, a sign rarely found in older age groups. Very rarely there are complaints of constipation, diarrhea, or abdominal pain. In general, stage 1 lasts about 1 wk but may be as long as 3 wk. If a tubercle ruptures into the subarachnoid space, stage 1 may be so brief as to be overlooked entirely and the patient may rapidly progress into stage 3.

Stage 2 is marked by the appearance of neurologic signs, which result from an exudate that forms over the cerebral convexities. Inflammation of the meninges produces nuchal rigidity and positive Kernig and Brudzinski signs. As time progresses, a thick gelatinous infiltrate and an exudate develop at the base of the brain, producing signs of cranial nerve and brain stem involvement consisting of strabismus, ptosis, sluggish pupils, visual disturbances, and variable, but often brisk, deep tendon and absent superficial reflexes.

Blood vessels of the meninges and cortex may become involved in the process, resulting in arteritis and vasculitis. These changes and the accompanying inflammation cause cerebral edema, which produces symptoms and signs of encephalitis, consisting of confusion, disorientation, slurred speech, grimacing, changes in consciousness, athetoid movements, and tremors of the extremities. With time, hemiparesis and tache cérébrale may develop.

The child now rapidly passes into stage 3, manifested by unresponsiveness, opisthotonos, decerebrate rigidity, and papilledema.

Obviously, the diagnosis of tuberculous meningitis should be established as early as possible. History of exposure to tuberculosis is useful. The tuberculin skin test is nearly always positive, and roentgenograms may show a pulmonary lesion. Lumbar puncture will invariably show abnormal spinal fluid. White blood cells are usually fewer than 350/mm^3 and consist primarily of mononuclear cells, but on occasion the count may rise up to 1000/mm^3, with a predominance of polymorphonuclear leukocytes. The spinal fluid glucose level is depressed early in the course of disease to levels below 40 mg/dl. Protein concentration is normal or slightly elevated early, but in time may increase to 300 mg/dl or more. A test formerly thought to be specific was a decrease in chloride concentration of spinal fluid. This change reflects levels of serum chloride which are depressed because of inappropriate antidiuretic hormone secretion or, more rarely, because of protracted vomiting. If an aliquot of spinal fluid is allowed to stand undisturbed for several hr, a pellicle may form. Organisms are most readily seen within the matrix of the pellicle and can also be easily cultured from this material.

Two major factors determine prognosis: the age of the patient and the stage of disease at which treatment is begun. In general, children under 2 yr of age have considerably higher mortality rates and a higher incidence of neurologic sequelae. In stage 1, a cure rate of 100%, with a low incidence of permanent nervous system damage, is expected. Even with optimal therapy, stage 2 is associated with a 15% mortality and a 75% incidence of neurologic sequelae. In stage 3, a 50% mortality is expected; the incidence of neurologic residua is more than 80% among survivors.

The most common neurologic sequelae are developmental retardation, cranial nerve palsies, hydrocephalus, optic atrophy, deafness, paralysis, continuing stupor or coma, convulsions, and pituitary disturbances.

Serous Meningitis

This unusual entity is in itself quite harmless. The clinical picture cannot be distinguished from that of early tuberculous meningitis or tuberculomas involving the brain or spinal cord, although spinal fluid glucose levels are usually normal. This process resolves spontaneously. However, because the condition is not readily distinguished from the clinical picture of more serious disease, the patient should be treated as a case of tuberculous meningitis until the diagnosis of serous meningitis is firmly established, a differentiation which may prove very difficult to accomplish.

Tuberculoma of the Central Nervous System

This consists of single or multiple tuberculomas of the brain or spinal cord, a syndrome apparently found more commonly in the Orient than in other parts of the world. A lesion may occur at any time during the course of tuberculosis and present as a slowly expanding mass lesion. The process, therefore, greatly resembles the clinical picture produced by an intracranial tumor and, while the presence of a tuberculoma may be suspected because of disease in other organs and a positive tuberculin test, the diagnosis is usually established when the patient is subjected to surgical exploration in order to remove the mass.

If a tuberculoma of the central nervous system is encountered at surgery, it is probably best not to attempt to excise or to evacuate it. Appropriate antituberculous therapy is begun, but it generally requires many yr for healing to take place. On occasion, a tuberculoma ruptures into the subarachnoid space, producing tuberculous meningitis of sudden onset.

Urogenital Tuberculosis

Organisms reach the genitourinary tract during the initial phase of tuberculous bacteremia but, for reasons which are poorly understood, manifestations of disease tend to be delayed for several yr and thus are seen more commonly in adolescents and adults than in young children.

The early course is usually asymptomatic; its only manifestation may be pyuria with sterile cultures on routine media. Eventually, the mycobacteria may invade the bladder, producing dysuria, frequency, and urgency. At this stage, urinalysis generally shows persistent proteinuria and microscopic hematuria in addition to pyuria. In male patients the process may spread to the epididymis and prostate.

Unfortunately, organisms are difficult to find in the urine and may be recognized only by culture or guinea pig inoculation. Intravenous pyelography is useful to delineate the extent of disease. Cystoscopy and other manipulations of the urinary tract should be preceded or promptly followed by the administration of appropriate antituberculous therapy to prevent dissemination of infection.

Once the process has produced considerable parenchymal damage, normal renal function is rarely restored. However, specific antimycobacterial therapy does arrest the disease promptly and relapses occur infrequently. Because of the possible late appearance of ureteral strictures, producing hydronephrosis with additional renal damage, it is necessary to follow patients annually with intravenous pyelograms for a period of at least a decade.

Tuberculous orchitis is rare in children as well as in adults. Tuberculosis of the female genital organs is also rare but may be found in adolescents. Most common is involvement of the fallopian tubes, often associated with endometritis. This process frequently results in generalized or localized tuberculous peritonitis; therefore, the symptoms of peritoneal involvement may mask those of salpingitis. On occasion, tuberculous salpingitis is mistaken for acute appendicitis, with the correct diagnosis established only at surgery.

Tuberculosis of the Skin

This organ may become involved in 3 ways: the skin may be inoculated directly, the process may follow hematogenous spread, or the lesion may represent a cutaneous manifestation of an underlying focus of active infection, such as osteomyelitis or adenitis (scrofuloderma). Direct inoculation of tubercle bacilli into the skin usually produces a painless ulcer or papule which may be overlooked until significant enlargement of the regional lymph nodes occurs. These lesions may slowly progress but quite commonly show a pattern of spontaneous healing followed by recurrence at about the time that the regional adenitis begins a few wk later.

Papulonecrotic tuberculids are typically associated with hematogenous spread and their presence is considered an important clinical manifestation of disseminating disease. They bear a superficial resemblance to the papules and pustules of chickenpox but tubercle bacilli can be demonstrated on biopsy. Much rarer manifestations of hematogenous spread are lichen scrofulosus and erythema induratum.

Tuberculosis of the Eye

In those rare instances in which the conjunctiva is directly inoculated with tubercle bacteria, severe, usually bilateral inflammation occurs, readily mistaken for a viral or bacterial infection. Progressive enlargement of the preauricular and anterior cervical lymph nodes invariably follows, and, quite frequently, small single ulcerative lesions may be found on the palpebral conjunctivae. If such an ulcer is scraped and the material appropriately stained, tubercle bacilli are readily demonstrable.

Phlyctenular conjunctivitis (Sec 25.10) results from a nonspecific hypersensitivity reaction and is manifested by a jelly-like mass appearing on the limbus.

Deeper structures of the eye may also be involved. Tubercles of the choroid occurring during the course of miliary tuberculosis are most common. Involvement of the retina or the uvea in children is very rare.

Tuberculosis of the Abdominal Cavity

Gastrointestinal tuberculosis most commonly follows ingestion of mycobacteria. Formerly, most cases were due to the consumption of infected cow's milk, a phenomenon which has virtually disappeared from most parts of the world. At present, most infection occurs when patients with pulmonary disease swallow their own sputum. The symptoms are nonspecific and consist of abdominal pain, diarrhea (sometimes alternating with constipation), and weight loss. Secondary anemia is common. The process is occasionally mistaken for regional ileitis. The frequency of intestinal tuberculosis is not well established, but is undoubtedly very low in children.

Abdominal lymph nodes may become involved either

from hematogenous spread or from local intestinal tuberculosis. The symptoms are similar to those described for gastrointestinal disease; additional findings are related to compression or involvement of adjacent structures, which may result in intestinal obstruction.

Occasionally, a node ruptures into the peritoneal cavity, producing peritonitis with effusion. This same syndrome may occur rarely following hematogenous spread of tuberculous salpingitis. Tuberculous peritonitis can usually be diagnosed by appropriate examination of peritoneal fluid. With time, massive adhesions may develop, producing generalized intestinal obstruction and death.

Tuberculosis of the Heart and Pericardium

Tuberculous pericarditis is a rare complication of childhood tuberculosis. Signs and symptoms are generally nonspecific, and the disease may vary from minimal to extensive. The clinical picture does not differ from pericarditis of any other cause, and diagnosis is usually established when a pericardiocentesis produces fluid containing mycobacteria or a pericardial biopsy shows appropriate histologic changes. Prognosis for complete recovery is excellent if the diagnosis is made early and appropriate therapy administered. Chronic adhesive pericarditis may develop in neglected patients.

Tuberculosis of the Endocrine and Exocrine Glands

Rarely, initial infection may occur in the lacrimal, salivary, and mammary glands; otherwise, tuberculosis of the endocrine-exocrine systems is generally a result of hematogenous dissemination. Disease usually occurs only after a very lengthy interval following initial infection, averaging 6–15 or more yr, and thus is exceedingly rare in children.

Bone and Joint Tuberculosis

This is discussed in Sec 23.3 and 23.6.

Tuberculosis in Newborn Infants

Since the portal of entry in the newborn infant may be different and the host and environment distinctive, tuberculosis in this age group is unique. Intrauterine infection is caused by hematogenous dissemination during the latter stages of the mother's pregnancy. The infecting organisms may penetrate directly into the fetal circulation after granulomas have formed in the placenta, or a tuberculous endometritis may develop with subsequent aspiration of infected amniotic fluid. Thus, infection can occur directly via the bloodstream of the fetus, with the initial site of infection being the liver, followed by the lymph nodes of the porta hepatis and

the spleen. Infection may then proceed via the ductus venosus through the heart into the lungs. On the other hand, aspiration of infected amniotic fluid results in direct infection of the respiratory tree, an event which might also occur immediately after birth by exposure to a mother with "open" tuberculosis or following resuscitation by a tuberculous individual.

The most common manifestations of congenital tuberculosis are jaundice, anemia, failure to thrive, cyanosis, enlargement of the spleen, and diffuse pneumonia, often associated with thrombocytopenia. The tuberculin test may remain negative until the 2nd–3rd mo; apparently the infant's cells fail to respond to the stimulus with the appropriate delayed hypersensitivity. Diagnosis is most commonly made by the history of maternal tuberculosis, occasionally by finding tubercle bacilli in gastric washings, or by discovery of granulomas and organisms in liver or lung biopsy specimens. Chemotherapy with isoniazid and rifampin produces excellent results; however, extensive calcification of the lesions usually occurs.

THERAPY OF TUBERCULOUS INFECTION AND DISEASE

Because of the unique properties of mycobacteria, the nature of the pathologic lesions, and the influence of various host factors on the course of tuberculous infection, appropriate management involves not only the application of a number of general principles but also the use of specific drug therapy. Unlike nearly all other types of infectious disease, management of tuberculosis involves months and years of effort, occasionally extending throughout the entire life span of the patient. Specifically, it is essential that parents understand the peculiar problems presented by the disease; when children are old enough to look after their own needs, they too must be appropriately educated about factors which aid or diminish the possibilities of progressive illness.

General Management

Once the diagnosis has been established, whether or not hospitalization is necessary for optimal management must be decided. Circumstances requiring hospitalization include (1) extensive or life-threatening disease, such as miliary, pericardial, renal, extensive pulmonary, osseous, or meningeal tuberculosis; (2) tuberculosis in a young infant; (3) need for isolation or for cultures or biopsies in order to arrive at a diagnosis; (4) need for surgical intervention or corticosteroid therapy; and (5) family or social circumstances such that appropriate management cannot be achieved in the home environment.

While the child is in the hospital, efforts should be made to identify, isolate, and appropriately manage the contact from whom the infection was acquired.

The great majority of children with initial tuberculosis do not require hospitalization but can be managed adequately at home. The patient should be encouraged to lead as normal a life as possible; specifically, there is no need to restrict activity, encourage bed rest, or, unless nutritional disturbances are present, prescribe a special diet. Parents should know that the child does not have to be protected from other individuals and is not contagious to playmates or family members. Once appropriate antituberculous therapy has been started, there is no need to withhold the usual childhood immunizations. When the patient is febrile because of intercurrent infection or the tuberculosis, bed rest should be considered only if the child wishes it. If he or she feels well enough out of bed to pursue normal activities, this should be encouraged. Throughout management, the excellent prognosis of appropriately treated tuberculosis should be re-emphasized to the parents, schoolteachers, or anyone else with frequent contact with the family, to diminish as much as possible those anxieties and concerns often found among people exposed to the popular or cultural myths concerning human tuberculosis.

Chemotherapy of Tuberculosis

Response to appropriate antituberculous therapy is slow and recovery is prolonged. The slow evolution of healing is usually not due to ineffective therapy or lack of patient compliance but is an essential feature of the disease. Ideally, the selection of therapeutic agents should be based on appropriate susceptibility studies of organisms isolated from the patient or, failing that, from the contact from whom the disease was acquired. Often this is not possible and choice of therapy must be either empiric or based on knowledge of the general susceptibility patterns of mycobacteria found in the specific geographic area where the patient resides or acquired the disease. It is not wise to accept sweeping statements of generalized drug resistance without detailed evidence that such is the case. In developing countries, it is often assumed on the basis of observed "therapeutic failures" that widespread resistance to isoniazid, rifampin, or other drugs is present when, in fact, treatment failures are due to lack of compliance of patients with the prescribed regimen.

Therapeutic agents are most active when the mycobacteria are multiplying rapidly; thus, as the disease becomes quiescent and bacterial multiplication slows, the efficacy of agents sharply diminishes. Prolonged therapy is therefore required to eliminate all bacteria, a goal which may not be achievable in some patients despite years of effort.

Antituberculous drugs are generally administered singly or in double or triple combinations. Combination therapy is not necessarily used to increase efficacy but rather to prevent the development of resistant strains of mycobacteria. For example, the incidence of naturally occurring resistance to isoniazid is about 1 in 10^5 bacilli. Similarly, assuming that spontaneous resistance to rifampin occurs once in 1 in 10^6 organisms, then the chance of resistance developing in 1 organism to both drugs is in the range of 1 in 10^{11} organisms. In general, since patients with acute and severe infections harbor larger numbers of organisms than those with more

established and chronic disease, the former group might be treated with 2 or even 3 drugs while the latter group might be given 1 or 2. Finally, data indicate that in those individuals who are infectious to others, the possibility of spread can be reduced more rapidly by the use of combined therapy.

Antituberculous Drugs. A considerable number of agents with antituberculous activity are available (Table 10–32) but differ in their degree of usefulness. Only 2 medications can be considered truly outstanding: isoniazid (INH) and rifampin (RMP). All other drugs are inferior in efficacy or have sufficiently high toxicity to prevent optimally effective use.

Isoniazid is an established drug which is rapidly absorbed and penetrates readily into all tissues and bodily fluids, including the central nervous system. The drug is excreted primarily through the kidney. Children tolerate and can be given substantially larger doses than adults on a weight or surface area basis. The hepatotoxicity and peripheral neuropathy occasionally observed in adults are rarely encountered in children. In fact, toxicity in the pediatric age group is so unusual that liver function need not be monitored except in those patients with pre-existing hepatic disease. Furthermore, there is no need for concurrent pyridoxine administration unless diet is inadequate. There is some suggestion that pyridoxine may diminish the efficacy of isoniazid.

Rifampin is available in the United States only as an oral drug but is so well absorbed that there is little need for a parenteral preparation. It penetrates well into tissues and spinal fluid. Because of inhibition of absorption by the concurrent administration of food, the drug should be given at least 1 hr before or 2 hr after a meal, a precaution which is not necessary with isoniazid.

A warning label required of the manufacturer in the United States notes that few data exit on its use in patients under 5 yr of age, but widespread experience indicates that rifampin is effective and safe in small children. As with isoniazid, the drug appears to be less toxic to children than to adults, liver damage occurring far less commonly in children.

Rifampin is never used alone for the treatment of tuberculosis but is always employed in combination with isoniazid or another drug such as ethambutol, streptomycin, or para-aminosalicylic acid (PAS).

Ethambutol (EMB) is a highly effective antituberculous agent which has replaced PAS almost entirely among adults. It is far cheaper than rifampin, and in areas of the world where the latter drug is excessively expensive, recent studies have shown that, for most purposes, excluding perhaps tuberculous meningitis, ethambutol can be safely substituted. However, its use in children remains quite limited because adequate toxicity data do not exist for patients under 13 yr of age; therefore, appropriate conditions for use are not well established. It is probably contraindicated in children less than 6 yr of age (unless rifampin is not available) because in this age group its major toxic effect (optic neuritis) cannot be adequately monitored by visual acuity and color discrimination tests.

Streptomycin (SM) is useful only parenterally because it is poorly absorbed when given orally. However,

Table 10–32 MAJOR ANTITUBERCULOUS DRUGS FOR CHILDREN

DRUG	TOTAL DAILY DOSE	ROUTE AND FREQUENCY OF ADMINISTRATION	MOST FREQUENT ADVERSE REACTIONS	MAJOR INTERACTIONS WITH OTHER DRUGS	COMMENTS
Isoniazid (INH)	10–20 mg/kg (max. 600 mg)	Oral; given in 1 or 2 doses per day	Hypersensitivity: rash, fever; peripheral or optic neuritis;*† hepatotoxicity†	Diphenylhydantoin: INH may enhance toxicity; antacids containing aluminum salts may inhibit absorption	Tablets of 50, 100, and 300 mg and syrup (10 mg/ml) available; tablets are preferred because of occasional erratic syrup stability or absorption
Rifampin (RMP)‡	10–20 mg/kg (max. 600 mg)	Oral; given in 1 or 2 doses per day, 1 hr before or 2 hr after meals	Dyes body fluids red; hepatotoxicity;† leukopenia; thrombocytopenia; G.I. upset	Coumarin derivatives: decreased anticoag. effect; oral contraceptives: decreased cardiac contractility, efficacy; glucocorticoids: decreased steroid effect; probenecid: increased RMP toxicity	300 mg capsules; pharmacist should prepare smaller doses for suspension in flavoring medium by parents just prior to use
Ethambutol (EMB)§	10–15 mg/kg (max. 1500 mg)	Oral; 1 dose daily	Hypersensitivity: rash, fever joints; optic neuritis;¶ G.I. upset; Neurologic: confusion, dizziness	No information available	Tablets of 100 and 400 mg (scored)
Streptomycin (SM)	20–40 mg/kg (max. 1 gm)	Intramuscularly; given in 1 or 2 doses per day	Ototoxicity: vestibular or hearing loss; hypersensitivity: rash, fever, joints	Increased nephrotoxicity with cephalosporins, increased ototoxicity with diuretics, esp. ethacrynic acid; neuromuscular block with curariform drugs	Ampules: dry — 1 gm and 5 gm; prediluted: 1 gm/2 ml
Aminosalicylic acid (PAS)	200–300 mg/kg (max. 12 gm)	Oral; given in 2, 3, or 4 doses per day	G.I. upset, anorexia; hypersensitivity: fever, rash	Probenecid: increases PAS toxicity; aspirin: concomitant use may produce salicylism	Very unstable in aqueous solution, or when tabs are in humid environment or light; only 1 month's supply should be dispensed; parent should mix preweighed powder with flavoring just prior to use

*Pyridoxine supplement not necessary unless patient is malnourished and will continue to receive inadequate diet while on INH therapy.
†Hepatotoxicity occurs very rarely in children. Monitoring of liver function indicated only on clinical evidence of hepatic dysfunction or if patient has history of previous liver disease.
‡Manufacturer's warning: Inadequate dosage data for children under 5 yr of age. See text.
¶Optic toxicity should be monitored by pretherapy visual acuity and visual field determinations and tests for color discrimination. Test should be repeated monthly while on therapy.
§Manufacturer's warning: Not recommended for children under 13 yr since conditions for use have not been established.

because of the existence of more effective and potentially safer drugs, the use of streptomycin is limited to the treatment of miliary or meningeal disease when the use of a 3rd drug is considered necessary.

The toxic effects of streptomycin are primarily on the vestibular and the cochlear portions of the 8th cranial nerve; generally, vertigo and ataxia are noted before hearing loss occurs. Streptomycin appears to be less toxic in children than in adults, but, in general, its use should be restricted to a 4 wk course because a longer period of administration increases the likelihood of damage.

Aminosalicylic acid (para-aminosalicylic acid, PAS) is an oral drug closely related to aspirin and commonly employed with INH. As an antituberculous agent it is not very effective, but it does have the property of diminishing the opportunity for development of resistance to other drugs, especially isoniazid. The major side effect of PAS is gastric and intestinal irritation; frequent occurrence of gastritis manifested by nausea, abdominal pain, and vomiting may prevent the administration of PAS and other oral medications and diminish the child's food intake, which, in poorly nourished patients, may have a detrimental effect on the course of disease. If PAS is administered with meals in a somewhat lower dosage which is then gradually increased, the incidence of gastritis and intestinal toxicity

is significantly reduced. Unfortunately, the stability of PAS powder is poor, especially in humid environments, and the liquid preparation is likely to deteriorate quickly. Thus, this drug should be prescribed in small amounts and, if liquid preparations are required in small children, parents should be instructed to make these up from measured aliquots of powder just prior to administration. Because of its close pharmacologic and chemical resemblance to aspirin, parents should be warned not to administer the latter drug if the child develops fever from intercurrent infection; to do so might result in acute salicylism.

In addition to the 1st-line drugs already mentioned, a number of other pharmacologic agents are useful primarily when mycobacteria have been shown to be resistant to isoniazid or rifampin or when other drugs are not available. Unfortunately, experience with these medications in children has been relatively limited; only kanamycin has been studied to any extent.

Kanamycin, viomycin, and *capreomycin* are probably equally efficacious and are somewhat similar in toxic effects, the major one being their effect on the auditory portion of the 8th nerve, with subsequent loss of vestibular function. Viomycin induces hypersensitivity and a variety of electrolyte abnormalities; capreomycin is more nephrotoxic than the other 2 drugs. These agents are rarely useful and then only in place of streptomycin

Table 10–33 INDICATIONS FOR USE OF SINGLE-DRUG THERAPY OR PROPHYLAXIS IN CHILDHOOD TUBERCULOSIS*

INDICATIONS	DURATION OF USE
Close contact with active case of tuberculosis	3 mo if tuberculin test remains negative and no evidence of disease; otherwise, 1 yr
Tuberculin-positive child or adolescent	
With known recent skin test conversion	1 yr
Prior conversion or skin test not previously treated	1 yr
Receiving glucocorticoid or immunosuppressive medication	For duration of immunosuppressive therapy
Receiving rubeola vaccine	1 mo
With rubeola, pertussis, or influenza	1 mo
Undergoing surgery with general anesthesia	1 mo

*Preferably isoniazid; alternative drug is rifampin.

when the organism in question has been shown to be resistant to the latter agent.

Cycloserine is occasionally useful in older children and in adolescents when these patients cannot tolerate PAS or ethambutol. It is given in a dose of 10 mg/kg/24 hr, not to exceed a maximum of 500 mg/24 hr. Generally, the dose is divided into 2 equal portions given at about 12 hr intervals. The drug has a variety of adverse effects on the central nervous system, and hypersensitivity to it develops quite rapidly.

Ethionamide is occasionally used when tubercle bacilli are resistant to other agents. Recommended dosage is 12–15 mg/kg/24 hr, divided into 3 equal doses, with a maximum daily dose of 750 mg/24 hr. The drug may

Table 10–34 CHEMOTHERAPY OF TUBERCULOUS DISEASE

DISEASE	ANTITUBERCULOUS DRUG THERAPY*	DURATION†	OTHER DRUG THERAPY	COMMENTS
1. Chest				
a. Initial infection with demonstrated pulmonary disease	INH, 10–20 mg/kg/24 hr, *and* RMP, 10 mg/kg/24 hr; *or* INH plus EMB; *or* INH plus PAS	12 mo	None	INH dose of 20 mg/kg/24 hr may be used for 3–4 wk in more severe disease
b. Locally progressive pulmonary disease	INH, 20 mg/kg/24 hr *and* RMP (? plus SM)‡	12 mo	None	SM given for 4 wk only; INH may be reduced to 10 mg/kg/24 hr after 4–12 wk
c. Endobronchial	Same as 1b	12 mo	Prednisone, 1–2 mg/kg/24 hr for 4–6 wk if severe symptoms of compression occur (i.e., dyspnea or cyanosis)	Same as 1b
d. Chronic (reactivation) pulmonary disease	Same as 1b	12 mo	None	Same as 1b
e. Pleurisy and/or pericarditis	Same as 1a	12–18 mo	When effusion present, prednisone, 1–2 mg/kg/24 hr, may increase rate of resorption	Fluid should be removed for diagnosis or relief of symptoms; thoracotomy tube not indicated
2. Miliary				
a. Acute	Same as 1b	18–24 mo	Prednisone, 1–2 mg/kg/24 hr, for 4–6 wk if severe dyspnea	Examine CSF weekly for 3–4 wk
b. Protracted	Same as 1b	18–24 mo		
3. Central nervous system				
a. Meningitis	Same as 1b	18–24 mo	See Comments	Prednisone probably decreases mortality but increases neurologic sequelae, may be used in impending CSF block; monitor fluid and electrolytes; provide adequate nutrition and active physical therapy even when comatose
b. Tuberculoma with or without meningitis	Same as 1b	18–24 mo	See Comments	
c. Serous meningitis	Same as 1a	12 mo	None	See text
4. Nonpulmonary primary disease	Same as 1a	12 mo	None	Same as 1a
5. Skeletal	Same as 1a	12–18 mo	None	Same as 1a; immobilize until healing established; abscesses should be curetted and drained
6. Superficial lymph node	Same as 1a	12–18 mo	None	Surgical excision if node is caseous
7. Urinary tract	Same as 1a	24 mo	None	Repeat IVP and voiding cystourethrogram every 6 mo while on therapy and every yr for 10 yr; see text
8. Miscellaneous: skin, endocrine, abdominal, upper respiratory tract, ocular, etc.	Same as 1a	12–18 mo	None	Same as 1a

*INH: isoniazid; RMP: rifampin; EMB: ethambutol; PAS: aminosalicylic acid; SM: streptomycin.
†Evidence has been presented that shorter courses may be adequate in adult patients, but whether this applies in children is presently unknown.
‡It has not been clearly established that a regimen of INH *and* RMP *and* SM produces better clinical rsults than INH *and* RMP. (See text.)

cause severe gastrointestinal irritation and induce hypersensitivity.

Pyrazinamide is a very potent agent which possesses marked hepatotoxicity and consequently cannot usually be given for periods in excess of 5–6 mo. No good data on dosage exist for children. In general, this drug is probably too hazardous for use.

Single-Drug Therapy. Under certain circumstances, the use of a single-drug regimen is indicated (Table 10–33). The preferred drug is isoniazid, which is administered for periods of time ranging from 1 yr in patients with minimal evidence of disease to 1 mo in children previously treated but found in situations favorable to reactivation of disease (as for example during the administration of measles vaccine or during illness with measles or pertussis). The medication is also useful in the treatment of household contacts of known infectious cases even if the contact's tuberculin skin test is still negative; it is known that early treatment prior to the stage of hematogenous dissemination (when hypersensitivity has not yet developed) will promptly eradicate infecting organisms and thus eliminate the focus of infection. Under these circumstances, skin tests may never become reactive.

Double- and Triple-Drug Therapy. For most forms of tuberculous disease, regimens utilizing 2 drugs are employed (Table 10–34). The generally most useful combination is isoniazid and rifampin, but when the latter drug is not available or excessively expensive, similar results can be achieved with isoniazid and ethambutol or, in younger children to whom ethambutol cannot be given, with isoniazid and PAS. In patients with severe, potentially fatal disease such as miliary, meningeal, locally progressive, and chronic cavitary tuberculosis, triple therapy is generally recommended (Table 10–34), usually consisting of isoniazid, rifampin, and streptomycin (for 1 mo). However, there is some evidence suggesting that therapy with isoniazid and rifampin may be as effective as regimens which add streptomycin to these 2 drugs.

Corticosteroids. Glucocorticoid preparations have limited usefulness in the treatment of tuberculosis. They are known to reactivate otherwise latent disease and, in the absence of appropriate antituberculous therapy, to spread the infection. However, because of their antiinflammatory effect, they may be useful in pleural and pericardial disease because reabsorption of fluid is promoted. These drugs also diminish respiratory problems in miliary disease with massive pulmonary involvement. Despite their frequent use in tuberculous meningitis and endobronchial disease, there is no convincing evidence that corticosteroids contribute to a better prognosis, improve effectiveness of therapy, or promote more rapid healing.

Surgery. Surgical intervention is rarely required in children. Biopsies may be necessary for diagnosis, and, in cases of tuberculosis of a cervical lymph node, excision of the affected structure may reduce the need for prolonged therapy and promote local healing. Bronchoscopy is sometimes required to diagnose various forms of pulmonary tuberculosis and to manage a few patients with endobronchial tuberculosis. In renal tuberculosis in which massive parenchymal destruction is evident and the disease is unilateral, excision of the kidney is occasionally indicated.

When any type of surgery is contemplated in a child who has a positive tuberculin test, it is generally advised that INH be administered beginning a few days prior to surgery and continuing for 1 mo if the procedure requires the use of general anesthesia. In emergency cases INH should be started as soon as possible after surgery and continued for 1 mo.

HEINZ F. EICHENWALD

Akbani Y, et al: Control of streptomycin and isoniazid in malnourished children treated for tuberculosis. Acta Pediatr Scand 66:237, 1977.

American Academy of Pediatrics: The tuberculin test. Pediatrics 54:650, 1974.

American Thoracic Society: BCG vaccines for tuberculosis. Am Rev Resp Dis 112:478, 1975.

British Medical Research Council: Clinical trial of six month and four month regimens of chemotherapy in the treatment of pulmonary tuberculosis. Am Rev Resp Dis 119:579, 1979.

Cawson RA: Tuberculosis of the mouth and throat. Br J Dis Chest 54:40, 1960.

Difenbach WCL: Tuberculosis of the heart. Am Rev Tuberc 62:390, 1950.

Dubos RJ: Biological and social aspects of tuberculosis. Bull NY Acad Med 27:351, 1951.

Edwards PQ: Tuberculin testing of children. Pediatrics 54:628, 1974.

Ehrlich RM, Lattimer JK: Urogenital tuberculosis in children. J Urol 105:461, 1971.

Glassroth J, Robins AG, Snider DE Jr: Tuberculosis in the 1980's. N Engl J Med 302:1441, 1980.

Hsu KHK: Isoniazid in the prevention and treatment of tuberculosis; a 20 year study of the effectiveness in children. JAMA 229:526, 1974.

Lincoln EM: Tuberculous meningitis in children with special reference to serous meningitis. II. Serous meningitis. Am Rev Tuberc 56:95, 1947.

Lincoln EM, Sewell EM: Tuberculosis in Children. New York, McGraw-Hill, 1963.

Lincoln EM, et al: Tuberculous pleurisy with effusion in children. A study of 202 children with particular reference to prognosis. Am Rev Tuberc 77:271, 1958.

Lorber B, et al: Failure of isoniazid to cure localized BCG infection. JAMA 238:55, 1977.

Pauker M, et al: Conservative treatment of a BCG osteomyelitis of the femur. Arch Dis Child 52:330, 1977.

Sbarbaro JA: Skin test antigens: An evaluation whose time has come. Am Rev Resp Dis 118:1, 1978.

Sifontes JE: Rifampin in tuberculous meningitis. J Pediatr 87:1015, 1975.

Strumf IJ, et al: Re-evaluation of sputum staining. Am Rev Resp Dis 119:599, 1979.

Sumaya CV, et al: Tuberculosis in children during the isoniazid era: J Pediatr 87:43, 1975.

Thompson NJ, et al: The booster phenomenon in serial tuberculin testing. Am Rev Resp Dis 119:587, 1979.

Udani PM, et al: Neurologic and related syndromes in CNS tuberculosis; clinical features and pathogenesis. J Neurol Sci 14:341, 1971.

Visudiphan P, Chiemchanya S: Evaluation of rifampin in the treatment of tuberculosis meningitis in children. J Pediatr 87:983, 1975.

Wasz-Hockert O, et al: Late prognosis in tuberculous meningitis. Acta Pediatr Scand 51:(Suppl. 141):1, 1963.

TUBERCULOSIS DURING PREGNANCY

The potential hazards of ionizing radiation and antituberculosis chemotherapy for the pregnant woman and her unborn child have modified the diagnostic and therapeutic approach to tuberculosis during pregnancy. Initial screening relies heavily on tuberculin skin testing with limited use of a roentgenographic examination, and therapeutic decisions require an understanding of the indicated drugs and their potential for producing serious untoward sequelae in the mother and her infant.

Tuberculosis Screening. Pregnancy has no inhibitory effect on cutaneous reactivity to tuberculin; thus all women should be skin tested during their 1st antenatal visit except for those with a previous history of a positive reaction. A positive skin test (greater than 10 mm induration with 5 TU PPD) warrants further investigation of the patient, family members, and close contacts to diagnose active disease. In asymptomatic women with a positive skin test and normal physical findings, roentgenographic examination of the chest is deferred until completion of the 1st trimester of pregnancy. When roentgenograms are obtained during pregnancy, shielding the abdomen and avoiding portable equipment with its excessive scattered radiation minimize the risk to the developing infant. Skin test positive patients with symptoms compatible with active disease and/or an abnormal physical examination should have an immediate roentgenogram of the chest.

Chemoprophylaxis. Pregnancy is considered a contraindication for isoniazid prophylaxis because of the hepatotoxicity of isoniazid and the possible adverse effects of this drug on the developing fetus. Thus asymptomatic pregnant women with positive skin tests and with chest roentgenograms showing no active disease should not begin isoniazid prophylaxis until completion of pregnancy.

Chemotherapy. Women who at any time during pregnancy are symptomatic and/or have roentgenographic evidence suggesting active disease should be hospitalized. Sputum and gastric aspirates should be collected, stained for acid-fast microorganisms, and cultured for *M. tuberculosis*. Women with sputum positive for acid-fast bacilli should begin immediate treatment with isoniazid, ethambutol, and pyridoxine. If stained smears fail to reveal microorganisms but the clinical history and roentgenograms are suggestive of active disease, treatment should begin after sputum and gastric aspirates have been cultured. If cultures fail to reveal mycobacteria after 8 wk of incubation, treatment should be discontinued; however, close follow-up and repeated evaluation should continue throughout pregnancy and the immediate postpartum period.

Infants Born to Mothers with Active Tuberculosis

Approximately 50% of infants born to mothers with active pulmonary tuberculosis develop disease within the 1st yr of life. Therefore, prophylaxis is recommended for them. There is controversy, however, whether such treatment should consist of BCG immunization or isoniazid administration. The advantages of BCG administration include probable effectiveness, lack of toxicity, and the need for a single injection. The latter eliminates problems of noncompliance and loss of follow-up examination. The disadvantages of immunoprophylaxis with BCG include variability of response in immunized individuals, limited value of subsequent tuberculin testing, and a necessary period of post-immunization separation of mother and infant prior to skin test conversion and protection. Chemoprophylaxis of newborn infants with isoniazid has proved efficacious and permits continued use of tuberculin skin testing to document subsequent infection. The major disadvantages of isoniazid prophylaxis in the newborn

Table 10–35 MANAGEMENT OF INFANTS OF MOTHERS WITH QUESTIONABLE OR ACTIVE TUBERCULOSIS

MOTHER	MANAGEMENT OF INFANT
Tuberculin-reactive (including recent converter)	No immediate prophylaxis necessary; tuberculin test every 3 mo for 1 yr
Asymptomatic	If positive, rule out active tuberculosis If active disease, begin therapy If no active disease, begin isoniazid prophylaxis* If negative tuberculin, retest annually
Past history of treated active tuberculosis, presumably asymptomatic	Same as above
X-ray consistent with questionable or minimally active disease†	Rule out congenital tuberculosis If present, begin therapy If not present, BCG‡ vaccination or isoniazid prophylaxis
Advanced pulmonary or extrapulmonary tuberculosis, or disseminated infection	Rule out congenital tuberculosis If present, begin triple therapy If not present, isoniazid for 1 yr, or isoniazid for 3 mo followed by chest x-ray and tuberculin; if both negative, give BCG; if tuberculin reactive and chest negative, give isoniazid; if chest positive, begin total therapy for 1 yr

*Isoniazid prophylaxis: 15–20 mg/kg/day given as a single dose.
†Mothers with active disease should be treated and separated from their infants until noncontagious.
‡BCG is recommended when noncompliance and/or loss to follow-up examination is considered likely in situations in which the infant will be exposed to endemic tuberculosis in the environment. Immunization requires that 0.05 ml of BCG be injected superficially over the deltoid or triceps muscle. The infant is separated from the mother or other potentially contagious individuals until tuberculin positive (6–8 wk); if persistently negative, a 2nd dose of BCG is given. BCG should not be given during isoniazid prophylaxis because isoniazid inhibits multiplication of BCG. (After Weinstein L, Murphy T: Clin Perinatol 1:395, 1974.)

are noncompliance in prophylactic medication and the lack of information on the pharmacology of isoniazid in the neonatal period. A combined prophylactic approach, e.g., BCG immunization and isoniazid administration until skin test conversion, is not recommended as it has not been adequately evaluated. However, the recent development of an isoniazid-resistant vaccine strain of *M. bovis* makes such an approach an attractive possibility.

The management approach outlined in Table 10–35 should be individualized for the newborn infant, taking into consideration the home environment and subsequent availability of the treated infant for follow-up evaluation.

WILLIAM T. SPECK

Editorial: Antituberculosis drugs in pregnancy. Lancet 2:1285, 1980.
Weinstein L, Murphy T: The management of tuberculosis during pregnancy. Clin Perinatol 1:395, 1974.

10.53 NONTUBERCULOUS MYCOBACTERIAL INFECTIONS

Organisms with biologic characteristics similar to *Mycobacterium tuberculosis* can produce clinical lesions closely resembling those caused by that pathogen. These organisms, variously called nontuberculous, unclassified, anonymous, or atypical mycobacteria, are, however, much less virulent, and the disease is thus more localized and indolent. From a clinical standpoint, part of the problem presented by this group of bacteria is the fact that they are readily confused with *M. tuberculosis*.

Etiology and Epidemiology. The organisms consist of species and strains of the family Mycobacteriaceae and thus have identical staining and morphologic characteristics. They differ from tubercle bacilli by rate of growth, temperature for optimal growth, pigment formation, type of colony, and enzymatic activity. Unlike tubercle bacilli, their natural habitat is soil, water, and vegetable matter; the preferred habitat differs from species to species. Nontuberculous mycobacteria are ubiquitous and worldwide in distribution, though certain species living in soil prefer warm, moist environments. In North America, infection is most commonly encountered in the southern United States, especially in the area near the Gulf of Mexico. Only fragmentary information exists about the distribution of disease in other parts of the world.

In general, the route of infection to humans remains unknown. Logically, one would expect the respiratory tract to be a portal of entry, but it is possible that the gastrointestinal system may also be involved. On occasion, the organism may infect the skin after being introduced through an abrasion, but this lesion then remains localized. Because of the ubiquitous distribution, it is likely that human beings are continuously exposed. The relative rarity with which disease occurs suggests that illness is due to some temporary or permanent diminution of host defense mechanisms or to an unusually virulent strain. Person-to-person transmission of the infection has not been demonstrated.

Cattle may become infected with nontuberculous mycobacteria and show positive reactions to appropriate skin test reagents. Swine develop a lymph-node form of disease. Guinea pigs are highly resistant to these organisms; usually only a small granuloma forms at the site of inoculation, while *M. tuberculosis* will produce widespread disease.

Pathology. The histologic appearances of the pathologic lesions caused by tuberculous and nontuberculous mycobacteria are remarkably similar and often indistinguishable. With the latter group of organisms, there is a greater predilection for lymphoid tissue; in fact, the process may remain entirely localized to lymph nodes. Tissue changes may resemble "nonspecific" inflammation more than typical granuloma formation and the lesion, instead of caseating, may liquefy quite quickly. Nevertheless, it is usually difficult to distinguish lesions produced by *M. tuberculosis* from those caused by mycobacteria, and it is, therefore, often necessary to culture the organism in appropriate media and to determine its exact nature by suitable tests.

Classification of Mycobacteria. Nontuberculous mycobacteria are generally divided into 4 classes (Table 10–36), depending on pigment formation, colony type, and growth. These differentiations are of some importance since the groups differ in their susceptibility to various antituberculous agents.

Group 1 (the photochromogens, *M. luciflavum*, *M. kansasii*): Most strains grow rapidly and reach maturity in about 2–3 wk. The colonies are generally rough, dry, and creamy white in the dark. When exposed to light, they turn yellow to orange.

Group 2 (the scotochromogens): These organisms grow more rapidly than group 1, maturing in 1–2 wk and forming moist and spreading colonies. An orange-to-red pigment forms in the dark as well as in light.

Group 3 (the nonphotochromogens, Battey bacillus):

Table 10–36 CLASSIFICATION OF MYCOBACTERIA, ANTIGENS, AND DISEASE PRODUCED*

ANTIGEN† — ORGANISM	RUNYON CLASSIFICATION	PIGMENTATION AT 37° C AND GROWTH CHARACTERISTICS	DISEASE PRODUCED
PPD-A *M. avium*	III	Nonphotochromogen, off-white to ivory; slow grower	Children: lymph nodes
PPD-B Battey bacilli	III	Nonphotochromogen; intermediate grower	Child, adult: lymph nodes; rare pulmonary, disseminated disease

PPD-F
  M. fortuitum
  M. ulcerans
  M. nanae
	IV	No pigmentation; rapid grower	Child, adult: very rare; lymph nodes, skin, eye

PPD-G (Gauss)
  M. scrofulaceum
  M. aquae
  M. gordonae, flavescens
	II	Scotochromogens (yellow-orange in dark); intermediate grower	Child, adult: lymph nodes; rare pulmonary, disseminated disease

PPD-S *M. tuberculosis*	None	None to light beige; slow grower	Human: pulmonary, lymph nodes, disseminated disease

PPD-Y
  M. kansasii
  M. marinum
    (*M. balnei*)
	I	Photochromogens (yellow pigment in light); intermediate grower	Child: rarely pulmonary, disseminated disease; granulomatous, nodular, ulcerative skin lesions.

*Courtesy of Dr. Andrew W. Margileth.
†Strength is 5 TU or 0.0001 mg/0.1 ml.

These grow at about the same rate as organisms from Group 2, but form small, discrete, nonpigmented colonies. Exposure to light does not result in pigment formation.

Group 4: The organisms from this group have the characteristic of very rapid growth rate, producing well-formed colonies in 2–7 days.

Clinical Manifestations. The most frequent disease caused by nontuberculous mycobacteria is infection of the cervical lymph glands. Involvement is commonly confined to a single group on 1 side. The nodes tend to liquefy early; if the patient remains untreated, sinus formation with chronic discharge occurs, resembling the classic scrofula of tuberculosis. The organisms involved are generally from groups 1, 2, or 3.

In unusual instances, nontuberculous mycobacterial disease may involve a bone or a joint. The lesion is clinically indistinguishable from that produced by *M. tuberculosis;* any bone may be involved, although there is some predilection for the vertebrae.

The skin is a fairly common site for disease. Outbreaks of "swimming pool" granuloma have been reported from various parts of the United States. This is due to *M. marinum (balnei),* which grows in the water and along the sides of swimming pools and is apparently inoculated when a swimmer abrades the skin. The lesion consists of a slowly progressive, sometimes linear granuloma which eventually ulcerates. The ulcers are quite superficial, but have thick and irregular borders and sparse serosanguineous or seropurulent drainage.

Pulmonary involvement is probably quite rare but is significant when it occurs because it can readily be mistaken for tuberculosis. Lung lesions apparently occur more frequently among adults than among children. They tend to remain localized, undergoing cavitation with some fibrosis. Only very unusually do they spread to other areas of the lung. Symptoms are relatively nonspecific and include low grade fever, cough, and modest general malaise. Occasionally, there is some hemoptysis. The diagnosis is most commonly suspected when the patient with pulmonary disease fails to respond to seemingly appropriate antituberculous therapy.

Only in children who have severe immunologic defects or are receiving immunosuppressive agents do nontuberculous mycobacteria produce life-threatening disseminated disease. Clinical manifestations are extremely diverse, and diagnosis nearly always depends on the fortuitous isolation and identification of the bacterium. In the absence of such generalized involvement, meningeal lesions or central nervous system invasion is exceedingly rare.

Diagnosis. Most commonly, disease with nontuberculous mycobacteria is diagnosed because a characteristic swimming pool granuloma is recognized or a patient presents classic cervical lymph node infection. In suspected cases appropriate skin tests may be useful to demonstrate that the patient probably has had an infection with 1 or another of these organisms. Appropriate interpretation of results depends on an understanding of the mechanisms involved. In children, a heterologous skin reaction occurs, with overlap between that caused by antigens derived from nontuberculous mycobacteria and from *M. tuberculosis.* When the infection is due to nontuberculous mycobacteria, the skin reaction is usually weaker to standard tuberculin (PPD-S) than one would anticipate were the infection due to *M. tuberculosis.* As a result, it has been suggested that when a tuberculin test causes a reaction but produces induration less than 5–9 mm in diameter, the test be repeated. Should the same results be obtained, simultaneous testing with tuberculin and skin testing antigens from the more common nontuberculous mycobacteria is advisable. If this produces a small tuberculin reaction but a considerably larger area of induration to antigen from the unclassified mycobacteria, one can assume that the patient has experienced an infection (but not necessarily disease) with nontuberculous mycobacterium. Table 10–36 lists the skin test reagents for the various groups of organisms; unfortunately, the availability of these reagents is limited.

Considerable cross-reaction exists among the 4 groups of nontuberculous mycobacteria. Skin testing is useful primarily in differentiating nontuberculous mycobacterial infection from tuberculosis and, more rarely, in demonstrating that a specific lesion is due to nontuberculous mycobacteria.

Therapy. Only overt disease should be treated; no prophylactic therapy should be given to asymptomatic children with positive skin tests to nontuberculous mycobacteria and no evidence of tuberculous infection. Most information concerning the chemotherapy of nontuberculous mycobacterial disease is derived from individual case reports and uncontrolled observation. It is likely that within each of the 4 groups considerable variation in susceptibility to antituberculous drugs exists. Whenever possible, therefore, the isolation of an organism should be followed by appropriate in vitro tests to provide information about the regimen most likely to be effective. Completion of such studies may require 6 wk or more. Meanwhile, a provisional regimen may be tried, which most commonly consists of isoniazid (8–10 mg/kg/24 hr) or ethambutol (15 mg/kg/24 hr), to which is added rifampin (15 mg/kg/24 hr) or, when the patient is acutely ill, streptomycin (20 mg/kg 3 times weekly). None of these drugs are as effective against nontuberculous mycobacteria as they are against the tubercle bacillus. If there is no clinical response or if in vitro susceptibility tests suggest that other drugs might be useful, the latter may be substituted, but only in serious disease because of their toxicity. Among them are ethionamide (10–20 mg/kg/24 hr), cycloserine (10 mg/kg/24 hr), capreomycin (20 mg/kg 3 times weekly), and kanamycin (15 mg/kg intramuscularly 3 times weekly).

For the most common manifestations of nontuberculous mycobacterial disease, surgical intervention is the most effective and immediate form of therapy. Local surgical excision of the affected nodes, along with an oval of skin if sinuses are present, is usually curative. Pre- or postoperative chemotherapy is unnecessary. With a swimming pool granuloma, local excision is probably all that is required, though recurrences are known. The organism most commonly responsible for these lesions (*M. marinum*) is usually quite susceptible to rifampin. A 6 mo course should be adequate to prevent local recurrence or extension of the process following surgical excision.

HEINZ F. EICHENWALD

Altman RP, Margileth PM: Cervical lymphadenopathy from atypical mycobacteria: Diagnosis and surgical treatment. J Pediatr Surg 10:419, 1975.

Arnold JH, et al: Specificity of PPD skin tests in childhood tuberculin converters. Comparison with mycobacterial species from tissue and secretions. J Pediatr 76:512, 1970.

Biackin G, et al: Pulmonary infection with Mycobacterium kansasii. Am J Dis Child 101:739, 1961.

Feldman RA, Hershfield E: Mycobacterial skin infections by an unidentified species. Ann Intern Med 80:445, 1974.

Lincoln EM, Gilbert LA: Disease in children due to mycobacteria other than Mycobacterium tuberculosis. Am Rev Respir Dis 105:683, 1972.

Mandell F, Wright PF: Treatment of atypical mycobacterial cervical adenitis with rifampin. Pediatrics 55:39, 1975.

McCracken GH, Reynolds RC: Primary lymphopenic immunologic deficiency: Disseminated Mycobacterium kansasii infection. Am J Dis Child 120:143, 1970.

Saphyakhajon P, et al: Mycobacterium kansasii arthritis of the knee joint. Am J Dis Child 131:573, 1977.

Smith DT, Johnston WW: New aspects of mycobacterial skin tests. 1. Tuberculin reactions due to organisms other than Mycobacterium tuberculosis. Arch Environ Health 10:699, 1966.

Van Dyke JJ, Lake KB: Chemotherapy for aquarium granuloma. JAMA 233:1380, 1975.

10.54 LEPROSY

Leprosy is a complex of clinical syndromes which represents a spectrum of reactions to infection with *Mycobacterium leprae*. Peripheral nerves are the primary site of infection, but the organisms also affect skin and less commonly other organs such as the eyes, muscles, testes, and mucosa of the upper respiratory tract. The infection is characterized by a long and variable incubation period, chronic clinical course, and unclear epidemiologic pattern.

The World Health Organization estimates that there are 15 million patients with leprosy throughout the world; only 25% have had access to any specific therapy. Endemic foci occur in Africa, South and Southeast Asia, and South America. There are more than 2 billion people living in areas with high risk of mycobacterial transmission, and 1 million new patients may be expected every 5 yr. However, transmission of M. leprae also occurs in other areas, such as North America, where approximately 200 cases are reported yearly.

Leprosy can occur at any age; young children are at extreme risk, but it is rare in infants. In endemic areas such as Madras, India, 20% of leprosy patients are under the age of 10 compared to 3% in the southern United States. Contact with infected patients seems to play a crucial epidemiologic role; in Hawaii over one half of new cases were children below 15 yr who were born to families with an active leprosy case. Only 20% of new cases occurred in children of families with no infected individuals.

Etiology. *Mycobacterium leprae* is an acid- and alcohol-fast organism. It is consistently recovered from patients with leprosy, although only 1 of many deliberate attempts to infect man with M. leprae has succeeded. The organism has not yet been reproducibly cultured in vitro. The organisms multiply very slowly. They can be killed by boiling or autoclaving and usually die within 2–7 days outside the body. The reservoirs of M. leprae and its mode of transmission and entry into humans are not known. It is assumed that bacterial dissemination originates from patients with lepromatous leprosy. As the 1st clinical lesion is almost always in the skin, it is thought that M. leprae gains entry through dermal tissues. Other modes of transmission such as droplet infection, swallowing, or breast milk may, however, be equally important.

Epidemiology. Although leprosy has been known as a cause of human disease for many yr, its epidemiology is still not fully understood. Man is the only known source and reservoir of infection, although the discovery of naturally infected armadillos suggests the possibility of animal reservoirs. Transmission occurs in sporadic as well as epidemic forms. Bacilli are shed continuously from patients with lepromatous leprosy and can be found in abundant numbers in their peripheral blood. Biting insects as well as tattooing have been suggested to play a role in transmission.

Pathology and Pathogenesis. Leprosy bacilli probably gain entry to the body through the skin where the earliest clinical lesions can be seen. Infection of the nerve fibers in the skin is nearly simultaneous. Organisms are taken up by the histiocytes and Schwann cells of the skin and terminal nerve endings, respectively. The earliest clinical lesion is a small macule. These lesions, classified as indeterminate leprosy, heal spontaneously or develop into 1 of the clinically recognized forms of leprosy. In *tuberculoid leprosy*, the infection and its sequelae are arrested at local sites through the host's cellular immune response as manifested by a positive lepromin test. Few organisms are found, and a cellular infiltration containing macrophages, epithelioid cells, and lymphocytes occurs in the skin. The cutaneous nerve endings within the cellular infiltrate are involved, and larger nerves become swollen. Nerve lesions are usually solitary. At the other end of the spectrum, *lepromatous leprosy* represents both local and systemic dissemination of mycobacteria and failure of the host response to stop their spread. The lepromin test is negative, and bacilli can be recovered in enormous numbers from the skin, nasal mucosa, Schwann cells, and other sites. Skin lesions show a disorganized pathologic response to the infection. Macrophages fail to change into epithelioid cells and teem with mycobacteria. The lesions are characteristically multiple with a striking bilateral symmetry. They can be found not only in nerves but also in other organs such as the eyes, smooth and striated muscles, bones, testes, and lymph nodes. Between these 2 extreme patterns several intermediate stages have been described which represent a balance between the invading organisms and host cellular immunity. *Borderline leprosy* is at the midpoint in this spectrum, with skin lesions characterized by macrophages that differentiate into epithelioid cells but fail to destroy mycobacteria; a lack of localization; an abundance of acid-fast bacilli; and a negative lepromin test. Most patients with leprosy do not fit into any of these rigid clinicopathologic categories, and accurate classification depends on histologic examination of skin and nerve lesions. Acute inflammations known as *leprosy reactions* may be superimposed on the classic manifestations of disease. These may be due to changes in cellular (Type 1) or humoral (Type 2) hypersensitivity.

Clinical Manifestations. The incubation period between implantation of *M. leprae* and the earliest manifestations of clinical disease varies widely; 2–4 yr is considered the average, but extremes as short as 3 mo and as long as 40 yr have been recorded. Disease due to *M. leprae* infection is characteristically insidious in onset and may pass unnoticed for long periods.

The outcome of *M. leprae* infection in man depends on the host response to the organisms. Infection is currently thought to be acquired at an early age; most individuals have an asymptomatic course while a small proportion develop chronic sequelae of disease. The existence of subclinical infections has recently been confirmed: fluorescent leprosy antibody absorption tests showed that in Okinawa, Japan, the rate of subclinical infection in school children was 0.7%; this is approximately 200 times higher than the incidence rate of clinical leprosy in this area. Several host factors may determine which of the different clinical syndromes of leprosy is expressed. These include age (children are more susceptible than adults), sex (males are more commonly infected), and race (Caucasians are more susceptible than non-Caucasians).

The spectrum of clinical disease in symptomatic patients varies from tuberculoid leprosy, where the disease is localized to 1 or few sites in the skin and large peripheral nerves, to lepromatous leprosy (Fig 10–5), where infection disseminates locally and by the bloodstream to other organs. The factors which determine the outcome of infection with *M. leprae* are not yet fully understood; the level of host cellular immune responses and the genetic constitution of the individual may be involved.

Indeterminate leprosy is the 1st symptomatic stage

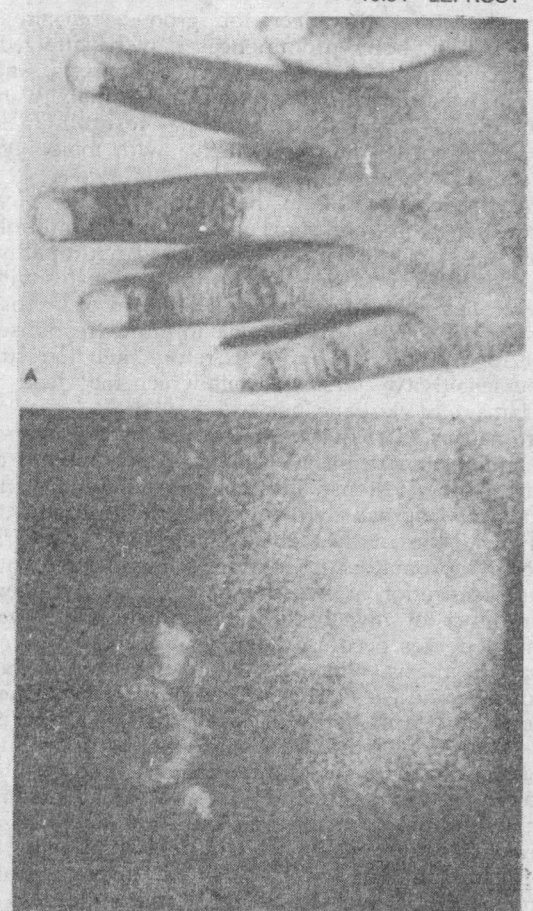

Figure 10–6 Tuberculoid leprosy. *A*, Early tuberculoid leprosy of finger: a hypopigmented anesthetic macule which had been present for 6 mo. *B*, Tuberculoid leprosy on buttock. The well defined, anesthetic hypopigmented macule had been present for a yr; the satellite lesions were of shorter duration. (Courtesy of Dr ABA Karat, India.)

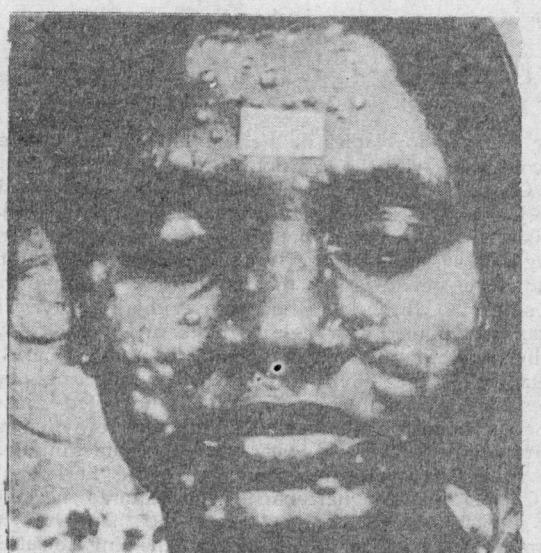

Figure 10–5 Lepromatous leprosy in an adolescent girl. Nodules are extensive, especially on exposed parts. The lepromin skin test result was negative.

following infection. Patients develop ill-defined macules which are hypopigmented in dark-skinned and erythematous in light-skinned individuals, and which measure a few cm in diameter. The lesions are commonly found on the face, trunk, or extensor surfaces of limbs and are associated with normal sensation, sweating, and hair growth. Approximately 75% of individuals who develop indeterminate leprosy demonstrate spontaneous healing of the lesions and do not develop clinically significant disease.

Tuberculoid leprosy is usually characterized by a lack of dissemination, infrequency of *leprosy reactions*, and a tendency to spontaneous healing. The most common skin manifestation is a single lesion with a raised papular edge and a hypopigmented surface (Fig 10–6). These are anesthetic, hairless, and dry. Tuberculoid skin lesions may be multiple, but all have the characteristic raised progressing edge and flat central part. Bacilli are never found in the nasal mucosa and only rarely in skin lesions. Nervous system involvement usually occurs in the form of enlargement of solitary peripheral nerves; the most common location is the ulnar nerve above the olecranon groove, but other nerves lying on bony prominences may be affected. Nerve enlargement leads to tenderness, paresis, and finally paralysis. Facial nerve palsy causes inability to close the eyelids; trigeminal lesions may result in anesthesia of the cornea and conjunctiva with major eye complications.

Borderline leprosy falls in the middle of the clinical spectrum; symptoms and signs are a mixture of multiple symmetrical skin lesions and widespread neuropathy. Invasion of nasal mucosa, eyes, bones, and testes with *M. leprae* does not usually occur. This form of leprosy reflects the instability of cellular immune responses against the mycobacteria and is therefore likely to result in hypersensitivity *leprosy reactions* which may lead to rapid damage of skin and nerves.

Lepromatous leprosy is characterized by persistence of the indeterminate macule and the development of papular or other lesions. These macules are shiny and erythematous, spread symmetrically, and usually do not involve skin in the axillae and groin. The early macules of lepromatous leprosy are not associated with decreased sensation or sweating and contain a tremendous number of mycobacteria. Destruction of small peripheral nerves occurs gradually and leads to symmetrical anesthesia, which begins on the extensor surfaces of arms and legs and slowly spreads to include the trunk and face. If the disease progresses, the affected skin becomes thickened and waxy with production of the characteristic leonine facies. Infection also extends to the mucosa of the nose and throat (causing stuffiness and ulcerations), eyes, bones, and testes.

Leprosy reactions result in symptoms and signs of acute inflammation in leprosy patients. The major manifestations include swelling, redness, and tenderness of skin lesions. These are often associated with functionally significant nerve lesions. Two types of hypersensitivity are recognized: Type 1 (cellular) is usually seen in patients with borderline disease; Type 2 (humoral) occurs at the lepromatous end of the spectrum and may involve deposition of antigen-antibody complexes.

Diagnosis. This is based on finding at least 2 of the 3 major clinical manifestations of anesthesia, thickened nerves, and/or skin lesions. Definitive bacteriologic diagnosis can be made in patients with lepromatous and borderline lesions by demonstrating *M. leprae* in slit skin smears. Skin biopsy may be helpful in doubtful cases and is necessary for accurate classification.

Treatment. Therapy of uncomplicated leprosy involves the oral administration of dapsone (2 mg/kg/24 hr). Patients with lepromatous leprosy are usually treated throughout life; those with other forms of the disease may need 3–10 yr of therapy. Compliance can become a problem because of the duration of therapy. Other antimycobacterial drugs such as thiambutosine, clofazimine, and rifampin may also be useful, particularly in patients with lepromatous leprosy. These individuals should be started on dapsone with rifampin or clofazimine; therapy is continued with dapsone alone. Social, psychologic, surgical, and anti-inflammatory therapy may be needed for the different complications encountered.

Control. This approach is based on identification and treatment of clinically manifest cases and observation of their contacts. BCG vaccination may be protective if given during the 1st 6 mo of life.

ADEL A. F. MAHMOUD

Abe M, Minagawa F, Yoshino Y, et al: Fluorescent leprosy antibody absorption (LFA-ABS) test for detecting sub-clinical infection with *Mycobacterium leprae*. Int J Leprosy 48:109, 1980.
Bryceson A, Pfaltzgraff RO: Leprosy. Edinburgh, Churchill Livingstone, 1979, p 1.
Bullock WE: Immunology and the therapeutics of leprosy. Ann Intern Med 91:482, 1979.

TREPONEMATOSES

10.55 SYPHILIS

Etiology. Syphilis is a systemic, communicable infection caused by *Treponema pallidum*, a long, slender, tightly coiled, motile spirochete with finely tapered ends belonging to the family Spirochaetaceae and the genus *Treponema*. The pathogenic members of this genus include *T. pallidum* (syphilis), *T. pertenue* (yaws), and *T. carateum* (pinta). Because these microorganisms stain poorly, detection in clinical specimens requires darkfield microscopy and/or immunofluorescent staining techniques. Unlike many nonpathogenic spirochetes, *T. pallidum* cannot be cultured in vitro and laboratory isolation has traditionally required animal inoculation; however, recent reports suggest successful propagation in tissue culture.

History and Epidemiology. The first European epidemic and initial description of syphilis as a distinct clinical entity occurred in Naples in the late 1400's. This outbreak was coincident with the invasion of that city by the French king, Charles VIII, who after a brief occupation withdrew his forces to France when confronted by a coalition of Italian and Spanish armies. The dispersal of Charles' mercenaries throughout Western Europe was responsible for the rapid spread of this new disease, "the great pox" (as distinguished from smallpox), throughout Europe over the next 3 yr. This illness, accompanied by a high morbidity and mortality, was initially labeled by the French as the "Italian disease" and by the Italians as the "French disease." The true origin was suggested by contemporary physicians who noted unusual cutaneous lesions on members of Columbus' crew after their return from the New World a year before the Naples outbreak. It was suggested that the European origin of the "new plague" was Charles' Spanish mercenaries who acquired the illness from contacts with Columbus' crew, who themselves had become infected in Haiti. Accordingly, the English labeled this illness the "Spanish disease."

Although the signs, symptoms, and venereal transmission of syphilis were recognized by the 1700's, early writers failed to distinguish between syphilis and gonorrhea. This confusion was perpetuated by John Hunter, the famous English physician, who in 1767 attempted to prove the distinct identity of gonorrhea by inoculating himself with purulent exudate obtained from a patient with gonorrhea. Unfortunately, the patient was simultaneously infected with syphilis, and Hunter's postinoculation signs and symptoms (he ultimately died of syphilitic heart disease) convinced generations of physicians of the unity of these 2 diseases. However, Ricord in 1838, reporting on his observations of more than 2500 human inoculations, convinced the scientific community of the separate nature of syphilis and gonorrhea. The early 1900's introduced the age of modern syphilis management with the almost simultaneous isolation of *Treponema pallidum*, the development of a serologic test for syphilis, and the introduction of arsenic and fever therapy. In the late 1930's and during World War II, major government programs to combat syphilis were initiated. These programs and the availability of penicillin in the 1940's were responsible for eventual control of the infection. Reported cases decreased from 106,000 in 1947 to 6500 cases a decade later. The incidence of syphilis has subsequently increased; a total of 27,204 cases were reported to the Center for Disease Control in Atlanta during 1980. Congenital infections, however, are not common, e.g., 277 cases reported in 1980.

Congenital (fetal) syphilis results from transplacental transmission of spirochetes; infant contact with a maternal chancre may rarely lead to postnatal infection. The risk of transplacental transmission varies with the stage of maternal illness. Thus, untreated pregnant women with primary and secondary syphilis and a high incidence of spirochetemia are more likely to transmit infection to their unborn infants than women with latent infection. However, infected infants have been delivered of women with latent infection. The risk also varies with the gestational age of the unborn infant, the likelihood of transmission being greatest during the later portions of pregnancy. Transmission can occur, however, throughout pregnancy, and congenital syphilis may be acquired during the 1st trimester. Untreated infection is associated with significant perinatal mortality and morbidity. Thus, congenital syphilis results in intrauterine death in 25% of pregnancies and postnatal death in 25% of infected live-born infants. Although treatment during the later stages of pregnancy results in the birth of an uninfected infant, clinical findings of intrauterine infection may be present.

Acquired syphilis is caused by sexual contact, transfusion of fresh blood, or accidental direct inoculation by needle stick. It is more common in the sexually active (15–30 yr), nonwhite, urban population. An unusually high number of cases occur among homosexuals.

Clinical Manifestations. Congenital syphilis has traditionally been divided into early and late findings. The former appear during the 1st 2 yr of life as a result of active infection, whereas the latter appear years after birth and result from hypersensitivity phenomena and/or residual scarring. *Early congenital syphilis* is analogous to the secondary stage of acquired syphilis, and, accordingly, clinical manifestations are varied and protean. The infected neonate may be normal during the 1st few wk or mo of life, or generalized symptoms such as fever, anemia, failure to gain weight, restlessness, and irritability may be present at birth without the "classic" skin and/or mucous membrane lesions, or local mucocutaneous lesions may be present in an infant who appears well.

The mucocutaneous lesions of congenital syphilis are varied. The 2 most characteristic cutaneous abnormalities include a vesicular or bullous eruption and/or an erythematous maculopapular rash. Both rashes are initially more common on the hands and feet but may become generalized, darken, and eventually desquamate. Wart-like moist lesions at the mucocutaneous junction of the mouth, anus, and external genitalia (analogous to the condylomata lata of acquired infection) have also been observed in congenital infection. The cutaneous lesions are highly infectious, often recur over a period of weeks or months, and eventually disappear. Mucous membrane involvement may be extensive, involve the nasal mucous membranes, and appear (10%) as a profuse, purulent, and blood-tinged nasal discharge ("snuffles") containing viable *T. pallidum*. This lesion appears during the 2nd wk of life, is often associated with excoriation of the nasal structures and upper lip, and heals spontaneously.

Hepatosplenomegaly is common (30%) in congenital syphilis. Histologically, liver involvement includes bile stasis, fibrosis, and extramedullary hematopoiesis. Hyperbilirubinemia and elevated liver enzymes are common. Lymphadenopathy (5%) tends to be diffuse and resolve spontaneously.

Bone involvement is also common (25%). Roentgenographic abnormalities include multiple sites of osteochondritis at the wrists, elbows, ankles, and knees; periostitis of the long bones and rarely the skull; widened and serrated epiphyseal lines; and, on occasion, separation of the epiphysis. The osteochondritis is painful, may be asymmetric, and often results in irritability and refusal to move the involved extremity (pseudoparalysis of Parrot). Osteochondritis of the hand (syphilitic dactylitis) resembles the hand-foot syndrome of sickle cell disease.

Histologic abnormalities involving 1 or all of the cellular elements of the bone marrow are common in congenital syphilis (20%). Thrombocytopenia is often associated with platelet trapping in an enlarged spleen. A Coombs-negative, hemolytic anemia is characteristic of congenital infection and may suggest blood group incompatibility. Leukocytosis is also observed, may be extreme and present as a leukemoid reaction, and, on rare occasions, may include only monocytes.

Renal dysfunction is secondary to glomerulonephritis and/or the nephrotic syndrome (5%). Clinical abnormalities appear within the 1st few mo of life and may include hypertension, hematuria, proteinuria, hypoproteinemia, hypercholesterolemia, and hypocomplementemia. They appear related to glomerular deposition of circulating immune complexes. Less common clinical manifestations of early congenital syphilis include gastroenteritis, peritonitis, pancreatitis, pneumonia, eye involvement (glaucoma and chorioretinitis), and testicular masses.

The manifestations of *late congenital syphilis* have decreased in frequency since the availability of penicillin. They result from either chronic inflammation or a hypersensitivity reaction. Skeletal changes due to persist-

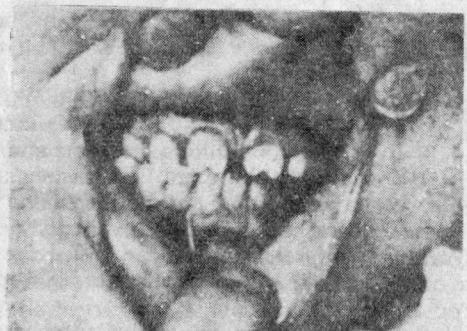

Figure 10–7 Hutchinson teeth in congenital syphilis.

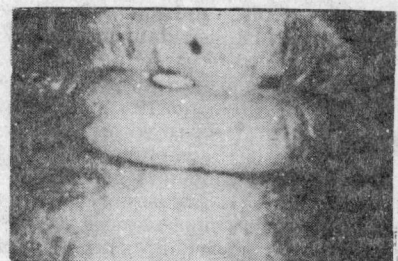

Figure 10–9 Rhagades as long-term residua of congenital syphilis.

ent or recurrent periostitis and associated thickening of bone include frontal bossing (87%), a bony prominence of the forehead ("olympian brow") to involvement of the supraorbital ridge; unilateral or bilateral thickening of the sternoclavicular portion of the clavicle (39%), referred to as Higouménakis sign; saber shins (5%), or anterior bowing of the mid-portion of the tibia; and scaphoid scapula (1%), a convexity along the vertebral border of the scapula. A short maxilla (80%) with or without a high arched palate may result from destruction of the maxilla during the neonatal period; a perforated palate may be an associated abnormality. Hutchinson teeth (63%) are the peg- or barrel-shaped upper central incisors that erupt during the 6th yr of life. Abnormal enamel results in the appearance of a notch along the biting surface (Fig 10–7). Mulberry molars (65%) refer to the abnormal 1st lower (6 yr) molar characterized by a small biting surface and an excessive number of cusps. Defects in their enamel formation lead to repeated caries and eventual tooth destruction.

A saddle nose (75%) results from a depression of the nasal root (Fig 10–8) due to syphilitic rhinitis and destruction of adjacent bone and cartilage. A perforated nasal septum is an associated abnormality. Rhagades (5%) are uncommon linear scars that extend in a spoke-like pattern from previous mucocutaneous lesions of the mouth, anus, and genitalia (Fig 10–9). Juvenile paresis is extremely uncommon and represents a latent meningovascular syphilitic infection which typically presents during adolescence with behavioral changes, focal seizures, and/or loss of intellectual function. Juvenile tabes with spinal cord involvement has also been

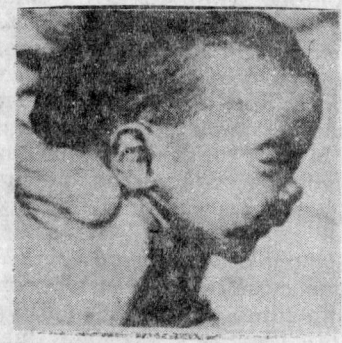

Figure 10–8 Saddle nose in early syphilis.

reported. Cardiovascular syphilis with aortitis has been described in children with congenital syphilis but is extremely rare.

Additional clinical manifestations of late congenital syphilis may represent a delayed hypersensitivity phenomenon. Unilateral or bilateral interstitial keratitis (10%) may appear at any age with symptoms such as intense photophobia and lacrimation, followed within weeks or months by corneal opacification and complete blindness. Less common ocular manifestations include choroiditis, retinitis, vascular occlusion, and optic atrophy. Eighth nerve deafness (2%) may be unilateral or bilateral, appears at any age, presents initially with vertigo and high tone hearing loss, and progresses to eventual deafness. Deafness, interstitial keratitis, and deformities of the teeth have been referred to as "Hutchinson triad." Clutton joint (1%) refers to a unilateral or bilateral synovitis involving the lower extremities which presents as painless joint swelling with sterile synovial fluid; spontaneous remission occurs after a period of several wk. Further rare hypersensitivity phenomena associated with late onset congenital syphilis include formation of soft tissue gummas (identical to those seen in acquired disease) and paroxysmal cold hemoglobinuria.

Acquired syphilis is divided into various stages which include incubating, primary, secondary, latent, and late syphilis. *Primary syphilis* begins with the appearance of a single painless papule at the site of inoculation 3–6 wk following contact. The papule becomes indurated and eventually erodes leaving a shallow, clean based, painless ulceration with a firm raised border—the chancre. Chancres appear at the site of inoculation (most often the external genitalia) and may be multiple but may go unrecognized. Sites of involvement include the cervix, mouth, rectum, and perineum. The primary chancre is often associated with bilateral, firm, painless, movable, nonsuppurative lymph nodes. In untreated patients the chancre spontaneously heals within 3–6 wk leaving behind a thin, atrophic scar.

Secondary syphilis begins 6–8 wk following the primary chancre. Clinical manifestations include a flu-like illness with low-grade fever, headache, malaise, anorexia, weight loss, sore throat, myalgias, arthralgias, and generalized lymphadenopathy. The initial cutaneous manifestation is an erythematous macular rash that begins on the trunk and upper portions of the extremities. This eruption subsequently progresses to a generalized, nonpruritic, copper-colored, macular rash with a predilection for the palms and soles. The initial rash may evolve into a maculopapular eruption which may involve hair follicles and result in localized alopecia. Pustule formation (pustular syphilis) is uncommon. In warm, moist areas of the body (e.g., axilla, perineum, breast) papules may enlarge, coalesce, and erode to produce plaque-like lesions or **condylomata lata.** Similar lesions may develop on mucous membranes (mucous patches) and appear as oval, slightly raised erosions, covered with a grayish membrane and surrounded by a red areola. The cutaneous lesions of secondary syphilis are all highly infectious. Noncutaneous manifestations also occur and result from multiple organ system involvement. Thus patients may present with meningitis (half of all patients with secondary syphilis have cerebrospinal fluid pleocytosis and elevated spinal fluid protein), hepatitis, glomerulonephritis (with or without nephrosis), bursitis, and/or periostitis. Laboratory abnormalities are common and reflect diffuse organ involvement.

Latent syphilis is defined as that stage following secondary syphilis in which a specific antitreponemal antibody test (FTA-ABS or TPI) is positive in a patient without clinical manifestations and there is normal cerebrospinal fluid, a normal chest roentgenogram, and a history of either prior untreated syphilitic disease, exposure, and/or the birth of a child with congenital infection. Early latent syphilis refers to the 1st yr of latency during which relapses and infectivity may occur (25% of patients will have 1 or more cutaneous relapses and 85% of these will occur within the 1st 2 yr). Patients with late latent syphilis have no signs or symptoms of active disease but remain seropositive; such patients are noninfectious and resistant to reinfection. Approximately 60% of untreated patients with late latent syphilis will remain asymptomatic, while 40% will progress to late or tertiary syphilis.

Late syphilis is a slowly progressive inflammatory disease of adults which can affect any organ system. This stage of syphilis may be associated with gumma formation and the development of neurosyphilis and/or cardiovascular disease.

Diagnosis. Serologic tests for syphilis are either nonspecific nontreponemal (or "reagin") tests or specific antitreponemal tests. The former detect IgG and IgM antibody against a nonspecific lipoidal antigen of obscure origin, and the latter measure antibody specific for *T. pallidum.* In many laboratories the traditional nontreponemal Venereal Disease Research Laboratory (VDRL) slide test and Kolmer test have been replaced by the more sensitive nontreponemal rapid plasma reagin card test (RPR) or the automatic reagin test (ART). The latter 2 tests in addition to being rapid and inexpensive offer the advantage of being quantifiable and, therefore, capable of determining the level of disease activity; titers rise during active disease (including treatment failure or reinfection) and fall in adequately treated patients (Fig. 10–10). The rate of fall is dependent on both the time interval before initiation of therapy and severity of the illness. Serum usually becomes nonreactive within 1 yr of adequate therapy of primary syphilis and within 2 yr of adequate treatment for secondary disease. However, a small number of adequately treated patients retain positive serology

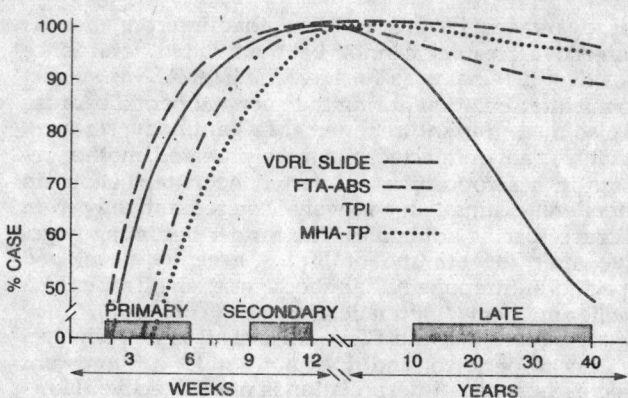

Figure 10–10 Serologic response in untreated syphilis.

("chronic persistent" or "sero-fast"). A major disadvantage of the nontreponemal tests, particularly the VDRL, is that they are not specific for active infection and may be falsely positive, particularly in the presence of immunologic stimulation such as infection, immunization, collagen vascular disease, pregnancy, and drug addiction. These "biologic false-positive tests" for syphilis are often low titered and their true nature verified by obtaining a negative specific antitreponemal test. Unfortunately, many conditions associated with false-positive nontreponemal tests also yield borderline positive antitreponemal tests, e.g., drug addiction, collagen vascular disease. Despite their value as screening tests for primary and secondary syphilis, the various nontreponemal tests may be used improperly in the diagnosis of congenital syphilis. For example, maternal antibody crosses the placenta, and accordingly a false-positive VDRL can occur in an uninfected infant delivered to a VDRL-positive mother. Passively acquired antibody is suggested when neonatal titers are significantly less (4-fold or less) than maternal titers and can be verified when they convert to negative by 3 mo. False-negative results may occur in congenital infections in infants who acquire infections late in pregnancy. Such infants are often seronegative or possess low titers at birth which rise in the postnatal period.

Two specific or anti-treponemal tests capable of detecting antibody to *T. pallidum* are available. The Treponema pallidum immobilization test (TPI), against which all other antitreponemal tests are compared, measures the ability of test serum (antibody) plus complement to immobilize *T. pallidum.* Few laboratories maintain the viable spirochetes necessary for this test. The principal antitreponemal antibody test in clinical use is the fluorescent treponemal antibody-absorption (FTA-ABS) test. This is an indirect immunofluorescence test which utilizes fixed *T. pallidum* as the antigen to measure serum antitreponemal antibodies. This test is both sensitive and specific. The antibodies are detected early in infection and remain detectable in latent or late infections (Fig. 10–10). False positives are uncommon but do occur in a small number of normal individuals during pregnancy and in patients with various diseases such as lymphoproliferative disorders, cirrhosis, collagen vascular disease, and drug addiction. The major

732 10 · INFECTIOUS DISEASES   TREPONEMATOSES

disadvantages of this test are that interpretation is subjective, results cannot be quantitated, and once positive, it remains so for life. The FTA-ABS is subject to misinterpretation during the neonatal period because it also measures antitreponemal IgG antibody; seropositivity in an uninfected adequately treated mother results in a seropositive uninfected neonate. Follow-up titers will distinguish passively acquired antibody from disease-specific antibodies, the former becoming negative after the 6th mo of life. A recently developed specific antitreponemal antibody test, the Treponema pallidum hemagglutination assay (TPHA-TP), may prove superior to the FTA-ABS test. It is inexpensive, is easy to perform, and does not require a fluorescent microscope; also, interpretation is not subjective. However, the test appears less sensitive than the FTA-ABS test.

The significance of cerebrospinal fluid serology in both acquired and congenital syphilis remains controversial. Cerebrospinal fluid (CSF) antibodies, both "reagin" and treponemal, result from local production within the nervous system as well as passive diffusion from serum. Thus, the CSF VDRL may be positive in congenital or in primary and secondary stage acquired syphilis in the absence of a central nervous system infection. However, because of the propensity to develop symptomatic illness, most authorities feel that a positive CSF serology (FTA-ABS or CSF-VDRL), even in the absence of neurologic findings, warrants treatment for neurosyphilis. Recent data demonstrating passive diffusion of various maternal IgG antibodies across the placenta into the neonatal CSF suggest that congenital neurosyphilis also cannot be diagnosed solely on the basis of positive CSF serology.

Darkfield microscopic examination of scrapings from primary lesions and moist freshly scraped or swabbed congenital or secondary lesions will reveal motile T. pallidum and often permits a definitive diagnosis prior to the development of seropositivity. Antibiotics and antiseptics interfere with treponemal motility and accordingly interfere with the accuracy of darkfield examination. This technique is of limited value in detecting T. pallidum in oral lesions since nonsyphilitic saprophytic spirochetes (T. microdentium) may contaminate the lesion and cannot be distinguished microscopically from T. pallidum. Placental examination by gross and microscopic techniques is a useful adjunct in the diagnosis of congenital syphilis. These disproportionately large placentas are characterized histologically by focal proliferative villitis, endovascular and perivascular arteritis, and focal or diffuse immaturity of placental villi.

Treatment. T. pallidum is extremely sensitive to penicillin, and there is no evidence of increasing penicillin resistance. Studies have determined that a serum concentration greater than 0.03 µg/ml of penicillin is needed to assure killing of spirochetes, that microorganisms will regenerate if subinhibitory concentrations of penicillin (less than 0.0025 µg/ml) persist for more than 24 hr, that inhibitory levels of penicillin must be maintained for at least 7 days to assure complete cure, and that increasing the dose of penicillin does not increase the efficacy of the treatment regimen. Table 10-37 presents appropriate therapeutic regimens for syphilis.

Incubating syphilis may be effectively treated with the currently recommended regimens for gonorrhea (Sec 10.26). Because of the high risk of acquiring infection, "prophylactic treatment" should be given to anyone exposed to infectious syphilis within the preceding 3 mo regardless of serology. Follow-up serologic studies should be obtained in exposed seronegative individuals to confirm the diagnosis and/or determine the adequacy of treatment.

Syphilis in Pregnancy. Routine serology for syphilis should be obtained during the 1st trimester and prior to delivery in high-risk patient populations. When clinical findings and/or serology suggest active infection or the diagnosis of active syphilis cannot be excluded with

Table 10-37 TREATMENT OF SYPHILIS

STAGE	CHOICE	DOSAGE	ALTERNATIVES
Early (primary, secondary or latent less than 1 yr)	Penicillin G benzathine *or*	2.4 million U IM (30,000 U/kg)	Tetracycline HCl (500 mg oral qid × 15 days)
	Penicillin G procaine	600,000 U/day, IM for 8 days	Erythromycin (500 mg oral qid × 15 days)
Late (more than 1 yr duration)	Penicillin G procaine *or*	600,000 U/day IM for 15 days	Tetracycline HCl (500 mg oral qid × 30 days)
	Penicillin G benzathine	2.4 million U IM weekly for 3 doses	Erythromycin (500 mg oral qid × 30 days)
Neurosyphilis	Penicillin G crystalline *or*	2–4 million U/day, IV for 10 days	Tetracycline HCl (500 mg oral qid × 30 days)
	Penicillin G procaine *or*	600,000 U/day, IM for 15 days	Erythromycin (500 mg oral qid × 30 days)
	Penicillin G benzathine	2.4 million U/weekly IM for 3 doses	
Congenital CSF normal	Penicillin G benzathine *or*	50,000 U/kg IM for 1 dose	
	Penicillin G procaine	50,000 U/kg/day for 10 days	
CSF abnormal	Penicillin G crystalline *or*	50,000 U/kg/day, IM or IV for 14–21 days	
	Penicillin G procaine	50,000 U/kg/day, IM daily for 14–21 days	

certainty, treatment is indicated. Women who have been adequately treated in the past do not require additional therapy unless quantitative serology suggests evidence of reinfection (4-fold increase in titer). Congenital syphilis has been reported in infants of pregnant women with syphilis treated with recommended doses of erythromycin. Therefore, infants born to mothers treated with a nonpenicillin regimen should be considered untreated. The cephalosporins may be an effective alternative to erythromycin for pregnant women allergic to penicillin; however, experience with these agents is limited. Chloramphenicol and tetracycline should not be utilized during pregnancy.

Congenital Syphilis. Adequate maternal therapy eliminates the risk of congenital syphilis. However, follow-up of all such infants should continue until nontreponemal serologic tests are negative. The risk of giving penicillin to a newborn is minimal; therefore, treatment should not be withheld in any child born to a mother who received inadequate penicillin therapy or treatment with antibiotics other than penicillin or whose treatment status cannot be ascertained. An acute systemic febrile reaction, *Jarisch-Herxheimer reaction,* with exacerbation of lesions will occur in 15–20% of patients with either acquired or congenital syphilis who are treated with penicillin. The etiology of this reaction is unknown (it may be related to sudden lysis of treponemes and release of endotoxin); however, it does not constitute an indication for the discontinuation of penicillin therapy.

Curtis AC, Philpott DS: Prenatal syphilis. Med Clin North Am 48:707, 1964.
Fiumara PJ, Lessell S: Manifestations of late congenital syphilis: An analysis of 276 patients. Arch Derm 102:78, 1970.
Jaffe HW: The laboratory diagnosis of syphilis: New concepts. Ann Intern Med 83:846, 1975.
Oppenheimer EH, Hardy JB: Congenital syphilis in the newborn infant: Clinical and pathological observations in recent cases. Johns Hopkins Med J 129:63, 1971.

10.56 BEJEL
(Endemic Syphilis, Nonvenereal Childhood Syphilis)

This is a nonvenereally transmitted infection caused by a *Treponema pallidum* (often referred to as *T. pallidum II* or *T. pallidum endemicum*). Bejel is limited to children, occurs exclusively in the warm semi-arid regions of Africa, the Middle East, Southeast Asia, and Australia, and follows penetration of the infecting spirochete through traumatized skin and/or mucous membranes. In experimental infections a primary papule is observed at the inoculation site after the incubation period of 3 wk; however, in human infection a primary lesion is almost never visualized. The initial clinical manifestations of the secondary stage of bejel are confined to the skin and mucous membranes and consist of highly infectious mucous patches on the oral mucosa and condyloma-like lesions on the moist areas of the body, especially the axilla and anus. These mucocutaneous lesions resolve spontaneously over a period of several mo; however, recurrences are common. The secondary

stage is followed by a variable latency period before the onset of late or tertiary bejel. This late stage is characterized by gumma formation of skin, subcutaneous tissue, and bone resulting in painful, destructive ulcerations, swelling, and deformity. Diagnosis is suspected on epidemiologic and clinical grounds and confirmed by darkfield examination of skin and mucous membrane lesions and serologic testing (positive VDRL, TPI, and TBA-ABS). Differentiation from syphilis is extremely difficult in nonendemic areas and requires animal inoculation studies. Bejel can be suspected by the absence of a primary chancre and lack of involvement of the central nervous system and cardiovascular system during the late stage. Treatment during the initial stage consists of a single dose of benzathine penicillin (1.2 million units); late infection is also treated with benzathine penicillin, 1.2 million units given in 3 doses each separated by an interval of 7 days.

10.57 YAWS

Yaws is a chronic relapsing nonvenereally transmitted disease caused by *Treponema pertenue,* a spirochete which cannot be differentiated microscopically or serologically from *T. pallidum*. It is primarily a disease of children living in rural areas of Africa, Southeast Asia, Australia, and South America.

Infection follows the penetration of the causative organism through abraded skin. After an incubation period of several wk an initial lesion ("the mother yaw") appears at that inoculation site as a localized maculopapular rash, a small cluster of papules, or a large exudative papilloma. This lesion ulcerates before healing spontaneously leaving behind a small hypopigmented scar. Following a period of weeks to months, a generalized papular eruption appears, often associated with generalized lymphadenopathy, anorexia, and malaise. Individual papules may enlarge and coalesce forming large papillomas and condylomas, disappear spontaneously, and/or ulcerate, each ulceration covered with a yellowish exudate containing treponemes. This polymorphic secondary eruption heals spontaneously without scarring; however, relapses are common and may extend over several yr. These exacerbations are often associated with bone pain and underlying periostitis and/or osteomyelitis. Following the initial period of clinical activity the patient enters a long period of latency. This is followed by the appearance of tertiary lesions at puberty, which are often solitary and destructive. Such lesions present as painful papillomas on the hands and feet, gummatous skin ulcerations, and/or osteitis of underlying bone. Bony destruction and deformity are common in tertiary yaws. Juxta-articular nodules, depigmentation, and painful hyperkeratosis (crab yaws) of the palms and soles are common sequelae.

Diagnosis depends on the clinical manifestations of the disease in an endemic area. Darkfield examination of cutaneous lesions and serologic tests for syphilis (VDRL, TPI, and FTA-ABS) are confirmatory. Treatment consists of a single intramuscular injection of long acting penicillin, which cures the lesions of active yaws, renders them immediately noninfectious, and prevents relapse. Eradication of yaws from endemic foci can be accomplished with penicillin treatment of entire populations.

10.58 PINTA

Pinta is a chronic nonvenereally transmitted infection caused by *Treponema carateum*, a spirochete morphologically and serologically indistinguishable from other human treponemes. The disease is endemic in regions of Central and South America (Mexico, Venezuela, Colombia, Peru, and Equador), the West Indies (Haiti and Cuba), and areas of Africa and the South Pacific. Infection follows the direct inoculation of the causative organism through abraded skin. Following a variable incubation period of days, a primary lesion appears at the inoculation site as a small erythematous papule resembling localized psoriasis or eczema. The regional lymph nodes are often enlarged, and spirochetes can be visualized on darkfield examination of skin scrapings and/or the involved lymph nodes. After an initial period of enlargement the primary lesion disappears. Secondary lesions follow (within 6–8 mo) and consist of small macules and papules localized to the face, scalp, and exposed portions of the body. These pigmented lesions are nonpruritic and scaly and may coalesce to form large plaque-like elevations resembling psoriasis. The late stage of pinta is associated with the development of atrophic and depigmented lesions on the hands, wrists, ankles, feet, face, and scalp. Hyperkeratosis of palms and soles is uncommon. Diagnosis depends on the clinical manifestations in patients from endemic areas and is confirmed by darkfield examination of early lesions and serologic test for syphilis. Treatment consists of a single injection of long-acting penicillin (600,000 units of benzathine penicillin).

10.59 LEPTOSPIROSIS

Etiology. Leptospirosis is a generalized infection of man and animals caused by spirochetes of the genus *Leptospira*. The pathogenic leptospires all belong to a single species, *L. interrogans*, which contains more than 130 distinct serotypes arranged in 16 serogroups pathogenic for man and animals. In the United States the serogroups most often responsible for human infection include canicola, icterohaemorrhagiae, pomona, autumnalis, grippotyphosa, hebdomidis, and australis. Although some correlation exists between clinical manifestations, severity of illness, and the specific serotype, e.g., Weil disease and *L. icterohaemorrhagiae*, a single serotype may produce a variety of distinct syndromes and a single clinical manifestation, e.g., aseptic meningitis, may be caused by multiple serotypes.

Epidemiology. Leptospirosis is a zoonosis of worldwide distribution. *Leptospira* infect many species of wild and domestic animals and have been isolated from birds, fish, and reptiles. The rat is the principal source of human infection; other important infective reservoirs in the United States include dogs, livestock, wild ani-

mals, and cats. Animal infection varies from inapparent to fatal; once infected, animals can excrete spirochetes in urine for extended periods of time. Survival of these organisms outside the human host is dependent upon the moisture content, temperature, and pH of the soil and/or water into which they are shed. *Leptospira* enter humans through moist and preferably abraded skin or exposed mucous membranes. On a worldwide basis the majority of human cases of leptospirosis result from occupational exposure to rat-contaminated water or soil. In the United States the major animal reservoir is the dog. Infection is common in women and children from urban and suburban settings, and contact with spirochetes (principally *L. canicola*) frequently follows bathing or other outdoor recreational activities during summer months.

Pathophysiology. Following penetration of the skin, *Leptospira* enter the bloodstream and are carried to all organs of the body. After an incubation period of 7–12 days, an initial asymptomatic "septicemic" phase begins, and *Leptospira* can be isolated from the blood, cerebrospinal fluid, and other tissues. Initial symptoms which last approximately 2–7 days are followed by a brief period of well-being and then a 2nd or "immune" phase. With the appearance of circulating antibody during the immune phase, organisms are cleared from the blood and cerebrospinal fluid but may persist in the kidney, urine, and aqueous humor.

Clinical Manifestations. Most cases of human leptospirosis are subclinical; inapparent infection is particularly common in high-risk occupational groups such as sewer workers or farmers. Symptomatic infection may present as an acute febrile illness with nonspecific signs and symptoms (70%), as meningitis (20%), or as hepatorenal dysfunction (10%). Clinical manifestations typically have a sudden onset, and the illness tends to follow a biphasic clinical course (Fig 10–11).

Anicteric Leptospirosis. The initial septicemic phase of leptospirosis presents with the abrupt onset of fever, shaking chills, headache, malaise, nausea, vomiting, and severe and often debilitating muscular pain. Prostration and circulatory collapse are uncommon. Physical examination during this phase typically reveals a lethargic child with mild to moderate dehydration. Most affected children have a sinus tachycardia and a normal blood pressure; however, bradycardia and hypertension are not uncommon. Additional physical findings include extreme muscle tenderness (most prominent in the lower extremities, the lumbosacral spine, and abdomen), conjunctival suffusion (associated with photophobia, orbital pain, and the absence of chemosis and purulent exudate), generalized lymphadenopathy, and hepatosplenomegaly. Cutaneous manifestations are common in children (50%) and usually consist of a truncal erythematous macular or maculopapular rash. Urticarial, petechial, purpuric, and desquamating skin lesions have also been described. A mild febrile illness with a macular or maculopapular rash localized in the pretibial area, *pretibial or Fort Bragg fever*, has been associated with infection due to *L. autumnalis*. Less common abnormalities include pharyngitis, pneumonitis, arthritis, carditis, cholecystitis, parotitis, orchitis, and otitis media.

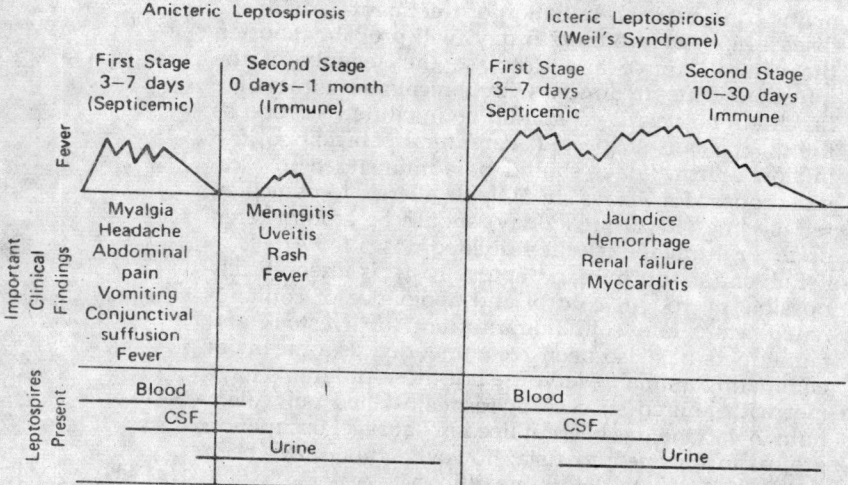

Figure 10–11 Stages of anicteric and icteric leptospirosis. Correlation between clinical findings and presence of leptospires in body fluids. (Reprinted with permission from Feigin RD, Anderson DC: CRC Crit Rev Clin Lab Sci 5:413, 1975. Copyright The Chemical Rubber Co., CRC Press, Inc.)

The immune phase of leptospirosis follows a brief asymptomatic interlude and is characterized by the recurrence of fever. Aseptic meningitis is the hallmark of this phase. Despite abnormal cerebrospinal fluid profiles in 80% of children with leptospirosis, only 50% have meningeal signs and/or symptoms. Spinal fluid abnormalities include a modest elevation in pressure, a mononuclear pleocytosis rarely exceeding 500 cells/mm³ (polymorphonuclear leukocytes predominate early), normal or slightly elevated protein, and a normal glucose. Encephalitis, cranial and peripheral neuropathies, papilledema, and paralysis are uncommon. Symptoms referable to the central nervous system resolve spontaneously within 1 wk. Uveitis may occur during this phase of leptospirosis, can be unilateral or bilateral, is usually self-limited, and rarely results in permanent visual impairment.

Icteric Leptospirosis (Weil Disease). This is the most severe form of leptospirosis and is present in fewer than 10% of affected children. Originally reported in infections due to *L. icterohaemorrhagiae,* it is now apparent that this syndrome is not species specific. The initial manifestations are similar to those previously described for anicteric leptospirosis. However, the immune phase is distinctive and characterized by clinical and laboratory evidence of hepatic and renal dysfunction. In fulminating cases, hemorrhagic phenomena and cardiovascular collapse are also observed. Hepatic abnormalities include right upper quadrant pain, hepatomegaly, direct and indirect hyperbilirubinemia, and elevated serum levels of liver enzymes. Renal manifestations are common, may dominate the clinical picture, and are the principal cause of death in fatal cases; all patients have abnormal urinalysis (hematuria, proteinuria, and casts), and azotemia is common and often associated with oliguria or anuria. Clinical evidence of cardiovascular dysfunction (congestive heart failure) is uncommon; however, abnormal electrocardiograms are present in 90% of affected children. Hemorrhagic manifestations are rare but when present may include epistaxis, hemoptysis, and gastrointestinal and adrenal hemorrhage. Thrombocytopenia and hypoprothrombinemia also occur.

Diagnosis. Silver impregnation and fluorescent antibody techniques permit identification of *Leptospira* in infected tissue or body fluids. Direct examination of clinical specimens by phase-contrast or darkfield microscopy may also demonstrate leptospires; however, the skill required for these techniques and the high frequency of artifacts limit their value. Unlike other pathogenic spirochetes, *Leptospira* are easily cultured on commercially available media. Thus, these pathogens can be recovered from the blood and/or cerebrospinal fluid of infected children during the 1st 10 days of illness and from the urine after the 2nd wk. However, because of the small number of *Leptospira* present in clinical specimens and their slow growth rate in artificial media, it is recommended that multiple cultures be obtained and incubated for 5–6 wk.

The laboratory diagnosis is most often made by serologic testing. A macroscopic slide agglutination test utilizing killed antigen is the most useful screening test. However, a microscopic slide agglutination test with a live antigen is used for the determination of antibody titer and tentative identification of the infecting serotype. Agglutinins are most often identified in the serum (CSF, urine, and bile may also be utilized), usually appear by the 12th day of illness, and reach a maximum titer by the 3rd wk of infection. Following recovery, low titers may persist for years. Approximately 10% of infected individuals have no detectable agglutinins against standard strains, presumably because currently available antisera do not identify all *Leptospira* serotypes.

Thus, a definitive diagnosis of leptospirosis depends on isolating the infecting organism from clinical specimens and/or a 4-fold rise in antibody titer in the presence of clinical symptoms compatible with leptospirosis. A presumptive diagnosis is made in symptomatic children with a stable titer of 1:100 or greater in 2 or more specimens or in asymptomatic children with evidence of exposure and a seroconversion, i.e., a 4-fold rise in antibody titer in specimens obtained 2 or more wk apart.

Treatment and Prevention. Despite the in vitro sensitivity of *Leptospira* to penicillin and tetracycline and the efficacy of these agents in experimental infection,

their use in the treatment of human leptospirosis remains controversial. Initiation of treatment early in the
disease, i.e., before the 7th day, will probably shorten
the clinical course and decrease the severity of the
infection. Thus, treatment with penicillin or tetracycline
(in children over 12 yr) should be instituted as soon as
the diagnosis is suspected. Parenteral penicillin G, 6–8
million units/M²/day, should be administered in 6 divided doses for 7 days. In patients allergic to penicillin,
tetracycline (10–20 mg/kg/day) should be administered
orally or intravenously in 4 divided doses for 7 days.

Prevention of human leptospirosis is theoretically
possible by rodent control and avoidance of contaminated water and soil. Immunization of livestock and
family pets has also been recommended as a means of
eliminating animal reservoirs, but these programs have
met with limited success. A formalin-killed polyvalent
human vaccine has been utilized in "at risk" occupation
groups in Europe and Asia; however, there have been
no clinical trials to determine efficacy.

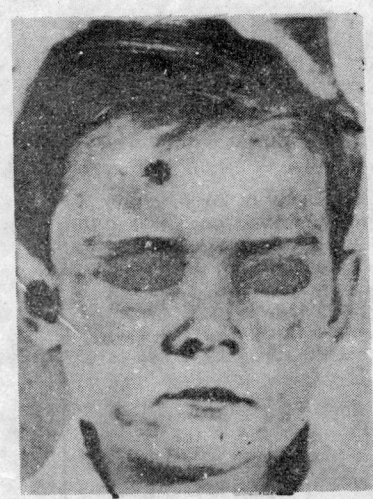

Figure 10–12 Sodoku: chancre-like indurated ulcer at bite site on
forehead; secondary macular eruption of face.

Edwards GA, Domm BM: Human leptospirosis. Medicine 39:117, 1960.
Feigin RD, Anderson DC: Human leptospirosis. CRC Crit Rev Clin Lab Sci 5:413,
1975.
Heath CW Jr, Alexander AD, Galton MM: Leptospirosis in the United States.
Analysis of 483 cases in man, 1949–1961. N Engl J Med 273:857, 1965.
Wong ML, Kaplan S, Dunide LM, et al: Leptospirosis: A childhood disease. J
Pediatr 90:532, 1977.

10.60 RAT BITE FEVER

Rat bite fever is an acute infectious disease caused by
Spirillum minor or *Streptobacillus moniliformis*. The illness
usually follows the bite or scratch of a rat; however,
cases have been reported in the absence of a history of
rodent exposure. Isolated case reports and several epidemics also have been described following the ingestion
of raw milk contaminated by rats (*Haverhill fever*). The
illness has a worldwide distribution, with a higher
incidence reported in urban settings with poor sanitation and large rat populations; it is more common in
children than adults and occurs in approximately 10%
of children bitten by wild rats.

SPIRILLARY RAT-BITE FEVER
(Sodoku)

This form of the disease is caused by *Spirillum minor*,
a short, tightly coiled, gram-negative spirochete, which
can be recovered from the saliva in 10% of healthy wild
and laboratory rats. This microorganism cannot be
grown consistently in commercially available media,
and laboratory isolation requires inoculation of mice
and guinea pigs. However, it can be visualized by direct
darkfield examination of infected lymph obtained from
the inoculation site (preferably during the ulcerative
phase) or adjacent lymph nodes. In addition, the spirochete also may occasionally be visualized on peripheral blood smears from infected individuals.

Clinical Manifestations. The initial inoculation of
spirochetes is followed by a long asymptomatic incu-

bation period of 14–18 days. Subsequently, the wound
becomes erythematous and indurated and eventually
undergoes suppuration and eschar formation (Fig.
10–12). During this phase of infection localized lymphangitis and lymphadenitis are observed in 50% of
affected children. The patient simultaneously develops
fever, chills, severe myalgias, and a reddish-brown or
purple macular rash (80%), which typically begins at
the inoculation site before spreading to involve the
entire body. In untreated children the fever persists for
3–4 days. Following normalization of body temperature,
the constitutional symptoms subside, the rash disappears, and the inoculation site heals. This asymptomatic
period persists for several days and is followed by a
2nd cycle of fever, rash, and constitutional symptoms.
This relapsing pattern of illness may continue for
months or years; however, the disease is eventually
self-limiting. Fatalities are uncommon (1%), and the
only life-threatening complication is infective endocarditis.

Diagnosis. In patients with a history of a rat bite,
the major differential diagnosis involves infection with
either *S. moniliformis* or *S. minor*. The long incubation
period; the prompt initial healing of the primary wound
followed by induration, ulceration, and eschar formation; and the absence of joint involvement suggest *S.
minor* infection. The laboratory diagnosis depends on
negative blood and joint fluid cultures for *S. moniliformis*, the presence of spirochetes on direct darkfield
examination of tissue specimens, and recovery of spirochetes following animal inoculation.

Treatment. *S. minor* is extremely sensitive to penicillin; however, because this illness is often confused
with rat bite fever due to *S. moniliformis*, which is more
penicillin resistant, and because dual infection with
both organisms has been described, most authorities
recommend treatment with large doses of procaine
penicillin, i.e., 600,000 units of procaine penicillin G
every 12 hr for 10 days. In patients allergic to penicillin,
tetracycline is a satisfactory alternative treatment in
children over 12 yr of age.

STREPTOBACILLARY RAT-BITE FEVER
(Haverhill Fever)

This form of rat-bite fever is caused by *Streptobacillus moniliformis*, an aerobic, nonmotile, pleomorphic, unencapsulated gram-negative bacillus, which can be isolated from the nasopharynx of 50% of healthy wild and laboratory rats. *S. moniliformis* can be grown on commercially available artificial media. The morphologic characteristics of the pathogen, including the formation of L-forms devoid of cell wall and resistant to penicillin, vary with the age of the inoculum and the components of the culture medium. Thus, Giemsa or Gram stain may reveal short rods, long chains, and/or long tangled filaments with fusiform swellings.

Clinical Manifestations. The incubation period is short and rarely exceeds 7 days. The illness begins with an abrupt onset of fever and chills. Associated symptoms include severe myalgias, weakness, headache, and upper respiratory symptoms, most notably pharyngitis. A generalized rash and joint involvement appear within several days after the onset of fever. The rash may be maculopapular, petechial, and/or urticarial; however, it most often appears as a diffuse morbilliform rash involving the palms and soles. Joint involvement is common and consists of a polyarticular, occasionally migratory arthritis with a predilection for the small joints of the hands and feet. The initial inoculation site heals without suppuration, and lymphangitis and lymphadenitis are uncommon. In untreated patients the symptoms spontaneously resolve after several days, whereupon the illness assumes a relapsing course with paroxysms of fever, rash, and arthritis occurring at irregular intervals for several mo; the illness is eventually self-limiting, and the mortality rarely exceeds 10%. Life-threatening complications include endocarditis and pneumonitis.

Diagnosis. In patients with a history of a rat bite or rodent contact, the major differential diagnosis involves the 2 forms of rat bite fever. In the streptobacillary form of infection the incubation period is short, the inoculation site heals without suppuration or eschar formation, lymphangitis and lymphadenitis are uncommon, and the responsible pathogen can be readily cultured from blood and joint fluid.

Treatment. Initial therapy consists of 600,000 units of procaine penicillin G every 12 hr for 7–10 days. Streptomycin is effective in the treatment of infections due to penicillin-resistant strains of *S. moniliformis* and should be considered as an alternative therapeutic regimen in children allergic to penicillin. Tetracycline has been used effectively in penicillin allergic children over 12 yr of age.

10.61 RELAPSING FEVER
(Recurrent Fever, Louse-Borne Fever, Tick-Borne Fever)

Relapsing fever is an uncommon arthropod-borne infection of man characterized by recurrent episodes of fever caused by spirochetes of the genus *Borrelia*. These fastidious microorganisms have a worldwide distribution and are transmitted to man by lice or ticks.

Etiology and Epidemiology. Epidemic relapsing fever is caused by *B. recurrentis* and is transmitted from man to man by the human body louse (*Pediculus humanus*). Following ingestion of an infective blood meal by the louse, the spirochetes penetrate the midgut, migrate to and multiply within the hemolymph, and remain viable throughout the life span of the infected vector (several wk). Human infection occurs following crushing or damage of lice during periods of scratching, cutaneous contamination with infected hemolymph, and spirochetal penetration of skin or mucous membranes. Louse-borne disease typically occurs in epidemics, often in association with typhus. It is more common during the winter and occurs under circumstances which favor dissemination of body lice, e.g., overcrowding and poor hygiene. Widespread epidemics have occurred during both world wars, and disease continues to be observed in central Africa (Ethiopia).

Endemic relapsing fever is caused by several species of *Borrelia* and transmitted to man by ticks (genus *Ornithodoros*). Following ingestion of an infective blood meal, spirochetes invade all tissues of their arthropod hosts including the salivary glands and the reproductive tract. The latter permits transovarial passage of infected spirochetes, thereby perpetuating arthropod infection in nature. Human infection occurs when saliva, coxal gland fluid, and/or excrement is released by the tick during feeding, thereby permitting spirochetes to penetrate skin and mucous membranes. *Ornithodoros* have a worldwide distribution (including the western United States), prefer warm humid environments and high altitudes, and are routinely found in rodent burrows, caves, and other nesting sites. Rodents are the preferred hosts and the principal reservoirs for these species of *Borrelia*. Infected ticks passively gain access to human dwellings on rodent host. Human contact is accidental and often unnoticed as these ticks are nocturnal feeders, have a painless bite, and detach immediately following a short blood meal.

Pathophysiology. The cyclic nature of relapsing fever is explained by the ability of *Borrelia* to continually undergo minor antigenic (phase) variation; spirochetes isolated during the primary febrile episode differ antigenically from isolates recovered during a subsequent relapse. During fevers spirochetes enter the bloodstream, promote the development of specific IgM and IgG antibody, and undergo agglutination, immobilization, lysis, and phagocytosis. During remission *Borrelia* disappear from the bloodstream, and antigenic variants sequestered in the reticuloendothelial system and brain increase in number. The number of relapses in untreated patients is dependent upon the number of possible antigenic variants of the infecting strain.

Clinical Manifestations. Louse-borne disease has a longer incubation period, longer periods of pyrexia, fewer relapses, and longer remission periods than tick-borne disease. Both illnesses are associated with the sudden onset of high fever, headache, photophobia, nausea, vomiting, myalgia, and arthralgia. Additional symptoms include abdominal pain, a productive cough, and mild respiratory distress. Bleeding manifestations are common and include epistaxis, hemoptysis, hematuria, and/or hematemesis. Physical examination often reveals a lethargic, febrile child with a diffuse, erythematous, macular, and/or petechial rash over the trunk and shoulders. This rash is more common in louse-borne fever (25%), is of 1–2 days' duration, and occurs almost exclusively during the end of the primary febrile episode. Hepatomegaly and splenomegaly are common. Pneumonia, jaundice, and lymphadenopathy are not uncommon. Central nervous system abnormalities are often present in tick-borne illness and may be the principal feature of the late relapses. Neurologic manifestations include lethargy, stupor, meningismus, convulsions, peripheral neuritis, focal neurologic deficits, and cranial nerve paralysis. Myocarditis and hepatitis are not uncommon in relapsing fever and are often responsible for the patient's demise. The initial symptomatic period characteristically ends with a crisis marked by an abrupt diaphoresis, hypothermia, hypotension, bradycardia, profound muscle weakness, and prostration. In untreated patients subsequent relapses become shorter, symptoms are milder, and the afebrile remission period lengthens.

Treatment and Prognosis. Oral or parenteral tetracycline, chloramphenicol, and erythromycin are the drugs of choice for louse-borne and tick-borne relapsing fever. In children under 12 yr of age chloramphenicol (50 mg/kg/24 hr) or erythromycin (50 mg/kg/24 hr) for a total of 10 days is recommended. For older children and young adults, tetracycline (500 mg every 6 hr) for 10 days has been effective in promoting a prompt defervescence and preventing relapse. Recent clinical trials have demonstrated the efficacy of single dose treatment with chloramphenicol or tetracycline (a single 500 mg oral dose) in adult louse-borne disease, but experience with single drug regimens in children is limited. Resolution of each febrile episode either by natural crisis or as a result of antimicrobial treatment is usually accompanied within 2 hr by the Jarisch-Herxheimer reaction, which is associated with clearing of the spirochetemia. Attempts to control this reaction by prior treatment with corticosteroids, antipyretics, and/or penicillin have met with limited success.

With adequate therapy the mortality rate for relapsing fever is below 5%. No vaccine is available, and disease control requires avoidance or elimination of the arthropod vectors. In epidemics of louse-borne disease, dissemination can be prevented by good personal hygiene and delousing of persons, dwellings, and clothing with DDT or other commercially available insecticides.

WILLIAM T. SPECK
PHILIP TOLTZIS

10.62 CHLAMYDIA

History. Trachoma, an eye disease caused by *Chlamydia*, was first described in 1500 B.C. The occurrence of neonatal conjunctivitis caused by maternal genitourinary tract infection with *Chlamydia* was reported in 1908 by a Viennese ophthalmologist. The organisms causing psittacosis and lymphogranuloma venereum were isolated in 1930, but the closely related *Chlamydia* causing trachoma was not successfully cultured until 1957. The spectrum of disease caused by these organisms was extended in 1977 by the description of a distinctive syndrome of pneumonia in young infants.

Etiology. *Chlamydia* organisms are obligate intracellular parasites with discrete cell walls similar in many ways to those of gram-negative bacteria. They contain both RNA and DNA, are inhibited by some antibiotics, multiply by binary fission, and are nonmotile spheroids about 0.3–1.0 μ in diameter. The organisms cannot be stained by Gram stain. Giemsa staining reveals typical cytoplasmic inclusion bodies lying close to the nucleus.

The genus *Chlamydia* is divided into 2 subgroups. Group A contains *Chlamydia trachomatis* and the agent of lymphogranuloma venereum. Both infect mainly humans and usually produce local disease. Group B includes the agents of psittacosis/ornithosis and Reiter syndrome as well as those of feline pneumonitis, bovine encephalomyelitis, and sheep polyarthritis. Typically, disease due to agents in group B is widespread in the body. Both groups have a common complement-fixing antigen, but microimmunofluorescence testing is species- and subclass-specific.

Epidemiology. *Chlamydia* is worldwide in distribution. Infection in adults is spread venereally as nonspecific nongonococcal urethritis and lymphogranuloma venereum and from eye to hand to eye in trachoma. Infection of the newborn occurs during passage through the infected maternal cervix.

Trachoma is associated with crowded and unsanitary living conditions. It has become less common in the United States and Europe but is still a problem in American Indians living on reservations. It is the leading cause of acquired blindness in the world.

Chlamydiae are etiologic in about 40% of cases of nonspecific nongonococcal urethritis. A syndrome of acute salpingitis and perihepatitis (Fitz-Hugh–Curtis syndrome), formerly attributed to gonococcal infection, can be caused by *Chlamydia*. Lower abdominal pain frequently precedes the sudden onset of right upper quadrant pain.

About 4% of pregnant women are infected with chlamydiae. Infection is more common in younger women of lower socioeconomic class with a history of venereal disease. Babies born through an infected cervix have a 35% incidence of conjunctivitis; 20% develop pneumonia. Fifty per cent of exposed babies are culture positive for *Chlamydia* and 70% show seroconversion. It is estimated that the incidence of *Chlamydia* infection is

28/1000 live births. A quarter of all babies under 6 mo old admitted to the hospital with lower respiratory disease and three fourths of all infants with afebrile pneumonia are infected with *Chlamydia*.

Chlamydia has been isolated from the lower respiratory tract of adults with disease ranging from severe bronchitis to diffuse interstitial pneumonia. Most of these patients were immunocompromised.

Psittacosis/ornithosis is transmitted by contact with infected birds such as parrots, parakeets, pigeons, turkeys, and ducks. Disease is usually seen in adults as an occupational hazard of working with these birds but may be seen in children who purchase infected birds as pets. Person-to-person transmission has been documented in medical personnel caring for infected patients.

10.63 CHLAMYDIAL CONJUNCTIVITIS AND PNEUMONIA IN INFANTS

Clinical Manifestations. *Conjunctivitis* usually begins in the 2nd wk of life but may occur after 3 days or as late as 5–6 wk. Infants typically are afebrile and alert but develop purulent discharge from 1 or both eyes, swollen lids, and pseudomembranes. Bacterial cultures are negative. If untreated, the conjunctivitis subsides after 2–3 wk, but chronic mild infection is common. Response to appropriate topical antibiotics is prompt, but relapse is frequent.

A distinctive syndrome of *pneumonia* has been reported in infants infected with *Chlamydia*. These patients are usually seen at 3–16 wk of age but frequently have been sick for several wk. The babies appear well and are afebrile but develop increasing tachypnea, with prominent cough but no whoop, leading to vomiting and cyanosis. Physical examination shows rales but little wheezing. Conjunctivitis is present in about 50% of these infants.

Chest roentgenogram shows hyperinflation and diffuse interstitial or patchy infiltrates. Moderate eosinophilia is common. pO_2 is decreased in arterial blood, but pCO_2 is normal. IgM and IgG are increased, sometimes to 2–4 times normal for age.

Mortality has not been reported. Organisms have been isolated from lung tissue obtained by biopsy. Light microscopy shows necrotic bronchioles with alveolar and bronchiolar consolidation. Several infants with pneumonia and documented infections with *Chlamydia* have also been infected with cytomegalovirus. Illness in these babies has not been clinically different.

Patients improve gradually without treatment, but symptoms and positive cultures for *Chlamydia* persist for weeks or months. No permanent residua have been described.

Diagnosis and Differential Diagnosis. *Chlamydia* can be isolated in specially treated McCoy hamster, kidney, or HeLa cell lines. Testing for complement-fixing and microimmunofluorescent antibody is possible but is not generally available. If conjunctivitis is present, the palpebral conjunctiva should be scraped with a blunt curette; loosened epithelial cells are fixed on glass slides and stained with Giemsa stain. Intracytoplasmic inclusions are easily seen. The diagnosis is usually made by a high index of suspicion in a patient with a compatible illness.

Chlamydia conjunctivitis must be differentiated from chemical conjunctivitis due to silver nitrate drops, which usually is seen while the infant is still in the nursery. Bacterial conjunctivitis caused by gonococcus or other bacterial organisms can be identified by Gram stain and culture.

Pneumonia may be caused by a variety of bacteria or viruses. Bacterial pneumonia usually has an increased white blood cell count without eosinophilia. Blood cultures or lung taps are frequently positive for bacteria. Viral agents can be isolated with appropriate tissue culture techniques.

Treatment. *Conjunctivitis* responds to topical preparations of tetracycline or sulfonamides. Therapy should be continued for 2–3 wk. Relapses are common. A controlled study comparing the efficacy of oral therapy of erythromycin, 40 mg/kg/24 hr, with topical erythromycin showed no difference in response or recurrence. Nasopharyngeal carriage of *Chlamydia* was eliminated by oral therapy.

Pneumonia associated with chlamydial infection appears to respond to erythromycin in dosage of 40 mg/kg/24 hr or sulfisoxazole (150 mg/kg/24 hr). Improvement is seen in 5–7 days and is associated with conversions of nasopharyngeal cultures to negative. Treatment should be continued for 3 wk.

Since neonatal infection with *Chlamydia* is caused by cervical infection in the mother, the disease could be averted by prevention or treatment of maternal disease. One gm of erythromycin daily for 14 days during the 3rd trimester is effective in eradicating the infection in the mother. Similar treatment of the sexual partner is also necessary. Eye prophylaxis of all newborns with a topical preparation effective against both gonococci and chlamydiae is another possible way to prevent conjunctivitis.

10.64 PSITTACOSIS/ORNITHOSIS

This disease was originally considered to be transmitted only by psittacine birds. It is now known that it can be carried by other species and thus the name ornithosis is preferred.

Onset of illness is usually abrupt, with fever, headache, malaise, sore throat, myalgias, cough, and, occasionally, production of blood-streaked sputum. Temperatures may reach 40.5° C (105° F). Nausea and vomiting are prominent symptoms, and mental confusion may be present.

Examination of the lungs may show rales, and the chest roentgenogram frequently shows diffuse interstitial pneumonia. Hepatosplenomegaly, endocarditis, myocarditis, and pericarditis may occur. The patient may remain quite ill for 3 wk with gradual improvement after that time.

Pneumonia caused by other agents, such as mycoplasma, influenza, and other viral agents, may present a similar clinical picture. Diagnosis usually is based on a history of employment in the poultry industry or in pet stores. Contact with a sick bird is suggestive. Total white blood count and differential are not helpful. Isolation of *Chlamydia* from blood or sputum is possible. A 4-fold rise in complement-fixing antibody is diagnostic.

Chlamydial infections are relatively infrequent in wild birds. Crowding during shipment to the United States is mainly responsible for the widespread infection of imported birds. These birds are held in quarantine on arrival in the United States, and chlortetracycline is added to their feed for prophylactic treatment. However, this program is not well administered, and animals have been shown to be still infected when released from quarantine.

Tetracycline (30 to 40 mg/kg/24 hr) is the drug of choice for treatment. Penicillin in a dose of 3–4 million units/24 hr may also be used. Treatment should be continued for 7–10 days. Control of fever and adequate oxygenation are important.

Beem MO, Saxon E: Respiratory tract colonization and a distinctive pneumonia syndrome in infants infected with *Chlamydia trachomatis*. N Engl J Med 296:306, 1977.

Beem MO, Saxon E, Tipple MA: Treatment of chlamydial pneumonia of infancy. Pediatrics 63:198, 1979.

Chandler JW, et al: Ophthalmia neonatorum associated with maternal chlamydial infections. Tr Am Acad Ophthalmol Otolaryngol 83:302, 1977.

Hieber JP: Infections due to *Chlamydia*. J Pediatr 91:864, 1977.

Schachter J: Chlamydia infections. N Engl J Med 298:428, 490, 540, 1978.

Schachter J, Holt J, Goodner E, et al: Prospective study of chlamydial infection in neonates. Lancet 2:377, 1979.

Wolner-Hanssen P, Westrom L, Mardh PA: Perihepatitis and chlamydial salpingitis. Lancet 1:901, 1980.

10.65   LYMPHOGRANULOMA VENEREUM
(Lymphogranuloma Inguinale)

Lymphogranuloma venereum (LGV) is usually sexually transmitted, and in the majority of children the transmission occurs from an infected adult. The causative agent is related to *Chlamydia trachomatis* but differs because it is more invasive in vivo and is lethal to mice when injected intracerebrally.

Epidemiology. Lymphogranuloma venereum has been reported worldwide. It is relatively uncommon in the United States, most cases being seen in Southeast Asia and Central and South America. The reported incidence is much higher in males, reaching 20:1 in some series. The disease is usually more obvious in males, with fever, toxicity, and inguinal lymphadenopathy. Women present more frequently with complications such as rectal stricture.

Pathology. Pathologic characteristics of the primary lesion are not specific and therefore do not help in establishing the diagnosis. Primary genital ulcers have an exudate of fibrin and contain cellular debris and polymorphonuclear leukocytes. The periphery of the ulcer contains large mononuclear cells and plasma cells as well. Lymph nodes draining the infected area show characteristic changes with stellate triangular abscesses, the centers of which contain polymorphonuclear leukocytes and some macrophages. Older, healing lesions tend to contain scars and sinus tracts.

Clinical Manifestations. The incubation period varies from 3–30 days if a primary genital lesion is considered the end point. If such a lesion is missed, the period from sexual contact to the development of adenopathy may be much longer.

The 1st manifestation is a small erosion, a pustule, or a papule. In men it is usually present on the coronal sulcus, frenulum, prepuce, glans, or shaft of the penis or on the scrotum. In women the most common sites are the posterior vaginal wall, cervix, or fourchette. Because the primary lesion is small and asymptomatic, it is frequently missed. Rare extragenital primary lesions have been reported but can usually be related to direct contact with infected genitals.

The secondary lesion, inguinal adenitis, develops 1–4 wk after the appearance of the primary lesion and is unilateral in two thirds of cases. The nodes are initially firm and tender but are movable. Later they become fixed to one another and to the overlying skin, which then first becomes erythematous and cyanotic, then scaly and edematous preceding rupture of the nodes. When nodes rupture, whether spontaneously or through surgical intervention, a chronic sinus tract tends to develop and drain for many wk or longer. Alternatively, the nodes may resolve without treatment over a period of several mo. Relapses of acute adenitis are common.

In women the anatomic site of the primary lesion determines the clinical picture of the disease. Lesions of the upper third of the vagina and on the cervix drain to nodes between the external and internal iliac arteries; those of the middle third of the vagina to nodes between the rectum and internal iliac arteries; those of the lower third of the vagina to the pelvic and inguinal nodes.

Rectal drainage of blood, mucus, or pus secondary to rupture of perirectal nodes also occurs. This may lead to fibrosis, scarring, and rectal stricture. The latter may result in periodic rectal bleeding and thin stools. Such symptoms are especially common in homosexual males.

Untreated cases may develop elephantiasis of the genitalia and attendant soft tissue infections.

Like so many other sexually transmitted infections, lymphogranuloma venereum is a systemic disease and may be associated with fever, malaise, headache, anorexia, and other nonspecific symptoms. Rare cases of meningoencephalitis have been reported and the infectious agent recovered from spinal fluid.

Hypergammaglobulinemia due to elevation of IgA and IgG is frequent. Autoimmune serum factors such as cryoglobulins, rheumatoid factor, antinuclear factor, positive Coombs test, and anticomplementary serum factors are present in most cases. Likewise a false-positive serologic test for syphilis is common.

Diagnosis and Differential Diagnosis. Lymphogranuloma venereum must be considered in patients with the typical primary lesions; in those with enlarged, matted, and tender inguinal lymph nodes; and in patients with proctitis, draining inguinal or perianal fistulas, and rectal strictures. It may mimic any cause of inguinal adenopathy, such as pyrogenic infections, plague, tularemia, cat-scratch disease, chancroid, granuloma inguinale, syphilis, and rectal neoplasms. Direct examination of the tissues may reveal the somewhat characteristic pathologic lesions but may also demonstrate the organisms within the cytoplasm of the cells. These appear as blue inclusions in specimens treated with Giemsa stain. Aspirates from lymph nodes should be cultured.

The diagnosis is made by recognition of the clinical syndrome, isolation of the organism from infected lymph nodes, and an increase in complement-fixing antibody or microimmunofluorescent testing. The Frei test (a skin test dependent on delayed hypersensitivity) is unreliable.

Serologic tests, such as the complement-fixation reaction, are carried out with heat-stable group antigens. If a test is positive in a patient with a suspicious clinical history and findings, the diagnosis is strongly supported. The indirect immunofluorescence (IF) test is more sensitive but less available.

Prevention. All measures applicable to prevention of sexually transmitted diseases would be effective in prevention of lymphogranuloma venereum. However, the general lack of success of such measures must be acknowledged. There is no available vaccine.

Treatment. Tetracyclines are effective in lymphogranuloma venereum; sulfonamides or chloramphenicol may also be used. Treated patients tend to have a shorter duration of the lesions, less occurrence of sinus tract formation, fewer relapses, and a decline in the complement-fixation titer. Any patient who shows a rise in titer after therapy should be retreated. The course of treatment should be 3–4 wk. Surgical excision or drainage is contraindicated because of the possibility of formation of sinus tracts. Response to therapy, although variable, is better in acute cases.

CAROL F. PHILLIPS

Banou L Jr: Rectal lesions of lymphogranuloma venereum in childhood. Am J Dis Child 83:860, 1952.
Becker LE: Lymphogranuloma venereum. Int J Dermatol 15:26, 1976.
Hieber JP: Infections due to Chlamydia. J Pediatr 91:864, 1977.
Jawetz E: Chemotherapy of chlamydial infections. Adv Pharmacol Chemother 7:235, 1969.
McLelland BA, Anderson PC: Lymphogranuloma venereum: outbreak in a university community. JAMA 235:56, 1976.

10.66 MYCOPLASMAL INFECTIONS

Mycoplasma pneumoniae is the only mycoplasma species known to be pathogenic for humans. It is now recognized as a major cause of respiratory infections in school-aged children and young adults, among whom it is responsible for 40–60% of cases of pneumonia during epidemic periods.

The incidence of illness due to *Mycoplasma pneumoniae* varies greatly with the age of the patient and the epidemicity of the organism. Clinically significant disease is unusual before the age of 4–5 yr; the peak incidence occurs in children between the ages of 10–15 yr. The quantitative role of the organism as a cause of nonpneumonic disease is not known.

Etiology. *Mycoplasma pneumoniae*, originally thought to be a virus and called the Eaton agent, was found to be a mycoplasma in the early 1960's. Mycoplasmas have no cell wall and are intermediate in size—larger than certain viruses, smaller than others. They can be grown on lifeless media and are, thus, the smallest free-living microorganisms known. *Mycoplasma pneumoniae* has a filamentous shape and a specialized tip at 1 end which allows attachment to ciliated epithelial cells in the respiratory tract. Methods for isolation, propagation, and specific identification have been well described but are highly technical and are performed routinely in only a few laboratories.

Epidemiology. *Mycoplasma pneumoniae* infections are found worldwide. In contrast to the acute, short-lived epidemics caused by some other respiratory agents, such as respiratory syncytial and influenza viruses, *Mycoplasma pneumoniae* epidemics are long-lasting and smoldering in character. They occur at irregular intervals but have a tendency to begin in the fall.

The occurrence of illnesses due to *Mycoplasma pneumoniae* is dictated at least in part by the age and antibody status of the patient. Overt illnesses are unusual under 4–5 yr of age, but younger children appear to have frequent mild or subclinical infections; reinfections appear to be common. In adults, previous infections, as demonstrated by the presence of circulating antibodies, prevent or ameliorate infections; that is, patients with high antibody levels tend to have fewer or milder illnesses than do patients with low or absent titers.

Infections with *Mycoplasma pneumoniae* are not highly communicable in that infections in contacts within families occur at a very slow rate. However, most susceptible family members will become infected over a period of weeks or months.

Pathology, Immunology, and Pathogenesis. Little information is available on the histopathologic features of *Mycoplasma pneumoniae* disease in humans because it is rarely fatal. Peribronchiolar infiltrates of mononuclear and plasma cells and the intraluminal accumulation of polymorphonuclear leukocytes and sloughed epithelial cells are a part of a picture of interstitial pneumonia and acute bronchiolitis.

Electron microscopic studies of infected hamster lungs and exfoliated cells from human cases have demonstrated the attachment of *Mycoplasma pneumoniae* by the specialized tip to ciliated epithelial cells. The organisms attach to cell surfaces and burrow down between cells, resulting in eventual sloughing of the cells, but intracellular organisms have not been found.

A variety of serologic responses occur following *Mycoplasma pneumoniae* infections. Nonspecific cold hemagglutinins are usually the 1st antibodies detected and the 1st to disappear but are not present at any time in some patients. Both the frequency of cold hemagglutinins and the height of the titer correlate with the severity of the illness. Specific immunologic reactions can be measured by a variety of techniques and persist for long periods of time. Complement-fixing antibody tests, in which commercially available antigen is used, are satisfactory for usual diagnostic purposes and can be run in most hospital laboratories.

Although the presence of circulating antibodies in humans can be correlated with protection against *Mycoplasma pneumoniae* infections, studies in the hamster have shown that circulating antibody alone, in the absence of other forms of immunity, is incompletely protective. Hamster studies have shown that most of the peribronchiolar mononuclear cells are laden with antibody. However, ablation of the T cell system using antithymocyte serum completely prevents the development of pneumonia. Thus, the disease produced by *Mycoplasma pneumoniae* is very complex; the immunologic response of the host is responsible for the disease itself or for protection against it, depending on the qualitative and quantitative balance of humoral and cellular immunity.

Clinical Manifestations. Respiratory and nonrespiratory sites are involved in *Mycoplasma pneumoniae* infections, but the lung is the primary site. The incubation period is thought to be 2–3 wk. The onset of illness is gradual and characterized by headache, malaise, and fever; cough is a prominent finding, and sore throat is frequent. The severity of symptoms is usually greater than the physical signs that appear later in the disease. Rales, which are often musical and resemble those heard in asthma and bronchiolitis, are the most prominent sign, but dullness to percussion and sputum production occur frequently. *Mycoplasma pneumoniae* can usually be isolated from the upper respiratory tract or sputum for several wk to mo after recovery.

Involvement of parts of the respiratory tract other than the lungs also occurs, including undifferentiated upper respiratory tract infections, pharyngitis, croup, tracheobronchitis, and bronchiolitis. In addition, otitis media and bullous myringitis have been described.

Nonrespiratory sites of involvement include the skin, central nervous system, blood, heart, and joints. In contrast to the proved and constant relationship between *Mycoplasma pneumoniae* and involvement of the respiratory tract, the association with nonrespiratory sites is unusual or tenuous. Skin lesions include maculopapular rashes, erythema nodosum, and the Stevens-Johnson syndrome. Meningoencephalitis and the Guillain-Barré syndrome have been reported. Hemolytic anemia is the most common hematologic disorder encountered, but thrombocytopenia and coagulation defects have been described. Myocarditis, pericarditis,

and a rheumatic fever–like syndrome have been reported.

In general, *Mycoplasma pneumoniae* illnesses are mild and hospitalization is infrequent. Fatal infections are rare. Complications following *Mycoplasma pneumoniae* infections are unusual; bacterial superinfection is not common.

There is nothing diagnostic about the roentgenographic findings. Pneumonia is usually described as interstitial or bronchopneumonic, and involvement is most common in the lower lobes. Pleural fluid is unusual; its presence in significant amounts would suggest another diagnosis in most instances.

The peripheral blood leukocyte and differential counts are usually normal. Cultures of the throat or sputum on special medium may demonstrate *Mycoplasma pneumoniae*. Cold hemagglutinins may be determined in acute-phase serum. A specific antibody rise in convalescent-phase serum obtained in 10 days–3 wk is diagnostic. Rapid diagnosis by fluorescent antibody or electron microscopic studies of exfoliative cells is still a research procedure.

Diagnosis. No specific clinical, epidemiologic, or laboratory observations allow a definite diagnosis of illnesses due to *Mycoplasma pneumoniae* early in their course. Certain observations are suggestive of the presence of infection due to this organism, however, and can be helpful to the practicing physician. Pneumonia in school-aged children and young adults, especially if cough is a prominent finding, is always suggestive of *Mycoplasma pneumoniae* disease. Cold hemagglutinins in a titer of 1:64 or greater support the diagnosis. The diagnosis can be confirmed by the isolation of the organism and identification of the development of specific antibodies. If the presence of *Mycoplasma pneumoniae* in a community can be confirmed in a few patients, the probability of other *Mycoplasma pneumoniae* illnesses is greatly increased.

Prevention. Efforts have been made to develop *Mycoplasma pneumoniae* vaccines, but these have met with variable success. At present no vaccine has been licensed for commercial use.

Treatment. *Mycoplasma pneumoniae* shows exquisite in vitro sensitivity to erythromycin and the tetracyclines; because of the absence of a cell wall in mycoplasmas, the organism is quite resistant to the penicillins. The effectiveness of both erythromycin and the tetracyclines in shortening the course of *Mycoplasma pneumoniae* illnesses has been demonstrated in several population groups. Erythromycin is the drug of choice in small children because of the toxic effects of the tetracyclines in this group; it should be given in full therapeutic doses for several days after defervescence, usually a total of 7–10 days. In spite of the efficacy of these drugs in ameliorating the clinical course, the organism is not eradicated.

Symptomatic treatment, including bed rest, analgesics and antipyretics, maintenance of fluid intake, and increased humidity, is indicated.

FLOYD W. DENNY

Collier AM, Clyde WA Jr: Appearance of *Mycoplasma pneumoniae* in lungs of experimentally infected hamsters and sputum from patients with natural disease. Am Rev Resp Dis 110:765, 1974.

Denny FW, Clyde WA Jr, Glezen WP: *Mycoplasma pneumoniae* disease: Clinical spectrum, pathophysiology, epidemiology, and control. J Infect Dis 123:74, 1971.

Fernald GW: Role of host response in *Mycoplasma pneumoniae* disease. J Infect Dis 127:S55, 1973.

Fernald GW, Clyde WA Jr: Pulmonary immune mechanisms in *Mycoplasma pneumoniae* disease. In: Kirkpatrick CH, Reynolds HY (eds): Immunologic and Infectious Reactions in the Lung. New York, Marcel Dekker, 1976.

Fernald GW, Collier AM, Clyde WA Jr: Respiratory infections due to *Mycoplasma pneumoniae* in infants and children. Pediatrics 55:327, 1975.

Foy HM, Grayston JT, Kenny GE: Epidemiology of *Mycoplasma pneumoniae* infection in families. JAMA 197:859, 1966.

Steinberg P, White RJ, Fuld SL, et al: Ecology of *Mycoplasma pneumoniae* in Marine recruits at Parris Island, South Carolina. Am J Epidemiol 89:62, 1969.

VIRAL INFECTIONS AND THOSE PRESUMED TO BE CAUSED BY VIRUSES

10.67 MEASLES
(Rubeola)

Measles is an acute communicable disease characterized by 3 stages: (1) an incubation stage of approximately 10–12 days with few, if any, signs or symptoms; (2) a prodromal stage with an enanthem (Koplik spots) on the buccal and pharyngeal mucosa, mild to moderate fever, slight conjunctivitis, coryza, and an increasingly severe cough; and (3) a final stage with a maculopapular rash erupting successively over the neck and face, body, arms, and legs and accompanied by high fever.

Etiology. Measles is an RNA virus classified in the family Paramyxoviridae, genus Morbillivirus. There is only 1 antigenic type known; it is similar in structure to the viruses of mumps and parainfluenza. It is present in the nasopharyngeal secretions, blood, and urine, at least during the prodromal period and for a short time after the rash appears. It can remain active for at least 34 hr at room temperature.

Measles virus may be isolated in primary cultures of human embryonic or rhesus monkey kidney tissue. Cytopathic changes, usually visible in 5–10 days, consist of multinucleated giant cells with intranuclear inclusions. Circulating antibody is detectable at the time of appearance of the rash.

Infectivity. Maximal dissemination of virus occurs by droplet spray from the respiratory tract during the prodromal period (catarrhal stage). Transmission to susceptible contacts often occurs before the diagnosis of the original case has been established. An infected person becomes infective for others by the 9th–10th day after exposure (beginning of the prodromal phase), in some instances as early as the 7th day. Isolation precautions to prevent spread, especially in hospitals or other institutions for children, should be maintained from the 7th day after exposure until about 5 days after the rash has appeared.

Epidemiology. Measles is endemic over most of the world. In the past, epidemics tended to occur irregularly, appearing in large cities at 2–4 yr intervals as new groups of susceptible children were exposed. Measles is very infectious; approximately 90% of susceptible family contacts acquire the disease. It is rarely subclinical. Prior to the use of measles vaccine, the age of peak incidence was 5–10 yr; most adults were immune. Since the widespread use of vaccine, most cases are seen in adolescents or young adults who did not receive vaccine, received inactivated vaccine, or were immunized when under 15 mo of age. There is no evidence that a carrier state exists, nor has any other mode of interepidemic transmission been established. During an epidemic the airborne route appears to be the most common mode of spread, although direct contact and spread by droplet spray are important means of cross-infection.

Infants acquire immunity transplacentally from mothers who have had measles. This immunity is usually complete for the 1st 4–6 mo of life and disappears at a varying rate. Although maternal antibody levels are generally undetectable in the infant by usual tests after 9 mo of age, protection persists in some children since fewer children immunized at that age will develop measurable antibody compared with children immunized at 15 mo or later. Infants of susceptible mothers have no such immunity and may contract the disease with the mother before or after delivery.

Pathology. The essential lesion of measles is found in the skin; in the mucous membranes of the nasopharynx, bronchi, and intestinal tract; and in the conjunctivae. Serous exudate and proliferation of mononuclear cells and a few polymorphonuclear cells occur around the capillaries. There is usually hyperplasia of lymphoid tissue, particularly in the appendix, where multinucleated giant cells up to 100 μ in diameter (Warthin-Finkeldey reticuloendothelial giant cells) may be found. In the skin the reaction is particularly notable about the sebaceous glands and hair follicles. Koplik spots consist of serous exudate and proliferation of endothelial cells similar to those in the skin lesions. There is a general inflammatory reaction of the buccal and pharyngeal mucosa which extends into the lymphoid tissue and the tracheobronchial mucous membrane. Interstitial pneumonitis due to measles virus takes the form of Hecht giant cell pneumonia. Bronchopneumonia may be due to secondary bacterial infection.

In fatal cases of encephalomyelitis there is perivascular demyelinization of areas of the brain and spinal cord. In Dawson subacute sclerosing panencephalitis (SSPE), degeneration of the cortex and white matter with intranuclear and intracytoplasmic inclusion bodies has been described.

Clinical Manifestations. The incubation period is approximately 10–12 days if the 1st symptoms are selected as the time of onset or approximately 14 days if the appearance of the rash is selected; rarely it may be as short as 6–10 days. A slight rise in temperature may occur 9–10 days from the date of infection and then subside for 24 hr or so.

The prodromal phase, which usually lasts 3–5 days, is characterized by low-grade to moderate fever, a slight hacking cough, coryza, and conjunctivitis. These almost always precede Koplik spots, the pathognomonic sign of measles, by 2–3 days. An enanthem or red mottling is usually present on the hard and soft palates. **Koplik spots** are grayish white dots, usually as small as grains of sand, with slight, reddish areolae; occasionally they are hemorrhagic. They tend to occur opposite the lower molars but may spread irregularly over the rest of the buccal mucosa. Rarely they are found within the midportion of the lower lip, on the palate, and on the lacrimal caruncle. They appear and disappear rapidly, usually within 12–18 hr. As they fade, there may remain red, spotty discolorations of the mucosa. The conjunctival inflammation and photophobia lead one to suspect measles before Koplik spots appear. In addition, a transverse line of conjunctival inflammation, sharply demarcated along the eyelid margin, may be of diagnostic assistance in the prodromal stage. As the entire conjunctiva becomes involved, the line disappears.

Occasionally the prodromal phase may be severe, being ushered in by sudden high fever, at times with convulsions and even pneumonia. Usually the coryza, fever, and cough are increasingly severe up to the time the rash has covered the body.

The temperature rises abruptly as the rash appears and often reaches 40–40.5° C (104–105° F). When the rash appears on the legs and feet, within about 2 days, the symptoms subside rapidly in uncomplicated cases. The patient up to this point may appear desperately ill and yet within 24 hr after the drop in temperature, which is usually abrupt, appear essentially well.

The rash usually starts as faint macules on the upper lateral parts of the neck, behind the ears, along the hairline, and on the posterior parts of the cheek. The individual lesions become increasingly maculopapular as the rash spreads rapidly over the entire face, neck, upper arms, and upper part of the chest within approximately the 1st 24 hr (Fig 10–13 [p. xxxiii] and 10–14). During the succeeding 24 hr it spreads over the back, abdomen, entire arms, and thighs. As it finally reaches the feet on the 2nd–3rd day, it is beginning to fade on the face. The fading of the rash proceeds downward in the same sequence as that of its appearance. The severity of the disease is directly related to the extent and confluence of the rash. In mild measles the rash tends not to be confluent, and in very mild cases there are few, if any, lesions on the legs. In severe measles the rash is confluent, the skin being completely covered, including the palms and soles, and the face is swollen and disfigured.

The rash is often slightly hemorrhagic; in severe cases with a confluent rash, petechiae may be present in large numbers, and there may be extensive ecchymoses. Itching is generally slight. As the rash fades, branny desquamation and brownish discoloration occur and then disappear within 7–10 days.

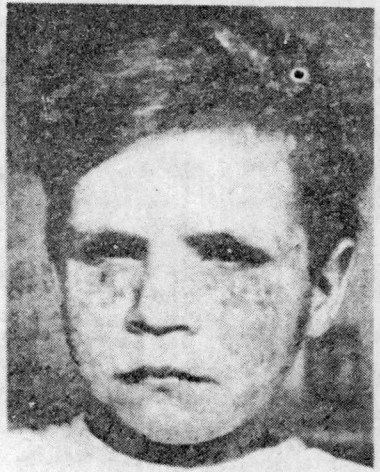

Figure 10–14 Purpuric rash of measles.

The rash may vary markedly. Infrequently a slight urticarial, a faint macular, or a scarlatiniform rash may appear during the early prodromal stage and disappear in advance of the typical rash. Complete absence of rash is rare except in patients who have received human antibodies during the incubation period and possibly in infants under 8 mo of age who have appreciable levels of maternal antibody. Occasionally, death may occur before the rash has appeared. In the hemorrhagic type of measles **(black measles)** bleeding may occur from the mouth, nose, or bowel. In mild cases the rash may be less macular and more nearly pinpoint, somewhat resembling that of scarlet fever.

Lymph nodes at the angle of the jaw and in the posterior cervical region are usually enlarged, and slight splenomegaly may be noted. Mesenteric lymphadenopathy may cause abdominal pain. Characteristic pathologic changes of measles in the mucosa of the appendix may cause obliteration of the lumen and symptoms of appendicitis. Changes of this type tend to subside with the disappearance of Koplik spots. Otitis media, bronchopneumonia, and gastrointestinal symptoms, such as diarrhea and vomiting, are more common in infants and small children than in older children.

Diagnosis. This is usually made from the typical clinical picture; laboratory confirmation is rarely needed. During the prodromal stage multinucleated giant cells can be demonstrated in smears of the nasal mucosa. Virus can be isolated in tissue culture, and diagnostic rises in antibody titer can be detected between acute and convalescent sera. The white blood cell count tends to be low with a relative lymphocytosis. Lumbar puncture in patients with measles encephalitis usually shows an increase in protein and a small increase in lymphocytes. The glucose level is normal.

Differential Diagnosis. The rash of rubeola must be differentiated from exanthem subitum, rubella, infections due to echo-, coxsackie-, and adenoviruses, infectious mononucleosis, toxoplasmosis, meningococcemia, scarlet fever, rickettsial diseases, serum sickness, and drug rashes.

Koplik spots are pathognomonic for rubeola, and the diagnosis of unmodified measles should not be made in the absence of cough.

Roseola infantum (exanthem subitum) is distinguished from measles because the rash appears as the fever disappears. The rashes of rubella and of enteroviral infections tend to be less striking than that of measles, as do the degree of fever and severity of illness. Although cough is present in many rickettsial infections, the rash usually spares the face, which is characteristically involved in measles. Headache is a more prominent feature of rickettsial infections. The absence of cough and the history of injection or ingestion of a drug usually serve to identify serum sickness or drug rashes. Meningococcemia may be accompanied by a rash somewhat similar to that of measles, but cough and conjunctivitis are usually absent. The diffuse, finely papular rash of scarlet fever, a confluent erythema with a "gooseflesh" texture most marked on the abdomen, is relatively easy to differentiate.

The milder rash and the clinical picture of measles modified by gamma globulin, by partial immunity induced by measles vaccine, or in infants by maternal antibody may be difficult to differentiate.

Complications. The chief complications of measles are otitis media, pneumonia, and encephalitis. Noma of the cheeks may occur in rare instances if the disease is severe. Gangrene elsewhere appears to be secondary to purpura fulminans or disseminated intravascular coagulation following measles.

Pneumonia (Sec 12.67) may be caused by the measles virus itself; the lesion is interstitial. Bronchopneumonia is more frequent, however; it is due to secondarily invading bacteria, particularly the pneumococcus, streptococcus, staphylococcus, and *Hemophilus influenzae.* Laryngitis, tracheitis, and bronchitis are common and may be due to the virus alone.

One of the potential dangers of measles is exacerbation of an existing *tuberculous process.* There may also be a temporary loss of hypersensitivity to tuberculin.

Myocarditis is an infrequent serious complication; transient electrocardiographic changes are said to be relatively common.

Neurologic complications are more common in measles than in any of the other exanthems. The incidence of *encephalomyelitis* is estimated to be 1–2/1000 reported cases of measles. There is no correlation between the severity of the measles and that of the neurologic involvement or between the severity of the initial encephalitic process and the prognosis. Rarely, encephalitis has been reported in association with measles modified by gamma globulin and by the use of live attenuated measles virus vaccine. In a few instances encephalitic involvement is manifest in the pre-eruptive period, but more often the onset is 2–5 days after the appearance of the rash. The cause of measles encephalitis remains controversial. It is suggested that when encephalitis occurs early in the course of the disease, viral invasion plays a large role, although measles virus has rarely been isolated from brain tissue; encephalitis which occurs later is predominantly demyelinating in nature and may reflect an immunologic reaction. In this demyelinating type of reaction the symptoms and course do not differ from those of other parainfectious encephalitides. Fatal encephalitis has been reported in children immunosuppressed for treatment of malignancies. Other central nervous system complications, such as Guillain-Barré syndrome, hemiplegia, cerebral thrombophlebitis, and retrobulbar neuritis, occur rarely.

Dawson subacute sclerosing panencephalitis (SSPE) (Sec 21.16) is due to measles virus. This is a progressive, fatal neurologic disease seen mainly in late childhood. Boys are affected 3 times more commonly than girls. Frequently the child has a history of having had measles before 2 yr of age. Rarely the disease occurs in patients who have received measles vaccine, but the risk of developing SSPE appears to be about 10 times less in children who receive vaccine compared with those who have had clinical measles.

A possible etiologic role of measles virus in multiple sclerosis has been suggested but not proved. Several studies have shown higher serum and CSF antibodies against measles in patients with multiple sclerosis compared with matched controls.

Prognosis. Case fatality rates in the United States have decreased in recent yr to low levels for all age groups, in large part because of improved socioeconomic conditions but also because of effective antibacterial therapy for the treatment of secondary infections.

When measles is introduced into a highly susceptible population, the results may be disastrous. Such an occurrence in the Faroe Islands in 1846 resulted in the deaths of about one fourth, nearly 2000, of the total population regardless of age. At Ungava Bay, Canada, where 99% of 900 persons had measles, the mortality rate was 7%.

Prophylaxis. Quarantine is of little value because of the high communicability of the disease during its prodromal stage, when its presence is usually not suspected.

Active Immunization. This can be achieved by use of live attenuated measles vaccine. The 1st live vaccine used was the Edmonston B strain. Further attenuation of the Edmonston strain led to the development and widespread use of Schwartz and Moraten strains. The incidence of fever and rash is about 10% with these vaccines; gamma globulin is not required and should not be given with them. The virus is grown in chick embryo fibroblast cultures, lyophilized, reconstituted at the time of immunization, and given by subcutaneous injection. The vaccine virus is heat- and light-sensitive; therefore, the vaccine should be stored in the refrigerator at 4° C and used as soon as it is reconstituted. About 95% of susceptible children and adults develop antibody.

Some infants under 15 mo of age fail to produce antibody to the vaccine, apparently because of persisting but unmeasurable maternal antibody. Therefore, it is recommended that routine measles vaccination not be given before age 15 mo. In a community where measles is endemic or in an undeveloped country where the disease is frequent in infants, the vaccine may be given at age 12 mo. Gamma globulin may be preferable to prevent measles in young infants exposed to the disease. Adults who receive measles vaccine do not have an increased incidence of reactions. The level of antibody produced by vaccine is about 20% of that developed by natural disease, but it is long lasting and protective. Subclinical infections in recipients of vaccine frequently result in boosts in titer of antibody. When a large percentage of a population has received measles vaccine, any outbreak of measles which develops will include a relatively large number of cases in children who have been vaccinated. However, repeated investigations of such outbreaks have shown a vaccine efficacy of 90% or more.

Since the vaccine virus is grown in chick fibroblast culture rather than in eggs, it can be given safely to children who are allergic to egg protein.

The estimated incidence of severe reactions, including neurologic involvement, following vaccination with live virus vaccine is about 1:1,000,000. Regional lymphadenopathy, thrombocytopenic purpura, and pneumonia have been recorded, as have febrile convulsions.

The response to live measles vaccine is unpredictable if immune globulin has been administered in the 3 mo preceding immunization. Anergy to tuberculin may develop and persist for 1 mo or longer after administration of live attenuated measles vaccine. A child with active tuberculous infection should be receiving antituberculosis treatment when live measles vaccine is administered. A tuberculin test prior to or concurrent with active immunization against measles is desirable.

Use of live measles vaccine is not recommended for pregnant women or for children with untreated tuberculosis. Live vaccine is contraindicated in children with leukemia and in those receiving immunosuppressive drugs because of the risk of persistent, progressive infection such as giant cell pneumonia. After exposure of susceptible children to measles, measles immune globulin (human) should be given intramuscularly in a dose of 0.25 ml/kg as soon as possible. A larger dose may be advisable in children with acute leukemia, even those in remission. Measles vaccine can be given following exposure to the disease. Reactions are not increased, and measles may be prevented.

The use of inactivated (killed) virus vaccine is not recommended, and none has been used since 1968 in the United States. Antibody response may be poor and short lived and does not include secretory IgA against measles; secretory antibody is present in respiratory tract secretions after the natural disease or use of live virus vaccine. Unusual local or systemic reactions have occurred in recipients of killed virus vaccine who were later exposed to natural measles or were vaccinated with live attenuated virus. Such reactions to live virus vaccine have included severe local tenderness, swelling, erythema, heat, and hemorrhagic or vesicular lesions accompanied by malaise, fever, and regional lymphadenopathy. Exposure to natural measles has resulted in a severe, atypical form of measles, with high fever, edema, pneumonia, and toxicity. Pleural effusions and enlarged hilar nodes can occur. Occasionally, pulmonary nodules develop which can persist for many mo. The rash, which may be petechial, vesicular, or urticarial, begins on the feet and extends upward but is concentrated largely on the extremities. Such reactions do not seem to follow repeated inoculations of the attenuated live virus vaccine in children. Combined measles-mumps-rubella and measles-rubella vaccines are available and effective.

Passive Immunization. Passive immunization with pooled adult serum, pooled convalescent serum, placental globulin, or gamma globulin of pooled plasma is effective for prevention and attenuation of measles. Measles can be prevented by the use of immune serum globulin (gamma globulin) in a dose of 0.25 ml/kg given intramuscularly within 5 days after exposure but preferably as soon as possible. Complete protection is indicated for infants, for children with chronic illness, and for contacts in hospital wards and children's institutions. Attenuation may be accomplished by the use of gamma globulin in a dosage of 0.05 ml/kg. Gamma globulin, including that now prepared in the United States from placental blood, is approximately 25 times as potent in antibody titer as pooled adult serum, and it avoids the risk of hepatitis. Attenuation is variable, and the modified clinical patterns may vary from those with few or no symptoms to those with little or no modification. Encephalitis may follow measles modified by gamma globulin.

After the 7th–8th day of incubation the amounts of antibody administered must be increased greatly for any degree of protection. If the injection is delayed until the 9th, 10th, or 11th day, slight fever may already have started and only slight modification of the disease may be expected.

Treatment. Sedatives, antipyretics for high fever, bed rest, and an adequate fluid intake are indicated. Humidification of the room may be necessary for laryngitis or an excessively irritating cough, and it is best to keep the room comfortably warm rather than cool. The patient should be protected from exposure to strong light during the period of photophobia. The complications of otitis media and pneumonia require appropriate antimicrobial therapy.

With complications such as encephalitis, subacute sclerosing panencephalitis, giant cell pneumonia, and disseminated intravascular coagulation, each case must be assessed individually. Good supportive care is essential. Gamma globulin, hyperimmune gamma globulin, and steroids are of limited value. Currently available antiviral compounds are not effective.

Aicardi J: Acute measles encephalitis in children with immunosuppression. Pediatrics 59:232, 1977.

Brem J: Koplik spots for the record: An illustrated historical note. Clin Pediatr 11:161, 1972.

Cherry JD: The 'new' epidemiology of measles and rubella. Hosp Pract 15:49, 1980.

Enders JF, et al: Studies on an attenuated measles virus vaccine (series of papers). N Engl J Med 263:159, 1960.

Jabbour JT, et al: Subacute sclerosing panencephalitis. JAMA 220:959, 1972.

Kamin PB, Fein BT, Britton HA: Use of live, attenuated measles virus vaccine in children allergic to egg protein. JAMA 193:1125, 1965.

Landrigan PJ, Witte JJ: Neurologic disorders following measles vaccination. JAMA 223:1459, 1973.

Laptook A, Wind E, Nussbaum M, et al: Pulmonary lesions in atypical measles. Pediatrics 62:42, 1978.

McCormick JB, Halsey NA, Rosenberg R: Measles vaccine efficacy determined from secondary attack rates during a severe epidemic. J Pediatr 90:13, 1977.

Modlin JF: Epidemiologic studies of measles, measles vaccine, SSPE. Pediatrics 59:505, 1977.

Panum PL: Observations Made During the Epidemic of Measles on the Faroe Islands in the Year 1846. Translated by AS Hatcher. New York, Delta Omega Society, American Public Health Association, 1940.

Payne FE, Baublis JV, Itabashi HH: Isolation of measles virus from cell cultures of brain from a patient with subacute sclerosing panencephalitis. N Engl J Med 281:11, 1969.

Ruuskanen O, Salmi TT, Halonen P: Measles vaccination after exposure to natural measles. J Pediatr 98:43, 1978.

Scott TF, Bonanno DF: Reactions to live measles-virus vaccine in children previously inoculated with killed-virus vaccine. N Engl J Med 277:248, 1967.

Starr S, Berkovich S: The effect of measles, gamma globulin modified measles and attenuated measles vaccine on the course of treated tuberculosis in children. Pediatrics 35:97, 1965.

Stokes J Jr, Weibel RE, Villarejos VM, et al: Trivalent combined measles-mumps-rubella vaccine. Findings in clinical-laboratory studies. JAMA 218:57, 1971.

Wilkins J, Wehrle PF: Measles vaccine in infants less than 12 months. J Pediatr 94:865, 1979.

Yeager AS: Measles immunizations. JAMA 237:347, 1977.

10.68 RUBELLA
(German or Three-Day Measles)

Rubella is a common communicable disease of childhood characterized ordinarily by mild constitutional symptoms, a rash similar to that of mild rubeola or scarlet fever, and enlargement and tenderness of the postoccipital, retroauricular, and posterior cervical lymph nodes. In older children and adults the infection may occasionally be severe, with such manifestations as joint involvement and purpura.

Rubella in early pregnancy may cause severe congenital anomalies in the newborn infant. The congenital rubella syndrome may also be an active contagious disease with multisystem involvement, a wide spectrum of clinical expression, and a long postnatal period of active infection with shedding of virus.

Etiology.   Rubella is caused by a pleomorphic, RNA-containing virus. It has been difficult to classify but is currently listed in the family Togaviridae, genus Rubivirus. Isolation of the virus is usually done in tissue culture. The presence of rubella virus is demonstrated by the ability of rubella-infected African green monkey kidney (AGMK) cells to resist challenge with enterovirus. During clinical illness the virus is present in nasopharyngeal secretions, blood, feces, and urine. Virus has been recovered from the nasopharynx 7 days before exanthem and 7–8 days after its disappearance. Patients with subclinical disease are also infectious.

Epidemiology.   Humans are the only natural host of rubella virus. Spread is accomplished by oral droplet or transplacentally in congenital infection. Prior to the institution of the rubella vaccine program, the peak incidence of the disease occurred in children 5–14 yr of age. Now most cases occur in teenagers and young adults. Maternal antibody is protective for the 1st 6 mo of life. Boys and girls are equally affected. In closed populations, such as institutions and military barracks, almost 100% of susceptible individuals may become infected. In family settings the spread of the virus is less: 50–60% of family members acquire the disease. Many infections are subclinical, with a ratio of 2:1 inapparent to overt disease. Rubella usually occurs during the spring. It can be very difficult to diagnose clinically since enteroviral and other rashes may produce a similar appearance. A single attack usually confers permanent immunity. Epidemics occurred every 6–9 yr before vaccine was available. Serologic studies done prior to the development and use of rubella vaccine showed that about 80% of the adult population in the United States and other large continental land masses had antibody to rubella. Island populations, such as those of Trinidad and Hawaii, had detectable antibody in only 20% of the adults screened.

In the congenital rubella syndrome, virus can be isolated from nasopharyngeal washings, stool, blood, urine, spinal fluid, and other involved organs of the newborn infant. Virus shedding continues for periods as long as 12–18 mo, making the infant a source of infection for older children who are not immune and nonimmune adults, including pregnant women and nursery personnel. The risk of malformations among the infants of women who contract rubella in the 1st weeks of pregnancy approaches 100%; 40% during the 2nd mo; 10% in the 3rd mo; and 4% in the 2nd–3rd trimesters.

Clinical Manifestations.   The incubation period for rubella is generally 14–21 days. The prodromal phase of mild catarrhal symptoms is shorter than that of measles and may be so mild as to go entirely unnoticed. The most characteristic sign is retroauricular, posterior cervical, and postoccipital adenopathy. No other disease causes the tender enlargement of all these nodes to the same extent as rubella. An enanthem may appear just before the onset of the skin rash. It consists of discrete rose spots on the soft palate which may coalesce into a red blush and may extend over the fauces.

Lymphadenopathy is evident at least 24 hr before the *rash* appears and may be present for 1 wk or more. The exanthem is more variable than that of rubeola. It begins on the face (Fig 10–15 [p. xxxiii]) and spreads quickly. Its evolution is so rapid that the rash on the face may be fading by the time it appears on the trunk. Discrete maculopapules are present in large numbers, but there are also large areas of flushing which spread rapidly over the entire body, usually within 24 hr. The rash may be confluent, particularly on the face. During the 2nd day the rash may assume a pinpoint appearance, especially over the trunk, resembling that of scarlet fever. Mild itching may occur. The eruption usually clears by the 3rd day. Any residual pigmentation disappears in a few days; desquamation is minimal. Rubella without a rash has been described.

The pharyngeal mucosa and the conjunctivae are slightly inflamed. In contrast to rubeola, there is no photophobia. Fever is slight or absent. When present, it occurs at the height of the rash and persists for 1, 2, or occasionally 3 days. The temperature seldom exceeds 38.4° C (101° F). Anorexia, headache, and malaise are not common in rubella. The spleen is often slightly enlarged. The white blood cell count is normal or slightly reduced; thrombocytopenia is relatively rare, with or without purpura. Especially in older girls and women, polyarthritis may occur with arthralgia, swelling, tenderness, and effusion but usually without any residuum. Its duration is usually several days to 2 wk; rarely it persists for months. Paresthesia also has been reported. In 1 epidemic, testalgia was reported in about 8% of infected college-aged males.

The congenital rubella syndrome is discussed in Sec 7.70. Subclinical intrauterine infection is common. The infant may appear normal at birth, but virus can usually be recovered from the nasopharynx or urine. Rubella-specific IgM is present. These infants are infectious to nonimmune contacts. Some infants appear to do well for several mo before developing severe illness characterized by interstitial pneumonia, rash, diarrhea, hypogammaglobulinemia, disorders of B and T cells, severe neurologic involvement, and death. This syndrome appears to be associated with circulating immune complexes containing rubella antigen. Histopathology shows diffuse vasculitis. Abnormalities such as hearing loss, psychomotor retardation, perceptual and motor impairment, and diabetes mellitus may not be apparent until the child is several yr old.

Progressive panencephalitis has been reported in several adolescents with congenital rubella syndrome. These children had been functioning well prior to the onset of the panencephalitis. Symptoms of seizures, ataxia, spasticity, and increasing mental deficiency developed. Rubella virus was isolated from the brain of 1 child.

Differential Diagnosis. Since similar symptoms and rashes can occur with many other viral infections (Sec 10.11), rubella is a difficult disease to diagnose clinically unless the patient is seen during an epidemic. A history of having had rubella or rubella vaccine is unreliable; immunity should be determined by testing for antibodies. Particularly in its more severe forms, rubella may be confused with the mild types of scarlet fever and rubeola. *Roseola infantum* (exanthem subitum) is distinguished from rubella by the height of the fever and by the appearance of the rash at the end of the febrile episode rather than at the height of the signs and symptoms. *Drug rashes* may be extremely difficult to differentiate from rubella. The characteristic enlargement of the lymph nodes would support the diagnosis of rubella. In *infectious mononucleosis* a rash may occur which resembles that of rubella, and enlargement of the lymph nodes in both diseases may lead to confusion. The hematologic findings in infectious mononucleosis should be sufficient to distinguish the 2 diseases. Enteroviral infections which are accompanied by a rash can be differentiated by their shorter incubation period and the absence of suboccipital adenopathy.

Diagnostic tests include isolation of virus from various tissues and serologic tests such as neutralization, complement-fixation, hemagglutination-inhibition (H1), and fluorescent-antibody studies. Rubella-specific IgM is present in the blood of affected newborn infants.

Complications and Prognosis. Complications are relatively uncommon in childhood rubella. Neuritis and arthritis occur occasionally. Resistance to secondary bacterial infection is not altered significantly. Encephalitis similar to that seen with rubeola occurs rarely. The prognosis of childhood rubella is good; that of congenital rubella varies with the severity of the infection. The mortality of infants with rubella-associated neonatal thrombocytopenic purpura is about 35% in the 1st 18 mo of life but tends to result from general debility, sepsis, and heart failure rather than from bleeding. Only about 30% of infants with encephalitis appear to escape residual neuromotor deficits, including an autis-

tic syndrome. Spontaneous abortion occurs in about one third of women who acquire rubella in the 1st trimester of pregnancy.

Prevention. In a susceptible person **passive protection** from or attenuation of the disease may or may not be afforded by intramuscular injection of immune serum globulin (ISG), given in large dosage (0.25–0.50 ml/kg, or 0.12–0.20 ml/lb) within the 1st 7–8 days after exposure. The effectiveness of immune globulin is not predictable, depending apparently upon the antibody content of the blood product used or upon factors as yet undetermined. The value of ISG has been questioned also because in some instances rash was prevented and clinical manifestations were absent or minimal though viable virus was demonstrable in the blood. There is no indication for prevention of rubella except in nonimmune pregnant women.

For **active immunization** against rubella the vaccines in current use are live virus vaccines prepared in tissue cell cultures: HPV-77-DE-5 (duck embryo) and RA 27/3 (human embryonic lung fibroblasts of the WI-38 line). RA 27/3 vaccine has many advantages over other rubella vaccines including HPV-77 since it produces nasopharyngeal antibody and a wide variety of serum antibodies, provides better protection against reinfection, and more closely resembles the protection provided by natural infection. The vaccine virus is heat and light sensitive; therefore, the vaccine should be stored in the refrigerator at 4° C and used as soon as it is reconstituted. Vaccine is administered as a single subcutaneous injection.

Antibody develops in about 95% of those vaccinated. While virus may persist, especially in the nasopharynx, and shedding occurs from 18–25 days after vaccination, communicability does not appear to be a problem.

The duration of persistence of rubella antibody following vaccination is uncertain. One study showed that one third of children had responded to rubella vaccine with low levels of antibody. On retesting 5 yr later, 26% of those who had originally developed low levels of antibody were without detectable rubella antibody of any type. Another study reported 36% of children with documented rubella immunization had HI titers of less than 8 when retested an average of 4.7 yr after vaccination. Both of these studies were done before RA 27/3 was available in the United States.

The rubella vaccine program in the United States calls for immunization of all boys and girls between the age of 15 mo and puberty and of nonpregnant postpubertal females who have been demonstrated to have a negative hemagglutination-inhibition test and can reasonably be relied upon not to become pregnant within 3 mo of immunization. Vaccination of infants under 15 mo is not recommended since persisting maternal antibody may interfere. This policy has successfully interrupted the usual epidemic cycle of rubella in the United States and decreased the reported incidence of congenital rubella syndrome. However, it has not resulted in a decrease in the percentage of women of childbearing age who are susceptible to rubella.

Some European countries have adopted a policy of immunizing only girls routinely at age 12 or older if they are found to be unprotected. This policy has not prevented epidemics of rubella but does appear to be increasing the level of immunity in women.

Pregnant women should not be given live rubella virus vaccine. Other contraindications include immune deficiency states, severe febrile illness, hypersensitivity to vaccine components, and therapy with antimetabolites, steroids, and steroid-like substances.

Clinical manifestations which may follow rubella immunization include fever, typical lymphadenopathy, rash, and arthritis and arthralgia. The last two occur more frequently in older girls and adult women and may last for weeks. Two unusual syndromes have been reported in association with rubella vaccine: one with paresthesia of the hand or arm that occurs at night lasts for up to 1 hr and may recur frequently during the night; the other is manifested by pain behind the knee and limitation of motion. Symptoms are worst in the morning, diminishing during the day. They may last for up to 5 wk. Both syndromes may recur.

Measles-mumps-rubella, measles-rubella, and mumps-rubella combined vaccines are also available and effective.

Management of Pregnant Women Exposed to or Acquiring Rubella. Preventive measures are of the greatest importance for the protection of the fetus. It is especially important that girls have immunity to rubella before the child-bearing age, either by contracting the natural disease or by active immunization. The immune status can be evaluated by appropriate serologic tests.

Pregnant women, especially early in pregnancy but also during the entire gestational period, should avoid exposure to rubella regardless of history of the disease during childhood or of history of active immunization. Exposure of pregnant women to infants with congenital rubella syndrome should be especially guarded against because of prolonged shedding. Risk of damage to the fetus is less after the 14th wk of gestation.

Since approximately 80% of women in the child-bearing age are immune to rubella as a result of the natural infection or immunization, women at risk to become pregnant should have their immune status to rubella determined by the hemagglutination-inhibition (HI) technique. Women should be actively immunized under certain conditions (see above).

If a pregnant woman of unknown immune status is exposed to rubella, an HI test should be performed *immediately and as an emergency measure.* If determined to be immune, she can be reassured that the pregnancy can be continued without added risk. If found to be susceptible and therapeutic abortion is unacceptable or unavailable to her, passive immunization with immune serum globulin (ISG), 20–30 ml intramuscularly, should be attempted immediately. Active immunization of pregnant women is not advised since the virus has been isolated from at least 1 fetus aborted after active immunization of a nonimmunized woman at a time when she did not know she was pregnant; no malformations were identified in that fetus.

If exposure to rubella occurs in a susceptible pregnant woman to whom abortion is available and desirable because of significant potential hazard to the fetus, it is probably advisable to withhold ISG, and observe her carefully, and repeat the rubella HI. If rubella then develops at a stage of pregnancy at which she feels the risk is greater than she wants to take or if serial antibody tests show that subclinical infection has occurred, abortion may be induced.

Reinfection. The incidence of reinfection on exposure of individuals serologically immune to wild virus is 3–10% among those demonstrating serologic immunity without a history of immunization, 14–18% among those immunized with RA 27/3 vaccine, and 40–100% among those immunized with HPV-77 or Cendehill vaccine. Infection has been demonstrated among the fetuses of reinfected pregnant women as well as among pregnant women receiving rubella vaccine. The importance of reinfection of serologically immune pregnant women in the production of congenital malformations remains to be determined but is of obvious significance in the planning of large-scale immunization programs against rubella. The effectiveness of "herd immunity" in preventing rubella-induced malformations remains controversial. Until these questions are answered, *all* pregnant women should make every effort to avoid exposure to rubella.

Treatment. Unless bacterial complications occur, treatment is symptomatic. Adamantanamine hydrochloride (amantadine) has been reported to be effective in vitro in inhibiting early stages of rubella infection in cultured cells. An attempt to treat a child with congenital rubella with this drug was unsuccessful. It is possible that the drug may be effective prophylactically or in the early incubation period of rubella, but no studies have been done. Since amantadine is not recommended for pregnant women, its usefulness would be very limited.

Alford CA Jr, Neva FA, Weller TH: Virologic and serologic studies on human products of conception after maternal rubella. N Engl J Med 271:1275, 1964.
Balfour HH, Amren DP: Rubella measles and mumps antibodies following vaccination of children. Am J Dis Child 132:573, 1978.
Chang TW: Rubella reinfection and intrauterine involvement (editorial). J Pediatr 84:617, 1974.
Clark, M et al: Effect of rubella vaccination programme on serological status of young adults in United Kingdom. Lancet 1:1224, 1979.
Desmond MM, et al: Congenital rubella encephalitis: Course and early sequelae. J Pediatr 71:311, 1967.
Desmond MM, et al: The early growth and development of infants with congenital rubella. In: Woolman DH (ed): Advances in Teratology, Vol 4. New York, Academic Press, 1970, p 39.
Forrest JM, et al: High frequency of diabetes mellitus in young adults with congenital rubella. Lancet 2:332 1971.
Gregg NM: Congenital cataract following German measles in the mother. Tr Ophthalmol Soc Austr 3:35, 1941.
Gregg NM, et al: The occurrence of congenital defects in children following maternal rubella during pregnancy. Med J Austr 2:122, 1945.
Horstman DM: Rubella: The challenge of its control. J Inf Dis 123:640, 1971.
Horstman DM: Controlling rubella: Problems and perspectives. Ann Intern Med 83:412, 1975.
Horstman DM, et al: Rubella. Reinfection of vaccinated and naturally immune persons exposed in an epidemic. N Engl J Med 283:771, 1970.
Krugman S: Commentary. Rubella immunization: Present status and future perspectives. Pediatrics 65:1174, 1980.
Lawless MR, Abramson JS, Harlan JE, et al: Rubella susceptibility in 6th graders: Effectiveness of current immunization practice. Pediatrics 65:1086, 1980.
Plotkin SA, et al: Hypogammaglobulinemia in an infant with congenital rubella syndrome; failure of L-adamantanamine to stop virus excretion. J Pediatr 69:1085, 1966.
Rawls WE, et al: Persistent virus infection in congenital rubella. Arch Ophthalmol 77:430, 1967.
Rawls WE, Desmyter J, Melnick JL: Serologic diagnosis and fetal involvement in maternal rubella. JAMA 203:627, 1968.
Rudolph AJ, et al: Transplacental rubella infection in newly born infants. JAMA 191:843, 1965.

Tardieu M, Grospierre B, Durandy A, et al: Circulating immune complexes containing rubella antigens in late-onset rubella syndrome. J Pediatr 97:370, 1980.
Townsend JJ: Progressive rubella panencephalitis: Late onset after congenital rubella. N Engl J Med 292:990, 1975.
Weil ML: Chronic progressive panencephalitis due to rubella virus simulating subacute sclerosing panencephalitis. N Engl J Med 292:994, 1975.
Weiss DI, Cooper LZ, Green RH: Infantile glaucoma: A manifestation of congenital rubella. JAMA 195:105, 1966.
Wilkins J: Reinfection with rubella virus despite live vaccine-induced immunity. Am J Dis Child 118:275, 1969.

10.69   EXANTHEM SUBITUM
(Roseola Infantum)

Exanthem subitum is an acute, probably viral disease of infants and young children, usually occurring sporadically but occasionally in epidemics. It is unique in that the diagnostic rash and clinical improvement occur almost simultaneously. The disease is characterized by a period of high fever lasting 1–5 but usually 3–4 days, during which time there are insufficient clinical findings to explain the hyperpyrexia, and by an abrupt termination with a precipitous drop of the temperature to normal and the appearance of a generalized eruption, which fades quickly.

Etiology. Available evidence supports viral origin. Serum, heparinized blood, and throat washings obtained from patients on the 3rd day of fever and also on the 1st day of the rash have been shown to be infective for susceptible infants and for monkeys. Typical disease resulted after an incubation period of 9–10 days in infants and 4–5 days in monkeys. All attempts to isolate the etiologic agent have failed. No serologic tests are available, and nothing is known of the pathologic changes of the disease.

Epidemiology. The degree of contagiousness is not known. There is a tendency for the disease to occur in the spring and fall. It attacks both sexes equally. In the rare epidemics described, the incubation period was estimated to be from 7–17 days, usually about 10 days. The epidemiologic pattern is not clear. The sporadic occurrence of exanthem subitum in early life, with rare epidemics in older age groups, suggests the possibility of an endemic spread through most of the population in early infancy and childhood with production of permanent immunity. Most of the cases occur from 6–18 mo of age. It is rare beyond 3 yr, but the disease does occur infrequently in older children and even in adults.

Clinical Manifestations. The onset is sudden, with fever which rises abruptly as high as 39.4–41.2° C (103–106° F); convulsions may occur at this time or later. Although the pharyngeal mucosa is slightly inflamed at times and there may be slight coryza, there are no typical signs. The outstanding feature is the absence of physical findings sufficient to explain the fever. Usually the child looks quite well despite the height of the temperature. The diagnosis is suspected chiefly by exclusion of other possible infections, particularly those which at this age are the most common causes of high fever and in which the diagnosis may not be evident, such as otitis media, acute pyelonephritis, pneumonia, meningitis, and pneumococcal bacteremia.

During the 1st 24–36 hr of fever the white blood cell count may be as high as 16,000–20,000/mm^3 with an increase in neutrophils. By the 2nd day leukopenia becomes evident, with counts from 3000–5000 on the 3rd–4th day of fever. There is an absolute neutropenia with a relative lymphocytosis, which may be as high as 90%. Occasionally, a large number of monocytes are present. The cerebrospinal fluid is normal.

The fever falls by crisis on the 3rd–4th day. Just before or shortly after the return of the temperature to normal, a macular or maculopapular eruption appears over the body, starting on the trunk and spreading to the arms and neck, with slight involvement of the face and legs. The rash soon fades, rarely remaining as long as 24 hr. Desquamation is rare, and no pigmentation remains. In the rare epidemic outbreaks cases without a rash may be suspected, but a definite diagnosis cannot be made. Clemens described an enanthem on the soft palate consisting of small erythematous spots and streaks. Slight periorbital edema has also been described. Occasionally, the lymph nodes, especially in the cervical area, may be enlarged, but not to the extent that they are in rubella. When present, postoccipital lymphadenopathy can be a helpful diagnostic sign in differentiating roseola infantum from pneumococcal bacteremia.

Differential Diagnosis. The principal difficulty in differential diagnosis is with *rubella*, from which exanthem subitum is distinguished chiefly by the prodromal period of high fever. *Rubeola* and *dengue* can be distinguished primarily by the time of appearance of their rash in relation to fever and other clinical findings. In measles, though there is usually a fever of variable degree for 3–4 days just before the rash, the temperature becomes abruptly elevated to 39.4–40° C (103–104° F) at the time of appearance of the rash and remains elevated for the next 2 days or so. The lack of Koplik spots, severe coryza, conjunctivitis, and cough also helps to distinguish exanthem subitum from rubeola. *Pneumococcal bacteremia* may present with high fever, a well-looking child, and no physical findings. The white blood count is frequently elevated. Blood culture is positive for pneumococcus. As a rule, distinction from entero- and adenoviral diseases does not present a problem. Certain allergic rashes, e.g., those resulting from sensitivity to drugs, may be difficult to distinguish from exanthem subitum, particularly if the patient is receiving penicillin.

Prognosis. This is good except in the rare patient who has extreme hyperpyrexia or persistent seizures.

Prophylaxis and Treatment. There are no known methods for shortening the course of the disease or for prophylaxis. In infants and young children who are prone to convulsions, the administration of a sedative at the appearance of the sharp febrile onset of exanthem subitum may be effective as prophylaxis against such seizures. An antipyretic may be of help in partially reducing the fever and in allaying restlessness.

Berenberg S, Wright S, Janeway CA: Roseola infantum (exanthem subitum). N Engl J Med 241:253, 1949.

Burnstine RC, Paine RS: Residual encephalopathy following roseola infantum. Am J Dis Child 98:144, 1959.

Clemens HH: Exanthem subitum (roseola infantum): A report of eighty cases. J Pediatr 26:66, 1945.

Hellström B, Vahlquist B: Experimental inoculation of roseola infantum. Acta Paediatr 40:189, 1951.

Kempe CH, Shaw EB, Jackson JR, et al: Studies on the etiology of exanthem subitum (roseola infantum). J Pediatr 37:561, 1950.

Letchner A: Roseola infantum: A review of fifty cases. Lancet 2:1163, 1955.

McEnery JT: Postoccipital lymphadenopathy as a diagnostic sign in roseola infantum (exanthem subitum). Clin Pediatr 9:512, 1970.

Veeder BS, Hempelmann TC: A febrile exanthem occurring in childhood (exanthem subitum). JAMA 77:1787, 1921.

Zahorsky J: Roseola infantum. JAMA 61:1446, 1913.

10.70 ERYTHEMA INFECTIOSUM (Fifth Disease)

Erythema infectiosum is a moderately contagious exanthematous disease affecting mainly children. It is frequently called fifth disease because it was the 5th illness described with a somewhat similar rash. The first 4 diseases were rubella, measles, scarlet fever, and Filatov-Dukes disease. The last of these is now considered a mild atypical form of scarlet fever.

Etiology. A viral etiology has been postulated. In 1 epidemic approximately 10% of the patients studied had evidence of rubella infection. A strain of rubella virus isolated from 1 of these patients produced an exanthem resembling erythema infectiosum in adult volunteers. However, study of 2 recent epidemics failed to show any association with rubella virus, and previous rubella vaccination did not decrease the incidence of erythema infectiosum. In most patients studied, no laboratory evidence for a viral disease could be detected.

Pathology. Biopsy of the skin lesion shows edema and a nonspecific inflammatory infiltrate of lymphocytes.

Epidemiology. Infants and adults are affected infrequently. There is no sex predilection. The incubation period has been estimated from family studies to range from 7–28 days (average, 16 days). Community epidemics involving mainly school-age children have been described. Distribution is worldwide.

Clinical Manifestations. There are usually no prodromal symptoms. Fever is absent or low grade. The characteristic rash appears in 3 stages. The illness usually begins with the sudden appearance of livid erythema of the cheeks which gives the child a "slapped-cheek" appearance. An erythematous maculopapular rash then appears on the trunk and extremities. However, the body rash may precede the facial rash. The rash fades with central clearing, giving a lacy or reticulated appearance (Fig 10–16 [p. xxxiii]), which is the most distinctive part of the disease. The rash lasts from 2–39 days (mean, 11 days). It is frequently pruritic. It resolves without desquamation, but periodic recrudescences may occur with exercise, warm baths, rubbing of the skin, or emotional upset. Constitutional symptoms such as headache, pharyngitis, coryza, and gastrointestinal disturbance are more frequent and more severe in adults.

Laboratory Data. There are no confirmatory laboratory tests.

Diagnosis. Erythema infectiosum must be differentiated from rubella, enteroviral diseases, systemic lupus erythematosus, atypical measles, and drug rashes.

Complications. Complications are rare. Arthritis, hemolytic anemia, pneumonitis, and encephalopathy have been reported.

Treatment. No treatment is indicated. Isolation is not required. Since the duration of the rash may be prolonged and the illness is mild, children with this disease should be allowed to attend school.

Balfour H: Fifth disease: Full fathom five. Am J Dis Child 130:239, 1976.

Balfour H, et al: Erythema infectiosum: Recovery of rubella virus and echovirus 12. Pediatrics 50:285, 1972.

Hall CB, et al: Encephalopathy with erythema infectiosum. Am J Dis Child 131:65, 1977.

Lauer BA, et al: Erythema infectiosum: An elementary school outbreak. Am J Dis Child 130:252, 1976.

10.71 HERPES SIMPLEX

Herpesvirus hominis (HVH) is a common parasite of man with a variety of clinical manifestations involving the skin, mucous membranes, eye, central nervous system, and genital tract. It also causes generalized systemic disease. Two strains of virus (HVH-1 and HVH-2) have differing biologic and serologic properties, HVH-1 commonly infecting skin and mucous membranes, HVH-2 infecting primarily the genitalia.

Two forms of infection are recognized: (1) Primary: this is the susceptible host's 1st experience with the virus, which results in most instances in a subclinical infection; the remainder of patients usually have local superficial lesions (see below) accompanied by varying degrees of systemic reaction. In newborn infants and severely malnourished infants, a fatal systemic infection, often without superficial lesions, may occur. Circulating antibodies develop in nonfatal cases. (2) Recurrent herpetic lesions are the result of reactivation of a latent infection in an immune host with circulating antibodies. Reactivation follows such nonspecific stimuli as changes in the external milieu (e.g., cold, ultraviolet light) or the internal milieu (e.g., menstruation, fever, or emotional stress). The lesions are localized and, generally, not associated with systemic reaction.

CLINICAL PATTERNS

Systemic Infection

In the Newborn Infant. Most neonatal herpes is caused by HVH-2 virus acquired by passage of the infant through an infected birth canal or ascension of virus into the uterine cavity after rupture of membranes. Occasionally HVH-1 infection occurs, possibly due to transplacentally or postnatally acquired infection. The true incidence of neonatal herpetic disease is not known. Since most of the early reports were based on autopsy material, it was originally believed that the disease had a very high mortality. With improved techniques for viral isolation, a number of mild cases have been diagnosed.

Mothers of infected babies are frequently young primiparas. Most have no symptoms of genital herpes at the time of delivery although genital lesions may be present. Many do not have a history of recurrent herpes infections. Infected infants are often premature. Respiratory distress or bacterial infections frequently occur before the onset of symptoms of herpes disease, which usually appear in the 1st–2nd wk of life. Infection can be disseminated and involve many organs, such as liver, lung, and brain, or be localized in the CNS, skin, eye, or mouth. Progression from only skin lesions to disseminated disease is common. Mortality is high with disseminated or CNS disease, and residual morbidity such as seizures, mental retardation, blindness, chorioretinitis, deafness, microcephaly, diabetes insipidus, and spasticity is common in all forms of the disease. Recurrences of skin lesions can be seen for 1 yr or longer. Some infants recover after a mild infection characterized only by a vesicular eruption and low-grade fever.

There are no generally accepted rules for handling babies in the nursery who have been exposed to herpes. Spread of herpes infection is probably caused by contact; droplet spread has not been established. Babies should be placed in an Isolette or in a bassinet separated from the other infants. Those caring for the baby should wear gown and gloves. The baby may go to the mother for feeding but probably should not room-in. The mother should wear a clean gown and wash her hands carefully before handling the infant. If labial lesions are present, she should wear a mask and avoid kissing the child.

Nursery personnel with labial herpes should wear a mask and scrub their hands well or wear gloves when handling infants.

HVH has been implicated as a cause of congenital malformations resembling those caused by rubella and cytomegalovirus. More studies are necessary to confirm this observation.

In Severely Malnourished Infants. The primary infection in infants who have severe protein malnutrition, often in their 2nd yr, may be generalized and fatal. The clinical and pathologic findings are similar to those in the newborn.

Lesions of the Skin and Mucous Membranes

Herpes Labialis, Facialis, Febrilis

Primary infection may, uncommonly, result in a generalized vesicular eruption in which the lesions are small and may continue to appear over a period of 2–3 wk. If the systemic manifestations are mild, the infection must be differentiated from varicella; if severe, from variola.

Clinical lesions of recurrent herpes infection occur on the skin or mucous membranes. On the skin the lesion consists of aggregates of thin-walled vesicles on an erythematous base. These rupture, scab, and heal within 7–10 days without leaving a scar except after repeated attacks or secondary bacterial infections; temporary depigmentation occurs in Blacks. The local lesions may be preceded by mild irritation or burning at the local site or by severe neuralgic pain in the region. In children the vesicles often become secondarily infected, introducing *impetigo contagiosa* into the differential diagnosis. The lesions tend to occur at mucocutaneous junctions but may occur anywhere. They tend to recur at the same site. The sites most commonly affected are also those where lip cancer occurs most commonly.

Traumatic lesions of the skin can be readily infected by the ubiquitous herpesvirus. Primary lesions can also occur on apparently unbroken skin, as, for example, on the chin of a drooling infant with herpetic stomatitis, in whom scattered isolated vesicles appear (contrast the grouped vesicles of recurrent attacks). When the skin of a limb is infected, vesicles appear in 2–3 days at the site of trauma. There is often centripetal spread along lymph channels causing enlargement of regional lymph nodes and scattered vesicles on the intervening undamaged skin. The final clinical picture may be mistaken for that of *herpes zoster*, especially if accompanied by neuralgic pain, unless the lesions are recognized as not being confined to a dermatome. The lesions heal slowly, often taking 3 wk; recurrences at the site of local trauma are common and may assume a bullous nature. Wrestlers and medical personnel are prone to herpetic infections of superficial abrasions (herpes gladiatorum and herpetic whitlow). In the latter, infection of minor trauma about the nails leads to extremely painful, deep-seated spreading lesions with vesicles which resolve spontaneously in 2–3 wk. Similar lesions occur on the fingers of thumb suckers who are suffering from herpetic gingivostomatitis. Treatment is symptomatic only; the lesions should not be incised.

Eczema Herpeticum
(Kaposi Varicelliform Eruption; Juliusberg Pustulosis Vacciniformis Acuta)

This, the most serious manifestation of "traumatic herpes," results from a widespread and usually primary infection of the eczematous skin with herpesvirus. The severity of the complication varies; the attacks may be so mild as to be overlooked without a high index of suspicion and adequate laboratory facilities, or they may be fatal. In a typical severe primary attack, vesicles develop abruptly in large numbers over the area of eczematous skin. They continue to appear in crops for as long as 7–9 days. Isolated at first, they later become grouped and may occur on adjoining areas of normal skin (Fig 10–17). Wide denudation of the epidermis may occur. Scabs eventually form, and epithelization occurs. The systemic reaction varies, but temperatures of 39.4–40.6° C (103–105° F) for 7–10 days are not uncommon. Recurrent attacks develop on chronic atopic skin lesions. The systemic reaction, presumably hypersensitivity, is usually less than in primary infection. Death may occur as the result of profound physiologic disturbances from loss of fluid, electrolytes, and protein

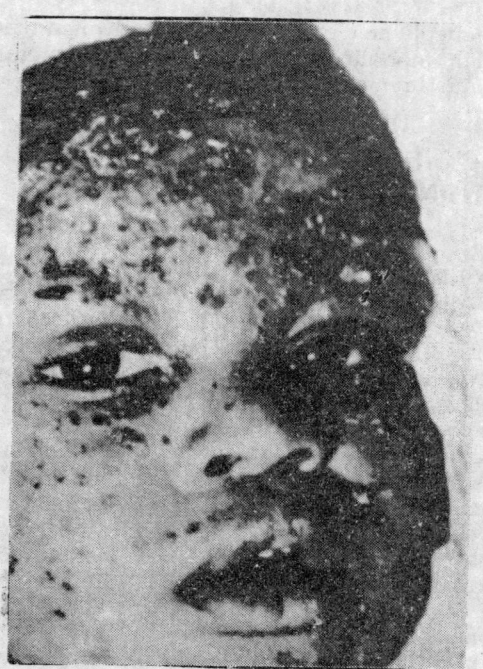

Figure 10–17 Eczema herpeticum. Note similarity of umbilicated vesicular lesions on face to those of eczema vaccinatum.

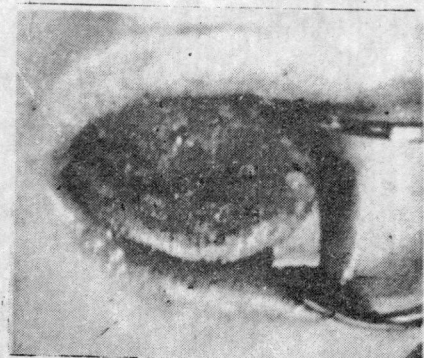

Figure 10–18 Lesions of herpetic stomatitis on the tongue.

through the skin, from dissemination of the virus to the brain and other organs, or from secondary bacterial invasion. A differentiation from *eczema vaccinatum* can usually be made clinically by determining with reasonable certainty that the child has not been exposed to vaccinia and by the occurrence of crops of vesicles in herpes. The diagnosis can be established quickly and accurately by examination of vesicular fluid with the electron microscope. Herpes simplex virus cannot be differentiated from varicella-zoster by this method but can easily be distinguished from vaccinia and variola.

Acute Herpetic Gingivostomatitis
(Acute Infectious Gingivostomatitis; Aphthous Stomatitis; Catarrhal Stomatitis; Ulcerative Stomatitis; Vincent Stomatitis)

This primary infection is probably the common cause of stomatitis in children 1–3 yr of age. It can occur in adults. The symptoms may appear abruptly, with pain in the mouth, salivation, fetor oris, refusal to eat, and fever, often as high as 40–40.6° C (104–105° F). The onset may be insidious, fever and irritability preceding the oral lesions by 1–2 days. The initial lesion is a vesicle (Fig 10–18), seldom seen because of its early rupture. The residual lesion is 2–10 mm in diameter and is covered with a yellow-gray membrane (Fig 10–19). When this membrane sloughs, a true ulcer remains. Although the tongue and cheeks are most commonly involved, no part of the oral lining is exempt. Except in edentulous infants, acute gingivitis is characteristic of the disease and may precede the appearance of mucosal vesicles. Submaxillary lymphadenitis is common. The acute phase lasts 4–9 days and is self-limited. Pain tends to disappear 2–4 days before healing of the

ulcers is complete. In some instances the tonsillar regions are involved early, and acute tonsillitis of bacterial origin or herpangina may be suspected. Failure of the lesion to respond to antibiotic therapy differentiates a bacterial infection, and the spread of the vesiculation to the buccal mucosa rules out herpangina.

Recurrent Stomatitis

Localized lesions may occur on the palate in association with a febrile illness or on the mucosa adjacent to a lesion on the lip; recurrent aphthous ulcers, however, are not caused by herpesvirus. In some persons a generalized stomatitis recurs consistently 7–10 days after a recurrent herpetic lesion of the lip or elsewhere and is often accompanied by skin lesions of erythema multiforme; this lesion is a hypersensitivity reaction to virus protein.

Genital Herpes

Genital infections with herpesvirus occur most commonly in adolescents and young adults, are usually due to HVH-2, and are spread venereally. Five–10% of cases are caused by HVH-1. When the patient has no antibody to either type of herpes (approximately 30% of cases), systemic symptoms such as fever, regional adenopathy, and dysuria are more likely to occur. In adult women, the vulva and vagina may be involved (Fig 10–20), but the cervix is the primary site of infection.

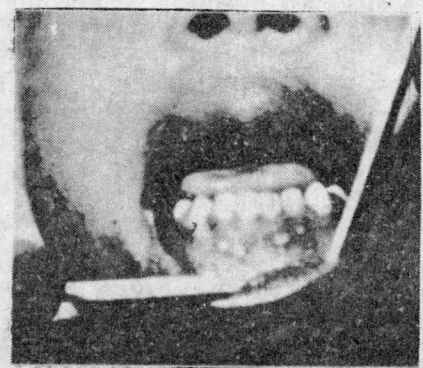

Figure 10–19 Herpetic stomatitis.

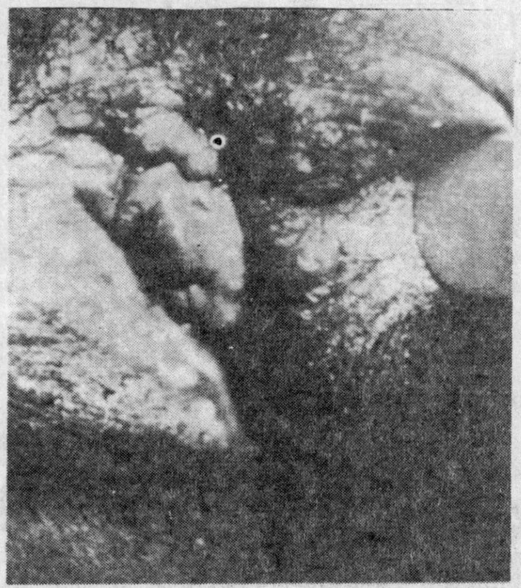

Figure 10–20 Primary herpetic vulvovaginitis. Note the similarity of the lesions to those of herpetic gingivostomatitis. (From Scott, Coriell, Blank, Burgoon: J Pediatr Vol 41.)

Recurrence is common. Recurrent disease involving only the cervix is frequently subclinical, an important point since active disease in the cervix can easily infect an infant during passage through the birth canal.

In males herpetic vesicles or ulcers are usually seen on the glans penis, prepuce, or shaft of the penis. The scrotum is less frequently involved.

Evidence suggests that HVH-2 may be a possible factor in the etiology of carcinoma of the cervix.

Lesions of the Eye

Conjunctivitis and keratoconjunctivitis may occur as manifestations of either a primary or a recurrent infection. The conjunctiva appears congested and swollen with little, if any, purulent discharge. In primary infection the preauricular node is enlarged and tender. Cataracts, uveitis, and chorioretinitis have been described in newborn infants.

Corneal lesions may be superficial, in the form of a dendritic ulcer, or deep, as a disciform keratitis. The diagnosis is suggested by the presence of herpetic vesicles of the lids and established by the isolation of the virus. The highly contagious *epidemic keratoconjunctivitis* (shipyard conjunctivitis) due to any of several serotypes of adenovirus must be considered in the differential diagnosis.

Meningoencephalitis

(See also Sec 10.19.) Herpes encephalitis is seen in all age groups. HVH-2 is the usual cause in newborns, HVH-1 in older patients. The pathogenesis is unknown, but it can occur in patients who already possess antibody against herpes simplex. It is the most common type of nonepidemic encephalitis in the United States, has a high mortality rate, and frequently produces severe sequelae in survivors.

GENERAL FEATURES OF HERPETIC INFECTIONS

Etiology. *Herpesvirus hominis* (HVH) is a DNA-containing virus. The virus readily infects rabbits, guinea pigs, hamsters, and mice; suckling mice are especially susceptible. It produces pocks on the chorioallantoic membrane of the embryonated hen's egg and characteristic cytopathic changes in a variety of cells growing in monolayer tissue cultures. Two strains are recognized from biologic and antigenic characteristics: type 1, which commonly infects skin and mucous membranes, and type 2, which infects primarily the genitalia.

Epidemiology. This virus is a parasite of man which has developed an extremely compatible relationship with its host. In about 85% of instances the infection is subclinical; even when clinical manifestations are present, the host is only rarely disabled or killed. Under exceptional circumstances the primary infection may lead to institutional or family outbreaks of stomatitis. The incubation period is 2–12 days (average, 6 days). *The spread of infection appears to be determined in large measure by 2 factors: trauma and close bodily contact.* Prior to the onset of symptoms there is often a history or implication of trauma to the site such as teething or a break in the skin.

The higher incidence of HVH antibody in lower socioeconomic groups correlates with crowded living conditions. The epidemiology differs for the 2 types of HVH. Detailed serologic studies have been done only in low income groups. In these groups most infants show transplacental antibody for about the 1st 6 mo of life. From 1–4 yr there is a sharp rise in antibodies to type 1; a much slower rate of acquisition is seen from 5–14 yr. After 14 there is again a sharp rise in antibodies to HVH—mostly to type 2. By adult life HVH antibodies are seen in 80–100% of the population of lower socioeconomic groups. Antibodies to type 2 are seen in up to 60% of adults in these groups. The incidence of type 2 antibody in higher socioeconomic groups is about 10% and in nuns about 3%.

Once infected, the majority of people continue to carry the virus in a latent state and maintain an almost constant level of circulating antibodies. It has been shown that the initial level of antibodies reached after a primary infection may fall, and that several subclinical reinfections may occur before a stable antibody level is established. Carriers may distribute virus without any manifest lesion. Herpes simplex virus can be isolated from the pharynx in about 5% of asymptomatic adults.

Pathology. The pathologic changes vary with the tissue infected. In general, a specific lesion is characterized by the presence of intranuclear inclusion bodies. These are homogeneous masses lying in the midst of a severely disorganized nucleus in which the basichromatin has marginated to the nuclear membrane. In the area of the specific lesion there is always evidence of an acute inflammatory reaction. In the skin and mucous membranes the typical lesion is a unilocular vesicle. In the skin the vesicle is tense. Ballooned epithelial cells containing intranuclear inclusions can best be seen at the margins of the vesicle. The vesicular fluid contains infected epithelial cells, including multinucleated "virus" giant cells and leukocytes. In the corium there is no necrosis, but capillaries are dilated, and there is infiltration with mononuclear and polymorphonuclear cells. In the mucous membrane, because of maceration, there is early leakage of the vesicular fluid resulting in a collapsed vesicle, mainly filled with fibrin. The edematous roof cells form a gray membrane over the lesion.

In normal persons the lesions are confined to the skin and mucous membranes; viremia has been described only rarely. Bloodstream spread of the virus with resultant widely disseminated disease is seen mainly in the newborn, in severely malnourished children, in persons with skin diseases such as eczema, and in those with defects in cell-mediated immunity. In these patients the virus spreads from the portal of entry by a primary viremia, and infection of most susceptible organs occurs. Virus increases within these organs, and secondary viremia occurs with evidence of extensive cell destruction. Healing begins with clearing of the viremia and decrease in the production of virus within the cells.

There is evidence that the method of spread to the central nervous system is different for type 1 and type 2 herpesvirus. It is probable that most cases of HVH-1 encephalitis in patients other than newborns are caused by neurogenic spread of the virus to the brain; HVH-2 is usually bloodborne.

Laboratory Data. Microscopic examination of properly fixed and stained scrapings from lesions (Tzanck stain) reveals multinuclear giant cells and intranuclear inclusions. Immunofluorescent techniques applied to these specimens can be useful in diagnosing herpes infection and in differentiating the 2 types of herpes. Virus can be isolated from vesicles, conjunctival swabs, and cerebrospinal fluid from infected newborns. Cerebrospinal fluid is rarely positive in older children with encephalitis; brain biopsy is required for a definitive diagnosis. Such cultures are usually positive in 1–4 days. Serologic tests are less helpful except for tests to determine herpes-specific IgM in the newborn infant.

There is moderate polymorphonuclear leukocytosis in acute herpetic gingivostomatitis, eczema herpeticum, and meningoencephalitis. In the last of these there are frequently red cells in the cerebrospinal fluid and an increase in lymphocytes, usually fewer than 100 but occasionally up to 1000/mm³; the protein level is elevated, and the sugar is within the normal range.

Diagnosis. The diagnosis is based on any 2 of the following: (1) a typical clinical pattern; (2) isolation of the virus; (3) development of specific neutralizing antibodies; (4) demonstration of characteristic cells or histologic changes in scrapings or biopsy material.

Course and Prognosis. Primary infection with the herpesvirus is a self-limited disease, usually lasting 1–2 wk. Fatalities may occur in the newborn infant, in older infants with severe malnutrition, and in patients with meningoencephalitis or severe eczema herpeticum; oth-

erwise, the prognosis is usually good. There may be frequent recurrent attacks, but they seldom cause more than temporary inconvenience except in the eye, where they may eventually cause scarring of the cornea and blindness.

Treatment. Since it is believed that most neonatal herpes is acquired during passage through an infected birth canal, cesarean sections have been advocated in women with genital herpes close to term. If the membranes have been ruptured for longer than 4 hr, there is an increased risk for ascending infection, and cesarean section is unlikely to protect the infant.

Many types of topical therapy for both labial and genital herpes have been advocated. In well controlled studies none has been shown to be effective. The psychologic effect of treatment is very strong; in 1 study of topical ether treatment of cold sores, 75% of treated and 77% of placebo controls reported reduction in the severity and duration of lesions. Topical 5-iodo-2'-deoxyuridine (IDU), adenine arabinoside (vidarabine, ara-A), ether, and 2-deoxy-D glucose have not been shown to be effective. Topical acyclovir (acycloguanosine; 9-[-2-hydroxyethoxymethyl] guanine) may decrease the period of viral shedding but has little effect on symptoms. Oral treatment with levamisole or lysine has not been shown to be effective.

Topical IDU or adenine arabinoside (vidarabine, ara-A) is usually effective in treatment of herpetic keratitis but does not reduce the rate of recurrence. Topical corticosteroids may cause increased ocular involvement and should not be used.

Adenine arabinoside given intravenously in a dose of 15 mg/kg/24 hr for 10 days can be effective in proven herpes encephalitis and local and disseminated neonatal disease. The drug is well tolerated; bone marrow depression occurs infrequently. Best results are obtained when treatment is started early. Patients who are lethargic when therapy is started are more likely to have intact survival than those already in coma. Patients under 30 have a better prognosis than older patients. Acyclovir is being evaluated for therapy of herpes encephalitis. Preliminary studies are encouraging. The drug is given intravenously and is excreted through the kidney; mild elevation of BUN is seen occasionally.

Many types of immunizing agents have been tried without success. Several inactivated herpes simplex vaccines have been developed, and some studies have shown that they are useful in preventing recurrent infections, particularly those due to type 1. The possibility that herpesvirus may be oncogenic even when inactivated limits the usefulness of these vaccines.

Hyperimmune gamma globulin against type 1 or type 2 herpes simplex is not available. Treatment of infected newborns with high doses of gamma globulin has been recommended but has not proved helpful.

Symptomatic and supportive therapy is of great importance. In infants especially, eczema herpeticum and stomatitis may lead to severe dehydration, shock, and hypoproteinemia, requiring replacement of fluids, electrolytes, and proteins.

Care of the mouth demands cleanliness by oral lavage; Ceepryn 1:4000 or Zephiran 1:1000 may be useful. Local analgesics, such as viscous lidocaine or benzocaine lozenges, may allay pain and enable the older child to eat. Labial lesions may be helped by application of drying agents such as calamine lotion or glycerine with carbamine peroxide. Analgesics should be used systemically as required. Antibiotics are useful only in the treatment of secondary bacterial infections.

The intake of food and fluid will be facilitated by acquiescing to the child's whims. Ice-cold fluids or semisolids are often accepted when other food is refused. Recurrences are often due to emotional stress, which must be recognized and treated.

Melnick J, Rawls W: Herpesvirus type 2 and cervical carcinoma. Ann NY Acad Sci 174:993, 1973.
Nahmias AJ, Roizman B: Infection with herpes-simplex viruses 1 and 2. N Engl J Med 289:667, 719, 781, 1973.
Selby PJ, Jameson B, Watson JG, et al: Parenteral acyclovir therapy for herpes virus infections in man. Lancet 2:1267, 1979.
Whitley RJ, Nahmias AJ, Soong SJ, et al: Vidarabine therapy of neonatal herpes simplex virus infection. Pediatrics 66:495, 1980.
Whitley RJ, Nahmias AJ, Visintine AM, et al: The natural history of herpes simplex virus infection of mother and newborn. Pediatrics 66:489, 1980.

10.72 VARICELLA AND HERPES ZOSTER

Herpes zoster and chickenpox are different clinical manifestations of the same causative agent.

Etiology. The common causative agent is now designated as *Herpesvirus varicellae*. The structure of viral particles as seen under the electron microscope is indistinguishable from that of *Herpesvirus hominis*. The agent can be grown in a variety of primary cultures of human and simian tissues. Serum antibodies in patients recovering from varicella react equally with the agents derived from varicella and herpes zoster vesicles.

The reasons for different clinical manifestations of the 2 diseases are not understood. It seems probable that varicella is the primary response of a susceptible host, whereas herpes zoster may be the response of partial immunity when a latent infection is activated by some exogenous factor, e.g., stress, trauma, malignancy, or radiation.

Pathology. The *skin lesions* of both diseases are identical, characteristic of the herpesvirus group, and cannot be distinguished histologically from those of *Herpesvirus hominis* (herpes simplex). Although not usual in cases of average severity, necrosis with hemorrhage can be found in the mucous membranes of the mouth, trachea, esophagus, and intestine.

Internally the lesions vary somewhat in the 2 diseases. In fatal cases of *varicella* intranuclear inclusions can be found in the endothelium of the blood vessels; the vessel walls may undergo necrosis. Intranuclear inclusions have also been found in most organs of the body, including the salivary glands and the nervous system, and in the cells of the myenteric plexus of the stomach and intestine. In the brain, perivenous demyelination is similar to that of other postinfectious en-

cephalitides; necrosis of nerve cells and leptomeningitis have been described.

In *herpes zoster* the characteristic lesions are in the nervous system, particularly in the dorsal root ganglia. Early in the disease the cells of the dorsal ganglia of the affected dermatome contain intranuclear inclusions. Shortly thereafter the ganglia show only necrosis of cells, sometimes associated with hemorrhage. As the disease progresses, evidence of inflammation and degeneration is found in the posterior roots and in the peripheral portions of the nerves. Unilateral and segmental necrosis of the nerve cells in the posterior horn may be found (cf. poliomyelitis, which involves the nerve cells of the anterior horn). Leptomeningitis occurs in the region of the involved nerves. Intranuclear inclusions have been found in the sympathetic ganglia, in the neurilemma cells of the nerve twigs in the corium, in the myenteric plexus, and in the walls of the bladder and other viscera.

VARICELLA
(Chickenpox)

Varicella is characterized by the appearance on the skin and mucous membranes of successive crops of typical vesicles, generally accompanied by a mild constitutional reaction.

Epidemiology. Varicella is a highly contagious disease. Ninety per cent of reported patients are under 10 yr of age. The peak age of incidence is 5–9 yr, but the disease may occur at any age, including the neonatal period. Secondary attack rates among susceptible household contacts is about 90%. About 96% of adults in the United States are immune. The disease is seen mainly from January to May. It is spread by direct contact or by droplet. An epidemic of chickenpox in a hospital was shown to be caused by airborne transmission. Infectious virus is present in the vesicles but, unlike the smallpox virus, is not contained in the crusts. Patients are infectious from about 24 hr before the appearance of the rash until all lesions are crusted (usually 6–7 days after the eruption). Epidemics of chickenpox have been initiated by exposure to herpes zoster. Second attacks are rare.

Clinical Manifestations. The incubation period varies from 11–21 days but is 13–17 days in the majority of instances. At the end of the incubation period, prodromal symptoms, except in the mildest cases, precede the characteristic rash by 24 hr. There may be slight fever, malaise, or anorexia, accompanied at times by a scarlatiniform or morbilliform rash. It is characteristic of the specific rash to appear rapidly. Typically, it begins as crops of small, red papules which almost immediately develop into clear, often oval, "tear-drop" vesicles on an erythematous base. These vesicles are usually not umbilicated. The contents become cloudy within about 24 hr. The vesicles are easily broken and become scabbed. Occasionally, they dry before becoming cloudy. Except for the mildest cases, in which few lesions occur, crops of widely scattered vesicles continue to erupt for 3–4 days, starting on the trunk and later spreading to the face and scalp, with minimal, if any, involvement of distal parts of the 'extremities. There is some tendency for the lesions to be concentrated in areas of skin pressure or irritation but not to the same extent as in smallpox. Characteristically, at the height of the disease the eruption consists of papules, early and late vesicles, and crusts present at the same time (Fig 10-21 [p. xxxiii]). Rarely, in severe disease, the lesions appear as hard, pearly lumps (mostly at the same stage of development) and resemble those of smallpox. Pruritus is a constant and annoying characteristic of the rash. Vesicles on the mucous membranes, particularly those of the mouth, rapidly become macerated. The top of the lesion sloughs to form a shallow ulcer. Less commonly, lesions are found on the genital mucous membranes and on the conjunctiva and the cornea, where they are potentially dangerous to sight. Laryngeal involvement is rare. There may be generalized lymphadenopathy.

The severity of the disease varies from a few lesions with little evidence of systemic illness to many hundreds of lesions and extreme toxicity with temperatures ranging from 39.4–40.6° C (103–105° F). Systemic manifestations occur only during the 1st 3–4 days when the rash is erupting.

Infrequently, the rash beomes hemorrhagic in association with a mild to severe thrombocytopenia. The more severe thrombocytopenia usually occurs with other complications, such as pneumonia, or in patients receiving immunosuppressive therapy. Purpura fulminans, which occurs about the end of the 1st wk and is associated with gangrene, probably represents a Shwartzman-like reaction.

Varicella bullosa is an uncommon variant, seen mainly in children under 2 yr of age, in which many of the lesions appear as bullae instead of vesicles. The course of the disease is not changed.

Congenital varicella may be manifest at birth or appear within a few days in infants whose mothers have an active infection. Such infections have a mortality rate of about 20%; in contrast, infections acquired postnatally by young infants are usually mild.

Laboratory Data. There may be a mild leukocytosis. Virus giant cells can be demonstrated in scrapings from the floors of fresh vesicles. The virus can be isolated in a variety of human tissue culture cell lines.

Diagnosis. Most important is the distinction between chickenpox and smallpox, which may be exceedingly difficult in patients with mild smallpox or severe chickenpox. The following clinical points are helpful: (1) The rash of chickenpox begins on the trunk and spreads toward the periphery, whereas that of smallpox tends to spread from the periphery toward the trunk. (2) The lesions of smallpox tend to be most frequent in areas of pressure or tightness of the skin, as over the bridge of the nose, on the wrist, or at the belt line, whereas those of chickenpox do not have this tendency to the same extent. (3) The lesions of chickenpox are more superficial and are not umbilicated, whereas the lesions of smallpox tend to be deeper, more "shotty" to the touch, and usually umbilicated. (4) The lesions of chickenpox are present in all stages of development at a given time, whereas those of smallpox are more or less in the same stage at each phase of the disease. (5) The prodromal symptoms of chickenpox are short (1–2 days) and usually mild; those of smallpox are longer (3–4 days) and may be severe, with high fever which drops with the appearance of the rash.

Material from vesicles can be examined by electron microscopy; varicella-zoster virus can be easily distinguished from variola virus by its morphologic appearance.

Complications. *Secondary bacterial infection* of the skin lesions is the most common complication. *Thrombocytopenia* with hemorrhage into the skin and mucous membranes may occur; internal hemorrhage from ulcerations or into an adrenal may be fatal.

Varicella *pneumonia* is uncommon in children, but 20–30% of adults with chickenpox have clinical or roentgenographic signs of lung involvement. Recovery is usually prompt, but roentgenographic changes may persist for 6–12 wk in the more seriously ill. Fatalities have been reported. *Purpura fulminans* (Sec 14.74) is most frequently seen following chickenpox. Lesions on the larynx may cause edema severe enough to produce respiratory distress. Myocarditis, pericarditis, endocarditis, hepatitis, glomerulonephritis, arthritis, and acute myositis of the limb muscles have been described. Keratitis and vesicular conjunctivitis are rare and usually benign. About 10% of cases of *Reye syndrome* are associated with chickenpox. Congenital malformations have been described in infants whose mothers had varicella during the 1st trimester of pregnancy. The babies have been small for gestational age, with scarring of the skin, muscular atrophy, chorioretinitis or other ocular abnormalities, seizures, mental retardation, and an unusual susceptibility to infection.

The most common central nervous system complication is postinfectious *encephalitis*. Cerebellar signs such as ataxia, nystagmus, and tremors are common. Encephalitis presenting mainly with cerebellar signs has a much better prognosis than cerebral symptoms of convulsions and coma. Overall mortality rates vary from 5–25%. About 15% of survivors have permanent sequelae of seizures, mental retardation, or behavior disturbances. Other central nervous system complications include Guillain-Barré syndrome, transverse myelitis, facial nerve palsy, optic neuritis with transient loss of vision, and the hypothalamic syndrome with obesity and recurrent fever. In contrast to herpes zoster, in which virus has been isolated from the cerebrospinal fluid, no virus has been isolated from the central nervous system of patients dying with chickenpox.

Children receiving corticosteroids or antimetabolites are at risk for severe, often fatal, chickenpox. The greatest risk appears to be in children with leukemia, but deaths have occurred in children receiving steroids for acute rheumatic fever or nephrosis.

Prevention. A live attenuated varicella vaccine has been developed and tested in Japan. The vaccine was well tolerated, produced measurable levels of varicella antibody, and was protective if given before or immediately after exposure to a contagious patient. This experimental vaccine was given without complications to children receiving corticosteroids. Because all herpesviruses produce latent disease and untoward effects may appear decades after the vaccine is given, great thought needs to be given to administering live herpesvirus vaccines, especially since varicella is generally a mild disease of childhood. Large-scale immunizations with this vaccine are not indicated at present, but the vaccine may be useful in susceptible individuals at risk for life-threatening varicella (e.g., those with leukemia).

Passive immunity can be induced by use of zoster immune globulin (ZIG). ZIG is a gamma globulin fraction of plasma with high titer of antibody obtained from patients recovering from herpes zoster infection. It is effective in preventing chickenpox when given within 72 hr of exposure. The recommended dose is at least 5 ml given intramuscularly. Most studies of ZIG have been done in susceptible normal children, and doses as small as 2 ml have been effective in preventing infection. However, prophylaxis is indicated only in susceptible patients at high risk for developing severe varicella: those with immunodeficiency diseases, leukemia, or other malignancies or those on immunosuppressive drugs. Because these children are not protected by ZIG as completely as are normal children, larger quantities of high-titer ZIG are required. ZIG should also be given to a newborn whose mother develops varicella just prior to or soon after delivery. Serum obtained from patients convalescing from herpes zoster has also been used. It appears to be less effective than ZIG and carries the added risk of transmitting hepatitis.

Treatment. Symptomatic treatment should be directed to alleviating itching by the use of local and systemic antipruritic agents and sedation as required. The effects of scratching should be minimized by having the patient wear mittens and keeping the nails short. Daily changes of clothes and linen and antiseptic baths will reduce the incidence of secondary bacterial infection. If secondary infection occurs, systemic antibiotic therapy is indicated. Recent data suggest that the use of aspirin in children with varicella may increase the risk of development of Reye syndrome. Until this matter is fully evaluated it will be necessary to use another agent when symptomatic relief is necessary.

Treatment of varicella pneumonia is usually supportive. Antibiotics are indicated only if secondary bacterial infection occurs. Steroids and immune serum gamma globulin are not helpful.

Adenine arabinoside (vidarabine), a purine nucleotide, has been shown to have activity in vitro against viruses of the herpes group. Success has been reported when this drug has been used to treat patients with severe varicella pneumonia. When used in dosages of 15 mg/kg/24 hr, the drug does not appear to have significant bone marrow toxicity or to depress immune responses. Acyclovir (acycloguanosine, 9-[2-hydroxyethoxy methyl] guanine) is a new investigational antiviral compound currently being tested in patients with severe disease due to herpes simplex and varicellazoster. Preliminary results are encouraging with minimal side effects.

Children hospitalized with varicella should be isolated in rooms where the air pressure is negative in relation to the hall. The room should have an air exhaust unit that prevents recirculation of air into the hospital, and the hall door should be kept closed.

Prognosis. The prognosis is usually good; fatalities occur from the complications.

HERPES ZOSTER
(Shingles)

Herpes zoster is an acute infection characterized by crops of vesicles, usually confined to a dermatome, and by neuralgic pain in the area of the affected dermatome.

Epidemiology. Herpes zoster is relatively uncommon under 10 yr of age, after which its incidence increases steadily with each succeeding decade. Second attacks are rare, fewer than 1% in 1 study of 206 patients. The patient with herpes zoster usually has a history of having had varicella. When this is not the case, the possibility must be considered that a mild case of varicella may have been misdiagnosed or that there had been exposure in the neonatal period which resulted in clinically unrecognized disease. There is an increased incidence of the disease in patients with malignancies and in those receiving immunosuppressive drugs. The severity of herpes zoster increases with age. There is no sex, race, or seasonal predilection. The factors which initiate an attack are not understood.

Clinical Manifestations. Herpes zoster has a preeruptive and a posteruptive phase. The illness usually starts with pain and tenderness along the involved dermatome, often accompanied by generalized malaise and fever. Within a few days groups of red papules appear, distributed along 1 or 2 adjacent dermatomes; the individual lesions quickly vesiculate (Fig 10-22), become pustular, dry up, and scab in the course of 5-10 days. The lesions tend to erupt first at a point nearest the central nervous system. Successive crops appear for 1-4 days. Occasionally they continue to appear for 7 days, extending along the course of the nerve. The eruption clears in 7-14 days in most patients under 20 yr of age, but when vesicles continue to appear for 7 days, healing may be delayed up to 5 wk. The lesions, except in rare instances, are unilateral. Fever, pain, and tenderness usually continue throughout the period of

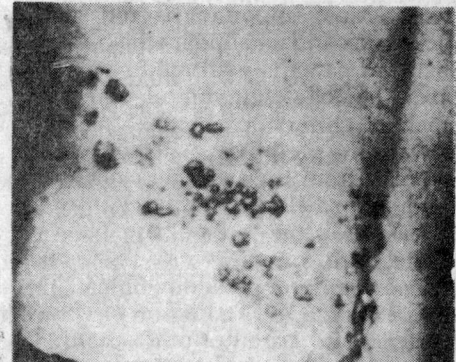

Figure 10-22 Herpes zoster. (Courtesy of Dr. Carroll S. Wright.)

progression. The regional lymph nodes are invariably enlarged. Although the dermatomes of the 2nd dorsal to the 2nd lumbar nerves are the most common sites under the age of 20 yr, cephalic zoster and infection of the sacral nerves, producing lesions of the leg and genitalia, do occur in children. Transient paralysis of the affected part is a rare complication.

With infection of the 5th cranial nerve, any or several of its branches may be affected. With involvement of the ophthalmic branch, lesions may occur on the forehead with local loss of hair, on the nasal tip, and on the cornea (Fig 10–23 [p. xxxii]); over the cheek and the homolateral palate with infection of the maxillary branch; and over the homolateral mandible and tongue when the mandibular branch is affected. Infection of the 7th nerve or the geniculate ganglion results in the *Ramsay Hunt syndrome* of paralysis of the facial nerve and vesicles in the external ear canal.

A generalized rash may accompany herpes zoster; this tends to occur in elderly patients but may occur in children who have had a mild attack of varicella in early infancy. Occasionally the 1st vesicles of varicella in children may be distributed along a dermatome.

Laboratory Data. Examination of the cerebrospinal fluid often reveals a mild lymphocytosis. Scrapings of the floors of vesicles in their initial stage contain virus giant cells.

Diagnosis. Diagnosis may be difficult before development of the rash; the pain may resemble that of pleural, cardiac, or peritoneal origin, depending on the site of the lesion. Once the rash has appeared, its distribution and characteristics along with the pain make the diagnosis relatively simple. Occasionally, herpes simplex may simulate the distribution of herpes zoster.

Complications. Postherpetic pain does not occur in children, and ocular complications are rare. Keratitis and uveitis may follow 5th nerve involvement in adults. Secondary bacterial infection is possible in any of the lesions.

Prophylaxis. The possibility that herpes zoster may follow exposure to chickenpox should be kept in mind. Conversely, since chickenpox can follow exposure to herpes zoster, it is unwise to admit to an open ward a child suffering from the latter disease.

Treatment. Treatment is symptomatic. Soaks and calamine or other drying lotions may be helpful. Pain is seldom a problem in children. Aspirin is usually effective in control of pain, but whether it may alter the risk of Reye syndrome in patients with herpes zoster is unknown (see Varicella, above). Corticosteroids have been shown to be useful in adults in diminishing the amount and duration of postherpetic neuralgia without affecting the rate of healing of the skin lesions or increasing the number of complications.

Vidarabine (adenine arabinoside) has been used successfully in the treatment of patients with severe or disseminated zoster. Acyclovir, an investigational drug, has been shown to be effective in controlled studies. Treatment or prophylaxis with zoster immune globulin is not effective.

Course and Prognosis. In children the course is usually mild, and the ultimate prognosis is good.

Aronson MD, et al: Successful treatment of severe herpesvirus infections with vidarabine. JAMA 235:1339, 1976.
Asano Y, et al: Protective efficacy of vaccination in children in four episodes of natural varicella and zoster in the ward. Pediatrics 59:8, 1977.
Brunell P, Gershon A: Passive immunization against varicella-zoster infections and other modes of therapy. J Infect Dis 127:415, 1973.
Griffith J, et al: The nervous system diseases associated with varicella. Acta Neurol Scand 46:279, 1970.
Leclair JM, Zaia JA, Levin MJ, et al: Airborne transmission of chickenpox in a hospital. N Engl J Med 302:450, 1980.
McKendry JDJ, Bailey JD: Congenital varicella associated with multiple defects. Can Med Assoc J 108:66, 1973.
Meyers JD: Congenital varicella in term infants: Risk reconsidered. J Infect Dis 129:215, 1974.
Triebwasser J, et al: Varicella pneumonia in adults. Medicine 46:409, 1967.
Whitley RJ, et al: Ara-A treatment of herpes zoster in the immunosuppressed. NIAID Collaborative Antiviral Study. N Engl J Med 294:1193, 1976.

10.73 SMALLPOX
(Variola)

Smallpox is an acute, communicable viral disease characterized by a papulovesicular, pustular rash and usually by severe systemic symptoms.

Etiology. There appear to be 2 stable types of virus, variola major and variola minor, which can usually be distinguished by the severity of the disease they cause. They can be dried under relatively unfavorable conditions and remain viable for months, e.g., in house dust. The nucleic acid is DNA. The virus grows on a variety of mammalian cells in tissue culture; it grows readily on the chorioallantoic membrane, where it produces small pocks similar to those of herpes simplex. In 1958 the World Health Organization (WHO) began a campaign to eliminate smallpox from the world. This was considered feasible because (1) humans are the only natural host for smallpox; (2) there are no subclinical carriers; (3) close contact appears to be necessary, in most cases, for spread of the disease, but although airborne spread in hospital has been documented, smallpox is not as contagious as measles or influenza; and (4) an effective vaccine was available. When this campaign was started, there were about 250,000 cases of smallpox reported yearly. Massive organization, tireless efforts to investigate every suspected case and vaccinate susceptible contacts, and unprecedented cooperation between nations resulted in a remarkable achievement. The last endemic case of smallpox occurred in Somalia in October, 1977; in May, 1980, the WHO formally declared the world to be free of smallpox.

The only remaining source of possible disease is laboratory accident; the last reported case of smallpox occurred in England in 1978 in this way. Seven laboratories in the world currently have stocks of variola virus. These laboratories are carefully controlled. The WHO plans to stockpile large amounts of freeze-dried vaccine as insurance against a future outbreak of smallpox.

Pathology. The virus first infects the bronchiolar and upper respiratory tract epithelium and multiplies locally. A primary viremia then occurs with dissemination to the reticuloendothelial system. A 2nd and more intense viremia follows, with spread to the skin and other organs producing a rash and systemic signs of illness. Specific changes are found in the skin, mucous membranes, upper digestive tract, kidneys, testes, bone marrow, and other organs.

Clinical Manifestations. The incubation period is usually 12–14 days but may be as long as 21 days in previously vaccinated persons and in variola minor.

Variola Major. In a typical case the prodromal symptoms are severe and usually start abruptly with headache, chills, aching of the back and limbs, and fever, which mounts rapidly to 41.2–41.8° C (106–107° F). In children there may also be vomiting, drowsiness, convulsions, and coma. Often delirium occurs, and the patient is prostrated.

During the 1st 2 days transient rashes are common and may resemble scarlet fever or measles or may be petechial. They tend to be most prominent over the upper thighs and buttocks and disappear rapidly by the 3rd–4th day, when the raised macules of the typical cutaneous lesion begin to appear over the face. Widespread prodromal rashes and the early appearance of macules presage a severe attack.

There is usually diminution in severity of symptoms as the rash becomes papular, and the temperature may even become normal and remain so until the pustular stage. The individual lesions appear in a single crop and progress at the same rate. Initially the papules are 2–4 mm in diameter and are firm and "shotty." Within about 24 hr the size of the papules increases and vesicles appear. They tend to be umbilicated in the early and again in the late stages. Some of the vesicles are superficial, others deeper and less readily recognized. A small red areola encircles each vesicle (Fig 10–24).

About the 5th–6th day of the disease the vesicles become cloudy and the pustular stage begins. The individual lesion is greenish or grayish-yellow and has an elevation slightly greater than its diameter. About the 9th day the lesions begin to dry and the areolae disappear. They are usually crusted over by the end of the 2nd wk, and the scabs drop off about the end of the 3rd–4th wk leaving scars which are permanent in about 50% of survivors. The scabs persist longest on the palms and soles, where they are known as "seeds," and may have to be enucleated with a needle.

The cutaneous areas chiefly involved in the early stages are those where the skin is tight, such as the wrists and the prominences of the face; the more exposed extensor surfaces of the forearms and upper arms are then involved, leaving the more protected flexor surfaces and the axillae relatively free. The rash then spreads to the chest. In severe cases the abdomen and legs are heavily covered; in milder cases they may be only slightly involved. Concurrently with the skin lesions, the mucous membranes of the mouth, eyes, and often the larynx become affected.

A striking feature of the disease, in contrast to chickenpox, is the profusion of lesions on the face, including the lips, and the presence of a relatively large number of lesions on the palms and soles. When the lesions become confluent, there is such severe edema of the face that there is difficulty in closing the eyes and mouth. The lesions on the mucous membranes also tend to be confluent. Scarring, greatest on the face, results from necrosis of sebaceous glands and is not greatly influenced by secondary infection. Intense pigmentation of the skin persists for a variable time after the scabs have fallen. In fatal cases death usually occurs during the 2nd wk of the disease.

Hemorrhagic smallpox may occur in 2 forms: *vesicular hemorrhagic smallpox*, in which hemorrhages occur in the corium after the development of vesicles, and *true hemorrhagic* or *black smallpox*, in which a diffuse hemorrhagic rash begins on the 2nd–3rd day of prodromal symptoms, followed by ecchymoses and hemorrhages into the mucous membranes. In the latter form the temperature may be subnormal although the symptoms are severe. Death may occur before the characteristic rash of smallpox develops.

Variola Minor (Alastrim). Variola minor is a much milder disease than variola major.

Modified Smallpox (Varioloid). Previously vaccinated persons with partial immunity may develop a modified illness. The prodrome is usually unchanged, but the rash evolves more rapidly, and the lesions are fewer and more superficial. Fatalities are rare. Since the disease may be quite atypical, diagnosis and isolation are frequently delayed. Such patients are capable of transmitting severe smallpox to susceptible contacts and have been the source of extensive outbreaks of smallpox.

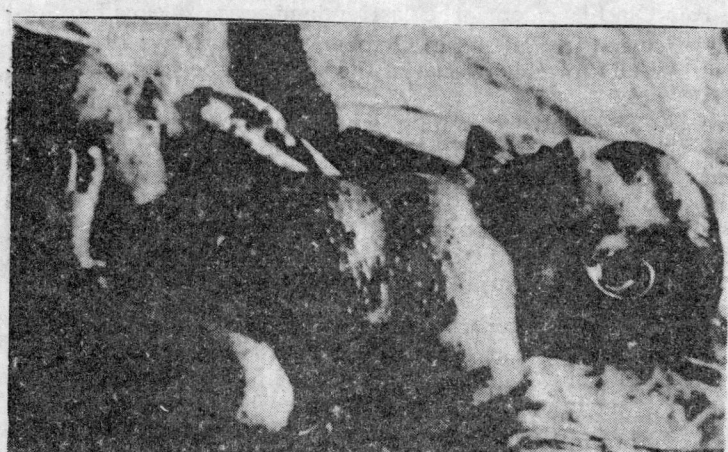

Figure 10–24   Variola in an unvaccinated infant. (Courtesy of Dr. Roger Feldman.)

Abortive Type. In persons who have been vaccinated shortly before exposure to smallpox, a condition known as *variola sine eruptione* may occur. Macules or papules may involute with great rapidity, or there may be no eruption at all, and the patient has only a mild, febrile illness. In this form, variola is not contagious.

Laboratory Data. Neutropenia is characteristic of the early stages of the disease. In hemorrhagic smallpox this may be associated with a reduction of platelets. Large lymphocytes are characteristically present in small numbers. During the pustular stage polymorphonuclear leukocytosis occurs. There is prolongation of the prothrombin time and a decrease in fibrinogen associated with the hemorrhagic type, probably dependent on extensive liver damage.

Diagnosis. The typical case of smallpox is readily diagnosed, but mild cases may be misdiagnosed as chickenpox or missed altogether. In a doubtful case the patient should be isolated and viral studies obtained.

Complications. *Pyogenic infections* of the skin and bacteremia may occur. An enanthem of the larynx may lead to *edema of the glottis* and perichondritis of the laryngeal cartilages. *Bronchopneumonia* is relatively common. *Viral osteomyelitis* occurs occasionally in children and usually appears between the 10th–20th days of the disease. Multiple joints as well as bones are commonly infected, but severe systemic symptoms are not related to this involvement. Serious deformities such as flail joints, ankylosis, malformed bones, and cessation of bone growth are common sequels. Central nervous system involvement is rare.

Prognosis. The case fatality rate varies with the type of the disease and the age of the patient. The rate during epidemics of variola minor is less than 1%, whereas an overall rate of about 10% may be expected in epidemics of variola major. The case fatality rate is considered to be about 5–6% in discrete smallpox, 60% in confluent smallpox, and 80% or over in hemorrhagic smallpox. Mortality is greatest in children under 5, pregnant women, and persons over 45 yr of age.

Treatment. No effective specific therapy is available once the disease has developed. Marboran is effective in prophylaxis (see below) but does not appear to be useful in treatment of established disease. Symptomatic treatment and nursing care are of extreme importance. The patient's room should be light and well ventilated; some odor-killing device is desirable. Severe cases of confluent and hemorrhagic smallpox should be treated for shock and dehydration by proper use of intravenous fluids, blood, and plasma. Appropriate antibiotics in therapeutic doses should be used in severe disease when secondary bacterial infection is identified or suspected. Nutrition should be maintained. Lesions of the eyes require frequent irrigation; this therapy should be supervised by an ophthalmologist. Sedation should be given as indicated. In the milder cases the general methods of treatment as outlined in Sec 10.72 are adequate.

Prophylaxis. Vaccination (Sec 10.74) is almost totally protective against acquiring variola major for 3 yr and variola minor for 7 yr; it reduces the severity of the disease for up to 20 yr. A primary vaccination given within 3–4 days of exposure to smallpox gives some protection. Revaccination of a previously immunized person is effective in preventing the disease if given within 7–8 days of exposure. Hyperimmune vaccinia gamma globulin given at the time of vaccination raises the protection rate 4-fold; Marboran (N-methylisatin β-thiosemicarbazone) raises it 16-fold. The drug is given orally as a 10–20% suspension in syrup in an initial dose of 200 mg/kg followed by 50 mg/kg every 6 hr for 8 doses. There may be nausea and vomiting if the drug is not given after meals.

Patients should be strictly isolated until all the crusts have dropped off. Fomites, books, letters, and the like must be sterilized, preferably by heat.

In the public health management of a smallpox epidemic the following steps, scrupulously enforced, can usually be relied on to control the spread of the disease without mass vaccination: (1) listing of contacts; (2) surveillance of contacts for 3 wk for any evidence of illness; (3) vaccination of contacts, preferably within 24 hr of exposure. Vaccination must produce reliable evidence of a take and must be repeated if negative or doubtful.

Bauer DJ, St. Vincent L, Kempe CH, et al: Prophylactic treatment of smallpox contacts with N-methylisatin β-thiosemicarbazone. Lancet 2:494, 1963.

Bras G: The morbid anatomy of smallpox. Docum Med Geog et Trop 4:303, 1952.

Dixon CW: Smallpox. London, J & A Churchill, 1962.

Kempe CH, et al: The use of vaccinia hyperimmune gamma globulin in the prophylaxis of smallpox. Bull WHO 25:41, 1961.

10.74 VACCINATION AGAINST SMALLPOX

The use of cowpox virus for vaccination against smallpox was the 1st successful development of a method for the protection of human beings against a serious epidemic disease. Dr. Edward Jenner in 1798 conclusively proved that the inoculation of human beings with material from cowpox led to immunity to smallpox. Cowpox and variola belong to the "pox" group of viruses which affect many species of animals, each animal having its own specific pox infection which, as a rule, is not transmissible to another host. Cowpox, however, is so closely related to the human "pox" virus, variola, that it can and does affect people with a specific disease of the skin of the hands on close contact. The stable pox virus of vaccinia may have been derived from hybridization between variola and cowpox viruses. In the laboratory such hybrids resemble the virus of vaccinia and could have occurred from documented early accidental contamination of vaccine virus batches with variola virus. The great diversity of vaccine strains that exist may also be the result of the past practice of mixing different strains of vaccinia virus in order to produce an effective vaccine.

For many yr vaccination against smallpox was a routine procedure for healthy children in the United States; most states required evidence of vaccination before entrance into school. In 1971 that policy was changed because the risk of acquiring smallpox in the

United States was very small, no cases having been reported since 1949, compared to the considerable risk of primary vaccination with a mortality rate of 1–2/ million primary vaccinations. Since smallpox has now been declared extinct, there is no medical reason for routine vaccination. Nevertheless, many countries still require proof of vaccination from visitors entering the country, and the military still routinely vaccinates American troops.

Type of Vaccine. The usual vaccine is obtained from the pulp of vesicles of vaccinated calves, which is diluted 1:5 in 50% glycerin-saline solution containing 1% phenol. It is distributed in capillary glass tubes. The vaccine is not completely free of bacteria. It is considered potent for 3 mo if kept below 5° C; it deteriorates rapidly at room temperature. Avianized vaccine prepared from vaccinia-infected chorioallantoic membranes of embryonated hens' eggs is equally effective. Lyophilized dried vaccine, which is stable at room temperature, is advisable in the tropics or where refrigeration facilities are inadequate.

Site of Vaccination. Vaccination should be performed on the skin over the insertion of the deltoid muscle or on the posterior axillary fold.

Method of Vaccination. Although there is good evidence that there is direct correlation between protection against the disease and the number and extent of the vaccination scars, the present policy is to make only 1 inoculation. After exposure, 2–4 sites of inoculation are advocated. The technique is as follows:

The skin should be cleansed with a volatile antiseptic, e.g., ether or acetone, care being taken to avoid making abrasions in which the virus could "take." The tube of lymph should be removed from the freezing section of the refrigerator only at the moment of use, the ends broken off after filing, and the contents expressed on the skin by means of a small rubber bulb. Introduction of the virus can be accomplished by the *multiple pressure method*, which is generally recommended in the United States. The needle is held almost parallel with the skin and the point pressed up and down against the skin through a drop of lymph in such a way that the surface cells are picked off, thus exposing the deeper-growing cells of the epidermis to the virus. Two–3 pressures over an area of about ⅛–¼ inch in diameter are usually sufficient for primary vaccination after the age of 6 mo. For revaccination, 30 pressures are recommended. The area should become erythematous, but should not bleed. The lymph is rubbed into the site with the shaft of the needle, the excess wiped off, and the remainder allowed to dry.

Type of Reaction. The reaction to smallpox vaccination is due to hypersensitivity as well as to the necrotizing action of vaccinia virus on infected cells. The usual reactions vary according to the degree of host sensitivity and are classified as primary, accelerated or vaccinoid, "early" reaction, or no visible reaction.

Primary Reaction. This is the reaction of the non-immune unsensitized person. There is little reaction at the site except a fading erythema until the 3rd–5th day, when a red, slightly itching papule appears. This rapidly vesiculates within about 24 hr and becomes surrounded by a red areola. The vesicle grows in size, becomes umbilicated and pearly gray, and is surrounded by an increasing area of erythema and induration. The reaction reaches its height about the 9th–10th day, when the area is hot and tender, the regional lymph nodes are enlarged and painful, and the spleen may be enlarged. There is usually some systemic reaction, which may be mild, with low-grade fever, malaise, and headache, or severe, with temperatures of 40° C (104° F) or higher for 3–4 days. There is little change in the leukocyte count. After the peak of the reaction the vesicle undergoes desiccation and becomes covered with a dark scab which is shed about the 21st day. The pink, pitted scar, which slowly fades to white, remains as the only evidence that successful vaccination has been performed.

Vaccinoid or Accelerated Reaction. This is the reaction of the partially sensitized person. The lesion goes through the same general stages as does the primary take but more rapidly. The greater the sensitization, the more rapid is the evolution. A papule may become vesiculated within 2 days and reach the peak of its reaction in less than 1 wk. The size of the reaction is smaller than with the primary take, and there are few, if any, general signs or symptoms.

"Early" Reaction. This reaction consists of a small area of redness and induration maximal at 8–72 hr; a vesicle may or may not be present. It occurs in highly sensitized persons and usually, but not always, indicates immunity. Nevertheless, a similar lesion can be produced by inactivated vaccine in such persons; therefore they should be revaccinated with a known potent vaccine if exposed to smallpox.

No Reaction. Poor technique or the use of inactivated virus may explain some of these failures. Such persons should be vaccinated several times with potent vaccine and by an approved technique before it is assumed that they have been immunized. Laboratory tests for neutralizing antibodies will provide definite proof of immunization.

Revaccination. Revaccination must be performed whenever there is contact with a case of smallpox. Under these circumstances a positive "take" is of such importance that at least 2 "insertions" should be made. Local skin immunity to vaccination can exist without systemic immunity; hence, the site of revaccination should be other than the original one; the forearm appears to be particularly sensitive.

Care of Site of Vaccination. Dryness and free flow of air about the vesicle are essential. Shields should never be used. If the vesicle ruptures because of excessive tension or trauma, the area should be sponged with alcohol 3–4 times daily and loosely covered with a piece of gauze attached to the skin above and below by adhesive tape placed well outside the indurated area. When the dressing is changed, it should be cut off and the fresh one taped over the original adhesive tapes, which should not be removed until the inflammation has subsided, to avoid secondary lesions in the adhesive-abraded areas.

Complications

Pyogenic Infections. As a result of scratching or neglect, the vaccination site can become contaminated with various bacterial pathogens, such as staphylococci and streptococci, giving rise to cellulitis, scarlet fever, or septicemia. The size of the scar is always increased by such contamination. Vaccine lymph can be contaminated with tetanus spores; however, tetanus has occurred only in the presence of a tight shield or other occlusive dressing.

Abnormal Distribution of Virus. *Local.* Transfer of infection to other parts of the body can result from scratching the primary lesion. In those autoinoculated, the secondary lesions heal, usually without scarring, at the same time as the primary lesion. When the lesion occurs at a potentially harmful site, e.g., the eye, specific treatment should be given (see below). A susceptible person can be infected by contact with the primary lesion of another person.

General. *Eczema vaccinatum* (Fig 10–25 [p. xxxii]) or vaccinia superimposed upon eczematous skin can result from autoinoculation, from infection of eczematous skin, or from contact with a vaccinated person. There is probably spread of virus via bloodstream and lymphatics in addition to local inoculation. The eczematous skin is covered with umbilicated vesicles which involute like the primary ones. Infants are seriously ill; the mortality is in the range of 30–40%. The condition is distinguished from eczema herpeticum chiefly by history of exposure. Patients with eczema or those who have contact with them should not be vaccinated.

Abnormal Host Response. *Antibody Formation.* In patients with defective immune mechanisms (e.g., decreased globulins, thymic dysplasia) or receiving corticosteroids, immunosuppressive drugs, or roentgen therapy, progressive vaccinia may develop as follows: (1) *Satellite* or *widespread vaccinal lesions,* which usually persist, along with the original lesion, for days or weeks beyond the normal time of healing until antibodies are eventually formed and all lesions heal together. Generalized vaccinia is sometimes mistakenly diagnosed when a coincidental skin eruption, e.g., varicella or impetigo, occurs in a child who has been vaccinated. Generalized vaccinia can be excluded if the original vaccination site is progressing normally without satellite lesions. (2) *Prolonged progressive vaccinia* or *vaccinia gangrenosa.* There is spreading necrosis at the site of the primary inoculation which eventually destroys the area, and metastatic necrotic lesions occur throughout the body, including the bones. The mortality is high.

Hypersensitivity Reactions. A variety of rashes which can be included under the general term "erythema multiforme" occur at 7–11 days in about 1 of 5000 vaccinations. They are commonly mild and maculopapular ("roseola vaccinosa"), papulovesicular, or urticarial. Less frequently, there is a severe, generalized, bullous rash which may also involve the mucous membranes of the mouth, anus, and genitalia (erythema multiforme pluriorificialis).

Central Nervous System. Postvaccinal encephalomyelitis is one of the allergic encephalitides. It usually appears 11–14 days after vaccination but often earlier in infants. The clinical signs and symptoms include fever, meningismus, seizures, coma, paralysis, polyneuritis, myasthenia, transverse myelitis, and signs of increased intracranial pressure. The cerebrospinal fluid may show pleocytosis and increased protein. It occurred in approximately 1 of 100,000 vaccinations in the United States; the case fatality rate is approximately 50%.

Treatment of Complications. Bacterial complications should be treated with appropriate antibiotic agents. Delay of antibody production leading to generalized vaccinia can be overcome by administration of hyperimmune vaccinia gamma globulin in a dose of 0.6 ml/kg, which can be repeated as required. Lesions due to autoinoculation or heteroinoculation in potentially dangerous sites should be treated with a similar dose of hyperimmune globulin except when the cornea is affected. Serotherapy aggravates this, and IDU drops should be used locally (Sec 10.71 and 10.72). For *eczema vaccinatum,* 2 administrations may be required. For *progressive vaccinia* the administration must be repeated every wk or 2 until healing is proceeding favorably and until vaccinia virus can no longer be demonstrated in the lesions. N-methylisatin β-thiosemicarbazone (Sec 10.73) has been effective in some patients in whom serotherapy has failed. The therapy for encephalitis is supportive; there is no reason to give hyperimmune gamma globulin because the normal development of antibodies is indicated by normal healing of the vaccinal lesion.

CAROL F. PHILLIPS

Galasso G, et al: A clinical and serologic study of four smallpox vaccines comparing variations of dose and route of administration. J Infect Dis 135:131, 1977.

Kempe CH: The end of routine smallpox vaccination in the United States. Pediatrics 49:489, 1972.

10.75 CYTOMEGALOVIRAL INFECTION

Cytomegaloviral infections may be inapparent or may cause cytomegalic inclusion disease when acquired before, during, or after birth. They are the most common of congenital infections. When acquired after birth, they may induce an illness resembling infectious mononucleosis and are frequently pathogenic among patients with impaired cellular immunity.

Etiology. Cytomegalovirus is a species-specific agent with the physicochemical and electron microscopic characteristics of herpesviruses. At least 2 serologic prototypes are demonstrable in cross-neutralization tests.

Epidemiology. Cytomegaloviral infections are worldwide in distribution. The incidence of congenital acquired infection is generally higher among populations with a lower standard of living. At least half of the women of childbearing age have serologic evidence of previous cytomegaloviral infection. Excretion of the virus in the urine can be demonstrated in 4–5% of pregnant women; cervical shedding occurs in 10%, and 5–15% excrete cytomegalovirus in their milk. The prevalence of congenital infection has been found to vary from 0.4–7.4%. In Japan, the majority of children become seropositive during infancy as opposed to 10% in the United States.

Cytomegalovirus is not readily transmitted from 1 person to another. When transmission does occur, it usually follows intimate contact and is associated with inapparent infection. Epidemics have not been described. When infection is introduced into a household, however, it is likely that every susceptible family member will develop infection eventually, usually in the absence of recognizable disease. Transmission to the fetus may occur following both primary and secondary or recurrent infection in the mother. Recent evidence indicates that congenital infection is not uncommon among fetuses of women known to be seropositive prior to pregnancy and that it can occur in consecutive pregnancies. Acquired infection may result from contact with cytomegalovirus in cervical secretions during the 2nd stage of labor. Since virus is present in saliva, the upper respiratory tract, spermatozoa, leukocytes, milk, and feces as well as urine, it is probable that contact with any of these infected sources can result in transmission of infection. Blood transfusion–associated cytomegaloviral mononucleosis has been described. Infection occurs more often in sexually promiscuous individuals. Most patients undergoing immunosuppressive therapy following renal homotransplantation develop active cytomegaloviral infection, which is more likely to be symptomatic if the recipient was seronegative prior to surgery. The virus may be present in the donor kidney even though it may show no histologic evidence of cytomegaloviral infection.

Pathology. The electron microscopic appearance of the cytomegalovirus particle is similar to that of varicella-zoster, Epstein-Barr, and herpes simplex virus particles. Light microscopy reveals large intranuclear inclusion bodies, especially in tissues with a high titer of virus. The large size of the intranuclear inclusions in cells from lung, liver, kidney, urine sediment, and so on is sufficiently distinctive to permit a specific diagnosis of cytomegaloviral infection, but tissue culture is a far more sensitive method for detection of cytomegalovirus.

Clinical Manifestations. *Congenital Infection.* Over 90% of infected newborns are asymptomatic, and observed illness varies in severity. Few infants are dangerously ill; death is rare. In approximate order of decreasing frequency, the most prominent manifestations include hepatosplenomegaly, jaundice, purpura, microcephaly, cerebral calcifications, and chorioretinitis. Any of these abnormalities may occur alone. Frequently there are no signs related to the central nervous system in the neonatal period. A petechial rash on the 1st day of life, particularly in association with splenomegaly, suggests cytomegaloviral infection. Some infants simply fail to thrive or show increased irritability. Isolated congenital anomalies such as clubfoot, strabismus, high-arched palate, deafness, and microcephaly occur more often in symptomatic infants with congenital infection. Although congenital heart lesions have also been described in congenital cytomegaloviral infection, there is no firm evidence that this association is more than coincidental. Infants with major multiple congenital anomalies are not likely to have cytomegalic inclusion disease as the cause.

Involvement of the central nervous system is the most common and important manifestation of fetal cytomegaloviral infection. Both symptomatic and asymptomatic infants may fail to attain optimal psychomotor potential when evaluated several yr after birth. In contrast, extraneural involvement of the liver, spleen, lungs, and kidney is usually reversible with relatively little chance of permanent malfunction. Visual loss has been reported rarely in association with chorioretinitis involving the macular area and severe optic atrophy. Cytomegalovirus-associated hearing loss is much more common; it appears to be a major etiologic factor in congenital deafness. Spasticity and hypotonia are seen in more severely affected children. Central nervous system dysfunction may range from diminished IQ with increased probability of school failure to severe brain damage precluding normal psychomotor development beyond early infancy.

Acquired Infection. As in congenital infection, cytomegaloviral infection acquired after birth is usually inapparent. There is evidence that some infants come in contact with maternal virus during the 2nd stage of labor and begin to excrete virus in the urine several wk later. Although infants acquiring infection under the cover of maternally acquired antibody usually do not have symptoms, the virus has been recovered in early infancy from patients with pneumonia, paroxysmal cough, petechial rash, hepatomegaly, and splenomegaly. The central nervous system is occasionally vulnerable to cytomegaloviral infection acquired after birth. Infantile spasms have not been implicated as a cytomegalovirus-induced abnormality. It is possible, however, that infectious polyneuritis has the same relationship to cytomegaloviral infection that it does to Epstein-Barr virus infection in patients with infectious mononucleosis. Chorioretinitis has been associated with acquired cytomegaloviral infection in immunosuppressed patients but otherwise is a rare manifestation of acquired disease.

In older children and adults, mononucleosis due to cytomegalovirus is the most common manifestation recognizable to the physician. There is considerable variation in clinical presentation, but usually malaise, sore throat, cervical or other regional adenopathy, myalgia, headache, anorexia, abdominal pain, hepatomegaly, and splenomegaly are noted. Abnormal liver function tests are common. Pharyngeal edema, usually without exudate, is seen, but the anginal symptoms generally are not striking. Fatigue can be extreme as well as extraordinarily persistent. Some patients require 12–15 hr of sleep/day. Fever and chills may last for 2 or more wk with daily spikes to levels of 40° C (104° F) or higher. Atypical lymphocytosis is a consistent and early feature.

When blood products, particularly multiple units of fresh whole blood, are administered to seronegative recipients, post-transfusion cytomegaloviral mononucleosis may occur 2–4 wk later. Cytomegalovirus has been demonstrated in donor white blood cells. Administration of blood to preterm infants is frequently associated with gray pallor, respiratory distress, splenomegaly, atypical lymphocytosis, and cytomegaloviruria.

If ampicillin is administered, a maculopapular rash similar to that seen in infectious mononucleosis patients has been observed. Abnormal serologic reactions, including cold agglutinins, antinuclear antibody, and cryoimmunoglobulins, have been described in both infectious mononucleosis and cytomegaloviral mononucleosis.

Although there is little evidence that cytomegalovirus is an important cause of chronic hepatitis, the virus has been isolated from children and young adults with mildly abnormal liver function tests and from some with hepatomegaly, chronic hepatitis, granulomatous hepatitis, or cirrhosis of the liver. It is possible in some instances that patients with severe disease were more susceptible to the infection because of steroids administered to ameliorate chronic liver disease.

Diagnosis and Differential Diagnosis. *Congenital Infection.* The diagnosis of congenital infection may be made by the isolation of virus within 1 wk after birth or by the demonstration of large inclusion-bearing cells in the tissues or urine at birth. However, since most infants do not have symptoms in the newborn period, the above tests are not usually performed. If any infant followed for several mo has a sustained complement-fixing, hemagglutination-inhibiting, or fluorescent antibody titer (IgG or IgM), strong evidence of congenital cytomegaloviral infection exists. Passively acquired antibody from the mother should be in a titer of less than 1:8 by 6 mo of age. An IgM level of 20 mg/dl or more in the cord serum suggests, but does not prove, that congenital infection is present. The presence of IgA antibody in the cord serum is also suggestive of congenital infection.

Congenital cytomegaloviral infection must be distinguished from toxoplasmosis, rubella, herpes simplex, and bacterial sepsis.

TOXOPLASMOSIS. Cytomegaloviral disease in the neonate may resemble toxoplasmosis in striking detail. Toxoplasmosis, however, is more likely to be associated with microphthalmia, scattered cerebral cortical calcifications, hydrocephalus, and chorioretinitis. The demonstration of specific toxoplasmal antibody titers persisting beyond 6 mo of age or the presence of toxoplasmal IgM antibody in early infancy is tantamount to isolation of the organism.

RUBELLA. Congenital cytomegaloviral infection may be difficult to distinguish from congenital rubella in the neonatal period. Both may be associated with a purpuric rash, jaundice, microcephaly, and deafness. The presence of central cataracts is strong presumptive evidence for rubella. If these are associated with a congenital heart lesion, the probability of rubella is high. Specific laboratory tests for rubella virus or rubella IgM antibody or serial hemagglutination-inhibition antibody tests are required for a definitive diagnosis. The marked increase in the incidence of rubella in recent yr makes this diagnosis much less likely than that of cytomegaloviral infection.

HERPES SIMPLEX NEONATORUM. Herpes simplex infection is usually transmitted to the infant during labor and has its onset 5–10 days after birth. The disease is often fulminant in character and may occur as a meningoencephalitis, pneumonitis, or undiagnosed vesicular rash. The virus is readily isolated from vesicular lesions in a variety of tissue culture systems.

BACTERIAL SEPSIS. Infants with bacterial sepsis usually are more acutely ill than infants with cytomegalic inclusion disease and usually do not have a petechial rash. Although the diagnosis of sepsis rests on a positive blood culture, the decision to treat with antibiotic drugs must be made on the basis of the early clinical findings.

Acquired Infection. The diagnosis of cytomegaloviral infection in a patient with mononucleosis-like symptoms can be established by viral isolation as described above. Serologic determinations, such as the presence of specific immunofluorescent IgM antibody or a 4-fold rise or decline in complement-fixing antibody, must be interpreted with more caution than in the newborn period. In the fluorescent antibody tests for IgM, cross-reactions with other cell-associated herpesviruses, such as Epstein-Barr virus, occur. In addition, cytomegaloviral complement-fixing antibody may fluctuate widely in some normal subjects, making interpretation of this serologic test difficult. Patients with cytomegaloviral mononucleosis are heterophil antibody–negative.

INFECTIOUS MONONUCLEOSIS. Cytomegaloviral mononucleosis may be difficult to distinguish from heterophil antibody–negative infectious mononucleosis because both conditions occur in young adults with atypical lymphocytosis, sore throat, abnormal liver function tests, splenomegaly, and fever. The cytomegaloviral IgM fluorescent antibody test is positive in both cytomegaloviral and infectious mononucleosis, presumably because EB virus and cytomegalovirus share common antigens. A patient with cytomegaloviral mononucleosis generally sheds virus in the urine and upper respiratory tract. Virus is also recoverable from peripheral leukocytes. EB virus antibody can be measured by an indirect immunofluorescence technique. The complement-fixation tests for EB virus and cytomegalovirus do not cross-react.

HEPATITIS A AND B. A jaundiced patient with cytomegaloviral mononucleosis may clinically resemble one with hepatitis A or B. A serum glutamic oxaloacetic transaminase level above 800 units is unusual for cytomegaloviral infections at any age but common in icteric hepatitis A. Both conditions may be associated with mild atypical lymphocytosis. Jaundice in an adult is more unusual in cytomegaloviral infections than in infections with the hepatitis viruses; history of recent contact with a jaundiced person favors the diagnosis of hepatitis A. Australian or hepatitis B surface antigen may be detected in the serum of many, but not all, patients with serum hepatitis. The latter virus may be transmitted in ways other than parenteral inoculation, including sexual and transplacental transmission.

Prevention. There is evidence that acquisition of cytomegaloviral infection may be prevented in specific situations, such as by using seronegative donors for kidney transplants or by avoiding the use of fresh blood, especially when multiple transfusions are required. Usually, however, prevention is not possible; virtually everyone acquires this infection by the 3rd decade of life. A vaccine is not available. A major concern is the capacity of some individuals to become reinfected even in the presence of existing humoral and cellular immunity. Congenital infection is rather common among infants of mothers seropositive prior to pregnancy. It will be important to learn whether the long-term sequelae in infants born to mothers experiencing primary infections during pregnancy are different quantitatively and qualitatively from those in infants born to mothers with evidence of infection *prior* to pregnancy.

Treatment.   A number of antiviral agents have been used in the treatment of congenital and acquired cytomegaloviral infections, including deoxyuridine, floxuridine, cytosine arabinoside, adenine arabinoside, and acyclovir. Although virus excretion has been temporarily halted in some instances, no role in the treatment of these infections has been established for these agents. Furthermore, they are all potentially toxic, and their use has not been approved by the U.S. Food and Drug Administration for this purpose. Corticosteroids, interferon, interferon inducers, and transfer factor have either not been adequately studied or not been shown to affect the clinical course.

Prognosis. *Congenital.*   If an infant has recognizable symptoms of cytomegaloviral infection at birth, the prognosis is fair for survival but guarded for normal psychomotor development. Approximately 90% of such infants will have some form of central nervous system sequelae such as low IQ, deafness, hypotonia, hypertonia, cerebral palsy, microcephaly, and so on. Asymptomatic infants with viruria at birth may have diminished intelligence, hearing loss, and school failure.

Acquired.   The prognosis is excellent for most patients with cytomegaloviral mononucleosis. Rarely, however, individuals have had extraordinary fatigue, recurrent sore throats, and intermittent low-grade fever lasting as long as 2–3 yr. Patients with postperfusion and renal allograft–associated cytomegaloviral infections usually do well. A small number of patients develop severe pneumonitis, hemolytic anemia, or hepatitis which may seriously impede recovery. A fatal outcome is not usually due to cytomegaloviral infection alone. Individuals with increased susceptibility to infections, such as those with Hodgkin disease and lymphomas, may have generalized cytomegaloviral infections terminally.

JAMES BARRY HANSHAW

Benyesh-Melnick M: Cytomegaloviruses. *In:* Lennette EH, Schmidt NJ (eds): Diagnostic Procedures for Viral and Rickettsial Infections. Ed 4. New York, American Public Health Association, 1969.
Hanshaw JB: Cytomegalovirus infections. Pediatr Rev 2:245, 1981.
Hanshaw JB, Scheiner AP, Moxley AW, et al: School failure and deafness after "silent" congenital cytomegalovirus infection. N Engl J Med 295:468, 1976.
Jordan MC, Rousseau WE, Stewart JA, et al: Spontaneous cytomegalovirus mononucleosis: Clinical and laboratory observations in nine cases. Ann Intern Med 79:153, 1973.
Plummer G: Cytomegaloviruses in man and animals. *In:* Melnick JL (ed): Progress in Medical Virology. Basel, S Karger, 1973.

Weller TH: The cytomegaloviruses: Ubiquitous agents with protean clinical manifestations. N Engl J Med 285:203, 267, 1971.

10.76   INFECTIOUS MONONUCLEOSIS

Infectious mononucleosis is a disease resulting from an infection of the lymphatic system by the Epstein-Barr (EB) virus of the herpes group. In its full-blown form the illness is characterized by malaise, fever, sore throat, lymphadenopathy, hepatosplenomegaly, atypical lymphocytes in the peripheral blood, and a heterophil antibody response. The infection is often mild or even inapparent, but occasionally severe complications may be observed.

Etiology.   The agent that causes infectious mononucleosis is indistinguishable morphologically from herpes simplex. It was originally observed by electron microscopy in cells cultured from specimens of Burkitt lymphoma, a neoplastic disease that occurs predominantly in central Africa. The original cultures were established by Epstein and Barr.

So far it has been possible to transmit EB virus only to lymphocytes, which may be productively infected (virus particles produced) or abortively infected (viral antigens only produced). Although most of the atypical lymphocytes found in infectious mononucleosis are T lymphocytes, the EB virus replicates in B lymphocytes. Infection of lymphocytes in vitro with EB virus enables them to grow indefinitely in culture (immortalization). With rare exceptions, only lymphocytes from individuals previously infected with EB virus produce cell lines in culture; therefore the process of immortalization is one which may also occur in vivo.

Epidemiology.   The epidemiology of infectious mononucleosis is related to the epidemiology of EB virus. Infection with EB virus occurs early in life in developing countries. In central Africa almost all children are infected by 3 yr of age, and in that environment typical infectious mononucleosis is practically unknown. In western countries the age at which EB virus infection occurs is related to socioeconomic group. Young adults are 60–80% seropositive, the more affluent being less likely to have been infected. Seropositivity increases with age until in the United States nearly all adults are positive. The seroconversion is particularly high during the high school and college years: at Yale University 15% of susceptibles developed antibodies to EB virus each yr, and 65% of those infected had clinical infectious mononucleosis. Infectious mononucleosis occurs at all ages but only rarely under the age of 2 yr, when most EBV infections remain silent, or over the age of 40 yr, when most individuals are already immune. The overall incidence is approximately 50:100,000 persons/yr, but in young adults the incidence rises to about 1:1000/yr.

Transmission of infectious mononucleosis takes place by exchange of saliva from child to child on contaminated objects or during kissing by young adults. Nonintimate contact does not lead to spread of EB virus. EB virus is excreted in the saliva in the cell-free state, particularly before and during the clinical disease, but also commonly for 6 mo after recovery and frequently longer. Healthy individuals with serologic evidence of past EB viral infection excrete virus in 10–20% of cases, probably intermittently. Immunosuppressed patients who are seropositive often reactivate EBV, and about 60% shed virus. The source of virus may be parotid gland cells.

Clinical Manifestations. The incubation period of infectious mononucleosis in young adults is 30–50 days. In children it may be shorter, but solid data are lacking. The onset is usually insidious and vague. The patient may complain of malaise, fatigue, headache, nausea, or abdominal pain. This prodromal period may last 1–2 wk. The complaints of sore throat and fever gradually increase until the patient seeks medical care. The sore throat is often accompanied by moderate to severe pharyngitis with marked tonsillar enlargement and even with exudates (Fig 10–26 [p. xxxiii]). The throat may resemble that of streptococcal pharyngitis, and the throat culture may be positive, but this phenomenon reflects the ubiquity of inapparent streptococcal infection in normal populations. An enanthem consisting of petechiae at the junction of hard and soft palate is frequently seen. Fever is present in about 85% of patients and is usually in the moderate range, about 39° C (102° F).

The characteristic signs, aside from sore throat, are lymphadenopathy and hepatosplenomegaly. The posterior cervical nodes are most often enlarged, but other groups are also affected. Epitrochlear lymphadenopathy is particularly consistent with infectious mononucleosis. The liver is enlarged in only about a third of patients, but elevations of enzymes signifying anicteric hepatitis occur in 80%; frank jaundice, much less common, is seen in only about 5%. Splenomegaly is found in about half of patients, though extension to 2–3 cm below the costal margin, rather than massive enlargement, is the rule. On the other hand, splenic enlargement may be rapid enough to cause left upper quadrant discomfort and tenderness, which may be the presenting complaint.

Other clinical findings include edema of the eyelids and rashes. Rashes are usually maculopapular and have been reported in from 3–15% of patients. An interesting facet of the skin manifestations is that 80% of patients with infectious mononucleosis will develop a rash if treated with ampicillin. The reason for this phenomenon is unknown.

The severe symptoms usually last 2–4 wk, followed by gradual recovery. Fatigue, malaise, and some disability are common complaints for several mo. Chronic infectious mononucleosis with persistently elevated EB virus antibody titers has been described, but fatigue without evident explanation is more common. Second attacks of infectious mononucleosis caused by EB virus have not been serologically documented. The prognosis for complete recovery is excellent if none of the severe complications described below ensue.

Symptomatic infection with EB virus is more common in children than is generally believed. The disease may be clinically quite similar to that in older individuals, including development of heterophil antibodies. On the other hand, identification of current infections by viral serology (see below) has demonstrated that children may show less specific symptoms, such as tonsillitis, fever of unknown origin, or acute undifferentiated respiratory disease. The younger the child, the less typical the symptoms are likely to be, particularly hepatosplenomegaly and lymphadenopathy. Atypical lymphocytes are usually present. Occasionally, EB virus antibodies may develop late; therefore rises in titer may need to be shown by collection of convalescent sera. Because heterophil antibody titers tend to be lower under the age of 5 yr, slide agglutination tests may be negative. Under the age of 2 yr the great majority of primary EBV infections remain silent.

Oncogenic Activity of EB Virus. EB virus is almost certainly a cofactor in the induction of Burkitt lymphoma (BL) in Africa and nasopharyngeal carcinoma (NPC) in Chinese populations. BL is found in restricted areas of tropical Africa, below certain elevations that correspond with the distribution of malarial parasites. It is a type of lymphoma, often of the jaw, that has a median onset age of 5 yr. A large prospective study in Uganda revealed that children who later developed BL had high preceding titers of anti–EB virus viral capsid antigen (VCA) antibodies.

NPC is mainly a disease of adults in which the involved cells are nasopharyngeal epithelium; it occurs at a very high rate only in Southeast Asia and among Eskimos. Cases also occasionally occur in children 10–18 yr old. Despite the fact that environmental cofactors for BL and NPC undoubtedly are necessary in addition to infection, the demonstration of EB virus genome in BL and NPC tumor cells and the induction of lymphomas by EB virus in New World monkeys provide compelling evidence that EB virus is a cause of certain cancers.

Complications. The most feared complication of infectious mononucleosis is splenic rupture, which is said to occur most frequently during the 2nd wk of the disease. Rupture is commonly related to trauma, often mild, including medical palpation. Swelling of the tonsils and pharynx may be so severe as to cause respiratory occlusion. Use of corticosteroids in impending obstruction may avert the need for tracheostomy. Neurologic involvement is more common than usually appreciated, and more serious. Convulsions, ataxia, and nuchal rigidity may be the 1st signs of disease. There may be meningitis with mononuclear cells in the cerebrospinal fluid, Bell palsy, transverse myelitis, encephalitis, or Guillain-Barré syndrome. The latter may produce complete paralysis and death, at times in the absence of other signs of infectious mononucleosis. Perceptual distortions of space and size, referred to as the "Alice in Wonderland" syndrome, may be a presenting symptom. Myocarditis and interstitial pneumonia are common complications, both resolving in 3–4 wk. A hemolytic anemia, often with a positive Coombs test and with cold agglutinins specific for red cell antigen i, may occur late in the illness. Thrombocytopenic purpura and even aplastic anemia may develop and confuse the diagnosis. Rare complications include pancreatitis, parotitis, and orchitis. Hepatitis is so common that it is considered part of the disease. Reye syndrome may occur in the wake of the disease. Severe, persistent, and sometimes fatal EB virus infection has been identified in patients with familial, genetic disorders of the lymphoid system. These patients die either of disseminated lymphoproliferation (perhaps an exaggerated T-cell response) involving multiple organs or of malignant lymphomas. Rare cases of fatal disseminated infection have also been reported in previously immunocompetent hosts who develop lymphopenia during the disease.

Diagnosis. Confirmation of the diagnosis of infectious mononucleosis by laboratory means has now become more precise.

Originally, the diagnosis could be made only on the basis of atypical lymphocytosis. Indeed, in more than 90% of cases there is leukocytosis of 10,000–20,000 cells/mm³, of which at least two thirds are lymphocytes; atypical forms usually account for 20–40% of the total number. The atypical cells are large with irregular shape and staining properties. They are T cells, apparently responding to the presence of infected B cells. Mild thrombocytopenia (50,000–200,000/mm³) occurs in no fewer than 50% of patients, but only the rare case has values low enough to cause purpura.

The well-known serologic test for infectious mononucleosis has been the Paul-Bunnell-Davidsohn test for sheep red blood cell agglutination. This test is based on the fact that numerous abnormal antibodies are found in persons with infectious mononucleosis, including those directed against antigens from animal tissues. The antibody specific for infectious mononucleosis is in the IgM class. In order to distinguish the heterophil antibodies of infectious mononucleosis from others, serum is tested for sheep red blood cell agglutination before and after absorption with ox red blood cells or guinea pig kidney cell suspension. In infectious mononucleosis the antibody titers to sheep red blood cells remain after guinea pig kidney absorption but disappear after ox cell absorption. Titers greater than 1:28 or 1:40 (depending on the dilution system used) after absorption with guinea pig cells are considered positive. Many laboratories prefer to use horse rather than sheep red blood cells because of greater sensitivity.

Other popular tests for heterophil antibodies use formalin-treated horse or sheep red blood cells for a rapid slide agglutination with commercially produced reagents. When the clinical situation is atypical, the slide test should be confirmed by the differential heterophil tube agglutination test.

Whereas the sheep red blood cell agglutination test is likely to be positive only for several mo, the horse red blood cell agglutination test may be positive for as long as 2 yr. The accuracy of heterophil tests in children has been a subject of controversy. In fact, mild or inapparent EB virus infections in adults may be heterophil negative, and it is perhaps on this basis, rather than inability of children to produce heterophil antibody, that heterophil tests may be negative. Children with typical infectious mononucleosis will have positive tests, but those under age 5 are more likely to be negative or to have lower titers than adults, and sensitive tests for heterophil antibodies are necessary for optimal results.

With the discovery that EB virus causes infectious mononucleosis, specific tests became available to diagnose the disease even in the absence of heterophil antibodies. The serologic tests for EB virus must be understood in the context of the structure of the virus particle. Replication of complete particles begins in the nucleus of infected cells, and virions then pass into the cytoplasm. The viral nucleocapsid can be detected by immunofluorescence. If a patient's serum is applied to fixed-cell smears of lymphoblastoid cell lines infected with EB virus, followed by exposure to fluorescein-conjugated, antihuman IgG or antihuman IgM, antibodies of either class may be determined by fluorescent staining of the infected cells. IgG antibody to VCA is usually present in a titer greater than 1:160 at the time of acute disease. In addition, VCA-specific IgM antibodies are present in all cases when tested at the appropriate time, but may occasionally be missed since the IgM response is not long lasting. IgM antibody remains in evidence for 2–3 mo.

Some lymphoblast lines do not produce viral capsid antigen or early antigens, but if these lines are superinfected with EB virus, antigens are produced in the nucleus and cytoplasm by abortive infection. These have been termed early antigens because during lytic infection they precede synthesis of viral particles. Antibodies to early antigens are found during the acute stage of infectious mononucleosis in about 80% of cases. Curiously, the "D," or diffuse-staining, pattern is found predominantly in infectious mononucleosis, whereas another staining pattern ("R," or restricted to the cytoplasm) is present in high titer in many sera from patients with Burkitt lymphoma and also at low titers during primary infection in infants below the age of 2 yr whose infection is silent. Antibody to the D component of early antigens is a marker of current infection and disappears after several mo in infectious mononucleosis. It may also be found in patients with nasopharyngeal carcinoma or some lymphomas, including Burkitt lymphoma.

The last serologic test useful at present for diagnosis is that for EBNA (EB nuclear antigen) antibodies. EB nuclear antigen is produced in every lymphoblast carrying EB viral genomes and is detected only by anticomplement immunofluorescence. Antibody will attach to the antigen and fix complement, which can then be detected by fluorescent antibody to complement. Antibody to EB nuclear antigen is the last to appear in

Table 10–38 EB VIRUS ANTIBODIES IN VARIOUS SITUATIONS

	Anti-VCA-IgG	Anti-VCA-IgM	Anti-EA(D)	Anti-EBNA
No previous infection	0	0	0	0
Acute infection	+	+	+/0	0
Recent infection	+	±	+/0	±
Past infection	+	0	0	+

0 = <10 or <2 for EBNA; + = ≥10 or ≥2 for EBNA; EA(D) = early antigen diffuse-staining; EBNA = Epstein-Barr nuclear antigen; VCA-IgG = viral capsid antigen immunoglobulin G; VCA-IgM = viral capsid antigen–specific immunoglobulin M.

infectious mononucleosis; thus, its absence when other antiodies are present implies recent infection, while its presence implies infection at least several wk previously. Table 10–38 and Fig 10–27 summarize the combinations of antibodies that would be expected in various situations.

EB virus can be demonstrated in the nasopharyngeal secretions of patients by its capacity to transform cord blood lymphocytes in vitro, a test which requires so much time that isolation is not clinically useful.

Differential Diagnosis. The patient with atypical lymphocytosis, lymphadenopathy, hepatosplenomegaly, and a positive heterophil test presents no problems in diagnosis. If a clinical picture suggestive of infectious mononucleosis is present but the heterophil tests are negative, 4 conditions should be given 1st consideration: EB virus infection without heterophil antibody response, cytomegaloviral infection, toxoplasmosis, and infectious hepatitis (hepatitis A). All 4 can be identified by serologic tests, including those for EB virus, and virus isolation. Cytomegalovirus is a particularly common cause of infectious mononucleosis–like illness with negative heterophil tests.

Other conditions which occasionally cause confusion are mumps, adenoviral disease, rubella, and streptococcal sore throat because of facial edema, lymphadenopathy, rash, and positive throat culture, respectively.

Throat cultures for streptococci may be positive in infectious mononucleosis but no more so than in any random population. Failure of a patient with "strep throat" to improve within 48 hr should evoke suspicion of infectious mononucleosis.

The most serious problem in diagnosis arises in the occasional case with low white blood cell counts, moderate thrombocytopenia, and even hemolytic anemia. In these cases bone marrow examination and hematologic consultation are warranted to rule out leukemia. Atypical lymphocytes may be found in cytomegaloviral infection, toxoplasmosis, infectious hepatitis, malaria, tuberculosis, typhoid, and mycoplasmal infection.

Treatment. There is no specific treatment for infectious mononucleosis, although the antiviral acyclovir is currently being studied. Short courses (under 14 days) of corticosteroids are useful in the event of pharyngotonsillar edema threatening to obstruct the airway, in hepatitis, or in severe abdominal pain due to splenomegaly or lymphadenopathy. Longer courses may be tried in hemolytic anemia or Guillain-Barré syndrome, but steroids should not be used in the average case of infectious mononucleosis.

Withdrawal from athletic activity is indicated while splenomegaly is present, but bed rest is necessary only when the patient is toxic. As soon as there is definite improvement, the patient should be allowed to begin resuming normal activities.

If group A streptococci are found in the throat, penicillin is the drug of choice except when there has been an allergic manifestation or a history of allergy.

Prognosis. If the rare occurrence of splenic rupture, severe central nervous system complications, or severe hemolytic anemia does not cause death in the acute period, the prognosis is uniformly good for recovery. Recrudescence of illness during the 1st yr does occur, and fatigue is often present for months after the acute illness. On the whole, however, the patient should be strongly reassured of eventual complete recovery.

STANLEY A. PLOTKIN
WERNER HENLE

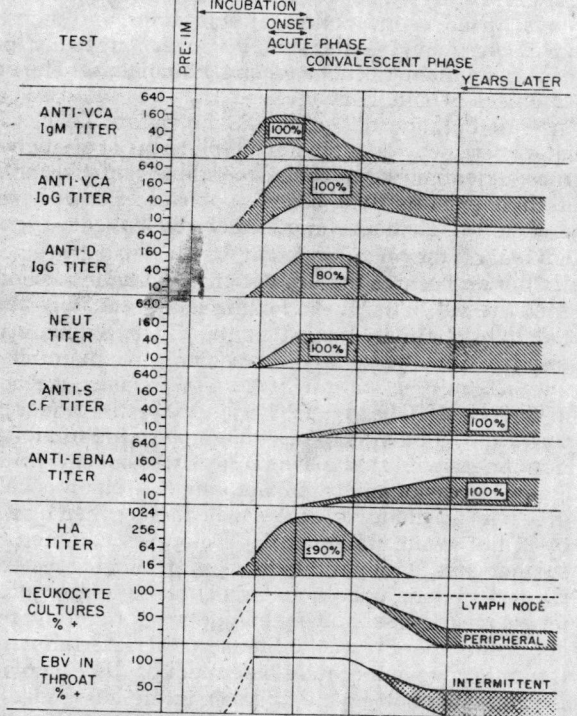

Figure 10–27 Scheme of antibody responses, leukocyte cultures, and EB virus assays in throat washings during the course of infectious mononucleosis. C.F. = complement fixing; D = diffuse-staining early antigen; EBNA = Epstein-Barr nuclear antigen; EBV = Epstein-Barr virus; H.A. = heterophile antibody; IM = infectious mononucleosis; NEUT. = neutralizing antibody; S = soluble complement-fixing antigen (probably identical with EBNA); VCA = viral capsid antigen.

Biggar RJ, Henle G, Böcker J, et al: Primary Epstein-Barr virus infections in African infants. II. Clinical and serological observations during seroconversion. Int J Cancer 22:244, 1980.

Evans AS, Niederman JC, Cenabre LC, et al: A prospective evaluation of heterophile and Epstein-Barr virus–specific IgM antibody titers in clinical and subclinical infectious mononucleosis: Specificity and sensitivity of the tests and persistence of antibody. J Infect Dis 132:546, 1975.

Fleisher G, Lennette ET, Henle G, et al: Incidence of heterophil antibody responses in children with infectious mononucleosis. J Pediatr 94:723, 1979.

Henle G, Henle W: The virus as the etiologic agent of infectious mononucleosis. In: Epstein AM, Achong BG (eds): The Epstein-Barr Virus. New York, Springer Verlag, 1979, p 61.

Henle W, Henle G, Horwitz CA: Epstein-Barr virus–specific diagnostic tests in infectious mononucleosis. Hum Pathol 5:551, 1974.

Miller G: Epstein-Barr herpesvirus and infectious mononucleosis. Prog Med Virol 20:84, 1975.

Naegele RF, Champion J, Murphy S, et al: Nasopharyngeal carcinoma in American children: Epsteen-Barr virus–specific antibody titers and prognosis. Int J Cancer 29:209, 1982.

Niederman JC, Evans AS, Subramanyan MS, et al: Prevalence, incidence and persistence of EB virus antibody in young adults. N Engl J Med 282:361, 1970.

10.77 MUMPS
(Epidemic Parotitis)

Mumps is an acute, contagious, generalized viral disease in which painful enlargement of the salivary glands, chiefly the parotids, is the usual presenting sign.

Etiology. The viral origin was firmly established by Johnson and Goodpasture in 1934. The virus is a member of the paramyxovirus group. In addition to mumps this group includes the parainfluenza and Newcastle disease viruses. The virus particle contains single-stranded RNA enclosed in an envelope of protein and lipid. The envelope contains a hemagglutinin, a neuraminidase, and a hemolysin. There is only 1 known serotype. Primary cultures of human or monkey kidney cells are used for viral isolation. Sometimes cytopathic effect is observed, but hemadsorption is the most sensitive indicator of infection. Virus has been isolated from saliva, cerebrospinal fluid, blood, urine, brain, and other infected tissues of patients with mumps.

Epidemiology. Mumps is endemic in most urban populations; the virus is spread from a human reservoir by direct contact, airborne droplet nuclei, fomites contaminated by infectious saliva, and, possibly, by urine. It has a worldwide distribution and affects both sexes equally; 85% of the infections occur in children under the age of 15 yr. Epidemics occur at all seasons of the year, although they are slightly more frequent in the late winter and spring. The source of infection may be difficult to trace because 30–40% of infections are subclinical.

It is uncertain how long a patient may be infectious, but virus has been isolated from saliva as long as 6 days before and up to 9 days after the appearance of salivary gland swelling. Under usual conditions, however, transmission does not seem to occur longer than 24 hr before the appearance of the swelling or later than 3 days after it has subsided. Virus has been isolated from the urine from the 1st–14th day after the onset of salivary gland swelling.

Lifelong immunity is usually produced by any type of clinical or subclinical infection, although 2nd infections have been documented occasionally. Transplacental antibodies seem to be effective in protecting infants during the 1st 6–8 mo of life. Infants born to mothers who have mumps in the week prior to delivery may have clinically apparent mumps at birth or develop illness in the neonatal period. Severity ranges from mild parotitis to severe pneumonia. The serum neutralization test is the most reliable method for determination of immunity but is cumbersome and expensive. A complement-fixing antibody test is available (see Diagnosis). The presence of V antibodies alone suggests previous mumps infection.

A mumps skin test antigen is no longer available commercially; it was of questionable value.

Pathogenesis. After entry and initial multiplication in the cells of the respiratory tract, the virus is bloodborne to many tissues, of which salivary and other glands seem to be the most susceptible. The swelling of the infected structures is probably the result of a hypersensitivity reaction to the locally multiplying virus.

Pathology. Little information is available about the lesions caused by mumps in the human patient. In a parotid from which the virus was isolated 70 hr after onset of the disease, the acini were well preserved, but there was periductal edema and lymphocytic infiltration extending slightly into the connective tissue. The main damage occurred in the ducts, ranging from slight epithelial swelling with a few polymorphonuclear cells in the lumen to complete desquamation of the epithelium and dilated lumens choked with debris. Cytoplasmic swelling was observed in some epithelial cells, but only rarely did one contain a large basophilic inclusion body. Other studies of parotid glands from patients with clinical mumps without viral isolation confirmed these general findings, although in some instances damage to the acini was observed. Changes in testes, when biopsies were taken within a day or 2 after onset of pain, have varied from mild interstitial edema and no disturbance of spermatogenesis in the majority of instances to focal destruction of epithelium with extensive perivascular lymphocytic cuffing. The basic injury appeared to be vascular; irregular hemorrhages occurred in the more severe infections. Even in these, however, areas of normal germinal epithelium could be seen.

Clinical Manifestations. The incubation period ranges from 14–24 days, with a peak incidence at 17–18 days. In children prodromal symptoms and signs are rare, but may be manifest by fever, muscular pain, especially in the neck, headache, and malaise. The onset of illness is usually characterized by pain and swelling in 1 or both parotid glands. The parotid swells in a characteristic way; it begins by filling the space between the posterior border of the mandible and the mastoid and then extends in a series of crescents downward and forward, being limited above by the zygoma. Edema of the skin and soft tissues usually extends further and obscures the limit of the glandular swelling with the result that the swelling is more readily appreciated by sight than by palpation. The swelling may proceed extremely rapidly, reaching a maximum size within a few hr, although the peak is usually reached in 1–3 days. The swollen tissues push the ear lobe upward and outward, and the angle of the mandible is no longer visible. The swelling slowly subsides within 3–7 days; occasionally it lasts longer. Usually swelling of 1 parotid gland precedes that of the other by a day or 2, but swelling limited to 1 gland is common. The swollen area is tender and painful, pain being especially elicited by tasting sour liquids such as lemon juice or vinegar. Redness and swelling are commonly noted about the opening of the Stensen duct. Accompanying the parotid swelling may be edema of the homolateral pharynx and soft palate, displacing the tonsil medially; acute edema of the larynx has been described. Edema over the manubrium and upper chest wall may be found, probably due to lymphatic obstruction. The parotid swelling is usually accompanied by moderate fever, but normal temperatures are common (20%) and temperatures of 40° C (104° F) or over are rare; no correlation exists between extent of swelling and degree of fever.

Although the parotid glands alone are affected in the majority of patients, swelling of the submandibular glands occurs frequently and usually accompanies or closely follows that of the parotid glands. In 10–15% of patients, however, only the submandibular gland(s) may be swollen. This swelling follows 2 patterns: the more common is an ovoid enlargement extending forward and downward from the angle of the mandible; in the other, the enlargement extends more directly downward in a half-egg shape. The deep portion of the gland is only rarely affected. Little pain is associated with the submandibular infection, but the swelling subsides more slowly than that of the parotids. Redness and swelling at the orifice of the Wharton duct frequently accompany swelling of the gland.

Least commonly the sublingual glands are infected, usually bilaterally; the swelling is evident in the submental region and in the floor of the mouth.

Complications. Viremia early in the infection probably accounts for the widespread complications, which are mainly manifestations of mumps infection in organs other than the salivary glands.

Meningoencephalomyelitis. This is the most frequent complication in childhood. The true incidence is hard to estimate because subclinical infection of the central nervous system, as evidenced by pleocytosis in the cerebrospinal fluid, has been reported in over 65% of patients with parotitis. Clinical manifestations have been reported in over 10% of patients. The reported incidence of mumps meningoencephalitis is approximately 250/100,000 cases; 10% of these cases occurred in patients over 20 yr old. The mortality rate is about 2%. Males are affected 3–5 times as frequently as females. Mumps is one of the most common causes of aseptic meningitis.

The pathogenesis of mumps meningoencephalitis has been described as both a primary infection of neurons by virus and a postinfectious encephalitis with demyelination. In the 1st type, parotitis frequently appears at the same time or following the onset of encephalitis. In the latter type, encephalitis follows parotitis by an average of 10 days. Parotitis may, in some cases, be absent. Mumps has been implicated as a possible etiologic agent in the production of aqueductal stenosis and hydrocephalus in children. Injection of mumps virus into suckling hamsters has produced similar lesions.

Meningoencephalitis begins typically with a rise in temperature, headache, vomiting, irritability, and, occasionally, a convulsion. This clinical picture is indistinguishable from meningoencephalitis of other origins. Moderate stiffness of the neck is seen, but the remainder of the neurologic examination is usually normal. Occasionally neck, shoulder, and leg weakness, resembling paralytic poliomyelitis, occurs. The CSF usually contains fewer than 500 cells/mm³, although occasionally the count may exceed 2000. The cells are almost exclusively lymphocytes, in contrast to enteroviral aseptic meningitis, in which polymorphonuclear leukocytes often predominate early in the disease. The CSF glucose level is normal. Protein is slightly elevated. Mumps virus can be isolated from the CSF early in the illness.

Orchitis, Epididymitis. These lesions rarely occur in prepubescent boys but are common (14–35%) in adolescents and adults. The testis is most often infected with or without epididymitis, or epididymitis may occur alone. Rarely, there is a hydrocele. The orchitis usually follows parotitis within 8 days but sometimes is delayed, and it may occur without evidence of salivary gland infection. In about 30% of patients with orchitis, both testes are affected. The onset is usually abrupt, with a rise in temperature, chills, headache, nausea, and lower abdominal pain; when the right testis is implicated, appendicitis may appear to be a diagnostic possibility. The affected testis becomes tender and swollen and the adjacent skin edematous and red. The average duration is 4 days. As the swelling subsides, the testis loses its normal turgor; approximately 30–40% of affected testes atrophy. Impairment of fertility is estimated to be about 13%, but absolute infertility is probably rare.

Oophoritis. Pelvic pain and tenderness are noted in about 7% of postpubertal female patients. There is no evidence of impairment of fertility.

Pancreatitis. Severe involvement of the pancreas is rare, but mild or subclinical infection may be more common than is recognized. It may be unassociated with salivary gland manifestations and be misdiagnosed as gastroenteritis. Epigastric pain and tenderness are suggestive; these may be accompanied by fever, chills, vomiting, and prostration. An elevated serum amylase value is characteristically present in any patient with mumps, with or without clinical manifestation of pancreatitis. Serum lipase determination may be helpful. The possibility that diabetes mellitus may be an infrequent sequel is being investigated.

Nephritis. Viruria has been reported frequently. In 1 study of adults, abnormal renal function was observed at some time in every patient, and viruria was present in 75%. The frequency of renal involvement in children is unknown. Fatal nephritis, occurring 10–14 days after parotitis, has been reported.

Thyroiditis. Although uncommon in children, a diffuse, tender swelling of the thyroid may occur about 1 wk after the onset of parotitis and has been followed by the development of antithyroid antibodies.

Myocarditis. Serious cardiac manifestations are extremely rare, but mild infection of the myocardium is probably more common and overlooked. In 1 series of adults, electrocardiographic tracings revealed changes, mostly depression of the S-T segment, in 13%. Such involvement could explain the precordial pain, bradycardia, and fatigue sometimes noted among adolescents and adults with mumps.

Mastitis. This is an uncommon occurrence in both male and female patients.

Deafness. Unilateral, or rarely bilateral, nerve deafness may occur after mumps; although the incidence is low (1:15,000), mumps is considered a leading cause of unilateral nerve deafness. The onset may be sudden or gradual. Hearing loss may be transient or permanent.

Ocular Complications. These include *dacryoadenitis,*

painful swelling of the lacrimal glands, which is usually bilateral; *optic neuritis (papillitis)* with symptoms varying from loss of vision to mild blurring and with recovery in 10–20 days; *uveokeratitis,* usually unilateral, with photophobia, tearing, rapid loss of vision, and recovery within 20 days; *scleritis; tenonitis* with resultant exophthalmos; and *central vein thrombosis.*

Arthritis. Arthralgia associated with swelling and redness of the joints is an infrequent complication which appears 12–14 days after the onset of parotitis; complete recovery is the rule.

Thrombocytopenic purpura follows mumps on occasion, as it does other infections.

Mumps Embryopathy. There is no firm evidence that maternal infection with mumps leads to any damage to the developing fetus; a possible relation to endocardial fibroelastosis has been postulated but not established. Mumps in early pregnancy increases the chance of spontaneous abortion.

Diagnosis. The diagnosis of mumps parotitis is usually readily apparent from the symptoms and physical examination. When the clinical manifestations are limited to those of 1 of the less common lesions, the diagnosis is not so clear but may be suspected, especially during an epidemic. The routine laboratory tests are nonspecific; there is usually leukopenia with relative lymphocytosis, but complications often result in polymorphonuclear leukocytosis of moderate degree. An elevation of serum amylase is found in most patients with mumps; the rise, paralleling the parotid swelling, reaches its peak in 1 wk and generally returns to normal over the course of the next 2 wk. The etiologic diagnosis depends on isolation of the virus from the saliva, urine, spinal fluid, or blood or the demonstration of a significant rise in circulating CF antibodies during convalescence. Serum antibodies to the S antigen reach their peak early in about 75% of patients and are detectable at the time of the presenting symptoms. They gradually disappear within 6–12 mo; antibodies against the V or viral antigen usually reach a peak titer in about 1 mo, remain stationary for about 6 mo, and then slowly decline over the ensuing 2 yr to a low level, at which they persist. The presence of a high anti-S titer and a low anti-V titer during the acute stage of an otherwise undiagnosed meningoencephalitis, for example, would be strongly suggestive of a mumps infection, which would be confirmed if a convalescent serum (taken 14–21 days later) revealed a 4-fold rise of anti-V antibodies with little change in the titer of anti-S antibodies.

Differential Diagnosis. This includes *parotitis* of other origin, as in the rare instances of coxsackievirus A and lymphocytic choriomeningitis infections, which can be distinguished only by specific laboratory tests; *suppurative parotitis,* in which pus can often be expressed from the duct; *recurrent parotitis,* a condition of unknown origin, but possibly allergic in nature, which has frequent recurrences and a characteristic sialogram; *salivary calculus,* obstructing either a parotid or, more commonly, a submandibular duct, in which the swelling is intermittent; *preauricular* or *anterior cervical lymphadenitis* from any cause; *lymphosarcoma* or other rare *tumors* of the parotid; *orchitis due to infections other than mumps,* e.g., the rare infections by coxsackievirus A or lymphocytic choriomeningitis viruses; and *parotitis due to cytomegalovirus* in immunocompromised children.

Treatment. This is entirely symptomatic. Bed rest should be guided by the patient's needs; there is no statistical evidence that it prevents complications. The diet should be adjusted to the ability of the patient to chew. The headache of meningoencephalitis may be relieved by a lumbar puncture. Orchitis should be treated with local support and bed rest.

Prophylaxis. Passive. Hyperimmune mumps gamma globulin is available but is not effective in preventing mumps or decreasing complications.

Active. A live, attenuated mumps virus vaccine has been developed (Mumpsvax [Merck, Sharp & Dohme]). It is given subcutaneously to children over the age of 15 mo. Vaccinated children usually do not develop fever or other detectable clinical reactions. They do not excrete virus and are not contagious to susceptible contacts. Rarely, parotitis can develop 7–10 days after vaccination. The vaccine induces antibody in about 96% of seronegative recipients. The antibody level produced is about one fifth of that achieved after natural infection, but a protective efficacy of about 97% against natural mumps infection has been demonstrated. The protection afforded by the vaccine appears to be long lasting. In 1 outbreak of mumps, several children who had been immunized with mumps vaccine in the past developed an illness characterized by fever, malaise, nausea, and a red papular rash involving the trunk and extremities but sparing palms and soles. The rash lasted about 24 hr. No virus was isolated from these children, but antibody titer rises to mumps were demonstrated.

CAROL F. PHILLIPS

Bistrian B, et al: Fatal mumps meningoencephalitis. JAMA 222:478, 1972.
Brunell PA, et al: Ineffectiveness of isolation of patients as a method of preventing the spread of mumps. Failure of the mumps skin-test antigen to predict immune status. N Engl J Med 279:1357, 1968.
Quast U, Hennessen W, Widmark RM: Vaccine induced mumps-like disease. Develop Biol Standard 43:269, 1979.

10.78 · INFLUENZA VIRAL INFECTIONS

Although influenza had the dubious distinction of having, in 1 epidemic, the greatest morbidity and mortality of all time, its role in pediatric infections is frequently given less attention than that of other respiratory viruses. This pediatric complacency in regard to influenza viral infections is unfortunate because the morbidity and mortality in children are significant and the spectrum of illness is protean.

Influenza Viruses. Influenza viruses are relatively large RNA viruses classified as *orthomyxoviruses.* There are 3 broad serologic types (A, B, and C), determined by the complement-fixing property of the ribonucleo protein component (S antigen) of the virus. The outer (glycoprotein) surface of influenza viruses contain spikelike projections which are responsible for antigenic characteristics that determine subtypes. On influenza A and B viruses the spikelike projections contain specific hemagglutinins and neuraminidase. The neuraminidase antigen has not been found on type C viral strains. Type A viruses were originally classified in 1933 on the basis of differences in their hemagglutinins. In 1972 a revised nomenclature system was put into use which more completely identified influenza A strains by the serologic study of both hemagglutinin and neuraminidase antigens. This system included a description of ribonucleoprotein (A, B, or C); the host of origin if isolated from nonhuman animals (equine, avian, swine); geographical origin, strain number, year of isolation; and, for influenza A strains, an index describing hemagglutinin and neuraminidase subtypes. By this classification the following hemagglutinin-neuraminidase subtypes were associated with human disease: Hsw1N1, H0N1, H1N1, H2N2, H3N2. In addition, various combinations of 9 hemagglutinins and 7 neuraminidases have been noted in nonhuman animal infections. In 1980 the hemagglutinin-neuraminidase classification system was again revised because Hsw1, H0, and H1 subtypes were found to be sufficiently related to be grouped together. The new nomenclature lists 12 hemagglutinins (H1 to H12) and 9 neuraminidases (N1 to N9) without indicating animal source. Although antigenic variation occurs among influenza B viruses, formal subclassification utilizing neuraminidase antigens has not been done. Influenza A viruses are subject to 2 types of change: frequent minor antigenic changes are called antigenic "drift"; less frequent major changes are referred to as antigenic "shift." The most recent sustained shift in influenza A virus occurred in 1968 when A/Hong Kong/68 (H3N2) appeared. Since 1968 several drifts in the antigenic character of the virus have been observed (A/England/72, A/Port Chalmers/74, A/Victoria/75, A/Texas/77, and A/Bangkok/79). Studies done during the 1960's and early 1970's suggested that major changes (shifts) in influenza A viruses causing human disease were cyclic; when a shift occurred, the previous viral subtype disappeared from circulation. Serologic evidence indicated that H3N2 viruses similar to those prevalent today were previously in circulation from 1902–1917. Viruses of the H2N2 make-up were prevalent from 1890–1901 and 1957–1968. If the pattern of cyclic recurrence were to continue, the next antigenic shift would lead to the circulation of H1N1 viral subtypes similar to those prevalent from 1918–1956.

In the late fall of 1977 the apparently expected shift of the influenza A subtype apparently occurred. In early 1978 epidemics of influenza due to an H1N1 serotype (A/USSR/77) occurred in many areas of the world. However, in contrast to predictions based upon past experiences, H3N2 influenza serotypes did not disappear but continued to cause epidemic disease. Since 1977 both H1N1 and H3N2 viral serotypes have remained in human circulation and have caused epidemic disease.

Antigenic drift is the result of point mutation. Selective pressure in an immune population results in the emergence of mutant viral strains with altered antigenic determinants; this drift allows a growth advantage in the presence of antibody. Considerable evidence suggests that antigenic shift may arise by recombination between human and animal influenza viruses during chance simultaneous infections.

Influenza B strains undergo antigenic drift; antigenic shift has not been demonstrated.

Epidemiology. Severe pandemic influenza A resulting from antigenic shift occurs every 10–40 yr. Once a pandemic involving a new subtype of influenza A has occurred, epidemics of generally lesser intensity occur every 2–3 yr in association with antigenic drift. Major outbreaks of influenza B are more variable but tend to occur at 4–7 yr intervals. Antibody studies reveal that virtually all children have experience with influenza C virus by age 10 yr. However, epidemiologic patterns of this virus have not been determined. In a large urban area there is generally some influenza viral activity each yr.

Influenza viruses have no geographic restrictions. In temperate climates epidemics usually occur at times of cooler weather; in the tropics epidemic disease usually occurs during the rainy season.

Following the appearance of a new subtype of influenza A, the highest incidence of disease occurs in children 5–14 yr old, with an attack rate approaching 50%. In subsequent outbreaks with variants (drifts) of the same subtype, the attack rate in children of similar age drops to about 15%. In outbreaks of influenza B, the attack rate is generally higher in children than in adults.

Respiratory secretions of infected children contain large amounts of virus, and infection is transmitted directly from person to person by the airborne route. Virus shedding and presumably transmissibility correlate directly with the severity of illness.

Pathology. Data are limited about uncomplicated influenza in children. The main site of cellular involvement is the mucous membrane of the respiratory tract, showing extensive destruction of the ciliated epithelium. Influenza uncomplicated by secondary bacterial infection reveals marked desquamation of the tracheal epithelium as early as the 1st day after onset of symptoms. Cellular infiltration with lymphocytes, histiocytes, plasma cells, eosinophils, and polymorphonuclear leukocytes occurs but to a lesser degree than might be expected on the basis of the extensive epithelial necrosis. Repair of the epithelium begins between the 3rd–5th days, as indicated by mitoses in the surviving basal cells. A pseudometaplastic response of undifferentiated epithelium up to 8 cell layers thick occurs and reaches its maximum 9–15 days after onset of the infection. After 15 days cilia and mucus production reappear. With secondary bacterial involvement there is extensive inflammatory cell infiltration and destruction of the basal cell layer and basement membrane, with consequent delay in regeneration of the ciliated epithelium.

In children dying of pneumonia the pulmonary findings have included peribronchiolar lymphocytic infiltration with mucus and cellular debris plugging the small bronchioles, necrosis of bronchiolar epithelium, and marked lymphocytic infiltration of the alveolar walls and interstitial lung tissue.

Although the main pathology in influenza lies in the

respiratory tract, the heart, brain, and lymphoid tissues are occasionally involved in fatal cases. Toxic, focal, and diffuse forms of myocarditis have been noted. Cerebral edema has been the most common central nervous system finding at autopsy. The lymph nodes of the tracheobronchial tree show extensive changes, including necrosis and disorganization of the germinal follicles.

Pathogenesis and Immunity. The usual incubation period is 2–3 days. The common distribution of the virus occurs in the respiratory tract, but in unusual instances viremia, viruria, and isolation of virus from other extrapulmonary tissues have been noted. Immunity has been shown to correlate better with secretory (IgA) nasal antibody than with circulating antibody, but high titers of serum antibody are usually protective.

Following natural infection with an influenza A virus, protection against reinfection and illness with the particular viral subtype, even though antigenic drift may have occurred, lasts for several yr. However, subclinical reinfections are common; these tend to broaden the antibody coverage and allow continued protection from disease.

When antigenic shift occurs with an influenza A virus, the previous influenza A antibody which a child may have is of no protective benefit. The duration of immunity to influenza B infections is less well known but appears quite variable. Although cell-mediated immune mechanisms can be repeatedly demonstrated in association with influenza infections, their role in protection against and recovery from influenza viral infection is not known.

Clinical Manifestations. The predominant manifestations of influenza viral infections are respiratory, although systemic complaints are usually an integral part of the picture. With a few notable exceptions the

Table 10–39 RELATIVE FREQUENCY OF SYMPTOMS AND SIGNS DURING CLASSIC INFLUENZA IN OLDER CHILDREN AND ADOLESCENTS

	Occurrence*
Symptoms	
Chilly sensation	+ + + +
Cough	+ + +
Headache	+ + +
Sore throat	+ + +
Prostration	+ +·
Nasal stuffiness	+ +
Diarrhea	+ +
Dizziness	+
Eye irritation or pain	+
Vomiting	+
Myalgia	+
Signs	
Fever	+ + + +
Pharyngitis	+ + +
Conjunctivitis (mild)	+ +
Rhinitis	+ +
Cervical adenitis	+
Pulmonary rales, wheezes or rhonchi	+

* + + + + = 76% to 100%; + + + = 51% to 75%; + + = 26% to 50%; and + = 1% to 26%.

characteristics of illness with influenza A and B viruses are similar. The clinical manifestations of influenza viral infections can be divided into 2 groups based upon age. In school-age children and adolescents classic influenza (similar to the disease in adults) is the usual picture; the manifestations of infection in young children are much more varied.

The symptoms and signs of classic influenza in older children and adolescents are presented in Table 10–39. The onset of illness is abrupt with fever and associated flushed face, chills, headache, myalgia, and malaise. The temperature range is 39–41° C (102–106° F) with a general inverse correlation with age; the severity of systemic symptoms generally correlates directly with age. Dry cough and coryza are also early manifestations of influenza but go unobserved by the patient because of the severity of the systemic manifestations. Sore throat occurs in over one half of cases and is usually associated with a not otherwise remarkable nonexudative pharyngitis. Ocular symptoms include tearing, photophobia, and burning and pain on eye movement.

The reporting of diarrhea in influenza has varied markedly. Extensive studies during Asian influenza outbreaks in 1957 indicated that diarrhea was uncommon. More recent observations during influenza B and influenza A (H1N1) outbreaks note diarrhea in about one third of the children and adolescents afflicted.

In uncomplicated influenza the fever usually persists for 2–3 days but may last up to 5 days. A biphasic temperature pattern may occur even without apparent secondary bacterial complications. By the 2nd–4th day, respiratory symptoms become more prominent, and the systemic complaints begin to subside. The cough is dry and hacking and usually persists for 4–7 days. Occasionally cough, in association with some degree of general malaise, will persist for 1–2 wk after the rest of the illness has subsided. Illness due to influenza B virus tends to be associated with more prominent nasal and eye complaints and less prominent systemic findings, such as dizziness and prostration, than do influenza A infections.

In uncomplicated classic influenza the leukocyte count is usually normal, but leukopenia (<4500 cells/mm³) has been noted in about 25% of cases. The differential cell count is of no diagnostic value. Approximately 10% of older children and adolescents have clinical signs and roentgenographic evidence of pulmonary involvement.

In younger children the manifestations of influenza viral infections are frequently similar to those resulting from other respiratory viruses (parainfluenza, respiratory syncytial, rhinovirus, and adenovirus) (Table 10–40). Laryngotracheitis, bronchitis, bronchiolitis, pneumonia, and the common cold all occur. Clinical descriptions of these illnesses are presented in Sec 12.54–12.67. Laryngotracheitis resulting from influenza A infection is frequently severe in association with a thick tenacious exudate in the trachea. A greater percentage of children with croup due to influenza A virus will require tracheostomy than children with similar illness resulting from other viral infections.

Illness in the younger child is ushered in with a striking fever, an appearance of moderate toxicity, and

Table 10–40 RELATIVE FREQUENCY OF CLINICAL MANIFESTATIONS OF INFLUENZA VIRAL INFECTIONS IN CHILDREN LESS THAN 5 YEARS OF AGE

	Occurrence*
Major Clinical Category	
Upper respiratory illness	+ + + +
Laryngotracheitis	+
Bronchitis	+
Bronchiolitis	+
Pneumonia	+
Symptoms	
Cough	+ + + +
Anorexia	+ +
Coryza	+ +
Vomiting	+ +
Diarrhea	+
Sore throat	+
Signs	
Fever	+ + + +
Pharyngitis	+ + +
Cervical adenitis	+ +
Otitis media	+ +
Convulsions	+
Exanthem	+
Generalized adenitis	+

* + + + + = 76% to 100%; + + + = 51% to 75%; + + = 26% to 50%; and + = 1% to 25%.

a clear nasal discharge. Febrile convulsions are common, and a surprising number of children will have vomiting. Mild diarrhea occurs in about 15% of cases; otitis media is noted in almost one fourth, and fleeting erythematous, macular, or maculopapular discrete rashes occur frequently.

In the neonate with influenza viral infection, the sudden occurrence of fever is suggestive of bacterial sepsis. However, nasal discharge and other respiratory symptoms appear early so that the viral etiology can be suspected.

Acute myositis, which particularly involves the gastrocnemius and soleus muscles, has been noted in association with influenza B viral infections in children. The myositis has occurred about 1 wk after onset of respiratory symptoms, usually after a brief period of clinical improvement. Acute parotitis has also been noted in association with influenza A viral infection.

Illness due to influenza C viral infection in children has only occasionally been observed. Common cold–like illnesses and typical influenza have been noted.

Diagnosis and Differential Diagnosis. The etiologic diagnosis of a sporadic influenza viral respiratory infection is frequently difficult, but during epidemics it should not be difficult. The main point to consider in separating epidemic influenza from other epidemic respiratory viral infections is that, with influenza, all age groups are clinically involved with febrile illnesses during outbreaks. With other agents, such as respiratory syncytial and parainfluenza viruses, illness in adults is only sporadic and not generally associated with fever.

In properly equipped laboratories the virologic confirmation of influenza viral infection is easy and relatively rapid. The standard method of influenza virus isolation is the inoculation of embryonated eggs and monkey kidney tissue cultures, which frequently allows a result in 72 hr. The direct use of fluorescent antibody procedures on respiratory secretions may provide a diagnosis within 24 hr. Retrospective diagnosis can also be made by study of paired serum samples by complement-fixation or hemagglutination-inhibition antibody techniques.

Complications. Complications occur frequently in influenza viral infections. Many so-called complications are, in actuality, variations of primary viral infection and have been considered above as clinical manifestations (myositis, parotitis, severe croup, etc.). Of most importance from the therapeutic point of view are secondary or superimposed bacterial infections. Otitis media, purulent sinusitis, and pneumonia are common. These complications vary greatly in both prevalence and specific bacterial agents involved from 1 epidemic to another. The common etiologic agents in superinfections are *Streptococcus pneumoniae*, *Hemophilus influenzae*, *Streptococcus pyogenes*, and *Staphylococcus aureus*.

Complications relating directly to the primary viral infection include hemorrhagic pneumonia, encephalitis and other neurologic syndromes, myocarditis, sudden infant death syndrome, and myoglobinuria. Reye syndrome (acute encephalopathy and fatty degeneration of the liver) is most commonly associated with epidemic influenza B viral infection, but recently many cases have occurred after influenza A (H1N1) infections. The pathogenesis is unknown.

Prevention. Immunization with potent and antigenically up-to-date inactivated influenza viral vaccines is safe and effective. However, routine immunization of normal children or adults has not been the recommended policy but has been reserved for persons known to be at particularly high risk for complications. These include the elderly and children with cardiovascular disorders such as rheumatic, congenital, or hypertensive heart disease; with chronic bronchopulmonary disease such as tuberculosis, cystic fibrosis, asthma, and bronchiectasis; with chronic metabolic diseases such as diabetes mellitus; with chronic glomerulonephritis and nephrosis; and with chronic neurologic disorders, especially those associated with weak or paralyzed respiratory muscles. Since the mortality and morbidity of influenza are significant in childhood and children are major contributors to the spread of virus in the community, it may be time to reconsider this approach to immunization. However, there are few data available on the nature of subsequent naturally acquired influenza among children in whom the primary antigenic exposure was to inactivated virus vaccine. Perhaps a more promising approach to the prevention of influenza is the development and use of live vaccines which could be administered by the respiratory route; several candidate live vaccines have been successfully used in adults, and a limited trial in children has shown some promise. Long-term studies which assess risks and benefits of more comprehensive immunization programs involving all segments of the population are needed.

The synthetic antiviral agent amantadine hydrochloride works prophylactically when taken prior to exposure to influenza A viruses. Although this drug is available for use in children, there are only minimal published data supporting its pediatric efficacy and safety. The dose for children 1–9 yr of age is 4 mg/kg/24 hr with a maximum daily dose of 150 mg. For pediatric patients over 9 yr of age, the dose is 200 mg/24 hr.

Treatment. Amantadine hydrochloride is specifically active against influenza A viruses and has been shown to provide therapeutic benefit in adult subjects when given early in the course of illness. The dose is the same as that for prophylaxis mentioned above.

Since morbidity from influenza is frequently the result of cardiorespiratory problems, it is prudent to encourage bed rest in all but the mildest cases. Since pulmonary abnormalities resulting from infection may persist for a greater period of time than fever and other symptoms, it is also wise to insist upon restricted physical activity during convalescence.

Fluid intake should be ensured; antipyretics are indicated for excessive fever. Parents should be advised to use caution when administering aspirin to children with influenza, however, because statistical study has suggested that there may be an association between salicylates and the occurrence of Reye syndrome. During convalescence the judicious use of codeine at bedtime will relieve cough. Although bacterial superinfections are common, prophylactic administration of antibiotics should be discouraged, but vigorous antibiotic therapy following appropriate culture is indicated at the 1st sign of bacterial infection.

Prognosis. Influenza viral infections are common, and the outcome is generally good. The prognosis must be guarded in children with underlying problems which place them in the high-risk category. Anoxia associated with severe laryngotracheitis or pneumonia can result in brain damage. Neurologic complications are frequently but not invariably associated with a poor prognosis.

Brocklebank JT, Court SDM, McQuillin J, et al: Influenza-A infection in children. Lancet 2:497, 1972.

Delorme L, Middleton PJ: Influenza A virus associated with acute encephalopathy. Am J Dis Child 133:822, 1979.

Dykes AC, Cherry JD, Nolan CE: A clinical, epidemiologic, serologic and virologic study of influenza C virus infection. Arch Intern Med 140:1295, 1980.

Eason RJ, Sage MD: Deaths from influenza A, subtype H1N1, during the 1979 Auckland epidemic. NZ Med J 91:129, 1980.

Farrell MK, Partin JC, Bove KE: Epidemic influenza myopathy in Cincinnati in 1977. J Pediatr 96:545, 1980.

Glezen WP: Consideration of the risk of influenza in children and indications for prophylaxis. Rev Inf Dis 2:408, 1980.

Glezen WP, Paredes A, Taber LH: Influenza in children; relationship to other respiratory agents. JAMA 243:1345, 1980.

Hall CB, Douglas RG, Gieman JM, et al: Viral shedding patterns of children with influenza B infection. J Inf Dis 140:610, 1979.

Horn MEC, Brain E, Gregg I, et al: Respiratory viral infection in childhood. A survey in general practice. Roehampton 1967–1972. J Hyg (Camb) 74:157, 1975.

Howard JB, McCracken GH Jr, Luby JP: Influenza A₂ virus as a cause of croup requiring tracheotomy. J Pediatr 81:1148, 1972.

Kim HW, Brandt CD, Arrobio JO, et al: Influenza A and B virus infection in infants and young children during the years 1957–1976. Am J Epidemiol 109:464, 1979.

LaMontagne JR: Summary of a workshop on influenza B viruses and Reye's syndrome. J Inf Dis 142:452, 1980.

Meibalane R, Sedmak GV, Sasidharan P, et al: Outbreak of influenza in a neonatal intensive care unit. J Pediatr 91:974, 1977.

Price DA, Postlethwaite RJ, Longson M: Influenza A₂ infections presenting with febrile convulsions and gastrointestinal symptoms in young children. Clin Pediatr 15:361, 1976.

Wright PF, Ross KB, Thompson J, et al: Influenza A infections in young children. Primary natural infection and protective efficacy of live vaccine-induced or naturally acquired immunity. N Engl J Med 296:829, 1977.

General

Boyer KM, Cherry JD: Influenza viruses. In: Feigin RD, Cherry JD (eds): Textbook of Pediatric Infectious Diseases. Philadelphia, WB Saunders, 1981.

Cherry JD: Newer respiratory viruses: Their role in respiratory illnesses of children. Adv Pediatr 20:225, 1973.

Kilbourne ED (ed): The Influenza Viruses and Influenza. New York, Academic Press, 1975.

10.79 PARAINFLUENZA VIRAL INFECTIONS

Parainfluenza viruses are common causes of respiratory illnesses in children and adults. They are of particular importance to the pediatrician because of their prominent association with croup.

Parainfluenza viruses are relatively large RNA viruses belonging to the paramyxovirus group. Their outer surfaces consist of lipoprotein envelopes with hemagglutinin spikes. Four serologic types cause disease in humans.

Epidemiology. By the age of 5 yr over 90% of children have been infected with parainfluenza type 3 virus and the majority have also been infected with types 1 and 2. Most infections with types 1, 2, and 3 are symptomatic, but there are marked variations in severity of illness. Infection with type 4 virus is common, but apparently most infections are asymptomatic. Symptomatic reinfections with types 1, 2, and 3 are common.

Infections with parainfluenza type 1 virus are frequently cyclic, with epidemics in the fall every 2nd yr. Endemic patterns of occurrence also may be noted. Infection with type 2 virus also tends to occur in fall epidemics. However, the pattern is more sporadic than with type 1, and type 2 virus may be absent from a particular community for several yr.

In contrast to parainfluenza viral types 1 and 2, type 3 infection characteristically is endemic, with illness noted throughout the year.

There are no geographic limitations associated with parainfluenzal infections, which are most common in young children but also frequent in adults. Serious illness, at least in association with type 1 infections, is more common in boys than in girls.

Infection is transmitted directly from person to person, by direct exposure to infected secretions through large airborne droplets, or through other inoculation.

Pathology. The hallmark of parainfluenza viral infection is replication of virus in the respiratory epithelium, usually without deeper invasion or systemic involvement. Only limited pathologic data are available, obviously obtained from cases representing the severe end of the spectrum of illness. In laryngotracheitis a marked inflammatory response of the glottic and tracheal surfaces has been noted. In children dying of pneumonia the spectrum of pulmonary pathology has included peribronchiolar lymphocytic infiltration with plugging of small bronchioles by mucus and cellular debris, necrosis of bronchiolar epithelium, and marked lymphocytic infiltration of the alveolar walls and interstitial lung tissue.

Pathogenesis and Immunity. Experimental infections have been initiated by intranasal viral administration. Under experimental conditions the incubation period is 2–4 days. Although viremia may occur, symptomatology is mainly related to the direct involvement of the ciliated cells of the respiratory epithelium. Parainfluenza type 3 viral infections frequently occur in early life when transplacentally acquired specific serum antibody is present, and reinfection in older children and adults regularly occurs despite measurable serum antibody. Immunity has been shown to correlate best with the presence of specific IgA nasal antibody, but high levels of serum antibody also reduce the risk of reinfection. The role of cell-mediated factors in parainfluenza viral infections is unknown. However, the observation of a fatal giant cell pneumonia in children with cell-mediated defects suggests that T cell function may be important in clinical recovery from parainfluenza viral infections. Although reinfection is common, illness is virtually always mild and upper respiratory in nature.

Clinical Manifestations. The predominant manifestations of parainfluenza viral infections are respiratory, although systemic signs and symptoms also occur. About 10–20% of all pediatric respiratory illnesses are due to parainfluenza viral infections, and 80% of all parainfluenza viral infections are upper respiratory in nature. In children hospitalized because of severe respiratory illnesses, parainfluenza viruses account for about 50% of the cases of laryngotracheitis and about 15% each of the cases of bronchitis, bronchiolitis, and pneumonia. Parainfluenza type 1 virus is the most frequent cause of laryngotracheitis, whereas parainfluenza type 3 virus is the most common agent in bronchitis, bronchiolitis, and pneumonia.

Clinical descriptions of laryngotracheitis, bronchitis, bronchiolitis, and pneumonia are presented in Sec 12.54–12.67. Other findings in parainfluenza viral infections are listed in Fig 10–28. Cough is the most common manifestation of parainfluenza viral infections, and rhinorrhea is frequent. Sore throat occurs in about 40% of cases but is a more common complaint in the older child. It is surprising to note that fever is observed in only 20% of cases and that its height is inversely related

to age and almost certainly determined by whether the infection is primary or secondary in nature. In children under age 3 yr who are experiencing primary infections, fever is usual.

Otitis media has been noted in about 10% of documented parainfluenza viral infections. It is probable that otitis media in these cases is due to secondary bacterial infection resulting from the pathologic changes in the respiratory mucous membranes caused by the viral infection. Rash has been noted on numerous occasions. In most instances the exanthem is erythematous, maculopapular, discrete, and of short duration.

The duration of illness in primary infections is quite variable, with an average of about 5 days. The persistence of fever for more than 5 days invariably indicates a secondary, usually bacterial, complication such as otitis media or pneumonia.

Parainfluenza viral types 1 and 3 have also been noted in association with acute parotitis. The clinical illnesses were indistinguishable from those due to mumps viral infections. A type 3 parainfluenza viral strain was isolated from the cerebrospinal fluid of an adolescent with Guillain-Barré syndrome. Reye syndrome has occurred in association with parainfluenza viral infections, and parainfluenza viruses have been recovered from victims of the sudden infant death syndrome. In most instances parainfluenza virus type 4 has been associated with only mild upper respiratory illness, which is usually afebrile.

Diagnosis and Differential Diagnosis. The clinical diagnosis of the etiology of respiratory illness in an individual case is difficult. However, if the epidemiologic patterns and clinical manifestations of the common respiratory viruses are considered, a parainfluenza viral etiology can be predicted with some certainty. Types 1 and 2 are the most likely etiologic agents when laryngotracheitis is epidemic in a community, particularly in the fall. Type 3 should be considered in sporadic instances of bronchiolitis or pneumonia in children under 1 yr of age.

The main differential diagnostic considerations in young children include influenza A virus in severe laryngotracheitis, respiratory syncytial virus in bronchiolitis, influenza A virus in bronchitis, and respiratory syncytial, influenza, and adenoviruses in pneumonia. In mild upper respiratory illnesses all the common respiratory viruses need to be considered (rhinoviruses, coronaviruses, adenoviruses, respiratory syncytial virus, influenza viruses, and selected enteroviruses); in the older patient *Mycoplasma pneumoniae* infection is a further possibility.

The most important clinical differential diagnostic consideration is that of laryngotracheitis from other acute upper airway obstructive diseases such as acute epiglottitis, angioneurotic edema, and foreign body.

The virologic confirmation of parainfluenza viral infections is relatively easy in properly equipped laboratories provided proper attention is paid to the collection and transportation of the specimens for culture. Swabs containing respiratory secretions are best maintained in a small amount of broth or other transport media; they should be refrigerated and transported to the laboratory, without exposure to sunlight, within 4 hr of

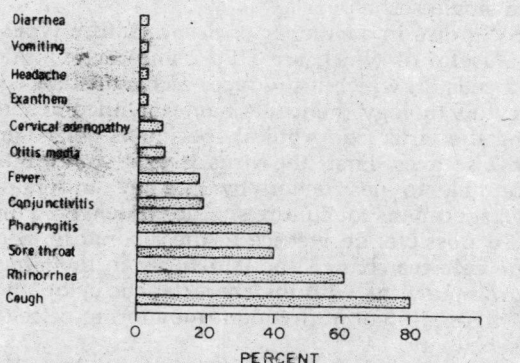

Figure 10–28 Signs and symptoms associated with parainfluenza viral infections.

collection. Parainfluenza viruses are isolated in monkey kidney tissue cultures with results available within 1 wk in the majority of instances. The use of fluorescent antibody procedures on respiratory secretions frequently provides a diagnosis within 24 hr. Retrospective diagnosis can also be made by the study of paired serum samples by complement-fixation, hemagglutination-inhibition, or neutralizing antibody techniques. However, caution must be observed in interpreting serologic results because of cross-reactions among agents in the paramyxovirus group.

Complications. Complications are relatively infrequent in parainfluenza viral infections. Secondary bacterial infections are of most concern; otitis media and pneumonia are easily recognized and treated. Bacterial secondary infections in laryngotracheitis occur occasionally. These infections usually manifest as extensive tracheitis, bronchitis, and pneumonia. Progressive viral pneumonia has occurred in the immunocompromised host.

Prevention. Although experimental inactivated parainfluenza viral vaccines have been widely tried and found to produce serum antibody, they have not offered protection against natural challenge, apparently because secretory nasal antibody is not produced following immunization. A more promising approach is development of a live viral vaccine which could be administered by the respiratory route; trials with candidate live viral vaccines are in progress.

Since the severity of illness with parainfluenza viruses is inversely related to age, it is prudent, whenever possible, to discourage group care of infants and, when possible, to reduce unnecessary exposure of young children to respiratory infections of older children and adults.

Treatment. No specific therapy for parainfluenza viral infections exists, but careful attention to symptomatic care is important in the management of severe laryngotracheitis, bronchiolitis, and pneumonia (Sec 12.54–12.67). Since the exclusion of a bacterial etiology in parainfluenza viral pneumonia and severe bronchitis is often impossible, it is reasonable to administer antibiotics when there is concern. Therapy with ampicillin or amoxicillin is usually adequate because the common bacteria that would cause confusing primary infections or superinfections in pneumonia are *Hemophilus influenzae*, *Streptococcus pneumoniae*, and *Streptococcus pyogenes*. Secondary infections in laryngotracheitis may be caused by *Staphylococcus aureus* in addition to *H. influenzae*, *S. pneumoniae*, and *S. pyogenes*, and therefore require therapy with oxacillin or nafcillin.

In parainfluenza viral upper respiratory illnesses, the prophylactic use of antihistamines, decongestants, and antibiotics should be discouraged as they are expensive and of unproven effectiveness.

Prognosis. Parainfluenza viral infections are exceedingly common and the outcome with rare exceptions is good. Anoxia associated with severe laryngotracheitis or pneumonia can result in brain damage. Rare deaths are due to cardiorespiratory arrest.

JAMES D. CHERRY

Cooney MK, Fox JP, Hall CE: The Seattle virus watch. VI. Observations of infections with and illness due to parainfluenza, mumps and respiratory syncytial viruses and *Mycoplasma pneumoniae*. Am J Epidemiol 101:532, 1975.

Downham MAPS, Gardner PS, McQuillin J, et al: Role of respiratory viruses in childhood mortality. Br Med J 1:235, 1975.

Glezen WP, Loda FA, Denny FW: The Parainfluenza Viruses. *In:* Evans AS (ed): Viral Infections of Humans: Epidemiology and Control. New York, Plenum Medical Book Co, 1976.

Hall CB, Geiman JM, Breese BB, et al: Parainfluenza viral infections in children: Correlation of shedding with clinical manifestations. J Pediatr 91:194, 1977.

Klein JD, Collier AM: Pathogenesis of human parainfluenza type 3 virus infection in hamster tracheal organ culture. Infect Immunol 10:883, 1974.

Powell HC, Rosenberg RN McKellar B: Reye's syndrome: Isolation of parainfluenza virus. Arch Neurol 29:135, 1973.

Roman G, Phillips CA, Poser CM: Parainfluenza virus type 3 isolation from CSF of a patient with Guillain-Barré syndrome. JAMA 240:1613, 1978.

Zinserling A: Peculiarities of lesions in viral and mycoplasma infections of the respiratory tract. Virchow's Arch (Pathol Anat) 356:259, 1972.

Zollar LM, Mufson MA: Acute parotitis associated with parainfluenza 3 virus infection. Am J Dis Child 119:147, 1970.

General Reference

Hall CB: Parainfluenza viruses. *In:* Feigin RD, Cherry JD (eds): Textbook of Pediatric Infectious Diseases. Philadelphia, WB Saunders, 1981.

10.80 INFECTIONS DUE TO RESPIRATORY SYNCYTIAL VIRUS (RSV)

Since 1957 when respiratory syncytial virus (RSV) was isolated from a number of young children with lower respiratory tract disease, it has become recognized as the major cause of bronchiolitis and pneumonia in infants under 1 yr of age. It is the most important respiratory tract pathogen of early childhood.

Etiology. RSV is a medium-sized membrane-bound RNA virus which develops in the cytoplasm of infected cells and matures by budding from the plasma membrane. It belongs to the family *Paramyxoviridae*, along with parainfluenza and mumps viruses, but is classified in a separate genus, the pneumoviruses, because the diameter of its ribonucleoprotein helix is smaller. In addition, unlike myxoviruses and most paramyxoviruses, it contains no detectable hemagglutinin or neuraminidase, and it does not grow in embryonated eggs.

Although different strains of RSV show some antigenic heterogeneity, this variation is not detectable with human sera, and the virus behaves in the human host like a single serotype.

RSV grows in a number of tissue culture types, the most useful of which are HEp-2 and some strains of HeLa cells, in which it produces a characteristic syncytial cytopathology (hence its name). Difficulties in culturing the virus from clinical specimens derive mainly from 2 sources. First, the virus is heat-labile and very susceptible to destruction by freezing and thawing. Thus, specimens for culture should be delivered rapidly and, if possible, on wet ice to the laboratory. Second, tissue cultures change spontaneously in their capacity to grow the virus with the characteristic cytopathology and therefore require frequent monitoring of cell lines for sensitivity.

Epidemiology. Two aspects of the epidemiology of respiratory syncytial virus are of paramount importance and, in combination, are unique among human viruses: the occurrence of annual outbreaks and the high incidence of infection during the 1st months of life.

RSV is distributed worldwide and appears in yearly epidemics. In temperate climates these epidemics occur each winter and last 4–5 mo. During the remainder of the year infections are sporadic and uncommon. Epidemics usually peak in January, February, or March, but peaks have been recognized as early as December and as late as June. At these times hospital admissions for bronchiolitis and pneumonia in infants under 1 yr of age increase and decrease in proportion to the number of RSV infections in the community. In the tropics outbreaks coincide either with the rainy season or, as in India, with religious festivals at which large numbers of children and adults congregate.

Placentally transmitted antibody, which is universal, has little or no protective effect. Thus, the age at which an infant undergoes the 1st infection depends primarily on the opportunities for exposure. It is estimated that in an urban setting about half the susceptible infants undergo primary infection in each epidemic. Thus infection is almost universal by the 2nd birthday. Reinfection occurs at a rate of 10–20%/epidemic throughout childhood; the frequency is lower in adults. In situations of high exposure such as day care centers, attack rates are higher: nearly 100% for young infants and 60–80% for older infants.

Estimates of the severity of primary infections have emerged from studies of outbreaks in nurseries and institutions. Under these circumstances asymptomatic infection is rare. Most infants develop coryza and pharyngitis, usually with fever and occasionally with otitis. In 10–40% the lower respiratory tract is involved to a varying degree. Bronchitis, bronchopneumonia, and bronchiolitis all occur.

Institutional studies probably overestimate the true frequency of lower respiratory tract disease due to RSV. Calculations based on hospital admissions in the United States and Britain yield a ratio of 1–3 hospitalized infants with bronchiolitis or pneumonia for every 100 primary infections with the virus. It is likely that the older a child is at 1st infection, the milder the illness.

Reinfection may occur as early as a few wk after recovery but usually takes place during subsequent annual outbreaks. The severity of illness during reinfection is probably as much influenced by age as by prior experience with this virus, older children being generally less ill. Nevertheless, several instances of severe RSV bronchiolitis occurring twice in succession have been recorded.

The most common clinical diagnosis in infants hospitalized with RSV infection is bronchiolitis. This syndrome is, however, often not clearly distinguishable from RSV pneumonia in infants, and, indeed, the 2 frequently coexist. All RSV diseases of the lower respiratory tract (excluding croup) have their highest incidence in the 2nd mo of life and decrease in frequency thereafter. The syndrome of bronchiolitis becomes uncommon after the 1st birthday; acute infective wheezing attacks after that age are often termed "wheezy bronchitis," "asthmatoid bronchitis," or, simply, asthma attacks. Viral pneumonia, on the other hand, is a persistent problem throughout childhood, although RSV becomes less prominent as the etiologic agent after the 1st yr. It is estimated in different series that RSV is responsible for 45–75% of cases of bronchiolitis, 15–25% of childhood pneumonias, and 6–8% of cases of croup.

Bronchiolitis and pneumonia due to RSV are more common in boys than in girls by a ratio of about 1.5:1. Racial factors make little difference. Lower respiratory tract disease, however, occurs more often and earlier in life in low socioeconomic groups and under crowded living conditions.

The incubation period from exposure to 1st symptoms is about 4 days. The virus is excreted for variable periods, probably depending on severity of illness and immunologic status. Most infants with lower respiratory tract illness shed virus for 5–12 days after hospital admission. Excretion for 3 wk and longer has been documented. Spread of infection occurs primarily by the respiratory route, but transmission on skin surfaces has been suspected in hospital outbreaks. RSV is probably introduced into most families by school children undergoing reinfection. Typically, in the space of a few days older siblings and 1 or both parents develop colds, while the infant becomes more severely ill with fever, otitis, or lower respiratory tract disease.

Recent studies have drawn attention to the problem of hospital cross-infection during epidemics due to RSV. Not only do children infect one another, but also symptomatic infected adults have been implicated in the spread of the infection.

Pathology and Pathogenesis. The microscopic pathology of bronchiolitis is characterized by virus-induced necrosis of the bronchiolar epithelium, hypersecretion of mucus, and round cell infiltration and edema of the surrounding submucosa. These changes result in formation of obstructing mucous plugs with consequent hyperinflation or collapse of the distal lung tissue. In interstitial pneumonia, infiltration is more generalized, and epithelial necrosis may extend to both the bronchi and the alveoli. In both diseases, but most commonly in bronchiolitis, infants are particularly apt to develop signs and symptoms of small airway obstruction because of the small size of the normal bronchioles.

Several facts argue for immunologic injury as a factor in the pathogenesis of bronchiolitis due to RSV: (1) autopsy studies of infants dying of bronchiolitis have shown both immunoglobulin and virus in the injured bronchiolar tissues; (2) children who received a highly antigenic, inactivated, parenterally administered RSV vaccine developed, on subsequent exposure to wild RSV, more severe and more frequent bronchiolitis than did their age-matched controls; and (3) in older infants bronchiolitis merges into asthma, and RSV is a frequently recognized cause of acute asthma attacks in children 1–5 yr old. However, studies have failed to substantiate a direct, age-independent relationship between severity of disease and level of placentally transmitted IgG antibody. Epidemiologic studies have also largely refuted the theory that presensitization (i.e., a prior asymptomatic RSV infection) may be required in the pathogenesis of bronchiolitis. Therefore, despite continuing suspicion, a proven immunopathologic mechanism in bronchiolitis remains to be established.

All the pathologic processes outlined above can be attributed to the destructive effect of the virus and the attendant host response. It is not clear what additional role is played by superimposed bacterial infection. In most infants with bronchiolitis, with or without interstitial pneumonia, clinical experience suggests that bacteria play an insignificant role. In severe cases or in infants with consolidative pneumonia, the possibility of pathogenic bacterial superinfection is somewhat greater.

Clinical Manifestations. The 1st signs of infection of the infant with respiratory syncytial virus are rhinorrhea and pharyngitis. Cough may appear simultaneously but more often after an interval of 1–3 days. At that time there may also be sneezing and a low-grade fever. Soon after the cough has developed, the child begins to wheeze audibly. If the disease is mild, the symptoms may not progress beyond this stage. Auscultation often reveals diffuse rhonchi, fine rales, and wheezes at this point. Rhinorrhea usually persists throughout the illness with intermittent fever. Roentgenograms of the chest are frequently normal.

If the illness progresses, cough and wheezing increase, and air hunger and evidence of hyperexpansion of the chest and of intercostal and subcostal retraction occur. The respiratory rate increases, and cyanosis occurs. Signs of severe, life-threatening illness are central cyanosis, tachypnea over 70/min, listlessness, and apneic spells. At this stage the chest may be greatly hyperexpanded and almost silent to auscultation because of poor air exchange.

Chest roentgenograms of infants hospitalized with RSV bronchiolitis are normal in about 10% of cases; air-trapping or hyperexpansion of the chest occurs in about 50%. Peribronchial thickening or interstitial pneumonia (readings which are considered interchangeable by some and in which disagreement among observers is common) is seen in 50–80%. Segmental consolidation occurs in 10–25%. Pleural effusion is rarely, if ever, seen.

In some infants the course of the illness may be more like that of pneumonia. In these instances, the prodromal rhinorrhea and cough are followed by dyspnea, poor feeding, and listlessness with a minimum of wheezing and hyperexpansion. Although the clinical diagnosis is pneumonia, wheezing is often present intermittently and the chest roentgenogram may show air-trapping. In some infants the cough may be so severe and paroxysmal that the illness may mimic the pertussis syndrome.

Fever is an inconstant sign in RSV infection. Rash and conjunctivitis each occur in a few cases. In young infants, particularly those who were born prematurely, periodic breathing and apneic spells have been distressingly frequent signs, even with relatively mild bronchiolitis. Finally, it is likely that a small portion of deaths included in the category of sudden infant death syndrome (Sec 26.1) are due to RSV infection.

Routine laboratory tests offer little helpful information in most cases of bronchiolitis or pneumonia due to respiratory syncytial virus. The white cell count is normal or elevated, and the differential count may be normal or shifted either to the right or left. Bacterial cultures usually grow normal flora. Hypoxemia is frequent and tends to be more marked than anticipated on the basis of the clinical findings. When it is severe, it is frequently accompanied by hypercapnia and acidosis.

Diagnosis. Bronchiolitis is a clinical diagnosis. The involvement of respiratory syncytial virus in any particular child's disease can be suspected with varying degrees of certainty from the season of the year and the presence of a typical outbreak at the time. Other features which may be helpful are the age of the child (aside from RSV, the only virus which attacks infants frequently during the 1st few mo of life is parainfluenza virus type 3) and the family epidemiology (colds in siblings and parents).

The diagnostic dilemma of greatest import is the question of possible bacterial or chlamydial involvement. When bronchiolitis is mild or when infiltrates are absent by roentgenogram, there is little likelihood of a bacterial component. In infants 1–4 mo of age, interstitial pneumonitis may be caused by *Chlamydia trachomatis* (Sec 10.62). In this instance there may be a history of conjunctivitis, and the illness tends to be of subacute onset. Coughing is prominent; wheezing is not. There may also be eosinophilia. Fever is usually absent.

Consolidation without other signs or with pleural effusion is considered of bacterial origin until proved otherwise. Other signs pointing to bacterial pneumonia are depression of the white cell count in the presence of severe disease, ileus or other abdominal signs, high fever, and circulatory collapse. In such instances there is rarely any doubt about the need for antibiotics.

Definitive diagnosis of RSV infection is based on virus isolation. The specimen should be taken directly to the laboratory and inoculated onto susceptible cell monolayers. Nasopharyngeal or throat swabs are probably of equal value. Still better, however, is an aspirate of mucus from the child's nasal cavity. Direct examination of nasal epithelial cells using fluorescent antibody techniques has proved of great value in the precise and rapid diagnosis of RSV infection.

Examination of acute and convalescent sera for a rise in antibody to RSV is often unrewarding, particularly in infants.

Prognosis. The mortality of hospitalized infants with RSV infection of the lower respiratory tract is about 2%. The prognosis is clearly worst in infants with underlying disease of the neuromuscular, pulmonary, cardiovascular, or immunologic systems.

For decades it has been recognized that many children with asthma give a history of bronchiolitis in infancy. There is recurrent wheezing in 33–50% of children with typical RSV bronchiolitis in infancy. The likelihood of recurrence is increased in the presence of an allergic diathesis (eczema, hay fever, or a family history of asthma). In bronchiolitis over the age of 1 yr there is an increasing probability that, though it may be virus-induced, this is the 1st of multiple wheezing attacks which will later be called asthma.

Treatment. In uncomplicated cases of bronchiolitis, treatment is symptomatic. Humidified oxygen is usually indicated for hospitalized infants since most are hypoxic. Many infants are slightly to moderately dehydrated; therefore fluids should be carefully administered in somewhat greater than maintenance amounts. Often intravenous or tube feeding is helpful when sucking is difficult. Most infants seem to breathe better when propped up at an angle of 10–30 degrees.

Bronchodilators should not be routinely used. However, a trial of epinephrine should be made in wheezing children over 1 yr of age and bronchodilators administered if it is beneficial. Corticosteroids are not indicated except as a last resort in critical cases. Sedatives are rarely necessary.

In most instances antibiotics are not useful, and their indiscriminate use in presumably viral bronchiolitis and pneumonia should be discouraged. Interstitial pneumonia in infants 1–4 mo old may be chlamydial, and erythromycin (40 mg/kg/24 hr) may therefore be beneficial. When infants with interstitial pneumonia are older, or when consolidation is found, parenteral ampicillin (150–200 mg/kg/24 hr) may be used. In the critically ill child antibiotics are likewise indicated, though cultures or Gram stains may indicate the use of those other than ampicillin to cover staphylococci or ampicillin-resistant *H. influenzae*.

Prophylaxis. Attempts to develop a useful inactivated vaccine have been unsuccessful. Several attenuated vaccines have been tested using the respiratory route of inoculation, but none has proved useful. Indeed, the insufficiency of protection following natural RSV infection diminishes the likelihood that an attenuated vaccine will prevent subsequent disease. Breast milk, which contains antibody to RSV, may have some protective effect, but definitive proof is lacking to date.

KENNETH MCINTOSH

Aherne W, Bird T, Court SDM, et al: Pathological changes in virus infections of the lower respiratory tract in children. J Clin Pathol 23:7, 1970.
Hall CB, Douglas RG Jr, Geiman JM, et al: Nosocomial respiratory syncytial virus infections. N Engl J Med 293:1343, 1975.
Henderson FW, Collier AM, Clyde WA Jr, et al: Respiratory-syncytial-virus infections, reinfections and immunity: A prospective, longitudinal study in young children. N Engl J Med 300:530, 1979.
Kapikian AZ, Bell JA, Mastrota FM, et al: An outbreak of febrile illness and pneumonia associated with respiratory syncytial virus infection. Am J Hyg 74:234, 1961.
Kim HW, Arrobio JO, Brandt CD, et al: Epidemiology of respiratory syncytial virus infection in Washington, DC. I. Importance of the virus in different respiratory tract disease syndromes and temporal distribution of infection. Am J Epidemiol 98:216, 1973.
Kim HW, Arrobio JO, Brandt CD, et al: Safety and antigenicity of temperature sensitive (ts) mutant respiratory syncytial (RS) virus in infants and children. Pediatrics 52:56, 1973.
Loda FA, Clyde WA, Glezen WP, et al: Studies on the role of viruses, bacteria and M. pneumoniae as causes of lower respiratory tract infections in children. J Pediatr 72:161, 1968.
McIntosh K: Bronchiolitis and asthma: Possible common pathogenetic pathways. J Allergy Clin Immunol 57:595, 1976.
Parrott RH, Kim HW, Arrobio JA, et al: Epidemiology of respiratory syncytial virus infection in Washington DC. II. Infection and disease with respect to age, immunologic status, race and sex. Am J Epidemiol 98:289, 1973.
Rooney JC, Williams HE: The relationship between proved viral bronchiolitis and subsequent wheezing. J Pediatr 79:744, 1971.
Simpson W, Hacking PM, Court SDM, et al: Radiological findings in respiratory syncytial virus infection in children. II. The correlation of radiological categories with clinical and virological findings. Pediatr Radiol 2:155, 1974.

10.81 ADENOVIRAL INFECTIONS

Human adenoviruses cause 5–8% of acute respiratory disease in infants and children, including pneumonia, and are the cause of pharyngoconjunctival fever, follicular conjunctivitis, and epidemic keratoconjunctivitis. Only a third of the 33-plus serotypes have been associated with disease. Fatal infections are very rare.

Etiology. Adenoviruses are DNA viruses of intermediate size; they share a common group-specific complement-fixing antigen. They are best recovered from clinical specimens by inoculating human embryonic kidney, HEp-2, or HeLa cells and observing for a typical cytopathic effect. ELISA and fluorescent antibody methods can detect adenovirus antigen prior to evident cytopathic effect. Most adenoviruses agglutinate rat or rhesus monkey erythrocytes, the basis for serotyping in many laboratories; testing with the group complement-fixing antigen is a practical way to detect a sero-response to adenovirus.

The association of various serotypes with clinical syndromes is shown in Table 10–41. Adenovirus types 1, 2, 3, and 5 are highly prevalent in infants and children and are associated with rhinopharyngitis and exudative tonsillitis. Type 3 is typically associated with pharyngoconjunctival fever. Several of the childhood types can induce follicular conjunctivitis. Types 4 and 7, which cause 50–70% of acute respiratory disease in military recruits, are rarely found in children. A newly recognized 7b genome type has been associated with severe, epidemic illness in infants in England and Sweden. Most of the childhood types have been found as "latent" or "persistent" agents in surgically removed enlarged tonsils and adenoids. Whether their presence plays a part in the enlargement is speculative. The childhood types may be associated with nonfatal pneumonia in young children. Adenoviruses have been reported as causative or provocative agents in a pertussis-like syndrome, hemorrhagic cystitis, mesenteric lymphadenitis, and intussusception.

Epidemiology. Adenoviral infections are worldwide in distribution. They occur year-round but are most prevalent in the spring or early summer and again in midwinter in temperate climates. Over 60% of school-age children have antibodies against the more common types. Almost all adults have serum antibody against types 1–7. In Washington, D.C., the more common serotypes recovered in children were as follows: type 1, 26%; type 2, 34%; type 3, 10%; type 5, 10%. Infection with types 1 and 2 tends to occur early in childhood, with types 3 and 5, a bit later. Types 4 and 7 tend to infect young adults brought together suddenly, particularly in military settings. Spread occurs by the respiratory and fecal-oral routes. Experimental infection has been accomplished by conjunctival inoculation, which may also be a natural means of infection, especially for conjunctivitis.

Pathogenesis and Pathology. Many observations suggest the following pathogenesis of adenoviral infection: (1) The oropharyngeal and perhaps nasopharyngeal mucous membranes are the primarily affected tissues in early acute infection, but only for a limited

Table 10–41 CLINICAL SYNDROMES ASSOCIATED WITH VARIOUS SEROTYPES OF ADENOVIRUS

	SYNDROME	ASSOCIATED SEROTYPES*
Frequent Association	Pharyngitis-rhinitis (children)	1, 2, 3, 5 (6, 7)
	Exudative tonsillitis	1, 2, 3, 5
	Pneumonia	1, 3 (2, 5, 7, 18, 21)
	Acute respiratory disease (military)	4, 7 (3, 11, 14, 21)
	Enlarged tonsils and adenoids (latent infection)	1, 2, 5, 6
	Pharyngoconjunctival fever	3 (1, 4, 7, 14)
	Follicular conjunctivitis	1, 3, 4, 5
	Epidemic keratoconjunctivitis	8 (4, 10, 11, 19)
Infrequent or Questionable Association	Hemorrhagic cystitis	11, 21
	Pertussis-like disease	1, 2, 3, 5, 12
	Intussusception (mesenteric lymphadenitis)	1, 2, 3, 5, 7
	Gastroenteritis	3, 7 and possibly nonculturable types demonstrable by electron microscopy

*Serotypes in parentheses rarely or infrequently associated.

time. (2) Later, and often intermittently for periods of days to years, virus replication presumably is supported and virus released from tissues of the lower gastrointestinal tract. (3) Adenovirus serotypes 1–7 can be etiologic agents in acute respiratory tract illness, but illness certainly does not accompany every adenoviral infection. The simultaneous presence of adenovirus in throat and anal specimens tends to indicate acute, overt infection, while the finding of adenovirus only in an anal specimen from a patient who is not ill might represent either inapparent infection or, more likely, a postinfection carrier state. (4) Adenoviral serotypes numbered above type 7, except for types 14 and 21, probably pass to the lower gastrointestinal tract with minimal or no oropharyngeal invasion since they are rarely recovered from oropharyngeal swabs. Whether they produce any illness remains speculative.

An ocular route of entry may favor conjunctival illness. Viremia can occur, which could account for the access to the bladder in the reported cases of hemorrhagic cystitis. There is direct and indirect evidence that adenovirus infection induces type-specific protective immunity, probably serum IgG-mediated.

Pathologic changes in the respiratory epithelium include acidophilic nuclear inclusions, basophilic masses of cells, rosette formation, a mononuclear cell infiltrate, and focal necrosis of mucous glands.

Clinical Manifestations. The symptoms of most of the clinical syndromes associated with adenoviral infection are localized to the pharynx, respiratory tract, and conjunctivae, although there are several reports of gastrointestinal symptoms.

Pharyngoconjunctival Fever. This is a clinically distinct and unique syndrome, occurring particularly in association with type 3 adenoviral infection. Its clinical features include fever, sore throat with pharyngitis, conjunctivitis, cervical adenopathy, and rhinitis. Fever is present in 90% of affected persons, is high, even in adults, and lasts 4–5 days. About 75% of patients have enlargement and erythema of lymphoid tissue on the posterior pharynx and on the anterior pillars of the tonsillar fauces. Nonpurulent conjunctivitis occurs in 75% and is manifested by inflammation of both the bulbar and palpebral conjunctivae of 1 or both eyes. The cervical lymphadenopathy is predominantly posterior in distribution. In general, conjunctivitis persists

beyond the period of fever, and cervical lymphadenopathy is evident for several wk after defervescence and subsidence of acute illness. Half of the patients have rhinitis with little rhinorrhea. Headache, malaise, and weakness are relatively common, and there is considerable lethargy after the acute stage.

Pharyngitis. Cases of rhinitis and pharyngitis with or without fever are not particularly distinct clinically. On the other hand, pharyngitis is probably among the most common clinical manifestations of adenoviral infection. Pharyngitis has been found primarily in association with types 1, 2, 3, and 5; these adenoviruses are also found in a large proportion of children with exudative tonsillitis.

Conjunctivitis. Both epidemic keratoconjunctivitis, a problem primarily of adults, and acute follicular conjunctivitis may be caused by adenoviruses. Also, adenoviruses can be found frequently in conjunctival scrapings or eye washings of patients with various eye diseases, including trachoma.

Pneumonia. A number of cases of severe and fatal pneumonia in infants have been caused by adenoviruses. In most of these cases intranuclear inclusions have been present in the respiratory epithelial tissue; other described changes apparently are similar to those seen in tissue cultures infected with adenoviruses. Seven–9.5% of hospitalized cases of pneumonia in infants and children have been adenovirus-associated, primarily with the lower numbered serotypes.

Diarrhea. Systematic studies of acute diarrhea have not frequently indicated cultivatable adenoviruses as etiologic agents. On the other hand, these viruses are found in the feces, and outbreaks of diarrhea have been reported with types 3 and 7 adenovirus infection. Electron microscopy of fecal samples from patients with gastroenteritis has uncovered adenoviruses which grow poorly if at all in cell culture and which appear to cause diarrhea, particularly in infants. These "enteral" adenoviruses were found in 5.2% of sporadic enteritis in hospitalized infants and children in Washington, D.C. They fit into certain RNA patterns by electrophoresis and are not among the serotypes commonly found in childhood respiratory disease.

Intussusception, Mesenteric Lymphadenitis. The pathogenesis of intussusception is thought by many to include enlarged lymph nodes as an initiating factor.

Adenoviruses have been recovered from mesenteric lymph nodes and also from a higher percentage of children with intussusception than from controls. Thus an etiologic role in some cases of intussusception has been postulated. Adenoviruses have been visualized in the appendix of a child with intussusception and also the appendix of children with appendicitis. Whether these findings represent acute etiologic relationships or manifestations of a protracted intestinal latency is not clear.

Pertussis-like Syndrome. The common childhood adenoviruses have been found in cases simulating pertussis, both in the absence and the presence of *Bordetella pertussis* infection. Whooping cough may be a manifestation of adenoviral infection, but this is probably uncommon. The finding of adenovirus in some cases may represent activation of a latent agent.

Hemorrhagic Cystitis. This is a syndrome with sudden onset of bacteriologically sterile hematuria, dysuria, frequency, and urgency; the process subsides in 1–2 wk. Infection with adenovirus types 11 and 21 has been found in some children and young adults with this clinical picture.

Diagnosis and Differential Diagnosis. Pharyngoconjunctival fever is clinically distinct, but most of the other syndromes of adenoviral infection are so indistinct as to frustrate precise etiologic diagnosis.

Complications, Prevention, and Treatment. Some infants with adenoviral pneumonia have subsequently had bronchiectasis or lobar collapse. Immunization with no resulting illness has been effected following the administration of unattenuated adenovirus types 4 and 7 in enteric capsules in military personnel. Such preparations are not available against the common childhood types of adenovirus. There is no specific treatment.

Brandt CD, Kim HW, Jeffries BC, et al: Infections in 18,000 infants and children in a controlled study of respiratory tract disease. II. Variation in adenovirus infections by year and season. Am J Epidemiol 95:218, 1971.

Fay HM, Grayston JT, Evans AS: Viral Infections of Humans. New York, Plenum Medical Books, 1976, pp 53–69.

Gary GW Jr, Herholzer JC, Black RE: Noncultivable adenoviruses associated with diarrhea in infants: A new subgroup of human adenoviruses. J Clin Microbiol 10:96, 1979.

Jackson GG, Muldoon RL: Viruses causing common respiratory infection in man. IV. Reoviruses and adenoviruses. J Infect Dis 128:811, 1973.

Nelson KE, Gavitt F, Batt MD, et al: The role of adenoviruses in the pertussis syndrome. J Pediatr 86:335, 1975.

Numazaki Y, Kumasaka T, Yano N, et al: Further study on acute hemorrhagic cystitis due to adenovirus type H. N Engl J Med 289:344, 1973.

Wadell G, Varsanyi TM, Lord A, et al: Epidemic outbreak of adenovirus 7 with special reference to the pathogenicity of adenovirus genome type 7b. Am J Epidemiol 112:619, 1980.

10.82 RHINOVIRAL INFECTIONS

Rhinoviruses, collectively the most common cause of the "common cold" in adults, have a less prominent role in young children because of the frequency and importance of other viral infections of the respiratory tract. Also rhinoviral infections in young children often do not produce respiratory illness. However, rhinoviruses readily spread and produce illness in nursery and other school groups, and school children provide a major link in their spread in a family.

Etiology. There are up to 111 serologically distinct rhinoviruses, all members of the picornavirus family of small RNA viruses. They are best recovered by inoculating nasal secretions from infected individuals into human embryonic kidney or human diploid cell cultures and observing for a cytopathic effect produced by an acid-labile agent. Routine serologic testing for acquisition of antibody is not practical because of the multiplicity of types and infrequency of their cross-reactivity.

Several cross-sectional studies indicate that a low percentage of control children or children with diarrhea (1% in our studies) yield rhinoviruses at the time of sampling; similarly, only 2.2% of children with respiratory tract illness yield rhinoviruses. In longitudinal studies, however, 75% of pediatric rhinovirus infection is associated with illness. Rhinoviruses are associated with a proportion of the rhinitis, pharyngitis-bronchitis syndrome in young children as well as in adults. Rarely, rhinoviruses have been reported in adults and children in connection with serious lower respiratory tract disease. They may precipitate asthma in children and chronic bronchitis in adults and have been associated with abnormalities of pulmonary function for up to 6 mo in normal adults and those with chronic bronchitis.

Epidemiology. Rhinoviruses have a worldwide distribution with no predictable pattern of infection by serotype. Multiple types may be present in a community at 1 time.

In temperate climates the incidence of rhinoviral infection peaks in September and again in April or May, but some rhinoviral infection occurs year-round. The peak incidence in the tropics occurs during the rainy season. Thermal cold alone does not explain this pattern, nor is it shown to be important in pathogenesis.

Rhinoviruses are recovered in highest titer in nasal secretions, and experimental infection is most easily accomplished by nasal or conjunctival instillation. Infection via aerosol is less efficient. Virus persists for several hr in secretions on hands or other surfaces. Most transmission probably occurs by spread of nasal secretions to nose or eye by hand, occasionally by cough or sneeze. Thus children are especially likely to introduce these viruses into the home.

Pathogenesis. The peak of nasal inflammatory response occurs when virus growth is at its greatest, 2–4 days after experimental infection. The immune response includes specific nasal IgA and serum IgG antibody; both may play a part in modifying illness and limiting viral shedding. Interferon and a nonspecific factor induced by infection with a heterotypic rhinovirus may be a part of the resistance mechanism. Usually the inflammatory response is limited to the nose, throat, and upper bronchial passages, but pneumonia has been reported.

Clinical Manifestations. The primary clinical response to rhinoviral infection, like that of most respiratory viral infections, is the "common cold." There is an incubation period of 2–4 days; then sneezing, nasal obstruction and discharge, and sore throat ensue. Cough and a hoarse voice occur in 30–40% of cases. Headache and other systemic symptoms are not as common as in influenza. Fever is neither so frequent nor so high as in primary infections with respiratory syncytial virus, parainfluenza virus, or adenovirus. Symptoms are at their worst in the first 2–3 days of illness and last for 1 wk in a majority of patients. Symptoms persist for over 14 days in 35% of young children, compared with 20% of adults.

Complications. Complications of rhinoviral infection are those of any infection which causes edema and inflammation in the nasopharyngeal area. They include obstructive otitis media, sinusitis, local spread down the respiratory tract, and bacterial superinfection.

Diagnosis and Differential Diagnosis. In view of the fact that other viral agents and β-hemolytic streptococci can produce such a picture, a clinical diagnosis can be only presumptive. Laboratory diagnosis is not practical under ordinary circumstances. If any question exists, bacterial cultures should be taken to exclude streptococcal infection.

Treatment and Prevention. There is no specific preventive or ameliorative treatment. Although attempts at immune prophylaxis have been made, there are so many rhinoviral serotypes that this approach is impractical. Careful handwashing and avoidance of manual nose and eye manipulation might be the best approach to reducing spread. For relief of acute symptoms, a mild analgesic and saline or decongestant nose drops may be used for a short time.

ROBERT H. PARROTT

Bloom HH, Forsyth BR, Johnson KM, et al: Relationship of rhinovirus infection to mild upper respiratory disease. JAMA 186:144, 1963.
Chanock RM, Parrott RH: Acute respiratory disease in infancy and childhood: Present understanding and prospects for prevention. Pediatrics 36:21, 1965.
Gwaltney JM: In: Evans AS (ed): Viral Infections of Humans. New York, Plenum Medical Books 1976, p 383.
Jackson GG, Muldoon RL: Viruses causing common respiratory infections in man. J Infect Dis 127:328, 1973.
Ketler A, Hall CE, Fox JP, et al: The Virus Watch Program: A continuing surveillance of viral infections in metropolitan New York families. VIII. Rhinovirus infections: Observations of virus excretion, intrafamilial spread and clinical response. Am J Epidemiol 90:244, 1969.

10.83   HEPATITIS

Hepatitis is a major health problem in the United States, where there are estimated to be more than 70,000 cases yearly.

The observation that serum of an Australian aborigine reacted to form a precipitin line in agar with serum obtained from multiply transfused patients led to the discovery of Australia antigen. Further studies revealed that this line represented the reaction between an antigen of hepatitis B virus and antibody against this virus. Subsequently, the virus of hepatitis A and at least 2 other viruses that cause hepatitis that is neither A nor B have been identified. Other as yet unidentified viruses may also cause hepatitis. In addition, cytomegalovirus, Epstein-Barr virus, rubella virus, and enteroviruses may cause hepatitis.

Etiology. *Hepatitis A (HA).* HA virus (HAV or enterovirus 72) can be demonstrated in human stool by a variety of immunologic techniques. Antibody against HA virus (anti-HA) can be measured; radioimmunoassay is commonly employed. Anti-HA appears soon after the development of icterus and can be identified in serum for many yr following infection. Laboratory strains of HAV have been propagated in tissue culture.

Hepatitis B (HB, Hepadnavirus 1). This infection was first recognized by the detection of a viral antigen—Australia antigen—in the blood of a hepatitis carrier. Electron microscopy initially revealed that the blood of carriers contained spherical and tubular particles of a similar diameter (22 nm). These structures subsequently were recognized to constitute the surface of the virion; hence, the structures originally designated Australia antigen are now referred to as hepatitis B surface antigen or HB_sAg; antibody directed against HB_s is designated anti-HB_s. A number of subtypes have been described for the HB_s antigen, referred to as a, y, w, d, r, and others. These have been useful in epidemiologic studies.

Dane observed virus-like particles 42 nm in diameter in the serum of some patients with hepatitis B. This particle, now known to represent the virion, was referred to as the Dane particle. The inner component or core of the virus is approximately 27 nm in diameter and is designated hepatitis B core antigen or HB_c. Antibody directed against HB_c is designated anti-HB_c.

The virus contains DNA. DNA polymerase is found in the sera of some patients with hepatitis B, often in association with the HB_e antigen. There appear to be 3 serotypes of HB_eAg. Antibody against HB_e is designated anti-HB_e (Table 10–42). HB_sAg has been identified in the liver of some infected patients and used to detect antibody against this antigen (anti-HB_s) in the serum.

Hepatitis Viruses Other than HA or HB (Non-A–Non-B Virus). The existence of at least 1–2 additional viruses which produce hepatitis, strongly inferred by epidemiologic studies, has now been confirmed by the demonstration that hepatitis can be produced in chim-

Table 10–42   COMPONENTS OF HEPATITIS B VIRUS (HBV)

ANTIGENS	ABBREVIATION	ANTIBODIES DIRECTED AGAINST HBV ANTIGENS
Hepatitis B surface antigen	HB_sAg	Anti-HB_s
— subtypes	HB_sAg/ayr; HB_sAg/adr; etc.	
Hepatitis B core antigen	HB_cAg	Anti-HB_c
Hepatitis B$_e$ antigen	HB_eAg	Anti-HB_e
Hepatitis B$_s$ antigen	HB_sAg	Anti-HB_s
Deoxyribonucleic acid polymerase	DNA polymerase	

panzees inoculated with blood from patients with non-A–non-B hepatitis. One virus that is 27 nm in diameter has been identified.

Viruses Which May Cause Hepatitis Incidentally. The liver is frequently involved in infectious mononucleosis and in newborns infected with cytomegalovirus or herpesviruses. Cytomegalovirus may cause a syndrome of hepatitis with prolonged fever and development of atypical lymphocytes in young adults. Newborns with encephalomyocarditis due to coxsackievirus B usually have hepatic and pancreatic involvement. Coxsackieviruses have also been associated with a syndrome of hepatitis with myocarditis seen most commonly during adolescence. Fatal adenoviral pneumonia in infants has also been found to involve the liver. Hepatitis is common in congenital rubella and may occur in rare instances as a complication of varicella, mumps, measles, and other common infections. Newborns infected with echovirus 11 may develop fatal hepatitis.

Epidemiology. That different agents cause hepatitis with characteristic incubation periods and different modes of transmission was recognized long before the development of the laboratory techniques necessary to study these diseases.

Hepatitis A (Infectious Hepatitis). This disease is highly contagious. It is transmitted from person to person and occasionally by ingestion of contaminated food or water. It occurs most commonly in childhood, with a high rate of subclinical illness. Anicteric hepatitis is estimated to occur in over 80% of those infected under 2 and in about half of 3–4 yr olds who are infected. As with most viral infections, the illness tends to be more severe in adults. Most infants appear to be protected by maternal antibody during the early mo of life.

The incubation period is approximately 4–6 wk from exposure until the appearance of jaundice. The highest titers of HAV in stool are found prior to onset of the rise in bilirubin. Although virus can be identified in the stool for several days following the onset of icterus, contagiousness during this period has not been delineated.

Infection with hepatitis A has no seasonal predilection. Seven yr cycles of peak incidence have been described. Infection appears to occur at an earlier age under conditions of poor hygiene; the disease is endemic in underdeveloped areas. Several common-source outbreaks from contaminated water or infected food or food handlers have been reported. Infection has also been contracted from primates. Spread occurs readily between homosexuals and in day care centers. Personnel in day care centers and household contacts of attendees are at increased risk for HAV infection.

Hepatitis A in women during pregnancy or at the time of delivery does not appear to result in clinical disease in the newborn, in teratogenic effects, or in increased risk of abortion.

Hepatitis B (Serum Hepatitis). The term *serum hepatitis* alludes to the most common method by which transmission occurs. Percutaneous or mucous membrane inoculation may also result in infection. Transmission has been documented between sexual partners

and under the conditions of institutional living. A higher rate of infection is found, for instance, among children with Down syndrome in institutions than among those living at home with their families. Hepatitis B surface antigen (HB$_s$Ag) can be demonstrated in saliva, feces, and other body secretions. Attempts to infect susceptible primates by oral feedings of HBV, however, have been unsuccessful.

The major mechanism of transmission is by inoculation with blood of carriers, which may have enormous amounts of virus. Even a prick with a needle contaminated with a minute amount of blood from a carrier of hepatitis B virus can transmit infection; shared needles probably account for the high frequency of infection among drug users. Transfusion of infected blood carried a considerable risk of serum hepatitis prior to screening of blood donors and conversion from paid to volunteer donors. Patients who required frequent transfusions, e.g., those with hemophilia or thalassemia, had a high rate of infection as did those undergoing renal dialysis. There is an increased incidence of hepatitis B in families of patients on dialysis or receiving blood frequently.

Of particular interest has been the transmission of hepatitis B from pregnant carriers of its surface antigen (HB$_s$Ag) to their infants. The presence of HB$_e$Ag in maternal carriers appears to be highly correlated with transmission of hepatitis B infection to their offspring. Investigation of the older siblings of affected infants, moreover, reveals a high rate of HB$_s$ and HB$_e$Ag positivity. There is no increased risk of abortion or malformations following hepatitis during the 1st trimester of pregnancy, but some evidence suggests that mothers positive for HB$_s$Ag tend to deliver prematurely.

HB$_s$Ag has been demonstrated inconsistently in the breast milk of infected mothers. Breast feeding by infected mothers does not appear to confer a greater risk of hepatitis on their offspring than does artificial feeding despite the possibility that cracked nipples may result in the ingestion of contaminated maternal blood by the nursing infant.

Reports of HB$_s$Ag in cord blood but not in blood obtained from the same infant a few days post partum suggest that the HB$_s$Ag may represent contamination with maternal blood. It is of no prognostic significance. Hepatitis B antigen is not usually demonstrable in the blood of infants born to affected mothers until several wk after delivery. The appearance of antigenemia at this time suggests that transmission occurred at the time of delivery; virus contained in amniotic fluid or in maternal feces or blood may be the source of infection. Although most infants become antigenemic from 2–5 mo of age, some infants of HB$_s$Ag positive mothers are not affected until later in the 1st or even the 2nd yr of life.

Infection with hepatitis B virus generally occurs later in life than with hepatitis A virus. Hepatitis B tends to be relatively milder in infants and children and probably is frequently unrecognized. Some infected patients, particularly newborns, become chronic carriers. Antigenemia can be readily demonstrated in these individuals. The carrier and HB$_e$Ag positivity rates appear to be higher in certain Asian and African groups.

The incubation period of hepatitis B from exposure to the onset of jaundice is 2–5 mo. There is no seasonal prevalence.

Pathology. The acute response of the liver to viral injury of either hepatitis A or B is similar regardless of etiology. Initial responses are balloon degeneration and necrosis of single or groups of parenchymal cells, starting in the center of the lobules. These are followed by infiltration of the parenchyma and portal areas with ·lymphocytes and macrophages as well as some plasma cells, eosinophils, and neutrophils. In the later stages, lymphocytes predominate. Regeneration of parenchymal cells is evidenced by the presence of cells or clusters of cells containing mitotic figures. Later there are striking changes in the periportal areas, with widening due to infiltration of inflammatory cells, proliferation of bile ducts, and biliary stasis. In fulminating hepatitis there is total destruction of parenchyma with only the reticular framework of the liver remaining. The newborn infant responds to hepatic injury by forming giant cells.

By 3 mo after onset of clinical illness, liver morphology is generally normal. Persistence of significant histologic changes beyond that time in patients with hepatitis B usually indicates the development of chronic liver disease.

The changes in *chronic persistent hepatitis* and *chronic active hepatitis* are discussed in Sec 11.96 and 11.97, respectively. Cirrhotic changes are sometimes found.

Other organ systems are affected in hepatitis. Biopsies of small intestinal tissue obtained during the course of infectious hepatitis show changes in villous structure. Renal, joint, and skin involvement is believed to result from circulating immune complexes. A hypoplastic bone marrow may result in aplastic anemia.

Pathogenesis. Jaundice results from both obstruction of biliary flow and damage to parenchymal cells. Elevations of both direct and indirect serum bilirubin are found. Intrahepatic obstruction to the flow of bile may result in acholic stools. Resumption of flow may lead to delivery of normal or increased amounts of bilirubin to the duodenum. Urobilinogen, a metabolite of bilirubin produced in the intestine, is normally reabsorbed. Damaged liver parenchymal cells may be unable to re-excrete this material which subsequently appears in the urine. More subtle evidence of biliary obstruction is the finding of elevated serum alkaline phosphatase, 5′-nucleotidase, or γ-glutamyl transpeptidase.

Damage to hepatic cells results in both the release of cellular contents into the circulation and derangement of the metabolic functions of the cells. The release of cellular enzymes from damaged liver cells into blood provides a convenient source for determining the extent and duration of injury. The serum transaminases are used for this purpose; serum glutamic-pyruvic transaminase (SGPT) provides a more specific indicator of liver cell injury than does serum glutamic-oxaloacetic transaminase (SGOT); injury to other cells such as erythrocytes, skeletal muscle cells, or myocardial cells may also cause rises in the SGOT. In severe liver injury, as in fulminating hepatitis, transaminases may fall to extremely low levels; this is interpreted to indicate total destruction of parenchymal cells. Other enzymes, e.g.,

lactic dehydrogenase (LDH), have also been used to detect the presence of injury to the parenchymal cells.

Damage to liver cells may be reflected by aberrations in their normal functions. Increased prothrombin time may result from the inability of liver cells to synthesize proteins required for clotting, with decreased absorption of vitamin K, or with both. Obstruction to biliary flow reduces the flow of bile salts to the intestine; these normally facilitate the absorption of fats, including lipid-soluble vitamin K.

Liver injury may result in changes in carbohydrate, ammonia, and drug metabolism; in hepatitis, drugs metabolized by the liver must be used judiciously.

Inflammation and response to the viral infection are commonly manifested by an elevation of the sedimentation rate in hepatitis A but not in hepatitis B. Elevation of immunoglobulins, particularly IgM, in hepatitis A is frequent. There is generally a modest leukopenia during the 1st 2 wk of infection.

Clinical Manifestations. In adolescents and older children hepatitis tends to resemble the more severe disease seen in adults. Hepatitis A tends to be acute in onset, hepatitis B, insidious. Hepatitis A classically is heralded by systemic complaints of fever, malaise, and digestive complaints, e.g., nausea, emesis, anorexia, intolerance of food and tobacco, and some abdominal discomfort. Dull right upper quadrant pain or epigastric fullness may be exaggerated by exercise or jolting of any kind. Manifestations of hyperbilirubinemia appear subsequent to the onset of systemic symptoms. These include dark urine as well as icteric skin and mucosal surfaces. Jaundice may be so subtle that it can be detected only by laboratory tests, or it may last overtly as long as 2–3 wk. Light or clay-colored stools may result from obstruction of biliary flow. A characteristic psychologic depression and feeling of general discontent are probably responsible for the cliché "a jaundiced view of life." During convalescence, which may last several wk, there is gradual return of appetite, exercise tolerance, and a feeling of well-being.

Hepatitis B may be heralded by arthralgia or skin eruptions, e.g., urticarial, purpuric, macular, or maculopapular rashes. The course tends to be insidious and lasts somewhat longer than that of hepatitis A. In a few patients hematuria or proteinuria may appear during convalescence.

On physical examination icteric skin and mucous membranes are found. In addition to the sclera, the mucosa under the tongue may be yellow. The liver is usually enlarged and tender to palpation. When the liver is not palpable below the costal margin, tenderness can be demonstrated by striking the rib cage over the liver gently with a closed fist. Splenomegaly and lymphadenopathy are common.

Asymptomatic hepatitis A and B are common, particularly in the very young. Although many exchange transfusions using blood contaminated with the virus of hepatitis B must have been performed, hepatitis was rarely reported as a sequela. Of the infants born to mothers with hepatitis B who develop demonstrable antigenemia and elevated transaminases, few have clinical evidence of hepatitis.

The prodrome described in adults with hepatitis A is often mild or unnoticed in children. Frequently, the 1st sign of liver disease is the observation of jaundice or dark urine. Children also tend to have less disability from hepatitis A; their convalescence is usually shorter. Anorexia, nausea, abdominal pain, malaise, and fever are found to varying degrees. Constipation resulting from poor fluid intake is more common than diarrhea. Emesis may occur as a result of parental urging of food on an anorectic, nauseated child. In young infants cessation of weight gain has been observed during hepatitis. One of the manifestations of hepatitis B infection which appears to be peculiar to children is papular acrodermatitis of childhood, referred to as the *Gianotti-Crosti syndrome.*

Diagnosis. A history of jaundice in family contacts, schoolmates, day care centers, or friends or travel to an endemic area may suggest the diagnosis. Accidental inoculation with blood of an infected person also should arouse suspicion of hepatitis B; a high rate of infection is found among drug users and homosexuals. Prior to mandated screening of donated blood for HB$_s$Ag, transfusion of multiple units of blood following cardiac surgery or operations for trauma was a major source of infection with the virus of hepatitis B. Patients who receive frequent transfusions of blood or blood products, e.g., fibrinogen, factor VIII, or factor IX particularly, and those with hemophilia or thalassemia are at high risk. Most hepatitis which follows transfusion is of the non-A–non-B type. Children undergoing dialysis are commonly infected with hepatitis B virus. Although hepatitis B is transmitted most commonly by parenteral exposure, intimate nonparenteral exposure can result in infection. Members of families of patients on dialysis or with leukemia, for instance, are at higher risk. Infants whose mothers are chronic carriers of HBV or have histories of jaundice during pregnancy should be suspected. Infants of certain Asian and African mothers are at increased risk.

Historic information and physical findings compatible with the diagnosis may be substantiated by *laboratory data* which indicate injury to the liver. Hyperbilirubinemia may occur in patients without clearly discernible jaundice. Both direct and indirect serum bilirubin levels are elevated, the conjugated portion more so during the early stage of disease. Later, excretion of conjugated bilirubin resumes, and there is a relative increase of indirect bilirubin. Conjugated bilirubin is metabolized in the intestine to urobilinogen, which is then reabsorbed; the inability of damaged liver cells to excrete urobilinogen into the bile results first in increased serum levels and, subsequently, in increased urinary levels during this stage of the disease.

Rises in serum transaminases, reflecting injury to hepatic cells, precede the onset of jaundice and can be detected into convalescence. A single enzyme test will usually suffice to demonstrate hepatocellular injury; a battery of such tests is ordinarily unnecessary. In hepatitis A the transaminases usually reach a higher peak, often exceeding 1000 units, and decline more rapidly. Although peak transaminase levels tend to be lower in hepatitis B, the duration of elevated levels usually exceeds that found in hepatitis A. Prolonged intermit-

tent elevations are found in non-A–non-B hepatitis. With severe liver injury the prothrombin time is usually elevated. Mild leukopenia with a relative lymphocytosis and atypical lymphocytes may be observed during the 1st 2 wk of illness. IgM values may be elevated, particularly in hepatitis A. Biliary obstructive disease as manifested by elevated alkaline phosphatase, 5'-nucleotidase, or γ-glutamyl transpeptidase can be demonstrated. The sedimentation rate is usually elevated in hepatitis A and is often used as a method of following the course of the disease. Bromsulphalein (BSP) retention, because of its great sensitivity, is useful in determining the duration of liver injury. Newer roentgenographic techniques, including thermography and the use of radionuclides, have been employed to demonstrate hepatic injury.

Acute and convalescent sera can be tested for the presence of anti-HA. IgM anti-HA is usually present at the onset of jaundice and is detectable for at least 6–8 wk. This test is often useful in detecting subclinical cases among contacts. IgG anti-HAV appears a few wk after onset and persists indefinitely. Hepatitis A virus can be demonstrated in stools for several days prior to and for up to 1 wk following the onset of jaundice.

A variety of antigen-antibody systems for confirming the diagnosis of hepatitis B are available. In testing patients for hepatitis B, the physician must understand the temporal sequence of appearance of the various antigens and antibodies. HB$_s$Ag (Table 10–43) appears early in the disease and may have disappeared before the disappearance of jaundice. In carriers, however, HB$_s$Ag may persist indefinitely. Anti-HB$_c$ is usually present soon after the onset of jaundice and then persists indefinitely. DNA polymerase and HB$_e$Ag appear early, prior to the onset of icterus. Anti-HB$_e$ and then anti-HB$_s$ may appear during convalescence. During exacerbations of hepatitis, rises in anti-HB$_c$ are often observed (Table 10–43). Serial samples tested simultaneously are often desirable for precise laboratory confirmation of hepatitis B.

HB$_e$Ag in a patient's serum denotes an increased risk of transmission of HBV infection. Donors or pregnant women who are HB$_s$Ag positive are more likely to transmit hepatitis B if they are also HB$_e$Ag positive. Determination of the HB subtypes, e.g., w, y, r, d, and so on, is useful in epidemiologic investigations.

Differential Diagnosis. Physiologic jaundice is usually easily distinguished from hepatitis. In the fullterm infant it is maximal at 3–4 days; in the premature infant, it may occur several days later and last longer. Rapidly rising or high levels of serum bilirubin, particularly in an infant who is lethargic and not feeding well, suggest hemolytic disease or infection (Sec 7.47). After the immediate newborn period, infection remains an important cause of hyperbilirubinemia, but other causes must be considered, e.g., galactosemia, hypothyroidism, and congenital defects in metabolism of bilirubin, as well as biliary atresia, hepatitis associated with alpha$_1$-antitrypsin deficiency, and choledochal cysts. The introduction of pigmented vegetables into the infant's diet may result in carotenemia, which may be mistaken for jaundice.

In later infancy and childhood hemolytic-uremic syn-

Table 10–43 TESTS FOR INFECTION WITH HEPATITIS B VIRUS

Test	Preicteric	Icteric	Convalescent	Carriers
HB$_s$	+ + + +	+ +	+	+ +
Anti-HB$_s$		±	+ +	−
Anti-HB$_c$		+ +	+ + +	+
Anti-HB$_e$			+ +	+ or −
Bilirubin		+ + +		+ or −
Transaminase	+ + + +	+ + +	+ +	+ or −
DNA polymerase	+ + +	±		+ or −

drome may be mistaken initially for hepatitis. The renal and red blood cell findings should facilitate differentiation. Reye syndrome is associated with cerebral changes that characterize the disease, but liver or muscle biopsy or measurement of serum levels of urea cycle components may sometimes be necessary to distinguish it from acute fulminating hepatitis. Jaundice may also occur with severe infection in older children, particularly in those with malignant disorders. Malaria, leptospirosis, or brucellosis may also cause hepatitis. In adolescents as well as in children with chronic hemolytic processes, gallstones may obstruct biliary drainage and cause jaundice. Cirrhosis, which may be associated with Wilson disease, cystic fibrosis, Banti syndrome, and other causes, may sometimes appear to present as hepatitis. The liver may be involved in collagen diseases, e.g., lupus erythematosus.

A variety of *medications* given to infants and children may produce jaundice; e.g., acetaminophen in excessive doses may cause liver damage, or other drugs may cause increased hemolysis, cholestasis, or hepatitis. Drugs well tolerated in normal children may cause problems in children with certain illnesses. Aspirin given to children with rheumatoid arthritis, for instance, is more likely to result in adverse effects on the liver.

Complications. Although most children recover uneventfully from hepatitis, a few may suffer serious complications of an acute or chronic nature.

Acute Fulminating Hepatitis. Some children develop a progressive course characterized by a rising serum bilirubin with peak levels exceeding 20 mg/dl, encephalopathy, bleeding, edema, and ascites. Transaminase levels may rise into the thousands and then return to normal or very low values. The full-blown disease may develop relentlessly over 1–2 wk or be more insidious. Liver biopsy is performed with reluctance because of bleeding problems. When hepatic tissue is examined, "bridging necrosis" is a characteristic finding; areas of parenchymal necrosis cross limiting plates and may extend from the central vein of 1 lobule to another.

A progressive encephalopathy often develops, characterized by drowsiness followed by stupor and then deep coma. *Asterixis* ("flapping tremor") may occur. Clonus and hyper-reflexia may be replaced later by loss of deep tendon reflexes. Late in the course pupillary and corneal reflexes may be lost. Hypothermia and hyperpnea are often seen. Blood ammonia is elevated and is often used as a guide to therapy. The electroencephalogram is usually abnormal.

Interference with the synthesis of clotting factors and absorption of vitamin K leads to an abnormal prothrombin time. Parenteral administration of vitamin K does not correct the abnormal clotting tests as the damaged liver cells are incapable of synthesizing proteins normally. Gastrointestinal bleeding, with melena, is common. Epistaxis, bleeding gums, and ecchymoses occur; bleeding is usually sufficient to cause anemia.

Edema and ascites frequently develop and are often severe enough to require diuretic therapy and administration of albumin. Hyponatremia, hypokalemia, and hypoalbuminemia are frequent.

Acute fulminating hepatitis appears to be more frequently associated with hepatitis A or non-A–non-B hepatitis than with hepatitis B. The reported mortality varies but is 33% or more. Death from bacterial or fungal sepsis is not unusual. Treatment should be aimed at sustaining the patient conservatively while providing the time for regeneration of hepatic cells. The compromised state of hepatic function should be considered when administering drugs metabolized by the liver.

Chronic Active Hepatitis (CAH). These children have jaundice. Although the onset may appear to be acute, careful questioning often reveals a more insidious course. Frequently, a history of anorexia, nausea, emesis, and weight loss of several wk duration is elicited. The disease occurs more commonly in girls and during the 2nd decade but may be seen in girls as young as 3 yr of age.

The spleen as well as the liver is usually enlarged. Low-grade fever and joint complaints are frequent. Menstrual difficulties may be reported in adolescents. Less frequent associated findings include erythema nodosum, parotitis, colitis, thyroiditis, diabetes mellitus, or hematuria. As the course progresses, digital clubbing and ascites may develop.

Along with evidence of hepatic dysfunction, there is usually hypergammaglobulinemia, with the development of abnormal antibodies. Antinuclear, antiglomerular, antimitochondrial, and anti–smooth muscle antibodies and a positive Coombs test are often found. The presence of these antibodies, together with hypergammaglobulinemia, suggests an autoimmune etiology. HB$_s$Ag is rarely found in children. Anemia and moderately elevated levels of both direct and indirect bilirubin are common. Transaminases are elevated and provide a useful parameter for following response to therapy. Thrombocytopenia and prolongation of the prothrombin time are frequently found. The bleeding diathesis poses a problem in liver biopsy, which is desirable for diagnosis and assessment of progress. The characteristic findings at liver biopsy are discussed in Sec 11.81.

Aplastic Anemia. Leukopenia normally occurs during the 1st wk or 2 of hepatitis. The onset of ecchymoses at this time, however, is an ominous sign that blood abnormalities characteristic of aplastic anemia may develop several wk after the onset of hepatitis, at which time hepatic function and architecture may have returned to normal. The bone marrow shows various stages of aplasia. Terminally, the marrow is replaced by fat. The prognosis of aplastic anemia associated with hepatitis has generally been poor.

Other. Nephrosis has developed in children with HBV infection. Renal biopsy has revealed membranous glomerulonephritis with deposition of complement and HB_sAg in glomular capillaries. Studies in Asia and Africa reveal an association of HB_sAg in mothers with the development in their offspring of hepatocellular carcinoma during young adulthood.

Prevention. *Hepatitis A.* Hospitalized patients with hepatitis A who are incontinent of stool or who are in diapers should be treated with enteric precautions including isolation. Patients are considered contagious for about 1 wk following onset of jaundice, even though it is often difficult to demonstrate virus in stool for more than a few days after jaundice has appeared. There is no need to isolate older children, but their stool and fecally contaminated materials should be treated with precautions, and handwashing should be strictly enforced.

Household contacts should receive 0.02 ml/kg of immune globulin (IG) as soon as the diagnosis is made. IG is singularly effective in preventing clinical hepatitis. It has been demonstrated that many recipients have rises in transaminase, indicating that the infection is probably modified rather than prevented. Immune globulin is not routinely recommended for sporadic nonhousehold exposure, e.g., protection of hospital personnel or schoolmates. It is possible to test for anti-HAV to establish immune status. Testing may be desirable where repeated exposure is anticipated. Mass immunization of school children has been used when epidemics have been school centered. HAV infection in pregnancy does not appear to affect the newborn. When a single case of hepatitis occurs in a day care center or in 2 families of children attending day care centers, IG should be administered to all children and personnel. It may also be advisable to immunize family members of the children in diapers. Handwashing after changing diapers should be stressed at all times in day care centers.

Prophylactic administration of immune serum globulin is recommended for those traveling for extended periods in areas where hepatitis A is endemic; e.g., a person planning to work in a rural Mexican village for 2 mo should be given immune serum globulin, but an individual spending a few days touring Mexico City should not. A dose of 0.05 ml/kg intramuscularly is recommended for those planning prolonged stays in endemic areas. This larger dose will provide protection for a longer period, obviating the need to find a local health care provider who can administer IG.

The propagation of HAV in cultured cells has made

the development of a vaccine feasible. Work toward this end is in progress.

Hepatitis B. Isolation of hospitalized patients is not mandatory, but the careful handling of blood and of needles and instruments contaminated with the blood of infected patients is essential.

The greatest advance in the control of hepatitis B has been change in blood transfusion practices. Indiscriminate use of blood products or blood transfusion should be avoided. Only donated blood which by testing is shown to be free of HBV should be used for transfusion. Purchased blood, even though screened for hepatitis B virus, confers a greater risk of transmission of hepatitis than does blood donated by volunteers; at present, most cases of hepatitis resulting from transfusion are due to non-A–non-B virus. A risk still exists for transmitting hepatitis B with fibrinogen, factor IX concentrate, and antihemophilic globulin.

HBIG is recommended for individuals who are injected with or have ingested HB_sAg-contaminated blood. A dose of 0.05 ml/kg should be given as soon as possible.

If the inoculated or ingested blood is positive for HB_sAg, the dose should be repeated in 1 mo. The risk of this type of exposure is about 1:20. If the blood is from a high-risk patient, e.g., a patient with hepatitis or Down syndrome, or someone of Asian or African descent, or a patient on dialysis, the risk is about 1:200. The blood should be tested for HB_sAg and if the results will be available within 1 wk, IG (0.05 ml/kg) should be given immediately. If the test is negative, nothing more need be done; if positive for HB_sAg, HBIG should be given immediately and repeated in 1 mo. If results of testing will not be available within 1 wk, a clinical judgment should be made as to whether IG or HBIG is immediately indicated. When the results become available, a decision can be made about the need for a dose of HBIG at 1 mo. For individuals not in the high-risk category or for ingestion or injection of blood from an unknown source, the physican may give IG or do nothing.

Deinstitutionalized children with a tendency to bite others should be tested for HB_sAg. If positive, measures may be needed to prevent infection of persons who might be bitten.

Infants whose mothers have hepatitis during the 3rd trimester of pregnancy or who are chronic carriers of HB_sAg should be immunized against HBV. Although infants of mothers who are also HB_eAg positive are at a greater risk of infection, infants born to all HB_sAg-positive women should be immunized. However, routine screening of all pregnant women for HB_sAg is not indicated. Certain women at increased risk (e.g., those of Asian or sub-Sahara origin, frequent recipients of blood products, intravenous drug users, those with frequent exposure to individuals with liver disease or those who have liver disease) should be tested for HB_sAg during pregnancy. Although infants of HB_sAg-positive mothers need not be isolated, it should be appreciated that the maternal blood which may be on their skin at delivery may contain HBV and should be removed by thorough washing. Breast-fed infants of HB_sAg-positive mothers do not have a higher rate of infection than those who are formula fed.

Infants whose mothers are HB$_s$Ag positive should receive 0.5 ml of HBIG in the delivery room. At 2 mo of age they should be tested for HB$_s$Ag. About 10% may have been infected in utero (and will be HB$_s$Ag positive), and no further prophylaxis is indicated for these infants. The rest should receive 0.5 ml of HBIG at 3 and 6 mo of age; hepatitis B vaccine, 10 µg, should also be given at 3, 4, and 9 mo of age. At the 15 mo visit infants should be tested for anti-HB$_s$Ag. The rare individual who might be negative should be tested for HB$_s$Ag.

A vaccine against HBV has been tested and found to be very effective. Three doses are given, the 2nd 1 mo and the 3rd 6 mo after the 1st. The vaccine is prepared by detergent treatment of purified HBV obtained from the blood of carriers. Its cost is a major deterrent to its widespread use. However, this vaccine is indicated for high-risk individuals prior to exposure, for frequent recipients of blood or blood products, for homosexuals, for household or institutional contacts of HB$_s$Ag-positive individuals, for patients recieving hemodialysis, and for health care personnel likely to come into frequent contact with blood. A synthetic vaccine containing 16 amino acids is under investigation. It is expected to cost 1/100 as much as the blood-derived virus vaccine.

The effectiveness of IG for prophylaxis of non-A–non-B hepatitis is unclear. There is some evidence to support its use in a dose similar to that used for prophylaxis of HBV infection.

Treatment. There is no specific therapy for *uncomplicated hepatitis.* Treatment is supportive. Patients often find that a diet low in fat is more acceptable. Parents should be prepared to be tolerant of the child's anorexia. Many patients will prefer limited activity, but there is no evidence that rigid restriction of physical activity will speed recovery.

Occasionally, severe anorexia or emesis may necessitate intravenous therapy to prevent dehydration. If possible, antiemetic preparations should be avoided since most are metabolized in the liver. If they are required, a minimal dose should be tried first and intervals between doses adjusted to the individual patient. Great care should be exercised in prescribing any medication metabolized by or having a potentially toxic effect on the liver; generally, such drugs should be avoided entirely.

Corticosteroids are not needed in the management of uncomplicated hepatitis. Although there is some evidence that steroid therapy quickens return of blood chemistries to normal values, it does not have an appreciable effect on clinical recovery or reduce the occurrence of chronic liver disease. The role of steroids in acute fulminating hepatitis has been studied with conflicting results, possibly because of the heterogeneous nature of the patients in the study groups. When liver biopsy may be contraindicated by a bleeding diathesis, the presence of hyperglobulinemia and abnormal autoimmune antibodies, e.g., antinuclear, anti–smooth muscle, and others, may help identify patients with *chronic active hepatitis.* These patients may respond to steroid therapy with prednisone, in alternate-day dosage if possible, using the minimal dose required to keep serum transaminase levels below 100 units/ml of serum. Azathioprine is sometimes used as an adjunct to steroid therapy.

The management of *acute fulminating hepatitis* is complicated and unsatisfactory at present. The conventional strategy is to manage the patient's acute problems while awaiting the restoration of hepatic function. These problems include encephalopathy, bleeding, fluid retention and electrolyte disturbances, maintenance of adequate nutrition, and others. They must be managed so as not to complicate 1 facet while trying to deal with another.

The encephalopathy is believed due to accumulation of toxic substances ordinarily metabolized by the liver. Efforts are directed at reducing blood ammonia levels. Measures include the feeding of lactulose, a nonabsorbed sugar metabolized by intestinal bacteria into acidic compounds which facilitate ammonium excretion. The diarrhea produced by lactulose feeding, however, may aggravate electrolyte problems. Bowel "sterilization" by administration of neomycin has been used, but absorption of this antibiotic over a long period of time may be sufficient to cause renal damage. A reduction in protein intake will decrease ammonia production, but sufficient amino acid substrate must be available for normal maintenance and for repair of damaged liver cells. Attempts have been made to monitor blood amino acids and to feed only those which are decreased and also essential.

A variety of methods have been used to remove ammonia and toxic substances. Exchange transfusion occasionally produces dramatic results, but the effects are usually short-lived, and the effect on long-term survival is uncertain. A variety of experimental perfusion techniques, including "total body washout," have also been attempted.

Electrolyte abnormalities may contribute to the encephalopathy. Low potassium levels are common; these may be aggravated by the use of diuretics. Metabolic alkalosis associated with hypokalemia may enhance ammonia diffusion into brain cells, thus potentiating the encephalopathy. Diuretics should be used with caution because of their tendency to cause hypovolemia and their effect on potassium. It is essential that adequate intake of potassium be provided. Adrenal steroids, which may be poorly metabolized by damaged liver cells, increase potassium excretion. Removal of ascites by paracentesis is indicated only when the fluid compromises pulmonary ventilation. Administration of serum albumin is sometimes required when low serum protein levels result in severe edema.

Bleeding may be serious enough to cause significant anemia. In addition, bacterial breakdown of blood in the gastrointestinal tract may increase blood ammonia levels. The choice of packed cells or whole blood for transfusion will depend on the need to provide serum proteins. Vitamin K is generally ineffective in correcting prothrombin time, even when given parenterally. In uncontrollable bleeding, treatment with fresh frozen plasma may be required.

PHILIP A. BRUNELL

Alter HJ, et al: Type B hepatitis: The infectivity of blood positive for e antigen and DNA polymerase after accidental needlestick exposure. N Engl J Med 295:909, 1976.

Alter HJ, et al: Transmissible agent in non-A, non-B hepatitis. Lancet 1:459, 1978.

Athreya BH, Gorske AL, Myers AR: Aspirin-induced abnormalities of liver function. Am J Dis Child 126:638, 1973.

Beasley RP, Stevens CE, Shiao IS, et al: Evidence against breast-feeding as a mechanism for vertical transmission of hepatitis B. Lancet 2:740, 1975.

Blum AL, et al: A fortuitously controlled study of steroid therapy in acute viral hepatitis. Am J Med 47:82, 1969.

Derso A, et al: Transmission of HB₅Ag from mother to infant in four ethnic groups. Br Med J 1:949, 1978.

Dubois RS, Silverman A: Treatment of chronic active hepatitis in children. Postgrad Med J 50:386, 1974.

Gregory PB, Knauer CM, Kempson RL, et al: Steroid therapy in severe viral hepatitis: A double-blind, randomized trial of methylprednisolone versus placebo. N Engl J Med 294:681, 1976.

Hadler SC, et al: Hepatitis in day-care centers: A community-wide assessment. N Engl J Med 302:1222, 1980.

Hoofnagle JH, Gerety RJ, Thiel J, et al: The prevalence of hepatitis B surface antigen in commercially prepared plasma products. J Lab Clin Med 88:102, 1976.

Levy RN, Sawitsky A, Florman AL, et al: Fatal aplastic anemia after hepatitis. N Engl J Med 273:1118, 1965.

Magnius LO, Lindholm A, Lundin P, et al: A new antigen-antibody system: Clinical significance in long-term carriers of hepatitis B surface antigen. JAMA 231:356, 1975.

Okada K, et al: E antigen and anti-e in the serum of asymptomatic carrier mothers as indicators of positive and negative transmission of hepatitis B virus to their infants. N Engl J Med 294:746, 1976.

Provost PJ, Hilleman MR: Propagation of human hepatitis A virus in cell culture in vitro (40422). Proc Soc Exp Biol Med 160:213, 1979.

Reesink HW, et al: Prevention of chronic HB₅Ag carrier state in infants of HB₅Ag-positive mothers by hepatitis B immunoglobulin. Lancet 2:436, 1979.

Repsher LH, Freebern RK: Effects of early and vigorous exercise on recovery from infectious hepatitis. N Engl J Med 281:1393, 1969.

Rizzetto M, et al: δ agent: Association of δ antigen with hepatitis B surface antigen and RNA in serum of δ-infected chimpanzees. Proc Natl Acad Sci USA 77:6124, 1980.

Schenker S, Breen KJ, Hoyumpa AM: Hepatic encephalopathy: Current status. Gastroenterology 66:121, 1974.

Schumacher HR, Gall EP: Arthritis in acute hepatitis and chronic active hepatitis: Pathology of the synovial membrane with evidence for the presence of Australia antigen in synovial membranes. Am J Med 57:655, 1974.

Seeff LB, Hoofnagle JH: Immunoprophylaxis of viral hepatitis. Gastroenterology 77:161, 1979.

Siegel M: Congenital malformations following chickenpox, measles, mumps, and hepatitis. JAMA 226:1521, 1973.

Siegel M, Fuerst HT: Low birth weight and maternal virus diseases: A prospective study of rubella, measles, mumps, chickenpox, and hepatitis. JAMA 197:680, 1966.

Steinberg SC, Alter JH, Leventhal BG: The risk of hepatitis transmission to family contacts of leukemia patients. J Pediatr 87:753, 1975.

Stevens CE, et al: Viral hepatitis in pregnancy: Problems for the clinician dealing with the infant. Pediatr Rev, 2:121, 1980.

Szmuness W, et al: Distribution of antibody to hepatitis A antigen in urban adult populations. N Engl J Med 295:755, 1976.

Szmuness W, et al: Hepatitis B vaccine: Demonstration of efficacy in a controlled clinical trial in a high-risk population in the United States. N Engl J Med 303:15, 833, 1980.

Takekoshi Y, et al: Free "small" and IgG-associated "large" hepatitis B e antigen in the serum and glomerular capillary walls of two patients with membranous glomerulonephritis. N Engl J Med 300:814, 1979.

US Public Health Service: Hepatitis B vaccine. Morbidity and Mortality Weekly Report 30:423, 1981.

Villarejos VM, Visona KA, Gutierrez A, et al: Role of saliva, urine and feces in the transmission of type B hepatitis. N Engl J Med 291:1375, 1974.

Villarejos VM, et al: Evidence for viral hepatitis other than type A or type B among persons in Costa Rica. N Engl J Med 293:1350, 1975.

Weiss TD, et al: Skin lesions in viral hepatitis: Histologic and immunofluorescent findings. Am J Med 64:269, 1978.

10.84 ENTEROVIRUSES

Enteroviruses—coxsackieviruses, echoviruses, and polioviruses—are responsible for significant and frequent human illnesses with protean clinical manifestations. Enteroviruses are a subgroup of picornaviruses.

Etiology. Enteroviruses are small viruses (18–30 nm) with a ribonucleic acid core. The classification of human enteroviruses is shown in Table 10–44. Enteroviruses are relatively stable in that they retain activity for several days at room temperature and can be stored indefinitely at ordinary freezer temperatures ($-20°$ C). They are rapidly inactivated by heat ($>56°$ C), formaldehyde, chlorination, and ultraviolet light. Satisfactory systems for the primary recovery of enteroviruses from clinical specimens include rhesus or African green monkey kidney and WI38 (diploid, human embryonic lung fibroblasts) tissue cultures and the intraperitoneal and intracerebral inoculation of suckling mice under 24 hr old. Although there are some minor serologic cross reactions between several coxsackievirus and echovirus types, there are no common group enteroviral antigens of diagnostic importance.

Epidemiology. Man is the only natural host of human enteroviruses. They are spread from person to person by fecal-oral and possibly oral-oral (respiratory) routes. Enteroviruses have been recovered from trapped flies, and it is probable that this carriage contributes to the spread of human infections, particularly in lower socioeconomic populations that have poor sanitary facilities.

Children are immunologically susceptible, and their unhygienic habits facilitate spread. Transmission occurs from child to child (via feces to skin to mouth) and then within family groups. Recovery of enteroviruses is inversely related to age, and prevalence of specific antibodies is directly related to age. The incidence of infections and the prevalence of antibodies do not differ between boys and girls.

In temperate climates there is a marked peak of viral infection in August, September, and October, although some viral activity does occur during the winter months. In contrast, no seasonal pattern is evident in the tropics. Infection and acquisition of postinfection immunity occur with greater frequency and at earlier ages among crowded, economically deprived populations.

Although there are presently 68 identified enteroviral types, most illness in the United States from 1967–1976 was due to just 13 nonpolio enteroviral types. Recently, the most prevalent enteroviral types have been echoviruses 4, 6, and 9 and coxsackieviruses A9 and B4. Although the use of live polioviral vaccine has virtually eliminated epidemic poliomyelitis in the United States, in 1970 polioviruses accounted for 6% of all enteroviral isolations from patients with neurologic illnesses. More than one third of the enteroviral isolations in 1962 from similar patients were polioviruses. Studies of specimens from sewage and asymptomatic children during the present vaccine era reveal that the number of polioviral isolations (presumably vaccine strains) is greater than the number of nonpolio enterovirus isolations. This prevalence of vaccine viruses has apparently not had an effect on the seasonal epidemiology of other enteroviruses.

Pathogenesis. Fig 10–29 shows a schematic diagram of the events of pathogenesis. Following initial acquisition of virus by the oral or respiratory route, implantation occurs in the pharynx and the lower alimentary tract. Within 1 day the infection extends to the regional lymph nodes. On about the 3rd day minor viremia

Table 10–44   HUMAN ENTEROVIRUSES; ANIMAL AND TISSUE CULTURE SPECTRUM*

VIRUS	ANTIGENIC TYPES†	CYTOPATHIC EFFECT (CPE)		ILLNESS AND PATHOLOGY	
		Monkey Kidney Tissue Culture	Human Tissue Culture	Suckling Mouse	Monkey
Polioviruses	1–3	+	+	–	+
Coxsackieviruses, group A	1–24‡	–	–	+	–
Coxsackieviruses, group B	1–6	+	+	+	–
Echoviruses	1–34§	+	±	–	–

*Many enteroviral strains that do not conform to these categories have been isolated.

†New types, beginning with type 68, are now assigned enterovirus type numbers instead of coxsackievirus or echovirus numbers. Types 68 through 71 have been identified.

‡Type 23 found to be the same as echovirus 9.

§Echovirus 10 reclassified as a reovirus; echovirus 28 reclassified as a rhinovirus.

Modified from Cherry JD, In: Remington, JS, Klein JO (eds): Infectious Diseases of the Fetus and Newborn Infant. Philadelphia, WB Saunders, 1976.

occurs, resulting in involvement of many secondary infection sites. Multiplication of virus in these sites coincides with the onset of clinical symptoms. Illness can vary from minor infections to fatal ones. Major viremia occurs during the period of multiplication of virus in the secondary infection sites, usually lasting from the 3rd–7th day of infection. In many enteroviral infections central nervous system involvement occurs at the same time as other secondary organ involvement, but the occasional delay of central nervous system symptoms suggests that seeding occurred later in association with the major viremia or by another pathway

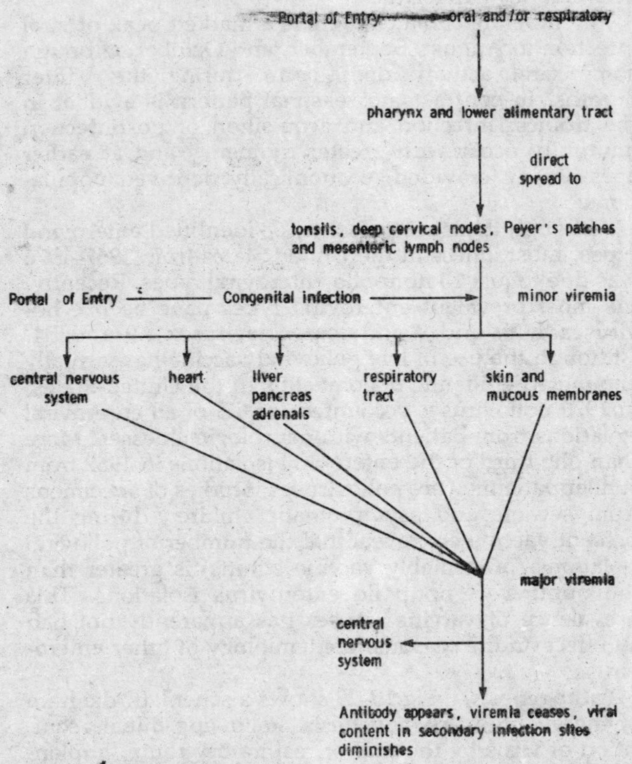

Figure 10–29 The pathogenesis of enteroviral infections. (Modifed from Cherry JD, In: Remington JS, Klein JO (eds): Infectious Diseases of the Fetus and Newborn Infant. Philadelphia, WB Saunders, 1976.)

such as autonomic nerve fibers. Cessation of viremia correlates with the appearance of serum antibody. The viral concentration in secondary infection sites begins to diminish on about the 7th day. However, infection continues in the lower intestinal tract for prolonged periods.

Pathology. The great variation in the clinical signs of enteroviral infections reflects wide variations in pathology. Since pathologic material is generally available only from patients with fatal illnesses, the discussion in this section will consider only the more severe manifestations. These fatal infections account for only a small portion of all enteroviral infections. The pathologic findings in children with milder infections such as nonspecific febrile illness have not been described.

Polioviruses. The *neuropathy* of poliomyelitis is usually pathognomonic; only certain cells and areas of the neuraxis are susceptible to the virus. Neuronal damage is due directly to virus multiplication, but not all affected neurons are killed. The injury may be reversible, and restoration of function may occur within 3–4 wk after onset. There is little histologic evidence of meningeal reaction. Perivascular cuffing and some interstitial glial infiltration are present. Histologic sections generally reveal more widespread lesions than would be estimated from the clinical findings. Considerable destruction of scattered neurons may occur without clinical disability.

The regions in which neuronal lesions occur are (1) spinal cord (anterior horn cells chiefly and to a lesser degree the intermediate and dorsal horn and dorsal root ganglia); (2) medulla (vestibular nuclei, cranial nerve nuclei, and the reticular formation which contains the vital centers); (3) cerebellum (nuclei in the roof and vermis only); (4) midbrain (chiefly the gray matter, but also the substantia nigra and occasionally the red nucleus); (5) thalamus and hypothalamus; (6) the pallidum; and (7) cerebral cortex (motor cortex). The viruses spare the following areas: (1) the entire cerebral cortex *except* the motor area; (2) the cerebellum except the vermis and deep midline nuclei; and (3) the white matter of the spinal cord. This distribution of lesions permits a histologic diagnosis of poliomyelitis.

Extraneural pathology is usually a secondary phenomenon. Bronchopulmonary changes may occur, e.g., aspiration pneumonia, atelectasis, and purulent bronchitis, due to impairment of cough and decreased thoracic movements. The cardiovascular changes may result in hypertension, cardiac failure, and pulmonary edema. Prolonged immobilization leads to negative nitrogen and calcium balances, with urinary lithiasis, renal failure, hypertension with encephalopathy, and convulsions. Treatment itself may cause untoward complications, such as urinary tract infection (following catheterization), decubitus ulcers, and psychotic disturbances. Ulcerations in the alimentary tract may result in serious bleeding and occasional perforation. Respiratory failure results in respiratory acidosis and anoxic changes.

Coxsackieviruses A. Records of severe illnesses associated with coxsackieviruses A are rare, and no distinctive pathology has been described.

Coxsackieviruses B. The most common findings have been myocarditis or meningoencephalitis or both. Involvement of the adrenals, pancreas, liver, and lungs has also been noted. The *heart* is usually enlarged, with dilatation of the chambers or flabby musculature. The pericardium frequently contains some inflammatory cells; thickening, edema, and focal infiltrations of inflammatory cells may be found in the endocardium. The myocardium is congested and contains infiltrations of a wide range of inflammatory cells. The involvement of the myocardium is often patchy and focal but occasionally diffuse. The muscle shows loss of striation as well as edema and eosinophilic degeneration. Frequently, muscle necrosis without extensive cellular infiltration is present. Lesions in *the brain and spinal cord* are focal rather than diffuse but frequently involve many different areas. The lesions consist of areas of eosinophilic degeneration of cortical cells, clusters of mononuclear and glial cells, and perivascular cuffing. The meninges are congested, edematous, and occasionally mildly infiltrated with inflammatory cells.

There are frequently areas of mild focal *pneumonitis* with peribronchiolar cellular infiltrations. The *liver* is often engorged and occasionally contains isolated foci of liver cell necrosis and mononuclear cellular infiltrations. In the *pancreas* occasional focal degeneration of the islet cells occurs. Congestion has been observed in the *adrenals*, with mild to severe cortical necrosis and inflammatory cell infiltrates.

Echoviruses. Hepatic necrosis has been observed in infections with echoviruses 6, 9, 11, 14, and 19. Other rare findings include adrenal and renal hemorrhage and interstitial pneumonitis.

Clinical Manifestations. *Poliovirus Infections.* When a susceptible person has had effective contact with poliovirus, 1 of the following responses may occur in this order of frequency: (1) asymptomatic infection, (2) abortive poliomyelitis, (3) nonparalytic poliomyelitis, (4) paralytic poliomyelitis. A mild response may blend into a more severe form and result in a biphasic course ushered in by a minor febrile illness, then a symptom-free interlude of a few days succeeded by symptoms and signs referable to the nervous system.

ABORTIVE POLIOMYELITIS. A brief febrile illness occurs with 1 or more of the following symptoms: malaise, anorexia, nausea, vomiting, headache, sore throat, constipation, and unlocalized abdominal pain. Coryza, cough, pharyngeal exudate, diarrhea, and localized abdominal tenderness and rigidity are uncommon. The fever seldom exceeds 39.5° C (103° F), and the pharynx shows little despite the frequent complaint of sore throat.

NONPARALYTIC POLIOMYELITIS. The symptoms are those enumerated for abortive poliomyelitis, except that headache, nausea, and vomiting are more intense, and there is soreness and stiffness of the posterior muscles of the neck, trunk, and limbs. Fleeting paralysis of the bladder is not uncommon, and constipation is frequent. Approximately two thirds of the children have a short symptom-free interlude between the 1st phase (minor illness) and the 2nd phase (central nervous system or major illness). This 2-phase course is less common in adults, in whom the evolution of symptoms is more insidious. Nuchal and spinal rigidity is a necessity for the diagnosis of nonparalytic poliomyelitis during the 2nd phase.

Physical examination reveals nuchal-spinal signs and changes in superficial and deep reflexes. With cooperative patients the nuchal-spinal signs are first sought by active tests. The child is asked to sit up unassisted. If this causes undue effort, if the knees flex upward and the patient writhes a bit from side to side in sitting up and uses hands on the bed for the tripod supporting position, there is unmistakable spinal rigidity (Fig 10–30). Still sitting, the patient is asked to flex chin to chest and observed for nuchal rigidity. Alternatively, from the supine position, with knees held down gently, the patient is asked to sit up and kiss his or her knees

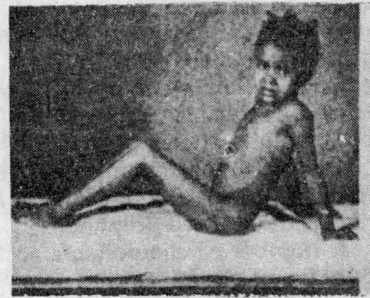
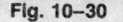
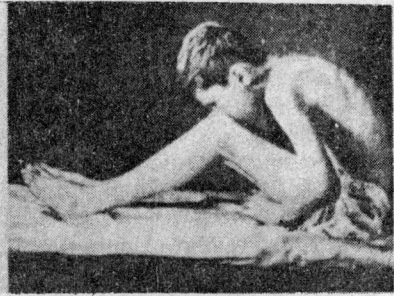

Fig. 10–30   Fig. 10–31

Figure 10–30 Tripod sign: characteristic position associated with stiffness of the spine. (From Steigman AJ: Pediatr Clin North Am, Vol 1, No 1A.)

Figure 10–31 Kiss-the-knee test: ability to complete the maneuver only by flexing the knee. Note tense appearance of the hamstrings. (From Steigman AJ: Pediatr Clin North Am, Vol 1, No 1A.)

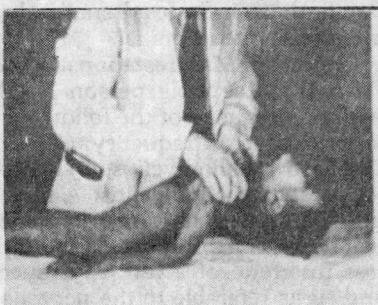
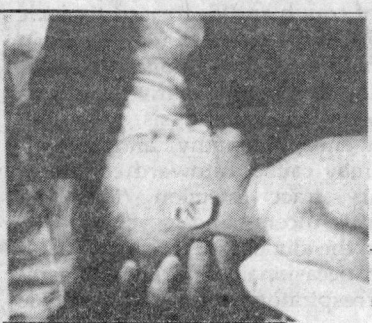

Fig 10–32   Fig 10–33

Figure 10–32   Head-drop sign: the head fails to continue in the plane of the body when the shoulders are elevated. This child had nonparalytic poliomyelitis. Tripod and head-drop signs appear in nonparalytic and paralytic poliomyelitis. (From Steigman AJ: Pediatr Clin North Am, Vol 1, No 1A.)

Figure 10–33   Testing nuchal rigidity in uncooperative, struggling infant: Place the shoulders at the edge of the table, supporting the occiput manually. Flex anteriorly. Only true involuntary rigidity persists. (From Steigman AJ: Pediatr Clin North Am, Vol 1, No 1A.)

(Fig 10–31). If the knees draw up sharply or if the maneuver cannot be adequately completed, there is stiffness of the spine due to muscle spasm. If the diagnosis is still uncertain, attempts should be made to elicit Kernig and Brudzinski signs. Gentle forward flexion of the occiput and neck will elicit nuchal rigidity, which may precede spinal rigidity. Head drop may be demonstrated by placing the hands under the patient's shoulders and raising the trunk (Fig 10–32). Normally the head follows the plane of the trunk, but in poliomyelitis it often falls backward limply. The frequency of the head-drop sign, even in nonparalytic poliomyelitis, with no subsequent residuals indicates that it is not due to true paresis of the neck flexors. In struggling infants it may be difficult to distinguish voluntary resistance from clinically important involuntary nuchal rigidity. One may place the infant's shoulders flush with the edge of the table, support the weight of the occiput in the hand, and then flex the head anteriorly (Fig 10–33). Nuchal rigidity that persists during this maneuver may be interpreted as involuntary. When not closed, the anterior fontanel also may be tense or bulging as in meningitis.

In the early stages the reflexes are normally active and remain so unless paralysis supervenes. Changes in reflexes, either increase or depression, may precede weakness by 12–24 hr; hence, it is important to detect them, especially in nonparalytic patients managed at home. The superficial reflexes, i.e., cremasteric and abdominal and the reflexes of the spinal and gluteal muscles, are usually the first to be diminished. The spinal and gluteal reflexes are elicited by tapping segmentally downward on each side of the spine and buttocks. These reflexes may disappear before the abdominal and cremasteric ones. Changes in the deep tendon reflexes, whether exaggerated or depressed, generally occur 8–24 hr after depression of superficial reflexes and indicate impending paresis of the extremities. There is absence of tendon reflexes with paralysis. Sensory defects do not occur in poliomyelitis.

PARALYTIC POLIOMYELITIS.   The manifestations are those enumerated for nonparalytic poliomyelitis plus weakness of 1 or more muscle groups, either skeletal or cranial. These symptoms may be followed by a symptom-free interlude of several days and then a recurrence of symptoms culminating in paralysis. Bladder paralysis of 1–3 days' duration occurs in approximately 20% of patients, and bowel atony is common, occasionally to the point of paralytic ileus. In some patients muscular paralysis may be the initial presentation.

Flaccid paralysis is the most obvious clinical expression of the neuronal changes. The ensuing muscular atrophy is due to denervation plus the atrophy of disuse. The pain, spasticity, nuchal and spinal rigidity, and hypertonia early in the illness are probably due to lesions of the brain stem, spinal ganglia, and posterior columns. Respiratory and cardiac arrhythmias, blood pressure and vasomotor changes, and the like are reflections of damage to vital centers in the medulla.

On physical examination the distribution of paralysis is characteristically spotty. To detect mild muscular weakness, it is often necessary to apply gentle resistance in opposition to the muscle group being tested. In the *spinal form* there is weakness of some of the muscles of the neck, abdomen, trunk, diaphragm, thorax, or extremities. In the *bulbar form* there is weakness in the motor distribution of 1 or more cranial nerves with or without dysfunction of the vital centers of respiration and circulation. Components of both the preceding forms occur together in *bulbospinal poliomyelitis*. In the *encephalitic form* of the disease irritability, disorientation, drowsiness, and coarse tremors not explained by inadequate ventilation are noted. Even during poliomyelitis epidemics this form can be recognized only if some peripheral or cranial nerve paralysis coexists or ensues. Hypoxia and hypercapnia due to inadequate ventilation from respiratory insufficiency may produce disorientation without true encephalitis.

A number of components acting together may produce insufficiency of ventilation (Table 10–45). The most serious consequences are hypoxia and hypercapnia, which may produce profound effects on many other systems. Respiratory insufficiency should be detected early in order to diminish its widespread effects, and since the situation may shift rapidly, continued clinical

Table 10-45 COMMON SOURCES OF HYPOXIA AND HYPERCAPNIA IN POLIOMYELITIS

1. Cranial nerves IX to XII involved, with
   a. Pharyngeal paralysis and pooling of secretions
   b. Laryngeal involvement — either spasm of laryngeal muscles or paralysis of vocal cords
   c. Lingual paralysis
   d. Tracheal accumulation of secretions due to inability to cough
   e. Aspiration of vomitus
2. Vital center involvement with
   a. Inefficient, irregular respiration
   b. Cardiovascular disturbance
   c. Hyperpyrexia causing increased oxygen consumption
3. Cervical and spinal cord involvement causing paresis of the primary and accessory muscles of respiration
4. Pulmonary complications, viz., pneumonia, atelectasis, edema
5. Contributory factors
   a. Panic
   b. Gastric dilatation
   c. Sedation
   d. Inadequate equipment, viz., small-bore tracheostomy tubes, unsuitable respirator settings, and the like

evaluation is essential. Despite weakness of the respiratory muscles, the patient may respond with so much respiratory effort that normal alveolar ventilation is maintained. In fact, the increased effort (associated with anxiety and fear) may actually produce overventilation at the outset, resulting in respiratory alkalosis. Such effort is fatiguing and soon leads to respiratory failure.

For clarity, certain terms characterizing patterns of disease need definition: (1) *Pure spinal poliomyelitis with respiratory insufficiency* refers to tightness, weakness, or paralysis of respiratory muscles (chiefly the diaphragm and intercostals) without discernible clinical involvement of cranial nerves or vital centers. The cervical and thoracic spinal cord segments are chiefly involved. (2) *Pure bulbar poliomyelitis* refers to paralysis of motor cranial nerve nuclei with or without involvement of the vital centers which control respiration, circulation, and body temperature. Involvement of the 9th, 10th, and 12th cranial nerves is most important since this results in paralysis of the pharynx, tongue, and larynx with consequent airway obstruction. (3) *Bulbospinal poliomyelitis with respiratory insufficiency* refers to involvement of the respiratory muscles with coexisting bulbar paralysis.

The clinical findings resulting from involvement of the respiratory muscles are (1) anxious expression; (2) inability to speak without frequent pauses, resulting in short, jerky, "breathless" sentences, which can be demonstrated by asking the child to count numbers serially; (3) increased respiratory rate; (4) movement of the alae nasi and of the accessory muscles of respiration; (5) inability to cough or sniff with full depth; (6) paradoxical abdominal movements due to diaphragmatic immobility from spasm or weakness of 1 or both leaves; (7) relative immobility of the intercostal spaces, which may be segmental, unilateral, or bilateral. When the arms are weak, and especially when deltoid paralysis occurs, it is well to beware of impending respiratory paralysis since the phrenic nerve nuclei are in adjacent areas of the spinal cord. Observing the patient's capacity for thoracic breathing while the abdominal muscles are splinted manually will indicate minor degrees of pa-

resis. Light manual splinting of the thoracic cage will help to assess the effectiveness of diaphragmatic movement.

The clinical findings of *bulbar poliomyelitis* with respiratory difficulty (other than paralysis of extraocular, facial, and masticatory muscles) include (1) nasal twang to the voice or cry due to palatal and pharyngeal weakness (hard-consonant words such as "cookie" or "candy" bring this out best); (2) inability to swallow smoothly, resulting in accumulation of saliva in the pharynx and indicating partial immobility (holding the larynx lightly and asking the patient to swallow will confirm immobility); (3) accumulated pharyngeal secretions which may cause irregular respiration since each inspiration must be "planned" and cannot be "subconscious" in view of the risk of aspirating; the respirations may thus appear interrupted and abnormal even to the point of falsely simulating intercostal or diaphragmatic weakness; (4) the impossibility of effective coughing, with resultant constant fatiguing efforts to clear the throat; (5) nasal regurgitation of saliva and fluids due to palatal paralysis, with inability to separate the oropharynx from the nasopharynx during swallowing; (6) deviation of the palate, uvula, or tongue; (7) involvement of vital centers, manifest by irregularity in rate, depth, and rhythm of respiration; by cardiovascular alterations which include blood pressure changes (especially increased), alternate flushing and mottling of the skin, and cardiac arrhythmias; and by rapid changes in body temperature; (8) paralysis of 1 or both vocal cords causing hoarseness, aphonia, and ultimately asphyxia unless recognized by laryngoscopy and managed by immediate tracheostomy; (9) the "rope sign," an acute angulation between the chin and larynx due to weakness of the hyoid muscles (the hyoid bone is pulled posteriorly, narrowing the hypopharyngeal inlet).

Nonpolio Enterovirus Infections (Table 10-46). Coxsackieviral and echoviral infections are exceedingly common, and their spectrum of disease is protean. Many of the clinical-virologic associations listed in Tables 10-46, 10-47, and 10-48 are based upon a limited number of cases. Because enteroviruses are frequently carried asymptomatically in the gastrointestinal tract for relatively long periods of time, some of the observed illnesses and concomitantly recovered viruses may not have a cause and effect relationship. However, repeated observations throughout the last 25 yr have confirmed many virus-illness associations even though their occurrence has been sporadic.

ASYMPTOMATIC INFECTION. Based upon the knowledge that 90–95% of persons infected by polioviruses are asymptomatic, the assumption has been made that the majority of infections with other enteroviruses also occur asymptomatically. This opinion is also strengthened by the fact that coxsackieviruses and echoviruses can frequently be recovered from the stools of well children. However, there are relatively few data on the rate of asymptomatic infection with nonpolio enteroviruses. The isolation of enteroviruses from the stool should not be equated with asymptomatic infection because illness, if it occurs, happens shortly after virus acquisition and is of short duration; a particular infec-

Table 10–46 CLINICAL MANIFESTATIONS OF NONPOLIO ENTEROVIRUSES

CLINICAL CATEGORIES	VIRUS TYPES		
	Coxsackieviruses A	Coxsackieviruses B	Echoviruses and Enteroviruses
Nonspecific febrile illness	All types	All types	All types
Respiratory			
Common cold	Mainly 21. 24; rarely other types	Mainly 1–5; rarely 6	Mainly 2, 20; rarely other types
Pharyngitis (pharyngitis, tonsillitis, tonsillopharyngitis, and nasopharyngitis)	Probably all types; mainly 9	Probably all types; mainly 1–5	Probably all types; mainly 2, 4, 6, 9, 11, 16, 19, 25, 30
Herpangina	1–10, 16, 22	1–5	6, 9, 16, 17, 25
Lymphonodular pharyngitis	10		
Stomatitis and other lesions in the anterior mouth	5, 9, 10, 16	2, 5	9, 11, 20, 71
Parotitis	Coxsackievirus A not typed	3, 4	
Croup	9	4, 5	4, 11, 21
Bronchitis		1, 4	8, 12–14
Bronchiolitis and asthmatic bronchitis	Many types	Many types	Many types
Pneumonia	9, 16	1–5	6, 7, 9, 11, 12, 19, 20, 30
Pleurodynia	1, 2, 4, 6, 9, 16	1, 2, 3, 5, 6	1–3, 6–9, 11, 12, 14, 16, 18, 19, 23
Gastrointestinal			
Nausea and vomiting	9, 16	2–5	2, 4, 6, 9, 11, 16, 19, 20, 22, 30
Diarrhea	9, 16	2–5	3, 4, 6, 7, 9, 11–14, 16–22, 25, 30
Constipation	9	3–5	4, 6, 9, 11
Abdominal pain	9, 16	2–5	4, 6, 9, 11, 19, 30
Pseudoappendicitis			1, 8, 14
Peritonitis		1	
Mesenteric adenitis		5	7, 9, 11
Appendicitis		2, 5	
Intussusception		3	7, 9
Hepatitis	4, 9, 10, 20, 24	1–5	1, 4, 6, 9, 11, 14
Reye syndrome	2	4	14, 22
Pancreatitis	9	3–5	
Diabetes mellitus		1, 2, 4	
Acute hemorrhagic conjunctivitis	24		70
Pericarditis and myocarditis	1, 2, 4, 5, 7–10, 16	1–5	1, 4, 6–9, 11, 14, 17, 19, 22, 25, 30
Genitourinary			
Orchitis and epididymitis		1–5	6, 9, 11
Nephritis		4	6, 9
Hemolytic-uremic syndrome	4, 9	2–5	
Pyuria, hematuria, or proteinuria		5	1, 6, 9
Myositis and arthritis	2, 9		9, 24
Exanthem	2, 4, 5, 7, 9, 10, 16	1–5	1–7, 9, 11, 13, 14, 16–19, 22, 25, 30, 32, 33, 71
Neurologic manifestations			
Aseptic meningitis	1–11, 14, 16–18, 22, 24	1–6	1–9, 11–23, 25–27, 30–33, 71
Encephalitis	2, 4–7, 9, 10, 16	1–5	2–9, 11, 12, 14, 15, 17–20, 22, 23, 25, 30, 33, 71
Paralysis (lower motor neuron involvement)	2, 4–7, 9–11, 14, 21	1–6	1–4, 6, 7, 9, 11, 14, 16–19, 30, 70, 71
Guillain-Barré syndrome and transverse myelitis	2, 4–6, 9, 16	1–4	6, 7, 19, 22, 70
Cerebellar ataxia	4, 7, 9	3, 4	6, 9, 16
Peripheral neuritis			9

tion may have been associated with nonspecific illness 1–3 mo prior to collection of a stool specimen. In general, the more carefully clinical symptomatology is sought, the less the percentage of truly asymptomatic infections. Clinical expression is also inversely related to age and varies by viral type. Overall, probably fewer than 50% of all infections are asymptomatic.

NONSPECIFIC FEBRILE ILLNESS.   This is the most common manifestation of coxsackieviral and echoviral infections. All viral types cause this clinical presentation, but the frequency varies considerably among the individual viruses. The onset of illness is usually abrupt without prodrome. In young children the initial finding is fever and associated malaise. In older children headache is usually also noted. The temperature ranges from 38.5–40° C (101–104° F) and has a mean duration of 3 days. In some instances the fever is biphasic; it occurs for 1 day, is absent for 2–3 days, and then recurs for

Table 10–47 CLINICAL EXANTHEMATOUS MANIFESTATIONS OF NONPOLIO ENTEROVIRUSES

Clinical Feature	Associated Viral Agents and Prevalence of Manifestation			
	Virus Subgroup	Common	Occasional	Rare
Macular rash	Coxsackievirus A		1, 2, 5	
	" B			
	Echovirus and enterovirus		2, 4, 5, 13, 14, 17, 19, 30	18, 71
Maculopapular rash	Coxsackievirus A	9	2, 4, 5, 10, 16	6, 7
	" B		1–5	
	Echovirus and enterovirus	4, 9	2, 5–7, 11, 16–19, 25, 30, 71	1, 3, 13, 14, 22, 27, 33
Vesicular rash	Coxsackievirus A	5, 16	8–10	4, 7
	" B			1–3
	Echovirus and enterovirus		11	6, 9, 17, 71
Petechial or purpuric rash	Coxsackievirus A	9	4	
	" B		2–5	
	Echovirus	9	4, 7	3
Urticarial rash	Coxsackievirus A	9	16	
	" B		4, 5	
	Echovirus		11	
Erythema multiforme or Stevens-Johnson syndrome	Coxsackievirus A		9	10, 16
	" B			4, 5
	Echovirus			6, 11
Exanthem and meningitis	Coxsackievirus A		2, 9	7
	" B		1, 2, 4, 5	
	Echovirus and enterovirus	4, 9	6, 11, 17, 18, 25, 30	3, 14, 33, 71
Exanthem and pneumonia	Coxsackievirus A		9	7
	" B			1
	Echovirus			9, 11
Hand, foot, and mouth syndrome	Coxsackievirus A	16	5, 10	7
	" B			1, 3, 5
	Echovirus and enterovirus			71
Hemangioma-like lesions	Coxsackievirus A			
	" B			
	Echovirus			25, 32
Herpangina and exanthem	Coxsackievirus A		4	9
	" B			2
	Echovirus		16, 17	
Roseola-like illness	Coxsackievirus A			6, 9
	" B		5	1, 2, 4
	Echovirus		16, 25	9, 11, 27, 30
Anaphylactoid purpura	Coxsackievirus A			4
	" B			
	Echovirus			9, 18
Zoster-like rash	Coxsackievirus A			
	" B			5, 6
	Echovirus			
Pityriasis-like rash	Coxsackievirus A			
	" B			
	Echovirus			6
Chronic or recurrent rash	Coxsackievirus A	16		
	" B			
	Echovirus			11

Modified from Cherry JD. *In:* Feigin RD, Cherry JD (eds): Textbook of Pediatric Infectious Diseases. Philadelphia, WB Saunders, 1981.

an additional 2–4 days. In many young children the only manifestation of illness is fever, and its presence is discovered quite by chance by a parent. Malaise and anorexia are often related to the degree of temperature elevation as is headache in older patients. The complaint of sore throat is common, but an inflamed pharynx is not seen on examination. Nausea and vomiting occasionally occur at the onset of illness as does mild abdominal discomfort. A few mildly loose stools may be noted. Generalized myalgia is also noted, and children complain of a scratchy feeling in the throat. Physical examination is generally benign. There may be minimal conjunctivitis, injection of the pharynx, and cervical lymphadenitis. The duration of illness varies from 24 hr–6 days with an average of 3–4 days. The white blood count is normal.

RESPIRATORY MANIFESTATIONS (Table 10–46). Coxsackievirus A21 is the only enterovirus which clearly

Table 10–48 MANIFESTATIONS OF NEONATAL NONPOLIO ENTEROVIRAL INFECTIONS

SPECIFIC INVOLVEMENT	COMMON	RARE
Inapparent infection		Cox* B2, B5
	Echo† 22	Echo 5, 9, 11, 14, 20, 31
Mild nonspecific febrile illness	Cox B5	Cox B1–B4, A9, A16
	Echo 5, 11, 33	Echo 4, 9, 17
Sepsis-like illness	Cox B2–B5	Cox B1, A9
	Echo 5, 11, 16	Echo 2–4, 6, 9, 14, 19, 21, 22
Respiratory illness (general)		Cox B1, B4, B5, A9
	Echo 11, 22	Echo 9, 17
Herpangina		Cox A5
Coryza		Cox A9
		Echo 11, 17, 19, 22
Pharyngitis		Cox B4
		Echo 11, 17, 18
Laryngotracheitis or bronchitis		Cox B1, B4
		Echo 11
Pneumonia		Cox B4, A9
		Echo 9, 11, 17, 22, 31
Gastrointestinal		
Vomiting or diarrhea		Cox B1, B2, B5
	Echo 5, 17, 18	Echo 4, 6, 8, 9, 11, 16, 19, 21, 22
Hepatitis		Cox B1, B4
	Echo 11, 19	Echo 6, 9, 14
Pancreatitis		Cox B4, B5
Necrotizing enterocolitis		Cox B2, B3
Cardiovascular		
Myocarditis	Cox B1–B4	Cox B5
		Echo 11, 19
Skin	Cox B5	Cox B1
	Echo 5, 17, 22	Echo 4, 9, 11, 16, 18
Neurologic		
Aseptic meningitis	Cox B2–B5	Cox B1
	Echo 3, 9, 11, 17	Echo 1, 14
		Entero‡ 71
Encephalitis	Cox B1–B4	Cox B5
		Echo 9
Paralysis		Cox B2
Sudden infant death		Cox B3, A4, A5, A8
		Echo 22

*Cox = coxsackievirus.
†Echo = echovirus.
‡Entero = enterovirus.
Modified from Cherry JD, In: Feigin RD, Cherry JD (eds): Textbook of Pediatric Infectious Diseases. Philadelphia, WB Saunders, 1981, p 1347.

qualifies as a *common cold* virus. This agent has produced epidemics of mild respiratory illness in military populations. Epidemic disease has not been observed in children. Other viruses which have been associated with the common cold syndrome are listed in Table 10–45.

Pharyngitis, tonsillitis, tonsillopharyngitis, and *nasopharyngitis* are common clinical manifestations of coxsackieviral and echoviral infections. It is probable that all enteroviruses on occasion cause mild pharyngitis. Pharyngitis in coxsackievirus and echovirus infections is frequently associated with other clinical findings such as meningitis, pleurodynia, or exanthem. Although evidence of pharyngeal involvement is present at the time of disease onset, the initial complaint is most often fever. The temperature usually ranges from 38.5–40° C (101–104° F), but higher temperatures are not unusual. In general, fever tends to be more pronounced in younger patients, who also have malaise and anorexia. School age children complain of headache and myalgia. Sore throat, coryza, and vomiting and/or diarrhea may also be noted. Examination of the tonsils and pharynx reveals varying degrees of erythema. In some cases injection is noted, while in others severe pharyngitis with patches of exudate will be seen. The usual duration of uncomplicated enteroviral pharyngitis is 3–6 days. Routine laboratory study is of minimal value; the total white blood cell count may be normal or slightly elevated with a normal differential count.

The onset of *herpangina* is characterized by the sudden awareness of fever. The initial temperature can be quite variable with a range from normal to 41° C (106° F). In general, the temperature tends to be higher in younger patients. Older children frequently complain of headache and backache. Vomiting occurs in about 25% of children under the age of 5 yr. In the majority of instances of herpangina, the oropharyngeal lesions are present on the 1st examination at the time or shortly after fever is observed (Fig 10–34 [p. xxxii]). The characteristic lesions are small, 1–2 mm vesicles and ulcers. These lesions start as papules, become vesicular, and then ulcerate in a short but variable time period. They are usually discrete with an average of 5/patient; some patients will have only 1–2 lesions; in others 14 or more may be noted. When seen early, the vesicular lesions are observed to enlarge over a 2–3 day period from 1–2 mm to 3–4 mm in size. Each vesicular and ulcerative lesion is surrounded by an erythematous ring which varies in size up to 10 mm in diameter. The major site of the lesions is the anterior tonsillar pillars. They also occur on the soft palate, uvula, tonsils, pharyngeal wall, and occasionally the posterior buccal surfaces. Aside from the specific lesions, the remainder of the throat appears either normal or minimally injected and/or erythematous. Although occasionally noted in association with aseptic meningitis or other more severe enteroviral illness, most cases of herpangina are mild and without complication. The usual duration of signs and symptoms is 3–6 days.

Pleurodynia (Bornholm disease) is an epidemic disease, but sporadic cases do occur. Following an incubation period of about 4 days, there is sudden onset of fever and pain. The typical pain is located in the chest or upper abdomen, is muscular in origin, and is of variable intensity. Occasionally, the pain occurs in other areas of the body. It is often excruciatingly severe and sudden and associated with profuse sweating. The patient may appear pale and shock-like. The pain is spasmodic with durations varying from a few min to several hr. Most commonly, the spasmodic periods last about 15–30 min. During spasms, the respirations are usually rapid, shallow, and grunting, suggesting pneumonia or pleural inflammation. Pleural friction rubs may be noted on auscultation, and they may appear and disappear with the coming and going of the pain episodes. Coughing, sneezing, or deep breathing makes the pain worse. In older children and adults the pain is described as stabbing or knife-like. The older person often fears that a heart attack is occurring. When pain is localized to the abdomen, it is frequently crampy and suggests colic in the younger child. The child may double over and refuse to walk or move. Occasionally, the abdominal pain in association with a pale, sweaty, shock-like appearance suggests acute intestinal obstruction. Splinting and guarding of the abdomen also leads to a consideration of appendicitis and peritonitis. Tenderness to some degree is present in areas of pain, but frank myositis with muscle swelling is not observed. Fever and pain usually last 1–2 days. Frequently, however, the illness is biphasic; after the initial febrile period the patient is asymptomatic for several days; then pain and fever recur. Rarely patients will have several recurrent episodes over a period of a few wk. In these cases fever is less prominent during the recurrences.

In epidemics both children and adults are afflicted, with the majority of cases occurring in persons under 30 yr of age. Most children have other signs of enteroviral infection such as anorexia, nausea, vomiting, headache, and sore throat. Routine laboratory study is not very helpful. The white blood count is variable, but an increased percentage of polymorphonuclear neutrophils and band forms is frequent. The erythrocyte sedimentation rate is also inconsistent, with normal to extremely high values observed. The chest roentgenogram is most often normal.

Complications in pleurodynia are uncommon. Aseptic meningitis has been noted in some patients, and adult males have experienced orchitis. Cardiac involvement—myocarditis and pericarditis—may also complicate pleurodynia.

The major etiologic agents in epidemic pleurodynia are coxsackieviruses B3 and B5. Other viruses associated with epidemic disease include coxsackieviruses B1 and B2 and echoviruses 1 and 6. Agents associated with sporadic occurrences are listed in Table 10–46.

A variety of nonpolio enteroviruses have been associated with sporadic instances of *parotitis, croup, bronchitis, bronchiolitis, asthmatic bronchitis,* and *pneumonia* as well as outbreaks of *lymphonodular pharyngitis, stomatitis,* and other lesions in the anterior mouth. Specific etiologic agents are noted in Table 10–45. *Acute lymphonodular pharyngitis* is a unique enanthem associated with coxsackievirus A10 infection. The lesions have the typical distribution of herpangina; they are papular, discrete, 3 mm in diameter, and surrounded by a zone of erythema. They are whitish to yellowish and persist for 6–10 days.

GASTROINTESTINAL MANIFESTATIONS (Table 10–45). Gastrointestinal manifestations are common in enteroviral infections. In a 4 yr review of World Health Organization virus reports, the main clinical sign or symptom was gastrointestinal in 12% of coxsackieviral and 6.8% of echoviral infections; in a 20 yr survey in Wisconsin, gastrointestinal symptoms occurred in about one third of all patients from whom nonpolio enteroviruses were recovered.

Vomiting is a common manifestation of infections with many coxsackieviral and echoviral types, but it is rarely the major complaint of the patient or the parent. Except for coxsackievirus A16 hand, foot, and mouth syndrome in which vomiting is an uncommon complaint, this manifestation occurs in about 50% of all cases in epidemic enteroviral disease. Vomiting is most common in meningitis and least common in pleurodynia and uncomplicated exanthematous disease. *Diarrhea* occurs commonly in coxsackieviral and echoviral infections (Table 10–46) as 1 of many manifestations of the systemic illness. It is rarely severe. In most instances loose stools occur for a 2–4 day period. The stools are rarely watery and never bloody and number at most 6–8/day. *Abdominal pain* is a common complaint in many enteroviral infections. About 10% of patients with coxsackievirus A16 hand, foot, and mouth syndrome have abdominal pain as a complaint. Coxsackievirus and echovirus meningitis is associated with abdominal pain in about 25% of the cases. The severity of abdominal pain in enteroviral infections is quite variable. For example, in aseptic meningitis, headache and other neurologic complaints overshadow the abdominal symptoms. In other situations fever and abdominal pain are diagnostically troublesome because of the possibility of a surgical abdomen. The pain is most often periumbilical; it may be either constant or colicky. The fever is most often greater than 38.3° C (101° F).

As noted in Table 10–46, nonpolio enteroviruses have been associated with a variety of other gastrointestinal and abdominal complaints. In most situations the findings are just 1 manifestation of a more typical enteroviral illness. The possible relationship with juvenile diabetes is based on observations of higher titers of serum antibody to coxsackievirus B4 within 3 mo of onset of disease than in controls, the recovery of coxsackievirus B4 from the pancreas of a previously healthy 10 yr old boy who died following diabetic coma, and serologic evidence of coxsackievirus B infections in patients at the time of onset of diabetes mellitus.

ACUTE HEMORRHAGIC CONJUNCTIVITIS. Although conjunctivitis has been noted as a frequent occurrence in nonpolioenteroviral illnesses for 25 yr, its occurrence as a dominant complaint has been observed only during the last 10 yr. In the majority of epidemics, enterovirus 70 has been the etiologic agent. Similar epidemics in Singapore in 1970 and Hong Kong in 1971 were due to a variant of coxsackievirus A24. Acute hemorrhagic conjunctivitis has a sudden onset with severe eye pain and associated photophobia, blurred vision, lacrimation, erythema and congestion of the eye, and edematous and chemotic lids. There are subconjunctival hemorrhages of varying size and frequently a transient punctate epithelial keratitis, conjunctival follicles, and preauricular lymphadenopathy. Eye discharge is initially serous but becomes mucopurulent with secondary bacterial infection. Systemic symptoms including fever are rare. Occasionally, a picture suggestive of pharyngoconjunctival fever has occurred. A small number of patients have had a polyradiculomyeloneuropathy following enterovirus 70 acute hemorrhagic conjunctivitis. The highest attack rate is in the 20–50 age group with children less involved. The disease has not occurred in the Americas, and most epidemics have occurred in coastal areas of tropical countries toward the end of hot rainy periods. Epidemics are explosive with spread mainly by the eye-hand-fomite-eye route.

PERICARDITIS AND MYOCARDITIS. These manifestations have been noted in association with 27 different nonpolio enteroviruses (Table 10–46). The group B coxsackieviruses have been most frequently implicated in heart disease; B5 has been the most common causative agent, but types B2, 3, and 4 have also been frequently implicated. Of the echoviruses, type 6 has been most frequently associated with cardiac involvement, but there have been few descriptions of the clinical findings with this agent. Cardiac disease, hepatitis, pneumonia, nephritis, meningitis, and orchitis have been occasional associated findings with coxsackievirus B. The mortality resulting from acute coxsackieviral and echoviral heart disease is unknown, but it is significant. In nonfatal cases recovery is usually complete without residual disability. Occasionally, constrictive pericarditis occurs as well as other sequelae.

GENITOURINARY MANIFESTATIONS (Table 10–46). Group B coxsackieviruses are second only to mumps as causative agents of *orchitis*. Coxsackievirus B5 is the most commonly associated virus, but B2 and B4 have also been implicated on many occasions. In almost all instances the orchitis is a secondary event, most commonly associated with pleurodynia. The illness is frequently biphasic with fever and pleurodynia or meningitis, then apparent recovery followed by orchitis about 2 wk after onset. Many patients also have *epididymitis*. In epidemics of disease due to group B coxsackieviruses, the occurrence of testicular involvement is quite variable. Generally, orchitis is infrequent, but in 1 coxsackievirus B2 outbreak, 17% of the postpubertal males had orchitis and 7% also had epididymitis. Other genitourinary manifestations of nonpolio enteroviral infections include acute glomerulonephritis; mesangiolytic glomerulonephritis in an infant with immune deficiency; hemolytic-uremic syndrome; acute renal failure; pyuria, hematuria, or proteinuria; hemorrhagic cystitis; and vaginal ulcerative lesions.

MYOSITIS AND ARTHRITIS (Table 10–46). Since group A coxsackieviruses routinely cause myositis in suckling mice, it is reasonable to suspect a similar clinical manifestation in humans. Myalgia is a common complaint in illnesses due to many coxsackieviruses and echoviruses. However, there is almost no direct evidence (demonstration of virus in muscle) or indirect evidence (muscle enzyme elevations) of muscle involvement in routine enteroviral illnesses. Coxsackievirus A2 has been associated with myositis, and coxsackievirus A9 and echovirus 18 have been associated with polymyositis. A dermatomyositis-like syndrome has been associated with immune deficiency and enteroviral infection. Arthritis has occurred rarely in enterovirus infection.

SKIN MANIFESTATIONS (Tables 10–46 and 10–47). Nonpolio enteroviruses are a common cause of a variety of skin manifestations. In the summer and fall they are the leading cause of exanthems. There is a marked variation in the exanthem clinical expression rate among the various viral types and also among different age groups of the host. In general, the expression is inversely related to the age of the infected patient. The major exanthematous manifestations and syndromes of coxsackieviruses and echoviruses are presented in Table 10–47.

Coxsackievirus A16 is the major cause of the *hand,*

foot, and mouth syndrome, which has a typically enteroviral pattern, with a short incubation period (4–6 days) and a summer and fall seasonal pattern. The clinical expression rate of the enanthem-exanthem complex is high, being close to 100% in young children, 38% in school children, and 11% in adults. In adults rash with coxsackievirus A16 is more common than with any of the other enteroviral agents. Illness is ushered in with a mild prodromal fever, anorexia, malaise, and frequently a sore mouth. Enanthem occurs 1–2 days after the onset of fever and then the exanthem appears. Oral lesions are more consistently present than those of the skin. Therefore, illness, particularly in adults, is often mistakenly identified as aphthous stomatitis (canker sores) or herpes simplex infection. The intraoral lesions are ulcerative and average about 4–8 mm in size. The tongue and buccal mucosa are most frequently involved. The hands are more commonly involved than the feet. Buttock lesions are also common, but these do not usually progress to vesiculation. The lesions on the hands and feet are usually vesicular and vary in size from 3–7 mm; they are generally more common on the dorsal surfaces but frequently occur on the palms and soles as well. They clear by absorption of the fluid in about 1 wk. Coxsackievirus A16 is frequently associated with subacute, chronic, and recurring skin lesions.

Echovirus type 9 is the most prevalent nonpolio enterovirus, and *exanthem* is a common clinical manifestation. Nonspecific febrile illness and aseptic meningitis are the usual major manifestations of echovirus 9 infection. Exanthem occurs in about one third of the cases; 57% of children under 5 yr of age have rash, whereas only 6% of those over 10 yr of age have similar cutaneous findings. The rash is most frequently rubelliform, but in addition or as the sole manifestation, petechiae frequently occur. Rash and fever usually appear at about the same time, and frequently the illness closely mimics meningococcemia. The rash usually lasts 3–5 days.

NEUROLOGIC MANIFESTATIONS (Table 10–46). *Aseptic meningitis* due to enteroviruses occurs in epidemics and as isolated cases. Epidemics have been most common with coxsackievirus B5 and echoviruses 4, 6, 9, and 30. In general, illness is more common in children, but if a specific outbreak is large, adults will also be involved. Virtually all patients have fever and pharyngitis; other respiratory manifestations are also common. Rash is common but varies with the specific viral agents. From 30–50% of all patients with echovirus 9 meningitis will have exanthem. Except for the occurrence of rash, herpangina, pleurodynia, or myocarditis, there is little clinically that helps in identifying the etiology in a sporadic case of aseptic meningitis. Initial symptoms include fever, headache, malaise, nausea, and vomiting. Headache is most often frontal or generalized; adolescents and adults frequently note retrobulbar pain. Pain in the neck, back, and legs is common. Abdominal pain occurs in about one fifth of patients, but this symptom varies with the specific etiologic viral type. Photophobia is common.

Physical examination reveals a temperature in the range from 38–40° C (100.4–104° F). The exanthem is most commonly erythematous, maculopapular, and discrete. Frequently, particularly with echovirus 9 infection, it is petechial and thus suggests meningococcemia. Pharyngitis is common. Generalized muscle stiffness or spasm is usually observed, although the degree varies considerably; Kernig and Brudzinski signs are positive in fewer than half the cases. Deep tendon reflexes are usually normal.

Cerebrospinal fluid examination reveals considerable variations among cases and in the same case with repeated examination. Cerebrospinal fluid leukocyte counts vary from a few cells to a few thousand/mm³; the median is in the 100–500 cells/mm³ range. The percentage of neutrophils also varies greatly. Initial examinations frequently reveal a predominance of neutrophils but rarely over 90% as seen in bacterial disease. Repeated cerebrospinal fluid examinations will demonstrate an increasing percentage of mononuclear cells. The cerebrospinal fluid protein is usually mildly elevated, and the glucose concentration is most often normal; rarely, hypoglycorrhachia occurs. Other routine laboratory studies such as the white blood cell count are occasionally abnormal but not helpful diagnostically.

The duration of illness is variable. In the majority of instances the temperature returns to normal within 4–6 days and disability due to neurologic involvement lasts 1–2 wk. Occasionally, a biphasic illness pattern occurs. In these cases there is an initial period with fever, headache, nausea, vomiting, and muscle aches and pains of a few days' duration followed by general recovery; then the same symptoms return with more pronounced neurologic involvement.

On the average there are about 2500 cases of *encephalitis* in the United States/yr reported to the Center for Disease Control. Of this group only about 2% are demonstrated to have an enteroviral etiology. However, the seasonal pattern of disease and the absence of arboviral activity in many geographic locations would suggest that 500–1000 cases of enteroviral encephalitis severe enough to be reported actually occur each yr in the United States. Echovirus type 9 is the most common cause of enteroviral encephalitis. Other commonly associated enteroviral types are echoviruses 4, 6, 11, and 30 and coxsackievirus B5. In general the prognosis in encephalitis due to enteroviral infections is good, but fatalities occur; the following viral types have been isolated from the brain or cerebrospinal fluid in fatal cases: coxsackieviruses B3 and B6, echoviruses 2, 9, 17, and 25, and enterovirus 71.

Paralysis on the basis of anterior horn cell disease occasionally results from infection with nonpolio enteroviruses. In contrast with poliovirus prevalence, which in the prevaccine era resulted in epidemic paralytic disease, paralysis due to nonpolio enteroviruses is most often a sporadic event. Many coxsackieviruses and echoviruses have been associated with the *Guillain-Barré syndrome*. In general, specific viral types are not associated with the disease. Rather, the disease occurs sporadically in association with prevalent enteroviral types. *Cerebellar ataxia* has been noted in association with coxsackieviruses A4, A7, A9, B3, and B4 and echoviruses 6, 9, and 16. *Peripheral neuritis* with echovirus 9 infection has been reported, and coxsackievirus

A9 has been noted in association with a *focal encephalitis and acute hemiplegia* on 2 occasions.

NEONATAL INFECTIONS. Nonpolio enteroviral infections in neonates result in a wide variety of clinical manifestations ranging from asymptomatic infection to fatal encephalitis and myocarditis. An overview by illness category and prevalence is presented in Table 10–48.

Mild, nonspecific febrile illness occurs most commonly in full term babies following uneventful pregnancies and deliveries without complications. Illness can occur anytime during the 1st mo of life. When the onset occurs after 7 days of age, a careful history will frequently reveal a trivial illness in a family member. The onset of illness is characterized by mild irritability and fever. The temperature is usually in the 38–39° C (100.4–102.2° F) range, but occasionally higher recordings are observed. Poor feeding is frequently observed. One–2 episodes of vomiting and/or diarrhea may occur in some babies. The usual duration of illness is 2–4 days. Routine laboratory study is not helpful, but cerebrospinal fluid examination may reveal an increased protein concentration and leukocyte count indicative of aseptic meningitis.

The major diagnostic problem in neonatal enteroviral infections is the differentiation of bacterial from viral disease producing a *sepsis-like* illness. Even in the infant with mild nonspecific fever, bacterial disease must be strongly considered. The sepsis-like illness is characterized by fever, poor feeding, abdominal distention, irritability, rash, lethargy, and hypotonia. Other findings include diarrhea, vomiting, seizures, shock, hepatomegaly, jaundice, and apnea. The onset of illness is marked by irritability, poor feeding, and fever followed within 24 hr by other manifestations. The duration of fever varies from 1–8 days but is usually 3–4 days. White blood counts are not helpful because the total count, the number of neutrophils, and the number of band form neutrophils are elevated in the majority of instances. The majority of mothers will have evidence of a recent, febrile, viral-like illness. In addition, other factors often associated with bacterial sepsis, such as prolonged rupture of membranes, prematurity, and low Apgar scores, are unusual in enteroviral infections.

In contrast with enteroviral cardiac disease in children and adults where pericarditis is common, neonatal disease virtually always involves the heart muscle. Most cases of *neonatal myocarditis* are due to coxsackievirus B infections, and nursery outbreaks have occurred on several occasions. The illness is most commonly abrupt in onset, with listlessness, anorexia, and fever. A biphasic pattern is noted in about a third of the patients. Progression is rapid, and signs of circulatory failure appear in a 2 day period. If death does not occur, recovery is occasionally rapid but usually gradual over an extended period. Most patients will have cardiac findings such as tachycardia, cardiomegaly, electrocardiographic changes, and transitory systolic murmurs. Many patients show signs of respiratory distress and cyanosis. About one third of the infants will have signs suggesting neurologic involvement.

The initial clinical findings in *neonatal meningitis or meningoencephalitis* are similar to those in nonspecific febrile illness or sepsis-like illness. Most often the child is normal and then is noted to be febrile, anorectic, and lethargic. Jaundice is frequently noted in newborns, and vomiting occurs in neonates of all ages. Less common findings include apnea, tremulousness, and general increased tonicity. Seizures occasionally occur. Cerebrospinal fluid examination reveals considerable variation in protein, glucose, and cellular values. Findings are frequently similar to those observed in bacterial disease. Hypoglycorrhachia is noted in about 10% of newborns with enteroviral meningitis.

Diagnosis. The clinical differentiation of enteroviral disease is frequently thought to be an impossible task. Although it is true that treatable bacterial illnesses should always be considered and treated first, it is also true that, when all the circumstances of a particular illness are considered, enterovirus diseases can be suspected on clinical grounds. The most important factors in clinical diagnosis are season of the year, geographic location, exposure, incubation period, and clinical symptoms. In temperate climates enteroviral prevalence is distinctly seasonal; therefore, disease is usually seen in the summer and fall and unlikely to be seen in the winter. In the tropics enteroviruses are prevalent throughout the year; season is therefore not helpful diagnostically. As with all infectious illnesses, the knowledge of exposure and incubation time is important. A careful history of maternal illness is vitally important in neonatal disease. For example, nonspecific mild febrile illness in a mother that occurs in the summer and fall should suggest the possibility of severe neonatal illness. Specific findings (i.e., aseptic meningitis, paralysis, pleurodynia, herpangina, pericarditis, myocarditis) should alert the clinician to enteroviral illnesses. The short incubation period of enterovirus infections should be taken into consideration. Poliovirus infection should be considered in any unimmunized or incompletely immunized child with nonspecific febrile illness, aseptic meningitis, or paralytic disease.

Most viral diagnostic laboratories have facilities for the recovery of the majority of enteroviruses that cause illness. Tissue culture systems allow the isolation of polioviruses, group B coxsackieviruses, echoviruses, and some group A coxsackieviruses (i.e., coxsackievirus A9 and A16). A complete diagnostic isolation spectrum can be obtained using suckling mouse inoculation. Specimens for virus isolation should be obtained from the throat and rectum (feces) and any other clinically involved site (cerebrospinal fluid, biopsy material, etc.). Virus isolation from all sites except the feces can usually be considered causally related to a specific illness. Because enteroviruses are carried for long periods in the lower gastrointestinal tract, fecal isolates may or may not be causally related to the illness being studied. The demonstration of a neutralizing antibody titer rise to a virus recovered from the feces indicates recent infection and tends to indicate a causal role for the isolated virus. Serum should be collected and stored frozen as soon as possible after the onset of illness and then again 2–4 wk later. Contrary to popular belief, tissue cultural evidence of enteroviral growth takes only a few days in many cases and less than 1 wk in most.

After isolation of an enterovirus, its identification as to type is conventionally done by neutralization, which frequently takes an extended period of time.

Differential Diagnosis. The differential diagnosis of enteroviral infections depends upon the clinical manifestations. In general, the most important considerations relate to bacterial diseases such as those commonly associated with pharyngitis, pneumonia, pericarditis, meningitis, and septicemia. Other viruses also must be considered in upper respiratory illness, gastrointestinal infection, rashes, meningitis, encephalitis, and neonatal illness.

Paralytic Poliomyelitis. Conditions causing muscular weakness include the following: (1) Infectious neuronitis (Guillain-Barré syndrome) is the most common and difficult differential problem in this group. Generally, the fever, headache, and meningeal signs are less notable. Characteristically, there are few cells but elevated globulin content in the cerebrospinal fluid. Paralysis is characteristically symmetrical. Sensory changes and pyramidal tract signs are common but are absent in poliomyelitis. (2) Peripheral neuritis—postinjectional, toxic (lead, avitaminosis, and so forth), paralytic cranial herpes zoster, postdiphtheritic neuropathy—is excluded by history, sensory examination, and related findings. (3) Arthropod-borne viral encephalitis, rabies, and tetanus have been confused with bulbar poliomyelitis. (4) Botulism may closely simulate bulbar poliomyelitis; nuchal-spinal rigidity and pleocytosis are absent. (5) Demyelinizing types of encephalomyelitis are associated with or follow the exanthems and other infections or occur as an untoward sequel of antirabies vaccination. (6) Tick-bite paralysis is uncommon; meningeal signs are absent, and removal of the tick is followed by swift recovery. (7) Neoplasms originating in and around the spinal cord may rarely have a fairly abrupt onset. (8) Familial periodic paralysis, myasthenia gravis, and acute porphyria are uncommon causes of weakness. (9) Hysteria and malingering are rare in children.

Conditions causing pseudoparalysis do not present with nuchal-spinal rigidity or pleocytosis and include the following: (1) Unrecognized trauma from contusions, sprains, fractures, and epiphyseal separation is a common cause of diagnostic confusion. (2) Nonspecific (toxic) synovitis produces a limp, usually unilaterally; the hip and the knee are the most common sites. There may be low grade fever for several days. (3) Acute osteomyelitis has a more septic course; there is polymorphonuclear leukocytosis, with localized signs, positive blood culture, and, later, roentgenographic changes. (4) In acute rheumatic fever the clinical pattern is usually diagnostic. (5) Scurvy is revealed by history of inadequate intake of vitamin C and by roentgenographic changes in the bones. (6) Congenital syphilitic osteomyelitis of the acute painful type is found only in early infancy.

Other Enteroviral Illnesses. The differential diagnosis of other enteroviral syndromes (respiratory, pericarditis/myocarditis, exanthems, meningitis/encephalitis, and so forth) is presented in the respective sections of this book relating to the clinical category.

Complications. Paralytic Poliomyelitis. Melena severe enough to require transfusion may result from single or multiple superficial erosions; perforation is rare. *Acute gastric dilatation* may occur abruptly during the acute or convalescent stage, causing further embarrassment of respiration; immediate gastric aspiration and external application of ice bags are indicated. In the hypoxic patient, atropine should be administered prior to aspiration in order to avoid a potentially fatal vagal reflex. Mild *hypertension* of a few days' or weeks' duration is common in the acute stage, probably related to lesions of the vasoregulatory centers in the medulla and especially to underventilation. In the later stages, because of immobilization, hypertension may occur along with hypercalcemia, nephrocalcinosis, and vascular lesions. Dimness of vision, headache, and a light-headed feeling in association with hypertension should be regarded as premonitory of a frank *convulsion*. Anticonvulsive therapy and a program of increased mobilization should be instituted. *Cardiac irregularities* are uncommon; they **vary** from unexplained tachycardias (which may yield to digitalization) to cardiac arrest, for which measures to restore cardiac action are indicated. Electrocardiographic abnormalities indicative of myocarditis are not rare. *Acute pulmonary edema* occurs occasionally, particularly in patients with arterial hypertension. *Pulmonary embolism* is uncommon despite the immobilization. Skeletal decalcification begins soon after immobilization and results in *hypercalciuria*, which in turn predisposes to *calculi*, especially when urinary stasis and infection are present. A high fluid intake is the only effective prophylactic measure. The patient should be mobilized as much and as early as possible.

Other complications of enteroviral infections such as those associated with myocarditis or encephalitis are presented in other sections of this text.

Prevention. In the United States and other industrialized countries poliomyelitis has been virtually eliminated through the widespread use of either inactivated (IPV) or oral polio vaccines. However, endemic and epidemic poliomyelitis is still a problem in many areas of the world. Immunization of children is discussed in Sec 4.1. Attenuated viral vaccines for enteroviruses other than polioviruses are not available. However, passive protection with pooled human immune globulin (0.2 ml/kg intramuscularly) may be useful in preventing disease. In practice, however, this is worthwhile only in sudden and virulent nursery outbreaks. For example, if several cases of myocarditis occurred in a nursery, it would seem wise to administer immune globulin to all babies in the nursery. Pooled human immune globulin in most instances can be expected to contain antibodies against coxsackievirus types B1–B5 and would offer protection to those infants without transplacentally acquired specific antibody who had not yet become infected.

Treatment. *Poliomyelitis.* The broad principles of management are to allay fear, to minimize ensuing skeletal deformities, to anticipate and meet complications in addition to the neuromusculoskeletal ones, and to prepare the child and family for the prolonged treatment which may be required and for permanent disability when this seems likely. Patients with the nonparalytic and mildly paralytic forms may be treated at home. No antibiotics are effective against poliovirus,

and human immune globulin is ineffective after the onset of illness.

For the **abortive form** simple analgesics, sedatives, an attractive diet, and bed rest until the child's temperature is normal for several days suffice. Avoidance of exertion for the ensuing 2 wk is desirable, and there should be a careful neuromusculoskeletal examination 2 mo later to detect any minor involvement.

Treatment for the **nonparalytic form** is similar to that for the abortive one, relief being indicated in particular for the discomfort of muscle tightness and spasm of the neck, trunk, and extremities. Analgesics alone are not so effective as when combined with the application of hot packs for 15–30 min every 2–4 hr. Hot tub baths are sometimes useful. A firm bed is desirable and is improvised at home by placing table leaves or a sheet of plywood beneath the mattress. A footboard should be used to keep the feet at a right angle with the legs. Muscular discomfort and spasm may continue for some wk, even in the nonparalytic form, necessitating hot packs and gentle physical therapy. Such patients should also be carefully examined 2 mo after apparent recovery to detect minor residuals which might cause postural problems in later yr. Most patients with the **paralytic form** require hospitalization. A calm atmosphere is desired. Suitable body alignment is necessary to avoid excessive skeletal deformity. A neutral position with the feet at a right angle, knees slightly flexed, and hips and spine straight is achieved by use of boards, sandbags, and, occasionally, light splint shells. Active and passive motions are indicated as soon as the pain has disappeared. Opiates and sedatives are permissible only if no impairment of ventilation is present or impending. Constipation is common, and fecal impaction should be prevented. When bladder paralysis occurs, a parasympathetic stimulant such as bethanechol (Urecholine), 5–10 mg orally or 2.5–5.0 mg subcutaneously, may induce voiding in 15–30 min; some patients do not respond, and others have nausea, vomiting, and palpitation. Bladder paresis rarely lasts more than a few days. If Urecholine fails, manual compression of the bladder and the psychologic effect of running water should be tried. If catheterization must be performed, strict asepsis is essential. An interesting diet and a relatively high fluid intake should be started at once unless there is vomiting. Additional salt should be provided if the environmental temperature is high or if the application of hot packs induces sweating. Anorexia is common initially. An indwelling polyethylene gastric tube may be necessary to ensure adequate dietary and fluid intake. The orthopedist and the physiatrist should see these patients as early in the illness as possible and assume responsibility before fixed deformities develop. The management of *pure bulbar poliomyelitis* consists essentially in maintaining the airway and avoiding all risks of inhalation of saliva, food, or vomitus. Gravity drainage of accumulated secretions is favored by the head-low (foot of bed elevated 20–25 degrees) prone position with the face to 1 side. Aspirators with rigid or semirigid tips are preferred for direct oral and pharyngeal use, and soft flexible catheters may be used for nasopharyngeal aspiration. Fluid and electrolyte equilibrium is best maintained by intravenous infusion since tube or oral feeding in the 1st few days may incite vomiting. After the 1st few days an indwelling polyethylene gastric tube may be used, and sips of sterile water may be given from a spoon with increments as indicated by ability to swallow. In addition to close observation for respiratory insufficiency, the blood pressure should be taken at least twice daily. Hypertension is not uncommon and occasionally leads to hypertensive encephalopathy. Patients with pure bulbar poliomyelitis may require tracheostomy because of vocal cord paralysis or constriction of the hypopharynx. The majority of patients with pure bulbar poliomyelitis who recover have little residual impairment; some patients exhibit mild dysphagia and occasional vocal fatigue with slurring of speech.

Impaired ventilation must be recognized early; mounting anxiety, restlessness, and fatigue are early indications for prompt intervention. Tracheostomy is indicated for some patients with pure bulbar poliomyelitis, spinal respiratory muscle paralysis, and bulbospinal paralysis. Unlike other patients for whom tracheostomy is performed, these patients are generally unable to cough, sometimes for many mo. Frequent and swift endotracheal aspiration under aseptic conditions is necessary. Mechanical respirators are often needed. The choice of equipment is determined by that with which the nursing and medical personnel are most familiar. These include whole-body-enclosing (tank) respirators, thoracic-enclosing (cuirass) respirators, and those operated in conjunction with a tracheostomy. Patients are fully conscious and aware; terrifying procedures are best carried out in an outward atmosphere of calm. Explaining the procedure and having parents on hand may be very helpful. Reduction in thoracic compliance occurs early, and higher than expected pressure gradients may be required in order to achieve adequate ventilation. Weaning a patient from dependency on respiratory assistance is a tortuous process, as is total musculoskeletal rehabilitation. Motivation of the patient and of the team of personnel is of paramount importance.

Nonpolio Enteroviruses.   No specific therapy for any enterovirus infection is commonly recognized. In severe, catastrophic, and generalized neonatal infection, it is likely that the baby received no specific antibody for the particular virus from his mother. In this situation, it is probably advisable to administer immune globulin to the infant, but there is no evidence that this therapy is beneficial. However, it can be expected to stop further organ seeding secondary to continued viremia. Corticosteroids should not be given during acute severe enterovirus infections, such as neonatal myocarditis or encephalitis, although some authors believe this therapy has been beneficial to coxsackievirus myocarditis. These agents have deleterious effects in experimental coxsackievirus infections of mice. Since the possibility of bacterial sepsis cannot be ruled out in many instances of enteroviral infections, antibiotics should frequently be administered for the most likely potential pathogens. Therapy of myocarditis and meningoencephalitis is discussed in Sec 13.74 and 10.19.

Prognosis.   Mortality in large urban epidemics of poliomyelitis in the United States in the prevaccine era was 5–7%. Most deaths occur within the 1st 2 wk after onset. Mortality and the degree of disability are greater after the age of puberty. In general, the more extensive the paralysis in the 1st 10 days of illness, the more severe the ultimate disability. Unexpected improvement may appear soon after defervescence and again about 6 wk after onset, a time which corresponds to functional restoration of temporarily inactive neurons. The degree of functional recovery also depends upon the adequacy and promptness of therapy as related to proper body positioning, active motion, use of assistive devices, and, of great importance, the psychologic motivation to return to as full and normal a life as possible.

The prognosis in nonpolio enteroviral infections is in the vast majority of instances excellent. Morbidity and mortality are related almost entirely to cardiac and neurologic disease in older children and these same diseases with general disseminated infection in neonates.

JAMES D. CHERRY

General

Cherry JD: Nonpolio enteroviruses: Coxsackieviruses, echoviruses, and enteroviruses. In: Feigin RD, Cherry JD (eds): Textbook of Pediatric Infectious Disease. Philadelphia, WB Saunders, 1981, p 1316.
Cherry JD: Enteroviruses. In: Remington JS, Klein JO (eds): Infectious Diseases of the Fetus and Newborn Infant. Philadelphia, WB Saunders, 1976, p 366.
Horstmann DM: Poliovirus (poliomyelitis). In: Feigin RD, Cherry JD (eds): Textbook of Pediatric Infectious Diseases. Philadelphia, WB Saunders, 1981, p 1386.
Melnick JL: Enteroviruses. In: Evans AS (ed): Viral Infections of Humans; Epidemiology and Control. New York, Plenum Medical Book Co, 1976, p 163.

Specific

Bodian D, Horstmann DM: Poliomyelitis. In: Horsfall FL, Tamm I (eds): Viral and Rickettsial Infections of Man. Ed 4. Philadelphia, JB Lippincott, 1965.
Center for Disease Control: Aseptic Meningitis Surveillance, annual summary, 1976. Atlanta Ga., US Dept HEW, issued January 1979.
Lake AM, Lauer BA, Clark JA, et al: Enterovirus infections in neonates. J Pediatr 89:787, 1976.
Linnemann CC Jr, Steichen J, Sherman WG, et al: Febrile illness in early infancy associated with ECHO virus infection. J Pediatr 84:49, 1974.
Morens DM: Enteroviral disease in early infancy. J Pediatr 92:374, 1978.
Morens DM, Zweighaft RM, Bryan JM: Non-polio enterovirus disease in the United States, 1971–1975. Intl J Epidemiol 8:49, 1979.
Nightingale EO: Recommendations for a national policy on poliomyelitis vaccination. N Engl J Med 297:249, 1977.

10.85 RABIES
(Hydrophobia)

Rabies is a viral infection of the central nervous system usually transmitted by contamination of a wound with saliva from a rabid animal and virtually 100% fatal once symptoms develop. It is a worldwide public health problem and a source of considerable terror for both exposed patients and their physicians.

Etiology.   Rabies virus belongs to the rhabdovirus group. The viral particles resemble striated bullets. Inside the cylinder is the RNA-containing nucleocapsid.

Antibodies to the nucleocapsid can be detected in infected animals, but only antibodies to the surface glycoproteins are neutralizing and protective. The surface carries a fringe of glycoprotein spikes which have hemagglutinating activity when present on the whole virion.

Epidemiology. Rabies is a widespread infection of warm-blooded animals. In North America the principal vectors for humans are skunks, foxes, raccoons, and bats. In Central and South America dogs are the usual source of exposure. Vampire bats, which bite cattle, are an important part of the cycle of rabies in Latin America. Europe has had an epizootic of fox rabies, with many humans bitten as a result. In Asia and Africa the principal problem is the rabid dog. Countries such as India, the Philippines, and Indonesia have large numbers of stray dogs, but social factors limit efforts at control of this important vector.

Recently the concept of rabies-free land areas has been promulgated. This permits health authorities in places like New York and Philadelphia to omit vaccination after most dog bites on the grounds that terrestrial rabies has been unknown in those cities for years. Whereas practically every state reported some animal rabies in 1975, only 25 reported canine rabies. The extent of the bat problem is attested to by the demonstration of rabies in bats from 42 states. Many islands, such as the United Kingdom, Australia, and Hawaii, are rabies-free.

Information concerning the local epidemiology of rabies is essential to the physician contemplating treatment of a human exposure. Unprovoked bites by bats or other wild animals will almost always require immunization; decisions regarding bites from domestic or pet animals should be made after discussion with public health veterinarians.

Pathogenesis and Pathology. The means by which rabies virus goes from the wound to the brain are only partially understood. Since the virus attaches to and penetrates cells rapidly in vitro, it is inconceivable that it remains dormant in the wound for long periods of time. Moreover, although the virus has been shown to ascend axons from the periphery to the spinal cord, the speed of spread (3 mm/hr) is far too rapid to explain the long incubation period of the disease.

The key to the pathogenesis of rabies probably lies in the observation that in animals the virus multiplies first in striated muscle. It may be hypothesized that antibody, interferon, and other host factors act on the virus as it leaves striated muscle; if these factors are insufficiently protective, virus eventually attaches to the nerve. From then on, rabies may be inevitable. The possibility that the virus must overcome another barrier in passing from the 1st infected neuron to other neurons is indicated by electron microscopic studies of the brain which demonstrate viral passage from cell to contiguous cell.

The basic lesion in the brain is neuronal destruction in the brain stem and medulla. The cerebral cortex is usually normal in the absence of prolonged anoxia before death. The hippocampus, thalamus, and basal ganglia often show neuronal destruction and glial infiltrates. The most severe pathology is evident in the pons

and the floor of the 4th ventricle. A proposed explanation for the inspiratory muscle spasms that result in the striking symptom of hydrophobia is that the virus destroys brain stem neurons inhibitory to the neurons of the nucleus ambiguus, which control inspiration. Hydrophobia does not occur in other diseases since only rabies combines brain stem encephalitis with intact cortex and maintenance of consciousness.

The Negri body, long the pathologic hallmark of rabies, is a cytoplasmic inclusion found in neurons; it consists of clumped viral nucleocapsid. The absence of Negri bodies does not exclude rabies; fluorescent antibody stains of brain sections or smears may be positive in their absence.

Transmission. In animals as well as in humans rabies produces encephalitis as the principal symptom. After establishment of the encephalitis, however, the virus spreads down nerves from the brain. It multiplies in many organs but those important to transmission are the salivary glands. Not all rabid animals have virus in the saliva, and even when it is present, the quantity is variable. Skunks are particularly likely to have large amounts of virus in saliva. Dogs are unlikely to have virus in saliva more than 5 days before the onset of symptoms. The variability of virus in saliva explains the fact that only about half of untreated bites by proven rabid animals will result in rabies.

Scratches by the claws of rabid animals are dangerous because animals lick their claws. Saliva applied to a mucosal surface such as the conjunctiva may be infectious.

Bat excreta contain enough rabies virus to pose danger of rabies to those who enter infested caves and inhale aerosols created by the bats. Aerosols of rabies virus inadvertently produced in laboratories are dangerous to laboratory workers.

In general, if a biting animal does not die within 10 days, rabies is unlikely, although rarely a rabid terrestrial animal will recover from rabies. Bats, on the contrary, are often infected for long periods without showing symptoms.

Since the dog is the most important vector of rabies for people throughout the world, this description by Blattner of rabies in the dog may be helpful:

In the dog symptoms may be considered under 2 general types, although it is not possible to separate them completely.

1. The "furious" type results from increased excitation of the central nervous system, with fever, hyperesthesia, and lack of appetite. The evidences of disease depend to a great extent upon the nature and training of the dog. The more aggressive dog will begin to snap and become excited and dangerous early in the course of the disease. The gentle dog in the early stages will more frequently seek seclusion and refuse food or will become excessively affectionate, after which it becomes agitated and restless. This is usually followed by irritability and snapping at strangers and a little later by snarling or snapping at imaginary objects and chasing and biting other animals. Finally, if free, it will run for miles, snapping at or biting all living things in its path until it falls paralyzed to the ground.

2. The "dumb" or paralytic type, despite its frequency (approximately 20%), is rarely recognized by the dog's owners, primarily because no agitation or excitement is seen. The

course is far more rapid, paralysis occurring in any group of muscles, but particularly in the lower jaw and in the muscles of deglutition. In such cases the tongue hangs out of the mouth, continuously dripping saliva; sympathetic persons, suspecting a foreign body in the dog's throat, may expose their hands to the infective saliva in an effort to relieve the dog. Rapidly extending paralysis soon results in death; occasionally dogs die suddenly without signs of illness, and encephalitis with Negri bodies is found at autopsy.

Recently, transmission of rabies by corneal transplant from a patient with encephalitis of unknown etiology to a healthy recipient was recorded.

Clinical Manifestations. The incubation period of rabies is extremely variable. Exceptionally long incubation periods of 1 yr have been seen. On the other hand, an incubation period of only 9 days has followed severe exposure. The great majority of cases have an incubation period of 20–180 days with the peak at 30–60 days. The length is related to the site of the bite: shortest for bites on the head, longest for bites on the legs. It also tends to be shorter in children and in vaccinated individuals who nevertheless develop rabies.

There is usually a prodromal phase of rabies, lasting 2–10 days. Common nonspecific symptoms include fever, malaise, headache, anorexia, and vomiting. The patient may be troubled by ill-defined anxiety. A characteristic symptom at this stage is pain or paresthesia at the site of the wound.

The illness then enters an acute neurologic phase, of either the furious or paralytic variety. In the former, hydrophobia is a pathognomonic sign. Attempts to swallow liquids, including saliva, result in spasms of the pharynx and larynx and aspiration into the trachea. Eventually a psychologic component exacerbates the spasms, and even the sight of water evokes terror. "Aerophobia" may be present and is considered by some also to be pathognomonic of rabies. Aerophobia is elicited by fanning a current of air across the face, which causes violent spasms of the pharyngeal and neck muscles.

The neurologic picture in the typical case may consist of bursts of hyperactivity, disorientation, and bizarre combative behavior, alternating with periods of lucidity. One of the most disturbing aspects of rabies to medical attendants is that during the patient's lucid periods he may be aware of what is happening to him and be able to articulate his fears. The facial expression of the patient is one of grim hopelessness.

Patients may also complain of pharyngeal pain, difficulty in swallowing, and hoarseness. Seizures are common, perhaps on the basis of hypoxia compounded by hyperventilation.

Some rabid patients develop meningismus or even opisthotonos. The cerebrospinal fluid may reflect meningeal irritation, with varying elevations of cells (predominantly lymphocytes) and protein, or may be normal. The peripheral white blood count often shows a polymorphonuclear leukocytosis.

In about 20% of patients, an ascending symmetric paralysis with flaccidity and decreased tendon reflexes dominates the entire acute phase. This course is particularly common after vampire bat bites. In the remainder of cases paralysis develops toward the end of the acute neurologic phase, which lasts from 2–10 days.

If the patient does not die of cardiorespiratory arrest during the acute stage, he or she slips into coma. With modern intensive care, life may be prolonged, but numerous complications occur during coma. Most significant is myocarditis, manifested by hypotension and arrhythmias. Rabies virus has been recovered from the heart which shows inflammation at autopsy. Also prominent is pituitary dysfunction expressed as either diabetes insipidus or inappropriate secretion of antidiuretic hormone. As the patient continues in coma, the complications of intensive hospital care appear. Unless recovery begins within 2 wk the outcome will be fatal, although patients can be kept alive for months.

Diagnosis and Differential Diagnosis. When a patient has a history of having been bitten by an animal, paresthesias at the wound site, and hydrophobia, a clinical diagnosis of rabies is not difficult. Any disease in which there is encephalitis may occasionally cause confusion, such as those caused by arboviruses, enteroviruses, and *Herpes simplex*. However, if one finds signs of brain stem involvement in a patient whose sensorium is basically clear and who has no signs of a space-occupying lesion, other diagnoses can usually be set aside.

Paralytic rabies may be misdiagnosed as *Guillain-Barré syndrome, poliomyelitis*, or *postrabies vaccine encephalomyelitis*. Careful neurologic examination and analysis of the cerebrospinal fluid will often help rule out these diagnoses.

The spasms of *tetanus* may cause momentary diagnostic confusion, but trismus is not seen in rabies, and hydrophobia is not seen in tetanus. Botulism (wound or ingestion) will cause paralysis, but the absence of sensory changes should exclude rabies.

Perhaps the most confusing differential problem is *hysteria* in an individual who thinks he or she has rabies. Normal blood gases and the absence of variation in bizarre behavior will suggest pseudorabies.

Laboratory diagnosis is now possible before death. The virus may be demonstrated by fluorescent antibody stain of smears of corneal epithelial cells or sections of skin from the neck at the hairline. These tests are positive because virus migrates down the nerves from the brain; both the cornea and hair follicles are richly innervated. Autopsy examination of the brains of patients with fatal encephalitis in rabies-endemic areas should include fluorescent antibody tests for rabies.

Serologic diagnosis is also possible if the patient survives beyond the acute period. Neutralizing antibodies develop in both serum and cerebrospinal fluid and rapidly rise to extremely high levels, e.g., >100 International Units (IU). Vaccination, even with potent vaccine, is unlikely to raise titers above 20 IU, and after duck embryo vaccine (DEV) the titers are often <2 IU.

Prognosis. The recovery of a child who developed rabies after a bat bite raised optimism that survival in rabies might be possible with intensive care. Two more patients have now survived rabies, but optimism seems unjustified. Many other patients have been treated intensively but have nevertheless died after prolonged courses. The severity of brain stem encephalitis determines the outcome; if too many neurons are destroyed, the patient does not survive.

Prevention of Rabies

Pre-exposure Prophylaxis. Vaccination of domestic dogs and elimination of strays have resulted in eradication of terrestrial rabies from many areas. If dog control were properly practiced, rabies could be suppressed in much of the world.

Those who are expected to be at risk, such as veterinarians, laboratory workers, and children going to rabies-enzootic areas, can be preimmunized. The new cell culture vaccine (see below) will produce virtually 100% response with 3 doses given at 0, 7, and 21 days. A titer of 0.3 IU has been accepted as protective, although some observations suggest the need for a higher titer.

Post-exposure Prophylaxis. First a decision must be made as to whether rabies prophylaxis is necessary. In many areas of the United States, rabies in mammals has been unknown for years. In those areas only bat bites call for treatment. Otherwise, the unprovoked bite of a wild animal should be considered rabid if the animal belongs to a species known to be a rabies host, such as a skunk, fox, raccoon, bat, or coyote. Rodents are very rare carriers of rabies in the United States.

If a domestic animal such as a dog or cat is the offender, consideration must be given to the question of provocation, to the clinical appearance of the animal if apprehended, and to the rabies vaccination status of the animal. Difficulty in making decisions arises when the biting animal has run away after a seemingly unprovoked attack. Whether the animal was rabid or merely ill-tempered is often impossible to decide. When the animal is under observation, rabies treatment can be withheld as long as it acts normally. However, a wild animal should be killed immediately and its brain examined for rabies antigen by the fluorescent-antibody technique.

Table 10–49 may help in making the often difficult decision whether to treat or not to treat.

If rabies prophylaxis is to be given after exposure, prevention depends on 3 complementary means of reducing the risk. Local treatment (see below) is designed to kill the virus by mechanical and virucidal action. Passive antibody (see below) then provides immediate blockage of attachment of virus to the nerve endings. However, passive antibody ultimately disappears and must be replaced by the active response provided by vaccine. The number of vaccine doses administered depends on its antigenic mass. The vaccine must not only produce a primary antibody response but also overcome the depressive effect of passive antibody on the immune response. In general, the latter requirement necessitates a booster 21 days or later after the administration of the passive antibody.

Local Treatment. The chief requirement of local treatment is that it be prompt and thorough. Simple mechanical removal by soap and water should be the 1st step, using copious amounts of solution. Catheters should be inserted for irrigation of puncture wounds. If the mechanical trauma of the local treatment is painful, procaine-type anesthetics may be used to infiltrate the area without adding risk.

The mechanical removal of virus should be followed by application of a virucidal solution such as 1% ben-

Table 10–49 POSTEXPOSURE ANTIRABIES TREATMENT GUIDE

ANIMAL	EVALUATION OF ANIMAL AT TIME OF EXPOSURE*	TREATMENT OF EXPOSED HUMAN
Wild Skunk Fox Raccoon Coyote Bat	Regard as rabid	HRIG + V†
Domestic Dogs and Cats	Healthy	None‡
	Escaped (unknown)	HRIG + V§
	Rabid or suspect rabid	HRIG + V†

*An exposure is considered to be by bite, by scratch with claws, or by contamination with saliva of mucosal surfaces or skin that has been cut or abraded.

†Discontinue vaccine if fluorescent antibody tests of animal are negative.

‡Begin HRIG + V at first sign of rabies in biting dog or cat during holding period (10 days).

§In a rabies enzootic area, treat; in a rabies free area, no treatment may be indicated. V = Rabies vaccine; HRIG = Human rabies immune globulin.

These recommendations are only a guide. They should be used in conjunction with knowledge of the animal species involved, circumstances of the bite or other exposure, vaccination status of the animal, and presence of rabies in the region.

Modified from Public Health Service Advisory Committee Recommendations, Ann Intern Med *86*:452, 1977.

zalkonium chloride made from concentrated Zephiran, 1% povidone-iodine, or 70% alcohol. In an emergency, any alcoholic liquor of 86 proof or higher may be used. However, some authorities eschew antisepsis and depend on soap and water irrigation.

Passive Antibody. Passive antibody is available in the form of equine antiserum (Lederle) or human rabies immune globulin (Cutter). The latter avoids serum sickness reactions to equine protein which occur in about 25% of recipients of the animal product. The dose for equine antirabies serum is 40 IU/kg. Up to half of the dose should be infiltrated subcutaneously at the site of bite or scratch; the remainder is injected intramuscularly into the arm or buttocks. The dose for human rabies immune globulin is 20 IU/kg delivered in the same manner.

Passive immunization should be performed regardless of the interval between rabies exposure and treatment. Anaphylaxis is a possibility with the equine antiserum, and tests for hypersensitivity should be carried out in the usual manner (consult package insert). Steroids should be avoided in the treatment of reactions since they cause activation of rabies virus in experimental situations.

Active Immunization. Until 1980, two vaccines were available in the United States—duck embryo vaccine (DEV) and human diploid cell vaccine (HDCV).

Duck embryo vaccine (DEV) had been used since the late 1950's. Its low antigenicity and frequent allergic reactions were problems. When DEV was used together with antiserum, as many as 23% of recipients failed to develop an antibody response. Reactions to DEV included rare neurologic problems (about 1 in 35,000 persons vaccinated), anaphylaxis in 0.9%, and systemic symptoms in 33%.

Human diploid cell vaccine (HDCV) has had 6 yr of commercial use in Europe and has withstood the challenge of severe exposures to confirmed rabid animals in Iran, West Germany, and France. HDCV has also had extensive prelicensing testing in the United States; it is now the only vaccine used widely for the prevention of rabies.

HDCV appears to be about 10-fold more antigenic than DEV; accordingly, the number of doses can be reduced. The schedule which has been used in Europe for postexposure vaccination consists of 6 doses (1 ml intramuscularly) at 0, 3, 7, 14, 30, and 90 days. However, the current American recommendation is 5 doses at 0, 3, 7, 14, and 28 days. For pre-exposure vaccination of high-risk groups, inoculations are given at 0, 7, and 21 days.

Reaction rates have been low, and neurologic reactions have been rare. Although greater numbers of vaccinated persons are needed to verify safety, it is comforting that no nerve tissue is present in the cell culture used to grow the virus. Allergic reactions have occurred in less than 0.1%, and systemic symptoms such as malaise and fever in only 5–15%, perhaps because of the absence of nonhuman protein in the vaccine.

Treatment of Clinical Rabies. Large doses of interferon and antirabies serum have been advocated, but it is doubtful that these substances can affect rabies that has already spread to the brain. Intensive supportive care may allow an occasional patient to survive.

STANLEY A. PLOTKIN

Anderson LJ, Sikes RK, Langkop CW, et al: Prophylactic immunization: Postexposure trial of a human diploid cell strain rabies vaccine. J Infect Dis 142:133, 1980.

Bhatt DR, Hattwick MAW, Gerdsen R, et al: Human rabies—diagnosis, complications, and management. Am J Dis Child 127:862, 1974.

Hattwick MAW, Rutin RH, Music S, et al: Postexposure rabies prophylaxis with human rabies immune globulin. JAMA 227:407, 1974.

Plotkin SA: Rabies vaccine prepared in human cell cultures: Progress and perspectives. Rev Infect Dis 2:433, 1980.

Plotkin SA, Clark HF: Committee on Immunization—prevention of rabies in man. J Infect Dis 123:227, 1971.

Public Health Service Advisory Committee on Immunization Practices: Rabies: Risk, management, prophylaxis, and immunization. Ann Intern Med 86:452, 1977

Turner GS: A review of the world epidemiology of rabies. Tr R Soc Trop Med Hyg 70:175, 1976.

Warrell DA: The clinical picture of rabies in man. Tr R Soc Trop Med Hyg 70:188, 1976.

Wiktor TJ, Hattwick MAW: Rhabdoviruses: Rabies and rabies-related viruses. In: Kurstak E, Kurstak C (eds): Comparative Diagnosis of Viral Diseases. New York, Academic Press, 1977.

10.86 SLOW REACTIONS OF THE HUMAN NERVOUS SYSTEM TO VIRUSES
(Slow Virus Infections)

As a result of evidence accumulated in recent yr, it has become clear that viruses are the causes of a group of central nervous system diseases that were previously regarded as degenerative or hereditary. These diseases are described as slow virus infections because the interaction between virus and host tissues that eventuates in disease takes place over a period of at least months and usually years. Once clinically manifest, these conditions progress rapidly and unremittingly, and are eventually fatal. Slow, therefore, is a term more descriptive of their long incubation period than of their course once clinical manifestations appear. Although viral replication occurs in various body organs, pathologic changes are seen only in the central nervous system. The viruses involved have been categorized into 2 groups: *conventional viruses* and *unconventional viruses*. The conventional viruses that sometimes produce slow infections (measles [rubeola], rubella, and papovaviruses) possess the usual structural and biologic properties of viruses. The unconventional viruses are quite different from all other viruses in that they possess no nucleic acid cores, protein coats, or lipid envelopes and are, therefore, not recognizable as viruses by electron microscopy. They cannot be detected by cell culture techniques and induce no immunologic or inflammatory changes in the host. They are also unusually resistant to physicochemical inactivation. The only evidence suggesting that these unconventional agents are viruses is that they pass through bacterial filters of small pore size and replicate in the reticuloendothelial system and later in the brains of experimental animals after parenteral inoculation. The possibility must be considered that they constitute a new class of infectious agents.

Slow Infections with Unconventional Viruses

The concept of slow virus infections of the nervous system of animals was proposed by Sigurdsson in 1954 as a result of his investigations of *scrapie*, a progressive degenerative and fatal neurologic disease of sheep and goats that, as the name suggests, causes the animals to rub and scratch. Infection with the scrapie agent, an unconventional virus, can be transmitted to small animals and serves as a model for slow virus infections associated with severe progressive neurologic disease in humans. Another animal disease in this category is transmissible mink encephalopathy.

Spongiform Encephalopathies. The histopathology of scrapie and transmissible mink encephalopathy closely resembles that seen in *kuru* and *Creutzfeldt-Jakob disease*, 2 degenerative neurologic diseases of humans caused by unconventional viruses. The pathologic changes are those of a progressive spongiform encephalopathy, so called because of the intracytoplasmic vacuoles that develop in neurons and astrocytes. The affected neurons degenerate and astrocytic gliosis ensues.

Kuru. This heredofamilial degenerative disease of the central nervous system presents as a trembling ataxia (kuru means "trembling with fear") with progressive incapacity and death. It is confined to an area of the eastern highlands of Papua, New Guinea, inhabited by the Fore tribe. By Fore custom the dead, including those dying of kuru, are eaten by female relatives. Participants in this practice of ritual cannibalism probably become infected by self-inoculation of infected brain tissue into dermal abrasions or mucosal surfaces. Because men do not participate, kuru occurs predominantly in women and in young children of both sexes who probably become inoculated with infected tissue by close association with their mothers during the ritual meal. With the decline in the practice of this custom, kuru has almost disappeared.

Several thousand cases have been documented in New Guinea. Some have occurred years later in persons who have migrated out of the endemic area. Kuru may appear in young children or after an incubation period of up to 18 yr. Brain tissue from subjects with kuru, when inoculated into chimpanzees, reproduces the disease after a latent period of 20 mo.

Creutzfeldt-Jakob Disease. This presenile dementia is predominantly a disease of older adults, although some affected patients in their 20's have been reported. It begins with vague psychic disturbances that progress within a few mo to dementia accompanied by pyramidal and extrapyramidal tract signs, cerebellar dysfunction, and rigidity. Death soon occurs. As in kuru, the brain shows noninflammatory spongiform changes and gliosis; however, Creutzfeldt-Jakob disease has a worldwide distribution. The prevalence rate in Europe and North and South America is estimated to be 1–2/million population.

The disease has been transmitted to primates and subprimates by intracerebral and parenteral inoculation with brain tissue from affected humans. Direct human-to-human transmission was first observed when a cornea collected post mortem from a patient retrospectively diagnosed as having the disease was transplanted to a normal individual who developed the disease 18 mo later. Since then, cases have been connected with neurosurgical procedures, such as the insertion of electrodes sterilized with ethanol and formaldehyde into the brain. The agent, as is true of kuru and of the viruses of scrapie and mink encephalopathy, withstands usual methods of sterilization. Neurosurgeons, neuropathologists, and others may be at special risk of acquiring the disease. Tissues from patients with Creutzfeldt-Jakob disease, therefore, should be handled with caution to prevent careless contamination of personnel and the environment. Equipment that has come in direct contact with tissues or blood from these patients should be autoclaved for 1 hr before being discarded or prepared for reuse. The natural route of transmission of this disease is unknown. Because it occurs in both a sporadic and familial form, it has been speculated that in some families there may be a genetic susceptibility to this slow virus infection.

Slow Infections with Conventional Viruses

These diseases are unusual late sequelae of commonly occurring infections with conventional viruses. The acute phase of these infections is not unusual. After a period of months or years, however, a neurologic illness appears that is usually progressive and fatal. These slow reactions to viruses are distinct from the early neurologic complications that sometimes occur during or shortly after the acute phase of viral infections (e.g., measles encephalitis).

Subacute Sclerosing Panencephalitis (SSPE). SSPE is a rare complication of infection with measles virus that appears 5–6 yr after the acute disease or immunization with live measles vaccine virus. The illness begins with insidious changes in personality, behavior, and intellect. After a period of weeks or months the steadily progressive course is characterized by dystonic and myoclonic movements, by convulsions, and terminally by decorticate rigidity. The estimated incidence of SSPE is 1/100,000 cases of natural measles and 1/1–2 million doses of attenuated measles vaccine. Mean age of onset is 7–8 yr, but cases have been reported in children less than 2 and in adults over 20. The disease occurs 3–4 times more frequently in boys than in girls.

The brain shows marked proliferation of astrocytes and microglial cells (hence the term sclerosing) along with demyelinization and intranuclear inclusion bodies. Perivascular cuffing and diffuse mononuclear infiltration of the gray and white matter are also observed. The isolation of a measles-like virus from the brain and the presence of high titers of measles virus antibody in the cerebrospinal fluid and serum are the basis for assuming that SSPE results from an unusual reaction between measles virus and the central nervous system. Cofactors appear to be involved, however, since the disease has a rural prevalence and occurs with increased frequency in underdeveloped countries. No cellular or humoral immune deficiencies have been identified in affected persons. The incidence of SSPE has declined as the use of measles vaccine has increased.

Progressive Rubella Panencephalitis (PRP). PRP is a chronic, progressive inflammatory disorder of the central nervous system that occurs as a late complication of either congenitally or postnatally acquired rubella. The onset in most cases is in the 2nd decade, and the disease follows a protracted course over a period of several yr. Patients exhibit slowly progressive cerebellar ataxia, spasticity, convulsions, and mental deterioration. PRP should not be confused with the encephalitis that frequently occurs as a component of the congenital rubella syndrome. The latter condition is either present at birth or develops during the 1st few mo of life. Although this early form of encephalitis follows a variable course, the child's neurologic status usually stabilizes by or during the 2nd yr of life. PRP, in contrast, occurs many yr later. The brain shows perivascular accumulations of lymphocytes and plasma cells, diffuse loss of neurons, and gliosis. Blood vessels of the central nervous system contain amorphous deposits similar to those seen in the blood vessels of children dying with congenital rubella. High titers of antibody against rubella virus are present in the serum and cerebrospinal fluid, and rubella virus has been isolated from the brain. No immunodeficiencies have been detected in patients with PRP. Rubella virus has an affinity for the central nervous system, and congenitally acquired infection can persist in certain tissues for months to years. The mechanisms by which this virus produces a progressive neurologic disease many yr after initial exposure, however, are unknown.

Progressive Multifocal Leukoencephalopathy (PML). The neuropathologic changes that occur in PML consist of noninflammatory foci of demyelination and loss of oligodendroglia throughout the white matter. The oligodendroglia at the periphery of these foci contain intranuclear inclusion bodies that are filled with papovavirus-like particles, and 2 strains of this group of viruses have been isolated from the brains of affected patients. Most patients with PML are adults who have pre-existing disorders associated with secondary immunodeficiency. The presenting neurologic signs depend upon the location of the foci of demyelinization. As these foci enlarge or coalesce, neurologic disability increases, and death usually occurs within 1 yr from onset of symptoms.

Although PML is a rare disease, asymptomatic infections with papovaviruses are widespread. Seroepidemiologic studies have shown that by adult life most persons have acquired this infection. Apparently when immune function is depressed by disease, an unusual reaction, manifest as PML, develops between brain tissue and papovaviruses in some infected persons. It is not known, however, whether PML results from activation of persistent central nervous system infection acquired earlier in life, or whether this disease represents the response of an immunodepressed host to 1st contact with these agents.

Slow Infections with Other Viruses. The slow virus infections that have been recognized are rare. Because of the potential for prevention, it is important to determine if slow infections with viruses play an etiologic role in other chronic diseases of higher prevalence such as multiple sclerosis, the dementias, and certain forms of cancer.

ALFRED D. HEGGIE

Chen TT, Watanabe I, Mealey J Jr: Subacute sclerosing panencephalitis: Propagation of measles virus from brain biopsy in tissue culture. Science 163:1193, 1969.

Duffy P, Wolf J, Collins G, et al: Person to person transmission of Creutzfeldt-Jakob disease. N Engl J Med 290:692, 1974.

Gadjusek DC: Unconventional viruses and the origin and disappearance of kuru. Science 197:943, 1977.

Gadjusek DC, Gibbs CJ Jr, Asher DM, et al: Precautions in medical care of, and in handling materials from, patients with transmissible virus dementia (Creutzfeldt-Jakob disease). N Engl J Med 297:1253, 1977.

Gibbs CJ Jr: Virus-induced subacute degenerative disease of the central nervous system. Ophthalmology 87:1208, 1980.

Horta-Barbosa L, Hamilton R, Wittig R, et al: Subacute sclerosing panencephalitis: Isolation of suppressed measles virus from lymph node biopsies. Science 173:840, 1971.

Johnson RT: Progressive rubella encephalitis. N Engl J Med 292:1023, 1975.

Kimerlin RH (ed): Slow Virus Diseases of Animals and Man. Amsterdam, North Holland Publishing, 1976.

Lebon P, Lyon G: Non-congenital rubella encephalitis. Lancet 2:468, 1974.

Meulen V ter, Hall WW: Slow virus infections of the nervous system: Virological, immunological, and pathogenetic considerations. J Gen Virol 41:1, 1978.

Modlin JF, Jabbour JT, Witte JJ, et al: Epidemiologic studies of measles, measles vaccine, and subacute sclerosing panencephalitis. Pediatrics 59:505, 1977.

Modlin JT, Halsey NA, Herrmann KL: Infantile onset of subacute sclerosing panencephalitis. J Pediatr 91:168, 1977.

Narayan O, Penney JB Jr, Johnson RT, et al: Etiology of progressive multifocal leukoencephalopathy. Identification of papovavirus. N Engl J Med 289:1278, 1973.

Nathanson N: Slow viruses and chronic disease: The contribution of epidemiology. Pub Health Rep 95:436, 1980.

Sutton RNP: Slow viruses and chronic disease of the central nervous system. Postgrad Med J 55:143, 1979.

Townsend JJ, Baringer JR, Wolinsky JS, et al: Progressive rubella panencephalitis. Late onset after congenital rubella. N Engl J Med 292:990, 1975.

Townsend JJ, Wolinsky JS, Baringer JR: The neuropathology of progressive rubella panencephalitis of late onset. Brain 99:81, 1976.

Weil ML, Habashi HH, Cremer NE, et al: Chronic progressive panencephalitis due to rubella virus simulating SSPE. N Engl J Med 292:994, 1975.

Arboviral Diseases

10.87   YELLOW FEVER

Yellow fever is an acute viral infection transmitted to man through bites of culicine mosquitos. Because of the availability of a highly protective vaccination, yellow fever is becoming a disease of limited clinical significance; but control measures should not be relaxed as recent experiences in West Africa showed that transmission can quickly reach epidemic dimensions.

Etiology. Man acquires yellow fever infection through bites of mosquitos of the various species of *Aedes* and less commonly *Haemagogus*. The insects inoculate into the bite site the yellow fever virus, a group B arbovirus. This single-stranded RNA virus appears in the peripheral blood of infected individuals within 1 wk and remains in the circulation for approximately 6 days. During this period of viremia, infection can be transmitted to mosquitos if they suck a blood meal. The insect vector becomes capable of transmitting the infection within 2–3 wk and remains so for the rest of its life (2–3 mo).

Epidemiology. Two patterns of yellow fever transmission occur in endemic areas. The urban form involves man–mosquito–man and is therefore dependent on domestic breeders such as *A. aegypti*. In the jungle form of yellow fever, the pattern of transmission is forest animals–mosquito–forest animals. The most commonly affected animals are primates, and the vectors are *Aedes* species other than *A. aegypti* or *Haemagogus*. Jungle yellow fever is transmitted to man accidentally, either through visits to forests or by infection of other vectors which transiently inhabit areas visited by man.

In endemic areas infection is maintained through young children or nonimmune visitors. Adults in these areas acquire some degree of resistance to yellow fever. Epidemics occur if this balance is upset by introduction of suitable nonimmune hosts in the presence of infective reservoirs and efficient insect vectors.

The geographic distribution of yellow fever is confined to northern parts of South America and West and Central Africa. Infection is rarely encountered in Central America, although it has appeared in some Caribbean islands. No yellow fever cases have ever been reported from Asia.

Clinical Manifestations. Infection with the yellow fever virus is usually mild and may pass unnoticed. In symptomatic patients sudden onset of fever, nausea, vomiting, myalgia, and headache is the characteristic clinical presentation. Symptoms begin approximately 3–6 days following viral inoculation, but the incubation period may last up to 2 wk. Symptoms are associated with viral dissemination which results in necrotizing lesions in almost all organs. In a small proportion of symptomatic patients, severe manifestations such as a bleeding tendency (particularly in the gastrointestinal tract), proteinuria, and jaundice may occur; disease usually progresses to hepatorenal failure and death in these individuals. Mortality in endemic areas does not exceed 5%; during epidemics, however, mortality rates as high as 40% have been reported.

Diagnosis and Treatment. Yellow fever should be suspected when recent visitors (within the previous 2 wk) or residents of endemic areas present with nausea, vomiting, or myalgias. Definitive diagnosis can be obtained only by demonstrating a rise in antibody titer or by isolation of the virus. None of the available antiviral agents has a known effect on yellow fever virus. Management is therefore supportive, with particular attention being paid to bleeding tendencies and kidney function.

Control. The single most important measure in achieving control of yellow fever is wide-scale vaccination of individuals in endemic areas and of those visiting or moving there. The recommended vaccine is a live attenuated virus prepared from the 17 D strain. It is administered as a single subcutaneous injection of the reconstituted vaccine. Children below 5 yr should be given 0.2 ml; older children, 0.5 ml. Protection, as demonstrated by the development of specific antibodies, begins 10 days after vaccination, lasts for 10 yr, and probably has an effect for the lifetime of the individual. The risk of encephalitis is very small, significantly less than with other live vaccines prepared in chick embryos. Yellow fever vaccination is regulated by international law; individuals going to or arriving from known endemic areas should carry a valid certificate.

ADEL A. F. MAHMOUD

Downs W: Arboviruses. *In* Evans AS (ed): Viral Infections of Humans. Plenum Medical Book Co, 1982, pp 95–126.
Yellow fever epidemic—The Gambia, 1978–1979. Morbidity and Mortality Weekly Report 28:351, 1979.

10.88 DENGUE FEVER AND DENGUE-LIKE DISEASE

Dengue fever is a benign syndrome, caused by several arthropod-borne viruses, characterized by biphasic fever, myalgia or arthralgia, rash, leukopenia, and lymphadenopathy.

History. Epidemic dengue-like disease was described by David Bylon in Java in 1779 and a year later in Philadelphia by Benjamin Rush. Epidemics were common in temperate areas of the Americas, Europe, Australia, and Asia until early in the 20th century. Dengue fever and dengue-like disease are now endemic in tropical Asia, Africa, and Central and South America. Extensive epidemics of dengue occurred in Oceania in 1971–1972 and 1974–1975. Sporadic cases occurred in the United States in 1980.

Etiology. There are at least 4 distinct antigenic types of dengue virus. In addition, 3 other arthropod-borne (arbo) viruses cause similar or identical febrile diseases with rash (Table 10–50).

Epidemiology. Dengue viruses are transmitted by mosquitoes of the Stegomyia family. *Aedes aegypti*, a daytime biting mosquito, is the principal vector. All 4 virus types have been recovered from naturally infected *Aedes aegypti*. In most tropical areas *Aedes aegypti* is highly urbanized, breeding in water stored for drinking or bathing or in rain water collected in any container. Dengue viruses have been recovered also from *Aedes albopictus*, and outbreaks in the Pacific area have been attributed to *Aedes scutellaris*. These species breed in water trapped in vegetation; *Aedes albopictus* frequently breeds in bamboo stumps. In Malaysia, dengue may be maintained in a cycle involving canopy-feeding jungle monkeys and *Aedes niveus*, which feeds on both monkeys and man.

Dengue outbreaks in urban areas infested with *Aedes aegypti* may be explosive; up to 70–80% of the population may be involved. Because *Aedes aegypti* has a limited range, spread of an epidemic occurs mainly through viremic human beings and follows main lines of transportation. Sentinel cases may infect household mosquitoes, with a large number of nearly simultaneous secondary infections giving the appearance of a contagious disease. Where dengue is endemic, children and susceptible foreigners may be the only persons to acquire overt disease, adults having become immune.

Dengue-like diseases may occur in epidemics. Epidemiologic features depend upon the vectors and their geographic distribution (Table 10–50). Chikungunya virus is widespread in the most populous areas of the world. In Asia *Aedes aegypti* is the principal vector; in Africa other Stegomyia may be important vectors. In Southeast Asia, dengue and chikungunya outbreaks occur concurrently. Outbreaks of O'nyong-nyong and West Nile fever usually involve villages or small towns, in contrast to the urban outbreaks of dengue and chikungunya.

Table 10–50 VECTORS AND GEOGRAPHIC DISTRIBUTION OF DENGUE-LIKE DISEASES

TOGAVIRUS GENUS	VIRUS AND DISEASE	VECTOR	GEOGRAPHIC DISTRIBUTION
Alphavirus	Chikungunya	*Aedes aegypti* *Aedes africanus*	Africa, India, Southeast Asia
Alphavirus	O'nyong-nyong	*Anopheles funestus*	East Africa
Flavivirus	West Nile fever	*Culex molestus* *Culex univittatus*	Africa, Middle East, India

Pathology. Insufficient pathologic material has been obtained from virologically confirmed cases of dengue fever to permit a comprehensive description. Fatalities are rare with chikungunya and West Nile infections; those recorded have been ascribed to viral encephalitis, hemorrhage, or febrile convulsions (Sec 10.89).

Clinical Manifestations. Biphasic fever and rashes are the most characteristic features of dengue. Manifestations vary with age and from patient to patient. In infants and young children the disease may be undifferentiated or characterized by a 1–5 day fever, pharyngeal inflammation, rhinitis, and mild cough. In outbreaks a majority of patients have most of the findings described below.

After an incubation period of 1–7 days there is a sudden onset of fever which rapidly rises to 39.4–41.1° C (103–106° F), usually accompanied by frontal or retro-orbital headache. Occasionally, back pain precedes the fever. A *transient*, macular, generalized rash which blanches under pressure may be seen during the 1st 24–48 hr of fever. The pulse rate may be slow relative to the degree of fever. Myalgia or arthralgia occurs soon after onset and increases in severity. Involvement of the knee may be particularly severe in patients with chikungunya or O'nyong-nyong infection. From the 2nd–6th day of fever, nausea and vomiting are apt to occur, and generalized lymphadenopathy, cutaneous hyperesthesia or hyperalgesia, taste aberrations, and pronounced anorexia may develop.

One–2 days after defervescence a generalized, morbilliform, maculopapular rash appears, which spares the palms and soles. It disappears in 1–5 days; desquamation may occur. Rarely there is edema of the palms and soles. About the time of appearance of this 2nd rash the body temperature, which has previously fallen to normal, may become slightly elevated and establish the biphasic temperature curve.

Epistaxis, petechiae, and purpuric lesions are uncommon but may occur at any stage of the disease. Swallowed blood from epistaxis, vomited or passed by rectum, may be erroneously interpreted as bleeding of gastrointestinal origin. Convulsions may occur during high fever, especially with chikungunya fever.

After the febrile stage prolonged asthenia, mental depression, bradycardia, and ventricular extrasystoles are common in adults but occur infrequently in children.

Laboratory Data. Pancytopenia may be found on the 3rd–4th day of illness; neutropenia may persist or reappear during the latter stage of the disease and may continue into convalescence. White blood cell counts as low as 2000/mm³ have been recorded. Platelets rarely fall below 100,000 cells/mm³. Venous clotting, bleeding and prothrombin times, and plasma fibrinogen values are within normal ranges. The tourniquet test infrequently is positive. Mild acidosis, hemoconcentration, increased transaminase values, and hypoproteinemia may occur during primary dengue virus infections, particularly in infants. Sinus bradycardia, ectopic ventricular foci, flattened T waves, and prolongation of the P-R interval may be observed electrocardiographically.

Diagnosis and Differential Diagnosis. *Clinical diagnosis* derives from a high index of suspicion and a knowledge of the geographic distribution and environmental cycles of causal viruses. Activities of the patient prior to the onset of illness may give a clue to the possibility of infection.

Differential diagnosis includes a number of viral respiratory and influenza-like diseases and the early stages of malaria, scrub typhus, hepatitis, and leptospirosis. Abortive forms of these latter diseases modified by therapy or vaccine may never evolve beyond a dengue-like stage.

Three arboviral diseases have dengue-like courses but without rash: Colorado tick fever, sandfly fever, and Rift Valley fever. Colorado tick fever occurs sporadically among campers and hunters in the Western United States; sandfly fever in the Mediterranean region, and Middle East, southern Russia, and parts of the Indian subcontinent; and Rift Valley fever in North, East, Central, and South Africa.

Because clinical findings vary and possible causative agents are many, the term "dengue-like disease" should be used until a specific diagnosis is provided by the laboratory. *Etiologic diagnosis* can be made by serologic study or by isolation of the virus from blood monocytes or serum. Blood for comparative antibody and viral studies should be obtained during the febrile period, preferably early, and during the convalescent phase, 14–21 days after onset. The acute phase serum or plasma may be frozen, optimally at −65° C or colder. Leukocytes should be refrigerated, not frozen. *Serologic diagnosis* depends on a 4-fold or greater increase in antibody titer in paired sera by hemagglutination-inhibition, complement-fixation, or neutralization test. It may not be possible to distinguish the infecting virus by serologic methods alone, particularly when there has been prior infection with another member of the same arbovirus group. For this reason, isolation of the virus should be attempted. Virus can be recovered from tissue culture or after intrathoracic inoculation of appropriate mosquitoes.

Prevention and Control. An attenuated vaccine for dengue type 1 and a killed vaccine for chikungunya are efficacious but not available for general use. Prophylaxis consists in avoiding mosquito bite by use of insecticides, repellents, body-covering with clothing, screening of houses, and destruction of *Aedes aegypti* breeding sites. If water storage is mandatory, a tight-fitting lid or a thin layer of oil may prevent egg-laying or hatching. A larvicide, such as Abate [O,O'-(thiodi-p-phenylene) O,O,O',O'-tetramethyl phosphorothioate], available as a 1% sand-granule formation and effective at a concentration of 1 part/million, may be added safely to drinking water. Ultra-low volume spray equipment effectively dispenses the adulticide malathion from truck or airplane for rapid intervention during an epidemic. Only personal antimosquito measures are effective against mosquitoes in the field, forest, or jungle.

Treatment. Treatment is supportive. Bed rest is advised during the febrile period. Antipyretics or cold sponging should be used to keep body temperature below 40° C (104° F). Analgesics or mild sedation may be required to control pain. Fluid and electrolyte replacement is required when there are deficits due to sweating, fasting, thirsting, vomiting, or diarrhea.

Prognosis. Primary infections with dengue fever and dengue-like diseases are usually self-limited and benign. Fluid and electrolyte losses, hyperpyrexia, and febrile convulsions are the most frequent complications in infants and young children, particularly in tropical countries. The prognosis may be adversely affected by passively acquired antibody or by prior infection with a closely related virus (Sec 10.89).

Dengue in the Caribbean, 1977. Scientific Publication No. 375. Washington, D.C., Pan American Health Organization, 1979.

Schlesinger RW: Dengue Viruses. Virology Monograph 16. New York, Springer Verlag, 1977.

10.89   DENGUE HEMORRHAGIC FEVER/DENGUE SHOCK SYNDROME
(Philippine, Thai, or Singapore Hemorrhagic Fever; Hemorrhagic Dengue; Acute Infectious Thrombocytopenic Purpura)

Definition. Dengue hemorrhagic fever is a severe, often fatal, febrile disease caused by dengue viruses. It is characterized by capillary permeability, abnormalities of hemostasis, and, in severe cases, a protein-losing shock syndrome. It is currently thought to have an immunopathologic basis.

History. Hammon in 1956 established the causative relation of dengue infection to dengue hemorrhagic fever, which may have occurred in Australian children as early as 1897. Recent epidemics have involved most of Southeast Asia and Cuba.

Etiology. At least 4 distinct types of dengue virus (types 1–4) have been isolated from patients with hemorrhagic fever.

Epidemiology. Dengue hemorrhagic fever occurs where multiple types of dengue virus are simultaneously or sequentially transmitted. It is almost exclusively a disease of children. It is endemic in tropical Asia, where warm temperatures and the practice of water storage in homes result in large, permanent populations of *Aedes aegypti*. Under these conditions infections with dengue viruses of all types are common, and 2nd infections with heterologous types are frequent. Ninety per cent of patients with typical severe hemorrhagic fever have a secondary rise of antibody against dengue virus, indicative of a previous infection with a closely related virus. Dengue hemorrhagic fever may occur during primary dengue infections, most frequently in infants whose mothers prove to be immune.

Nonimmune foreigners, adults or children, exposed to dengue virus during outbreaks of hemorrhagic fever have classic dengue fever or even milder disease. The differences in clinical manifestations of dengue infections between natives and foreigners are probably re-lated more to immunologic status than to racial susceptibility.

In 1981 a large outbreak of dengue hemorrhagic fever occurred in Cuba. More than 10,000 children and adults were hospitalized with dengue shock syndrome, and 158 died. The outbreak was caused by dengue 2, which had been preceded by an island-wide epidemic of dengue 1 in 1977. Severe cases occurred in individuals experiencing 2nd infections.

Pathology. Usually no pathologic lesions are found to account for death. In rare instances, death may be due to gastrointestinal or intracranial hemorrhages. Minimal to moderate hemorrhages are seen in the upper gastrointestinal tract, and petechial hemorrhages are common in the interventricular septum of the heart, on the pericardium, and on the subserosal surfaces of major viscera. Focal hemorrhages are occasionally seen in the lungs, liver, adrenals, and subarachnoid space. The liver is usually enlarged, often with fatty changes. Yellow, watery, at times blood-tinged effusions are present in serous cavities in about three fourths of patients. Retroperitoneal tissues are markedly edematous.

Microscopically, there is perivascular edema in the soft tissues and widespread diapedesis of red blood cells. There may be maturational arrest of megakaryocytes in bone marrow, and increased numbers of them are seen in capillaries of the lungs, in renal glomeruli, and in sinusoids of the liver and spleen. Proliferation of lymphocytoid and plasmacytoid cells, lymphocytolysis, and lymphophagocytosis occur in the spleen and lymph nodes. In the spleen the germinal centers of the malpighian corpuscles are active and often necrotic. The thymus is depleted of lymphocytes. The liver shows varying degrees of fatty metamorphosis, focal midzonal necrosis, and hyperplasia of the Kupffer cells; there are non-nucleated cells with vacuolated acidophilic cytoplasm, resembling Councilman bodies, in the sinusoids. There is a mild proliferative glomerulonephritis. Biopsies of the rash reveal swelling and minimal necrosis of endothelial cells and subcutaneous deposits of fibrinogen. Dengue viral antigen has been found in extravascular mononuclear cells; on blood vessel walls; in Kupffer cells; in splenic, thymic, and lung macrophages; and in skin histiocytes.

Dengue virus is almost invariably absent in tissues at the time of death, with rare isolations reported from lymphatic tissues.

Pathogenesis. The pathogenesis of shock and hemorrhage in human dengue is incompletely understood. It is possible that prior exposure may promote cellular infection and thus paradoxically enhance severity of the disease. Dengue viruses demonstrate enhanced growth in cultures of human mononuclear phagocytes prepared from dengue-immune donors or in cultures supplemented with non-neutralizing dengue antibody. Since biopsy and autopsy evidence from humans suggests that dengue virus infects macrophages, it has been proposed that the number of infected mononuclear phagocytes in individuals with naturally or passively acquired antibody may exceed that in nonimmunes and that increased production of phlogistic molecules by infected cells may contribute to shock. Early in the acute stage of secondary dengue infections, there is rapid activation of the complement system. During shock, blood levels of C1q, C3, C4, C5-8, and C3 proactivator are depressed and C3 catabolic rates elevated. The blood clotting and fibrinolytic systems are activated and levels of factor XII (Hageman factor) depressed, though there is no evidence of involvement of the kinin system. Shock may be mediated by histamine released from mast cells by the peptides C3a and C5a. As yet, however, no specific mediator of vascular permeability in dengue hemorrhagic fever has been identified. A mild degree of disseminated intravascular coagulation, liver damage, and thrombocytopenia may produce hemorrhage synergistically. Capillary damage allows fluid, electrolytes, protein, and, in some instances, red blood cells to leak into extravascular spaces. This internal redistribution of fluid, together with deficits due to fasting, thirsting, and vomiting, results in hemoconcentration, hypovolemia, increased cardiac work, tissue hypoxia, metabolic acidosis, and hyponatremia.

Clinical Manifestations. The incubation period of dengue hemorrhagic fever is presumed to be that of dengue fever. The course is characteristic in the severely ill child. A relatively mild 1st phase with abrupt onset of fever, malaise, vomiting, headache, anorexia, and cough is followed after 2–5 days by rapid clinical deterioration and collapse. In this 2nd phase the patient usually has cold, clammy extremities, a warm trunk, flushed face, diaphoresis, restlessness, irritability, and midepigastric pain. Frequently, there are scattered petechiae on the forehead and extremities; spontaneous ecchymoses may appear, and easy bruisability and bleeding at sites of venipuncture are common. A macular or maculopapular rash may appear, and there may be circumoral and peripheral cyanosis. Respirations are rapid and often labored. The pulse is weak, rapid, and thready and the heart sounds faint. The pulse pressure is frequently narrow (20 mm Hg or less); the blood pressure may be low or unobtainable. The liver may enlarge to 4–6 cm below the costal margin and is usually firm and somewhat tender. Fewer than 10% of patients have gross ecchymosis or gastrointestinal bleeding, usually following a period of uncorrected shock.

After a 24–36 hr period of crisis, convalescence is fairly rapid in the children who recover. The temperature may return to normal before or during the stage of shock. Bradycardia and ventricular extrasystoles are common during convalescence. Infrequently, there is residual brain damage due to prolonged shock or occasionally to intracranial hemorrhage.

In contrast to the fairly characteristic pattern in the severely ill child, secondary dengue infections are relatively mild in the majority of instances, ranging from an inapparent infection through an undifferentiated upper respiratory or dengue-like disease to an illness similar to that described above but without apparent shock.

Laboratory Data. The most common hematologic abnormalities during clinical shock are a 20% or greater increase in hematocrit over the recovery value, thrombocytopenia, mild leukocytosis (seldom exceeding 10,000/mm^3) with 1–5% of Türk cells, prolonged bleeding time, and moderately decreased prothrombin level

(seldom to less than 40% of control). Particularly after prolonged periods of shock and metabolic acidosis, fibrinogen levels may be subnormal and fibrinogen split-products elevated. The tourniquet test gives a positive result early in the illness except in the moribund child.

Other abnormalities include moderate elevations of the serum transaminases, mild metabolic acidosis with hyponatremia, and, at times, hypochloremia, slight elevation of serum urea nitrogen, and hypoalbuminemia. Roentgenograms of the chest reveal bronchopneumonia and pleural effusions in not quite 50% of patients.

Diagnosis and Differential Diagnosis. In areas endemic for dengue, hemorrhagic fever should be suspected in children with a febrile illness who exhibit hemoconcentration, thrombocytopenia, and hemorrhagic manifestations with or without shock. Since many rickettsial diseases, meningococcemia, and other severe illnesses caused by a variety of agents may produce a similar clinical picture, the diagnosis should be made only when epidemiologic or serologic evidence suggests the possibility of dengue fever. Hemorrhagic manifestations have been described in other diseases of viral or presumed viral origin, including the clinically distinguishable hemorrhagic fevers described in Sec 10.90.

In secondary dengue infections, there is a rapid and pronounced rise of both hemagglutination-inhibiting (HI) and complement-fixing (CF) antibodies to dengue antigen. The characteristic IgG antibody response establishes the diagnosis of secondary infection. There are usually high titers of HI antibody (1:640 or greater) and CF antibody (1:32 or greater) in both acute and convalescent serums.

Prevention. Preventive measures are described in Sec 10.88. The possibility exists that dengue vaccination may sensitize a recipient so that ensuing dengue infection may result in hemorrhagic fever. Vaccination with yellow fever 17D strain has no effect on dengue illness.

Treatment. Management requires immediate evaluation of vital signs and degrees of hemoconcentration, dehydration, and electrolyte imbalance. Close monitoring is essential for at least 48 hr since shock may occur or recur precipitously early in the disease. Patients who are cyanotic or have labored breathing should be given oxygen. Rapid intravenous replacement of fluids and electrolytes can frequently sustain patients until spontaneous recovery occurs. When elevation of the hematocrit persists after replacement of fluids, plasma or plasma colloid preparations are indicated. Care must be taken to avoid overhydration, which may contribute to cardiac failure. Transfusions of fresh blood or of platelets suspended in plasma may be required to control bleeding; they should not be given during hemoconcentration but only after evaluation of hemoglobin or hematocrit values. Salicylates are contraindicated because of their effect on blood clotting.

Paraldehyde or chloral hydrate may be required for children who are markedly agitated. Use of pressor amines, α-adrenergic blocking agents, and aldosterone has not resulted in a significant reduction of mortality over that observed with simple supportive therapy.

Heparin may be used with caution in patients with intractable bleeding, especially with objective evidence of severe disseminated intravascular coagulation. The general experience is that steroids do not shorten the duration of disease or improve prognosis in children receiving careful supportive therapy.

Hypervolemia during the fluid reabsorptive phase may be life threatening. This is heralded by a fall in hematocrit with wide pulse pressure. Diuretics, such as furosemide, should be administered; digitalization may be necessary.

Prognosis. Death has occurred in 40–50% of patients with shock, but with adequate intensive care should fall to less than 2%. Survival is directly related to early and intense management.

Bokisch VA, Top FH Jr, Russell PK, et al: The potential pathogenic role of complement in dengue hemorrhagic shock syndrome. N Engl J Med 289:996, 1973.

Cohen SN, Halstead SB: Shock associated with dengue infection. I. The clinical and physiological manifestations of dengue hemorrhagic fever in Thailand, 1964. J Pediatr 68:448, 1966.

Halstead SB: Dengue hemorrhagic fever, a public health problem and a field for research. Bull WHO 58:1, 1980.

Halstead SB: Immunological parameters of togavirus syndromes. In: Schlesinger RW (ed): Togaviruses. New York, Academic Press, 1980.

Halstead SB, O'Rourke EJ: Antibody-enhanced dengue virus infection in primate leukocytes. Nature 266:739, 1977.

Technical Guides for Diagnosis, Treatment, Surveillance, Prevention and Control of Dengue Haemorrhagic Fever. Geneva, World Health Organization, 1980.

10.90 OTHER VIRAL HEMORRHAGIC FEVERS

Viral hemorrhagic fevers are a loosely defined group of clinical syndromes in which hemorrhagic manifestations are either common or especially notable in severe illness. Both the etiologic agents and clinical features of the syndromes differ, but disseminated intravascular coagulation may be a common pathogenetic feature. A list of the more important viral hemorrhagic fevers is given in Table 10–51. Since overt hemorrhagic manifestations and abnormal hemostasis are relatively common in many viral diseases, the designation "viral hemorrhagic fever" should not be regarded as restrictive.

Etiology. Six of the viral hemorrhagic fevers are caused by arthropod-borne (arbo) viruses (Table 10–51). Four are togaviruses of the flavivirus group (KFD, OHF, DHF, and YF), and 2 are bunyaviruses (Congo and RVF). Junin (AHF), Machupo (BHF), and Lassa (LF) are arenaviruses, a morphologic and ecologic viral group. Ebola (EHF) and Marburg viruses are enveloped, filamentous RNA viruses, sometimes branched, unlike any other known virus. Hemorrhagic fever with renal syndrome (HFRS) is due to Hantaan virus, a bunyavirus.

Epidemiology. With rare exceptions, the viruses causing viral hemorrhagic fevers are initially transmitted through a nonhuman agency. Since a specific ecosystem is required for viral survival, these are diseases of place. Although it is commonly thought that all viral hemorrhagic fevers are arthropod-borne, 8 may be contracted from environmental contamination caused by animals or animal cells or from infected humans (RVF, AHF, BHF, CHF, LF, Marburg disease, EHF, and HFRS). To establish a diagnosis of hemorrhagic fever the physician must first show that the patient has had an appropriate geographic or ecologic exposure. Laboratory and hospital infections have occurred with many of these agents. This occupational hazard should be considered during any diagnostic evaluation. Lassa fever and Argentine and Bolivian hemorrhagic fevers are reportedly milder in children than in adults. Dengue hemorrhagic fever (Sec 10.89) and yellow fever (Sec 10.87) are well-established pediatric problems. Features of the more common viral hemorrhagic fevers are summarized below.

Tick-Borne Hemorrhagic Fevers. CONGO-CRIMEAN HEMORRHAGIC FEVER (CHF). Sporadic human infection in Africa provided the original virus isolation. Natural foci are recognized in Bulgaria, western Crimea, and the Rostov-on-Don and Astrakhan regions; a somewhat similar disease occurs in Kazakstan and Uzbekistan. In 1976 index cases were followed by nosocomial transmission in Pakistan and Baluchistan. In the Soviet

Table 10–51 OTHER VIRAL HEMORRHAGIC FEVERS

MODE OF TRANSMISSION	DISEASE	VIRUS
Tick-borne	Congo- Crimean HF (CHF)*	Congo
	Kyasanur Forest disease (KFD)	Kyasanur Forest disease
	Omsk HF (OHF)	Omsk
Mosquito-borne†	Dengue HF (DHF)	Dengue (4 types)
	Rift Valley fever (RVF)	Rift Valley fever
	Yellow fever (YF)	Yellow fever
Infected animals or materials to humans	Argentine HF (AHF)	Junin
	Bolivian HF (BHF)	Machupo
	Lassa fever (LF)*	Lassa
	Marburg disease*	Marburg
	Ebola HF (EHF)*	Ebola
	Hemorrhagic fever with renal syndrome (HFRS)	Hantaan

*Patients may be contagious; nosocomial infections are common.

†Chikungunya virus (Sec 10.88) is associated at low frequency with petechiae, petechial hemorrhages, and epistaxis. More severe hemorrhagic manifestations have been reported in some studies.

Union the vectors are *Hyaloma marginatum* and *H. anatolicum*, which, along with hares and birds, may serve as a viral reservoir since transovarial transmission is likely. Disease occurs from June to September, largely among farmers and dairy workers.

KYASANUR FOREST DISEASE (KFD). Human cases occur chiefly in adults in an area of Mysore State, India. The main vectors are 2 Ixodidae ticks, *Haemaphysalis turturis* and *H. spinigera*. Monkeys and forest rodents may be amplifying hosts. Laboratory infections are common.

OMSK HEMORRHAGIC FEVER (OHF). The disease occurs throughout the south central Soviet Union and in northern Rumania. Vectors of Omsk hemorrhagic fever virus may include *Dermacentor pictus* and *D. marginatus*, but direct transmission from moles and muskrats to humans seems well established. Human disease occurs in a spring-summer-autumn pattern, paralleling the activity of vectors. Omsk hemorrhagic fever occurs most frequently in persons with outdoor occupational exposure. Laboratory infections are common.

Mosquito-Borne Hemorrhagic Fevers. DENGUE HEMORRHAGIC FEVER AND YELLOW FEVER (DHF AND YF). See Sec 10.87 and 10.89.

RIFT VALLEY FEVER (RVF). The etiologic agent, first isolated in 1930, is responsible for epizootics involving sheep, cattle, buffalo, certain antelopes, and rodents in North, Central, East, and South Africa. The virus is transmitted to domestic animals by *Culex theileri* and several *Aedes* species. An epizootic in Egypt in 1977–78 was accompanied by thousands of human infections, principally among veterinarians, farmers, and farm laborers. Humans are most often infected during the slaughter or skinning of sick or dead animals. Laboratory infection is common.

Hemorrhagic Fever Transmitted Through Environmental Contamination. ARENAVIRAL DISEASE. The 1st described arenavirus was that of lymphocytic choriomeningitis (a non-HF); this virus establishes a persistent, tolerated infection in the young of the common house mouse, *Mus musculus*, which excretes virus continuously throughout life, contaminating food and fluids and creating a risk of airborne infection. There is evidence that Machupo and Junin viruses have similar host-parasite relationships with South American rodents as has Lassa virus with African rodents.

ARGENTINE HEMORRHAGIC FEVER (AHF). First recognized in 1955, hundreds to thousands of cases occur annually from April through July in the maize-producing area northwest of Buenos Aires that reaches to the eastern margin of the Province of Cordoba. Junin virus has been isolated from the rodents *Mus musculus*, *Akodon arenicola*, and *Calomys laucha laucha*. It infects migrant laborers who harvest the maize and who inhabit rodent-contaminated shelters.

BOLIVIAN HEMORRHAGIC FEVER (BHF). The recognized endemic area consists of the sparsely populated province of Beni in Amazonian Bolivia. Sporadic cases occur in farm families who raise maize, rice, yucca, and beans. In the town of San Joaquin a disturbance in the domestic rodent ecosystem may have led to an outbreak of household infection caused by *Calomys callosus*, ordinarily a field rodent. Mortality rates are high in young children.

LASSA FEVER (LF). First recognized in 1969 among American missionaries in Nigeria, Lassa virus has shown an unusual potential for human-to-human spread in many small epidemics in Nigeria, Sierra Leone, and Liberia. Medical workers in Africa and the United States have contracted the disease. Patients with acute Lassa fever have been transported by international aircraft, necessitating extensive surveillance among passengers and crews. Virus is probably maintained in nature in a species of African house rat, *Mastomys natalensis*. Rodent-to-rodent transmission and infection of humans probably operate via mechanisms established for other arenaviruses.

MARBURG DISEASE. Until recently, the world experience has been limited to 26 primary and 5 secondary cases in Germany and Yugoslavia in 1967 and to small outbreaks in Zimbabwe in 1975 and Kenya in 1980. Transmission occurred by direct contact with tissues of the African green monkey, with infected blood, or with human semen. The reservoir and mode of transmission of the virus in nature are unknown.

EBOLA HEMORRHAGIC FEVER. Ebola virus was isolated in 1976 from a devastating epidemic involving small villages in northern Zaire and southern Sudan. Smaller outbreaks have occurred since then. Outbreaks initially have been nosocomial. Attack rates have been highest in the 0–1 yr and 15–50 yr age groups. The virus resembles Marburg virus. Vertebrate reservoir and mode of transmission to man are unknown.

HEMORRHAGIC FEVER WITH RENAL SYNDROME. (Synonyms: epidemic hemorrhagic fever; Korean hemorrhagic fever.) The endemic area includes Japan, Korea, Far eastern Siberia, north and central China, European and Asian Russia, Scandinavia, Czechoslovakia, Rumania, and Bulgaria. Although the incidence and severity of hemorrhagic manifestations and mortality are lower in Europe than in northeast Asia, the renal lesion is the same. Cases occur predominantly in the spring and summer. There appears to be no age factor in susceptibility, but because of occupational hazards, young adult men are most frequently attacked. Rodent plagues or evidences of rodent infestation have accompanied endemic and epidemic occurrences. Hantaan virus has been detected in lung tissue and excreta of *Apodemus agrarius coreae*. A similar agent has been detected in laboratory rats and in urban rat populations around the world. *Rodent-rodent and rodent-man transmission presumably occurs via the respiratory route.*

Clinical, Pathologic, and Laboratory Features. OMSK HEMORRHAGIC FEVER AND KYASANUR FOREST DISEASE. After an incubation period of 3–8 days, both diseases begin with sudden onset of fever and headache. In Omsk hemorrhagic fever there is moderate epistaxis, hematemesis, and a hemorrhagic enanthem but no profuse hemorrhage; bronchopneumonia is common. Kyasanur forest disease is characterized by severe myalgia, prostration, and bronchiolar involvement; it often presents without hemorrhage, but occasionally with severe gastrointestinal bleeding. Severe epistaxis is regarded by some observers as a good prognostic sign. Severe leukopenia and thrombocytopenia occur in both diseases. In many patients recurrent febrile illness may follow an afebrile period of 7–15 days. This 2nd phase takes the form of a meningoencephalitis.

Pathologic and pathophysiologic studies are scant. In Kyasanur forest disease acute degeneration of renal tubules may correlate with the urinary changes noted. There may be focal liver damage. In both diseases vascular dilatation, increased vascular permeability, gastrointestinal hemorrhages, and subserosal and interstitial petechial hemorrhages occur.

CRIMEAN HEMORRHAGIC FEVER. The incubation period of 3–12 days is followed by a febrile period of 5–12 days and a prolonged convalescence. Illness begins suddenly with fever, severe headache, myalgia, abdominal pain, anorexia, nausea, and vomiting. After a day or more fever may subside until the patient develops an erythematous facial or truncal flush, injected conjunctivae, and a 2nd febrile period of 2–6 days, with a hemorrhagic enanthem on the soft palate and a fine petechial rash on the chest and abdomen. Less frequently, there are large areas of purpura and bleeding from gums, nose, intestine, lungs, or uterus. Hematuria and proteinuria are relatively rare. During the hemorrhagic stage there is usually tachycardia with weak heart sounds, and in some cases hypotension occurs. The liver is usually enlarged, but there is no icterus. In protracted cases central nervous system signs may include delirium, somnolence, and progressive clouding of consciousness. In convalescence there may be hearing and memory loss. Mortality ranges from 2–50%. Early in the disease leukopenia with relative lymphocytosis, progressively worsening thrombocytopenia, and gradually increasing anemia occur.

RIFT VALLEY FEVER (RVF). Most recorded infections have been in adults, in whom disease is dengue-like. Onset is acute with fever, headache, prostration, myalgia, anorexia, nausea, vomiting, conjunctivitis, and lymphadenopathy. The fever lasts 3–6 days and is often biphasic. Convalescence is often prolonged. In the 1977–78 outbreak, many patients died with severe hemorrhagic signs, including purpura, epistaxis, hematemesis, and melena. At autopsy there was extensive eosinophilic degeneration of the parenchymal cells of the liver.

ARGENTINE AND BOLIVIAN HEMORRHAGIC FEVER AND LASSA FEVER. The incubation period is commonly 7–14 days; the acute illness lasts for 2–4 wk. Clinical illnesses range from undifferentiated fever to the characteristic severe illness. Lassa fever is most often clinically severe in Caucasian subjects. Onset is usually gradual, with increasing fever, headache, diffuse myalgia, and anorexia. During the 1st wk there are frequently a sore throat, dysphagia, cough, oropharyngeal ulcers, nausea, vomiting, diarrhea, and pains in chest and abdomen. Pleuritic chest pain may persist into the 2nd–3rd wk of illness. In Argentine and Bolivian hemorrhagic fevers and less frequently in Lassa fever, a petechial enanthem appears on the soft palate 3–5 days after onset and at about the same time on the trunk. The tourniquet test may be positive.

In 35–50% of all patients the disease may become severe, with persistent high fever, increasing toxicity, swelling of face or neck, microscopic hematuria, and frank hemorrhages from the stomach, intestines, nose, gums, and uterus. A syndrome of hypovolemic shock is accompanied by pleural effusion and renal failure. Respiratory distress due to outlet obstruction, pleural effusion, or congestive heart failure may occur. Ten–20% of patients develop late neurologic involvement characterized by intention tremor of the tongue and associated speech abnormalities. In severe cases there may be intention tremors of the extremities, seizures, and delirium. The cerebrospinal fluid is normal. Prolonged convalescence is accompanied by alopecia and in Argentine and Bolivian hemorrhagic fevers by signs of autonomic nervous system lability, such as postural hypotension, spontaneous flushing or blanching of the skin, and intermittent diaphoresis.

Laboratory studies reveal marked leukopenia, mild to moderate thrombocytopenia, proteinuria, and, in Argentine hemorrhagic fever, moderate abnormalities in blood clotting proteins, decreased fibrinogen, increased fibrinogen split-products, and elevated serum transaminases. Pathologically, there is focal, often extensive, eosinophilic necrosis of liver parenchyma, focal interstitial pneumonitis, focal necrosis of the distal and collecting tubules, and partial replacement of splenic follicles by amorphous eosinophilic material. Usually bleeding occurs by diapedesis with little inflammatory reaction. Mortality is 10–40%.

MARBURG DISEASE AND EBOLA HEMORRHAGIC FEVER. After an incubation period of 4–7 days, illness begins abruptly with severe frontal headache, malaise, drowsiness, lumbar myalgia, vomiting, nausea, and diarrhea. Five–7 days later a papular eruption begins on the trunk and upper arms; becomes generalized, often hemorrhagic, and maculopapular; and exfoliates during convalescence. The exanthem is accompanied by a dark red enanthem on the hard palate, conjunctivitis, and scrotal or labial edema. Gastrointestinal hemorrhage occurs as the severity of illness increases. Late in the illness the patient may become tearfully depressed with marked hyperalgesia to tactile stimuli. In fatal cases, patients become hypotensive, restless, and confused and lapse into coma. Convalescent patients may develop alopecia and have paresthesias of the back and trunk. There is a marked leukopenia with necrosis of granulocytes. Disseminated intravascular coagulation and thrombocytopenia are universal and correlate with severity of disease; there are moderate abnormalities in clotting proteins and elevated serum transaminases and amylase. The mortality of Marburg disease is 25%; that of Ebola hemorrhagic fever, 50–90%.

HEMORRHAGIC FEVER WITH RENAL SYNDROME (HFRS). In most cases HFRS is characterized by fever, petechiae, mild hemorrhagic phenomena, and mild proteinuria, followed by relatively uneventful recovery. In 20% of recognized cases the disease may progress through 4 rather distinct phases. The *febrile phase* is ushered in with fever, malaise, and facial and truncal flushing, lasts 3–8 days, and ends with thrombocytopenia, petechiae, and proteinuria. The *hypotensive phase* of 1–3 days follows defervescence. Loss of fluid from the intravascular compartment may result in marked hemoconcentration. Proteinuria and ecchymoses increase. The *oliguric phase,* usually 3–5 days in duration, is characterized by a low output of protein-rich urine, with increasing nitrogen retention, nausea, vomiting, and dehydration. Confusion, extreme restlessness, and hypertension are common. The *diuretic phase,* which may last for days or weeks, usually initiates clinical improvement. The kidneys show little concentrating ability, and rapid loss of fluid may result in severe dehydration and shock. Potassium and sodium depletion may be severe. Fatal cases manifest abundant protein-rich retroperitoneal edema and marked hemorrhagic necrosis of the renal medulla. Mortality is 5–10%.

Diagnosis. Diagnosis rests upon a high index of suspicion in endemic areas. In nonendemic areas histories of recent travel, recent laboratory exposure, or exposure to an earlier case may evoke suspicion of viral hemorrhagic fever.

In all viral hemorrhagic fevers except HFRS, the viral agent circulates in the blood at least transiently during the early febrile stage. The diagnostic specimens required for togaviruses and bunyaviruses are as described in Sec 10.88 for dengue fever. The principles for etiologic diagnosis of Argentine and Bolivian hemorrhagic fevers are similar. Acute phase blood or throat washings from patients can be inoculated intracerebrally into guinea pigs, infant hamsters, or infant mice. Lassa virus may be isolated from the same specimens by inoculation into tissue cultures. In arenavirus infections, group-reactive complement-fixing antibodies and specific neutralizing antibodies appear in convalescent serum 3–4 wk after onset of illness. For Marburg disease and EHF, acute-phase throat washings, blood, and urine may be inoculated into tissue culture, guinea pigs, or monkeys. The virus is readily visualized by electron microscopy, its filamentous structure differentiating it from all other known agents. Specific complement-fixing and immunofluorescent antibodies appear during convalescence. The virus of HFRS is recovered from acute phase serum or urine by inoculating susceptible *Apodemus agrarius coreae* and identifying antigen in lung tissues by use of fluorescent antibody from convalescent serum.

Handling of blood and other biologic specimens is hazardous and must be left to specially trained personnel. Blood and autopsy specimens should be placed in tightly sealed metal containers, wrapped in absorbent material inside a sealed plastic bag, and shipped on dry ice to laboratories with biocontainment level 4 facilities. Even routine hematologic and biochemical tests should be done with extreme caution.

Differential Diagnosis. Mild cases of hemorrhagic fever may be confused with almost any self-limited systemic bacterial or viral infection. More severe cases may suggest typhoid fever, epidemic, murine, or scrub typhus, leptospirosis, or a rickettsial spotted fever, for which, with the exception of leptospirosis, effective chemotherapeutic agents are available. Many of them may be acquired in geographic or ecologic locations similar to those that may provide exposure to a viral hemorrhagic fever.

Prevention. A form of inactivated mouse brain vaccine is said to be effective in preventing Omsk hemorrhagic fever. A similar vaccine for Kyasanur Forest disease was produced experimentally but is no longer available. Inactivated Rift Valley fever vaccines are widely used to protect domestic animals and laboratory workers. Prevention of transmission by ticks includes careful examination of the skin after exposure with removal of any vectors found. Tight-fitting clothing which fully covers the extremities is helpful as is the use of tick repellents. Disease transmitted from a rodent-infected environment can be prevented through methods of rodent control; elimination of refuse and breeding sites is particularly successful in urban or suburban areas. Congo-Crimean hemorrhagic fever, Lassa fever, Marburg disease, and Ebola hemorrhagic fever may be transmitted in hospital settings. Patients should be isolated until virus-free or for 3 wk following illness. Patients' urine, sputum, blood, clothing, and bedding should be disinfected. Disposable syringes and needles should be used. Prompt and strict enforcement of barrier nursing may be lifesaving. Case fatality among medical workers contracting these diseases is presently 50%.

Treatment. The principle involved in all these diseases, especially hemorrhagic fever with renal syndrome, is the careful reversal of dehydration, hemoconcentration, renal failure, and protein, electrolyte, or blood losses. Disseminated intravascular coagulation (DIC) has been said to occur in all viral hemorrhagic fevers, but the contribution of DIC to the hemorrhagic manifestations has not been well established and the management of hemorrhage should be individualized. Heparin should be used only if severe DIC can be shown. Transfusions of fresh blood and platelets are frequently given. Good results have been reported in a few cases following the administration of clotting factor concentrates. The efficacy of steroids, ε-aminocaproic acid, pressor amines, or α-adrenergic blocking agents has not been established. Sedatives should be selected with regard to the possibility of kidney or liver damage. The successful management of hemorrhagic fever with renal syndrome may require renal dialysis. Dramatic improvement in some cases of Lassa fever has been reported following administration of Lassa immune serum free of infectious virus.*

SCOTT B. HALSTEAD

Casals J, Henderson BE, Hoogstraal H, et al: A review of Soviet viral hemorrhagic fevers, 1969. J Infect Dis 122:437, 1970.
International symposium on arenaviral infections of public health importance, 14–16 July 1975. Bull WHO 52:381, 1975.
Johnson KM, Halstead SB, Cohen SN: Hemorrhagic fevers of Southeast Asia and South America, a comparative appraisal. Prog Med Virol 9:106, 1967.
Lee HW, Lee MC, Cho LS: Management of Korean hemorrhagic fever. Med Prog Sept:15, 1980.
Monath TP: Lassa fever and Marburg virus disease. WHO Chron 28:212, 1974.
Pattyn SR: (ed): Ebola Virus Haemorrhagic Fever. Amsterdam, Elsevier/North Holland, 1978.
Simpson DIH: Viral haemorrhagic fevers of man. Bull WHO 56:819, 1978.

*Serum or immune serum globulin and information concerning dosage schedules may be obtained from the Center for Disease Control, Atlanta, Georgia, or the World Health Organization, Geneva, Switzerland.

10.91 CAT SCRATCH DISEASE
(Cat Scratch Fever, Felinosis, Benign Lymphoreticulosis)

Cat scratch disease is a self-limited, suppurative lymphadenitis of children and young adults. The etiology is unknown. Circumstantial evidence, however, suggests that a *Chlamydia*-like microorganism may be responsible.

Pathology. The microscopic appearance of the involved lymph nodes, although not diagnostic, is sufficiently characteristic to suggest cat scratch disease. Three pathologic states have been described, progressing from reticulum cell hyperplasia to tubercle-like granuloma, which often contains Langerhans giant cells, and finally to microabscess formation; all stages may occur within a single node.

Epidemiology. Eighty per cent of the diagnosed cases occur in patients under 20 yr of age; 95% have a history of a cat scratch or contact. The disease also has been reported following the scratch or bite of dogs and monkeys. In temperate climates 80% of cases occur between September–February. This illness is limited to man; involved cats have no apparent illness, fail to yield an infectious agent, and have negative Hanger-Rose skin test. Person-to-person transmission has not been reported.

Clinical Manifestations. A primary skin lesion develops at the scratch site in 50% of patients approximately 10 days (range 7–56 days) following inoculation. This painless, nonpruritic erythematous papule may pustulate before healing without scar formation. Regional lymphadenopathy occurs within 2 wk (range 7–61 days) of the primary lesion. The involved nodes, which are superficial and may reach 8–10 cm in diameter, are painful during the early stages of the disease. The axillary and epitrochlear nodes are the most often involved (45%), followed by lymph nodes of the head and neck (25%), and the lower extremity (20%). Suppuration of involved nodes occurs in 30% of cases. Within 4–6 wk the involved nodes become less tender, and regression occurs within 8 wk in the majority of cases. Constitutional symptoms appear during the period of regional lymphadenopathy in half of the affected individuals and include malaise, anorexia, fatigue, and low grade fever. Laboratory studies are often normal; however, mild elevations in the erythrocyte sedimentation rate and the absolute eosinophil count have been reported. Atypical presentations may include unilateral swelling of the preauricular lymph node (Perinaud oculoglandular fever) or parotid gland, erythema nodosum, thrombocytopenia purpura, and encephalitis.

Diagnosis. The diagnosis in a child with regional lymphadenopathy is based on satisfying 3 of the following 4 criteria: (1) a history of animal (usually a cat) contact, scratch, bite, and/or primary cutaneous lesion; (2) aspiration of sterile pus from an involved node; (3) a positive Hanger-Rose skin test; and (4) characteristic histopathologic changes in an involved lymph node. The skin test antigen is not commercially available but can be prepared from purulent material obtained from patients with cat scratch disease. The bloodless pus is diluted, 1 part in 4 parts normal saline; cultured for bacteria, mycobacteria, and fungi; and incubated for 72 hr at 60° C to inactivate hepatitis virus. The antigen may be refrigerated ($-20°$ C) for several mo without loss of potency. The skin test is performed by injecting 0.1 ml of the antigen intradermally. A positive test is defined as 5 mm or more of induration or 10 mm or more of erythema at 48 hr. Positive skin tests have been observed in 90% of patients with cat scratch disease and in 5% of unaffected controls. Skin tests remain positive for years. Rarely, skin testing may produce an exacerbation of the disease with worsening of systemic symptoms and transient enlargement of involved nodes.

Differential Diagnosis. Cat scratch disease must be differentiated from pyogenic, fungal, and tuberculous adenitis, atypical mycobacterial infection, brucellosis, plague, tularemia, lymphogranuloma venereum, rat bite fever, sarcoidosis, and lymphoma.

Treatment and Prognosis. This benign illness has an excellent prognosis. Aspiration may be indicated to resolve symptoms when the involved nodes become large, fluctuant, and extremely painful.

WILLIAM T. SPECK

10.92 RICKETTSIAL DISEASES

The rickettsiae are microorganisms which commonly inhabit the alimentary canal of certain insects and may be associated with disease in humans. Stained preparations appear under the ordinary microscope as pleomorphic coccobacilli 0.3–0.5 μ in diameter. Most species are retained by bacterial filters, and all require the presence of living cells for multiplication. Biologically, the rickettsiae have some characteristics of bacteria and some of viruses.

The rickettsial diseases of humans, with the exception of Q fever, are febrile illnesses with rashes. They may be separated into 4 groups on the basis of clinical characteristics, insect vectors, etiologic agent, and epidemiology (Table 10–52).

Epidemic typhus and endemic typhus are almost identical clinically and pathologically. The causative agents are so similar antigenically that cross-reactions occur in *Proteus* or rickettsial agglutination tests. The 2 forms of the disease may be distinguished by specific complement-fixation tests and by the inability of epidemic typhus to produce a scrotal reaction in guinea pigs. Brill disease is a recrudescence of epidemic typhus. *R. canada*, a member of the typhus fever group, has recently been associated with human illness clini-

Table 10–52   RICKETTSIAL DISEASES OF MAN: SUMMARY OF PERTINENT INFORMATION

Group	Disease	Causative Agent	Arthropod Vector	Animal Host	Proteus Aggluti- nation*	Geographic Distribution
Typhus	Epidemic typhus	R. prowazekii	Body louse	None	OX19	Worldwide; rarely United states
	Brill disease	R. prowazekii	None		OX19	Eastern coastal cities of United States; Israel
	Murine typhus	R. mooseri	Rat flea, louse	Rat	OX19	Worldwide; southern states of United States
Spotted fever	Rocky Mountain spotted fever	R. rickettsii	Tick	Rodents, mammals	Variable OX2 or OX19	North and South America; related diseases worldwide
	Rickettsial pox	R. akari	Mite	House mice	None	Reported from eastern United States
Tsutsugamushi fever	Scrub typhus	R. orientalis (tsutsugamushi)	Mite	Rodents	OXK	Far East
Q fever	Q fever	R. burnetti (Coxiella burnetii)	Rarely ticks?	Ticks, cattle, sheep, goats	None	Worldwide; western United States

*Specific serologic procedures using rickettsial antigens in complement-fixation, agglutination, or neutralization tests are more reliable.

cally indistinguishable from Rocky Mountain spotted fever.

There are many related strains of rickettsiae which cause spotted fever of variable severity in different parts of the world. The list includes boutonneuse fever of the Mediterranean regions; São Paulo, Tobia, and pinta fevers of South America; Kenya or Nigeria fever of Africa; and many others. Rickettsialpox is included in the spotted fever group because of antigenic relations of Rickettsia akari to the causative agent of Rocky Mountain spotted fever.

Tsutsugamushi fever, or scrub typhus, is known in certain areas of Japan and among the populations of India, Australia, Indonesia (Dutch East Indies), and Malaya. Effective vaccines are not available, and scrub typhus continues to be a hazard to those who enter endemic areas.

Q fever differs clinically, histologically, and epidemiologically from the other diseases listed and is classified with them only because it is caused by a rickettsia.

Rocky Mountain spotted fever and Q fever are the 2 rickettsial infections diagnosed with greatest frequency in the United States; however, rapid air travel and the presence of indigenous reservoirs have also resulted in cases of murine typhus, Brill disease, rickettsialpox, scrub typhus, and boutonneuse fever.

The immunity, pathology, methods for making a laboratory diagnosis, and manner of treatment of each of the rickettsial diseases in humans are so similar that these topics are discussed together before the individual diseases are described.

Immunity.   Prolonged immunity to specific rickettsial agents follows recovery from disease. In experimentally infected laboratory animals, immunity has been proved by unsuccessful attempts to reinfect. A significant degree of cross-immunity to related organisms may result from infection with 1 member of a group, i.e., the individual who has had Rocky Mountain spotted fever is protected against other tick-borne spotted fe-

vers; immunity to epidemic and murine typhus is linked, but an attack of scrub typhus that confers good homologous immunity protects only transiently against heterologous strains of R. orientalis. Chronic or recurrent infections with rickettsiae may occur. Brill disease is the well-known example, but exacerbations of scrub typhus with repeated isolation of the same strain of R. orientalis have been observed. Cell-mediated immune mechanisms appear to play an important role in limiting the intracellular persistence of rickettsiae.

Pathology.   The lesion of the arthropod-borne rickettsial diseases is sufficiently distinctive to be diagnostic in patients with a history of an exanthem. The main changes involve the small blood vessels, chiefly of the skin, subcutaneous tissue, kidneys, and central nervous system. The endothelial cells swell and occlude the small blood vessels; thrombosis results. The occluded vessels are surrounded by cuffs of mononuclear cells, plasma cells, and macrophages. Rickettsiae localize in the endothelium of capillaries and extend via the intima into larger vessels. Rocky Mountain spotted fever may be distinguished histologically from other rickettsial diseases by the presence of rickettsiae in the smooth muscle cells of the media. This results in severe destruction of blood vessels and may explain the occurrence of necrosis of skin in sites such as the ear lobes, fingers, toes, and scrotum.

The symptomatology of vector-transmitted rickettsial diseases correlates with the degree of involvement and the location of affected vessels. For example, fall in blood pressure, an outstanding clinical feature of rickettsial disease, is the result of changes in the peripheral vessels. Perivascular reactions in the lung may result in atelectasis and pneumonia. Vascular changes in the brain may produce central nervous system symptoms.

Q fever, which is not accompanied by a rash and does not require an insect vector, differs pathologically from the other rickettsial diseases. The principal, and usually the only, lesions occur in the lungs, where there is a patchy interstitial pneumonitis with copious exudate composed of fibrin and mononuclear cells. Alveolar walls, alveolar ducts, and terminal bronchioles are infiltrated by large mononuclear cells.

Diagnosis. The diagnosis of a human rickettsial infection is most readily established early by the demonstration of specific rickettsial antigen in specimens of involved skin obtained by biopsy. Retrospective or late diagnosis can be made by serologic tests employing either cross-reactive *Proteus* antigens or specific rickettsial reagents.

Immunofluorescent Demonstration of Rickettsia. A typical petechial rickettsial lesion included in a skin biopsy is frozen, sectioned, and stained with fluorescein isothiocyanate labeled antibody to *R. rickettsii.* Fluorescent coccobacillary forms are clearly visible in positive preparations. Appropriate controls are included with each test. The immunofluorescent method has high specificity and reasonably good sensitivity. False negatives may occur if a vascular lesion is not included in the biopsy or if the patient has been treated with broad-spectrum antibiotics for 24 hr or longer. Antibiotic treatment should be started if the test is positive; if it is negative, the decision on treatment remains a clinical judgment.

Serologic Diagnosis. During etiologic studies of typhus fever, Felix isolated a strain of *Proteus vulgaris* from the urine of a patient. This strain (OX19) was not the causative agent of typhus but had sufficient antigenic similarity to *Rickettsia prowazekii* so that serum from patients convalescent from typhus fever contained high titers of OX19 agglutinin. Additional strains of *Proteus* antigenically related to the causative agents of tsutsugamushi (OXK) and Rocky Mountain spotted fever (OX2) were also discovered. These easily prepared antigens are used for agglutination tests in patients' serums (the *Weil-Felix* reaction).

In epidemic typhus fever the agglutination to OX19 usually reaches a titer greater than 1:160 during the 2nd wk of illness; the OX2 and OXK titers remain low. The agglutinin pattern observed with murine typhus is similar to that of epidemic typhus. Patients with Rocky Mountain spotted fever differ in the type and degree of response they provoke in the *Proteus* agglutination test; most show a rise in antibody to OX19 to 160 or greater, some develop a high OX2 titer and little response to OX19, and others have persistently negative Weil-Felix tests. *Proteus* OXK agglutinin titers are high after tsutsugamushi disease. Convalescent serum from patients with Q fever or rickettsialpox does not agglutinate to significant titer the *Proteus* strains used in the Weil-Felix reaction. *Proteus* titers do not persist and are usually below a significant level within 3 mo after the illness.

Serologic procedures using rickettsial antigens in complement-fixation, agglutination, or neutralization tests are more sensitive and specific than the Weil-Felix reaction and should be used to confirm the diagnosis of rickettsial infections. Unfortunately, the serologic confirmation of a rickettsial infection is usually not possible until day 9–14 of the illness. A single titer of 1:160 or greater with *Proteus* antigen or a rickettsia

complement fixation titer of at least 1:16 or a 4-fold rise in titer by either test supports the diagnosis.

Culturing of Rickettsiae. Rickettsiae may be propagated by inoculating susceptible experimental animals or developing chick embryos, but the culturing of rickettsiae in the laboratory is extremely hazardous and has been the source of infection for many investigators. This is a task for a special laboratory with proper facilities and immunized personnel.

Prognosis. In general, there is a relationship between age and mortality from rickettsial disease; children do better than adults or the aged. Epidemics of typhus in the 19th century had an average mortality rate of 20%, ranging from less than 3% in the pediatric age group to 50% in those in their 5th decade of life. The range was similar in severe outbreaks of scrub typhus or Rocky Mountain spotted fever. Mortality rates are diminished by prompt use of antibiotics; in the United States approximately 5–7% of patients with Rocky Mountain spotted fever die. Murine typhus, Q fever, and rickettsialpox are relatively mild diseases with low mortality rates even when untreated.

Treatment. Tetracycline or chloramphenicol is usually curative if begun in adequate dosage on or before the 6th day of disease. The penicillins and other antibiotics are without effect, and the sulfonamides may make the patient worse by enhancing rickettsial replication. Final eradication of the microorganism depends upon the immune processes of the host.

The recommended dose of tetracycline is 40–50 mg/kg/24 hr given in 4 divided doses orally or intravenously. Chloramphenicol in a dose of 100 mg/kg/24 hr administered every 6 hr is the alternative form of treatment. The latter agent is preferable in patients with poor renal function. Antimicrobial therapy should continue until the patient has been afebrile 4–5 days, usually for a total course of 8–12 days.

Early diagnosis and the proper use of antimicrobial agents are all that is necessary in the management of most rickettsial infections. Vigorous supportive therapy, parenteral fluids, transfusions, sedation, and oxygen are necessary for the severely ill patient.

10.93 TYPHUS FEVER (Epidemic Typhus; Louse-Borne Typhus)

History. Typhus fever has been associated with misery since man donned clothing. Typhus was probably responsible for the plague of Athens, 430 B.C.; it existed during the Middle Ages and was associated with each of the serious famines in England. Typhus was spread through Europe by louse-infected soldiers and was often the most important factor in determining the outcome of battles or the survival of nations.

In more recent yr large outbreaks of typhus have not occurred. Louse-borne epidemic typhus has not been reported in the United States for many decades, but the existence of endemic areas within a few hr of travel and the demonstration that flying squirrels trapped in the southeastern United States may act as reservoirs make the occurrence of typhus a possibility.

Etiology and Transmission.   Humans have been the sole reservoir of *Rickettsia prowazekii*, the causative agent of epidemic typhus. The body or head louse may become infected by feeding upon the blood of a person with rickettsemia. The ingested organisms multiply within the cells lining the alimentary tract of the insect and are eliminated in the feces.

Contaminated feces may be introduced into a susceptible human host through abrasions or perforations in the skin or by way of the conjunctival sac or upper respiratory tract. Inhalation of dried, infected louse excreta present in the clothing, bedding, or furniture of a typhus patient is probably an important source of infection.

Pathology.   See Section 10.92.

Clinical Manifestations.   Typhus fever is a milder disease in children than in adults. The clinical manifestations may include fever, transient rash, and only a few constitutional symptoms; therefore recognition of the disease is often difficult.

The incubation period is usually less than 14 days and is followed classically by an abrupt onset with severe frontal headache, weakness, malaise, generalized aches and pains, chills, and fever of 40° C (104° F) or more. Four–7 days later the rash appears. The clinical course is similar to that of Rocky Mountain spotted fever.

Brill disease is an unusual phenomenon in which a patient with a history of typhus suffers a recrudescence of the illness. It has been observed among immigrants from eastern Europe in the coastal cities of the United States and, more recently, in Israel. The strains of rickettsiae isolated from such patients are indistinguishable from those of epidemic typhus. It is presumed that organisms have persisted in the tissues of the host for years, and then, for reasons not understood, they increase in number and produce clinical symptoms. A patient with Brill disease can infect lice and is a potential point of origin for a typhus epidemic when the vector is present. Brill disease is not a problem in children.

Differential Diagnosis.   Meningococcemia, typhoid, measles, or smallpox may be confused with typhus, but the history, clinical course, and laboratory data usually permit a proper diagnosis.

Control.   The immediate destruction of vectors with an insecticide that has persisting effect such as DDT is an important measure in the control of an epidemic. Dust containing excreta from infected lice is also capable of transmitting typhus, and care must be taken to prevent its inhalation. This usually requires washing the patient's clothing, bedding, and other possessions with hot water and a disinfectant after they have been dusted with DDT.

Treatment.   See Sec 10.92.

10.94   MURINE TYPHUS
(Endemic Typhus)

Etiology and Transmission.   Endemic typhus is fairly common in the United States, particularly in Texas and the southeastern states, and has been seen in most regions of this country. It usually occurs in the summer and fall, in contrast to typhus, which is characteristically a disease of winter and spring.

Murine typhus is a disease of rats caused by *Rickettsia mooseri*. It is usually transmitted from rat to rat by the rat louse or flea. In both the rat and the insect vectors murine typhus is a mild disease with no apparent effect on their life span. The eggs laid by infected fleas or lice do not transmit *R. mooseri* to the next generation. Man usually acquires murine typhus when bitten by an infected rat flea but can also be infected by inhaling or possibly ingesting infected excreta of fleas.

Clinical Manifestations.   Murine typhus is a mild, seldom fatal illness that can be distinguished from epidemic typhus only by special laboratory procedures.

The incubation period is usually about 8 days. Prodromal symptoms such as headache, arthralgia, and backache are followed by a gradually increasing temperature which may reach 41.1° C (106° F) in children and last 9–14 days. Any time from the 1st to the 8th day of fever, most often by the 5th day, the rash appears. The eruption begins on the trunk and spreads to the periphery, rarely involving the face, palms, or soles. Initially, the skin lesion is a dull red macule with ill-defined margins which becomes slightly papular as it matures. It persists for a much shorter period than the rash of epidemic typhus and rarely, if ever, becomes purpuric. Twenty per cent or more of children may have no rash or such a transient one that it is not noted. Central nervous system symptoms are uncommon, as are peripheral vascular collapse and other complications.

Diagnosis.   See Sec 10.92.

Control.   Control of murine typhus requires elimination of the rat reservoir or the insect vector, or both.

Treatment.   See Sec 10.92.

10.95   SCRUB TYPHUS
(Tsutsugamushi Fever; Mite Typhus)

Etiology and Transmission.   *Rickettsia tsutsugamushi*, also known as *R. orientalis*, causes scrub typhus. The vectors which carry the agent are the larval forms of the chigger or trombiculid mites. The larvae feed on rats or other rodents and when not feeding are present on low-lying vegetation, whence they can attack man. *Rickettsia tsutsugamushi* has been isolated from many species of rodents, and it seems likely that both mites and rodents serve as reservoirs of rickettsiae. Scrub tyhphus is mainly a disease of persons whose occupations bring them into contact with infected mites.

Clinical Manifestations.   The symptomatology of scrub typhus, although showing some distinctive features, is similar to that of other rickettsial infections. The mite bite usually results in a local skin lesion, which begins as an asymptomatic, pink papule, increases in size, and becomes either an eschar, consisting of a central, black scab 4–8 mm in diameter surrounded by a red areola, or, in moist areas (axilla, perineum), a punched-out shallow ulcer. By the end of the 1st wk of illness a maculopapular rash develops on the chest and abdomen and gradually spreads to involve the entire body but rarely the hands and face. Diffuse, tender adenopathy, greater in the region of the primary lesion, is common. The mortality rate when antibiotics are administered early is less than 5%.

Protective clothing and early treatment with broad-spectrum antibiotics are the most useful aids to prevention of death from scrub typhus.

Treatment. See Sec 10.92.

10.96 ROCKY MOUNTAIN SPOTTED FEVER

History. Rocky Mountain spotted fever is an exanthem of man first recognized in the Rocky Mountain region of the United States. Ricketts inoculated monkeys and guinea pigs with infected human blood and was able to transmit the infection and demonstrate the causative agent. He later showed that the disease is spread by the wood tick. Close to 1000 cases occur annually. More than half of these are reported from a group of states in the Southeast including North and South Carolina, Virginia, Tennessee, and their neighbors. Fewer than 5% originate in the Rocky Mountain area.

Etiology and Transmission. The causative agent of Rocky Mountain spotted fever, *Rickettsia rickettsii,* is maintained in nature by many hosts, including the ground squirrel, jack rabbit, chipmunk, wood rat, meadow mouse, and weasel; the animal hosts do not become ill. Transmission among animals and from animal to man occurs most commonly via the wood tick. *Dermacentor andersoni,* or the dog tick, *Dermacentor variabilis.*

A history of contact with ticks is helpful in reaching a diagnosis of Rocky Mountain spotted fever, but such information has been obtained in only 50–60% of reported cases. An additional 25% may have been exposed to possibly tick-infected woods or dogs, but 15–20% can identify no possible source of infection. Most cases in the United States, however, occur from April–September when outdoor living and tick activity are maximum.

Pathology. See Sec 10.92.

Clinical Manifestations. The incubation period in children varies from 1–8 days. The disease usually begins with such nonspecific symptoms as headache, fever, anorexia, and restlessness. There may be a his-

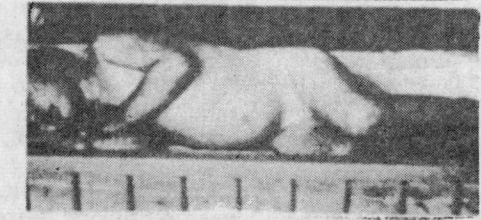

Figure 10–35 Patient with Rocky Mountain spotted fever. Note the greater concentration of skin lesions on the ankles, wrists, and lower legs. (Courtesy of William H. Wood, M.D., Cleveland.)

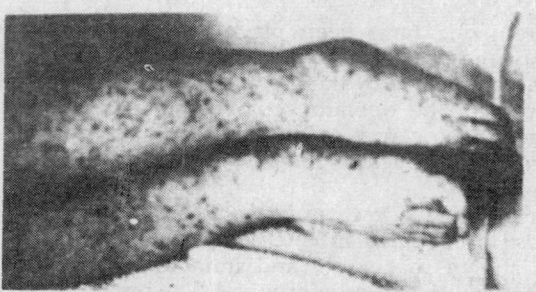

Figure 10–36 Ninth day of rash in Rocky Mountain spotted fever, showing hemorrhagic nature of rash and puffy edema of feet. (Courtesy of William H. Wood, M.D., Cleveland.)

tory of tick bite or of exposure to tick-infested dogs or woods. Local reaction at the site of the bite is uncommon. Discrete, pale, rose-red macules or maculopapules appear 1–5 days after the onset of illness; rarely, there may be little or no rash. The rash characteristically begins peripherally on the ankles, wrists, or lower legs (Fig 10–35) and then spreads, often rapidly, to involve the entire body, including the scalp, palms, and soles. Early, the rash fades with pressure, but after 1–2 days it becomes more purple, papular, and frequently petechial (Fig 10–36). Fever and headache persist; intense myalgia and malaise are frequent complaints. Splenomegaly is present in approximately 33% of patients and shock in 7–10%. Bizarre central nervous system symptoms, edema of the face, electrocardiographic evidence of myocarditis, renal involvement, peripheral collapse, and pneumonitis are the more severe manifestations. Thrombocytopenia is present in nearly half the patients and may be an important clue for early diagnosis. Patients with multiple coagulation disturbances (disseminated intravascular coagulation) constitute the group with highest risk of death. Fatality rates before the availability of antibiotics varied from 10–40%; in 1978 the case fatality rate was 3.7%. Recovery in uncomplicated cases occurs in the 3rd wk, initiated by a fall in temperature and gradual subsidence of symptoms.

Laboratory Data. The clinical laboratory findings are not specific. See prior pages for serologic tests.

Differential Diagnosis. Infectious mononucleosis, rubella, measles, especially atypical measles in children who have received killed vaccine, echovirus exanthems, meningococcemia, leptospirosis, and mucocutaneous lymph node syndrome (Kawasaki disease) are diseases frequently considered in patients with Rocky Mountain spotted fever. The spread of rash from distal portions of the extremities to the trunk and face, with involvement of palms and soles, is often the clue that leads to the diagnosis. Season of the year, negative blood cultures, and normal spinal fluid are additional aids in reaching a correct diagnosis.

Control. The reservoirs and vectors of spotted fever are so numerous and widespread that removal of the source of infection is not feasible. Protection from tick bite is best accomplished by the use of proper wearing apparel plus tick repellents or, optimally, the avoidance during the tick season of areas known to be infested.

Ticks rarely transmit infection until they have fed on the person for several hr; thus careful examination of children who have been playing in the woods and prompt removal of ticks may prevent disease. This is best accomplished by the use of gloves or forceps which will protect the operator from being infected by the crushed insect. Application of a coating of petrolatum to provoke the tick to remove its mouth parts is recommended.

An inactivated vaccine prepared from a strain of *R. rickettsii* propagated in chick embryo cell cultures has been shown to be safe and immunogenic. Trials in human volunteers are in progress. The previously available rickettsial vaccines were not of proven effectiveness and have been withdrawn from the market.

Treatment. See Sec 10.92.

10.97 FIÈVRE BOUTONNEUSE

This is a relatively benign rickettsial disease, limited almost exclusively to Europeans in the countries surrounding the Mediterranean. The natives in this area are infected early in life and develop long-lasting immunity. *Rickettsia conorii*, the causal agent, is transmitted by the dog tick, *Rhipicephalus sanguineus*. As in rickettsialpox or scrub typhus, a local lesion known as *tache noire*, or primary eschar, develops, followed by a diffuse, maculopapular rash which later becomes petechial. Severe systemic manifestations are uncommon. The diagnosis is usually made on the basis of the clinical symptoms in an exposed person with a primary skin lesion. Agglutinins to both OX19 and OX2 occur during the 2nd wk of the disease and may be used to confirm the diagnosis if the more specific complement-fixation test is not available. Treatment with broad-spectrum antibiotics is followed by rapid clinical improvement.

10.98 RICKETTSIALPOX

History. In 1946 an epidemic of an unusual febrile disease with varicelliform rash occurred in a New York City housing development. The disease was recognized as a new entity caused by a previously unknown rickettsia, *Rickettsia akari*, and transmitted by the mouse mite, *Allodermanyssus sanguineus*. The illness, named rickettsialpox, has continued endemic in New York, and isolated cases have been reported from Boston, Philadelphia, and Cleveland. The mite vector has been found in many cities of the United States.

Clinical Manifestations. Rickettsialpox is a mild illness characterized by an initial skin lesion followed by fever, chills, headache, and a papulovesicular rash.

The initial lesion, presumed to be the site of the mite bite, has been observed in more than 90% of cases. It may be located anywhere on the body, beginning as a nontender, nonitching, firm, red papule, 0.5–2.0 cm in diameter. A deeply entrenched vesicle develops in the center of the papule and ruptures after several days, leaving a crusted, pigmented lesion or eschar which may persist 3 wk or longer. Adjacent lymph nodes become enlarged and tender, but do not suppurate.

The initial lesion is followed in 2–7 days by fever, headache, chills, and sweats. Temperature ranges from 39–40° (C 102–105° F), but the patient remains oriented and does not appear severely ill.

Within 24–72 hr after the onset of fever, scattered erythematous maculopapules appear over the body, showing no preference of trunk, head, or extremity. The lesions enlarge, become more papular, and develop vesicles on the summit of each papule. The secondary lesions (rash) resemble the initial lesion except that they are smaller in size and heal, without leaving scars, in 4–7 days.

The duration seldom exceeds 7–10 days. Complications, sequelae, and fatalities are rare.

Differential Diagnosis. The rash of rickettsialpox may be confused with that of chickenpox. In the latter the vesicles are superficial, thin, dewdrop lesions which appear in successive crops beginning on the chest. These differ from the deeply seated, randomly distributed firm vesicles of the rickettsial disease. The initial lesion and the presence of chills and fever before the rash may also help in differentiation. Other diseases to be considered include infectious mononucleosis, meningococcemia, Rocky Mountain spotted fever, and typhus.

Control. Preventive measures should include the eradication of rodent reservoirs as well as the mite vector. A vaccine could be prepared if there were substantial need.

Treatment. See Sec 10.92.

10.99 Q FEVER

History. Q fever, a febrile disease without rash and often associated with an interstitial pneumonia, was originally observed among Australian abattoir workers in 1935. Since that time the disease has been reported from all parts of the world.

Etiology and Transmission. Q fever occurs naturally in cattle, sheep, goats, and many wild animals. The causative agent of Q fever, *Coxiella burnetii*, has been found in many species of ticks, in which it may pass from the adult through ova to progeny.

Experimentally, Q fever has been transmitted by insect bite and by inhalation. Careful studies of outbreaks of the disease in human beings have failed to incriminate insect vectors, although this mode of transmission may be important among animals. Person-to-person spread is rare but can occur. Studies suggest that excreta from infected animals or insects are the major source of infection. In the endemic areas of California, human infections are related to contact with sheep or dairy cows. The main route of infection is inhalation of contaminated material from domestic animals which may be present in dust, hay, wool, or hides.

Milk may be another source of infection for man. In a study of sporadic cases of Q fever in England, *Coxiella burnetii* was isolated from 10 of the 20 (raw) milk sources used by the patients; *Coxiella burnetii* may survive pasteurization temperatures.

Clinical Manifestations. Q fever is usually a mild disease diagnosed only in retrospect by serologic survey. As commonly recognized, it is a disease of moderate severity with a duration in children of 2–3 wk. The onset is characteristically sudden, but in some instances symptoms may increase slowly in intensity. Malaise, fever, chilliness, and generalized weakness appear early, but the most prominent symptom is severe frontal headache, often associated with pain upon movement of the eyes. There is no rash. Complaints referable to the respiratory tract are mild and infrequent. Cough may occur late in the 1st wk of illness, with production of small amounts of blood-streaked sputum, and chest pain may be associated with pneumonitis or infrequently with pleural effusion. Differential diagnosis in the immunologically competent individual includes the long list of agents associated with the atypical pneumonia syndrome such as mycoplasma, Epstein-Barr virus, psittacosis, and Legionnaires disease.

Pneumonitis is common; rales may be audible, but the pulmonary involvement is usually established roentgenographically. Pulmonary consolidation is usually patchy and in the peripheries of the lower lobes; hilar involvement is rare. Resolution is slow and may require 3–6 wk.

During the acute phase the temperature may reach 40–40.6° C (104–105° F), but may be remitting with wide daily swings. After 5–15 days the temperature gradually returns to normal and most symptoms disappear. Convalescence may be prolonged for several wk, but complications are rare. The mortality rate is less than 1%.

Routine hematologic data are not significant. Serologic tests for syphilis may give falsely positive results during the illness.

Control. Complete control of Q fever is not possible because of ignorance of the exact mode of spread. Recognition of the disease in livestock should alert communities to the risk of infection. Stockyard workers and others exposed to infected material might receive the formalinized vaccine, which at present is not generally available. Milk from infected herds must be pasteurized at temperatures sufficient to destroy the rickettsiae. Person-to-person spread of Q fever is not a problem, and special isolation measures are not necessary.

Treatment. See Sec 10.92.

ELI GOLD

Ascher MS, Oster CN, Harber PI, et al: Initial clinical evaluation of a new Rocky Mountain spotted fever vaccine of tissue culture origin. J Infect Dis 138:217, 1978.

Bradford WD, Hawkins HK: Rocky Mountain spotted fever in childhood. Am J Dis Child 131:1228, 1977.

D'Angelo LJ, Winkler WG, Bregman DJ: Rocky Mountain spotted fever in the United States, 1975–1977. J Infect Dis 138:273, 1978.

Fleisher G, Lennette ET, Honig P: Diagnosis of Rocky Mountain spotted fever by immunofluorescent identification of *Rickettsia rickettsii* in skin biopsy tissue. J Pediatr 95:63, 1979.

Hattwick MAW, O'Brien RJ, Hanson BF: Rocky Mountain spotted fever. Epidemiology of an increasing problem. Ann Intern Med 84:732, 1976.

Hechemy KE: Laboratory diagnosis of Rocky Mountain spotted fever. N Engl J Med 300:859, 1979.

Walker DH, Burday MS, Folds J: Laboratory diagnosis of Rocky Mountain spotted fever. South Med J 73:1443, 1980.

MYCOTIC INFECTIONS

10.100 BLASTOMYCOSIS

North American blastomycosis is an uncommon noncontagious granulomatous infection of the lungs, skin, bone, and genitourinary tract caused by a dimorphic saprophytic fungus *Blastomyces dermatitidis*. In infected tissue the yeast form of *B. dermatitidis* appears as spherical, multinucleated structures with thick, double refractile cell walls; each large daughter cell is attached to the parent by a broad-based neck. Blastomycosis occurs mainly in the southeastern United States and in the Mississippi, Ohio, and St. Lawrence River valleys. This endemic area includes the north central region of the United States and extends into Canada. Blastomycosis has also been reported in England, Africa, and India. Human infection occurs following inhalation of airborne spores from contaminated soil which reach the lower respiratory tract and after a long incubation period (30–45 days), during which they are converted to yeast forms, establish a primary pulmonary infection. In isolated epidemics the majority of patients are less than 20 yr old.

Pulmonary blastomycosis occurs as an asymptomatic infection. The lack of an effective skin test antigen prevents a true estimate of the incidence in this form of disease; however, proof of subclinical infection has been obtained from studies of epidemic blastomycosis. Primary pulmonary blastomycosis may also present as a mild self-limited lower respiratory tract infection, a progressive or fulminant life-threatening pneumonia with or without extrapulmonary manifestations, or chronic pneumonia. In mild cases the child presents with low grade fever, pleuritic chest pain, a nonproductive cough, and occasional hemoptysis. Roentgenographic examination reveals lobar consolidation and hilar adenopathy. In the progressive form of pneumonia, symptoms include high fever, night sweats, chills, anorexia, and dyspnea. Productive cough and hemoptysis are common. The physical examination reveals diffuse rales and signs of pulmonary consolidation. Roentgenographic examination demonstrates diffuse bilateral nodular basilar infiltrates. Cavitation and effusion are uncommon.

Disseminated blastomycosis is found most often in adults with chronic pulmonary infection. The skin is the principal site of extrapulmonary involvement and may be the presenting complaint in patients with asymptomatic or mild pulmonary disease. Solitary or multiple subcutaneous nodules of the face and trunk are characteristic of *cutaneous blastomycosis*. These appear initially as papules or pustules which over a period of weeks or months progress to verrucous granulomas with erythematous, indurated, raised serpentine borders. The lesions advance centripetally with central scarring; regional lymphadenopathy does not occur. Other extrapulmonary sites of involvement include bone, joints, genitourinary tract (prostate, epididymis, and testes) and, on rare occasions, central nervous system, adrenals, thyroid gland, and liver.

Blastomycosis should be considered in the differential diagnosis in a patient from an endemic area presenting with any combination of lung, skin, bone, or genitourinary disease. Skin tests and serologic techniques lack specificity. A presumptive diagnosis requires the identification of the yeast forms of *B. dermatitidis* using a histologic examination of biopsy material or a wet mount preparation (with 10% potassium hydroxide) of exudate from sputum or abscesses. Definitive diagnosis requires isolation of the infecting organism.

Pulmonary blastomycosis may be a mild, self-limited illness that requires no specific treatment. However, progressive pulmonary disease with or without extrapulmonary dissemination is often fatal, and immediate therapeutic intervention is indicated. Cutaneous or chronic pulmonary disease is fatal in 20–30% of cases. Amphotericin B is the treatment of choice for progressive, disseminated, or chronic blastomycosis. In children a cumulative dose of 100 mg/kg up to a maximum of 2 gm is effective in a majority of cases. If amphotericin fails, 2-hydroxystilbamidine has been used.

Cushey WK, Sarosi GA: Blastomycosis in children. Pediatrics 65:111, 1980.
Macher A: Histoplasmosis and blastomycosis. Med Clin North Am 64:447, 1980.
Sarosi GA, Davies SF: Blastomycosis. Am Rev Resp Dis 120:911, 1979.

10.101   CRYPTOCOCCOSIS
(Torulosis)

Cryptococcosis is an uncommon subacute or chronic fungal infection, often involving the central nervous system, caused by an encapsulated budding yeast, *Cryptococcus neoformans*. This fungus is uniquely surrounded by a polysaccharide capsule which contains antigenic determinants that permit the identification of 4 serotypes, A, B, C, and D.

Epidemiology.   *C. neoformans* has a worldwide distribution and exists in nature as a soil saprophyte. The roosting sites of birds, particularly pigeons, provide the necessary conditions for luxuriant growth, and high rates of positive skin tests occur in individuals with a history of heavy exposure to pigeons. Human disease results from inhalation of spores, which germinate in the pulmonary tissue and may disseminate via the bloodstream to brain, meninges, bone marrow, and skin. *Cryptococcus* occurs sporadically, without any occupational predisposition, and is rarely associated with historical or roentgenographic evidence of respiratory involvement. There is an increased incidence of infec-

tion in patients receiving corticosteroids and in those with lymphoreticular malignancies (especially Hodgkin disease), sarcoidosis, and insulin-dependent diabetes.

Pathology.   The characteristic lesion is a cyst-like cavity containing gelatinous material, presumably cryptococcal capsular polysaccharide. Microscopic examination reveals clumps of cryptococci within the cyst and an inflammatory response consisting of macrophages, giant cells, and lymphocytes. In pulmonary cryptococcosis the common finding is a subpleural granuloma. In central nervous system disease multiple cystic lesions occur throughout the brain, particularly in the cortical gray matter and basal ganglia. Mass lesions are extremely rare.

Clinical Manifestations.   *Pulmonary cryptococcosis* is uncommon in children, most often occurring in an immunosuppressed child as an influenza-like illness with low grade fever, cough, pleuritic chest pain, and minimal sputum production. Physical examination may reveal diffuse rales. The chest roentgenogram demonstrates a varied pattern which may include a single pulmonary granuloma, apical cavities, pulmonary masses, or interstitial pneumonitis. Routine laboratory studies are normal. Cultures of sputum and bronchial washings are occasionally positive, but invasive procedures may be needed to recover pathogens from tissues.

Cryptococcal meningitis is the most common form of life-threatening cryptococcal infection and has a subacute or chronic presentation. Symptoms include headache, 73%; mental changes, 45%; visual changes, 40%; nausea and vomiting, 33%; pain and stiffness of the neck and back, 33%; chills or fever, 30%; lethargy, weakness, and fatigue, 23%; ataxia, 20%; and aphasia or slurred speech, 13%. Physical examination may reveal papilledema, hearing loss, motor weakness, cerebellar signs, and coma. Laboratory findings include an elevated opening pressure and protein concentration in 90% of cases, hypoglycorrhachia in 55%, and a mononuclear pleocytosis rarely exceeding 300 cells/mm³. The mortality rate is 50%. Treatment failure and early death are associated with underlying lymphoreticular malignancy or corticosteroid therapy; cerebrospinal fluid findings consisting of a high opening pressure, a low glucose level, fewer than 20 leukocytes/mm³, and cryptococci seen in smear; cryptococci isolated from extraneural sites; and high titers of cryptococcal antigen in cerebrospinal fluid and serum. Forty per cent of survivors have residual neurologic deficits including visual loss, hearing defects, cranial nerve damage, motor impairment, personality change, and, on rare occasions, hydrocephalus.

Additional clinical manifestations of cryptococcosis include multiple papules, pustules, or small subcutaneous masses, most often located on the face or scalp, which eventually become necrotic and ulcerate. Osteomyelitis, septic arthritis, lymphadenitis, endocarditis, pericarditis, renal abscesses, and prostatitis have all been reported as rare complications.

Diagnosis.   Diagnosis of cryptococcosis depends on (1) histologic identification of the infecting organism in biopsy specimens or body fluids, (2) recovery of *C. neoformans* following appropriate cultures, and/or (3) serologic demonstration of cryptococcal antigen. Histologically, appropriately stained organisms are yeast-like with narrow based buds. The encapsulated yeast may be visualized in 50% of patients with cryptococcal meningitis after mixing sediment of the cerebrospinal fluid with an equal volume of India ink. Culture of *C. neoformans* from cerebrospinal fluid, sputum, blood, urine, and other sources results in creamy white mucoid colonies within 10 days of inoculation onto Sabouraud medium. Negative cultures of cerebrospinal fluid do not necessarily exclude the diagnosis of cryptococcal meningitis as the often small numbers of organisms present necessitate repeated cultures of large volumes of centrifuged specimens. The latex agglutination technique detects cryptococcal polysaccharide capsular antigen in cerebrospinal fluid or serum in more than 90% of patients with cryptococcal meningitis.

Treatment. The traditional treatment for life-threatening cryptococcal infection is amphotericin B, which is administered parenterally (0.3 mg/kg/24 hr) for a period of at least 6 wk or until repeated cultures have been negative for 1 mo. Despite relatively low levels of this agent in the cerebrospinal fluid, intrathecal, and/or intraventricular administration of amphotericin B is rarely indicated. Studies of the treatment of cryptococcal meningitis suggest that 5-fluorocytosine (200 mg/kg/24 hr) combined with amphotericin B is more efficacious than treatment with amphotericin alone. The role of 5-fluorocytosine in the treatment of extraneural cryptococcosis has not been studied.

Bennett JE, Dismukes WE, et al: A comparison of amphotericin B alone and combined with flucytosine in the treatment of cryptococcal meningitis. N Engl J Med 301:126, 1979.

Diamond RD, Bennett JE: Prognostic factors in cryptococcal meningitis. Ann Intern Med 80:176, 1974.

Goodman JS, Kaufman L, Loenig MG: Diagnosis of cryptococcal meningitis. N Engl J Med 285:434, 1971.

Lewis JC, Rabinovich S: The wide spectrum of cryptococcal infections. Am J Med 53:315, 1972.

10.102 MUCORMYCOSIS
(Phycomycosis, Zygomycosis)

Mucormycosis refers to a group of infections caused by dimorphic fungi of the class Zygomycetes and the order Mucorales. The principal human pathogens include *Rhizopus, Absidia,* and *Mucor.* These fungi have a worldwide distribution, commonly grow on fruit and other food (e.g., bread mold), and are easily isolated from soil. The Mucorales grow on a variety of laboratory media as fluffy white, gray, or brownish molds following incubation at 37° C. In appropriately stained clinical specimens thick-walled, nonseptate, irregular right-angle branching hyphae are easily visualized. Mucormycosis is an invasive disease that spreads across tissue planes.

Epidemiology. Exposure to spores of Mucorales is universal; however, disease is uncommon. Infection is sporadic and almost exclusively limited to children who have underlying disease, e.g., diabetes mellitus (especially with acidosis), leukemia, and lymphoma; who have undergone organ transplantation and immunosuppression; or who have burns, renal failure, or malnutrition. An unusual and recent epidemic of cutaneous mucormycosis was associated with use of Elastoplast bandages.

Clinical Manifestations. Mucormycosis follows inhalation or ingestion of spores which germinate and invade the nasal, tracheal, and/or gastrointestinal mucosa. *Rhinocerebral mucormycosis* is the most common form of disease and typically occurs in children with poorly controlled diabetes. Infection begins in the nasal turbinates or hard palate and presents as a black eschar. Hyphae gradually extend with involvement of the paranasal sinuses. Further extension through nerves, blood vessels, cartilage, and bone lead to involvement of the face, orbit, meninges, and brain. Initial symptoms of unilateral headache, nasal stuffiness, epistaxis, and facial numbness may progress to include periorbital cellulitis, with proptosis, loss of extraocular movements, and blindness. Intracranial extension may occur, resulting in occlusion of cerebral arteries and veins. Roentgenographic examination reveals diffuse clouding of the paranasal sinuses and extensive bony destruction; computed axial tomography delineates orbital involvement. Diagnosis is dependent on demonstration of hyphae in biopsy specimens; cultures are positive in only 15% of cases.

Pulmonary mucormycosis is an acute, life-threatening disease which occurs in immunosuppressed children with leukemia or lymphoma. Infection can occur in association with rhinocerebral mucormycosis or following inhalation of spores. In isolated pulmonary disease patients often present with a pulmonary infarction syndrome secondary to hyphal invasion and occlusion of pulmonary vessels, an acute onset of fever, pleuritic chest pain, and hemoptysis. Subsequent hematogenous dissemination with involvement of multiple organ systems is not uncommon. Roentgenographic examination is nonspecific and may reveal a number of abnormalities including patchy infiltrates, lobar consolidation, cavity formation, and pleural effusion. Nodule formation, fungus balls, and mass lesions have also been reported. Diagnosis requires an aggressive attempt to obtain tissue culture and histologic examination by transthoracic needle aspiration, transbronchial biopsy, and/or open lung biopsy.

Gastrointestinal mucormycosis is uncommon and in children is most often associated with malnutrition, kwashiorkor, or treatment with corticosteroids. Necrotic ulcers may involve the entire gastrointestinal tract, especially the stomach. Symptoms are acute and include bloody diarrhea, intestinal obstruction, and/or perforation.

Disseminated mucormycosis occurs in children with leukemia and lymphoma; is often associated with infections due to bacteria, viruses, and other pathogenic fungi; and is invariably fatal. Infection originates in the lung and disseminates to involve the brain and other organ systems. Neurologic manifestations are secondary to cerebrovascular invasion. Meningeal involvement is uncommon; however, cerebrospinal fluid abnormalities may include a mild pleocytosis with a predominance of polymorphonuclear leukocytes, an elevated protein, and a normal sugar. Cultures of blood and cerebrospinal fluid are invariably negative, and diagnosis depends on the demonstration of fungus in the biopsy material.

Cutaneous mucormycosis occurs as a secondary infection following extensive burns and/or surgical procedures. It presents as an erythematous papule which ulcerates, leaving a black necrotic center. Diagnosis depends on biopsy, culture, and histologic examination of suspicious skin lesions.

Miscellaneous infections reported with Mucoracea include endocarditis, bone marrow necrosis, and isolated renal infection.

Treatment. The treatment of mucormycosis must be aggressive and includes control of the underlying predisposing illness, reduction or elimination of immunosuppressive therapy, surgical resection of involved tissue, and intravenous administration of amphotericin B. The optimal dosage regimen for mucormycosis in children has not been established; however, in adults with extensive disease, treatment consists of 30–40 mg/kg/24 hr of amphotericin B given over a 2–3 mo period. In superficial infection of the skin, debridement and topical therapy with amphotericin B have proved successful; however, with evidence of deep hyphal invasion, systemic therapy with amphotericin B is indicated.

Lehrer RI, Howard DH, Sypherd PS, et al: Mucormycosis. Ann Intern Med 93:93, 1980.
Meyer RD, Rosen P, Armstrong D: Phycomycosis complicating leukemia and lymphoma. Ann Intern Med 77:871, 1972.
Meyers BR, Wormser G, Hirschman SZ, et al: Rhinocerebral mucormycosis—premortem diagnosis and therapy. Arch Intern Med 139:557, 1979.

10.103   SPOROTRICHOSIS

Sporotrichosis is an uncommon chronic fungal infection caused by a dimorphic fungus, *Sporothrix schenckii*. It has a worldwide distribution and exists in its saprophytic form in living, decaying, or dead vegetation. Disseminated infection is unusual and may follow inhalation or ingestion of spores. The cutaneous form of disease is more common and results from intradermal inoculation of spores following contact with contaminated vegetation, e.g., sphagnum moss, barberry, rosebushes, and various species of grass. Consequently, sporotrichosis is often an occupational disease of farmers, horticulturalists, and others in continual contact with soil and vegetation. Epidemic sporotrichosis has been reported in adults and children following contact with straw and hay heavily contaminated with spores of *S. schenckii*. Human-to-human transmission has not been reported.

Pathology. Histologically, sporotrichosis is characterized by noncaseating granulomas and microabscess formation. Oval or cigar-shaped forms may be visualized in biopsy material stained with methenamine silver or periodic acid–Schiff.

Clinical Manifestations. *Cutaneous sporotrichosis* is the most common form of disease in infants and children. Lymphocutaneous sporotrichosis, which accounts for more than 75% of reported cases, occurs after subcutaneous inoculation of spores. Following a variable and often prolonged incubation period (1–12 wk) an isolated, painless erythematous papule develops at the inoculation site, most often an extremity. The initial lesion enlarges and eventually ulcerates. Although infection may remain limited to the inoculation site, satellite lesions usually appear as multiple, painless, subcutaneous nodules extending along the lymphatic channels draining the initial lesion. These secondary nodules represent subcutaneous granulomas that attach to the overlying skin and ulcerate. Sporotrichosis does not heal spontaneously, and ulcerative lesions may persist for years unless appropriately treated. Systemic signs and symptoms are uncommon. Extracutaneous sporotrichosis is rare in children; however, pulmonary sporotrichosis, meningitis, osteomyelitis, septic arthritis, and disseminated disease have been reported in adults.

Diagnosis. Cutaneous sporotrichosis must be differentiated from the cutaneous forms of coccidioidomycosis, North American blastomycosis, histoplasmosis, tuberculosis, syphilis, anthrax, and tularemia. Histologic examination of biopsy material may demonstrate the organisms; however, a definitive diagnosis requires isolation of *S. schenckii* from infected tissue.

Treatment. Oral administration of potassium iodide is the treatment of choice for cutaneous sporotrichosis. The solution is given orally (1 gm/ml) beginning with 1–10 drops 3 times a day and increasing each dose by 1 drop/dose each day until a final dose of 10–40 drops 3 times a day is reached or until symptoms of iodism appear (skin eruptions, lacrimation, parotid swelling, nausea, vomiting). Treatment is continued for 1 mo after resolution of cutaneous lesions. Systemic administration of amphotericin B is required for extracutaneous infection and for cutaneous infection in patients sensitive to iodides.

Chandler JW, Kriel RL, Tosh FE: Childhood sporotrichosis. Am J Dis Child 115:368, 1968.
Dahl BA, Silberfarb PM, Sarosi GA, et al: Sporotrichosis in children. JAMA 215:1980, 1971.
Orr ER, Riley HD: Sporotrichosis in childhood: Report of ten cases. J Pediatr 78:951, 1971.

10.104   ASPERGILLOSIS

Aspergillosis refers to a group of diseases caused by a monomorphic fungus of the genus *Aspergillus (A. fumigatus, A. niger, A. flavus*, etc.). This mold has a worldwide distribution in soil and decaying vegetation. Although exposure to *Aspergillus* spores is frequent, disease is uncommon. Infection is most often acquired from inhalation of airborne spores which gain access to the paranasal sinuses or lower respiratory tract. Spores may also gain access to the body following ingestion, aspiration, or surgical instrumentation or following skin and wound contamination.

The pathologic manifestations of aspergillosis vary with the nature of the infection. Hyphae, easily visualized in tissue specimens stained with periodic acid–Schiff or methenamine silver, are 2–4 μ in diameter, septate, and dichotomously branched. On cross-section individual hyphae may be mistaken for spores; however, sporulation occurs only in infection confined to air-containing spaces.

Aspergillus species are capable of producing both pulmonary and nonpulmonary disease. Pulmonary aspergillosis may present as a hypersensitive pneumonitis, a noninvasive or saprophytic infection, or a life-threatening pneumonitis.

Hypersensitivity Syndromes

Atopic asthma may be precipitated by spores from *Aspergillus* species. Inhalation triggers an IgE-mediated response and an associated bronchospasm. The clinical manifestations are nonspecific and include the acute onset of wheezing in the absence of pulmonary infiltrates or fever.

Allergic alveolitis occurs in nonatopic individuals as a consequence of repeated exposure to organic dust. *Aspergillus* is 1 of many organic substances that lead to the development of this syndrome ("malt-workers lung"). The pathogenesis is unknown but may represent an immune-complex disease of lung tissue. The clinical manifestations include fever, cough, and dyspnea, which occur within 4–6 hr following exposure to the offending antigen. Physical examination reveals rhonchi in the absence of wheezing. Sputum and blood examinations are normal (e.g., no eosinophils), and the chest roentgenogram reveals diffuse interstitial infiltrates. Persistent exposure to the offending antigen gradually leads to irreversible pulmonary fibrosis.

Allergic bronchopulmonary aspergillosis often occurs in atopic children with a long history of asthma or other chronic pulmonary disease. The immune response to *Aspergillus* in these children is mediated by both IgG and IgE antibody directed against the fungus which colonizes the airways and produces a continued supply of antigen. This disorder is more common in children than adults. Symptoms include recurrent episodes of wheezing, pulmonary infiltrates, and eosinophilia. Additional features include immediate skin reactivity and precipitating antibodies to *Aspergillus fumigatus*, elevated total serum IgE concentrations, and central bronchiectasis. Other less common manifestations are expectoration of brown mucous plugs, positive sputum cultures for *Aspergillus* species, and the demonstration of hyphal elements in bronchial secretions. Treatment with steroids, often for extended periods of time, is effective in eliminating signs and symptoms and preventing bronchiectasis. Administration of systemic antifungal agents is of no proven value.

Noninvasive (Saprophytic) Syndromes

Otomycosis is a benign condition characterized by pain and otorrhea in which *Aspergillus* species (e.g., *A. niger*) grow on the cerumen and cellular debris within the external auditory canal. Resolution follows curettage and topical antifungal therapy.

Sinusitis secondary to *Aspergillus* species most often involves the maxillary sinuses and presents with fever and pain over the involved sinus. Roentgenographic examination typically reveals a fungus ball lying free or attached to the mucosa of a chronically infected sinus. Curettage and drainage are the treatment of choice.

Aspergilloma follows colonization of poorly drained bronchi, cysts, or cavitary lesions within the pulmonary parenchyma by *Aspergillus* species which proliferate a mass of hyphal elements (fungus ball). Aspergillomas occur primarily in the upper lobes of the lung and have been observed in pulmonary cavities of tuberculosis, histoplasmosis, and sarcoidosis. Mycelia may extend from the fungus ball into the wall of the cavity; however, extensive pulmonary invasion and hematogenous dissemination are uncommon. Affected children are often asymptomatic, although chronic cough and hemoptysis may occur. Diagnosis is established by roentgenographic demonstration of an air shadow outlining a pulmonary cavity which surrounds the fungus ball. The natural history of this saprophytic form of aspergillosis varies, and controversy surrounds the preferred therapeutic approach. Antifungal chemotherapy has little effect, and most clinicians follow asymptomatic patients, reserving surgical resection for those individuals with recurrent or life-threatening hemoptysis.

Invasive pulmonary aspergillosis is an acute life-threatening disease occurring almost exclusively in immunosuppressed or myelosuppressed patients. Leukemia is the most common predisposing illness in children, but it also occurs with lymphoreticular malignancies, during organ transplantation and treatment of collagen vascular disease, and/or in patients with abnormal granulocyte number or function. Illness typically begins as a pulmonary infection followed by hematogenous dissemination to the brain, heart, liver, other viscera, and skin. The overall mortality exceeds 80%. Clinical manifestations are nonspecific, are initially confined to the respiratory tract, and mimic acute bacterial pneumonitis. Thus, temperature elevation, a nonproductive cough, and dyspnea are common. Roentgenographic examination often reveals 1 or more areas of patchy consolidation which gradually increase in size and extend toward the periphery of the lung. There may also be lobar consolidation, cavitation, and miliary disease.

Cultures of blood, CSF, bone marrow, and urine are rarely positive in disseminated disease; however, sputum cultures yield aspergillosis species in 30% of autopsy-proven cases. Attempts to diagnose *Aspergillus* infections serologically have been unrewarding, although recent techniques for identifying circulating *Aspergillus* antigens in patients with disseminated disease are promising. Tissue obtained by transthoracic needle aspiration, transbronchial biopsy and brushings, and open lung biopsy should be immediately stained with both methenamine silver and periodic acid–Schiff and cultured on blood agar.

Successful treatment with amphotericin B (0.5 mg/kg/ 24 hr) is related to early initiation of therapy. Although synergism between amphotericin B and 5-fluorocytosine has been demonstrated for most *Aspergillus* species in vitro, there are limited data to support the combined use in clinical disease. Similarly, the efficacy of granulocyte transfusions as adjunct therapy in neutropenic patients is not established.

Miscellaneous nonpulmonary *Aspergillus* infections also occur in immunosuppressed or myelosuppressed children. Central nervous system involvement often presents as an acute focal neurologic deficit secondary to hyphal invasion and occlusion of cerebral blood vessels; meningitis and abscess formation are rare. Gastrointestinal and cutaneous ulcerations occasionally occur in children with leukemia or lymphoma and/or in those receiving long-term immunosuppressive therapy. Treatment is similar to that of invasive pulmonary infections.

WILLIAM T. SPECK
STEPHEN C. ARANOFF

Pennington JE: Aspergillus lung disease. Med Clin North Am 64:475, 1980.

Rosenburg M, et al: Clinical and immunologic criteria for the diagnosis of allergic bronchopulmonary aspergillosis. Ann Intern Med 86:405, 1977.

Wong JCF, et al: Allergic bronchopulmonary aspergillosis in pediatric practice. J Pediatr 94:376, 1979.

Young RC, et al: Aspergillosis—the spectrum of disease in 98 patients. Medicine 49:147, 1970.

10.105   COCCIDIOIDOMYCOSIS
(San Joaquin Fever; Valley Fever; Desert Rheumatism; Coccidioidal Granuloma)

Etiology.   Coccidioidomycosis is an infection caused by the fungus *Coccidioides immitis* found in the soil of the New World. The minute spores of its mycelial saprophytic phase are inhaled or, rarely, enter through injured skin. In the infected host they round up into spherules (sporangia) which develop endospores. Liberation of the latter leads to formation of new spherules. These spherules or endospores do not spread from person to person or from animal to person. Viable *C. immitis* does occur in pulmonary cavities, often in the mycelial as well as spherule form, but no cases of person-to-person infection have been discovered. As they occur naturally, however, and on surface cultures, the arthrospores (arthroconidia) of the saprophytic phase are highly infectious. Although isolation is unnecessary, precautions should be taken with dressings and casts over open lesions lest the mycelial arthrospores develop as they do on surface cultures. Within the arid endemic areas of California's San Joaquin Valley, in scattered regions in northern and southern

California, in central and southern Arizona, and even in southwestern Texas, many long-time residents have been infected, along with cattle, sheep, dogs, and wild rodents. Infection apparently confers permanent immunity; where the population is stable, coccidioidomycosis is a childhood infection.

Clinical Manifestations.   The human infection must be considered under 3 broad headings: (1) a benign, self-limited, primary infection (60% of infected persons show no clinical manifestations); (2) residual pulmonary lesions; and (3) a rare, disseminating, sometimes fatal disease. The disease tends to be milder in children; however, in those requiring medical attention, dissemination to bones and meninges is fairly common and approaches the incidence of these complications in adults. Infection acquired in utero has been reported.

Primary Coccidioidomycosis.   The incubation period varies from 1–4 wk, with an average of 10–16 days. Symptoms are influenzal in type; the onset may be insidious or abrupt with malaise, chills, and fever. Night sweats and anorexia are common. On occasion, there is a persistent dry cough with which there may be a painful throat. There may be headache, backache, and chest pain, which may vary from a mere sense of constriction to excruciating pleurisy.

A generalized, fine, macular erythema or urticarial eruption may appear within the 1st day or 2. It may be evanescent and present only in the groin. The most frequent dermatologic manifestation is erythema nodosum with or without erythema multiforme. These lesions develop at the time sensitivity to coccidioidin is maximal, 3–21 days after onset of symptoms. Skin lesions may occur, however, in persons otherwise asymptomatic. Other allergic manifestations, arthritis, and phlyctenular conjunctivitis may occur concomitantly.

Physical examination of the chest rarely discloses positive findings, even though roentgenography reveals extensive consolidation. Infrequently, dullness, a friction rub, or fine rales may be detected. Pleural effusions occur at times and may be so massive as to embarrass respiration. Like tuberculous pleural effusions, they may develop without preceding respiratory symptoms.

Residual Pulmonary Coccidioidomycosis.   Infrequently, a cavity may develop in an area of pulmonary consolidation during the primary infection and then regress. More often, however, after a variably prolonged period a persistent cavity may form. There are usually no symptoms related to it, and the diagnosis is made roentgenographically. Occasionally there is hemoptysis which, although it may recur and be alarming, is seldom so severe as to impair health. Rarely, fatal hemorrhage has occurred. Dissemination of the fungus from cavities to cause lesions in other areas is rare. Pulmonary residual "granulomas" sometimes persist. They are not harmful but do pose problems of differentiation from tuberculosis or neoplasms. Infrequently, a chronic progressive fibrocavitary pulmonary disease is seen.

Disseminated or Progressive Coccidioidomycosis (Coccidioidal Granuloma).   Certain persons lack ability to localize coccidioidal infection. Dissemination, which is rare and occurs mainly in males, especially in Filipinos and Blacks, usually follows the initial illness within 6 mo, often without any interlude. It is most closely analogous to progressive primary tuberculosis. Skin lesions and cold abscesses, both subcutaneous and osseous, occur. Meningitis is the most serious of the disseminated lesions, being clinically similar to tuberculous meningitis. In Whites it is not unusual for meningitis to be the only extrapulmonary lesion. Miliary dissemination and peritonitis may be distinguishable from tuberculosis only by demonstration of the causative agent, though coccidioidal peritonitis may present as a very mild disease. The case fatality rate of the untreated meningitis is practically 100% but is variable with other forms of disseminated coccidioidomycosis.

Diagnosis. Diagnosis of the disseminated infection may be established by biopsy or at autopsy. If histologic examination demonstrates the characteristic double-contoured spherules with endospores and without budding, the diagnosis is certain. Demonstration of the fungus by culture and by animal inoculation is also diagnostic. Sputum is generally so scanty in the primary infection that gastric lavage may be advisable, especially in children. The fungus will not withstand the concentration procedures usually used for tubercle bacilli. The material should be cultured or, after treatment with penicillin and streptomycin, chloramphenicol, or 0.05% copper sulfate, should be injected intraperitoneally into a mouse or intratesticularly into a guinea pig. Any suspicious fungus should be injected into a mouse or guinea pig to demonstrate diagnostic spherules. In vitro methods also may be used. Pure cultures can also be identified serologically ("exoantigen" test). Only especially qualified laboratories should undertake such hazardous procedures.

Skin Test. The test with coccidioidin or the newer spherulin is specific except for occasional cross-reactions in histoplasmosis and blastomycosis. A positive reaction does not distinguish between a recent or old infection unless preceded within a reasonably short time by a negative test result. *A negative skin test does not rule out coccidioidal infection.* Coccidioidin is administered intradermally as 0.1 ml of a 1:1000, 1:100, or even 1:10 dilution. The reaction generally reaches its peak at 36 hr and should be read at 24 and 48 hr. The criterion for a positive result is an area of induration more than 5 mm in diameter. Patients with suspected coccidioidal erythema nodosum are likely to be hypersensitive and should receive the 1:1000 dilution. Patients with disseminated infections are much less sensitive; on occasion, even a 1:10 dilution may not elicit a reaction. Dermal sensitivity to coccidioidin is less durable than to tuberculin. There is no danger of disseminating or activating a coccidioidal infection by a strong coccidioidin reaction, although there may be a systemic reaction as well as a local one. Coccidioidin does not evoke humoral coccidioidal antibodies in the human; therefore, the skin test may precede serologic tests and will provide information useful in their interpretation.

Blood and Cerebrospinal Fluid Tests. Serum precipitins and complement fixation antibodies may follow development of coccidioidin sensitivity and persist during periods of anergy associated with disseminated coccidioidomycosis. In general, the more severe the infection, the higher the complement fixation titer. Humoral antibodies are generally not demonstrable in asymptomatic acute infections. The sedimentation rate is rapid in both primary and disseminated infections and is helpful in evaluating clinical status. Eosinophilia is common. The cerebrospinal fluid findings are similar to those of tuberculous meningitis. Fixation of complement by cerebrospinal fluid occurs in 95% of patients with coccidioidal meningitis and is usually diagnostic. Occasionally, epidural coccidioidal lesions may also lead to complement fixation by the cerebrospinal fluid. Complement-fixing antibody may be detected in cisternal and lumbar fluid but be deceptively absent from the ventricular fluid. Complement-fixing antibodies do not pass the blood-brain barrier but are found in cord blood at the same titer as in the mother's blood. Passively transferred antibody in the infant disappears within 6 mo.

Roentgenography. During the primary infection roentgenograms of the chest may reveal no pulmonary changes, and those that occur are not diagnostic. Hilar adenopathy is frequent, and there may be single or multiple, sharply circumscribed or soft, feathery, small pulmonary densities or larger consolidated areas. Pulmonary cavities, when present, tend to be thin-walled. Pleural effusions are of variable extent. The osseous lesions, usually multiple and with a predilection for cancellous bone, often show considerable proliferation and are generally indistinguishable from those of tuberculosis.

Prevention. Avoidance of exposure to the spores is the only means for preventing infection. An available vaccine is of unproved value in humans.

Treatment. The treatment of primary coccidioidal infection consists of restriction of activity and symptomatic measures. Treatment should be continued until the sedimentation rate is returning to normal, precipitins have vanished, the complement-fixing titer of serum is regressing, and roentgenographic improvement is noted. Pulmonary cavities frequently close spontaneously. When a cavity persists or is located peripherally or there is recurrent bleeding or secondary infection, excision should be considered. Infrequently, bronchopleural fistulas or recurrent cavitation may occur as surgical complications; rarely, dissemination may result. When extensive thoracic surgery is required, therapy with amphotericin B may be desirable.

Amphotericin B, given parenterally, has been the mainstay of treatment of disseminated coccidioidomycosis. Its nephrotoxicity may result in diminished creatinine clearance, an elevation of the blood urea level, and at times depletion of potassium. Once the full dose is achieved, it can be administered every other day or 2–3 times/wk in the face of reduced renal function. Thrombophlebitis is common even with scrupulous care in intravenous administration. Anemia is expected during adequate administration of the drug but is effectively controlled by transfusions and terminates when treatment is stopped. Agranulocytosis is rare, but hepatic insufficiency develops occasionally, mainly in those with pre-existing liver damage. The drug should not be used in primary infections except when dissemination seems imminent. Although the response is occasionally dramatic in the disseminated form of the disease, generally treatment must be continued for months and, if possible, until improvement is demonstrated by a significant reduction in complement-fixing antibodies. An increase in sensitivity to coccidioidin is evidence of a favorable immunologic response. Immunologic reconstitution with leukocyte transfer factor (not yet fully evaluated) may be helpful in patients anergic to coccidioidin. Cold abscesses should be drained, infected synovial membranes removed, and, if osseous lesions are accessible, excision considered. In these cases intravenous and local amphotericin B may be used, depending on extent of involvement.

Amphotericin B does not pass the blood-brain barrier in therapeutic amounts, but it may mask meningitis during intravenous treatment. Early treatment of coccidioidal meningitis is important. Intrathecal administration of the drug in doses of 0.5 mg 2–3 times/wk (gradually increased from a dose of 0.025 mg) is usually necessary. Arachnoiditis and transverse myelitis are a hazard of intraspinal administration.

Treatment of coccidioidal meningitis should begin with both intravenous and intrathecal or intraventricular administration of amphotericin B. Intrathecal administration into the cisterna magna is preferred. Limited experience indicates that amphotericin in 10% glucose solution may be administered via the lumbar route with the patient's head tilted down at −30 degrees from the horizontal. Some, but not all, patients treated this way have escaped serious arachnoiditis. Intravenous therapy may be discontinued when the physician feels confident that meningitis is the only extrapulmonary involvement and when the patient appears clinically well and laboratory findings support the clinical impression of improvement. Treatment of coccidioidal meningitis should continue for at least 3 mo after the cerebrospinal fluid has normal cells, glucose, and protein and has become negative by complement-fixation test. Follow-up should include examination of the cerebrospinal fluid at intervals of 1–3 mo (and immediately if there is headache or any change in behavior or personality) for a period of at least 2 yr (Winn). Clinical surveillance should be continued for some years longer as relapses have been noted as late as 3–5 yr after return of the CSF to normal.

Miconazole, intravenously or intrathecally, has been successful in few adult patients and children. Ketoconazole given orally has shown promise in treatment of disseminated nonmeningeal coccidioidomycosis in adults. Experience with children is limited. The relative lack of toxicity of ketoconazole may permit its use in severe primary coccidioidal infections in which metapulmonary spread has not yet been demonstrated.

DEMOSTHENES PAPPAGIANIS

General

Ajello L (ed): Symposium on Coccidioidomycosis. Tucson, Ariz, University of Arizona Press, 1967. Also, Third Symposium, 1976.

Kafka JA, Catanzaro A: Disseminated coccidioidomycosis in children. J Pediatr 98:355, 1981.

Pappagianis D, Levine HB: The present status of vaccination against coccidioidomyocosis in man. Am J Epidemiol 102:30, 1975.

Restrepo A, Stevens DA, Utz J: First international symposium on ketoconazole. Rev Infect Dis 2:519, 1980.

Richardson HB, Anderson JA, McKay BM: Acute pulmonary coccidioidomycosis in children. J Pediatr 70:376, 1967.

Shafai T: Neonatal coccidioidomycosis in premature twins. Am J Dis Child 132:634, 1978.

Stevens DA (ed): Coccidioidomycosis: A Text. New York, Plenum Medical Book Co, 1980.

Winn WA: The treatment of coccidioidal meningitis. The use of amphotericin B in a group of 25 patients. Calif Med 101:78, 1964.

10.106   HISTOPLASMOSIS

Etiology. Histoplasmosis is a disease of man and animals caused by a dimorphic fungus *Histoplasma capsulatum*. The mycelial or saprophytic form of this fungus has been isolated from soil throughout the world. It grows on Sabouraud medium at room temperature (25° C) as white or tan fluffy colonies; small, budding, oval yeast forms, 2–4 µ in diameter, are found in the infected tissue and grow on enriched agar (cysteine glucose) at 37° C.

Epidemiology. Human histoplasmosis follows inhalation of airborne spores released by *H. capsulatum*. The saprophytic form grows best in soil heavily contaminated with avian and bat excreta. Birds, because of their high body temperature, are not infected but may carry the fungus on their feathers. However, bats, which have the lowest body temperature of mammals, may be infected and disseminate the microorganism in their excreta. Chicken, starling, or blackbird roosts and hollow trees as well as bat-infested caves, lofts, attics, and bridges may be heavily contaminated and serve as a reservoir for human infection. Histoplasmosis occurs throughout the United States, is endemic in the Mississippi, Ohio, and Missouri River valleys, and is most common in Kentucky and Tennessee, where up to 90% of the population have a positive histoplasmin skin test reaction by the age of 20. Additional areas of high prevalence, often very local, occur in South America, Asia, and Europe. Focal outbreaks of epidemic histoplasmosis have been reported following cave exploration, excavation, demolition, or other dust-raising activities in heavily contaminated areas. Histoplasmosis is not transmitted from person to person.

Pathogenesis and Pathology. Histoplasmosis usually occurs following inhalation of microconidia, which reach the alveoli and transform into small budding yeast. During an initial period of multiplication, there is both a local spread to adjacent lymph nodes and transient dissemination from the pulmonary focus to organs throughout the body. In most patients these primary lesions enlarge and undergo caseous necrosis, fibrosis, and subsequent calcification. In the lung, calcification of a primary focus and adjacent lymph nodes may resemble the Gohn complex of primary pulmonary tuberculosis. Multifocal "buckshot" areas of calcification may also occur throughout the lungs, lymphatic tissue, and spleen. Two forms of progressive histoplasmosis occur in a small proportion of infected patients. *Disseminated histoplasmosis* occurs in infants and debilitated adults and in patients with defects in cell-mediated immunity. Yeast-laden macrophages infiltrate the entire reticuloendothelial system with extensive involvement of the bone marrow, liver, spleen, lungs, heart, adrenals, and brain. *Chronic pulmonary histoplasmosis* typically occurs in adult males and is associated with yeast invasion and multiplication in pre-existing emphysematous cavities, producing a progressive fibronodular pneumonia characterized by cavity formation, large areas of caseous necrosis, and extensive fibrosis.

Clinical Manifestations. Acute pulmonary histoplasmosis is the most common form of disease due to *H. capsulatum* and is classified as primary (initial infection) or secondary (reinfection) according to previous exposure history. Primary pulmonary histoplasmosis is often an asymptomatic disease in infants and young children, a positive histoplasmin skin test being the only manifestation of infection. The incubation period is 10–23 days, and the severity of symptoms, when present, corresponds to the concentration of inhaled microconidia. Symptomatic acute pulmonary histoplasmosis presents as an influenza-like illness with abrupt onset of fever, malaise, myalgia, headache, and nonproductive cough. Physical examination is often normal; however, diffuse rales and mild hepatosplenomegaly have been described. Roentgenographic examination of the lungs during the acute illness reveals scattered patchy pneumonic infiltrates and hilar adenopathy. The illness is benign and self-limited in children, and abnormal signs and symptoms rarely persist more than 3 wk. However, abnormal chest roentgenograms may persist for several mo, showing small nodular residues that eventually calcify. Secondary, or reinfection type, pulmonary histoplasmosis has the onset of symptoms within 3 days of exposure. Symptoms are similar but less severe and of shorter duration. The roentgenographic findings following reinfection consist of uniformly distributed miliary nodules indistinguishable from miliary tuberculosis. These abnormalities resolve over a period of several mo without calcification.

Epidemic histoplasmosis has been reported in both endemic and nonendemic areas following massive exposure to dust heavily contaminated with spores of *H. capsulatum*. Clinical manifestations begin within 3–20 days following exposure and include an abrupt onset of high fever, chills, headache, malaise, and a nonproductive cough; pleuritic chest pain and dyspnea are common. Physical examination reveals diffuse rales often associated with minimal hepatosplenomegaly. Erythema nodosum and erythema multiforme appearing separately or together have been reported in young women during epidemics. Roentgenographic examination of the chest reveals pulmonary infiltrates, which may persist for several mo. The prognosis is excellent with spontaneous resolution of all signs and symptoms occurring within weeks. Epidemic illness has, on rare occasions, led to disseminated disease in infants and children.

Chronic pulmonary histoplasmosis, a disease of middle-aged white male smokers with a history of chronic obstructive pulmonary disease, has not been reported in children.

Disseminated histoplasmosis is an acute illness of infants, young children, and immunosuppressed patients with high morbidity and mortality. The illness begins as an acute pulmonary infection with fever, cough, and dyspnea and quickly progresses to involve multiple organ systems. These patients appear critically ill with persistent nausea, vomiting, abdominal pain, and diarrhea. Physical findings reveal generalized rales, diffuse lymphadenopathy, and hepatosplenomegaly. Roentgenographic abnormalities often include a diffuse interstitial pneumonitis. The clinical course in untreated patients is progressively downhill; death is secondary to respiratory failure, uncontrolled gastrointestinal bleeding, disseminated intravascular coagulation, and/or bacterial sepsis. Subacute and chronic forms of disseminated disease have been reported in adults and are often associated with oropharyngeal, nasopharyngeal, laryngeal, and gastrointestinal ulcerations; adrenal insufficiency; endocarditis; osteomyelitis; arthritis; and meningitis.

Histoplasmoma and *mediastinal collagenosis* are rare in children and represent an exaggerated immune response to infection. The former presents as an enlarging, solitary pulmonary nodule with concentrated layers of fibrous tissue and calcium surrounding a healed primary focus; these nodules may reach 3–4 cm in diameter and must be differentiated from neoplasms. The latter is associated with fibrocalcification originating in a mediastinal node and extending through the mediastinum resulting in entrapment and obstruction of mediastinal structures.

Diagnosis. Diagnosis of acute pulmonary histoplasmosis relied in the past on conversion of the histoplasmin skin test and more recently on seroconversion of the complement fixation assay or the immunodiffusion test. Sputum cultures are rarely positive in acute pulmonary histoplasmosis. The histoplasmin skin test resembles the tuberculin test and is considered positive if an area of at least 5 mm of induration is observed at 48 hr. A positive reaction indicates previous sensitization to *H. capsulatum* but is not diagnostic of active disease. However, conversion from a negative to positive reaction within a few wk or a positive reaction in an infant is suggestive of active infection. Skin testing has limited usefulness because of a large number of false negatives in patients with disseminated disease and late conversion following initial infection. Approximately 25% of patients with positive skin test will convert their histoplasmin serology from negative to positive after skin testing. Reactivity to histoplasmin antigen is relatively short lived, and conversion to a negative test occurs several yr after primary infection. Complement fixation titers are often helpful in diagnosing acute infection. An initial titer greater than 1:16 suggests active disease; only 25% of infected individuals will demonstrate a 4-fold increase between acute and convalescent titers. Cross-reaction with the serologic test for blastomycosis is common, and an initial titer of greater than 1:8 for *B. dermatitidis* in the absence of blastomycosis is therefore suggestive of acute infection with *H. capsulatum*. The immunodiffusion test with the

M antigen has fewer false negatives than the standard complement fixation assay. Definitive diagnosis requires demonstration of the infecting organism by culture or histology.

Treatment. Amphotericin B is the treatment of choice for all life-threatening infections due to *H. capsulatum*. In acute pulmonary histoplasmosis in older children and adults, treatment is not indicated since the disease is often benign and self-limited. However, symptomatic pulmonary histoplasmosis in infants and young children (under 2 yr) may progress to disseminated disease; therefore a short course of amphotericin B (2 wk) is recommended. In disseminated histoplasmosis treatment with amphotericin B is indicated. Although experience is limited in children, most authorities recommend a total dose of 30 mg/kg. Cultures often convert to negative within a few wk; however, relapses are not uncommon, and repeated cultures to monitor

the success or failure of chemotherapy are therefore indicated. In vitro studies have demonstrated synergistic killing of *H. capsulatum* when amphotericin B is combined with rifampin, but clinical experience with this combination is limited.

WILLIAM T. SPECK
STEPHEN C. ARANOFF

Goodwin RA, Des Prez RM: Histoplasmosis. Am Rev Resp Dis 117:929, 1978.
Goodwin RA, Shapiro JL, et al: Disseminated histoplasmosis: Clinical and pathologic correlations. Medicine 59:1, 1980.
Kauffman CA, Israel KS, et al: Histoplasmosis in immunosuppressed patients. Am J Med 64:923, 1978.
Macher A: Histoplasmosis and blastomycosis. Med Clin North Am 64:447, 1980.
Straus SE, Jacobson SE: The spectrum of histoplasmosis in a general hospital: A review of 55 cases diagnosed at Barnes Hospital between 1966 and 1977. Am J Med Sci 279:147, 1980.

10.107 PARASITIC INFECTIONS

Infectious diseases represent a major cause of morbidity and mortality in infants and children in most parts of the world. While, in general, infections due to viral, bacterial, or fungal agents are easily recognized and adequately investigated and managed, those due to protozoa and helminths have received relatively little attention. Such neglect of parasitic diseases contrasts with their global significance; malaria alone claims more than a million lives of African children annually and is increasingly imported to Europe and North America. Parasites are endemic in many parts of the world; although they are more common in hot climates, no specific geographic area is spared. Recognition of these infections and their proper management are therefore essential. The major parasitic infections and their estimated prevalence, mortality, and morbidity are presented in Table 10–53.

Parasitism in its widest sense is a specialized, dependent type of life which includes all infectious agents. The term "parasites" has been used historically and conventionally to refer only to those infectious organisms which belong to the animal kingdom, i.e., *proto-*

zoa, helminths, and *arthropods.* The distinction between bacteria, viruses, etc., and "parasites" implied by this definition, however, is artificial. Protozoa are unicellular organisms which multiply within their hosts and are therefore closely related to other infectious agents. In contrast, worms or helminths are multicellular and usually do not divide within the human host. These basic differences between protozoa and helminths have important epidemiologic, clinical, and therapeutic implications.

The host-parasite relationship in most of these infections has several unique features. Infection and disease due to these agents must be clearly distinguished. When a parasite invades a host, it may die at once or survive without causing harm to the host (infection). Alternatively, it may survive and produce morbidity (disease) and possibly kill the host. Survival of the phenomenon of parasitism suggests, in an evolutionary sense, that infection is much more common than disease. Parasites have adapted through various modifications to establish infections and allow the development of a symbiotic relationship with their hosts. In

Table 10–53 ESTIMATED WORLDWIDE PREVALENCE (IN THOUSANDS) OF THE MAJOR PARASITIC INFECTIONS IN RELATION TO ASSOCIATED MORBIDITY AND MORTALITY

INFECTION	PREVALENCE	MORBIDITY	MORTALITY
Protozoa			
Amebiasis	400,000	1500	30
Giardiasis	4000	1–2000	0.1
Malaria	800,000	150,000	1200
Trypanosomiasis, African	1000	10	5
Trypanosomiasis, American	12,000	1200	60
Toxoplasmosis	800,000	10	0.1
Leishmaniasis	12,000	12,000	5
Helminths			
Ascariasis	1,000,000	1000	30
Hookworms	900,000	1500	50–60
Filariasis	300,000	500	20–50
Schistosomiasis	300,000	150,000	1200

addition, these organisms have evolved evasive mechanisms against host immune or protective responses. In respect to the host's well-being, parasites may cause disease by their physical presence or by competition with the host for specific nutrients. Disease may also result from the host's attempts to destroy the invaders, e.g., the host pathologic reaction.

The sections on individual infections deal with the most important parasitic infections encountered in the pediatric age group. A deliberate attempt has been made to include only the most effective, reliable, and safe therapeutic agents.

Parasitic Zoonoses. WHO Tech Rep Series, No 637, 1979.
Walsh JA, Warren KS: Selective primary health. An interim strategy for disease control in developing countries. N Engl J Med 301:967, 1979.
Warren KS, Mahmoud AAF: Geographic Medicine for the Practitioner. Algorithms in the Diagnosis and Management of Exotic Diseases. Chicago, University of Chicago Press, 1978, p 1.

Protozoa

INTESTINAL PROTOZOA

Parasitic protozoan infections of the intestine cause a wide variety of clinical syndromes which range from asymptomatic carrier states to severe disease associated with pathologic lesions in the gastrointestinal tract or other organs (Table 10–54). *Entamoeba histolytica* and *Giardia lamblia* belong to this group and cause important and clinically well-defined pathologic lesions. Infections with less common organisms such as *Balantidium coli* and *Isospora hominis* are usually asymptomatic or associated with mild disease. Infection by any of the intestinal protozoa is usually acquired orally through fecal contamination of water or food. As a group, they are more endemic in countries with unsanitary water conditions. *G. lamblia*, however, has recently been recognized as a major cause of epidemics of waterborne diarrhea in North America.

10.108 AMEBIASIS

Human infection with *Entamoeba histolytica* is prevalent worldwide; endemic foci are particularly common in areas with low socioeconomic and sanitary standards. *E. histolytica* parasitizes the lumen of the gastrointestinal tract and causes few or no disease sequelae in most infected subjects. In a small proportion of individuals the organisms invade the intestinal mucosa or may disseminate to other organs, especially the liver.

Etiology. Infection with *Entamoeba histolytica* is established by ingestion of food or water contaminated with parasite cysts. These cysts measure 10–18 μm, contain 4 nuclei, and are resistant to environmental conditions such as low temperature and the concentra-

tions of chlorine commonly used in water purification; the parasite can be killed by heating to 55° C. Upon ingestion, the cyst wall is digested, and the nuclei double in number to form 8 trophozoites. These are large, actively motile organisms which colonize the lumen of the large intestine and may invade its mucosal lining. Trophozoites have an average diameter of 20 μm; the cytoplasm consists of an outer clear zone and an inner densely granular endoplasm. The latter contains a spherical nucleus which has a small central karyosome and fine granular chromatin material. The endoplasm also contains vacuoles where erythrocytes may be seen in cases of invasive amebiasis. Two other species of *Amoeba* may infect the human gastrointestinal tract: *E. coli* and *E. hartmanni*. As these are not pathogenic, it is important to recognize their characteristic features and distinguish them from *E. histolytica*.

Epidemiology. The prevalence of amebic infections varies from 5–81% in different parts of the world. Amebic dysentery due to invasion of the intestinal mucosa is found in approximately 1–17% of infected subjects. Dissemination of the parasites to internal organs such as the liver occurs in an even smaller fraction of infected individuals and is thought to be less common in children than in adults.

Man is the natural host and reservoir of *E. histolytica*; primates and laboratory animals may be infected. The outcome of amebic infection varies in different parts of the world. For example, infection acquired in India, Mexico, or Durban, South Africa, is more virulent than that from other locations. The definition of virulence, geographic strains, and pathogenicity of different amebae is not, however, clear.

E. histolytica infection is transmitted via contaminated food and drinks. Food handlers carrying amebic cysts

Table 10–54 IMPORTANT INTESTINAL PROTOZOAN INFECTIONS OF CHILDREN

INFECTION	ETIOLOGY	TRANSMISSION	MAJOR CLINICAL FEATURES	DIAGNOSIS
Amebiasis	*Entamoeba histolytica*	Fecal-oral	Diarrhea-dysentery	Trophozoites or cysts in stools
			Liver abscess	Serology
Giardiasis	*Giardia lamblia*	Fecal-oral Person-to-person	Diarrhea	Cysts in stools
			Malabsorption	Cysts or trophozoites in duodenal aspirate
Balantidiasis	*Balantidium coli*	Fecal-oral	Bloody diarrhea	Trophozoites or cysts in stools

may therefore play a role in spreading the infection. Direct contact with infected feces also may be responsible for person-to-person transmission.

Pathogenesis and Pathology. The parasite factors responsible for the pathologic changes are not known. Once E. histolytica trophozoites invade the intestinal mucosa, they produce tissue destruction (ulcers) with little local inflammatory response. The organisms multiply and spread laterally underneath the intestinal epithelium to produce the characteristic flask-shaped ulcers. These lesions are commonly seen in the cecum, transverse, and sigmoid colon. Amebae may produce similar lytic lesions if they reach the liver (these are commonly called abscesses although they contain no granulocytes). E. histolytica occasionally disseminates to other extraintestinal sites such as the lungs. The contrast between the extent of tissue destruction by amebae, the absence of a local host inflammatory response, and the demonstration of systemic humoral (antibody) and cell-mediated reactions against the organisms remain a major scientific puzzle.

Clinical Manifestations. Most infected individuals are asymptomatic; the only evidence of infection is the cysts found in their feces. Invasion of the host occurs in 2–8% of infected individuals and may be related to the strain of parasites or the nutritional status and intestinal flora of the host. The most common clinical manifestations of amebiasis are due to local invasion of the intestinal epithelium and dissemination to the liver.

Intestinal amebiasis may occur within 2 wk of infection or be delayed for months. The onset is usually gradual with colicky abdominal pains and frequent bowel movements (6–8 movements/24 hr). Diarrhea is frequently associated with tenesmus. Stools are blood stained and contain a fair amount of mucus with few leukocytes. Generalized constitutional symptoms and signs are characteristically absent. Acute amebic dysentery occurs in attacks lasting a few days to several wk; recurrence is very common in untreated individuals. Occasionally, amebic dysentery is associated with sudden onset of disease characterized by fever, chills, and severe diarrhea. This may result in dehydration and electrolyte disturbances. In a few patients complications such as ameboma, extraintestinal extension, or local perforation and hemorrhage may occur. The characteristic flask-shaped ulcers with healthy intervening mucosa which occur in most cases of amebic dysentery may be detected by sigmoidoscopy in 25% of patients.

Hepatic amebiasis is a very serious manifestation of disseminated infection. Diffuse liver enlargement has been associated with intestinal amebiasis, but the only well defined clinical entity is liver abscess, which occurs in fewer than 1% of infected individuals and may appear in patients with no clear history of intestinal disease. In children fever is the hallmark of amebic liver abscess. It is frequently associated with abdominal pain, distention, and an enlarged, tender liver. Changes at the base of the right lung, such as elevation of the diaphragm and parenchymal compression, may also occur. Laboratory examination shows a slight leukocytosis, moderate anemia, and no significant elevation of liver enzymes. Stool examination for amebae is negative in more than 50% of patients with documented amebic liver abscess. In most cases hepatic ultrasonography and isotope scans localize and delineate the size of the abscess cavity. Most patients have a single cavity in the right hepatic lobe. Amebic liver abscess may be associated with grave complications when diagnosis and therapy are delayed. The most common of these is rupture into the peritoneum or thorax or through the skin.

Diagnosis. Definitive diagnosis is based on detection of the organisms in stool samples or, rarely, in aspirates of a liver abscess. Demonstration of E. histolytica trophozoites or cysts requires examination of several fresh stool samples by an experienced person. It is therefore recommended that whenever amebiasis is suspected, an additional stool sample be preserved in polyvinyl alcohol for further identification and staining of the organisms. Material for microscopic examination may also be obtained by scraping the ulcerated areas of rectal mucosa. The indirect hemagglutination test may be helpful in cases of invasive intestinal amebiasis; a diagnostic titer of $\geq$1:128 has been reported in 98% of cases. This test is also positive in 100% of patients with amebic liver abscess.

Treatment. All individuals with E. histolytica trophozoites or cysts in their stools, whether symptomatic or not, should be treated to eradicate the infection. Diloxanide furoate is the drug of choice for asymptomatic cyst passers; it is most effective as a luminal amebicide. The recommended dose is 10 mg/kg/24 hr orally for 10 days. Toxicity is rare, but the drug should not be used in children under 2 yr of age. Invasive amebiasis of the intestine, liver, or other organs requires the use of tissue amebicidal drugs. Metronidazole is currently the drug of choice; it is administered orally in a daily dose of 50 mg/kg for 10 days. Side effects of this drug include nausea, diarrhea, metallic taste in the mouth, and leukopenia; these are uncommon and disappear on completion of therapy. Metronidazole is also a luminal amebicide but less effective than diloxanide furoate in this respect. Patients with invasive amebiasis should therefore receive an additional course of the latter drug following metronidazole therapy. If the case is severe or metronidazole cannot be used, dehydroemetine is the recommended alternative therapeutic agent. It is administered by the subcutaneous or intramuscular route (never intravenously) in a dose of 1 mg/kg/24 hr for 10 days. Patients should be hospitalized when this drug is given because cardiac or renal complications may occur. If tachycardia, T wave depression, arrhythmias, or proteinuria develops, use of the drug should be stopped. A course of diloxanide furoate is also recommended following completion of dehydroemetine therapy. Amebic liver abscesses are treated with specific therapy as outlined above; however, aspiration of large lesions may be necessary if rupture is imminent or if the patient shows poor clinical response 4–6 days after administration of amebicidal drugs. Stool examination should be repeated 2 wk following completion of antiamebic therapy as a test of cure.

Control of amebiasis, like that of most other water- and food-borne infections, can be achieved by exercising proper sanitary measures. Regular examination of food handlers and thorough investigation of diarrhea episodes may lead to identification of the source of infection in some communities. There is no prophylactic drug for amebiasis.

10.109 GIARDIASIS

Infection with *Giardia lamblia* has only recently been recognized as a common worldwide cause of infectious diarrhea. The infection is more prevalent in children than in adults and is particularly significant in those with malnutrition or immunodeficiencies or in those living in institutions.

Etiology. *Giardia lamblia* infects man through ingestion of food or water contaminated by its cysts. The mature cyst, which measures approximately 8–10 μm, is thick walled and oval and contains 4 nuclei. These organisms are passed in the stools of infected individuals and may remain viable in water for longer than 3 mo. Their viability is not affected by the normal concentrations of chlorine used to purify water for drinking. Epidemics in nurseries suggest that person-to-person transmission may also occur. Upon reaching the upper small intestine, each *Giardia* cyst liberates 4 trophozoites. This stage of the protozoa is piriform and measures $2-4 \times 14$ μ. The body of the trophozoite is divided longitudinally by 2 median rods and contains 2 oval nuclei anteriorly, a large sucking disc on the ventral surface, and a curved median body posteriorly. Each organism has 4 pairs of flagella, which help in its motility.

Epidemiology. *Giardia* is the most frequently identified intestinal parasite in North America; its prevalence in other parts of the world varies from 0.5–18%, and there has been an increase in epidemics of diarrhea due to giardiasis. Man was thought to be the primary reservoir of *G. lamblia*, but it is now believed that the human parasite may infect dogs as well. Man can also be infected by parasites obtained from beavers; the presence of these or other animal reservoirs may explain the sporadic nature of epidemics.

Giardiasis has been recognized as an important cause of chronic diarrhea in immunodeficient children for almost 2 decades. However, the relationship of the host immune system to susceptibility to infection and subsequent disease remains unclear.

Clinical Manifestations. Infection may occur in infants but is more common in older children. Symptoms occur in 40–80% of infected children; the most common presentation is diarrhea, weight loss, and failure to thrive. The clinical course of giardiasis varies. The onset of symptoms may be abrupt or gradual; the disease may be self-limited or produce severe protracted diarrhea and malabsorption. Alterations in the digestive function of the brush border are common in those with protracted symptoms. Malabsorption of sugars (such as xylose and disaccharides), fats, and fat-soluble vitamins occurs in more than half of patients who have nonspecific morphologic abnormalities of the small intestinal mucosa similar to those seen in other malabsorptive disorders.

Persistence of diarrhea and malabsorption may occur in children with compromised immune responses due to malignancy. Histologic abnormalities of the intestinal mucosa are more severe in these patients, but eradication of the parasite is associated with clinical improvement.

Diagnosis. *G. lamblia* trophozoites or cysts may be found in fecal samples obtained from infected children. As cyst excretion is irregular, examination of several fecal samples or duodenal contents may be needed. The Entero-test is an efficient, simple, and safe method for detection of *G. lamblia* in duodenal fluid of children.

Treatment. The efficacy of the 2 major anti-giardia agents has been evaluated in children. Metronidazole (25 mg/kg/24 hr for 5 days) and quinacrine (8 mg/kg/24 hr for 5 days) were compared in 160 infected children. Five positive stools were detected among 73 children who received quinacrine, while none was found in those treated with metronidazole. Tinidazole has also recently been introduced for treatment of infected children; a single oral dose of 1–1.5 gm resulted in a 90% cure rate.

The recent increase of epidemics of giardiasis dictates re-examination of sanitary practices. Water supply is the most important factor; its quality should be routinely monitored. The concentration of chlorine required for control, particularly in communities dependent on surface water with no sand filtration, needs to be determined. Spread of infection in institutions can be prevented by identification and proper treatment of asymptomatic carriers. There is no prophylactic medication against giardiasis.

OTHER INTESTINAL PROTOZOA

Infection of children with *Balantidium coli* or *Isospora hominis* may be associated with vague gastrointestinal complaints such as abdominal pain, distention, and diarrhea. *B. coli* may invade the intestinal mucosa, causing bloody diarrhea and ulcerations. Diagnosis of either infection is made by fecal examination. Therapy with metronidazole is recommended for symptomatic cases of balantidiasis; *Isospora* infections tend to be self-limited.

ADEL A. F. MAHMOUD

Amebiasis

Adams EB, MacLeod IN: Invasive amebiasis. I. Amebic dysentery and its complications. Medicine 56:315, 1977.

Adams EB, MacLeod IN: Invasive amebiasis. II. Amebic liver abscess and its complications. Medicine 56:325, 1977.

Harrison RH, Crowe PC, Fulginiti VA: Amebic liver abscess in children: Clinical and epidemiologic features. Pediatrics 64:923, 1979.

Krogstad DJ, Spencer HC, Healy GR: Current concepts in parasitology: Amebiasis. N Engl J Med 298:262, 1978.

Stamm WP: Amoebiasis: A neglected diagnosis. J Clin Pathol 29:83, 1976.

Welch JS, Rowsell BJ, Freedman C: Treatment of intestinal amebiasis and giardiasis. Efficacy of metronidazole and tinidazole compared. Med J Aust 1:469, 1978.

Giardiasis

Kavousi S: Giardiasis in infancy and childhood: A prospective study of 160 cases with comparison to quinacrine (atabrine) and metronidazole (Flagyl). Am J Trop Med Hyg 28:19, 1979.

Meyer EA, Jarroll EL: Giardiasis. Am J Epidemiol 111:1, 1980.
Rosenthal P, Liebman WM: Comparative study of stool examinations, duodenal aspiration and pediatric Entero-test for giardiasis in children. J Pediatr 96:278, 1980.
Stevens DP, Mahmoud AAF: Giardiasis: The rediscovery of an ancient pathogen. In Remington JS, Swartz MN (eds): Current Clinical Topics in Infectious Diseases. New York, McGraw-Hill Book Co, 1980, p 195.

SYSTEMIC PROTOZOAN INFECTIONS

10.110 MALARIA

Malaria results from invasion of erythrocytes by any of 4 species of protozoan parasites of the genus *Plasmodium*. It is characterized by high fever, which is often intermittent, and by anemia and splenic enlargement. Despite worldwide campaigns aimed at eradication of malaria through interruption of its life cycle in the intermediate mosquito host, the disease continues to be the principal health problem of warm climates; it is frequently imported to countries in the temperate zones where, in the summer mo, it may be spread locally by mosquitoes.

For clinical and diagnostic purposes, malaria may be regarded as 2 disease entities: the more dangerous one, caused by *Plasmodium falciparum* and formerly termed "subtertian" or "malignant tertian malaria," can produce a variety of acute clinical manifestations and may, if untreated, be fatal within a few days of onset; the other, caused by *P. vivax* (benign tertian malaria), *P. ovale* (a rarity resembling *P. vivax*), or *P. malariae* (quartan malaria), is more typically paroxysmal and almost never fatal. The latter 3 infections may recur weeks after apparent cure of a primary attack, in contrast to falciparum infections, which, except in the case of drug-resistant strains, rarely recrudesce after standard treatment.

Etiology.   Malaria is usually acquired from the bites of previously infected female anopheline mosquitoes. In other instances, malaria, particularly of the quartan type, has developed after the transfusion of infected blood, in which circumstance the pre-erythrocytic phase of the parasite's development in the liver is avoided. The usual evolution of the disease is as follows:

Pre-Erythrocytic Phase.   The *sporozoites* injected by the biting mosquito reach the sinusoids of the liver through the bloodstream and enter the cytoplasm of hepatic cells. Growth and nuclear division are rapid, and microscopic cysts *(schizonts)* are formed which contain *merozoites*. Most of these cysts of all species rupture at the end of 6–15 days of development, liberating thousands of merozoites which penetrate red blood cells, but a few *P. vivax* and *P. ovale* forms remain dormant in the liver for weeks or months, paving the way for relapses.

The incubation period (between the infecting mosquito bite and the presence of parasites in the blood) varies with the species; with *P. falciparum* it is 10–13 days; with *P. vivax* and *ovale*, 12–16; and with *P. malariae*, 27–37, depending on the size of the inoculum. Malaria transmitted by the transfusion of infected blood becomes apparent in a shorter time. Clinical manifestations of infection induced by any means may be suppressed for many mo by subcurative treatment, particularly in the cases of vivax and quartan malaria.

Erythrocytic Phase.   The merozoites which invade red blood cells appear first in stained smears as bluish rings or

(P. malariae) bands of cytoplasm, with 1 or occasionally 2 red dots of nuclear chromatin. The growing parasites are named *trophozoites*, and appearing with them in the red cells are granules of yellow-brown pigment which consist of hematin derived from the hemoglobin consumed by the parasite to meet its protein requirements. The shape of the organism varies during growth until it becomes round and, with the scattered or clumped pigment, almost fills the red blood cell, which in the case of *P. vivax* is enlarged and stippled.

The nucleus of the parasite now divides asexually several times, its cytoplasm is arranged around the new nuclei, and the pigment aggregates into large clumps; this segmenter, or mature *schizont*, contains a varying number of merozoites, depending on the species. The erythrocytes containing these merozoites rupture, and naked merozoites, pigment, and erythrocytic debris are freed in the plasma. Those merozoites that escape inactivation by immunoglobulins or phagocytosis enter fresh red blood cells. Thus, an asexual cycle is begun each time a new crop of merozoites invades red cells, and this cycle, the duration of which is of considerable clinical importance, lasts 48 hr in falciparum, vivax, and ovale malaria and 72 hr in quartan malaria. The malarial paroxysm does not take place until enough cycles have occurred to produce the amount of parasitic material, pigment, and red cell debris required to induce febrile or other reactions.

Certain of the growing parasites fail to divide, the nucleus remaining intact during the period of maturation. They are differentiated into male or female forms called *gametocytes*, which are of no clinical importance but are capable of infecting mosquitoes feeding on the patient.

Mixed Infections and Broods.   In mixed infections 1 species is usually responsible for the clinical pattern, with falciparum dominating vivax, and vivax dominating quartan; only when sufficient immunity is developed to the dominant strain does the other begin to produce clinical manifestations.

In an infection with a single species, distinct broods may develop. Since the merozoites in the liver are not released simultaneously and the erythrocytic schizonts do not all rupture at the same time, some groups of parasites begin their existence in red blood cells before or after the majority, often maturing in sufficient numbers to produce an independent clinical reaction. In vivax infections single broods will produce a febrile reaction every other day, whereas if 2 broods develop, there will be daily paroxysms; in falciparum malaria the classic picture of intermittent fever may likewise soon become disrupted.

Epidemiology.   Only in regions where the people have gametocytes in their blood can anopheline mosquitoes become infected. Children may be especially important in this respect. Transmission of malaria occurs in most tropical and some temperate zones; although the United States, Canada, and northern Europe are now free of indigenous malaria, focal outbreaks have occurred through infection of local mosquitoes by travelers coming from endemic areas.

Congenital malaria, caused by transfer of the causative agent across the placental barrier, is extremely rare. Neonatal malaria, on the other hand, is less uncommon and may result from mingling of infected maternal blood with that of the infant during the birth process.

Pathology.   The extent of destruction of red blood cells depends upon the duration and severity of the infection. Hemolysis often leads to an increase in the serum bilirubin, and in falciparum malaria it may be sufficiently intense to result in hemoglobinuria *(blackwater fever)*. In any malarial infection the degree of anemia is greater than that attributable solely to the destruction of cells by parasites. Autoantigenic changes produced in the red cell by the parasite probably contribute to hemolysis; these changes and increased osmotic fragility occur in all erythrocytes, whether infected or not. Hemolysis may also be induced by quinine or primaquine in persons with hereditary glucose-6-phosphate dehydrogenase deficiency.

The pigment extruded into the circulation upon red cell disintegration accumulates in the reticuloendothelial cells of the spleen, the follicles of which become hyperplastic and sometimes necrotic, in the Kupffer cells of the liver, and in the bone marrow, brain, and other organs. Deposition of sufficient pigment and of hemosiderin results in a slate-gray color of the organs.

The malignancy of falciparum malaria is peculiar to that species. The merozoites emerging from the liver are considerably more numerous than those of other species; there are as many in young children as in adults, so that children have a proportionately greater initial wave of infection. Young children are particularly prone to severe, often lethal, parasitemia.

Eight–18 hr after the parasite has entered the red blood cells, these cells become increasingly sticky and tend to adhere to the endothelial lining of blood sinuses and vessels, especially when the circulation is slow. The sticky cell is thus fixed and unable to return to the general circulation, although the parasite within it matures in the normal manner. As more cells adhere, flow within the vessel is progressively impeded, and occlusion or even rupture may occur.

The site and extent of this interference with vascular function, coupled with a selective localization of parasitized cells in various organs or systems, are responsible for the variety of symptoms from falciparum infections. Thus, pneumonitis, encephalitis, or enteritis may be manifest when the bulk of the infection is in the lungs, brain, or intestinal tract, respectively. In the pregnant woman damage to the placenta may result in death of the fetus or in premature birth; infants born at full term to infected women have lower birth weights than those of infants born to uninfected mothers living under similar conditions.

The release of merozoites where the circulation is slowed facilitates the invasion of nearby red blood cells, so that falciparum parasitemia may be heavier than that of other species in which the rupture of schizonts takes place in the active circulation. Whereas P. falciparum invades all erythrocytes irrespective of age, P. vivax attacks primarily reticulocytes, and P. malariae invades mature red cells, features which tend to limit parasitemia of the latter forms to less than 20,000 red cells/mm³. Falciparum infections in the nonimmune child may develop densities as high as 500,000 parasites/mm³; the prognosis is correspondingly grave.

Successful treatment stops the growth of parasites. Specific antibodies are associated with increased levels of immunoglobulin G in the serum of people repeatedly infected with a particular species. Antibody facilitates the phagocytosis of naked merozoites and of parasite-containing erythrocytes, which are ingested by reticuloendothelial cells, by large lymphocytes and neutrophils, and particularly by monocytes. These antibodies do not, however, interfere with development of the parasite in the liver. Passive immunity, effective in limiting the severity of attacks of malaria for several wk after birth, occurs in infants born to mothers who have the disease. The beneficial effect of this transplacental humoral immunity may be enhanced by persistence of fetal hemoglobin and by a diet limited to milk (low in PABA, hence inimical to growth of parasites). Certain hemoglobinopathies are also protective and tend to be genetically selective in endemic malarious regions. Plasmodium falciparum may fail to mature in children with the sickle cell trait and P. vivax, in those with thalassemia and enzyme deficiencies; P. falciparum is unable to attain high densities in children deficient in glucose-6-phosphate dehydrogenase.

Clinical Manifestations. Children who acquire malaria fall into 2 groups: those without previous contact with the disease have little or no immunity and become severely ill unless treated; those with repeated malarial infections since birth may survive early childhood to acquire a high degree of tolerance by about 10 yr of age, though growth and development may be impaired. In the partially immune child heavy parasitemia may occur with a few symptoms, or an intercurrent infection may initiate renewed activity of a quiescent malarial infection. Tolerance to malaria is most apparent among Africans and persons of African descent; it appears to be based on inherited factors that modify the severity of the disease.

In a nonimmune child clinical signs usually appear 8–15 days after infection and may not be distinctive. Behavioral changes such as fretfulness, anorexia, unusual crying, drowsiness, or disturbances of sleep may be observed. Fever may be absent or increase gradually for 1–2 days, or the onset may be sudden with temperature up to 40.6° C (105° F) or higher, with or without prodromal chill. After varying periods of time, the temperature falls to normal or below, and sweating occurs.

The febrile paroxysm may be extremely short or may last for 2–12 hr; its characteristic pattern is usually obscured in children less than 5 yr of age. Complaints may be made of headache, nausea, generalized aching, particularly of the back, and occasionally of pain in the abdomen, when the spleen has swollen quickly and is tender. In vivax and quartan infections dominated by a single brood the fever is the characteristic manifestation, occurring at intervals of 48 hr in the former and 72 in the latter. If convulsions occur, they abate when the fever falls. Herpetic lesions of the mouth are not uncommon. The red blood cell count and hemoglobin level may decrease rapidly; leukopenia is variable, but monocytosis is common.

In falciparum infections the fever is less characteristic and may even be continuous; it may be overshadowed by severe manifestations related to the cerebral, pulmonary, intestinal, or urinary systems. Cerebral complications are evidenced by convulsions or coma, with few localizing neurologic signs and (unless bacterial or viral infections of the central nervous system are superimposed) a normal cerebrospinal fluid. In cases of algid malaria, coma is preceded in the child by shock. Persistent nausea and vomiting, an enlarged and tender liver, and progressive jaundice may evolve into hepatic failure; severe diarrhea may occur; or occasionally the signs of acute appendicitis may be imitated.

The spleen is more commonly enlarged in vivax than in falciparum infections; perisplenitis, infarction, and even rupture may occur, and after repeated attacks the spleen may become very large and hard. "Idiopathic splenomegaly" (so-called big-spleen disease of Africa) may constitute an abnormal immune response to *P. malariae* in malnourished children in developing countries. Enlargement of the spleen is accompanied by lymphocytic infiltration of liver sinusoids and an elevated fluorescent antibody titer for malaria, with or without scanty parasitemia.

Disturbances of renal function are shown by oliguria, and anuria may supervene. The *nephrotic syndrome* is associated with *P. malariae* in children inhabiting endemic malarious areas; the prognosis is poor. *Blackwater fever*, now rarely seen, is associated with *P. falciparum*. Hemoglobinuria results from severe and sudden intravascular hemolysis, which may lead to anuria and to death from uremia.

Diagnosis. The diagnosis of malaria depends upon identification of parasites in the blood. In falciparum malaria, only ring forms are likely to be seen initially, crescents (gametocytes) joining them after 10 days; up to 20% of the erythrocytes may be infected. All stages of the other species of parasites appear in the blood, but less than 1% of red cells will contain them.

In the properly stained blood smear the parasites within the red cells have red chromatin and bluish cytoplasm. In some leukocytes, particularly monocytes, remnants of phagocytized parasites and pigment may be seen. The parasites should first be looked for in thick blood films, since in light infections it may not be possible to find plasmodia in the thin film; the latter is best used for species differentiation. As parasites may not be seen at the height of the fever, examinations should be repeated preferably at intervals of 12 hr. Of the various stains available, the most suitable is Giemsa diluted 1:25 with distilled water preferably buffered to pH 7.0–7.2. Wright stain may be used, 0.75 gm of the powder being repeatedly shaken for 2 days with 65 ml of pure methyl alcohol and 35 ml of pure glycerin.

A falsely positive Wassermann reaction will be found in many cases. The presence of species-specific antibodies associated with an elevated level of IgG, persisting for months or years after an acute attack, may be detected serologically, particularly by the indirect fluorescent antibody (IFA) test.

Prevention. Natural infection of humans does not occur where breeding of anopheline mosquitoes is prevented, where the adult mosquitoes are kept from contact with people by screens or bed nets, or where they are killed by natural enemies or insecticides before sporozoites have had time to mature. Children visiting endemic malarious areas should be screened from mosquitoes from dusk to dawn, but as this is rarely entirely effective, they should also be given 1 of the chemoprophylactic drugs *regularly* throughout their stay and for 6 wk thereafter. At least during this period, malaria should be suspected if febrile illness or chronic debility affects the child.

Chemoprophylactic drugs in common use are the following: the slightly bitter but extremely safe chlorguanide (proguanil), taken daily in amounts of 25 mg (to 2 yr), 50 mg (2–6 yr), or 100 mg (older than 6); the tasteless

but more toxic pyrimethamine (supplies of which should be particularly well guarded from inquisitive children), taken weekly in amounts of 6.25 mg (to 2 yr), 12.5 mg (2–6 yr), or 25 mg; and chloroquine or amodiaquine taken weekly in amounts of 37.5 mg of the base (to 1 yr), 75 mg (1–2 yr), 112.5 mg (2–6 yr), 150 mg (6–12 yr) or 300 mg. The bitterness of chloroquine diphosphate and sulfate may be disguised if the crushed tablet is mixed with a spoonful of jam or thick syrup, and syrups are available commercially; a tasteless product is the base preparation of amodiaquine (Basoquin).

Chlorguanide and pyrimethamine not only suppress the development of parasites in the red blood cells, as do chloroquine and amodiaquine, but also interfere with the pre-erythrocytic stage in the liver. Unfortunately cross-resistance of *P. falciparum* to the 1st 2 drugs is widely distributed, for which reason chloroquine and amodiaquine are generally preferred in prophylaxis. When resistance to the latter compounds also occurs, as in northern South America and southeast Asia, potentiating combinations of chlorguanide with dapsone (daily) or pyrimethamine with long-acting sulfonamides (weekly) may be ingested, but their use for periods longer than 6 mo is discouraged until more information becomes available concerning possible chronic toxicity.

Treatment. Therapy falls into 4 categories: (1) specific chemotherapy for the attack, whether fresh infection, recrudescence, or relapse; (2) supportive treatment and management of complications; (3) specific chemotherapy to prevent late relapse of vivax or ovale infections; (4) specific chemotherapy to destroy or sterilize gametocytes, and thus to protect the community if mosquitoes are present.

1. Any of the drugs listed in Table 10–55 will effect a clinical cure of all types of malaria and provide a radical cure of falciparum and quartan malaria, unless drug-resistant parasites are present. Children who have inhabited malarious regions and through previous infections have acquired some immunity may be cured by one half of the quantities listed. Treatment must be repeated if vomiting occurs within 30 min of ingestion of drugs; persistent vomiting is an indication for parenteral therapy.

Although specific treatment should not usually be undertaken until the diagnosis has been established, many experienced physicians, when confronted with a critically ill or comatose child whose history is suggestive of malaria or exposure thereto, would consider it advisable to administer quinine or chloroquine parenterally while awaiting the result of blood film examination.

Parenteral administration of chloroquine or quinine, although hazardous in children bordering on shock, is often essential for those who are vomiting persistently, who are in coma, or who cannot be induced to swallow the drugs even if the bitterness is concealed. Parenteral therapy with antimalarial drugs should be replaced by oral administration as soon as possible. Chloroquine may be given intravenously by slow drip in the quantity of 5 mg base/kg in 10 ml/kg of isotonic saline, infused over a 3–4 hr period, and should be repeated once, 6

Table 10–55 TREATMENT OF UNCOMPLICATED MALARIA ATTACK

DRUG (USP)	SCHEDULE	DOSAGE IN MG BASE (CHLOROQUINE AND AMODIAQUINE)* OR MG SALT (QUININE)				
		Age Under 1 Yr	Age 1–3 Yr	Age 3–6 Yr	Age 6–12 Yr	Older Children
Chloroquine or Amodiaquine	Day 1 — 1st dose	75	100	200	300	450
	6 hr later	75	75	150	150	300
	6 hr later	37.5	75	75	150	150
	Day 2 — 1st dose	37.5	75	75	100	150
	6 hr later	—	75	75	150	150
	Day 3 — 1st dose	37.5	75	75	—	150
	6 hr later	—	—	—	150	150
						150
Quinine	Daily†	167–250	250–333	333–583	583–1000	1000–2000

*Commercial tablets usually contain 250 mg of chloroquine diphosphate or sulfate, of which 150 mg is base; the quantity of base is stated on the label of the container, and should be prescribed as such. A formulation of amodiaquine more acceptable to children because of its reduced bitterness is marketed as "Basoquin."

†Given for 10 days in divided doses every 4 or 8 hr, as tolerated. Dosages indicated are multiples of the standard tablet containing 333 mg of quinine sulfate.

hr later, if treatment still cannot be given by mouth. The volume of saline should be adjusted to the state of hydration of the patient, dehydrated children requiring 20 ml/kg, and overhydrated children 5 ml/kg. Administration of chloroquine intramuscularly is not recommended in small children, as it has occasionally precipitated convulsions and aggravated shock and resulted in death. It should not be given subcutaneously because of slow absorption by that route. Quinine dihydrochloride is administered intravenously in a dose of 10 mg/kg and may be repeated 12 hr later; it should be given well diluted (1 mg/ml) and slowly (during 1 hr).

2. Supportive treatment includes that for hyperpyrexia. Particular attention should be paid to fluid and electrolyte needs (Sec 5.32).

Metabolic requirements of the parasite rapidly deplete the reserves of glucose, vitamins, and coenzymes as well as of hemoglobin. Vitamin B_1 may be given, and when the acute phase is passed, ferrous sulfate should be prescribed for a considerable time. Transfusion of packed red cells may be beneficial to children who have had longstanding infections and consequently severe anemia (hemoglobin 5 gm/dl or less).

It is essential that children with severe falciparum infections receive fluids intravenously if dehydrated or in shock. Rapid expansion of the circulating blood volume with whole blood is more satisfactory than with dextran, plasma, or glucose-saline solution. Renal failure, which may require dialysis, is a rare development. When it is present, no more than one third of the conventional doses of antimalarial drugs should be given until the child is hydrated, out of shock, and urinating; quinine and primaquine are contraindicated in the presence of hemoglobinuria. The judicious use of chloroquine or amodiaquine is indicated for heavy parasitemia.

In the comatose stage of cerebral malaria, in addition to specific parenteral antimalarial treatment, dextran-75 may be useful for the prevention of intravascular sludging. Convulsions may be controlled with paraldehyde or barbiturates.

The nephrotic syndrome associated with quartan malaria is managed by the regimen described in Sec 16.10, together with a course of chloroquine.

3. Late relapse of vivax or ovale malaria rarely occurs more than 5 yr after the primary attack and may be prevented by treatment of the child with primaquine. Because primaquine given at the height of symptoms increases the tendency to vomit and may be immunosuppressive, it should not be given until the 3rd day of the concomitant clinical curative course of chloroquine, amodiaquine, or quinine. Primaquine is given for 14 days in a daily dose of 0.3 mg base/kg; for fear of possible side reactions some authorities prefer not to administer this drug to children aged less than 3 yr (or to pregnant women), but treat the acute attack with chloroquine and then place the patients on a chemoprophylactic regimen for several mo.

Children receiving primaquine should be watched for toxic manifestations such as methemoglobinemia, hemolytic anemia, hemoglobinuria in children with G-6-PD deficiency, neutropenia, and renal dysfunction. Hemolytic anemia may be particularly severe in G-6-PD deficient children of eastern Mediterranean or Asian descent, for whom 2 approaches are available in respect of anti-relapse treatment: primaquine may be given once each wk for 8 wk in a dose of 0.9 mg base/kg, or the drug may be omitted entirely and chemoprophylaxis given for several mo following treatment of the acute attack with chloroquine. Quinacrine (mepacrine) should not be used simultaneously with primaquine, but since the former is obsolete as an antimalarial drug, the problem need not arise. Other synthetic antimalarial drugs are relatively nontoxic in therapeutic doses.

4. Gametocytes do not give rise to symptoms and disappear from the circulation soon after destruction of their asexual precursors by chloroquine, amodiaquine, or quinine. Gametocytes may be destroyed by a single dose of primaquine, 7.5 mg base for children aged 1–3 yr, 15 mg for those aged 4–6 yr, 30 mg for those aged 6 to 12 yr, and 45 mg for older children, or their further development in the mosquito inhibited by single doses of chlorguanide or pyrimethamine, provided the parasite is not resistant to these drugs.

Drug resistance is of growing concern. Many strains of *P. falciparum* are now resistant to chlorguanide and pyrimethamine, but a greater problem is posed by the spread in northern South America and in Southeast Asia of resistance by this species to chloroquine and amodiaquine; some strains are also tolerant to quinine. These strains are being introduced into North America, Europe, and Australia, where focal outbreaks may occur in the summer mo, and children may become infected. Should the malarial attack not respond to chloroquine or amodiaquine, quinine should be used immediately. If this has only a temporary effect, the course should be repeated with the addition of sulfadiazine, 35 mg/kg every 6 hr for 5 days, and pyrimethamine, each day for 3 days, 6.25 mg (to 2 yr of age), 12.5 mg (2–6 yr), or 25 mg. An effective alternative is the full course of quinine, together with tetracycline hydrochloride, 10 mg/kg every 6 hr for 7 days. Where they are obtainable, preparations containing sulfadoxine or sulfalene and pyrimethamine are generally effective as a single dose, the long-acting sulfonamide in the amount of 25 mg/kg and pyrimethamine 1.25 mg/kg. Rapidity of action is enhanced if quinine is also administered. A parenteral preparation is available, each ml containing 200 mg of sulfadoxine and 10 mg of pyrimethamine; children under 5 yr may be given 1 ml, those from 5–8 yr 2 ml, and older children 3 ml.

DAVID F. CLYDE

Center for Disease Control (USPHS), Atlanta Ga.: Chemoprophylaxis of malaria. Morbidity and Mortality Weekly Report 27:81, 1978.

Gilles HM: Malaria in children. Br Med J 2:1375, 1966.

Jelliffe DB (ed): Child Health in the Tropics. Ed 4. London, E Arnold, 1974.

MacGregor JD, Avery JG: Malaria transmission and fetal growth. Br Med J 2:433, 1974.

Young MD: Malaria. *In:* Hunter GW III, Swartzwelder JC, Clyde D (eds): Tropical Medicine. Ed 5. Philadelphia, WB Saunders, 1976.

10.111 AMERICAN TRYPANOSOMIASIS
(Chagas Disease)

This insect-transmitted infection is 1 of the major health problems of South America, largely because the primary infection, which occurs in children and young adults, usually passes unnoticed and is essentially untreatable. A conservative estimate of the prevalence of infection in South America in 1960 indicated that about 7 million people were infected and no fewer than 35 million exposed.

Trypanosoma cruzi infection in humans occurs in every country in South America and is particularly prevalent in Brazil, Argentina, Uruguay, Chile, and Venezuela. Human infections have also been found in Central America and in the Caribbean. Two cases have been reported in the United States, in Texans who had never left that state. No authenticated cases have been reported outside the Western Hemisphere. The intermediate host (reduviid) is a blood-sucking arthropod widespread in the endemic areas. In the United States reduviid bugs have been found in all southwestern states and most southeastern states as far north as Maryland. In these areas rates of infection of the insects with trypanosomes are high and comparable to those found in the endemic areas of South America.

Etiology. Human and animal reservoirs are infected while the insect vector takes a blood meal, during which the insect may take up to 0.35 ml of blood. The reduviid usually defecates after commencing to feed. The infective forms pass with the insect feces and penetrate the skin of the mammalian host. The length of the life cycle of *T. cruzi* varies because of marked differences among the various species of triatomine insects. In some species the cycle takes approximately 5 mo within the insect.

Trypanosoma cruzi is a protozoan parasite of the suborder Trypanosomatina, and is characterized by a variety of morphologic forms distinguished primarily by the site of origin of the single flagellum. Within the suborder the organisms are divided into groups of species based on several characteristics such as morphology, number of forms occurring in the life cycle, and the host-parasite relationship.

In humans *Trypanosoma cruzi* exists in several morphologic forms in the peripheral blood and in tissues. In the bloodstream trypanosomes may be slender or broad and are called trypomastigotes. They are 16–20 μ long with a large oval posterior kinetoblast and a single flagellum, which lies in the outer border of the undulating membrane and extends anteriorly beyond the body of the trypanosome. Division by binary fission takes place only intracellularly when the organisms invade the reticuloendothelial system and the striated and cardiac muscles. There they transform into amastigotes, rounded organisms 1.4–4.0 μ in diameter without a free flagellum. The multiplication of *T. cruzi* amastigotes within the host cells results in the formation of nestlike cysts which eventually destroy these cells.

The insect family Reduviidae contains the subfamily Triatominae, hematophagous insects responsible for the transmission of trypanosomiasis to animals or people. Triatomine bugs are variously known as wild bedbugs, cone-nose bugs, Mexican bedbugs, or assassin or kissing (based on a predilection to attack the face) bugs. After such an insect ingests infected blood, the organisms pass to its midgut, where the trypomastigote forms change to amastigotes and multiply; within 1–2 wk infective metacyclic forms appear in the rectum of the insect.

Epidemiology. *T. cruzi* infection originally occurred among wild mammals of the American continent and extended to humans only when the reduviid insect vectors adapted to human dwellings. The infection occurs principally in rural and low socioeconomic areas. The degree of adaptation of triatomine bugs to human habitation varies. Some species live in close contact with wild animals and seldom have contact with people; others are common visitors to human habitations; a few have adapted well to human dwellings, influenced by a variety of entomologic, anthropocentric, and environmental factors. Housing of adobe, mud, or cane with numerous cracks in the walls provides excellent shelter for reduviid bugs. Woodpiles near houses and the custom of keeping domestic animals near or within households shelter some species and provide easy access to human living quarters.

The efficacy of the insect as a vector depends on its ability to produce infective forms in feces, its aggressiveness, and the time between a blood meal and defecation. Not all North American triatomine species defecate during or immediately after feeding, and several South American species are potentially more efficient vectors because a higher percentage defecates within 2 min after feeding.

Dogs and cats are important domestic reservoirs of *T. cruzi*. One survey in Brazil showed that 28% of dogs and 20% of cats are infected. In Panama and Costa Rica *Rattus rattus* is the main domestic reservoir. Because of their habitat and its proximity to people, some of these animal reservoirs may play an important role in linking the wild and domestic cycles of the parasite.

In the United States the most important wild reservoirs are opossums and raccoons, with infection rates of 17% and 2%, respectively. The prevalence of infection in reduviids has been estimated at 20–25% in the Southwest. Serologic evidence of human infection has been found in southern Texas; 1.8% of 500 unselected individuals and 2.5% of 117 persons who had been bitten by the insects had significant titers of antibodies. The rarity of human infection in the United States may be due to low virulence of the organisms and inefficiency of the insect vector but more probably results from the better housing conditions of the human hosts.

Other mechanisms of transmission of *T. cruzi* to the human host are recognized, e.g., blood transfusion and damaged placenta. Accidental inoculation of laboratory workers has also occurred.

Pathogenesis and Pathology. Human infection is usually initiated by introduction of metacyclic trypanosomes through abraded or intact skin, mucous membranes, or conjunctiva. Trypomastigote forms can first be detected in the peripheral blood in 2–4 wk. On entering the host tissues, the organisms assume amastigote forms and multiply to fill a whole cell, forming the so-called parasite nest or pseudocyst. The trypanosomes have an unexplained predilection for cardiac, smooth, and striated muscle. Most infected individuals remain asymptomatic although serologically positive; few develop late complications of Chagas disease. During the phase of parasite multiplication and active inflammatory response in the heart and smooth muscles of the digestive tract of the host, muscle fibers and peripheral ganglia of the autonomic nervous system are damaged. Accumulation of macrophages and lymphocytes is commonly seen. Both humoral and cellular immune responses develop within a few wk of infection with *T. cruzi*. The extent to which the immune response of the host limits multiplication of the parasite or precipitates tissue injury is an area of active investigation.

The histopathology of acute cardiomyopathy due to *T. cruzi* is characterized by mononuclear cellular infiltration of the interstitial space and degeneration of the muscle fibers associated with the development of amastigote cysts. As the disease progresses to the chronic stage, marked deposition of fibrous tissue and myocardial degeneration predominate. Chronic inflammatory changes, associated with damage to the Auerbach plexus, may also be found in the smooth muscle layer of the intestinal wall. A reduction of the number of ganglia has been demonstrated in the hypertrophic dilated organs of patients with Chagas disease and may account for the organomegalic syndromes seen in chronic trypanosomiasis.

Clinical Manifestations. Initially the infection is largely asymptomatic. Only about 1% of those infected have clinical symptoms acute enough to attract attention. This acute stage is followed by a long silent period; the disease then progresses to the chronic stage, presenting mainly with cardiac or intestinal manifestations. There are differences in the clinical picture of Chagas disease as it occurs in different geographic localities; the etiology of these differences is unknown. In most endemic areas, however, the infection remains asymptomatic for decades, after which approximately 10% of all serologically positive persons manifest chronic sequelae of the disease.

Acute American Trypanosomiasis. This rare syndrome is seen only in children in endemic areas. Its clinical manifestations coincide with local multiplication of the parasites at the site of entry and their subsequent hematogenous dissemination approximately 10 days after infection. Initially, local inflammation with heat, swelling, and redness of the area of invasion predominates. While 25% of individuals with symptomatic acute trypanosomiasis will have no local reactions, half will present with unilateral swelling of the eye region (Romaña sign), and one fourth will develop a nodular skin lesion or a local tumor of the skin (chagoma). Enlargement of the local lymph nodes often accompanies these symptoms. The next stage coincides with hematogenous dissemination of the organism. Malaise, fever, muscular pain, and nontender enlargement of lymph nodes occur. A cutaneous morbilliform eruption, hepatosplenomegaly, and, less often, acute meningoencephalitis may be seen. About 40% of these patients show electrocardiographic abnormalities such as tachycardia and arrhythmias. Mortality from acute trypanosomiasis is difficult to assess but may be approximately 10% and is related to heart failure or meningoencephalitis.

Chronic American Trypanosomiasis. Approximately 10–20% of acute cases in the endemic areas go on to develop the chronic manifestations of Chagas disease. In endemic areas the cardiomyopathy of trypanosomiasis is the leading cause of both cardiac disease and sudden death. In a large study 82% of patients with chronic chagasic cardiomyopathy were 11–50 yr of age. Males are more frequently affected than females. Patients commonly present with symptoms and signs of congestive heart failure. The clinical course is one of gradually advancing myocarditis and cardiac failure with tachycardia, ventricular premature beats, enlargement of the heart, and various conduction defects. The most frequent electrocardiographic findings are partial or complete AV block and complete right bundle branch block. Signs of valvular damage and dysfunction are exceedingly rare.

The incidence of organomegaly differs in the various endemic areas; it is particularly common in Brazil. Any hollow muscular viscus may be involved but most commonly the esophagus and colon. In 80% of 820 cases dysphagia was the 1st symptom of megaesophagus. As dysphagia increases, nutritional impairment may be seen. Dilatation and enlargement of other hollow organs, such as the colon, ureters, or bronchi have been reported but are less frequent than dilatation of the esophagus.

Diagnosis. Chagas disease should be suspected in individuals who have lived in endemic areas and show suggestive symptoms and signs. A history of insect bites and their sequelae and the probable duration of infection are suggestive. The latter is of particular value with respect to the diagnostic techniques employed and the prognosis. *T. cruzi* can be demonstrated in the peripheral blood of infected individuals, particularly during the acute stages of the infection. A drop of blood pressed by a cover slip and microscopically examined under high power will reveal the motile trypanosomes. Giemsa-stained blood smears should be examined for the characteristic C-shaped organisms. Failure to demonstrate the trypanosomes in direct blood smears necessitates the use of a concentration method (add 10 ml of blood to 30 ml of a 0.87% solution of ammonium chloride, centrifuge, and examine the pellet for the trypanosomes). Continued failure to demonstrate the parasites suggests the need for a blood culture on diphasic blood agar medium or an injection of 1 ml of blood into 2 albino mice with examination of their blood for the parasites weekly for 1 mo. Xenodiagnosis, or feeding the patient's blood to laboratory-reared reduviid bugs and examining their rectal contents 30–60 days later, has been shown to be the most satisfactory diagnostic method, but the unavailability of suitable bugs in many areas precludes its wide diagnostic use.

Several serologic tests have been developed, e.g., precipitin, complement fixation, and more recently, a promising microenzyme-linked immunosorbent assay. These tests are of primary importance in cases of chronic Chagas disease in which parasitologic techniques usually fail to demonstrate the organisms. About 80% of patients with chagasic heart disease and 90% of those with megaesophagus have positive complement-fixation tests.

Treatment. Parasitologic cure of American trypanosomiasis is difficult to achieve as most patients present the chronic sequelae of the infection at a time when parasites cannot be easily demonstrated in their blood. There is no established and reliable therapeutic agent against *T. cruzi*. Lampit is a promising compound effective in eradication of parasitemia in acute and possibly chronic American trypanosomiasis, but it is associated with severe side effects and must be given for periods of up to 120 days. Symptomatic treatment is needed in patients with chronic Chagas disease; medical or surgical intervention may be necessary.

Control. This is based on education of people in endemic areas about the relation between bites from triatomine bugs and Chagas disease. Residual insecticides such as gammexane, dieldrin, or lindane are highly effective in controlling the bug population when sprayed inside buildings, but these insecticides do not destroy the bug ova and should therefore be sprayed repeatedly at 2–4 wk intervals. Razing of adobe houses which harbor the insects and replacement with adequately screened, more modern structures are indicated when feasible. Travelers should avoid sleeping in unscreened adobe houses in endemic areas. If this is unavoidable, bed nets should be used.

Andrade ZA, Andrade SG, Olviera GB, et al: Histopathology of the conducting tissue of the host in Chagas myocarditis. Am Heart J 95:316, 1978.
Fife EH Jr: *Trypanosoma* (schizotrypanum) *cruzi. In:* Krier JP (ed): Parasitic Protozoa, Vol I. New York, Academic Press, 1977, p 135.
Hoff R, Mott KE, Silva JF, et al: Prevalence of parasitema and seroreactivity to *Trypanosoma cruzi* in a rural population in Northeast Brazil. Am J Trop Med Hyg 28:461, 1979.
Spencer HC, Akain DS, Sulzer AJ, et al: Evaluation of the microenzyme-linked immunosorbent assay for antibodies to *Trypanosoma cruzi.* Am J Trop Med Hyg 29:179, 1980.
Texeira ARL: Chagas disease: Trends in immunological research and prospects for immunoprophylaxis. Bull WHO 57:697, 1979.

10.112 AFRICAN TRYPANOSOMIASIS
(Sleeping Sickness)

The trypanosomiases of tropical Africa are a group of diseases of great social and economic importance. Human infection with subspecies of the hemoflagellate *Trypanosoma brucei* has been responsible for significant mortality and much morbidity, while *nagana*, or trypanosomiasis in livestock, has restricted the ability of many African nations to produce enough animal protein for the well-being of their populations. Infection is transmitted to humans or domestic animals via species of tsetse flies of the genus *Glossina*.

Human infections are caused by 2 subspecies of *Trypanosoma brucei*, *T. b. rhodesiense* and *T. b. gambiense*. These subspecies are morphologically indistinguishable, but they differ markedly in their epidemiology and the disease syndromes they cause. Infection with *T. rhodesiense* usually results in acute syndromes that run a rapid and, if untreated, fatal course, whereas *T. b. gambiense* infections usually run a more chronic course, resulting in the typical syndrome of sleeping sickness.

Information on the distribution, prevalence, and mortality rate of African trypanosomiasis is unreliable. Political changes and the decline of surveillance and control measures have resulted in an ever-present threat of epidemics. Human trypanosomiasis in Africa occurs primarily in the region between latitudes 15° N and 15° S. This corresponds roughly to the area where the annual rainfall (500 mm or more) creates optimal climatic conditions for *Glossina* flies. The 2 subspecies of *Trypanosoma brucei* which infect man each have their own characteristic geographic distribution: *T. b. rhodesiense* infection is restricted to the eastern third of the endemic area in tropical Africa, stretching from Ethiopia to the northern boundaries of South Africa; *T. b. gambiense* occurs mainly in the western half of the continent's endemic region. The disease has been found in almost all West African countries, extending occasionally eastward into southern Sudan, Uganda, and Kenya.

Etiology. Human infection is initiated by insect bite or by organisms penetrating intact mucous membranes or skin. The infective metacyclic forms of the trypanosomes are 15 μ long and possess no free flagella. A minimum inoculum of 300–450 organisms is needed to establish infection with *T. b. rhodesiense* in humans. One–3 wk after a period of local multiplication in the skin, long and slender trypomastigote forms (12–42 μ) can be seen in the peripheral blood; intermediate and stumpy forms also occur. These are flagellated forms with a well developed undulating membrane. The proportion of trypomastigotes belonging to any specific form varies during the course of infection, but, as a rule, the thin slender forms predominate. They are the only blood forms that show an appreciable rate of binary division.

In the early stages of human infection, the organisms multiply rapidly in the blood and lymph nodes. They appear in waves in the peripheral blood, each wave being followed by a crisis when the organisms disappear. This phenomenon results from destruction of the trypomastigotes by host defense mechanisms. The reappearance of another population of organisms in the blood heralds the formation of a new antigenic variant, in response to which the host in turn forms a new "clone" of specific antibodies. *T. brucei* are capable of producing hundreds of antigenic variants. As the infection becomes chronic, fewer trypomastigotes are seen in the peripheral blood, but they can usually be recovered from lymph nodes. Invasion of the central nervous system occurs early in *T. b. rhodesiense* infections but late in the gambian form, in which organisms can be recovered from the cerebrospinal fluid.

The insect intermediate vectors are species of the tsetse flies of the genus *Glossina*. In the laboratory the rhodesian and gambian organisms are capable of infecting and developing inside a wide range of *Glossina*, but under natural conditions they are associated with only certain species. The specificity of human trypanosomes for particular *Glossina* species is determined by the epidemiologic pattern of each infection. Both sexes of *Glossina* feed on human blood, but in nature only a small proportion of the insect population is infected. Inside the flies the organisms localize in the posterior part of the midgut, where they transform in 3–4 days into a new trypomastigote form with a less pronounced undulating membrane. These flagellates multiply enormously in the lumen of the insect's intestinal tract for about 10 days, then gradually migrate anteriorly where they attach to the walls of the salivary ducts and complete the final stages of development into the infective metacyclic forms. These are similar to the short, stumpy forms in the blood, but typically they lack the free flagellum. The life cycle within the tsetse fly takes 15–35 days; each fly infected with rhodesian trypanosomes has been estimated to produce 40,000 infective organisms.

Direct transmission of African trypanosomiasis to humans has also been reported. It is accomplished either mechanically through contact with the contaminated mouth parts of tsetse flies during feeding or congenitally to infants via the placenta of infected mothers.

Epidemiology.   The interaction between the parasite and its arthropod and mammalian hosts, together with the geophysical nature of the endemic areas, determines the overall epidemiologic pattern for each of the 2 major African human trypanosomiases.

In formulating this epidemiologic pattern, the insect intermediate vector plays a major role. Several *Glossina* species transmit the infection in different parts of tropical Africa. *Glossina* captured in endemic foci show a low rate of infection, usually under 5%. This relative inefficiency of the insect vector determines some of the epidemiologic features of trypanosomiasis. In the rhodesian form, which usually runs an acute and often fatal course, chances of transmission to tsetse flies are drastically reduced. However, the ability of *T. b. rhodesiense* to multiply enormously in the bloodstream of humans and to infect other species of mammals helps maintain its life cycle. *T. b. rhodesiense* infections found in wild mammals (bushbuck and hartebeest) are mainly transmitted by the so-called game tsetse flies.

T. b. gambiense infections usually run a chronic protracted course with very low levels of parasitemia. Because of low rates of infection in tsetse flies and the absence of animal reservoirs, the gambian life cycle necessitates close and repeated contact between humans and insects to permit frequent biting. Important foci for transmission are therefore found where people habitually enter rivers to wash or to collect water.

Pathogenesis and Pathology.   The initial site of entry of the organisms soon develops into a hard, painful, red nodule, a "trypanosomal chancre." Histologically, it contains long, thin trypanosomes multiplying beneath the dermis and is surrounded by a lymphocytic cellular infiltrate. Dissemination of the organisms into the blood and lymphatic systems follows, with subsequent localization in the central nervous system. The histopathologic lesions in the brain are those of meningoencephalitis, with increased cellularity of the pia-arachnoid due to lymphocyte infiltration and perivascular cuffing of the blood vessels by the same cell type. In chronic cases the appearance of morular cells (large, strawberry-like cells, supposedly derived from plasma cells) is the most characteristic finding.

The pathogenesis of the disease remains unclear. Damage to host tissues may result from metabolic activities of the organisms or from the sequelae of immune complex formation. The release of pharmacologically active kinins and changes in the blood clotting system may explain in part the vascular changes, but the role of host immune responses is yet to be defined. Chronic trypanosomiasis is associated with impairment of the host immune response to other antigens. The concomitant state of immunosuppression, therefore, may explain the increased susceptibility of infected individuals to other viral, bacterial, and parasitic infections.

Clinical Manifestations.   The clinical presentations of the African trypanosomiases vary not only because of the 2 subspecies of organisms but also because of differences in host response in the indigenous population of endemic areas and in newcomers or visitors. Visitors usually suffer more from the acute symptoms and signs, but in untreated cases death is inevitable for natives and visitors alike. The clinical syndromes of African trypanosomiasis are best described as acute and chronic stages. Disease due to *T. b. rhodesiense* usually runs a more acute course, that due to *T. b. gambiense* a more protracted one. However, mild, chronic or asymptomatic rhodesian infection and acute, virulent gambian disease also occur.

Acute African Trypanosomiasis. The *site of the tsetse fly bite* may be the 1st presenting feature. A nodule or chancre develops in 2–3 days; within 1 wk it becomes a painful, hard, red nodule surrounded by an area of erythema and swelling. These nodules are commonly seen on the lower limbs but sometimes also on the head. The trypanosomal nodule usually passes unnoticed in the local population of endemic areas. These lesions subside spontaneously in about 2 wk leaving no permanent scar. The *most common presenting features* of acute African trypanosomiasis occur at the time of invasion of the bloodstream by the parasites, approximately 2–3 wk after the infection. Irregular episodes of fever, each lasting from 1–7 days, are the usual early feature. Attacks may be separated by free intervals of days or even weeks. Headache, sweating, and generalized lymphadenopathy are frequently encountered along with the fever. Enlargement of lymph nodes is 1 of the most constant signs, particularly in the gambian form. It most commonly affects the posterior cervical and supraclavicular groups. The lymphadenopathy is painless; the glands are moderately enlarged and are not matted together. The 3rd most common feature of trypanosomiasis in Caucasians is the presence of *blotchy, irregular, nonitching, erythematous macules* which may appear any time following the first febrile episode, usually within 6–8 wk. The majority of macules have a central normal skin area, giving the rash a circinate outline. This trypanosomal skin rash is seen mainly on the trunk and is evanescent, fading in 1 place only to appear at another site. Examination of the blood during this stage may show anemia, leukopenia with relative monocytosis, and elevated levels of IgM.

Neurologic symptoms and signs of acute African trypanosomiasis are generally nonspecific. They may precede invasion of the central nervous system by the organisms and present as irrational and inexplicable anxieties with frequent changes in mood. In untreated *T. b. rhodesiense* infections, invasion of the central nervous system occurs within 3–6 wk. It is associated with recurrent bouts of fever, weakness, and signs of acute toxemia. Tachycardia from myocarditis and neurologic symptoms such as irritability, insomnia, and personality or mood changes develop. Death occurs in 6–9 mo from secondary infection or cardiac failure.

Chronic African Trypanosomiasis. There is no precise time when cerebral symptoms begin in this disease. In the gambian form they can be expected to appear within 2 yr after the onset of acute symptoms, although a general increase in drowsiness during the day and insomnia at night reflect the continuous nature of the pathologic processes. Progress of the disease is characterized by increasing anemia, leukopenia, and wasting of body musculature. Patients with chronic gambian trypanosomiasis have an increased susceptibility to secondary infections.

Involvement of the central nervous system results in a chronic diffuse meningoencephalitis with no localizing symptoms, commonly known as *sleeping sickness*. Drowsiness and an uncontrollable urge to sleep are the major features of this stage of the disease and may become almost continuous in the terminal stages. Associated signs and symptoms also point to involvement of the basal ganglia. Tremor or rigidity with stiff and ataxic gait may occur. Psychotic changes occur in almost one third of untreated patients. Prior to the use of specific therapy both gambian trypanosomiasis and the rhodesian form were invariably fatal-conditions.

Diagnosis. Since the African trypanosomiases occur only in certain well defined areas of that continent, patients in other areas presenting with symptoms or signs of the disease should be questioned about their travel activities. Definitive diagnosis can be made during the early stages by examination of a fresh thick blood smear which will allow visualization of the motile active trypomastigote forms. Dried, Giemsa-stained smears should be examined for the detailed morphology of the organisms. If a thick blood smear is negative, a simple concentration method may be of help. Ten ml of heparinized blood is added to 30 ml of 0.87% ammonium chloride and the mixture centrifuged at 1000 g for 15 minutes. The sediment can then be examined fresh or by staining dried smears. Aspiration of an enlarged lymph node can also be used to obtain material for parasitologic examination. In every positive case a sample of CSF should also be examined for the organisms. In suspected cases when parasitologic diagnosis has failed, 2 rats should be inoculated intraperitoneally with 1 ml of blood; 2 wk later their blood should be examined for the parasites.

Treatment. The choice of chemotherapeutic agents for the treatment of clinical African trypanosomiasis depends on the stage of the infection and the causative organisms. The hematogenous forms of both rhodesian and gambian trypanosomiasis are susceptible to the action of suramin (Antrypol)* available as a 10% solution for intravenous administration. A test dose of 10 mg should first be administered intravenously to detect the rare idiosyncratic reactions of shock and collapse. The dose for subsequent injections is 20 mg/kg intravenously, repeated every 5–7 days for a total of 5 injections. Suramin is nephrotoxic; therefore urine should be examined before each injection. The presence of marked proteinuria, blood, or casts is a contraindication for the completion of therapy with suramin. In these rare circumstances therapy should be continued by initiation of a course of melarsoprol,* or, in early cases without central nervous system invasion, pentamidine* may be used. Pentamidine, like suramin, is effective only against the hematogenous forms of the trypanosomes; moreover, its activity may be less certain in the rhodesian form. It is administered intramuscularly as a 10% solution on alternate days for 5 doses. The dose for each injection is 3–4 mg/kg. Side effects of pentamidine are few; hypotension, faintness, and, occasionally, collapse may occur but can be reversed by administration of epinephrine.

If invasion of the central nervous system has oc-

---

*Available in the United States from the Parasitic Drug Service, Centers for Disease Control, Atlanta, Ga. 30333.

curred, melarsoprol should be used. Melarsoprol contains 18.8% arsenic and is formed from the original arsenical melarsen oxide by the incorporation of dimercaprol (BAL). The drug is effective against all stages of both gambian and rhodesian trypanosomiasis but because of its arsenic content is restricted to use in cases with central nervous system involvement. It is administered intravenously as a 3.6% solution beginning with 0.4 mg/kg. The drug is given in 3 courses, each consisting of an injection on each of 3 successive days with a 1 wk interval between courses. According to the tolerance of the patient, the dose should be increased gradually to reach a maximum of 3.6 mg/kg for the 3rd course. Slight reactions such as fever and pains in the chest or abdomen may occur immediately or very soon after an injection of melarsoprol, but they are generally rare. The most important and serious of its toxic effects is encephalopathy and, less commonly, exfoliative dermatitis.

Control. The control of trypanosomiasis in endemic areas of Africa depends on recognition and effective therapy of human infections and on control of the vector. In the early part of this century only 2 methods for control of tsetse flies had been used with success: the destruction of larger wild mammals on which the vector depends for feeding, and felling trees and brush to deprive tsetse flies of suitable habitats. Modern control emphasizes widespread spraying with residual insecticides. The control of African trypanosomiasis is complicated by the fact that it involves cattle and humans and by the logistics of applying the available preventive measures.

Pentamidine has been used successfully as a prophylactic drug. A single injection of 3–4 mg/kg will give protection against gambian trypanosomiasis for at least 6 mo. Its effect against the rhodesian form, however, is not certain. Chemoprophylaxis has been used as a method for the protection of individuals and for the control of trypanosomiasis in some countries in West Africa, but detailed evaluation is not available.

ADEL A. F. MAHMOUD

Baker JR: Epidemiology of African sleeping sickness. In: Trypanosomiasis and Leishmaniasis with Special Reference to Chagas' Disease. Ciba Foundation Symposium 20 (New Series). New York, Associated Scientific Publishers, 1974, p 29.
deRaadt P, Seed JR: Trypanosomes causing disease in man in Africa. In: Kreier JP (ed): Parasitic Protozoa. New York, Academic Press, 1977, p 175.
Greenwood BM, Whittle HC: The pathogenesis of sleeping sickness. Trans Roy Soc Trop Med Hyg 74:716, 1980.
Mulligan HW (ed): The African Trypanosomiases. New York, Wiley-Interscience Publishers, 1970.

10.113 TOXOPLASMOSIS

Infection with Toxoplasma gondii, an intracellular parasite, may result in the human disease toxoplasmosis. There are 2 forms of infection: congenital, transmitted in utero; and acquired, most often asymptomatic. Congenital toxoplasmosis is typically manifested by cho-rioretinitis, cerebral calcification, psychomotor retardation, hydrocephalus or microcephaly, and convulsions.

Etiology. T. gondii is a protozoon which is a coccidian of cats. Its trophozoites are oval or crescent-like and measure $2–4 \times 4–7$ μ; they are best stained with Giemsa or Wright stains. They multiply by endodyogeny, only in living cells. Tissue cysts containing hundreds of parasites, which appear to remain alive indefinitely, are produced early in infection. Toxoplasma can multiply in all tissues of mammals and birds except for non-nucleated erythrocytes. Its disease spectrum is expressed with remarkable similarity in different host species, perhaps because the parasite accommodates to an unparalleled variety of cells. Only 1 species is known, and all strains examined are serologically similar.

Only newly infected cats (and other Felidae) excrete Toxoplasma oocysts in their feces. The oocysts are infectious for all animals studied, including the chimpanzee (experimental) and humans (accidental). Toxoplasma are acquired by susceptible cats, presumably by eating infected meat. They multiply through schizogonic and gametogonic cycles in the distal ileal epithelium. Oocysts contain 2 sporocysts and are excreted. Under proper conditions of temperature and moisture, each sporocyst matures into 4 sporozoites. For about 2 wk the cat excretes oocysts, which, in a suitable environment, may retain their viability for 1 yr or more. Given proper temperature and humidity, oocysts sporulate in 1–5 days and become infectious. Ordinarily very resistant, oocysts are killed by drying, boiling, and exposure to some strong chemicals. Several isolations have been reported from soil and sand frequented by cats, but the role of this stage in the causation of human disease remains undefined. There is ample evidence for incriminating tissue cysts as a significant source of animal and human infections.

Epidemiology. Based upon serologic evidence, the incidence of Toxoplasma infections varies considerably among people and animals in different parts of the world. Significant titers of dye test and other antibodies have been detected in 50–80% of residents of some localities but in fewer than 5% in other areas. The higher frequencies are more often, but not always, noted in warmer, more humid climates. Similar variations have been observed in feral and domesticated animals and birds. The interpretation of positive serologic findings in older children and adults may be difficult unless changing titers are demonstrable in serial samples or the appearance and disappearance of IgM antibodies suggest recent infection.

Except for transmission by mother to fetus and, rarely, by organ transplant or transfusion, Toxoplasma are not communicated from person to person. The high incidence of subclinical infections in animals and humans makes it difficult to relate a human case to a specific animal. Desmonts found that institutionalized young children in Paris, France, acquired antibodies for Toxoplasma without exhibiting significant clinical symptoms at the rate of 4.8%/mo. The rate almost doubled when their diets were supplemented with additional feedings of undercooked beef and mutton. Freezing and thawing usually renders meat noninfectious. Contaminated meat may explain some human infections, but the sources of parasites for vegetarians and herbivorous animals remain undefined.

Two longitudinal studies among families residing in Cleveland and Syracuse demonstrated very few acquisitions of *Toxoplasma* infections and no clinical illness that could be ascribed to them. In the first study, only 4 serologic conversions were detected in a 10 yr period. On the other hand, high acquisition rates among Parisian women of childbearing age led to significant numbers of congenital infections.

Pathology. In both the acute congenital and acquired forms of toxoplasmosis, histologic changes may be found in almost all tissues. In the congenital form such changes are especially frequent in the central nervous system, the retina, and the choroid; choroid involvement occurs occasionally in acquired toxoplasmosis. *Toxoplasma* in tissues usually are seen as cysts, especially in muscle, often with little or no associated tissue reaction. In severe acute infections free trophozoites may be noted. Gross or microscopic areas of necrosis may be present in many tissues, especially in heart, lungs, skeletal muscle, liver, and spleen. Areas of calcification occur in the brain in the congenital form but not in acquired cases. Some pathologists believe that lymph node changes specific for toxoplasmosis can be identified. Parasites have been found in lymph nodes and tonsils even months after an acute infection. In congenital infection, tissue damage stabilizes early and tends not to progress, but parasites in tissue cysts may remain viable for the life of the host.

Clinical Manifestations. *Congenital Toxoplasmosis.* Fetal infections result only when the initial maternal *Toxoplasma* infection occurs during pregnancy. Maternal antibody acquired at any time prior to pregnancy is fully protective. Clinical severity may vary, and not all fetuses in the same pregnancy need be infected. Desmonts and Couvreur's prospective study provided data on the products of pregnancies in which susceptible women acquired toxoplasmosis. The maternal infections characteristically were asymptomatic, and their offspring, contrary to previous impressions, often were not infected at all. Thus, in 176 such pregnancies there were 30 infected, 110 uninfected, and 11 possibly infected babies. Most infections were subclinical. Among the 6 stillbirths or neonatal deaths in this group, 2 were proved to be the result of congenital toxoplasmosis and the remaining 4, "possible." The important finding is that 110 (63%) of these 176 pregnancies ended with uninfected offspring. Among the 55 infected offspring, injury was severe in 9, mild in 11, and absent in 35.

The severely affected fetus may be stillborn or born prematurely or at term. Illness may be apparent at birth or may not become evident for some days. Manifestations include poor feeding, fever, maculopapular rash, lymphadenopathy, hepatomegaly, splenomegaly, icterus, hydrocephalus, microcephaly, microphthalmia, and convulsions, singly or in combination. Cerebral calcification (often a single, semilunar line in the area of the striate body) and chorioretinitis may be present at birth or appear subsequently.

Active congenital infection may terminate fatally in days or weeks or become inactive with residuals of varying degrees and combinations of hydrocephalus or microcephaly, chorioretinitis, ocular palsies, psychomotor retardation, and convulsive disorders. The full impact of the infection upon development may not become evident until some wk or mo after its apparent cessation.

In a large series of cases of symptomatic congenital toxoplasmosis (Feldman), premature birth was common (31%), with a higher mortality rate (27%) than among infants born at term (12%). Chorioretinitis was noted in 99%, cerebral calcification in 63%, psychomotor retardation in 56%, and hydrocephalus or microcephaly in about half of these infants. Chorioretinitis was bilateral in 85%, but residual damage in some cases was as slight as a minute peripheral retinal scar or a single oculomotor palsy. Recurrent chorioretinitis, especially in early adolescence, which can be related to *Toxoplasma*, usually occurs in those with congenital infections.

The data of Desmonts and Couvreur suggest that the later in pregnancy the infection occurs, the lower the fetal infection rate and the less severe the manifestations. Though *Toxoplasma* may be responsible for premature birth, cerebral palsy, blindness, and mental retardation, it does not appear to be a prominent cause of any of them. Indeed, 86% of the pregnancies which were studied ended in either uninfected or asymptomatic offspring. Because the disease occurs in the offspring of only 1 pregnancy of a given mother, subsequent pregnancies may be undertaken without fear of its repetition. Parasitemia probably occurs in all cases and is the presumed route by which the fetus acquires infection from its mother. Except for occasional instances of lymphadenopathy, clinical evidence of maternal infection usually is not discernible.

Acquired Toxoplasmosis. Postnatally acquired toxoplasmosis is relatively common as an inapparent infection; clinically expressed disease is unusual.

When clinical manifestations are apparent in acquired toxoplasmosis, they may include almost any combination of malaise, fever, myalgia, maculopapular rash, generalized lymphadenopathy, hepatomegaly, encephalitis, pneumonia, and myocarditis. Chorioretinitis (usually unilateral) occurs in fewer than 1% of cases. The rash, when present, persists for about 3 days. Symptoms may be evident for a few days or for some wk; most patients recover spontaneously. The incubation period and mortality rate are unknown.

Generalized lymphadenopathy is said to be frequent in acquired toxoplasmosis in Denmark. Such cases may resemble infectious mononucleosis, Hodgkin disease, or other lymphadenopathies. The Paul-Bunnell test is negative, and splenomegaly is uncommon. The involved lymph nodes (most often posterior cervical) are generally firm and tender at the start but quickly become nontender. They do not suppurate. Because of the vagueness of this syndrome, the correct diagnosis is usually not considered until too late in its course to obtain serologic confirmation. Persistently negative serologic tests exclude the diagnosis.

Caution. Since the classical complement pathway has been found to be essential for the action of neutralizing antibody, it has been shown that sera naturally deficient in C2, C4, C5, C6, C7, or C8 cannot serve this function. Thus, individuals with any such deficiencies may be at greater risk of severe or fatal infections, whether congenital or acquired. Individuals known to have such deficiencies should be advised to eat only thoroughly cooked meat or that which has been well frozen and to avoid handling cat feces.

Laboratory Data. Congenital toxoplasmosis may be diagnosed in its active stage shortly after birth by demonstration of parasites in smears from cerebrospinal and ventricular fluid sediments. These may be xanthochromic and contain cells (sometimes eosinophils) and increased protein. Otherwise, identification depends upon isolation of the parasites in laboratory-reared mice. The inoculum should consist of unfrozen suspensions of fresh tissue or of sediment from body fluids. Organisms, especially cysts, may be found in sections of tissue.

The dye test is the most sensitive and reliable indicator of *Toxoplasma* antibody in human sera but requires live parasites, the classical complement pathway, and meticulous attention to detail. *Toxoplasma* antibodies identified by the dye test appear early in the course of infection and remain in high titer for months or years. Titers diminish gradually, but some antibody usually persists for life. In the sera of infants or young children with congenital disease and of their mothers, titers of 1:1000 to 1:16,000 are usual for at least some mo. If the infant's antibodies have been acquired only by passive transfer, there will be a sharp decline in titer by 3 mo of age and almost total disappearance by 6 mo.

The complement-fixation test may offer additional aid. It becomes positive more slowly so that early in the course there may be a strong positive dye but a negative complement-fixation reaction. The latter tends to decrease relatively quickly so that within months or 1–2 yr after the initial illness, there again may be a negative complement fixation and a positive dye reaction. An infant born with active disease and a positive dye titer may have a negative complement-fixation reaction even though the mother has high titers by both procedures.

The skin test has no clinical diagnostic value. The indirect hemagglutination test has some attractiveness because of its relative simplicity. Its results often parallel the dye test, but there are sufficient differences so that they cannot be substituted for each other. It is especially likely to be negative in newborns with active disease.

More recently, indirect fluorescent antibody (IFA) systems have been adapted to measure *Toxoplasma* antibodies of both the IgM and the IgG classes. The IgM has been used to identify acquired infections early. Screening cord bloods for elevated IgM levels may disclose cases of toxoplasmosis as well as other congenital infections, but about 75% of infants born with active toxoplasmosis will be negative by this test. If the diagnosis is suspected strongly, negative IgM test reactors should be restudied at 2–4 wk. Persisting antibodies of the IgG class also can be detected by IFA. This method most closely approaches the dye test in sensitivity and specificity.

Differential Diagnosis. Any manifestation of congenital toxoplasmosis may occur in other diseases, especially that caused by cytomegalovirus. Neither the cerebral calcification nor the chorioretinitis is pathognomonic. In our experience fewer than 50% of children under 5 yr of age with chorioretinitis satisfy the serologic criteria for congenital toxoplasmosis. Most of the other cases are the result of unknown causes. The clinical picture in the newborn infant also may be compatible with sepsis, syphilis, or hemolytic disease. In acquired cases primary lymphadenopathic disease must be separated from toxoplasmosis.

Prevention. Identification of the cat as a producer of infective oocysts has led to much interest in it as a source of infection for humans, especially the pregnant female. Those women who have antibodies prior to pregnancy are safe from further difficulty. Those who do not have such antibodies or who have not been tested should be guided as follows: eat only thoroughly cooked meat during pregnancy and avoid handling cat litter. This should be disposed of daily to prevent sporulation of any freshly excreted cysts. A cat known to have antibodies presents no problem. Cats kept indoors, maintained on prepared diets, and not fed fresh, uncooked meat also should present no problem. At its worst, the available data suggest the overall risk from this source to be very small for both mother and fetus.

Treatment. A combination of pyrimethamine (Daraprim) and sulfadiazine (or triple sulfonamides, but not sulfisoxazole) is superior to either drug alone in the treatment of experimental *Toxoplasma* infections. The combination also has been used in human patients. It has been effective in interrupting acute, acquired disease, but because of the variable natural course of toxoplasmosis, satisfactory evaluation of any therapeutic regimen is difficult. Sulfadiazine should be administered in usual therapeutic dosage and pyrimethamine, 1 mg/kg/24 hr, in divided doses. The total daily dose of pyrimethamine should not exceed 25 mg, except that twice the calculated daily dose is usually prescribed for the initial 24–48 hr. Treatment should be continued arbitrarily for 4 wk.

Because both pyrimethamine, an antifolic agent, and sulfonamide may produce severe leukopenia and/or thrombocytopenia, thrice weekly leukocyte counts should be performed. The hematologic complications induced by pyrimethamine may be alleviated by the simultaneous administration of leucovorin and fresh yeast cakes. Frenkel suggests that infants receive 1 mg of leucovorin and 100 mg of fresh baker's yeast daily. These substances will not interfere with the antiparasitic activity of the drug but will counteract its hematologic effects. Unfortunately, there is no evidence that the pyrimethamine-sulfonamide treatment affects intracellular or encysted organisms. In newborn infants with active disease, the best that can be hoped for is that further damage will be prevented, but its regression cannot be expected. While there is some experimental evidence that clindamycin may be quite effective, it is not licensed for such use in humans. This drug may present other toxicity problems.

HARRY A. FELDMAN

Couvreur J, Desmonts G, Girre JY: Congenital toxoplasmosis in twins. J Pediatr 89:235, 1976.

Desmonts G, Couvreur J: Congenital toxoplasmosis: A prospective study of 378 pregnancies. N Engl J Med 290:110, 1974.

Dorfman RF, Remington JS: Value of lymph node biopsy in the diagnosis of acute acquired toxoplasmosis. N Engl J Med 289:878, 1973.

Frenkel JK, Weber RW, Lunde MN: Acute toxoplasmosis. Effective treatment with pyrimethamine, sulfadiazine, leucovorin, calcium, and yeast. JAMA 173:1471, 1960.

Schreiber RD, Feldman HA: Identification of the activator system for antibody to toxoplasma as the classical complement pathway. J Infect Dis 141:366, 1980.

Symposium on toxoplasmosis. Bull NY Acad Med 50:107, 1974.

10.114   LEISHMANIASIS

Leishmaniasis in children includes 3 clinical entities: visceral leishmaniasis (kala-azar), cutaneous leishmaniasis (oriental sore, Aleppo boil, Biskra button, tropical ulcer), and naso-oral or mucocutaneous leishmaniasis (espundia, forest yaws, bouba braziliana, uta). Each has a defined clinical picture and geographic distribution, but all are caused by morphologically identical and possibly the same protozoal parasite of the genus *Leishmania*.

Etiology. Although various names have been assigned to the etiologic parasite for each clinical entity, e.g., *L. donovani* for kala-azar, *L. tropica* for cutaneous leishmaniasis, and *L. braziliensis* for naso-oral leishmaniasis, none of the strains can be differentiated from the others serologically or by light or electron microscopy. In humans and other reservoir mammals the parasite is observed as a round or ovoid intracellular organism, 2 to 4 μ in size, chiefly in reticuloendothelial cells of viscera or skin. With Leishman stain, lilac-colored chromatic masses of varying size are seen enclosed in cytoplasm having a faint blue tint about the periphery. In culture on NNN medium and in the intestinal tract of the insect vector, the parasite transforms into a 15–20 μ elongated flagellate (leptomonad).

Visceral Leishmaniasis
(Kala-Azar)

Kala-azar ("black sickness") is also known in India as tropical splenomegaly and sirkari disease or Dumdum fever, in Greece as ponos, and in Malta as mard el bicha. The usual characteristics of the disease are a long incubation period, an insidious onset, and a prolonged course during which the child has irregular fever, loss of weight, progressive enlargement of spleen and liver, leukopenia, and anemia. If it is untreated, mortality is high and death may occur within 2–24 mo.

Epidemiology. Kala-azar is endemic in India, particularly in the eastern states of Assam and Bengal and some areas of Madras. Small foci have been detected in Bombay. It also occurs in Ceylon and throughout Africa, particularly in the eastern region, especially the Sudan. It has been reported from China, Russia, many countries of Central and South America (Paraguay, Argentina, Brazil, Colombia, Venezuela, Guatemala, Mexico), and recently in the United States. In certain areas of the Mediterranean (Malta) it occurs mainly in infants and is termed infantile kala-azar. Epidemiologic studies in Brazil revealed that the majority of cases occurred in rural areas, in small towns, and in peripheral areas of the cities; 81% of those infected were children up to the age of 10 yr, and 75% of them were under the age of 5. The risk of infection was highest in those living in low socioeconomic conditions. In India and China the disease is confined to rural areas, especially alluvial plains; it is rare at elevations above 730 meters. Favorable climatic conditions include temperature of 20–45° C and a humidity of not less than 70%. Usually the disease is transmitted by the bites of sandflies, dogs, foxes, and jackals, which are important reservoirs of infection.

Pathogenesis. The bite of an infected sandfly introduces leptomonads into the skin, where they are engulfed by macrophages in which the parasites change into the leishmanial form. They then multiply in the spleen, bone marrow, and lymph glands. The presence of *Leishmania* in the cells of the reticuloendothelial system leads to great proliferation of macrophages, resulting in expansion of the red bone marrow and in progressive enlargement of the liver and spleen, which may fill the entire abdomen. The reticuloendothelial cells of the lymph nodes, lungs, intestines, and skin may also be heavily infected. Histologically, the main feature is distortion of the normal structure of involved tissues by the proliferation of macrophages. In the liver the parasites proliferate in Kupffer cells, and there is little fibrous tissue formation; the so-called leishmanial fibrosis of the liver is probably due to associated malnutrition. Anemia is due to chronic disease, dietary deficiency, reduced hematopoiesis because of myelophthisic bone marrow, reduced red cell survival, and hypersplenism.

Reza et al have studied several mouse strains after 130 days of infection with *L. donovani* and found that the protective immune response to *L. donovani* infection depended upon thymus-dependent lymphocytes, while the serum or the humoral factor did not confer immunity in the sensitive animals. However, it has been found that removal of the activated lymphocytes and replacement of lymphokine help the macrophages to destroy amastigotes of *Leishmania tropica major* in vitro; therefore, failure of lesions to heal may be due to the quantity of lymphokines and not only to a T cell defect. In chronic experimental leishmaniasis there is also altered immune response. Specific and nonspecific immunodepression accompanies heavy parasitization in experimental cutaneous leishmaniasis, and suppressor T cells play a role in these reactions.

Clinical Manifestations. Following a bite by an infected sandfly, the symptoms may develop during a period of 2 wk–2 yr or more. An unusually prolonged incubation period of 4 yr has been documented.

Infantile Kala-Azar. The majority of affected infants are 1–2 yr of age, but a patient of 4 mo has been reported. The onset is acute, with high fever, vomiting, and toxemia. The fever rises gradually to a peak in 1–2 wk, becomes remittent or continuous, and resolves by lysis. There is enlargement of lymph nodes, spleen, and liver; mild generalized edema; leukopenia; and anemia. If the disease is untreated, agranulocytosis develops; this may lead to cancrum oris, septicemia, pneumonia, and gastroenteritis, any of which may prove fatal. Sudden death may occur from hyperpyrexia, vomiting, intense dyspnea, or hemorrhage.

Congenital Kala-Azar. Rarely, cases of congenital kala-azar occur in infants whose mothers have been affected during pregnancy.

Chronic Kala-Azar. This form occurs chiefly in older children. The onset is insidious, and patients often seek treatment late. In the early stages lassitude, general ill health, weakness, and pallor occur. There is low-grade fever, rarely above 38.5° C (102° F), and often there are 2 remissions in a 24 hr period. The fever may be continuous in the first 2–6 wk of the disease; later there may be periods of low grade or no fever. The child develops abdominal distention and progressive enlargement of the spleen, which initially is soft and later very firm to hand. It may enlarge as rapidly as 2.5 cm/mo and may ultimately extend into the pelvis. Hepatic enlargement occurs a little later in the disease and in advanced cases the liver may be enormous. Neither organ is tender. Moderate lymphadenopathy occurs in patients in the Mediterranean areas and China but not in India. The skin becomes dry and rough and acquires an earthy gray pigmentation over the major bones, temples, hands, feet, and abdomen; hence the name kala-azar. There may be edema of the feet and puffiness of the face. The hair becomes sparse and brittle. Despite the state of chronic illness, the appetite is often good and the tongue clean but pale. Rare clinical presentations include hemorrhages, absence of fever in spite of other manifestations, hepatomegaly, and ascites.

There is marked leukopenia, usually below 400/mm³; neutrophils are mainly affected, and there is an associated mononucleosis. Neutropenia may progress to agranulocytosis, and this may lead to severe septic complications. Involvement of bone marrow and hypersplenism may lead to thrombocytopenia and progressive anemia. The sedimentation rate is high. The indirect bilirubin level may be increased. Serum protein levels are low, with reduction of albumin, increase in globulins, and reversal of the albumin-globulin ratio.

In advanced stages secondary bacterial infections may supervene. Gastroenteritis, dysentery, and pneumonia may cause death. Septic infection of the mouth may lead to cancrum oris and loss of the teeth. Purpura, gingivitis, and stomatitis are common.

Though patients with comparatively mild kala-azar may recover without treatment, the mortality of the untreated disease is very high, with death usually within 2 yr of onset.

Post–kala-azar Dermal Leishmaniasis. This is an important and not uncommon sequel of kala-azar in India but less frequent in China and the Sudan. It is due to the localization of the parasite in the skin, which occurs 1 yr or so after kala-azar has been cured by specific treatment. The skin lesions may take the form of erythematous patches on the face, particularly nose and cheeks, or of hypopigmented macules or nodules resembling those of leprosy on the face and trunk. Rarely, the nodules ulcerate. Ulcerative lesions may become secondarily infected and heal with scars. Cutaneous lesions in the form of nodular lymphangitis are seen in Senegal. When the nodular lesion affects the nose, the nasal mucosa may also be involved. Smears positive for *Leishmania* are more common in the ulcerative type. The diagnosis of post–kala-azar dermal leishmaniasis can be made from the history of kala-azar in the past and recovery of Donovan bodies from skin lesions.

Diagnosis. In endemic areas visceral leishmaniasis should be suspected in children who have fever, especially if it is long-term and irregular; anemia, especially with pancytopenia, or neutropenia with relative mononucleosis; splenomegaly; hepatic involvement with or without hepatomegaly; and alteration of the serum proteins with a reduction of albumin and marked increase of gamma globulin. The diagnosis is confirmed by detection of *Leishmania* in smears or cultures of peripheral blood or of material aspirated from bone marrow, spleen, or liver. Splenic puncture provides the highest percentage of positive results, viz., 95%. However, there is a risk of hemorrhage when anemia and a bleeding tendency are present. In smears of peripheral blood and of material obtained from lymph nodes, the organisms are less likely to be detected. A single negative bone marrow examination does not rule out the diagnosis of visceral leishmaniasis. In some instances diagnosis can be made with a fair degree of certainty because of contact with a proved case in the family.

The various serologic tests, though helpful, are nonspecific; they depend on marked increase in the globulin content of the serum. The formol-gel (aldehyde) test is performed by adding 2 drops of commercial formalin to 2 ml of the patient's serum in a test tube. The mixture is shaken and left to stand at room temperature. A positive reaction is indicated by opacity of the serum progressing in 20 min to a gel resembling boiled egg white. The test becomes positive within 1–2 mo of development of the disease and negative within 6 mo of successful treatment. It is also positive in other infections in which there is hypergammaglobulinemia. The Chopra antimony test is also useful in the diagnosis of chronic kala-azar. The complement fixation test (using an antigen from Kedrowsky acid-fast bacillus) is useful in diagnosis during the early stage of the disease. The immunofluorescent and micro-ELISA tests are the most sensitive and useful. The latter is positive in 80–100% of cases. It has been found to be useful even in cases of hepatosplenomegaly due to leishmaniasis when the bone marrow examination for *Leishmania* Donovan bodies and the aldehyde reaction are both negative. Moreover, the test is negative in children with hepatosplenomegaly due to malaria and trypanosomiasis.

Differential Diagnosis. In the early stage kala-azar may be confused with malaria, typhoid fever, and disseminated tuberculosis. Prolonged recurring fever may simulate protracted hematogenous tuberculosis (particularly abdominal tuberculosis with enlargement of liver and spleen), chronic active hepatitis, amebic abscess of the liver, brucellosis, leukemia, Hodgkin disease, rheumatoid arthritis, and disseminated lupus erythematosus. The chronic stage may be confused with Indian childhood cirrhosis, myeloid leukemia, tropical splenomegaly syndrome described in Uganda and New Guinea, and, rarely, the splenomegaly of extrahepatic portal hypertension.

The leishmanin skin test (Montenegro test) depends upon the delayed hypersensitivity reaction following intra-cutaneous injection of 0.5 ml of a suspension of lepto-monads in formolized saline. The test is read 48–72 hr after the injection. A local induration of more than 5 mm suggests a positive reaction and signifies immunity against reinfection with a homologous strain of leish-mania. The test is not meant for the diagnosis of active kala-azar, in which it is negative; it becomes positive within 2 mo of successful treatment and remains posi-tive for many yr thereafter. A positive leishmanin rate above 5% is suggestive of endemic kala-azar.

Treatment.   The susceptibility of kala-azar to specific drug therapy appears to vary considerably in different parts of the world. Three drugs are useful in its treat-ment: (1) pentavalent antimonial drugs, (2) aromatic diamidines such as pentamidine and stilbamidine, and (3) amphotericin B. Pentavalent antimonial drugs in-clude *sodium antimony gluconate* (sodium stibogluconate, Solustibosan, Stibatin, Pentostam), which is made up in solution ready for injection (100 mg/ml). Children tolerate this drug well in a daily intramuscular dose of 10 mg/kg (maximum 600 mg). For Indian kala-azar the total dose is 3.4 gm for children 5–15 yr and 1.2 gm for those below 5 yr. For kala-azar occurring in other parts of the world the total dose is 12 gm above 5 yr and 6 gm below 5 yr. The criteria for cure are absence of fever, regression of enlargement of spleen and liver, clearing of the hematologic signs of the disease, return of the serum proteins to normal, and negative serologic tests. If the patient fails to respond satisfactorily, a 2nd course of treatment should be tried. *Urea stibamine* is another pentavalent antimony compound successfully used in the treatment of kala-azar. It is given in solution in water on alternate days intravenously for 6–10 doses. The dose is 125 mg intravenously for children above 5 yr and 65 mg for children below 5 yr. Six doses are given for Indian kala-azar. During treatment with these compounds anaphylactic shock may rarely occur; epi-nephrine should be kept ready for injection. Aromatic diamidine drugs such as *hydroxystilbamidine isethionate* should be used when pentavalent antimony therapy has failed. Children under 15 yr should receive 150 mg daily, and under 5, 65 mg daily, intravenously for 10 days. A 2nd and a 3rd course should be given at 10 day intervals for complete cure. Since this compound produces a fall in blood pressure by release of hista-mine, antihistamine drugs should be given.

Amphotericin B is necessary when there is no im-provement with repeated courses of pentavalent anti-mony and diamidine drugs.

Intercurrent infections should be treated with appro-priate antibiotics. Nutrition should be improved through a diet adequate in calories and proteins. In children with severe neutropenia, anemia, and throm-bocytopenia, repeated blood transfusions may be re-quired. In addition to correcting malnutrition, oral hy-giene is necessary to prevent stomatitis and cancrum oris.

Cutaneous Leishmaniasis

Cutaneous leishmaniasis of the Old World (oriental sore) is a chronic ulcerative granuloma of the skin caused by *L. tropica* and occurring chiefly in Mediter-ranean countries, Asia, Africa, and parts of South America. It begins as a papule at the site of a bite from a sandfly and progresses successively to formation of a tubercle, a scab, and finally an ulcer on an exposed area of skin. Healing may be rapid and no treatment re-quired. Diagnosis is made by microscopic identification of *Leishmania* in tissue obtained from the margin of the ulcer or in culture of such tissue on NNN medium.

Treatment with metronidazole, 250 mg orally 3 times a day for 10 days, repeated twice with a 10 day interval between courses, has been given with conflicting results in clinical trials. Secondary bacterial infection should be treated locally and systemically with antibacterial agents suitable to the organisms isolated. In progressive cases pentavalent antimony drugs should be used as in vis-ceral leishmaniasis, in addition to 400–600 mg injected locally every 2nd day for 2–3 injections. In resistant cases 100 mg of mepacrine should be injected around the edge of the lesion daily for 3 days. Levamisole therapy in the dosage of 50 mg daily for 2 successive days each wk till the lesions heal appears encouraging; the drug has a stimulating effect on cellular immune mechanisms.

Cutaneous leishmaniasis of the New World is caused by either *L. braziliensis* or *L. tropica mexicana*. A form known as chiclero ulcer is seen chiefly in Central Amer-ica. It is often a self-limited disease, but if there is any evidence of spread in mucocutaneous regions, penta-valent antimony drugs or amphotericin B should be administered as in visceral leishmaniasis. In resistant cases pyrimethamine (Daraprim) should be used in dosage of 6.25 mg 3 times/day for 7 days for children under 5 yr of age. The dose is doubled for those over 5. In American cutaneous leishmaniasis, rifampin in a dose of 300–600 mg daily for 3–15 wk has produced more rapid complete or partial cicatrization of the le-sion.

Mucocutaneous Leishmaniasis

Mucocutaneous (naso-oral, nasopharyngeal) leish-maniasis is a disease of Central and South America caused by *L. braziliensis*. Ulcerative lesions of the nose and throat may result in widespread destruction of the tissues of the mouth, nose, and throat. Treatment is the same as that for visceral leishmaniasis and should be instituted as soon as the diagnosis is made. It is often necessary to resort to amphotericin B because of poor response to antimony compounds.

Prevention

Sandfly control is not difficult to achieve with insec-ticides and other measures. Early diagnosis and specific treatment of the human host have also helped to reduce the incidence of the disease. The adequate treatment of post–kala-azar dermal leishmaniasis is important since these patients are highly infectious. Destruction of infectious dogs in Crete was followed by a decrease in the incidence of kala-azar. A strain of leptomonad cultures of this protozoan obtained from ground squirrels has been used for mass inoculation of those exposed to infection in North Kenya. Animal strains of Leishmania are dermatotropic and capable of producing skin immunity without causing kala-azar. Some populations in East Africa have a high incidence of immunity to experimental infections with human strains of Leishmania, possibly due to previous exposure to nonhuman strains. Irradiated L. donovani vaccine is under trial in laboratory animals. The use of repellent cream, insecticidal sprays, and protective nets may help in personal prophylaxis against sandflies.

P. M. Udani

Abdel-Aai H, Morsy TA, Hawwary GH: Clinical forms of cutaneous leishmaniasis in Riyadh, Saudi Arabia. J Pak Med Assoc 25:239, 1975.

Adams ARD, Maegrith BDG: Clinical Tropical Diseases. London, Blackwell Scientific Publications, 1971.

Amato NV: Visceral leishmaniasis, a case of at least four years of incubation period. Rev Inst Med Trop S Paulo 20:312, 1978.

Arredondo B, Perez H: Alteration of the immune response with chronic experimental leishmaniasis. Infection Immunity. 25:(1)16, 1979.

Brito T De, Hoshinoo-Shimizu S, Amato Neto V, et al: Glomerular involvement in human kala-azar. Trop Med Hyg 24:9, 1975.

Butler PG: Levamisole therapy of chronic Leishmania tropica. J Trop Med Hyg 81:221, 1978.

Dourado HV, Borborema CT, Alecrim W, et al: American cutaneous leishmaniasis: Treatment with rifampicin. Rev Bras Clin Terapeut 4:1, 1975.

Hommel M, Peters W, Ranque J, et al: The micro ELISA technique in the serodiagnosis of visceral leishmaniasis. Ann Trop Med Parasit 72:213, 1978.

Ilardi A, Proietti AM: Immunization of hamsters against Leishmania donovani by means of an irradiated homologous strain. Parasitologia 10:143, 1974.

Manson-Bahr PEG: Manson's Tropical Diseases. London, Bailliere, Tindall and Cox, 1968.

Mattock NM, Peters W: The experimental chemotherapy of leishmaniasis. III. Detection of antileishmanial activity in some new synthetic compounds in a tissue culture model. Ann Trop Med Parasitol 69:449, 1975.

Muhlpfordt H: Comparative electron microscope studies on the labeling of Leishmania donovani, L. tropica, and L. braziliensis with ferritin. Trop Med Parasitol 26:385, 1975.

Nuernberger SP, Ramos CV, Custodio R: Visceral leishmaniasis in Honduras: Report of three proven cases and a suspected case. Trop Med Hyg 24:917, 1975.

Pedersen IK, Sawicki S: Metronidazole therapy for cutaneous leishmaniasis. Arch Dermatol 111:1343, 1975.

Prasad LSN, Savan R, Sells T: Micro plate enzyme linked immunosorbent assay of visceral leishmaniasis. J Trop Med Res 71:708, 1980.

Strobel M, M'Diaye BR, Renaud-Steens C, et al: Cutaneous leishmaniasis in the form of nodular lymphangitis. Bull Soc Med Afr 23:4, 370, 1978.

Swarup Mitra S, Choudhury AKR, Sarkar M: Inhibition of some erythrocytic enzymes in kala-azar. Ind J Med Res 69:571, 1979.

Zavoral JM, Paloucek JT, Yaeger RG: Kala-azar imported into USA. Pediatrics 50:471, 1972.

PNEUMOCYSTIS CARINII

See Sec 12.68.

10.115 PRIMARY AMEBIC MENINGOENCEPHALITIS

Amebic meningoencephalitis is an acute and usually fatal infection of the central nervous system in children and young adults with a history of swimming in fresh water and heated pools and ponds or lakes heavily contaminated with algae or bacteria.

Etiology and Epidemiology. Free-living amebae are ubiquitous in nature. The genera most often isolated from the central nervous system are Naegleria fowleri, Acanthamoeba, and, on rare occasions, "unidentified" amebae. Naegleria are motile freshwater amebae-flagellates, 10–20 μ in diameter, with a large nucleus, a prominent central karyosome, and large pseudopodia. Naegleria can be cultured on a number of laboratory media and on non-nutrient agar which has been seeded with bacteria, e.g., E. coli. Various species of Acanthamoeba are found free-living in nature and as part of the normal flora of the mouth and nasopharynx. They are morphologically similar to Naegleria, are 6–8 μ in diameter, and have a large nucleus with a central karyosome and an abundant cytoplasm. Acanthamoeba are less motile than Naegleria and in clinical specimens can be confused with macrophages.

Human infections with Naegleria were first reported in Australia and the United States in 1965. Human infection has been acquired through contact with tap water in Australia, thermally polluted water in Belgium, and swimming pools in Czechoslovakia. Most cases in the United States have occurred during summer months in children and young adults with a history of swimming, diving, or water skiing in fresh water ponds and lakes. Acanthamoeba infection of the central nervous system is less common, has a worldwide distribution, is not associated with previous aquatic activity, and occurs as an opportunistic infection in a debilitated and/or immunosuppressed patient.

Pathology. Naegleria gain access to the central nervous system through the nasal mucosa covering the cribriform plate and produce diffuse and extensive damage to the brain. Hemorrhagic necrosis of the olfactory nerves, the adjacent inferior frontal lobes, and the basilar surface of the cerebrum and cerebellum is common. Amebae mixed with neutrophils and macrophages can be found in the subarachnoid space, in the superficial substance, and in small perivascular spaces of the brain. The inflammatory response in the meninges is reflected in the spinal fluid by a large number of polymorphonuclear leukocytes, an elevated protein, and a low glucose level. Acanthamoeba reach the central nervous system following hematogenous dissemination. The histopathologic findings consist of a granulomatous encephalitis with foci of hemorrhagic necrosis in the occipital, parietal, temporal, and (less often) frontal lobes. The upper portion of the spinal cord may be involved, and visceral lesions (lung, kidney, adrenals, etc.) are not uncommon. The inflammatory response of the meninges is minimal and reflected in the cerebrospinal fluid by lymphocytic pleocytosis, an elevated protein, and a normal or borderline low glucose.

Clinical Manifestations. Naegleria meningoencephalitis is an acute and rapidly progressive illness presenting with fever, headache, neck rigidity, vomiting, and lethargy within 5 days of exposure to fresh water. Symptoms rapidly progress over the 1st 24 hr with increasing lethargy, convulsions, and eventually coma. The clinical course is one of rapid deterioration and death. The clinical course of acanthamoebic infection is that of a subacute or chronic meningoencephalitis with focal neurologic manifestations, e.g., hemiplegia, aphasia, visual disturbances, in debilitated or immunosuppressed patients who usually have no history of recent exposure to fresh water.

Diagnosis. The cerebrospinal fluid in *Naegleria* infection is similar to that observed with purulent bacterial meningitis. However, the Gram stain and culture fail to reveal bacteria, and motile amebae can be seen in a fresh wet-mount examination of uncentrifuged and nonrefrigerated cerebrospinal fluid. *Acanthamoeba* infection yields a cerebrospinal fluid consistent with aseptic meningitis; the amebae are not present in the cerebrospinal fluid and can be demonstrated only by brain biopsy.

Treatment. Most cases of *Naegleria* meningoencephalitis have been fatal, and numerous amebicides have been tried unsuccessfully. Two patients have been successfully treated with intravenous and intrathecal (1.5 mg at 12 hr intervals) amphotericin (1 was simultaneously treated with rifampin and miconazole). *Acanthamoeba* are more sensitive than *Naegleria* to antimicrobial agents including sulfanilamides, clotrimazole, and 5-fluorocytosine; amphotericin is ineffective. Though the sensitivity of these amebae to a number of therapeutic agents is obvious, sufficient information is not available to identify the drug(s) most efficacious in human infection.

—WILLIAM T. SPECK

Darby CP, Conradi SE, Holbrook TW, et al: Primary amebic meningoencephalitis. Am J Dis Child 133:1025, 1979.
Martinez AJ: Is *Acanthamoeba* encephalitis an opportunistic infection? Neurology 30:567, 1980.

Helminths

NEMATODES
(Roundworms)

INTESTINAL NEMATODES

Human infection with intestinal roundworms constitutes the largest incidence of helminthiasis of man. Although these infections are more prevalent in tropical and subtropical climates, temperate and cold regions are not spared. Children are generally more heavily infected than adults and are therefore more likely to suffer from the pathologic consequences of these infections. Intestinal nematodes may infect man either directly by ingestion of mature eggs or indirectly via larval penetration of skin. With the exception of *Strongyloides stercoralis*, the adult stages of all these nematodes live in the lumen of the intestinal tract, do not multiply in the human host, and are not associated with peripheral blood eosinophilia. Increased eosinophil counts occur only during the phase of infection when nematode larvae migrate through host tissues. The more prevalent intestinal roundworm infections of children will be discussed according to their final location in the gut: small intestine (*Ascaris lumbricoides*, *Ancylostoma duodenale*, *Necator americanus*, and *Strongyloides stercoralis*), cecum (*Enterobius vermicularis*), and large intestine (*Trichuris trichiura*) (Table 10–56).

10.116 Ascariasis

Infection with *Ascaris lumbricoides* is the most prevalent human helminthiasis with an estimated 1 billion cases worldwide. Infection is most common in preschool and young children. The distribution of ascariasis is ubiquitous with the greatest number of cases in countries with warmer climates. Nevertheless, there are approximately 4 million infected individuals, mainly children, in North America.

Etiology. The infective stage of *A. lumbricoides* is the mature larva-containing egg. It is broadly oval, has a thick shell with an outer mamillated covering, and measures approximately 40×60 μm (Fig 10–37). Eggs are passed in the feces of infected individuals and mature in 5–10 days under favorable environmental conditions to become infective. After ingestion by man, larvae are released from the eggs and penetrate the intestinal wall before migrating to the lungs via the

Table 10–56 IMPORTANT INTESTINAL NEMATODE INFECTIONS OF CHILDREN

INFECTION	ETIOLOGY	MODE OF TRANSMISSION	MAJOR CLINICAL FEATURES	DIAGNOSIS
Ascariasis	*Ascaris lumbricoides*	Eggs in soil	None, nutritional or obstructive lesions	Eggs in stools
Hookworms	*Ancylostoma duodenale*, *Necator americanus*	Larvae in soil	Anemia, hypoalbuminemia	Eggs in stools
Strongyloidiasis	*Strongyloides stercoralis*	Larvae in soil, autoinfection	Abdominal pain, diarrhea and malabsorption, dissemination	Larvae in stools or duodenal aspirate
Enterobiasis	*Enterobius vermicularis*	Fecal-oral, person-to-person, eggs in environment	Perianal itching	Eggs on perianal swabs
Trichuriasis	*Trichuris trichiura*	Eggs in soil	None	Eggs in stools

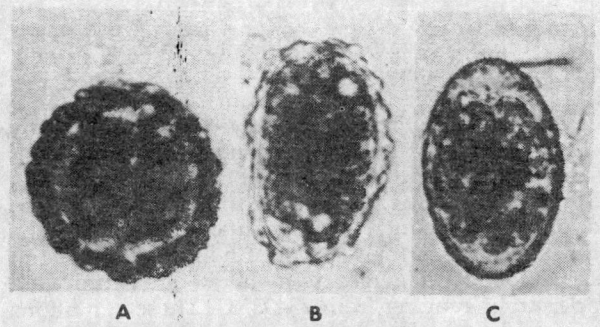

Figure 10–37 Fertilized (A) and unfertilized (B, C) eggs of *Ascaris lumbricoides*. (× 400.) The egg illustrated in C may be mistaken for that of a different nematode or of a trematode.

venous circulation. They then break through the pulmonary tissues, ascend the bronchial tree and trachea, and are reswallowed. Upon their arrival in the small intestine, the larvae develop into mature adult worms (males measure 15–25 cm × 3 mm and females 25–35 cm × 4 mm). Each female has a life span of 1–2 yr and is capable of producing 200,000 eggs/day.

Epidemiology. Ascariasis is a soil-transmitted infection dependent on dissemination of eggs into environmental conditions suitable for their maturation. Promiscuous defecation and use of human manure are the 2 most important unhygienic practices responsible for the endemicity of ascariasis. The mode of transmission to man is hand to mouth; the fingers are contaminated by soil contact. Alternatively, food items (particularly those commonly consumed raw) become infected by human fertilizers or by flies. Endemicity of *A. lumbricoides* is aided by the extremely high egg output of worms and their resistance to unfavorable environmental conditions. Eggs have been shown to remain infective in soil for months and may survive cooler weather (5–10° C) for 2 yr. Transmission of ascariasis may occur seasonally or throughout the year and is dependent on the suitability of soil conditions for maturation of eggs.

Clinical Manifestations. Although disease sequelae occur in only a small proportion of infected individuals, they amount to a significant clinical problem because of the high incidence of ascariasis. Morbidity may be manifested during migration of the larvae through the lungs or be associated with the presence of adult worms in the small intestine. The pathogenesis of pulmonary ascariasis is not known, although a hypersensitivity phenomenon may be involved. Adult worms may cause disease by obstruction of the gut or biliary tree and by their effects on host nutrition. The few controlled studies of the effects of ascariasis on the nutritional status of children are contradictory and relate more to the socioeconomic and nutritional background of the study population rather than to the effects of *Ascaris* infection per se.

Pulmonary ascariasis may occur following heavy exposure and is also common in individuals who live in areas with seasonal transmission of infection (seasonal pneumonitis). The most characteristic features are cough, blood-stained sputum, and eosinophilia. This Loeffler-like syndrome may be associated with transient pulmonary infiltrates. In children the differentiation of this syndrome from visceral larva migrans may be difficult, but abdominal symptoms or signs are very rare in pulmonary ascariasis.

The presence of adult *Ascaris* worms in the small intestine is associated with vague complaints such as abdominal pain and distention. There is, however, no definitive proof that these symptoms are related to the presence of the parasites. Examination of the nutritional status of Indian children with *Ascaris* infection showed that nitrogen excretion decreased after specific therapy. Steatorrhea and diminished vitamin A absorption have also been demonstrated in some *Ascaris*-infected children. A study of Colombian children with moderate infections (30–50 worms) showed that administration of anthelmintic drugs was followed by decreased fat and nitrogen excretion and improved xylose absorption.

Obstructive clinical syndromes due to ascariasis are extremely rare. Intestinal blockage due to a mass of worms occurs in heavily infected children; the peak incidence occurs in children 1–6 yr old. The onset is usually sudden with severe colicky abdominal pain and vomiting which may be bile stained; these symptoms may progress rapidly and follow a course similar to acute intestinal obstruction of any other etiology. Migration of *Ascaris* worms into the biliary tract has also been reported, particularly occurring in China and the Philippines; the likelihood of this condition increases in heavily infected children. The onset is acute with colicky abdominal pain, nausea, vomiting, and fever. Jaundice is rarely seen.

Diagnosis. Adult female *Ascaris* worms deposit eggs which can be detected by direct fecal smear examination. Quantification of eggs, if needed, can be performed by the Kato thick smear method. The morphology of eggs detected in the stools is important: bisexual infections result in the excretion of typical mature fertile eggs, whereas infertile eggs are seen in individuals infected with female worms only (Fig 10–37B and C). Diagnosis of pulmonary or obstructive ascariasis is based primarily on clinical data and a high index of suspicion.

Treatment. Several chemotherapeutic agents are effective against ascariasis; none of these drugs, however, is useful during the pulmonary phase of the infection. Treatment of children, particularly those with heavy infections, should be approached with caution. Piperazine salts (citrate, adipate, or phosphate) are administered orally in a daily dose of 50 mg/kg for 2 days. A single dose rather than 2 day regimens has proved effective in reducing worm loads in infected children. As piperazine results in necrosis of the worms, it is the drug of choice in cases of intestinal or biliary obstruction. Other drugs useful for treatment of uncomplicated intestinal ascariasis include mebendazole and levamisole. Rarely, surgical treatment may be needed in severe obstructive cases.

Control. Although ascariasis is the most prevalent worm infection worldwide, little attention has been given to its control, partly because of controversy concerning its clinical significance and also because of its unique epidemiologic features. Control attempts directed at reducing worm loads in humans by mass chemotherapy have shown some promise. Because of the high rate of reinfection, chemotherapy has to be repeated at 3–6 mo intervals. The feasibility and cost of such an undertaking will have to be evaluated before it can be widely accepted. Sanitary practices directed at treatment of human feces before use as fertilizer and the provision of hygienic sewage disposal facilities may be the most effective long-term preventive measures against ascariasis.

10.117 Hookworms

Three species of hookworms infect man: *Ancylostoma duodenale*, *Necator americanus*, and *Ancylostoma ceylonicum*. Infection is endemic in temperate, subtropical, and tropical areas of the world. Although there are no recent estimates of their prevalence, hookworms are thought to infect more than 900 million people. During the past few decades *A. duodenale* and *N. americanus* have become endemic in many tropical and subtropical countries.

Etiology. Hookworm larvae are usually found in warm damp soil and infect man by penetration of skin. Infection may also be acquired by drinking contaminated water. Larvae migrate to the venous circulation and are carried to the lungs, where they break into the alveolar spaces, migrate upward, and are then swallowed to reach their final habitat in the upper small intestine. Mature worms develop in 2–4 wk; they are grayish-white and slightly curved and measure 5–13 mm in length. The buccal cavity of *A. duodenale* has pointed clawed teeth and that of *N. americanus* has 2 chitinous plates. These buccal structures help the mature worms attach to the jejunal mucosa and suck blood. In 6–9 wk worms reach sexual maturity and start to deposit eggs, which are excreted in the feces. Mature *A. duodenale* female worms produce about 30,000 eggs/day; daily egg production by *N. americanus* is 9000. The mean life span of adult hookworms is 1–3 yr, although they may occasionally survive up to 9 yr. Hookworm eggs are ovoidal and thin shelled and measure approximately 36 × 58 μm (Fig 10–38). When freshly passed, these eggs contain 4 embryonic segments. These mature into 1st stage larvae that hatch in 1–2 days under favorable environmental conditions. Larvae live in the soil for 1–2 wk, molt twice, and

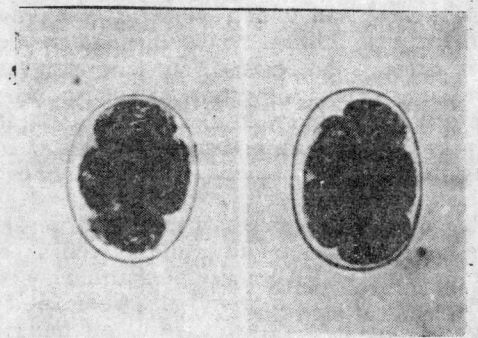

Figure 10–38 Eggs of hookworm, *Necator americanus*, in early cleavage as seen in freshly passed feces. (×400.)

change into infective larvae which are capable of penetrating human skin.

Epidemiology. Man is the primary host for the 3 species of hookworms. Endemicity of infection in any specific geographic location depends on suitability of environmental conditions for hatching of eggs and maturation of larvae, on fecal contamination of soil, and on human contact with contaminated soil. The optimal conditions for survival of hookworm larvae in soil include good aeration, moderate moisture, and temperatures ranging from 23–33° C. These conditions are found in many parts of agrarian tropical countries and also in the southeastern part of the United States.

The morbidity of hookworm infections in endemic areas is sustained primarily by children. In 1 study half of the children were infected before age 5; 90% were infected by 9 yr of age. Intensity of infection increases up to age 6–7, then stabilizes for a few yr. Newly infected children acquire a mean of 2 female worms; there is a net gain of 2.7 parasites/yr.

Pathology and Pathogenesis. Several factors may contribute to the morbidity of hookworm infection; these include worm burden, diet, race, and development of immunity in chronically infected individuals. Worm burden and diet seem to be the most significant of these factors in regard to anemia, the major pathologic manifestation of hookworm infection.

Pathologic lesions due to hookworm may occur during the migratory phase of infection or may be related to the presence of adult worms in the small intestine. Ground itch or dermatitis results from larval invasion of skin and the subsequent inflammatory response. Mild pulmonary lesions similar to those described in ascariasis may occur during lung migration of larvae. It is questionable whether a Loeffler-like syndrome occurs during hookworm infection. The presence of adult worms in the small intestine results in anemia and hypoalbuminemia. The pathogenesis of hookworm anemia is related to intensity of infection and host iron balance. Blood loss varies with hookworm species: in *A. duodenale* infection 0.16–0.34 ml/worm is lost daily; in *N. americanus* the corresponding figure is 0.03–0.05 ml.

Clinical Manifestations. Infections are usually asymptomatic; significant clinical disease occurs in a small percentage of children in whom symptoms follow the chronologic order of worm migration in the host. Exposure of skin for the 1st time to infective larvae may lead to pruritus. Skin reactions vary from erythematous papules on primary exposure which disappear within 1 wk to vesiculation and generalized edema on subsequent infections which may last 1–3 wk. Migration of the larvae through the lungs is associated with few, if any, specific symptoms or signs.

Symptoms of abdominal pain, loss of appetite, indigestion, postprandial fullness, and diarrhea have been attributed to the intestinal phase of hookworm infection. These clinical correlates are based primarily on observations of experimental infections in volunteers with heavy worm loads; there have been no adequately controlled community studies which document the occurrence of specific abdominal symptoms in natural hookworm infections. The significant disease sequelae of chronic hookworm infections include anemia, hypoalbuminemia, and edema. There is a statistically significant inverse correlation between intensity of infection and hematologic values; for example, only egg counts of >2000/ml feces in women and children or >5000/ml feces in men are associated with anemia. Hemoglobin concentrations under 5 gm/dl have been associated with heart failure and sudden death. Hypoalbuminemia in excess of that anticipated from whole blood loss may also occur; the attendant decrease in plasma oncotic pressure may lead to edema.

Diagnosis. Direct examination of fecal smears for hookworm eggs provides a qualitative assessment of infection. The Kato thick smear offers a simple technique for quantitation of infection, but since hookworm eggs disappear within 1 hr of preparation, prompt examination of these smears is mandatory. Eggs of *A. duodenale* and *N. americanus* are morphologically indistinguishable; the only way to differentiate the species is to allow the eggs to hatch and examine the released larvae.

Treatment. Evaluation of intensity of infection and severity of anemia should precede therapy. In children with severe anemia (hemoglobin concentration under 5 gm/dl) iron therapy should be given before anthelmintic drugs. Elemental iron is administered orally at a dosage of 2 mg/kg 3 times/day until anemia is corrected. In cases of life-threatening anemia with signs of heart failure, diuretics followed by slow transfusion of packed red cells may be indicated. Mebendazole (100 mg orally twice a day for 2 days) or tetrachlorethylene (single dose of 0.1 ml/kg) will eradicate or reduce the hookworm load.

Control. Eradication or control of hookworm infection depends on sanitation and mass chemotherapy. To allow cost-effective application of these 2 principles, the rate of worm acquisition, its life span, and the rate at which infection is lost have to be determined. Seasonal variations in transmission and the hookworm species must also be taken into consideration. Eradication has been achieved in the southeast United States.

10.118 Strongyloidiasis

Infection with the nematode *Strongyloides stercoralis*, unlike that with other worms, may cause autoinfection with massive parasite invasion of the host and eventual death. The incidence of this complication is increased in malnourished or immunosuppressed children. *S. stercoralis* infection is widely distributed throughout tropical and temperate regions, though it is less common than infection by other intestinal roundworms. Infection is more prevalent in institutionalized children, perhaps because of person-to-person transmission.

Etiology. Infected individuals pass larvae in their stools; these parasites may develop into free-living adults in the soil or change into infective filariform larvae. These latter forms penetrate human skin, pass via the bloodstream to the lungs, and follow a pathway similar to hookworm and *Ascaris* larvae until they reach their final habitat in the upper small intestine. Mature female worms, which are larger than males (2.2 mm vs

0.7 mm in length), burrow into the intestinal mucosa and begin releasing eggs approximately 4 wk after infection. *S. stercoralis* eggs hatch rapidly, and small larvae (225 × 16 μm) are passed in feces. The larvae must undergo morphologic changes in soil to become infective, but these changes may also be accomplished as they are being discharged from the body of infected individuals. Larvae are then capable of infecting the same individual by penetration of the intestinal wall or perianal skin. This unique feature of the *Strongyloides* life cycle allows the parasite to survive for many yr inside the same host and occasionally to cause overwhelming infection.

Epidemiology. Man is the primary host of *S. stercoralis*. Transmission of infection and its endemicity depend on suitable soil and climatic conditions and poor sanitary habits. Close contact and poor personal hygiene may be important as the prevalence of infection is much higher in institutions for the mentally retarded. Host factors such as nutrition and immune status may play a crucial role in the development of the hyperinfection syndrome.

Pathology and Pathogenesis. The initial penetration of skin by infective larvae usually produces no apparent pathologic lesions. Repeated skin invasion may, however, result in dermatitis; in cases in which autoinfection is established through the skin, a more extensive skin lesion called larva currens may occur. A Loeffler-like syndrome with eosinophilia may be seen during migration of the larvae through the lungs. Eosinophilia may also occur when adult females burrow into the intestinal mucosa. Disseminated strongyloidiasis is a complex pathologic entity due to larval invasion of internal organs and complicating gram-negative bacteremia.

Clinical Manifestations. Signs and symptoms of strongyloidiasis occur in only a small percentage of infected individuals or in those with the hyperinfection syndrome. Pulmonary symptoms and skin lesions due to larval invasion are usually mild and generally pass unnoticed. Pruritus with a papular erythematous rash may occur. Larva currens, a condition due to repeated skin invasion by larvae, is characterized by the presence of large erythematous urticarial lesions with rapidly moving edges. These are usually localized to an area within 30 cm of the anus and have a tendency to recur. The typical symptoms of strongyloidiasis, which include abdominal pain, vomiting, and diarrhea, are caused by adult worms in the upper small intestine. These symptoms occur with uncertain frequency and may have an abrupt onset with periodic recurrences. Abdominal pain is often epigastric and may be burning, colicky, or dull in nature. Diarrhea with passage of mucus may alternate with periods of constipation. Chronic strongyloidiasis may result in a malabsorption-like syndrome with protein-losing enteropathy and weight loss. Blood eosinophilia is usually associated with and is often the only indication of the intestinal phase of infection.

Disseminated strongyloidiasis occurs in children with predisposing factors such as malnutrition or defects in cell-mediated immunity (lymphomas, Hodgkin disease, etc.). The onset is usually sudden with generalized abdominal pain, distention, fever, and shock due to gram-negative septicemia. Massive invasion of internal organs by the parasite larvae causes extensive tissue destruction. Although leukocytosis may occur in these patients, eosinophilia is often absent.

Diagnosis. Intestinal strongyloidiasis is diagnosed by examination of feces or duodenal fluid for the characteristic larvae. Several stool samples should be examined either by direct smear or by a concentration method such as formaldehyde-ether or that of Baermann. Alternatively, duodenal fluid obtained by the pediatric Entero test or aspiration may provide samples for definitive diagnosis. In children with hyperinfection syndrome larvae may be found in sputum, gastric aspirates, or, rarely, in small intestinal biopsies. Strongyloidiasis should also be suspected in immunosuppressed patients who suddenly develop signs and symptoms consistent with disseminated infection.

Treatment. The only available and effective therapeutic agent against strongyloidiasis is thiabendazole. Treatment of infected children should aim at eradication of infection, and therefore subsequent stool examination is essential. Thiabendazole is administered orally in a dose of 25 mg/kg twice daily for 2 days. Courses of up to 2 wk may be needed in those with the hyperinfection syndrome.

Control. Sanitary practices designed to prevent soil and person-to-person transmission of strongyloidiasis are the most effective control measures. As the infection is uncommon, case detection and treatment are also advised. Individuals who will be subjected to immunosuppressive therapy should have a screening examination for *S. stercoralis* and, if infected, be treated with thiabendazole.

10.119 Enterobiasis
(Pinworm)

Infection with *Enterobius vermicularis* occurs in all areas of the world. Enterobiasis or pinworm infection affects individuals of all ages but is especially common in children; it occurs in all socioeconomic groups. Living in congested districts, institutions, or families with pinworm infections predisposes to enterobiasis. The infection is essentially harmless and causes social more than medical problems in affected children and their families.

Etiology. Man is infected by ingestion of embryonated eggs which are usually carried on fingernails, clothing, bedding, or house dust. In the stomach the eggs hatch and larvae migrate to the cecal region where they mature into adult worms. *E. vermicularis* are small (1 cm) white worms; the gravid females migrate by night to the perianal region to deposit masses of eggs. Pinworm ova are asymmetric, are flattened on 1 side, and measure 30 × 60 μm (Fig 10–39). After a 6 hr maturation period a single-coiled larva can be seen within each ovum. These larvae may remain viable for 20 days.

Epidemiology. Irritation of the perianal region during the act of oviposition by female *E. vermicularis* worms induces scratching. Eggs carried under the fingernails are transmitted directly or disseminated in the

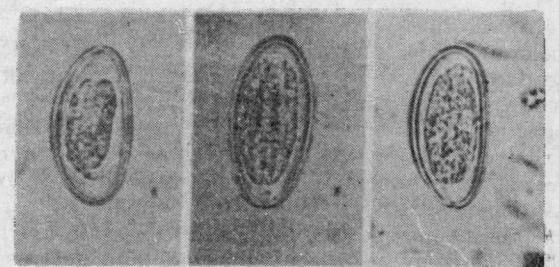

Figure 10–39 Eggs of *Enterobius vermicularis* in early developmental stages recovered from feces. (×400.) One side of the shell is somewhat flat, but when viewed from above (center) it appears to be symmetrical and may be mistaken for a different species. When found in human feces, which is unusual, pinworm eggs contain a tadpole-stage embryo, whereas eggs recovered on a perianal swab contain a coiled larva which is more than twice the length of the egg.

environment to infect others. Man is the only natural host of *E. vermicularis*. The prevalence and intensity of infection are low in infants and young children and reach a peak in the 5–14 yr old age group. Infection decreases in prevalence in adulthood because of either reduced exposure or acquisition of immunity.

Clinical Manifestations. Many local and systemic signs and symptoms have been ascribed to *Enterobius* infection; however, a controlled study of infected children 2–12 yr old failed to document specific syndromes due to *E. vermicularis*. Symptomatic individuals most commonly complain of nocturnal anal pruritus and sleeplessness. The etiology and incidence of perianal and perineal irritation are unknown but may be related to the intensity of infection, to the psychiatric profile of the infected individual and his or her family, or to an allergic reaction to the parasite. As tissue invasion does not occur in most cases of enterobiasis, eosinophilia is not observed. In a few cases, however, *E. vermicularis* has been recovered from ectopic sites such as the appendix, female genital tract, and peritoneal cavity.

Diagnosis. Definitive diagnosis is established by either finding the parasite eggs or examining recovered worms. Eggs can easily be detected on adhesive cellophane tape pressed against the perianal region early in the morning. Repeated examinations may be necessary, and in certain situations examination of all family members may be advised. If a worm is seen in the perianal region, it should be preserved in 75% ethyl alcohol until microscopic examination can be performed.

Treatment. Drug therapy should be given to all infected and symptomatic individuals; mebendazole (single oral dose of 100 mg) is recommended. Piperazine salts or pyrvinium pamoate may also be used. While personal cleanliness is a useful general recommendation, there is no proof that it plays a significant role in control of enterobiasis.

10.120 Trichuriasis

Trichuris trichiura is the cause of 1 of the most common worm infections of man; approximately half a billion cases are estimated to occur worldwide. Infection is more common in warm climates but does exist in North America. In spite of its prevalence, *T. trichiura* infection

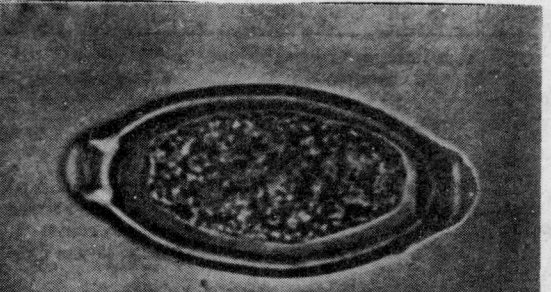

Figure 10–40 Egg of *Trichuris trichiura*, as seen in freshly passed feces. (×1000.)

is not associated with any specific clinical manifestations.

Etiology. Man is infected by ingestion of mature parasite eggs (Fig 10–40). These are passed in the stools of infected individuals and mature in 2–4 wk if moisture and temperature conditions of the soil are optimal. Upon ingestion by man *Trichuris* eggs hatch, and larvae penetrate the small intestinal villi where they remain for 3–10 days before slowly moving down the bowel and maturing to adult worms. The final habitat of these organisms is the cecum and ascending colon. *T. trichiura* are called whipworms because of their characteristic shape. The body is divided into an anterior whip-like portion and a posterior bulky part and measures approximately 40 mm in length. The worms remain in the gut by anchoring the anterior portion of their body to the intestinal mucosa. Egg deposition by maturing females begins 1–3 mo after infection.

Epidemiology. Trichuriasis is most common in poor rural communities where sanitary facilities are lacking. Man is the primary host; the highest prevalence and intensity of infection are in children. Transmission of embryonated eggs occurs by contamination of hands, food, or drink. Eggs may also be carried by flies and other insects.

Clinical Manifestations. Most infected individuals are asymptomatic; however, vague abdominal complaints, colic, and distention have been associated with infection. Adult *Trichuris* suck approximately 0.005 ml of blood/worm/day. However, only heavy infections in children may produce mild anemia, bloody diarrhea, or, rarely, rectal prolapse.

Diagnosis and Treatment. Direct examination of stool smears reveals the characteristic eggs of *T. trichiura*. An oral course of mebendazole (100 mg twice a day for 3 days) produces a cure rate of 70–90% and reduces egg output by 90–99%.

ADEL A. F. MAHMOUD

Ascariasis

Jandoes MF, Cornet P, Thienpont D: Mass control of ascariasis with single oral doses of levamisole. Trop Geogr Med 31:111, 1979.
Louw JH: Abdominal complications of *Ascaris lumbricoides* infestation in children. Br J Surg 53:510, 1966.

Spillman RK: Pulmonary ascariasis in tropical communities. Am J Trop Med Hyg 24:791, 1975.
Stephenson LS, Crompton DWT, Latham MC, et al: Relationship between *Ascaris* infection and growth of malnourished preschool children in Kenya. Am J Clin Nutr 33:1165, 1980.

Hookworms

Miller TA: Hookworm infection in man. Adv Parasitol 17:315, 1979.
Nawalinski T, Schad GA, Chowdhury AB: Population biology of hookworms in children in rural West Bengal. I. General parasitological observations. Am J Trop Med Hyg 27:1152, 1978.
Nawalinski T, Schad GA, Chowdhury AB: Population biology of hookworms in children in rural West Bengal. II. Acquisition and loss of hookworms. Am J Trop Med Hyg 27:1162, 1978.

Strongyloidiasis

Burke JA: Strongyloidiasis in childhood. Am J Dis Child 132:1130, 1978.
Scowden EB, Schaffner W, Stone WJ: Overwhelming strongyloidiasis. Medicine 57:527, 1978.
Smith JD, Goette DK, Odom RB: Larva currens: Cutaneous strongyloidiasis. Arch Dermatol 112:1161, 1976.

Enterobiasis

Boyer A, Berdknikoff IK: Pinworm infestation in children; the problem and its management. Can Med Assoc J 86:60, 1962.
Weller TH, Sorensen CW: Enterobiasis: Its incidence and symptomatology in a group of 505 children. N Engl J Med 224:131, 1941.

Trichuriasis

Blumenthal DS: Intestinal nematodes in the United States. N Engl J Med 297:1437, 1977.
Jung RC, Beaver PC: Clinical observations on *Trichocephalus trichiurus* (whipworm) infestation in children. Pediatrics 8:548, 1951.

TISSUE NEMATODES

Tissue-dwelling nematodes infect over 800 million people worldwide. Although morbidity from these helminths primarily afflicts the population of tropical and developing countries, inhabitants of regions with temperate climates may also be affected. These parasites have a complex life cycle which in most instances includes an intermediate invertebrate host. Disease in children results mainly when they act either as an incidental host in whom the helminth does not undergo its normal development (*Toxocara sp.*, *Dirofilaria sp.*) or as the definitive host (filariae, *Dracunculus medinensis*). Those infections which are particularly common in the pediatric age group (visceral larval migrans) will be presented first and will be followed by a discussion of tissue nematodes which cause disease in individuals of all ages (cutaneous larva migrans, *Trichinella spiralis*, *D. medinensis*) or primarily in adults (human and animal filariae). The major characteristics of these infections are outlined in Table 10–57.

10.121 Visceral Larva Migrans
(Toxocariasis)

Visceral larva migrans is caused by infection with larvae of *Toxocara sp.* The clinical syndrome associated with infection occurs most frequently in children under the age of 10 yr and is characterized by fever, hepatomegaly, pulmonary disease, and eosinophilia.

Etiology. *Toxocara canis*, *T. cati*, and *Toxascaris leonina* are common parasites of dogs and cats which infect

Table 10–57   TISSUE NEMATODE INFECTIONS OF CHILDREN

INFECTION	ETIOLOGY	MODE OF TRANSMISSION	MAJOR CLINICAL SYNDROMES	DIAGNOSIS
Visceral larva migrans	Toxocara canis, T. cati	Eggs in soil	Wheezing and cough, hepatomegaly; many infections asymptomatic	Serology, clinical
Ocular toxocariasis	Toxocara canis, T. cati	Eggs in soil	Decreased visual acuity	Serology, clinical
Trichinosis	Trichinella spiralis	Larvae in undercooked meat	Myalgias, fever, diarrhea	Serology and larvae in muscle biopsy
Dracunculosis	Dracunculus medinensis	Larvae in freshwater crustaceans	Skin ulceration	Clinical, larvae in ulcer
Filariases	Brugia malayi and Wuchereria bancrofti	Mosquitoes and flies	Acute: lymphangitis; chronic: elephantiasis	Microfilariae in blood or tissues
	Onchocerca volvulus	Mosquitoes and flies	Dermatitis, blindness	Microfilariae in blood or tissues
	Loa loa	Mosquitoes and flies	Calabar swelling	Microfilariae in blood or tissues
Tropical pulmonary eosinophilia	Filariae of unknown type	Mosquito	Asthma, fever	Chest x-ray, eosinophilia, serology
Animal filariae	Dirofilaria immitis, D. tenuis, Brugia beaveri	Mosquito	Pulmonary coin lesions, subcutaneous nodules	Identification of parasite in tissue sections

man when eggs of the helminth are ingested. Adult worms of *Toxocara sp.* reside in the gastrointestinal tract of these animals and release large numbers of eggs which are passed in the feces. Ingestion of these infective eggs by man is followed by larval penetration of the gastrointestinal tract and migration to liver, lung, and occasionally other sites (central nervous system, eye, kidney, and heart). *Toxocara* larvae do not develop beyond this stage in the human host.

Epidemiology. Visceral larva migrans is most common in young children 1–4 yr of age, particularly those who engage in pica and have close contact with dogs and cats; ocular toxocariasis occurs most frequently in older children. Potential sources of infection are widely distributed in the canine and feline population (it has been estimated that 20% of dogs in the United States excrete *Toxocara* eggs). These animals often defecate in areas where children play (24% of 800 soil samples taken from public parks in Great Britain were found to contain *Toxocara* eggs).

Pathology. *Toxocara* larvae usually elicit a granulomatous response characterized by large numbers of eosinophils, mononuclear cells, and tissue necrosis. These lesions are found in liver, lung, and other organs in which the helminth migrates. The inflammatory reaction to the parasite is much less intense in the eye, where lesions consist mainly of mononuclear cells and a few eosinophils.

Clinical Manifestations. Major symptoms of visceral larva migrans include fever (80%), cough with wheezing (60–80%), and seizures (20–30%). Respiratory distress may be severe enough to warrant hospitalization. Abdominal pain has been noted in occasional patients. Physical findings include hepatomegaly (65–87%), rales and/or rhonchi (40–50%), papular or urticarial skin lesions (20%), and lymph node enlargement (8%). These symptoms and signs subside over a period of several mo. Scattered patchy infiltrates are often seen on chest roentgenograms.

Patients with ocular toxocariasis most commonly present with decreased visual acuity (three fourths of cases) and occasionally with strabismus or periorbital edema. In 1 study unilateral blindness was noted in 6 of 17 patients. Most children do not have concurrent signs and symptoms of visceral disease. Funduscopic examination of the eye usually reveals solitary granulomatous lesions situated in the retina near the optic disc or macula. These may be mistaken for retinoblastomas and have led to inappropriate enucleation. Peripheral retinal lesions with vitreous bands and involvement of the iris have been documented in a few cases.

Diagnosis. The diagnosis of toxocariasis is made on the basis of the symptoms and signs described above and serologic testing. The only reliable and specific test currently available is an enzyme-linked immunosorbent assay (ELISA) which utilizes infective eggs of *T. canis* as antigen. This assay is positive (serum antibody titer ≥1:32) in 78% of cases of visceral larva migrans and in 45% of individuals with a clinical diagnosis of ocular toxocariasis. Eosinophilia (>500/mm³ blood) occurs in nearly all subjects with the visceral syndrome but is much less common with ocular disease. Nonspecific findings associated with *Toxocara* infection include elevations in serum gamma globulins and isohemagglutinins. Although larvae may be found upon examination of tissue sections, biopsy of liver or other organs is generally not indicated as clinical and laboratory data provide enough evidence to make the diagnosis.

Treatment. Therapeutic intervention is not required in the majority of cases since the signs and symptoms are usually mild and subside over a period of weeks to months. When significant hypoxemia secondary to pulmonary disease occurs, however, the administration of anti-inflammatory drugs (prednisone, 5 mg/kg/24 hr until respiratory function improves) is beneficial. When larvae lodge in critical locations, such as the eye, or disease is severe, the use of drugs with possible larvicidal activity (diethylcarbamazine, 0.5 mg/kg/24 hr for 3 days, increased gradually to 3 mg/kg/24 hr for 21 days) has been advocated. There is disagreement about this approach, however, as dying larvae theoretically may incite an inflammatory response which produces more tissue damage than encapsulated, dormant parasites.

Control. Transmission of *Toxocara* infection may be prevented by requiring children to wash their hands after playing with pets and instructing them to avoid areas where these animals defecate, particularly children with the habit of pica. Periodic deworming of dogs, especially puppies below the age of 6 mo, also decreases the likelihood of infection.

10.122 Cutaneous Larva Migrans
(Creeping Eruption)

Cutaneous larva migrans is caused by several larval nematodes not usually parasitic for man. *Ancylostoma braziliense* (a hookworm of dogs and cats) is the most common of these helminths, but other animal hookworms (*A. caninum, Uncinaria stenocephala,* and *Bunostomum phlebotosum*) and human parasites (*Necator americanus, Ancylostoma duodenale,* and *Strongyloides stercoralis*) may produce the disease. These organisms are widely distributed throughout tropical and subtropical areas of the world. In the United States infections are most prevalent in the South. Eggs of the parasite are deposited in the feces of animals and hatch to form infective larvae in warm moist areas, such as near vegetation on beaches or under porches. Man is infected when the skin comes in contact with these larvae.

Clinical Manifestations. After penetrating the skin, larvae localize at the epidermal-dermal junction and migrate in this plane, moving at a rate of 1–2 cm/day. The response to the parasite is characterized by raised, erythematous, serpiginous tracks which occasionally form bullae (Fig 10–41 [p. xxxii]). These lesions may be single or multiple and are usually localized to an extremity, although any area of the body may be affected. As the organism migrates, new areas of involvement may appear every few days. Intense localized pruritus may be associated with the lesions.

Diagnosis and Treatment. Cutaneous larva migrans is diagnosed on the basis of clinical examination of the skin. Patients are often able to recall the exact time and location of exposure as the larvae produce intense itching at the site of penetration. If left untreated, the larvae die and the syndrome resolves within a few wk to several mo.

10.123 Trichinosis

Human infection with *Trichinella spiralis* is fairly common worldwide. Infection is transmitted to man by ingestion of pork or other meat carrying the parasite. Recent sporadic epidemics have occurred in North America following ingestion of bear meat.

Etiology. Man is infected with *Trichinella spiralis* when flesh contaminated with viable larvae is eaten. This stage of the parasite excysts in the stomach and matures to form adult worms within the small intestine. Female *T. spiralis* release large numbers of newborn larvae which penetrate the gut wall and migrate to striated muscles or occasionally to other sites such as the central nervous system and heart. Larvae which enter muscle cells eventually become encysted and may remain viable for years. The life cycle in nature is maintained by hogs or other animals which ingest garbage containing carcasses of infected rodents.

Epidemiology. *T. spiralis* is found in all areas of the world except Australia and some islands in the South Pacific. Although infection with this helminth was common in the United States in the past (4% of diaphragms examined post mortem in 1968 contained viable larvae), recent cases in North America have been related to outbreaks from ingestion of undercooked homemade sausage, other pork products, or meat of bears, wild pigs, and walruses. Larvae are destroyed by cooking meat until there is no trace of pink fluid or flesh (this occurs at 55° C) or by storage in a freezer at −15° C for 3 wk. Smoked or salted meat may still contain viable parasites.

Pathology and Pathogenesis. Adult worms of *T. spiralis* are localized in the upper gastrointestinal tract and induce a mucosal inflammatory reaction characterized by a reduced villous:crypt ratio and the presence of eosinophils, neutrophils, and mononuclear cells. This response reaches its peak within the 1st wk of infection, then gradually subsides as adult worms are expelled. In muscle cells migratory larvae elicit a host pathologic reaction which consists of large numbers of eosinophils and mononuclear cells. These lesions may eventually calcify.

Clinical Manifestations. The signs and symptoms of *T. spiralis* infection appear only in heavily infected individuals. Within the 1st wk adult worms in the upper gastrointestinal tract produce gastroenteritis and diarrhea associated with abdominal discomfort. Next, during larval invasion of muscle, periorbital or facial edema (80% of cases), and myalgias occur. Pain is associated with muscle activity; it is most common in the masseters, diaphragm, and intercostals. These signs and symptoms are first noted 10–14 days after infection and last for another 2–3 wk. Heart failure and arrhythmias may occur in patients with exceptionally heavy infections.

Diagnosis. The findings of periorbital edema, myalgias, fever, and eosinophilia in an individual who gives a history of eating undercooked meat make the diagnosis of trichinosis likely. A history of similar illness in those sharing the food should be sought. Serologic studies such as the bentonite flocculation test (titer of 1:5 or greater) are confirmatory. Biopsy of muscle, usually the deltoid, may reveal larvae upon microscopic examination 3–4 wk after infection. Muscle enzymes such as creatine phosphate kinase and lactate dehydrogenase are elevated in 50% of patients.

Treatment. There is no therapy for the clinical syndrome related to larval invasion of muscles. Thiabendazole (25 mg/kg/24 hr for 1 wk) is active only against adult worms and should therefore be given only to those rare individuals who were known to acquire the infection in the preceding 1–7 days. Corticosteroids may be used in critically ill patients, such as those with myocarditis or central nervous system damage, but evidence for their beneficial effect is equivocal.

10.124　Dracunculosis
(Guinea Worm Infection)

Dracunculosis occurs in all areas of the tropics and is especially common in India and West Africa. The parasite, *Dracunculus medinensis*, infects man when he swallows larval-containing microscopic crustaceans (copepods) living in communal water sites. Adult worms grow to a length of 1 meter or more and migrate through the subcutaneous tissues of the lower extremities (or occasionally other sites). An ulcer is produced when they penetrate the skin. The diagnosis is confirmed by identification of larvae contained in washings from the base of the lesion. Administration of niridazole (12.5 mg/kg/24 hr for 2 days) or thiabendazole (25 mg/kg/24 hr for 2 days) diminishes the local inflammatory response and permits removal of the helminth. Infection may be prevented by avoiding ingestion of water that humans walk in or use for bathing. Boiling or chlorination kills the organism.

10.125　Filariases

Filariae are thread-like nematodes which may cause significant human morbidity. Disease due to infection with these organisms usually becomes evident years after exposure; it is thus uncommon for children to have clinically significant filariasis.

10.126　Malayan and Bancroftian Filariasis

Infection with *Brugia malayi* or *Wuchereria bancrofti* results in similar clinical syndromes characterized in the early stages by acute lymphangitis and lymphadenitis and later by lymphatic obstruction with hydrocele and elephantiasis. It is estimated that over 200 million people in developing countries are infected with these parasites.

Etiology.　Filarial larvae are introduced into man in secretions of biting mosquitoes. Over several mo to 1 yr this stage of the helminth develops into adult worms which reside in the lymphatics. Sexually mature adult female worms release large numbers of microfilariae which circulate in the bloodstream. The life cycle of the parasite is completed when mosquitoes ingest these organisms in a blood meal.

Epidemiology.　Although as much as 80% of the population of endemic areas may be infected, fewer than 10–20% of these subjects have clinically significant morbidity. Individuals most at risk are those who work in areas where there is repeated and chronic exposure to larvae-containing mosquitoes, such as in crowded urban areas with poor sanitation. *W. bancrofti* infection is distributed throughout tropical and subtropical Africa, Asia, and South America, while infection with *B. malayi* is restricted to the South Pacific and Southeast Asia.

Clinical Manifestations.　The acute stage of infection is characterized by episodes of fever, lymphangitis of an extremity, headaches, and myalgias which last a few days to several wk. This syndrome is most frequently observed in young people 10–20 yr old. Chronic manifestations of disease, such as hydrocele and ele-phantiasis, occur mostly in those over 30 and are a direct result of lymphatic fibrosis and obstruction to lymph flow. The presence of larvae (microfilariae) in the blood is not thought to have any pathologic consequences.

Diagnosis and Treatment.　The demonstration of microfilariae in the blood is the only way to diagnose lymphatic-dwelling filariasis. Ten ml of blood obtained at a time of day when the number of parasites in the circulation is expected to be highest (this varies with the geographic strain of filaria) should be filtered and examined for the organisms.

The use of antifilarial drugs must be individualized. Older patients with chronic lymphatic obstruction and those who remain in endemic areas will not benefit from specific therapy. Younger individuals with acute lymphangitis should be given a course of diethylcarbamazine (50 mg on day 1, 50 mg 2 and 3 times on days 2 and 3, respectively, then 10 mg/kg on days 4–21).

10.127　Onchocerciasis, Loiasis, and Tropical Pulmonary Eosinophilia

Infection with *Onchocerca volvulus* (onchocerciasis, river blindness) is a major cause of blindness in West Africa and Central America. The parasite is introduced into man by blackflies of the genus *Simulium* which breed in rapidly running water; people who live or work near waterways are thus most likely to be infected. Most individuals with onchocerciasis are asymptomatic. Subjects with chronic and heavy infections (usually men over 30 yr old) may suffer from pruritic dermatitis and eye disease (punctate keratitis, corneal pannus formation, chorioretinitis). These lesions are due to the presence of microfilariae in subcutaneous and ocular tissues. Firm, nontender subcutaneous nodules containing adult parasites may also be palpable. *O. volvulus* infection is diagnosed by demonstration of parasites in skin snips removed from the buttocks or extremities or by visualization with a slit lamp of microfilariae in the cornea or anterior chamber of the eye. Patients with skin and eye disease should be treated with diethylcarbamazine as described for lymphatic filariasis and observed carefully for eye reactions (decreased visual acuity and iritis), increased pruritus with desquamation, and fever. If these reactions appear, corticosteroids should be administered.

Loa loa infection occurs in the rain forest of West and Central Africa; the parasite is transmitted to man by tabanid flies. Adult worms migrate in the subcutaneous tissues and produce painful transient areas of localized edema known as calabar swellings. These tend to appear around the joints of the legs and arms. The parasite occasionally may be directly visualized in the conjunctiva, where it produces an intense inflammatory reaction. Microfilariae of *L. loa* are present in highest concentrations in the peripheral circulation between 10 AM–2 PM; identification in blood samples is diagnostic. Symptomatic individuals should be given gradually increasing doses of diethylcarbamazine as described for onchocerciasis. Therapy should be discontinued and corticosteroids administered if fever, headache, or joint swelling occurs.

Tropical pulmonary eosinophilia (TPE) is a syndrome caused by infection with microfilariae of unspecified types. It occurs only in subjects who have lived for at least several mo in endemic areas of bancroftian or malayan filariasis and is most common in Southeast Asia and the South Pacific. Although TPE has been observed in children, 20–30 yr old men are most likely to be affected. Patients present with paroxsymal non-productive cough, occasional episodes of dyspnea, fever, weight loss, and fatigue. Rales and rhonchi are found on auscultation of the chest; roentgenographic examination may occasionally be normal but usually reveals increased bronchovascular marking, discrete opacities in the middle and basal regions of the lung, or diffuse miliary lesions 1–3 mm in diameter. Recurrent untreated episodes may result in interstitial fibrosis and chronic respiratory insufficiency. In children hepatosplenomegaly and generalized lymphadenopathy are often seen. Eosinophilia (>2000/mm^3 blood) with the appropriate history and symptoms suggests the diagnosis. Increased serum IgE levels (>1000 units/ml) and high titers of antimicrofilarial antibodies in the absence of blood-borne helminths should also be documented. Although microfilariae may be found in sections of lung or lymph node, biopsy is unwarranted in most patients. The clinical response to diethylcarbamazine (5 mg/kg/24 hr for 10 days) is the final criterion for diagnosis. In the majority of patients symptoms improve with this therapy. If they recur, a 2nd course of the drug should be administered. Subjects presenting with chronic symptoms are less likely to show improvement than those who have been ill for a short time.

10.128 Infection with Animal Filariae

Humans may be infected with 3 types of animal filariae. *Dirofilaria immitis*, the heartworm, is found on all continents and is a common parasite of dogs in many parts of the United States. *D. tenuis*, *Brugia beaveri*, and other unclassified *Brugia sp.* have also been reported to infect man. These worms may be introduced into man by the bite of mosquitoes containing 3rd-stage larvae. The organisms, however, do not undergo normal development in the human host. *D. immitis* are trapped in the lung parenchyma after migration in the subcutaneous tissues for several mo. The pulmonary response consists of granulomas with eosinophils, neutrophils, and tissue necrosis. *D. tenuis* does not leave the subcutaneous tissues, while *B. beaveri* eventually localizes to superficial lymph nodes.

Most human infections with *D. immitis* are discovered incidentally when the chest roentgenogram reveals a solitary pulmonary nodule 1–3 cm in diameter. Definitive diagnosis and cure depend on surgical excision and identification of the nematode within the surrounding granulomatous response. *D. tenuis* and *B. beaveri* infections present as painful, rubbery 1–5 cm diameter nodules in the skin of the trunk, extremities, and orbit. Patients often report engaging in activities suggestive of exposure to infected mosquitoes, such as working in swampy areas. Diagnosis and management of these infections are similar to those of *D. immitis*.

JAMES W. KAZURA

Toxocariasis

Huntley CC, Costas MC, Lyerly A: Visceral larva migrans syndrome: Clinical characteristics and immunologic studies in 51 patients. Pediatrics 36:623, 1965.
Schantz PM, Glickman LT: Toxocaral visceral larva migrans. N Engl J Med 298:436, 1978.
Zinkham WH: Visceral larva migrans. A review and reassessment indicating two forms of clinical expression: Visceral and ocular. Am J Dis Child 132:627, 1978.

Filariasis

Grove DI, Valeza FS, Cabrera BD: Bancroftian filariasis in a Philippine village: Clinical, parasitological, immunological and social aspects. Bull World Health Org 56:975, 1978.
Grove DI, Warren KS, Mahmoud AAF: Filariasis. *In:* Warren KS, Mahmoud AAF (eds): Geographic Medicine for the Practitioner. Chicago, University of Chicago Press, 1978, p 85.
Neva FA, Ottesen EA: Tropical (filarial) eosinophilia. N Engl J Med 298:1129, 1978.

TREMATODES
(Flukes)

Parasitic trematodes form a group of important and prevalent human infections. Trematodes are characterized by their complex life cycle; sexual reproduction of adult worms in the definitive host is followed by asexual multiplication by the larval stages in the intermediate host. This phenomenon, called alternation of generations, requires that flukes parasitize more than 1 host (often 3) to complete their life cycle. Trematode infections are endemic worldwide but are more prevalent in the less developed parts of the world. The most important infections of man are outlined in Table 10–58. Discussion of each trematode infection will be presented according to the site of final habitat in the definitive host.

BLOOD FLUKES

10.129 Schistosomes

Three main schistosome species infect man; these are *Schistosoma haematobium*, *S. mansoni*, and *S. japonicum*. Schistosomiasis infects more than 200 million people, mainly children and young adults. With the necessity of developing irrigation projects, the infection is spreading as more suitable habitats for the snail intermediate host are created. *S. haematobium* is prevalent in Africa and the Middle East; *S. mansoni* in Africa, the Middle East, Caribbean, and South America; and *S. japonicum* in China, the Philippines, and Indonesia, with some sporadic foci in Japan and other parts of Southeast Asia. Infection with any of the schistosome species is not endemic in North America or Europe; however, as many as half a million infected individuals (mainly Puerto Ricans) are believed to live currently in the United States.

Etiology. Man is infected upon contact with water contaminated with cercariae, the infective forms of the parasite. These motile, forked-tail organisms emerge from infected snails and are capable of penetrating intact human skin within a few min. In the subcutaneous tissues cercariae change into another larval stage

Table 10-58 IMPORTANT TREMATODE INFECTIONS OF CHILDREN

INFECTION	ETIOLOGY	MODE OF TRANSMISSION	MAJOR CLINICAL SYNDROMES	DIAGNOSIS
Schistosomiasis	Schistosoma haematobium	Cercariae in fresh water	Hematuria, dysuria, and obstructive uropathy	Eggs in urine
	S. mansoni, S. japonicum	Cercariae in fresh water	Hepatosplenomegaly, portal hypertension	Eggs in feces
Clonorchiasis	Clonorchis sinensis	Metacercariae in freshwater fish	Mainly asymptomatic	Eggs in feces
Opisthorchiasis	Opisthorchis felineus and O. viverrini	Metacercariae in freshwater fish	Mainly asymptomatic	Eggs in feces
Fascioliasis	Fasciola hepatica	Metacercaria on aquatic vegetation	Early: fever, hepatomegaly, and eosinophilia Late: mainly asymptomatic	Eggs in feces
Fasciolopsiasis	Fasciolopsis buski	Metacercaria on aquatic plants	Mainly asymptomatic	Eggs in feces
Paragonimiasis	Paragonimus westermani	Metacercaria in freshwater crayfish or crabs	Hemoptysis, productive cough, and eosinophilia	Eggs in sputum or feces

(schistosomula) and migrate to the lungs and finally the liver. The pathway of migration is still controversial, but in 2–4 wk maturing adult worms appear in the portal circulation. Once they reach sexual maturation, adult worms migrate to specific anatomic sites characteristic of each schistosome species: *S. haematobium* adults are found in the vesical plexus, *S. mansoni* in the inferior mesenteric, and *S. japonicum* in the superior mesenteric veins. Adult schistosome worms (1–2 cm in length) are different from most other flukes in that they exist as separate sexes; the female, however, accompanies the male in a groove formed by the lateral edges of its body. Upon fertilization, female worms begin oviposition in the small venous tributaries. The eggs of each schistosome species have characteristic morphologic features: *S. haematobium*, terminal spine; *S. mansoni*, lateral spine; and *S. japonicum*, smaller size with a short curved spine (Fig 10–42). Eggs force themselves out of the blood vessels through surrounding tissues to reach the lumen of urinary tract or intestines, where they are carried to the outside. *S. haematobium* eggs are usually seen in urine and those of the other 2 species in feces of infected individuals. A certain proportion of the schistosome eggs may fail to reach the outside, get trapped in the host tissues, and elicit most of the pathologic lesions associated with schistosomiasis. Eggs which reach the outside environment hatch if deposited in fresh water. Motile miracidia emerge; they infect specific fresh water snail intermediate hosts and divide asexually. In 4–6 wk the infective cercariae are released in the water.

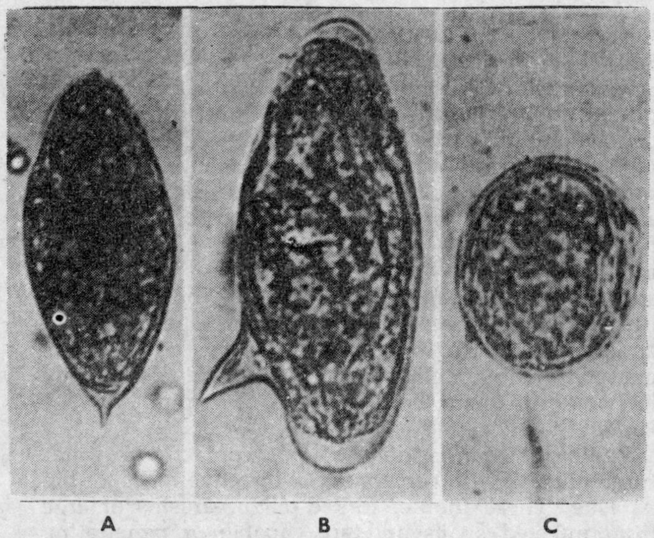

Epidemiology. Man is the definitive host for the 3 clinically important species of schistosomes, although *S. japonicum* may infect some animals such as dogs and cattle. Transmission of schistosomiasis depends on several factors, including disposal of excreta, the presence of specific intermediate snail hosts, and the patterns of water contact and social habits of the population. The distribution of infection in endemic areas shows that incidence increases with age to a maximum in the 10–20 yr age group, after which it declines. Furthermore, measurement of intensity of infection (by egg count in urine or feces) demonstrates that most infected individuals have light infections; the smaller proportion of patients with heavy worm loads is usually found in the younger age groups. Schistosomiasis, therefore, is most prevalent and severe in children and young adults who are at maximal risk of suffering from its disease sequelae. The explanation of this pattern may relate to immunologic, ecologic, or genetic factors.

Pathology and Pathogenesis. The major pathologic lesions due to schistosomiasis are associated with retention of eggs in the host tissues during the chronic stages of infection. Eggs may be trapped at sites of deposition (urinary bladder, ureters, intestine) or be carried by the bloodstream to other organs, most commonly the liver but less often the lungs and central nervous system. The host response to these eggs involves local as well as systemic manifestations. Granulomas composed of lymphocytes, macrophages, and eosinophils surround the trapped eggs and add significantly to the size of tissue destruction. It has been shown that these granulomas are due to cell-mediated responses in *S. haema-*

Figure 10-42 Eggs of *Schistosoma hematobium* (A), *Schistosoma mansoni* (B), and *Schistosoma japonicum* (C). (×320.)

tobium and *S. mansoni* infections; their origin in schistosomiasis japonica remains unclear, however. Granuloma formation in the bladder wall and at the ureterovesical junction leads to the major disease manifestations of schistosomiasis hematobia: hematuria, dysuria, and obstructive uropathy. Intestinal as well as hepatic granulomas underlie the pathologic sequelae of the other 2 schistosome infections: ulcerations and fibrosis of intestinal wall, hepatosplenomegaly, and portal hypertension due to presinusoidal obstruction of blood flow. Fibrosis usually follows the granulomatous process and adds to pathophysiologic changes. Granuloma formation undergoes modulation in chronically infected individuals with a decrease in size and diminution in pathologic sequelae, a phenomenon perhaps related to some of the systemic host responses (antibody, immune complexes, suppressor cells) which ultimately function as ameliorating factors. The development of protective immunity against schistosomiasis has been conclusively demonstrated in some animal species but not in man. The decrease in the prevalence and intensity of infection in the older age groups in endemic areas may be related to the development of immunity or to decreased water exposure.

Clinical Manifestations. Most infected individuals suffer from no apparent ill health; symptomatology occurs mainly in heavily infected individuals. Cercarial penetration of human skin may result in a papular pruritic rash (swimmer's itch). It is more pronounced in previously exposed individuals and involves edema and massive cellular infiltrates in the dermis and epidermis. Katayama fever may occur, particularly in heavily infected individuals 4–8 wk after exposure, and is a serum sickness–like syndrome manifest by the acute onset of fever, chills, sweating, lymphadenopathy, hepatosplenomegaly, and eosinophilia. Its pathogenesis is unknown but may be due to immune complex formation.

Symptomatic children with chronic schistosomiasis haematobia usually complain of frequency, dysuria, and hematuria (often terminal). Urine examination shows erythrocytes, parasite eggs, and occasional leukocytes. Intravenous pyelography demonstrates the extent of granulomatous lesions in the ureters and bladder and the consequences of obstructive uropathy. In most endemic areas extensive pathologic lesions have been demonstrated in the urinary tract of more than half of infected children. The extent of disease is correlated to intensity of infection, but significant morbidity may occur even in lightly infected children. The terminal stages of schistosomiasis haematobia are associated with chronic renal failure, secondary infections, and cancer of the bladder in some endemic areas.

Children with chronic schistosomiasis mansoni or japonica may have intestinal symptoms; colicky abdominal pain and bloody diarrhea are the most common. The intestinal phase may, however, pass unnoticed, and the syndrome of hepatosplenomegaly, portal hypertension, ascites, and hematemesis may be the initial presentation. Liver disease in either form of schistosomiasis is due to granuloma formation and subsequent fibrosis; there is no appreciable liver cell injury, and hepatic function may be preserved for a long time.

Schistosome eggs may escape into the pulmonary vasculature causing hypertension and cor pulmonale. Furthermore, *S. japonicum* worms may migrate to the brain vasculature and produce seizures.

Diagnosis. Schistosome eggs are found in the excreta of infected individuals; quantitative procedures should be used as they give an indication of intensity of infection. Urine should be collected around midday (time of maximal egg excretion) and 10 ml filtered through a nucleopore membrane for diagnosis of *S. haematobium* infection. Stool examination by the Kato thick smear procedure is the method of choice for diagnosis and quantification of *S. mansoni* and *S. japonicum* infections.

Treatment. Management of children with schistosomiasis should be based on intensity of infection and extent of disease. The drug of choice for *S. haematobium* infection is metrifonate given orally in a dose of 7.5 mg/kg to be repeated twice at 2 wk intervals. For *S. mansoni* infection, oxamniquine in a single oral dose of 20 mg/kg is effective; individuals infected in Africa may need higher doses (up to 60 mg/kg). Treatment of schistosomiasis japonica has benefited from the recent introduction of praziquantel; it is given orally (30 mg/kg, twice daily).

Control. Transmission of schistosomiasis in endemic areas may be decreased by reduction of the parasite load in the population. The availability of oral, single dose, effective chemotherapeutic agents may facilitate achievement of this goal. Other measures, particularly sanitary, socioeconomic, and focal application of molluscicides, are adjunct tools in attempts to contain the infection.

10.130 LIVER FLUKES

Clonorchiasis

Infection of bile passages with the Chinese or Oriental fluke *Clonorchis sinensis* is endemic in China, other parts of Southeast Asia, and Japan. Man acquires infection with *C. sinensis* by ingestion of raw or inadequately cooked freshwater fish carrying the encysted metacercariae of the parasite under its scales or skin. These metacercariae excyst in the duodenum and pass through the ampulla of Vater to the common bile duct and bile capillaries, where they mature into hermaphroditic adult worms (3 × 15 mm). *C. sinensis* worms deposit small operculated eggs (14 × 30 μm), which are discharged via the bile duct to the intestine and feces (Fig 10–43). The eggs mature and hatch, releasing motile miracidiae. If these are ingested by specific snails, numerous cercariae develop, which may escape and encyst under the skin or scales of freshwater fish.

Most *C. sinensis*–infected individuals, particularly those with light infections, are asymptomatic. Localized obstruction of a bile duct and thickening of its walls may be the result of repeated local trauma and inflammation in heavily infected individuals. In these cases cholangitis and cholangiohepatitis may lead to liver enlargement and jaundice. In Hong Kong cholangiocarcinoma in the Chinese population is associated with *C.*

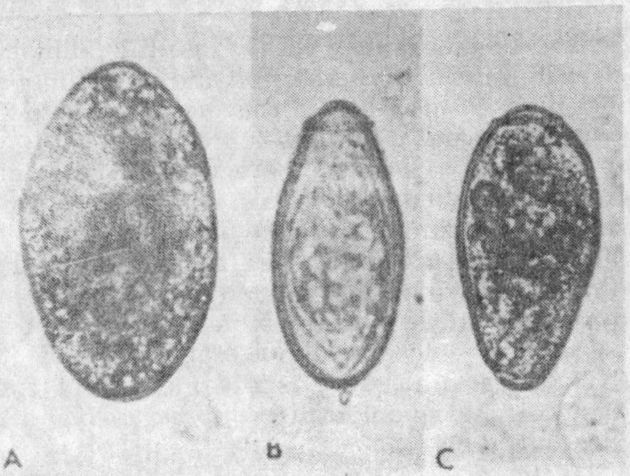

Figure 10–43 Eggs of liver flukes and a lung fluke. A, *Fasciola hepatica* (×400). B, *Clonorchis sinensis* (×1000). C, *Paragonimus westermani* (×400).

sinensis infection. Diagnosis of clonorchiasis may be made by examination of feces or duodenal aspirates for the parasite eggs. Praziquantel has recently been reported to be effective against clonorchiasis.

Opisthorchiasis

Infections with species of *Opisthorchis* are clinically similar to clonorchiasis. *O. felineus* and *O. viverrini* are common liver flukes of cats and dogs which may occasionally infect man through ingestion of metacercariae in freshwater fish. Infection with *O. felineus* is endemic in eastern Europe and Southeast Asia, and *O. viverrini* is found mainly in Thailand. Most individuals are asymptomatic; liver enlargement, relapsing cholangitis, and jaundice may be seen in heavily infected individuals. Adenocarcinoma of bile ducts has been described, but its causal relationship to opisthorchiasis is not clear. Diagnosis is based on recovery of eggs from stools or duodenal aspirates. Praziquantel is the drug of choice.

Fascioliasis

The sheep liver fluke *Fasciola hepatica* infects cattle, other ungulates, and occasionally man. Human infection has been reported from different parts of the world, particularly South America, Europe, Africa, China, and Australia. Although *F. hepatica* is enzootic in North America, human cases are extremely rare. Man is infected by ingestion of metacercariae attached to vegetations, especially wild watercress. In the duodenum the parasites excyst; penetrate the intestinal wall, liver capsule, and parenchyma; and wander for a few wk before entering the bile ducts where they mature. Adult *F. hepatica* (1 × 2.5 cm) commence oviposition approximately 12 wk after infection; the eggs are large (75 × 140 μm) and operculated, pass to the intestines with bile, and leave the body in the feces (Fig 10–43). On reaching fresh water, the eggs mature and hatch into miracidia, which infect specific snail intermediate hosts

to multiply into many cercariae. Cercariae emerge from infected snails and encyst on aquatic grasses and plants.

Clinical manifestations of fascioliasis usually occur either during the liver migratory phase of the parasites or after their arrival at their final habitat in bile canaliculi. The 1st phase is characterized by fever, right upper quadrant pain, and hepatosplenomegaly. Peripheral blood eosinophilia is usually marked. As the worms enter bile ducts, most of the acute symptoms subside. On rare occasions, patients may suffer from obstructive jaundice or biliary cirrhosis. *F. hepatica* infection is diagnosed by finding the characteristic eggs in fecal smears or duodenal aspirates. Praziquantel or bithionol may be used for treatment.

10.131   INTESTINAL FLUKES

Several wild and domestic animal intestinal flukes, such as *Fasciolopsis buski* and *Heterophyes heterophyes*, may accidentally infect man. The clinical significance of most of these infections is doubtful and not fully understood. *Fasciolopsis buski* is endemic in the Far East. Man is infected by ingestion of metacercariae encysted on aquatic plants. They hatch and produce large flukes (1 × 5 cm) which inhabit the duodenum and jejunum. Mature worms produce operculated eggs that pass with feces; the organisms, like *F. hepatica*, completes its life cycle through specific snail intermediate hosts. Individuals with *F. buski* infection are usually asymptomatic; heavily infected subjects complain of diarrhea and abdominal pain and show signs of malabsorption. Diagnosis of fasciolopsis is made by fecal examination for eggs. As in other fluke infections, praziquantel is the drug of choice.

10.132   LUNG FLUKES
(Paragonimiasis)

Human infection by the lung fluke *Paragonimus westermani* occurs throughout the Far East, in localized areas of West Africa, and in several parts of Central and South America. A recent report of an epidemic of pulmonary paragonimiasis showed a maximal incidence in the age group 11–15 yr. Although *P. westermani* is found in many carnivora, human cases are relatively rare and seem to be associated with specific dietary habits such as eating raw freshwater crayfish or crabs. These crustaceans contain the infected metacercariae in their tissues; they excyst in the duodenum, penetrate the intestinal wall, and migrate to their final habitat in the lungs. Adult worms (5 × 10 mm) encapsulate within the lung parenchyma and deposit brown operculated eggs (60 × 100 μm), which pass into the bronchioles and are coughed up (Fig 10–43). Ova can be detected in the sputum of infected individuals or in their feces. If eggs reach fresh water, they hatch and undergo asexual multiplication in specific snails. The cercariae encyst in the muscles and viscera of crayfish and freshwater crabs.

Most individuals infected with *P. westermani* harbor

low or moderate worm loads and are asymptomatic. In symptomatic infected children hemoptysis occurs in 98% of cases; other pulmonary symptoms include cough and production of rusty-colored sputum. There are no characteristic physical findings, but laboratory examination usually demonstrates marked eosinophilia. Chest roentgenogram often reveals small patchy infiltrates or radiolucencies in the mid-lung fields; however, the roentgenogram may be normal in one fifth of infected individuals. In rare circumstances lung abscess, pleural effusion, or bronchiectasis may be demonstrable. Extrapulmonary localization of *P. westermani* in the brain, peritoneum, intestines, or pleura may rarely occur. Cerebral paragonimiasis is seen primarily in individuals with heavy infections in highly endemic areas of the Far East. The clinical presentation of *P. westermani* infection in the brain resembles jacksonian epilepsy or cerebral tumors. Definitive diagnosis of paragonimiasis is made by finding eggs in fecal or sputum smears. The treatment of choice is praziquantel (25 mg/kg) given orally 3 times for 1 day.

Schistosomiasis

Domingo EO, Tiu E, Peters PA, et al: Morbidity in schistosomiasis japonica in relation to intensity of infection: Study of a community in Leyte, Philippines. Am J Trop Med Hyg 29:858, 1980.
Mahmoud AAF: Schistosomiasis. *In:* Wyngaarden JB, Smith LH Jr (eds): Cecil Textbook of Medicine. Ed 16. Philadelphia, WB Saunders, 1982.
Siongok TKA, Mahmoud AAF, Ouma JH, et al: Morbidity in schistosomiasis mansoni in relation to intensity of infection: Study of a community in Machakos, Kenya. Am J Trop Med Hyg 25:273, 1976.
Warren KS, Mahmoud AAF, Muruka JF, et al: Schistosomiasis haematobia in Coast Province Kenya. Am J Trop Med Hyg 28:864, 1979.

Other Flukes

Drugs for parasitic infections. Medical Letter 24:5, 1982.
Fischer GW, McGrew GL, Bass JW: Pulmonary paragonimiasis in childhood. JAMA 243:1360, 1980.
Seah SKK: Digenetic trematodes. Clin Gastroenterol 7:87, 1978.
Straus WG: Clinical manifestations of clonorchiasis. A controlled study of 105 cases. Am J Trop Med Hyg 11:625, 1962.

CESTODES
(Tapeworms)

Man serves as the main definitive host of some of the cestodes, the segmented or tapeworms; other worms of this class parasitize lower animals, human infection occurring only incidentally. In the most common cestode infections of man, adult worms parasitize the gastrointestinal tract and cause little or no clinical morbidity except when they interfere with host nutrition. Major clinical syndromes may occur, however, when man is infected with the larval stages of some cestodes which disseminate and can cause disease in any internal organ. The common cestode infections of children are outlined in Table 10–59.

10.133 TENIASIS AND DIPHYLLOBOTHRIASIS
(Giant Tapeworms)

There are 3 giant tapeworms which may cause infection in man. All 3 infections may be acquired by ingesting animal flesh which contains the larval stage of the parasites. *T. saginata* is found in all parts of the world and is particularly common in East Africa; in North America it is estimated to infect 23 persons/100,000 population. The exact prevalence of *T. solium* is not known but is reportedly less than that of *T. saginata*; the infection is most endemic in India, China, South Africa, Central Europe, and some parts of South America. Teniasis solium is not endemic in North America. *D. latum* is endemic in countries with cold lakes such as Scandinavia, Northern Europe, Siberia, China, and North and South America. Parasitized fish may also be found in lakes at high altitudes in tropical areas, such as Uganda, Zaire, and Central Africa.

Etiology. Man is infected by ingestion of raw or undercooked flesh. Infective larvae of *T. saginata* are found in beef, those of *T. solium* in pork, and those of *D. latum* in freshwater fish. The cysticerci of taeniae (5 × 10 mm) or the plerocercoids of *D. latum* (3 × 20 mm) start their development upon reaching the human small intestine and mature in several mo. Adult tapeworms consist of ribbon-like segments, approximately 1000 in *T. solium*, 2000 in *T. saginata*, and 4000 in *D. latum*. Mature worms vary in length from 4–10 meters. Identification of the particular tapeworm species is made by microscopic examination of mature segments which may passively (*T. solium*) or actively (*T. saginata*) find their way out of the intestinal tract through the anus. Taenia eggs are rarely seen in stools. They are small

Table 10–59 IMPORTANT CESTODE INFECTIONS OF CHILDREN

INFECTION	ETIOLOGY	MODE OF TRANSMISSION	MAJOR CLINICAL SYNDROMES	DIAGNOSIS
Teniasis	*Taenia saginata*	Cysticerca in beef	Passage of segments through anus	Microscopy of segments
	T. solium	Cysticerca in pork	Mainly asymptomatic	Microscopy of segments
Cysticercosis	*T. solium*	Ingestion of eggs	Space occupying lesion in brain, muscles, etc.	Clinical and serology
Diphyllobothriasis	*Diphyllobothrium latum*	Plerocercoid in freshwater fish	B$_{12}$ deficiency	Eggs in feces
Hymenolepiasis	*Hymenolepis nana*	Ingestion of eggs	Mainly asymptomatic	Eggs in stool
Echinococcosis	*Echinococcus granulosus*	Ingestion of eggs	Cysts in liver, lungs, brain, or bones	Clinical and serology

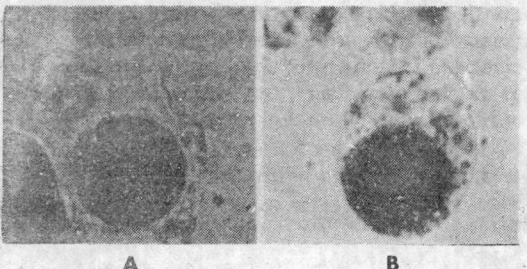

Figure 10–44   Eggs of *Taenia saginata* recovered from fresh feces. (×400.) The cellular structure in which the egg develops while in the proglottid, more evident in *B* than in *A*, may be retained around the dark prismatic egg-membrane which contains the larva. Usually evident in the larva are 3 pairs of hooklets *(A)* which occasionally may be seen in motion.

(35 μm in diameter) and yellowish brown and contain hooklets in their center (Fig 10–44). In contrast to *Taenia sp.*, *D. latum* segments usually deposit their eggs within the intestinal lumen. Therefore, the eggs can be easily seen in fecal smears of infected individuals. They are operculate and measure 45 × 75 μm (Fig 10–45). When eggs of *Taenia sp.* are ingested by the appropriate host, they are digested and embryos emerge. This stage of the helminth penetrates the intestinal wall, disseminates throughout the tissues, and develops into mature infectious cysticerci. The cysticercus stage of *T. saginata* can be formed only in cattle. Ingestion of *T. solium* eggs by man may, however, occasionally lead to the development of cysticercosis. Further development of *D. latum* eggs takes place in fish and crustacea; the infective forms finally lodge in the tissues of freshwater fish.

Epidemiology.   Human infection by any of the giant tapeworms is most common in adults. Transmission is primarily related to nutritional habits, fecal disposal practices, and the methods used to feed domestic animals. Thorough cooking or freezing destroys the infective stages of these parasites. Adult worms may live for decades; human infection is usually due to only 1 worm and has no adverse effects. Infection with many worms or with the larval stage of *T. solium* may, however, produce serious clinical manifestations.

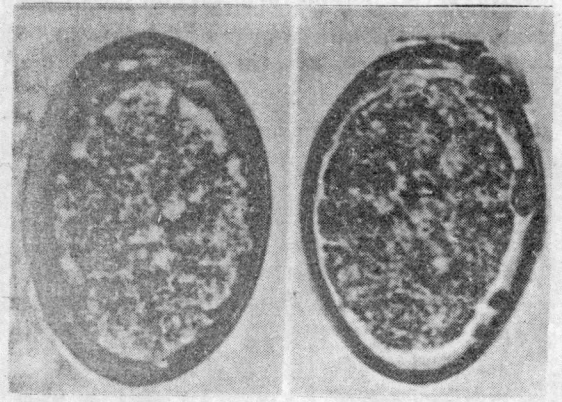

Figure 10–45   Eggs of *Diphyllobothrium latum* as seen in fresh feces. (×400.) The operculum is usually evident.

Clinical Manifestations.   Infection with adult *T. saginata* or *T. solium* is almost always asymptomatic. These parasites do not compete to any significant degree for host nutrients. The most frequent symptom in teniasis saginata is passage of motile segments through the anus. While a host of abdominal symptoms have been associated with tapeworm infections, none of these clinical observations have been based on properly controlled studies. Similar vague abdominal complaints have been associated with *D. latum* infection. The most important clinical sequela of this infection is vitamin B_{12} deficiency. Adult worms absorb the vitamin at a fast rate and may cause megaloblastic anemia in infected individuals. In Finland it was estimated that 0.1% of an infected population developed anemia. Typical morphologic changes in the bone marrow and subacute cord degeneration may be seen.

Human infection with the cysticercus stage of *T. solium* may be asymptomatic. However, heavy infection with localization of larvae in important anatomic areas, principally the brain, may lead to such manifestations of cysticercosis as generalized or focal seizures and raised intracranial pressure. Eosinophilia is variable in patients with cysticercosis.

Diagnosis.   Infection with *Taenia* worms is diagnosed by identification and morphologic characterization of adult segments; proper handling and preparation of the segments for microscopic examination are essential. *D. latum* infection is usually identified by direct smear examination of feces. Cysticercosis may be diagnosed by a combination of clinical presentations, roentgenographic examination to detect calcified cysts in brain or soft tissues, and serology. Hemagglutination titers are significantly elevated in 85% of individuals with cysticercosis.

Treatment.   All 3 giant tapeworm infections are treated with a single oral dose of niclosamide (2 tablets [1 gm] for children weighing 11–34 kg and 3 tablets [1.5 gm] for those above 34 kg). Patients with megaloblastic anemia due to *D. latum* infection should be given vitamin B_{12} and observed for neurologic complications. Symptomatic patients with cysticercosis are treated by palliative measures directed at control of their neurologic manifestations.

10.134 HYMENOLEPIASIS
(Dwarf Tapeworms)

Infection with *Hymenolepis nana* is most common in children living in warm climates; the prevalence ranges from 0.3–2.9% in North America. Although most children harbor light infections that are not associated with specific symptoms or signs, young children are more likely to develop heavy worm loads, possibly secondary to autoinfection, and may present with abdominal pain or diarrhea.

Infection is acquired by ingestion of eggs passed in feces of parasitized individuals. *H. nana* eggs are spherical or ovoid, measure 40 × 50 μm, and contain embryos with characteristic hooklets (Fig 10–46). The ova hatch in the intestinal lumen and liberate embryos that mature into adult worms (1 × 40 mm); these usually

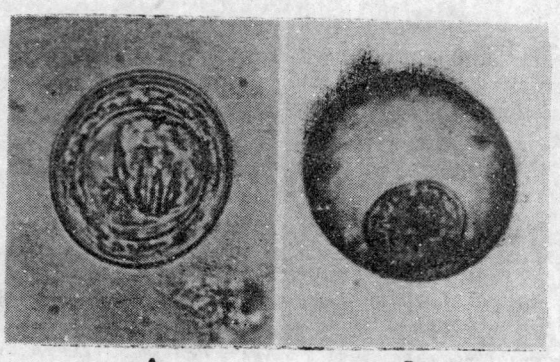

Figure 10–46 Eggs of *Hymenolepis nana* (A) (×575) and *Hymenolepis diminuta* (B) (×400).

reside in the ileum and begin oviposition in a few wk. The eggs are carried to the outside via feces but may hatch inside the same host (autoinfection) and increase the intensity of infection. *H. diminuta*, a parasite of rodents, occasionally infects man. Adult worms are larger than *H. nana*, the life cycle is similar, and eggs are identical in shape but slightly greater in size (diameter of 70 μm).

The characteristic eggs of *H. nana* and *H. diminuta* may be found on fecal examination by direct smear or by concentration methods such as formol-ether. Patients may be treated with niclosamide (same dose as for tapeworms). Praziquantel has recently been found to be highly effective; a single dose of 25 mg/kg cured 94% of infected children.

10.135 ECHINOCOCCOSIS
(Hydatid Disease)

Human infection with the larval stage of the canine tapeworm *Echinococcus granulosus* occurs worldwide but is most prevalent in countries where sheep and cattle are raised. Endemic areas include Australia, South America, South Africa, the Soviet Union, and the Mediterranean region. Clinical disease occurs when hydatid cysts present as space-occupying lesions; these are most common in the liver, but other tissues, such as the lungs, brain, and bones, may also be affected.

Etiology. Domesticated dogs acquire the infection by eating parasitized viscera of sheep and cattle. Man incidentally acquires infection with *E. granulosus* by ingestion of parasite eggs which are discharged in the feces of infected dogs or wolves. Embryos escape from the eggs in the duodenum, penetrate its wall, and pass to the liver where they are usually trapped. If the embryos escape from the liver, they may seed the lungs or travel to other organs via the systemic circulation. Wherever the parasite embryos are trapped, they may be destroyed by the host response or develop into hydatid cysts. These cysts can grow in size up to 20 cm in diameter and are lined on the inside by a germinal layer, which forms multiple larval scolices and daughter cysts. *E. granulosus* infection in man cannot maintain the life cycle of the parasite as it is dependent on the death of the intermediate host and ingestion of larvae by dogs and wolves. The life cycle in nature is maintained between carnivorous and various herbivorous animals.

Epidemiology. *E. granulosus* transmission to man is most common in regions of the world with major livestock industries. Infection is usually acquired by direct contact with dogs but may also occur by ingestion of contaminated soil, vegetables, and water. The prevalence of infection is highest in children; clinical manifestations, however, occur several yr later. Another cycle of transmission to man occurs in North America, particularly in some areas of Alaska and Canada. The strain of *E. granulosus* endemic in these regions is found in the wolf, and larvae are found in large deer such as moose, reindeer, or caribou.

Clinical Manifestations. Most individuals with hydatid cysts are asymptomatic; clinical disease appears in a small proportion and is usually the result of the space-occupying nature of the parasite cysts. When they occur in the liver, symptoms and signs develop only when a cyst reaches large dimensions and presses on adjacent tissues and structures or is located in an area which obstructs blood flow, such as the porta hepatis. Since it takes several yr for hydatid cysts to grow, clinical morbidity is usually detected in middle-aged or elderly patients. Symptoms occur earlier when the cysts are located in less well-supported tissues like the brain and lung, where there is also an increased risk of rupture into adjacent structures. Dissemination of the daughter cysts may lead to serious infections in the peritoneal or pleural cavities. In a recent large study approximately two thirds of hydatid cysts were found in the liver and one quarter in the lungs. In contrast to liver lesions, pulmonary hydatid cysts are commonly seen in children. These patients may present with hemoptysis, cough, or dyspnea. The cysts may rupture into the bronchial tree and spread by discharging their contents in respiratory secretions. Hydatid disease in the brain usually presents as space-occupying lesions; the most common presentation in bone is invasion with erosion and spontaneous fracture.

In some parts of North America, Europe, and Asia, another species of canine tapeworm, *E. multilocularis*, is found in foxes as well as domestic cats and dogs. Human infection with this parasite leads to the so-called malignant hydatid. Many small cysts occur in organs such as the liver; they multiply, spread quickly, and destroy adjacent normal tissues. The prognosis is grave as measures to stop the spread of the infection are not yet available. Surgical intervention is hazardous.

Diagnosis and Treatment. Some cases of hydatid cyst may be discovered on routine roentgenographic examination of the chest or abdomen. Children in endemic areas with suggestive symptoms and signs should undergo roentgenographic and ultrasonic examination. The benign nature of the cyst may be confirmed by angiography. Serology, either by indirect hemagglutination or bentonite flocculation assay, may be helpful. These tests are positive in approximately 85% of individuals with liver cysts. Antibody titers are significantly elevated in fewer than one half of individuals with pulmonary cysts. Diagnosis of hydatid disease may, therefore, have to be made on the basis of history and clinical presentation.

Once a presumptive diagnosis is made, the extent of disease must be assessed. Small or calcified liver cysts should be left alone. Enlarging or symptomatic cysts in the liver should be removed surgically. In patients with pulmonary or bone cysts, surgical removal is also recommended. Care should be taken during the operative procedure not to disseminate the infection. It is therefore advisable to inject aqueous iodine or a concentrated salt solution into the cyst before its removal to kill the contained embryos. Recently several reports have claimed that long-term therapy with mebendazole resulted in cessation of cyst growth and diminution of its size in some patients. If these observations are confirmed, administration of this drug may provide an alternative to surgical intervention in many patients, particularly those with liver cysts.

ADEL A. F. MAHMOUD

Pawlowski Z, Schultz MG: Taeniasis and Cysticercosis. Adv Parasitol 10:269, 1972.
Saidi F: Surgery of Hydatid Disease. Philadelphia, WB Saunders, 1976.
Schenone H: Praziquantel in the treatment of *Hymenolepis nana* infection in children. Am J Trop Med Hyg 29:329, 1980.
von Bonsdorff B: Diphyllobothriasis in Man. London, Academic Press, 1977, p 189.
Williams JF: Recent advances in the immunology of cestode infections. J Parasitol 65:337, 1979.

10.136   ARTHROPODS AND DISEASE

The role of arthropods (i.e., insects and their allies) in the production of disease is 4-fold: (1) certain arthropods elaborate venoms which they introduce into the human body; (2) some are blood-sucking ectoparasites; (3) others are tissue invaders; and (4) many arthropods are mechanical transmitters of pathogenic microorganisms, and others are obligate incubators and transmitters of disease-producing microorganisms.

VENENATING ARTHROPODS

This group of arthropods includes centipedes, scorpions, spiders, ticks, mites, and several species of insects.

Centipedes. These animals have a pair of hollow jaws which serve as fangs to introduce into the skin toxic substances elaborated in their heads. The venom is relatively weak, and, at most, even in an infant, will produce an inflammatory reaction at the puncture site and mild lymphangitis. The affected areas may be treated with local compresses and an antiseptic.

Scorpions. Many species of scorpions, including the dangerous ones in the southwestern United States, Latin America, many areas in Africa, southern Europe, Israel, and India, have potent venom. This is elaborated in the swollen caudal segment and is introduced through the sharp, caudal sting into the skin of a person who accidentally steps on the animal or otherwise makes contact with it.

The venom of some species produces only local tissue reaction (swelling at the puncture site is distinctive), while that of other species is primarily neurotoxic in its action. The latter type of venom contains several fractions, including hemolysins, endotheliolysins, and neurotoxins. In addition to an intense aching pain and numbness radiating from the site of the injury and lymphadenitis, there is typically an ascending motor paralysis, with convulsions resembling those observed in strychnine poisoning, a rapid weak pulse, excessive salivation, extreme thirst, and dysuria; at times there is evidence of acute pancreatitis. Deaths from scorpion stings occur particularly in children under 4 yr of age.

Initially, spread of venom from the site of the sting may be retarded by prompt application of a temporary tourniquet and (without incision) prolonged, but not excessive, cooling with ice packs. In most countries where the more dangerous species are common, standardized species-specific or group-specific antivenin is available for intramuscular administration.* Supportive treatment consists initially of infiltrating into the puncture wound a 2% solution of procaine containing 1:1000 epinephrine to relieve pain, then parenteral administration of glucose and amino acid solutions. Shock should be treated with parenteral solutions, including blood plasma. Morphine and its derivatives are contraindicated because they synergistically increase the toxicity of scorpion venom as much as 7-fold. Effective control can be achieved with phenobarbital; for irrational patients and those with convulsions, 6 mg/kg of sodium phenobarbital may be given as an initial parenteral dose in infants and children; subsequent doses of similar amounts are given at intervals of 20–30 min up to 4–5 administrations.

The application of creosote and oil as repellents or of residual sprays of available insecticides such as DDT, BHC, lindane, or malathion to hiding places around homes and outbuildings will reduce the number of scorpions and the risk of stings.

Spiders. Nearly all spiders produce venoms to stun or kill their prey, but relatively few species have powerful enough fangs or potent enough venom to endanger human beings as does the black widow spider of the United States, *Latrodectus mactans*. This is a black spider with a red ventral spot and variable red dorsal spots, attaining a body length of 13 mm and a leg spread of 40 mm. The spider may bite on chance contact or attack when her web is touched, striking with a pair of anterior fangs. There is an immediate sharp pain at

---

*For sources of scorpion antivenins, contact the Information Officer, U.S.P.H.S. Center for Disease Control, Atlanta, Ga. 30333 (tel. 404–329–3311) or the nearest Poison Control Center.

the site, with a burning, swollen, inflamed area around the puncture wound. The venom enters the bloodstream and in about 30 min produces dizziness, weakness, tremors, abdominal cramps, and, typically, a spastic contraction of the muscles, particularly those of the abdomen, simulating acute abdominal conditions and sickle cell crisis. Concomitant symptoms are rapid shallow respiration, tachycardia, and high arterial blood pressure. Acute nephritis may develop as a result of the intoxication. Hemoglobinuria has been reported in small children. The double fang markings at the site of inoculation may provide a diagnostic clue, but diagnosis is usually made from the clinical history.

Treatment consists of intramuscular injection of standardized species- or group-specific antivenin.* Pain can be reduced by intramuscular or slow intravenous injection of a 10% solution of calcium gluconate, 0.05–0.1 ml/kg repeated as necessary, or by subcutaneous morphine sulfate, alone or with intramuscular phenobarbital. Prolonged hot baths are also effective. Barbiturates may be needed to allay muscle spasm and pain. Neostigmine bromide, USP, may also be used to reduce spasms of smooth muscle. Acute symptoms usually abate after 24 hr, but there may be a long convalescence. Most deaths occur within 36 hr and are due to delay in supportive treatment or administration of antivenin.

Species of the genus *Loxosceles*, which are domestic in their habitats, produce necrotic arachnidism. *Loxosceles laeta* and *L. rufipes* in South America cause topical necrosis and, at times, systemic hemolysis. In the central and southern United States, *L. reclusa*, brown recluse spiders and related species (body 7–12 mm long, leg spread 30–40 mm; yellowish to reddish brown with 6 eyes and a dark, violin-shaped mark dorsally between the legs), inhabit dry cellars, closets, and outbuildings. They are not aggressive, but when crushed or entangled in clothing, both the male and the female bite, causing severe local pain, with rapid development of an indurated wheal which transforms into a large violaceous sloughing ulcer, leaving a deep granulating base. Healing occurs very slowly over a period of weeks if the lesion is not excised. Systemic reactions vary but may include restlessness, fever, and sometimes a scarlatiniform rash; rarely, deaths have been reported. The venom contains a powerful necrotoxin. Parenteral administration of corticotropin to victims of *Loxosceles* bites will hasten healing of the wound.

Contact insecticides, such as lindane in kerosene sprayed on the spider's web, are lethal to *Latrodectus* and to *Loxosceles*.

Ticks and Mites. Ticks are macroscopic and mites microscopic arthropods with unsegmented flat or swollen bodies and 6–8 legs. Ticks are brown or gray, whereas mites may be colorless, reddish, or dark. Many species of ticks and several species of mites cause serious local irritation at the sites on the skin which they pierce to feed on blood or (chiggers) tissue fluid. The mites most irritating to children are chiggers ("red bugs") and rat or bird mites. Red bugs, encountered in grass, weeds, or undergrowth, produce intensely prur-

itic, gross, and hemorrhagic papular lesions which are frequently grouped in areas where clothing is snug. Rat and bird mites, invading rooms from nests, cause less prominent, widely dispersed lesions resembling mosquito bites. The local lesion at the site of attachment can be effectively treated by applying phenolated camphor solution in pure mineral oil or Quotane ointment containing dimethisoquin hydrochloride, or by coating chigger bites with collodion or nail polish. Dusting sulfur into socks and pants or rubbing dimethyl phthalate on the ankles and legs will usually prevent infestation with chiggers; repellents containing toluamide are effective for ticks as well. Nonparasitic mites may be involved in house-dust allergy (*Dermatophagoides* spp. and others) and, infrequently, in contact dermatitis (grain-itch, cheese, and produce mites).

Tick Paralysis. Certain ticks, including the Rocky Mountain wood tick and Eastern dog tick, after being attached for a number of days, introduce toxic saliva that may cause a flaccid ascending motor paralysis which usually begins in the legs. The entire body should be thoroughly searched for a tick that may be hidden in skin crevices or hair. Recovery is usually rapid and complete if the tick is removed promptly, but if it is allowed to remain, death may result from respiratory paralysis. The application of petrolatum or heat to induce the tick to detach will avoid the risk of leaving the imbedded mouth parts in the skin through forceful removal.

Lyme Arthritis. See Sec 9.80.

Insects. These include bees, wasps, ants, blister beetles, moth caterpillars, and many bloodsucking insects. The honeybee worker, unlike bumblebees and wasps, may leave the stinger imbedded in the skin; it should be scraped off carefully to avoid pressure on the attached poison sac. The venoms of bees, wasps, and ants are complex mixtures of peptides, proteins, and amines, including histamine and hyaluronidase. Hypersensitive people who go into shock require prompt use of epinephrine and then should be gradually desensitized (Sec 9.55) to minimize subsequent reactions.

Blister beetles produce a painful blister when their juices are brought into contact with the skin. Ammonia will partly neutralize the blister fluid, and a corticosteroid ointment will ease the pain. Certain caterpillars elaborate venom in nettling hairs which, on contact with the skin or mucous membranes, produce an intense stinging sensation and a painful burn which heals slowly. Prompt washing with soap and water or alcohol is advisable, and a palliative such as calamine lotion may be applied. The pain is partially eased by a corticosteroid ointment, but systemic effects (e.g., from the puss caterpillar), which may be severe during the 1st day or longer, sometimes require sedation and bed rest.

Blood-Sucking Insects. Insects such as mosquitoes, gnats, deerflies, stable flies, fleas, lice, and assassin bugs introduce saliva into the skin while taking a blood meal. This foreign protein produces allergic manifestations in many persons. Antihistamines topically or orally may be palliative for insect bites and stings; specific desensitization may alleviate hypersensitivity. *Papular urticaria* in children may result from sensitivity to insect bites, particularly of fleas or bedbugs in the

---

*Antivenin *Latrodectus mactans* (Merck Sharp and Dohme) is specific.

home, and requires appropriate control or protective measures. Repellents applied to exposed skin provide temporary protection out of doors; indoors, flying insects can be killed by household fly sprays or dichlorvos (DDVP)-impregnated plastic strips. For *pediculosis*, see Sec 24.30.

TISSUE-INVADING ARTHROPODS

Among the arthropods which invade tissues the following are important: the itch mite (*Sarcoptes scabiei*), which produces scabies; the chigoe (*Tunga penetrans*); and the maggots or larval stage of many species of filth flies and their relatives, which cause myiasis.

Scabies. See Sec 24.30.

Chigoe Infestation. *Tunga penetrans*, a flea, is a common skin parasite of dogs, pigs, and barefooted persons in the American tropics and tropical Africa. The most common sites of human infestation are the spaces between the toes, into which the fleas burrow. The females swell to the size of a pea and produce painful, festering lesions. The gravid fleas should be removed with a sterile needle and the wound painted with tincture of iodine to kill the remaining fleas and eggs. Since infestation is usually acquired from direct contact between the bare foot and dust or dirt harboring fleas from dogs or pigs, well shod feet practically guarantee safety from attack.

Myiasis. This results from invasion of tissues and organs by the larvae (maggots or grubs) of various species of flies, which may be specific obligate parasites or semispecific or accidental facultative parasites. Myiasis may affect the skin, connective tissue, eye, nasopharynx, ear, intestines, or urethra; the clinical effects range from benign intestinal infestations or localized lesions to severe mutilation and even death from deep penetration into vital organs. Children are particularly vulnerable to myiasis through either outdoor exposure or the ingestion of fly-contaminated food. The larvae are active, whitish, headless, segmented, and wormlike and are diagnostic when found imbedded in tissues or in freshly passed stools that have been protected from contamination by flies.

In specific myiasis the gravid fly deposits eggs or larvae on skin, hair, mucous membranes, or (tropical warble fly) carrier arthropods. The natural hosts are animals, and infestation of man is incidental. Individual larvae of the tropical warble fly (*Dermatobia hominis*) and fox, mink, and rodent parasites (*Wohlfahrtia* and *Cuterebra* species) produce furuncular lesions; horse bots (*Gasterophilus* species), a cutaneous creeping eruption; sheep bots (*Oestrus ovis*), conjunctival invasion; and cattle bots (*Hypoderma* species), deep migratory invasion; multiple larvae of the primary screwworm (*Cochliomyia hominivorax*) burrow deeply and destructively into the skin or head.

Semispecific and accidental myiasis may result from attraction of saprophagous flies to open lesions or soiled skin or from ingestion of food containing eggs or larvae of flies. Blowflies (species of *Calliphora, Lucilia, Phaenicia,* and *Cochliomyia macellaria*) and flesh flies (*Sarcophaga*

species) are semispecific and most frequently involved, while other species, including the house fly (*Musca domestica*), are rare accidental intestinal parasites.

Maggots burrowing into tissues or breeding in wounds should be removed as soon as possible. The lesions should be irrigated, treated with a bactericidal ointment, and covered with a sterile dressing. In intestinal myiasis frequent saline purgation and enemas may be helpful. Young children, particularly those around stock farms, should be protected from flies by screening or mosquito netting, and any discharges from the eyes, nares, or skin lesions should not be allowed to accumulate since these attract myiasis-producing flies. Fly-control measures should be applied, especially around domestic animals and fur-breeding farms.

ARTHROPODS AS TRANSMITTING AGENTS OF DISEASE

Arthropods serve in 2 ways to transmit disease-producing microorganisms to humans: mechanically or directly; and indirectly as essential biologic hosts or incubators of pathogens.

Mechanical Transmitters. The most important mechanical transmitters are the filth flies, including the common housefly, the lesser houseflies, stable flies, greenbottles, bluebottles, blowflies, flesh flies, and fruit flies. During epidemics or times of gross pollution with human excreta of food and water, they are often responsible for the transmission of typhoid and other salmonella infections, shigellosis, cholera, and amebiasis. Evidence is less conclusive that they play a conspicuous role in the spread of poliomyelitis and epidemic conjunctivitis. Cockroaches may also transmit enteric organisms to food.

Essential Transmitters. Arthropods which are biologic vectors of pathogens include (1) ticks (spotted fever, Q fever, Colorado tick fever, hemorrhagic fever, relapsing fever, and tularemia); (2) red mites (scrub typhus) and rat and mouse mites (murine typhus and rickettsial pox); (3) lice (epidemic typhus, trench fever, and relapsing fever); (4) fleas (plague, murine typhus, and several other infections); (5) mosquitoes (malaria, yellow fever, dengue, a number of viral encephalitides, filariasis, and tularemia); (6) sandflies (kala-azar, cutaneous and mucocutaneous leishmaniasis, Oroya fever, and pappataci fever); (7) *Glossina* (tsetse) flies (African trypanosomiasis); (8) black gnats (onchocerciasis); and (9) assassin bugs (Chagas disease).

Children are particularly susceptible to all of these diseases. In some instances protection can be afforded by vaccine, as in yellow fever, Rocky Mountain spotted fever, and typhus fever. In some, individual prophylaxis consists of avoiding endemic territory or the use of repellents or screens against the vectors. In certain diseases the only practical safeguard consists of dusting the exposed person's clothing with DDT, malathion, or lindane, as in louse-borne typhus fever, or using these or other insecticides as residual sprays, as in areas of rodent plague. Another method of attack is the destruction of the reservoir host (rats in the case of plague and murine typhus). Vector arthropods constitute one of mankind's most serious challenges.

ALBERT MILLER

Baker EW, et al: A Manual of Parasitic Mites. New York, National Pest Control Association, 1956.
Blattner RJ: Necrotic arachnidism. J Pediatr 53:377, 1958.
DeBusk FL, O'Connor S: Tick toxicosis. Pediatrics 50:328, 1972.
Frazier CA: Diagnosis and treatment of insect bites. Clin Symp (Ciba) 20:75, 1968.
Frazier CA: Insect Allergy: Allergic and Toxic Reactions to Insects and Other Arthropods. St. Louis, WH Green, 1969.
Goldman L, et al: Investigative studies of skin irritation from caterpillars. J Invest Dermatol 34:67, 1960.
Haller JS, Fabara JA: Tick paralysis. Case report with emphasis on neurological toxicity. Am J Dis Child 124:915, 1972.
Horen WP: Insect and scorpion stings. JAMA 221:894, 1972.
Horsfall WR: Medical Entomology. Arthropods and Human Disease. New York, Ronald Press, 1962.
James JA, et al: Reactions following suspected spider bite. Am J Dis Child 102:395, 1961.
James MT: The Flies That Cause Myiasis in Man. Washington DC, US Department of Agriculture. Misc Publ No 631, 1947.
James MT, Harwood RF: Herm's Medical Entomology. Ed 6. London, Macmillan, 1969.
Mallis A: Handbook of Pest Control. Ed 5. New York, MacNair-Doland, 1969.
Maretic Z, Stanic M: The health problem of arachnidism. Bull WHO 11:1007, 1954.
O'Rourke FJ: The toxicity of black widow spider venom. In: Venoms. Washington DC, American Association for the Advancement of Science, Publ 44, 1956.
Reed HB Jr, et al: Variation in severity of loxoscelism. J Tenn Med Assoc 61:1097, 1968.
Stahnke HL: Scorpions. Tempe, Arizona, Arizona State College Bookstore, 1956.
Vorse H, et al: Disseminated intravascular coagulopathy following fatal brown spider bite (necrotic arachnidism). J Pediatr 80:1035, 1972.
Wand M: Necrotic arachnidism: A new entity in the Northwest. Northwest Med 71:292, 1972.

THE DIGESTIVE SYSTEM 11

THE ORAL CAVITY

The condition of the oral cavity is important to the physical and psychologic health and sense of well being of each child. Timely diagnosis and treatment require close cooperation between physicians and dentists. Although many older children have regular dental examinations, oral problems of infants are recognized primarily through routine visits to physicians and subsequently require dental referral.

All children should receive a dental examination by 2 yr of age; an examination when a child's 1st teeth erupt is ideal. This provides an excellent opportunity to discuss dental disease when parental interest is high, to counsel about avoiding harmful practices, and to initiate measures to prevent dental caries. At this age, because oral disease is rare, any symptoms generally indicate an unusual situation that should be evaluated. Parents can be given advice that may dramatically reduce the incidence of further oral lesions. However, regular professional surveillance is necessary throughout childhood since changes in oral conditions may occur suddenly. If neglected, discomfort and permanent disability may result.

11.1 DEVELOPMENTAL ABNORMALITIES IN JAWS AND TEETH

DEVELOPMENT OF THE JAWS

The cranial structures mature rapidly in early childhood, but the lower face, including the jaws, develops at a slower rate comparable to that of the body as a whole. As a result the teeth and their supporting structures undergo a prolonged sequence of adjustments.

The maxillary bone is formed in utero from a fusion of the maxilla and premaxilla; the latter contains the upper incisors and anterior portion of the palate. Sutures are formed with the adjoining maxillary, zygomatic, frontal, and palatine bones. The inclination of the sutures follows the direction of enlargement of the maxillary bone. Growth of the vomer bone and these sutures permits the forward and downward movement of the maxilla in relation to the base of the cranium. Remodeling and appositional bone growth result in the maxillary sinuses, alveolar ridges, and mature facial contours. Transverse growth is achieved by prolifera-

tion of bone at the median palatal suture and at the outer surface of the maxilla. Bony union occurs, and growth terminates during adolescence.

The mandible arises both from centers of ossification and from bony replacement of portions of Meckel cartilage. Longitudinal growth is accomplished by interstitial bone growth at the condyles. The ramus maintains its configuration through resorption on the anterior border and deposition of bone on the posterior border. The body of the mandible also undergoes appositional growth at the alveolar ridges and inferior border. Condylar growth normally stops with adolescence, but the potential for further growth remains.

11.2 HYPOPLASIA OF THE MANDIBLE

Pierre Robin Syndrome. This abnormality consists of micrognathia with associated pseudomacroglossia, glossoptosis, and high-arched or cleft palate. Posterior displacement of the attachment of the genioglossus muscle to the hypoplastic mandible prevents the normal anchorage of the tongue. Under the influence of gravity the tongue assumes a retruded position, obstructing the pharynx. A postalveolar cleft of the hard and soft palates is a common but not constant feature, and in some instances the palate is high-arched.

Though the tongue is usually of normal size, the floor of the mouth is foreshortened and the buccal cavity reduced in size. The lack of space further contributes to the glossoptosis. Obstruction of the air passages may occur, particularly on inspiration, and usually requires treatment to avoid suffocation. The infant should be placed in the prone or partially prone position so that the tongue falls forward to relieve respiratory obstruction. Temporarily suturing the ventral surface of the tongue to the lower lip or tracheostomy is usually not necessary since sufficient mandibular growth generally takes place within a few mo to relieve the glossoptosis. A variety of splints and traction devices designed to pull the mandible forward have been unsuccessful. The feeding of infants with mandibular hypoplasia requires great care and patience but can usually be accomplished without resort to gavage. Often the growth of the mandible will progress so that an essentially normal profile is achieved within 4–6 yr. A variety of dental anomalies usually require individual treatment.

Mandibulofacial Dysostosis (Treacher Collins or Franceschetti-Klein Syndrome). In this syndrome there is less severe micrognathia than in the Pierre

Robin syndrome. The facial appearance is characterized by palpebral fissures sloping downward toward the outer canthi, colobomas of the lower eyelids, sunken cheekbones, blind fistulas opening between the angles of the mouth and the ears, deformed pinnas, atypical hair growth extending toward the cheeks, receding chin, and large mouth. Facial clefts, abnormalities of the ears, and deafness are common. The disorder is a dominant trait, but expression is often incomplete. The mandible is almost always hypoplastic; the undersurface is often pronouncedly concave, the ramus may be deficient, and the coronoid and condyloid processes are flat or even aplastic. The palatal vault may be either high or cleft. Infrequently, unilateral or bilateral macrostomia, or failure of embryonic fusion of the maxillary and mandibular processes, may occur. Dental malocclusions are frequent due to poor maxillary development and palatal deformity. The teeth may be widely separated, hypoplastic, or displaced or have an open bite. Orthodontic and routine dental treatments are indicated.

Unilateral hypoplasia of the mandible is sometimes part of an anomaly that includes partial paralysis of the facial nerve, macrostomia, blind fistulas between the angles of the mouth and the ears, and deformed ear lobes. Severe facial asymmetry and malocclusion develop because of the absence or hypoplasia of the mandibular condyle on the affected side. Congenital condylar deformity tends to increase with age. Early plastic surgery may be indicated to minimize the deformity.

Facial asymmetries resulting from excessive molding of the cranium or from displacement of the mandible during breech or face presentations are common and are usually self-correcting. Facial asymmetry due to injury of the growing cartilage or fracture of the condylar head during birth, infancy, or early childhood may be permanent. Traumatic injuries may occur during birth from placing obstetric forceps over the area or may result from blows on the chin during infancy and childhood.

Injuries, acute infections, or arthritis of the growing condylar cartilage may result in partial (fibrous) or complete (bony) **ankylosis of the temporomandibular joint** and failure of that side of the mandible to grow. The normal side, meanwhile, continues to grow and pushes the midline toward the affected side. The midline deviation is exaggerated during mouth opening. Roentgenograms of the affected side reveal an increased preangular notch or displaced condylar head. Bilateral injuries to the growing cartilage result in failure of the mandible and chin to grow downward and forward, causing the entire mandible to be considerably smaller than normal and retruded.

11.3 DEVELOPMENT OF THE TEETH

Initiation. The primary teeth form in dental crypts which arise from a band of epithelial cells incorporated into each developing jaw. Prior to the calcification of the maxilla and mandible a ribbon of epithelial cells grows from the oral epithelium into the underlying mesenchyme. By the 12th wk of fetal life these epithelial bands, the dental lamina, each have 5 areas of rapid growth on each side of the maxilla and the mandible, which result in rounded, budlike enlargements. An accompanying organization of the mesenchyme adjacent to each area of epithelial growth takes place, and the 2 elements together constitute the beginning stages of a tooth.

The *permanent teeth* form in 2 groups. After the formation of the primary crypts a bandlike extension of the dental lamina proliferates lingually from each side to form another generation of tooth buds for the permanent incisors, cuspids, and premolars, which erupt into sites previously occupied by primary teeth. This process takes place from about the 5th gestational mo for the central incisors to about 10 mo of age for the 2nd bicuspids. The permanent molars, on the other hand, arise from a backward extension of the dental lamina beyond the site of initiation of the 2nd primary molars. Budlike enlargements for each of the 3 permanent molars form sequentially at approximately 4 mo of gestation, 1 yr, and from 4–5 yr, respectively.

Histodifferentiation-Morphodifferentiation. As the epithelial bud proliferates, the deeper surface invaginates, and a mass of mesenchyme becomes partially enclosed. Beginning with the crown, the epithelial cells assume the shape of the tooth they represent and lay down the organic matrix for calcification of dentin. The vascular, nerve, and lymph structures (the *dental pulp* of the mature tooth) are confined in the mesenchyme of the hollow central portion of the tooth bud.

Calcification. The deposition of the inorganic mineral crystals of mature enamel and dentin takes place after the organic matrix has been laid down; all teeth form from several sites of calcification which later coalesce. The characteristics of the inorganic portions of a tooth can be altered by (1) disturbances in formation of the matrix, (2) decreased availability of 1 or more of the minerals involved, and (3) the incorporation of foreign materials. Disturbances at this time affect the color, texture, and thickness of the tooth surface.

Eruption. At the time of tooth bud formation each tooth begins a continuous movement outward in relation to the bone. The full chronology of human dentition is given in Table 2–4; the relative times of eruption and shedding of the primary teeth and the times of eruption of the permanent teeth are listed in Tables 11–1 and 11–2. The mandibular teeth usually erupt before the maxillary teeth and those of girls generally earlier than those of boys.

11.4 ANOMALIES ASSOCIATED WITH TOOTH DEVELOPMENT

Both failures and excesses of tooth initiation are observed. **Anodontia,** or absence of teeth, occurs when no tooth buds form. Total anodontia often occurs with ectodermal dysplasia. Partial anodontia results from disturbance of a normal site of initiation, e.g., the area of a palatal cleft, or from genetic failure (frequently familial) to code the formation of specific teeth. The 3rd molars, maxillary lateral incisors, and mandibular 2nd

Table 11–1   TIME OF ERUPTION AND SHEDDING OF THE PRIMARY TEETH

	ERUPTION		SHEDDING	
	Lower	Upper	Lower	Upper
	Age (Months)		Age (Years)	
Central incisor	6	7½	6	7½
Lateral incisor	7	9	7	8
Cuspid	16	18	9½	11½
First molar	12	14	10	10½
Second molar	20	24	11	10½
Incisors	Range ± 2 mo		Range ± 6 mo	
Molars	Range ± 4 mo			

From Massler and Schour: Atlas of the Mouth. Chicago, American Dental Association.

premolars are the teeth that most commonly fail to form. If the dental lamina produces more than the normal number of buds, **supernumerary teeth** occur, most often in the area of the maxillary central incisors. Since they tend to disrupt the position and eruption of the adjacent normal teeth, their identification as supernumerary teeth by roentgenographic examination is important. **Natal teeth**, present at birth or erupting shortly thereafter, may be part of the normal primary dentition, but they must be differentiated from supernumerary teeth, which should be removed.

Disturbances during differentiation may result in gross alterations in dental morphology, such as **macrodontia**, large teeth, and **microdontia**, small teeth. The maxillary lateral incisors may assume a slender, tapering shape ("peg-shaped laterals").

Twinning, in which 2 teeth are joined together, is most often observed in the mandibular incisors of the primary dentition. It may result from gemination, fusion, or concrescence. *Gemination* is the result of division of 1 tooth germ to form a bifid or cloven crown on a single root with a common pulp canal; an extra tooth is then present in the dental arch. *Fusion* is the joining of incompletely developed teeth that, under pressure of trauma or crowding, continue to develop as 1 tooth. Fused teeth are sometimes joined through their entire length; in other instances a single wide crown is supported on 2 roots. *Concrescence* is the attachment of the roots of closely approximated adjacent teeth by an excessive deposit of cementum. This type of twinning, unlike the others, is found most often in the maxillary molar region.

Table 11–2   TIME OF ERUPTION OF THE PERMANENT TEETH

	LOWER AGE (YEARS)	UPPER AGE (YEARS)
Central incisors	6–7	7–8
Lateral incisors	7–8	8–9
Cuspids	9–10	11–12
First bicuspids	10–12	10–11
Second bicuspids	11–12	10–12
First molars	6–7	6–7
Second molars	11–13	12–13
Third molars	17–21	17–21

From Massler and Schour: Atlas of the Mouth. Chicago, American Dental Association.

Dens in dente, a "tooth in a tooth," is a roentgenographic finding in which the outline of a 2nd dental structure is seen within a tooth of normal outward appearance. It results from an invagination in the lingual surface, usually of a maxillary incisor, at the site of fusion between separate sites of calcification in the same tooth; an enamel-lined hollow space results.

Amelogenesis imperfecta, a dominant genetic trait, results in faulty production of the organic matrix. The teeth are covered by only a thin layer of abnormally formed enamel through which the yellow coloration of the underlying dentin is seen, giving a darkened appearance to the dentition. Usually both primary and permanent teeth are affected. Although susceptibility to caries is low, the enamel is subject to destruction from abrasion. Complete coverage of the crown may be indicated for protection and improved appearance. **Dentinogenesis imperfecta,** or hereditary opalescent dentin, is an analogous condition in which the odontoblasts fail to differentiate normally and poorly calcified dentin results. The junction between the enamel and dentin is altered, the enamel has a tendency to flake away, and the exposed dentin is then susceptible to abrasion. The teeth are opaque and pearly, and the pulp chambers are obliterated by calcification. Both primary and permanent teeth are usually involved. Unless the crowns of these teeth are covered early and completely, the abrasion of chewing often reduces them to the level and contour of the supporting alveolar bone.

Localized disturbances of calcification which correlate with periods of illness or malnutrition are frequent; they are analogous to the growth disturbance lines often seen in the long bones. An example is the *neonatal line* commonly observed on all the primary teeth and on the permanent central incisors and tips of cuspids at coronal levels consistent with the stage of calcification present at birth. Two general disturbances of the surface of the enamel are also seen. Discoloration of the smooth surface, usually a more opaque white patch, is referred to as *hypocalcification.* A more severe disturbance, *hypoplasia,* may be manifest as pitting, or areas devoid of covering enamel. Hypoplasia is uncommon in the primary dentition because of the relative infrequency of intrauterine stress as opposed to the frequent occurrence of illness or malnutrition during early infancy when the enamel of the outer third of the permanent incisors, cuspids, and 1st molars is forming. Dental restoration of such areas is desirable to eliminate the sensitivity of exposed dentin, to prevent caries, and to improve the appearance.

Mottled enamel is found in persons whose early life is spent in areas where the fluoride content of the drinking water is greater than 2.0 parts/million (ppm) and is probably due to ameloblastic dysfunction. It varies from small inconspicuous white patches to severe, brownish discoloration and hypoplasia; the latter changes are usually seen with fluoride concentrations over 5 ppm.

Disturbances due to mineral deficiency are rare, but irregular dentin and enlarged pulp chambers have been observed with vitamin D–resistant rickets and hypoplasia with vitamin D–deficient rickets.

Discolored teeth may result from incorporation of foreign substances into developing enamel. The hemolysis accompanying erythroblastosis fetalis may produce blue to black discoloration of the primary teeth, beginning at the neonatal line; the tips of the permanent 1st molars may also be affected. All of the tetracyclines are extensively incorporated into bones and teeth and may result in brownish yellow discoloration and even hypoplasia of the enamel if administered during the period of formation of enamel. This period extends from about the 4th mo of gestation to the 10th mo of life for the primary teeth and from about the 4th mo to the 16th yr of life for permanent teeth. The enamel is completely formed on all but the 3rd molars by about 8 yr of age. Therefore, if possible, tetracyclines should not be prescribed for pregnant women or for children under 8 yr of age. Fluorescence of the teeth under ultraviolet light is diagnostic.

As the teeth penetrate the gums, inflammation and sensitivity sometimes occur, a condition referred to as **teething.** The child may become irritable, and salivation may increase markedly. Bacterial invasion through a break in the tissue or under a gingival flap covering the teeth may be responsible. A blunt, firm object for the infant to bite usually provides some relief; incision of the gums is seldom indicated. There is no definite evidence to support claims of accompanying temporary systemic disturbances, such as low-grade fever, facial rashes, and mild diarrhea.

Delayed eruption of all teeth may indicate systemic or nutritional disturbances such as hypopituitarism, hypothyroidism, cleidocranial dysostosis, and rickets. Local causes such as malpositioning of teeth, supernumerary teeth, cysts, or retained primary teeth may be responsible for failure of eruption of single or small groups of teeth. Early loss of primary predecessors is the most common cause of *premature eruption* of teeth. If the entire dentition is advanced for age and sex, an endocrine disorder, such as hyperpituitarism, must be considered.

Natal teeth are erupted teeth observed in approximately 1:2000 newborn infants; usually there are 2 in the position of the mandibular central incisors. Their attachment is generally limited to the gingival margin, with little root formation or bony support; such teeth should not be considered supernumerary until so identified roentgenographically. A natal tooth may be a prematurely erupted primary tooth which suggests that early dental eruption may be expected.

The presence of teeth at birth may result in pain secondary to looseness and movement. They may also produce maternal discomfort due to abrasion or biting of the nipple during nursing. There is danger of detachment with subsequent aspiration of the tooth. Since the tongue lies between the alveolar processes during birth, it may become lacerated, and occasionally the tip is amputated (Riga-Fede disease). The decision to extract prematurely erupted primary teeth must be made on an individual basis; it should be performed by carefully dissecting away the gingival attachment to prevent tearing of the tissue and excessive hemorrhage.

Exfoliation failure occurs when a primary tooth fails to exfoliate prior to the eruption of its permanent successor. The primary tooth should be extracted if the erupting permanent tooth becomes visible. This occurs most commonly in the mandibular incisor region.

11.5 DISORDERS OF THE TEETH ASSOCIATED WITH OTHER CONDITIONS

Osteogenesis imperfecta is usually accompanied by hereditary opalescent dentin, also termed dentinogenesis imperfecta. Treatment is usually not indicated.

In *cleidocranial dysostosis* there are a number of oral-facial variations. Frontal bossing, mandibular prognathism, and a broadened base of the nose may be seen. Eruption of teeth is characteristically delayed. The primary teeth are abnormally retained, and the permanent teeth may remain unerupted. The presence of supernumerary teeth is common, especially in the premolar area. Erupted teeth are free of hypoplasia, but variations in size and shape are frequent. The primary dentition and those permanent teeth which do erupt should be restored if they become carious. Extraction of a primary tooth rarely results in the eruption of its permanent successor. The removal of the unerupted permanent teeth is also contraindicated. Their roots are usually crooked and curved, often leading to fracture during attempted removal.

In *ectodermal dysplasia* the teeth are totally or partially absent. Since alveolar bone does not develop in the absence of teeth, the alveolar processes are usually either totally or partially absent, and the resulting overclosure of the mandible causes the lips to protrude. Facial development is otherwise not disturbed. Teeth, when present, are small and conical in form. Aplasia of the buccal and labial mucous glands, leading to dryness and irritation of the oral mucosa, has also been observed. Persons with ectodermal dysplasia need either partial or full dentures. The vertical height between the jaws is thus restored, improving the position of the lips and facial contours. Masticatory function is restored, and eating habits are thereby improved.

Congenital syphilis affects differentiation of permanent teeth, resulting in screwdriver-shaped incisors, often with central notches in their incisive edges (Hutchinson incisors), and mulberry molars, with lobular occlusal surfaces and narrow, pinched crowns.

11.6 DISEASES OF THE JAW

Caffey Disease (Infantile Cortical Hyperostosis). See Chapter 23.

Osteomyelitis (Sec 10.14 and 23.1). In the newborn infant osteomyelitis tends to occur in the area of the premaxillary suture, but during childhood the mandible is the more common location. The infection is marked by swelling and redness of the oral mucosa or skin, associated with pain, fever, and lymphadenopathy. Drainage should be established and the exudate cultured so that an appropriate antibiotic may be administered. Large sequestra may require surgical removal.

Reticuloendotheliosis (Histiocytosis X) (Sec 26.5). Oral lesions may occur in any of the syndromes and may be an early manifestation. Lesions of the jaws may produce pain, swelling, loosening of teeth, and fetid breath. Healing is often delayed after dental extraction.

Neoplasms. *Benign Tumors.* OSSIFYING FIBROMA. This is the most common benign tumor of the jaws. Prior to puberty its growth is rapid, after which it may slow or cease. Since the lesion is painless, a unilateral soft tissue swelling is usually the 1st sign. Most patients do not require treatment, but if the lesion is extensive, curettage or further surgical correction may be required.

CYSTS OF JAW. *Multiple basal cell nevoid syndrome* (Sec 24.8).

Malignant Tumors. The malignant tumors of the jaws that occur in children include Burkitt sarcoma, osteogenic sarcoma, lymphosarcoma, and, more rarely, fibrosarcoma.

DISEASES OF THE TEETH

11.7 DENTAL CARIES

Dental caries, or tooth decay, is a progressive, destructive lesion of the calcified dental tissues. It is the principal oral problem of children. Untreated, dental caries eventually results in total destruction of involved teeth.

Etiology. The susceptibility to dental caries is influenced by several interrelated circumstances. The organisms initiating the disease process are principally streptococci; they produce extracellular polysaccharides that begin the formation of a gelatinous "plaque" over the tooth to which many organisms adhere. Fermentable carbohydrates, especially sucrose, are the main substrate for the production of metabolic acids by the enmeshed bacteria. The acids first decalcify the enamel, which has variable rates of dissolution, and then cause lysis of the protein of the organic matrix producing total destruction of the involved portions of tooth structure.

Factors Influencing Caries. *Age.* Caries is primarily a disease of childhood and adolescence. When diet and oral hygiene are unfavorable, the periods of greatest carious activity are ages 4–8 yr in the primary dentition and 12–18 yr in the permanent dentition.

Fluoride. The incorporation of fluoride into the enamel surface increases its resistance to acid dissolution. The presence of fluoride also reduces acid production by microorganisms and aids in the remineralization of partially demineralized areas. Children living in communities where the drinking water contains 1.0 ppm or more of fluoride have on the average 60% fewer carious lesions than those in areas where the fluoride content is under 0.5 ppm. The maximal reduction in dental caries occurs when the drinking water contains the optimal amount of fluoride for the climatic conditions of that community. If the fluoride content is 2.0–2.5 ppm or more, mottling of the enamel becomes evident. Supplemental fluorides and surface fluoride applications are effective in reducing dental caries, both in communities with suboptimal fluoride levels in the water supplies and, to a lesser extent, in optimally fluoridated communities.

Diet. An important factor contributing to caries is the ingestion between meals of foods or fluids containing sugars, particularly sucrose, in forms that cling, such as taffy, or promote prolonged contact with the teeth, such as lollipops and lozenges. Such ingestion provides the substrate for production of tooth-destroying acid by the bacteria adherent to the teeth. Sugars ingested at mealtime are less injurious because of the reduced frequency, the detergent action of some foods, and the buffering capacity of other foods and saliva, which tends to neutralize the acids.

The practice of putting small children to sleep with a bottle of milk or other sweetened fluids results in an accumulation of sugar within the oral cavity. The acids produced by bacterial action on this substrate frequently result in early, rampant caries, **milk-bottle caries;** a prominent diagnostic feature is the progression of the destruction from the maxillary anteriors to the posterior teeth, with the lower anteriors relatively protected by the nipple and tongue. This practice is probably the most common cause of severe caries in children under 3 yr of age.

Oral Hygiene. Lack of oral hygiene (rinsing and brushing, particularly after meals) permits the accumulation of plaque and food debris. The primary purpose of brushing and the use of dental floss is removal of the bacteria-laden plaque, thereby reducing the quantity of oral microorganisms and exposing the tooth surfaces to the remineralizing components of saliva. For prevention of caries and the early stages of periodontal disease, children need the assistance of parents to demonstrate and supervise oral hygiene procedures.

State of Health. In chronic debilitating diseases both the quantity and the bacteriostatic quality of saliva may be reduced. Oral hygiene after each meal is even more important than for the healthy person. Prevention is especially important for children who are unable to receive regular dental care because of disabilities.

Clinical Manifestations. Caries originates in areas where plaque may accumulate, such as in the pits and fissures on the grooves of occlusal surfaces of the posterior teeth, between the teeth, and along the gingival margins at the necks of the teeth. The lesions may penetrate rapidly through the substance of the tooth, or their progress may be intermittent and slow. Rapidly invading caries is characteristic in children; the slow intermittent type predominates in middle age. A visible defect on an exterior tooth surface is frequently a sign of more extensive interior invasion. The dentin inside is less mineralized and more rapidly destroyed than the exterior enamel substance.

Prevention. The most effective preventive measure against dental caries is natural or artificial fluoridation of the water supply. If an optimal amount of fluoride (approximately 1.0 ppm) is not present in the water supply, supplemental fluorides can provide some of the benefits. Children exposed to water fluoride below 0.3 ppm should be given 0.25 mg/24 hr of fluoride starting at age 6 mo and 0.5–1.0 mg/24 hr of fluoride (1.1–2.2 mg of sodium fluoride) after 1 yr of age.

Reduced dosages are recommended for 0.3–1.0 ppm fluoride levels in the water supply. A beneficial effect is obtained with oral fluoride preparations even after teeth have erupted. This is probably derived from topical incorporation of fluoride into the surface enamel and direct antimicrobial action. Oral retention for surface contact is necessary for optimal benefits. Therefore, when liquid preparations containing fluoride are given, the dose should be deposited into the buccal area with the head tilted slightly sideways; in general, chewable tablets should be prescribed. Such fluoride preparations are not recommended for areas where the water supply contains fluoride in excess of 0.7 ppm until after 6 yr of age.

The prescription of fluoride supplements is not a substitute for fluoridation of community water supplies since the latter ensures availability of adequate fluoride and includes all children in the area at considerably lower cost. There is no conclusive evidence that the administration of fluoride to the pregnant woman reduces the incidence of caries in the child.

After dental eruption biannual topical applications of fluoride to the teeth increase the concentration of fluoride in the surface enamel, where decay begins. Such applications are beneficial whether the fluoride content in the community water supply is adequate or not.

Less frequent eating and avoidance of sucrose-containing snacks, candies, or drinks between meals can markedly reduce the incidence of new carious lesions. The small child's "bedtime bottle" of milk should be avoided. If the habit has become established, substitution of a cup of milk for the bottle before brushing the teeth at bedtime is more desirable than gradual withdrawal.

The elimination of active lesions by restoration of primary as well as permanent teeth reduces the bacterial population in the oral cavity and the hazard to uninvolved teeth. When a child exhibits the rapid appearance and progression of new carious lesions, dental examinations at intervals of 3 rather than 6 mo may be appropriate.

The mechanical removal of plaque and debris from tooth surfaces by brushing and dental floss is the primary method of preventing caries. Small children can be held in the lap; 1 hand can retract the lips while brushing is accomplished with the other. Brushing should be initiated on eruption of the 1st primary teeth. Dental floss is required to cleanse all areas where teeth are in direct contact and therefore cannot be brushed. The child who is properly instructed will eventually accomplish the procedure routinely without help.

11.8 MALOCCLUSION

The oral cavity can be viewed as a masticatory machine. The cusps of the opposing posterior teeth interdigitate and slide across each other to reduce foodstuffs to a soft, moist bolus. The cheeks and tongue force the food onto the areas of tooth contact. The incisal edges of the anterior teeth are opposed by mandibular manipulation for the purpose of biting off increments of larger food items.

The masseter and temporal muscles are the main forces of mandibular closure. Acting in conjunction with the internal pterygoid muscles, they produce high pressures on contact of opposing teeth. If a number of teeth meet simultaneously, the force is distributed over a large area of bone to tooth attachment. In malocclusion, when only a few teeth touch, the same force is exerted over a much smaller area. In adulthood occlusal deformities are a leading cause of loss of teeth. For this reason preventive measures in childhood should be directed at establishing proper relations between upper and lower dental arches for physiologic as well as cosmetic reasons.

Variations in growth patterns are classified into 3 main types of occlusion (Fig 11–1). The occlusal relation is determined by observing the positions of the teeth when the jaws are closed and the heads of the mandibular condyles are in the most posterior position within the glenoid fossa of the temporal bone. In class I (normal) the cusps of the posterior mandibular teeth interdigitate ahead of and inside the corresponding cusps of the opposing maxillary teeth. This jaw relationship provides a normal facial profile. In class II the cusps of the posterior mandibular teeth are behind and inside the corresponding cusps of the maxillary teeth. This is the most common occlusal discrepancy; about 45% of the population exhibits this condition to some degree. An increased space between upper and lower anterior teeth encourages sucking and tongue-thrust habits. The appearance of a receding chin accompanies the retrognathia. In class III the cusps of the posterior mandibular teeth interdigitate a tooth or more ahead of their opposing maxillary counterparts. The anterior teeth are directly opposed, or the mandibular incisors are protruded beyond the maxillary incisors; a protruding chin is exhibited with the prognathia.

Cross Bite. Normally the mandibular teeth are in a position just inside the maxillary teeth so that the outside mandibular cusps or incisal edges meet the central portion of the opposing maxillary teeth. A reversal of this relation is referred to as a cross bite.

Open and Closed Bites. If the posterior mandibular and maxillary teeth contact each other but the anterior ones are still apart, the situation is termed an open bite. With the posterior teeth together, if the mandibular anterior teeth fit inside the maxillary anterior teeth in an overclosed position, the situation is referred to as a closed bite. If the overclosure is extreme, the mandib-

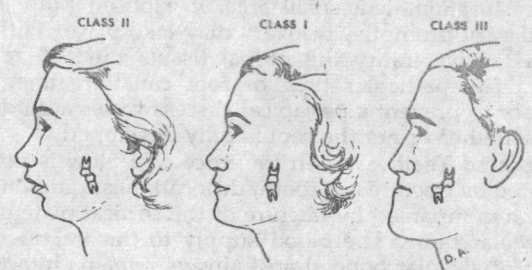

Figure 11–1 Angle classification of occlusion. The typical correspondence between the profile and molar relationship is shown. (Moyers RE: Handbook of Orthodontics. Ed 2. Chicago, Year Book Medical Publishers, 1963.)

ular incisors may strike and injure the mucosa behind the maxillary incisors.

Genetic factors are the most common cause of malocclusion. Malocclusion may also result from other circumstances leading to abnormal growth; for example, the mandibular protrusion seen with acromegaly leads to class III malocclusion. Habits such as thumb sucking and tongue thrusting may become important causative factors. Injuries to the mandibular condyles also disrupt mandibular growth.

The severity of the malocclusion is the principal factor that determines the timing of treatment. Many cross bites, open and closed bites, and a few mild class II malocclusions can be corrected as early as they are diagnosed. Most class II and class III malocclusions are more easily correctable after the eruption of all the permanent dentition except the 3rd molars.

The congenital absence or extraction of teeth also may cause occlusal discrepancies. These may be corrected either by prosthetic replacement of the missing tooth or teeth or by moving other teeth to close the vacant space. Early roentgenographic appraisal is important in establishing a plan for treatment.

11.9   DENTAL INJURIES

The risk of accidental damage to the teeth is exaggerated with the protruding anterior teeth of class II malocclusions or protrusions of maxillary incisors from finger sucking or tongue thrusting; protruding teeth should be moved into a less vulnerable position as soon as possible after the eruption of the permanent incisors. Sports are responsible for many dental injuries. Individually fitted protective mouthpieces are available and should be used. When injury does occur, prompt treatment of a fracture or displacement improves the prognosis for retaining the teeth and for subsequent alignment. Emergency dental therapy usually should precede soft tissue treatment to preserve the periodontal membrane.

Fractured Incisors.   Blows on the mouth usually strike the maxillary incisors since they are the most anteriorly located hard structures. Fractures of the crowns and roots of these teeth are therefore frequent. If the cleavage of the crown does not include a portion of the pulpal cavity, treatment is limited to covering any exposed dentin followed by placement of an esthetic restoration. If a small area of exposed pulp is covered very promptly, recovery may take place. With more extensive injury the pulpal tissue must be removed. The particular type of root canal treatment necessary to prevent a periapical abscess varies according to whether or not the root is fully developed.

Dislocated Teeth.   When the force of a blow is not dissipated by fracture of a tooth, dislocation is common, usually accompanied by fracture of the cortical plate of the alveolar bone. The blood supply to the fractured portion of alveolar bone almost always remains intact, and healing is complete in 3–4 wk. On the other hand, because the alveolar ridge acts as a fulcrum, the apex of a tooth may be forced out of position, frequently severing the pulpal blood vessels and nerve which enter

through the small apical foramen. Dislocated teeth should be promptly repositioned and splinted. After 1 wk, if the sensitivity of the tooth to stimuli like heat and cold has not returned, it is likely nonvital and root canal therapy is indicated to prevent abscess formation.

Avulsed Teeth.   Completely avulsed teeth should be reimplanted immediately at the scene of the accident. If that is not possible, they should be placed in saline or milk and taken immediately to a dentist for reimplanting. The devitalized tooth usually becomes firmly attached once again, but retention may be limited, varying from 6–12 yr. Breakdown of the periodontal membrane leads to osteoclastic resorption of the root surface from the alveolar bone. However, reimplantation increases the success of ultimate prosthetic replacement because it allows adjacent dental structures to mature normally.

Habits Injurious to the Teeth.   The positions of the teeth significantly determine the contour of the alveolar bone and the shape of the face. The positions of the teeth, in turn, are dependent on a balance of forces. Normal pressure from the tongue is opposed by buccal and labial pressures; the force of eruption offsets the depression of mastication. Alteration in equilibrium between these forces can change the position of teeth, disturb the interarch relations, and, with time, change facial appearance.

Tongue Thrust.   Since swallowing occurs about once every 2 min during the waking hours, the common oral habit of thrusting the tongue forward against the teeth instead of upward against the palate during swallowing produces almost continuous lingual pressure on the teeth. Anterior inclination of the incisors with frequent anterior open bite and a tight, protruding upper lip may result. Pursing of the lips during swallowing is common with the habit. The placement on the palate of an appliance with a guard-reminder section is useful. Tongue exercises directed by a speech therapist may also be effective in treatment.

Finger Sucking.   Sucking thumb, fingers, or a pacifier between feedings is common in infants. Many children continue this habit well beyond infancy, frequently in response to stress. Weaning from a pacifier is usually less difficult than from a thumb or fingers. The outward push, particularly of thumb sucking, may produce a forward movement of the primary maxillary incisors and, in turn, may induce the associated alveolar bone to shift anteriorly. The permanent incisors then erupt in a more forward position. If the habit persists during eruption of these permanent teeth, they are frequently directed into a protruding inclination. Finger sucking should be terminated by 5 yr of age to prevent the displacement of permanent teeth when they erupt.

After the age of 4 yr finger sucking is usually self-correcting in response to social pressures. Persuasion by the pediatrician or dentist may furnish the motivation to stop. If the habit is very strong, an appliance with a guard in the region of the anterior palate may be successful. With the guard a palatal vacuum is unattainable, and interest in sucking is lost. A nighttime wrapping of the appropriate elbow with an elastic bandage has also proved helpful. An emotional problem usually underlies only severely protracted cases.

DEVELOPMENTAL ABNORMALITIES OF THE PALATE AND SOFT TISSUES OF THE MOUTH

The functions of the oral cavity depend in large part on the ability to form a closed and hollow compartment. Labial and palatal competence are required for this closure. Either anatomic or functional deficiencies disrupt normal speech, fluid ingestion, and mastication.

11.10 CLEFT LIP AND CLEFT PALATE

Incidence and Epidemiology. The incidence of the cleft lip (harelip) or cleft palate ranges from 1:600–1:1250 births. Genetic factors are of more importance in cleft lip with or without cleft palate than in cleft palate alone. The incidence of cleft lip with or without cleft palate is about 1:1000 births; the incidence of cleft palate alone is about 1:2500 births. Cleft lip with or without cleft palate is more frequent in males; cleft palate alone is more frequent in females. There is an increased incidence of associated congenital malformations and of intellectual impairment among children with cleft defects; both are more common with cleft palate alone. These findings are partially explained by an increased incidence of hearing impairment in children with cleft palate and by the frequency of cleft defects among children with chromosomal abnormalities. The risks of recurrence of cleft defects within families are enumerated in Chapter 6.

Animal studies suggest that nongenetic influences may also be responsible for clefts in a susceptible host at a critical period of organogenesis. Associated malformations are especially frequent in structures derived from the 1st branchial arch.

Clinical Manifestations. *Cleft lip* may vary from a small notch in the vermilion border to a complete separation extending into the floor of the nose. Clefts may be unilateral (more often on the left side) or bilateral and usually involve the alveolar ridge. Deformed, supernumerary, or absent teeth are associated anomalies. The nasal alar cartilage clefts of the lip are frequently associated with a deficiency of the columella and elongation of the vomer, producing a protrusion of the anterior aspect of the cleft premaxillary process (Fig 11–2).

Clefts of the palate may occur alone or in association with cleft lip. Isolated cleft palate occurs in the midline and may involve only the uvula or extend into or through the soft and hard palates to the incisive foramen. When associated with cleft lip, the defect may involve the midline of the soft palate and extend into the hard palate on 1 or both sides, exposing 1 or both of the nasal cavities as a unilateral or bilateral cleft palate.

Treatment. The immediate concerns for the infant with a cleft lip or palate are provision of adequate nutrition and prevention of aspiration and infection. Management for most infants consists of feeding in an upright position and using softened nipples with slightly enlarged openings. In some instances medicine

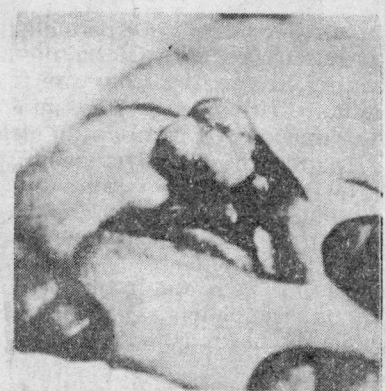

Figure 11–2 Double cleft lip and cleft palate in an infant 2 mo of age. Note the intermaxillary process between the clefts.

dropper or gavage feedings may be indicated. Special cleft palate nipples and plastic palatal coverings are usually not necessary but may be helpful for some infants.

Surgical closure of a cleft lip is usually performed at 1–2 mo of age after the infant has shown satisfactory weight gain and is free of any oral, respiratory, or systemic infection. Z-plasty, the most commonly used technique, involves a staggered suture line to minimize notching of the lip from retraction of scar tissue. A *Logan clamp* (a wire bow attached by adhesive to the cheeks) is applied immediately after the operation to take tension off the suture line. The initial repair may be revised at 4–5 yr of age. In most instances corrective surgery on the nose should be delayed until adolescence. Cosmetic results depend on the extent of the original deformity, absence of infection, and the skill of the surgeon.

Since clefts of the palate vary considerably in size, shape, and degree of deformity, the timing of surgical correction should be individualized. Criteria such as width of the cleft, adequacy of the existing palatal segments, the morphology of the surrounding areas (such as width of the oropharynx), and the neuromuscular function of the soft palate and pharyngeal walls affect the decision. The goals of surgery are the union of the cleft segments, intelligible and pleasant speech, and avoidance of injury to the growing maxilla. The optimal time for palatal surgery varies from 6 mo–5 yr of age, depending on the need to take advantage of the palatal changes that occur with growth. When surgical correction is delayed beyond the 3rd yr of age, a contoured speech bulb can be attached to the posterior of a maxillary denture so that contraction of the pharyngeal and velopharyngeal muscles can bring tissues into contact with the bulb to accomplish occlusion of the nasopharynx and help the child develop intelligible speech. Almost always the cleft crosses the alveolar ridge and interferes with the formation of teeth in the area. The missing elements of the dentition must be replaced by prosthetic devices; alterations in the positions of teeth may also be necessary.

Pre- and Postoperative Management. Even the suspicion of infection is a contraindication to operation. If the child is in good nutritional state and in fluid and electrolyte balance, feeding may be permitted to within 6 hr of the operation (Sec 5.31). During the immediate postoperative period special nursing care is essential. Gentle aspiration of the nasopharynx minimizes the chances of the common complications of atelectasis or pneumonia. The primary considerations in postoperative care are maintenance of a clean suture line and avoidance of strain on the sutures. For these reasons the infant is fed with a medicine dropper and the arms are restrained with elbow cuffs. A fluid or semifluid diet is maintained for 3 wk, and feeding is done with a dropper or spoon. The patient's hands as well as toys and other foreign bodies must be kept away from the palate.

Complications.   Recurrent otitis media and hearing loss are frequent. Excessive dental decay is not unusual and requires a special care. Displacement of the maxillary arches and malpositions of the teeth usually require orthodontic correction.

Speech defects may be present even after good anatomic closure of the palate. Such speech is characterized by emission of air from the nose and by a hypernasal quality when certain sounds are made. The speech defect before and, at times, after palatal surgery is due to inadequacies in function of the palatal and pharyngeal muscles. The muscles of the soft palate and the lateral and posterior walls of the nasopharynx constitute a valve which functions to separate the nasopharynx from the oropharynx during swallowing and in the production of certain sounds. If the valve does not function adequately, it is difficult to build up enough pressure in the mouth to make such explosive sounds as p, b, d, t, h, g or the sibilants s, sh, and ch, and such words as "cats," "boats," and "sisters" are not intelligible. After operation or the insertion of a speech appliance speech therapy may be necessary.

A *complete program of habilitation* for the child with a cleft lip or palate may require years of special treatment by a team consisting of pediatrician, plastic surgeon, otolaryngologist, pedodontist, prosthodontist, orthodontist, speech therapist, medical social worker, psychologist, child psychiatrist, and public health nurse. Ideally, however, the child's physician should be responsible for parental counseling, coordination of specialists, and guidance.

11.11   PALATOPHARYNGEAL INCOMPETENCE

The speech disturbance characteristic of the child with a cleft palate can also be produced by other osseous or neuromuscular abnormalities characterized by an inability to form an effective muscular seal between oropharynx and nasopharynx during swallowing or phonation. The anomaly may be in the body structures of the palate or pharynx or in the muscles attached to these structures. In a child who previously spoke normally an adenoidectomy may precipitate the speech defect when there is an unrecognized submucous cleft palate. It is assumed that the adenoids had a static function as a mass protruding into the epipharynx which facilitated a seal when the elevated soft palate

made contact with it. This becomes impossible after removal of the adenoids. If there is sufficient reserve neuromuscular function, compensation in palatopharyngeal movement may take place and the speech defect disappear, although often some symptoms of palatopharyngeal incompetence may persist. In other instances slow involution of the adenoids may allow for gradual compensation in palatal and pharyngeal muscular function. This may explain why a speech defect does not become apparent in some children who have a submucous cleft palate or similar anomaly predisposing to palatopharyngeal incompetence. *Adenoidectomy should be avoided when there is a submucous cleft palate or a potential palatopharyngeal incompetence.*

Clinical Manifestations.   The symptoms of palatopharyngeal incompetence are similar to those of a cleft palate, although clinical signs vary. There may be hypernasal speech especially noted in the articulation of pressure consonants, such as p, b, d, t, h, v, f, and s; conspicuous constricting movement of the nares during speech; inability to whistle, gargle, blow out a candle, or inflate a balloon; loss of liquid through the nose when drinking with the head down; and otitis media and hearing loss. Oral inspection may reveal a cleft palate or a relatively short palate with a large oropharynx; absent, grossly asymmetric, or minimal muscular activity of the soft palate and pharynx during phonation or gagging; or a *submucous cleft.* The latter is suggested by a bifid uvula, a translucent membrane in the midline of the soft palate revealing lack of continuity of muscles, a palpable notching in the posterior border of the hard palate instead of a posterior nasal spinous process, and forward or V-shaped displacement or grooving on the soft palate during phonation or gagging.

Palatopharyngeal incompetence may also be demonstrated roentgenographically. The head should be carefully positioned to obtain a true lateral view; 1 film is obtained with the patient at rest and another during continuous phonation of the vowel "u" as in "boom." The soft palate contacts the posterior pharyngeal wall in normal function, while in palatopharyngeal incompetence such contact is absent.

Treatment.   In selected cases the palate may be repositioned or a pharyngoplasty performed utilizing a flap of tissue from the posterior pharyngeal wall. Dental speech appliances have also been used successfully.

11.12   PERIODONTAL DISEASE

The roots of teeth are somewhat conical in shape. Their retention and stability depend on the integrity of the surrounding alveolar bone and on a healthy periodontal membrane, with its fibers running from the root surface to the bone. Apart from the normal events of eruption, either trauma or an underlying systemic condition is likely to be responsible for looseness or exfoliation. The differential diagnosis of noneruptive loss of teeth in children includes scurvy, osteomyelitis of the jaw, juvenile periodontitis, dysplasia of dentin, leukemia, acrodynia, vitamin D deficiency, vitamin D–refractory rickets, hypophosphatasia, Papillon-Lefèvre syndrome (hyperkeratosis of palms and soles and disintegration of alveolar bone), and reticuloendotheliosis.

Poor oral hygiene may set the stage for more severe periodontal breakdown. Inflammation of the gingival margins may lead to irreversible changes in the capillary vessels. The inflammatory response results from plaque accumulations in the gingival sulci and the toxic products of bacterial growth. When the epithelial barrier to invasion is damaged, more severe infections destroy portions of the periodontal membrane or the alveolar bone. Plaque control measures may effectively ameliorate the condition.

Periapical Infection (Alveolar Abscess).   Teeth may lose their internal blood supply as a result of deep caries or trauma and become nonvital with or without accompanying pain. Grayish discoloration, looseness, and sensitivity on mastication are frequent symptoms. Localized tissue swelling and redness are most commonly due to infection around the roots of nonvital teeth, which may also lead to chronically draining fistulas visible in the alveolus at the level of the apex of the root. Periapical infections of primary teeth may cause defects in underlying permanent teeth. Infectious exudates may cause decalcification of the enamel of the underlying teeth. The roots of infected primary teeth may not follow the normal pattern of resorption, thus inducing abnormalities in eruption.

Chronic periapical infections from nonvital teeth have the potential for becoming acute infections if not treated and should be referred promptly to a dentist. Surveillance for these conditions should be routine during pediatric physical examinations. Root canal therapy can be carried out on primary teeth and is especially valuable in the retention of permanent teeth. The reduction of acute symptoms is advised before the involved tooth is extracted to reduce the accompanying bacteremia and further local tissue invasion.

Impacted Teeth.   Impaction of teeth is a common dental problem in children. Previously erupted permanent teeth with limited space available may prevent the subsequent eruption of another tooth that must occupy the same area of the alveolar bone. The teeth most frequently involved are the maxillary canines and the mandibular 3rd molars. The impacted tooth becomes lodged against the one impeding its eruption. Ectopic eruption or resorption of the offending tooth may result. Pain is common. Unless there are unique contraindications, all impacted teeth should be extracted. When retained for any length of time impacted teeth should be monitored by periodic roentgenographic examinations to avoid complications.

Dentigerous Cysts.   Impacted teeth retained in alveolar bone for longer periods of time are the source of dentigerous cysts or of cystic degeneration of the enamel epithelium around the crown. The teeth most frequently involved are the mandibular 3rd molars and the maxillary canines. Roentgenographically, the crown of the unerupted tooth is surrounded by a well demarcated radiolucent zone. A dentigerous cyst may dislodge the tooth with which it is associated, e.g., to the inferior border of the mandible or to the floor of the nasal cavity. The lesion requires enucleation or curettage; cysts arising from enamel epithelium have the

potential of becoming ameloblastomas. Marsupialization may be used where immediate extraction is likely to result in complications.

11.13   DISEASES OF THE ORAL MUCOSA AND GINGIVA

Bednar Aphthae (Pterygoid Ulcer).   Abrasions of the palatal membrane of the newborn infant, resulting from efforts to clear the mouth of debris, are termed Bednar aphthae. Superficial trauma denudes a region of the posterior hard palate over which a grayish necrotic membrane forms, typically on either side of the midline just anterior to the junction with the soft palate.

Epstein Pearls (Bohn Pearls).   Epithelial retention cysts may appear on either side of the median raphe of the palate of the newborn infant. They disappear within a few wk.

Mucocele (Mucous Cysts).   At any age small mucus-containing cysts may occur in salivary gland-bearing areas of the oral cavity. They have a circumscribed, translucent, bluish appearance. Though usually elevated, they may be deep seated and mobile on palpation. The cysts form after traumatic rupture of the excretory ducts of minor salivary glands. They are usually lined by granulation tissue, rarely by epithelium. Surgical removal of the cyst and the superficially located gland is recommended since recurrence is frequent with drainage alone.

Fordyce Granules.   Almost 80% of adults have multiple, yellowish white granules in clusters or plaquelike areas on the oral mucosa, most commonly on the buccal mucosa or lips. Histologically, normal sebaceous glands are seen in the lamina propria and submucosa. The glands are present at birth, but they hypertrophy and first appear as discrete yellowish papules during the preadolescent period in approximately 50% of children. No treatment is necessary.

Epulis.   This term is commonly used for any tumor-like growth of the gums, many of which are reactive rather than neoplastic. They are pedunculated or sessile growths which may recur after removal but do not metastasize.

Oral Moniliasis (Thrush).   Oral infection with the fungus *Candida albicans* is common in the newborn infant. The organisms are regular inhabitants of skin and of oral, vaginal, and intestinal mucosa and are spread to the infant during birth. The oral lesions in children are white, flaky plaques covering all or part of the tongue, lips, gingiva, and buccal mucous membranes. They are removable, leaving a brightly inflamed base. Discomfort may interfere with food ingestion. The condition is likely to be acute in newborn infants and chronic in infants and young children with nutritional deficiencies and other debilitating conditions. Alterations in the oral flora due to antibiotic therapy also may be responsible. The diagnosis can usually be confirmed by direct microscopic examination and culture of scrapings from mucous membranes.

Though the infection in the newborn infant is usually self-limited, treatment with 1 ml of a solution of nystatin

(100,000 units/ml) 4 times a day at intervals of 6 hr will limit spread within the nursery and avoid the occasional protracted infection. The solution should be slowly and gently instilled in the mouth so that there is an opportunity for it to be widely distributed throughout the oral cavity before it is swallowed.

Topical application of 1% aqueous gentian violet is also effective, but it is temporarily disfiguring and stains clothing and bed linen (stains can be removed with a paste of sodium bicarbonate). Applications should be made on individual lesions, and care should be taken to avoid an excess of the solution, which may be irritating when swallowed. The latter complication can be lessened if the infant is placed face downward after the application so that saliva containing the drug will drain outward.

Of primary importance in the chronically ill or malnourished infant or child with oral moniliasis is correction of the underlying disturbance.

Herpangina.   See Sec 10.84.

Herpetic Stomatitis.   See Sec 10.71.

Aphthous Ulcers (Canker Sores).   These are painful lesions found commonly and recurrently on the oral mucosa, including the tongue and palate. An initial erythematous macule ruptures to form a highly sensitive crater surrounded by an indurated zone of inflammation. The lesions, which somewhat resemble those of herpetic stomatitis but are more localized, occur singly and may multiply, usually following situations of stress. Topical applications of tincture of benzoin are of value in the control of pain. The ulcer usually heals in 1–2 wk without scar formation.

Necrotizing Ulcerative Gingivitis (Vincent Infection; Vincent Angina).   This lesion is characterized by formation of a gray necrotic membrane and small ulcers localized upon painful hyperemic gingivae. Fever, malaise, and a prominent fetid odor are common. The infection usually represents a decrease in resistance of gingival tissue to infection with the usual oral flora and with an especially heavy overgrowth of fusiform bacilli and spirochetes. Such infections are largely limited to chronically ill, malnourished children. The acute stage of the infection responds dramatically, usually within 48 hr, to thorough cleansing of the mouth with oxidizing sprays or mouth rinses; hourly rinses with half-strength (3%) hydrogen peroxide while the child is awake are also helpful.

Since necrotizing ulcerative gingivitis is extremely rare in childhood except in areas of extreme poverty, the diagnosis should be made with caution. Herpetic stomatitis and the oral manifestations of acute leukemia and the reticuloendothelioses may be similar and should be excluded.

Noma (Gangrenous Stomatitis; Cancrum Oris; Infective Gangrene of the Mouth).   Noma is a rare progressive gangrene of the buccal mucosa which results in a perforating ulcer of the cheek. It is caused by invasion of the buccal tissues by fusospirochetal organisms and other bacteria in children whose resistance has been lowered by concurrent disease or nutritional deficiency. The lesion usually begins as a small ulcer with few constitutional symptoms but soon results in a gangrenous, greenish-black area on the gums, buccal mucosa, or mucocutaneous borders. The gangrenous area spreads slowly but inexorably until the cheeks are perforated and the jaws denuded.

Intensive antibacterial therapy should be instituted as soon as the diagnosis is made and continued until all necrotic tissue, whether soft tissue or bone, has sloughed. Since malnutrition is frequent in these patients, an adequate diet should be introduced gradually, with special emphasis on adequate amounts of protein and vitamins. Plastic surgical procedures may be indicated when healing is complete.

Chemical Burns.   In addition to accidental ingestion of acids, alkalis, or other caustic substances, incorrect self-medication may cause burns of the oral mucosa, which usually appear as white lesions. The most common example is holding an aspirin tablet locally against a painful tooth or gingival area so that the tablet dissolves slowly. The result is a white, irregular patch of coagulated tissue. Camphor held in the mouth is another frequent cause of oral burns. The only treatment required is elimination of the practice; healing is spontaneous.

Dilantin Hyperplasia.   A generalized enlargement of the gingiva occurs in about 10–30% of patients who receive diphenylhydantoin sodium (Dilantin) for control of seizures. The affected gingiva is pale, firm, and granular and may hypertrophy to the point of covering the crowns of the teeth. Superimposed trauma, infection, or poor oral hygiene may cause inflammation and discomfort. Careful oral hygiene helps to avoid discomfort and reduce the occurrence. Alternative anticonvulsants should be prescribed where possible.

Fibromatosis Gingivae.   This is a rare familial idiopathic gingival hyperplasia which resembles Dilantin hyperplasia. It may be associated with other developmental defects such as mental deficiency and hypertrichosis. The firm, smooth-surfaced, generalized enlargement of the gingiva consists of collagen covered by stratified squamous epithelium. The swelling may produce protrusion of the lips and migration of the teeth. The only effective treatment is surgical removal of the excess gingiva, but recurrence is common. Particular attention to oral hygiene to prevent irritation and stimulation of further gingival overgrowth is required.

11.14   DISEASES OF THE LIPS AND TONGUE

DISEASES OF THE LIPS

Prominent Labial Frenum.   The labial frenum may appear prominent and thick. The fibers also may pass between the maxillary central incisors rather than attach to the labial mucosa. This may appear to cause spacing, or diastema, of deciduous or permanent incisors.

A space between the primary maxillary incisors is common. If a wide band of the frenum with an attachment to the lingual side of the alveolar ridge persists after eruption of the permanent canines, the frenum may be suspected as the cause of a diastema. In most cases the downward growth of the alveolar bone raises the attachment, and the lateral force of the erupting canines closes any existing space. When necessary, the attachment can be raised surgically, and a simple appliance can be used to bring the incisors together.

Cheilitis. Dryness of the lips followed by scaling and cracking and accompanied by a characteristic burning sensation is common in children. It is usually caused by sensitivity to contact substances (from toys and foods) plus photosensitivity to the sun's rays. It is aggravated by the habit of alternate wetting with the tongue and drying by the wind, especially in cold weather. Cheilitis also often occurs in association with fever. Frequent application of a bland ointment permits healing and is also preventive.

Angular Fissures. Maceration and fissuring at the angles of the mouth may be caused by an infection with *Candida albicans*. It usually causes no constitutional symptoms or pain and extends inside the mouth. Treatment with a mold antiseptic is successful.

When fissuring is caused by a nutritional deficiency, it is termed **cheilosis.** Cheilosis is an early sign in riboflavin deficiency and is often accompanied by moniliasis. Fissuring also occurs in mentally deficient children who drool (rhagades in the Down syndrome).

Herpes Simplex (Herpes Labialis; Cold Sore; Fever Blister). Herpes simplex (Sec 10.71) is an aggregate of small transparent vesicles on an inflammatory base and is accompanied by itching or burning. It usually affects the mucocutaneous junction but may affect the skin of the face or the mucous membrane of the mouth. It is self-limited, disappearing in 8–14 days.

Allergic Eruptions. Certain substances, such as lipsticks and toothpastes, may produce eruptions where they come in contact with the lips. The lesions may be vesicular or elevated reddish wheals (*urticaria*), and there may be a glossitis. There is usually a history of other allergic manifestations.

Angioedema (Sec 9.51) is a variety of urticaria which may be responsible for a sudden diffuse swelling of short duration (1–2 days) in children with allergic tendencies. It often itches but is seldom painful. There is no erythema, the tissues appear normal in color and firm, and they do not pit.

Mucous Retention Cysts. These are single teatlike projections covered by a thinned-out mucous membrane and filled with a clear fluid. They are caused by occlusion of the orifice of a labial or buccal mucous gland, resulting in retention of the secreted fluid.

Postanesthetic Trauma. Local anesthetic blockage for dental procedures or minor surgery may leave a portion of the lips temporarily senseless. Young children will occasionally traumatize the area with their teeth; swelling results, frequently accompanied by ulceration. Spontaneous remission usually occurs in 2–3 days, but antibiotic therapy is occasionally necessary to control secondary infection.

DISEASES OF THE TONGUE

In certain instances the tongue may assume an unusual appearance without undue clinical significance, and the patient is often not aware of any problem.

Ankyloglossia (Tongue-Tie). Occasionally, the lingual frenum extends to near the tip of the tongue and interferes with its free protrusion; if the attachment reaches the anterior border, a notch may be visible. It is not advisable to clip the lingual frenum at birth because bleeding or infection may result and because it usually stretches with time. Should the rare surgical correction be necessary, it should be done after 8–10 mo of age.

Fissured Tongue. The pattern may be foliaceous (leaflike) or cerebriform. The tongue may also be somewhat enlarged and show imprints of the teeth at the sides. Fissured (scrotal) tongue is usually congenital, but may be acquired, especially in Down syndrome. Occasionally, fissuring may follow certain diseases such as scarlet fever, syphilis, or typhoid fever.

Black Hairy Tongue (Lingua Nigra). This condition is characterized by an elongation of the filiform papillae into hairlike projections as long as 0.5–1 inch. It is generally concentrated in a triangular area in front of the V-shaped line of circumvallate papillae and associated with debris accumulation in that region. The patch may vary from brown to black. The condition is usually chronic but often disappears with regular dorsal cleansing. A similar condition also occurs in association with chronic intraoral hemorrhage, as in purpura and hemophilia. The filiform papillae become hypertrophied and colored dark brown by the blood pigments. There is always a characteristic *fetor ex ore* due to the presence of blood in the mouth.

Hairy tongue may occur during prolonged antibiotic therapy, especially with oral troches. Disturbances in the normal oral microbial flora are significant contributing factors.

Geographic Tongue (Wandering Rash). This benign lesion is characterized by 1 or more smooth, bright red patches, often showing a yellowish, grayish, or whitish membranous margin upon the dorsum of an otherwise normally roughened tongue. The patches are areas in which the filiform papillae have become completely desquamated, leaving a smooth, slick surface. The patches may be single or multiple, discrete or confluent (maplike). They travel by an extension of desquamation of the papillae at 1 edge and regeneration of the normal papillae at the other. The condition is usually chronic, and a single cycle may last 2–7 days.

Temporary smooth red patches on the dorsum of the tongue simulating geographic tongue are frequent in children with low-grade fevers, particularly those accompanying the common cold and chronic systemic infections. Treatment is contraindicated.

Macroglossia. The tongue in infants occasionally appears proportionately larger than the other oral structures because it grows at a relatively faster rate and is not confined by the teeth. In stocky infants the tongue is sometimes so large and unconfined that it protrudes from the mouth and may be mistaken for a manifestation of hypothyroidism. As the infant grows, the other oral structures gradually catch up and confine the tongue so that its relative size is decreased.

A true hypertrophy of the tongue is rare but may exist congenitally as a diffuse lymphangioma or as a muscular hypertrophy (rhabdomyoma). The tongue may reach such a size that it cannot be retained in the mouth, with the result that nursing and, later, speech are difficult. In such cases the teeth are pushed into a malocclusion by the action of the tongue.

Treatment is surgical, although some relative adjustment usually occurs as the child grows older.

Hemangiomas and cysts may be responsible for diffuse or localized enlargement of the tongue. Enlargement is also present in cretinism, acromegaly, Beckwith syndrome, and, occasionally, gargoylism.

White-Coated Tongue.   The accumulation of food debris and bacteria among hypertrophied filiform papillae causes a moist *white-coated tongue*. The filiform papillae are present at birth but are much shorter than even the fungiform papillae until about 5 yr of age so that the tongue appears smooth. Thus, in the young child the cause should be sought for any coating of the tongue.

The condition of *dry furry tongue* (hypertrophied filiform papillae) is seen early in states of mild dehydration and low-grade fever.

A transitional stage from the white-coated tongue to the raw red tongue is known as the *white strawberry tongue*. The appearance is that of an unripe strawberry. The engorged and enlarged fungiform papillae appear prominently above the level of the white, desquamating, filiform papillae. It is seen early in scarlet fever and other acute febrile states.

Raw Red Tongue (Glossitis).   This condition occurs when the filiform papillae of the white strawberry tongue or coated tongue are shed, leaving the engorged fungiform papillae raised above the smooth, denuded surface of the tongue. It is also known as red raspberry or red strawberry tongue and is seen often in the later stages of febrile states and about the 6th–7th day of scarlet fever.

When the papillae become flattened and edematous (mushroom-shaped) but not atrophied or shed, the *raw pebbly tongue* results. The color is a characteristic purplish red (magenta) instead of pink. Edema of the tongue is common, and the indentations of the teeth can easily be seen. As the edges of the tongue often become denuded and raw, there is a burning, painful sensation. Fissuring is common. Such lesions occur in *ariboflavinosis* in association with cheilosis, photophobia, and lacrimation.

Complete atrophy of both the filiform and fungiform papillae results in a *smooth atrophic tongue*. The desquamated surface is usually dry and extremely sensitive (glazed tongue). **Atrophic glossitis** with a fiery red (scarlet) coloration of the tongue is characteristic of niacin deficiency (pellagrous glossitis), especially when accompanied by infection. Atrophic glossitis with a pale salmon coloration of the tongue (*Hunter glossitis*) occurs in pernicious anemia, sprue, achlorhydria, and hypochromic anemia.

Taste buds may be reduced or absent in the tongue in familial dysautonomia (Riley-Day syndrome).

Trauma.   Accidental biting of the tongue, irritation by carious teeth, injuries by sharp objects placed in the mouth, and burns by hot foods occur frequently in children. Such injuries may result in a simple blister or ulcer which disappears in a few days, but even superficial ulcers are painful. In extreme cases the tongue may become swollen and edematous. Ice may be used to reduce the swelling. The food should be cool and in liquid form; it may be necessary to feed young infants through a nasal tube. A mild antiseptic mouthwash such as 1% tincture of iodine in physiologic saline solution may be used.

Accidental injuries and burns resulting from ingestion of poisons are not uncommon in young children. Immediate care is determined by the poison ingested and the extent of the injury (Sec 28.4). In severe cases particular attention should be given to adequacy of the airway; occasionally, tracheostomy is essential as a lifesaving measure.

Ulcerations of the frenum and the margins of the tongue are usually aphthous ulcers; those limited to the frenum may be secondary to biting the tongue during paroxysms of coughing in pertussis. Such ulcers have also been observed in association with familial dysautonomia.

11.15   SALIVARY GLANDS

Salivary excretions originate from 3 pairs of glands: the parotid, submaxillary, and sublingual. The parotid fluid is serous and contains amylase and secretory immunoglobulin (IgA); that of the submaxillary glands is a mixed seromucoid fluid; and that of the sublinguals is a mucoid viscous fluid. The volume and composition of the mixed saliva are a function of the degree of secretory stimulation to each of the 3 pairs of glands and are subject to many local and systemic influences.

With the exception of mumps (Sec 10.77) disease of the salivary gland is rare in children. Bilateral enlargement of the submaxillary glands may occur in cystic fibrosis, in malnutrition, and, transiently, during acute asthmatic attacks. Chronic vomiting and aspiration, as in achalasia, may also be accompanied by enlargement of the parotids.

Infants exhibit salivary discharge or **drooling** until muscular reflexes that initiate swallowing and lip closure are developed. Later, the irritation of teething in conjunction with the accompanying increase in oral activity may also lead to drooling. In some children with mental retardation drooling is never overcome. Excessive secretion of saliva occurs as a reflex to anticipated feeding or pain, from irritative lesions in the mouth, in conjunction with nausea, after administration of mercurial compounds, and in certain nervous afflictions, such as encephalitis and chorea.

If salivary flow rates are decreased by medications, disease, or irradiation, an increase in dental decay usually follows. In addition to the obvious washing action, saliva also appears to furnish the materials from which the cell-free film which covers dental enamel is formed. This film influences the surface equilibria between enamel and bathing fluids; its absence is accompanied by a pronounced increase in caries. Fluoride-containing artificial saliva rinses are advisable.

Xerostomia (Dry Mouth).   Temporary dryness of the mouth occurs with fever, dehydration, and the ingestion of drugs such as the phenothiazine derivatives, atropine, and other anticholinergic substances. In *con-*

genital xerostomia the mouth becomes glazed, dry, and filled with debris. This condition responds to the administration of pilocarpine.

Recurrent Parotitis. Recurrent idiopathic swelling of the parotid gland may occur in otherwise healthy children. The swelling is usually unilateral, but both parotid glands may be involved simultaneously or alternately. Up to 10 or more recurrences may be observed in an individual child. There is little pain associated with the swelling, which is limited to the gland and usually lasts 2–3 wk. Subsidence is spontaneous and may be complete or partial. The incidence appears to be higher in the spring.

Suppurative Parotitis. This is most often due to *Staphylococcus aureus* and may occur as a primary disease or as a complication of parotitis due to another cause. It is usually unilateral and may be accompanied by fever; the gland becomes swollen, tender, and painful.

Recurrent parotitis requires no treatment, but it may be confused with suppurative parotitis, which responds to appropriate antibacterial therapy based on culture of the purulent discharge from Stensen duct or of pus obtained by infrequently required surgical drainage. Radiotherapy appears to shorten the attacks of recurrent parotitis and to decrease the number of recurrences. Because of the potential hazards of radiation to the growing child, it should be considered only in severe or prolonged cases.

Mikulicz Disease. This refers to idiopathic, bilateral, painless enlargements of the parotid and lacrimal glands, usually associated with dryness of the mouth and an absence of tears. The manifestations may also occur in diseases such as tuberculosis, leukemia, and lymphosarcoma.

Ranula. Because of resemblance to the appearance of a frog's belly, a cyst associated with 1 of the major salivary glands in the sublingual area is termed a ranula. The large, soft, mucus-containing swelling occurs in the floor of the mouth and may be seen at any age, including infancy. The cyst should be excised and the severed duct exteriorized.

LAWRENCE A. FOX

Braham RL, Morris ME: Textbook of Pediatric Dentistry. Baltimore, Williams & Wilkins, 1980.

Finn SB: Clinical Pedodontics. Ed 4. Philadelphia, WB Saunders, 1973.

Gorlin RJ, Pindborg JJ: Syndromes of the Head and Neck. New York, McGraw-Hill Book Company, 1964.

Kraus BS, Jordan RE: The Human Dentition Before Birth. Philadelphia, Lea & Febiger, 1965.

McDonald RE: Dentistry for the Child and Adolescent. Ed 4. St. Louis, CV Mosby, 1978.

Moyers RE: Handbook of Orthodontics. Ed 3. Chicago, Year Book Medical Publishers, 1972.

Newbrun E: Fluorides and Dental Caries. Ed 2. Springfield II, Charles C Thomas, 1975.

Nowak A: Dentistry for the Handicapped. St Louis, CV Mosby, 1976.

Rapp R, Winter GB: Color Atlas of Clinical Conditions in Pedodontics. Chicago, Year Book Medical Publishers, 1979.

THE GASTROINTESTINAL TRACT

11.16 NORMAL DIGESTIVE TRACT PHENOMENA

The continuing maturation of the digestive system is reflected in changing patterns of function during childhood. These normal developmental phenomena should not be mistaken for manifestations of significant disease.

The processes involved in *ingestion of food* are well developed and coordinated at birth. The suckling infant initially encounters difficulties with solid foods, thrusting them forward with the tongue rather than back to the pharynx, but practice quickly corrects the problem. The relatively short frenulum has no effect on ingestion. During suckling, infants swallow air; unlike older children they must be stimulated to burp during the course of feeding. Otherwise, gaseous gastric distention can interfere with intake. A sense of taste probably develops by 1 mo of age, after which sweet and salty foods seem to be preferred. Primary teeth begin to erupt from 6–10 mo of age (Sec 11.3).

Regurgitation of gastric content is very common in infants before 9–12 mo, when children normally become upright for much of the day. This incompletely understood phenomenon may accompany or follow several feedings each day; it usually resolves with time. If general health and development are unaffected and the complications of aspiration or esophagitis do not develop, there is no need for detailed investigation of these patients.

The *pattern of food intake* and *appetite* of children at different ages often seem bizarre to those who regularly consume 3 meals a day. Particularly distressing to parents, but normal, is the toddler's habit of gorging him- or herself after refusing to consume the daily requirements for a few days. Appetite fluctuates enormously. In periods of rapid growth during infancy and adolescence, appetite is usually voracious, while during the intervening years some children appear to eat almost nothing while growing and gaining weight normally.

The *number, color, and consistency of bowel actions* vary greatly in the same infant and between infants of similar age regardless of diet or environment. After birth the 1st stools consist of meconium, a dark, viscous, gum-like material. When milk feedings begin, meconium is replaced by green-brown transition stools, often containing curds, and then in 4–5 days by yellow-brown milk stools. Stool frequency may vary from 1–7/day in babies who are otherwise perfectly well. Color of the stool is of little significance unless, of course, blood is present. Some children are 2–3 yr of age before they have formed stools. Breast-fed infants tend to have infrequent yellow stools of loose consistency. Later, the husks of vegetables like corn and peas and the black "worm-like" threads from the surface of the peeled banana may appear in stools after these foods have been eaten.

Abdominal findings in a normal young child sometimes give rise to unnecessary concern. During the 1st 3–4 yr of life the abdominal musculature is relatively weak, the abdominal organs relatively large, and the lower spine lordotic so that the belly is protuberant but soft. Up to 2 yr a soft liver edge will be palpable as far as 2 cm below the right costal margin. Although the spleen is not usually palpable, a soft tip may be felt in the course of an acute infection.

Blood loss from the digestive tract is never normal, but swallowed blood can easily be misinterpreted as enteric hemorrhage. Maternal blood may be ingested at the time of birth or later by the breast-fed baby when there is bleeding near the mother's nipple. Children may also swallow their own blood from an epistaxis or some other source in the nasopharynx.

Jaundice occurs in about 20% of all newborn term infants; the more prematurely born the baby, the higher the incidence of jaundice. In most newborn infants jaundice results not from a specific disease but from a limited capacity of the immature liver to conjugate the large quantities of hemoglobin breakdown products presented to it during the early wk of life (Sec 7.44).

11.17   MAJOR SYMPTOMS AND SIGNS OF DIGESTIVE TRACT DISORDERS

An understanding of the pathogenesis of major symptoms is particularly important in dealing with childhood gastroenterologic disorders because in so many cases the cause is unknown and specific or curative treatment not available. The mechanisms underlying the important clinical manifestations of gastrointestinal diseases are briefly summarized below.

Disordered Ingestion. Abnormalities at several sites in the upper digestive tract can significantly compromise dietary intake.

Transfer Dysphagia. Impaired capacity to deliver food to the upper esophagus suggests a disorder involving the mouth or pharynx. A complex sequence of neuromuscular events is involved in the delivery of foods to the upper esophagus. Suckling requires the lips to form a tight seal about the nipple while the tongue is displaced posteriorly. As the glottis closes to guard the airway, the soft palate raises to close the nasopharynx, the cricopharyngeal muscles relax, and food passes to the back of the pharynx. Solids similarly require a coordinated series of actions, and when they are consumed in large pieces, jaw movement and teeth become factors to consider. Salivary secretions, stimulated by the anticipation and act of ingestion, lubricate

foods as they pass through the mouth. Although severe structural, dental, and salivary abnormalities are relatively common, ingestion seems to proceed relatively well in the hungry child despite these potential handicaps. It is abnormalities of the muscles involved in the ingestion process (in their innervation, strength, or coordination) that usually cause transfer dysphagia in infants and children. In such cases, the oral-pharyngeal problem is almost always part of a more generalized neurologic or muscular problem. Occasionally, painful oral lesions, such as an acute viral stomatitis or trauma, will temporarily interfere with ingestion. If the nasal air passage is seriously obstructed, the need for air will cause severe distress when suckling.

Dysphagia, Regurgitation. The motor function of the esophagus is largely self-regulated with high pressure zones acting as sphincters at its upper and lower ends. The act of swallowing is normally well coordinated at birth: primary peristaltic waves, initiated by swallowing, proceed down the length of the esophagus, while secondary waves which appear to empty the esophagus of residue are initiated by distention. Regurgitation can occur if swallowing is completely or partially obstructed by an intrinsic lesion in the body of the esophagus or an extrinsic lesion, in which case possible compression of the trachea will lead to stridor and cough. Primary motility disorders causing impaired peristaltic function and dysphagia are rare in children.

The lower esophageal sphincter (LES) helps to prevent reflux of gastric contents into the esophagus (Sec 11.20). In general, if lower esophageal sphincter pressure is abnormally reduced, flow of gastric content in a retrograde direction will be encouraged with a loss of nutrients and eventually malnutrition. However, in very young symptomatic patients there is a poor correlation between sphincter function and the severity of gastroesophageal reflux. Hiatus hernia (Sec 11.20) is probably not an important determinant of gastroesophageal reflex in many instances.

Continued exposure of the lower esophageal mucosa to gastric juice can cause esophagitis and, as a consequence, dysphagia and chronic blood loss. The chance of aspirating gastric juice is enhanced by underlying motility problems in the esophagus, particularly dysfunction of the upper esophageal sphincter.

Anorexia. Hunger and satiety centers in man are probably located in the hypothalamus, and numerous pathways exist by which gastrointestinal diseases might depress appetite. Particularly important are afferents to the hypothalamus from the gut. Satiety is stimulated, for example, by distention of the stomach or upper small bowel, the signal transmitted by sensory efferents which are especially dense in the upper gut. Chemoreceptors in the intestine, influenced by the presence and assimilation of nutrients, also affect afferent flow to the appetite centers. Impulses also reach the hypothalamus from higher centers possibly influenced by pain or the emotional disturbance of an intestinal disease. Further control comes from circulating factors including hormones and plasma glucose, which in turn are affected by intestinal function.

Vomiting. Vomiting results from a violent descent of the diaphragm and constriction of the abdominal muscles, forcing gastric content back up the esophagus.

In man a vomiting center in the cerebral medulla causes vomiting when stimulated. Also, there are probably cerebral chemoreceptors which influence this center and respond to circulating factors. Consequently, diseases affecting almost any system, but particularly the brain, may cause vomiting.

Obstructions of the digestive tube at the pylorus or beyond cause vomiting, probably mediated by visceral afferents reaching the vomiting center. If obstruction occurs below the 2nd part of the duodenum, emesis is often bile stained. Lesions of the digestive tract other than those that obstruct can also cause vomiting; most diseases of the upper bowel, pancreas, liver, or biliary tree are capable of provoking emesis. Furthermore, metabolic derangements such as those occurring in hepatocellular failure of Reye syndrome may lead to severe, even fulminant cerebral edema and, as a result, severe persistent emesis.

Rarely, violent vomiting itself may cause mucosal tears and bleeding at the gastroesophageal junction (Mallory-Weiss syndrome).

Diarrhea. Diarrhea is defined as the excessive loss of fluid and electrolyte in stool (Sec 5.24 and 10.12). Water movement across intestinal membranes is passive and determined by both active and passive fluxes of solutes, particularly sodium, chloride, and glucose. The basis for all diarrhea, therefore, is disturbed intestinal solute transport. In most clinical situations epithelial abnormalities are the major known determinants of diarrhea; hypermotility is rarely a significant factor, and little is known about the roles of blood and lymphatic flow to the gut. Normally, all but a final small percentage of water absorption occurs in the small bowel, and it is small bowel disease that tends to cause voluminous diarrhea. Colonic diarrhea is usually less voluminous and characterized by alternating loose and formed or hard stools.

Disease may disturb intestinal transport causing diarrhea by damaging the bowel wall or by elaborating secretagogues, which reach the epithelium via the circulation or from the bowel lumen. When the mucosa is damaged, not only is absorptive surface area diminished but often the function of the remaining cells is severely compromised. For example, in rotavirus enteritis, glucose transport is defective, disaccharidase and Na^+-K^+ATPase activities are reduced, and glucose-stimulated Na^+ transport is impaired in the small bowel epithelium.

Bacterial secretagogues have no effect on absorptive surface area or on the structure of the intestinal epithelium. For example, the very potent secretagogue choleragen, produced in the gut lumen by *V. cholerae*, binds to the small intestinal brush border and, via adenylate cyclase activity, stimulates cyclic AMP accumulation in the epithelium. The result is a massive watery diarrhea characterized by brisk chloride secretion, impaired NaCl absorption, but preservation of the glucose-stimulated Na^+ absorption and Na^+-K^+ATPase activity that are defective in viral enteritis. Other secretagogues cause cyclic GMP accumulation but a similar result, e.g., circulating hormones, gastrin, and vasoactive intestinal peptide (VIP). Some intraluminal fatty acids and bile salts can also cause the colonic mucosa to secrete,

although the mechanism is unknown. This phenomenon may explain the diarrhea occurring with steatorrhea and with bile salt malabsorption secondary to resection of the distal ileum.

Constipation. Excessively infrequent and dry stools can arise from defects in filling or, more commonly, in emptying the rectum. Defective rectal filling occurs when colonic peristalsis is ineffective, e.g., in cases of hypothyroidism or opiate use, and when there is bowel obstruction caused either by a structural anomaly or by Hirschsprung disease. The resultant stasis leads to excessive drying of stool and a failure to initiate reflexes from the rectum that normally trigger evacuation. Emptying the rectum by spontaneous evacuation depends on a defecation reflex initiated by pressure receptors in the rectal muscle. Stool retention therefore may also result from lesions involving these rectal muscles, the sacral spinal cord afferent and efferent fibers, and the muscles of the abdomen and pelvic floor or from problems preventing relaxation of the anal sphincter.

Unfortunately, constipation tends to be self-perpetuating whatever its cause. Hard, large stools in the rectum become difficult and even painful to evacuate so that more retention occurs and a vicious cycle ensues. Distention of the rectum and colon lessens the sensitivity of the defecation reflex and the effectiveness of peristalsis. Eventually, watery content from the proximal colon may percolate around hard retained stool and pass per rectum unperceived by the child. This fecal soiling, *encopresis*, is involuntary and frequently mistaken for diarrhea. Constipation per se does not have deleterious systemic organic effects, although the problem itself and the attendant anxiety may have a marked impact on the child's emotional health. There may also be associated urinary tract stasis in severe longstanding cases.

Abdominal Pain. Individuals differ greatly in their tolerance and response to painful intra-abdominal events, but abdominal pain should always be assumed to be real. Although a specific cause is often difficult to determine, the nature and location of a pain-provoking lesion can usually be determined from the clinical description of the pain. Two types of nerve fibers transmit painful stimuli in the abdomen. In skin and muscle, A fibers mediate sharp localized pain, and C fibers from viscera, peritoneum, and muscle transmit poorly localized, dull pain. These afferent fibers have their cell bodies in the dorsal root ganglia, and some axons cross the mid-line and ascend to the medulla, mid-brain, and thalamus. Pain is perceived by the cortex of the postcentral gyrus, which therefore can receive impulses arising from both sides of the body.

Visceral pain tends to be experienced in the dermatome from which the affected organ receives innervation. Painful stimuli originating in liver, pancreas, biliary tree, stomach, or upper bowel are felt in the epigastrium; pain from the distal small bowel, cecum, appendix, or proximal colon is felt at the umbilicus; and pain from distal large bowel, urinary tract, or pelvic organs is usually suprapubic. When pain is referred to remote areas supplied by the same neurosegment as the diseased organ, the phenomenon usually means an increased intensity of the provoking stimulus. Parietal impulses travel in C fibers with peripheral nerves corresponding to dermatomes T6 to L1 and tend to be more localized and intense than visceral pain.

In the digestive tract the major provoking stimulus is tension or stretching. Inflammatory lesions probably lower the pain threshold, but the mechanisms producing inflammatory pain are not clear. Tissue metabolites released near nerve endings probably account for the pain caused by ischemia. Obviously, perception of these painful stimuli can be modulated by input from both cerebral and peripheral factors. Psychologic factors are particularly important in this regard.

Gastrointestinal Hemorrhage. Bleeding may occur at any site in the digestive tract, but the most common sites are the lower esophagus, stomach, duodenum, and colon. Usually, it is an erosion of the mucosa down to the vasculature that leads to hemorrhage, but vessel malformations or raised portal pressure also causes hemorrhage. It is rare for clotting defects to cause gastrointestinal bleeding except in hemorrhagic diseases of the newborn. When bleeding originates in the esophagus, stomach, or duodenum, it may appear in vomitus and is termed **hematemesis.** When exposed to gastric or intestinal juices for any time, blood darkens to resemble coffee grounds; therefore, the more massive and proximal the bleeding, the more likely it is to be red. Red blood in stools, **hematochezia,** signifies either a distal bleeding site or massive hemorrhage above the distal ileum. Moderate to mild bleeding from sites above the distal ileum tends to cause blackened stools of tarry consistency, **melena,** but major hemorrhages in the duodenum or above can cause melena.

Gastrointestinal bleeding can be significant yet invisible. Children may develop iron deficiency anemia from enteric blood loss but not demonstrate even occult blood in stools on random testing. Bleeding into the gut rarely, in itself, causes gastrointestinal symptoms, although brisk duodenal or gastric bleeding may lead to nausea and vomiting. The breakdown products of intraluminal blood may tip the patient into hepatic coma if liver function is already compromised.

Abdominal Distention and Abdominal Masses. Enlargement of the abdomen can result from diminished tone of the wall musculature or from increased content—fluid, gas, or solid. Fluid accumulation in the peritoneal cavity, ascites, distends the abdomen both in the flanks and anteriorly. Usually, the fluid is a transudate with a low protein concentration resulting from reduced plasma colloid osmotic pressure of hypoalbuminemia, raised portal venous pressure, or both. In cases of portal hypertension the fluid leak probably occurs from lymphatics on the liver surface and from visceral peritoneal capillaries, but ascites does not usually develop until the serum albumin level falls. For unknown reasons sodium excretion in the urine decreases greatly as the ascitic fluid accumulates so that additional dietary sodium goes directly to the peritoneal space, taking with it more water. Ascitic fluid may also be an exudate, in which case it is usually a response to either an inflammatory or a neoplastic process. When fluid has accumulated in the peritoneal cavity, it can transmit vibrations from 1 side of the abdomen to another. Significant ascites formation, therefore, can

usually be detected by attempting to elicit a fluid thrill transmitted across the abdomen or a shifting area of dullness to percussion. Fluid accumulation confined to the lumen of the gut will not produce these physical signs.

When the gut distends with fluid, either obstruction or a disturbance of the balance between absorption and secretion should be suspected. Frequently, the factors causing fluid accumulation in the bowel lumen also cause gas to accumulate. The result may be audible gurgling noises. The source of gas is usually swallowed air, but the small amount normally produced by endogenous flora may increase considerably in malabsorptive states where substrate reaches the lower intestine. Gas in the peritoneal cavity, which may cause a tympanic percussion note over even solid abdominal organs like the liver, signals impending disaster since it indicates a perforated viscus.

An abdominal organ may enlarge diffusely or be affected by a discrete mass. In the digestive tract these discrete masses may occur in the lumen, in the wall, or in the mesentery. In the constipated child, mobile, nontender fecal masses are often easily palpable. The wall of the gut can be affected by anomalies, cysts, or inflammatory disease, but, fortunately, neoplasms are extremely rare in children. The liver may enlarge diffusely in response to many disorders. Discrete liver masses may be islands of normal regenerating liver tissue occurring in a cirrhotic liver, but inflammatory and neoplastic processes also occur.

Jaundice (Sec 7.44). Jaundice means yellow staining of tissues, and it is caused by a dipyrrol pigment, bilirubin, formed from the breakdown of heme. Excessive production of bilirubin occurs in clinical states causing excessive heme breakdown. If the load exceeds hepatocyte capacity to transport bilirubin, serum and tissue levels of unconjugated bilirubin rise. Bilirubin is taken up from plasma into the hepatocyte, bound to specific ligands, and conjugated with UDP glucuronide to form bilirubin diglucuronide. If the conjugation mechanism is defective or if the cytoplasmic binding ligands are defective, unconjugated bilirubin accumulates in serum and tissues. This unconjugated bilirubin is insoluble and in serum largely albumin bound; therefore, it is not filtered by glomeruli and it does not stain the urine. Normally, the excretion of relatively water-soluble conjugated bilirubin from the hepatocyte into canaliculi is rapid; it is this pigment that gives the yellow-green color to bile. After it is concentrated by the gallbladder, bile normally reaches the intestinal lumen where bilirubin remains conjugated until bacteria of the terminal ileum and colon deconjugate it. Urobilinogen is also produced in the terminal ileum, from which it can be reabsorbed and excreted both in the urine and in bile. Defects in bilirubin excretion may occur in the hepatocyte itself or in the intrahepatic or extrahepatic collecting systems. The clinical manifestations of these excretory defects will include a rise in serum and tissue levels of conjugated bilirubin, the appearance of this soluble pigment in urine, and, depending on the degree of obstruction, a loss of pigmentation of stool and disappearance of urobilinogen from urine.

Berman NF, Holtzapple PG: Gastrointestinal hemorrhage. Pediatr Clin North Am 22:885, 1975.

Borison HL, Wong SC: Physiology and pharmacology of vomiting. Pharmacol Rev 5:193, 1953.

Dobbins WJ, Binder HJ: Pathophysiology of diarrhea: Alterations in fluid and electrolyte transport. Clin Gastroenterol 10:605, 1981.

Fitzgerald JF: Difficulties with defecation and elimination in children. Clin Gastroenterol 6:283, 1977.

Gupta JM: Neonatal jaundice. Med J Aust 1:745, 1977.

Hall RJC: Normal and abnormal food intake. Gut 16:744, 1975.

Hamilton JR: Infectious diarrhea in children. Aust Pediatr J 15:25, 1979.

Lumsden K, Holden WS: The act of vomiting in man. Gut 10:173, 1969.

Pope CE II: The esophagus: Physiology. In: Sleisenger MH, Fordtran JS (eds): Gastrointestinal Disease. Ed 2. Philadelphia, WB Saunders, 1978.

11.18   IMPORTANT CAUSES OF DIGESTIVE TRACT SYMPTOMS

In children gastrointestinal symptoms and signs may be caused by non-digestive-tract disorders (Table 11–3). Particular note should be taken of cerebral and urinary tract diseases as causes of gastrointestinal symptoms since in infants and young children the clinical manifestations of these conditions may be subtle.

Important gastroenterologic causes of digestive tract symptoms are summarized in Table 11–4. This table deals with conditions likely to be encountered in North America and includes a few conditions in which digestive tract dysfunction is secondary to pathologic processes elsewhere.

J. RICHARD HAMILTON

THE ESOPHAGUS

11.19   DEVELOPMENT AND FUNCTION OF THE ESOPHAGUS

The esophagus develops from the primitive foregut, with the trachea separated from the ventral aspect. The lateral walls of 2 laryngotracheal grooves fuse and separate the primitive esophagus from the trachea in front.

The function of the esophagus is to transport fluids and solids to the stomach and to prevent their regurgitation. The esophagus appears capable of peristalsis in the smallest of prematures, and in infants of 1500 gm sucking and swallowing seem coordinated. At birth the full term infant has short bursts of sucking followed by swallows, but in a few days (weeks in prematures) the infant has prolonged bursts of sucking during which he or she swallows and breathes in a coordinated rhythmic manner.

Swallowing is a complex act initiated by sudden elevation of the posterior portion of the tongue which thrusts the contents of the posterior pharynx into the esophagus. There is a simultaneous anterior displacement of the laryngeal orifice, which is further protected by the epiglottis, closure of the nasopharynx by the soft palate, and relaxation of the cricopharyngeal muscle that facilitates entrance of food into the esophagus.

Table 11–3   COMMON NON-DIGESTIVE-TRACT CAUSES OF GASTROINTESTINAL SYMPTOMS

Anorexia
  Systemic disease (infection, neoplasm, etc.)
  Iatrogenic—drug therapy, unpalatable therapeutic diets
  Depression
  Anorexia nervosa
Vomiting
  Increased intracranial pressure (CNS infection, tumor, hematoma)
  Infection (e.g., urinary tract)
Diarrhea
  "Parenteral" infection, (e.g., respiratory, urinary infection)
  Uremia
Constipation
  Hypothyroidism
  Dehydration (e.g., diabetes insipidus, renal tubular lesions)
Abdominal pain
  Pyelonephritis, hydronephrosis, renal colic
  Pneumonia
  Pelvic inflammatory disease
  School phobia
Abdominal mass
  Ascites (e.g., nephrotic syndrome, neoplasm, heart failure)
  Discrete mass (e.g., Wilms tumor, hydronephrosis, neuroblastoma)
  Pregnancy
Jaundice
  Hemolytic disease

Peristaltic waves are initiated to transport the bolus of food along the esophagus. Three types of esophageal pressure waves are described. A primary wave is a zone of increased esophageal pressure initiated by a swallow that proceeds along the esophagus; secondary waves are usually initiated by distention of the esophagus and serve to empty it of residual food or gastric contents. These waves empty the esophagus as one does a tube of toothpaste, by neatly rolling the tube from 1 end. Tertiary waves in the esophagus are nonpropulsive, nonperistaltic contractions likened to squeezing a tube of toothpaste in the middle; when present in large numbers they are abnormal. The distal 1–3 cm of the esophagus contains a specialized segment of circular musculature, the lower esophageal sphincter, where the intraluminal pressure is normally higher than that in the more proximal esophagus or stomach. This sphincter prevents gastroesophageal reflux and relaxes during deglutition to allow food to enter the stomach.

The common symptoms of esophageal disease are cough or choking with swallowing, vomiting, dysphagia, complete inability to swallow, pain on swallowing, and hematemesis. Each can be attributed to 1 or more defects in the complex coordination of the sequence just described and may require further diagnostic evaluation. A conventional barium swallow outlines the mucosa and may demonstrate a mass impinging on the lumen or gastroesophageal reflux. Evaluation of the dynamics of swallowing and abnormalities that are present only fleetingly requires fluoroscopy. Quantitative measurements may be obtained with esophageal manometry, inserting and slowly withdrawing pressure-sensitive catheters from the stomach. The pressure in the lower esophageal sphincter is often decreased in patients with reflux, especially if esophagitis is present; in achalasia pressures are elevated with poor relaxation after a swallow (Fig 11–3B). Measurement of intraluminal esophageal pH with a flexible 2 mm diameter pH

Table 11–4   IMPORTANT GASTROENTEROLOGIC DISORDERS CAUSING DIGESTIVE TRACT SYMPTOMS

	INFANTS	OLDER CHILDREN
Dysphagia	Neuromuscular dysfunction (i.e., cerebral palsy) Esophageal atresia	Corrosive and foreign body damage Peptic esophagitis Achalasia
Regurgitation	Gastroesophageal reflux Feeding problem	Gastroesophageal reflux
Anorexia	Stomatitis Gastroesophageal reflux Intestinal infection Celiac disease	Hepatitis Inflammatory bowel disease Celiac disease
Vomiting	Congenital obstruction Pyloric stenosis Intestinal atresia Intussusception Intestinal infection Celiac disease	Acute abdomen Appendicitis Pancreatitis Intestinal infection, food poisoning Intestinal obstruction—adhesions, volvulus Inflammatory bowel diseases Hepatitis Reye syndrome
Diarrhea	Intestinal infection Necrotizing enterocolitis Celiac disease Cystic fibrosis	Intestinal infection Inflammatory bowel diseases
Constipation	Bowel obstruction Atresia Hirschsprung disease Meconium ileus	"Functional" constipation Meconium ileus equivalent
Abdominal pain	Infantile colic Intestinal infection Intussusception Volvulus	Appendicitis Intestinal infection Inflammatory bowel diseases Lactose intolerance Peptic ulcer Pancreatitis Cholecystitis Recurrent abdominal pain syndrome
Hematemesis		Gastritis (aspirin ingestion) Esophagitis Esophageal varices Peptic ulcer Stress ulcer
Hematochezia or melena	Bacterial infection Necrotizing enterocolitis Anal fissure Meckel diverticulum Intussusception	Intestinal infection (bacterial, parasitic) Inflammatory bowel diseases Peptic ulcer Meckel diverticulum Colonic polyp Anal fissure
Abdominal mass Intestine	Distal bowel obstruction (Hirschsprung disease) Necrotizing enterocolitis Intestinal infection Celiac disease Cystic fibrosis Hernia (inguinal or umbilical)	Functional constipation Aerophagia Bowel obstruction Celiac disease Cystic fibrosis Intestinal infection
Peritoneum	Chylous ascites Peritonitis (bowel perforation)	Ascites Peritonitis
Hepatomegaly	Pancreatitis Cirrhosis Storage disease Neoplasm	Hepatitis Cirrhosis Passive congestion
Jaundice (hyperbilirubinemia) Unconjugated Mixed (conjugated, unconjugated)	Breast feeding Perinatal infections Metabolic disorders Galactosemia Tyrosinemia α_1-Antitrypsin deficiency Biliary atresia	Gilbert disease Hepatitis (A, B, non-A–non-B) Chronic active hepatitis Drug reactions Metabolic disorders Wilson disease α_1-Antitrypsin deficiency Choledochal cyst

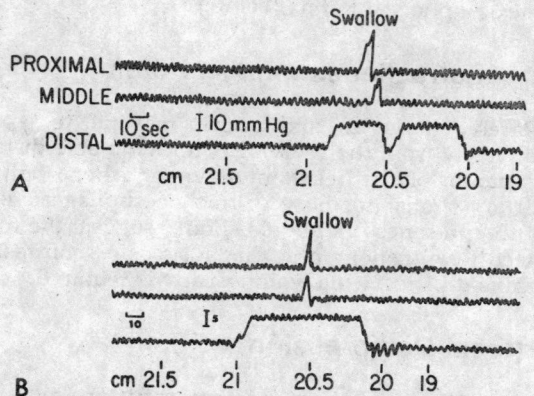

Figure 11–3 *A,* Pressures in the esophagus of a normal infant as recorded with a triple lumen catheter with recording tips 2.5 cm apart. When the distal recording tip was 21.5 cm from the gum line, it was within the lower esophageal sphincter. A swallow initiates a primary peristaltic wave. The pressure wave is detected first in the more proximal catheter and then the more distal one. A relaxation in the lower esophageal sphincter allows the food to enter the stomach. *B,* Abnormal esophageal manometry in a patient demonstrating simultaneous pressure in the 2 proximal recording tips, characteristic of tertiary esophageal wave. There is no relaxation of the lower esophageal sphincter. Such a pattern is seen in patients with achalasia.

probe in the distal esophagus is the most sensitive method to detect reflux of acid gastric contents into the esophagus. Esophagoscopy is especially useful in visualizing lesions on the mucosal surface and in detecting and removing foreign bodies. Flexible fiberoptic endoscopes permit direct examination and biopsy of the esophagus without general anesthesia in most cases.

11.20   DISORDERS OF THE ESOPHAGUS

Atresia and Tracheoesophageal Fistula

Esophageal atresia occurs in 1:3000–4500 live births; about one third of these infants are premature. In more than 75% of cases a fistula between the trachea and distal esophagus accompanies the atresia (Fig 11–4A). Less commonly, the 2 lesions coexist in a different anatomic relationship. Either atresia or tracheoesophageal fistula also can occur alone. These anomalies are thought to arise from defective differentiation as the

primitive trachea separates from the esophagus; defective growth of entodermal cells leads to atresia, and incomplete fusion of the lateral walls of the foregut leads to incomplete closure of the laryngotracheal tube and a fistula, usually at the level of tracheal bifurcation. Genetic factors are unimportant in the pathogenesis of these defects.

Clinical Manifestations. Atresia of the esophagus should be suspected if (a) a history of maternal polyhydramnios exists; (b) the catheter used at birth for resuscitation cannot be inserted into the stomach; (c) the infant has excessive oral and pharyngeal secretions; or (d) if choking, cyanosis, or coughing occurs with an attempt at feeding. Unfortunately, the diagnosis is often missed until the baby has been fed, and although suctioning of secretions from the mouth and pharynx frequently results in improvement, symptoms quickly recur. Since a fistula often connects the trachea and the distal esophagus, the abdomen is usually tympanitic and may be so distended as to interfere with breathing. If the fistula connects the proximal esophagus to the trachea, the 1st attempt at feeding may lead to massive aspiration. Infants with atresia but no fistula have scaphoid, gasless abdomens. In the rare situation of fistula without atresia (Fig 11–4C) the usual symptom is recurrent aspiration pneumonia, and diagnosis may be delayed for days or even months. Although aspiration of pharyngeal secretions is an almost constant finding in patients with esophageal atresia, it is the aspiration of gastric contents via a distal fistula that causes a much more severe life-threatening chemical pneumonitis.

Additional congenital anomalies, many of them in themselves life-threatening, occur in at least 30% of infants with esophageal atresia. Cardiovascular anomalies are the most common, but other digestive tract, urinary, vertebral, and central nervous system defects are found.

Diagnosis. Diagnosis must be early, preferably in the delivery room, since pulmonary aspiration is a major determinant of prognosis. Once esophageal atresia is suspected, an inability to pass a catheter into the stomach confirms the diagnosis. Usually the catheter stops abruptly 10–11 cm from the upper gum line and roentgenograms show a coiled catheter in the upper esophageal pouch (Fig 11–5). Occasionally, plain roentgenograms of the chest show the typical appearance of an esophagus dilated with air. The presence of air in the abdomen indicates a fistula between the trachea and the distal esophagus. If contrast material is used,

Figure 11–4 Diagrams of the 5 most commonly encountered forms of esophageal atresia and tracheoesophageal fistula, in order of frequency.

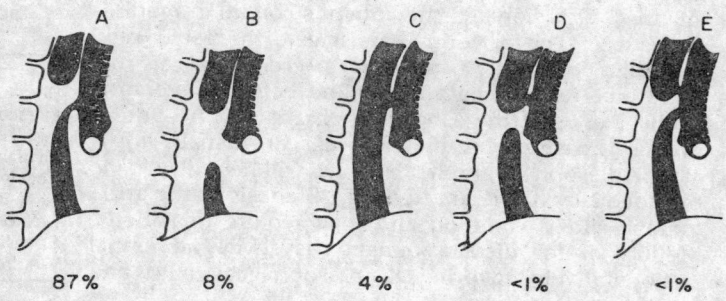

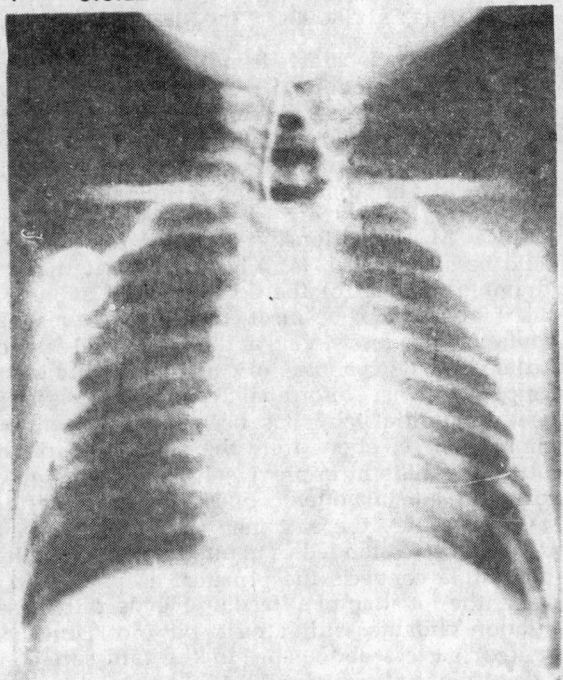

Figure 11–5 Roentgenogram of newborn infant with esophageal fistula. The coiled catheter outlines the upper blind pouch. The presence of air in the abdomen indicates a fistula to the distal esophagus.

it should be water soluble; less than 1 ml given under fluoroscopic control is sufficient to outline the blind upper pouch. The material should then be withdrawn to prevent overflow into the lungs and chemical pneumonitis. Some fistulas without atresia, the so-called H-type (Fig 11–4C), can be demonstrated with difficulty by cineradiography taken while the esophagus is filled with water-soluble contrast material. The tracheal orifice of this type of fistula may be readily detectable at bronchoscopy.

Treatment. Esophageal atresia is a surgical emergency. Preoperatively, the patient should be placed prone to decrease the opportunity for gastric contents to reach the lungs, and the contents from the upper esophageal pouch should be drained constantly by suction in an effort to keep the proximal esophagus empty. Careful attention to temperature control and respiratory function is important. Bronchoscopic aspiration may be required preoperatively as well as postoperatively for atelectasis. Associated congenital anomalies are common and are often a major cause of fatalities. Occasionally, the patient's condition requires that surgery be performed in stages, the 1st usually being ligation of the fistula and insertion of a gastrostomy tube for feeding and the 2nd being anastomosis of the 2 ends of the esophagus. Eight–10 days after a primary anastomosis, oral feedings are usually tolerated. An esophagograph at 10 days will help determine the adequacy of the anastomosis. Stenosis at the anastomotic site is common and may require dilatations. Motility of the distal esophagus is always abnormal postoperatively, favoring gastroesophageal reflux and

aspiration, esophagitis, and stricture formation (see Gastroesophageal Reflux, below).

Laryngotracheoesophageal Cleft

Rarely, the larynx and trachea may fail to separate completely from the esophagus for a variable distance. Symptoms of the resultant laryngotracheoesophageal cleft are similar to those of tracheoesophageal fistula, but the presence of aphonia should suggest the former defect. Roentgenographic diagnosis using contrast material is difficult; usually endoscopy is required.

External Compression

Masses impinging on the esophagus are most commonly lymph nodes in the subcarinal area, enlarged because of tuberculosis, histoplasmosis, other forms of pulmonary suppuration, or lymphoma. Partial obstruction of the esophagus may also be caused by extrinsic pressure from vascular anomalies in the mediastinum, such as anomalous aortic arch (Sec 13.62).

Esophageal duplication cysts may also cause esophageal compression and are usually diagnosed with barium esophagographs. Their epithelium may come from any portion of the intestine, and they do not communicate with the esophagus unless there is ulceration from gastric mucosa in the cyst. Two thirds are on the right side of the esophagus. Rarely, duplication cysts may extend through the diaphragm and communicate with the intestine. *Neurenteric cysts* are esophageal duplication cysts that contain glial elements; vertebral anomalies usually accompany these cysts.

Congenital Stenosis and Web

Congenital webs and stenoses are rare, but their embryonic development is probably similar to that of atresia. Dysphagia usually occurs when solids are introduced into the diet. The treatment is similar to that of the much more common strictures caused by peptic esophagitis from which they must be distinguished (Sec 11.22).

Dysphagia Due to Neuromuscular Diseases

The many systemic, neurologic, and muscular disorders, listed in Table 11–5, that may give rise to esophageal symptoms are discussed elsewhere (see Index).

Table 11–5   NEUROMUSCULAR DISORDERS THAT MAY CAUSE DYSPHAGIA

Cerebral palsy (more common)
Dermatomyositis
Infections—diphtheria, poliomyelitis, tetanus
Muscular dystrophy (more common)
Myasthenia gravis
Polyneuritis
Riley-Day syndrome
Scleroderma
Specific cranial nerve defects
Werdnig-Hoffmann disease

Cricopharyngeal Dysfunction

Spasm of the cricopharyngeal muscle or achalasia of the superior esophageal sphincter causes intermittent dysphagia. Eventually, increased pressure in the pharynx and upper esophagus may lead to development of a posterior pharyngeal diverticulum. Diagnosis of this idiopathic disorder is made by demonstrating with cineradiography or manometry a failure of the superior esophageal sphincter to relax during deglutition. Myotomy of the cricopharyngeal muscle, similar to the procedure used in hypertrophic pyloric stenosis (Sec 11.23), relieves symptoms.

Cricopharyngeal Incoordination of Infancy

Cricopharyngeal incoordination of infancy is usually evident soon after birth. Sucking is normal, but the patients tend to choke and aspirate with deglutition. Generally, these infants have small jaws that open poorly. On cineradiography there is repetitive to and fro movement of the contrast medium in the posterior pharynx. Careful spoon or gavage feedings are required until approximately 6 mo of age when symptoms abate. The cause of this disorder is not known.

Bulbar Palsy

Bulbar palsy, supranuclear or lower motor neuron, may cause dysphagia. Sucking is poor, the child chews and swallows solid food with difficulty, the jaw jerk is exaggerated, and usually signs of generalized cerebral palsy with spasticity develop. Lower motor neuron disease with flaccid bulbar palsies and facial diplegias constitute the Moebius syndrome.

Paralysis of the Superior Laryngeal Nerve

This has been reported in neonates with dysphagia, diminished esophageal motility, a preference to lie with the head turned to 1 side, and, in some, unilateral facial weakness. The syndrome is thought to be caused by an unusual intrauterine position in which the nerve is compressed between the thyroid cartilage and the hyoid bone. Spontaneous recovery occurs during the 1st yr of life.

Transient Pharyngeal Muscle Dysfunction

This is often associated with palatal dysfunction and may be due to delayed normal development, or it may be associated with cerebral palsy. Choking during feeding and dribbling of formula are the main symptoms. Paralysis of pharyngeal constrictors and a flaccid soft palate are noted in cineroentgenographic studies. Gavage feeding may prevent aspiration, the main complication, and may be required for only a few days or for weeks. As the child develops, other nervous system dysfunctions often occur.

Achalasia
(Megaesophagus)

Achalasia, a lack of relaxation of the lower esophageal sphincter with swallowing, causes a relative obstruction that is made worse by a lack of peristaltic waves in the esophagus (Fig 11–3B). It is primarily a condition of adults; children under age 4 yr constitute fewer than 5% of all patients. The disease has been reported in siblings. Ganglion cells are frequently decreased in number and surrounded by inflammatory cells. A heightened response of esophageal muscles to metacholine has been interpreted as evidence of a denervation hypersensitivity, but only in Chagas disease has the etiology been documented.

Clinical Manifestations and Diagnosis. Symptoms include difficult swallowing, regurgitation of food, cough from overflow of fluids into the trachea, and failure to gain weight. The diagnosis is usually made roentgenographically by demonstrating a persistently narrowed cardioesophageal junction and absence of propulsive peristaltic waves in the esophagus. If obstruction at the gastroesophageal junction persists, esophageal dilatation may become massive and air-fluid levels are often seen on an upright roentgenogram. Pulmonary infections, even bronchiectasis, may result from constant overflow of esophageal contents. In advanced cases retention of fluid and food in the esophagus may cause esophagitis.

Treatment. Acute symptoms may be relieved temporarily by dilating the cardioesophageal junction with an esophagoscope or mercury bougie, but permanent relief may require an operation in which the muscles of the cardioesophageal junction are divided (Heller procedure). Unfortunately, a procedure that relieves obstruction may allow gastroesophageal reflux, esophagitis, and rarely stricture formation. In older children permanent relief may be obtained by careful dilatation with a pneumatic bag placed in the cardioesophageal junction under fluoroscopic control.

Hiatal Hernia
(Partial Thoracic Stomach)

Herniation of part of the stomach into the thorax through the esophageal hiatus is paraesophageal in some patients, sliding in others (Fig 11–6). In the paraesophageal hernia, the gastroesophageal junction is positioned normally, but a portion of the stomach herniates into the chest through a patent esophageal hiatus. Fullness after eating and upper abdominal pain are the usual symptoms; infarction of the herniated stomach is a rare complication.

In the sliding variety the gastroesophageal junction and a portion of the stomach lie within the chest. The condition is usually congenital in children and frequently associated with symptomatic gastroesophageal reflux. There is an association with other congenital malformations and evidence of genetic factors. It is unknown whether the common occurrence of hiatal hernias in adults represents a lesion acquired in later

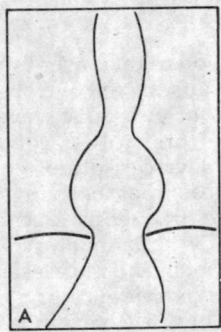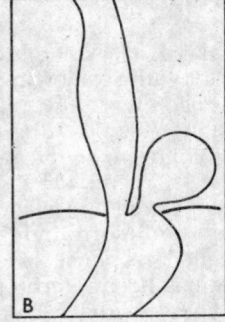

Figure 11–6 Types of esophageal hiatal hernia. *A*, Sliding hiatal hernia, the most common type; *B*, paraesophageal hiatal hernia.

life or one present since infancy. Treatment is directed not at the hernia but at the gastroesophageal reflux.

Gastroesophageal Reflux
(Chalasia)

When the lower esophageal sphincter is not competent, excessive reflux may cause significant symptoms. In the United States the term chalasia is frequently used to describe this condition; in Europe the terms partial thoracic stomach or hiatal hernia are often used.

Etiology. Factors important in the development of gastroesophageal reflux in children differ from those in adults. Hiatal hernia is frequently associated with reflux in children. Pressure in the lower esophageal sphincter is consistently decreased in adults with reflux, while in children the data are much less clear cut. Several factors appear to maintain lower esophageal sphincter integrity; some may be more important in children than in adults. For example, although increased pressure is important, the intra-abdominal position of a portion of this high pressure zone may help ensure competency in a child, as may the gathering of the mucosa within the sphincter and the angle of insertion of the esophagus into the stomach.

Clinical Manifestations. The signs and symptoms relate directly to the exposure of the esophageal epithelium to refluxed gastric contents. Excessive vomiting occurs in 85% of patients during the 1st wk of life, and an additional 10% have symptoms by 6 wk. Without treatment (Fig 11–7), symptoms abate in 60% by age 2 as the child assumes a more upright position and eats solid foods, but the remainder continue to have symptoms until at least 4 yr of age.

Vomiting may be forceful because of pylorospasm due to a reflex initiated by esophageal irritation. Aspiration pneumonia affects about one third of cases in infancy, but in those that persist until later childhood chronic cough, wheezing, and recurrent pneumonia are common. There may be rumination (see below). Growth and weight gain are adversely affected in about two thirds of cases since repeated vomiting can lead to inadequate retention of nutrients. The major manifestation of esophagitis is hemorrhage from the esophagus causing hematemesis in some children, but rarely melena. Iron deficiency anemia affects about 25% of all patients, and often the associated blood loss is occult. Substernal pain is rare, but dysphagia may contribute to diminished food intake in advanced cases. Rarely, esophagitis may progress to stricture formation.

Diagnosis. In mild cases a careful clinical assessment may be sufficient for diagnosis, which is confirmed by assessing the response to therapy. In severe or complex cases the diagnosis can be confirmed with barium esophagogram done under fluoroscopic control. The presence of gastric folds above the diaphragm is 1 way of detecting the presence of a hiatal hernia (Fig 11–8); in children these folds are more readily detected in a collapsed than in a full esophagus. Since gastro-

Symptoms present by age 3 months (98%)	Symptom-free by age 2	60–65%
	No improvement on solid foods, symptoms present > 4 years, no stricture	30%
	Esophageal stricture	5%
	Death (aspiration and innutrition)	<5%

Figure 11–7 Natural history of gastroesophageal reflux in untreated patients. (Adapted from Carre KJ: Arch Dis Child 34:344, 1959.)

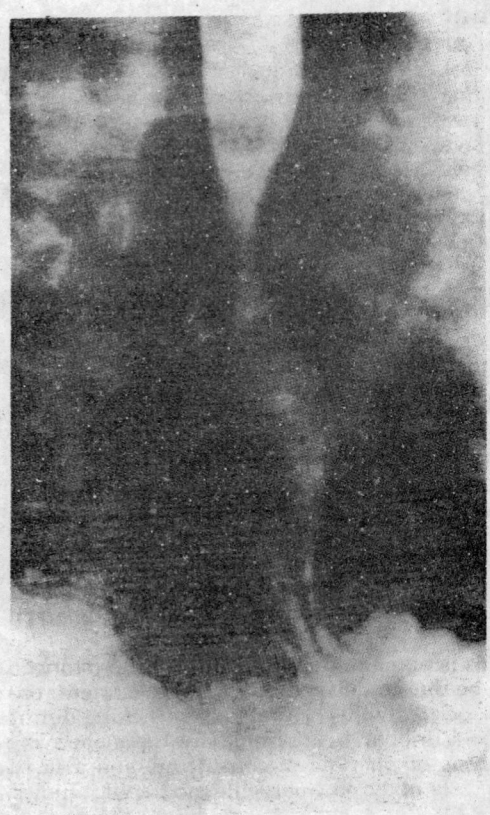

Figure 11–8 Barium esophagogram demonstrating free gastroesophageal reflux. A stricture due to peptic esophagitis is present. Longitudinal gastric folds above the diaphragm indicate the presence of an associated hiatal hernia.

esophageal reflux is an episodic event, significant reflux is not demonstrated roentgenographically in approximately 10% of cases. In such cases reflux may be detected during repeated examination or by demonstrating reflux of gastric acid with a pH probe placed in the esophagus. A volume of barium that approximates a normal meal should be administered and the patient examined in a head down position and during abdominal compression. Any child may have a small amount of reflux that is quickly cleared from the esophagus, but recurrent reflux is definitely abnormal beyond 6 wk of age. Strictures are easily demonstrated with barium esophagograms. Although severe esophagitis may be suspected because of a ragged mucosal outline on roentgenogram, esophagoscopy is a superior diagnostic technique for this disorder.

Treatment. In children treatment is directed at the reflux with the expectation of success. The results of medical therapy are better in infants than in older children. In mild, uncomplicated cases propping the child upright during and for 1 hr after feeding and careful attention to burping are enough. In severe cases positional therapy should be continued for 24 hr a day. The child sitting down or lying on the back should be propped at an angle of about 50°. If the child is prone, 30° is adequate (Fig 11–9). Thickened foods are often helpful. If esophagitis is present, the use of antacids between feedings is recommended. The response to intensive medical therapy may not be noticeable for 2 wk; increased weight is often the 1st sign of improvement. One study has demonstrated that bethanechol, in a dose of 8.7 mg/m²/day given 3 times a day prior to meals, can lessen vomiting and improve weight gain.

If symptoms do not respond to a 6 wk trial of intensive medical therapy, operative treatment is indicated; the trial may be shortened with recurrent aspiration and apnea. Stricture with reflux esophagitis is an indication for operation without a trial of positional therapy. Bouginage of strictures can provide temporary relief of dysphagia, but unless reflux can be prevented, the stricture will recur. If reflux is controlled, repeated bouginage is usually not needed. The Nissen fundopli-

cation or a variation of it is most often used in children; reflux is controlled in over 90% of cases. When the esophagus is severely shortened, an intrathoracic Nissen procedure is favored. Occasionally, stricture formation is so extensive that a colonic interposition is required to replace a portion of the esophagus.

Rumination
(Mercyism)

Rumination is an uncommon but serious form of chronic regurgitation which may cause growth failure usually presenting during the latter half of the 1st yr of life. The etiology is unknown. In some patients psychologic factors may be of prime importance. Often there are abnormalities in the mother-child relationship. There may be an inability of the mother to develop a mature marital or parental role. It is thought by some that the rumination is a repetitive self-stimulatory pattern of the infant which substitutes for the lack of appropriate external stimuli. In some cases such infants have been left for protracted intervals without soothing tactile, visual, or auditory stimulation. In other patients abnormalities of esophageal function, especially severe gastroesophageal reflux, are the major abnormalities, and in most infants abnormal esophageal function at least facilitates the development of rumination movements. Chewing movements and mouthing of the fingers and regurgitated material often precede or accompany the regurgitation. Careful observation may disclose that the infant actively gags him- or herself with the tongue or fingers. The large loss of nutrient may appear deceptively small; the infant lies continuously in a small pool of regurgitated liquid. A barium study will usually demonstrate easy reflux or a hiatal hernia and aid in ruling out other intestinal lesions such as esophageal stricture, achalasia, or duodenal ulcer.

Treatment. In those cases in which a warm intensive relationship with the mother is lacking, all efforts should be expended to achieve this. The establishment of regular eye contact is often associated with decreased regurgitation. Positional therapy for gastroesophageal reflux is indicated. If the patient does not improve, surgery for gastroesophageal reflux regularly stops rumination and initiates weight gain.

Esophagitis

Peptic Esophagitis

Peptic esophagitis with pain, blood loss, and possibly stricture formation is the most common form of esophagitis. It is caused by reflux of gastric contents into the esophagus.

Infection

Retroesophageal abscess is usually caused by extension of a retropharyngeal abscess downward to the retroesophageal component of this single, potential space; other causes are esophageal perforations, foreign

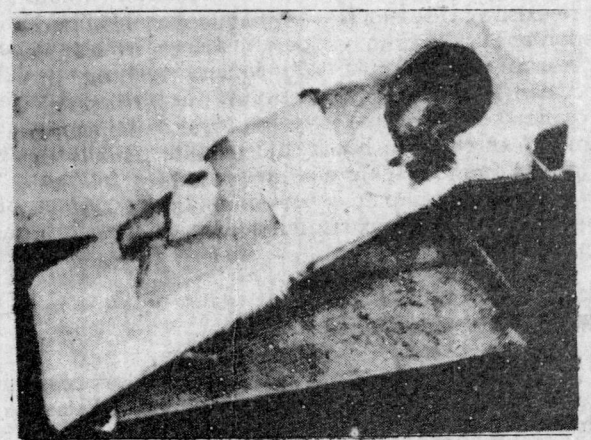

Figure 11–9 Child receiving positional treatment for gastroesophageal reflux. The child straddles a padded peg in the board and is thus kept in position.

bodies, spinal osteomyelitis, pleuritis, pericarditis, ulceration from an intubation or tracheostomy tube, diphtheria of the pharynx, or suppurating mediastinal lymph nodes. The abscess forms behind and around the esophagus and often displaces it to 1 side, while at the same time it compresses the more firmly seated trachea.

The symptoms are dyspnea, brassy cough, dysphagia, and, as the trachea is pushed forward, swelling of the neck. Pain and tenderness on palpation of the neck and cervical emphysema may be present. The increased retrotracheal space can be demonstrated on lateral roentgenograms of the neck without the use of contrast medium; if the abscess is due to esophageal perforation, barium is contraindicated.

Prognosis. The abscess may rupture into the pleura, trachea, or lung. Death may result from pressure of the abscess upon the trachea with consequent asphyxia or from an erosion into the great vessels of the neck with exsanguinating hemorrhage.

Treatment. Prompt surgical drainage is indicated. If the abscess is high, the retroesophageal space may be opened in the neck along the anterior border of the sternocleidomastoid muscle. Drainage here is effective to the level of the 4th dorsal vertebra. For retroesophageal abscesses occurring below this point a posterior mediastinotomy is generally indicated. Appropriate antibiotic therapy is indicated, but it should be recognized that such therapy may mask an advancing mediastinal infection and that only repeated lateral roentgenograms of the neck and chest will indicate the situation in the post-tracheal area.

Esophageal moniliasis usually occurs in patients on chemotherapy for hematologic or neoplastic diseases. Oral moniliasis may be absent. Pain and difficulty in swallowing are prominent. A barium esophagogram demonstrates a shaggy mucosal outline or numerous round filling defects, and esophagoscopy shows a friable mucosa with overlying whitish plaques. Treatment consists of oral nystatin, 200,000 units every 2 hr, or parenteral amphotericin B. If other antibiotics are being administered, they should be stopped if possible. Prognosis is determined by the underlying disease.

Diphtheria may involve the esophagus with extension of the membrane from the oropharynx. Therapy is the same as for diphtheria itself (Sec 10.23).

Tuberculosis rarely affects the esophagus; when it does, it usually extends directly from the larynx or contiguous lymph nodes.

Herpes simplex infections may cause acute esophagitis. Fever is common and pain on swallowing often so severe that no nutrients can be taken. Inspection usually shows typical vesicular lesions in the pharynx; endoscopy demonstrates the same lesions in the esophagus. The illness often lasts only a few days. Viscous 2% lidocaine, 2–3 ml every 4 hr, offers symptomatic relief. In severe cases wih underlying diseases the use of adenine arabinoside may be considered.

Corrosive Esophagitis

The most common cause of corrosive esophagitis and subsequent stricture is ingestion of household cleaning products. Hydrochloric and sulfuric acid, bleaches, and strong bases in products used to clean ovens or unclog drains are the most common offenders. A history of access to the substances and chemical burns of the hands, mouth, or other parts of the body strongly suggests the possibility of corrosive ingestion. The acute swelling and dysphagia clear in 2–4 wk. An asymptomatic period of weeks or even months may occur before an insidious formation of strictures leads to esophageal obstruction and the symptoms of dysphagia and vomiting.

Treatment. Prevention is the only effective treatment. Parents should be educated about the danger of many household chemicals and encouraged to keep corrosive compounds beyond the reach of children. Emergency management involves ingestion of large quantities of fluid to flush away and neutralize the chemical. Gastric lavage is contraindicated (Sec 28.4). Edema of the pharnyx may require a tracheostomy to preserve an airway. Esophagogastroscopy should be performed within 48 hr to determine the presence and severity of esophageal burns since the absence of oral or pharyngeal lesions does not ensure against esophageal lesions. Rarely, the corrosive material may be transported to the stomach with few or no esophageal burns and cause severe gastritis and perforation or late stricture formation. If no burns are detected, further therapy is unnecessary. If esophageal burns are detected, ampicillin and prednisone (2 mg/kg/24 hr in divided doses) are usually administered for 10 days. Prednisone may decrease subsequent stricture formation. Early detection and dilatation of developing strictures are an important part of continuing care. Occasionally, there is complete obliteration of the esophageal lumen, or stricture formation is so severe that dilatation is impossible. In such cases the involved portion of the esophagus is replaced at operation with a section of colon or a tube fashioned from the stomach.

Esophageal Perforation

Perforation is usually caused by instrumentation for pre-existing disease. The esophagus may also perforate spontaneously from sudden increases in esophageal pressure, for example, with violent retching, in auto accidents, or even compression in the birth canal. Perforation occurs on the left side of the distal esophagus in 95% of children but in the neonate usually on the right. Common symptoms are vomiting followed by severe substernal pain, cyanosis, and shock. An esophagogram showing extraluminal water-soluble contrast material is diagnostic.

Mallory-Weiss Syndrome

Violent retching can tear the esophageal mucosa and submucosa, causing hematemesis (Mallory-Weiss syndrome). Esophagoscopy should differentiate this disorder from other more serious forms of upper gastrointestinal bleeding. Blood replacement is usually sufficient treatment for this self-limited disease in children.

Esophageal Varices

Esophageal varices may occur in children as a complication of portal hypertension. The principal signs are recurrent, profuse, bright red hematemesis and tarry stools with signs of intravascular volume depletion. In children with esophageal varices and gastrointestinal bleeding, the source of bleeding will not be the varices in over 50% of patients. Roentgenographic studies with barium may outline the varices, but esophagoscopy is a more precise technique for diagnosis. Treatment of portal hypertension and acute gastrointestinal bleeding is discussed in Sec 11.102.

Foreign Bodies in the Esophagus

Children may swallow a variety of objects that can pass through the intestinal tract without complications. Objects that become lodged in the esophagus usually do so in 1 of 3 areas of physiologic narrowing: below the cricopharyngeal muscle, at the level of the aortic arch, or just above the diaphragm. Lodgement of material in other areas should alert one to coexisting esophageal disease.

Clinical Manifestations. The swallowing of a foreign body may provoke an attack of coughing and choking. Foreign bodies in the esophagus will usually cause pain, dysphagia (especially solid foods), and occasionally dyspnea owing to compression of the larynx. After an initial symptom-free period edema and inflammation produce symptoms of esophageal obstruction. Pain, fever, and shock develop with perforation.

Diagnosis. Radiopaque foreign bodies are easily diagnosed. Flat objects such as coins will usually be seen on edge in a lateral film. Recognition of plastic and glass objects is often difficult, but their presence can be detected with a barium swallow. The use of barium-soaked cotton to demonstrate the position of a foreign body is unnecessary and only complicates therapy.

Treatment. The usual treatment is removal of the object under direct vision esophagoscopy. A roentgenogram should be repeated just prior to the procedure to make sure the foreign body has not passed into the stomach or been vomited. For blunt objects such as coins an alternative procedure has been proposed: a Foley catheter is inserted beyond the foreign body under fluoroscopic visualization. The balloon is inflated and catheter and foreign body are removed together, care being taken that the object is not aspirated. Under no circumstance should attempts be made to force the foreign object into the stomach. After removal of the foreign body the patient should be observed for 24 hr for signs of obstruction or perforation.

JOHN J. HERBST

Esophageal Anomalies

Berdon WE, Baker DH: Vascular anomalies and the infant lungs: Rings, slings and other things. Semin Roentgenol 7:39, 1972.
Grossfeld JL, O'Neill JA, Clatworthy HW Jr: Enteric duplications in infancy and childhood: An 18 year review. Ann Surg 172:83, 1970.
Holder TM, Cloud DT, Lewis JE Jr, et al: Esophageal atresia and tracheoesophageal fistula. A survey of its members by the surgical section of the American Academy of Pediatrics. Pediatrics 34:542, 1964.

Hiatal Hernia and Gastroesophageal Reflux

Carre IJ: The natural history of the partial thoracic stomach (hiatus hernia) in children. Arch Dis Child 34:344, 1959.
Friedland GW, Dodds WJ, Sunshine P, et al: The apparent disparity in incidence of hiatal herniae in infants and children in Britain and the United States. Am J Roentgenol Radium Ther Nucl Med 120:305, 1974.
Jolley SG, Herbst JJ, Johnson DG, et al: Surgery in children with gastroesophageal reflux and respiratory symptoms. J Pediatr 96:194, 1980.

Rumination

Fleisher DR: Infant rumination syndrome. Report of a case and review of the literature. Am J Dis Child 133:266, 1979.
Herbst JJ, Friedland GW, Zboralske FF: Hiatal hernia and "rumination" in infants and children. J Pediatr 78:261, 1971.
Richmond JB, Eddy E, Green M: Rumination: A psychosomatic syndrome of infancy. Pediatrics 22:49, 1958.

Achalasia

Azizkhan RG, Tapper D, Eraklis A: Achalasia in childhood: A 20-year experience. J Pediatr Surg 15:452, 1980.
Westley CR, Herbst JJ, Goldman S, et al: Infantile achalasia inherited as an autosomal recessive disorder. J Pediatr 87:243, 1975.

Swallowing and Dysphagia

Illingworth RS: Sucking and swallowing difficulties in infancy: Diagnostic problems of dysphagia. Arch Dis Child 44:655, 1969.
Utian HL, Thomas RG: Cricopharyngeal incoordination in infancy. Pediatrics 43:402, 1969.
Wolff PH: The serial organization of sucking in the young infant. Pediatrics 42:943, 1968.

Corrosive Esophagitis

Holinger PH: Management of esophageal lesions caused by chemical burns. Ann Otolaryngol 77:819, 1968.
Viscomi GJ, Beekhuis GJ, Whitten CF: An evaluation of early esophagoscopy and corticosteroid therapy in the management of corrosive injury of the esophagus. J Pediatr 59:356, 1961.

Foreign Bodies

Alexander WJ, Kadish JA, Dunbar JS: Ingested foreign bodies in children. In: Kaufmann JH: Progress in Pediatric Radiology, Vol II. Chicago, Year Book Publishers, 1969.
Brown LP: Blind esophageal coin removal using a Foley catheter. Arch Surg 96:931, 1968.

The Stomach and Intestines

11.21 NORMAL DEVELOPMENT, STRUCTURE, AND FUNCTION OF THE STOMACH AND INTESTINE

Development.   In its gross and microscopic structure the gut matures relatively early in fetal life. Recognizable in the 4 wk, 3 mm embryo, the primitive fore- and hindgut form a simple tube which rotates counterclockwise around the umbilical artery as the stomach and cecum become distinct. The tube then elongates quickly and protrudes into the umbilical cord. At 8 wk the caudal end becomes continuous with the rectum which has evolved from the cloaca, and at 10 wk the bowel rapidly re-enters the abdomen. Later, the colon extends to achieve its mature conformation. Most structural anomalies are attributable to a delay or an aberration in this complex series of steps.

In the stomach the pyloric musculature is seen by the 3rd mo of gestation, but even at birth the muscle layers are relatively thin. Parietal and chief cells appear by 14 wk. During fetal life the intestinal-type cells found in the gastric mucosa gradually disappear. Relatively mature villi are seen along the intestine by 12 wk, and by 20 wk the crypts are deep and the enterocytes columnar with relatively sparse microvilli. Blood vessels and the nerve supply to the gut are fully developed by 12–13 wk. The intramural ganglia appear first at the top end so that if their development is delayed, the effect will be seen in the distal regions. Peristalsis has been recognized as early as 8 wk, but motility is usually not fully coordinated until near term. Peyer patches are well developed by 20 wk.

In general, an intestine of relatively mature appearance is present in even the smallest premature baby. Function also develops relatively early in the fetal gut, but, unlike structure, some functions continue to mature even in postnatal life. For example, gastric acid secretion increases dramatically in the 1st 24 hr after birth. Although there is some uncertainty, acid secretion probably peaks during the 1st 10 days and decreases from 10–30 days; the response of acid secretion to secretagogues is probably low, however, until about 3 mo of age, when it approaches the lower limit of adult normals. Maximum pepsin secretion seems to parallel that for acid. Intrinsic factor secretion rises slowly during the 1st 2 wk of life, but circulating gastrin levels, on the other hand, are inexplicably 2–3-fold higher in newborn infants at term than in adults.

Small intestinal functional development also continues to mature during pre- and postnatal life. Epithelial glucose transport is detectable in the jejunum of the human embryo by 20 wk, but adult capacity may not be achieved for years. Disaccharidase activities are measurable in the human fetus at 12 wk; sucrase and maltase achieve maximum activities by the 24th and 32nd wk, respectively; but lactase activity rises later, reaching maximum levels by 36 wk (Fig 11–10). In many children, particularly of black and oriental races, intestinal lactase activity begins to decline by 3 yr of age.

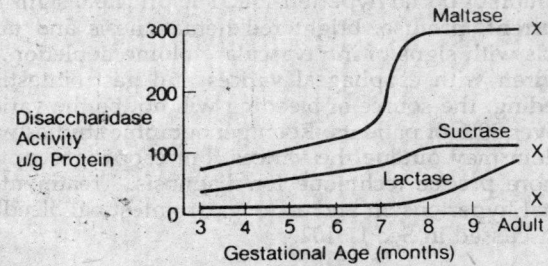

Figure 11–10 Pre- and postnatal development of disaccharidase activities in man. Lactase activity develops relatively late in gestation and falls off to a low level in the adult. (Based on data of Aurichio S, et al: Pediatrics 35:944, 1965.)

The fetal intestine is involved in the daily turnover of a large amount of amniotic fluid and there is significant Na^+-K^+-ATPase activity in 10 wk old human fetal gut. Thus, with respect to solute transport, a major determinant of diarrheal disease, small intestine function is probably adequate but marginal in term and even premature infants. Therefore, in very young children relatively severe functional disturbances in response to small intestinal diseases can be anticipated, while older children can be expected to have mature gut function. On the other hand, a relatively high incidence of intolerance to dietary lactose can be expected in older children, particularly among black and oriental populations.

Fat absorption is less efficient in term babies than in older children and even less efficient in premature infants than in those at term. One factor contributing to these age-related changes is lower bile salt transport and synthesis rates in early life.

During the 1st days of life the human gut is capable of transporting small quantities of intact protein. The entry of potential protein antigens through the mucosal barrier in early life may play a role in later food- and microbe-induced symptoms, although the phenomenon has not yet been clearly elucidated.

Normal Structure.   The bowel wall consists of several layers, each serving an important purpose and each subject to disease. The serosal layer is an extension of the peritoneum that extends distally as far as the rectum. There are 2 muscle layers, outer longitudinal fibers and inner circular ones; in the colon the longitudinal fibers form bands, or taeniae. The submucosa is a matrix for lymph and vascular plexuses, containing lymphoid cells and macrophages and, in the duodenum, Brunner glands. The mucosa of the small bowel is well designed to absorb nutrients since its surface area is expanded to an area similar to that of a tennis court by a multitude of constantly moving villi which extend into the lumen. In children these villi tend to be leaflike rather than finger-shaped projections; thus, the functioning surface area of the small intestine probably increases with age. The colonic mucosal surface is flat with numerous tubular crypts opening into the surface, but in the rectum the surface becomes smooth. The lamina propria, a cellular layer just beneath the epithelium containing cells capable of phagocytosis and immunoglobulin synthesis, provides a connective tissue core for the epithelium and its vascular supply. Lymphoid tissue is concentrated in Peyer patches, which become more frequent in the distal small bowel. There are 4 types of columnar epithelial cells in the small intestine. The dominant cell type is the absorptive cell, concerned primarily with a host of complex absorptive functions; goblet cells presumably secrete mucus, and endocrine cells secrete certain intestinal hormones; in the crypts there are Paneth cells, whose function is unknown. The columnar absorptive cell is polarized with a microvillus "brush" border at the luminal surface to which a glycocalyx or "fuzz coat" is tightly adherent. All the enterocytes divide in the crypts. The absorptive cells mature as they migrate up to the tips of the villi, from which they are shed into the lumen. The jejunal epithelium is completely renewed in 5–6 days, providing a mechanism for rapid repair after injury, but in the very young infant the process may be slower. The epithelium over Peyer patches is not villose in contour and appears to contain specialized "M" cells that may have an antigen sampling role. The colonic columnar cell differs from its small bowel counterpart in that its microvilli are shorter and fewer; the lower 2 cm segment of the rectum is lined by stratified squamous epithelium.

Normal Function. The stomach is primarily a reservoir that delivers liquefied, blended, but minimally digested portions of the diet to the intestine. It also secretes intrinsic factor, essential for the assimilation of vitamin B_{12} in the ileum. The small intestine must process not only ingested nutrients but also a large volume of water and shed epithelial cells which reach the gut lumen. In adults the total water load to the gut is at least 7 times the amount ingested.

Intraluminal ingestion depends largely on the exocrine pancreas. Synthesis and secretion of bicarbonate and digestive enzymes are stimulated by secretin and cholecystokinin, which are released by the upper intestinal mucosa in response to various intraluminal stimuli, among them components of the diet. Digestion, an efficient, fast process, is usually completed in the most proximal intestinal segment. Sugars and starches arrive at the microvillose surface of the bowel as disaccharides and monosaccharides, protein as peptides and amino acids, and triglycerides as monoglycerides and fatty acids. Bile salts in the lumen facilitate digestion and are essential for the efficient delivery of products to the absorptive surface of the epithelium. Emulsification aids digestion, and long chain monoglycerides and fatty acids usually reach the epithelium in the form of mixed micelles with conjugated bile acids and phospholipid. Sterols such as vitamin D are particularly dependent on these micelles for their absorption; therefore, diseases such as biliary atresia cause particular difficulties with vitamin D assimilation; medium chain triglycerides available in certain specially designed therapeutic diets, on the other hand, do not require micelles, emulsification, or hydrolysis for their absorption.

Carbohydrate, protein, and fat are normally absorbed by the upper half of the small intestine, although the distal segments represent a vast reserved absorptive capacity. Most of the sodium, potassium, chloride, and water is also absorbed from the lumen of the gut in the small bowel. Bile salts and vitamin B_{12} are selectively absorbed in the distal ileum and iron in the duodenum and proximal jejunum. In general, these metabolic and transport functions of the intestinal epithelium are more active in the mature villose cells than in the crypts.

At the surface of the epithelium disaccharides are hydrolyzed by specific disaccharidases located on the outer surface of the microvillus membranes, and resultant monosaccharide moieties are then actively transported across the cell to be taken away, primarily by portal venous drainage. Dipeptides and probably larger peptides can be hydrolyzed at the brush border surface, but they may also enter the cell intact before they contact peptidases. The small bowel has active transport pathways for specific groups of amino acids, similar to those seen in the renal tubule. Monoglycerides and fatty acids enter the epithelium intact; triglycerides are resynthesized, incorporated with phospholipid and lipoprotein into chylomicrons, and released into lymphatics. Since medium chain triglycerides, unlike normal dietary long chain triglycerides, may be taken up intact and released into the portal stream, these specially prepared dietary fats have definite theoretical advantages for patients with defective fat absorption. The entry of sodium with a protein carrier into the epithelial cell across the brush border is facilitated by glucose, but the active sodium pump is located in the basolateral cell membrane and associated with the Na^+-K^+-ATPase system.

The major function of the colon is to extract more water from the luminal contents in order to render the stools partially or completely solid. Then the stools can be stored in the rectum until distention triggers a defecation reflex which, when assisted by voluntary relaxation of the external sphincter, permits evacuation.

J. RICHARD HAMILTON

Grand RJ, Watkins, JB, Torti FM: Development of the human gastrointestinal tract; a review. Gastroenterology 79:790, 1976.
Gryboski JD: Gastrointestinal function in the infant and young child. Clin Gastroenterol 6:253, 1976.
Watkins JB: Mechanisms of fat absorption and the development of gastrointestinal function. Pediatr Clin North Am 22:721, 1975.

11.22 ULCER DISEASE

The exact incidence of ulcer disease is unknown, but in Erie County, New York, where careful records were kept, the annual incidence in children under 15 was 3.5/100,000, rising to 3.7/100,000 in boys at age 15 and 3.9/100,000 in girls. In comparison with the incidence in adults, ulcer disease is rare in children, and many large childrens' hospitals have only 2–4 new cases of paptic ulcer disease/yr. Although treatment, methods of diagnosis, and biologic factors are similar, it is convenient to discuss peptic ulcer disease and stress ulcers separately.

PEPTIC ULCER DISEASE

Peptic ulcers occur mainly in the duodenum and less commonly in the stomach. In the 1st yr or 2 of life gastric and duodenal ulcers occur with a similar frequency, but after 7 yr most ulcers occur in the duodenal bulb.

Pathology and Pathophysiology. The etiology of peptic ulcer disease is uncertain, but a number of factors are important. A familial incidence and the frequent history of ulcer disease in siblings or parents indicate the importance of genetic factors. Blood type and secretory status have also been shown to be associated with ulcer disease in adults.

The presence of gastric acidity is of major importance in the development of ulcer disease. Both adults and children with duodenal ulcer disease have increased acid secretion as a group, but there is a large overlap with normals, and acid secretion studies do not correlate with ulcer size and length of symptoms. In gastric ulcer disease acid output is often normal or low. Pepsinogen may be important in ulcer formation, possibly by digestion of the mucosa. Tissue resistance is an important variable in preventing ulcer formation; factors that affect resistance include anoxia, poor perfusion, and drugs. Salicylates and other factors are known to interfere with integrity of the mucosa and allow back diffusion of acid and ulcer formation with normal or even low gastric acid output. The rate of cell turnover and type and the amount of mucus secretion are also thought to be important. In general, acid-related factors are most important in duodenal ulcers, and tissue resistance appears to be of greater importance in gastric ulcers.

Histologically, the ulcer may be very superficial, may erode deeply into the mucosa and submucosa, may penetrate a blood vessel and cause hemorrhage, or may cause perforation. It is usually surrounded by an infiltration of acute and chronic inflammatory cells. If the ulcer is very shallow, it is considered an abrasion. If inflammation and edema are extensive, acute or chronic gastric outlet obstruction may occur. Occasionally, a red granular duodenal mucosa is seen on endoscopy; it is often diagnosed as duodenitis and treated as a developing ulcer. The relation of this lesion to symptoms or eventual ulcer formation is unknown. Most duodenal ulcers occur in the posterior part of the bulb, and most gastric ulcers occur on the lesser curve or the antral area. Malignant gastric ulcers in children are exceedingly rare.

Clinical Manifestations. The manifestations of peptic ulcer disease are variable and often nonspecific but include vomiting, gastrointestinal blood loss, pain, and a strong familial incidence. In adults with dyspepsia thought to be compatible with ulcer disease, about 15% will have ulcers on investigation; the frequency of abdominal pain in children and the infrequent diagnosis of ulcer disease suggest a similar situation. The symptoms can be easily confused with those of gallbladder disease, inflammatory bowel disease, esophagitis, renal disease, or pancreatitis. The last of these can occasionally occur as a complication of a penetrating duodenal ulcer.

In spite of the variability of symptoms, certain presentations are more common at different ages and may be related to the child's ability to communicate symptoms. In the 1st mo of life gastrointestinal hemorrhage and perforation are the 2 main presentations. Most of these ulcers will be stress ulcers (see below), and other disorders such as sepsis, heart disease, or respiratory distress will usually be present. It is likely that many ulcers with symptoms less demanding of diagnosis go undiagnosed. Beyond the neonatal period until 2 yr of age, recurrent vomiting, slow growth, and gastrointestinal hemorrhage are the 3 major presentations. In the preschool period atypical pain that is periumbilical and worse after eating is often elicited. Recurrent vomiting and intestinal hemorrhage are also common.

Beyond 6 yr of age the clinical presentation is similar to that in adults, with a predilection for males, dyspepsia, acute or chronic gastrointestinal blood loss, and a strong family history of ulcer disease. In patients with dyspepsia the pain is often described as dull or aching in character rather than sharp or burning as in adults. It may last from minutes to hours, and there are frequent periods of exacerbations and remissions lasting from weeks to months. Relief with antacids is often equivocal. Ulcer disease cannot be differentiated from functional abdominal pain or symptoms alone. In patients with acute or chronic blood loss or penetration of the ulcer into adjacent organs or into the abdominal cavity, symptoms of shock, anemia, pancreatitis, or peritonitis may occur.

Diagnosis. An upper gastrointestinal roentgenographic examination is the most useful regularly available test. Approximately 25% of children with duodenal ulcers will not be detected on the 1st examination. A duodenal bulb is often difficult to examine in infants because of its high posterior position. The ulcer crater should be demonstrated in multiple spot films, preferably in a distended bulb so as not to be confused by barium caught in mucosal folds in normal children. True deformity of the bulb is a good sign of past ulcer disease but does not assure that the current symptoms are due to ulcer disease or that an ulcer is present. Spasm of the bulb that relaxes and allows filling of the bulb is common in normal patients, and radiographic interpretations such as "duodenitis," "irritability of the bulb," and "pylorospasm" should not be interpreted as ulcer disease.

Gastroduodenoscopy should be used to diagnose an ulcer if the roentgenographic examination is equivocal or if, in selected patients, incapacitating pain or evidence of chronic blood loss makes immediate diagnosis of ulcer disease important. In patients with acute upper gastrointestinal hemorrhage, if gastric lavage can clear the stomach of obscuring blood and clots, endoscopy is the diagnostic procedure of choice. Although direct visualization of the upper intestine has dramatically increased precision of diagnosis of intestinal bleeds, there is no evidence that the increased accuracy has decreased mortality from hemorrhage.

Gastric acid analysis is not a useful routine test since the overlap observed in normal and abnormal patients is large. In patients with recurrent severe ulcers or patients with multiple ulcers, serum gastrin should be measured to detect the patient with Zollinger-Ellison syndrome.

In patients with active, severe upper intestinal bleeding, selective abdominal angiography may be indicated early in the diagnostic evaluation. Leakage of dye into the lumen from a bleeding ulcer can demonstrate the ulcer, and infusion of Pitressin into vessels just proximal to the bleeding site may control bleeding or allow for positioning of the catheter for therapeutic embolization of the bleeding vessels.

Treatment. The goal of therapy is to hasten healing of the ulcer, relieve pain, and prevent complications. Since acid plays a central role in ulcer formation and propagation, control of gastric acidity has centered on alterations in diet, use of antacids to buffer gastric acid, avoidance of factors that help stimulate acid secretion, and use of agents that inhibit acid secretion. Drugs that predispose to ulcer formation or hemorrhage should also be avoided. Because manipulation of the diet has not been shown to decrease acid secretion, the patient should eat a normal diet avoiding only those foods which cause discomfort. Use of a bland diet or avoidance of cola drinks, coffee, or spiced foods has not been shown to decrease acid secretion. Aspirin should be avoided since it inhibits mucosal resistance. Tobacco smoking is associated with delayed healing. Recent studies in adults suggest that corticosteroids do not predispose to ulcers but that an increased incidence may be related to the underlying illness.

Antacids are the main method of medical control of gastric acidity. Large doses hasten healing of duodenal ulcers in adults. The buffering ability of the antacids varies greatly, and the liquid form is much more efficient than the tablet form, which must be thoroughly chewed for maximal efficiency. A quantity of antacid capable of buffering 100 mEq of stomach acidity/M^2 should be administered 1–3 hr after meals and at bedtime. A bedtime snack should not be substituted since food will stimulate acid secretion during the night. Intensive therapy with antacids should continue for 4–6 wk.

Most antacids are a mixture of magnesium hydroxide, magnesium trisilicate, and aluminum hydroxide. The magnesium compounds are more effective but cause catharsis while aluminum hydroxide tends to cause constipation. If diarrhea becomes a problem, intermittent use of antacids containing mainly aluminum hydroxide is warranted. Aluminum antacids do bind with dietary phosphates and interfere with absorption. If large doses of aluminum hydroxide without phosphate are used over a prolonged period of time, especially in patients with renal disease, it is possible to develop complications of phosphate depletion including anorexia, osteomalacia, and osteoporosis. Calcium antacids can cause increased acid secretion after their buffering effect has stopped. Sodium bicarbonate is a very effective acid buffer, but is not suitable for chronic use because of the large systemic alkaline and sodium load.

Cimetidine, a potent histamine H_2-receptor antagonist, blocks the secretion of gastric acid. The usual recommended dose in children is 300 mg/M^2 before meals and at bedtime. Side effects are unusual but include gynecomastia and, on rare occasions, coma. This drug has not been shown to be more effective against gastric acidity than antacids, but it can hasten the healing of ulcers.

Anticholinergic drugs can inhibit gastric acid secretion but are effective only when side effects of dry mouth or slightly blurred vision occur. It is often difficult to monitor these changes in children; therefore, they are not recommended as primary therapy.

Surgery is indicated in patients with perforation of the intestine, intractable pain, chronic bleeding, or loss of over one third of the blood volume in 48 hr during an acute bleed. In severe continuing hemorrhage, selective abdominal angiography can identify the site of bleeding when endoscopy is impossible because of continuing bleeding. After visualization of the bleeding site, hemorrhage can often be stopped with local infusion of Pitressin or embolization therapy with Gelfoam or other material. These methods may allow time for improvement in the hemodynamic status or avoid the need for surgery. Surgery is indicated if gastric outlet obstruction caused by edema and fibrosis around a chronic ulcer is not improved after 72 hr of nasogastric drainage. Vagotomy and either pyloroplasty or antrectomy are the procedures most used in children.

STRESS ULCERS

Stress erosions and ulcers are usually seen in association with physical trauma, burns, sepsis, hemorrhagic shock, or critical illness. These ulcers are usually acute; there is a lack of chronic inflammation and debris in the crater, and there are often multiple lesions. Ulcers or erosions related to head injury tend to be located more in the distal stomach and duodenum; ulcers in the more proximal stomach are likely to be associated with other conditions. Stress ulcers related to burns are more likely to penetrate and tend to involve duodenum and proximal stomach.

Acute massive painless bleeding is frequently the 1st and only clinical manifestation of the ulcer. Partially because of the associated severe underlying disease, mortality is high even if bleeding is controlled. Antacids or cimetidine can decrease the incidence of stress ulcers in adults who are at high risk. Therefore, measures to control gastric acidity during periods of acute stress in children are recommended, especially in patients with massive burns or head injuries. Most ulcers that occur in the neonatal period and in the 1st 5 yr of life are stress ulcers.

The treatment for stress ulcers is similar to that for chronic peptic ulcer, especially in regard to antacid therapy. Often bleeding will stop with iced-saline lavage. Blood replacement, avoidance of aspirin, and correction of coagulation defects in the acutely ill patient are critical features of treatment. As noted previously, selective intra-arterial infusion of Pitressin or embolization therapy may control bleeding or at least allow stabilization of these very sick patients prior to surgery. Suture ligature of the bleeding sites combined with a vagotomy and pyloroplasty is usually the recommended surgical procedure.

ZOLLINGER-ELLISON SYNDROME

This rare syndrome can cause multiple recurrent duodenal and jejunal ulcers and is occasionally associated with diarrhea. Gastric secretion is markedly increased in volume and acidity, and hypertrophy of gastric folds is often noted on radiography. Islet cell tumor or hypertrophy causes massive elevation in serum gastrin–like activity which stimulates secretion of acid; occasionally, other hormones which cause diarrhea may also be secreted. Chronic cimetidine therapy may control gastric acid secretion and reduce the need for complete gastrectomy. Symptoms can be controlled for longer periods even if these slow-growing tumors cannot be entirely removed.

JOHN J. HERBST

Christie DL, Ament ME: Diagnosis and treatment of duodenal ulcer in infancy and childhood. Pediatr Ann 5(11):10, 1976.

Filtston HC, Jackson DC, Johnsrude IS: Arteriographic embolization for control of recurrent severe gastric hemorrhage in a ten year old boy. J Pediatr Surg 14:276, 1979.

Fordtran JS: Placebos, antacids and cimetidine for duodenal ulcer. N Engl J Med 298:1081, 1978.

Ippoliti A, Walsh J: Newer concepts in the pathogenesis of peptic ulcer disease. Surg Clin North Am 56:1479, 1976.

Peterson WL, Sturdevant RAL, Frankl HD, et al: Healing of duodenal ulcer with an antacid regimen. N Engl J Med 297:341, 1977.

Priebe JH, Skillman JJ, Bushnell LS, et al: Antacid versus cimetidine in preventing acute gastrointestinal bleeding. N Engl J Med 302:426, 1980.

Robb JDA, Thomas PS, Orszulok J, et al: Duodenal ulcer in children. Arch Dis Child 47:688, 1972.

Sultz HA, Schlesinger ER, Feldman JG, et al: The epidemiology of peptic ulcer in childhood. Am J Public Health 60:492, 1970.

CONGENITAL AND PERINATAL ANOMALIES OF THE GASTROINTESTINAL TRACT AND INTESTINAL OBSTRUCTION

Many congenital and perinatal anomalies of the gastrointestinal tract may be responsible for partial or complete obstruction. The majority of the obstructions involve the rectum and anus; the remainder are predominantly in the small intestine. The important anomalies are as follows:

Pyloric stenosis
Duodenal atresia or stenosis (with or without annular pancreas)
Jejunal or ileal atresia or stenosis
Malrotation with or without volvulus neonatorum
Meconium ileus
Hirschsprung disease (aganglionic megacolon)
Imperforate anus
Duplications and diverticula

11.23 CONGENITAL HYPERTROPHIC PYLORIC STENOSIS

Pyloric stenosis affects approximately 1:150 male and 1:750 female infants; some believe it occurs more frequently in 1st-born male infants. Familial incidence is observed in about 15% of patients, but a specific pattern of inheritance is not established.

Etiology. The cause of pyloric stenosis is not known. Favoring a congenital origin are its high incidence in both of monovular twins, in contrast to relative infrequency in both of binovular twins, and a slight association with hiatal hernia and esophageal atresia. However, an undetermined, acquired factor involved in the pathogenesis of the lesion appears probable. High levels of serum gastrin have been observed in these infants, but it is not known whether this is a cause or a result of the condition.

Pathology and Pathophysiology. A diffuse hypertrophy and hyperplasia of the smooth muscle of the antrum of the stomach narrows to a fine channel and easily becomes obstructed. The antral region is elongated, is thickened to as much as twice its normal size, and is of cartilaginous consistency. The muscular thickening is never confined to the isolated band of circular muscle fiber called the pyloric sphincter but extends well proximally into the antrum, ending distally quite abruptly where the duodenum begins. In response to outflow obstruction and vigorous peristalsis the stomach musculature becomes uniformly hypertrophied and dilates. Gastritis with bleeding may occur after prolonged stasis. As a result of vomiting the patient may become dehydrated and develop hypochloremic alkalosis.

Clinical Manifestations. Initially there is only regurgitation or occasional nonprojectile *vomiting*. The onset rarely occurs before 1 wk of age, usually the 2nd–3rd wk, and is seldom delayed until the 2nd–3rd mo. The vomiting becomes projectile, usually within 1 wk after onset, and generally occurs during or shortly after feeding but at times as much as several hr later. In some instances there is vomiting after each feeding; in others it is intermittent. The infant is hungry and will take another feeding immediately. The vomitus consists only of gastric contents but may be blood-tinged; it is not bile-stained. The stools may become very small and infrequent, depending on the amount of food that reaches the intestinal tract.

Physical examination shows varying degrees of dehydration and lethargy depending on the metabolic state of the infant. Weight loss may occur. In advanced cases the baby may appear moribund and weight may decrease to a level below that at birth. Decreased elasticity of the skin and loss of subcutaneous tissue may occur. The eyes may be sunken and the fat pads of the cheeks lost so that the infant has a wrinkled, "old man" appearance.

Visible peristalsis, proceeding from the left upper quadrant toward the pylorus in the right upper quadrant of the abdomen, is most prominent immediately after feeding or just before vomiting (Fig 11–11). The infant may appear uncomfortable, but distress is not prominent. Successful palpation of the abdomen requires patience since it depends on a totally relaxed anterior abdominal wall and an empty stomach. Continuous gentle gastric suction with a #10 nasogastric tube while simultaneously feeding the baby warm sugar solution will facilitate palpation of the "tumor." Palpation is best done from the infant's left side, and if the

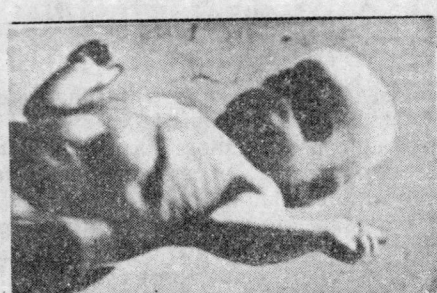

Figure 11–11 Gastric peristaltic waves of pyloric stenosis in an infant 3 wk of age. (Courtesy of Dr. Carl Wagner, Cincinnati.)

baby has pyloric stenosis, a mass can be felt in the epigastrium to the right of the midline, deep to the right rectus muscle, and under the edge of the liver. The tumor is hard, mobile, and nontender and feels like an acorn or olive; it is often best felt immediately after the baby has vomited. There is no need for barium studies once the tumor has been palpated; if the diagnosis of pyloric stenosis cannot be established after several examinations, roentgenograms to look for other causes of the projectile vomiting are indicated. The diagnosis is essentially a clinical one, confirmed by palpating the mass. No surgeon should undertake to operate for pyloric stenosis unless he or she has personally palpated and definitively identified the tumor.

When a barium study is necessary, the appearance of hypertrophic pyloric stenosis is characteristic. There is a vigorously peristaltic stomach with delayed or no gastric emptying, a fine elongated pyloric canal seen as a single ("string sign") or sometimes a double line of barium, and an umbrella-shaped duodenal cap stretched out over the hypertrophied pylorus. Just proximal to the canal a curious diverticulum may be seen (Fig 11–12).

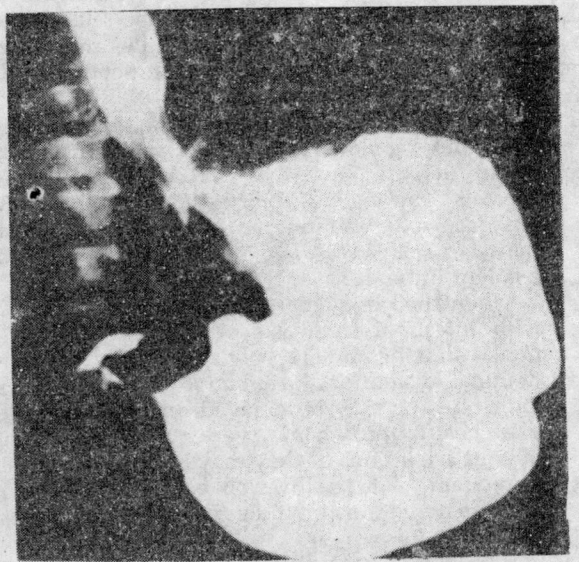

Figure 11–12 Barium in the stomach of an infant with projectile vomiting. The attenuated pyloric canal is typical of congenital hypertrophic pyloric stenosis.

Two–9% of these infants will have jaundice; the hyperbilirubinemia is thought to result from glucuronyl transferase deficiency or an increased enterohepatic circulation of bilirubin. It usually disappears within 72 hr of operative treatment.

Metabolic Alterations. Extensive and protracted vomiting in pyloric stenosis, as in other forms of high intestinal obstruction, may lead to critical deficits of potassium and sodium, which may be reflected by low values in the serum. Much more striking are the decrease in chloride concentration and increases in pH and in carbon dioxide content, which constitute the characteristic serum chemical changes of *hypochloremic alkalosis* (Sec 5.25). Correction of these chemical changes requires replacement of both sodium and potassium. The intravenous administration of ammonium chloride solution is contraindicated. Intravenous administration of 5% glucose in isotonic sodium chloride solution, to which potassium chloride is added (to a concentration of 3–5 mEq/dl, or 30–50 mEq/l), will gradually and satisfactorily replace the calculated deficits of potassium, chloride, and sodium. This will also avoid the danger of hyponatremia, which may ensue if hypotonic electrolyte solutions are used for replacement of fluid and electrolytes in dehydrated infants who have had protracted vomiting. The serum chloride level, which may vary from nearly normal to as low as 70 mEq/l, may be used as a rough index of potassium deficit; if the serum chloride is normal, the potassium deficit may be minimal and care should be taken not to overload the infant with this ion. Maintenance fluids should be given following correction of dehydration.

Differential Diagnosis. The usual case can be diagnosed by the characteristic clinical pattern and the identification of a pyloric mass. Infants who are exceptionally reactive to external stimuli, those fed by inexperienced or anxious caretakers, or those for whom an adequate maternal-infant bonding relationship has not been established may vomit frequently in the early weeks of life. Such infants may come to resemble infants with pyloric stenosis; the vomiting may be persistent and even projectile. Gastric waves are occasionally visible in small, emaciated infants who do not have pyloric stenosis. Chalasia of the esophagus and hiatal hernia usually result in vomiting in the 1st wk of life and can be differentiated from pyloric stenosis by roentgenographic studies. Adrenal insufficiency may simulate pyloric stenosis, but the absence of a palpable tumor and the metabolic acidosis and elevated serum potassium and urinary sodium concentrations of adrenal insufficiency aid in differentiation. Vomiting with diarrhea suggests gastroenteritis, although occasionally a patient with pyloric stenosis will have diarrhea. Infrequently, gastroesophageal reflux with or without a hiatal hernia may be confused with pyloric stenosis. Very rarely, a pyloric membrane or pyloric duplication may result in projectile vomiting, visible peristalsis, and, in the case of a duplication, a palpable mass.

Treatment. Surgical relief of the pyloric obstruction as soon as the diagnosis is established and the metabolic imbalances have been corrected is the treatment of choice. Well hydrated infants without evidence of electrolyte imbalance may be operated on without delay; delays of 24–36 hr for replacement therapy without oral intake are indicated in severely dehydrated infants. At operation, after the stomach has been emptied by catheter, the seromuscular layer of the gastric antrum and pylorus is incised and the muscle split with a blunt instrument, allowing the mucosa to bulge between the split muscle (Fredet-Ramstedt pyloromyotomy). Four–6 hr postoperatively, oral feedings are begun in small amounts and increased gradually. An acceptable regimen is to give 4 ml of 5% glucose in saline solution hourly for 4 feedings. If no vomiting develops, 8 ml is given hourly for the next 4 feedings; then a 4 hr schedule can be initiated with increasing volumes and formula gradually substituted for clear fluid until normal feedings are achieved, usually within 48 hr. If the infant is breast fed, it is advisable to continue by placing the infant on each breast for 1 min for the 1st postoperative feeding, thereafter increasing the time on each breast with each subsequent feeding. An alternative regimen is to maintain the administration of intravenous fluids postoperatively, giving the infant nothing orally for 24 hr. Full feeding is then started. If vomiting occurs after feedings are begun, oral feedings are withheld for 4 hr, and the regimen is reinstituted from the beginning. Persistence of vomiting suggests an incomplete pyloromyotomy or possibly concomitant hiatal hernia or chalasia; occasional episodes of vomiting are not uncommon after operation, probably as the result of persisting gastritis. During an initial period of small feedings, intravenous administration of fluids is often required, depending on the fluid and electrolyte balance of the infant. Vomiting persisting for 3–5 days after operation suggests an incomplete division of the hypertrophied pyloric muscle and may require exploratory laparotomy. Complete cessation of vomiting is the rule after operation, even though postoperative roentgenographic studies have shown that the pyloric canal may remain narrow for many mo in the asymptomatic infant. Usually hospitalization is not required beyond 48 hr postoperatively.

Nonsurgical Treatment.   The slowness of improvement (2–8 mo), the higher case fatality rate, and the current high cost and probable adverse effect on emotional development of prolonged hospitalization have led to a virtual abandonment of nonsurgical treatment for pyloric stenosis. If, for some reason, medical rather than surgical management is necessary, slow improvement will usually take place on a regimen of small, frequent feedings thickened with cereal, maintenance of a semi-upright position for 1 hr or so after feedings, sedation, administration of a cholinergic blocking agent, and parenteral administration of fluids as required. Emptying of the stomach by lavage when there is epigastric distention before a feeding may likewise decrease the chance of vomiting.

Prognosis.   When the diagnosis is made early in the course of the disease and the infant is properly prepared for operation, the operative fatality rate is less than 1%. Medical therapy has a higher mortality rate. Severe and prolonged undernutrition may have an untoward effect on subsequent development.

11.24 CONGENITAL INTESTINAL OBSTRUCTION

General Considerations.   Intestinal obstruction is observed in approximately 1:1500 newborn infants. The cardinal signs are vomiting, abdominal distention, and failure to pass feces. Since a number of days may go by prior to full certainty that the infant has an obstructive lesion, early diagnosis depends on appreciation of the significance of vomiting and distention. *High intestinal obstruction* is characterized by vomiting, which tends to be persistent even when feedings have been stopped; distention may be absent. *Low obstruction* is characterized principally by distention, and vomiting may be only a later manifestation. When the obstruction is in the duodenum, symptoms may become manifest within a few hours; if it is in the large intestine, symptoms may be delayed for more than 24 hr.

From an anatomic standpoint congenital obstructive lesions of the intestines can be viewed as *intrinsic*, e.g., atresia, stenosis, meconium ileus, and aganglionic megacolon, or *extrinsic*, e.g., malrotation, constricting bands, intra-abdominal hernias, and duplications. An attempt should be made to locate the lesion preoperatively in order to guide the surgical approach.

When the obstruction is *complete*, there should be little difficulty in clinical recognition, but when it is *incomplete*, there may be considerable difficulty. Polyhydramnios is frequently an accompaniment of high intestinal obstruction, as it is of esophageal atresia. When polyhydramnios has been noted, the infant's stomach should be aspirated immediately after birth. Aspiration of 10–15 ml or more of gastric fluid, especially if it is bile-stained, is suggestive of a high intestinal obstruction.

Meconium stools may be passed initially if the obstruction is in the upper part of the small intestine.

Obstruction in the duodenal area may cause epigastric distention and, at times, gastric waves similar to those of pyloric stenosis. The distention may not be persistent, however, since it may be relieved by vomiting. The vomiting may be projectile, and the vomitus will usually contain bile if the obstruction is below the ampulla of Vater, as it usually is.

Obstructions in the lower ileum, colon, or rectum cause more generalized distention, often with bulging of the flanks. When the liver dullness is obliterated, there is a strong possibility that intestinal perforation has occurred. Vomiting with lower bowel obstruction may be delayed a day but eventually may become feculent in type.

When the obstruction is *incomplete*, as, for example, with intestinal stenosis, constricting bands, duplications, and incomplete volvulus, signs (vomiting, abdominal distention, obstipation) may appear shortly after birth or may be delayed an indeterminate time. They may approach in severity those of a completely obstructive lesion, or they may be sufficiently mild and infrequent as to be overlooked until either an acute episode or diagnostic studies disclose the lesion. Incomplete obstruction may constitute a surgical emergency as much as complete obstruction.

Valuable information on the location of congenital obstructive lesions in the intestine may often be obtained from flat and upright roentgenograms of the abdomen without ingestion of contrast media. With completely obstructive lesions there will be distention of the bowel above the obstruction, and there may be a series of fluid levels with superimposed gas in the distended loops. Pneumoperitoneum may be seen with free air in the subphrenic regions. Calcification within the peritoneal cavity will indicate meconium peritonitis. A characteristic "ground glass" appearance in the right lower quadrant with trapped bubbles of air within the obstructing meconium may be seen in patients with meconium ileus. A study of the colon with an enema containing radiopaque material may provide additional localizing information, especially in respect to the possibility of a misplaced cecum with malrotation of the intestine. Under usual circumstances air is demonstrable roentgenographically in the stomach of the normal infant immediately after birth. Within 1 hr air may be observed in the proximal portion of the small intestine and segments of the colon. Air may be visible in the distal parts of the colon as early as the 3rd hr or as late as 18 hr.

Prognosis. If a complete obstruction is not relieved promptly, the clinical course progresses rapidly. Vomiting is persistent; dehydration, loss of weight, and prostration become severe, and the infant dies within a few days. When the obstruction is not complete, the infant may survive for weeks; minor obstructions may be compatible with life even without treatment. Recovery from both complete and incomplete obstructions can be expected in many instances with early diagnosis and appropriate management.

Treatment. Not every obstructive lesion is amenable to surgery, but infants can withstand massive resection of the small intestine when the lesion necessitates it. Preoperative preparation, including constant gastric aspiration, and postoperative care are of the greatest importance, especially in relation to the correction of dehydration and electrolyte deficits and to the maintenance of fluid balance and nutrition by parenteral means (Sec 5.31 and 7.16).

11.25 ATRESIA AND STENOSIS

Atresia (complete occlusion) and, less commonly, *stenosis* (partial occlusion) of the gastrointestinal tract account for about one third of cases of intestinal obstruction. The obstructive lesion (excluding anorectal lesions) is most frequently in the ileum (50%) and duodenum (25%), less frequently in the jejunum, rarely in the colon, and almost never in the stomach. There is an increased incidence of duodenal atresia as well as of imperforate anus in infants with Down syndrome. About 15% of intestinal atresias are multiple. The types of atresia are (1) a diaphragm-like occlusion of the lumen, (2) a blind end not in continuity with a distal segment, and (3) segments of bowel with cordlike connections.

11.26 CONGENITAL DUODENAL OBSTRUCTION

Etiology. Delayed vacuolization of the embryonic intestinal lumen is thought to account for both mucosal diaphragms within the duodenum and duodenal atresia. Atresia may also develop secondary to vascular insufficiency.

Pathology. The atretic duodenum usually ends blindly just distal to the ampulla of Vater. Twenty–30% of these infants have Down syndrome, and in 20% the common bile duct drains into the distal bowel, beyond the site of atresia. Rarely, bile enters the bowel both proximal and distal to the site of the obstruction, especially when a duodenal diaphragm is present. Incomplete rotation of the midgut, with the duodenum becoming obstructed by the misplaced peritoneal reflections of the preduodenal cecum, is 2nd to duodenal atresia as a cause of congenital duodenal obstruction. Volvulus neonatorum is a serious complication of malrotation and requires prompt relief. An annular pancreas, encircling the 2nd portion of the duodenum, may compress and obstruct it partially or completely; this condition is almost always associated with an underlying duodenal stenosis. A **duodenal web**, mucosal diaphragm, or "windsock" may coexist in patients with malrotation and should always be sought. Rarely, a preduodenal portal vein may compress the anterior wall of the 1st part of the duodenum and obstruct it.

Clinical Manifestations. Vomiting of bile-stained material may occur shortly after birth or be delayed, especially with incomplete obstruction. Early, the epigastrium may be full with peristalsis observed, although there may be no abdominal distention. Down syndrome may be present, and a history of maternal hydramnios may be obtained. With prolonged vomiting a metabolic alkalosis with profound dehydration and electrolyte imbalance ensues. If the duodenum is atretic proximal to the ampulla of Vater, the vomitus will not contain bile. Any cause of duodenal obstruction other than atresia may result in an incomplete obstruction with delay in the onset of symptoms beyond the neonatal period. Thus, a patient with duodenal stenosis may remain well for several mo, and chronic duodenal ileus in association with malrotation may be encountered even later in life.

Diagnosis. The diagnosis of duodenal obstruction may be made by studying the air pattern in supine and erect roentgenograms of the abdomen. Classically, a "double bubble" will be seen on the upright film as the air in the stomach and the distended duodenum rises to the top of each viscus and the contained gastric fluid and duodenal contents form a level line at the fluid-air interface (Fig 11–13). With complete atresia no gas will be seen in the rest of the abdomen. A similar appearance may occur with malrotation, annular pancreas, and duodenal atresia or severe stenosis. If there is roentgenographic evidence of duodenal obstruction, a barium enema should be done as an emergency to determine whether a malrotation is present. If the cecum is undescended, it must be assumed that the duodenal obstruction is due to Ladd bands in associa-

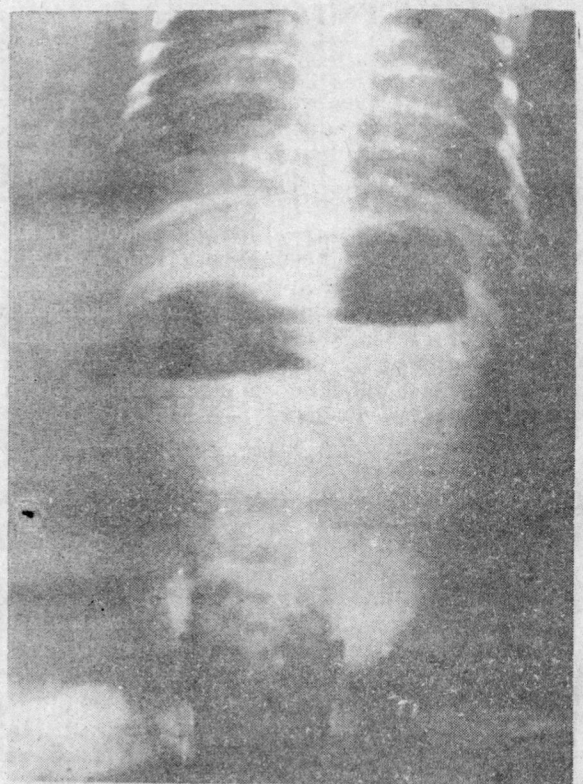

Figure 11–13 Abdominal roentgenogram of a newborn infant held upright. Note the "double bubble" gas shadow above and the absence of gas in the distal bowel in this case of congenital duodenal atresia.

tion with malrotation and that a coexisting volvulus neonatorum of the entire midgut may be also present.

Treatment. In duodenal atresia or stenosis the surgical procedures of choice are duodenoduodenostomy or duodenojejunostomy to bypass the obstruction. If obstruction is due to Ladd bands with malrotation, emergency operation is necessary. After division of the abnormal peritoneal folds or bands, the entire large intestine is placed on the left within the abdomen, with the small bowel on the right—the fetal position of nonrotation. Malrotation may also coexist with an intrinsic duodenal obstruction, such as a membrane or stenosis; this may be identified by passing a nasogastric balloon-tipped catheter into the jejunum below the site of obstruction, inflating the balloon, and slowly withdrawing the catheter. Annular pancreas is best treated by duodenoduodenostomy without dividing the pancreas, leaving as short a defunctioned loop as possible. If a duodenal diaphragm obstruction is present, a duodenoplasty is the treatment of choice.

11.27 ANOMALIES OF ROTATION (Malrotation)

Incomplete rotation, or *malrotation of the intestine,* represents a failure of the bowel to rotate and become

fixed normally. The normal embryologic sequence is: (1) the cecum rotates around the superior mesenteric artery, which acts as an axis, counterclockwise from a position in the middle of the abdomen just below the stomach; (2) the colon, which lies on the left side of the abdomen, follows as the cecum rotates into the right upper quadrant and finally into the right lower quadrant; (3) when rotation is completed, the ascending and descending mesocolons fuse to the back of the abdomen, anchoring the mesentery from the ligament of Treitz obliquely downward to the cecal area. In some instances rotation may be complete, but the mesentery is incomplete so that there is abnormal mobility of the midgut and colon.

Most often in malrotation the cecum fails to move into the right lower quadrant, and the bands fixing it to the posterior abdominal wall cross over and may obstruct the duodenum (Fig 11–14). The narrow mesenteric stalk which suspends the small intestine in the area of the superior mesenteric vessels is liable to volvulus, resulting in intermittent or acute obstruction that may progress to strangulation. Obstruction occurs first at the upper portion of the duodenum, then at the lower end of the loop. Volvulus is present in more than half of the patients operated on for intestinal obstruction when the cecum is in the right upper portion of the abdomen. This problem usually presents symptoms of acute or recurrent intestinal obstruction at birth or in the 1st yr of life. Occasionally, a child with malrotation presents the clinical picture of celiac disease, which is relieved by surgical repair. Nonrotation is associated with midgut volvulus, gastroschisis, omphaloceles, and hernia through the foramen of Bochdalek. Malrotation may be present with an annular pancreas and congenital atresia or stenosis of the duodenum.

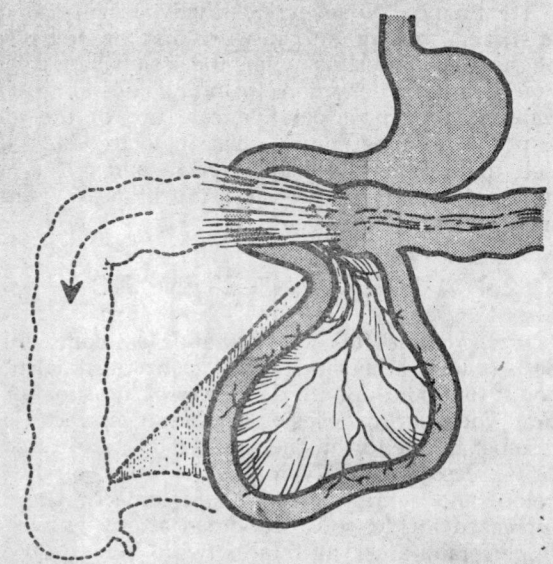

Figure 11–14 The mechanism of intestinal obstruction with incomplete rotation of the midgut (malrotation). The dotted lines show the course the cecum should have taken. Failure to rotate has left obstructing bands across the duodenum, and a narrow pedicle for the midgut loop, making it prone to volvulus. (From Nixon HH, O'Donnell B: The Essentials of Pediatric Surgery. Philadelphia, JB Lippincott, 1961.)

Roentgenograms of the abdomen may show an abnormal colonic gas pattern, and barium enema confirms the abnormal position of the cecum. In acute obstruction, diagnosis occurs at laparotomy, and only an upright film of the abdomen is taken in order to disclose the gas and fluid shadows.

Management includes fluid therapy to combat shock and disturbance of body fluids and electrolytes, followed by laparotomy, at which the volvulus is unwound, transduodenal bands are divided, and the large intestine is straightened and placed in the left side of the abdomen with all the small bowel on the right.

11.28 JEJUNAL OR ILEAL OBSTRUCTION

These obstructions may result from atresia or stenosis, meconium ileus, Hirschsprung disease, intussusception, Meckel diverticulum, intestinal duplication, or strangulated hernia.

Pathology. The bowel in *ileal* or *jejunal atresia* ends blindly proximal and distal to an interruption in its continuity; there may even be a gap in the mesentery. With stenotic or "windsock" obstructions the bowel and mesentery are in continuity. The large size of the proximal obstructed loop of bowel contrasts greatly with that of the collapsed distal bowel. Rarely, atretic segments are multiple; this form has a familial incidence. Atresias, including reabsorption of gangrenous bowel, have been experimentally produced by intrauterine ligation of mesenteric vessels of fetal bowel.

Meconium ileus occurs in newborn infants with cystic fibrosis, but only 10% of patients with this disease develop meconium ileus. The last 20–30 cm of ileum are collapsed and filled with pellets of pale-colored stool, above which a dilated loop of varying length appears obstructed by meconium with the consistency of thick syrup or glue. Peristalsis fails to project this very viscid material through the ileum, where it impacts. Volvulus, atresia, or perforation of the bowel may accompany meconium ileus. If the bowel perforates in utero, meconium peritonitis results. Intraperitoneal meconium can cause dense adhesions leading postnatally to adhesive intestinal obstruction.

In 3% of patients with *Hirschsprung disease* the aganglionic segment involves not only the entire colon but also a segment of terminal ileum. This condition causes a dilated small intestine with ganglionated but somewhat hypertrophied walls, a funnel-shaped transitional hypoganglionic zone, and a collapsed distal aganglionic bowel.

Clinical Manifestations. A history of hydramnios may be elicited with high jejunal atresias, and in fibrocystic disease there is a familial incidence. The obstructed patient may be born with abdominal distention from loops of meconium-filled bowel, or obstruction may develop shortly after birth and progress as the result of swallowed air. Distention often results from meconium peritonitis due to intrauterine perforation and leakage of meconium into the peritoneal cavity, where it may rapidly become calcified. The site of perforation usually seals in utero so that operative intervention after birth is seldom necessary, but if the

perforation is still patent, increasing abdominal distention with free intraperitoneal air develops after birth, and an operation is required. Vomiting may occur early, with vomitus bilirubin-stained in color. Infants with ileal or jejunal atresia may pass several surprisingly large meconium stools, but with meconium ileus there is usually no stool. A pneumoperitoneum should be suspected if abdominal distention increases rapidly within the 1st 24 hr of life, the liver is less dull to percussion, or free fluid is evident within the abdomen.

Diagnosis. In meconium ileus, plain films of the abdomen show a typical "ground glass" appearance or haziness in the right lower quadrant. Radiolucent areas made by small bubbles of gas trapped in meconium are dispersed within this area. Furthermore, because of their viscid contents, moderately dilated loops of bowel do not have the fluid levels usually seen roentgenographically on the erect projection. Gastrografin enemas should be used with caution in the diagnosis and treatment of meconium ileus because their hyperosmolality may result in dehydration and undue pressure may result in perforation. If there is meconium peritonitis, patchy calcification may be noted, usually in the flanks. If a pneumoperitoneum is present, the free air is most readily seen between liver and diaphragm on an upright roentgenogram of the abdomen, but if there is a large amount of free air, the entire abdomen may look like a football from distention with air; the ligamentum teres is sometimes clearly visible in the midline.

If plain roentgenograms are nonspecific, a barium or Gastrografin study of the colon may be needed to distinguish small from large intestine obstructions. A small colon, "microcolon," suggests disuse and the presence of obstruction proximal to the ileocecal valve. It is impossible consistently to distinguish small bowel from large bowel by studying plain roentgenograms of the abdomen in newborn babies and infants.

Treatment. Patients with small bowel obstruction should be stable and in adequate fluid and electrolyte balance before operation or roentgenographic attempts at disimpaction. Infections should be treated with appropriate antibiotics. Prophylactic antibiotics are indicated.

Ileal or jejunal atresia requires resection of the dilated proximal portion of the bowel, followed by end-to-end anastomosis. If a simple mucosal diaphragm is present, a jejuno- or ileoplasty with partial excision of the web is an acceptable alternative to resection of a loop. An attempt to reduce obstruction from meconium ileus with a Gastrografin enema is usually indicated. The material should be allowed to flow around the pellets of stool in the terminal ileum and into the dilated proximal small bowel containing the obstructing meconium, where it will result in an outpouring of fluid from the bowel wall, dilution of the viscid meconium, and subsequent diarrhea. This enema may have to be repeated after an interval of 8–12 hr. Resection after reduction is not needed if there have been no ischemic complications.

About 50% of patients with meconium ileus cannot be successfully treated by a Gastrografin enema and will need laparotomy. A simple small ileotomy is done within a purse-string suture just large enough to allow the insertion of a #10 or #12 French catheter. The catheter is used to irrigate and remove the viscid contents of the bowel, using acetylcysteine as a mucolytic agent in concentrations of less than 5%. Once the contents have been aspirated, the purse-string suture is tied and a small drain placed near the ileostomy, making resections and anastomoses unnecessary.

Laparotomy for pneumoperitoneum may necessitate a colostomy or ileostomy at the site of perforation, but if the perforation is in the stomach, duodenum, or upper jejunum, primary closure is the procedure of choice. Total parenteral nutrition may be required.

11.29 CONGENITAL MEGACOLON
(Hirschsprung Disease)

This is the most common cause of intestinal obstruction of the colon and accounts for about 33% of all neonatal obstructions, although it is rare in premature infants. Occasionally there is a familial incidence of megacolon. *Atresia* of the colon is extremely rare.

Etiology. There may be failure of migration of the cells of the embryonic neural crest into the bowel wall or failure of the myenteric and submucous plexuses to progress in a craniocaudal direction within the bowel wall.

Pathology. This disease results from absence of ganglion cells in the bowel wall, extending proximally from the anus for a variable distance. The aganglionic segment is limited to the rectosigmoid in 80% of patients; in 15% the colon is aganglionic as far proximally as the hepatic flexure; while in 3% the entire colon lacks ganglion cells.

Incomplete parasympathetic innervation in the aganglionic segment of bowel results in abnormal peristalsis, constipation, and a functional intestinal obstruction. Proximal to the transition zone between normally and abnormally innervated bowel, muscular hypertrophy causes thickening of the intestinal wall. The intestine also becomes enormously dilated with large quantities of retained feces and gas.

Clinical Manifestations. Early symptoms of megacolon vary from complete acute obstruction in the neonate to chronic constipation in the older child. Often the patient fails to thrive, and sometimes there is diarrhea.

In newborn infants the symptoms may be present at birth, with failure to pass meconium, or may appear during the 1st wk and be those of partial or even complete intestinal obstruction with vomiting, abdominal distention, and failure to pass stools. Temporary relief of symptoms may occur after a rectal examination, which is characteristically followed by an explosive discharge of feces and gas. Bile-stained and even feculent vomiting may occur, and the infant may lose weight and become dehydrated. Diarrhea may be a prominent symptom in the neonatal period and occur in association with symptoms of intestinal obstruction. Hypoproteinemia and edema may develop in association with protein-losing enteropathy.

Episodes of constipation and diarrhea may alternate with periods of apparent normality. The diarrhea may develop into a fulminant enterocolitis, causing a profound dehydration and shock with fluid and electrolyte loss into the lumen of the bowel but without isolation of any specific bacteria. Unless energetically treated, the condition tends to recur and may be fatal within 24 hr. This complication seems to be precipitated by gaseous and fecal colonic distention.

Hirschsprung disease in the older child causes chronic constipation and abdominal distention. The history often reveals increasing difficulty with the passage of stools, starting in the 1st few wk of life. A large fecal mass is palpable in the left lower portion of the abdomen, but on rectal examination the rectum is not dilated and is usually empty of feces. The stools, when passed, may consist of small pellets, be ribbon-like, or have a fluid consistency; the large stools and fecal soiling of patients with functional constipation are absent. In mild cases the nutrition may not be greatly disturbed; in severe cases there is likely to be loss of subcutaneous tissue and failure to grow. The wasted extremities and large, protruding abdomen of such patients create a typical appearance but one which may be confused with some of the *malabsorption syndromes* (Sec 11.45), especially when diarrhea is present. Hypochromic anemia may be present. Intermittent attacks of intestinal obstruction from retained feces may be associated with pain and fever. This condition has to be distinguished from the more common acquired megacolon (Fig 11–15) of colonic inertia, chronic idiopathic constipation, obstipation, and so on (Table 11–6).

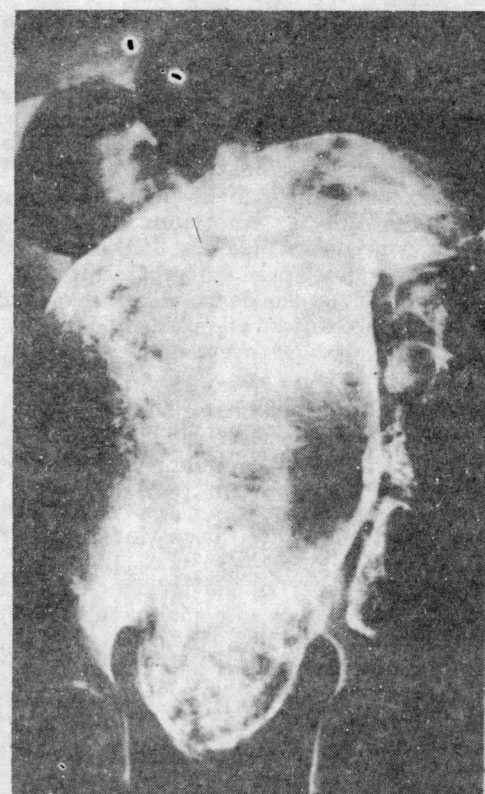

Figure 11–15 Barium enema in a 14 yr old boy with severe constipation. The enormous dilatation of rectum and distal colon is typical of acquired megacolon.

Table 11–6 COMPARATIVE CHARACTERISTICS OF ACQUIRED MEGACOLON AND HIRSCHSPRUNG DISEASE

	HIRSCHSPRUNG DISEASE	AQUIRED MEGACOLON
History		
From birth	Always	Never
Enterocolitis	Possible	None
Rectal bleeding	None	Possible
Coercive bowel training	Absent	Usually present
Encopresis (fecal soiling)	Never	Always
Size of stool	Normal small	Huge
Examination		
Malnutrition	Possible	Absent
Abdominal distention + wide subcostal angle	Usual	Absent
Feces palpable abdominally	Usually	Often
Anal fissure	Never	Possible
Anal tone	Tight	Patulous
Feces in ampulla	Never	Packed with stool
Barium Enema		
Empty segment of rectum	Usually	Absent
Fecaloma in rectal ampulla	Absent	Always present
Delay in evacuation of barium	Usually	Absent
Biopsy		
Ganglion cells in plexuses	Absent	Present

Note: Ultrashort-segment Hirschsprung disease may have clinical features of acquired megacolon.

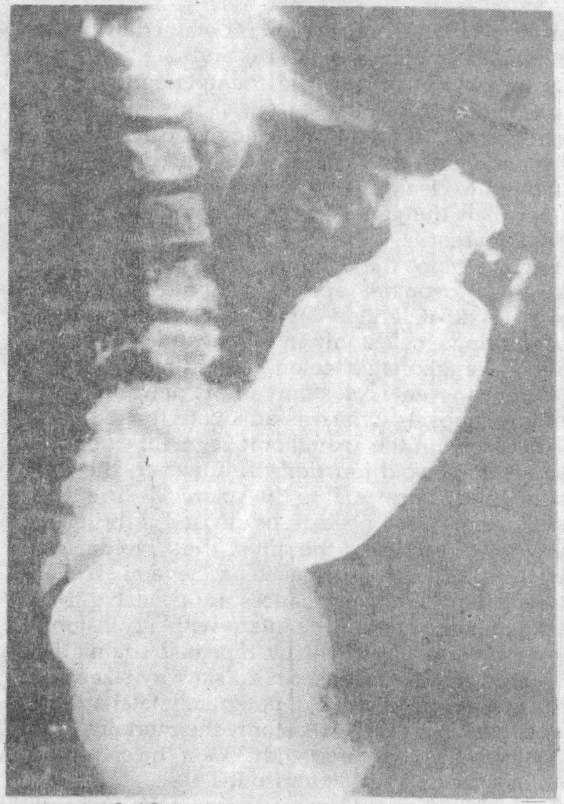

Figure 11–16   Lateral view of barium enema in a 3 yr old girl with Hirschsprung disease. The aganglionic distal segment is narrow with distended normal ganglionic bowel above it.

Rarely, a variant of megacolon may be encountered, the ultrashort-segment Hirschsprung disease, with the aganglionosis confined to the internal anal sphincter and immediately adjacent anal canal and rectum. Such patients may have encopresis, and unless a particularly low biopsy is done, ganglion cells may be found and the patient presumed to be normal.

Diagnosis. Rectal biopsy by the punch or suction method, demonstrating absent ganglion cells in the submucosa and intermuscular nerve plexuses with or without increased numbers of nerve fibers, is the only conclusive means of diagnosing megacolon. Because of the diminishing numbers of ganglion cells normally found in the more distal rectum and anal canal, biopsies should be taken no closer than 2 cm to the pectinate line.

Roentgenographic studies in the young infant with intestinal obstruction due to aganglionic megacolon show dilated loops of bowel throughout the abdomen on anteroposterior films taken in the erect position. In lateral erect films, rectal air, which is usually visible in the presacral area, is absent. The diagnostic findings on barium enema are (1) an abrupt change in caliber between the ganglionic and aganglionic sections of bowel (Fig 11–16); (2) irregular "sawtooth" contractions of the aganglionic segment; (3) parallel transverse folds in the dilated proximal colon; (4) a thickened, nodular, edematous proximal colon characteristic of protein-losing enteropathy; and (5) failure to evacuate the barium. In infants only a small amount of contrast material should be injected slowly through a small catheter, the tip of which is inserted barely beyond the anal sphincter, while the patient, in an oblique position, is being observed under the fluoroscope; the characteristic abrupt transition in caliber may be missed if the lower colon is flooded with too much barium.

In the newborn infant with intestinal obstruction due to megacolon a barium enema will not always show the classic features of the disease as there may not have been time for the disparity in size to develop between the dilated proximal colon and the empty distal aganglionic bowel. The roentgenographic appearances are even less typical when the entire colon lacks ganglion cells, although usually evacuation of the barium from the colon is delayed on a 24 hr roentgenogram.

Anorectal manometry, measured by distention of a balloon placed within the rectal ampulla, shows a fall of pressure in the internal anal sphincter in normal individuals but a striking rise in pressure in patients with megacolon. The accuracy of this diagnostic test is over 90%. In the neonate, however, the test is less reliable.

In the older child the diagnosis will usually be made by the history of constipation since birth and the finding of an empty rectum. Confirmation is obtained by studying the barium enema (Fig 11–16) and the results of anal manometry. However, the roentgenographic appearance of megacolon may be misleading in terms of the diagnosis and the level of aganglionosis. When a barium enema is to be done in a suspected case, it is important not to cleanse the bowel so that the disparity in size between the ganglionic and aganglionic bowel is readily apparent.

Treatment. Once the diagnosis is unequivocally established in a neonate, operation is indicated. It is preferable to do a limited laparotomy with multiple biopsies, placing a colostomy in the most distal portion of normally ganglionated colon. Some surgeons perform a right transverse colostomy in the newborn without multiple biopsies, which is adequate for the usual type of disease with the aganglionic segment extending up to the rectosigmoid junction. If, however, the transition zone is at or proximal to the splenic flexure, then such a colostomy may need to be revised to bring the transverse colon down to the anus, thus avoiding excision of the intervening normal colon. Several excellent disposable infant stoma appliances are available to facilitate the management of the infant with a colostomy.

Nonoperative management by repeated colonic irrigations until the infant reaches a satisfactory size is not justified because of the risk of a potentially fatal episode of enterocolitis. With early colostomy the mortality from enterocolitis is 4%, compared with 33% if the colostomy is done after the onset of enterocolitis.

When the infant is 6–12 mo of age a definitive pull-through operation is done using the Swenson, Duhamel, or modified Soave procedure. Surgical management consists of excising the aganglionic segment and pulling the ganglionic intestine down through the anus, anastomosing it to the anal canal within 2.5 cm of the pectinate line.

In most older children a preliminary colostomy is also advisable, with its retention after the Swenson and Duhamel types of operation.

Ultrashort Segment Hirschsprung Disease. If the aganglionic segment is so short as to give rise to a clinical and roentgenographic picture almost indistinguishable from acquired megacolon, major surgery is unnecessary. Excision of a strip of internal anal sphincter (internal anal myectomy) is all that is usually required if nonoperative management is unsuccessful.

Total Colon Aganglionosis. When the entire colon is aganglionic, often together with a length of terminal ileum, ileal-anal anastomosis is the treatment of choice because of the degree of continence attained, but it may result in appalling excoriation of the perianal skin and buttocks which may resist treatment for many mo.

Prognosis. Results of treatment of Hirschsprung disease are generally satisfactory, with a great majority of patients achieving fecal continence. Because most cases are diagnosed and treated in the neonatal period, immediate postoperative continence is impossible to assess. Toilet training is usually delayed, and for several yr intermittent incontinence with diarrhea may occur; with time most children develop continence. Loperamide is very useful in the management of diarrhea.

11.30 DIVERTICULA AND DUPLICATIONS

These lesions consist of abnormal tissue, usually intestinal, in close relation to a part of the alimentary tract. In many there is ectopic gastric, pancreatic, duodenal, ileal, or colonic mucosa. These congenital anomalies may be due to an abnormal formation of a part of an organ or duct or a failure of obliteration of one. If a diverticulum is anywhere but on the antimesenteric border, it is considered a dorsal enteric remnant.

With the exception of a Meckel diverticulum, congenital and acquired single and multiple diverticula of the intestinal tract are extremely rare in children. *Diverticulosis*, the presence of multiple outpouchings of the intestinal tract, usually in the colon, and *diverticulitis*, or inflammation of diverticula, are essentially diseases of adult life.

Meckel Diverticulum

Two–3% of people have a Meckel diverticulum; the most common complication is bleeding from the alimentary tract. Other complications are rare.

In the embryo the intestine is linked to the yolk sac by the vitellointestinal duct. If this duct does not become completely atretic, it may persist in the form of a Meckel diverticulum. There may also be persistence of a fibrous cord from the Meckel diverticulum to the umbilicus, with cystic structures contained within the cord anywhere between the diverticulum and the peritoneal surface of the umbilicus. If the entire embryonic duct remains patent (persistence of the omphalomesenteric duct), there will be an enterocutaneous fistula; if the ileal end is closed, there is only mucoid secretion. A fibrous remnant of the vitelline artery may also persist as a band with the potential of resulting in intestinal obstruction.

Pathology. The Meckel diverticulum is usually 50–75 cm proximal to the ileocecal junction on the antimesenteric side of the intestine. The mucosal lining is the same as that of the adjacent ileum, but in at least 35% there is ectopic gastric or pancreatic tissue near the tip. This ectopic acid or pepsin-secreting mucosa can cause an ulcer in the adjacent basal portion of the diverticulum or in the ileum to which it is attached. The erosion of the mucosa results in hemorrhage which may be massive. Much less frequently, the diverticulum is the site of inflammation; this diverticulitis occurs usually without demonstrable cause, although rarely a foreign body may be found. Diverticulitis may progress to perforation and fecal peritonitis. Sometimes, the lesion is turned inside out and may become the apex of an ileoileal intussusception. A *Littre hernia* is seen when the Meckel diverticulum is contained within an indirect inguinal hernia. The diverticulum itself may undergo volvulus, or a band attached to it may cause a volvulus of loops of small intestine, leading to gangrene.

Clinical Manifestations. Symptoms and signs from Meckel diverticulum can arise at any age but occur more frequently in the 1st 2 yr of life.

Painless rectal bleeding is the most common sign in children. There may be periodicity to the bleeding as with peptic ulcer; usually it is acute, but exsanguinating hemorrhage is rare. Blood is often passed without stool; it is usually dark red in color, but, if bleeding is brisk, it may be bright red. With mild recurrent bleeding a chronic iron deficiency anemia may develop and be refractory to iron therapy. Repeatedly positive tests for occult blood in the stool in an anemic young child suggest Meckel diverticulum.

Abdominal pain, when it occurs, may be acute and due to diverticulitis, with a clinical picture resembling that of acute appendicitis, or it may be vague and recurrent. Referral of the (ileal) pain to the umbilicus may suggest the true diagnosis. Perforation of an ulcer in the diverticulum may be responsible for peritoneal bleeding or inflammation. A Meckel diverticulum may become the leading point of an intussusception with associated clinical manifestations. The signs may also be those of an incarcerated hernia, volvulus, appendicitis, or intestinal obstruction. A child, other than a newborn infant, who has intestinal obstruction without having had a previous operation and who does not have an intussusception most likely has a Meckel diverticulum or a fibrous remnant.

Diagnosis. In infancy the Meckel diverticulum with ectopic gastric tissue will often be symptomatic and require rapid and accurate preoperative evaluation. The diverticulum cannot be demonstrated reliably by barium studies. However, an accurate preoperative diagnosis is possible, based on the fact that ^{99m}technetium is excreted by gastric mucosa; a negative scan is also useful because of its high correlation with the absence of a Meckel diverticulum. Patients with Meckel diverticulitis may be misdiagnosed preoperatively as having acute appendicitis but correctly diagnosed and treated at surgery. A patent vitellointestinal duct and its communication with a loop of bowel will be shown by injection of radiopaque material into the fistula.

Treatment. Excision of the diverticulum is the treatment of choice. If there is a peptic ulcer in the adjacent ileum, it will be necessary to excise the involved bowel together with the diverticulum.

Non-Meckelian Diverticula

These may occur in the duodenum, jejunum, ileum, or colon and are usually incidental roentgenographic or necropsy findings. Rarely, they may result in a clinical problem by causing mechanical pressure, becoming inflamed or ulcerated, or perforating.

Duplications

Dorsal Enteric Remnants

Duplication may result from a failure of normal regression of embryonic diverticula, persistence of transitory intestinal diverticula, median septum formation, errors of recanalization of epithelial plugs, or traction between adhering neural tube ectoderm or notochordal

mesoderm and intestinal endoderm. The latter theory would account for the frequent association of a band extending from the duplicated intestine through the diaphragm and posterior mediastinum, gaining an attachment to the thoracic or cervical spine; this is often associated with vertebral anomalies, such as hemivertebrae or anterior spina bifida.

Pathology. Duplications are saccular or tubular structures, which have a smooth muscle wall and mucous membrane similar to some parts of the gastrointestinal tract. They are found on the mesenteric side of any segment of intestine and vary widely in size and shape. Their blood supply is the same as that of the adjacent bowel, precluding selective excision of the duplication. If saccular, the duplication is not lined by gastric mucosa; nor does it communicate with the lumen of normal bowel; thus peptic erosion of the intestine does not occur. The duplication may be so large that the intestine is stretched out over it and thereby obstructed. Less commonly, the duplication forms the apex of an intussusception.

Tubular duplications have a gastric mucosal lining and are in communication with the adjacent bowel by one or more foramina. Acid secretion gains ready access to the normal unprotected small bowel and may cause a peptic ulcer that may bleed or perforate.

Clinical Manifestations. Symptoms and signs usually arise during infancy and early childhood and include (1) obstruction of adjoining intestine by compression; (2) intestinal bleeding from peptic ulceration secondary to gastric mucosa in the lining of a duplication that communicates with the intestine; (3) pain from secretory distention of a noncommunicating duplication; (4) gangrene of the bowel from obstruction of segmental vasculature; and (5) a movable abdominal mass palpated on routine examination of the abdomen. Duplications are most frequent in the ileum, ileocecal region, and esophagus but may occur in any part of the gastrointestinal tract. Duplications in the thorax are usually of the esophagus or the stomach and only rarely communicate with either. They are evident through dysphagia and respiratory symptoms produced by esophageal and pulmonary compression and are demonstrable roentgenographically. Associated anomalies of vertebrae are not uncommon and often are at a higher level than the intrathoracic mass. Some intrathoracic duplications are of duodenal or jejunal origin.

Roentgenographic studies may show stenosis or compression of the intestinal lumen but more frequently are normal. An intrathoracic duplication is usually visible as a mediastinal mass in roentgenograms of the chest. Very rarely barium studies may fill a communicating duplication.

Cystic Remnants of the Tail Gut

These lesions are found between the anus and the sacrum or coccyx and may be derivatives of that portion of the primitive archenteron extending caudal to the cloaca. Others consider these lesions to be duplications of the rectum or even teratoma. Symptoms are produced by the presence of a mass, which, if large, may obstruct the rectum.

11 · THE DIGESTIVE SYSTEM THE GASTROINTESTINAL TRACT

Bilateral Duplications of Colon and Rectum

These are rare anomalies ("partial twinning") consisting of doubling of the alimentary tract from where a Meckel diverticulum would be found down to the anus. There may also be doubling of the vagina or penis and bladder, and even the sacrum and lumbar vertebrae may be doubled.

INTRA-ABDOMINAL HERNIAS

An intra-abdominal hernia occurs when loops of intestine are trapped by an anomalous fold of peritoneum created by malrotation or malfixation of the duodenum or colon to the posterior abdominal wall. Loops of intestine also may herniate through congenital defects of the mesentery, particularly near the terminal ileum. The symptoms and signs are those of intermittent or acute intestinal obstruction. Gangrene of the intestine can occur if there is compression of the vasculature. Surgical reduction of the hernia and repair of the anomaly in order to prevent recurrence require great care and a knowledge of embryologic anatomy because of the danger of interference with intestinal blood supply.

EXTRA-ABDOMINAL HERNIAS

See Sec 7.53 and 11.75.

11.31 ACQUIRED INTESTINAL OBSTRUCTION

Paralytic ileus is an important cause of acquired intestinal obstruction. It is likely to occur as a complication of acute infections, electrolyte imbalance, or uremia. Pneumonia is probably the most frequent cause of paralytic ileus in infants; peritonitis, especially as a complication of perforated appendicitis, is the most frequent in older children. Ileus is likely to present as distention, with absence of bowel sounds and minimal pain.

Incarcerated inguinal hernias, complications of a Meckel diverticulum, and intussusception are the most frequent *mechanical causes* of intestinal obstruction in infants. Intestinal obstruction may also result from postoperative adhesions, or those produced by recovery from acute peritonitis, and from chronic peritonitis, e.g., tuberculous peritonitis. Other causes are duplications; foreign bodies in the intestine, including fecal concretions and inspissated meconium in the newborn infant; late obstruction by intraluminal contents in cystic fibrosis (pseudomeconium ileus); and masses of roundworms. Tumors of the bowel, including mesenteric cysts and polyps, may also be obstructive. Although vomiting and abdominal distention may occur with mechanical obstruction or ileus, severe colicky periumbilical pain and hyperactive, sometimes tinkling, bowel sounds are almost invariably found in the former.

Huge amounts of electrolyte-rich fluid are secreted into the lumen of the bowel in infants and children with intestinal obstruction. This may lead to severe imbalances of fluid and electrolytes and to distention that compromises the circulation of a segment of intestine. With prolonged stasis this fluid becomes secondarily infected, often with putrefactive organisms, and the patient may have feculent vomiting which should not be confused with true fecal vomiting that occurs with gastrocolic fistula or in coprophagy. A palpable distended single ("closed") loop and unexplained temperature, leukocytosis, and anemia, together with abdominal tenderness, are ominous signs signifying strangulation. However, the presence of gangrenous intestine may be insidious.

11.32 INTUSSUSCEPTION

An intussusception occurs when a portion of the alimentary tract is telescoped into a segment just caudad to it. It is the most common cause of intestinal obstruction from 2 mo–6 yr of age; it is rare under 3 mo and decreases in frequency after 36 mo. Although a small proportion of intussusceptions may reduce spontaneously, most, if left untreated, result in death.

Etiology and Epidemiology. The cause of most intussusceptions is unknown. There is a seasonal incidence, with peaks occurring in spring and autumn. Correlation with adenovirus infections has been noted, and the condition may complicate gastroenteritis. The greater frequency of Peyer patches in the ileum may be relevant; the swollen patch of lymphoid tissue may stimulate intestinal peristalsis in an attempt to extrude the mass, thus causing an intussusception. At the peak age of incidence of this condition the infant's alimentary tract is also being introduced to a variety of new materials. In about 5% of patients recognizable causes for the intussusception are found, such as inverted Meckel diverticulum, an intestinal polyp, duplication, or lymphosarcoma. Uncommonly, the condition will complicate Henoch-Schönlein purpura with an intramural hematoma acting as the apex of the intussusception. Rarely, a postoperative intussusception will be diagnosed; these are always ileoileal.

Pathology. Most intussusceptions are ileocolic and ileoileocolic, less commonly cecocolic, and, rarely, exclusively ileal. Very rarely an intussusception of the appendix forms the apex of the lesion. The upper portion of bowel, the intussusceptum, invaginates into the lower, the intussuscipiens, dragging its mesentery along with it into the enveloping loop. Initially, there is a constriction of the mesentery obstructing the venous return. Engorgement of the intussusceptum occurs with edema and bleeding from the mucosa, resulting in a bloody stool, sometimes containing mucus. The apex of the intussusception may extend into the transverse, descending, or sigmoid colon—even to the anus in neglected cases. After reduction of an idiopathic intussusception the portion of the bowel that had formed the apex of the intussusceptum is edematous and thickened, often with a dimple visible on the serosal surface that represents the origin of the lesion. Most intussusceptions do not strangulate the bowel within the 1st 24 hr but may lead subsequently to intestinal gangrene and shock.

Clinical Manifestations. In typical cases there is sudden onset of severe paroxysmal pain in a previously well child, which recurs at frequent intervals and is accompanied by straining efforts and loud outcries. Initially, the infant may be comfortable and play normally between the paroxysms of pain, but if the intussusception is not reduced, the infant becomes progressively weaker and lethargic. Eventually a shock-like state may develop with an elevation of body temperature to as high as 41° C (106° F). The pulse becomes weak and thready, the respirations shallow and grunting, and the pain may be manifested only by moaning sounds. Vomiting occurs in most instances and is usually more frequent at the beginning. In the later phase the vomitus becomes bile-stained. Fecal matter of normal appearance may be evacuated during the 1st few hr of symptoms. After this time fecal excretions are small or more often do not occur, and little or no flatus is passed. Blood generally is passed in the 1st 12 hr, but at times not for 1–2 days and infrequently not at all; 60% of infants will pass a stool containing red blood and mucus, the *currant jelly stool.* Some patients have only irritability and alternating or progressive lethargy.

Palpation of the abdomen usually reveals a slightly tender, sausage-shaped mass, sometimes ill defined, which may increase in size and firmness during a paroxysm of pain and is most often in the right upper portion of the abdomen with its large axis directed cephalocaudally. If it is felt in the epigastrium, the long axis is directed transversely. About 30% of patients do not have a palpable mass. It is more readily located by bimanual rectal and abdominal palpation between paroxysms of pain. The presence of bloody mucus on the finger as it is withdrawn after rectal examination supports the diagnosis of intussusception. Abdominal distention and tenderness develop as intestinal obstruction becomes more acute. On rare occasions the advancing intestine prolapses through the anus. This prolapse can be distinguished from prolapse of the rectum by the separation between the protruding intestine and the rectal wall, which does not exist in prolapse of the rectum.

Ileoileal intussusception may have a less typical clinical picture, the symptoms and signs being chiefly those of small intestinal obstruction. *Recurrent intussusception* is uncommon. *Chronic intussusception*, in which the symptoms exist in milder form at recurrent intervals, is more likely to occur with or following acute enteritis and may arise in older children as well as in infants.

Diagnosis. The clinical history and physical findings are usually sufficiently typical for diagnosis. Roentgenographically, abdominal scout films may show a masslike density in the area of the intussusception. The film after a barium enema will show a filling defect or cupping in the head of barium as its advance is obstructed by the intussusceptum (Fig 11–17). A central linear column of barium may be visible in the compressed lumen of the intussusceptum, and a thin rim of barium may be seen trapped around the invaginating intestine in the folds of mucosa within the intussuscipiens (coil-spring sign), especially after evacuation. Retrogression of the intussusceptum under the pressure of the enema and gaseous distention of the small

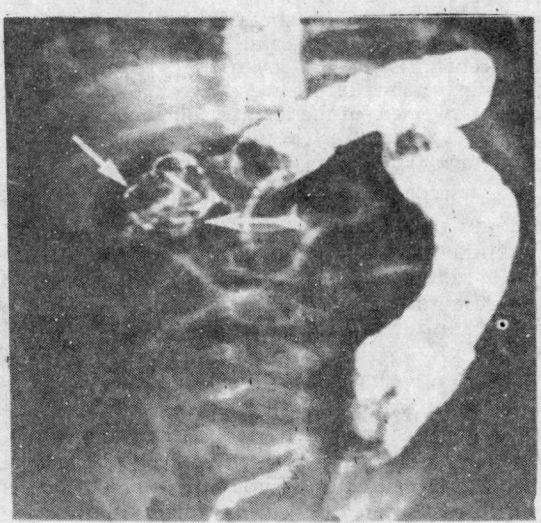

Figure 11–17 Intussusception in an infant. The obstruction is evident in the proximal transverse colon. Contrast material between the intussusceptum and the intussuscipiens is responsible for the coilspring appearance.

intestine from obstruction are also useful roentgenographic signs. Ileoileal intussusception is usually not demonstrable by barium enema but is suspected because of gaseous distention of the intestine above the intussusception.

Differential Diagnosis. It may be particularly difficult to diagnose intussusception in a child who already has *gastroenteritis;* a change in the pattern of illness, character of pain, and nature of vomiting or the onset of rectal bleeding should alert the physician. Bloody bowel movements and abdominal cramps accompanying *enterocolitis* can usually be differentiated from intussusception because the pain is less severe and less regular and because the infant is recognizably ill between pains from the time of onset with an intussusception. Bleeding from *Meckel diverticulum* is usually painless. The intestinal hemorrhage of *anaphylactoid purpura* is usually, but not invariably, accompanied by joint symptoms or purpura elsewhere, and the colicky pain may be similar. However, since intussusception may be a complication of this disorder, a barium enema may be required.

Treatment. Reduction of the intussusception is an emergency procedure to be carried out immediately after diagnosis and after rapid preparation for operation with fluids and blood for shock and for water and electrolyte replacement. In over 75% of cases of short duration, when there are no signs of prostration, shock, or peritoneal irritation, it is possible to reduce the intussusception by hydrostatic pressure under fluoroscopic guidance and with the consultation and close proximity of a surgeon.

A nonlubricated Foley bag catheter is placed in the rectum and inflated. The buttocks are compressed tightly and taped with adhesive plaster. A barium solution is then allowed to flow by gravity into the colon from a height of not more than 3 ft above the fluoroscopic table. The abdomen is *not touched* during the procedure. The column of barium advances slowly in a proximal direction with progressive simultaneous movement of the filling defect in the same direction. Reduction of the intussusception is manifest by free filling of the small intestine, disappearance of the mass, passage of flatus or feces, and improvement in the infant's condition. If there is any doubt about the completeness of the reduction, an exploratory operation is performed immediately.

If there is clinical evidence of intestinal obstruction with abdominal distention, especially for 48 hr or longer, roentgenographic reduction of the intussusception should not be attempted because of the risk of perforating the intussuscipiens. In an ileoileal intussusception a barium enema is usually not diagnostic and reduction by the hydrostatic technique may not be effective. Such intussusceptions may also develop insidiously as a complication of a laparotomy and require resection. A right-sided transverse paraumbilical incision gives ready access to the ascending colon. If manual operative reduction is impossible or the bowel is not viable, resection of the intussusception will be necessary with end-to-end anastomosis to reconstitute continuity of the intestine.

Prognosis.   Untreated intussusception in infants is nearly always fatal; the chances of recovery are directly related to the duration of intussusception before reduction. The majority of infants will recover if the intussusception is reduced within the 1st 24 hr, but the mortality rate rises rapidly after this time, especially when reduction is deferred to the 3rd day. Spontaneous reduction during transport or preparation for operation is not uncommon.

The recurrence rate following barium enema reduction of intussusceptions at The Hospital for Sick Children, Toronto, is about 10%; following surgical reduction about 2–5% recur; and none have recurred after surgical resection. It is extremely unlikely that an intussusception caused by a lesion, such as lymphosarcoma, polyp, or inverted Meckel diverticulum will be successfully reduced by barium enema. With adequate surgical management, operative reduction carries a very low mortality rate in early cases.

Colonic Polyps

These lesions rarely cause obstruction and only when they constitute the lead point of a colocolic intussusception. Usually, they cause painless rectal bleeding. Consisting largely of granulation tissue and cystic spaces, they normally have relatively narrow pedicles; 80% of colonic polypi in children are single and within reach of a standard sigmoidoscope. There is no record that a juvenile polyp ever became malignant. Most disappear spontaneously, presumably undergoing necrosis from twisting of the polyp pedicle. If within reach of the sigmoidoscope, a polyp is easily removed by intussuscepting it out of the anus, transfixing its base, and excising it. If beyond visualization by sigmoidoscopy, the mucosal lesions can be demonstrated by a double air/barium contrast study of the colon; if still present after prolonged observation by annual barium studies, lesions should be removed by use of a colonoscope. This approach is preferable to laparotomy and colo-

tomy, but the latter may be necessary if the polyp has a broad sessile base.

11.33   FOREIGN BODIES IN THE STOMACH AND INTESTINES

If ingestion of a foreign body is suspected, plain roentgenograms of the abdomen and chest are indicated; if an object is visible above the diaphragm, esophagoscopy or bronchoscopy may be needed to retrieve it (Sec 11.20). An object that reaches the stomach will, in most instances, pass through the gastrointestinal tract without causing injury. Certain types of foreign bodies, however, are potentially dangerous. Needles, hairpins, or bobby pins pass easily through the esophagus on their long axis, but may be unable to round the turns of the duodenum, where they become fixed and eventually perforate the intestine. Such potentially dangerous foreign bodies can usually be removed gastroscopically. If safety pins are small, they will probably pass without difficulty, whether open or closed. If they are large, either closed or open, peroral removal is safe and is indicated.

If the foreign body has passed through the pylorus into the intestine, its progress should be observed by means of roentgenograms and every stool examined for its presence. The stool can be placed in a fine-meshed sieve and disintegrated by allowing water to run through the sieve with some force. If serial roentgenograms show the foreign body moving progressively down the intestinal tract, perforation is not likely. If it remains stationary for several wk or is long or sharp, it should be removed either under fluoroscopy by a magnetized nasogastric tube or by laparotomy because of the dangers of ulceration and perforation of the bowel. If at any time such signs of perforation as tenderness, rigidity, pain, nausea, or vomiting develop, surgery is indicated immediately. The diet should be normal, with no change from that to which the child has been accustomed. Bizarre roughage, wool, or cotton diets are valueless and may be dangerous. Laxatives are contraindicated since the accelerated activity of the intestine increases the danger of perforation.

Bezoars

Occasionally, infants and children, particularly if emotionally disturbed or mentally retarded, acquire the habit of swallowing hair from their heads or from dolls or brushes, or they may swallow fur, wool, or cotton from wearing apparel or blankets. This material is usually passed through the intestines, but when the habit is persistent, there may be an accumulation in the stomach with formation of the so-called *hairball* or *trichobezoar*. The symptoms are indefinite, but indigestion and gastric distress may be present. The tumor mass is often palpable and may give a soft crackling sensation on palpation. A bald spot or sparse hair may be apparent. A roentgenogram after administration of barium may disclose a mass outlined by barium. A portion of the bezoar may be dislodged and subsequently become impacted in the intestine and cause obstruction. The diagnosis may be suspected from observation of the stool or of the child in the act of swallowing these materials. Surgical removal is indicated, and the child's mental and psychologic status should be evaluated.

Phytobezoars are accumulations of fibrous or mucilaginous materials as found in persimmons and various tar products. The accumulation is usually rapid compared with that of the hairball.

11.34 MOTILITY DISORDERS

This group of conditions includes disorders of unknown etiology leading to functional obstruction, usually of a chronic nature. As a result, management is less than satisfactory.

Chronic Duodenal Ileus, Superior Mesenteric Artery Syndrome, Cast Syndrome

This syndrome is associated with intermittent functional obstruction of the duodenum and is thought by some to result from compression of the 3rd part of the duodenum between the superior mesenteric artery and the aorta (though the left renal vein curiously escapes this vise). Others consider it to result from loss of supporting fat to the 2nd and 3rd parts of the duodenum with normal or exaggerated lumbar lordosis effectively occluding the duodenum. Some cases of chronic duodenal obstruction occur as the result of incomplete rotation of the intestine.

Usually the patient is a tall, asthenic, visceroptotic teenage female. A history of "bilious attacks" or other forms of episodic vomiting may be elicited. A barium study typically shows megaduodenum and rapid, churning, to-and-fro peristaltic movements. The dilatation of the duodenum usually ends abruptly just to the right of the midline. The stomach may also be hugely dilated. If malrotation is suspected, a barium enema should be done to determine the position of the cecum.

If patients can be nourished and the duodenum rested, most of them will be relieved of their obstruction. The simplest form of treatment consists of a prone knee-elbow position after meals, which allows the duodenum to fall away from the retroperitoneal structures which may be causing obstruction. Nasojejunal intubation and jejunal feeding for a period of several wk or total parenteral nutrition may allow periduodenal fat to accumulate, increasing the support of the duodenum and lessening the kinking at the duodenojejunal flexure. Metoclopramide has been reported helpful in management. If there is no relief despite energetic and prolonged conservative treatment, operation may become necessary. A Ladd procedure is the operation of choice; duodenojejunostomy is less satisfactory.

Pseudo-Obstruction

With increasing survival of infants with gastroschisis, more cases of intestinal pseudo-obstruction are being encountered. In these children innervation is normal, but the bowel seems unable to respond to the stimulation of distention with a normal propagated wave of pressure. Treatment consists of complete rest of the bowel, using total parenteral nutrition. A gastrostomy may be necessary to prevent swallowed air from being ingested. Esophageal manometric studies may also demonstrate abnormal motility.

At least 15 cases of *congenital segmental dilatation* of the ileum, jejunum, or colon have been reported. A localized short segment of the small intestine is dilated and ineffective in propelling its contents into the adjacent normal distal bowel. The innervation of the bowel in the segment is normal. The condition may cause acute neonatal intestinal obstruction or chronic obstruction with great dilatation of the small bowel in an older child. Local resection of the dilated loop of bowel is effective treatment.

Intestinal pseudo-obstruction may also occur in the colon, with barium or Gastrografin studies demonstrating inertia of a segment of bowel. Treatment with parasympathomimetic drugs is not effective.

A colonic obstructive condition has also been described in which the roentgenographic appearances are those of Hirschsprung disease but ganglion cells are present. If a colostomy results in relief, then excision of the roentgenographically abnormal segment may be indicated. Some newborn infants of diabetic mothers develop manifestations of bowel obstruction called *immature left colon syndrome;* a barium enema shows an appearance typical of extensive megacolon with the apparently aganglionic segment extending up to the splenic flexure or even beyond. Anal manometric studies and rectal biopsy are normal. The condition usually requires no specific treatment.

11.35 ANORECTAL MALFORMATIONS

Congenital anomalies of the anus and rectum are relatively common. Minor abnormalities occur in about 1:500 live births, major anomalies in 1:5000 live births. A variety of anomalies are associated with those of the rectum, including malformations of the urinary tract, esophagus, and, less commonly, the duodenum. The most useful clinical classification separates "low" and "high" lesions in accordance with whether the rectum does or does not pass through the puborectalis muscle, which is a major portion of the levator ani muscle of defecation.

Embryology and Pathogenesis. The anus and rectum develop from the dorsal portion of the hindgut or cloacal cavity when lateral ingrowths of mesenchyme form the urorectal septum in the midline, separating the rectum and anal canal dorsally from the bladder and urethra ventrally. There is a small communication, the cloacal duct, between the 2 systems, which is closed by the 7th wk of gestation by a downgrowth of the urorectal septum. An ingrowth of mesoderm divides the cloacal membrane into the urogenital membrane ventrally and the anal membrane dorsally. During the 7th wk the urogenital portion of the original cloaca has acquired an external opening, but the anal membrane does not open until later. The anus develops by a fusion of the anal tubercles and an external invagination known as the proctodeum, which deepens toward the rectum but is separated by the anal membrane. This membrane ruptures by the 8th wk of gestation.

Interference with the development of anorectal structures at varying stages gives rise to a variety of anomalies that range from anal stenosis and incomplete rupture of the anal membrane or anal agenesis (the "low" types) to complete failure of descent of the upper portion of the cloaca and failure of invagination of the proctodeum (the "high" types). The persistence of the communication between the urinary and rectal portions of the cloaca is responsible for fistulas, which are more common in the male. In the female, fistulas connect the rectum with the vagina more commonly than with the urinary system.

Since the muscle of the external anal sphincter is derived from exterior mesoderm, it is usually intact and not involved with the obstructive lesions of the anus and rectum.

Pathology. Supralevator "high" anomalies occur almost exclusively in males, and there is usually a rectourethral fistula between the rectum, ending blindly proximally, and the prostatic urethra. The bowel ends proximal to the puborectalis muscle with absence of functional internal and external anal sphincters; the puborectalis muscle is relatively ineffectual in sustaining rectal continence. Associated maldevelopment of the sacrum, with absence of all or part of it, interferes with innervation of both anal and urethral musculature and also with the development of continence. When these supralevator anomalies occur in girls, there is usually a fistulous communication between the rectum and the posterior vaginal fornix. **Rectal atresia** occurs when the proctodeum (anal canal) develops normally but fails to communicate with the rectum; the rectum may be separated by a substantial gap, or there may be only a mucosal diaphragm. There is no fistula. In rectocloacal anomalies the urethra opens anteriorly into a common cloacal (vaginal) channel and the rectum communicates posteriorly with the same channel. There is thus a single (cloacal) orifice on the perineum with neither rectum nor urethra visible. **Cloacal exstrophy** is a complex mixture of exstrophy of the bladder, imperforate anus, maldevelopment or absence of the colon, and grossly malformed external genitalia. There may be an associated small omphalocele.

In translevator "low" anomalies the hindgut has transversed the levator ani muscle and the internal and external anal sphincters are present and well developed with normal function. In males there is a covering of skin or membrane over the anus (a so-called "covered anus") with an anteriorly placed fistulous opening onto the skin in the midline anterior to where the anus would be. This opening may be on the perineum, scrotum, or even the under surface of the penis. In females the anus is ectopic; it may be perineal, vestib-

ular, or even (low) vaginal in location. An intermediate type of translevator anomaly with rectourethral fistulas may also occur.

Diagnosis. Evaluation of the newborn infant with an anorectal malformation should be directed toward establishing whether a low or high lesion is present since initial treatment, definitive treatment, and prognosis differ for these 2 lesions.

Stenosis of the anorectal canal may occur at any point or extend its entire length. The constriction can be identified by digital and endoscopic examination. An *imperforate anal membrane* is readily identified as a thin translucent membrane which becomes progressively distended by the meconium just behind it.

More than 90% of the other low anomalies are associated with an external fistula to the perineum or vestibule. These fistulas may not be apparent at birth, but peristalsis will gradually force meconium through the fistula. Repeated meticulous examinations during the 1st 24 hr of life will, in most cases, eventually reveal a tiny speck of meconium at the opening of the fistula. In males, if meconium is seen at or anterior to the anus, a low anomaly is present. Folds of skin ("buckethandles") may be encountered in high or low atresias. The presence of *perineal pearls*, cystic accumulations of inspissated mucus anywhere in the midline anterior to the anus and even extending onto the scrotum, always connotes a covered anus. In females it is usually possible to insert a feeding tube into the ectopic anus to establish its presence and the direction of the anal canal and rectum. The presence of a dimple at the site of the anus does not indicate a low lesion. Roentgenograms employing contrast media injected through a tiny catheter inserted into the fistula will confirm the diagnosis.

A poorly developed anal dimple, a rounded perineum, or vertebral anomalies suggest a high lesion. Passage of meconium in the urine is diagnostic of a rectourinary fistula and a rectal pouch ending above the puborectalis muscle. In most cases a lateral roentgenogram in the upside down position (Fig 11–18) should be obtained after clinical distention is evident or after 18–24 hr of life. The infant should be held upside down for several min before the film to allow the gas in the bowel to displace the meconium and proceed as far distally as possible. Stephens has suggested that the level of the levator ani muscle is represented by a line joining the symphysis pubis with the last segment of the sacrum; if the gas bubble is proximal to this line, the anomaly is a high one. Other methods of estimation involve the comparison of the level of the gas bubble with a comma-shaped ischium. A retrograde urethrocystogram will usually demonstrate the rectourethral fistula.

If none of these measures clearly identifies the level of the rectal pouch, it is safest to assume the infant has a high lesion. Blind exploration of the perineum in hopes of finding a low lying rectal pouch should not be done.

Associated anomalies are common in these babies. Significant urinary tract and vertebral abnormalities occur in about 50% of patients with high anorectal malformation and 25% of those with low types. Excretory urography should be done in all cases and should

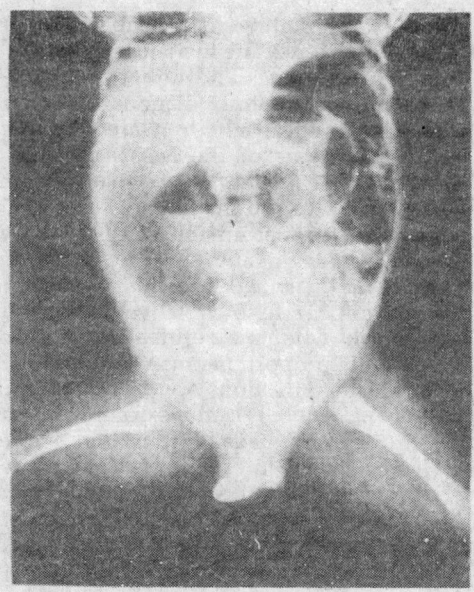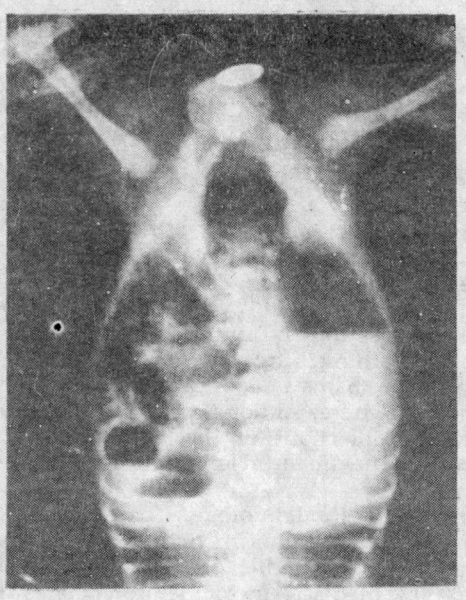

A   B

Figure 11–18 Wangensteen-Rice roentgenographic technique for demonstration of the position of the blind colonic pouch in the case of an imperforate or absent rectum. The infant is held head downward, causing the intestinal gas to rise to the blind end of the gut. *A*, Roentgenogram of child in upright position, showing transverse level of gas. The level of the obstruction is not demonstrated. *B*, The level of the obstruction is apparent when the roentgenogram is taken with the child in the inverted position. The site of the anus is marked by a lead disk.

precede definitive therapy in high lesions. The anatomy of the bony pelvis may reveal sacral anomalies which may be important to later bowel or urinary functions. Meconium or flatus may be passed with urine, confirming a rectourethral fistula.

Treatment. Anal stenosis can generally be treated by digital or instrumental dilatations. All other forms of imperforate anus should be surgically corrected.

In the low types in females, since the bowel has the proper levator relationship, repair can be managed from below. These patients are perfectly continent unless ill-advised operations are performed. There is no evidence that an anus placed 1 cm or so anterior to its normal position results in either urinary or genital infections or major problems with parturition. Rarely, the anus will have to be transplanted dorsally when there is a true low rectovaginal fistula. The "covered anus" in males and infrequently the vestibular ectopic anus in females will need a cut-back operation, in which the coverings of the anus are incised in a dorsal direction and the mucosa sutured to the margins of the newly created anus. Postoperative regular dilatations for 1–2 mo may be necessary.

The high types are best treated by a preliminary transverse colostomy followed by a definitive repair in 6–12 mo. Careful positioning of the anus in the region of the external sphincter and anatomic positioning of the bowel in the puborectalis sling are essential. Fistulas are also eliminated.

The higher the blind pouch and the more extensive the operation, the more difficulty encountered in the postoperative period. Significant sacral anomalies are usually associated with deficient neurologic control of defecation. With continuing care through the period of toilet training a satisfactory functional solution can usually be expected. In a few instances there will be continuing problems due to stenosis, poor anal control, or poor guidance. In the postoperative period constipation rather than incontinence is the principal problem. The lack of sensation of fecal material in the rectum leads to fecal impactions with paradoxic or overflow diarrheal stools and gives rise to the acquired type of megacolon. Early attention to ensure regular evacuations will prevent massive fecal impactions. As a rule, the child should be taught to defecate at a given time of day rather than await the urge. In some instances a daily enema may be needed.

Prognosis. All patients with a low type of anorectal malformation should be continent. Patients with a high anomaly, on the other hand, will rarely be perfectly continent; most are left with what is, in effect, a perineal colostomy. This form of incontinence, however, is infinitely preferable to an abdominal colostomy in children and adolescents.

BARRY SHANDLING

INFLAMMATORY DISEASES OF THE INTESTINE

11.36 INFECTIONS

See Sec 10.12.

Diarrheal illness, most of it attributable to enteric infection, was estimated to have resulted in the death of at least 20 million African, Asian, and Latin American children under the age of 4 yr in 1975. Where populations have access to good nutrition and sanitary living conditions, death rates are very much lower, but infectious diarrhea remains a major cause of illness in young children everywhere. Although the term "gastroenteritis" persists, infections of the gastrointestinal tract usually affect the small or large intestine but not the stomach.

Etiology and Epidemiology. The major known causes of enteric infection in children are summarized in Table 11–7. No specific pathogen is identified in about 20–30% of cases. In temperate climates human rotavirus (HRV) accounts for about 50% of cases and up to 80% of all severe cases in infants during the winter mo; in the tropics a similar incidence probably occurs in the rainy seasons. Some parvo-like agents have caused severe community outbreaks of acute diarrhea (Norwalk, Hawaii, Montgomery County), and cytomegalovirus, on rare occasions, has been shown to infect the colon.

Table 11–7 CAUSES OF INTESTINAL INFECTION IN CHILDREN

Viruses
  Human rotavirus
  Norwalk-like viruses
  Cytomegalovirus
  Others—adenovirus, etc.*
Bacteria
  Enteroinvasive
    Shigellae
    Salmonellae—*S. typhosa*, others
    Yersinia enterocolitica
    Campylobacter jejuni
    E. coli
    Tubercle bacillus
  Enterotoxigenic
    E. coli
    V. cholerae
    Clostridium perfringens
Protozoa
  Giardia lamblia
  Entamoeba histolytica
  Balantidium coli
Helminths
  Ascariasis (roundworm)
  Enterobiasis (pinworm)
  Trichuriasis (whipworm)
  Toxocariasis (visceral larva migrans)
  Ancylostomiasis (hookworm)
  Trichinosis
  Cestodiasis (tapeworm)
Mycoses
  Candida albicans (Monilia)

*Several other viruses have been associated with acute infantile diarrhea, but none is yet a proven pathogen.

Bacterial pathogens probably cause 10–15% of intestinal infections. The incidence of bacterial infection rises in warm climates and under poor sanitary conditions. The most commonly diagnosed bacterial pathogens in North American children are *Campylobacter jejuni* and various strains of the *Salmonella* and *Shigella* species. *Yersinia enterocolitica* is also relatively common, particularly in Eastern Canada and Europe. Certain strains of *E. coli*, a normal inhabitant of the distal bowel, can be pathogenic, causing sporadic cases of acute enteritis, epidemic diarrhea, and *traveler's diarrhea*. These infections appear to be relatively uncommon in children except in epidemic outbreaks. Cholera is a problem of epidemic proportions in Asia (Sec 10.33).

Parasitic infections are discussed in Sec 10.107. *Entamoeba histolytica* infections occur in all parts of the world, but they are usually found in subtropical climates. *Giardia lamblia* infestation is endemic in the tropics but is now a common cause of enteric infection in children everywhere. *Balantidium coli* infection is common in Latin America but rare in North America. *Ascaris* (the roundworm), *Enterobius vermicularis* (pinworm), and *Toxocara (canis* or *cati)* are common in North America. *Trichuris trichiura* (whipworm) and hookworms *(Necator americanus, Ancylostoma duodenale,* and *Ancylostoma ceylonicum)* are confined to warm climates.

Fungi, like bacteria, are normal inhabitants of the human gut. *Candida albicans* may cause local enteric disease and serve as a reservoir for disseminated infection in debilitated or immune-deficient patients.

Pathogenesis. Most known pathogens disturb intestinal function and cause diarrhea either by invading the bowel wall or by elaborating an enterotoxin in the lumen. The capacity of an organism to bind to the intestinal surface appears to be an important determinant of its pathogenicity. Of the enterotoxins, choleragen, produced by *V. cholerae*, has been the most intensively studied. It binds to the epithelial surface and activates the adenylate cyclase system provoking intracellular accumulation of cyclic AMP, impaired absorption of sodium and chloride, and secretion of chloride; glucose-stimulated sodium absorption at the brush border remains intact (Sec 10.33). The heat-labile strain of *E. coli* enterotoxin acts similarly to cholera toxin, but it is likely that cyclic GMP mediates the secretory response to the heat-stable *E. coli* enterotoxin (Sec 10.29).

Human rotavirus invades the upper intestinal epithelium causing defective sodium and chloride transport in the upper bowel; glucose-stimulated sodium transport and glucose absorption are impaired, and intracellular cyclic AMP levels are normal (Sec 10.12). Diarrhea occurs not as a direct response of the epithelial cell to viral damage but as a failure of the epithelium to differentiate as it migrates to repair the regions damaged by virus. Much less is known about the pathogenesis of diarrhea caused by invasive bacteria. Some invasive salmonellae appear capable of activating an enterotoxin-like response.

Sodium and chloride concentrations in acute enterotoxigenic diarrhea approach those of plasma (130–140 mEq/l) and are much higher than those typical of invasive viral enteritis (30–50 mEq/l). Although glucose transport in acute viral enteritis is defective and disaccharidase activities reduced, large quantities of sugar are rarely found in stools during the acute disease since unabsorbed sugar is broken down by enteric bacteria.

The intestine possesses effective mechanisms to clear unwanted organisms in addition to the body's immunologic defenses. Diarrhea itself promotes flushing out of infecting agents, and microbes that are lodged in enterocytes are quickly shed into the lumen as the epithelium undergoes constant renewal. Consequently, the enteric infections are usually self-limited. However, infection may persist in the gut because of a source of reinfection, special properties of the organism involved, or a defect in the hosts' defenses.

Clinical Manifestations. In North America most intestinal infections are acute, self-limited diseases. Diarrhea begins suddenly, accompanied usually by vomiting and low grade fever. In severe cases the stools are so loose that they can be easily mistaken for urine. The patient is irritable and cries as if in pain. Vomiting and fever usually resolve quickly, but diarrhea persists for 3-4 days, then gradually improves over another 4-5 days. Physical examination discloses hyperactive bowel sounds and, in some cases, abdominal distention. Rectal examination may cause a rush of pooled secretions and thus reveal a severe disorder not previously suspected. Usually, it is not possible to distinguish between bacterial and viral disease on clinical grounds (Table 10-16) unless contact with a diagnosed case is known or blood and pus are present to suggest an invasive bacterial or amebic infection of the colon. The child's fluid and acid-base status should be quickly assessed as death from shock, dehydration, and acid-base and electrolyte imbalance may be sudden. When *Yersinia enterocolitica* causes chronic diarrhea, there is usually periumbilical pain, right lower quadrant tenderness, and often erythema nodosum and arthritis. *Campylobacter jejuni* may cause chronic bloody diarrhea with severe crampy lower abdominal pain.

Treatment. See discussion of specific agents in Chapter 10.

Gall DG, Hamilton JR: Infectious diarrhea in infants and children. Clin Gastroenterol 6:431, 1977.
Hamilton JR: Infectious diarrhea in children. Aust Pediatr J 15:25, 1979.
Schreiber DS, Trier JS, Blacklow NR: Recent advances in viral gastroenteritis. Gastroenterology 73:174, 1977.

NONINFECTIVE INFLAMMATORY BOWEL DISEASE

11.37 Idiopathic Ulcerative Colitis

This chronic condition of unknown etiology affects the distal large bowel extending proximally within the colon to a varying extent in different patients; in some cases the entire colon may be affected. There is diffuse inflammation characterized by an infiltrate of neutrophils with crypt abscesses, but the lesion rarely extends beyond the mucosa into deeper layers. In its typical form, therefore, this process is quite distinct from the lesion that characterizes Crohn disease.

Epidemiology. Ulcerative colitis is relatively common in Jews and rare in black and oriental people. There is an unexplained concentration of cases in Europe and North America. The disease is relatively common among 1st degree relatives of patients, in patients with ankylosing spondylitis, and in individuals with the histocompatibility antigen HLA-B27.

Clinical Manifestations. The disease begins before the age of 20 yr in about 15% of patients. Symptoms may start in the newborn period, but the onset usually does not occur until the preadolescent years. The common symptoms are chronic diarrhea with fresh blood, fecal urgency, tenesmus, and lower abdominal cramps, particularly just before defecation. In most patients the onset is gradual; as diarrhea persists, anorexia develops, leading to weight loss. At times, the initial course is fulminant with high fever and progression to peritonitis and even perforation within days. If the symptoms are prolonged, particularly when nutrient intake has been poor, delayed maturation and growth occur. Postmenarchal girls may cease to menstruate. The general impact of the disease on the child is often reflected in the child's attendance and performance both at school and at extracurricular activities.

There will usually be clinical signs of chronic ill health at the time of diagnosis. The abdomen is tender, particularly along the left side, and bowel sounds are increased. There may be abdominal distention and tenderness on rectal examination. In fresh stools blood is usually present and there are always masses of leukocytes and mucus. There may be anal fissures, but perianal fistulas and abscesses are less common than in Crohn disease.

Extraintestinal manifestations of colitis are less common in children than in adults, but signs of arthritis are seen in about 10% of patients. Usually, large joints such as the knees, hips, or shoulders are tender, swollen, warm, and red. Rarely, the hands and feet are affected. Spondylitis is more likely to coexist with colitis than in noncolitic patients. but it is rare in children. Usually, but not always, arthritic activity parallels colitic activity. However, joint signs may be quite severe in the presence of very subtle colitic activity. Erythema nodosum, consisting of characteristic discrete, painful, raised red lesions over the legs, occurs in fewer than 5% of cases, usually when the colitis is active. Pyoderma gangrenosum, a necrotic lesion of the skin, is also associated with ulcerative colitis but is very rare. Iritis is also rare and develops relatively late in the course of the disease. It is characterized by pain, conjunctival hyperemia in a perilimbal distribution, cells in the aqueous, deposits on the back of the cornea, and congestion of the iris. Coexisting hepatitis, also rare in children, usually causes a mixed hyperbilirubinemia with an enlarged firm liver. Unlike other extraintestinal disorders, the activity of this hepatitis tends not to be related to the activity of the colonic disease. Finger clubbing is seen in fewer than 10% of patients and is always associated with extensive disease. Peripheral edema (from excessive enteric protein loss), phlebitis, and hemolytic anemia are also associated with ulcerative colitis but are rare in childhood cases.

In the clinical assessment of these patients particular attention should be paid to their psychologic status.

Table 11–8 CHRONIC INFLAMMATORY DISORDERS OF THE INTESTINE

Infections
  Salmonella
  Yersinia enterocolitica
  Campylobacter jejuni
  Tuberculosis
  Cytomegalovirus
  Entamoeba histolytica
  Trichuriasis
Others
  Particularly in infants
    Necrotizing enterocolitis
    Hirschsprung enterocolitis
    "Allergic" colitis
  All ages
    Idiopathic ulcerative colitis
    Crohn disease
    Anaphylactoid purpura
    Hemolytic-uremic syndrome
    Pseudomembranous (antibiotic-associated) enterocolitis
    Eosinophilic gastroenteritis

Although emotional problems do not appear to cause or to have a direct impact on the course of the disease, they clearly exacerbate the severity of the child's symptoms. If the child and family are carefully evaluated initially, they can be better supported through the course of a serious, chronic illness for which satisfactory drug therapy is unavailable.

Differential Diagnosis. The incidence of specific disorders causing chronic intestinal inflammation (Table 11–8) varies in different regions, but infections are by far the most common causes. A careful search for infectious contacts and microbiologic studies should be completed before a diagnosis of idiopathic ulcerative colitis is made. Infections that cause a chronic colitis with pus and blood in stools include *Shigella, Salmonella, Yersinia enterocolitica, Campylobacter,* and *Entamoeba histolytica.* Ulcerative colitis is rare in infants, but dietary protein, particularly cow's milk, is capable of causing colitis, and Hirschsprung disease may be complicated by colitis in this age group. In older children Crohn disease is characterized by its segmental distribution, frequent small bowel disease, and involvement of all layers of the gut by a granulomatous inflammatory lesion. Intestinal involvement with anaphylactoid purpura or hemolytic-uremic syndrome may precede other manifestations of these diseases, but evidence of a widespread vasculitis becomes apparent in time. Pseudomembranous colitis with a typical sigmoidoscopic lesion is usually associated with prior antibiotic use.

Diagnosis. Clinical evaluation will usually point to a possible diagnosis of an inflammatory bowel lesion, but further studies will be needed to define the specific diagnosis. Microbiologic studies should be guided by knowledge of possible contacts. If *Entamoeba histolytica* is suspected, serology is indicated as well as appropriate stool examinations. Longstanding infections with *Yersinia enterocolitica, Campylobacter jejuni,* and some *Salmonella* species may cause elevated serum antibody titers. *Clostridium difficile* enterotoxin assays should be carried out if antibiotic-associated colitis is suspected.

Sigmoidoscopic examination demonstrates the typical diffuse inflammatory lesion of the rectum and distal colon in idiopathic ulcerative colitis. The mucosa is inflamed, granular, and extremely friable; ulcers are rarely seen in children. In the typical case biopsy shows an inflammatory lesion characterized by polymorphonuclear infiltration and crypt abscesses. A barium enema may be normal initially, but usually the examination shows a diffuse distal lesion; the process may extend proximally to involve the entire colon. None of these roentgenographic, endoscopic, and biopsy abnormalities is specific for idiopathic ulcerative colitis.

Treatment. Curative medical therapy is not available, but medications can reduce the activity of the inflammatory process and prevent recurrences.

Supportive measures are particularly important. Within the limits of their capacity to understand, the child and his or her parents must be given insight into the nature of the disease. In general, dietary restrictions have little place in treatment as long as a nutritious, balanced diet is provided. Some patients become seriously malnourished because of an inability to tolerate sufficient nutrient intake. Total parenteral nutrition is a very effective technique for restoring nutritional status, but it usually does not affect the inflammatory process in the bowel. Emphasis should be placed on encouraging the patient to live as full a life as possible. In general, mood-altering drugs and appetitic stimulants should not be used in the treatment of these patients.

Controlled studies in adults show that *sulfasalazine* reduces the likelihood of exacerbation when taken on a chronic basis, even years after the onset of the disease. Used in a dose of 0.5 gm/15 kg/24 hr (maximum 4 gm) it rarely has side effects; anorexia or nausea can usually be reduced by using the enteric coated form of the drug. Occasionally, neutropenia or a hypersensitivity reaction necessitates discontinuing the medication. A high incidence of reversible toxic effects on semen with oligospermia and infertility has been associated with long term use of the drug. Nevertheless, the drug should be used on a regular, continuing basis for patients in whom the diagnosis of idiopathic ulcerative colitis is proved.

Corticosteroids are most effective for treating active disease. For mild cases, particularly those with disease confined to the distal colon, soluble hydrocortisone or prednisolone may be used as an enema, 100 mg hydrocortisone or its equivalent, given slowly at bedtime to an adolescent for 6 wk, daily for the 1st 3 wk and then on alternate nights. If the patient deteriorates or does not improve over 10 days, oral prednisone should be added. Prednisone, 1–2 mg/kg/24 hr to a maximum daily dose of 60 mg/24 hr, is used for moderate to severe cases and those which fail to respond to enema therapy. Occasionally, with fulminant disease, the patient may be too ill to tolerate oral medication and will require an equivalent intravenous dose of hydrocortisone. Once begun, a 3–4 mo course of systemic medication should be given, in a full dose for 6 wk, then tapered by 5 mg/24 hr each wk. The changes in facial appearance and acne that occur in children receiving this medication vary in severity but are universally dreaded by young patients. Additional complications are cataracts, systemic hypertension, and growth retardation. Alternate-day administration of prednisone may avoid suppression of the patient's adrenals but is usually inadequate to suppress active disease.

Other medications have been tried but are not of proven benefit. Sodium cromoglycate given by mouth in large doses has provided symptomatic relief to some patients. Azathioprine has also been used in conjunction with prednisone in an attempt to control disease activity on a reduced steroid dose.

The disease can be cured by *surgical resection* of the entire colon. Colectomy may be indicated on an emergency basis because of actual or impending perforation, massive hemorrhage, or the development of a carcinoma in the diseased bowel. Prolonged or debilitating symptoms, particularly growth or maturational delay in the face of an extended trial of medical therapy, are the common indications for operative treatment of a child with ulcerative colitis. A very difficult therapeutic decision arises when the young patient is found to have active colitis 10 yr after onset of the disease. Because of the risk of carcinoma in the diseased colon most authorities advise colectomy for these patients, particularly if the disease is extensive. Semiannual colonoscopy with multiple biopsies is necessary for effective early tumor recognition.

For children the usual primary operative procedure is subtotal colectomy, leaving the rectal stump in situ. This limited resection has the advantages of being less traumatic, of allowing for improvement in general health (growth, etc.), and of preserving the option for a 2nd stage procedure. Although the patient's general condition usually improves after partial colectomy, active disease invariably persists in the retained rectal stump. At a 2nd operation the stump can be removed. Preliminary reports suggest success with a pull-through anastomosis that removes diseased mucosa but preserves bowel continuity and continence. If continuity of the intestine is not restored after colectomy, a permanent conventional ileostomy may be maintained or a continent Koch pouch may be fashioned. Encouraging results have been obtained in limited numbers of patients with this latter procedure, which allows the patient to drain an internal surgically created reservoir and eliminates the need for an ileostomy appliance.

Prognosis. Most cases beginning in childhood are severe in terms of both disease activity and extent of involved colon. Occasionally, fulminant disease progresses to perforation of the colon before a diagnosis is made. The usual course is one of initial improvement on medication followed by recurrent exacerbations. Occasionally, blood loss can be massive and life threatening, but the most serious acute complication is toxic megacolon, a massive dilatation of the colon which signals impending perforation. Ulcerative colitis predisposes the patient to cancer; the risk is only 3% in the 1st decade and rises 20%/decade subsequently.

Ament M: Inflammatory disease of the colon: Ulcerative colitis and Crohn's colitis. J Pediatr 86:322, 1975.

Davidson M, Bloom AA, Kugler MM: Chronic ulcerative colitis of childhood: An evaluative review. J Pediatr 67:471, 1965.

Devroede GJ, Taylor WF, Saver WG, et al: Cancer risk and life expectancy in children with ulcerative colitis. N Engl J. Med 285:17, 1971.

Edwards FC, Truelove SC: The course and prognosis of ulcerative colitis. III. Complications. Gut 5:1, 1964.

Ein SH, Lynch MJ, Stephens CA: Ulcerative colitis in children under one year: A twenty year review. J Pediatr Surg 6:264, 1975.

Gadacz TR, Kelly KA, Phillips SF: The continent ileal pouch: Absorptive and motor features. Gastroenterology 72:1287, 1977.

Hamilton JR, Bruce GA, Abdourhaman M, et al: Inflammatory bowel disease in children and adolescents. Adv Pediatr 26:311, 1980.

Martin LW, LeCoultre C, Schubert WK: Total colectomy and mucosal proctectomy with preservation of continence in ulcerative colitis. Ann Surg 186:477, 1977.

Toovey S, Hudson E, Hendry WF, et al: Sulphasalazine and male infertility: Reversibility and possible mechanism. Gut 22:445, 1981.

11.38 CROHN DISEASE
(Regional Enteritis, Granulomatous Enterocolitis)

Crohn disease is a segmental transmural intestinal disease that may involve 1 or more segments of the gut from the mouth to the anus; the distal ileum and colon are commonly affected. The inflammatory process consists of noncaseating granulomas with regional lymphatic involvement. There is also a tendency to fistula formation between loops of bowel or from bowel to neighboring structures such as the skin or urinary tract. Early in the course biopsied tissue may not reveal granulomas and may be identical to the mucosa of a child with ulcerative colitis. Crohn disease and ulcerative colitis are the major causes of "nonspecific" *inflammatory bowel disease* (IBD), a term often used to refer to either of these entities.

An increase in incidence of Crohn disease has occurred in Western Europe and North America in the past decade. The cause of Crohn disease is unknown, but the disease is relatively common among Jews, 1st degree relatives of patients, and patients with ankylosing spondylitis and the histocompatibility antigen, HLA-B27.

Clinical Manifestations. Eighteen–30% of cases of Crohn disease begin before the age of 20 yr, but most childhood cases appear in preadolescence or adolescence. Onset in infancy is extremely rare. Usually, the onset is subtle; many mo pass between the 1st symptoms and the establishment of a correct diagnosis. Crampy abdominal pain is the most common initial complaint, followed by diarrhea. Rather than suffer intestinal complaints, as in the onset of ulcerative colitis, about half of these patients will initially be troubled by nonintestinal problems such as fever, anorexia, growth failure, general malaise, and joint symptoms. Any teenager with chronic malaise or persisting growth problems, particularly with fever, should be suspected of having this condition. Chronic perianal lesions, even when there are no reasons to suspect primary bowel disease, may be another early sign.

In time, most children with active Crohn disease develop abdominal pain and diarrhea. Pain from small intestinal disease is often periumbilical or in the right lower quadrant rather than confined to the lower abdomen, as in ulcerative colitis. Stools are less explosive than in ulcerative colitis, and there is less tenesmus except when the distal segment is involved. Blood is seen in stools less frequently than in ulcerative colitis, but bleeding can be massive.

Extraintestinal manifestations are similar to those occurring in ulcerative colitis, but they occur more often in Crohn patients. Arthritis, usually affecting large joints, was reported in 18% of 1 pediatric series. Erythema nodosum, iritis, hepatitis, and phlebitis are rare; they tend to exacerbate and remit with the activity of the intestinal lesion. Finger clubbing is much more common than in ulcerative colitis, occurring in about a third of patients with Crohn disease.

Differential Diagnosis. The usual causes of inflammatory bowel lesions are summarized in Table 11–8. Infections that are particularly likely to be confused with Crohn disease are those that involve the distal small bowel, e.g., *Yersinia enterocolitica*, which is common, and tuberculosis, which is quite rare in North America. *Yersinia* and anaphylactoid purpura may cause small intestinal abnormalities in barium studies similar to those found in Crohn disease. The most important feature distinguishing Crohn disease from ulcerative colitis is the segmental distribution of the Crohn lesion while that of ulcerative colitis is diffuse and confined to the colon.

Diagnosis. A careful clinical evaluation will usually suggest a diagnosis of an inflammatory bowel lesion. Laboratory evidence to support an active inflammatory process includes an erythrocyte sedimentation rate which is raised in more than 75% of patients at diagnosis. Hemoglobin levels are mildly depressed and serum albumin reduced in about a third of cases.

If an inflammatory lesion is suspected and microbiologic studies exclude a specific infection, barium contrast roentgenograms of the small and large bowel are needed to define the segments involved. Crohn involvement is often characterized by irregular mucosa or a cobblestone-like pattern, thickened bowel, and enteric fistulas, but it is the lesion's segmental distribution that is diagnostic. Detail may be better seen in the small bowel by injecting barium directly by tube into the duodenum and into the colon by using a double air-contrast technique.

Biopsies of rectal mucosa may show typical granulomas even if there is no gross evidence of distal segment involvement on sigmoidoscopy. Because involvement of the colon is often proximal, a sigmoidoscope may not reach the diseased area. Colonoscopy, which allows visualization of the proximal colon from below, has been useful in further defining the limits of colonic Crohn lesions.

Treatment. Curative medical therapy is not available, and in contrast to treatment of ulcerative colitis, operative resection is less likely to be feasible and is not curative. A 30 yr recurrence rate of over 90% is reported in Crohn disease.

Since medications are palliative at best, supportive measures are very important. The child and family must be helped to attain insight into the nature of this disease and its very troublesome symptoms. Therapy should be directed at enabling the patient to live as full a life as possible and creating an atmosphere in which the child does not consider himself or herself an invalid. For example, undue fatigue should be avoided but exercise encouraged. Usual household discipline should be exercised. In general, a full nutritious diet should be encouraged; appetite stimulants and mood-altering drugs are unlikely to be helpful. Some guidance for the use of anti-inflammatory medications has come recently from a multi-center treatment study. *Prednisone* is indicated to treat acute exacerbations. For active small bowel disease 1–2 mg/kg/24 hr (maximum 60 mg) of prednisone should be given at full dosage for 6 wk, after which gradual tapering of the dose should be attempted over a further 4–8 wk. If the disease reactivates with decreased doses, the drug should be continued at higher levels for a longer period. Alternate-day therapy is rarely effective in maintaining a remission. In some difficult cases the concomitant use of azathioprine, 2 mg/kg/24 hr, permits the reduction of steroid dose, but azathioprine should be used for no more than 1 yr with careful monitoring of the patient's white blood count. Sulfasalazine does not have the same beneficial effect on Crohn disease that is seen in ulcerative colitis. Available data support the use of sulfasalazine (0.5 gm/15 kg/24 hr up to 4 gm/24 hr) for colonic Crohn disease, but the drug does not increase long-term recurrence rates or enhance the effect of corticosteroid.

Because of high recurrence rates and in some cases extensive small bowel involvement, surgical resection has less to offer to the Crohn patient than to the child with ulcerative colitis. Recurrence rates are lowest when resection of diseased bowel is complete and undertaken when disease activity is extremely low. Massive hemorrhage, intestinal perforation, or bowel obstruction that persists will necessitate operative intervention as a lifesaving procedure; these emergencies are rare in children with Crohn disease. The question of operative resection usually arises around the issue of persisting debility, particularly when growth and maturation are delayed. Although recurrence appears to be inevitable, resection frequently allows for an interval of good health, growth, and a return to full activity. The decision to operate will be based on the severity and duration of debility, the patient's age and potential for growth, and the response of the patient and family to the disease. Every effort should be made to do an elective resection at a time when the patient's nutritional status is satisfactory and the inflammatory process is inactive.

Prognosis. In general, the inflammatory activity of Crohn disease tends to remit and exacerbate through life without a consistent pattern. In many cases the region involved remains constant; when extension occurs, it often appears to be a postoperative event. The natural course of this inflammatory process is to develop scar tissue resulting in bowel obstruction. Eventual obstructive problems are almost inevitable for ileal disease, but usually this complication develops a decade or more after onset of the disease. The incidence of intestinal cancer is increased in patients with longstanding Crohn disease but not nearly to the degree seen in ulcerative colitis.

Ament M: Inflammatory disease of the colon. Ulcerative colitis and Crohn's colitis. J Pediatr 86:322, 1975.
Gryboski JD, Spiro HM: Prognosis in children with Crohn's disease. Gastroenterology 74:807, 1978.

Hamilton JR, Bruce GA, Abdourhaman M, et al: Inflammatory bowel disease in children and adolescents. Adv Pediatr 26:311, 1980.

Kelts DG, Grand RJ, Shen G, et al: Nutritional basis of growth failure in children and adolescents with Crohn's disease. Gastroenterology 76:720, 1979.

Kirschner BS. Voinchet O, Rosenberg IH: Growth retardation in inflammatory bowel disease. Gastroenterology 75:504, 1978.

Miller RC, Larson E: Regional enteritis in early infancy. Am J Dis Child 122:301, 1971.

11.39 NEONATAL NECROTIZING ENTEROCOLITIS (NEC)

This serious disease of the newborn is of unknown etiology and characterized by necrosis of the intestine. No particular race or sex is unduly susceptible to the disease (see also Sec. 7.45). Incidence ranges from 1–8% of admissions to neonatal intensive care units. Since the very small ill newborn infant is particularly susceptible to NEC, a rising incidence in recent yr may reflect improved survival of this high-risk group of patients. The disease does occur occasionally in term babies.

Pathology and Pathogenesis. Many factors may contribute to the development of a necrotic segment of intestine, the gas accumulation in the submucosa of the bowel wall, and progression of the necrosis leading to perforation, sepsis, and death. The distal ileum and proximal colon are involved most frequently. Some form of perinatal stress, especially asphyxia or hypothermia, is thought to predispose the infant to ischemia of the intestine. A variety of other factors may contribute to mucosal injury and subsequent infection leading to bowel necrosis. Endothelial injury may lead to thrombosis. Intestinal distention, umbilical catheters, and low flow states have also been suggested as contributing factors. Breast milk probably does not protect the infant from NEC.

Clinical Manifestations. Onset usually occurs in the 1st 2 wk but can be as late as 2 mo of age. Meconium is passed normally, and the 1st signs are abdominal distention with gastric retention. Obvious bloody stools are seen in 25% of patients. The onset is often insidious, and sepsis may occur before an intestinal lesion is suspected. Once affected, the child usually deteriorates rapidly, becoming lethargic and acidotic; shock and disseminated intravascular coagulation may develop.

Diagnosis. A very high index of suspicion in managing infants at risk is essential. Plain roentgenograms may demonstrate pneumatosis intestinalis, a finding that is diagnostic of NEC in the newborn infant; 50–75% of patients have pneumatosis when treatment is started. Portal vein gas is an ominous sign of severe disease, and pneumoperitoneum indicates a perforation.

The differential diagnosis of NEC includes specific infections (systemic or intestinal), obstruction, and Hirschsprung disease. Cultures and roentgenograms may be diagnostic. An antecedent history of distal bowel obstruction is suggestive and a rectal biopsy abnormality diagnostic of Hirschsprung disease. Barium enemas are contraindicated in these patients because of the risk of bowel perforation.

Treatment. Intensive therapy is advisable for suspected as well as for diagnosed cases. Cessation of feeding, nasogastric decompression, and intravenous fluids with careful attention to acid-base and electrolyte balance are very important. Once cultures are taken of blood, urine, and cerebrospinal fluid, systemic antibiotics (Sec 10.1) should be started. When present, umbilical catheters should be removed, and ventilation should be assisted if distention is contributing to hypoxia and hypercapnia.

The patient's course should be monitored by frequent abdominal roentgenograms looking for pneumatosis intestinalis and by hematocrit, platelet, electrolyte, and acid-base determinations. A falling platelet count suggests intestinal gangrene.

A surgeon should be consulted early in the course of treatment. Evidence of perforation or a soft intra-abdominal mass suggesting a walled-off perforation is usually an indication for resection of necrotic bowel. Peritoneal drainage may be helpful for the patient in extremis with peritonitis who is unable to withstand bowel resection.

Prognosis. Medical management fails in about 50% of patients in whom there is pneumatosis intestinalis at diagnosis; of these, at least half die. Strictures develop at the site of the necrotizing lesion in fewer than 10% of patients. No long term problems with intestinal function have been noted as a sequel of NEC unless a massive resection is necessary.

Jarik JS. Ein SH: Peritoneal drainage under local anaesthesia for necrotizing enterocolitis (NEC) perforation: A second look. J Pediatr Surg 15:565, 1980.

Scintulli TV, Schillinger MD, Heird WC, et al: Acute necrotizing enterocolitis in infants. A review of 64 cases. Pediatrics 55:376, 1975.

Stevenson DK, Graham CB, Stevenson JK: Neonatal necrotizing enterocolitis: 100 new cases. Adv Pediatr 27:319, 1981.

11.40 ANTIBIOTIC-ASSOCIATED (PSEUDOMEMBRANOUS) ENTEROCOLITIS

This rare but serious small and large bowel disorder may present a spectrum of illness ranging from diarrhea associated with antibiotic administration to pseudomembranous enterocolitis. The common etiologic factor is an enterotoxin-producing strain of *Clostridium perfringens* in the lumen of the distal bowel.

Within 1 wk of starting antibiotic therapy the patient develops diarrhea. The drug has usually been given orally. Many different agents cause the problem, but clindamycin and ampicillin have been incriminated most often. The disease may run a fulminant course with increasing severity of diarrhea, bloody stools, and abdominal distention. Often, in the severe form of the disease, sigmoidoscopy reveals a typical pseudomembranous lesion, a patchy cream-white exudate, resembling a membrane, adherent to normal mucosa. Preceding abdominal surgery and underlying vascular disease, such as periarteritis nodosa, increase the likelihood of a fulminant course. Enterotoxin-producing clostridia are found in the stools in these severe cases. However, in less severely ill children with diarrhea but no visible pseudomembrane formation after antibiotic therapy, the same organisms are found.

Florid pseudomembranous enterocolitis requires emergency treatment. The possible offending antibiotics and all oral intake should be stopped, nasogastric suction begun, intravenous fluid and nutrients provided, and vancomycin given by mouth. Use of an appropriate antibiotic shortens the course in most cases and allows for the return to oral intake within 1 wk. For mildly affected children with some diarrhea, stopping the causative antibiotic is usually sufficient. In the moderately severe case it is best to err on the aggressive side in therapy for this potentially fatal disease.

Bartlett JG, Moon N, Chang TW, et al: Role of *Clostridium difficile* in antibiotic-associated pseudomembranous colitis. Gastroenterology 75:778, 1978.
Buts JP, Weber AM, Roy CC, et al: Pseudomembranous enterocolitis in childhood. Gastroenterology 73:823, 1977.
Keating JP, Frank AL, Barton LL, et al: Pseudomembranous colitis associated with ampicillin therapy. Am J Dis Child 128:369, 1974.
Tedesco FJ, Stanley RJ, Alpers DH: Diagnostic features of clindamycin-associated pseudomembranous colitis. N Engl J Med 290:84, 1974.

11.41   GASTROINTESTINAL SYMPTOMS IN ANAPHYLACTOID PURPURA

Two thirds of patients with anaphylactoid (Henoch-Schönlein) purpura have abdominal symptoms (Sec 9.65). Crampy abdominal pain may be very severe and precede any other manifestations of the disorder. The pain results from submucosal and subserosal hemorrhages and may precede small or large amounts of blood in the stools and intussusception. In the acute disease barium contrast roentgenograms may show large filling defects in the bowel wall, suggestive of Crohn disease or a neoplasm. Diagnosis is made when the characteristic purpuric rash and urinary tract manifestations develop.

Silver DL: Henoch-Schönlein syndrome. Pediatr Clin North Am 19:1061, 1972.

11.42   GASTROINTESTINAL PROBLEMS IN HEMOLYTIC-UREMIC SYNDROME

See Sec 16.22.

This potentially fatal disorder may present as an intestinal inflammatory disorder. Bloody diarrhea is frequently the 1st symptom. Barium contrast roentgenograms show transient early filling defects, but the lesions may progress to stenosis. Diagnosis depends on the recognition of acute renal failure, hemolytic anemia, and thrombocytopenia, none of which may be apparent in the early stages.

Kaplan BS: The hemolytic-uremic syndrome. Pediatr Clin North Am 23:761, 1976.
Sawaf H, Sharp MJ, Youn KJ, et al: Ischemic colitis and stricture after hemolytic-uremic syndrome. Pediatrics 61:315, 1978.
Tachen ML, Campbell JR: Colitis in children with hemolytic-uremic syndrome. J Pediatr Surg 12:213, 1977.

11.43   DIETARY PROTEIN INTOLERANCE

Adverse reactions in the child's intestine can be a direct result of exposure to specific dietary proteins. Although in many cases these reactions appear allergic, proof for a true allergic response is often lacking; therefore, the term *intolerance* seems appropriate. Because specific laboratory diagnostic criteria are not available, diagnosis is based on clinical responses to withdrawal and challenge with the potential dietary agent. Most cases are recognized in infants, and cow milk is the most commonly incriminated food.

COW MILK PROTEIN INTOLERANCE

Because of uncertain diagnostic criteria, accurate incidence statistics are difficult to determine; in Sweden estimates range from 0.5–1.5%. In North America estimates are much lower than 0.5%.

Clinical Manifestations.   Several clinical syndromes are attributed to cow milk, and the incidence of allergic diseases (e.g., eczema, asthma) is increased in these patients and their family members.

Acute Vomiting and Diarrhea.   In young infants the usual onset is acute and characterized by vomiting and watery diarrhea which is often bloody, suggesting colitis. In its most fulminant form there is glottic swelling and anaphylactic shock, which, if untreated, can be fatal. The cellular exudate in stools often contains many eosinophils in addition to erythrocytes.

Chronic Diarrhea and Malabsorption.   The clinical response of some children consists of chronic diarrhea and general ill health, leading to slow gain and eventually to growth retardation. This chronic syndrome tends to occur in older infants and is associated with small bowel dysfunction (mild steatorrhea and malabsorption of d-xylose). Small intestine biopsies have shown patchy mucosal lesions of varying severity. In general, the lesion is characterized by shortening of villi, elongation of crypts, and an increase in intraepithelial lymphocytes and lamina propria cellularity. Single suction biopsy specimens may be normal. Most patients with this chronic syndrome have been reported from European centers.

Excessive Enteric Protein and Blood Loss.   This syndrome has been reported mainly in older infants presenting with generalized edema, hypoproteinemia, and iron deficiency anemia. There may be diarrhea or no intestinal symptoms. These children show excessive enteric loss of protein and blood that terminates after withdrawal of milk. Often, the syndrome is associated with the change in feeding from milk formula to ordinary fresh dairy milk.

Diagnosis. Milk protein intolerance is diagnosed by clinical characteristics. Acute symptoms should subside within 48 hr and chronic within 1 wk of complete withdrawal of milk. Caution and judgment must be exercised in rechallenging these patients with milk. In a young infant, particularly if an acute response is anticipated, the challenge should be carried out under observation, beginning with 1–5 ml of milk and increasing the dose progressively over a few days provided a response does not occur. Skin tests, circulating antibody titers, complement assays, and coproantibody titers are not of diagnostic value. In children with chronic symptoms some centers use mucosal biopsy to evaluate the response to challenge. It is important to rule out other conditions that may cause similar symptoms such as enteric infections, lactose intolerance, and other forms of nonspecific inflammatory bowel disease.

The syndromes described for cow milk intolerance may occur also in response to **soy protein.** Some series estimated that up to 50% of children intolerant to cow milk are intolerant to soy. Since soy is not a commonly used food, most will not be exposed to soy unless they are first found intolerant to cow milk. The approach to diagnosis is the same as that described for cow milk.

Treatment. Prolonged breast feeding reduces the likelihood of later cow milk intolerance. Treatment consists of removing the offending food from the diet. For the young infant the non-milk-containing dietary formulas consist of various soy feedings and meat base formulas. Some infants who cannot tolerate milk formulas can be successfully fed hydrolyzed milk protein feedings. Many children with the enteric protein loss syndrome will benefit by changing from fresh milk to processed (i.e., evaporated, powdered) milk. For rare causes of intolerance to many foods, oral sodium cromoglycate has been reported to suppress intestinal symptoms and permit continued ingestion of the food.

Prognosis. In most cases, food protein intolerances are transitory. About 50% of patients have recovered within 1 yr and most of the remainder within 2 yr.

Ament ME, Rubin CE: Soy protein—another cause of the flat intestinal lesion. Gastroenterology 62:227, 1972.
Fontaine SL, Navarro J: Small intestinal biopsy in cow's milk protein allergy in infancy. Arch Dis Child 50:357, 1975.
Goldman AS, Anderson DW, Sellers WA, et al: Milk allergy. Oral challenge with milk and isolated milk protein in allergic children. Pediatrics 32:425, 1963.
Powell GK: Milk and soy-induced entercolitis of infancy. J Pediatr 93:558, 1978.
Savilahti E, Kuitunen P, Visakorpi JK: Cow's milk allergy. In Lebenthal E (ed): Textbook of Gastroenterology and Nutrition. New York, Raven Press, 1981.
Waldman TA, Wochner RD, Laster L, et al: Allergic gastroenteropathy: A cause of excessive gastrointestinal protein loss. N Engl J Med 276:761, 1967.

11.44 EOSINOPHILIC GASTROENTERITIS

A rare form of inflammatory involvement of the intestine is characterized by infiltrates of eosinophils.

Usually, the stomach and the upper small bowel are involved, but esophageal and distal intestinal lesions also occur.

The lesions normally cause abdominal pain, vomiting, diarrhea, and delayed growth and weight gain. Often, there are other atopic symptoms, such as rhinitis and asthma, suggesting an allergic basis for the disorder. A peripheral eosinophilia and excessive enteric protein loss may cause reduced serum albumin and immune globulin levels. Endoscopy may reveal an inflammatory lesion in the stomach and duodenum; eosinophilic congestion of the lamina propria and patchy villus shortening are found in biopsies.

Rarely, eosinophils infiltrate more deeply to cause bowel wall thickening and granuloma formation. The disease usually runs a chronic debilitating course with sporadic severe exacerbations. A few patients are helped by elimination diets, but most require systemic corticosteroids to suppress disease activity.

Katz AJ, Golman H, Grand RJ: Gastric mucosal biopsy in eosinophilic (allergic) gastroenteritis. Gastroenterology 73:705, 1977.
Klein NC, Hargrove RL, Sleisenger MN, et al: Eosinophilic gastroenteritis. Medicine 49:299, 1970.

11.45 MALABSORPTIVE DISORDERS

Because they result in defective assimilation of ingested nutrients, a number of gastrointestinal diseases with a wide range of clinical features are termed malabsorptive disorders. Those that cause maldigestion or malabsorption of many nutrients tend to share certain clinical manifestations: abdominal distention; pale, foul, bulky stools; wasting of muscles, particularly the proximal muscle groups; and retarded growth and weight gain (Fig 11–19). *Celiac syndrome* or *malabsorption syndrome* is used to describe these diseases. There are also many chronic nongastroenterologic diseases capable of causing significant malnutrition and growth problems. For example, children with chronic renal disease or intracranial lesions may develop clinical manifestations very similar to those of a child with a malabsorptive state. Over the years specific digestive tract disorders have been identified as causes of this *celiac syndrome*. One of these, a specific *gluten-induced enteropathy*, is called *celiac disease* or *celiac sprue*. Major causes of generalized defects in absorption or digestion are summarized in Table 11–9, where those diseases that tend to occur relatively frequently in North America and Europe are separated from the less common disorders.

Congenital disorders have also been identified that affect only a single specific intestinal transport process. The clinical manifestations of these diseases are often very different from those of a generalized malabsorptive state. Some cause intestinal symptoms, particularly diarrhea, but others may be associated with only a nutritional deficiency and no gastrointestinal symptoms. In Table 11–10 the known specific absorptive pathway defects are listed; only some of this latter

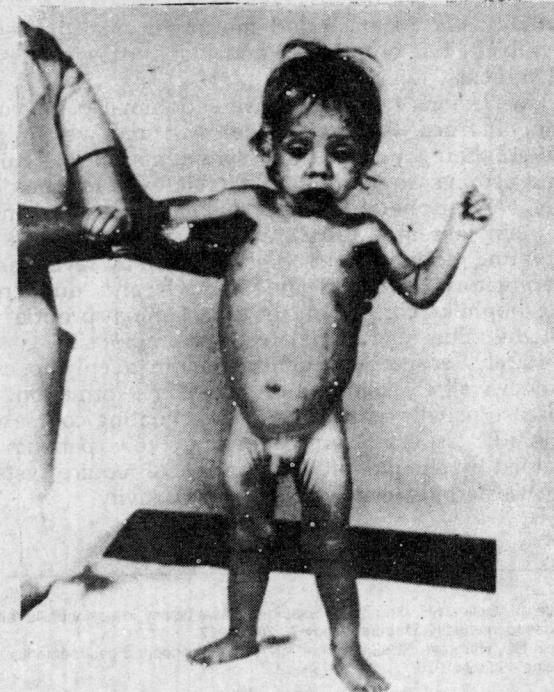

Figure 11–19 An 18 mo old boy with active celiac disease. Note the loose skin folds, marked proximal muscle wasting, and full abdomen. The child looks ill.

group cause gastrointestinal symptoms, and all except the acquired disaccharidase deficiencies are rare.

EVALUATION OF PATIENTS SUSPECTED OF HAVING INTESTINAL MALABSORPTION

Success in distinguishing those children with true malabsorptive diseases from patients with chronic non-specific diarrhea or nongastrointestinal diseases causing small stature depends primarily upon clinical findings. Descriptions of the known malabsorptive diseases are presented in subsequent sections with their specific diagnostic features; elements in the history and physical examination of many of these entities are presented in this section for special emphasis.

Clinical Manifestations. Because diseases of many systems may produce clinical manifestations such as failure to thrive and abdominal distention suggestive of a malabsorptive state, a complete history is essential.

Disorders of the central nervous system and urinary tract deserve particular attention. Since many of the gastrointestinal diseases are genetically determined, the family history often suggests the diagnosis. Because most congenital lesions cause symptoms early in infancy, attention should be focused on the timing of the onset of symptoms. Specific intestinal transport defects affect specific nutrients, and celiac disease is caused by a general response of the mucosa to dietary glutens; therefore the relationship between symptom onset and diet consumption should be determined.

Some aspects of the history that tend to be offered in great detail are of limited value. Description of stools tends to be a highly subjective matter, and although quantity is of obvious interest, color, odor, and consistency are often of relatively little diagnostic significance. Similarly, the relationship between diet and diarrhea must be logical to be meaningful. For example, if lactose is responsible for diarrhea, then 1 lactose-containing food should be as great a provoking factor as the next when the quantities ingested are equivalent.

The impact of symptoms on the child's general health is best assessed in terms of body weight and growth. If possible, measurements should be related to earlier measurements and family patterns. Signs of malnutrition such as muscle wasting, edema, mouth sores, smooth tongue, and excessive bruising should be interpreted in the light of estimated nutrient intake. In cases of diarrhea parents and physicians may limit the child's nutrient intake for prolonged periods, thereby inducing malnutrition which may be erroneously assumed to result from malabsorption.

A rectal examination is the most important step in the initial examination of children suspected of having intestinal malabsorption. In addition to assessing the anus and rectum, this procedure provides immediate access to stool for gross, microscopic, and, in some cases, chemical analysis. If they are receiving a complete diet, children with pancreatic insufficiency will have excessive triglyceride and undigested meat fibers in their stools; those with intestinal malabsorption will have crystalline aggregates of monoglyceride and fatty acid.

Laboratory Manifestations. *Absorptive Function.*

Table 11–9 GENERALIZED MALABSORPTIVE STATES IN CHILDHOOD

	MORE COMMON	LESS COMMON
Exocrine pancreas	Cystic fibrosis Chronic protein-calorie malnutrition	Schwachman-Diamond syndrome Chronic pancreatitis
Liver, biliary tree	Biliary atresia	Other cholestatic states
Intestine		
Anatomic defects	Massive resection Stagnant loop syndrome	Congenitally short gut
Chronic infection (± immune deficiency)	Giardiasis Coccidiosis	
Miscellaneous	Celiac disease Postenteritis malabsorption	Dietary protein intolerance (milk, soy) Tropical sprue Intestinal Whipple disease Idiopathic diffuse mucosal lesions

Table 11–10 SPECIFIC DEFECTS OF DIGESTIVE-ABSORPTIVE FUNCTION OCCURRING IN CHILDREN

	DISEASE
Intestinal	
Fat	Abetalipoproteinemia
Protein	Enterokinase deficiency
	Amino acid transport defects (cystinuria, Hartnup disease, methionine malabsorption, blue diaper syndrome)
Carbohydrate	Disaccharidase deficiencies (congenital: sucrase-isomaltase, lactase; developmental: lactase; acquired: generalized glucose-galactose malabsorption)
Vitamin	Vitamin B_{12} malabsorption (juvenile pernicious anemia, transcobalamin II deficiency, Immerslund syndrome)
	Folic acid malabsorption
Ions, trace elements	Chloride-losing diarrhea
	Acrodermatitis enteropathica
	Menkes syndrome
	Vitamin D–dependent rickets
	Primary hypomagnesemia
Drug-induced	Salazosulfapyridine (folic acid malabsorption)
	Cholestyramine (Ca, fat malabsorption)
	Dilantin (Ca)
Pancreatic	Specific enzyme deficiencies
	Lipase
	Trypsinogen

Net *fat* absorption can be quantitated by a *fecal fat balance* in which total losses are related to estimated dietary fat intake. If the patient is consuming appreciable quantities of fat (>20 gm/day) and total collections are carried out for at least 4 days, excretion should not exceed 15% of intake in an infant and 10% in an older child. To avoid the unpleasant and time-consuming task of stool analysis, many screening tests have been developed to assess absorption and to detect steatorrhea. The simplest of these is to measure *serum carotene* concentration in the fasting state. In the presence of adequate dietary intake a result of <50 mg/dl suggests fat malabsorption and >100 mg/dl normal absorption. However, a significant number of false-positive and negative results occur with this screening test. In skilled hands, stool microscopy to assess directly the fat content of random stools compares favorably with other screening procedures for steatorrhea.

Carbohydrate absorption cannot be quantitated by simple balance procedures because sugars are broken down in the intestinal lumen by enteric bacteria. No more than a trace of sugar is found in normal stools except for those passed by breast-fed infants. Finding of excess sugar in fresh stool suggests sugar intolerance, but a lack of excess sugar does not exclude the diagnosis. Random stool samples can be tested for reducing substance quickly and easily using commercially available tablets.* A result of >0.5% indicates abnormal absorption if the diet contains significant amounts of a reducing sugar. Most dietary sugars, except for sucrose, are reducing sugars; if sucrose is to be tested, it must first be hydrolyzed by heating the stool sample with HCl. Usually fresh stool of a patient with sugar intolerance will also have a pH of less than 6.0 because of

*Clinitest, Ames Co.

the organic acids produced in the lumen by bacterial action on the unabsorbed sugar. The indirect method for measuring carbohydrate absorption is the *oral tolerance test.* An oral dose (0.5 mg/kg body weight) of the sugar to be tested is given to the fasting patient and plasma concentration of glucose is measured at 15, 30, 60, and 120 min. A rise of at least 20 mg/dl glucose should occur normally after lactose and sucrose are given and at least 50 gm/dl when glucose is given. However, many variables apart from digestion and absorption can affect the results, e.g., rates of gastric emptying and glucose utilization. *Hydrogen concentrations in expired air* may also be measured after an oral dose of sugar (2 gm/kg body weight to 50 gm maximum). If the sugar being tested is not absorbed in the upper small bowel, it reaches the distal small bowel and colonic lumen, where enteric bacteria act on it to produce hydrogen gas, which is quickly absorbed and expired quantitatively. A rise in breath hydrogen greater than 10 ppm during the 1st 2 hr is abnormal. Patients taking antibiotics and about 2% of the normal population do not have hydrogen-producing enteric flora.

Protein absorption cannot be accurately quantitated in routine clinical practice. Balance studies do not necessarily reflect assimilation because of endogenous sources of fecal protein, but *fecal nitrogen* can be measured as a rough guide. *Enteric protein loss* can be quantitated using an intravenous injection of $^{51}CrCl$ followed by measurement of the fecal excretion of the label in a 4 day collection of stool. A result exceeding 0.8% of the injected dose indicates excessive loss. *Fecal clearance of* α_1-*antitrypsin* also reflects enteric protein loss; experience with this latter technique is limited, but a result measured on a 48 hr stool collection exceeding 15 ml/day is excessive.

Other nutrients may be measured in the blood in the presence of apparent adequate intake and a depressed circulating concentration of them taken as a reflection of inadequate absorption. These nutrients include iron, the level of which will depend on the transferrin concentration as well as absorption; folic acid, the red cell concentration being a more accurate reflection of nutritional status than is serum concentration; serum calcium and magnesium; vitamin D and its metabolites; vitamin A; and vitamin B_{12}. It may take years to deplete stores of vitamin B_{12} after absorption is impaired.

Certain absorptive studies are helpful in localizing the site of an intestinal lesion. Iron and *d-xylose*, a pentose minimally metabolized in man, are absorbed by the upper small bowel. A blood concentration of less than 25 mg/dl xylose 1 hr after a 14.5 gm/M^2 body surface (up to 25 gm) oral dose of the sugar usually indicates a proximal intestinal mucosal lesion, although some false-negative and false-positive results are obtained using this technique. In the distal bowel, vitamin B_{12} is absorbed and bile salts are reabsorbed. *Vitamin B_{12} absorption* can be measured directly using the *Schilling test*, in which, after body stores of the vitamin are saturated, a tracer dose of radioactive B_{12} is given by mouth, with or without intrinsic factor, and urinary excretion measured over the next 24 hr. Defective absorption is shown by urinary excretion of less than 5% of the dose; this occurs when an extensive length of distal ileum is resected or diseased.

Diagnostic Procedures. MICROBIOLOGIC. The only common primary infection causing chronic malabsorption is giardiasis (Sec 10.109). The trophozoite or its cysts may be identified in duodenal contents or the duodenal mucosa. When enteric clearing of bacteria is impaired, either from stasis of luminal contents or impaired immune function, colony counts from bacterial cultures of proximal intestinal juice may be very high.

HEMATOLOGIC. Routine blood smears may demonstrate an iron deficiency pattern. A megaloblastic smear suggests deficiency and therefore malabsorption of folic acid or vitamin B_{12}. Acanthocyte transformation of erythrocytes occurs in abetalipoproteinemia. A blood smear may also suggest a lymphocyte defect or a neutropenia associated with Shwachman syndrome.

IMAGING PROCEDURES. These procedures are used primarily to identify localized lesions in the abdomen. In children with malabsorptive disorders **plain roentgenograms** and **barium contrast** studies may suggest a site and cause of intestinal stasis. For example, the most common anomaly causing incomplete bowel obstruction is intestinal malrotation, a condition difficult to exclude without a barium enema to localize the cecum. In general, large quantities of nonflocculating barium should be used to examine the small intestine. Although flocculation of normal barium and dilated bowel with thickened mucosal folds have been attributed to diffuse malabsorptive lesions such as celiac disease, these abnormalities are nonspecific and of little diagnostic value. **Technetium (^{99}Tc) scan** is an accurate technique with which to detect aberrant gastric mucosa such as might be present in a duplication or Meckel diverticulum, but these lesions rarely cause malabsorption. **Ultrasound scans** are capable of detecting alterations in pancreatic mass, biliary tree abnormalities, and stones, even in infants with malabsorption. **Retrograde studies of the pancreatic and biliary tree** using contrast injection via endoscopy are reserved for rare and difficult cases requiring careful delineation of the biliary tree and pancreatic ducts.

SMALL BOWEL BIOPSY. Perioral suction biopsy of the small intestinal mucosa has become an important diagnostic tool in studying children with malabsorptive states. The demonstration of a typical diffuse mucosal lesion is a prerequisite for diagnosing celiac disease, and a specific abnormality is seen in children with abetalipoproteinemia. Microscopic abnormalities may also be seen in the mucosa of patients with giardiasis, lymphangiectasia, gamma globulin deficiencies, viral enteritis, tropical sprue, and cow milk or soy milk intolerance and in some infants with idiopathic diffuse mucosal lesions.

Disaccharidase assays may be carried out on mucosa. If there is diffuse mucosal disease, these assays will be depressed, but specific congenital abnormalities may also be detected. Biopsy specimens maintained in organ culture may also be challenged with gluten in vitro to assist in the diagnosis of celiac disease.

DISEASES CAUSING GENERALIZED MALDIGESTION OR MALABSORPTION

Cystic Fibrosis
(Fibrocystic Disease of the Pancreas, Mucoviscidosis)

See Sec 11.78 and 12.110.

Shwachman-Diamond Syndrome
(Pancreatic Hypoplasia with Neutropenia)

See Sec 11.78.

11.46   THE DIGESTIVE TRACT IN CHRONIC MALNUTRITION

Exocrine pancreatic function is much more susceptible to protein-calorie malnutrition than the intestine, and suppression of digestive enzyme secretion may occur relatively early in patients with primary malnutrition (Sec 11.78). In developed countries where primary malnutrition is rare, chronic gastrointestinal disorders and their treatment are significant causes of malnutrition; undoubtedly, some degree of compromised pancreatic function develops. This phenomenon might be a particular hazard to children since their nutritional reserves are relatively meager. Because 90% of functioning exocrine tissue must be lost before significant digestive problems develop in patients who are otherwise well, malnutrition is usually prolonged before pancreatic insufficiency causes clinically apparent digestive defects. Nevertheless, where severe chronic malnutrition is prevalent, exocrine pancreatic insufficiency is most often attributable to the malnutrition, not to a primary pancreatic disease.

The intestine is remarkably resistant to the effects of protein-calorie malnutrition. Patients with *kwashiorkor* may have a severely flattened small intestinal villus structure, but these abnormalities probably are attributable to coexisting infections and infestations. In *marasmus* the villus structure is preserved, but some microvillus changes and intracellular electron microscopic abnormalities have been observed. Chronic malnutrition can lead to impaired immune function (Sec 11.78), and the enteric microflora differs from normal in malnourished children.

Recent findings in experimental animals may be clinically relevant. When oral intake is completely withheld, intestinal mucosal mass and absorptive function diminish even when nutrient balance is maintained by the intravenous route. These intestinal changes can be reversed by small amounts of oral nutrient. Therefore, there is a theoretical advantage in delivering nutrients via the gut rather than by vein. Also, because mucosal epithelial repair may be delayed in chronic malnutrition, convalescence from acute self-limited mucosal diseases such as viral enteritis may be prolonged in the malnourished state and shortened when adequate nutrients are provided.

Little is known about the effect of *specific nutritional deficiencies* on the pancreas or intestine; apart from potassium depletion causing ileus and severe dehydration causing constipation, available data suggest a relatively minor clinical effect of a wide range of specific deficiencies. Iron deficiency is associated with enhanced iron uptake at the mucosa and, in a few severe cases, occurrence of mucosal flattening. Deficiencies of vitamin B_{12} and folic acid may cause distortion of enterocyte morphology but no known serious functional abnormalities. Some hypocalcemic states may be accompanied by steatorrhea and even iron and water secretion, but this poorly understood relationship is not constant.

11.47 LIVER AND BILIARY DISORDERS

Steatorrhea occurs secondary to hepatobiliary disorders if bile flow to the duodenum is interrupted. When intraluminal bile salt concentrations fall below the critical micellar concentration, dietary fat cannot be efficiently assimilated. Because sterol absorption is especially dependent on bile formation, bone lesions secondary to vitamin D malabsorption are particularly likely to occur in these patients unless large supplements of the vitamin are given. In general, steatorrhea is associated with severe obstructive jaundice such as occurs in biliary atresia, but, on occasion, other types of severe cholestasis cause steatorrhea.

11.48 INTESTINAL INFECTIONS CAUSING MALABSORPTION

Malabsorption is a rare consequence of primary intestinal infection. Only parasites with a propensity to chronic infestation cause malabsorption in the host who is not immunologically compromised. *Giardia lamblia* infestation is common in children, particularly toddlers, but a very small proportion of the infected patients develop malabsorption (Sec 10.109). Children with immune deficiencies are particularly susceptible to *Giardia*, but even in these patients malabsorption affecting fat and sometimes disaccharides is mild. *Coccidiosis* caused either by *Isospora belli* or *I. hominis* is uncommon but distributed widely in warm climates of the Southern Hemisphere. It can invade human small intestine causing malabsorption and diarrhea (Sec 10.107). *Intestinal hookworm*, although associated, is not thought to cause malabsorption.

11.49 IMMUNE DEFICIENCY STATES AND THE INTESTINE

See also Sec 9.14.

Gastrointestinal symptoms are common in children with certain immune deficiency states, but the mechanisms for disturbed intestinal function in these children are not clear. Some patients are predisposed to infection with *Giardia lamblia*; others with measurable abnormalities of intestinal function or structure do not have clearcut evidence of a specific enteric infection; yet it seems likely that defective resistance to enteric microflora lies behind their intestinal disorder. Diagnostic evaluation of these patients is complicated since some intestinal diseases may cause secondary immune deficiency due to excessive enteric losses of immunoglobulins and lymphocytes.

Congenital Sex-Linked Panhypogammaglobulinemia (Bruton). Mild intermittent diarrhea usually begins early and improves after 2 yr of age. Giardiasis is relatively common. Crypt abscesses may be seen in rectal biopsies of these patients; yet they rarely experience colitic symptoms.

Hypogammaglobulinemia. Diarrhea is more common and more severe in children with these acquired disorders than in those with the congenital sex-linked deficiency. By late childhood about 50% have diarrhea and many have steatorrhea. In some patients a patchy shortening of jejunal villi is seen, but generalized disaccharidase deficiency may occur without a marked structural abnormality. Nodular lymphoid hyperplasia, detected on barium roentgenograms or by mucosal biopsy, is common but asymptomatic.

Isolated IgA Deficiency. Although it is the most common primary immune deficiency, this specific defect rarely causes intestinal symptoms. Giardiasis, ulcerative colitis, Crohn disease, and celiac disease all occur more frequently in patients with selective IgA deficiency than in the general population. The basis for these associations is unclear.

Severe Combined Immunodeficiency (Swiss Type). Severe diarrhea and generalized malabsorption beginning early in life contribute substantially to the early death of many of these patients. Disaccharidase deficiencies are common, and on microscopic examination of the small bowel partial villous atrophy and PAS-positive macrophages are seen in the lamina propria. These children may harbor organisms like the human rotavirus in their intestines for months.

Chronic Granulomatous Disease. Granulomas, characterized by multinucleated giant cells and lipid histiocytes, may occur throughout the intestine of patients with this sex-linked defect and cause diarrhea, malabsorption, and obstructive phenomena.

11.50 STAGNANT LOOP SYNDROME
(Blind Loop Syndrome)

These terms describe conditions in which there is stasis of small intestinal contents, particularly in the upper regions. The cause of such stasis is usually incomplete bowel obstruction, either congenital (malrotation with duodenal bands, intestine stenosis, a diverticulum) or acquired (postoperative intestinal adhesions, longstanding Crohn disease). Significant stasis can also result from neuromuscular dysfunction causing disordered intestinal motility (intestinal pseudo-obstruction, hollow viscus myopathy). Whatever the cause, the sequence of pathophysiologic events is similar. Enteric bacteria, incompletely cleared by peristalsis, colonize the upper small bowel. These bacteria deconjugate intraluminal bile salts and thus contribute to inefficient intraluminal processing of dietary fat and steatorrhea; they bind vitamin B_{12}, interfering with absorption of the vitamin; and they may damage the surface of the microvillus brush border membrane, diminishing disaccharidase activities.

In addition to symptoms of chronic incomplete bowel obstruction such as distention, pain, and vomiting, the patient may have pale, foul, bulky stools suggesting steatorrhea, a megaloblastic anemia from vitamin B_{12} deficiency, and even diarrhea from disaccharidase deficiency. Often, the clinical manifestations do not suggest chronic intestinal obstruction, but laboratory investigations show the functional abnormalities described above in addition to bacterial colonization of the upper intestine and deconjugated bile salts in the upper intestinal juice after a fatty meal. Barium contrast roentgenograms may not reveal the existence or cause of obstruction.

Definitive therapy is operative correction of incomplete bowel obstruction. However, the administration of a small oral dose of an antimicrobial such as trimethoprim-sulfamethoxazole may be sufficient to control the problem temporarily.

11.51 SHORT SMALL INTESTINE (Short Gut Syndrome)

Congenital. The small bowel is congenitally short, probably because it fails to elongate in utero. The defect has been associated with intestinal malrotation and, in some cases, atresia. When the anomaly is severe, diarrhea and malabsorption begin at birth. Barium studies show a malrotated colon and a markedly shortened small bowel, but the villus structure is relatively mature. If the infant survives the early mo, intestinal function improves in later yr.

Massive Intestinal Resection. Throughout life, acute illnesses can occur that necessitate removal of large portions of the small intestine, but the newborn period is a particularly hazardous time in this regard. Even in young infants intestinal reserves are sufficient to tolerate the loss of the colon or short segments of small intestine, but problems in maintaining fluid and nutrient balance should be anticipated if more than 25% of the 200–300 cm of the newborn infant's small bowel is removed. Now that total parenteral nutrition is widely available to provide nutritional support for extended periods, survival is feasible even when all but 20 cm is resected. Spontaneous improvement in absorptive and digestive function in the young infant can be expected over a 2 yr period after intestinal resection.

In general, loss of distal small bowel is more serious than loss of the proximal segment. The jejunum is relatively incapable of compensating for ileal loss since the ileum is the sole site for absorption of bile salts and vitamin B_{12}. Preservation of the ileocecal sphincter is advantageous to infants who have had extensive bowel resections; the sphincter impedes retrograde flow of colonic flora and lengthens the time of contact with the mucosa of the remaining small bowel.

A variety of complications occur after massive resection. Gastric acidity and bacterial contamination of the intestinal lumen are both common after large proximal resections and may compromise absorptive function. Hyperacidity is usually transient under these circumstances. If the terminal ileum is resected, excessive bile salt losses lead to malabsorption of dietary fats and fat-soluble vitamins. Unabsorbed bile salts reaching the colon may also provoke increased water and electrolyte secretion. If the resection includes the mid and distal jejunum as well as the ileum, the patient may be unable to maintain positive fluid balance. Hyperoxaluria may occur after distal small bowel resections in which the colon is preserved, but resultant nephrolithiasis is rare during early childhood. Cell-mediated immunity is normal although circulating immunoglobulin concentrations may be reduced after massive resection.

Often an oral diet cannot be tolerated until weeks after resection. In the interval the patient can be supported by intravenous nutrition. The particular diet offered should depend on the patient's age and functional deficit. Initially, liquids or liquid formulas should be isotonic and given in frequent small amounts. Excessive water intake should be avoided, particularly at times when solids are being taken. When there is severe steatorrhea, long chain fats should be restricted and medium chain triglycerides substituted for them. Initially, dietary glucose may be better tolerated than disaccharides, but the concentration should not exceed 5 gm/dl in order to maintain relative isotonicity of the feeding. Vitamin supplements are usually needed, and serum concentrations of calcium, magnesium, potassium, and phosphorus should be monitored and supplements given as required. If a large portion of the ileum is resected, monthly injections of 100 μg of vitamin B_{12} must be given for life, but it usually takes 2 yr or more for a deficiency to develop in the face of even a severe absorptive defect. Large doses of vitamin D may be necessary to prevent rickets. Prothrombin time should also be monitored as a basis for vitamin K supplementation. Antidiarrheal agents are rarely helpful in the management of massive bowel resection. Cholestyramine may reduce fecal water and sodium losses in infants with relatively short ileal resections by binding bile acids before they reach the colon, but if ileal resection is massive and steatorrhea severe, cholestyramine is likely to aggravate the problem. Theoretically, antacids should benefit infants with hyperacidity, but their value in this situation is unproved. Patients with bacterial contamination and blind loop syndrome will derive temporary benefits from oral antibiotics, but they may require additional surgery.

Successful management of young infants after massive resection requires a coordinated team approach. Along with the essential measures to maintain nutrient intake a concerted effort should be made to encourage mother-child bonding and to stimulate development. Studies suggest impressive preservation of intellectual function even in the most severely affected patients with early profound, prolonged malnutrition.

11.52 CELIAC DISEASE
(Celiac Sprue, Gluten-Induced Enteropathy, Nontropical Sprue)

The inability to tolerate wheat and rye gluten, celiac disease, was first recognized by Dicke in 1950 as an important cause of the celiac syndrome in children. The incidence ranges from 1:300 (in the west of Ireland) to 1:2000; accurate statistics are not available in North America, where the disease occurs as frequently as 1:2000 in some regions but much less frequently in other areas.

The intestinal damage is caused by a *permanent* intolerance to the gliadin fraction of gluten, a protein found in wheat and rye grains. There is controversy as to whether oats and barley are also injurious, but in most patients moderate intakes of these latter grains are well tolerated. One theory of pathogenesis argues that the mucosal lesion of celiac disease is due to an inborn mucosal enzyme defect which permits undigested toxic components of the gluten molecule to accumulate in the mucosa. A 2nd theory attributes the intestinal damage to immune-based reactions.

A predisposition to the disease is inherited; the most likely pattern is mendelian dominant with incomplete penetrance. About 80% of celiac patients carry the HL-B8 antigen compared with 22% of the normal population. Celiac disease and diabetes mellitus are significantly more common among 1st degree relatives of patients than among controls.

Clinical Manifestations. The clinical features of celiac disease range from generalized severe intestinal malabsorption to normal or near normal health. Major manifestations are summarized in Table 11–11. The typical pattern is one of irritability, anorexia, and chronic diarrhea beginning late in the 1st yr. The stools are pale and foul, the child underweight and perhaps short, with wasted muscles, particularly in the proximal groups. Additional physical signs may include mouth sores, a smooth tongue, excessive bruising, finger clubbing, and peripheral edema. However, the range of clinical findings among patients with celiac disease is extraordinarily wide so that a "textbook" appearance should not always be expected. At least 30% of patients are neither irritable nor anorexic; as many have problems with vomiting as with diarrhea, and some are even constipated. The most constant features are decreased rates of weight gain and growth which may persist throughout childhood without obvious gastrointestinal symptoms. However, some patients apparently with the same disease remain perfectly well throughout childhood only to develop typical symptoms in adult life.

Laboratory Manifestations. Anemia is common; usually the patient is iron deficient, but blood and serum folate levels may also be low. Vitamin B_{12} deficiency is seen only in severe, longstanding disease. Hypoalbuminemia and reduced circulating gamma globulin levels may occur as the result of poor intake, reduced absorption, and excessive loss.

Most affected children have steatorrhea if they are eating significant amounts of fat. Based on a 4 day balance, fat excretion exceeding 10% of dietary intake indicates steatorrhea in a child beyond 6 mo of age. Stool microscopy usually reveals an excess of crystalline aggregates of fatty acid. There may also be a reduced fasting serum carotene level (<50 mg/dl); low serum 25-OH vitamin D, calcium, and vitamin A levels; and prolonged prothrombin times. These latter findings may be normal in the presence of proven steatorrhea and celiac disease.

Reflecting diffuse small bowel mucosal damage, the oral glucose tolerance test is usually flat, and the blood xylose concentration does not exceed 25 mg/dl after an oral load in children with active celiac disease. However, false-negative and false-positive results are obtained sufficiently often to make these tests unreliable.

In barium contrast studies the small bowel is usually dilated and the mucosal folds coarse. Because these findings are nonspecific and inconsistent, roentgenograms are not indicated in the diagnostic evaluation of a suspected case unless a localized lesion is suspected. Bone films often show osteoporosis, but rickets is rare.

Pathology. The typical diffuse lesion of the upper small intestinal mucosa that characterizes celiac disease can be seen in a perioral suction biopsy specimen (Fig 11–20A). Short, flat villi, deepened crypts, and irregular vacuolated surface epithelium with lymphocytes in the epithelial layer are seen by light microscopy. Similar abnormalities occur in other conditions, none of which is likely to be confused with celiac disease. Invasive infections such as rotavirus enteritis, *Giardia lamblia,* or tropical sprue can cause villus flattening and elongated crypts but not the marked abnormalities of enterocytes. Some cases of cow milk protein or soy protein intolerance are associated with lesions similar to those of celiac disease in children. In immune deficiency and eosinophilic gastroenteritis, villi can be partially shortened. Infants with familial enteropathy have flattened villi, but the crypt dimensions are normal.

Diagnosis. This is based on finding the characteristic duodenal or jejunal mucosal lesion in a mucosal suction biopsy; a clinical and laboratory response to a gluten-free diet; and the reappearance of the lesion after

Table 11–11 ACTIVE CHILDHOOD CELIAC DISEASE—42 CASES

SYMPTOMS	NO. OF PATIENTS
Failure to thrive	36
Diarrhea	30
Instability	30
Vomiting	24
Anorexia	24
Foul stools	21
Abdominal pain	8
Excessive appetite	6
Rectal prolapse	3

SIGNS	NO. OF PATIENTS
Height <25%	30
Body weight <25%	37
Wasted muscles	40
Abdominal distention	33
Edema	14
Finger clubbing	11

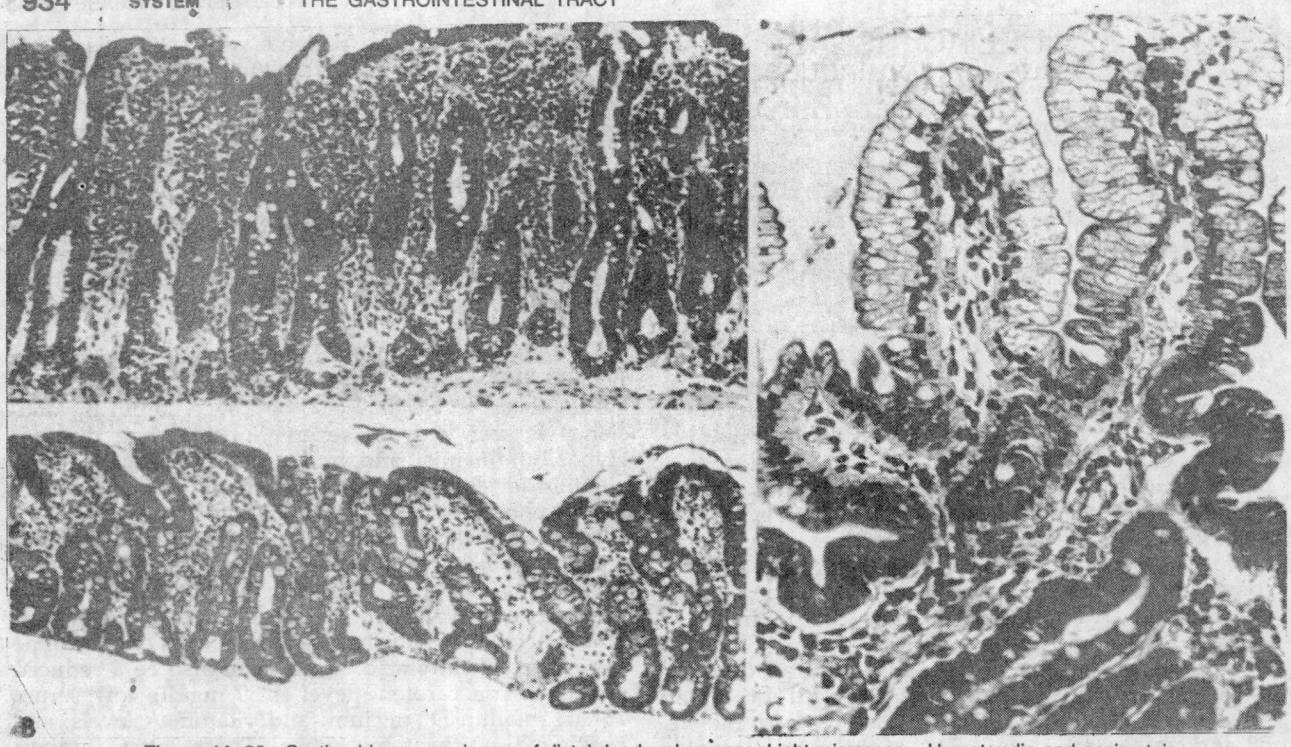

Figure 11–20 Suction biopsy specimens of distal duodenal mucosa. Light microscopy. Hematoxylin and eosin stain. *A,* Celiac disease (×160). There is a loss of the normal villus structure with elongation of crypts. The surface epithelium is flattened, irregular, and infiltrated with lymphocytes. The lamina propria contains increased numbers of cells. *B,* Familial enteropathy (×160). Although the villus structure is lost, the crypts are not elongated and the mucosa is very thin. The surface epithelium is less distorted than is seen in celiac disease. *C,* Abetalipoproteinemia (×400). Two villi are seen at greater magnification than the above sections to show the normal villus contour and extreme vacuolation of columnar epithelial cells. These vacuoles contain triglyceride.

gluten challenge. The final test may not be appropriate in some patients because of the risk from exacerbation of the disease. If gluten is reintroduced, the challenge should not be given until at least 2 yr after therapy has been started to allow for mucosal healing. It may take 2 yr for the mucosal lesion to reappear in a patient with true celiac disease. Furthermore, once the mucosa has healed, moderate quantities (1–2 slices of bread/day) can be taken for months by many children without obvious symptoms. Gluten has been shown to injure celiac mucosa in organ culture, and this procedure may eventually be helpful diagnostically.

Children on a Gluten-Free Diet in Whom a Specific Diagnosis Has Not Been Established. If a child improves after gluten-free diet is prescribed without a definite biopsy-proven diagnosis, the question arises whether the improvement was spontaneous or actually a response to therapy. The child can be returned to a full gluten-containing diet and the response observed. Assuming celiac disease is a possible diagnosis, a perioral intestinal biopsy can be done when symptoms of malabsorption develop or when 2 yr have passed, at which time the diagnosis can be based on the development of a typical mucosal lesion. If the initial illness strongly suggests celiac disease, a gluten challenge should be deferred until the patient is at least 4 yr old and should be roughly equivalent to 1 slice of bread/day.

Treatment. All wheat and rye should be eliminated from an otherwise full diet. Most patients tolerate oats, at least in moderation. Although disaccharidase activities in the mucosa are diminished during active celiac disease, significant disaccharide intolerance is rare. A small proportion of patients who have definite lactose deficiency will benefit from a short period of disaccharide restriction. During the early mo of therapy extra fat-soluble vitamins are advisable, and for those who are iron or folate deficient appropriate supplements should be given. Lifelong dietary treatment is a major undertaking and best carried out with the help of an experienced nutritionist and ample written instructions and recipes.

Prognosis. The clinical response to a gluten-free diet of a child with celiac disease is gratifying. Improvement of mood and appetite is followed by lessening of diarrhea. In most cases changes occur within 1 wk of starting therapy, but the response may occasionally be delayed. Older patients and very ill patients tend to respond slowly, but once in remission the celiac child should be treated as a well child. The extra dietary care makes these patients particularly healthy. During preadolescence and adolescence children with proven celiac disease seem to tolerate considerable quantities of dietary gluten without symptoms although the typical abnormalities reappear in their mucosa. No complications from long term gluten-free diet treatment are recognized. In adult patients the incidence of intestinal malignancy is somewhat higher than in the normal population; the scant data available do not indicate that diet therapy prevents the development of malignancy.

11.53   POST-ENTERITIS MALABSORPTION

The majority of children with chronic diarrhea and mild absorptive defects do not suffer from any of the specific diseases listed in Tables 11–9 and 11–10. These patients, usually infants and toddlers, are rarely seriously ill but suffer from persistent small intestine symptoms after an initial acute acquired illness which often resembles an enteric infection.

Since the normal small intestine possesses mechanisms for rapid repair after acute damage, persisting malfunction suggests either continuing damage or a failure of the repair process. The damage could result from persisting infection or some other injury. However, except for *Giardia lamblia*, most enteric pathogens are quickly shed after invading the mucosa unless the host has an immunodeficiency syndrome. Sugars, if inadequately assimilated, may accumulate in the lumen and ferment to produce organic acids which can injure the mucosa. Proteins, particularly milk protein, are capable of causing immunologically mediated mucosal damage. This is particularly likely to develop after an acute injury, when the repair process may be impaired by many factors including malnutrition and antibiotics.

Clinical Manifestations.   In children from 6 mo–3 yr of age there is usually an acute onset of watery diarrhea with or without fever and vomiting followed by persistent loose stools. The patient's general health is good and nutritional status adequate unless severe dietary restrictions have been imposed. Diarrhea tends to worsen if the sugar intake is high; the stools contain excess sugar and organic acid, and the buttocks are excoriated. Usually there is diminished disaccharidase activity, but if the damage is severe, glucose and ion transport are affected and there may be mild steatorrhea.

Treatment.   Specific measures to accelerate healing of the bowel are not available. Therefore, it is important that natural healing not be delayed by inappropriate measures. Excessive investigations may upset the child and accentuate parental anxiety. Inadequate nutrition may delay growth and may, secondarily, impair digestive tract repair and function (Sec 11.45). Antidiarrheal medications may improve stool appearance in mild chronic cases, but they may also contribute to bowel stasis and, perhaps, persistent infection.

These patients and their parents need reassurance. Sugar intake, particularly in the form of fruit juices which are hyperosmolar, should be limited, diluted in half with water; when lactose intolerance occurs, milk intake should be limited or eliminated for a brief period. Adequate nutrition should be maintained using foods relatively low in sugar such as meats and cereals.

DIETARY PROTEIN INTOLERANCE

See Sec 11.43.

11.54   TROPICAL SPRUE

This syndrome of unknown and perhaps multiple etiologies is confined to certain tropical areas; it occurs in the Caribbean but not Jamaica and in Africa but not the southern half of the continent. It is characterized by generalized malabsorption associated with a diffuse lesion of the small intestinal mucosa.

Clinical Manifestations.   Epidemics affect all ages but usually adults first. Fever and malaise precede the onset of watery diarrhea. Then, in a few days, the acute features subside and are followed by chronic malabsorption, intermittent diarrhea, and anorexia eventually leading to severe malnutrition. Malnutrition may be manifest as night blindness, glossitis, stomatitis, cheilosis, cutaneous and mucosal pigmentation, and edema. There is marked muscle wasting, and the abdomen is often distended.

Laboratory studies usually demonstrate malabsorption of fat, sugars, and vitamin B_{12}. Biopsies of the small intestinal mucosa show varying degrees of villus shortening, increased crypt depth, round cell infiltration of the lamina propria, and irregularity and mild shortening of the surface epithelial cells. These pathologic changes are nonspecific and in their mild form are seen in healthy people in the same communities.

Treatment.   Therapy consists of antidiarrheal agents and nutritional supplements. Folic acid and vitamin B_{12} supplements combined with oral broad spectrum antibiotics may result in rapid improvement of the intestinal lesion. The findings and the response to treatment suggest that enteric flora are involved in the pathogenesis of this syndrome.

11.55   WHIPPLE DISEASE

This rare disease has been reported only once in a child. A rod-shaped bacillus may be the etiologic agent. The disease may involve many organ systems, but the small intestine is always affected, and malabsorption results. Common findings are arthralgia, fever, and polyserositis. Duodenal biopsy shows focal accumulation of PAS-positive macrophages, and bacilli may be seen in the lamina propria. Patients improve dramatically on antibiotics, but long term therapy is necessary.

11.56   INTESTINAL LYMPHANGIECTASIA

This congenital generalized defect of the lymphatic system can involve the intestine extensively, causing steatorrhea, protein-losing enteropathy, edema, and lymphocytopenia. Usually, there is slight if any disturbance of bowel habit, and edema is the major clinical manifestation. Absorptive function, except long chain fat assimilation, is usually intact. Reduction of dietary long chain fats may reduce enteric protein loss; medium chain triglycerides can be substituted in the diet since they are transported by the portal stream.

11.57   WOLMAN DISEASE

This rare lethal lipidosis leads to lipid accumulation in many organs including the small intestine. In addition to vomiting and hepatosplenomegaly there may be steatorrhea as the result of lymphatic obstruction.

11.58   IDIOPATHIC DIFFUSE SMALL INTESTINAL MUCOSAL LESIONS

Some infants continue to be seen with severe chronic malabsorptive states that do not fit into a recognized disease pattern. Two idiopathic syndromes have been associated with lesions of the small intestine mucosa.

Infants with *familial enteropathy* are affected from birth by global malabsorption causing severe diarrhea and malnutrition. Unable to sustain adequate nutritional balance with oral feeding, they are dependent on total parenteral nutrition. Irrespective of nutrient intake, duodenal mucosal biopsy shows a profoundly flattened villus structure (Fig 11–20B). Unlike celiac disease, the crypts are not elongated and mitotic activity seems depressed. In most cases there is a familial incidence of the condition, which appears to be a defect in intestinal epithelial renewal. In spite of aggressive supportive treatment and steroids most of these patients have eventually died without improvement in intestinal function.

A 2nd rare idiopathic syndrome of *persistent villus damage* causes serious chronic malabsorption in young infants. Affected infants develop severe generalized malabsorption after a few mo of apparently normal health. Initially, an acute illness such as an infection is suspected, but the problem persists for months, even years. Dietary restrictions do not alter the course. The mucosal lesion is characterized by shortened villi, but, as in celiac disease, the crypts may be elongated and mitotic figures are plentiful. Corticosteroids may be beneficial.

Malabsorption Syndromes

General Reviews

Ament ME: Malabsorption syndromes in infancy and childhood. J Pediatr 81:685, 867, 1972.
Anderson CM: Malabsorption in children. Clin Gastroenterol 6:355, 1977.
Hamilton JR: Diarrhea and malabsorption in children. In: Sleisenger MH, Fordtran JS (eds): Gastrointestinal Disease. Ed 2. Philadelphia, WB Saunders, 1978, p 336.
Wilson FA, Dietschy JM: Differential diagnostic approach to clinical problems of malabsorption. Gastroenterology 61:911, 1971.

Diagnostic Investigations

Barr RG, Levine MD, Watkins JB: Recurrent abdominal pain of childhood due to lactose intolerance. N Engl J Med 300:1449, 1979.
de Silva M: Radiological investigation of small bowel disease in children. Med J Aust 1:819, 1971.
Drummey GD, Benson JA Jr, Jones CM: Microscopical examinations of the stool for steatorrhea. N Engl J Med 264:85, 1961.
Hill RE, Cutz E, Cherian G, et al: An evaluation of d-xylose absorption measurements in children suspected of having small intestinal disease. J Pediatr 99:245, 1981.
Hill RE, Hercz A, Corey MD, et al: Fecal clearance of alpha-1-antitrypsin. A reliable measure of protein loss in children. J Pediatr 99:416, 1981.
Katz AJ, Grand RJ: All that flattens is not sprue. Gastroenterology 76:375, 1979.
Kerry KR, Anderson CM: A ward test for sugar in the faeces. Lancet 1:981, 1964.
Magnus EM: Low serum and red cell folate activity in adult celiac disease. Am J Dig Dis 11:314, 1966.

McIntyre PA, Hahn R, Conley CL: Genetic factors in predisposition to pernicious anemia. Bull Johns Hopkins Hosp 104:309, 1959.
Shmerling DH, Farrer JCW, Prader A: Fecal fat and nitrogen in healthy children and in children with malabsorption or maldigestion. Pediatrics 46:690, 1970.
Townley RRW, Barnes GL: Intestinal biopsy in childhood. Arch Dis Child 48:480, 1973.

The Digestive Tract in Chronic Malnutrition

Barbesat GO, Hansen JDL: The exocrine pancreas and protein-calorie malnutrition. Pediatrics 42:77, 1968.
Brunser O: Effects of malnutrition on intestinal structure and function in children. Clin Gastroenterol 6:341, 1977.
Suskind RM: Gastrointestinal changes in the malnourished child. Pediatr Clin North Am 22:873, 1975.

Liver and Biliary Disorders

Atkinson M, Nordin BEC, Sherlock S: Malabsorption and bone disease in prolonged obstructive jaundice. Quart J Med 25:299, 1956.
Hadorn B, Hess J, Troesch V, et al: Role of bile acids in the activation of trypsinogen by enterokinase: Disturbance of trypsinogen activation in patients with intrahepatic biliary atresia. Gastroenterology 66:548, 1974.
Kooh SW, Jones G, Reilly BJ, et al: Pathogenesis of rickets in chronic hepatobiliary disease in children. J Pediatr 94:870, 1979.

Short Small Intestine

Congenital

Hamilton JR, Reilly BJ, Morecki R: Short small intestine associated with malrotation. A newly described cause of intestinal malabsorption. Gastroenterology 56:124, 1969.

Acquired

Bohane TD, Haka-Ikse K, Biggar WD, et al: A clinical study of young infants after small intestinal resection. J Pediatr 94:552, 1979.
Wilmore DW: Factors correlating with a successful outcome following extensive intestinal resection in newborn infants. J Pediatr 80:88, 1972.
Young WF, Swain VAJ, Pringle EM: Long term prognosis after major resection of small bowel in early infancy. Arch Dis Child 44:465, 1969.

Stagnant Loop Syndrome

Bayes BJ, Hamilton JR: Blind loop syndrome in children. Acta Dis Child 44:76, 1969.
Jonas A, Krishnan C, Forstner G: Release of disaccharidases from brush border membranes by extracts of bacteria obtained from intestinal blind loops of rats. Gastroenterology 75:791, 1978.
Soderlund S: Anomalies of midgut rotation and fixation. Clinical aspects based on sixty-two cases in childhood. Acta Pediatr 51:135, 1966.

Infections Causing Malabsorption

Ament ME: Diagnosis and treatment of giardiasis. J Pediatr 80:663, 1972.
Brandborg LL, Goldberg SB, Breidenbach WC: Human coccidiosis—a possible cause of malabsorption. N Engl J Med 283:1306, 1970.

Immune Deficiency States and the Intestine

Ament ME: Immunodeficiency syndromes and gastrointestinal disease. Pediatr Clin North Am 22:807, 1975.
Brown WR, Butterfield D, Savage D, et al: Clinical, microbiological and immunological studies in patients with immunoglobulin deficiencies and gastrointestinal disorders. Gut 13:441, 1972.
Katz AJ, Rosen F: Gastrointestinal complication of immunodeficiency syndromes. In: Immunology of the Gut. Ciba Foundation Symposium 46:243, 1977.
Walker WA, Hong R: Immunology of the gastrointestinal tract. J Pediatr 83:517, 711, 1973.

Celiac Disease

Anderson CM, Gracey M, Burke V: Celiac disease—some still controversial aspects. Arch Dis Child 47:292, 1972.
Barry RE, Read AE: Celiac disease and malignancy. Quart J Med 42:665, 1973.
Hamilton JR, McNeil LK: Childhood celiac disease: Response of treated patients to a small uniform daily dose of wheat gluten. J Pediatr 81:885, 1972.
Hamilton JR, Lynch MJ, Reilly BJ: Active celiac disease in childhood. Quart J Med 38:135, 1969.
Katz AJ, Falchuk ZM: Definitive diagnosis of gluten-sensitive enteropathy. Use of an in vitro organ culture model. Gastroenterology 75:695, 1978.
Young WF, Pringle EM: 110 children with celiac disease, 1950 to 1969. Arch Dis Child 46:421, 1971.

Postenteritis Malabsorption

Gribbin M, Walker-Smith JA, Wood CBS: Delayed recovery following acute gastroenteritis. Acta Paediatr Belg 29:167, 1976.
Lifshitz F: Carbohydrate problems in paediatric gastroenterology. Clin Gastroenterol 6:415, 1977.
Manuel PD, Walker-Smith JA, Soeparto P: Cow's milk sensitive enteropathy in Indonesian infants. Lancet 2:1365, 1980.

Tropical Sprue

Klipstein FA, Baker SJ: Regarding the definition of tropical sprue. Gastroenterology 58:717, 1970.
Santiago-Borrero PJ, Maldanado N, Horta E: Tropical sprue in children. J Pediatr 76:470, 1970.

Whipple Disease

Aust CH, Smith EB: Whipple's disease in a 3-month old infant. Am J Clin Pathol 37:66, 1962.

Intestinal Lymphangiectasia

Strober W, Wochner RD, Carbone PP, et al: Intestinal lymphangiectasia: A protein-losing enteropathy with hypogammaglobulinemia, lymphocytopenia and impaired homograft rejection. J Clin Invest 46:1643, 1967.
Waldman TA, Wochner RD, Strober W: The role of the gastrointestinal tract in plasma protein metabolism. Am J Med 46:275, 1969.

Wolman Disease

Queloz JM, Capitanio MA, Kirkpatrick JA: Wolman's disease. Radiology 104:357, 1972.

Idiopathic Diffuse Small Intestinal Mucosal Lesions

Candy DCA, Larcher VF, Cameron DJS, et al: Lethal familial protracted diarrhea. Arch Dis Child 56:15, 1981.
Davidson GP, Cutz E, Hamilton JR, et al: Familial enteropathy. A syndrome of protracted diarrhea from birth, failure to thrive and hypoplastic villus atrophy. Gastroenterology 75:793, 1978.

DEFECTS OF SPECIFIC ENZYMES OR TRANSPORT PROCESSES INVOLVED IN DIGESTION OR ABSORPTION

11.59   ABETALIPOPROTEINEMIA
(Bassen-Kornzweig Syndrome)

This relatively rare congenital disease, probably autosomal recessive, is characterized by fat malabsorption, acanthocytosis of erythrocytes, ataxic neuropathy, and retinitis pigmentosa. The underlying defect is not fully defined, but in the small bowel there is an absence of low density lipoproteins resulting in an inability to form normal chylomicrons and defective release and transport of triglycerides from the enterocyte.

Clinical Manifesations. These patients are normal at birth but usually fail to thrive during the 1st yr. The stools are pale and bulky and the abdomen distended. In most patients intellectual development is also slightly retarded. After 10 yr of age central nervous system problems may develop. Ataxia, loss of deep tendon reflexes and the sense of position and vibration, and intention tremors reflect involvement of cerebellum, posterolateral columns, peripheral nerves, and basal ganglia. In adolescence pigmentary degeneration (atypical retinitis pigmentosa) develops in the retina.

Diagnosis rests on finding acanthocytes in the peripheral blood, very low serum levels of cholesterol (20–80 mg/dl), absent or minute levels of β-lipoprotein, and the typical marked lipid accumulation in villus enterocytes in the fasting duodenal mucosa (Fig 11–20C). Usually, there is steatorrhea in younger patients, but apart from defects in absorption of fat and fat-soluble vitamins other processes of assimilation are intact.

Treatment. Specific therapy is not available, but large supplements of the fat-soluble vitamins A, D, E, and K, should be given. Massive doses of vitamin E (100 mg/kg/24 hr) may arrest progression of neurological degeneration. Limiting long chain fat intake may alleviate intestinal symptoms; medium chain triglycerides can be used to supplement the fat intake.

11.60   ENTEROKINASE DEFICIENCY

Congenital deficiency of this small intestine enzyme has been reported in a few children. The disease results in a complete absence of pancreatic proteolytic activity since enterokinase is an essential activator of pancreatic trypsinogens. Affected patients are ill from very early life with severe diarrhea and failure to thrive. Hypoproteinemia is common and may lead to edema. In duodenal juice tryptic activity is missing while lipase and amylase are normal; in vitro tryptic activity of the juice can be restored by the addition of enterokinase. Malabsorption of protein is the major defect, although mild steatorrhea has been reported. Pancreatic enzyme replacements restore normal digestive function.

11.61   AMINO ACID TRANSPORT DEFECTS

In several of the specific congenital disorders of amino acid transport (Chapter 8) defective intestinal amino acid transport occurs. Amino acid uptake into the intestinal mucosa is defective in *cystinuria*, but these patients have no gastrointestinal symptoms. In *Hartnup disease* there is malabsorption of tryptophan leading to ataxia, intellectual deterioration, and a pellagra-like skin rash. *Methionine malabsorption* is associated with episodes of diarrhea in fair-complexioned, retarded children whose urine has a sweet odor and contains excess α-hydroxybutyric acid. In the *blue diaper syndrome* tryptophan absorption is defective. *Lysine malabsorption* is reported in a case of hyperlysinuria.

11.62   DISACCHARIDASE DEFICIENCIES

The disaccharidases are located on the brush border membrane surface of the small bowel. At different fetal and postnatal ages different developmental enzyme patterns are seen (Fig 11–10). Occasionally, congenital deficiencies occur, but if disaccharidase activities are abnormal, they have most often been affected secondarily by some diffuse lesion of the intestinal epithelium such as infection or celiac disease.

The response of the patient to significant disaccharidase deficiency, disaccharide intolerance, is similar whatever its cause or the enzymes involved. If disaccharide hydrolysis at the brush border is incomplete, the sugar accumulates in the intestinal lumen. In the distal regions the intraluminal flora is presented with this substrate, and organic acids and hydrogen gas are produced. The excess intraluminal sugar and organic acids draw water into the lumen, leading to watery diarrhea with stools that are frothy, loose, and of low pH (<pH 6.0); contain excess sugar; and tend to excoriate the buttocks. There may be bloating and borborygmi, but steatorrhea is rare. In some children, particularly those beyond infancy, gas production causing crampy abdominal pain rather than diarrhea is the dominant problem.

If the disaccharide involved is a reducing sugar, e.g., lactose, the standard Clinitest procedure* will be 1+ or greater in most cases. Oral tolerance tests using the potential offending sugar have been employed for the clinical diagnosis of disaccharide intolerance, but these tests are unreliable. Disaccharidase activities can be assayed in mucosal biopsy specimens. Breath hydrogen excretion after an oral sugar load is a useful test for detecting disaccharide intolerance in children beyond the age of 4 yr who can cooperate for breath collection.

Lactase Deficiency. *Congenital* absence of lactase has been reported in a very few cases. The usual primary mechanism for lactose intolerance relates to the *developmental* pattern of lactase activity. Because lactase activity rises relatively late in fetal life and begins to fall after the age of 3 yr, intolerance to lactose can be anticipated in very premature infants and in older children and adults. This decrease in lactase activity in childhood is very common in Blacks and Orientals and less common in Whites. Since lactase activity in the mucosa is somewhat marginal, this enzyme is particularly likely to be depleted *secondary to diffuse mucosal diseases* (Sec 11.58).

The clinical manifestations of lactase deficiency occur in response to ingestion of lactose, the sugar in milk. Watery diarrhea may result. More recently, a common syndrome of recurrent, vague, crampy abdominal pain has been attributed to lactose intolerance. School and preschool age children develop episodic mid-abdominal pain. Usually, their general health is unaffected, and there is often no obvious relationship of pain to milk ingestion or to diarrhea. (See also Sec 11.43.)

Treatment consists of removal of milk from the diet. In most cases the elimination need not be total; stopping milk ingestion as a beverage is important. A lactase preparation is now available which for some children allows asymptomatic consumption of modest quantities of milk incubated with the added enzyme.

Sucrase-Isomaltase Deficiency. The only congenital deficiency of disaccharidase activities occurring with significant frequency is a combined deficiency of sucrase and isomaltase. Symptoms usually begin when a sucrose-containing diet is started. There may also be some intolerance to starch, but since isomaltase acts only on the branch points of the starch molecule, isomaltase deficiency itself is relatively asymptomatic. The symptoms are bloating, watery diarrhea, and buttocks excoriation. Recurrent abdominal pain has not been attributed to sucrose-isomaltose intolerance. Since sucrose is not a reducing sugar, its presence will not be detected in stool by Clinitest unless the specimen is first hydrolyzed with HCl. The morphology of the small intestine mucosa is normal, but enzyme assays show specific deficiencies of sucrase and isomaltase with normal levels of lactase and maltase. Breath testing usually demonstrates increased H_2 after sucrose ingestion. These patients improve quickly after sucrose is reduced to minimal amounts in their diets.

Glucose-Galactose Malabsorption. This rare congenital transport defect in brush border membrane glucose transport is inherited as an autosomal recessive trait. It also affects renal tubular epithelium to a mild degree. Acute viral enteritis and severe chronic diffuse mucosal damage also may impair the glucose-galactose carrier sufficiently to cause intolerance to these sugars. Usually, if mucosal damage is severe enough to impair glucose transport, other absorptive processes are affected.

The symptomatic response to sugar ingestion is similar whether the defect is congenital or secondary. Watery stools follow the ingestion of glucose, breast milk, or conventional formulas since most diet sugars are polysaccharides or disaccharides with glucose and/or galactose moieties. The patient may be bloated, and, if diarrhea persists, dehydration and acidosis can be severe. The stools are acidic and contain sugar. Glucose and galactose tolerance curves are flat. Patients with a congenital defect tolerate fructose normally; their small bowel function is normal in all other aspects as are mucosal structure and disaccharidase activities.

Treatment consists of rigorous restriction of glucose and galactose and provision of a fructose-containing formula. Later in life limited amounts of glucose or sucrose may be tolerated.

11.63 VITAMIN B₁₂ MALABSORPTION

Several rare congenital defects may affect assimilation of vitamin B_{12}. In *juvenile pernicious anemia* intrinsic factor production in the stomach is defective. Although gastric structure and function are otherwise normal, vitamin B_{12} malabsorption results, leading to megaloblastic anemia and growth failure.

Transcobalamin II deficiency is an inherited defect of intestinal transport of vitamin B_{12} in which a transporting protein for the vitamin is lacking. The result is severe megaloblastic anemia, diarrhea, and vomiting.

A different selective malabsorption of vitamin B_{12} has been described by *Immerslund* in which ileal absorption of the vitamin is defective. In these patients ileal structure and function are otherwise normal. Megaloblastic anemia develops toward the end of the 1st yr. A common associated finding is proteinuria.

Treatment of these disorders is to administer vitamin B_{12} by injection: 1000 μg/wk for transcobalamin II deficiency, 100 μg/mo for the others.

---

*Ames Company.

11.64 CONGENITAL MALABSORPTION OF FOLIC ACID

A few patients are described with folic acid deficiency occurring in infancy as the result of a specific defect in folic acid assimilation. In addition to megaloblastic anemia, they have had cerebral degeneration.

11.65 CHLORIDE-LOSING DIARRHEA

This rare specific congenital defect of ileal chloride transport is associated with maternal polyhydramnios. The dominant symptom is severe watery diarrhea beginning at birth, the result of the accumulation of chloride ion in the intestinal lumen. Watery diarrhea persists, leading to dehydration and severe systemic electrolyte imbalance characterized by hypokalemia, hypochloridemia, and alkalosis, a most unusual pattern for a patient with chronic diarrhea. Other aspects of intestinal absorption are normal. Stools contain chloride in excess of the sum of sodium and potassium. Adequate treatment is not available. Potassium supplements and some restriction of chloride intake are advisable.

11.66 VITAMIN D–DEPENDENT RICKETS

In this autosomal recessive disorder a specific defect in the metabolism of vitamin D causes malabsorption of calcium (Sec 23.20). Intestinal function is otherwise normal.

11.67 PRIMARY HYPOMAGNESEMIA

A specific intestinal transport defect affects magnesium transport and causes severe hypomagnesemia and, secondarily, hypocalcemic tetany in infancy. Other aspects of intestinal function are normal. The findings are reversed by large supplements of magnesium, which must be continued indefinitely.

11.68 ACRODERMATITIS ENTEROPATHICA

The cause of this unusual constellation of clinical findings is zinc deficiency secondary to zinc malabsorption. Early in life the patient develops skin rashes around mucocutaneous junctions and in the extremities. There is alopecia, chronic diarrhea, and sometimes steatorrhea. Untreated, the patient fails to thrive. Serum zinc concentrations are very low. Intestinal mucosal biopsies show Paneth cell inclusions that disappear after treatment. An oral supplement of zinc sulfate heptahydrate, 150 mg/24 hr, causes rapid healing of the skin lesions and improvement of diarrhea.

11.69 MENKES (KINKY HAIR) SYNDROME

This rare recessively inherited disorder is characterized by growth retardation, abnormal hair, cerebellar degeneration, and early death. Its pathogenesis is unclear, but there is a widespread defect in cellular copper transport that affects the intestine in addition to other tissues. Serum copper and ceruloplasmin levels are low, but cellular copper content is increased.

11.70 DRUG-INDUCED ABSORPTIVE DEFECTS

Some drugs have a diffuse impact on the small intestinal epithelium. For example, methotrexate can cause arrest of enterocyte mitoses and result in a mucosal lesion; large doses of neomycin also affect mucosal structure. *Sulfasalazine* interferes with folic acid absorption. *Cholestyramine* binds bile salts and calcium in the intestinal lumen to cause hypocalcemia and steatorrhea. *Phenytoin* interferes with calcium absorption and can cause rickets.

J. RICHARD HAMILTON

Abetalipoproteinemia

Isselbacher KJ, Scheig R, Plotkin ER, et al: Congenital β-lipoprotein deficiency. An hereditary disorder involving a defect in the absorption and transport of lipid. Medicine 43:347, 1964.
Lee RS, Ahren E Jr: Fat transport in a β-lipoproteinemia. N Engl J Med 284:1261, 1969.
Lloyd JE: Lipoprotein deficiency disorders. Clin Endocrinol 2:127, 1973.

Enterokinase Deficiency

Hadorn B, Tarlow M, Lloyd JD, et al: Intestinal enterokinase deficiency. Lancet 1:812, 1969.

Amino Acid Transport Defects

Drummond KN, Michael AF, Ulstrom RA, et al: The blue diaper syndrome: Familial hypercalcemia with nephrocalcinosis and indicanuria. Am J Med 37:928, 1964.
Hooft G, Timmermand J, Snoeck J, et al: Methionine malabsorption syndrome. Ann Pediatr 205:73, 1965.
Milne MD: Hartnup disease. Biochem 111:3, 1969.
Morin CL, Thompson MW, Jackson SH, et al: Biochemical and genetic studies in cystinuria: Observations on double heterozygotes of genotype I/II. J Clin Invest 50:1961, 1971.
Whelan DT, Scriver CR: Hyperdibasicaminoaciduria: An inherited disorder of amino acid transport. Pediatr Res 2:525, 1968.

Disaccharidases

Ament ME, Perera DR, Esther L: Sucrase-isomaltase deficiency: A frequently misdiagnosed disease. J Pediatr 83:721, 1973.
Auricchio S, Rubino A, Murset G: Intestinal glycosidase activities in the human embryo, foetus and newborn. Pediatrics 35:344, 1965.
Barr RG, Levine MD, Watkins JB: Recurrent abdominal pain of childhood due to lactose intolerance. N Engl J Med 300:1449, 1979.
Gray GM: Carbohydrate digestion and absorption. Role of the small intestine. N Engl J Med 292:1225, 1975.
Harrison M, Walker-Smith JA: Reinvestigation of lactose intolerant children: Lack of correlation between continuing lactose intolerance and small intestinal morphology, disaccharidase activity and lactose tolerance tests. Gut 18:48, 1977.
Kretchmer N: Lactose and lactase. Sci Am 221:70, 1972.
Lifshitz F: Carbohydrate problems in paediatric gastroenterology. Clin Gastroenterol 6:415, 1977.

Glucose-Galactose Malabsorption

Lindqvist B, Meeuwisse GW, Melin K: Glucose-galactose malabsorption. Lancet 2:666, 1962.

Meeuwisse G: Glucose-galactose malabsorption. Studies on renal glucosuria. Helvet Paediatr Acta 25:13, 1970.

Schneider AJ, Kinter WB, Stirling CE: Glucose-galactose malabsorption. N Engl J Med 274:305, 1966.

Vitamin B$_{12}$ Malabsorption

Hall CA: Congenital disorders of Vitamin B$_{12}$ transport and their contribution to concepts. Gastroenterology 65:684, 1973.

Hitzig WH, Dohmann V, Pluss HJ, et al: Hereditary transcobalamin 11 deficiency: Clinical findings in a new family. J Pediatr 85:622, 1974.

Imerslund O: Idiopathic chronic megaloblastic anaemia in children. Acta Paediatr 49: Suppl 119, 1960.

MacKenzie IL, Donaldson RM, Trier JS, et al: Ileal mucosa in familial selective vitamin B$_{12}$ malabsorption. N Engl J Med 286:1021, 1972.

Folate Malabsorption

Lanzkowsky P: Congenital malabsorption of folate. Am J Med 48:580, 1970.

Chloride-Losing Diarrhea

Bieberdorf FA, Gorden P, Fordtran JS: Pathogenesis of congenital alkalosis with diarrhea. Implications for the physiology of normal ileal electrolyte absorption and secretion. J Clin Invest 51:1958, 1972.

Perheentupa J, Eklund J, Kojo N: Familial chloride diarrhoea ('congenital alkalosis with diarrhoea'). Acta Paediatr Scand (Suppl) 159:119, 1965.

Vitamin D–Dependent Rickets

Hamilton R, Harrison J, Fraser D, et al: The small intestine in vitamin D dependent rickets. Pediatrics 45:364, 1970.

Primary Hypomagnesemia

Paunier L, Radde IC, Kooh SW, et al: Primary hypomagnesemia with secondary hypocalcemia in an infant. Pediatrics 41:385, 1968.

Stromme JH, Nesbakken R, Normann T, et al: Familial hypomagnesemia. Acta Paediatr Scand 58:433, 1969.

Acrodermatitis Enteropathica

Bohane TD, Cutz E, Hamilton JR, et al: Acrodermatitis enteropathica, zinc and the Paneth cell. Gastroenterology 73:587, 1977.

Moynahan EJ: Acrodermatitis enteropathica: A lethal inherited human zinc-deficiency disorder. Lancet 2:399, 1974.

Menkes Syndrome

Danks DM, Stevens BJ, Campbell PE, et al: Menkes' kinky-hair syndrome. Lancet 1:110, 1972.

Drug-Induced Malabsorption

Franklin JL, Rosenberg HH: Impaired folic acid absorption in inflammatory bowel disease: Effects of salicylazosulfapyridine (Azulfidine). Gastroenterology 64:517, 1973.

Morijiri Y, et al: Factors causing rickets in institutionalized handicapped children on anti-convulsant therapy. Arch Dis Child 56:446, 1981.

Rogers AI, Vloedman DA, Bloom EC, et al: Neomycin-induced steatorrhea. JAMA 197:185, 1966.

Trier JS: Morphologic alterations induced by methotrexate in the mucosa of human proximal intestine. I. Serial observations by light microscopy. Gastroenterology 42:295, 1962.

11.71   IRRITABLE BOWEL SYNDROME
(Recurrent Abdominal Pain Syndrome)

The irritable bowel syndrome is a common gastrointestinal condition of childhood presenting with intermittent episodes of watery stools or crampy abdominal pain. A majority of children with recurrent abdominal pain have this problem rather than a specific organic lesion such as lactose intolerance, nonorganic constipation, or a specific psychiatric disease.

Etiology and Epidemiology. The cause of this condition is unknown. An increase in intestinal motility after stimulation suggests that a local lowered intestinal threshold to stimuli or an altered neurohumoral control mechanism may be present. It often occurs in several family members. Physical and emotional stresses are frequently observed to act as precipitating events, and infantile colic is retrospectively reported in some children with the irritable bowel syndrome. There is no sex difference until adolescence, when the incidence in females is higher than in males.

Clinical Manifestations. In the infant and toddler recurrent diarrhea is the common presentation with bouts of watery stools over a number of days. The 1st stool of the day may have some form but is followed by 3 or more watery bowel movements which are malodorous, runny, and irritating to the buttocks. Affected children usually have an intense thirst but do not become dehydrated from the fluid loss or lose weight unless their dietary intake is markedly restricted. The diarrhea appears to follow periods of intensive stimulation, travel, or holidays. The physical examination is usually normal except for occasional fluctuating abdominal distention and increased bowel sounds. The children not only appear healthy but show intense vigor and activity. Laboratory tests of intestinal function and general health are normal. When these children are hospitalized for study, their diarrhea almost always stops.

The school-aged child usually presents with recurrent abdominal pain which is variable in time of occurrence, intensity, and duration. Usually, the pain has no obvious relationship to eating, bowel movements, or a particular experience. It is frequently localized in the epigastric or periumbilical areas, although location can also be quite variable. At times, it may suggest acute appendicitis. Constipation may occur but is usually not protracted. The stools may at times be pellet-like and at other times unformed. There may be loud borborygmus and frequent passage of flatus. In some children fecal incontinence or episodes of soiling may be the pervasive symptom. Dysuria or urinary frequency also occurs in the absence of any changes in the urine. Headaches, facial pallor, dizziness, and blurred vision are common and suggest some disturbance of autonomic function. On deep palpation of the abdomen there is often vague tenderness without muscle guarding, more frequently in the right and left lower quadrants and the epigastrium. The sigmoid colon may be tender to palpation, which may reveal a row of stool balls. On proctoscopy the mucosa is pale with localized areas of hyperemia, prominent vascular markings, lymphoid hyperplasia, and a dilated rectal vault.

The clinical course may vary directly with stressful events, such as family crises, deaths, illness, and other events that threaten the child's sense of security. The child with irritable bowel syndrome commonly exhibits heightened sensitivity, lowered self-image, and an exaggerated concern for friends and family suggesting his or her feelings of insecurity. Such children often appear older than their years and relate exceedingly well to adults and younger children. Occasionally, school phobia with poor learning performance is an associated finding.

Treatment. Discussion with the child may help him or her to attain a new adaptation toward well-being. At times, hospitalization may be useful in demonstrating that symptoms usually abate. Studies of the urinary and gastrointestinal systems may be necessary to help a worried family and child, even when negative results are expected. The pain should be accepted as real and not belittled. Exploration of factors influencing the pain may be helpful. A strong, empathic relationship of the physician with the child and family may be most helpful in ameliorating the condition. Antispasmodics may benefit some children. A full nutritious diet with adequate fiber should be provided.

The prognosis is variable; in some instances the pain may continue into adulthood. Counseling often enables these children to learn to tolerate the pain and to lead effective lives in spite of occasional episodes which may persist into adult life.

GIULIO J. BARBERO
R. JAMES McKAY

Apley J: The Child with Abdominal Pain. Ed 2. Oxford, Blackwell, 1975.
Christensen ML, Morlinsen O: Long-term prognosis in children with recurrent abdominal pain. Arch Dis Child 50:110, 1975.
Davidson M, Wasserman R: The irritable colon of childhood (chronic non-specific diarrhea syndrome). J Pediatr 69:1027, 1966.
Galler JR, Neustein S, Walker WA: Clinical aspects of recurrent abdominal pain in children. Adv Pediatr 27:31, 1980.
Stone RT, Barbero GJ: Recurrent abdominal pain in childhood. Pediatrics 45:732, 1970.

11.72 ACUTE APPENDICITIS

Acute appendicitis is the most common disease requiring abdominal surgery in childhood, and along with traumatic visceral injury, intussusception, adhesive bowel obstruction, and lesions of the ovary it is one of the few indications for emergency surgery in a child over 2 yr of age. However, diagnosis in children can be difficult; more often in children than in adults appendicitis is permitted to progress to perforation by a physician who has failed to recognize it. Preventable deaths of children from appendicitis still occur.

Epidemiology. The true incidence of acute appendicitis is unknown, but there are about 4 appendectomies performed annually in every 1000 children under the age of 14. A busy physician is likely to see 2–3 cases each yr, and an active pediatric emergency service receives about 3–4 each wk. Males predominate in most series. Although appendicitis does occur in infancy and has been reported in the neonatal period, it is unusual under age 2 and rare under 1 yr. The incidence peaks in the teenage and young adult years. The frequency increases in autumn and spring.

Etiology. Acute appendicitis is almost always caused by obstruction of the lumen, but the mechanism of obstruction varies. Hard concretions and appendiceal fecaliths are frequently discovered at the site of the obstruction in inflamed appendices. The proximal portion of the vermiform appendix may be bound to the cecum by a congenital peritoneal fold (Jackson membrane), forming a sharp kink and obstruction where the organ emerges from beneath the free border of this fold. The appendiceal mesentery can be so narrow that the distal portion of the appendix, with the mesentery, undergoes torsion, producing acute ischemic necrosis. Appendiceal obstruction has also been attributed to hyperplasia of the submucosal lymphoid tissue, presumably as a result of intercurrent infection. Although many resected appendices, both normal and diseased, contain pinworms, parasites have never been proved to cause appendicitis. Fibrous stenosis resulting from an earlier inflammation or a carcinoid tumor (argentaffinoma) may also predispose to appendicitis by narrowing the lumen.

Nonobstructive appendicitis is rare; some reported cases are probably due to fecaliths that have dislodged. Both the clinical manifestations and the tissue changes are less severe in the nonobstructive form of appendicitis, and resolution without perforation may occur in some instances.

Bacteriologic studies generally show a mixed growth of intestinal organisms. Anaerobes are particularly important causes of intraperitoneal abscesses after perforation or surgery. Associated disease may delay the diagnosis of appendicitis and increase the risk of perforation, but it is doubtful that systemic infections predispose to or cause appendicitis.

Pathology. In the younger child the progression of the disease is generally so rapid that the 1st of 3 pathologic stages usually passes before medical attention is sought. First, when acute obstruction of the appendix occurs, the intraluminal pressure increases because the mucosal cells continue to elaborate mucus. Compression of mucosal vessels causes ischemia, death of cells, and ulceration. Second, bacterial invasion and infection of the appendiceal wall occur readily once the mucosa ulcerates. Inflammatory infiltrate appears within all layers, and fibrinous exudate is deposited in the serosa. Even before perforation is visible, organisms can usually be cultured from the serosal surface of the appendix. Third, necrosis of the appendiceal wall results in perforation and fecal contamination of the abdomen. Perforation usually occurs at the tip or near the base where a fecalith has eroded through the wall.

In the older child the omentum and adjacent ileum usually adhere to the inflamed appendix prior to perforation and prevent widespread fecal spillage. The result is a localized abscess, usually in the right iliac fossa but occasionally low in the pelvis. Multiple foci of intraperitoneal sepsis and pleural empyema resulting from general peritonitis rarely occur now because diagnoses are made early when treatment is more effective. There may be an associated paralytic ileus or a degree of mechanical bowel obstruction, or the abscess may rupture, usually into an adjacent loop of intestine to which it is adherent rather than into the general peritoneal space. Spontaneous recovery follows rupture of the abscess into the bowel lumen. In an infant or younger child appendicitis can progress quickly to perforation and general peritonitis since at this age the omentum is small and ineffective in localizing the infection.

Clinical Manifestations.   Pain is invariably present. Initially, when the pathology is confined to the mucosa and muscular layers of the appendix, it is crampy and located in the periumbilical region. The colicky nature of the pain may reflect appendicular peristalsis directed at extruding the obstructing agent. When the visceral and the parietal peritoneal layers are involved in the inflammation, however, the pain is localized to the area immediately overlying the appendix. Thus, it is commonly located in the right iliac fossa but may even be felt in the hypogastrium or within the pelvis, if pelvic, and in the loin, if retrocolic. Movement such as jumping and driving over bumps in a car aggravates the pain. At this stage there is severe tenderness over the appendix, fever, tachycardia, and leukocytosis. Unfortunately, although some older children may give the classic history described above, others describe pain in the right iliac fossa throughout the illness. A young child will often hold his hand over his navel when asked to show where it hurts. In infancy, general irritability and a tendency to lie quietly with hips flexed may be the only indication of pain. The cramps of appendiceal obstruction are rarely severe. In fact, if an older child cries because of abdominal pain, he probably does not have appendicitis. The pain of peritoneal inflammation is made worse by any movement, such as a cough or a sudden turn. A patient who winces when jostled probably has peritoneal irritation.

Vomiting is almost always noted after the onset of the pain; it is not copious or frequent and is less common in older than in younger children. Anorexia is almost invariably present.

In children the duration of appendicitis before rupture is usually so short that there is insufficient time for constipation to develop. Although diarrhea suggests that cramps are due to gastroenteritis, loose stools can also result from irritation of the colon by an adjacent, acutely inflamed appendix. Similarly, pelvic appendicitis can cause urinary frequency and urgency by irritating the bladder.

Sometimes a child with an acute retrocecal or retroiliac appendicitis will walk with an exaggerated lumbar lordosis and a slightly flexed hip due to spasm of the right psoas muscle.

Many children with acute appendicitis have previously had milder, self-limited attacks of a similar nature.

In getting the history, it is helpful to observe the patient for pallor, flushing, physical activity, and abdominal movement. Pulse rate and rectal temperature should be obtained in advance. During the history taking, jiggling the bed or gently shaking the child's thigh by a hand placed casually on the leg can suggest appendiceal inflammation if pain in the right lower abdomen results. Throughout the interview and examination it is important to proceed slowly, never threatening with a sudden movement and whenever possible distracting the child with jokes and tricks.

The physician should proceed directly to the specific abdominal examination leaving the remainder of the examination until later. First, the abdomen should be inspected for visible swelling and movements. If the child is old enough, compliance with a request to cough or to move the abdominal wall in and out will produce pain over any site of peritoneal inflammation. Palpation in younger children may be initiated by using a stethoscope as a light palpating instrument. The pressure on the abdomen with the instrument is gradually increased, and later the hand replaces the stethoscope. There should also be an attempt to elicit increased muscle tone, pressing gently in each quadrant, observing as well as feeling the resistance. Palpation must be gentle since voluntary splinting is the response to pain and involuntary tone cannot be assessed. The site of maximum tenderness is important; in the older child it is often well localized to the McBurney point, the junction between the lateral and middle thirds of the line joining the right anterior superior iliac spine and the umbilicus. In younger children localization to the right iliac fossa is usually all that can be detected. Pain produced in the appendiceal area by pressure elsewhere in the abdomen is a valuable sign in an anxious child. Rebound tenderness is a needlessly painful sign; eliciting it serves only to destroy the carefully built up relationship between the examiner and the child. It is also often falsely positive or negative. Bowel sounds may be depressed in appendicitis.

Atypical positioning of the appendix causes difficulty in diagnosis. If it lies up the gutter, lateral to the cecum, the tenderness will be in the flank. A pelvic appendix may be reached only by rectum. Retroiliac appendicitis usually causes very poorly localized pain so that the diagnosis is unlikely to be made before perforation occurs. A posteriorly situated appendix lying on the psoas muscle will cause hip flexion, and pain may be produced by passive extension of the hip with the child lying on the left side (psoas sign). The single most important physical sign is a constant, localized, significant degree of tenderness. The site of tenderness must not vary from examination to examination or from examiner to examiner. An acutely inflamed but unruptured appendix should not give rise to tenderness of the entire hemiabdomen, nor should there be bilateral tenderness. The finding of an unduly extensive area of tenderness should call into question the diagnosis of appendicitis.

After the abdominal assessment the general examination is completed, leaving until last the essential rectal examination. A mild hypnotic, such as one of the barbiturates, is sometimes indicated to facilitate the examination of a child who is particularly upset, but, if at all possible, hypnotics or sedatives should be avoided. Patience and gentle persistence are more effective aids to facilitate the examination of an apprehensive child. In difficult cases re-evaluation of the patient in 4-6 hr is helpful since the course of appendicitis is usually sufficiently rapid in children that 6 hr produces enough change to make the diagnosis. Even under ideal circumstances, 15% of operations for presumed acute appendicitis in children lead to the removal of noninflamed appendices.

Laboratory Data.   A high white blood cell count suggests acute suppurative disease. Usually, there is neutrophilia with a shift to the left and absence of eosinophils. The teenager with early appendicitis is unlikely to have a count higher than 15,000/mm³, but the infant may show a leukocyte response of 20,000/mm³ or more even before perforation. Occasionally, the white count is depressed. Pyuria usually suggests urinary tract infection, particularly if there are bacteria in a fresh specimen, but an inflamed appendix lying across the ureter or irritating the bladder can also cause pyuria. Other hematologic or biochemical tests are not useful in establishing a diagnosis but may be important in assessing a patient's general state.

Roentgenograms may be helpful to detect intestinal obstruction, calcified appendicolith, or pneumonia. Scoliosis concave to the right can be caused by an inflamed appendix, and a degree of paralytic ileus may be noted. Nevertheless, the indications for surgery should be based, in almost all instances, on abdominal physical findings and not on roentgenograms.

Differential Diagnosis. The diffuse crampy pain and diarrhea of enteric infection usually distinguish it from appendicitis, but appendicitis may occur in a child who has had gastroenteritis for several days. The enteritis caused by *Yersinia enterocolitica*, an acute flare-up of *Crohn disease* or regional ileitis, and, infrequently, intussusception in an older child may produce right lower abdominal symptoms highly suggestive of appendicitis. Occasionally, Crohn disease may begin by mimicking appendicitis. Inflammation rarely complicates a *Meckel diverticulum*, but when it does, the clinical findings may be identical to those of appendicitis. Many children with pain and tenderness in the appendiceal area are seen with an infection and are assumed to have *mesenteric adenitis*. However, ileocecal lymphadenopathy causing appendicitis-like symptoms is rare. Many generalized *viral infections* cause abdominal pain, which is usually midabdominal, worse upon eating, and associated with neutropenia. Early fever, headache, and chills favor a systemic infection, even if abdominal pain is noted later. *Pneumonia* involving the right lower lobe with diaphragmatic irritation may result in enough right-sided abdominal muscular rigidity and referred pain that appendicitis is suspected. Abdominal pain occasionally accompanies acute *streptococcal tonsillitis* or *pharyngitis* and can mimic appendicitis very closely, but these disorders may also occur with true appendicitis. *Acute rheumatic fever* can also cause abdominal pain in its early stages. *Urinary tract infections* occasionally cause abdominal pain and tenderness; there should always be a careful urinary tract evaluation prior to appendectomy. *Diabetic ketoacidosis* frequently causes abdominal pain and vomiting, and in the undiagnosed diabetic can be confused with appendicitis. Urinalysis should lead to the correct diagnosis and must never be omitted prior to emergency surgery. *Bleeding from the right ovary*, a graafian follicle, or a persisting corpus luteum can also simulate appendicitis. Primary peritonitis is discussed in Sec 11.105.

Abdominal pain is a common symptom of many hematologic disorders. It is associated with leukemia, especially in relapse. However, appendicitis also occurs in leukemia and may be masked by immunosuppressant drugs. One should also suspect the diagnosis of appendicitis in a hemophiliac patient with abdominal pain, although in most instances it is due to hemophilia.

Sickle cell disease and anaphylactoid purpura (Henoch-Schönlein purpura) frequently cause very severe abdominal pain (Sec 9.65 and 14.18).

Treatment. Emergency appendectomy is the treatment for early acute appendicitis. Only under the most extreme circumstances should operation be delayed more than a few hr. Recovery is rapid and the child active in 3–4 days. Most surgeons recommend that the child with a localized appendiceal abscess receive adequate external drainage after appropriate preoperative correction of any fluid and electrolyte problems. However, at The Hospital for Sick Children, Toronto, only supportive care is provided until spontaneous drainage of the abscess occurs into an adjacent loop of a bowel, a process that rarely takes longer than 1 wk. Then 8–12 wk later appendectomy is carried out. In most centers primary surgical drainage of the abscess is preferred.

The child with generalized peritonitis due to appendiceal rupture requires intravenous hydration and correction of any electrolyte disturbance before surgery because of substantial fluid loss into the abdominal space from an inflamed peritoneum. The amount of fluid given is directly related to the degree of hydration. If there are no clinical signs of dehydration, Ringer lactate solution should be administered at a volume of 5% of the body weight. Half of the calculated deficit should be given in the 1st 1–2 hr, followed by the rest during and after the operation. If there are signs of dehydration, a volume equivalent to 7% of the body weight is administered; half of the deficit should be given preoperatively. For severe cases of dehydration 10–15% of the body weight is required as a replacement volume. An adequate urinary output should be established before surgery.

It is essential that antibiotics be given before the operation when the appendix has ruptured to ensure adequate blood and tissue levels of the drugs used. Triple intravenous therapy using an aminoglycoside, ampicillin, and clindamycin or 1 of the more recent cephalosporins is the treatment of choice. Appendectomy is necessary to limit continued fecal contamination of the peritoneum. After surgery a normal fluid and electrolyte balance should be maintained, and the stomach and bowel should be kept decompressed by effective nasogastric suction until intestinal activity returns.

Prognosis. The prognosis is excellent provided an appendectomy is performed before perforation has occurred, but even after perforation the prognosis is good. In 550 children with generalized peritonitis from ruptured appendix operated on at The Hospital for Sick Children, Toronto, 3 deaths (0.5%) occurred.

Complications. The most common postoperative complication is infection, usually of the wound. However, pelvic, subphrenic, or other intra-abdominal suppuration is especially likely to develop after operation on a gangrenous, perforated appendix. Ultrasound is a useful diagnostic aid at this stage. There is no urgent need for the surgeon to reoperate because of the development of intra-abdominal suppuration. Almost all pelvic abscesses will rupture into an adjacent loop of bowel and spontaneously resolve. It is virtually never necessary to drain these by the rectum. Subphrenic suppuration requires surgical drainage.

Prolonged paralytic ileus is often seen following generalized peritonitis; it may be aggravated by premature attempts at oral feedings.

Intestinal obstruction may occur as a postoperative complication. If this happens within 30 days of the appendectomy, nonoperative management is advisable. If obstruction occurs more than 30 days later and there is no evidence of ischemia of the bowel, nasogastric compression may be attempted for a short period (48 hr); if this is unsuccessful, a laparotomy will be necessary. A volvulus may be present with gangrenous bowel caused by a single adhesion in the right lower quadrant. This complication may occur many yr after the appendectomy. Pelvic peritonitis due to a ruptured appendix may result in obstruction to the uterine tubes with consequent sterility.

The Appendix and Chronic Abdominal Pain. Obstruction of the vermiform appendix, whether by fibrous band, worms, or fecalith, used to be considered an important cause of recurrent or chronic abdominal pain, and many children were subjected to elective appendectomy for this reason. Although some children may have been helped, most continued to have pain and were belatedly diagnosed as having urinary tract pathology, gastrointestinal malfunction unrelated to the appendix, or psychologically induced pain. Recurrent appendiceal obstruction is a rare cause of chronic or intermittent abdominal pain; an operation should be considered only after careful evaluation of these other possibilities. It is doubtful that chronic inflammation of the appendix ever occurs.

Acute Mesenteric Lymphadenitis. This ill-defined entity is frequently associated with an acute infection of the upper respiratory tract that may initially simulate acute appendicitis. Both acute and chronic involvement of the mesenteric lymph nodes may also be associated with infections of the appendix and the intestine.

JAMES C. FALLIS
BARRY SHANDLING

Apley J: The Child with Abdominal Pains. Ed 2. Oxford, Blackwell Scientific Publications, 1975.
Bartlett RH, Eraklis AJ, Wilkinson RH: Appendicitis in infancy. Surg Gynecol Obstet 130:99, 1970.
Johnson W, Borella L: Acute appendicitis in childhood leukemia. J Pediatr 67:595, 1965.
Raffensperger JG, Seeler RA, Moncada R: The Acute Abdomen in Infancy and Childhood. Chapters 10 and 12. Philadelphia, JB Lippincott, 1970.
Shandling B, Ein SH, Simpson JS, et al: Perforating appendicitis and antibiotics. J Pediatr Surg 9:79, 1974.

11.73   DISEASES OF ANUS, RECTUM, AND COLON

Close inspection of the anal area is usually of greater value than a digital examination in infants and children. Suspected fissures can be best identified by having the mother hold the infant's hips in acute flexion for the examiner to separate the patient's buttocks, using both thumbs, gently stretching the anus and everting the lining to expose the fissure. However, in all cases of constipation, especially when an intrinsic or extrinsic rectal obstruction is possible, a digital rectal examination is indicated. Properly done, this should cause little or no discomfort to the patient. A well lubricated finger is passed over the anus a few times to accustom the patient to the unusual sensation. Then the pulp of the index finger is pressed against the anus with increasing flexion of the interphalangeal joints and the finger slips easily and painlessly into the anal canal.

ANAL FISSURE

A small slit or crack at the mucocutaneous line is a common acquired lesion in infancy and an uncommon lesion in the school-aged child. Most anal fissures occur in the sagittal plane, usually dorsally in the midline. The cause is often not evident but may be trauma secondary to overzealous cleaning, constipation with passage of large hard stools, scratching induced by irritation from *Enterobius vermicularis* or eczema, or other perianal conditions.

Clinical Manifestations. Pain on defecation and, frequently, refusal to defecate are the principal manifestations. Bright red blood on the surface of the stool or on toilet paper and sometimes bleeding following defecation may be observed. The diagnosis is usually made by inspection of the anal area while the child is straining. The skin at the peripheral end of the fissure becomes swollen and forms a "tag." A history of prolapse of some tissue suggests a rectal polyp rather than a tag. Fissures also occur with Crohn disease.

Treatment. Most fissures will heal spontaneously if the local irritation is lessened or eliminated. The pain is the result of spasm of the lower fibers of the internal sphincter. The administration of laxatives to keep the stool fluid affords only temporary relief as eventually a more substantial stool must be passed with recurrence of the pain. If the patient is passing very hard stools, a mild stool softener may be useful, but the aim should not be to render the stools fluid. The addition of natural bran to the diet (1–3 tablespoons depending on the child's age) is of great value in softening the stool. Although anesthetic ointment is traditionally prescribed, it is often not helpful since it is most effective when applied 30 min before a bowel movement, which is impossible to predict in an infant. In contrast, dilatation by the mother with a well lubricated index finger inserted into the infant's anus twice daily for 1–2 wk will cure most anal fissures. A well formed but not hard stool makes an excellent dilator of the anal canal and is attended by less psychic trauma than anal digital dilatation. Sitz baths may be a useful adjunct. Often the entire perianal skin is excoriated and inflamed, and sometimes multiple superficial anal fissures occur. In such cases an ointment or cream with a triamcinolone base is useful.

If there is no response to medical management or if the fissure has been present a long time, a minor operation may be indicated since excessively prolonged symptoms from a fissure may result in the development of acquired megacolon with fecal impaction and encopresis. The operation is done under general anesthesia and may consist of stretching the anus, excision of the fissure, internal anal sphincterotomy, or a combination of the 3 procedures. Minimal postoperative discomfort occurs; recurrence is unusual.

ANORECTAL ABSCESS

A perianal abscess may occur in young infants, often starting as a small perianal pustule from an infected diaper rash. The infection usually gains entrance to the ischiorectal fossa through the anal crypts and the preformed spaces and soon extends into the subcutaneous tissues and develops into a nodule, usually within 1.5 cm of the anus. The symptoms are pain and swelling. Defecation is painful, and the child is unable to sit comfortably. The temperature is usually not elevated unless the perirectal space is infected. A painful swelling overlies the ischiorectal fossa, with redness, heat, induration, and fluctuation. Treatment consists of immediate incision and drainage under anesthesia. In contrast to cervical lymphadenopathy, it is not necessary to wait for fluctuation to develop before surgical drainage. Hot sitz baths are helpful postoperatively. Antibiotics are not efficacious in the treatment of perianal abscess. Often, after drainage a persistent or intermittent discharge of purulent material continues from the site of drainage, indicating an anal fistula.

Ischiorectal suppuration is occasionally seen in the older child or teenager and should suggest the possibility of Crohn disease or ulcerative colitis. The causative organism in this condition, as with most perianal abscesses, is usually *E. coli*. The treatment is prompt surgical drainage.

ANAL FISTULA

Fistulas originating in the anus or rectum may be congenital or acquired and rarely may extend to and communicate with the urinary bladder, urethra, vagina, or perianal skin. Acquired fistulas are residuals of an abscess and usually open on the skin surface. There is frequently a history of 1 or more incisions into the abscess, of neglect, or of antibiotic treatment of the abscess.

Clinical Manifestations. The symptoms of an acquired fistula are those of a painful swelling which recurs intermittently followed by a purulent discharge. Diagnosis is based on the presence of an opening into the skin beside the anal orifice into which a probe may be introduced.

Treatment. No fistulas close spontaneously. Simple incision and unroofing of the fistulous tract is always effective. Care must be taken not to injure the anal sphincter and cause incontinence.

HEMORRHOIDS

Hemorrhoids are uncommon in infants and children. When they are encountered, an underlying cause may be present, such as a venacaval or mesenteric obstruction, cirrhosis, portal hypertension, or other reasons for venous obstruction. Occasionally, chronic constipation, fecal impaction, and straining at stool result in hemorrhoids. Operation is rarely indicated except for an acute external thrombus. The hemorrhoids generally subside when the primary condition is corrected.

PRURITUS ANI

Anal itching in childhood is generally secondary to enterobiasis, anal fissures, and other local inflammatory lesions and to coarse or moist undergarments. Nocturnal itching is perhaps the most frequent evidence of pinworm infestation. Treatment consists of eradication of the underlying cause and cleansing the anal area with a mild soap and drying it with a soft cloth or tissue. Powders or solutions such as witch hazel may be used. In small infants exposure to sunlight or dry heat for as long as possible is helpful when the anal area is inflamed.

PROLAPSE AND PROCIDENTIA OF THE RECTUM AND SIGMOID

Prolapse is abnormal descent of the mucous membrane of the rectum with or without protrusion through the anal orifice; *procidentia* is abnormal descent of all the coats of the rectum or sigmoid with or without protrusion through the anus. These conditions are most common from 3–5 yr of age. The infantile rectum lies on a lower plane than the other pelvic organs; this anatomy, combined with the effect of the nearly vertical infantile sacrum, predisposes to prolapse. Any factor causing suddenly increased intra-abdominal pressure, such as straining at bowel movements after prolonged sitting with the hips and knees flexed, may precipitate abnormal descent of the bowel wall. Malnutrition with absorption of ischiorectal fat is a contributory factor. Children with chronic malabsorption, particularly cystic fibrosis, are prone to develop prolapse. Protrusion at stool initially recedes spontaneously but later requires manual replacement. Bleeding and the passage of mucus may occur. The protruding mass varies from bright to dark red; it may be as much as 6 in long. In prolapse the striations or furrows radiate from the center of the anal aperture in contrast to the concentrically arranged rosette of procidentia. Both conditions must be differentiated from an intussusception with the apex presenting at the anus.

Treatment should be directed to dietary correction of constipation, to proper toilet training, and to the elimination of any underlying disturbance, such as parasitic infection, diarrhea, or polyps. Oral administration of mineral oil, modification of the defecatory position by having the child empty his bowels with his feet off the floor, and strapping the buttocks together with adhesive tape, having first placed a cotton ball over the anal area, may be helpful.

Reduction of protrusion is aided by pressure with warm compresses. An easy method of reduction is to cover the finger with a piece of toilet paper, introduce it into the lumen of the mass, and gently push it into the rectum. The finger is then immediately withdrawn. The toilet paper adheres to the mucous membrane, permitting release of the finger; the paper, when softened, is later expelled. For intractable cases perineal operation may, on rare occasion, be indicated. Submucosal injection of sclerosants into the rectal ampulla is an effective means of preventing prolapse when prolonged attempts at medical therapy have failed. In procidentia of the rectum and sigmoid, abdominal sigmoidopexy is required.

POSTANAL DIMPLE

A postanal dimple is seen relatively frequently in normal babies, located behind the anus, close to the upper limit of the natal cleft. It almost never requires treatment except when it is very deep and becomes the site of minor recurrent infections. If simple hygienic measures are inadequate, excision of the dimple may be necessary.

A dermal sinus is present when there is a communication between a postanal dimple and the sacrum or coccyx. Such a tract may be attached to the dural linings of the spinal canal. This lesion requires meticulous excision to prevent the development of postoperative meningitis.

A *pilonidal sinus* is an acquired condition which is not a sequel to or a complication of a postanal dimple. It consists of 1 or several pits dorsal to the anus and is usually seen in hairy youths. The physician is consulted when infection supervenes. A pilonidal sinus results from shed hairs piercing the skin in the natal cleft. This may follow undue friction of the buttocks, and during World War II it was called "jeep driver's disease." A similar condition is seen in the interdigital webs on the hands of barbers. The sinus tract may become obstructed forming a *pilonidal cyst* or abscess.

Pilonidal cysts and sinuses do not cause symptoms unless infected. Swelling, heat, redness, tenderness, and fluctuation over the sacrococcygeal region are characteristic of an infected sinus. Purulent material may be discharged from 1 or more openings. If infection occurs, total excision or drainage should be performed.

BARRY SHANDLING

11.74 TUMORS OF THE DIGESTIVE TRACT IN CHILDREN

See also Sec 15.17.

Juvenile Colonic Polyp. This is the most common tumor of the bowel seen in childhood. It is hamartomatous and has no potential for malignancy. The lesion usually appears after the 1st yr and rarely persists beyond the age of 15. Approximately 80% are found in the distal segment of the large bowel within reach of a sigmoidoscope, and all but 10% are distal to the splenic flexure. Rarely, multiple colonic juvenile polyps occur in families; these lesions are identical to those described above and are also without malignant potential.

The typical *clinical manifestation* is painless rectal bleeding. Blood may be on the stool or mixed with it,

but the amount is usually modest. Losses may not become visible; an iron deficiency anemia from blood loss may be the initial problem. There may be crampy pain if the lesion causes the bowel to intussuscept or if a polyp prolapses. Most polyps infarct and pass spontaneously.

The *differential diagnosis* includes other forms of polyposis, particularly the familial types, Meckel diverticulum, fissure in ano, and inflammatory problems including infection, Crohn disease, and other forms of colitis.

Diagnosis may be made by rectal examination. About one third of these polyps are within reach of the examining finger, although they are difficult to feel. Most are visible on sigmoidoscopy as smooth, pedunculated lesions containing gray-white cysts. An air contrast barium enema may show lesions above the level of sigmoidoscopic examination. Fiberoptic colonoscopy, which allows for the visualization of at least the descending colon and often the transverse and proximal segments, is the preferred diagnostic procedure. When a polyp is observed at endoscopy, it should be biopsied to confirm its hamartomatous nature.

Treatment is conservative for this self-limited, nonmalignant problem except in rare cases in which hemorrhage is life-threatening. If the polyp can be reached with forceps, it can be removed per rectum using a speculum. Experience with removing more proximal polyps via colonoscopy is increasing, but the use of the technique is not widespread. Laparotomy for polyp removal is recommended only for multiple proximal polyps if they cannot be adequately assessed and treated by colonoscopy.

Familial Polyposis Syndromes. The rare familial syndromes associated with intestinal polyposis are important because they represent premalignant states which raise the fear of cancer in the patient or family.

Familial Adenomatous Polyposis Coli. This dominant premalignant condition with reduced penetrance is characterized by large numbers of adenomatous lesions in the distal large bowel. Although earlier lesions are reported, the usual onset is late in the 1st decade of life or during the teens. Initially, the polyps are asymptomatic and in many cases remain so. When symptomatic, they cause diarrhea, then blood loss, and, occasionally, crampy pain. Malignancy may develop during the teens.

The diagnosis should be suspected from the family history, but no technique is available for prediction of the disorder in a young child of a proven case. Diagnosis is made by showing filling defects in a double contrast barium enema and finding various sized polyps on sigmoidoscopy or colonoscopy. The polyps are usually numerous; biopsies show that they are adenomatous without the inflammatory and cystic findings of the juvenile polyp.

Treatment consists of a careful family survey, genetic counseling, and, for diagnosed cases, pancolectomy. This approach has meant an ileostomy, but recently developed anastomotic procedures may permit restoration of bowel continuity for preserving the muscle and serosal layers of the rectum.

Peutz-Jeghers Syndrome. This rare dominantly inherited syndrome is characterized by mucosal pigmentation of the lips and gums and hamartomas of the stomach and small bowel. The polyps are not premalignant. Deeply pigmented discrete freckles are usually seen at birth or appear during infancy in the lips, buccal mucosa, and even around the mouth. Later evidence of intestinal lesions may come from bleeding, crampy pain associated with obstruction, and even intussusception.

Treatment is directed at family studies and genetic counseling. Relatives may be found with either partial or complete manifestations of the syndrome. Intestinal lesions that are causing significant symptoms should be excised; involvement is usually too extensive to remove all the polyps.

Gardner Syndrome. This rare, dominantly inherited disorder is characterized by multiple intestinal polyps and tumors of the soft tissue and bone, particularly the mandible. The soft tissue lesions and osteomas may appear during childhood, but intestinal polyps usually do not become apparent until early adult life. These polyps may develop anywhere along the digestive tract and are premalignant. Therefore, aggressive surgical treatment of the intestinal lesions is indicated.

Hemangioma of the Intestine. These rare benign lesions can cause massive, even fatal intestinal hemorrhage. The usual clinical manifestation is painless bleeding beginning in childhood. The blood loss can be subtle and chronic, but it may be sudden and large in amount. Usually, there are no additional intestinal symptoms, but, if intussusception occurs, there will be obstructive symptoms. About 50% of patients have cutaneous hemangiomas and, in some, a family history of similar lesions. About half of these lesions are in the colon, where they may be seen by colonoscopy. During a period of bleeding selective mesenteric arteriography may be useful in identifying a lesion.

Leiomyoma. This rare benign tumor occurs most commonly in stomach and jejunum. It remains asymptomatic for long periods, but, if it extends into the lumen, it may cause intussusception and abdominal pain.

Carcinoma. The fact that epithelial tumors of the digestive tract are extremely rare in children argues against an aggressive diagnostic approach to many gastrointestinal symptoms in this age group. Several conditions predispose the patient to developing adenocarcinoma of the gut: familial polyposis, Gardner syndrome, idiopathic ulcerative colitis, and, to a lesser extent, Crohn disease and disorders associated with chromosomal breaks. In these disorders tumors are not usually seen until adult life.

The usual site of the lesion is the colon. Symptoms are general ill health, abdominal pain, a palpable abdominal mass, and, less frequently, hemorrhage. When these tumors do develop, they are often relatively undifferentiated and highly malignant.

Lymphosarcoma of the Intestine. Malignancies of the digestive tract are very rare in children; most of them are lymphosarcomas (Sec 15.5). The usual site is the lower small intestine. Manifestations are those of general ill health, abdominal pain, and anemia. Adults with longstanding celiac disease have a relatively high incidence of lymphosarcoma; a beneficial effect of dietary treatment on the basis of this relationship has been suggested but not proved.

Carcinoid Tumors (Sec 15.10). These tumors of the enterochromaffin cells of the intestine usually occur in the appendix in children and have very low grade malignancy. They cause symptoms similar to those of appendicitis and do not recur after resection, even when the tumor has extended to the muscularis and lymphatics.

Usually, carcinoid tumors outside the appendix metastasize, and the metastatic lesions give rise to the carcinoid syndrome. This syndrome, the result of pharmacologically active secretions produced by the tumor, is characterized by episodic intestinal hypermotility and diarrhea, vasomotor disturbances, and bronchoconstriction. The most important active substance is serotonin. The diagnosis is usually made by finding high urinary levels of its metabolite 5-hydroxyindoleacetic acid. These functioning neoplasms are very rarely seen in children.

Abrahamson J, Shandling B: Intestinal hemangiomata in childhood and a syndrome for diagnosis: A collective review. J Pediatr Surg 8:487, 1973.
Bartholomew LG: Peutz-Jeghers syndrome. JAMA 183:901, 1963.
Berry CL, Keeling JW: Gastrointestinal lymphoma in childhood. J Clin Pathol 23:459, 1970.
Cohen SB, Pavlidos GP, Krush AJ, et al: Familial polyposis coli. Md State Med J 27:64, 1978.
Gardner EJ, Richards RC: Multiple cutaneous and subcutaneous lesions occurring simultaneously with hereditary polyposis and osteomatosis. Am J Hum Genet 5:130, 1953.
Holgerson LO, Miller RE, Zintel HA: Juvenile polyps of the colon. Surgery 69:288, 1971.
Mazier WP, Bowman HE, Ming Sun K, et al: Juvenile polyps of the colon and rectum. Dis Colon Rectum 17:523, 1974.
Mestel DL: Lymphosarcoma of small intestine in infancy and childhood. Am Surg 149:87, 1949.
Postlethwait RW: Gastrointestinal carcinoid tumors—a review. Postgrad Med 40:445, 1966.
Recalde M, Holyoke ED, Elias EG: Carcinoma of the colon, rectum and anal canal in young patients. Surg Gynecol Obstet 139:909, 1974.

Functioning Tumors Causing Diarrhea. Certain hormone-producing tumors may cause an increase in secretion leading to severe chronic diarrhea. The most common of these rare functioning tumors are those arising from the neural crest. *Neuroblastoma* or *ganglioneuroma* occurs most often in the adrenal gland but may develop anywhere along the sympathetic chain (Sec 18.28). A diarrhea syndrome probably mediated by vasoactive intestinal peptide (VIP), a secretagogue produced by the tumor, is associated with about 10% of these lesions. The resultant diarrhea may fluctuate in intensity but is usually massive, causing systemic fluid and electrolyte imbalance. Diagnosis is made by identifying the tumor and its secretory products, which include catecholamines and their metabolites. Pheochromocytomas do not cause diarrhea. Severe diarrhea is seldom associated with the rare *Zollinger-Ellison syndrome* in children (Sec 11.22); in this disorder the clinical manifestations are attributed to a gastrin-secreting pancreatic islet tumor. Rare non-gastrin-secreting pancreatic *islet tumors* may also cause diarrhea; the secretagogue may also be a VIP.

Buchta RM, Kaplan JM: Zollinger-Ellison syndrome in a nine-year old child: A case report and review of this entity in childhood. Pediatrics 47:594, 1971.

Hamilton JR, Radde IC, Johnson G: Diarrhea associated with adrenal ganglioneuroma. New findings related to the pathogenesis of diarrhea. Am J Med 44:473, 1968.

Mitchell CH, Sinatra FR, Crast FW, et al: Intractable watery diarrhea, ganglioneuroblastoma and vasoactive intestinal peptide. J Pediatr 89:593, 1976.

Rambaud JC, Modigliani R, et al: Pancreatic cholera: Studies on tumor secretions and pathophysiology of diarrhea. Gastroenterology 69:110, 1975.

Verner JV, Morrison AB: Islet cell tumor and a syndrome of refractory watery diarrhea and hypokalemia. Am J Med 25:374, 1958.

Nodular Lymphoid Hyperplasia. Lymphoid follicles in the lamina propria of the gut normally aggregate in Peyer patches. These areas appear as submucosal nodules which may be visible on barium contrast roentgenograms and mistaken for an abnormality. Peyer patches are much more frequent in the lower than the upper small bowel. In some patients lymphoid follicles become hyperplastic. The hyperplasia may occur in the colon or extend to the small bowel. Small bowel lesions are seen in cases of immunoglobulin deficiency with and without *Giardia lamblia* infestation. Symptoms are mild. There may be rectal bleeding, diarrhea, and abdominal cramps beginning usually by 3 yr of age.

The major importance of this entity is the similarity of its manifestations to more serious disorders. Lymphoid hyperplasia resolves spontaneously and requires no specific treatment.

J. RICHARD HAMILTON

Hodgson JR, Hoffman HN, Huizenga KA: Roentgenologic features of lymphoid hyperplasia of the small intestine associated with dysgammaglobulinemia. Radiology 88:883, 1967.

Poley JR, Smith EI: Benign lymphatic hyperplasia of the rectum. South Med J 65:420, 1972.

TUMORS OF THE SACROCOCCYGEAL REGION

See Chapter 15.

11.75   HERNIAS

A hernia is a protrusion of the contents of a body compartment through the wall that normally encloses it. Hernias or "ruptures" and hydroceles (Sec 16.61) are the most common significant anomalies of children. The most common hernia of the groin in infancy and childhood is the indirect (congenital, infantile) inguinal hernia. Femoral and direct inguinal hernias are rare in children. Congenital posterolateral diaphragmatic hernias and esophageal hiatal hernias are discussed in Sec 11.105 and 11.20, respectively. Omphaloceles and umbilical hernias are covered in Sec 7.53.

INDIRECT INGUINAL HERNIAS

Pathology and Pathogenesis. During the later stages of fetal development the processus vaginalis, an outpouching of peritoneum originating at the internal ring, extends medially down each inguinal canal. Leaving the canal at the external ring, the process turns inferiorly in the male into the scrotum, where it invests the developing testicle. Its lumen normally obliterates completely before birth except for the portion enveloping the testicle. This part remains as a potential sac, the tunica vaginalis. In the developing female the process extends from the external ring into the labia majora. The proximal part of the processus vaginalis may fail to close, producing a potential hernial sac, into which an abdominal viscus may herniate. The patent portion extends inferiorly a variable distance, sometimes into the scrotum, where it may be continuous with the tunica vaginalis, forming a complete hernia.

Inguinal hernias are particularly common in premature infants, presumably because there was less time for intrauterine development, hence for the entire process of closure. When the testicle fails to descend (cryptorchid), there is usually a large hernial sac, probably because something has arrested both testicular descent and closure of the peritoneal process. Children with multiple congenital anomalies, particularly those involving the lower abdomen, pelvis, or perineum, often have inguinal hernias as part of the complex.

Clinical Manifestations. Usually, a swelling is noted at the external ring, but it may extend for a variable distance downward into the scrotum or labium majus. The lump may be present always, or it may be apparent only with raised intra-abdominal pressure, such as when an infant cries or strains at stool. In the older child the mass typically appears at the end of an active day or with vigorous coughing. A hernia usually disappears when a baby relaxes with a bottle or when an older child lies down. The diagnosis of inguinal hernia in infancy and childhood may be made from history alone even if significant physical findings are absent when the child is seen by the doctor so long as the typical swelling is described by a competent observer. Usually, however, it is preferable that the surgeon see and feel the lump for himself to rule out the possibility of a retracted testis or another etiology.

Uncomplicated inguinal hernias in children rarely cause pain; pain in the groin is much more likely to be caused by hip disease than by a hernia. Occasionally, a baby will cry constantly when the hernia protrudes, but usually the hernia is protruding because the child is crying.

The older child with a hernia may have had a hydrocele in early infancy.

The observation of an inguinal or inguinoscrotal mass which reduces either spontaneously or with manipulation is diagnostic. If the hernia is not present on initial inspection, inducing the baby to cry while the abdomen is firmly compressed is very likely to force it out. In the older child the hernia can usually be demonstrated by having the patient strain down when in the standing position as the examiner manually compresses the abdomen. If these maneuvers fail to demonstrate a suspected hernia, the diagnosis may be supported by palpation of a thickened spermatic cord on the side in question. Occasionally, the examiner may feel a silken sensation as he gently rolls the spermatic cord back and forth over the pubis with 1 finger ("silk glove sign"); this sensation is produced by the 2 peritoneal layers of the sac rubbing on each other. Introducing a finger into the external ring to detect a peritoneal impulse is of no value since the ring may be so large and the canal so short that an impulse is often readily palpable in the absence of herniation. Occasionally, a full bladder may occlude the internal inguinal ring and prevent elicitation of the physical findings of the hernia; having the child urinate will enable the hernia to be demonstrable.

Treatment. The treatment of choice for inguinal hernia in infancy and childhood is surgical repair. For the older child this is carried out at the earliest convenient time. In a young infant an inguinal hernia should be repaired on an urgent basis when the patient's general condition is satisfactory in order to remove the risk of incarceration. Except in the 1st few wk of life or in the older teenager, surgical repair is best done on an outpatient basis, provided appropriate facilities for surgery of ambulatory patients are available.

Supports and trusses designed to keep the abdominal contents from protruding into a hernial sac are not indicated.

Any inguinal hernia that cannot be reduced needs emergency surgical repair. Resection may be required if strangulation of bowel has occurred but is almost never necessary.

Although a bleeding tendency is generally a contraindication to surgery, the child with hemophilia should have his hernia repaired. Replacement therapy should be instituted prior to surgery and carried out after operation.

When associated with prematurity, a hernia should be repaired only after the infant gains strength and weight in the hospital. During this time the hernia should be carefully watched and manually reduced as necessary. When the baby is big enough to go home, the hernia should be operated upon in a facility accustomed to caring for small infants.

Complications. A hernia is incarcerated when its contents cannot be reduced and the contained bowel is obstructed. A hernia may seem irreducible on initial examination but prove to be reducible when the manipulation is carried out by a more experienced physician. Incarceration of an inguinal hernia is most likely to occur at the external inguinal ring and, with time, produces obstruction of the venous return from the herniated bowel. This results in edema and progresses to venous infarction. The risk of incarceration is greatest in the youngest children. When the circulation to bowel

has become compromised, the hernia is said to be strangulated. Redness, edema, and tenderness of the lump indicate strangulation and impending necrosis. Cramps, bilious vomiting, and distention will occur with incarceration of bowel as the picture of intestinal obstruction develops. Irritability may be the only symptom of incarcerated hernia in an infant, and the diagnosis may be missed if the infant is not examined completely undressed.

A *Richter hernia* is a rare form of incarceration in which only a part of the bowel's circumference is pinched off within the hernia and intestinal obstruction does not develop. Venous infarction of the testicle is also a common result of hernial incarceration as the spermatic cord is readily compressed between the margin of the external ring and the hernial contents.

Inguinal Hernias in Girls. About 10% of inguinal hernias in children occur in girls. In an infant girl the ovary is the organ most likely to herniate into the inguinal canal, where it is usually easily palpable as a movable almond-sized nodule. Although uncommon, infarction of the herniated ovary may occur because of torsion or compression of the pedicle. The inflamed abscess-like lesion which then develops in the groin is easily mistaken for inguinal lymphadenitis if one forgets that there are no lymph nodes in the anterior abdominal wall immediately above the inguinal ligament. In about 1% of operations on apparent "girls" for inguinal hernial repair, a testicle is discovered in the canal, abdomen, or labia majora. Closer examination reveals completely normal external genitalia although the vagina is a little shorter than usual. Laparotomy in such instances reveals the absence of female internal genital organs. The absence of chromatin bodies on buccal smear confirms the diagnosis of testicular feminization (Sec 18.46).

Prognosis. The prognosis following surgical repair of an inguinal hernia in an infant or child is excellent. The complication rate is low and recurrences should be fewer than 1% following surgery.

JAMES C. FALLIS

Hendren WH, Crawford JD: The child with ambiguous genitalia. Curr Probl Surg 1–64, Nov, 1972.
Mustard WT, Ravitch MM, Snyder WH, et al (eds): Pediatric Surgery. Ed 2. Chicago, Year Book Medical Publishers, 1969, Chapter 46.

The Exocrine Pancreas

11.76 DEVELOPMENT AND FUNCTION OF PANCREAS

Development. The pancreas appears at 5 wk of embryonic life as 2 outpouchings of the duodenum, ventral and dorsal. By 7 wk these pouches have rotated and fused to take up their established positions to the left of the duodenum, with the ventral derivative form-

ing the posterior and lower portion of the pancreatic head drained by the duct of Wirsung and the dorsal derivative the body and the tail of the pancreas drained by the duct of Santorini. A variety of patterns arise from fusion of the 2 duct systems. The duct of Wirsung usually maintains its connection with the bile duct during rotation and opens into the papilla of Vater as the major excretory duct of the pancreas. The duct of Santorini most commonly fuses with and enters the major pancreatic duct but in 10% of people drains into the duodenum independently. The main pancreatic duct and the bile duct may also enter separately.

Exocrine and endocrine cells develop at the tips of the bifurcating duct systems, gradually filling the mesenchymal space between them. The exocrine cells form acinar glands, each drained by a small ductule connected through larger channels with the major duct system. Endocrine cells form nests in the interstices between acini. Zymogen granules containing pancreatic enzymes are present in exocrine cells at the 4th mo of gestation, but acinar growth is not complete until the age of 1–2 yr. Enzyme output is therefore relatively low during infancy although generally sufficient to provide adequate intraluminal digestion even in premature infants.

Function. Acinar cells secrete a variety of enzymes which degrade the macromolecular constituents of food to simpler compounds suitable for digestion and absorption by the intestine. α-Amylase splits the extended oligosaccharide chains of starch and other polysaccharides by cleaving α-1,4 glucosidic bonds and forming maltose, isomaltose, and small molecular weight dextrins with α-1,6 branch points. Proteolytic endopeptidases, trypsin, chymotrypsin, and elastase attack peptide bonds within proteins, producing a variety of smaller peptides that are ultimately degraded by aminopeptidases of the intestinal surface. The exopeptidases, carboxypeptidases A and B, cleave terminal amino acids from some of these peptides. Each of the proteolytic enzymes is secreted as an inactive proenzyme blocked in its function by a terminal peptide segment. Activation depends on the collision of the trypsin proenzyme, trypsinogen, with the intestinal brush border endopeptidase, enterokinase, which releases the blocking segment and permits trypsin to attack and activate the proenzymes of the remaining proteases. In this way proteolytic activity is reserved for nutrients in the intestinal lumen and is absent within the pancreas and its ducts, where autodigestion of pancreatic tissue might occur. A phospholipase which might also digest pancreatic tissue is secreted similarly as an inactive precursor and activated by trypsin. Lipase, which hydrolyzes triglycerides to monoglycerides and fatty acids, is secreted as an active enzyme.

The exocrine pancreas also secretes fluid and electrolytes. The daily volume is approximately 1500 dl in the adult. Sodium and potassium concentrations are similar to those of the plasma. Bicarbonate originates in the cells lining the smaller pancreatic ducts and rises to several times the concentration of plasma as pancreatic flow increases.

Secretion is under both hormonal and neurogenic control. Two hormones are elaborated by the epithelium of the upper intestine, cholecystokinin-pancreozymin, which primarily stimulates enzyme secretion, and secretin, which stimulates fluid and bicarbonate secretion. Cholecystokinin-pancreozymin also stimulates the release of enterokinase from the brush border of the intestinal epithelium into the lumen, enhancing the opportunity for contact of this activating enzyme with trypsinogen. Hormone secretion responds to food products and acid in the duodenum and is therefore closely regulated by requirements for the digestion of nutrients.

Pancreatic secretion is also mediated by visceral efferent fibers of the vagus, which mimic cholecystokinin-pancreozymin in their effects.

Zoppi et al studied pancreatic secretion in response to cholecystokinin-pancreozymin and secretin in premature and full-term infants. Trypsin and lipase secretion at birth was approximately the same in both groups, but amylase secretion was 5-fold greater in the full-term infants. In childhood, secretion of trypsin and lipase was 10-fold greater than in the full-term newborn infant. Normally, enzyme levels rise gradually during infancy, but Zoppi showed that mature concentrations could be induced within 1 mo by high protein diets. Amylase secretion, comparatively much lower in infants, rises 300- to 500-fold by early childhood, but this enzyme adapts sluggishly to a starch diet. However, starch intolerance due to maldigestion is extremely rare; therefore, amylase output seems generally to be adequate for infant requirements.

Pancreatic function can be assessed by measuring the secretion of enzymes, fluid, and bicarbonate in response to exogenous hormones (exogenous response) or in response to food, fat, or amino acid in the intestine (endogenous response). For this purpose a tube must be placed in the duodenum under fluoroscopic control to collect pancreatic juice. Exogenous and endogenous responses are not always equal, particularly when the intestinal mucosa is damaged and the cells are incapable of producing endogenous cholecystokinin-pancreozymin and secretin. A more quantitative assessment of total pancreatic secretory capacity can be achieved by perfusing the duodenum with fluid containing a nonabsorbable marker substance while stimulating secretory activity with an intravenous infusion of hormone. A 2nd tube must be placed in the stomach to siphon off gastric contents to prevent their mixing with pancreatic secretions.

A less direct evaluation of pancreatic function can be obtained by examining stool under the microscope for unhydrolyzed neutral fat droplets and muscle fibers which accumulate when digestive enzymes are missing. The measurement of stool proteases, usually trypsin and chymotrypsin, is useful when coupled with a 3 or 5 day stool collection since enzyme activity in stool is usually quite low in pancreatic insufficiency. *Enterokinase deficiency*, a rare but important cause of infantile malnutrition and diarrhea, can be detected by examining duodenal juice for its ability to activate trypsinogen.

Borgstrom B, Lindquist B, Lundh G: Enzyme concentration and absorption of protein and glucose in the duodenum of premature infants. Am J Dis Child 99:338, 1960.

Hadorn B: The exocrine pancreas. In: Anderson CM, Burke V (eds): Paediatric Gastroenterology. London, Blackwell Scientific Publications, 1975.

Go V, Hofmann A, Summerskill WH: Pancreozymin bioassay in man based on pancreatic enzyme secretion: Potency of specific amino acids and other digestive products. J Clin Invest 49:1558, 1970.

Zoppi G, Andreotti G, Pajano-Ferrara F, et al: Exocrine pancreas function in premature and full term neonates. Pediatr Res 6:880, 1972.

11.77 ANOMALIES OF THE PANCREAS

Annular Pancreas. This rare anomaly occurs when a portion of the embryonic ventral pancreas remains behind as the rest of the organ rotates posteriorly during the 6th embryonic wk and thereafter completes the fusion of a complete pancreatic ring around the duodenum.

The clinical manifestations depend on the extent to which the duodenum is obstructed. Maternal polyhydramnios, complete or partial duodenal obstruction in the newborn period, symptoms of obstruction arising later in childhood and adult life, or no symptoms may be seen. Occasionally, an obstructed bile duct causes episodes of biliary colic or pancreatitis. Roentgenograms are typical of an obstructing lesion in the 2nd part of the duodenum. Treatment is surgical bypass of the obstruction; the pancreas must not be dissected or divided.

Annular pancreas is often associated with other anomalies including Down syndrome, intestinal atresia, obstructive diaphragms, malrotation, and imperforate anus.

Congenital cysts of the pancreas are usually multiple. They are asymptomatic and are frequently associated with polycystic involvement of other organs.

Ectopic pancreatic tissue (*pancreatic rests*) can occur in the stomach or small intestine. Usually asymptomatic, these lesions can cause hemorrhage, ulceration, and obstruction or even, in rare instances, can serve as a lead point for an intussusception.

PANCREATIC INSUFFICIENCY—CYSTIC FIBROSIS

See Sec 12.110.

11.78 PANCREATIC INSUFFICIENCY NOT DUE TO CYSTIC FIBROSIS

Pancreatic Insufficiency with Neutropenia, Short Stature, and Bone Abnormalities (Shwachman Syndrome). This entity is 100 times less common than cystic fibrosis, but it is still the 2nd most common pancreatic cause of malabsorption in children. The etiology is unknown. There is an associated defect in the migration of peripheral polymorphonuclear leukocytes in response to chemotactic stimuli. An autosomal recessive inheritance pattern best fits the cases in which more than 1 sibling in a family is affected, but sporadic cases appear to be frequent.

Pancreatic acini are usually replaced by fat without fibrosis and with little damage to ducts or islets. Glandular loss must be more variable than the scarce pathologic specimens suggest since some patients are able to digest and absorb fat quite effectively, particularly as they grow older. After stimulation with cholecystokinin and secretin, pancreatic enzyme output is invariably low, but in contrast to symptoms of cystic fibrosis, water and bicarbonate secretion are well preserved. Neutropenia may be severe or mild, constant, episodic, or cyclic. Thrombocytopenia and a hypoplastic anemia are common but rarely of concern. In the bone marrow a maturation arrest in the granulocyte line and a reduction in committed granulocyte stem cells may occur but

are not constant. In about 50% of patients bone roentgenograms reveal metaphyseal dyschondroplasia; the femoral head is often affected initially, but any metaphysis may be involved. Abnormally short ribs with flared anterior ends are a striking feature in some patients. In a small number of patients the thoracic cage is sufficiently narrow at birth to interfere with respiration. Linear growth rates are normal in the absence of severe malnutrition, although 80% of patients are shorter than the 3rd percentile for height. Bone age is appropriate for height.

The diagnosis is usually made in infancy, when patients suffer most severely from recurrent infections and malabsorption. A normal sweat chloride readily distinguishes Shwachman patients from those with cystic fibrosis. Other causes of malabsorption are usually excluded easily by documenting pancreatic insufficiency and neutropenia. Occasionally, a patient with severe malnutrition will develop secondary pancreatic insufficiency and may have a relatively low leukocyte count. Shwachman syndrome can be excluded in these patients only by documenting the return of pancreatic function as malnutrition improves. Leukocyte mobility is impaired in malnutrition as well as in Shwachman syndrome.

There is no specific treatment. Pancreatic supplements are necessary in infancy but may not be required later in the absence of malabsorption. Most patients survive infancy, and their subsequent course is often surprisingly mild.

Congenital Enterokinase Deficiency. Sec 11.45.

Specific Pancreatic Enzyme Deficiencies. Rare cases are reported in which specific pancreatic enzymes appear to be deficient on a congenital basis, but their documentation is incomplete. The children reported as having lipase deficiency may actually have had pancreatic hypoplasia (Shwachman syndrome). Reported cases of trypsinogen deficiency may be examples of enterokinase deficiency.

Secondary pancreatic insufficiency occurs in malnourished infants as noted above and in patients with a severe enteropathy. In malnutrition the packaging of pancreatic enzymes may be compromised by the inability to support sustained protein synthesis, or secretory failure may result from decreased elaboration of stimulatory hormones. Enteropathy produces pancreatic insufficiency in the latter manner by destroying the cells which produce secretin and cholecystokinin-pancreozymin. In celiac disease, for example, patients are fully capable of producing a pancreatic response to exogenous hormone while unable to respond to the presence of acid or digestive products in the duodenum.

Anomalies

Barbosa JJ de C, Dockerty MB, Waugh JM: Pancreatic heterotopia: Review of the literature and report of 41 authenticated cases of which 25 were clinically significant. Surg Gynecol Obstet 2:527, 1946.

Montgomery RC, Poindexter MH, Hall GH, et al: Report of a case of annular pancreas of the newborn in two consecutive siblings. Pediatrics 48:148, 1971.

Ravitch MM: The pancreas in infants and children. Surg Clin North Am 55:377, 1975.

Pancreatic Insufficiency Not Due to Cystic Fibrosis

Aggett PJ, Cavanagh NPC, Matthew DJ, et al: Shwachman's syndrome. Arch Dis Child 55:331, 1980.

Bodian M, Sheldon W, Lightwood R: Congenital hypoplasia of the exocrine pancreas. Acta Pediatr Scand 53:282, 1964.

Burke V, Colebatch JH, Anderson CM, et al: Association of pancreatic insufficiency and chronic neutropenia in childhood. Arch Dis Child 42:147, 1967.

Schmerling DH, Prader A, Hitzig WH, et al: The syndrome of exocrine pancreatic insufficiency, neutropenia, metaphyseal dysostosis and dwarfism. Helv Paediatr Acta 24:547, 1969.

Schussheim A, Choi SJ: Exocrine pancreatic insufficiency with congenital anomalies. J Pediatr 89:782, 1976.

Shwachman H, Diamond LK, Oski FA, et al: The syndrome of pancreatic insufficiency and bone marrow dysfunction. J Pediatr 65:645, 1964.

11.79 PANCREATITIS

Etiology. The pancreas is particularly susceptible to inflammation because its glands contain an arsenal of potentially destructive proenzymes which, when activated, rapidly digest pancreatic tissue. Activating enzymes are found in leukocytes, serum, and bacteria; therefore, any condition which produces a local inflammatory response or causes retrograde infection of the pancreatic ducts may initiate a cascade of autodigestion. The causes of pancreatitis in children are listed in Table 11–12. The majority of cases occur after the age of 10 and are acute illnesses which can be attributed to drugs, toxins, trauma, and viral illnesses. The typical traumatic injury is a fall onto the handlebars of a bicycle, but any blunt trauma or abdominal operation will suffice. The incident may be trivial and the onset of pancreatitis somewhat delayed so that the association with trauma is easily missed without a careful history. Mumps is the most common cause of viral pancreatitis. Symptoms usually occur in association with other signs of the disease and are rather mild. Elevated amylase is present

Table 11–12 ETIOLOGY OF PANCREATITIS IN CHILDHOOD

Idiopathic
Drugs and toxins
  Thiazides
  Prednisone
  Alcohol
  Azathioprine
  Valproic acid
Trauma
Viral illnesses
  Mumps
  Reye syndrome
  Hepatitis A and B
  Rubella
  Coxsackie B
  Influenza A
Disease and anomalies of the bile and pancreatic ducts
  Cholelithiasis
  Ascaris lumbricoides
  Choledochal cyst
  Duplication cysts
  Anomalous insertion of the common bile duct
  Nonfusion of dorsal and ventral pancreas
Cystic fibrosis
Systemic illnesses
  Lupus erythematosus
  Periarteritis nodosa
  Hyperlipidemia, type I, IV, and V
  Hypercalcemia (hyperparathyroidism, etc.)
Hereditary pancreatitis

in approximately 50% of cases of Reye syndrome, often for a surprisingly prolonged period. However, pancreatitis is rarely the dominant feature of the disease. In about 1 case in 5 no cause is apparent.

Recurrent attacks of pancreatitis are relatively infrequent but create major diagnostic and therapeutic difficulties. Cholelithiasis and developmental anomalies of the biliary-pancreatic duct system are frequently found. Recurrent or chronic relapsing pancreatitis is also a feature of hereditary pancreatitis, a rare autosomal dominant condition; approximately 281 cases have been reported in 18 kindreds, chiefly in Whites from the United States. Cystic fibrosis is less well recognized as a cause of acute and recurrent pancreatitis, but both forms may occur in patients with sufficient pancreatic tissue to support normal absorption.

Clinical Manifestations. The dominant symptom is abdominal pain, epigastric, steady, and possibly radiating to the back. Usually nausea and vomiting occur. The child lies on his or her side and is very still. The abdomen is full, tender, and quiet, and in some cases a mass is palpable. If the lesion is hemorrhagic, blue discoloration about the umbilicus may be seen. In severe cases a pleural effusion and ascites may be found. Loss of large amounts of plasma into the pancreas and surrounding tissue may cause shock. High fever is an ominous sign associated with extensive pancreatic necrosis or abscess formation. In most instances symptoms improve gradually over 3–10 days. Prolonged abdominal discomfort or repeated attacks of pain over several wk may be associated with the development of a pancreatic pseudocyst, which is sometimes palpable. Very rarely, the appearance of an unexplained abdominal mass is the initial sign of pancreatitis.

Laboratory Manifestations. The serum amylase level is usually elevated within 12 hr of the onset but may return to normal within 24 hr. If ascitic or pleural fluid is obtained, it too will have a high amylase concentration. The ratio of the urinary clearance of amylase to that of creatinine is elevated, usually above 4.0, and is helpful in excluding nonpancreatic causes of hyperamylasemia such as mumps parotitis or macroamylasemia. There may be transient hyperglycemia and glycosuria. A low serum calcium concentration is a late and serious finding but rarely occurs in children. Plain roentgenograms of the abdomen may show dilated segments of small intestine (the sentinel loop) in the vicinity of the pancreas or generalized ileus. Calcification of the pancreas is rare in children except in hereditary pancreatitis. Roentgenograms of the stomach and duodenum may delineate large retroperitoneal pseudocysts which distort the duodenal loop or press forward against the stomach and into the lesser sac. Pancreatic ultrasonography is particularly helpful in detecting pseudocysts. It is also a sensitive technique for confirming the diagnosis of pancreatitis since the pancreatic density decreases while the organ is inflamed and returns to normal with improvement. Endoscopic retrograde cholangiopancreatography (ERCP) may demonstrate obstructing stones, ductal narrowing or tortuosity, and unusual anatomic alignments. It is, therefore, an essential part of the investigation of patients with recurrent attacks of pancreatitis. Steatorrhea is an extremely rare consequence of chronic recurrent pancreatitis in children but may be seen after corrective surgery or in some cases of hereditary pancreatitis.

Treatment. The main goals of therapy are to put the pancreas at rest and to support the patient. The vigor with which these efforts are made should depend on the seriousness of the illness, but in general it is best to err on the safe side. Oral feedings should be stopped, constant nasogastric suction begun, and intravenous fluids and electrolytes given. In some patients total parenteral nutrition may be needed; in others blood or albumin is necessary to combat shock. Demerol should be used for severe pain. The efficacy of anticholinergic agents and antibiotics is less certain, but they continue to be used with enthusiasm in most centers. Oral feedings can be started very slowly once symptoms have subsided but should be discontinued if pain recurs. A pseudocyst can be treated conservatively with prolonged parenteral nutrition in the early acute stage in the hope that it will spontaneously resorb. Cysts which continue to enlarge or persist for 6 wk will usually require surgical drainage. When ductal abnormalities have been outlined by ERCP, patients often benefit from a variety of surgical techniques directed at improving pancreatic drainage.

THE PANCREAS IN SYSTEMIC DISEASE

Acute and chronic changes in the pancreas are often associated with a variety of systemic diseases without producing symptoms that would lead to clinical recognition of pancreatic involvement. Infiltration of the pancreas by leukemia, Hodgkin disease, and other lymphogranulomatous conditions is common. Severe congenital syphilis involving the pancreas causes widespread fibrosis. Fibrotic changes with extensive atrophy of acinar tissue result from chronic passive congestion of the pancreas produced by longstanding cardiac decompensation. Miliary abscesses occur in association with septicemia and tubercles with miliary tuberculosis. Neoplasms of the pancreas in childhood are rare.

—GORDON FORSTNER

Pancreatitis

Craighead JE: The role of viruses in the pathogenesis of pancreatic disease and diabetes mellitus. Prog Med Virol 19:161, 1975.
Hendren WH, Greep JM, Patton AS: Pancreatitis in childhood: Experience with 15 cases. Arch Dis Child 40:132, 1965.
Jordan SC, Ament ME: Pancreatitis in children and adolescents. J Pediatr 91:211, 1977.
Kattwinkel J, Lapey L, di Sant'Agnese PA, et al: Hereditary pancreatitis: Three new kindreds and a critical review of the literature. Pediatrics 51:55, 1973.
Mallory A, Kern F: Drug-induced pancreatitis: A critical review. Gastroenterology 78:813, 1980.

Pseudocysts of the Pancreas

Bradley EL, Gonzalez AC, Clements JL: Acute pancreatic pseudocysts: Incidence and implications. Ann Surg 184:734, 1976.
Pena SDJ, Medovy H: Child abuse and traumatic pseudocyst of the pancreas. J Pediatr 83:1026, 1973.

LIVER AND BILIARY SYSTEM

11.80 DEVELOPMENT OF LIVER STRUCTURE AND FUNCTION

Anatomic and Cellular Morphogenesis. The embryology and anatomy of the liver and biliary tract provide the basis for understanding the physiology and pathophysiology of the liver and of congenital lesions of the bile ducts caused by abnormal organogenesis.

The liver, bile ducts, and gallbladder originate from a cluster of cells capping a ventral diverticulum in the primitive foregut. From day 18–22 of gestation the diverticulum is segmented into buds (Fig 11–21, 3 mm embryo), the solid cranial one evolving into the liver (pars hepatis) and the hollow caudal one (pars cystica) developing into the gallbladder, cystic duct, and common bile duct.

Epithelial cords and tubules extending from the cranial bud establish contact with blood vessels in the adjoining mesenchymal septum transversum (Fig 11–21, 5 mm embryo). The network of primitive hepatocytes, sinusoids, and septal mesenchyme establishes the basic architectural pattern of the adult liver lobule from 5–6 wk of gestation (Fig 11–21, 7 mm embryo).

Interlobular bile ducts differentiate from the intrahepatic ducts at points of contact with the connective tissue investing the branching portal vein. Terminal ductules (cholangioles) develop from vesicles which appear in hepatocytes around the smallest branches of

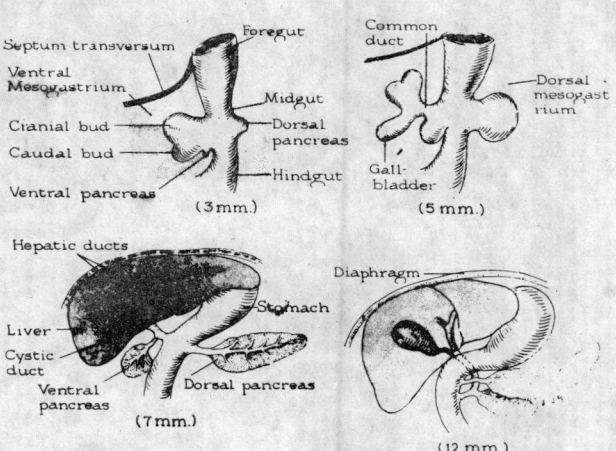

Figure 11–21 Stages in the embryonic development of the liver, bile ducts, and gallbladder. (Courtesy of Dr. Harold Lindner.)

the portal vein. Canaliculi, the specialized portions of the liver cell surface concerned with biliary secretion, appear as small vesicles between hepatocytes in the 6 wk embryo.

The gallbladder and common bile duct arise from the caudal portion of the hepatic diverticulum, elongating to form the cystic duct at 4 wk (Fig 11–21, 12 mm embryo). Initially, the gallbladder and hepatic ducts are hollow, but proliferation of the epithelial lining temporarily blocks the lumen. The obstructing epithelium is removed by vacuolization around the 7th wk. First, the common bile duct recanalizes and then the cystic duct, which expands distally to form the definitive gallbladder.

In the fully differentiated organism the hepatic terminal of the biliary system consists of intercellular canaliculi emptying into the smallest ductules. These unite to form interlobular bile ducts which follow the terminal branches of the portal vein (Fig 11–22). Larger ducts arise from the converging interlobular ducts until their coordination with the portal vein branches is lost at the hilum of the liver, where the intrahepatic and extrahepatic bile ducts meet. The right and left lobar ducts continue outside the liver as the hepatic ducts which join to form the common hepatic duct in front of the portal vein. The common bile duct is formed from the merger of the common hepatic duct and cystic duct. It runs distally along the right edge of the lesser omentum, terminating as the intramural papilla of Vater on the left side of the duodenum, where the duct unites with the major pancreatic duct to form the ampulla of Vater. The sphincter of Oddi invests the intraduodenal portion of the common bile duct, the pancreatic duct (in 80% of individuals), and the ampulla. The sphincter complex of smooth muscle fibers regulates the flow of bile into the intestine, prevents entry of bile into the

pancreatic duct, and inhibits reflux of intestinal contents into the ducts.

The initial lobulation of the liver early in gestation results from the branchings of the bile ducts and their associated radicles of the hepatic artery and portal vein. Eventually, liver cords formed by rows of hepatocytes separated by sinusoids converge toward the tributaries of the hepatic vein located in the center of the lobule, while bile flows through canaliculi toward ductules and interlobular ducts. Products secreted by the liver, such as the plasma proteins, are transported from afferent vessels (portal vein and hepatic artery) through sinusoids to the systemic circulation (central vein); biliary components move through a series of enlarging channels from the canaliculi to the common bile duct and finally to the intestine.

Functional Development. The mature liver is the main organ for maintenance of a stable internal environment. The liver absorbs raw materials which it transforms into metabolically useful compounds or unusable end products; it selectively secretes the former into blood or bile and the latter exclusively into bile. These activities are facilitated by the structural arrangement of hepatocytes in rows (cords) bordered by channels in which blood and bile flow in directions perpendicular to each other.

The maternal liver via the placenta provides calories, biotransformation reactions, and elimination of metabolic end products for the fetus. The fetal liver is relatively inactive in glycogenolysis, formation of bile acids, and processes of elimination. However, the fetal liver is devoted initially to the production of plasma proteins adapted to the special requirements of an evolving vascular system and rapidly proliferating tissues; it later produces and stores essential nutrients needed during the immediate postnatal period.

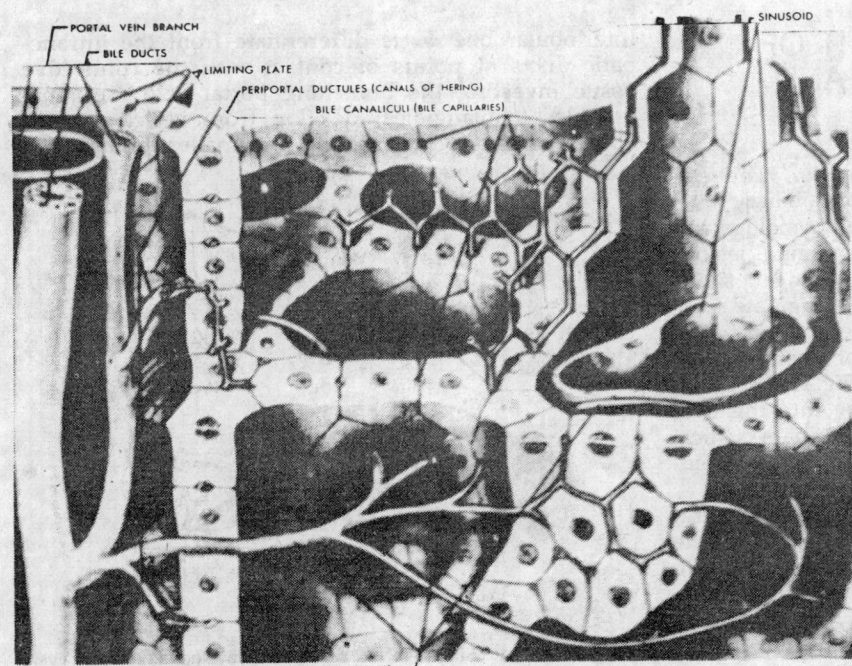

Figure 11–22 Structural features of the intrahepatic biliary drainage system. (Courtesy of Dr. Hans Elias and Ciba Pharmaceutical Company.)

Before birth the portal circulation is shunted through the, ductus venosus bypassing the liver. After birth, when oral feeding is initiated, the portal circulation begins to carry nutrients. The ductus venosus closes, and the nutrients absorbed from the intestine are delivered to the hepatic parenchyma, accelerating the synthesis of bile acids, triggering microsomal biotransformation pathways, and promoting bile flow.

Supply of Energy. The liver stores carbohydrate as glycogen, a polymer readily degraded to monomeric glucose. The newborn depends entirely on hepatic glycogen to maintain the supply of glucose suddenly interrupted at delivery. The liver acquires the ability to synthesize glycogen from the 9th wk of gestation, but hepatic glycogen accumulates rapidly only near term, gaining 20 mg/gm liver/day until the day of birth. The human fetal liver at term contains 2–3 times as much glycogen as adult liver. At least 90% of the stored glycogen is released from the liver within the 1st 2–3 hr after birth in response to the sudden interruption of the placental circulation. The remaining glycogen is gradually depleted during the next 48 hr, and accumulation begins only during the 2nd postnatal wk. Hepatic glycogen stores reach adult levels by the 3rd wk in a full term, normally fed infant. Likewise, the human liver begins to store fat early in gestation and accelerates the storage process near term. The accumulated lipid is gradually released during the 1st few days after birth.

Production of Proteins. The liver is the main source of proteins in the circulation, including plasma proteins, enzymes, and clotting factors. In the fetus, production of plasma and tissue must compete with the extremely high synthesis rates of nuclear and cytoplasmic structural components necessitated by the explosive growth of the liver near term. The albumin fraction is present in plasma of the 8 wk human fetus and increases from less than 2 gm/100 ml to near-adult values at term, when the alpha globulins, containing alpha fetoprotein, decrease markedly. At 3–4 mo, fetal liver slices incorporate amino acids into all serum protein fractions and fibrinogen as well as into transferrin and low density lipoproteins. From the 11th wk onward, human fetal plasma contains all major plasma proteins but at concentrations considerably below adult values (e.g., ceruloplasmin, low density lipoproteins, haptoglobin). Further, the fetal mammalian liver, like the mature liver, may be capable of synthesizing additional reactant proteins in response to stress.

During postnatal development certain proteins reach adult values within days and others in 1–2 yr. Lipoproteins of all classes rise abruptly in the 1st 3–4 days after birth to levels which display little variation until puberty, while albumin reaches adult levels after several mo. Ceruloplasmin and complement factors increase slowly from very low to normal adult levels during the 1st yr. In contrast, transferrin levels are in the adult range at birth, decline during the subsequent 3–5 mo, and rise to adult values thereafter.

Biotransformation and Elimination of Metabolites. THE MONOXYGENASE SYSTEM. The oxidative, reductive, hydrolytic, and conjugative reactions concerned with biotransformation are microsomal, i.e., located in the hepatic smooth endoplasmic reticulum (SER). Although the neonatal liver contains little SER and activities of microsomal enzymes are either undetectable or extremely reduced at birth, the major electron transport components of the monooxygenase system (cytochrome P-450, cytochrome b_5, NADPH–cytochrome c reductase, NADPH cytochrome P-450 reductase) have been demonstrated in human fetal liver microsomal preparations as early as the 7th wk of gestation. Fetal cytochrome P-450 and NADPH–cytochrome c reductase activities are approximately 25% and 50%, respectively, of adult values.

Measurements of metabolites in urine of infants treated with a variety of common therapeutic agents (diazepam, caffeine, phenobarbital, diphenylhydantoin) after birth indicate a low capacity for oxidative drug metabolism in fullterm newborns and nearly none in premature infants. Similarly, the biologic half-lives of drugs catalyzed by the cytochrome P-450–dependent monoxygenase system are generally longer in infants than in adults; the half-lives of tolbutamide, diphenylhydantoin, and amobarbital are 2–5 times longer in infants than in their mothers.

The presence of monoxygenase activity in the human fetal liver results in the capacity for conversion of drugs to potentially toxic metabolites by the fetal liver during the 1st trimester and the possibility that agents administered to the mother early in pregnancy may interfere with normal development of the liver or other organs. Conversely, the relative inefficiency of biotransformation reactions at birth may produce exaggerated or prolonged responses to a variety of drugs administered to newborn infants. Maturation of the monoxygenase system proceeds rapidly after birth.

CONJUGATION REACTIONS. Conjugation reactions involving the conversion of a metabolite or end product to a form which can be eliminated in bile are catalyzed by hepatic microsomal enzymes. The fetal liver is almost entirely devoid of bilirubin glucuronyl transferase activity responsible for conversion of toxic unconjugated bilirubin to an excretable glucuronide conjugate. The transferase increases after birth, but there is severe limitation of bilirubin conjugation at birth. The mechanisms responsible for induction of bilirubin conjugation after birth are not fully understood. The human newborn develops transient hyperbilirubinemia during the 1st wk after birth, presumably reflecting relative deficiency of bilirubin glucuronyl transferase. Cord blood is devoid of conjugated bilirubin. Monoconjugates of bilirubin appear during the 1st 24–48 hr in a distinct sequence, and the disconjugate follows on the 3rd day. In contrast to the cord blood of normal newborns, that of infants with prenatal hyperbilirubinemia due to blood group incompatibility contains both mono- and diglucuronide conjugates of bilirubin; thus, bilirubin glucuronyl transferase activity can be prematurely induced in utero in the presence of chronically elevated concentrations of the pigment substrate.

Microsomal glucuronyl transferase activities for bilirubin and other substrates can be stimulated by drugs, such as the barbiturates, which are also inducers of P-450 and other components of the monoxygenase system. Such agents may act on microsomal activities by altering the properties of the membranes in which these activities are located.

Bile Acid Metabolism.   Bile acids are steroids which facilitate formation of mixed micelles with cholesterol and phospholipids in aqueous environments. The hydrophobic core and hydrophilic exterior of micelles form a vehicle for solubilization and intestinal absorption of hydrophobic compounds such as lipids, fatty acids, and fat-soluble vitamins. The 2 primary bile acids, cholate and chenodeoxycholate, are synthesized in the liver, conjugated with the amino acids glycine and taurine, and excreted in bile. Conjugation of bile acids interferes with their absorption in the jejunum, maintaining the bile acid concentration in the upper small intestine above the critical concentration necessary for micelle formation. After dietary lipids are absorbed, conjugated bile acids are reabsorbed from the terminal ileum by a specific transport process, shunted back to the liver, and re-excreted in bile. This *enterohepatic circulation* occurs after each meal, and its efficiency is reflected in reabsorption of 90–95% of the bile salt pool secreted during each cycle.

Bile acids which escape ileal absorption are dehydroxylated to secondary bile acids by the action of colonic bacteria. Cholic acid is converted to deoxycholic acid, and chenodeoxycholic acid is converted to lithocholic acid. Normal bile contains about 50% cholate, 30% chenodeoxycholate, 15% deoxycholate, and 5% lithocholate. The newborn mammal is relatively deficient in the production, intestinal reabsorption, and hepatic clearance of bile acids. In addition, because bile acids in the intestinal lumen of neonates are frequently below concentrations required for micelle formation (1–2 mM), absorption of dietary fats is inefficient. The fetal liver produces considerable amounts of 31-hydroxy-Δ5-cholenoic acid, a bile acid which can induce cholestasis. This monohydroxy bile acid gradually decreases in concentration as gestation progresses.

In the human neonate the bile acid pool is reduced by about 50% compared with that of adults, and the intraluminal bile acid concentration is correspondingly lowered. These findings, combined with evidence of increased fecal bile acid losses and of total pool size per day, are consistent with deficient intestinal reabsorption of bile acids in newborns. Studies in premature infants indicate an even greater degree of inadequacy leading to intraluminal bile acid concentrations clearly below the critical micellar concentration. That the enterohepatic circulation may be further limited in newborns by inefficient biliary secretory or hepatic clearance mechanisms is suggested by significant delay in disappearance of conjugated cholic acid from plasma of infants 2 hr after a meal (postprandial bile acid test).

The cumulative effects of immature biliary functions and kinetics in newborns include excessive fecal losses of bile salts, inefficient absorption of dietary lipids and lipophilic components, and a tendency toward cholestasis.

11.81   DIAGNOSTIC ASSESSMENT OF LIVER DISEASE

The diagnostic investigation of liver disease in all age groups rests on the following: (1) proper assessment of symptoms and signs from the history and physical examination, (2) judicious selection of useful functional indices, (3) appropriate application and interpretation of liver biopsy and specimens, and (4) careful selection and interpretation of visualization procedures.

Symptoms and Signs.   The family history is especially important in liver disease presenting in early infancy. The liver and biliary tract are affected by heritable disorders and congenital malformations which become manifest within days or weeks after birth and may lead to chronic or fatal liver disease unless recognized and treated promptly.

Jaundice, the earliest and often the only sign in most liver disorders of infants, requires urgent evaluation since the pigment may be of the toxic unconjugated type, may reflect sepsis, may be a sign of a treatable metabolic disorder such as galactosemia, or may be due to a congenital malformation of the bile ducts requiring surgical repair. A history of jaundice in the mother before or during pregnancy suggests the possibility that hepatitis B infection has been transmitted to the infant. Jaundice in an older child is most likely due to hepatitis A infection. Other conditions, such as chronic active hepatitis, Wilson disease, or α_1-antitrypsin deficiency, must also be considered if the jaundice proves persistent or other suggestive physical findings are observed (Table 11–13).

Hepatomegaly is another very frequent sign of liver disease (Table 11–13). The examination for liver size, shape, and consistency should include a determination of liver span. The liver edge is normally palpable at 2–3 cm below the right costal margin in infants and at 1–2 cm in children. Displacement of the liver by adjoining organs or masses can create an erroneous impression of enlargement. Percussion of the upper margin should be performed and the liver span measured as the distance between the lower edge of the liver and the margin of dullness at the right midclavicular line. While the span varies with age and body weight, the upper margin should be located within 1 cm of the 5th intercostal space in the right midclavicular line. If these measures fail to delineate liver size, a nuclear scan of the liver should be obtained (ultrasonograms are less precise for this purpose). The examination of the liver includes a determination of tenderness and auscultation of the liver surface for bruits and concludes with careful palpation of the abdomen for a detectable spleen, other masses, and areas of tenderness. Pertinent extrahepatic physical findings in conditions associated with liver disease are listed in Table 11–14.

Functional Indices of Liver Disease.   Since the liver has multiple functions, many tests have been developed to enhance the specificity, sensitivity, and reliability of laboratory adjuncts to diagnosis. The situation is rare, however, when information obtained from routinely available liver function tests can be significantly improved upon with additional determinations. The short list of established tests includes total and conjugated (direct) serum bilirubin, serum aspartate transaminase (SGOT) and alanine transaminase (SGPT), alkaline phosphatase, serum albumin, prothrombin time, and gamma globulin determinations. In infants and children α_1-antitrypsin should also be determined in the investigation of jaundice and hepatomegaly, and blood ammonia should be measured in the diagnostic evaluation

Table 11–13

A. Liver Diseases Presenting with Jaundice

Newborns and young infants
  Infections (congenital and acquired)
    Bacterial—sepsis (*E. coli*, etc.)
    Viral—cytomegalovirus, hepatitis B, rubella, coxsackievirus, echovirus, herpes simplex
    Parasitic—syphilis, toxoplasmosis
  Metabolic disorders
    Inherited—α_1-antitrypsin deficiency, galactosemia, hereditary fructose intolerance, cystic fibrosis, tyrosinosis, Niemann-Pick disease
    Acquired—cholestasis and liver disease associated with total parenteral nutrition; "insipissated bile syndrome" associated with severe erythroblastosis
  Idiopathic disorders: Neonatal hepatitis (giant cell hepatitis), familial cirrhosis (Byler disease), hereditary lymphedema with cholestasis
  Malformations of the bile ducts
    Atresias and hypoplasias—extrahepatic biliary atresia, intrahepatic biliary hypoplasia (asyndromatic), Watson-Alagille syndrome (arteriohepatic dysplasia)
    Cystic malformations—choledochus cysts, cystic dilatation of the major intrahepatic bile ducts (Caroli disease), congenital hepatic fibrosis, polycystic disease of liver and kidneys
Children and adolescents
  Chronic hepatitis—persistent hepatitis, chronic active hepatitis
  Inherited disorders—Wilson disease (hepatolenticular degeneration), cystic fibrosis, hepatic porphyrias
  Malignancies—leukemia, lymphoma, liver tumors (cholangioma)
  Chemicals—hepatotoxic agents, toxins (insecticides, hydrocarbons, organophosphates, hypervitaminosis A)
  Parasitic infections—schistosomiasis, leptospirosis, visceral larva migrans
  Idiopathic or secondary lesions—inflammatory bowel disease (ulcerative colitis), rheumatoid arthritis

B. Liver Diseases Presenting with Hepatomegaly

Congenital hepatic fibrosis
Congestive heart failure
Storage disorders
  Acute—Reye syndrome (fat)
  Chronic—glycogenoses, mucopolysaccharidoses, Gaucher disease, Niemann-Pick disease, gangliosidosis, cholesterol storage disease, Wolman disease
Nutritional problems: total parenteral alimentation (caloric overload), kwashiorkor, diabetes
Infiltrative disorders: leukemia, lymphoma, histiocytosis X, granulomas (sarcoidosis, tuberculosis)
Tumors
  Primary—hepatoblastoma, hematoma, hemangioendothelioma, hematoma
  Metastatic—neuroblastoma, Wilms tumor, gonadal tumors

of Reye syndrome, hepatocellular failure, and hepatic encephalopathy.

The *fractionated serum bilirubin* permits rapid distinction between hepatic and hemolytic varieties of jaundice, provides a relatively sensitive index of minimal hepatocellular or biliary excretory dysfunction, and is liver specific. A rapid increase in the serum bilirubin with a concomitant decrease in the direct to indirect ratio may be a grave prognostic sign in conditions associated with severe hepatocellular failure (e.g., fulminant hepatitis).

The *transaminases* are sensitive indices of minimal hepatocellular damage and are therefore useful for detecting anicteric forms of liver disease, for monitoring patients on hepatotoxic drugs, for estimating progression or response to therapy in chronic liver disease, and for determining the rate of cellular damage. SGPT is almost exclusively liver specific and remains constant throughout childhood; SGOT is derived from several sources and declines modestly with age. While these advantages of SGPT appear to limit the usefulness of SGOT, in practice both are often measured since useful information can be derived from their relative rise or fall in acute viral hepatitis and fulminant hepatitis.

The *alkaline phosphatase* reflects obstructive or inflammatory processes involving the biliary tract. The enzyme is usually strikingly elevated in children with intrahepatic biliary hypoplasia or paucity of the intrahepatic bile ducts, especially when compared with normally modest elevations of serum transaminases. A small rise in alkaline phosphatase (up to 1.5 × normal) is difficult to interpret in growing children since the values may reflect enzyme derived from bone. Determination of isoenzyme patterns or measurement of 5'nucleotidase, gamma glutamyl transferase, or leucine aminopeptidase activity may facilitate the interpretation of elevated alkaline phosphatase values.

The *serum albumin* and *prothrombin time* reflect synthetic functions of hepatocytes. Thus, albumin measurement, with a half-life of 20–25 days, may be useful in estimating the status of a progressive liver disorder such as chronic active hepatitis where a decline in albumin with a rise in gamma globulin levels may indicate advancing cirrhosis. In contrast, a prolonged prothrombin time, indicating a decline in prothrombin may occur within hours in such acute disorders as Reye syndrome or massive hepatic necrosis due to drug toxicity. Failure of vitamin K to reduce the prothrombin time is an indication of extensive hepatocellular destruction in patients in hepatic coma or precoma. However, unlike the decline of albumin, prolonged prothrombin time is not liver specific.

Percutaneous Liver Biopsy. This is a most valuable diagnostic tool in pediatric hepatology. The information obtained is often essential for characterization of inborn errors of metabolism by tissue analysis of enzymes (e.g., urea cycle defects, glycogenoses, hereditary fructose intolerance), metals (e.g., copper in Wilson disease), and stored metabolites (e.g., glycogen, sphingomyelin). The histologic appearance of the liver

Table 11–14 PHYSICAL FINDINGS ASSOCIATED WITH LIVER DISEASES

Infants
Microcephaly—congenital cytomegalovirus, rubella, toxoplasmosis
Characteristic facies—arteriohepatic dysplasia (Watson-Alagille syndrome)
Telangiectasia—hereditary hemorrhagic telangiectasia
Cataracts—galactosemia
Retinal pigmentation and posterior embryotoxin—arteriohepatic dysplasia
Abnormal ausculation of lungs—cystic fibrosis
Neuromuscular abnormalities (tremors, flaccidity)—lipid storage disease
Children
Pruritus—chronic cholestasis
Hemangiomas—hemangiomatosis of the liver
Carotenemia—hypervitaminosis A
Kayser-Fleischer rings—Wilson disease
Glossitis—cirrhosis
Enlarged kidneys—congenital hepatic fibrosis or polycystic disease
Neuromuscular abnormalities—Wilson disease
Arthritis and erythema nodosum—liver disease with chronic inflammatory bowel disease

determines the diagnosis and course of action in chronic active hepatitis, Reye syndrome, Dubin-Johnson syndrome, intrahepatic biliary hypoplasia, congenital hepatic fibrosis, severe portal hypertension, and extrahepatic biliary atresia. Finally, biopsies are used to monitor the results or complications of prolonged treatment such as steroid and antimetabolite therapy in chronic active hepatitis, iron overload in β-thalassemia, hepatotoxicity due to chemotherapy in leukemia, and recurrent cholangitis in patients with surgically repaired malformations of the biliary tree.

The safety record of percutaneous liver biopsy is excellent, without a single mortality and few complications reported among thousands of children ranging in age from 1 wk–15 yr who underwent biopsy with the Menghini needle. The 2 prerequisites for safe performance are an operator experienced with biopsies in infants and children and a carefully selected patient. Contraindications include prolongation of the prothrombin time beyond 16 sec, platelet counts below 40,000, evidence that a vascular or infectious lesion may lie in the path of the biopsy needle, and severe ascites.

Imaging Procedures. The indications for visualization of the liver and bile ducts with radiologic and radioisotopic procedures are similar in children and adults. However, these techniques present special problems when applied to infants.

Ultrasonography is the most useful of the imaging procedures for detection of choledochal cysts, dilated bile ducts, and gallstones in infants and children.

Radionuclide scanning is indicated for accurate estimation of liver size and detection of vascular malformations. The widely used ^{131}I rose bengal scan has limited value in the investigation of infants with obstructive jaundice and may be replaced by newer cholephilic isotopes. Such scans are frequently overinterpreted to indicate extrahepatic biliary atresia when the label cannot be detected over the intestinal region within 24 hr after injection. This finding may reflect the presence of severe cholestasis of either parenchymal or biliary origin. Intestinal labeling may not be observed in infants with acholic stools, and pigment may reappear in stools of infants recovering from severe neonatal hepatitis several days before labeled ^{131}I rose bengal becomes detectable over the intestinal area. The introduction of high intensity imaging with agents such as ^{99m}Tc-PIPIDA (paraisopropyliminodiacetic acid) combined with priming of bile flow in cholestatic infants with phenobarbital administered for 7 days before the scan is performed, may improve the reliability and sensitivity of scintigraphy in the evaluation of infants with cryptogenic cholestasis.

CT (computed tomography) scanning of the liver is technically difficult in infants, who may require general anesthesia for immobilization. It is the procedure of choice for delineating a tumor prior to surgery. CT scans will detect cystic malformations and ductile dilatations with definition superior to ultrasound, but this advantage should be weighed against the difficulties in performance and increased costs. Occasionally, in the investigation of isolated hepatomegaly a CT scan may replace the need for a liver biopsy since a fatty liver can be reliably distinguished from a liver rich in glycogen by the low radiologic density of the former and the high density of the latter.

Transhepatic and Endoscopic Cholangiography. Imaging procedures requiring direct injection of contrast media into the biliary tract are generally not applicable to infants for technical reasons. Percutaneous transhepatic cholangiography using a "skinny" needle inserted through the abdominal wall into the liver parenchyma can produce diagnostic images in children with dilated bile ducts but is impractical in infants because of the small diameter of their intrahepatic bile ducts and constriction of these structures by scar tissue in intra- and extrahepatic infantile cholestasis. Endoscopic retrograde cholangiopancreatography (ERCP) has been successfully applied to visualization of the entire biliary and pancreatic duct system in patients with malformations of the pancreatic duct, but presently available instrumentation limits its application to children at least 3 yr old. Smaller fiberoptic endoscopes with improved optics may extend this useful procedure to younger patients.

11.82 CHOLESTATIC LIVER DISEASE IN INFANCY

SPECIAL FEATURES OF LIVER DISEASE IN NEWBORN AND YOUNG INFANTS

Liver diseases in infants differ from those in older patients in clinical evolution, in histopathology, and in prognosis. Genetic endowment, intrauterine and postnatal factors (maternal disease and drug intake, hypoxia, hypoglycemia, endocrine status), and gestational age influence the expression of teratogenic and destructive agents in fetuses and newborns. Microorganisms and metabolic derangements which spare the liver in children and adults may produce fatal liver disease in infants. Infections with rubella, syphilis, toxoplasmosis, and herpes simplex and errors of metabolism such as α_1-antitrypsin deficiency, galactosemia, and hereditary fructose intolerance cause severe cholestasis only during the 1st months after birth. Conversely, the major cause of acute parenchymal liver disease in children, hepatitis A, does not affect the infant liver.

The immature liver displays a unique tendency to form giant cells. These large syncytial membrane-bound structures observed in association with every disease process causing cholestasis in early infancy may themselves contribute to hepatic excretory deficiency during the 1st 4 mo after birth. In addition, proliferative phenomena such as rapid deposition of connective tissue and formation of pseudoducts and pseudoacini frequently complicate the interpretation of hepatic lesions in young infants. The clinical and pathologic peculiarities of liver disease in infants are difficult to describe meaningfully in terms coined for fully differentiated cellular elements. Thus, neonatal hepatitis, a term often confused with viral hepatitis in older patients, actually describes idiopathic parenchymal disorders (in contrast to bile duct lesions) for which a viral causative agent has never been identified. The term "cholestatic syndromes of infancy" is used by some as a label for all neonatal hepatobiliary disorders of unknown origin.

Cirrhosis is an intractable disease due to processes of necrosis, fibrosis, and regeneration. In young infants the lobule contains several plates of actively dividing hepatocytes that can be mistaken for regenerative nodules, and young connective tissue grows rapidly, distorting the lobular architecture. While this appearance may resemble cirrhosis in adults, the immature liver is endowed with remarkable capacities for resorption of connective tissue and restoration of portal structures. For example, in galactosemia and biliary atresia lesions consistent with cirrhosis in adults may completely disappear after treatment. Thus, features subsumed under the term cirrhosis in adults may not have the same grave connotations when observed in young infants.

DIFFERENTIAL DIAGNOSIS AND MANAGEMENT OF CHOLESTATIC LIVER DISEASE IN INFANCY

The diagnosis of hepatobiliary disease in early infancy requires a systematic approach as outlined in Fig 11–23. Infants with parenchymal cholestatic liver disease are clinically indistinguishable from those with biliary lesions, nor do standard liver function tests discriminate among these types. Transhepatic cholangiography and endoscopic retrograde cholangiography are currently impractical in infants. Ultrasonography is an excellent procedure for detection of cysts but cannot delineate the fine structures in the porta hepatis. Isotope scans provide an impression of the severity of cholestasis but cannot determine whether intrahepatic or extrahepatic interruption of bile flow is involved.

Specific metabolic causes of cholestatic liver disease can be detected with serum α_1-antitrypsin, urinary galactose and sweat chloride determinations and urinary amino acid screen. Infections may be diagnosed with viral cultures or antibody titers, HB_sAg, and VDRL. However, at least 80% of the remaining infants with cholestatic jaundice fall into the cryptogenic category.

The investigation of cryptogenic infantile cholestasis is initially directed toward separation of intrahepatic (parenchymal and ductile) from extrahepatic (ductile) forms. The presence of bile pigment in stools indicates that the disorder is intrahepatic since the connection between liver and intestine is preserved. An ultrasonogram is obtained to evaluate the possibility of intrahepatic cystic malformations and choledochal cysts, and a percutaneous liver biopsy is performed. The biopsy will reveal the severity of the disease process and the presence or absence of cholangitis. In addition, the biopsy will demonstrate whether the predominant lesion is extensive giant cell transformation ("neonatal hepatitis"), hypoplasia of the interlobular bile ducts, or a proliferative response of the terminal bile ducts to a distal obstruction. α_1-Antitrypsin deficiency may be suggested by the presence of PAS-positive granules (Fig 11–24), cytomegalovirus infection identified from characteristic cytoplasmic inclusions (Fig 11–25), and cystic fibrosis suspected from mucous plugs and fibrotic formations in portal zones. Infections may occasionally be clarified by culture of liver tissue obtained at biopsy.

The infant with *acholic stools* may have extrahepatic atresia. Therefore, the patency of the biliary passages between liver and intestine must be evaluated, preferably by estimation of bile flow to the intestine. Measurement of ^{131}I rose bengal fecal excretion provides the most sensitive and accurate index of bile flow. Stools and urine are collected separately for 72 hr after intravenous injection of 3 microcuries of ^{131}I rose bengal/kg, the same dose as employed for scanning. The radioactivity excreted in stools is measured and expressed as a percentage of the radioactivity administered. Excretion of less than 5% of the injected radiolabeled dye over a 3 day period is evidence of total interruption of bile flow. Abdominal scans are obtained at 24 and 48 hr after injection of labeled dye. The stool collection is discontinued if the label appears at any time over the intestinal region.

A less sensitive but simpler method for demonstration of biliary patency is aspiration of intestinal secretions by nasogastric tube placed in the duodenum. Gallbladder contraction is stimulated by administration of fluids and the aspirate examined for bile pigment. A positive result rules out biliary atresia; a negative indicates severe cholestasis consistent with but not pathognomonic of biliary atresia.

Other procedures aimed at evaluation of the extrahepatic biliary passages employ scanning of the liver and abdomen after injection of 1 of the newer short-lived isotopes designed to improve definition of biliary structures. The diagnostic accuracy of imaging biliary outflow with such radionuclides (e.g., ^{99m}technetium-PIPIDA) may be enhanced by prior treatment with phenobarbital to increase bile secretion. The sensitivity and specificity of these approaches remain to be firmly established. Indirect measures of biliary excretory efficiency include red cell peroxidation, lipoprotein X determination before and after cholestyramine treatment, and serum IgA levels. Such procedures reflect the degree but not the site of cholestasis.

Operative cholangiography through the gallbladder is indicated in infants in whom liver biopsy and radioactive rose bengal excretion indicate extrahepatic biliary obstruction. Demonstration of continuity between the major intrahepatic bile ducts and the duodenum rules out biliary atresia. When the gallbladder is absent or malformed, the porta hepatis is carefully explored. Choledochal cysts or bile-containing remnants of the left or right bile ducts are anastomosed to the small intestine, preferably the jejunum. If patent biliary structures are not present, a hepatic portoenterostomy (Kasai procedure) is performed.

CHOLESTATIC PARENCHYMAL DISORDERS IN EARLY INFANCY

11.83 Idiopathic Neonatal Hepatitis

This idiopathic parenchymal disorder accounts for 35–45% of all cholestatic liver disease in infancy. Statistics show a 2:1 incidence of males over females, a higher

(Text continues on page 964)

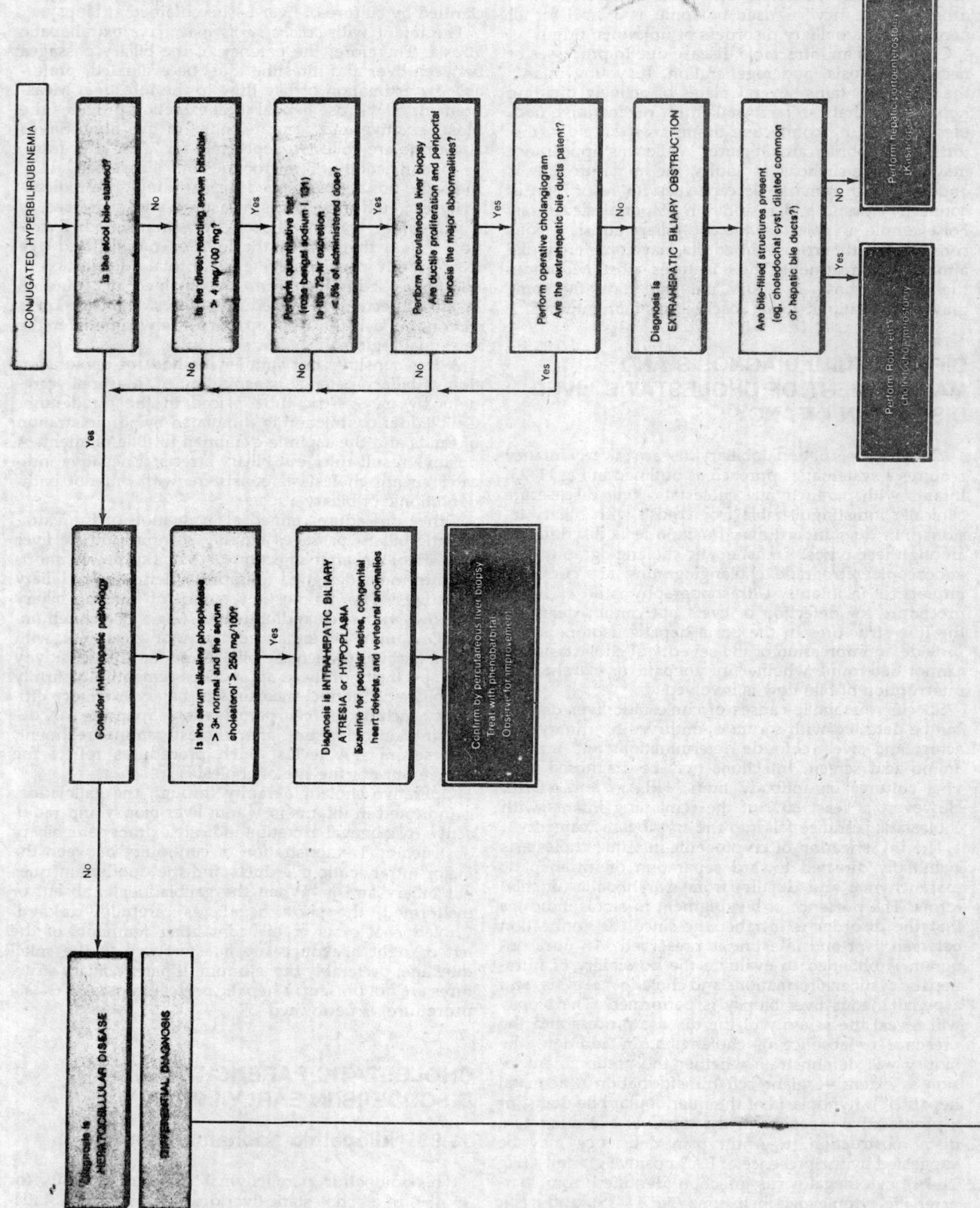

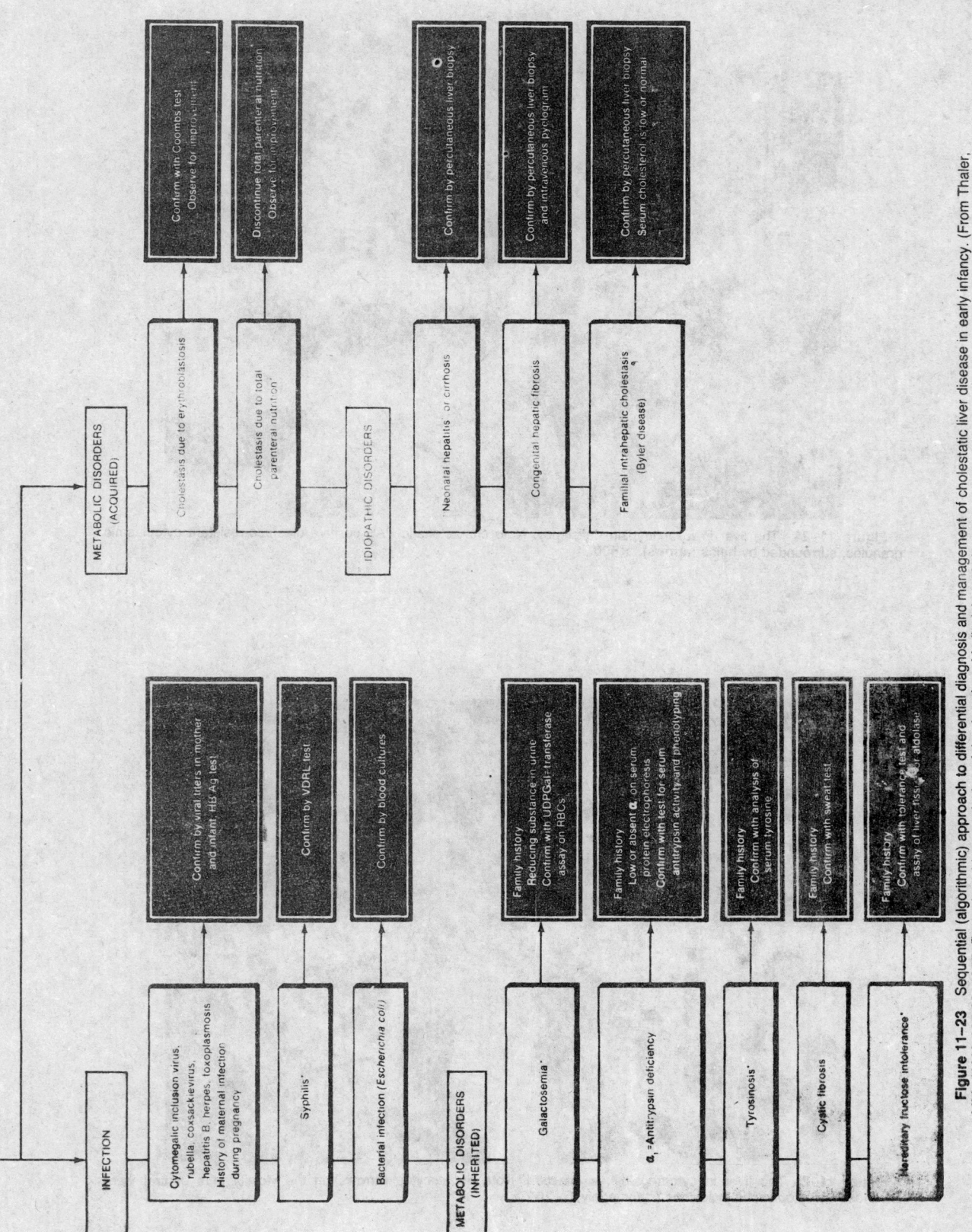

Figure 11-23 Sequential (algorithmic) approach to differential diagnosis and management of cholestatic liver disease in early infancy. (From Thaler, MM. JAMA 237:60, 1977. Reproduced by permission of the American Medical Association.)

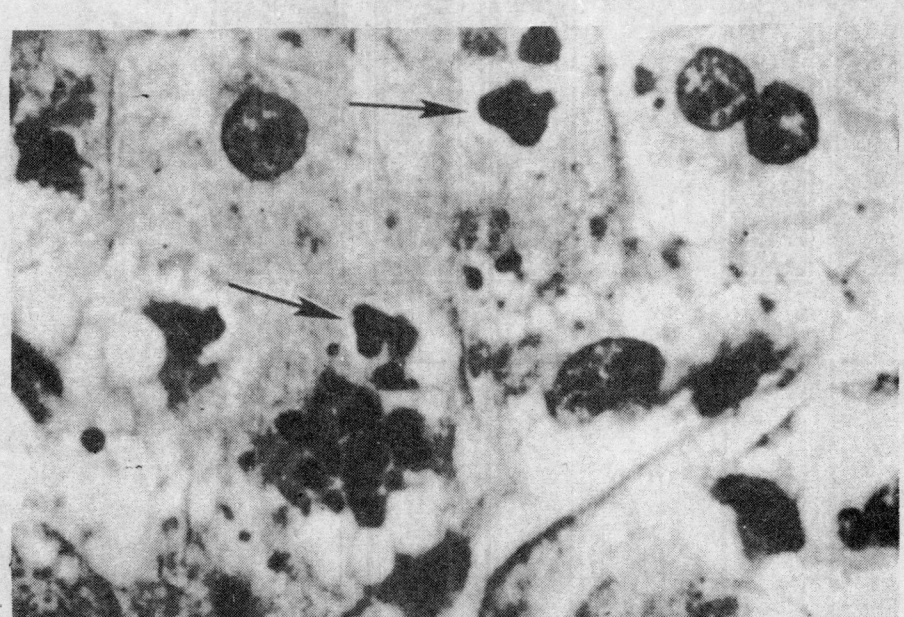

Figure 11–24 The liver in α_1-antitrypsin deficiency. Note characteristic PAS-positive diastase-resistant cytoplasmic granules, surrounded by halos (arrows). ×400.

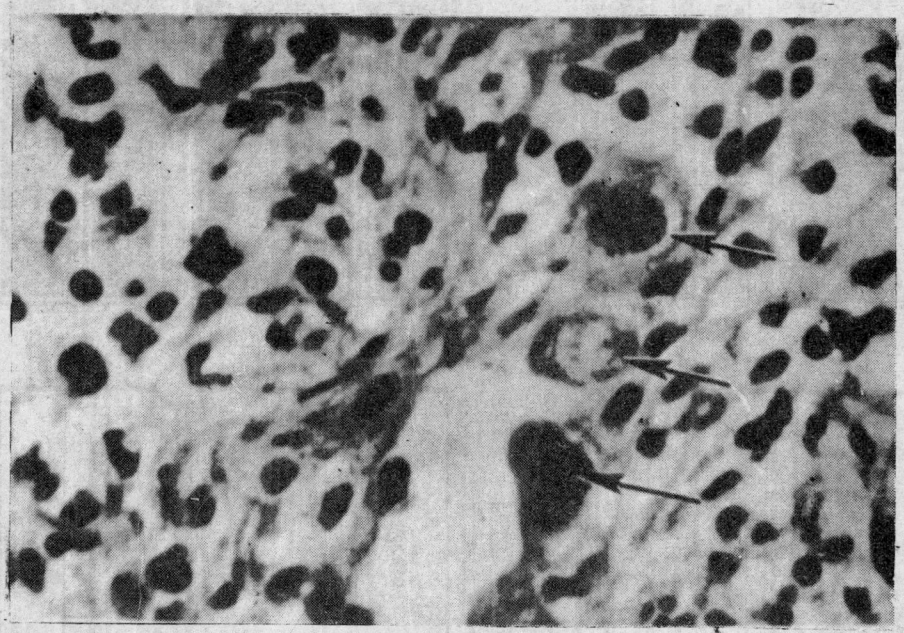

Figure 11–25 The liver in cytomegalovirus infection. Note hepatocytes (arrows) in the vicinity of a central vein, expanded by cytoplasmic inclusions (cytomegaly). ×100.

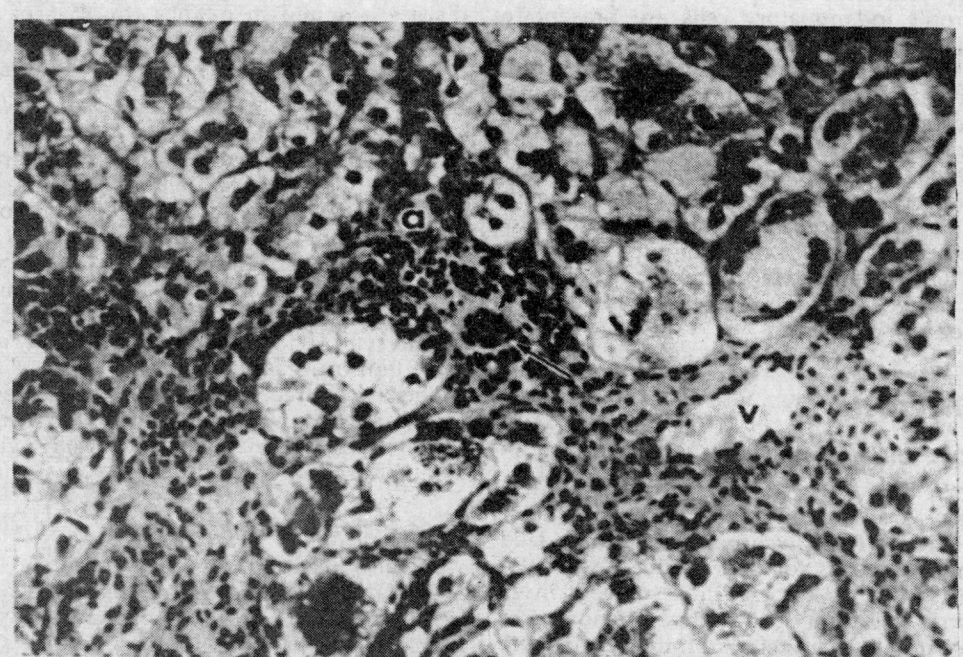

Figure 11–26 The liver in "neonatal hepatitis" (giant cell hepatitis). Extensive giant cell formation impinges on structures in the portal zone. Note inflammatory cells surrounding an inconspicuous bile duct (arrow), portal vein (v), and hepatic arteriole (a). The presence of pericholangitis and fibrosis suggests evolution toward chronic liver disease. × 100.

frequency among premature infants, and a familial incidence consistent with either an autosomal recessive inheritance or a common environmental etiologic factor.

Clinical Manifestations. Jaundice due to conjugated hyperbilirubinemia is usually noted during the 1st wk after birth (80%) but may appear at any time up to 3 mo. Jaundice is usually the only complaint, but mild anemia, poor feeding, and vomiting are occasionally encountered. Dark urine and intermittent loss of pigment from stools suggest intrahepatic cholestasis. Hepatomegaly with a smooth, firm liver edge occurs in nearly every patient; 50% have splenomegaly.

Pathology. Lobular architecture is distorted by massive giant cell transformation. Giant cells predominate in centrilobular zones. Severe cholestasis during the acute illness is indicated by inspissated bile pigment in giant cells and canalicular bile plugs. In 1 of 5 cases, acute and chronic inflammatory cells are present in portal zones (Fig 11–26).

Laboratory Findings. Serum bilirubin ranges from 8–12 mg/dl with >60% direct-reacting pigment. Transaminase values may rise as high as 400 IU but are extremely variable. Alkaline phosphatase is usually modestly elevated, serum albumin and gamma globulin are normal, and prothrombin time is slightly prolonged.

Treatment. There is no specific therapy; corticosteroids are not effective.

Prognosis. Complete recovery occurs in 75% of patients by 1 yr of age; 25% suffer chronic liver disease due to micronodular cirrhosis.

Metabolic Disorders

11.84 α_1-Antitrypsin Deficiency

See also Sec 12.87.

α_1-Antitrypsin is an inhibitor of trypsin and other proteolytic activities. This glycoprotein is synthesized by the liver and accounts for 80% of the α_1 globulin fraction of the serum. α_1-Antitrypsin is present in 24 phenotypic forms in serum. The normal phenotype of the P_i (protease inhibitor) system is M; the type associated with liver disease is Z. Intermediate types MS, MZ, and SZ may also cause liver disease. The incidence of the Z phenotype is estimated at 1:2000–1:4000, inherited as an autosomal codominant gene.

Clinical and Laboratory Manifestations. Cholestatic jaundice and hepatomegaly are the presenting features in infants under 3 mo of age. In addition to nonspecific elevations in serum bilirubin, transaminases, and alkaline phosphatase, serum α_1-antitrypsin activity levels are 10–20%, and there is a missing α_1 globulin peak on serum protein electrophoresis. The definitive diagnostic test is identification of the P_i phenotype by specialized immunoelectrophoretic typing procedures.

Pathology. Periportal fibrosis and cholestasis are constantly present. PAS-positive diastase-resistant granules confined to periportal hepatocytes initially and eventually enlarging and spreading to the midzone are characteristic of the disease (Fig 11–24). These granules, anomalous α_1-antitrypsin, are retained in the liver presumably because they are relatively insoluble. Other histologic features are variable, including bile duct hypoplasia, periportal inflammation, giant cells, and formation of pseudoductules.

Treatment. Only supportive therapy is available.

Prognosis. Cirrhosis develops in most affected children. In adults with α_1-antitrypsin deficiency and liver disease acquired in infancy, the risk of hepatic carcinoma is considerably increased.

11.85 Cystic Fibrosis

See also Sec 12.110.

The liver is involved in 20–40% of patients at autopsy; usually there is focal biliary cirrhosis secondary to biliary obstruction with thickened secretions. Occasionally, cystic fibrosis in neonates presents with cholestatic jaundice and hepatomegaly and nonspecific abnormalities in liver function tests. The initial clinical manifestation is usually jaundice, which clears spontaneously after several wk. Patients may eventually develop portal hypertension years later.

There is no treatment for infantile cholestasis. In later childhood, complications of multifocal biliary cirrhosis and portal hypertension, especially gastrointestinal hemorrhage, may require a portacaval shunt.

11.86 Galactosemia

See also Sec 8.19.

This autosomal recessive disorder is caused by a deficiency of galactose-1-phosphate uridyl transferase, which results in liver disease, cataracts, and mental retardation. Toxicity is due to accumulation of galactose-1-phosphate.

Clinical and Laboratory Manifestations. The damage caused by this defect is initiated in utero and exacerbated after birth upon introduction of a lactose-rich diet (milk). Vomiting, diarrhea, and failure to thrive are rapidly followed by cholestatic jaundice, hepatomegaly, ascites, hypoglycemia, and seizures. Unless intake of dietary galactose is discontinued, death from liver failure may occur in a few wk. The diagnosis should be suspected from the finding by Benedict test of a reducing substance (galactose) in the urine of an infant with cholestatic jaundice. The definitive diagnosis is established by an assay of galactose-1-phosphate uridyl transferase activity in red blood cells.

Pathology. Pseudoacinar formation of hepatocytes is common in galactosemia but also occurs in other metabolic disorders. In addition to cholestasis and steatosis, copious scar tissue forms and distorts the lobular architecture.

Treatment. A galactose-free diet of casein or soy protein formula is indicated. Later, a rigid regimen of galactose and lactose exclusion should be prescribed. Cataracts may require surgery.

Prognosis. Exclusion of galactose from the diet of the newborn is dramatically effective: signs of liver disease disappear, even if advanced to scarring, and ascites clears within a few days. Cataract formation is arrested or reversed. Effects on mental status may be minimal.

11.87 Hereditary Fructose Intolerance

See also Sec 8.19.

This autosomal recessive disease is due to deficiency of fructose-1-phosphate aldolase (common) or fructose-1,6-diphosphatase (rare); the toxic metabolite is presumed to be fructose-1-phosphate. Infants develop toxic manifestations (vomiting, diarrhea, hypoglycemia, seizures) and cholestatic jaundice upon introduction into the diet of sucrose and fructose. The liver enlarges, and ascites develops; subsequently, cirrhosis and liver failure occur in infancy unless fructose is excluded from the diet. Laboratory findings include proteinuria, fructosuria, hypoglycemia, and hypophosphatemia after an intravenous fructose tolerance test and increased urinary excretion of uric acid.

The liver biopsy is characterized by steatosis, edematous parenchyma, pseudoacinar formation, cholestasis, and extensive periportal fibrosis. Diagnosis may be confirmed by assay of liver tissue for the aldolase and diphosphatase.

When a strict fructose exclusion regimen is instituted, liver pathology resolves, and patients can lead normal lives. Patients develop a strong distaste for sweets.

11.88 Hereditary Tyrosinemia

See also Sec 8.3.

This autosomal recessive disorder affects the liver, kidneys, and pancreas. It is endemic in northern Quebec. There is a deficiency of parahydroxyphenylpyruvic (PHPPA) acid oxidase, the enzyme converting PHPPA to homogentisic acid.

Clinical and Laboratory Manifestations. Hereditary tyrosinemia occurs in 2 forms. In the acute form the disease progresses to liver failure with a high fatality rate during infancy. In the chronic form the course is slowly progressive to nodular cirrhosis, vitamin D–resistant rickets, failure to thrive, and Fanconi syndrome in childhood. Patients with the chronic form have a high incidence of hepatoma. Tyrosine and methionine are elevated in plasma, and urinary excretion of tyrosine and its metabolites is increased. These findings are nonspecific; tyrosinemia should be suspected when infants treated for galactosemia or hereditary fructose intolerance respond poorly to their respective diets.

Treatment. A diet low in phenylalanine and tyrosine is indicated. The diet improves the renal lesion but has no effect on the liver disease.

11.89 Neonatal Hepatitis with Cortisol Deficiency

This condition affects infants with hypopituitarism or congenital adrenal hypoplasia. The onset occurs before 3 mo of age and is typical of cryptogenic infantile cholestasis. The pathogenesis appears related to cortisol deficiency.

The course is characterized by hypoglycemia and cholestatic jaundice in addition to manifestations of the associated disorder. The diagnosis is established on the basis of reduced serum cortisol, associated with low growth hormone levels in patients with hypopituitarism. Liver pathology includes extensive giant cell transformation, minimal inflammation, and absence of fibrosis. Cortisol replacement therapy results in clinical improvement and complete recovery of liver functions.

11.90 Infections

The main infectious agents affecting the liver in newborns and young infants include hepatitis B virus, cytomegalovirus, herpes simplex, rubella, coxsackievirus B and echoviruses 14 and 19, congenital syphilis, and toxoplasmosis. Special features of each infection are described here although these organisms are covered primarily in Chapter 10.

Hepatitis B virus may be acquired in utero, during delivery, or postnatally by maternal contact. The virus is usually transmitted by a mother who is an asymptomatic hepatitis B carrier positive for the "e" antigen or who develops B-positive acute viral hepatitis within 2 mo before or after delivery. The course of perinatal hepatitis B infection is generally not associated with clinical signs. In the typical case the infant becomes HB_sAg positive at 2–3 mo and retains positivity for years thereafter. A small number display transaminase elevations associated with mild inflammatory changes in the portal zones on liver biopsy. In rare instances of fulminant hepatitis, severe jaundice develops rapidly and progresses to hepatic coma within a few days; a fatal outcome can be expected in 60–80% of patients. Adults exposed to hepatitis B virus in infancy may be at risk for hepatocellular carcinoma as a late sequela.

Effective protection of infants against vertically transmitted hepatitis B virus is provided with injections of hepatitis B immune globulin (HBIG) within 48 hr after birth (effectiveness declines sharply thereafter) and at regular intervals for 6 mo (Sec 10.83).

Cytomegalovirus hepatitis can be contracted after birth from ingested milk or saliva or in utero. Clinical and laboratory findings are those of cryptogenic infantile cholestasis. The diagnosis can be confirmed with urinary cultures and demonstration of rising titers of specific IgG and IgM antibodies. Rarely, direct evidence of infection can be obtained from liver biopsies when the characteristic cytoplasmic inclusions in bile and liver ducts and liver cells are observed (Fig 11–25). Cytomegalovirus causes a severe inflammatory reaction in the liver followed by extensive fibrosis and distortion of lobular architecture. Cirrhosis and portal hypertension are the usual outcome.

Congenital infections with *herpes simplex virus, coxsackievirus B*, and *echovirus 14 and 19* involving the liver are usually fatal. All produce massive necrosis and rapidly progressive liver failure. There is no treatment. *Congenital rubella* infection can cause a hepatitis the clinical manifestations of which are typical of cryptogenic infantile cholestasis. Hepatic histology shows cholestasis, mild periportal fibrosis, and focal necrosis. Recovery of liver functions is usually complete, but chronic liver disease in association with the rubella syndrome (cardiac lesions, cataracts, mental retardation) has been described.

E. coli sepsis may present with jaundice as its only manifestation (Sec 7.59). Clotting abnormalities are usually present and are a contraindication to liver biopsy. When obtained, biopsy reveals foci of necrosis throughout the lobule, periportal inflammation due to polymorphonuclear cells, and occasional small abscesses. The course and prognosis are related to the systemic infection and its treatment.

Congenital syphilis hepatitis is rare (Sec 10.55). Jaundice is the usual 1st sign and diagnosis is established by VDRL. Liver biopsy reveals intralobular fibrosis with pericentral mononuclear infiltrates. Recovery of liver function is expected after treatment with penicillin.

Congenital toxoplasmosis hepatitis resembles sepsis in its presentation. Jaundice is variable and relatively mild. A positive Sabin-Feldman dye test confirms the diagnosis. The liver histology reveals nonspecific periportal inflammation and, rarely, the presence of histiocytes filled with toxoplasma. See Sec 10.113 for treatment.

CONDITIONS ASSOCIATED WITH MALFORMATIONS OF THE BILE DUCTS

It is often not possible to distinguish between developmental (teratogenic) and acquired malformations of the biliary ducts. The developmental nature of the malformations can be inferred when associated anomalies exist in the kidneys, as in congenital hepatic fibrosis and polycystic disease of liver and kidneys. However, the commonly encountered intrahepatic and extrahepatic atresias, hypoplasias, and dilatations of the biliary passages represent anomalies of complex and obscure origin. Although these dysmorphic lesions are often congenital, i.e., present at birth, this fact does not establish their origin. Inflammatory or toxic processes beginning as early as the 4th mo of gestation may produce secondary deformations due to interference with primordial morphogenic events. Sluggish or obstructed bile flow through either malformed or deformed bile ducts causes cholestatic jaundice, gallstone formation, pruritus, cholangitis, hepatocellular damage, and/or cirrhosis. Nevertheless, distinctions between developmental and acquired lesions are of clinical impor-

tance since surgical correction of authentic malformations may be lifesaving, whereas operations on lesions produced by progressive inflammatory, infectious, or metabolic processes may be ineffective or contraindicated.

The following outline of biliary anomalies provides a basis for diagnosis and management of these difficult therapeutic problems. With the exception of certain cystic malformations (congenital hepatic fibrosis and polycystic disease of liver and kidneys), anomalies of the biliary passages interfere with bile flow, resulting in obstructive jaundice.

11.91   Atresias and Hypoplasias

Atretic lesions of the extrahepatic and major intrahepatic bile ducts are the most common malformations of the biliary passages. The incidence of extrahepatic biliary atresia is 5–10 cases/100,000 live births or 3–15/100,000 infant hospital admissions. In comparison, the incidence of choledochal cysts, the next most common biliary anomaly, is 0.5/100,000 hospital admissions.

Atresias of the extrahepatic bile ducts may now be grouped empirically into operable or correctable types, treated by choledochojejunostomy, and previously "inoperable" variants that may currently be considered for radical hepatic portoenterostomy (direct anastomosis of the intestine to the decapsulated and incised surface of the liver in the porta hepatis or Kasai procedure). The origin of atretic lesions of the extrahepatic biliary passages is not clear. The passage of bile-stained meconium by newborns with extrahepatic biliary atresia and observation of normally formed biliary structures engulfed by inflammatory cells (Fig 11–27A) or scarred remnants of bile ducts in areas where inflammation is no longer present (Fig 11–27B) are consistent with the possibility of an acquired insult to previously normal structures.

The characteristic histologic features of extrahepatic biliary atresia are periportal fibrosis and proliferation of interlobular bile ducts (Fig 11–28). These findings, when supported by quantitative evidence of interrupted bile flow, such as fecal ^{131}I rose bengal excretion of less than 5% in 3 days, are an indication for operative cholangiography to visualize the type of atresia.

Without treatment the average survival of infants with extrahepatic atresia not correctable by choledochojejunostomy is 1.5–2.5 yr. All develop portal hypertension, ascites, and gastrointestinal hemorrhage. Treatment for these complications and maintenance of adequate nutrition is described in Sec 11.101. Approximately 40–50% of the total number of patients with radical anastomoses have been reported to survive for 5 yr or longer, but a large proportion eventually develop chronic cholangitis and/or severe portal hypertension. Successful outcome correlates directly with the diameter of the biliary structures at the site of transection in the porta hepatis.

The encouraging results of the Kasai operation are drastically reduced when performed on infants over 2 mo of age. The necessity to operate as early as possible represents a potential danger as operative cholangiography and visual inspection may fail to detect the thin,

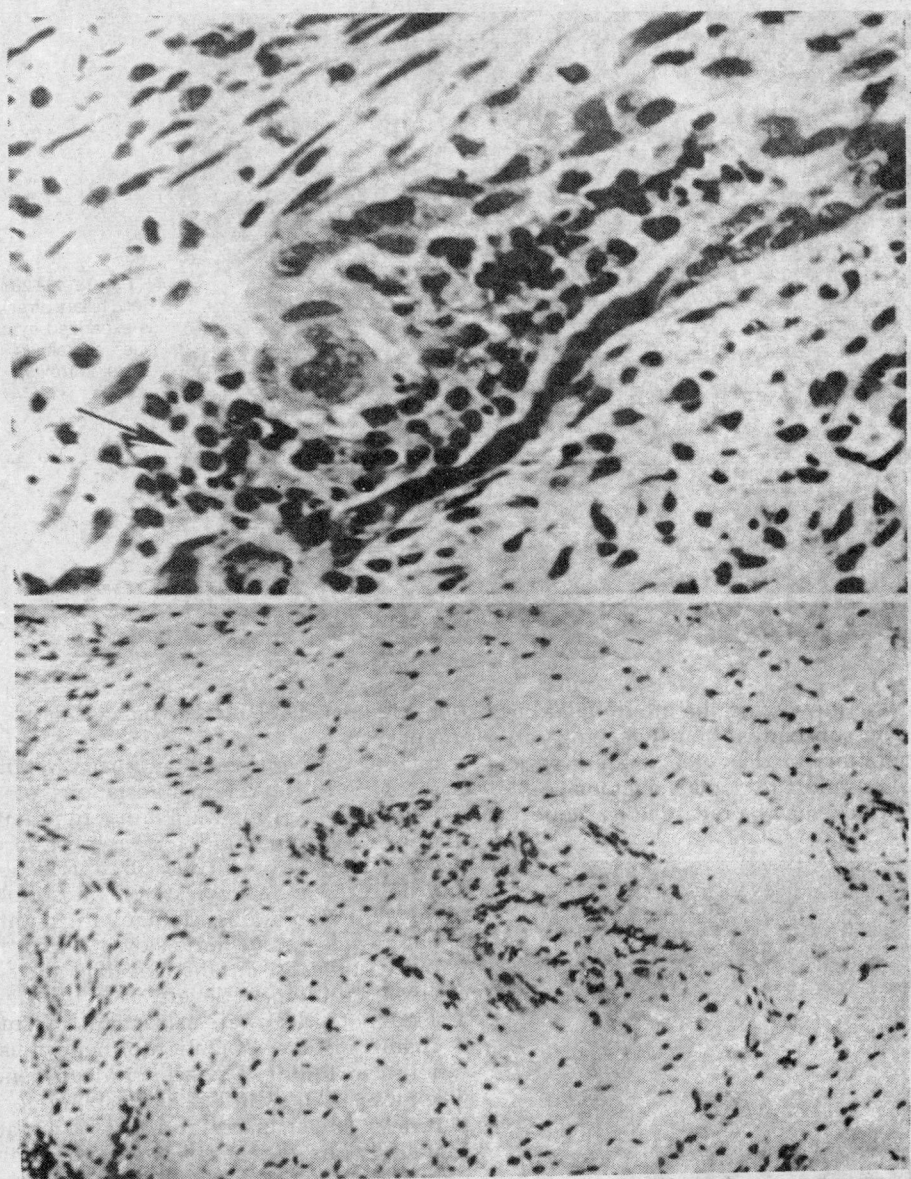

Figure 11–27 *A*, Major branch of hepatic bile duct coursing through fibrous tissue in the porta hepatis. The lumen is filled with acute and chronic inflammatory cells which appear to penetrate the duct wall and invade the surrounding parenchyma (arrow). Surgical specimen obtained at portoenterostomy in an 8 wk old infant. ×100. *B*, Sclerosed branch of hepatic bile duct in region of liver-to-gut anastomosis in the porta hepatis. Note absence of inflammatory elements compared with *A*. Autopsy specimen obtained from the same infant as in *A* at 10 mo of age. ×100.

collapsed, but patent bile ducts present during the acute shutdown phase of neonatal hepatitis and other parenchymal cholestatic conditions. Such "hypoplastic" but functional structures have been transected under these circumstances and infants provided with an unnecessary portoenterostomy. Moreover, the results of the Kasai procedure in infants over 2 mo old parallel the overall results obtained with types of atresia treated with choledochojejunostomy. The Kasai procedure may succeed only when performed prior to permanent closure of the passages in the porta hepatis. Thus, hepatic portoenterostomy may be effective only in hypoplasia of the bile ducts evolving toward atresia. It is not known whether this form of intervention arrests the sclerosing process.

Intrahepatic biliary atresia or hypoplasia or paucity of the intrahepatic bile ducts is a major cause of severe, chronic cholestasis beginning in early infancy. A significant proportion of infants with this disorder have associated facial, cardiac, and vertebral anomalies, the Watson-Alagille syndrome (Fig 11–29). Liver biopsies obtained during the 1st mo after birth frequently reveal

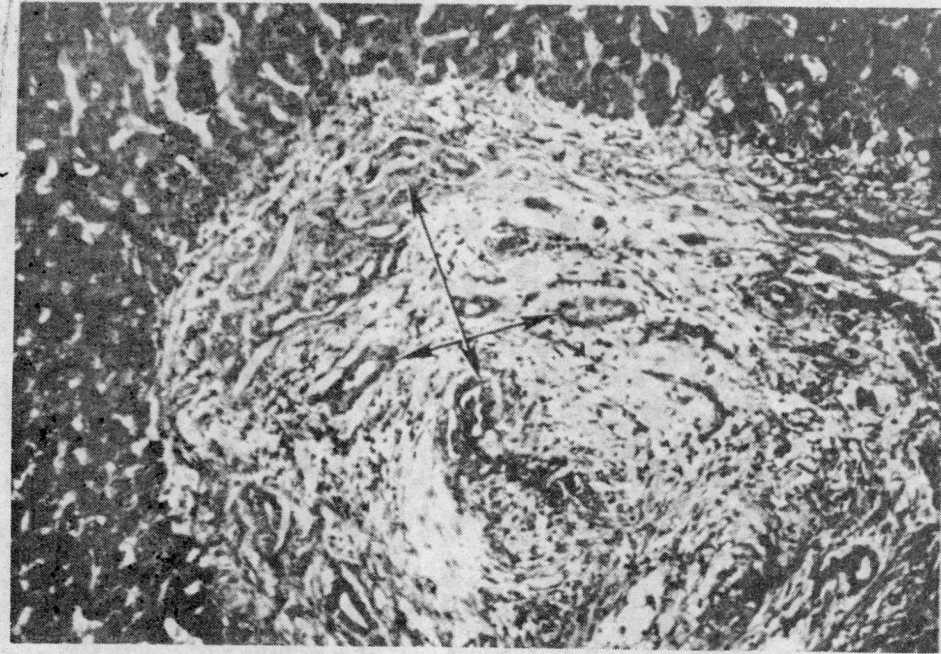

Figure 11–28 Liver in extrahepatic biliary atresia. The portal zone is expanded by copious fibrous tissue containing proliferating bile ducts (arrows). Trichrome stain. × 100.

an inflammatory process involving the interlobular bile ducts. This recedes on subsequent biopsy leaving variable reductions in number or diameter of these structures (Fig 11–30). Thus, most hypoplastic anomalies of the intrahepatic bile ducts may be regarded as sequelae

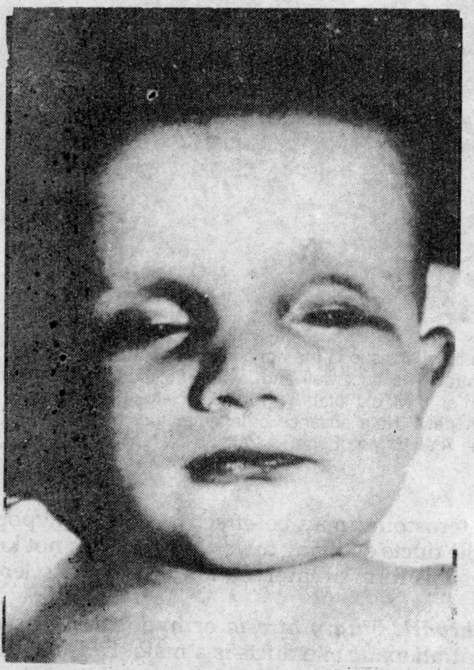

Figure 11–29 Typical facies of Alagille-Watson syndrome (arteriohepatic dysplasia). Constant features include prominence of frontal skull development, hypertelorism, anti-mongoloid ocular slant, flat nasal bridge, and small pointed chin. Note scratch marks over right clavicular area. The patient also had pulmonary artery stenosis and defects of the anterior vertebral arches.

of a sclerosing cholangitis which terminates during early infancy.

Infants with intrahepatic biliary hypoplasia usually present with clinical manifestations of jaundice and hepatomegaly during the 1st mo. In infants with severe disease there are rapid increases in serum transaminases, alkaline phosphatase (5–20-fold normal values), and lipid fractions (cholesterol, phospholipids, triglycerides); corresponding changes in infants with extrahepatic atresia occur more slowly. Accordingly, infants with hypoplastic intrahepatic bile ducts consistently develop xanthomas. Severe pruritus, steatorrhea, and a bleeding tendency are also common clinical problems. A characteristic combination of neuromuscular complications, including absence of deep tendon reflexes, weakness of upward gaze, inability to walk due to paresis of lower limbs, and loss of vibratory sense, is frequently observed in children with intrahepatic biliary hypoplasia after 6 yr of age. These abnormalities may reflect anterior horn lesions due to severe vitamin E deficiency and may be reversible if blood levels of the vitamin are maintained within the normal range.

Treatment should include a low fat, high protein diet supplemented with medium chain triglycerides if biliary insufficiency is severe. Special attention should be given to providing adequate intake of fat-soluble vitamins as these are frequently malabsorbed when cholestyramine is added to the regimen. Vitamins A, D, E, and K are provided as water-soluble preparations. There are no advantages in administration of 25-hydroxy vitamin D rather than vitamin D itself. Vitamin E deficiency may require oral supplementation with up to 1000 IU of vitamin E/24 hr; in certain patients no significant absorption from the intestine is apparent even at these doses. In such patients intramuscular injections of vitamin E (experimental use) are effective in maintaining blood vitamin E concentrations within the normal

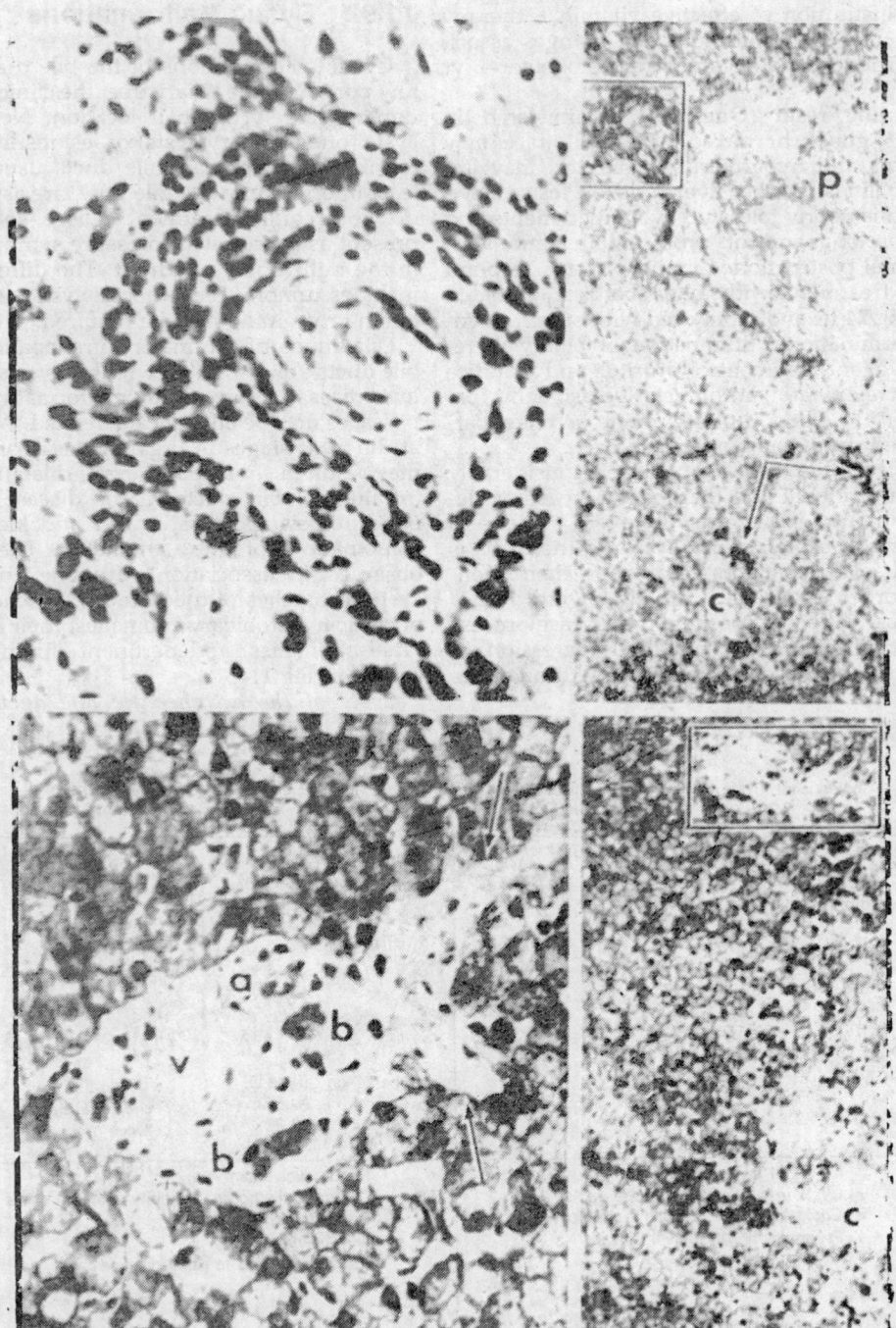

Figure 11–30 *A*, The liver in intrahepatic biliary hypoplasia. Biopsy obtained at 7 wk of age from the infant shown in Fig 11–29 at 8 mo of age. *Right panel*, Liver lobule, displaying a greatly expanded portal zone (p), a central vein (c), and erythropoietic elements (arrows). ×60. The framed area is shown at higher magnification in the left panel. *Left panel*, Interlobular bile duct lined by thickened epithelium showing degenerative changes. The duct is surrounded by concentric layers of connective tissue and inflammatory cells (pericholangitis). ×200. *B*, Liver biopsy obtained at 2 yr of age from the infant shown in Fig 11–29. *Right panel*, Portal zone in framed area is reduced in size (compare with *A*). There is no evidence of inflammation, necrosis, or fibrosis. Central vein (c) is at lower right. ×60. *Left panel*, Area framed in right panel, at higher magnification. Note hypoplastic and atrophied bile ducts (b) and absence of inflammatory elements. A branch of the portal vein (v) and a hepatic arteriole (a) are also present in this portal area, distorted by stellate extensions of fibrous strands (arrows). ×200.

range. Early institution of effective vitamin E therapy is important since the neuromuscular changes associated with deficiency may become irreversible by 6–8 yr of age.

Cholestyramine resin (Questran) administered in doses of 8–16 gm/24 hr mixed with fruit juice may reduce pruritus and hyperbilirubinemia and may improve abnormalities in other liver function tests. However, the resin is poorly tolerated by many patients and may cause prolongation of prothrombin time and, rarely, intestinal obstruction. Certain patients respond favorably to treatment with phenobarbital, initiated with 3–5 mg/kg/24 hr and monitored with serum phenobarbital determinations. Stimulation of biliary secretion with this agent may control pruritus and jaundice and reduce or eliminate xanthomas. Occasionally, patients refractory to either cholestyramine or phenobarbital may benefit from combined therapy.

The *prognosis* in this disorder has been considerably improved by nutritional and therapeutic measures designed to counteract the effects of severe cholestasis and malabsorption of lipids. Survival into the teens is expected, and several patients are alive in their twenties. The disorder progresses slowly toward biliary cirrhosis in most patients. In others the disease process appears to stabilize without notable progression of hepatic fibrosis or alterations of blood flow through the liver.

11.92 Cystic Malformations

Cystic malformations of the bile ducts may occur in any portion of the biliary tree; the clinical manifestations depend largely on their location. Noncommunicating cysts (often solitary cysts) or lesions involving only the terminal (interlobular) bile ducts usually produce the least interference with bile flow, are asymptomatic, and do not require treatment. Large solitary cysts may present as a mass with pressure symptoms, most often in the right upper quadrant. The differential diagnosis includes tumors, echinococcal cysts, and abscesses; excision or draining may be required.

Dilatations of the major intrahepatic or extrahepatic bile ducts are associated with bile stasis and progressive liver disease. Many cystic malformations of the biliary passages may be etiologically related. An identical insult at different stages in organogenesis or in different loci may result in choledochal cysts, dilatations of the major intrahepatic bile ducts (Caroli disease), congenital hepatic fibrosis, polycystic liver and kidney disease, or combinations of these anomalies. They have all been observed in association with one another and with cystic anomalies of the kidneys. A schematic summary of cystic hepatobiliary anomalies, their relationship with renal anomalies, and pertinent clinical aspects is presented in Fig 11–31.

Cysts of the extrahepatic bile ducts may occur as

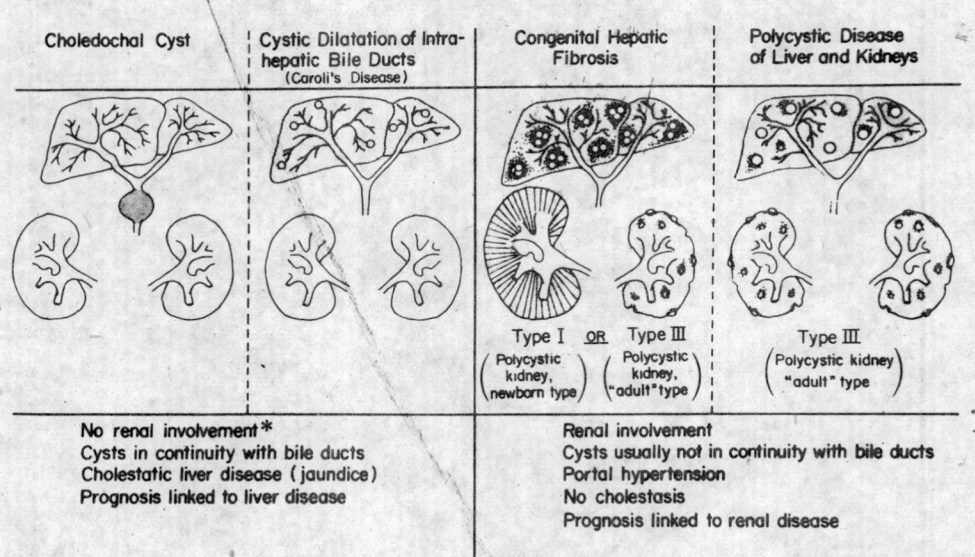

| Choledochal Cyst | Cystic Dilatation of Intra-hepatic Bile Ducts (Caroli's Disease) | Congenital Hepatic Fibrosis | Polycystic Disease of Liver and Kidneys |

Type I OR Type III   Type III
(Polycystic   (Polycystic   (Polycystic kidney)
kidney,   kidney,   "adult" type
newborn type) "adult" type)

No renal involvement*   Renal involvement
Cysts in continuity with bile ducts   Cysts usually not in continuity with bile ducts
Cholestatic liver disease (jaundice)   Portal hypertension
Prognosis linked to liver disease   No cholestasis
                                         Prognosis linked to renal disease

Figure 11–31 Cystic malformations involving the liver and bile ducts occur in 2 main categories: (1) Choledochal cysts and cystic dilatations of the main branches of the intrahepatic bile ducts (Caroli disease). (2) Congenital hepatic fibrosis and polycystic disease of the liver and kidneys. Category 1 malformations interfere with biliary drainage through major passages, causing chronic or recurrent cholestasis, cholangitis, and progressive liver disease. Prognosis of category 1 lesions reflects extent of hepatic involvement and complications, since the kidneys are only rarely affected (the asterisk indicates that ectasia of the renal tubules has been occasionally reported in cases of Caroli disease which overlap with congenital hepatic fibrosis). Category 2 malformations are patchy and are either noncommunicating with the biliary passages or confined to the terminal interlobular bile ducts. The predominant features of these anomalies are heavy deposits of fibrous tissue and a striking association with polycystic kidneys. Fibrous tissue is more prominent in congenital hepatic fibrosis, denoted by dark stippling surrounding the cysts. Patients with congenital fibrosis and polycystic liver and kidney disease do not suffer from cholestasis and have normal liver functions. Apart from portal hypertension in congenital hepatic fibrosis, their prognosis is linked to the renal manifestations. Types I and III of polycystic kidneys are classified according to Potter; respectively, they represent medullary ("sponge") kidneys and polycystic kidneys of the adult as seen in infants.

diverticula or fusiform dilatations of the common bile duct, common hepatic duct, or gallbladder, or as a choledochocele of the intraduodenal portion of the common duct. They are most common along the free portion of the duct (choledochus cyst). This type of cyst is associated in 33–100% of cases with a premature union of the common bile duct and the pancreatic duct before their entry into the sphincter of Oddi. Because of the higher pressures in the pancreatic duct, reflux of pancreatic juice into the common bile duct may occur, causing inflammation, stenosis, and weakening of the duct wall.

The lesion may remain undetected until biliary obstruction develops because of gallstones within the cyst or until cholangitis occurs. The obstruction is usually intermittent and results in jaundice, pain, and a mass. Thus, few patients with choledochal cyst are diagnosed under 1 yr of age, and approximately 50% of all cases are discovered after 10 yr of age. The symptoms are usually chronic (1–5 mo) and consist of pain in the right upper quadrant, vomiting, and fever. Abdominal ultrasound scan is especially useful in infants who generally do not manifest the classic clinical triad of jaundice, pain, and mass. The diagnosis should also be suspected when there is prolonged obstructive jaundice with serum alkaline phosphatase levels of 200–300 IU or when a liver biopsy reveals findings consistent with extrahepatic biliary obstruction and there is bile pigmentation in duodenal drainage or stools. Diagnosis can usually be established by roentgenographic examination of the upper intestinal tract, intravenous cholangiogram, or computed tomography.

The treatment is primary excision of the cyst or choledochocystojejunostomy with cholecystotomy. Recurrent cholangitis, stricture of the anastomotic site, progressive liver disease, and intestinal obstruction may continue to plague these patients.

Cystic dilatation of the intrahepatic bile ducts (Caroli disease) is characterized by berrylike cysts lined with normal cuboidal epithelium in continuity with the primary branches of the main intrahepatic bile ducts. Thus, among cystic malformations of the biliary tree Caroli disease occupies an intermediate position between choledochal cysts and the dilatations of interlobular and intralobular ducts observed in congenital hepatic fibrosis. That this disease has been associated with both of these other conditions would be consistent with a common prenatal origin for all 3 types of cystic malformation, with variability in expression reflecting temporal and hereditary as well as teratogenic factors.

The major *clinical manifestations* of Caroli disease are gallstone formation within the saccular dilatations of the intrahepatic bile ducts, recurrent bouts of cholangitis, and abscess formation. Patients usually present as children or as young adults, although the disease may manifest itself at any age. Fever, pruritus, mild icterus, a tender liver which is usually only slightly enlarged, and modestly elevated values of serum bilirubin, transaminases, and alkaline phosphatase are observed during acute episodes. The *diagnosis* may be suspected when an ultrasonogram reveals multiple opacities within the liver parenchyma. Definitive evidence can be obtained with percutaneous transhepatic cholangiography. A liver biopsy may reveal associated congenital hepatic fibrosis, and intravenous pyelography may demonstrate the presence of renal tubular ectasia.

Treatment consists of antibiotics, which often fail to control cholangitis adequately. Disease involving a single lobe has been treated successfully by partial hepatectomy. Repeated laparotomies to remove affected canaliculi from the accessible portions of the biliary tree have also been attempted. The *prognosis* is unpredictable, and fatalities due to liver abscess, sepsis, cholangiocarcinoma, and amyloidosis are not uncommon.

Congenital hepatic fibrosis is an inherited (autosomal recessive) disorder characterized by hamartomatous lesions involving the interlobular bile ducts. The portal triads are surrounded by thick deposits of fibrous tissue in which are embedded distorted structures lined with biliary epithelium. Additional multiple small cystic formations are usually observed lining the outer boundaries of the fibrous plaques in contact with the liver parenchyma. The cystic structures usually are not in communication with the biliary ductule system and do not interfere with bile flow except in rare cases which are indistinguishable from Caroli disease. The parenchyma is well preserved and free from inflammatory elements.

The disease is usually discovered in late childhood when hepatosplenomegaly is noted or when upper gastrointestinal bleeding due to portal hypertension intervenes. Liver function tests are usually normal or only mildly disturbed while thrombocytopenia due to hypersplenism may be severe. In 60–80% of childhood cases congenital hepatic fibrosis is associated with cystic dilatations of renal collecting tubules demonstrable by intravenous pyelography.

Treatment requires control of bleeding from esophageal varices. Splenectomy may become necessary to control thrombocytopenia and to eliminate displacement of neighboring organs by the greatly enlarged spleen. A splenorenal shunt is performed at the time of splenectomy to provide relief from portal hypertension. The prognosis is often excellent provided normal renal function is preserved.

Polycystic liver disease is a rare disorder of unknown origin which is distinguished from congenital hepatic fibrosis by absence of excessive connective tissue deposits within the liver parenchyma. The cysts range in size from microscopic vesicles to cavernous structures several cm in diameter, but they are not in continuity with the biliary passages. The hepatic parenchyma is well preserved, and its functions are not disturbed. The liver is not tender but may be irregular to palpation because of the presence of large subcapsular cysts. Ultrasonography or computed axial tomography may indicate the presence of fluid-filled cavities in the liver and kidneys.

Polycystic kidney disease is present in at least 50% of all patients with hepatic cysts. In most the symptomatology is due to the renal lesion, which may cause severe or fatal renal insufficiency. Occasionally, the anomaly is discovered after the rupture of a large cyst or after an intracystic hemorrhage which requires surgical intervention, but most cases are asymptomatic and are found only incidentally at autopsy. No treatment is necessary, and cysts should be left undisturbed even if found unexpectedly at laparotomy performed for other reasons.

11.93 CHOLESTASIS AND LIVER DISEASE ASSOCIATED WITH TOTAL PARENTERAL NUTRITION (TPN)

Liver dysfunction is the most common metabolic complication of parenteral alimentation. Up to 80% of patients receiving this form of therapy display elevations of serum SGOT and SGPT, and jaundice develops frequently in these infants, with the highest incidence (40–50%) being recorded in the smallest newborns. A distinction must be made between benign reversible hepatic dysfunction associated with TPN and overt, potentially irreversible liver disease precipitated or exacerbated by TPN. Table 11–15 lists factors which predispose to liver dysfunction and destructive pathology in patients receiving TPN. Prematurity, duration of treatment, and nature of the underlying disorder are the major factors responsible for development of cholestasis in infants on TPN. TPN extended for more than 2 wk carries a high probability of cholestasis, but this type of isolated cholestasis is generally completely reversible after cessation of TPN. The mechanism responsible for TPN-associated cholestasis is not established but may be related to interference with formation or secretion of bile by certain amino acids, essential fatty acid deficiency, and interference with hepatic membrane transport.

Liver disease, as distinct from dysfunction, develops rarely but can be a life-threatening complication. Sepsis, abdominal surgery, and necrotizing enterocolitis may predispose to inflammatory and fibrosing lesions of the liver in infants on long term TPN. Infants with these disorders who become jaundiced while receiving TPN should be investigated with percutaneous liver biopsies. If periportal inflammation, necrotic lesions, and fibrotic changes are observed, a trial of enteral alimentation with elemental formulas is indicated. Such formulas (Vivonex, Travasorb, Pregestimil) may be tolerated if administered by continuous drip through a nasogastric tube; supplementation by glucose administered through a peripheral vein also may be required.

Hepatomegaly with mild elevation of transaminase in the absence of cholestasis is occasionally encountered in infants on TPN receiving more than 100 kcal/kg/24 hr. In most such instances lipid deposition is responsible for liver enlargement. Fatty liver due to excessive caloric intake is readily reversible in nearly all instances by reduction of the total calories administered. The carbohydrate/protein ratio may also play a role in development of fatty liver, but optimal ratios appear to vary with the underlying disorder and nutritional status at initiation of TPN.

Hepatic complications of TPN tend to be less frequent and relatively less severe in patients beyond infancy. However, abnormal liver function tests are not uncommon in patients maintained on home hyperalimentation for months or years. Those with chronic intestinal conditions complicated by infection or bacterial overgrowth are particularly susceptible to hepatic complications. In most of these patients, elevated serum transaminase levels can be reversed by instituting partial enteral alimentation. However, when alkaline phosphatase or gamma glutamyl transferase levels are also elevated, liver disease may be present and should be evaluated by liver biopsy.

11.94 DRUG-INDUCED LIVER INJURY

As the main organ responsible for drug metabolism, the liver is particularly susceptible to injury from drugs and environmental toxins. The possibility of liver damage is increased when 2 agents are administered together since 1 drug may inhibit or induce hepatic microsomal enzymes necessary for the metabolism of the other. In addition, predictable dose dependent or unexpected dose independent (idiosyncratic) drug reactions may affect the liver. Potentially hepatotoxic agents are listed in Table 11–16.

The *dose dependent* type of injury is due to compounds that are directly hepatotoxic because they disrupt the liver cell, produce microsomal and mitochondrial injury, and damage the canalicular apparatus. These hepatotoxins produce their undesirable effects by competitive inhibition, by diversion of essential metabolites, or by other interference with the metabolic or secretory activities of the liver cell. Drugs such as the antimetabolites and acetaminophen cause hepatocellular necrosis manifested by variable degrees of hepatic decompensation. Chronic liver disease, ranging from fibrosis and portal inflammation to frank cirrhosis, may also be a consequence of direct hepatotoxicity.

Dose independent liver damage is produced indirectly

Table 11–15 HEPATIC COMPLICATIONS ASSOCIATED WITH TOTAL PARENTERAL NUTRITION

LIVER DYSFUNCTION	
Predisposing Factors	Predominant Manifestations
Prematurity	Cholestasis
Duration of total parenteral alimentation	Cholestasis
Nutrient imbalance	
Excessive amino acids	Cholestasis
Inadequate amino acids	Fatty liver (kwashiorkor)
Caloric overload	Fatty liver

LIVER DISEASE	
Predisposing Factors	Predominant Manifestations
Systemic infections	Cholangitis
Gastrointestinal disorders	Cholangitis and fibrosis
Necrotizing enterocolitis	
Inflammatory bowel disease	
Abdominal surgery	Cholangitis and fibrosis
Intestinal atresias	
Gastroschisis	
Hepatotoxic agents	Necrosis and fibrosis

Table 11-16 HEPATOTOXIC AGENTS

DRUG	MECHANISM OF TOXICITY*	PREDOMINANT CLINICAL PATTERN†
Analagesics		
Acetaminophen (Tylenol, paracetamol)	Direct	A, CAH, F
Acetylsalicylic acid (aspirin)	Direct	A
Propoxyphene (Darvon)	Indirect	Ch
Anesthetics		
Halothane (Fluothane)	Indirect	A, F
Antibiotics		
Erythromyoinestolate	Indirect (direct)	Ch
Griseofulvin	Indirect (direct)	Ch
Isoniazid	Indirect (direct)	A, CAH, F
Nitrofurantoin (Furadantin)	Indirect	Ch
Oxacillin (Prostaphlin)	Indirect	Ch
Quinacrine (Atabrine)	Indirect	A, F
Rifampin	Indirect (direct)	Ch
Sulfonamides	Indirect (direct)	A, CAH, F
Tetracyclines	Direct	CAH
Anticonvulsants		
Diphenylhydantoin (Dilantin)	Indirect	A, Ch, F
Phenacemide (Phenurone)	Indirect	A, Ch
Trimethadione (Tridione)	Indirect	A
Diuretic agents		
Chlorothiazide (Diuril)	Indirect	Ch
Methyldopa (Aldomet)	Indirect (direct)	A, CAH
Quinethazone (Hydromox)	Indirect	Ch
Cytotoxins and Immunosuppressants		
Azathioprine (Imuran)	Direct	A
Chlorambucil (Leukeran)	Indirect	A
6-Mercaptopurine	Direct	A, F, C
Methotrexate	Direct	C
Urethane	Direct	A, F, C
Hormones and metabolic agents		
Androgens		
Methyltestosterone	Direct	Ch, A
Norethandrolone	Direct	Ch, A
Estrogens		
Ethinyl estradiol	Direct	Ch, A
Methylestranolone	Direct	Ch, A
Progestins		
Norethindrone (Norlutin)	Direct	A
Antithyroid agents		
Methimazole (Tapazole)	Indirect	Ch
Propylthiouracil	Indirect	A
Thiouracil	Indirect	Ch, A, F
Thiourea	Indirect	A
Hypoglycemic agents		
Carbutamide	Indirect	A
Chlorpropamide (Diabinese)	Indirect (direct)	Ch
Metahexamide (Euglycin)	Indirect	Ch, A, CAH
Tolbutamide (Orinase)	Direct (indirect)	Ch
Psychopharmacologic agents		
Phenothiazines		
Chlorpromazine (Thorazine)	Direct (indirect)	Ch
Mepazine (Pactal)	Indirect (direct)	Ch
Perphenazine (Trilafon)	Indirect (direct)	Ch
Prochlorperazine (Compazine)	Indirect	Ch, A, CAH
Promazine (Sparine)	Indirect	Ch
Thioridazine (Mellaril)	Indirect	Ch
Monoamine oxidase inhibitors		
Iproniazid (Marsalid)	Indirect	A, CAH
Isocarboxazid (Marplan)	Indirect	A
Other psychopharmacologic agents		
Chlordiazepoxide (Librium)	Indirect	Ch
Diazepam (Valium)	Indirect	Ch
Ethchlorvynol (Placcidyl)	Indirect	Ch
Imipramine (Tofranil)	Indirect	Ch, A
Meprobamate (Equanil)	Indirect	Ch
Miscellaneous		
Topical copper sulfate	Direct	A
Ferrous sulfate	Direct	A, CAH
Trimethobenzamide (Tigan)	Indirect	Ch
Tripelennamine (Pyribenzamine)	Indirect	Ch

*Direct—dose dependent liver damage. Indirect—dose independent liver damage due to idiosyncratic response.

†A = acute hepatitis; CAH = chronic active hepatitis; F = fulminant hepatitis; Ch = cholestasis; C = cirrhosis.

Adapted from H. Zimmerman.

in a small percentage of patients receiving a drug. It is an expression of an individual's susceptibility due to hypersensitivity or to formation of abnormal metabolites. Covalent linkage with tissue macromolecules and subsequent antibody response may be the common initiating mechanisms. The characteristic features of drug hypersensitivity are present, including a "sensitization" period of 1–4 wk, recurrence of liver dysfunction when the drug is readministered, a high incidence of allergic manifestations (rash, fever, eosinophilia, and granuloma formation in the liver), and an incidence of less than 1%. The morphologic changes produced by idiosyncratic reactions include pure cholestasis, invasion of the liver parenchyma by mononuclear cells and eosinophils, diffuse hepatocellular degeneration, and necrosis. In the cholestatic form the serum transaminases undergo a mild increase compared with striking elevations in alkaline phosphatase. Conversely, hepatocellular degeneration and necrosis are associated with high transaminase values compared with alkaline phosphatase and with hypoprothrombinemia.

Idiosyncratic reactions due to formation of hepatotoxic metabolites are less common. The morphologic and biochemical features are similar to those of hypersensitivity reactions. Clinically, the latent period is more variable (2–52 wk), and allergic symptoms are minimal or absent. Examples of this type are reactions to iproniazid and isoniazid.

The *diagnosis* of drug toxicity is based on a history of exposure to the drug and a syndrome compatible with the ingestion of certain drugs. Fever, rash, and eosinophilia are suggestive in a patient with abnormal liver function tests. Recurrence of symptoms and hepatic dysfunction after a test dose of the drug are supportive evidence of toxicity. This type of test should be performed only in patients in whom the drugs must be continued.

Treatment consists primarily of withdrawal of the offending drug. A high caloric (80–100 calories/kg/24 hr), high protein (2.0 gm/kg/24 hr), high carbohydrate diet helps recovery unless hepatic decompensation develops. Liver failure should be treated as described in Sec 11.101. Cholestasis without hepatocellular failure may be treated with cholestyramine (8–16 gm/24 hr) or phenobarbital (3–5 mg/kg/24 hr) to alleviate pruritus and jaundice. Specific therapy with cysteamine for acetaminophen poisoning is discussed in Sec 28.5.

Early withdrawal of the toxic agent and the extent of initial hepatic injury determine the *prognosis*. In most cases symptoms subside within days, the biochemical abnormalities resolve within weeks, and the hepatic lesion heals without sequelae. In more advanced injuries initial improvement may be followed by development of portal hypertension. Fulminant hepatitis is a relatively rare complication.

11.95 REYE SYNDROME

See also Sec 21.20.

Reye syndrome is an acute illness which may develop in the course of a nonspecific viral infection (upper respiratory, gastrointestinal) and occurs frequently in association with varicella, influenza B, and influenza A infections. Cases have also been reported in children with aflatoxin poisoning from Thailand and warfarin poisoning from Israel. Jamaican vomiting sickness, an illness which resembles Reye syndrome, is produced by ingestion of hypoglycin A (methylenecyclopropane-acetic acid) contained in the unripe fruit of the akee tree.

Epidemiology and Etiology. The illness affects infants and children of all ages but is more frequent around ages 6–9 and 11–14. Both sexes are affected equally. An association with antipyretic use has been noted. Mortality has gradually decreased from 50% to under 30% during the past decade.

The cause of Reye syndrome is unknown. The leading hypothesis implicates mitochondrial dysfunction as the underlying lesion on the basis of ultrastructural changes in mitochondria (swelling, pleomorphism, and loss of intramitochondrial dense bodies), although these alterations may reflect primary or secondary events. An underlying inherited or acquired predisposition toward development of this metabolic disorder may be triggered by a virus, toxin, drug, or endogenous factor. The basic defect has been postulated to be an abnormality in the intramitochondrial portion of the urea cycle involving a complex of 2 enzymes, carbamyl phosphate synthetase and ornithine transcarbamylase, the 1st catalyzing the conversion of ammonia to carbamyl phosphate, the 2nd reacting with carbamyl phosphate and ornithine to produce citrulline. Interference with these steps would cause hyperammonemia and may lead to the formation of orotic acid. Since orotic acid interferes with lipoprotein synthesis, the fatty liver observed in Reye syndrome could result from liver cells lacking in lipoprotein.

Clinical and Laboratory Manifestations. The typical presentation is a previously well child who develops severe nausea and vomiting in the course of an unremarkable viral illness. Within hours to days the patient begins to display hyperactive or combative behavior, followed by decreased responsiveness, somnolence, stupor, loss of deep tendon reflexes, decorticate posturing, convulsions, and coma. The liver is soft and usually moderately enlarged. Coma may persist for an unpredictable period before recovery or death intervenes. Average duration of illness in nonsurvivors is 4–5 days. Most survivors recover completely, but serious neurologic sequelae may occur in infants under 2 yr of age and in older children requiring prolonged intensive care during the acute illness.

The characteristic profile of liver functions consists of rapidly rising transaminases, prolonged prothrombin time, elevated blood ammonia early in the course, and serum bilirubin values within normal limits. Creatinine phosphokinase values are also consistently elevated. Hypoglycemia is a feature in younger children and infants. The severity of changes in these indices has little prognostic significance. Respiratory alkalosis frequently precedes metabolic acidosis due to lactic acid accumulation. The differential diagnosis includes inherited urea cycle disorders, salicylate poisoning, hepatic coma, carnitine deficiency, lead intoxication, and certain organic acidurias.

Pathology. There are characteristic microvesiculated fatty deposits in hepatocytes in the absence of inflammatory, necrotic, or fibrotic changes (Fig 11–32). Similar but less extensive fatty changes are present in proximal renal tubules, myocardium, and pancreas. Pancreatitis is not infrequent but is often detected at postmortem only. The brain reveals severe edema, neuronal degeneration, and a striking absence of inflammatory ele-

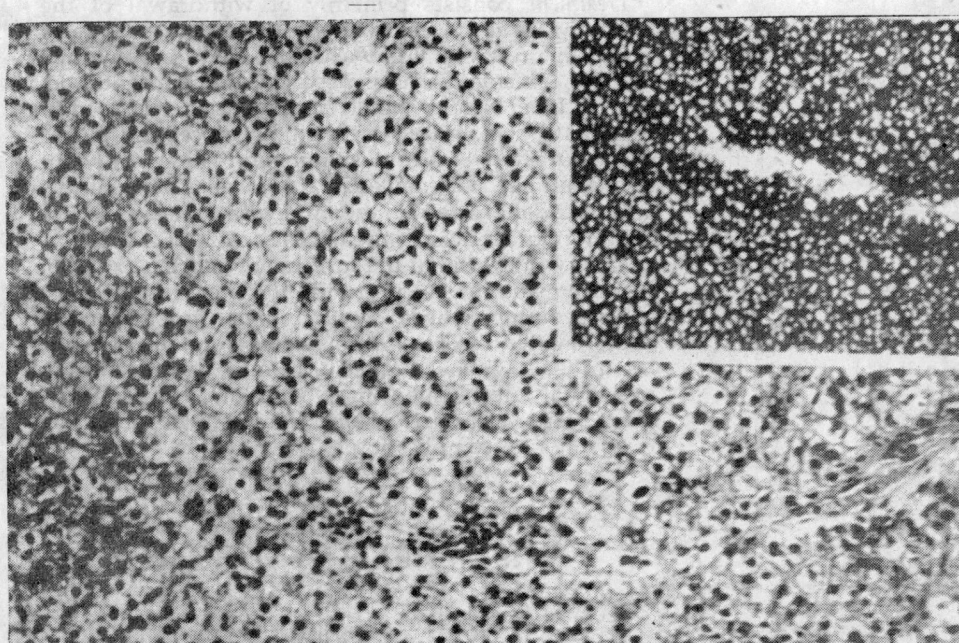

Figure 11–32 The liver in Reye syndrome. Note uniform microvesiculation of hepatocytes and absence of inflammation or necrosis. Hematoxylin and eosin stain. ×100. *Inset*, Frozen section of the same specimen, stained with Giemsa to highlight fine droplets of neutral fat deposited in every hepatocyte. Clear horizontal area is the central vein. ×200.

Table 11–17 STAGES OF REYE SYNDROME

STAGE	CRITERIA
I	Lethargy, vomiting, indifference
II	Delirium, combativeness, hyperventilation
III	Decorticate posturing, light coma, hypoventilation, intact pupillary responses
IV	Decerebrate posture, deep coma, loss of spontaneous ventilation, fixed dilated pupils
V	Seizures, flaccidity, respiratory arrest

After Lovejoy et al.

ments. Electron microscopic examination shows extensive deposition of fine droplets of fat in the cytoplasm of hepatocytes, swollen and distorted mitochondria, hyperplastic smooth endoplasmic reticulum, and large numbers of peroxisomes.

Treatment. All patients suspected of having Reye syndrome should be admitted to an intensive care unit even if awake and responsive. Supportive care is provided and the stage of illness assessed (Table 11–17). Arterial and central venous pressure lines, a urinary catheter, and a nasogastric tube are inserted. Fever is controlled with a cooling blanket, and intravenous fluids are administered at two thirds maintenance using 15% glucose solution. Prothrombin time is corrected with intramuscular vitamin K (5 mg), and neomycin is administered by nasogastric tube or enema to reduce blood ammonia.

When the patient's condition deteriorates to stage III (Table 11–17), mechanical ventilation through an endotracheal tube is provided and an intracranial pressure monitor (catheter or bolt) is placed. The intracranial pressure (ICP) is monitored continuously and maintained at or below 2 mm Hg with intravenous injections of an osmotic agent such as mannitol and controlled hyperventilation to maintain pCO_2 at 25–30 mm Hg (Sec 21.20). Mannitol is initially infused at 0.25 gm/kg over 10 min using a 20% solution. This dose may be increased stepwise up to 2.0 gm/kg if the ICP remains above 20 mm Hg and infused continuously to maintain serum osmolality at 320 mOsm/l. When ICP remains below 20 mm Hg but spikes on occasion, these sudden elevations can be treated with bolus injections of mannitol at 0.25 gm/kg over 10 min. Other agents employed for this purpose are 30% urea or glycerol.

If ICP cannot be controlled by osmotherapy, coma may be induced with phenobarbital although the benefits and risks of this experimental therapy have not been evaluated for patients with Reye syndrome. Phenobarbital is administered intravenously, initially at 5 mg/kg, then 2.5 mg/kg every 4 hr, until a blood level of 3–5 mg/dl is achieved. When ICP returns to normal for 12–24 hr or when complications intervene, pentobarbital levels should be reduced gradually. The most serious complications of barbiturate therapy are declines in arterial pressure and in cardiac output and hypoxia.

CHRONIC LIVER DISORDERS AND CIRRHOSIS

CHRONIC HEPATITIS

In adults with hepatitis, chronicity is usually defined as liver disease persisting longer than 6 mo. Chronicity in children with hepatitis is more difficult to define since the usual course of illness is milder than that of adults. Moreover, hepatitis A, which is prevalent in childhood, neither persists nor progresses to chronic liver disease (Sec 10.83). The relationship between acute viral infection and chronic hepatitis is not entirely clear. Few patients with chronic inflammatory liver disease have a history of previous acute illness, and carriers of hepatitis B virus rarely develop chronic hepatitis (Sec 10.83). However, hepatitis B infection may persist for months or years after an acute attack. The relationship between acute hepatitis B and chronicity is illustrated in Fig 11–33.

The course of illness and outcome in chronic hepatitis are determined by the aggressiveness of the inflammatory process in the liver parenchyma. Two distinct

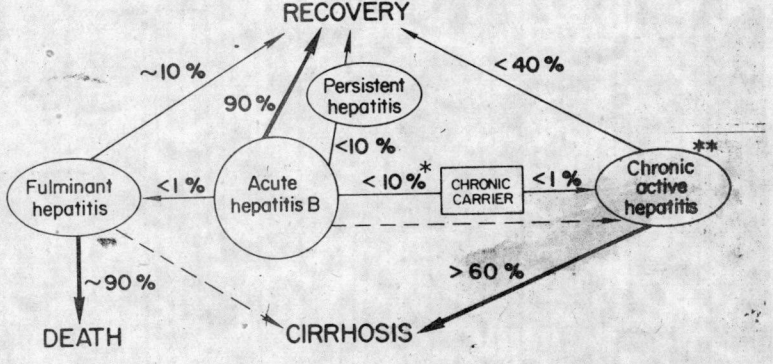

Figure 11–33 Relationships between acute hepatitis B and persistent hepatitis, chronic active hepatitis, and fulminant hepatitis.

* Newborns infected with hepatitis B virus by vertical transmission become carriers almost without exception.

** Very few pediatric cases of chronic active hepatitis are positive for hepatitis B surface antigen. The recovery/cirrhosis ratio is considerably more favorable (8:1) in the predominant B-negative "lupoid" variety.

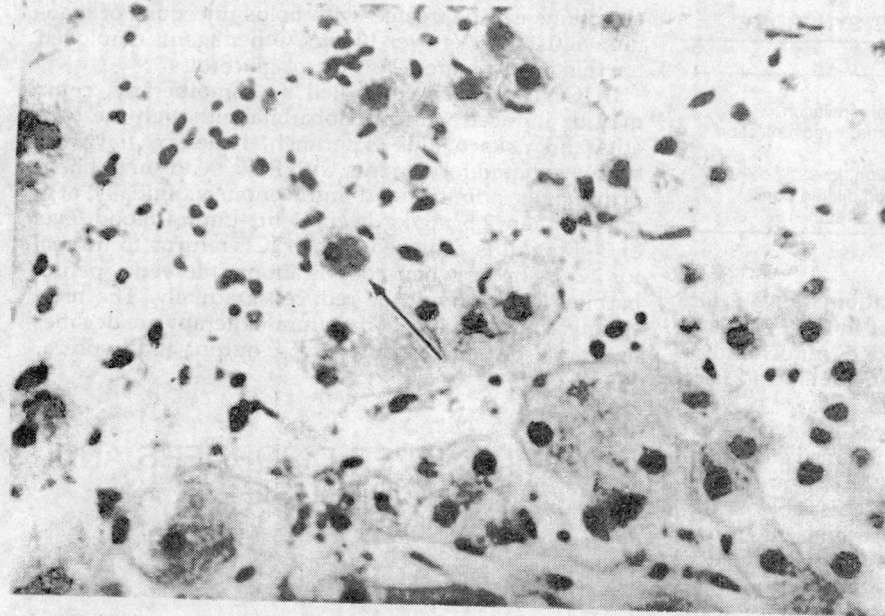

Figure 11–34 The liver in persistent hepatitis. Hepatocytes lack uniformity, displaying differences in staining cell size and shape, but the arrangement of hepatic cords is preserved. Inflammatory cells (mostly lymphocytes) are concentrated in the lobular periphery at upper left. Councilman bodies (arrow) are often seen in persistent hepatitis. There is no fibrosis or piecemeal necrosis in evidence. ×200.

categories of chronic inflammatory liver disease are based on histologic criteria observed in liver biopsy specimens: persistent hepatitis and chronic active hepatitis. The characteristic features of each are described in legends to Fig 11–34 and 11–35.

11.96   Chronic Persistent Hepatitis

Clinical and Laboratory Manifestations.   The majority of patients present with vague complaints of abdominal tenderness (not necessarily over the liver), fatiga-

bility, weight loss due to poor appetite, and malaise. These are often ignored or ascribed to a nonspecific viral illness. Mild scleral icterus is occasionally present. The liver is often tender to palpation but is rarely enlarged.

Laboratory investigations reveal mildly elevated serum bilirubin in about 50% of cases and fluctuating but consistently elevated transaminase values. Alkaline phosphatase, serum albumin and globulin, and prothrombin time are nearly always within normal limits. Tests for HB$_s$Ag are positive in fewer than 10%, mostly in adolescents. In the remainder, detection of serum

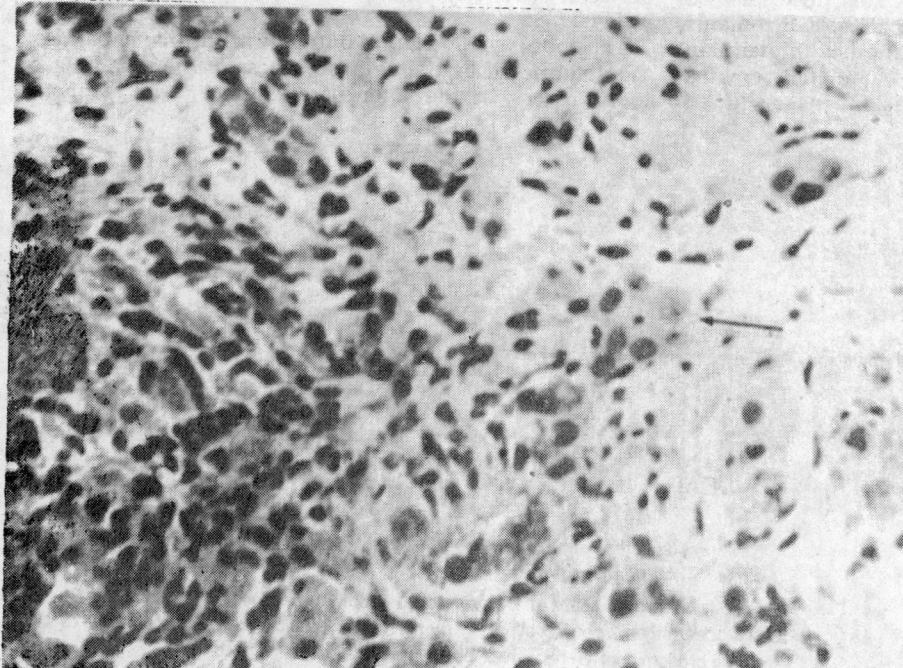

Figure 11–35 The liver in chronic active hepatitis. The portal area at lower left displays disorganized architecture, with the limiting plate breached by fibrous septa, lymphocytes, and plasma cells, and filled with entrapped, dying hepatocytes (piecemeal necrosis). Other features include pseudoacinar formation (arrow), ballooning of the hepatocytes, and fibrous strands extending into the parenchyma causing disruption of sinusoidal pattern. ×200.

Table 11–18 FEATURES OF CHRONIC ACTIVE HEPATITIS

	HB$_s$AG NEGATIVE	HB$_s$AG POSITIVE
Age	5–16 years	17 years or older
Sex	Female predominance (4:1)	Male predominance (>2:1)
Autoimmune disease	Usual	Very rare
Corticosteroid therapy	Excellent results (>75% remission)	Largely ineffective
Serum gamma globulin	2 to 4 times normal	Less than 2 times normal
Antinuclear antibody	Positive (60–80%)	
Smooth muscle antibody	High titer	Low titer
Serum hepatitis B surface antigen	Negative	Positive
Serum hepatitis B surface antibody	Negative	Often positive
Direct Coombs test	Positive (~70%)	Negative
LE cells	Positive (~50%)	Negative

IgM anti-hepatitis A antibody may indicate a recent infection; the presence of the IgG antibody merely confirms past exposure to the virus.

Diagnosis. Persistence of symptoms and abnormal liver function tests for 3 mo is an indication for a percutaneous liver biopsy to rule out quiescent chronic active hepatitis or other unsuspected liver disorders (Fig 11–34).

Treatment. The most important therapeutic measures are to reassure the entire family, withhold or remove any form of drug therapy, and allow a regular diet, with exercise as tolerated. Careful observation with evaluation of liver function tests every 3 mo is indicated.

Prognosis. This is excellent with eventual full recovery.

11.97 Chronic Active Hepatitis

Clinical Manifestations. The disease in children is primarily (>95%) the hepatitis B surface antigen negative variety, frequently called "lupoid" (Table 11–18). In contrast with the B positive variety, lupoid hepatitis predominates in females and is most prevalent among preadolescents. Extreme variability of symptoms and signs is characteristic at the onset. Fluctuating jaundice, fatigue, and loss of appetite are common, but symptoms may be as mild as those observed with persistent hepatitis. Hepatosplenomegaly is present in 50–80%. Pyrexia, gastrointestinal bleeding, edema, and arthralgia may develop rapidly during exacerbations and suggest incipient hepatic failure. Other organs are frequently involved in the "lupoid" form of chronic active hepatitis (glomerulonephritis, colitis, thyroiditis, etc). Control of these manifestations may require aggressive therapy since the mortality in chronic active hepatitis during the 1st 3 yr after onset reflects these complications as well as liver-related problems.

Laboratory Findings. Liver function tests reveal consistent and often striking elevations of the transaminases, mild to severe hyperbilirubinemia (2–30 mg/dl) with more than 60% of the pigment direct reacting, and serum gamma globulin greater than 2.0 gm/dl in nearly all patients. The prothrombin time is generally prolonged, while alkaline phosphatase and serum albumin are near the normal range, except in cases advancing to cirrhosis. Nonspecific autoimmune abnormalities are frequently detectable in chronic active hepatitis, including antinuclear antibodies (80%), LE cells (40%), and lesser percentages of antibodies to smooth muscle and mitochondria.

Diagnosis. Since the differential diagnosis includes Wilson disease and α_1-antitrypsin deficiency, the appropriate tests to rule out these conditions should be performed during the initial evaluation. A careful history of drug intake during the preceding 3 mo should also be obtained to eliminate the possibility of superimposed damage from hepatotoxic agents. The biopsy of chronic active hepatitis is presented in Fig 11–35.

Treatment. Controversy exists about the use of corticosteroids in hepatitis B positive chronic active hepatitis. In the B negative type with predominantly autoimmune features ("lupoid" hepatitis) the benefits of corticosteroids in controlling the morbidity and prolonging life have been firmly established. Since the large majority of pediatric cases are of the latter variety, prognosis of chronic active hepatitis in children and adolescents (especially females) is better than in adults.

A suggested treatment approach is illustrated in Table 11–19. Therapy is initiated with prednisone or prednisolone at 2 mg/kg/24 hr to a maximum total of 60 mg daily. This dosage level is maintained until transaminase values decline below twice normal (remission) or

Table 11–19 CORTICOSTEROID THERAPY OF CHRONIC ACTIVE HEPATITIS

Induction
  Obtain baseline liver biopsy
  Prednisone, 2 mg/kg/day, in 2 divided doses, to a maximum of 60 mg/day
  Monitor at monthly intervals with transaminase determinations (SGOT or SGPT)
  Continue at this dosage until transaminase values decline to near normal or until serious complications intervene (severe obesity, osteoporosis, hypertension, growth arrest, diabetes)
Remission
  Obtain follow-up liver biopsy; if histology returns to normal or indicates persistent (benign) hepatitis, reduce dosage of prednisone by 5 mg/wk to 15 mg/day, then reduce by 5 mg every 2 wk and discontinue
Serious complications
  Administer maximum dose (2 mg/kg or 60 mg total)
  Monitor at monthly intervals with transaminases
No remission or relapse at reduced dosages
  Maintain on prednisone at 20 mg/day, with the addition of azathioprine (50 to 100 mg/day)
  Monitor white blood cells and platelets weekly and transaminases monthly
  Continue on combined regimen indefinitely unless remission or serious complications occur

until serious complications of hormone therapy develop. In remission, dosage is reduced by 5 mg/wk to a maintenance dose of 10–15 mg/24 hr. Should complications such as retardation of growth, diabetes, osteoporosis, hypertension, or obesity occur before remission, the maximum dose is administered on an alternate day basis (e.g., 40 mg every other day if the previous schedule called for 40 mg daily). While the evidence in adults suggests that alternate day therapy may be ineffective, control of the disease process can be maintained in prepubertal children with every other day regimens. In many patients treated in this manner, growth is resumed and the cushingoid appearance greatly diminished. If remission cannot be obtained with alternate day therapy or relapses occur at less than 20 mg prednisone daily, azathioprine (50–100 mg daily) is added to the regimen and maintained continuously until remission occurs or serious complications intervene. Combined therapy must be monitored at weekly intervals with differential blood cell and platelet counts. Corticosteroid therapy is monitored monthly with liver function tests, and a follow-up biopsy is obtained when the transaminase values return to the normal range. If resolution of the characteristic lesion (piecemeal necrosis) has occurred or the tissue has the appearance of persistent hepatitis, the maintenance dose of prednisone is reduced by 5 mg every 2 wk until the hormone is discontinued.

Prognosis.   The beneficial effects of corticosteroid therapy are often dramatic during the 1st 3 yr. The autoimmune extrahepatic complications are most common during this initial period and often respond rapidly to immunosuppressive therapy. Long term remissions in children can be expected in at least 70% of those receiving corticosteroid therapy. In certain cases corticosteroid therapy must be continued for several yr since attempts at withdrawal are followed by exacerbation of clinical and biochemical abnormalities. Cirrhosis develops in a few instances, including a relatively high percentage of hepatitis B positive cases. In these patients the complications of chronic liver disease (portal hypertension, ascites, gastric hemorrhage, and liver failure) must be treated as they arise.

11.98   Wilson Disease

See also Sec 21.17.

This autosomal recessive disorder is an important cause of progressive liver disease in children and young adults. The lesions are presumed to be due to excessive accumulation of copper in the liver, brain, kidneys, and cornea caused by a defect in biliary copper excretion. The possibility of Wilson disease should be considered in every child with chronic liver disease because of the importance of early diagnosis to the patient and siblings.

Pathogenesis.   The molecular basis for defective biliary copper excretion in Wilson disease is unknown. In addition to ceruloplasmin, the liver and other organs contain metallothionein, a sulfur-rich protein with an affinity for copper. Metallothionein may play a role in intracellular copper transport, compartmentation, and utilization, but its relationship to ceruloplasmin-mediated copper transport is unclear. The normal fetal and newborn liver is rich in metallothionein and copper, while serum ceruloplasmin and copper levels are relatively low throughout infancy, a pattern resembling Wilson disease. Nevertheless, infants do not accumulate copper in extrahepatic tissues, nor do they exhibit the abnormalities attributed to copper toxicity in Wilson disease. Development of stable copper, ceruloplasmin, and hepatic metallothionein levels is achieved by 2 yr of age. Phenotypic expression of the Wilson trait begins at around 4 yr of age, the age by which a control mechanism responsible for copper homeostasis and biliary excretion after infancy should have matured. Along with this theory of maturational failure, other hypotheses concerning defective biliary copper excretion include anomalous metallothioneins, a lysosomal defect, and a regulatory gene defect resulting in perpetuation of fetal copper metabolism.

Clinical Manifestations.   The classic presentation of Wilson disease is the triad of neurologic abnormalities, Kayser-Fleischer rings, and cirrhosis associated with low serum copper and ceruloplasmin levels. However, the initial findings may be extremely variable, as demonstrated in a recent series of 26 patients ranging in age from 8–20 yr: 24% had normal transaminase levels, 24% had normal ceruloplasmin levels, Kayser-Fleischer rings were not visible in 24%, and only 50% had cirrhosis.

The earliest signs of liver involvement include, in sequence, hepatomegaly, splenomegaly, jaundice, and anorexia. Edema and ascites may develop suddenly, or gastrointestinal hemorrhage may be the initial sign of disease. Occasionally, the disease begins with a hemolytic crisis due to the toxic effects of copper on erythrocytes. At onset the clinicopathologic picture may resemble acute viral hepatitis, fulminant hepatitis, established cirrhosis, or, most frequently, chronic active hepatitis. Frank cirrhosis develops eventually in all untreated patients.

The advent of neurologic manifestations may be insidious or precipitous. Intention tremors, dysarthria, and dystonia are common. A proximal renal tubular defect due to copper deposition results in urinary losses of glucose, amino acids, phosphate, uric acid, and renal tubular acidosis.

Laboratory Findings.   In addition to abnormal liver function tests indistinguishable from those observed in chronic active hepatitis, serum copper and ceruloplasmin are reduced and urine copper excretion (24 hr) is consistently elevated in the majority of patients. The most reliable indication of Wilson disease is liver tissue copper content greater than 400 µg/gm dry weight. This is in excess of values observed even in the most advanced cases of chronic active hepatitis. In patients unable to tolerate a liver biopsy, pulse injection of ^{64}Cu produces a characteristic pattern of radioactivity reflecting the failure of ceruloplasmin bound radiocopper to enter the bloodstream.

Pathology.   A liver biopsy is indicated in every patient suspected of having Wilson disease. A specimen is obtained for analysis of liver copper and a portion of the specimen examined by a pathologist. The liver lesions are not specific but are strongly supportive of the diagnosis in combination with the clinical and laboratory findings. Extensive irregular scarring or an established macronodular cirrhosis is seen in advanced cases, while fatty cellular degeneration, empty nuclei ("glycogen nuclei"), and alcoholic hyalin (Mallory bodies) are commonly observed in the acute stages.

Treatment. Therapy is based on removal of excess tissue copper by chelation with D-penicillamine forming a complex readily eliminated in urine. The chelator is administered before meals, up to a total daily intake of 1500 mg, and continued on a permanent basis even after the urinary copper excretion is in the normal range. Normality of urinary copper is reached in most patients within 6–12 mo and corresponds to marked improvement of neurologic and hepatic functions and disappearance of Kayser-Fleischer rings.

Untoward reactions to penicillamine are rare in patients with Wilson disease. Aplastic anemia and membranous glomerulonephritis are the most serious, while leukopenia, fever, rash, and lymphadenopathy are much more common. Treatment of complications consists of discontinuing the drug until the complication resolves, then reinitiating penicillamine therapy with gradually increasing doses. Corticosteroids administered with penicillamine in this manner help prevent recurrence of most complications. Patients on penicillamine should receive vitamin supplementation, especially vitamin B_6. Children and adolescents in school may benefit from counseling or special classes as their handwriting and general performance improve. Physiotherapy may accelerate recovery of gait and body movements.

Prognosis. All untreated patients die from the neurologic, hepatic, renal, or hematologic complications of Wilson disease. The prognosis in patients receiving penicillamine depends on early treatment and individual responsiveness to chelation therapy. Optimal results are obtained in siblings of affected patients who are asymptomatic at the time of diagnosis. Expression of the disease can be permanently prevented in such patients. In symptomatic patients, outcome is related to type of presentation. Children with acute liver failure or severe neuromuscular involvement are usually refractory to therapy, while those with established chronic active liver disease respond poorly and progress to cirrhosis and its complications.

11.99 Indian Childhood Cirrhosis

This familial disease of early childhood is especially prevalent on the Indian subcontinent but is also seen in the Middle East, West Africa, and Central America. The highest incidence occurs in children of both sexes from 1–5 yr of age. The inheritance pattern is still uncertain, and the pathogenesis may reflect environmental factors superimposed on inherited susceptibility.

Clinical and Laboratory Manifestations. The onset is usually insidious but may be rapidly progressive. Silent hepatomegaly is the usual presenting sign, followed by signs of acute viral hepatitis such as fever, anorexia, pale stools, and darkly colored urine with or without jaundice. The disease may evolve rapidly toward cirrhosis and liver failure or may be arrested spontaneously at any point in the course. The standard liver function tests are abnormal, but the only findings specific to this disorder are striking elevations of serum immunoglobulins.

Pathology. Biopsies taken serially during the course reveal progression from an acute inflammatory process resembling viral hepatitis to piecemeal necrosis and scarring characteristic of chronic active hepatitis. In rapidly progressive cases (malignant hepatitis) the predominant process is necrosis, cellular degeneration, and lobular collapse. Mallory bodies are often seen within dying hepatocytes surrounded by inflammatory cells. The necrotic areas heal by scarring, resulting in micronodular cirrhosis. Orcein stains reveal heavy cytoplasmic deposits of copper, predominantly in lyso-

Treatment. No specific therapy is available. Corticosteroids as administered for chronic active hepatitis may provide prolonged or permanent remission.

Prognosis. The disease is fatal within 1 yr in the majority of children. Survivors usually have a quiescent cirrhosis.

11.100 Liver Disease Associated with Chronic Inflammatory Bowel Disease

Abnormalities of liver function are frequently observed in patients with ulcerative colitis or granulomatous enterocolitis (Crohn disease). The type of liver pathology observed ranges from fatty liver to carcinoma of the bile ducts. However, the most frequently encountered hepatic disorders are chronic active hepatitis and sclerosing cholangitis. Colitis is a frequent complication of chronic active hepatitis of the hepatitis B negative ("lupoid") variety in cases where manifestations of liver disease precede evidence of intestinal involvement. This type of colitis responds to corticosteroid therapy and may not recur if the systemic autoimmune process remains under control. In other patients the chronic intestinal disorder persists for years before chronic liver disease becomes apparent. Eventually, cirrhosis becomes established and predominates over the manifestations of colitis.

Sclerosing cholangitis is the most clearly delineated liver lesion occurring in association with chronic inflammatory bowel disease. Nearly 80% of patients with this type of cholangitis have ulcerative colitis. The etiology of this association is unknown, although portal vein toxemia and bacteremia have been implicated. The entire biliary tract from terminal interlobular bile ducts to the common bile duct and gallbladder is involved in a progressive inflammatory process which eventually destroys portions of the biliary tree. In percutaneous biopsy specimens the interlobular bile ducts are surrounded by chronic inflammatory cells and fibrous tissue similar in appearance to intrahepatic biliary hypoplasia of infancy in its early phase of evolution. Copper accumulates in hepatocytes with time. Whether the inflammatory exudate is a reaction to or the cause of the sclerosing process is unclear.

Sclerosing cholangitis predominates in males but affects both sexes. The disease usually becomes manifest in the early twenties but has been observed in older children and teenagers. The initial presentation ranges from typical signs of cholangitis (fever, jaundice, right upper quadrant pain, anorexia, weight loss, pruritus) to portal hypertension. Cirrhosis may be incidentally discovered. Laboratory investigations reveal elevated alkaline phosphatase and serum immunoglobulin (IgM) with variable serum bilirubin levels. The diagnosis of sclerosing cholangitis is made by endoscopic retrograde cholangiography, which reveals beading and irregularity of portions of the intra- and extrahepatic bile ducts. Carcinoma of the bile ducts is a difficult exclusion diagnosis in certain cases.

The prognosis depends on the extent of the sclerosing lesion and complications of portal hypertension. Usually, the course is slowly progressive with a fatal termination within 10 yr. Treatment is unsatisfactory. Corticosteroid therapy is ineffective. Treatment with D-penicillamine is under trial to determine whether removal of accumulated hepatocellular copper may arrest progression of the parenchymal lesions.

11.101 CIRRHOSIS AND LIVER FAILURE

Chronic liver damage may occur in a number of diseases. Chronic active hepatitis, galactosemia, cystic fibrosis, Wilson disease, and structural abnormalities of the biliary passages (biliary atresia and choledochal cyst) are conditions associated with cirrhosis for which effective preventive therapy is available. No specific therapy is available for cirrhosis that follows various forms of acute liver disease (neonatal hepatitis, neonatal sepsis, viral hepatitis, and toxic hepatitis) and some cases that are without discernible antecedents. Therapeutic measures in these cases should be directed against the destructive process and toward the prevention of complications. Serious complications, such as gastrointestinal hemorrhage or hepatic coma, must be treated promptly because they may threaten life if not arrested.

Management. The most important aspect of the management of cirrhotic patients is a planned program of follow-up visits at which times the liver can be evaluated by physical examination, function tests, and percutaneous biopsy at appropriate intervals. After each examination advice should be given concerning nutrition and the relative amounts of activity and rest required by the patient. Strenuous physical exercise should be avoided. The importance of trauma, intercurrent infection, and various hepatotoxic drugs as aggravating factors in liver disease should also be carefully explained to parents and older children. Drugs to be avoided are long acting sulfonamides, tetracyclines, novobiocin, the lauryl sulfate salts of erythromycin (Ilosone), the anticonvulsants trimethadione and diphenylhydantoin, phenothiazines, phenacetin, and acetaminophen. The use of anabolic hormones in patients who are refractory to dietary therapy should also be limited because of potential hepatotoxicity.

The general aim in all cases of advanced liver disease uncomplicated by ascites or coma is the provision of a diet with sufficient calories and essential nutrients to maintain growth and to prevent the development of specific deficiencies. Such a diet must be tailored to individual needs, although usually it is rich in protein. The consumption of a normal daily diet containing at least 1.5 gm of protein/kg is usually sufficient. Although fat malabsorption, which in adults is probably due to pancreatitis associated with alcoholic cirrhosis, is not a common problem in children, supplements of fat-soluble vitamins are provided, especially in patients with biliary atresia. In these patients and in those with prothrombin deficiency a single dose of a water-soluble analogue of vitamin K (2–4 mg), subcutaneously or intramuscularly, should return the prothrombin time to nearly normal levels within 1–2 days. Hypofibrinogenemia may require infusions of fresh frozen plasma if clot formation is deficient.

Pruritus. Severe pruritus, which may become a problem in infants with intra- and extrahepatic atresia, can be controlled with large doses of cholestyramine resin (Questran). Unfortunately, this material frequently produces diarrhea. Doses should be increased to maximal tolerance (up to 16 gm daily). Since severe vitamin E deficiency is a common finding in these patients, provision of up to 1000 IU/24 hr of a water-soluble preparation (Aquasol E) may be required to maintain serum vitamin E within the normal range. Additional supplementation of vitamin D or 25-hydroxy D should also be provided for children on cholestyramine.

Major Complications. The 3 major complications of chronic liver disease are bleeding from esophageal varices, ascites, and hepatic coma. Portal hypertension is an important factor in all of these problems. However, shunting procedures for relief of portal hypertension due to cirrhosis do not improve hepatic function and may precipitate the development of portal systemic encephalopathy. Furthermore, the small caliber of veins in young children often prevents successful anastomosis. Emergency procedures are accompanied by high mortality rates, while prophylactic portacaval anastomoses do not increase chances of survival.

Transthoracic ligation of varices may be a useful temporizing procedure in small children, but in adults the cumulative mortality rate accompanying ligation followed by elective portacaval anastomosis exceeds the mortality rate following emergency portacaval anastomosis alone. Therefore, in the presence of liver disease, it is preferable to treat the complications of portal hypertension instead of resorting to definitive surgical procedures unless hemorrhage cannot be otherwise controlled.

Hemorrhage. Gastrointestinal bleeding in cirrhotic patients is complicated not only by their debilitated general condition but also by impaired synthesis of clotting factors, by thrombocytopenia due to hypersplenism, and by the presence of circulating fibrinolysins. There may also be excessive reabsorption of ammonia from the breakdown of blood in the intestine and electrolyte abnormalities, such as hyponatremia, hypokalemia, and severe metabolic alkalosis. Correction of these abnormalities has a direct bearing on prevention of coma and eventual survival and, therefore, must be considered as an integral part of the emergency management of bleeding.

An adequate airway should be maintained and oxygen administered when necessary. Transfusions of fresh whole blood are given to maintain blood volume, to ensure adequate tissue perfusion, and to elevate levels of circulating coagulation factors and platelets. Stored blood and transfusions of platelets can be used when fresh blood is unavailable. Fluid and electrolyte balance should be managed parenterally, as should the administration of vitamin B complex and K. Venous pressure should be measured frequently, and a catheter inserted into the urinary bladder may be necessary for close surveillance of urinary output. Measures for the prevention of hepatic coma should be instituted in all cases of gastrointestinal bleeding in the presence of severe hepatic decompensation. Cathartics and enemas are administered repeatedly to remove blood from the colon and thus eliminate the absorption of ammonia from this source. Blood can also be aspirated from the stomach through a lavage tube. Liquid neomycin is given orally, 2–4 gm/24 hr, or by enema in an effort to suppress the production of ammonia by bacterial enzymes.

A patient with advanced liver disease may bleed at sites other than esophageal varices. Because the treatment of hemorrhage from peptic ulcers or gastritis or other lesions differs from the aggressive procedures employed in intractable esophageal bleeding, the site of bleeding should be located as soon as the patient has been given transfusions. Endoscopic examination of the upper gastrointestinal tract is the best means of doing so. The diagnosis can be established with a high degree of accuracy, especially if the varices continue to ooze blood.

In preparation for endoscopy the stomach is lavaged with ice water. This procedure occasionally slows or stops esophageal bleeding. When bleeding esophageal varices are demonstrated, vasopressin (or posterior pituitary extract) is administered intravenously, over a period of 10 min in doses of 10–20 units in 25 ml of saline, to reduce portal venous pressure. Effective pharmacologic dosages are evidenced by an increase in blood pressure and diarrhea. If the response is positive, the treatment can be repeated at hourly intervals.

When all else fails and massive life-threatening bleeding continues, the use of a balloon tube (Sengstaken-Blakemore tube) is necessary. The gastric balloon is inserted and then inflated to at least 300 ml volume in older children (smaller volumes may be sufficient in infants), fitted against the esophageal hiatus, and held in position with the use of foam rubber under the nose. Additional traction is usually not required. If venous compression at the cardioesophageal junction controls the bleeding, inflation of the esophageal balloon may not be necessary. Otherwise, the esophageal balloon is inflated to approximately 30 mm Hg and monitored with a manometer. The administration of antibiotics and cathartics as well as removal of blood from the stomach can be accomplished through the tube. There are great hazards involved in the use of the tube, especially the danger of massive pulmonary aspiration of vomitus, suffocation by an improperly positioned balloon, and damage to the esophageal mucosa. Fatal complications in up to 20% of intubated patients have been reported from medical centers experienced in the use of the tube.

Although bleeding from esophageal varices can be controlled in most cases with these measures, elective portal shunting may become necessary in some survivors. Measures such as injection of esophageal varices with sclerosing solutions or transhepatic variceal sclerosing with Gelfoam or bucrylate can be effective temporizing procedures in patients who cannot tolerate shunt surgery. However, in the long term, these procedures are relatively unrewarding.

Ascites. A combination of hypoalbuminemia, hyperaldosteronism, and renal failure associated with impairment of liver function may result in retention of sodium and total body water. Portal hypertension appears to be mainly responsible for the localization of the excess fluid in the abdomen. Despite better understanding of some mechanisms involved in the production of ascites, it is not known whether this condition represents a physiologic adjustment or a pathologic state. Therefore, the mildest therapeutic measures are employed in order to limit dangerous accumulations of fluid. Therapeutic paracenteses should be avoided unless acute dyspnea develops. Approximately 50 ml of fluid may be withdrawn for diagnostic purposes, especially to rule out peritonitis.

Sudden ascites can be precipitated during the course of chronic liver illness by intercurrent infections, hemorrhage, or surgery. Obviously, these stresses are best avoided, and infections should be treated rapidly. Acute ascites is often reversed by limiting daily dietary sodium to 300–500 mg. It is important that growing children on such a diet receive an adequate caloric and protein intake.

"Chronic" ascites, which is a reflection of progressive liver decompensation and portal hypertension, gradually results in discomfort, dyspnea, and severe limitation of physical activity. In addition to dietary management, successful diuresis in these patients requires combinations of diuretic agents (thiazides, furosemide, and ethacrynic acid) and inhibitors of sodium-potassium exchange (spironolactone and triamterene).

Treatment is initiated in hospital. Daily sodium intake should be less than 0.5 gm, or 1–2 mEq/kg. Fluid intake is not restricted in patients with adequate renal water clearance but should not exceed 1 l/24 hr. Protein intake is also limited to 1 gm/kg/24 hr in children with advanced cirrhosis to minimize the potential danger of hepatic coma and to restrict intake of salt contained in most protein-rich foods. A dietitian can be very helpful in prescribing salt-depleted proteins, starches, and vitamin supplements in combinations which augment caloric intake and make the diet palatable. Serum sodium and potassium are measured daily during the initial period of therapy, and urinary electrolytes are determined at least once every 2 days. A urinary sodium excretion of greater than 15 mEq/24 hr and weight loss of at least 250 mg daily are desirable goals of sodium restricted dietary therapy. A negative sodium balance of 100–150 mEq will assist in the elimination of approximately 1 liter of water. Maintenance of blood potassium levels is occasionally a problem necessitating supplementation with potassium chloride (up to 90 mEq/24 hr). These dietary control measures should induce a successful diuresis in up to 50% of initial episodes of ascites.

Refractory cases require management with diuretics, using the least toxic agents in the most effective combinations. Spironolactone, 75–100 mg, is given in 3 divided doses as the agent of choice. Weight loss and urinary sodium are monitored for the next 4 days. If the response is not satisfactory (i.e., less than 1 kg lost and urinary sodium excretion remaining below 15 mEq/24 hr), a thiazide diuretic is added to the regimen. Furosemide, 60–80 mg/24 hr, should produce a net water loss well below the rate of reabsorption of ascitic fluid. Since fluid is absorbed from the peritoneal cavity at about 700 ml/24 hr, a net loss of 300 ml water daily in a nonedematous patient is safe and effective.

Contraction of plasma volume and renal azotemia may occur if water is lost from the circulation more rapidly than from ascitic and edema fluid. Albumin (1 mg/kg) can be infused over 3 hr to expand circulatory volume rapidly and dosage of furosemide adjusted to maintain diuresis well below the maximum rate of ascitic fluid absorption. The urinary potassium concentration must be monitored closely to prevent severe hypokalemia induced by the action of thiazides on the renal tubule. Enteric coated potassium chloride tablets should be avoided because of the danger of ulcerative obstructive lesions of the small bowel. If hypokalemia persists despite these measures, triamterene can be substituted or used with spironolactone because the effect of these agents on potassium retention is additive.

Several wk in the hospital are often required for relief of ascites and establishment of a suitable maintenance regimen. Ascites can then be controlled at home with a low sodium diet and intermittent diuretic therapy when weight gain becomes excessive. Children with chronic active hepatitis often require steroid therapy and potassium supplementation during exacerbations of the underlying pathologic process.

Most patients with ascites can be returned to normal water and electrolyte balance. An occasional case of hepatic decompensation may be complicated by relative hyponatremia due to expansion of the vascular space by retained water or by hypokalemia that is difficult to correct with potassium supplements. Renal failure may intervene spontaneously or as a result of intestinal hemorrhage. Diuretic therapy is contraindicated in such cases. Protein intake is reduced to counteract the rising level of blood urea nitrogen, fluid intake is restricted because of oliguria and water retention, and potassium intake is limited in the presence of hyperkalemia. The prognosis is extremely grave, and coma frequently develops. Such patients are candidates for portosystemic shunts or the LeVeen shunt, which moves fluid mechanically from peritoneal cavity to jugular vein.

Coma. This condition can be precipitated in a cirrhotic patient by infection, fluid imbalance, diuretic therapy, surgery, hemorrhage, sedatives, tranquilizers, and protein intoxication. Appropriate measures include antibiotics, correction of over- or underhydration, removal of diuretics and other hepatotoxic drugs, avoidance of surgery, and prevention of hemorrhage.

When the deleterious effects of ammonia were recognized, the management of hepatic encephalopathy shifted from the use of high protein diets to avoidance of excessive protein intake. Nevertheless, the exact role of ammonia in inducing hepatic coma is still controversial, and controlled clinical trials involving factors such as dietary protein, antibiotic therapy, and the possible toxicity of diuretics have not been published.

A therapeutic dilemma arises because protein restriction may spare the brain but further endanger the liver. Current therapy of hepatic coma is based on efforts to diminish production of ammonia by elimination of protein intake during the comatose period and use of poorly absorbed antibiotics, such as neomycin, to control intestinal ammonia producing bacteria. A daily oral dose of 2–4 gm of neomycin is given during the acute period. For maintenance, lactulose, 10–15 ml 3 times daily, can be substituted for neomycin.

Lactulose, a nonabsorbable synthetic disaccharide, inhibits colonic organisms active in formation of ammonia. It may also exert its suppressive effect on blood ammonia by lowering colonic pH which favors conversion of ionized ammonia to nonionized ammonium ($NH_3^+ \rightarrow NH_4$). Ammonium is not absorbed by the intestine and may be utilized by fecal bacteria as a source of nitrogen. The dose of lactulose is 45 ml/24 hr in 3 divided portions. The dose is subsequently adjusted to avoid diarrhea secondary to lactic acid production and an excessive osmotic load in the colon. In comatose patients lactulose enemas may be used as an adjunct to neomycin therapy for rapid control of intestinal sources of ammonia and other absorbable bacterial products. Other measures include control of renal ammonia by maintenance of normal potassium levels and avoidance of diuretics.

During the precoma phase all intake of protein is stopped. When coma develops, avoidance of overhydration and hyponatremia is essential. Urinary sodium levels are used to monitor tolerance to intravenous sodium, and simultaneous measurements of serum and urine osmolality permit assessment of hydration. Maintenance fluids with 10% glucose are supplemented with carefully monitored sodium and potassium replacements. Fresh frozen plasma or fresh whole blood is used to correct defective clotting when the prothrombin time is unresponsive to vitamin K injections (10 mg). Systemic antibiotic coverage is provided with a broad-spectrum antibiotic (e.g., ampicillin) unless bacterial cultures yield a specific organism.

Calories are administered exclusively from glucose to the maximum tolerated in order to minimize muscle breakdown and production of ammonia. Insulin may be added to promote utilization of glucose if hyperglycemia is excessive. During the recovery phase, protein is reintroduced in 0.5 gm/kg increments by frequent small meals and tolerance monitored with blood ammonia determinations. The goal is to raise protein intake to 1.5 gm/kg/24 hr over several days.

Exchange blood transfusions and corticosteroid therapy are not of benefit in treatment of hepatic coma. Among experimental therapies, extracorporeal hemoperfusion with activated charcoal and dialysis through porous acrylonitrile membranes continue to be investigated. The benefits of ketoanalogues of essential amino acids appear promising in selected cases with reasonable preservation of liver function.

Patients with uncomplicated chronic liver disease usually recover when treated in the foregoing manner, but those with progressive liver disease, renal failure, or encephalopathy that develops after a shunt anastomosis usually do not recover.

TUMORS OF THE LIVER

See Sec 15.88.

M. MICHAEL THALER

Development of Liver Structure and Function

Short CR, Kinden DA, Stith R: Fetal and neonatal development of the microsomal monooxygenase system. Drug Metabol Rev 5:1, 1976.
Thaler MM: Liver function and maturation in the perinatal period. *In:* Lebenthal E (ed): Textbook of Gastroenterology and Nutrition in Infancy. New York, Raven Press, 1981, Vol I.
Watkins JB, Perman JA: Bile acid metabolism in infants and children. Clin Gastroenterol 6:201, 1977.

Diagnostic Assessment of Liver Disease

Alagille D, Odievre M: Liver and Biliary Tract Disease in Children. New York, John Wiley and Sons, 1977.
Andres JM, Mathis RK, Walker AW: Liver disease in infants, I and II. J Pediatr 90:686, 964, 1977.
Biello DR, Levitt RG, Wiegel BA, et al: Computed tomography and radionuclide imaging of the liver: Comparative evaluation. Radiology 127:159, 1978.
Brough AJ, Bernstein J: Liver biopsy in the diagnosis of infantile obstructive jaundice. Pediatrics 43:519, 1969.
Glasgow JFT: Evaluation of hepatic function. *In:* Chandra RK (ed): The Liver and Biliary System in Infants and Children. Edinburgh, Churchill Livingstone, 1975.
Korobkin M, Goldberg HI: Computed tomography of the hepatobiliary system. Ann Rev Med 30:181, 1979.
Majol M, Reba RC, Altman RP: Hepatobiliary scintigraphy with ^{99m}Tc-PIPIDA in the evaluation of neonatal jaundice. Pediatrics 67:140, 1981.
Roy CC, Silverman A, Cozzetto FJ: Pediatric Clinical Gastroenterology. Ed 2. St Louis, CV Mosby, 1975.

Differential Diagnosis and Management of Cholestatic Liver Disease in Infancy

Mowat AP, Psacharopoulos HT, Williams R: Extrahepatic biliary atresia versus neonatal hepatitis: Review of 137 prospectively investigated infants. Arch Dis Child 51:763, 1976.
Poley JR, Magnani HN: Cholestatic jaundice in infancy. Diagnosis, differential diagnosis and treatment. Aust Paediat J 12:134, 1976.
Thaler MM: Jaundice in the newborn: Algorithmic diagnosis of conjugated and unconjugated hyperbilirubinemia. JAMA 237:58, 1977.
Thaler MM, Gellis SS: Studies in neonatal hepatitis and biliary atresia. I. Long-term prognosis of neonatal hepatitis. II. The effect of diagnostic laparotomy on long-term prognosis of neonatal hepatitis. III. Progression and regression of cirrhosis in biliary atresia. IV. Diagnosis. Am J Dis Child 116:257, 1968.

Idiopathic Neonatal Hepatitis (Giant Cell Hepatitis)

Alagille D: Clinical aspects of neonatal hepatitis. Am J Dis Child 123:287, 1972.
Brent RL: Persistent jaundice in infancy. J Pediatr 61:111, 1962.
Danks DM, Campbell PA, Smith AL, et al: Prognosis of babies with neonatal hepatitis. Arch Dis Child 52:368, 1977.
Thaler MM, Gellis SS: Studies in neonatal hepatitis and biliary atresia. Am J Dis Child 116:257, 1968.

Metabolic Disorders

Cystic Fibrosis

Oppenheimer EH, Esterly JR: Hepatic changes in young infants with cystic fibrosis: Possible relation to focal biliary cirrhosis. J Pediatr 86:683, 1975.
Valman HB, France NE, Wallis PG: Prolonged neonatal jaundice in cystic fibrosis. Arch Dis Child 116:262, 1968.

α_1-Antitrypsin Deficiency

Sharp HL: The current status of α-1-antitrypsin, a protease inhibitor, in gastrointestinal disease. Gastroenterology 70:611, 1976.
Sveger T: Liver disease in alpha-1-antitrypsin deficiency detected by screening 200,000 infants. N Engl J Med 294:1316, 1976.

Galactosemia

Applebaum MN, Thaler MM: Reversibility of extensive liver damage in galactosemia. Gastroenterology 69:496, 1975.
Monk AM, Mitchell AJM, Milligan DWA, et al: The diagnosis of classical galactosemia. Arch Dis Child 52:943, 1977.

Hereditary Fructose Intolerance

Odievre M, Gentil C, Gantier M, et al: Hereditary fructose intolerance in childhood: Diagnosis, management and course in 55 patients. Am J Dis Child 132:605, 1978.

Neonatal Hepatitis with Cortisol Deficiency

Leblanc A, Odievre M, Hadchouel M, et al: Neonatal cholestasis and hypoglycemia: Possible role of cortisol deficiency. J Pediatr 99:577, 1981.

Infections

Neonatal Hepatitis B Infection

Jhaveri R, Rosenfeld W, Salazar D, et al: High titer multiple dose therapy with HBIG in newborn infants with HB$_s$Ag positive mothers. J Pediatr 97:305, 1980.

Neonatal Cytomegalovirus Infection

Reynolds DW, Stegnos S, Hasty TS, et al: Maternal cytomegalovirus excretion and perinatal infection. N Engl J Med 289:1, 1973.

Other Neonatal Viral, Bacterial, and Parasitic Infections

Brightman VJ, Scott TFM, Westphal M, et al: An outbreak of coxsackie B5 virus infection in a newborn nursery. J Pediatr 69:179, 1966.
Desmonts G, Couvreur J: Congenital toxoplasmosis. A prospective study of 378 pregnancies. N Engl J Med 290:1110, 1974.
Hamilton JR, Sass-Kortsak A: Jaundice associated with severe bacterial infection in young infants. J Pediatr 63:121, 1963.
Krous HF, Dietzman D, Ray G: Fatal infections with echovirus types 6 and 11 in early infancy. Am J Dis Child 126:842, 1973.
Nahmias AJ: The TORCH complex. Hosp Pract 1974, p 65.
Oppenheimer EH, Hardy JB: Clinical syphilis in the newborn infant. Johns Hopkins Med J 129:63, 1976.
Stevens CE, Bernstein J: Neonatal hepatitis in congenital rubella. Arch Pathol 86:317, 1968.

Atresias and Hypoplasias

Alagille D, Odievre M, Gautier M, et al: Hepatic ductular hypoplasia associated with characteristic facies, vertebral malformations, retarded physical, mental and sexual development and cardiac murmur. J Pediatr 86:63, 1975.
Altman RP: The portoenterostomy procedure for biliary atresia: A 5-year experience. Ann Surg 188:351, 1978.
Kasai M, Watanabe I, Ohi R: Follow-up studies of long-term survivors after hepatic portoenterostomy for "non-correctable" biliary atresia. J Pediatr Surg 10:173, 1975.
Thaler MM: Biliary disease in infancy and childhood. *In:* Sleisenger MH, Fordtran JS (eds): Gastrointestinal Disease. Ed 2. Philadelphia, WB Saunders, 1978.

Cystic Malformations

Hermansen MC, Starshak RJ, Werlin SL: Caroli disease: The diagnostic approach. J Pediatr 94:879, 1979.
Kerr NS, Harrison CV, Sherlock S, et al: Congenital hepatic fibrosis. Quart J Med 30:91, 1961.
Scholtz FJ, Carrera GF, Larsen CR: The choledochocele: Correlation of radiological, clinical and pathological findings. Radiology 118:25, 1976.
Thaler MM, Ogata ES, Goodman JR, et al: Congenital fibrosis and polycystic disease of liver and kidneys. Am J Dis Child 126:374, 1971.
Trout HH, Longmire WP Jr: Long-term follow-up study of patients with congenital cystic dilatation of the common bile duct. Surgery 69:776, 1971.

Cholestasis and Liver Disease Associated with Total Parenteral Alimentation

Beale EF, Nelson RM, Bucciarelli RL, et al: Intrahepatic cholestasis associated with parenteral nutrition in premature infants. Pediatrics 64:342, 1980.

Postuma R, Trevenen CL: Liver disease in infants receiving total parenteral nutrition. Pediatrics 63:110, 1979.
Sondheimer JM, Bryan H, Andrews W, et al: Cholestatic tendencies in premature infants on and off parenteral nutrition. Pediatrics 62:984, 1978.

Drug-Induced Liver Injury

Zimmerman H: Hepatotoxicity. The Adverse Effects of Drugs and Other Chemicals on the Liver. New York, Appleton-Century-Crofts, 1979.

Reye Syndrome

Crocker JFS (ed): Reye's Syndrome. II. New York, Grune and Stratton, 1978.
Pollack JD (ed): Reye's Syndrome. New York, Grune and Stratton, 1974.
Reye RDK, Morgan G, Baral J: Encephalopathy and fatty degeneration of the viscera: A disease entity in childhood. Lancet 2:749, 1963.
Thaler MM, Bruhn FW, Applebaum MN, et al: Reye's syndrome in twins. Clinical course and ultrastructural studies. J Pediatr 77:638, 1970.

Chronic Active Hepatitis in Children

Arasu THS, Wyllie R, Hatch TF, et al: Management of chronic aggressive hepatitis in children and adolescents. J Pediatr 95:501, 1979.
Roy CC, Silverman A, Cozzetto FJ: Pediatric Clinical Gastroenterology. Ed 2. St Louis, CV Mosby, 1975.

Wilson Disease

Slovis TL, Dubois RS, Rodgerson DO, et al: The varied manifestations of Wilson's disease. J Pediatr 78:578, 1971.
Werlin SL, Grand RJ, Perman JA, et al: Diagnostic dilemmas of Wilson's disease: Diagnosis and treatment. Pediatrics 62:47, 1978.

Indian Childhood Cirrhosis

Nayak NC, Ramalingaswami V: Indian childhood cirrhosis. Clin Gastroenterol 4:333, 1975.

Liver Disease Associated with Chronic Inflammatory Bowel Disease

Kern F: Hepatobiliary disorders in inflammatory bowel disease. In: Popper H, Schaffner F (eds): Progress in Liver Diseases, Vol 5. New York, Grune and Stratton, 1976, p 575.

Cirrhosis

Sherlock S: Diseases of the Liver and Biliary System. Ed 6. Oxford, Blackwell Scientific Publ, 1981.

Tumors of the Liver

Ishak KG, Glunz PR: Hepatoblastoma and hepatocarcinoma in infancy and childhood: Report of 47 cases. Cancer 20:396, 1967.
Keeling JW: Liver tumors in infancy and childhood. J Pathol 103:69, 1971.
Leonidas JC, Strauss L, Beck AR: Vascular tumors of the liver in newborns. Am J Dis Child 125:507, 1973.

11.102 PORTAL HYPERTENSION AND VARICES

Etiology. Extrahepatic portal venous obstruction causes 50–70% of portal hypertension in children, but in about two thirds of these patients no specific cause can be found. In many patients it develops gradually after birth, and umbilical vein catheterization and infusion are associated factors in about one third of cases. Lymphatic spread of infection from the umbilicus to the ductus venosus may cause portal vein thrombosis. Sludging of venous flow at the time of normal closure of the umbilical vein and ductus venosus is another suggested mechanism. In older children, abdominal trauma, pancreatitis, and tumors or inflammatory masses adjacent to the portal vein have occasionally led to portal hypertension. In Gaucher disease, arteriovenous fistulas may develop in the spleen, resulting in portal hypertension. Rarely in children, hepatic vein thrombosis, the Budd-Chiari syndrome, causes raised portal venous pressure.

Cirrhosis may also cause portal hypertension; the intrahepatic scarring and collapse distort hepatic vasculature and raise vascular resistance (Sec 11.101). Most survivors of surgically corrected biliary atresia and all nonoperated cases develop portal hypertension. Many of the remaining known causes of childhood cirrhosis are insidious in onset and often do not progress to portal hypertension until relatively late in childhood. Examples of these conditions are α_1-antitrypsin deficiency, Wilson disease, cystic fibrosis, trypsinemia, and chronic active hepatitis. Congenital hepatic fibrosis may also lead to portal hypertension. The portal pressure may also rise following right hepatic lobectomy as the entire portal flow encounters greater resistance from the reduced vascular bed.

Pathology. The liver is normal in patients with extrahepatic portal obstruction. Some portal blood does reach the liver through collateral channels in the suspensory ligaments, the diaphragmatic veins, and hepatorenal and hepatocolic veins. With intrahepatic obstruction there is no blood flow to the liver other than via the partially obstructed portal vein. A cavernomatous transformation of the portal vein is encountered in some children, with the normal vein being replaced by a number of thin-walled tortuous veins. Whether this is the result or the cause of the portal obstruction is unknown, but the portal venous pressure exceeds the pressure within the inferior vena cava by at least 150 mm of saline. Portal systemic shunts open up and lead to dilatation and varicosities in otherwise unimportant veins. Such anastomoses are found in the region of the esophagogastric junction, the retroperitoneal veins, the internal hemorrhoidal plexus in the distal rectum, and around the ligamentum teres at the umbilicus. The varicosities in the lower esophagus and cardia of the stomach are especially prone to erosion with consequent massive hemorrhage. Hypersplenism may complicate the picture in any patient with portal obstruction.

Clinical Manifestations. Massive hematemesis is usually the initial symptom of portal hypertension in children. The blood passed per rectum will vary from bright red with severe bleeding to melena. The underlying disease will determine the patient's age when seen; younger infants tend to present ascites rather than hematemesis. Physical examination may reveal jaundice if the obstruction is hepatic. A cluster of diverging, dilated veins with centrifugal flow from the umbilicus, the caput medusae, may occur. Internal anal hemorrhoids are uncommon in children.

Diagnosis. Roentgenographic demonstration of varicosities in the esophagus is relatively noninvasive and usually accurate; a barium paste is used to adhere to the esophageal mucous membrane. In children, peptic ulcer disease rarely coexists with portal hypertension. The varicosities have an unmistakable appearance when visualized directly by fiberoptic gastroesophagoscopy. Liver function should be evaluated. The portal vein may be demonstrated by retrograde umbilical vein catheterization, splenoportography, or selective angiography. Splenoportography also allows the measurement of splenic pulp and portal pressures and indicates the flow within the splenic and portal veins. Selective angiography does not demonstrate the portal vein as well as splenoportography, but it allows assessment of the size of the superior mesenteric vein. If the bleeding is not from varices, this investigation may demonstrate sites of hemorrhage not associated with portal hypertension, e.g., traumatic hemobilia. It may also be useful therapeutically as a means of introducing vasopressor substances selectively into the portal system.

Treatment. Hematemesis from esophageal varices in children usually stops spontaneously without measures other than blood transfusion. A nasogastric tube should be inserted as a guide to the amount and rate of hemorrhage and is *not* contraindicated by a risk of precipitating or aggravating hemorrhage from varices. In many patients the bleeding is from varices at the cardia of the stomach and not the esophagus. A central venous pressure measurement may be helpful in assessing the rate of blood volume replacement required. Vital functions must be measured frequently, including pH, arterial oxygen saturation, and electrolytes. Incipient hepatic failure from cirrhosis made worse by hemorrhage is rarely seen in children. If cirrhosis is present, these patients require terminal care unless hepatic transplantation is anticipated; Wilson disease is an exception. Intravenous and local administration of *posterior pituitary extract* may be of use by causing splanchnic vasoconstriction with resultant diminished blood flow to the bleeding varices. Cooling the stomach is probably of no value, and if bleeding persists, the passage of the triple lumen Sengstaken-Blakemore tube to produce balloon tamponade may be required. In many instances only the distal gastric balloon needs to be inflated and with traction on the tube, bleeding is controlled. Unfortunately bleeding often recurs on deflation of the balloon(s).

It is rarely necessary to operate upon pediatric patients with portal hypertension as an emergency to stop bleeding. There is no ideal operation, but 2 types of procedures are currently employed: those that attack the varices directly and those that divert portal blood to the systemic circulation (Sec 11.100).

There are many methods of diverting the portal blood flow to the systemic circulation. Splenorenal shunts offer excellent means of controlling portal hypertension in children. Siguira has also documented good results following a thoracoabdominal operation in which as many as 80 varicose veins or their tributaries are ligated within the thorax. The esophagus is transected and then anastomosed to interrupt the intramural varicosities. Within the abdomen the veins related to the upper stomach are all ligated. This procedure has been used on several children with no recurrences of bleeding, and we believe that the Siguira procedure is preferable to shunt operations.

11.103 FATTY INFILTRATION

Fatty infiltration of the liver results from deposition of dietary or mobilized tissue fat in the hepatic cells. Fat is deposited in normal liver cells and, in larger amounts, in damaged liver cells in a variety of clinical conditions. Fatty infiltration of the liver occurs in many metabolic disorders such as obesity, starvation, galactosemia, diabetes mellitus, and familial hyperlipemia. It is encountered frequently in chronic tuberculosis and osteomyelitis and occasionally after pneumonia. It may occur rapidly during corticosteroid therapy. Large fatty livers occur in poisoning with phosphorus, phlorhidzin, chloroform, alcohol, arsenic, and mushrooms and in severe anemic states, presumably from anoxia. It is also a common secondary condition in childhood.

Fatty infiltration of the liver should not be confused with *fatty degeneration* of hepatic cells, in which preexistent cell lipids are altered chemically and become visible as fat droplets. In fatty infiltration the normal lipid content of the liver (3–5%) may increase to 40%. In fatty degeneration there is an alteration in the normal proportion between hepatic cholesterol and other hepatic lipids but no absolute increase of liver fat. Occasionally, with hyperlipidemia, the Kupffer cells of the liver will phagocytize fat droplets and become swollen.

Clinical Manifestations. Infiltration of the liver by fat is usually not directly responsible for symptoms or abnormalities in hepatic function. When hypoglycemia and ketosis are present, the hepatomegaly may be confused with glycogen storage disease. The usual clinical finding is hepatic enlargement, which may be extreme in some instances.

Treatment. Reduction of fat intake with a liberal allowance of protein is indicated. Beneficial effects have been described after administration of choline and its analogues (betaine) but are difficult to evaluate. Reduction of corticosteroid dosage or improved control of the hyperglycemia in diabetes will result in decreased lipolysis and clearing of the fat from the liver in some instances.

11.104 CHOLECYSTITIS

This disease is rare in children. In teenage girls a history of current or past pregnancy is possible.

Etiology. *Noncalculous cholecystitis* is associated with acute systemic diseases, including streptococcal septicemia with or without glomerulonephritis, typhoid fever, erysipelas, salmonella infections, giardiasis, ascariasis, leptospirosis, and anaerobic diphtheroid infections. There is also an association with severe dehydration or malnutrition. The condition has been reported in a neonate with associated amnionitis and has also been found in association with Kawasaki disease.

Cholelithiasis (gallstones) is a common cause of cholecystitis in older teenagers. It is rare in males and in Blacks. The stones are composed primarily of cholesterol and are of small diameter. It is rare for choledocholithiasis to be present, but cholelithiasis may complicate a choledochal cyst. Despite the relative frequency of hemolytic disease in children, pigment stones are uncommon, occurring in less than 10% of cholecystectomies in childhood.

Anomalies of the cystic duct may be an important factor in the genesis of biliary disease in infants and children. Such anomalies have included complete or partial obstruction of the common bile duct and choledochal cysts with secondary cholangitis.

Clinical Manifestations. Symptoms and signs of biliary tract inflammation in childhood are similar to those seen in the adult, although a history of indigestion, flatulence, or food intolerance is seldom obtained. Fever, tenderness in the right upper quadrant, and a palpable mass are usual. The pain is usually localized fo the right upper quadrant or epigastrium, with or without radiation to just below the right scapula. If cholangitis is present, the patient may have shaking chills. Jaundice is present more often in children than in adults.

Diagnosis. Cholecystography is the investigation of choice in the absence of jaundice; if a nonfunctioning

gallbladder is found, the tests should be repeated. If still no function is demonstrable, an intravenous cholangiogram will show the gallbladder provided the cystic duct is not obstructed. A ^{99m}technetium pyrrodoxylidine glutamate scan is recommended when there is jaundice.

Treatment. Cholecystectomy is the usual treatment for cholecystitis. The patient undergoing cholecystectomy may need an operative cholangiogram to demonstrate whether common bile duct exploration and drainage are necessary. In acute noncalculous cholecystitis (acute hydrops) cholecystostomy alone, with preservation of the gallbladder, is an alternative though most pediatric surgeons favor cholecystectomy.

BARRY SHANDLING

11.105   PERITONEUM AND ALLIED STRUCTURES

MALFORMATIONS OF THE PERITONEUM

Congenital peritoneal bands may be responsible for intestinal obstruction; numerous other anomalies may occur in the course of the development of the peritoneum but are rarely of clinical importance. Intra-abdominal herniations infrequently occur through ringlike formations produced by anomalous peritoneal bands. Absence of the omentum or duplications of it are rare anomalies. Omental cysts and torsion of the omentum are unusual causes of acute abdominal crises leading to laparotomy.

ASCITES

The term ascites indicates an accumulation of fluid in the peritoneal cavity, but it is usually applied to accumulations of serous fluid. Renal, especially nephrotic, and cardiac conditions are most often responsible for ascites. It may represent an accumulation of fluid secondary to chronic adhesive pericarditis, or it may be part of a polyserositis in Pick syndrome. Other causes include obstruction of the portal circulation due to hepatic cirrhosis (Sec 11.101) or to enlarged lymph nodes, tumors, thrombosis, chronic tuberculous peritonitis, rheumatic peritonitis, or obstruction of the splenic vein.

The abdomen is distended; when distention is great, there is flattening or pouting of the umbilicus. Fluctuation can be detected on palpation; a wavelike impulse is obtained by sharp tapping on 1 side of the abdominal wall while the other hand is placed on the opposite side of the abdomen and an assistant's hand compresses it in the midline; shifting percussion dullness can often be demonstrated.

Ascites must be differentiated from other conditions that cause distention of the abdomen. These include

gaseous distention of the intestine; fecal distention as in megacolon; tumor masses, including cysts of the mesentery; acute or chronic peritonitis; peritoneal hemorrhage; extreme distention of the bladder; and simple obesity.

The course, prognosis, and treatment of ascites depend entirely upon the cause.

CHYLOUS ASCITES

The accumulation of chyle is an uncommon form of ascites which may occur at any age of childhood and is occasionally congenital in origin. True chylous ascites is caused by some anomaly, injury, or obstruction of the thoracic duct within its abdominal portion. In the case of anomalies the condition is present at birth or shortly thereafter. There may be an associated chylothorax (Sec 7.30 and 12.101). Obstructions may be produced by enlarged lymph nodes or neoplasms. The fluid has the appearance of milk because of its high fat content. In chronic peritonitis, peritoneal fluid may have a somewhat similar color from degeneration of inflammatory products.

The prognosis of chylous ascites is unfavorable, but recovery may occur. The accumulation of chyle can be reduced by providing a diet containing medium-chain triglycerides which are absorbed directly into the portal circulation. Since there is a loss of considerable protein in this fluid, high protein diets should be prescribed. Abdominal exploration may be justified to search for the site of the leak if a trial of dietary management is unsuccessful.

PERITONITIS

Acute infections of the peritoneum are arbitrarily designated as *primary* when the focus is outside the abdominal cavity and the infection is blood- or lymph-borne. The infection is termed *secondary* when it is disseminated by extension from or rupture of an intra-abdominal viscus or of an abscess of 1 of the solid organs.

Peritonitis in the neonatal period may arise from a transplacental infection in utero; more frequently it is the result of infection acquired during or shortly after birth. It may be a manifestation of septicemia, a direct extension from an umbilical infection, perforation of the intestine, or, rarely, the sequel of a ruptured appendix. Meconium peritonitis is described in Sec 7.43.

ACUTE PRIMARY PERITONITIS

Etiology. Primary peritonitis is a bacterial infection of the peritoneal cavity without a demonstrable intra-abdominal source. Despite the decreasing incidence of this entity, presumably due to the availability of effective antimicrobial therapy, it continues to occur in children with ascites secondary to nephrosis or cirrhosis and, occasionally, in otherwise healthy children. The pneumococcus and the group A streptococcus are the predominant pathogens recovered in these children; however, gram-negative bacteria are often involved (*E. coli*). Both sexes are equally affected, and most cases occur before 6 yr of age.

Clinical Manifestations. The onset may be insidious or rapid and is characterized by fever, abdominal pain, and vomiting. Diarrhea is common and extreme prostration may occur. The child may appear toxic or anxious. In very ill patients, especially young infants, the temperature may be normal or subnormal. The pulse may be rapid, small, and compressible, and the respirations rapid and shallow because of the pain that abdominal respiration produces. There is usually distention of the abdomen, moderate diffuse tenderness, and a doughy resistance. Examination often reveals signs of active nephrosis or cirrhosis, including ascites. Palpation may demonstrate rebound tenderness and rigidity. Auscultation reveals hypoactive or absent bowel sounds.

Diagnosis and Treatment. Laboratory studies reveal leukocytosis with 85–95% polymorphonuclear cells. An abnormal urinalysis with proteinuria is present in children with active nephrosis. Roentgenographic examination of the abdomen reveals dilatation of the large and small intestines, with edema of the small intestinal wall as evidenced by an increased distance between adjacent loops of gas-filled small bowel. In most cases the clinical presentation is indistinguishable from appendicitis, with or without perforation, and the diagnosis of primary peritonitis can be made only at laparotomy. However, in a child with active nephrosis or cirrhosis whose physical findings are compatible with diffuse peritonitis, an attempt should be made to establish the diagnosis of primary peritonitis by evaluation of peritoneal fluid obtained with a short beveled needle. Cytologic and chemical analyses of the exudate are helpful. Infected ascitic fluid usually contains an elevated protein concentration and more than 300 leukocytes/mm$_3$, more than 25% of which are polymorphonuclear. Microscopic examination of Gram-stained

ascitic fluid characteristically reveals 1 species of gram-positive bacteria or, less often, gram-negative microorganisms; in this situation antibiotic therapy with intravenous ampicillin and gentamicin is indicated. Subsequent changes in the antibiotics depend upon sensitivity testing. Although resolution of all signs and symptoms characteristically occurs within 48 hr, parenteral antibiotic therapy should be continued for a minimum of 7 days. Surgical exploration is indicated if after 48 hr of parenteral antibiotic therapy either the child's clinical condition fails to improve or the physical findings persist and show localization.

Cross RE (ed): Primary peritonitis. *In:* The Surgery of Infancy and Childhood. Philadelphia, WB Saunders, 1953.
Speck WT, Dresdale SA, MacMillan RW: Primary peritonitis and the nephrotic syndrome. Am J Surg 127:267, 1974.

ACUTE SECONDARY PERITONITIS

This type of peritonitis is most often due to the entry of enteric bacteria into the peritoneal cavity through a necrotic defect in the wall of the intestines or other viscus as a result of obstruction and infarction. In children, peritonitis is primarily associated with an inflamed appendix but may occur with intussusception, volvulus, incarcerated hernias, or rupture of a Meckel diverticulum. Peritonitis may also occur as a complication of intestinal mucosal disease, including peptic ulcers, ulcerative colitis, and pseudomembranous enterocolitis. Peritonitis in the neonatal period most often occurs as a complication of necrotizing enterocolitis but may be associated with meconium ileus or spontaneous rupture of the stomach or intestines. The bacteria involved are the normal flora of the gastrointestinal tract, which includes many species of aerobic and anaerobic bacteria.

Clinical Manifestations. The early clinical manifestations of secondary peritonitis are a reflection of the underlying disease process. Fever, diffuse abdominal pain, nausea, and vomiting are characteristic. Physical examination reveals signs of peritoneal inflammation, including rebound tenderness, abdominal wall rigidity, and hypoactive or absent bowel sounds. These early findings may be followed by signs and symptoms of shock due to the loss of large quantities of protein-rich fluid from the vascular compartment into the peritoneal cavity and bowel lumen and an associated intravascular volume depletion.

The manifestations of shock from a ruptured viscus or the early symptoms of acute appendicitis may merge with those of peritonitis and may be followed by an increasing toxemia, as evidenced by greater restlessness and irritability, by a higher temperature, often 39.5° C or more (103–105° F), by an increase in the pulse rate, and, at times, by chills or convulsions. In extreme situations, and especially in early infancy, the temperature may be normal or subnormal. Constipation is marked.

Laboratory studies reveal an elevated blood leukocyte count in excess of 12,000/mm^3 with a predominance of polymorphonuclear forms. Roentgenograms of the abdomen (supine, upright, or lateral decubitus) may reveal free air in the peritoneal cavity, evidence of ileus or obstruction, peritoneal fluid, and obliteration of the psoas shadow.

Treatment. The main principle of therapy is to stabilize the patient by correcting fluid and electrolyte deficiencies with parenteral fluids, alleviating intestinal obstruction with nasal suction, and controlling the peritoneal infection with broad-spectrum antibiotics. Numerous antibiotic regimens have been advocated depending on the presence or absence of previous illness. In the absence of previous chemotherapy, a regimen consisting of ampicillin, gentamicin, and chloramphenicol is indicated. A satisfactory alternative antibiotic regimen includes gentamicin in combination with clindamycin. Surgery should be performed at the earliest time consistent with good preparation of the patient in order to repair the damaged viscus. Cultures taken during surgery will determine whether a change in the antibiotic regimen is indicated.

ACUTE SECONDARY LOCALIZED PERITONITIS
(Peritoneal Abscess)

Etiology. A single localized pyogenic abscess, most often secondary to perforation of an inflamed appendix, is somewhat less common in children than in adults. The poor ability of young children to localize a peritoneal infection of appendiceal origin has been attributed to lower general resistance and to a relatively smaller omentum. Though localized peritoneal abscesses occur most often in the appendiceal region, they may be at any site, originating from various sources; or appendiceal infections may gravitate to other areas, notably the pelvis. An abscess in the subdiaphragmatic area may originate from an appendiceal or other intra-abdominal infection or, rarely, from an empyema. Diagnostic ultrasound or CT scan may be helpful in localizing an abscess.

Clinical Manifestations. The general symptoms of *peritoneal abscess* are continued fever or recurrences of it, poor appetite, and vomiting following ingestion of food. The white blood cell count is increased, with a predominance of polymorphonuclear cells. With *appendiceal abscess*, tenderness in the right lower quadrant is observed, and there is often a palpable mass.

A *pelvic abscess* is suggested by abdominal distention, rectal tenesmus with or without the passage of small stools containing mucus, or bladder irritability. Rectal examination may reveal a tender mass anteriorly.

A *subphrenic abscess* is evidenced by physical signs at the base of the lung, usually on the right, due to elevation of the diaphragm and frequently to the presence of pleural fluid. The diagnosis can often be established roentgenographically. The diaphragm is elevated and the liver depressed if the infection is on the right side, and there is frequently a pocket of air just below the diaphragm due to production of gas by bacteria.

Treatment. The abscess should be drained and appropriate antibiotic therapy provided. Initial broad-spectrum coverage should be modified, if indicated, by the results of sensitivity tests of the bacteria obtained from cultures. If the appendix cannot be removed at the initial operation, an appendectomy should be performed subsequently within 3 mo.

TUBERCULOUS PERITONITIS

See Sec 10.52.

INGUINAL HERNIA

See Sec 11.75.

HYDROCELE

See Sec 16.61.

EPIGASTRIC HERNIA

Epigastric hernias occur in the midline between the umbilicus and the lower end of the sternum. They are not common and, except for their location, are similar to umbilical hernias. They may become acutely painful and tender when a bit of preperitoneal fat becomes incarcerated. They should be repaired surgically.

INCISIONAL HERNIA

Postoperative hernias should be repaired as soon as the local condition of the wound and the general condition of the child warrant it. Incisional hernias tend to enlarge and may also become incarcerated.

DIAPHRAGMATIC HERNIA

Diaphragmatic hernias may be congenital (Fig 11–36) or acquired. Acquired hernias are usually traumatic in origin and are not considered here. Congenital herniation of abdominal contents into the thoracic cavity may be responsible for serious embarrassment of respiration and usually constitutes a medical-surgical emergency in the immediate neonatal period. There may be an association between the delayed presentation of a right diaphragmatic hernia and group B streptococcal infection. Infrequently there is little or no respiratory embarrassment, and the hernia may not be detected until later in infancy or childhood. In addition to herniation through a defect in the diaphragm (see below), there may be partial herniation of the stomach through the esophageal hiatus (Sec 11.20), phrenic paralysis with displacement of abdominal contents upward but not herniated (Sec 7.25), and eventration of the diaphragm. *Eventration is not a herniation* but is also an upward

12.4 RESPIRATORY ANATOMY, PHYSIOLOGY, AND PATHOPHYSIOLOGY

12.5 AIRWAY OBSTRUCTION

Narrowing of the airway lumen may be the result of (1) the presence of intraluminal material (secretions, tumor, or foreign matter), (2) mural thickening (edema and hypertrophy of glands or muscle), (3) contraction of the bronchial smooth muscle (spasm), and (4) extrinsic compression. These mechanisms are rarely found in pure form except in very acute situations, and all impair the normal mechanisms of tracheobronchial hygiene and interfere with air flow.

Since resistance to air flow is inversely proportional to the 4th power of the radius of a tube, small decreases in the lumen of bronchioles or bronchi or in the laryngeal area may significantly decrease airflow. Even a small degree of airflow obstruction can induce an obstructive process in young children. It is not surprising then that wheezing is a common reason for admission of infants and toddlers to the hospital.

In partial airway obstruction the flow of air and drainage of bronchial secretions still take place but are impaired. In complete obstruction neither airflow nor drainage of the secretions can occur; complete obstruction of a lobar bronchus leads to lobar atelectasis after the residual gas diffuses into the pulmonary circulation.

Partial airway obstruction can be divided into 2 types: bypass valve or check valve, depending on the degree of narrowing of the bronchial lumen and on the nature of the pathologic process producing it. In the bypass type of obstruction the lumen is narrowed; though resistance to the flow is increased, air can still flow in during inspiration and out during expiration. With the check valve type of airway obstruction air entry is possible, but during expiration the lumen is completely occluded so that escape of air is trapped behind (distal to) the point of obstruction. For bypass valve obstructions air trapping is a result of the changes in the diameter of the airways' lumen that accompany inspiration and expiration: during inspiration the chest enlarges, creating negative intrathoracic pressure and causing enlargement of the lungs and bronchial tree and widening of the bronchial lumen; during expiration the increase in intrathoracic pressure causes narrowing of the lumen. If expiration is forceful and a positive pressure is produced, this narrowing and air trapping will be even more marked. Thus, alveolar overdistention may occur with either type of partial obstruction but especially with the check valve type.

HIGH AIRWAY OBSTRUCTION

High obstruction occurs above the level of the secondary bronchi and in general interferes more with inspiration than expiration. If it is complete and above the bifurcation of the trachea, asphyxia and death result. Partial high airway obstruction may result in intense dyspnea. A small increase in respiratory rate and a marked increase in respiratory effort may occur, particularly in inspiration. A harsh, low-pitched inspiratory sound called *stridor* is produced. Increased inspiratory effort results in more negative intrathoracic pressure and retraction of the skin and muscles over the suprasternal notch, the supraclavicular space, and the intercostal spaces. Violent contraction of the diaphragm often pulls in the ribs at the site of attachment of the diaphragm (subcostal retractions).

Cough provides a mechanism for removal of a nonfixed high airway obstruction. However, the depth and effectiveness of the cough are often limited by the poor inspiratory air flow. The air that is expelled during cough in high obstruction flows through a narrowed large tube, giving it a characteristic sound. If the obstruction is adjacent to the larynx, the cough is croupy or barking. If the obstruction is in the trachea or major bronchi, the cough is brassy. In most cases of high obstruction the cough is nonproductive.

LOW AIRWAY OBSTRUCTION

Peripheral obstructive lesions of the respiratory tract are generally diffuse in their distribution and primarily involve airways less than 3 mm in diameter. The lumen of these bronchi and bronchioles can be narrowed by spasm of their encircling smooth muscle, accumulation of secretions, edema of the mucous membrane, extrinsic compression, or any combination of these. With complete obstruction of these peripheral airways, patchy areas of atelectasis occur. Rarely are such atelectatic changes sufficient to produce obvious clinical manifestations.

Though peripheral obstructive lesions interfere with inspiration, the primary manifestations are expiratory. Expiration is prolonged. The passage of air through bronchi narrowed by compression changes from a laminar flow to a turbulent flow resulting in the wheezing expiratory sound. The excursion of the chest is diminished, and less air flow is heard on auscultation. In most cases accumulation of secretions and inflammation result in a cough which is usually hacking, ineffective, and repetitive.

The marked increase in airway resistance during exhalation rapidly results in overinflation. The chest is held in an inflated position with an increased anteroposterior (AP) diameter and spreading of the intercostal spaces. Percussion over the chest elicits hyperresonance; depression of the diaphragm can be detected by percussion over the middle of the back.

If the obstruction is marked, the accessory muscles of respiration are used. Although inspiratory retractions and use of accessory inspiratory muscles may be prominent, expiration is even more labored. Bulging of soft tissues above the clavicle or between the ribs and violent contraction of the abdominal muscles are often obvious. If ventilation is severely impaired, dyspnea results, often with associated orthopnea. In most cases the individual is limited in exercise tolerance and, with severe obstruction, may sit or lie and concentrate solely on breathing. Cyanosis indicates severe peripheral obstruction and impending death.

Chest roentgenogram reveals increased radiolucency from hyperinflation. Coarse bronchovascular markings may be associated with accumulated secretions, hypertrophied mucous glands, inflammation and edema of the bronchial walls, or peribronchial infiltrates. The increased AP diameter, depression of the diaphragm, and narrow, elongated heart shadow are all indicative of the overinflated state of the lungs.

12.6 RESPIRATORY FUNCTION AND MECHANISMS OF DEFENSE

The upper airway includes the nose, paranasal sinuses, and pharynx. The lower airway consists of the remainder of the system from the larynx peripherally. The nose has a relatively large surface area lined with a richly vascular, ciliated epithelium. By the time the air column reaches the bifurcation of the trachea, up to 75% of the warming and humidification of the inspired air has occurred. During exhalation, heat and moisture are removed from the air stream. Gross filtering of particles greater than 10–15 μm is achieved by the coarse hairs at the nasal orifices, and most inhaled particles greater than 5 μm are impacted on the nasal surface.

The larynx is relatively narrow and is ringed with cartilage. It is therefore relatively susceptible to obstruction, particularly by inflammation in young children, since the resultant swelling of tissues rapidly encroaches on the lumen. Obstruction at this level in the airway is primarily inspiratory and produces inspiratory stridor.

The trachea and bronchi are lined with pseudostratified, ciliated, columnar epithelium and occasional goblet cells. Mucous glands occupy approximately one third the thickness of the airway wall and for the most part lie between the epithelial surface and the cartilage. The trachea is supported by incomplete rings of cartilage with a muscular membrane posteriorly. Irregular plates of cartilage support the bronchi, especially at bifurcations. These diminish and finally disappear in the smallest bronchi. The goblet cells and principally the submucosal glands secrete the mucous layer, which is 2 to 5 μm in depth and rests on the tips of the cilia. It is estimated that an adult airway produces 100 ml of mucus daily. Each ciliated cell has about 275 cilia; movement results from action by microtubules within each cilium. The cilia beat within a periciliary fluid layer at about 1000 beats/min, moving the mucous blanket toward the pharynx at a rate of approximately 10 mm/min in the trachea. In the respiratory portion of the lung the surface cells gradually become cuboidal and then flat; ciliated cells and goblet cells ordinarily are absent.

The final 25% of warming of the inspired airstream and the accompanying obligatory humidifying occur in the trachea and large bronchi. Any failure of humidification permits dry air to reach the more distal parts of the conducting airway. Particles 5–1 μm in size sediment out on the tracheobronchial mucous blanket so that only particles of 1 μm or less reach the respiratory bronchioles and airspaces, where some may deposit and many will be exhaled.

Respiratory tract secretions are primarily derived from mucous (glycoproteins) and serous cells of the submucosal glands that empty onto the surface epithelium; from goblet cells and Clara cells, the special secreting cells in the surface epithelium of bronchi and bronchioles, respectively; from transudation from the vascular space; and from alveolar fluid, which contributes most of the phospholipid found in tracheobronchial mucus. This mucus contains about 95% water, 2% glycoproteins (mucins), 1% carbohydrate, and less than 1% lipid, DNA, and other substances.

Beyond infancy, collateral alveolar ventilation can occur increasingly with development of the pores of Kohn (10–15 μm) between alveoli. They provide a means for gas to pass from 1 lobule to another, perhaps even between segments of lung. Bronchiolar-alveolar communications (approximately 30 μm in diameter), known as the canals of Lambert, are also found. These anatomic connections may be helpful in preventing or delaying the occurrence of atelectasis.

The respiratory tract distal to the larynx is normally sterile. The defenses of the respiratory system which protect the lung include the filtering of large particles in the upper airway and smaller particles in the lower airway, the warming and humidification of inspired air, and the absorption of noxious fumes and gases by the vascular upper airway. The temporary cessation of breathing, reflexly shallow breathing, laryngospasm, or even bronchospasm limits the depth and amount of penetration of foreign matter. Spasm or decreased breathing can provide only brief protection. Aspiration of food, secretions, and foreign bodies is prevented by an intact swallowing mechanism and closure of the epiglottis.

CLEARANCE OF PARTICLES

Particles deposited in conducting airways are cleared within hours by the mucociliary mechanism, while clearance of those reaching the alveoli may take several days to months. The latter may be phagocytized by alveolar macrophages and removed from lungs by the mucociliary system or carried into the interstitium for clearance by the lymphocytes into regional nodes or the blood. Some particles penetrate into the interstitium without phagocytosis. Mucociliary clearance may be aided by cough, which provides an effective means by propelling excess mucus up the airways at pressures of up to 300 mm Hg and at flows of up to 5–6 l/sec. Mucus raised by the cough mechanism is usually swallowed by young children but may be expectorated.

DEFENSE AGAINST MICROBIAL AGENTS

Phagocytosis and mucociliary clearance may not be sufficient protection from living agents, such as bacteria and viruses. Additional factors include cellular killing of organisms and immune responses to assist in the phagocytosis-killing process. Alveolar and interstitial macrophages, derived from monocytes, are an essential component of the defense system of the lung. These high energy cells are rich in hydrolases such as lysozyme, acid phosphatase, and cathepsin which help digest bacteria and neutralize substances. The engulfment and killing of living particles by these macrophages may be enhanced by opsonins or by small lymphocytes. The principal antibody in respiratory secretions is secretory immunoglobulin A (IgA) which is produced, by plasma cells in the submucosa of the airways. Two molecules of IgA combine with a polypeptide (secretory component) produced by the respiratory epithelium to yield secretory IgA, which is highly resistant to digestion by proteolytic enzymes released after lysis of bacteria and dead cells. IgA can neutralize certain viruses and toxins and help in the lysis of bacteria. Although serum levels of IgA remain low during early childhood, pulmonary secretory IgA is reported to reach adult levels in the 1st mo of life. IgA may also prevent antigenic substances from penetrating the epithelial surfaces. IgG and IgM are also found in the secretions when lung inflammation occurs.

Other proteins such as lysozyme, lactoferrin, and interferon may also play a defense role in respiratory secretions. A small fraction of the antibodies of the respiratory surface is made up of immunoglobulin E (IgE), which is attached to mast cells and relatively concentrated in respiratory mucosa; it plays an important role in allergic reactions (Sec 9.43).

IMPAIRMENT OF DEFENSE MECHANISMS

The phagocytic ability of alveolar macrophages and, in most cases, the mucociliary mechanism can be impaired by ethanol ingestion, cigarette smoke, hypoxemia, starvation, chilling, corticosteroids, nitrogen dioxide, ozone, increased oxygen concentration, narcotics, and some anesthetic gases. The antibacterial killing capacity of the macrophages can be decreased by acidosis, azotemia, and recent acute viral infections, especially rubeola and influenza. Beryllium and asbestos, organic dust from cotton and sugar cane, and gases such as sulfur, nitrogen dioxide, ozone, chlorine, ammonia, and cigarette smoke are toxic to epithelial cells.

Mucociliary clearance can be reduced by hypothermia, hyperthermia, morphine, codeine, and hypothyroidism. Inhalation of dry gas by mouthbreathing during periods of nasal obstruction, after placement of a tracheostomy, or during use of poorly humidified oxygen results in drying of the mucous membrane and slowing of the ciliary beat. Cold air may irritate the tracheobronchial tree.

Damage to the respiratory epithelium may be reversible with rhinitis, sinusitis, bronchitis, bronchiolitis, acute respiratory infections associated with high levels of air pollution, the epithelial shedding that can occur in asthma or with some irritants, bronchospasm, edema, congestion, and perhaps mild surface ulceration. However, severe ulceration, bronchiectasis, bron-

chiolectasis, squamous cell metaplasia, and fibrosis represent serious injury and permanent impairment of the normal clearance mechanism. Other events that can alter metabolism of the lung or the release of biologically active substances by the lung include hyperventilation, alveolar hypoxia, pulmonary thromboembolism, pulmonary edema, hypersensitivity reactions, and certain drugs such as salicylates.

12.7 METABOLIC FUNCTIONS OF THE LUNG

The lung has a heterogeneous cell population with over 40 separate cell types. Among the many cells, the type I and II pneumocytes, the alveolar macrophage, and the Clara cell are unique to the lung. The lung can synthesize lipids and proteins, including glycoproteins, secretory antibodies, interferon, proteolytic and fibrinolytic enzymes and activators, collagen, and elastin. Tissue factors such as thromboplastin are found in higher concentration in the lung than in any other organ. Megakaryocytes are concentrated in the lung.

Since the lung has the only capillary bed through which the entire blood flow must pass in the normal state, the pulmonary capillary circulation is ideally positioned to have a controlling influence on circulating vasoactive hormones (Table 12–1). Angiotensin II, up to 50 times more active than its precurser, is converted from angiotensin I during 1 passage through the pulmonary circulation. Other vasoactive materials, including serotonin, bradykinin, ATP, and prostaglandins E_1, E_2, and F_2, are almost completely removed or inactivated by 1 passage through the pulmonary circulation while others, such as epinephrine, prostaglandin A_1 and A_2, angiotensin II, and vasopressin, may be minimally affected. Norepinephrine and histamine are taken up to a moderate degree. Failure of inactivation or periodic release of potent substances such as serotonin, bradykinin, histamine, and so on may be important in the pathogenesis of some pulmonary disease or as a mediator of secondary effects.

Table 12–1 BIOLOGICALLY ACTIVE SUBSTANCES AND THE LUNG

Substances secreted and/or released by lung cells
- Histamine
- Slow reactive substance of anaphylaxis (SRS-A)
- Eosinophil chemotactic factor
- Platelet aggregation factor
- Prostaglandins E and F
- Angiotensin II
- Bradykinin, kallidin
- Serotonin
- Endocrine substances?

Substances degraded during passage through the lung
- Angiotensin I (80%/pass)
- Serotonin (65–95%/pass)
- Prostaglandins E and F (92%/pass)
- Bradykinin (80%/pass)
- Norepinephrine (20–40%/pass)

Fishman AP: Non-respiratory functions of the lung. Chest 72:84, 1977.

Fishman AP, Pietra GG: Handling of bioactive materials by the lung. N Engl J Med 291:884, 1974.

Green GM: In defense of the lung. Am Rev Resp Dis 102:691, 1970.

Kendig EL (ed): Disorders of the Respiratory Tract in Children. Philadelphia, WB Saunders, 1977.

Loosli CG, Potter EL: Pre- and post-natal development of the respiratory portion of the human lung. Am Rev Resp Dis 80 (suppl):5, 1959.

Lough MD, Doershuk CF, Stern RC (eds): Pediatric Respiratory Therapy. Chicago, Year Book Medical Publishers, 1979.

Proctor DF: The upper airways. I. Nasal physiology and defense of the lungs. Am Rev Resp Dis 115:97, 1977.

Said SI: The lung as a metabolic organ. N Engl J Med 279:1330, 1968.

Said SI: The lung in relation to vasoactive hormones. Fed Proc 32:1972, 1973.

Scarpelli M (ed): Pulmonary Physiology of the Fetus, Newborn and Child. Philadelphia, Lea & Febiger, 1975.

Thurlbeck WM: Postnatal growth and development of the lung. Am Rev Resp Dis 111:803, 1975.

12.8   PULMONARY FUNCTION

See also Sec 12.19.

VENTILATION

Normal ventilation provides for maintenance of arterial oxygen, carbon dioxide, and pH at the least level of work. The alveolar-capillary membrane is so thin that normally there is no discernible difference in oxygen tension between the alveolar gas and pulmonary venous blood or in arterial or alveolar carbon dioxide tensions. At sea level the oxygen tension of ambient, relatively dry air is about 150 mm Hg, and this is reduced to 100–105 mm Hg in the alveolus, in part because CO_2 and water vapor are also present (Fig 12–2). The normal pressure of oxygen in the aorta (PaO_2) at sea level is 90–100 mm Hg, while that for carbon dioxide ($PaCO_2$) is about 38–42 mm Hg. The slight further drop in pO_2 (4–5 mm Hg) observed between alveoli and arterial blood is due to diffusion and shunting from the bronchial arterial circulation and coronary venous blood. Hypoventilation (or hypercapnia) is defined as a $PaCO_2$ greater than 45 mm Hg and hyperventilation (hypocapnia) as a $PaCO_2$ less than 35 mm Hg.

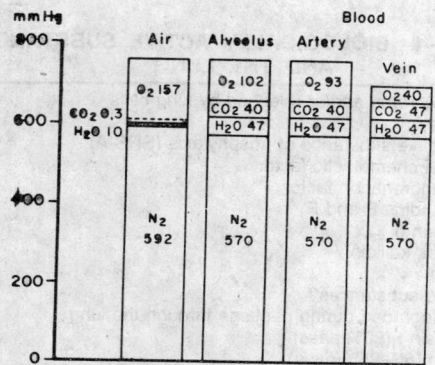

Figure 12–2 Partial pressures of oxygen, carbon dioxide, water vapor, and nitrogen in ambient air and in the body at sea level. Partial pressure = 760 mm Hg.

VENTILATION-PERFUSION RELATIONSHIPS

For the lung as a whole, the ratio of alveolar ventilation at rest ($\dot{V}_A$ = 4 l/min) to pulmonary perfusion ($\dot{Q}$ = 5 l/min) is 0.8. However, the pattern of ventilated air does not uniformly follow the pattern of distribution of blood flow through the lung. In the erect position the lung apices are underventilated with respect to their volume and are underperfused to an even greater extent (high $\dot{V}_A/\dot{Q}$) than the lung bases, which receive proportionately more blood flow than ventilated air (low $\dot{V}_A/\dot{Q}$). With disease this matching may be sufficiently deranged so that regional imbalances lead to an early decrease in arterial oxygen tension. At the same time, minimal overall alveolar hyperventilation can maintain the carbon dioxide tension at normal levels or lower until much later in the disease process because of the greater ease of diffusion of carbon dioxide across the alveolus.

CAUSES OF HYPOXEMIA

Ventilation-perfusion abnormalities are the most frequent cause of arterial hypoxemia. Shunts (intracardiac or intrapulmonary), diffusion problems, and primary hypoventilation (for example, due to central nervous system depression, upper airway obstruction, or neuromuscular problems) also cause arterial hypoxemia. Primary hypoventilation also results in a parallel hypercapnia; however, the other 3 causes of hypoxemia result in hypercapnia only late in disease, when overall alveolar ventilation is reduced to the extent that CO_2 retention (greater than 45–50 mm Hg) occurs.

LUNG VOLUMES

The standard terminology for lung volume and its various subdivisions is diagrammed in Fig 12–3.

Some gas is moved with each breath, and some, the residual volume (RV), always remains in normal lungs. Most lung subdivisions are measured from the resting end-tidal midposition where the retractive lung forces are balanced by the thoracic forces which tend to expand the chest and lungs. The volume of gas remaining in the lungs at this point is the functional residual capacity (FRC), which comprises the expiratory reserve volume (ERV) plus residual volume (RV). The FRC is normally about 50% of the total lung capacity (TLC), and the residual volume is normally about 25% of the TLC and increases somewhat with age. In an average adult the tidal volume is about 500 ml. Approximately two thirds of each tidal volume enters the alveoli and one third remains in the conducting airways per breath (the anatomic dead space).

The volume changes and certain flow rates are measured by use of a spirometer or a system that integrates flow through a flowmeter or pneumotachometer. Functional residual capacity is measured by a closed circuit

Figure 12-3 Lung volumes and forced vital capacity. MMF = maximal midexpiratory flow rate, i.e., mean flow rate calculated over mid-one half of forced expiratory curve. FEV = forced expiratory volume in a given time, such as 1 sec. Air is almost completely expelled within 3 sec in the normal, but emptying is delayed with obstruction. (From Doershuk CF, Lough MD, *In* Lough MD, Doershuk CF, Stern RC (ed): Pediatric Respiratory Therapy. Courtesy Year Book Medical Publishers, Chicago, 1974.)

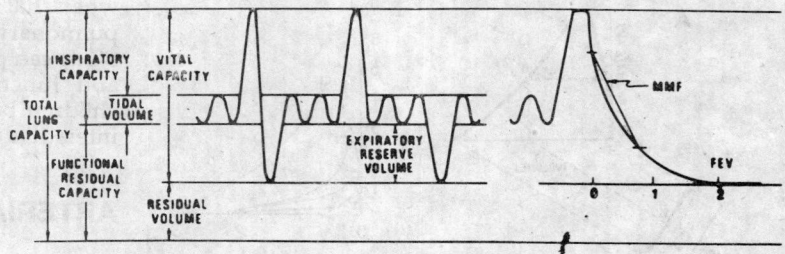

helium dilution method, by an open circuit nitrogen washout method, or by use of the total body plethysmograph to measure the volume of thoracic gas (V_{TG}). RV and TLC are calculated from the spirometer data and the FRC; for example, RV = FRC − ERV and TLC = FRC + IC (inspiratory capacity). The lung volumes are affected by changes in position and disease (Sec 12.19).

Pulmonary function tests do not usually result in an etiologic diagnosis except, perhaps, when a response to a bronchodilator suggests a reversible airways problem consistent with bronchospasm and bronchial asthma. Rather, they permit recognition of 2 main categories of pulmonary involvement: obstruction and restriction. The *obstruction* pattern, which is encountered most often in childhood diseases, includes loss of vital capacity, principally ERV, while the FRC increases. The combined effect of these changes is an even greater increase in residual volume than in FRC. TLC is usually somewhat increased in obstructive disease, but the RV/TLC ratio will be increased even more. Flow rates are generally decreased. Bronchiolitis, bronchial asthma, and cystic fibrosis are the most common conditions that produce a pattern of airways obstruction in children.

The typical pattern of *restriction* includes a decrease in vital capacity and total lung capacity while the flow rates remain relatively unimpaired until VC and TLC fall below approximately 50% of predicted normal. The slight decrease of RV results in an apparent increase in the RV/TLC ratio, suggesting obstruction. When the TLC is decreased, no attempt should be made to interpret the RV/TLC ratio. Any condition causing stiffening of the chest or lungs, deformity of the spine, abnormality of the respiratory muscles, neurologic impairment of the diaphragm or other respiratory muscles, or anything acting to decrease the volume of the lungs (tumor, hydrothorax, pneumothorax) will produce a restrictive type of abnormality. Kyphoscoliosis and neuromuscular conditions are the most commonly encountered causes of a restrictive abnormality in childhood. Some conditions, such as cystic fibrosis, advanced tuberculosis, and asthmatic bronchitis, may have a combination of both obstructive and restrictive elements.

The lung volumes and capacities increase with body growth and in the normal child can best be related to body size, particularly to length in the infant and young child studied supine and to height in older patients studied in the erect position. There is a relatively wide range of normal for lung volumes and capacities—up to ± 20%; results from test to test in the same individual can vary by as much as 5%.

MECHANICS OF RESPIRATION

The mechanical factors in lung expansion include (1) the flow-resistive or dynamic properties, which include airway resistance and tissue viscous resistance and which combine to make up total pulmonary resistance, and (2) the elastic or static properties, expressed as compliance. Determining the dynamic forces requires both flow and pressure change measurements; determining the static forces of breathing requires both volume and pressure change measurements.

Flow rate measurements can be used to assess flow resistance since all portions of the lung do not expand or retract at the same rate. Flow resistance is monitored inferentially by determining fractional portions of the forced expiratory volume (FEV), expiratory flow rates from the maximal expiratory flow volume (MEFV) curve (Sec 12.19 and Fig 12-4), and maximal breathing capacity (MBC) or maximal voluntary ventilation (MVV). These tests are dependent upon the size or overinflation of the lung and are not specific measures of resistance since compliance also enters into the results. The mean flow rate in liters/sec calculated over the middle half of the forced expiratory volume achieved is useful early in the course of obstructive disease.

The determinants of airway resistance (R_{AW}) during the usually predominant laminar flow that occurs in the airways during tidal breathing are the viscosity of gas and the length and radius of the bronchi and bronchioles. R_{AW} is inversely related to lung volume since airway caliber is affected by increases and decreases in lung size. Although the smallest airways offer the highest resistance, the tremendous increase in total cross-sectional area of the airways toward the periphery means that the peripheral airways contribute less than 20% of the airway resistance, and it is thought that peripheral R_{AW} plays a prominent role in children only up to age 4-5 yr. Considerable peripheral airways disease thus may be present before significant alterations in R_{AW} are apparent.

The elastic characteristic of the respiratory system, **compliance**, is expressed as volume/cm H_2O pressure. Since determination of pressure change requires a balloon positioned in the esophagus, compliance is not frequently measured during childhood. The lungs of infants are less compliant than those of older children and young adults, but when the effect of lung size at FRC is considered (specific compliance), no differences are observed. In disease states, altered lung elasticity and surface characteristics, areas of atelectasis or consolidation, or increased airway resistance will alter the pressure-volume characteristics of the lung.

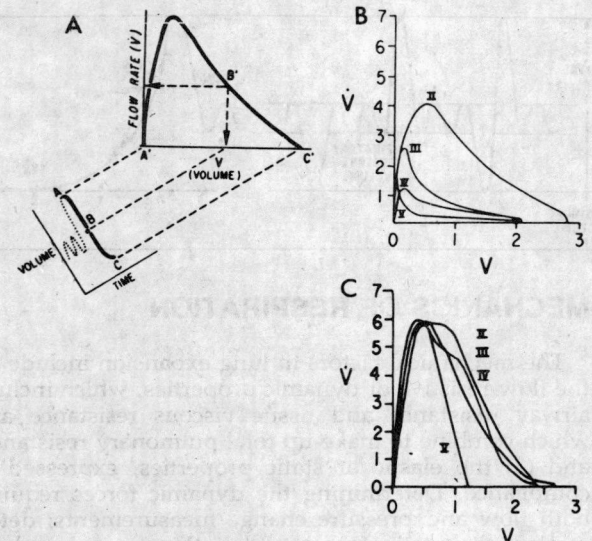

Figure 12–4 *A,* A standard spirogram (points A, B, and C) is compared with the expiratory flow-volume (FV) curve in a normal subject. In the FV curve, expiration proceeds from peak lung inflation at A'along A'B' to the forced expiratory position at C'. Flow rate at a given lung volume may be determined by drawing a tangent at any point in the spirogram. Such measurements are subject to error. By contrast, the flow rate at the same lung volume can be read directly at point B on the FV curve. (V̇, flow rate in liters/sec; V, expiratory volume in liters from the total lung capacity.) *B,* Flow-volume curves in obstructive lung disease. Four classes of obstructive disease of increasing severity are shown. The curves in classes III, IV, and V were selected from patients of the same sex and height who had approximately the same forced vital capacities. As obstructive disease becomes more severe, the curve becomes more convex to the volume axis. A universal finding in class V is a sudden drop in flow soon after the onset of expiration. This phenomenon occurs even at low intrathoracic driving pressures. *C,* The flow-volume curve in pulmonary parenchymal fibrosis is characterized by a high peak flow rate and small forced vital capacity. In class V, with marked decrease in vital capacity, the high, peaked curve is distinctive. (From Lord GP, et al: Am J Med 46:73, 1969. Courtesy American Journal of Medicine.)

WORK OF BREATHING

The work of breathing meets the energy requirements to overcome inertia, surface active forces, air flow and elastic resistance, and tissue viscous resistance. In general, the rate and depth of breathing are adjusted so that alveolar ventilation is maintained at a minimum of total respiratory work. At all ages it appears that approximately 1% of the total basal metabolism is expended on the work of breathing in normal circumstances.

DIFFUSION

Diffusion of oxygen and carbon dioxide depends upon the thickness of the alveolar-capillary membrane, the capillary transit time, uptake of oxygen by the blood, and total surface area of the capillary bed in relation to that of the alveolar membrane. Because of its high diffusing capacity (20 times greater than that of oxygen), carbon dioxide levels are rarely abnormal in diffusion problems. When the inspired oxygen percentage is reduced to 14%, arterial hypoxemia is increased in a diffusion problem. The hypoxemia can be corrected

when 100% oxygen is breathed. Measurement of the pulmonary diffusing capacity (D_L) using carbon monoxide can provide a useful index of pulmonary structure and function. Primary diffusion defects are rare in children but are met in conditions resulting in diffuse interstitial fibrosis.

ARTERIAL BLOOD GASES

In primary hypoventilation, such as central nervous system depression or muscle paralysis, a decrease in arterial pO_2 will be paralleled by an increase in $PaCO_2$. Diffusion abnormalities, shunt problems, and especially the ventilation-perfusion inequalities occurring in conditions such as bronchial asthma, bronchiolitis, and cystic fibrosis also result in arterial hypoxemia. A decrease in PaO_2 is the earliest observation, usually accompanied by a *decrease* in $PaCO_2$ due to the overall increase in ventilation. When the condition deteriorates to overall alveolar hypoventilation, the $PaCO_2$ returns toward normal. Subsequently, CO_2 retention greater than 45–50 mm Hg indicates respiratory failure.

Acute respiratory failure results in the elevation of $PaCO_2$ and decrease in pH; the bicarbonate (HCO_3^-) remains normal. When the kidneys have had 1–2 days to compensate by HCO_3^- retention, the pH is restored toward normal and compensated respiratory acidosis results. When improvement in ventilation then results in reduction of the carbon dioxide, there is again a slower fall in HCO_3^-, resulting in metabolic alkalosis for several days.

Bates DV, Macklem PT, Christie RV (eds): Respiratory Function in Disease. Philadelphia, WB Saunders, 1971.
Briscoe WA, Dubois AB: The relationship between airway resistance, airway conductance, and lung volume in subjects of different ages and body size. J Clin Invest 37:1279, 1958.
Comroe JH, et al (eds): The Lung. Chicago, Year Book Medical Publishers, 1962.
Comroe JH: Physiology of Respiration. Chicago, Year Book Medical Publishers, 1965.
DeMuth GR, Howatt WF, Hill G: The growth of lung function. Pediatrics 35:162, 1965.
Doershuk CF, Lough MD: Pulmonary function testing and interpretation. *In:* Lough MD, Doershuk CF, Stern RC (eds): Pediatric Respiratory Therapy. Chicago, Year Book Medical Publishers, 1979.
Lord GP, et al: Flow-volume curves in lung disease. Am J Med 46:73, 1969.
Murray JF: The Normal Lung. Philadelphia, WB Saunders, 1976.
Nelson NM: Neonatal pulmonary function. Pediatr Clin N Am 13:769, 1966.
West JB: Respiratory Physiology. Baltimore, Williams & Wilkins, 1974.

12.9   REGULATION OF RESPIRATION

CENTRAL NERVOUS SYSTEM

Breathing appears to be coordinated in the brain stem by 2 components of the pons and 2 components of the medulla which together compose the respiratory center. Conscious control can also be imposed from the cerebral cortex—cough, sniff, speech, cry, laugh, breathholding, and voluntary hyperventilation.

The inherent rhythmicity of the medullary center

results from the interaction of its inspiratory and expiratory components so that there is reciprocal inhibition, with the inspiratory component being dominant. Nonspecific stimuli from pain, cold, and other nearby nonrespiratory-related nervous system activity probably help maintain the local rhythmicity of this portion of the brain stem. The medullary area appears to be modulated by the 2 pontine components, the apneustic and the pneumotaxic, and by afferent fibers from the vagus, which also has fibers to the pontine area. The apneustic component located in the middle and caudal pons has an inspiratory activity that can be inhibited by the pneumotaxic component or by vagal afferent fibers. The pneumotaxic area located in the superior pons inhibits inspiratory activity of the lower components, either through the apneustic component or by direct effect on the medullary areas.

PULMONARY VENTILATION

The inherent rhythmicity of the reticular formation of the medullary portion of the respiratory center is played upon by the pontine area and by 2 feedback mechanisms whose coordinated systematic interaction regulates pulmonary ventilation and provides the best respiratory pattern for any metabolic level. The 2 feedback mechanisms are the proprioceptive reflexes from the chest wall and lungs and the humoral system involving chemical factors (H^+, PaO_2, and $PaCO_2$).

A number of **proprioceptive reflexes** in the chest wall and lungs affect respiration, mostly by afferent pathways in the vagus nerves. In the *Hering-Breuer reflex*, impulses from distention of lung or airways inhibit inspiration by action on the apneustic component of the pons. The *paradoxic reflex of Head* receptors are located in the lung parenchyma and produce an inspiratory stimulus beyond an initial inspiration in infants when the vagus is inactivated. The *deflation reflex* increases the force and frequency of inspiration effort as the lungs are deflated via receptors located in the bronchioles and bronchi, but it is not involved in normal breathing. The *muscle spindle efferent (gamma) system* of respiratory muscles influences the excitability of local spinal motor neurons, thus affecting the tone and strength of the muscles of breathing, and may be important to voluntary control of the respiratory muscles for functions such as speech. Changes in pulmonary and systemic blood pressure, mechanical stimulation of the upper airway, chemical stimulus of the lower airway, and the presence of substances such as serotonin and antihistamines also affect ventilation.

Both peripheral and central chemoreceptors sense the chemical composition of the blood and thus influence the activity of the respiratory center. The peripheral receptors are the carotid bodies, located near the bifurcation of the common carotid artery and supplied by the glossopharyngeal nerve, and the aortic body, found in the ascending arch of the aorta and supplied by the vagus nerve. Hypoxemia (decreased PaO_2) is the major stimulus to these bodies and results in an increased rate and depth of breathing. Hypercapnia and acidosis potentiate the response of these bodies to hypoxemia. The central chemoreceptors are located in the ventrolateral areas of the medulla and stimulate ventilation in response to local changes in pH caused by increased arterial pCO_2.

Patients with obesity-hypoventilation (Pickwickian syndrome), hypothyroidism, starvation, and familial dysautonomia (Riley-Day syndrome) may be less responsive to $PaCO_2$ and PaO_2 changes than normal children, presumably because of a central defect in either or both of the chemoreceptors and their reticular formation. Athletes also exhibit decreased responsiveness to hypoxia, and there may be familial patterns of decreased responsiveness to increasing carbon dioxide tensions. Conversely, increased responsiveness to carbon dioxide and hyperventilation occur in pregnancy and in the luteal phase of the menstrual cycle because of the increased level of progesterone. Exogenous progesterone given to healthy males also produces hyperventilation by increasing responsiveness to carbon dioxide.

FETAL-NEWBORN PERIOD

See Chapter 7 for discussion of fetal and neonatal respiration.

CARL F. DOERSHUK

Cherniak NS: The clinical assessment of the chemical regulation of ventilation. Chest 70:274, 1976.

Chernick V (ed): Onset and control of fetal and neonatal respiration. Semin Perinatol 1:321, 1977.

Cunningham DJC, Lloyd BB (eds): The regulation of human respiration. *In*: Proceedings of the JS Haldane Centenary Symposium. Philadelphia, FA Davis, 1963.

Davis JN: Spinal control. *In*: Campbell EJM, Agostoni E, Davis JN (eds): The Respiratory Muscles. Philadelphia, WB Saunders, 1970.

Dejours P: Chemoreflexes in breathing. Physiol Rev 42:335, 1962.

Dejours P: Respiration. New York, Oxford University Press, 1966.

Mitchell RA, Berger AJ: Neural regulation of respiration. Am Rev Resp Dis 111:206, 1975.

Negus V: The Biology of Respiration. Baltimore, Williams and Wilkins, 1965.

Severinghaus JW: Chemical regulation of ventilation: Who needs it? N Engl J Med 295:895, 1976.

Slonim NB, Hamilton LW: Respiratory Physiology. St Louis, CV Mosby, 1976.

Wang SC, Nagel SH: General organization of central respiratory mechanisms. *In*: Fenn WO, Rahn H (eds): Handbook of Physiology, Vol. 1. Washington DC, American Physiologic Society, 1964.

12.10   DIAGNOSTIC PROCEDURES IN PULMONARY MEDICINE

12.11   RADIOGRAPHIC TECHNIQUES

An appropriate, properly performed and interpreted roentgenogram can be one of the most useful diagnostic tools available to the pediatrician. However, with faulty technique or interpretation it can be confusing or misleading. To minimize radiation exposure, proper collimation and gonadal shielding should be employed, and films must be limited to the area of clinical concern. Roentgenograms should be taken in the radiology department whenever possible rather than with portable equipment. The area of greatest interest should generally be placed closest to the film, and the patient should be properly positioned and gently immobilized if necessary. Exposure time should be short to minimize motion artifact, particularly in infants.

Chest Roentgenograms

A posterior-anterior and a lateral view, upright and at full inspiration, should be obtained in most circumstances. Films taken during expiration are often misinterpreted by the inexperienced as showing pulmonary infiltrates or other abnormalities. Comparison of expiratory and inspiratory films may reveal a mediastinal shift, helpful in the evaluation of possible bronchial obstruction (as with foreign body), but fluoroscopy is usually more informative. Decubitus films are indicated if there is suspicion of pleural fluid. Recumbent films may be difficult to interpret in the presence of free fluid, either within the pleural space or in a cavity. Oblique views may be helpful to evaluate the hilum and the area behind the heart, while the apices are best seen in a lordotic view.

Tomograms, Computed Tomography

For detailed investigation of specific lesions of the hilum, tomograms may be indicated. However, the radiation exposure is much higher than with plain films and good patient cooperation is necessary. Computed tomography (CT scan) of the chest is more useful in the evaluation of mediastinal than parenchymal lesions.

Lateral Neck Films

A lateral view of the neck can yield invaluable information in patients with upper airway obstruction, especially about the retropharyngeal space, supraglottic area, and subglottic space. Knowledge of the phase of respiration during which the film was taken is often essential for accurate interpretation. Patients with severe airway obstruction must not be sent unattended to the radiology department.

Xerography

Xerography gives exceptionally good soft tissue detail but results in much higher doses of radiation (especially to the thyroid) and should not be used routinely.

Sinus, Nasal Films

Roentgenographic examination of the sinuses is indicated when sinus disease is suspected. Because of the small size and slow development of the frontal and maxillary sinus cavities in children, transillumination is not as successful in documenting sinus disease as are roentgenograms. The need for examination of the nasal passages in children is unusual and occurs most often in the neonate with obstruction when tumor or occult foreign body is suspected. Instillation of a small amount of barium or other liquid contrast material may facilitate the demonstration of choanal stenosis or atresia.

Fluoroscopy

Fluoroscopic techniques with image intensification have markedly reduced the radiation exposure for dynamic studies. Fluoroscopy is especially useful for evaluation of stridor and abnormal movement of the diaphragm or mediastinum. Many procedures such as needle aspiration or biopsy of a peripheral lesion are also best accomplished with the aid of fluoroscopy. Video tape recording does not increase radiation exposure, an advantage over cine roentgenograms, and its use may even decrease exposure by allowing detailed study, through "replay" capability, of a brief exposure to fluoroscopy.

Contrast Studies

Barium Swallow. This study is indicated in the evaluation of patients with recurrent pneumonia, persistent coughs of undetermined etiology, and stridor or persistent wheezing. A barium swallow should be done with fluoroscopy, and spot films should also be obtained. In the search for an "H" type of tracheoesophageal fistula, a simple barium swallow is often inadequate; the barium may have to be injected through a catheter placed at several locations in the esophagus. The barium may thus be forced through a normally closed fistulous tract which would not otherwise be demonstrable. If esophageal atresia is suspected, no more than 0.5 ml of barium should be injected into the esophagus through a soft catheter with great care to avoid aspiration into the trachea. The barium swallow is also useful in the evaluation of abnormal swallowing mechanics and for the diagnosis of gastroesophageal reflux, both of which can lead to aspiration and recurrent pneumonias.

Bronchograms. Air contrast is usually insufficient for delineation of airways smaller than main stem bronchi, except in the presence of parenchymal consolidation. A study of smaller bronchi may be performed by instilling a contrast material directly into the airway. In small children bronchograms are usually performed through an endotracheal tube under general anesthesia. In older children and adults sedation and topical anesthesia may be sufficient. The contrast material is placed into the airways with a catheter passed transnasally, through the endotracheal tube or through a fiberoptic bronchoscope. Care should be taken to use the smallest amount of contrast material necessary to coat (not fill) the airways. The procedure should be performed with fluoroscopy so that the contrast material can be placed selectively in the areas and in the quantity desired. In general, bronchograms are indicated only when pulmonary surgery may be considered. Specific indications include recurrent hemoptysis, recurrent pneumonia in the same area, chronic productive cough with persistent localized physical findings, and previously demonstrated bronchiectasis unresponsive to therapy.

Pulmonary Arteriograms. These studies are indicated for detailed evaluation of the pulmonary vasculature and are helpful in the diagnosis of suspected congenital anomalies such as lobar agenesis, unilateral hyperlucent lung, and vascular rings and sometimes in evaluation of solid or cystic lesions.

Aortograms. Thoracic aortograms may be used to define the systemic (bronchial) pulmonary circulation, especially in suspected pulmonary sequestration. Although most hemoptysis is from the bronchial arteries, bronchial arteriography is seldom helpful in the diagnosis or treatment of intrapulmonary bleeding in children.

Pneumoperitoneum, Pneumothorax. In selected situations it may be advantageous to inject a small amount of air into the pleural or peritoneal cavity to provide air contrast and thus outline the limits of the diaphragm or pleural surfaces as in the evaluation of diaphragmatic eventration. The air is rapidly absorbed and causes no functional impairment.

Radionuclide Lung Scans. The usual scan employs intravenous injection of material (macroaggregated human serum albumin) that will be trapped in the pulmonary capillary bed. The distribution of radioactivity is proportional to *pulmonary capillary blood flow* and is useful in the evaluation of pulmonary embolism and congenital cardiovascular and pulmonary defects. Acute changes in the distribution of pulmonary perfusion may reflect alterations of pulmonary ventilation.

The distribution of *pulmonary ventilation* may be determined by scanning following the inhalation of a radioactive gas such as xenon-133. A useful technique for evaluation of both pulmonary perfusion and ventilation is the intravenous injection of xenon-133 dissolved in saline, followed by continuous recording of the rate of appearance and disappearance of the xenon over the lung. Appearance of xenon in the early phase after injection is a measure of perfusion, while the rate of washout during breathing is a measure of ventilation.

12.12 ENDOSCOPY

Laryngoscopy

Direct inspection of the glottis is often necessary in the evaluation of stridor and local abnormalities. In infants and small children direct laryngoscopy is usually necessary and requires general anesthesia. Indirect (mirror) laryngoscopy is useful in older children and adults but is rarely possible in infants. A newer technique for direct laryngoscopy, which can be done with topical anesthesia and mild sedation, is to pass a small flexible fiberoptic bronchoscope through the nose; this allows the glottis to be seen without the anatomic distortion that may be introduced by a laryngoscope blade, and it is more comfortable for the patient. It is especially useful for the evaluation of the dynamics of the larynx and upper airway.

Bronchoscopy

Indications for bronchoscopy include the evaluation of recurrent pneumonia or atelectasis, possible foreign bodies, unexplained and persistent wheezes and infiltrates, hemoptysis, and suspected congenital anomalies or mass lesions. The bronchoscope is used for visual examination, for biopsy of mass lesions or for transbronchial lung biopsy, and for aspiration of secretions for culture and microscopic examination. Therapeutic applications include removal of foreign bodies and mucus plugs, as well as bronchial toilet and bronchopulmonary lavage. An open tube bronchoscope should be used for patients with massive pulmonary bleeding, for removal of foreign bodies, or for other operative procedures. Small flexible fiberoptic bronchoscopes are now available for diagnostic (and some therapeutic) procedures in infants and children; their advantages include ease of insertion, greater peripheral range, a lower incidence of complications, and the avoidance of general anesthesia. Recent development of high resolution glass rod telescopes of small diameter (Stortz-Hopkins) has also greatly improved the open tube bronchoscope for pediatric use.

Complications of bronchoscopy depend on the instrument used and the procedure performed. Transient hypoxia, cardiac arrhythmias, laryngospasm, and bronchospasm are most common, and infection, bleeding, pneumomediastinum, or pneumothorax may occur. After open tube bronchoscopy the patient must be carefully observed for airway obstruction resulting from trauma to the subglottic space. This is much less common after use of a flexible bronchoscope because of its relatively small size. Postbronchoscopy croup is treated with oxygen, mist, vasoconstrictor aerosols (racemic epinephrine), and corticosteroids as necessary.

12.13 THORACENTESIS

Fluid may be removed from the pleural space by needle puncture for diagnostic or therapeutic purposes. The site of puncture is chosen to maximize the yield of fluid and minimize the risk. The procedure is usually done with the patient sitting, and the needle is most often inserted through the inferior aspect of the 7th or 8th intercostal space in the mid or posterior axillary line. Local anesthetic is first injected, using a 1.5 in, 22 gauge needle passed just *above* the rib margin to avoid the neurovascular bundle. The pleura may be identified by feel or by withdrawing an initial volume of pleural fluid. A larger needle is then inserted to the same depth. It is often advantageous to pass a plastic catheter through the needle into the pleural space and then withdraw the needle. This procedure allows the operator to move both catheter and patient, thereby often collecting more fluid, and reduces the possibility of puncture or laceration of the lung. In general, as much fluid as possible should be withdrawn and an *upright* chest roentgenogram obtained after the procedure.

Complications of thoracentesis include infection, pneumothorax, and bleeding. Thoracentesis on the right may be complicated by puncture or laceration of the capsule of the liver (and on the left, the spleen). Specimens obtained by thoracentesis should always be cultured and examined microscopically for evidence of bacterial infection. Diagnostic evaluations should include, as a minimum, total protein and total and differential cell counts. Lactic acid dehydrogenase, glucose, cholesterol, and amylase determinations may be useful. If malignancy is suspected, cytologic examination is imperative.

Transudates result from mechanical factors influencing the rate of formation or reabsorption of pleural fluid and generally require no further diagnostic evaluation. *Exudates* result from inflammation or other disease of the pleural surface and underlying lung and require a more complete diagnostic evaluation. In general, transudates have a total protein of less than 3 gm/dl or a ratio of pleural protein to serum protein under 0.5, a total leukocyte count of fewer than 2000 with a predominance of mononuclear cells, and low lactic acid dehydrogenase levels. Exudates have high protein levels and a predominance of polymorphonuclear cells (although malignant or tuberculous effusions may have a higher percentage of mononuclear cells). Tuberculous effusions may have low glucose and high cholesterol content.

12.14   PERCUTANEOUS LUNG TAP

This is the most direct method of obtaining bacteriologic specimens from the pulmonary parenchyma and the only technique other than open lung biopsy not associated with a relatively high risk of contamination by oral flora. The technique is very similar to that for thoracentesis. A 20 or 22 gauge, 1.5 in needle attached to a 10 ml syringe containing approximately 1 ml of sterile saline is inserted, with aseptic technique and after local anesthesia, through the inferior aspect of an intercostal space in the area of interest. The needle is rapidly advanced into the lung, the saline injected and reaspirated, and the needle withdrawn, all as quickly as possible. This procedure usually yields a few drops of "lung juice," which should be cultured and examined microscopically.

Indications for lung tap include roentgenographic infiltrates of undetermined etiology, especially if unresponsive to therapy and particularly in immunosuppressed patients susceptible to unusual organisms. Complications are the same as for thoracentesis, although the incidence of pneumothorax is higher and somewhat dependent on the nature of the underlying disease process. In patients with poor pulmonary compliance, as with pneumocystis pneumonia, the rate may approach 30%, with 5% requiring chest tubes. In most patients with bacterial pneumonia the rate of pneumothorax is much lower.

12.15   LUNG BIOPSY

Lung biopsy may be the only way to establish a diagnosis, especially in protracted noninfectious disease. In infants and small children an open surgical biopsy is the procedure of choice and in expert hands is associated with an extremely low morbidity; it assures that an adequate specimen is obtained, and the surgeon is able to inspect the lung surface and choose the site of biopsy. In older patients transbronchial biopsies can be performed, using flexible forceps through an endotracheal tube or a bronchoscope, usually with fluoroscopic guidance. This technique is most appropriate in older patients with diffuse lung diseases, such as pneumocystis pneumonia, and is associated with the least morbidity and complications. However, because of the small specimens obtained (1 × 1.5 mm) the diagnosis may be more easily missed than with an open biopsy.

12.16   TRANSILLUMINATION OF THE CHEST WALL

In infants up to at least 6 mo of age a pneumothorax may often be diagnosed by transillumination of the chest wall with a fiberoptic light probe. The presence of free air in the pleural space will often result in a larger than usual halo of light in the skin surrounding the probe. This test is unreliable in older patients or in those with subcutaneous emphysema.

12.17   MICROBIOLOGY

The specific diagnosis of infection in the lower respiratory tract depends on the proper handling of an adequate specimen obtained in an appropriate fashion. Although specimens should be obtained from as near the source of infection as possible, this is often impractical. Nasopharyngeal or throat cultures are often used but may not correlate with cultures obtained by more direct techniques. Sputum specimens are preferred and can often be obtained by deep throat swab immediately after coughing from patients who do not expectorate. Specimens also may be obtained directly from the tracheobronchial tree by nasotracheal aspiration (usually heavily contaminated), by transtracheal aspiration through the cricothyroid membrane (useful in adults and adolescents but hazardous in children), and in infants and children by a sterile catheter inserted into the trachea during direct laryngoscopy or through an endotracheal tube. A percutaneous lung tap or an open biopsy is the only way to ensure a specimen free of oral flora.

Examination of Secretions

A specimen obtained by direct expectoration is usually assumed to be of tracheobronchial origin, but often it is not. The presence of alveolar macrophages is the hallmark of tracheobronchial secretions. Alveolar macrophages are large, mononuclear cells (occasionally multinucleated but never polymorphonuclear) with abundant cytoplasm which stains blue on Wright-stained smears. They are easily distinguished from the "fried egg" appearance of squamous cells. Both nasopharyngeal and tracheobronchial secretions may contain ciliated epithelial cells, although they are more common in sputum. Nasopharyngeal and oral secretions often contain large numbers of squamous epithelial cells. Sputum may contain both, having picked up oral contents during expectoration.

During sleep, tracheobronchial secretions continue to be brought to the pharynx by mucociliary transport, where they are swallowed. Because of the low gastric motility and acidity during sleep, an early morning gastric aspirate will often contain material from the tracheobronchial tract which is suitable for smear and culture for acidfast bacilli.

The absence of polymorphonuclear leukocytes in a Wright-stained smear of sputum containing adequate numbers of macrophages is significant evidence against a bacterial infectious process in the lower respiratory tract, assuming the patient has normal neutrophil function. The presence of more than an occasional eosinophil is suggestive of allergic disease. Iron stains may reveal hemosiderin granules within macrophages, suggesting the diagnosis of pulmonary hemosiderosis. Specimens should also be examined for bacterial flora with a Gram stain. Squamous epithelial cells are usually covered with bacteria, which should be ignored. Bacteria within or near macrophages and neutrophils are more significant in the evaluation of inflammatory processes in the lungs. Viral pneumonia may be accompanied by intranuclear or cytoplasmic inclusion bodies, which may be seen on Wright-stained smears, and fungal forms may be identified on Gram stains.

SWEAT TESTING

See Sec 12.110.

12.18 BLOOD GAS ANALYSIS

An arterial blood gas analysis is probably the single most useful test of pulmonary function as arterial levels of oxygen and carbon dioxide reflect the result of ventilation, perfusion, and gas exchange, and the test may be performed on patients of any age, with or without their cooperation. Preferably, specimens of arterial blood are obtained from the umbilical, radial, brachial, or temporal arteries, although other vessels are sometimes used. If multiple samples are to be drawn over a relatively short time, an indwelling arterial line may be placed; constant perfusion of the arterial line with heparinized saline (1 unit/ml, 3–5 ml/hr) may prevent thrombus formation.

Arterial punctures are painful and often result in hyperventilation. Use of local anesthesia can result in more patient comfort and more accurate data. The artery should be entered with a 21 or 23 gauge straight or scalp vein needle at an angle of approximately 45°. The arterial blood specimen is best collected in a heparinized glass syringe. Only enough heparin solution should be used to displace the air from the syringe, and no air should be permitted to enter the syringe during collection. The syringe should be sealed, placed in ice, and carried to the laboratory for immediate analysis.

Arterialized capillary blood may be used if tissue perfusion is good and great care is taken in the collection and handling of the specimen. Under ideal conditions there is good correlation between arterialized capillary and arterial samples. Local vasodilation is produced in the finger, heel, or ear lobe by warming or by application of nitroglycerin or nicotinic acid cream. When the site has become flushed, blood is collected into a capillary tube from a free-flowing stab wound.

Noninvasive techniques may also be employed for estimation of arterial blood gas values. An ear oximeter can give a continual measure of peripheral oxygen saturation and generally correlates well with simultaneous arterial saturation. Direct-reading transcutaneous oxygen electrodes can provide continuous monitoring of oxygen and carbon dioxide tension. Both these techniques are dependent upon tissue perfusion as well as the partial pressure of the gases in arterial blood. End-tidal pCO_2 may be monitored and usually correlates well with arterial pCO_2 unless there is a very uneven distribution of ventilation.

Venous blood may be used for determination of pH and pCO_2, and samples should be drawn without venous stasis. Venous pCO_2 averages 6–8 mm Hg higher than arterial pCO_2, and pH is slightly lower. Such samples are more useful in management of acid-base disturbances than acute respiratory disease.

12.19 PULMONARY FUNCTION TESTING

See also Sec 12.8.

Ventilation, perfusion, and gas exchange may all be quantified, but in clinical practice measurements of ventilation are the most commonly performed "pulmonary function test."

Measurement of Ventilatory Function

Volume displacement *spirometers* record changes in the volume of gas the subject breathes into and out of a closed container. Electronic spirometers integrate flow through a pneumotachometer to determine volume. A spirometer is used to measure vital capacity and its subdivisions and expiratory (or inspiratory) flow rates (Fig 12–3 and 12–4). Peak flow rates are measured with either an electronic spirometer or a special peak flow meter. A body *plethysmograph* is used to measure functional residual capacity (FRC), from which are calculated (with spirometric data) the total lung capacity (TLC) and residual volume (RV). The pressure plethysmograph is an airtight box in which the subject sits; pressure changes in the box and at the mouth are measured during respiratory efforts against a closed shutter in a mouthpiece. The technique is simple for the patient, rapid, and accurate. *Gas dilution tests* can also measure FRC by allowing the subject to breathe to equilibrium into a closed volume which initially contained a known concentration of marker gas (usually helium). The equilibrium volume (box + lungs) is calculated from the initial concentration, box volume, and the final concentration. This method is less useful in children than the plethysmograph because of the long times required to reach equilibrium. A simple *manometer* may be used to measure the maximal inspiratory and expiratory force a subject can generate, which is normally at least 30 cm H_2O. This is useful in the evaluation of the neuromuscular component of ventilation.

Lung volumes usually measured include vital capacity (VC), FRC, TLC, and RV. The last 3 require gas dilution or a plethysmograph. Expected normal values are obtained from prediction equations based on body height.

Flow rates measured by spirometry usually include the volume expired in the 1st sec (FEV$_1$) and the maximal midexpiratory flow rate (MMEF). More information results from a maximal expiratory flow-volume curve (MEFV), in which expiratory flow rate is plotted against expired lung volume (expressed in terms of either VC or TLC). Flow rates at lung volumes less than about 75% VC are relatively independent of effort. Expiratory flow rates at low lung volumes (less than 50% VC) are influenced much more by small airways than flow rates at high lung volumes (FEV$_1$). The flow rate at 25% VC (V_{25}) is a useful index of small airway function. Low flow rates at high lung volumes associated with normal flow at low lung volumes are indicative of upper airway obstruction.

Airway resistance (R_{AW}) is measured in a plethysmograph and is expressed as cm H_2O/l/sec. Alternatively, the reciprocal of R_{AW}, *airway conductance* (G_{AW}), may be used. Because airway resistance measurements vary with the lung volume at which they are taken, it is convenient to use specific airway resistance, SR_{AW} (SR_{AW} = R_{AW} × lung volume), which is nearly constant in subjects older than 6 yr (normally less than 7 sec/cm H_2O).

Measurement of Gas Exchange

The *diffusing capacity for carbon monoxide* (D_LCO) is measured by rebreathing from a container with a known initial concentration of CO or by a single breath technique. Decreases in D_LCO reflect decreases in effective alveolar capillary surface area or decreases in diffusibility of the gas across the alveolar-capillary membrane.

This test is rarely used in pediatric practice as primary diffusion abnormalities are unusual in children. Estimation of *regional gas exchange* may be conveniently performed with the perfusion/ventilation xenon scan (Sec 12.11). An *arterial blood gas* determination will also give a measure of the effectiveness of alveolar gas exchange.

Measurement of Perfusion

Pulmonary blood flow may be measured by cardiac catheterization or by a technique employing the uptake of nitrous oxide. The distribution of blood flow may be studied in a pulmonary arteriogram or with radioisotope scans.

Other Tests of Lung Function

Other available tests include measurements of compliance, distribution of ventilation, dead space, elastic recoil, closing volume, and others. Pulmonary function tests performed before and after exercise may be useful in detection of exercise-induced bronchospasm. Sufficient exercise should be performed to elevate the pulse to 160–170/min for 5–6 min. Testing should be done 10 min after the end of the exercise period. There is poor correlation between the results of objective exercise testing and subjective evaluation of exercise tolerance by patient or parent.

Clinical Use of Pulmonary Function Testing

Pulmonary function testing rarely results in an etiologic diagnosis but is helpful in defining the type of process (e.g., obstruction, restriction) and the degree of functional impairment, in following the course of disease and its treatment, and in estimating prognosis. It is also useful in preoperative evaluation and to confirm the presence of functional impairment in patients with subjective complaints in whom physical examination is normal. In most patients with obstructive disease a repeat test following the administration of a bronchodilator is warranted.

Most tests require some degree of cooperation and understanding on the part of the subject. Their interpretation is greatly facilitated if the test conditions and behavior of the subject during the test are known. Accurate testing of children aged 3–6 yr requires great patience and training of the subject, while most children aged 6 yr or older can be tested reliably without excessive difficulty. Infants and young children may be studied by gas dilution and plethysmographic methods for measurement of FRC and R_{AW} but may require sedation for the procedure.

ROBERT E. WOOD

Caffey J: Pediatric X-ray Diagnosis. Ed 6. Chicago, Year Book Medical Publishers, 1972.

Comroe JH, Forster RE, Dubois AB, et al: The Lung, Clinical Physiology and Pulmonary Function Tests. Ed 2. Chicago, Year Book Medical Publishers, 1962.
Hochschild TJ, Cremin BJ: Technique in infant chest radiography. Radiography 41:21, 1975.
Hughes WT: Pediatric Procedures. Philadelphia, WB Saunders, 1964.
Kendig EL, Chernick V: Disorders of the Respiratory Tract in Children. Ed 3. Philadelphia, WB Saunders, 1977.

Klein JO: Diagnostic lung puncture in the pneumonias of infants and children. Pediatrics 44:456, 1969.
Mustard WI, Ravitch MM, Snyder WH, et al: Pediatric Surgery. Ed 2. Chicago, Year Book Medical Publishers, 1969.
Sackner MA: Bronchofiberoscopy. Am Rev Resp Dis 111:62, 1975.
Tuft L, Mueller HL: Allergy in Children. Philadelphia, WB Saunders, 1970.
Wood RE, Sherman JM: Pediatric flexible bronchoscopy. Ann Otol Rhinol Laryngol 89:414, 1980.

12.20   SPECIAL TREATMENT IN PEDIATRIC PULMONARY DISEASE

Treatment of specific infections should be given priority in most pediatric pulmonary diseases. Such treatment is usually more effective when combined with measures known to assist the impaired normal defense mechanisms that are the cause or result of infection.

HUMIDIFICATION OF INSPIRED AIR

Many pediatric pulmonary diseases seriously impair the normal humidification of inspired air. This occurs whenever the nose is bypassed with a tracheostomy or is obstructed by lesions such as viral or bacterial upper respiratory tract infections, allergic rhinitis, or choanal atresia. The failure of the nose to humidify inspired air results in bronchorrhea and an impairment of mucociliary clearance (slowing of ciliary beat and/or increased viscosity of the dehydrated mucus secretions).

Nebulization therapy (mist therapy) can provide humidification of inspired air and add water to pulmonary secretions. Complete humidification of inspired air at 37° C requires 44 mg of H_2O/l of air, 25% of which is usually provided in the trachea and large bronchi. For upper airway disease the mist particles should be 6–10 μm in diameter to ensure their deposition in the diseased area. For tracheostomized patients or patients with peripheral airway disease, an ultrasonic nebulizer should be used to produce a small particle size (1–0.5 μm) in a dense mist in the air flow over the tracheostomy, in a tent (cooled), or in a large bore tube connected to a mask or, preferably, a mouthpiece. Some patients with hypersensitive bronchi and peripheral airway obstruction due to asthma or cystic fibrosis do not tolerate nebulization therapy.

Although the beneficial effects of humidification are unproved, it is generally accepted that nebulization is helpful in the treatment of croup, laryngotracheobronchitis, and tracheostomized patients. For patients with asthma, bronchitis, and cystic fibrosis, variable, often adverse, effects have been observed. If used, such therapy should be evaluated and humidification provided only when it is beneficial. Whenever a nebulizer is used to provide humidification, it must be cleaned and sterilized frequently and only sterile solutions, to which the patient does not have an adverse reaction, nebulized. Simple humidification of inspired air is beneficial during administration of oxygen or other compressed gases and for treating patients who have been intubated or tracheostomized or who are suffering from post-thermal respiratory injury. Warming and humidifying inspired air also may prevent exercise-induced asthma.

INTERMITTENT AEROSOL THERAPY

The chief purpose of this form of nebulization therapy is to deposit medications directly on the mucosa of the bronchial tree. Because most of these medications are potent, they are nebulized either in small quantities of water, usually 2 ml, or as a dry powder. Such therapy may be administered every 3–4 hr.

To decrease mucosal edema and promote the removal of secretions in patients with bronchitis, a solution of 9 parts of 0.125% *phenylephrine hydrochloride* plus 1 part USP *propylene glycol* may be used as an aerosol before segmental postural drainage (Sec 12.110).

Racemic epinephrine (vaponephrine solution, 2.25% epinephrine base diluted 1:8 with water) administered as an aerosol is effective for the treatment of laryngotracheobronchitis (Sec 12.54), but, though beneficial effects are seen immediately after inhalation, recurring symptoms frequently necessitate repeated inhalations every 2–4 hr. This type of therapy should be limited to a closely monitored hospital setting and is contraindicated in children with epiglottitis.

Intermittent therapy with *sympathomimetic* or *beta-agonist* aerosol agents may be used for the treatment of bronchospasm. Epinephrine, isoproterenol, isoetharine, terbutaline, metaproterenol, fenoterol, and salbutamol are all capable of improving pulmonary mechanics by dilating airway smooth muscle and facilitating mucociliary transport. Epinephrine stimulates alpha and both beta-adrenergic receptors and isoproterenol stimulates both beta-adrenergic receptors; only isoetharine and metaproterenol are specifically $beta_2$-adrenergic agents. To relieve bronchospasm, 1% isoetharine (0.1–0.5 ml of Bronkosol in 1.5 ml of sterile distilled water or 0.5 normal saline) can be administered by aerosol every 3–4 hr. Because it acts specifically on the $beta_2$ receptors, it produces a significantly longer bronchodilator effect than does isoproterenol, with fewer cardiovascular side effects (Sec 9.45).

The side effects only occasionally observed with inhaled $beta_2$ agents are tremor and excitation. Tolerance, arrhythmias, and mortality have not been reported in children. The administration of such agents by metered aerosols is appropriate in older children, but for those too young to coordinate inhalation with activation of the metered aerosol unit, solutions of the $beta_2$ agonists should be nebulized over a period of several min using a mask or preferably a mouthpiece that depresses the tongue and enhances deposition in more peripheral airways. In patients with cystic fibrosis intermittent inhalation of a beta$_2$ agonist may be effective both because of its bronchodilating effect on those with bronchial hyperactivity and its speeding up of mucociliary clearance velocity. In all cases the patient's pulmonary function response to the aerosols should be determined before their repeated use is initiated.

Anticholinergic drugs may be effective bronchodilators when given by aerosol. The bronchodilating effects of SCH1000 (ipratropium bromide) is seen within 15–30 min and lasts for 4 hr (0.02–0.04 mg administered by 1–2 inhalations of a metered aerosol). Several investigators have reported it to be more effective in patients with bronchitis than the sympathomimetics. Because of its relatively slow onset of action and the availability of more effective agents, it should not be used during an acute asthma attack.

Many aerosolized *mucolytic agents* have been used in an attempt to treat effectively the obstructive lesion of cystic fibrosis. N-acetylcysteine decreases mucus viscosity in vitro but in vivo can act as a mucosal irritant causing bronchial constriction and deterioration of pulmonary function. Its routine long term use should be discouraged. Other mucolytic agents such as pancreatic dornase, urea, and L-arginine appear to be ineffective. *Aerosolized corticosteroids* and *cromolyn sodium* are valuable in the treatment of both steroid and nonsteroid dependent children with asthma (Sec 9.45). Although there is no evidence available to support *antibiotic aerosol therapy,* some pediatric pulmonary specialists feel it may be useful to supplement parenteral antibiotic therapy in selected cases.

OXYGEN THERAPY

Because both inadequate ventilation and ventilation-perfusion imbalances result in hypoxemia early in most pediatric pulmonary diseases, oxygen therapy is frequently indicated. In rare patients with hypercapnia, if a low PaO$_2$ is the primary stimulus for respiration, oxygen administration, by removing this stimulus, may depress ventilation and result in further elevation of the PaCO$_2$. In such situations administration of supplemental oxygen must be carefully monitored and controlled.

In all cases in which supplemental oxygen is prescribed, its potential toxicity must be considered. Experiments show that early effects of oxygen toxicity include decreases in mucociliary function and mucus secretion and destruction of type I alveolar epithelial cells with replacement by proliferating type II granular pneumocytes. In premature infants fibroblasts proliferate around alveolar ducts, squamous metaplasia occurs in the bronchial lining, and a necrotizing bronchiolitis may develop (Sec 7.30). The earliest pulmonary function alteration in older children is a reduction in vital capacity associated with the morphologic findings of tracheobronchitis, alveolitis, and alveolar hemorrhage. The patient complains of substernal pain and paresthesias.

In general, oxygen should always be prescribed with a specific dose response in mind and with appropriate monitoring of blood gases aimed at obtaining a specific inspiratory oxygen concentration (FiO$_2$). It is also important that a method be used that will provide the prescribed oxygen concentration without causing discomfort or harm to the patient. In infants this requires use of an incubator, hood, oxygen tent, or nasal prongs. In older patients a nasal cannula, catheter or prongs, a tracheostomy mask, or an oxygen tent can be used. Venturi masks are very helpful in providing predictable oxygen concentrations of from 24–50% for older children. Care also must be taken to select oxygen administration equipment of the proper size and design for use in children. In neonates specifically designed Silastic nasal prongs that extend only 1 cm into the nares facilitate the tongue's serving as a physiologic blow-off valve via the unrestricted mouth. This arrangement permits the use of nasal continuous positive airway pressure (CPAP) with less danger of pneumothorax or interstitial emphysema. The older child in need of oxygen may have associated upper respiratory disease that results in mouthbreathing and greatly decreases the effectiveness of oxygen administration via a nasal cannula or catheter. Abdominal distention or even intestinal rupture may result from the use of a nasal catheter in a child with epiglottitis or an impaired epiglottal reflex. Because comatose infants and children vomit frequently, they should be given oxygen by a method that will not impede the outflow of vomitus.

Pulmonary atelectasis is another hazard of oxygen therapy. Nitrogen is washed out of the lungs by oxygen breathing, and the oxygen trapped behind an obstructed airway is then rapidly absorbed by perfusing blood; atelectasis of the involved segment follows.

Another form of oxygen therapy for the ambulatory treatment of conditions that produce chronic hypoxemia is low flow O$_2$ via a nasal cannula or Venturi mask. The latter is recommended because it delivers a known concentration of oxygen. Such therapy via nasal prongs can be effective if the flow rates are varied to meet O$_2$ needs for rest and exercise.

AIRWAY MAINTENANCE

In the treatment of all types of pediatric pulmonary disease, the maintenance or establishment of an adequate airway is vital. When an endotracheal or tracheostomy tube is indicated, the proper size and length should be used (Table 12–2) and the position of the tube in the airway confirmed by roentgenogram. Though cuffed tubes are usually too large for use in children under 3 yr of age, they can be used in older patients.

MECHANICAL VENTILATION

Successful mechanical ventilation depends upon experienced personnel and close clinical and laboratory monitoring. Most ventilators available for infants and children generate positive pressure and are controlled

Table 12-2 DATA FOR DETERMINATION OF INSIDE DIAMETER AND LENGTH OF PEDIATRIC ENDOTRACHEAL TUBES

Age	French Size	Internal Diameter	Oral Length	Nasal Length (cm)	15 mm Adapter (mm Internal Diameter)
Premature	14–16	3.0–3.5	8	11	3
Newborn–14 days	16	3.5	8.5	13	4
2–24 wk	16–18	3.5–4.0	10	15	4
6–12 mo	18–20	4.0–4.5	12	16	4–5
12–18 mo	20–22	4.5–5.0	13	16	5
18–24 mo	22–24	5.0–5.5	14	17	5–6
2–4 yr	24–26	5.5–6.0	15	18	6
4–7 yr	26–28	6.0–6.5	16	19	6–7
7–10 yr	28–30	6.5–7.0	17	21	7
10–12 yr	30–32	7.0–7.5	20	23–25	7–8

by (1) volume delivered or (2) pressure generated. The former determine the pattern of flow into the lungs, the volume delivered and the pressure required to deliver it being determined by the compliance of the lungs. Pressure-controlled generators regulate the pressure pattern; the resultant flow and volume patterns depend on the characteristics of the lungs. Ventilators also differ in their controlling cycles and may be time, pressure, volume, or flow cycled, or use a combination of these modes. A machine that can be used for both controlled and assisted ventilation is advisable.

For children under 3 yr of age a ventilator with a variable inspiratory flow rate (50–200 ml/sec) that is volume or time cycled and pressure limited, such as the Bourns pediatric unit, is preferred. For older patients the machine should have a variable flow rate of from 10–100 l/min, a maximum pressure of 80 cm of water, a cycling rate that can be adjusted from 6–100 breaths/min, and tidal volumes that can be varied from 10–200 ml/breath, such as the Bennett MA-1. The inspiratory/expiratory (I/E) ratio and the flow pattern are more physiologic in these machines because they are determined by the variable flow rate.

SEGMENTAL POSTURAL DRAINAGE

Bronchial or postural drainage and breathing exercises may be indicated when clinical examination reveals excessive fluid in the bronchi. Both are physical means for assisting the normal clearance mechanisms. Segmental postural drainage consists of carefully positioning the patient to use gravitational forces to facilitate airway secretion drainage. Twelve positions can be used to drain the major bronchi, and these are generally combined with chest cupping (1–2 min) and vibration of the treated segment for 5 exhalations. Combined with cough instruction and breathing exercises, such therapy is generally accepted, though not yet proved, as an effective way of facilitating the drainage of secretions from the bronchial trees of patients with cystic fibrosis, bronchitis, asthma, bronchiectasis, and impaired coughs as a result of muscle weakness or postoperative pain or endotracheal intubation. Preferably, such therapy should be performed after intermittent aerosol treatment. The technique can be taught to parents, and older patients can effectively treat themselves using positioning, a mechanical percussor, and effective coughing. Some forms of acute atelectasis in young infants that have been resistant to intermittent positive pressure breathing (IPPB) may respond to chest percussion and vibration. Because endotracheal tubes interfere with normal cough mechanisms, intubated patients are frequently suctioned with a sterile catheter after such physical therapy; the volumes of secretion aspirated are significantly increased by chest percussion and vibration.

PHYSICAL ACTIVITY

Physical activity vigorous enough to result in deep breathing often results in significant expectoration. In children with chronic pulmonary disease a regular exercise program may not only help with clearance of mucus secretions but also maintain thoracic muscle mass and ventilatory ability.

LeRoy W. Matthews

Boat TF, Kleinerman JI, Fanaroff AA: Toxic effects of oxygen on cultured human neonatal respiratory epithelium. Pediatr Res 7:607, 1973.

Block AJ: Low flow oxygen therapy. Am Rev Resp Dis 110:71, 1974.

Caldwell PRB, Weibel ER: Pulmonary oxygen toxicity. In: Fishman AP (ed): Pulmonary Diseases and Disorders. New York, McGraw-Hill, 1980, Ch 67.

Chen WY, Horton DJ: Heat and water loss from the airways and exercise-induced asthma. Respiration 34:305, 1977.

Chernick V, Avery ME: Hazards of high oxygen mixtures. In: Kendig EL (ed): Pulmonary Disorders, Vol I. Philadelphia, WB Saunders, 1972.

Doershuk CF, Matthews LW, et al: Evaluation of jet-type and ultrasonic nebulizers in mist tent therapy for cystic fibrosis. Pediatrics 41:723, 1968.

Doershuk CF, Stern RC: Cystic fibrosis, pulmonary therapy. In: Gillis SS, Kagan BM (eds): Current Pediatric Therapy. Philadelphia, WB Saunders, 1980, p 218.

Lough MD, Doershuk CF: Respiratory therapy. In: Lough MD, Doershuk CF, Stern RC (eds): Pediatric Respiratory Therapy. Chicago, Year Book Medical Publishers, 1979.

Lough MD, Schuchardt B: Mechanical ventilation. In Lough MD, Doershuk CF, Stern RC (eds): Pediatric Respiratory Therapy. Chicago, Year Book Medical Publishers, 1979.

Leifer KN, Wittig HJ: Beta-2 sympathomimetic aerosols in the treatment of asthma. Ann Allergy 35:69, 1975.

Matthews LW, Dearborn DG, Tucker AS: Cystic fibrosis. In: Fishman AP (ed): Pulmonary Diseases and Disorders. New York, McGraw-Hill, 1980, Ch 50.

McFadden ER Jr: Aerosolized bronchodilators and steroids in the treatment of airway obstruction in adults. Am Rev Resp Dis 122:89, 1980.

Tabachnik E, Levison H: Clinical application of aerosols in pediatrics. Am Rev Resp Dis 122:97, 1980.

12.21   DISEASES OF THE RESPIRATORY SYSTEM

GENERAL CONSIDERATIONS

The patterns of respiratory tract disease in childhood relate to several modifying factors: age, sex, seasonal variation, geography, socioeconomic conditions, and race. Intrauterine acquisition of viral infections, such as cytomegalovirus, may result in neonatal pneumonia; cytomegalovirus, ureaplasma, or *Chlamydia trachomatis* respiratory infection may be acquired during descent through the birth canal; and immediately after birth tuberculosis can be transmitted to the newborn and present after several wk of life as a severe pneumonitis. Lung immaturity and certain events related to the perinatal period predispose to hyaline membrane disease. Beyond the newborn period a lack of specifically directed antibodies against common viral pathogens results in an increased incidence of respiratory tract infections; this peaks at 1 yr of age. Pneumococcal lobar pneumonia is uncommon in small children, and pneumonia due to mycoplasma infection is uncommon during the 1st 3–4 yr of life. Another peak in the incidence of respiratory tract infection occurs during the 1st 2–3 school years because of increased exposure to respiratory infections against which children have not yet developed specific immunity.

The anatomic distribution of respiratory tract disease may also change with age. Group A β-hemolytic streptococcal infections are commonly located in the nasopharynx in young children but in the tonsillar and lower pharyngeal areas of older children. A relatively short and open eustachian tube in infants and young children allows easy access of pharyngeal organisms to the middle ear cavity and is in part responsible for the higher incidence of otitis media in this group. The small size of bronchial and bronchiolar lumina in the 1st 2 yr of life is an important determinant in the incidence of bronchiolitis from respiratory syncytial and other virus infections in children. Aspiration during the 1st yr of life most often causes lung changes in the upper lobes because during the feeding and postfeeding periods the infant is often recumbent; thereafter most aspirations take place when children are upright, and the lung changes occur more often in the right lower lobe.

There is little variation in the incidence or severity of respiratory tract disease on the basis of *sex*. Lower respiratory tract infections are slightly more common in boys than in girls under 6 yr of age; thereafter the infection rates are equal. Noninfectious pulmonary diseases of childhood usually have an equal sex incidence, with the exception of several rare sex-linked recessive disorders such as chronic granulomatous disease and a form of severe combined immunodeficiency.

Seasonal variations in the incidence of respiratory tract infections and bronchial asthma are clinically important. The most common respiratory tract viral pathogens appear in epidemics during the winter and spring months. However, mycoplasma infections occur more commonly in autumn and early winter. With asthma, pollen-related symptoms occur more often in the spring, summer, and early fall; symptoms due to house dust and molds may be more common when children are confined to the house during the cold weather months. Infection-related asthma also occurs more frequently during the cold weather months.

Certain fungal respiratory tract infections, such as coccidioidomycosis and histoplasmosis, have well-defined *geographical distributions* in the United States, but the incidence of common viral, mycoplasmal, and bacterial respiratory tract infections varies little with geographic location. In addition, areas with high levels of air pollution predispose to frequent respiratory tract infections and episodes of asthma, and at high altitudes hypoxemia and cor pulmonale may play an earlier or more prominent role in the natural history of chronic lung disease, as in cystic fibrosis.

Although frequency is not different, the severity of lower respiratory tract illness is generally less in middle class than in lower class families. This may reflect the difference in availability of medical care for these groups.

Cystic fibrosis largely affects Caucasians, especially those of central and northern European extraction; the incidence in Blacks in the United States is approximately 10% of that in Whites, and it is even less in oriental populations. Lung infections and infarctions attending sickle cell disease are almost exclusively seen in black populations.

THOMAS F. BOAT
CARL F. DOERSHUK
ROBERT C. STERN

Ferguson CF, Kendig EL (eds): Disorders of the Respiratory Tract in Children. Vol II, Pediatric Otolaryngology. Philadelphia, WB Saunders, 1972.
Glezen WP, Denny FW: Epidemiology of acute lower respiratory disease in children. N Engl J Med 288:498, 1973.
Kendig EL (ed): Disorders of the Respiratory Tract in Children. Vol I, Pulmonary Disorders in Children. Philadelphia, WB Saunders, 1972.
Miller ME: Natural defense mechanisms: Development and characterization of imnate immunity. In: Stiehm RE, Fulginiti VA (eds): Immunologic Disorders in Infants and Children. Philadelphia, WB Saunders, 1973.
Wood RE, Boat TF, Doershuk CF: Cystic fibrosis: State of the art. Am Rev Resp Dis 113:833, 1976.

12.22   ACUTE RESPIRATORY FAILURE

Acute respiratory failure may be defined as the development of hypercapnia during an acute illness.

Etiology.   Frequently, acute respiratory failure occurs in patients who are known to have mild to moderately severe chronic pulmonary disease with normal arterial carbon dioxide tension. During an intercurrent acute illness (e.g., influenza), such a patient may deteriorate rapidly and develop hypercapnia. Previously well children also may develop acute respiratory failure as a result of pneumonia, epiglottitis or other cause of upper airway obstruction, status asthmaticus, aspiration (including near-drowning), and certain poisonings. Patients with cystic fibrosis or severe scoliosis often develop acute respiratory failure following surgery. Acute central nervous system disease may cause respiratory failure by interfering with the central control of breathing. Severe muscle disease and thoracic abnormalities may result in respiratory failure because of inadequate alveolar ventilation. Occasionally, congenital heart lesions with large right-to-left shunts cause respiratory failure when pulmonary perfusion is too low to allow adequate excretion of carbon dioxide.

Clinical Manifestations. The patient is hyperpneic and cyanotic. Patients with airway disease will show obvious use of the accessory muscles of respiration; most will sit up and lean forward to provide the best possible leverage for the accessory muscles and to allow easy diaphragmatic movement. Symptoms and signs of the underlying disease are also present. Hypercapnia may cause central depression with impaired consciousness and confusion. A $PaCO_2$ of over 40 mm Hg should suggest the possibility of developing acute respiratory failure, and a $PaCO_2$ of 50 mm Hg or higher should suggest its imminence. Most patients with acute hypercapnia also will have a PaO_2 below 55 mm Hg in room air, suggesting that the oxygen content of the blood may be inadequate to meet the normal oxygen needs of the vital organs.

Acute hypoxemia and hypercapnia result in dilatation of the cerebral blood vessels and increased blood flow, often accompanied by severe headache. The sudden increased work of the accessory muscles of breathing may result in severe lower back pain. Although moderate to severe hypercapnia can cause peripheral vasodilatation, mild to moderate hypoxemia can cause peripheral vasoconstriction and the patient may complain of cold extremities. Other symptoms of hypoxia include restlessness, dizziness, and impaired thought.

Treatment. Patients with early respiratory failure should receive maximum therapy aimed at relieving the underlying disease. If these measures fail to reduce arterial carbon dioxide, mechanical ventilation with control of the airway is needed. If the patient is apneic or gasping, 100% oxygen is administered by bag and mask, followed immediately by endotracheal intubation. When there is less urgency and reason to believe that several days of mechanical assistance will be required, nasotracheal intubation is preferable. Immediately following intubation, auscultation of the chest is important to ensure that the tube is not obstructing one of the main stem bronchi and that there is adequate air exchange. A chest roentgenogram should be obtained to confirm proper tube placement. Patients with upper airway obstruction may not require any treatment other than intubation. For the vast majority of intubated children, continuous positive airway pressure (CPAP) is useful to prevent alveolar collapse.

The goal of therapy is to achieve adequate oxygen saturation and normal arterial carbon dioxide tension using the least pressure and lowest possible concentration of inspired oxygen (FiO_2). Once artificial ventilation is undertaken, the patient must be monitored closely, both clinically and by arterial blood gas determinations, to ensure that ventilation is adequate. An indwelling arterial catheter is very helpful. Maintaining adequate tissue oxygenation is of paramount importance since devastating effects of transient severe hypoxemia may persist after restoration of pulmonary function; this usually requires maintaining a PaO_2 of at least 45–50 mm Hg and, preferably, 50–55 mm Hg. On the other hand, as the patient improves, the inspired oxygen concentration should be decreased as rapidly as possible to reduce the risks of oxygen toxicity. The risk of direct oxygen toxicity to the airways is markedly increased at FiO_2 levels between 70–100%.

Bedside measurements of tidal volume, vital capacity, and negative inspiratory force are very helpful in predicting when the patient has a good chance of successful extubation. Ventilator assistance is then terminated and the patient extubated. Management of children with acute respiratory failure is best undertaken in a pediatric intensive care unit.

Prognosis. Survival should be expected in previously normal children who develop respiratory failure with an acute illness. When acute respiratory failure is superimposed upon underlying chronic illness, the prognosis is related to the nature of the chronic illness and the severity and duration of the acute process. Many of these patients can regain their previous status.

Burke RH, George RB: Acute respiratory failure in chronic obstructive pulmonary disease. Arch Intern Med 132:865, 1973.
Downes JJ, Fulgencio T, Raphaely RC: Acute respiratory failure in infants and children. Pediatr Clin North Am 19:423, 1972.
Kumar A, Falke KJ, Geffin B, et al: Continuous positive pressure ventilation in acute respiratory failure. Effects on hemodynamics and lung function. N Engl J Med 283:1430, 1970.
Nicodemus HF: Respiratory failure and airway management in congenital cardiovascular diseases. Clin Pediatr 12:259, 1964.
Pontoppidan H, Geffin B, Lowenstein E: Acute respiratory failure in the adult. N Engl J Med 287:690, 743, 799, 1972.
Rogers RM, Juers JA: Physiologic considerations in the treatment of acute respiratory failure. Basics of RD 3 (No 4):1, 1975.

12.23 IATROGENIC AND DRUG-INDUCED PULMONARY DISEASE

Any patient who has had mechanical manipulation of the airway, mechanical ventilation, or prolonged drug therapy and then develops chronic respiratory symptoms or recurrent respiratory infection may have an iatrogenic disease. Prolonged use of high oxygen concentrations and pressure ventilators can cause bronchopulmonary dysplasia (Sec 7.34). Overtransfusion or excessive doses of plasma expanders may cause pulmonary edema. Anesthetic gases may have direct pulmonary toxicity, and atelectasis may occur as a result of both anesthetic agents and decreased deep breathing and coughing secondary to postoperative pain. Prolonged intubation has resulted in tracheal granulomas and other sequelae.

Cancer Therapy

Complex treatment programs based on multiple drug protocols combined with radiation therapy are used frequently in the common childhood malignancies. The increased survival time, together with the increasing total dose of many chemotherapeutic agents and radiation, has been associated with a variety of pulmonary complications (Chapter 15).

Radiation injury in children probably is mediated primarily by 2 pathophysiologic mechanisms: First, the radiation may stimulate inflammation, in part because of cellular debris in the airways, which ultimately leads to progressive fibrosis. Second, in children radiation has a profound long term retarding effect on the growth of pulmonary parenchyma. Occasionally, scoliosis occurs as a result of radiation, and this further compromises pulmonary status. Radiation-induced reduction in chest wall growth also may secondarily limit growth of the lung. Since children rarely receive extensive thoracic radiation without chemotherapy, the effects of each may be difficult to distinguish.

Oncologic chemotherapeutic drugs may cause progressive pulmonary disease and limit lung size even when used without radiation therapy. Pulmonary complications have occurred following administration of bleomycin, cyclophosphamide, busulfan, methotrexate, carmustine (BCNU), and procarbazine. Vincristine, 6-mercaptopurine, and 5-fluorouracil have not been reported to cause pulmonary injury in patients who did not receive other drugs with known pulmonary toxicity. The symptoms usually begin after a substantial duration of therapy and even after the drug has been discontinued. There appears to be a total dose-risk relationship for bleomycin and busulfan but not for methotrexate. Early symptoms include dry cough, dyspnea, and, occasionally, fever. Physical findings include cyanosis, tachypnea, and rales. Pulmonary function testing reveals decreased diffusing capacity for carbon monoxide, evidence of restriction, and hypoxemia. Chest roentgenograms show linear interstitial densities in most cases, but a fine nodular pattern or an alveolar filling process has also been reported. Lung tissue shows fibrosis, interstitial infiltrates, and abnormal alveolar epithelial cells. In the case of busulfan, bizarre type II pneumocytes are a common finding. Excessive use of oxygen appears to predispose the patient to and aggravate bleomycin toxicity. It may be possible to predict the risk of pulmonary toxicity with carmustine (BCNU). These drugs also may predispose the patient to developing a new pulmonary malignancy.

Diagnosis. The principal diagnostic dilemma is to differentiate chemotherapy-induced pulmonary disease from a pneumonia or *Pneumocystis carinii* infestation and, more rarely, from diffuse tumor infiltration. Bronchoscopy and lung biopsy may be needed for definitive diagnosis.

Treatment and Course. The natural history of the pulmonary lesion is not known. In critically ill patients treatment with antibiotics and trimethoprim-sulfamethoxazole may be justified on an empirical basis even when lung injury from chemotherapy is strongly suspected. Patients recover occasionally even if the suspected drug is continued. On the other hand, some patients have progressed to death from respiratory failure even though chemotherapy was promptly discontinued with the advent of pulmonary symptoms. Adrenal corticosteroids have been used with varying success. Supportive treatment with oxygen and mechanical ventilation may be necessary.

Other Drug-Induced Pulmonary Disease

Nitrofurantoin can cause an acute or chronic pulmonary complication. The more common acute reaction is characterized by fever, dyspnea, cough, and, occasionally, chest pain and cyanosis. Eosinophilia may occur transiently. Histologic findings include eosinophilia, proteinaceous edema in the air spaces, and perivasculitis. Chronic pulmonary fibrosis also occurs with prolonged nitrofurantoin treatment. Dyspnea on exertion and nonproductive cough are the most prominent symptoms. Pulmonary function testing reveals restriction and decreased carbon monoxide diffusing capacity, and the chest roentgenogram shows a diffuse interstitial pattern. Patients usually improve following discontinuation of nitrofurantoin treatment. Corticosteroids have been advocated, but there is little evidence for their effectiveness.

Gold therapy (*chrysotherapy*) of rheumatoid arthritis results in interstitial fibrosis with dyspnea and rales. The pulmonary symptoms may be ascribed to rheumatoid lung disease. Discontinuation of gold treatments is indicated, after which some amelioration of symptoms can be expected. The pathogenesis may involve a drug-induced defect in cell-mediated immunity.

Although chronic *alcohol abuse* may have its onset during adolescence, its pulmonary sequelae (airway obstruction, decreased diffusion capacity, and alteration of ventilation-perfusion adjustment secondary to cirrhosis) will not usually be seen until adult years. The acute pulmonary toxicity of alcohol includes depression of ciliary motion (at high ethanol levels) and of pulmonary macrophage function and interference with production of surfactant. Although these changes usually do not result in clinical pulmonary problems in otherwise healthy individuals, children with chronic pulmonary disease may be at increased risk from infection.

Aspirin intolerance may be associated with nasal polyps and asthma. Pulmonary fibrosis has been reported to result from chronic use of *penicillamine* and *methysergide*. The *aminoglycosides* and *polymyxin* group of antibiotics (including colistin) can cause neuromuscular blockade with paralysis of the diaphragm and other muscles of respiration. This is a rare but potentially fatal toxicity, particularly in patients with pre-existing severe pulmonary disease.

ROBERT C. STERN

Aronin PA, Mahaley MS Jr, Rudnick SA, et al: Prediction of BCNU pulmonary toxicity in patients with malignant gliomas. N Engl J Med 303:183, 1980.

Epler GR, Snider GL, Gaensler EA, et al: Bronchiolitis and bronchitis in connective tissue disease: A possible relationship to the use of penicillamine. JAMA 242:528, 1979.

Heinemann HO: Alcohol and the lung: A brief review. Am J Med 63:81, 1977.

Jacoby I: Drug-induced pulmonary disease: Confusion with infections of the lungs. Inf Dis Pract 1:1, 1978.

McCormick J, Cole S, Lahirir B, et al: Pneumonitis caused by gold salt therapy: Evidence for the role of cell-mediated immunity in its pathogenesis. Am Rev Resp Dis 122:145, 1980.

Rachelefsky GS, Coulson A, Siegel SC, et al: Aspiring intolerance in chronic childhood asthma: Detected by oral challenge. Pediatrics 56:443, 1975.

Samter M: Intolerance to aspirin. Hosp Pract 8:85, 1973.

Slauson DO, Hahn FF, Benjamin SA, et al: Inflammatory sequences in acute pulmonary radiation injury. Am J Pathol 82:549, 1976.

Sostman HD, Matthay RA, Putman CE: Cytotoxic drug-induced lung disease. Am J Med 62:608, 1977.

Weiss RB, Muggia FM: Cytotoxic drug-induced pulmonary disease: Update 1980. Am J Med 68:259, 1980.

Winterbauer RH, Wilske KR, Wheelis RF: Diffuse pulmonary injury associated with gold treatment. N Engl J Med 294:919, 1976.

Wohl MEB, Griscom NT, Traggis DG, et al: Effects of therapeutic irradiation delivered in early childhood upon subsequent lung function. Pediatrics 55:507, 1975.

12.24 Upper Respiratory Tract

The nose provides initial warming and humidification of inspired air. In the anterior nares turbulent air flow and coarse hairs enhance the deposition of large particulate matter; the remaining nasal airways filter out particles as small as 6 μm in diameter. In the turbinate region the air flow becomes laminar and the air stream is narrowed; thus particle deposition, warming, and humidification are enhanced. Nasal air flow contributes about 50% of the total resistance of breathing. The nasal mucosa is relatively more vascular, especially in the turbinate region, than that of the lower airways; however, the surface epithelium is similar, with ciliated cells, goblet cells, submucosal glands, and a covering blanket of mucus. Mucus flows toward the nasopharynx, where the air stream widens, the epithelium becomes squamous, and secretions are wiped away by swallowing; replacement of the mucous layers occurs about every 10 min. In addition to mucous glycoproteins, which provide viscoelastic properties, the nasal secretions contain lysozyme and secretory IgA, both of which have antimicrobial activity.

The *paranasal sinuses* develop as a group of air spaces in the bones of the face. They are lined with ciliated, mucus-secreting epithelium, and their ostia drain into the middle and superior meatuses of the nose. Development of the sinuses—maxillary, frontal, ethmoid, and sphenoid—occurs largely after birth, with the maxillary sinuses being earliest and the ethmoid sinuses being roentgenographically visible by 1–2 yr of age. The frontal sinuses usually begin their ascent into the frontal bone by the 2nd yr but, along with the sphenoid sinuses, are not readily visible roentgenographically until 5–6 yr of age or later. Growth of the sinuses, which may be unequal from side to side, continues through adolescence. Thickening of the epithelial lining and a diffuse haziness detected by roentgenogram suggest sinusitis, which can occur alone or in association with other conditions such as cystic fibrosis, Kartagener syndrome, or immunoglobulin deficiency.

The adenoids on the posterior nasopharyngeal wall and the tonsils at the base of the tongue are directly in line with the mucociliary flow and the air stream. These positions enhance their protective capabilities. The eustachian tubes, also lined with mucus-secreting, ciliated epithelium, enter the nasopharynx on the lateral walls.

12.25 CONGENITAL DISORDERS OF THE NOSE

Congenital structural nasal abnormalities are uncommon in contrast to acquired malformations. Occasionally, nasal bones are congenitally absent so that the bridge of the nose fails to develop; the result is nasal hypoplasia. Congenital absence of the nose, complete or partial duplication, or a single centrally placed nostril occasionally occurs but usually as a part of malformation syndromes incompatible with life. Rarely, supernumerary teeth may be found in the nose, or teeth may grow into it from the maxilla. If teeth are supernumerary, they may be absent from their normal site.

Hypertelorism is a common defect resulting from overdevelopment of the lesser wings of the sphenoid. The most prominent physical manifestation is widening of the base of the nose with the eyes widely separated.

On occasion, nasal bones are sufficiently malformed to produce severe narrowing of the nasal passages. Often such narrowing is associated with a high and narrow hard palate. Children with these defects may suffer from chronic or recurrent infections of the nasal and paranasal passages. Rarely, the alae nasi may be sufficiently thin and poorly supported to result in inspiratory obstruction.

Choanal atresia, the most common congenital anomaly of the nose, consists of a unilateral or bilateral bony or membranous septum between the nose and the pharynx. There is a strong familial tendency. Nearly 50% of infants with choanal atresia have other congenital anomalies. Since most, but not all, newborn infants are obligate nosebreathers, the obstruction does not produce the same symptoms in every infant. When only 1 side is affected, the infant usually does not have severe symptoms at birth and may be asymptomatic for a prolonged period, often until the 1st respiratory infection, when the diagnosis may be suggested by unilateral nasal discharge or disproportionately severe nasal obstruction.

Usually, infants with bilateral choanal atresia who are unable to mouthbreathe will make vigorous attempts to inspire with sucking in of their lips or become apneic immediately after birth and then develop cyanosis requiring resuscitation to avoid asphyxia; those who are able to mouthbreathe at once will experience difficulty when sucking and swallowing, becoming cyanotic when they attempt to nurse. Persistent mouthbreathing and cyanosis when the mouth is closed (which is relieved when the infant cries) are additional manifestations.

Diagnosis is established by inability to pass a firm catheter through each nostril 3–4 cm into the nasopharynx. Occasionally, it may be necessary to instill contrast material and obtain roentgenograms in the supine position to show the area of obstruction.

Treatment consists of promptly providing an oral airway or maintaining the mouth in an open position. Once an oral airway is established, the infant can be fed by gavage until breathing and eating without the assisted airway is learned, usually in 2–3 wk. Tracheostomy is rarely indicated. Subsequently, elective operative correction can be done weeks, months, or even years later in patients who adapt well to the obstruction. Some surgeons advise immediate surgical correction for bilateral choanal atresia. Operative correction of unilateral obstruction should be deferred until infection is controlled and the infant is in a satisfactory condition.

Congenital defects of the nasal septum, such as *perforation* or *deviation,* are rare. Perforation can be developmental or secondary to infection, such as syphilis or tuberculosis, and to trauma. Septal deviation can be congenital but more commonly results from trauma and may, in rare instances of obstruction, require surgical correction; it is best deferred until 14–15 yr of age to avoid external deformities of the nose. Abnormal formation of the nasal bones is infrequent unless other malformations are also present, such as cleft lip or palate. *Encephalocele* protruding through a defect in the cribriform plate into the nasal cavity is a rare anomaly that must be differentiated from polyps and tumors of extracranial origin. Poor development of the paranasal sinuses is associated with recurrent or chronic upper airway infection in Down syndrome.

12.26 ACQUIRED DISORDERS OF THE NOSE

Foreign Body

Foreign bodies, such as food, crayons, small toys, pieces of plastic, erasers, paper wads, beads, and stones, are frequently introduced into the nose by children. Initial symptoms are local obstruction, sneezing, relatively mild discomfort, and, rarely, pain. Irritation results in mucosal swelling, and, because some foreign bodies are hygroscopic and increase in size as water is absorbed, signs of local obstruction and discomfort may increase with time. Infection usually follows and gives rise to a purulent, malodorous, or bloody discharge. Tetanus is a rare complication in nonimmunized children. *Unilateral nasal discharge and obstruction should suggest the presence of a foreign body,* which can often be seen upon examination with a speculum or nasoscope. The object is usually situated anteriorly at first, but through unskilled attempts at removal it may be forced deeper into the nose. Removal should be carried out promptly to minimize the danger of aspiration and to prevent local tissue necrosis. In most children removal can be performed with topical anesthesia, using either forceps or nasal suction apparatus. Infection usually clears promptly upon removal of the object, and generally no further therapy is necessary.

Epistaxis

Nosebleeds are rare in infancy, are common in childhood, and decrease in incidence after puberty. Epistaxis, when it does occur, is often transient and not very severe; the bleeding often stops spontaneously or with minimal pressure. These isolated episodes of bleeding require no diagnostic evaluation or specific treatment. However, some children develop recurrent epistaxis with mild or moderate bleeding.

Etiology. Trauma, including picking the nose and foreign bodies, is the most common cause. There is frequently a family history of childhood epistaxis, and susceptibility is increased during respiratory infections and in the winter months. Epistaxis is also associated with adenoidal hypertrophy, allergic rhinitis, sinusitis, polyps, and a variety of acute infections. Diseases with paroxysmal and forceful cough, such as cystic fibrosis, may also foster epistaxis. Severe bleeding may be encountered with congenital vascular abnormalities, such as telangiectasias or varicosities, and in children with thrombocytopenia, deficiency of clotting factors, hypertension, renal failure, or venous congestion. Adolescent girls may have epistaxis at the time of menarche.

Clinical Manifestations. Epistaxis usually occurs without warning, with blood flowing slowly but freely from 1 nostril or occasionally both. In children with nasal lesions, bleeding may follow physical exercise. When bleeding occurs at night, the blood may be swallowed and may become apparent only when the child vomits or passes blood in his stools. The source of the bleeding is usually the vascular plexus on the anterior septum (Kiesselbach plexus) or the mucosa of the anterior portions of the turbinates.

Treatment. Most nosebleeds stop spontaneously in a few min, but if bleeding continues, the nares should be compressed and the child kept as quiet as possible, in an erect position with the head tilted forward to avoid blood trickling posteriorly into the pharynx, until hemostasis. If these measures do not stop the bleeding, local application of a solution of epinephrine (1:1000) with or without topical thrombin may, on occasion, be useful. If bleeding persists, an anterior nasal pack should be inserted; if bleeding originates in the posterior nares, combined anterior and postchoanal packing is necessary. After bleeding has been controlled, and if a bleeding site is identified, its obliteration by cautery with silver nitrate may prevent further difficulties.

In patients with severe or repeated epistaxis, blood transfusions may be necessary. Otolaryngologic evaluation is indicated for these children and for those with bilateral bleeding or with hemorrhage that does not arise from the Kiesselbach plexus. Replacement of deficient clotting factors may be required for patients who have an underlying hematologic disorder (Sec 14.54). If a patient lives in a dry environment, a room humidifier may be useful to prevent epistaxis.

12.27 INFECTIONS OF THE UPPER RESPIRATORY TRACT

General Considerations. Upper respiratory tract infections are those primarily affecting the structures of the respiratory tract above the larynx. Most respiratory illnesses affect the upper and lower portions of the tract simultaneously or sequentially, but some predominantly involve specific portions of the respiratory tree.

Large numbers of different microorganisms (chiefly viruses) are capable of causing primary upper respiratory tract disease. The same organism may cause inapparent infection or clinical symptoms or syndromes of differing severity and extent in accordance with such host factors as age, sex, previous contact with the agent, allergy, nutritional status, and the like (Sec 10.10–10.19). For example, among different members of the same family a single virus may simultaneously produce typical colds in the parents, bronchiolitis in the infant, croup in a somewhat older child, pharyngitis in another, and a subclinical infection in another.

Etiology. Most acute respiratory tract infections are caused by viruses and mycoplasma. Exceptions are acute epiglottitis and the pneumonias of lobar distribution. Various streptococci and the diphtheria organism are the only bacterial agents capable of causing primary pharyngeal disease; even in cases of acute tonsillopharyngitis, most illnesses are of nonbacterial origin. Though considerable overlapping exists, some microorganisms are more likely to produce a given respiratory syndrome than others, and certain agents have a greater tendency than others to produce severe disease. Some viruses (e.g., rubeola) may be associated with varying amounts of upper and lower respiratory tract symptomatology as part of a general clinical picture involving other organ systems.

The **respiratory syncytial virus** (RSV) is the principal single cause of bronchiolitis, accounting for about one third of all cases. It is a common cause of pneumonia, croup, and bronchitis, as well as of undifferentiated febrile disease of the upper respiratory tract (Sec 10.80).

The **parainfluenza viruses** account for the majority of cases of the croup syndrome, but may also produce bronchitis, bronchiolitis, and febrile upper respiratory tract disease (Sec 10.79). The **influenza viruses** do not play a large part in the various respiratory syndromes except during epidemics. In infants and children, influenza viruses account for more disease of the upper than the lower respiratory tract. Croup severe enough to require tracheostomy is occasionally seen during influenza epidemics.

The **adenoviruses** account for fewer than 10% of respiratory illnesses, many of which are mild. A large proportion may be asymptomatic. Pharyngitis and pharyngoconjunctival fever are the most common clinical manifestations in children. However, adenoviruses and respiratory syncytial viruses occasionally cause severe lower respiratory tract infection (Sec 10.80 and 10.81).

The **rhinoviruses** and **coronaviruses** usually produce disease limited to the upper tract, most commonly the nose. They account for a significant proportion of the "common cold" syndromes (see Chapter 10 and Sec 12.28).

The **Coxsackie A and B viruses** produce primarily disease of the nasopharynx (Sec 10.84). **Mycoplasma** can produce both upper and lower respiratory tract illness, including bronchiolitis, pneumonia, bronchitis, pharyngotonsillitis, myringitis, and otitis media (Sec 10.66).

THOMAS F. BOAT
CARL F. DOERSHUK
ROBERT C. STERN
ALFRED D. HEGGIE

12.28 ACUTE NASOPHARYNGITIS
(The "Common Cold")

In children this inflammatory infectious syndrome differs from that in adults in that it is more extensive and involves the accessory paranasal sinuses more often and usually the middle ear as well as the nasopharynx. Acute nasopharyngitis is the most common infectious condition of children, but its importance depends primarily upon the relative frequency with which complications occur.

Etiology. The illness is caused by many different viruses (Sec 10.80 and 10.81) although the principal agents may be rhinoviruses (Sec 10.82). The period of infectivity lasts from a few hr prior to the appearance of symptoms to 1–2 days after the illness has appeared. Invasion of tissue by potentially pathogenic bacteria may occur during the course of the infection and be responsible for complications in the sinuses, ears, mastoids, lymph nodes, and lungs. The bacteria most frequently involved are group A streptococci, pneumococci, *H. influenzae*, and staphylococci, the last 2 principally in young children. These bacterial conditions may respond to appropriate antibiotics, but bacteria play no role in the course of uncomplicated infection or in the pathogenesis of symptoms.

Epidemiology. Susceptibility to agents causing acute nasopharyngitis is universal but for poorly understood reasons varies in the same person from time to time. Although infections occur throughout the year, in the northern temperature zone there are peaks: (1) in September about the time school opens, (2) in late January, and (3) toward the end of April. Children have 3–6 infections/yr, but some have a greater number, especially during the 2nd–3rd yr of life. The frequency of acute nasopharyngitis varies directly with the number of exposures and may be virtually epidemic in nursery schools.

Unknown predisposing events and/or the infection itself usually produce vasomotor effects; initial vasoconstriction of the nasal mucous membranes is followed by vasodilatation and, on occasion, nasal irritation and discharge. Susceptibility seems to be increased by poor nutrition, and malnutrition increases the incidence of purulent complications.

Pathology. The 1st changes are edema and vasodilatation in the submucosa. A mononuclear cell infiltrate follows, which, within 1–2 days, becomes polymorphonuclear. The superficial epithelial cells separate and may slough, and there is profuse production of mucus, at first thin, later thicker and usually purulent.

Clinical Manifestations. Colds are more severe in the young child than in the older child and adult. In general, children from 3 mo–3 yr have fever early in the course of infection, occasionally a few hr before localizing signs have appeared. Younger infants are usually afebrile; older children may have low grade fevers. Purulent complications occur with increased frequency and severity in inverse relation to age. Persistent sinusitis, however, is more common in the older child, occurring rarely in infants. In the latter, however, acute ethmoiditis may occur.

The initial manifestations in infants more than 3 mo of age are the sudden onset of fever (39–49° C), irrita-

bility, restlessness, and sneezing. Nasal discharge begins within a few hr, quickly leading to nasal obstruction, which may interfere with nursing; in small infants
with relatively greater dependency on nose breathing
signs of moderate respiratory distress may occur. During the 1st 2–3 days the eardrums are usually congested
and fluid may be noted behind the drum, whether or
not purulent otitis media subsequently occurs. A few
infants may vomit and some have diarrhea. The febrile
phase lasts from a few hr to 3 days; fever may recur
with purulent complications.

In older children characteristically the initial symptoms are dryness and irritation in the nose and at times
in the pharynx. These are followed within a few hr by
sneezing, chilly sensations, muscular aches, a thin nasal
discharge, and sometimes cough. Headache, malaise,
anorexia, and low grade fever may be present. The
secretions become thicker, usually within a day, and
eventually purulent. The discharge is irritating, particularly during the purulent phase. Nasal obstruction
leads to mouth breathing, and this, through drying of
the mucous membranes of the throat, increases the
sensation of soreness. The acute phase lasts 4–10 days.

Differential Diagnosis. Nasopharyngitis occurs
early in the course of many contagious and acute
infectious diseases in children. One must also consider
acute exacerbations of chronic upper respiratory tract
infections such as adenoiditis, allergies, vasomotor responses to colds, diphtheria, and streptococcal infection.

The initial manifestations of measles and pertussis
and, to a lesser extent, of poliomyelitis, hepatitis, and
mumps are those of nasopharyngitis. A persistent nasal
discharge, particularly if it is bloody, suggests a foreign
body or diphtheria and, in the 1st wk of life, choanal
atresia or congenital syphilis.

Allergic rhinitis (Sec 9.48) differs from infectious rhinitis in that it is not accompanied by fever, the nasal
discharge usually does not become purulent, and there
is usually persistent sneezing, with itching of the eyes
and nose. The nasal mucous membranes in allergic
rhinitis are usually pale rather than inflamed, and nasal
smears will often contain many eosinophils rather than
the polymorphonuclear leukocytes associated with infection. Antihistamines may produce rapid and relatively complete disappearance of signs and symptoms;
in infectious rhinitis their effect is slight.

Complications. These are primarily due to the invasion of the paranasal sinuses and other portions of
the respiratory tract with bacteria. The cervical lymph
nodes may also become involved and occasionally suppurate. The most common complication is otitis media,
seen most frequently in the small infant. Although it
may occur early in the course of a cold, it usually
appears after the initial acute phase of nasopharyngitis
is past. It can, therefore, be suspected if fever recurs.
Complications in the lower respiratory tract such as
laryngitis, bronchitis, and pneumonia occur much less
frequently but are more common in the infant than in
the older child.

Prevention. Effective vaccines are not available.
Gamma globulin does not reduce the frequency or
severity of infections, and its use is not recommended.

Because of the ubiquity of the common cold, it is not
possible to isolate children from this condition. However, since in the very young infant complications may
be relatively serious, some attempt should be made to
protect infants from contact with potentially infected
persons, particularly other children.

Treatment. There is no specific therapy. Antibiotics
do not affect the course of the illness or reduce the
incidence of bacterial complications. Bed rest is generally recommended, but there is no evidence that it
shortens the course of the illness or has any effect on
the outcome. Aspirin is usually helpful in reducing
irritability, aching, and malaise for the 1st 1–2 days of
infections, but excessive use should be avoided.

Most of the distress is related to nasal obstruction.
Attempts should be made to relieve this condition as
relief will permit the child to sleep better and take more
fluids and food. Nasal instillation of medications is the
most consistently effective method to relieve nasal obstruction. Ephedrine or epinephrine in isotonic salt
solutions in concentrations approximately one half to
one third of those used in adults are effectively and
relatively harmless. Phenylephrine (0.25–0.50%) is
widely used in the United States. The more potent,
longer acting nose drops useful in adults tend to be
irritating for use in infants and occasionally are associated with the development of hyperexcitability or sedation. Nose drops in oily vehicles should be avoided
because they are readily aspirated. The addition of
antibiotics, corticosteroids, or anthistamines to nose
drops increases their expense and adds nothing to their
effectiveness.

Nose drops are best administered 15–20 min before
feeding and at bedtime. One–2 drops are instilled in
each nostril while the child is lying on his or her back
with the neck extended. Since this will usually produce
shrinkage only of the anterior mucous membranes,
ideally an additional 1–2 drops should be instilled 5–10
min later. Introducing nasal decongestant by cotton-
tipped applicators is not generally recommended in
infants and small children, although this method is
useful in the older child if the cotton pledget is inserted
beyond the anterior nares.

Bottles of nose drops should be used by only 1 person
and for only 1 illness since they usually become quickly
contaminated with bacteria. Only older children should
use a nasal spray under supervision since such applications tend to be overused. In general, no medication
instilled into the nose should be used for more than
4–5 days; after this time any drug may become irritating
and produce a chemically induced nasal congestion
mimicking acute nasopharyngitis.

Nasal obstruction is most difficult to treat in infants.
Various types of apparatus for suction of secretions
from the nose have been used but are relatively ineffective and sometimes dangerous. However, they are
occasionally essential to clear the nasal passage sufficiently to permit the young infant to nurse. The best
drainage can usually be obtained by placing the infant
in the prone position, if this does not further embarrass
respirations. A highly humidified environment such as
that provided by an efficient vaporizer usually provides
substantial benefit.

Orally administered decongestants are also widely employed in the belief that they result in shrinkage of engorged nasal mucosa, thereby relieving stuffiness and preventing otitis media. Most available preparations combine antihistamines and a phenylephrine-like agent. In many patients the atropine-like action of the antihistaminic causes some drying of the mucous membranes; little evidence exists that mucus shrinking is produced in a majority of children or that otitis media is prevented.

If the child is coughing but has a profuse nasal discharge, potent antitussives should be avoided. Depressing the cough reflex may greatly increase the danger of aspiration of material from the nasopharynx.

Most children with acute nasopharyngitis have decreased appetite, but there is no advantage in compelling them to take nourishment. Fluids of the child's choice should be offered at frequent intervals. Transient constipation is common but does not require treatment and rapidly disappears when the child returns to a normal diet.

After the acute phase of the illness, the child's contact with other children should be limited for a few days because there may be an increased susceptibility to the acquisition of potentially pathogenic bacteria and other viruses.

12.29 ACUTE PHARYNGITIS

This term refers to all acute infections of the pharynx, including tonsillitis and pharyngotonsillitis. The presence or absence of tonsils does not affect the frequency, the course or complications of the illness, or susceptibility to it. Pharyngeal involvement is part of most upper respiratory tract infections and is also found with various acute generalized infections (Chapter 10). However, in the strict sense "acute pharyngitis" refers to conditions in which the principal involvement is in the throat. The disease is uncommon under 1 yr of age. The incidence then increases to a peak from 4–7 yr but continues throughout later childhood and adult life. In diphtheria (Sec 10.23), herpangina (Sec 10.84), and infectious mononucleosis (Sec 10.76) pharyngeal involvement may be prominent.

Etiology. Acute pharyngitis, whether febrile or not, is generally caused by viruses (Sec 10.78). Group A beta-hemolytic streptococcus (Sec 10.21) is the only common bacterial causative agent, and except during epidemics it accounts for probably fewer than 15% of cases. Other bacteria may proliferate during acute viral infections and may therefore be cultured in large numbers from the pharynx of an affected person.

Clinical Manifestations. These differ somewhat, depending on whether streptococci or viruses are the cause. There is, however, much overlapping in signs and symptoms, and it is often impossible to distinguish clinically 1 form of pharyngitis from another.

Viral pharyngitis is generally a disease of relatively gradual onset, which usually has as early signs fever, malaise, and anorexia with moderate throat pain. Sore throat may be present initially but more commonly begins a day or so after onset of symptoms and reaches its peak by the 2nd–3rd day. Hoarseness, cough, and rhinitis are also common. Even at its peak, pharyngeal inflammation may be relatively slight; but on occasion it is severe, and small ulcers may form on the soft palate and the posterior pharyngeal wall. Exudates may appear on lymphoid follicles of the palate and tonsils and be indistinguishable from those encountered with streptococcal disease. The cervical lymph nodes are usually moderately enlarged and firm and may or may not be tender. Laryngeal involvement is common, but the trachea, bronchi, and lungs are rarely involved. White blood cell counts range from 6000 to above 30,000, an elevated count (16,000–18,000) with predominance of polymorphonuclear cells being common in the early phase of illness. Leukocyte counts are therefore of little value in differentiating viral from bacterial disease. The entire illness may last less than 24 hr and usually does not persist more than 5 days. Significant complications are rare.

Streptococcal pharyngitis in a child over 2 yr often begins with complaints of headache, abdominal pain, and vomiting. These symptoms may be associated with a fever as high as 40° C (104° F); occasionally a temperature elevation is not noted for 12 hr or so. Hours after the initial complaints, the throat may become sore, and in approximately one third of patients tonsillar enlargement, exudation, and pharyngeal erythema are found. The degree of pharyngeal pain is inconstant and may vary from slight to sufficiently severe to make swallowing difficult. Two thirds of patients may have only mild erythema, with no particular enlargement of the tonsils and with no exudate. Anterior cervical lymphadenopathy usually occurs early, and the nodes are often tender. Fever may continue for 1–4 days; in very severe cases the child may remain ill for as long as 2 wk. The physical findings most likely to be associated with streptococcal disease are diffuse redness of the tonsils and tonsillar pillars, with a petechial mottling of the soft palate whether or not lymphadenitis or follicular exudations are found. These features, although common in streptococcal pharyngitis, are not diagnostic and occur with some frequency in viral pharyngitis.

Conjunctivitis, rhinitis, cough, and hoarseness occur rarely with proven streptococcal pharyngitis, and the presence of 2 or more of these signs or symptoms suggests the diagnosis of viral infection.

The term **streptococcosis** refers to systemic variations in the presentation of acute streptococcal infections which are believed to be related to earlier infection with the beta-hemolytic streptococcus. In infants they may take the form of an acute, usually mild episode lasting less than 1 wk characterized by variable fever (under 39° C [102° F]), mucoserous nasal discharge, and pharyngeal infection. Children between 6 mo–3 yr of age are usually more severely ill. Coryza with postnasal discharge, diffusely reddened pharynx, fever, vomiting, and loss of appetite occur early. Usually for a few days there is fever of 38–39.5° C (100–103° F) which continues irregularly for 4–8 wk, gradually becoming normal. Within a few days of onset cervical nodes begin to enlarge and become tender; typically the course of the adenopathy parallels that of the fever. Focal complications are common during the course.

Differential Diagnosis. Throat culture is the only reliable method to differentiate viral from streptococcal pharyngitis. However, since normal children may carry group A streptococcus in their throats, even a positive culture may not be conclusive.

A syndrome of purulent nasal discharge, pharyngitis, and fever may also be associated with positive pharyngeal cultures for pneumococci or *H. influenzae*. Although this syndrome is probably a complication of viral pharyngitis, some of these patients respond to antibiotics.

When a membranous exudate is present on the tonsils or pharynx, specific culture for diphtheria is indicated even if the clinical course does not suggest this diagnosis. The membranous exudate of infectious mononucleosis closely resembles that found in the partially immunized child with a diphtheritic infection. Herpangina (Sec 10.84) is not usually associated with tonsillar exudates, but rather with many vesiculoulcerative lesions on the anterior pillars, fauces, and soft palate.

Agranulocytosis often is first manifested by symptoms of acute pharyngitis. The tonsils and posterior pharyngeal wall may be covered by a yellowish or dirty white exudate. The mucous membranes under this exudate will usually become necrotic, and ulceration will extend into the mouth and tongue. The lesions are very painful and dysphagia is severe. Enlargement of cervical lymph nodes commonly occurs, as do mucosal hemorrhages.

Pharyngoconjunctival fever is discussed in Sec 10.81.

Complications. With viral infections the complication rate is low, although purulent bacterial otitis media may occur. In debilitated children both viral and streptococcal infections may lead to large, chronic ulcers in the pharynx. With streptococcal disease, peritonsillar abscess occasionally occurs, as do sinusitis, otitis media, and, rarely, meningitis. Since acute glomerulonephritis (Sec 16.14) and rheumatic fever (Sec 9.58) may follow streptococcal infections, children with proven streptococcal disease should be re-examined 2–3 wk after illness.

Mesenteric adenitis is occasionally associated with pharyngitis of either viral or bacterial origin. This may result in abdominal pain with or without vomiting which may closely simulate appendicitis.

Treatment. Following an examination, culture for beta-hemolytic streptococcal infection and, if indicated, *Corynebacterium diphtheriae* should be done.

Since even exudative tonsillitis is usually of viral origin, for which there is no specific therapy, the use of antibiotics shoud be deferred pending the results of culture, unless there are strong clinical and epidemiologic grounds to suspect a streptococcal infection. Streptococcal pharyngitis is best treated orally with penicillin (200,000–250,000 units of penicillin G 3–4 times daily for 10 days). This usually produces prompt clinical response with defervescence within 24 hr. Erythromycin is a satisfactory alternative if the patient is allergic to penicillin.

Most children prefer to remain in bed during the acute phase of the disease. When throat pain is severe, aspirin is often helpful as are hot or cold compresses to the neck, depending on the patient's preference. Gargles of warm saline solution offer some symptomatic relief for throat pain in children old enough to cooperate; in younger children the inhalation of steam occasionally produces similar effects. Because of pain on swallowing, cool bland liquids such as ginger ale are usually more acceptable to the child than solids or hot foods. No attempt should be made to force the child to eat.

The child with a streptococcal infection is noninfectious to others within a few hr after penicillin therapy has begun. Children with viral disease remain infectious for several days. It is not possible to prevent viral pharyngitis, but in children who require protection against streptococcal disease, such as those with past history of rheumatic fever, antibiotic prophylaxis is indicated and effective (Sec 9.58).

RICHARD E. BEHRMAN

12.30 CHRONIC RHINITIS AND NASOPHARYNGITIS

One of the difficult problems of pediatric practice is that of the child with persistent or recurring upper respiratory tract infection with or without associated chronic bronchial involvement. Children with such chronic infections cannot be placed in any 1 category; each must be studied to determine, if possible, the underlying factor or factors.

The greatest incidence of respiratory infection occurs from the latter part of the 1st yr of life to 6–7 yr. During this time it can be expected that the average child will have 3–6 "colds" a year. Recovery should occur after each attack, and the child should appear healthy between episodes. In the chronic cases the child seems to recover from 1 acute attack only to enter another, or there is more or less persistent rhinitis and cough and a general failure to do well. Such patterns may reflect familial or individual susceptibility or repeated exposure to respiratory infection within the home.

Chronic Rhinitis. Chronic nasal discharge, with or without a tendency to acute exacerbations, may be a reflection of an underlying disturbance, such as nasal polyps, chronic sinusitis, chronically infected adenoids, cystic fibrosis, allergy, foreign bodies, deviated septum, various congenital malformations, nasal diphtheria, or syphilis. In addition, the possibility of a chronic debilitating infection or some nutritional, immunologic, or metabolic (as of the thyroid) deficiency must be considered.

Clinical Manifestations. Symptoms vary, but chronic nasal discharge is common to all cases. In the persistent cases the odor may be foul, and there may be excoriation of the anterior nares and upper lip. Bloody discharge is common in syphilitic and diphtheritic lesions and with foreign bodies but may also occur in other conditions, especially if there is persistent picking of the nose. Disturbances of taste and smell are frequent. During exacerbations or superimposed infections, fever is common but is otherwise usually absent.

Persistent **allergic rhinitis** is relatively common and may be seasonal (Sec 9.48). The mucous membrane tends to be pale; the soft tissues are swollen and resistant to pressure.

Chronic rhinitis also may be the result of prolonged or excessive use of nasal decongestants (rhinitis medicamentosa).

Atrophic rhinitis is uncommon; it is usually associated with some general debilitating condition, or it may be a sequel to long-continued nasal infection. The sense of smell is impaired. There may be little or no discharge but considerable crusting and a sense of dryness in the nose and throat. In some instances there is a profuse, excessively foul nasal discharge (ozena).

Treatment. The frequent application of a lanolin, silicone, or petrolatum-base ointment protects against excoriation. Otherwise treatment is directed toward the underlying disturbance. Particular emphasis must be placed upon eradicating foci of infection in sinuses, ears, adenoids, or tonsils and upon the removal of or desensitization to known allergens. Attention should be given to nutritional status, rest, and prevention of exposure to reinfection. In an attempt to provide symptomatic relief, it is often difficult to avoid the use of such mucosa-shrinking solutions as phenylephrine and related compounds. However, their use is not without danger, and they may cause further damage. The use of antibiotics locally should be avoided, but systemic administration may be indicated in selected cases.

Chronic Pharyngitis. Chronic pharyngitis is rare. It is a secondary condition resulting from chronic infections of the sinuses, adenoids, or tonsils, although on occasion there is no evidence of infection other than hypertrophied lymphoid tissue on the posterior pharyngeal wall and on the base of the tongue. The latter type of involvement occurs with frequency only in children whose faucial tonsils have been removed; some of these children may have infected tonsillar tags.

Clinical Manifestations. There are likely to be repeated acute exacerbations; in the intervals there are complaints of discomfort in the throat such as dryness and raspy irritation. Frequent efforts to clear the throat and an irritative cough are common. The mucous membrane is usually inflamed, though on occasion it is pale, and the blood vessels are prominent. The pharyngeal wall is frequently covered with a mucopurulent secretion, and the lymphoid tissue is often hypertrophied and has a pebbled appearance.

Treatment. This should be directed toward any disturbance in the sinuses, nose (deformities), adenoids, and tonsils. Attention should also be given to the general nutrition and hygiene of the child.

12.31   RETROPHARYNGEAL ABSCESS

During early childhood the potential space between the posterior pharyngeal wall and the prevertebral fascia contains several small lymph nodes which usually disappear during the 3rd–4th yr of life. The lymphatic channels that communicate with these nodes drain portions of the nasopharynx as well as the posterior nasal passages. With purulent infections of these areas the nodes may become infected; this may, in turn, progress to breakdown of the nodes and to suppuration.

Etiology. Retropharyngeal abscess may be a complication of bacterial pharyngitis. Less commonly, it occurs after extension of infection from vertebral osteomyelitis or by wound infection following a penetrating injury of the posterior pharynx. *Staphylococcus aureus* and group A hemolytic streptococci are the most common pathogens.

Clinical Manifestations. The patient usually has a history of an acute nasopharyngitis or pharyngitis, and the clinical features of the earlier illness may still be present. There is generally an abrupt onset of high fever with difficulty in swallowing, refusal of feeding, severe distress with throat pain, hyperextension of the head, and noisy, often gurgling respirations. Respirations become increasingly labored, and secretions accumulate in the mouth and cause drooling due to the difficulty in swallowing.

A bulge in the posterior pharyngeal wall is usually readily apparent. Sometimes the abscess is located in an area of the nasopharynx where it may cause nasal obstruction and a bulging forward of the soft palate. A digital examination to determine whether or not the abscess is fluctuant must be performed with the patient in the Trendelenburg position and with provision for adequate suction in case the abscess ruptures. Retropharyngeal abscesses may not be detectable by simple inspection, but a lateral film of the nasopharynx or neck will reveal the retropharyngeal mass.

If left untreated, the abscess may rupture into the pharynx spontaneously, resulting in aspiration of pus. The process may also dissect laterally and present externally on the side of the neck or burrow into the esophagus, mediastinum, or auditory canal. Sudden death may occur if the abscess presses on the larynx, produces edema of the glottis, or erodes into major blood vessels.

Differential Diagnosis. Pressure on the larynx may result in stridor, making retropharyngeal abscess 1 of the differential diagnostic possibilities in patients with high fever and croup. Many patients have hyperextension of the neck, and this may be mistaken for meningismus. Nonfluctuant lymphadenitis may produce a tender bulge in the retropharyngeal space. Tuberculous caries of the cervical spine may on occasion produce a lateral retropharyngeal abscess; in this condition considerable rigidity of the neck and other signs of spinal involvement are usually present.

Treatment. If the condition is recognized in the prefluctuant stage, intensive treatment with parenteral penicillin G (100,000–250,000 units/kg/24 hr) or a semisynthetic penicillin (to cover penicillinase-producing *Staphylococcus aureus*) may prevent suppuration and abscess formation. Analgesic drugs may be needed for pain. As soon as fluctuance is present, the abscess should be incised and antibiotics started; the operation is best performed under general anesthesia. Before incision is made, the mass should be aspirated to see whether retropharyngeal hemorrhage may not also be present from erosion of blood vessels. If no blood is obtained, an incision is made where the abscess is pointing, and the pus is carefully aspirated. If there is serious bleeding, ligation of the carotid artery may be necessary. If properly treated, the prognosis is good.

12.32　LATERAL PHARYNGEAL ABSCESS

This condition occurs later in childhood than a retropharyngeal abscess. The process is usually so extensive that the entire pharyngeal wall is displaced medially, including the tonsil, the soft palate, and the uvula.

The patient usually has high fever, appears acutely ill, and complains of severe pain and difficulty on swallowing. The bulge in the lateral pharyngeal wall is obvious. Cervical adenitis is usually present and nuchal rigidity due to muscular spasm is common.

Treatment is identical to that of retropharyngeal abscess.

12.33　PERITONSILLAR AND RETROTONSILLAR ABSCESSES

Both peritonsillar and retrotonsillar abscesses are uncommon in childhood. Since these diseases rarely appear in patients who have had a tonsillectomy, the tonsil apparently represents the initial focus from which the process develops. The abscesses are almost always caused by group A beta-hemolytic streptococci, rarely by *Staphylococcus aureus* or *H. influenzae*.

Clinical Manifestations.　The abscesses are usually preceded by an attack of acute pharyngotonsillitis. There may be an afebrile interval of several days, or the fever of the primary infection may not subside. The patient complains of severe throat pain, has progressive difficulty in opening the mouth because of spasm of the pterygoid muscles, and often refuses to swallow or speak. Occasionally, there is sufficient spasm of the homolateral muscles of the neck to produce torticollis. The fever may be septic and reach 40.5° C (105° F). The affected tonsillar area is markedly swollen and inflamed; the uvula is displaced to the opposite side. In untreated patients the abscess becomes fluctuant within a few days and usually points in the region of the anterior faucial pillar. If the abscess is not incised, spontaneous rupture will occur.

Treatment.　See *retropharyngeal abscess* (above). Subsequent attacks of peritonsillar abscess should be prevented by removal of the tonsils 3–4 wk after inflammation has subsided.

12.34　SINUSITIS

See also Sec 12.24.

The maxillary antrums and the anterior and posterior ethmoid cells are present at birth and are usually of sufficient size to harbor infection. The frontal sinus is rarely a site of significant infection until the 6th–10th yr. When there is severe ethmoidal disease in the 1st few yr of life, the development and pneumatization of the frontal sinuses may be curtailed or even completely prevented. The sphenoidal sinus usually does not assume clinical significance until the 3rd–5th yr of life.

The paranasal sinuses are probably involved in an exudative process in practically all acute nasal infections, but, as a rule, the sinus involvement does not persist after the nasal infection has subsided unless there has been a preexisting sinus infection. The incidence of both acute and chronic sinus infections increases in the latter part of childhood. Unrecognized allergic factors, poor sinus drainage such as might occur with septal deviation, constitutitional factors, and environmental factors may increase the possibility of sinus infection. The maxillary and anterior and posterior ethmoids are most frequently involved.

Acute Purulent Sinusitis

In addition to involvement of the sinuses during acute nasal infections, there may be acute empyema of 1 or more sinuses, signs or symptoms of which often appear 3–5 days following the acute rhinitis.

Clinical Manifestations.　The symptoms of acute purulent sinusitis are fever, localized pain or a sense of fullness, localized tenderness to pressure or direct percussion, headache, and, at times, edema over the affected sinus. So-called sinus headaches, which tend to involve the region of the affected sinus, may assist in localization. In sphenoidal sinusitis the headache may be in the suboccipital region; in anterior ethmoidal sinusitis, in the region of the temples and over the eyes; and in posterior ethmoidal sinusitis, over the distribution of the trigeminal nerve, especially over the mastoid area. In maxillary sinusitis there may be aching or tenderness on tapping of the underlying teeth. Unless the sinal ostia are obstructed, there is a purulent discharge which can be observed directly through a nasoscope. Pus in the middle meatus suggests involvement of the maxillary, frontal, or anterior ethmoid sinuses; pus in the superior meatus suggests involvement of the sphenoid or posterior ethmoid cells. Postnasal discharge may result in sore throat or cough, especially at night. Recurrent colds, particularly with purulent secretions, may really be recurrences of sinusitis requiring more intensive therapy.

In acute ethmoiditis, especially in infants and small children, periorbital cellulitis with edema of the soft tissues and redness of the skin is a common manifestation.

Diagnosis.　A frontal or maxillary sinus filled with pus is roentgenographically opaque; markedly thickened sinus membranes also indicate bacterial infection. Transillumination may be helpful in older children but not in young ones. In children it is rarely necessary to puncture a sinus simply to establish a diagnosis. There may be clouding of the ethmoid cells on the roentgenogram in acute and chronic ethmoiditis. Direct smear of the secretions usually reveals mostly neutrophils and may aid in detecting associated allergy if many eosinophils are present. Nasal swab cultures do not correlate well with cultures of sinus aspirates, which most often grow *S. pneumoniae* or *H. influenzae*. Anaerobic organisms are also frequently identified. Complications are otitis media, meningitis, cavernous sinus thrombosis, optic neuritis, orbital cellulitis and abscess, and nephritis.

Treatment.　Treatment is essentially that of the rhinitis. Shrinkage of the nasal mucous membranes will often facilate drainage from the sinus. Phenylephrine nose drops or spray, 0.25–0.125% 4 times a day, can be used for 5 day periods. Systemic decongestants may provide additional relief. Antihistamines may be useful with associated allergic rhinitis. Gentle suction or aspiration may be used but may be more annoying than helpful, especially in infants. Drainage of a sinus is rarely necessary but may be justified if local and systemic manifestations are persistent. Appropriate antibiotic therapy, usually consisting of ampicillin, should be used.

Chronic Sinusitis

Even though it is a common ailment of persons living in harsh climates, chronic infection of the paranasal sinuses should suggest the possibility of a local or generalized disturbance that facilitates persistence of the infection. Search should be made for nasal deformities, polyps, or infected and hypertrophied adenoids which might cause obstruction, for infected teeth as a source of maxillary sinusitis, for a sinus polyp or mucocele, and for such general disturbances as allergy, cystic fibrosis, and immotile cilia. Chronic or recurrent sinusitis is common in patients with absence of secretory antibodies and in other immunodeficiency states.

Clinical Manifestations. Symptoms of chronic sinusitis vary considerably. Fever, when present, is low grade. Malaise, easy fatigability, difficulty in mental concentration, and anorexia frequently occur. Nasal discharge, which may be bilateral or unilateral, varies from day to day and may be greater during a certain portion of the day. Frequently there is sufficient swelling of the middle turbinates to cause complete nasal obstruction. Postnasal discharge or drip is common and, in the absence of infected adenoids or acute upper respiratory tract infection, is virtually diagnostic. Headaches are frequent, and pain or tenderness to palpation or percussion is helpful in localization. There are frequent attacks of sneezing; when there is an associated watery nasal discharge, the possibility of allergic rhinitis must be considered.

Constant pharyngeal irritation or inexplicably persistent mouthbreathing suggests sinusitis. Any of the complications of acute sinusitis may occur with chronic sinusitis, but probably the most frequent association is chronic bronchial infection. The term *sinobronchitis* is occasionally used to designate the relationship; children with this condition may have cystic fibrosis, immunodeficiency, or immotile cilia as the underlying disease.

Treatment. Therapy is similar to that for acute sinusitis. Repeated courses of decongestants and antibiotics may be required as guided by the symptoms, physical findings, and culture results. Nasopharyngeal cultures are not useful; the offending organism can be accurately identified only by culturing aspirates from the involved sinus. There is little agreement about the organisms most commonly involved in children; prominently mentioned are staphylococci, pneumococci, and *H. influenzae*. Anaerobic infection is more common than previously recognized.

Antibiotics are of no proven benefit, but some claim they may be efficacious when used for extended periods. Locally obstructive nasal deformities should be corrected, if possible, and infected or hypertrophic adenoid tissue should be removed.

Shrinkage of the mucous membranes by ephedrine or related compounds with the head positioned to facilitate entrance of the solution into the sinuses, may help, particularly if followed 2–3 times a day by exposure of the sinus areas to local heat. Such therapy should be administered several times a day for about 2 wk.

Every effort should be made to avoid operative procedures, but if there is persistence of chronic purulent sinusitis in spite of all nonoperative measures, surgical drainage may be indicated.

12.35 NASAL POLYPS

Etiology. Nasal polyps are benign pedunculated tumors formed from edematous, usually chronically inflamed nasal mucosa. They usually originate in the region of the upper turbinates and from the maxillary and ethmoid sinus ostia. Occasionally, they appear within the maxillary antrum. Very large or multiple polyps may completely obstruct the nasal passage.

Cystic fibrosis is probably the most common childhood cause of nasal polyposis; as many as 15% of patients develop polyps at some point in their lifetime. Every child with nasal polyposis should be tested for cystic fibrosis, even in the absence of typical respiratory and digestive symptoms. Nasal polyposis is also associated with chronic sinusitis of other etiologies, chronic allergic rhinitis, and asthma.

Clinical Manifestations. Obstruction of nasal passages with nasal phonation and mouthbreathing is prominent. Profuse mucoid or mucopurulent rhinorrhea may also result. Examination of the nasal passages shows glistening, gray, grape-like masses squeezed between the nasal turbinates and the septum. Polyps can be readily distinguised from the well-vascularized turbinate tissue, which is pink or red. Prolonged presence of polyps may widen the bridge of the nose and erode adjacent osseous structures.

Treatment. Local or systemic decongestants are usually not effective in shrinking the polyps. Similarly, improvement is not usual from the use of corticosteroid sprays in the nose, although a trial is warranted in recurrent cases. Polyps should be removed surgically if complete obstruction, uncontrolled rhinorrhea, or deformity of the nose appears. Unfortunately, if the underlying pathogenic mechanism cannot be eliminated (e.g., cystic fibrosis), the polyps may soon return. Antihistamines may be helpful in delaying recurrence due to allergic causes.

12.36 TONSILS AND ADENOIDS

The term tonsils is used in its commonly accepted sense of indicating the 2 faucial tonsils; the term adenoids refers to the pharyngeal tonsil. The tonsils and adenoids are part of the lymphoid tissues that circle the pharynx and are known collectively as *Waldeyer ring*.

This consists of the lymphoid tissue on the base of the tongue (lingual tonsil), the 2 faucial tonsils, the adenoids (pharyngeal tonsil), and the lymphoid tissue on the posterior pharyngeal wall. This tissue serves naturally as a defense against infection; when its defense mechanism is overcome, it may become a site of acute or chronic infection.

The principal disturbances of the tonsils and adenoids are infection and hypertrophy. The latter is in most instances temporary and secondary to infection. The most important medical issue is if and when they are to be removed. Though both tonsils and adenoids are usually removed at the same operation, there are good reasons for making the decisions for tonsillectomy and adenoidectomy separately, especially in children under 4–5 yr of age. Tonsillar disturbances are uncommon in infancy.

Neoplasms of the Tonsils

Neoplasms of the tonsils are rare, although papilloma, lipoma, angioma, teratoma, fibroma, plasmocytoma, and lymphosarcoma have been reported.

Acute Tonsillitis

Acute infections of the tonsils are considered as acute pharyngitis and are discussed in Chapter 10 and in Sec 12.29.

Chronic Tonsillitis
(Chronically Hypertrophic and Infected Tonsils)

The management of tonsillitis is of particular concern in pediatric practice because of the frequency of chronic tonsillar involvement and the potential importance of this tissue to the normal development of the immune system.

Clinical Manifestations. These vary considerably; the more significant features are recurrent or persistent sore throat and obstruction to swallowing or breathing; the latter is most often due to adenoids. There may be a sense of dryness and irritation in the throat, and the breath may be offensive. Constitutional symptoms are neither characteristic nor, as a rule, striking. Rarely, hypertrophied tonsils and adenoids obstructing the upper airway are associated with respiratory distress and the development of pulmonary hypertension.

Indications for Tonsillectomy. Parents often attribute frequent respiratory infections, allergic bronchitis, mouthbreathing, recurrent purulent or serous otitis, poor appetite, failure to gain weight, or recurrent or chronic fever to chronic tonsillitis. However, there is no evidence that tonsillectomy and adenoidectomy decrease the incidence of these problems during childhood. Until better means are available to identify those children who may truly benefit from tonsillectomy and adenoidectomy, it seems prudent to avoid surgery in most cases. Physician awareness that hospital charts were being monitored routinely by others to identify the stated indications for tonsillectomy and adenoidectomy has resulted in a marked decrease in the frequency of these operations.

Decision for removal of tonsils should be based on symptoms and signs directly related to the tonsils and to disturbances in closely related structures. Local indications for removal are symptomatic hypertrophy, associated with signs and symptoms of obstruction, and chronic infection. Tonsillectomy should be considered only in those children who have 4 or more culture-proved episodes of group A streptococcal pharyngitis associated with tonsillitis in a year and in whom immunologic development is adequate; it should rarely be considered in a child under 2 yr of age. Since the frequency with which episodes of acute pharyngitis or tonsillitis occur is not decreased by tonsillectomy, "frequent sore throat" is not a valid indication. *Furthermore, most tonsils considered to be hypertrophic actually are normal in size; the misinterpretation results from failure to appreciate that normally tonsils are relatively larger during childhood than in later years.*

Tonsils may virtually meet in the midline in some children who are asymptomatic, and tonsils of average size are projected toward the midline when the child is gagged and may be interpreted as being hypertrophic. On the other hand, infection does not always produce hypertrophy, and chronically infected tonsils may be small and embedded behind the faucial pillars. There is no certain way to demonstrate by direct observation whether tonsils are harboring chronic infection. The consistency or size of the tonsils and the presence of cheesy material within the crypts are not reliable guides. Persistent hyperemia of the anterior pillars is a more reliable sign, and enlargement of the cervical lymph nodes is supporting evidence. Persistent enlargement of the node just below and slightly in front of the angle of the jaw is especially significant. In contrast to the difficulty in determining the presence of chronic infection, hypertrophy sufficient to obstruct swallowing or breathing is readily detectable. Such tonsils practically meet in the midline when the throat is examined without gagging the patient. However, before tonsillectomy is recommended, it should be ascertained that the hypertrophy is chronic and not the result of a recent acute infection. Tonsils can increase in size greatly during an acute infection and recede after its subsidence.

Among the disturbances in adjacent tonsillar structures, peritonsillar (and retrotonsillar) abscess is the only definite indication for tonsillectomy. The removal of tonsils is of no value in the prevention or treatment of acute or chronic sinusitis. Perhaps in some instances of recurrent sinusitis removal of the adenoids is indicated, but even in this instance the benefits achieved are usually minor. This is also probably true in cases of chronic otitis media and of middle ear deafness. There is no evidence to indicate that the removal of tonsils is justified for infections in the lower respiratory tract, although such conditions are not a contraindication if there are other reasons for tonsillectomy.

No systemic disturbance in itself is an indication for tonsillectomy. This applies to children with rheumatic fever or glomerulonephritis as well as to those with other infections in which the tonsils may be removed in a blind search for a focus of infection or as a remedy for undernutrition or slow growth.

Tonsillectomy in Relation to Age of Child. When, on rare occasions, it seems advisable to recommend tonsillectomy for a child of 2–3 yr of age, every attempt should be made to postpone the operation. Frequently when the operation is postponed for reasons of age, the apparent need for it disappears within the next yr or so. In the 1st few yr of life the indications for adenoidectomy, though infrequent, are present more often than those for tonsillectomy. Neither procedure should be performed as a prophylaxis against the "common cold" at any age.

Tonsillectomy in Relation to Active Infection. Tonsillectomy should be postponed until 2–3 wk after subsidence of an infection, except in rare instances of acute respiratory obstruction with pulmonary arterial hypertension and cor pulmonale.

Type of Operation. Careful removal by dissection should be carried out to ensure that all the tonsillar tissue is removed without destruction of adjacent tissues. Too frequently, small amounts of tonsillar tissue are allowed to remain which later become infected and hypertrophied, or there is removal of adjacent tissue from the lateral pharyngeal wall, from the soft palate and even at times from the uvula. Aspiration of the throat during the operation will lessen the chances of pulmonary abscess or pneumonia. Bleeding should be completely controlled, and the child should not leave the operating room until he has dry tonsillar fossae.

Preoperative Preparation. A careful preoperative evaluation frequently uncovers unsuspected underlying conditions, recognition of which explains the apparent indication for the surgery and at the same time contraindicates it. The medical history should include questions related to recent infection, to exposure to contagious diseases, and to bleeding tendencies in the patient and family. A thorough physical examination should include observation for loose or carious teeth, which should be removed or repaired before tonsillectomy. Bleeding and clotting times are usually obtained, but a careful history of bleeding tendencies is a more effective screening method. The child should be told of the operation and the procedure explained, preferably by informed parents. Though food is withheld for at least 6 hr before the operation, feeding should be adequate up to this time. In children who are undernourished or readily susceptible to ketosis, preoperative intravenous administration of glucose is indicated.

Postoperative Care. The child should be kept in bed for the remainder of the day and at rest for several more; it is wise to encourage eating and drinking as soon as the nausea from the anesthetic has disappeared. Acetaminophen may be prescribed for discomfort. Avoidance of contact with infection is of the greatest importance. The membrane that forms at the operative site is at times interpreted as being diphtheritic. Fusiform bacilli (Vincent organisms) may be cultured from it with considerable regularity, but this by itself is not an indication for treatment.

Complications. Complications are not particularly frequent, but postoperative hemorrhage, lung abscess, pneumonia, and septicemia do occur. Hemorrhage is the most frequent problem and should be controlled by packing or, in the case of severe bleeding, by ligation. Transfusion may be necessary to prevent hemorrhagic shock and death if bleeding is extensive or prolonged.

Results to Be Expected from Tonsillectomy. No reduction in the incidence of respiratory infections is to be expected. Obstructive symptoms due to hypertrophied tonsils can be relieved. Nasal allergy is not affected, nor is the incidence of initial or recurrent attacks of rheumatic fever. The incidence of cervical lymphadenitis may be decreased. In rare instances nutrition may be improved after tonsillectomy. This may be due to psychologic factors or to removal of a focus of infection. Care should be taken, however, in making predictions in this respect.

Adenoidal Hypertrophy
(Hypertrophy of Pharyngeal Tonsil; "Adenoids")

Disturbances of the lymphoid tissue of the nasopharynx (adenoids) tend to parallel those of the faucial tonsils. Hypertrophy and infection may occur separately but often occur together; infection is usually primary. The soft adenoid structure, which is normally widespread in the nasopharynx; especially on the posterior wall and the roof, undergoes hypertrophy, and masses of varying size, up to 2–3 cm, are formed. These masses may almost fill the vault of the nasopharynx, interfere with the passage of air through the nose, and obstruct the eustachian tubes.

Clinical Manifestations. Mouthbreathing and more or less persistent rhinitis are the most characteristic symptoms. Mouthbreathing may be present only during sleep, especially when the child lies supine; in this position snoring is also likely to occur. With severe adenoid hypertrophy the mouth is kept open during the day as well, and the mucous membranes of the mouth and lips are dry. Chronic nasopharyngitis may be constantly present or recur frequently. The voice is altered with a nasal, muffled quality. The breath is offensive, and taste and smell are impaired. A harassing cough may be present, especially at night, resulting from irritation of the larynx by inspired air which has not been warmed and moistened by passage through the nose. Impaired hearing is common. Chronic otitis media may be associated with infected, hypertrophied adenoids and blockage of the eustachian tube orifices.

A small number of young children with marked adenoidal (also tonsillar) enlargement are incapable of mouthbreathing during sleep. They snort and snore loudly and often display signs of respiratory distress, such as intercostal retractions and nasal flaring. These children are at risk for respiratory insufficiency (hypoxemia, hypercapnia, acidosis) during sleep. While apneic spells occasionally may result, more often some of these children develop pulmonary arterial hypertension and, ultimately, cor pulmonale. Lymphoid tissue enlargement of the upper airway with consequent cor pulmonale has been reported to be related to cow's milk hypersensitivity in a number of preschool-aged children. Very obese children (e.g., Prader-Willi syndrome) and children with a large or posteriorly placed tongue (e.g., Pierre Robin syndrome) may also develop upper airway obstruction in sleep, mimicking the adenoidal hypertrophy syndrome.

Diagnosis. During 1st yr or 2 of life, the size of adenoids can be assessed by digital palpation. Indirect visualization with a pharyngeal mirror is possible in older, cooperative children. Alternatively, the fiberoptic bronchoscope can be used for visualization of the nasopharynx. Lateral pharyngeal roentgenograms are also helpful for detection of nasopharyngeal air column obliteration. Otherwise, the presence of adenoid hypertrophy can be suspected from such symptoms as mouthbreathing, snoring, and persistent rhinitis with or without chronic otitis media.

An abscess in the adenoid tissue is uncommon but may be a cause of protracted fever. Identification and drainage of the abscess have been achieved by digital expression.

Treatment. Adenoidectomy may be indicated with symptoms such as persistent mouthbreathing, nasal speech, adenoid facies, repeated attacks of otitis media (especially when accompanied by a conductive hearing loss), deafness, and persistent or recurring nasopharyngitis, when these seem to be related to infected hypertrophied adenoid tissue. Tonsillectomy should not be routinely done for such problems. Chronic serous otitis media may improve after adenoidectomy in some patients. The same precautions for complete removal and control of bleeding points as in tonsillectomy should be observed; for this reason, removal under direct vision is preferable to the use of the adenotome.

THOMAS F. BOAT
CARL F. DOERSHUK
ROBERT C. STERN
ALFRED D. HEGGIE

Alfaro VF: Nasal sinus disease in children. Pediatr Clin North Am 9:1061, 1962.

Boat TF, Polmar SH, Whitman V, et al: Hyperreactivity to cow milk in young children with pulmonary hemosiderosis and cor pulmonale secondary to nasopharyngeal obstruction. J Pediatr 87:23, 1975.

Cain WA, Amman AJ, Hong R, et al: IgE deficiency associated with chronic sinopulmonary infections. J Clin Invest 48:12A, 1969.

Dingle JH, Badger GF, Jordan WS: Illness in the Home. A Study of 25,000 Illnesses in a Group of Cleveland Families. Cleveland, Press of Western Reserve University, 1964, p 129.

Evans FO, Snyder JB, Moore WEC, et al: Sinusitis of the maxillary antrum. N Engl J Med 293:735, 1975.

Fox JP, Cooney MK, Hall CE: The Seattle virus watch. V. Epidemiologic observation of rhinovirus infections. Am J Epidemiol 101:122, 1975.

Greenwald HM, Messeloff CR: Retropharyngeal abscess in infants and children. Am J Med Sci 177:767, 1929.

Gwaltney JM, Hendley JO, Simon G, et al: Rhinovirus infections in an industrial population. III. Number and prevalence of serotypes. Am J Epidemiol 87:158, 1968.

Haynes RE, Cramblett HG: Acute ethmoiditis: Its relationship to orbital cellulitis. Am J Dis Child 114:261, 1967.

Hendley JO, Wenzel RP, Gwaltney JM: Transmission of rhinovirus colds by self-inoculation. N Engl J Med 288:1361, 1973.

Johnson F: Bleeding factors and tonsils and adenoid surgery. Arch Otolaryngol 86:584, 1967.

Kaye HS, Marsh HB, Dowdle WR: Seroepidemiologic survey of coronavirus (strain OC43) related infections in a children's population. Am J Epidemiol 94:43, 1971.

Knight V: Coxsackieviruses and echoviruses. In Knight V (ed): Viral and Mycoplasmal Infections of the Respiratory Tract. Philadelphia, Lea and Febiger, 1973, p 153.

Lough M, Boat T, Doershuk C: The nose. Resp Care 20:844, 1975.

Maresh MM: Paranasal sinuses from birth to late adolescence. Am J Dis Child 60:55, 1949.

Paradise JL, Bluestone CD, Backman RZ, et al: History of recurrent sore throat as an indication for tonsillectomy. N Engl J Med 298:410, 1978.

Schwachman H, Kulczycki LL, Mueller HL, et al: Nasal polyposis in patients with cystic fibrosis. Pediatrics 30:389, 1962.

12.37   THE EAR

Diseases of the ear constitute 1 of the most frequently encountered morbid conditions of childhood. Ability to recognize their presence, adequate knowledge of the most efficacious treatment, and skills to prevent complications and sequelae are imperative for every clinician caring for children.

12.38   SIGNS AND SYMPTOMS

Eight prominent signs and symptoms are associated primarily with diseases of the ear and temporal bone. **Otalgia** is most commonly associated with inflammation of the external and middle ear but may also arise from the temporomandibular joint, teeth, or pharynx. In young infants, pulling at the ear or general irritability, especially when associated with fever, may be the only sign of ear pain. Purulent **otorrhea** is a sign of otitis externa, otitis media with perforation of the tympanic membrane, or both. Bloody discharge may be associated with acute or chronic inflammation, trauma, neoplasm, or blood dyscrasias. Clear drainage suggests a perforation of the drum with a serous middle ear effusion or cerebrospinal fluid otorrhea draining through a defect in the external auditory canal or through the tympanic membrane from the middle ear.

Hearing loss results from disease of either the external or middle ear (conductive hearing loss) or from pathology in the inner ear, retrocochlea, or central auditory pathways (sensorineural hearing loss). **Swelling** about the ear is most commonly the result of inflammation (e.g., external otitis, perichondritis, or mastoiditis), trauma (hematoma), or, on rare occasions, neoplasm.

Vertigo is not a common complaint in children. The most frequent cause is eustachian tube–mastoid disease, but vertigo also may be due to labyrinthitis; perilymphatic fistula between the inner and middle ear from a congenital defect, trauma, or cholesteatoma; vestibular neuronitis; benign paroxysmal positional vertigo; Meniere disease; or disease of the central nervous system. Older children may describe a feeling of spinning or turning, while younger children may manifest the disequilibrium only by falling, stumbling, or clumsiness. Unidirectional, horizontal, or jerk **nystagmus,** usually associated with vertigo, is vestibular in origin. **Tinnitus,** though infrequently described by children, is common, especially in patients with eustachian tube–middle ear disease or conductive or sensorineural hearing loss.

Facial paralysis is an infrequent but frightening condition for both child and parents. When due to disease within the temporal bone in children, it most commonly occurs as a complication of acute or chronic otitis media, but it may also be idiopathic (Bell palsy) or the result of temporal bone fracture or neoplasm or, on rare occasions, herpes zoster oticus. Other signs and symptoms of conditions that may be associated with ear disease may also be present, e.g., symptoms of upper respiratory allergy associated with otitis media.

12.39 DIAGNOSTIC METHODS

Adequate examination of the entire child, with special attention to the head and neck, can lead to the identification of a condition which may predispose to or be associated with ear disease. The appearance of the child's face and the character of his speech may be important clues to the possibility of his or her having an abnormal ear. Many of the craniofacial anomalies, e.g., mandibulofacial dysostosis (Treacher-Collins syndrome) and trisomy 21 (Down syndrome), are associated with disorders of the ear. Mouth breathing and hyponasality may indicate intranasal or postnasal obstruction, while hypernasality is a sign of velopharyngeal insufficiency. Examination of the oropharyngeal cavity may uncover an overt cleft palate or a submucous cleft, both of which conditions predispose the infant to otitis media with effusion. A bifid uvula is also associated with an increased incidence of middle ear disease. Examination may also reveal posterior nasal or pharyngeal inflammation and discharge. Polyposis, severe deviation of the nasal septum, or a nasopharyngeal tumor may also be associated with otitis media.

Examination of the ear itself is the most critical part of the assessment of the patient. The auricle and external auditory meatus should be examined first as the presence or absence of signs of infection in these areas may aid later in the differential diagnosis or evaluation of complications of otitis media. For instance, eczematoid external otitis may result from acute otitis media with discharge, or inflammation of the postauricular area may be indicative of a periosteitis or subperiosteal abscess which has extended from the mastoid air cells.

The otoscopic examination, the most important part of physical assessment, is then undertaken. However, before adequate visualization of the external canal and tympanic membrane is possible, obstructing cerumen must be removed from the canal either with an otoscope with a surgical head and a wire loop or a blunt cerumen curette or by gentle irrigation of the canal with warm water. In the newborn the external canal is filled with vernix caseosa, which disappears shortly after birth.

Proper assessment of the tympanic membrane and its mobility is accomplished by use of the *pneumatic otoscope*. Assessment of the light reflex is of limited value. The normal tympanic membrane should be in the neutral position, in contrast to a drum that is bulging. The latter condition may be due to increased middle ear air pressure, an effusion within the middle ear, or both; the visualization of the malleus handle and short process is obscured by a bulging drum. Retraction of the tympanic membrane usually indicates the presence of middle ear negative pressure; however,

it may also result from previous disease and subsequent fixation of the ossicles and ligaments. When retraction is present, the short process of the malleus is prominent and the long process is foreshortened.

The normal tympanic membrane has a ground glass appearance; a blue or yellow color usually indicates a middle ear effusion. A red membrane may not alone indicate pathology since the blood vessels of the drum head may be engorged as the result of crying, sneezing, or blowing the nose. The normal tympanic membrane is also translucent: the observer should be able to look through the drum and visualize the middle ear landmarks—incudostapedial joint, promontory, round window niche, and frequently the chorda tympani nerve. If a middle ear effusion is present medial to a translucent drum, an air-fluid level or bubbles of air mixed with the fluid may be visible. Inability to visualize the middle ear structures indicates opacification of the drum, which is usually the result of thickening of the tympanic membrane, a middle ear effusion, or both.

Abnormal middle ear pressure is reflected in the pattern of tympanic membrane mobility when first positive and then negative pressure is applied to the external canal, using a pneumatic otoscope. Pressure is applied by first obtaining an adequate seal between the external auditory canal and the ear speculum and then applying slight pressure on the rubber bulb (positive pressure) followed by release of the bulb (negative pressure). The presence of a liquid or abnormal pressure (positive or negative) within the middle ear can markedly restrict the movement of the eardrum; it will not move at all when the middle ear–mastoid cavity is completely filled with a liquid.

Aspiration of the middle ear is the definitive method of verifying the presence and type of a middle ear effusion. Diagnostic tympanocentesis is performed by inserting, through the inferior portion of the tympanic membrane, an 18-gauge spinal needle attached to a syringe. Alcohol cleansing and culturing of the ear canal should precede tympanocentesis and culture of the middle ear aspirate. The canal culture helps to determine whether cultured organisms are contaminants from the external canal or pathogens from the middle ear.

Tympanometry with an electroacoustic impedance bridge can be helpful in identifying middle ear effusions, disarticulation or fixation of the ossicular chain, and other pathology that cannot be definitively diagnosed with an otoscope. Tympanometry is also useful when the otoscopic diagnosis is equivocal or difficult to obtain and is valuable in screening for otitis media with effusion. *Audiometry* measures hearing. Usually, in patients older than 2–3 yr of age, behavioral audiometry, which is a subjective assessment of hearing, is possible; in the young infant or in children who are difficult to test, objective audiometry is necessary (e.g., auditory brainstem response audiometry or the acoustic reflex obtained with an electroacoustic impedance bridge) (Sec 2.77). *Roentgenographic assessment* of the ear and temporal bone is frequently helpful. When the tympanic membrane is not intact (as a result of perforation or insertion of a tympanostomy tube), *assessment of the ventilatory function of the eustachian tube* by pressure-flow studies may be an additional diagnostic aid. *Assessment of labyrinthine function* is essential in evaluation of a child with a vestibular disorder (Chapter 21).

12.40   CONGENITAL MALFORMATIONS

The external and middle ear, which are derived from the 1st and 2nd branchial arches and grooves, continue to grow through puberty, but the inner ear, which develops from the otocyst, reaches adult size and shape by the middle of fetal development. Malformed external and middle ears may be associated with serious renal anomalies, mandibulofacial dysostosis, and many other craniofacial malformations. Severely deformed external and middle ears may be associated with malformations of the inner ear.

Severe malformations of the external ear are rare, but minor deformities are common. A pitlike cutaneous depression just in front of the helix and above the tragus may represent a cyst or an epidermis-lined fistulous tract; these are common but do not require surgical removal unless they become recurrently infected. Accessory skin tags on narrow pedicles about the ear may be removed by ligation, but if the pedicle is broad-based or contains cartilage, the defect should be corrected surgically. The unusually prominent or "lop" ear is the result of a lack of bending of the cartilage that creates the antihelix; it may be improved cosmetically by otoplasty after the auricle has sufficiently developed (at about the age of 5 yr). Microtia includes cases of rudimentary auricles which, besides being abnormally small in size, are often more anterior and inferior in placement than normal auricles. In rare instances the auricle may be totally absent (anotia).

Congenital stenosis or atresia of the external auditory canal may be associated with malformation of the auricle and middle ear. Audiometric, tympanometric, and roentgenographic assessment are essential in the diagnosis and management of these conditions. Reconstructive middle ear surgery for atresia is restricted to patients (1) above 5 yr of age, (2) with bilateral deformities or unilateral lesions in which there is a deformity only of the middle ear ossicles, resulting in a significant conductive hearing loss, (3) with significant bilateral conductive hearing loss, (4) with roentgenographic evidence of an adequate middle ear cleft and mastoid, and (5) with a normally positioned facial nerve. A congenital perilymphatic fistula of the oval or round window membrane may present as rapid onset, fluctuating, or progressive sensorineural hearing loss with or without vertigo and should be repaired to prevent possible spread of infection from the middle ear to the labyrinth, hearing loss, or both.

Congenital malformations of the inner ear are rare but usually result in severe sensorineural hearing loss. The bony deformities are frequently associated with central nervous system malformations.

Congenital cholesteatoma is a congenital rest of epithelial tissue that may appear as a white cystlike structure medial to an intact tympanic membrane. It is unrelated to infections of the middle ear and should be surgically removed promptly since it will invariably enlarge and cause irreversible structural change.

12.41   INFLAMMATORY DISEASES

External Otitis

In the infant the outer two thirds of the ear canal is cartilaginous and the inner one third bony, whereas in the older child and adult only the outer one third is cartilaginous. The highly viscid secretions of the sebaceous glands and the watery, pigmented secretions of the apocrine glands in the outer portion of the canal combine with exfoliated surface cells of the skin to form a protective, waxy, water-repellent coating. The normal flora of the external canal consists of *Staphylococcus epidermidis*, *Corynebacterium* (diphtheroids), *Micrococcus sp.*, and occasionally *Staphylococcus aureus* and *Streptococcus viridans*. Excessive wetness (swimming, bathing, or increased environmental humidity) or dryness (previous infection, dermatoses, or insufficient cerumen) and trauma (digital or foreign body) make the skin of the canal vulnerable to infection. Once the preinflammatory stage has been set, endogenous bacteria assume pathogenic characteristics or virulent exogenous bacteria may propagate in the canal.

Etiology. External otitis is most commonly caused by *Pseudomonas aeruginosa*, *Enterobacter aerogenes*, *Proteus mirabilis*, *Klebsiella pneumoniae*, streptococci and *S. epidermidis*, and fungi such as *Candida* and *Aspergillus*. The condition known as "swimmer's ear" results from loss of protective cerumen and chronic irritation and maceration from excessive moisture in the canal, with *Pseudomonas sp.* being the most common bacteria isolated. The viral infections involving the auricle and canal are primarily herpesvirus hominis and varicella-zoster.

Clinical Manifestations. The predominant symptom in diffuse otitis externa is pain in the ear, accentuated by manipulation of the pinna and especially by pressure on the tragus. The severity of the pain and tenderness may be out of proportion to the apparent degree of inflammation since the skin of the external ear canal is attached to the perichondrium and periosteum. Itching is a frequent precurser of the pain and is usually characteristic of chronic inflammation of the canal. Conductive hearing loss may be present as a result of edema of the skin and tympanic membrane, serous or purulent secretions, or the progressive meatal skin thickening associated with longstanding external otitis. Edema of the canal, erythema, and greenish otorrhea make up the prominent signs of the acute disease.

Frequently, the canal is so tender and swollen that adequate visualization of the entire ear canal and tympanic membrane is not possible, in which instance complete otoscopic examination should be withheld until the acute swelling subsides. If the tympanic membrane can be visualized, it may be either normal or opaque in appearance, mobility of the drum may be normal or, when the drum is thickened, reduced to both applied positive and negative pressure.

Periauricular edema and fever often result from a combined infection with *Pseudomonas sp.* and *Streptococcus pyogenes* or from *S. aureus*. When there is such secondary infection, lymphadenitis, with tender nodes anterior to the tragus or in the postauricular region, may also occur.

Differential Diagnosis. Diffuse external otitis may be confused with furunculosis, otitis media, and mastoiditis. A furuncle usually causes a localized swelling of the canal limited to 1 quadrant, whereas acute diffuse external otitis is associated with concentric swelling. In otitis media, the eardrum may be perforated, severely retracted, or bulging and immobile, and hearing is usually impaired. Pain on manipulation of the auricle and lymphadenitis are not features of middle ear disease. In some patients with acute diffuse external otitis, the periauricular edema is so extensive that the auricle is pushed forward, creating a condition that could be confused with acute mastoiditis with subperiosteal abscess; however, in mastoiditis the postauricular fold is obliterated, while in external otitis the fold is maintained. In addition, when the edema over the mastoid process is due to mastoiditis, there is usually a history of otitis media and hearing loss, and tenderness is noted over the mastoid antrum or tip and not upon movement of the auricle, as in external otitis. Sagging of the posterior external canal wall may also be present with acute mastoiditis.

Treatment. Topical otic preparations containing neomycin (active against gram-positive organisms and also some gram-negative organisms, notably *Proteus sp.*) with either colistin or polymyxin (active against gram-negative bacilli, notably *Pseudomonas sp.*) and corticosteroids are effective in the treatment of most forms· of acute diffuse external otitis. In marked canal edema a cotton or selvedged-gauze wick should be inserted into the outer third of the ear canal and the medication applied as frequently as possible for 24–48 hr; the wick can then be removed and the otic medication instilled 3–4 times a day. Acetic acid preparations (2%), with or without corticosteroids, or half-strength Burow solution (aluminum acetate, 1:20) are probably equally effective. When the pain is severe, analgesics (salicylates, codeine) and dry heat may be necessary.

As the inflammatory process subsides, cleaning the canal with cotton-tipped applicators or, more effectively, irrigation with 2% acetic acid to remove the debris will enhance the effectiveness of the topical medications. In subacute and chronic infections, periodic cleansing of the canal is essential. In severe, acute, diffuse external otitis associated with fever and lymphadenitis from which sensitive bacteria have been cultured, oral and, on occasion, parenteral antibotics are indicated; the choice of drug depends upon the antibiotic susceptibility of the organism. A fungal infection (otomycosis) of the external auditory canal may be treated by application of metacresylacetate. Prevention of diffuse external otitis may be necessary in those individuals susceptible to recurrent bouts, especially in children who swim frequently. The most effective prophylaxis is instillation of dilute alcohol or acetic acid immediately following swimming or bathing.

Furunculosis is due to *S. aureus* and is seen only in the hair-containing outer third of the ear canal. It is treated with incision and drainage and systemic penicillin or one of the penicillinase-resistant penicillins, depending upon the antibiotic susceptibility of the organism.

Acute cellulitis may invade the auricle and external auditory canal and is usually caused by *S. pyogenes*, occasionally by *S. aureus*. The skin is red, hot, and indurated without a sharply defined border. Fever may be present with little or no exudate in the canal. Parenteral administration of penicillin G or a penicillinase-resistant penicillin is the therapy of choice.

Dermatoses (seborrheic, contact, infectious eczematoid, atopic, or neurodermatoid) are common causes of inflammation of the external canal and can be precursors of acute diffuse external otitis due to scratching and the introduction of infecting organisms. *Seborrheic dermatitis* is characterized by the presence of greasy scales which flake and crumble as they are detached from the epidermis; associated changes in the scalp, forehead, cheeks, brow, postauricular areas, and the concha are usual. *Contact dermatitis* may be caused by topical otic medications such as neomycin, polymyxin, and colistin, which may produce erythema, vesiculation, edema, and weeping. Poison ivy, oak, and sumac may also be responsible for this type of dermatitis. *Infectious eczematoid dermatitis* is caused by a purulent infection of the external canal, middle ear, or mastoid; the purulent drainage infects the skin of the canal, auricle, or both. The lesion is weeping, erythematous, or crusted. *Atopic dermatitis* occurs in children with familial or personal histories of allergy; the auricle, particularly the postauricular fold, becomes thickened, scaly, and excoriated. *Neurodermatitis* is recognized by the intense itching and erythematous, thickened epidermis localized to the concha and orifice of the meatus. Treatment of these dermatoses depends on the type but should include application of the aural medication described for external otitis, elimination of the source of infection or contactant when identified, and management of any underlying dermatologic problem.

Herpes simplex may appear as vesicles on the auricle and lips, which eventually become encrusted and dry up, and may be confused with impetigo. Topical application of a 10% solution of carbamide peroxide in anhydrous glycerol is symptomatically helpful.

Herpes zoster oticus (Ramsay Hunt syndrome) is a vesicular eruption on the posterior canal wall with facial paralysis. Spontaneous recovery is usual.

Bullous myringitis is commonly associated with an acute upper respiratory infection. The ear is very painful, and there are hemorrhagic or serous blebs on the membrane. The disease is difficult to differentiate from acute otitis media since early in the course of acute otitis the drum may appear to have bullae. The organisms involved are probably the same as those causing an acute middle ear effusion. Treatment consists of antibiotic therapy of the type usually given for acute otitis media. Incision of the bullae, although not necessary, will promptly relieve the pain.

Otitis Media

Inflammation of the middle ear, or otitis media, is the most prevalent disease of childhood after respiratory tract infections. Acute or chronic otitis media with effusion is frequent, and the complications and sequelae of otitis media represent significant health hazards in children. Acute otitis media is usually thought of as being suppurative or purulent, but serous effusions may also have an acute onset. There are many terms for chronic otitis media with effusion, such as serous, secretory, catarrhal, mucoid, nonsuppurative, or allergic otitis media. It is often difficult to determine the specific variety without a diagnostic aspiration of the middle ear effusion.

Epidemiology and Pathogenesis. Infants and young children appear to be at highest risk for otitis media; incidence rates are 15–20%, with peaks occurring from 6–36 mo and 4–6 yr of age. Children who develop otitis media with effusion in the 1st years of life have an increased risk of recurrent acute or chronic disease. A study of 2565 children followed for the 1st 3 yr of life found that only 29% of infants failed to develop at least 1 attack of otitis media, whereas about 33% had 3 or more episodes. In addition, after the 1st episode, 40% of children had a middle ear effusion that persisted for 4 wk and 10% had an effusion which was still present at 3 mo. The incidence of the disease tends to decrease as a function of age after the age of 6 yr. The incidence is high in males, lower socioeconomic groups, Alaskan natives, American Indians, and children with cleft palate and other craniofacial anomalies and higher in Whites than in Blacks. The incidence is also higher in winter and early spring.

The eustachian tube protects the middle ear from nasopharyngeal secretions, provides drainage into the nasopharynx of secretions produced within the middle ear, and permits equilibration of air pressure with atmospheric pressure in the middle ear with replenishment of the oxygen which has been absorbed. Mechanical or functional obstruction of the eustachian tube can result in middle ear effusion. Intrinsic mechanical obstruction can result from infection or allergy and extrinsic obstruction from obstructive adenoids or nasopharyngeal tumors. Persistent collapse of the eustachian tube during swallowing can result in functional obstruction related to decreased tubal stiffness or an inefficient active opening mechanism. Functional obstruction is common in infants and younger children since the amount and stiffness of the cartilage support of the tube are less than in older children and adults; marked age differences in the craniofacial base render the tensor veli palatini muscle (the only active opener of the tube) less efficient prior to puberty. All infants with unrepaired palatal clefts have chronic otitis media with effusion due to functional obstruction of the eustachian tube.

Eustachian tube obstruction results in negative middle ear pressure and, if persistent, in a sterile transudative middle ear effusion. Drainage of the effusion is inhibited by impairment of the mucociliary transport system and sustained negative pressure. When the eustachian tube is not mechanically totally obstructed, contamination of the middle ear space from nasopharyngeal secretions may occur by reflux (especially when the tympanic membrane has a perforation or when a tympanostomy tube is present), by aspiration (from high negative middle ear pressure), or by insufflation during crying, nose blowing, sneezing, and swallowing when the nose is obstructed. Rapid alterations in am-

bient pressure or barotrauma during deep water diving or flying can also result in acute middle ear effusion which may be hemorrhagic.

Acute Otitis Media

Clinical Manifestations. In the usual course a child suffering an upper respiratory infection for several days suddenly develops otalgia, fever, and hearing loss. Examination with the pneumatic otoscope reveals a hyperemic, opaque, bulging tympanic membrane of poor mobility. Purulent otorrhea may be present. However, earache and fever are not invariably present. Children with diminished or absent mobility and opacification of the tympanic membrane should be suspected of having bacterial otitis media with effusion. Any child with a "fever of undetermined origin" must also be evaluated for a middle ear infection.

Diagnosis. When the diagnosis of acute otitis media is in doubt or identification of the causative agent is desirable, aspiration of the middle ear should be performed. Tympanocentesis should also be considered for children who are seriously ill or appear toxic; for unsatisfactory response to antibiotic therapy; for onset of otitis media in a patient who is receiving antibiotic agents; for suppurative aural, intratemporal, or intracranial complications; and for otitis in the newborn, the very young infant, or the immunologically deficient patient, in each of whom unusual organisms may cause infection.

Treatment. Therapy depends upon the bacterial cause of the disease and sensitivity testing. *S. pneumoniae* has been cultured from at least 40% of the effusions and is the most common causative agent in all age groups; *Hemophilus influenzae* causes approximately 20% of cases, but this proportion declines with increasing age; group A beta-hemolytic streptococcus, *S. aureus*, and *Branhamella catarrhalis* each account for about 5%. In about 25% of cases the effusion is sterile. In neonates approximately 20% of effusions may contain gram-negative enteric bacilli. Since the causative organism is rarely known before starting therapy, oral ampicillin, 50–100 mg/kg/24 hr in 4 divided doses for 10 days, is recommended as it is usually effective against the 2 most commonly encountered bacteria. Amoxicillin, 20–40 mg/kg/24 hr, is equally effective and can be given in 3 divided doses. An increasing percentage of *H. influenzae* strains have become beta-lactamase producing and therefore ampicillin-resistant. When a resistant organism is cultured from a middle ear aspirate or when the patient fails to improve clinically after initial treatment with ampicillin or amoxicillin (probably because of an ampicillin-resistant *H. influenzae*) and if a tympanocentesis/myringotomy is not performed, the initial antimicrobial should be changed. Erythromycin, 50 mg/kg/24 hr, in combination with a sulfonamide (100 mg/kg/24 hr of triple sulfonamides or 150 mg/kg/24 hr of sulfisoxazole) in 4 divided doses, or trimethoprim-sulfamethoxazole, 8–40 mg/kg/24 hr in 2 divided doses, or cefaclor, 40 mg/kg/24 hr in 3 divided doses, may be appropriate choices. If the patient is allergic to the penicillins, the combination of oral erythromycin and triple sulfonamides or sulfisoxazole is an alternative.

The combination of trimethoprim and sulfamethoxazole also can be given initially to penicillin-sensitive individuals, but its effectiveness in the treatment of acute otitis media due to *S. pyogenes* is uncertain.

Additional supportive therapy, including analgesics, antipyretics, and local heat, is usually helpful. Meperidine hydrochloride may also be required for sedation. An oral decongestant, pseudoephedrine hydrochloride, may relieve some nasal congestion, and antihistamines may help patients with known or suspected nasal allergy. However, the efficacy of antihistamines and decongestants in the treatment of acute otitis media has not been proved.

No patient should be considered cured until there has been complete resolution of both symptoms and signs of otitis media. If the patient continues to have appreciable pain or fever or both after 24–48 hr, tympanocentesis and myrinogotomy should be performed as diagnostic and therapeutic procedures. In patients with unusually severe earache, myringotomy may be performed initially to provide immediate relief. When therapeutic drainage is required, a myringotomy knife should be used and the incision should be large enough to allow for adequate drainage of the middle ear.

All patients should be re-evaluated approximately 2 wk after the institution of treatment, when there should be some otoscopic evidence of resolution, such as decrease in inflammation and return of mobility of the tympanic membrane. However, complete clearing of the effusion may take 6 wk or longer. Within 2–3 mo the tympanic membrane should be entirely normal. Periodic follow-up is indicated for patients who have had recurrent episodes. If the middle ear fluid is persistent, the patient should be treated as described below under Chronic Otitis Media with Effusion.

Recurrent Acute Otitis Media

It is not uncommon for an infant to have recurrent bouts of acute otitis media. Some children develop an acute episode with almost every respiratory tract infection, have more or less dramatic symptoms, respond well to therapy, and have fewer episodes with advancing age. Others have persistent middle ear effusion and suffer recurrent episodes of acute otitis media superimposed on the chronic disorder. The child with recurrent acute otitis media who completely clears between episodes may be managed as previously outlined. However, if the bouts are frequent and close together, further treatment similar to that described for patients with chronic otitis media with effusion is indicated. In many of these children the underlying cause is not evident, but myringotomy with insertion of middle ear ventilation tubes is frequently helpful. Prophylactic antibiotics (a daily dose of amoxicillin or sulfonamides) have been advocated as an alternative to myringotomy and ventilating tubes in children with recurrent acute otitis media who are free of effusion between attacks. The preventive efficacies of myringotomy with tympanotomy tube insertion, chemoprophylaxis, hyposensitization, and adenoidectomy are not established.

Chronic Otitis Media with Effusion

Chronic middle ear effusions may be serous (thin), mucoid (thick), or purulent in character. Frequently either a retracted or convex tympanic membrane is seen. The membrane is usually opaque, but when it is translucent, an air-fluid level or air bubbles may be seen and an amber or sometimes bluish fluid may be apparent in the middle ear. The mobility of the ear drum is almost always impaired. Occasionally, even when there is no effusion, the tympanic membrane is retracted and its mobility impaired, usually because of negative middle ear air pressure, which, when extreme, is termed "atelectasis of the tympanic membrane." The auditory acuity is usually decreased, and, although systemic symptoms are usually absent, there may be behavioral disturbances due to the child's inability to communicate adequately. A feeling of fullness in the ear, tinnitus, and even vertigo may be present. Audiometry may be helpful in establishing the diagnosis but is not reliable because some patients, even with thick middle ear effusions, have fairly good hearing. Tympanometry is more reliable.

A patient with chronic otitis media with effusion who has not received prior antibiotic therapy should be treated initially as a case of acute otitis media since bacteria are frequently present. However, the efficacy of antibiotics, decongestants, antihistamines, and corticosteroids has not been established. Occasionally, attempts at middle ear inflation by the Valsalva or Politzer method are successful. In most children the effusions are self-limited. If the effusion persists for 3 mo or longer or if there have been frequent recurrences of episodes of acute otitis media, the patient requires further evaluation for respiratory allergy, adenoid tissue obstructing the nose and nasopharynx, an immunologic disorder (if other organs are involved), or abnormalities such as submucous cleft palate or a tumor of the nasopharynx.

For patients in whom medical management (including a trial with an appropriate antibiotic) has failed, myringotomy with aspiration of the middle ear fluid is indicated if the effusion has persisted for 3 mo. Frequently, insertion of a ventilation or tympanostomy tube may be necessary to allow the middle ear mucous membrane to return to normal and to prevent subsequent accumulation of effusion. Myringotomy and insertion of ventilation tubes may also be helpful in patients with atelectasis of the tympanic membrane when pain, hearing loss, vertigo, or tinnitus is present. Ventilation tubes may prevent permanent structural damage and cholesteatoma if a deep retraction pocket develops in the posterosuperior quadrant or in the attic (pars flaccida) portion of the tympanic membrane. Occasionally, troublesome otorrhea develops after the insertion of tympanostomy tubes, which can usually be treated successfully with ear drops containing neomycin, polymyxin, or colistin with hydrocortisone. Since these medications may be ototoxic, some physicians advocate the use of systemic antibiotics without the aural drops. In selected cases allergic hyposensitization and adenoidectomy may be beneficial; the efficacy of these has not been fully assessed. Tonsillectomy has not been shown to alter the course of otitis of any type and should not be performed for these conditions.

Complications and Sequelae of Otitis Media

The intracranial suppurative complications of otitis media are relatively uncommon except in neglected cases. However, those that occur within the aural cavity and adjacent structures of the temporal bone are more common, and awareness of them is essential in management of children with otitis media. The aural and intratemporal complications and sequelae of otitis media are hearing loss, perforation of the tympanic membrane with or without suppuration, acquired cholesteatoma, mastoiditis, petrositis, adhesive otitis media, tympanosclerosis, ossicular discontinuity, facial paralysis, and labyrinthitis.

Hearing loss is the most prevalent complication and morbid outcome of otitis media and may be caused by 1 or more of the intratemporal complications. To a varying degree, fluctuating or persistent loss of hearing is usually associated with acute or chronic middle ear effusions or high negative pressure within the middle ear in the absence of an effusion. The audiogram usually reveals a mild to moderate conductive loss. However, there may be a sensorineural component, generally attributed to the effect of increased tension and stiffness of the round window membrane. This hearing loss is usually reversible with resolution of the effusion, but permanent conductive hearing loss can result from irreversible changes secondary to recurrent acute or chronic inflammation, e.g., adhesive otitis, tympanosclerosis, or ossicular discontinuity. Irreparable sensorineural loss may also occur, presumably as the result of spread of infection through the round or oval window membrane. Although persistent or episodic conductive hearing loss may result in impairment of cognitive, language, and emotional development of children, the degree and duration of the hearing loss required to produce such deficits have not been defined (Sec 2.77).

Perforation of the tympanic membrane most frequently occurs with spontaneous rupture of the central portion of the eardrum during a bout of acute otitis media. If persistent purulent otorrhea follows, a culture should be obtained, if possible from the middle ear, and appropriate antibiotics administered. Antibiotic-cortisone otic medication may also be helpful. Healing of the tympanic membrane frequently follows cessation of the suppurative process. A central perforation that fails to heal spontaneously despite a dry middle ear and good eustachian tube function may be closed with a graft, tympanoplasty. However, if the otorrhea persists or if the drainage seems to be coming from an apparent posterosuperior or attic (pars flaccida) defect, then a cholesteatoma should be suspected. Aural polyps, which appear as red friable masses, may protrude through one of these defects, indicating the presence of a cholesteatoma. **Chronic suppurative otitis media with mastoiditis** may also be associated with a perforation or a cholesteatoma in which there is a persistent or episodic purulent discharge; the most common pathogenic organisms are the gram-negative bacilli, e.g., *Bacillus proteus* and *P. aeruginosa*.

Acquired cholesteatoma is a saclike structure lined by keratinized, stratified, squamous epithelium with accumulation of desquamating epithelium or keratin within the middle ear. White, shiny, greasy debris accompanied by a foul-smelling discharge may be observed. Tympanomastoid surgery is indicated, and if it is delayed, the disease can invade and destroy other structures of the temporal bone and spread to the intracranial cavity.

Mastoiditis or inflammation of the mastoid air cell system frequently accompanies acute and chronic otitis media with effusion. Roentgenographic examination reveals a cloudy mastoid. The process is usually reversible as the effusion resolves with appropriate medical management. Occasionally, a severe acute otitis media is accompanied by mastoiditis in which there is pain, tenderness, edema, and erythema of the postauricular area. The pinna is displaced inferiorly and anteriorly, and swelling or sagging of the posterosuperior canal wall may also be present; this is the stage of mastoid periostitis. It requires immediate tympanocentesis, myringotomy, and systemic ampicillin, with possible later adjustment of medication according to the antibiotic susceptibility of the organism. If the condition progresses to the stage of rarefying osteitis, the infectious process may break through the cortex of the mastoid to form a subperiosteal abscess. The infection may also break through the mastoid tip into the neck (Bezold abscess) or fistulize into the external ear canal. When osteitis is present, mastoid surgery is required to prevent further intratemporal or intracranial complications. **Petrositis** may result from acute or chronic infections of the pneumatized apical and perilabyrinthine cells of the temporal bone. The triad of otitis media with effusion, paralysis of the external rectus muscle, and pain in the homolateral orbit or retro-orbital area with headache constitutes petrous apicitis, i.e., *Gradenigo syndrome*.

Adhesive otitis is the result of healing reaction following chronic inflammation of the middle ear. The mucous membrane is thickened by proliferation of fibrous tissue, which frequently impairs the movement of the ossicles and thus results in an irreversible conductive hearing loss. **Tympanosclerosis** is a complication of chronic middle ear inflammation characterized by the presence of whitish plaques in the tympanic membrane and nodular deposits in the submucosal layers of the middle ear. There is hyalinization with deposition of calcium and phosphate crystals, and conductive hearing loss may result from the ossicles imbedding in the deposits. Prevention is the only successful means of controlling this disease and adhesive otitis media. **Ossicular discontinuity** is the result of rarefying osteitis secondary to chronic middle ear inflammation. The long process of the incus is commonly involved, but the crural arch of the stapes, the body of the incus, or the manubrium of the malleus may also be eroded. The conductive hearing loss that frequently results can be corrected surgically.

Facial paralysis may occur during an episode of acute otitis media because of exposure of the facial nerve from a congenital bony dehiscence within the middle ear. When it occurs as an isolated complication, a myringotomy should be performed and parenteral antibiotics administered. The paralysis will usually improve rapidly without requiring further surgery (i.e., facial nerve decompression). Mastoidectomy is not indicated unless mastoid osteitis is present. However, immediate surgical intervention is indicated when a facial paralysis develops in a child who has chronic suppurative otitis media with or without cholesteatoma.

Suppurative labyrinthitis may occur during an episode of acute otitis media from the direct invasion of bacteria through the round or oval windows. When chronic otitis media is present, the infection may penetrate the windows or enter through a pathologic fistula of the bony horizontal semicircular canal. There may be vertigo, nystagmus, tinnitus, hearing loss, nausea, and vomiting. Treatment consists of intensive parenteral antibiotic therapy; however, labyrinthectomy may be indicated to prevent spread to the intracranial cavity.

The **intracranial suppurative complications** of acute and chronic otitis media are meningitis, focal encephalitis, brain abscess, sinus thrombophlebitis, extradural abscess, subdural abscess, and otitic hydrocephalus. These complications occur more often in association with chronic suppurative otitis and mastoiditis, with or without cholesteatoma, than with acute otitis media. Infection spreads from the middle ear and mastoid to the intracranial structures by vascular channels (osteothrombophlebitis), direct extension (osteitis), or preformed pathways: for instance, round window, previous skull fracture, and congenital or surgically acquired bony dehiscences. Any child with an acute or chronic otitis media who develops 1 or more of the following signs or symptoms, especially while receiving medical treatment, should be suspected of having a suppurative intracranial complication: persistent headache, severe otalgia, onset of fever, nausea, vomiting, stiff neck, focal seizures, ataxia, blurred vision, hemiplegia, intention tremor, papilledema, diplopia, pastpointing, dysdiadochokinesia, aphasia, or hemianopsia. Conversely, children with intracranial infection (recurrent meningitis or brain abscess) should have middle ear–mastoid disease ruled out as the origin.

Inner Ear

The inner ear may be affected by viral or bacterial infections. Congenital rubella, cytomegalovirus, and mumps are causes of severe sensorineural deafness. Labyrinthitis may result as a complication of acute or chronic otitis media and mastoiditis but also may follow bacterial meningitis as a result of organisms entering the labyrinth through the internal auditory meatus, the endolymphatic duct, vascular channels, or the perilymphatic duct.

12.42 TRAUMATIC INJURIES OF THE EAR AND TEMPORAL BONE

Auricle and External Auditory Canal

Hematoma, or accumulation of blood between the perichondrium and the cartilage, may follow trauma to the pinna. Immediate needle aspiration or, when the

hematoma is extensive, incision and drainage and a pressure dressing are necessary to prevent perichondritis, which can result in a **cauliflower ear** deformity. **Frostbite** of the auricle should be managed by rapidly rewarming the exposed pinna with warm irrigations or warm compresses. **Foreign bodies** in the external canal are a common occurrence in childhood; removal can usually be accomplished without general anesthesia: (1) if the child is informed of the procedure (if old enough to understand it), (2) if the child is properly restrained, (3) when an adequate headlight or surgical head otoscope is used for visualization of the object, and (4) when an alligator forceps, wire loop, or blunt cerumen curette is used, depending on the shape of the object. Irrigation is sometimes helpful. General anesthesia and the otomicroscope are necessary for the more difficult foreign bodies, especially those that are deeply imbedded in the canal just lateral to the tympanic membrane. Following removal of an external canal foreign body, the tympanic membrane should be carefully inspected for possible traumatic perforation or a pre-existing middle ear effusion. If the foreign body has resulted in acute inflammation of the canal, treatment as described for acute diffuse external otitis should be instituted.

Tympanic Membrane and Middle Ear

Traumatic perforation of the tympanic membrane in children usually occurs as the result of either a sudden external compression (e.g., a slap) or penetration by a foreign object (e.g., a stick or cotton-tipped applicator). The perforation may be either linear or stellate and is most frequently in the anterior portion of the pars tensa when the result of compression; it may be in any quadrant of the tympanic membrane when caused by a foreign object. Spontaneous healing usually occurs, but if the drum does not heal within 2–3 mo, tympanoplastic surgery is indicated. Systemic antibiotics and topical otic medications are not required unless suppurative otorrhea is present. However, otorrhea may occur at any time during periods of upper respiratory tract infection since the middle ear air cushion is lost, permitting reflux of nasopharyngeal secretions into the middle ear cavity. Perforations resulting from penetrating foreign bodies are less likely to heal than those caused by compression. Implantation of epithelium from a traumatic perforation of the tympanic membrane can result in a cholesteatoma.

Immediate surgical exploration is indicated if the injury is accompanied by 1 or more of the following: vertigo, nystagmus, severe tinnitus, moderate to severe hearing loss, or cerebrospinal fluid otorrhea. Exploratory tympanotomy is necessary to inspect the ossicles, especially the stapes, which may have been dislocated.

Perilymphatic fistula may occur following sudden barotrauma or increase in cerebrospinal fluid pressure. This condition is probably more common than generally appreciated and should always be suspected in a child who develops a sudden or fluctuating sensorineural hearing loss or vertigo or both following physical exertion, deep water diving, flying in an airplane, playing a wind instrument, or any other activity that suddenly increases the pressures within the middle ear or the intracranial-labyrinthine system. Characteristically, the leak is either at the oval or the round window, which may be congenitally abnormal, and immediate repair of the fistula is essential since the hearing loss may become irreversible.

Temporal Bone Fractures

Children are particularly prone to basilar skull fractures, which usually involve the temporal bone. Most temporal bone fractures are longitudinal and are commonly manifested by bleeding from a laceration of the external canal and tympanic membrane or, if the drum is intact, by a hemotympanum; conductive hearing loss resulting from the laceration of the tympanic membrane, hemotympanum, or ossicular injury; delayed onset of facial paralysis (which usually improves spontaneously); and temporary cerebrospinal fluid otorrhea. Transverse fractures of the temporal bone have a graver prognosis than longitudinal fractures and are associated with immediate facial paralysis, which may not improve without surgical intervention; severe sensorineural hearing loss, vertigo, nystagmus, tinnitus, nausea, and vomiting associated with complete loss of cochlear and vestibular function; hemotypanum and, rarely, external canal bleeding; and cerebrospinal otorrhea, seen either in the external auditory canal or behind the tympanic membrane, which may come through the nose via the eustachian tube.

Vigorous removal of external auditory canal blood clots, tympanocentesis, and application of otic preparations are not indicated, but prophylactic parenteral administration of antibiotics when cerebrospinal otorrhea is present has been advocated. Surgical intervention is reserved for those children who require tympanoplastic repair of the perforated tympanic membrane (that fails to heal spontaneously) or who have suffered dislocation of the ossicular chain or who need decompression of the facial nerve. Sensorineural hearing loss can also occur following a blow to the head without an obvious fracture of the temporal bone (labyrinthine concussion).

Acoustic trauma results from exposure to high intensity sound (e.g., fireworks, gunfire, rock music) and is manifested by a depression at 4000 Hz on the audiometric examination. The loss may be temporary but may become permanent if the noise exposure is chronic. Avoiding chronic exposure to loud noise and ear protection for unavoidable exposure are preventive measures.

12.43 TUMORS OF THE EAR AND TEMPORAL BONE

Benign tumors of the external canal include osteoma and monostotic and polyostotic fibrous dysplasia. Osteomas present as bony masses in the canal and require removal only if hearing is impaired or external otitis results. *Eosinophilic granuloma* of the middle ear should be suspected when there is otalgia, otorrhea, hearing loss, and roentgenographic findings of a sharply delineated destructive lesion of the temporal bone. *Rhabdomyosarcoma* originating in the middle ear should be considered when there is bleeding from the ear or otorrhea associated with paralysis of the facial nerve. *Reticulum cell sarcoma* and *leukemia* may also present in the middle ear. Although primary neoplasms of the middle ear are relatively uncommon, the initial signs and symptoms of the more common nasopharyngeal neoplasms (e.g., angiofibroma, rhabdomyosarcoma, epidermoid carcinoma) may be associated with the insidious onset of a chronic otitis media with effusion.

12.44 DISEASES OF THE BONY LABYRINTH

Otosclerosis can cause a fixation of the stapes, resulting in progressive hearing loss in older children and teenagers. It is an autosomal dominant disease for which a hearing aid may be necessary. Corrective surgery is more successful and permanent in adults than in children. *Osteogenesis imperfecta* may involve both the middle and inner ears. If the hearing loss is severe enough, a hearing aid is preferable as an alternative to surgical correction of the fixed stapes since the disease is progressive. *Osteoporosis* may involve the middle ear resulting in a moderate to severe hearing loss. A hearing aid may be necessary for rehabilitation.

CHARLES D. BLUESTONE

Special References

American Academy of Otolaryngology, Self-Instruction Package from the Committee on Continuing Education in Otolaryngology. Neely JB: Treatment of the Uncomplicated Aural Cholesteatoma (Keratoma), 1977; Part I, Aural Complications (1978); Part II, Intracranial Complications (1979), Rochester, Minn.

Basser LS: Benign paroxysmal vertigo of childhood (a variety of vestibular neuronitis). Brain 87:141, 1964.

Bergstrom L, Hemenway WG, Downs MP: A high risk registry to find congenital deafness. Otolaryngol Clin North Am 4:369, 1971.

Bluestone CD, Cantekin EI, Beery QC, et al: Function of the eustachian tube related to surgical management of acquired aural cholesteatoma in children. Laryngoscope 88:1155, 1978.

Bluestone CD, Cantekin EI, Douglas GS: Eustachian tube function related to the results of tympanoplasty in children. Laryngoscope 89:450, 1979.

Bluestone CD, Cantekin EI: Eustachian tube dysfunction. In: English GM (ed): Otolaryngology, Vol 1. Hagerstown, Md., Harper and Row, 1980.

Cantekin EI, Beery QC, Bluestone CD: Tympanometric patterns found in middle ear effusions. Ann Otol Rhinol Laryngol, Suppl 41, 86:16, 1977.

Fria TJ: The auditory brainstem response: Background and clinical applications. Monographs in Contemporary Audiology, Educational Publications Division, Maico Hearing Instruments, Minneapolis, Minn., Vol 2, No 2, 1980.

Gates G: Vertigo in children. EENT Journal 59:358, 1980.

Grundfast KM, Bluestone CD: Sudden or fluctuating hearing loss and vertigo in children due to perilymph fistula. Ann Otol Rhinol Laryngol 87:761, 1978.

Harford ER, Bess FH, Bluestone CD, et al: Use of acoustic impedance measurement in screening for middle ear disease in children. Ann Otol Rhinol Laryngol 87:288, 1978.

Hicks TW, Wright JW, Wright JW: Cerebrospinal fluid otorrhea. Laryngoscope, Suppl 25, 90:1, 1980.

Holm VA, Kunze LH: Effect of chronic otitis media on language and speech development. Pediatrics 43:833, 1969.

Hough JVD, Stuart WD: Middle ear injuries in skull trauma. Laryngoscope 78:899, 1968.

Howie VM, Ploussard JH: The "in vivo sensitivity test"—bacteriology of middle ear exudate. Pediatrics 44:940, 1969.

Jahn AJ, Snell GE: Otogenic intracranial complications. J Otolaryngol 9:184, 1980.

Konigsmark BW: Hereditary deafness in man. N Engl J Med 281:713, 774, 827, 1969.

Linthicum FH: Evaluation of the child with sensorineural hearing impairment. Otolaryngol Clin North Am 8:69, 1975.

Makishima K, Sobel SF, Snow JB: Histopathologic correlates of otoneurologic manifestations following head trauma. Laryngoscope 86:1303, 1976.

Manning JT, Adour K: Facial paralysis in children—diagnosis and treatment. Pediatrics 49:102, 1972.

Maynard JE, Fleshman JK, Tschopp CF: Otitis media in Alaskan Eskimo children: Prospective evaluation of chemoprophylaxis. JAMA 219:597, 1972.

Paparella MM, Oda M, Hiraida F, et al: Pathology of sensorineural hearing loss in otitis media. Ann Otol Rhinol Laryngol 81:632, 1972.

Paparella MM, Winter LE: Sensorineural deafness in childhood. Trans AAOO 72:782, 1968.

Paradise JL, Smith C, Bluestone CD: Tympanometric detection of middle ear effusion in infants and young children. Pediatrics 58:198, 1976.

Perrin JM, Charney E, MacWhinney JB Jr, et al: Sulfisoxazole chemoprophylaxis for recurrent otitis media. A double-blind crossover study in pediatric practice. N Engl J Med 291:667, 1974.

Powers WH, Britton BH: Nonotogenic otalgia: Diagnosis and treatment. Am J Otolaryngol 2:97, 1980.

Proctor C: Diagnosis, prevention and treatment of hereditary sensorineural hearing loss. Laryngoscope 87:Suppl 7, 1977.

Pulez JL, Freedman HM: Management of congenital middle ear abnormalities. Laryngoscope 88:420, 1978.

Riding KH, Bluestone CD, Michaels RH, et al: Microbiology of recurrent and chronic otitis media with effusion. J Pediatr 93:739, 1978.

Sarno CN, Clemis JD: A workable approach to the identification of neonatal hearing impairment. Laryngoscope 90:1313, 1980.

Schiff M, Poliquin JF, Catanzaro A, et al: Tympanosclerosis. Ann Otol Rhinol Laryngol Suppl 70, 89:1, 1980.

Schuknecht HF: Mondini dysplasia: A clinical and pathological study. Ann Otol Rhinol Laryngol Suppl 65, 89:1, 1980.

Simmons FB: Patterns of deafness in newborns. Laryngoscope 90:448, 1980.

Suehiro S, Sando I: Congenital anomalies of the inner ear. Ann Otol Rhinol Laryngol Suppl 59, 88:1, 1979.

Valvassori GE, Buckingham RA: Tomography and Cross Sections of the Ear. Philadelphia, WB Saunders, 1975.

General References

Bluestone CD (ed): Workshop on tonsillectomy and adenoidectomy. Ann Otol Rhinol Laryngol, Suppl 19, 1975.

Bluestone CD, Shurin PA: Middle ear disease in children: Pathogenesis, diagnosis and management. Pediatr Clin North Am 21:379, 1974.

Bluestone CD, Stool SE (eds): Pediatric Otolaryngology. Philadelphia, WB Saunders Company, 1981, Chapters 16–18.

Hanson DG, Ulvestad RF (eds): Otitis media and child development: Speech, language, and education. Ann Otol Rhinol Laryngol 88:Suppl 60, 1979.

Northern JL, Downes MP: Hearing in Children, Ed 2. Baltimore, Williams and Wilkins, 1978.

Paparella MM, Shumrick DA: The ear. In: Otolaryngology, Vol II. Ed 2. Philadelphia, WB Saunders, 1980.

Paradise JL: Otitis media in infants and children. Pediatrics 65:917, 1980.

Schuknecht HE: Pathology of the Ear. Cambridge, Mass., Harvard University Press, 1974.

Senturia BH, Bluestone CD, Lim DJ (eds): Recent advances in otitis media with effusion. Ann Otol Rhinol Laryngol 89:Suppl 68, 1980.

Senturia NH, Marcus MD, Lucente FE (eds): Diseases of the External Ear: An Otologic-Dermatologic Manual. Ed. 2. New York, Grune and Stratton, 1980.

Shambaugh GE Jr, Glasscock ME III: Surgery of the Ear. Ed. 3. Philadelphia, WB Saunders, 1980.

Wiet RJ, Coulthard SW: Otitis Media, Proceedings of the Second National Conference on Otitis Media. Columbus, Ohio, Ross Laboratories, 1979.

12.45   Lower Respiratory Tract

CONGENITAL ANOMALIES

12.46   CONGENITAL LARYNGEAL ANOMALIES

Complete **atresia of the larynx** is incompatible with life; only rarely can an infant in whom the diagnosis is made at birth be saved by an immediate tracheostomy. Subsequent successful surgical restoration of a completely functional upper airway has not been reported. Many patients with laryngeal atresia have other congenital defects which also may be incompatible with life. **Laryngeal webs** are uncommon defects which result from incomplete separation of the fetal mesenchyme between the 2 sides of the larynx. Immediate diagnosis is essential if the web is complete or almost complete to prevent asphyxiation of the newborn infant. Respiratory distress with severe stridor may be present and the cry weak and abnormal in character. Often the obstruction is not complete, with only mild stridor and dyspnea. Direct laryngoscopy is required for prompt diagnosis and treatment. Thin supraglottic webs can be incised, but many infants with thicker subglottic or intralaryngeal webs require initial incision, excision, and subsequent dilations, which may be unsuccessful because of reformation of the web. An external approach to divide and excise the web with insertion of silicone or metal is often required. Many patients need a tracheostomy for a prolonged period after surgery.

Laryngotracheoesophageal cleft is a very rare congenital lesion in which there is a long connection between the airway and the esophagus, sometimes extending to the level of the carina. The lesion involves failure of dorsal fusion of the cricoid, which normally is completed by the 8th wk of gestation. Symptoms of chronic aspiration with pneumonia and gagging during feeding are similar to those in H-type tracheoesophageal fistula but are usually more severe and associated with abnormalities in voice. Diagnosis is extremely difficult, but careful roentgenographic studies of swallowing will show aspiration of contrast material into the trachea and indicate the need for endoscopic examination of the airway and perhaps the esophagus. Successful repair has been reported, but prolonged tracheostomy is always necessary.

12.47   CONGENITAL LARYNGEAL STRIDOR
(Laryngomalacia and Tracheomalacia)

Stridor persisting or appearing after the 1st few days of life usually results from disturbances in or adjacent to the larynx. The most common of these, **laryngomalacia** and **tracheomalacia,** are congenital deformities or flabbiness of the epiglottis and supraglottic aperture and weakness of the airway walls, leading to collapse and some airway obstruction with inspiration. Males are affected twice as often as females. The embryologic origin of the defect is unknown.

Clinical Manifestations.   Noisy, crowing respiratory sounds, usually associated with inspiration, are relatively common during the neonatal period and the 1st yr of life. Stridor is usually present from birth but may not appear until 2 mo in some patients. Symptoms can be intermittent and are worse when the infant lies on his or her back. Some infants merely have noisy breathing, whereas others have a laryngeal "crow," hoarseness or aphonia, dyspnea, and inspiratory retractions in the supraclavicular, intercostal, and subcostal spaces. When retractions are severe, deformity of the thorax may result, and infants with severe dyspnea may have difficulty nursing, with undernutrition and poor weight gain. The stridor may persist for several mo to 1 yr after birth, occasionally becoming slightly worse in the 1st few wk of life and then gradually disappearing with growth and development of the airway.

Diagnosis. Most cases of laryngomalacia can be diagnosed by direct laryngoscopy. In the 1st few days of life, distinguishing between a congenital laryngeal disturbance and neonatal tetany or laryngeal edema secondary to trauma or aspiration at birth may be difficult. The differential diagnosis includes malformations of the laryngeal cartilages or vocal cords, intraluminal webs, generalized severe chondromalacia of the larynx and trachea, tumors of the larynx, mucus retention cysts, branchial cleft cysts, thyroglossal duct remnants, hypoplasia of the mandible, macroglossia, hemangioma, lymphangioma, Pierre Robin syndrome, congenital goiters, and vascular anomalies.

Treatment. Usually no specific therapy is indicated; the condition resolves spontaneously though there may be difficulty in feeding. In 1 review, only 4 of 1415 patients required tracheostomy. Parents should be reassured about the ultimate resolution and counseled to provide slow, careful feedings. A small nipple or dropper or, infrequently, gavage may be required. Most patients seem more comfortable or less noisy lying prone. Severe symptoms may require nasotracheal intubation or, rarely, tracheostomy.

Other Anomalies. Bifid epiglottitis, resulting from cleavage of two thirds or more of the epiglottis, is a rare condition which may not compromise swallowing. It usually does require treatment, however, and is associated with other laryngeal anomalies and with polydactyly. Total absence of the epiglottis is extremely rare.

Burroughs N, Leape LL: Laryngotracheoesophageal cleft; Report of a case successfully treated and review of the literature. Pediatrics 53:516, 1974.
Landing BH: State of the art: Congenital malformations and genetic diseases of the respiratory tract (larynx, trachea, bronchi, and lungs). Am Rev Resp Dis 120:151, 1979.
Maze A, Bloch E: Stridor in pediatric patients. Anaesthesiology 50:132, 1979.
McGill TJI, Healy BG: Congenital and acquired lesions of the infant larynx. Clin Pediatr 17:584, 1978.
McSwiney PF, Cavanagh NPC, Languth P: Outcome in congenital stridor (laryngomalacia). Arch Dis Child 52:215, 1977.
Tucker JA, Tucker G, Vidic B: Clinical correlation of anomalies of the supraglottic larynx with the staged sequence of normal human laryngeal development. Ann Otol Rhinol Laryngol 87:636, 1978.

TRACHEOESOPHAGEAL FISTULA

The majority of tracheoesophageal fistulas are associated with esophageal stenosis and become symptomatic in the newborn period (Sec 11.20). Occasionally, a patient with an H-type fistula will present at a later age with a long history of problems "handling mucus," respiratory symptoms after feeding (particularly with fluid), and recurrent pneumonia.

VASCULAR RING

Abnormal configuration of the great vessels, often including remnants of normally lost branchial arteries, can cause extrinsic pressure on the trachea and compromise respiration (Sec 13.58).

12.48 AGENESIS/HYPOPLASIA OF THE LUNG

Bilateral pulmonary agenesis or hypoplasia is rare and incompatible with life; the latter may be associated with anencephaly, diaphragmatic hernias, urinary tract abnormalities, deformities of the thoracic spine and rib cage (thoracic dystrophy), and pleural effusions. Unilateral agenesis or hypoplasia may have few symptoms and nonspecific findings such that only one third of the cases are diagnosed during life. In unilateral agenesis the entire pulmonary parenchyma and supporting structures and airways are absent below the level of the carina. In pulmonary hypoplasia there is a small unexpandable lung. Persistent fetal circulation is often present when pulmonary hypoplasia presents in the newborn period.

There is no specific treatment. Supportive measures including mechanical ventilation and supplemental oxygen may allow sufficient pulmonary parenchymal development to permit survival (25% of the infants in 1 series). Older patients should be given antibiotics for pulmonary infection and receive yearly influenza vaccine. Prognosis in those patients who survive infancy is extremely variable and largely dependent on the presence of associated anomalies. Death may occur from overwhelming pulmonary infection or from complications of pulmonary hypertension associated with congenital heart disease.

Maltz DL, Nadas AS: Agenesis of the lung. Presentation of eight new cases and review of the literature. Pediatrics 42:175, 1968.
Reale FR, Esterly JR: Pulmonary hypoplasia: A morphometric study of the lungs of infants with diaphragmatic hernia, anencephaly, and renal malformation. Pediatrics 51:91, 1973.
Swischuk LE, Richardson CF, Nichols MM, et al: Primary pulmonary hypoplasia in the neonate. J Pediatr 95:573, 1979.

LOBAR EMPHYSEMA

See Sec 12.86.

12.49 PULMONARY SEQUESTRATION

A mass of nonfunctioning embryonic and cystic pulmonary tissue which has no connection to the functioning airways and which receives its entire blood supply from the systemic circulation is known as a sequestration. Both intralobar and extralobar sequestration arise through the same pathoembryologic mechanism as a remnant of a diverticular outgrowth of the esophagus.

Intralobar sequestration is generally found in a lower lobe. These patients usually present with infection. In older patients hemoptysis is fairly common. Chest roentgenogram, during a period when there is no active infection, reveals a mass lesion; an air-fluid level may be present. During infection the margins of the lesion may be blurred. There is no difference in the incidence of this lesion in each lung. Treatment is surgical removal of the lesion, a procedure which usually requires excision of the entire involved lobe. Occasionally, a segmental resection will suffice.

Extralobar sequestration is much more common on the left. This lesion is strongly associated with diaphragmatic hernia. Most of these patients are asymptomatic when the mass lesion is discovered by routine chest roentgenogram taken for another reason. Surgical resection of the involved area is recommended.

Physical findings in patients with sequestration include an area of dullness to percussion and decreased breath sounds over the lesion. During infection rales may also be present. A continuous or purely systolic murmur may be heard over the back. If routine chest roentgenograms are consistent with the diagnosis, other procedures are indicated prior to surgical intervention. Bronchography reveals a mass of intrathoracic tissue without connection to the airways. Aortography should be performed in all such patients; this procedure allows definitive diagnosis by demonstration of systemic blood supply from an anomalous aortic artery. The elucidation of blood supply is necessary prior to surgery to prevent inadvertent severing of this systemic artery, which accounted for much of the intraoperative mortality in the past.

Gottrup F, Lund C: Intralobar pulmonary sequestration: A report of 12 cases. Scand J Resp Dis 59:21, 1978.

Iwai K, Shindo G, Hajikano J, et al: Intralobar pulmonary sequestration, with special reference to developmental pathology. Am Rev Resp Dis 107:911, 1973.

Pryce DM: Lower accessory pulmonary artery with intralobar sequestration of lung: Report of seven cases. J Pathol Bacteriol 58:547, 1946.

Sperling DR, Finck EJ: Intralobar bronchopulmonary sequestration: Association with a murmur over the back in a child. Am J Dis Child 115:362, 1968.

Telander RL, Lennox C, Sieber W: Sequestration of the lung in children. Mayo Clin Proc 51:578, 1976.

12.50 BRONCHOGENIC CYSTS

These cysts are originally lined with ciliated epithelium and usually occur close to a midline structure (e.g., trachea, esophagus, carina). Once infected, the ciliated epithelium may be lost, and accurate pathologic diagnosis is then impossible. Cysts are rarely demonstrable at birth. Later, some cysts become symptomatic either by becoming infected or by enlarging in size and compromising the function of an adjacent airway. Fever, chest pain, and productive cough are the most common presenting symptoms. Chest roentgenogram reveals the cyst, which may contain an air fluid level. Treatment for symptomatic cysts is surgical excision following appropriate antibiotic management. An asymptomatic cyst discovered incidentally by chest roentgenogram taken for another reason may not require treatment.

12.51 BRONCHOBILIARY FISTULA

This rare anomaly usually presents life-threatening problems during early infancy, but, occasionally, diagnosis has been delayed until after 2 yr of age. Pathologically, there is a fistulous connection between the right middle lobe bronchus and the left hepatic ductal system. All patients have recurrent severe bronchopulmonary infection and atelectasis starting in early infancy. Definitive diagnosis requires endoscopy and bronchography or exploratory surgery. Treatment is surgical excision of the entire intrathoracic portion of the fistula.

Weitzman JJ, Cohen SR, Woods LO Jr, et al: Congenital bronchobiliary fistula. J Pediatr 73:329, 1968.

12.52 CONGENITAL PULMONARY LYMPHANGIECTASIS

This disease is characterized by greatly dilated lymphatic ducts throughout the lung and is usually symptomatic with dyspnea and cyanosis in the newborn. Chest roentgenograms reveal both punctate and reticular densities. Respiration is compromised because of the space-occupying nature of the lesion and, possibly, because pulmonary compliance is reduced, increasing the work of breathing. Two forms of the disease—1 in which the abnormality is limited to the lung and 1 in which the pulmonary lymphangiectasis is secondary to pulmonary venous obstruction—are always symptomatic in the neonatal period. A 3rd form, in which the pulmonary lymphangiectasis is part of a generalized disease involving other organ systems (e.g., intestine), is associated with milder pulmonary disease and survival to midchildhood and beyond. Definitive diagnosis requires lung biopsy. There is no specific treatment.

Felman AH, Rhatigan RM, Pierson KK: Pulmonary lymphangiectasis. Am J Roent 116:548, 1972.

Noonan JA, Walters LR, Reeves JT: Congenital pulmonary lymphangiectasia. Am J Dis Child 120:314, 1970.

12.53 CYSTIC ADENOMATOID MALFORMATION

In this disease a single lobe of 1 lung is enlarged and often cystic. This lobe compresses the remainder of the ipsilateral lung and causes a shift of the mediastinum and compression of the other lung. There is slight male predominance. The genesis of this lesion is unknown, but it probably results from an embryologic insult before the 50th day of gestation. The involved lobe contains many glandular structures and very few areas of normal lung. Cysts are common but not universally present. A morphologic classification of this lesion which may be helpful prognostically has been proposed by Stocker et al. The majority of patients become symptomatic and die in the newborn period although a few survive after emergency surgery. Other patients may be asymptomatic until midchildhood, when brief episodes of recurrent or persistent pulmonary infection or relatively acute chest pain occur. Breath sounds may be diminished with mediastinal shift away from the lesion on physical examination. Chest roentgenograms reveal a cystic mass with mediastinal shift. Occasionally, an air-fluid level suggests a lung abscess. The lesion may be confused with diaphragmatic hernia in the newborn. Surgical excision of the affected lobe is indicated. Long-term survival after surgery in the newborn period and in later childhood has been reported.

Moncrieff MW, Cameron AH, Astley R, et al: Congenital cystic adenomatoid malformation of the lung. Thorax 24:476, 1969.
Stocker JT, Madewell JE, Drake RM: Congenital cystic adenomatoid malformation of the lung: Classification and morphologic spectrum. Hum Pathol 8:155, 1977.

ACQUIRED DISEASE

ACUTE INFECTIONS OF THE LARYNX AND TRACHEA

General Considerations. Acute infections of the larynx and trachea are of great importance in infants and small children because the younger child has a smaller airway which is predisposed to greater narrowing with the same degree of inflammation.

Croup is a generic term encompassing a heterogeneous group of relatively acute infectious conditions characterized by a peculiarly brassy ("croupy") cough, which may or may not be accompanied by inspiratory stridor, hoarseness, and signs of respiratory distress due to varying degrees of laryngeal obstruction. When there is sufficient involvement of the larynx to produce symptoms, the laryngeal part of the clinical picture is likely to overshadow other manifestations.

The infection in infants and small children is rarely limited to a single area of the respiratory tract, usually affecting in varying degrees the larynx, trachea, bronchi, and even the upper respiratory portion. Thus, although an exact classification of these infections is not possible, identification of several clinical varieties is justified:

Acute diphtheritic laryngitis (Sec 10.23)
Infectious croup (acute nondiphtheritic infections)
  Epiglottitis
  Laryngitis
  Laryngotracheobronchitis
  Spasmodic laryngitis

12.54 INFECTIOUS CROUP
(Acute Nondiphtheritic Infections)

Etiology and Epidemiology. Viral agents account for nearly all croup except that associated with diphtheria

and acute epiglottitis. The parainfluenza viruses account for approximately two thirds of all cases with the adenoviruses, respiratory syncytial, influenza, and measles viruses causing most of the remaining cases for which an agent can be identified. Although *H. influenzae* type b is almost always the cause of acute epiglottitis, the group A streptococcus, the pneumococcus, and the staphylococcus are occasionally implicated. Viral epiglottitis is extremely rare, but a milder and superficially similar picture from inflammation of the supraglottic area is probably caused by viruses.

The majority of patients with viral croup are between the ages of 3 mo–5 yr, whereas croup due to *H. influenzae* and *C. diphtheriae* is more common from 3–7 yr of age. The incidence of croup is higher in males. The disease occurs most commonly during the cold season of the year. Approximately 15% of patients have a strong family history of croup, and laryngitis tends to recur in the same child.

Clinical Manifestations. With progressive compromise of the upper airway, a characteristic sequence of symptoms and signs occurs. At first, there is only a mild brassy cough with intermittent respiratory stridor; the latter is sometimes preceded by 1–2 days of mild upper respiratory symptoms. As obstruction increases, hypoventilation worsens, causing hypoxemia and, eventually, hypercapnia. Stridor becomes continuous and is associated with dyspnea reflected in nasal flaring and use of the accessory muscles of respiration. Suprasternal, and infrasternal, and intercostal retractions become evident, and the child prefers to sit up in bed or be held upright. Agitation and crying greatly aggravate the symptoms and signs.

With further compromise of the airway, air hunger and restlessness occur briefly and then are superseded by severe hypoxemia and weakness with decreased air exchange and stridor, increasing pulse, and eventual death from hypoventilation. Most patients with croup progress only as far as stridor and slight dyspnea, then start recovery within a few hr. In the hypoxic child who may be cyanotic, pale, or obtunded, any manipulation of the pharynx, including use of a tongue depressor, may result in sudden cardiorespiratory arrest. This examination, therefore, should be deferred and oxygen administered until transfer to a hospital, where optimal management of the airway and shock is possible.

Acute Epiglottitis. This form of croup is a severe, life-threatening, rapidly progressive infection of the epiglottis and surrounding areas. It usually has an abrupt onset, preceded by a minor respiratory illness in only about 25% of children. The illness rarely lasts more than 2–3 days, and respiratory distress frequently is the 1st manifestation. Often the child, particularly the younger patient, is apparently well at bedtime but awakens later in the evening with a high fever, aphonia, drooling, and moderate to severe respiratory distress with stridor. Usually no other family members are ill with acute upper respiratory disease. The older child often complains initially of sore throat and dysphagia. Severe respiratory distress may ensue within minutes or hours of the onset, with inspiratory stridor, hoarseness, brassy cough, irritability, and restlessness. Drooling and dysphagia are common. The young child may assume a position of hyperextension of the neck, although other signs of meningeal irritation are absent. The older child may prefer a sitting position, leaning forward, with mouth open and tongue somewhat protruding. Some children may progress rapidly to a shock-like state characterized by pallor, cyanosis, and impaired consciousness.

Physical examination discloses moderate to severe respiratory distress with inspiratory and sometimes expiratory stridor, flaring of the alae nasi, and inspiratory retractions of the suprasternal notch, supraclavicular and intercostal spaces, and subcostal area. The pharynx is inflamed, and there is an abundance of mucus and saliva, which may also result in rhonchi. With progression of airway obstruction, stridor and breath sounds may be diminished as the patient tires. A brief period of air hunger with restlessness and agitation may be followed by rapidly increasing cyanosis, coma, and death. This sequence of events may occur in airway obstruction from any form of croup but may be very rapid in epiglottitis.

The diagnosis requires depressing the tongue to see a large, swollen cherry red epiglottis. If the diagnosis is probable on other clinical grounds, visualization in a seriously ill child should be deferred until complete cardiorespiratory support is available and definitive treatment can be carried out since some patients may have reflex laryngospasm, aspiration of secretions, and cardiorespiratory arrest following examination of the pharynx. Laryngoscopy reveals intense inflammation of the epiglottis and surrounding area: arytenoids and arytenoepiglottic folds, vocal cords, and subglottic regions. If epiglottitis is thought to be a reasonable possibility, however remote, in a patient with croup, the patient should have a lateral roentgenogram of the nasopharynx and upper airway prior to physical examination of the pharynx (Fig 12–5). If a roentgenogram shows a normal epiglottis or if the patient is unlikely to have croup by history and other physical findings, examination of the epiglottis may be performed when

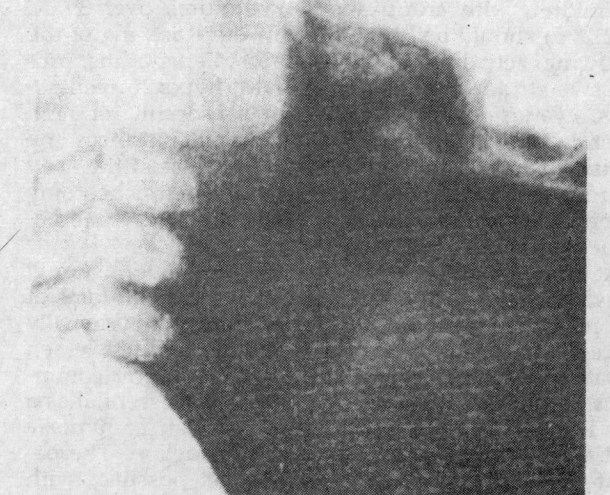

Figure 12–5 Epiglottitis. Lateral roentgenogram of upper airway reveals swollen epiglottis.

appropriate equipment and personnel are present to control the airway and provide ventilatory support. Patients with suspected epiglottitis should be accompanied by a physician and intubation equipment at all times, including the trip to and from the radiology department.

There is usually a striking polymorphonuclear leukocytosis, and throat and blood cultures are positive for *H. influenzae* type b.

Acute Infectious Laryngitis. Laryngitis is a common illness; except for diphtheria nearly all cases are caused by viruses. The onset is usually characterized by an upper respiratory tract infection during which sore throat, cough, and croup appear. The illness is generally mild; respiratory distress is unusual except in the young infant. In severe cases, however, hoarseness is marked, and the patient may present severe inspiratory stridor, retractions, dyspnea, and restlessness. As the process progresses, air hunger and fatigue become evident, and the child alternates between periods of agitation and exhaustion. Physical examination is usually not remarkable except for evidence of pharyngeal inflammation and, with respiratory distress, evidence of high respiratory obstruction. Inflammatory edema of the vocal cords and subglottic tissue may be demonstrated laryngoscopically. The principal site of obstruction is usually the subglottic area.

Acute Laryngotracheobronchitis. This is the most common form of croup and is caused primarily by viruses. Secondary bacterial infection is rare. Most patients have an upper respiratory tract infection for several days before the brassy cough, inspiratory stridor, and respiratory distress become apparent. As the infection extends downward to involve the bronchi and bronchioles, respiratory difficulty increases and the expiratory phase of respiration also becomes labored and prolonged. The child often appears extremely restless and frightened. The temperature may be only slightly elevated or as high as 39–40° C (102–104° F). There are usually bilaterally diminished breath sounds, rhonchi, and scattered rales. Symptoms characteristically appear worse at night and often recur with decreasing intensity for several days. The children are usually not seriously ill and often have associated rhinitis, conjunctivitis, or both. Other family members may have mild respiratory illness. Occasionally, the pattern of severe laryngotracheobronchitis may be difficult to distinguish from epiglottitis despite the usually more explosive onset and rapid course of the latter; it also requires similar precautions. Roentgenographic examination of the nasopharynx and upper airway may be helpful. The duration of illness ranges from several days to several wk, and recurrences are frequent from 3–6 yr of age, decreasing with growth of the airway.

Acute Spasmodic Laryngitis. Spasmodic croup most often occurs in children 1–3 yr of age and is clinically similar to acute laryngotracheobronchitis except that findings of infection in the patient and family are frequently absent. The etiology is viral in most instances, but allergic and psychologic factors appear important in some cases. The anxious and excitable child is more prone to this syndrome, and in some instances there is a familial predisposition.

Spasmodic croup occurs most frequently in the evening or night with a sudden onset, usually preceded by mild to moderate coryza and hoarseness. The child awakens with a characteristic barking, metallic cough, noisy inspiration and respiratory distress and appears anxious and frightened. Breathing is slow and labored, the pulse accelerated, and the skin cool and moist. The patient is usually afebrile. Dyspnea is aggravated by excitement, and there may be intermittent episodes of cyanosis. Usually the severity of the symptoms diminishes within several hr, and the following day the patient often appears well except for slight hoarseness and cough. Similar, but usually less severe, attacks without extreme respiratory distress may occur for another night or 2 with eventual complete recovery. Such episodes often recur several times.

Differential Diagnosis. These 4 syndromes must be distinguished from one another and from a variety of other entities that may present upper airway obstruction. *Diphtheritic croup* (Sec 10.23) is usually preceded by an upper respiratory tract infection for several days; symptoms develop more slowly although respiratory obstruction may occur suddenly; a serous or serosanguineous nasal discharge is occasionally present; and pharyngeal examination reveals the typical gray-white membrane. *Measles croup* almost always coincides with the full manifestations of systemic disease (Sec 10.67), and the course may be fulminant.

Sudden onset of respiratory obstruction may be due to *aspiration of a foreign body.* The child is generally between 6 mo–2 yr of age. Choking coughing occurs suddenly, usually without signs of inflammation. A *retropharyngeal abscess* may also present as respiratory obstruction; palpation of the posterior pharyngeal wall usually reveals a fluctuant mass. Roentgenographic examination of the upper airway and chest is essential in evaluating these possibilities as well as possible causes of *extrinsic compression* of the airway, such as a hematoma from trauma and *intraluminal obstruction* from masses, e.g., cysts or tumors.

Croup is also occasionally associated with *angioedema* of the subglottic areas as part of anaphylaxis and generalized allergic reactions, edema following *endotracheal intubation* for general anesthesia or respiratory failure, *hypocalcemic tetany, infectious mononucleosis*, trauma, and tumors or malformations of the larynx. A croupy cough may be an early sign of *asthma.*

Complications. Complications occur in approximately 15% of patients with viral croup. The most common one is extension of the infectious process to involve other regions of the respiratory tract, such as the middle ear, the terminal bronchioles, or the pulmonary parenchyma. Interstitial pneumonia may occur, but it is difficult to distinguish from patchy areas of atelectasis secondary to obstruction. Bronchopneumonia is unusual unless aspiration of stomach contents has occurred during a period of severe respiratory distress. Secondary bacterial pneumonias are rarely found; suppurative tracheobronchitis is an occasional complication of laryngotracheobronchitis.

Pneumonia, cervical lymphadenitis, otitis, and, rarely, meningitis and septic arthritis may occur during the course of epiglottitis. Mediastinal emphysema and pneumothorax are the most common complications of tracheotomy.

Prognosis. In general, the length of hospitalization and the mortality increase as the infection extends to involve a greater portion of the respiratory tract—except in epiglottitis, in which the localized infection itself may prove fatal. Most deaths from croup are due to laryngeal obstruction or to the complications of tracheotomy. Untreated epiglottitis has a mortality rate of up to 25% in some series, but if the diagnosis is made and appropriate treatment initiated before the patient is moribund, the prognosis is excellent. The outcome of acute laryngotracheobronchitis, laryngitis, and spasmodic croup is also excellent.

Treatment. Therapy for infectious croup consists primarily in maintaining or providing for adequate respiratory exchange and depends in part on the primary location of the disease and its cause. In the bacterial forms antibiotic therapy is also important.

Sleeping with a humidifier near the bedside, but out of reach, is thought by some to reduce the likelihood of development of spasmodic croup in children known to be susceptible to it.

Most afebrile children with *acute spasmodic croup* or febrile patients with mild *laryngotracheobronchitis* can usually be safely and effectively managed at home. Use of steam from a hot shower or bath in a closed bathroom, hot steam from a vaporizer, or "cold steam" from a nebulizer (which has a safety advantage) often terminates acute laryngeal spasm and respiratory distress within minutes. The same effect has been noted by many parents as they take their child out into the cold night air on the way to the physician's office. Induction of vomiting, either by coughing or by syrup of ipecac, may also break the laryngeal spasm. However, although vomiting occasionally appears to break the laryngeal spasm, there is no objective evidence for the effectiveness of ipecac, and respiratory distress may be complicated by vomiting.

Once laryngeal spasm has been broken, its return may sometimes be prevented by use of warm or cool humidification near the child's bed until the cough has subsided, usually after 2–3 days.

Children with croup and temperatures over 39° C (102.2° F) should be hospitalized if there are any of the following: actual or strongly suspected epiglottitis, progressive stridor, respiratory distress, hypoxia, restlessness, cyanosis, pallor, depressed sensorium, or high fever in a toxic-appearing child. In all instances the decision for hospitalization is made because of the need for reliable observation and relatively safe tracheotomy or nasotracheal intubation, should either of these become necessary.

At home or in the hospital, the croup patient should be watched carefully for intensification of symptoms of respiratory obstruction. The hospitalized child is usually placed in an atmosphere of high cold humidity to lessen irritation and drying of secretions. Frequent or continuous monitoring of the respiratory rate is essential as a rapid and rising rate may be the 1st sign of hypoxia and approaching total respiratory obstruction. The patient should be disturbed as little as possible; with moderate to severe respiratory distress, parenteral fluids should be given to lessen physical exertion and vomiting with its potential for aspiration. Sedatives are usually contraindicated since restlessness is used as 1 of the principal clinical indices of the severity of obstruction and the need for tracheotomy or nasotracheal intubation. Rarely, when the patient is extremely agitated and frightened, chloral hydrate (5–10 mg/kg) or paraldelhyde (0.1 mg/kg) may be administered since they do not depress respirations or dry secretions. Oxygen should be used to alleviate hypoxia and apprehension but, since it reduces cyanosis, which is an indication for tracheotomy or nasotracheal intubation, these patients must be observed particularly closely. Expectorants, bronchodilating agents, and antihistamines are not helpful. Opiates are contraindicated because they may depress respirations and dry secretions.

Laryngotracheobronchitis and *spasmodic croup* do not respond to antibiotics, and antibiotics are not indicated to prevent suprainfection. The use of corticosteroids remains controversial; their efficacy is unproved. Unnecessary tests should be delayed in view of increased symptoms associated with agitation and anxiety. Racemic epinephrine by aerosol (2.25% solution diluted 1:8 with water in doses of 2–4 ml over 15 min) with or without positive pressure may result in transient relief of symptoms; usually close observation and repeated treatments are necessary. Rarely, there is sufficient obstruction to warrant tracheotomy or nasotracheal intubation.

Epiglottitis, if diagnosed by inspection of the epiglottis or by roentgenographic examination (Fig 12–5) or if strongly suspected clinically in a severely ill child, should be treated immediately with an artificial airway; untreated patients have a substantial mortality even when observed in the hospital with appropriate intubation equipment nearby. Ampicillin (200 mg/kg/24 hr) and chloramphenicol (50 mg/kg/24 hr) should be given parenterally pending culture and sensitivity reports because of the increasing possibility of ampicillin-resistant strains of *H. influenzae* type b. All patients should receive oxygen en route to the operating room unless it is contraindicated by the increased agitation caused by the mask. Racemic epinephrine and corticosteroids are ineffective, do not avert the need for an artificial airway, and may dangerously delay definitive treatment. After insertion of the artificial airway, the patient should improve immediately with disappearance of respiratory distress and cyanosis and return of normal or near normal blood gases. Patients usually fall asleep. The epiglottitis resolves after a few days of antibiotics, and the patient can be weaned from the tracheostomy or nasotracheal tube; antibiotics should be continued for 7–10 days.

Acute laryngeal swelling on an allergic basis responds to epinephrine (1:1000 dilution in dosage of 0.01 ml/kg to a maximum of 0.3 ml/dose) administered subcutaneously, and isoproterenol (1:200 dilution in dosage of 0.01 ml to a maximum of 0.3 ml/dose) by aerosol. Following recovery, the patient and parents should be instructed in emergency administration of these drugs at home. Corticosteroids are frequently required (50–100 mg of hydrocortisone every 6 hr).

Reactive mucosal swelling, severe stridor, and respi-ratory distress unresponsive to mist therapy may follow endotracheal intubation for general anesthesia in children. Intermittent use of racemic epinephrine aerosols or, occasionally, corticosteroids may be helpful.

TRACHEOTOMY AND NASOTRACHEAL INTUBATION. With the introduction of routine tracheotomy for epiglottitis, mortality in a reported series dropped to almost zero. Nasotracheal intubation has also been reported to be very effective in those hospitals with special interest in and appropriate facilities for the care of intubated children. Both procedures should always be done in an operating room if time permits; prior intubation and general anesthesia greatly facilitate doing a tracheotomy without complications.

Tracheotomy or nasotracheal intubation is required for patients with epiglottitis, but it is required only for those with severe laryngotracheobronchitis and for those with spasmodic croup or laryngitis who have increasing signs of respiratory failure secondary to obstruction despite appropriate treatment. Severe forms of laryngotracheobronchitis that required tracheostomy in a high proportion of patients have been reported during severe measles and influenza A virus epidemics. Assessment of the need for these procedures requires experience and judgment. They should not be delayed until cyanosis and extreme restlessness have developed; a pulse rate over 150/min and rising, and an elevated pCO_2 especially in a tiring child, are indications of impending respiratory failure.

The tracheostomy or nasotracheal tube must remain in place until edema and spasm have subsided and the patient is able to handle secretions satisfactorily. They should always be removed as soon as possible, usually within a few days. There is some evidence that hydrocortisone (50–100 mg/24 hr) and racemic epinephrine may be used to facilitate extubation or to treat croup associated with extubation.

Epiglottitis

Battaglia JD, Lockhart CH: Management of acute epiglottitis by nasotracheal intubation. Am J Dis Child 120:334, 1975.
Cohen SR, Chai J: Epiglottitis: Twenty-year study with tracheostomy. Ann Otol Rhinol Laryngol 87:1, 1978.
Faden HS: Treatment of *Haemophilus influenzae* type b epiglottitis. Pediatrics 63:402, 1979.
Margolis CZ, Ingram DL, Meyer JH: Routine tracheotomy in *Hemophilus influenzae* type b epiglottitis. J Pediatr 81:1150, 1972.
Molteni RA: Epiglottitis: Incidence of extraepiglottic infection: Report of 72 cases and review of the literature. Pediatrics 58:526, 1976.
Rapkin RH: The diagnosis of epiglottitis: Simplicity and reliability of radiographs of the neck in differential diagnosis of the croup syndrome. J Pediatr 80:96, 1975.

Laryngotracheobronchitis

Adair JC, Ring WH, Jordan WS, et al: A ten year experience with IPPB in the treatment of acute laryngotracheobronchitis. Anesth Analg 50:649, 1971.
Gardner HG, Powell KR, Roden VJ, et al: The evaluation of racemic epinephrine in the treatment of infectious croup. Pediatrics 52:52, 1973.
Jordan WS, Graves CL, Elwyn RA: New therapy for postintubation laryngeal edema and tracheitis in children. JAMA 212:585, 1970.
Leipzig B, Oski FA, Cummings CW, et al: A prospective randomized study to determine the efficacy of steroids in treatment of croup. J Pediatr 94:194, 1979.
Singer OP, Wilson WJ: Laryngotracheobronchitis: 2 years' experience with racemic epinephrine. Can Med Assoc J 115:132, 1976.
Tunnessen WW Jr, Feinstein AR: The steroid-croup controversy: An analytic review of methodologic problems. J Pediatr 96:751, 1980.

12.55   FOREIGN BODIES IN THE LARYNX, TRACHEA, AND BRONCHI

The air passages of children are frequent sites for the lodgment of foreign bodies; the carelessness of adults is occasionally an important contributing factor. The changes produced by foreign bodies depend upon their nature, location, and the degree of obstruction of the air passage. A sharp or irritating object lodged in the larynx will produce severe edema and later suppurative perichondritis, whereas an obstructive object in the bronchus will produce atelectasis and later bronchiectasis, pulmonary abscess, or empyema.

The vast majority of foreign bodies aspirated into the respiratory tract are probably expelled immediately by reflex cough and never require medical attention. However, if an object too large to be eliminated by mucociliary clearance is aspirated and is not expelled by coughing, respiratory symptoms inevitably result. A large foreign body that can occlude the upper airway completely is an immediate threat to life. Smaller objects that lodge in 1 of the main stem or lobar bronchi cause more chronic and usually less severe symptoms.

After the initial symptoms, which may have been forgotten, there is often a symptom-free interval which may last for hours, days, or weeks. On occasion, dysphagia may occur from the swelling that results from a foreign body in the region of the larynx, and foreign bodies in the upper esophagus may cause symptoms referable to the air passages by compression or by the overflow of food or secretions into the larynx.

Laryngeal Foreign Body

Clinical Manifestations. A foreign body in the larynx causes hoarseness, a cough which soon becomes croupy, and aphonia. Hemoptysis, dyspnea with wheezing, and cyanosis may occur. Obstruction resulting from the foreign body or the combination of it and the inflammatory reaction may prove fatal if the signs of high respiratory tract obstruction are not promptly recognized and appropriate treatment given.

Diagnosis. Roentgenographic and direct laryngoscopic examinations reveal the presence of a foreign body in the larynx (Fig 12–6). An opaque foreign body in the neck will be clearly demonstrated on a lateral roentgenogram. When it is lodged anteriorly, it is obviously in the larynx; when it is behind the soft tissue shadows of the larynx, it is in the hypopharynx or the cervical esophagus. The plane in which the foreign body lies is another differential point in its localization. If it lies in the sagittal plane, it is probably in the larynx. If it is in the coronal plane, it is probably in the esophagus. Even if the foreign body is not opaque, indirect evidence of its presence may be seen on the roentgenogram. Films should always be taken from both the lateral and the anteroposterior projections. In some instances administration of a small amount of opaque material may be helpful. Direct laryngoscopy will confirm the diagnosis and provide access for instrumental removal of the foreign body. When there is

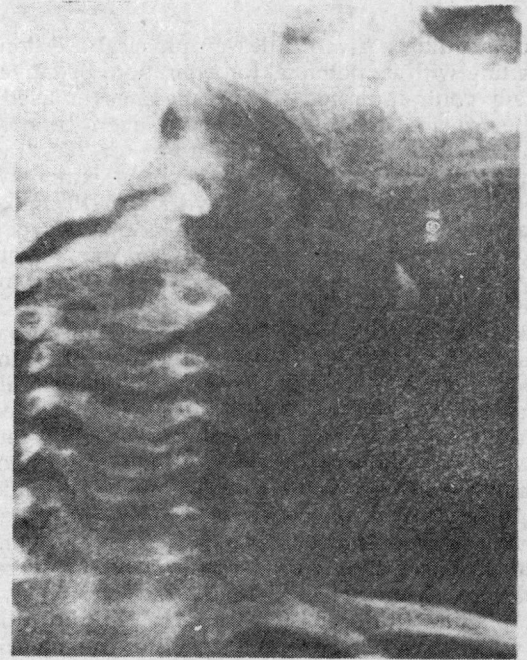

Figure 12–6 Foreign body (fragment of sea shell) in larynx of a 2 yr old child treated for "croup" 6 days before it was suspected. Fortunately tracheotomy was not required despite the presence of moderately severe laryngeal edema.

a severe degree of dyspnea, it may be advisable to do a tracheotomy before the laryngoscopic examination.

Tracheal Foreign Body

Though a foreign body in the trachea may be responsible for cough, hoarseness, dyspnea, and cyanosis, the characteristic signs are the audible slap and palpable thud due to momentary expiratory impaction at the subglottic level and the asthmatoid wheeze. The diagnosis of tracheal foreign body may occasionally be made from the symptoms, physical signs, and roentgenogram of the chest, but in most instances a definite diagnosis can be made only by bronchoscopy.

Bronchial Foreign Body

Clinical Manifestations. The initial symptoms are usually similar to those of foreign bodies in the larynx or trachea. Cough, blood-streaked sputum, and metallic taste with metallic foreign bodies also may be produced by bronchial foreign bodies. The degree of obstruction and the stage in which the patient is seen are the determining factors in the symptomatology as well as in the pathologic changes. A nonobstructive, nonirritating foreign body may produce few symptoms even after a prolonged time in the lung. An obstructive foreign body quickly produces symptoms and signs and pathologic changes. When there is only a slight (bypass valve) obstruction which allows passage of air or fluid in both directions with only slight interference, a wheeze will be noted. When obstruction is of greater degree, obstructive emphysema or obstructive atelectasis will be produced; if either is allowed to persist, chronic bronchopulmonary disease may ensue.

Most often, the object is aspirated into the right lung. There is usually an immediate episode of choking, gagging, and paroxysmal coughing, which may lead to medical consultation. If this acute episode is missed or its importance underestimated by the parents, a relatively long latent period may pass with only occasional cough or slight wheezing; then the patient may develop recurrent lobar pneumonia or intractable "asthma," often with bilateral wheezing and many episodes of "status asthmaticus." Occasionally, chronic wheezing starts immediately after the aspiration. Rarely, a foreign body will cause hemoptysis. Detailed history may reveal a forgotten episode of choking while eating or while playing with small objects. Physical examination may reveal a tracheal shift. Breath sounds are decreased on the side of the obstruction, but this sign may not be obvious if there is diffuse wheezing.

When both main bronchi are obstructed, there may be severe dyspnea and even asphyxia. If the foreign body is vegetal, e.g., a peanut, a severe condition known as *vegetal* or *arachidic bronchitis* will result. This is characterized by cough, a septic type of fever, and dyspnea. Chronic pulmonary suppuration may be expected when a bronchial foreign body has been present for a long time.

Diagnosis. The possibility of a foreign body must be considered in acute or chronic pulmonary lesions whether or not there is a history of a foreign body accident. The physical signs of bronchial obstruction from foreign bodies include limited expansion, decreased vocal fremitus, impaired (atelectasis) or hyperresonant (overinflation) percussion note, and diminished breath sounds distal to the foreign body. When there is complete obstruction, with a "drowned lung" or with atelectasis, there is absence of vocal resonance and vocal fremitus, which may lead to an erroneous diagnosis of empyema. Varying degrees of tympany may be noted over areas of obstructive emphysema. Rales are more likely to be on the uninvaded side than on the invaded one.

If the lumen is obstructed by an object that causes complete obstruction in the expiratory phase but allows air to pass in the inspiratory phase, air will enter the distal portion of the lung on inspiration, but little or none will escape during expiration (*check valve*). This type of obstruction produces obstructive overinflation (Fig 12–7). Complete blockage of the bronchus due to the object in itself or in combination with the inflammatory swelling of the bronchial mucosa results in a *stop valve* obstruction, and the air in the distal portion of the lung is soon absorbed, leaving an area of atelectasis (Fig 12–8).

These phenomena are readily appreciated by fluoroscopy. In a check valve type of obstruction, the obstructive emphysema makes it possible to localize a bronchial foreign body. The obstructed lung will remain expanded during expiration, while the heart and the mediastinum will shift to the opposite side as the unobstructed lung empties. The diaphragm is low, flattened, and fixed on the obstructed side; its excursion will be free and exaggerated on the unobstructed side. The differences between the lungs are much more evident on expiration than on inspiration. With complete obstruction of the bronchus producing obstructive atelectasis, the heart and the mediastinum are drawn toward the obstructed side and remain there during both phases of respiration. The diaphragm on the obstructed side remains high, while that on the unobstructed side moves normally. Films taken at the end of inspiration and of expiration will show only a slight difference resulting from the filling and emptying of the unobstructed lung.

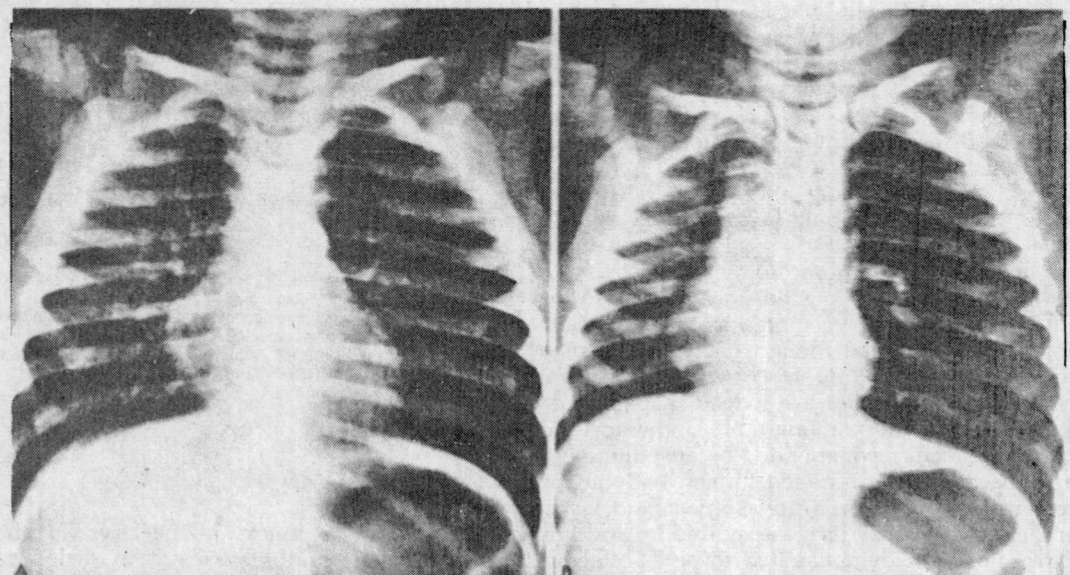

Figure 12–7 Obstructive emphysema (overinflation) due to peanut fragment in left main bronchus. Inspiratory film (*A*) appears relatively normal except for slight mediastinal shift to the right. In expiration (*B*) the left lung remains overaerated (check valve mechanism), and the mediastinum moves far to the right.

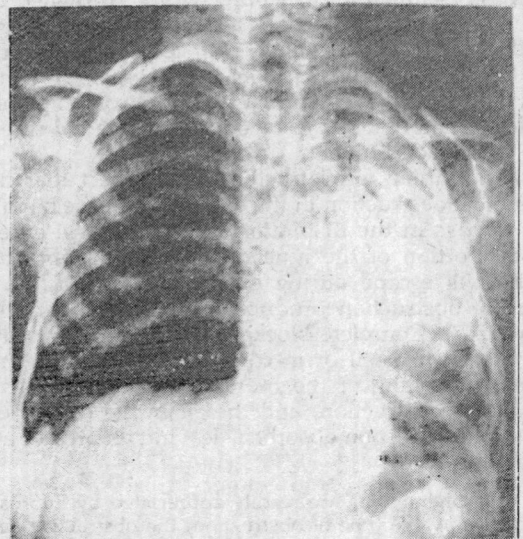

Figure 12–8 Foreign body lodged in left main bronchus, producing atelectasis of left lung. Note that the heart is drawn completely into the left side of the chest.

Prognosis. Foreign bodies lodged in the air passages prove almost invariably fatal if not removed. However, if brought to medical attention, almost all can be removed safely by a skilled bronchoscopist, and almost all patients recover completely.

Prevention. Foreign body aspiration can be prevented by keeping small objects out of reach of children who are too young to obey restrictions; by not giving small pieces of candy, nuts, or similar food to children too young to chew them; and by not giving toys containing small or loosely attached parts to children who are still putting such objects into their mouths. Beads, button boxes, and coins should not be given to toddlers as playthings. Safety pins should always be closed and not left near a baby or in reach of small children. Balloons are also underestimated as potential foreign bodies.

Treatment. Endoscopy and removal of the foreign body under direct vision should be performed as soon as possible. Although the success rate is extremely high, in a very rare patient a thoracotomy is necessary to "milk" the object into a position where it can be removed by bronchoscopy. Occasionally, especially with long duration vegetal foreign bodies, lobectomy may be necessary. Biplane fluoroscopy may be helpful when opaque foreign bodies are lodged in peripheral bronchi. Treatment with pulmonary physiotherapy and bronchodilators is not recommended because there is a risk that impaction of a dislodged foreign body at the subglottic area may result in acute asphyxia; a delay in instituting endoscopy may increase morbidity, and this method has not been demonstrated to be as effective as endoscopy. Treatment of complicating conditions is important in obtaining a good outcome. Secondary infections should be treated with appropriate antibiotics. The outcome of the aspiration of a *large foreign body* that may be immediately life-threatening depends on proper and prompt action taken at the scene of the accident.

Emergency treatment of local upper airway obstruction, as described below, is part of the "basic rescuer course" in cardiopulmonary resuscitation (CPR) of the American Heart Association. The recommendations for treating infants and young children differ slightly from those for treating teenagers and adults. The repetitive use of 4 back blows and 4 chest thrusts is recommended. The back blows are delivered while holding the infant with the head lower than the trunk. Four blows are delivered with the heel of the hand between the scapulae. The purpose of this maneuver is to loosen the foreign body. After the back blows, the patient is turned and 4 chest thrusts are delivered using the same technique and hand positioning as is used for closed cardiac compression (i.e., over the mid-sternum for infants and slightly lower for older children). The purpose of this maneuver is to increase intrathoracic pressure which causes explusion of the foreign body. Blind finger sweeps (as recommended for unconscious adult victims) should not be used in infants and young children. Instead, after the administration of the 4 chest thrusts, the mouth should be opened and a visualized foreign body grasped and removed. Following each sequence of back blows, chest thrusts, and visual attempt to remove foreign body, rescue breathing should be attempted for the unconscious patient. If unsuccessful, the sequence described above is repeated. Although there is controversy concerning the precise technique to be used in total upper airway obstruction by a foreign body, pediatricians should provide up-to-date information in these techniques to parents and should urge parents to expect that their babysitters (including teenagers) be familiar with the symptoms and emergency treatment of foreign body aspiration.

Abdulmajid OA, Ebeid, AM, Motaweh MM, et al: Aspirated foreign bodies in the tracheobronchial tree: Report of 250 cases. Thorax 31:635, 1976.

Blazer S, Naveh Y, Friedman A: Foreign body in the airway: A review of 200 cases. Am Rev Dis Child 134:68, 1980.

Ferguson CF, Kendig EL: Pediatric Otolaryngology. Philadelphia, WB Saunders, 1972.

Gann DS: Emergency management of the obstructed airway. JAMA 243:1141, 1980.

Heimlich JH: A life-saving maneuver to prevent food-choking. JAMA 234:398, 1975.

Hollinger PH, Andrews AH Jr, Anison GC: Pulmonary complications due to endobronchial foreign bodies. Ill Med J 93:19, 1948.

Law D, Kosloske AM: Management of tracheobronchial foreign bodies in children: A reevaluation of postural drainage and bronchoscopy. Pediatrics 58:362, 1976.

Standards and guidelines for cardiopulmonary resuscitation (CPR) and emergency cardiac care (ECC). JAMA 244:453, 1980.

12.56   TRAUMA TO THE LARYNX

Birth Trauma. Injury of the larynx during birth is not infrequent and may result in dislocation of the cricothyroid or cricoarytenoid articulations. Hoarseness and at times wheezing or fluttering respiratory sounds are heard. The diagnosis is made by direct laryngoscopic examination. Treatment by direct laryngoscopic manipulations, using a laryngeal dilator, may occasionally be effective, but tracheotomy should be done when there is evidence of hypoxia.

Unilateral or bilateral *recurrent laryngeal nerve paralysis* may also be produced by birth trauma, especially during forceps delivery. When only 1 cord is paralyzed, there may be only hoarseness and slight stridor without dyspnea. In bilateral paralysis there is dyspnea with stridor. Direct laryngoscopic examination will establish the diagnosis. Tracheotomy is usually necessary for bilateral paralysis. The older child may wear a valvular cannula, or a laryngoplasty with lateral fixation of 1 vocal cord may be done to improve the airway and permit decannulation if breathing through the larynx has not improved spontaneously.

Postnatal Trauma. Any trauma, such as that brought about by a fall against a hard object, may produce acute or chronic stenosis of the larynx, as may high tracheotomy and prolonged intubation. Clinically important laryngeal injury is rare in children. Penetrating injuries are usually obvious and require treatment by an otolaryngologic surgeon. Serious nonpenetrating injuries may be deceptive since substantial edema and even a compressing hematoma may give surprisingly few external clues. Laryngoscopy and, occasionally, surgical exploration may be indicated in patients with relatively normal physical findings but a history compatible with substantial blunt neck trauma. Most patients with serious laryngeal or upper tracheal injuries require tracheostomy as part of their management; if there are signs of high obstruction, the need may be urgent. Similarly, severe thermal injury (e.g., following accidental inhalation of steam or smoke) is often best managed with tracheostomy.

Acute *overuse of the voice* (e.g., prolonged screaming at a concert or athletic event) may cause transient hoarseness. With cessation of this stress, the voice returns to normal without other treatment. The roles of resting the voice (whispering or no use of speech at all) or mist in accelerating recovery are not clear. Acute laryngitis is fairly common in older children during mild viral respiratory infections; spontaneous recovery is the rule, and the importance of steam and other therapeutic maneuvers is not known. Occasionally, a teenager may develop chronic laryngitis from heavy cigarette smoking. The differential diagnosis of persistent hoarse voice includes vocal nodules ("singer's" or "screamer's"), papillomas, and serious tumors such as rhabdomyosarcoma. A laryngeal abscess is a rare cause of persistent hoarseness. All are diagnosed by laryngoscopy and may require surgical treatment, which may be followed by voice training. Otolaryngologic consultation is indicated for any child with unexplained continuous hoarseness longer than 1 wk.

12.57   ACUTE LARYNGEAL STENOSIS

Acute stenosis may result from any acute infection responsible for edema of the subglottic region or epiglottis and arytenoids; from inflammation secondary to the inspiration of a vegetal foreign body, and especially after instrumentation for the removal of such an object; from edema of an allergic reaction; or from a foreign body lodged in the larynx. Treatment consists of immediate provision of an airway by intubation or tracheotomy, followed by appropriate medical therapy.

12.58   CHRONIC LARYNGEAL STENOSIS

This is a frequent sequela of high tracheotomy in which damage of the 1st tracheal ring or cricoid cartilage results in perichondritis and subsequent overgrowth of cartilage or fibrous tissue. Chronic stenosis may also result from laryngeal diphtheria, syphilis, tuberculosis, radiation burns, and external trauma. The clinical manifestations may include dyspnea with audible stridor and suprasternal, supraclavicular, and intercostal retractions or may be limited to inability to decannulate a patient's tracheostomy or remove a laryngeal tube. The diagnosis is made by direct laryngoscopy, palpation of the larynx, and roentgenographic examination. Scarring and stenosis usually develop in the subglottic region, occasionally with necrosis of cartilage.

Milder cases can be treated by replacement of the tracheostomy cannula with a smaller one and closure of this tube, at first partial and then complete, with a cork, thus re-educating the patient to mouthbreathe and permit removal of the cannula. If this method is unsuccessful, dilation through a direct laryngoscope may help but should not be done too frequently. In some patients external surgery with or without the use of an indwelling mold may be necessary. The prognosis for eventual cure is good, but treatment may require months or years.

Fearon B: Acute airway obstruction. *In*: Ferguson CF, Kendig EL Jr (eds): Disorders of the Respiratory Tract, Vol 2, Pediatric Otolaryngology. Philadelphia, WB Saunders, 1972.
Proctor DF: The upper airways: II. The larynx and trachea. Am Rev Resp Dis 115:315, 1977.

12.59   NEOPLASMS OF THE LARYNX

Papilloma is the most common tumor of the larynx in childhood; it rarely becomes malignant and often disappears after puberty. The pink, warty tumors may grow profusely from any portion of the larynx though usually from the vocal cords. The initial symptom is hoarseness, but dyspnea is likely if the condition is allowed to persist. Asphyxia has occurred. Direct laryngoscopy accomplishes both diagnosis (confirmed histologically) and treatment as the papilloma can be easily removed by forceps. Care should be taken not to damage normal tissue. Cure is ultimately assured, although at first rapid recurrence is usual. Tracheostomy may be required because of recurrences and the threat of aspiration. Cryosurgery and laser surgery have been advocated as adjuvant therapy. Radical excision and radiation are contraindicated. Patients with laryngobronchial papillomatosis who fail to respond to usual treatment may improve after receiving systemic bleomycin.

Vocal nodules or small tumors may occur in children at the junction of the anterior and middle thirds of the cords. They are usually bilateral and produce slight hoarseness. Spontaneous regression may occur if strenuous use of the voice is avoided, or they may be removed under direct laryngoscopic view.

Mehta P, Herold N: Regression of juvenile laryngobronchial papillomatosis with systemic bleomycin therapy. J Pediatr 97:479, 1980.

12.60 TRACHEAL AMYLOIDOSIS

Primary amyloidosis of the the trachea is an extremely rare but potentially treatable lesion. Symptoms are caused by gradual reduction in the tracheal lumen secondary to progressive deposition of amyloid. Cough, dyspnea, and wheezing occur early in the course of the disease. Recurrent infection and hemoptysis are late complications. Expiratory wheezing, cough, and signs of respiratory distress may be present. Chest roentgenogram may be normal. Diagnosis is made by bronchoscopy, which reveals a narrowed tracheal lumen with friable tissue lining the airways; biopsy allows confirmation of the diagnosis. Treatment is repeated bronchoscopy for removal of amyloid until an adequate airway is restored, but improvement may be only temporary, and repeated bronchoscopic treatments are often necessary.

Gottlieb LS, Gold WM: Primary tracheobronchial amyloidosis. Am Rev Resp Dis 105:425, 1972.
Prowse CG: Amyloidosis of the lower respiratory tract. Thorax 13:308, 1958.

12.61 ACUTE BRONCHITIS

Though the diagnosis of "acute bronchitis" is frequently made, this condition may not exist in children as an isolated clinical entity. Rather, bronchitis occurs in association with a number of other conditions of the upper and lower respiratory tracts, and the trachea is nearly always involved. The term "capillary bronchitis" (bronchiolitis) is an entirely different illness (Sec 12.64).

Asthmatic bronchitis, a form of asthma with obscure pathogenesis, is often confused with acute bronchitis. With a variety of upper respiratory tract infections, some children have bronchial spasm and exudation similar to signs in older children with asthma.

Acute tracheobronchitis is most commonly found in association with an upper respiratory tract infection such as nasopharyngitis but is also associated with influenza, pertussis, measles, typhoid fever (and other salmonelloses), diphtheria, and scarlet fever. An acute, primary, undifferentiated tracheobronchitis also occurs, most commonly in older children and adolescents. It is likely that, except for the bacterial diseases mentioned, acute tracheobronchitis is of viral origin. Pneumococci,

staphylococci, *H. influenzae*, and various hemolytic streptococci may be isolated from the sputum, but their presence does not imply a bacterial origin, and antibiotic therapy does not appreciably alter the course of the illness. Some children appear to be far more susceptible to acute tracheobronchitis than others. The reasons are unknown, but allergy, climate, air pollution, and chronic infections of the upper respiratory tract, particularly sinusitis, may be contributing factors.

The syndrome *bronchiolitis obliterans* may begin with an episode of acute bronchitis, bronchiolitis, or bronchopneumonia and then progress over several wk to severe chronic pulmonary disease characterized by bronchiolar and bronchial obliteration and bronchiectasis.

Clinical Manifestations. Acute bronchitis is usually preceded by a viral upper respiratory infection. Secondary bacterial infection with *S. pneumoniae* or *Hemophilus influenzae* may occur. Typically, the child presents a frequent, dry, hacking, unproductive cough of relatively gradual onset, beginning 3–4 days after the appearance of rhinitis. Low substernal discomfort or burning anterior chest pain is often present and may be aggravated by coughing. As the illness progresses, the patient may be bothered by whistling sounds during respiration (probably rhonchi), soreness of the chest, and occasionally shortness of breath. Coughing paroxysms or gagging on secretions is occasionally associated with vomiting. Within several days the cough becomes productive, and the sputum changes from clear to purulent. Usually within 5–10 days the mucus thins and the cough gradually disappears. The considerable malaise often associated with the illness may continue for 1 wk or more after acute symptoms have subsided.

Physical findings vary with the age of the patient and the stage of the disease. Initially, the child usually is afebrile or has low grade fever, and there are signs of nasopharyngitis, conjunctival infection, and rhinitis. Later, auscultation reveals roughening of breath sounds, coarse and fine moist rales, and rhonchi which may be high pitched, resembling the wheezing of asthma.

In otherwise healthy children complications are few, but in undernourished children or those in poor health, otitis, sinusitis, and pneumonia are common.

Treatment. There is no specific therapy; most patients recover uneventfully without any treatment. In small infants pulmonary drainage is facilitated by frequent shifts in position. Older children are more comfortable in high humidity, but there is no evidence that this shortens the duration of illness. Irritating and paroxysmal coughing may cause considerable distress and interfere with sleep. Although suppression of cough may increase the possibility of suppuration, judicious use of cough suppressants (including codeine) may be appropriate for symptomatic relief. Antihistamines, which dry secretions, should not be used, and expectorants are not helpful. Antibiotics do not shorten the duration of the viral illness or decrease the incidence of bacterial complications, although the fact that patients with recurrent episodes may occasionally improve with such treatment suggests that some secondary bacterial infection is present.

Children with repeated attacks of acute bronchitis should be carefully evaluated for the possibility of anomalies of the respiratory tract, foreign bodies, bronchiectasis, immune deficiency, tuberculosis, allergy, sinusitis, tonsillitis, adenoiditis, and cystic fibrosis.

12.62 CHRONIC BRONCHITIS

There is considerable doubt whether chronic bronchitis as an isolated clinical entity exists in children, and it should rarely be accepted as a final diagnosis. A chronic or frequently recurring productive cough usually indicates an underlying pulmonary or systemic disease; affected patients should be evaluated for immune deficiencies, anatomic abnormalities, allergic disorders, environmental disease, upper airway infection with postnasal discharge, cystic fibrosis, immotile cilia syndrome, and bronchiectasis. Cough and wheezing are common, often suggesting an allergic basis. Rarely, bronchial irritation may be secondary to the chronic inhalation of dust or noxious fumes.

Air Pollution and Cigarette Smoking. There is a significant association between high levels of air pollution and an elevated incidence of chronic pulmonary disease including bronchitis, but a direct causal relationship has not been established. Air pollutants also aggravate pre-existent pulmonary disease and decrease pulmonary function in exercising children and teenagers. Children and their parents should be advised of these relationships. An increased incidence and exacerbations of bronchitis and other forms of acute and chronic lung disease are associated with cigarette smoking. In addition, there is increased morbidity from respiratory infections in teenagers who smoke, as reflected in school and work absences as well as in functional and pathologic evidence of small airway abnormalities. Smoking parents, and especially those whose children have chronic lung disease, should be advised that they are subjecting their children's lungs to significant amounts of "2nd hand" cigarette smoke in the home; they should be urged to stop smoking.

Clinical Manifestations. The chief symptom is cough, with or without expectoration. The child will usually also complain of soreness of the chest; characteristically these signs and symptoms are worse at night; wheezing may also be prominent, and physical findings are similar to those of acute bronchitis.

Course and Prognosis. Both the course and the prognosis depend upon appropriate management or eradication of any underlying illness. Complications will be those of the underlying illness.

Treatment. When an underlying cause for chronic bronchitis has been found, this should receive appropriate management. Allergic management may be helpful on occasion even when no underlying cause can be discovered. Autogenous vaccines or inhalation of antibiotics is not effective.

Doyle NC: The facts about second hand cigarette smoke. American Lung Association Bulletin, Mar 1974.

Doctors could dissuade youth from smoking. Pediatr News 4:24, 1970.
Goldsmith JR: Health effects of air pollution. Basics Resp Dis 4:1, 1975.
Lebowitz MD, Bendheim P, Cristea G, et al: The effect of air pollution and weather on lung function in exercising children and adolescents. Am Rev Resp Dis 109:262, 1974.
Niewoehner DE, Kleinerman J, Rice DB: Pathologic changes in the peripheral airways of young cigarette smokers. N Engl J Med 291:755, 1974.
White JR, Froeb HF: Small-airways dysfunction in nonsmokers chronically exposed to tobacco smoke. N Engl J Med 203:720, 1980.

12.63 IMMOTILE CILIA SYNDROME
(Dyskinetic Cilia Syndrome; Kartagener Syndrome)

In the respiratory tract the majority of the lining mucosal cells are ciliated (about 275 cilia per cell). Each cilium is anchored to the apical cytoplasm by a basal body and contains 2 central and 9 peripheral microtubules which traverse its entire length and are loosely bound to one another by radial spokes. It is the movement of these microtubules with relation to the others which causes the typical 1000 cycle/min beat of the cilia. The chemical basis for this movement involves an ATPase located within the cilia and visible ultrastructurally as dynein arms.

Kartagener initially described a group of patients all of whom had situs inversus, chronic sinusitis, and chronic bronchitis with bronchiectasis. Situs inversus is also seen commonly in men with infertility secondary to sperm immotility. These observations led Afzelius to postulate that these patients have a generalized disorder of ciliary motility, some of them lacking the ATPase-containing dynein arms necessary for ciliary movement. The disease appears to be transmitted as an autosomal recessive with an incidence of about 1:4000 persons.

Clinical Manifestations. The symptoms of this disease reflect the wide distribution of cilia throughout the body. Relentless ciliary activity of embryonal tissues may be responsible for the characteristic direction of the rotation of the gut. Impairment of ciliary movement and thus of intestinal rotation could produce situs inversus, a very common but not universal finding in the immotile cilia syndrome. Absence of ciliary clearance from the middle ears, eustachian tubes, and sinus cavities results in an increased incidence and greater severity of chronic otitis media and sinusitis in childhood. Sterility results from inadequate spermatozoal movement. Abnormal mucociliary clearance in children results in chronic bronchitis, usually without bronchiectasis. Bronchiectasis is a relatively late complication, usually not present until early adult years. Wheezing is common, perhaps due in part to inadequate clearance of antigen from the airways.

Diagnosis. The disease should be suspected in children who have chronic sinusitis and otitis media in addition to bronchitis. If such a patient has situs inversus, the diagnosis is a virtual certainty, but definitive testing (see below) should be done. Chronic wheezing, a family history of bronchiectasis in young adults, and/or male infertility would be important additional clinical support for this diagnosis.

Decreased ciliary movement may be observed at bronchoscopy. Another preliminary screening test involves scraping the nasal mucosa above the 1st turbinate with an ear curette, brush, or swab; immediate suspension of mucosal cells in Hank saline; and examination by light microscope for evaluation of ciliary activity. Absence of ciliary activity on more than 2 occasions when the patient does not have an acute upper respiratory infection justifies more definitive testing. Definitive diagnosis depends on electron microscopic examination of cilia, obtained either by brushing of the trachea at bronchoscopy or by nasal mucosal biopsy. Spermatozoa can also be examined in older patients. Absence of dynein arms is probably the most common form of the disease, but other morphologic abnormalities with the same phenotypic expression (i.e., decreased or absent ciliary movement) are also possible.

Treatment. Treatment is symptomatic and includes close medical supervision with early and aggressive antibiotic treatment of pulmonary infection, chest physiotherapy, and bronchodilators. Early infection involves the pneumococcus and *Hemophilus* organisms primarily. Treatment of serous otitis and sinusitis is also important.

Prognosis. The average life expectancy is unknown, but there is considerable morbidity due to bronchiectasis and other problems. The effects of early aggressive therapy are unknown. The dangers of smoking and of exposure to industrial fumes should be explained to the patient and appropriate vocational guidance supplied.

Afzellius B: A human syndrome caused by immotile cilia. Science 193:317, 1976.
Eliasson R, Mossberg B, Camner P, Afzelius BA: The immotile cilia syndrome. N Engl J Med 297:1, 1977.
Fischer TJ, McAdams JA, Entis GN, Cotton R, Ghory JE, Ausdenmoore RW: Middle ear ciliary defect in Kartagener's syndrome. Pediatrics 62:443, 1978.
Pedersen H, Mygind N: Absence of axonemal arms in nasal mucosa cilia in Kartagener's syndrome. Nature 242:494, 1976.
Rooklin AR, McGeady SJ, Mikaelian DO, Soriano RZ, Mansmann HC: The immotile cilia sydrome: A cause of recurrent pulmonary disease in children. Pediatrics 66:526, 1980.
Sturgess JM, Chao J, Wong J, Aspin N, Turner JAP: Cilia with defective radial spokes: A cause of human respiratory disease. N Engl J Med 300:53, 1979.

12.64　ACUTE BRONCHIOLITIS

Acute bronchiolitis is a common disease of the lower respiratory tract of infants resulting from inflammatory obstruction of the small airways. It occurs during the 1st 2 yr of life, with a peak incidence at approximately 6 mo of age, and in many localities is the most frequent cause of hospitalization of infants. The incidence is highest during the winter and early spring mo. The illness occurs both sporadically and epidemically.

Etiology and Epidemiology. Acute bronchiolitis is a viral illness. The respiratory syncytial virus is the causative agent in over 50% of cases; the parainfluenza 3 virus, mycoplasma, some adenoviruses, and occasionally other viruses produce the remaining cases. Adenovirus may be associated with long-term complications, including bronchiolitis obliterans and unilateral hyperlucent lung syndrome (Swyer-James syndrome). There is no firm evidence that bacteria cause this condition. Occasionally, bacterial bronchopneumonia may be confused clinically with bronchiolitis.

The source of the viral infection is usually a family member with minor respiratory illness. Older children and adults can tolerate bronchiolar edema better than infants and thus escape developing the clinical picture of bronchiolitis even though their small airways are infected by the virus.

Pathophysiology. Acute bronchiolitis is characterized by bronchiolar obstruction due to edema and accumulation of mucus and cellular debris and by invasion of the smaller radicles of the bronchial tree by virus. Since resistance to airflow in a tube is inversely related to the cube of the radius, even minor thickening of the bronchiolar wall in infants may produce a profound effect on airflow. Airway resistance in the small air passages is increased during both the inspiratory and expiratory phases, but since the radius of an airway is smaller during expiration, the resulting ball valve respiratory obstruction leads to early air trapping and overinflation. Atelectasis may occur when obstruction becomes complete and trapped air is absorbed.

The pathologic process impairs the normal exchange of gases in the lung. Diminished ventilation of the alveoli results in hypoxemia which may occur early in the course. Carbon dioxide retention (hypercapnia) usually does not occur except in severely affected patients. Generally, the higher the respiratory rate, the lower the arterial oxygen tension. Hypercapnia is usually not found until respirations exceed 60/min; it then increases in proportion to the tachypnea.

Clinical Manifestations. Most affected infants have a history of exposure to older children or adults with minor respiratory diseases within the week preceding onset of illness. The infant is first noted to have a mild upper respiratory tract infection with serous nasal discharge and sneezing. These symptoms usually last several days and may be accompanied by fever of 38.5 to 39° C (101–102° F) and diminished appetite. There is then the gradual development of respiratory distress characterized by paroxysmal wheezy cough, dyspnea, and irritability. Bottle feeding may be particularly difficult since the rapid respiratory rate may not permit time for sucking and swallowing. In mild cases symptoms disappear in 1–3 days. On occasion, in the more severely affected patients, symptoms may develop within several hr, and the course is protracted. Other systemic manifestations, such as vomiting and diarrhea, are usually absent. The infant is commonly afebrile, has only a low grade fever, or may be hypothermic.

Examination reveals a tachypneic infant, often in extreme distress. Respirations range from 60–80/min; severe air hunger and cyanosis may be present. There is flaring of the alae nasi, and use of the accessory muscles of respiration results in intercostal and subcostal retractions, which are shallow because of the persistent distention of the lungs by the trapped air. The liver and the spleen may be palpable several cm below the costal margins as a result of depression of the diaphragm due to overinflation. Widespread fine rales may be heard at the end of inspiration and in early expiration. The expiratory phase of breathing is prolonged, and wheezes are usually audible. In the most severe cases, breath sounds are barely audible when bronchiolitic obstruction is nearly complete.

Roentgenographic examination reveals hyperinflation of the lungs and an increased anteroposterior diameter on lateral view. Scattered areas of consolidation are found in about one third of patients and are due either to atelectasis secondary to obstruction or to inflammation of the alveoli. Early bacterial pneumonia cannot be excluded on radiographic grounds alone.

The white blood cell and differential counts are usually within normal limits. Lymphopenia, commonly associated with many viral illnesses, is usually not found. Nasopharyngeal cultures reveal normal flora. Virus may be demonstrated in nasopharyngeal secretions by immunofluorescence, in a rise in blood antibody titers, or in culture.

Differential Diagnosis. The condition most commonly confused with acute bronchiolitis is bronchial asthma. Asthma occurs uncommonly in the 1st yr of life, but frequently after this period. The presence of 1 or more of the following favors the diagnosis of asthma: a family history of asthma, repeated attacks in the same infant, sudden onset without preceding infection, markedly prolonged expiration, eosinophilia, and an immediate favorable response to the administration of a single small dose of epinephrine (0.01 ml/kg of 1:1000 dilution subcutaneously). Repeated attacks represent an important differential point: fewer than 5% of recurrent attacks of clinical bronchiolitis have viral infections as a cause. Other entities that may be confused with acute bronchiolitis are congestive heart failure, foreign body in the trachea, pertussis, organic phosphorus poisoning, cystic fibrosis, and bacterial bronchopneumonias associated with generalized obstructive emphysema.

Course and Prognosis. The most critical phase of illness occurs during the 1st 48–72 hr after the onset of cough and dyspnea. During this period the infant appears desperately ill, apneic spells occur in the very small infant, and respiratory acidosis is likely to be noted. After the critical period improvement occurs rapidly and often dramatically. Recovery is complete in a few days. The case fatality rate is below 1%; death may result from prolonged apneic spells, severe uncompensated respiratory acidosis, or profound dehydration secondary to loss of water vapor from tachypnea and the inability to drink fluids. Infants with such complications as congenital heart disease or cystic fibrosis have a higher mortality. Bacterial complications, such as bronchopneumonia or otitis media, are uncommon. Cardiac failure during bronchiolitis is rare.

It has been reported that a significant proportion of infants with bronchiolitis have asthma during later childhood, but the relation of these 2 entities, if any, is not understood. Similarly, the suggestion in some recent studies that even a single episode of bronchiolitis may result in very long term small airway abnormality requires further investigation.

Treatment. Infants with respiratory distress should be hospitalized, but only supportive treatment is indicated. It is common practice to place the patient in an atmosphere of cold humidified oxygen to relieve hypoxemia and reduce insensible water loss from tachypnea. This serves not only to relieve the dyspnea and cyanosis but also to allay anxiety and restlessness. Sedatives should be avoided whenever possible because of potential depression of respiration. When a sedative must be given, paraldehyde or chloral hydrate is preferred. The infant is usually more comfortable sitting at a 30–40° angle or with head and chest slightly elevated in such a way that the neck is somewhat extended. Tachypnea has a dehydrating effect, and oral intake must often be supplemented or replaced by parenteral fluids. In the event of respiratory acidosis, electrolyte balance and pH should be adjusted by suitable intravenous solutions.

Since acute bronchiolitis is a viral illness, antibiotics have no therapeutic value unless there is secondary bacterial pneumonia. The low incidence of bacterial complications is not made lower by antibiotic therapy. Corticosteroids have not proved to be beneficial in bronchiolitis and may, under certain conditions, be harmful. On the other hand, corticosteroids have not been evaluated in patients with severe adenovirus bronchiolitis in whom long term severe sequelae (necrotizing lesions) might be more likely. Bronchodilating drugs may be contraindicated since they increase restlessness and cardiac output. Epinephrine or other alpha-adrenergic agents, which have a theoretical basis for use, have not been adequately tested. Because the obstruction occurs at the bronchiolar level, tracheostomy is not beneficial and involves substantial risks which are not justified in these acutely ill infants. Occasional patients may progress rapidly to respiratory failure requiring ventilatory assistance.

Aherne W, Bird T, Court SDM, et al: Pathological changes in viral infection of the lower respiratory tract in children. J Clin Pathol 23:7, 1970.
Becroft DMO: Bronchiolitis obliterans, bronchiectasis and other sequelae of adenovirus type 21 infection in young children. J Clin Pathol 24:72, 1971.
Henderson FW, Clyde WA, Collier AM, et al: The etiologic and epidemiologic spectrum of bronchiolitis in pediatric practice. J Pediatr 95:183, 1979.
Hogg JC, Williams J, Richardson JB, et al: Age as a factor in the distribution of lower-airway conductance and in the pathologic anatomy of obstructive lung disease. N Engl J Med 282:1283, 1970.
Wohl MEB, Chernick V: State of the art: Bronchiolitis. Am Rev Resp Dis 118:759, 1978.

12.65 BRONCHIOLITIS OBLITERANS

In this disease, the bronchioles and occasionally some of the smaller bronchi are partially or completely obliterated by nodular masses, which are found on histologic examination to contain granulation and fibrotic tissue. In adults some cases can be clearly related to exposure to the oxides of nitrogen or other chemicals. In children most cases can be temporally related to pulmonary infection. No other precipitating illness or environmental event is known to lead to this condition, but measles, influenza, adenoviral infection, and pertussis have all been reported to precede its development.

Initially, cough, respiratory distress, and, possibly, cyanosis occur and may be followed by a brief period of apparent improvement. The disease then progresses as reflected by increasing dyspnea, cough, sputum production, and wheezing. The pattern may resemble bronchitis, bronchiolitis, or pneumonia. The chest roentgenogram often suggests miliary tuberculosis. A more nonspecific diffuse infiltrate also may be seen. Bronchography shows obstruction of the bronchioles, with little or no contrast material reaching the periphery of the lung. The disease can then be confirmed by lung biopsy.

There is no specific treatment. Since the pathology suggests a progressive fibrotic picture which could theoretically be delayed by corticosteroid treatment, these agents are almost universally used, but there are no data as to their efficacy. Some patients deteriorate rapidly and die within weeks of the onset of initial symptoms; others run a much more chronic course; and a few may go on to develop the unilateral hyperlucent lung syndrome.

Azizirad H, Polgar G, Borns PF, et al: Bronchiolitis obliterans. Clin Pediatr 14:572, 1975.
Becroft DMO: Bronchiolitis obliterans, bronchiectasis and other sequelae of adenovirus type 21 infection in young children. J Clin Pathol 24:72, 1971.
Wohl MEB, Chernick V: State of the art: Bronchiolitis. Am Rev Resp Dis 118:759, 1978.

BRONCHIAL ASTHMA

See Sec 9.49.

PNEUMONIA

The various clinical forms of pneumonia are often classified by their anatomic distribution—lobar, lobular, interstitial, bronchopneumonia—or by the agents which cause them, such as viral, bacterial, or aspiration pneumonia. Fig 12–9 depicts the lobes of the lung by their roentgenographic location. Many etiologically unclassified infections occur in infancy and are probably of viral origin. Most bacterial infections are susceptible to antibiotic therapy whereas viral infections usually are not.

Certain lesions are commonly produced by specific causative agents. For example, the pneumococcus produces an inflammatory lesion of the mucosa and an alveolar exudate, usually without destruction of mucosal cells or extensive involvement of interstitial tissues. The gross lesion is a consolidation of all or part of a lobe in the lobar variety or of scattered lobules in the bronchopneumonic variety. In contrast, viral agents, H. influenzae, and certain strains of the viridans group of streptococci invade or destroy the mucous membrane and may produce principally bronchiolitis, peribronchiolitis, and interstitial lesions. Both staphylococcus and Klebsiella tend to destroy tissue and to produce multiple small abscesses.

The following classification is helpful in considering pneumonias in children:

I. BACTERIAL INFECTIONS
   Pneumococcus
   Streptococcus
   Staphylococcus
   H. influenzae
   Klebsiella
   Tubercle bacillus

II. VIRAL OR PROBABLE VIRAL INFECTIONS
   Interstitial pneumonitis and bronchiolitis
   Giant cell pneumonia
   Influenza
III. OTHER INFECTIONS
   Pneumocystis carinii pneumonia
   Q fever (Sec 10.99)
   Mycoplasma pneumoniae pneumonia (Sec 10.66)
   Treponema pallidum
   Nocardiosis
   Actinomycosis
   Chlamydia
   Ornithosis
   Psittacosis
IV. MYCOTIC INFECTIONS
   Aspergillosis
   Coccidioidomycosis
   Histoplasmosis
   Blastomycosis
   Mucormycosis
   Sporotrichosis
   Thrush
V. ASPIRATION OF:
   Amniotic contents (fetal anoxia)
   Food
   Foreign bodies
   Zinc stearate
   Dust
   Hydrocarbons
   Lipoid substances
VI. LÖFFLER SYNDROME
VII. HYPOSTATIC PNEUMONIA

12.66 BACTERIAL PNEUMONIA

General Considerations. Primary infection of the parenchyma of the lung (pneumonia) is much less common than secondary bacterial infection complicating the acute bronchitis that occurs during minor upper respiratory infection. Bacterial pneumonia during childhood and recurrent pneumonia in the absence of an underlying chronic illness, such as cystic fibrosis or immunologic deficiency, is quite unusual. In infants and young children with infection of the lower respiratory tract, signs and symptoms of pulmonary involvement are often nonspecific, and findings on physical examination may be surprisingly few. Accordingly, roentgenographic evidence of pneumonia is frequently found in infants who clinically appear to have only upper respiratory tract infections or only tachypnea and fever without physical findings that suggest pulmonary involvement.

The most common event disturbing the defense mechanisms of the lung (Sec 12.6) is a viral infection which alters the properties of normal secretions, inhibits phagocytosis, modifies the bacterial flora, and may temporarily disrupt the normal epithelial layer of the respiratory passages. A viral respiratory disease often precedes the development of bacterial pneumonia by a few days. Once pneumonia has occurred, a series of intricate mechanisms brings about resolution of infection and recovery.

Children with defects in defense mechanisms or in the chain of events involved in recovery from infection, experience recurrent pneumonias or failure to resolve

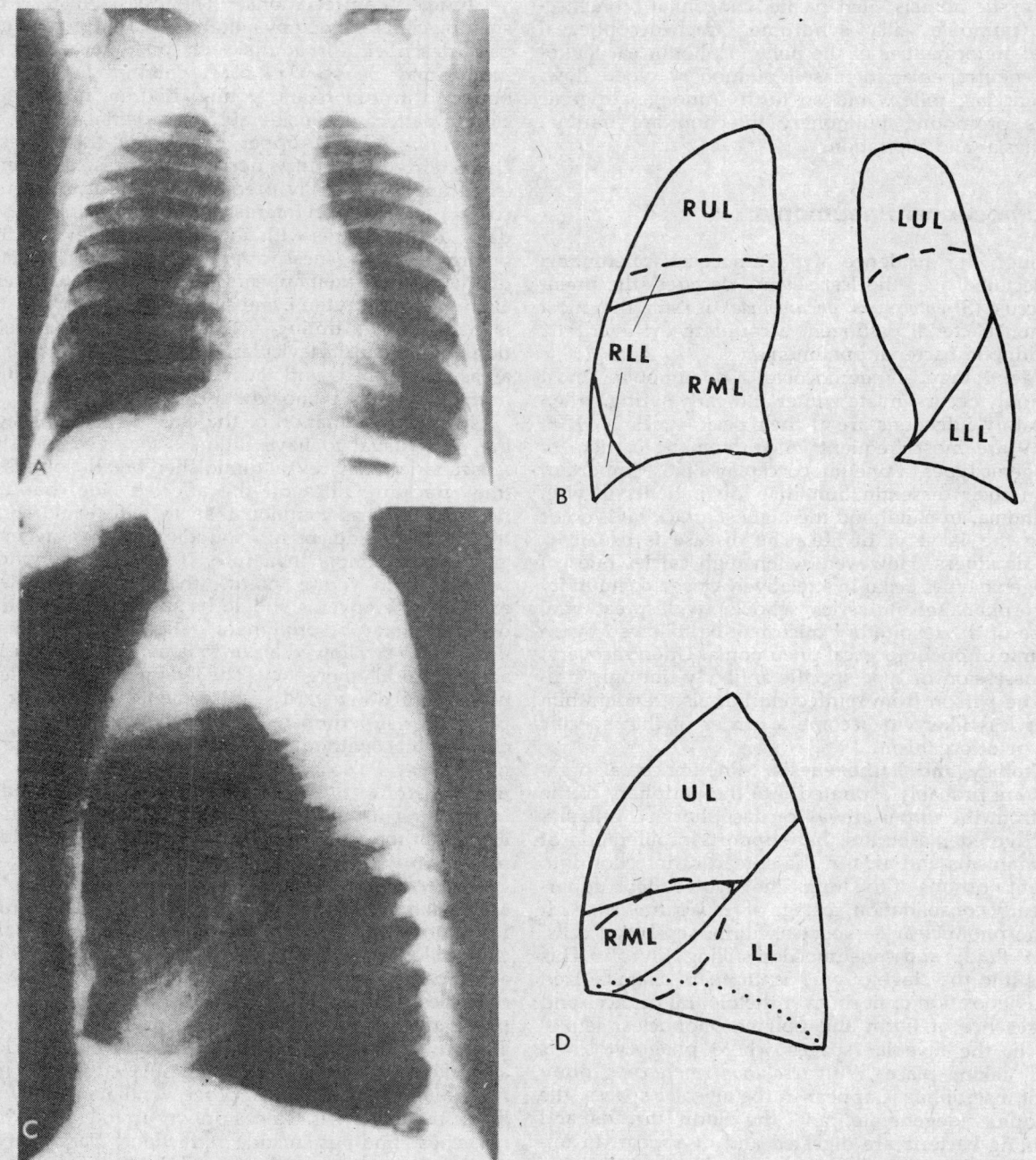

Figure 12–9 *A,* Posterior-anterior chest film of a 12 mo old boy with a history of sudden onset of cough and wheezing. Physical examination revealed decreased breath sounds and wheezes on the left. The film was made in full inspiration, and shows only some hyperinflation. The film of the same patient taken in expiration showed that the right lung emptied more completely than the left, and appeared denser. The mediastinum was shifted to the right, similar to the shift seen in Fig 12–7*B.* A peanut was found at bronchoscopy.

B, Line drawing to demonstrate lobar distribution in the posterior-anterior projection. The right middle lobe overlies most of the right lower lobe. Lesions in the lingula and the right middle lobe often result in a loss of definition of the heart borders, but frequently the lateral view is necessary to accurately locate a roentgenographic lesion. RUL, right upper lobe; RLL, right lower lobe; RML, right middle lobe; LUL, left upper lobe; LLL, left lower lobe.

C, Lateral chest film of the same patient. The diaphragms are quite flat, indicating hyperinflation. The film appears otherwise normal.

D, Line drawing to demonstrate lobar distribution in the lateral projection. The normal contour of the diaphragm is shown as a dotted line, and the outline of the heart as a dashed line. The left upper lobe occupies the equivalent position of both the right upper and middle lobes; the lingular portion of the left upper lobe corresponds to the right middle lobe. UL, upper lobes; RML, right middle lobe; LL, lower lobe.

the disease completely. These defects occur with abnormalities of antibody production (agammaglobulinemia), cystic fibrosis, cleft palate, congenital bronchiectasis, immotile cilia syndrome, tracheoesophageal fistula, abnormalities of the polymorphonuclear leukocytes, neutropenia, increased pulmonary blood flow, deficient gag reflex, and so forth. Among iatrogenic factors promoting pulmonary infection are trauma, anesthesia, and aspiration.

Pneumococcal Pneumonia

Though the incidence of pneumococcal pneumonia has declined over the last several decades, the pneumococcus (Streptococcus pneumoniae) is still the most common bacterial pathogen, accounting for over 90% of childhood bacterial pneumonia.

Epidemiology. Pneumococcal pneumonia most commonly occurs in late winter and early spring, when respiratory infections are at their peak; types 14, 1, 6, and 19 are most frequent. Asymptomatic carriers of pathogenic types of pneumococci play a more important role in their dissemination than do patients ill with pneumonia. In childhood the highest attack rates occur during the 1st 4 yr of life. The disease is usually a sporadic illness. However, when high carrier rates of pathogenic types occur in a relatively closed community (e.g., orphanages, nurseries, schools), widespread viral disease of the respiratory tract may be followed by an epidemic of pneumococcal pneumonia. Upon recovery, the possession of type-specific antibody not only protects the person from reinfection but also renders him or her less likely to become a carrier of that specific serotype of organism.

Pathology and Pathogenesis. Pneumococcal organisms are probably aspirated into the periphery of the lung from the upper airway or nasopharynx. Initially, a reactive edema occurs that supports proliferation of the organisms and aids in the spread of infection into adjacent portions of the lung. The involved lobe undergoes early consolidation, a stage of *red hepatization*, with polymorphonuclear leukocytes, fibrin, red blood cells, edema fluid, and pneumococci filling alveoli. This passes into the stage of *gray hepatization*, characterized by the deposition of fibrin over the pleural surfaces and the presence of fibrin and polymorphonuclear leukocytes in the alveolar spaces where phagocytosis is rapidly taking place. With *resolution*, increasing numbers of macrophages appear in the alveolar spaces, the neutrophils degenerate, and the fibrin threads and remaining bacteria are digested and disappear. In untreated cases a clinical crisis occurs about the 7th day of illness, and resolution and re-expansion require an additional 1–3 wk. Antibiotics given in the 1st several days of illness interrupt the course, and the characteristic stages are not seen.

Usually 1 or more lobes, or parts of lobes, are involved, leaving the remaining bronchopulmonary system uninvolved. However, this pattern of lobar pneumonia is often not present in infants. They may have a more patchy and diffuse disease that follows a bronchial distribution and is characterized by many limited areas of consolidation around the smaller airways. Permanent injury is rare.

Clinical Manifestations. The classic history of a shaking chill followed by a high fever, cough, and chest pain described for adults with pneumococcal pneumonia may be seen in older children but is rarely observed in infants and young children, in whom the clinical pattern is considerably more variable.

Infants. A mild upper respiratory tract infection characterized by stuffy nose, fretfulness, and diminished appetite usually precedes the onset of pneumococcal pneumonia in infants. This mild illness of several days' duration ends with abrupt onset of fever of 39° C or higher, restlessness, apprehension, and respiratory distress. The patient appears ill with moderate to severe air hunger and often cyanosis. The respiratory distress is manifest by grunting, flaring of the alae nasi, retractions of the supraclavicular, intercostal, and subcostal areas, tachypnea, and tachycardia. Cough is unusual initially but may be noted later.

Physical examination of the chest is often unrevealing. It is usual to have dullness localized to 1 lobe. Auscultation may reveal diminished breath sounds and fine, crackling rales on the affected side, but these findings are less common than in older children. On the opposite side, breath sounds may be exaggerated and almost tubular in nature. If dullness is found on percussion in young infants, the presence of pleural effusion or empyema should be suspected. Abdominal distention may be prominent, reflecting gastric distention due to swallowed air or to ileus; it may suggest an acute surgical emergency. The liver may appear enlarged because of downward displacement of the right diaphragm or superimposed congestive heart failure. Nuchal rigidity without meningeal infection (meningismus) may also be prominent, especially with involvement of the right upper lobe. Physical findings in the lung usually change little during the course of illness, although moist rales may become audible during resolution.

Children and Teenagers. The signs and symptoms are similar to those of adults. After a brief, mild, upper respiratory infection there is often onset of a shaking chill followed by fever as high as 40.5° C. This is accompanied by drowsiness with intermittent periods of restlessness, rapid respirations, a dry, hacking, unproductive cough, anxiety, and occasionally delirium. There may be circumoral cyanosis, and many children are noted to be splinting on the affected side to minimize pleuritic pain and improve ventilation; they may lie on their side with knees drawn up to chest. Abnormal chest findings include retractions, flaring of alae nasi, dullness, diminished tactile and vocal fremitus, diminished breath sounds, and fine and crackling rales on the affected side. On the 1st day of illness, dullness over the affected lobe is usually not evident, and the suppression of breath sounds on the affected side may lead to misinterpretation of the exaggerated breath sounds in the opposite lung as tubular breathing.

The physical findings undergo change during the course of illness. Classic signs of consolidation are noted on the 2nd–3rd day of illness and are characterized by dullness, increased fremitus, tubular breath sounds, and the disappearance of rales. As resolution occurs, moist rales are heard, and the signs of consolidation disappear. The initial dry, hacking cough loosens and becomes productive of large amounts of blood-tinged mucous material.

The development of a pleural effusion or empyema may cause a visible lag in respiration on the affected side, with exaggerated excursion on the opposite side. Examination usually reveals dullness over the area of the effusion, with diminished fremitus and breath sounds. Tubular breathing is often noted immediately above the fluid level and on the unaffected side.

Laboratory Findings. The white blood cell count is usually elevated to 15,000–40,000 cells/mm³, with a preponderance of polymorphonuclear cells. White blood cell counts below 5000/mm³ are often associated with a grave prognosis. The hemoglobin value is usually normal or only slightly diminished. Arterial blood samples usually show hypoxemia without hypercapnia.

In most patients pneumococci can be isolated from the nasopharyngeal secretions, but this finding cannot be considered proof of a causative relation; the isolation of pneumococci should be attempted from secretions obtained upon deep coughing, from gentle tracheal aspiration, from blood, or from pleural fluid obtained at thoracentesis. Bacteremia is found in about 30% of cases of pneumococcal pneumonia. Countercurrent immunoelectrophoresis of blood, pleural fluid, and/or urine may be helpful in establishing the diagnosis.

Roentgenographic Findings. The roentgenographic changes in pneumococcal pneumonia do not always correspond to the clinical observations. Consolidation may be demonstrated by roentgenography before it is detectable by physical examination, and resolution of the infiltrate may not be complete until several wk after the child is clinically well. Lobar consolidation is not as common in infants and young children as in the older child. Pleural reaction with the presence of fluid is not uncommon; it may be seen early in the course of illness and, even in the untreated patient, is not necessarily indicative of developing empyema. It is extremely important that roentgenographic demonstration of complete resolution be obtained 3–4 wk after disappearance of all symptoms. Persistence of infiltrate suggests an underlying process, such as a foreign body or immunologic deficiency. If clinical response is slow, serial roentgenograms are indicated.

Differential Diagnosis. Pneumococcal pneumonia cannot be differentiated from other bacterial and viral pneumonias without suitable microbiologic studies. Conditions possibly confused with pneumonia are bronchiolitis, allergic bronchitis, congestive heart failure, acute exacerbations of bronchiectasis, aspiration of a foreign body, sequestered lobe, atelectasis, pulmonary abscess, and endotracheal tuberculosis with secondary bacterial pneumonia.

An older child with right lower lobe pneumonia may have diaphragmatic irritation with pain referred to the right lower quadrant of the abdomen. Since ileus may accompany pneumonia, right lower quadrant pain and absent bowel sounds may be misinterpreted as acute appendicitis.

When meningismus is severe and presents opisthotonos or positive Kernig and Brudzinski signs, it can be differentiated from meningitis only by examination of the spinal fluid.

Complications. With the use of antibiotic therapy, complications of bacterial pneumonia have become unusual. Although concomitant infection in other locations with pneumococci (e.g., otitis media) may be present prior to the onset of the symptoms of pneumonia, metastatic infection after the initiation of antibiotic treatment is infrequent. Local complications such as empyema and lung abscess are uncommon. Empyema results from extension of infection to the pleural surfaces and occurs most commonly in the young infant who has received medical attention late in the course of illness or who has been inadequately treated. Persistent pneumatoceles may also occur and usually do not require treatment.

Prognosis. In the preantibiotic era the mortality rate from pneumococcal pneumonia in infants and small children ranged from 20–50% and in older children from 3–5%. Furthermore, the incidence of chronic empyema with altered pulmonary function was relatively high. With appropriate antibiotic therapy instituted early in the course of the illness, the mortality rate during infancy and childhood is now less than 1%, and long-term morbidity is correspondingly low.

Treatment. The drug of choice is penicillin since most pneumococci are exquisitely sensitive to this agent. The recent emergence of penicillin-resistant pneumococci in certain areas of the world suggests that alternative antibiotic therapy may be indicated pending the results of antibiotic sensitivity testing. In infants and young children initial therapy should be parenteral penicillin G in a dosage of 50,000 units/kg/24 hr. In older children a single intramuscular injection of procaine penicillin, 600,000 units, followed by oral penicillin, is usually adequate outpatient treatment. If the child is not vomiting, initial therapy with oral penicillin V (50,000 units/kg/24 hr) may be appropriate, particularly for older children. In patients allergic to penicillin, a cephalosporin may be used, such as cefazolin (50 mg/kg/24 hr). Treatment is given for 7–10 days in uncomplicated cases.

The majority of older children with pneumococcal pneumonia can be treated at home; the decision to hospitalize depends on the severity of illness, the physical adequacy of the home, and the ability of the family to supply good nursing care. Pneumonia in the young infant is best treated in the hospital since fluids and antibiotics may have to be administered intravenously. Furthermore, the course of illness in young infants is more variable and complications more common. Patients with pneumonia associated with pleural effusion or empyema should also be hospitalized. Liberal oral intake of fluids and the administration of aspirin for high fever are the principal adjuncts to therapy. Oxygen administered promptly to patients with significant respiratory distress will greatly reduce the need for sedatives and analgesics; it should be given before the patient becomes cyanotic.

Polyvalent pneumococcal polysaccharide vaccine has

proved efficacious in certain patient populations such as patients with sickel cell anemia. However, its routine use in healthy children is not indicated.

Streptococcal Pneumonia

Group A streptococci most commonly cause disease limited to the upper respiratory tract, but the organisms may spread to other areas of the body, including the lower respiratory tract. Streptococcal pneumonia and tracheobronchitis are uncommon, but certain viral infections, particularly the exanthems and epidemic influenza, predispose to these diseases, which are most frequently encountered in children 3–5 yr of age and very rarely in infants. Group B streptococcal pneumonia is discussed in Sec 10.21.

Pathology. Streptococcal infections of the lower respiratory tract result in tracheitis, bronchitis, or interstitial pneumonia. Lobar pneumonia is uncommon. Lesions consist of necrosis of the tracheobronchial mucosa with the formation of ragged ulcers and large amounts of exudate, edema, and localized hemorrhage. The process may extend to the interalveolar septa and involve lymphatic vessels. Infection may spread by way of the lymphatics to the mediastinal and hilar lymph nodes or may proceed in a retrograde direction in occluded vessels and reach the pleural surfaces. Pleurisy is relatively common; the effusion is often large and serous, occasionally serosanguineous, or thinly purulent, with less fibrin than the exudate of pneumococcal pneumonia.

Clinical Manifestations. The signs and symptoms of streptococcal pneumonia are similar to those of pneumococcal pneumonia. The onset may be sudden, characterized by high fever, chills, signs of respiratory distress, and, at times, extreme prostration. However, on occasion it may be more insidious as is often the case with *H. influenzae* pneumonia, and the child appears only mildly ill with cough and low grade fever. If an exanthem or influenza precedes the pneumonia, the onset may be seen only as an increasingly severe clinical course of the viral illness. The clinical findings may be less impressive than the disseminated interstitial infiltration noted on roentgenogram. Pleurisy, which commonly occurs, may be evidenced by clinical findings and pleural effusion.

Laboratory Manifestations. Leukocytosis occurs as in pneumococcal pneumonia. A rise in serum antistreptolysin titer is supportive diagnostic evidence. The disease may be suspected if large amounts of group A β-hemolytic streptococci are isolated from throat swab, nasopharyngeal secretions, bronchial washings, or sputum, but definitive diagnosis rests on recovery of the organism from pleural fluid, blood, or lung aspirate. Bacteremia occurs in about 10% of patients.

Chest roentgenograms usually show diffuse bronchopneumonia, often with a large pleural effusion. Occasionally, there is hilar adenopathy. Final roentgenographic resolution should be demonstrated but may not be complete for up to 10 wk.

Differential Diagnosis. The clinical course and roentgenographic findings of streptococcal pneumonia with purulent pleurisy are often similar to those of staphylococcal pneumonia. Pneumatoceles may occur in both conditions. The roentgenographic changes of uncomplicated streptococcal pneumonia may be indistinguishable from other interstitial pneumonitides, including those caused by *Mycoplasma pneumoniae*.

Complications. Bacterial complications and long-term morbidity are common in the untreated patient but rare after antibiotic treatment is begun. Empyema occurs in 20% of children, and occasionally septic foci develop in other areas, such as the bones or joints; otherwise extension of the disease is uncommon. Acute glomerulonephritis occurs rarely.

Treatment. The drug of choice in streptococcal pneumonia is penicillin G (100,000 units/kg/24 hr). Parenteral penicillin is used initially, and a 2–3 wk course may be completed orally after clinical improvement has begun in the hospital. If empyema develops, a thoracentesis should be performed for diagnostic purposes and for removal of fluid. On occasion, repeated thoracenteses or closed drainage with indwelling chest tubes may be required if the fluid reaccumulates. Intrathoracic administration of antibiotics or enzymes to liquefy pus or dissolve fibrin is ineffective.

Staphylococcal Pneumonia

Pneumonia caused by *S. aureus* is a serious and rapidly progressive infection which, unless recognized early and treated appropriately, is associated with prolonged morbidity and high mortality. It occurs less frequently than pneumococcal or viral pneumonia and is more common in infants than in children (Sec 7.60 and 7.67).

Epidemiology. The majority of cases occur from October–May, and, as with other bacterial pneumonias, staphylococcal pneumonia is frequently preceded by a viral upper respiratory tract infection. Although it may occur at any age, 30% of all patients are under 3 mo of age and 70% under 1 yr. Boys are affected more commonly than girls.

Although *S. aureus* is commonly found on normal skin and mucous membranes, serious disease is comparatively rare. Nearly 90% of normal infants become nasal carriers in the neonatal period. This declines to about 20% during the 1st 2 yr of life and then rises to the adult rate of 30–50% by age 4–6 yr.

The occurrence of epidemics of staphylococcal disease in nurseries is usually associated with specific pathologic strains that are commonly resistant to many antibiotics. Even during these outbreaks most of the colonized infants and hospital personnel or family contacts remain free of disease, although they may serve to spread the infection to others. The infant may exhibit disease within a few days after colonization or not until weeks later. Viral respiratory infections may play a significant role in promoting dissemination of the staphylococcus among infants and in converting colonization to disease.

Pathogenicity and Pathology. *Staphylococcus aureus* produces a variety of toxins and enzymes, such as hemolysin, leukocidin, staphylokinase, and coagulase.

Coagulase interacts with a plasma factor to produce an active principle that converts fibrinogen to fibrin and thereby causes clot formation. A good correlation exists between coagulase production and virulence; coagulase-negative staphylococci rarely produce serious disease.

Staphylococci cause confluent bronchopneumonia which is often unilateral or more prominent on 1 side than the other and is characterized by the presence of extensive areas of hemorrhagic necrosis and irregular areas of cavitation. The pleural surface is usually covered by a thick layer of fibrinopurulent exudate. Multiple abscesses occur, containing clusters of staphylococci, leukocytes, erythrocytes, and necrotic debris. Rupture of a small subpleural abscess may result in a pyopneumothorax, which in turn may erode into a bronchus, producing a bronchopleural fistula. Septic thrombi may form in pulmonary veins in regions of extensive destruction and inflammation.

Clinical Manifestations. Most commonly, the patient is an infant under 1 yr of age, often with a history of staphylococcal skin lesions in him- or herself or in a family member and with signs and symptoms of an upper or lower respiratory tract infection for several days to 1 wk. Abruptly, the infant's condition changes, with the onset of high fever, cough, and evidence of respiratory distress. Signs and symptoms include tachypnea, grunting respirations, sternal and subcostal retractions, nasal flaring, cyanosis, and anxiety. If left undisturbed, the infant is lethargic but upon arousal is irritable and appears toxic. Severe dyspnea and a shock-like state may be present. Some infants have associated gastrointestinal disturbances characterized by vomiting, anorexia, diarrhea, and abdominal distention secondary to a paralytic ileus. A rapid progression of symptoms is characteristic.

Physical findings depend on the stage of pneumonia. Early in the course of illness diminished breath sounds, scattered rales, and rhonchi are commonly heard over the affected lung. With the development of effusion, empyema, or pyopneumothorax, dullness on percussion is noted, and breath sounds and vocal fremitus are markedly diminished. A lag in respiratory excursion often occurs on the affected side. Physical examination may, however, be misleading, particularly in the young infant with meager findings disproportionate to the degree of tachypnea.

Laboratory Manifestations. In the older infant and child a leukocytosis of 20,000 or more cells/mm³ usually occurs, with the increase primarily among the polymorphonuclear cells; in the young infant the white blood cell count may remain within the normal range. As in other forms of bacterial infection, a count below 5000 cells/mm³ is a poor prognostic sign. Mild to moderate anemia is common.

Material for diagnostic cultures should be obtained by tracheal aspiration or pleural tap; Gram stain frequently reveals gram-positive cocci. The finding of staphylococci in the nasopharynx is of no diagnostic value, but blood culture may be positive. Pleural fluid reveals an exudate with polymorphonuclear cell counts ranging from 300–100,000/mm³, protein above 2.5 gm/dl, and low glucose level relative to the blood level.

Roentgenographic Findings. Most patients with staphylococcal pneumonia have roentgenographic evidence of nonspecific bronchopneumonia early in the illness. The infiltrate may soon become patchy and limited in extent or be dense and homogeneous and involve an entire lobe or hemithorax. The right lung alone is involved in about 65% of cases; bilateral involvement occurs in fewer than 20% of patients. A pleural effusion or empyema will be noted during the course in most patients; pyopneumothorax occurs in about 25%. Pneumatoceles of varying size are common.

Though no roentgenographic change can be considered diagnostic, progression over a few hr from bronchopneumonia to effusion or pyopneumothorax with or without pneumatoceles is highly suggestive of staphylococcal pneumonia. Chest films should be obtained at frequent intervals if the diagnosis of early staphylococcal pneumonia is suspected. Clinical improvement usually precedes roentgenographic clearing by days or weeks, and pneumatoceles may persist in an asymptomatic patient for months.

Differential Diagnosis. The recognition of early staphylococcal pneumonia in the infant is often difficult. Abrupt onset and rapid progression of symptoms of pneumonia should be considered due to staphylococci until proved otherwise. A history of furunculosis, a preceding viral upper respiratory tract infection, a recent hospital admission, or maternal breast abscess should also alert the physician to the possibility of this diagnosis in the infant. Other bacterial pneumonias that cause empyema or pneumatoceles and may thus be readily confused with staphylococcal disease include streptococcal, *Klebsiella*, *H. influenzae*, and pneumococcal pneumonias and primary tuberculous pneumonia with cavitation. Occasionally, the aspiration of a nonradiopaque foreign body followed by pulmonary abscesses may lead to a similar clinical and radiologic picture.

Complications. Since empyema, pyopneumothorax, and pneumatoceles are so commonly seen with staphylococcal pneumonia, they are considered part of the natural course of the illness and not complications. Septic lesions outside the respiratory tract occur rarely except in the young infant, in whom staphylococcal pericarditis, meningitis, osteomyelitis, and multiple metastatic abscesses in soft tissue may occur. Metastatic infection after the initiation of appropriate antibiotic therapy is rare.

Prognosis. Survival has improved substantially with present-day management, but mortality still ranges from 10–30% and varies with the length of illness prior to hospitalization, age of patient, adequacy of therapy, and the presence of other illness or complications. Children who do not have demonstrable underlying disease have an excellent prognosis for complete recovery with normal growth and development, normal pulmonary function, and no increased susceptibility to pulmonary infections. The course is usually prolonged, with hospitalizations of from 6–10 wk. All infants with staphylococcal pneumonia should be tested for cystic fibrosis and screened for immunodeficiency disease.

Treatment. Therapy consists of appropriate antibiotics and drainage of collections of pus. The infant should be given oxygen and placed in a semireclining position to relieve cyanosis and anxiety. During the acute phase intravenous hydration and nutrition are indicated, and if the patient is severely anemic, blood transfusion may be benefical. Assisted ventilation may occasionally be needed.

A semisynthetic, penicillinase-resistant penicillin should be administered intravenously immediately after culture while reports are pending (e.g., methicillin 200 mg/kg/24 hr). Patients receiving these drugs should be closely monitored for possible nephrotoxicity. If the cultures subsequently demonstrate an organism sensitive to penicillin G, then this agent should be used in dosages of 100,000 units/kg/24 hr instead of the initial drug. Some advise initially administering both drugs concurrently until the antibiotic sensitivity is known, when 1 can be discontinued. There is no evidence that this practice increases the efficacy of treatment, but it may increase the frequency of adverse reactions. In patients allergic to penicillin, a cephalosporin may be used, such as cefazolin, 50 mg/kg/24 hr. Three–4 wk of therapy is usually adequate, but the clinical response may indicate a need for longer therapy.

Although patients with staphylococcal pneumonia may occasionally recover completely without chest tube drainage, it is recommended even if only a small effusion or empyema is present in order to reduce the chance of bronchopleural fistula and the necessity for repeated pleural taps. Generally, pus reaccumulates so rapidly and becomes so viscous or loculated that closed drainage with a chest tube of the largest possible caliber is required. The appearance of pyopneumothorax is another indication for immediate insertion of a catheter into the pleural space. It is often necessary to use several chest tubes when loculation occurs. Once the infant begins to improve and the lung has re-expanded, the tubes may be removed, even if they are still draining small amounts of pus; in general, tubes should not remain in the chest more than 5–7 days.

Instillation of antibiotics or enzymes into the chest cavity has no beneficial effect and is associated with an increased incidence of pneumothorax and systemic toxic reactions.

Ammann AJ, Addiego J, Wara DW, et al: Polyvalent pneumococcal-polysaccharide immunization of patients with sickle-cell anemia and patients with splenectomy. N Engl J Med 297:897, 1977.
Ceruti E, Contreras J, Neira M: Staphylococcal pneumonia in childhood. Long-term follow-up including pulmonary function studies. Am J Dis Child 122:386, 1971.
Honig PJ, Pasquariello PS Jr, Stool SE: H. influenzae pneumonia in infants and children. J Pediatr 83:215, 1973.
Jay SJ, Johanson WG Jr, Pierce AK: The radiographic resolution of Streptococcus pneumoniae pneumonia. N Engl J Med 293:798, 1975.
Klein JO, Mortimer EA: Use of pneumococcal vaccine in children. Pediatrics 61:31, 1978.
Michaels RH, Poziviak CS: Countercurrent immunoelectrophoresis for the diagnosis of pneumococcal pneumonia in children. J Pediatr 88:72, 1975.
Rebban AW, Edwards HE: Staphylococcal pneumonia. Review of 329 cases. Can Med Assoc J 82:513, 1960.

Pneumonias Caused by Gram-Negative Organisms

A small percentage of pneumonias of infants and children after the neonatal period are caused by gram-negative organisms. However, the number has been increasing in recent yr, perhaps because of the widespread use of antibiotics, the contamination of hospital equipment, the increasing use of immunosuppressive agents in the treatment of malignant disorders, and the increasing survival of children with chronic pulmonary disease such as cystic fibrosis. The organisms most commonly encountered are H. influenzae type b, Klebsiella pneumoniae, and Pseudomonas aeruginosa. The morbidity and mortality rates of these infections are high as a result of the pathogenicity of the bacteria and the altered host resistance in many of these patients (Chapter 10).

Hemophilus influenzae Pneumonia. H. influenzae type b is a frequent cause of serious bacterial infection in infants and children. Nasopharyngeal infection precedes almost all clinical varieties of localized H. influenzae disease, such as otitis media, epiglottitis, pneumonia, and meningitis.

Hemophilus influenzae pneumonias are lobar in distribution; occasionally, 2 or more lobes are involved. Disseminated pulmonary disease and bronchopneumonia have also been described. Males are affected slightly more often than females. Pathologically, involved areas show a polymorphonuclear or lymphocytic inflammatory reaction with extensive destruction of the epithelium of smaller airways, interstitial inflammation, and marked, often hemorrhagic, edema.

Although the disease may be difficult to distinguish clinically from pneumococcal pneumonia, it is more often insidious in onset, and the course is usually prolonged over several wk. Many patients are already receiving treatment for otitis media at the time of diagnosis. Although chloramphenicol and ampicillin (see below) are recommended for treatment of Hemophilus influenzae pneumonia, a clinical response to penicillin G is common and does not exclude this diagnosis. Cough is almost always present but may not be productive, and the patient is febrile and often tachypneic with nasal flaring and retractions. There may be localized dullness to percussion and rales and tubular breath sounds; empyema is often present on roentgenogram in the young infant.

The diagnosis is established by isolation of the organism from the blood, particularly in the young infant, or from pleural fluid, lung aspirate, or bronchoscopic washings. There is usually moderate leukocytosis with a relative lymphopenia. Counterimmunoelectrophoresis on tracheal secretions, blood, urine, and pleural fluid may be helpful in making an early diagnosis. If atelectasis is present, bronchoscopy is indicated to rule out a foreign body.

Complications are frequent, particularly in the young infant, and include bacteremia, pericarditis, cellulitis, empyema, meningitis, and pyarthrosis.

Treatment consists of the same symptomatic and supportive measures utilized in pneumococcal and staphylococcal pneumonias. When *H. influenzae* is suspected as the causative agent, chloramphenicol (100 mg/kg/24 hr) is the antibiotic agent of choice until it is known whether the organism produces penicillinase; if the strain is sensitive, ampicillin (200 mg/kg/24 hr) should be administered. The child should be hospitalized and both drugs administered intravenously. Empyema and pyarthrosis may require drainage. If the initial response to therapy is good, oral treatment can be instituted to complete a 10–14 day course. Roentgenographic demonstration of complete resolution should be obtained 2–4 wk later.

Klebsiella pneumoniae (Friedländer Bacillus) Pneumonia. This organism is found in the respiratory and gastrointestinal tracts of approximately 5% of normal persons. It is known to cause pneumonia in debilitated or immunosuppressed patients and frequently occurs as a secondary invader in the lungs of patients with chronic bronchiectasis, influenza, or tuberculosis. Primary *K. pneumoniae* infection is unusual in infants and young children; it may occur, rarely, in nursery epidemics or as a sporadic case in neonates. During epidemics many infants will carry the organism in their nasopharynges without signs of clinical illness; only an occasional baby will have severe disease. Contaminated fomites, including nursery equipment, and humidification apparatus are the primary source of nosocomial infection with the organism.

Pneumonia due to *K. pneumoniae* may be difficult to distinguish clinically from pneumonia due to other causes. In nursery epidemics, diarrhea and vomiting may be the presenting symptoms; the onset of respiratory difficulty is often abrupt. The disease may have a fulminant course characterized by copious, thick, purulent secretion and the formation of pulmonary abscesses and cavitations. A lobar infiltrate with bulging fissures on roentgenogram is suggestive of the diagnosis (Fig 12–10). Complications are common and include bacteremia, empyema, and residual parenchymal damage. The fatality rate in sporadic cases is about 50%, but it is lower during epidemics.

Isolation of the organism from purulent tracheal secretions, blood, or lung aspirate establishes the diagnosis. Supportive treatment is similar to that of other bacterial pneumonias; drainage of empyema and abscesses may be necessary. Kanamycin (15–20 mg/kg/24 hr, intramuscularly every 8 hr for 10–14 days) is the agent of choice; however, gentamicin may be employed initially if local sensitivity testing indicates a high degree of kanamycin resistance among *Klebsiella* isolates. In older children and adults the cephalosporins have also proved efficacious in treating these infections.

Pseudomonas aeruginosa Pneumonia (Sec 10.34). *Pseudomonas aeruginosa* produces a severe, progressive, usually fatal, necrotizing bronchopneumonia. It is rarely a primary infection of the lung but occurs with chronic debilitating illnesses, such as cystic fibrosis and malignant disorders; with altered immunologic function; during prolonged antibiotic therapy; and in premature infants exposed to contaminated hospital equipment. In cystic fibrosis a fulminant course is uncommon. Ticarcillin administered alone or in combination with an aminoglycoside represents the most effective therapy.

Asmar BI, Slovis TL, Reed JO, et al: *Hemophilus influenzae* type b pneumonia in 43 children. J Pediatr 93:389, 1978.

Morgan HR: The enteric bacteria. *In*: Dubos R, Hirsch J (eds): Bacterial and Mycotic Infections of Man. Ed 4. Philadelphia, JB Lippincott, 1965.

Nyhan WL, Rectanus DR, Fousek MD: *Hemophilus influenzae* type b pneumonia. Pediatrics 161:31, 1955.

Riley HD, Bracken EC: Empyema due to *Hemophilus influenzae* in infants and children. Am J Dis Child 110:24, 1965.

Thaler MM: *Klebsiella-Aerobacter* pneumonia in infants. Pediatrics 30:206, 1962.

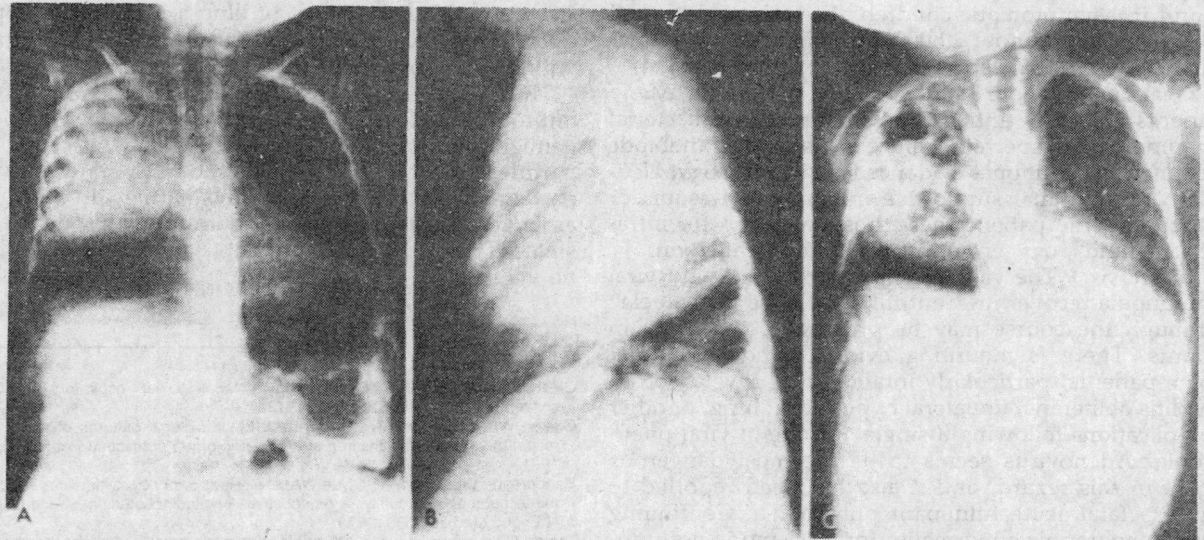

Figure 12–10 Klebsiella pneumonia in an 8 mo old infant admitted with complaints of cough, fever, and dyspnea. Roentgenograms (*A, B*) demonstrated pulmonary consolidation with characteristic bulging of fissure. Multiple pneumatoceles and abscesses appeared within 48 hr (*C*). Recovery occurred with kanamycin therapy.

12.67   PNEUMONIAS OF VIRAL ORIGIN

Etiology.   Many viruses are capable of causing lower respiratory tract disease in children, principally bronchiolitis and interstitial lesions. The type and severity of the illness are influenced by several factors including age, sex, season of the year, and crowding. Viral pneumonia is most commonly caused by respiratory syncytial virus, one of the parainfluenza viruses, adenovirus, or enterovirus. Less commonly, rhinovirus, influenza virus, herpes simplex virus, and others have also been recovered from children with pneumonia. Local epidemics may skew incidence figures for a given year or location. Respiratory syncytial virus causes a more serious disease during infancy, when it is the agent most commonly recovered.

Clinical Manifestations.   Most viral pneumonias are preceded by several days of respiratory symptoms, including rhinitis and cough. Often, other family members are ill. Although cough and fever are prominent, temperatures are generally lower than in bacterial pneumonia. Dyspnea with retractions and nasal flaring is more common in younger children and infants. Physical examination may be surprisingly unrevealing although rales are present late in the illness. The viral pneumonias cannot be definitely differentiated from mycoplasmal disease on purely clinical grounds and may, on occasion, be difficult to distinguish from bacterial pneumonias.

Diagnosis.   The chest roentgenogram is characterized by a diffuse infiltrate, especially in the perihilar areas. In some patients transient lobar infiltrates may also be present or even dominate the picture. Hyperinflation is common. Effusion may occur. Serologic studies may allow retrospective diagnosis by demonstrating a rise in antibody titer. Respiratory viruses, including parainfluenza virus, respiratory syncytial virus, and, less commonly, adenovirus, are occasionally found in asymptomatic children. The white blood cell count is usually under 20,000/mm^3. Platelets may occasionally be slightly depressed.

Treatment.   There is no specific treatment. Many patients are given antibiotic agents initially if bacterial pneumonia is suspected. Failure to respond to antibiotic treatment is additional evidence for viral etiology. Usually, only minimal supportive measures are required, although some patients need hospitalization for intravenous fluids, oxygen, or even assisted ventilation.

Prognosis.   The vast majority of children with viral pneumonia recover uneventfully and have no sequelae although the course may be prolonged, especially in infants. There is mounting evidence, however, that some patients, particularly infants, may develop bronchiolitis obliterans, unilateral hyperlucent lung, or other complications following a single episode of viral pneumonia. Adenovirus seems to be the most dangerous agent in this regard, and it also has been reported to cause a fatal acute fulminant pneumonia. Continuing roentgenographic abnormality for 6–12 mo is not unusual. See Chapter 10 for discussion of specific immunization procedures for the viruses most often implicated in serious lower tract respiratory disease.

Primary Atypical Pneumonia

See Sec 10.66.

Giant Cell Pneumonia
(Hecht Pneumonia)

Giant cell pneumonia is an uncommon interstitial pneumonitis of infancy and childhood. A definitive diagnosis depends on histologic demonstration of characteristic multinuclear giant cells with intranuclear and intracytoplasmic inclusion bodies in the lung. Also present are a mononuclear infiltrate, squamous metaplasia of the bronchial and bronchiolar epithelium, proliferation of the alveolar lining cells, and the occasional occurrence of giant cells in organs other than the lungs. Patients often develop giant cell pneumonia after measles. Rubeola virus has also been recovered from the lung tissue of patients with giant cell pneumonia who had no clinical evidence of measles or had leukemia complicated by measles infection. The giant cell formation seen in Hecht pneumonia and in cystic fibrosis is not, on the other hand, a histologic feature of the pneumonia commonly encountered with clinical measles. In the former group the process of giant cell formation originates in or near terminal bronchioles or alveoli, whereas in the latter the origin is bronchial. Hecht pneumonia may also follow immunization with attenuated measles vaccine in children who have leukemia or lymphomas and in patients with deficiency of cell-mediated immunity.

Clinically, patients with giant cell pneumonia have moderate to severe respiratory distress manifested principally by tachypnea and dyspnea. Inspiratory and early expiratory rales and musical sounds are heard, but dullness is rarely present. Some patients continue to excrete rubeola virus from the upper respiratory tract for weeks after the onset of illness. Roentgenographically, there are usually generalized, patchy infiltrates with areas of overinflation.

The course of illness may be several wk; clinical improvement may occur days to weeks prior to roentgenographic improvement. Occasionally, bacterial superinfection may occur. The mortality rate is high, particularly in patients with debilitating diseases such as leukemia, cystic fibrosis, and immunologic deficiency states. Treatment is symptomatic; gamma globulin is of no value.

Glezen WP, Denny FW: Epidemiology of acute lower respiratory disease in children. N Engl J Med 288:498, 1973.

Glezen WP, Loda FA, Clyde WA, et al: Epidemiologic patterns of acute lower respiratory disease of children in a pediatric group practice. J Pediatr 78: 397, 1971.

Henderson FW, Collier AM, Clyde WA, et al: Respiratory-syncytial-virus infections, reinfections and immunity: A prospective, longitudinal study in young children. N Engl J Med 300:530, 1979.

James AG, Lang WR, Liang AY, et al: Adenovirus type 21 bronchopneumonia in infants and young children. J Pediatr 95:530, 1979.

Malatzky AJ, Cooney MK, Luce R, et al: Epidemiology of viral and mycoplasmal agents associated with childhood lower respiratory illness in a civilian population. J Pediatr 78:407, 1971.

PNEUMONIAS OF MISCELLANEOUS CAUSES

12.68 Pneumocystis carinii Pneumonia
(Interstitial Plasma Cell Pneumonia)

Epidemiology. *Pneumocystis carinii* organisms, ubiquitous protozoans, are found only in the peripheral respiratory airways of man and a variety of other animals, including rodents. In the human, infection with this parasite is associated with immunosuppressed or chronic debilitated states or with prematurity or severe neonatal illness. Most cases in the United States occur in patients with primary immunodeficiency diseases or with immunosuppression induced by malignancy or its treatment. As the treatment of malignancy has become more sophisticated and patients survive longer, the incidence of this complication has increased. In a recent series 4% of over 1200 children with malignancies had proven pulmonary pneumocystis infestation (Sec 10.45).

Pathogenesis and Pathology. In newborn infants an incompletely developed immunologic responsiveness and exposure to a humidified atmosphere contaminated with the parasite may interact synergistically to produce sporadic or epidemic disease in the nursery. In some infants intensive treatment of a respiratory tract infection with antibiotics may produce activation of a latent pneumocystic infection. Infants with cytomegalic inclusion disease or children with lymphoreticular malignancies treated with cytotoxic agents, corticosteroids, or prolonged antibiotic therapy are particularly susceptible to *P. carinii* pneumonia. Infection produces a characteristic intra-alveolar exudate of lacelike appearance which contains histiocytes, lymphocytes, plasma cells, and cysts. Plasma cells are diminished or absent in agammaglobulinemia and hypogammaglobulinemia. In the alveolar septa are varying degrees of edema, inflammation, and fibrosis.

Clinical Manifestations. Onset in infants is usually at 3–5 wk of life, and it may be seen at any age in patients with immune deficiency syndromes or acquired temporary or permanent loss of host resistance. In infants the disease usually begins insidiously with cough and proceeds over a period of 1–4 wk to be characterized by low grade fever, tachypnea, and severe respiratory distress. Nasal flaring, cyanosis, and suprasternal, infrasternal, and intercostal retractions usually occur, but rales may be absent or few. In older children the onset is more abrupt with fever, tachypnea, and cough followed rapidly by retractions, nasal flaring, and cyanosis. Rales are not usually present. Fever and cough, particularly in infants, also may be absent. There is a relative paucity of pulmonary findings for the severity of distress.

The roentgenogram characteristically consists of hyperexpanded lung fields, a generalized granular pattern, and bilateral pulmonary infiltrates which originate at the hilus, extend peripherally, and eventually create a nearly solid appearance. Overaeration is most pronounced in the periphery. Arterial oxygen is reduced, but hypercapnia is uncommon.

Pneumocystis carinii pneumonia usually lasts from 3–6 wk but may continue over many mo.

Diagnosis. Definitive diagnosis is made by demonstrating the presence of the organism in the lung by appropriate staining of tracheal or lung aspirates, bronchial washings, or lung biopsies; sputum samples or tonsillar smears may occasionally be satisfactory. A complement fixation test may show conversion after 2–3 wk if the patient's immune system is sufficiently functional. The presence of pneumocystis antigen in 15% of patients with cancer but without pneumonitis suggests that the disease is not always an acute severe illness.

Treatment. Untreated, the disease is often fatal; patients with cellular immune deficiency or extensive malignancy usually die within 3 wk of onset of the typical roentgenographic features. Treatment with *pentamidine isothionate* (4 mg/kg/24 hr intramuscularly for 2 wk) has allowed over 50% of patients to recover even without restoration of immunocompetence; serious side effects of this drug include azotemia. Currently, *trimethoprim* (20 mg/kg/24 hr) and *sulfamethoxazole* (100 mg/kg/24 hr) are the treatment of choice. In very ill patients, supplemental oxygen with or without ventilator assistance may be needed.

Preventive treatment with trimethoprim (5 mg/kg/24 hr) and sulfamethoxazole (20 mg/kg/24 hr) may be useful in children who are at high risk for this disease.

Hughes WT: Current concepts. *Pneumocystis carinii* pneumonia. N Engl J Med 297:1381, 1977.
Hughes WT, Price RA, Kim HK, et al.: *Pneumocystis carinii* pneumonitis in children with malignancies. J Pediatr 82:404, 1973.
Walzer PE, Schultz MG, Western KA, et al: *Pneumocystis carinii* pneumonia and primary immune deficiency diseases of infancy and childhood. J Pediatr 82:416, 1973.

Mycotic Pulmonary Infections

See also Sec 10.100 to 10.106.

Thrush Pneumonia
(Pulmonary Candidiasis)

Pulmonary infections with *Candida albicans* are rare in children despite the relatively high incidence of oral thrush (Sec 11.13) in early infancy. This fact has been attributed to a natural resistance of columnar epithelium to invasion by the fungus. In 17 infants under 8 wk of age, all of whom had respiratory distress, about half had oral thrush, but there was no clinical or roentgenographic characteristic to suggest it as the cause of pulmonary infection. Amphotericin B and 5-fluorocytosine, although toxic, are the only effective therapeutic agents.

Emanuel B, Lieberman AD, Glodin M, et al: Pulmonary candidiasis in the neonatal period. J Pediatr 61:44, 1962.

12.69 Aspiration Pneumonia

See also Sec 7.36 and 7.37.

Aspiration of Food and Vomitus. Infants with obstructive lesions, such as tracheoesophageal fistula and duodenal obstruction, weak and debilitated infants and children with no obstructive lesions, patients with familial dysautonomia, and patients with impaired consciousness may aspirate, or aspirate and then regurgitate, an amount of food and vomitus sufficient to cause a chemical pneumonia. Aspiration may rarely be an immediate cause of death by asphyxiation. More frequently, following aspiration of gastric contents, there is a relatively brief latent period before the onset of signs and symptoms of pneumonia. Over 90% of patients have symptoms within 1 hr, and almost all patients have symptoms within 2 hr. Fever, tachypnea, and cough are common. Apnea and hypotensive shock also occur.

Physical examination reveals diffuse rales and wheezing, and many patients are cyanotic. Chest roentgenograms reveal alveolar and, occasionally, reticular infiltrates which may be localized but often are more extensive and frequently are bilateral. The irritated mucous membrane may also subsequently become the site for bacterial invasion and pneumonia.

Prophylaxis is of the greatest importance. Care should be taken to avoid amounts of feedings that will overdistend the stomach, especially in infants who are fed by gavage. After being fed, the infant should be placed on the abdomen or right side. When the infant is supine, the head should not be lower than the rest of the body. While the infant is lying face down, however, drainage from the lungs may be materially aided by lowering the head of the bed.

Immediate suctioning of the airway and administration of oxygen are indicated for aspiration. Endotracheal intubation with suctioning and mechanical ventilation is often required in severe cases. Although prophylactic use of antibiotics and corticosteroids is advocated by some for patients who have aspirated gastric contents, evidence of their benefit is lacking. Some data suggest that corticosteroid treatment may predispose the patient to pneumonia due to gram-negative organisms.

Prognosis depends partly on the severity of aspiration and partly on the underlying disease. The majority of patients demonstrate clearing of infiltrates within 2 wk; mortality before clearing of aspiration infiltrates is about 25%. Over half the patients develop a secondary infection with either gram-positive or gram-negative organisms, including *Proteus, Pseudomonas, E. coli,* and *Klebsiella.*

Bynium LJ, Pierce AK: Pulmonary aspiration of gastric contents. Am Rev Resp Dis 114:1129, 1976.

Wolfe JE, Bone RC, Ruth WE: Effects of corticosteroids in the treatment of patients with gastric aspiration. Am J Med 83:719, 1977.

Aspiration of Zinc Stearate. Aspiration pneumonia resulting from inhalation of zinc stearate powder has become rare with decreased use of the product and safer containers for it. Severe respiratory distress almost immediately follows inhalation. Generalized obstructive emphysema with an expiratory type of dyspnea occurs as a result of an inflammatory reaction caused by zinc stearate powder. Following inhalation, it is almost immediately drawn into the finer bronchioles because of its extreme lightness; for this reason bronchoscopic aspiration is useful, if at all, only to remove the secretions that may subsequently accumulate in the larger air passages. Immediate treatment is oxygen therapy in an atmosphere of high humidity.

Pneumonitis from Other Chemicals. Many chemicals, particularly if inhaled at high concentrations, may cause an inflammatory reaction with edema and cellular infiltrations and acute respiratory distress. Prolonged exposure to lower concentrations of these same agents or other chemicals may cause chronic interstitial pneumonitis characterized by granuloma formation. For example, shellac, polyvinylpyrrolidone (found in hair spray), gum arabic, beryllium, mercury vapors, and chlorine may cause this reaction. Corticosteroids may reduce the inflammatory reaction and prevent fibrosis.

12.70 Hydrocarbon Pneumonia

Etiology. Hydrocarbons, such as furniture polish, kerosene, charcoal lighter fluid, and gasoline, are occasionally accidentally ingested by young children, causing a secondary pneumonitis. Gasoline may be aspirated by teenagers attempting to siphon gasoline (Sec 28.9).

Pathogenesis. Although controversy over the route of hydrocarbon entry to the lungs persists, evidence favors that they reach the lung by aspiration during swallowing, vomiting, or gastric lavage. The low viscosity of hydrocarbons allows them to flow from the hypopharynx into the larynx. Therefore, gastric lavage after the ingestion of hydrocarbons is usually contraindicated. The pulmonary changes observed in animals after hydrocarbon aspiration are edema, inflammation, and hemorrhage.

Clinical Manifestations. Coughing and vomiting follow ingestion almost immediately. Within hours there may be an elevation of temperature (38–40° C), and the child may be drowsy or comatose. However, with less extensive aspiration the onset of pulmonary symptoms and inflammation may be delayed 12–24 hr. The pulmonary findings may include dyspnea, diminished resonance on percussion, suppressed or tubular breath sounds, and rales. Pneumonic involvement is disclosed more frequently by roentgenographic examination than by physical findings. Occasionally, roentgenograms may show minimal changes a few hr after ingestion only to progress rapidly after that time with extensive infiltrates. In spite of what may be a stormy clinical course, which averages 2–5 days, recovery occurs in most instances.

Complications. Pneumothorax, subcutaneous emphysema of the chest wall, and pleural effusion, including empyema, have occurred. After the 1st wk pneumatoceles may develop in areas of extensive consolidation. There may be secondary infection with bacteria or viruses.

Treatment. Patients must be observed closely even if they are asymptomatic when seen by the physician because symptoms and lung infiltrates may be delayed. Observation may be done at home if parents are instructed to bring the child to the hospital for any respiratory symptom. If the history suggests a large amount of ingested material or the agent is particularly toxic (e.g., furniture polish), the child should be admitted for observation. No pulmonary therapy is indicated prior to symptoms.

Following ingestion of small to moderate amounts of hydrocarbons, induction of vomiting or gastric lavage is contraindicated because of the risk of aspiration, especially if several hr have elapsed. If a large volume of hydrocarbon is thought to be in the stomach, nasogastric suction performed with great care to avoid aspiration may be necessary to reduce the other dangers of hydrocarbon poisoning, including central nervous system toxicity. The risk of aspiration during gastric lavage or suctioning can be minimized if an endotracheal tube with a balloon cuff can be inserted without inducing vomiting prior to lavage. If there is dyspnea or cyanosis or if chemical pneumonitis develops, supportive measures including oxygen, physiotherapy, and, if necessary, continuous positive airway pressure or other forms of ventilatory assistance are important components of therapy. A cathartic is usually indicated.

The routine use of antibiotics is not recommended; the occurrence of secondary infection of the affected lung can usually be readily detected by the reappearance of fever on the 3rd–5th day following ingestion and can then be suitably treated with penicillin G and kanamycin. Corticosteroids have no beneficial effect on the course of the illness and may, on occasion, be harmful. Pneumatoceles, when they occur, rarely rupture and do not require treatment. Parents must be reminded to keep cleaning fluids and kerosene in locked cabinets out of reach of children or out of the home.

Prognosis. Although most children survive without complications or sequelae, some progress rapidly to respiratory failure and death. Prognosis depends on a variety of factors, including the volume of the ingestion or aspiration, the specific agent involved, and the adequacy of medical care. Long-term pulmonary function studies several yr later are inconclusive, but if lasting damage does occur, the small airways seem to be at greatest risk.

Bergeson PS, Hales SW, Lustgarten MD, et al: Pneumatoceles following hydrocarbon ingestion. Report of three cases and review of the literature. Am J Dis Child 129:49, 1975.
Bratton L, Haddow J: Ingestion of charcoal lighter fluid. J Pediatr 87:633, 1975.
Brown J III, Burke B, Dajani AS: Experimental kerosene pneumonia: Evaluation of some therapeutic regimens. J Pediatr 84:396, 1974.
Guruntz D, Kattan M, Levison H, et al: Pulmonary function abnormalities in asymptomatic children after hydrocarbon pneumonitis. Pediatrics 62:789, 1978.
Taussig LM, Castro O, Landau LI, et al: Pulmonary function 8–10 years after hydrocarbon pneumonitis. Clin Pediatr 16:57, 1977.

12.71 Lipoid Pneumonia

Lipoid pneumonia is a chronic, interstitial, proliferative inflammation resulting from aspiration of lipoid material; it occurs principally in debilitated infants.

Pathogenesis. The factors that may be responsible for aspiration of oil include (1) intranasal instillation of medicated oils; (2) any condition that interferes with the swallowing act, such as cleft palate, debilitation, or a horizontal position during feeding; and (3) forced feeding, and especially the administration of cod liver oil, castor oil, or mineral oil to crying children.

The severity of the pulmonary reaction depends upon the kind of oil inhaled. Vegetable oils, such as olive, cottonseed, and sesame, are generally the least irritating and produce no inflammation; however, chaulmoogra, also a vegetable oil, produces extensive damage. Animal oils, owing to their high fatty acid content, are the most damaging. Cod liver oil belongs in this category. Liquid petrolatum is chemically inert and not as irritative as some of the other oils but does act as a foreign body.

The reaction within the lung begins as an interstitial proliferative inflammation with which there may be an exudative pneumonia. In the 2nd stage there is diffuse, chronic, proliferative fibrosis and sometimes superimposed acute infectious bronchopneumonia. In the 3rd stage there are multiple localized nodules, tumor-like paraffinomas. There are numerous macrophages in the involved areas, with giant cell formation of the foreign body type. The lipoid substance is both intracellular and extracellular. The oil-laden cells may be carried to the hilar lymph nodes.

Clinical Manifestations. There are no characteristic signs or symptoms; a cough is most common, and in severe cases there may be dyspnea. Unless there is superimposed infection, there is usually no fever or physical sign, although with extensive involvement there may be some impairment to percussion and change in voice and breath sounds. Secondary bronchopneumonic infections are common.

The roentgenographic appearance is characteristic. With mild involvement there is an increase in density and in the extent of the hilar shadows. With increasing involvement there is greater density of the perihilar shadows with widening in all directions (Fig 12–11). Pulmonary changes may be limited to the right lung, and in the infant who is recumbent most of the time the changes may be mainly in the right upper lobe.

Prognosis. The prognosis is guarded. It depends upon the extent of pulmonary damage, the discontin-

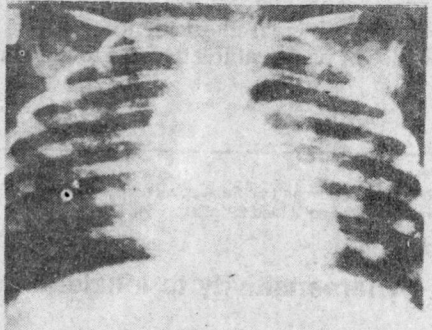

Figure 12–11 Roentgenogram showing increased density radiating from the hilus of each lung in an infant 13 mo of age after intranasal application of liquid petrolatum 3 times a day for 5 mo.

uation of oil inhalation, the general condition of the patient, and the avoidance of intercurrent infections.

Prevention. Intranasal medications in an oily vehicle should not be used. Concentrated preparations of vitamins A and D in water-miscible vehicles should be substituted for cod liver oil. Administration of mineral oil and castor oil should be avoided. Infants who regurgitate or vomit frequently should be placed on their abdomens to lessen the likelihood of aspiration.

Treatment. There is no specific therapy other than elimination of further exposure. The infant's position should be changed frequently to lessen the chances of hydrostatic pneumonia.

12.72   Silo Filler's Disease

This rare condition is an acute interstitial pneumonia which occurs following the inhalation of nitrogen dioxide, a gas generally encountered only in freshly filled silos. Cough and dyspnea occur immediately after exposure. An asymptomatic phase of several days follows, but then the patient suddenly experiences chills and fever associated with progressive cough, dyspnea, and cyanosis. There are rales throughout both lung fields and widespread pulmonary infiltration on roentgenogram. The interalveolar septa are widened, edematous, and filled with accumulated mononuclear cells and fibroblasts, and the epithelium is hyperplastic. The disease usually progresses rapidly to death. Corticosteroids have been used, but there is no known effective treatment.

12.73   Paraquat Lung

Paraquat, a dipyridilium compound used as a weed killer, is highly toxic, causing death from respiratory failure a few days to weeks after ingestion. The pulmonary lesion is secondary to systemic absorption through the gastrointestinal tract or skin and consists of proliferative bronchiolitis, alveolitis, hemorrhage causing intra-alveolar hyaline membranes, and fibrosis. Gas exchange is impaired. It is a corrosive that also causes painful lesions of the mouth and esophagus, renal tubular damage, azotemia, and hematuria. There is no treatment except for general supportive measures. Animal experiments suggest oxygen may increase pulmonary toxicity. Increased incidence may be due to large scale use of paraquat in attempts to kill marihuana plants.

Copland GM, Kolin A, Shulman HS: Fatal pulmonary intra-alveolar fibrosis after paraquat ingestion. N Engl J Med 291:290, 1964.

12.74   Hypersensitivity to Inhaled Materials

Repeated inhalation of organic dusts may result in chronic pneumonitis which progressively worsens with continued exposure to the antigen. Although the syn-

drome is most common in adults, it has been reported frequently in children. Unlike those of asthma, the symptoms of this hypersensitivity syndrome are almost entirely unrelated to bronchospasm (Sec 9.45). Symptoms may result from inhalation of small particles from moldy hay (farmer's lung), maple bark (maple bark stripper's disease), sugar cane fiber (bagassosis), redwood tree bark, pigeon droppings and feathers (pigeon breeder's disease), cheese, desiccated pituitary powder, dusty output from air conditioners, and a fungus or mold associated with the specific material to which the patient is exposed.

Clinical Manifestations. The signs and symptoms are similar in all of these diseases. Within several hr following exposure cough, dyspnea, chest pain, and sometimes fever occur with few physical findings though occasional wheezes and moist rales may be audible. Roentgenography may show minimal emphysema but is usually normal. If no further exposure occurs, the symptoms abate over a period of several days; but if contact with the responsible antigen continues, symptoms progress to severe dyspnea and cyanosis associated with diffuse, fine, interstitial or nodular densities with peripheral alveolar infiltrates on chest roentgenogram and occasionally irreversible loss of pulmonary function. The disease should be suspected in children with relatively mild symptoms including cough, fever, and occasional dyspnea, particularly if bronchopneumonia persists despite appropriate treatment with antibiotics.

Pathology. Histologically, the infiltrate consists of subacute granulomatous inflammation with accumulation of plasma cells, lymphocytes, epithelioid cells, and giant cells of the Langhans type. With continued exposure inflammatory lesions may be replaced by fibrosis.

Diagnosis. There may be moderate to marked leukocytosis, particularly with acute attacks, elevated serum immunoglobulins (IgG, IgM, and IgA fractions), precipitin lines when the patient's serum is diffused against a suspected organic antigen, and a primary restrictive pattern on pulmonary function tests. Arterial blood gas analysis reveals moderate or marked hypoxemia, usually without hypercapnia. Skin testing with the suspected antigen may cause a vigorous delayed hypersensitivity response and is especially useful if an Arthus reaction can be demonstrated histologically by skin biopsy of the test site. Lung biopsy reveals a diffuse fibrotic or granulomatous response. If the antigen is available in purified form, an inhalation challenge may be of diagnostic importance.

Treatment. Optimal therapy requires the complete elimination of exposure to the suspected (or proven) antigen. The administration of adrenal corticosteroids (e.g., prednisone in initial dosage of 1–1.5 mg/kg/24 hr) usually results in prompt remission of symptoms; continued use for 1–6 mo may prevent the subsequent development of pulmonary fibrosis in cases of chronic exposure. Corticosteroid therapy may be slowly tapered down following evidence of recovery of lung function or several wk after exposure to a known antigen has stopped. If hypersensitivity pneumonitis is strongly suspected on clinical grounds but the antigen remains unknown, long-term use of corticosteroid therapy, perhaps on an alternate day regimen, may be indicated. The patient should be cautioned that re-exposure to the antigen is extremely dangerous even long after apparent complete recovery. Even if treatment is optimal and the exposure is eliminated, some fatalities occur, and a substantial percentage of patients do not completely regain their previous pulmonary status.

Allen DH, Williams GV, Woolcock AJ: Bird breeder's hypersensitivity pneumonitis. Progress studies of lung function after cessation of exposure to the provoking antigen. Am Rev Resp Dis 114:555, 1976.

Cunningham AS, Fink JN, Schlueter DP: Childhood hypersensitivity pneumonitis due to dove antigen. Pediatrics 58:436, 1976.

Katz RM, Knicker WT: Infantile hypersensitivity pneumonitis as a reaction to organic antigen. N Engl J Med 288:233, 1973.

Stiehm ER, Reed CE, Tooley WH: Pigeon breeder's lung in children. Pediatrics 39:904, 1967.

12.75 Pulmonary Aspergillosis

See Sec 9.48 and 10.104.

A variety of species of the fungal genus *Aspergillus* are potentially pathogenic for man. The spectrum of pulmonary manifestations is great and depends upon the nature of the exposure and the condition of the host. A hypersensitivity reaction with bronchospasm is most common. The majority of these cases of *allergic bronchopulmonary aspergillosis* have occurred in children with chronic pulmonary diseases. In some patients the immunologic response which results in allergic aspergillosis appears to be genetically determined. *Aspergillomas* (fungus balls) typically occur in an ectatic bronchus or old tuberculous cavity. Affected patients are generally asymptomatic. There have been, however, isolated case reports of parenchymal invasion by aspergillus in normal children, but *invasive aspergillosis* generally occurs in immunosuppressed patients, and any organ may be involved.

Clinical Manifestations. Allergic aspergillosis should be suspected in an immunosuppressed or chronically ill child who presents relatively acute onset of cough, wheezing, and low-grade fever. The cough may be productive, and, occasionally, brown plugs are expectorated which on microscopic examination are found to contain hyphae. Aspergillus can be recovered from this material on culture.

Many patients have multiple precipitin lines on diffusion of serum against aspergillus antigen. The immediate skin test reaction is often strongly positive, and a type III hypersensitivity (Arthus) reaction can usually be demonstrated after skin testing. Chest roentgenograms show transient, occasionally extensive, infiltrates. Peripheral eosinophilia occurs in almost every patient. Serum levels of immunoglobulin E are elevated, and specific immunoglobulin E antibody to aspergillus has been demonstrated. Aspergillus organisms are frequently recovered from cultures of respiratory tract secretions of patients with chronic pulmonary disease who do not have symptoms of allergic aspergillosis. The recovery of these organisms without typical symptoms and serologic evidence of hypersensitivity is not an indication for treatment.

Treatment. Therapy of allergic aspergillosis should be directed at eradication of the organism. Unfortunately, the best approach to treatment is not clear. Systemic amphotericin B (0.25–1.0 mg/kg/24 hr intravenously) or 5-fluorocytosine (50–150 mg/kg/24 hr) may be effective. Aerosolized amphotericin or direct instillation of amphotericin into the trachea also has been recommended, but correct dosage is not established. Symptomatic treatment with systemic and aerosolized bronchodilators and corticosteroids may also often be necessary (Sec 9.49). Disodium cromoglycate is not useful.

Aspergillomas may respond to specific antifungal chemotherapy. However, surgical resection with local instillation of amphotericin is considered the treatment of choice. The prognosis, whatever the treatment, is heavily dependent on the underlying chronic illness. Invasive aspergillosis may be so fulminant that antifungal chemotherapy is not efficacious. Treatment generally consists of amphotericin B combined with 5-fluorocytosine. Treatment should be continued for 2–3 wk.

Bardana EJ, Sobti KL, Cianciulli FD, et al: Aspergillus antibody in patients with cystic fibrosis. Am J Dis Child 129:1164, 1975.

Berger I, Phillips WL, Shenker IR: Pulmonary aspergillosis in childhood. Clin Pediatr 11:178, 1972.

Graves TS, Fink JN, Patterson R, et al: A familial occurrence of allergic bronchopulmonary aspergillosis. Ann Int Med 91:378, 1979.

Katz RM, Kniker WT: Infantile hypersensitivity pneumonitis as a reaction to organic antigens. N Engl J Med 288:233, 1973.

Slavin RG, Laird TS, Cherry JD: Allergic bronchopulmonary aspergillos's in a child. J Pediatr 76:416, 1970.

Strelling MK, Rhaney K, Simmons DAR, et al: Fatal acute pulmonary aspergillosis in two children of one family. Arch Dis Child 41:34, 1966.

Varkey B, Rose HD: Pulmonary aspergilloma: A rational approach to treatment. Am J Med 61:626, 1976.

12.76 Löffler Syndrome
(Eosinophilic Pneumonia)

This syndrome is characterized by widespread transitory pulmonary infiltrations, which roentgenographically vary in size but may resemble those of miliary tuberculosis, and by a blood eosinophilia that may be as high as 70%. The clinical course is usually not severe and ranges from a few days to several mo. There are usually paroxysmal attacks of coughing, dyspnea, pleurisy, and little or no fever. There may be associated hepatomegaly, especially in infants and young children, and biopsy sections of the liver have revealed multiple focal areas of necrosis, granuloma formation, and eosinophilic infiltration. These children have hyperglobulinemia, presumably as the result of hepatic dysfunction and in response to parasitic invasion of tissue. Autopsy studies have revealed evidences of eosinophilic infiltrations in the lungs and in other organs. Localized pneumonic consolidation with an associated eosinophilia may occur.

Löffler syndrome may be an unusual allergic manifestation of a variety of antigens and not a distinct clinical entity. In children it is most often a manifestation of helminthic infections. Perhaps the most common pathogen in this country is the larva of the dog ascarid, *Toxocara canis,* and less often of the cat ascarid, *Toxocara cati* (Sec 10.121). Other roundworms may also be responsible for the syndrome; these include *Ascaris lumbricoides* (usually responsible for transient pulmonary lesions), *Strongyloides stercoralis,* and hookworms. So-called tropical eosinophilia may be manifest as Löffler syndrome and is probably caused by a number of different helminths. Paragonimiasis caused by a lung fluke (Sec 10.132) may produce the syndrome as well as extrapulmonary manifestations. A drug reaction may also result in this syndrome; aspirin, penicillin, sulfonamides, and imipramine are among those implicated.

Beaver P: Wandering nematodes as a cause of disability and disease. Am J Trop Med Hyg 6:433, 1957.
Leitch AG: Pulmonary eosinophilia. Basics Resp Dis 7 (No 5):1, 1979.
Zuelzer WW, Apt L: Disseminated visceral lesions associated with extreme eosinophilia: Pathologic and clinical observations on a syndrome of young children. Am J Dis Child 78:153, 1949.

12.77   Pulmonary Involvement in Collagen Diseases

Pulmonary manifestations are rarely the dominant feature of periarteritis, systemic lupus erythematosus, scleroderma, polymyositis, or dermatomyositis. However, recurrent infection and progression to bronchiectasis may occur in scleroderma. Diffusion abnormalities are common when the lungs are involved by this group of diseases. Hemoptysis may occur. Pleural effusions and pleuritic pain are fairly common in systemic lupus. Corticosteroid treatment may ameliorate some of these problems. Patients who are chronically immunosuppressed as a part of the therapy of these diseases are at risk to develop *Pneumocystis carinii* pneumonia.

Rheumatic pneumonia is a usually fatal, but rare, complication of acute rheumatic fever, characterized clinically by extensive pulmonary consolidation and rapidly progressive functional deterioration and pathologically by alveolar exudate, inflammatory interstitial infiltrates, and necrotizing arteritis. Physical findings are unexpectedly minimal; frequently there are no rales. Chest roentgenograms reveal transient areas of infiltrate that resemble pulmonary edema. There is no specific treatment; these patients do not respond to corticosteroids, to treatment of congestive heart failure with diuretics and digitalis, or to the antibiotic treatment of presumed infection. If the lesion is diagnosed by lung biopsy, treatment with immunosuppressive agents theoretically may be of value but has not been reported to be effective.

Park S, Nyhan WL: Fatal pulmonary involvement in dermatomyositis. Am J Dis Child 129:723, 1975.
Rajani KB, Aschbacher LV, Kinney TR: Pulmonary hemorrhage and systemic lupus erythematosus. J Pediatr 93:810, 1978.
Serlin SP, Rmisza ME, Gay JH: Rheumatic pneumonia: The need for a new approach. Pediatrics 56:1075, 1975.
Singsen BH, Bernstein BF, Kornreich HK, et al: Mixed connective tissue disease in childhood: A clinical and serologic survey. J Pediatr 90:893, 1977.

12.78   Desquamative Interstitial Pneumonitis

This disease of unknown etiology is characterized pathologically by massive proliferation and desquamation of alveolar cells and thickening of the alveolar walls. The degree of desquamation is far greater than the degree of alveolar wall thickening. In most children there is a history of preceding upper respiratory infection, although the relationship of the desquamative pneumonitis to this infection of probable viral origin has not been firmly established. Circulating immune complexes and alveolar deposition of IgG and complement suggest an immune basis for the disease.

Clinical Manifestations.   Symptoms usually develop slowly. As alveolar function is compromised, tachypnea and dyspnea occur, and with progression of the disease there is a nonproductive cough, anorexia, and weight loss. Cyanosis eventually results; clubbing is not a constant feature, and fever is unusual. Physical findings include tachypnea, nasal flaring, and, occasionally, fine rales. Use of the accessory muscles of respiration is not as prominent as one would expect in obstructive diseases with an equal amount of hypoxemia.

Laboratory Manifestations.   Chest roentgenograms reveal a diffuse, hazy, ground glass appearance, particularly at the lung bases, along with poorly defined hilar densities. Viral and bacteriologic cultures and acute and convalescent sera analyses are not helpful diagnostically. Arterial blood samples show hypoxemia; most patients seek medical care prior to the advent of hypercapnia. Definitive diagnosis requires open lung biopsy.

Treatment.   Patients with desquamative interstitial pneumonitis often recover without specific treatment. Those suspected of having the disease can occasionally be simply observed if their respiratory symptoms are not too severe. With worsening pulmonary status or rapidly deteriorating chest roentgenogram, open lung biopsy is important to establish a definitive diagnosis. These patients usually respond to corticosteroid therapy with rapid resolution of symptoms and gradual improvement on roentgenogram. Occasional corticosteroid-resistant patients are reported, and a variety of other treatments, including immunosuppression, have been proposed. Supportive treatment including supplemental oxygen is often necessary. Corticosteroid therapy without lung biopsy diagnosis is hazardous; chronic viral pneumonitis can present with a similar clinical picture and may be worsened by corticosteroid depression of host defenses. Relapses are reported with premature cessation of therapy.

Buchta RM, Park S, Giammona ST: Desquamative interstitial pneumonia in a 7 week old infant. Am J Dis Child 120:341, 1970.
Dreisin RB, Schwartz MI, Theofilopoulus AN, et al: Circulating immune complexes in the idiopathic interstitial pneumonias. N Engl J Med 298:353, 1978.
Rosenow EC, O'Connell EJ, Harrison EG: Desquamative interstitial pneumonia in children. Am J Dis Child 120:344, 1970.
Stillwell PC, Norris DG, O'Connell EJ, et al: Desquamative interstitial pneumonitis in children. Chest 77:155, 1980.

12.79 Hypostatic Pneumonia

Hypostatic pneumonia occurs after prolonged passive pulmonary congestion and may occur in any marantic state. Lying for a long time in 1 position favors its development. There is dependent congestion, edema, and pneumonia. The symptoms are not characteristic. There is neither dyspnea nor fever unless these symptoms are secondary to another disorder. The physical signs are principally slight dullness on percussion, feeble respiratory sounds, and the presence of moist rales. Hypostatic congestion is usually a terminal event. There is no specific treatment. Prophylaxis is of the greatest importance; the position of any immobile patient should be changed frequently.

12.80 RESPIRATORY BURNS AND SMOKE INHALATION

Thermal and chemical injury to the lung, systemic toxicity of inhaled gases—particularly carbon monoxide—and asphyxia are important causes of morbidity and mortality in children who have been exposed to fire; they should be considered in the initial treatment whether or not there are surface burns. Excessive heat may injure the respiratory mucosa, especially above the trachea. A variety of noxious gases may be generated by fires, including oxides of sulfur and nitrogen, hydrochloric acid, acetaldehyde, corrosive acids and alkalis, and carbon monoxide. Fine particles of soot carried deep within the lung may cause thermal burns or have toxic gases adsorbed on them.

Although there is usually a history of being trapped in a smoke-filled room or evidence of superficial burns around the face or singed nasal vibrissae, serious respiratory damage may occur in the absence of any of these. The onset of clinical manifestation of respiratory distress may be immediate or delayed several hr. Roentgenographic changes may be delayed from hours to days.

Signs of central nervous system injury from hypoxemia due to asphyxia may vary from irritability to depression. Carbon monoxide poisoning may be mild (<20% HbCO) with slight dyspnea and decreased visual acuity and higher cerebral functions; moderate (20–40% HbCO) with irritability, nausea, dimness of vision, impaired judgment, and rapid fatigue; or severe (40–60% HbCO) producing confusion, hallucination, ataxia, collapse, and coma.

Direct measurement of carboxyhemoglobin (HbCO) is important for diagnosis and prognosis as it reflects the degree of tissue hypoxia caused by the combination of carbon monoxide and hemoglobin and the change in the shape and position of the oxygen dissociation curve. PaO_2 may be normal and the oxyhemoglobin saturation values misleading because HbCO is not detected by the usual tests of saturation. Thermal injury may lead to edema, exudate, and necrosis with desquamation of tissue, obstruction, and atelectasis. Respiratory insufficiency may occur from asphyxia, carbon monoxide poisoning, airway obstruction due to edema and necrotic material in the airways, or bronchoconstriction.

Children who have been in fires should be hospitalized for at least 24 hr of careful observation. If there is any suspicion that carbon monoxide poisoning may have occurred, humidified 100% oxygen should be administered.

After thermal injury, respiratory complications follow a fairly predictable timetable. From 1–12 hr after exposure acute respiratory distress secondary to bronchospasm, laryngeal edema, and/or lung consolidation may occur. Laryngeal obstruction, characterized by a prolonged inspiratory phase and virtually absent breath sounds, is uncommon; endotracheal intubation followed by tracheostomy is necessary in these patients. Bronchospasm, characterized by wheezing and prolonged expiration, responds best to a large intravenous bolus of corticosteroid. Usual bronchodilator treatment is ineffective. Lung consolidation is an ominous development; in 1 series 80% of affected patients died within 36 hr. Pulmonary edema occurs usually 6–72 hr after exposure. Although fluid overload may account for some of these cases, the majority are directly due to the injury itself. Treatment includes fluid restriction and diuretics. Ventilatory assistance may be required. Cervical eschar formation with constriction of the airway may occur from 60–120 hr after exposure in patients with circumferential full-thickness burns of the neck; treatment consists of vertical division of the burn crust and immediate endotracheal intubation. Bronchopneumonia may complicate the patient's course, especially following the 4th day. At first *Staphylococcus aureus* is the most common pathogen, but by the 8th day *Pseudomonas aeruginosa* and *Klebsiella pneumoniae* are the dominant organisms recovered. Treatment includes encouraging cough, nasotracheal suctioning, and, on occasion, bronchoscopic suctioning. Specific antibiotic treatment based on culture results is important. Early and continuous use of intravenous corticosteroids contributes to a poor prognosis in these patients. Respiratory therapy equipment is the source of the infecting organisms in some patients.

Children with respiratory burns account for the vast majority of fatalities following survival of exposure to fire (Sec 5.28). Careful observation and specific therapy as complications develop are extremely important. Supportive care, including postural draining and encouragement of cough, are important.

Mellins RB, Park S: Respiratory complications of smoke inhalation in victims of fires. J Pediatr 87:1, 1975.
Pietak SP, Delahaye DJ: Airway obstruction following smoke inhalation. Can Med Assoc J 115:329, 1976.
Stone HH: Pulmonary burns in children. J Pediatr Surg 14:48, 1979.

12.81 PULMONARY HEMOSIDEROSIS

The term "pulmonary hemosiderosis" is used to describe a number of rare conditions characterized by an abnormal accumulation of hemosiderin in the lungs. Hemosiderin deposits follow diffuse alveolar hemorrhage and may occur either as a primary disease of the lungs or secondary to cardiac or systemic vascular disease. In children primary hemosiderosis occurs more frequently than the secondary varieties. There appear to be 4 types of primary pulmonary hemosiderosis: an idiopathic form, a form associated with cow's milk hypersensitivity (Heiner syndrome), a form occurring in association with myocarditis, and a form associated with progressive glomerulonephritis (Goodpasture syndrome). Three types of secondary pulmonary hemosiderosis are recognized: 1 occurs with mitral stenosis and chronic left ventricular failure of any cause; 1 is associated with collagen diseases; and 1 with hemorrhagic diseases.

Idiopathic Primary Pulmonary Hemosiderosis.   The cause of this illness is unknown. However, rarely reported familial incidence suggests a genetic basis for some cases. Onset usually occurs in childhood, rarely later than early adult life. Most of the clinical features are related to blood in the alveoli and to the effects of chronic blood loss. Symptoms are those of recurrent or chronic pulmonary disease and include cough, hemoptysis, dyspnea, wheezing, and occasional cyanosis associated with fatigue and pallor. The cough may be productive of bloody sputum, or the infant or child may simply vomit large quantities of blood. During acute attacks, which usually last 2–4 days, the child may be febrile.

The usual clinical features of fever, tachycardia, tachypnea, leukocytosis, respiratory distress, and abnormal roentgenographic findings may suggest bacterial pneumonia, and only prolonged follow-up will reveal the correct diagnosis. In some children, however, the early manifestations of illness are related to chronic iron deficiency anemia, which is often refractory to therapy, and the characteristic pulmonary symptoms do not appear until much later. Paradoxically, the child may have severe pulmonary manifestations without roentgenographic abnormalities, or the roentgenographic picture may be abnormal before pulmonary symptoms have occurred.

The anemia is typically microcytic and hypochromic; serum iron concentrations are low, and there may be elevations in bilirubin, urobilinogen, and reticulocyte count. The stool usually contains occult blood, presumably swallowed. Hemosiderin can usually be demonstrated in macrophages in smears of sputum or material obtained from tracheal or gastric aspirates. Roentgenographic changes range from minimal infiltrates resembling pneumonia to massive pulmonary involvement with secondary atelectasis, emphysema, and hilar lymphadenopathy. The findings may suggest tuberculosis or pulmonary edema, and significant changes may be seen from day to day. Open lung biopsy may be required to establish the diagnosis by histologic demonstration of intra-alveolar hemorrhage, large numbers of hemosiderin-laden macrophages, alveolar epithelial hyperplasia, interstitial fibrosis, and sclerosis of small vessels. Closed biopsy by needle has been followed by serious complications.

Approximately half the patients die within 1–5 yr, usually from acute pulmonary hemorrhage and progressive respiratory failure. A milk-free diet is indicated pending analysis of serum for precipitins and also serves as a diagnostic test for cow's milk–related pul-

monary hemosiderosis. Corticosteroids (prednisone, 1 mg/kg/24 hr) may produce remission in some patients and be of no benefit to others. Maintenance corticosteroid therapy has been used between attacks with variable results. Immunosuppressant drugs and deferoxamine have not been adequately evaluated.

Primary Pulmonary Hemosiderosis with Hypersensitivity to Cow's Milk (Heiner Syndrome).   These children have the typical picture of idiopathic hemosiderosis, unusually high serum titers of precipitins to multiple constituents of cow's milk, and positive intradermal skin tests to various cow's milk proteins. They may also have chronic rhinitis, recurrent otitis media, gastrointestinal symptoms, and growth retardation. The symptoms improve when cow's milk is removed from the diet and return with its reintroduction. Some patients fail to improve at all on a milk-free diet, and others without multiple serum precipitins have improved. Some of these patients with high titers of milk precipitins and pulmonary hemosiderosis develop cor pulmonale secondary to hypertrophied nasopharyngeal lymphoid tissue. These patients should also have a tonsilloadenoidectomy. In general, patients with hemosiderosis and precipitins to cow's milk have a better prognosis than do those with other forms of the disease, and they may eventually lose their sensitivity to milk. Corticosteroids may be useful, at least during acute bleeding episodes.

Primary Pulmonary Hemosiderosis with Myocarditis.   Some patients have varying degrees of inflammation of the myocardium associated with pulmonary hemosiderosis, and, if significant myocardial disease is present when pulmonary symptoms are first noted, it may be impossible to determine whether the hemosiderosis is a primary or secondary phenomenon. The clinical picture does not differ from that of the idiopathic disease except that the heart may be enlarged and there may be electrocardiographic signs compatible with myocarditis.

Primary Pulmonary Hemosiderosis with Glomerulonephritis (Goodpasture Syndrome).   This is a disease primarily of young adult males and is rarely observed in children. Initially, the presentation of the disease may be similar to idiopathic pulmonary hemosiderosis with hemoptysis and iron deficiency anemia, but careful study at the time of the initial attack will usually reveal a proliferative or membranous glomerulonephritis. Patients most often have progressive renal disease with hypertension and eventual renal failure and death. The pulmonary disease has improved following bilateral nephrectomy in a few patients but not in others.

Secondary Pulmonary Hemosiderosis.   Heart disease producing a chronic increase in pulmonary capillary pressure, such as mitral stenosis, can lead to intrapulmonary hemorrhage and secondary hemosiderosis. Collagen vascular diseases may present clinical manifestations of pulmonary hemosiderosis. Occasionally, the vascular changes of polyarteritis are initially limited to the lungs. Other diseases, such as rheumatoid arthritis, may also produce pulmonary hemosiderosis as an effect of generalized diffuse vasculitis. A few patients with anaphylactoid purpura or thrombocytopenic purpura have similarly had hemosiderosis secondary to intrapulmonary hemorrhage.

Beckerman RC, Taussig LM, Pinnas JL: Familial idiopathic hemosiderosis. Am J Dis Child 133:609, 1979.

Boat TF, Polmar SH, Whitman V, et al: Hyperreactivity to cow milk in young children with pulmonary hemosiderosis and cor pulmonale secondary to nasopharyngeal obstruction. J Pediatr 87:23, 1973.

Case records of the Massachusetts General Hospital (case 30–1979). N Engl J Med 301:201, 1979.

Gilman PA, Zinkham WH: Severe idiopathic pulmonary hemosiderosis in the absence of clinical or radiologic evidence of pulmonary disease. J Pediatr 75:118, 1969.

Heiner DC, Sears JW, Kniker WT: Multiple precipitins to cow's milk in chronic respiratory disease. A syndrome including poor growth, gastrointestinal symptoms, evidence of allergy, iron deficiency anemia and pulmonary hemosiderosis. Am J Dis Child 103:634, 1962.

12.82 PULMONARY ALVEOLAR PROTEINOSIS

In children pulmonary alveolar proteinosis is a rare disease of unknown etiology. Occasionally there are families with 2 affected children; such occurrences suggest an underlying genetic basis.

Clinical Manifestations. The 1st symptoms are usually cough and dyspnea. Fever is present in about a third of the patients. Most clinical findings result from hypoxia and include weakness, fatigue, weight loss, and cyanosis. Physical findings are relatively few unless hypoxia is severe, but roentgenographic changes generally are characteristic and consist of a fine, diffuse infiltrate radiating from the hilus to the periphery, often in a "butterfly" distribution (Fig 12–12). Some patients demonstrate bilateral lower lobe infiltrates, while others initially show nodular densities progressing to complete lobar consolidation. Pulmonary function testing reveals a restrictive pattern, and arterial blood gases show marked hypoxemia, usually with normal CO_2 tensions.

The diagnosis of pulmonary alveolar proteinosis must be confirmed by biopsy, although a sputum examination revealing a large amount of PAS-positive material with few or no inflammatory cells is suggestive of the disease. There is a progressive accumulation in the alveoli of amorphous lipid-protein complex. Whether this material accumulates because of an accelerated rate of transport from the serum or because of defective clearance is unknown. Tissue sections show alveoli distended by fine, granular, eosinophilic material which stains positively with PAS stain.

Various immunologic deficiency states, including thymic alymphoplasia, have been found in some children with this disease. Not surprisingly, therefore, various fungal and bacterial superinfections also may be associated with the disease.

No effective treatment exists. Corticosteroids do not alter the relentless, progressive course of the illness. Aerosols with N-acetylcysteine or proteolytic enzymes have been reported effective, but the mainstay of treatment is repeated pulmonary lavage to clear out the alveoli. With improving techniques, including the use of the fiberoptic bronchoscope, this procedure can be accomplished without anesthesia and often with tran-

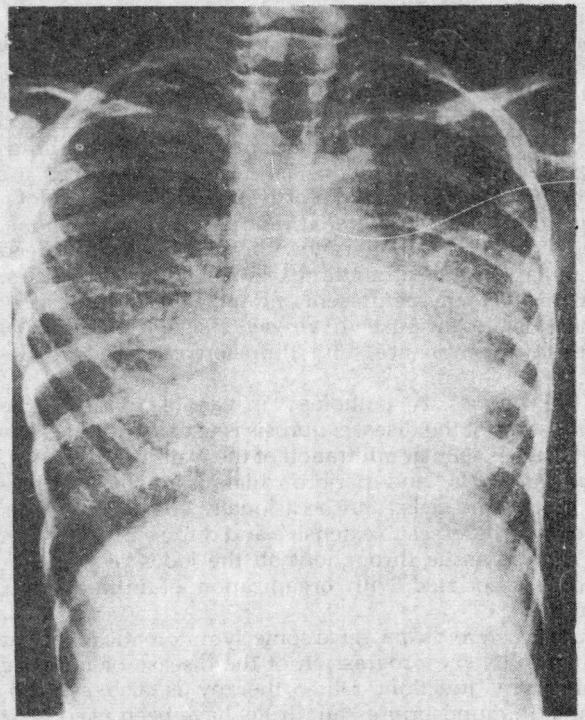

Figure 12–12 Alveolar proteinosis. PA view of chest shows diffuse alveolar infiltrate.

sient dramatic improvement; eventually, reaccumulation forces another series of lavages. Infection plays a relatively minor role in the progression of symptoms, and antibiotic therapy should be used conservatively. Survival has improved greatly with the introduction of modern bronchoscopic techniques. The adult form of pulmonary alveolar proteinosis has a much more favorable prognosis.

Bell DY, Hook GER: Pulmonary alveolar proteinosis: Analysis of airway and alveolar proteins. Am Rev Resp Dis 110:979, 1979.

Mazyck EM, Bonner JT, Herd HM, et al: Pulmonary lavage for childhood pulmonary alveolar proteinosis. J Pediatr 80:839, 1972.

Rosen SH, Castelman B, Liebow AA: Pulmonary alveolar proteinosis. N Engl J Med 258:1123, 1958.

Wilkinson RH, Blanc WA, Hagstrom JWC: Pulmonary alveolar proteinosis in three infants. Pediatrics 41:510, 1968.

12.83 IDIOPATHIC DIFFUSE INTERSTITIAL FIBROSIS OF THE LUNG
(Hamman-Rich Syndrome)

This is a rare, chronic, usually fatal disorder of unknown origin, ordinarily observed in adults but occasionally in infants and children. In vitro data suggest that the disease may have an immunologic basis. The clinical pattern is characterized by progressive pulmonary insufficiency resulting from interstitial fibrosis and alveolar-capillary block. Onset is usually insidious, with dyspnea generally the 1st symptom, initially occurring only with exercise but later present even at rest. A dry cough is frequent and may be productive of blood. The patient is usually afebrile. As the disease progresses, anorexia, weight loss, and fatigability occur, and finally cyanosis, clubbing of the fingers, cor pulmonale, and evidence of right-sided cardiac failure. Usually the lungs are clear on auscultation, but occasionally rales are present. Most children die of respiratory failure following 1 of the frequent intercurrent pulmonary infections. Serial roentgenograms show progressive widespread granular or reticular mottling or small nodular densities. Hypoxemia may be present and increase with exercise. There is no increase in airway resistance, and vital capacity, compliance, and diffusion capacity are decreased.

The pulmonary pathology is variable. During the early stage of the disease, fibrosis is usually not present, but there is cellular infiltration of the walls of the alveoli, alveolar ducts, and peribronchial tissue by lymphocytes, plasma cells, and occasionally eosinophils. This usually progresses to extensive and diffuse proliferation of fibrous tissue throughout all the lobes of the lung and is associated with organization of intra-alveolar exudate.

Corticosteroids may give some symptomatic relief but do not alter the progression of the disease or improve pulmonary function. Other therapy is also symptomatic. Immunosuppressant drugs have been used with benefit in some adults.

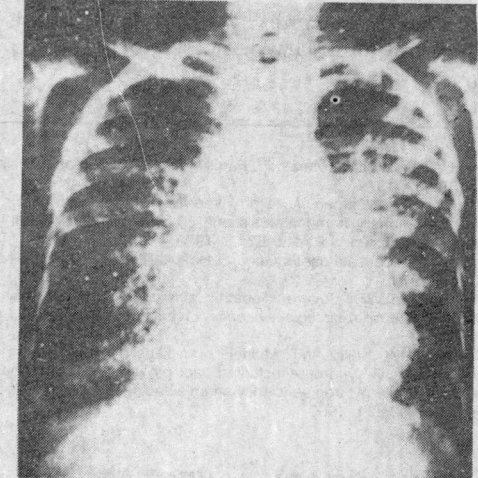

Figure 12–13 Roentgenogram of chest of a 7 yr old boy with pulmonary alveolar microlithiasis. (From Clark RB III, Johnson FC: Pediatrics 28:650, 1961.)

and parents should be counseled that future children are also at risk to develop the disease. Children with alveolar microlithiasis require prompt treatment of respiratory infection and should be advised about the dangers of smoking and exposure to industrial fumes. Immunization to measles and pertussis should be completed and yearly influenza vaccine given.

Bradley CA: Diffuse interstitial fibrosis of the lungs in children. J Pediatr 48:422, 1956.
Brown CH, Turner-Warwick M: The treatment of cryptogenic fibrosing alveolitis with immunosuppressant drugs. Quart J Med 40:289, 1971.
Ivemark BI, Wallgren CG: Diffuse interstitial pulmonary fibrosis (Hamman-Rich syndrome) in an infant. Report of a case with histologic and respiratory studies. Acta Paediatr 51 (Suppl 135):97, 1962.
Kravis TC, Ahmed A, Brown TE, et al: Pathogenic mechanisms in pulmonary fibrosis. J Clin Invest 58:1223, 1976.
Rubin EH, Lubliner R: The Hamman-Rich syndrome: Review of the literature and analysis of 15 cases. Medicine 36:397, 1957.

12.84   PULMONARY ALVEOLAR MICROLITHIASIS

This rare disease of unknown etiology often has its onset during childhood, but the clinical manifestations may be delayed until later years. It is characterized by widely disseminated intraalveolar calculi, which create a characteristic pattern on the roentgenogram (Fig 12–13). Frequently, the disease is recognized when the roentgenogram is taken for an unrelated illness or when symptoms are still minimal. Definitive diagnosis requires lung biopsy.

The familial incidence strongly suggests a genetic basis, but no specific metabolic abnormalities have been identified. Serum calcium and phosphorus are normal. No treatment is available, and patients eventually die during the middle years of adulthood of slowly progressive cardiorespiratory failure, often with superimposed infection. Following diagnosis, other family members should be screened by chest roentgenograms,

Caffrey PR, Altman RS: Pulmonary alveolar microlithiasis occurring in premature twins. J Pediatr 66:758, 1965.
Kino T, Kohara Y, Tsuji S: Pulmonary alveolar microlithiasis: A report in two young sisters. Am Rev Resp Dis 105:105, 1972.
Saputo V, Zocchi M, Mancoso M, et al: Pulmonary alveolar microlithiasis. Helv Paediat Acta 34:245, 1979.

EOSINOPHILIC GRANULOMA OF THE LUNG

See Sec 26.5.

12.85   ATELECTASIS

Congenital atelectasis and hyaline membrane disease are discussed in Sec 7.33 and 7.34.

Acquired Atelectasis

Etiology.   Atelectasis, the imperfect expansion or the collapse of air-bearing tissue of the lung, is relatively common in infants and children. Collapse may be produced by any factor that completely obstructs the intake of air into the alveolar sacs and persists sufficiently long to permit absorption of alveolar air into the bloodstream. In general, the causes may be divided into 3 groups: (1) external pressure directly upon the pulmonary parenchyma or a bronchus or bronchiole,

(2) intrabronchial or intrabronchiolar obstruction, and (3) any factor responsible for a continuously decreased amplitude of respiratory excursion or for respiratory paralysis. Bronchoconstriction and increased bronchosecretion due to allergy or other stimuli including embolus and chest wall trauma may also be contributing factors. Exudate formation may be responsible for atelectasis as in patients with cystic fibrosis.

ATELECTASIS FROM EXTERNAL PRESSURE

External factors may be operative in 1 of 2 ways: (1) direct interference with expansion of lungs (pleural effusion, pneumothorax, intrathoracic tumors, diaphragmatic hernia); and (2) external compression of a bronchus completely obstructing ingress of air (enlarged lymph node, tumors, cardiac enlargement).

ATELECTASIS FROM INTRABRONCHIAL OR INTRABRONCHIOLAR OBSTRUCTION

See also Sec 12.55.

Complete intraluminal obstruction of a bronchus may be produced by a foreign body; by a neoplasm; by granulomatous tissue, as in tuberculosis; or by secretions (including mucous plugs), as with cystic fibrosis, bronchiectasis, pulmonary abscess, allergy, chronic bronchitis, or acute laryngotracheobronchitis.

Obstruction of 1 or more bronchioles in a given area may be produced by any of the conditions mentioned, but widespread bronchiolar obstruction is most often produced by bronchiolitis or interstitial pneumonitis and by asthma. Generalized obstructive overinflation is the initial result of such bronchiolar obstructions; but as the pathologic changes progress, some of the bronchioles may become completely obstructed, and there are then interspersed small areas of atelectasis and emphysema. Patchy atelectasis is relatively common in acute bronchiolitis or asthma and is probably always present in advanced chronic diffuse infections, such as the pulmonary infection associated with cystic fibrosis.

ATELECTASIS FROM REDUCED AMPLITUDE OF RESPIRATORY EXCURSION OR FROM RESPIRATORY PARALYSIS

This may result from (1) interference with the movements of the thoracic cage (neuromuscular abnormalities as in cerebral palsy, poliomyelitis, spinal muscular atrophy, myasthenia gravis, osseous deformities caused by rickets, scoliosis, kyphosis, scleroderma, overly restrictive casts, and surgical dressings); (2) defective movement of the diaphragm (paralysis of phrenic nerve, increased abdominal pressure); or (3) voluntary restriction of respiratory effort because of postoperative pain.

Pathology. The atelectatic areas are airless, congested, deep red, firm in consistency, and depressed below the neighboring healthy or emphysematous lung. When there is extensive atelectasis of 1 or more lobes, there is usually compensatory expansion of the airbearing lung.

Clinical Manifestations. Symptoms vary with the cause and extent of the atelectasis. A small area of atelectasis is likely to be asymptomatic. When a large area of the lung becomes atelectatic, and especially when it does so suddenly, dyspnea with rapid shallow respirations, tachycardia, and often cyanosis occur. If the obstruction is removed, the symptoms disappear rapidly. Even atelectasis of an entire lobe may not be responsible for changes in the percussion note because there is compensatory expansion of the adjacent lung tissue. Breath and voice sounds are decreased or absent over extensive atelectatic areas.

Diagnosis. The diagnosis can usually be established by roentgenographic examination (Fig 12–14). Small areas may be indistinguishable from pneumonic consolidations, but those that involve as many as several lobules of a lobe can usually be identified by the contraction of the area. When 1 or more lobes are atelectatic, the roentgenographic findings are those of massive collapse. Bronchoscopic examination will reveal a collapsed main bronchus when the obstruction is at the tracheobronchial junction and may also disclose the nature of the obstruction.

Prognosis. If the obstruction disappears spontaneously or is removed, the atelectasis usually disappears unless there is secondary infection. The atelectatic area is more susceptible to infection because mucociliary clearance is impaired and cough is ineffective. In persistent cases bronchiectasis is a frequent complication and pulmonary abscess an occasional one.

Treatment. Bronchoscopic examination is immediately indicated if atelectasis is the result of a foreign body or any other bronchial obstruction that may be relieved. It is also indicated when an isolated area of atelectasis persists for several wk. Usually, it is advisable to suction the orifice of the involved bronchus; occasionally, a mucous plug can be removed, with prompt re-expansion. If no anatomic basis for atelectasis is found and no material can be obtained by suctioning, the introduction of a small amount of saline followed by suctioning will allow recovery of bronchial secretions for culture and, possibly, cytologic examination. Frequent changes in the child's position and deep breathing may be beneficial. Oxygen therapy is indicated when there is dyspnea. Morphine and atropine are contraindicated.

If the atelectasis is unchanged or only partially helped by bronchoscopy, postural drainage and, occasionally, antibiotics are indicated. In some situations, such as asthma, bronchodilator and, possibly, corticosteroid treatment may accelerate clearing of the atelectasis. Intermittent positive pressure breathing, incentive inspirometry, and blow bottles have been recommended, but their efficacy remains unproved. Repeated bronchoscopies may be needed. Postural drainage should be continued at home. Lobectomy should not be considered unless chronic infection poses a threat to the remainder of the lung, bronchiectasis is demonstrated by bronchography, or systemic symptoms, such as anorexia or fatigue, are persistent. Occasionally, the atelectatic area becomes completely fibrosed; in this case no further treatment is needed.

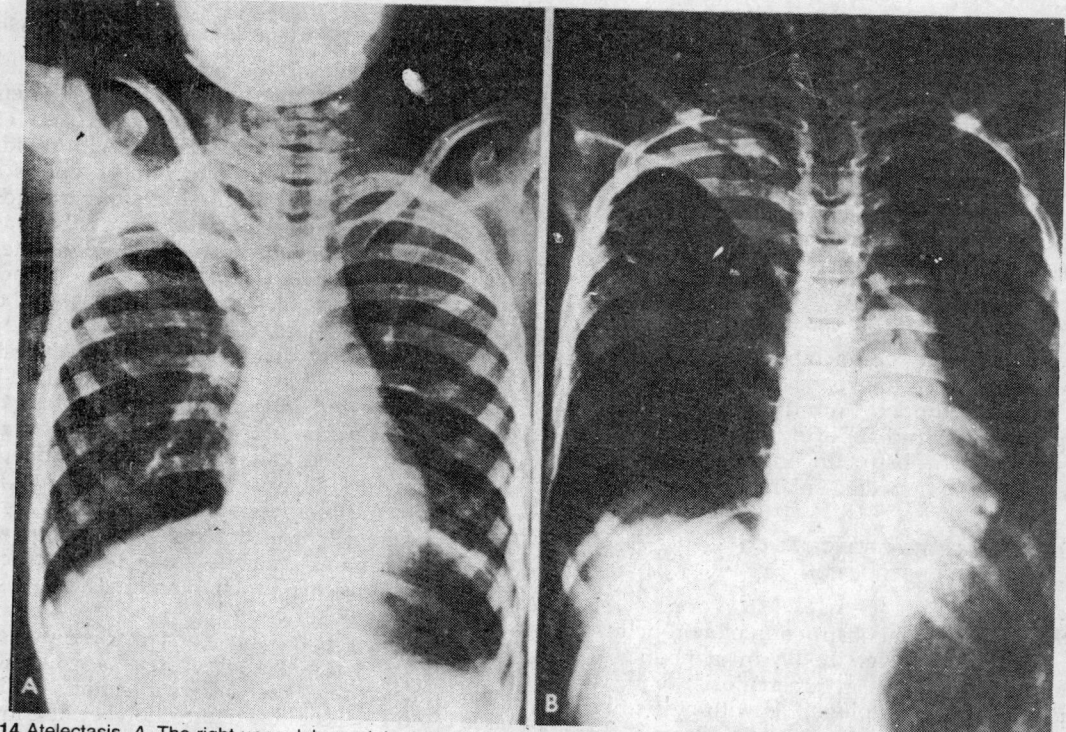

Figure 12–14 Atelectasis. *A,* The right upper lobe and the left lower lobe are collapsed. The atelectasis of the left lower lobe is demonstrated on the overpenetrated film (*B*). The atelectasis occurred postoperatively and disappeared spontaneously.

Massive Pulmonary Atelectasis

Massive collapse of 1 or both lungs is most often a postoperative complication but occasionally results from other causes, such as trauma, asthma, pneumonia, tension pneumothorax, the aspiration of foreign material (either a solid object large enough to obstruct a main stem bronchus or liquids such as water or blood), or paralysis, as in diphtheria or poliomyelitis. Massive atelectasis is usually produced by a combination of factors: immobilization or decreased use of the diaphragm and the respiratory muscles, obstruction of the bronchial tree, and abolition of the cough reflex.

Clinical Manifestations. The onset in postoperative cases usually occurs within 24 hr after operation, but may not occur for several days, with dyspnea, cyanosis, and tachycardia. The child is extremely anxious, prostration is likely, and the patient, if old enough, complains of chest pain. The temperature may be as high as 39.5–40° C (103–104° F).

The physical signs are characteristic. The chest appears flat on the affected side, where there is also decreased respiratory excursion, dullness to percussion, and feeble or absent breath and voice sounds. Lower lobes are more frequently involved than upper ones. The heart and the mediastinum are displaced toward the affected side. Roentgenograms show the collapsed lung, elevation of the diaphragm, narrowing of the intercostal spaces, and displacement of the mediastinal structures and heart toward the affected side (Fig 12–15).

Prognosis. Bilateral massive collapse is usually rapidly fatal, although prompt bronchoscopic aspiration and artificial respiration may be lifesaving. In the unilateral cases the prognosis is usually good.

Prevention. Prophylaxis is of the greatest importance. The incidence of postoperative atelectasis can be reduced by adequate ventilation during anesthesia. After operation the child's position in bed should be changed frequently, and collections of secretions in the oropharynx should be aspirated; when consciousness returns, the child should be encouraged to breathe deeply. Tight thoracic or abdominal binders should be avoided.

Treatment. When there is bilateral atelectasis, bronchoscopic aspiration should be performed immediately. When there is only unilateral atelectasis, the child should be placed on the unaffected side. Forced coughing or crying while the child is lying on the unaffected side may also be helpful, as is positive pressure ventilation. When these measures are not successful, bronchoscopic aspiration should be performed.

Relapses are not infrequent, and the child should be kept under constant observation.

12.86   EMPHYSEMA AND OVERINFLATION

Pulmonary emphysema is a distention with irreversible rupture of the alveoli. It may be generalized or localized and involve part or all of a lung. Overinflation is a reversible distention without alveolar rupture.

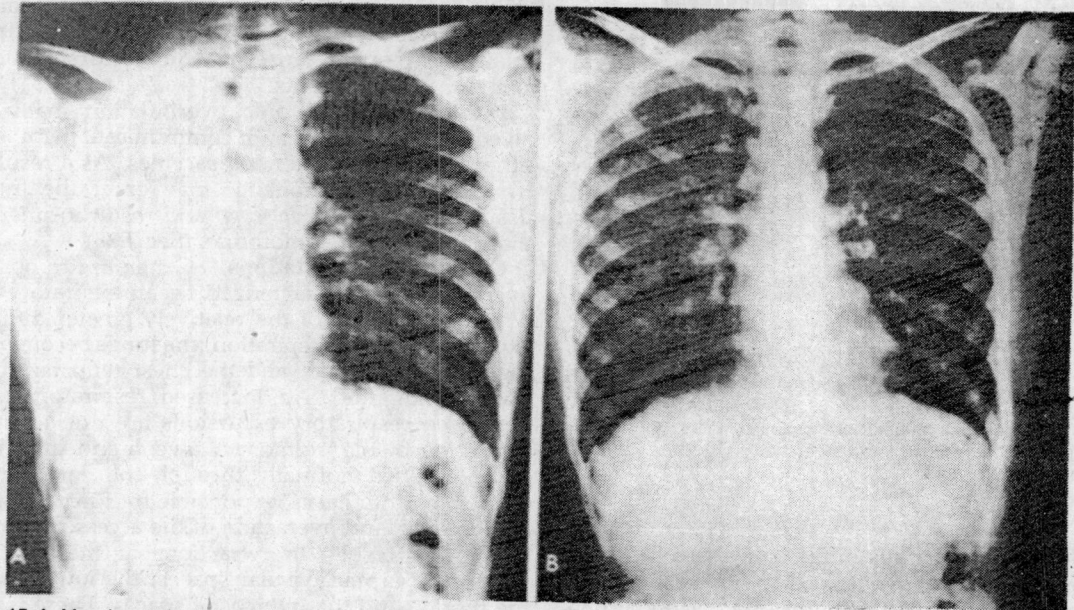

Figure 12–15 *A*, Massive atelectasis of the right lung. *B*, Comparison study after reaeration following bronchoscopic removal of a mucous plug from the right stem bronchus. The patient is asthmatic. The heart and the other mediastinal structures are shifted to the right during the atelectatic phase.

Compensatory overinflation may be either acute or chronic. It occurs in normally functioning pulmonary tissue when for any reason a sizable portion of the lung is partially or completely airless, as may occur with pneumonia, atelectasis, empyema, and pneumothorax.

Obstructive overinflation results from partial obstruction of a bronchus or bronchiole when getting air out of the alveoli becomes more difficult than getting it in; under such circumstances there is a gradually increasing accumulation of air distal to the obstruction, the so-called bypass or check valve type of obstruction. Such obstructions may be intrabronchial or extrabronchial (Sec 12.5 and 12.55).

Localized Obstructive Overinflation

When a bypass type of obstruction partially occludes the main stem bronchus, the entire lobe becomes overinflated; only individual lobules are affected when the obstruction is that of a secondary bronchus. Localized obstructions that may be responsible for overinflation include foreign bodies and the inflammatory reaction to them, intrabronchial tuberculosis or tuberculosis of the tracheobronchial lymph nodes, and intrabronchial or mediastinal tumors. When most or all of a lobe is involved, the percussion note will be hyperresonant over the area and the breath sounds decreased in intensity. The distended lung may extend across the mediastinum into the opposite hemithorax. Fluoroscopically, during expiration the overinflated area does not decrease in size, and the heart and the mediastinum shift to the opposite side.

Unilateral hyperlucent lung may occur in association with a variety of cardiac and pulmonary diseases of children, but in some patients it occurs without easily demonstrable underlying active disease. Over half of the reported cases have followed 1 or more episodes of pneumonia; in several patients a rising titer to adenovirus has been documented. Patients may present signs and symptoms of pneumonia, but some are discovered only when a chest roentgenogram is taken for an unrelated reason. A few patients have hemoptysis initially. Physical findings may include hyperresonance and decreased breath sounds over the involved area. Chest roentgenogram reveals unilateral hyperlucency and an apparently small lung with the mediastinum shifted toward the more abnormal lung. Some patients will show mediastinal shift away from the lesion with expiration. Bronchiectasis may be demonstrated on bronchography. There is markedly decreased perfusion on the affected side. In some patients previous chest roentgenograms have been normal or have shown only an acute pneumonia, suggesting that hyperlucent lung is an acquired lesion. No specific treatment is known; it may become less symptomatic with time.

Congenital obstructive lobar emphysema may cause severe respiratory distress in early infancy. Symptoms usually become apparent in the neonatal period but may be delayed for as much as 5–6 mo in 5% of the patients. Occasional patients remain undiagnosed until school age or beyond. A part, but usually all, of a lobe may be involved; the left upper lobe is most often affected. In some instances the obstruction is not demonstrable, but it is assumed to be produced by a check valve type of mechanism. Such obstructions have been attributed to defective or overly compliant cartilage in the bronchi, mucosal folds which create a valve-like obstruction, bronchial stenosis, and external compression by aberrant vessels or tumors. A radiolucent lobe and a mediastinal shift are often present on roentgenographic examination. When the distention is consid-

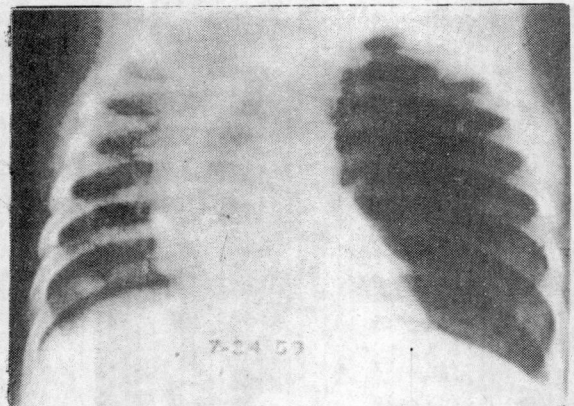

Figure 12–16 Congenital left upper lobe emphysema. Note extension of emphysematous lobe into left lower lobe and its displacement of the mediastinum toward the right.

erable, the emphysematous lung compresses the unaffected lung below or above it and the opposite lung by extending across the mediastinum (Fig 12–16). Immediate surgery and excision of the lobe may be lifesaving when cyanosis and severe respiratory distress are present. However, some patients have responded to medical treatment.

Overinflation of all 3 lobes of the right lung has been produced by anomalous location of the left pulmonary artery, which partially constricts the right main bronchus. A number of neonates have developed lobar overinflation while being treated for hyaline membrane disease with assisted ventilation, suggesting an acquired etiology. Medical management, sometimes with selective intubation, has occasionally been successful and lobectomy avoided.

Cumming GR, Macpherson RI, Chernick V: Unilateral hyperlucent lung syndrome in children. J Pediatr 78:250, 1971.
Dickman GL, Short BL, Krauss DR: Selective bronchial intubation in the management of unilateral pulmonary interstitial emphysema. Am J Dis Child 131:365, 1977.
Eigen H, Lemen RJ, Waring WW: Congenital lobar emphysema: Long-term evaluation of surgically and conservatively treated children. Am Rev Resp Dis 116:823, 1976.
Guzowski J, Duvall A: Swyer-James syndrome: A cause of hyperlucent lung. Ann Otol Rhinol Laryngol 84:657, 1975.
McBride JT, Wohl MEB, Strieder D, et al: Lung growth and airway function after lobectomy in infancy for congenital lobar emphysema. J Clin Invest 66:962, 1980.
Shannon DC, Todres ID, Moylan FMB: Infantile lobar hyperinflation: Expectant treatment. Pediatrics 59:1012, 1977.

Generalized Obstructive Overinflation

Acute overinflation of the lung depends upon widespread involvement of the bronchioles and is reversible. It occurs more commonly in infants than in children and may be secondary to a number of clinical conditions, including respiratory infections associated with cystic fibrosis of the pancreas, acute bronchiolitis, interstitial pneumonitis, atypical forms of acute laryngotracheobronchitis, aspiration of zinc stearate powder, chronic passive congestion secondary to a congenital cardiac lesion, and miliary tuberculosis. Asthma is a relatively frequent cause in older children but an uncommon one in infants.

Pathology. In chronic overinflation many of the alveoli are ruptured and communicate with one another, producing distended saccules. As a result of the rupture of the alveoli, air may enter the interstitial tissue (*interstitial emphysema*) and result in pneumomediastinum and pneumothorax (Sec 7.38).

Clinical Manifestations. Generalized obstructive overinflation is characterized by an expiratory type of dyspnea. Because of the relatively greater difficulty in expiration than in inspiration, the lungs become increasingly overdistended, and the chest remains expanded during expiration. An increased respiratory rate and decreased respiratory excursions are due to the overdistention of the pulmonary alveoli and their inability to be emptied normally through the narrowed bronchioles. Air hunger is responsible for forced respiratory movements, and overaction of the accessory muscles of respiration results in retractions at the suprasternal notch, the supraclavicular spaces, the lower margin of the thorax, and the intercostal spaces. There is scarcely any reduction in size of the overdistended chest during expiration, in contrast to the flattened chest during both inspiration and expiration when there is laryngeal obstruction. There is no hoarseness or stridor as with laryngeal obstruction. Cyanosis is common in the severe cases. The percussion note is hyperresonant, and on auscultation the inspiratory phase is usually less prominent than the expiratory phase, which is prolonged and roughened. Fine or medium rales may be present.

Roentgenographic and fluoroscopic examinations of the chest are a great help in establishing the diagnosis. Both leaves of the diaphragm are low and flattened, the ribs are farther apart than usual, and the lung fields are less dense (Fig 12–17). There is restriction in the movement of the diaphragm, best demonstrated by fluoroscopic examination. The normal "doming" of the diaphragm during expiration is decreased, and the excursion of the low, flattened diaphragm in the severe cases is barely discernible. Retention of air in the lungs during expiration is also increased by a paradoxical increase in the horizontal diameters of the chest during this phase.

Bullous Emphysema

Bullous emphysematous blebs or cysts (**pneumatoceles**) result from overdistention and rupture of alveoli during birth or shortly thereafter, or they may be sequelae of pneumonia and of other infections. They have been observed in tuberculous lesions while the patient was being treated with specific antibacterial therapy. These emphysematous areas presumably result from rupture of distended alveoli so that a single or multiloculated cavity is formed. The cysts may become large (Fig 12–10). They may contain some fluid, and an air-fluid level may be demonstrated on the roentgenogram. They must be differentiated from pulmonary abscesses. In most instances the cysts disappear spontaneously within a few mo, although they may persist for 1 yr or so.

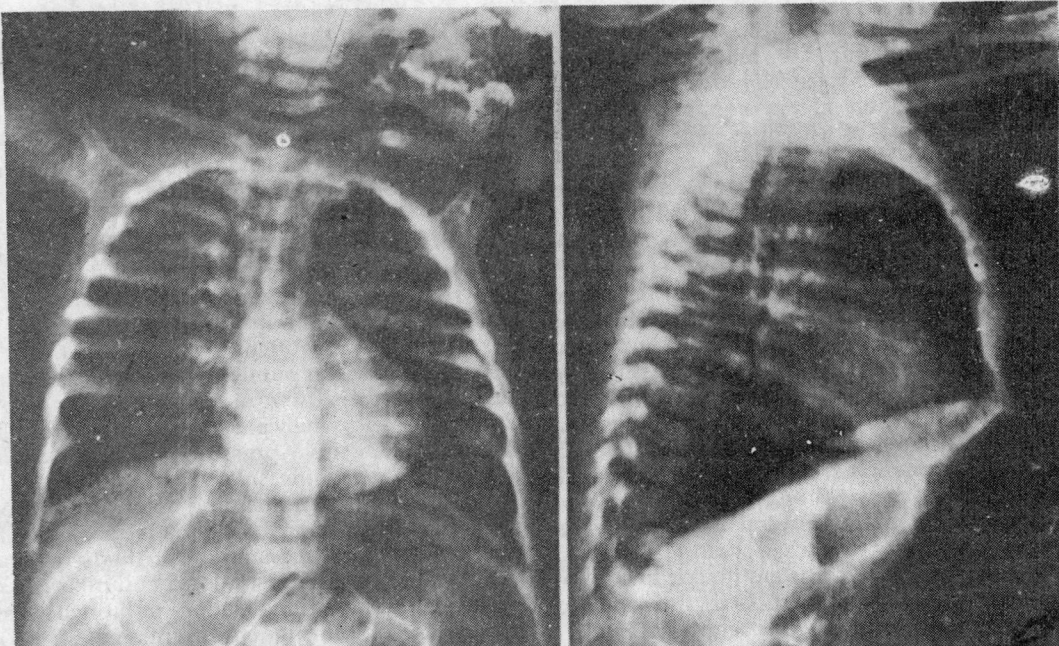

Figure 12–17 Generalized obstructive emphysema (overinflation); dorsal projections of thorax in inspiratory and expiratory phases of respiration. Notice the relative failure of the lungs to empty in the expiratory phase. The left lung is less obstructed than the right (empties to a greater degree in the expiratory phase). This difference between the lungs is not apparent from a study of the diaphragm, which moves very little during respiration; it is evident, however, in the upper portions of the left lung space.

There is almost never any indication for aspiration or surgery unless there is severe respiratory and cardiac embarrassment.

Subcutaneous Emphysema

This occurs whenever free air finds its way into the subcutaneous tissue. It may be a complication of fracture of the orbit permitting free air to escape from the nasal sinuses. In the neck and thorax, emphysema may follow tracheotomy, deep ulcerations in the pharyngeal region, esophageal wounds, or any perforating lesion of the larynx or trachea. It is an occasional complication of thoracentesis, of asthma, or of abdominal surgery. Air may also be formed in the subcutaneous tissues by gas-producing bacteria.

The problem is usually self-limited and requires no specific treatment. Resolution occurs by resorption of subcutaneous air following elimination of its source. Rarely, dangerous compression of the trachea by air in the surrounding soft tissue requires surgical intervention.

Caffey J: Pediatric X-Ray Diagnosis. Ed 4. Chicago, Year Book Medical Publishers, 1961.

Kress MB, Finklestein AH: Giant bullous emphysema occurring in tuberculosis in childhood. Pediatrics 30:269, 1962.

Nelson WE, Smith LW: Generalized obstructive emphysema in infants. J Pediatr 26:36, 1945.

12.87 Alpha₁-Antitrypsin Deficiency and Emphysema

Homozygous deficiency of alpha₁-antitrypsin characterized by the early onset of severe panacinar emphysema is a rare cause of pulmonary disease in children. Alpha₁-antitrypsin and other serum antiproteases are thought to be important in the inactivation of proteolytic enzymes released from dead bacteria or leukocytes in the lung. Deficiency leads to accumulation of these enzymes, proteolytic destruction of pulmonary tissue, and development of emphysema. The type and concentration of alpha₁-antitrypsin are inherited as a series of codominant alleles; the inferred genotype is referred to as the "pi-type." Normal persons are pi-type MM. Type ZZ and, to a lesser exent, other abnormal pi-types such as SZ have been associated with early onset emphysema and a characteristic form of infantile cirrhosis (Sec 11.101). The evidence that individuals who are the MZ pi-type are also at risk to develop chronic pulmonary disease is not conclusive; if pulmonary disease is associated with the MZ pi-type, it seems to be relatively mild.

The concentration of proteases (e.g., elastase) in the patients' leukocytes may be an important factor in determining the severity of clinical pulmonary disease with a given level of alpha₁-antitrypsin.

Most patients who have pi-type ZZ have had little or no detectable pulmonary disease during childhood. A few have had very early onset of chronic pulmonary symptoms, including dyspnea, wheezing, and cough, and panacinar emphysema has been documented by lung biopsy. Physical examination may reveal growth failure, an increased anteroposterior diameter of the chest with a hyperresonant percussion note, rales if there is active infection, and clubbing. Severe emphysema may depress the liver and spleen, making them more easily palpable. Chest roentgenogram reveals overinflation with depressed diaphragms. Serum has a low trypsin inhibitory capacity, and immunoassay confirms the low level of alpha₁-antitrypsin.

No specific treatment is available. Every effort to minimize the presence of proteases in the lung is important. Thus prompt use of antibiotics is indicated for pulmonary infection, and postural drainage may be useful. Influenza vaccine should be administered yearly. The same measures are probably also indicated for other members of the family found to be pi-type ZZ even if they are asymptomatic. The clinical significance of other pi-types, especially SZ and MZ, is unknown, but a similar treatment seems reasonable. All persons with low levels of serum antiprotease should be warned that the eventual development of emphysema may be partially related to environmental factors, including exposure to industrial fumes and cigarette smoking.

Dunand P, Cropp GJA, Middleton E Jr: Severe obstructive lung disease in a 14 year old girl with alpha₁-antitrypsin deficiency. J Allergy Clin Immun 57:615, 1976.
Hall WJ, Hyde RW, Schwartz RH, et al: Pulmonary abnormalities in intermediate alpha-1-antitrypsin deficiency. J Clin Invest 58:1069, 1976.
Kidokoro Y, Kravis TC, Moser KM, et al: Relationship of leukocyte elastase concentration to severity of emphysema in homozygous alpha₁-antitrypsin deficient persons. Am Rev Resp Dis 115:793, 1977.
Moore JO: Alpha₁-antitrypsin deficiency. N Engl J Med 299:1045, 1099, 1978.
Sveger T: Alpha₁-antitrypsin deficiency in early childhood. Pediatrics 62:22, 1978.

12.88 PULMONARY EDEMA

Etiology. Pulmonary edema results from the transudation of fluid from the pulmonary capillaries into the alveolar spaces and the bronchioles. It is usually associated with circulatory or neurocirculatory collapse and consequently is often a terminal event in a variety of diseases. Though pulmonary edema may vary in severity, even in its mildest stages it is an ominous finding. It is a common manifestation of left ventricular failure, the edema resulting from a rise in pulmonary venous pressure, or it may be due to hypervolemia from too rapid or too large an intravenous infusion. It may also be a manifestation of acute or chronic nephritis or, rarely, of pneumonic and other infections with substantial degrees of toxicity. Poisoning by such substances as barbiturates, morphine, epinephrine, and alcohol may be responsible for the development of pulmonary edema, as may the inhalation of toxic gases, such as illuminating gas, ammonia, and nitrogen dioxide, or the ingestion and consequent aspiration of highly volatile hydrocarbons, such as lighter fluid.

Clinical Manifestations. The onset is variable but rapid in most instances. The child often complains of difficulty in breathing or a sense of oppression or pain in the chest. Cough is usually present and often pro-

duces a frothy, pink-tinged sputum. There is tachypnea, and the pulse is rapid and feeble. The child is usually very pale and may be cyanotic. On physical examination, dullness to percussion and moist, bubbly rales are heard in the lower portions of the chest. Chest roentgenogram shows a diffuse perihilar infiltrate (butterfly distribution). Occasionally, 1 lung is more affected than the other. If the pulmonary edema is superimposed on another pulmonary process (e.g., pneumococcal pneumonia, left heart failure in cystic fibrosis), the clinical and roentgenographic findings of the primary illness may obscure those of pulmonary edema.

Treatment. Treatment is directed at the primary disease causing the pulmonary edema. The administration of oxygen is often useful in relieving some of the chest pain, and when possible is best accomplished by intermittent positive pressure. Dyspnea can often be relieved by morphine sulfate, in a dosage of 0.15 mg/kg, and oxygen. Antifoaming agents and atropine are not useful. If pulmonary edema is secondary to excessive parenteral administration of fluids or blood or to cardiac failure, administration of diuretics, e.g., furosemide (1 mg/kg), digitalization, or bronchodilators, the application of tourniquets or inflated blood pressure cuffs to the extremities, or the withdrawal of blood may be lifesaving.

High Altitude Pulmonary Edema

This disease characteristically affects young people at altitudes above 2700 meters (8860 ft). In 1 series, 29 of 32 patients were under 21 yr of age and 14 were under 10. The pathogenesis is unknown. Cough, shortness of breath, vomiting, and chest pain are the most common symptoms and occur within hours of high altitude exposure. Not all persons are affected, and even affected persons may not develop symptoms after every exposure. Chest roentgenogram reveals bilateral patchy pulmonary infiltrates. Oxygen is indicated. Bed rest, diuretics, antibiotics, and corticosteroids have been used, but their efficacy has not been established. Recovery occurs within 48 hr, and further residence at high altitude is then tolerated without symptoms. The disease may recur, however, following return to high altitude after even a brief visit to lower levels.

Scoggin CH, Hyers TM, Reeves JT, et al: High-altitude pulmonary edema in the children and young adults of Leadville, Colorado. N Engl J Med 297:1269, 1977.

12.89 PULMONARY EMBOLISM AND INFARCTION

Pulmonary embolism is rare in infants and children. Emboli most often arise from thrombi in the femoral and pelvic veins and are usually postoperative complications. Scoliosis surgery, in particular, may predispose to deep vein thrombosis and pulmonary embolization. Embolization may also occur following prolonged inactivity or as a complication of intravenous infusions. Intrapulmonary thrombosis also may occur in sickle cell anemia; the subsequent infarction is often difficult to differentiate from pneumonia. Fat emboli are most likely to be derived from fractured bones; on occasion they stem from necrotic tissue in the bone marrow of patients with sickle cell disease. Multiple pulmonary infarcts resulting from small emboli may be associated with severe dehydration in diarrheal disease, cyanotic heart disease, bacterial endocarditis, ventriculoatrial shunts for the treatment of hydrocephalus, and long-standing nutritional deficiencies.

Clinical Manifestations. The clinical pattern is apt to be interpreted as a pneumonic process, and the diagnosis is usually made at autopsy. Emboli carrying bacteria may be responsible for multiple pulmonary abscesses.

Embolism of the pulmonary artery or its larger branches has a characteristic clinical picture. There is sudden pulmonary pain, usually substernal, but it may be pleural and radiate to the shoulder. Dyspnea, tachycardia, and signs of collapse are seen. Though there are often no physical signs, if the infarct is sufficiently large, there may be impaired resonance and a pleural friction rub. Breath sounds may be distant or absent, and there may be moist rales. Expectorated material, which may be profuse, often contains blood. The case fatality rate is high, but recovery may occur even when the area of infarction is relatively large. Secondary infection may result in abscess formation.

Massive, potentially fatal pulmonary thrombosis may occur after bronchography of patients with sickle cell anemia. This procedure should be performed with great caution, if at all, in these patients.

Chronic showers of emboli from **ventriculoatrial shunts** may cause gradual obliteration of the pulmonary vascular bed and eventual pulmonary hypertension. Clinical findings are those of pulmonary hypertension and may include accentuation of the pulmonic component of the 2nd heart sound and the development of pulmonary or tricuspid insufficiency. In severe cases, exercise intolerance and right-sided heart failure occur indicating that substantial compromise of lung function has already taken place. Serial electrocardiograms that show increasing right ventricular hypertrophy may give an early clue to continuing chronic embolization. Diagnosis may be confirmed by right heart catheterization and determination of pulmonary arterial blood pressure. If chronic embolization is suspected, the shunt should be removed.

Treatment. Embolization of the larger branches of the pulmonary artery is a medical emergency. The initial objective in management is to support cardiovascular function and prevent circulatory collapse and pulmonary insufficiency through cardiotonic drugs, oxygen, and ventilatory assistance. After stabilization and definitive diagnosis, efforts should be made to prevent further embolization. Recurrent pulmonary emboli arising in patients with deep vein thrombosis may be prevented by immediate anticoagulation with intravenous heparin given by continuous infusion or intermittently (50–100 units/kg given every 4 hr) to maintain the clotting time at 2–2.5 times the baseline level. Heparinization is usually followed by chronic oral anticoagulation with 1 of the coumarin drugs (sodium warfarin or bishydroxycoumarin). Anticoagulation is usually discontinued after 6 mo.

Bashour TT, Lindsay J: Hemoglobin S-C disease presenting as acute pneumonitis with pulmonary angiographic findings in two patients. Am J Med 58:559, 1975.
Bromberg PA: Pulmonary aspects of sickle cell anemia. Arch Int Med 133:652, 1974.
Friedman S, Zita-Gozum C, Chatten J: Pulmonary vascular changes complicating ventriculovascular shunting for hydrocephalus. J Pediatr 64:305, 1964.
Noonan JA, Ehmke DA: Complications of ventriculovenous shunts for control of hydrocephalus. Report of three cases with thromboemboli to the lungs. N Engl J Med 269:70, 1963.
Uden A: Thromboembolic complications following scoliosis surgery in Scandinavia. Acta Orthrop Scand 50:175, 1979.

PULMONARY SUPPURATION

12.90 Bronchiectasis

Bronchiectasis refers to dilatation of the bronchi associated with inflammatory destruction of bronchial and peribronchial tissue, accumulation of exudative material in dependent bronchi, and, in some instances, distention of dependent bronchi.

Etiology. Some patients may have *congenital bronchiectasis* possibly due to an arrest in bronchial development leading to cyst formation, and when the cysts become infected there is apt to be destruction of the bronchial wall. Alternatively, there may be defective development of the bronchial cartilaginous supports. *Tracheobronchomegaly* is a rare congenital condition in which the distal trachea and main bronchi are grossly dilated; a similar condition may be associated with recurrent pneumonia.

The majority of instances of bronchiectasis are acquired after birth, usually the result of chronic pulmonary infection, but the mechanisms involved are poorly understood. Obstruction of the bronchial tree followed by infection is 1 likely cause. Measles, pertussis, and pneumonia, once regarded as frequent antecedent infections, are rare causes of bronchiectasis. Cystic fibrosis is the most common underlying disease in children with generalized bronchial involvement. Other predisposing factors include aspiration of a foreign body, often a nonopaque one, enlarged bronchopulmonary nodes due to tuberculosis, recurrent and chronic lung infections, sarcoidosis, neoplasm, lung abscess, localized cysts, emphysema with compression of the other lung parenchyma, allergy, asthma, and, rarely, extreme forms of pectus excavatum or scoliosis. Patients with immune deficiency syndromes may have bronchiectasis, usually after repeated attacks of bacterial pneumonia and bronchitis. Recurrent aspiration pneumonitis in familial dysautonomia frequently leads to bronchiectasis. The immotile cilia syndrome (Sec 12.63) results in chronic pulmonary infection which eventually leads to bronchiectasis. Bronchiectasis and sinusitis frequently coexist, as in the immotile cilia syndrome, but their interrelationship is not always clear. Gastroesophageal reflux with chronic aspiration may be a cause of bronchiectasis.

Reversible bronchiectasis or pseudobronchiectasis occurs commonly after pertussis as well as with lobar and interstitial pneumonias. Shortly after or during these illnesses the bronchi may appear cylindrically dilated on bronchography, but if these studies are repeated some mo later, the changes have disappeared.

Pathology. The 1st destructive change is a loss of ciliated epithelium, which is regenerated as cuboidal and squamous epithelium. Concurrently the elastic tissue within the bronchial walls disappears and thickening occurs, due to interstitial edema, fibrosis, and round cell infiltration, together with involvement of adjacent parenchymal and peribronchial tissue. In these peribronchial areas multiple abscesses may develop, and there usually is characteristic obstructive endarteritis of the small pulmonary vessels. Generally, bronchiectasis follows a segmental distribution, except in cystic fibrosis. The areas involved depend somewhat on the cause; most frequently affected are the right middle lobe segments, the basal segments of the lower lobes, and the lingular segments of the left upper lobe. The right lower lobe is commonly involved in aspiration of a foreign body, whereas the right middle lobe is most frequently affected by hilar lymphadenopathy.

Clinical Manifestations. In symptomatic cases cough is invariably present and produces copious mucopurulent sputum during acute respiratory infections. The sputum is generally swallowed by young children. Physical activity or change in position, particularly while reclining, will often initiate a bout of coughing.

Recurring infections of the lower respiratory tract are common; they tend to persist and are difficult to control. Anorexia, irritability, and poor weight gain are common. Fever is much less common. Later in the course, during acute exacerbations, hemoptysis may occur, varying in severity from streaking of the sputum to exsanguinating hemorrhage. Bronchiectasis characteristically follows an intermittently improving and relapsing course.

The **middle lobe syndrome** may occur, which consists of subacute or chronic pneumonitis, bronchial obstruction, and atelectasis, and is generally caused by extrinsic compression of the middle lobe bronchus by hilar nodes, followed by peribronchitis and chronic infection. Bronchiectasis may result. On occasion this syndrome is related to asthma or congenital anomalies of the bronchi.

Physical findings are absent or few. Clubbing of the fingers may be present if the patient has been symptomatic for over 1 yr. Moist or musical rales may be heard or elicited by cough; during acute exacerbations physical signs of atelectasis or diffuse pneumonitis are often present. The usual roentgen examination is never pathognomonic, although such predisposing factors as mediastinal lymph nodes or radiopaque foreign bodies may be demonstrated, as well as suggestively increased bronchovascular markings near the hilus of the lung. Atelectasis is relatively common.

With extensive bronchiectasis there is persistent dyspnea, and physical development is retarded. Ventilatory and diffusion studies may reveal more widespread or severe pulmonary involvement than suspected otherwise.

Every patient with suspected or proved bronchiectasis should be evaluated for the presence of such possible causative factors as sinusitis, immotile cilia, agammaglobulinemia, tuberculosis, asthma or other respiratory allergy, and cystic fibrosis. If such a diagnosis cannot be made, these patients should have bronchoscopy to exclude bronchial stenosis, strictures, tumors, and foreign bodies and then bronchography to document the bronchiectasis and determine its extent and severity. A familial deficiency of bronchial cartilage has also been proposed as an explanation of some cases of bronchiectasis in childhood and may be suggested by marked dilatation of the 2nd–4th order bronchi with inspiration and apparent collapse during expiration. Bronchoscopic washings and sputum samples should be cultured for routine pathogens and for mycobacteria and fungi, and a tuberculin skin test should be done.

Therapy. Treatment includes elimination of all foci of infection in the respiratory tract, effective postural drainage, and, when indicated, antibiotic therapy. Postural drainage must be carried out intensively as long as secretions are being formed and is 1 of the most important aspects of management.

Systemic antibiotic therapy is usually administered only during acute exacerbations in short courses of 5–7 days or up to 2 wk. Patients with cystic fibrosis require more prolonged therapy (Sec 12.110). Prolonged treatment for most other patients, however, increases the risk of acquisition of resistant flora and reactions to the drugs employed. The appropriate drug is selected on the basis of the tested antibiotic susceptibility of bacteria isolated from sputum or at bronchoscopy. If cultures contain only normal flora, antibiotics should not be used. The administration of antibiotics by aerosol inhalation immediately following appropriate postural drainage may also be helpful but should not be continued for excessively long periods of time, since this will encourage the establishment of a drug-resistant bacterial flora. *Pseudomonas* is particularly troublesome.

In the infrequent instances when localized severe disease progresses despite adequate medical management, segmental or lobar resection should be considered, even though the long-term results are often discouraging. Some patients with lobar bronchiectasis, especially those with the right middle lobe syndrome, do very well postlobectomy. Surgery may also be indicated when an intrinsic anatomic obstruction of the bronchus is found or when suppurative lesions exist due to aspiration of fragmented foreign bodies, especially such vegetal objects as grass fibers or fragments of peanut which elude bronchoscopic removal.

Becroft DMO: Bronchiolitis obliterans, bronchiectasis and other sequelae of adenovirus type 21 infection. J Clin Pathol 24:72, 1971.

Camner P, Mossberg B, Afzelius BA: Evidence for congenitally non-functioning cilia in tracheobronchial tract in two subjects. Am Rev Resp Dis 112:807, 1975.

Clark NS: Bronchiectasis in childhood. Br Med J 1:80, 1963.

Dees SC, Spock A: Right middle lobe syndrome in children. JAMA 197:8, 1966.

Field CE: Bronchiectasis: Third report of a follow-up study of medical and surgical cases from childhood. Arch Dis Child 44:551, 1969.

Miller RD, Divertie MB: Kartagener syndrome. Chest 62:130, 1972.

Mitchell RE, Bury RG: Congenital bronchiectasis due to deficiency of bronchial cartilage (Williams-Campbell syndrome): Case report. J Pediatr 87:230, 1975.

Pederson H, Mygind N: Absence of axonemal arms in nasal mucosa cilia in Kartagener's syndrome. Nature 262:494, 1976.

Williams H, O'Reilly RN: Bronchiectasis in children: Its multiple clinical and pathological aspects. Arch Dis Child 34:192, 1959.

12.91 Pulmonary Abscess

A lung abscess is a suppurative process resulting in destruction of the pulmonary parenchyma with formation of a cavity containing purulent material. Lung abscesses in children most often result from the *aspiration of infected material* when the local defense mechanisms are overwhelmed by a large number of virulent microorganisms or compromised by such factors as alcohol, drug abuse, recent surgery (particularly tonsillectomy or adenoidectomy), or systemic disease. Aspirated material reaches the most dependent portions of the lung and contains bacteria which are normal inhabitants of the naso- and oropharynx. Thus, the posterior segments of the upper lobes and the superior segments of the lower lobes are involved most frequently, and anaerobic bacteria including bacteroides, *Fusobacterium,* and anaerobic streptococci are commonly isolated. Occasionally *pneumonia* caused by aerobic pyogenic microorganisms (*Staphylococcus aureus* and *Klebsiella*) or *bronchial obstruction* due to a tumor or foreign body may be complicated by abscess formation. *Metastatic lung abscess* secondary to septic emboli from right-sided bacterial endocarditis and septic thrombophlebitis is uncommon in pediatric patients. Rare causes in children also include amebic abscess of the lung and infections with *Nocardia*, actinomyces, and mycobacteria.

Pathology. Abscesses of the lung occur when pulmonary parenchyma becomes obstructed, infected, and then suppurative and necrotic. Initial inflammatory changes are followed by suppuration and thrombosis of the local blood vessels, which result in necrosis and liquefaction. Granulation tissue forms around the periphery of the abscess and may succeed in walling off the area, but more commonly the abscess ruptures into a bronchus. Contents of the abscess may then be coughed up or aspirated into other parts of the pulmonary tree with additional abscess formation. Sputum is usually fetid, may separate into layers, and often contains elastic fibers. Peripheral abscesses may involve the adjacent pleura, with development of an associated pleural effusion. Abscesses may rupture into the pleural cavity and produce empyema.

Clinical Manifestations. The onset is generally insidious, with fever, malaise, anorexia, and weight loss. Cough, often associated with hemoptysis and producing copious amounts of foul-smelling or purulent sputum, is characteristic about 10 days after the onset in untreated patients. Lung abscess secondary to staphylococcal and *Klebsiella* pneumonia produces the acute signs and symptoms described for bacterial pneumonia. There may be respiratory distress, spiking fevers, chest pain, and marked leukocytosis. The diagnosis of lung abscess is generally made by roentgenographic examination when a cavity with or without a fluid level surrounded by alveolar infiltration is demonstrated. Gram stain of the sputum may reveal numerous polymorphonuclear leukocytes and findings consistent with

anaerobic microorganisms, such as pleomorphic, slender, gram-negative bacilli (bacteroides, *Fusobacterium*); gram-negative rods with tapered ends (*Fusobacterium*); large gram-positive bacilli (clostridium); and tiny to small cocci (anaerobic streptococci). Sputum cultures characteristically yield a mixture of anaerobic bacteria.

Treatment. If a predominant aerobic organism is identified, appropriate antibiotic therapy is initiated. However, if lung abscess is secondary to aspiration and the Gram stain is compatible with anaerobic bacteria, treatment with penicillin (100,000 U/kg/24 hr) for an extended period of time (4–6 wk) is the treatment of choice pending the results of anaerobic sputum culture. This drug is effective even in patients infected with penicillin-resistant strains of *Bacteroides fragilis*. Alternative treatment in children allergic to penicillin is chloramphenicol. Clindamycin and metronidazole have also been used in adult patients with lung abscess; however, experience with these drugs in children is limited. Appropriate investigation for dental disease should also be done in older children and adolescents.

Serial roentgenograms of the chest show gradual diminution in the size of the abscess cavity over a period of several wk or mo. Most patients are afebrile within 1 wk of institution of appropriate antibiotic therapy. Delayed closure is common. Bronchoscopy is indicated only to identify and remove a foreign body. The routine use of bronchoscopy to facilitate drainage or to obtain culture material is controversial. Surgical drainage of a lung abscess is almost never indicated, and resection should be considered only in children with recurrent hemoptysis, repeated episodes of infection, or suspicion of malignancy.

The overall prognosis for complete recovery from primary lung abscess is excellent. In patients with secondary lung abscess, the prognosis is heavily dependent on the underlying disease.

Bartleh JG, Gorbach SL, Tally FP et al: Bacteriology and treatment of primary lung abscess. Am Rev Resp Dis 109:510, 1974.

Brook I, Finegold JM: Bacteriology and therapy of lung abscess in children. J Pediatr 94:10, 1979.

Levine MM, Ashman R, Heald F: Anaerobic (putrid) lung abscess in adolescence. Am J Dis Child 130:77, 1976.

McCracken GH: Lung abscess in childhood. Hosp Prac 13:35, 1978.

12.92 Pulmonary Gangrene

Gangrene of the lung is extremely rare. It occasionally follows measles and is seen in persons with severe immunologic deficits. The onset is usually sudden and is associated with early pulmonary hemorrhage; there is rapid development of pneumothorax and putrid empyema, and death may occur quickly. Treatment consists of adequate pleural drainage and intensive antibiotic therapy.

12.93 HERNIA OF LUNG

Protrusion of the lung beyond its normal thoracic boundaries may be a complication of pulmonary disease in which there is frequent coughing with generation of high intrathoracic pressure, such as cystic fibrosis or asthma, or may result from a congenital weakness of the suprapleural membrane or the musculature of the neck. Over half of congenital lung hernias and almost all acquired lung hernias are cervical. Paravertebral or parasternal hernias are usually due to rib anomalies (Sec 12.97). The presenting complaint is usually the presence of a mass in the neck with straining or coughing. Occasionally, transient pain is noted in the region of the hernia. Physical examination is normal except during a Valsalva maneuver when a soft bulge is noted in the neck. In most cases no treatment is necessary. Occasionally a surgical procedure is justified for cosmetic purposes. In patients with severe chronic pulmonary disease in whom coughing is present daily and cough suppression is contraindicated, permanent surgical correction may not be achieved.

Bronsther B, Coryllos E, Epstein B, et al: Lung hernias in children. J Pediatr Surg 3:544, 1968.
Jones JG: Cervical hernia of the lung. J Pediatr 76:122, 1970.

12.94 PULMONARY NEOPLASMS

Metastatic lesions, such as Wilms tumor, osteogenic sarcoma, and hepatoblastoma, are the most common forms of pulmonary malignancy in childhood (Chapters 15 and 16). A great variety of primary malignant tumors have been reported, but all are extremely rare. Patients with symptoms, or with roentgenographic or other laboratory findings suggesting pulmonary malignancy, should be searched carefully for a tumor at another site before surgical excision is done. Pulmonary tumors may present with fever, hemoptysis, wheezing, cough, pleural effusion, dyspnea, or recurrent or persistent pneumonia or atelectasis. Isolated primary lesions and isolated metastatic lesions discovered long after the primary tumor has been removed are best treated by excision. Prognosis is variable and depends on the type of tumor involved.

ROBERT C. STERN

Case records of the Massachusetts General Hospital (Case 4–1976). N Engl J Med 294:210, 1976.
Emory WB, Mitchell WT Jr, Hatch HB Jr: Mucous gland adenoma of the bronchus. Am Rev Resp Dis 108:1407, 1973.
Owenby D, Lyon G, Spock A: Primary leiomyosarcoma of the lung in childhood. Am J Dis Child 130:1132, 1976.
Wellons HA Jr, Eggleston P, Golden GT, Allen MS: Bronchial adenoma in childhood: Two case reports and review of the literature. Am J Dis Child 130:301, 1976.

12.95 AN APPROACH TO RECURRENT OR PERSISTENT LOWER RESPIRATORY TRACT SYMPTOMS IN CHILDREN

Respiratory tract symptoms such as cough, wheeze, and stridor may occur frequently or persist for long periods of time in a substantial number of children; in others there may be persistent and recurring lung infiltrates with or without symptoms. Determining the cause of these chronic findings can be very difficult since symptoms may be due to a rapid succession of unrelated acute respiratory tract infections or to a single pathophysiologic process, and there is a paucity of easily performed, specific diagnostic tests for many chronic respiratory conditions. Pressure from the affected child's family for a quick remedy because of concern over symptoms related to breathing may complicate diagnostic and therapeutic efforts.

A systematic approach to the diagnosis and treatment of children with chronic or recurrent lower respiratory tract symptoms consists of (1) determining whether the symptom is the manifestation of a minor problem or a life-threatening process; (2) establishing or hypothesizing the most likely underlying pathogenic mechanism; (3) selecting the simplest effective therapy for the underlying process, which may often be only symptomatic therapy; (4) carefully evaluating the effect of therapy to verify the correctness of the diagnosis and to determine whether additional therapy is required.

Judging the Seriousness of Chronic Respiratory Complaints

Several signs and symptoms which suggest that a respiratory tract illness may be life-threatening or associated with the potential for chronic disability are listed in Table 12–3. If none of these are detected, the chronic respiratory process is usually benign. For example, infants who are active, well nourished, and growing appropriately may present with intermittent noisy breathing but no other physical or laboratory abnormalities. Only symptomatic treatment and reassurance are necessary. Initially benign-appearing but persistent symptoms occasionally may be the harbinger of a serious lower respiratory tract problem and, conversely, a few children (e.g., with infection-related asthma) may have acute recurrent life-threatening episodes but few or no symptoms in the interval. For these reasons repeated examinations over an extended period of time, both when the child appears healthy and when the child is symptomatic, may be required.

Differential Diagnostic Features

Recurrent or Persistent Cough. Cough is a reflex response of the lower respiratory tract to stimulation of irritant or cough receptors in the tracheobronchial mu-

Table 12–3 EVIDENCE OF SERIOUS CHRONIC LOWER RESPIRATORY TRACT DISEASE IN CHILDREN

Persistent fever
Restriction of activity
Failure to grow
Failure to gain weight appropriately
Clubbing of the digits
Persistent tachypnea and labored ventilation
Persistent hyperinflation
Substantial hypoxemia
Roentgenographic infiltrates
Persistent pulmonary function abnormalities

Table 12–4 DIFFERENTIAL DIAGNOSIS OF RECURRENT AND PERSISTENT COUGH IN CHILDREN

Recurrent cough
Increased bronchial reactivity, including asthma
Drainage from upper airways
Occasional aspiration (as in pharyngeal incoordination)
Frequently recurring respiratory tract infections
Idiopathic pulmonary hemosiderosis

Persistent cough
Postinfection hypersensitivity of cough receptors
Asthma
Asthmatic bronchitis
Bronchitis, tracheitis due to chronic infection, smoking (in older children)
Bronchiectasis, including cystic fibrosis
Immotile cilia syndrome
Foreign body aspiration
Frequent aspiration due to pharyngeal incompetence, tracheolaryngoesophageal cleft, tracheoesophageal fistula, gastroesophageal reflux
Pertussis syndrome
Extrinsic compression of the tracheobronchial tract (vascular ring, neoplasm, lymph node, lung cyst)
Endobronchial or endotracheal tumors
Endobronchial tuberculosis
Habit cough
Hypersensitivity pneumonitis
Fungal infections

cosa. Specific stimuli include excessive secretions, aspirated foreign material, inhaled dust particles or noxious gases, and an inflammatory response to infectious agents or allergic processes. Some of the conditions responsible for chronic cough are listed in Table 12–4. A common cause of chronic cough in children, presenting without other respiratory tract signs and symptoms, is hyperreactive airways (asthma).

Some characteristics of cough that may aid in distinguishing its origin are presented in Table 12–5. Additional information required to determine the etiology may include (1) a history of atopic conditions (asthma, eczema, urticaria, allergic rhinitis), a seasonal or environmental variation in frequency or intensity of cough, and a strong family history of atopic conditions, all suggesting an allergic etiology; (2) symptoms of malabsorption or family history indicative of cystic fibrosis; (3) symptoms related to feeding, suggesting aspiration;

Table 12–5 CHARACTERISTICS OF A CHRONIC COUGH AND THEIR ETIOLOGIC SIGNIFICANCE

TYPE OF COUGH	LIKELY RESPONSIBLE CONDITION
Loose (discontinuous), productive	Bronchitis, asthmatic bronchitis, cystic fibrosis, other bronchiectasis
Brassy	Tracheitis, habit cough
Croupy	Laryngitis
Paroxysmal (with or without gagging and vomiting)	Cystic fibrosis, pertussis syndrome, foreign body
Staccato	Chlamydia pneumonitis
Nocturnal	Upper and/or lower respiratory tract allergic reaction, sinusitis
Most severe on awakening in morning	Cystic fibrosis, other bronchiectasis, chronic bronchitis
With vigorous exercise	Exercise-induced asthma, cystic fibrosis, other bronchiectasis
Disappears with sleep	Habit cough, mild hypersecretory states as in cystic fibrosis and asthma

(4) a choking episode, suggesting foreign body aspiration; (5) a smoking history in older children and adolescents.

Considerable information pertaining to the etiology of chronic cough can be obtained at physical examination. Posterior pharyngeal drainage coupled with a nighttime cough suggests chronic nasopharyngeal drainage. An overinflated chest suggests chronic airway obstruction, as in asthma or cystic fibrosis. An expiratory wheeze strongly suggests asthma or asthmatic bronchitis, but may also be consistent with a diagnosis of cystic fibrosis, vascular ring, aspiration of foreign material, or pulmonary hemosiderosis. Careful auscultation during forced expiration may reveal expiratory wheezes which are otherwise undetectable and which are the only indication of underlying hyperreactive airways. Coarse rales suggest bronchiectasis, including cystic fibrosis, but may attend an acute or subacute exacerbation of asthma. Clubbing of the digits is seen in most patients with bronchiectasis, but in only a few with other respiratory conditions with chronic cough. Tracheal deviation suggests foreign body aspiration or a mediastinal mass.

Sufficient time during the examination to observe the presence or absence of spontaneous cough is essential. If cough is not spontaneous, most children by 4–5 yr of age will cough on request. A helpful maneuver is to ask the child to take a maximal breath and forcefully exhale several times in succession. This usually induces a cough reflex. Children who cough as often as several times a minute with regularity are likely to have a habit (tic) cough. If the cough is loose, every effort should be made to obtain sputum; most older children can comply. It is sometimes possible to pick up small bits of sputum with a throat swab quickly placed into the lower pharynx while the child coughs with the tongue protruding. Clear mucoid sputum is most often associated with an allergic reaction or asthmatic bronchitis. Cloudy (purulent) sputum suggests a respiratory tract infection, but may also reflect increased cellularity (eosinophilia) due to an asthmatic process. Very purulent sputum is characteristic of bronchiectasis. In cystic fibrosis the sputum, even when purulent, is rarely foul smelling.

Laboratory tests may be helpful in evaluation of a chronic cough. Only sputum specimens containing alveolar macrophages should be used for study of lower respiratory tract processes. Sputum eosinophilia suggests asthma, asthmatic bronchitis, or hypersensitivity reactions of lung, while a polymorphonuclear cell response indicates the likelihood of infection; if sputum is not available, the detection of eosinophilia in nasal secretions also suggests the presence of atopic diseases. If most of the cells in sputum are macrophages, postinfectious hypersensitivity of cough receptors should be suspected. Sputum macrophages can be stained for hemosiderin content, diagnostic of pulmonary hemosiderosis. Children with a cough persisting longer than 6 wk should have a sweat chloride test. Sputum culture is helpful but not specific since throat flora may contaminate the sample.

Hematologic assessment may reveal anemia which is the result of pulmonary hemosiderosis, eosinophilia which accompanies asthma and other hypersensitivity reactions of the lung, or a deficiency of polymorphonuclear leukocytes or lymphocytes, indicating a phagocytic or immune deficiency state. Infiltrates on the chest roentgenogram of a patient with a primary complaint of chronic cough may suggest cystic fibrosis, bronchiectasis, foreign body, hypersensitivity pneumonitis, or tuberculosis. When asthma equivalent cough is suspected, a trial of bronchodilator therapy may be diagnostic. After the initial evaluation, especially if the cough does not respond to initial therapeutic efforts, more specific diagnostic procedures may be indicated, including an immunologic or allergic evaluation, paranasal sinus roentgenograms, esophagograms, special microbiologic studies, evaluation of ciliary morphology and function, and bronchoscopy with or without bronchograms.

Recurrent or Persistent Wheeze.   Wheezing is a relatively frequent and particularly troublesome manifestation of obstructive lower respiratory tract disease in children. The site of obstruction may be anywhere from the lower trachea to the small bronchi or large bronchioles. Children under 2–3 yr of age are especially prone to wheezing, as bronchospasm, mucosal edema, and accumulation of excessive secretions have a relatively greater obstructive effect on their smaller airways. With growth, wheeze often becomes a less frequent or severe manifestation of lower respiratory tract disease. Isolated episodes of acute wheezing, such as may occur with bronchiolitis, are not uncommon, but wheezing which recurs or persists for longer than 4 wk suggests other diagnoses (Table 12–6). Most recurrent or persistent wheezing in children is the result of hyperreactive airways disease.

Frequently recurring or persistent wheezing starting

Table 12–6   CAUSES OF RECURRENT OR PERSISTENT WHEEZING IN CHILDREN

Hyperreactive airways disease
  Asthma
  Exercise-induced asthma
  Salicylate-induced asthma and nasal polyposis
  Asthmatic bronchitis
  Other hypersensitivity reactions:
    Hypersensitivity pneumonitis
    Tropical eosinophilia
    Visceral larva migrans
    Allergic aspergillosis
Aspiration
  Foreign body
  Food, saliva, gastric contents
  Laryngotracheoesophageal cleft
  Tracheoesophageal fistula, H-type
  Pharyngeal incoordination or neuromuscular weakness
Cystic fibrosis
Immotile cilia syndrome
Cardiac failure
Bronchiolitis obliterans
Extrinsic compression of airways
  Vascular ring
  Enlarged lymph node
  Mediastinal tumor
  Lung cysts
Tracheobronchomalacia
Endobronchial masses
Gastroesophageal reflux
Pulmonary hemosiderosis
Sequelae of bronchopulmonary dysplasia

Table 12–7   CAUSES OF RECURRENT OR PERSISTENT STRIDOR IN CHILDREN

RECURRENT	PERSISTENT
Allergic croup	Laryngeal obstruction
Respiratory infections in a child with otherwise asymptomatic anatomic narrowing of the large airways	Laryngomalacia
	Papillomas, other tumors
	Cysts and laryngoceles
Laryngomalacia	Laryngeal webs
	Bilateral abductor paralysis of the cords
	Foreign body
	Tracheobronchial disease
	Tracheomalacia
	Subglottic tracheal webs
	Endotracheal, endobronchial tumors
	Subglottic tracheal stenosis
	Congenital
	Acquired
	Extrinsic masses
	Mediastinal masses
	Vascular ring
	Lobar emphysema
	Bronchogenic cysts
	Thyroid enlargement
	Esophageal foreign body
	Tracheoesophageal fistulas
	Other
	Macroglossia, Pierre Robin syndrome
	Cri du chat syndrome
	Hysterical stridor

at or soon after birth suggests a variety of other diagnoses, including congenital structural abnormalities involving the lower respiratory tract. Wheezing that attends cystic fibrosis is most common in the 1st yr of life. Sudden onset of severe wheezing in a previously healthy child should raise the suspicion of foreign body aspiration.

Repeated examination may be required to verify a history of wheezing in a child with episodic symptoms and should be directed toward assessment of air movement, ventilatory adequacy, and evidence of chronic lung disease, such as fixed overinflation of the chest, growth failure, and digital clubbing. Clubbing suggests chronic lung infection and is rarely prominent in uncomplicated asthma. Tracheal deviation secondary to mediastinal shift from foreign body aspiration should be sought. It is essential to rule out wheezing secondary to congestive heart failure. Allergic rhinitis, urticaria, eczema, or evidence of ichthyosis vulgaris suggests asthma or asthmatic bronchitis. The nose should be examined for polyps, which may be present in either allergic conditions or cystic fibrosis.

Presence of sputum eosinophilia, elevated serum IgE levels, and response to bronchodilators may be especially helpful in identifying allergic reactions.

Frequently Recurring or Persistent Stridor.   Stridor is a harsh, medium-pitched, inspiratory sound associated with obstruction of the laryngeal area or trachea. It is often accompanied by a croupy cough and hoarse voice. Most commonly stridor is observed in children with croup; foreign bodies and trauma may also cause acute stridor. However, a small number of children develop recurrent stridor or have persistent stridor from the 1st days or wk of life (Table 12–7). Most congenital anomalies of large airways leading to stridor are symptomatic soon after birth. Increase of stridor when a child is supine suggests laryngomalacia or tracheomalacia. An accompanying history of hoarseness or aphonia suggests involvement of the vocal cords.

Physical examination for recurrent or persistent stridor is usually unrewarding, although the severity and the changes in the intensity of stridor with position should be assessed. Anteroposterior and lateral roentgenograms of the laryngeal and tracheal areas may demonstrate focal narrowing of the air column or extrinsic pressure on the tracheobronchial airways. Occasionally a specific lesion, such as a laryngocele, can be identified, especially with the aid of tomography. However, in most cases direct observation is indicated to make a diagnosis. Undistorted views of the larynx are best obtained with a fiberoptic bronchoscope positioned in the pharynx.

Recurrent and Persistent Lung Infiltrates. Roentgenographic lung infiltrates due to acute pneumonia usually resolve within 1–3 wk. However, a substantial number of children, particularly infants, fail to clear infiltrates within a 4 wk period. These children may be either febrile or afebrile and may present a wide range of respiratory symptoms and signs. Determining the cause of these persistent infiltrates often requires considerable diagnostic skill and effort. Recurring infiltrates also present a diagnostic challenge (Table 12–8).

Symptoms associated with chronic lung infiltrates during the 1st several wk of life (but not related to neonatal respiratory distress syndrome) suggest infection acquired in utero or during descent through the birth canal. Early appearance of chronic infiltrates may also be associated with cystic fibrosis or congenital anomalies, which may result in aspiration or airway obstruction. A history of recurrent infiltrates, wheezing, and cough may reflect asthma, even in the 1st yr of life.

One uncommon but characteristic syndrome appearing in the 1st yr of life includes recurrent lung infiltrates due to pulmonary hemosiderosis related to cow's milk hypersensitivity. Children with a history of bronchopulmonary dysplasia frequently have recurrent episodes of respiratory distress attended by wheezing and new lung infiltrates. Recurrent pneumonia in a child with frequent otitis media, nasopharyngitis, adenitis, or dermatologic manifestations suggests an immunodeficiency state, complement deficiency, or phagocytic defect. A history of paroxysmal coughing in an infant suggests pertussis syndrome or cystic fibrosis. Persistent infiltrates, especially with loss of volume, in a toddler should suggest foreign body aspiration.

A thorough chest evaluation is mandatory. Evidence of overinflation suggests cystic fibrosis or chronic asthma. A "silent chest" with infiltrates should arouse suspicion of alveolar proteinosis, *Pneumocystis carinii* infection, desquamative interstitial pneumonitis, or tumors. Growth should be carefully assessed to determine whether the lung process has had systemic effects, indicating substantial severity and chronicity as in cystic

Table 12–8 DISEASES ASSOCIATED WITH RECURRENT OR PERSISTENT LUNG INFILTRATES BEYOND THE NEONATAL PERIOD

Recurrent or migrating infiltrates
  *Asthma
  *Chronic aspiration
  Hypersensitivity pneumonitis
  *Pulmonary hemosiderosis
  Foreign body
  *Immunodeficiency, phagocytic deficiency
  Sickle cell disease
  *Cystic fibrosis
Persistent infiltrates
  *Congenital infection
    Cytomegalovirus
    Rubella
    Syphilis
  Acquired infection
    *Cytomegalovirus
    *Tuberculosis
    *Chlamydia
    *Other viruses
    *Mycoplasma, ureaplasma
    *Pertussis
    Fungal organisms
    *Pneumocystis carinii
    Inadequately treated bacterial infection
  Congenital anomalies
    *Lung cysts
    Pulmonary sequestration
    Bronchial stenosis
    Vascular ring
    Congenital heart disease with large left to right shunt
  Aspiration
    *Pharyngeal incompetence (e.g., cleft palate)
    *Laryngotracheoesophageal cleft

    *Tracheoesophageal fistula
    *Gastroesophageal reflux
    Foreign body
    Lipid aspiration
  Immunodeficiency, phagocytic deficiency
    *Humoral, cellular, combined immunodeficiency states
    *Chronic granulomatous disease and related phagocytic defects
    *Complement deficiency states
  Allergy-hypersensitivity
    *Pulmonary hemosiderosis (cow's milk-related, other)
    Asthma
    Hypersensitivity pneumonitis (allergic alveolitis)
  *Cystic fibrosis
  Immotile cilia syndrome (Kartagener), deficiency of bronchial cartilage, right middle lobe syndrome, other bronchiectasis
  Sarcoidosis
  Neoplasms (primary, metastatic)
  *Interstitial pneumonitis and fibrosis
    Usual (Hamman-Rich)
    Desquamative
  Alveolar proteinosis
  *Pulmonary lymphangiectasia
  α_1-Antitrypsin deficiency
  Drug-induced, radiation-induced inflammation and fibrosis
  Collagen-vascular diseases
  Eosinophilic pneumonias
  Visceral larva migrans
  Histiocytosis
  Leukemia

*Conditions that often cause chronic lung infiltrates in infants.

fibrosis or alveolar proteinosis. The presence of cataracts, retinopathy, or microcephaly suggests 1 of the infections acquired in utero. Chronic rhinorrhea may be associated with atopic disease, cow's milk intolerance, cystic fibrosis, or congenital syphilis. The absence of tonsils and cervical lymph nodes suggests a combined immunodeficiency state.

Diagnostic studies should be done selectively, based on information obtained from history and physical examination and on a thorough understanding of conditions listed in Table 12–7. Cytologic evaluation of bronchial secretions may be helpful. In patients unresponsive to antibiotics, needle aspiration of the involved area may demonstrate a pathogenic organism. Bronchography, as a rule, is most helpful in identifying surgically approachable focal bronchiectasis and should not be undertaken for routine evaluation of chronic lung infiltrates. Bronchoscopy is indicated for detection of foreign bodies, congenital or acquired anomalies of the tracheobronchial tract, and obstruction by endobronchial or extrinsic masses. If all appropriate studies have been completed and the condition remains undiagnosed, lung biopsy may yield a definitive diagnosis.

Optimal medical or surgical treatment of chronic lung infiltrates frequently depends on a specific diagnosis. However, chronic conditions responsible for these infiltrates may be self-limiting, e.g., severe and prolonged viral infections in infants; in these instances symptomatic therapy may maintain adequate lung function until spontaneous improvement occurs. Helpful measures include inhalation and physical therapy for excessive secretions, antibiotics for secondary bacterial infections, supplementary oxygen for hypoxemia, and maintenance of adequate nutrition. With symptomatic or specific measures, normal lung function ultimately may be achieved despite a severe pulmonary insult during infancy, since the lung of a young child has remarkable recuperative potential.

THOMAS F. BOAT

Beem ME, Saxon EM: Respiratory tract colonization and a distinctive pneumonia syndrome in infants infected with *Chlamydia trachomatis*. N Engl J Med 296:306, 1977.
Cloutier MM, Loughlin GM: Chronic cough in children: A manifestation of airway hyperreactivity. Pediatrics 67:6, 1981.
Danus O, Casar C, Larrain A, et al: Esophageal reflux—an unrecognized cause of recurrent obstructive bronchitis in children. J Pediatr 89:220, 1976.
Eliasson R, Mossberg B, Camner P, et al: The immotile cilia syndrome. N Engl J Med 297:1, 1977.
Kendig EL (ed): Disorders of the Respiratory Tract in Children. Ed 3. Philadelphia, WB Saunders, 1977.
Stagno S, Brasfield DM, Brown MB, et al: Infant pneumonitis associated with cytomegalovirus, chlamydia, pneumocystis, and ureaplasma: A prospective study. Pediatrics 68:322, 1981.
Williams HE: Chronic and recurrent cough. Aust Paediatr J 11:1, 1975.
Wood RE, Boat TF, Doershuk CF: State of the art: Cystic fibrosis. Am Rev Resp Dis 113:833, 1976.

DISEASES OF THE PLEURA

12.96 PLEURISY

The most common cause of pleural effusion in children is pneumococcal pneumonia, with metastatic intrathoracic malignancy being the 2nd. Tuberculous effusion has become much less common with improved screening procedures and chemotherapy. A variety of other diseases, including lupus erythematosus, aspiration pneumonitis, uremia, and rheumatoid arthritis, account for the remainder of the cases. Males and females are equally affected. The incidence of effusion is probably lower for infants with lobar pneumococcal pneumonia than for older children.

Inflammatory processes in the pleura are usually divided into 3 general types: dry or plastic, serofibrinous or serosanguineous, and purulent pleurisy or empyema.

Dry or Plastic Pleurisy

Dry or plastic pleurisy may be associated with acute bacterial pulmonary infections or develop during the course of an acute upper respiratory tract illness. The condition also is associated with tuberculosis and with mesenchymal diseases, such as rheumatic fever.

Pathology. The process is usually limited to the visceral pleura. There are usually small amounts of yellow serous fluid which clots rapidly upon removal. Adhesions between the pleural surfaces develop rapidly, particularly in tuberculosis, in which thickening of the pleura often occurs. Occasionally fibrin deposition and adhesions may be sufficiently severe to produce a fibrothorax which markedly inhibits the excursions of the lung.

Clinical Manifestations. Signs and symptoms are often overshadowed by the primary disease. The principal symptom is pain, which is exaggerated by deep breathing, coughing, and straining. Occasionally, however, pleural pain is described as a dull ache; this type of pain is less likely to vary with breathing. Often the pain is not only localized over the chest wall but also may be referred to the shoulder or the back. Pain with breathing is responsible for grunting and guarding of respirations, the child often lying on the affected side in an attempt to decrease respiratory excursions. Early in the illness a leathery, rough, to-and-fro friction rub may be audible, but this usually disappears rapidly. Occasionally, increased dullness on percussion and suppressed breath sounds are heard when the layer of exudate is thick. On occasion, pleurisy is asymptomatic and is detected only on roentgenography; a diffuse haziness at the pleural surface or a dense, sharply demarcated shadow may be noted. The latter finding may be indistinguishable from small amounts of pleural exudate. Chronic pleurisy is occasionally encountered with such conditions as atelectasis, pulmonary abscess, mesenchymal diseases, and tuberculosis.

Differential Diagnosis. Plastic pleurisy must be distinguished from other diseases, such as epidemic pleurodynia or trauma to the rib cage, particularly fracture of a rib, and from lesions of the dorsal root ganglia, tumors of the spinal cord, herpes zoster, gallbladder disease, and trichinosis. Even if evidence of pleural fluid is not found on physical or roentgenographic examination, a pleural tap in suspected cases will often result in the recovery of small amounts of exudate, which, when cultured, will usually reveal the underlying bacterial cause in cases associated with an acute pneumonia. When pleurisy and pneumonia continue for more than 1 wk, tuberculosis should be considered.

Treatment. Therapy should be aimed at the underlying disease. In the presence of pneumonia neither immobilization of the chest with adhesive plaster nor therapy with drugs capable of suppressing the cough reflex should be undertaken. If pneumonia is not present, or is under good therapeutic control, strapping of the chest to restrict expansion may afford relief from pain.

Serofibrinous Pleurisy

Serofibrinous pleurisy is most commonly associated with infections of the lung or with inflammatory conditions of the abdomen or mediastinum. Less commonly it is found with such mesenchymal diseases as lupus erythematosus, periarteritis, or rheumatic fever. On occasion it is seen with primary or metastatic neoplasms of the lung, pleura, or mediastinum; tumors are, however, more commonly associated with a hemorrhagic pleurisy.

Clinical Manifestations. Since serofibrinous pleurisy is often preceded by the plastic type, the early signs and symptoms may be those of the latter illness. As fluid accumulates, pleuritic pain may disappear and the patient becomes asymptomatic (so long as the effusion remains small), or there may be only the signs and symptoms of the underlying disease. If a large amount of fluid collects, there may be cough, dyspnea, retractions, tachypnea, orthopnea, or cyanosis. Physical findings depend to some degree on the amount of effusion. Dullness to flatness may be found on percussion. There is a decrease or absence of breath sounds, a diminution in tactile fremitus, a shift of the mediastinum away from the affected side, and, on occasion, fullness of the intercostal spaces. If the fluid is not loculated, these signs may shift with changes in position. In infants, physical signs are less definite; sometimes, instead of decreased or absent breath sounds, bronchial breathing will be heard. If extensive pneumonia is present, rales and rhonchi may also be audible. Friction rubs are usually present only during the early or late plastic stage. The process is usually unilateral.

Roentgenographic examination shows a more or less homogeneous density obliterating the normal markings of the underlying lung. Small effusions may cause only obliteration of the costophrenic or cardiophrenic angles or a widening of the interlobar septa. Examination should be performed both in the supine and in the upright positions to demonstrate a shift of the effusion with change in position. The decubitus position may also be helpful. Ultrasound examinations may be useful.

Differential Diagnosis. Thoracentesis should be done when pleural fluid is known to be present or is suspected unless the effusion is very small and the patient has a classic lobar pneumococcal pneumonia. Examination of the fluid is essential to identify acute bacterial infections and may disclose tubercle bacilli. Furthermore, thoracentesis can differentiate between serofibrinous pleurisy, empyema, hydrothorax, hemothorax, and chylothorax. In hydrothorax the fluid has a low specific gravity, below 1.015, and only a few mesothelial cells rather than leukocytes. Chylothorax and hemothorax usually have fluid distinctive in appearance. It is not possible to differentiate serofibrinous from purulent pleurisy without bacterial examination of the fluid. The fluid of serofibrinous pleurisy is clear or slightly cloudy and contains relatively few white cells and, occasionally, some red cells. Protein levels greater than 3 gm/dl indicate an exudate and are likely to be associated with an infectious process. Similarly, pleural fluid lactic dehydrogenase values higher than 200 IU/l suggest an exudate. Serofibrinous fluid may rapidly become purulent; its nature may depend on when thoracentesis is performed during the course of the illness.

Course. Unless the fluid becomes purulent, it usually disappears relatively rapidly, particularly with bacterial pneumonias. It persists somewhat longer with mesenchymal diseases and tuberculosis and may remain or recur for a long time with neoplasms. As the effusion is absorbed, adhesions usually develop between the 2 layers of the pleura, but no functional impairment results. Pleural thickening may develop and is occasionally mistaken for small quantities of fluid or for pulmonary infiltrates. Residual pleural thickening may persist for a long time. In general, however, the process disappears, leaving no residua.

Treatment. Therapy is that of the underlying diseases. When a diagnostic thoracentesis is done, as much fluid as possible should be removed for therapeutic purposes. If the underlying disease is adequately treated, there is usually no necessity for further drainage, but if sufficient fluid reaccumulates to embarrass the patient's respiration, repeated thoracentesis or chest tube drainage should be performed. Patients with pleural effusions may need analgesia, particularly after thoracentesis or insertion of chest tube. Those with acute pneumonia often need supplemental oxygen in addition to antibiotic treatment.

Gryminski J, Krakowka P, Lypacewicz G: The diagnosis of pleural effusion by ultrasonic and radiologic techniques. Chest 70:1, 1976.
Light RW, MacGregor I, Luchsinger PC, et al: Pleural effusions: The diagnostic separation of transudates and exudates. Ann Int Med 77:507, 1972.
Wolfe WG, Spock A, Bradford WD: Pleural fluids in infants and children. Am Rev Resp Dis 98:1027, 1968.

Purulent Pleurisy
(Empyema)

Purulent pleurisy, or empyema, is an accumulation of pus in the pleural spaces. The condition is most often associated with pneumonia due to staphylococci, less frequently with pneumococci (especially types 1 and 3) and *H. influenzae*. In pediatric practice, empyema is most frequently encountered in infants and preschool children.

The disease may be produced also by rupture of a

lung abscess into the pleural space, by contamination introduced from trauma or thoracic surgery, or, rarely, by mediastinitis or by the extension of intra-abdominal abscesses.

Pathology. Most commonly, purulent pleurisy is an extensive process, consisting of a series of loculated areas involving a large portion of 1 or both pleural cavities. Thickening of the parietal pleura occurs. If the pus is not drained, it may dissect through the chest wall and into lung parenchyma, producing bronchopleural fistulas and pyopneumothorax, or into the abdominal cavity. Pockets of loculated pus may eventually develop into thick-walled abscess cavities, or, as the exudate organizes, the lung may collapse and be surrounded by a thick, inelastic envelope.

Clinical Manifestations. Since most purulent pleurisy occurs early in the course of bacterial pneumonia, the initial signs and symptoms are primarily those of the underlying disease. Patients treated inadequately or with inappropriate antibiotic agents may have an interval of a few days between the clinical phase of pneumonia and the evidence of empyema. Most patients are febrile. In infants, manifestations of the disease may consist only of moderate exacerbation of respiratory distress. The older child is apt to appear more toxic and in greater respiratory difficulty. Physical and roentgenographic findings may be identical to those described for serofibrinous pleurisy and the 2 conditions differentiated only by thoracentesis, which should always be performed when empyema is suspected. (See Serofibrinous Pleurisy, above.) The roentgenographic finding of no shift of fluid with change of position indicates a loculated empyema. The maximum amount of pus obtainable should be withdrawn. The appearance of pus produced by different organisms is not distinctive; cultures must always be obtained and Gram-stained smears examined for the presence of microorganisms. Staphylococci are usually numerous; pneumococci and *H. influenzae* occasionally are present only in small numbers, particularly if antibiotic therapy has been given previously. In the latter instance countercurrent immunoelectrophoresis may be more useful than culture. Leukocytosis and an elevated sedimentation rate may occur.

Complications. With staphylococcal infections, bronchopleural fistulas and pyopneumothorax commonly develop. Other local complications include purulent pericarditis, pulmonary abscesses, peritonitis secondary to rupture through the diaphragm, osteomyelitis of the ribs, and such septic complications as meningitis, arthritis, and osteomyelitis. With staphylococcal empyema, septicemia occurs infrequently; it is often encountered in *H. influenzae* and pneumococcal infections.

Treatment. If pus is obtained by thoracentesis, closed drainage should be instituted immediately and controlled either by an underwater seal or by continuous suction. A catheter with the largest possible internal diameter should be inserted into the site where accumulation of pus is suspected; sometimes several tubes are required to drain loculated areas. Closed drainage is usually necessary only for 1 wk or so, even though small amounts of material will continue to drain after this time; this material is usually formed in response to the presence of the tube in the pleural cavity. When it is time to withdraw the tube, it should be removed all at once.

The instillation of fibrinolytic agents or proteolytic enzymes into the pleural cavity commonly produces severe systemic reactions in small children and does not promote drainage. If the chest tube is of sufficient caliber and is kept clear, a free flow of pus is obtained. Antibiotics should not be instilled into the pleural cavity since they do not improve results obtained with systemic antibiotic therapy alone and are associated with local reactions. No attempt should be made to control empyema by multiple aspirations of the pleural cavity rather than by closed continuous drainage.

Systemic antibiotic therapy is required; the selection of the antibiotic should be based on the in vitro sensitivities of the responsible organism. Staphylococcal empyema in infancy is best treated by parenteral routes with methicillin or, when applicable, with penicillin G. Pneumococcal infection usually responds to penicillin, and *H. influenzae* to ampicillin or chloramphenicol. There is no advantage in the use of multiple antibiotic agents. With staphylococcal infections, resolution of the process is slow, and systemic antibiotic therapy is required for 3–4 wk. In patients with inadequately treated empyema, extensive fibrinous changes may take place over the surface of the collapsed lungs; these may require decortication at a future date. If pneumatoceles form, no attempt should be made to treat them surgically, or by aspiration, unless they reach sufficient size to embarrass respiration or become secondarily infected. The long term prognosis for adequately treated empyema is excellent.

Bechamps GJ, Lynn HB, Wenzl JE: Empyema in children. Mayo Clin Proc 45:43, 1970.
Middlekamp JN, Purterson ML, Burford TH: The changing pattern of empyema thoracis in pediatrics. J Thorac Cardiov Surg 47:165, 1964.
Murphy D, Lockhart CH, Todd JK: Pneumococcal empyema. Am J Dis Child 134:659, 1980.
Ravitch MM, Fein R: The changing picture of pneumonia and empyema in infants and children. A review of the experience at the Harriet Lane Home from 1934 through 1958. JAMA 175:1039, 1961.
Riley HD Jr, Bracken EC: Empyema due to *Hemophilus influenzae* in infants and children. Am J Dis Child 110:24, 1965.
Siegel JD, Gartner JC, Michaels RH: Pneumococcal empyema in childhood. Am J Dis Child 132:1094, 1978.

12.97 PNEUMOTHORAX

Pneumothorax in the neonatal period is discussed in Sec 7.38. In staphylococcal pneumonia in infancy the incidence of pneumothorax is relatively high, but aside from the accidental introduction of air into the pleural cavity during thoracentesis, pneumothorax is uncommon during childhood. Pneumothorax may occur in pneumonia, usually in connection with empyema; it may also be secondary to pulmonary abscess, gangrene, infarct, rupture of a cyst or an emphysematous bleb (as in asthma), foreign bodies in the lung, and external thoracic trauma or surgical procedures. It is found in about 5% of hospitalized asthmatic children and usually resolves without treatment. Pneumothorax is a serious complication in cystic fibrosis (Sec 12.110). In association with mediastinal emphysema it is an occasional complication of tracheotomy. Spontaneous pneumothorax occasionally occurs in teenagers and young adults, most frequently in males. Occasional families have been described in which many members have had spontaneous pneumothoraces with onset ranging from birth to adulthood. Patients with collagen synthesis defects such as Ehlers-Danlos disease and Marfan syndrome are also unusually prone to develop pneumothorax.

Pneumothorax may be associated with a serous effusion (*hydropneumothorax*) or a purulent effusion (*pyopneumothorax*). Bilateral pneumothorax is rare.

Clinical Manifestations. The onset is usually abrupt and the severity of symptoms usually depends upon the extent of the lung collapse and the amount of pre-existing lung disease. When the pneumothorax is extensive, there may be pain, dyspnea, and cyanosis. In infancy symptoms and physical signs may be difficult to recognize. If the pneumothorax is only moderate in extent, there may be little displacement of intrathoracic organs and few or no symptoms. The severity of pain usually does not directly reflect the extent of the collapse.

Usually respiratory distress, retractions, and markedly decreased breath sounds over the involved lung are present. The percussion note over the involved area is tympanitic. Larynx, trachea, and heart may be shifted toward the unaffected side. When fluid is present, there is usually a sharply limited area of tympany above a level of flatness to percussion. It is important to determine whether the pneumothorax is under tension (*tension pneumothorax*) since this will limit expansion of the contralateral lung and may compromise cardiovascular function. The presence of amphoric breathing or of gurgling sounds synchronous with respirations when fluid is present in the pleural cavity is suggestive of an open fistula connecting with air-bearing tissues. Confirmatory evidence is provided when the pneumothorax fills rapidly after it has been aspirated. The diagnosis can usually be established by roentgenographic examination (Fig 12–18).

Differential Diagnosis. Pneumothorax must be differentiated from localized or generalized emphysema, from an extensive emphysematous bleb, from large pulmonary cavities or other cystic formations, from diaphragmatic hernia, and from gaseous distention of the stomach. In most instances a chest roentgenogram will differentiate these entities; expiratory views accentuate the contrast between lung markings and the clear area of the pneumothorax. In the case of diaphragmatic hernia, however, a small amount of barium may be necessary to demonstrate that a portion of the gastrointestinal tract is in the thoracic cavity.

Treatment. Therapy varies with the extent of the collapse and the nature and severity of the underlying disease. A small or even moderately sized pneumothorax in an otherwise normal child may resolve without specific treatment, usually within 1 wk or so. A small (less than 5%) pneumothorax complicating asthma may also spontaneously resolve. Administration of 100% oxygen may hasten resolution by increasing

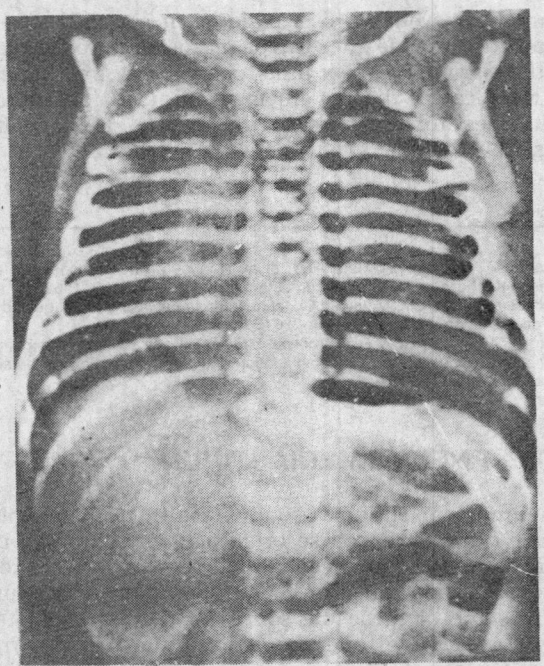

Figure 12–18 Pneumothorax in a newborn infant. The air in the left pleural cavity has resulted in partial collapse of the left lung and shift of the heart and mediastinal structures to the right.

the nitrogen pressure gradient between the pleural air and the blood. Patients with chronic hypoxemia should be monitored closely during administration of supplemental oxygen. Pleural pain deserves analgesic treatment. Codeine may be justified, but its respiratory depressant effect should be considered. Occasionally, morphine or meperidine is needed. If there is more than 5% collapse or if the pneumothorax is recurrent or under tension, definitive treatment is necessary. Pneumothoraces complicating cystic fibrosis frequently recur, and definitive treatment may be justified with the 1st episode even with less than 5% collapse.

Closed thoracotomy (simple insertion of a chest tube) and drainage of the trapped air through a catheter, the external opening of which is kept in a dependent position under water, will be adequate to re-expand the lung in almost all patients. To induce the formation of strong adhesions between the lung and chest wall when there have been many repeated pneumothoraces, and thus prevent future recurrences, a sclerosing procedure such as the introduction of tetracycline or silver nitrate into the pleural space (chemical pleurodesis) may be used. Open thoracotomy through a limited incision; with plication of blebs, closure of fistula, stripping of the pleura (usually in the apical lung where the surgeon has direct vision), and basilar pleural abrasion is also an effective treatment of recurring pneumothorax. Postoperative pain is comparable to chemical pleurodesis with silver nitrate, but the chest tube can usually be removed within 24–48 hr, as opposed to the usual 72 hr minimum for closed thoracotomy and pleurodesis.

Treatment of the underlying pulmonary disease should begin on admission. When open thoracotomy is planned for cystic fibrosis patients, it should be done as soon as possible after the patient is admitted. Delaying the surgery to allow time for antibiotic treatment is contraindicated; the patient may gradually deteriorate as the chest tube interferes with postural drainage and physical activity.

Bernhard WF, Malcolm JA, Berry RW, et al: A study of the pathogenesis and management of spontaneous pneumothorax. Dis Chest 42:403, 1962.

Kattwinkel J, Taussig LM, McIntosh CL, et al: Intrapleural instillation of quinacrine for recurrent pneumothorax. JAMA 226:557, 1973.

Youmans CR Jr, Williams RD, McMinn MR, et al: Surgical management of spontaneous pneumothorax by bleb ligation and pleural dry sponge abrasion. Am J Surg 120:644, 1970.

12.98 PNEUMOMEDIASTINUM

Pneumomediastinum usually results from alveolar rupture during the course of an acute or chronic pulmonary disease. However, a diverse group of nonrespiratory entities can also cause pneumomediastinum, and in some of these the source of the air is not the lung. For example, pneumomediastinum has been reported following dental extractions, pneumoencephalography, obstetric delivery, diabetes mellitus with ketoacidosis, acupuncture, and acute gastroenteritis. Pneumomediastinum can also result from esophageal perforation and penetrating chest trauma.

Following intrapulmonary alveolar rupture, air can dissect through the perivascular sheaths and other soft tissue planes toward the hilum and enter the mediastinum. Pneumomediastinum is rarely a major problem in older children since the mediastinum can be depressurized by escape of air into the neck or abdomen. In the newborn, however, the rate at which air can leave the mediastinum is quite limited, and pneumomediastinum can lead to dangerous cardiovascular compromise or to pneumothorax (Sec 7.41). Acute asthma is the most common cause of pneumomediastinum in older children and teenagers. Simultaneous pneumothorax is unusual in these patients.

The principal symptom of pneumomediastinum is transient stabbing pains in the chest which may radiate to the neck. However, isolated abdominal pain and sore throat also occur. The patient may complain of dyspnea, but it is difficult to know if this is really a separate symptom or if it is related to the chest pain. Pneumomediastinum is often difficult to detect by physical examination alone. Subcutaneous emphysema, if present, is virtually diagnostic. Although cardiac dullness may be decreased, many of these patients are chronically overinflated and it is unlikely that the clinician will be sure of this finding. A mediastinal "crunch" is occasionally present but is easily confused with a friction rub. The diagnosis is made easily by chest roentgenogram; the cardiac border, highlighted by the mediastinal air, is more distinct than normal, and on the lateral projection the posterior mediastinal structures are also clearly defined. Subcutaneous air, seen roentgenographically, confirms the pneumomediastinum.

Treatment is directed primarily at the underlying obstructive pulmonary disease. Analgesics are occasionally needed for chest pain. Rarely, subcutaneous emphysema can cause sufficient tracheal compression to justify tracheotomy; the tracheotomy also decompresses the mediastinum.

Church JA, Richards W: Air leak syndromes as complications of respiratory disease in infancy and childhood. Ann Allergy 39:393, 1977.

Girard DE, Carlson V, Natelson EA, Fred HL: Pneumomediastinum in diabetic ketoacidosis: Comments on mechanism, incidence, and management. Chest 60:455, 1971.

Munsell WP: Pneumomediastinum: A report of 28 cases and review of the literature. JAMA 202:689, 1967.

Sandler CM, Libshitz HI, Marks G: Pneumoperitoneum, pneumomediastinum and pneumopericardium following dental extraction. Radiology 115:539, 1975.

Tsai FY, Lee KF: Pneumopericardium and pneumomediastinum: Rare complications of pneumoencephalography. Radiology 112:95, 1974.

12.99 HYDROTHORAX

In hydrothorax the fluid is noninflammatory and has a lower specific gravity (1.015) than that of a serofibrinous exudate. It contains less protein and fewer cells and is usually associated with an accumulation of fluid in other parts of the body, such as the peritoneal cavity and the subcutaneous tissues. Hydrothorax is most often associated with cardiac or renal disease, although on occasion it may be a manifestation of severe nutritional edema, and, rarely, it results from venous obstruction by neoplasms, enlarged lymph nodes, or adhesions. Hydrothorax is usually bilateral in renal disease and in nutritional edema and may be in myocardial disease, although in this instance it may be limited to the right side or greater on the right than on the left side. The physical signs are those described under Serofibrinous Pleurisy, but there is more rapid shifting of the level of dullness with changes of position. The treatment is that of the primary disorder; aspiration may be necessary when pressure symptoms are notable.

Berger HW, Rammohan G, Neff MS, et al: Uremic pleural effusion. A study in 14 patients on chronic dialysis. Ann Int Med 82:362, 1975.

12.100 HEMOTHORAX

Extensive bleeding into the pleural cavity may result from erosion of a blood vessel in association with such inflammatory processes as tuberculosis and empyema, but it is rare in children. It is also an occasional manifestation of intrathoracic neoplasms and blood dyscrasias and may be the result of thoracic trauma. Rupture of an aneurysm is not likely during childhood. When a pleural hemorrhage occurs in association with a pneumothorax, it is termed *hemopneumothorax*. The diagnosis of a hemothorax can be made only by thoracentesis. In every instance an effort must be made to determine and treat the cause. Surgical intervention may be required to control active bleeding, and transfusion is necessary when loss of blood is excessive. Inadequate removal of blood in extensive hemothorax may lead to substantial restrictive disease secondary to deposition and organization of fibrin. A decortication procedure may then be necessary.

Block LF: Pleural disease. Basics Resp Dis 6 (May 1978):1, 1978.
Kilman JS, Charnock E: Thoracic trauma in infancy and childhood. J Trauma 9:863, 1969.

12.101 CHYLOTHORAX

Chylothorax results from the escape of chyle from the thoracic duct into the thoracic cavity. The incidence of chylothorax has increased as cardiac surgery is performed on more complex congenital abnormalities; about 50% of these cases are now operative complications resulting from rupture of the thoracic duct. Most of the remainder are associated with traumatic chest injury or with primary or metastatic intrathoracic malignancy as a result of the pressure of enlarged lymph nodes or tumor. A variety of even less common causes are known and include lymphangiomatosis, restrictive pulmonary diseases, thrombosis of the duct or the subclavian vein, and congenital anomalies of the duct system. In some patients no specific etiology is identified. Chylothorax is rarely bilateral, usually being on the left side.

The symptoms and signs are those related to the presence of fluid in the thoracic cavity. The diagnosis is established when thoracentesis demonstrates a chylous effusion, a milky fluid containing fat, protein, lymphocytes, and other constituents of chyle. In newborn infants who have not yet been fed, the fluid may be clear. A pseudochylous milky fluid has been reported in cases of serous effusion, in which the fatty material was thought to arise from degenerative changes within the fluid and not to be due to the presence of lymph. This type of fluid may be distinguished from one containing chyle by shaking it with alkalis or ether; the fluid containing chyle tends to become clear. A more definitive test is the quantitation of fluid triglyceride (elevated in chylous fluid) and fluid cholesterol (which may be elevated in chronic serous effusions).

Spontaneous recovery has occurred in over half of the reported cases in infants under 1 yr of age. Repeated aspirations may be required to relieve the symptoms of pressure. However, chyle reaccumulates quickly, and repeated thoracenteses may cause considerable loss of calories and protein as well as large numbers of lymphocytes. Immunodeficiencies including hypogammaglobulinemia and abnormal cell-mediated immune responses have been reported associated with repeated thoracenteses for chylothorax. Attempts to prevent these problems by intravenous infusion of pleural contents are technically difficult and dangerous and of doubtful benefit.

Treatment should begin in most cases with a brief period of observation on a low fat (or medium chain triglyceride), high protein diet. For most patients, bed rest, salt restriction, diuresis, and digitalis are also indicated. The total caloric intake should be above the average requirement, and several times the daily requirements of the various vitamins, especially the fat-soluble vitamins A and D, should be added. If fluid continues to reaccumulate over 1–2 wk, a more aggressive attempt to locate and ligate the thoracic duct may be indicated. Many successful ligations have now been reported in patients with nontraumatic chylothoraces (Sec 7.30).

Berberich FR, Bernstein ID, Ochs HD, et al: Lymphangiomatosis with chylothorax. J Pediatr 87:941, 1975.
Brodman RF, Zavelson TM, Schiebler GL: Treatment of congenital chylothorax. J Pediatr 85:516, 1974.
Kirkland I: Chylothorax in infancy and childhood. A method of treatment. Arch Dis Child 40:186, 1965.
Macfarlane JR, Holman CW: Chylothorax. Am Rev Resp Dis 105:287, 1972.

NEUROMUSCULAR AND SKELETAL DISEASES AFFECTING PULMONARY FUNCTION

12.102 PECTUS EXCAVATUM

Pectus excavatum ("funnel chest") is usually an isolated skeletal anomaly. This midline narrowing of the thoracic cavity may result in demonstrable restrictive pulmonary disease, but rarely if ever does the degree of restriction have any clinical consequence. Pectus excavatum may be associated with segmental bronchomalacia, especially involving the left main stem bronchus. In some patients, cardiac function may be adversely affected. Surgical correction of this lesion is not beneficial for the vast majority of patients, although for some patients with extreme deformity operative intervention may be indicated for functional or cosmetic reasons (Sec 23.8).

Beiser GD, Epstein SE, Stampfer M, et al: Impairment of cardiac function in patients with pectus excavatum, with improvement after operative correction. N Engl J Med 287:267, 1972.
Godfrey S: Association between pectus excavatum and segmental bronchomalacia. J Pediatr 96:649, 1980.
Orzaleski MM, Cook CD: Pulmonary function in children with pectus excavatum. J Pediatr 66:898, 1965.

12.103 ASPHYXIATING THORACIC DYSTROPHY

Thoracic dystrophy is 1 manifestation of a generalized abnormality of skeletal growth and usually causes life-threatening respiratory difficulties in the newborn period or early infancy. Some patients with less severe disease have survived into their school years. The disease appears to be an autosomal recessive defect. A variety of associated congenital malformations have been reported. Most patients have respiratory distress or infection before 1 yr of age. Older children are occasionally brought to the physician when parents note abnormality in the appearance of the chest. Physical examination reveals constriction of the thorax and, usually, short extremities. There is no specific treatment. Progressive renal failure occurs frequently among older children with this disease. Respiratory infections should be treated promptly with antibiotics and, perhaps, physical therapy. Influenza vaccine should be administered yearly.

Hanissian AS, Riggs WW, Thomas DA: Infantile thoracic dystrophy—variant of the Ellis–van Creveld syndrome. J Pediat 71:855, 1967.
Herdman RC, Langer LO: Thoracic asphyxiant dystrophy and renal disease. Am J Dis Child 116:192, 1968.
Oberklaid F, Dantes DM, Mayne V, et al: Asphyxiating thoracic dysplasia. Clinical, radiological, and pathological information on 10 patients. Arch Dis Child 52:758, 1977.

12.104   RIB ANOMALIES

The absence or malformation of 1–2 ribs usually has no substantial effect on pulmonary function and does not require treatment. Absence of multiple ribs is associated with vertebral anomalies and, ultimately, scoliosis. In addition, a portion of lung can herniate through the defect in the chest wall; these hernias are most frequent at the level of the 1st–5th ribs and are usually anterior. Minor abnormalities of muscle caused by loss of their normal attachments are also associated with this lesion. Most rib anomalies are discovered as incidental findings on chest roentgenograms obtained as part of a work-up for another illness; absence of underlying ribs may result in a hernia of lung presenting as a soft, easily reducible, usually nontender swelling. When the defect is large and associated with lung hernia, rib splitting and strutting techniques can provide both functional and cosmetic improvement.

Bronsther B, Coryllos E, Epstein B, et al: Lung hernias in children. J Pediatr Surg 3:544, 1968.
Rickham PP: Lung hernia secondary to congenital absence of ribs. Arch Dis Child 34:14, 1959.

12.105   NEUROMUSCULAR DISEASES WITH HYPOVENTILATION

A variety of acute (e.g., poliomyelitis, Guillain-Barré syndrome, spinal cord injury) and chronic (e.g., muscular dystrophy, progressive spinal muscular atrophy, myasthenia gravis) neuromuscular diseases can cause respiratory problems. (See Chapter 22.)

Clinical Manifestations. Alveolar hypoventilation with hypoxemia and respiratory failure is easily recognized, and the need for emergency measures, including artificial ventilation, is obvious. Arterial blood gas determinations and lung volume measurements confirm its presence and are necessary for proper management. Some of these patients cannot handle secretions and may need a cuffed endotracheal tube or tracheostomy (Sec 12.30).

Chronic, slowly progressive, neuromuscular weakness is more likely to cause the insidious onset of respiratory abnormalities that may ultimately become incapacitating and often life-limiting. With progression of weakness the patients cannot generate sufficient intrathoracic pressure for effective coughing, or they cannot hold the glottis closed well enough to allow sufficient pressure build-up in the lung. In addition, although tidal volumes may continue to be normal, the progressive decrease in vital capacity also compromises the effectiveness of the cough. Multiple minor episodes of aspiration occur as laryngeal muscles become weaker. Finally, with loss of adequate sigh and decreased ability of the diaphragm to prevent compromise of the thoracic volume by the abdominal organs, patchy microscopic atelectasis occurs with a ventilation-perfusion abnormality and hypoxemia. Recurrent or chronic infection then results and further restricts vital capacity. The increased viscosity of infected secretions also aggravates already impaired mucociliary clearance. Progressive loss of pulmonary tissue from the fibrosis associated with chronic infection and the chronic and worsening hypoxemia eventually may lead to pulmonary arterial hypertension and, ultimately, to right heart failure.

Treatment. All patients with chronic or progressive muscular weakness require close surveillance for, and early treatment of, respiratory complications. Prompt antibiotic treatment of upper respiratory infections is indicated. Most patients intermittently require respiratory physical therapy, including postural drainage with chest percussion, and parents should be instructed in these techniques; postural drainage is often effective when used throughout each acute respiratory illness. In some patients, an artificial cough can be accomplished by application of sudden external pressure to the thorax. Influenza vaccine should be administered yearly. Pneumococcal vaccine may be indicated.

A permanent tracheostomy to allow better access to the airway for suctioning can be very helpful. A small tracheostomy can be plugged when suctioning is not being performed and the patient can then breathe and talk around the tube. Patients with substantial diaphragmatic weakness may benefit from a mechanical rocking bed to reduce alveolar collapse. Intermittent positive pressure breathing has also been proposed for this purpose. Once pulmonary hypertension and overt right heart failure are present, the prognosis is grave, and treatment with supplemental oxygen and other symptomatic measures allows only temporary improvement. Tolazoline is not effective.

Bergofsky EH: State of the art: Respiratory failure in disorders of the thoracic cage. Am Rev Resp Dis 119:643, 1979.
Greenberg M, Edmonds J: Chronic respiratory problems in neuromyopathic disorders. Their nature and management. Pediatr Clin North Am 21:927, 1974.

12.106   KYPHOSCOLIOSIS

Scoliosis, including idiopathic adolescent scoliosis, is discussed in Sec 23.6. With mild or moderately severe scoliosis, the chest cage is usually not restricted enough to have a serious effect on pulmonary function. Severe scoliosis, however, can dangerously impair function and may be associated with respiratory failure, cor pulmonale, or both. In addition to their restrictive lesion, these patients may also have a diffusion abnormality that aggravates hypoxemia. Minor respiratory infections may be life threatening. There is an age-related worsening of pulmonary function, but acute respiratory failure is rare below 20 yr of age. Even patients with moderate scoliosis may have unexpected severe pulmonary problems immediately after fusion procedures because pain and use of a body cast restrict and interfere with coughing. Patients with severe scoliosis, especially males, may have abnormalities of breathing during sleep. The resultant periods of hypoxemia may contribute to the eventual development of hypertension.

Patients in these categories should be treated as if they had life-threatening pulmonary disease. Influenza vaccine should be given yearly. Careful pulmonary function evaluation is essential prior to elective surgical procedures, especially before fusion. If pulmonary function is marginal (e.g., vital capacity of less than 40-50% of predicted), the patient should receive instruction in, and get experience with, positive pressure breathing prior to surgery. The possibility that the patient may awake on assisted ventilation with an endotracheal tube should be discussed prior to surgery. If possible the patient should actually see the mechanical ventilator and understand how and why it might be used. For patients with marginal pulmonary function, careful monitoring of blood gases postoperatively is essential. An occasional patient with extremely severe restrictive disease should have a tracheostomy completed prior to surgery. Scoliosis surgery may predispose to deep thrombosis formation and pulmonary embolus.

Kafer ER: Idiopathic scoliosis: Gas exchange and the age dependence of arterial blood gases. J Clin Invest 48:825, 1976.
Mezon BL, West P, Israels J, et al: Sleep breathing abnormalities in kyphoscoliosis. Am Rev Resp Dis 122:617, 1980.
Uden A: Thromboembolic complications following scoliosis surgery in Scandinavia. Acta Orthop Scand 50:175, 1979.
Weber B, Smith JP, Briscoe WA, et al: Pulmonary function in asymptomatic adolescents with idiopathic scoliosis. Am Rev Resp Dis 111:389, 1975.

12.107   OBESITY

Extreme obesity occasionally causes respiratory embarrassment with somnolence, dyspnea, cyanosis, and, possibly, right heart failure. Chest and diaphragmatic excursions are limited, resulting in rapid shallow breathing, and alveolar ventilation is decreased, resulting in hypoxemia. Ventilation-perfusion abnormalities also contribute to arterial desaturation. Some of these patients appear to have a diminished ventilatory response to hypoxic drive. In the Prader-Willi syndrome, an abnormal ventilatory response to carbon dioxide has been demonstrated in family members who are otherwise normal suggesting that the abnormal ventilatory control adds to the respiratory problems caused by the obesity rather than results from them.

Weight loss is the primary goal of treatment and, if successful, it alone will reduce the pulmonary problems. Some children with hypoventilation and right heart failure secondary to the extreme obesity of Prader-Willi syndrome may be benefited by treatment with progesterone.

Orenstein DM, Boat TF, Owens RP, et al: The obesity hypoventilation syndrome in children with the Prader-Willi syndrome: A possible role for familial decreased response to carbon dioxide. J Pediatr 67:765, 1980.
Orenstein DM, Boat TF, Stern RC, et al: Progesterone treatment of the obesity hypoventilation syndrome in a child. J Pediatr 90:477, 1977.
Riley DJ, Santiago TV, Edelman NH: Complications of obesity-hypoventilation syndrome in childhood. Am J Dis Child 130:671, 1976.
Zwillick CW, Sutton FD, Pierson DJ, et al: Decreased hypoxic ventilatory drive in the obesity-hypoventilation syndrome. Am J Med 49:343, 1975.

12.108   PRIMARY FAILURE OF RESPIRATORY REGULATION
(Ondine's Curse)

Primary failure of central nervous system regulation of breathing may also occur in nonobese persons and has been infrequently reported in children. The principal abnormality in these patients is an insensitivity to hypercapnia. Hypoventilation occurs more severely or exclusively during sleep. This disease is a serious threat to life. Suggested therapeutic measures include bilateral phrenic nerve pacing or tracheostomy with assisted ventilation during sleep. Although preliminary success has been reported with both these approaches, the long-term prognosis is unknown.

Deonna T, Arczynska W, Torrado A: Congenital failure of automatic ventilation (Ondine's curse). J Pediatr 84:710, 1974.
Hyland RH, Jones NL, Powles ACP, et al: Primary alveolar hypoventilation treated with nocturnal electrophrenic respiration. Am Rev Resp Dis 117:165, 1978.
Shannon DC, Marsland EW, Gould JB, et al: Central hypoventilation during quiet sleep in two infants. Pediatrics 57:342, 1976.

12.109   COUGH SYNCOPE

Cough syncope has been infrequently reported in children. During a coughing paroxysm in which high intrathoracic pressures are generated, venous obstruction, characterized by redness of the face, is followed by decreased venous return and, ultimately, decreased cardiac output, which results in transient cerebral hypoxia and syncope. Convulsive movements and incontinence are rare. Asthma is the most frequent precipitating disease. There is no specific treatment.

ROBERT C. STERN

Katz RM: Cough syncope in children with asthma. J Pediatr 77:48, 1970.

12.110   CYSTIC FIBROSIS

Cystic fibrosis is a multisystem disorder of children and adults, characterized chiefly by chronic obstruction and infection of airways and by maldigestion and its consequences. This condition is the most common, life-threatening genetic trait in the Caucasian population. Dysfunction of exocrine glands appears to be the predominant pathogenetic mechanism and is responsible for a broad, variable, and sometimes confusing array of presenting manifestations and subsequent complications.

Cystic fibrosis is an important pediatric problem for a number of reasons. It is the major cause of severe chronic lung disease of children. It is responsible for most exocrine pancreatic insufficiency during early life. It is also responsible for many cases of childhood nasal polyposis, pansinusitis, rectal prolapse, and hyperglycemia unrelated to diabetes mellitus. In addition, cystic fibrosis may present as failure to thrive and occasionally as cirrhosis or other forms of hepatic dysfunction. Therefore, this disorder enters into the differential diagnosis of many pediatric conditions. Investigators and clinicians have been intrigued by the elusive basic defect in cystic fibrosis, by problems relating to prenatal diagnosis and heterozygote detection, and by the challenge of designing therapies to combat the broad range of manifestations.

History.   Medieval German folk literature noted a relationship between salty-tasting skin and early death. However, description of the syndrome was delayed until the late 1930's when several investigators published accounts of exocrine pancreatic insufficiency in early childhood, associated with severe, chronic respiratory tract symptoms. In 1938, Anderson reported a pathologic and clinical description of cystic fibrosis and used the name cystic fibrosis of the pancreas. In 1944, Farber noted that inspissation of secretions in gland ducts and acini of many organs, including the pancreas, intestinal tract, biliary system, airways, and salivary glands, was a general pathologic feature. He suggested that diminished clearance of mucus was the common pathophysiologic event and in 1945 proposed the name mucoviscidosis to reflect this generalized obstruction. In 1953, Di Sant'Agnese investigated salt depletion in children with cystic fibrosis during a summertime heat wave, astutely concluded that excessive loss of salt must occur via the sweat, and documented that sodium and chloride levels in sweat are elevated in virtually all individuals with cystic fibrosis. Measurement of chloride concentrations in sweat became the standard diagnostic test for this disorder. The introduction of comprehensive and aggressive approaches to the care of patients by Matthews and others in 1964 has been accompanied by a steadily increasing longevity despite the failure to identify the underlying abnormality.

Epidemiology.   Cystic fibrosis is recognized in approximately 1:2000 and 1:17,000 live births in white and black populations of the United States, respectively. The estimated incidence worldwide varies from 1:620 in a confined population with Dutch ancestry in southwest Africa to 1:90,000 in an Oriental population of Hawaii. Generally, the cystic fibrosis gene is most prevalent in Northern and Central Europeans and individuals who derive from these areas.

Cystic fibrosis is most probably inherited as an auto-somal recessive trait. Multiple allelic determinants cannot be excluded, but there is no convincing evidence for more than a single mutant allele. Chromosomal location of the affected gene(s) is unknown. There appears to be no correlation with major HLA loci or with other genetic disorders. In Caucasian populations, 4–5% of individuals are carriers of the cystic fibrosis gene. These individuals have no clinical stigmata of cystic fibrosis. Although a number of chemical or biologic alterations of body fluids or cells from obligate heterozygotes have been described, these alterations can be identified only on a statistical basis. There is no test which reliably identifies heterozygotes for genetic counseling. The high frequency of the cystic fibrosis gene in Caucasians suggests that an undefined reproductive advantage is conferred by the heterozygous state. It has been suggested that the relatively low frequency in populations living in tropical and semitropical geographic locations is related to adverse consequences in the past of excessive salt loss in heterozygotes as well as homozygotes.

Pathogenesis.   The basic defect in cystic fibrosis has not been identified, and none of the postulated abnormalities explains all aspects of the syndrome. Following Farber's report of widespread mucous obstruction, a search was initiated for abnormal mucous glycoproteins, which are high molecular weight secretory components that determine the viscoelastic properties of mucus. Although cystic fibrosis mucins may be more highly sulfated than normal, the relationship of sulfation to altered behavior of mucus is unclear. Activities of enzymes which remove specific sugars from these mucous glycoproteins are normal or near normal. There is currently little evidence that uninfected cystic fibrosis mucus has abnormal chemical properties.

While basal rates of mucous secretion are appropriate in cultured cystic fibrosis airways and intestinal epithelium, the regulation of secretion in vivo may be disturbed. Patients with cystic fibrosis are hyperresponsive to cholinergic and α-adrenergic drugs and are hyporesponsive to β-adrenergic effects, perhaps due to a disturbance of coupling of the β-adrenergic receptor and adenylate cyclase, a membrane enzyme which generates the intracellular messenger, cyclic AMP. In addition, the blood of patients contains unidentified mucus-stimulating substances.

Mucus secretions in cystic fibrosis are relatively deficient in water. Inadequate secretion of water may explain the excessively tenacious mucus and plugging of gland ducts and acini which are characteristic of cystic fibrosis. Studies of patients who have some residual pancreatic function indicate that water and bicarbonate secretion are more severely disturbed than enzyme secretion.

Water secretion is linked secondarily to altered electrolyte transport across exocrine epithelia. High levels of sodium and chloride in cystic fibrosis sweat (and to a lesser extent in salivary secretions) appear to result from inhibition of sodium reabsorption by duct cells as the primary secretory fluid passes from acinar regions to the skin surface. It has been postulated that the inhibitor interacts specifically with the amiloride-sensitive sodium transporter at the luminal membrane of duct epithelium. Although calcium has received considerable attention as a pathophysiologic factor, its levels are, for the most part, appropriate for the protein or glycoprotein content of secretions in this disorder. There is little evidence for a generalized disturbance of membrane function in cystic fibrosis.

Infection, especially with *S. aureus* and *P. aeruginosa*, plays a major role in the pathogenesis of lung disease in cystic fibrosis. Infection is confined to the lung, and the determinants of lung infection appear to be expressed selectively at the airway surface. Humoral and cellular immunity, as well as complement activity, are generally normal, although functional deficits may occur in cellular immunity and in the alternative pathway of complement as lung infection progresses to an advanced stage. Pulmonary alveolar macrophages display normal phagocytic properties unless exposed to cystic fibrosis serum. However, acquired phagocytic dysfunction in vitro seems to occur only in the presence of sera from individuals who have been infected with *Pseudomonas*. A predisposition to bacterial colonization of airways may reflect delayed mucociliary clearance, which has been documented in some patients with cystic fibrosis. Alternatively, it may be the result of an unrecognized biochemical disturbance which unfavorably alters the interactions of bacteria with surface secretions or the epithelial cell membranes.

Some have claimed that the syndrome of cystic fibrosis, including growth failure, chronic obstructive respiratory tract disease, and sweat electrolyte abnormalities, can be attributed to fatty acid deficiency. However, people with cystic fibrosis who retain exocrine pancreatic function do not develop fatty acid deficiency. Evidence suggests that the 10–15% of individuals with cystic fibrosis and substantial pancreatic function have statistically lower sweat chloride values and delayed onset of chronic lung disease. However, preservation of pancreatic function does not preclude development of the typical features.

A number of circulating "CF factors" have been described, including those that disrupt ciliary motility, inhibit debrancher enzyme, and stimulate the release of mucus. Only the last of these appears to relate directly to the pathogenesis of cystic fibrosis. None of these factors has been isolated or completely characterized, and the assay systems employed do not yield consistent results from 1 laboratory to the next. Absence of protease (arginine esterase) activity in cystic fibrosis serum and secretions has also been reported from several laboratories. However, the potential effects of pancreatic insufficiency and administration of exogenous pancreatic enzymes on endogenous proteolytic activities has not been assessed systematically. Quantitation of protease activity in amniotic fluid may distinguish some cystic fibrosis fetuses from those who carry a single cystic fibrosis gene or none at all. The usefulness of this or other tests for prenatal diagnosis has not been established.

Cultured fibroblasts from patients with cystic fibrosis, when compared with control cells, contain less protein and more glycogen, grow more slowly after 7 or more doublings, accumulate metachromatic substances in granules, sequester calcium in mitochondria, fail to process hydrolytic enzymes normally, and have increased resistance to the toxic effects of a number of drugs including dexamethasone and ouabain. Some of these observations have not been confirmed. In addition, it is not clear that the basic defect in cystic fibrosis is directly expressed in fibroblasts.

Pathology. Striking changes are characteristically observed in the organs which secrete mucus. Eccrine sweat glands and parotid salivary glands, including ducts, are not involved pathologically in spite of abnormalities in the electrolyte content of their secretory product.

The lung usually has a normal macroscopic and microscopic appearance at birth. With the development of symptoms, goblet cell hyperplasia and gland hypertrophy with extensive intraluminal accumulation of mucus occur in the bronchial airways secondary to infection. Another early lesion is acute and chronic peribronchiolar inflammatory cell infiltration (bronchiolitis), followed by plugging of small airways with inspissated secretions as goblet cell metaplasia of bronchiolar epithelium develops. Bronchiolar stenosis is a frequent consequence. Infection, the chief cause of progression of the lung involvement, leads to destruction of the airway walls, creating bronchiolectasis and bronchiectasis. Bronchiectatic cysts and abscesses are prominent features of advanced pulmonary disease. Squamous metaplasia of ciliated epithelium may occur. As the airways involvement advances, peribronchial inflammatory disease becomes more extensive and areas of fibrosis develop. Bronchitis and bronchiolitis are potentially reversible with treatment but subsequent changes are essentially irreversible.

Distention of air spaces is an early finding but little alveolar wall destruction (emphysema) is observed. Areas of segmental or even lobar pneumonitis may attend acute exacerbations of pulmonary disease. Subpleural blebs often develop, and their rupture is responsible for most episodes of pneumothorax. Bronchiectasis results in the development of a rich vascular network in peribronchial granulation tissue. This network shunts blood from bronchial to pulmonary arteries, compounding the problem of uneven ventilation-perfusion distribution. Bronchial arteries enlarge and become tortuous.

The paranasal sinuses are uniformly filled with secretions and the lining contains hyperplastic and hypertrophied secretory elements.

The pancreas is usually small, occasionally cystic, and often difficult to find at postmortem examination. The extent of involvement is variable at birth. In infants, the acini and ducts often are distended and filled with eosinophilic material. The acinar epithelium is attenuated. In 85–90% of patients the lesion progresses to complete or nearly complete disruption of acini and replacement of exocrine pancreas with fibrous tissue and fat. Infrequently, foci of calcification may be seen on roentgenograms of the abdomen. The islets of Langerhans contain a normal number of β cells, although they may begin to show some evidence of architectural disruption by fibrous tissue during the 2nd decade of life.

The intestinal tract shows only minimal changes.

Esophageal and duodenal glands are often distended with mucus secretions. Goblet cells may be hyperplastic in surface epithelium, especially in the colon and appendix. Concretions may form in the appendiceal lumen or cecum. Rectal biopsies uniformly show dilated crypt lumina and inconsistently show increased numbers of goblet cells.

Focal biliary cirrhosis secondary to blockage of intrahepatic bile ducts is uncommon in early life, although it is responsible for occasional cases of prolonged neonatal jaundice. This lesion becomes more prevalent and extensive with age and is found at postmortem examination in 25% or more of patients. Infrequently this process proceeds to symptomatic multilobular biliary cirrhosis, with a distinctive pattern of large irregular nodules and contracted bands of fibrous tissue. In addition, percutaneous biopsy shows that approximately 30% of patients have fatty infiltration of the liver, a change which occurs in spite of apparently adequate nutrition. At autopsy, hepatic congestion secondary to cor pulmonale is frequently observed. The gallbladder may be hypoplastic and filled with mucoid material and not infrequently contains stones. The epithelial lining often displays extensive mucous metaplasia. Atresia of the cystic duct has been observed.

Mucus-secreting salivary glands are usually enlarged and display focal plugging and dilatation of ducts.

The reproductive organs show several changes. Glands of the uterine cervix are distended with mucus, and copious amounts of mucus collect in the cervical canal. In males, the body and tail of the epididymis, the vas deferens, and the seminal vesicles are obliterated or atretic.

Clinical Manifestations. Expression of the cystic fibrosis gene defect results in a highly variable and wide range of pathologic involvement of the lung and pancreas.

Lung Disease. Cough is the most constant symptom of pulmonary involvement. At first the cough may be dry and hacking, but eventually it becomes loose and then productive. Characteristically in older patients, the cough is most prominent on arising in the morning or after activity. Expectorated mucus is usually purulent and if green may indicate airways colonization by *P. aeruginosa*. Some patients remain asymptomatic for long periods of time or seem to have only prolonged acute respiratory infections. Others develop a chronic cough within the 1st months of life and/or repeatedly develop pneumonia. Extensive bronchiolitis is attended by wheezing, a not infrequent symptom during the 1st years of life. As lung disease progresses, exercise intolerance, shortness of breath, and failure to gain weight or grow are noted. Exacerbations of lung symptoms eventually require hospitalization for effective treatment. Finally, respiratory failure, cor pulmonale, and death supervene.

Early physical findings include increased anteroposterior diameter of the chest, generalized hyperresonance, scattered or localized rales, and digital clubbing. High-pitched expiratory rhonchi may be heard, especially in young children. Cyanosis is a late sign. Common pulmonary complications include atelectasis, hemoptysis, pneumothorax, and cor pulmonale. These complications usually appear in the 2nd or 3rd decade of life as the lung lesion progresses.

Acute sinusitis is infrequent. Nasal obstruction and rhinorrhea are common, due either to inflamed, swollen mucous membranes or in some cases to nasal polyposis.

Intestinal Tract. In nearly 10% of newborns with cystic fibrosis, the ileum is completely obstructed by meconium (meconium ileus). Evidence for obstruction, including abdominal distention, emesis, and failure to pass meconium, appears within the 1st 24–48 hr of life. Abdominal roentgenograms (Fig 12–19) show dilated loops of bowel with air fluid levels and frequently a collection of granular, "ground glass" material in the lower central abdomen. Rarely, meconium peritonitis results from intrauterine rupture of the bowel wall and can be detected roentgenographically by the presence of peritoneal or scrotal calcifications. Meconium plug syndrome may occur more commonly in infants with cystic fibrosis than in other infants. Ileal obstruction with fecal material (meconium ileus equivalent) occasionally occurs in older patients, causing cramping abdominal pain and abdominal distention.

More than 85% of children with cystic fibrosis show evidence of maldigestion due to exocrine pancreatic insufficiency. Symptoms include frequent, bulky, greasy stools and failure to gain weight even when food intake appears to be large. Characteristically, stools contain readily visible droplets of fat. A protuberant abdomen, decreased muscle mass, poor growth, and delayed maturation are typical physical signs. Excessive flatus may be a problem.

Less common gastrointestinal manifestations include intussusception, fecal impaction of the cecum or appendix with an asymptomatic right lower quadrant mass, and epigastic pain due to duodenal inflammation. The occurrence of rectal prolapse is relatively frequent. Occasionally, hypoproteinemia with anasarca appears in infancy, especially if children are fed protein-poor formulas such as soy-base preparations. Deficiency of fat-soluble vitamins is occasionally symptomatic. For example, hypoprothrombinemia due to vitamin K deficiency may result in a bleeding diathesis.

Biliary Tract. Biliary cirrhosis becomes symptomatic in only 2–3% of patients. Manifestations may include icterus, ascites, hematemesis from esophageal varices, and evidence of hypersplenism. Biliary colic secondary to cholelithiasis may occur in the 2nd decade of life.

Pancreas. In addition to exocrine pancreatic insufficiency, evidence for hyperglycemia and glucosuria including polyuria and weight loss may appear, especially after 10 yr of age. In most cases, ketoacidosis does not occur and the other complications of diabetes mellitus are infrequently observed. Recurrent acute pancreatitis occasionally occurs in those adolescents and young adults who have residual exocrine pancreatic function and may be exacerbated by diet and/or tetracycline.

Genitourinary Tract. Sexual development is often delayed, but only by an average of 2 yr. More than 95%

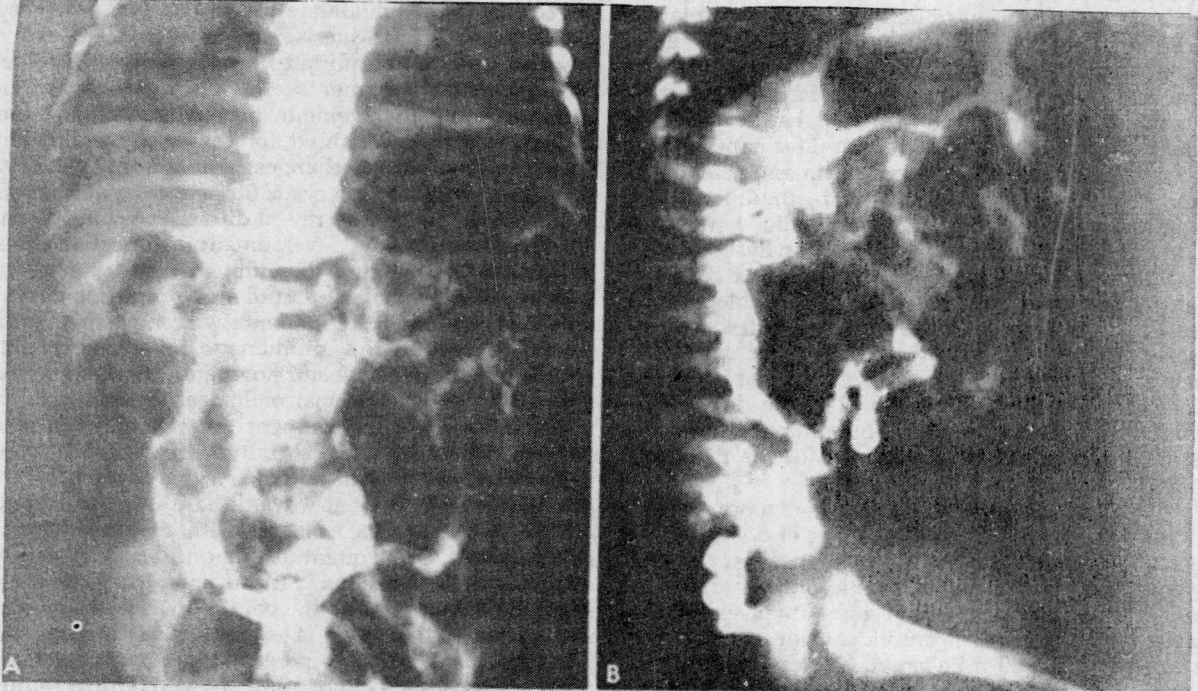

Figure 12-19 *A, B,* Contrast enema in a newborn infant with abdominal distention and failure to pass meconium. Note the small diameter of the sigmoid and ascending colon and dilated, air-filled loops of small intestine. Several air-fluid levels in small bowel are seen on the upright lateral view.

of males with cystic fibrosis are azoospermic because of failure of development of wolffian duct structures, but sexual function is generally unimpaired. The incidence of inguinal hernia, hydrocele, and undescended testicle appears to be higher than expected. Adolescent females may experience secondary amenorrhea, especially with exacerbations of pulmonary disease. Cervicitis and accumulation of tenacious mucus in the cervical canal have been noted. The female fertility rate is unknown, but is probably lower than expected. Pregnancy is generally tolerated well by women with good pulmonary function but may cause progression of pulmonary disease and even death in those with moderate or advanced lung problems.

Sweat Glands. Excessive loss of salt in the sweat predisposes young children to salt depletion episodes, especially at the time of gastroenteritis with vomiting and/or diarrhea. These children present with hypochloremic alkalosis. This complication appears to be more common in warm-weather zones. Frequently, parents note salt "frosting" of the skin or a salty taste when they kiss the child.

Diagnosis. The diagnosis of cystic fibrosis should be based on a positive sweat test in conjunction with 1 or more of the following: typical chronic obstructive pulmonary disease, documented exocrine pancreatic insufficiency, or a positive family history. In rare instances, the sweat test may be in the intermediate range (40-60 mEq/l), and a normal range sweat test has been

reported in a patient thought to have typical clinical manifestations of cystic fibrosis.

Sweat Testing. The sweat test, using pilocarpine iontophoresis to collect sweat and chemical analysis of its chloride content, is the best diagnostic test (Table 12-9). Modifications of the test, using variations of the Wheatstone bridge to determine conductivity or an ion-specific electrode to measure chloride concentrations,

Table 12-9 INDICATIONS FOR SWEAT TESTING*

Pulmonary	Gastrointestinal
Chronic or productive cough	Meconium ileus
Recurrent or chronic pneumonia or infiltrates	Steatorrhea, malabsorption
Recurrent bronchiolitis	Rectal prolapse
Atelectasis	Childhood cirrhosis, portal hypertension, bleeding esophageal varices
Hemoptysis	
Infection with *Pseudomonas* (mucoid)	Hypoprothrombinemia beyond newborn period
Staphylococcal pneumonia	
Other	
Family history of cystic fibrosis	
Failure to thrive	
Salty taste when kissed	
Nasal polyps	
Heat prostration with unexplained hypochloremic alkalosis	
Pansinusitis	
Aspermia in mature males	

*Individuals with cystic fibrosis may initially present with any of these signs or symptoms.

have resulted in both false-positive and false-negative results. Pilocarpine iontophoresis with quantitative chloride analysis requires care and accuracy throughout. A 3 milliamp electric current is used to carry pilocarpine into the skin of the forearm and locally stimulate the sweat glands. After washing the arm with distilled water, sweat is collected on filter paper which has been placed on the stimulated skin and covered to prevent evaporation. After 30–60 min, the filter paper is removed, weighed, and eluted in distilled water. A chloridometer is recommended for the analysis of chloride in these samples. The amount of sweat collected should be measured and reported. For reliable results, at least 50 and preferably 100 mg of sweat should be collected. In infants, it may be necessary to use the upper back to obtain enough sweat. Reliable testing may be difficult in the 1st wk or 2 of life due to low sweat rates. Positive tests should be confirmed; negative tests should be repeated if suspicion of the diagnosis remains.

Up to the age of approximately 20 yr, more than 60 mEq/l of chloride in sweat is diagnostic of cystic fibrosis when 1 or more other criteria are present. Values between 40–60 mEq/l suggest cystic fibrosis and have been reported in cases with typical involvement. In normal adults, the sweat chloride values increase so that a level up to 80 mEq/l may be normal. Chloride concentrations in sweat are somewhat lower in individuals with cystic fibrosis who retain exocrine pancreatic function but remain within the diagnostic range.

Few other conditions are associated with elevated concentrations of sweat electrolytes. These include untreated adrenal insufficiency, ectodermal dysplasia, hereditary nephrogenic diabetes insipidus, glucose-6-phosphatase deficiency, hypothyroidism, mucopolysaccharidoses, fucosidosis, and malnutrition. Most of these conditions can be distinguished easily from cystic fibrosis by clinical criteria.

Pancreatic Function. Although most patients with cystic fibrosis have exocrine pancreatic insufficiency, it is important to document this defect. Qualitative stool fat examination may be suggestive, but a 3 day collection with controlled fat intake is required for documentation of steatorrhea. Duodenal intubation, with the addition of pancreozymin-secretin stimulation, may help in diagnosis of borderline cases but should not be used routinely. Quantitation of trypsin and chymotrypsin activity in a fresh stool sample is an easy and fairly reliable test to screen for pancreatic insufficiency. Pancreatic isoamylase in serum is either absent or markedly diminished in patients with pancreatic insufficiency. Stool enzyme and serum pancreatic isoamylase analyses are widely accepted and reliable.

Radiology. Radiologic findings may suggest the diagnosis of cystic fibrosis. Generalized hyperinflation alone by chest roentgenogram occurs early and may be overlooked in the absence of infiltrates or streaky markings. Bronchial thickening and plugging, especially in the upper lobes, and irregular hyperinflation are frequently encountered as symptoms develop. More diffuse patchy areas of atelectasis and infiltration, hilar adenopathy, and more hyperinflation with depression of the diaphragms, anterior bowing of the sternum,

and increased anterior-posterior diameter of the chest are common with moderate to advanced disease. Segmental or lobar atelectasis, cyst formation, extensive bronchiectasis and infiltrates, pneumothorax, dilated pulmonary artery segments, and/or cardiac enlargement all indicate late involvement. Bronchoscopy and bronchograms are not required for diagnostic evaluation. Typical progression of changes is shown in Fig 12–20.

In older children with cystic fibrosis, roentgenograms of the paranasal sinuses reveal diffuse pansinusitis and failure of frontal sinus development in almost all cases.

Pulmonary Function. Routine pulmonary function studies cannot be obtained until 4–6 yr of age, by which time most undiagnosed patients will show the typical pattern of obstructive pulmonary involvement with decreased vital capacity and flow rates, increased residual volume, and a normal or increased total lung capacity. The earliest involvement occurs in the peripheral airways, affecting the distribution of ventilation and increasing the alveolar-arterial oxygen difference. The finding of obstructive airways disease unresponsive to a bronchodilator is consistent with the diagnosis of cystic fibrosis. Subsequent testing once or twice yearly, or more often if needed, can be used to evaluate the effect of therapy and the course of the pulmonary involvement. The latter is extremely variable as suggested in Fig 12–21. An increasing number of patients are reaching adolescent or adult life with normal routine tests and without evidence of overinflation.

Screening—Heterozygote Detection—Prenatal Diagnosis. There is no widely accepted routine screening test for cystic fibrosis. Some feel that the study of meconium for albumin content and a blood test for immunoreactive trypsin are effective screening procedures. At best, both miss patients without pancreatic function, and there is a moderately frequent occurrence of false-positive results. Likewise, there is no established test for heterozygote detection or for prenatal diagnosis.

Treatment. The treatment plan should be comprehensive as well as individualized. At the time of diagnosis most individuals have some pulmonary involvement.

General Approach to Care. Because of the serious prognosis, we almost always recommend a period of hospitalization for accurate diagnosis, overall baseline assessment, initiation of treatment, optimal clearing of the pulmonary involvement, and education of the patient and parents. The patient is hospitalized for as long as is necessary to control the pulmonary involvement and achieve steady weight gain. Follow-up outpatient visits are scheduled every 4–8 wk because many aspects of the condition require careful monitoring. The interval history and physical examination should be obtained at such visits. A sputum sample or, if that is not available, a deep throat swab taken during or after a forced cough is obtained for culture and susceptibility studies. Even apparently asymptomatic patients may produce sputum after forced exhalations or pharyngeal stimulation with a swab. Since progressive and irreversible loss of pulmonary function from low grade infection can occur very gradually, without acute symptoms, emphasis is placed on the pulmonary history including any change

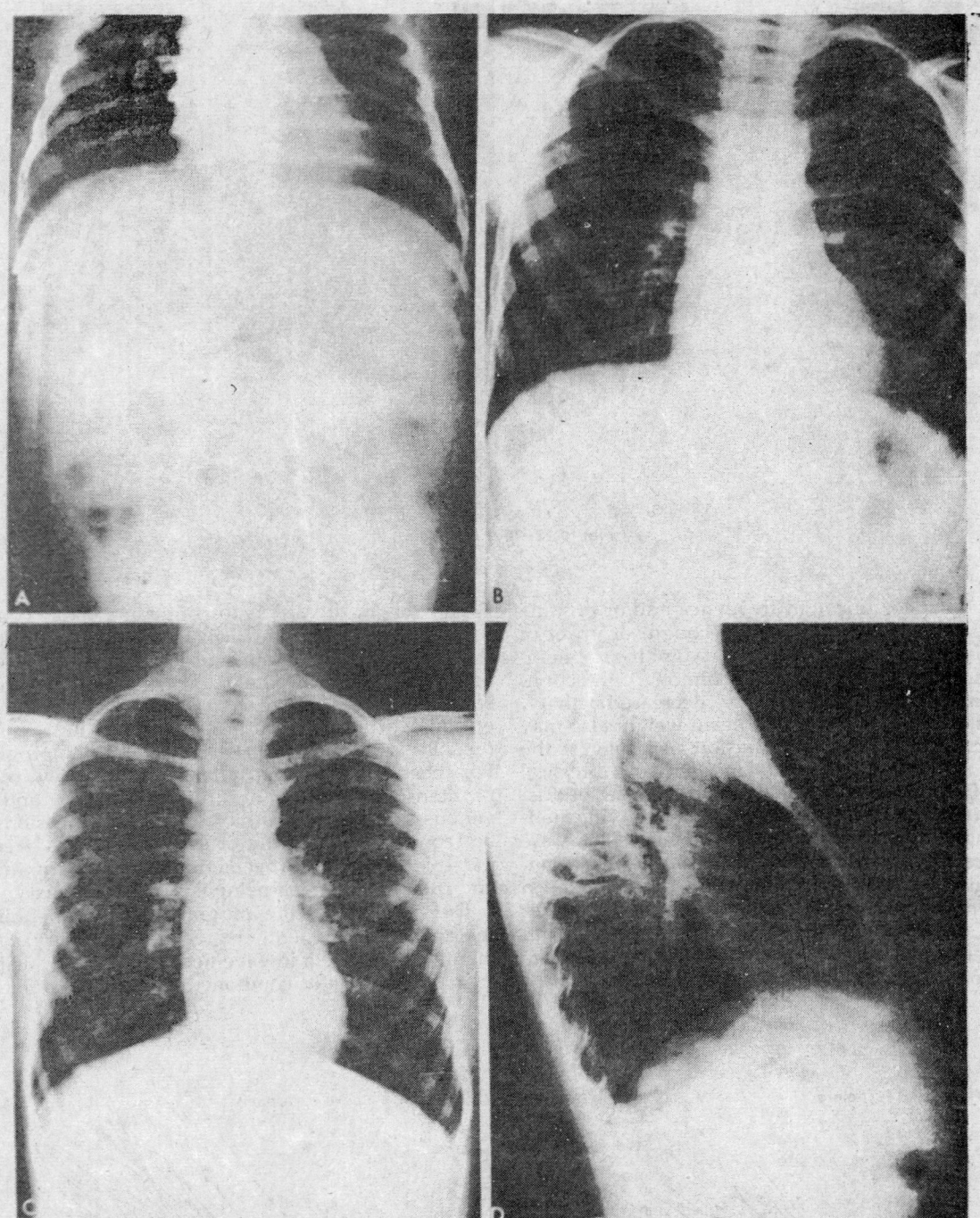

Figure 12–20 Roentgenographic progression of cystic fibrosis lung disease from diagnosis in infant to 17 yr of age. *A*, Admitted with cough and wheezing at 2 mo of age. Note the mild increase in bronchovascular markings especially in the upper lobe areas. *B*, At age 4 yr cough was minimal. Mild increase in bronchovascular markings was present with some improvement in the upper lobes. The wheeze never recurred. *C, D*, At age 13 yr, there was minimal cough and occasional sputum production. The bronchovascular markings were generally further increased with early bronchiectatic changes in the right upper lobe. The lateral view does not suggest overinflation. *E, F*, Age 18 yr. During adolescence, cough and sputum production increased even though outpatient antibiotic therapy was intensified. Small volume hemoptysis, occasional paroxysms of cough, and weight loss as well as increased nodular infiltrates (especially in the right upper lobe and hyperinflation, as seen on the lateral view) led to the 1st hospitalization since infancy. Height and weight were maintained in the 25th–50th percentile.

Illustration continued on following page

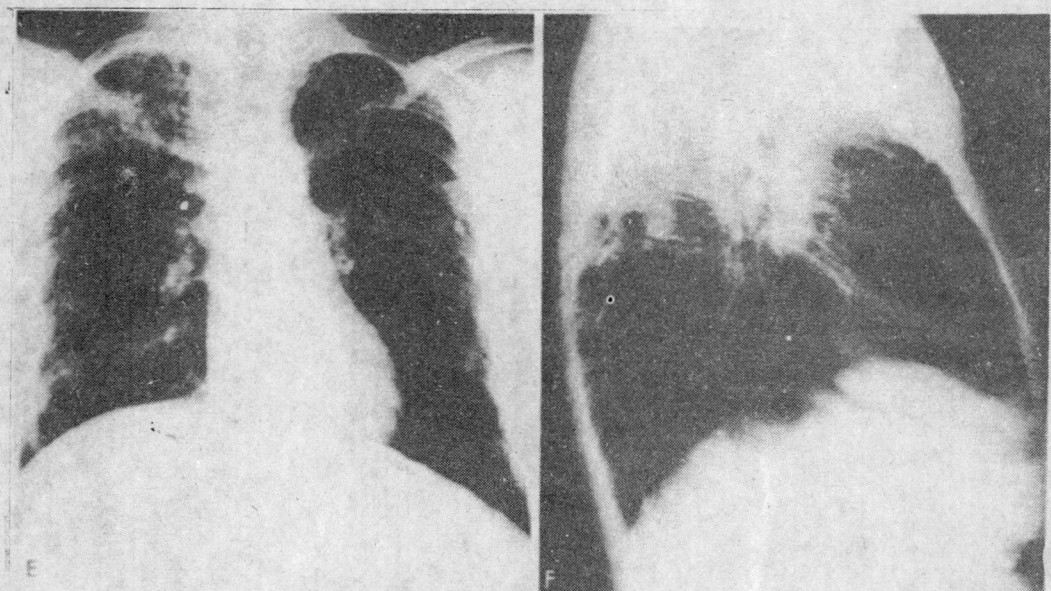

Figure 12–20 *(Continued)*

in cough. Changes in cough frequency and/or productivity, the appearance of nocturnal cough, or onset of paroxysmal cough with or without vomiting or hemoptysis indicates exacerbation of pulmonary infection. The appearance of rales, irritability, decreased activity, decreased appetite, and failure to gain weight also may reflect increased pulmonary infection. All suggest the need for altered or increased antibiotic and physical therapy. Immunoprophylaxis against rubeola, pertussis, and influenza is recommended. When specific medical, financial, school, emotional or other problems are encountered, a nurse, therapist, social worker, dietitian, psychologist or other specialists should participate in the care program until the problem is resolved or under control. Considerable understanding, education, and encouragement are required to maintain an adequate level of home care.

The goal of therapy is to maintain a stable condition for long periods of time. This can be accomplished for the majority of patients with interval evaluation and adjustments of the home treatment program. However, some patients never reach a stable condition but have episodic acute or low grade chronic lung infection (usually with *Pseudomonas aeruginosa*) that progresses. For these patients, rehospitalization for 2 wk or more of intensive inhalation and physical therapy and intravenous antibiotics is indicated. Such admissions may be required infrequently or as frequently as every 2–3 mo. Significant improvement in pulmonary function and the patient's well-being is usually achieved.

The basic daily care program varies depending on the age of the patient, degree of pulmonary involvement, other system involvement, and time available for therapy. The major components of this care are diges-

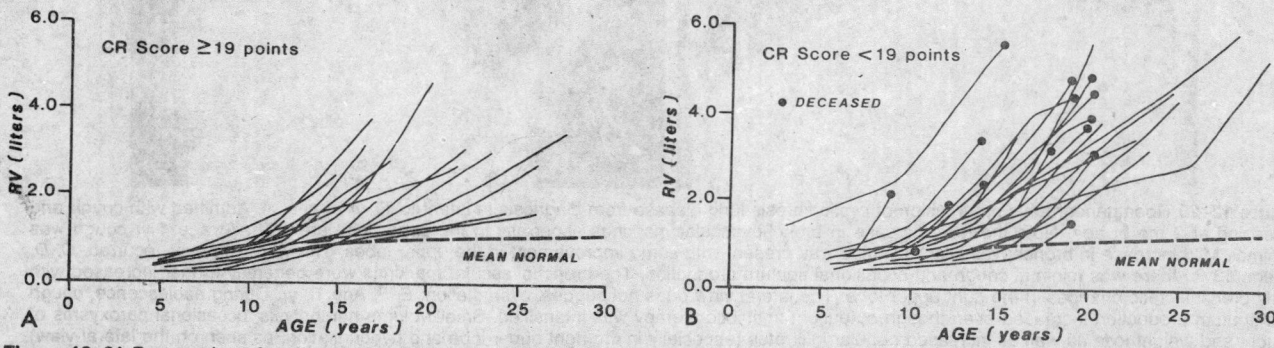

Figure 12–21 Progression of residual volume (RV) changes in patients with cystic fibrosis evaluated over several yr. An increasing RV reflects overinflation due to obstruction of airways. The patients were classified by their best chest roentgenogram (CR) score achieved during the 1st yr of treatment. A score of 25 points is maximum so that 19 or more is within normal limits. Although not all are shown, there are 30 patients in each group, *A*, Several in the group with high roentgenogram scores during the 1st yr developed an RV of 4 or more L by 15–20 yr of age. However, 13 of 30 had a normal RV throughout follow-up and none died. *B*, In the group with an initial CR score <19 points, 15 of 30 died in the follow-up period. Many developed an RV of 4 or more L and several approached 6 L.

tive therapy and pulmonary therapy. Measures to control or combat the pulmonary obstruction and infection play a major role and are the most time-consuming and/or expensive.

Pulmonary Therapy (Sec 12.20). This is empirical and/or symptomatic. The objective is to clear secretions from airways and to control infection. There is a divergence of opinion about various aspects of therapy. However, the effectiveness of the overall approach to therapy, including close supervision, continuity of care, aggressive intervention, and an optimistic outlook, is more important than minor variations in the use of individual measures. When an individual patient is not doing well, every potentially useful aspect of therapy should be evaluated; each measure may not be effective for all patients. Because of the large numbers of medications used, iatrogenic symptoms are frequent and deserve full consideration.

INTERMITTENT AEROSOL THERAPY. Intermittent aerosol therapy (5–10 min duration) is used to deliver medications and/or water to the lower respiratory tract. It can be given before or after segmental postural drainage or both. Intermittent positive pressure breathing does not improve delivery of the aerosol and may aggravate the obstructive lesion. The basic aerosol solution consists of 2 ml of 0.125% phenylephrine in 10% USP propylene glycol or of 0.45% saline and is administered 2–4 times daily, usually before chest physiotherapy. In patients with hyperreactive airways, isoetharine or isoproterenol can be added. When secretions are very thick and difficult to clear, a mucolytic agent such as N-acetylcysteine may be useful. Two ml of 20% N-acetylcysteine in 2 ml of basic aerosol solution can be used prior to postural drainage. Because of the potential for irritation of respiratory epithelium, the duration of use should be limited.

When the bacteria are resistant to oral antibiotics or when the infection is difficult to control at home, aerosolized antibiotics administered after postural drainage may reduce symptoms, especially those referable to tracheitis or bronchitis. Twenty–40 mg of colistimethate, gentamicin, or tobramycin in 2 ml of saline has been used 2–4 times daily in home therapy and also in the hospital in conjunction with intravenous therapy. Carbenicillin (1 gm) and ticarcillin (0.5 gm) have also been used in aerosol. Sensitization or resistance to antibiotics may occur as a result of this use.

A small compressor which drives a nebulizer, such as the Bennett twin-jet, is useful for home nebulization therapy. Daily cleaning of the nebulizer should be followed by rinsing and air drying. As soon as the patient can reliably breathe through the mouth and not through the nose, mouth-breathing inhalation therapy should be encouraged with occasional breath-holding following deep inspiration in an effort to increase deposition. The patient's position should not restrict diaphragmatic breathing during aerosol therapy. Nebulization therapy can provoke irritation or intolerance; if either is suspected, the therapy should be discontinued.

MIST INHALATION THERAPY. When thick or copious secretions are difficult to mobilize, some patients benefit from direct inhalation from an ultrasonic nebulizer for 10–20 min prior to postural drainage; one fourth isotonic saline solution is usually well tolerated. Mist tent therapy used overnight to enhance humidification and deposit water droplets in the lower respiratory tract may be beneficial for selected patients. Either a pneumatic-type nebulizer or an ultrasonic nebulizer can be used to generate mist with a mean particle size of 1–2 microns. Ultrasonic units are quiet and have a large water output. They are more difficult to maintain and more easily contaminated by *Pseudomonas*. A relatively small tent should be used to achieve a relatively dense mist. For ultrasonic units, the solutions most commonly nebulized are 5% USP propylene glycol by volume in distilled water, a one fourth isotonic saline solution, or distilled water. In pneumatic units, 10% USP propylene glycol by volume in distilled water is used. The solution should be sterile and free from organic matter to minimize bacterial growth. Nebulizers should be washed every other day with A-33 or 2% acetic acid solution followed by rinsing and thorough drying. Gas sterilization is preferable in the hospital.

CHEST PHYSICAL THERAPY. Also see Sec 12.20. This form of therapy is most effective when used in conjunction with inhalation and antibiotic therapy. Postural drainage therapy can be initiated even in the young infant. When old enough to cooperate, children are encouraged to extend exhalations using pursed-lip breathing to prevent airway collapse and to permit better emptying of the lungs. Because localized mucous plugging has been described even in patients with little or no clinical evidence of active pulmonary infection, a minimum of 1 aerosol treatment followed by 20–30 min of postural drainage is recommended daily for every patient. Young infants with pulmonary symptoms receive this therapy 3–4 times a day. Flare-ups of the pulmonary infection or periods of acute respiratory illness require additional treatment periods. Although infants and children can be treated effectively on the lap, the use of a tilt board or folding therapy table facilitates this treatment for older individuals. Effective coughing should be encouraged after each segment is clapped. For those positions which are quite productive, the clapping and vibrating should be repeated. Older individuals are encouraged to do their own therapy, which can be facilitated by the use of mechanical percussors or vibrators. On occasion chest physical therapy may contribute to hemoptysis and may need to be discontinued or modified temporarily. Physical activity and forced deep breathing frequently result in significant expectoration of mucus and should be encouraged. A regular program of exercise appears to maintain a feeling of general well-being.

ANTIBIOTIC THERAPY. The goal of antibiotic therapy is to reduce the intensity of pulmonary infection and to minimize or delay the inflammatory reaction and progressive lung damage. While some organisms such as *S. aureus* can be eradicated temporarily from sputum, others such as *P. aeruginosa* are rarely eliminated, even for short periods. Patients vary considerably in their past history, in the type and quantity of organisms present in their respiratory tract secretions, and in the amount of damage already incurred. Differentiation of colonization from infection is a recurring problem, and the usual guidelines for acute infections such as fever, tachypnea, or chest pain are often absent. Consequently, all aspects of the patient's history and examination must be utilized to guide the frequency and duration of antibiotic therapy. Antibiotic treatment varies from intermittent short courses of 1 antibiotic, e.g., a semisynthetic penicillin for a 2 wk period, to continuous treatment with 1 or more antibiotics for weeks at a time. Dosages are often 2–3 times the amount recommended for minor infections because patients with cystic fibrosis have proportionately more lean body mass and higher clearance rates for many antibiotics than do other individuals. In addition, it is difficult to achieve effective drug levels of many antimicrobials in respiratory tract secretions.

Outpatient Antibiotic Therapy. Many patients require at least 2 wk of some antibiotic therapy during each 6–8 wk interval. Indications include the presence of symptoms, e.g., cough, and identification of pathogenic organisms in respiratory tract cultures. The most frequent organisms are *S. aureus* and *P. aeruginosa,* but many patients harbor the common repiratory tract agents such as pneumococcus and *H. influenzae.* When acute symptoms develop, initial antibiotic selection should include appropriate therapy for all these organisms. For patients with acute symptoms, treatment usually should be continued for 2 wk or more after the symptoms have abated. If improvement is not observed in 5–7 days, the antibiotic therapy should be adjusted. If symptoms reappear after successful therapy, the course of antibiotic therapy should be repeated. Some recommend continuous semisynthetic penicillin therapy in full dosage from the time of diagnosis in an effort to prevent or minimize staphylococcal infection. Low-dosage, continuous antibiotic therapy is not recommended because achievement of adequate airway levels is difficult and because *Pseudomonas* and other organisms tend to develop resistance.

Patients in good condition may have cultures of only *S. aureus, H. influenzae,* or even normal flora. Sputum of those with more advanced involvement usually contains *P. aeruginosa,* including the mucoid form. A number of other forms of *Pseudomonas,* notably *maltophilia* or *cepacia,* have been recovered. These organisms along with some of the *P. aeruginosa* may develop resistance to most or all available antibiotics. Whenever possible, choice of antimicrobials should be guided by in vitro sensitivity testing. Often sulfisoxazole or trimethoprim-sulfamethoxazole are the only agents which appear effective. Chloramphenicol succinate can be extremely valuable in cases in which symptoms are uncontrolled by other agents. These agents may be effective even when the cultured organisms are not sensitive in vitro. Tetracyclines should be avoided in children under 9 yr of age. Young children may be colonized with *Pseudomonas* relatively early. If they seem to be doing well clinically, antibiotic therapy should be directed at the other organisms that are present. However, if symptoms are not controlled, every effort is made to treat the *Pseudomonas* as well.

Inpatient Antibiotic Therapy. For the patient who has progressive or unrelenting symptoms or signs despite intensive measures at home, hospitalization for intravenous antibiotic therapy is indicated. Although many patients improve within 7 days, it is usually advisable to extend the hospital treatment period to at least 14 days. Even then some patients have a relapse of symptoms after discharge and require further intensive hospital therapy. The use of the "heparin lock" with a 21-gauge scalp vein needle and a resealing cap or an indwelling intravenous cannula permits frequent infusions with minimal discomfort to the patient and freedom for activities between infusions. The scalp vein needle can be maintained for periods up to 10–14 days with rare evidence of local phlebitis or infection. The heparin lock system is flushed and filled between infusions with a solution containing 10 units of heparin/ml of normal saline. In some cases requiring chronic home antibiotic therapy, a Broviac catheter has been surgically placed and used for periods up to 2 yr without complications.

Antibiotics should be selected on the bases of sputum culture and susceptibility studies. A combination of ticarcillin, 200–400 mg/kg/24 hr, or carbenicillin, 300–800 mg/kg/24 hr, administered every 4 hr, and tobramycin or gentamicin is frequently used against *Pseudomonas.* The aminoglycosides have a relatively short half-life in many patients with cystic fibrosis. The initial dose is 8 mg/kg/24 hr, generally given every 8 hr. After blood levels have been determined, the total daily dose should be adjusted appropriately to minimize the risk of toxicity. Trough levels should be kept below 2.0 mg/l. Frequently an antistaphylococcal antibiotic is added even if the organism is not cultured, especially in those with hemoptysis or a poor response. Changes in therapy should be guided by culture results and by lack of improvement. In patients who do not improve, other possibilities should be considered, such as heart failure, hyperreactive airways, *Aspergillus fumigatus,* or, rarely, mycobacteria.

BRONCHODILATOR THERAPY. Reversible airway obstruction occurs in up to one third of patients with cystic fibrosis, often in conjunction with frank asthma or acute bronchopulmonary aspergillosis. Reversible obstruction is suggested by improvement of 15% or more in flow rates or indices of hyperinflation after inhalation of a bronchodilator aerosol. Treatment may include regular use of bronchodilator aerosol, oral sympathomimetic agents, and/or sustained-release oral theophylline, with the dosage adjusted after blood levels are obtained. In some cases aerosol or systemic steroid is required, at least briefly.

ENDOSCOPY AND LAVAGE. Treatment of obstructive airways disease sometimes includes tracheobronchial suctioning or lavage, especially if atelectasis or mucoid impaction is present. Bronchoscopy can also be used for the investigation of hemoptysis. The flexible fiberoptic bronchoscope has simplified and increased the acceptance of endoscopy, although it has limitations in smaller patients because it decreases ventilatory space. Bronchopulmonary lavage may be performed by the instillation of small volumes of saline or mucolytic agent through a fiberoptic bronchoscope or by the introduction of several liters of solution through a Carlin double lumen tube under general anesthesia. Antibiotics (usually gentamicin or tobramicin) may also be directly instilled at lavage, transiently achieving a much higher endobronchial concentration than can be obtained using intravenous therapy. There is no evidence for sustained benefit of endoscopic or lavage procedures.

EXPECTORANTS. Systemic drugs that effectively assist with physical removal of secretions from the respiratory tract are not available. This includes the frequently used iodides and glyceryl guaiacolate, which in recommended doses do not increase water secretion into the respiratory tract, change the rheologic properties of the secretions, or provide clinical improvement. Goiter formation with prolonged use of iodides has occurred.

Treatment of Pulmonary Complications. A number of pulmonary complications require extra attention or special measures.

ATELECTASIS. Lobar atelectasis occurs relatively infrequently. It may be asymptomatic and noted only at the time of routine chest roentgenogram. Aggressive intravenous therapy with antibiotics is warranted and increased chest physical therapy directed at the affected lobe. If there is no improvement in 7–10 days, bronchoscopy may be indicated for possible removal of a mucous plug. If the atelectasis does not resolve, the patient should be discharged with continued intensive home therapy to the involved lobe. There should be no early decision for lobectomy since the atelectasis may resolve over a period of weeks or months. Even if the lobe does not expand, it may not be a source of symptomatic infection. However, lobectomy should be considered if the patient has progressive difficulty from fever, anorexia, unrelenting cough, or sputum production. Lobectomy should be performed only after a period of hospitalization for intensive therapy to improve the status of all remaining portions of the lung.

HEMOPTYSIS. With increasing numbers of older patients, hemoptysis has become a relatively frequent complication. When small amounts (~20 ml) of blood are lost, postural drainage should be continued and the antibiotic regimen reviewed to be certain that coverage is adequate. When the hemoptysis is persistent or increases in severity, hospital admission is indicated. Massive hemoptysis, defined as total blood loss of 250–500 ml or more within a 24 hr period, requires close monitoring, including a fresh sputum culture and a blood sample for cross-match. Intravenous antibiotic therapy should be instituted. Chest physical therapy is often discontinued until 12–24 hr after the last bleeding episode and then gradually reinstituted. Patients should receive vitamin K in the event that they have an abnormal prothrombin time. During hemoptysis the patient may require a great deal of reassurance that the bleeding will stop. Hemoptysis may be aggravated in the recumbent position and require a semi-erect sitting position. Blood transfusion is not indicated unless there is hypotension or the hematocrit is significantly reduced. Drugs such as ticarcillin may interfere with platelet function and may aggravate hemoptysis. Bronchoscopy has been used in an effort to localize the site of bleeding. However, usually no bleeding site is found. Lobectomy should be avoided if possible because functioning lung must be preserved and because it is difficult to be absolutely certain of the bleeding site. Bronchial artery catheterization and embolization may control persistent, significant hemoptysis in some cases.

PNEUMOTHORAX. This is encountered with increasing frequency, especially in older patients, and may be life threatening. The episode may be asymptomatic but is often attended by chest and shoulder pain, shortness of breath, or hemoptysis. Even mild symptoms should be taken seriously and a chest roentgenogram obtained. If the pneumothorax is smaller than 5–10%, the patient is admitted and observed. A pneumothorax greater than 10% or under tension requires rapid, definitive treatment. Because of frequent delayed closure of the air leak and a high rate of recurrence when closed thoracotomy treatment alone is performed, an open thoracotomy through a small incision with plication of blebs, apical pleural stripping, and basal pleural abrasion is recommended with the 1st occurrence and within 24 hours of the diagnosis. This procedure has been well tolerated even in cases of advanced lung disease. Intravenous antibiotics are begun on admission. The thoracotomy tube is removed as soon as possible, usually by the 2nd or 3rd postoperative day. The patient then can be mobilized and full postural drainage therapy resumed. Recurrences, intraoperative complications, and deaths are extremely rare as a result of this procedure. Closed thoracotomy in conjunction with a sclerosing agent continues to be used by some specialists. Rarely, bilateral simultaneous pneumothorax is encountered; in this case, control of the air leak must be achieved rapidly, at least on 1 side. Both sides can be treated surgically through a split-sternum approach.

ALLERGIC ASPERGILLOSIS. This complication may present with wheezing, increased cough, and/or shortness of breath or marked hyperinflation on pulmonary function testing. In some patients there are new, focal infiltrates on chest roentgenogram. The presence of brown sputum, recovery of *Aspergillus* from the sputum, several serum precipitin bands to *Aspergillus fumigatus* extract, or the presence of eosinophils in fresh sputum samples supports the diagnosis. The IgE level may be high or within normal limits. Treatment is directed at controlling bronchospasm with bronchodilators. In most cases systemic corticosteroid therapy and, possibly, aerosol corticosteroid should also be used. This is usually a self-limited illness and will subside with several wk of therapy. Remissions should be similarly treated. For refractory cases, aerosolized amphotericin B or systemic 5-fluorocytosine may be required.

HYPERTROPHIC OSTEOARTHROPATHY. This complication causes elevation of the periosteum of the distal portions of long bones and bone pain, edema, and joint effusions. Acetaminophen or ibuprofen may provide relief. Control of lung infection may be most helpful. Some medications may aggravate symptoms.

ACUTE RESPIRATORY FAILURE. Acute respiratory failure (Sec 12.22) is rarely encountered and is usually the result of a severe viral illness such as influenza. Since patients with this complication usually regain their previous status, intensive therapy is indicated. In addition to the aerosol, postural drainage, and intravenous antibiotic treatment, oxygen is required to raise the arterial pO_2 above 50 mm Hg. A rising pCO_2 may require intermittent positive pressure breathing or ventilatory assistance. Endotracheal or bronchoscopic suction may be necessary and can be repeated daily. Right heart failure may occur. Recovery is often slow and does not begin until after the acute illness has subsided. Intensive intravenous antibiotic therapy and postural drainage should be continued for 1–2 wk after the patient has regained baseline status.

CHRONIC RESPIRATORY FAILURE. Patients develop chronic respiratory failure either as a result of incomplete recovery from an acute exacerbation or from prolonged slow deterioration. Although this can occur at any age, it is more frequently seen in adolescent and adult patients. Because a longstanding arterial pO_2 of less than 45–50 mm Hg promotes the development of right heart failure, these patients usually benefit from low-flow oxygen therapy to raise the arterial pO_2 to 50–55 mm Hg. Increasing hypercapnia may prevent the use of optimal FiO_2. These patients do not benefit from continuous ventilator assistance or tracheostomy. Most patients will improve somewhat with intensive antibiotic and pulmonary therapy measures and can be discharged again from the hospital after gradual weaning from supplemental oxygen. In some cases it is necessary to provide low-flow oxygen therapy at home. These patients nearly always display cor pulmonale. They should be maintained on a reduced salt intake and should be watched for edema, increasing shortness of breath, or fatigue. Rehospitalization for intensive care may result in further slow improvement.

RIGHT HEART FAILURE. Some patients develop right heart failure as the result of a complication such as an acute viral infection or pneumothorax. Individuals with longstanding, advanced pulmonary disease, especially those with severe hypoxemia (PaO_2 below 50 mm Hg), often develop chronic right heart failure. Some combination of cyanosis, increased shortness of breath, increased liver size with tender margin, ankle edema, jugular venous distention, an unusual weight gain, increased heart size by chest roentgenogram (Fig 12–22), and/or evidence for right heart enlargement by electrocardiogram or echocardiography helps to confirm the diagnosis. Furosemide, 1 mg/kg administered intravenously, may result in a good diuresis and confirm the suspicion of fluid retention. Repeated doses may be required at 24–48 hr intervals in the initial period to reduce fluid accumulation and accompanying symptoms. Concomitant use of spironolactone or triamterene guards against potassium depletion. These agents also are useful for long-term diuretic therapy. Digitalis is not effective in cases of pure right-sided failure, but it may be useful when there is associated left-sided failure. The arterial pO_2 should be maintained above 50 mm Hg if at all possible. Loss of respiratory drive may occur during the initial phases of oxygen therapy, and repeat arterial blood gases or noninvasive monitoring is required to assure the continuation of adequate respiration. Intensive pulmonary therapy including intravenous use of antibiotics is most important. Initially the salt intake should be limited to 2 gm sodium/day; carbenicillin may be hazardous because of its relatively high sodium content. Fluid overload should be avoided. Tolazoline, 1 mg/kg/dose every 12 hr by slow intravenous injection, has been reported to be effective in refractory cases studied at high altitude. However,

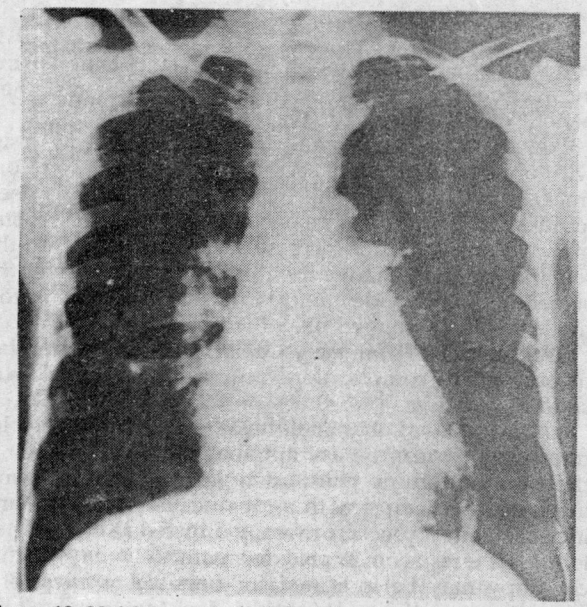

Figure 12–22 Advanced pulmonary disease with cardiac enlargement (cor pulmonale) in a 26 yr old. Diffuse infiltrates, bronchiectasis, and prominent pulmonary artery segments are present. The cardiac shadow is enlarged from previous studies, but this is not readily apparent because of marked overinflation.

when a large group of patients was treated at sea level, no clear-cut long-term benefit could be discerned. In the past, cardiac failure usually meant death within 1–2 mo. In recent years the prognosis has been improving, and a number of older patients have survived 3–5 yr after an initial episode of cardiac failure.

Gastrointestinal Therapy. Up to 85–90% of patients require digestive therapy, which includes diet adjustment, pancreatic enzyme replacement, and vitamin supplements.

DIET. In the past, a low fat, high protein and caloric diet was generally recommended. With the advent of the microsphere enzyme product, the fat intake is decreased only for symptoms, e.g., cramps or frequent, oily stools. A good protein source is required. When young infants with cystic fibrosis who present with wheezing respirations are fed soy protein formula, they do not utilize this protein well and may develop hypoproteinemia and anasarca within 4 wk.

PANCREATIC ENZYME REPLACEMENT. Extracts of animal pancreas given with ingested food reduce but do not fully correct stool fat and nitrogen losses. Adjustment of enzyme dosage and product should be individualized for each patient. The introduction of pH-sensitive enteric-coated enzyme microspheres (Pancrease, Cotazym-S) has been a major advance in patient care. One–3 capsules/meal is sufficient for most patients; infants may need only one third or one half capsule or may do better with pancreatin powder (Cotazym). The microsphere preparations usually are sufficiently effective to permit a liberal diet, which may include homogenized milk. Some patients develop episodes of rhinitis, watery eyes, or bronchospasm on repeated administration of hog pancreatin extracts, a problem which is less frequent with the use of coated microspheres. Enzyme preparations containing bile salts are infrequently needed. A cherry-flavored enzyme is more readily accepted by some children. The dose of enzymes required seems to increase with age initially, but some teenagers and young adults have noted a decrease in their requirement. Enzyme replacement therapy is best distributed throughout the meal but may be sufficiently effective when taken either right after or in some cases just before eating.

VITAMIN SUPPLEMENTATION. Because pancreatic insufficiency results in malabsorption of fat-soluble vitamins (A, D, E, and K), vitamin supplementation is recommended. Vitamins A and D can be supplied by 1 of several multivitamin preparations. Vitamin E deficiency is usually corrected with daily doses of 100 units. Vitamin K is needed only sporadically (i.e., in the newborn period) and during periods of hemoptysis, intense antimicrobial therapy, or surgery. The usual dose is 5 mg orally given daily or every other day. Those with cheilosis may benefit from extra riboflavin (5–10 mg daily), from additional B vitamins, or from local corticosteroid-antifungal applications.

NUTRITIONAL SUPPLEMENTATION. If pancreatic replacement therapy is used and enough calories are provided, nutrition should be adequate unless the cachexia of chronic pulmonary infection intervenes. Anorexia secondary to pulmonary infection cannot be consciously overcome by the patient. Attempts to force the child to consume more calories will be unsuccessful and lead to unnecessary friction. However, some children, especially teenagers, fail to eat properly, and efforts to increase caloric intake will result in weight gain. Medium chain triglycerides (MCT) are more readily absorbed without digestion than long chain triglycerides and provide a ready source of calories. Most patients find them unpalatable although infant formulas containing MCT are occasionally useful. A number of artificial diets have been proposed. However, cost and taste factors usually lead most patients to abandon such diets after a short period.

MECONIUM ILEUS. When meconium ileus is suspected, a nasogastric tube is placed for suction and the infant is hydrated and prepared for surgery. However, in a number of cases Gastrografin enemas with reflux of contrast material into the ileum have resulted in passage of a meconium plug and clearing of the obstruction. Use of this hypertonic solution requires careful replacement of water losses into the bowel. Patients with an atretic segment of the ileum require resection and anastomosis. Individuals who survive surgery generally have a prognosis similar to that of other patients. Infants with meconium ileus should be treated as having cystic fibrosis until adequate sweat testing can be carried out, usually after 1–2 wk of life.

MECONIUM ILEUS EQUIVALENT, INTUSSUSCEPTION, AND OTHER CAUSES OF ABDOMINAL PAIN. Despite appropriate pancreatic enzyme replacement, some patients accumulate fecal material in the terminal portion of the ileum and in the cecum. Ileal accumulation may result in intermittent or complete obstruction (meconium ileus equivalent). For intermittent obstruction, pancreatic enzyme replacement should be continued or even increased and laxative and/or stool softeners (milk of magnesia, Colace, mineral oil) given. Increased fluid intake is also recommended. When there is complete obstruction, a Gastrografin enema, accompanied by large amounts of intravenous fluids, can be therapeutic. If the enema reaches the terminal ileum, this hypertonic material will draw water into the bowel and loosen the inspissated fecal material. Intussusception and volvulus also must be considered in the differential diagnosis. Intussusception, usually ileocolic, occurs at any age and often follows a 1–2 day history of "constipation." If an intussusception is present, it often can be both diagnosed and reduced by a Gastrografin enema. If a nonreducible intussusception or a volvulus is present, a laparotomy is required. Repeated episodes of intussusception may be an indication for cecectomy. Once or twice daily dosages of mineral oil (1 tablespoon) may prevent repeated episodes of meconium ileus equivalent.

Chronic appendicitis with or without periappendiceal abscess occurs occasionally in patients on long-term antibiotic therapy and may present with recurrent or persistent abdominal pain. Lack of acid buffering in the duodenum appears to promote duodenitis and ulcer formation in some children.

RECTAL PROLAPSE. This occurs frequently in infants with cystic fibrosis and less commonly in older children. It is usually related to steatorrhea, malnutrition, and repetitive cough. The prolapsed rectum usually can be replaced manually by continuous gentle pressure with the patient in the knee-chest position. Sedation may be helpful. To prevent an immediate recurrence, the buttocks can be taped closed. Adequate pancreatin replacement, decreased fat and roughage in the diet, and control of pulmonary infection result in improvement. An infrequent patient may continue to have rectal prolapse and require surgery (a rectal sling of Silastic placed around the rectum just below the skin).

BILIARY CIRRHOSIS. Portal hypertension with esophageal varices, hypersplenism, and/or ascites is the most common complication of biliary cirrhosis. The acute management of bleeding esophageal varices includes nasogastric suction and cold saline lavage. Intravenous or celiac artery infusion of Pitressin may be of help. An episode of significant bleeding is an indication for portal-systemic shunting. Splenectomy and splenorenal anastomosis decrease portal pressure and also effectively treat hypersplenism when it is present. Adequate pressure and vessel size are necessary for successful shunt. This procedure has proved satisfactory in many cases. Portacaval anastomosis may also be used. Ascites is best managed conservatively, with a low-sodium diet and diuretics as necessary. These patients may also require a shunt for long-term management.

Obstructive jaundice occurs infrequently in newborns with cystic fibrosis and requires no specific therapy. Rarely, biliary cirrhosis proceeds to hepatocellular failure, which should be treated as in other patients with hepatic failure (Sec 11.101).

PANCREATITIS. Pancreatitis is usually precipitated by fatty meals, alcohol ingestion, or tetracycline therapy. Serum amylase and lipase levels may remain elevated for long periods of time. Treatment is symptomatic and includes analgesia, intravenous fluids, and nasogastric suctioning. An occasional patient may have mild symptoms and improve with several days of clear liquids. Once the pain diminishes, the patient can be returned to oral intake. Potential precipitating factors should be avoided.

HYPERGLYCEMIA. Onset can occur at any age and is not related to the severity of the disease. Ketoacidosis is rarely encountered. If blood glucose levels are only moderately elevated and urine glucose losses are small, no treatment is necessary. With more marked elevation of blood glucose, calorie and water losses into the urine become significant and insulin treatment should be instituted. Oral antidiabetic agents are usually not effective in these patients. Exocrine pancreatic insufficiency and malabsorption make strict dietary control of hyperglycemia virtually impossible. The development of significant hyperglycemia does not appear to change the prognosis significantly; however, it is at least a nuisance and may precipitate psychologic problems.

Other Therapy. NASAL POLYPS. These occur in 15–20% of patients with cystic fibrosis and in some become a recurrent problem. Corticosteroid and decongestant nasal sprays occasionally provide relief. Allergy skin testing and possible hyposensitization may be helpful in those with allergic symptoms. When the polyps completely obstruct the nasal airway or rhinorrhea becomes constant, surgical removal is indicated. Polyps may recur promptly after surgical removal but frequently do not grow to the point of obstruction for long periods. Patients with many recurrences inexplicably may stop developing polyps.

SALT DEPLETION. Sweat salt losses can be high on hot summer days. Infants and, less frequently, older patients may present with hyponatremic hypochloremic dehydration and require 10–15 ml/kg of normal saline to re-establish an adequate circulating volume. Children should have free access to salt, and precautions against overdressing infants in hot weather should be observed.

MATURATION. Delayed sexual maturation, often associated with short stature, occurs fairly frequently in association with cystic fibrosis. Although many have severe pulmonary infection and/or poor nutrition, delayed puberty also occurs in patients with otherwise mild disease and is not well explained. Adolescents with cystic fibrosis have the same developmental concerns as other adolescents. They should receive specific counseling concerning sexual development and potential reproductive problems through their developing years.

SURGERY. Minor surgical procedures, including dental work, should be performed under local anesthesia if possible. Patients with good or excellent pulmonary status can tolerate general anesthesia without any intensive pulmonary measures prior to the surgery. Those, however, with moderate or severe pulmonary infection are usually better off with a 1–2 wk course of intensive antibiotic treatment prior to surgery. If this is impossible, prompt intravenous antibiotic therapy is indicated once it is recognized that major surgery will be required. An aerosol and postural drainage treatment immediately prior to the anesthesia and surgery is advisable. Total anesthesia time should be kept to a minimum. After induction, tracheal suctioning is useful and should be repeated at least at the end of the operation. When necessary, even patients in respiratory failure and/or right heart failure can undergo anesthesia and major surgery without intraoperative or postoperative mortality. Such patients require frequent monitoring of their blood gases and may require ventilatory assistance in the immediate postoperative period. Tracheostomy has not been necessary.

After major surgery, cough should be encouraged and postural drainage treatments should be reinstituted as soon as possible, usually within 24 hr, and gradually intensified until full treatments are completed. For those with significant pulmonary involvement, intravenous antibiotics are continued for a minimum of 14 postoperative days. Early ambulation and intermittent deep breathing are important, and an incentive spirometer can also be helpful. Following open thoracotomy for treatment of pneumothorax or lobectomy, the chest tube is the greatest single obstacle to effective pulmonary therapy and should be removed as soon as possible so that full postural drainage therapy can resume.

Prognosis. Cystic fibrosis remains a life-limiting disorder, although survival has improved dramatically during the past 25 yr. Occasionally infants with severe lung disease succumb. Most children survive this difficult period and are relatively healthy into adolescence or adulthood. However, the slow progression of lung disease eventually reaches disabling proportions. National life table data now indicate a median cumulative survival of approximately 20 yr. Male survival is somewhat better than female survival for reasons that are not readily apparent. Survival beyond 20 years of treatment exceeds 90% at some centers if cystic fibrosis is diagnosed before substantial lung damage, as assessed by chest roentgenogram, has occurred.

For the most part, children with cystic fibrosis have good school attendance records and can be unrestricted in their activities. A high percentage eventually attend and graduate from college. Most find satisfactory employment and an increasing number marry.

With increasing life span, a new set of psychosocial considerations has emerged, including dependence-independence issues, self-care, peer relationships, sterility, educational and vocational planning, financial burdens, and psychologic reactions to anxiety. Many of these issues are best addressed during childhood and early adolescence, prior to the onset of psychosocial dysfunction. With appropriate medical and psychosocial support, children and adolescents with cystic fibrosis generally cope well. Achievement of an independent and productive adulthood is a realistic goal for many.

CARL F. DOERSHUK
THOMAS F. BOAT

Chase HP, Long MA, Lavin MH: Cystic fibrosis and malnutrition. J Pediatr 95:337, 1979.

Davis PB, diSant'Agnese PA: Assisted ventilation for patients with cystic fibrosis. JAMA 239:1851, 1978.

Denning CR, Huang NN, Cuasay LR, et al: Cooperative study comparing three methods of performing sweat tests to diagnose cystic fibrosis. Pediatrics 66:752, 1980.

Doershuk CF, Reyes AL, Regan A, et al: Anesthesia for cystic fibrosis patients. Anes Anal 51:413, 1972.

Esterly JR, Oppenheimer EH: Cystic fibrosis of the pancreas: Structural changes in peripheral airways. Thorax 23:670, 1968.

Handwerger S, Roth J, Gorden P, et al: Glucose intolerance in cystic fibrosis. N Engl J Med 261:451, 1969.

Levine SB, Stern RC: Sexual function in cystic fibrosis: Relationship to overall health status and pulmonary disease severity in 30 married patients. Chest 81:422, 1982.

Orenstein DM, Boat TF, Stern RC, et al: The effect of early diagnosis and treatment in cystic fibrosis; a seven-year study of 16 sibling pairs. Am J Dis Child 131:973, 1977.

Stern RC, Boat TF, Abramowsky CF, et al: Intermediate range sweat chloride concentration and pseudomonas bronchitis: A cystic fibrosis variant with preservation of exocrine pancreatic function. JAMA 239:2676, 1978.

Stern RC, Boat TF, Doershuk CF, et al: Course of ninety-five patients with cystic fibrosis. J Pediatr 89:406, 1976.

Stern RC, Boat TF, Matthews LW, et al: Treatment and prognosis of massive hemoptysis in cystic fibrosis. Am Rev Resp Dis 117:825, 1978.

Stern RC, Borkat G, Hirschfeld SS, et al: Heart failure in cystic fibrosis: Treatment and prognosis of cor pulmonale with failure of the right side of the heart. Am J Dis Child 134:267, 1980.

Stowe SM, Boat TF, Mendelsohn H, et al: Open thoracotomy for pneumothorax in cystic fibrosis. Am Rev Resp Dis 111:611, 1975.

Taussig L (ed): Cystic Fibrosis. New York, Thieme-Stratton Inc, 1982.

Wood RE, Boat TF, Doershuk CF: State of the art: Cystic fibrosis. Am Rev Resp Dis 113:833, 1976.

THE CARDIOVASCULAR SYSTEM 13

EVALUATION OF THE CARDIOVASCULAR SYSTEM

13.1 HISTORY AND PHYSICAL EXAMINATION

The importance of the history and physical examination cannot be overemphasized in the evaluation of infants and children with suspected cardiovascular disorders. After this assessment, patients may require further laboratory evaluation and eventual treatment, or the family may be reassured that no significant problem exists.

There are a number of areas of special interest in taking a *history* for a potential cardiac abnormality. Cyanosis is often overlooked by parents who are observing their children on a day-to-day basis; cyanosis may be considered merely a "deep coloring," a normal individual variation. Blueness during exercise is more often noted as an abnormal finding by observant parents. Eliciting a history of fatigue in an older child requires specific questions about activity including stair-climbing, walking various distances, bicycle riding, etc.; information should also be obtained regarding more severe manifestations such as orthopnea and nocturnal dyspnea. The history obtained from the parents of a young infant, however, should focus on the feeding process. The baby with congestive heart failure will often take less volume per feeding, become dyspneic while sucking, and perhaps perspire profusely. After falling into an exhausted sleep, the baby, inadequately fed, will awaken for the next feeding after a brief period of time. This cycle continues around the clock and must be carefully differentiated from colic or other feeding disorders.

Physical examination begins with an assessment of growth and development. Severe cardiac disease may lead to failure to thrive manifested by poor weight gain while length remains relatively unaffected. For example, an infant with severe congestive heart failure may appear long and undernourished in contrast to an infant with cyanotic heart disease unaccompanied by cardiac decompensation who may display normal height and weight. The physician should search specifically for signs of heart failure such as pulmonary rales, peripheral edema, and enlargement of the liver and spleen. Failure to thrive, tachypnea, and liver enlargement in a baby who appears to be ill are the major manifestations of heart failure on physical examination. Cyanosis may be too subtle for early detection, and clubbing of the fingers and toes is not usually manifested until late in the 1st yr of life even in the presence of severe arterial oxygen desaturation. Blueness is best observed over the nail beds, lips, and mucous membranes. Circumoral cyanosis or blueness about the forehead may be the result of prominent venous plexuses in these areas rather than decreased arterial oxygen saturation.

The *cardiac rate* of newborn infants is rapid and subject to wide fluctuations (Table 13–1). The average rate ranges from 120–140 beats/min and may increase to 170 or more during crying and activity or drop to 70–90 during sleep. As the child grows older, the average pulse rate becomes slower, as low as 40/min in athletic adolescents. Persistent tachycardia (over 200/min in neonates, 150/min in infants, or 120/min in older children), bradycardia, or irregular heartbeat other than sinus arrhythmia may require investigation to exclude pathologic arrhythmias.

Careful evaluation of the *character of the pulses* is an important early step in physical diagnosis of congenital heart disease. A wide pulse pressure with bounding pulses may suggest an aortic runoff lesion such as patent ductus arteriosus, aortic insufficiency, or various arterial-venous communications. Diminished pulses are associated with severe congestive heart failure, pericardial tamponade, or cardiomyopathy.

The *blood pressure* should be measured in the arms as well as in the legs, the latter on at least 1 occasion to be certain that coarctation of the aorta is not overlooked. Palpation of decreased femoral and/or dorsalis pedis pulses is not reliable to diagnose a coarctation. In older children a mercury sphygmomanometer with a cuff that covers approximately two thirds of the upper arm or leg may be utilized for measurement. A cuff that is too small will invariably result in falsely high readings, while a cuff that is somewhat too large will record slightly decreased pressures. Three, 5, 7, 12, and 18 cm cuffs should be available to accommodate the large

Table 13–1   AVERAGE PULSE RATES AT REST

AGE	LOWER LIMITS OF NORMAL		AVERAGE		UPPER LIMITS OF NORMAL	
Newborn	70/min		125/min		190/min	
1–11 mo	80		120		160	
2 yr	80		110		130	
4 yr	80		100		120	
6 yr	75		100		115	
8 yr	70		90		110	
10 yr	70		90		110	
	Girls	Boys	Girls	Boys	Girls	Boys
12 yr	70	65	90	85	110	105
14 yr	65	60	85	80	105	100
16 yr	60	55	80	75	100	95
18 yr	55	50	75	70	95	90

spectrum of pediatric patient sizes. The 1st Korotkoff sounds indicate the systolic pressure. As the cuff pressure is slowly decreased, the sounds usually become muffled before they disappear. The diastolic pressure may be recorded when the sounds are muffled (preferred) as well as when they disappear; the former is usually higher and the latter lower than the true diastolic pressure. For lower extremity blood pressure determination the stethoscope is placed over the popliteal artery. Ordinarily, the pressure recorded in the legs with the cuff technique is about 10 mm Hg higher than in the arms.

In infants the blood pressure can be obtained by auscultation, by palpation, or by the *flush method*. The last is most feasible in a restless infant. A cuff of appropriate size is placed around the upper arm or thigh. The distal limb is squeezed and the cuff rapidly inflated so that blanching is noted. The cuff is then gradually deflated. At the point at which the limb flushes, the blood pressure reading obtained corresponds to a systolic value slightly below what would be found by the direct arterial or auscultatory methods. Also available are ultrasonic (Doppler) devices, which provide accurate measurements in infants as well as children.

The blood pressure varies with the age of the child and is closely related to height and weight. Significant increases occur during adolescence, and there are many temporary variations before the more stable levels of adult life are attained. Exercise, excitement, coughing, and straining may raise the systolic pressure of children as much as 40–50 mm above their usual levels. Variability of blood pressure among children of approximately the same age and body build should be expected, and serial measurements should always be obtained in the evaluation of a patient with hypertension (Fig 13–1 and 13–2).

In cooperative children inspection of the regular venous pulse wave provides information about the *venous pressure* and right atrial pressure. The veins should be inspected with the patient sitting at a 90° angle. Under these conditions the external jugular vein should not be visible above the clavicles unless there is elevation of venous pressure. Increased venous pressure transmitted to the internal jugular vein may appear as venous pulsations without visible distention; such pulsation does not occur in normal children reclining at an angle of 45°.

The normal *jugular phlebogram* or direct tracings from the superior vena cava show 3 positive components corresponding to each cardiac cycle; they are termed "a," "c," and "v," respectively (Fig 13–3). The "a" wave is synchronous with atrial systole, the "v" wave with atrial diastole, and the "c" wave with early ventricular systole. Since the great veins are in direct communication with the right atrium, changes of pressure and volume of the chamber are transmitted to the veins. For example: (1) In congestive cardiac failure the increased right atrial pressure is transmitted to the cervical veins. The main pulsation at the upper part of distribution of these veins occurs in late diastole. (2) Cardiac compression by pericardial effusion or constriction increases the jugular pressure, but the amplitude

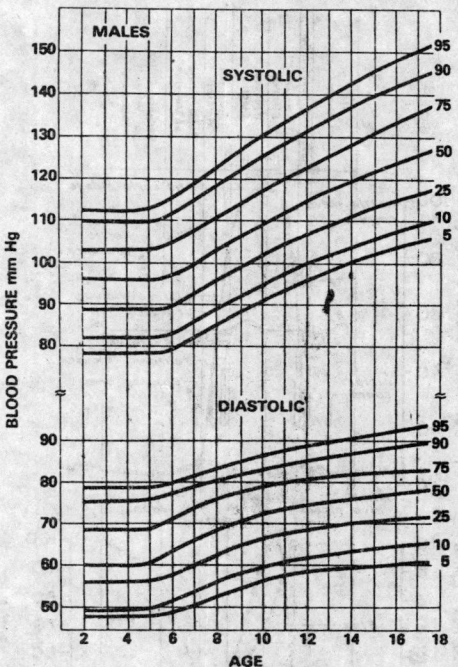

Figure 13–1 Percentiles of blood pressure in seated males. (From Report of the Task Force on Blood Pressure Control in Children, National Heart, Lung, and Blood Institute. Pediatrics (Suppl) 59:803, 1977. Copyright American Academy of Pediatrics.)

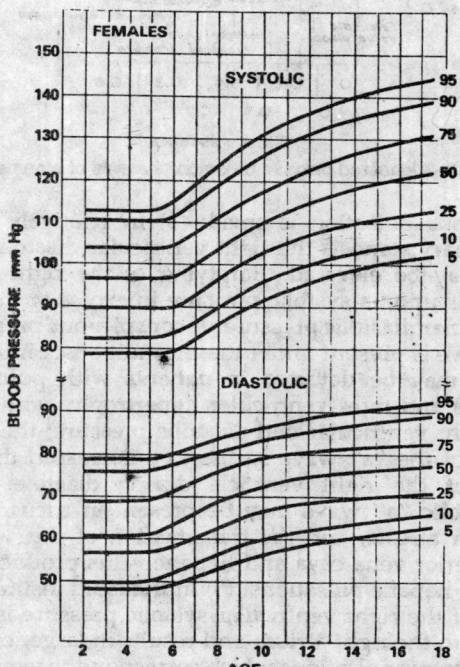

Figure 13–2 Percentiles of blood pressure in seated females. (From Report of the Task Force on Blood Pressure Control in Children, National Heart, Lung, and Blood Institute. Pediatrics (Suppl) 59:803, 1977. Copyright American Academy of Pediatrics.)

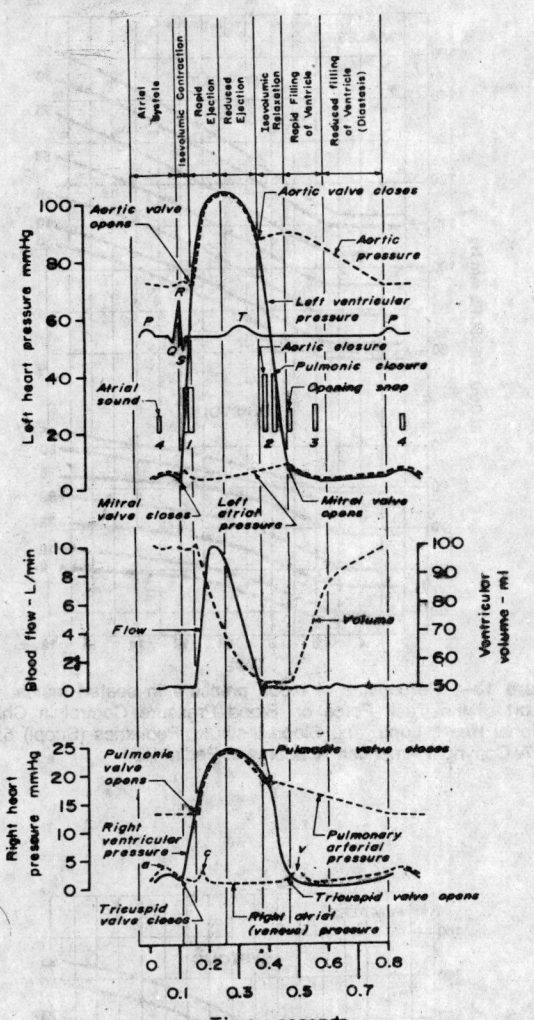

Figure 13-3 Idealized diagram of temporal events of a cardiac cycle.

of venous pulsation is small. (3) In relatively severe pulmonary stenosis the right ventricular diastolic pressure may be elevated. Emptying of the right atrium depends upon a systolic pressure in excess of the right ventricular diastolic pressure. A conspicuous presystolic "a" wave is present under these conditions. Similar "a" waves may be detected in patients with pulmonary stenosis and right ventricular hypertrophy with a normal right ventricular end-diastolic pressure; the mechanism of the "a" wave is due to a decreased distensibility of the right ventricle during diastole. (4) A presystolic "a" wave may be present in tricuspid stenosis or atresia, and the transmission of this wave to the inferior vena cava and hepatic veins produces presystolic hepatic pulsations. (5) In tricuspid insufficiency some of the right ventricular systolic pressure is transmitted to the right atrium and results in large, conspicuous venous pulsations which correspond to ventricular systole and produce a fusion of the "c" and "v" waves. (6) In complete heart block the occurrence of cervical venous pulsations depends on the position of the tricuspid valve at the time of atrial systole. If the right

atrium contracts when the tricuspid valve is closed, a large venous pulsation will occur. (7) In superior vena caval obstruction the jugular venous pressure is increased, but the veins do not pulsate.

Cardiac Examination. The heart should be examined in a systematic manner concentrating on the meaning of each manifestation. Much can be learned prior to auscultation. A precordial bulge to the left of the sternum with increased precordial activity suggests cardiac enlargement. A substernal thrust indicates the presence of right ventricular enlargement; an apical heave is noted with left ventricular hypertrophy. Both manifestations may be present. A "hyperdynamic" precordium suggests a volume load like that found with a large left to right shunt. In contrast, a silent precordium with a barely detectable apical impulse suggests pericardial effusion or severe cardiomyopathy. The relationship of the apex beat to the midclavicular line with the child prone is also helpful in the estimation of cardiac size; the apex beat moves laterally with enlargement of the left ventricle. Thrills are palpable murmurs which should always correlate with areas of maximum intensity of the auscultatory murmurs. It is important to palpate the suprasternal notch and neck for aortic bruits, which may indicate the presence of aortic stenosis or, when less prominent, pulmonary stenosis. Rough lower sternal border and apical systolic thrills are characteristic of ventricular septal defect and mitral insufficiency, respectively. Diastolic thrills are palpable in the presence of atrioventricular valvular stenosis. The timing and localization of thrills should be carefully noted.

Auscultation is an art which can be improved upon with practice and determination. The diaphragm of the stethoscope is placed firmly on the chest for high-pitched sounds; a lightly placed bell is optimal for low-pitched sounds. The physician should listen for 1 component at a time, concentrating initially on the characteristics of the individual heart sound and, later, on the murmurs. He or she must listen for the special characteristics of each heart sound and murmur. The 1st heart sound is caused by the closure of the atrioventricular valve (mitral and tricuspid); the 2nd sound is due to closure of the semilunar valves. During inspiration and increased filling of the right heart, right ventricular ejection time increases and pulmonary valve closure is delayed; the variable normal splitting is thus related to respirations (Fig 13-4). The 1st heart sound is best

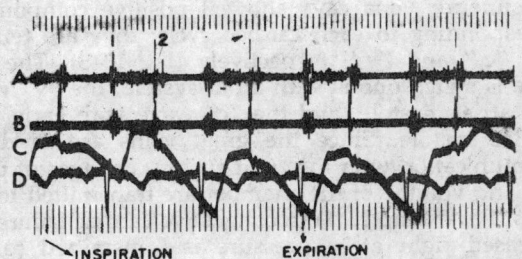

Figure 13-4 Physiologic splitting of 2nd heart sound in a 5 yr old child with an innocent systolic murmur. Tracings from above are (A) phonocardiogram at pulmonary area, (B) phonocardiogram at apex, (C) carotid pulse, (D), electrocardiogram. Time lines 0.04 sec. 1, First heart sound; 2, 2nd heart sound.

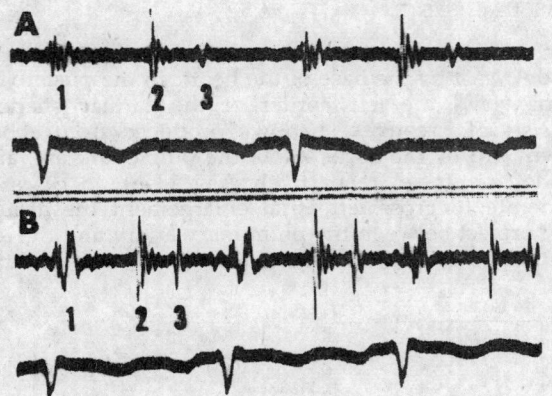

Figure 13–5 A, Phonocardiogram at pulmonary area. B, Phonocardiogram apex. Numbers indicate heart sounds.

heard at the apex, while the 2nd sound should be evaluated at the left upper sternal border. The patient should be supine, lying quietly, and breathing normally. The 2nd sound is split just beyond the height of inspiration and closes with expiration. The presence of splitting is more important than the intensity. The latter varies according to the age of the patient, the thickness of the chest wall, and the cardiac output. The presence of a normally split 2nd sound is strong evidence against the diagnosis of an atrial septal defect, defects associated with pulmonary artery hypertension, severe pulmonary valve stenosis, and numerous other conditions.

The 3rd heart sound is best heard with the bell at the apex in mid diastole (Fig 13–5). A 4th sound, occurring in conjunction with atrial contraction, may be heard just prior to the 1st heart sound in late diastole. The 3rd sound may be normal in an adolescent with a relatively slow heart rate, but in a patient with the clinical signs of congestive heart failure and tachycardia it may be heard as a gallop rhythm and may merge with a 4th heart sound. A gallop rhythm is attributed to poor compliance of the ventricle with an exaggeration of the normal 3rd sound associated with ventricular filling.

Ejection clicks which are heard in early systole are related to dilatation of or hypertension in the aorta and pulmonary artery. They are heard so close to the 1st heart sound that they may be mistaken for a split 1st sound. Aortic systolic clicks are best heard at the left lower sternal border and are constant. They occur in conditions in which the aorta is dilated (e.g., aortic stenosis, tetralogy of Fallot, truncus arteriosus). Pulmonary ejection clicks associated with pulmonary stenosis are best heard at the left mid sternal border and vary with respiration, disappearing with inspiration. A mid systolic click which is heard at the apex preceding a late systolic murmur suggests prolapse of the mitral valve.

Murmurs should be described as to their intensity, pitch, timing (systolic or diastolic), area of maximal intensity, and transmission. Systolic murmurs are classified as ejection, pansystolic, or late systolic according to the timing of the murmur in relation to the 1st and 2nd heart sounds. Ejection systolic murmurs start after a well heard 1st heart sound, increase in intensity, peak, and then decrease in intensity; they usually end before the 2nd sound. However, in patients with severe aortic or pulmonary stenosis, the murmur may extend beyond the 1st component of the 2nd sound, thus obscuring it. Pansystolic murmurs begin almost simultaneously with the 1st heart sound and continue throughout systole, on occasion becoming gradually decrescendo. In general, significant ejection murmurs imply increased flow or stenoses across a semilunar valve, whereas pansystolic murmurs are heard with ventricular septal defects or A-V valve (mitral or tricuspid) insufficiency. A "continuous murmur" is a systolic murmur which continues or "spills" into diastole. This should be differentiated from a to and fro murmur, which indicates that the systolic component of the murmur ends at or before the 2nd sound and the diastolic murmur begins after semilunar valve closure. A late systolic murmur is a bruit which begins well beyond the 1st heart sound and continues until the end of systole. Such murmurs may be heard after a mid systolic click in the presence of mitral valve prolapse.

Several types of diastolic murmurs can be identified: (1) A high-pitched blowing diastolic murmur along the left sternal border beginning with S2 is associated with aortic insufficiency or, if pulmonary pressure is high, pulmonary valve insufficiency. (2) Early short lower pitched protodiastolic murmurs along the left mid and upper sternal border are heard with pulmonary valvular insufficiency. These murmurs are typically noted after surgical repair of the pulmonary outflow tract in defects such as tetralogy of Fallot. (3) Early diastolic murmurs at the left mid and lower sternal border may be due to increased flow across the tricuspid valve, or less often, stenosis of this valve. (4) Rumbling mid diastolic murmurs at the apex follow the 3rd heart sound and are due to increased left ventricular flow in conditions with large right to left shunts. (5) Long diastolic rumbling murmurs at the apex, accentuated at the end of diastole (presystolic), indicate anatomic mitral stenosis.

Many murmurs are not associated with significant hemodynamic abnormalities. These are referred to as functional, accidental, insignificant, or innocent (preferred). During routine random auscultation, over 30% of children may have an innocent murmur; this percentage increases when auscultation is carried out under nonbasal circumstances (high cardiac output due to fever, infection, anxiety, etc.). The most common innocent murmur is a medium-pitched, vibratory, relatively short systolic ejection murmur which is heard best along the left lower and mid sternal border and has no significant radiation to the apex, base, or back. The short systolic ejection murmurs at the base and the continuous sound of a venous hum are other examples of common but insignificant bruits heard in childhood. The common innocent murmur (Still murmur) is heard most frequently from 3–7 yr. The murmur occurs during ejection and is musical, frequently sounding like the vibration of a tuning fork; it is brief in duration, may be attenuated in the sitting position, and is intensified by fever, excitement, or exercise. Innocent pulmonic murmurs are also common in children and adolescents and originate from the normal turbulence during ejection into the pulmonary artery. They are high pitched, blowing, brief, early systolic murmurs, grades 1–3/6 in intensity, and best detected in the 2nd left parasternal space with the patient in the supine position. The venous hum is another example of a common insignificant bruit heard during childhood. This is produced by turbulence of blood in the jugular venous system; it has no pathologic significance and may be heard in the neck or anterior portion of the upper chest. It consists of a soft humming sound heard in both systole and diastole which can be exaggerated or made to disappear by varying the position of the head or by light compression over the jugular venous system in the neck. These simple maneuvers are sufficient to differentiate a venous hum from the murmurs produced by organic cardiovascular disease, particularly patent ductus arteriosus.

The significance of an innocent murmur should be discussed with the parents. It is important to offer complete reassurance because lingering doubts about the importance of a cardiac murmur may have profound effects on child-rearing practices, most often in the form of overprotectiveness. An underlying fear that a cardiac abnormality is present may negatively affect a child's self-image and subtly influence personality development. The physician should explain that the innocent murmur is simply a "noise" and does not indicate the presence of a significant cardiac defect. At times, additional studies will be necessary to support this conclusion.

13.2 ROENTGENOGRAPHIC EXAMINATION

The chest roentgenogram provides information about cardiac size and shape as well as other features which directly relate to the status of the cardiovascular system. Variations are due to differences in body build, the phase of respiration or cardiac cycle, abnormalities of the thoracic cage, position of the diaphragm, or pulmonary disease.

The most frequently used measurement of cardiac size is the maximal width of the cardiac shadow in a midinspiration posteroanterior film: a vertical line is drawn down the middle of the sternal shadow and perpendicular lines from the sternal line to the extreme right and left borders of the heart; the sum of the lengths of these lines is the *maximal cardiac width*. The *maximal chest width* is obtained by drawing a horizontal line between the right and left inner borders of the rib cage at the level of the top of the right diaphragm. When the cardiac width is more than half the maximal chest width, the heart is usually enlarged. This *cardiothoracic ratio* is a *less* accurate index of cardiac enlargement in infancy than in subsequent yr because the horizontal position of the heart may increase the ratio to more than half in the absence of true enlargement. In children with vertical hearts the cardiothoracic ratio will tend to give an erroneously low impression of the true heart size.

In infants the thymic shadow may overlap the shadow cast by the base of the heart. In the posteroanterior view, the left border of the cardiac shadow consists of 3 convex shadows produced from above downward by the aortic knob, the pulmonary arc, and the left ventricle, respectively (Fig 13–6). In cases of moderate to gross left atrial enlargement the atrium may project between the pulmonary artery and the left ventricle. The outflow tract of the right ventricle or the

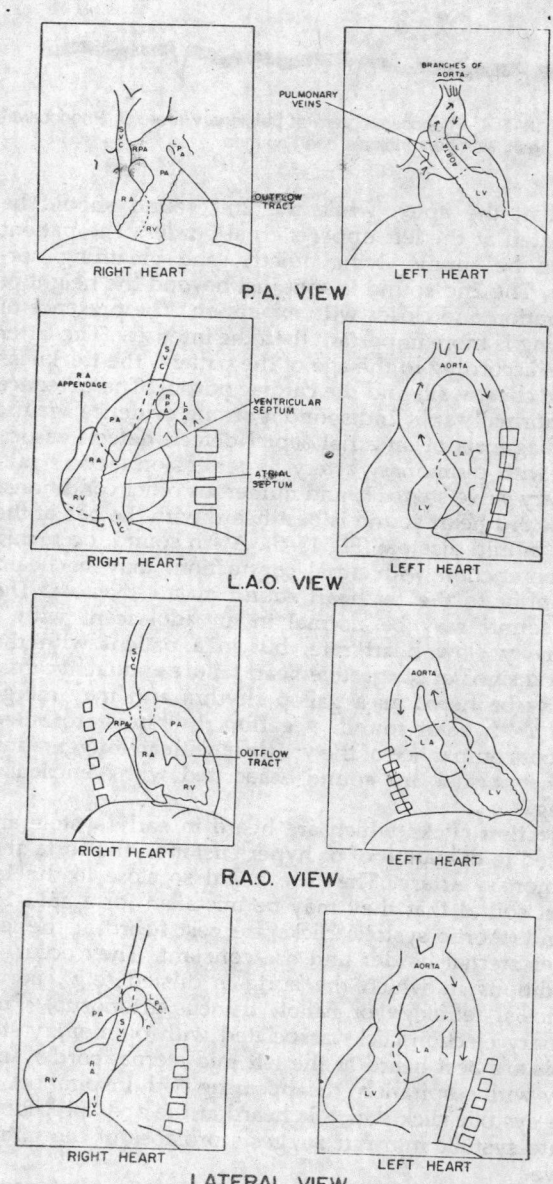

Figure 13–6 Idealized diagrams showing the normal position of the cardiac chambers and great blood vessels. P.A., posteroanterior; L.A.O., left anterior oblique; R.A.O., right anterior oblique; S.V.C., superior vena cava; R.A., right atrium; R.V., right ventricle; P.A., pulmonary artery; R.P.A., right pulmonary artery; L.P.A., left pulmonary artery; L.A., left atrium; L.V., left ventricle; I.V.C., inferior vena cava. (Adapted and redrawn from Dotter and Steinberg: Radiology, 53:513, 1949.)

pulmonary conus does not contribute to the shadows formed by the left border of the heart (Fig 13–6). The aortic knob is not as easily seen in infants and children as in adults. Three structures also contribute to the right border of the cardiac silhouette; from above downward they are the superior vena cava, the ascending aorta, and the right atrium. It is also of fundamental importance to assess the degree of pulmonary vascularity as represented by the intrapulmonary shadows. Angiocardiographic studies have shown that the hilar shadows are mainly vascular. Pulmonary overcirculation is usually associated with left to right shunts and undercirculation with stenosis or atresia of the outflow tract of the right ventricle or of the pulmonary valve.

Interpretation of atrial or ventricular enlargement in infants and children by roentgenographic means is difficult. Displacement of a normal chamber by a hypertrophied ventricle gives a false impression of ventricular enlargement. Thus, posterior displacement of a normal left ventricle by a hypertrophied right ventricle may cause the roentgenographic picture to resemble that of biventricular enlargement. Therefore, the roentgenographic findings should be complemented by an electrocardiogram which is a more sensitive and accurate index of ventricular enlargement.

The esophagus is closely related to the great vessels, and visualization with barium helps to delineate these structures in selected situations such as coarctation of the aorta and vascular ring. However, echocardiographic examination best defines specific intracardiac chamber enlargement. Thus, routine esophagrams and fluoroscopy (even with image intensification and video tape or cine recording) are not necessary for the evaluation of most cardiac abnormalities.

13.3   THE ELECTROCARDIOGRAM (ECG)

The hemodynamic load of the heart is usually reflected in the electrocardiogram of the full term infant. Since vascular resistances in the pulmonary and systemic circulations are nearly equal in the fetus at term, the intrauterine work of the heart results in virtually equal mass of both the right and left ventricles. After birth, systemic vascular resistance rises when the placental circulation is eliminated, and pulmonary vascular resistance falls when the lungs expand. These changes are effected over a period of hours or days. The electrocardiogram demonstrates these anatomic and hemodynamic features principally by changes in the QRS and T wave morphology. During the 1st days of life right axis deviation, large R waves, and upright T waves in the right precordial leads (V_3R or V_4R and V_1) occur (Fig 13–7). When pulmonary resistance decreases and right ventricular pressure reaches its normal level, the right precordial T waves become negative. In the great majority of instances they do so within the 1st 48 hr of life.

In the frontal plane leads of the standard ECG, the mean QRS axis normally lies in the range of +110 to +180°. The right-sided chest leads reveal a larger pos-

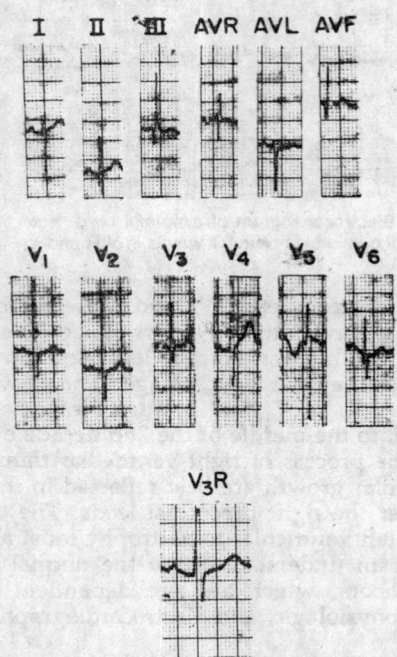

Figure 13–7 Electrocardiogram in a normal neonate less than 24 hr of age. Note the dominant R wave and upright T waves in leads V_3R and V_1. (V_3R paper speed = 50 mm/sec.)

itive (R) than negative (S) wave and may do so for months or years since the voltage recorded by the right precordial leads is influenced to a greater extent by right ventricular depolarization. Left-sided leads (V_5 and V_6) also reflect right-sided dominance in the early neonatal period when the RS ratio may be less than 1. However, since left precordial leads are in direct proximity to the left ventricle, a dominant R wave reflecting left ventricular forces quickly becomes evident within the 1st few days of life (Fig 13–8). Over the years, the QRS axis gradually shifts leftward and right ventricular forces slowly regress. As the left ventricle becomes dominant, the ECG evolves to the characteristic pattern of the older child (Fig 13–9), and finally the typical adult electrocardiogram emerges (Fig 13–10).

With the growth of the infant there is slow regression of right ventricular dominance and an increase in left

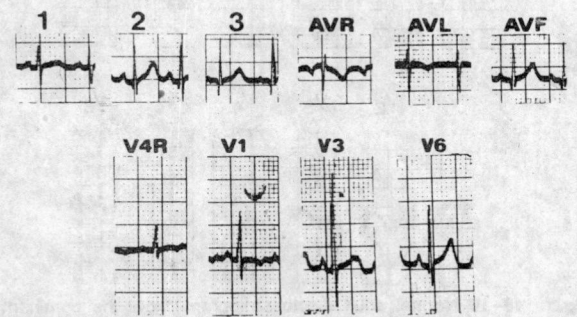

Figure 13–8 Electrocardiogram of a normal infant. Note the tall R and small S waves in V_4R and V_1, and the inverted T wave in these leads. There is also a dominant R wave in V_6.

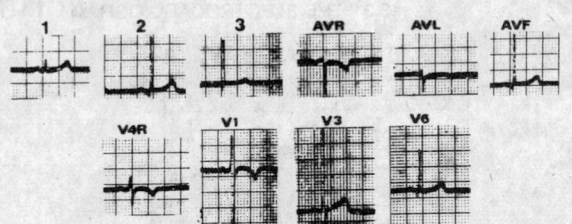

Figure 13–9 Electrocardiogram of a normal child. Note the relatively tall R waves and inversion of the T waves in V₄R and V₁.

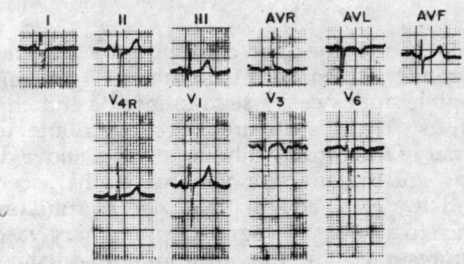

Figure 13–11 Electrocardiogram and vectorcardiogram of infant with right ventricular hypertrophy (tetralogy of Fallot). Note the tall R waves in the right precordium and deep S waves in V₆. The positive T waves in V₄R and V₁ are also characteristic of right ventricular hypertrophy.

ventricular forces. Leads V₁ and V₄R will display a prominent R wave until 6 mo–8 yr of age. The majority of children will have an RS ratio less than 1 in lead V₄R by the time they are 4 yr of age. The T waves are inverted in V₄R, V₁, V₂, and V₃ during infancy and may remain so into the middle of the 2nd decade of life and beyond. The process of right ventricular thinning and left ventricular growth are best reflected in the QRS T pattern over the right precordial leads. The diagnosis of right or left ventricular hypertrophy must always be made with an understanding of the normal states of these chambers, which are age dependent from an anatomic, physiologic, and electrocardiographic standpoint.

Ventricular hypertrophy may result in increased voltage in the R and S waves in the chest leads. However, the height of these deflections is governed by the proximity of the exploring electrode to the surface of the heart, by the sequence of electrical activation through the ventricles, which causes various degrees of cancellation of forces, and by the hypertrophy of the myocardium. Since the chest wall in infants and children as well as in adolescents may be relatively thin, the diagnosis of ventricular hypertrophy should not be based on voltage changes alone during childhood.

The diagnosis of pathologic right ventricular hypertrophy is difficult in the 1st wk of life. Serial tracings are often necessary to determine whether marked right axis deviation and abnormal right precordial forces or T waves, or both, will persist (Fig 13–11). An adult ECG pattern seen in a neonate suggests left ventricular

enlargement (Fig 13–10). The premature infant, however, may display a more "mature" ECG than his or her full term counterpart (Fig 13–12) as a result of lower pulmonary resistance secondary to underdevelopment of the medial muscular layer of the pulmonary arterioles. Thus, the electrocardiogram may simulate that of the older child with left ventricular dominance manifested by a more mature R wave progression across the precordium (qR in V₆, R/S ratio in V₄R, and V₁ equal to or less than 1). Some premature infants display a pattern of generalized low voltage across the precordium.

The P Wave. Tall, narrow, and spiked P waves are seen in congenital pulmonary stenosis, Ebstein anomaly of the tricuspid valve, tricuspid atresia, and sometimes cor pulmonale. These abnormal waves are probably due to right atrial hypertrophy, are usually taller than 2.5 mm, and are most obvious in standard lead II and leads V₄R, V₃R, and V₁ (Fig 13–13A). Similar waves are sometimes seen in thyrotoxicosis. Widened P waves, commonly bifid, indicate left atrial enlargement (Fig 13–13B). They are seen in some patients with large ventricular septal defects, with communications between the aorta and pulmonary circulation, and with severe mitral stenosis. Flat P waves may be found in hyperkalemia. Inverted P waves are seen in junctional rhythm as well as in atrial inversion, which occurs in dextrocardia with situs inversus.

Right Ventricular Hypertrophy. Right ventricular surface leads of infants and children differ from those of adults, and tracings of the right side of the chest (V₄R or V₃R) are essential in young children. In infants

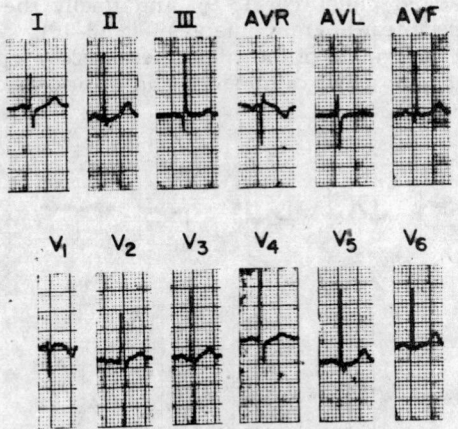

Figure 13–10 Normal adult electocardiogram. Note the dominant S wave in lead V₁. This pattern in an infant would indicate the presence of left ventricular hypertrophy.

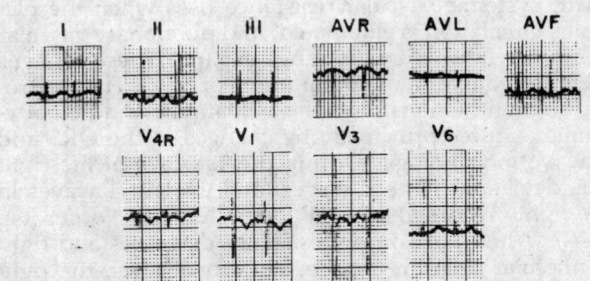

Figure 13–12 Electrocardiogram of premature infant (weight 2 kg and age 5 wk at time of tracing). The cardiovascular system was clinically normal. Left ventricular dominance is manifest by R wave progression across the chest simulating tracings obtained from older children. Compare with normal fullterm infant tracing, Fig 13–8.

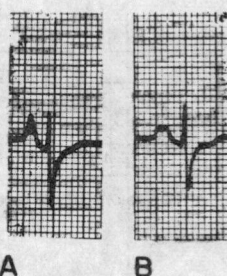

Figure 13–13 Atrial enlargement. *A,* Peaked narrow P waves characteristic of right atrial enlargement. *B,* Wide bifid M-shaped P waves typical of left atrial enlargement.

with known **right ventricular hypertrophy** the following changes may occur singly or in combination (Fig 13–11): (1) a qR pattern in the right ventricular surface leads; (2) a positive T wave in leads V_4R through V_3 after the 1st 48 hr of life; (3) a monophasic R wave in V_4R, V_3R, or V_1; (4) rsR' in right precordial leads with a tall secondary R wave usually exceeding 10 mm (this pattern is frequently associated with volume overload and hypertrophy of the right ventricular outflow track); (5) age-related voltage criteria in V_3R and $V_1(R)$, and/or $V_{6-7}(S)$; (6) marked right axis deviation (>120°); (7) a complete reversal of the normal adult precordial RS pattern; and (8) right atrial enlargement. At least 2 of these changes should be present to diagnose right ventricular hypertrophy. In general, since a pattern of right ventricular hypertrophy exists in the newborn and young infant, a persistence of this finding into early childhood suggests that right ventricular hypertrophy may be present. In contrast, the small infant who displays the pattern of a "normal" electrocardiogram for an older child may have left ventricular hypertrophy.

Abnormal hemodynamics can be correlated with abnormal electrocardiographic patterns. Obstruction to right ventricular and pulmonary flow (e.g., pulmonary stenosis) is associated with a systolic overload pattern characterized by an increasingly tall pure R wave in the right precordial leads. In these leads the T wave is initially upright and later becomes inverted. In contrast, diastolic overload of the right ventricle (e.g., with atrial septal defect) is characterized by an rsR' pattern and right ventricular conduction delay (Fig 13–14). However, there are many instances of overlap, e.g., in patients with mild to moderate pulmonary stenosis (systolic overload) who exhibit an rsR' in the right precordial leads; others with excessive right ventricular volume may show signs of systolic overload.

The following features are consistent with **left ventricular hypertrophy** (Fig 13–15): (1) depression of the S-T segments and inversion of T waves and left precordial surface leads (V_5, V_6, and V_7), a left ventricular strain pattern; (2) increase in magnitude of initial forces to the right (i.e., deep Q in left precordial leads); (3) voltage criteria in V_3R and V_1. It is important to emphasize that evaluation of ventricular hypertrophy should not be based on voltage criteria alone. The concepts of systolic and diastolic overload, although not always consistent, are also useful in evaluating left ventricular enlargement. Systolic overload of the left ventricles is suggested by depression of the S-T segments and inverted T waves over the left precordial leads; diastolic overload may result in tall R waves, a large Q wave, and normal T waves over the left precordium.

Bundle Branch Block. Complete right bundle branch block may occur as a congenital finding or be acquired after open heart surgery, especially when a right ventriculotomy has been carried out. Congenital left bundle branch block is rare; this pattern is occasionally seen with cardiomyopathy.

The Q-T Interval. The duration of the Q-T interval varies with the cardiac rate; a corrected Q-T interval can be calculated by dividing the measured Q-T in-

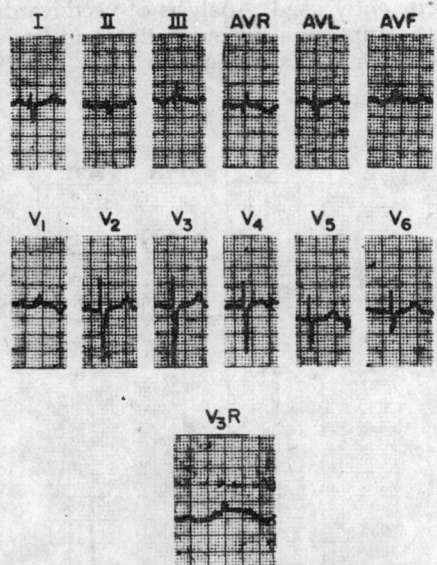

Figure 13–14 Electrocardiogram showing right ventricular conduction delay characterized by a vsr' pattern in V_1 and a deep S wave in V_6. (V_3R paper speed = 50 mm/sec.)

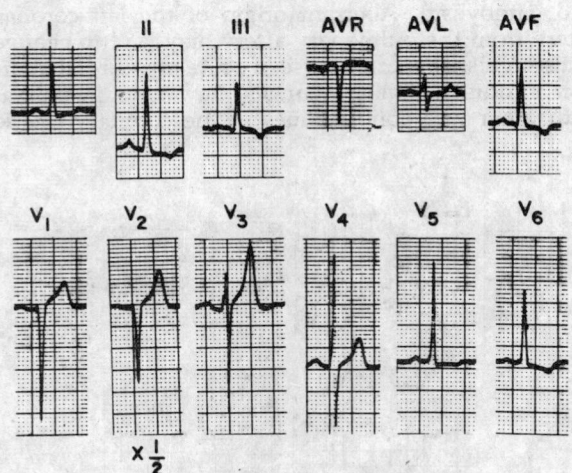

Figure 13–15 Electrocardiogram showing left ventricular hypertrophy in a 12 yr old child with aortic stenosis. Note the deep S wave in V_1–V_3 and tall R in V_5. Also, T wave inversion is present in 2, 3, AVF and V_6.

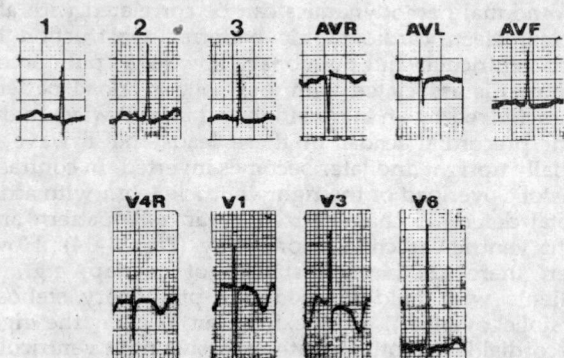

Figure 13–16 Electrocardiogram in hypocalcemia and hypokalemia (serum calcium 1.8 mEq/l; serum potassium 2.2 mEq/l at time of tracing). Note prolongation of electrical systole owing to long S-TU segment. This graph also shows left ventricular hypertrophy.

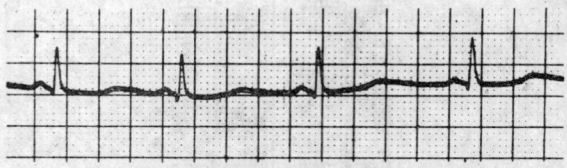

Figure 13–18 Prolonged QT intervals.

terval by the square root of the cycle length of the R-R interval. The normal Q-TC should be less than 0.45 sec. It is often lengthened in children with hypokalemia and hypocalcemia; in the former instance a U wave may be noted at the end of the T wave (Fig 13–16 and 13–17). Prolonged Q-T intervals (Fig 13–18) may be seen in children who are at risk for ventricular arrhythmias and sudden death (Jervel–Lange-Nielson syndrome with hearing loss or Romano-Ward syndrome).

S-T Segment and T Wave Abnormalities. Elevation of the S-T segment in normal teenagers is attributed to early repolarization of the heart. In generalized pericarditis, superficial epicardial involvement may cause elevation of the S-T segment followed by abnormal T wave inversion as healing progresses. Administration of digitalis is associated with sagging of the S-T segment and abnormal inversion of the T wave. Depression of the S-T segment may also occur in conditions that produce myocardial damage, e.g., anemia, carbon monoxide poisoning, endocardial sclerosis, aberrant origin of the left coronary artery from the pulmonary artery, glycogen storage disease of the heart, myocardial tumors, and gargoylism. Aberrant origin of the left coronary artery from the pulmonary artery may lead to changes indistinguishable from those of acute myocardial infarction in adults. Similar changes may occur in patients with other rare abnormalities of the coronary arteries

and with cardiomyopathy without anatomic abnormalities of the coronary arteries.

In any form of carditis simple inversion of the T wave may occur. Hypothyroidism may produce flat or inverted T waves in association with generalized low voltage. In hyperkalemia the T waves are commonly of high voltage and are tent-shaped (Fig 13–19).

13.4 VECTORCARDIOGRAPHIC DISPLAY

The spread of depolarization and repolarization through the heart is a succession of innumerable instantaneous electrical forces. The average of these forces determines a direction of electrical depolarization beginning with the ventricular septum and spreading to the free wall of the myocardium over both ventricles. The recording of the average direction magnitude and orientation of the individual vectors in a single curve constitutes the vectorcardiographic loop. The P wave and T waves are similarly inscribed. Reference lead systems have been devised to record the vectorcardiogram in 3 planes: horizontal, sagittal, and frontal. Furthermore, distorting factors of proximity, resistivity, and variations in thorax size are "corrected" by the lead systems currently used. Analysis of vectorcardiograms is helpful in supplemental evaluation and understanding of the scalar electrocardiogram.

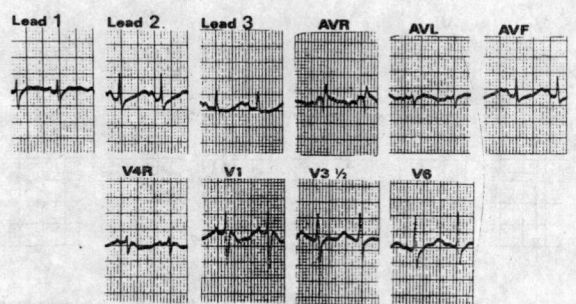

Figure 13–17 Electrocardiogram in hypokalemia (serum potassium 2.7 mEq/l; serum calcium 4.8 mEq/l at time of tracing). Note the prolongation of electrical systole as evidenced by a widened TU wave; also depression of the S-T segment in V₄R, V₁, and V₆.

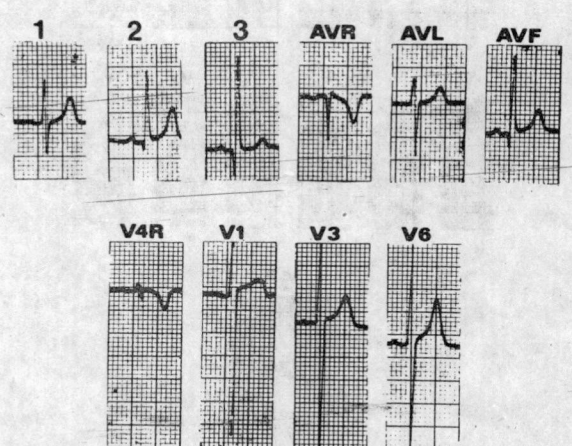

Figure 13–19 Electrocardiogram in hyperkalemia (serum potassium 6.5 mEq/l; serum calcium 5.1 mEq/l). Note the tall, tent-shaped T waves, especially in leads I, II, and V₆.

13.5 HEMATOLOGIC DATA

Evaluation of hematologic findings in infancy as part of the assessment of the cardiovascular system should be carried out with an awareness of the normal variations in infancy. Persistent polycythemia after the 1st mo of life is frequently noted in patients with right to left shunts and cyanosis. Patients with marked polycythemia have a delicate balance between intravascular thrombosis and a bleeding diathesis; this abnormal hemostasis should be recognized and treated prior to any surgical procedure. The most frequent abnormalities are accelerated fibrinolysis, thrombocytopenia, abnormal clot retraction, hypofibrinogenemia, prolonged prothrombin time, and prolonged partial thromboplastin time or thromboplastin generation time. These abnormalities occur singly or in combination and appear to be related to the severity of the polycythemia. Abnormal coagulation may be related to the effects of hypoxia and polycythemia on platelet production and consumption combined with the effects of chronic liver dysfunction on procoagulants and fibrinolysis. Since there are surgical palliative or corrective procedures for the majority of patients with cyanotic heart disease, the child with severe cyanosis and polycythemia is less frequently encountered than previously.

The preparation of cyanotic polycythemic patients for elective surgery such as dental extraction includes evaluation for and treatment of abnormal coagulation. Accelerated fibrinolysis has been suppressed with epsilon-aminocaproic acid. Thrombocytopenia and hypofibrinogenemia may be improved by phlebotomies. Repeated phlebotomies have also been used for symptomatic relief of headache, fatigue, and extreme dyspnea which frequently accompany longstanding polycythemia. This procedure, however, is not without risk, especially in polycythemic patients with extreme elevation of pulmonary vascular resistance. Because these patients do not tolerate wide fluctuations in circulating blood volume, the phlebotomy should be performed in the same way as an exchange transfusion; blood is replaced with fresh frozen plasma or albumin. Usually, the ideal level of hematocrit cannot be predicted; the frequency of phlebotomy is determined by improvement of symptoms and by the patient's sense of well-being as well as a hematocrit level above 65%. Initially, these patients require frequent phlebotomies (often weekly) until the hematocrit is more or less stabilized at the desired level (± 60%). Subsequently, phlebotomies may be necessary at only 3–5 wk intervals.

Iron deficiency anemia is poorly tolerated by cyanotic patients with right to left shunts, especially by infants and toddlers. Such children have more frequent hypercyanotic spells, more severe attacks of dyspnea, and greater increase in heart size. Iron therapy produces improvement, but surgical treatment of the cardiac anomaly is often required.

Because of high viscosity of polycythemic blood, infants with cyanotic congenital heart disease are at risk to develop vascular thrombosis, especially of cerebral veins. Polycythemic infants with iron deficiency are at even greater risk for cerebrovascular accidents, probably because thrombosis is enhanced by a decrease in velocity of blood flow as well as by altered deformability of the red cells.

13.6 ECHOCARDIOGRAPHY

Echocardiography (ultrasonography) has become an extremely important technique in the diagnosis of congenital and acquired cardiac disease in infants and children. Furthermore, it can be used to evaluate cardiac performance in a variety of circumstances, such as cardiac effects of drug toxicity, where there are secondary influences on myocardial function.

Echocardiography utilizes pulsed ultrasound with frequency above the audible range. These waves travel through fluid in a straight line but are reflected at the interface of substances of differing densities. They return in echoes from the strike zones (interfaces) of different acoustic impedance with a constant transit time. The distance can then be measured between the transducer on the skin and the interface from which the echoes are returned. Because there are no known risks to diagnostic ultrasound, this method can be used repeatedly in individual patients.

The reflected ultrasound display on an oscilloscope appears as dots. The horizontal axis of the oscilloscope relates to time, the vertical axis to the depth of tissues. The dots that are moving in the vertical axis because of cardiac contractions are swept across the oscilloscope to produce the motion mode (*M-mode*). The method is used to define the presence or absence of individual anatomic structures and their relationship to one another (Fig 13–20 and 13–21) and to evaluate cardiac function (Table 13–2). The development of cross section or *2 dimensional echocardiography* has greatly enhanced the ability to visualize spatial relationships of the cardiac structure (Fig 13–22). With this technique the image of the contracting heart is displayed in 2 dimensions by means of a number of different views which emphasize individual structures (valves, septa, hypertrophied muscle, etc.). Two dimensional echocardiographic studies display images similar to those seen by angiocardiogram, and they are interpreted in much the same manner (Fig 13–22). Motion mode and 2 dimensional echocardiography complement each other. The former is most important for evaluating cardiac function, whereas the latter allows specific visualization of structures and spatial relationships.

Used along with other clinical and/or laboratory methods, echocardiography facilitates a more rigorous selection process for cardiac catheterization and helps to improve the timing of hemodynamic studies. Echocardiography has also proved useful in the evaluation of congestive heart failure, pericardial fluid accumulation, atrial or ventricular septal defects, cardiac valve problems, vegetations due to infective endocarditis, intracardiac tumor or hematoma, cardiotoxic agents, and ductus arteriosus in premature infants. It also can monitor the results of surgical or medical intervention.

Contrast Echocardiography. The rapid injection of fluid (e.g., the patient's blood, saline, or other substances) produces microbubbles at the site of injection;

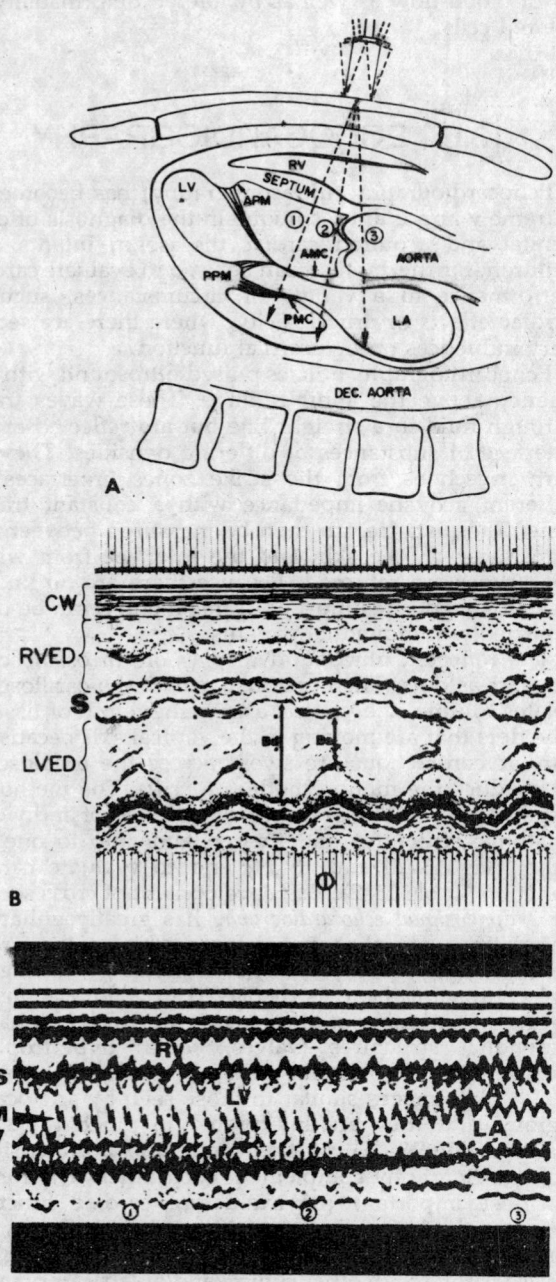

Figure 13–20 Normal echocardiograms. *A,* Diagram of sagittal section of heart showing structures traversed by echo beam in positions (1), (2), and (3). AMC, anterior mitral cusp; APM, anterior papillary muscle; Dec. aorta, descending aorta; LA, left atrium; LV, left ventricle; PMC, posterior mitral cusp; PPM, posterior papillary muscle; RV, right ventricle. *B,* Echocardiogram from transducer position (1); this is the best view to evaluate interventricular septum (S) and for measurement of right ventricular dimension (RVED) as well as of the left ventricular dimension (LVED) in end diastole (Bd) and end systole (Bs). CW, chest wall. *C,* Normal septal aortic and mitral aortic relationships obtained when transducer is swept from positions (1) through (3) of *A.* A, aortic valve; LA, left atrium; LV, left ventricle; MV, mitral valve; RV, right ventricle; S, interventricular septum. Note continuity of anterior mitral leaflet with posterior wall of aorta and of the ventricular septum with anterior wall of aorta.

these are harmless to the patient and travel in a bolus, from the site of infection in a vein or right atrium, through the chambers of the heart. This bolus is manifested by a cloud of echoes which can be visualized both by M-mode and 2 dimensional echocardiograms. The technique has great value in revealing flow patterns through various structures and in detecting intravascular shunts in the preoperative and immediate postoperative periods (Fig 13–23).

13.7 EXERCISE TESTING

The normal cardiorespiratory system adapts to the extensive demands of exercise with a several-fold increase in oxygen consumption and in cardiac output. Since there is a large reserve capacity for exercise, significant abnormalities of cardiovascular performance may exist without symptoms at rest or during ordinary activities. Generally, patients are evaluated in a resting state during which significant abnormalities of cardiac function may not be appreciated or, if detected, their implications about the quality of life may not be recognized. Permission for children with cardiovascular disease to participate in various forms of physical activity is frequently based on subjective criteria. Exercise testing plays an important role in evaluating symptoms, quantitating the severity of the cardiac abnormality, and assisting in the management of these patients.

As the child grows, the capacity for work increases with body size and skeletal muscle mass. All indices of cardiopulmonary function, however, do not increase in a uniform manner (Fig 13–24). A major response to exercise is an increase in cardiac output, principally as a result of increased heart rate, but stroke volume, systemic venous return, and pulse pressure are also increased. Systemic vascular resistance is greatly decreased by immediate vasodilatation. As the child becomes older and larger, the response of the heart rate to exercise remains prominent, but the cardiac output increases because of growing cardiac volume. Similarly, stroke volume is affected by both body size and sex. The larger the child, the larger the stroke volume; and, for any given body surface area, boys have a larger stroke volume than girls. At rest in the upright position the gravity effect results in venous pooling in the legs; with exercise, venous return increases and contributes to an increase in stroke volume.

In normal children an electrocardiogram during exercise shows a decrease in the R-R interval commensurate with the level of exercise. This decrease is primarily due to shortening of the T-P and Q-T intervals. S-T segmental depression may reflect changes in myocardial perfusion so that subendocardial ischemia may occur during exercise in children with a hypertrophied left ventricle. The exercise electrocardiogram is considered abnormal if S-T segmental depression is equal to or greater than 1 mm and extends for at least 0.06 sec after the J point (onset of S-T segment) in conjunction with a horizontal, upward, or downward sloping S-T segment. About 10% of normal children (more com-

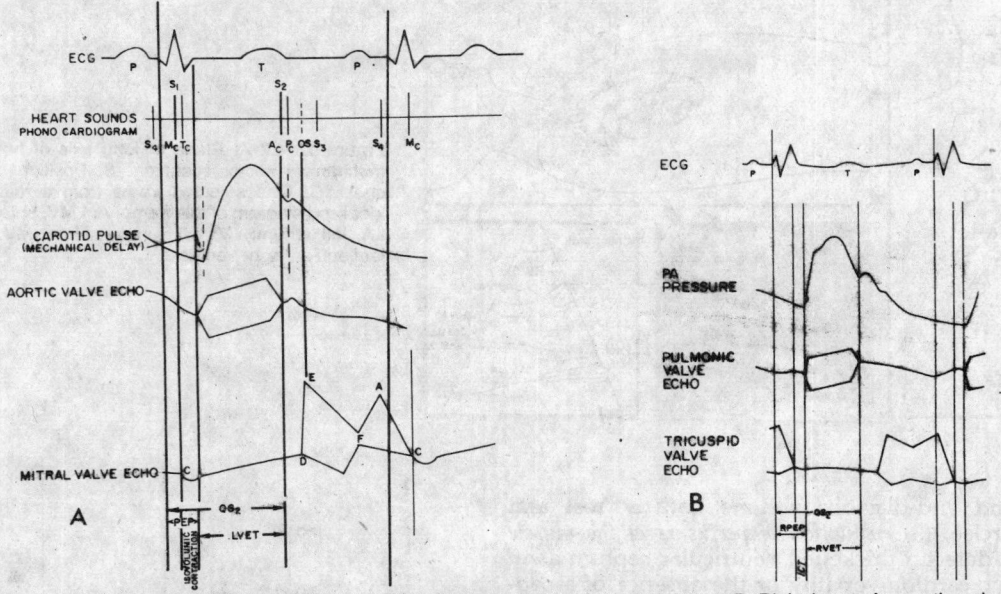

Figure 13–21 Temporal events of cardiac cycle determined by echocardiography. *A*, Left heart. *B*, Right heart. Ac, aortic valve closure; ECG, electrocardiogram; LVET, left ventricular ejection time; Mc, mitral valve closure; OS, opening snap; Pc, pulmonary valve closure; PEP, pre-ejection period; QS₂, total electromechanical systole; RVET, right ventricular ejection time; S₁, S₂, S₃, and S₄, 1st, 2nd, 3rd, and 4th heart sounds, respectively; Tc, tricuspid valve closure.

Table 13–2 ECHOGRAPHIC MEASUREMENT OF CARDIOVASCULAR PERFORMANCE

1. Per cent shortening = $\dfrac{LVED-LVES}{LVED} \times 100$ (see Fig 13–20*A*)

   LVED = left ventricular end diastolic dimension; LVES = left ventricular end systolic dimension. (*Normal*, 28–38%.)

2. Mean VCF = $\dfrac{LVED-LVES}{LVED \times ET}$

   VCF = mean velocity of circumferential fiber shortening (expressed as circumference [circ] per second); LVED and LVES as in (1) above; ET = ejection time. (*Normal values:* neonates, 1.51 ± 0.04 (SE) circ/sec; children (5–15 yr), 1.34 ± 0.03 (SE) circ/sec.)

3. Left ventricular volumes in end diastole (LVEDV) and systole (LVESV) may be derived from the following regression equation: LVEDV and LVESV = −19.2 + 14.58 Dd + 0.62 (Dd)³ when Dd or Ds = dimension in diastole or systole, respectively.

4. Ejection fraction (EF) $\dfrac{B_{es}}{B_{ed}} = \dfrac{\sqrt{1-EF}}{\sqrt{\dfrac{A_{es}}{A_{ed}}}}$

   B_{es} = end systolic dimension; B_{ed} = end diastolic dimension; A_{es} and A_{ed} represent the long axis of the left ventricle in systole and diastole, respectively, and are assumed to be 10%.

5. Stroke volume. SV = LVEDV−LVESV (abbreviations as in (3) above) or SV = LVEDV × EF (EF = ejection fraction).

6. Systolic time intervals (a) $\dfrac{LPEP}{LVET}$ (normal ranges are between 0.3–0.39; average, 0.35). LPEP = left ventricular pre-ejection period. LVET = left ventricular ejection time. (b) $\dfrac{RPEP}{RVET}$

   (normal ranges are between 0.16–0.30; average, 0.24). These ratios are increased by increased afterload, decreased preload, decreased contractility, electromechanical delay; they are decreased by decreased afterload, increased preload, enhanced contractility.

7. Isovolumic contraction (ICT) (Fig 13–21) may be derived from the following regression equation: ICT = 53 − .22 × heart rate (S.E. ± 7.3). ICT increased in left ventricular myocardial disease and decreased in aortic runoff (e.g., patent ductus arteriosus).

monly girls than boys) have depression of the S-T segment during exercise; this is frequently recorded in only 1 lead (usually V₅). The significance of this change is unknown. Arrhythmias are rarely recorded during or within 20 min after exercise in normal children.

Established indications for exercise testing include (1) left ventricular outflow obstruction, such as valvular, subvalvular, and supravalvular aortic stenosis, hypertrophic cardiomyopathy, and coarctation of the aorta; (2) chronic volume overload of the left or right ventricles, such as atrioventricular or semilunar valve incompetence and left to right shunts; (3) arrhythmias; and (4) hypertension.

A physician should be present during the exercise test to supervise its performance. Indications for its termination are (1) failure or inadequacy of the electrocardiographic monitoring; (2) onset of serious arrhythmias, such as ventricular or supraventricular tachycardia; (3) arrhythmias (more than 25% of beats) precipitated or aggravated by exercise; (4) development of heart block; (5) precipitation of pain, headache, dizziness, or syncope; (6) S-T segmental depression or elevation of 3 mm or more; (7) inappropriate hypertension (systolic pressure >230 mm Hg or diastolic pressure >120 mm Hg); (8) inappropriate fall of blood pressure; or (9) development of cutaneous vascular insufficiency (e.g., pallor).

13.8 RADIOACTIVE TRACERS

Advances in pediatric nuclear cardiology include (1) *radionuclide angiography* to detect and quantify shunts (Fig 13–25); (2) *hemodynamic measurements*, such as of cardiac output, stroke volume, left ventricular ejection

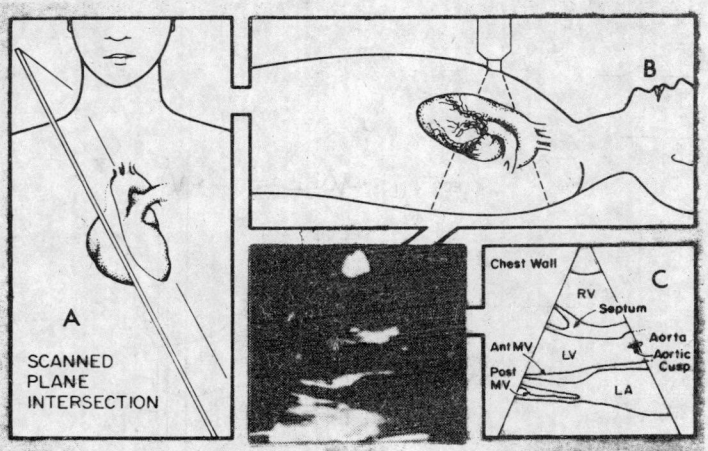

Figure 13–22 A, Plane of long axis of heart examined by mechanical sector scanning. B, Position of transducer on chest. C, One selected frame from a real-time study and idealized diagram of this frame. Ant MV, anterior mitral leaflet; LA, left atrium; LV, left ventricle; Post MV, posterior mitral leaflet; RV, right ventricle.

fraction, and end-diastolic volume both at rest and during exercise; (3) *evaluation of perfusion of the muscle mass:* (a) to detect a thickened ventricular septum as in hypertrophic cardiomyopathy or the absence of a septum (single ventricle); (b) to differentiate pulmonary arterial origin of the left coronary artery from dilated cardiomyopathy; (c) to recognize myocardial dysfunction in the stressed neonate; (d) to identify focal areas of myocardial ischemia; (4) *mapping of alterations in regional pulmonary blood flow* to aid in differentiating the combination of pulmonary arterial and venous hypertension (in which there is a relative increase of blood flow to the lung apices) from pulmonary arterial hypertension per se and to analyze the distribution of blood flow to each lung.

These advances reflect developments of gamma computer systems, short-lived radionuclides, and portable equipment that can be taken to the bedside of the seriously ill patient. The techniques impose little discomfort to the patient, and the radiation exposure is remarkably low, especially when compared to that of

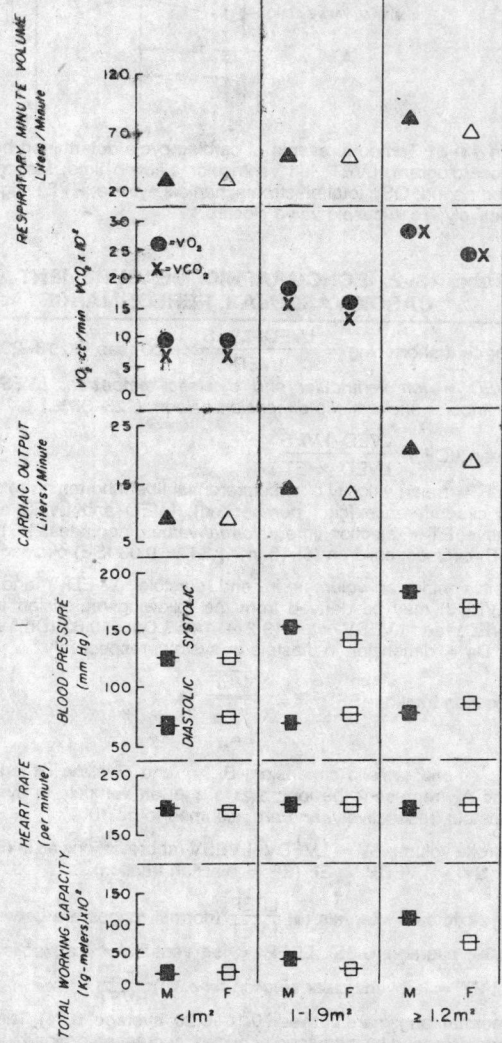

Figure 13–24 Cardiorespiratory changes at *maximal* exercise in normal children. The 3 columns refer to body surface area of <1 m², 1–1.19 m², and ≥ 1.2 m². In each column M refers to males and F to females. Total working capacity, heart rate, and blood pressure plotted as mean ± 2 standard errors. VO₂ = oxygen consumption, VCO₂ = carbon dioxide production.

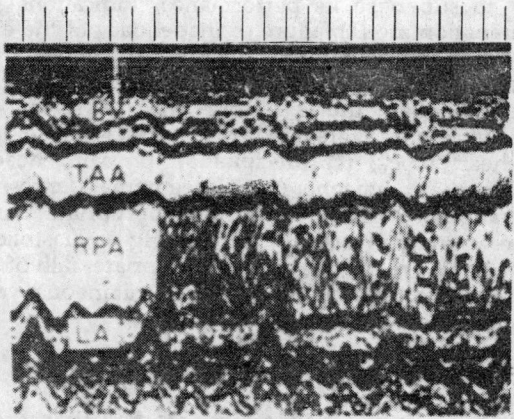

Figure 13–23 Contrast echocardiogram obtained after injection of 1 ml of blood in inferior vena cava of 3 day old infant with aortic atresia. Moment of injection indicated by arrow. Transducer in suprasternal notch identifies the small transverse aortic arch (TAA), the large right pulmonary artery (RPA) filled with a cloud of echocontrast soon after injection, and the small left atrium (LA). Time lines 40 msec.

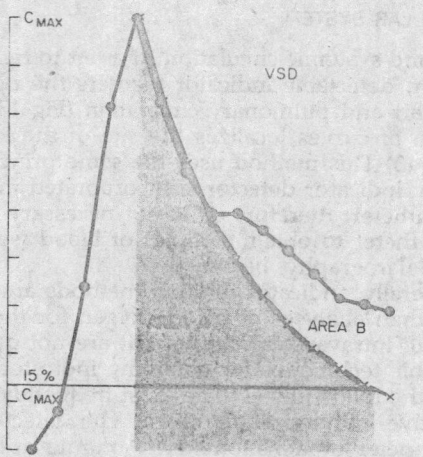

Figure 13–25. Estimation of left to right shunt from a pulmonary time activity curve obtained after injection of a bolus of ⁹⁹ᵐtechnetium. The method uses a Stewart-Hamilton extrapolation of the downslope of the curve. On the vertical axis is the course of radionuclide material from the area of interest in the lung. On the horizontal axis is time measured in sec. The line joined by dots represents the time activity curve of a patient with a ventricular septal defect. In the presence of a left to right shunt the exponential decline is interrupted by early recirculation. The line joined by Xs represents the idealized exponential decline in the absence of shunting and is extrapolated to a minimum value of 15% of the maximum radionuclide count (C_{max}). Thus the region beyond the peak is divided into 2 areas: A and B. From the ratio of area B to area A, an approximation of the shunt size can be made. Gamma function fitting of the pulmonary activity curve can be used as an alternative method for shunt estimation.

angiocardiography. Serial studies are thus possible when required for proper management. Isotope images obtained from radionuclide angiography do not provide the fine anatomic detail generally required to plan repair of intracardiac anomalies.

13.9 CARDIAC CATHETERIZATION

Cardiac catheterization remains the major tool of the pediatric cardiologist in the diagnosis of congenital heart disease. With this technique the various chambers of the heart, great vessels, and veins may be entered and blood samples obtained for measurement of oxygen saturation. Pressures are measured and contrast and indicator materials may be injected as required. Cardiac catheterization is essentially a presurgical diagnostic test and should be utilized only when there is a reasonable expectation that an operation will be required. Its use for purposes of reassurance when the clinical picture clearly indicates that no significant heart disease is present should be avoided. Although the risks are low, cardiac catheterization is an invasive test involving risk for the patient and should not be used without an opportunity for benefit. In many instances echocardiographic and radionuclide studies may be utilized in lieu of multiple cardiac catheterizations in individual patients who require careful monitoring of their hemodynamic status.

Cardiac catheterization should be carried out with the patient in a basal state; this is often not possible with children. Children are routinely sedated during these studies, but anesthesia is avoided if possible since depression of cardiovascular function by various anesthetic agents may distort the calculations of hemodynamic measurements, including cardiac output, pulmonary and systemic resistance, and shunt ratios.

If cardiac catheterization is performed on a critically ill infant with congenital heart disease, a surgical team should be alerted in the event that an operation is required immediately afterward. The complication rate of cardiac catheterization and angiography is greatest among critically ill infants; they must be studied in a thermally neutral environment and treated quickly for complications, including hyperthermia, acidemia, or excess blood loss. Development of soft, flow-directed balloon-tipped catheters has greatly decreased the frequency of complications from catheter manipulation, such as severe arrhythmias, cardiac perforations, and intramyocardial injection of contrast material.

In most instances catheterization involves both the left and right heart. The catheter is passed into the heart under fluoroscopic guidance via a percutaneous entry point in the femoral vein. The left heart is usually entered by passing the catheter across the former foramen ovale to the left atrium and left ventricle. The left heart is also catheterized by passing the catheter retrograde through the femoral artery and the aorta and across the aortic valve. The catheter is manipulated through abnormal intracardiac defects or into malpositioned great vessels. Complete hemodynamics can be calculated (Table 13–3) through data obtained at catheterization: cardiac output, intracardiac shunts, and systemic and pulmonary resistances.

Indicator Dilution and Appearance Techniques. If a bolus of indicator material is injected intravenously or into the right side of the heart, it traverses the pulmonary circulation and enters the left side of the heart and then the arterial circulation. This indicator material may then be detected in the arterial blood. A continuous record of the circulation of indicator in normal subjects shows 2 peaks (Fig 13–26). The time between the instant of injection and the detection of the indicator in arterial blood is known as the appearance time and is a measure of circulation time. The 1st peak of the indicator curve is due to the passage of indicator past the arterial detectors, the 2nd, to recirculation through the systemic arterial and venous systems, the pulmonary circulation, and reappearance in the arterial tree. If the concentration of circulating indicator is known, cardiac output can be computed.

Localization of intracardiac and extracardiac shunts may be facilitated by these methods. Curves obtained after the injection of indicator at or upstream from the site of a **right to left shunt** show a short appearance time because of the escape of indicator across the defect (Fig 13–26). This initial curve is followed by a 2nd peak produced by the indicator which has traversed the longer normal pathway through the lungs. In contrast, curves obtained from injection of an indicator downstream from the site of a right to left shunt show a normal appearance time.

Table 13–3 NORMAL VALUES AND FORMULAS FOR DETERMINATION OF HEMODYNAMICS IN CARDIAC CATHETERIZATION

1. Cardiac index 3.1 ± 0.4 l/min/M²
2. Arteriovenous oxygen difference 4.5 ± 0.7 ml/dl
3. Oxygen consumption 140–160 ml/M²/min
4. Arterial oxygen saturation 94–100%
5. Difference in oxygen content between venae cavae and right atrium < 1.9 vol %
6. Difference in oxygen content between right atrium and right ventricle < 0.9 vol %
7. Difference in oxygen content between right ventricle and pulmonary artery < 0.5 vol %
8. Normal mean left atrial pressure 4–8 mm Hg
9. Pulmonary arteriolar resistance 50–150 dyne sec cm⁻⁵ (1 unit = 80 dynes)
10. Cardiac output ml/min =

$$\frac{O_2 \text{ intake (ml/min)}}{\left\{ \begin{array}{l} O_2 \text{ content of arterial blood (vols \%)} \\ \text{minus } O_2 \text{ content of mixed venous blood} \end{array} \right.} \times 100$$

11. Cardiac index = cardiac output (l/min)/M² of body surface area
12. Pulmonary artery flow =

$$\frac{O_2 \text{ intake (ml/min)}}{\left\{ \begin{array}{l} O_2 \text{ content of pulmonary venous blood (vols \%)} \\ \text{minus } O_2 \text{ content of pulmonary arterial blood (vols \%)} \end{array} \right.} \times 100$$

If a pulmonary venous sample is not available, it is assumed to be saturated to 95% of capacity

13. Systemic flow =

$$\frac{O_2 \text{ intake (ml/min)}}{\left\{ \begin{array}{l} \text{systemic arterial } O_2 \text{ content (vols \%)} \\ \text{minus arterial venous } O_2 \text{ content (vols \%)} \end{array} \right.} \times 100$$

14. Effective pulmonary artery flow =

$$\frac{O_2 \text{ intake (ml/min)}}{\left\{ \begin{array}{l} \text{pulmonary venous } O_2 \text{ content (vols \%)} \\ \text{minus mixed venous } O_2 \text{ content (vols \%)} \end{array} \right.} \times 100$$

15. Total left to right shunt = pulmonary artery flow minus effective pulmonary artery flow
16. Total right to left shunt = systemic flow minus effective pulmonary artery flow
17. Pulmonary arteriolar resistance $R = \dfrac{PA - PC}{PF}$

   Where R = pulmonary arteriolar resistance (resistance units)
   PA = mean pulmonary artery pressure in mm Hg
   PC = mean pulmonary "capillary" pressure in mm Hg
   PF = pulmonary flow in l/min/M²

In the presence of left to right shunts some of the indicator has a normal transit time to the detection site while the remaining indicator recirculates through the lungs in a prolonged transit time. Curves recorded from systemic arterial blood have normal appearance times, reduced peak concentration, and prolonged disappearance times (Fig 13–26). Similar curves may be obtained in the presence of valvular regurgitation. Left to right shunts may be localized by the following methods: (1) Indicator is injected upstream or downstream from the site of the shunt and curves are recorded from a systemic arterial detector. Downstream injections result in normal curves. If indicator is injected at or upstream to the site of shunt, the curve is as described above. (2) This method requires 2 cardiac catheters. The 1st is placed in the distal pulmonary artery or left side of the heart for injection of indicator. The 2nd is placed in the lesser circulation for sampling of blood containing indicator from the vena cava, right atrium, right ventricle, or pulmonary artery. After injection of the indicator into the distal pulmonary artery, it traverses the pulmonary circulation and appears in the left side of the heart and systemic circulation. If a left to right shunt is present, detectable indicator reenters the right side of the heart and pulmonary circulation (Fig 13–26); comparison of curves localizes the site of the left to right shunt. (3) This method uses the same principle as (2), but the indicator detector is incorporated into the cardiac catheter; therefore, it is not necessary to insert a 2nd catheter to obtain samples of blood (see Ascorbic Acid Polarography, below).

Generally, indicator dilution methods are more sensitive than analyses of blood oxygen for the detection of small intravascular shunts but are not quantitative. Available techniques for obtaining indicator curves include the following: (1) The most frequently used indicator dye is indocyanine green. The detector is either an oximeter or densitometer. Accurate application of this method usually requires the continuous withdrawal of blood for the inscription of the dye dilution curve. (2) Ascorbic acid polarography consists of anodically polarized platinum electrodes which are depolarized by certain readily oxidizable substances such as ascorbic acid to generate a current. This technique has a particular advantage in infants and children because the platinum detector is placed intravascularly; it is not necessary to withdraw blood for the inscription of the ascorbate dilution curve. The platinum electrode may be inserted intra-arterially for localization of right to left shunts and incorporated in the wall of the catheter for detection of left to right shunts. (3) Radioactive gases such as krypton-85 have also been used for the localization of left to right shunts by principles similar to those described under (4).

(4) A platinum electrode capable of sensing hydrogen is incorporated onto the tip of a cardiac catheter which is inserted intravascularly or into the cardiac chambers (usually right). The detection and localization of left to right shunts depend on the fact that the electrode develops a potential in the presence of blood which has been exposed to hydrogen in the lungs, the patient having taken a breath of hydrogen. The instant the hydrogen appears in the nasal passages may be timed with another hydrogen electrode mounted in a flexible tube which has been brought into contact with the mucosa of the nose (airway signal). Some prefer to use an arterial hydrogen electrode for timing. Thus, it is possible to time accurately the inhalation of hydrogen and its subsequent appearance in any part of the circulatory system. For example, in patients with ventricular septal defect and left to right shunt, the hydrogen appearance time will be normal in the venae cavae and right atrium. However, curves obtained from the right ventricle and pulmonary artery will show an early appearance time because left heart blood containing hydrogen has been shunted across the ventricular defect.

(5) Thermodilution estimates cardiac output by measurement of forward systemic venous flow. A known change in heat content of the blood is induced at 1 point in the circulation (usually the right atrium or inferior vena cava), and the resultant change in temperature is detected at a point downstream (usually the pulmonary artery). The injectate is iced or room temperature saline. This method of measuring cardiac out-

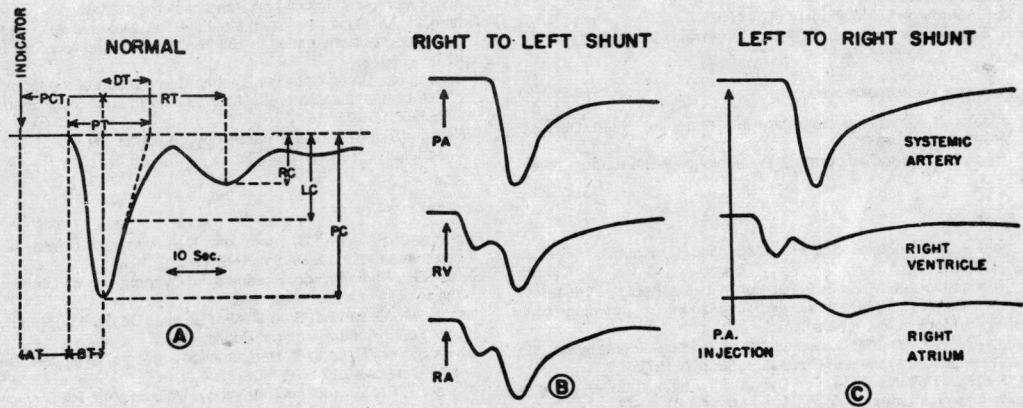

Figure 13–26 Idealized diagrams of indicator dilution curves. *A,* Normal curve showing time and concentration components. Instant of indicator injection in right side of heart shown by arrow at top left. Curve obtained from indicator detector in a systemic artery. AT, appearance time; BT, build-up time; DT, disappearance time; LC, least concentration; PC, peak concentration; PCT, peak concentration time; PT, passage time; RC, maximal recirculation concentration; RT, recirculation time. Extrapolation of declining slope of concentration is easier if the curve is plotted on a logarithmic scale. Cardiac output may be computed by the formula $\frac{601}{c(PT)}$, where 1 = amount of indicator, c = mean concentration of indicator, PT = passage time. *B,* Localization of *right to left shunt.* Instant of injection of indicator shown by arrows. Example illustrates shunt at ventricular level. Site of injection: PA, pulmonary artery; RA, right atrium; RV, right ventricle. Indicator detector in systemic artery in all instances. PA injection (i.e., downstream from shunt level) shows normal appearance time. RV and RA injections (i.e., at and upstream from shunt level) show early appearance times. *C,* Localization of *left to right shunt.* Example illustrates shunt at ventricular level. Indicator injected into distal pulmonary artery (PA) in all instances. In upper tracing indicator detector is in a systemic artery, and curve shows prolonged disappearance time. Middle curve is from indicator detected in right ventricle and shows an early appearance time because of ventricular septal defect. Right atrial curve shows normal appearance time.

put can be useful in planning therapy immediately after cardiac surgery and in caring for the critically ill infant or child with suspected low cardiac output (e.g., septic or traumatic shock). It is also of value in measuring cardiac output in the catheterization laboratory in patients without shunts (e.g., aortic stenosis or coarctation of the aorta). When combined with the dye dilution technique, it is also used to measure the volume of regurgitant flow across diseased mitral or aortic valves.

Angiocardiography. The great blood vessels and individual cardiac chambers may be seen by selective angiocardiography, i.e., injection of contrast material into specific cardiac chambers or great vessels. This method allows identification of specific abnormalities without interference from the superimposed shadows of normal chambers. Serial roentgenograms may be obtained in 2 planes at a rate of 6–14/sec.

Photofluorography with image intensification has made possible simultaneous cardiac catheterization and selective angiocardiography. The preferred method is a combination of photofluorography with closed-circuit television to monitor the fluoroscopic screen and allow visualization of the cardiac silhouette and the cardiac catheter. After the cardiac catheter is introduced into the chamber to be studied, a small amount of contrast medium is rapidly injected and moving pictures are exposed at 60 frames/sec. Biplane cineangiocardiography allows detailed evaluation of specific cardiac chambers and blood vessels in 2 planes with the injection of a single bolus of contrast material. Various angle views are utilized to best display anatomic features in individual lesions. These techniques require sophisticated radiographic equipment including special tables and flexibly placed x-ray units.

The rapid injection of contrast medium under pressure into the circulation is not without risks, and each injection should be carefully planned. Contrast agents consist of hypertonic solutions containing organic iodides which can cause complications including nausea, a generalized burning sensation, central nervous system symptoms, and allergic rashes. Intramyocardial injection, generally avoided by careful placement of the catheter prior to injection, can lead to transient nausea, vomiting, and a generalized or localized burning sensation. Hypertonicity of the contrast media may result in transient myocardial depression, a drop in blood pressure, tachycardia, increase in cardiac output, shift of fluid into the circulation with aggravation of cardiac failure, and dehydration from subsequent diuresis.

"Idealized" diagrams of the normal angiocardiogram are shown in Fig 13–6. The indications for this study are outlined under the individual congenital lesions.

General

Friedman WF, Lesch M, Sonnenblick EH: Neonatal Heart Disease. New York, Grune & Stratton, 1972 and 1973.

Keith JD, et al: Heart Disease in Infancy and Childhood. Ed 3. New York, Macmillan, 1978.

Kidd BS, Keith JD: The Natural History and Progress in Treatment of Congenital Heart Defects. Springfield, Ill., Charles C Thomas, 1971.

Moss AJ, Adams FH, Emmanouilides GC: Heart Disease in Infants, Children and Adolescents. Ed 2. Baltimore, Williams & Wilkins, 1977.

Nadas AS, Fyler DC: Pediatric Cardiology. Ed 3. Philadelphia, WB Saunders, 1972.

Rudolph AM: Congenital Diseases of the Heart. Chicago, Year Book Medical Publishers, 1974.

Cardiac Sounds and Phonocardiography

Baragan J, Fernandez F, Thiron JM, et al (eds): Dynamic Auscultation and Phonocardiography. Bowie, Md., Charles Press Publishers, 1979.

Caceres CA, Perry LW: The Innocent Murmur: A Problem in Clinical Practice. Boston, Little, Brown, 1966.
Leatham A: Systolic murmurs. Circulation 17:601, 1958.
Mills P, Craige E: Echophonocardiography. Prog Cardiovasc Dis 20:337, 1978.

Electrocardiogram and Vectorcardiogram

Ellison RC, Restieaux NJ: Vectorcardiography in Congenital Heart Disease. Philadelphia, WB Saunders, 1972.
Guntheroth WG: Pediatric Electrocardiography. Philadelphia, WB Saunders, 1965.

Echocardiography

Baker ML, Dalrymple GV: Biologic effects of diagnostic ultrasound: A review. Radiology 126:479, 1978.
Feigenbaum H: Echocardiography. Ed 3. Philadelphia, Lea & Febiger, 1981.
Goldberg SJ, Allen HD, Sahn DJ: Pediatric and Adolescent Echocardiography. Chicago, Year Book Medical Publishers, 1975.
Henry WL, Maron BJ, Griffith JM: Cross-sectional echocardiography in the diagnosis of congenital heart disease. Circulation 56:267, 1977.
Kisslo JA, von Ramm OT, Thurstone FL: Dynamic cardiac imaging using a focused, phased-array ultrasound system. Am J Med 63:61, 1977.
Meyer RA: Pediatric Echocardiography. Philadelphia, Lea & Febiger, 1977.
Sahn DJ, Allen HD, Goldberg SJ, et al: Mitral valve prolapse in children. A problem defined by real-time cross-sectional echocardiography. Circulation 53:651, 1976.
Silverman NH: Newer noninvasive methods in pediatric cardiology: Echocardiography, isotope angiography. In: Barness LA (ed): Advances in Pediatrics, Vol 23. Chicago, Year Book Medical Publishers, 1976, p 357.
Williams RG: Echocardiographic Diagnosis of Congenital Heart Disease. Boston, Little, Brown, 1977.

Exercise Testing

Astrand P, Rodahl K: Textbook of Work Physiology. New York, McGraw-Hill, 1970.
Cumming GR, Everatt D, Hastman L: Bruce treadmill test in children: Normal values in a clinical population. Am J Cardiol 41:69, 1978.
Epstein SE, Beiser GD, Goldstein RE, et al: Hemodynamic abnormalities in response to mild and intense upright exercise following operative correction of an atrial septal defect or tetralogy of Fallot. Circulation 47:1065, 1973.
Fortuin NJ, Weiss JL: Exercise stress testing. Circulation 56:700, 1977.
Godfrey S: Exercise Testing in Children. Philadelphia, WB Saunders, 1974.

James FW, Glueck CJ, Fallat RW, et al: Maximal exercise stress testing in normal and hyperlipidemic children. Atherosclerosis 25:85, 1976.
Rozanski JJ, Dimich I, Steinfeld L, et al: Maximal exercise stress testing in evaluation of arrhythmias in children: Results and reproducibility. Am J Cardiol 42:951, 1979.
Truccone NJ, Steeg CN, Dell R, et al: Comparison of the cardiocirculatory effects of exercise and isoproterenol in children with pulmonary or aortic valve stenosis. Circulation 56:79, 1977.
Willerson JT (ed): Nuclear cardiology. In: Brest AN (ed): Cardiovascular Clinics. Philadelphia, FA Davis, 1979.

Radioactive Tracers

Friedman WF, Sahn DJ, Hirschklau MS: A review: Newer, noninvasive cardiac diagnostic methods. Pediatr Res 11:190, 1977.
Gates GF: Radionuclide Scanning in Cyanotic Heart Disease. Springfield, Ill., Charles C Thomas, 1974.
Serafini AN, Gilson AJ, Smoak WM: Nuclear Cardiology, Principles and Methods. New York, Plenum Medical Books, 1977.
Treves S, Fogl R, Lang P: Radionuclide angiography in congenital heart disease. Am J Cardiol 46:1247, 1980.
Willerson JT (ed): Nuclear Cardiology. Philadelphia, FA Davis, 1979.

Cardiac Catheterization

Bargeron LM, Elliot LP, Soto B, et al: Axial cineangiography in congenital heart disease. Circulation 56:1075, 1977.
Braunwald E, Swan HJC: Cooperative Study on Cardiac Catheterization. Am Heart Assoc Monograph No 20, New York, 1968.
Elliott LP, Bargeron LM, Bream PR, et al: Axial cineangiography in congenital heart disease. Circulation 56:1048, 1977.
Freed MD, Keane JF: Cardiac output measured by thermodilution in infants and children. J Pediatr 92:39, 1978.
Martin EC, Olson AP, Steeg CN, et al: Radiation exposure to the pediatric patient during cardiac catheterization and angiography. Circulation 64:153, 1981.
Rushmer RF: Cardiovascular Dynamics. Ed 4. Philadelphia, WB Saunders, 1976.
Schwartz DC, Kaplan S: Cardiac catheterization and selective angiography in infants with a new flow-directed catheter. Cath Cardiovasc Diag 1:59, 1975.
Stanger P, Heymann MA, Tarnoff H, et al: Complications of cardiac catheterization of neonates, infants, and children: A three year study. Circulation 50:595, 1974.
Wood EH: Diagnostic applications of indicator dilution technics in congenital heart disease. Circ Res 10:531, 1962.
Yang SS, Bentivoglio LG, Maranhao V, et al: From Cardiac Catheterization Data to Hemodynamic Parameters. Ed 2, Philadelphia, FA Davis, 1978.

13.10   FETAL AND NEONATAL CIRCULATION

Fetal Circulation.   Most of the information concerning fetal circulation has been derived from studies of lambs and monkeys. Although there may be some species differences, the human fetal circulation and its adjustments after birth are probably similar. Oxygenated blood from the placenta flows to the fetus through the umbilical vein at an average rate of 175 ml/kg with a pressure close to 12 mm Hg and a pO_2 of about 30 mm Hg. Approximately 50% of the umbilical venous blood bypasses the liver and flows through the ductus venosus into the inferior vena cava, where it mixes with the remainder of the blood returning from the caudal part of the body and enters the right atrium from the inferior vena cava. It preferentially passes across the foramen ovale to the left atrium, flows into the left ventricle, and is ejected into the ascending aorta. The coronary and cerebral arteries and those of the upper extremities are thus perfused with blood having a higher pO_2 than that perfusing other parts of the body, except for the liver. The superior vena caval blood which is considerably less oxygenated, traverses the tricuspid valve and flows primarily to the right ventricle and pulmonary arterial trunk. The major portion of this blood (which has a pO_2 of 19–22 mm Hg) bypasses the lungs and flows through the ductus arte-

riosus into the descending aorta to perfuse the caudal part of the body as well as the placenta via the umbilical arteries. The effective fetal cardiac output, i.e., the sum of the left ventricular output and the ductal flow, amounts to about 220 ml/kg/min. Approximately 65% of this blood returns to the placenta; the remaining 35% perfuses the fetal organs and tissues (Fig 13–27). See also Sec 7.4 and 7.7.

Since the fetal ventricles work in parallel rather than in series, the distribution of their ejected blood depends on resistance and flow and the fact that the large ductus arteriosus equalizes aortic and pulmonary arterial pressures. The high pulmonary vascular resistance diverts pulmonary arterial blood from the lungs to the ductus arteriosus and descending aorta. The mechanisms that result in pulmonary arteriolar constriction are not completely understood. Fetal alveoli filled with fluid and the tortuous and kinked small blood vessels of the unexpanded lung both retard blood flow. It is generally agreed, however, that the level of pO_2 of the blood perfusing the lung has the greatest influence on pulmonary vascular resistance; when pulmonary arterial pO_2 exceeds about 35 mm Hg, pulmonary vascular resistance falls and pulmonary flow increases.

Neonatal Circulation.   Dramatic changes occur as

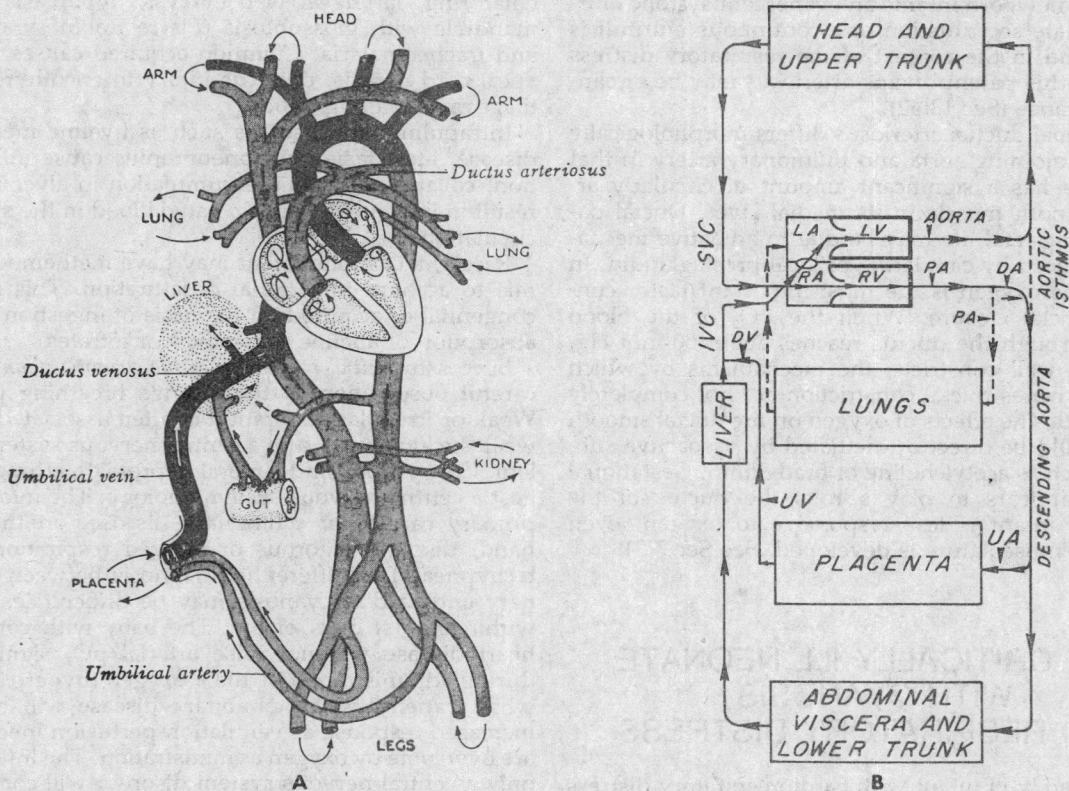

HEAD

ARM

ARM

Ductus arteriosus

LUNG

LUNG

LIVER

Ductus venosus

Umbilical vein

KIDNEY

GUT

PLACENTA

Umbilical artery

LEGS

A

HEAD AND
UPPER TRUNK

SVC

IVC

LA   LV   AORTA

RA   RV   PA   DA

AORTIC
ISTHMUS

PA

DV

LIVER

LUNGS

DESCENDING AORTA

UV

PLACENTA

UA

ABDOMINAL
VISCERA AND
LOWER TRUNK

B

Figure 13–27 A, Plan of the human circulation before birth (partly after Dawes). Colors show the quality of the blood, and arrows indicate its direction of flow (Arey). B, In the fetus a large fraction of the umbilical venous blood enters the ductus venosus (DV) and bypasses the liver. This relatively well-oxygenated blood flows across the foramen ovale to the left heart, which preferentially perfuses the head and upper trunk. Superior vena caval blood (SVC) is ejected by the right heart into the pulmonary artery (PA) and ductus arteriosus (DA). This blood circulates to the placenta as well as to the abdominal viscera and lower trunk. Interrupted lines indicate a low pulmonary blood flow and the flow from the ascending aorta across the aortic isthmus is also diminished. DA, ductus arteriosus; DV, ductus venosus; IVC, inferior vena cava; LA, left atrium; LV, left ventricle; PA, pulmonary artery; RA, right atrium; RV, right ventricle; SVC, superior vena cava. (From Kaplan S, Assali NS: Pathophysiology of Gestation, 1972).

the fetal circulation adapts to extrauterine life and gas exchange is transferred from the placenta to the lung of the newborn infant. These changes do not occur instantaneously but are effected over hours or days. After an initial fall there is a progressive rise in systemic blood pressure, and the heart rate slows as a result of an increase in systemic vascular resistance when the placental circulation is eliminated. The average central aortic pressure in the neonate is 75/50 mm Hg. With the onset of ventilation a marked increase in pulmonary blood flow occurs because of the dilatative effect of oxygen on the constricted pulmonary blood vessels. Pulmonary venous return is thus increased and consequently left ventricular output. In the normal neonate, ductal closure and fall of pulmonary vascular resistance result in a fall of pulmonary arterial and right ventricular pressures. The major decline of pressure from the high fetal levels to the low "adult" levels in the human infant at sea level usually occurs within the 1st 2–3 days but may be prolonged for 7 days or more.

Significant differences between the neonatal circulation and that of older infants may be summarized as follows: (1) right to left shunting may persist across the patent foramen ovale; (2) continued patency of the ductus arteriosus may allow left to right, right to left, or bidirectional shunting; (3) the neonatal pulmonary vasculature retains the ability to constrict vigorously in response to hypoxemia, hypercapnia, and acidosis; (4) the muscular mass of the left and right ventricles is almost equal; (5) the neonate has a lower systemic arterial pressure and an unusual tolerance to hypoxemia; and (6) newborn infants at rest have a relatively high oxygen consumption which is associated with their relatively high cardiac output. A high percentage of fetal hemoglobin may interfere with delivery of oxygen to the tissues since there is reduced binding of 2,3-diphosphoglycerate in fetal hemoglobin. Under these conditions an increased cardiac output would be required for adequate delivery of oxygen to the tissues. See also Sec 7.31.

After birth the foramen ovale, ductus arteriosus, and ductus venosus are no longer needed, but their closure proceeds gradually. The foramen ovale is functionally closed by the 3rd mo of life, though it is possible to pass a probe through the overlapping flaps in 25% of adults. Functional closure of the ductus arteriosus is usually complete by 10–15 hr in the normal neonate. During the periods of adjustment there are rarely physical signs of patency of these structures. However, in premature newborn infants an evanescent systolic murmur with late accentuation or a continuous murmur is audible, and in the context of the respiratory distress syndrome this patent ductus arteriosus may be of clinical importance (Sec 13.42).

The normal ductus arteriosus differs morphologically from the adjoining aorta and pulmonary artery in that the ductus has a significant amount of circularly arranged smooth muscle in its medial layer. Ductal patency during fetal life may be due to an active mechanism produced by circulating or local prostaglandin. In the neonate oxygen is the most important factor controlling ductal closure. When the pO_2 of the blood passing through the ductus reaches about 50 mm Hg, the ductal wall constricts; the mechanisms by which oxygen activates ductal constriction are not completely understood. The effects of oxygen on the ductal smooth muscle could be direct or mediated by vasoactive substances such as acetylcholine or bradykinin. Gestational age also appears to play a role; the ductus of the premature infant is less responsive to oxygen, even though its musculature is developed. See Sec 7.31.

THE CRITICALLY ILL NEONATE WITH CYANOSIS AND RESPIRATORY DISTRESS

The severely ill infant with cardiorespiratory distress and cyanosis presents a diagnostic challenge which is especially amenable to systematic evaluation based on the mechanism of the oxygenation defect. Cyanosis on a cardiac basis occurs secondary to right to left intracardiac or intraductal shunting. The neonate with primary pulmonary disease will be cyanotic on the basis of ventilation-perfusion inequalities or hypoventilation. In addition, the baby with severe central nervous system disease or upper airway obstruction will be cyanotic secondary to hypoventilation.

Cardiac Disease. Congenital heart disease is responsible for cyanosis when obstruction to right ventricular outflow causes intracardiac right to left shunting or when complex anatomic defects, unassociated with pulmonary stenosis, cause admixture of pulmonary and systemic venous return in the heart. In addition, right to left shunts across the foramen ovale and ductus arteriosus due to pulmonary vascular obstruction also occur in neonates (Sec 13.12).

Central Nervous System. Irregular shallow breathing, secondary to central nervous system depression, results in reduced alveolar ventilation and an abnormally low alveolar oxygen tension. Arterial pCO_2 is elevated. Intracranial hemorrhage accounts for most cases of this type of cyanosis.

Pulmonary Disease. Upper airway obstructions result in cyanosis by the same basic mechanism responsible for central nervous system cyanosis, e.g., alveolar hypoventilation due to reduced pulmonary ventilation. Obstruction may occur from the nares to the carina, and the important diagnostic possibilities among the

congenital abnormalities include choanal atresia, vascular ring, laryngeal web or cyst, hypoplasia of the mandible with glossoptosis (Pierre Robin syndrome), and tracheomalacia. Common acquired causes include vocal cord paresis, obstetric injury to cricothyroid cartilage, and a foreign body.

Intrapulmonary diseases such as hyaline membrane disease, atelectasis, and pneumonitis cause inflammation, collapse, and fluid accumulation in alveoli which result in incompletely oxygenated blood in the systemic circulation.

Rarely, a cyanotic infant may have methemoglobinemia to account for arterial desaturation. This may be congenital or acquired on the basis of ingestion or skin absorption of analine derivatives or nitrates.

Successful *initial evaluation of the cyanotic infant* lies in careful observation of the infant's breathing pattern. Weak or irregular respiration is often associated with a weak sucking reflex and a central nervous system problem. Convulsions and general depression strongly suggest a central nervous system etiology. The infant with primary cardiac or pulmonary disease, on the other hand, displays vigorous or labored respirations with tachypnea. The differential diagnosis between pulmonary and cardiac cyanosis may be difficult, especially within the 1st days of life. The baby with congenital heart disease will not raise arterial pO_2 significantly during administration of 100% oxygen (hyperoxia test), while patients with pulmonary disease will have an increased response as ventilation-perfusion inequalities are overcome by oxygen administration. The infant with only a central nervous system disorder will completely normalize arterial pO_2 during artificial ventilation. If the arterial pO_2 rises above 150 torr during 100% oxygen administration, an anatomic shunt can generally be excluded.

A significant heart murmur suggests a cardiac basis for cyanosis. However, several of the more severe cardiac defects do not manifest a murmur. The chest roentgenogram may be helpful in the differentiation of pulmonary from cardiac disease and, in the latter, will indicate whether pulmonary blood flow is increased, normal, or decreased. This distinction is important in the differentiation of various congenital heart lesions which cause cyanosis in the neonate.

Echocardiography is extremely helpful in determining whether congenital heart disease is present in situations in which cardiac and pulmonary disease both appear to be present. The information obtained by this technique can help avoid unnecessary cardiac catheterization and angiography in the absence of a cardiac defect.

13.11 NEONATAL PULMONARY HYPERTENSION

Persistent pulmonary hypertension in the newborn occurs under a variety of different circumstances and as a result of a number of different underlying mechanisms. Pulmonary vasoconstriction and hypertension following hypoxemia can result in right to left patent foramen ovale and ductus arteriosus shunting in what appears to be a primary syndrome (persistent fetal circulation). In addition, pulmonary hypertension may be a secondary feature of a variety of cardiac and pulmonary diseases. Furthermore, decreased numbers of arterial vessels in the lungs of infants with congenital or acquired pulmonary hypoplasia result in a similar syndrome of high pulmonary vascular resistance and right to left shunting via the fetal channels.

The numerous disease entities which result in pulmonary hypertension should be classified on the basis of anatomic and physiologic causes in order to formulate a rational approach to diagnosis and management. Pulmonary hypertension may occur secondary to (1) pulmonary venous hypertension, (2) functional obstruction of pulmonary vascular blood flow, (3) pulmonary vascular constriction with or without increased pulmonary vascular smooth muscle, or (4) decreased pulmonary vascular bed, or (5) it may be associated with systemic right ventricle or single ventricle without pulmonary stenosis (Table 13–4). The term **persistent pulmonary hypertension** is applied to all of these cases but is not a specific diagnosis.

Pulmonary venous hypertension may occur in infants with a variety of congenital defects which cause pulmonary venous obstruction in the 1st day or 2 of life. These include stenosis of the pulmonary veins, cor triatriatum, congenital mitral stenosis, and supervalvular webs. Infants with left ventricular failure because of a well defined cardiac lesion also have pulmonary artery hypertension. Coarctation of the aorta, aortic valve disease, and cardiomyopathy (such as endocardial fibroelastosis) are included in this group. Infants with transient left ventricular dysfunction secondary to hypoxia also have congestive heart failure and pulmonary artery hypertension.

Hyperviscosity syndrome occurs in patients with polycythemia which may be due to maternal-fetal or fetal-fetal transfusion or may be secondary to perinatal hypoxemia.

The patient with pulmonary vascular constriction (with or without increased pulmonary vascular smooth muscle) and no parenchymal pulmonary disease or

Table 13–4 PERSISTENT PULMONARY HYPERTENSION IN THE NEWBORN INFANT: CLINICAL CLASSIFICATION

Pulmonary venous hypertension
  Pulmonary venous, left atrial, mitral obstruction
  Left ventricular failure; cardiac lesion present
  Transient left ventricular dysfunction (H)*
Functional obstruction of pulmonary vascular bed
  Hyperviscosity (H)
Pulmonary vascular constriction (with or without increased pulmonary
    vascular smooth muscle)
  Persistent of the fetal circulation (PFC syndrome) (H)
  Secondary to pulmonary disease (H)
  Premature ductal closure
Decreased pulmonary vascular bed
  Pulmonary hypoplasia, congenital
  Pulmonary hypoplasia, secondary
Systemic right ventricle or single ventricle without pulmonary stenosis
  Cardiac lesions

*Hypoxia.

cardiac lesion should be diagnosed as having *persistence of the fetal circulation*. However, infants with both a pulmonary vascular constrictive component and pulmonary parenchymal disease, although also having an oxygenation defect induced in part by hypoxemia, should be classified according to the basic disease entity, e.g., meconium aspiration with pulmonary vascular constriction and right to left shunting.

A decreased pulmonary vascular bed leads to elevated pulmonary resistance and persistent pulmonary hypertension of the newborn. This may occur with *congenital pulmonary hypoplasia* but is also seen secondary to *diaphragmatic hernia*, space-occupying *intrathoracic masses*, and other diseases. Once hypoxia occurs in these patients, the resulting pulmonary vascular constriction may add to the pulmonary resistance and exacerbate the cyanosis.

Infants with *systemic right ventricles* or *single ventricles* as a result of complex congenital heart lesions without pulmonary stenosis have pulmonary hypertension. Such infants also develop medial muscular hypertrophy of small pulmonary vessels.

Perinatal hypoxemia associated with anatomic and physiologic abnormalities results in persistent pulmonary hypertension of mixed etiologies. For example, infants with diaphragmatic hernia have ipsilateral pulmonary hypoplasia and contralateral pulmonary vasoconstriction, both of which contribute to high pulmonary resistance, hypertension, and right to left shunting. Some preterm infants with severe respiratory distress syndrome may also be cyanotic on the basis of pulmonary vasoconstriction, pulmonary hypertension, and right to left ductus arteriosus and foramen ovale shunting on the 1st day or 2 of life. Later in the neonatal period ventilation-perfusion inequalities result in cyanosis, and large ductal left to right shunting may occur as pulmonary resistance falls.

13.12 PERSISTENCE OF THE FETAL CIRCULATION (PFC)

In this condition the hemodynamics of fetal life are maintained, in part, after birth; the pulmonary vascular bed remains constricted, and the blood entering the right heart shunts away from the lungs into the systemic vascular bed via the foramen ovale and ductus arteriosus. The etiology for persistent constriction of the pulmonary vascular bed is not always known, but in many cases the clinical pattern strongly implicates perinatal hypoxemia.

Pathophysiology. Table 13–5 outlines the relevant multiple effects of perinatal hypoxemia in the newborn that result in the clinical manifestations of the PFC syndrome. Hypoxemia and acidemia lead to pulmonary arteriolar constriction and hypertension, perhaps in the presence of increased pulmonary vascular smooth muscle. However, hypoxemia may also lead to left or right ventricular dysfunction and transient cardiac failure. These manifestations may occur together in various combinations accounting for the variable clinical presentations. Some infants with PFC have echocardi-

Table 13–5 CARDIOPULMONARY EFFECTS OF PERINATAL HYPOXEMIA*

Effect	Physiologic Manifestations	Pulmonary Artery Hypertension (PAH)	Disease
Pulmonary arteriolar constriction (? prenatal hypertrophy of pulmonary vascular smooth muscle)	PAH ↓ PaO$_2$ R → L shunt (PFO and PDA) ↑ Hct ↓ Glucose ↓ Ca^{++}	+	PFC syndrome (persistent fetal circulation)
LV dysfunction	LV Failure	+	Transient LV myocardial ischemia syndrome
RV dysfunction	RV failure	–	Transient RV myocardial dysfunction (tricuspid insufficiency syndrome)
Combination of above effects	All of above (with CNS, renal, GI manifestations)	+	The asphyxiated newborn

*Any or all may occur with concomitant cardiac or pulmonary parenchymal disease.

ographic findings of left ventricular dysfunction with large hearts and congested lung fields; others have clear lung fields but large right ventricles and physical signs of tricuspid insufficiency. In the most severely hypoxic infants many of these manifestations are present along with central nervous system, renal, and gastrointestinal effects of asphyxia. Any or all of these effects may be superimposed on concomitant cardiac or pulmonary parenchymal disease.

Clinical Manifestations. The typical patient is a full term infant who is observed to be cyanotic virtually from birth with varying degrees of respiratory distress. In approximately 80% of patients there is a history consistent with perinatal hypoxemia. Apgar scores are often low, and resuscitative measures may have been required to stabilize the condition of the newborn infant. Physical examination may also reveal a murmur at the left sternal border consistent with tricuspid regurgitation. An unusually high hematocrit should suggest hyperviscosity as a basis for elevated pulmonary vascular resistance. The electrocardiogram, similar to those of many patients with congenital heart disease, shows right ventricular hypertrophy which is physiologic for age. Cardiac size and pulmonary vascularity on roentgenograms of the chest are not diagnostic. Echocardiographically, the right ventricular pre-ejection period/right ventricular ejection time ratios are consistent with pulmonary artery arterial hypertension but are not specific for PFC syndrome. Administration of oxygen does not initially improve the arterial oxygen saturation significantly in most cases; lack of improvement indicates the presence of true right to left shunt and does not exclude cyanotic heart disease.

The clinical course of infants with PFC is highly variable. Mortality is significant, in the range of 10–30%. Most survivors improve steadily over a few days and are normal by the end of the 1st wk of life.

Differential Diagnosis. Since the syndrome of PFC results in true right to left shunt, the hemodynamics are similar to those in infants with cyanotic heart disease, and the differential diagnosis includes (1) severe left heart failure, (2) obstruction of the mitral valve within the left atrium or of the pulmonary veins, and (3) marked pulmonary vascular constriction secondary to a recognized pathologic process. The major differ-

ential diagnosis among congenital cardiac lesions is transposition of the great arteries. In both this condition and PFC, the patient is most often a term infant who is markedly cyanotic, does not have a striking murmur, and has a nondiagnostic electrocardiogram and chest roentgenogram. Echocardiography is very helpful in establishing a diagnosis.

In infants with pulmonary disease or central nervous disturbances the oxygenation defect is due to hypoventilation or ventilation-perfusion inequality, and these infants can usually be differentiated from those with PFC of the primary type on the basis of the clinical features and arterial blood gas analysis in response to oxygen administration. However, PFC may be responsible for a component of cyanosis in a number of entities.

Treatment. The major goal of therapy is to keep the infant well oxygenated until the natural course of the illness leads to spontaneous improvement. Oxygen administration and mechanical ventilation should be utilized as indicated by blood gas measurement. Some centers advocate hyperventilation. The hemoglobin should be followed carefully and severe polycythemia treated with appropriate exchanges of blood for plasma. Sodium bicarbonate is administered for metabolic acidosis. Many infants will have severe hypoglycemia or hypocalcemia, which should be corrected.

The vasodilator *tolazoline* has been utilized for treatment of PFC syndrome with encouraging but inconclusive results; pulmonary vascular dilatation may be minimal in the most severely ill infants. The administration of this agent acutely increases pulmonary blood flow and raises arterial pO$_2$. Pulmonary arterial pressure may remain elevated initially but with improved oxygenation falls toward normal levels. However, even when tolazoline is injected directly into the pulmonary artery, there is a marked systemic effect. The lowering of systemic resistance may result in low systemic blood pressure and shock. The drug should be given carefully, first as a bolus (0.5–1.0 mg/kg) over a period of about 1 min, followed by an infusion of 2–5 mg/kg/hr. Monitoring of arterial pressure is essential, and the infant should also be carefully observed for spontaneous gastrointestinal hemorrhage, which also has been noted during tolazoline therapy.

CONGENITAL HEART DISEASE

Incidence. Congenital heart disease occurs in approximately 8/1000 live births. Among infants born with cardiac defects there is a spectrum of severity; about 2–3/1000 infants with congenital heart disease will be symptomatic in the 1st yr of life. Since palliative and surgical techniques have evolved, the percentage of individuals who survive with various lesions has changed; complex, severe defects now account for a larger number of patients. For example, transposition of the great arteries, a defect rarely seen in its natural state after 1 yr of age, is relatively common since surgical repair of this defect. Table 13–6 summarizes the incidence of specific congenital defects in different age groups.

Most congenital defects are well tolerated during fetal life. It is only after the maternal circulation is eliminated and the cardiovascular system must be independently sustained that the impact of an anatomic and subsequent hemodynamic abnormality becomes apparent. The infant's circulation continues to change after birth, and later changes affect the hemodynamic impact of cardiac lesions. For example, as pulmonary vascular resistance falls over the 1st weeks of life, left to right shunts may become more apparent. The relative importance of various defects also changes with growth; the large ventricular septal defect may become a relatively small communication later. Aortic or pulmonary valve stenosis which is relatively mild may become worse if the orifice of the valve does not grow with the patient. The physician should be aware of both the spectrum of severity for the various malformations and their evolution with time, both decreasing and increasing in severity depending on the circumstances.

Etiology. The cause of congenital heart disease is rarely known in individual cases. Multifactorial inheritance patterns are responsible for most lesions; single gene syndromes are rare (Sec 6.1). Several chromosomal abnormalities are associated with severe congenital heart disease, but these represent fewer than 5% of the total. In most instances there is a combination of genetic and environmental influences. The incidence of congenital heart disease among siblings of probands is approximately twice that of the reported general incidence, occasionally reaching 5%. It has been reported that the same lesion or a variant is most likely to be repeated in siblings.

With some exceptions, environmental influences during pregnancy have rarely been found to explain congenital cardiac defects in man. Pregnant women who contract German measles in the 1st 2 mo of pregnancy may give birth to infants with cardiac lesions, including patent ductus arteriosus, branch pulmonary stenosis, and less often other defects. Limited evidence suggests a relationship of maternal cytomegalovirus, coxsackievirus B, and herpesvirus hominis B with congenital cardiovascular abnormalities. There is an increased incidence of patent ductus arteriosus among infants born at high altitudes; seasonal variations have also been described.

Associated noncardiac malformations are common, especially in the context of certain syndromes (Table 13–7); Turner syndrome, Noonan disease, Marfan syndrome, Ellis–van Creveld syndrome, and numerous other less common multisystem diseases have congenital heart disease as a major or minor component of a spectrum of anomalies. Renal anomalies, cleft palate, and abnormalities of the arm and hand may occur with associated cardiac lesions. Congenital heart disease was observed in about 10% of children with the thalidomide syndrome; folic acid antagonists are also cardiovascular teratogens. Maternal therapy with anticonvulsant agents, especially diphenylhydantoin and trimethadione, is associated with a relatively high incidence of congenital heart disease. Dextroamphetamine, lithium chloride, alcohol, progesterone/estrogen, and warfarin are suspected to be teratogenic agents. Overexposure of the pregnant woman to radiation is potentially teratogenic and has caused some congenital heart disease. Although animal studies suggest that there are other cardiovascular teratogens, clear associations to human disease have not been established in most instances.

Genetic Counseling. Parents who have had a child with congenital heart disease should be told that the incidence of a 2nd infant with a cardiac malformation, although higher than in the general population, is still quite low (2–5%). They should generally be supported if they desire to have another child. When 2 siblings have congenital heart disease, the incidence in a 3rd pregnancy may reach 20–25%.

The incidence of atrial or ventricular septal defects among siblings of a child with either anomaly varies from 1–4%; patent ductus arteriosus, truncus arteriosus, primary pulmonary hypertension, and aortic stenosis have been observed in siblings. The incidence of coarctation of the aorta in siblings is low, but that of pulmonary stenosis is probably highest of any congenital heart lesion. A relatively high incidence of consanguinity of parents has been reported with situs inversus.

Since a large number of patients with congenital heart

Table 13–6 PERCENTAGE INCIDENCE OF CONGENITAL CARDIOVASCULAR MALFORMATIONS AMONG AFFECTED PERSONS IN THREE DIFFERENT AGE GROUPS (EXCLUDING NEONATES)

	INFANTS	CHILDREN	OLDER CHILDREN AND ADULTS
Ventricular septal defect	28.3	24	15
Patent ductus arteriosus	12.5	15	15.5
Atrial septal defect	9.7	12	16
Coarctation	8.8	4.5	8
Transposition	8	4.5	2
Fallot tetralogy	7	11	15.5
Pulmonary stenosis	6	11	15
Aortic stenosis	3.5	6.5	5
Truncus	2.7	0.5	—
Tricuspid atresia	1	1.5	1
All others	12.5	9.5	7
Total	100.0	100.0	100.0

Adapted from Campbell M, *In*: Watson H (ed): Paediatric Cardiology. London, Lloyd-Luke, Ltd., 1968, Chap 5.

Table 13–7 CARDIOVASCULAR INVOLVEMENT IN VARIOUS SYNDROMES

CHROMOSOMAL ABNORMALITIES
Autosomal Chromosomal Abnormalities

Trisomies		Deletions	
Trisomy 21	VSD, ECD, ASD	4p–	VSD, AS, PDA
Trisomy 18	VSD, PDA, PS	5p– (Cri du chat)	VSD, PDA, ASD
Trisomy 13	VSD, DORV, PDA, ASD	13q–	VSD
		18q–	VSD

Sex Chromosomes

XXXXY	PDA, ASD	Turner XO	Coarct, AS, ASD

HERITABLE AND POSSIBLE HERITABLE SYNDROMES AND DISORDERS

Syndrome	Involvement
Apert	VSD
Carpenter	PDA
Cockayne	Atherosclerosis
Congenital hypertrophic subaortic stenosis	Obstructive cardiomyopathy
Conradi	VSD, PDA
Crouzon	PDA, Coarct
Cutis laxa	Pulmonary hypertension, PA stenosis
Ellis–van Creveld	Single atrium (other defects in 30%)
Familial deafness	Occasionally arrhythmia, sudden death
Familial dwarfism and nevi	Cardiomyopathy
Familial elfin facies, mental retardation, infantile hypercalcemia	Supravalvular AS, PA branch stenosis
Forney	MI
Holt-Oram	ASD (other defects common)
Jarvell-Lange-Nielsen	Prolonged Q-T, sudden death
Kartagener	Dextrocardia
Laurence-Moon-Biedl	Variable, including T of F
Leopard (lentiginosis)	PS, + Q-T interval
Mucolipidosis III	Aortic valve disease
Neurofibromatosis	PS, pheo, coarct
Neurologic and muscular diseases:	
Friedreich ataxia	Cardiomyopathy
Muscular dystrophy	Cardiomyopathy
Refsum	Arrhythmia, sudden death
Riley-Day	Episodic hypertension, postural hypotension
Noonan	PS, ASD, cardiomyopathy
Progeria	Accelerated atherosclerosis
Rendu-Osler-Weber	Arteriovenous fistula (lung, liver, mucous membranes)
Romano-Ward	+ Q-T interval, sudden death
Rubinstein-Taybi	PDA
Scimitar	Hypoplasia of right ventricle, anomalous PV return to IVC
Seckel	VSD, PDA
Smith-Lemli-Opitz	VSD, PDA
Thrombocytopenia and absent radius (TAR)	ASD, T of F
Treacher Collins	VSD, ASD, PDA
Tuberous sclerosis	Myocardial rhabdomyoma
von Hippel–Lindau	Hemangiomas, pheochromocytomas
Weill-Marchesani	PDA
Werner	Vascular sclerosis, cardiomyopathy

INBORN ERRORS OF METABOLISM

Alcaptonuria	Atherosclerosis, valvular disease
Homocystinuria	Pulmonary arterial and aortic dilatation, intravascular thrombosis, flushing of skin
Pompe disease	Glycogen storage disease of heart

CONNECTIVE TISSUE DISORDERS

Arterial calcification of infancy	Calcinosis of coronary arteries
Ehlers-Danlos	Arterial dilatation
Hurler-Hunter	Multivalvular and coronary artery disease
Marfan	Aortic dilatation with aortic incompetence, mitral incompetence, dilatation of PA
Morquio-Ulrich	Aortic incompetence
Osteogenesis imperfecta	Aortic incompetence
Pseudoxanthoma elasticum	Peripheral arterial disease
Scheie	Aortic incompetence

AS = aortic stenosis
ASD = atrial septal defect
Coarct = coarctation
DORV = double outlet right ventricle
ECD = endocardial cushion defect
IVC = inferior vena cava
MI = mitral insufficiency
Q-T = Q-T interval of electrocardiogram
T of F = tetralogy of Fallot
VSD = ventricular septal defect
PA = pulmonary artery
PDA = patent ductus arteriosus
PS = pulmonic stenosis
Pheo = pheochromocytoma
PV = pulmonary valve

disease have had corrective surgery, there is an increasing likelihood that affected women will become pregnant; the incidence of congenital heart disease among offspring is 2–5%. Decisions regarding an attempt to carry a fetus to term are usually oriented toward the mother's cardiovascular status. There are definite risks that a woman with marginal cardiac function will deteriorate in the final trimester of pregnancy. Furthermore, the incidence of spontaneous abortion is high, especially among cyanotic women. It is important to discuss various methods of birth control with afflicted young women.

Congenital Cardiac Disease with Cyanosis
(Dominant Right to Left Shunt)

13.13 TETRALOGY OF FALLOT

The combination of (1) obstruction to right ventricular outflow (pulmonary stenosis), (2) ventricular septal defect, (3) dextroposition of the aorta, and (4) right ventricular hypertrophy constitutes the tetralogy of Fallot. Obstruction to pulmonary arterial flow is usually at the right ventricular infundibulum and pulmonary valve. The pulmonary arterial trunk may be smaller than usual, and there may be branch stenosis.

Pathology. The pulmonary valve may have a small ring, is often bicuspid, and, occasionally, is the only site of stenosis. Hypertrophy of the crista supraventricularis contributes to the infundibular stenosis and results in an infundibular chamber of variable size and contour. Occasionally, the right ventricular outflow tract is completely obstructed (pulmonary atresia); under these circumstances the anatomy of the pulmonary arteries is extremely variable. The ventricular septal defect is generally large, just below the aortic valve, and related to the posterior and right aortic cusps. The normal continuity of the mitral and aortic valves is maintained. The aorta arches to the right in about 20% of instances; it is large and straddles the ventricular septal defect so that a varying proportion of it originates in the right ventricle.

Pathophysiology. Systemic venous return to the right atrium and right ventricle is normal. When the right ventricle contracts in the face of pulmonary stenosis, blood is shunted across the ventricular septal defect into the aorta. Persistent arterial unsaturation and cyanosis result. The pulmonary blood flow, when severely restricted by the obstruction to right ventricular outflow, may be supplemented by bronchial collateral circulation and occasionally by a patent ductus arteriosus. The peak systolic and diastolic pressures in each ventricle are usually similar, as are the mean pressures in the atria. A measurable gradient of pressure, due to the pulmonary stenosis, is almost always detected across the outflow of the right ventricle. When obstruction to right ventricular outflow and the ventricular septal defect exist without right to left shunt, the anomaly is termed acyanotic Fallot.

Clinical Manifestations. *Cyanosis,* one of the most obvious manifestations of tetralogy, may not be present at birth. Right ventricular outflow obstruction may not be severe, and the infant may present with a large left to right shunt and even congestive heart failure. However, with time there is increasing hypertrophy of the infundibulum, and as the child grows, the obstruction is further exaggerated. Later in the 1st yr cyanosis occurs, most prominently on the mucous membranes of the lips and mouth and in the fingernails and toenails. In severe cases cyanosis occurs in the neonatal period. With severe cyanosis the skin surface has a dusky blue color, and the sclerae, gray with engorged blood vessels, suggest mild conjunctivitis (Sec 13.1). Clubbing of the fingers and toes becomes apparent by 1–2 yr of age.

Dyspnea occurs on exertion. Infants and toddlers will play actively for a short time and then sit or lie down. Older children may be able to walk a block or so before stopping to rest. The severity of the cardiac lesion is often reflected by the intensity of the cyanosis. Characteristically, children assume a *squatting* position for the relief of dyspnea due to physical effort; the child is usually able to resume physical activity within a few min.

Paroxysmal dyspneic attacks (anoxic "blue" spells) are a particular problem during the 1st 2 yr of life. The infant becomes dyspneic and restless, cyanosis increases, gasping respirations ensue, and syncope may follow. The spell occurs most frequently in the morning. Temporary disappearance or decrease in intensity of the systolic murmur is usual. The spells may last from a few min to a few hr and are occasionally fatal. Short episodes are followed by generalized weakness and sleep. Severe spells may progress to unconsciousness and, occasionally, to convulsions or hemiparesis. The onset is usually spontaneous and unpredictable. The spells are associated with a reduction of an already compromised pulmonary blood flow, which results in hypoxia and metabolic acidosis. The disappearance or attenuation of the systolic murmur and reduction of arterial oxygen saturation and pulmonary arterial pressure suggest that blue spells are associated with a further increase in resistance at the right ventricular outflow tract, transient decrease in systemic resistance, or both. Hyperpnea may precipitate an attack by increasing systemic venous return. In the presence of fixed or decreased pulmonary blood flow the right to left shunt is increased. The resultant arterial hypoxia, metabolic acidosis, and increased pCO_2 further stimulate the respiratory mechanism to maintain hyperpnea. Depending on the frequency and severity of the attacks, 1 or more of the following procedures should be tried,

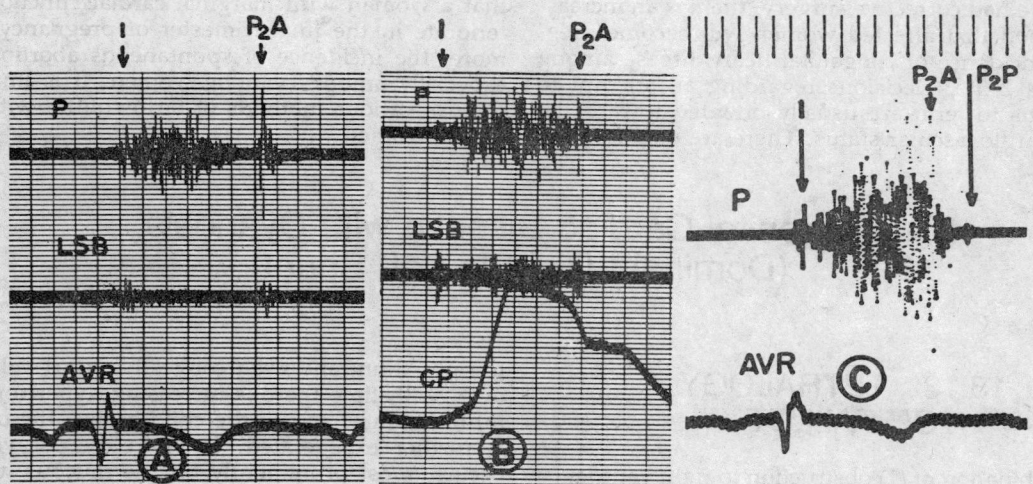

Figure 13–28 Phonocardiograms illustrating the variability of auscultatory findings in cyanotic tetralogy of Fallot. AVR, electrocardiogram; CP, carotid pulse; LSB, left sternal border; P, pulmonary area; P₂A, aortic component of 2nd heart sound; P₂P, pulmonic component of 2nd heart sound; 1, 1st heart sound. The systolic murmur may be early (*A*), or when long (*B*) or accentuated in late systole (*C*), it ends at P₂A. The 2nd heart sound is single, owing to aortic valve closure (*A* and *B*) or split with a delayed soft pulmonic component (*C*). Time lines 0.04 sec.

if needed, in sequence: (1) placement of the infant on the abdomen in the knee-chest position making certain that there is no constricting clothing; (2) administration of oxygen; and (3) injection of morphine subcutaneously in a dose not in excess of 0.1 mg/kg. Since metabolic acidosis develops when the arterial pO_2 is below 40 mm Hg, rapid correction (within several min) is necessary if the spell is severe and there is lack of response to the foregoing therapy. This may be accomplished with intravenous administration of sodium bicarbonate. Recovery from the spell is rapid once the pH has returned to normal. Repeated blood pH measurements are necessary because rapid recurrence of acidosis is common. Beta-adrenergic inhibition by intravenous administration of propranolol (0.1 to a maximum of 0.2 mg/kg) has been used successfully in some patients with severe spells, especially spells accompanied by tachycardia. Drugs that increase systemic vascular resistance, such as intravenous methoxamine and phenylephrine, will decrease the right to left shunt and thus improve the symptoms; but their use has been limited.

Growth and development may be delayed in severe untreated tetralogy of Fallot. Stature and nutritional status are usually below averages for age, and muscles and subcutaneous tissues are flabby and soft. Puberty is delayed.

The *pulse* is usually normal, as are the venous and arterial pressures. The left anterior hemithorax may bulge forward. The heart is usually normal in size, and the apical impulse is tapping. A *systolic thrill* is felt in 50% of cases along the left sternal border in the 3rd and 4th parasternal spaces.

The *systolic murmur* is frequently loud and harsh; it may be transmitted widely but is most intense at the left sternal border. The murmur may be either ejection or pansystolic (Fig 13–28) and may be preceded by a click. The systolic murmur is due to turbulence over the right ventricular outflow tract and tends to be less prominent with severe obstruction and large right to left shunts. The 2nd heart sound is single and is

produced by closure of the aortic valve. Infrequently, the systolic murmur is followed by a diastolic murmur; this continuous murmur may be audible in any part of the chest, anteriorly or posteriorly; it is produced by enlarged bronchial collateral vessels or rarely by persistence of a patent ductus arteriosus. This finding is frequent with pulmonary atresia.

Diagnosis. *Roentgenographically,* the typical configuration as seen in the anteroposterior view consists of a narrow base, concavity of the left border in the area usually occupied by the pulmonary artery, and normal heart size. The rounded apical shadow situated rather high above the diaphragm is produced chiefly by the hypertrophied right ventricle. The cardiac silhouette has been likened to that of a wooden shoe (**coeur en sabot**) (Fig 13–29). In the lateral projection the anterior

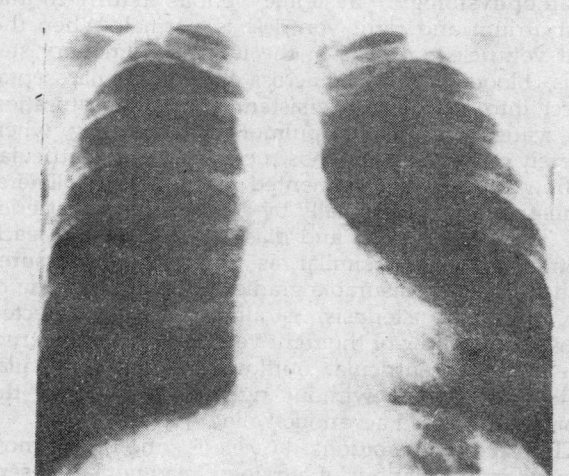

Figure 13–29 Roentgenogram of an 8 yr old boy with tetralogy of Fallot. Note the normal heart size, some elevation of the cardiac apex, concavity in the region of the main pulmonary artery, right aortic arch, and diminished pulmonary vascularity.

clear space may or may not be encroached upon by the hypertrophied right ventricle.

The aorta is usually large, and its position is important. In about 20% of instances the aorta arches to the right instead of to the left; this may result in an indentation of the leftward positioned air-filled tracheobronchial shadow in the anteroposterior view or may be confirmed by displacement of the barium-filled esophagus to the left. In the left oblique view a right aortic arch may indent the esophagus.

The hilar areas and lung fields are relatively clear, probably because of diminished pulmonary blood flow, an important diagnostic sign.

Variations from the typical roentgenographic picture include poststenotic dilatation of the pulmonary artery, which suggests valvular pulmonary stenosis. Occasionally, pulmonary vascularity is made prominent by collateral bronchial circulation which radiates from the hilus of the lungs. Localized proximal infundibular stenosis with an infundibular chamber may produce a bulge at the upper left cardiac border in the frontal projection; it is distinguished from stenosis of the pulmonary artery because it remains prominent in the right anterior oblique view.

The *electrocardiogram* reveals evidence of right axis deviation and right ventricular hypertrophy. The latter, without which the diagnosis of tetralogy of Fallot is unlikely, is found in the right precordial chest leads where the configuration of the QRS complex is Rs, R, qR, qRs, rsR', or RS. In these leads the T wave may be positive, further evidence of right ventricular hypertrophy. The P wave is tall and peaked or sometimes bifid (Fig 13–11).

Echocardiography *(M-mode)* demonstrates the aortic override (Fig 13–30), large aorta, and thick anterior right ventricular wall, but the stenotic pulmonary valve may be difficult to record. Normal continuity maintained between the anterior mitral leaflet and the posterior

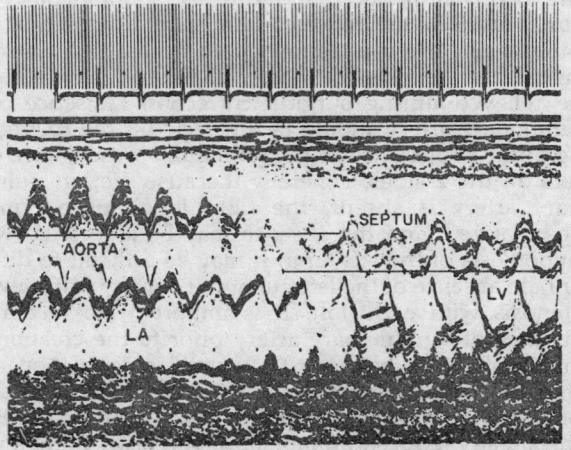

Figure 13–30 Echocardiographic sweep from left ventricle (LV) to aorta to demonstrate aortic override in a patient with tetralogy of Fallot. LA, left atrium. Arrows point to anterior mitral leaflet which is continuous with posterior aortic wall. The normal continuity between the septum and anterior wall of the aorta is lost because the aorta is anterior and overrides the septum. This relationship is emphasized by the 2 horizontal lines which in the normal form 1 straight continuous line.

aortic wall distinguishes tetralogy of Fallot from the double outlet right ventricle, subaortic conus, and pulmonary stenosis. The left atrium is normal in size, in contrast to its large size in truncus arteriosus. Two dimensional echocardiography demonstrates that the aorta is displaced anteriorly and to the right, confirming the presence of aortic override.

Cardiac catheterization and angiocardiography are essential to elucidate the anatomic abnormalities and to exclude other defects which may mimic the tetralogy of Fallot, especially double outlet right ventricle with pulmonary stenosis and arterial transposition with pulmonary stenosis.

Cardiac catheterization reveals systolic hypertension in the right ventricle equal to systemic pressure, with a marked decrease in pressure as the catheter enters the infundibular chamber or pulmonary artery. Serial pressure determinations taken from the region of stenosis of the right ventricular outflow tract *may* differentiate valvular and subvalvular stenosis. In valvular stenosis the change in pressure from the pulmonary artery to the right ventricle is abrupt, whereas in infundibular stenosis 2 pressure differentials are recorded as the catheter tip is withdrawn from the pulmonary artery to the infundibular chamber and right ventricle.

The mean pulmonary arterial pressure is commonly 5–10 mm Hg; the right atrial pressure is usually normal. The aorta may be easily entered from the right ventricle through the ventricular septal defect. The level of arterial oxygen saturation depends on the magnitude of the right to left shunt; at rest it is usually 75–85%. Samples of blood from the venae cavae, right atrium, right ventricle, and pulmonary artery are frequently similar in oxygen content and thus indicate absence of a left to right shunt. In many patients, however, a left to right shunt is demonstrated at the ventricular level. Angiography and/or indicator dilution curves localize the site of right to left or bidirectional shunt at the ventricular level.

Selective right ventriculography is of great diagnostic value. The contrast medium outlines the heavily trabeculated right ventricle. The infundibular stenosis varies in length, width, contour, and distensibility (Fig 13–31). An infundibular chamber may also be demonstrated. The pulmonary valve may be normal, but frequently the leaflets are thickened and domed, and the valve ring is small. Nearly simultaneous opacification of the aorta and pulmonary artery is usual. The size of the pulmonary trunk varies considerably. In severe cases it is small or hypoplastic, and localized or multiple areas of stenosis may be seen in the branches of the pulmonary artery. The subaortic ventricular septal defect is usually large, and the aorta is well opacified.

Among patients with severe tetralogy (pulmonary atresia) the anatomy of the pulmonary vessels is extremely complex. There may be a central confluence of the left and right artery with a smaller or absent main pulmonary artery. In some instances, only peripheral arteries are seen with blood entering these vessels from a patent ductus, mammary arteries, or collateral arteries arising separately or together from the descending aorta. Often, there are parallel collateral arteries which, like the true pulmonary artery, branch into the periph-

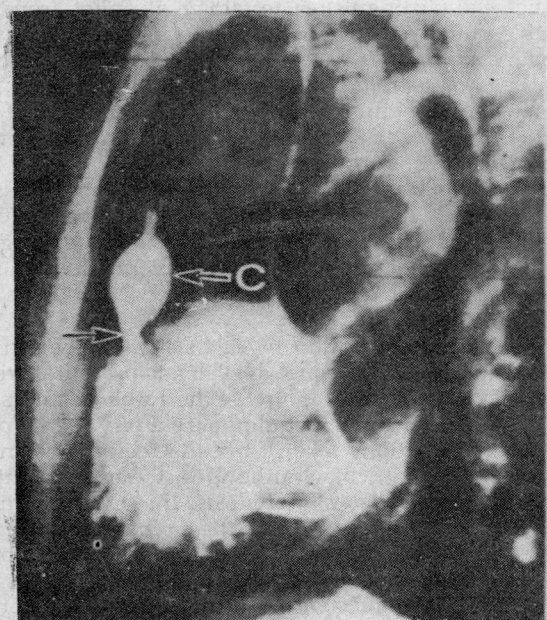

Figure 13–31 Lateral view of selective right ventriculogram in patient with Fallot tetralogy. Arrow points to infundibular stenosis which is below the infundibular chamber (C).

ery of the lung. These vessels may have long segments of stenosis as they arrive from the descending aorta. Complete and accurate information regarding the anatomy of the pulmonary arteries is very important in evaluating these children as surgical candidates.

Left ventriculography demonstrates the size of the ventricle, the position of the ventricular septal defect, and the overriding aorta; it also confirms mitral-aortic continuity and rules out double outlet right ventricle. *Aortography* excludes associated aortic valvular disease and outlines the course of the coronary arteries. In a few instances a large coronary artery crosses over the right ventricular outflow tract; this artery must be preserved during surgical repair.

Complications. *Cerebral thromboses,* usually occurring in the cerebral veins or dural sinuses and occasionally in the cerebral arteries, are more common in the presence of extreme polycythemia. They may also be precipitated by dehydration. Thromboses are more frequent under the age of 2 yr. These patients most often have iron deficiency anemia, frequently with hemoglobin and hematocrit levels in the normal range. Therapy includes adequate hydration, especially in the comatose patient. Phlebotomy and volume replacement with fresh frozen plasma are indicated in the rare extremely polycythemic patient. Heparin is of little value since it does not influence blood viscosity and may not prevent extension of venous thrombosis; it is contraindicated in hemorrhagic cerebral infarction. Physical therapy to the affected extremities should be instituted as early as possible.

Brain abscess is less common than cerebral thrombosis. Patients are usually over the age of 2 yr. The onset of the illness is often insidious with low grade fever. There may be localized skull tenderness, and the erythrocyte sedimentation rate and white cell count may be elevated. In some patients there is acute onset of symptoms, which may develop after a recent history of headache, nausea, and vomiting. Epileptiform seizures may occur; localized neurologic signs depend on the site and size of the abscess and the presence of increased intracranial pressure. Computed axial tomography and radionuclide brain scans have facilitated making this difficult diagnosis. Massive antibiotic therapy may help to keep the infection localized, but surgical drainage of the abscess is almost always necessary (Sec 21.19).

Bacterial endocarditis occurs in unoperated patients but is more common in children who have had a palliative shunt procedure during infancy. Prophylaxis, preferably with penicillin, is essential during all surgical procedures since the patient is at risk for developing bacteremia and subsequently endocarditis.

Congestive heart failure may occur in the infant with pulmonary atresia and large collateral blood flow. This almost invariably regresses during the 1st months of life, and the patient becomes cyanotic with decreased pulmonary blood flow.

Associated Cardiovascular Anomalies. Patent foramen ovale and patent ductus arteriosus are frequent during infancy. Recognition of the drainage of a persistent left superior vena cava into the coronary sinus is important prior to surgical correction since temporary occlusion of systemic venous return is essential prior to cardiotomy. Failure to close defects in the atrial septum during corrective surgery may result in cyanosis from a right to left shunt due to high venous pressure in the immediate postoperative period. Absence of the pulmonary valve produces a distinct syndrome; cyanosis is mild or absent, the heart is large and hyperdynamic, and loud to and fro murmurs are present. Aneurysmal dilatation of the pulmonary artery often produces wheezing respiration and recurrent pneumonitis from bronchial compression. This syndrome may be lethal in the neonatal period but improves spontaneously in survivors. The incidence of stenosis of a branch of the pulmonary artery is estimated to be as high as 25%; significant stenosis of major pulmonary arteries must be relieved during surgical correction. Absence of a pulmonary artery should be suspected if the roentgenographic appearance of the pulmonary vasculature differs on the 2 sides; generally, because the left pulmonary artery is absent, the right lung appears more vascularized; and the absence may be associated with hypoplasia of the left lung. It may be difficult to differentiate absence of the left pulmonary artery from severe stenosis with occlusion. It is important to recognize absence of a pulmonary artery prior to the creation of an anastomosis between the systemic circulation and the single remaining pulmonary artery since occlusion of the latter during operation seriously compromises the already reduced pulmonary blood flow. Right aortic arch occurs in approximately 20% of cases of tetralogy of Fallot, and other anomalies of the pulmonary artery and aortic arch may also be seen. Muscular ventricular septal defects are also important associated anomalies.

Treatment. Although tetralogy of Fallot often presents insidiously during the 1st yr with gradually increasing cyanosis, there are patients with severe tetralogy who require medical treatment and palliative surgical intervention in the neonatal period. Therapy is aimed at providing an immediate increase in pulmonary blood flow to prevent the sequela of severe hypoxia. The infant should be transported to a medical center adequately equipped to evaluate and treat neonates under optimal conditions. It is critical that oxygenation and normal body temperature be maintained during the transfer. Prolonged, severe hypoxia may lead to shock, respiratory failure, and intractable acidosis and will significantly reduce the chances of survival from cardiac catheterization and surgery, even when surgically amenable lesions are present. Infants with markedly reduced pulmonary blood flow deteriorate rapidly because the ductus arteriosus does not stay sufficiently patent to provide adequate pulmonary blood flow after birth. The administration of prostaglandin E_1, a potent and specific relaxant of ductal smooth muscle, causes dilatation of the ductus arteriosus, allowing adequate pulmonary blood flow to occur until a surgical procedure can be carried out in neonates with severe tetralogy of Fallot and other lesions which benefit from ductal patency. This agent is administered intravenously when the clinical diagnosis is made and continued through cardiac catheterization and surgery. Postoperatively, the infusion may be continued to augment the palliative shunt or forward flow through a surgical valvulotomy. However, it is not used as a long term therapy.

Infants with tetralogy of Fallot who are stable and awaiting surgical intervention require careful observation. The prevention or prompt treatment of dehydration is important to avoid hemoconcentration and possible thrombotic episodes. Paroxysmal dyspneic attacks in infancy may be precipitated by a relative iron deficiency; iron therapy may decrease their frequency and also improve exercise tolerance and general well-being. The hematocrit should be maintained at 55–65%. Oral propranolol (1 mg/kg every 6 hr) has been used to decrease the frequency and severity of dyspneic spells, but it is preferable to go ahead with surgical treatment if spells occur.

Controversy exists regarding the type of surgical intervention required and the timing of the procedure. In general, infants presenting with symptoms and severe cyanosis in the 1st months of life have marked obstruction of the right ventricular outflow tract or pulmonary atresia. In such infants a systemic to pulmonary artery shunt procedure should be carried out to augment pulmonary artery blood flow. Corrective open heart surgery in early infancy is rarely advisable in such patients. Later in the 1st yr of life, open correction is a reasonable alternative when the usual single high ventricular septal defect is present, pulmonary arteries are of sufficient size, and no other complicating great vessel abnormalities are present. In general, older patients should have open heart correction of the defect regardless of whether an earlier palliative shunt procedure was carried out.

The Blalock-Taussig shunt is the most useful shunt procedure and is created by anastomosis of a subclavian artery to the homolateral branch of the pulmonary artery. This operation was previously impractical for the neonate because of technical problems in achieving an unobstructed connection. However, with the advent of microvascular surgery, the operation can now be successfully performed in these infants. Less frequently performed procedures are side to side anastomosis of the ascending aorta and right pulmonary artery (Waterson) and anastomosis of the upper descending aorta and left pulmonary artery (Potts); these procedures have a higher frequency of complicating congestive heart failure and late onset pulmonary hypertension as well as greater technical difficulties in closing the shunt during subsequent corrective surgery. Recently, small conduits from the aorta to a pulmonary artery have been utilized for early palliation.

Usually, the postoperative course of patients with a successful anastomosis is relatively untroubled. However, in addition to the usual postoperative complications following a thoracotomy, chylothorax, diaphragmatic paralysis, and Horner syndrome may occur. Chylothorax may require repeated thoracocentesis and, on occasion, reoperation in order to ligate the thoracic duct. Diaphragmatic paralysis due to injury to the recurrent laryngeal nerve may result in a more difficult postoperative course. More prolonged respiratory support and vigorous physical therapy may be required, but diaphragmatic function will return in 1–2 mo unless the nerve was completely divided. Horner syndrome is usually temporary and does not require treatment. Postoperative cardiac failure may be due to the large size of the anastomosis; its treatment is described later. Vascular problems are rarely seen in the upper extremity supplied by the subclavian artery used for the anastomosis.

After a successful shunt procedure, cyanosis and clubbing diminish. The development of a machinery-type murmur after the operation indicates a functioning anastomosis. However, this may not be heard for several days after surgery. The duration of symptomatic relief is variable. As the child grows, more pulmonary blood flow is needed and the shunt may eventually become inadequate. If the anatomy is such that a corrective operation can be carried out, then it should be undertaken. However, if it is not possible or the 1st shunt lasts only a brief period in a small infant, a 2nd anastomosis may be undertaken on the opposite side. Infective endocarditis is a threat in any patient with a systemic to pulmonary artery shunt; appropriate prophylactic measures should be taken (Sec 13.71).

The preferred surgical therapy is relief of the obstruction to the right ventricular outflow track and closure of the ventricular septal defect by direct vision intracardiac surgery with a pump oxygenator. When there is a previously established systemic-pulmonary shunt, it must be obliterated prior to cardiotomy. The surgical risk of **total correction** is currently under 10%. Factors that have contributed to increasing success of this approach include optimal total body perfusion, adequate myocardial protection during bypass, relief of right ventricular outflow obstruction, prevention of air embolism, and meticulous postoperative care. The presence of a previous Blalock-Taussig anastomosis does not increase the operative risk. Increased bleeding in the immediate postoperative period is common in polycythemic patients but should not seriously affect the outcome. The operative risks are higher in small infants because more complicated anatomy is likely to be encountered.

Prognosis. After successful total correction the patients are generally asymptomatic and able to lead unrestricted lives. The long term effects of isolated, surgically induced pulmonary valvular incompetence are unknown, but this lesion is common when a right ventricular outflow patch is utilized and is generally well tolerated. Patients who have a significant left to right shunt postoperatively or obstruction to right ventricular outflow have moderate to marked cardiac enlargement. A right ventricular outflow aneurysm may also be present at the site of the ventriculotomy or outflow patch. Reoperation is usually necessary in such patients, but this condition is now rarely seen.

Follow-up of patients 5–15 yr after operation indicates that the marked improvement in symptomatology is generally maintained. In many instances, however, young and active patients have an abnormal response during exercise study; their working capacities, maximal heart rates, and cardiac outputs are lower than those of controls. These abnormal findings may be less frequent when surgery is undertaken at an early age.

Conduction disturbances are also frequent after operation. The atrioventricular node and the bundle of His and its divisions are in close proximity to the ventricular septal defect and may be injured during surgery. Permanent complete heart block following surgery is now rare. When present, it should be treated by placement of a permanently implanted pacemaker. Bifascicular block, due to injury to the anterior fascicle of the left bundle (manifested as postoperative left axis deviation) and of the right bundle (manifested as complete right bundle branch block), occurs in about 10% of patients; the long term significance is uncertain, but in most instances there are no clinical manifestations. The additional finding of transient complete heart block in the immediate postoperative period, however, appears to be associated with an increased incidence of late onset complete heart block and sudden death. Unexpected cardiac arrest may also occur many yr after surgery in patients without postoperative bifascicular block or transient complete heart block. Some of these patients have multiple premature ventricular contractions at rest, and it is hypothesized that sudden cardiac arrest may be preceded by ventricular tachyrhythmias. These arrhythmias may be documented by continuous ambulatory monitoring (Holter) or unmasked by exercise; they are treated with quinidine, propranolol, Dilantin, or combinations of these drugs.

13.14 PULMONARY ATRESIA WITH VENTRICULAR SEPTAL DEFECT

This condition is an extreme form of tetralogy of Fallot. The pulmonary valve is atretic, rudimentary, or absent, and the pulmonary trunk is atretic or hypoplastic. The entire ventricular output is ejected into the aorta. Pulmonary blood flow is dependent on a patent ductus arteriosus and/or bronchial collaterals.

Clinical Manifestations. These are similar to those of the tetralogy with the following exceptions: cyanosis usually appears within a few days after birth in contrast to later in the 1st yr; the systolic murmur is absent or soft; the 1st heart sound is frequently followed by an ejection click; the 2nd sound at the base is moderately loud and single; and continuous murmurs of a patent ductus arteriosus or bronchial collateral flow may be heard anywhere in the chest, anteriorly or posteriorly, but are usually most prominent under the clavicles.

The presentation of these infants in the neonatal period is variable. Some patients have congestive heart failure due to increased pulmonary blood flow via collateral vessels; others are severely cyanotic and require urgent prostaglandin E_1 infusion and surgical intervention; and some infants have adequate pulmonary blood flow and can be managed like an uncomplicated less severe tetralogy patient.

The *roentgenogram* may reveal an enlarged heart, a concavity at the position of the pulmonary arterial segment, and the reticular pattern of bronchial collateral flow. The *electrocardiogram* shows right ventricular hypertrophy. The *echocardiogram* identifies the aortic override and the thick right ventricular wall but not the pulmonary valve. The best diagnostic study is *right ventriculography*. The large aorta is opacified immediately by passage of the contrast medium through the septal defect; the pathway of pulmonary blood flow from the aorta is also demonstrated. (See cardiac catheterization, Sec 13.13.)

Treatment. Since hypercyanotic spells and increasing hematocrit are frequent and commonly occur during infancy, systemic pulmonary artery anastomosis may be indicated for the patient with pulmonary arteries of reasonable size. Some centers advocate an open heart bypass from the right ventricle directly to the pulmonary artery either by "unroofing" the outflow tract or, indirectly, by implanting a conduit. This type of bypass may stimulate the growth of the pulmonary arteries and allow the patient to become a candidate for future open heart repair which would include closure of the ventricular septal defect. The corrective operation for pulmonary atresia and a ventricular septal defect also includes insertion of a valve-containing conduit from the right ventricle to the pulmonary artery and the elimination of previous systemic to pulmonary anastomoses (Fig 13–32). Unfortunately, many patients have malformations of the primary divisions of the pulmonary arteries in the form of hypoplasia, multiple branch stenoses, absence of a pulmonary artery, and large bronchial collaterals. These patients are difficult to treat surgically even with anastomotic procedures.

Acquired total obstruction (stenosis) of the right ventricular outflow tract may occur after a systemic-pulmonary anastomosis for tetralogy of Fallot. Some time after operation there may be a return of symptoms due to total obstruction at the infundibulum or pulmonary valve. The systolic murmur due to pulmonary stenosis is attenuated or disappears; the completeness of outflow obstruction is confirmed by right ventriculography. Corrective surgery is similar to that for tetralogy of Fallot.

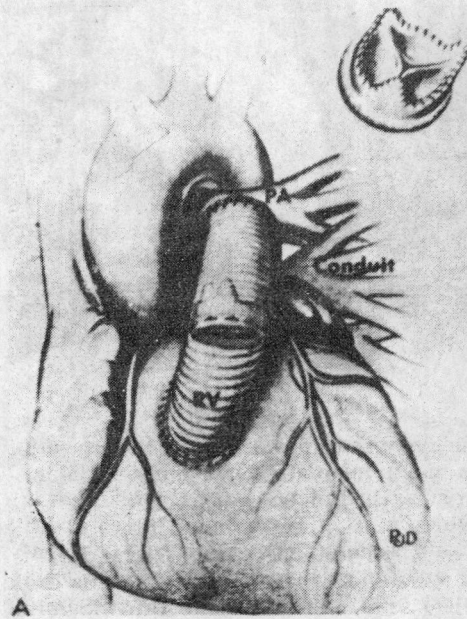

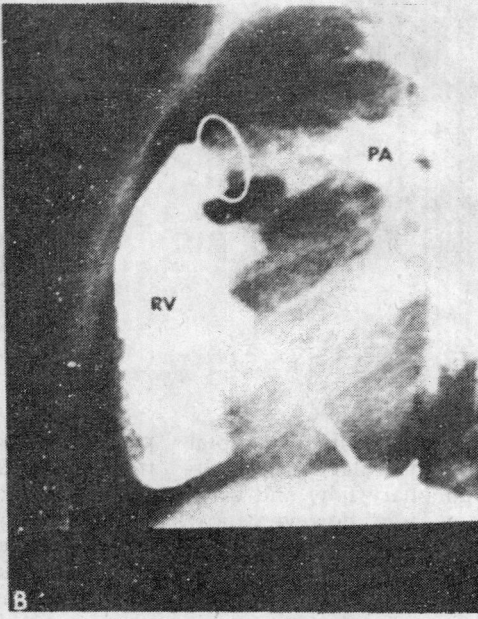

Figure 13–32 *A,* Artist's sketch of valve-containing conduit utilized in repair of pulmonary atresia. The porcine valve is portrayed in the inset. *B,* A right ventricular angiogram (lateral view) in a patient with pulmonary atresia and ventricular septal defect after repair with a valve-containing conduit.

WITH INTACT VENTRICULAR SEPTUM

In this anomaly the pulmonary valve leaflets are completely fused and the right ventricular outflow tract is atretic. In some instances the right ventricle is large. Since there is no egress of blood from the right ventricle, right atrial blood is shunted into the left atrium via the foramen ovale, mixes with pulmonary venous blood, and enters the left ventricle. The combined left and right ventricular output is pumped by the left ventricle into the aorta. Pulmonary blood flow occurs via a patent ductus arteriosus. In addition, among patients with small right ventricular cavities, sinusoidal channels connect the blood from within the right ventricle to the coronary arterial circulation retrograde to the aorta. Patients with intermediate-sized or large ventricular cavities also may have tricuspid insufficiency which serves to decompress the right ventricle.

Clinical Manifestations. As the ductus arteriosus closes in the 1st days of life, infants with pulmonary atresia and intact ventricular septum become markedly cyanotic. Untreated, most patients die within the 1st wk of life. Physical examination reveals severe cyanosis and respiratory distress. The 2nd heart sound is single, and most often there are no murmurs.

The electrocardiogram is helpful in that the frontal QRS axis almost always lies between 0 and +90°. The tall, spiked P waves indicate right atrial enlargement. The electrocardiogram is consistent with left ventricular dominance or hypertrophy; right ventricular forces are markedly decreased. Occasionally, with large right ventricular cavities, right ventricular hypertrophy is seen. The chest *roentgenogram* shows the heart to be variable in size with markedly decreased pulmonary vascularity. The *echocardiogram* is useful in helping to estimate the right ventricular dimensions and the size of the tricuspid valve. *Cardiac catheterization* demonstrates right atrial and ventricular hypertension. Ventriculography reveals the size of the ventricular cavity, the atretic right ventricular outflow tract, the degree of tricuspid regurgitation, and the intramyocardial -sinusoids filling the coronary vessel.

Treatment. The prognosis for this lesion has improved with urgent medical and surgical management. Infusion of prostaglandin E is usually effective in keeping the ductus open prior to intervention (Sec 13.13), thus reducing hypoxemia and acidemia during cardiac catheterization, angiography, and surgery. Pulmonary valvotomy is carried out to relieve outflow obstruction whenever possible, but in order to preserve adequate pulmonary blood flow, a systemic-pulmonary arterial anastomosis is carried out during the same procedure. Some groups have reported success by unroofing the outflow tract and patch grafting. The aim of surgery is to encourage growth in the right ventricular chamber by allowing forward flow while utilizing the shunt to be certain that pulmonary blood flow is adequate. Later, when possible, a more extensive valvotomy is carried out and the shunt taken down (Fig 13–33).

13.15 TRICUSPID ATRESIA

In tricuspid atresia there is no outlet from the right atrium to the right ventricle, and the entire systemic venous return enters the left heart by means of the foramen ovale. Pulmonary blood flow depends on the size of the ventricular septal defect or patent ductus arteriosus, the only means by which the pulmonary circulation is perfused. If the ventricular septum is intact, the right ventricle is hypoplastic and pulmonary

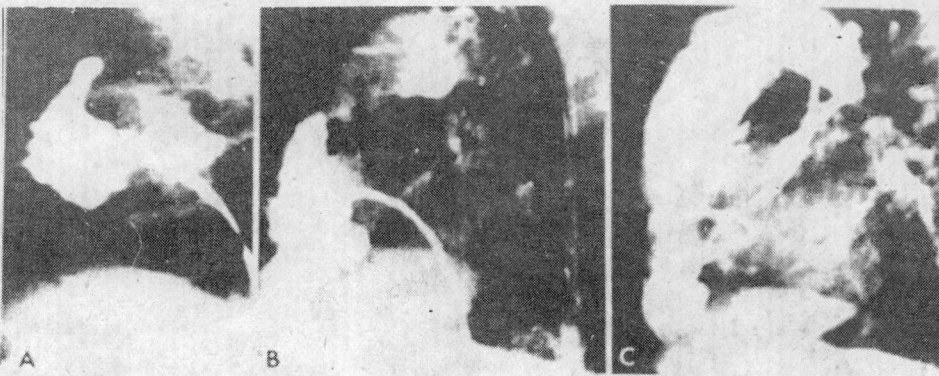

Figure 13–33 Growth of right ventricle in pulmonary atresia and intact ventricular septum (lateral views). *A*, Right ventricular angiogram prior to surgery at 2 days of life. Note the small ventricular chamber and atretic pulmonary outflow tract. The pulmonary artery is not visualized. *B*, At age 2 yr, after valvotomy and systemic pulmonary artery shunt. Normal-sized pulmonary artery fills across narrow outflow tract. The right ventricle is larger, but is trabeculated and hypertrophied. *C*, Normal right ventricle after repair at age 6 yr.

atresia is present. Rarely, a large ventricular septal defect in the absence of right ventricular outflow obstruction can lead to high pulmonary flow and early congestive heart failure. By and large, however, most patients with tricuspid atresia present in the early months of life with decreased pulmonary blood flow and cyanosis.

Clinical Manifestations. Cyanosis, polycythemia, easy fatigability, exertional dyspnea, and occasional hypoxic episodes develop as a result of compromised pulmonary blood flow. Clubbing and cyanosis are noted on physical examination, and there is a heaving left ventricular apical impulse. The majority of patients have pansystolic murmurs audible along the left sternal border; the 2nd heart sound is single.

Roentgenographic studies show pulmonary undercirculation. Left axis deviation and left ventricular hypertrophy are almost invariably present on the *electrocardiogram* except when there is transposition of the great arteries. In the right precordial leads the normally prominent R wave is replaced by rS complex. The left precordial leads show a QR complex followed by a normal flat diphasic or inverted T wave. RV_6 is normal or tall and SV_1 generally deep. Although the P waves may be normal, they are usually diphasic with the initial component tall and spiked. The *echocardiogram* identifies the absence of a tricuspid valve, the small right ventricle, and the large left ventricle and aorta.

Cardiac catheterization shows normal or elevated right atrial pressure with a prominent "a" wave. With selective angiography there is immediate opacification of the left atrium from the right atrium followed by left ventricular filling and visualization of the aorta (Fig 13–34). Absence of flow to the right ventricle results in a filling defect between the right atrium and the left ventricle. In early films in frontal projection the small right ventricle is opacified via a ventricular septal defect. Rarely, the pulmonary arteries are filled only through a patent ductus arteriosus. The absence of associated transposition of the great vessels and pulmonary stenosis is demonstrated by selective left ventriculography.

Treatment. Symptomatic neonates require a surgical shunt procedure to increase pulmonary blood flow. In severe cases adequate pulmonary blood flow may be temporarily ensured by maintaining ductal patency with infusion of prostaglandin. The Blalock-Taussig

procedure is the preferred anastomosis. Patients with tricuspid atresia may remain stable for many yr. Eventually, left ventricular dysfunction may occur since it is this chamber which must provide blood flow to both the pulmonary and systemic circulation. In older patients the Glenn anastomosis (right superior vena cava to right pulmonary artery) is utilized to provide more physiologic blood flow of unoxygenated systemic venous blood directly to the lungs. This type of shunt also does not increase the volume work of the left ventricle.

The Fontan operation is another approach to surgical management. This procedure is carried out by anastomosing the right atrium to the pulmonary artery either directly or through a conduit insertion. The atrial septal defect or foramen ovale is closed. If the right ventricle is of adequate size, a modification of this procedure may be utilized in which a valve-containing conduit is placed between the right atrium and right ventricle closing the ventricular and atrial septal defects (Fig 13–35). A 4-chambered, 4-valved heart is the result. Early evaluation of this procedure is encouraging, but

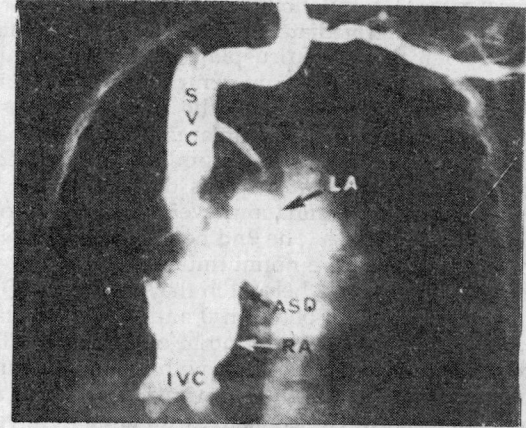

Figure 13–34 Angiocardiogram demonstrates the course of the circulation in tricuspid atresia with underdeveloped right ventricle. Systemic venous blood flows from the right to the left atrium. Absence of right ventricular opacification is due to tricuspid atresia. ASD, interatrial communication through atrial septal defect; IVC, inferior vena cava; LA, left atrium; RA, right atrium; SVC, superior vena cava.

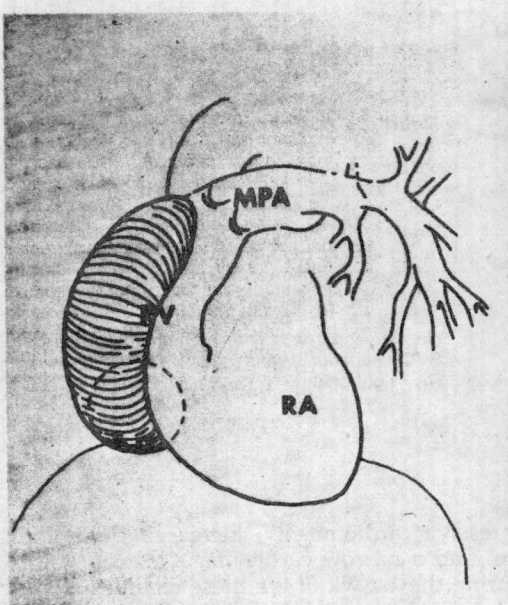

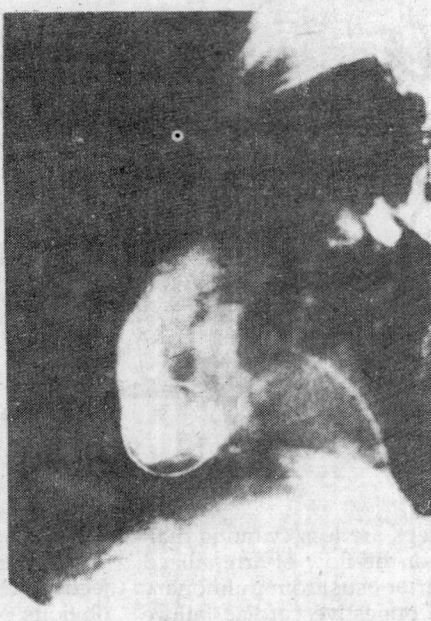

Figure 13–35 Modified Fontan operation.

the long term performance of these types of anastomoses is not known.

13.16   ORIGIN OF BOTH GREAT VESSELS FROM THE RIGHT VENTRICLE, WITH PULMONARY STENOSIS

This anomaly is often clinically indistinguishable from tetralogy of Fallot. The aorta and pulmonary artery arise from the right ventricle, and the only outlet for the left ventricle is the ventricular septal defect. The aortic and mitral valves lose their normal continuity, and the ventricular defect is inferior to the crista supraventricularis. The history, physical examination, electrocardiogram, and roentgenograms are similar to those described in Sec 13.13. The echocardiographic demonstration of lack of mitral-aortic continuity suggests the diagnosis. Selective angiocardiography shows that the aortic and pulmonary valves lie in the same horizontal body plane and that the anteriorly displaced aorta arises exclusively from the right ventricle. The angiocardiographic differentiation from tetralogy may be difficult because the aorta may also be in a markedly anterior position. Surgical correction consists of creating an intraventricular channel so that the left ventricle ejects blood through the ventricular septal defect into the aorta. The pulmonary obstruction is relieved with or without a valved conduit. In small infants palliation with an aortic pulmonary shunt provides symptomatic improvement.

13.17   TRANSPOSITION OF THE GREAT ARTERIES (TGA)

In this anomaly the aorta arises from the right ventricle and the pulmonary artery from the left ventricle. The systemic veins return to the right atrium, the pulmonary veins to the left atrium. Thus, the blood from the right heart passes to the aorta; the pulmonary venous blood is returned to the lungs. The 2 independent circuits allow survival because the foramen ovale and/or the ductus arteriosus remains open or a ventricular septum is present to permit some mixture of blood (Fig 13–36A). TGA accounts for the majority of deaths in infants under the age of 1 yr with cyanotic congenital heart disease. It occurs predominantly in males.

The aorta is usually, but not invariably, anterior and to the right of the pulmonary trunk. The pulmonary valve is continuous with the mitral valve. (Normally, the mitral and aortic valves are continuous.) Defects of the ventricular septum occur in about 50%. Generally, the right coronary artery arises above the posterior sinus of Valsalva, the left, above the left sinus. (The right coronary artery normally arises above the right sinus.) The hemodynamics vary in relation to the presence or absence of associated defects.

Clinical Manifestations.   Cyanosis, congestive cardiac failure, dyspnea, tachypnea, and retardation of growth dominate the clinical picture, but the pattern of presentation depends on the associated defects. Cyanosis usually appears shortly after birth or in the 1st weeks of life and is progressive in intensity. Polycythemia and arterial unsaturation are usual in older infants. Occasionally, cyanosis of moderate intensity appears late in patients who have a torrential pulmo-

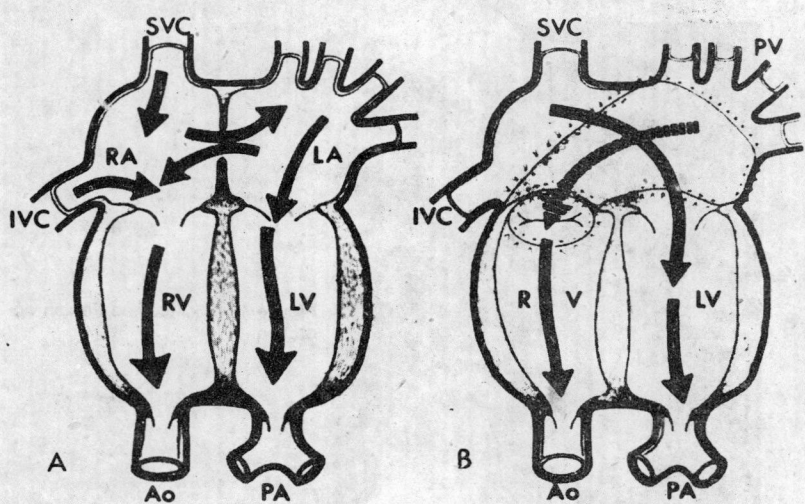

Figure 13–36 *A*, In transposition of the great arteries the circulation is in parallel. Mixing of the pulmonary and systemic circulation must occur in order to sustain life. The diagram shows bidirectional shunting at the atrial level. *B*, After intra-atrial repair (Mustard procedure), systemic venous return is routed to the left ventricle and pulmonary artery, and pulmonary venous blood reaches the systemic circulation via the right ventricle. AO = aorta, PA = pulmonary artery, LV = left ventricle, RV = right ventricle, IVC = inferior vena cava, SVC = superior vena cava, LA = left atrium, RA = right atrium.

nary flow. Infrequently, the legs are less cyanotic than the rest of the body because of the flow of arterialized blood across a patent ductus arteriosus from pulmonary artery to descending aorta. Congestive cardiac failure occurs when there is an associated ventricular septal defect; it is frequent in the neonatal period and usually occurs before the age of 4 mo. Cardiomegaly with a hyperactive precordium and a right ventricular thrust is usual, especially after the 1st mo of life. The 2nd heart sound is single or narrowly split.

With pulmonary vascular obstruction and reduced pulmonary blood flow, cyanosis is intense but heart failure minimal. Clubbing is marked in older children. Signs of pulmonary hypertension are obvious on auscultation and include a systolic ejection click, a booming 2nd heart sound, a short systolic ejection murmur, and sometimes an early diastolic murmur of pulmonary incompetence.

Diagnosis. The typical *roentgenogram* (Fig 13–37) re-

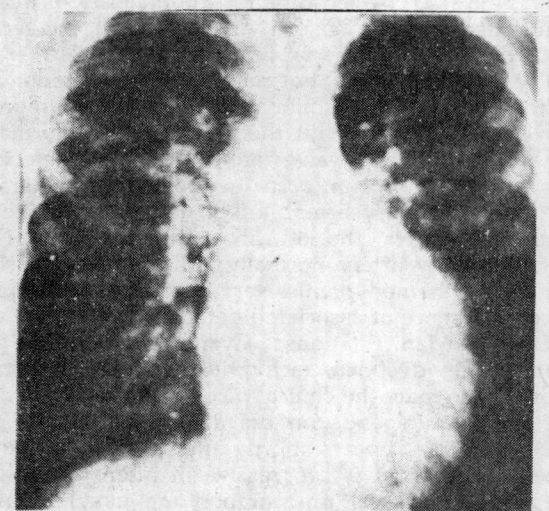

Figure 13–37 Roentgenogram in complete transposition of the great arteries with intact ventricular septum, showing cardiomegaly, gross pulmonary overcirculation, and a narrow cardiac base.

veals progressive cardiomegaly, increased pulmonary vasculature, and a narrow cardiac base in frontal projection. During the 1st wk of life these changes are not obvious. Progressive generalized cardiomegaly develops rapidly, however, and is much more striking if pulmonary blood flow is excessive. The narrow cardiac base in frontal projection is due to superimposition of the shadows of the aorta and pulmonary trunk; it may be obscured by a large thymic shadow. With pulmonary vascular obstruction, cardiomegaly is only mild to moderate, and the pulmonary vessels, prominent in the hilar areas, appear narrow peripherally.

The *electrocardiogram* characteristically shows right axis deviation, right ventricular hypertrophy, and, frequently, P pulmonale. In patients with a large pulmonary flow the axis is usually to the right of normal; there may be biventricular hypertrophy or dominance of the left ventricle. In the newborn the electrocardiogram may initially be normal.

There are characteristic *echocardiographic features:* (1) An anterior (aortic) semilunar valve echo is medial to that of the posterior (pulmonary) root. (2) The posterior root echo is more lateral than usual. (3) Real-time 2-dimensional echograms identify the aorta anterior to the pulmonary artery and usually to the right of it (Fig 13–38*B*). Occasionally, the great arteries are superimposed, and, infrequently, the aorta is to the left. (4) The ratios of the systolic time interval are reversed in patients with normal left ventricular pressure; in normal infants the ratio of the ejection time of the left ventricle to that of the right ventricle is 0.80 and the ratio of left pre-ejection time to right pre-ejection time, 1.25. (5) Contrast echocardiography with a suprasternal notch transducer shows that the aorta is visualized soon after injection of echocontrast material.

13.18 ISOLATED (SIMPLE) TRANSPOSITION OF THE GREAT ARTERIES

In this anomaly the ventricular septum is intact, and mixing of the systemic and pulmonary circulations

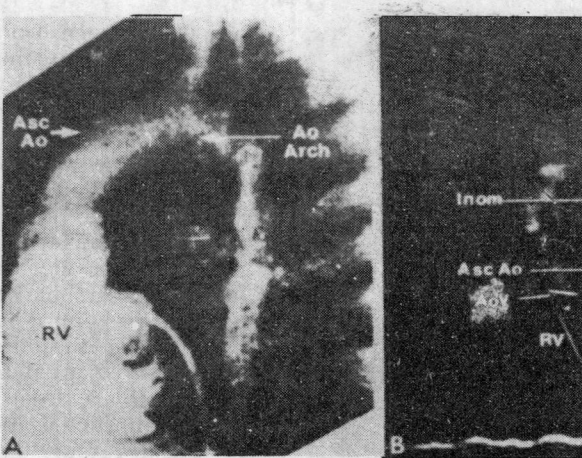

Figure 13–38 Transposition of the great arteries. *A,* Ascending aorta (Asc Ao) arising from the right ventricle (RV). *B,* Aorta (Asc Ao) is anterior to pulmonary artery (LPA). Inom = innominate vein; AoV = aortic valve; RV = right ventricle; DA = ductus arteriosus; LPA = left pulmonary artery; MPA = main pulmonary artery.

occurs from bidirectional shunting across the foramen ovale.

Clinical Manifestations. Cyanosis and tachypnea generally appear within the 1st days. If the foramen ovale is large, significant mixing may occur so that cyanosis may be delayed for a few wk or mo. *The neonate of normal weight in whom cyanosis and tachypnea are unexplained should be suspected of having the anomaly; it constitutes a medical emergency.* In the 1st days of life there may be hepatomegaly, but cardiomegaly is unusual and murmurs usually absent.

Diagnosis. *The electrocardiogram* shows normal neonatal right-sided dominance. *Roentgenograms* of the chest may be entirely within normal limits or may show cardiomegaly, a narrow cardiac waist, and increased pulmonary arterial and venous circulation. The arterial pO_2 value is low and does not rise appreciably after the patient breathes 80–100% oxygen. *Echocardiography* is useful in confirming the suspected diagnosis. The size of the intra-atrial communication can be visualized by apical and subxiphoid 2-dimensional scanning.

Cardiac catheterization shows right ventricular hypertension. The catheter enters the aorta directly from the right ventricle; it also passes across the foramen ovale or an atrial septal defect into the left heart chambers and out the pulmonary artery. The blood in the pulmonary artery has a higher oxygen content than that in the aorta. Systemic venous unsaturation is usual; the degree of arterial desaturation is variable and can be extreme. The left ventricular and pulmonary arterial pressures are also variable and are usually less than 50% of systemic pressures. A pressure gradient across the atrial septum is usual, with the left atrial pressure exceeding that of the right. *Right ventriculography* demonstrates the origin of the anteriorly placed aorta from the right ventricle, the intact ventricular septum, the closure of the ductus arteriosus, and the aortic valve cephalad to the pulmonary valve (reverse of normal). The origin of the coronary arteries is also shown. *Left ventriculography* shows that the pulmonary artery arises exclusively from the left ventricle and that the ventricular septum is intact (Fig 13–39).

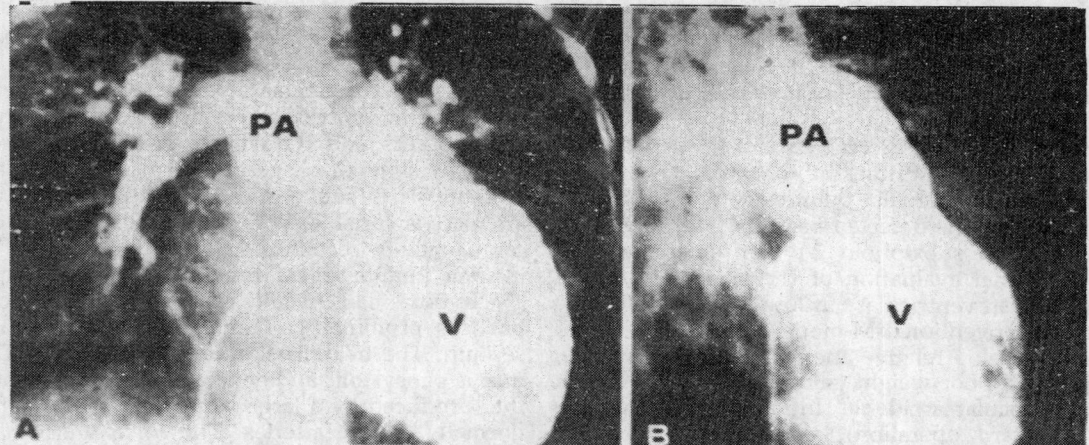

Figure 13–39 Transposition of great vessels Injection of contrast medium into a smooth-walled posterior (left) ventricle. The pulmonary artery arises exclusively from the posterior ventricle, and the interventricular septum is intact. *A,* Anteroposterior view; *B,* lateral view. PA, pulmonary artery; V, posterior (left) ventricle.

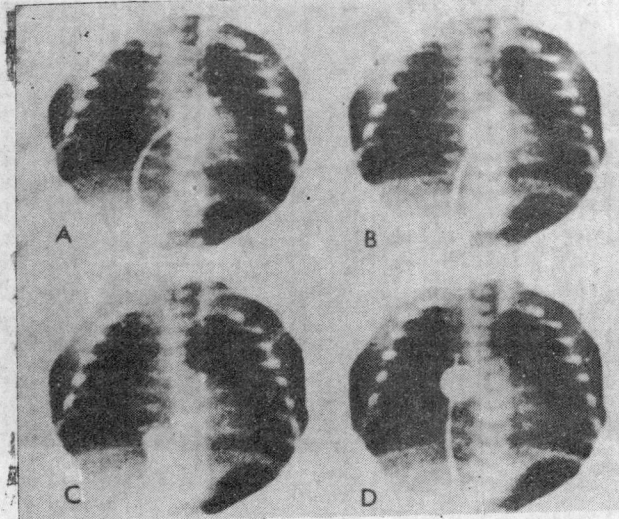

Figure 13–40 Balloon septostomy (Rashkind). Four frames from a continuous cinema that show the creation of an atrial septal defect in a hypoxemic newborn infant with transposition of the great arteries and intact ventricular septum. *A*, Balloon inflated in left atrium. *B*, Catheter is jerked suddenly so that balloon ruptures the foramen ovale. *C*, Balloon in inferior vena cava. *D*, Catheter advanced to right atrium to deflate balloon. Time from *A* to *C* less than 1 sec.

Prognosis. The prognosis for untreated infants is extremely poor; about 50% die in the 1st wk of life and most of the remainder within the 1st yr.

Treatment. Particular attention must be paid to maintaining normal body temperature; hypothermia intensifies the metabolic acidosis resulting from hypoxemia. Prompt correction of acidosis and hypoglycemia is essential. Prostaglandin E_1 may be useful to prolong ductal patency and mixing of the pulmonary and systemic circulations. After the diagnosis has been confirmed by an emergency catheterization, a large interatrial communication is created by the balloon atrial septostomy technique of Rashkind (Fig 13–40). After an adequate septostomy, mixing of the blood occurs at the atrial level, significant elevation of atrial oxygen saturation occurs, and tachypnea is relieved because of reduction of pulmonary venous pressure. Although the infants remain cyanotic, they are no longer acidotic and begin to feed well.

In some infants there is recurrence of severe cyanosis due to inadequate shunting at the atrial level or to development of subvalvular pulmonary stenosis. These complications can be detected by serial echocardiography. Apical and subxiphoid 2-dimensional scanning allows sequential evaluation of the size of the atrial septal defect; left ventricular outflow obstruction can be detected by conventional M-mode tracings. These patients may develop relative anemia, effort intolerance, irritability, and poor weight gain, and they are at risk for cerebrovascular accidents. Intra-atrial surgical correction (Mustard operation) is carried out in these infants at any age.

Surgical correction is recommended between the ages of 6–12 mo even if only moderate cyanosis is present. In the Mustard operation an atrial baffle is developed that directs systemic venous blood to the mitral valve and posterior (left) ventricle. Pulmonary venous blood flows through the tricuspid valve to the anterior (right) ventricle (Fig 13–36*B*). Thus, systemic venous blood is ejected by the left ventricle to the lungs for oxygenation, and arterialized pulmonary venous blood is pumped by the right ventricle into the aorta. Symptomatic improvement after this operation is dramatic with disappearance of cyanosis and marked increase in effort tolerance, but careful follow-up is necessary for many yr because of potential complications. Arrhythmias are common and are primarily atrial in origin; they consist of brady-tachyrhythmia, atrial tachycardia with block, atrial flutter, and junctional rhythm. Recurrence of cyanosis may be due to rupture of the baffle with resultant bidirectional atrial shunting. Obstruction by the baffle may interfere with entry of blood into the atria from the superior and inferior vena cava, from the pulmonary veins, or from both. Development of tricuspid valve incompetence, with or without right ventricular dysfunction, may result in an increase in left atrial pressure and in pulmonary edema and congestive cardiac failure. Some surgeons use the Senning type of interatrial procedure for management of transposition of the great vessels. Anatomic correction (the Jatene switch operation) is also being investigated. This involves switching the great arteries and reimplanting the coronary vessels. A pulmonary artery banding is done initially to increase left ventricular pressure so that this ventricle will not be forced to generate high pressures suddenly after having pumped blood at low pressure into the low resistance pulmonary circulation. This initial step is not required if a large ventricular septal defect is present.

13.19 TRANSPOSITION OF THE GREAT ARTERIES WITH VENTRICULAR SEPTAL DEFECT

If the septal defect is small, the clinical manifestations, laboratory findings, and treatment are similar to those described above. Many of the small defects close spontaneously.

When the ventricular septal defect is large and nonrestrictive to ventricular ejection, significant mixing of blood occurs and the *clinical manifestations* are dominated by signs of congestive cardiac failure. The onset of cyanosis is subtle and frequently delayed, and its intensity is variable. With careful observation, cyanosis can usually be recognized within the 1st mo of life, but in some infants several mo elapse before it is apparent. The hypoxemia is usually associated with polycythemia but less prominently than in patients with an intact septum. The heart is significantly enlarged. The murmur is pansystolic and generally indistinguishable from that produced by a large ventricular septal defect with normally related arteries. The *electrocardiogram* shows prominent P waves, isolated right ventricular hypertrophy, or biventricular hypertrophy. Usually, the QRS axis is to the right, but sometimes it is normal or even to the left. Occasionally, isolated dominance of the left ventricle is present. The cardiomegaly, narrow cardiac waist, and significant pulmonary vascularity are demonstrated *roentgenographically*. Pulmonary blood flow can also be assessed by *echocardiography*. (Increased flows are associated with enlargement of the left atrium and ventricle.) Serial measurements of the systolic time interval ratios from the pulmonary valve are useful in determining the progression of pulmonary hypertension. The diagnosis is confirmed by *cardiac catheterization* and angiocardiography. Right and left ventriculography indicates the presence of arterial transposition and demonstrates the site and size of the ventricular septal defect. The catheter may cross the ventricular septum from the right ventricle and enter the pulmonary artery. Peak systolic pressures are equal in the 2 ventricles, the aorta, and the pulmonary artery. The ventricular end diastolic pressures are elevated in the presence of cardiac failure.

At the time of cardiac catheterization a balloon septostomy is performed to decompress the left atrium even though adequate mixing occurs at the ventricular level. Elective but urgent surgical therapy is advised in selected cases since congestive heart failure and failure to thrive are difficult to manage and pulmonary vascular disease develops rapidly. Patients with this combination of defects almost always also require maintenance digitalis and diuretic therapy.

The *prognosis* is poor; the majority of patients succumb in the 1st yr of life because of congestive cardiac failure, hypoxemia, and pulmonary hypertension. Some survive infancy with medical therapy and without surgical intervention. The clinical picture and treatment of these patients are almost identical to those described in Eisenmenger syndrome (Sec 13.26) with a large ventricular septal defect. *Surgical palliation* with a Mustard operation has been successful in relieving the hypoxemia of intensely cyanotic patients, but the pulmonary vascular disease is not affected.

There is a lack of unanimity concerning the appropriate *surgical therapy*; the case fatality rates are higher than with simple transposition. To date most experience has been with pulmonary artery banding, with or without atrial septectomy, during infancy followed by debanding and correction after the age of about 1 yr. Direct early repair without initial banding has also been advocated. The method of repair consists of intra-atrial correction of venous return and patch closure of the ventricular septal defect. Mortality remains high. Another approach to correction is placement of a ventricular prosthesis so that the left ventricle ejects into the aorta and establishment of right ventricular-pulmonary artery continuity with a valved prosthesis (Rastelli). This is done later in childhood; there is little experience during infancy. Closure of the ventricular septal defect and anatomic correction of the great arteries so that the aorta carries left ventricular blood and the pulmonary artery carries blood from the right ventricle have also been carried out in infants with this lesion. The coronary arteries are implanted into the great vessel arising from the left ventricle. It is too early to evaluate results.

13.20 TRANSPOSITION OF THE GREAT ARTERIES WITH A LARGE PATENT DUCTUS ARTERIOSUS

In the neonate with TGA a large patent ductus arteriosus may be of benefit. Persistent patency beyond the 1st weeks of life, however, aggravates the situation since the dominant flow across the duct runs from aorta to pulmonary artery, further increasing the pulmonary blood flow. This clinical picture is dominated by signs of congestive cardiac failure; cyanosis may not be obvious. After effective palliation with balloon atrial septostomy, many of these infants remain in uncontrollable congestive cardiac failure and require surgical closure of the duct and an intra-atrial correction of TGA.

13.21 TRANSPOSITION OF THE GREAT ARTERIES WITH PULMONARY STENOSIS

This combination of anomalies may mimic tetralogy of Fallot. The site of obstruction is either valvular or subvalvular and may be associated with a hypoplastic pulmonary arterial trunk. A ventricular septal defect may or may not be present. It is important to recognize that subvalvular obstruction may be acquired after successful atrial septostomy or pulmonary arterial banding.

The onset of *clinical manifestations* varies from soon after birth to late infancy and includes cyanosis, hypercyanotic (paroxysmal dyspneic) episodes, decreased exercise tolerance, and poor physical development. Congestive heart failure is not common in infancy but may occur in later yr. The manifestations are similar to those described under tetralogy of Fallot. The cyanosis is usually more intense, however, and the heart may be enlarged. The pulmonary vasculature as seen on *roentgenogram* is normal or somewhat diminished but in some instances may be increased, especially if the pulmonic stenosis is not severe. The *electrocardiogram* usually shows right axis deviation, right and left ventricular hypertrophy, and sometimes tall, spiked P waves. *Echocardiography* is useful in sequential evaluation of the degree and progression of the pulmonic obstruction. Narrowing of the left ventricular outflow tract is produced by a thickened ventricular septum. Other echographic features that may be present include premature closure of the pulmonary valve, reduction of the systolic time interval ratio from the pulmonary valve, and systolic anterior motion of the mitral valve.

Cardiac catheterization shows that the pulmonary arterial pressure is low and that the oxygen saturation exceeds that of the aorta. Selective right and left ventriculography demonstrates the origin of the aorta from the right ventricle, the origin of the pulmonary artery from the left ventricle, the ventricular defect, and the pulmonary stenosis.

The preferred *treatment* in hypoxemic infants is establishment of a systemic-pulmonary arterial shunt, with or without an atrial septectomy. In children beyond the age of 2–5 yr the Rastelli procedure is usually undertaken. After this procedure the left ventricle ejects into the aorta via the ventricular septal defect and the right ventricle, through a valved conduit into the pulmonary artery. This approach has been successful in the majority of cases. Surgical correction by the Mustard operation with simultaneous closure of the ventricular septal defect and relief of left ventricular outflow obstruction has been done successfully but is associated with a high risk if the subvalvular obstruction is long and narrow and if the main pulmonary artery is hypoplastic.

13.22   TRANSPOSITION OF THE GREAT ARTERIES WITH TRICUSPID ATRESIA

If arterial transposition is associated with tricuspid atresia and pulmonary stenosis, the syndrome is similar to that described under Tricuspid Atresia. If pulmonary stenosis is absent, however, and pulmonary flow excessive, cyanosis is mild. Tachypnea, feeding difficulties, poor weight gain, recurrent respiratory infections, and heart failure are usual. Increased venous pressure may result in presystolic pulsations of a large liver and a prominent "a" wave in the jugular venous pulse. Cardiac enlargement is moderate to excessive. Systolic ejection murmurs of varying intensity are usual, and the 2nd heart sound is loud and single. Although the electrocardiogram may show prominent P waves, left axis deviation, and left ventricular hypertrophy, many patients have right axis deviation. Cardiac enlargement is confirmed roentgenographically; increased pulmonary vascularity is usual. The diagnosis is confirmed by selective left ventriculography, which delineates a large left ventricle, small right ventricle, arterial transposition, and the relative sizes of the pulmonary artery and aorta. Generally, the prognosis is poor, especially when the aorta is hypoplastic and pulmonary flow torrential. Surgical palliation is achieved with pulmonary arterial banding, which is most effective when the aortic root is near normal in size. Variations of the Fontan concept (right atrium–pulmonary artery connection) may be utilized in selected patients.

13.23   EBSTEIN DISEASE

This anomaly consists of downward displacement of an abnormal tricuspid valve into the right ventricle. The anterior cusp of the valve retains some attachment to the valve ring, but the other leaflets are attached to the wall of the right ventricle. The latter chamber is divided into 2 parts by the abnormal valve; the 1st is continuous with the cavity of the right atrium; the 2nd is a thin-walled ventricle. The right atrium is huge, and the tricuspid valve may or may not be competent. The effective output from the right side of the heart is decreased because of the small size of the functioning right ventricle and possible obstruction produced by the large, sail-like, anterior tricuspid leaflet. Variable amounts of right to left shunting occur at the atrial level via the foramen ovale, resulting in mild to severe cyanosis.

Clinical Manifestations.   The severity of symptoms depends on the degree of displacement of the tricuspid valve. In many patients, symptoms are mild and the only complaint is fatigue. Cardiac dysrhythmias are frequent, the most common being numerous extrasystoles or attacks of paroxysmal tachycardia, usually supraventricular. If the foramen ovale is open or an interatrial defect is present, a right to left shunt is responsible for cyanosis and polycythemia. The venous pressure is normal or increased if there is associated tricuspid insufficiency. On palpation the precordium is quiet. A systolic murmur, sometimes accompanied by a thrill, is audible over most of the anterior left side of the chest. Gallop rhythm is common as is a diastolic murmur at the left sternal border. This murmur is superficial and may mimic a pericardial friction rub. A series of systolic ejection clicks and an opening snap of the tricuspid valve may also be audible.

Although some patients may be asymptomatic until well into adult life, newborn infants with Ebstein disease may present with cyanosis, massive cardiomegaly, and long systolic murmurs. The case fatality rate is high because of cardiac failure and hypoxemia. Spontaneous and rapid improvement occurs in some and has been attributed to a decrease in pulmonary vascular resistance.

Diagnosis.   The *electrocardiogram* shows right bundle branch block, normal or tall and broad P waves, and normal or prolonged P-R interval. Sometimes the pattern of the Wolff-Parkinson-White syndrome is present.

On *roentgenographic examination* the heart size varies from normal to massive cardiomegaly because of great enlargement of the right atrium and ventricle. The amplitude of cardiac pulsations is decreased, the intrapulmonary vasculature is normal or decreased, and the aorta is small.

Echocardiography shows delayed closure and an increased amplitude of the tricuspid valve. Abnormal septal motion, retardation of the E-F slope of the tricuspid valve, and a dilated right atrium may also be recorded. The atrialized portion of the right ventricle and the abnormal tricuspid valve can be visualized with 2-dimensional ultrasound.

Cardiac catheterization and selective angiocardiography confirm the presence of a large right atrium and demonstrate the right to left shunt at the atrial level, if this exists. The right atrial pressure may be normal, but it is frequently elevated as is the right ventricular diastolic pressure. Simultaneous intracardiac electrocardiograms and pressures are of great value when the following are recorded: (1) right ventricular pressure with a right ventricular intracavity electrocardiogram; (2) from the atrialized portion of the right ventricle, atrial pressure curve with a right ventricular intracavity electrocardiogram; and (3) from the right atrium, atrial pressure curve and atrial intracavity electrocardiogram. There is a significant risk of arrhythmia during catheterization and angiographic studies.

Prognosis.   This is extremely variable; many patients survive into adult life.

Treatment.   Control of hypoxemia and supraventricular dysrhythmias is of primary importance. Surgical treatment is seldom necessary in childhood. In deeply cyanotic patients, anastomosis of the superior vena cava to the right pulmonary artery (Glenn) has resulted in symptomatic improvement. Replacement of the abnormal tricuspid valve with a prosthesis or tricuspid valvuloplasty with closure of the atrial septal defect, however, is preferred for the deeply cyanotic patient.

13.24 TRUNCUS ARTERIOSUS

In this anomaly a single arterial trunk leaves the ventricular portion of the heart and supplies the systemic, pulmonary, and coronary circulations. A ventricular septal defect is always present, and the number of semilunar valve cusps varies from 2–6. In the majority of instances the pulmonary arteries arise from the ascending portion of the truncus proximal to the origin of the innominate artery. The pulmonary arteries may arise as a single vessel from the truncus or as 2 separate arteries. In some instances the pulmonary arteries and ductus are absent; the pulmonary blood flow then is derived from collateral vessels, often bronchial. Usually there is a remnant of main and/or left and right pulmonary arteries which may carry blood flow from the aorta via a ductus arteriosus. This condition is considered by some to be pulmonary atresia with ventricular septal defect (Sec 13.14), occasionally referred to as pseudotruncus.

Hemodynamics. Both ventricles empty their blood at systemic pressure into the truncus. When the pulmonary vascular resistance approximates normal, the blood flow to the lungs is greatly increased, the arteriovenous oxygen difference is small, and cyanosis is minimal or absent. When the pulmonary resistance rises, the pulmonary circulation is inadequate and cyanosis intense. The truncal valve is occasionally incompetent.

Clinical Manifestations. These vary because of the extremely variable hemodynamics. In the majority of infants, pulmonary blood flow is torrential and the clinical picture dominated by dyspnea, fatigue, heart failure, recurrent respiratory infections, and poor physical development. Cyanosis is minimal or absent. This situation closely simulates that produced by an isolated large ventricular septal defect. The runoff of blood from the truncus to the pulmonary circulation may result in a wide pulse pressure. The heart is usually enlarged, and the precordium is hyperdynamic. A systolic ejection murmur, sometimes accompanied by a thrill, is usual along the left sternal border. The murmur is frequently preceded by an ejection click. The 2nd heart sound is loud and generally single, though it may be split. A mid-diastolic apical rumbling murmur is audible. In older children with restricted pulmonary blood flow, progressive cyanosis, polycythemia, and clubbing develop. When pulmonary arteries are hypoplastic, cyanosis and dyspnea are present from infancy; cardiomegaly is moderate, and there are continuous murmurs.

Diagnosis. The *electrocardiogram* is variable and shows right, left, or combined ventricular hypertrophy. There is considerable variation in the roentgenographic appearance of the chest. Cardiac enlargement is due to prominence of both ventricles. The truncus may produce a prominent shadow which follows the normal course of the ascending aorta and aortic knob; it arches to the right in almost 50% of patients. Sometimes a high bulge, left of the aortic knob, is produced by the main or left pulmonary artery. The pulmonary vascularity is increased in the presence of normal pulmonary resistance; it decreases as the resistance rises. *Echocardiography* demonstrates the large, overriding (Fig 13–30), and usually anterior truncal artery and the mitral-aortic continuity. Since there is no pulmonary valve, differentiation from pulmonary atresia with ventricular septal defect or severe tetralogy of Fallot may be difficult. A helpful sign in truncus arteriosus is delineation of a large left atrium which reflects the increased pulmonary blood flow.

The diagnosis is confirmed by *cardiac catheterization* and by selective right ventriculography. The catheter may enter the pulmonary arteries from the truncus. A left to right shunt is demonstrated at the ventricular level, and the systolic pressures in both ventricles and the truncus are similar. Selective angiocardiography reveals the large truncus arteriosus and the origin of the pulmonary arteries. Injection of contrast medium into the truncus just above the truncal valve is essential since the abnormal valves have varying degrees of incompetence.

Prognosis. This is variable, but the majority of patients succumb during the 1st 2 yr of life. If pulmonary blood flow is restricted by development of pulmonary hypertension, the patient may survive well into adult life.

Treatment. Treatment is not standardized. Radical surgical treatment has been accomplished successfully, even in infants. The ventricular septal defect is closed, the pulmonary arteries are amputated from the truncus, and continuity is established between the right ventricle and the pulmonary arteries with a valved conduit. Immediate surgical results are remarkable if the preoperative pulmonary vascular resistance is not greatly increased. Long term results are not known, but the conduit must be replaced as the child grows. The other option is banding of the pulmonary arteries followed by surgical correction in later yr; morbidity and mortality associated with banding, however, are high. In patients with pulmonary vascular obstruction or hypoplastic pulmonary arteries, surgical treatment is contraindicated.

13.25 SINGLE VENTRICLE

With a single ventricle, both atria empty through a common valve or 2 separate atrioventricular valves into a single ventricular chamber from which the aorta and pulmonary artery arise. Associated cardiac anomalies are usual and vary considerably. The more frequent ones are arterial transposition, rudimentary outlet chamber from which the aorta arises, and pulmonary stenosis.

Clinical Manifestations. The hemodynamics and clinical picture are extremely variable because they depend on the associated intracardiac anomalies and the degree of pulmonary blood flow. If a single ventricle is associated with pulmonary stenosis, cyanosis is present in infancy and increases in intensity during childhood, when clubbing and polycythemia also appear. Dyspnea and fatigue are frequent, and paroxysmal dyspneic spells may occur. Cardiomegaly is mild or moderate, a left parasternal lift is palpable, and a systolic thrill is common. The systolic ejection murmur is usually loud; an ejection click may be audible, and the 2nd heart sound is single and loud. When a single ventricle is associated with an unobstructed pulmonary outflow tract, pulmonary blood flow is torrential. These patients have tachypnea, dyspnea, poor physical development, recurrent pulmonary infections, and congestive heart failure. Cyanosis is only mild or moderate. Cardiomegaly is generally marked, and a left parasternal lift is palpable. The systolic ejection murmur is generally not intense, and the 2nd heart sound is loud and closely split. A 3rd heart sound is frequent and may be followed by a short mid-diastolic murmur. The development of pulmonary vascular disease may restrict pulmonary blood flow so that cyanosis increases in intensity, heart size decreases, and signs of cardiac failure appear to improve.

Diagnosis. The *electrocardiogram* is nonspecific. P waves are normal, spiked, or bifid. The precordial lead pattern suggests right ventricular hypertrophy, combined ventricular hypertrophy, or sometimes left ventricular dominance. The initial QRS forces are usually to the left and anterior. *Roentgenographic examination* confirms the degree of cardiomegaly. The rudimentary systemic outflow chamber may produce a bulge on the upper left border of the cardiac silhouette in the posteroanterior projection. In the absence of pulmonary stenosis, pulmonary vasculature is increased with prominence of the major branches of the pulmonary artery. Attenuation of the size of the peripheral pulmonary arteries occurs with the development of obstructive pulmonary hypertension. Absence of the ventricular septal echo is the principal *echographic* sign. If there are 2 atrioventricular valves (double inlet), the mitral valve is posterior and the tricuspid to the right. If a single atrioventricular valve is present, it occupies the entire ventricle. With transposition of the great arteries, the mitral valve is in continuity with the pulmonary artery.

Cardiac catheterization reveals a left to right shunt at the ventricular level. The arterial oxygen saturation is decreased in the presence of severe pulmonary stenosis or obstructive pulmonary hypertension but is near normal when pulmonary blood flow is increased. The pressure in the single ventricle is high; a gradient may be demonstrated between it and the rudimentary outflow tract or the pulmonary artery in the presence of pulmonary stenosis. Severe pulmonary hypertension is present in the absence of pulmonary stenosis. Selective ventriculography is diagnostic and demonstrates the single ventricle and the positions and relation of the pulmonary artery and aorta.

Prognosis. Some patients succumb during infancy from congestive heart failure and superimposed pulmonary infection. Others may survive to adolescence and early adult life but finally succumb to the effects of pulmonary hypertension. Patients with moderate pulmonary stenosis have the best prognosis.

Treatment. If pulmonary stenosis is present, a systemic-pulmonary arterial anastomosis can result in improvement, but some patients suffer heart failure months after the operation. Pulmonary artery banding is advised for patients with a large pulmonary flow. Definitive repair has been accomplished by inserting an artificial septum in single ventricles with a double inlet. Success has been limited with this approach. Recently, the Fontan operation has been utilized in patients whose pulmonary pressure and resistance are low.

13.26   EISENMENGER SYNDROME

The term Eisenmenger syndrome refers to the combination of pulmonary hypertension with reversed or bidirectional shunt through either a ventricular or atrial septal defect or a patent ductus arteriosus (or other communication between the aorta and lesser circulation). The principal physiologic abnormality is elevation of the pulmonary vascular resistance. In normal neonates, within a few wk, the structure of the pulmonary arteriole changes to that of the adult with a thin wall and a large lumen, and the pulmonary vascular resistance falls to normal adult levels. In the Eisenmenger syndrome the pulmonary vascular resistance either remains high or falls during early infancy and rises thereafter because of increased shear stress on pulmonary arterioles. The phenomenon is the result of prolonged elevated pulmonary pressure.

Clinical Manifestations. Symptoms may not occur until the 2nd or 3rd decade of life, although less often a more fulminant course is seen. Irreversible pulmonary vascular obstruction results in high pulmonary vascular resistance. Intra- or extracardiac communications which normally would shunt left to right allow right to left shunting as pulmonary resistance exceeds systemic resistance. Cyanosis becomes apparent, and dyspnea, fatigue, and tendency toward dysrhythmias begin to occur. In the late stages of the disease, congestive heart failure, chest pain, syncope, and hemoptysis may be seen. Physical examination reveals a right ventricular heave and a loud, narrowly split 2nd heart sound. Only a soft ejection systolic murmur is audible along the left sternal border. Pulmonary artery pulsation may be palpable at the left upper sternal border. Various degrees of cyanosis may be observed depending on the stage of the disease. Functional incompetence of the pulmonary valve may result in a blowing diastolic murmur along the left sternal border (Graham Steell murmur).

Diagnosis. *Roentgenographically*, the heart varies in size from normal to greatly enlarged. Larger hearts are seen with atrial defects. Small cardiac silhouettes are noted with ventricular defects and patent ductus arteriosus (Fig 13–41), but there is a large overlap. The pulmonary artery is usually enlarged. The pulmonary vessels are enlarged in the hilar areas and diminish in caliber in the peripheral branches. The right ventricle and atrium are prominent. The *electrocardiogram* fre-

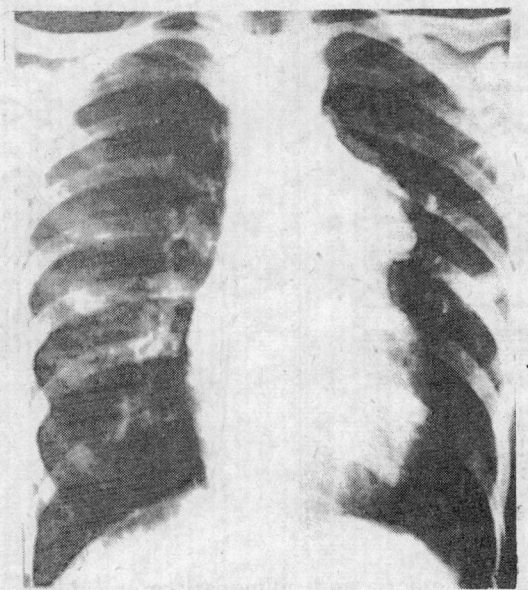

Figure 13–41 Roentgenogram in Eisenmenger syndrome due to a patent ductus arteriosus. The heart size is normal, the pulmonary artery segment is dilated, and the pulmonary vascularity is normal or slightly increased.

quently shows right ventricular hypertrophy, occasionally associated with incomplete right bundle branch block. The P wave may be tall and spiked. Sometimes the electrocardiogram is balanced, with signs of biventricular hypertrophy. The *echocardiogram* shows a thick-walled right ventricle, and the chamber dimension is frequently increased. The right side systolic time interval shows a significant increase in the ratio of preejection period to ejection time because of the increased pulmonary vascular resistance.

Cardiac catheterization usually shows a bidirectional shunt at the site of the defect. The systolic pressures are usually equal in the systemic and pulmonary circulations. There is a definite decrease in arterial oxygen saturation when there is only a right to left shunt. The catheter frequently traverses the defect, especially with a patent ductus arteriosus or atrial septal defect. The pulmonary vascular resistance is elevated. Indicator dilution curves demonstrate the bidirectional shunts or the unidirectional right to left one. Selective angiocardiography is helpful in locating the site of the shunt. With patent ductus arteriosus, contrast medium enters the descending aorta from the pulmonary artery.

Treatment. Surgical closure of the defect is contraindicated. Pulmonary hypertension with increased pulmonary blood flow but without a right to left shunt, however, is not the Eisenmenger syndrome, and surgery may be lifesaving. Medical treatment of the Eisenmenger syndrome is entirely symptomatic. Older children and adolescents with significant polycythemia may be improved by cautious, repeated venesections with volume replacement.

13.27 HYPOPLASTIC LEFT HEART SYNDROME

The term hypoplastic left heart syndrome is used to describe varying degrees of underdevelopment of the left side of the heart. The anomalies include underdevelopment of the left atrium and ventricle, stenosis or atresia of the aortic or mitral orifices, and hypoplasia of the ascending aorta. Associated defects include endocardial fibroelastosis of the left ventricle and atrial and ventricular septal defects. The left ventricular cavity is small, but the wall may be thick if obstruction to left ventricular outflow is associated with mitral stenosis. If aortic atresia and mitral atresia coexist, the left ventricular cavity is minute.

Since the left ventricle is virtually nonfunctional, the right ventricle maintains both pulmonary and systemic circulations. Pulmonary venous blood passes through an atrial defect or dilated foramen ovale from the left to the right side of the heart, where it mixes with systemic venous blood. If the ventricular septum is intact, all the right ventricular blood is ejected to the pulmonary arteries; the systemic circulation is supplied via the ductus arteriosus. With a ventricular septal defect and a patent but small aortic orifice, right ventricular blood is ejected to the small left ventricle and ascending aorta as well as to the pulmonary artery. The major hemodynamic abnormalities are inadequate maintenance of the systemic circulation and pulmonary venous hypertension.

Clinical Manifestations. Signs of heart failure appear within the 1st weeks of life and include dyspnea and hepatomegaly. All peripheral pulses are weak or absent. Although cyanosis may not be obvious in the 1st 48 hr of life, a grayish blue color of the skin is soon apparent. Differential cyanosis may be noted if the aortic valve has a small opening. In these patients oxygenated blood from the left ventricle enters the ascending aorta and innominate artery and gives normal color to the right arm and right side of the head and neck, but contrasting cyanosis is seen in the rest of the body. Cardiac enlargement is usual, with a palpable right ventricular parasternal lift. Murmurs, if present, are short and midsystolic.

Diagnosis. *Roentgenographically*, the heart is variable in size in the 1st days of life, but moderate or gross cardiomegaly develops rapidly and is associated with increased pulmonary vascularity. The *electrocardiogram* may show only the normal right ventricular dominance initially, but later P waves become prominent and right ventricular hypertrophy is usual.

Echocardiograms are diagnostic (Fig 13–42). They show absence or gross distortion of the normal mitral valve echo, absent or small aortic root, a small posterior ventricle, a large anterior ventricle, and an easily identifiable tricuspid valve. Contrast echocardiography (Fig 13–23) with the transducer in the suprasternal notch identifies the small transverse aortic arch and left atrium. These findings are so characteristic that the diagnosis of aortic atresia can be made without cardiac catheterization. The hypoplastic ascending aorta is best

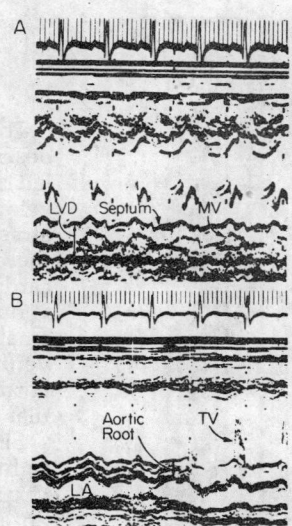

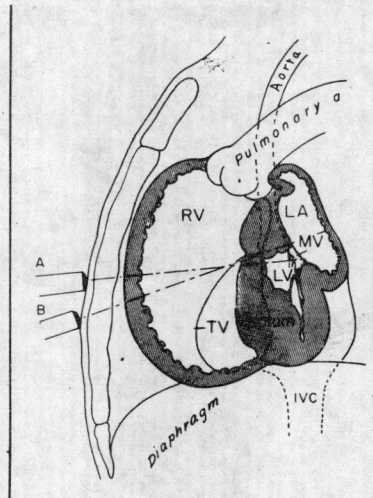

Figure 13–42   Echocardiogram from neonate with aortic valve atresia. Idealized diagram on right shows the small left ventricle and aorta. Echogram A (from transducer position A) shows minute left ventricular dimension (LVD) containing a small mitral valve (MV).

demonstrated by aortography, which may also show the coronary arterial system.

Prognosis.   Most patients succumb during the 1st mo of life, usually during the 1st wk.

Treatment.   Therapy is symptomatic. Surgical procedures have been attempted to decompress the left atrium by septectomy, to maintain systemic flow by creation of a systemic-pulmonary shunt, and to prevent pulmonary vascular disease by banding both pulmonary arteries. These are formidable procedures in critically ill infants. The immediate mortality is high, and the long term prognosis is not known.

13.28   ABNORMAL POSITIONS OF THE HEART: DEXTROCARDIA AND LEVOCARDIA

An approach to the classification and diagnosis of abnormal cardiac position has been suggested by Van Praagh et al. *Atrial localization* is facilitated by roentgenographic demonstration of the position of the abdominal organs and of the tracheal bifurcation for recognition of the situs of the right and left bronchi. Atrial situs is related to the visceral situs; if the viscera are in normal position, the atria have a normal position. Abdominal situs inversus is associated with the left atrium to the right and right atrium to the left. If the abdominal situs cannot be determined, as with a centrally located liver and asplenia or rudimentary spleen, atrial localization is difficult. *Localization of the ventricles and great arteries* depends on the direction of development of the embryonic cardiac loop. Initial protrusion to the right (d-loop) carries the future right ventricle to the right, and the left ventricle remains on the left. Protrusion to the left (l-loop) carries the future right ventricle to the left, and the left ventricle is on the right. With each type of loop the relations of the great arteries may be normal or transposed. Angiographic demonstration of the rela-

tions of the aorta and pulmonary artery indicates the type of cardiac loop and the relative location of the ventricle. The clinical manifestations of abnormal cardiac position are dominated by the associated cardiovascular anomalies.

Dextrocardia with or without Situs Inversus.   Dextrocardia without situs inversus is virtually always complicated by severe malformations that include various combinations of single ventricle, arterial transposition, pulmonary stenosis, ventricular and atrial septal defects, complete atrioventricular canal, anomalous pulmonary venous return, tricuspid atresia, and pulmonary arterial hypoplasia or atresia. When abdominal heterotaxia is present, the cardiac anomalies are associated with polysplenia or asplenia. Surveys of older children and adults indicate that dextrocardia with situs inversus and with normally related great arteries (so-called mirror-image dextrocardia) is most often associated with a functionally normal heart.

Abnormalities of the lung, diaphragm, and thoracic cage may result in displacement of the heart to the right, mimicking dextrocardia. Hypoplasia of a lung may be accompanied by anomalous pulmonary venous return from that lung. The *electrocardiogram* is helpful in diagnosis but frequently difficult to interpret. Inversion of the P wave in lead I is indicative of atrial inversion. Q waves produced by right ventricular hypertrophy may make interpretation of ventricular dominance difficult. Deep Q waves or QS in V_1, V_2, and aV_L are seen in patients with dextrocardia and normally related great arteries.

Levocardia with Varying Degrees of Visceral Heterotaxia   (Partial or Complete Situs Inversus).   This combination is usually associated with severe cardiovascular defects, frequently of the cyanotic type. These include combinations of abnormal systemic venous return (bilateral superior vena cava; absence of inferior vena cava with venous drainage of the lower part of the body into the azygous system), anomalous pulmonary venous return, arterial transposition, pulmonary stenosis or atresia, atrial or ventricular septal defect, common atrioventricular canal, single ventricle, and patent ductus arteriosus. These patients have a high incidence of asplenia or rudimentary spleen, which may be suspected when Howell-Jolly bodies (nuclear remnants) or Heinz bodies (precipitated hemoglobin) are seen in the red blood cells.

Treatment of abnormal cardiac position is determined by the underlying defect. Cyanotic infants with pulmonic stenosis and ventricular septal defect as a part of the malformation improve after anastomosis of the systemic and pulmonary blood supplies. Lesions such as atrial or ventricular septal defect and tetralogy of Fallot have been repaired successfully.

13.29 PULMONARY ARTERIOVENOUS FISTULA

Fistulous vascular communications in the lungs may be large and localized or multiple, scattered, and small. They may be a manifestation of the Rendu-Osler-Weber syndrome (hereditary hemorrhagic telangiectasia) with angiomas of the nasal and buccal mucous membranes, gastrointestinal tract, or liver. A rare variant is a direct communication between the pulmonary artery and left atrium.

Venous blood in the pulmonary artery is shunted through the fistula into the pulmonary vein without exposure to alveolar air, enters the left heart, and results in systemic arterial unsaturation. The shunt across the fistula is at low pressure and resistance so that pulmonary arterial pressure is normal; cardiomegaly is unusual, and heart failure is rare.

The clinical picture depends on the magnitude of shunt. Dyspnea, cyanosis, clubbing, and polycythemia occur with large fistulas. Hemoptysis is rare, but may be massive. Features of the Rendu-Osler-Weber syndrome occur in about 50% of patients (or other members of their family) and include recurrent epistaxis and gastrointestinal bleeding. Transitory dizziness, diplopia, aphasia, motor weakness, or convulsions may result from cerebral thrombosis, abscess, or paradoxic emboli. Soft systolic or continuous murmurs may be audible over the site of the fistula.

The *electrocardiogram* is normal. *Roentgenographic examination* of the chest (Fig 13–43) may show opacities produced by large fistulas; multiple small fistulas may be visualized by fluoroscopy (abnormal pulsations) or tomography. Selective *pulmonary arteriography* demonstrates the site, extent, and distribution of the fistulas (Fig 13–44).

Excision of solitary or localized lesions by lobectomy or wedge resection results in complete disappearance of symptoms. If the fistulas are widely distributed, extensive pulmonary resection may be followed by postoperative growth of smaller fistulas and recurrence of symptoms. If there is a direct communication between the pulmonary artery and left atrium, it is obliterated by division and suture.

13.30 ECTOPIA CORDIS

This is a rare malformation in which the heart is in an abnormal location. In the most common thoracic form the sternum is split and the heart protrudes outside the chest. In others the heart protrudes through the diaphragm into the abdominal cavity or may be situated in the neck. Associated intracardiac anomalies are common. Death occurs in the 1st days of life in the majority of instances, usually from infection, cardiac failure, or hypoxemia. Surgical objectives are to cover the heart with skin without compromising venous return or ventricular ejection. Palliation of associated defects is also usually necessary. Occasional patients with the abdominal type have survived to adulthood.

13.31 DIVERTICULUM OF THE LEFT VENTRICLE

In this rare anomaly a diverticulum of the left ventricle protrudes into the epigastrium. The lesion may be isolated or associated with complex cardiovascular

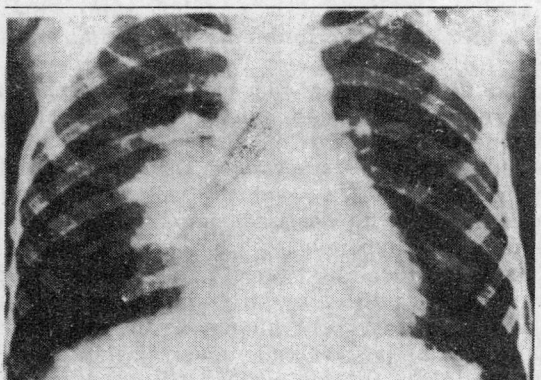

Figure 13–43 Roentgenogram of patient with pulmonary arteriovenous fistula, showing a localized increase in pulmonary vascularity in the right lung.

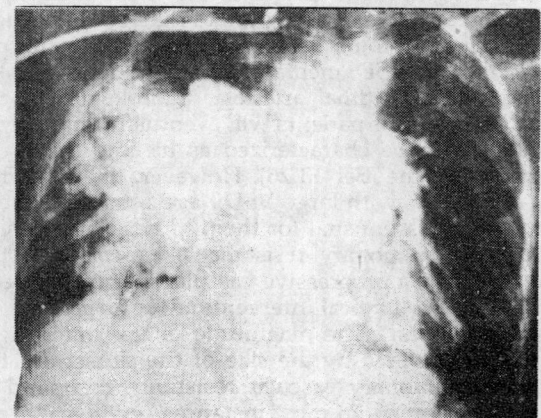

Figure 13–44 Angiocardiogram of patient with pulmonary arteriovenous fistula. (Same patient as Fig 13–43.) The contrast medium has delineated the extent of the fistula in the right lung.

anomalies. A pulsating mass is visible and palpable in the epigastrium. Systolic or systolic-diastolic murmurs produced by blood flow in and out of the diverticulum may be audible over the lower sternum and the mass. The *electrocardiogram* shows a pattern of complete or incomplete left bundle branch block. *Roentgenograms* of the chest may or may not show the mass. Associated abnormalities include defects of the sternum, abdominal wall, diaphragm, and pericardium. Surgical treatment of the diverticulum and associated cardiac defects may be considered in the presence of uncontrollable heart failure or hypoxemia.

Congenital Heart Disease with Little or no Cyanosis (Dominant Left to Right Shunt or No Shunt)

13.32 VENTRICULAR SEPTAL DEFECTS (VSD)

Ventricular septal defect is the most common cardiac malformation accounting for 25% of congenital heart disease. The majority of defects are of the membranous type in a posteroinferior position, anterior to the septal leaflet of the tricuspid valve. Defects between the crista supraventricularis and the papillary muscle of the conus may be associated with pulmonary stenosis and the other manifestations of tetralogy of Fallot. Defects superior to the crista supraventricularis are less common; they are found just beneath the pulmonary valve and may impinge on an aortic sinus, causing aortic insufficiency. Defects involving the inflow portion of the ventricular septum or apical area are muscular in type and may be single or multiple.

Pathophysiology. If the defect is small, the cardiac chambers and pulmonary vascular bed are normal. Large defects produce significant left to right shunt and result in left ventricular volume overload as well as right ventricular and pulmonary artery hypertension. The left atrium and ventricle are enlarged because of the large left to right shunt. The pulmonary arterial trunk is large. After birth, in the presence of a large VSD, pulmonary resistance may remain higher than in a normal infant and left to right shunt may be limited. However, within a few wk there is relatively normal involution of muscular media of the small pulmonary arteries and arterioles. A large left to right shunt ensues, and clinical symptoms become apparent. In some patients with large VSD, medial thickness remains present and, with time, intimal arteriolar pathologic changes occur; this group of patients will eventually shunt right to left and can be characterized as having the Eisenmenger syndrome (Sec 13.26). However, the great majority of patients with large VSD have a massive left to right shunt; it is unusual for them to have progressive increases in pulmonary resistances, especially in the present era when progressive vascular disease has been limited by early surgical intervention for large VSD.

Hemodynamics. The magnitude of the left to right shunt is determined by the size of the defect and the degree of pulmonary vascular resistance compared to systemic resistance. In most instances, even at 2–3 mo of age when the shunt is maximal, pulmonary resistance is only slightly elevated. However, the major contribu-

tion to pulmonary hypertension is the extremely large blood flow through the right heart and pulmonary artery. When a small communication is present, the defect is restrictive and right ventricular pressure measurements are normal. Pulmonary artery hypertension with VSD may be related to either flow or resistance, or both. The infant with a large left to right shunt is considered to have hyperkinetic pulmonary artery hypertension, whereas the child or young adult with Eisenmenger syndrome has pulmonary hypertension based on pulmonary vascular obstruction. In the former the right ventricular output is supplemented by left ventricular blood, and pulmonary arterial blood flow is increased as is the return of pulmonary venous blood to the left atrium and ventricle. Left ventricular diastolic overload and left ventricular dilatation result. Depending on left ventricular performance, the filling pressure of the ventricle will be variable.

Clinical Manifestations. These vary according to the size of the defect and the pulmonary blood flow and pressure. Small defects with trivial left to right shunts and normal pulmonary arterial pressures are the most frequent. The patients are asymptomatic, and the cardiac lesion is usually found during routine physical examination. Characteristically, there is a loud, harsh, or blowing left parasternal pansystolic murmur, heard best over the lower left sternal border and frequently accompanied by a thrill. In a few instances the murmur ends well before the 2nd sound, presumably because of closure of the defect during late systole (Fig 13–45). The left to right shunt is limited in the neonate, and the systolic murmur may be inaudible during the 1st days of life. In premature infants the murmur may be audible early since pulmonary vascular resistance appears to decrease more quickly. *Roentgenograms* are usually normal, although minimal cardiomegaly and borderline increase in pulmonary vasculature may be observed. The *electrocardiogram* is usually normal but may suggest left or combined ventricular hypertrophy.

Large defects with excessive pulmonary blood flow and pulmonary hypertension are responsible for dyspnea, feeding difficulties, poor growth, profuse perspiration, recurrent pulmonary infections, and episodes of cardiac failure from early infancy. Cyanosis is absent, but a duskiness is sometimes noted during infections or crying. In the absence of heart failure, arterial and venous pulses are normal. Prominence of the left precordium and sternum is common, as are cardiomegaly,

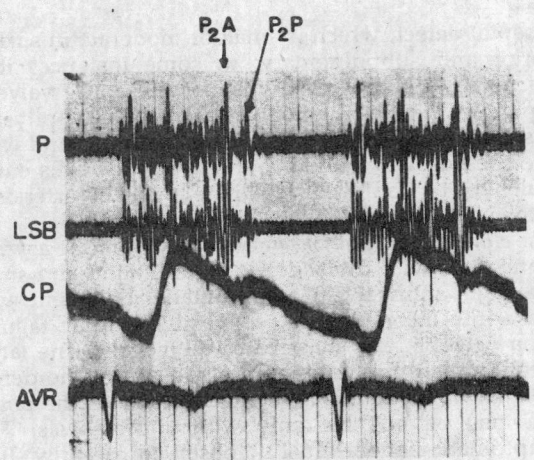

Figure 13–45 Phonocardiograms (P, pulmonary area; LSB, left sternal border) to illustrate auscultatory findings in moderate-sized ventricular septal defect with normal pulmonary arterial pressure. Long pansystolic murmur is evident. AVR, electrocardiogram; CP, carotid pulse; P_2A, aortic components of 2nd sound; P_2P, pulmonary component of 2nd sound.

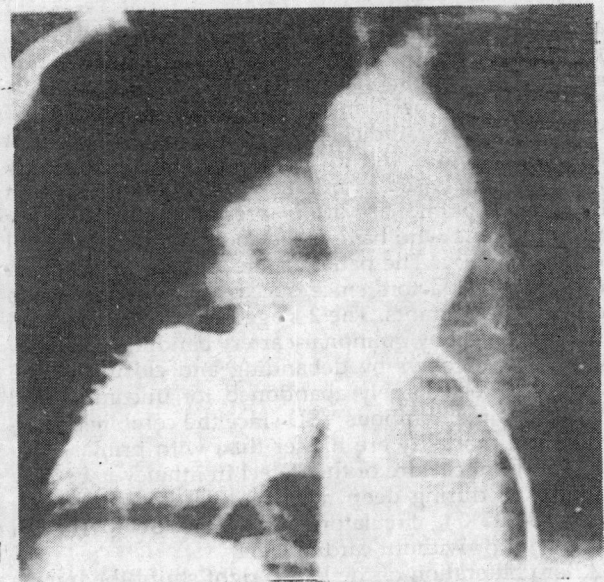

Figure 13–46 Left ventricular angiogram in a child with ventricular septal defect. Note the jet of contrast material across a high membranous defect with early filling of the pulmonary artery.

a palpable parasternal lift, an apical thrust, and a systolic thrill. The systolic murmur may be similar to that of smaller defects, but the sound of pulmonary valvular closure is louder, and the 2nd sound is only narrowly split. The presence of an apical diastolic murmur indicates an appreciable left to right shunt. *Roentgenographically*, gross cardiomegaly is present with prominence of both ventricles, the left atrium, and pulmonary artery. The *electrocardiogram* shows biventricular hypertrophy; P waves may be notched or peaked. The *echocardiogram* shows volume overload of the left atrium and ventricle; the extent of their increased dimensions reflects the size of the left to right shunt. Most small or moderate-sized defects cannot be visualized, but there may be a gap in septal echoes at the site of large shunts.

Diagnosis. The effects of a VSD on the circulation may be documented by cardiac catheterization. However, this diagnostic procedure is not required when it is clear that an isolated small defect is present. Since oxygenated blood passes across the defect from the left ventricle, blood from the right ventricle is higher in oxygen than that from the right atrium; this increase is occasionally apparent only in pulmonary arterial blood. Small shunts may not result in a detectable increase in oxygen content of blood from the right ventricle but may be demonstrated by indicator dilution tests, hydrogen or indocyanine green (Fig 13–26). Small defects are associated with normal right heart pressure and pulmonary vascular resistance. Pulmonary and systemic blood flows in patients with large defects with nearly equal pulmonary and systemic pressures are determined primarily by the resistances of the pulmonary and systemic circuits. The location and number of ventricular defects are demonstrated by left ventriculography. Contrast medium passes across the defect(s) to opacify the right ventricle and pulmonary artery (Fig 13–46).

Prognosis and Complications. The natural course of VSD includes the following: (1) A significant number (estimated to be approximately 50%) of small defects close spontaneously, most frequently during the 1st yr of life. It is less common for moderate or large defects to close spontaneously. (2) A large number of children remain asymptomatic without evidence of increase in heart size, pulmonary arterial pressure, or resistance. (3) Infective endocarditis occurs in fewer than 1%. (4) A significant number of infants with large defects have repeated episodes of respiratory infection and congestive heart failure. (5) Pulmonary hypertension occurs as a result of high pulmonary blood flow. A few patients will develop elevated pulmonary vascular resistance with time if the defect is not repaired. (6) A small number acquire pulmonary stenosis, which serves as a protection to the pulmonary circulation. In these patients the clinical picture changes from VSD with large left to right shunt to VSD with pulmonary stenosis.

Treatment. Parents should be reassured of the benign nature of the small defect, and the child should be encouraged to live a normal life. Surgical repair is not recommended. As a protection against infective endocarditis the integrity of primary and permanent teeth should be carefully maintained; antibiotic prophylaxis should be provided for dental surgery, tonsillectomy, adenoidectomy, and other oropharyngeal surgical procedures as well as for instrumentation of the genitourinary and lower intestinal tracts.

The medical management of infants with a large VSD is primarily aimed at the control of congestive cardiac failure. These patients may show signs of chronic pulmonary disease and often fail to thrive. If early treatment is successful, the shunt may diminish in size with spontaneous improvement, especially during the 1st yr of life. Since surgical mortality has decreased significantly, medical management should not be pursued in symptomatic infants after a suitable trial. Furthermore, progression of pulmonary vascular disease is unlikely when surgery is performed in the 1st 2 yr of life.

Surgery is contraindicated in patients with significant right to left shunts and trivial left to right shunts. Early correction is advised in infants with moderate to high elevation of pulmonary artery pressures and large left to right shunts who have failed to respond to maximal medical therapy. The patient's age and size should not be prohibitive factors since successful surgery can be performed on infants. The 2-stage repair for an isolated subaortic defect by pulmonary artery banding in infancy followed in later yr by debanding and closure of the defect has been largely abandoned for uncomplicated large single membranous VSD since the combined morbidity and mortality are higher than with primary closure. Surgical closure of the defect in infancy is usually undertaken during deep hypothermia (body temperatures 18–20° C), circulatory arrest, or low perfusion rates, with or without cardioplegia.

After obliteration of the left to right shunt the hyperdynamic heart becomes quiet, cardiac size decreases toward normal (Fig 13–47), thrills and murmurs are abolished, and pulmonary artery pressures begin to approach normal. In some instances after successful operation, systolic ejection murmurs of low intensity persist for months. The long term prognosis after surgery is good. Surgery only rarely leads to late-onset complications such as heart block or ventricular tachyrhythmias.

13.33 VENTRICULAR SEPTAL DEFECT WITH AORTIC INSUFFICIENCY

In this syndrome the VSD is complicated by prolapse of the aortic valve and aortic insufficiency. Frequently, the septal defect, which is small or moderate in size, is anterior and subpulmonary; in some instances it is infracristal. The prolapsed cusp of the aortic valve is the right or at times the noncoronary one. The physical signs of aortic insufficiency (diastolic murmur and wide pulse pressure) are added to those of VSD. This entity should not be confused with patent ductus arteriosus or other defects associated with aortic runoff.

The *clinical manifestations* vary widely from the asymptomatic child with trivial aortic regurgitation and small left to right shunt to the symptomatic adolescent with florid aortic incompetence, congestive cardiac failure, angina pectoris, and massive cardiomegaly. The latter patients urgently require surgical closure of the defect and relief of aortic incompetence. Repair of the aortic valve may be possible only with a prosthesis. The asymptomatic patient must be observed carefully. It is doubtful that aortic insufficiency is affected by closure of the septal defect; but aortic valvular reconstructive procedures are available for patients with moderate incompetence, and they are recommended prior to the development of severe insufficiency and left ventricular dysfunction.

13.34 VENTRICULAR SEPTAL DEFECT WITH LEFT VENTRICULAR–RIGHT ATRIAL SHUNT

Ventricular defects may be associated with an abnormal septal leaflet of the tricuspid valve. During left ventricular systole, arterialized blood is ejected through the defect into the right atrium. The physical signs are those of VSD or ostium primum defect. High right atrial pressure is manifest as a large systolic venous pulsation in the neck. Cardiac catheterization reveals a left to right shunt at the atrial level and may result in the misdiagnosis of atrial septal defect. The diagnosis may

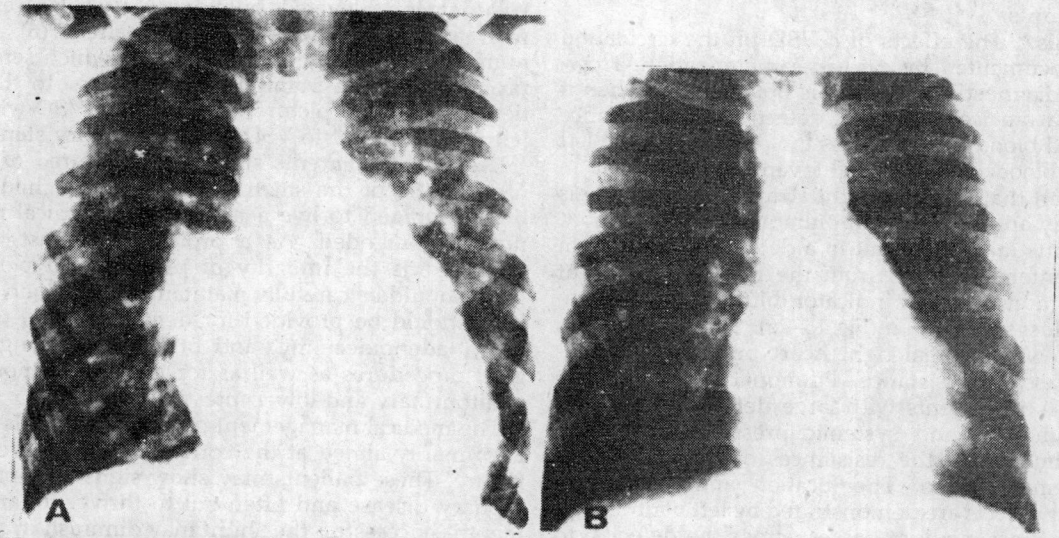

Figure 13–47 *A,* Preoperative roentgenogram in ventricular septal defect with large left to right shunt and pulmonary hypertension. Significant cardiomegaly, prominence of the pulmonary arterial trunk, and pulmonary overcirculation are evident. *B,* Three yr after surgical closure of defect. There is marked decrease in heart size, and the pulmonary vasculature is normal.

be confirmed by left ventriculography; the right atrium opacifies immediately after delivery of contrast medium to the left ventricle. Treatment is surgical closure of the ventricular defect.

13.35 ORIGIN OF BOTH GREAT ARTERIES FROM THE RIGHT VENTRICLE
(Double Outlet Right Ventricle)

In this anomaly (also known as double outlet right ventricle) both the aorta and the pulmonary artery arise from the right ventricle. The only outlet from the left ventricle is a ventricular septal defect. The clinical picture closely simulates that of an uncomplicated VSD with a large left to right shunt and pulmonary hypertension. The *electrocardiogram* usually shows a superior, counterclockwise frontal loop (left axis deviation) and biventricular hypertrophy. *Echocardiography* is diagnostic since it shows discontinuity of the mitral and aortic valves. The condition may also be recognized by *left ventriculography*, which demonstrates the position of the VSD and its relation to the crista supraventricularis, visualizes the outlet from the left ventricle, confirms mitral aortic discontinuity, and shows the high position of the aortic valve which is at the same level as the pulmonary valve. It is important to differentiate this condition from simple VSD. Surgical correction is accomplished with an intraventricular repair which funnels the ejection of left ventricular blood via the VSD into the aorta without obstructing right ventricular outflow. Pulmonary artery banding may be required in infancy, followed by surgical correction during the preschool years. Natural pulmonary stenosis is not infrequent (Sec 13.16).

In **double outlet right ventricle with transposition of the great arteries** the VSD is supracristal and subpulmonary **(Taussig-Bing complex)** or related to both pulmonary and aortic valves (doubly committed). These patients develop cyanosis early in life and have poor physical development, pulmonary hypertension, and cardiac failure. Cardiomegaly is usual, and there is a parasternal ejection systolic murmur, sometimes preceded by an injection click and a loud closure of the pulmonary valve. Left-sided obstructive lesions are frequently associated; they include aortic coarctation, interruption of the aortic arch, and a small VSD that is restrictive to left ventricular ejection. The *electrocardiogram* shows right axis deviation and right, left, or biventricular hypertrophy. The *roentgenogram* documents the cardiomegaly, the large left atrium, and prominence of the pulmonary trunk and vasculature. The anatomic features of the anomaly and associated abnormalities are best demonstrated by selective right and left ventriculography. Treatment is difficult because of the early onset of pulmonary vascular disease. This can be palliated by pulmonary artery banding in infancy to permit surgical correction at a later age, which may be accomplished by a Rastelli procedure (Sec 13.19) or by closure of the VSD coupled with a Mustard procedure to allow egress of the left ventricle blood to the pulmonary artery.

13.36 L-TRANSPOSITION OF THE GREAT ARTERIES
(Corrected Transposition)

This malformation consists of *ventricular inversion* and transposition of the great arteries. Systemic blood is returned to a normal right atrium, from which it passes through a bicuspid atrioventricular valve into a right-sided ventricle that has the internal appearance of a normal left ventricle. The venous blood is then ejected into the pulmonary artery. Pulmonary venous blood returns to a normal left atrium, passes through a tricuspid valve into the left ventricle, which has the internal structure of a normal right ventricle, and is ejected into the aorta. The pulmonary artery and ascending aorta are parallel, and the former is medial. The course of the blood and the hemodynamics are normal in patients with uncomplicated corrected transposition. In the majority of instances, however, associated anomalies coexist; the common ones are VSD, abnormalities of the left atrioventricular valve (tricuspid) with or without incompetence, pulmonary valvular stenosis, and atrioventricular conduction disturbances, frequently with complete atrioventricular dissociation.

Symptoms and signs are dominated by the associated lesions. Posteroanterior chest *roentgenograms* may suggest the abnormal position of the great arteries; the ascending aorta occupies the upper left border of the cardiac silhouette. In addition to atrioventricular conduction disturbances, *electrocardiograms* may show abnormal P waves; absent QV_6; initial Q waves in leads III, aVR, aVF, and V_1; and upright T waves across the precordium.

Surgical treatment of the associated anomalies, most often the VSD, is complicated by the position of the bundle of His, which may be injured at the time of surgery; such an injury may cause heart block. Mapping of the conduction system at surgery has been an important step in eliminating this sequela in those patients who were initially in sinus rhythm.

13.37 OTHER DEFECTS ASSOCIATED WITH VENTRICULAR SEPTAL DEFECT

To plan surgical treatment for VSD the surgeon must know whether associated cardiovascular malformations are present and, if so, include them in the overall management plan.

Patent Ductus Arteriosus. During cardiopulmonary bypass for repair of ventricular defects, arterialized blood from the heart-lung apparatus is returned to the ascending aorta. If there is a patent ductus arteriosus, blood leaks into the pulmonary artery, floods the surgical field, and contributes to postoperative pulmonary complications. In most infants with large defects the signs of the VSD dominate so that the murmur of the patent ductus is inaudible. In such cases the passage of the cardiac catheter from the pulmonary artery through the ductus and into the descending aorta is diagnostic (as is the aortic angiogram). The ventricular defect and the patent ductus are closed during the same operation.

Multiple Ventricular Septal Defects. In some instances there are multiple defects involving the ventricular septum. Generally, these patients have signs of a large left to right shunt and pulmonary hypertension in infancy. Multiple defects cannot be detected clinically. A left ventriculogram in the left anterior oblique view shows the septum in profile and permits identification of the number and location of the defects. Exploration of the entire ventricular septum is indicated during open cardiotomy to ensure that all defects have been treated. A surgical approach from the left ventricle may sometimes be required with apical muscular defects because they are more easily reached and the smooth left septal surface allows defects to be more easily identified. However, this approach increases the risk of surgery. Because the postoperative period can be hazardous if significant left to right shunts and pulmonary hypertension persist, it is preferable to carry out pulmonary artery banding in infancy with debanding and closure of the defects in the preschool years.

Atrial Septal Defect. In patients with a ventricular defect and an ostium secundum atrial defect the physical signs are usually dominated by the ventricular defect. The clinical picture is similar to that of moderate-sized or large VSD. This combination of defects may result in congestive heart failure in infancy and should be suspected during cardiac catheterization if left to right shunts are demonstrated at both the atrial and ventricular levels. During right ventriculotomy or atriotomy for closure of ventricular defects the atrial septum is easily explored; if both defects are present, they can be repaired during the same procedure.

Coarctation of the Aorta. The signs of coarctation of the aorta are clear (Sec 13.52), but those of the ventricular defect may be confused with the signs produced by the collateral circulation secondary to the coarctation. It is usually necessary to repair these lesions at separate surgical procedures.

Persistent Left Superior Vena Cava. This condition cannot be diagnosed clinically. It is identified by catheterization when the catheter enters the persistent left superior vena cava from the coronary sinus. Surgical treatment of ventricular defects with cardiopulmonary bypass requires occlusion of the venous inflow; if the left superior vena cava is not occluded, large volumes of venous blood enter the heart during cardiotomy. The persistent left superior vena cava in itself does not require treatment.

Complete Heart Block. This arrhythmia is rare in patients with VSD, although systolic murmurs of varying intensity are not unusual in patients with complete heart block; the association was once considered common. The murmurs are produced by the turbulence associated with the large stroke volume. Any patients with VSD and complete heart block should be suspected of having corrected transposition of the great vessels. The presence of this anomaly does not contraindicate closure of the ventricular defect, but surgical treatment may be more complicated (Sec 13.69).

13.38   ATRIAL SEPTAL DEFECT
(Patent Foramen Ovale)

An isolated patent foramen ovale is of no clinical significance. If the right atrial pressure is increased (e.g., secondary to pulmonary stenosis or pulmonary hypertension), venous blood may be shunted across the patent foramen ovale into the left atrium and result in cyanosis. Shunting of venous blood across the foramen ovale may also occur in the immediate postcardiotomy period. It is thus preferable to close the foramen during operation for pulmonary stenosis to eliminate this potential complication.

Because of the anatomic structure of a patent foramen ovale, blood cannot be shunted from the left atrium to the right atrium. An isolated patent foramen ovale does not require treatment.

13.39   OSTIUM SECUNDUM DEFECT

This defect in the region of the fossa ovalis is associated with normal atrioventricular valves at birth. Late myxomatous changes in the mitral valve have been described. The defects may be multiple, and in symptomatic older children openings of 2 cm or more in diameter are not unusual. Large defects may extend inferiorly toward the inferior vena cava and ostium of the coronary sinus, superiorly toward the superior vena cava, or posteriorly.

Hemodynamics. A considerable shunt of oxygenated blood flows from the left to the right atrium. This blood is added to the usual venous return to the right atrium and is pumped by the right ventricle to the lungs. Pulmonary blood flow is usually 2–4 times systemic flow. Although the left atrial pressure may exceed that of the right atrium by a few mm Hg, the principal factor which determines the direction of shunt is the diastolic compliance of the chambers of the right heart. The greater distensibility of the right atrium and ventricle and the low pulmonary vascular resistance allow a torrential left to right shunt. The paucity of symptoms in infants with atrial septal defects has been related to the structure of the right ventricle in early life when its muscular wall is thick and less compliant, thus limiting the left to right shunt. As the infant becomes older, the right ventricular wall becomes thinner and the left to right shunt across the atrial defect increases. The large blood flow through the right side of the heart results in enlargement of the right atrium and ventricle and dilatation of the pulmonary artery. In spite of the large pulmonary blood flow, the pulmonary arterial pressure is usually normal or only moderately elevated. The left ventricle and aorta are normal in size. Cyanosis is extremely rare; it is seen occasionally in adults with the complicating features of pulmonary vascular disease.

Clinical Manifestations. A child with an ostium secundum defect is often asymptomatic, and the lesion is discovered during a physical examination. It rarely produces heart failure in infancy; in older children varying degrees of exercise intolerance may be noted.

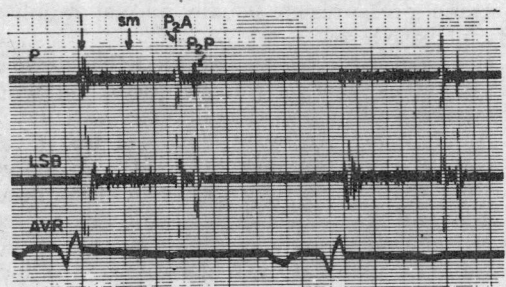

Figure 13–48 Phonocardiograms (P, pulmonary area; LSB, left sternal border) to illustrate auscultatory findings in ostium secundum atrial septal defect. AVR, electrocardiogram; P_2A, aortic component of 2nd sound; P_2P, pulmonary component of 2nd sound; sm, systolic murmur; 1, 1st heart sound. Note wide splitting of 2nd sound. This splitting persisted in all phases of respiration. Time lines 0.04 sec.

The pulse is normal, and the venous pressure is normal unless there is associated tricuspid insufficiency or heart failure. The heart may be normal in size or enlarged. A right ventricular systolic lift is usually palpable from the left sternal border to the midclavicular line. The systolic murmur, ejection in type, soft, and seldom accompanied by a thrill, is best heard at the upper left sternal border; it is produced by the increased flow into the pulmonary artery. The murmur is preceded by a loud 1st heart sound and sometimes by a pulmonic ejection sound. In most patients the 2nd heart sound at the upper left sternal edge is widely split and fixed in all phases of respiration. This auscultatory finding is characteristic (Fig 13–48). A mid-diastolic murmur produced by the high blood flow across the tricuspid valve may be audible at the lower left sternal edge.

Diagnosis. *Roentgenograms* show varying degrees of enlargement of the right ventricle and atrium; the left ventricle and aorta are small. The pulmonary artery is large, and the pulmonary vascularity greatly increased. These signs vary and may not be conspicuous in mild cases.

The *electrocardiogram* shows diastolic overload of the right ventricle with right axis deviation and right ventricular hypertrophy (usually rsR′ in right precordial leads); the diagnosis should be doubted if these signs are absent. Infrequent electrocardiographic abnormalities include tall P waves, prolonged P-R intervals, dysrhythmias (e.g., atrial fibrillation and complete heart block), Wolff-Parkinson-White syndrome, complete right bundle branch block, and left axis deviation. Occasionally, the electrocardiogram is normal.

The *echocardiogram* shows findings characteristic of right ventricular volume overload: (1) increased right ventricular end-diastolic dimension; (2) abnormal motion of the ventricular septum (The normal septum moves posteriorly during systole and anteriorly during diastole. With right ventricular overload and normal pulmonary vascular resistance, the septal motion is reversed, i.e., anterior movement in systole, or the motion is intermediate so that the septum remains straight); and (3) real-time 2-dimensional scans from the apical position identify the location and size of the atrial defect.

The diagnosis may be confirmed by *cardiac catheterization.* The oxygen content of blood from the right atrium is much higher than that from the superior vena cava. This feature is not diagnostic since it may occur with anomalous pulmonary venous return to the right atrium, with ventricular septal defect with tricuspid insufficiency, with ventricular septal defects associated with left ventricular–right atrial shunts, and with aortic–right atrial communications (e.g., ruptured sinus of Valsalva). The physical signs produced by these anomalies generally differ greatly from those of atrial septal defects, and their presence can usually be confirmed by selective angiocardiography. In a few patients, mixing of blood is incomplete in the right atrium; the principal site of shunt appears, therefore, to be at the ventricular level.

The catheter frequently enters the left atrium from the right atrium. Indicator dilution curves may be used to demonstrate the site of the left to right shunt and the presence of anomalous pulmonary veins. Streaming of inferior vena caval blood across the defect to the left atrium may occur with uncomplicated atrial septal defects. This minute right to left shunt may be demonstrated by indicator dilution curves but does not result in significant arterial unsaturation or cyanosis. The pressures in the right side of the heart are frequently normal, but there may be moderate right ventricular and pulmonary hypertension. Pressure gradients may be measured across the right ventricular outflow in the absence of organic pulmonary stenosis and are probably due to functional stenosis related to the excessive blood flow. The pulmonary arteriolar resistance is almost always normal. The shunt is also variable, but it is usually considerable (as high as 20 l/min/M²).

Prognosis and Complications. Secundum atrial septal defects are well tolerated during childhood; symptoms usually appear in the 3rd decade or later. Pulmonary hypertension, atrial dysrhythmias, tricuspid incompetence, and heart failure are uncommon in infancy and more so in childhood. Infective endocarditis is rare. The principal guides to prognosis are the presence or absence of symptoms and of continuing cardiac enlargement.

Secundum atrial septal defects are usually isolated, although they may be associated with partial anomalous pulmonary venous return, pulmonary valvular stenosis, ventricular septal defect, pulmonary arterial branch stenosis, and persistent left superior vena cava.

Treatment. Direct vision, open-heart surgery during cardiopulmonary bypass allows accurate closure. The mortality rate from surgery is less than 1%, and surgery is advised even in asymptomatic patients prior to entry into school. It is preferred during childhood because the surgical mortality is higher in adults, especially in those with pulmonary hypertension, cardiac failure, tricuspid incompetence, or atrial arrhythmias.

The results after operation in children with large shunts are gratifying in most instances. Symptoms disappear rapidly, and physical development frequently appears to be enhanced. The heart size decreases to normal, and the electrocardiogram shows decreased right ventricular forces. Late complications are rare.

13.40 DEFECT OF THE SINUS VENOSUS

The defect is situated in the upper part of the atrial septum in close relation to the entry of the superior vena cava. One or more pulmonary veins (usually from the right lung) drain anomalously into the superior vena cava. Sometimes the superior vena cava straddles the defect; some systemic venous blood is then able to enter the left atrium. The abnormal hemodynamics are similar to those of secundum atrial septal defect consisting primarily of a volume overload of the right ventricle. The clinical picture, electrocardiogram, and roentgenogram are similar to those of secundum atrial defect. Generally, the anomalous pulmonary veins are not recognized by routine roentgenography, although a bulge of the superior vena caval shadow may suggest the diagnosis. During cardiac catheterization the catheter may enter the pulmonary veins from the superior vena cava. Anatomic correction usually requires the insertion of a patch to ensure the entry of anomalous veins into the left atrium; surgical results are generally good; atrial arrhythmias occur occasionally, possibly from surgical injury to the sinus node.

13.41 OSTIUM PRIMUM DEFECT AND COMMON ATRIOVENTRICULAR CANAL
(Endocardial Cushion Defects)

These abnormalities are grouped together because they have a common embryologic relation and the clinical patterns may be similar.

The *ostium primum defect* is situated in the lower portion of the atrial septum and overlies the mitral and tricuspid valves. In the majority of instances there is a cleft in the anterior leaflet of the mitral valve. The tricuspid valve is usually normal, although some thickening of the septal leaflet may be present. The ventricular septum is usually intact functionally, but its proximal part is anatomically deficient.

Common atrioventricular canal consists of an interatrial and interventricular defect with an atrioventricular valve. The valve, common to both ventricles, consists of an anterior and a posterior leaflet related to the ventricular septum with a lateral leaflet in each ventricle. The lesion is relatively common among children with Down syndrome; other congenital heart defects may also occur in this syndrome.

Transitional varieties of these defects also occur. They include ostium primum defects with clefts in the anterior mitral and septal tricuspid valve leaflets, and, less commonly, ostium primum defects with normal atrioventricular valves. In others the atrial septum is intact, but the ventricular septal defect simulates that found in common atrioventricular canal. These defects are also associated with deformities of the atrioventricular valves.

Hemodynamics. In *ostium primum defects* the basic abnormality is the combination of a left to right shunt across the atrial defect with mitral incompetence. The shunt is usually moderate or large. The degree of mitral incompetence is ordinarily mild or moderate. Pulmo-nary arterial pressures are usually normal or only moderately increased.

In *common atrioventricular canal* the left to right shunt is transatrial as well as transventricular. Pulmonary hypertension and increased pulmonary vascular resistance are common. Atrioventricular valvular incompetence results in regurgitation of blood from the ventricles to the atria. Some right to left shunting occurs at both atrial and ventricular levels. Although it is usually small in volume, it may result in significant arterial unsaturation. Pulmonary vascular disease will increase the right to left shunt so that more severe cyanosis may develop.

Clinical Manifestations. Many children with *ostium primum defect* are asymptomatic, and the anomaly is discovered during a general physical examination. In patients with moderate shunts and trivial mitral incompetence, the physical signs are similar to those of atrial defect of the secundum type; there may also be an apical systolic murmur and a characteristic electrocardiogram.

A history of effort intolerance, easy fatigability, and recurrent pneumonitis may be obtained, especially in patients with large left to right shunts and severe mitral incompetence. In these patients cardiac enlargement is moderate or massive, a precordial bulge is common, a hyperdynamic parasternal right ventricular lift is palpable, and a left ventricular apical heave suggests significant mitral incompetence. The auscultatory signs produced by the left to right shunt include a normal or accentuated 1st sound, wide, fixed splitting of the 2nd sound, a pulmonary ejection systolic murmur sometimes preceded by a click, and a rumbling early diastolic murmur at the lower left sternal edge. Mitral incompetence is usually manifested by an apical pansystolic murmur which radiates to the left axilla; it is variable in nature and may be short or musical.

With *common atrioventricular canal*, congestive heart failure and intercurrent pulmonary infection usually appear in infancy. During these episodes minimal cyanosis may be evident. The jugular venous pressure may be increased because of pulmonary hypertension, congestive heart failure, or incompetence of the atrioventricular valve. Cardiac enlargement is moderate or massive, and a systolic thrill is frequently palpable. The 1st heart sound is normal or accentuated and is followed by a widely distributed, harsh systolic murmur. The 2nd heart sound is widely split if pulmonary flow is massive; if severe pulmonary hypertension develops, the width of splitting may not be striking, but pulmonary valve closure is loud. A low-pitched early diastolic murmur is audible at the lower left sternal edge, and a pulmonic systolic ejection murmur is produced by the large pulmonary flow.

Diagnosis. *Roentgenograms* of children with endocardial cushion defects confirm the cardiac enlargement due to prominence of both ventricles and the right atrium. The pulmonary artery is large, and pulmonary vascularity is increased. The aorta is small or normal in size.

The *electrocardiogram* of children with endocardial cushion defects is unusual and diagnostic. The principal abnormalities are (1) superior orientation of the mean frontal QRS axis with left axis deviation or occasional extreme right axis deviation; (2) counterclockwise inscription of the superiorly oriented QRS vector loop; (3) signs of biventricular hypertrophy or, sometimes, isolated right or left ventricular hypertrophy; (4) normal or tall P waves; and (5) occasional prolongation of the P-R interval (Fig 13–49).

The *echocardiogram* is characteristic and shows signs of right ventricular enlargement with encroachment of the mitral valve echo on the left ventricular outflow; this corresponds to the angiographic "gooseneck" deformity. In the common atrioventricular canal, the ventricular septal echo is fragmented, and the mitral valve echo appears to pass through the ventricular septum. When the defect of the ventricular septum is large, the common atrioventricular valve occupies the canal defect and crosses the plane of the ventricular septum (Fig 13–50).

Cardiac catheterization and *angiocardiography* confirm the diagnosis. These studies demonstrate the magnitude of the left to right shunt, the severity of pulmonary hypertension, the degree of elevation of increased pulmonary vascular resistance, and the amount of incompetence of the atrioventricular valve. The shunt is usually demonstrable at the atrial level; in some patients with inadequate mixing of blood it appears to be principally at the ventricular level. The arterial oxygen saturation is normal unless severe pulmonary hypertension is present. In these patients a small right to left shunt may be demonstrable. Patients with ostium primum defects usually have normal or only moderate elevation of the pulmonary arterial pressure. Nevertheless, common atrioventricular canal is usually associated with right ventricular and pulmonary hypertension as well as with a moderate increase in pulmonary vascular resistance. The cardiac catheter enters the chambers of the left side of the heart with ease from the right side, especially if there is a common atrioventricular canal.

Selective left ventriculography is extremely helpful in diagnosis of endocardial cushion defects. The deformity of the mitral or common atrioventricular valve and the distortion of the outflow of the left ventricle, the gooseneck deformity, are demonstrated. The abnormal ante-

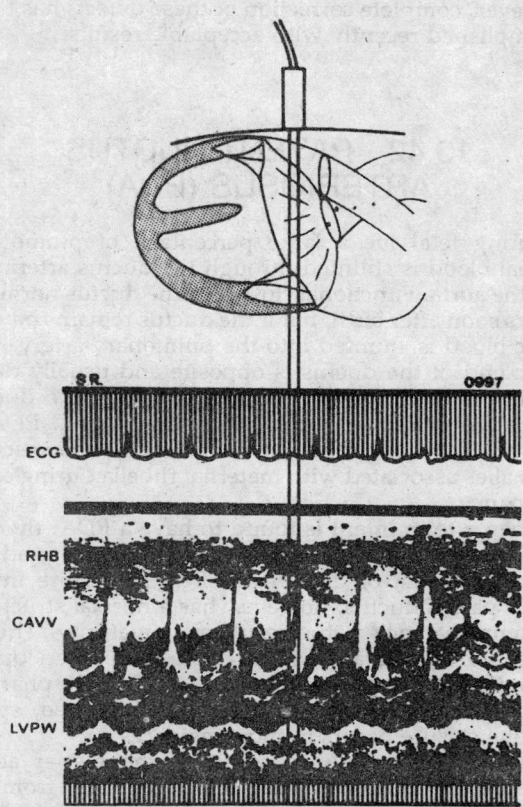

Figure 13–50 Echocardiographic study in an infant with atrioventricular canal showing a single AV valve (CAVV) with a large diastolic excursion that traverses the entire heart from the left ventricular posterior wall (LVPW) to the anterior right heart border (RHB). (Williams RG, Tucker CR: Echocardiographic Diagnosis of Congenital Heart Disease. Boston, Little, Brown, 1977.)

rior leaflet of the mitral valve is serrated, and mitral incompetence may be demonstrable. A large left ventricular–right atrial shunt is frequently present.

Prognosis. The prognosis of endocardial cushion defects depends on the magnitude of the left to right shunt, the degree of pulmonary vascular resistance, and the severity of mitral incompetence. Death from congestive cardiac failure during infancy is not unusual with common atrioventricular canal, but many patients with ostium primum defects are asymptomatic or have only minor, nonprogressive symptoms until they reach the 3rd–4th decade of life.

Treatment. Direct vision intracardiac surgery with an artificial heart-lung machine permits correction of endocardial cushion defects. Ostium primum defects are approached from an incision in the right atrium. The cleft in the mitral valve is located through the atrial defect and is repaired by direct suture. The defects in the atrial and ventricular septa are usually closed by insertion of a patch prosthesis; prosthetic valves are rarely required. The surgical mortality rate for primum defects is low. Surgical treatment for common atrioventricular canal is more difficult, especially in infants with congestive cardiac failure and pulmonary hypertension. Pulmonary arterial banding has been successful in patients with dominant shunts at the ventricular level.

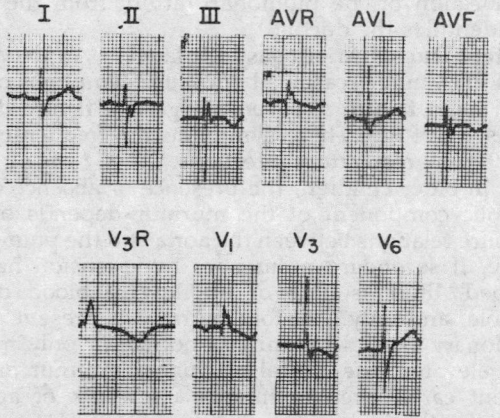

Figure 13–49 Electrocardiogram from a child with atrioventricular canal. Note the QRS axis of −60°, and the RV conduction delay; RSR' in V₁. (V₃R paper speed = 50 mm/sec.)

However, complete correction of these defects has been accomplished recently with acceptable results.

13.42   PATENT DUCTUS ARTERIOSUS (PDA)

During fetal life a large percentage of pulmonary arterial blood is shunted through the ductus arteriosus into the aorta. Functional closure of the ductus normally occurs soon after birth, but if the ductus remains patent, aortic blood is shunted into the pulmonary artery. The aortic end of the ductus is opposite and usually distal to the origin of the left subclavian artery; the ductus enters the pulmonary artery at its bifurcation. PDA is one of the most common congenital cardiovascular anomalies associated with maternal rubella during early pregnancy.

When a term infant is found to have a PDA, there is deficiency of both the mucoid endothelial layer and the muscular media of the ductus. The premature infant with a patent ductus, however, has a normal structural anatomy; patency is the result of immaturity. Thus a PDA in a term infant will rarely close spontaneously, while in the premature baby, in whom early pharmacologic or surgical intervention is not indicated, spontaneous closure occurs in most instances.

Hemodynamics. As a result of the higher aortic pressure, blood flow through the ductus goes from the aorta to the pulmonary artery. The extent of shunt depends on the size of the ductus and the pressure gradient between aorta and pulmonary artery. In extreme cases 50–65% of the left ventricular output may be shunted through the ductus to the pulmonary circulation. The pressures within the pulmonary artery, the right ventricle, and the right atrium are usually normal, but they may be elevated moderately or even to systemic levels (Sec 13.11). There is a wide pulse pressure due to runoff of blood into the pulmonary artery during diastole. The total blood volume is increased; it returns to normal limits after surgical closure of the ductus.

Clinical Manifestations. There are usually no symptoms, but they may develop at any age and include slowly progressive exertional dyspnea, followed by left ventricular or congestive cardiac failure. Retardation of physical growth may be a major manifestation.

A large PDA will result in striking physical signs attributable to the wide pulse pressure. These include water-hammer radial pulsations and conspicuous arterial Corrigan pulsations in the neck. The heart is normal in size when the ductus is small but moderately or grossly enlarged in cases with a large communication. The apical impulse is normal or left ventricular and, with cardiac enlargement, is heaving. A thrill, maximal in the 2nd left interspace, is often present and may radiate toward the left clavicle, down the left sternal border, or toward the apex. It is usually systolic in time, often extends into diastole, and, in some instances, may be palpated throughout the cardiac cycle. The classic murmur has been variously described as machinery, humming top, millwheel, or rolling thunder in quality. It begins soon after onset of the 1st sound, reaches maximum intensity at the end of systole, and wanes in late diastole. It may be localized to the 2nd left intercostal space or radiate down the left sternal border or to the left clavicle. The murmur is harsh and uneven with a "clicky" quality. Infrequently, there are atypical murmurs; e.g., when there is pulmonary hypertension, the murmur is only systolic in time. In patients with a large left to right shunt a low-pitched mitral diastolic murmur may be audible; it is due to the large blood flow across the mitral valve.

The *electrocardiogram* is usually normal. If the ductus is large, left ventricular hypertrophy is present. The diagnosis of uncomplicated PDA is untenable when there is evidence of isolated right ventricular hypertrophy.

Roentgenographic studies commonly show a prominent pulmonary artery with increased intrapulmonary vascular markings. The cardiac size depends on the degree of left to right shunt; it may be normal, or moderately to grossly enlarged. The chambers involved are the left atrium and ventricle. The aortic knob is normal or prominent and pulsates vigorously. Rarely, there may be calcification in the wall of the ductus.

The *echocardiogram* is normal if the ductus is small. Left atrial and ventricular dimensions are increased, and isovolumic contraction time is decreased with large shunts. Real-time 2-dimensional scanning from the suprasternal notch allows visualization of the ductus.

The clinical pattern is sufficiently distinctive to allow an accurate diagnosis in the majority of patients. In patients with atypical murmurs, further confirmatory studies are indicated.

Cardiac catheterization reveals normal or increased pressures in the right ventricle and pulmonary artery. The presence of oxygenated blood in the pulmonary artery confirms a left to right shunt, as do hydrogen and indicator dilution curves. Samples of blood from the venae cavae, right atrium, and right ventricle have comparable oxygen contents. With pulmonary valvular insufficiency there may be an increased oxygen content in the right ventricular blood. The catheter may pass through the ductus into the descending aorta. Injection of contrast medium into the ascending aorta shows opacification of the pulmonary artery from the aorta and identifies the ductus.

Patent Ductus Arteriosus in Infancy. An uncomplicated PDA may occasionally produce symptoms of left-sided heart failure or severe congestive failure during the 1st yr of life. These symptoms are frequently precipitated by respiratory infections.

As in older children, the presence or absence of the diastolic component of the murmur depends on the pressure relations between the aorta and the pulmonary artery. If secondary pulmonary hypertension has developed, there is little or no flow of blood during diastole, and only a systolic murmur is present. If the pulmonary arterial pressure is normal or only moderately elevated, the typical machinery murmur may be present early, even in infants a few wk of age. In addition, the pulse pressure is wide and the heart enlarged.

The diagnosis of symptomatic uncomplicated PDA in infancy is important because surgical treatment is indicated in all symptomatic patients regardless of age.

Differential Diagnosis. The diagnosis of uncomplicated PDA is usually not difficult. There are other conditions, however, which, in the absence of cyanosis, produce systolic and diastolic murmurs in the pulmonic area and may be misinterpreted.

The characteristics of a *venous hum* are described in Sec 13.1. An aorticopulmonary septal defect may be clinically indistinguishable from a patent ductus, although in most cases the murmur is only systolic and is loudest at the right upper sternal border rather than at the left. Similarly, there may be difficulty in diagnosis of a *sinus of Valsalva that has ruptured into the right side of the heart or pulmonary artery* and of *coronary arteriovenous fistulas.* In these 3 conditions the dynamics are those of an arteriovenous fistula with a machinery murmur and a wide pulse pressure. Sometimes the murmur is not maximal in the pulmonary area but is heard along the lower left sternal border. *Truncus arteriosus* with torrential pulmonary flow may also be difficult to differentiate, especially in infancy. *Pulmonary branch stenosis* is associated with systolic and diastolic murmurs, but the pulse pressure is normal. *Arteriovenous fistulas* of medium-sized intrathoracic vessels, e.g., the internal mammary, also produce signs which may be indistinguishable from those of patent ductus.

Ventricular septal defect with aortic insufficiency and *combined rheumatic aortic and mitral insufficiency* may be confused with PDA, but the murmurs should be differentiated by their to and fro rather than continuous timing. Careful auscultation and the absence of pulmonary overcirculation are usually adequate for differentiation.

A large PDA and pulmonary hypertension may produce a clinical picture resembling a large ventricular septal defect. When a widely patent ductus is associated with a ventricular septal defect, a wide pulse pressure may suggest the presence of the ductus; cardiac catheterization is indicated for clarification.

Prognosis and Complications. Patients with a small PDA live a normal span with little or no cardiac embarrassment; however, a sufficient number have clinically manifest complications to make it clear that the lesion is not innocuous. Spontaneous closure of the ductus after infancy is extremely rare.

Congestive cardiac failure, which may be preceded by attacks of left ventricular failure, may occur at any age but is most common in the 3rd decade of life. Cardiac failure is an urgent indication for operation when the patient's condition permits.

Infective endarteritis, the most frequent complication in late childhood, may occur at any age. Pulmonary and/or systemic emboli may occur. Treatment with appropriately selected antibiotics should be followed by surgical closure of the ductus about 3 mo after apparent cure of the infective process.

Rarer complications include aneurysmal dilatation of the pulmonary artery or the ductus, calcification of the ductus, noninfective thrombosis of the ductus with embolization, paradoxic emboli, and acquired rheumatic heart disease. PDA with pulmonary hypertension (Eisenmenger syndrome) has been described.

Treatment. Irrespective of age, patients with a PDA or similar shunt will derive great benefit from surgical closure of the abnormality. If congestive cardiac failure develops, surgical treatment should not be postponed too long after adequate medical therapy has been instituted, even if some signs of failure persist.

Because the case fatality rate with surgical treatment is less than 1% and the risk without it is greater, ligation and division of the ductus are indicated in the asymptomatic patient, preferably between the ages of 2–4 yr. Pulmonary hypertension is not a contraindication to operation at any age if it can be demonstrated that the shunt goes from aorta to pulmonary artery and not the opposite direction.

Surgical closure is achieved by ligation or by division and suture of the ductus; the latter is preferred if technically feasible.

After closure, symptoms of frank or incipient cardiac failure rapidly disappear. If the patient was physically stunted, there is usually an improvement in physical development within months. The pulse and blood pressure return to normal, and the machinery murmur disappears. A systolic murmur over the pulmonary area may occasionally persist; it may represent turbulence in a persistently dilated pulmonary artery or, rarely, an unsuspected associated ventricular or atrial septal defect. The roentgenographic signs of cardiac enlargement and pulmonary overcirculation disappear (Fig 13–51), and the electrocardiogram becomes normal. Pulmonary hypertension, if present preoperatively, also recedes.

PATENT DUCTUS ARTERIOSUS IN LOW BIRTH WEIGHT INFANTS

See also Sec 7.16.

Virtually all infants whose birth weight is less than 1750 gm have a PDA in the 1st 24 hr of life. Beyond that time the number of infants with continued patency is greater in the lower birth weight groups. In a significant number of neonates with respiratory distress syndrome clinical symptoms, and a considerable morbidity and mortality, can be related to the presence of a large left to right shunt via the ductus arteriosus. The clinical features of a large left to right shunt through the ductus arteriosus in a preterm infant appear characteristically on the 4th–5th day of life but may be earlier in severe cases. The diagnosis may be made clinically in some instances on the basis of bounding peripheral pulses and a continuous murmur along the infraclavicular region and left upper sternal border. Occasionally, only a systolic murmur or no murmurs may be audible. *Chest roentgenograms* demonstrate pulmonary plethora in the great majority of patients. Cardiac enlargement is observed in approximately one third. An *echocardiographically* determined left atrial/aortic root ratio increase or absolute enlargement of the left atrium is helpful in deciding whether a premature baby with respiratory distress syndrome has a large left to right shunt via a PDA regardless of whether physical signs are diagnostic. Contrast echocardiography with injection of saline into the aortic root, although nonquantitative, may be

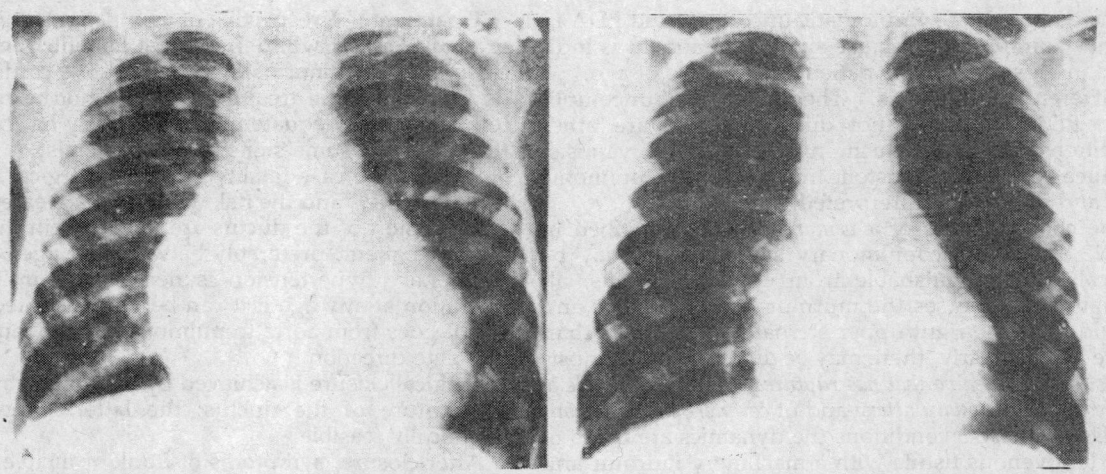

Figure 13–51   Preoperative (A) and 3 yr postoperative (B) roentgenograms of a child with patent ductus arteriosus. Preoperative roentgenogram shows cardiac enlargement, prominent aorta and pulmonary artery, and increased pulmonary vascularity. The decrease in heart size and degree of pulmonary vasculature is evident in the postoperative roentgenogram.

helpful in establishing the diagnosis in patients whose only manifestation may be the necessity for continued ventilator support after the 3rd–4th day of life, a time when respiratory distress syndrome should be improving.

In uncomplicated cases the ductus closes spontaneously within the 1st weeks or months of life. When a large symptomatic PDA is present, general treatment may include fluid restriction, correction of anemia, digitilization, and diuretic therapy. Oxygen is administered so that the PaO$_2$ is kept between 50–70 mm Hg. Continuous positive airway pressure (CPAP) and positive pressure ventilation may be required. If medical management fails and the infant cannot be weaned from the ventilator, surgical or pharmacologic closure of the ductus should be carried out.

Delayed closure should be differentiated from patency. The former is to be expected in the premature infant, while the latter occurs as a pathologic entity in a full term infant. Ductus arteriosus patency is mediated through the prostaglandins, and the ductus arteriosus in preterm infants with respiratory distress syndrome can be constricted and closed by administration of inhibitors of prostaglandin synthesis such as indomethacin (Sec 7.34). Indomethacin administration early in the course of respiratory distress syndrome associated with large ductal left to right shunts appears as effective as surgery in limiting mortality and morbidity in premature infants with this syndrome.

Untoward effects of indomethacin include oliguria, increases in blood urea nitrogen and serum creatinine, and substantial reduction in urinary sodium concentration. Platelet function may also be altered by indomethacin; the drug should not be used if there is evidence of a coagulation disorder.

13.43 AORTICOPULMONARY SEPTAL DEFECT

This defect is a communication between the ascending aorta and main pulmonary artery. The presence of

pulmonary and aortic valves and an intact ventricular septum distinguishes this anomaly from truncus arteriosus. Symptoms resembling those of a large ventricular septal defect may appear at any age and include recurrent pulmonary infections, congestive heart failure, and, occasionally, minimal cyanosis. In the absence of severe pulmonary hypertension, physical signs are a wide pulse pressure, cardiac enlargement, and a right and left upper sternal border systolic murmur, which may occasionally be continuous. The electrocardiogram shows either left, right, or biventricular hypertrophy. Roentgenographic studies confirm the cardiac enlargement and demonstrate prominence of the pulmonary artery and intrapulmonary vasculature.

This condition may simulate a patent ductus arteriosus. Cardiac catheterization reveals a left to right shunt at the level of the pulmonary artery as well as hyperkinetic pulmonary hypertension since the defect is almost always large. Selective aortography with injection of contrast medium into the ascending aorta demonstrates the lesion, but manipulation of the catheter from the main pulmonary artery to the ascending aorta and brachiocephalic vessels is also diagnostic.

Aorticopulmonary defects can be corrected surgically. In virtually all instances the defect occurs in the intracardiac portion of the aorta, and cardiopulmonary bypass is necessary during surgery.

13.44 CORONARY ARTERY FISTULA

A congenital fistula may exist between a coronary artery and vein, or a coronary artery may empty directly into the heart, usually into the right ventricle. In each defect the signs are similar to those of patent ductus arteriosus, but the machinery murmur may be more diffuse. With the *coronary arteriovenous fistula*, arterialized blood enters the coronary veins, which in turn empty into the coronary sinus. In such cases the right atrial blood has a higher oxygen content than that in the cavae. When a *coronary artery empties directly into the right ventricle*, there is a left to right shunt at the ventricular level. The anatomic abnormality is demonstrable by injection of contrast medium into the ascending aorta. Treatment consists of surgical abolition of the fistula.

13.45 RUPTURED SINUS OF VALSALVA

When 1 of the sinuses of Valsalva of the aorta is weakened by congenital or acquired disease, an aneurysm may form and rupture, usually into the right atrium or ventricle. This condition is extremely rare in early childhood. The clinical manifestations are similar to those of patent ductus arteriosus, but often the murmurs are to and fro rather than continuous. Cardiac catheterization demonstrates the left to right shunt at the atrial or ventricular level. Aortography with injection of contrast medium into the ascending aorta demonstrates the site of aneurysm and rupture. Surgical obliteration of the shunt during cardiopulmonary bypass is usually necessary.

13.46 PULMONARY VALVULAR STENOSIS WITH INTACT VENTRICULAR SEPTUM

Various forms of right ventricular outflow obstruction with intact ventricular septum exist. The most common is valvular pulmonary stenosis. In this entity the valve cusps are deformed so that a dome-like obstruction occurs during systole. The cusps are thickened, and there is an eccentric outlet. The ventricular septum is intact. Isolated infundibular stenosis, supravalvular pulmonary stenosis, and branch pulmonary artery stenosis. are less often encountered. In some instances when pulmonary valve stenosis is the dominant lesion, a small associated ventricular septal defect is present, but this problem is better classified as pulmonary stenosis than as tetralogy of Fallot. In addition, patients are seen with pulmonary stenosis and atrial septal defect or patent foramen ovale.

Hemodynamics. The obstruction to outflow from the right ventricle to the pulmonary artery results in increased systolic pressure and hypertrophy of the right ventricle. The severity of these abnormalities depends on the size of the restricted valvular opening. In severe cases right ventricular pressure may be much higher than systemic systolic pressure, whereas in milder obstruction right ventricular pressure is only slightly elevated. Pulmonary artery pressure is normal or decreased. Arterial oxygen saturation is normal except in severe cases, when a combination of poor right ventricular compliance and intra-atrial communication leads to right to left shunting at the atrial level. This is seen most often in the neonate.

Clinical Manifestations. With mild or moderate stenosis there are usually no symptoms. If the stenosis is severe, there may be dyspnea on effort or exercise intolerance. When obstruction is critical in infancy, there are signs of right ventricular failure and cyanosis. Growth and development are most often normal, and usually patients with pulmonary stenosis appear to be especially well developed and healthy. Pulmonary stenosis with valve dysplasia is the common cardiac abnormality of *Noonan syndrome* (Sec 18.32).

With stenosis of a mild degree the venous pressure and pulse are normal. The heart is not enlarged; the apical impulse is normal, and the right ventricle is not palpable. A relatively short pulmonary systolic ejection murmur is maximally audible over the pulmonic area. The murmur is usually preceded by a pulmonic ejection sound which is heard best during expiration. The 2nd heart sound is split with a delayed pulmonary element of normal intensity (Fig 13–52). The *electrocardiogram* is normal or characteristic of minimal right ventricular hypertrophy. The only abnormality demonstrable *roentgenographically* is poststenotic dilatation of the pulmonary artery. Real-time *echocardiographic* scanning shows the domed stenotic valve.

In moderate stenosis the venous pressure may be slightly elevated with an intrinsic "a" wave noted in the jugular pulse. A right ventricular sternal lift may be

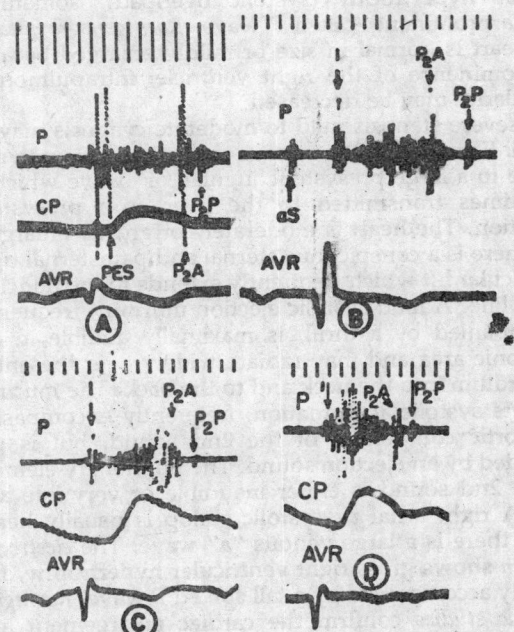

Figure 13–52 Phonocardiograms to illustrate auscultatory findings in valvular pulmonary stenosis of varying severity. AS, atrial sound; AVR, electrocardiogram; CP, carotid pulse; P, pulmonary area; PES, pulmonic ejection sound; P₂A, aortic component of 2nd sound; P₂P, pulmonary component of 2nd sound. Time lines 0.04 sec.

A, Mild pulmonary stenosis. Ejection sound followed by midsystolic murmur. Second sound split with delayed, diminished pulmonic component. *B, Severe pulmonary stenosis.* Systolic murmur accentuated in late systole and extends beyond P₂A, P₂P delayed and diminished. *C, Severe pulmonary stenosis (preoperative).* Compare with B, D. Same patient as in C, 1 wk postoperative. Murmur is now in early systole and midsystole. P₂P more accentuated and closer to P₂A. Compare with A.

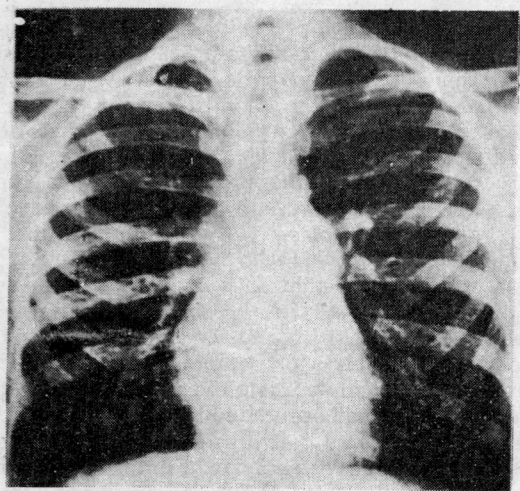

Figure 13–53 Roentgenogram in valvular pulmonary stenosis with normal aortic root. The heart size is within normal limits, but there is poststenotic dilatation of the pulmonary artery.

palpable. The systolic ejection murmur is accentuated in later systole, and a pulmonic ejection sound may or may not be present. The 2nd heart sound is split, with a delayed and diminished pulmonary component. The *electrocardiogram* reveals varying degrees of right ventricular hypertrophy (systolic overload), sometimes with a prominent spiked P wave. *Roentgenographically,* the heart is normal in size or mildly enlarged because of prominence of the right ventricle; intrapulmonary vascularity may be decreased.

In severe stenosis mild to moderate cyanosis may be noted. Elevation of the venous pressure is common and is due to a large presystolic jugular "a" wave which is sometimes transmitted to the liver as a presystolic pulsation. The heart is moderately or greatly enlarged, and there is a conspicuous sternal and parasternal right ventricular lift which frequently extends to the midclavicular line. A loud systolic ejection murmur, frequently accompanied by a thrill, is maximally audible in the pulmonic area and may radiate widely over the entire precordium into the neck and to the back. The murmur has late systolic accentuation, frequently encompasses the aortic component of the 2nd sound, but is not preceded by an ejection sound. The pulmonary element of the 2nd sound is either inaudible or very late and soft. A right atrial presystolic gallop is usually heard when there is a large venous "a" wave. The *electrocardiogram* shows gross right ventricular hypertrophy, frequently accompanied by a tall spiked P wave. *Roentgenographic studies* confirm the cardiac enlargement and prominence of the right ventricle and atrium. Prominence of the pulmonary artery segment is due to poststenotic dilatation (Fig 13–53). The intrapulmonary vascularity is decreased.

Cardiac catheterization demonstrates an abrupt gradient of pressure across the pulmonary valve. The pulmonary arterial pressure is normal or low. The right ventricular systolic pressure is 30–50 mm Hg in mild cases, 50–100 mm in moderate cases, and in severe cases frequently higher than the systemic systolic pressure unless cardiac

output is low. In severe and in some moderate cases the right atrial pressure shows a prominent, frequently giant, "a" wave. *Selective right ventriculography* clearly demonstrates the obstruction. The flow of contrast medium through the stenotic valve in ventricular systole produces a jet of dye which fills the dilated pulmonary artery. The abnormal pulmonary valve is frequently visible. Subvalvular hypertrophy which may intensify the obstruction may also be present (Fig 13–54). This study also indicates whether the ventricular septum is intact.

Complications.   Congestive cardiac failure, the most common complication, occurs only in severe cases and most often during the 1st mo of life. The development of cyanosis from a right to left shunt across a foramen ovale is seen in infancy when stenosis is very severe. Infective endocarditis is not common.

Course and Prognosis.   Children with mild stenosis can lead a normal life, as can many with moderate stenosis, but their progress should be evaluated at regular intervals. Progression of obstruction to right ventricular outflow is indicated by change in the systolic murmur with the development of late systolic accentuation. Progressive electrocardiographic signs of right ventricular hypertrophy also indicate increasing obstruction to right ventricular outflow. In severe stenosis the course is rapidly downhill with the development of congestive cardiac failure. Infants with severe stenosis require urgent surgical treatment.

Treatment.   In contrast to children with mild and many with moderate stenosis who need no specific therapy, all patients with severe isolated pulmonary stenosis require surgical therapy (pulmonary valvotomy). During cardiopulmonary bypass the valve is approached through pulmonary arteriotomy. The valve leaflets are separated by incisions at the fused commis-

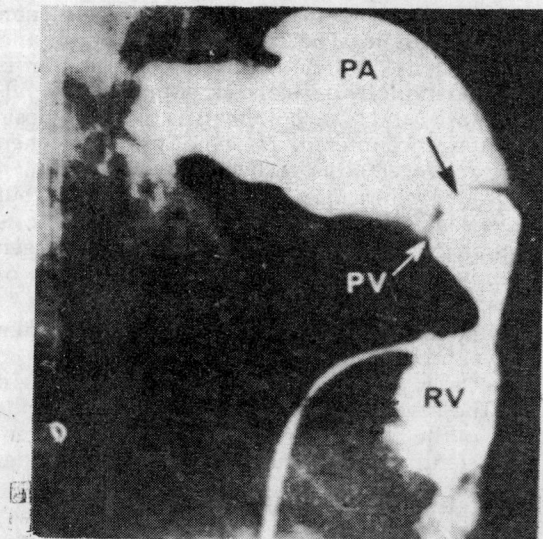

Figure 13–54 Lateral projection of selective right ventriculogram in severe valvular pulmonary stenosis. Arrow points to jet of contrast medium through minute opening of pulmonary valve. Subvalvular infundibular hypertrophy is also present. PA, poststenotic dilatation of pulmonary artery; PV, thickened pulmonary valve; RV, right ventricle.

sures. Emergency closed valvotomy for the neonate is also utilized in some cases.

Good results should be obtained in the majority of instances. The gradient across the pulmonary valve is reduced or abolished. A pulmonary diastolic murmur due to surgically created pulmonary valvular incompetence is not unusual; it is not clinically significant.

13.47 INFUNDIBULAR STENOSIS

This condition is due to muscular or fibrous obstruction in the outflow tract of the right ventricle. The site of obstruction may be close to the pulmonary valve or well below it; an infundibular chamber may be present between the right ventricular cavity and the pulmonary valve. In some cases a ventricular septal defect may have been present initially and later closed spontaneously. When the pulmonary valve is abnormal (combined valvular and infundibular stenosis), the infundibular stenosis is frequently due to hypertrophy of the right ventricular outflow tract secondary to pulmonary valvular stenosis. Such cases are primarily classified as valvular stenosis.

The *hemodynamics* and *clinical manifestations* are similar to those described under simple valvular pulmonary stenosis (Sec 13.46) with the following exceptions: (1) The systolic thrill and murmur are frequently maximal in the 3rd and 4th left parasternal spaces but radiate widely. The murmur is long and seldom preceded by an ejection sound. (2) Poststenotic dilatation of the pulmonary artery may be present but is not usual. (3) With an infundibular chamber and valvular pulmonary stenosis 2 pressure gradients may be noted during cardiac catheterization: between the right ventricle and the infundibular chamber and between the latter and the pulmonary artery. (4) Selective angiocardiography is diagnostic in the majority of instances. When contrast material is injected into the right ventricle, the site of the infundibular stenosis is demonstrated, the presence of an infundibular chamber is evident, and associated abnormalities of the pulmonary valve are shown. It is important to prove that the ventricular septum is intact because the clinical picture of isolated infundibular stenosis closely mimics that of acyanotic tetralogy of Fallot.

The complications, course, and prognosis are similar to those of simple valvular pulmonary stenosis (Sec 13.46).

In severe cases surgical treatment is indicated. The infundibular stenosis is relieved under direct vision and a pulmonary valvuloplasty performed if there is associated pulmonary stenosis. After operation the pressure gradients are reduced or abolished.

13.48 PULMONARY STENOSIS WITH LEFT TO RIGHT SHUNT

Valvular or infundibular pulmonary stenosis, or both, may be associated with a left to right shunt across an atrial septal defect, a ventricular septal defect, or a patent ductus arteriosus. The clinical features depend on the degree of stenosis and the magnitude of the left to right shunt.

Pulmonary Stenosis and Atrial Septal Defect. In patients with dominant valvular pulmonary stenosis and a small atrial left to right shunt, the clinical picture is indistinguishable from that of simple valvular pulmonary stenosis. If the shunt is large and the pulmonary stenosis slight, the clinical manifestations are similar to those of atrial septal defect (Sec 13.38), but the systolic murmur is harsh and may be accompanied by a thrill. The diagnosis is made during cardiac catheterization; a left to right shunt is demonstrated at the atrial level, and the pulmonary stenosis is demonstrated by a pressure gradient across the valve. Selective angiocardiography shows the presence of pulmonary stenosis and the left to right shunt across the atrial defect.

Pulmonary Stenosis and Ventricular Septal Defect. When the ventricular septal defect is dominant and the pulmonary stenosis is minimal, the clinical picture is limited to that of ventricular septal defect. During cardiac catheterization, however, a gradient is demonstrated across the pulmonary valve as well as the left to right shunt at the ventricular level. The recognition of a small ventricular septal defect with dominant valvular or infundibular pulmonary stenosis is also difficult. Rarely, in patients with ventricular septal defects, progressive ventricular hypertrophy may result in the development of infundibular pulmonary stenosis that obscures the presence of the septal defect. Even during cardiac catheterization the small shunt across the ventricular defect may not be demonstrated. Selective left ventriculography proves whether the ventricular septum is intact.

Pulmonary Stenosis and Patent Ductus Arteriosus. In addition to the signs of pulmonary stenosis, a machinery-type murmur is audible over the pulmonary area. This rare combination of anomalies is suspected in patients with signs of patent ductus arteriosus and right ventricular hypertrophy. Pulmonary atresia is excluded by the absence of cyanosis and the presence of poststenotic dilatation of the pulmonary artery.

Treatment. These anomalies are treated by direct vision surgery. Defects in the atrial or ventricular septa are closed, and the pulmonary stenosis is relieved by infundibular resection or pulmonary valvuloplasty. The patent ductus is divided during the same procedure. Surgery for the pulmonary stenosis is recommended only for severe or progressive cases.

13.49 PULMONARY STENOSIS WITH RIGHT TO LEFT SHUNT

With Atrial Septal Defect or Patent Foramen Ovale. As indicated above, patients with moderate or severe valvular or infundibular stenosis have right ventricular systolic hypertension. If, in addition, right ventricular compliance is decreased (secondary to hypertrophy) or right ventricular diastolic pressure is elevated (in right heart failure), the right atrial pressure increases, and a right to left shunt results across the atrial septal defect; cyanosis also occurs. A similar sequence of events occurs if the foramen ovale is patent.

Cyanosis may be present at birth or appear later, during adolescence, in the rare unoperated patient and is accompanied by clubbing of the digits and polycythemia. The jugular venous pressure is increased in many instances and is manifested by an intrinsic "a" wave. Other physical signs and technical data are similar to those of severe valvular pulmonary stenosis. The right to left shunt produces arterial oxygen unsaturation.

Right to left shunting at the atrial level in pulmonary stenosis always indicates severe obstruction. Surgical therapy is required in all cases; it consists in valvotomy and closure of the atrial septal defect.

13.50   PULMONARY ARTERIAL BRANCH STENOSIS

Single or multiple constrictions may occur anywhere along the major branches of the pulmonary artery and may be mild, extensive, localized, or multiple. Frequently, this defect is associated with other types of congenital heart disease, especially pulmonary valvular stenosis, tetralogy of Fallot, patent ductus arteriosus, ventricular septal defect, atrial septal defect, and supravalvular aortic stenosis. A familial tendency has been recognized in some patients with peripheral stenosis. A high incidence has been found in infants with the congenital rubella syndrome. Supravalvular aortic stenosis with pulmonary arterial branch stenosis has also been observed with idiopathic hypercalcemia of infancy.

With a mild constriction there is little effect on the pulmonary circulation. With multiple severe constrictions there is an increase in pressure in the right ventricle and in the pulmonary artery proximal to the site of obstruction. When the anomaly is isolated, the diagnosis is suspected by the presence of murmurs in widespread locations over the chest, anteriorly or posteriorly. These murmurs are usually systolic but may be continuous. They are occasionally heard in newborn infants and will eventually disappear; therefore mild branch stenosis in this age group may be transient. Frequently, the physical signs are dominated by the associated anomaly, e.g., tetralogy of Fallot. If the stenosis is severe, there is electrocardiographic evidence of right ventricular and right atrial hypertrophy.

Cardiomegaly and prominence of the main pulmonary artery are present in severe cases. Generally, the pulmonary vasculature is normal; in some cases small intrapulmonary vascular shadows are seen which may be shown by pulmonary arteriography to be areas of poststenotic dilatation. Pressure gradients across the areas of obstruction are demonstrable by cardiac catheterization. These gradients may not be easily identified if right ventricular outflow obstruction coexists since the pressure in the main pulmonary artery is normal or low in such patients. Severe obstructions of the main pulmonary artery and its primary branches should be resected, especially during corrective surgery for tetralogy of Fallot or valvular pulmonary stenosis. Multiple intrapulmonary obstructions are not amenable to surgical management.

13.51   PULMONARY VALVULAR INSUFFICIENCY

Pulmonary valvular insufficiency usually accompanies other cardiovascular diseases, especially those that result in severe pulmonary hypertension. Incompetence of the valve is also frequent after surgery for right ventricular outflow obstruction, e.g., pulmonary valvotomy and infundibular resection. Isolated congenital incompetence of the pulmonary valve is rare and usually asymptomatic since the incompetence is mild. The prominent abnormal sign is a diastolic murmur at the upper left sternal border which has a lower pitch than the murmur of aortic insufficiency. Roentgenograms of the chest show prominence of the main pulmonary artery. The electrocardiogram is normal or shows minimal right ventricular hypertrophy. The diagnosis is confirmed by cardiac catheterization which demonstrates a low pulmonary arterial diastolic pressure. Selective pulmonary arteriography shows the incompetent valve. Isolated pulmonary valvular incompetence is usually well tolerated and does not require surgical treatment.

Absence of the pulmonary valve is usually associated with other defects, especially tetralogy of Fallot and ventricular septal defect. In infancy the pulmonary arteries become widely dilated and compress the bronchi, thus causing recurrent episodes of wheezing, pulmonary collapse, and pneumonitis. Florid pulmonary valvular incompetence is not well tolerated, and death may occur from bronchial compression and heart failure. In older patients a valved conduit may be inserted at the time of correction of the ventricular defect and the infundibular stenosis.

13.52   COARCTATION OF THE AORTA

Constrictions of varying length may occur at any point from the arch to the bifurcation of the aorta, but 98% of them occur just below the origin of the left subclavian artery. The anomaly occurs twice as often in males as in females. Coarctation of the aorta occurs frequently in Turner (XO) syndrome.

Hemodynamics. Obstruction of the aorta usually causes the development of extensive collateral circulation, chiefly from the branches of the subclavian, the superior intercostal, and the internal mammary arteries. The thoracic and subscapular branches of the axillary artery may also enlarge as collateral channels. These vessels unite with the intercostal branches of the descending aorta and inferior epigastric branches of the femoral artery to create a channel for arterial blood to bypass the area of coarctation. The vessels contributing to the collateral circulation become markedly enlarged and tortuous by early adulthood.

The blood pressure may be elevated in the vessels that arise proximal to the coarctation; below it the amplitude of pulsation is diminished, and the pressure below the constriction is lower. The basis for the hypertension is not clear. It is not due to the mechanical obstruction alone.

Clinical Manifestations. Although symptoms are not usual during the 1st decade of life, they may develop at any age and are the result of the hypertensive state, decreased myocardial performance, or a deficient circulation in the legs. Hypertension may result in epistaxis and throbbing headache as well as left ventricular or congestive cardiac failure. Cerebral hemorrhages can occur. Deficient circulation to the legs may be evidenced by cold feet and, occasionally, by fatigue.

The classic sign of coarctation of the aorta is the disparity in pulsations and blood pressures of the arms and legs. The femoral, popliteal, posterior tibial, and dorsalis pedis pulsations are weak and delayed or absent in contrast with the bounding pulses of the arms and carotid vessels. In normal persons the systolic blood pressure in the legs as obtained by the cuff method is 10–20 mm Hg higher than that in the arms. In coarctation of the aorta the blood pressure in the legs is much lower than that in the arms; frequently, it cannot be obtained. There is also a rise of systemic blood pressure in response to exercise. It is essential to determine the blood pressure in each arm; a difference of more than 30 mm between the right and left arms suggests involvement of the left subclavian artery in the area of coarctation.

The collateral arterial circulation may give rise to systolic murmurs, especially in the back between the scapulae and at their angles. These signs are usually more striking after the 1st decade of life, as is cardiac enlargement with a left ventricular apical impulse. Murmurs are variable in location, intensity, and quality and are not diagnostic. The common murmur is systolic in time, ejection in nature, and maximal over the base of the heart; it radiates down the sternum to the apex and to the interscapular area and frequently is loudest in the back. The murmur may be produced by the coarctation, by tortuous collateral vessels, by abnormalities of the aortic valve, or by associated structural anomalies of the heart such as septal defects. Occasionally, there is also a diastolic element which may be due to associated congenital aortic insufficiency; it is heard best over the base of the heart and down the left sternal border. A continuous murmur over the pulmonary area radiating to the left clavicle suggests an associated patent ductus arteriosus. Rarely, a diastolic murmur is heard in the back, and a rumbling, apical diastolic murmur suggesting a mitral valve deformity may also be present.

Diagnosis. The findings on *roentgenographic examination* depend on the age of the patient and on the effects of hypertension and collateral circulation. In infancy there are usually no changes except cardiac enlargement if congestive cardiac failure develops. During childhood the findings are not striking unless the left ventricle is prominent. After the 1st decade the heart tends to be mildly or moderately enlarged because of left ventricular prominence. The enlarged left subclavian artery commonly produces a prominent shadow in the left superior mediastinum. Notching of the inferior border of the ribs from pressure erosion by enlarged collateral vessels is common by late childhood except in the upper and lower 2–3 ribs. Rarely, erosion is unilateral and is due to 1 of the subclavian arteries arising below the area of coarctation. In the majority of instances there is an area of poststenotic dilatation of the descending aorta. This may be demonstrated by displacement of the barium-filled esophagus and by discontinuity of the lateral margin of the aorta below the arch (Fig 13–55). Prominent serrations on the posterior aspect of the barium-filled esophagus suggest the presence of large intercostal arteries entering the aorta below the coarctation. Occasionally, scalloping in the soft tissues may be seen retrosternally; it is due to dilated internal mammary arteries.

The *electrocardiogram* is usually normal in children but may reveal evidences of left ventricular hypertrophy and of occasional left bundle branch block. In scalar tracings, right ventricular hypertrophy may be erroneously diagnosed because of prominence of primary or secondary R waves in the right precordium. This finding is related to the rightward and posterior maximum QRS vector and is probably the result of hypertrophy of the posterobasal portion of the left ventricle.

Most often, the diagnosis can be made simply by careful evaluation of the pulse in all major accessible peripheral arteries and by comparative blood pressure determinations in the arms and legs. The segment of coarctation can be visualized by 2-dimensional real-time *echographic scanning;* associated anomalies of the aortic valve can also be demonstrated. *Cardiac catheterization* with selective left ventriculography and aortography is advocated for coarctation in selected cases with additional anomalies.

Associated Abnormalities. Abnormalities of the

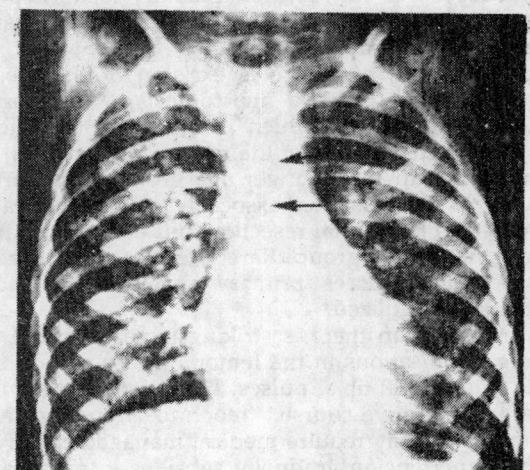

Figure 13–55 Roentgenogram of a 6 yr old boy with coarctation of the aorta. The barium-filled esophagus shows indentations produced by the aortic knob and left subclavian artery (upper arrow) and poststenotic dilatation (lower arrow). These 2 indentations produce the E sign. The left ventricle is prominent; there is no evidence of notching of the ribs.

aortic valve are present in a majority of patients. Bicuspid aortic valves are common but usually do not produce signs unless aortic incompetence or stenosis develops. The association of patent ductus arteriosus and coarctation of the aorta is common. Ventricular and atrial septal defects may be suspected by signs of left to right shunt.

Severe neurologic damage or even death may occur from associated cerebrovascular disease. Subarachnoid or intracerebral hemorrhage may result from rupture of congenital aneurysms in the circle of Willis, of other vessels with defective elastic and medial tissue, or of normal vessels; these accidents are secondary to the hypertensive state. Abnormalities of the subclavian arteries may include involvement of the left subclavian artery in the area of coarctation, stenosis of the orifice of the left subclavian artery, and anomalous origin of the right subclavian artery.

Prognosis and Complications. The majority of untreated patients with coarctation of the aorta succumb between the ages of 20–40 yr; some live well into middle life without serious handicap. Symptoms may appear in infancy and are nearly always present by the age of 25 yr. The common serious complications are related to the hypertensive state, which may result in congestive cardiac failure or intracranial hemorrhage. Heart failure is frequently related to complicating anomalies, e.g., aortic stenosis or insufficiency. Infective endocarditis or endarteritis is a frequent complication that most commonly involves abnormal aortic valves. Rupture of the aorta may be related to defective elastic and medial tissue. Aneurysms of the descending aorta or of the enlarged collateral vessels are not unusual.

Treatment. Patients with significant coarctation of the aorta should be treated surgically. The optimal age for operation is 3–6 yr; the mortality rate at this age is less than 1%. After the 2nd decade the operation may be more hazardous because of decreased left ventricular function and degenerative changes. Nevertheless, if cardiac reserve is sufficient, satisfactory repair is possible well into midadult life. Associated valvular lesions increase the hazards of surgery.

The operation of choice is excision of the area of coarctation and primary anastomosis. A subclavian turndown procedure, which incorporates the subclavian artery into the wall of the repaired coarctation, has been utilized in the younger age group. This vertical incision may be less often associated with recoarctation compared to horizontal resection and end-to-end anastomosis in this age group. Rarely, if the length of aortic constriction precludes primary anastomosis, Dacron grafts may be utilized.

After operation there is striking increase in the amplitude of pulsations in the femoral artery and dorsalis pedis and arterial tibial pulses. However, in the immediate postoperative course, "rebound" hypertension is common and may require medical management. Eventually, hypertension gradually subsides in most cases. Residual murmurs are common and may be due to associated cardiac anomalies, to flow across the repaired area, and/or to collateral blood flow. Repair of coarctation in the 2nd decade of life or beyond may be associated with a higher incidence of premature cardiovascular disease, even in the absence of residual cardiac abnormalities. There may be recurrence or early onset of adult hypertension, which has been shown to occur even in patients with adequately resected coarctation. However, most follow-up studies involve young adults who were operated on several decades earlier, and the excellence of the original repair has not been documented. Most centers now advocate repair of coarctation early in the 1st decade of life; it remains to be seen whether there will be premature cardiovascular disease in these patients during adult life. In patients with normal blood pressure following repair at 3–4 yr of age, late hypertension, early atherosclerosis, and dissecting aneurysm, all of which have been reported in the older age group, should be less likely to occur.

Although restenosis in a patient who had an adequate coarctectomy is extremely rare, a significant number of infants with end-to-end anastomoses carried out urgently in the 1st months of life require revision later in childhood. However, follow-up of patients who had subclavian turndown procedures in this age group suggests that restenosis is much less likely. All patients should be followed carefully for an indefinite period after repair of coarctation of the aorta.

13.53 THE POSTCOARCTECTOMY SYNDROME

Postoperative mesenteric arteritis may be associated with hypertension and abdominal pain in the immediate postoperative period. The pain varies in severity and may be associated with anorexia, nausea, vomiting, leukocytosis, and even signs of small bowel obstruction. Relief is usually obtained with antihypertensive drugs and intestinal decompression; corticosteroids may help to alleviate the symptoms and thus avoid surgical exploration for bowel obstruction. This syndrome has been seen much less frequently in recent yr.

13.54 COARCTATION IN INFANCY

Coarctation occurs in infancy associated with other cardiovascular anomalies, including patent ductus arteriosus, ventricular septal defect, severe aortic valvular disease, transposition of the great arteries, and variations of single ventricle. Severe coarctation may also be associated with endocardial sclerosis and mitral valve disease. The clinical pattern in this age group depends on the effects of the associated malformations as well as of the coarctation itself. Both anatomic and physiologic classifications have been utilized to describe all existing abnormalities and their contributions to the clinical manifestations of coarctation in infancy. These depend on the site and length of coarctation, the site of the aortic opening of the ductus, and the size of the aorta proximal to the coarctation. The direction of blood flow across the ductus depends on position, severity of obstruction at the site of the coarctation, and pulmonary vascular resistance. Virtually all coarctations are juxtaductal rather than in the pre- and postductal positions referred to in the early literature.

In patients in which the ductus is relatively unobstructed distal to the coarctation, right ventricular blood is ejected through the ductus to the descending aorta. Systemic flow to the lower body is dependent on right ventricular output. In this situation femoral pulses are palpable, and differential blood pressures are not helpful in the diagnosis. Such infants will have severe pulmonary hypertension and high pulmonary vascular resistance. Cyanosis, failure to thrive, and heart failure are prominent. Because the descending aorta is supplied with venous blood, differential cyanosis may be noted, but this is not a conspicuous sign. The heart is large, and there is a systolic murmur heard along the left sternal border with a loud 2nd heart sound. The electrocardiogram shows right ventricular hypertrophy, and the chest roentgenogram shows cardiac enlargement and prominent vascularity. In coarctation with a large right to left shunt across the ductus arteriosus the prognosis is often poor, but some cases respond well to medical management and surgical excision of the coarctation. On the other hand, the occasional infant with coarctation and a large left to right shunt through the ductus arteriosus has a much better outlook. In some of these infants, surgical repair may be delayed if response to digitalization and diuretic therapy is good.

Coarctation of the aorta associated with severe mitral and aortic valve disease should be considered within the context of hypoplastic left heart syndrome. Such patients have a long segment narrow arch with or without isolated coarctation at the site of the entrance of the ductus into the aorta. Coarctation of the aorta with transposition of the great arteries or single ventricle may be repaired alone or in combination with other palliative measures.

13.55 COARCTATION WITH VENTRICULAR SEPTAL DEFECT IN INFANCY

Isolated coarctation of the aorta is rarely a cause of congestive heart failure during infancy. However, coarctation in the presence of ventricular septal defect results in both increased preload and afterload on the left ventricle, and patients with this combination of defects will present in the 1st mo of life, often with intractable cardiac failure. The clinical picture is that of a seriously ill infant with tachypnea, failure to thrive, and typical findings of heart failure. Often, there is not a marked difference in blood pressures between the upper and lower extremities since cardiac output may be low. These infants present earlier in a more severely ill state than those with either ventricular septal defect or coarctation alone. Although medical management may be helpful initially, early surgery is necessary to the patient's survival. In the majority of cases coarctation is the major anomaly which is causing the severe symptoms, and resection of the coarcted segment will result in marked improvement. Some centers will not band the pulmonary artery, and a number of patients will improve sufficiently so that further surgery is not required during infancy. Later repair of the ventricular

septal defect is carried out in some patients. However, if there is difficulty in managing the patient after surgery, open repair of the ventricular septal defect is done in infancy. When it is determined that a complicated ventricular septal defect is present (multiple, muscular), pulmonary artery banding can be done at the time of coarctation repair to avoid infant open heart surgery for complex ventricular septal abnormalities.

13.56 ANOMALOUS PULMONARY VENOUS RETURN

Abnormal development of the pulmonary veins may result in anomalous partial or complete drainage into the systemic venous circulation. The abnormal point of entry may be the right atrium, the superior or inferior vena cava or one of their major tributaries, or a persistent left superior vena cava which opens into the coronary sinus. The pulmonary veins may join a common trunk which enters the venous circulation below the diaphragm (portal vein, ductus venosus, or inferior vena cava). An associated atrial septal defect is frequently present.

Partial Anomalous Pulmonary Venous Return. A varying number of pulmonary veins may enter the systemic venous circulation or the right atrium and produce a left to right shunt of oxygenated blood, which is increased if there is an associated atrial septal defect. Partial anomalous pulmonary venous return usually involves some or all of the veins of only 1 lung, more frequently the right. An associated sinus venosus type of atrial septal defect usually is present (Sec 13.40). The history, physical signs, electrocardiogram, and roentgenographic findings are indistinguishable from those of atrial septal defect (ostium secundum). Occasionally, an anomalous vein draining into the inferior vena cava is visible roentgenographically as a crescentic shadow of vascular density along the right border of the cardiac silhouette (scimitar syndrome); an atrial septal defect is usually not present.

During *cardiac catheterization* the catheter may enter the anomalous pulmonary vein from the superior vena cava or right atrium or may traverse the associated atrial septal defect. The site of left to right shunt depends on the point of entry of the pulmonary veins and may be in the superior vena cava or right atrium. Frequently, the oxygen content and saturation of the caval and right atrial blood are indistinguishable from those associated with atrial septal defect. Indicator dilution curves are valuable to demonstrate the presence of anomalous pulmonary veins. They may also be demonstrated by *selective pulmonary arteriography*.

The prognosis is excellent, similar to that for atrial septal defect (ostium secundum). When a large left to right shunt is present, surgical therapy is indicated during cardiopulmonary bypass. An associated atrial septal defect should be closed in such a way as to direct the pulmonary venous return to the left atrium.

Total Anomalous Pulmonary Venous Return. There is no venous connection with the left atrium, and all blood returning to the heart (the systemic and pulmonary venous blood) enters and mixes in the right atrium. Some of the blood passes into the right ventricle and pulmonary artery, and the remainder passes through an atrial septal defect or patent foramen ovale to the left atrium.

Usually, the pulmonary veins form a single trunk before entering the systemic venous circulation at 1 of the following sites: left superior vena cava (43%), coronary sinus (19%), right atrium (14%), and right superior vena cava (12%). The remainder enter the circulation below the diaphragm.

Three types of *clinical patterns* have been described for this lesion. Some infants present in the neonatal period with severe obstruction to venous return. This is most often prevalent in the infradiaphragmatic group. Cyanosis is prominent, and there is severe tachypnea. There may be no murmurs present on physical examination.

Another group of patients also presents with congestive heart failure in early life, but in these infants a large left to right shunt is present; obstruction to pulmonary venous return is only mild or moderate. Since pulmonary artery hypertension is present, the infants will be severely ill. Systolic murmurs along the left sternal border are audible, and there may be a gallop rhythm. A continuous murmur is occasionally heard along the left upper sternal border over the pulmonary area. Cyanosis is mild.

The 3rd clinical group of patients with total anomalous venous return are those in whom pulmonary venous obstruction is not present. In this situation there is a large left to right shunt, but pulmonary hypertension is absent and the patients are unlikely to be symptomatic during infancy or early childhood. Cyanosis is virtually never apparent.

The *electrocardiogram* demonstrates right ventricular hypertrophy (usually a qR pattern in V_{4R} and V_1, and the P waves are frequently tall and spiked. *Roentgenograms* are pathognomonic in older children if the pul-

monary veins enter the innominate vein and persistent left superior vena cava (Fig 13–56). There is a large supracardiac shadow with a **figure 8** or **snowman** appearance. The supracardiac shadow is produced by the dilated left superior vena cava, left innominate vein, and right superior vena cava. If the pulmonary veins drain elsewhere, the heart is enlarged, the pulmonary artery and right ventricle are prominent, and the pulmonary vascularity is increased. In these patients cyanosis is severe; the chest roentgenograms reveal pulmonary edema with a small heart and thus commonly cause confusion with the respiratory distress syndrome.

The *echocardiogram* reflects the right ventricular overload and an intermediate or reversed ventricular septal motion. The left ventricular dimension is 50–65% of normal; the waveform of the mitral valve echo is normal, and the aortic root is smaller than normal. The common venous channel into which the pulmonary veins drain may be visualized if it lies directly behind the left atrium.

Cardiac catheterization shows that the oxygen saturations of blood in both atria, both ventricles, and the aorta are more or less similar and higher than those of peripheral systemic venous blood. In older patients the pulmonary arterial and right ventricular pressures may be only moderately elevated, but in infancy pulmonary hypertension is usual. *Selective pulmonary arteriography* shows the anatomy of the pulmonary veins and their point of entry into the systemic venous circulation (Fig 13–57).

Untreated, the prognosis for total anomalous pulmonary venous return is usually poor, and survival beyond infancy is unusual in the presence of pulmonary hypertension. Death is due to congestive heart failure. Patients who survive beyond 2 yr of age do not have pulmonary arterial hypertension and may have surprisingly few symptoms. Surgical treatment during cardiopulmonary bypass is indicated. The common pulmonary venous trunk is anastomosed to the left atrium, the atrial septal defect is closed, and the connection to

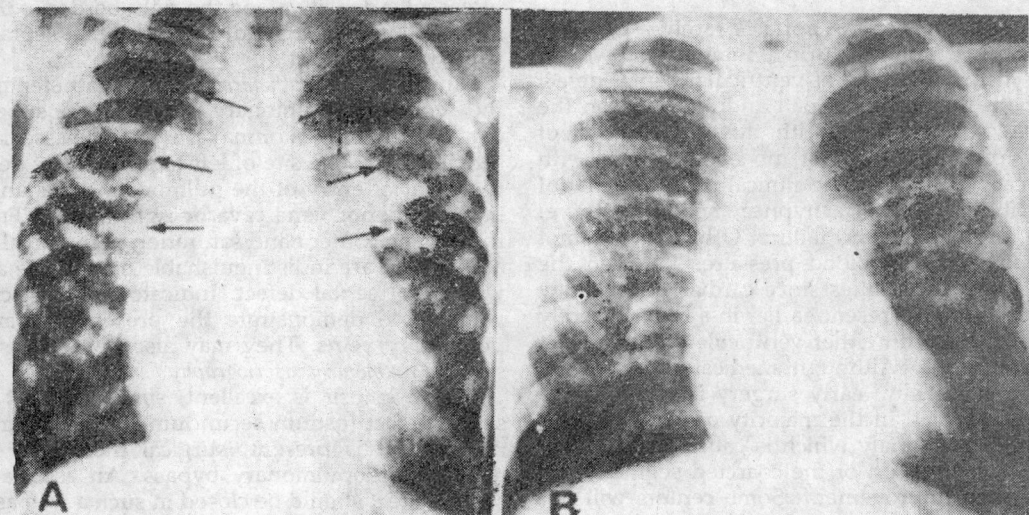

Figure 13–56   Roentgenograms in total anomalous pulmonary venous return to the left superior vena cava. *A,* Preoperative. Arrows point to the supracardiac shadow, which produces the snowman or figure # 8 configuration. Cardiomegaly and increased pulmonary vascularity are evident. *B,* Postoperative, showing decrease in size of the heart and supracardiac shadow.

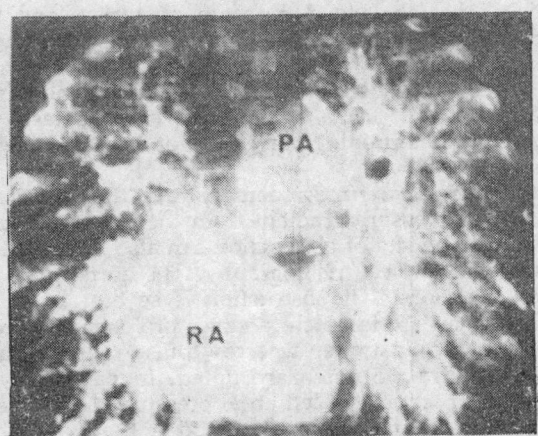

Figure 13–57 Total anomalous pulmonary venous return to the coronary sinus. Injection of contrast medium into the pulmonary artery (PA) opacifies the pulmonary arterial tree. The contrast medium returns to the coronary sinus, which drains into the densely opacified right atrium (RA).

the systemic venous circuit is obliterated. The surgical results have been good, even in symptomatic infants, and if the postoperative hemodynamics are normal, the prognosis appears to be excellent.

13.57 CONGENITAL AORTIC STENOSIS

Congenital aortic stenosis accounts for about 5% of cardiac malformations in childhood, but an abnormality of the aortic valve (frequently bicuspid with trivial stenosis) is the most common congenital heart lesion recognized in adults. Stenosis is more common in males (3:1). In the majority of instances the stenosis is valvular, the leaflets are thickened, and the commissures fused to varying degrees. In others the stenosis is subvalvular (subaortic) with a discrete fibrous or muscular obstruction to the left ventricular outflow below the aortic valves. In rare instances the stenosis is supravalvular. This lesion may be sporadic, familial, or associated with a syndrome of mental retardation and a typical facies (full face, broad forehead, flattened bridge of nose, long upper lip, and rounded cheeks). Idiopathic hypercalcemia of infancy (Sec 23.26) has been associated with this syndrome (Fig 13–58).

Clinical Manifestations. Symptomatology among patients with aortic stenosis depends on the severity of the obstruction. When aortic stenosis is critical, the patient presents in early infancy with severe left ventricular failure. However, most children with aortic stenosis, even with a relatively large degree of stenosis, will be asymptomatic and display a normal growth and development pattern. The murmur is usually discovered during routine physical examination. It is rare to see an older child with severe obstruction to left ventricular outflow with fatigue, angina, dizziness, or syncope. Sudden death has been reported with aortic stenosis but usually occurs in patients with severe left ventricular outflow obstruction manifested by electrocardiographic changes and a large gradient across the aortic valve, in whom surgical relief has been delayed.

The pulse is usually normal but has a small volume and may be anacrotic when obstruction is critical. The heart size and apical impulses are usually normal. In severe cases the heart may be enlarged with a left ventricular apical thrust. A coarse, rasping systolic ejection murmur, usually accompanied by a thrill, is audible maximally in the aortic area and radiates to the neck and down the left sternal border and toward the apex; in some patients it may be maximal down the left sternal border or even at the apex. In valvular aortic stenosis the murmur is usually preceded by an aortic ejection click best heard at the apex and left sternal edge (Fig 13–59). Clicks are unusual in discrete subaortic stenosis. Diastolic murmurs are frequent, especially when the obstruction is subvalvular.

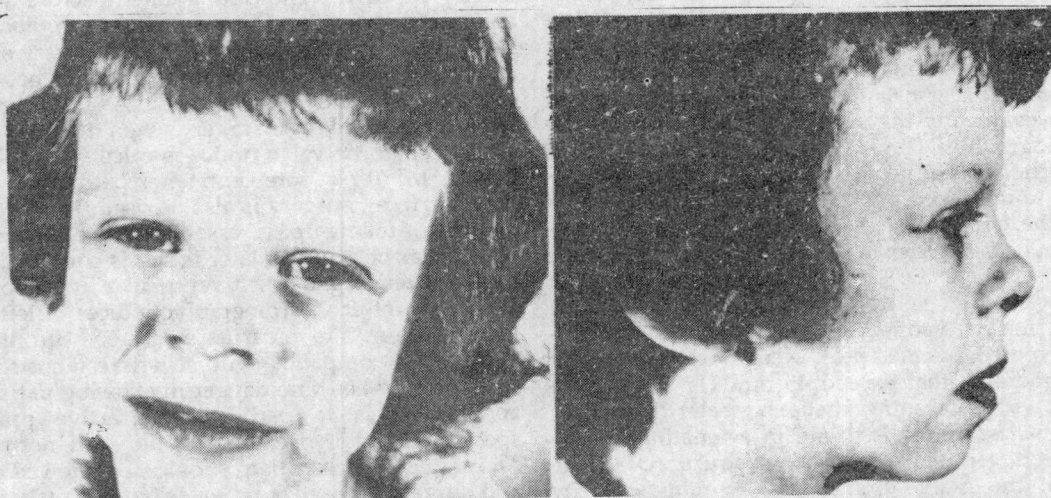

Figure 13–58 Patient with documented hypercalcemia during infancy who had supravalvular aortic stenosis relieved surgically at age 8. The upper lip is prominent, the bridge of the nose is flat, the nose is short and upturned, and hypertelorism is present.

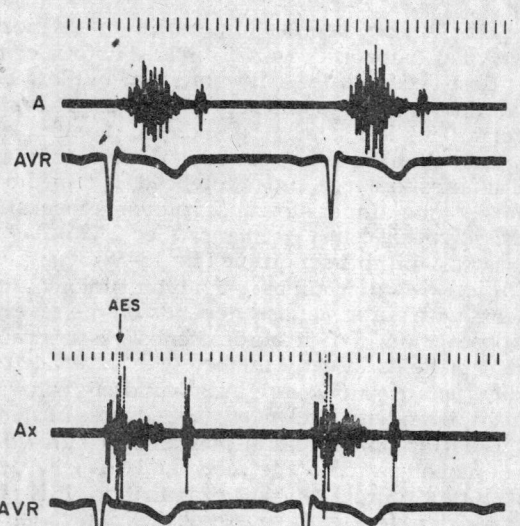

Figure 13–59 Phonocardiogram to illustrate auscultatory findings in congenital aortic valvular stenosis. At the aortic area the systolic murmur is ejection in type. At the apex the systolic murmur is initiated by an aortic ejection sound. A, aortic area; AES, aortic ejection sound; AVR, electrocardiogram; Ax, apex.

Concomitant aortic insufficiency produces an aortic blowing diastolic murmur. Occasionally, an apical mid-diastolic rumbling murmur is audible even in the presence of a normal mitral valve. The normal splitting of the 2nd heart sound is present in mild cases. In patients with severe obstruction, aortic valve closure is diminished, or the 2nd sound may be split paradoxically. A prominent 4th heart sound is audible, especially when the obstruction is severe.

Diagnosis. If the gradient of pressure across the aortic valve is small, the *electrocardiogram* is normal. It may also be normal with severe obstruction, but evidence of left ventricular hypertrophy and strain is usual. Children with severe obstruction and a normal electrocardiogram may have vectorcardiographic signs of left ventricular hypertrophy. *Roentgenograms* may show signs of left ventricular enlargement. The ascending aorta is frequently prominent, but the aortic knob is normal. Valvular calcification has been noted even in children. *Echocardiography* identifies the anomaly and is helpful in evaluating the severity of obstruction. Anatomic echographic M-mode features include multiple diastolic echoes of the aortic valve, eccentric aortic valve closure, and increased thickness of the ventricular septum and the free wall of the left ventricle. Real-time 2-dimensional studies visualize the domed stenotic aortic valve and estimate the size of the valvular orifice. In the absence of left ventricular failure the shortening fraction of the left ventricle is increased since the ventricle is hypercontractile. Peak systolic left ventricular outflow gradients that exceed 45 mm Hg are usually associated with shortening fractions greater than 40%.

Graded exercise testing is useful in evaluating the severity of left ventricular outflow obstruction. As the severity of the gradient increases, working capacity decreases, systolic blood pressure fails to rise ade-quately, diastolic blood pressure may rise, and S-T segmental depression occurs. Since patients with severe aortic stenosis may deny symptoms and have normal electrovectorcardiograms and chest roentgenograms, serial echocardiograms and graded exercise tests are valuable in determining the timing of cardiac catheterization.

Left cardiac catheterization demonstrates the magnitude and site of pressure gradient from the left ventricle to the aorta. The site of obstruction can also be identified by selective left ventriculography. The aortic pressure curve is abnormal if obstruction is severe; an early-appearing anacrotic notch, a slow, prolonged and delayed systolic upstroke, a narrow pulse pressure, and a delayed dicrotic notch are noted. In patients with severe obstruction, the left atrial pressure is increased.

Prognosis. The outcome is good in the majority of children; however, in a small number sudden death has occurred. In such instances there is usually, but not always, evidence of gross left ventricular hypertrophy. The prognosis is also affected by associated malformations, including ventricular and atrial septal defects, coarctation of the aorta, and pulmonary stenosis. Infants who die from congestive heart failure frequently have endocardial fibroelastosis of the left ventricle and atrium and of the mitral valve.

Treatment. Surgery is indicated in symptomatic patients, in those with electrocardiographic evidence of gross left ventricular hypertrophy, and in those with severe obstruction. Obstructions to left ventricular outflow are repaired during cardiopulmonary bypass.

Aortic valvular stenosis is usually treated by valvotomy, but a minority of patients may require valve replacement. Discrete subaortic stenosis can usually be resected without damage to the aortic valve, anterior leaflet of the mitral valve, or the conduction system. Relief of supravalvular stenosis can be achieved if the area of obstruction is discrete and is not associated with a hypoplastic aorta. Postoperative evaluation is difficult, especially when aortic insufficiency is produced or aggravated by surgery. Surgery is not indicated in the absence of definitive evidence of left ventricular hypertrophy or of a significant gradient across the aortic valve. The definition of a "significant gradient" is difficult, but it is generally agreed that surgery should be advised when the peak systolic gradient between the left ventricle and aorta exceeds 70 mm Hg at rest, although some advise surgery when it is ≥45 mm Hg. When the aortic valve orifice is calculated at less than 0.7 cm^2/M^2 (0.7 square centimeter per square meter of body surface), surgery is also advised.

Careful follow-up is essential since recurrence of ventricular obstruction later in life is common. Electrocardiographic signs of left ventricular hypertrophy, deterioration of echocardiographic indices of left ventricular function, and recurrence of signs during graded exercise are compatible with severe restenosis.

There may be some danger in allowing patients with aortic stenosis to participate in active competitive sports, but otherwise they should lead normal lives. The status of each patient should be reviewed annually and surgery advised if progression of signs is definite. Prophylaxis against infective endocarditis is essential.

13.58 CONGENITAL MITRAL STENOSIS

This relatively rare anomaly can be isolated or associated with other defects; the most common are patent ductus arteriosus, aortic stenosis, and coarctation of the aorta. The mitral valve is funnel shaped, its leaflets are thickened, and the chordae tendineae are shortened and deformed.

Symptoms usually appear within the 1st 2 yr. The infants are underdeveloped and usually have obvious dyspnea; cyanosis and pallor are common as are episodes of pulmonary edema and congestive heart failure. Heart enlargement is common and is due to dilatation and hypertrophy of the right ventricle and left atrium. Most patients have rumbling diastolic murmurs followed by a loud 1st sound, but the lesion may be relatively quiet. The 2nd sound is loud and split. An opening snap of the mitral valve may be present. The *electrocardiogram* reveals right ventricular hypertrophy with normal, bifid, or spiked P waves. *Roentgenograms* usually show left atrial and right ventricular enlargement and pulmonary congestion. *Echocardiograms* are typical and show thickened mitral valve leaflets, diminished E-F slope, and an enlarged left atrium with a normal or small left ventricle. The ratio of the right side systolic-time intervals (RPEP/RVET) is elevated. Real-time 2-dimensional examinations in the short axis show a significant reduction of the mitral valve orifice in diastole; the size of the mitral valve orifice can be measured. At *cardiac catheterization* there is an increase in right ventricular, pulmonary arterial, and wedge pressures, and associated anomalies such as patent ductus arteriosus may be demonstrated. *Angiocardiography* may show delayed emptying of the left atrium.

The prognosis is usually poor; the majority of children succumb during the 1st 2 yr of life. The results of surgical treatment have been variable; a mitral valve prosthesisis is required.

13.59 CONGENITAL MITRAL INSUFFICIENCY

This anomaly can be isolated or associated with patent ductus arteriosus, coarctation of the aorta, ventricular septal defect, corrected transposition of the great vessels, anomalous origin of the left coronary artery from the pulmonary artery, endocardial fibroelastosis, or Marfan syndrome. It is frequently associated with congestive cardiomyopathy. Mitral incompetence is an integral part of many endocardial cushion defects.

In isolated mitral insufficiency the mitral valve annulus is usually dilated; the chordae tendineae are short and may insert anomalously; the valve leaflets are deformed; and endocardial sclerosis of varying degree is usual. When mitral incompetence is clinically significant, the left atrium enlarges to accommodate the regurgitant flow; the left ventricle becomes hypertrophied and dilated, and thus the degree of mitral incompetence is increased; the pulmonary venous pressure is increased and ultimately results in right ventricular and atrial hypertrophy and dilatation. Mild lesions produce no symptoms; the only abnormal sign is the murmur of mitral incompetence. In the majority of instances, however, regurgitation results in symptoms that can appear at any age. These include poor physical development, frequent respiratory infections, fatigue on exertion, and episodes of pulmonary edema or congestive heart failure. Some degree of cardiac enlargement is usual, as is the typical apical pansystolic murmur of mitral insufficiency. An associated apical mid-diastolic or late diastolic rumbling murmur is frequent. The pulmonary component of the 2nd heart sound is accentuated in the presence of pulmonary hypertension. The *electrocardiogram* usually shows bifid P waves, signs of left ventricular hypertrophy, and sometimes signs of right ventricular hypertrophy. *Roentgenographic examination* shows enlargement of the left atrium, which at times is massive. The left ventricle is prominent, the aorta small, and the pulmonary vascularity normal or increased. *Echocardiograms* demonstrate the enlarged left atrium and ventricle. Although motion of the mitral valve is excessive with a steep E-F slope, this sign is not diagnostic.

Cardiac catheterization shows an elevated left atrial pressure and at times pulmonary hypertension. Selective left ventriculography reveals the presence of mitral regurgitation. *Mitral valvuloplasty* has resulted in striking improvement in symptoms and heart size, but in some patients installation of a mitral valve may be necessary. Prior to surgery, associated anomalies must be identified. In children beyond 3–4 yr it may be difficult to exclude rheumatic fever as the cause of mitral insufficiency.

13.60 MITRAL VALVE PROLAPSE

This distinctive syndrome results from an abnormal mitral valve mechanism which allows billowing of 1 or both mitral leaflets, especially the posterior cusp, into the left atrium toward the end of systole. The abnormality is almost always congenital but may be associated with complications of rheumatic or viral myocarditis or secundum atrial septal defect. The syndrome is more common in girls and may affect siblings. The dominant abnormal signs are auscultatory. The apical murmur is late systolic in timing and may be preceded by a click, but these signs vary in the same patient so that at times only the click is audible. In the standing position the click appears earlier in systole and the murmur is longer. Arrhythmias, primarily unifocal or multifocal premature ventricular contractions, may occur.

The *electrocardiogram* may be normal, but characteristically it shows diphasic T waves, especially in leads II, III, VF, and V_6; the T waves may vary in the same patient so that the electrocardiogram may sometimes be normal. The *chest roentgenogram* is normal. The *echocardiogram* shows a characteristic posterior movement of the posterior mitral leaflet during mid- or late systole or pansystolic prolapse of both anterior and posterior mitral leaflets. These M-mode echographic findings must be interpreted cautiously since improper technique may record mitral prolapse in normal children. Two-dimensional real-time echocardiography appears to be more accurate; both the free edge and the body of the mitral leaflets move posteriorly in systole toward the left atrium. The lesion is not progressive in childhood, and specific therapy is not indicated. The patient is at risk to develop infective endocarditis. Antibiotic prophylaxis is recommended during surgery and dental procedures (see Table 13–10).

13.61 PULMONARY VENOUS HYPERTENSION

A variety of lesions may result in pulmonary venous hypertension which may be followed by pulmonary arterial hypertension and congestive heart failure. These include congenital mitral stenosis, mitral insufficiency, some varieties of total anomalous pulmonary venous return, left atrial myxomas, cor triatriatum (stenosis of the common pulmonary vein), individual pulmonary venous stenosis, and supravalvular stenosing ring of the left atrium. In these conditions early symptoms can be confused with chronic pulmonary disease as there may be no specific cardiac findings on physical examination. However, subtle signs of pulmonary hypertension may be present. The *electrocardiogram* shows right ventricular hypertrophy with spiked P waves. *Roentgenographic studies* show cardiac enlargement and prominence of pulmonary veins, the right ventricle and atrium, and the main pulmonary artery; the left atrium is normal in size or only slightly enlarged. *Echocardiograms* may demonstrate a lesion in the left atrium, such as myxomas, cor triatriatum, or a supravalvular stenosing ring. Associated pulmonary hypertension is suggested by the increased right-sided, systolic, time-interval ratio. *Cardiac catheterization* excludes the presence of a shunt and demonstrates pulmonary hypertension with an elevated pulmonary arterial wedge pres-

sure. The left atrial pressure is normal if the lesion is proximal. Selective pulmonary arteriography may delineate the anatomic lesion. It is important to recognize this clinical pattern since cor triatriatum, left atrial myxoma, and some cases of supravalvular stenosing ring can be cured surgically.

13.62 ANOMALIES OF THE AORTIC ARCH

Right Aortic Arch. In this abnormality the aorta curves to the right, and, if it descends on the right side of the vertebral column, it is usually associated with other cardiac malformations. It is found in about 20% of cases of tetralogy of Fallot and is common in truncus arteriosus. A right aortic arch without another anomaly is not associated with symptoms. Right aortic arch can be visualized on roentgenograms. The barium-filled esophagus is indented on its right border at the level of the aortic arch.

Vascular Rings. Congenital abnormalities of the aortic arch and its major branches result in the formation of vascular rings around the trachea and esophagus with varying degrees of compression. The following are the more common anomalies: (1) double aortic arch (Fig 13–60 and 13–61), (2) right aortic arch with left ligamentum arteriosum, (3) anomalous right subclavian artery arising as the last major thoracic branch of a normally placed aorta, (4) anomalous innominate artery arising further to the left on the arch than usual, (5) anomalous left carotid artery arising further to the right than usual and passing anterior to the trachea, and (6) anomalous left pulmonary artery (vascular sling). This abnormal vessel arises from an elongated main pulmonary artery or from the right pulmonary artery. It courses between and compresses the trachea and esophagus.

The clinical patterns are extremely variable. In some instances, especially with anomalous right subclavian artery, the condition is asymptomatic. If the vascular ring produces compression of the trachea and esophagus, symptoms are frequently present during infancy.

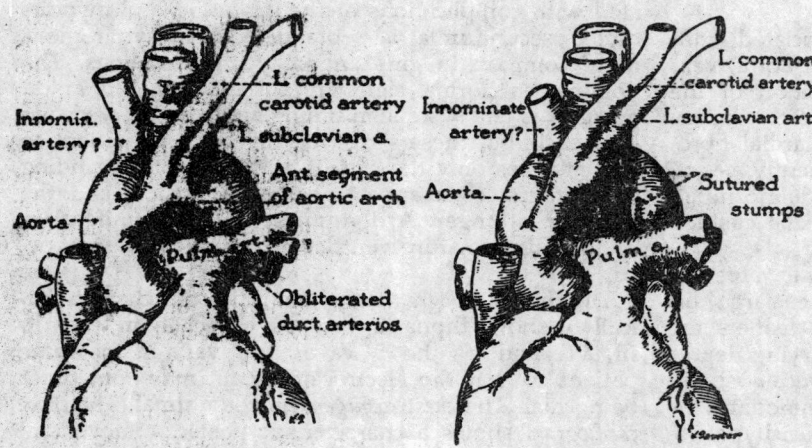

Figure 13–60 Double aortic arch. *A,* Small anterior segment of double aortic arch (most common type). *B,* Operative procedure for release of vascular ring. (Courtesy of Dr. Willis J. Potts.)

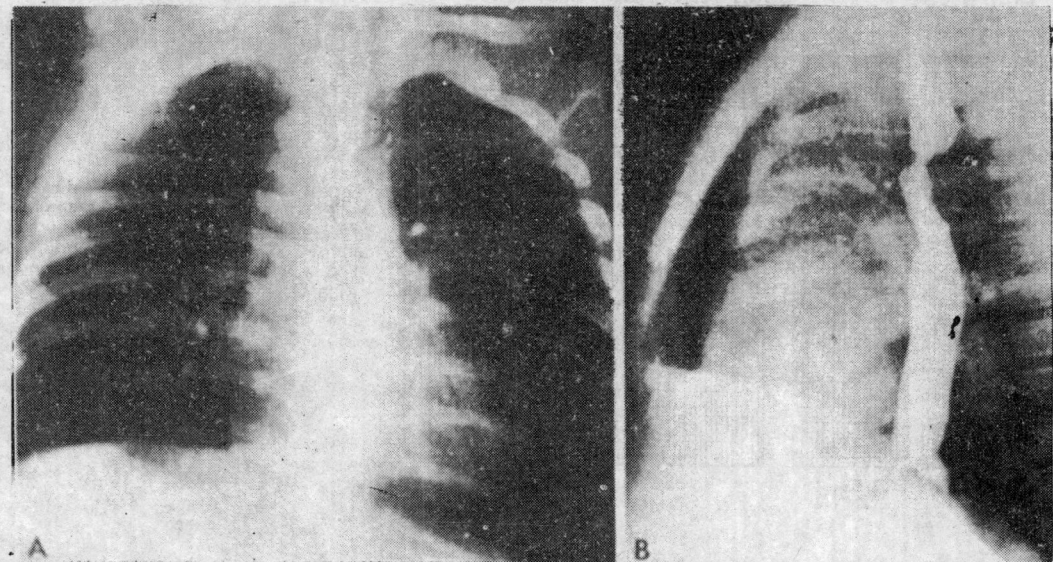

Figure 13–61 Double aortic arch in an infant aged 5 mo. *A,* Anteroposterior view. The barium-filled esophagus is constricted on both sides. *B,* Lateral view. The esophagus is displaced forward. The anterior arch was the smaller and was divided at operation. (Courtesy of Drs. Eugene Saenger, Frederick Silverman, and Edward McGrath.)

Respirations are wheezing and are aggravated by crying, feeding, and flexion of the neck. Extension of the neck tends to relieve the noisy respiration. Vomiting is frequent. There may be a brassy cough, and pneumonia is common. Roentgenographic examination of the barium-filled esophagus and aortography identify the anomaly (Fig 13–61).

Surgery is advised for symptomatic patients who have roentgenographic evidence of tracheal or esophageal compression. The anterior vessel is usually divided in patients with double aortic arch (Fig 13–60). Compression produced by a right aortic arch and left ligamentum arteriosum is relieved by division of the latter. An anomalous right subclavian artery is divided at its origin from the aorta. Anomalous innominate or carotid arteries cannot be divided; the tracheal compression is relieved by attaching the adventitia of these vessels to the sternum. Anomalous left pulmonary artery is corrected during cardiopulmonary bypass by division at its origin and reanastomosis to the main pulmonary artery after it has been brought in front of the trachea. Severe tracheomalacia may be associated and result in a poor prognosis.

13.63 ANOMALOUS ORIGIN OF CORONARY ARTERIES

Anomalous Origin of the Left Coronary Artery from the Pulmonary Artery. In this condition the blood supply to the left ventricular myocardium is compromised. Soon after birth, as the pulmonary arterial pressure falls, the perfusion pressure to the left coronary artery becomes inadequate; myocardial infarction and fibrosis may result. In some instances interarterial collateral anastomoses develop between the right and left coronary arteries. Blood flow in the left coronary artery is then reversed, and it empties into the pulmonary artery. The left ventricle becomes dilated and somewhat hypertrophied, and there may be patchy fibrosis and microscopic deposition of calcium. Mitral incompetence is a frequent complication secondary to infarction of papillary muscle. Localized aneurysms may also develop in the left ventricle.

In the majority of instances, evidence of congestive heart failure is apparent within the 1st months and is often precipitated by respiratory infection. Recurrent attacks of discomfort, restlessness, irritability, sweating, dyspnea, and pallor with or without mild cyanosis could be interpreted as due to angina pectoris. Cardiac enlargement is moderate to massive. Gallop rhythm is common. Murmurs may be absent, nonspecific, ejection in type, or regurgitant because of mitral incompetence. Older patients with abundant intercoronary anastomoses may have continuous murmurs and little or no left ventricular dysfunction.

Roentgenographic examination confirms the cardiomegaly, but the contour and pulsations are not specific unless there is a complicating ventricular aneurysm. The *electrocardiogram* resembles the pattern described in anterior myocardial infarction in adults. A QR pattern followed by inverted T waves is seen in leads I and aVL. The left ventricular surface leads (V_5 and V_6) show deep, wide Q waves and may also exhibit elevated S-T segments and inverted T waves (Fig 13–62). *Aortography* is diagnostic; there is immediate opacification of only the right coronary artery. Generally, this vessel is large and tortuous. After filling of the intercoronary anastomoses, the left coronary artery and the pulmonary artery are in turn opacified. Selective pulmonary arteriography may opacify the anomalous left coronary artery. Selective left ventriculography in the infantile type reveals a dilated left ventricle which empties poorly.

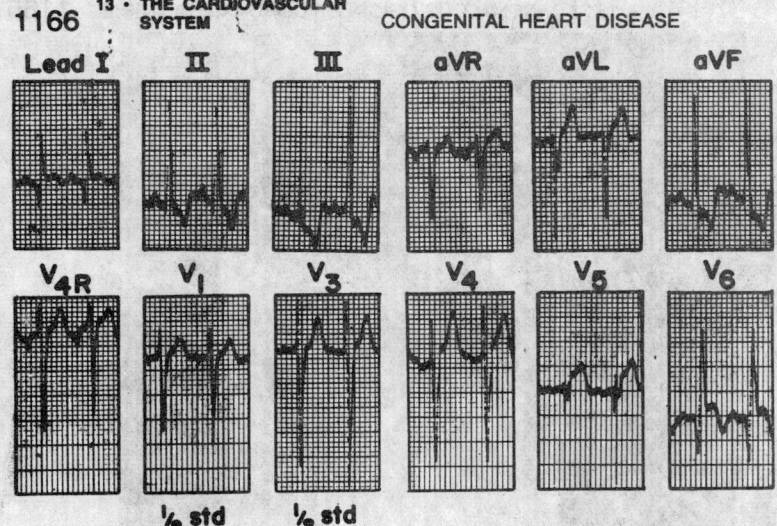

Figure 13–62   Electrocardiogram of a 3 mo old child with anomalous origin of the left coronary artery from the pulmonary artery. Anterolateral myocardial infarction is present as evidenced by abnormally large and wide Q waves in leads 1, V_5 and V_6, elevated S-T segment in V_5 and V_6, and inversion of TV_6.

In the majority of instances death from heart failure occurs within the 1st 6 mo. Those who survive usually have abundant intercoronary anastomoses.

Treatment is not standardized. In older patients the anomalous left coronary artery can be detached from the pulmonary artery and attached to the ascending aorta to establish normal arterial perfusion. The seriously ill infant who does not respond to anticongestive measures presents a difficult therapeutic problem. Ligation of the anomalous left coronary artery at its origin has been advised to prevent runoff from the coronary circuit and possibly to increase myocardial perfusion by collateral circulation. This operation, however, is of variable effectiveness, and attempts to transplant the anomalous artery in infancy may be warranted.

Anomalous Origin of the Right Coronary Artery from the Pulmonary Artery. This is a rare anomaly which rarely produces signs or symptoms in childhood.

13.64   PRIMARY PULMONARY HYPERTENSION

Primary pulmonary hypertension is a disease of unknown origin; it is characterized by hypertension of the lesser circulation and right-sided heart failure. It may occur at any age and may be clinically recognizable during childhood and adolescence. The pulmonary hypertension is associated with precapillary obstruction of the pulmonary vascular bed due to hyperplasia of the muscular and elastic tissues and the thickened intima of the small pulmonary arteries and arterioles. Atherosclerotic changes may be found in the larger pulmonary arteries. Other causes of pulmonary heart disease (chronic cor pulmonale) are absent, and there is no evidence of emphysema, pancreatic fibrosis, or kyphoscoliosis. Recurrent pulmonary emboli may produce the same clinical picture, but this disease is rare in childhood. Severe pulmonary hypertension may result from myriads of minute microemboli from an indwelling intravascular catheter inserted for hyperalimentation.

Pulmonary hypertension may also result from persistent obstruction of the upper airway, e.g., by gross enlargement of the tonsils and adenoids; it may also be an accompaniment of extreme obesity, as in the Prader-Willi syndrome.

Hemodynamics. Pulmonary hypertension places a mechanical burden on the right ventricle and pulmonary artery with resultant right ventricular hypertension and dilatation of the pulmonary artery. Frequently, the cardiac output is decreased. Right-sided heart failure may develop.

Clinical Manifestations. The predominant symptoms include effort intolerance and fatigability; occasionally, there is precordial chest pain, dizziness, or syncope. Peripheral cyanosis may be present and is associated with cold extremities and a normal arterial oxygen saturation. If right-sided heart failure has supervened, the jugular venous pressure is elevated and hepatomegaly and edema are present. Jugular venous "a" waves are present, and when there is functional tricuspid insufficiency, a conspicuous jugular "c" wave and systolic hepatic pulsations are manifest. The heart is moderately enlarged, and there is a right ventricular apical tap. The 1st heart sound is frequently followed by a pulmonic ejection click. The systolic murmur is soft and short and is sometimes followed by a blowing diastolic murmur due to pulmonary incompetence. The 2nd heart sound is closely split, loud, sometimes booming, and frequently palpable. A presystolic gallop rhythm may be audible down the left sternal border.

Roentgenograms reveal a prominent pulmonary artery and right ventricle (Fig 13–63). The pulmonary vascularity in the hilar areas may be prominent and contrast with the peripheral lung fields, which are clear. The *electrocardiogram* shows right ventricular hypertrophy with spiked P waves.

Diagnosis. At cardiac catheterization this condition must be differentiated from Eisenmenger syndrome and from left-sided lesions which result in pulmonary venous hypertension. In the latter conditions the pulmonary arterial wedge pressure is significantly elevated. The risks of cardiac catheterization may be high in severely ill patients with primary pulmonary hyperten-

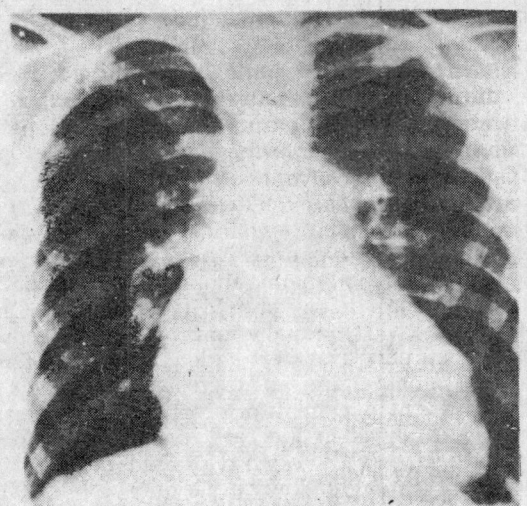

Figure 13–63 Roentgenogram in primary pulmonary hypertension; note the moderate cardiac enlargement, dilatation of the pulmonary artery, and relative pulmonary undervascularity in the outer two thirds of the lung fields. A similar roentgen pattern may also be seen in valvular pulmonic stenosis with a normal aortic root.

sion, and syncope or death may occur after pulmonary artery angiography (which should rarely be done in the most severely ill individuals).

Prognosis. Primary pulmonary hypertension is pro-

gressive, and there is no specific treatment. The terminal event may be related to right ventricular failure and is most often sudden, possibly related to severe arrhythmias.

13.65 MARFAN SYNDROME: CARDIOVASCULAR MANIFESTATIONS

Congenital malformations of the heart occur with Marfan syndrome (Sec 6.32). The most progressive lesion is dilatation of the aorta, beginning at the aortic valve and usually confined to the ascending portion. The valve ring is stretched, and the resultant aortic insufficiency may be pronounced. Left ventricular failure occurs with or without angina pectoris. Dissecting aneurysm of the aorta with medial cystic necrosis is a common terminal event or may result in the development of aortic valvular incompetence. Cardiac symptoms may occur as early as the 5th yr of life but frequently do not appear until adult life. Mitral insufficiency is even more common than aortic involvement and results from redundant cusps and chordae tendineae. Infective endocarditis may be a complication. Other congenital cardiac malformations have been reported occasionally in association with the Marfan syndrome.

13.66 PRINCIPLES OF TREATMENT OF CONGENITAL HEART DISEASE

The majority of patients with mild congenital heart disease require no treatment. It should be pointed out to the parents and child that a normal life is expected and that no restriction of the child's activities is necessary. Overprotective parents may use the presence of a mild congenital lesion or even a functional heart murmur as a means to control the child's activities. Although he or she may not express fears overtly, the child may become quite anxious regarding early death or debilitation, especially when an adult member of the family develops symptomatic heart disease. The family may have an unexpressed fear of sudden death, and the rarity of this manifestation should be emphasized in discussions directed at improving their understanding of the child's congenital heart defect. The difference between congenital heart disease and degenerative coronary disease in adults should be outlined. General management, including a well balanced diet, prevention of anemia, and the usual immunization program, should be encouraged.

Even patients with moderate to severe heart disease need not be markedly restricted in physical activities. Physical education should be modified appropriately to the child's capacity to participate. Rough, competitive sports should be discouraged. Patients with severe heart disease with decreased exercise tolerance will tend

to limit their own activities. Transportation to school may be helpful so that fatigue will not interfere with classroom activities. Dyspnea, headache, and fatigability in cyanotic patients may be a sign of increasing hypoxemia and may require some limitation of activities among those for whom specific medical or surgical treatment is not available.

Bacterial infections should be treated vigorously, but the presence of congenital heart disease is not an appropriate reason to utilize antibiotics indiscriminately. Prophylaxis against infective endocarditis should be carried out during extensive dental procedures, during instrumentation of the urinary tract, and prior to lower gastrointestinal manipulation. Treatment of iron deficiency anemia is especially important in cyanotic patients who will improve their exercise tolerance and general well being with adequate hemoglobins. However, these patients should also be carefully observed for polycythemia. Cyanotic patients should avoid situations in which dehydration may occur. High altitudes and sudden changes in thermal environment should be avoided. Patients with severe congenital heart disease or a history of rhythm disturbance should be carefully monitored during anesthesia for even routine surgical procedures. Women should be counseled on the dangers of child-bearing and the use of contraceptives and tubal ligation. Pregnancy is an extremely high risk for such patients and rarely results in normal delivery at term. However, women with mild to moderate heart disease and many of those who have had corrective surgery can have normal pregnancies.

The treatment for congestive heart failure is described in Sec 13.77, for paroxysmal dyspneic attacks in Sec 13.13, and for cardiac arrhythmias in Sec 13.67. Appropriate surgical procedures for specific cardiac lesions are discussed in the relevant sections of this chapter.

The Postoperative Period. (Sec 5.40). After successful direct vision open heart surgery, the postoperative course depends on numerous factors. The type of congenital defect operated upon, the age and condition of the patient prior to surgery, the events in the operating room, and the quality of the postoperative care will influence the patient's course following surgery. Many patients will have a benign postoperative period without complications, but others may be in a precarious state for hours or days after the operation.

Postoperative care should be initiated in the intensive care unit by a staff experienced with the unique problems encountered after open heart surgery. The function of the patient's critical organ systems must be carefully supported and the environment controlled until cardiac function has significantly improved. Physicians and nurses must be in constant attendance to act promptly upon monitored physiologic data. A femoral arterial catheter placed prior to open heart surgery allows direct arterial pressure measurements and arterial samplings for blood gas determinations. A 2nd catheter positioned in the inferior vena cava via the saphenous or femoral vein is utilized for measurement of central venous pressure. Functional failures in 1 system may cause profound physiologic and biochemical changes in another. Respiratory insufficiency, for example, will lead to hypoxia, acidosis, and hypercarbia, which in turn will compromise cardiac and renal function. The latter problems cannot be managed successfully until adequate ventilation is re-established. Thus, it is essential that the primary source of each postoperative problem be identified and treated.

Respiratory failure is probably the major postoperative complication encountered after open heart surgery. Cardiopulmonary bypass carried out in the presence of pulmonary congestion results in decreased lung compliance, copious tracheal and bronchial secretions, atelectasis, and increased breathing efforts. Since fatigue and subsequently hypoventilation and acidosis may rapidly ensue, mechanical positive pressure endotracheal ventilation is instituted immediately following open heart surgery. This is continued for a minimum of several hr in relatively stable patients and up to 2–3 days or more in severely ill infants.

Cardiac rhythm disorders must be diagnosed quickly since a prolonged untreated arrhythmia may add a severe burden to the myocardium in the critical early postoperative period. Injury to the conduction system of the heart during surgery may cause postoperative *complete heart block.* This complication is treated with surgically placed pacing wires which are later removed. Occasionally, heart block will become permanent, requiring insertion of an implanted pacemaker, but in most instances this rhythm pattern is transient, and temporary pacing wires may be utilized.

The *electrocardiogram* should be monitored continuously during the postoperative period. A change in the heart rate may be the 1st indication of a serious complication, such as hemorrhage, hypothermia, hypoventilation, or congestive heart failure.

Congestive heart failure following cardiac surgery may be secondary to respiratory failure, serious arrhythmias, myocardial injury, blood loss, hypervolemia, or significant residual hemodynamic abnormality. Specific treatment related to etiology should be instituted. Cardiac performance will gradually improve if corrective or palliative surgery has been adequate. Isoproterenol, dopamine, dobutamine, and digoxin are the drugs most useful in the management of heart failure, low cardiac output, and shock in the early postoperative period; diuretic therapy is also often required (Sec 5.7).

Acidosis secondary to low cardiac output, renal failure, or hypovolemia must be prevented or promptly corrected. An arterial pH below 7.30 may result in a decrease in cardiac output with increase in lactic acid production and may be the forerunner of a series of arrhythmias or cardiac arrest.

Kidney function may be compromised by congestive heart failure and further impaired by prolonged cardiopulmonary bypass. Persistent anuria or oliguria indicates the presence of poor cardiac function, hypokalemia, and/or acute renal failure. Blood and fluid replacement and/or a cardiotonic regimen will rapidly re-establish normal urine flow in patients with hypovolemia or cardiac failure, but renal failure secondary to tubular injury will require more prolonged management.

The *postcardiotomy syndrome* may occur toward the end of the 1st postoperative wk or sometimes weeks or months after operation. This febrile illness is characterized by pericarditis and pleurisy with or without fluid. In most patients the condition is benign. When pericardial fluid accumulates, the potential danger of cardiac tamponade should be recognized. Symptomatic patients usually respond to salicylates or indomethacin and bed rest. If there is no response, a corticosteroid may be used. Some patients have a tendency for the condition to recur.

Hemolysis of probable mechanical origin may occur after treatment of endocardial cushion defects or the insertion of an artificial prosthetic valve. It may be associated with jets of blood at high pressure since it tends to occur with residual mitral incompetence after treatment of an ostium primum defect. Jets of blood may impinge on the plastic prosthesis used to close the defect. Intravascular hemolysis may also be seen after insertion of an artificial valve, especially if the valve is incompetent. Reoperation may be necessary in patients with severe and progressive hemolysis who require frequent blood transfusions.

Infection. Sepsis with infective endocarditis is a serious complication, especially when prosthetic patches or valves are used (Sec 13.71).

Prognosis. Patients who have had palliative procedures for extremely complex heart disease may lead limited but productive lives. Such patients require careful follow-up and various restrictions depending on the severity of their disease. Other lesions generally result in excellent cardiac function and a markedly improved prognosis but may be associated with late complications or require reoperation; such patients should be followed at intervals with appropriate laboratory tests (e.g., Holter monitors, exercise studies, echocardiograms, radionuclide studies, and, when indicated, cardiac catheterizations). The need for special studies should be decided upon after careful clinical evaluation, electrocardiogram, and chest roentgenogram. After successful repair of simple lesions with no evidence of residual abnormalities, such as patent ductus arteriosus, atrial septal defect, or valvular pulmonary stenosis, patients require very little specific follow-up and should be encouraged to lead active and full lives.

The Neonatal Circulation

Dawes GS: Fetal and Neonatal Physiology. Chicago, Year Book Medical Publishers, 1968.
Gersony WM: Evaluating cyanosis in the newborn. Hosp Prac 4:43, 1969.
Gersony WM, Duc GV, Sinclair JC: "PFC" syndrome (persistence of the fetal circulation). Circulation 40:111, 1969.
Heymann MA, Rudolph AM: Effects of congenital heart disease on fetal and neonatal circulations. Prog Cardiovasc Dis 15:115, 1972.
Kaplan S, Assali NS: Disorders of circulation. In: Assali NS (ed): Pathophysiology of Gestation, Vol 3. New York, Academic Press, 1972.

Incidence and Etiology

Nora JJ: Etiologic factors in congenital heart diseases. Pediatr Clin North Am 18:1059, 1971.
Warkany J: Congenital Malformations. Chicago, Year Book Medical Publishers, 1971.

Tetralogy of Fallot and Pulmonary Atresia

Barratt-Boyes BG, Neutze MJ: Primary repair of tetralogy of Fallot in infancy using profound hypothermia with circulatory arrest and limited cardiopulmonary bypass. Ann Surg 178:406, 1974.
Garson A, Nihill MR, McNamara DG, et al: Status of the adult and adolescent after repair of tetralogy of Fallot. Circulation 59:1232, 1976.
Gersony WM, Batthany S, Bowman FO Jr, et al: Late followup of patients evaluated hemodynamically after total correction of tetralogy of Fallot. J Thorac Cardiovasc Surg 66:209, 1973.
Guntheroth WG, Morgan BC: Physiologic studies of paroxysmal hyperpnea in cyanotic congenital heart disease. Circulation 31:70, 1965.
Kirklin JW, Karp RB: The Tetralogy of Fallot: From a Surgical Viewpoint. Philadelphia, WB Saunders, 1970.
Malm JR, Bowman FO Jr, Hayes CJ, et al: Results of surgical treatment of pulmonary atresia with intact ventricular septum. In: Advances in Cardiology, Vol II. Basel, Karger, 1974.
Olin CL, Ritter DG, McGoon OC, et al: Pulmonary atresia: Surgical considerations and results in 103 patients undergoing definitive repair. Circulation 54 (suppl III):35, 1976.
Rocchini AP: Hemodynamic abnormalities in response to supine exercise in patients after operative correction of tetralogy of Fallot after early childhood. Am J Cardiol 48:325, 1981.
Rosing DR, Borer JS, Kent KM, et al: Long-term hemodynamic and electrocardiographic assessment following operative repair of tetralogy of Fallot. Circulation 58 (Suppl):209, 1978.
Sunderland CO, Matarazzo RG, Lees MH, et al: Total correction of tetralogy of Fallot in infancy: Postoperative hemodynamic evaluation. Circulation 48:398, 1973.

Transposition of the Great Vessels

Duncan WJ, Freedom RM, Rowe RD, et al: Echocardiographic features before and after the Jatene procedure (anatomical correction) for transposition of the great vessels. Am Heart J 102:227, 1981.
Freedom RM, Culham JA, Olley PM, et al: Anatomical correction of transposition of the great arteries: Pre- and postoperative cardiac catheterization with angiocardiography in five patients. Circulation 63:905, 1981.
Gillette PC, Kugler JD, Gutgesell HP, et al: Mechanisms of cardiac arrhythmias after the Mustard operation for transposition of the great arteries. Am J Cardiol 45:1225, 1980.

Hagler DJ, Ritter DC, Mair DD, et al: Clinical, angiographic, and hemodynamic assessment of late results after Mustard operation. Circulation 57:1214, 1978.
Mustard WT, Keith JD, Trusler GA, et al: The surgical management of transposition of the great vessels. J Thorac Cardiovasc Surg 48:593, 1965.
Rashkind WJ, Miller WW: Creation of an atrial septal defect without thoracotomy: A palliative approach to complete transposition of the great vessels. JAMA 196:991, 1966.
Rastelli GC, McGoon DC, Wallace RB: Anatomic correction of transposition of the great arteries with ventricular septal defect and subpulmonary stenosis. J Thorac Cardiovasc Surg 58:545, 1969.
Yacoub M, Bernhard A, Lange P, et al: Clinical and hemodynamic results of the two-state anatomic correction of simple transposition of the great arteries. Circulation 62 (Suppl):190, 1980.

Eisenmenger Syndrome

Wood P: Pulmonary hypertension. Mod Conc Cardiovasc Dis 28:513, 1959.

Tricuspid Atresia

Bowman FO Jr, Malm JR, Hayes CJ, et al: Physiological approach to surgery for tricuspid atresia. Circulation 58(Suppl):83, 1978.
Fontan F, Baudet E: Surgical repair of tricuspid atresia. Thorax 26:240, 1971.
Gale AW, Danielson GK, McGoon DC, et al: Fontan procedure for tricuspid atresia. Circulation 62:91, 1980.

Ebstein Disease

Genton E, Blount SG: The spectrum of Ebstein's anomaly. Am Heart J 73:395, 1967.
Kumar AE, Fyler DC, Miettinen OS, et al: Ebstein's anomaly. Am J Cardiol 28:84, 1971.

Atrial Septal Defect and Atrioventricular Canal

Cohn LH, Morrow AG, Braunwald E: Operative treatment of atrial septal defect: Clinical and haemodynamic assessments in 175 patients. Br Heart J 29:725, 1967.
Evans JR, Rowe RD, Keith JD: Clinical diagnosis of atrial septal defect in children. Am J Med 30:345, 1961.
Mair DD, McGoon DC: Surgical correction of atrioventricular canal during the first year of life. Am J Cardiol 40:66, 1977.
Rastelli GC, Kirklin JW, Titus JL: Anatomic observations on complete form of persistent common atrioventricular canal, with special reference to atrioventricular valves. Proc Mayo Clin 41:296, 1966.
Wallace RB, McGoon DC, Danielson GK: Complete atrioventricular canal. Repair and results. Adv Cardiol 11:26, 1974.

Ventricular Septal Defect

Edwards JE: The pathology of ventricular septal defect. Semin Radiol 1:2, 1966.
Kirklin J: Current status of corrective surgery for ventricular septal defect. In: Rowe RD, Kidd BSL (eds): The Child with Congenital Heart Disease After Surgery. Mount Kisco N.Y., Futura Publishing, 1976.
Levin AR, et al: Intracardiac pressure-flow dynamics in isolated ventricular septal defects. Circulation 35:430, 1967.
Ritter DG, Feldt RH, Weidman WH, et al: Ventricular septal defect. Circulation 32 (Suppl 3):42, 1965.
Sigman JM, Perry BL, Behrendt DM, et al: Ventricular septal defect: Results after repair in infancy. Am J Cardiol 39:66, 1977.
Tatsuno K, Konno S, Ando M, et al: Pathogenetic mechanisms of prolapsing aortic valve and aortic regurgitation associated with ventricular septal defect. Anatomic, angiographic, and surgical considerations. Circulation 48:1028, 1973.
Weidman WH, Blount SG Jr, DuShane JW, et al: Clinical course in ventricular septal defect. Circulation 56:156, 1977.
Weidman WH, Gersony WM, Nugent EW, et al: Indirect assessment of severity in ventricular septal defect. Circulation 56 (Suppl): 24, 1977.

Pulmonary Stenosis with Normal Aortic Root

Abrahams DG, Wood PH: Pulmonary stenosis with normal aortic root. Br Heart J 13:519, 1951.
Ellison RC, Freedom RM, Keane JF, et al: Indirect assessment of severity in pulmonary stenosis. Circulation 56 (Suppl):14, 1977.
Leatham A, Weitzman D: Auscultatory and phonocardiographic signs of pulmonary stenosis. Br Heart J 19:303, 1957.
Nugent EW, Freedom RM, Nora JJ, et al: Clinical course in pulmonary stenosis. Circulation 56 (Suppl):38, 1977.
Stone FM, Bessinger FB Jr, Lucas RV Jr, et al: Pre- and postoperative rest and exercise hemodynamics in children with pulmonary stenosis. Circulation 49:1102, 1974.

Anomalous Pulmonary Venous Return

Cooley DA, Hallman GL, Leachman RD: Total anomalous pulmonary venous drainage. Correction with the use of cardiopulmonary bypass in 62 cases. J Thorac Cardiovasc Surg 51:88, 1966.

Delisle G, Masahiko A, Calder AL, et al: Total anomalous pulmonary venous connection: Report of 93 autopsied cases with emphasis on diagnostic and surgical considerations. Am Heart J 91:99, 1976.

Duff DG, Nihill MR, McNamara DG: Infradiaphragmatic total anomalous pulmonary venous return. Review of clinical and pathological findings and results of operation in 28 cases. Br Heart J 39:619, 1977.

Gersony WM, Bowman FO Jr, Steeg CN, et al: The management of total anomalous pulmonary venous drainage in early infancy. Circulation 43:1, 1971.

Turley K, Tucker WY, Ullyot DJ, et al: Total anomalous pulmonary venous connection in infancy: Influence of age and type of lesion. Am J Cardiol 45:92, 1980.

Whight CM, Barratt-Boyes BG, Calder AL, et al: Total anomalous pulmonary venous connection. Long-term results following repair in infancy. J Thorac Cardiovasc Surg 75:52, 1978.

Aortic Stenosis

Freedom RM, Dische MR, Rowe RD: Pathologic anatomy of subaortic stenosis and atresia in the first year of life. Am J Cardiol 39:1035, 1977.

Friedman WF, Pappelbaum SJ: Indications for hemodynamic evaluation and surgery in congenital aortic stenosis. Pediatr Clin North Am 18:1207, 1971.

Doyle EF, Arumugham P, Lara E, et al: Sudden death in young patients with congenital aortic stenosis. Pediatrics 53:481, 1974.

Edmunds LH, Wagner HR, Heyman MA: Aortic valvulotomy in neonates. Circulation 61:421, 1980.

Kelly DT, Wulfsberg E, Rowe RD: Discrete subaortic stenosis. Circulation 46:309, 1972.

McCue CM, Spicuzza TJ, Robertson LW, et al: Familial supravalvular aortic stenosis. J Pediatr 73:889, 1968.

Sandor GG, Olley PM, Trusler GA, et al: Long-term follow-up of patients after valvotomy for congenital valvular aortic stenosis in children: A clinical and actuarial follow-up. J Thorac Cardiovasc Surg 80:171, 1980.

Wagner HR, Ellison RC, Keane JF, et al: Clinical course in aortic stenosis. Circulation 56(Suppl):47, 1977.

Wagner HR, Weidman WH, Ellison RC, et al: Indirect assessment of severity in aortic stenosis. Circulation 56 (Suppl):20, 1977.

Mitral Valve Anomalies

Barlow JB, Bosman CK: Aneurysmal protrusion of the posterior leaflet of the mitral valve. Am Heart J 71:166, 1966.

Bisset GS, Schwartz DC, Meyer RA, et al: Clinical spectrum and long-term follow-up of isolated mitral valve prolapse in 119 children. Circulation 62:423, 1980.

Daoud G, Kaplan S, Perrin EV, et al: Congenital mitral stenosis. Circulation 27:185, 1963.

John S, Krishnaswami S, Jairaj PS, et al: The profile and surgical management of mitral stenosis in young patients. J Thorac Cardiovasc Surg 69:631, 1975.

Reed GE, Pooley RW, Moggio RA: Durability of measured mitral annuloplasty: Seventeen year study. J Thorac Cardiovasc Surg 79:321, 1980.

Sahn DJ, Allen HD, Goldberg SJ, et al: Mitral valve prolapse in children. A problem defined by real-time cross-sectional echocardiography. Circulation 53:651, 1976.

Dextrocardia and Levocardia

Liberthson RR, et al: Levocardia with visceral heterotaxy-isolated levocardia: Pathologic anatomy and its clinical implications. Am Heart J 85:40, 1973.

Van Praagh R: Malposition of the heart. In: Moss AJ, Adams FH (eds): Heart Disease in Infants, Children and Adolescents. Baltimore, Williams & Wilkins, 1968.

Principles of Treatment

Benzing G, Kaplan S: Late complications of cardiac surgery. Pediatr Clin North Am 18:1225, 1971.

Engle MA, Zabriskie JB, Senterfit LB, et al: Immunologic and virologic studies in the postpericardiotomy syndrome. J Pediatr 87:1103, 1975.

Gersony WM, Hayes CJ: Perioperative care of the infant with congenital heart disease. Prog Cardiovasc Dis 15:213, 1975. Also In: Friedman WF, Lesche M, Sonnenblick EH (eds): Neonatal Heart Disease. New York, Grune and Stratton, 1972, p 149.

Gersony WM, Krongrad E: Evaluation and management of patients after surgical repair of congenital heart disease. Progr Cardiovasc Dis 18:39, 1975. Also In: Rosenthal EH, Sonnenblick EH, Lesch M (eds): Postoperative Congenital Heart Disease. New York, Grune and Stratton, 1975, p 145.

Kaplan MH: Symposium on immunity and the heart. Am J Cardiol 24:459, 1969.

13.67   DISTURBANCES OF RATE AND RHYTHM OF THE HEART

Sinus arrhythmia represents a variation in impulse discharges from within the sinus node. The variations in the sinus rate may be considerable and are usually related to respiration; there is slowing during inspiration and acceleration during expiration. Occasionally, if the sinus rate becomes slow enough there will be an escape beat from the atrioventricular junctional region (Fig 13–64). This pattern is entirely physiologic and it should not be mistaken for an abnormality of cardiac rhythm. Irregularities of sinus rhythm are commonly seen in premature infants, especially in those with periodic apnea. Sinus arrhythmia is exaggerated during convalescence from febrile illness and by drugs which increase vagal tone, such as digitalis; it is usually abolished by exercise or by atropine. Some children have great variation in rate during sinus arrhythmia, which should not be confused with a significant rhythm disorder.

Sinus bradycardia is due to slow discharge of impuls-

es from the sinus node. The sinus rate varies mildly during childhood, and the lower limit of the normal rate is determined empirically. In general, a sinus rate under 90/min in neonates and under 60–75 thereafter is considered to be sinus bradycardia. Sinus bradycardia is commonly seen in athletic individuals; it causes no symptoms, and in healthy individuals it is without significance. It may occur in systemic disease, e.g., myxedema, and will resolve when the disorder is under control. It must be differentiated from sinoatrial and A-V blocks. Disappearance of bradycardia with exercise is expected. *Low birth weight infants* display great variation in sinus rate. Sinus bradycardia is common and may be associated with junctional escape beats. Premature atrial contractions are frequent. These rhythm changes, especially bradycardia, appear more commonly during sleep and are not associated with symptoms. No therapy is necessary.

Wandering atrial pacemaker (Fig 13–65) is a shift in

Lead 2

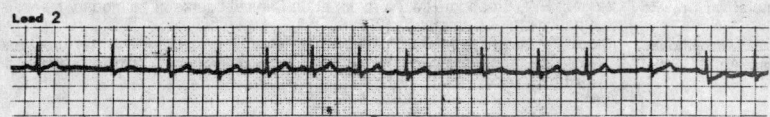

7 yrs.

Figure 13–64 Sinus arrhythmia with junctional escape beat: note the variation in P-P interval with little change in P morphology or P-R interval. When the sinus rate is slow enough the atrioventricular junction takes over, producing escape beats. This rhythm is normal.

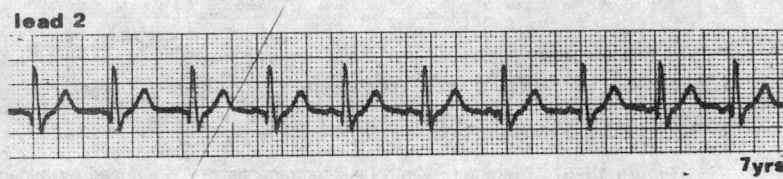

Figure 13–65 Wandering atrial pacemaker: note the change in P wave configuration in the 7th, 9th, and 10th beats. The 7th P wave may represent a fusion between the sinus P and the ectopic atrial pacemaker seen in the 10th beat.

the controlling pacemaker from the sinus node to another part of the atrium. It is common in childhood and a normal variant.

Extrasystoles are produced by the discharge of an ectopic focus that may be situated anywhere in atrial, junctional, or ventricular tissue. In the majority of instances extrasystoles are of no clinical or prognostic significance. Under certain circumstances premature beats may be due to organic heart disease, e.g., acute carditis, or they may occur many yr after cardiac surgery. Drugs, especially digitalis, may also produce extrasystoles.

Premature atrial complexes are not uncommon in childhood, even in the absence of cardiac disease. Depending on the degree of prematurity and the preceding cycle length, some premature atrial complexes result in a normal QRS configuration. In other instances they may be conducted to the ventricle while the specialized ventricular conducting system is partially refractory and result in an abnormal QRS configuration (Fig 13–66), which then must be distinguished from premature ventricular systoles. Careful scrutiny of the electrocardiogram for a premature P wave, preceding the QRS, that has a different contour from sinus P waves is essential for diagnosis.

Premature ventricular complexes may arise in any region of the ventricles. They are characterized by premature, widened, bizarre QRS complexes which are not preceded by a P wave (Fig 13–67). When they have identical contours and coupling intervals, they are thought to be unifocal in origin and due to a re-entry mechanism. When they vary in contour and in coupling interval, they are designated as multifocal.

Extrasystoles are usually followed by a compensatory pause as they interfere with the next sinus beat. In the majority of instances extrasystoles disappear during the tachycardia of exercise. If they remain or become exaggerated during exercise, the arrhythmia may have greater significance. Extrasystoles produce a smaller stroke and pulse volume than normal and, if very premature, may not be audible with a stethoscope or palpable at the radial pulse. Extrasystoles may assume a definite rhythm, e.g., alternating with normal beats (pulsus bigeminus) or occurring after 2 normal beats

(pulsus trigeminus). This rhythmicity may be seen in digitalis intoxication.

Most patients are unaware of premature contractions, although some may be aware of a "skipped beat" or a sudden "turnover" or "tickle" over the precordium. This is due to the increased cardiac output from the normal beat following a compensatory pause. Anxiety, a febrile illness, or ingestion of various drugs or stimulants causes premature ventricular beats. The basis of therapy is convincing reassurance that the arrhythmia is not the result of structural heart disease. Sedatives or suppressive agents may be used in selected cases.

13.68 TACHYARRHYTHMIAS

SUPRAVENTRICULAR TACHYARRHYTHMIAS

Paroxysmal Atrial Tachycardia. Re-entry within the A-V node is thought to be the most common mechanism of paroxysmal atrial tachycardia. The tachycardia is initiated by a premature atrial beat which is conducted with delay through the A-V node.

In older children paroxysmal atrial tachycardia is characterized by abrupt onset and cessation; the attack may be precipitated by an acute infection. If an attack is not witnessed, its occurrence may be elicited by an accurate history. Attacks may last from a few sec to several wk but usually persist for a few hr, seldom for more than 2–3 days. The cardiac rate usually exceeds 180/min and occasionally may be as rapid as 300/min. The only complaint may be awareness of the rapid cardiac rate. Many children tolerate these episodes extremely well, and it is unlikely that short paroxysms are a danger to life. If the rate is exceptionally rapid or if the attack is prolonged, precordial discomfort and congestive cardiac failure may supervene.

In young infants the diagnosis may be more obscure since the cardiac rate at this age is normally rapid and increases greatly with crying. A persistent tachycardia during quiet periods or sleep suggests the diagnosis. The cardiac rate during paroxysms is frequently in the

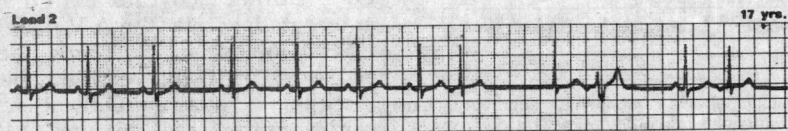

Figure 13–66 Premature atrial contraction (PAC): QRS complexes, the 8th, 10th, and final, in this strip are preceded by a P wave, which is inverted, denoting an ectopic origin of atrial depolarization. Note that the 8th and final QRS complexes resemble those of sinus origin, whereas the 10th is aberrantly conducted. This is a function of the preceding cycle length that influences the refractory period of the bundle branches. Note that the pause after the PAC is longer than 2 P-P intervals, implying that the premature atrial depolarization has invaded and discharged the sinus node, and reset it, so that it fires later.

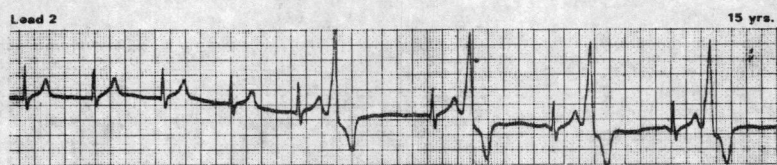

Figure 13–67 Premature ventricular contractions (PVC) induced by hyperventilation: note that the premature beat is wide and has a completely different morphology from that of the sinus beat. The premature beat is not preceded by a P wave, and the pause following it is fully compensatory, i.e., the P-P interval containing the PVC equals 2 sinus cycles; this indicates that the sinus mechanism has not been disturbed by the premature beats.

range of 300/min, and signs of congestive cardiac failure will eventually supervene. If the attack lasts 6–24 hr or more, the infant becomes acutely ill, has an ashen, slightly cyanotic color, and is restless and irritable. Tachypnea and hepatomegaly are the prominent signs of cardiac failure, and there may be fever and leukocytosis. Intrauterine tachycardia can cause severe cardiac failure and be responsible for hydrops fetalis (Fig 13–68).

Treatment. Vagal stimulation by a simple procedure, such as unilateral carotid sinus massage, may abort the attack. Older children may be taught a vagotonic maneuver to abolish the paroxysm, such as straining, the Valsalva maneuver, breath-holding, drinking ice water, or the adoption of a particular posture. When these measures fail and the child is symptomatic enough to warrant treatment, several alternatives are available. In urgent situations when congestive heart failure is a prominent presenting sign, electrical cardioversion is recommended as initial management. Pharmacotherapy should be considered as the initial approach under other circumstances. In the past digoxin has been the mainstay of therapy for patients with supraventricular tachycardia. It slows conduction within the A-V node and interrupts the re-entrant circuit. Digoxin is effective in 95% of instances but often requires from several hr to a day to take effect. In infants, digoxin should be used even if the paroxysm has been abolished by vagal stimulation since the recurrence rate is high; therapy should be maintained for 3–6 mo or longer.

Other drugs which have been used to abolish the paroxysms include infusions of phenylephrine (Neo-Synephrine), edrophonium (Tensilon), diphenylhydantoin (Dilantin), and oral administration of quinidine sulfate or propranolol. More recently a new class of agents, the calcium channel blockers, has been used in the initial treatment of paroxysmal supraventricular tachyarrhythmias in infants and children. Verapamil (Isoptin, Cordan) is the agent in this class currently available. When administered intravenously 92–96% of infants and children converted to normal sinus rhythm within 5 min of an initial 0.1–0.2 mg/kg dose. No side effects were experienced by patients whose supraventricular tachycardias were due to re-entrant mechanisms, but hypotension responsive to intravenous calcium chloride was observed in 2 children with ectopic tachycardia. Thus verapamil may be useful for the initial treatment of supraventricular tachyarrhythmias due to re-entrant mechanisms. For maintenance therapy digoxin remains the treatment of choice for most patients, but rapid digitalization may no longer be necessary.

In most instances of paroxysmal atrial tachycardia there is no underlying structural cardiac disease. If cardiac failure supervenes during the paroxysms, cardiac function rapidly returns to normal after cessation of the attack.

Between attacks some children may exhibit the electrocardiographic changes of the *Wolff-Parkinson-White (pre-excitation) syndrome;* these are a short P-R interval and slow upstroke of the QRS—the so-called delta wave (Fig 13–69). This syndrome is usually present in an otherwise normal heart; it may, however, occur with Ebstein anomaly, corrected transposition (ventricular inversion), and cardiomyopathy. The syndrome is the prototype of re-entrant tachycardia. The anatomic substrate comprising the re-entrant circuit is the A-V node and an accessory pathway, a muscular bridge connecting atrium to ventricle; it is usually on the right or left lateral cardiac border (Fig 13–70). During sinus rhythm the impulse is carried over both the A-V node and the accessory pathway; it produces some degree of fusion of the 2 depolarization fronts that results in an abnormal QRS. During tachycardia an impulse is usually carried anterogradely over the A-V node, resulting in a normal QRS complex, and in retrograde fashion through the accessory pathway, reaching the atrium and perpetuating the tachycardia. Only after cessation of the tachycardia are the typical features of Wolff-Parkinson-White syndrome recognized (Fig 13–69). Increasing numbers of cases are reported in which the accessory pathway can conduct only retrogradely. This situation is indistinguishable from other supraventricular tachycardias be-

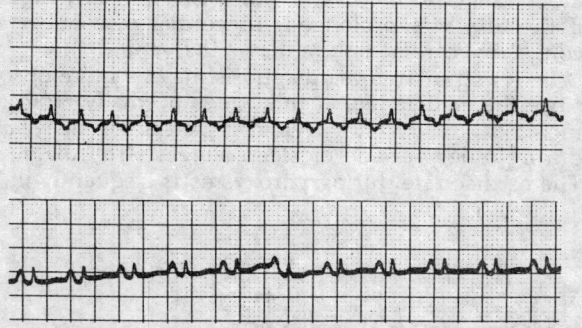

Figure 13–68 Upper tracing shows paroxysmal supraventricular tachycardia ("pat") with a ventricular rate of 230/min. The lower tracing shows sinus rhythm after D-C cardioversion. Note that during the tachycardia, the T wave is deformed by an inverted, presumably retrograde, P wave. The QRS morphology is unchanged during the tachycardia. Low voltage is due to peripheral edema in a 1 day old infant with intrauterine tachycardia and hydrops fetalis.

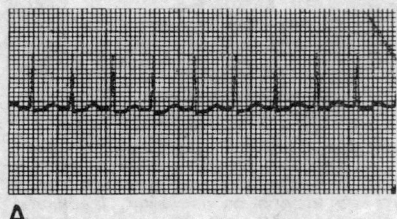

A

B

Figure 13–69 *A,* PAT in a child with Wolff-Parkinson-White (WPW) syndrome. Note the normal QRS complexes during the tachycardia. *B,* Later the typical features of WPW are apparent (short P-R interval, delta wave, and wide QRS).

cause conduction occurs anterograde only over the A-V node and can be diagnosed only by invasive electrophysiologic studies. When rapid antegrade conduction occurs through the pre-excitation pathway during tachycardia, the risks of deterioration in the patient's condition are greater.

Ectopic atrial tachycardia is an uncommon tachycardia in childhood. It is characterized by a variable rate (seldom greater than 200), identifiable P waves with abnormal frontal plane axis, and chronicity in either a sustained or intermittent tachycardia. It is usually more difficult to control pharmacologically than the more common reciprocal tachycardias. Suppression of the ectopic atrial focus is difficult; therapy should, therefore, be directed to slowing atrioventricular conduction with digitalis and perhaps with propranolol before using drugs that suppress atrial automaticity, such as quinidine and disopyramide. In some cases no treatment is necessary.

Chaotic or multifocal atrial tachycardia is characterized by 2 or more ectopic P waves with 2 or more different ectopic P-P cycles, frequent blocked P waves, and varying P-R intervals of conducted beats. This arrhythmia usually occurs in the absence of cardiac disease and usually terminates spontaneously after weeks or months. If the patient is asymptomatic, no treatment is necessary. Digitalis may be used to control the ventricular rate.

Accelerated junctional tachycardia is an arrhythmia in which the junctional rate exceeds that of the sinus node so that atrioventricular dissociation results. This arrhythmia is not infrequent after cardiac surgery or during acute rheumatic fever. It is an important sign of digitalis intoxication. Usually, no treatment is necessary. When arrhythmia is associated with digitalis, the drug should be discontinued.

Atrial flutter is due to rapid and regular but abnormal atrial contractions. These contractions may be due to a circus movement in the atria and produced by an irritable focus in the atrial muscle similar to that responsible for paroxysmal atrial tachycardia and atrial extrasystoles. The rate of atrial beats ranges from 250–400/min. Because the atrioventricular node cannot transmit such rapid impulses, the ventricles respond to every 2nd–4th atrial beat. Occasionally, the response will be variable and the rhythm appear to be irregular.

Atrial flutter is not common in children but may sometimes complicate myocarditis of any cause. It may also occur during acute infectious diseases and in patients with large stretched atria, such as those with longstanding mitral or tricuspid insufficiency. It has also been recognized and has persisted after palliative or corrective intra-atrial surgery, e.g., for transposition of the great arteries, ostium secundum defect, or total anomalous pulmonary venous return. Atrial flutter should be suspected in patients with a regular tachycardia that is not influenced by effort, emotion, or posture. Atrial flutter may precipitate congestive cardiac failure. Carotid sinus pressure frequently produces a temporary slowing of the cardiac rate. The diagnosis is confirmed by electrocardiography which demonstrates the rapid and regular atrial flutter or "f" waves.

Digitalis slows the ventricular response in atrial flutter by prolonging conduction time through the A-V node. In many instances the rhythm will then convert to atrial fibrillation. After full digitalization, quinidine may be added if necessary to convert to sinus rhythm. Atrial flutter usually responds to cardioversion, which has become an important method for treatment.

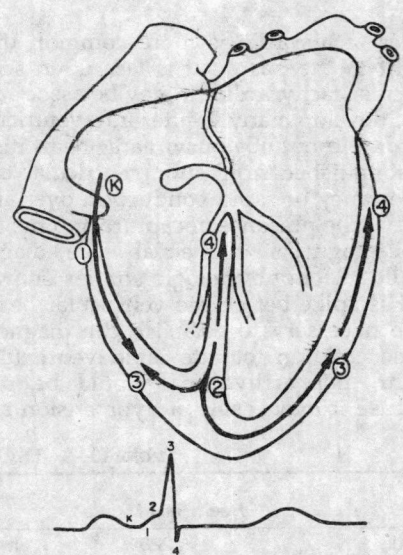

Figure 13–70 Schematic presentation of a heart with a right-sided anomalous pathway (type B), indicated by K. Arrows indicate the direction of spread of excitation; the circled numbers designate the relative time sequence in which the activation wavefronts are initiated. In the electrocardiogram, the time of activation of the anomalous pathway is labeled K; the numbers 1–4 denote when the various activation wave fronts are initiated. (Moore EN, Spear JF, Boineau JD: N Engl J Med 289:956, 1973. Reproduced by permission.)

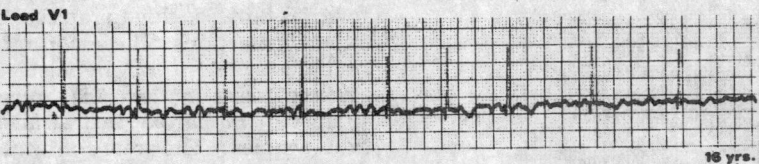

Figure 13–71 Atrial fibrillation, characterized by absence of P waves; presence of fibrillatory waves, which are grossly irregular, rapid undulations; and an irregular ventricular response. Fibrillatory waves may not be visible in all leads, and should be carefully sought in every tracing with irregular R-R intervals. (The coexisting qR in V₁ is diagnostic of right ventricular hypertrophy in this patient with Eisenmenger syndrome.)

Atrial fibrillation is produced by a mechanism similar to that causing atrial flutter; the atrial excitation is irregular and more rapid (300–500/min). The arrhythmia occurs most frequently in older children with rheumatic mitral valve disease. It has been reported as a complication of atrial septal defect, after intra-atrial surgery (e.g., Mustard operation), and with left atrial enlargement secondary to left atrioventricular valve incompetence.

The rhythm is grossly irregular (Fig 13–71) and is associated with a pulse deficit. Atrial fibrillation may complicate or precipitate congestive cardiac failure.

Treatment is digitalization, which restores the ventricular rate to normal, although the rhythm remains irregular. Normal sinus rhythm may then be restored with quinidine sulfate or electrical cardioversion. Maintenance of sinus rhythm is not usual in the patient whose atrial fibrillation is associated with florid mitral valve disease and cardiomegaly. Continuation of prophylactic therapy with digitalis and quinidine is usually required in these patients.

VENTRICULAR TACHYARRHYTHMIAS

Ventricular tachycardia is more common than had been thought in the past, but is less often seen than supraventricular tachycardia. It may be associated with myocarditis, develop many yr after intraventricular surgery, or occur without obvious organic heart disease. It must be distinguished from supraventricular tachycardia with aberrancy or rapid conduction over an accessory pathway. The presence of capture and fusion beats confirms the diagnosis. In their absence, diagnosis is more difficult. Electrophysiologic studies showing absence of a His spike before the ventricular depolarization may be necessary to establish the diagnosis. Although some children tolerate rapid ventricular rates for many hr, this arrhythmia should be promptly treated because it may result in hypotension and may

deteriorate into ventricular fibrillation. Lidocaine and cardioversion are methods of choice for rapid treatment. Quinidine, procainamide, and propranolol are useful for chronic therapy.

Ventricular fibrillation results in death unless an effective ventricular beat is restored. A thump on the chest sometimes restores sinus rhythm. Usually external cardiac massage with artificial ventilation and electrical defibrillation is necessary.

Differential Diagnosis of Tachyarrhythmias. It is important from the standpoint of prognosis and treatment to identify accurately the type of tachyarrhythmia which is present according to heart rate, presence and configuration of the P wave, duration of the QRS deflection, and rhythmicity (Table 13–8). Often the diagnosis is clear cut on a clinical and electrocardiographic basis, but in some instances differential diagnosis may be difficult.

First, it should be determined whether the patient is actually in sinus tachycardia. Time for treating an infection, acute anemia, or other illness which results in sinus tachycardia may be lost while a tachyarrhythmia is being considered, wrongly diagnosed, or even treated. Heart rates greater than 225/min are too rapid for sinus tachycardia, but rates in the 140–220 range could signify either an arrhythmia or a sinus tachycardia. Ventricular tachycardia is almost invariably slower than supraventricular tachycardia.

Second, the configuration of the P waves should be evaluated. Although it is possible to have a supraventricular tachycardia with P waves of normal configuration (upright in leads I, II, and AVF), in most instances P waves will be abnormal. Unfortunately, in many cases of supraventricular tachycardia with rapid ventricular response, the P wave will not be visible on the standard electrocardiogram, and it may be necessary to obtain Lewis-Golub leads (exploring right chest electrodes) or an esophageal lead to identify obscure P waves. The distinctive saw-toothed atrial waves produced by atrial flutter are best recognized in lead V₁. During atrial

Table 13–8 DIAGNOSIS OF TACHYARRHYTHMIAS

	Heart Rate/Minute	ELECTROCARDIOGRAPHIC FINDINGS		
		P Wave	QRS Duration	Regularity
Sinus tachycardia	<225	Always present Normal axis	Normal	Rate varies with respiration
Atrial tachycardia	180–320	Present—50% Superior axis common	Normal or prolonged (RBBB pattern)	Regular
Atrial fibrillation	120–180	Fibrillatory waves	Normal or prolonged (RBBB pattern)	Irregularly irregular
Atrial flutter	Atrial: 250–400 Ventricular response variable: 100–320	Sawtoothed flutter waves	Normal or prolonged (RBBB pattern)	Regular ventricular response (e.g., 2:1, 3:1, 3:2, etc.)
Ventricular tachycardia	120–240	Absent	Usually prolonged	Slightly irregular

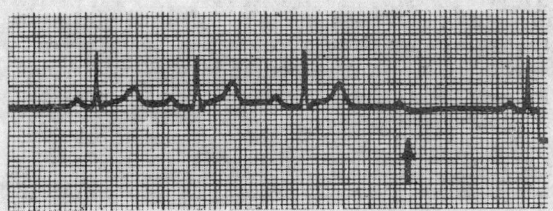

Figure 13–72 Wenckebach phenomenon (Mobitz I). The P-R interval gradually lengthens until the 4th P wave in the cycle is not conducted to the ventricle (arrow). The ensuing P-R interval is once again normal.

fibrillation atrial activity is represented by a chaotic baseline. During ventricular tachycardia the P wave is either absent or noted to be out of phase with the QRS deflections.

Third, an extremely narrow QRS suggests that the rhythm comes from either the supraventricular area or the region of the A-V node. However, prolonged QRS duration may be seen with a QRS aberrancy in the face of a supraventricular tachycardia as well as with ventricular arrhythmias. In the former the QRS morphology is almost always of the right bundle branch block type.

Finally, the rhythmicity should be determined. In sinus tachycardia the rate will vary every few sec and will gradually slow with vagotonic maneuvers only to speed up again when they are discontinued. Atrial tachycardia is extremely regular, except at the onset or just prior to ending, whereas ventricular tachycardia displays slight beat-to-beat variations. Either atrial flutter will be regular or, with block, the ventricular response will consistently be some multiple of the interval between the flutter waves. In atrial fibrillation the ventricular response will be irregularly irregular.

13.69 BRADYARRHYTHMIAS (Heart Block)

Sinus arrest and sinoatrial block may cause a sudden pause in the heart beat. The former is presumed to be due to failure of impulse formation within the sinus node, the latter, to a block between the sinus impulse and the surrounding atrium. These arrhythmias are rare in childhood except as manifestations of digitalis intoxication.

Atrioventricular block may be divided into *1st degree block*, in which the P-R interval is prolonged; *2nd degree block*, in which some impulses are conducted to the ventricle; and *3rd degree block*, in which no impulses from the atria reach the ventricles. In a variant of 2nd degree block, known as the *Wenckebach type* (also called Mobitz Type 1), the P-P interval remains constant, the P-R interval increases until a P wave is not conducted,

and, in the cycle following the pause, the P-R is again shorter (Fig 13–72).

Congenital complete atrioventricular block in children is probably the result of a congenital defect in the main stem of the bundle of His. The arrhythmia is occasionally suspected in the fetus. In an international study of almost 600 patients with congenital complete heart block, about 70% had no other evidence of heart disease. At greatest risk were infants with associated congenital heart disease who, in the 1st weeks of life, were in congestive cardiac failure, with atrial rates exceeding 150/min and ventricular rates less than 55. The most frequently associated cardiac malformations were "corrected" transposition of the great arteries (ventricular inversion), single ventricle, and patent ductus arteriosus. Isolated ventricular septal defect was seldom associated with complete heart block.

In older children with otherwise normal hearts the condition is commonly asymptomatic, although attacks of syncope may occur. The peripheral pulse is of the water-hammer type as a result of the large ventricular stroke volume and the peripheral vasodilatation; the systolic blood pressure is elevated. Jugular venous pulsations occur irregularly and may be large when the atrium contracts against a closed tricuspid valve (cannon wave). The 1st cardiac sound has varying intensity, and isolated atrial contractions may be audible along the left sternal border or at the apex. Exercise and atropine produce an acceleration of 10–20 beats/min or more in the child. Systolic murmurs are frequent along the left sternal border, and apical mid-diastolic murmurs are not unusual. Heart block in itself results in cardiac enlargement.

The diagnosis is confirmed by electrocardiogram; the P waves and QRS complexes have no constant relation (Fig 13–73). The QRS duration may be prolonged or may be normal if the heart beat arises high in the His bundle.

The prognosis for congenital heart block is usually favorable; patients who have been observed to the age of 30–40 yr have lived normally active lives. However, some patients have episodes of dizziness with or without syncope (Stokes-Adams attacks); this complication requires the implantation of a permanent pacemaker. Acquired heart block is discussed in Sec 13.69.

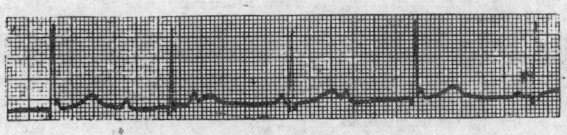

LEAD II

Figure 13–73 Complete atrioventricular block: the ventricular rate is regular at 53/min. The atrial rate varied from 65–95/min (probably sinus arrhythmia). The QRS morphology is normal, which is usual in congenital A-V block.

13.70 BRADYCARDIA-TACHYCARDIA SYNDROME

The bradycardia-tachycardia syndrome (sick-sinus syndrome) is a collection of functional disorders of the atria, sinus node, and A-V junctional tissues as outlined

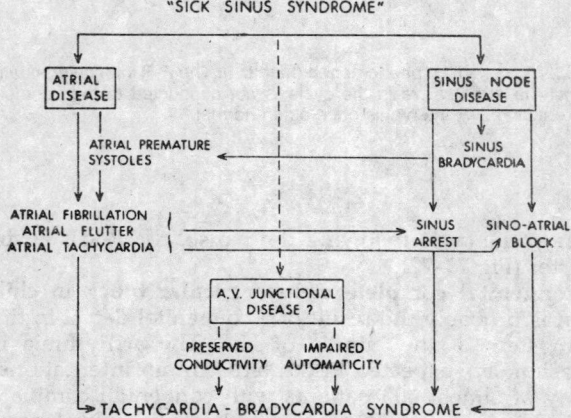

Figure 13–74 Factors resulting in bradycardia-tachycardia syndrome. (Kaplan BM, Langendorf R, Lev M, et al: Am J Cardiol 31:497, 1973. Reproduced by permission of Technical Publishing Company.)

in Fig 13–74. This syndrome may occur in the absence of congenital heart disease and has been reported in siblings, but it is most commonly seen after surgical correction of congenital heart defects, especially the Mustard procedure for transposition of the great arteries. Clinical presentation depends on the underlying arrhythmia. Dizziness and syncope are usually due to periods of marked sinus slowing with failure of junctional escape (Fig 13–75). Supraventricular tachycardias with rapid ventricular response may cause complaints of palpitations, exercise intolerance, and/or dizziness. Treatment must be individualized. In general, aside from digitalis, drug therapy to control tachyarrhythmia (e.g., propranolol, quinidine, procainamide) may sup-press sinus and atrial ventricular nodal function to the degree that symptomatic bradycardia may be produced. Therefore, an insertion of a demand ventricular pacemaker in conjunction with drug therapy is necessary for symptomatic patients.

Bigger JT Jr, Goldmeyer BN: The mechanism of supraventricular tachycardia. Circulation 42:673, 1970.

Gillette PC: The mechanism of supraventricular tachycardia in children. Circulation 54:133, 1976.

Gillette PC: Concealed anomalous cardiac conduction pathways: A frequent cause of supraventricular tachycardia. Am J Cardiol 40:848, 1977.

Gillette PC, Garson A: Electrophysiologic and pharmacologic characteristics of automatic ectopic atrial tachycardia. Circulation 56:571, 1977.

Gillette PC, Garson A, Kugler JD: Wolff-Parkinson-White syndrome in children: Electrophysiologic and pharmacologic characteristics. Circulation 60:1487, 1979.

Gillette PC, Kugler JD, Garson A, et al: Mechanisms of cardiac arrhythmias after the Mustard operation for transposition of the great vessels. Am J Cardiol 45:1225, 1980.

Greenwood RD, Rosenthal A, Sloss LJ, et al: Sick sinus syndrome after surgery for congenital heart disease. Circulation 52:208, 1975.

Michaelson M, Engle MA: International cooperative study of congenital complete heart block. In: Engle MA (ed): Cardiovascular Clinics: Pediatric Cardiology. Philadelphia, FA Davis, 1972.

Morgan BC, Bloom RS, Guntheroth WG: Cardiac arrhythmias in premature infants. Pediatrics 35:658, 1965.

Pickoff AS, Zies L, Ferrer PL, et al: High-dose propranolol therapy in the management of supraventricular tachycardia. J Pediatr 94:144, 1979.

Porter CJ, Gillette PC, Garson A Jr, et al: Effects of verapamil on supraventricular tachycardia in children. Am J Cardiol 48:487, 1981.

Porter CJ, Gillette PC, McNamara DG: Twenty-four hour ambulatory ECG's in the detection and management of cardiac dysrhythmias in infants and children. Pediatr Cardiol 1:203, 1980.

Roberts NK, Gelband H: Cardiac Arrhythmias in the Neonate, Infant and Child. New York, Appleton-Century-Crofts, 1977.

Rocchini AP, Chun PO, Dick M: Ventricular tachycardia in children. Am J Cardiol 47:1091, 1981.

Shahar E, Barzilay Z, Frand M: Verapamil in the treatment of paroxysmal supraventricular tachycardia in infants and children. J Pediatr 98:323, 1981.

Soler-Soler J, Sagrista-Sauleda J, Cabrera A, et al: Effect of verapamil in infants with paroxysmal supraventricular tachycardia. Circulation 59:876, 1979.

13.71   INFECTIVE ENDOCARDITIS

The term infective endocarditis includes the entities referred to as acute and subacute bacterial endocarditis as well as infections of nonbacterial endocarditis such as those caused by viruses, fungi, and other agents. The disease remains a significant cause of morbidity and mortality among children and adolescents despite the advances in the management and prophylaxis of the disease with antimicrobial agents. The inability to eradicate infective endocarditis by prevention or early treatment stems from several factors: the nature of the infecting organism has changed over the years; physicians, dentists, and the public are not sufficiently aware of the threat of infective endocarditis and the preventive measures which are available; diagnosis may be difficult when delayed; and special risk groups have emerged which include an increasing number of narcotics abusers, survivors of cardiac surgery, and patients with lower resistance to infection who require intravascular catheters.

Etiology. *Streptococcus viridans* is responsible for ap-

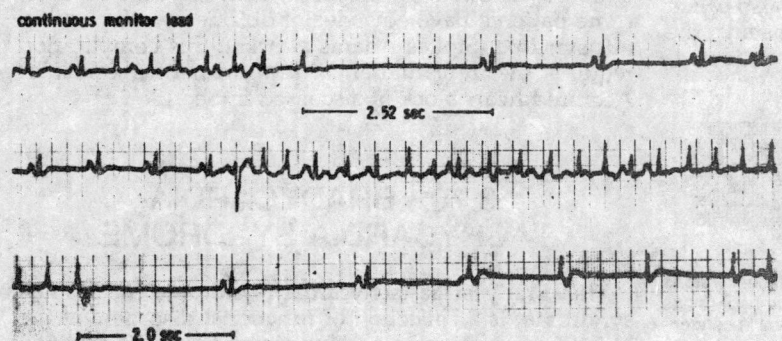

Figure 13–75 Bradycardia-tachycardia syndrome (sick-sinus syndrome): note the bursts of supraventricular tachycardia, probably multifocal in origin, followed by long periods of sinus arrest and by sinus bradycardia.

proximately 50% of cases of infective endocarditis. However, its predominance has been decreasing in recent yr. Staphylococcal endocarditis has become more common over the past 2 decades and is now estimated to be responsible for almost one third of the cases. Other organisms cause endocarditis less frequently, and in approximately 10% of cases blood cultures are negative. No relationship exists between the infecting organism and the type of congenital defect, duration of the illness, or age of the child. However, staphylococcal endocarditis is more common in patients who do not have underlying heart disease.

Epidemiology. Infective endocarditis is most often seen as a complication of congenital or rheumatic heart disease but can also occur in children who do not have a cardiac malformation. Recently, congenital heart disease has become the overwhelming predisposing factor. The disease is extremely rare in infancy.

Patients with a lesion which is associated with a high velocity of blood injected into a chamber or vessel are most susceptible to the infection. Vegetation is usually formed at the site of the endocardial or intimal erosion which results from the turbulent flow (Fig 13–76). Thus, children with ventricular septal defect, left-sided valvular disease, and systemic pulmonary arterial communications are at the highest risk for developing infective endocarditis, while a very low incidence is reported in secundum atrial septal defect, a lesion characterized by low velocity flow across the interatrial defect. The postoperative pediatric patient with a palliative systemic-to-pulmonary artery shunt is most at risk for infective endocarditis. However, the increasing use of valve replacement and valve conduit repairs in children with complex heart disease may lead to a larger number of cases of infective endocarditis among these patients.

In approximately 30% of patients with infective endocarditis a predisposing factor is recognized. A surgical or dental procedure can be implicated in approximately two thirds of the cases in which the potential source of bacteremia is identified. Furthermore, poor

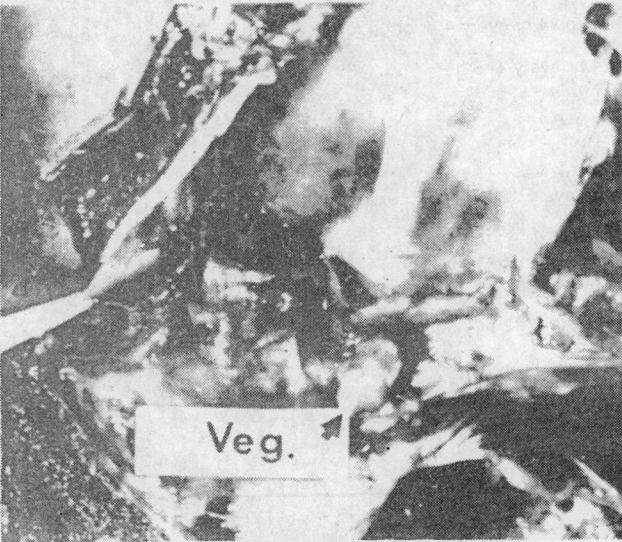

Figure 13–76 A large vegetation (arrow) is noted in the right ventricle just beneath the pulmonary valve. Veg. = vegetation.

dental hygiene in children with cyanotic heart disease results in a greater risk for contamination of blood and eventually of the endocardium. Recurrence of infective endocarditis directly following cardiac catheterization or heart surgery is relatively low. However, on the basis of frequency of the performance of these procedures, cardiac surgery and, to a lesser extent, cardiac catheterization rank high on the list of significant antecedent events which are reported prior to the onset of infective endocarditis.

Clinical Manifestations. The early symptoms and signs of the disease are usually mild, especially when *Streptococcus viridans* is the infecting organism. Prolonged fever, without other manifestations (except occasionally weight loss), persisting for as long as several mo may often be the only medical history which can be elicited. Alternatively, the onset may be acute and severe, with high, intermittent fever and prostration. Usually, however, the onset and course vary within a range between these 2 extremes. The symptoms are usually nonspecific and consist of low-grade fever with afternoon elevations, fatigue, myalgia, arthralgia, headache, and at times chills, nausea, and vomiting. Depending on the virulence of the agent the clinical findings may include signs of embolization and changes in the cardiac examination. Splenomegaly is relatively common, and petechiae may occur. New or changing heart murmurs are common, especially when there is destruction of valves and when there is associated congestive heart failure.

Serious neurologic complications, such as emboli, cerebral abscesses, mycotic aneurysms, and hemorrhage, that are manifested by meningismus, increased intracranial pressure, altered sensorium, and focal neurologic signs are often associated with staphylococcal disease.

Myocardial abscesses may also occur with staphylococcal disease and may rupture into the pericardium. Pulmonary and other systemic emboli are infrequent except with fungal disease. Many of the classic skin manifestations develop late in the course of the disease; hence, they are seldom seen in the appropriately treated patient. These are *Osler nodes* (tender pea-sized intradermal nodules in the pads of the fingers and toes), *Janeway lesions* (painless small erythematous or hemorrhagic lesions on the palms and soles), and *splinter hemorrhages* (linear lesions beneath the nails). These lesions probably represent vasculitis produced by circulating antigen-antibody complexes.

The identification of infective endocarditis will most often be based on a high index of suspicion in the evaluation of an infection in a child with an underlying contributory factor.

Laboratory Data. *The critical information for appropriate treatment of infective endocarditis is obtained from cultures of the blood.* All other laboratory data are secondary in importance. Mild to moderate leukocytosis can be expected; the erythrocyte sedimentation rate is commonly elevated, and a mild hemolytic anemia (hemoglobin value seldom <9 gm/dl) is not unusual. Microscopic hematuria, when present, is usually a manifestation of immune complex glomerulonephritis. Autoantibodies may develop as the disease progresses, and rheumatoid factors (antiglobulins), the Kahn reaction, and/or cryoglobulins may be demonstrable at times.

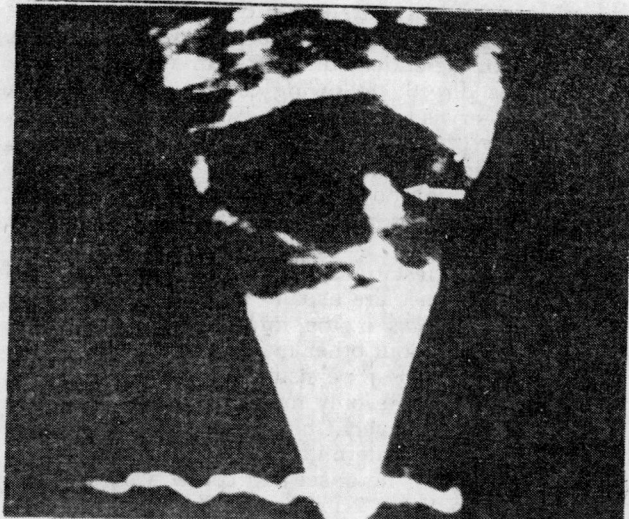

Figure 13–77 Two-dimensional echocardiogram obtained from a child with bacterial endocarditis. Arrow indicates the presence of a large vegetation in the left atrium attached to the mitral valve.

Blood cultures must be obtained as promptly as possible in each child in whom infective endocarditis is considered a diagnostic possibility. These must be drawn even if the child feels well and has no other physical findings.

Three separate blood collections should be obtained after careful preparation of the phlebotomy site. Contamination presents a special problem since bacteria found on the skin may themselves cause infective endocarditis. The timing of collections is not important because bacteremia can be expected to be relatively constant. In 90% of cases of endocarditis the etiologic agent is recovered from the 1st 2 blood cultures. Therefore, further blood drawings may be deferred for 2–3 days until the results of the initial cultures are known.

Echocardiography has been utilized to document the presence and specific location of vegetations (Fig 13–77), but this modality is not always helpful in the early stages of the disease. The effects of mitral and aortic valvular incompetence on left ventricular performance can also be evaluated by ultrasound techniques.

Prognosis and Complications. In the preantibiotic era infective endocarditis was a fatal disease. After a marked improvement in the 1950's the percentage of survivals continues to increase but at a slow rate. Mortality remains at 20–25%. Complications occur in 50–60% of children with documented infective endocarditis; the most common is cardiac failure due to vegetations involving the aortic or mitral valve. Myocardial abscesses and toxic myocarditis may also lead to congestive heart failure but without characteristic changes in auscultatory findings.

Superimposed on left heart or aortic lesions, systemic

Table 13–9 TREATMENT OF INFECTIVE ENDOCARDITIS

ETIOLOGIC AGENT	DRUG	DOSAGE	ROUTE	DURATION OF THERAPY
Streptococcus viridans	Penicillin G	300,000 units/kg/24 hr every 4 hr or up to 20 million units*	IV	4–6 wk
	+ Streptomycin†	30 mg/kg/24 hr every 12 hr	IM	2 wk
Streptococcus faecalis	Penicillin G	300,000 units/kg/24 hr every 4 hr or up to 20 million units*	IV	6 wk
	or Ampicillin	200 mg/kg/24 hr every 4 hr	IV	6 wk
	+ Gentamicin	4–6 mg/kg/24 hr every 8–12 hr	IV	6 wk
Staphylococcus aureus Penicillin sensitive	Penicillin G	300,000 units/kg/24 hr every 4 hr or up to 20 million units*	IV	6–8 wk
Penicillin resistant	Oxacillin or Nafcillin or Methicillin‡	200 mg/kg/24 hr every 4–6 hr	IV	6–8 wk
	+ Rifampin§	10 mg/kg/24 hr every 12 hr—not to exceed 600 mg/24 hr	PO	6–8 wk
	or Gentamicin†	4–6 mg/kg/24 hr every 8–12 hr	IV	2 wk
Methicillin resistant	Vancomycin	50 mg/kg/24 hr every 6 hr	IV	6–8 wk
	+ Rifampin§	10 mg/kg/24 hr every 12 hr—not to exceed 600 mg/24 hr	PO	6–8 wk
Unknown agent	Penicillin G	300,000 units/kg/24 hr every 4 hr or up to 20 million units*	IV	6–8 wk
	+ Oxacillin	200 mg/kg/24 hr every 4–6 hr	IV	6–8 wk
	+ Gentamicin	4–6 mg/kg/24 hr every 8–12 hr	IV	6–8 wk

*For relatively resistant organisms.
†Addition of aminoglycoside advocated by some centers.
‡Least preferred.
§Addition of rifampin advocated by some centers.
IV = intravenous; IM = intramuscular; PO = oral.

emboli, often with central nervous system manifestations, are a major threat in patients with infective endocarditis. Pulmonary emboli are most often recognized in children with ventricular septal defect or tetralogy of Fallot, although massive life-threatening pulmonary embolization is extremely rare. Mycotic aneurysms, ruptured sinus of Valsalva, obstructive valve disease secondary to large vegetations, acquired ventricular septal defect, and heart block as a result of involvement of the specialized conduction system have all been reported as a result of infective endocarditis.

Treatment. Antibiotic therapy should be instituted immediately on diagnosis of infective endocarditis. When virulent organisms are responsible, small delays may result in progressive endocardial damage and a greater likelihood of severe complications. The choice of antibiotics, method of administration, and length of treatment are outlined in Table 13–9. High serum bactericidal levels must be maintained long enough to eradicate organisms that are growing in relatively inaccessible avascular vegetations. From 5–20 times the minimum in vitro inhibiting concentration must be produced at the site of infection to destroy bacteria growing at the core of these lesions. Several wk are required for a vegetation to organize completely; thus, therapy must be continued through this period so that recrudescence can be avoided. A total of 4–6 wk of treatment is recommended, with serumcidal levels by tube dilution of at least 1:8 prior to administration of a subsequent dose of antibiotic. Depending on the clinical and laboratory responses, antibiotic therapy may require modification, and in some instances more prolonged treatment is required. With highly sensitive *Streptococcus viridans* infections, shortened regimens including oral penicillin have been recommended.

Bed rest should be instituted and should be extended if congestive heart failure occurs. Similarly, digitalis, restriction of sodium, and diuretic therapy should be utilized when indicated.

Surgical intervention during the course of infective endocarditis is an integral part of management in cases in which severe aortic or mitral valve involvement leads to intractable heart failure. Rarely, a mycotic aneurysm or a rupture of an aortic sinus requires emergency operation. Although antibiotic therapy should be administered for as long as possible prior to surgical intervention, active infection is not a contraindication if the patient is critically ill as a result of severe hemodynamic deterioration from infective endocarditis. Removal of vegetations and, in some instances, valve replacement may be lifesaving, and sustained antibiotic administration will most often prevent reinfection. Successful late surgical intervention has been reported in children with infective endocarditis who have been unresponsive to treatment and in patients who have shown evidence of continued embolic phenomena. Replacement of infected prosthetic valves carries a higher risk but is necessary in refractory cases.

Fungal endocarditis is difficult to manage and has a poor prognosis regardless of treatment. It is most often encountered after cardiac surgery or in the immunosuppressed patient. The drug of choice is amphotericin B, but surgery to excise infected tissue is occasionally attempted with limited success.

Prevention. Antimicrobial prophylaxis prior to and after various procedures, including tooth extractions and other forms of dental manipulation, reduces the incidence of infective endocarditis in susceptible patients. Proper general dental care and oral hygiene further decrease the risk of infective endocarditis in susceptible individuals. Vigorous treatment of sepsis and local infections and careful asepsis during cardiac surgery and catheterization will also reduce the incidence of infective endocarditis.

Recommendations for specific antibiotic regimens for prevention of infective endocarditis under various circumstances are listed in Table 13–10.

13.72 RHEUMATIC CARDITIS

Rheumatic involvement of the valves and endocardium is the most important manifestation of rheumatic fever (Sec 9.81). The lesions begin as small verrucae composed of fibrin and blood cells along the borders of any of the valves; the mitral valve is affected most often. The aortic valve is next in frequency; right heart manifestations are rare. As the inflammation subsides, the verrucae tend to disappear and leave scar tissue. With each repeated infection new verrucae form near the previous ones, and the mural endocardium and chordae tendineae become involved.

Clinical Patterns of Valvular Disease. *Mitral Insufficiency.* Insufficiency of the valve is the result of structural changes that usually include some loss of valvular substance and shortening and thickening of the chordae tendineae. During acute rheumatic fever with severe cardiac involvement, congestive heart failure is most often due to severe mechanical mitral insufficiency coupled with inflammatory disease which may involve the pericardium, myocardium, endocardium, and epicardium. Because of the high volume load

and inflammatory process the left ventricle becomes large and inefficient. The left atrium dilates as blood regurgitates into this chamber. Increased left atrial pressure results in pulmonary congestion and symptoms of left heart failure. In patients with severe chronic mitral insufficiency the pulmonary artery pressure becomes elevated, and enlargement of the right ventricle and atrium and subsequent right heart failure will occur. In most cases mitral insufficiency is mild or moderate; even in those patients in whom incompetence is severe at the onset, there is spontaneous improvement in time. The resultant chronic lesion is most often mild or moderate in severity, and the patient will be asymptomatic.

The principal physical signs of mitral insufficiency include a heaving apical left ventricular precordial impulse with a pansystolic murmur at the apex radiating to the axilla and the sternal edge. However, with severe mitral insufficiency, signs of chronic congestive heart failure, including fatigue, weight gain, weakness, and dyspnea on exertion, may be noted. The heart is en-

Table 13–10 RECOMMENDATIONS FOR PREVENTION OF BACTERIAL ENDOCARDITIS

For Dental Procedures and also for Tonsillectomy, Adenoidectomy, and Bronchoscopy

I. For most patients: **PENICILLIN**	a) *Intramuscular* plus *Oral* *Adults:* 600,000 units of procaine penicillin G mixed with 1,000,000 units of aqueous crystalline penicillin G intramuscularly 30–60 min prior to procedure, followed by 500 mg penicillin V orally every 6 hr for 8 doses. *Children:* 30,000 units aqueous penicillin G/kg mixed with 600,000 units of procaine penicillin intramuscularly (not to exceed adult dose). For children less than 60 lb the dose of penicillin V is 250 mg every 6 hr for 8 doses. b) *Oral only* *Adults:* 2.0 gm of penicillin V 30–60 min prior to procedure and then 500 mg every 6 hr for 8 doses. *Children less than 60 lb:* 1.0 gm of penicillin V orally 30 min–1 hr prior to procedure and then 250 mg orally every 6 hr for 8 doses.
II. For those allergic to penicillin (may also be selected for those receiving oral penicillin as continuous rheumatic fever prophylaxis): **ERYTHROMYCIN**	*Adults:* 1.0 gm orally 1½–2 hr prior to procedure and then 500 mg every 6 hr for 8 doses (or Regimen IV). *Children:* 20 mg/kg orally 1½–2 hr prior to procedure and then 10 mg/kg (not to exceed adult dosage) every 6 hr for 8 doses (or Regimen IV).
III. For those patients at higher risk of infective endocarditis (especially those with prosthetic heart valves) who are not allergic to penicillin: **PENICILLIN** plus **STREPTOMYCIN**	*Adults:* IM penicillin as outlined above in I.a, plus streptomycin, 1.0 gm IM, both given 30–60 min before procedure; then penicillin V, 500 mg orally every 6 hr for 8 doses. *Children:* Timing of doses is same as for adults. Aqueous penicillin dose is 30,000 units/kg mixed with 600,000 units procaine penicillin. Streptomycin dose is 20 mg/kg (not to exceed adult dosage). For children less than 60 lb the dose of penicillin V is 250 mg every 6 hr for 8 doses.
IV. For higher risk patients (especially those with prosthetic heart valves) who are allergic to penicillin: **VANCOMYCIN** intravenously and **ERYTHROMYCIN** orally	*Adults:* Vancomycin, 1 gm IV over 30–60 min, begun 30–60 min before procedure; then erythromycin, 500 mg orally every 6 hr for 8 doses. *Children:* Timing of doses is same as for adults. Dose of vancomycin is 20 mg/kg. Dose of erythromycin is 10 mg/kg every 6 hr for 8 doses (not to exceed adult dose).

For Gastrointestinal and Genitourinary Tract Surgery and Instrumentation And Also For Any Surgery of Infected Tissues

I. For most patients: **PENICILLIN** or **AMPICILLIN** plus **STREPTOMYCIN** or **GENTAMICIN**	*Adults:* 2 million units of aqueous penicillin G IM or IV or 1.0 gm ampicillin IM or IV *plus* gentamicin 1.5 mg/kg (not to exceed 80 mg) IM or IV or streptomycin 1.0 gm IM. This should be given 30–60 min before procedure. Repeat every 8 hr for 2 additional doses if gentamicin is used, or every 12 hr for 2 additional doses if streptomycin is used. *Children:* Same timing of medications as adult schedule. Dosages are aqueous penicillin G, 30,000 units/kg, or ampicillin, 50 mg/kg; gentamicin, 2.0 mg/kg (not to exceed adult dosage).
II. For patients allergic to penicillin: **VANCOMYCIN** plus **STREPTOMYCIN**	*Adults:* 1.0 gm vancomycin IV given over 30–60 min *plus* 1.0 gm streptomycin IM, each given 30–60 min before procedure. Doses may be repeated in 12 hr. *Children:* Timing as above. Doses are vancomycin, 20 mg/kg, and streptomycin, 20 mg/kg (not to exceed adult dosage).

Note: in patients with significantly compromised renal function, antibiotic dosages may need to be modified. Intramuscular injections may be contraindicated in patients receiving anticoagulants.

Adapted from: The Report of the Committee on Rheumatic Fever and Bacterial Endocarditis, American Heart Association, 1977.

larged with an apical systolic thrill. The 1st heart sound is normal; the 2nd heart sound may be accentuated if pulmonary hypertension is present. A 3rd heart sound is prominent. In addition to the pansystolic murmur a short diastolic rumble follows the 3rd sound; it is due to increased blood flow from the left atrium across the left mitral valve that results from the massive insufficiency. This murmur is associated with mitral incompetence and does not mean that mechanical mitral stenosis is present. The latter lesion is characterized by a diastolic murmur of greater length with presystolic accentuation.

The *electrocardiogram* and *roentgenograms* are normal if the lesion is mild. With more severe lesions the electrocardiogram shows prominent bifid P waves, signs of left ventricular hypertrophy, and sometimes associated right ventricular hypertrophy. Roentgenographically, there is prominence of the left atrium and ventricle. When pulmonary hypertension or congestive heart failure supervenes, the pulmonary artery segment and right heart chambers are prominent. Signs of pulmonary venous hypertension may also be evident. Calcification of the mitral valve is rare in children. *Echocardiography* shows enlargement of the left atrium and ventricle with an increased velocity of diastolic closure of the anterior mitral leaflet in moderate or severe regurgitation. The signs of mitral valve prolapse are usually absent.

Cardiac catheterization and *left ventriculography* are undertaken *only* if there is rapid progression of the disease and surgical treatment is contemplated. The cardiac output is normal or decreased in severe lesions. The left atrial pressure is frequently but not always increased. The pulse curve of the left atrium shows a steep rise in early systole to the peak of the "v" wave and is followed by a rapid "y" descent. A diastolic gradient may be measured across the mitral valve even in the absence of mitral stenosis. The left ventricular end-diastolic pressure rises during exercise or in the presence of left ventricular failure. Left ventriculography results in opacification of the left atrium. The degree of opacification is used as a qualitative assessment of the severity of incompetence.

A frequent problem is evaluation of an apical systolic murmur without other signs in patients who have had a mild attack of rheumatic fever or a history of recurrent upper respiratory tract infections. Though many of these patients are considered to have organic mitral insufficiency, the diagnosis is often incorrect. In some the murmur is an innocent one with transmission to the apex.

COMPLICATIONS. Severe mitral incompetence may result in cardiac failure that may be precipitated by progression of the rheumatic process, the onset of atrial fibrillation with rapid ventricular response, or infective endocarditis. Right-sided heart failure may be accompanied by tricuspid or pulmonary incompetence. Occasional atrial or ventricular extrasystoles are well tolerated. First-degree heart block may persist for years after the original rheumatic infection or be due to digitalis therapy. Atrial fibrillation is more common when mitral incompetence is associated with a large left atrium.

TREATMENT. In the majority of patients with mitral insufficiency, prophylaxis against recurrences of rheumatic fever is all that is required since the lesions are mild and well tolerated. (See Sec 9.81 for management of acute and convalescent stages of the disease and for prophylactic therapy.) The treatment of complicating heart failure, dysrhythmias, and infective endocarditis is described elsewhere in this chapter. Surgical treatment is indicated in patients who, despite adequate medical therapy, suffer from recurrent episodes of heart failure, extreme dyspnea with moderate activity, and progressive cardiomegaly, often with pulmonary hypertension. Although annuloplasty gives good results in some children and adolescents, valve replacement may be required. Many children with murmurs suggestive of mitral insufficiency lose all evidence of cardiac disease after some years. Untold harm may be done if the patient's activities are reduced on the basis of the presence of a murmur alone.

Mitral Stenosis. Congenital mitral stenosis has been described in Sec 13.58.

Organic mitral stenosis is nearly always rheumatic in origin and results from fibrosis of the mitral ring, commissural adhesions, and contracture of the valve leaflets, chordae, and papillary muscles. It may take 2 yr or more for the lesion to become fully established, although the process may occasionally be accelerated. Mitral stenosis is seldom encountered prior to adolescence.

Mitral stenosis of critical degree is considered to exist if the valvular orifice is reduced to 25% or less of the expected normal. Such reductions result in increased pressure and hypertrophy of the left atrium. The increased pressure causes pulmonary venous hypertension, increased pulmonary vascular resistance, and pulmonary hypertension. Right ventricular and atrial dilatation and hypertrophy ensue and are followed by right-sided heart failure.

Generally, there is a good correlation between symptoms and severity of obstruction. Patients with mild lesions are asymptomatic. More severe degrees of obstruction are associated with effort intolerance and dyspnea. Critical lesions can result in orthopnea, paroxysmal nocturnal dyspnea, and overt pulmonary edema. These symptoms may be precipitated by uncontrolled tachycardia, atrial fibrillation, or pulmonary infections. Congestive heart failure is usually associated with moderate or severe pulmonary hypertension. Right ventricular dilatation may result in functional tricuspid incompetence, hepatomegaly, ascites, and edema. Hemoptysis due to ruptured bronchial or pleurohilar veins and, occasionally, pulmonary infarction may occur. Blood-streaked sputum occurs during episodes of pulmonary edema.

With severe lesions, cyanosis and a malar flush are seen. The jugular venous pressure is increased in the presence of congestive heart failure, tricuspid valve disease, or severe pulmonary hypertension. The heart size is normal with minimal disease. Moderate cardiomegaly is usual with severe mitral stenosis and sinus rhythm, but cardiac enlargement can be great, especially when atrial fibrillation and heart failure supervene. The apical impulse is brief and tapping, and a parasternal right ventricular lift is palpable when pulmonary pressure is high. The principal auscultatory findings are a loud 1st heart sound, an opening snap of the mitral valve, and a long, low-pitched, rumbling mitral diastolic murmur with presystolic accentuation. Severe obstruction is present when (1) the diastolic murmur is long (in the absence of mitral incompetence), (2) the Q-1 interval is long (i.e., time between the Q wave of the electrocardiogram and the 1st heart sound), and (3) the 2-OS interval is short (i.e., time between aortic valve closure and the opening snap). The mitral diastolic murmur may be absent in congestive heart failure. An apical systolic murmur may be audible even in the absence of mitral incompetence; in some instances it is due to complicating tricuspid incompetence. In the presence of pulmonary hypertension, pulmonary valvular closure is accentuated. An early diastolic murmur is usually due to associated aortic incompetence; pulmonary valvular incompetence is not as common.

Electrocardiograms and *roentgenograms* are normal if the lesion is mild; as severity increases, there are prominent and notched P waves and varying degrees of right ventricular hypertrophy. Moderate or critical lesions are associated with roentgenographic signs of left atrial enlargement, prominence of the pulmonary artery and right heart chambers, and a normal or small aorta and left ventricle (Fig 13–78). Severe obstruction is associated with a redistribution of pulmonary blood flow so that the apices of the lung have a greater perfusion (i.e., reverse of normal). Septal lines at the costophrenic angles may also be present. *Echocardiography* shows distinct slowing of the diastolic closure of the anterior

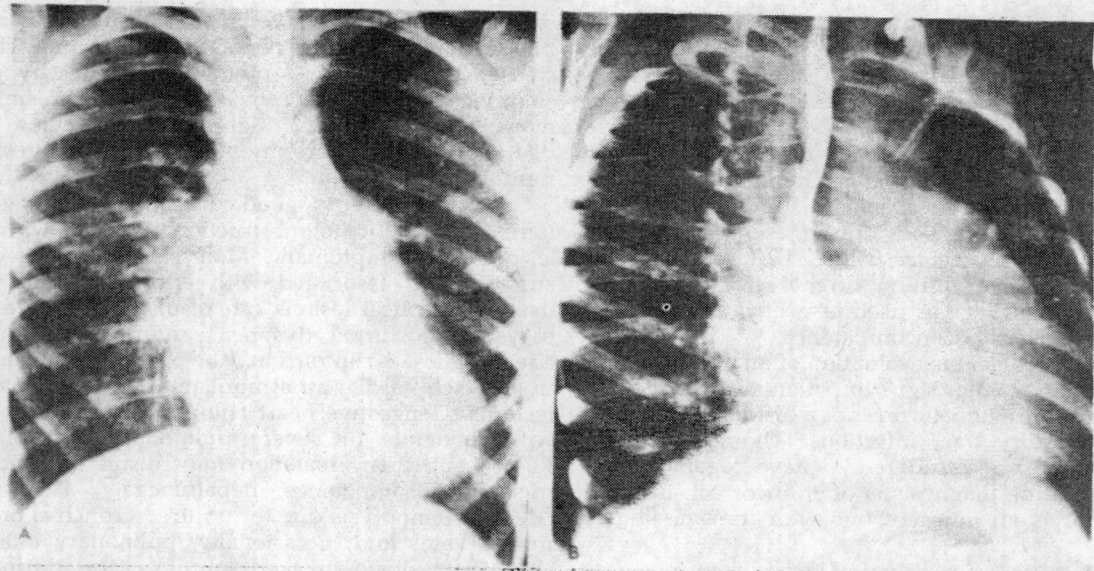

Figure 13–78 Roentgenograms in isolated rheumatic mitral stenosis. *A,* Posteroanterior view showing cardiomegaly and prominent main pulmonary artery. Vascular shadows in lungs are due to prominent pulmonary arteries and veins. *B,* Right anterior oblique view showing indentation of esophagus by large left atrium. This patient required valvotomy at age 8 yr.

mitral leaflet, left atrial enlargement, and increased right-sided systolic time interval ratios in the presence of pulmonary hypertension. *Cardiac catheterization* quantitates the diastolic gradient across the mitral valve and the degree of pulmonary hypertension.

TREATMENT. Surgical treatment is undertaken when there are clinical signs and hemodynamic evidence of severe obstruction. Since extreme valvular distortion and calcification are rare in children, mitral valvotomy generally yields good results.

Aortic Insufficiency. In chronic rheumatic aortic insufficiency, sclerosis of the aortic valves results in distortion and retraction of the cusps. Regurgitation of blood results in a volume overload with dilatation and hypertrophy of the left ventricle. Secondary mitral incompetence may follow progressive left ventricle dilatation. Left ventricular failure results in left atrial hypertension. Congestive cardiac failure may occur insidiously or be preceded by bouts of pulmonary edema.

Symptoms are unusual except in gross aortic incompetence. The large stroke volume and forceful left ventricular contractions may result in palpitations. Excessive sweating and heat intolerance are related to vasodilatation. Dyspnea on effort progresses to orthopnea and pulmonary edema. Angina pectoris may occur during heavy exertion. In adolescents with severe incompetence, nocturnal attacks with nightmares, sweating, tachycardia, chest pain, and hypertension may occur. It is now rare to encounter patients with the classic clinical picture of florid mitral or aortic disease.

Because of the reflux of blood through the aortic valve during diastole and the associated vasodilatation, the radial and carotid arterial pulsations are, respectively, water-hammer and Corrigan in type. Associated signs of severe aortic insufficiency include capillary pulsations in the lips or fingernails, an audible systolic shock over the peripheral arteries (pistol shot), and systolic and

diastolic murmurs over the femoral arteries if pressure is applied to the artery just distal to the stethoscope (Duroziez sign). The systolic blood pressure is elevated, the diastolic lowered.

In severe aortic insufficiency, the heart is enlarged and has a left ventricular apical heave. There may be a diastolic thrill. The typical murmur begins immediately with the 2nd heart sound and continues until late in diastole. The murmur is heard over the upper and middle left sternal border with radiation to the apex and to the aortic area. Characteristically, it has a hollow, high-pitched blowing quality. Generally, the murmur is more easily audible in full expiration, with the diaphragm of the stethoscope placed firmly on the chest and the patient leaning forward. Occasionally, it may be louder in the recumbent position. A systolic ejection murmur sometimes preceded by a click is frequent and is produced by the large stroke volume. An apical presystolic murmur (Austin Flint) resembling that of mitral stenosis is sometimes heard.

The *echocardiogram* shows a large left ventricle and diastolic mitral valve flutter or oscillation, at a frequency of 30–40 cycles/sec.

Roentgenograms show prominence and exaggerated pulsations of the left ventricle and aorta. The *electrocardiogram* may be normal but in severe cases reveals signs of left ventricular hypertrophy with prominent P waves.

Cardiac catheterization is seldom necessary and is undertaken only when surgery is contemplated because of a progressive lesion. The degree of elevation of left ventricular end-diastolic, left atrial, and pulmonary arterial pressures is established, and ascending aortography demonstrates the regurgitant flow across the aortic valve into the left ventricle.

Mild and moderate lesions are well tolerated. Many adolescents with severe regurgitation are symptom-free and tolerate advanced lesions into the 3rd–4th decades. Unfavorable signs are the onset of congestive heart failure, recurrent episodes of pulmonary edema, or development of angina pectoris.

Treatment in most cases consists of prophylaxis against the recurrence of acute rheumatic fever and occurrence of infective endocarditis as well as encouragement to lead as active and normal a life as possible. Surgical treatment (usually valve replacement) is undertaken when there is progressive cardiomegaly or deterioration from heart failure, pulmonary edema, or angina pectoris.

Tricuspid Valvular Disease. Tricuspid involvement is rare following rheumatic fever. *Tricuspid insufficiency* secondary to right ventricular dilatation resulting from severe left-sided lesions is usually functional. The signs produced by tricuspid insufficiency include prominent pulsations of the jugular veins with a "c-v" wave, systolic pulsations of the liver, and blowing systolic murmur in the 4th and 5th left parasternal spaces that increases in intensity during inspiration. Concomitant signs of mitral or aortic valvular disease, with or without atrial fibrillation, are frequent. Signs of tricuspid incompetence decrease or disappear when heart failure produced by the left-sided lesions is successfully treated.

Acquired tricuspid stenosis is rare, especially in childhood; it is usually associated with rheumatic mitral or aortic valvular disease. The signs are increased jugular venous pressure with prominence of the "a" wave, presystolic hepatic pulsation, and a rumbling diastolic murmur in the 4th and 5th left parasternal spaces.

Hepatomegaly, edema, and ascites are present with severe lesions. Cardiac catheterization shows a gradient of pressure across the tricuspid valve.

Pulmonary Valvular Disease. Pulmonary insufficiency is rarely due to organic disease but occasionally occurs on a functional basis secondary to pulmonary hypertension or dilatation of the pulmonary artery. Occasionally, it complicates severe mitral stenosis (Graham Steell murmur). The murmurs are similar to those of aortic insufficiency, but the peripheral arterial signs are absent in pulmonary insufficiency. Pulmonary stenosis is not seen with rheumatic diseases.

Arnett EN, Roberts WC: Prosthetic valve endocarditis. Am J Cardiol 38:281, 1976.

Bisno SL, Dismukes WE, Durack DT, et al: Treatment of infective endocarditis due to viridans streptococci. Circulation 63:730A, 1981.

Gersony WM, Hayes CJ: Bacterial endocarditis in patients with pulmonary stenosis, aortic stenosis, or ventricular septal defect. Circulation 56(Suppl):84, 1977.

Gersony WM, Hordoff AH: Infective endocarditis and diseases of the Pericardium. Pediatr Clin North Am 25:831, 1978.

Johnson DH, Rosenthal A, Nadas A: A forty-year review of bacterial endocarditis in infancy and childhood. Circulation 51:581, 1975.

Kaplan EL, Rich H, Gersony WM, et al: A collaborative study of endocarditis in the 1970's. Circulation 59:327, 1979.

Weinstein L, Schlesinger JJ: Pathoanatomic, pathophysiologic and clinical correlation in endocarditis. N Engl J Med 291:832, 1122, 1974.

Wilson WR, Nichols DR, Thompson RL, et al: Infective endocarditis: Therapeutic considerations. Am Heart J 100:689, 1980.

13.73 DISEASES OF THE MYOCARDIUM

13.74 CONDITIONS CAUSING MYOCARDIAL DAMAGE

The status of the myocardium is a critical factor in the prognosis of cardiac disease. If, in spite of congenital cardiac malformations, acquired valvular disease, or arrhythmias, the myocardium is able to provide satisfactory circulation of blood, the child will be able to maintain adequate nutrition, growth, and activity. The myocardium may be affected by infections, mesenchymal diseases, endocrine disorders, metabolic and nutritional diseases, neuromuscular diseases, blood diseases, tumors, hypertension, and congenital anomalies.

Bacterial Infections. In **diphtheria** the toxin of the bacillus may produce peripheral circulatory failure or toxic myocarditis. These complications occur in all types of diphtheria, including the cutaneous form. Peripheral circulatory failure occurs within the 1st 2 wk of the disease and is associated with a rapid, thready pulse; cold, pale, and clammy skin; and hypotension. In addition to therapy for diphtheria (Sec 10.23), treatment for cardiogenic shock is essential.

Toxic myocarditis is characterized by the development of arrhythmia in the form of atrioventricular block, bundle branch block, or extrasystoles. Congestive cardiac failure occurs later and is associated with cardiac enlargement and gallop rhythm. In addition to the arrhythmia, the electrocardiogram shows S-T segment depression and T wave inversion in most leads. The

immediate prognosis is grave (about 50% mortality). Treatment (Sec 10.23) includes strict bed rest until all signs of myocarditis have disappeared. Digitalis is reserved for patients with frank congestive heart failure but must be used with care because of the possibility of increased sensitivity.

In **typhoid fever,** toxic myocarditis may be inferred if there is electrocardiographic evidence of T wave inversion in most leads. This sign may be transient, however, and by itself is of no clinical significance. Cardiac failure is rare, and peripheral circulatory failure is no longer common.

In **other bacterial infections,** circulatory involvement is manifested as peripheral circulatory collapse or toxic myocarditis. The incidence of toxic myocarditis is difficult to gauge because its diagnosis frequently depends on minor pathologic evidence such as cloudy swelling or fatty degeneration. Toxic myocarditis as evidenced by tachycardia, gallop rhythm, and cardiac enlargement may complicate pneumonia, infective endocarditis, and septicemia. The prognosis depends on control of the primary infection.

Rickettsial Diseases. Rocky Mountain spotted fever, in particular, may be complicated by hypotension and peripheral vascular collapse. This complication has been attributed to the general vasculitis characteristic of the disease, but acute myocarditis may be a contributing factor.

Viral Infections. A viral etiology has been implicated in many patients with acute myocarditis. The viral agents include among others those of coxsackievirus A and B, echovirus, rubella, varicella, and influenzal infections. However, in many instances in which a viral infection is suspected, a virus cannot be identified. Acute myocarditis may occur in conjunction with diseases of other systems, especially of the central nervous system; on occasion, the myocarditis may be masked by the other involvement.

The clinical spectrum of viral myocarditis varies widely from that of a rapidly fatal disorder, especially in the newborn infant, to that of a mild disease with apparent complete recovery. Between these 2 extremes is a range of clinical patterns; a chronic course characterized by cardiomegaly with mitral incompetence that progresses to chronic congestive cardiac failure is not unusual.

Parasitic and Fungal Infections. Lesions in the myocardium have been described in association with *histoplasmosis, coccidioidomycosis, toxoplasmosis,* and *trichinosis.* In these conditions the cardiac lesion seldom produces clinical signs of myocarditis. *Actinomycosis* may involve the pericardium and myocardium by direct contiguity to, for example, a pulmonary abscess. *Hydatid cysts* of the pericardium may be found on routine roentgenograms of the chest and usually produce symptoms only when they rupture. *Schistosomiasis* may produce pulmonary hypertension and cor pulmonale. *Cruz trypanosomiasis* (Chagas disease) may produce acute or subacute myocarditis and sudden death.

Mesenchymal Diseases. *Rheumatic carditis* is described in Sec 13.72, and *rheumatic carditis* and the cardiovascular manifestations of *rheumatoid arthritis, disseminated lupus erythematosus, periarteritis nodosa, dermatomyositis, and scleroderma* are described in Chapter 9.

Endocrine Disorders. *Hyperthyroidism* produces tachycardia, vasodilatation, wide pulse pressure, cardiac enlargement, and, rarely, atrial fibrillation. *Cretinism* seldom produces gross cardiac involvement, but the electrocardiogram is characterized by bradycardia, low voltage of all complexes—especially of the P and T waves, left axis deviation, and prolonged electrical systole. These signs may disappear within 1 mo after initiation of adequate thyroid therapy.

Metabolic and Nutritional Diseases. Among vitamin deficiency diseases, *beriberi* (Sec 3.23) causes the most conspicuous cardiac damage. In patients with malnutrition the deficiencies are often multiple, and it is difficult to separate the cardiac lesion of 1 nutritional disease from that of another. (See iron deficiency disease below and Sec 14.11.)

Neuromuscular Diseases. In the original description of *Friedreich ataxia,* heart disease was noted in 5 of 6 cases. In most instances cardiac symptoms are masked by the basic disease, which limits physical activities. In some patients effort intolerance, chest pain, and heart failure have been the presenting symptoms. These are due to primary myocardial disease which affects chiefly the left ventricle and results in congestive or obstructive cardiomyopathy. The electrocardiogram shows generalized T wave inversion or signs of left ventricular hypertrophy. Arrhythmias may also occur and consist of atrial tachycardia or fibrillation or extrasystoles. Varying degrees of cardiomegaly, left ventricular promi-

nence, and pulmonary congestion are demonstrable roentgenographically. (See Sec 21.17.)

In *progressive muscular dystrophy* (Sec 22.6) 50% of children have postmortem evidence of myocardial involvement similar to that of the striated muscle. Cardiac symptoms, however, are not common, but the electrocardiogram is frequently abnormal and may reveal tachycardia, abnormalities of the P waves, short P-R interval, and abnormal Q and T waves. Minimal evidence of right or left ventricular hypertrophy also may be noted, and some patients have congestive heart failure.

Blood Diseases. In infants and children anemia is the most common blood disease associated with cardiac involvement, as, for example, in leukemia, hemolytic anemias, severe iron deficiency, and hemorrhage. Although cardiac output must increase when the hemoglobin is below about 7 gm/dl, cardiac enlargement in infants with or without congestive heart failure occurs only with an extreme reduction in hemoglobin, to 3–4 gm or less. The heart rate is rapid, the pulse pressure widened, and the venous pressure increased. A systolic murmur at the apex and/or along the left sternal border is usual; diastolic murmurs may occur in the same areas, and gallop rhythm is common. The electrocardiographic changes include depressed S-T segments and flat T waves. Occasionally, minimal signs and symptoms are present when extreme states of anemia have developed gradually.

Treatment is directed toward the cause of the anemia. If blood transfusions are indicated in the presence of cardiomegaly or cardiac failure, small volumes (4–5 ml/kg) of packed cells are preferred. (See Sec 14.11 and 14.35.)

Glycogen Storage Disease. Cardiac as well as skeletal muscle is affected in the generalized form of glycogen storage disease known as Type II or Pompe disease (Sec 8.21). The clinical pattern is dominated by skeletal muscle weakness, macroglossia, and hepatomegaly. Cardiomegaly is massive, but murmurs are insignificant. Pulmonary atelectasis with secondary infection is common and is related to compression by the large heart. The *electrocardiogram* is characteristic and shows prominent P waves, short P-R interval, massive QRS voltage, signs of isolated left or biventricular hypertrophy, and intraventricular conduction defects. *Roentgenograms* confirm the striking cardiomegaly with prominence of the left ventricle. The prognosis is poor, and the majority of infants succumb before the age of 2 yr. Effective therapy is not available.

Hurler Syndrome (Sec 23.18). The lesion in the heart and great vessels is the same as that in the connective tissue elsewhere in the body. The most pronounced lesions are found in the valves and coronary arteries, but abnormalities in the pericardium and aorta are not uncommon. The heart may be moderately enlarged, with electrocardiographic signs of left ventricular hypertrophy. Cardiac murmurs may result from incompetence and stenosis of the mitral and aortic valves. Sometimes the pulmonary and tricuspid valves are also involved. Coronary arterial disease may result in angina and perhaps explain the frequent occurrence of sudden death. The prognosis is poor, and many children succumb before the age of 10 yr with heart failure and pulmonary infection.

Calcinosis of the Coronary Arteries. This is a rare disease of infancy. Familial aggregation has been recorded. The coronary arteries are tortuous and calcareous, and the ventricles, especially the left, are hypertrophied. Other blood vessels may be similarly involved. The onset of cardiac failure is sudden; death usually occurs in infancy.

Adriamycin (Doxorubicin Hydrochloride) Cardiotoxicity. Severe, dose-dependent cardiomyopathy occurs in about 30% of patients when the total cumulative dose of Adriamycin exceeds 550 mg/M². Cardiomegaly is due principally to left ventricular and left atrial enlargement. If congestive cardiac failure develops, the case fatality rate is 30–50%. T wave flattening or inversion is nonspecific evidence of cardiac involvement; early cardiac changes may be detected by serial echocardiograms which show progressive decrease in myocardial contractility, even in asymptomatic patients.

13.75 ENDOCARDIAL FIBROELASTOSIS (EFE)

This condition has been described under a variety of names, including fetal endocarditis, endocardial fibrosis, prenatal fibroelastosis, elastic tissue hyperplasia, and endocardial sclerosis.

It is classified into 2 general types: primary and secondary. In primary EFE there is no apparent predisposing valvular lesion or other congenital abnormality. In the secondary type severe congenital heart disease of the left-sided obstructive type (e.g., aortic stenosis or atresia, other forms of hypoplastic left heart, and severe coarctation of the aorta) is present. In secondary EFE the ventricular cavity is often contracted, whereas in the primary disease a dilated left ventricular chamber is seen in the infant. However, in young adults a primary contracted type of EFE has been observed.

No etiology for primary EFE has been established. Proposed possibilities include inflammation or infection before or after birth, maldevelopment, and inadequate blood supply to the endocardium. The endocardial changes could also be secondary to myocardial disease which, resulting in cardiac dilatation and in stretching of the endocardium, initiates fibroelastic proliferation. The disease has occurred in siblings.

Pathologically, there is a white, opaque fibroelastic thickening of the endocardium, especially of the left side of the heart, which frequently obscures the trabeculation of the inner surfaces of the cardiac chamber. The lesion may spread to involve the valves, especially the aortic and mitral ones. Microscopically, the lesion consists of a fibroelastic thickening of the endocardium which follows the course of the trabecular sinusoids and may result in subendocardial degeneration or necrosis of muscle with vacuolation of muscle fibers. The involved valve leaflets are characterized by a myxomatous proliferation with an increase in collagenous elements.

The *clinical manifestations* are variable. Infants, usually less than 6 mo of age, who apparently have been in good health develop severe congestive cardiac failure, often precipitated by a respiratory infection. The prognosis is poor unless there is a significant response to therapy for cardiac failure. Other infants have similar milder symptoms with periods of remission. At some time during the 1st 2 yr of life, affected infants may manifest some dyspnea, refusal to feed, failure to gain weight adequately, and recurrent pulmonary infections. There are repeated episodes of congestive cardiac failure, which in many instances can be controlled by digitalis and diuretics. Most eventually succumb. Infants in whom valvular lesions or associated congenital cardiovascular defects are predominant expire in the 1st months of life.

During episodes of congestive cardiac failure the infant with primary EFE is acutely ill with dyspnea, cough, and anorexia. Cyanosis is infrequent but occurs sometimes in the terminal phase or as a sign of associated congenital cardiovascular defects. The jugular venous pressure is elevated, the liver greatly enlarged, and edema of the extremities, sacral area, or face may be present. Rales and rhonchi in the lung fields are due to intercurrent pulmonary infection and congestion. The heart is moderately or greatly enlarged and has a normal or left ventricular impulse. Murmurs of mitral incompetence are frequent; some patients have a grade I or II blowing systolic murmur down the left sternal border.

Roentgenograms confirm the cardiac enlargement (Fig 13–79). There may be signs of intercurrent pulmonary infection. The *electrocardiogram* is usually abnormal, with changes indicative of left atrial and ventricular hypertrophy and strain. The *echocardiogram* shows a dilated, poorly functioning left ventricle.

The short term *prognosis* has improved because of the availability of more potent diuretics and more effective management of cardiac failure in infants. In patients who have survived, it should be recognized that the clinical diagnosis is inferential since it is not possible to

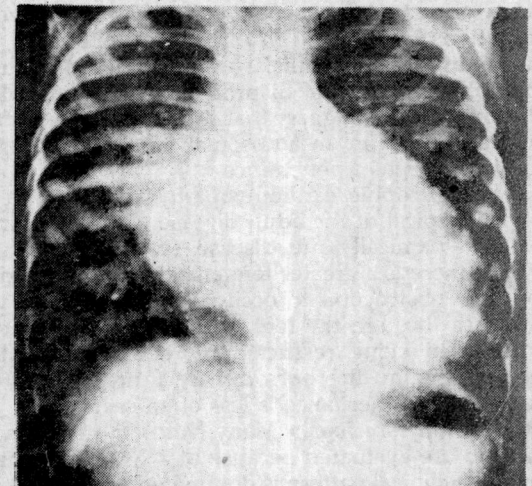

Figure 13–79 Roentgenogram of a 7 mo old girl with endocardial sclerosis. Note enlargement of the heart, without a distinctive contour.

be certain that the original cardiac involvement was that of EFE or of another myocardial lesion.

Treatment is directed toward alleviation of congestive cardiac failure and prevention of intercurrent infections.

13.76 CARDIOMYOPATHY

Heart muscle disease of unknown origin has been classified into hypertrophic, congestive, restricting, and obliterative types. The 1st 2 are relatively common in North American children and adolescents.

Hypertrophic Cardiomyopathy. This condition is also known as *idiopathic hypertrophic subaortic stenosis* and *asymmetrical septal hypertrophy*. Massive ventricular hypertrophy with principal involvement of the ventricular septum characterizes the disease, but all portions of the left ventricle and sometimes of the right are affected. Varying degrees of myocardial fibrosis are also present. The mitral valve is displaced anteriorly by the hypertrophy of papillary muscle, and the left ventricular cavity is distorted by the massive generalized hypertrophy. Microscopically, patchy areas of abnormally thick and short muscle fibers are arranged in circular collections and interspersed among normal as well as hypertrophied muscle fibers. Electron microscopy shows disarray of myofibrils and myofilaments.

Hemodynamics. The hypertrophic, fibrosed, stiff muscle has a decreased distensibility so that there is resistance to left ventricular filling, but systolic pumping function remains good until late in the course of the disease. Obstruction to left ventricular outflow may develop and is due to apposition of the abnormally placed anterior mitral leaflet against the hypertrophied septum. Peak systolic pressure gradients across the left ventricular outflow are variable. They may never or only intermittently be demonstrable, or they may be permanent. Varying degrees of mitral valve regurgitation are common.

Epidemiology. The disease has been recognized in all age groups, even in neonates, and may occur in many members of the same family, although overt manifestations are present in only about one third of affected individuals. Familial studies, including echocardiographic evidence of disproportionate ventricular septal hypertrophy, suggest that in some patients disease is transmitted in an autosomal dominant pattern with a high degree of penetrance.

Often hypertrophic cardiomyopathy occurring in a child is not typical of the adult disease, although clinically and dynamically the disease seems similar. In childhood, there is a greater tendency for right ventricular outflow obstruction to occur; the disease may be more diffuse through the left ventricular muscularity, as opposed to being restricted more or less to the ventricular septum; the pure disease form with autosomal dominant inheritance is less often seen.

Clinical Manifestations. Many children are asymptomatic and are evaluated because of a heart murmur. In others the clinical pattern is dominated by weakness, fatigue, dyspnea on effort, palpitations, angina pectoris, dizziness, and syncope. There is risk of sudden death even in asymptomatic children. The pulse is brisk because of the early systolic ejection of blood from the ventricle. The heart is enlarged, with a prominent left ventricular lift and double apical impulse. The 1st and 2nd heart sounds are usually normal; paradoxical splitting of the 2nd sound is associated with a large gradient. The rarity of systolic ejection clicks helps to differentiate valvular aortic stenosis. A 3rd sound is not common, but a 4th sound may be audible. The systolic murmur is ejection in type and of medium intensity; it is heard maximally at the left sternal edge and apex. The *electrocardiogram* shows left ventricular hypertrophy with or without S-T segment depression and T wave inversion. The Wolff-Parkinson-White syndrome and other intraventricular conduction defects may be manifested. *Roentgenograms* show cardiomegaly with prominence of the left and sometimes the right ventricle. The ascending aorta and aortic knob are usually normal. The *echocardiogram* shows asymmetric ventricular septal hypertrophy, systolic anterior motion of the anterior leaflet of the mitral valve, and premature closure of the aortic valve.

Cardiac catheterization data are variable since obstruction may or may not be present. When a systolic gradient is present, it is variable even during a relatively short study. The obstruction may be intensified by digitalis glycosides, isoproterenol, amyl nitrite, and nitroglycerin. The gradient may increase shortly after exercise is discontinued, during the Valsalva maneuver, or during assumption of the erect position. Left ventriculography shows encroachment on the left ventricular cavity by the hypertrophied muscle, especially by the interventricular septum. During systole the anterior mitral leaflet is drawn into the left ventricular outflow. Mitral regurgitation is common. It is extremely important to rule out a discrete obstruction with secondary muscular hypertrophy in patients with left ventricular outflow gradients.

The prognosis is unpredictable, especially in the asymptomatic patient.

Treatment. This is not standardized. Competitive sports and strenuous physical activity should be discouraged. Digitalis should be used with extreme caution; in most patients it is contraindicated. Brisk diuresis or the infusion of isoproterenol should also be avoided. Beta-adrenergic blocking agents (propranolol) have been used with apparent success, but obliteration of an LV-AO gradient does not necessarily affect prognosis. Surgical incision or resection of the left ventricular outflow tract has been successfully accomplished in some patients, especially in those with disabling angina or syncope and in some with severe obstruction at rest (a gradient exceeding 70 mm Hg).

Congestive Cardiomyopathy. This is characterized by massive cardiomegaly as a result of the extensive dilatation of the ventricles, especially of the left. Associated ventricular hypertrophy is mild to moderate. The etiology is unknown and is probably multifactorial; a remote history of viral disease in some patients suggests that the disease may be a sequel of a previous myocarditis. Myocardial performance is poor as evidenced by reduced stroke volume, low ejection fraction, and increased systolic and diastolic volumes. All age groups are affected, even infants. Usually the onset is insidious, but sometimes symptoms of congestive cardiac failure occur suddenly. Irritability, anorexia, cough due to pulmonary congestion, and dyspnea with mild exertion are common. When the disease is fully established, the skin is cool and pale; the arterial pulse volume is small; the pulse pressure is reduced, and tachycardia is usual. Jugular venous pressure is increased, hepatomegaly is usual, and ankle edema is common. The heart is enlarged, and pansystolic murmurs of mitral and tricuspid incompetence are frequent. Gallop rhythm is usual.

The *electrocardiogram* shows a combination of atrial enlargement, varying degrees of left ventricular hypertrophy, and nonspecific T wave abnormalities. The *roentgenogram* confirms the cardiomegaly; evidences of pulmonary congestion and edema are frequent, and pleural effusions may be present. The *echocardiogram* shows the inordinate dilatation of the left ventricle, which has a thin free wall and poor septal contraction; the enlarged left atrium; and the displaced mitral valve.

The course of the disease is unpredictable, but it is frequently downhill. Vigorous treatment for heart failure may result in remissions, but relapses are common, and in time patients tend to become resistant to therapy. Complications include arrhythmias (premature atrial and ventricular complexes and later atrial fibrillation) and systemic emboli from intracardiac thrombi.

Restrictive Cardiomyopathy. Poor ventricular compliance is the major abnormality and is responsible for inadequate filling of the ventricular cavities during diastole. This results in a clinical pattern which closely simulates that of constrictive pericarditis. In its overt form restrictive cardiomyopathy results in dyspnea, edema, ascites, hepatomegaly, increased venous pressure, and pulmonary congestion. The heart is mildly or moderately enlarged, and murmurs are nonspecific. The electrocardiogram shows prominent P waves, frequently normal QRS voltage, S-T segment depression, and T wave inversion. Roentgenographic examination shows slight or moderate cardiomegaly with poor cardiac pulsations. Differential diagnosis from constrictive pericarditis is important since the latter can be treated surgically with dramatic success. The prognosis is generally poor. Treatment is directed toward relief of edema with diuretics.

Obliterative Cardiomyopathy. In a variety of conditions the cavity of the left ventricle is encroached upon by abnormal tissue, as, for example, by fibrosis with additional thrombus in endomyocardial fibrosis or by masses of tissue heavily infiltrated with eosinophils. Recurrent episodes of heart failure are characteristic.

13.77 CONGESTIVE HEART FAILURE

Clinical Manifestations. In children the signs and symptoms of congestive heart failure are similar to those in adults. Fatigue, effort intolerance, anorexia, abdominal pain, and cough are frequent. In addition to breathlessness at rest, the systemic venous pressure is ele-

vated, as gauged by clinical assessment of the jugular venous pressure, and the liver is enlarged and tender. Orthopnea and basal rales are commonly present, edema is usually present in dependent portions of the body, or anasarca may be present. Cardiomegaly is invariably noted. Auscultatory findings are those produced by the basic lesion; gallop rhythm is common.

In infants congestive heart failure may be more difficult to identify. Symptoms are dominated by tachypnea, feeding difficulties, poor weight gain, excessive perspiration, irritability, weak cry, and noisy, labored respiration with costal and subcostal retractions as well as flaring of the alae nasi and sternal retractions. Pulmonary congestion may be indistinguishable from bronchospasm. Pneumonitis with or without atelectasis of part of the lung is common. Hepatomegaly nearly always occurs, and cardiomegaly is invariably present. In spite of pronounced tachycardia, gallop rhythm can be recognized frequently. The other auscultatory signs are those produced by the cardiac lesion which resulted in heart failure. A clinical assessment of the jugular venous pressure in infants may be difficult because of the shortness of the neck and the difficulty of securing a relaxed state. Although weight loss after diuretic therapy is common, edema, especially in infants, is frequently not detectable clinically. When present, the edema may be generalized, involving the eyelids as well as the sacrum, legs, and feet.

Treatment. The underlying cause of cardiac failure must be removed or alleviated if possible. If it is a congenital cardiovascular anomaly amenable to surgery, medical treatment is indicated for a time before the surgical procedure and should usually be continued in the immediate postoperative period. For some diseases, such as hyperthyroidism, hypothyroidism, anemia, and beriberi, specific therapy is available, but in the majority of instances only general measures are adaptable. Results will vary with the underlying etiology.

Bed rest in a comfortable position is essential. Some patients prefer to lie flat, but breathing is easier for most in a semireclining position. Initially, sedation may be necessary to produce complete relaxation; the most frequently used drug is morphine (0.05 mg/kg).

A *low sodium diet* is indicated in the treatment of cardiac edema and paroxysmal cardiac dyspnea. The oral intake of sodium should be reduced to as low as 0.5 gm daily; the diet may be made more palatable with a salt substitute. Formulas with a low sodium content are available for infants. However, unpalatable low sodium diets may result in a reduced appetite and thus decreased caloric intake and growth. Excessive restriction may also lead to hyponatremia.

Fluid restriction is indicated. In severely ill infants it is preferable to withhold oral feedings and to restrict intravenous fluids to 75 ml/kg/24 hr while administering diuretics. With clinical improvement, fluid intake is increased slowly, and oral feedings are begun. In older children restriction of fluid intake is balanced with diuretic therapy. Generally, balancing estimated fluid loss and intake suffices, especially when diuretics are prescribed.

Oxygen administered by any method which is effective and comfortable for the patient will help to relieve dyspnea and cyanosis.

Metabolic abnormalities are common, especially in infants; intravenous infusions may be required for hypoglycemia, hypocalcemia, hypomagnesemia, or acidemia as indicated.

Diuretics. Diuretics are utilized to relieve the edema and pulmonary congestion of heart failure. Available diuretics have a wide range of potency; those most frequently used are furosemide, ethacrynic acid, and thiazides.

Furosemide and **ethacrynic acid** are extremely potent diuretics that are effective when given orally or parenterally. They act in the renal tubules by inhibiting sodium transport and by interfering with diluting mechanisms. A redistribution of blood into the venous pool precedes the diuresis induced by furosemide. With parenteral therapy the induction of diuresis is rapid (within 30 min) and the action short-lived (about 4 hr). The usual parenteral dose of either drug is 1 mg/kg, although in resistant patients doses up to 3 mg/kg have been used. One parenteral dose/24 hr usually suffices, although early in the course of therapy the dose can be repeated 2–3 times in 24 hr if clinical improvement is inadequate. Because furosemide may be administered intramuscularly or intravenously, it is more convenient than ethacrynic acid, which must be given intravenously. It is important to measure serum electrolytes during therapy since hypokalemia or hypochloremic alkalosis can be induced with these potent diuretic agents. Potassium supplementation is advisable because hypokalemia exaggerates signs of digitalis toxicity. The efficacy of therapy is gauged by measuring the urinary volume and by comparing daily body weights. When a constant weight is reached, it should be maintained. Decreases in venous pressure, hepatic size, dyspnea, and edema parallel the diuresis.

Once cardiac failure is compensated, the diuretic may be given orally. The usual oral dose of furosemide or ethacrynic acid is 1 mg/kg 1–2 times daily or every other day. In exceptional instances, 2–3 mg/kg has been used without apparent ill effect.

Thiazides are moderately potent diuretic agents. Since they can be given orally (e.g., chlorothiazide syrup), they are useful in the long term management of cardiac failure. They act by increasing renal excretion of sodium and chloride with an accompanying volume of water. The usual dose of oral chlorothiazide (Diuril) is 20–40 mg/kg/24 hr. Patients maintained on chlorothiazide should also be given potassium to supplement the usual dietary intake.

Infants with refractory heart failure may have secondary hyperaldosteronism which contributes to retention of fluid. It may be suspected when parenteral furosemide therapy does not result in weight loss, diuresis, and natriuresis. The aldosterone antagonist **spironolactone** (Aldactone) (1 mg/kg/dose, 3 times daily) should be considered in these patients in addition to other anticongestive measures. The diuretic effect with natriuresis may not be noted until 2–4 days after initiation of spironolactone therapy. Potassium excretion is decreased by this drug.

Cardiac failure which is resistant to therapy or becomes worse after breakdown of response to previously successful management may be due to (1) deterioration of myocardial function; (2) reactivation of rheumatic fever, superimposed infective endocarditis, or infections of the lungs or of the urinary tract; (3) electrolyte imbalance, especially hypokalemia, hypochloremic alkalosis, or hyponatremia; (4) development of arrhythmia such as atrial fibrillation with rapid ventricular response; (5) inadequate digitalization or digitalis toxicity; or (6) pulmonary embolism, a rare complication in children. If ascites or pleural effusions produce discomfort, fluid should be removed by paracentesis.

Digitalis. This drug is useful in the management of most forms of cardiac failure. The most satisfactory response is obtained in failure due to rheumatic heart disease, paroxysmal tachycardia, and myocardial diseases. In general, patients with primary left ventricular failure respond better than those with primary right-sided failure. The response of patients with congestive cardiac failure due to cyanotic congenital cardiovascular disease is unpredictable because hypoxia, acidosis, and hypoglycemia may complicate the situation.

Many preparations of digitalis are available, but familiarity with only a few is necessary. The dose of digitalis (Table 29–2) and the rapidity of administration depend on the weight of the patient, the severity of congestive cardiac failure, the type of preparation, and, subsequently, the response of the patient.

Digoxin is the form of digitalis used most frequently in pediatric practice because of its availability in oral and parenteral forms, its fast action, and its relatively rapid excretion. The maximal effect of digoxin occurs about 4 hr after administration; it is excreted within 48–72 hr. For *fullterm newborn infants* the total digitalizing dose is 0.03–0.05 mg/kg (30–50 μg/kg), with a daily maintenance dose of about 0.01 mg/kg (10 μg/kg). *Premature infants* should be treated with extreme caution. Some cardiologists prefer to initiate therapy with daily maintenance doses of 0.005–0.010 mg/kg (5–10 μg/kg) and rely principally on diuretic therapy and fluid restriction. Others use a total digitalizing dose of 0.03–0.035 mg/kg (30–35 μg/kg) followed by 0.005–0.010 mg/kg (5–10 μg/kg) as daily maintenance. For *infants beyond the neonatal period but under 2 yr of age* the total *oral* digitalizing dose is 0.05–0.06 mg/kg (50–60 μg/kg) with a daily maintenance dose of about 0.01–0.015 mg/kg (10–15 μg/kg). The *parenteral* digitalizing dose is 75% of the oral dose. For *children over 2 yr of age* the oral digitalizing dose is 0.04–0.05 mg/kg (40–50 μg/kg) with a daily oral maintenance dose of 0.01–0.015 mg/kg (10–15 μg/kg). In this age group the parenteral digitalizing dose is also 75% of the oral dose. In older children the total digitalizing dose should not exceed 2.0 mg.

Half of the digitalizing dose is given initially, followed by one fourth of the total dose in 6–8 hr, and the remaining fourth is given in another 6–8 hr. Alternatively, 3 one third doses are used, or oral maintenance is begun without a loading dose, depending in part on the nature of the indication for the use of digitalis. The daily maintenance dose may be started 12 hr later and is given preferably in 2 equally divided doses.

It cannot be overemphasized that *any dosage schedule of any digitalis preparation is only a guide* because of the significant individual differences in response and toxicity among patients. The dose may need to be modified after part or all of the calculated digitalizing dose has been given. Fullterm and premature newborn infants have a distinct intolerance for digitalis preparations. In these patients, digitalization should be controlled by careful and repeated physical examination, supplemented by electrocardiography. In some infants the only reliable guide to digitalis intoxication is electrocardiographic evidence of arrhythmia.

The digitalizing dose is effective if the cardiac rate is reduced, the venous pressure and liver size are decreased, dyspnea is relieved, and diuresis occurs. Electrocardiographic evidence of digitalis effect includes shortening of electrical systole, depression of the S-T segment with T wave inversion, and lengthening of the P-R interval. In many patients the difference between an adequate and a toxic dose of digitalis is small.

Serum digoxin levels reflect the higher dosages used in infants. In older children and adolescents the serum level is about 1.3 ng/ml when the above dosage schedule is used and frequently exceeds 2.0 ng/ml when signs of toxicity are present. In infants the serum level is about 2.8 ng/ml when the above dosage schedule is used and frequently exceeds 4.0 ng/ml when toxicity is manifested. The diagnosis of digitalis toxicity should not depend on measurements of serum levels; rather, it depends principally on the clinical and electrocardiographic signs described below. Knowledge of serum digoxin levels, however, is helpful in confirming the clinical evidence of toxicity, managing accidental ingestion, monitoring patients with renal disease, and confirming the compliance of patients on long term therapy.

The signs of digitalis toxicity include anorexia, nausea, vomiting, diarrhea, visual symptoms, dizziness, headache, and arrhythmias. However, in pediatric patients clinical signs are often absent, arrhythmias being the critical manifestation of toxicity. Virtually every form of rhythm disturbance may be seen. The arrhythmias include atrial and ventricular extrasystoles, paroxysmal atrial tachycardia with block, atrial flutter or fibrillation, bundle branch block, ventricular tachycardia, and intra-atrial block. Atrial arrhythmias are most likely among infants. If signs of digitalis toxicity occur, the drug must be discontinued and an infusion of potassium administered if there is hypokalemia. Diphenylhydantoin is frequently helpful in management of arrhythmias due to digitalis toxicity, especially supraventricular tachycardia. However, other agents may be equally efficacious. Lidocaine is utilized for ventricular ectopy. Electrical cardioversion may be necessary for ventricular flutter or fibrillation; but it should be emphasized that these severe disturbances can be produced following cardioversion for less dangerous arrhythmias in the presence of digitalis toxicity. Sinus bradycardia usually responds to atropine but, in occasional patients with a high degree of atrioventricular block, temporary artificial ventricular pacing may be necessary. Manifestations of digitalis toxicity may persist for many days despite discontinuance of the drug.

Other Inotropic Agents. These agents are reserved for emergency situations when cardiac output is low (Sec 5.1 and 13.47). Isoproterenol (0.05–0.2 μg/kg/min) is useful, but its effectiveness is limited because of the associated severe tachycardia and primary augmentation of blood flow to skin and skeletal muscle. *Dopamine*, the precursor of norepinephrine, has been used in a dose of 5–10 μg/kg/min, but doses as high as 30 μg/kg/min have sometimes been necessary. This drug is useful when depression of arterial pressure and cardiac output are moderate; it is not always effective in the presence of severe hypotension.

Vasodilators. These agents have been reserved for patients with intractable heart failure who are unresponsive to conventional therapy, but their range of use has now been broadened. In patients with congestive cardiac failure, cardiac dilatation and elevated systemic vascular resistance increase the afterload on the left ventricle. In this situation vasodilation increases cardiac output and reduces myocardial oxygen consumption. Observations in children have shown a salutary effect from infusion of nitroprusside (0.5–8 μg/kg/min) in severe heart failure. Since this drug is also a potent venodilator, it is essential to monitor pulmonary artery diastolic pressure as well as systemic blood pressure, cardiac output, and thiocyanate blood levels (Sec 5.1 and 13.47). In some instances epinephrine is used at the same time as nitroprusside. Chronic oral vasodilator therapy with prazosin or hydralazine is being evaluated in children. These agents appear to be most helpful in patients with severe cardiomyopathy.

The convalescent care of children who have suffered congestive cardiac failure is important. As the child improves, greater freedom of activity may be permitted, and schoolwork may be resumed.

13.78 CARDIOGENIC SHOCK

See also Sec 5.46.

Cardiogenic shock may occur as a complication of (1) severe cardiac dysfunction, often following surgery; (2) septicemia; (3) severe burns; (4) immunologic disease; (5) severe debilitation; and (6) acute central nervous system disorders. It is characterized by low cardiac output and hypotension resulting in inadequate tissue perfusion.

Treatment of shock is aimed at reinstitution of adequate cardiac output and peripheral perfusion to prevent the untoward effects of prolonged ischemia to vital organs. Under normal conditions, the cardiac output is most reliably increased by increasing heart rate with positive chronotropic agents such as isoproterenol and epinephrine. However, in the presence of marked tachycardia a further increase in heart rate will not be useful and may decrease cardiac output by decreasing diastolic filling time. Cardiac output may also be increased by increasing stroke volume. If fluid administration is increased, the Starling mechanism results in increased stroke volume by increasing central venous pressure and ventricular filling pressure (preload). When central venous pressure is low, infusion of volume will reliably increase cardiac output. Optimal filling pressure is variable and depends on a number of extracardiac factors including ventilatory support with high positive end-expiratory pressure, peak inspiratory pressure, and intra-abdominal pressure. The increased pressure necessary to fill relatively noncompliant right ventricles should also be considered, particularly in post-open heart patients. If incremental fluid administration does not result in improved cardiac output, abnormal myocardial contractility and/or high afterload must be implicated as the cause of low cardiac output.

Myocardial contractility will improve when treatment of the basic cause of shock is instituted, hypoxia eliminated, and acidosis corrected. Isoproterenol, dopamine, epinephrine, and dobutamine are catecholamines which will also improve cardiac contractility, increase heart rate, and ultimately increase cardiac output. The major differences among these agents lie in their effects on the peripheral vascular bed. Isoproterenol has pure beta-adrenergic action and will decrease peripheral vascular resistance throughout the therapeutic dosage range. Dopamine has no significant peripheral beta effects on vascular resistance at dosage of 2–4 μg/kg/min. However, at higher doses (>10 μg/kg/min) it causes significant dose-dependent increases in systemic vascular resistance via alpha receptors similar to those seen with norepinephrine. Dopamine also has specific effects on the renal vascular system and increases renal blood flow out of proportion to other vascular beds. In addition, at high doses dopamine may cause an increase in pulmonary vascular resistance, particularly in patients with extremely reactive pulmonary vascular circulations. Epinephrine will also cause a dose-dependent increase in systemic vascular resistance via the alpha-adrenergic receptors. All of these agents may cause tachycardias and, particularly in the presence of hypoxia and/or acidosis, may be arrhythmogenic. A major advantage of the catecholamines is their very short half-lives; therefore, positive inotropic effects are virtually immediate, and untoward effects can be reversed quickly by discontinuation of the drug. Dobutamine has "pure" central beta effects similar to those of isoproterenol with fewer peripheral vascular effects than the other catecholamines at equivalent therapeutic doses. Along with dopamine, dobutamine has less chronotropic effect than isoproterenol and is more advantageous when a marked tachycardia is pres-

ent prior to initiation of an inotropic agent. These drugs may be used in various combinations.

The use of cardiac glycosides to treat acute low cardiac output states should be approached with caution. Digoxin is less effective than the catecholamines in that action begins slowly, even with intravenous administration. In addition, adverse effects may result from larger doses, and toxicity is less predictable, depending on myocardial and serum potassium and calcium levels. Since it is quite common for patients with cardiovascular shock to have compromised renal perfusion, the administration of digoxin may result in high persistent blood levels because it is excreted in the kidneys. When digoxin is required for such patients, a lower dosage scale should be used and serum digoxin levels frequently monitored.

Patients with cardiogenic shock may have a marked increase in systemic vascular resistance resulting in high afterload and poor peripheral perfusion. If high systemic vascular resistance is persistent and the administration of positive inotropic agents alone does not result in improved tissue perfusion, the use of afterload reducing agents may be appropriate, e.g., nitroprusside used in combination with dopamine.

Sequential evaluation and management of cardiovascular shock is mandatory (Sec 5.46). Table 13–11 provides an outline for the treatment of acute cardiac circulatory failure under most circumstances. The treatment of infants and children with low cardiac output syndrome following cardiac surgery requires specific management dependent on the nature of the operative procedure and the patient's status after surgery. (See Sec 13.16.)

Awan NA, Miller RR, Mason DT: Comparison of effects of nitroprusside and prazosin on left ventricular function and the peripheral circulation in chronic refractory congestive heart failure. Circulation 57:152, 1978.
Benzing G III, Helmsworth JA, Schreiber JT, et al: Nitroprusside after open-heart surgery. Circulation 54:467, 1976.
Black-Schaffer B: Infantile endocardial fibroelastosis: A suggested etiology. Arch Pathol 63:281, 1957.
Chatterjee K, Parmley WW: The role of vasodilator therapy in heart failure. Prog Cardiovasc Dis 19:301, 1977.
Dungan WT, Doherty JE, Harvey C, et al: Tritiated digoxin XVIII. Studies in infants and children. Circulation 46:983, 1972.

Table 13–11   TREATMENT OF CARDIOGENIC SHOCK

Goal—to improve peripheral perfusion by increasing cardiac output

Cardiac output = Heart rate × stroke volume

| | DETERMINANTS OF STROKE VOLUME | | |
	Preload	Contractility	Afterload
Parameters measured	CVP, PCWP	CO, BP	CO, BP
Abnormal physiologic manifestations	Low CVP and/or PCWP ↓ CO ↓ BP	Elevation of CVP and/or PCWP ↓ CO ↓ BP	Elevation of CVP and/or PCWP ↓ CO → ↑ BP
Treatment to improve cardiac output	Volume expansion 　Plasma 　Whole blood	Catecholamines 　Isoproterenol, 0.05–2 µg/kg/min 　Dopamine, 5–20 µg/kg/min 　Dobutamine, 2.5–10 µg/kg/min	Vasodilatation 　Nitroprusside, 0.5–8 µg/kg/min 　Hydralazine, 0.2 mg/kg

CVP	= Central venous pressure.	↓	= Decreased.
PCWP	= Pulmonary capillary wedge pressure.	→	= Normal.
CO	= Cardiac output.	↑	= Increased.
BP	= Blood pressure.		

Goodwin JF: Prospects and predictions for the cardiomyopathies. Circulation 50:210, 1974.

Goroodischer R, Jusko WJ, Yaffe SJ: Tissue and erythrocyte distribution of digoxin in infants. Clin Pharmacol Ther 19:256, 1976.

Greenwood RD, Nadas AS, Fyler DC: The clinical course of primary myocardial disease in infants and children. Am Heart J 92:549, 1976.

Harris LC, Nghiem QX: Cardiomyopathies in infants and children. Prog Cardiovasc Dis 25:255, 1972.

Hayes CJ, Butler VP Jr, Gersony WM: Serum digoxin studies in infants and children. Pediatrics 52:561, 1973.

Hernandez A, Burton RM, Pagtakhan RD, et al: Pharmacodynamics of ^{3}H-digoxin in infants. Pediatrics 44:418, 1969.

Lang D, von Bernuth G: Serum concentration and serum half-life of digoxin in premature and mature infants. Pediatrics 59:902, 1977.

13.79 DISEASES OF THE PERICARDIUM

Major diseases that involve the pericardium include bacterial, tuberculous, fungal, and parasitic infections; acute rheumatic fever; rheumatoid arthritis; systemic lupus erythematosus; uremia; radiation injury; thalassemia; trauma; pericardial cysts; congenital malformations; postpericardiotomy syndrome; and chronic constrictive disease. In some instances the involvement of the pericardium is only 1 manifestation of a more generalized illness, and the prominence of the pericardial component will vary depending on the disease entity.

Hemodynamics. Pericardial inflammation results in an accumulation of fluid in the pericardial space. The nature of the fluid varies according to the etiology of the pericarditis; it may be serous, fibrinous, purulent, or hemorrhagic. Cardiac tamponade occurs when the amount of pericardial fluid reaches a level which causes cardiac function to be compromised. In a healthy child there is 10-15 mm of fluid in the pericardial space, whereas in an adolescent with pericarditis an excess of 1000 mm of fluid may accumulate. For every increment of fluid accumulation there is an increase in pericardial pressure. With small amounts of fluid the pressure rises slowly, but once a critical level is reached, there is a rapid rise in pressure culminating in severe cardiac compression. Inhibition of ventricular filling during diastole, elevated systemic and pulmonary venous pressures, and, if untreated, eventual compromised cardiac output and shock occur.

Clinical Manifestations. The 1st symptom of pericardial disease is often precordial pain. The major complaint is a sharp, stabbing sensation of the left shoulder; the chest, shoulder, and back pain which occurs may be exaggerated by lying and relieved by sitting, especially leaning forward. Since there is no sensory innervation of the pericardium, the pain is probably referred pain from diaphragmatic and pleural irritation. Cough and fever may also occur. The presence of symptoms or signs associated with other organs and systems depends on the basic etiology of the pericarditis.

On physical examination, many of the findings relate to the degree of fluid accumulation in the pericardial sac. The presence of a friction rub is helpful but may be a late sign in acute pericarditis, becoming apparent only after the effusion is reduced. Narrow pulses, quiet precordium, distant heart sounds, neck vein distention, and a paradoxical pulse suggest significant fluid accumulation.

Greater than 20 mm Hg of *paradoxical pulse* in a child with pericarditis is a reliable indicator of the presence of cardiac tamponade; 10-20 mm Hg change is equivocal. There is normally a slight decrease in systolic arterial pressure during inspiration. With cardiac tamponade this normal phenomenon is exaggerated, probably because of decreased left heart filling with the inspiratory phase of respiration. In order to determine the degree of pulsus paradoxus, one first measures the exact systolic blood pressure during normal expiration. The manometer is then slowly allowed to fall. The point when the systolic pressure is heard equally well during inspiration and expiration is then recorded. The difference between the 2 determinations represents the degree of paradox. Significant pulsus paradoxus may also be present with severe dyspnea of any origin and is not infrequent in patients who have emphysema or asthma or who are being ventilated with a positive pressure respirator. In these patients the paradoxical pulse is due to a marked increase in intrathoracic pressure. Determination of the etiology of paradoxical pulse in a child on a ventilator after cardiac surgery may be difficult to assess since in this situation more than 1 potential mechanism is possible.

Laboratory Data. The specific laboratory findings in pericarditis depend on the underlying disease. The effects of pericarditis on the *electrocardiogram* are multiple. Low voltage of the QRS complexes results from a damping effect of pericardial fluid. Pressure on the myocardium by fluid or exudate produces a current of injury that results in mild elevation of S-T segments. Generalized T wave inversion occurs as a consequence of associated myocardial inflammation. The S-T segment and T wave changes with pericarditis are more generalized than those seen with myocardial infarction, and the S-T segment elevations tend to precede the T wave changes. There may be an interval when the ECG is in a transitional phase and appears to be normal. This may occur during the acute phase of the illness prior to diagnosis. In some instances clear cut abnormalities are never identified.

A relatively large pericardial effusion must be present to cause an enlarged cardiac shadow with the usual "water-bottle" configuration on *chest roentgenogram* (Fig 13-80). In most instances the lung fields are clear. With constrictive disease the heart is relatively small and calcification may be present.

The *echocardiogram* is a sensitive technique for evaluation of the size and progression of pericardial effusions. Normally, the pericardium is closely adherent to the epicardium, and the 2 layers can be only narrowly separated by the ultrasound beam. In patients with pericardial effusion a clear echo-free space is recorded between the epicardium and pericardium. A posterior effusion is recorded behind the left ventricular epicar-

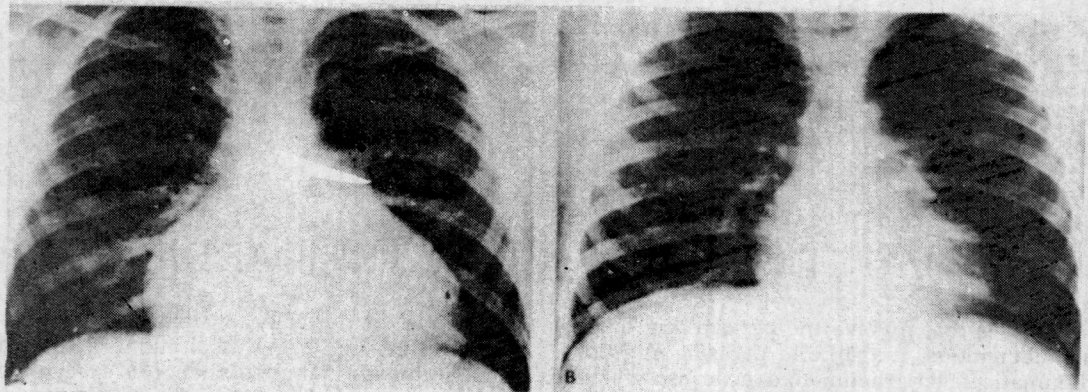

Figure 13–80   Roentgenograms in acute nonspecific pericarditis. *A*, Increase in cardiopericardial shadow due to pericardial effusion. *B*, One mo later after complete recovery.

dium and ends at the junction of the left ventricle and left atrium. An anterior effusion will be recorded between the chest wall and the anterior right ventricular wall. The presence of both an anterior and posterior effusion generally indicates that a large collection of fluid is present. False positives are rare in the hands of experienced echocardiographers.

Differential Diagnosis. *Viral and Acute Benign Pericarditis.* These entities are considered to be synonymous since most episodes of acute benign pericarditis follow or coincide with viral illness. Viruses recognized to cause pericarditis include coxsackievirus B, influenza, echovirus, and adenovirus. The pathogenesis is unclear but may be related to a hypersensitivity reaction to a viral disease. However, pericardial inflammation is not necessarily the precursor of a generalized inflammatory process. Most cases are mild, and recovery occurs within several wk. However, in rare instances the patient will be severely ill, and cardiac tamponade may ensue. Thus, the term "benign" may not be appropriate.

For most patients, only symptomatic therapy is indicated and the disease is self-limiting. However, there are patients in whom a chronic relapsing illness occurs. The differential diagnosis between these patients and those with collagen vascular disease may be difficult. These patients respond dramatically to anti-inflammatory therapy with corticosteroids. Milder forms may be controlled with aspirin. The clinical course may vary from months to 1–2 yr, during which time the patients are dependent on drug therapy for suppression of the pericarditis. Ultimately, the patients improve and the prognosis is good.

The clinical differential diagnosis between acute pericarditis and myocarditis may be difficult. Indeed, in patients with pericarditis there is usually a myocardial inflammatory component, and the reverse is also true. However, management of these conditions is quite different; anti-inflammatory treatment and urgent response to cardiac tamponade are appropriate in the former, and therapy for congestive heart failure is required in the latter. The echocardiogram is useful in the differential diagnosis as it will demonstrate large pericardial effusions and can also indicate the presence of myocardial dysfunction.

Purulent Pericarditis. This is most often associated with bacterial infections such as pneumonia, epiglottitis, meningitis, or osteomyelitis. Initially, the diagnosis of pericardial involvement may be accompanied by signs and symptoms of the primary infection. However, once the purulent process is established, the course is fulminant, terminated by acute cardiac tamponade and death. Open pericardial drainage is mandatory, along with appropriate intravenous antibiotics. Although closed pericardial aspiration provides exudate for diagnostic purposes and may be lifesaving in the face of severe cardiac compression, it should not be considered final therapy. Without open drainage, tamponade will recur because with large effusions only a small reaccumulation of pericardial fluid may markedly increase intrapericardial pressure. Management with open pericardial drainage has significantly increased survival in patients with this disease. The most common organisms implicated in purulent pericarditis are *Staphylococcus aureus, Hemophilus influenzae* type b, and *Neisseria meningitidis.* Tuberculous pericarditis rarely occurs in children outside of underdeveloped countries. Extensive treatment with antituberculous chemotherapy is required, and late constriction may occur.

Acute Rheumatic Fever. Pericarditis occurs in acute rheumatic fever as a component of pancarditis. Rheumatic pericarditis occurs with acute valvulitis, and a murmur of mitral and/or aortic regurgitation will be audible. If there is no evidence of acute valvulitis, another cause should be considered. Pericarditis, along with the other manifestations of acute rheumatic pancarditis, appears to respond to therapy with steroids. Cardiac tamponade is extremely rare.

Rheumatoid Arthritis. Pericarditis is not an uncommon manifestation of rheumatoid arthritis in children. Most often, pericardial inflammation is associated with the other signs of rheumatoid arthritis. However, rarely, pericarditis may be the only manifestation of rheumatoid arthritis and precede the onset of arthritis by months or even years. Differentiation of rheumatoid pericarditis from that seen with other collagen vascular disease, particularly lupus erythematosus, may be difficult. Treatment consists of steroids or salicylates, which may be needed on a long term basis to suppress the disease process.

Uremia. Uremic pericarditis occurs only in the presence of prolonged severe renal failure and results from chemical irritation of the pericardium secondary to the metabolic abnormalities. It has been a feature primarily of end-stage chronic renal disease and in most instances is an incidental part of the clinical picture. However, with the advent of chronic hemodialysis, uremic pericarditis has been recognized as a more chronic problem, culminating in cardiac tamponade. Pericardial effusion has also been implicated in the etiology of recurrent hypotension during hemodialysis. If adequate relief of uremic pericarditis does not occur with hemodialysis, pericardiectomy is recommended.

Neoplastic Disease. Neoplastic pericardial effusion is seen in patients with Hodgkin disease, lymphosarcoma, and leukemia and results from direct neoplastic invasion of the pericardium. Cardiac tamponade may occur late in the course of the illness. Rarely, pericardial infiltration is the initial manifestation of neoplastic disease, and the diagnosis can be made by examination of the pericardial fluid for neoplastic cells.

In addition to showing signs of direct invasion of the pericardium, patients with malignancy may develop pericarditis as a result of radiation therapy to the mediastinum. This manifestation may be related to the radiation dose and to the technique utilized.

Postpericardiotomy Syndrome. Postpericardiotomy syndrome is characterized by fever, chest pain, pleural and pericardial effusion, and fluid retention. It is seen 1–2 wk following open heart surgery in approximately 15% of postoperative patients. The syndrome is a nonspecific hypersensitivity reaction to trauma to the pericardium and epicardial surface of the heart. High titers of anti-heart antibody have been reported to correlate with clinical signs of the syndrome.

In most patients, postpericardiotomy syndrome is a relatively short illness, and affected children will generally respond well to anti-inflammatory therapy with aspirin or corticosteroids. Treatment is maintained for 1–3 mo, but recurrences may be seen as long as 1 yr postoperatively and require reinstitution of therapy.

Constrictive Pericarditis. This represents a special problem in terms of both the clinical picture and the differential diagnosis. Predisposing pericardial diseases include purulent pericarditis, tuberculous pericarditis, acute benign or viral pericarditis, mediastinal irradiation for intrathoracic malignancy, neoplastic invasion of the pericardium, and trauma. In most instances constriction occurs months or years after the initial insult but occasionally may be an acute, rapidly progressive process. Despite the numerous known etiologies, constrictive pericarditis most often occurs without a preceding illness or generalized systemic disease.

The clinical manifestations of this disease occur as a result of impairment of diastolic ventricular filling, compromise of myocardial contractility, and resultant depression of cardiac function. Hepatomegaly and ascites may appear to be out of proportion to the other signs and symptoms and thus suggest chronic liver disease. However, liver function studies are only mildly abnormal, and careful physical examination will reveal other sometimes subtle findings of constriction including neck vein distention, narrow pulses, quiet precordium, distant heart sounds, faint pericardial friction rub, and paradoxical pulse. Typical findings become apparent gradually and thus may be easily overlooked. The auscultatory presence of an early pericardial knock and the appearance of calcification of the pericardium on chest roentgenogram are the more obvious manifestations which become apparent when the disease is well established. Protein-losing enteropathy with hypoproteinemia and lymphopenia may be seen in association with constriction.

Constrictive pericarditis may be difficult to distinguish from chronic constrictive cardiomyopathy. Impairment of myocardial function occurs with both conditions. However, the myocardial disease of constrictive pericarditis is almost always reversible with pericardiectomy. At times, despite all efforts at differentiation a definite diagnosis can be made only by exploratory thoracotomy and direct examination of the pericardium.

Surgical intervention is the only therapy for constrictive pericarditis. The surgical procedure of choice is radical pericardiectomy with decortication of the pericardium over a wide area of the heart to include the systemic and pulmonary veins. In most patients surgical intervention elicits a rapid response characterized by increased cardiac output and prompt diuresis.

Benzing G III, Kaplan S: Purulent pericarditis. Am J Dis Child 106:289, 1963.
Gersony WM, Hordof AH: Infective endocarditis and diseases of the pericardium. Pediatr Clin North Am 25:831, 1978.
Gersony WM, McCracken GH: Purulent pericarditis in infancy. Pediatrics 40:224, 1967.

13.80   DISEASES OF THE BLOOD VESSELS

13.81   ANEURYSMS AND FISTULAS

Aneurysms are not common in children and occur most frequently in the aorta in association with coarctation of the aorta, patent ductus arteriosus, and Marfan syndrome and in intracranial vessels (Sec 21.21). They may also occur secondary to an infected embolus; infection contiguous to a blood vessel; trauma; congenital abnormalities of structure, especially of the medial coat; and arteritis, e.g., periarteritis nodosa and Takayasu arteritis (Sec 9.70). Aneurysm of the coronary arteries with thrombosis and myocardial infarction may complicate the mucocutaneous lymph node syndrome (Sec 9.68).

Arteriovenus fistulas may be limited to small cavernous hemangiomas or may be extensive (Sec 21.21 and 24.7). The most common sites for arteriovenous fistulas in infants and children are intracranial, hepatic, and pulmonary (Sec 13.29) and the extremities. They have also been described in other parts of the body, especially in vessels in or near the thoracic wall. The fistulas, though usually congenital, may follow trauma or be a manifestation of hereditary hemorrhagic telangiectasia (Rendu-Osler-Weber syndrome).

Cardiovascular manifestations occur only in association with large communications when arterial blood flows into a low pressure venous system, increasing local venous pressure and decreasing arterial flow beyond the fistula. Systemic arterial resistance falls because of the runoff of blood through the fistula. Compensatory mechanisms include tachycardia and increased stroke volume so that cardiac output rises. Blood volume is also increased. Cardiac failure may develop with large arteriovenous fistulas.

The clinical manifestations of arteriovenous fistulas appear to depend primarily on the size of the shunt across the fistula and the associated vasodilatation. Discoloration of the skin, prominence of the superficial vessels, and local edema may occur at the site of the fistula or involve the entire extremity. Prominent arterial pulsations and a continuous machinery bruit may be heard over the site of the lesion, especially over one of traumatic origin. The venous pressure is elevated in an affected extremity, the temperature of the skin may be higher at the site of the lesion than elsewhere, and the venous oxygen saturation distal to the fistula is higher than that of venous blood taken from the comparable site on the unaffected side. In extensive fistulas, left ventricular hypertrophy and dilatation, a widened pulse pressure, and congestive heart failure occur. Arteriograms after injection of contrast material into an artery proximal to the fistula confirm the diagnosis.

Intracranial arteriovenous fistulas are described in Sec 21.21.

Hepatic arteriovenous fistulas may be localized or generalized in the liver. The fistula may be located between the hepatic artery and ductus venosus or portal vein. Congenital hemorrhagic telangiectasia may also be associated with hepatic fistula. Large arteriovenous fistulas are associated with a large cardiac output and heart failure. Hepatomegaly is usual, and systolic or continuous murmurs may be audible over the liver.

Peripheral arteriovenous fistulas usually involve the extremities. These lesions are associated with disfigurement, swelling of the extremity, and visible hemangiomas. Since only a small minority result in large arterial runoff, cardiac failure is not common.

Treatment. Surgical removal of a large arteriovenous fistula is often not possible, especially in the most severe cases with large arterial runoffs, such as intracranial and hepatic types. Medical management of congestive heart failure is initially helpful in the neonate with these conditions; with time the size of the shunt may diminish and symptoms spontaneously regress. Hemangiomas of the liver often completely disappear with time. This abnormality is occasionally treated by steroid administration and/or local radiation, but the beneficial effects of this management have not been established; individual patients display marked variations in clinical course without treatment. Surgical removal of a large fistula may be indicated in the presence of severe cardiac failure and the lack of improvement with medical treatment. However, surgical treatment may be unsuccessful when the lesion is extensive and diffuse or is located in a position where adjoining tissue may be injured during the surgery or related procedures, e.g., extubation.

13.82   COLD INJURY

See also Neonatal Cold Injury, Sec 7.54.

Frostbite.   Frostbite may occur especially in the face or extremities from exposure to cold. The mechanism of cellular injury is related to intravascular thrombosis or ice crystal formation in the tissues. The skin initially becomes red and then pale or, rarely, cyanotic as the arterioles remain in spasm in an effort to preserve body heat. During thawing, hyperemia occurs, and blisters may form on the skin. Gangrene may occur if early relief is not obtained.

Treatment consists of rapidly rewarming the skin of the affected area that is still white. Analgesics are usually necessary. Massage of the damaged area or rubbing with snow or ice is contraindicated. Other therapeutic measures which have yielded equivocal results include anticoagulants (especially heparin), low molecular weight dextran, and sympathectomy. Meticulous local care to the injured area is essential. Recovery of an extremity from apparent severe frostbite can be striking and, in the absence of infection, amputation or excision of tissue should be postponed as long as possible to make certain that it is necessary.

Chilblains (Pernio).   This form of cold injury, presumably vascular in origin, consists of a (sometimes blistering) localized erythema which itches, may be painful, and frequently results in swelling and in scabbing ulcerations of the affected areas. The mechanism is unknown, but it is probably related to prolonged constriction of peripheral arterioles, which is manifested by pallor and coldness of the subsequently affected areas during cold, particularly damp, weather.

The tops of the ears and tips of the fingers and toes are most frequently affected; the exposed legs of girls wearing skirts and no stockings may also be involved. Without further exposure the lesions usually clear in 1–2 wk but may persist longer.

Avoidance of prolonged chilling or the protection of susceptible areas with woolen caps, gloves, and stockings can be preventive. Therapeutic measures include dermal corticosteroid preparations for itching and antibiotics for infection.

13.83   EMBOLISM

Emboli, consisting of bacteria and fibrinous material, usually arise from mural thrombi or vegetations in the heart or large blood vessels, as, for example, in infective endocarditis. Within weeks after bacteriologic cure of infective endocarditis, sterile embolization to major vessels may occur; this does not necessarily indicate reactivation of infection. Other rarer causes of emboli include fat (secondary to trauma) and foreign material such as air introduced accidentally into the vascular system during therapeutic procedures. Large systemic emboli are common in patients with left atrial myxomas. In patients with atrial or ventricular septal defects, emboli arising in the systemic venous system may pass across the defect and enter the systemic arterial system (paradoxic embolus).

When emboli lodge in an artery, the blood flow through the vessel is compromised. If the collateral circulation is inadequate, necrosis or gangrene supervenes; if the collateral circulation is adequate, the emboli may be silent. Thus, an embolus to the arteries of the forearm may not give rise to symptoms and is detected only if the radial or ulnar pulse disappears.

The manifestations of arterial emboli depend on their location: e.g., an embolus to the middle cerebral artery may result in hemiparesis; an embolus to the femoral artery may result in ischemia with or without gangrene in the leg. If the emboli are infected, an abscess may form locally.

Treatment consists of eradicating the source of the emboli, e.g., infective endocarditis, and increasing the collateral circulation to the affected area. Surgical therapy such as embolectomy, sympathectomy, and amputation may be indicated in specific instances.

Pulmonary embolism is not as frequent in children as in adults. Thrombosis of the calf veins with secondary pulmonary embolism is rare in children. Pulmonary emboli may arise secondary to infective endocarditis in patients with a left to right shunt and have also occurred in association with ventriculocardiovascular shunts for hydrocephalus. Occasionally, pulmonary embolism is seen in older children with chronic rheumatic heart disease and atrial fibrillation. Multiple small pulmonary emboli are described in Sec 13.64.

13.84 THROMBOSIS

Frequently arterial thrombosis in children is associated with polycythemia secondary to severe cyanotic congenital heart disease. A frequent site for such thrombi is the brain, but they may occur anywhere in the body. They may be precipitated by dehydration.

Venous thrombosis may occur in veins used for prolonged intravenous therapy or in an area surrounding an infective process. The inflammation in the vein (phlebitis) is usually local; the thrombi seldom give rise to emboli.

Any severe illness associated with intense dehydration may be complicated by venous thrombosis. This complication is relatively frequent in infants with severe diarrhea or septicemia and in children with cyanotic congenital heart disease and polycythemia who become dehydrated. The common sites for thrombosis are the sagittal sinus of the brain and the renal vein with extension into the inferior vena cava (Sec 21.21 and 16.49).

WELTON M. GERSONY

13.85 SYSTEMIC HYPERTENSION

Hypertension, which occurs in approximately 30% of the adult population, places affected individuals at increased risk for heart disease, stroke, and renal failure. The incidence of hypertension in the neonatal intensive care nursery is about 2.5%. In children the incidence is 1–2%, in adolescents approximately 10%, and in black young adults 25–30%. Thus hypertension is at least as common in childhood as congenital heart disease, and because of its incidence and potential morbidity, blood pressure measurement should be part of every routine pediatric physical examination. In preadolescents hypertension is almost always secondary in nature, and morbidity usually relates to the underlying cause of the hypertension. In black adolescents and adolescent white males 80%–100% of the hypertension is "essential" and the morbidity relates to those who, if untreated, will go on to develop chronic fixed adult hypertension with its attendant risks.

Definition. In identifying hypertension it is important that standardized methods be used to measure blood pressure. The bladder of the pressure cuff should encircle the upper arm without either a gap or overlap and should cover at least two thirds of the length of the arm. Diastolic measurements should be read at the 4th Korotkoff sound, and the pressure measurement should be made with the patient seated and in as relaxed a setting as possible. In infants and young children instruments which utilize the Doppler technique are quite reliable. Initially, elevated values must be assessed against repeated measurements; blood pressure values generally fall over 3–4 successive measurements before reaching a consistent level. Pressure consistently above the 95th percentile for age should be considered abnormal. Fig 13–1 and 13–2 show standard percentiles for seated boys and girls.

Etiology. Tables 13–12 and 13–13 list the causes of hypertension in children. Table 13–14 lists conditions associated with transient hypertension. In general when considering the etiology of hypertension, children can be divided into 2 groups. In the 1st group are patients with overt symptoms who usually have diastolic blood pressures above 100–110 mm Hg regardless of age; these patients have secondary hypertension and an underlying disease is found in 63–94% of cases. Those in the 2nd group are found incidentally to have elevated blood pressure and are most often asymptomatic; 95% of the patients within this group have essential hypertension.

Table 13–12 POTENTIALLY CURABLE FORMS OF HYPERTENSION IN CHILDREN

Renal
Unilateral dysplastic kidney
Unilateral hydronephrosis
Unilateral pyelonephritis
Traumatic damage, e.g., constrictive perirenal hematoma
Renal tumors and isolated cysts (including Robertson-Kihari syndrome)
Unilateral multicystic kidney
Unilateral ureteral occlusion
Ask-Upmark kidney
Vascular
Coarctation of the thoracic or abdominal aorta
Abnormalities of the renal artery (stenosis, arteritis, fibromuscular dysplasia, thrombosis, neurofibromatosis, fistula, aneurysm)
Renal vein thrombosis
Postumbilical catheterization
Adrenal
Neuroblastoma, ganglioneuroma
Pheochromocytoma
Cortical hyperplasia (adrenogenital syndrome)
Cushing disease
Primary aldosteronism (hyperplasia or adenoma)
Adrenal carcinoma
Miscellaneous
Vascular or unilateral renal parenchymal abnormalities from irradiation
Ingestion of excessive amounts of licorice
Administration of glucocorticoids
Administration of oral contraceptives

Approximately 75–80% of patients with **secondary hypertension** have a renal abnormality (Chapter 16). Chronic pyelonephritis is found in 25–50% of these patients, although the pathophysiologic relationship is unclear. Chronic loss of renal tissue may result in hypertension because of salt retention, diminution of vasoactive substances secreted by the kidneys, and elevated renin-angiotensin levels. A proportion of children with pyelonephritis do not develop hypertension until they become azotemic. Hypertension per se may predispose to recurrent urinary tract infection, and pyelonephritis may simply unmask essential hypertension. On the other hand, both infection and the hypertension may be a function of underlying renal disease.

Table 13–13 SOME CONDITIONS ASSOCIATED WITH INCURABLE FORMS OF CHRONIC HYPERTENSION IN CHILDREN

Renal
Chronic glomerulonephritis (all forms including those due to connective tissue diseases)
Bilateral congenital dysplastic kidneys
Chronic bilateral pyelonephritis
Bilateral hydronephrosis
Polycystic kidneys
Medullary cystic disease
Postrenal transplantation (rejection damage)
Vascular
Surgically irremediable abnormalities of the renal artery
Surgically irremediable coarctation of the aorta
Generalized hypoplasia of the aorta
Miscellaneous
Essential hypertension
Renal parenchymal damage from irradiation
Lead nephropathy (late)
Dexamethasone suppressible hypertension
ACTH-dependent hypertension

Table 13–14 CONDITIONS ASSOCIATED WITH TRANSIENT OR INTERMITTENT HYPERTENSION IN CHILDREN

Renal
Acute poststreptococcal glomerulonephritis
Hemolytic-uremic syndrome
Anaphylactoid purpura with nephritis
After renal transplant (immediate and during episodes or rejection)
After blood transfusion in patients with azotemia
Anephric hypervolemia
Vasomotor nephropathy (acute tubular necrosis)
Miscellaneous
Administration of corticosteroids (including DOCA and ACTH)
Administration of oral contraceptives
Preeclamptic toxemia of pregnancy
Elevated intracranial pressure (any cause)
After surgery, especially of genitourinary tract
During traction on legs, e.g., for reduction of a fracture
Hypercalcemia
Burns
Guillain-Barré syndrome
Poliomyelitis
Leukemia
Hypernatremia
Stevens-Johnson syndrome
Familial dysautonomia
Acute intermittent porphyria
Mercury poisoning
Amphetamine overdosage
Postcoarctation syndrome
Polycythemia
After renal biopsy or administration of sympathomimetics (nose drops, decongestants, cold preparations)
Phencyclidine
Drug withdrawal hypertension (clonidine, propranolol, Aldomet)

Acute and chronic glomerulonephritis, cystic disease of the kidney, renal dysplasia, renal tumors, and traumatic injury are other renal causes of hypertension. Wilms tumor may be associated with marked hypertension secondary either to renovascular compression or to secretion of a pressor substance.

Renovascular lesions occur in approximately 12% of secondary cases. Because of the stenosis, renin production is increased, elevated levels of angiotensin result in vasoconstriction, and aldosterone-mediated salt and water retention occurs. Neurofibromatosis, trauma, and fibromuscular hyperplasia are common causes. Some neonates with umbilical artery catheters (highly placed) have also been found to be hypertensive; renovascular disease occurs in a large proportion of these cases.

Approximately 2% of secondary hypertension in childhood is due to coarctation of the aorta. The consequences of delayed detection of coarctation may include persistent hypertension despite surgical correction, severe left heart dysfunction, intermittent claudication, and cerebral hemorrhage. Coarctation is especially common in Turner syndrome and neurofibromatosis.

Pheochromocytoma (Sec 18.28) is a cause of hypertension in approximately 0.5% of secondary cases; about one third of children have extra-adrenal tumors and another one third have multiple tumors. Unlike adults, children with pheochromocytoma tend to have persistent elevation of blood pressure. The tumor is seen in 5% of children with neurofibromatosis. Neuroblastoma and ganglioneuroma can also cause hypertension because of excess circulating catecholamines.

Other factors cause less than 10% of secondary hypertension. Of special interest are the adrenocortical causes of hypertension. Defects in 17- and 11-hydroxylation result in increased ACTH stimulation and consequent mineralocorticoid excess. Salt and water retention, hypokalemia, and hypertension result (Sec 18–21 and 18–25). Cushing syndrome with hypertension in children is most often secondary to adrenal tumor. The excessive glucocorticoids have mineralocorticoid effects, increase vascular reactivity, and may produce increased plasma renin substrate.

Oral contraceptives are the most common cause of secondary hypertension in adolescent females; up to 15% become hypertensive while taking them. The hypertension may persist for as long as 12 mo after stopping the contraceptives. Possible mechanisms include stimulation of the renin-angiotensin aldosterone system, direct effect of estrogen on salt and water retention, and sensitization of vascular smooth muscle to angiotensin II.

Patients with **essential hypertension** are rarely symptomatic; the diastolic blood pressures are almost always below 120 mm Hg and tend to hover just above the 95th percentile for age. The vast majority of hypertensive adolescent males have essential hypertension; Blacks are at greatest risk and show a dramatic postpubertal increased incidence. Approximately 30–40% of this group will have essential hypertension as adults. Risk factors include borderline blood pressure itself, genetic predisposition to hypertension, obesity, and high salt intake. Other associated factors include hyperuricemia, abnormal response to glucose loading, persistent tachycardia, and low urine kallikrein excretion.

Hemodynamically, children with essential hypertension progress from a high cardiac output, normal systemic vascular resistance state to the adult pattern of normal cardiac output with elevated systemic vascular resistance. Adolescent hypertensives show echographic evidence of increased contractility compared to normotensive controls suggesting high catecholamine output and a hyperdynamic circulation in the juvenile form of essential hypertension.

Clinical Manifestations. In general, elevated blood pressure per se produces few, if any, signs or symptoms in childhood until sustained at high levels (diastolic >120 mm Hg). In cases of secondary hypertension the clinical manifestations of the underlying disease most frequently draw attention to the hypertension. Table 13–15 summarizes the clinical and diagnostic characteristics of some of the curable causes of secondary hypertension. Elevated blood pressure may, however, produce significant symptomatology such as headaches, dizziness, and changes in vision. In infants and children there may also be a history of irritability and frequent wakefulness at night. If hypertensive encephalopathy is imminent or present, vomiting, hyperpyrexia, ataxia, seizures, stupor, posturing, and coma are prominent features. Cerebral hemorrhage, although uncommon, may result in focal signs. Facial paralysis as the sole manifestation of hypertension is sufficiently common to warrant blood pressure measurement. The sudden progressive increase in previously stable hypertension,

accelerated hypertension, may result in necrotizing renal arteriolitis, hypertensive encephalopathy, or heart failure. Arrhythmia and myocardial infarction may occur secondary to prolonged left ventricular strain. In *malignant hypertension* changes in the fundi may include papilledema, peripheral arterial spasm, hemorrhage, and exudates.

Diagnosis. A careful history and physical examination together with relatively few simple laboratory studies identify the majority of secondary causes of hypertension. Screening tests should include height, weight, urinalysis, complete blood count, serum electrolytes, blood urea nitrogen, creatinine, and uric acid. Fasting cholesterol and triglycerides should also be obtained in older children. Urine culture should be done even if the sediment is normal in all hypertensive females and in males with evidence of underlying renal disease. Chest roentgenograms and ECG are relatively unproductive as screening tests but should still be performed. If these tests are negative, further evaluation is warranted.

The standard intravenous pyelogram (IVP) has potential value in renovascular disease (delayed calyceal appearance) and in delineation of renal size and anatomy, and may suggest the presence of an intra- or extrarenal mass. However, up to 40% of IVPs may be normal in proven renal or renovascular disease. Biopsy should be reserved for those patients with evidence of glomerulonephritis.

Indications for renal angiography include IVP evidence of renovascular disease, increased plasma renin activity, severe hypertension, and previous history of umbilical artery catheterization. Approximately 55% of patients with renovascular disease have an abdominal bruit, but up to 40% of children with normal arteriography can have an abdominal bruit. Renal vein renins should be obtained at the time of arteriography.

Plasma renin activity standardized to sodium intake should be obtained. Supine and upright samples obtained 2–4 hr apart are most reliable. The results may not be reliable if the patient is taking contraceptives or hypertensive medication. Levels of aldosterone must also be standardized for urinary sodium. In most patients with adrenocortical disease or pheochromocytoma, history and physical examination indicate the need for urinary catechols, 17-OH steroids, and 17-ketosteroids. If pheochromocytoma is diagnosed, sequential blood sampling along the inferior vena cava should be done to help localize an extra-adrenal tumor; this must be done cautiously and under alpha-adrenergic blockade.

Essential hypertension is suggested by patient age, race, level of blood pressure, obesity, and paucity of symptomatology. There may also be a family history of hypertension or coronary artery disease and excessive salt intake.

Course and Prognosis. These depend upon the nature of the underlying disease. Previously grim statistics on survival, especially in patients with renal etiologies, may have been improved by the widespread use of dialysis, renal transplant, and aggressive pharmacologic management. In renovascular disease renal vein renin ratios of greater than 1.5 are predictive of successful

Table 13–15 SOME CLINICAL AND LABORATORY MANIFESTATIONS OF CURABLE FORMS OF HYPERTENSION IN CHILDREN

Cause of Hypertension	History	Physical Examination	Readily Available Laboratory Data	Other Studies Which May Be Indicated
Coarctation of aorta Thoracic	Nonspecific, Turner neurofibromatosis	Femoral pulses decreased or delayed; higher BP in arms than legs; systolic murmur	ECG-LVH; chest x-ray, rib notching	Cardiac catheterization
Abdominal	Nonspecific	Abdominal bruit may be present; femoral pulses may or may not be normal; there may or may not be a significant pressure differential between arms and legs	ECG	Abdominal angiogram
Renovascular disease	History of trauma to abdomen or flank; pain; hematuria (aneurysm); symptoms of aldosteronism may be present	Bruit in abdomen or flank; café-au-lait spots or other manifestations of neurofibromatosis	Nonspecific unless secondary aldosteronism is present (low K, high CO_2; Na may be normal); fast sequence intravenous pyelogram may be abnormal	Abdominal angiogram; measurement of plasma renin activity from each renal vein
Trauma	Trauma to back or abdomen; hematuria after trauma; closed renal biopsy	May have abdominal bruit or mass	Hematuria; intravenous pyelogram may be helpful	Abdominal angiogram may show fistula or other abnormality
Unilateral renal parenchymal disease	Symptoms of recurrent urinary tract infection; unexplained fever; history of trauma to abdomen or flank; growth retardation	Enlarged kidney, if present, may be helpful; costovertebral angle tenderness with acute infection	Urinalysis may be abnormal; intravenous pyelogram abnormal	Abdominal angiogram may demonstrate stenosis of renal artery associated with, for example, dysplastic kidney; measurement of plasma renin activity from each renal vein; ultrasound examination of the kidney
Neuroblastoma	Dependent on site of abdominal mass found by parent; cough, chest pain, dyspnea; spinal cord compression with neurologic signs and symptoms	Abdominal or other masses palpable	Anemia; abnormal cells in marrow; lytic bone lesions; abnormal intravenous pyelogram	Measurement of catecholamines and their metabolites in the urine; ultrasound and body CT scan
Wilms tumor	Mass found by parent; fever; abdominal pain; hematuria; rarely seizures	Palpable abdominal mass (usually does not cross midline)	Abnormal intravenous pyelogram	Ultrasound and body CT scan
Pheochromocytoma	Episodes of sweating, flushing, or mottling; palpitations or rapid heart beat; episodic headache; weight loss; personality change; polyuria and polydipsia; family history of pheochromocytoma or neurofibromatosis	Tachycardia; flushing; pallor; fever; excess perspiration; palpable tumor; postural hypotension	Hyperglycemia; glucosuria; anemia or polycythemia; leukocytosis; intravenous pyelogram usually not helpful	Measurement of catecholamines and their metabolites in the urine; angiography; measurement of blood catecholamines at various levels in vena cava; pharmacologic tests (e.g., Regitine, histamine, tyramine, glucagon) of limited use
Primary aldosteronism	Periodic muscular weakness; paresthesias; tetany; polyuria; polydipsia; no edema	Muscular weakness; tetany; positive Chvostek or Trousseau sign	Serum Na high, K low, CO_2 high; ECG shows hypokalemia; intravenous pyelogram not usually helpful	Abdomen angiography sometimes helpful; measurement of plasma renin activity, aldosterone (urine and/or blood); renin suppression test; adrenal venography, adrenal imaging
Cushing disease	Retardation of growth and development; weakness; weight gain; easy bruising; change in body habitus	Truncal obesity; buffalo hump; moon facies; hirsutism; red or purple striae	Glucosuria; hyperglycemia; eosinopenia; abnormal dexamethasone suppression test; intravenous pyelogram usually not helpful	Increased plasma cortisol and increased excretion of 17-OHCS in urine; adrenal arteriogram

surgical outcome. Neonates with renovascular disease can be successfully treated medically and the majority weaned from medication within a matter of months. Earlier recognition and surgery in coarctation of the aorta have decreased late morbidity and mortality. Although 90% of children with untreated malignant hypertension die within 1 yr of diagnosis, aggressive drug therapy can prolong their lives. Similarly, *accelerated hypertension* can be arrested with vigorous prompt drug therapy.

Thirty per cent of adolescents with untreated essential hypertension progress to become adult hypertensives. Treatment of moderate and severe essential hypertension in adults reduces morbidity and mortality. Patient risk is directly related to the mean pressure levels. Morbidity and mortality may also be reduced by treating even mild hypertension. Concerns about the effects of antihypertensive medication on growth are gradually being dispelled by reports of normal growth in children followed 2–10 yr.

Treatment. Surgery is the treatment of choice for many of the causes of secondary hypertension such as unilateral renal disease, renovascular disease, coarctation, and both secretory and nonsecretory tumors.

In essential hypertension reduction of salt intake and weight may be all that is required to normalize blood pressure, and these measures should always be initiated. Other nonpharmacologic regimens such as moderate exercise programs, meditation, and biofeedback have not been extensively studied but may result in moderate blood pressure reduction in highly motivated subjects. In patients with positive family histories and elevated fasting lipids, cholesterol should be reduced to less than 300 mg/day; saturated fats should provide less than 10% and dietary fat less than 30% of total daily calories. Smoking should be discontinued.

The pharmacologic approach to hypertension is based upon carefully titrating single agents until either control or dosage maximums are achieved before adding another drug. Table 13–16 summarizes the dosages,

Table 13–16 ANTIHYPERTENSIVE DRUGS

Agent	Mechanism of Action	Starting Dose	Maximum Therapeutic Response	Maximum Dose	Adverse Effects
Diuretic agents					
Chlorothiazide	Diuresis; may have mild immediate vasodilator effects	10 mg/kg/24 hr	14 days	20 mg/kg/24 hr up to 2 gm total	Hypokalemia and hyperuricemia
Hydrochlorothiazide	Diuresis; possible vasodilator effects	1 mg/kg/24 hr	14 days	2 mg/kg/24 hr up to 200 mg total	Hypokalemia and hyperuricemia
Chlorthalidone	Diuresis	1 mg/kg/24 hr	14 days	2 mg/kg/24 hr up to 200 mg total	Hypokalemia and hyperuricemia
Furosemide	Diuresis; possible immediate vasodilator effects	0.5 mg/kg/24 hr	14 days	?	Hypokalemia, ototoxicity, and contraction alkalosis
Spironolactone	Potassium sparing	1 mg/kg/24 hr	14 days	2 mg/kg/24 hr up to 200 mg total	Gynecomastia and amenorrhea
Agents acting on the adrenergic system					
Propranolol*	Beta-adrenergic blockade— central, juxtaglomerular and cardiac	0.5 mg/kg/24 hr	3–5 days	?	Bradycardia, congestive heart failure, bronchospasm, hypoglycemia, rebound hypertension
Methyldopa	Production of "false" neurotransmitter; direct vasodilator, central vasomotor inhibition	10 mg/kg/24 hr	7 days	40 mg/kg/24 hr up to 2 gm total	Rebound hypertension, sedation, positive Coombs, lupus reaction, and sexual dysfunction
Guanethidine	Depletion of norepinephrine at nerve endings; blocks neurotransmitter release	0.2 mg/kg/24 hr	14 days	?	Postural hypotension and sexual dysfunction
Reserpine	Depletes catecholamine stores	0.02 mg/kg/24 hr	7 days	0.07 mg/kg/24 hr up to 2.5 mg total	Sedation, emotional lability, depression, nasal congestion, gastrointestinal tract hypersecretion
Clonidine*	Inhibition of central vasomotor center	3 μg/kg/24 hr	5–7 days	2.4 mg/24 hr	Rebound hypertension
Phenoxybenzamine	Alpha-adrenergic blockade	2 mg/24 hr	5–7 days	?	
Phentolamine	Alpha-adrenergic blockade	0.1 mg/kg/dose	Minutes	5 mg	
Vasodilators					
Hydralazine	Direct arterial dilatation	1 mg/kg/24 hr	3–4 days	Up to 200 mg/24 hr	Postural hypotension, reflex tachycardia, lupus-like syndrome
Diazoxide	Relaxation of smooth muscle	2 mg/kg/dose	Minutes	10 mg/kg/dose	Inhibition of insulin secretion, hyperglycemia
Nitroprusside	Direct arterial and venous dilatation	0.5 μg/kg/min	Minutes	10 μg/kg/min	Cyanide toxicity, platelets
Prazosin*	Alpha-adrenergic blockade— arterial and venous dilatation	(?) 10 μg/kg/dose	3–4 days	?	"1st dose" hypotension
Minoxidil	Potent arterial vasodilator	0.02 mg/kg/24 hr		1 mg/kg/24 hr up to 5 mg total	Hypertrichosis
Captopril†	Inhibits conversion of angiotensin I to angiotensin II		Minutes (acute IV); 1–3 mo (chronic PO)		Skin rash, altered taste, proteinuria

*Not approved by FDA for use in children.
†Approved for use only as the "last resort."

modes of action, and prominent side effects of currently used drugs.

Volume-dependent hypertension should respond maximally to diuretic therapy within 2 wk. If an additional agent is added, the diuretic should be continued since most other agents cause secondary salt and water retention. In non-volume-dependent hypertension a diuretic alone will be only moderately effective in less than 40% of the cases, and another agent should be included initially. In children, elevated serum uric acid levels have correlated with serum thiazide levels. Salt restriction should accompany diuretic therapy since excessive dietary salt intake will limit the effectiveness of many diuretics. Since thiazides do not work when the glomerular filtration rate is less than 20–25 ml/min, furosemide is the diuretic of choice with impaired renal function. Spironolactone is ineffective as a single agent. Chlorothiazide has the advantage of coming in a liquid oral preparation, and chlorthalidone has the advantage of single daily dosing.

The beta-adrenergic blockade of propranolol causes reduction in blood pressure by decreasing heart rate and contractility, by reducing beta-stimulated juxtaglomerular secretion of renin, and possibly by inhibiting the central vasomotor center. Considering the hemodynamic profile of adolescent and young adult essential hypertension, propranolol may be the agent of choice for these patients. Caution must be used when treating diabetics, and the drug is contraindicated in asthma, hypoglycemic metabolic disease, and congestive heart failure.

Although reserpine can provide smooth control of blood pressure without postural symptoms, side effects can be severe. Severe depression occurs in 25% of patients taking the drug. Death from asphyxiating nasal congestion has occurred in breast-feeding neonates of mothers receiving the drug, and gastrointestinal hypersecretion has resulted in hemorrhage and perforation. Phentolamine is used for acute hypertensive crises associated with pheochromocytoma; phenoxybenzamine may provide smooth control of pheochromocytoma-related hypertension.

Diazoxide causes inhibition of insulin secretion and has a markedly variable duration of action. Nitroprusside therapy should be titrated in an intensive care setting with continuous monitoring of blood pressure;

with normal liver and kidney function cyanide toxicity almost never occurs at infusion rates of less than 3 μg/kg/min. Minoxidil is a very potent agent for patients who fail to respond to aggressive multidrug therapy.

Captopril inhibits conversion of angiotensin I to angiotensin II, thus effecting immediate vasodilatation and sustained reduction of aldosterone despite very high renin activity. The drug has value not only in chronic hypertension but also in acute hypertensive encephalopathy and accelerated hypertension. In combination with powerful new vasodilators this drug or others like it may virtually eliminate the need for bilateral nephrectomy in severe drug-resistant hypertension.

Hypertensive emergencies include hypertensive encephalopathy, intracranial hemorrhage, dissecting aneurysms, acute congestive failure and/or myocardial infarction, pheochromocytoma, catheterization pressor crises, postcoarctectomy abdominal crises, and eclampsia. These situations should be treated in an intensive care unit where therapy can be instituted safely and rapidly and drugs titrated while continuously monitoring vital signs.

STEPHEN R. GUERTIN

Case DH, Atlas SA, Sullivan PA, et al: Acute and chronic treatment of severe and malignant hypertension with the oral angiotensin-converting enzyme inhibitor captopril. Circulation 64:765, 1981.

Goldring D, Hernandez A, Choi S, et al: Blood pressure in a high school population. II: Clinical profile of the juvenile hypertensive. J Pediatr 95:298, 1979.

Loggie JMH (ed): Symposium on Hypertension in Childhood and Adolescence. Pediatr Clin North Am 25 (1): February, 1978.

Messerli FH, Frohlich ED, Suarez DH, et al: Borderline hypertension: Relationship between age, hemodynamics and circulating catecholamines. Circulation 64:760, 1981.

Moser M: Less severe hypertension: Should it be treated? Am Heart J 101:465, 1981.

New MI, Baum CJ, Levine L: Nomograms relating aldosterone excretion to urinary sodium and potassium in the pediatric population: Their application to the study of childhood hypertension. Am J Cardiol 37:658, 1976.

Oberfield S, Case DB, Levine L, et al: Use of the oral angiotensin I–converting enzyme inhibitor (captopril) in childhood malignant hypertension. J Pediatr 95:641, 1979.

Report of the Task Force on Blood Pressure Control in Children. Pediatrics 59:797, Supplement 1977.

Sinaiko AR, Mirkin BL: Management of severe childhood hypertension with minoxidil: A controlled clinical study. J Pediatr 91:138, 1977.

13.86   HYPERLIPIDEMIA IN CHILDREN

The hyperlipidemias may cause morbidity and mortality in childhood and adolescence as well as atherosclerotic heart disease presenting in adulthood. The precursors of atherosclerosis, fatty streaks and intimal involvement of arteries with fibrous plaque formation, have been documented in early infancy and may be fully developed in some by the 3rd or 4th decades. The potential, although unproven, benefits of programs directed at preventing or retarding the development of atherosclerosis and coronary disease in children with hyperlipidemia make their identification and management increasingly important.

Etiology and Epidemiology.   The pattern of inheritance of the hyperlipoproteinemias is unclear in most situations, although a homozygous or heterozygous autosomal dominant transmission may be identified in type IIa. However, in the heterozygous state the degree of expression varies from an essentially normal individual to one with a markedly elevated cholesterol and severe symptoms. The genetic control involves the synthesis, breakdown, and possibly transfer of diverse lipids and carbohydrates suggesting that many gene loci must be involved. Individual family trees often demonstrate multiple phenotypes with variability from generation to generation.

Cholesterol is the major blood lipid implicated in the

pathogenesis of atherosclerotic heart disease. It does not circulate in the free state but in combination with 1 of the lipoprotein fractions. For example, the increased cholesterol in conjunction with the increased low density lipoproteins (LDL) in type IIa hyperlipidemia results in an increase in LDL-cholesterol. The receptor theory, first proposed by Brown and Goldstein in 1974, helps to clarify understanding of the mechanisms for the transfer of LDL-cholesterol into cells and for the feedback system to control the production of endogenous cholesterol. Receptors are present on cell surfaces that are responsible for transport of lipoprotein-bound cholesterol into cells; there is an ionic interaction between the protein component and the cell surface. The receptors are specific for LDL-cholesterol and possibly for very low density lipoprotein (VLDL)-cholesterol but not for high density lipoprotein (HDL)-cholesterol. Transport of LDL-cholesterol into the cells leads to a reduction in the production of endogenous cholesterol and an increase in esterification of cholesterol. Patients with familial homozygous hypercholesterolemia (type IIa) have reduced numbers of receptors, and those with heterozygous type IIa have numbers of receptors in between those of the homozygotes and normals. However, LDL receptors, although present on numerous cell types, have not been demonstrated on hepatic cells which are responsible for the majority of endogenously produced cholesterol. Further, the relationship between the receptor theory and the pathogenesis of atherosclerosis remains unclear.

Screening. An appreciation of the normal patterns of serum lipids is a prerequisite to identifying those children with elevated levels. Normal values for children between the ages of 5–18 are presented in Table 29–11*A, B,* and *C.* Reliable normal data for younger children are not yet available. The levels tend to be constant from 6–11 yr; cholesterol begins to drop from ages 11–12 to 15 and then rises again thereafter. Females have higher cholesterol and triglycerides than males. Blacks have higher mean cholesterol and lower mean triglycerides than Whites. Triglycerides behave in an inverse fashion to cholesterol during adolescence. Between the ages of 8–15 yr serial lipid values in individual children correlate significantly with each other over a 5 yr period, although there is some decrease in the general level.

Cord blood screening is not indicated since values for serum cholesterol and triglycerides are unreliable over the 1st years of life. The identification of LDL receptors on lymphocytes may eventually prove useful for accurate identification of patients with homozygous familial hypercholesterolemia. However, at present the method does not distinguish between normals and heterozygotes. Receptors are present even on the lymphocytes of preterm infants.

Screening for hyperlipidemia in the general childhood and young adult population for whom normal values are established is also not indicated. The costs of the tests are high; the tests are not reliable and have high false-positive and false-negative rates; and the effectiveness of treatment is not proved. Alternatively, the identification of affected subjects by screening high risk populations is warranted. The yield is high and treat-ment of patients from families with a history of frequent and severe disease is indicated, despite questions about efficacy, because of their high risk. By defining a high risk population as one in which a 1st degree relative has known coronary artery disease or hyperlipidemia prior to the age of 50, some abnormality (elevated cholesterol, triglycerides, or decreased HDL-cholesterol) may be identified in 60% of the remaining family members.

Risk Factors for Atherosclerosis. Several risk factors correlate positively with the development of atherosclerotic heart disease. These include an elevated total cholesterol, smoking, obesity, and hypertension. The relationship of cholesterol to the type of lipoprotein with which it circulates in vivo is also a factor in identifying the risk of coronary artery disease. Elevated HDL-cholesterol is associated with a reduced risk of developing coronary artery disease while elevated LDL-cholesterol is associated with increased risk. However, it is uncertain whether the protective effect of HDL affects survival.

Clinical Manifestations and Classification. The hyperlipidemias are classified by a combination of clinical and biochemical findings. The 6 known phenotypes are summarized in Table 13–17, which may serve as a guide to the diagnosis and management of the hyperlipidemia. The frequent overlap of clinical and biochemical findings often makes it difficult to identify the phenotype exactly. Family history may be helpful; however, the lack of data on deceased relatives, the paucity of clear genetic definition of most of the disorders, and the variability of the age of onset may make the diagnosis difficult. Nevertheless, it is generally possible to classify an individual's disorder accurately enough to determine the basis for a therapeutic plan.

Treatment. A summary of specific recommendations for the therapy of each type of hyperlipidemia is presented in Table 13–17.

Diet. This remains the most important modality of treatment, either singularly or in conjunction with pharmacologic intervention. The basic principles are: (1) Reduce the total fat content with a specific emphasis on increasing the polyunsaturated/saturated fat (P:S) ratio. Since cholesterol is exclusively an animal product and unsaturated fats also predominate in animals, this diet requires increasing the intake of vegetables, and, to a lesser degree, fish and chicken and reducing the intake of beef and dairy products. The intentional addition of polyunsaturated fats is not recommended. (2) Calorie intake should be reduced to achieve weight loss where indicated. (3) Family counseling is essential to implementing such a dietary regimen, and the emphasis must be placed on involvement of all family members whether affected or not. A low fat, low cholesterol diet is safe for all.

Drugs. Colestipol *(Colestid)* is the most effective cholesterol-lowering agent available. It is not absorbed from the gastrointestinal tract and acts as a bile acid sequestrant binding cholesterol and leading to its increased excretion in the stool. Side effects are not systemic, are usually mild, and are limited to the gastrointestinal tract (constipation, nausea, vomiting, and flatulence). Colestipol is safe and effective in children, and it has been

Table 13–17. CLINICAL MANIFESTATIONS, CLASSIFICATION, AND TREATMENT OF HYPERLIPIDEMIAS

	TYPE I	TYPE IIA	TYPE IIB	TYPE III	TYPE IV	TYPE V
Lipoprotein electrophoretic pattern	Heavy band at origin	Increased density of B band	Increased density of B and pre-B bands	Broad B band (merging of B and pre-B bands)	Increased pre-B band	Heavy band at origin and increased pre-B band
Lipoprotein abnormality	Chylomicrons present	Increased LDL; normal VLDL	Increased LDL and VLDL	LDL and VLDL increased and of abnormal composition	Increased VLDL; LDL not increased	Increased chylomicrons, increased VLDL
Plasma cholesterol	Normal or slightly increased	Elevated	Elevated	Elevated	Normal to slightly increased	Elevated
Plasma triglyceride	Markedly elevated	Normal	Moderately elevated	Moderately to markedly elevated	Markedly elevated	Markedly elevated
Biochemical defect	Lipoprotein lipase deficiency	Possible lack of nonhepatic LDL cell receptors	Unknown	Problem with conversion to LDL	Unknown	Unknown; normal lipoprotein lipase
Onset in childhood	2/3 before age 10	Can be detected in young children; ? at birth	Yes	No	No	No
Atherosclerotic heart disease	No	Yes	Yes	Yes	Questionable	Questionable
Signs and symptoms	Xanthoma, lipemia retinalis, abdominal pain, pancreatitis	1. Nothing to severe coronary heart disease 2. Xanthomas, tendinitis	Same as type IIa	Palmar, planar, and tendinous xanthoma	Obesity, diabetes, usually asymptomatic	Same as type I
Treatment	Low fat diet; unresponsive to presently available drugs	Low fat diet; drugs include colestipol, nicotinic acid, probucol	Same as type IIa; weight loss if obese	Low fat diet, weight loss, clofibrate	Low fat diet, weight loss, clofibrate	Low fat diet; ? clofibrate

demonstrated to lower cholesterol 20–30% in conjunction with diet.

Clofibrate (Atromid-S) is the most effective agent in lowering the VLDL lipoprotein fraction and serum triglyceride. It is not an effective agent for lowering cholesterol and should not be used as a 1st line drug for type IIa disease, the most common of the hyperlipidemias. The mechanism of action is unknown. Liver toxicity is reported as well as an increased incidence of malignant neoplasms and gastrointestinal problems. Its efficacy and safety in children have not been established.

Other pharmacologic agents have been utilized to lower blood lipids including thyroxine, estrogens, neomycin, nicotinic acid, and Probucol (Lorelco). Of these the only useful additions may be the latter 2, although there is no information on the efficacy or safety of *Probucol* in children. *Nicotinic acid* is not generally useful alone, but its combination with colestipol is more effective than either drug alone. This has also been suggested as a means of raising HDL-cholesterol, but large trials are necessary before this can be recommended.

Surgical therapy including portacaval shunts and ileal bypass have been tried with little or no success. *Plasmapheresis* has also been utilized to lower plasma cholesterol in adults and children with at least short term improvement. It may prove useful in severely affected and otherwise unresponsive patients.

Moderate *alcohol* ingestion and *physical activity* are inversely related to coronary artery disease. Recent studies suggest that these effects may be secondary to an associated elevation of HDL-cholesterol, which itself reduces the risk of coronary artery disease.

Hyperlipidemia is a family problem with both short term and long range implications for children and their families. Pediatricians are frequently the physicians most involved with the entire family, and, using appropriate guidelines as discussed above, they should identify, treat as indicated, and work along with other health professionals to provide comprehensive management of this family problem.

I. BRUCE GORDON

Andersen GE, Johansen KB: LDL receptor studies in children with heterozygous familial hypercholesterolemia (FH): Measurement of sterol synthesis in blood lymphocytes. Acta Paediatr Scand 69:447, 1980.

Andersen GE, Johansen KB: LDL receptor studies in term and pre-term infants. Acta Paediatr Scand 69:577, 1980.

Andersen GE, Lous P, et al: Screening for hyperlipoproteinemia in 10,000 Danish newborns. Acta Paediatr Scand 68:541, 1979.

Breslow JL: Pediatric aspects of hyperlipidemia. Pediatrics 62:510, 1978.

Brown MS, Goldstein JL: Receptor-mediated control of cholesterol metabolism. Science 191:151, 1976.

Ellefsom KD, Elveback LR, Hodgson PA, et al: Cholesterol and triglycerides in serum lipoproteins of young persons in Rochester, Minnesota. Mayo Clin Proceed 53:307, 1978.

Enos WF, Holmer RH, Beyer J: Coronary disease among United States soldiers killed in action in Korea. JAMA 152:1090, 1953.

Frerichs RR, Srinivasan SR, et al: Serum cholesterol and triglyceride levels in 3446 children from a biracial community. The Bogalusa Heart Study. Circulation 54:302, 1976.

Gordon T, Castelli WP, et al: High density lipoprotein as a protective factor against coronary heart disease: The Framingham study. Am J Med 62:707, 1977.

Hennekens CH, Willett W, et al: Effects of beer, wine, and liquor in coronary deaths. JAMA 242:1973, 1979.

Ho YK, Brown MS, Bilheimer DW, et al: Regulation of low density lipoprotein receptor activity in freshly isolated human lymphocytes. J Clin Invest 58:1465, 1976.

Keys A: Alpha lipoprotein (HDL) cholesterol in the serum and the risk of coronary heart disease and death. Lancet 2:603, 1980.

King ME, Breslow JL, et al: Plasma-exchange therapy of homozygous familial hypercholesterolemia. N Engl J Med 302:1457, 1980.

Lauer RM, Connor WE, et al: Coronary heart disease risk factors in school children: The Muscatine Study. J Pediatr 86:607, 1975.

Morrison JA, deGrood I, et al: Plasma cholesterol and triglyceride levels in 6775 school children, ages 6–17. Metabolism 26:1199, 1977.

Morrison JA, et al: Parent-child associations at upper and lower ranges of plasma cholesterol and triglyceride level. Pediatrics 62:468, 1978.

ver Brervhet JP, Vercaemst R, et al: Evolution of lipoprotein patterns in newborns. Acta Paediatr Scand 69:593, 1980.

Willett W, Hennekens CH, et al: Alcohol consumption and high density lipoprotein cholesterol in marathon runners. N Engl J Med 303:1159, 1980.

DISEASES OF THE BLOOD 14

DEVELOPMENT OF THE HEMATOPOIETIC SYSTEM

As long as animals remained small and the cells of their bodies had direct access to the surrounding sea water, exchange of gas and nutrients was easily effected by simple diffusion. With the evolution of multicellular and terrestrial organisms came development of a vascular system and hemic fluid. Blood probably originated as a simple saline solution similar to sea water, cellular components with specialized functions coming soon thereafter. Among the principal functions of blood cells are transport of respiratory gases, hemostasis, and phagocytosis and other defense mechanisms. Most advanced organisms have separate lines of blood cells, each with specialized functions.

Blood formation in the human embryo can be recognized as early as the 3rd wk after conception. Large, primitive hematopoietic elements are then widely scattered through mesodermal tissues, intimately associated with developing vascular channels. By 2 mo active hematopoiesis is established in the liver, which is the main site of blood formation during the middle portion of fetal life. After about 6 mo hematopoiesis shifts gradually to the medullary spaces, and by birth most blood formation normally takes place in bone marrow.

Active hematopoietic tissue (red marrow) fills the medullary spaces of the bones of infants. During childhood fatty tissue (yellow marrow) gradually replaces hematopoietic tissue in the long bones, active blood formation in the older child and adult being concentrated in ribs, sternum, vertebrae, pelvis, skull, clavicles, and scapulas. The yellow marrow of the extremities can resume active hematopoiesis in response to certain severe hematologic stresses.

Study of the bone marrow provides valuable information in the evaluation of many hematologic diseases. Marrow aspiration is safe and technically simple. Although the marrow aspirate represents only a minute sample of the entire hematopoietic tissue, in most instances there is a striking uniformity of aspirates taken simultaneously from multiple sites. In the infant the preferred sites for aspiration are the proximal tibia and posterior iliac crest. In older children the posterior iliac crest provides a large marrow-bearing space which is not adjacent to major blood vessels or vital organs. Marrow biopsy using special instruments such as the Jamshidi needle permits more accurate assessment of marrow cellularity than is possible through simple aspiration. Biopsy is also useful for detecting focal involvement of marrow in metastatic or granulomatous processes. Table 14–1 lists the types and proportions of cells that occur in marrow of normal infants and children.

14.1 THE RED CELLS

Synthesis of red cells requires a constant supply of amino acids, iron, certain vitamins, and other trace nutrients. Production of red cells is regulated by a specific hormone—erythropoietin. The prohormone of erythropoietin is produced in the epithelial cells of the glomerular tuft and is activated by a serum factor to become biologically active erythropoietin. The process is stimulated by decreases in tissue oxygenation. The principal action of erythropoietin is to induce differentiation of stem cells into an erythrocytic sequence. The early erythrocyte precursors, erythroid-committed progenitor cells, then undergo successive cellular division. Studies of bone marrow in tissue culture have added to understanding of red cell development. After culture of small mononuclear, lymphocyte-like marrow cells in semi-solid media for 5–6 days, small numbers of erythropoietin sensitive precursors form recognizable clusters of red cells called colony-forming units, erythroid (CFUe). At 12–14 days larger burst-forming erythroid units (BFUe) appear, which are believed to be the most primitive committed erythroid precursors (no longer erythropoietin sensitive). Cellular differentiation as the red cell attains maturity includes condensation and

Table 14–1 DIFFERENTIAL COUNTS OF BONE MARROW DURING INFANCY AND CHILDHOOD

Age	Blasts %	Pro- Myelo- cytes %	Myelo- cytes and Meta- myelocytes %	Bands and Poly- morpho- nuclears %	Eosino- phils %	Lympho- cytes %	Nucleated Red Blood Cells %	Myeloid/ Erythroid (M:E) Ratio
Birth	1	2	5	40	1	10	40	1.2/1
7 days	1	2	10	40	1	20	25	2.1/1
6 mo–2 yr	0.5	0.5	8	30	1	40	20	2.0/1
6 yr	1	2	15	35	1	25	20	2.7/1
12 yr	1	2	20	40	1	15	20	3.2/1
Adult	1	2	21	44	2	10	20	3.5/1

extrusion of the nucleus and production of hemoglobin. Ninety per cent of the dry weight of the mature red cell is hemoglobin.

14.2 HEMOGLOBIN

The combustion that is essential to life requires that tissues receive a constant supply of oxygen. The evolutionary development of oxygen-carrying proteins, the hemoglobins, has increased the capacity of blood to give fluid transport to this gas. Further, the combination of oxygen with and its dissociation from hemoglobin are accomplished without expenditure of metabolic energy.

Hemoglobin is a complex protein consisting of iron-containing heme groups and the protein moiety, globin. A dynamic interaction between heme and globin gives hemoglobin its unique properties in the reversible transport of oxygen. The hemoglobin molecule is a tetramer made up of 2 pairs of polypeptide chains, each chain having a heme group attached. The polypeptide chains of various hemoglobins are of chemically different types. For example, the hemoglobin of the normal adult (Hgb A) is made up of alpha (α) and beta (β) polypeptide chains, 1 pair of each. Hemoglobin A can therefore be represented as $\alpha_2\beta_2$. Alpha and beta chains differ from each other in both the number and sequence of amino acids, and their synthesis is directed by separate genes.

Within the red cells of the embryo, fetus, child, and adult, 6 different hemoglobins may normally be detected: the embryonic hemoglobins, Gower 1, Gower 2, and Portland; the fetal hemoglobin, Hgb F; and the adult hemoglobins, Hgb A and A_2. The electrophoretic mobilities of hemoglobins vary with their chemical structures. The compositions of the polypeptide chains of human hemoglobins are listed in Table 14–2. The time of appearance and quantitative relations between these hemoglobins are determined by complex developmental processes. The relations are depicted in Fig 14–1. Two sets of genes for α polypeptide chains are located on human chromosome 16. β, γ, and δ genes are closely linked on chromosome 11.

Embryonic Hemoglobins. The blood of early human embryos contains 2 slowly migrating hemoglobins, Gower 1 and Gower 2, and Hgb Portland, which has Hgb F–like mobility. The zeta (ζ) chains of Hgb Portland and Gower 1 are structurally quite similar to α chains. Both Gower hemoglobins contain a unique type of polypeptide chain, the epsilon (ϵ) chain. Hgb Gower 1 has the structure $\zeta_2\epsilon_2$ and Gower 2, $\alpha_2\epsilon_2$. Hgb Portland has the structure $\zeta_2\gamma_2$. In embryos of 4–8 wk gestation the Gower hemoglobins predominate, but by the 3rd mo they have disappeared.

Fetal Hemoglobin. Hemoglobin F contains gamma polypeptide chains in place of the beta chains of Hgb A. Hgb F can be represented as $\alpha_2\gamma_2$. Its resistance to denaturation by strong alkali is usually used in its quantitation. After the 8th gestational wk Hgb F is the predominant hemoglobin; in the 6 mo old fetus it constitutes 90% of the total hemoglobin. Then a gradual decline occurs so that at birth Hgb F averages 70% of the total. Synthesis of Hgb F decreases rapidly postnatally, and by 6–12 mo of age only a trace is present. Less than 2.0% can be detected by alkali denaturation in older children and adults. Hgb F is heterogeneous because of 2 types of γ chains, whose synthesis is directed by 2 sets of genes. The chains differ at position #136 in the presence of either a glycine (Gγ) or an alanine (Aγ) residue. In the newborn the relative proportion or ratio of Gγ to Aγ chain is 3:1.

Adult Hemoglobins. Some Hgb A ($\alpha_2\beta_2$) can be detected in even the smallest embryos. Therefore, it is possible as early as 16–20 wk gestation to make a prenatal diagnosis of major β chain hemoglobinopathies, such as sickle cell anemia and thalassemia major. By the 6th mo of gestation there is about 5–10% of Hgb A present. A steady increase follows so that at term Hgb A averages 30%. By 6–12 mo of age the normal adult hemoglobin pattern appears. The minor adult hemoglobin component Hgb A_2 contains delta (δ) chains and has the structure of $\alpha_2\delta_2$. It is seen only when significant amounts of Hgb A are also present. At birth less than 1.0% of Hgb A_2 is seen, but by 12 mo of age the normal level of 2.0–3.4% is attained. Throughout life the normal ratio of Hgb A to A_2 is about 30:1.

Table 14–2 THE NORMAL HUMAN HEMOGLOBINS

HEMOGLOBIN NAME	FORMULA	COMMENT
Gower 1	$\zeta_2\epsilon_2$	Major embryonic hemoglobins Not present after 3rd mo of gestation
Gower 2	$\alpha_2\epsilon_2$	
Portland	$\zeta_2\gamma_2$	
Fetal (γ^G)	$\alpha_2\gamma_2^{136\ glycine}$	Predominant hemoglobin throughout fetal life, alkali-resistant
(γ^A)	$\alpha_2\gamma_2^{136\ alanine}$	
A_1	$\alpha_2\beta_2$	Major adult hemoglobin
A_2	$\alpha_2\delta_2$	Detectable postnatally

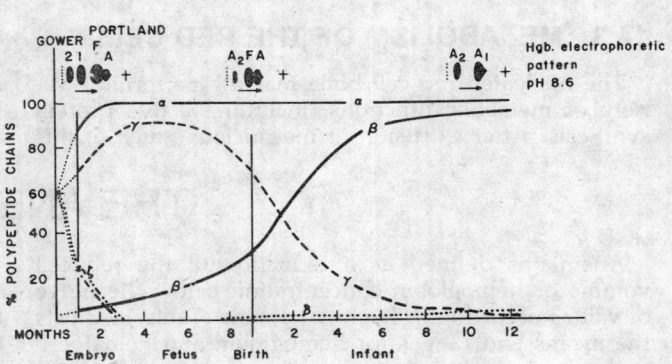

Figure 14–1 Proportions of the various human hemoglobin polypeptide chains through early life. The hemoglobin electrophoretic pattern typical for each period is also shown. (Modified from Pearson HA: J Pediatr 69:466, 1966.)

Normal Relations of the Various Hemoglobins. During fetal life and early childhood the rates of synthesis of gamma and of beta chains and the amounts of Hgb A and of Hgb F are inversely related. How this reciprocal relation is regulated is uncertain. By analogy with microbiologic genetics, a "switch mechanism" involving regulator genes has been postulated which during fetal life facilitates gamma chain synthesis while beta and delta chain production is repressed. After birth the "switch" is reversed so that fetal hemoglobin synthesis is inhibited and the adult hemoglobins accumulate. These regulatory mechanisms have not been clearly defined, nor has any therapeutic maneuver been able to switch on Hgb F synthesis postnatally. Were it possible to do so, the clinical courses of thalassemia major and sickle cell anemia could be dramatically modified. •

Alterations of the Hemoglobins by Disease. Since hemoglobins containing epsilon chains are normally present only very early in intrauterine life, they are largely of theoretic interest. Small amounts of the Gower hemoglobins have been detectable in a few newborn infants with 13–15 trisomy. Increased levels of Hgb Portland have been found in cord blood of stillborn infants with homozygous α-thalassemia.

Levels of fetal hemoglobin may be influenced by a variety of factors. In persons heterozygous for β-thalassemia (β-thalassemia trait) the postpartum decrease of Hgb F is retarded; about 50% of such persons have elevated levels of Hgb F (more than 2.0%) in later life. In homozygous thalassemia (Cooley anemia) and in hereditary persistence of fetal hemoglobin, large amounts of Hgb F are characteristically found. In patients with major beta chain hemoglobinopathies (Hgb SS, SC, and so on) Hgb F is usually elevated, particularly during childhood. Finally, moderate elevations of Hgb F may be seen in many diseases accompanied by hematologic stress, such as hemolytic anemias, leukemia, and aplastic anemia, because of the presence of a minor population of red cells which contain increased amounts of Hgb F, as can be demonstrated by the acid-elution staining technique of Kleihauer and Betke. Tetramers of γ chains (γ_4 or Hgb Bart's) or β chains (β_4, Hgb H) may be seen in α-thalassemia syndromes.

The normal adult level of Hgb A_2 (2.4–3.4%) is seldom altered. Levels of Hgb A_2 exceeding 3.4% are found in most persons with the β-thalassemia trait and in those with megaloblastic anemias secondary to vitamin B_{12} and folic acid deficiency. Decreased Hgb A_2 levels are found in iron deficiency anemia and α-thalassemia.

14.3 METABOLISM OF THE RED CELL

The nucleated red cell bone marrow performs a variety of metabolic functions, including active protein synthesis. After extrusion of the nucleus much of this metabolic capacity is lost, including ability to synthesize proteins. Loss of the nucleus makes the red cell a better vessel for oxygen transport, but it imposes upon the red cell a finite life span, for the cell cannot replace or repair its vital enzymatic proteins. The mature red cell contains more than 40 enzymes. Many of these are essential for cellular viability, but genetically determined deficiencies of others, such as catalase, do not interfere with normal survival.

The mature red cell is not metabolically inert. It has no mitochondria, however, and ATP generation cannot occur by oxidative phosphorylation in Krebs cycle reactions. Rather, glucose is utilized and lactic acid produced mostly by anaerobic glycolysis (Embden-Meyerhof pathway); about 10% of glucose is metabolized oxidatively through the pentose phosphate pathway. At least 5 functions for the ATP generated by glucose metabolism are essential for normal cell viability: (1) *Maintenance of electrolyte gradients.* The principal intracellular cation of the red cell is potassium, while that in plasma is sodium. Reversal of the constant tendency for sodium to enter the red cell and concomitantly for potassium to leak out, with preservation of normal ionic gradients, is accomplished by an energy (ATP)-dependent membrane mechanism, the cation pump. When the cation pump fails, sodium and water accumulate within the red cell, causing it to swell and ultimately to hemolyze. Energy is also utilized to maintain low intracellular levels of calcium ion. (2) *Initiation of energy production.* ATP is required for the initial reaction of glycolysis involving phosphorylation of glucose to glucose-6-phosphate. (3) *Maintenance of red cell membrane and shape.* Energy is required to maintain the complex phospholipid structure of the red cell membrane. Maintenance of the biconcave shape is probably also energy dependent. (4) *Maintenance of heme iron in the reduced (ferrous) form.* Oxidative potentials within the red cell may cause oxidation of the iron of hemoglobin. Hemoglobin containing ferric iron (methemoglobin) is ineffective in oxygen transport. Moreover, if peroxides and other oxidant substances are not inactivated, hemoglobin may be denatured and precipitated. Cells containing such denatured hemoglobin are rapidly removed from the circulation. Protection of the red cell from the detrimental effects of oxidation ultimately depends upon NADPH and NADH. These compounds are continually regenerated by activities of the glycolytic pathway and pentose shunt. In many genetically determined deficiencies of glycolytic and pentose pathway enzymes hemolytic states occur because the energy necessary to perform these vital functions cannot be generated. (5) *Maintenance of the levels of organic phosphates such as 2,3-diphosphoglycerate (2,3-DPG) and ATP within the red cells.* These compounds interact with hemoglobin and have profound effects upon oxygen affinity.

THE ANEMIAS

Anemia is defined as a reduction of the red cell volume or hemoglobin concentration below the range of values occurring in healthy persons. Table 14–3 lists the means and ranges for hemoglobin and hematocrit values by age groups of well nourished children. Recent extensive studies of American children suggest that there may be racial differences in hemoglobin levels. Black children appear to have levels which average

Table 14–3 HEMATOLOGIC VALUES DURING INFANCY AND CHILDHOOD

	Hemoglobin GM/DL		Hematocrit %		Reticulocytes %	Leukocytes WBC/MM.³		Differential Counts					
								Neutrophils %		Lymphocytes %	Eosinophils %	Monocytes %	Nucleated Red Cells
Age	Mean	Range	Mean	Range	Mean	Mean	Range	Mean	Range	Mean*	Mean	Mean	/100 WBC
Cord blood	16.8	13.7–20.1	55	45–65	5.0	18,000	(9–30,000)	61	(40–80)	31	2	6	7.0 (3–10)
2 wk	16.5	13.0–20.0	50	42–66	1.0	12,000	(5–21,000)	40		48	3	9	0
3 mo	12.0	9.5–14.5	36	31–41	1.0	12,000	(6–18,000)	30		63	2	5	0
6 mo–6 yr	12.0	10.5–14.0	37	33–42	1.0	10,000	(6–15,000)	45		48	2	5	0
7–12 yr	13.0	11.0–16.0	38	34–40	1.0	8000	(4500–13,500)	55		38	2	5	0
Adult													
Female	14	12.0–16.0	42	37–47	1.6	7500	(5–10,000)	55	(35–70)	35	3	7	0
Male	16	14.0–18.0	47	42–52									

*Relatively wide range.

about 0.5 gm/dl lower than those of white children of comparable age and socioeconomic status, possibly in part because of the relatively high incidence of α-thalassemia and nutritional anemias in Blacks.

Although reduction in amount of circulating hemoglobin decreases the oxygen-carrying capacity of the blood, few physiologic disturbances occur until the hemoglobin level falls below 7–8 gm/dl. Below this level pallor becomes evident in skin and mucous membranes. Physiologic adjustments to anemia include tachycardia, increased cardiac output, a shift in the dissociation curve which makes oxygen more readily available to the tissues, and a deviation of blood flow toward vital organs and tissues. In response to anemia or hypoxia the concentration of 2,3-DPG increases within the red cell. The resultant "shift to the right" of the oxygen dissociation curve, by reducing the affinity of hemoglobin for oxygen, results in more complete transfer of oxygen to the tissues. The same shift may also occur at high altitude in response to a decrease in oxygen content of inspired air. When moderately severe anemia develops slowly, surprisingly few symptoms or objective findings may be evident, but weakness, tachypnea, shortness of breath on exertion, tachycardia, cardiac dilatation, and congestive heart failure ultimately result from increasingly severe anemia, regardless of its cause.

Anemia is not a specific entity but an indication of an underlying pathologic process or disease. A useful physiologic (erythrokinetic) classification of the anemias of childhood divides them into 2 large groups: (1) those resulting primarily from decreased production of red cells or hemoglobin; and (2) those in which increased destruction or loss of red cells is the predominant mechanism. In Table 14–4 the important anemias of childhood are classified by these criteria. In addition, a morphologic classification is often used, the red cells being characterized by their mean corpuscular volume (MCV) as microcytic (MCV <75 fl), macrocytic (MCV >100 fl), or normocytic (75–100 fl). In every case of significant anemia it is essential to describe the morphologic characteristics of the red cells, to determine the relative importance of defective red cell production and of cell destruction in the genesis of the anemia, and, when possible, to identify the basic etiologic process.

Table 14–4 CLASSIFICATION OF THE ANEMIAS

Anemias resulting primarily from inadequate production of red cells or hemoglobin
  Decreased numbers of red cell precursors in the marrow
    "Pure red cell" anemias
      Congenital pure red cell anemia
      Acquired pure red cell anemias (TEC)
  Inadequate production despite normal numbers of red cell precursors
    Anemia of infection, inflammation, and cancer
    Anemia of chronic renal disease
    Congenital dyserythropoietic anemias
  Deficiency of specific factors
    Megaloblastic anemias
      Folic acid deficiency or malabsorption
      Vitamin B_{12} deficiency, malabsorption, or transport
      Orotic aciduria
    Microcytic anemias
      Iron deficiency
      Pyridoxine-responsive and X-linked hypochromic anemias
      Lead poisoning
      Thalassemia trait
Hemolytic anemias
  Intrinsic abnormalities of the red cell
    "Structural" defects
      Hereditary spherocytosis
      Hemolytic elliptocytosis
      Paroxysmal nocturnal hemoglobinuria
      Pyropyknocytosis
    Enzymatic defects (nonspherocytic hemolytic anemias)
      Enzymes of glycolytic pathway; pyruvate kinase, hexokinase, and others
      Enzymes of the pentose phosphate pathway and glutathione complex
    Defects in synthesis of hemoglobin
      Hgbs S, C, D, E, etc., alone and in combination
      Thalassemia
  Extrinsic (extracellular) abnormalities
    Immunologic disorders
      Passively acquired antibodies (hemolytic disease of the newborn)
        Rh isoimmunization
        A or B isoimmunization
        Other blood group families
      Active antibody formation
        Idiopathic autoimmune hemolytic anemia; cold agglutinin diseases
        Symptomatic—lupus, lymphoma
        Drug-induced
    Nonimmunologic disorders
      Toxic from drugs, chemicals
      Infections—malaria, clostridium

See also anemia in pancytopenias and leukemia.

Anemias Resulting from Inadequate Production of Red Cells

These anemias result when the bone marrow is unable to produce sufficient numbers of new red cells to replace those removed from the circulation. A slight reduction in the red cell life span may be present, but generally this is insufficient to cause anemia if hematopoiesis is adequate. Low reticulocyte counts are observed in most anemias of this group.

14.4 CONGENITAL PURE RED CELL ANEMIA

(Congenital Hypoplastic Anemia; Diamond-Blackfan Syndrome)

This rare condition usually becomes symptomatic in early infancy. The most characteristic diagnostic feature is a deficiency of red cell precursors in an otherwise normally cellular bone marrow.

Etiology. A genetic basis is suggested by several instances of familial occurrence. Males and females are affected in equal numbers. An ill-defined abnormality of tryptophan metabolism has been reported in some children. A consistent finding is low numbers of CFUe and BFUe in the bone marrow. High levels of erythropoietin are present in serum and urine.

Clinical Manifestations. About half of affected infants appear pale even in the 1st few days of life, but hematopoiesis must be generally adequate during intrauterine life. Profound anemia usually becomes evident by 2–6 mo of age, occasionally somewhat later. Unless blood transfusions are given, the anemia progresses to heart failure and death. The liver and spleen are not enlarged initially. A number of cases of pure red cell anemia have been associated with congenital anomalies, including triphalangeal thumbs. Some patients with pure red cell anemia have had the Turner syndrome phenotype but normal karyotypes.

Laboratory Data. The red blood cells are normochromic and macrocytic. Assay of red cell enzymes reveals a pattern characteristic of a "young" erythrocyte population. The level of Hgb F is increased for age; in more chronic cases the fetal membrane antigen i is found on the red cells. Thrombocytosis and occasionally neutropenia may also be present initially. The most important feature is the lack of evidence of erythropoietic activity in blood and bone marrow despite high levels of erythropoietin. Reticulocytes are diminished even when the anemia is severe. Red cell precursors are markedly reduced in the marrow, and myeloid-erythroid ratios are 10–200:1. In some cases a few pronormoblasts may be present but not more mature forms. A normal complement of other marrow elements is usually present. Serum iron levels are elevated, with a decrease in the iron-binding capacity. Red cell survival is normal. Bone marrow culture studies show markedly reduced numbers of CFUe and BFUe. In a few cases incubation of the marrow cells with T cell antibodies prior to culture has restored normal red cell maturation in vitro.

Differential Diagnosis. Congenital hypoplastic anemia must be differentiated from other anemias in which there are low peripheral reticulocyte counts. The anemia of the convalescent phase of hemolytic disease of the newborn may, on occasion, be associated with markedly reduced erythropoiesis. This terminates spontaneously at 5–8 wk of age, whereas congenital hypoplastic anemia is not usually recognized before this time. Aplastic crises characterized by reticulocytopenia and by decreased numbers of red cell precursors may complicate various types of hemolytic disease. These episodes are transient, and evidence of antecedent hemolytic disease is usually present.

The syndrome of transient erythroblastopenia in older children may be differentiated from Diamond-Blackfan syndrome by its relatively late onset as well as by biochemical differences in the circulating red cells (Sec 14.6).

Prognosis. Unless corticosteroid therapy produces remission of hypoplastic anemia, survival depends upon blood transfusions. By late childhood affected children may have had 100 or more transfusions, and hemosiderosis is an inevitable consequence. The liver and spleen enlarge, and secondary hypersplenism with leukopenia and thrombocytopenia may occur. Growth retardation is usual, and puberty may not occur. Diabetes mellitus due to hemosiderosis is common.

Death usually occurs in the 2nd decade. Chronic congestive heart failure due to ischemic and siderotic myocardial disease is a common terminal event.

Treatment. When anemia becomes severe, blood transfusions must be given. Corticosteroid therapy is frequently beneficial if begun early; the mechanism of its effect is unknown. Relatively large doses, 2–4 mg/kg, of prednisone or its equivalent are administered initially. One–3 wk after therapy is begun red cell precursors appear in bone marrow, and then a brisk peripheral reticulocytosis occurs. The hemoglobin may reach normal levels in 4–6 wk. The dose of corticosteroid may then be reduced gradually until the lowest effective dose is found. This is often a very small amount, such as 2.5 mg/24 hr of prednisone or less, which may produce no adverse side effects or growth suppression. Intermittent administration every other day or for 3–4 consecutive days each wk may also be effective. Therapy should be discontinued periodically to determine whether the child is still dependent upon steroids since many responsive cases ultimately outgrow the dependence on steroid therapy and maintain normal hemoglobin levels.

About 10–15% of patients do not respond to corticosteroid therapy, and transfusions at intervals of 4–8 wk are necessary to sustain life. Other therapies, including hematinics, cobalt, and testosterone, have had no beneficial effect. Splenectomy is usually of no value but may decrease the need for transfusion if hypersplenism or isoimmunization has developed. Since spontaneous remission occasionally occurs, children refractory to corticosteroid therapy should be maintained as long as possible by transfusions, preferably of freshly drawn, packed red cells. The use of chelating agents to induce excretion of excess iron is discussed with thalassemia major (Sec 14.25).

14.5 ACQUIRED PURE RED CELL ANEMIAS

A number of forms of acquired anemia with reticulocytopenia and reduced red cell precursors in the marrow have been described. The cause of most of them is uncertain. In some cases in adults remission has followed removal of a tumor of the thymus. Association with thymoma has been reported in a child. In other cases an erythropoietin-inhibiting antibody, antibodies to erythroblasts, or inhibitors of heme synthesis have been found in plasma. The presence of a complement-dependent antibody cytotoxic for erythroblasts in some adults has suggested their need for immunosuppressive therapy. The acquired pure red cell anemias may respond to therapy with corticosteroids, and a trial is indicated in any chronic case. Immunosuppressive therapy with cyclophosphamide or azathioprine may be given a trial if corticosteroids are ineffective.

Administration of large doses of chloramphenicol inhibits erythropoiesis. Reticulocytopenia, erythroid hypoplasia, and vacuolated pronormoblasts in the marrow are reversible pharmacologic effects of this drug (Sec 14.32).

Episodes of acute failure of erythropoiesis may follow a variety of viral infections. During these episodes a marked reduction in circulating reticulocytes (<0.1%) and an elevation of the serum iron level occur. Bone marrow aspiration shows markedly reduced numbers of erythrocytic precursors. These episodes are self-limited, lasting only 10–14 days, and are of no consequence to a child with a normal red cell survival. In a patient with a shortened red cell survival, however, profound anemia may ensue; this is the basis of the so-called *aplastic crises* of some hemolytic anemias.

14.6 TRANSIENT ERYTHROBLASTOPENIA OF CHILDHOOD (TEC)

A self-limited syndrome of severe aregenerative anemia is being increasingly recognized. Previously normal children, 6 mo–5 yr of age, slowly develop anemia with reticulocytopenia and decreased numbers of red cell precursors in the bone marrow. Serum iron is increased, with increased iron saturation. The level of Hgb F is normal, and the profile of red cell enzymes is consistent with an "old" red cell population. Marrow culture studies suggest varying pathogenetic mechanisms: in some cases, a serum inhibitor of erythroid stem cells and in others, abnormalities of erythroid stem cells, either in number or in responsiveness to erythropoietin. Spontaneous remission occurs; corticosteroid therapy is not necessary or indicated. Transfusions may be necessary until recovery occurs.

14.7 ANEMIAS OF CHRONIC INFECTION, INFLAMMATION, AND RENAL DISEASE

Anemia complicates a number of chronic systemic diseases associated with infection, inflammation, or tissue breakdown. Examples of such conditions include chronic pyogenic infections such as bronchiectasis and osteomyelitis; chronic inflammatory processes such as rheumatic fever, rheumatoid arthritis, and ulcerative colitis; and advanced renal disease. Despite diverse underlying causes the erythrokinetic abnormalities are similar. Red cell life span is moderately decreased, reflecting increased red cell destruction by a hyperactive reticuloendothelial system. This increased hemolysis is less important, however, than a relative failure of bone marrow response, reflecting both hypoactivity of marrow and an erythropoietin production inadequate for the degree of anemia. Further, there are abnormalities of iron metabolism including defective iron release from the tissues into the plasma. In renal failure accumulation of toxic nondialyzable substances in the blood can directly inhibit erythropoiesis.

Clinical Manifestations. Few symptoms are attributable to the usually moderate degree of anemia present; the important symptoms and signs are those of the underlying disease.

Laboratory Data. Hemoglobin concentrations usually range from 6–9 gm/dl. The proportionate decrease in the red blood cell count and hemoglobin and hematocrit levels results in a normochromic and normocytic anemia. Occasionally, a modest degree of hypochromia and microcytosis is observed. Reticulocyte counts are normal or low, and leukocytosis is common. Free erythrocyte protoporphyrin (FEP) levels are moderately elevated (>35 μg/dl whole blood). Serum iron is low, averaging 30 μg/dl; there is, however, no increase in total iron-binding capacity as in iron deficiency anemia. The iron-binding capacity averages 200 μg/ml, and saturation percentage may be low. This pattern of serum iron and iron-binding protein is a regular and valuable diagnostic feature. Serum ferritin is often elevated. The bone marrow has normal cellularity; the red cell precursors are adequate, and granulocytic hyperplasia may be present. Increased hemosiderin can often be seen in marrow.

Treatment and Prognosis. Since these anemias are secondary to other disease processes, they do not respond to iron or hematinics unless there is concomitant deficiency. Transfusions raise the hemoglobin concentration only temporarily and are rarely indicated. If the underlying systemic disease can be controlled, the anemia is spontanously corrected.

14.8 CONGENITAL DYSERYTHROPOIETIC ANEMIAS

These rare, recessively transmitted normocytic or macrocytic anemias display multinuclearity and abnormal chromatin patterns in red cell precursors. Four types have been distinguished, with considerable variation within each type and overlap among them. Type I (about 15% of cases) is defined by binuclearity of erythroblasts and megaloblastic morphology. Type II (more than 60% of cases) has erythroblastic multinuclearity and a positive acidified serum (Ham) test (but only with some normal serum added). Red cells in Type II are strongly agglutinated by anti-i antibody. Types I and II appear to be inherited as autosomal traits. Type

III (about 15% of cases) has pronounced multinuclearity and huge red cell precursors in marrow. It appears to be inherited as an autosomal dominant trait. Type IV is rare; it resembles Type II morphologically but does not have associated serologic abnormalities. In all types there are variable degrees of anemia (sometimes only in adults), ineffective erythropoiesis, and abnormal utilization of iron. Nonspecific findings of chronic hemolysis, such as intermittent jaundice, gallstones, and splenomegaly, are common. There is no treatment other than blood transfusion for anemia. Splenectomy has been advocated for patients with severe anemia requiring chronic transfusions.

14.9   PHYSIOLOGIC ANEMIA OF INFANCY

The normal newborn has higher hemoglobin and hematocrit levels than older children and adults. Within the 1st wk of life a progressive decline in hemoglobin level begins, which persists for approximately 6–8 wk. This decline is generally referred to as a physiologic anemia of infancy. The term is a misnomer, for at its nadir the hemoglobin level in the fullterm infant rarely falls below 9 gm/dl.

A number of factors are operative. First, there is an abrupt cessation of erythropoiesis with onset of respiration when arterial oxygen saturation rises from 45 toward 95%. Concomitantly, the high fetal levels of erythropoietin drop to undetectable levels. A shortened survival of the fetal red cell also contributes to the development of physiologic anemia. Further, the sizable expansion of blood volume that accompanies rapid weight gain during the 1st 3 mo of life creates a situation which has aptly been described as "bleeding into the circulation." Lack of stimulation of bone marrow by erythropoietin is the most important determinant of physiologic anemia. When the hemoglobin level has fallen to 10–11 gm/dl at 2–3 mo of age, erythropoiesis resumes. This "anemia" should be viewed as a physiologic adaptation to extrauterine life.

The premature infant also develops a physiologic anemia; the same factors are operative as in term infants, but they are exaggerated. The decline in hemoglobin level is both more extreme and more rapid. Minimal hemoglobin levels of 7–9 gm/dl commonly occur by 3–6 wk of age, and, in very small prematures, levels may be even lower.

The difference between term and premature infants is not due to their relative abilities to secrete erythropoietin but may rather be due to lower respiratory quotients and metabolic rates in premature infants. Further, when premature infants are transfused with adult blood containing Hgb A, the shift of the oxygen dissociation curve due to Hgb A facilitates delivery of oxygen to the tissues. Accordingly, the definition of anemia and the need for transfusion in the premature infant must be based not only upon hemoglobin level but also upon oxygen requirements and the affinity of the infant's circulating hemoglobin for oxygen.

The marginal erythropoietic equilibrium responsible for physiologic anemia can aggravate processes associated with increased hemolysis such as congenital he-

molytic states which may be associated with severe anemia in the early wk of life.

Dietary factors may also aggravate physiologic anemia. Deficiencies of folic acid or vitamin E superimposed upon the physiologic process may result in more severe anemia.

In the premature infant vitamin E has been shown to play an important role in red cell stability. Premature infants are born with a small reserve of vitamin E and frequently become deficient, with serum vitamin E levels falling to less than 0.5 mg/l during the 1st months of life. If the diet contains a high proportion of polyunsaturated fatty acids (as in many proprietary formulas), and especially if an iron supplement is given, a syndrome of hemolytic anemia, thrombocytosis, and edema may occur. Red cells include many bizarre acanthocytes (burr cells). Vitamin E prophylaxis, 5 mg/24 hr, should be considered for the small premature infant; therapeutic doses of vitamin E (50 mg) are indicated for established deficiency. The composition of most proprietary formulas is such that hemolysis does not occur even when iron supplementation at a concentration of 10–12 mg/qt is used. However, larger doses of medicinal iron are not indicated in the newborn. These may not only provoke hemolysis but also predispose to serious infections, particularly if parenteral iron preparations are employed. In patients with malabsorption of fat, vitamin E deficiency may lead to significant hemolytic anemia, as occurs in cystic fibrosis.

Infantile pyknocytosis, a self-limited hemolytic process with large numbers of acanthocytes in blood, probably represents vitamin E deficiency.

Unless there has been significant perinatal blood loss, iron deficiency should not be considered as a cause of anemia in the 1st 3 mo of life.

Treatment. As a developmental process, physiologic anemia usually requires no therapy other than seeing that the diet of the infant contains the essential nutrients for normal hematopoiesis, especially folic acid and vitamin E. A premature infant who is feeding well and growing normally rarely needs transfusion. Occasionally, very low hemoglobin levels (<6 gm/dl) or complicating medical conditions may necessitate small transfusions of packed red blood cells. If so, only enough blood should be given to raise the hemoglobin level to about 9 gm/dl. Larger transfusions may delay spontaneous recovery by suppressing normal erythropoiesis. Neither iron nor any other hematinic substance has any effect upon physiologic anemia.

14.10   MEGALOBLASTIC ANEMIAS

The megaloblastic anemias all have in common certain diagnostic abnormalities of red cell morphology and maturation. The red cells at every stage of development are larger than normal and have a peculiar open, finely dispersed arrangement of nuclear chromatin and an asynchrony between the maturation of nucleus and cytoplasm. Biochemically, there is an increased amount of RNA in proportion to DNA in megaloblastic tissues. Megaloblastic morphology may be seen in a number of conditions, but almost all instances in children result from a deficiency of folic acid, of vitamin B_{12}, or of both. Both substances are necessary cofactors in the synthesis of nucleoproteins. Megaloblastic anemias are uncommon in the United States.

Folic Acid Deficiencies

Megaloblastic Anemia of Infancy. This disease is caused by a deficient intake or absorption of folic acid. Dietary deficiency is usually compounded by rapid growth or infection, which may increase folic acid requirements. The normal daily requirement is small, estimated at 20–50 μg/24 hr. Human and cow milks provide adequate amounts of folic acid. Goat milk is clearly deficient; folic acid supplementation must be given when it is the main food. Unless supplemented, powdered milk may also be a poor source of folic acid. Ascorbic acid deficiency probably impairs the availability of dietary folic acid conjugates.

CLINICAL MANIFESTATIONS. Mild megaloblastic anemia has been reported in very low birth weight infants and routine folic acid supplementation advised. Megaloblastic anemia has its peak incidence at 4–7 mo of age, somewhat earlier than iron deficiency anemia. Besides having the usual features of severe anemia, affected infants are irritable, fail to gain weight adequately, and have chronic diarrhea. Thrombocytopenic hemorrhages occur in advanced cases. Concomitant signs and symptoms of scurvy may be present. Folic acid deficiency may accompany kwashiorkor or marasmus.

LABORATORY DATA. The anemia is progressive. The red blood cell count is disproportionately lower than the hematocrit; accordingly, the anemia is macrocytic (MCV >100 fl). Considerable variations in red cell shape and size are common (Fig 14–2C). The reticulocyte count is low, but nucleated red cells demonstrating megaloblastic morphology are often seen in the peripheral blood. Neutropenia and thrombocytopenia may be present. The neutrophils are large, with hypersegmented nuclei; more than 5% of the neutrophils will have 5 or more nuclear segments. Serum folic acid activity is measured by microbiologic assay or by isotopic techniques. Normal serum values are 5–20 ng/ml; deficiency is accompanied by levels of less than 3 ng/ml. Levels of red cell folate are a better indicator of chronic deficiency. The normal red cell folate level is 150–600 ng/ml of packed cells. Levels of iron and vitamin B_{12} in serum are normal or elevated. Formiminoglutamic acid is excreted in the urine, especially after an oral dose of histidine. Serum levels of lactic acid dehydrogenase (LDH) are markedly elevated. The bone marrow is hypercellular because of erythroid hyperplasia. Megaloblastic changes are prominent, though some normal red cell precursors may also be found. Large, abnormal neutrophilic forms (giant metamyelocytes) with cytoplasmic vacuolization are seen as well as hypersegmentation of the nuclei of megakaryocytes.

TREATMENT. Initially, folic acid may be administered parenterally in a dose of 2–5 mg/24 hr. Since a hematologic response can be expected within 72 hr, transfu-sions are indicated only when the anemia is severe or the child very ill. Folic acid therapy should be continued for 3–4 wk. Satisfactory responses have been obtained with doses of folic acid as low as 50 μg/24 hr. These "physiologic" doses have no effect on primary vitamin B_{12} deficiencies; a therapeutic test using such low amounts may be used, therefore, to differentiate between primary folic acid and vitamin B_{12} deficiencies. If there is a likelihood that juvenile pernicious anemia may be present or if the anemia recurs after therapy, the prolonged use of folic acid should be avoided since in pernicious anemia folic acid may produce a partial response of anemia without benefiting the neurologic abnormalities. If signs of scurvy are present, therapeutic doses of ascorbic acid should be given. Antibiotic therapy should be used for superimposed bacterial infection.

Megaloblastic Anemia of Pregnancy. Folate requirements markedly increase during pregnancy, in part because of the requirements of the fetus. Decreases in serum and red cell folate levels can be found in as many as 25% of pregnant women at term and may be aggravated by infection. Folate supplementation, 1 μg/day, is often advocated, particularly during the last trimester.

Folic Acid Deficiency of Malabsorption Syndromes. Folic acid is absorbed throughout the small intestine, and diffuse inflammatory or degenerative disease of the intestine may reduce intestinal polyglutamate deconjugase activity as well as markedly impair absorption. Celiac disease, chronic infectious enteritis, and enteroenteric fistulas may lead to folic acid deficiency and megaloblastic anemia. Measurement of serum folate is widely used to assess small intestinal absorptive functions in malabsorptive disorders. Oral folic acid supplements of 1 mg/day may be indicated in these states. (See also Chapter 11.)

Congenital Defect of Folic Acid Absorption. A specific congenital defect in the intestinal absorption of folic acid and an associated inability to transfer folate from the plasma to the central nervous system have been associated with megaloblastic anemia, convulsions, mental retardation, and cerebral calcifications. Treatment with oral folic acid, 15–50 mg/24 hr, was necessary to maintain normal hematologic values.

Folic Acid Deficiency Complicating Hemolytic Anemias. Folic acid is necessary for normal hematopoiesis, and it is possible that chronic hemolytic processes may increase the requirement for this vitamin, probably more often in adults than in children. Frank megaloblastic erythropoiesis may complicate hemolytic anemia, leading to more severe anemia and increased need for transfusion. The bone marrow should be examined for megaloblastic changes if there is an unexplained worsening of chronic anemia or increased transfusion requirements in chronic hemolytic states. Continuous folic acid supplementation is not ordinarily necessary for such patients if their diets are normal, at least during childhood.

Folic Acid Deficiency Associated with Anticonvulsants and Other Drugs. Many patients have low serum levels of folic acid during therapy with certain anticonvulsant drugs (e.g., phenytoin, primidone, or phenobarbital), but they usually have no anemia or symp-

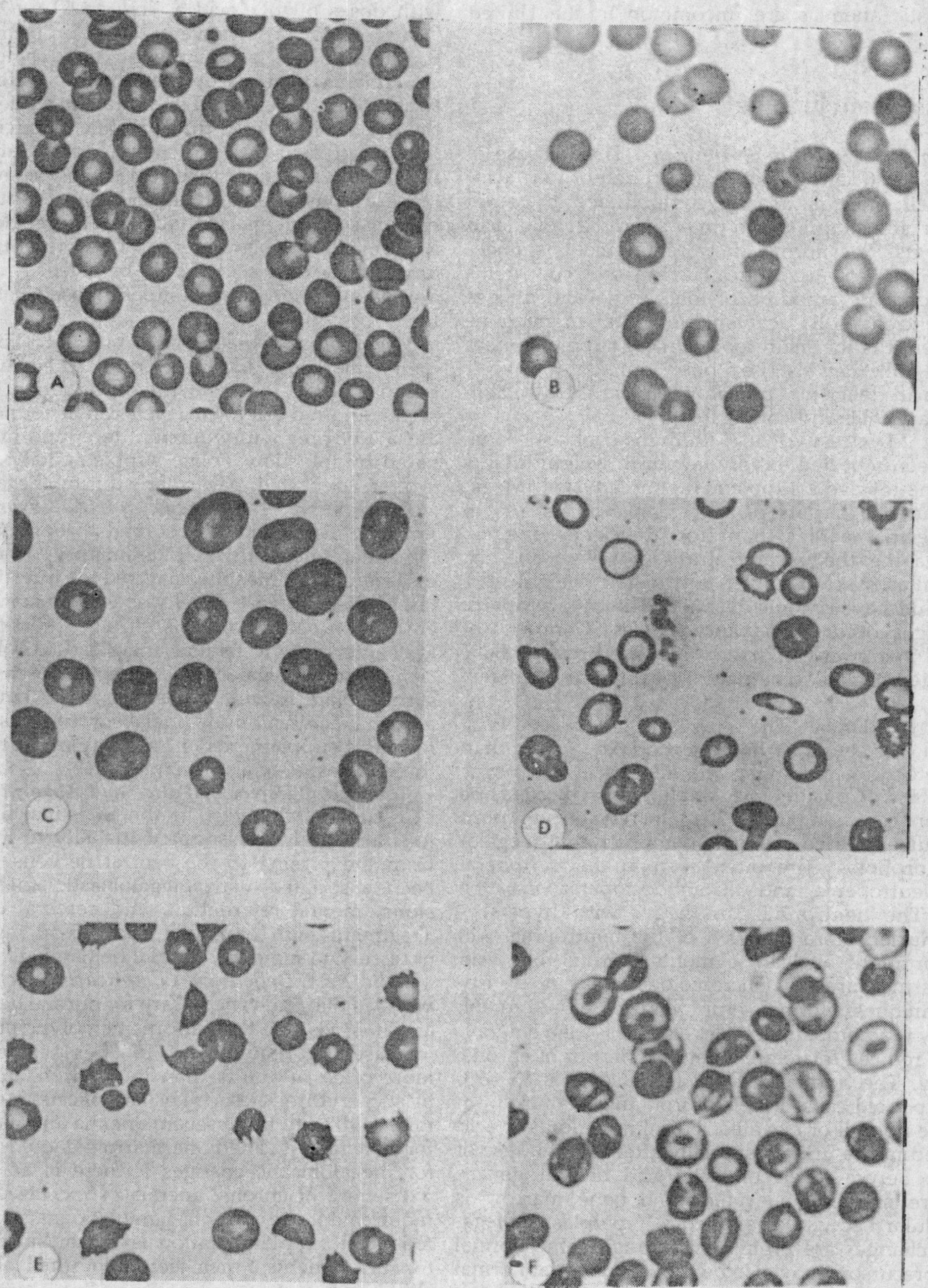

Figure 14–2 Morphologic abnormalities of the red cell. *A*, Normal. *B*, Spherocytes (hereditary spherocytosis). *C*, Macrocytes (folic acid deficiency). *D*, Hypochromic microcytes (iron deficiency). *E*, Schizocytes (hemolytic-uremic syndrome). *F*, Target cells (Hgb CC disease).

toms. Frank megaloblastic anemia is rare and responds to folic acid therapy even if administration of the offending drug is continued. Malabsorption of folic acid induced by anticonvulsant drugs is the probable mechanism; displacement by the drug of folate from its serum carrier has also been suggested. Megaloblastic anemia, probably due to folic acid malabsorption, has been seen in users of oral contraceptives.

A number of drugs have antifolic acid activity as their primary pharmacologic effect and will regularly produce megaloblastic anemia. Methotrexate and aminopterin prevent the utilization of folic acid by inhibiting its enzymatic reduction to active coenzymatic forms. Pyrimethamine (Daraprim), which is used in the therapy of toxoplasmosis, may induce folic acid deficiency and megaloblastic anemia. Trimethoprim-sulfamethoxazole, which is also being increasingly used for the treatment of urinary infections and pneumonia due to *Pneumocystis carinii*, also may cause megaloblastic anemia.

Vitamin B$_{12}$ Deficiencies

In order to be absorbed, dietary vitamin B$_{12}$ must combine with a glycoprotein (intrinsic factor) secreted by the parietal cells of the gastric fundus. The B$_{12}$–intrinsic factor complex passes to the terminal ileum, where specific absorptive sites exist. In the presence of intrinsic factor and ionic calcium, vitamin B$_{12}$ traverses the intestinal mucosa and enters the blood. Vitamin B$_{12}$ deficiency may therefore result from (1) inadequate intake, (2) lack of secretion of intrinsic factor by the stomach, (3) consumption or inhibition of the B$_{12}$–intrinsic factor complex, or (4) abnormalities involving the receptor sites in the terminal ileum.

Because vitamin B$_{12}$ is present in many foods, dietary deficiency is rare. It may be seen in extreme dietary restriction ("vegans") in which no milk, eggs, or animal products are consumed. B$_{12}$ deficiency is not commonly seen in kwashiorkor or infantile marasmus. Instances have been reported in breast-fed infants whose mothers had deficient diets or pernicious anemia. Since vitamin B$_{12}$ is so ubiquitous, most cases of deficiency stem from failure to absorb the vitamin.

Juvenile Pernicious Anemia. This rare disease is due to inability to secrete gastric intrinsic factor. It differs from the typical disease in adults in that the stomach secretes acid normally and is histologically normal. Consanguinity is common in parents of affected children, and a mendelian recessive inheritance pattern is suggested.

CLINICAL MANIFESTATIONS. The symptoms of juvenile pernicious anemia become prominent at 9 mo–5 yr of age. This interval is consistent with exhaustion of the stores of vitamin B$_{12}$ acquired in utero. As the anemia becomes severe, irritability, anorexia, and listlessness occur. The tongue is smooth, red, and painful. Neurologic involvement is manifested by ataxia, paresthesias, hyporeflexia, Babinski responses, clonus, and coma.

LABORATORY DATA. The anemia is macrocytic, with prominent macro-ovalocytosis of the red cells. The neutrophils are large and hypersegmented. In advanced cases neutropenia and thrombocytopenia are seen. Serum vitamin B$_{12}$, as measured by radioactive techniques or microbiologic assay, is below 100 pg/ml. Concentrations of serum iron and serum folic acid are normal or elevated. Levels of serum LDH are markedly increased, primarily because of the 1st and 2nd heat-stable isoenzymes. Moderate elevations (2–3 mg/dl) of serum bilirubin may be seen. Serum iron levels are elevated. Excessive excretion of methylmalonic acid in the urine constitutes a reliable and sensitive index of vitamin B$_{12}$ deficiency. In contrast to many adult cases, serum antibodies directed against parietal cells or intrinsic factor cannot be detected in children. Gastric acidity may be reduced initially but returns to normal when vitamin B$_{12}$ therapy is instituted. Biopsy reveals a normal gastric mucosa, but intrinsic factor activity is absent in the gastric secretion.

Absorption of vitamin B$_{12}$ is usually assessed by the Schilling test, using radioactive vitamin B$_{12}$. When a normal person ingests a small amount of vitamin B$_{12}$ into which ^{57}Co or ^{60}Co has been incorporated, the radioactive vitamin combines with the intrinsic factor in the stomach secretions and passes to the terminal ileum, where absorption occurs. As the absorbed vitamin is bound to blood proteins and tissues, none is normally excreted in the urine. If a large (1000 µg) dose of nonradioactive vitamin B$_{12}$ is then injected parenterally ("flushing dose"), from 10–30% of the previously absorbed radioactive vitamin will appear in the urine. Patients with pernicious anemia excrete 2% or less under these conditions. That malabsorption of vitamin B$_{12}$ is due to lack of intrinsic factor can be confirmed through a modification of the standard Schilling test: 30 mg of intrinsic factor is administered along with the radioactive vitamin. If absence of intrinsic factor is the basis of the B$_{12}$ malabsorption, normal amounts of radioactive vitamin should now be absorbed and flushed out. On the other hand, when vitamin B$_{12}$ malabsorption is due to disease of the ileal receptor sites or other intestinal causes, no improvement in absorption will be seen with intrinsic factor. The Schilling test result will remain abnormal in pernicious anemia even when therapy has completely reversed the hematologic and neurologic manifestations of the disease.

TREATMENT. A prompt hematologic response follows parenteral administration of vitamin B$_{12}$. The physiologic requirement for vitamin B$_{12}$ is 1–5 µg/24 hr, and hematologic responses have been observed with these small doses. If there is evidence of neurologic involvement, 1 mg should be injected intramuscularly daily for at least 2 wk. Maintenance therapy will be necessary throughout the patient's life; monthly intramuscular administration of 1 mg of vitamin B$_{12}$ is sufficient. Attempts at oral therapy are contraindicated.

Transcobalamin Deficiency. There are two major vitamin B$_{12}$ binding proteins in the plasma, designated transcobalamins I and II. Transcobalamin II is the principal transport vehicle for vitamin B$_{12}$; a congenital deficiency is inherited as an autosomal recessive condition associated with failure to absorb and transport vitamin B$_{12}$. Severe megaloblastic anemia occurs in early infancy; therapy requires massive parenteral doses of vitamin B$_{12}$.

Vitamin B₁₂ Deficiency in Older Children. In some cases of vitamin B_{12} malabsorption in late childhood atrophy of the gastric mucosa and achlorhydria have been seen; in others the stomach is normal. Malabsorption of vitamin B_{12} may also occur in combination with a familial syndrome of cutaneous moniliasis, hypoparathyroidism, and other endocrine deficiencies; the serum contains antibodies against intrinsic factor; the Schilling test result is abnormal but is corrected by addition of exogenous intrinsic factor. Parenteral vitamin B_{12} should be administered regularly to these patients to prevent the development of megaloblastic anemia. A case of megaloblastic anemia with a structurally abnormal intrinsic factor has been reported.

Vitamin B₁₂ Malabsorption Due to Intestinal Causes. A few cases have been reported of familial occurrence of a specific intestinal defect in the absorption of vitamin B_{12}, in some instances associated with proteinuria (Imerslund syndrome); histology of the stomach is normal, and intrinsic factor and acid are present in gastric secretions.

Surgical resection of the terminal ileum or such inflammatory diseases as regional enteritis or tuberculosis may also impair absorption of vitamin B_{12}. When the terminal ileum has been removed, lifelong parenteral administration should be considered if the Schilling test indicates that vitamin B_{12} is not absorbed. An overgrowth of intestinal bacteria within diverticula or duplications of the small intestine may cause vitamin B_{12} deficiency by consumption of or competition for the vitamin or by splitting of its complex with intrinsic factor. In these cases hematologic response may follow broad spectrum antibiotic therapy. Similar mechanisms may operate when the fish tapeworm *Diphyllobothrium latum* infests the upper small intestine. When megaloblastic anemia occurs in these situations, the serum vitamin B_{12} level is low, the gastric juice contains intrinsic factor, and the abnormal Schilling test result is not corrected by the addition of exogenous intrinsic factor.

Rare Megaloblastic Anemias

Orotic aciduria is a genetically determined defect in pyrimidine biosynthesis associated with a severe megaloblastic anemia, neutropenia, and crystalluria due to excretion of orotic acid. Physical and mental retardation may be frequently present. The anemia is refractory to vitamin B_{12} or folic acid, but responds promptly to administration of the nucleic acid precursor, uridine, or yeast. The basic defect appears to be a deficiency of orotate phosphoribosyl transferase and orotidine-5-phosphate decarboxylase, which involves many tissues. Inheritance is autosomal recessive. Megaloblastic anemia can also occur in the Lesch-Nyhan syndrome, in which regeneration of purine nucleotides is blocked.

Two instances of thiamine responsive and thiamine dependent megaloblastic anemia have been reported. Administration of thiamine, 100 mg/24 hr, produced a brisk reticulocyte response and a sustained increase in hemoglobin level. Sensorineural deafness and diabetes mellitus were associated. The pathogenesis of this disorder is unclear.

MICROCYTIC ANEMIAS

14.11   IRON DEFICIENCY ANEMIA

Anemia resulting from lack of sufficient iron for synthesis of hemoglobin is by far the most frequent hematologic disease of infancy and childhood. The prevalence of this deficiency is related to certain basic aspects of iron metabolism and nutrition. The body of the newborn infant contains about 0.5 gm of iron, whereas the adult content is estimated at 5.0 gm. In order to make up this 4.5 gm discrepancy, an average of 0.8 mg of iron must be absorbed each day during the 1st 15 yr of life. In addition to this growth requirement an additional small amount is necessary to balance normal losses through excretion of iron. Accordingly, to maintain an adequate positive iron balance in childhood, 0.8–1.5 mg of iron must be absorbed each day. Since less than 10% of iron in the diet is absorbed, a diet containing 8–15 mg of iron is necessary for optimal nutrition. Absorption of iron from human milk is much more efficient than from cow milk; breast-fed infants may, therefore, require less from other foods. During the 1st years of life, because relatively small quantities of iron-rich foods are taken, it is often difficult to attain these amounts. For this reason the diet should include such foods as infant cereals or cow milk formulas which have been fortified with iron. At best, the infant is in a precarious situation with respect to iron. Should the diet become inadequate or external blood loss occur, anemia ensues rapidly.

Etiology. A preponderance of the iron of the newborn is contained in the circulating hemoglobin. Low birth weight and significant perinatal hemorrhage are associated with a decreased neonatal hemoglobin mass and store of iron. As the high hemoglobin concentration of the newborn decreases during the 1st 2–3 mo of life, considerable iron is reclaimed and stored (Sec 14.9). These reclaimed stores are usually sufficient for blood formation for the 1st 6–9 mo of life; transplacental iron stores are exhausted by the time the birth weight approximately triples. In low birth weight infants or with perinatal blood loss, stored iron may be depleted earlier, and dietary sources become of paramount importance. Anemia due solely to inadequate dietary iron is unusual during the 1st 4–6 mo, but becomes common from 9–24 mo of age. Thereafter, it is relatively infrequent. The usual dietary pattern observed in infants with iron deficiency anemia is the consumption of large amounts of milk and of carbohydrates unsupplemented with iron.

Blood loss must be considered a possible cause in every case of iron deficiency anemia, particularly in the older child. Chronic iron deficiency anemia from occult bleeding may be due to a lesion of the gastrointestinal tract, such as peptic ulcer, Meckel diverticulum, polyp, or hemangioma. In some geographic areas hookworm infestation is an important cause. As many as one third of infants with severe iron deficiency in the United States have chronic intestinal blood loss induced by exposure to a heat labile protein in whole cow milk (Wilson, Lahey, and Heiner). Loss of 1–7 ml of blood in the stools each day can be shown which is not influenced by iron replacement or transfusion but can be prevented either by reducing the quantity of whole cow milk to 1 pint/day or less or by using heated or evaporated milk or a milk substitute. This gastrointestinal reaction is not related to enzymatic abnormalities in the mucosa, such as lactase deficiency, or to typical "milk allergy." Characteristically, involved infants develop anemia that is more severe and occurs earlier than would be expected simply from inadequate intake of iron.

Histologic abnormalities of the mucosa of the gastrointestinal tract are present in advanced iron deficiency anemia. The morphologic changes may be a direct manifestation of tissue deficiency of iron.

Clinical Manifestations. Pallor is the most important clue to iron deficiency. In mild to moderate iron deficiency (hemoglobin levels of 6–10 gm/dl), compensatory mechanisms, including increased levels of 2,3-DPG and a shift of the oxygen dissociation curve, may be so effective that few symptoms of anemia are noted. When the hemoglobin level falls below 5.0 gm/dl, irritability and anorexia are prominent. Tachycardia and cardiac dilatation occur, and systolic murmurs are often present.

The spleen is palpably enlarged in 10–15% of cases, and in longstanding cases widening of the diploë of the skull similar to that seen in congenital hemolytic anemias may occur. These changes resolve slowly with adequate replacement therapy. The child with iron deficiency anemia may be obese, or underweight with other evidences of undernutrition. Pica is sometimes prominent. The irritability and anorexia characteristic of advanced cases may reflect deficiency in tissue iron, for with iron therapy striking improvement in behavior frequently occurs before significant hematologic improvement.

Monoamine oxidase (MAO), an iron-dependent enzyme, plays a crucial role in neurochemical reactions in the central nervous system. MAO can also be measured in platelets. Catalase and peroxidase contain iron, but their biologic essentiality is not well established. It is not possible to measure easily and accurately in vivo the iron in the enzymatic compartment, and yet this is perhaps the most vital area of iron metabolism. In the past the intracellular enzyme iron component was held to be tenaciously maintained even in the face of marked depletion in the other iron compartments, including in severe anemia. This traditional view is being questioned. Iron deficiency produces decreases in the activities of enzymes such as catalase and cytochromes. Iron deficiency is increasingly regarded as involving multiple systems rather than just the hematologic.

Iron deficiency may also have effects on neurologic and intellectual function. Preliminary reports suggest that iron deficiency affects attention span, alertness, and learning of both infants and adolescents, even when the degree of anemia is not severe.

Laboratory Data. In progressive iron deficiency a sequence of biochemical and hematologic events occurs (Table 14–5). First, the tissue iron stores represented by liver and bone marrow hemosiderin disappear. It is possible to measure in the serum small amounts of

Table 14–5 SEQUENCE OF CHANGES IN IRON DEFICIENCY ANEMIA

1. Decrease in iron stores; decrease in hemosiderin content of liver and bone marrow
2. Decrease in levels of serum ferritin to less than 10 ng/ml
3. Decrease in level of serum iron; increase in total iron binding capacity; fall in per cent of saturation to less than 15%
4. Increase in levels of free erythrocyte protoporphyrins (FEP)
5. Anemia; progressive hypochromia and microcytosis
6. Decrease in activity of intracellular enzymes containing iron*

*Depletion of the enzyme compartment of iron is listed as the final stage of iron deficiency, but certain iron-containing enzymes may be significantly and functionally decreased even when the degree of anemia is relatively mild.

ferritin, the iron-binding protein of the tissues. The level of serum ferritin appears to provide a relatively accurate estimate of body iron stores. During infancy and childhood the mean level of serum ferritin is 35 ng/ml. Levels less than 10 ng/ml accompany iron deficiency. Next, there is a decrease in serum iron to less than 30 µg/dl. Concomitantly, the iron-binding capacity of the serum increases to more than 350 µg/dl and the per cent saturation falls below 15%. At a level of transferrin saturation of 15%, iron becomes rate-limiting for hemoglobin synthesis, and a moderate accumulation of heme precursors results; these are designated free erythrocyte protoporphyrins (FEP). Normal FEP levels are 1.9 ± 0.4 µg/gm Hgb (<35 µg/dl whole blood); a characteristic level in iron deficiency is 10.9 ± 6.2 µg/gm Hgb (>50 µg/dl whole blood).

As the deficiency progresses, the red cells become smaller than normal and their hemoglobin content decreases. The morphologic characteristics of red cells are best quantified by means of determination of mean corpuscular volume (MCV) and mean corpuscular hemoglobin (MCH). There are important developmental changes in MCV which require utilization of age-related standards for diagnosis of microcytosis (see Table 14–6). With increasing severity the red cells become deformed and misshapen and present characteristic microcytosis, hypochromia, and poikilocytosis (Fig 14–2D), without which a diagnosis of significant iron deficiency anemia is untenable. The reticulocyte count is normal or minimally elevated; nucleated red cells may occasionally be seen in the peripheral blood. White blood cell counts are normal. Thrombocytosis, sometimes of a striking degree (600,000–1,000,000/mm³) may occur. On the other hand, in a few cases significant thrombocytopenia may be present. The mechanism of these platelet abnormalities is not clear; they appear to be a direct consequence of iron deficiency, and they

Table 14–6 MEAN CORPUSCULAR VOLUME IN CHILDREN

AGE	MCV (fl[µ³]) MEAN (RANGE)
Birth	119 (110–128)
6–24 mo	77 (70–85)
2–6 yr	81 (75–90)
6–12 yr	85 (78–95)
Adult	90 (80–100)

After Koerper MA, Mentzer WC, Brecher G, et al: J Pediatr 89:580, 1976.

return to normal with iron therapy. The bone marrow is hypercellular with erythroid hyperplasia. The normoblasts have scanty, fragmented cytoplasm with poor hemoglobinization. Leukocytes and megakaryocytes are normal. Hemosiderin cannot be demonstrated in marrow specimens by the Prussian blue staining techniques. In about a third of cases occult blood can be detected in the stools.

Differential Diagnosis. Iron deficiency must be differentiated from other hypochromic microcytic anemias. In lead poisoning the red cells are morphologically similar, but coarse basophilic stippling of the red cells is prominent. Very marked elevations of blood lead, free erythrocyte protoporphyrins, and urinary coproporphyrins are seen. The blood changes of the thalassemia trait resemble those of iron deficiency, but characteristic elevations in the levels of Hgb A_2 and Hgb F are usually present, which do not occur in iron deficiency. Thalassemia major with its pronounced erythroblastosis and hemolytic component should present no diagnostic confusion. The red cell morphology of chronic inflammation and infection, though usually normochromic, may occasionally be microcytic, but in these conditions both serum iron and iron-binding capacity are reduced, and serum ferritin levels are normal or elevated.

Treatment. The regular response of iron deficiency anemia to adequate amounts of iron is an important diagnostic as well as therapeutic feature. Oral administration of simple ferrous salts (sulfate, gluconate, fumarate) provides inexpensive and satisfactory therapy. There is no evidence that addition of any trace metal, vitamin, or other hematinic substance significantly increases the response to simple ferrous salts. On the other hand, absorption of some iron chelates may be suboptimal. For routine clinical use the physician should familiarize himself with an inexpensive preparation of 1 of the simple ferrous compounds. The therapeutic dose should be calculated in terms of elemental iron; ferrous sulfate is 20% and ferrous gluconate is 10–12% elemental iron by weight. A daily total of 6 mg/kg of elemental iron in 3 divided doses provides an optimal amount of iron for the stimulated bone marrow to utilize. Doses of elemental iron in excess of 6 mg/kg/24 hr do not result in a more rapid hematologic response. Better absorption may result when medicinal iron is given between meals. Ingestion of large amounts of milk may significantly decrease absorption of iron. Intolerance to oral iron is extremely rare; malabsorption of oral iron is more frequently invoked than demonstrated. A parenteral iron preparation (iron-dextran) is an effective, reasonably safe form of iron when given in a properly calculated dose, but the response to parenteral iron is no more rapid or complete than that obtained with proper administration of iron orally; in most cases the indication for parenteral iron therapy is a social one.

While adequate iron medication is given, the family must be educated about the patient's diet, and the consumption of milk should be limited to a reasonable quantity, preferably to 500 ml (1 pt)/day or less. This reduction has a dual effect: the amount of iron-rich foods in the diet is increased; and gastrointestinal blood loss from intolerance to cow's milk proteins is prevented. When the re-education of child and parent is not successful, parenteral iron medication may be indicated.

The expected clinical and hematologic responses to iron therapy are described in Table 14–7.

Within 72–96 hr after administration of iron to the anemic child peripheral reticulocytosis is seen. The height of this response is inversely proportional to the severity of the anemia. Reticulocytosis is followed by a rise in the hemoglobin level, which may increase as much as 0.5 gm/dl/24 hr. Iron medication should be continued for 4–6 wk after blood values are normal. Failures of iron therapy occur when the child does not receive the prescribed medication, when it is given in a form that is poorly absorbed, or when there is continuing unrecognized blood loss. An incorrect original diagnosis of iron deficiency anemia may be revealed by therapeutic failure of iron medication.

Since a rapid hematologic response can be confidently predicted in typical iron deficiency, blood transfusion is indicated only when the anemia is very severe or when superimposed infection may interfere with the response. It is not necessary and may be dangerous to attempt rapid correction of severe anemia by transfusion because of associated hypervolemia and cardiac dilatation. Packed or sedimented red cells, which are relatively fresh or preserved in CPD anticoagulant to assure normal oxygen-hemoglobin affinity, should be administered slowly in an amount sufficient to raise the hemoglobin to a safe level at which the response to iron therapy can be awaited. In general, severely anemic children with hemoglobins under 4 gm/dl should be given only 2–3 ml/kg of packed cells at any 1 time. If there is evidence of frank congestive heart failure, a modified exchange transfusion employing fresh packed red cells should be considered. Furosemide may also be administered. Digitalis is usually unnecessary.

Sideroblastic Anemias

The sideroblastic anemias are a heterogeneous group of hypochromic microcytic anemias whose basic defects may be abnormalities of iron or heme metabolism. Serum iron levels are increased. In the bone marrow ringed sideroblasts are found; these are nucleated red cells with a perinuclear collar of coarse hemosiderin granules which represent iron-laden mitochondria.

A form of sideroblastic anemia transmitted as an X-linked recessive trait becomes symptomatic by late childhood. Splenomegaly is usually present. FEP levels

Table 14–7 RESPONSES TO IRON THERAPY IN IRON DEFICIENCY ANEMIA

12–24 hr:	Replacement of intracellular iron enzymes; subjective improvement; decreased irritability; increased appetite
36–48 hr:	Initial bone marrow response; erythroid hyperplasia
48–72 hr:	Reticulocytosis, peaking at 5–7 days
4–30 days:	Increase in hemoglobin level
1–3 mo:	Repletion of stores

are not elevated. In some cases an enzymatic deficiency of ALA synthetase has been postulated. A syndrome of refractory sideroblastic anemia with vacuolization of marrow precursor cells and exocrine pancreatic dysfunction has been reported in 4 infants. Acquired sideroblastic anemias occur in adults with a variety of inflammatory and malignant processes or with alcoholism.

Some cases of sideroblastic anemia are partially responsive to pyridoxine (vitamin B_6) given in doses of 200–500 mg/24 hr, though abnormalities of tryptophan metabolism may not occur and other findings of B_6 deficiency are not observed.

Lead Poisoning

See also Chapter 28.

Lead interferes with iron utilization and hemoglobin synthesis so that a hypochromic microcytic anemia is a prominent finding in chronic lead poisoning. The red cells are hypochromic and microcytic, with coarse basophilic stippling. Examination of the red cells with the ultraviolet microscope reveals intense fluorescence due to markedly increased levels of red cell porphyrins. Blood levels of FEP in excess of 150 μg/dl of erythrocytes and urinary excretion of large amounts of coproporphyrins are regularly seen in chronic lead poisoning.

Rare Types of Hypochromic Microcytic Anemia

Isolated cases are known of hypochromic microcytic anemia with other abnormalities of iron metabolism; some cases have had defects in iron mobilization or reutilization. Congenital absence of the iron-binding protein (atransferrinemia) is associated with hypochromic anemia.

Several patients have had refractory hypochromic anemia associated with lymphatic tumors or lymphoid hyperplasia. Correction of the anemia followed removal of the abnormal lymphatic tissue in these cases.

See also Thalassemia, Sec 14.23.

14.12   Hemolytic Anemias

The fundamental basis of the hemolytic anemias is a shortened survival time of the red blood cells. Red blood cells normally spend 100–120 days in the circulation; about 1% of red cells (senescent ones) are removed from the blood each day and are replaced by an equal number of new cells released from the bone marrow.

In response to a shortened peripheral survival of red cells, the activity of bone marrow increases. The peripheral reticulocyte count exceeds 2%. Sustained reticulocytosis in conjunction with an unchanging hemoglobin level is presumptive evidence of a hemolytic disorder. Hyperplasia of the erythropoietic marrow elements occurs, with lowering or reversal of the myeloid-erythroid ratio from the normal ranges of 2:1 to 4:1. In the chronic hemolytic processes of childhood, hypertrophy of the marrow may expand the medullary spaces and result in striking roentgenographic changes, particularly in the skull, metacarpals, and phalanges.

Elevations of unconjugated (indirect) bilirubin may accompany many hemolytic states, but overt jaundice is unusual if hepatic function is not impaired. Accelerated destruction of red cells increases the biliary excretion of heme pigments, which can be quantitated by measurement of fecal urobilinogen. Pigmented gallstones composed of calcium bilirubinate may be formed as early as the 4th yr of life. A chronic hemolytic process should be considered possible in any case of pigmentary cholelithiasis in childhood, but only about 15% of cases of gallstones in children are a consequence of hemolytic anemia. Plasma concentrations of hemoglobin increase in hemolytic anemias, and the free hemoglobin combines irreversibly with specific binding proteins called haptoglobins. The large haptoglobin-hemoglobin complex is cleared from the circulation by reticuloendothelial activity. Normal levels of serum haptoglobin are 20–200 mg/dl. In severe hemolytic states the loss of haptoglobin exceeds the synthetic capacity of the liver, and serum haptoglobin is decreased or absent. The level of hemopexin, another plasma protein that binds hemoglobin, is also reduced in hemolytic states. Catabolism of hemoglobin results in formation of carbon monoxide, and quantitation of CO in blood or expired air can provide a dynamic indicator of hemolysis. The assay is difficult, however, and not often employed clinically.

Besides these indirect indicators of hemolysis, isotopic techniques can estimate red cell survival directly. Sodium chromate ($Na_2^{51}CrO_4$) and diisofluorophosphate ($DF^{32}P$) are the radioactive compounds most often used as red cell "tags." After injection of ^{51}Cr-tagged red cells, blood radioactivity normally decreases to 50% of its initial level in 25–35 days (^{51}Cr T½ or half-life). A shortened red cell survival is likely when the ^{51}Cr T½ is reduced below 20 days. $DF^{32}P$ is expensive and more difficult to count but permits an actual measurement of red cell survival. In practice it is rarely necessary to use these techniques.

The stimulated normal bone marrow can ordinarily increase its output 6–8-fold. By such compensation red cell survival can theoretically be reduced to 15–20 days without producing anemia, but in childhood chronic hemolysis usually results in some degree of anemia. Patients with hemolytic anemias of whatever type may have transient episodes of bone marrow failure. These *aplastic crises* are characterized by reticulocytopenia and markedly decreased numbers of red cell precursors in the marrow. Occasionally, huge abnormal erythroid precursors ("gigantoblasts") are seen. Profound and life-threatening anemia may develop quickly because the shortened red cell survival is no longer even partially compensated. These episodes of acute marrow failure are self-limited and last 10–14 days. Aplastic crises are usually associated with infection and may occur within a few days in several affected members of a family. They constitute a potentially serious, life-threatening complication of any chronic hemolytic process.

The hemolytic anemias may be generally divided into 2 large classes: (1) those with premature destruction due to intrinsic abnormalities of the red cell and (2) those due to noxious extraerythrocytic factors. Table 14–4 lists the important hemolytic anemias of childhood. In hemolytic states associated with intrinsic defects red cell survival is short in normal persons receiving transfusions of the patient's red cells as well as in patients themselves. In contrast, red cells from patients with anemias due to extrinsic factors have an adequate life span when transfused to a normal recipient.

HEMOLYTIC ANEMIAS DUE TO INTRINSIC ABNORMALITIES OF THE RED CELL

14.13 HEREDITARY SPHEROCYTOSIS
(Congenital Hemolytic Anemia; Congenital Acholuric Jaundice)

This is the most common of the hereditary hemolytic states in which there is no abnormality of hemoglobin. The classic features are a congenital and familial hemolytic process associated with splenomegaly and with red cells which are spherical in shape. Cases have been reported in most ethnic groups, but the disease is most common among persons of northern European origin.

Etiology.   Hereditary spherocytosis is transmitted as an autosomal dominant trait; about 25% of cases are sporadic and presumably represent new mutations. The basic defect is thought to be an as yet undefined abnormality of the proteins or spectrins of the red cell membrane. Affected cells are unduly permeable to sodium and acquire the characteristic morphologic appearance. An increased concentration of intracellular sodium is believed to lead to an increased utilization of ATP to drive the "cation pump." Premature senescence and destruction of red cells are thought to result from metabolic overwork and loss of red cell membrane.

The spleen is intimately involved in the hemolytic process. The splenic circulation imposes a metabolic environment which is stressful to the spherocytic cell, and repeated passages through this unfavorable environment result in their sequestration and destruction. The spherocyte is relatively rigid and passes with difficulty · through the minute apertures between the splenic cords and sinuses. The hemolytic process abates after splenectomy, though the biochemical and morphologic abnormalities persist.

Clinical Manifestations.   The disease has its onset in infancy and may present in the neonatal period with anemia and hyperbilirubinemia severe enough to require phototherapy or exchange transfusions. The anemia varies considerably in severity during infancy and childhood but tends to be similar within families. Some patients with relatively severe anemia during the 1st 6–8 mo of life show more satisfactory compensation thereafter. Slight jaundice is usually present. Moderate expansion of the marrow cavity of the skull may occur but to a lesser extent than in thalassemia or the hemoglobinopathies. After infancy the spleen is almost always palpably enlarged. Although pigmentary gallstones have been reported as early as 4–5 yr of age, they usually do not develop until late childhood or adolescence. Approximately 50% of unsplenectomized patients will ultimately form gallstones. Aplastic crises are the most serious complications that occur during childhood.

Laboratory Data.   Evidences of hemolysis include reticulocytosis, anemia, and hyperbilirubinemia. The hemoglobin level usually ranges from 6–10 gm/dl and the reticulocyte count from 5–20%, averaging 10%. The characteristic spherocytic red cell is smaller than the normal erythrocyte and lacks the central pallor of the biconcave disk (Fig 14–2B). This morphologic change may be subtle, and only a relatively small proportion of the cells may be spherocytic. There is erythroid hyperplasia in marrow, but the red cell precursors are not spherocytic. There are no abnormal hemoglobins.

The basic abnormality of the red cell can be demonstrated by osmotic fragility studies. When red cells are placed in hypotonic saline solutions, water and sodium enter the cells, causing them to swell. The normal red cell of biconcave shape can increase its volume, but the spherical cell already contains the maximum volume for its surface area. Imbibition of small amounts of water causes the spherocyte to rupture. In 10–20% of cases of hereditary spherocytosis the abnormality may be demonstrated only if the blood is incubated at 37° C for 24 hr before determining osmotic fragility. The autohemolysis test is also useful in hereditary spherocytosis. When normal blood is incubated under sterile conditions for 48 hr at 37° C, fewer than 5% of the red cells hemolyze. Red cells of patients with hereditary spherocytosis have markedly increased rates of autohemolysis (15–45%). Abnormal autohemolysis can be corrected by the addition of small amounts of glucose to the blood before incubation.

Differential Diagnosis.   Hereditary spherocytosis must be differentiated from other congenital hemolytic states. The family history, blood smear, and studies of osmotic fragility and autohemolysis are of most diagnostic value. Acquired spherocytosis of the red cells is seen in autoimmune hemolytic anemias; here the spherocytosis is more noticeable than in hereditary spherocytosis, and the Coombs test result is usually positive. It may be difficult to differentiate hereditary spherocytosis in the newborn infant from hemolytic disease due to A or B incompatibility when an appropriate blood group incompatibility is coincidentally present. A period of observation may be necessary to clarify the diagnosis. Acquired spherocytosis may be seen in the thermal injury to red cells that occurs during extensive burns.

Treatment.   Splenectomy invariably produces a clinical cure. Splenectomy should be deferred whenever possible until the patient is 5–6 yr of age or older. If anemia is severe enough to impair growth or if aplastic crises are frequent, the operation may be considered earlier; an extended period of observation will be indicated before splenectomy can be justified in infancy. Splenectomy prevents gallstones and eliminates the threat of aplastic crises. Hemochromatosis and hepatic failure have been described in adults with hereditary spherocytosis who were not splenectomized. After splenectomy, jaundice and reticulocytosis rapidly disappear, and the hemoglobin level attains the normal range, though the spherocytosis and abnormal osmotic fragility become more pronounced. Thrombocytosis may occur in the immediate postoperative period, but anticoagulation therapy is not routinely indicated. Overwhelming sepsis after splenectomy is not a frequent threat to older patients with hereditary spherocytosis, but after splenectomy the febrile or infected child should be carefully evaluated and therapy initiated on the presumption of life-threatening infection (Sec 14.78).

14.14 HEREDITARY ELLIPTOCYTOSIS

Oval or elliptical shape of red cells occurs as a benign, dominantly inherited morphologic curiosity in about 1 in 2000 persons (Fig 14–3E). Elliptocytes may be seen in other conditions, such as thalassemia and iron deficiency anemia, but in these they are far fewer in number than in hereditary elliptocytosis. Hemolysis is usually mild or absent, but about 10% of patients have a significant hemolytic anemia.

Etiology. The cause is uncertain. Family studies of affected children usually reveal 1 parent with elliptocytosis without hemolysis, while the other parent is normal. A few cases may have represented homozygous inheritance. The gene for elliptocytosis is sometimes linked with the Rh locus. No biochemical abnormality of the red cell has been defined; a primary membrane abnormality has been suggested. Recent reports suggest a relationship between hemolytic elliptocytosis and pyropoikilocytosis.

Clinical Manifestations. Hemolytic elliptocytosis may produce jaundice in the neonatal period even though characteristic elliptocytosis may not be evident at that time; the blood of the affected newborn may show bizarre poikilocytosis and pyknocytosis. The usual features of a chronic hemolytic process are seen later as anemia, jaundice, splenomegaly, and osseous changes. Cholelithiasis may occur in later childhood, and aplastic crises have been reported.

Laboratory Data. The morphology of the red blood cells is the most important diagnostic feature (Fig 14–3F). Elliptical cells are prominent, but in cases with overt hemolysis many bizarre poikilocytes, microcytes, and spherocytes are also present. The reticulocyte count is increased. Erythroid hyperplasia is present in the bone marrow, but red cell precursors are not elliptical. There is no abnormal hemoglobin. The genes for abnormal hemoglobin, thalassemia, or G-6-PD deficiency do not interact with the gene for elliptocytosis to produce more severe disease.

Treatment. Splenectomy decreases the hemolytic component of this disease, although some degree of hemolysis may continue. It should be considered if there is significant chronic hemolysis. The red cell morphology is not corrected by the operation and may, in fact, be considerably more abnormal in the postoperative period.

14.15 OTHER STRUCTURAL DEFECTS

Paroxysmal Nocturnal Hemoglobinuria. Paroxysmal nocturnal hemoglobinuria is a rare chronic anemia with prominent intravascular hemolysis. The hemolysis is characteristically worse during sleep, and nocturnal and morning hemoglobinuria is a classic finding. The disease is not congenital; it results from an ill-defined intrinsic defect of the red cell membrane which renders it susceptible to hemolysis by serum complement. In addition to chronic hemolysis, there may be thrombocytopenia and/or leukopenia. Pyogenic infection, thrombosis, and thromboembolic phenomena are serious complications. Abdominal, back, and head pain may be prominent complaints. Since a number of cases have followed aplastic anemia, it has been suggested that the same agent causing aplastic anemia may predispose to paroxysmal nocturnal hemoglobinuria. The diagnosis is established by a positive result in the acid serum (Ham) or thrombin tests. The sucrose lysis test is also useful. Markedly reduced levels of red cell acetylcholinesterase activity are found. Splenectomy is not indicated. Prolonged anticoagulation therapy may be of benefit when thromboses occur. Since there is chronic loss of hemoglobin iron in the urine, iron therapy may be necessary.

Hereditary Stomatocytosis. Hereditary stomatocytosis is a rare morphologic abnormality in which the red cells are swollen and cup shaped; on stained smears they present a mouthlike slit in place of the usual circular area of central pallor. There may be hemolytic anemia. Extreme permeability of the red cell membrane to cations has been observed. Splenectomy has not been consistently effective but may be indicated in patients with severe hemolysis. Acquired stomatocytosis may be seen in a variety of conditions, especially liver disease.

Acanthocytosis. This rare defect of lipid metabolism is characterized by malabsorption, neuromuscular abnormalities, and retinitis pigmentosa. The distorted red cells have sharp projections (Fig 14–3C), but there is usually no significant hemolytic anemia. The striking morphologic changes presumably result from decreased levels of cholesterol and betalipoprotein in the serum. (See Abetalipoproteinemia in Chapters 8, 11, and 21.)

Pyropoikilocytosis. This anemia is rare, recessively transmitted, and hemolytic and is characterized by bizarre fragmented and poikilocytic red cells and spherocytes. Osmotic fragility is abnormal. These cells have reduced thermal stability. Splenectomy may be helpful; the morphologic abnormalities are more pronounced after the operation.

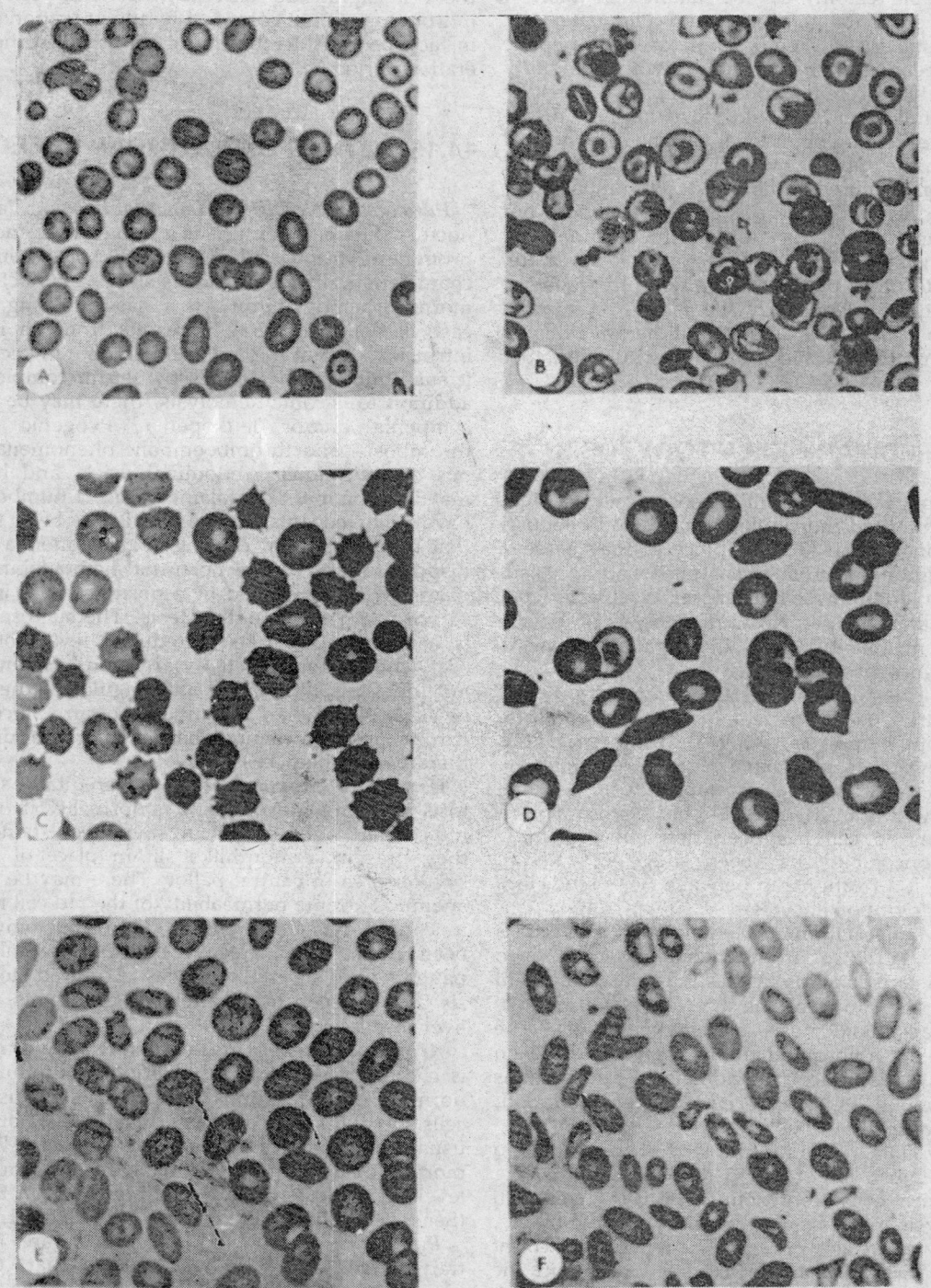

Figure 14–3 Morphologic abnormalities of the red cell. *A,* Thalassemia trait. *B,* Thalassemia major. *C,* Acanthocytes (abetalipoproteinemia). *D,* Sickle cells (Hgb SS disease). *E,* Elliptocytes (hereditary elliptocytosis). *F,* Bizarre elliptocytes (hemolytic elliptocytosis).

ENZYMATIC DEFECTS OF THE RED CELLS

Development of techniques for quantitating various red cell enzymes has permitted the identification of a number of specific entities within a group of diseases which have been identified collectively as congenital nonspherocytic hemolytic anemias because they lack spherocytosis and have normal osmotic fragility. Abnormalities of enzymes may involve the major pathways of glucose catabolism, the anaerobic Embden-Meyerhof pathway, or the oxidative pentose phosphate shunt. Disorders involving G-6-PD affect more than 100 million people throughout the world; patients with pyruvate kinase deficiency probably number in the thousands; all of the other reported red cell enzyme deficiencies probably affect not more than a few hundred individuals.

Biochemical criteria suggested for diagnosis of these diseases include demonstration of a markedly reduced level of enzyme activity in the patient's red cells by specific assay. In addition, there should be an increase in glycolytic intermediates which precede the enzyme block and a reduced level of substances dependent upon the enzyme for formation. Assays for the most important enzymes (i.e., glucose-6-phosphate dehydrogenase, pyruvate kinase) are widely available; several research laboratories in the United States are able to quantitate all glycolytic enzymes and intermediate compounds.

14.16 PYRUVATE KINASE DEFICIENCY

A congenital hemolytic anemia occurs in persons homozygous for an autosomal recessive gene which causes either a marked reduction in red cell content of pyruvate kinase or production of an abnormal enzyme with decreased activity. Generation of ATP within the red cell is impaired, and low levels of ATP, pyruvate, and NAD are seen. Concentrations of 2,3-DPG are increased. As a consequence of decreased ATP, potassium leaks from the red cell at a markedly increased rate and the cell's life span is considerably reduced.

Clinical Manifestations and Laboratory Data. The clinical manifestations vary from a severe, congenital hemolytic process to a mild, well-compensated one noted first in adulthood. Jaundice and anemia may occur in the neonatal period, and kernicterus has been reported. The later severity of the hemolytic component varies from patient to patient, but pallor, jaundice, and splenomegaly are usually present. A severe form of the disease has a relatively high frequency among the Amish of the midwestern United States.

Macrocytosis and polychromatophilia in peripheral blood reflect the elevated reticulocyte count. Spherocytes are uncommon, but a few spiculated pyknocytes are usually present. Nonincubated osmotic fragility is normal. Autohemolysis is moderately or markedly increased, but addition of glucose does not regularly correct the abnormality as it does in hereditary spherocytosis.

Diagnosis rests upon demonstration by spectrophotometric assay of marked reductions of pyruvate kinase activity in the red cells. Other red cell enzyme activities are normal or elevated. There are no abnormalities of hemoglobin. The white blood cells have normal pyruvate kinase activity. Heterozygous carriers usually have moderately reduced levels of pyruvate kinase activity.

Treatment. Exchange transfusions may be indicated for control of hyperbilirubinemia during the neonatal period. Transfusions of packed red cells are necessary for severe anemia or for aplastic crises. If the degree of anemia is consistently severe or if frequent transfusions are required, splenectomy should be performed after 5–6 yr of age. Although not curative, the operation may be followed by higher hemoglobin levels. The reticulocyte count may be strikingly high (30–60%) following splenectomy. Deaths due to overwhelming pneumococcal sepsis have followed splenectomy on rare occasions (Sec 14.78).

DEFICIENCIES OF OTHER GLYCOLYTIC ENZYMES

Congenital nonspherocytic anemias may stem from defects in hexokinase, glucose phosphate isomerase, phosphofructokinase, glyceraldehyde 3-phosphate dehydrogenase, triose phosphate isomerase, and 2,3-diphosphoglycerate mutase; these defects are transmitted as autosomal recessive traits. Phosphoglycerate kinase deficiency due to an X-linked defect has been described in a mentally retarded boy. In homozygous triose phosphate isomerase deficiency, progressive neurologic dysfunction, mental retardation, and cardiac abnormalities occur in infants surviving to more than a few mo of age.

In these conditions the red cell morphology is not strikingly abnormal except for polychromasia and macrocytosis. Nonincubated osmotic fragility is normal. Splenectomy has been of variable benefit and is indicated when the hemolytic process is severe.

In addition to these glycolytic enzymopathies, rare cases of hemolytic anemia due to pyrimidine-5' nucleotidase or ATPase have been reported as well as inherited deficiencies of a number of other red cell enzymes (lactic hydrogenase, methemoglobin reductase, catalase, and others) without hemolysis.

DEFICIENCIES OF ENZYMES OF THE PENTOSE PHOSPHATE PATHWAY AND RELATED COMPOUNDS

The most important function of the pentose pathway, through which about 10% of the glucose utilized by the red cell passes, is to provide the NADPH or reduced triphosphopyridine nucleotide (TPNH) necessary for conversion of oxidized to reduced glutathione. This is essential for the physiologic inactivation of oxidant compounds, such as hydrogen peroxide, that accumulate within the red cell. If glutathione or any of the compounds or enzymes necessary for maintaining it in the reduced state are decreased, hemoglobin may become denatured and precipitated into red cell inclusions called *Heinz bodies*. Once Heinz bodies have formed, the red cell is rapidly removed from the circulation; an acute hemolytic process may result from damage to the red cell membrane by the precipitated hemoglobin and the action of the spleen.

14.17　GLUCOSE-6-PHOSPHATE DEHYDROGENASE (G-6-PD) DEFICIENCY

G-6-PD deficiency, by far the most important disease in this group, is responsible for 2 clinical syndromes: an episodic hemolytic anemia induced by infections or certain drugs and a spontaneous chronic nonspherocytic hemolytic anemia. The deficiency is due to inheritance of any of a large number of abnormal alleles of the gene responsible for the synthesis of the G-6-PD molecule. The normal enzyme found in most populations is designated G-6-PD B+. A normal variant designated G-6-PD A+ is common in American Blacks. Nearly 100 distinct enzyme variants of G-6-PD have been found associated with a wide spectrum of hemolytic disease.

Drug-Induced Hemolytic Anemia Associated with G-6-PD Deficiency
(Primaquine Sensitivity)

Synthesis of red cell G-6-PD is determined by genes borne on the X chromosome. Diseases involving this enzyme occur, therefore, more frequently in males than in females. About 13% of American black males and 2% of black females have a mutant enzyme which results in a deficiency of red cell G-6-PD activity. Italians, Greeks, and other Mediterranean, Middle Eastern, African, and Oriental ethnic groups also have high frequencies ranging from 5–40%. The G-6-PD activity of the homozygous female or the heterozygous male is 5–10% of normal. The heterozygous female has an intermediate enzymatic activity and, as an example of random X chromosome inactivation (Lyon hypothesis), has 2 populations of red cells; 1 is normal, the other deficient in G-6-PD activity. The heterozygous female does not, however, have clinical hemolysis after exposure to oxidant drugs.

There is considerable variation in the defect among various racial groups; the defect in Blacks is less severe than in affected Caucasians. In Blacks, enzyme deficiency is associated with an electrophoretically distinct enzyme variant designated G-6-PD A− and 5–15% or less of normal enzyme activity. In addition, the enzyme is unstable in vivo, and the activity of the enzyme is decreased in the older red cells in the circulation. Affected Caucasians have a variant designated G-6-PD B− (G-6-PD Mediterranean). The activity of red cells containing this enzyme is very low, often under 1% of normal. A 3rd common mutant enzyme with markedly reduced activity (G-6-PD Canton) occurs in about 5% of Chinese. A number of other rare enzyme variants have

been associated with drug-induced hemolysis. The basic defect appears to be production of an unstable enzyme which becomes inactive much more rapidly than normal.

In the usual pattern of G-6-PD deficiency no evidence of hemolysis is apparent until 48–96 hr after the patient has ingested a substance which has oxidant properties. Drugs that have these properties include antipyretics, sulfonamides, antimalarials, and naphthaquinolones. The fava bean, a Mediterranean dietary staple, is also particularly potent, producing an acute and severe hemolytic syndrome called "favism." The degree of hemolysis varies with the agent, the amount ingested, and the severity of the enzyme deficiency in the patient. In severe cases hemoglobinuria and jaundice result, and the hemoglobin concentration may decrease 60–70%. Death may occur as a consequence of severe hemolysis. Even if administration of the responsible drug is continued, recovery is the rule, with evidence of a compensated hemolytic process. Infection may result in hemolysis. This defect is an important cause of neonatal hyperbilirubinemia and kernicterus in Greek and Chinese newborn infants with the G-6-PD Mediterranean and Canton enzyme variants. Significant hemolysis may occur even when no exposure to drugs can be documented. In the G-6-PD A− variant the hemolytic process after drug exposure is usually self-limited and mild because the younger red cells in the circulation have nearly normal enzyme activity and resist hemolytic destruction. In black newborns spontaneous hemolysis may occur in premature, but not term, infants with G-6-PD deficiency. When a pregnant woman ingests drugs such as sulfonamides or naphthalene, they may be transmitted to her G-6-PD–deficient fetus, and hemolytic anemia and jaundice may ensue after birth.

Laboratory Data. Hemoglobinemia and hemoglobinuria are manifest in severe acute cases, with falls in hemoglobin of 2–10 gm/dl. Unstained or supravital preparations of the red cell reveal the multiple small round inclusions called Heinz bodies, which are not visible on Wright-stained blood smears. Because cells containing these inclusions are rapidly removed from the circulation, they are not seen after the 1st 3–4 days of illness. Recovery is heralded by reticulocytosis and increase in hemoglobin concentration.

Diagnosis. Diagnosis depends upon direct or indirect demonstration of reduced G-6-PD activity in red cells. By direct measurement, enzyme activity in affected persons is 10% of normal or less, and the reduction of enzyme is more extreme in Caucasians and Orientals than in Blacks. Satisfactory screening tests are based upon decoloration of methylene blue and upon reduction of methemoglobin. Immediately after a hemolytic episode reticulocytes and young red cells predominate. These young cells have significantly higher enzyme activity than older cells; therefore, testing may have to be deferred for a few wk before a diagnostically low level of enzyme can be shown. The diagnosis can be suspected when the G-6-PD activity is within the low normal range in the presence of high reticulocyte count. G-6-PD variants can also be detected by electrophoretic analysis.

Treatment. Prevention of hemolysis constitutes the most important therapeutic measure. When possible, males belonging to ethnic groups in which there is a significant incidence of G-6-PD deficiency (Greeks, southern Italians, Sephardic Jews, Filipinos, southern Chinese, Blacks, and Thais) should be tested for the defect before drugs are given which are known to be oxidant. When hemolysis has occurred, supportive therapy may include blood transfusions. Spontaneous recovery is the rule.

Other Hemolytic Anemias Associated with Deficiencies of G-6-PD and Related Substances

In rare instances chronic hemolytic anemias have been associated with profound deficiencies of G-6-PD due to inheritance of enzyme variants particularly defective in quantity, activity, or stability. Occasionally and unaccountably, persons with G-6-PD B⁻ (Mediterranean) enzyme deficiency have chronic hemolysis. The anemia is inherited as an X-linked recessive, and many males of northern European origin have been affected. Chronic hemolytic anemia is maintained, and worsening of the hemolytic process may follow ingestion of oxidant drugs. Splenectomy is of little value. A mild, chronic nonspherocytic anemia has also been reported in association with a genetically determined deficiency of red cell glutathione. 6-Phosphogluconate dehydrogenase deficiency has been associated with drug hemolysis. Hyperbilirubinemia has been related to a deficiency of glutathione peroxidase in several newborn infants.

HEMOGLOBINOPATHIES

The molecular and biochemical characteristics of the hemoglobins are remarkably well known. The genes of their component polypeptide chains have been located on chromosomes No. 11 and No. 16, and the actual genes have been isolated and their DNA sequences determined. Alpha and beta chains consist of about 150 amino acids, and the precise sequence of these amino acids in the peptide chains has been defined. It is possible to identify and locate precisely the single amino acid substitutions which result in abnormal hemoglobins. (See also Chapter 8.)

The clinically important abnormal hemoglobin syndromes result from single amino acid substitutions in the α or β chains of adult hemoglobin. Many hemoglobin variants have been described; only a few of them are relatively prevalent. Hemoglobin variants are usually identified by electrophoresis.

14.18 SICKLE CELL HEMOGLOBINOPATHIES

The sickle cell hemoglobinopathies are superb models of molecular disease, from the levels of gene structure and action to the ultimate clinical syndrome in the patient. The basic defect resides in a mutant, autosomal gene which causes valine to be substituted for glutamic acid in the No. 6 position of a beta polypeptide chain ($\alpha_2\beta_2^{6val}$). This minor substitution has profound physiochemical consequences: deoxygenation now results in a change which facilitates stacking of deoxygenated sickle hemoglobin molecules into monofilaments; these aggregate into elongated crystals, distorting the red cell membrane and ultimately forming the sickled cell.

It is possible to make a prenatal diagnosis of sickle cell anemia as early as 16–20 wk of gestation. Fetal blood from aspiration of the placenta or of a fetal vein is incubated with ^{14}C-leucine to assess polypeptide chain synthesis by reticulocytes. In fetuses destined to have sickle cell anemia only α, γ, and βˢ polypeptide chains are synthesized. Techniques using recombinant DNA and endonuclease restriction enzymes have shown that the DNA segment bearing a Hgb S gene often differs from the segment bearing a Hgb A gene; this finding may permit the diagnosis of sickle cell anemia using fibroblasts from amniotic fluid. The possibilities of prenatal diagnosis may help in genetic counseling for the hemoglobinopathies.

Sickle Cell Trait

Heterozygous occurrence of the sickle gene usually has a benign clinical course. About 8% of American Blacks have the trait; there is a much greater incidence in parts of Africa. Typical cases also occur in other ethnic groups from Mediterranean and Mid- and Near-Eastern areas. Possession of a sickle gene is believed to confer a degree of resistance to falciparum malaria. The individual red cells of persons with the trait contain a mixture of normal and sickle hemoglobins (Hgb A and Hgb S). The Hgb S proportion varies from 35–45%. With these low proportions of Hgb S, sickling does not occur under physiologic conditions. Rarely, severe hypoxia resulting from shock or from flying at high altitudes in unpressurized aircraft may produce vaso-occlusive phenomena. Spontaneous hematuria, usually from the left kidney, and mild hyposthenuria may also occur; but anemia, hemolysis, or other clinical abnormalities are not attributable to the uncomplicated sickle trait. Sickle cell trait and various conditions will occur by chance in 8% of the black population. The sickle cell trait does not affect longevity. Carriers should avoid situations in which hypoxia may occur, but otherwise do not need to modify their life or activities.

Sickle Cell Anemia

Sickle cell anemia is a severe, chronic hemolytic anemia occurring in persons homozygous for the sickle gene. The clinical course is marked by episodes of pain due to occlusion of small blood vessels by spontaneously sickled red cells. These have traditionally been called "crises." Crises are of several varieties, however, and the "crisis" is not a specific diagnostic entity.

Clinical Manifestations. Manifestations of sickle cell disease do not usually appear until the latter part

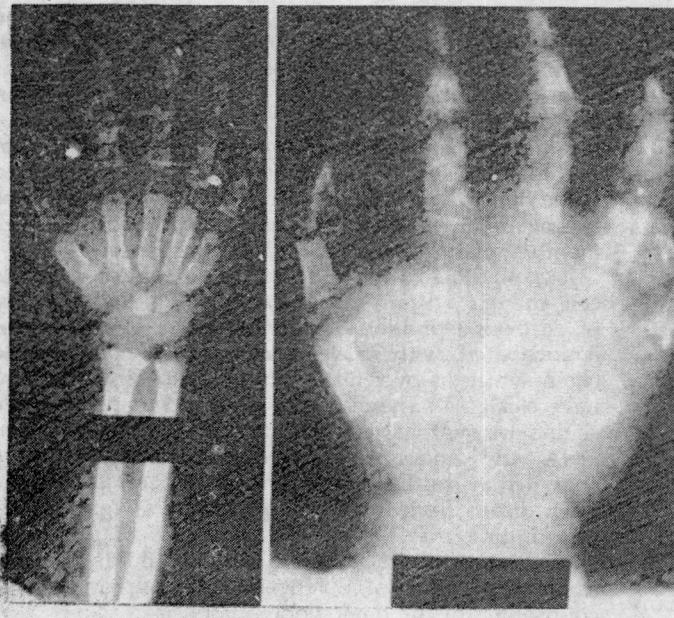

Figure 14—4 Roentgenograms of infant with sickle cell anemia. Note bony destruction.

of the 1st yr of life. The large amounts of Hgb F present in the red cells of young infants obscure the detection of small amounts of nonfetal hemoglobins. Use of specialized techniques such as agar gel electrophoresis at acid pH or microcolumn chromatography is necessary for precise diagnosis in early life. Coincidentally with the postnatal decrease in Hgb F, the concentration of Hgb S rises. Intravascular sickling and evidences of a hemolytic process are present by 6–8 wk of age, but clinical symptoms are unusual before 5–6 mo.

The painful or *vaso-occlusive crises*, the most frequent variety, with distal ischemia and infarction may be precipitated by infections or develop spontaneously in any or in many parts of the body. Symmetrical, painful swelling of the hands and feet (hand-foot syndrome or sickle cell dactylitis) caused by infarction in the small bones of the extremities may be the initial manifestation of sickle cell anemia in infancy. Striking bony destruction with periosteal reaction may be observed roentgenographically (Fig 14–4). In older patients the large joints and surrounding parts become painful and swollen. Severe abdominal pains, resembling those of an acute surgical condition of the abdomen, often accompany infarction in abdominal structures. Strokes due to cerebral occlusion are serious and, if not immediately fatal, may leave hemiplegias. Extensive pulmonary infarction is difficult to differentiate from pneumonia. Vaso-occlusive crises are not associated with pronounced changes in the usual hematologic picture.

A 2nd type of crisis, seen only in the young patient, is the so-called *sequestration crisis*. For unknown reasons large amounts of blood become acutely pooled in the liver and the spleen. The spleen becomes massively enlarged, and signs of circulatory collapse develop rapidly. If the patient is supported by hydration and by blood transfusion, much of the sequestered blood is remobilized. This sort of episode is a frequent cause of death in the infant with sickle cell disease and occurs

in older patients with sickle cell variants in whom splenomegaly persists into later life.

The 3rd well characterized type of crisis is the *aplastic crisis* previously described (Sec 14.5).

Hyperhemolytic crises are unusual but may result when a person with homozygous sickle cell disease, who coincidentally has G-6-PD deficiency, ingests an oxidant drug. They may also be precipitated by infection.

In addition to the acute crises, a wide variety of clinical signs and symptoms result from severe hemolytic anemia and chronic vaso-occlusive disease. Progressive impairment of liver function contributes to the visible jaundice these patients regularly demonstrate. Gallstones have occurred in patients as young as 3 yr of age. Central nervous system infarctions, manifested as "strokes," occur in 5–10% of children and may leave permanent sequelae such as hemiplegia. Renal function is progressively impaired by diffuse glomerular and tubular fibrosis; renal papillary necrosis and the nephrotic syndrome may occasionally occur.

The spleen is initially considerably enlarged, but the clinically enlarged spleen has markedly reduced phagocytic and reticuloendothelial functions, and there is functional hyposplenism. Later, because of repeated episodes of infarction, the spleen becomes small and fibrotic and is rarely palpably enlarged after 5–6 yr of age. Episodes of severe pulmonary involvement due to infarction occur with or without infection.

Persons with sickle cell anemia have a markedly increased susceptibility to pneumococcal meningitis and septicemia, like patients after splenectomy, especially in the 1st years of life. As many as 30% of children with sickle cell anemia develop sepsis and meningitis during the 1st 5 yr of life; mortality is as high as 25%. The increased risk stems from the functional hyposplenia and a deficiency of serum opsonins against pneumococci. A striking susceptibility to *Salmonella* osteomyelitis is also present.

By childhood most patients are underweight, and puberty is delayed, particularly in males. Chronic leg ulcers are common in adolescent and early adult life.

Laboratory Data. Hemoglobin concentrations range from 6–8 gm/dl. A peripheral blood smear usually contains irreversibly sickled cells (Fig 14–3D). Spontaneous sickling in capillary blood smears almost always indicates classic homozygous sickle cell disease; it is not observed with the trait and is infrequently present with the sickle cell variants. Target cells and poikilocytes are seen. The reticulocyte count ranges from 5–15%, and nucleated red cells and Howell-Jolly bodies are usually present. The total white blood cell count is elevated to 12,000–20,000/mm³ with a predominance of neutrophils. The platelet count is increased; the sedimentation rate is slow. Other changes include abnormal liver function test results, hyperbilirubinemia, and diffuse hypergammaglobulinemia. The bone marrow is markedly hyperplastic and shows erythroid predominance. Roentgenograms show expanded marrow spaces and osteoporosis.

Studies of the red cells and hemoglobin are essential to the diagnosis. A rapid, simple test for the presence of Hgb S is the sickle cell preparation, in which red cells are deoxygenated or exposed to reducing agents such as sodium metabisulfite. Virtually 100% of the red cells can be induced to sickle in both sickle disease and sickle trait, but sickling is more rapid and extreme in the disease state than with the trait. Under 100% of sickling occurs after transfusion or during early infancy. Rapid solubility tests are also available for detection of the presence of Hgb S in red cells, utilizing the principle that reduced Hgb S is insoluble and precipitates into a turbid solution. Neither sickling nor solubility tests are genetically definitive, both giving false positive and false negative test results. Electrophoretic examination of hemoglobin is conclusive. After infancy the red cells of patients with sickle cell anemia contain approximately 90% Hgb S, 2–10% Hgb F, and a normal amount of Hgb A₂. No Hgb A is present. Each parent has the sickle cell trait, 1 of the sickle variants, or thalassemia trait.

Differential Diagnosis. Sickle cell disease may be associated with a wide variety of clinical signs and symptoms. The presence of painful joints with the heart murmurs of anemia may suggest acute rheumatic fever or rheumatoid arthritis. Pneumonia, osteomyelitis, and leukemia are occasionally difficult to differentiate. Because of the varied signs and symptoms of sickle cell anemia, it is important to perform electrophoretic studies on black patients.

Treatment. No therapy is necessary except during acute episodes. Administration of extra quantities of vitamins or of hematinics is of no proven value, though some centers prescribe folic acid supplements. Iron therapy is not indicated unless iron deficiency can be established. No pharmacologic treatment of the painful crisis has proved safe or of consistent value, including the use of intravenous infusions of urea and of oral cyanate. Analgesics such as codeine and phenothiazines usually suffice for the discomfort and pain. Regular administration of narcotics should be avoided to prevent addiction. Dehydration and acidosis should be vigorously corrected by the intravenous route. Compli-

cating bacterial infections require appropriate antibiotic therapy. Blood transfusions are not necessary for the usual painful crises but are indicated for prolonged or extreme pain, for extensive involvement of lungs or central nervous system, in preparation for general anesthesia, and during the latter part of pregnancy. Transfusions of packed red cells are given to dilute the patient's red cells with normal ones. When the proportion of Hgb SS red cells can be reduced to less than 40% by transfusions, vaso-occlusive symptoms will generally abate. Partial exchange transfusion can rapidly lower the number of sickling cells. Transfusions are essential in sequestration and aplastic episodes. Splenectomy is not indicated unless sequestration crises have been recurrent or hypersplenism can be shown.

14.19 OTHER HEMOGLOBINOPATHIES

Hemoglobin C ($\alpha_2\beta_2^{6\,lys}$). Hemoglobin C occurs in about 2% of American Blacks. In the heterozygous state (Hgb AC) no anemia or disease is present, but increased numbers of target cells are seen in the peripheral blood. In the homozygous person (Hgb CC disease) a moderately severe hemolytic anemia with hemoglobin levels from 8–11 gm/dl, a reticulocytosis of 5–10%, and splenomegaly are regularly observed. The peripheral blood contains striking numbers of target cells and spherocytes (Fig 14–2).

Hemoglobin D. The hemoglobin Ds include several varieties of abnormal hemoglobin with electrophoretic mobilities similar to those of Hgb S, but with different biochemical and physical properties. Sickling does not occur in Hgb D syndromes. The homozygous state (Hgb DD) is characterized by a mild hemolytic anemia with splenomegaly.

Hemoglobin E ($\alpha_2\beta_2^{26\,lys}$). Hemoglobin E is prevalent in persons from Southeast Asia, particularly Thailand. Homozygous Hgb E disease is characterized by a mild hemolytic anemia, with target cells prominent, and microcytosis, with moderate to severe splenomegaly. The clinical and hematologic findings are similar to those associated with Hgb C.

Hemoglobin SC Disease. When the genes for both Hgb S and Hgb C are present in the same person, a moderately severe anemia with splenomegaly results. There are vaso-occlusive episodes, but these are usually less frequent and milder than those of sickle cell disease. Aseptic necrosis of the femoral head is an occasional complication, and severe retinal damage also occurs. The hemoglobin concentration averages 9–10 gm/dl. Target cells are numerous, but irreversibly sickled cells are usually not present in the peripheral blood. Hemoglobin electrophoresis reveals a nearly equal mixture of Hgb S and Hgb C, with slight elevation of Hgb F. Hgb SC disease does not usually affect growth and is compatible with extended survival into adult life. Aplastic and sequestration crises are potential threats to life.

14.20 UNSTABLE HEMOGLOBINS

With at least 50 varieties of abnormal hemoglobin, amino acid substitutions in either α or β chains cause molecular instability leading to denaturation and precipitation of hemoglobin within the red cell. The precipitated hemoglobin attaches to the red cell membrane, destroying the cell. These chronic hemolytic processes are characterized by intraerythrocytic inclusions (Heinz bodies) and sometimes by excretion of dark brown urine containing dipyrrolic compounds, especially pronounced after splenectomy. These anemias are transmitted as autosomal dominant states. Each variant is usually assigned the name of its city of origin (Hgb Zürich, Köln, Santa Ana, Bristol, etc.).

Hemolysis is usually evident 3–6 mo after birth with β variants. The severity ranges from a compensated mild anemia to a severe hemolytic process. Mean corpuscular hemoglobin concentration is characteristically reduced. Jaundice and splenomegaly are regularly found. The abnormal hemoglobin accounts for 30–40 % of the total. It may or may not be detected by electrophoresis, but heating of hemolysate at 50° C for 1 hr results in a heavy precipitate of the abnormal hemoglobin, whereas normal hemoglobin is not affected. Unstable hemoglobins may also be demonstrated by adding fresh hemolysate to a 17% buffered solution of isopropanol. Heinz bodies may be produced by incubation of whole blood for 48 hr prior to supravital staining with brilliant cresyl blue and appear in markedly increased numbers following splenectomy. In some variants (Hgb Zürich, Hgb Toronto) severe hemolysis is precipitated by ingestion of sulfonamides. Splenectomy appears sometimes to improve patients with moderately severe disease, but those with severe hemolysis derive little benefit.

14.21   HEMOGLOBINS CAUSING CYANOSIS (Hgb M)

A group of 5 abnormal hemoglobins designated as the hemoglobin Ms are associated with dominantly transmitted familial cyanosis due to the production of methemoglobinemia. Because the characteristic amino acid substitutions are strategically located near the attachments of heme groups, internal oxidation of heme iron to the trivalent (ferric) form occurs. The Hgb M diseases are characterized by cyanosis and mild polycythemia. With Hgb M variants resulting from β chain substitutions, such as Hgb M Saskatoon, cyanosis is not seen until 4–6 mo of age, whereas in α chain variants, such as Hgb M Boston, cyanosis is congenital. Hgb M disease has often been mistaken for cyanotic congenital heart disease.

Methemoglobinemias due to Hgb M can be distinguished from other forms of methemoglobinemia by characteristic changes in the spectral absorption patterns of hemoglobin solutions. Electrophoresis can demonstrate and quantitate the abnormal hemoglobin. No therapy is indicated; specifically, use of methylene blue or ascorbic acid is of no benefit (Sec 8.44).

14.22   HEMOGLOBINS WITH ALTERED OXYGEN AFFINITY

More than 20 abnormal hemoglobins are known to have a marked increase in their affinity for oxygen, as indicated by a shift to the left of the oxygen dissociation curve and a low P_{50} in the range of 12–18 mm Hg. Because of the increased affinity for hemoglobin there is decreased release of oxygen to the tissues, leading to tissue hypoxia. This causes increased production of erythropoietin and secondary polycythemia. Most of these variants can be demonstrated electrophoretically (Sec 14.30). Examples include Hgbs Chesapeake, Rainier, and Malmo.

Six hemoglobin variants with markedly reduced affinity for oxygen have been reported. These are associated with familial chronic cyanosis or "pseudoanemia." The oxygen dissociation curve is shifted to the right, with P_{50} values greater than 30 mm Hg. Examples include Hgbs Kansas and Providence.

14.23   THALASSEMIA

The thalassemias are a heterogeneous group of heritable hypochromic anemias of varying degrees of severity. Basic genetic defects include abnormalities of messenger RNA processing in some patients, deletion of genetic material in others. In either case, a deficient quantity of mRNA leads to deficient synthesis of hemoglobin polypeptide chains. Different types of thalassemia with different clinical and biochemical manifestations are associated with defects in each polypeptide chain (α, β, γ, δ). In contrast to the hemoglobinopathies, no basic chemical abnormality of hemoglobin species lies behind the thalassemias, although alterations in the amounts of Hgb A_2 and Hgb F may be seen. Tetrameric forms, such as Hgb H (β_4) and Hgb Bart's (γ_4), may be found in certain types of α-thalassemia (see below). Polypeptide chain synthesis may be totally absent, as in the β^0 type of β-thalassemia, or only partially deficient (β^+ type).

The most common genetic variety of thalassemia involves impaired production of beta chains (β-thalassemia). The gene is prevalent in ethnic groups from areas around the Mediterranean Sea, especially in Italy, in Greece, and on the Mediterranean islands. Foci of high prevalence are found also in India and Southeast Asia. From 3–8% of Americans of Italian or Greek ancestry and 0.5% of black Americans carry a gene for β-thalassemia. The incidence of β-thalassemia in most non-Mediterranean peoples is very low, but typical cases occur in many racial groups. Like the sickle cell gene, that of thalassemia appears to be associated with increased resistance to malaria, which may account for its incidence and geographic distribution. Most cases can be clinically classified as thalassemia major or minor, to correspond in general with homozygous or heterozygous genotype.

14.24   Thalassemia Minor
(β-Thalassemia Trait)

Heterozygous β-thalassemia is associated with mild anemia. The hemoglobin concentration averages 2–3 gm/dl lower than age-related normal values. The red cells are hypochromic and microcytic, with poikilocytosis, ovalocytosis, and often coarse basophilic stippling

(Fig 14–3A). Target cells are present but usually not prominent and should not be considered specific for thalassemia. The mean corpuscular volume (MCV) is low, averaging 65 fl. Mean corpuscular hemoglobin (MCH) is also low (< 26 pg). A mild decrease in red cell survival can be documented, but overt signs of hemolysis are usually absent. The serum iron level is normal or elevated.

Individuals with thalassemia trait are often misdiagnosed as having iron deficiency anemia and may be inappropriately treated with iron for extended periods of time. More than 90% of persons with β-thalassemia trait have diagnostic elevations of Hgb A$_2$ of 3.4–7.0%. About 50% of these persons also have slight elevations of Hgb F, from 2–6%. In a small number of otherwise typical cases, normal levels of Hgb A$_2$ with Hgb F levels ranging from 5–15% are found (the so-called high fetal or β-δ-thalassemia variant). The Lepore hemoglobin is a molecular variant which represents a combination of β and δ chains. Individuals heterozygous for Lepore hemoglobin have clinical and hematologic features of thalassemia minor.

Other than being mistaken for iron deficiency anemia, the important implication of thalassemia trait is genetic. When both mother and father have thalassemia trait, each pregnancy carries a 25% risk of thalassemia major. Techniques for fetal blood sampling permit prenatal diagnosis of thalassemia major. A small sample of fetal blood can be obtained at 16–20 wk of gestation by fetoscopy with direct aspiration from a placental vein. This blood is incubated with ^{14}C leucine, and the synthesis of α, β, and γ chains can be quantitated. Fetuses having homozygous β-thalassemia will demonstrate a marked reduction of β-chain synthesis. Endonuclease restriction enzyme analysis of DNA from amniotic fluid fibroblasts may permit diagnosis of affected fetuses in the future.

14.25 Thalassemia Major
(Cooley Anemia)

Homozygous β-thalassemia usually becomes symptomatic as a severe, progressive hemolytic anemia during the 2nd 6 mo of life. Regular blood transfusions are necessary to prevent profound weakness and cardiac decompensation due to anemia. Without transfusion life expectancy is only a few yr. In untreated cases or cases receiving infrequent transfusions at times of severe anemia and hemolysis, hypertrophy of erythropoietic tissue occurs in medullary and extramedullary locations. The bones become thin, and pathologic fractures may occur. Massive expansion of the marrow of the face and skull (Fig 14–5 and 14–6) produces a typical facies. Pallor, hemosiderosis, and jaundice combine to produce a greenish-brown complexion. The spleen and liver are enlarged by extramedullary hematopoiesis and hemosiderosis. In older patients the spleen may become so enlarged that it causes mechanical discomfort, and secondary hypersplenism. Growth is impaired in older children; puberty rarely occurs because of endocrine abnormalities. Diabetes mellitus due to pancreatic siderosis occurs often. Cardiac complications such as pericarditis and chronic congestive failure due to myocardial siderosis are common terminal events. In transfusion-dependent patients death usually occurs during the 2nd decade; only a few patients have survived to their 30's.

Laboratory Data. The red cell changes of thalassemia major are extreme. In addition to severe hypochromia and microcytosis (Fig 14–3B), many bizarre, fragmented poikilocytes and target cells are present. Large numbers of nucleated red cells circulate, especially after splenectomy. Intraerythrocytic precipitations thought to represent excess alpha chains are also seen after splenectomy. In the usual case the hemoglobin level falls progressively to less than 5 gm/dl unless transfusions are given. About 10% of patients with homozygous thalassemia can maintain hemoglobin levels of 6–8 gm/dl without transfusions (thalassemia in-

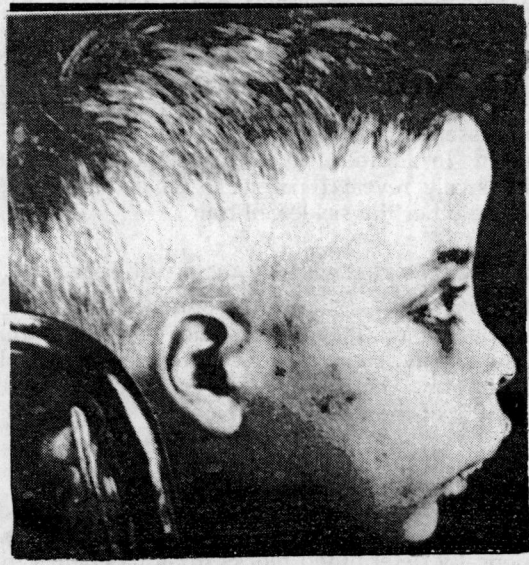

Figure 14–5 Appearance of patient with thalassemia major (Cooley anemia). Note the maxillary hyperplasia and resulting dental abnormality.

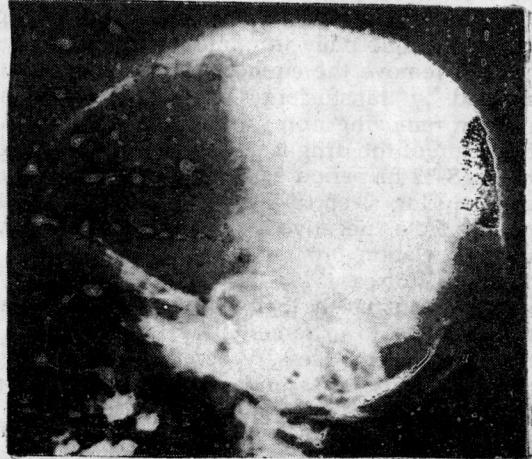

Figure 14–6 Roentgenogram of skull, showing overgrowth of the maxilla with opacification of the sinuses. The diploic spaces are widened, with prominent vertical trabeculae (hair on end).

termedia). The unconjugated serum bilirubin level is elevated. The concentration of serum iron is high, with saturation of the iron-binding capacity. LDH levels are also very high, reflecting ineffective erythropoiesis. A striking biochemical characteristic is the presence of large amounts of fetal hemoglobin in the red cells. The level of Hgb F is greater than 70% during the early yr of life but has a tendency to decline with increasing age. Quantitation of the actual level of fetal hemoglobin is imprecise because of frequent transfusions. Hemoglobin A_2 level is usually under 3%, but the ratio of Hgb A_2 to Hgb A is markedly increased. Dipyrrolic compounds render the urine dark brown, especially after splenectomy.

Treatment. Transfusions are given to maintain the hemoglobin level above 10 gm/dl. This "hypertransfusion" has striking clinical benefit: it permits normal activity with comfort; it prevents progressive marrow expansion that leads to cosmetic problems associated with facial bone changes; and it minimizes cardiac dilatation and osteoporosis. Transfusions of 15 ml/kg of packed cells are usually necessary every 4–5 wk. Even more vigorous transfusional programs have been advocated ("supertransfusion") to keep the hemoglobin level above 12 gm/dl and completely suppress erythropoiesis.

Careful cross-matching should be performed to forestall isoimmunization and prevent transfusion reactions. The use of packed red blood cells which are relatively fresh (less than 1 wk in CPD anticoagulant) is desirable. Even with meticulous care febrile reactions to transfusions are common. These may be minimized with the use of erythrocytes reconstituted from frozen blood, or leukocyte-poor red cell preparations, and by the administration of salicylates before transfusions.

Hemosiderosis is an inevitable consequence of prolonged transfusion therapy because each 250 ml of blood delivers to the tissues about 200 mg of iron which cannot be excreted by physiologic means. The cardiac complications which are the usual cause of death appear to be a direct consequence of myocardial siderosis. It may be possible to reduce this lethal iron burden by means of iron-chelating agents. The most promising of these is deferoxamine. The drug must be given parenterally. A single daily intramuscular injection usually does not remove the equivalent daily amount of iron delivered by transfusions. The efficiency of deferoxamine in removing iron can be markedly enhanced if 1.5–2.0 gm of the drug is administered subcutaneously over an 8–12 hr period using a compact battery-driven pump, during sleep, 5–6 nights/wk. In most patients over 7 yr old a "negative" iron balance is possible. Such chronic chelation programs may alter the poor prognosis of this disease.

Liberal transfusion therapy prevents massive splenomegaly due to extramedullary erythropoiesis. Splenectomy is often necessary because of the size of the organ or because of secondary hypersplenism, but has no effect on the basic hematologic disease. In some patients who have had splenectomy, severe, overwhelming sepsis may develop. For this reason the operation should be performed only for significant indications and should be deferred as long as possible.

The most important indication for splenectomy is an increased need for transfusions, indicating an element of hypersplenism. Immunization with pneumococcal polysaccharide vaccine is indicated and prophylactic penicillin therapy is advocated by some authorities (Sec 14.78).

14.26   OTHER THALASSEMIC SYNDROMES

THALASSEMIA INTERMEDIA

This term is often assigned to patients with thalassemia syndromes intermediate in severity between major and minor. Jaundice and moderate splenomegaly are present, and the hemoglobin level is 7–8 gm/dl. Transfusions are not regularly necessary to prevent severe anemia, but transfusion therapy may prevent marked cosmetic and other osseous abnormalities. Even without regular blood transfusions these patients absorb large amounts of iron, and hemosiderosis may occur. Tea, which markedly reduces iron absorption, has been advocated with meals. Splenectomy is often necessary.

These patients are heterogeneous: Some are apparently homozygous; others are heterozygous for thalassemia genes with genes for other thalassemia variants, such as $\beta\delta$ or Lepore traits.

HEMOGLOBIN S-THALASSEMIA

Combination of a thalassemia gene with that of an abnormal beta chain hemoglobin results in clinical disease more severe than with either trait alone. Hbg S-thalassemia is a moderately severe hemolytic anemia with mild to moderate vaso-occlusive symptoms and significant splenomegaly. When the β^+ thalassemia gene is present, the hemoglobin electrophoretic pattern shows a predominance of Hgb S, ranging from 60–80%, the remainder being Hgb F and Hgb A. In some instances, when the β^0 thalassemia gene is present, no Hgb A can be detected and the electrophoretic pattern is like that of sickle cell disease. In sickle cell anemia, however, the red cells are normocytic, whereas in Hgb S-thalassemia microcytosis with an MCV under 75 fl is present. In addition, in such instances family studies will usually reveal 1 parent to have thalassemia trait and the other the sickle cell trait.

HEMOGLOBIN C-THALASSEMIA AND D-THALASSEMIA

Hemoglobin C-thalassemia and hemoglobin D-thalassemia are mild hemolytic anemias with significant splenomegaly. Hemoglobin electrophoresis reveals that the abnormal hemoglobin, C or D, constitutes more than 60% of the total.

ALPHA-THALASSEMIA

A group of diseases especially prevalent in Southeast Asia and in China results from genetic deletions, with genetically determined blocks in alpha chain synthesis (α-thalassemia). Understanding of α-thalassemia syndromes is difficult because their genetic basis is complex. There appear to be 4 α chain genes. In Orientals 4 distinct thalassemia syndromes are noted: the silent carrier, α-thalassemia trait, Hgb H disease, and fetal hydrops. These are believed to result from increasing numbers of α-thalassemia genes from 1–4. No specific alterations in the proportions of the minor hemoglobins A_2 or F are seen in the 1st 2 states. Special techniques may reveal traces of hemoglobin tetramers lacking alpha chains. These are Hgb H (β_4) and Barts (γ_4). In the newborn period 3–6% of Hgb Barts is found in the blood. It does not persist after 6 mo, except occasionally in trace amounts. The most severe form of α-thalassemia, associated with 4 α-thalassemia genes, produces the clinical picture of hydrops fetalis. In these cases the predominant hemoglobin is Hgb Barts (γ_4). This variant has abnormal oxygen dissociation properties which make oxygen unavailable to the tissues under physiologic conditions.

α-Thalassemia is also involved in Hgb H syndromes. These moderately severe anemias resemble Cooley anemia but are characterized by an unstable hemoglobin component (Hgb H or β_4). In Blacks Hgb H disease is very rare, and the fact that fetal hydrops syndrome has not been reported suggests that α-thalassemia differs genetically in this ethnic group, as compared with Mediterraneans and Orientals. The combination of α-thalassemia with genes for beta chain hemoglobin abnormalities or β-thalassemia results in hematologic diseases that are no more severe than with either trait alone.

HEREDITARY PERSISTENCE OF HIGH FETAL HEMOGLOBIN

This interesting condition is associated with high levels of normal fetal hemoglobin but with no other abnormalities. It is thought to result from a genetic deletion which results in inability to convert from gamma to beta chain synthesis at the time of birth. The trait occurs most frequently in Blacks, Italians, and Greeks. In the heterozygous person the level of Hgb F is 15–30%. In Blacks the proportion of Hgb F is higher than that in Mediterraneans. There is an even distribution of fetal hemoglobin through the red cell population, in contrast to the thalassemias, in which Hgb F content shows variation from cell to cell. Instances of homozygosity for the high fetal gene have been observed. These patients' hemoglobin was completely Hgb F, but no significant anemia or manifestations of hematologic disease were found. When both the high fetal gene and the sickle genes are present in the same person, hematologic manifestations are very mild. The even distribution of a large amount of Hgb F through the red cell population prevents sickling.

HEMOLYTIC ANEMIAS DUE TO ABNORMALITIES OF THE RED CELL PRODUCED BY EXTRINSIC FACTORS

A number of agents with capacity to damage red blood cells may lead to their premature destruction.

Among the most clearly defined are antibodies associated with immune hemolytic anemias. These antibodies, directed against specific intrinsic antigens, so damage the red cell that viability is compromised and rapid destruction ensues in the reticuloendothelial tissues of the spleen and liver. The hallmark of this group of diseases is the positive result of the Coombs test, which detects a coating of immunoglobulin or components of complement on the red cell surface. The most important immune hemolytic disorder in pediatric practice is hemolytic disease of the newborn (erythroblastosis fetalis), caused by transplacental transfer of maternal antibody active against the red cells of the fetus (Sec 7.47).

14.27 AUTOIMMUNE HEMOLYTIC ANEMIAS ASSOCIATED WITH "WARM" ANTIBODIES

In the autoimmune hemolytic anemias, abnormal antibodies directed against red cells are produced by the patient. The pathogenic mechanism of these disorders is uncertain. One theory postulates the basic cause to be an autonomous proliferation of a forbidden clone of immunologically competent cells which do not recognize self-antigens. Alternative explanations suggest that drugs or infectious agents in some way alter the red cell membrane so that it becomes "foreign" or antigenic to the host.

Autoimmune hemolytic anemias associated with an underlying disease process such as lymphoma, lupus erythematosus, or immunodeficiency are said to be secondary or symptomatic. In other instances (idiopathic) no underlying cause can be found. In as many as 20% of cases of immune hemolysis, drugs may be implicated. A number of drugs, such as penicillin and cephalosporins, attach to the red cell membrane, changing antigenicity and evoking production of antibodies directed against the red cell–drug complex. Other drugs, such as phenacetin and quinidine, form immune complexes which become attached to the red cell, causing its destruction. Alpha-methyldopa produces an autoimmune hemolytic process by unknown mechanisms.

Clinical Manifestations. Autoimmune hemolytic anemias occur in 2 general clinical patterns. The 1st is an acute transient type which occurs predominantly in infants and younger children and is frequently preceded by an infection, usually respiratory. The onset is acute, with prostration, pallor, jaundice, pyrexia, and hemoglobinuria. The spleen is usually markedly enlarged. Underlying systemic disorders are unusual in this group. A consistent response to corticosteroid therapy, low mortality, and full recovery within 3 mo are characteristic of the acute form.

The 2nd type pursues a prolonged and chronic course. Hemolysis continues for many mo or yr. Abnormalities involving other blood elements are common, and the response to corticosteroids is variable and inconsistent. Mortality is about 10%, often attributable to an underlying systemic disease.

Laboratory Data. In many cases the anemia is profound, with hemoglobin levels under 6 gm/dl. Considerable spherocytosis and polychromasia are present.

More than 50% of the circulating red cells may be reticulocytes, and nucleated red cells may be present. In some cases an initially low reticulocyte count may reflect a process so acute that the bone marrow has not yet had time to respond. Leukocytosis is common. The platelet count is usually normal; occasionally, there is a concomitant immune thrombocytopenic purpura (*Evans syndrome*).

The direct Coombs test result is strongly positive, and free antibody can sometimes be demonstrated in the serum. These antibodies are active at 37° C ("warm" antibodies) and belong to the IgG class. They do not require complement for activity and may not produce agglutination in vitro. Antibodies from the serum and those eluted from the red cells react with many different red cells, including those of the patient. Although they have often been regarded as nonspecific panagglutinins, careful studies have revealed many to have specificity for certain red cell antigens, usually those of the Rh system. A number of such antibodies have had anti-e(hr″) specificity. Since more than 95% of the population have the red cell e antigen, the antibody might be considered a panagglutinin unless careful tests were performed. In other cases antibodies specific for the ubiquitous antigen LW are found. Sometimes spontaneous agglutination of the patient's own red cells occurs in all testing sera so that the patient may be mistakenly blood-typed as group AB Rh-positive. In many cases only complement is found on the red cells, chiefly the C3 and C4 components. A "broad spectrum" Coombs serum must be used to detect complement-coated red cells. In 80% of acute transient cases only complement-type positive Coombs tests are found, whereas in the chronic variety an IgG or mixed type of Coombs response occurs in over 80% of cases. Occasionally, the Coombs test is negative because of the limited sensitivity of the Coombs reaction (a minimum of 250–500 molecules of IgG is necessary on the red cell membrane to produce a positive reaction). Special tests are required to detect the antibody in cases of "Coombs test negative" autoimmune hemolytic anemia.

Treatment. Transfusions are usually of only transient benefit but may be required by the severity of the anemia. It may be extremely difficult to find compatible blood; blood in which the red cells give the least positive in vitro reaction by the Coombs technique should be chosen. The mainstays of therapy are the corticosteroids. Prednisone or its equivalent should be administered in a dose of 2.5 mg/kg/24 hr. In some cases with severe hemolysis doses up to 6 mg/kg/24 hr of prednisone may be required in order to reduce the rate of hemolysis. Treatment should be continued until the evidence of hemolysis decreases, and then the dose is gradually reduced. If relapse occurs, resumption of full dosage may be necessary. The disease tends to remit spontaneously within a few wk or mo. The Coombs test result may remain positive even after hemolysis has subsided. When hemolytic anemia remains severe despite corticosteroid therapy or if very large doses are necessary to maintain a reasonable hemoglobin level, splenectomy may be beneficial. Immunosuppressive agents have been of some benefit in chronic cases refractory to conventional therapy.

Course and Prognosis. The acute variety of idiopathic autoimmune hemolytic disease in childhood may be severe, but is self-limited. The disease may be fulminating; severe cases have been refractory to corticosteroids, immunosuppressive agents, splenectomy, and thymectomy. In immune hemolytic anemia secondary to lymphoma or lupus erythematosus the status of the basic disease determines the prognosis.

14.28 AUTOIMMUNE HEMOLYTIC ANEMIAS ASSOCIATED WITH "COLD" ANTIBODIES

Red cell antibodies that are more active at low body temperatures have been called "cold." They are of the IgM class and require complement for activity.

Cold Agglutinin Disease

Cold antibodies may be present in low levels in normal blood. Following viral infections or mycoplasmal pneumonia, the levels may increase considerably, and occasionally enormous increases may occur, titers of 1/30,000 or greater being recorded. The antibody has specificity for the i antigen and reacts poorly with human cord blood cells possessing the i antigen. Spontaneous agglutination and rouleaux formation are seen on the blood smear.

When very high titers of cold antibodies are present, severe episodes of intravascular hemolysis with hemoglobinemia and hemoglobinuria may follow exposure of the patient to cold.

Occasionally, patients with infectious mononucleosis develop acute immunohemolytic anemia. The antibodies in these cases have anti-i specificity.

Paroxysmal Cold Hemoglobinuria

This form of hemolytic anemia is associated with a specific type of cold antibody, the Donath-Landsteiner hemolysin, which has anti-P specificity. About one third of cases are associated with either congenital or acquired syphilis. Transfusions are given for severe anemia. Chilling of the patient should be avoided.

14.29 HEMOLYTIC ANEMIAS OF INTOXICATIONS AND INFECTIONS

In sufficiently large doses arsenic and phenylhydrazine produce hemolysis.

Hemolytic anemias may complicate a variety of infections. Direct red cell damage by microorganisms or their toxins may be the basis of hemolysis observed in septicemia. Actual parasitism of the red cell occurs in malaria and bartonellosis.

General

Miller DR, Pearson HA: Smith's Blood Diseases of Infancy and Childhood. Ed. 4. St. Louis, CV Mosby, 1978.
Nathan DG, Oski FA: Hematology of Infancy and Childhood. Ed 3. Philadelphia, WB Saunders, 1981.
Oski FA, Naiman, JL: Hematologic Problems of the Newborn. Ed 3. Philadelphia, WB Saunders, 1982.
Wintrobe MD: Clinical Hematology. Ed 7. Philadelphia, Lea and Febiger, 1972.

The Red Cells

Harris JW, Kellermeyer RW: The Red Cell. Ed 2. Cambridge, Mass., Harvard University Press, 1970.

Pure Red Cell Anemias

Alter BP: Childhood red cell aplasia. Am J Pediatr Hematol 2:121, 1980.
Diamond LK, Wang WS, Alter BP: Congenital hypoplastic anemia. Adv Pediatr 22:349, 1976.
Nathan DG, Clarke BJ, et al: Erythroid precursors in congenital hypoplastic (Diamond-Blackfan) anemia. J Clin Invest 61:489, 1978.
Wang WC, Mentzer WC: Differentiation of transient erythroblastopenia of childhood from congenital hypoplastic anemia. J Pediatr 88:784, 1976.

Anemias of Chronic Infections, Inflammation, and Renal Disease

Cartwright GE: The anemia of chronic disorders. Semin Hematol 3:351, 1966.
Douglas SW, Adamson JW: The anemia of chronic disorders: Studies of marrow regulation and iron metabolism. Blood 45:55, 1975.
Koerper MA, Stempel DA, Dallmar PR: Anemia in patients with juvenile rheumatoid arthritis. J Pediatr 91:878, 1978.

Physiologic Anemia of Infancy

O'Brien RT, Pearson HA: Physiologic anemia of infancy. J Pediatr 79:132, 1971.
Stockman JA, Garcia JF: The anemia of prematurity. Factors governing the erythropoietin response. N Engl J Med 296:647, 1977.
Williams ML, Shott RJ, O'Neal PL, et al: Role of dietary iron and fat in vitamin E deficiency of infancy. N Engl J Med 292:887, 1975.

Megaloblastic Anemias

Haggard ME, Lockhart LH: Megaloblastic anemia and orotic aciduria: an hereditary disorder of pyrimidine metabolism responsive to uridine. Am J Dis Child 113:733, 1967.
Hakami N, Neiman PE: Neonatal megaloblastic anemia due to inherited transcobalamin II deficiency in two siblings. N Engl J Med 285:1163, 1971.
Hoffbrand AV: Megaloblastic anaemia. Clin Haematol 5:52, 1976.
Lampkin BC, Shore NA, Chadwick D: Megaloblastic anemia of infancy secondary to maternal pernicious anemia. N Engl J Med 274:1168, 1966.
McIntyre OR, Sullivan LW, Jeffries GH, et al: Pernicious anemia in childhood. N Engl J Med 272:981, 1965.
Vrana MB, Carvalho RJ: Thiamine responsive megaloblastic anemia. Sensorineural deafness and diabetes mellitus: A new syndrome. J Pediatr 93:235, 1978.

Microcytic Anemia

Committee on Nutrition: Iron supplementation for infants. Pediatrics 58:765, 1976.
Dallman PR, Siimes MA, Stekel A: Iron deficiency in infancy and childhood. Am J Clin Nutr 33:86, 1980.
Piomelli S, Brickman A, Carlos E: Rapid diagnosis of iron deficiency by measurement of free erythrocyte porphyrins and hemoglobins. Pediatrics 57:136, 1976.
Pollit E, Leibel RL: Iron deficiency and behavior. J Pediatr 88:372, 1976.
Siimes MA, Addiego JE Jr, Dallman PR: Ferritin in serum: Diagnosis of iron deficiency and iron overload in infants and children. Blood 43:581, 1974.
Voorhess ML, Stuart MJ, Stockman JA, et al: Iron deficiency anemia and increased urinary norepinephrine excretion. J Pediatr 86:542, 1975.
Wilson JF, Lahey ME, Heiner DC: Studies on iron metabolism. V. Further observations on cow's milk induced gastrointestinal bleeding. J Pediatr 84:355, 1974.

Hemolytic Anemias

Dacie JV: The Haemolytic Anemias. Ed 3. New York, Grune and Stratton, 1970.

Hereditary Spherocytosis

Bellingham AJ, Prankerd TAJ: Hereditary spherocytosis. Clin Haematol 4:139, 1975.
Kruger HC, Burgert EO: Hereditary spherocytosis in 100 children. Mayo Clin Proc 41:921, 1966.

Trucco JT, Brown AK: Neonatal manifestations of hereditary spherocytosis. Am J Dis Child 113:263, 1967.
Valentine WN: The molecular lesion of hereditary spherocytosis: A continuing enigma. Blood 49:241, 1977.

Hereditary Elliptocytosis

Austin RF, Desforges JF: Hereditary elliptocytosis: An unusual presentation of hemolysis in the newborn associated with transient morphologic abnormalities. Pediatrics 44:196, 1969.
Jensson O, Jonasson T, Olafsson O: Hereditary elliptocytosis in Iceland. Br J Haematol 13:884, 1967.
Pearson HA: The genetic basis of hereditary elliptocytosis with hemolysis. Blood 32:972, 1968.

Paroxysmal Nocturnal Hemoglobinuria

Dacie JV, Lewis SM: Paroxysmal noctural hemoglobinuria: Clinical manifestations, hematology and nature of the disease. Ser Haematol 5:3, 1972.
Miller DR, Baehner RL, Diamond LK: Paroxysmal nocturnal hemoglobinuria in childhood and adolescence. Pediatrics 39:675, 1967.

Hereditary Stomatocytosis

Mentzer WC, Smith WB, Goldstone J, et al: Hereditary stomatocytosis: Membrane and metabolism studies. Blood 46:659, 1975.

Enzymatic Defects of the Red Cell

Beutler E: Abnormalities of the hexose monophosphate shunt. Semin Hematol 8:311, 1971.
Gilman PA: Hemolysis in the newborn resulting from deficiencies of red blood cell enzymes: Diagnosis and management. J Pediatr 84:625, 1974.
Jaffe ER: Hereditary hemolytic disorders and enzymatic deficiencies of human erythrocytes. Blood 35:116, 1970.
Tanaka KR, Paglia DE: Deficiency of pyruvate kinase. Semin Hematol 8:367, 1971.

Autoimmune Hemolytic Anemia

Buchanan GR, Boxer LA, Nathan DG: The acute and transient nature of idiopathic immune hemolytic anemia in childhood. J Pediatr 88:780, 1976.
Dacie JV, Worlledge SM: Autoimmune hemolytic anemias. Prog Hematol 6:82, 1969.
Garratty G, Petz LD: Drug induced immune hemolytic anemia. Am J Med 58:398, 1975.
Habibi B, Homberg JC, Schaison G, et al: Autoimmune hemolytic anemia in children. Am J Med 56:61, 1974.
Zuelzer WW, Mastrangelo R, Shulberg CS, et al: Autoimmune hemolytic anemia; natural history and viral-immunologic interactions in childhood. Am J Med 49:80, 1970.

Hemoglobinopathies

Bunn HF, Forgst BG, Ranney HM: Hemoglobinopathies. Major Probl Int Med 13:1, 1977.
Diggs LW: Sickle cell crises. Am J Clin Pathol 44:1, 1965.
Lehmann H, Huntsman RG: Man's Haemoglobins. Ed 2. London, North-Holland, 1974.
O'Brien RT, McIntosh S, Aspnes GT, et al: Prospective study of sickle cell anemia in infancy. J Pediatr 89:205, 1976.
Pearson HA, Diamond LK: Sickle cell disease crises and their management. In: Smith CA (ed): The Critically Ill Child. Ed 2. Philadelphia, WB Saunders, 1977.
Pearson HA, Spencer RP, Cornelius EA: Functional asplenia in sickle cell anemia. N Engl J Med 281:293, 1969.
Powers DR: Natural history of sickle cell disease—the first ten years. Semin Hematol 12:267, 1975.
Serjeant GR: The Clinical Features of Sickle Cell Disease. London, North-Holland, 1975.

Thalassemia

Alter BP: Prenatal diagnosis of hemoglobinopathies and other hematologic diseases. J Pediatr 95:701, 1979.
Cerami, A: "Proper" use of desferrioxamine. N Engl J Med 294:1456, 1976.
Orkin SH, Nathan DG: Current Concepts: The Thalassemias. N Engl J Med 295:710, 1976.
Pearson HA, O'Brien RT: Management of thalassemia major. Semin Hematol 12:255, 1975.
Problems of Cooley's anemia. Ann NY Acad Sci 119:371, 1964; 165:1, 1969; 232:1, 1974; 344:1, 1980.
Wetherall DJ, Clegg JB: The Thalassemia Syndromes. Ed 2. London, Blackwell Scientific Publications, 1972.

14.30 POLYCYTHEMIA
(Erythrocytosis)

Polycythemia exists when the red cell count, the hemoglobin and hematocrit levels, and the total red cell volume significantly exceed the upper limits of normal. In the older child the levels of hemoglobin and hematocrit that can be considered to represent polycythemia are 16 gm/dl and 55% respectively, corresponding to a total red cell mass exceeding 35 ml/kg. A decrease in plasma volume, such as occurs in acute dehydration and burns, may result in disproportionately high levels of hemoglobin and hematocrit, but these situations are more accurately designated hemoconcentration than relative polycythemia. The volume of red cell mass is not increased; expansion of the plasma volume or rehydration restores the hematocrit to normal levels.

Measurement of the total red cell volume by radioisotopic techniques is essential in the differential diagnosis of polycythemia. True polycythemia is characterized by increases of both the total red cell and total blood volumes.

SECONDARY POLYCYTHEMIA

Polycythemia may be present in any clinical situation associated with chronic arterial oxygen desaturation. Hypoxia of the kidney results in increased production of erythropoietin, which stimulates increased production of red cells and ultimately results in an expanded red cell mass. Cardiovascular defects involving right to left shunts and pulmonary diseases interfering with proper oxygenation are the most common causes of secondary polycythemia. Examples of such conditions are cyanotic congenital heart disease, emphysema, and bronchiectasis. Clinical findings usually include cyanosis, hyperemia of sclerae and mucous membranes, and clubbing of the fingers. The red blood cell count and hemoglobin and hematocrit values are all increased. The oxygen saturation of arterial blood is decreased. In children with cardiac lesions causing severe cyanosis, as the hematocrit rises above 65%, symptoms of hyperviscosity may require phlebotomy. On the other hand, such children may also have iron deficiency (as indicated by microcytosis and relatively low hemoglobin levels); the risk of intracranial thrombosis has been reported to be increased by such anemia, and iron therapy is indicated. Living at high altitudes also causes a secondary polycythemia; the hemoglobin level increases about 4% for each rise of 1000 meters in altitude.

More subtle forms of hypoxia may also cause polycythemia. Congenital methemoglobinemia due to a deficiency of NADH-reactive diaphorase may cause familial cyanosis and polycythemia. This condition is transmitted as an autosomal recessive. Dominantly transmitted cyanosis and polycythemia may be associated with the hemoglobins which have altered oxygen affinity (see above). Transient benign polycythemia is said to occur in otherwise healthy adolescents; this syndrome has not been studied sufficiently to determine its frequency or cause. In several families benign polycythemia seems to have been transmitted as dominant or recessive conditions, the bases of which are not known.

Polycythemia has also been associated with renal tumors and cysts and with vascular tumors of the cerebellum when these tumors have secreted erythropoietin.

When the hematocrit exceeds 65–70% there is a marked increase in blood viscosity, and periodic phlebotomies may be done, blood being replaced with plasma or saline solution.

POLYCYTHEMIA RUBRA VERA
(Erythremia)

This disorder, characterized by polycythemia, leukocytosis, thrombocytosis, and hyperplasia of the bone marrow, has been reported in only a few children. High leukocyte alkaline phosphatase activities and elevated serum vitamin B_{12} levels are characteristic. In contrast to those of normal persons, in vitro cultures of erythroid precursors of affected persons do not require added erythropoietin to stimulate growth.

PLETHORA OF THE NEWBORN

High levels of hemoglobin and hematocrit are usual in the newborn infant. The range of normal hemoglobin at birth is 14.7–21 gm/dl, and the hematocrit 45–65%. The blood volume of normal term newborns is 70–100 ml/kg, and the red cell volume 40–60 ml/kg. Occasionally, findings in newborn infants significantly exceed these ranges. Some of these plethoric infants have convulsions, respiratory distress, tachycardia, congestive heart failure, and hyperbilirubinemia. Hypoglycemia and hypocalcemia may contribute to morbidity of this syndrome. Monozygotic twins with placental vascular anastomosis may have unequal distribution of the circulation so that 1 twin is born with anemia and hypovolemia while the other twin is plethoric. On rare occasions maternofetal transfusion or congenital adrenal hyperplasia may be associated with neonatal polycythemia. Neonatal polycythemia has also been reported to have increased frequency in the Down and Beckwith syndromes and with intrauterine growth retardation in newborn infants small for gestational age. In most instances no cause can be discovered. When these infants have symptomatic difficulties, such as tachypnea, congestive heart failure, hypoglycemia, or jaundice, phlebotomy in aliquots of 10–15 ml/kg replaced with equal volumes of plasma or normal saline may be indicated to reduce red cell mass and hyperviscosity.

THE PANCYTOPENIAS

Aplasia of bone marrow, or replacement of its hematopoietic elements by other tissue, results in profound depression of all the formed elements of the blood. The clinical manifestations that result are anemia, thrombocytopenic hemorrhage, and decreased resistance to infection because of neutropenia. The pancytopenias have traditionally been classified with the anemias, but the consequences of the thrombocytopenia and the neutropenia are much more striking and serious than the anemias. The pancytopenias may be constitutional and genetically determined, may be acquired as a result of damage to the marrow by a variety of chemical or other agents, including viruses, or may result from invasion by abnormal tissue. In these conditions underproduction of blood cells is due to hypocellularity or replacement of marrow. Examination of an adequate sample of marrow obtained by needle or surgical biopsy is essential to diagnosis.

14.31 CONSTITUTIONAL APLASTIC PANCYTOPENIA
(Fanconi Syndrome)

The constitutional aplastic anemias are familial disorders, believed to be inherited as autosomal recessive conditions with variable penetrance, whose expression may be modified by other genetic and environmental factors. About two thirds of affected children have evident congenital anomalies; especially common are microcephaly, microphthalmia, and absence of the radii and thumbs (Fig 14–7); abnormalities of heart and kidney are also relatively common. Short stature is found in more than two thirds of cases as well as generalized hyperpigmentation of the skin. Some affected children have no serious anatomic defects.

Pancytopenia is not usually present at birth or during early infancy. The clinical onset occurs from 1½–22 yr, with an average of 6–8 yr. Bruising due to thrombocytopenia is noted first, followed by progressively severe anemia and leukopenia.

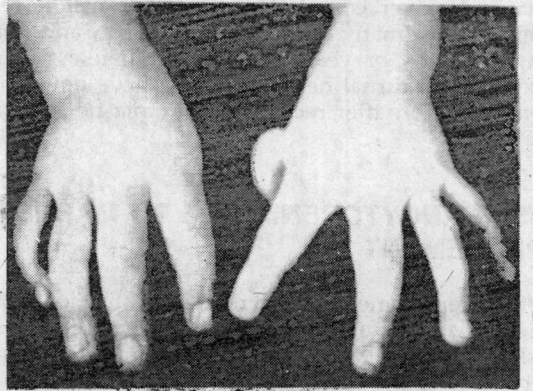

Figure 14–7 Hands of a child with constitutional aplastic pancytopenia. The thumb is absent on the right and rudimentary on the left.

Laboratory Data. Severe pancytopenia is evident in peripheral blood. The red cells are macrocytic, with MCV of 95–105 fl. The bone marrow is strikingly hypocellular, with depression of all cell types and an increase in fatty tissue. Reticulum, plasma, and mast cells are prominent. Cultures of bone marrow cells have shown markedly reduced numbers of myeloid and erythroid progenitors. A surgical or needle biopsy of the bone marrow is useful as an adjunct to aspiration, for it provides a large specimen in which to judge cellularity. There is an increase in the percentage of Hgb F of 5–15%, which may antedate development of marrow aplasia and cytopenia. A patchy distribution of Hgb F is shown by Kleihauer-Betke preparations. In vitro cultures of bone marrow show decreased numbers of precursors of both erythroid and granulocytic series. Chromosomal studies of blood lymphocytes reveal an abnormally high percentage (10–70%) of chromatid breaks, gaps, rearrangements, exchanges, and endoreduplications (changes seen in fewer than 10% of normal individuals); these changes also precede frank pancytopenia. The same changes are seen in tissue fibroblast cultures and offer the possibility of prenatal diagnosis by amniocentesis (not yet reported).

Treatment. In addition to symptomatic treatment with blood transfusions and antibiotics, therapy with androgenic steroids is beneficial. Testosterone propionate is given as sublingual tablets in a dose of 1–2 mg/kg/24 hr to a maximum of 60 mg/24 hr. Alternatively, 400–600 mg may be given as an intramuscular injection every 4 wk. Synthetic androgen derivatives such as oxymetholone and stanozolol are also effective. Relatively small doses of corticosteroids, such as 5–10 mg of prednisone or equivalent, are also given to reduce the tendency to bruising and bleeding and to retard acceleration of bone age. In a majority of instances a hematologic response becomes evident within 2–4 mo. The marrow develops greater cellularity, and the hemoglobin rises. The response of the neutrophils is usually less complete, and platelets may show only moderate increases in numbers. When the hemoglobin has reached normal levels, it is often possible to reduce the dose of androgen. But if the drug is too rapidly or drastically decreased, relapse occurs. Most patients require continuous therapy to maintain hematologic response, but many ultimately become refractory to androgen therapy.

These effective doses of androgen regularly produce signs and symptoms of masculinization, including acne, hirsutism, deepening of the voice, and enlargement of the penis or clitoris. Synthetic androgen derivatives have fewer of these side effects, but some degree of masculinization is probably inevitable. Some of the testosterone preparations have hepatic toxicity. Prior to the advent of testosterone therapy these patients usually died during late childhood of hemorrhage, infection, or the complications of multiple transfusions. Experience with androgen therapy is still too recent to show what the ultimate prognosis may now be. Hemorrhagic cysts of the liver (peliosis hepatis) and malignant hepatomas occur with increased frequency in patients receiving prolonged treatment with large doses of oral synthetic androgens. Bone marrow transplantation can be considered when a histocompatible sibling is available. Acute myelogenous leukemia (AML) develops in 5–10% of patients with Fanconi anemia, and their close relatives are at increased risk of AML.

Fanconi anemia must be differentiated from dyskeratosis congenita, a rare form of ectodermal dysplasia. Cutaneous hyperpigmentation, pancytopenia, and short stature occur in both conditions. Skeletal and renal anomalies do not regularly occur in dyskeratosis congenita.

14.32 ACQUIRED APLASTIC PANCYTOPENIAS

A number of physical, chemical, and infectious agents may severely damage the bone marrow and lead to severe pancytopenia. Some of these agents will produce marrow aplasia in any person who is exposed to them in a sufficient dose. Such obligate marrow depressants include ionizing radiation; chemotherapeutic drugs, such as nitrogen mustard, 6-mercaptopurine, and methotrexate; and certain organic solvents, especially benzene. A 2nd group of agents produces aplastic pancytopenia only in a small (often remarkably small) number of persons exposed to them. In these persons the adverse hematologic reactions must reflect idiosyncrasies. The drug most frequently associated with aplastic pancytopenia is chloramphenicol. It has been estimated that only 1 in 24,000–60,000 patients taking chloramphenicol suffers marrow aplasia; but this drug has been involved in more than 50% of drug-related aplastic pancytopenias. Other drugs associated with appreciable incidences of marrow aplasia are sulfonamides, phenylbutazone, and certain anticonvulsants. Severe infections may also produce severe marrow damage, but it is often difficult to decide whether the infection represents cause or effect. A number of cases of marrow aplasia have been described following instances of apparent infectious hepatitis, and it has been reported to follow infectious mononucleosis or appear as a complication of pregnancy. In about 50% of cases of aplastic pancytopenia no history of exposure to toxins or other agents can be elicited; these cases are usually called idiopathic, but the possibility of an environmental factor cannot be ruled out.

Clinical and Laboratory Data. Hemorrhage secondary to thrombocytopenia is usually the 1st clinical manifestation. The signs and symptoms of anemia and neutropenia become apparent subsequently. The spleen and lymph nodes are not enlarged. Profound decreases in red cells, platelets, and neutrophils are observed. The level of fetal hemoglobin may be increased. The marrow aspirate is scanty; the particles are fatty, and lymphocytes, plasma cells, and reticulum cells predominate. Culture of bone marrow reveals decreased numbers of progenitor stem cells of the erythroid and granulocytic series. Chromosome configuration is normal. Levels of Hgb F may be elevated above 2%; earlier reports that elevated levels of Hgb F indicate a good prognosis are not confirmed. T lymphocyte suppressor cells active against both erythroid and granulocytic colony growth have been described in certain patients with aplastic anemia.

Treatment. The patient must immediately be removed from contact with any potentially toxic drugs or agents. When the onset of the disease is acute, with massive hemorrhage and serious sepsis, aggressive therapy with platelet concentrates and antibiotics is necessary; choice of antibiotic should be based upon bacterial culture and sensitivity tests. Even with the best of supportive therapy the prognosis of severe aplastic pancytopenia is grave. As many as two thirds of patients succumb within 6 mo of diagnosis, and fewer than 10–20% recover. Reports of success with androgen and corticosteroid therapy in acquired aplastic pancytopenia have not been confirmed by more recent studies. Other forms of therapy are of dubious value.

Controlled studies indicate that bone marrow transplantation, when an HLA compatible sibling is available as a donor, is the therapy of choice. Siblings of patients with severe pancytopenia who have markedly hypocellular bone marrows should be examined for both HLA and MLC compatibility. If compatibility between patient and sibling is established, bone marrow transplantation, after suitable immunosuppression, is indicated. About 50% of transplanted patients will accept the donor marrow and have restoration of normal peripheral blood values. Graft-versus-host disease is common and may be severe.

Cases of apparent hematologic improvement in severe aplastic pancytopenia after unsuccessful marrow transplantation and intense immunosuppressive therapy indicate that some patients may have an immunologic basis for their bone marrow depression. Criteria to identify those patients who should be treated with immunosuppressive therapy alone have not been defined, but successful treatment with anti-thymocyte globulin (ATG) or high dose dexamethasone is being increasingly reported.

Course. Unless marrow engraftment is possible approximately a third of patients die very quickly as a result of uncontrollable hemorrhage and infection. *Pseudomonas* and staphylococcal septicemias are common causes of death. The remaining two thirds of children have a subacute clinical course. In some of these androgen therapy may be beneficial. Half of this group ultimately recover completely; the other half have a chronic course, many succumbing to sepsis and hemorrhage months or years after onset. Leukemia and paroxysmal nocturnal hemoglobinuria have developed in some children after recovery from aplastic pancytopenia.

14.33 PANCYTOPENIA DUE TO MARROW REPLACEMENT

Diffuse replacement of marrow space by nonhematopoietic tissue results in peripheral pancytopenia. *Neuroblastoma* is the childhood tumor which most frequently metastasizes to the bone marrow. *Osteopetrosis*, or marble bone disease, is frequently associated with anemia and thrombocytopenia because of marrow obliteration;

an element of hypersplenism may also be present. In these diseases the red cell morphology is frequently abnormal, showing teardrop formations and ovalocytes. Nucleated red cells are noted in the peripheral blood. Bone marrow transplantation has been used successfully in a small number of patients with severe osteopetrosis. *Acute leukemia* occasionally presents pancytopenia and a reticular appearance of the initially aspirated marrow. Adequate sampling or biopsy of the marrow from other sites will usually provide the proper diagnosis. A short trial of corticosteroid therapy, which results in rapid return of the blood counts to normal, favors a diagnosis of leukemia.

Myelofibrosis has occurred in a few infants and children, presenting as severe anemia with abnormal forms (teardrops, ovalocytes), nucleated red cells, and high white blood cell counts (leukoerythroblastic anemia) and with enlarged liver and spleen due to extramedullary erythropoiesis.

TRANSFUSIONS*

The most important indications for transfusions are to restore blood volume and treat shock following acute blood loss and to provide red cells for maintenance of the blood hemoglobin level. An individual component of blood, such as red cells, platelets, plasma, or specific plasma proteins, may often be used effectively in place of whole blood.

INDICATIONS FOR TRANSFUSION

14.34 ACUTE HEMORRHAGE

The signs and symptoms accompanying hemorrhage vary with the magnitude and rapidity of the blood loss. When 15–20% or more of the circulating blood volume is acutely lost, tachycardia, hypotension, and shock may develop, accompanied by weakness, restlessness, and syncope. Immediately after acute hemorrhage the hemoglobin or hematocrit level may be deceptively high, but hemodilution soon reduces this to a value reflecting the magnitude of the blood loss. Thrombocytosis and neutrophilia occur within a few hr and reticulocytosis within a few days of an acute bleeding episode. The most common causes of severe acute hemorrhage are trauma and gastrointestinal bleeding from peptic ulcers, Meckel diverticulum, and esophageal varices. In patients with defects of the hemostatic mechanism, exsanguinating hemorrhage may occur from nosebleeds or gastritis.

Severe bleeding in the perinatal period may result in the clinical picture of asphyxia pallida. Pallor, shock, tachycardia, and low venous pressures are seen. External hemorrhage may occur from the umbilicus or the gastrointestinal tract. The fetus may bleed before and during birth into the maternal circulation, and fetofetal transfusions between identical twins are not infrequent.

Laboratory Data. The anemia of acute blood loss is usually normochromic and normocytic. Depending upon the duration of the hemorrhage and timing of the tests, compensatory reticulocytosis and normoblastemia may be seen. In the newborn infant with hemorrhage the Coombs test result is generally negative and the level of serum bilirubin low. With loss of blood from fetus to mother, maternal blood will contain a minor population of red cells which contain Hgb F (Kleihauer-Betke technique).

*See Sec 7.47 for Exchange Transfusion.

Treatment. When possible, local measures to control the hemorrhage should be taken. Whole blood transfusions should be given to restore blood volume and treat shock; 20 ml/kg of blood should be administered initially. The need for additional blood will be determined by the clinical response and by physical and laboratory findings. Plasma or plasma expanders may be used to sustain the patient in shock until blood can be made available, but if the blood loss has been great, red cell replacement will be necessary.

14.35 CHRONIC ANEMIAS

With anemias that develop slowly and stabilize at levels of 6–9 gm/dl, the patient may experience remarkably few symptoms, and transfusions are not routinely indicated. When such anemias result from deficiency of a specific factor, such as folic acid or iron, a rapid response will follow replacement therapy. Transfusion is indicated only if the anemia is profound or if infections or other complications are present. No firm rule can be made as to the hemoglobin level at which transfusion is recommended. Some children with iron deficiency anemia may have hemoglobin levels of 4–5 gm/dl with few signs of clinical or cardiorespiratory distress. A reasonable estimate of the effect of transfusion of packed red cells is that the increase in hematocrit (%) will equal the ml/kg of packed cells given. For example, if 5 ml/kg of packed cells is given, the recipient's hematocrit will rise about 5%. The formula assumes a recipient blood volume of about 75 ml/kg and a hematocrit of about 75% for packed red cells.

In progressive refractory anemias such as thalassemia major and pure red cell anemias, transfusions are necessary to sustain life. Packed red cells, like leukocyte-poor or glycerol-frozen preparations, are preferred for the correction of such chronic anemias. The maximal dose of packed red cells to be given in 1 transfusion is 15 ml/kg; if signs suggestive of incipient congestive heart failure are present, considerably smaller amounts should be used. In extreme anemia with secondary heart failure, multiple small transfusions of 2–4 ml/kg of packed red cells may be helpful, and the simultaneous use of furosemide may be considered. If frank congestive heart failure is present, exchange transfusion should be considered, replacing the patient's blood isovolumetrically with packed red cells. Digitalis is of limited value.

14.36 PLATELET TRANSFUSIONS

Platelets may be transfused to attain temporary hemostasis in some patients with thrombocytopenic hemorrhage. The life span of transfused platelets is normally 9–10 days. Although administration of fresh whole blood produces inconsequential rises in the recipient's platelet count, clinical hemorrhage may be controlled. Use of platelet-rich plasma or platelet concentrates prepared from fresh blood drawn in plastic equipment permits attainment of more nearly normal platelet counts. While it is desirable to utilize platelets which are ABO and Rh compatible, it is frequently impossible to do so. The infusion of platelet concentrates from incompatible donors rarely produces problems, but since these concentrates contain red cells, those from Rh-positive donors should not be given to Rh-negative recipients. Transfusion of platelets that are HLA compatible does not readily evoke isoimmunization and results in more satisfactory platelet survival. Platelet transfusions are temporarily beneficial in thrombocytopenias due to inadequate production, such as hypoplastic pancytopenia and leukemia but are useless or of only transient value in states characterized by peripheral hyperdestruction of platelets such as idiopathic thrombocytopenic purpura. In addition, isoantibodies to platelet antigens are frequently formed after transfusions of platelets from multiple donors. With successive platelet transfusions, decreasing therapeutic responses are noted. Transfusion of 1 unit of platelet concentrate can be expected to produce an increment in platelet count of about $100,000/mm^3$ in the newborn and about $10,000 \ mm^3$ in the adult.

14.37 GRANULOCYTES

Because of the brief intravascular life span and low concentration of granulocytes in normal blood, transfusions of normal whole blood have no practical value for the supply of white blood cells. Transient clinical and hematologic benefit in neutropenias has been reported from use of donor blood from patients with chronic granulocytic leukemia who have very high total white blood cell counts. Extraction of large numbers of polymorphonuclear leukocytes from normal donors can be accomplished with continuous-flow blood separators employing differential centrifugation or nylon fiber filter systems. Double-flow plasmapheresis and continuous flow centrifugation techniques are also used to harvest large numbers of granulocytes from single donors. Administration of granulocytes lowers mortality in profoundly leukopenic patients with gram-negative sepsis. This has become accepted practice in the management of febrile and infected patients with severe potentially self-limited neutropenia resulting from cancer chemotherapy or bone marrow transplantation.

14.38 PLASMA AND PLASMA CONCENTRATES

In acute dehydration, when the plasma volume is decreased but the red cell mass is adequate, plasma can be used effectively to expand the blood volume and to restore circulation and renal blood flow. The usual dose of plasma is 10 ml/kg. The use of fresh plasma and of concentrates of plasma such as factor VIII and fibrinogen preparations for bleeding disorders is described elsewhere. The usual gamma globulin preparations cannot be administered intravenously because they form large reactive aggregates which may produce hypotension and shock. However, new preparations of gamma globulin have been introduced which can be safely and effectively administered by the intravenous route.

SPECIAL CONSIDERATIONS

14.39 CHOICE OF BLOOD FOR TRANSFUSION

Storage of blood at 4° C results in a decrease in red cell viability which is proportional to the length of storage time. When blood is given for acute hemorrhage, this is of no consequence, but for children who must receive transfusions repeatedly the blood selected should be as fresh as possible.

A citrate-phosphate-dextrose (CPD) mixture has supplanted ACD as the standard anticoagulant because it better maintains red cell viability and function.

Blood for transfusion should be of the same blood group (O, A, B, or AB) as the recipient's. The donor red cells should always be tested for compatibility with the recipient's plasma (major cross-match) by the Coombs technique. Compatibility for the Rh antigens between donor and recipient is desirable. Rh-negative (d/d) persons should never receive Rh-positive blood; the reverse is permissible. Though considerable battlefield experience indicates that the use of so-called universal donor blood (group O Rh-negative blood with a low titer of anti-A and anti-B isohemagglutinins) is safe, with adequate modern blood banking facilities this is rarely necessary except in an emergency.

14.40 RISKS OF BLOOD TRANSFUSION

Although modern technology has made blood transfusion a generally safe procedure, a definite risk is involved. Transfusions should be given, therefore, only when the benefit to the patient exceeds the inherent danger of the procedure. It has been estimated that 1 of every 2000 persons receiving a blood transfusion has a severe reaction as a result of the immediate procedure or its consequences. Problems may arise from:

Clerical Errors. The mislabeling or faulty identification of containers may lead to a patient's receiving the wrong blood. If a type O patient receives type A or B blood, fatal intravascular hemolysis may occur.

Red Cell Isoimmunization. In almost every blood transfusion the donor red cells have some antigen factor which the recipient does not possess. Many such factors are poor antigens, but some evoke intense antibody formation, the immunized persons being at increased risk if another transfusion is given.

Hepatitis. A small proportion of the normal population are asymptomatic carriers of the agents for serum hepatitis. Only about one-third of donors who can transmit serum hepatitis have demonstrable hepatitis B–associated antigen (Australia antigen, HB_sAg) in their blood. Currently, the most common cause of transfusional hepatitis is designated non-A–non-B; it has a variable incubation period and is usually clinically mild. There is no way to detect all carriers with certainty or to inactivate the agent in blood, the risk in pooled plasma being proportional to the number of donors to the pool. Use of frozen red blood cells is believed to reduce the risk of hepatitis. Syphilis, malaria, toxoplasmosis, and cytomegalovirus infection can also be transmitted by blood transfusion.

White Cell, Platelet, and Plasma Protein Immunization. White cells, platelets, and some of the serum proteins have polymorphic antigens; multiple transfusions may be associated with development of antibodies against these components.

Circulatory Overload. Patients with chronic anemia have expanded plasma volume and increased cardiac output; infusion of blood or plasma may precipitate congestive heart failure; rapid administration of large volumes of blood should be avoided.

Depletion of Labile Substances. Storage of blood is associated with loss of platelets and decreasing activities of the labile coagulation factors, such as factor VIII, 75% of which is lost after 7 days of storage. When massive or exchange transfusions of stored blood are given, a complex disturbance of hemostasis may ensue. Use of fresh blood will avoid these complications. As a general rule, when multiple transfusions are given in a short period of time, every 4th unit of blood should be fresh. Reconstitution of packed red cells with fresh frozen plasma is also effective. Acute citrate toxicity may occur.

Iron Overload. Each 500 ml of blood contains about 250 mg of iron. Patients with refractory anemias who require frequent transfusion ultimately have hemosiderosis. Iron is deposited in skin, liver, spleen, and other organs and may interfere with normal function (Sec 14.4).

14.41 REACTIONS TO BLOOD TRANSFUSION

Allergic Reactions. These occur in association with 1–2% of transfusions. The most common clinical manifestation is urticaria with itching; occasionally, wheezing and arthralgia occur. The mechanism of these reactions is not certain, but they may be due to allergenic substances or to antibodies in the donor plasma. The development of urticaria alone does not necessitate discontinuing the transfusion; therapy with antihistamines or corticosteroids is effective in treating or preventing this type of reaction.

Febrile Reactions. The use of disposable plastic equipment has eliminated most external pyrogenic substances. Sensitization to white cell antigens may produce febrile reactions characterized by shaking chills and an increase in temperature of 1–2° C (2–4° F) beginning during or shortly after the transfusion and lasting only a few hr. The use of washed, leukocyte-poor packed cells excluding the buffy coat, and liberal dosage of salicylates may reduce these reactions. Use of reconstituted frozen red cells may greatly ameliorate severe febrile reactions. Rarely, a unit of blood may be contaminated with bacteria. Severe febrile reactions, shock, and death may occur if infected blood is transfused. Because it is difficult to differentiate febrile from hemolytic reactions, blood transfusions must be promptly discontinued if fever and chills occur during their administration.

Hemolytic Transfusion Reactions. Hemolytic reactions result in massive intravascular destruction of red cells, manifested clinically by fever, chills, headache, and back pain. These symptoms do not appear when the patient is anesthetized. In severe reactions, shock and acute renal failure may ensue. Hemoglobinemia and hemoglobinuria are usually observed. When a hemolytic reaction is suspected, the transfusion should be *terminated immediately*. Diagnosis is proved by re-examining the blood types of donor cells and of the recipient, repeating the cross-match, and examining plasma and urine for free hemoglobin. A diuresis should be established by fluid therapy and administration of mannitol. The patient generally survives the initial acute episode; if a period of renal failure can be adequately managed, recovery is the rule.

Polycythemia

Michael AF Jr, Mauer AM: Maternal-fetal transfusion as a cause of plethora in the neonatal period. Pediatrics 28:458, 1961.
Naeye R: Human intrauterine parabiotic syndrome and its complications. N Engl J Med 268:804, 1963.
Natelson EA, Lynch EC: Polycythemia vera in childhood. Am J Dis Child 122:241, 1971.
Usher R, Shepard M, Lind J: The blood volume of the newborn infant and placental transfusion. Acta Paediatr Scand 52:497, 1963; 54:419, 1965.
Weinberger MM, Oleinick A: Congenital marrow dysfunction in Down's syndrome. J Pediatr 77:273, 1970.

The Pancytopenias

Alter BP, Potter NU: Classification and aetiology of the aplastic anemias. Clin Haematol 7:431, 1978.
Beard MEJ: Fanconi anemia. Congenital disorders of erythropoiesis. Ciba Foundation Symposium No 37 (new series). New York, Elsevier, Excerpta Medica, North-Holland, 1976.
Bloom GE, Warner S, Gerald PS, et al: Chromosome abnormalities in constitutional aplastic anemia. N Engl J Med 274:8, 1966.
Camitta BM, Nathan DG, Forman EN, et al: Posthepatic severe aplastic anemia—an indication for early bone marrow transplantation. Blood 43:473, 1974.
Camitta BM, Thomas ED, Nathan DG: Severe aplastic anemia: A prospective study of the effect of early marrow transplantation on acute mortality. Blood 48:63, 1976.
Ragab AH, Gilkerson E, Christ WM, et al: Granulopoiesis in childhood aplastic anemia. J Pediatr 88:790, 1976.
Williams DM, Lynch RE, Cartwright GE: Drug induced aplastic anemia. Semin Hematol 10:195, 1973.

Transfusions

Bove JR: Practical Blood Transfusion. Ed 2. Boston, Little, Brown, 1978.
Bucholz DM: Pediatric transfusion therapy. J Pediatr 84:1, 1974.
Herzig RH, Herzig GP, Graw RG, et al: Successful granulocyte transfusion therapy for gram-negative septicemia. N Engl J Med 296:701, 1977.
Mollison PL: Blood Transfusion in Clinical Medicine. Ed 6. London, Blackwell, 1979.
Race RR, Sanger R: Blood Groups in Man. Ed 6. London, Blackwell Scientific Publishers, 1975.

DISORDERS OF THE LEUKOCYTES

The leukocytes of the blood and their precursors in the bone marrow are easily studied, enumerated, and classified. The most important leukocyte functions are concerned with resistance to infection and disposal of products of cellular breakdown. Because characteristic changes occur in many diseases, the white blood cell and differential counts are important as general screening tests. Normal values are listed in Table 14–3.

The leukocytes are divided into 2 major classes: the granulocytes, consisting of neutrophils, eosinophils, and basophils, and the nongranulated lymphocytes and monocytes. White cells have cellular antigens different from those of the erythrocyte.

14.42 TYPES OF LEUKOCYTES

Neutrophils. Neutrophils are the predominating type of granulocyte. The nuclei of these cells have 1–5 segments and are thus designated as polymorphonuclear leukocytes. They have ameboid motility, chemotaxis, and the capacity for active phagocytosis. Their fine cytoplasmic granules have a light purple (neutrophilic) color when stained with Wright stain. These granules are lysosomes and contain digestive enzymes of several sorts, including proteases, cathepsins, and lysozymes. When bacteria or other particles are ingested by neutrophils, degranulation occurs as the enzymes of the granules are discharged into a vacuole formed about the ingested material. The phagocytic process is associated with a burst of metabolic activity and a considerable increase in oxygen consumption. The metabolic burst is associated with hydrogen peroxide formation and a marked increase in activity of the pentose phosphate pathway of glucose metabolism. Aberrations of the biochemistry of phagocytosis and intracellular digestion may result in markedly impaired resistance to disease.

The neutrophils occupy definable compartments or pools within the body. The *mitotic compartment* consists of myeloblasts, promyelocytes, and myelocytes of the bone marrow. The *maturation compartment* consists of metamyelocytes and band forms, which are relatively completely differentiated and have lost the capacity to divide but still reside within the marrow. The *marrow storage compartment* consists of a rapidly mobilizable reserve of mature neutrophils. It has been estimated that it takes 6–11 days for a cell to pass through the stages of differentiation from a myeloblast to a mature neutrophil emerging into the peripheral blood.

The neutrophils of the blood exist in 2 exchangeable pools of approximately equal size. The *circulating granulocytic compartment* is in equilibrium with a *marginal compartment* consisting of neutrophils sequestered in small blood vessels. Vigorous exercise or injection of epinephrine causes the marginal pool to be mobilized into the circulation. The half-time of granulocytes within the circulation is 6–9 hr, after which they enter the *tissue pool*, where they carry out their primary function of phagocytosis. Little is known of their survival in the tissues.

The intramedullary mitotic and maturation compartments are generally estimated by examining bone marrow tissue. Hypertrophy of the neutrophilic series is reflected in alterations of the ratio between myeloid and erythroid elements (M/E, or myeloid-erythroid, ratio). With chronic inflammatory processes the usual M/E ratio of 2–4:1 may be markedly increased to 5–10:1. Adequacy of the marrow storage compartment can be estimated from changes in the peripheral leukocyte count after intravenous injection of extracts of bacterial endotoxin or the steroid compound etiocholanolone. Normally a 2–4-fold increase in the numbers of circulating neutrophils results from such stimulated release of cells from the marrow storage compartment. In states of marrow hypoplasia or failure no increase occurs. Radioisotopic techniques can estimate the time required for maturation and release of neutrophils from the marrow or the rate of turnover of neutrophils in the blood.

Neutrophil formation and regulation can be assessed by the culture of cells in semisolid agar gel. Normal bone marrow contains a small number of colony-forming cells or units (CFU). In tissue culture, CFU form aggregates of granulocytes under stimulation of a hormone-like glycoprotein, which has been designated colony-stimulating factor (CSF) and is elaborated by blood monocytes or tissue macrophages. Measurements of CFU and CSF are being used increasingly in the study of diseases involving neutrophils, along with assessments of neutrophil mobility and chemotaxis. The Rebuck skin window method may be used to study leukocyte migration and mobility in vivo.

Eosinophils. Eosinophils are characterized by large coarse granules of a prominent red color with Romanowsky stains and by a nucleus with 1 or 2 segments. They normally account for fewer than 5% of the circulating leukocytes. Eosinophil counts are depressed by high levels of adrenocortical hormones and increased in parasitic and allergic disorders. Eosinophilia may also accompany Hodgkin disease. Mild increases in eosinophils may be seen during convalescence from viral infections. The most pronounced eosinophilia encountered in this country accompanies such diseases as visceral larva migrans and trichinosis, which involve invasion of the tissues by parasitic helminths. Familial, and presumptively genetic, eosinophilia has been described.

Basophils. These leukocytes are distinguished by coarse, deep blue granules which fill the cytoplasm and obscure the nucleus. They contain large amounts of heparin and histamine. They normally account for under 1% of the circulating leukocytes. Increases occur in chronic myelogenous leukemia and in generalized mast cell disease.

Lymphocytes. Lymphocytes constitute 30–60% of the blood leukocytes. Most are small cells measuring 9 μ in diameter, with a round, dark, blue-black nucleus and scanty blue cytoplasm. Other lymphocytes, probably younger forms, have more abundant blue cytoplasm. Lymphocytes are actively motile, but not phagocytic. The lymphocytes can be characterized as T or B lymphocytes on the basis of physical and immunologic properties (Chapter 9). A pronounced lymphocytosis is characteristic of pertussis and the syndrome of infectious lymphocytosis. In infectious mononucleosis atypical lymphocytes characteristically appear in large numbers. Thymic alymphoplasia is associated with profound lymphopenia and immunoglobulin deficiency (Chapter 9).

Monocytes. These large phagocytic cells are characterized by a large lobulated nucleus and an abundant gray cytoplasm containing fine azurophilic granules. They normally account for 1–5% of the circulating leukocytes; they are increased in such diseases as tuberculosis, systemic mycosis, bacterial endocarditis, and certain protozoan infections. Monocytes spend about 8 hr in the circulation before entering the tissues, where they become alveolar macrophages, Kupffer cells, and other tissue macrophages.

QUANTITATIVE DISORDERS OF THE NEUTROPHILS

Absolute neutrophil counts vary widely in normal subjects. The relative proportion of neutrophils and lymphocytes in the blood varies with age (Table 14–1). Neutrophils predominate at birth but decrease rapidly in the 1st few days of life. During infancy they constitute 30–40% of the circulating leukocytes. Parity between neutrophils and lymphocytes occurs by about 5 yr of age, but the approximately 70% predominance of neutrophils characteristic of the adult is not attained until puberty. In normal healthy children, therefore, from 30–70% of the total circulating white blood cells may be neutrophils. In absolute terms they number 2500–6000/mm³. Levels exceeding this range are designated neutrophilia or polymorphonuclear leukocytosis.

14.43 NEUTROPHILIA

Neutrophilia accompanies a wide variety of localized and generalized pyogenic infections as well as some noninfectious inflammatory processes. Both the total white blood cell count and the proportion of neutrophils increase. In addition, larger numbers of nonsegmented (band) neutrophils and even a greater number of cells that are more immature (metamyelocytes and myelocytes) may be seen ("shift to the left"). In general, younger children demonstrate more pronounced responses to infections than adults and manifest higher white cell counts with greater numbers of immature forms. When the total white cell count exceeds 40,000/mm³, a "leukemoid" blood picture is said to be present. A presumptive cause is usually evident for leukemoid reactions, such as infection, intoxication, and the like, but occasionally the blood picture may be difficult to differentiate from chronic myelogenous leukemia. The neutrophils in leukemoid reactions have elevated levels of alkaline phosphatase activity, whereas this enzyme is low in chronic myelocytic leukemia. The neutrophilia of infection or inflammation is acompanied by increased

activity and hypertrophy of the entire neutrophilic series. On the other hand, the transient neutrophilia accompanying acute stress reflects shifts of previously formed neutrophils between circulating and marginal pools rather than actual increased production and is not accompanied by changes in marrow.

14.44 NEUTROPENIA

Neutropenia is a reduction below normal of the numbers of circulating neutrophils. This occurs in a substantial number of congenital and acquired diseases and results from either underproduction or peripheral hyperdestruction of neutrophils. When the absolute neutrophil count is under 1500/mm³, the patient becomes unusually susceptible to bacterial infections, especially to those of the skin and respiratory tract. Buccal and rectal ulcerations are also frequently associated.

Infantile Lethal Agranulocytosis. This familial disease is characterized by the onset in early infancy of recurrent, severe pyogenic infections, especially of the skin and the lung. Neutrophils are totally absent in the blood or present in reduced numbers (<300/mm³); absolute monocytosis and eosinophilia are present. The platelets are normal, and primary anemia is absent. The bone marrow contains markedly decreased numbers of mature neutrophilic precursors. The neutrophilic series is represented by abnormally vacuolated promyelocytes and myelocytes. CFU and CSF are usually normal. Lymphocytes and plasmacytes are prominent. Erythrocytic and megakaryocytic elements are normal.

There is no effective therapy. Hematinics, corticosteroids, and splenectomy produce no beneficial effect. Antibiotics may be of temporary value, but death frequently occurs during infancy or the 1st years of life as a result of overwhelming sepsis. Family studies suggest an autosomal recessive transmission. The basic defect is unknown.

Chronic Neutropenias. This group of diseases usually produces relatively mild clinical manifestations and is differentiated from the preceding disorder by its relative mildness and sporadic occurrence. The child experiences recurrent pneumonia, skin infections, and mouth ulcerations. Because of the paucity of granulocytes at sites of inflammation, the usual indications of infection, including pus, may be minimal. The peripheral white blood cell count is decreased, and there is a striking paucity of neutrophils; absolute neutrophil counts range from 0–1000/mm³. There is usually no anemia, and the platelets are normal. Compensatory monocytosis and eosinophilia are usually present. Serum protein studies demonstrate diffuse hypergammaglobulinemia. In the bone marrow there is often maturation arrest at the myelocyte or metamyelocyte stage as well as plasmacytosis, but no alteration of the erythrocytic and megakaryocytic elements. Some affected patients appear able to mobilize a neutrophilic response in case of major pyogenic infection.

Infections can be controlled by appropriate antibiotic therapy. Attempts to stimulate granulopoiesis with corticosteroids or other therapy are usually ineffectual. Affected children tend to improve with age, and some undergo total remissions in late childhood. Familial patterns of occurrence have suggested both autosomal dominant and recessive transmission, and some cases appear to be sporadic. Bone marrow cultures from children with chronic neutropenia have revealed no consistent pattern; assay for colony-stimulating factor (CSF) is usually positive. Neutropenia may occur in patients with various immunodeficiencies. Immunoglobulin determinations are indicated.

Acquired Neutropenia. Decrease in the total white blood cell count and concomitant neutropenia occur in many viral infections, particularly roseola infantum, rubella, rubeola, and influenza. This is the most common type of neutropenia. Neutropenia is also characteristic of typhoid and paratyphoid infections and brucellosis. In severe pyogenic infections the observation of neutropenia is an ominous prognostic sign, often indicating the overwhelming nature of the disease. In some cases of rheumatoid arthritis and lupus erythematosus, neutropenia occurs; its pathogenesis in these diseases is uncertain but may represent peripheral sequestration or hyperutilization.

Acquired neutropenia may have an autoimmune basis. Serologic assays for antineutrophil antibodies may be positive. In such cases therapy with corticosteroids has been effective in increasing circulating neutrophil numbers.

A few cases of acquired infantile copper deficiency have been described with profound neutropenia and osseous abnormalities. Serum copper levels were very low, and hematologic responses occurred with oral copper therapy.

Neutropenia results from marrow insufficiency in leukemia, aplastic pancytopenia, and disseminated neoplasms such as neuroblastoma. In advanced megaloblastic anemia due to deficiency of vitamin B_{12} or folic acid, neutropenia regularly occurs, possibly because of ineffective leukopoiesis. On the other hand, an enlarged spleen may filter or sequester large numbers of neutrophils from the circulation. Ionizing radiation and such drugs or chemicals as nitrogen mustard, methotrexate, and benzene regularly cause marrow depression and neutropenia in any person receiving them in sufficient amounts.

Pancreatic Insufficiency and Neutropenia
(Bodian-Shwachman Syndrome)

This is a familial syndrome of severe, chronic neutropenia, with pancreatic insufficiency due to atrophy and fatty replacement (Sec 11.77). It can be differentiated from cystic fibrosis by the normal electrolyte levels in sweat and the absence of pulmonary disease. The peripheral blood count reveals decreased numbers of neutrophils and occasionally thrombocytopenia and anemia. Bone marrow is markedly hypocellular. Roentgenograms reveal metaphyseal dysostosis in some cases. The most prominent symptoms are related to pancreatic insufficiency, which produces malabsorption, diarrhea, and growth failure. This is to be differentiated from a syndrome of refractory sideroblastic anemia with vacuolated marrow precursors and fibrosis of the exocrine pancreas.

No therapy has been effective in improving the he-

matologic abnormalities; pancreatic enzyme replacements ameliorate the malabsorption.

14.45 DRUG-INDUCED NEUTROPENIA
(Malignant Agranulocytosis)

This syndrome is characterized by a profound reduction of neutrophils in the blood and of their precursors in the bone marrow, accompanied by severe systemic infection. It is usually self-limited but occasionally lethal.

Etiology. The drugs or agents which produce this condition do so in relatively small numbers of patients so that idiosyncrasies seem partly responsible. In some instances, such as in neutropenia associated with aminopyrine, an immunologic basis is probable. This drug acts as a hapten in combination with a protein of the neutrophil, forming an antigenic complex which stimulates formation of a leukocidal antibody. Recently, the drug most frequently producing neutropenia has been the aminopyrine derivative, dipyrone (Pyralgin); the use of this potentially dangerous drug for its symptomatic effect on fever is inappropriate. Neutropenia following the use of phenothiazines has been attributed to a toxic inhibition of nucleic acid synthesis. Administration of semisynthetic penicillins (oxacillin, methicillin) may in large doses produce agranulocytosis after 3–4 wk. Recovery occurs promptly when the drug is discontinued. Other drugs associated with a significant incidence of neutropenia include thiourea derivatives and sulfonamides. In many cases of neutropenia no cause can be discovered.

Clinical Manifestations. An abrupt onset with a racking rigor occurs in aminopyrine-induced neutropenia. In other cases the onset may be insidious. Ulcerations of the mouth and rectum, cutaneous infections, and pneumonia are common. The temperature curve is septic, with frequent high spikes, but purulent exudates are not formed so that the usual physical findings of pyogenic infections may not occur. Death results from overwhelming sepsis in the 1st wk of the disease in about 20% of cases unless antibiotic therapy is effective in treating bacterial infections. Intestinal perforations may occur.

Laboratory Data. The total white blood cell count is reduced. Circulating neutrophils are low (<1000/mm³), but a compensatory monocytosis and eosinophilia are frequently present. There is no anemia or thrombocytopenia. Bone marrow changes depend upon the stage of illness. At the height of the disease the marrow is cellular, with normal numbers of erythroid precursors and megakaryocytes, but neutrophilic precursors are reduced. Five–20% of the nucleated cells may be plasma cells. Recovery is presaged by a return of granulopoiesis in the marrow, which proceeds as a surge of maturation through the several stages of development. Bone marrow examination in this early recovery stage may be misinterpreted as showing a maturation arrest. Four–5 days after the return of precursors to the marrow, mature neutrophils reappear in the blood. Coincident with their reappearance prompt defervescence and clinical improvement usually ensue.

Treatment. The most important therapeutic measure is immediate discontinuation of any medications that may be causative. Infection should be treated with therapeutic doses of antibiotics, the choice of which should be determined by cultures and sensitivity studies; when feasible, bactericidal antibiotics should be used. Prophylactic use of antibiotics is not indicated. Corticosteroid therapy is not of significant value. Once a patient has acquired neutropenia after administration of a specific drug, that drug or closely related agents should not be administered again. White blood cell transfusions have been used for support during periods of profound neutropenia.

CYCLIC NEUTROPENIA

This ill-defined disease is characterized by periodic episodes of fever and oral ulcerations, with profound neutropenia. Onset usually occurs by 10 yr of age. Neutropenia persists from 5–10 days, after which the white blood cell count returns to normal and symptoms abate. Such episodes occur in cycles, generally of 19–21 days but ranging from 14–30 days. Bone marrow during periods of neutropenia shows diminished numbers of neutrophilic precursors or maturation arrest. Between episodes blood and marrow are normal. Monocytosis may precede the drop in neutrophil count. Therapy is symptomatic, with antibiotics for bacterial infections. The course is usually benign, but catastrophic complications, including intestinal perforations and peritonitis, may occur. A similar disorder, genetically determined, occurs in the gray collie dog.

TRANSITORY NEUTROPENIA OF THE NEWBORN

Neutrophilia is characteristic of the immediate postnatal period, but with severe infections, such as cytomegalic inclusion disease, toxoplasmosis, or bacterial sepsis, striking neutropenia may occur. Newborn infants have been described with familial neutropenia and bacterial infections; in some cases the mother has also been neutropenic, suggesting transmission of a humoral inhibitor or antibody from mother to infant. Maternal isoimmunization to fetal neutrophil antigens is analogous to Rh sensitization. Bacterial infections usually respond to vigorous antibiotic therapy. The duration of neutropenia is variable but usually 2–4 wk.

14.46 INHERITED ABNORMALITIES OF THE LEUKOCYTES

Ninety per cent of the neutrophils in the blood of normal persons have 2–4 segments. Only about 5% are unsegmented (bands), and fewer than 5% have 5 or more segments. An increase in unsegmented forms, or "shift to the left," usually indicates infection or inflammation, whereas hypersegmentation, or "shift to the

right," most commonly occurs in megaloblastic anemias due to folic acid or vitamin B_{12} deficiency.

Hereditary Hyposegmentation (Pelger-Huet Anomaly). This defect of neutrophil segmentation is inherited as an autosomal dominant trait. In heterozygous persons more than 90% of circulating neutrophils and eosinophils either are unsegmented or have only 2 lobes. Their phagocytic capacity is normal, and no predisposition to infection is associated. The homozygous state may be lethal.

Hereditary Hypersegmentation (Undritz Anomaly). This rare condition, inherited as an autosomal dominant trait, is characterized by predominance of neutrophils with 4 and 5 or more segments. No adverse clinical effects are associated.

May-Hegglin Anomaly. This rare, dominantly transmitted anomaly involves the neutrophils and platelets. A majority of the neutrophils contain irregular blue cytoplasmic inclusions similar to Döhle bodies. Döhle bodies consist of precipitated ribosomal material and are usually observed in patients with severe systemic infections. In patients with the May-Hegglin anomaly no infection need be present. There are abnormally large platelets and, at times, thrombocytopenia. The thrombocytopenia responds to splenectomy.

Alder Anomaly. In this condition, which is probably transmitted as an autosomal recessive trait, the neutrophilic granulations are larger and stain much more prominently than normal ones. The granules are distinctly lavender or blue and are thus easily differentiated from eosinophils. A small proportion of patients with mucopolysaccharidoses may show somewhat similar granulations in their neutrophils (Reilly bodies) or, more commonly, metachromic granules in the cytoplasm of lymphocytes (Mitwoch bodies).

QUALITATIVE ABNORMALITIES OF THE NEUTROPHILS

A number of syndromes with intracellular defects of the neutrophils display increased susceptibility to infections despite adequate numbers of these cells in the circulation.

14.47 Chronic Granulomatous Disease (CGD)

This disease is characterized by a metabolic defect which results in failure of intracellular killing of certain types of bacteria following their phagocytosis by the neutrophils (Sec 9.30).

14.48 Myeloperoxidase Deficiency

A few patients with increased susceptibility to pyogenic infections who have defective and delayed intracellular killing of bacteria have a defect of the enzyme myeloperoxidase (Sec 9.32).

14.49　Chédiak-Higashi Disease

See Sec 9.31.

14.50　Job Syndrome

This apt term describes patients with recurrent severe cold staphylococcal abscesses of the skin. Some patients may represent a variant of chronic granulomatous disease; in others the basis for infection is not clear. See Sec 9.36.

14.51　Disorders of Leukocyte Chemotaxis

Migration of leukocytes to areas of inflammation and infection depends in part upon the complement system; accordingly, in congenital or acquired deficiency of any of several of the phases of complement, impaired chemotaxis may result in infection. Isolated defects in chemotaxis as a result of cellular abnormalities have also been described (lazy leukocyte syndrome). See Sec 9.35.

General

Davidson WM: Inherited variations in leukocytes. Br Med Bull 17:190, 1961.
Robinson WA, Mangalik A: The kinetics and regulation of granulopoiesis. Semin Hematol 12:7, 1975.

Neutropenia

Al-Rashed R, Spangler J: Neonatal copper deficiency. N Engl J Med 285:841, 1971.
Boxer LA, Greenberg MS, Boxer GJ: Autoimmune neutropenia. N Engl J Med 293:748, 1975.
Leventhal JM, Silken AB: Oxacillin-induced neutropenia in children. J Pediatr 89:769, 1976.
Pearson HA, Lobel JF, Kocoshis SA, et al: A new syndrome of refractory sideroblastic anemia with vacuolization of marrow precursors and exocrine pancreatic dysfunction. J Pediatr 95:976, 1979.
Pincus SH, Boxer LA, Stossel TP: Chronic neutropenia in childhood. Am J Med 61:849, 1976.
Shwachman H, Diamond LK, Oski FA, et al: The syndrome of pancreatic insufficiency and bone marrow dysfunction. J Pediatr 65:645, 1964.

Qualitative Abnormalities

Baehner RL: Microbe ingestion and killing by neutrophils: Normal mechanisms and abnormalities. Clin Haematol 4:609, 1975.
Miller ME: Pathology of chemotaxis and random mobility. Semin Hematol 12:59, 1975.
Quie PG: Pathology of bactericidal power of neutrophils. Semin Hematol 12:143, 1975.

HEMORRHAGIC DISEASES

The blood is in dynamic equilibrium between fluidity and coagulation. This balance must be precisely maintained to assure that exsanguination does not follow trivial trauma or that spontaneous thrombosis does not occur. The hemostatic mechanism is complex: it involves local reactions of the blood vessels, the several activities of the platelet, and the interactions of specific coagulation factors which circulate in the blood. The vascular endothelium is the primary barrier against hemorrhage. When small blood vessels are transected, active vasoconstriction and local tissue pressure control minute areas of bleeding even without mobilization of the coagulation process, but the platelet is essential for maintenance of small blood vessels and of their endothelial stability. Hemostatic defects due to abnormalities of the vessels are manifested by small intracutaneous hemorrhages and petechiae. Hemorrhagic states related to the platelets and the soluble coagulation proteins are more dramatic and urgent.

14.52　SCHEMA OF COAGULATION

The classic schema of coagulation has pictured coagulation as proceeding in 3 phases: in phase I a hypothetical substance called thromboplastin is formed by interaction of plasma, platelets, and tissue juice; in phase II prothrombin is converted to thrombin in the presence of thromboplastin and calcium; and in phase III thrombin is converted by soluble fibrinogen into the visible fibrin clot. Although this simple scheme, involving only 6 substances, has been expanded so that a dozen factors have now been defined, retention of the concept of a basic 3-phase reaction has considerable merit. Table 14–8 lists the currently recognized coagulation factors and their common synonyms. A comprehensive schema of coagulation is depicted in Fig 14–8.

In phase I, in addition to an increased number of factors, intrinsic and extrinsic systems have been recognized. The intrinsic mechanism involves the succes-

Table 14–8　THE COAGULATION FACTORS

INTERNATIONAL NUMBERS	SYNONYMS	COMMENT
I	Fibrinogen	Number rarely used—congenital deficiency known (afibrinogenemia)
II	Prothrombin	Number rarely used—congenital deficiency known
III	Thromboplastin	No specific factor identified
IV	Calcium	Number rarely used
V	Labile factor, proaccelerin	Congenital deficiency known (parahemophilia, Owren disease)
VI	Activated labile factor, accelerin	No longer differentiated from V
VII	Stable factor, SPCA, proconvertin	Congenital deficiency known
VIII	Antihemophilic factor (AHF) or globulin (AHG)	Hemophilia A (classic hemophilia) results from congenital deficiency
IX	Christmas factor, plasma thromboplastin component (PTC)	Hemophilia B results from congenital deficiency
X	Stuart-Prower factor	Congenital deficiency known
XI	Plasma thromboplastin antecedent, PTA	Congenital deficiency known
XII	Hageman factor	No clinical symptoms associated with congenital deficiency
XIII	Fibrin stabilizing factor	Congenital deficiency known

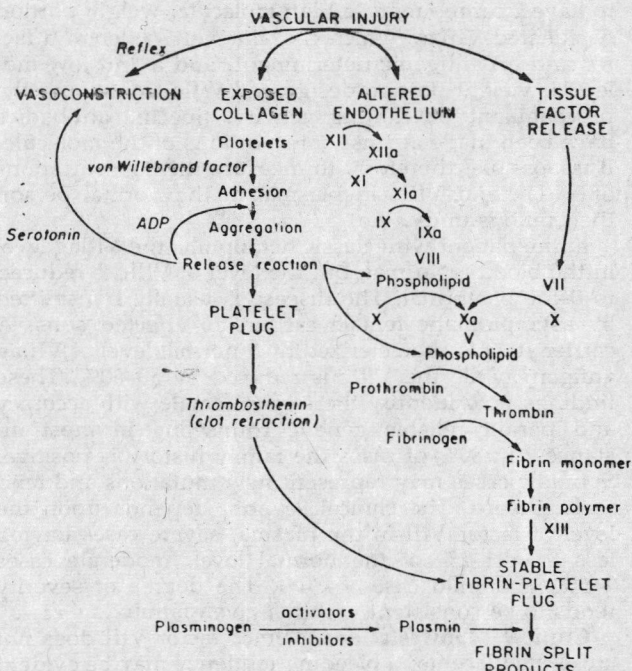

Figure 14—8 Diagrammatic representation of the hemostatic mechanism. (From Nathan DG, Oski FA: Hematology of Infancy and Childhood. Ed 2. Philadelphia, WB Saunders, 1981.)

sive enzymatic conversion of the inactive forms of factors XII, XI, and IX. Activated factor IX interacts with factor VIII, platelet factor 3, and calcium to activate factor X. Activated factor X interacts with factor V in generation of a plasma activity called prothrombinase that converts prothrombin to thrombin. The extrinsic mechanism involves the conversion of inactive factor VII to its active state by a substance (thromboplastin) derived from tissue fluid. In the extrinsic system active factor VII directly activates factor X.

Phase II of coagulation is concerned with the enzymatic cleavage of inactive prothrombin into smaller molecules, one of which is active thrombin. This step requires factor II as substrate as well as active factor X, factor V, and calcium.

Finally, in phase III thrombin splits 4 small peptides from the fibrinogen molecule, uncovering reactive sites in the fibrin monomer. These monomers then spontaneously polymerize, both side to side and end to end, to form fibrin. Factor XIII facilitates lateral bonding by specific peptide cross-links between fibrin strands to form a stable 3-dimensional clot. The coagulation mechanism interacts with other systems such as the kallikrein and fibrinolytic systems.

14.53 TESTS FOR EVALUATION OF THE HEMOSTATIC MECHANISM

Laboratory tests are of considerable value in the diagnosis of hemorrhagic disorders, but the importance of the history, including the family history, and of the physical examination cannot be overemphasized. Sig-

nificant congenital defects are almost invariably associated with histories of easy bruising or prolonged bleeding after minor injury.

The platelet count, tourniquet test, and bleeding time are used to assess the integrity of the small blood vessels. The *tourniquet test* is performed by inflating a blood pressure cuff to a point midway between the systolic and diastolic pressures for 5 min. Normally, this stress results in fewer than 5 petechiae on an area of skin on the forearm 2.5 cm square. A greater number of petechiae indicates thrombocytopenia, abnormally functioning platelets, or increased fragility or dysfunction of the small blood vessels. The *Ivy bleeding time* also assesses the vascular and platelet phases of hemostasis. A blood pressure cuff is applied to the arm and inflated to 40 mm Hg, and a stab incision 2 mm long and deep is made using a scalpel blade or utilizing a template. At 30-sec intervals drops of blood are blotted from the margin of the incision. Normally blood flow stops within 4–8 min. A *platelet count* or estimation is essential in the evaluation of any patient suspected of having a hemostatic disorder. When the platelet count is under 40,000/mm³, those tests that rely upon platelet function, such as the bleeding time and tourniquet test, usually give abnormal results. Platelet function tests include measurement of clot retraction, glass bead adhesion (Salzman test), and platelet aggregation.

The *whole blood clotting time* tests the entire coagulation mechanism. The interval for a firm blood clot to form in a glass test tube is normally 8–12 min; if a careful 3-tube technique is used, the upper limit of normal is 15–19 min. The clotting time is a crude assessment of the hemostatic mechanism; normal clotting times may accompany fairly severe defects. Capillary tube clotting time is unreliable.

The 3 phases of coagulation can be individually assessed by simple, reliable tests. In any hemorrhagic state the adequacy of phase III should be ascertained first. Unless adequate fibrinogen is present, the blood is incoagulable, and the other laboratory tests in which the formation of a visible clot is the end-point give, perforce, abnormal results. Phase III can be evaluated by the *thrombin time*, the time required for plasma to clot after the addition of bovine thrombin. The normal thrombin time is 15–20 sec. Prolongation indicates hypofibrinogenemia or a circulating anticoagulant. Fibrinogen can be measured also by chemical or immunologic methods.

Phase II in its entirety is assessed by the *prothrombin time*, the time taken for plasma to clot after the addition of thromboplastin and calcium. Normal prothrombin time is 12–14 sec. If phase III is intact, a prolonged prothrombin time indicates a deficiency involving factors II, V, VII, or X, alone or in combination. Specific assays for all these factors are available. The level of ionized calcium must be below 2.5 mg/dl (1.25 mmol/l) in order to impair blood coagulation.

Phase I, the most complex part of the coagulation mechanism, can be evaluated by several tests. The *activated partial thromboplastin time* (PTT) is the time required for clotting of plasma which has been activated by incubation with kaolin when calcium and platelets, or a lipid substitute for platelets (partial thromboplastin), are added. The normal partial thromboplastin time is 25–40 sec. The PTT is a simple, inexpensive, and reliable way to assess the adequacy of factors XII, XI, IX, and VII. The *prothrombin consumption time* is a standard prothrombin determination performed on serum instead of plasma. Because prothrombin is used up during coagulation, the serum normally contains little prothrombin and the serum prothrombin time is prolonged to 35 sec or more. Deficiencies of the phase I factors are associated with poor utilization of prothrombin. If the serum prothrombin time does not differ significantly from that obtained with plasma, deficiency of 1 of the phase I factors is likely.

The *thromboplastin generation* test is the most sensitive of all the tests of phase I. The thromboplastic activity of an incubated mixture of plasma, serum, and platelet substrate is estimated at regular intervals. A deficiency of any of the phase I factors will be reflected in an abnormal generation test result. This test can be modified to quantitate precisely factors VIII and IX.

There is considerable difference in sensitivity among these tests. For example, a plasma level of factor VIII which is only 1–2% of normal is sufficient for a normal clotting time. A level of factor VIII at 3–5% of normal produces a normal prothrombin consumption test. Results of PTT and thromboplastin generation tests become abnormal when the factor VIII level is 15–20% of normal or less.

If the PTT, prothrombin consumption, or thromboplastin generation test results are abnormal, the way in which they can be corrected identifies the specific deficiency. Normal plasma adsorbed with barium sulfate retains factors VIII and XI. Normal serum contains factors IX and XI. Accordingly, if an abnormal test result can be rectified by adsorbed plasma but not by serum, factor VIII deficiency is proved. If an abnormal result is corrected by serum but not by adsorbed plasma, factor IX deficiency is present. If both serum and plasma are corrective, factor XI deficiency may be present.

COAGULATION DISORDERS

PHASE I DISORDERS—THE HEMOPHILIAS

The hemophilias are the most common and serious of the congenital coagulation disorders. They are associated with genetically determined deficiencies of factors VIII, IX, or XI.

14.54 Factor VIII Deficiency
(Classic Hemophilia; Hemophilia A; Antihemophilic Factor (AHF) Deficiency)

About 80% of cases of hemophilia are caused by a gene carried on the X chromosome which results in a profound depression of the level of factor VIII (AHF) activity in the plasma. The factor VIII molecule appears to have 2 components: a high molecular weight portion designated VIIIag, which contains von Willebrand factor and an antigenic determinant, and a 2nd low molecular weight portion designated VIIIc, containing the procoagulant or clotting activity. Specific antibodies have been made against both portions of the molecule. It is possible, therefore, to measure the concentrations of VIIIag and VIIIc in plasma; in the normal person their ratio is unity.

In the patient with classic hemophilia the VIIIag level in the blood is normal, but the level of VIIIc is reduced to 0–5% of normal. The disease is usually transmitted by asymptomatic female carriers to affected sons. A carrier state is characterized by a normal level of VIIIag antigen, while the VIIIc is reduced by 50–60%. These findings now identify the carrier female with accuracy and permit reliable genetic counseling in most instances. In 80% of cases the family history is positive. Sporadic cases may represent new mutations and tend to be severe. The clinical severity depends upon the level of factor VIII in the plasma, severe cases having less than 1–2% of the normal level, moderate cases 2–5%, and mild cases 6–30%. The degree of severity tends to be consistent within a given family.

Clinical Manifestations.   Since factor VIII does not cross the placenta, a bleeding tendency may be evident in the neonatal period. Hematomas after injections and bleeding from circumcision are common, but many affected newborns exhibit no clinical abnormalities. As ambulation begins, excessive bruising occurs. Large intramuscular hematomas result from minor trauma. A relatively minor traumatic laceration, as of the tongue or lip, which bleeds persistently for hours or days is frequently the event that leads to diagnosis. Ninety per cent of patients with severe disease have had clear clinical evidence of increased bleeding by 3–4 yr of age.

The hallmark of hemophilia is hemarthrosis. Hemorrhages into the elbows, knees, and ankles cause pain and swelling and limit movement of the joint; these may be induced by relatively minor trauma but often appear to be spontaneous. Repeated hemorrhages may produce degenerative changes, with osteoporosis, muscle atrophy, and, ultimately, a fixed, unusable joint. Spontaneous hematuria is a troublesome but not usually serious complication. Intracranial hemorrhage and bleeding into the neck constitute life-threatening emergencies.

Patients with levels of factor VIII greater than 6% may not have severe spontaneous symptoms. These patients with "mild hemophilia" may experience only prolonged bleeding following tooth extractions, surgery, or injury.

Laboratory Data.   The only significant laboratory abnormalities occur in coagulation tests and are due to serious deficiency of factor VIII. The partial thromboplastin time (PTT) is greatly prolonged. Prothrombin consumption is so markedly impaired that the serum and plasma prothrombin times may be similar. The thromboplastin generation test result is grossly abnormal. The abnormal tests can be corrected by normal plasma adsorbed with barium sulfate but not by serum. In less severe cases only the PTT and thromboplastin generation test result may be abnormal.

Treatment. Prevention of trauma is an important aspect of care for the hemophilic child. During early life the crib and the playpen should be padded, and the child should be carefully supervised while learning to walk. As he becomes older, physical activities which do not entail a risk of trauma should be encouraged. It is important that a course between overprotection and permissiveness be followed. Aspirin and other drugs that affect platelet function may provoke severe hemorrhage and must be strictly avoided by hemophilic patients.

When bleeding episodes occur, replacement therapy is essential to prevent pain, disability, or life-threatening hemorrhage. The aim of therapy is to increase the level of factor VIII in the plasma to a level securing hemostasis. Presently, this can be done only by the intravenous infusion of fresh plasma or plasma concentrates (fresh or fresh-frozen plasma in a dose of 10–15 ml/kg every 12 hr). This regimen maintains a plasma level from 10–25% of normal. Because of danger of circulatory overload no more than 30 ml/kg of plasma should be administered in a 24-hr period.

Therapy of the hemophilic patient has been considerably facilitated by the development of factor VIII concentrates; these permit fairly precise estimation of the dosage necessary to attain hemostatic levels. By definition, 1 ml of normal plasma contains 1 unit of factor VIII. Because the plasma volume is about 45 ml/kg, it is necessary to infuse 45 units/kg of factor VIII to increase its level in the hemophiliac recipient from 0–100%. A dose of 25–50 units/kg of factor VIII is usually given to raise the recipient's level to 50–100% of normal. Because the half-life of factor VIII in the plasma is about 8–12 hr, repeated infusions can be given as necessary to maintain a desired level of activity.

Several factor VIII concentrates are available. The most inexpensive of these is cryoprecipitate, which can be prepared in the blood bank from fresh plasma. The yield from 250 ml of fresh plasma is 1 bag of cryoprecipitate, which usually contains 75–125 units of factor VIII; there may, however, be marked variability in the content of bags. One bag of cryoprecipitate/5 kg of body weight will raise the recipient's level to about 50% of normal.

Commercial preparations containing large amounts of relatively pure factor VIII are also available. These are dispensed as lyophilized powders in bottles of 250–500 units which can be reconstituted just prior to use; they have tremendous utility and convenience. Their potency and relatively low protein content permit rapid restoration of normal hemostatic levels with very small volumes.

Commercial factor VIII concentrates also contain anti-A and anti-B isohemagglutinins; when massive amounts of them are given to persons of blood group A or B, hemolysis may occur. Hyperfibrinogenemia due to the fibrinogen content of the concentrations may also result.

When the hemophilic child has significant bleeding, replacement therapy should be given promptly. Local measures should include application of cold and pressure, but these should not substitute for adequate replacement therapy. For ordinary hemarthroses, it is necessary to raise the factor VIII level to about 50% and to maintain it at least above 5% for 48–72 hr. A single infusion of 20–30 units/kg of factor VIII concentrate suffices, permitting the "1 shot" therapy of ordinary bleeding episodes. Immobilization is indicated initially, but passive exercise should be begun within 48 hr to prevent joint stiffness and fibrosis. The need for aspiration of blood from the joint is controversial. When the skin overlying the joint is very tense because therapy has been delayed, aspiration of blood, after adequate factor VIII has been given, may provide relief of pain. Replacement therapy is the most important part of management of hemarthrosis since equally good results have been obtained by some who routinely practice joint aspiration and by others who do not. Aggressive replacement therapy with factor VIII and careful orthopedic management of hemarthroses can prevent much severe deformity and crippling, which are now much less common than in the past. When hemorrhage occurs in vital areas such as the brain or neck or when major surgery is contemplated, intensive therapy using factor VIII concentrates is indicated to maintain the plasma level above 75% for 2 wk; a continuous infusion of factor VIII in a dose of 2 units/kg/hr can maintain a steady level of 50%. Epsilon-aminocaproic acid, 100 mg/kg every 6 hr, may be indicated in conjunction with replacement therapy for mucous membrane hemorrhage and dental extraction. Venipunctures should be performed only from superficial veins; aspiration from femoral or internal jugular veins is hazardous. Deaths have occurred following such ill-advised practice. There is compelling evidence that early treatment with factor VIII concentrates will reduce disability and deformity as well as the amount and duration of replacement treatment necessary for bleeding episodes. Parents, or even the older patient himself, can be trained to give intravenous infusions of concentrates at home, with substantial decreases in hospitalization and morbidity and with savings in costs.

The major obstacles to home treatment have been the unavailability and costs of concentrates and the reluctance of some health insurance programs to underwrite this kind of treatment. There is little doubt that home treatment with periodic assessment and counsel from the physician represents optimal management for the hemophilic child and family, and it is to be hoped that this enlightened management will permit the present generation of hemophilic children to enter adult life without major physical or psychologic crippling. On the other hand, some long term complications may result from modern therapy. Abnormalities of hepatic enzyme activities are found in 50% of patients. Instances of chronic active hepatitis and cirrhosis have occurred. These abnormalities probably result from repeated exposures to hepatitis viruses. Hypertension and renal disease with hematuria occur in many adult patients; their causes have not been defined.

Factor VIII Inhibitors. Five–10% of patients with hemophilia become refractory to factor VIII therapy because a circulating inhibitor or antibody develops. The development of inhibitors is not related to the number of plasma transfusions, and replacement therapy should not be withheld in hope of avoiding this.

These inhibitors are IgG globulins and are specifically active against factor VIII. The inhibitors may be of low titer and transient or of extremely high titer and very persistent. The "Bethesda unit" of inhibition is the amount of inhibitory activity in 1 ml of plasma that reduces the factor VIII level in 1 ml of normal plasma from 1 to 0.5 unit. It is virtually impossible to overpower a high titer inhibitor, but when hemorrhage occurs, massive doses of factor VIII concentrates or exchange transfusions with fresh blood should be given and may be of temporary benefit. Such replacement therapy should be limited to life-threatening hemorrhage. Immunosuppressive therapy has been of no value.

A novel approach to the therapy of the hemophilic child who has developed a factor VIII inhibitor has utilized certain factor IX concentrates (Konyne, Proplex), which apparently contain small amounts of activated factor VII and other coagulants. These activated coagulants enter the coagulation cascade distal to the level of factor VIII (Fig 14–8) and so bypass the effects of the inhibitor.

Prenatal Diagnosis. Each male fetus of a hemophilic carrier mother has a 50% risk of having the disease. Prenatal diagnosis is possible through examination of the blood of the (male) fetus, which can be obtained at fetoscopy. Fetal plasma is assayed for VIIIag and VIIIc; as in the older patient, a VIIIag level markedly higher than the VIIIc level will identify an affected male.

14.55   Factor IX Deficiency
(Christmas Disease; Hemophilia B)

About 15% of cases of hemophilia are due to a genetically determined deficiency of factor IX. This disease is clinically indistinguishable from factor VIII deficiency and is also transmitted as an X-linked recessive trait. The disease has a wide range of clinical severity, which in general corresponds to the level of factor IX in the serum.

Laboratory Data. The partial thromboplastin time (PTT), prothrombin consumption, and thromboplastin generation test results are usually abnormal. These in vitro abnormalities can be corrected by normal serum but not by plasma.

Treatment. Replacement therapy is accomplished by infusions of plasma. Ten–15 ml/kg should be given every 12–24 hr during bleeding episodes. The response to fresh or fresh-frozen plasma is superior to that obtained with stored plasma; cryoprecipitate and factor VIII concentrates are of no value.

Commercial concentrates containing factors II, VII, IX, and X (Konyne, Proplex) have excellent levels of factor IX—about 250 units/bottle—and can be given in dosage similar to that outlined for factor VIII. Because the half-life of factor IX is about 24 hr, administration may be less frequent. Some of the commercial concentrates are strongly contaminated with the agent for serum hepatitis and must be used with caution, particularly in patients with liver disease. Episodes of thrombosis have occurred following the administration of these concentrates, especially in postoperative patients, presumably because of their content of activated coagulants.

14.56   Factor XI Deficiency
(Plasma Thromboplastin Antecedent [PTA] Deficiency; Hemophilia C)

This usually mild bleeding disorder is inherited as an autosomal dominant or completely recessive trait. Typical cases are seen in both sexes. The usual clinical manifestations are mild, including nosebleeds; excessive hemorrhage and hemarthroses are rare. The PTT, prothrombin consumption, and thromboplastin generation test results are abnormal in the more severe cases. Normal plasma and serum correct the deficiency. Plasma therapy in a dose of 10–15 ml/kg every 12–24 hr should be given for significant clinical hemorrhage.

14.57   Factor XII Deficiency
(Hageman Factor Deficiency)

This interesting condition is due to homozygous occurrence of an autosomal gene which results in a profound deficiency of factor XII. Despite markedly abnormal test results of the 1st phase of coagulation (PTT and clotting times), affected persons have no clinical abnormalities.

14.58   Von Willebrand Disease
(Vascular Hemophilia)

This dominantly inherited disease is complex, characterized by a vascular abnormality producing a prolongation of bleeding time and by decreased levels of factor VIII. In contrast to classic hemophilia, there is no discrepancy between the levels of VIIIc and VIIIag; in von Willebrand disease both are depressed. The platelets in von Willebrand disease have decreased adhesiveness, and they do not aggregate when the antibiotic ristocetin is added to platelet-rich plasma, unlike platelets from normal individuals. This platelet defect is attributed to deficiency of a plasma factor necessary for normal platelet functioning (VW factor).

The clinical manifestations are nosebleeds, bleeding from the gums, menorrhagia, prolonged oozing from cuts, and increased bleeding after trauma or surgery. The bleeding time is usually prolonged. Fresh plasma infusions result in increases in the factor VIII level which are sustained for several days because of de novo synthesis, but they have an inconsistent effect on the bleeding time. Cryoprecipitate has been shown to correct the prolonged bleeding time and is probably the preferred form of replacement therapy for hemorrhage or of preparation for surgery. The recommended dose is 3–4 bags of cryoprecipitate/10 kg of body weight every 12 hr for 2 days and then 2 bags/10 kg/24 hr for 4–6 days.

PHASE II DISORDERS

Factors II, V, VII, and X are involved in the 2nd phase of coagulation and are designated the *prothrombin complex*. The factors are produced in the liver, and all except factor V require vitamin K for normal synthesis.

The laboratory diagnosis of these deficiencies depends upon a prolonged prothrombin time. Significant bleeding does not usually occur until the prothrombin time exceeds 20–25 sec, corresponding to a level of 10–15% of normal.

Genetically determined congenital deficiencies of factors II, V, and VII have been described, the most common of which is factor V deficiency (parahemophilia, Owren disease). The clinical manifestations of these deficiencies are mucocutaneous hemorrhages, bleeding into tissues, and hemorrhages after injury. Hemarthroses occur infrequently. These deficiencies are refractory to vitamin K therapy, and fresh plasma should be administered for active hemorrhage.

14.59 Hemorrhagic Disease of the Newborn

Hemorrhagic disease of the newborn is a self-limited bleeding disorder resulting from a deficiency of the coagulation factors dependent upon vitamin K.

The levels of factors II, VII, IX, and X are about 50% of normal in umbilical cord blood and decline rapidly to reach a nadir at 48–72 hr of life. In 0.25–0.5% of infants the decline is so extreme that severe hemorrhage may result. Thereafter the levels of these factors slowly increase but remain below adult values for several wk. The increase results from absorption of vitamin K from the diet. Cow milk contains a good level of vitamin K. Breast milk, on the other hand, has quite low levels, and symptomatic hemorrhagic disease of the newborn is much more common in breast-fed than formula-fed infants unless vitamin K prophylaxis is given.

Clinical Manifestations. In most instances hemorrhagic manifestations become evident on the 2nd–3rd day of life. Melena, bleeding from the navel, and hematuria are frequent signs of the disorder. The most serious complications are intracranial hemorrhagic and hypovolemic shock.

Treatment. Prophylactic administration of vitamin K_1 to the newborn prevents the postnatal decline of the factors of the prothrombin complex and virtually eliminates hemorrhagic disease of the newborn. Preparations of vitamin K_1 are indicated, for they do not have a hemolytic effect as do large doses of synthetic vitamin K_1 analogues. Vitamin K given to the mother may be beneficial, but a therapeutic effect is more certain if the drug is administered to the infant. As little as 25 μg of vitamin K prevents the postnatal decline of the prothrombin complex; the currently recommended dose of 1 mg of vitamin K_1 is safe and effective, given parenterally or orally. Larger doses do not increase the therapeutic effect.

In overt hemorrhagic disease 1 mg of vitamin K_1 should be given by intravenous or intramuscular injection. Clinical hemorrhage usually stops within 2 hr. If intracranial or other serious hemorrhage has occurred, an infusion of 10–15 ml/kg of fresh plasma will immediately correct the hemostatic defects. Profound anemia and shock may be corrected by infusions of fresh blood.

Premature infants may experience a complex hemorrhagic state involving several coagulation factors as well as platelet abnormalities. Vitamin K therapy is ineffective in correcting the abnormalities because of hepatic immaturity. Fresh plasma infusions are indicated if significant hemorrhage occurs.

Vitamin K deficiency rarely occurs after the neonatal period. Intestinal malabsorption of fats and prolonged administration of broad spectrum antibiotics may, however, result in vitamin deficiency, and cystic fibrosis and biliary atresia may be complicated by disorders of the prothrombin complex. Prophylactic administration of water-soluble vitamin K is indicated in these situations. In the past certain formulas based on meats or hydrolysates of protein were low in vitamin K, but this deficiency has been corrected. In advanced liver disease, synthesis of the factors of the prothrombin complex may be compromised by hepatocellular damage. Vitamin K therapy is not often effective in correcting the disorders if advanced liver disease is present. The anticoagulant properties of dicumarol and related anticoagulants depend on interference with synthesis of factors II, VII, and X. Vitamin K_1 is a specific antidote.

PHASE III DISORDERS

14.60 Congenital Afibrinogenemia

This rare hemorrhagic disorder is due to an autosomal recessive gene. Despite totally incoagulable blood these patients usually do not have severe spontaneous hemorrhages or hemarthroses, but trauma or surgery may be followed by severe bleeding. Therapy with 100 mg/kg of concentrated fibrinogen provides a hemostatic plasma level. Since the plasma half-life of fibrinogen is 5 days, frequent infusions are not necessary. A high risk of homologous serum hepatitis attends use of fibrinogen concentrates. Cryoprecipitate also contains fibrinogen and may be used effectively for therapy.

14.61 Congenital Dysfibrinogenemias

A number of abnormal fibrinogens with defective function may be associated with mild bleeding states. Inheritance is dominant. The thrombin time is prolonged, but chemical or immunologic methods reveal normal levels of fibrinogen.

14.62 Factor XIII Deficiency
(Fibrin Stabilizing Factor Deficiency)

A deficiency of factor XIII is the most recently recognized inherited hemorrhagic disease. Onset occurs most often in infancy, with bleeding after separation of the umbilical cord stump. Gastrointestinal, intracranial, and intra-articular hemorrhages have been the most common clinical manifestations. Routine coagulation studies are normal. Factor XIII deficiency is diagnosed by finding an abnormal solubility of the clot in 5 M urea solution and a short euglobulin lysis time.

Abildgaard CF: Current concepts in the management of hemophilia. Semin
    Hematol 12:223, 1975.
Abildgaard CF, Button M, Harrison J: Prothrombin complex concentrate (Konyne)
    in the treatment of hemophilic patients with factor VIII inhibitors. J Pediatr
    88:200, 1976.
Baehner RL, Strauss HS: Hemophilia in the first year of life. N Engl J Med
    275:524, 1966.
Bleyer WA, Hakami N, Shepard TH: The development of hemostasis in the
    human fetus and newborn infant. J Pediatr 75:838, 1971.

Glader BE, Buchanan GR: The bleeding neonate. In: Smith CA (ed): The Critically
    Ill Child—Diagnosis and Management. Ed 2. Philadelphia, WB Saunders, 1977.
Hathaway WE: The bleeding newborn. Semin Hematol 12:175, 1975.
Hilgartner MW: Hemophilic arthropathy. Adv Pediatr 21:139, 1974.
Perkins HA: Correction of the hemostatic defects of von Willebrand's disease.
    Blood 30:375, 1967.
Sutherland JM, Glueck H, Gliser G: Hemorrhagic disease of the newborn. Am J
    Dis Child 113:524, 1967.

14.63   The Purpuras

The purpuras are a group of diseases in which small hemorrhages occur into the superficial layers of the skin, producing areas of purple discoloration. Minute extravasations of blood about the small vessels are recognized as petechiae; more extensive hemorrhages cause ecchymoses. Bleeding may also occur from the mucous membranes and into other organs and tissues. The purpuras may be classified into 2 general groups according to platelet count. In *thrombocytopenic purpuras* the platelet count is reduced below 40,000/mm³, and hemorrhages are due to this quantitative deficiency. In *nonthrombocytopenic purpuras* bleeding results from defects in the small blood vessels or from defective platelet function despite their adequate numbers.

Platelets are non-nucleated, cellular fragments produced by the megakaryocytes of the bone marrow. The large size of the megakaryocyte reflects its polyploidy. As the megakaryocyte reaches maturity, fragmentation of the cytoplasm occurs and large numbers of platelets are liberated. They have a life span in the circulation of 7–10 days. The platelet has a number of intrinsic antigens, which are distinct from those of the red blood cell; some are shared by the leukocytes.

The platelets are intimately involved in both the vascular and the clotting aspects of hemostasis. They are necessary for integrity of the vascular endothelium; when small blood vessels are transected, platelets accumulate at the site of injury, forming a hemostatic plug. Platelet adhesion is initiated by contact with extravascular components such as collagen. Release of thromboxane (a prostaglandin derivative) and endogenous ADP causes firm aggregation. Serotonin and histamine liberated during these processes increase local vasoconstriction. Platelets have a phospholipid with partial thromboplastin activity, which makes an important contribution to coagulation. They also transport other blood coagulation factors through adsorption to the platelet surface. Finally, the platelet is necessary for normal clot retraction.

The *normal platelet count* is 150,000–400,000/mm³. Counts below this range indicate thrombocytopenia, due either to inadequate production or to excessive destruction or removal of platelets. Inadequate production is almost always due to marrow dysfunction, with decreases in the number of megakaryocytes. By contrast, in the thrombocytopenias due to increased destruction, the megakaryocytes are quantitatively normal or increased. The hypomegakaryocytic thrombocytopenias result from aplasia of the marrow or from its infiltration by abnormal or neoplastic tissue. Because of the grave prognosis of such disorders bone marrow aspiration is indicated in every case of significant unexplained thrombocytopenia. Bone marrow aspiration can usually be performed without serious bleeding even in patients with severe thrombocytopenia since thromboplastins in tissue juice will usually effect hemostasis.

14.64   NONTHROMBOCYTOPENIC PURPURAS

Purpura Associated with Normal Numbers of Platelets

The most common nonthrombocytopenic purpura is *anaphylactoid purpura*, or *Henoch-Schönlein syndrome* (Sec 9.65), an acute inflammatory process of unknown origin involving the small blood vessels of the skin, joints, gut, and kidney. The striking centrifugal distribution of the rash and involvement of the legs and buttocks are characteristic, particularly when combined with arthritis, nephritis, or gastrointestinal bleeding. The petechiae must be differentiated from those of early meningococcemia or septicemia due to other microorganisms. Septic emboli cause the petechiae observed in bacterial endocarditis. Toxic vasculitis may produce a hemorrhagic rash as a reaction to drugs such as arsenicals and iodides. Similar findings may occur during viral or rickettsial infections.

In *thrombasthenias*, or thrombocytopathic purpuras, quantitatively normal platelets have defective function. Abnormal function is reflected in petechiae and excessive bleeding. The abnormality of platelet function may also be revealed by defective clot retraction or by failure of the patient's platelets to support normal thromboplastin generation. Platelets in these diseases may be much larger than normal and have other abnormal morphology. A number of other congenital disorders of platelet function have been described, some with associated somatic defects; these have been summarized by Weiss.

Drug-Induced Abnormalities of Platelet Aggregation

Some drugs produce an irreversible reduction of prostaglandin synthesis within the platelet by inhibition of cyclooxygenase enzymes. This action prevents release of endogenous ADP and the prostaglandin derivative thromboxane, which are essential for platelet aggregation. This abnormality can be demonstrated most easily with a platelet aggregometer, by which an ablation of the so-called secondary wave of platelet aggregation can be demonstrated. The most important drug having this effect is aspirin. The effect is not dose-related. Abnormal platelet aggregation can be demonstrated in adults within 1 hr of ingestion of as little as 300 mg of aspirin. This abnormality persists for 4–6 days, until the platelets which have been exposed to the drug have been replaced. Under usual circumstances the effects of these drugs produce no clinical problems, though prolongation of the bleeding time is frequently seen. If, however, the patient has an underlying bleeding disorder such as hemophilia or undergoes a surgical operation, severe hemorrhage may occur. Aspirin or other drugs that inhibit platelet aggregation are contraindicated in these circumstances and should be replaced with other agents such as acetaminophen when indicated. Aspirin may have transplacental effects on platelet function in the newborn, producing neonatal hemorrhage; maternal aspirin consumption should be avoided during the last trimester of pregnancy. Transfusions of normal platelets are indicated if serious hemorrhage follows administration of aspirin.

THROMBOCYTOPENIC PURPURAS

14.65 IDIOPATHIC THROMBOCYTOPENIC PURPURA (ITP)

Acute idiopathic thrombocytopenic purpura (ITP), the most common of the thrombocytopenic purpuras of childhood, is associated with petechiae, mucocutaneous bleeding, and, occasionally, hemorrhages into tissues. There is a profound deficiency of circulating platelets despite adequate numbers of megakaryocytes in the marrow.

Etiology. The disease often appears to be related to sensitization by viral infections, for in about 70% of cases there is an antecedent disease such as rubella, rubeola, or viral respiratory infection. The interval between infection and onset of purpura averages 2 wk. By analogy with the disease seen in adults, it seems likely that an immune mechanism is the basis for the thrombocytopenia. Platelet antibodies can rarely be detected in acute cases with use of current methods; on the other hand, high levels of IgG have been found bound to platelets and may represent immune complexes adsorbed on the platelet surface.

Clinical Manifestations. The onset is frequently acute. One–4 wk after a viral infection or without antecedent illness, bruising and a generalized petechial rash occur. The bleeding is typically asymmetrical and may be most prominent over the legs. Hemorrhages in mucous membranes may be prominent, with hemorrhagic bullae of the gums and lips. Nosebleeds may be severe and difficult to control. The most serious complication is intracranial hemorrhage, which occurs in fewer than 1% of cases. The liver, spleen, and lymph nodes are not enlarged. Except for the signs of bleeding

the patient appears clinically well. The acute phase of the disease associated with spontaneous hemorrhages lasts for only 1–2 wk. Thrombocytopenia may persist, but spontaneous mucocutaneous hemorrhages subside. In some instances the onset is more insidious, with moderate bruising and few petechiae.

Laboratory Data. The platelet count is reduced below 20,000/mm³. The few platelets observed on blood smear are large in size (megathrombocytes) and reflect increased marrow production. Those tests that depend upon platelet function such as the tourniquet test and bleeding time and clot retraction give abnormal results. The white blood cell count is normal, and anemia is not present unless significant blood loss has occurred.

Bone marrow aspiration reveals normal granulocytic and erythrocytic series and frequently modest eosinophilia. Normal or increased numbers of megakaryocytes are seen. Some of the latter are immature, with deep basophilic cytoplasm; platelet budding may be scanty, but there is no pathognomonic or diagnostic megakaryocyte morphology. The changes seen reflect increased megakaryocytic turnover.

Differential Diagnosis. Idiopathic thrombocytopenic purpura must be differentiated by marrow examination from aplastic or infiltrative processes of the bone marrow. Marrow aplasia or replacement is unlikely if the physical examination is normal and the blood count is normal except for thrombocytopenia. On occasion, however, failure to perform a marrow examination may lead to diagnostic error and delay institution of correct therapy. Significant enlargement of the spleen will suggest primary liver disease with congestive splenomegaly, lipidosis, or reticuloendotheliosis. Thrombocytopenic purpura may be an initial manifestation of systemic lupus erythematosus or lymphoma, but this sequence is unusual in young children; in adolescents the possibility is greater, and serologic studies for systemic lupus erythematosus are indicated. Genetically determined thrombocytopenias must be considered in infants (particularly males) found to have low platelet counts.

Treatment. Idiopathic thrombocytopenic purpura has an excellent prognosis even when no specific therapy is given. Seventy-five per cent of patients recover completely within 3 mo, most within 8 wk. Severe spontaneous hemorrhages and intracranial bleeding are usually confined to the initial phase of the disease. After the initial acute phase, spontaneous manifestations tend to subside. Nine–12 mo after the onset about 90% of affected children have regained normal platelet counts, and relapses are unusual.

Fresh blood or platelet concentrates are of no value or of transient benefit because transfused platelets survive only briefly, but they should be administered when life-threatening hemorrhage occurs. Corticosteroid therapy is of great value; though it has not decreased the number of chronic cases, it does reduce the severity and shorten the duration of the initial phase.

When the disease is mild and hemorrhages of the retina or mucous membranes are not present, no specific therapy may be indicated. The affected child should be protected from falls or trauma. Bacterial infections should be treated with appropriate antibiotics. Vitamins

K and C have no therapeutic effect. Although infusions of plasma and, more recently, intravenous gamma globulin have been reported to be occasionally followed by sustained rises of platelet count, their efficacy is unproved. In more severe cases therapy with a corticosteroid, such as prednisone in a dose of 1–2 mg/kg or its equivalent, is indicated. The necessity for corticosteroid therapy in mild cases has been debated, though the platelet count returns to a hemostatic level more rapidly with such therapy. If the hemorrhagic manifestations are severe or if intracranial hemorrhage is suspected because of headache, meningismus, or other neurologic signs, larger doses of prednisone (5–10 mg/kg) should be used initially. This therapy is continued until the platelet count is normal or for 3 wk, whichever comes first. At this point, steroid therapy should be discontinued even if the platelet count remains low. Prolonged corticosteroid theapy is not indicated and may depress the bone marrow, in addition to producing cushingoid changes and growth failure. If thrombocytopenia persists for 4–6 mo, a 2nd short course of corticosteroid therapy may be given. Splenectomy should be reserved for chronic cases, defined by thrombocytopenia persistent for more than 1 yr, and for the severe ones that do not respond to corticosteroids. Considerable improvement can be expected in most instances. Only about 2% of cases of idiopathic thrombocytopenia purpura in children tend to be chronic and refractory. In these chronic cases therapy with immunosuppressive drugs (azathioprine, vincristine) may be attempted.

14.66 OTHER THROMBOCYTOPENIC PURPURAS

Drug-Induced Thrombocytopenias. A number of drugs may be associated with immune thrombocytopenia. Quinidine and apronalide (Sedormid) function as haptens which combine with proteins on the platelet surface and stimulate antibody formation. Administration of these drugs to sensitized persons is followed by severe thrombocytopenia. This syndrome is unusual in pediatric practice because the responsible drugs are rarely prescribed. In any case of thrombocytopenia, however, a careful search for any drug exposure should be made and the patient removed from contact with potential offenders.

Wiskott-Aldrich Syndrome and Other Inherited Thrombocytopenias. The Wiskott-Aldrich syndrome consists of cutaneous eczema, thrombocytopenic hemorrhage, and increased susceptibility to infection due to an immunologic defect that is transmitted as an X-linked recessive trait. Bloody diarrhea and hemorrhage during the 1st months of life are usually the initial clinical manifestations. The bone marrow contains a normal number of megakaryocytes, but many have bizarre nuclear morphology. Homologous platelets survive normally when transfused into these patients, but autologous platelets have a shortened life span and are small in size. Wiskott-Aldrich syndrome may represent an unusual circumstance in which thrombocytopenia results from abnormal platelet formation or release despite quantitatively adequate numbers of megakary-

ocytes. The immunologic defect is discussed in Sec 9.16. Splenectomy has often been followed by overwhelming sepsis and death. A recent report described significant improvement in thrombocytopenia after splenectomy in a group of patients. Prophylactic penicillin was used and considered very important postsplenectomy. A number of patients with Wiskott-Aldrich syndrome have developed lymphoreticular malignancies. A few cases have been reported to benefit from administration of transfer factor and from 1 marrow transplantation.

A number of other types of inherited thrombocytopenias have been described. Some are X-linked, and some have autosomal transmission. Responses to therapy, including splenectomy, have usually been disappointing. The inordinately high mortality of young males splenectomized for presumed idiopathic thrombocytopenic purpura suggests that, even without other stigmata, X-linked thrombocytopenia may represent a variant of Wiskott-Aldrich syndrome. Thus, the young thrombocytopenic male must be carefully studied before a diagnosis of ITP is made. A platelet survival study is indicated in such patients.

Thrombopoietin Deficiency. A single child has been described (Schulman) with chronic thrombocytopenia presumably resulting from a deficiency of a megakaryocyte maturation factor contained in normal plasma. Plasma infusions repeatedly produced a sustained peripheral rise in the platelet count. In a somewhat similar case episodic thrombocytopenia and microangiopathic hemolysis were reversed by infusions of plasma.

Thrombocytopenia with Cavernous Hemangioma (Kasabach-Merritt Syndrome). Some infants with large cavernous hemangiomas of the trunk, extremities, or abdominal viscera have severe thrombocytopenia and other evidence of intravascular coagulation. Histologic and isotopic studies indicate that platelets are trapped and destroyed within the extensive vascular bed of the tumor. The peripheral blood shows thrombocytopenia and red cell fragments, and the bone marrow contains adequate numbers of megakaryocytes. Spontaneous thrombosis within the tumor may lead to obliteration of the vascular channels and spontaneous recovery; radiation therapy in a single dose of 600–800 r may accelerate this process, but repeated courses may be necessary. When anatomically feasible, external compression or total excision may be attempted, but surgery may be associated with uncontrollable hemorrhage. Corticosteroids may hasten involution and warrant trial, especially in the young infant. Splenectomy is unnecessary and contraindicated.

14.67 NEONATAL THROMBOCYTOPENIA

Thrombocytopenia of the newborn has aspects which merit special consideration. Thrombocytopenia may reflect diseases primary in the infant's hematopoietic system or be due to transfer of abnormal factors from the mother.

Thrombocytopenias may occur in a variety of fetal and neonatal infections and may be responsible for serious spontaneous bleeding. These include viral infections (especially rubella and cytomegalic inclusion disease); protozoal infections such as toxoplasmosis; syphilis; and bacterial infections, especially those caused by gram-negative bacilli. Hemolysis is usually also present in infants with prominent anemia and jaundice. The liver and spleen are considerably enlarged. The bone marrow changes are variable, but reduced numbers of megakaryocytes may be seen.

Immune Neonatal Thrombocytopenia. About 30% of infants born of mothers with active idiopathic thrombocytopenic purpura have thrombocytopenia in the neonatal period due to transplacental transfer of antiplatelet antibodies. Rarely, infants with neonatal disease have been born of mothers with a remote history of idiopathic thrombocytopenic purpura who have normal platelet counts and whose disease has been inactive for many years. Petechiae are not present initially but appear in a generalized distribution within a few min after birth. Bleeding from bowel or kidney and intracranial hemorrhage may occur. In mild cases there may be few abnormal findings. Hepatosplenomegaly is not present. The duration of the thrombocytopenia is 2–3 mo. Although therapy is not strikingly successful, fresh blood, exchange transfusions, or platelet transfusions may be of temporary value in arresting acute bleeding. Corticosteroid therapy has not been proved beneficial but can be used when thrombocytopenia is severe (platelet counts below 20,000/mm³). Because of the self-limited nature of the disease, splenectomy is contraindicated. Corticosteroid therapy given to the mother 1 wk prior to delivery may reduce the severity of disease in the infant.

When the fetus has platelet antigens which the mother does not have, isoimmunization may occur. If maternal antibodies to fetal platelet antigens reach a sufficiently high titer, enough may cross the placenta to produce thrombocytopenia in the fetus. The disease may be familial, and 1st-born infants are frequently affected. The clinical signs include petechiae and other hemorrhagic manifestations. By use of sensitive tests involving complement fixation, antiplatelet antibodies can be demonstrated in about 50% of cases. The PLA-1 antigen is most frequently involved. Exchange transfusion is temporarily effective in stopping bleeding. If compatible platelets can be obtained (these are most easily procured by preparing washed platelet concentrates from the mother), they offer specific effective therapy. Infants born of successive pregnancies may be affected. Elective cesarean section has been advocated to spare the infant's head the trauma of delivery.

When the mother has drug-induced thrombocytopenia, both antibody and drug may cross the placenta and cause neonatal thrombocytopenia. Corticosteroid therapy and especially exchange transfusions should be considered when bleeding manifestations are severe.

Congenital Hypoplastic Thrombocytopenia with Associated Malformations (Thrombocytopenia Absent Radius [TAR] Syndrome). Severe thrombocytopenia has been described as a familial condition associated with aplasia of radii and thumbs and cardiac and renal anomalies. Severe hemorrhagic manifestations are evident in the 1st days of life. Hemoglobin levels are normal; leukocytosis and even leukemoid reactions

have been found in some cases. Megakaryocytes are absent from the bone marrow.

The anomalies in this disease are similar to those observed in Fanconi pancytopenia, in which the hematologic abnormalities are not usually observed until the 3rd–4th yr of life. Chromosomes do not here show the abnormalities found in Fanconi syndrome. No infants with congenital hypoplastic thrombocytopenia have been reported to develop full blown Fanconi syndrome, nor have both conditions been observed in the same family.

14.68 THROMBOCYTOSIS
(Thrombocythemia)

Platelet counts in excess of 750,000/mm³ may be designated as thrombocytosis. Markedly elevated counts may accompany hemorrhage, iron deficiency anemia, hemolytic anemias, and primary myeloproliferative disorders. Acute and chronic inflammatory states may be accompanied by elevated platelet counts. Platelet counts exceeding 600,000/mm³ are regularly observed in Kawasaki disease. After splenectomy for idiopathic thrombocytopenic purpura or hemolytic anemia the platelet count often rises precipitously and may exceed 1,000,000/mm³ 10–14 days postoperatively. In general, no specific therapy such as anticoagulation is necessary, for thrombosis is extremely rare. The use of aspirin (or dipyridamole), which inhibits platelet function, may be considered if there are factors predisposing to thrombosis.

A case of primary thrombocytosis associated with thrombotic episodes and myocardial infarction has been described.

Canales ML, Mauer AM: Sex-linked hereditary thrombocytopenia as a variant of Wiskott-Aldrich syndrome. N Engl J Med 277:899, 1967.
Glader BE, Buchanan GR: The bleeding neonate. In: Smith CA (ed): The Critically Ill Child—Diagnosis and Management. Ed 2. Philadelphia, WB Saunders, 1977.
Hall J, Levin J, Kuhn J, et al: Thrombocytopenia with absent radius (TAR). Medicine 48:411, 1969.
Imbach P, Barundune S, d'Apuzzo V: High dose gamma globulin for idiopathic thrombocytopenic purpura. Lancet 1:1228, 1981.
Karpatkin S: Autoimmune thrombocytopenic purpura. Blood 56:329, 1980.
Lightsey AL, Koenig HM: Platelet associated immunoglobulin G in childhood idiopathic thrombocytopenic purpura. J Pediatr 94:20, 1979.
McIntosh S, Pearson HA: Isoimmune neonatal purpura. J Pediatr 82:1020, 1973.
Schulman I, Pierce M, Lukens A, et al: Studies on thrombopoiesis. I. A factor in normal human plasma required for platelet production. Chronic thrombocytopenia due to its deficiency. Blood 16:943, 1960.
Simons SM, Main CA, Yarsh HM, et al: Idiopathic thrombocytopenic purpura in children. J Pediatr 87:16, 1975.
Spach MA, Howell DA, Harris JS: Myocardial infarction with multiple thrombosis in a child with primary thrombocytosis. Pediatrics 31:268, 1963.
Weiss HJ: Platelet physiology and abnormalities of platelet function. N Engl J Med 293:531, 1975.
Wolff JA: Wiskott-Aldrich syndrome: Clinical immunologic and pathologic observations. J Pediatr 70:221, 1967.
Zinkham WH, Osborn JE, Medearis DN Jr: Blood and bone marrow findings in congenital rubella. J Pediatr 67:985, 1965.

14.69 DISSEMINATED INTRAVASCULAR COAGULATION
(Consumption Coagulopathy)

Consumption coagulopathy is a unifying concept linking a large group of conditions associated with disseminated intravascular coagulation (DIC). Consequences of this process include widespread intravascular deposition of fibrin and may lead to tissue ischemia and necrosis, a generalized hemorrhagic state, and hemolytic anemia.

Etiology. A number of pathologic processes may incite episodes of disseminated intravascular coagulation, including hypoxia, acidosis, tissue necrosis, endotoxic shock, and endothelial damage. Accordingly, it is not surprising that a large number of diseases have been reported associated with disseminated intravascular coagulation. These include incompatible blood transfusions, cyanotic congenital heart diseases, sepsis (especially gram-negative), rickettsial infections, snakebite, purpura fulminans, giant hemangioma, malignancies, acute promyelocytic leukemia, and many other conditions.

Clinical Manifestations. Disseminated intravascular coagulation most frequently accompanies a severe systemic disease process. Bleeding frequently first occurs from sites of venipuncture or surgical incision, with associated petechiae and purpura. Tissue thrombosis may involve many organs and may be most spectacular as infarction of large areas of skin and subcutaneous tissue or of kidneys. Anemia due to hemolysis may develop rapidly.

Laboratory Data. There is no well defined sequence of events. The labile coagulation factors (II, V, and VII), fibrinogen, and platelets may be consumed by the ongoing intravascular clotting process, with prolongation of the prothrombin, partial thromboplastin, and thrombin times. Platelet count may be profoundly depressed. Blood contains fragmented burr and helmet-shaped red cells (schizocytes), changes referred to as microangiopathic. In addition, because the fibrinolytic mechanism is activated, fibrin split products (FSP) appear in the blood.

Treatment. The most important component of therapy is control or reversal of the process that initiated disseminated intravascular coagulation. Infection, shock, acidosis, and hypoxia must be treated promptly and vigorously. If the underlying problem can be controlled, bleeding quickly ceases, and there is improvement of the abnormal laboratory findings.

Infusions of platelets and fresh-frozen plasma may be considered as replacement therapy to support the child until the underlying disease can be controlled. The use of heparin in disseminated intravascular coagulation has become restricted because there is increasing evidence that it does not alter mortality or prognosis. Most authorities restrict its use to situations in which there is actual widespread thrombosis, as in purpura fulminans. If heparin is to be used, it should be given in doses of 100 units (1 mg)/kg intravenously every 4-6 hr. In the bleeding sick neonate with disseminated intravascular coagulation, exchange transfusion with fresh blood may be considered.

14.70　THROMBOPHLEBITIS

Symptomatic thrombophlebitis is uncommon in children. The most common precipitating factor is trauma of the lower extremities or pelvis. Stasis from immobilization increases the risk. Increased frequency of spontaneous thrombophlebitis has been reported in pregnancy, with the use of oral contraceptive agents, and in the nephrotic syndrome. Management commonly involves manipulation of the clotting mechanism.

Massive deep thrombophlebitis involving an entire lower extremity produces diffuse edema, pain, and cyanosis. Thrombophlebitis of the deep veins of the lower leg is accompanied by calf pain elicited by sharp dorsiflexion of the foot (Homan sign). A deep painful cordlike mass can sometimes be felt. When necessary, diagnosis can be corroborated by venography.

Venous thrombosis of the deep leg veins should be treated with bed rest, elevation of the leg, and heat. Heparin should be administered intravenously in a dose of 50-100 units/kg every 4 hr. Alternatively, continuous intravenous therapy can be accomplished by an initial injection of 50-75 units/kg of heparin to be followed in 2 hr by constant infusion of 10-20 units/kg/hr. The partial thromboplastin time should be maintained at 60-80 sec (twice its normal value). When the process appears to be resolving, the patient can be maintained with oral anticoagulation with sodium warfarin. The adolescent or young adult should receive a loading dose of 10 mg of warfarin (2.5-5.0 mg for smaller children). Daily dose is 1-5 mg, but adequacy of dosage should be assessed frequently by determinations of prothrombin time, which should be maintained between 20-30 sec. Therapy should be continued for 3-6 mo.

Pulmonary embolism may occur as a complication of deep vein thrombophlebitis; signs vary with the magnitude of the infarct. Chest roentgenogram and radionuclide perfusion studies are useful in diagnosis. Long-term anticoagulation is necessary.

Congenital deficiency of antithrombin III, an autosomal dominant trait, is associated with recurrent episodes of deep vein thrombosis and pulmonary embolism. Standard coagulation tests are normal, but antithrombin III levels are 25-50% of normal in affected individuals. Chronic therapy with warfarin has been suggested.

Bennett B, Mackie M, Douglas AS: Familial thrombosis due to antithrombin III deficiency: An extensive family study. Thromb Haemost 38:78, 1977.

14.71　THE FIBRINOLYTIC MECHANISM

Fibrinolysis, the process of dissolution of the clot, is a complex and essential physiologic mechanism. It comprises a number of fairly well-defined factors, the most important of which involves a fibrinolytic enzyme called plasmin and its inactive precursor plasminogen. Thrombin and a urokinase found in urine are particularly potent converters of inactive plasminogen to its active enzymatic form. The fibrinolytic system is activated at the same time that coagulation occurs, with the result that in disease associated with diffuse intravascular coagulation, increased fibrinolytic activity of the plasma and fibrin degradation products (fibrin split products, FSP) is also often found in the circulation. Increased fibrinolytic activity is demonstrated in the test tube by spontaneous dissolution of the clot on incubation of clotted blood or by a shortened euglobulin lysis time. Rarely, spontaneous fibrinolytic states may be associated with hemorrhagic symptoms. It may be difficult to differentiate these primary fibrinolytic states from consumption coagulopathies, in which fibrinolysis is a secondary phenomenon. In consumption coagulopathies factors I, II, V, and VIII and platelets are usually decreased, whereas in fibrinolytic states platelets are usually normal and the other factors inconstantly affected. Treatment with epsilon-aminocaproic acid (EACA) may be of value in fibrinolytic states, but it is not indicated in consumption coagulopathies.

14.72 HEMOLYTIC-UREMIC SYNDROME

See also Sec 16.22.

This acute disease of infancy and early childhood usually follows an episode of acute gastroenteritis. Shortly thereafter, signs and symptoms of hemolytic anemia, thrombocytopenia, and glomerulonephritis develop. Bilateral renal cortical necrosis may occur, and case fatality rates as high as 30% have been reported. Its sometimes epidemic occurrence suggests that an infectious agent may be involved.

Laboratory Data. The hemolytic anemia is associated with characteristically bizarre red cell morphology. Many of the red cells are contracted and distorted, with prominence of spherocytes, burr cells, and helmet-shaped forms (Fig 14–2E). A depressed platelet count despite normal numbers of megakaryocytes in marrow indicates excessive peripheral destruction. Tests of the coagulation mechanism are usually normal. Protein, red cells, and casts are present in the urinary sediment, and grave renal damage is reflected in oliguria and azotemia. Renal biopsy reveals fibrinoid deposits in small blood vessels and glomeruli, which may represent deposition of fibrin on a diffusely damaged endothelium.

Treatment. For management of uremia and anuria see Sec 16.22. Transfusions are indicated for severe anemia. Corticosteroid and heparin therapy do not appear to affect survival or prognosis.

14.73 THROMBOTIC THROMBOCYTOPENIC PURPURA

This rare and serious disease has many similarities to the hemolytic-uremic syndrome. Diffuse embolism and thrombosis of the small blood vessels of the brain are evidenced by shifting neurologic signs such as aphasias, blindness, and convulsions. The prognosis is grave. Laboratory findings include thrombocytopenia and a hemolytic anemia associated with distorted and fragmented red cells. Treatment has been of dubious success, but large doses of ACTH or corticosteroids and emergency splenectomy have been advocated. Anticoagulant therapy may also be used but is of uncertain value. Plasmapheresis has been reported as beneficial in some cases.

14.74 PURPURA FULMINANS

Purpura fulminans is an unusual disease which usually occurs in the convalescent phase of a bacterial or viral infection. Diffuse symmetrical hemorrhages occur, with prominent inflammatory vasculitis and necrosis of skin and subcutaneous tissues, particularly involving the buttocks and lower extremities. Systemic toxicity may be extreme, and mortality is high. In nonfatal cases large areas of gangrenous skin and muscle may slough, leaving areas requiring plastic surgical repair. The platelet count is normal or low. Fragmented red cells may be seen on blood smear. The levels of consumable coagulation factors, especially of fibrinogen, are decreased. Replacement therapy with fibrinogen and fresh plasma transfusions and high doses of corticosteroids have appeared to be helpful on occasion. Intravenous administration of heparin, 50–100 units/kg (0.5–1 mg/kg) every 4–6 hr or the use of dextran infusions may arrest the progression of the cutaneous lesions and correct the coagulation defects.

Allen DM: Heparin therapy of purpura fulminans. Pediatrics 32:211, 1966.
Corrigan JJ, Jordan CM: Heparin therapy in septicemia with disseminated intravascular coagulation. N Engl J Med 283:778, 1970.
Corrigan JJ, Kiernat JF: Effect of heparin in experimental gram-negative septicemia. J Infect Dis 131:138, 1975.
Hathaway WE: Disseminated intravenous coagulation. In: Smith CA (ed): The Critically Ill Child. Ed 2. Philadelphia, WB Saunders, 1977.
Liberman E: Hemolytic uremic syndrome. J Pediatr 80:1, 1972.
MacWhinney JB Jr, Packer JT, Miller G, et al: Thrombotic thrombocytopenic purpura in childhood. Blood 19:181, 1962.

14.75 THE SPLEEN

The spleen has excited speculations of man since antiquity. Pliny believed it to be the seat of mirth and laughter; Galen pronounced it an organ full of mystery. No unique cells or tissues occur within the spleen, but the particular arrangements and anatomic relations there are responsible for unique functions. The spleen is a large mass of lymphoid and phagocytic reticuloendothelial cells with a complex network of tortuous capillaries and fenestrated sinusoids. These impart the important properties of a biologic filter.

Functions. A number of functions can be assigned to the spleen, and some of these are germane to hematologic processes and diseases:

Reservoir Function. In lower animals the spleen is a contractile organ because considerable smooth muscle is present in the capsule and trabeculae. In man little muscle is present, and the reservoir function is normally not very great. The spleen does release both factor VIII and platelets following infusion of epinephrine. The normal spleen contains only about 25 ml of blood, but when the spleen enlarges for any reason, its content of blood increases. The sequestration crisis of sickle cell states is an exaggeration of reservoir function.

Hematopoiesis. The spleen is a site of active blood formation during fetal life, but by about 6 mo of gestation hematopoiesis disappears unless a condition such as hemolytic disease of the newborn is present. In a few exceptional diseases such as thalassemia and osteopetrosis, hematopoiesis persists or is resumed postnatally. The stimulus for this is not known.

"Culling." This term has been used to describe the ability of the spleen by virtue of its unique circulation and structure to remove damaged or abnormal blood cells from the circulation. This function is clearly demonstrated by the fact that red cells and platelets lightly coated by antibodies are selectively sequestered and destroyed by the spleen. The spleen's activity in destroying spherocytes is another example of culling.

"Pitting." The spleen has the ability to remove or "pit" intracytoplasmic inclusions such as Howell-Jolly bodies or siderotic granules from within the red cell without destroying the cell. The peripheral blood of a person with no spleen contains relatively large numbers of these intracellular inclusions.

Destruction of Old Red Cells. The spleen is probably the principal site of destruction of senescent red cells. This function is easily assumed by other portions of the reticuloendothelial system, however, and red cell life span is not significantly increased in the absence of spleen.

Membrane Effect. The normal spleen is postulated to have an ill-defined effect on the red cell membrane. When the spleen is absent, red cells are flatter and thinner than normal, increased numbers of target cells are seen, and osmotic fragility is decreased. Examination of the circulating blood by the technique of interference phase contrast microscopy shows membrane indentations resembling craters in 20% or more of the red cells of asplenic persons. Fewer than 1% of the red cells of individuals with a normal spleen have these depressions or "pocks," which may actually be small vesicles.

Filtering and Immunologic Functions. Because of the intimate relation of the circulating blood with lymphoid and reticuloendothelial elements within the spleen, this organ plays an important role in primary defense against bacteria which gain access to the circulation. The spleen is especially vital in the immature and nonimmune person, for it constitutes the primary site of clearance of organisms such as pneumococci in the absence of specific antibody. The spleen has a relatively minor role in overall antibody formation so long as the antigen is administered by intramuscular or subcutaneous routes, but the spleen is essential to antibody formation in response to small doses of particulate intravenous antigens.

The spleen participates in a major way in synthesis of IgM, properdin, and "tuftsin," a phagocytosis-promoting tetrapeptide (Sec 8.28). Levels of these humoral factors are depressed in the splenectomized child.

Hormonal Function. It has been postulated that the spleen produces a hormonal substance ("splenin") which exerts an effect on bone marrow activity. There is little evidence for such a hormone, and "hypersplenism" is better explained on the basis of excessive filtering or culling activities. The spleen can be functionally inactive despite clinical enlargement, as in young children with sickle cell anemia (functional hyposplenism).

Clinical Examination. Careful and gentle palpation of the relaxed abdomen provides reliable information about the size of the spleen. The tip can be felt at the left costal margin in 5–10% of normal children and in a higher proportion of children with viral infections. The spleen must be increased to 2–3 times average size before it can be regularly felt on physical examination. Lesser degrees of enlargement can be detected radiographically. An enlarged spleen must be differentiated from other masses in the left upper quadrant. Useful physical characteristics which aid in identifying the spleen include concealment of its upper margin by the rib cage, the presence of a palpable notch, and the absence of overlying bowel. When it is impossible to be certain of the identity of a mass, isotopic scanning studies are of value. Short-lived isotopes such as technetium-99m (^{99m}Tc) may be used to label gelatin sulfur colloid particles. Injected intravenously, this radioactive colloid is rapidly cleared by reticuloendothelial elements in the liver, spleen, and, to a lesser extent, bone marrow; scanning permits definition of the size and configuration of spleen and liver. This technique has proved of great value in demonstrating anatomic abnormalities of the spleen; it is noninvasive and involves a very low radiation exposure.

The spleen has vascular, lymphatic, and reticuloendothelial components; pathologic processes involving any of these systems may be manifested as splenomegaly. Table 14–9 lists important causes of splenic enlargement.

Table 14–9 SOME CAUSES OF SPLENOMEGALY IN CHILDREN

I. *Hematologic diseases*
Hemolytic anemias—due to extramedullary hematopoiesis and reticuloendothelial hyperplasia
   A. Congenital and acquired hemolytic anemias
   B. Hemoglobinopathies and thalassemia
II. *Infections*
   A. Bacterial: septicemias; typhoid; endocarditis
   B. Viral: Epstein-Barr, cytomegalovirus, etc.
   C. Protozoal: malaria, toxoplasmosis
III. *Congestive splenomegaly*
   A. Secondary to portal or splenic vein obstruction
   B. Secondary to intrahepatic disease—cirrhosis
   C. Chronic congestive heart failure
IV. *Infiltrations*
   A. Lipidoses—Niemann-Pick, Gaucher diseases
   B. Nonlipid reticuloendothelioses
V. *Cysts*
   A. Congenital—epidermoid cysts
   B. Acquired—pseudocysts
VI. *Neoplasms*
   A. Leukemia and lymphosarcoma
   B. Hodgkin disease
   C. Hemangioma and lymphangioma
VII. *Miscellaneous*
   A. Rheumatoid arthritis (Still disease)
   B. Lupus erythematosus

14.76 CONGESTIVE SPLENOMEGALY
(Banti Syndrome)

The venous outflow from the spleen may be obstructed within the liver or in the portal or splenic veins. This vascular obstruction produces congestion and ultimately splenomegaly. Liver diseases associated with parenchymal inflammation, fibrosis, and vascular constriction include postnecrotic cirrhosis, galactosemia, Wilson disease, cystic fibrosis, biliary atresia, α_1-antitrypsin deficiency, and microcystic disease of liver and kidney. Septic omphalitis, either primary or following umbilical vein cannulation, may progress to portal vein thrombophlebitis and thrombosis. Rarely, congenital or acquired anomalies of the splenic or portal veins may cause obstruction and secondary splenomegaly. In some areas of the world schistosomiasis and malaria are important causes of splenomegaly.

Clinical Manifestations. Observation or palpation of an enlarged spleen may be the initial indication of the disease process. The enlarged spleen may filter out and destroy excessive numbers of blood cells and platelets and thus cause thrombocytopenic hemorrhage and anemia. In response to portal vein obstruction, collateral circulation develops through the short gastric, esophageal, superficial abdominal, and hemorrhoidal veins. In some cases massive hemorrhage from ruptured esophageal varices is the 1st clinical manifestation of congestive splenomegaly.

Laboratory Data. Pancytopenia of varying degree is seen. The bone marrow shows active hematopoiesis with abundant megakaryocytes. Liver function tests may indicate hepatocellular disease. It is possible to measure portal venous pressure, and injection of radiopaque dyes into the spleen will permit radiologic visualization of the splenic and portal veins. This should usually be done under direct vision, for percutaneous needling may lacerate the splenic capsule. In cases secondary to hepatic fibrosis and cirrhosis, ^{99m}Tc scan may show a contracted liver with massive splenomegaly.

Treatment. The site of obstruction must be determined. If only the splenic vein is involved, splenectomy is curative. In cases in which the portal vein is extensively involved or in which intrahepatic obstruction is present, splenectomy will correct pancytopenia but will not relieve portal hypertension. On the other hand, because generalized bleeding or infection rarely results from thrombocytopenia or neutropenia, these hematologic findings do not mandate splenectomy. Portacaval anastomosis, which in general is preferred to splenorenal shunting in the young child, is indicated when portal hypertension is clearly shown or when repeated episodes of life-threatening hemorrhage have occurred. Successful relief of portal hypertension may result in decrease in splenic size and improvement of pancytopenia. It may also result in metabolic complications, especially hyperammonemia.

14.77 ANOMALIES AND TRAUMA

Splenic Cysts. Cysts of the spleen are of 2 general types: Epidermoid cysts are lined with stratified columnar epithelium. Pseudocysts, which are presumably of post-traumatic or postinfarction origin, have no epithelial lining and are filled with necrotic material and blood. Diagnosis is suggested by an asymptomatic smooth mass in the left upper quadrant which displaces the stomach medially. Isotopic scans with ^{99m}Tc gelatin colloid clearly indicate that the cystic mass is within the substance of the spleen. Ultrasonographic techniques and computed tomography (CT scan) effectively demonstrate splenic cysts.

Accessory Spleens. Multiple and accessory spleens are not uncommon. Of a group of 1413 children subjected to splenectomy, 229 (16%) had 1 or more accessory spleens (145 had only 1; 10 had 5 or more). Accessory spleens are usually located close to the hilum or adjacent to the tail of the pancreas. A congenital syndrome of polysplenism is characterized by left-sided visceral isomerism and congenital heart disease. Affected children have a high rate of intrahepatic biliary atresia.

Congenital Absence of the Spleen. Absence of the spleen occurs as part of an unusual group of anomalies, including complex abnormalities of the heart and great vessels with severe cyanotic congenital heart disease. Apparent dextrocardia and varying degrees of heterotopia of the abdominal viscera are seen (Ivemark syndrome). The condition can be suspected from examination of the blood: target cells, increased numbers of spherocytes, intraerythrocytic inclusions such as Howell-Jolly and Heinz bodies, and hemosiderin granules are easily demonstrated. The incidence of overwhelming sepsis is increased in congenital asplenia.

Hypersplenism. Hypersplenism is not a specific diagnosis but rather a descriptive term for a clinical complex which includes (1) depression of 1 or more of the cellular elements of the blood; (2) active formation of that element in the bone marrow; (3) an enlarged spleen, which may be due to a large number of causes (Table 14-9); and (4) correction of the hematologic abnormalities by splenectomy. A diagnosis of primary hypersplenism is difficult to establish; other causes of splenomegaly with secondary pancytopenia must be excluded.

Functional Hyposplenia. Occasionally, anatomically enlarged spleens may be devoid of reticuloendothelial system (RES) activity. This has been most clearly demonstrated in infants and young children with sickle cell anemia. In the great majority of these children, after 6–18 mo of age ^{99m}Tc scans fail to demonstrate RES activity of the anatomically enlarged organ. Howell-Jolly and Heinz bodies are seen in the blood. Young children with sickle cell anemia are 600 times more likely to develop pneumococcal meningitis and sepsis than their normal peers, and this propensity to infection is, in part, due to defective splenic function. Functional hyposplenia can be temporarily reversed with transfusion of normal red blood cells; after years, autoinfarction ultimately reduces the spleen to a siderofibrotic nubbin.

Rupture of the Spleen. Traumatic injury of the spleen may result from a hard, direct blow to the left flank or left side of the abdomen, such as may occur during automobile accidents or contact sports. If the tear in the splenic capsule is small, the symptoms may be moderate and include left upper quadrant or left shoulder pain and signs of peritoneal irritation due to blood. In more extreme cases shock may develop rapidly. When the spleen is pathologically enlarged, rupture may occur after relatively minor trauma. This occurs in the newborn infant with hemolytic disease and in the older child with infectious mononucleosis. Radionuclide and CT scanning are valuable in demonstrating lacerations and hematomas of the spleen.

Laparotomy and splenectomy are indicated when rupture leads to severe intra-abdominal bleeding and hypotension, but it has become increasingly evident that splenectomy is not always mandatory for splenic laceration. In the child, bleeding from the lacerated splenic surface often stops spontaneously. If the child's vital signs are stable or controlled with relatively small amounts of blood transfusion (<25 ml/kg) during the 1st 48 hr after splenic injury, nonoperative management may be safely attempted. This observational period requires a surgeon in attendance who can act rapidly if deterioration occurs. Several scans of spleen are needed to show that the splenic lesion is not expanding. The child should be watched carefully in the hospital for 10–14 days and maintained on restricted activities for several mo. Late rupture or splenic pseudocysts have not been observed; scans have shown complete healing of the lesion.

Nonoperative management is not indicated if other abdominal organs are damaged or if the patient develops severe shock. If laparotomy is necessary, it may be possible to repair the damaged spleen or to leave some splenic tissue in situ (see below).

Splenosis. Heterotopic autotransplantations of splenic tissue onto the surface of the peritoneum, with its subsequent growth, occur frequently after splenic injury requiring splenectomy. Changes in the circulating red blood cells (Howell-Jolly bodies, membrane craters) are not found in affected patients. 99mTc spleen scans show extrahepatic uptake of the radionuclide by small masses of recurrent splenic tissue. This regenerated splenic tissue may be to some degree protective against severe bacterial infections. The degree of protection may vary, however, with the amount of splenic tissue and its arterial blood supply; death from overwhelming infection has been observed in patients with splenosis.

14.78 SPLENECTOMY

Removal of the spleen is a common operation performed for a variety of indications. Primary surgical indications include (1) rupture of the spleen; (2) removal of tumors, cysts, or vascular anomalies involving the spleen; (3) need for adequate surgical exposure of the left upper portion of the abdomen; (4) certain shunting procedures; (5) relief of mechanical distress due to massive enlargement in thalassemia major or Gaucher disease; and (6) need for staging procedures for Hodgkin disease and other lymphoreticular malignancies (Sec 15.6 and 15.7).

Hematologic indications include (1) congenital hemolytic states, such as hereditary spherocytosis and elliptocytosis, and some cases of nonspherocytic ane-

mias, such as pyruvate kinase deficiency; (2) autoimmune hemolytic anemia when chronic and refractory to corticosteroid therapy; (3) chronic idiopathic thrombocytopenic purpura (ITP); and (4) hypersplenism.

Overwhelming Sepsis Following Splenectomy. Removal of the spleen alters host resistance, and overwhelming and often fatal meningitis and septicemia are seen with increased frequency in asplenic persons. The consequences and risks vary with the reasons for which splenectomy was done and especially with the age of the patient.

The risk of overwhelming sepsis is low (0.5–1%) when splenectomy is done for traumatic rupture, hereditary spherocytosis, or idiopathic thrombocytopenic purpura. A higher incidence of infection is seen when the indication is thalassemia major, histiocytosis, or lipidosis. The risk is high when there is an underlying disease which in itself has a predisposition to infection, such as the Wiskott-Aldrich syndrome. The risk is higher in all categories for younger infants and children. Sepsis has occurred at all ages and regardless of the indication for splenectomy or the interval after the operation. Severe infections after splenectomy, usually meningitis and septicemia, are characterized by an acute and fulminating course, death frequently occurring within 12–24 hr after onset of symptoms. In more than 60% of cases, pneumococci are the responsible agents; Hemophilus influenzae and meningococci are responsible for a smaller number of infections. Because of this risk, splenectomy should be performed only for clear indications, and when possible the operation should be deferred until after 5–6 yr of age or even longer if the condition of the patient is well compensated. Prophylactic use of penicillin has been advocated for the young child after splenectomy, and many centers use this routinely. There are no data adequately assessing the effectiveness of such management.

Immunization with polyvalent capsular polysaccharide antigens of pneumococci, H. influenzae, and meningococci should reduce the frequency of postsplenectomy infection but is generally ineffective before 18–24 mo.

In any case, patients whose spleens have been removed should know that splenectomy carries a risk of development at any time of a life-threatening infection, and that any febrile illness calls for immediate medical evaluation.

Crosby WH: Normal functions of the spleen relative to red-blood cells; a review. Blood 14:399, 1959.
Eraklis AJ, Feller RM: Splenectomy in childhood: A review of 1413 cases. J Pediatr Surg 7:382, 1972.
Likhite VV: Immunological impairment and susceptibility to infection after splenectomy. JAMA 236:1376, 1976.
Medical Letter: Prevention of serious infections after splenectomy. Med Let 19:2, 1977.
Pearson HA: The born again spleen. N Engl J Med 298:1373, 1978.
Pearson HA: Splenectomy, its risk and role, Hosp Pract Aug 1980, p 85.
Pearson HA, Spencer RP, Touloukian R: The binary spleen: A radioisotopic scan sign of splenic pseudocyst. J Pediatr 77:216, 1970.
Pearson HA, Spencer RP, Cornelius E: Functional asplenia in sickle cell anemia. N Engl J Med 281:923, 1969.
Sherman R: Perspective in management of trauma to the spleen. J Trauma 20:1, 1980.
Singer DB: Post-splenectomy sepsis. Perspect Pediatr Pathol 1:3, 1973.

14.79 THE LYMPHATIC SYSTEM

The lymphatic system includes the free lymphocytes of the blood and lymph as well as such organized lymphatic structures as lymph nodes, spleen, Peyer patches, appendix, and tonsils. The origin of lymphocytes is uncertain; some are believed to originate or be modified in the embryonic thymus, from which their progenitors migrate to populate other lymphatic tissues. Others may arise from such tissues as the lymphoid areas of the gastrointestinal tract, tonsillar area, or appendix.

The lymph vessels start as small capillaries between the cells of all organs except the brain and the heart. Small lymphatic capillaries join to form progressively larger channels which drain the extremities, trunk, and head. The largest of the lymphatic vessels is the thoracic duct, which discharges most of the central return of body lymph into the left subclavian vein.

The lymph channels are characteristically interrupted by lymph nodes. These well defined structures are networks of dilated sinusoids lined by reticuloendothelial elements and surrounded by masses of actively proliferating lymphocytes. The lymph nodes are located in groups, through which the lymphatic drainage of well defined anatomic areas passes. Because of their locations and structure the lymph nodes function as protective barriers to the spread of infections. They also filter particulate antigens, and the lymphocytes and plasma cells within lymph nodes actively participate in antibody formation.

The superficial lymph nodes are evaluated by palpation. Small nodes can normally be felt in the neck, axillae, and groin. Roentgenograms of the chest assess enlargement of the mediastinal lymph nodes. Lymphangiography permits evaluation of the size and structure of the pelvic and retroperitoneal lymph nodes.

The lymph is a clear fluid. It has a protein content intermediate between that of interstitial fluid and plasma and contains a substantial number of small lymphocytes.

14.80 DISEASES OF THE LYMPH VESSELS

Acute Lymphangitis. This is an inflammation of the lymphatics draining an area of acute infection, usually bacterial. It is manifested as red painful streaks radiating proximally from the infected site. Painful swelling of the regional nodes is also usually present.

Lymphedema. Lymphedema is a diffuse, permanent, pitting edema due to obstruction of the lymph drainage of an area, usually an extremity. Congenital lymphedema occurs in Milroy disease and as part of the syndrome of gonadal dysgenesis. Acquired lymphedema may result from inflammatory processes or from surgical or radiologic obliteration of lymph nodes or lymph channels.

14.81 DISEASES OF THE LYMPH NODES

Enlargement of the lymph nodes occurs in response to a wide variety of infectious, inflammatory, and neoplastic processes. Enlargement of a single node or group of nodes is most frequently due to an infection in the area it drains. Generalized lymphadenopathy occurs in many acute infections, especially rubella, rubeola, typhoid, tularemia, and infectious mononucleosis. Leukemia, lymphoma, and reticuloendotheliosis are sometimes accompanied by striking degrees of lymph node enlargement. Malignant tumors such as neuroblastoma sometimes metastasize to lymph nodes, and large numbers of lipid-bearing histiocytes may be present in the lymph nodes of Gaucher disease and other lipidoses.

14.82 ACUTE LYMPHADENITIS

As a result of cellulitis or other infections, bacteria and toxins and other byproducts of acute inflammation are carried in the lymph to regional lymph nodes where an acute inflammatory process occurs. Bacteria may cause abscess formation. Acute cervical adenitis secondary to acute pharyngitis and inguinal lymphadenopathy resulting from infections of the lower extremity are common. The involved nodes become swollen and painful, and the overlying skin is hot and red. Although the primary infectious process is usually obvious, the site of inoculation may not be apparent, as in cat-scratch disease. Mediastinal lymphadenitis secondary to pulmonary infections may produce obstructive symptoms and cough. Mesenteric lymphadenopathy may, on occasion, be associated with crampy abdominal pain simulating appendicitis.

Treatment. Antibiotic therapy which is appropriate for the primary infection will benefit the lymphadenitis. When suppuration occurs, needle aspiration or surgical drainage is necessary.

14.83 CHRONIC LYMPHADENITIS

Chronic infection or inflammation is frequently associated with hyperplasia of the lymph nodes. Tuberculous infections regularly result in regional lymphadenopathy. Scrofula, or chronic cervical lymphadenopathy, may be secondary to infection of the nasopharynx with bovine tuberculosis. This organism is uncommon in the United States, where chronic lymphadenopathy is more often due to infection by atypical acid-fast organisms. The organisms are trapped in the nodes, where granuloma and caseous necrosis occur. Affected nodes are hard, nontender, and frequently matted to adjacent tissues. Biopsy may be necessary to differentiate chronic infections from malignant processes.

HOWARD A. PEARSON

NEOPLASMS AND NEOPLASM-LIKE LESIONS 15

15.1 GENERAL CONSIDERATIONS

In the United States cancer causes more deaths than any other disease of children between the ages of 1–15 yr. The Third National Cancer Survey found the annual incidence rates for all malignant tumors in children under 15 yr of age to be 124.5/million Whites and 97.8/million Blacks. The rates for malignant neoplasms of the more commonly involved tissues are shown in Table 15–1. Rates differ not only for white and black children but also for various countries and ethnic groups. Wilms, tumor has a fairly stable rate and, therefore, provides a standard for comparison among different populations. Differences in incidence rates may provide important clues to factors involved in the etiology of childhood cancer. For example, the different rates for bone tumors in white and black children reflect the rare occurrence of Ewing sarcoma in Blacks in the United States. Ewing sarcoma is also rare among African Blacks; there may, therefore, be a genetically determined resistance to development of this form of bone cancer. On the other hand, Burkitt lymphoma, which is more frequent among black children in some parts of Africa, is not seen with increased frequency in black children in the United States. This observed difference would seem, therefore, most likely related to differing environmental exposures.

Little is known about the causes of cancer in children. Accordingly, the possibilities for prevention, which are a major concern of those who care for children, are limited. Efforts continue toward expanding our knowledge of the causes of childhood cancer.

Host Factors. Several conditions are associated with an increased risk of cancer during childhood. Four general classes of conditions have been identified: (1) Patients with such diseases as ataxia-telangiectasia and xeroderma pigmentosum, which are characterized by defects in repair of DNA, have an increased susceptibility to radiation. (2) Immunodeficiency states predispose to the development of lymphoma. (3) Specific congenital anomalies may carry with them an increased risk for certain tumors; e.g., children with aniridia or hemihypertrophy have a predisposition to the development of Wilms tumor or hepatoma. (4) Chromosomal abnormalities also may carry an increased risk of malignancy; the best known instance is the relationship of Down syndrome to the development of leukemia; another is the association of deletion of the long arm of chromosome 13 with the development of retinoblastoma. Some of the recognized associations between clinical conditions and increased risk of cancer in childhood are listed in Table 15–2.

Table 15–1 OCCURRENCE OF MALIGNANT NEOPLASMS IN CHILDREN UNDER 15 YEARS OF AGE (UNITED STATES DATA*)

NEOPLASM	RATE (PER MILLION/YEAR) White	Black
Leukemia	42.1	24.3
Central nervous system	23.9	23.9
Lymphoma	13.2	13.9
Sympathetic nervous system	9.6	7.0
Kidney tumor	7.8	7.8
Bone tumor	5.6	4.8
Soft tissue sarcoma	8.4	3.9
Retinoblastoma	3.4	3.0
Gonadal and germ cell	2.2	2.6
Liver tumor	1.9	0.4

*Results of The Third National Cancer Survey, modified from Young TL, Jr, Miller RW: J Pediatr 86:254, 1975.

Table 15–2 CONDITIONS ASSOCIATED WITH AN INCREASED RISK OF MALIGNANT NEOPLASIA DURING CHILDHOOD

CONDITION	ASSOCIATED NEOPLASM
Congenital anomalies	
Hemihypertrophy	Wilms tumor, hepatoma, adrenocortical carcinoma
Sporadic aniridia	Wilms tumor
Renal dysplasia	Wilms tumor
Visceral cytomegaly syndrome (Beckwith-Wiedemann syndrome)	Wilms tumor, hepatoma, adrenocortical carcinoma
Gonadal dysgenesis	Gonadal cancer
DNA repair defects	
Xeroderma pigmentosum	Skin cancer
Ataxia-telangiectasia	Lymphoma, leukemia
Immunodeficiency states	
Congenital X-linked immunodeficiency	Lymphoma, leukemia
Severe combined immunodeficiency	Lymphoma, leukemia
IgM deficiency	Lymphoma
Wiskott-Aldrich syndrome	Lymphoma
Chromosomal Anomalies	
Down syndrome	Leukemia
Klinefelter syndrome	Breast cancer
Fanconi anemia	Leukemia, hepatoma
Bloom syndrome	Leukemia
13q – syndrome	Retinoblastoma
Miscellaneous genetic diseases	
Neurofibromatosis	Fibrosarcoma, schwannoma, pheochromocytoma
von Hippel–Lindau syndrome	Pheochromocytoma
Multiple endocrine adenomatosis I (Wermer syndrome)	Schwannoma
Multiple endocrine adenomatosis II (Sipple syndrome)	Thyroid carcinoma, pheochromocytoma
Familial polyposis	Carcinoma of the colon

Preventive measures can be taken only in the instances of defects in repair of DNA, in which cases all efforts should be made to avoid the specific radiation to which the patient is vulnerable.

Some specific tumors are genetically determined; others occur sporadically. More than 160 traits now known or suspected to be hereditary are associated with benign or malignant neoplasia. Observations of the characteristics of sporadic and genetically determined tumors have led to a hypothesis that malignant transformation of a cell occurs by a 2-step process. For example, about half of the offspring of surviving patients with the heritable form of retinoblastoma will also have the disease, which is usually bilateral and multicentric in origin. In this form of the tumor the clinical evidence of disease appears early after birth. In patients with the sporadic form of retinoblastoma the time of appearance is later, and the tumors are unilateral. It is therefore postulated that in the genetically determined tumor a prezygotic mutation has involved all target cells. A single 2nd mutation is sufficient in any of this large number of susceptible cells to bring about malignant transformation, which is likely, therefore, to be multifocal and to have an early occurrence. In the patient who does not have the hereditary prezygotic defect both mutations must occur in the same cell before cancer can develop; in this case the tumors would be more likely unicentric and have longer latency to clinical appearance. Similar observations have been made in the case of Wilms tumor.

In some families there seems to be a predisposition to the development of cancer which is not always concordant as to the type of tumor. Soft tissue sarcomas may occur in children of families in which breast cancers are found in young women. Brain tumors and adrenocortical carcinomas have occurred among siblings in several families. For each child with cancer a careful family history should seek any possible indication of genetic predisposition.

Environmental Factors. Estimates have been made that from 60-90% of cancer in adults is caused by exposure to environmental carcinogens. Only a small proportion of childhood cancers are now known to be caused by environmental agents. Cancers in adults occur most frequently in organs which have exposed surfaces, such as skin, intestine, lung, and bladder, or are under endocrine regulation, such as breast and prostate. In children, by contrast, the predominant tumors are leukemia, brain tumors, lymphoma, neuroblastoma, Wilms tumor, and soft tissue sarcomas, none of which arise in organs exposed to the surface. Moreover, the peak incidences of lymphoblastic leukemia, Wilms tumor, neuroblastoma, liver cancer, and 2 of the brain tumors—ependymoma and medulloblastoma—are all found in children under 5 yr of age. These characteristics suggest that if environmental agents are instrumental in the development of cancer in childhood, the agents are likely to differ from those involved in cancer in adults. There also arises the suspicion that for some tumors exposure may be prenatal.

Oncogenic viruses have in the past received prime attention as possible inducers of cancer in children. Reports of "clusters" of childhood leukemia have suggested transmission of an infectious agent, but these have not been substantiated by careful epidemiologic studies. Attempts to identify viral particles or products within neoplastic cells have been unsuccessful. The strongest support for the involvement of a viral agent has been the consistent demonstration of serologic evidence of the Epstein-Barr virus in African children with Burkitt lymphoma.

Ionizing radiation is capable of inducing leukemia and some other forms of cancer in humans. Studies have implicated exposure in utero to diagnostic radiation in the development of leukemia but not of any other forms of childhood cancer. Irradiation to the mediastinal and cervical regions during infancy or early childhood is associated with an increased risk of thyroid cancer. Therapeutic radiation for 1 tumor can lead to a 2nd malignancy. This risk should be reduced by increasing knowledge about the optimal use of ionizing radiation in children.

Chemical and physical agents are also associated with the development of cancer. Intrauterine exposure to diethylstilbestrol carries an increased risk of clear cell adenocarcinoma of the vagina in the daughters of mothers given this drug for prevention of abortion. The period of fetal growth is presumed to be especially sensitive to teratogenic and carcinogenic agents. No chemicals other than diethylstilbestrol have so far been definitively identified as carcinogenic, but reports have indicated a possible relationship between in utero exposure to barbiturates and brain tumors and between the fetal hydantoin syndrome and neuroblastoma. Careful records must therefore be made of drugs given to mothers during pregnancy.

Treatment of aplastic anemia with anabolic androgenic steroids is associated with the development of hepatocellular carcinoma. Exposure to asbestos is linked to a rare tumor, mesothelioma. Children may be exposed to this agent if they live near asbestos mines or manufacturing plants or in the same households as asbestos workers.

With the increasing duration of survival for children with cancer, there is also an increasing incidence of 2nd malignant neoplasms. The cumulative risk for children cured of a 1st cancer to develop a 2nd neoplasm over a 25 yr period may be as high as 12%. In some instances, the 2nd malignant neoplasm occurs in a genetically predisposed host. In other instances, the irradiation or chemotherapy used for treating the primary tumor may play an etiologic role. There are now reports of malignancies occurring with increased frequency in patients treated for nonmalignant diseases with drugs also used for cancer chemotherapy.

The identification of additional environmental agents that cause cancer in children will require alert physicians and careful epidemiologic studies (Sec 4.3 and 28.16).

PRINCIPLES OF DIAGNOSIS

Although cancer is the leading cause of death among the diseases of childhood, it remains unusual for a general physician to have a child with cancer in his or her practice. Family physicians are estimated to encounter about 2 children with cancer during 40 yr in practice. Physicians must, therefore, be alert to the possible diagnosis of a rare but important disease. We have found the average delay in diagnosis of rhabdomyosarcoma of the head and neck to be 2 mo from onset of signs and symptoms. The diagnosis of cancer is too frequently avoided while treatment is pursued for more common conditions such as infections. Atypical courses of what appear to be common childhood conditions, prolonged and unexplained pain or fever, and unexplained and, especially, growing masses should initiate prompt and appropriate studies.

Delays in diagnosis are a particular problem in 3 clinical situations. Tumors of the nasopharynx or middle ear may mimic an infection. Therefore, prolonged unexplained ear pain, nasal discharge, retropharyngeal swelling, or trismus should be investigated as a possible malignancy. Cervical lymph node enlargement is common in children in response to upper respiratory tract infections. Cervical gland involvement is also common in children with Hodgkin and non-Hodgkin lymphoma. Hodgkin lymphoma is usually found in older children and adolescents at a time that enlarged cervical lymph nodes persisting for long times are unusual as a consequence of infection. Involved glands in non-Hodgkin lymphoma are characterized by progressive and usually painless enlargement. In either of these clinical situations, a diagnostic biopsy should be considered in the appropriate time. Finally, the bone tumors osteosarcoma and Ewing sarcoma usually occur during the 2nd decade of life, a time associated with physical activity. The cardinal symptom is the presence of localized and persistent pain which may be associated by the patient with an episode of trauma. Localized pain of greater severity and duration than can be accounted for by trauma should be investigated roentgenographically.

When a malignant neoplasm is suspected, the immediate goal is to determine its nature and extent. A tentative diagnosis can be obtained from an analysis of such clinical features as the presenting symptoms, location of the tumor, age of the child, and the location of metastases, if any. It is usually appropriate to complete the search for metastatic lesions before obtaining a biopsy for confirmation of the diagnosis. If the surgeon knows the likelihood of disseminated disease, he can exercise judgment in choosing between an attempt to complete resection and a more limited diagnostic biopsy. The studies appropriate for this preoperative review depend on the tentative diagnosis and will be discussed for each specific tumor. There are a large number of noninvasive techniques useful in the search for metastases. Their proper deployment depends on an understanding of the clinical course of each neoplasm.

At the time of diagnosis it is critical that the extent of disease be accurately defined; "staging" refers to this delineation. A system of staging must be designed for each tumor, depending on the experience that has been gained in relating the extent of disease at the time of diagnosis to the subsequent clinical course. Staging is necessary both for the design of a treatment regimen and for an assignment of prognosis. The extent of disease at diagnosis not only is related to the duration

of tumor growth but also reflects the biologic characteristics of a particular tumor, including proliferative activity and ability to metastasize.

In the United States staging systems designated by Roman numerals are in general use. Stage I describes a tumor which can be completely resected by the surgeon. Stage II usually indicates localized tumor which cannot be completely resected. Stages III and IV designate tumor which has extended beyond the site of origin or has become disseminated systemically. Specific staging systems will be described for each tumor type as appropriate. In Europe the predominant staging system classifies tumors by size, lymph node involvement, and presence of metastases: the TNM system (tumor, nodes, metastasis). Since it is more easily applied to carcinomas than to the sarcomas, which are the usual tumors of childhood, further experience will determine its applicability in pediatric oncology.

At the core of initial diagnostic studies is the determination of the histologic character of any tumor. The initial specimen of tumor tissue should be obtained under conditions that allow for the full range of pathologic studies which may be necessary to identify the tumor accurately.

The surgeon must search carefully at biopsy, excision, or exploration for evidences of regional dissemination to lymph node groups or to adjacent organs. If an attempt is made to remove the whole tumor or the organ containing the tumor, the pathologist will need to examine carefully the margins of resection to make sure that no microscopic residual tumor remains. The planning for subsequent treatment of the patient rests on this cornerstone of initial diagnostic studies, which must be done by physicians experienced in the care of children with cancer.

PRINCIPLES OF TREATMENT

Treatment of the child with cancer has 2 aspects: the *specific* and the *supportive*. For specific therapy the physician can offer surgical removal, irradiation, and chemotherapy. The majority of tumors in childhood have spread beyond the site of origin at the time of diagnosis and are not, therefore, amenable to complete surgical removal or to destruction by local irradiation. In most children with cancer a combination of these 3 modalities of therapy is necessary. The goal of all forms of treatment is the same: to remove or destroy all or as much tumor as possible with the least damage to normal cells.

Drugs for treatment of cancer are selected from several classes of agents, including hormones, antimetabolites, antibiotics, plant alkaloids, and the radiomimetic group of nitrogen mustard compounds. Initial studies in systems of cell culture select agents with apparent antitumor activity. The effects of active agents are then studied in animals for their efficacy in suppressing tumor growth and for toxicity. The few agents of promise are then studied in humans. The initial clinical (Phase I) studies are carried out in volunteer patients who have cancer no longer responsive to available treatment methods. The starting doses of a new drug to be tested are small, the dose increasing to the point of tolerance as the study progresses. The drug is then studied (Phase II) in patients with a wide variety of tumors to determine its range of effectiveness. For those tumors found to be responsive to the drug, further trials are designed (Phase III) in which the agent is incorporated into schedules with other active drugs and the new regimens compared for effectiveness. During each phase pharmacologic studies are made of drug action. Treatment regimens rarely involve single drugs; it is necessary, therefore, to evaluate a new agent in combination with other drugs. In design of specific treatment regimens the goal is complete control of the tumor.

Supportive measures are necessary for complications both of the disease and of therapy, which include problems of nutrition, bone marrow suppression, immunosuppression, and predisposition to infection. All chemotherapeutic regimens are capable of producing bone marrow suppression. Tumors which invade and replace the bone marrow can also result in pancytopenia. Anemia can be corrected by blood transfusions of packed red blood cells. Thrombocytopenia can be corrected by platelet infusions. Granulocytopenia poses a great risk of serious bacterial infections, particularly when the levels are less than $500/mm^3$. Febrile granulocytopenic patients must be carefully examined for clinical evidences of bacterial infections and appropriate cultures obtained. Upon clinical suspicion of a bacterial infection, treatment should be given with penicillinase-resistant forms of penicillin and with aminoglycosides in order to cover both gram-positive and gram-negative organisms. For the patient in whom granulocytopenia will be prolonged, transfusions of granulocytes may control infection until bone marrow recovery occurs.

Immunosuppression of variable degree is a consequence of some tumors and of some treatment regimens. Ordinary viral infections can become inordinately severe and prolonged, and viruses normally of low pathogenicity can produce serious disease. Patients receiving chemotherapy should not be given vaccines containing live virus. Fungal infections are common, particularly with *Candida*; such opportunistic organisms as *Pneumocystis carinii* can produce fatal disease. If severe degrees of immunosuppression are anticipated, prophylactic treatment against pneumonitis due to *Pneumocystis carinii* should be given with a combination of trimethoprim and sulfamethoxazole.

It is not uncommon for patients undergoing cancer therapy to lose 10% or more of body weight. Malnutrition in patients with cancer adds to immunosuppression. Special problems may arise with irradiation of the head and neck areas since a resulting mucositis may lead to marked difficulty in eating and swallowing. The dietitian can help patient and parents to design meals appropriate for maintenance of good nutrition. For some patients parenteral alimentation will be necessary to prevent severe weight loss during periods of intensive therapy.

A foremost consideration should be psychologic support for patient and family. An honest examination of the facts is the best policy in dealing with both parents and child. In practice the child should be told all that can be usefully understood. One of the major concerns of any patient is the unknown, and much anxiety can be alleviated if the expected clinical course and possible consequences of the disease and its therapy can be defined. Special problems, such as the need for amputation of a limb or of loss of hair during chemotherapy, must be anticipated and fully discussed, with ample opportunity for questions from patient and family.

Parents and child will need help in expressing feelings of anxiety, depression, guilt, and anger. These same feelings are shared by siblings, and parents must be helped to understand the needs of other children in the family. Since more than half of the children with cancer will achieve cures, it is important to maintain schooling to the best degree possible during the period of treatment (Sec 2.64 and 2.81).

Cancer drugs in common use with their major modes of action and important toxic side effects are listed in Table 15-3.

PROGNOSIS

The prognosis varies with the type of tumor and the extent of dissemination at diagnosis. For some types of tumor, prognosis depends heavily on histologic features as well as on some other biologic characteristics. For example, Hodgkin lymphoma can be divided into 4 histologic types in accordance with the cellular components and the amount of fibrosis. Each type has some specific clinical features as well as a different prognosis. For non-Hodgkin lymphoma, specific membrane surface markers indicating either T or B lymphocyte relationships are associated with special clinical features and differing responses to therapy. Prognosis in some tumors has an important relationship to age at diagnosis. This relationship, however, is not a consistent one. The prognosis in neuroblastoma is better under 1 yr of age. However, infants with acute leukemia under the age of 1 yr have a worse prognosis. The site of origin may influence expected prognosis. Rhabdomyosarcoma of the orbit or the genitourinary tract is associated with a better prognosis than the same tumor arising elsewhere.

Prognosis is also influenced by the promptness of diagnosis and treatment. The earlier the diagnosis, the more likely the tumor is to be caught at a time of least extension. The outcome of treatment for a cancer also depends to some degree upon the immunologic status of the patient. Deficiencies in cellular immune responses, as measured by skin tests and in vitro stimulation of lymphocytes, carry a tendency toward poor responses to therapy. Such observations, while statistically valid, are not sufficiently consistent to be applied to individual patients. Prognosis for most tumors is also greatly influenced by adequate treatment through a carefully designed program of surgery, radiotherapy, and/or chemotherapy.

DELAYED OR LATE CONSEQUENCES OF THERAPY

Late consequences of therapy may modify the expected long survival following successful treatment of cancer or result in serious morbidity. Successful surgical removal of a tumor may require the sacrifice of important functional structures. Following amputation of a leg for bone tumor, for example, careful attention must

Table 15-3 CANCER CHEMOTHERAPEUTIC AGENTS

DRUG	MAJOR MODE OF ACTION	IMPORTANT TOXICITIES
Methotrexate	Inhibits tetrahydrofolate synthesis	Marrow suppression, mucosal and gut ulceration, liver damage, leuko-encephalopathy
5-Fluorouracil	Inhibits thymidine synthetase	Marrow suppression, mucosal and gut ulceration
6-Mercaptopurine	Inhibits purine biosynthesis	Marrow suppression, mucosal and gut ulceration, liver damage
Cytosine arabinoside	Inhibits initiation of DNA synthesis and DNA polymerase	Marrow suppression, mucosal and gut ulceration, liver damage
Alkylating agents (nitrogen mustard, cyclophosphamide, phenylalanine mustard, chlorambucil and the nitrosureas)	Alkylation of DNA and RNA	Marrow suppression, immunosuppression, hemorrhagic cystitis (cyclophosphamide)
Procarbazine	Inhibits DNA and RNA synthesis	Marrow suppression, mucosal and gut ulceration, CNS toxicity
Bleomycin	DNA strand scission	Pulmonary fibrosis
Actinomycin D	Inhibits DNA-dependent RNA synthesis	Marrow depression, mucosal and gut ulceration, radiosensitization
Anthracyclines (doxorubicin, daunomycin)	Complex with DNA	Marrow suppression, radiosensitization, myocardial damage, mucosal and gut ulceration
Plant alkaloids (vincristine and vinblastine)	Microtubule disruption with metaphase block	Marrow suppression, paresthesias, loss of deep tendon reflexes, paresis, abdominal and jaw pain, constipation, inappropriate ADH secretion
Asparaginase	Induces asparagine deficiency, inhibits protein synthesis	Chills, fever, anaphylactic reactions, liver dysfunction, pancreatitis, hyperglycemia, immunosuppression
Epipodophyllotoxins (VM-26, VP-16)	Premitotic cell cycle delay	Myelosuppression, vomiting, fever, chills, hypotension

be given to rehabilitation with a functional prosthesis. Irradiation may produce irreversible damage to organs. The symptoms and degree of limitation will depend on the organ involved and the severity of injury. Irradiation of the lung may cause reduced pulmonary function. Irradiation of endocrine organs can cause abnormalities, e.g., hypothyroidism and sterility following thyroid and gonadal irradiation, respectively.

Chemotherapy also carries the risk of irreversible damage to organs depending upon the organ, the agent, the dose, and the duration of exposure. Agents such as actinomycin D and doxorubicin (Adriamycin) will have their toxicities potentiated by concomitant radiation.

THE LEUKEMIAS

The leukemias are the most common form of childhood cancer; they account for about one third of an estimated 7000 new cases of childhood cancer each year in the United States. The same kinds of leukemia are found in children and in adults except for chronic lymphocytic leukemia, of which only a few cases have been reported in children. The acute lymphocytic leukemias account for 76% of the total, with the acute nonlymphocytic leukemias and chronic myelocytic leukemias accounting for the remaining 21 and 3%, respectively. Chronic myelocytic and chronic lymphocytic leukemias are more common in adults.

Leukemia occurs in 42.1/million white and in 24.3/million black children/yr. The difference is ac-

counted for primarily by the lower frequency with which acute lymphocytic leukemia is seen in black children. The acute lymphocytic leukemia of childhood was the first form of disseminated cancer to respond completely to chemotherapy; it is, therefore, an important model around which concepts of chemotherapy for other malignancies have been developed.

A current classification for childhood leukemia is shown in Table 15–4. Subtypes of acute lymphocytic leukemia vary considerably with respect to clinical features and response to therapy; their classification in Table 15–4 is based on the characteristics of surface markers of the lymphoblasts.

Table 15–4 CLASSIFICATION OF CHILDHOOD LEUKEMIAS

TYPE	FAB* MORPHOLOGY
Acute lymphocytic leukemia (ALL)	
Common	L1, 2
T cell	L1, 2
B cell	L3
Nondifferentiated	L1, 2
Acute nonlymphocytic leukemia (ANLL)	
Myeloblastic, no maturation	M1
Myeloblastic with some maturation	M2
Hypergranular promyelocytic	M3
Myelomonocytic	M4
Monocytic	M5
Erythroleukemia	M6
Chronic myelocyctic leukemia	
Adult form	
Juvenile form	
Familial form	

*French-American-British.

The general clinical features of the leukemias are similar since all involve a severe disruption of bone marrow function. Specific clinical and laboratory features differ, however, and there are considerable differences in their responses to therapy and their prognoses.

15.2 ACUTE LYMPHOCYTIC LEUKEMIA (ALL)

The common ALL accounts for about 60% of leukemia in children and has a peak incidence at 3–4 yr of age. ALL occurs slightly more frequently in boys than in girls. Several reports of clusters of acute leukemia in children have suggested some common environmental factor, such as an infectious agent or chemical carcinogen, but careful statistical analyses have not supported this possibility.

Pathology. A bone marrow smear from a patient with ALL is illustrated in Fig 15–1. The variability of the cytologic appearance is so great, even within a single patient, that no completely satisfactory system has yet been devised for differentiation of the different forms of ALL by cytologic appearance alone. A French, American, and British FAB working group has devised a classification based on the appearance of bone marrow leukemic cells at diagnosis (SAB system). Three cytologic types are identified and called L-1, 2, and 3. L-1 lymphoblasts are predominantly small with little cytoplasm; in L-2 morphology more of the cells are larger and have greater amounts of cytoplasm, irregular nuclear membranes, and more prominent nucleoli. L-3 morphology with characteristic cytoplasmic vacuolization is uncommon and associated with blast cells having surface immunoglobulin. The distribution of the FAB subtypes in ALL is shown in Table 15–4.

Cytochemical characteristics which identify ALL blast cells are absence of peroxidase-positive and Sudan B black–positive granules in the cytoplasm and the frequent appearance of clumps of periodic acid–

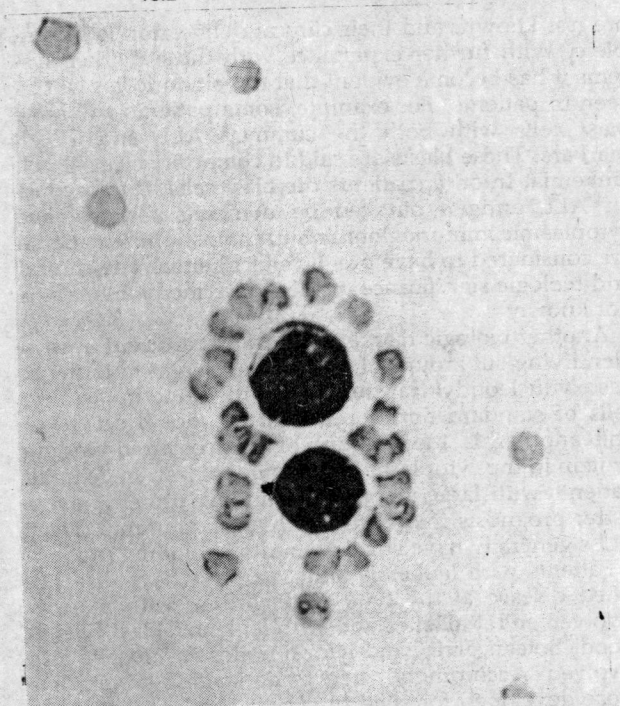

Figure 15–2 Lymphoblasts of a patient with acute lymphocytic leukemia showing rosette formation with sheep erythrocytes. These rosettes are stable at 4° and 37° C, as is characteristic of thymic lymphocytes. (From Mauer AM: Compr Ther 4:58, 1978.)

Schiff–positive material. The lymphoblasts also have a negative nonspecific esterase reaction.

The most useful classification of subtypes of ALL depends on cell membrane markers, of which 5 are of value. Four of the 5 markers indicate that the normal lymphocyte is the cell line of origin for the leukemic cell. The 1st marker identified with a specific subtype of ALL is the formation of rosettes with sheep erythrocytes which are stable at 4° and 37° C (Fig 15–2). This characteristic is found in T cell ALL and in lymphocytes derived from normal thymus. The T cell lymphoblast can also be identified by an antiserum which reacts with a thymus cell antigen other than the sheep erythrocyte receptor. T cell antisera will identify about twice as many T cell ALLs as will rosette formation with sheep erythrocytes. T cell ALLs comprise about 25% of patients with ALL.

Leukemic cells of B lymphocyte origin can be identified by immunofluorescent techniques which identify cell surface immunoglobulins. B cell ALLs comprise no more than 5% of the total.

The common ALL is characterized by cells which lack T and B cell markers; these leukemic lymphoblasts react with an antiserum directed specifically against them. They react also with a B cell antibody, which reacts as well with myeloblasts and monocytes. The nature of the antigen involved in this reaction is not known. This form of ALL accounts for about 75% of cases of ALL.

A small group of patients whose cells do not react with any of the above techniques are said to have nondifferentiated leukemias. Their cell lines of origin

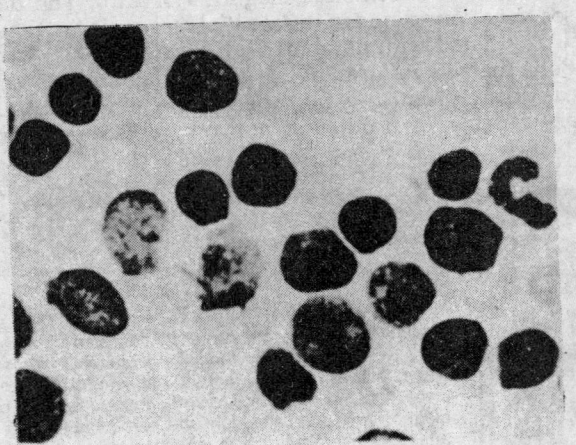

Figure 15–1 Bone marrow of a patient with acute lymphocytic leukemia. Virtually all normal marrow elements are replaced by a fairly uniform population of small cells with dense nuclei. These cells have minimal cytoplasm, and the nuclear chromatin pattern tends to be coarse and clumped. The membrane of the nucleus, where visible, is well defined.

are not known, and their clinical delineation is incomplete. With further experience with these marker systems it has become evident that transition forms can be seen in patients. For example, some patients will have blast cells with both the common ALL and T cell markers. These blasts are said to characterize pre–T cell leukemia. In other patients the blast cells have become an ALL antigen but can be demonstrated to have cytoplasmic immunoglobulin mu chains. These patients are considered to have pre–B cell leukemia. The clinical and biologic significance of these intermediate forms is not known.

Another biologic marker with potential usefulness in identifying subgroups of ALL is the increased terminal desoxynucleotidyl transferase activity found in the blast cells of standard and T cell ALL but not B cell ALL. Still another is the amount of corticosteroid-binding protein in the cytoplasm of the lymphoblast. In general, patients with large amounts of binding protein have a better prognosis than those with small amounts. T cell ALLs generally have small amounts of binding protein.

Patients with leukemia almost always have disseminated disease at the time of diagnosis, with marrow involvement at all sites and with leukemic blast cells in blood. Spleen, liver, and lymph nodes are usually also involved. Accordingly, there is no staging system like those developed for solid tumors. There are, however, clinical and laboratory features which predict the behavior of leukemia.

Clinical Manifestations. Children with ALL have a fairly consistent presentation. About two thirds will have had signs and symptoms of their disease for less than 6 wk at the time of diagnosis. The 1st symptoms are usually nonspecific; there may be a history of a viral respiratory infection or exanthem from which the child has not appeared fully to recover. Frequent early manifestations are anorexia, irritability, and lethargy. Progressive failure of normal bone marrow function leads to pallor, bleeding, and fever, which are usually the features that precipitate diagnostic studies.

On initial examination most of the patients are pale, and about 50% have petechiae or mucous membrane bleeding. About 25% have fever, which can sometimes be ascribed to a specific cause such as another respiratory tract infection. Lymphadenopathy is occasionally prominent, and splenomegaly (usually less than 6 cm

below the costal margin) can be demonstrated in about two thirds of patients. Hepatomegaly is less common and generally minimal. About one third of patients have bone tenderness due to periosteal invasion and subperiosteal hemorrhage. Bone pain and arthralgia are infrequently the major complaints leading to the diagnosis of ALL.

Sometimes signs of increasing intracranial pressure such as headache and vomiting may indicate leukemic meningeal involvement. Children with T cell leukemia are more likely to have significant lymphadenopathy and hepatosplenomegaly and initial leukemic infiltration of the central nervous system.

Diagnosis. Usually, the diagnosis of ALL is easily made on the finding of leukemic lymphoblasts in the blood smear. On initial examination most patients will have anemia; in only 25% will this be severe, with hemoglobin levels less than 6 gm/dl. Most patients will also have thrombocytopenia, though 25% may have platelet counts greater than 100,000/mm³. About 50% of children with ALL will have leukocyte counts under 3000/mm³; about 20% will have counts greater than 50,000/mm³.

The definitive study is an examination of bone marrow, which in almost all patients will be found to be completely replaced by leukemic lymphoblasts. Occasionally, patients in whom an aspirated specimen is hypocellular will require needle biopsy of the bone marrow to demonstrate the leukemic replacement.

A chest roentgenogram should be made to determine if there is a mediastinal mass, as is frequently the case in patients with T cell ALL (Fig 15–3). Bone roentgenograms may show altered medullary trabeculae, cortical defects, or subepiphyseal bone resorption, but these findings have no clinical or prognostic significance. Cerebrospinal fluid should be examined for leukemic cells since early central nervous system involvement has important prognostic implications.

Differential Diagnosis. History, physical examination, and studies of blood and bone marrow almost always permit a definitive diagnosis of ALL. The diseases to be considered in differential diagnosis are those also associated with bone marrow failure.

Bone marrow infiltration by other malignant cells can occasionally produce pancytopenia. In children the tumors capable of producing marrow replacement are

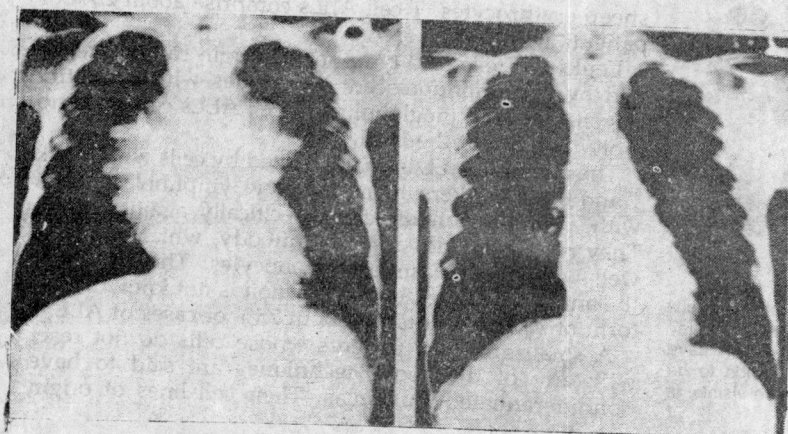

Figure 15–3 The chest roentgenograms of a patient with acute lymphocytic leukemia, whose lymphoblasts formed rosettes with sheep erythrocytes. On the left is the roentgenogram at time of diagnosis, and on the right the same patient after attaining a remission with induction chemotherapy. (From Mauer AM: Compr Ther 4:58, 1978.)

neuroblastoma, rhabdomyosarcoma, and retinoblastoma. Usually these cells are found in clumps scattered throughout normal marrow tissue, but occasionally there may be complete replacement of marrow. In such patients there is usually evidence of a primary tumor in some other site and of considerable destructive bone involvement on roentgenograms.

The bone marrow failure of ALL needs to be distinguished from the nonmalignant marrow failure associated with aplastic anemia. Patients with ALL who have marked leukopenia sometimes have no blast cells evident either on a blood smear or in aspirated marrow, the hypocellular marrow resembling that of aplastic anemia. An adequate bone marrow biopsy will distinguish marrow infiltration with leukemic cells from the marrow failure of aplastic anemia.

Infectious mononucleosis should only rarely be confused with ALL, though the former may present immature lymphocytes in the blood smear of a patient with fever, lymphadenopathy, hepatosplenomegaly, and the clinical findings associated with thrombocytopenia or anemia. There should be no difficulty, however, in identifying the cells in a blood smear as typical of infectious mononucleosis. If doubt should remain, a bone marrow aspirate will demonstrate a normal cell population.

Treatment. The treatment of ALL varies with the clinical risk features. A standard risk patient at diagnosis has a white blood count under 100,000/mm³, a normal mediastinum on chest roentgenogram, no evidence of leukemic central nervous system involvement, and blast cells which do not have B- or T-cell features. The basic components of treatment programs for standard risk ALL include an initial regimen for induction of remission, a 2nd phase of treatment of the central nervous system, where the initial regimen may not clear residual leukemic cells, and a final phase of continuation or maintenance therapy (Table 15–5).

A combination of prednisone, vincristine, and another agent such as daunomycin or L-asparaginase can be expected to produce a remission in about 95% of children with *standard risk ALL*. The addition of the 3rd agent to prednisone and vincristine does not improve the initial remission rate, but there is evidence that it prolongs the remission. For almost all patients a remission is achieved within 4 wk. For the residual 5–10% of patients who have not achieved remission by that time,

about two thirds can achieve a remission with additional therapy.

The central nervous system is the site of initial relapse in more than 50% of the patients who have not received some kind of treatment to that area. Evidence indicates that leukemic cells are present in the meninges at the time of diagnosis and that their survival is due to the lower drug concentrations achieved in the cerebrospinal fluid. The therapeutic invasion of this sanctuary area is achieved through irradiation of the cranium and intrathecal administration of methotrexate given over a 2.5 wk period (Table 15–5). Other forms of prophylaxis have been proposed, such as periodic intrathecal injections of methotrexate or attempts to achieve high drug levels in cerebrospinal fluid by giving large doses intravenously.

If no further treatment is given after induction of a remission, bone marrow relapse soon occurs, even if the regimen producing the induction was intensive. Continuation therapy is essential, therefore, to reduce the population of leukemic cells to minimal levels or to effect its eradication. The regimen shown in Table 15–5 for continuation therapy is effective for disease control and carries a minimal level of harmful side effects. The drugs used for treatment of leukemia have both short- and long-range complications. In most centers continuation treatment is stopped after 2.5–5 yr of continuous complete remission as there is no evidence that further therapy raises the proportion of patients achieving long-term disease-free control.

The treatment of patients with *T cell ALL* is at present unsatisfactory. A regimen similar to that for standard risk ALL will often achieve an initial remission; and prophylactic therapy to the central nervous system effectively prevents recurrence of the disease in that area. Most patients with T cell ALL will, however, relapse in bone marrow and blood during the period of continuation therapy after a median interval of about 1 yr. Various forms of intensification of treatment to such patients are under study but have not yet improved these results. The tumor cells seem to acquire drug resistance during the period of continuation therapy. Remission can be induced in some of these patients following their initial relapse, but the subsequent period of relief tends to be relatively brief. The few patients with L-3 morphology and surface immunoglobulin positive blast cells are best treated according to regimens designed for B-cell non-Hodgkin lymphoma.

In both standard and high-risk patients there are 2 important extramedullary areas of relapse. These are the central nervous system (CNS) and the testes. The common early manifestations of CNS leukemia are those of increasing intracranial pressure. Vomiting and headache (especially in the mornings), papilledema, and lethargy occur with progressive severity. Convulsions and nuchal rigidity are usually among the later manifestations, which may also include paresis of the 6th cranial nerve with diplopia and strabismus. Hypothalamic involvement is rare, but it must be suspected if excessive weight gain, behavioral disturbances, or hirsutism occurs. In most treatment centers periodic examination of the cerebrospinal fluid is routine. Accordingly, CNS involvement is often detected before

---

Table 15–5 EFFECTIVE TREATMENT REGIMENS FOR ACUTE LYMPHOBLASTIC LEUKEMIA (ALL)

Remission induction for 1 mo.
 Prednisone: 40 mg/M²/day orally for 28 days
 Vincristine: 1.5 mg/M²/wk intravenously for 4 wk
 Daunomycin: 25 mg/M²/wk intravenously for 4 wk
Central nervous system prophylaxis (beginning at 4 wk if remission is achieved)
 ⁶⁰Co cranial irradiation: for 2.5 wk
  Total dose: 1800 rads
 Intrathecal methotrexate: 12 mg/M² twice weekly for 2.5 wk
  during cranial irradiation: single dose limited to 15 mg
Continuation therapy for 30 mo
 6-Mercaptopurine: 50 mg/M²/24 hr, orally
 Methotrexate: 20 mg/M²/wk, intravenously

clinical signs appear. In almost all patients with leukemia involving the CNS, spinal fluid pressure is elevated; 85% of patients have a pleocytosis of the spinal fluid due to leukemic cells. When the cell count is not increased, leukemic cells may be found in the smears of spinal fluid specimens after centrifugation.

If CNS relapse occurs after preventive CNS therapy and during the initial hematologic remission, the patient should be given methotrexate intrathecally in a dose of ½ mg/M² (no more than 15 mg/injection) weekly for 4–6 wk. After at least 2 clear spinal fluid specimens have been obtained, the same dose of methotrexate is given monthly. If leukemic pleocytosis persists after the administration of methotrexate, then weekly intrathecal administrations of cytosine arabinoside (60 mg/M²) can be given for 6–12 wk. The development of active leukemic cell proliferation within the CNS is assumed to carry a risk of systemic spread of these cells. Accordingly, concurrent systemic chemotherapy with prednisone (40 mg/M² daily for 14 days) and vincristine (1.5 mg/M² weekly for 3 doses) is given routinely.

Preventive CNS therapy must be instituted for all patients in whom relapses have been found in bone marrow; the regimen uses intrathecal methotrexate and cytosine arabinoside. The cranial irradiation is not repeated.

Testicular relapse may be the 1st manifestation of leukemia in an extramedullary site, either during continuation therapy or after treatment has been discontinued. The clinical findings are painless swelling of 1 or both firm and nontender testes. Even if only 1 testis appears involved, biopsy must be made of both to look for leukemic cell infiltration; the apparently uninvolved testis will sometimes show early proliferation. Treatment for testicular involvement is irradiation with 2000 rads to the involved gonad. If the testes are the sole site of leukemic cell activity, then concurrent systemic chemotherapy must be given as described above for CNS involvement.

Prognosis. A number of clinical features have been identified as having prognostic importance for patients with ALL. Their significance was established for the most part before the recognition of the subtypes of ALL, and they are not as valuable as identification of the specific subtype. In general, a poor prognosis is associated with onset at an age under 2 yr or over 10 yr, with a white blood count greater than 100,000/mm³ at the time of diagnosis, with the presence of a mediastinal mass, with early involvement of the CNS, and with leukemia in a black patient. In all of these situations bone marrow relapse is likely to occur during the period of continuation therapy with an inability to achieve subsequent further long-term remission.

The identification of the specific subtypes of ALL permits clearer definition of prognostic categories. Common ALL has the most favorable prognosis, and it may be that with current therapy most affected patients can achieve long-term disease-free control. No more than a few of the patients with T cell ALL can expect long-term control; with current regimens the median duration of remission is only 1 yr. The few patients with B cell ALL have a response to therapy even less favorable than that of patients with T cell ALL. Experience with

nondifferentiated cell ALL is too meager to permit prognostic judgments. The FAB classification also permits some prognostic predictions. Those patients with L-1 morphology have a better prognosis as a group than do patients with L-2 morphology. Patients with L-3 morphology have the poor prognostic characteristics of B-cell leukemias and non-Hodgkin lymphomas.

There is now sufficient experience with patients having common ALL who have achieved long-term disease-free intervals after cessation of therapy to indicate that with current regimens a patient who has been in continuous complete remission for 6 yr or more has a very small likelihood of later relapse.

15.3 ACUTE NONLYMPHOCYTIC LEUKEMIA (ANLL)

This form of leukemia accounts for about 20% of all cases in children. It occurs with about the same frequency at all ages of childhood and equally in boys and girls. ANLL characteristically occurs in such predisposing conditions as Fanconi anemia and Bloom syndrome in which there is excessive chromosomal breakage.

Pathology. The several subgroups of ANLL are indicated in Table 15–4. They are distinguished on the basis of characteristic cytomorphology in Wright-stained smears of blood and bone marrow. The degree to which the predominant cell resembles a normal cell of bone marrow provides the designation of type. The most common form has a leukemic cell population resembling the myeloblast or the myelomonoblast. The proportion of admixture of cell types resembling myeloblasts or monoblasts makes the distinction between these 2 forms, which account for 90% of all ANLL. Although there are cytologic differences, the clinical presentations and responses to therapy are similar for these subgroups with 1 exception: when the predominant cell resembles a promyelocyte, there is a significant risk that bleeding symptoms will arise from disseminated intravascular coagulation during the course of an early response to therapy. This cytologic subtype occurs in about 5% of all ANLL patients.

Clinical Manifestations. The duration of symptoms and signs before the diagnosis is made in these patients is usually brief, 50% of the patients having less than 6 wk of illness. In a few patients, however, the history of symptoms or signs may indicate a probable onset up to 12 mo before definitive presentation; in such patients the usual complaints are fatigue and recurrent infections. The mounting symptoms or signs during the 2 wk immediately before diagnosis are likely to include pallor, fever, active bleeding, bone pain, gastrointestinal distress, or severe infection. It is not possible to distinguish between ALL and ANLL on the basis of prediagnostic findings. A finding relatively specific for ANLL is gingival swelling due to leukemic cell infiltration.

The initial physical findings do not differ greatly from those in ALL. The liver and spleen are enlarged in 60% of patients, but marked hepatosplenomegaly occurs in only 10–15%. In 20% there may be marked lymphadenopathy. A few patients may initially have joint pain mimicking arthritis, with a localized tumor mass (chloroma) that may produce such findings as proptosis or with neurologic manifestations of CNS leukemia.

Diagnosis. The variability of initial leukocyte and platelet counts is similar to that in patients with ALL. Initial hemoglobin levels can range from markedly decreased to normal, most patients having levels from 5–10 gm/dl. The suspected diagnosis is confirmed by examination of the blood smear and bone marrow. In patients in whom the cytology is consistent with acute promyelocytic leukemia, coagulation studies must be done at the time of diagnosis to detect any acceleration of intravascular coagulation and to provide baseline values for evaluation of the subsequent clinical course.

The same considerations for differential diagnosis of ALL apply to ANLL. Additionally, there may be megaloblastic features in the bone marrow in ANLL which may superficially mimic those of folic acid or vitamin B_{12} deficiency. The experienced cytologist can easily distinguish ANLL by the more striking defects in maturation, the greater degree of atypical morphology, and the greater proportion of blast cells seen in this disease.

Sometimes children with ANLL have a long antecedent period of progressive marrow failure. In this early phase the proportion of blast cells may be so small that the diagnosis of leukemia cannot be confirmed. Sometimes the diagnosis can be facilitated by the demonstration that these are clones of bone marrow cells having aneuploid karyotypes. In these patients the course of progressive marrow failure may be hastened rather than reversed by chemotherapy; accordingly, a period of observation is the best current management, there being no indication that early treatment is of any demonstrable benefit.

In most cases, standard Wright- or Giemsa-stained blood and bone marrow smears are adequate to differentiate between the 2 characteristic types of blast cells (see Fig 15–1 and 15–4). The cells in ANLL are usually positive for peroxidase and Sudan B black stains; and when their cytoplasm is positive for the periodic acid–Schiff stain, the reaction is diffuse rather than aggregated or clumped as in ALL. In monoblastic leukemia the cytoplasm will be positive with the nonspecific esterase stain. Even with all of these aids there are, occasionally, patients in whom the leukemic cells are so undifferentiated as to leave doubt about their specific cell line of origin. In most treatment centers these patients are treated for ALL because of the better prognosis expected with current therapy.

Treatment. There is currently no satisfactory treatment for patients with ANLL. Various combinations of drugs, including cytosine arabinoside, daunomycin, vincristine, 6-azauridine, 6-thioguanine, and 6-mercaptopurine, may induce remission in about 75% of these patients. The most effective regimens include cytosine arabinoside and daunomycin. As in ALL, the central nervous system can be a site of initial relapse in ANLL. The frequency of CNS relapse as the initial sign of reactivation of disease can be reduced by prophylaxis; however, because early blood and bone marrow relapse is so common, the prevention of CNS disease does not currently prolong survival for these patients.

For maintenance therapy several regimens are pro-

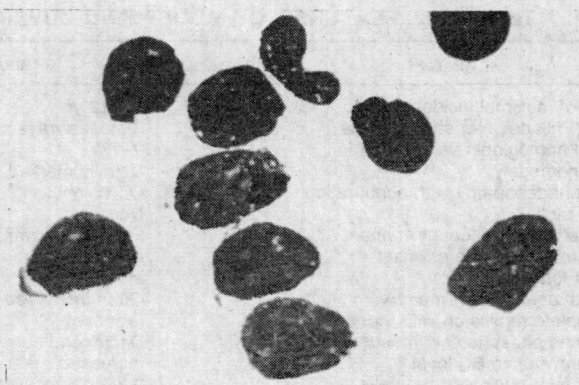

Figure 15–4 Bone marrow of a patient with acute nonlymphocytic leukemia. There are few normal marrow elements and virtually no differentiation of the leukemic myeloblasts. There tends to be more cytoplasm and a greater degree of nuclear irregularity than in leukemic lymphoblasts. Nucleoli are frequently seen and tend to be large and irregular. The nuclear chromatin pattern is fine and well dispersed. The nuclear membrane, where seen, is fine. Sometimes cytoplasmic granules representing a degree of differentiation are seen as well as rodlike structures called Auer bodies.

posed which may prolong a complete remission. None is as yet clearly superior. Some treatment regimens of nonspecific immunotherapy have used BCG, with or without allogeneic leukemic cells. As yet such immunotherapy has had neither adverse effects nor any clearly demonstrated benefits. The use of bone marrow transplantation in patients for whom suitable donors are available is currently under study.

In patients with acute promyelocytic leukemia, a regimen using cytosine arabinoside, daunomycin, and heparin during initial induction of remission has successfully managed the tendency to disseminated intravascular coagulation and bleeding. In some such patients long periods of disease-free survival may be achieved.

Prognosis. The prognosis for patients with ANLL has been so uniformly poor that it is difficult to discern specific prognostic signs. The initial cytologic appearance is not helpful in predicting outcome except for those patients with acute promyelocytic leukemia. Initial white blood cell counts under 10,000/mm³ at the time of diagnosis are favorable, as are platelet counts greater than 10,000/mm³. With current therapy regimens the median duration of remissions achieved has been from 1.5–2 yr. Fewer than 30% of patients achieve long-term continuous complete remissions; only rarely have patients achieved 5 yr of such remission.

15.4 CHRONIC MYELOCYTIC LEUKEMIA (CML)

This form of leukemia accounts for only 3% of cases in children. There are 2 basic types of chronic myelocytic leukemia. They share only the general characteristic of increased numbers of differentiating myeloid cells in the blood. In the adult form the pathognomonic Ph¹

Table 15–6 FEATURES OF ADULT AND JUVENILE TYPES OF CHRONIC MYELOCYTIC LEUKEMIA

FEATURE	ADULT TYPE	JUVENILE TYPE
Age of maximal incidence	10–12 yr	1–2 yr
Ph¹ (Philadelphia) chromosome	Almost always present	Never present
Fetal hemoglobin values	2–7%	30–70%
Splenomegaly	Usually marked	Mild to moderate
Lymphadenopathy with suppuration	Occasional	Frequent
Skin rash	None	Frequent eczematous rash of face
White blood cell count at onset	Frequently over 100,000/mm³	Rarely over 100,000/mm³
Thrombocytopenia at onset	Uncommon	Usually present
Blast forms in blood	Infrequent	Often present
Megakaryocytes in marrow	Often increased	Usually decreased
Complete remission with therapy	Frequent	Rare
Alkaline phosphatase in neutrophils	Decreased	Decreased or lower limit of normal
Serum vitamin B_{12} level	Increased	Increased
Maximum nucleated red cells	0.25–0.5 ($\times 10^3$/min³)	1–18 ($\times 10^3$/mm³)
Monocytes in blood	Normal to increased	Increased

(Philadelphia) chromosome is consistently found. In the juvenile form, leukemic cells may have variable chromosomal aneuploidy, but the Ph¹ chromosome is never found. The adult form of CML is usually found in older children but has occasionally been reported in infants; accordingly, any patient with CML must have a chromosomal analysis to determine the specific form. The clinical features differentiating these 2 forms are shown in Table 15–6.

CHRONIC MYELOCYTIC LEUKEMIA, ADULT TYPE

The onset of symptoms is generally insidious. The diagnosis may not be suspected until hepatosplenomegaly is found on a routine examination. Laboratory abnormalities are usually confined initially to the white blood cell count; anemia is minimal or absent, and the platelet counts are usually normal or increased at diagnosis. The white blood cell count is usually greater than 100,000/mm³, with all forms of myeloid cells being seen in the blood smear. There are no characteristic morphologic abnormalities of the cells, but eosinophilia and basophilia are present and may be striking. The bone marrow is hypercellular and presents normal myeloid cells in all stages of differentiation. Other helpful laboratory findings are increased levels of serum vitamin B_{12} and marked decreases in leukocyte alkaline phosphatase activity.

Treatment for this disease is busulfan given in doses of 4 mg/M² daily until the white blood cell count falls below 10,000/mm³; it can be resumed when the white blood cell count again rises to 15,000/mm³ or more. With this therapy reduction in hepatosplenomegaly and control of the disease can usually be maintained for months or even years.

The terminal phase of this disease is characterized by a gradual increase in the number of myeloblasts in the blood (blast crisis) and by the development of anemia and thrombocytopenia. With the onset of a blast crisis, the treatment program is changed to that for ANLL. In some of the patients in blast crisis the predominant cells resemble lymphoblasts, and some of these cells will have increased levels of terminal deoxynucleotidyl transferase. In such patients the usual form of therapy is an attempt at induction of remission with vincristine

and prednisone; some temporary remissions have been induced.

JUVENILE CHRONIC MYELOCYTIC LEUKEMIA

These patients usually have a history of an eczematoid rash, lymphadenopathy, and recurrent bacterial infections; accordingly, they may resemble patients with chronic granulomatous disease. By the time of diagnosis they have usually developed pallor, purpura, and moderate enlargement of both liver and spleen.

The consistent laboratory findings are anemia, thrombocytopenia, and an increased white blood cell count, usually about 50,000/mm³ with a range from 15,000 to almost 200,000/mm³. The blood smear is similar to that found in the adult form of CML and contains myeloid cells in all stages of differentiation. There may be a striking monocytosis, but eosinophilia and basophilia are not consistent findings. The bone marrow is usually cellular, with fewer megakaryocytes and erythroid cells than are found in the adult form of CML.

The leukocyte alkaline phosphatase may be either normal or reduced and is not a pathognomonic feature. The proportion of fetal hemoglobin ranges from 30–70%, and other characteristics of fetal erythropoiesis occur, such as fetal oxygen dissociation curves, hemoglobin A_2 level, antibodies against erythrocyte i antigen, and structure of the gamma chain.

Chemotherapy with either single or multiple agents is of limited or no value for inducing remission or prolonging survival. It may be possible to reduce the white blood cell count without significant improvement in hemoglobin or platelet levels.

During the course of juvenile CML the blast forms may increase, but there is no typical blast crisis as is seen in the adult form. There is progressive increase in organomegaly. Median survival is about 6 mo; a 2 yr survival is unusual. Death results from the complications of marrow failure.

FAMILIAL CHRONIC MYELOCYTIC LEUKEMIA

A small subgroup of patients with CML have a familial disease. The age of onset is 6 mo–4 yr and the clinical features are increasing lethargy, pallor, growth retardation, and massive hepatosplenomegaly. The blood findings are similar to those seen in the patients with juvenile CML. The leukocyte alkaline phosphatase levels are reduced; fetal hemoglobin levels may be increased or normal. The chromosome patterns in the leukemic cells are normal.

Patients with this condition have not responded to chemotherapy, but if there is evidence of accelerated blood cell removal, splenectomy can improve the anemia and thrombocytopenia. These patients are capable of long survival, and some eventually show spontaneous improvement. Their therapy should be supportive unless there are indications for splenectomy.

15.5 BONE MARROW TRANSPLANTATION AS THERAPY

Transplantation of bone marrow is recommended for patients with acute myeloblastic leukemia in 1st remission and acute lymphoblastic leukemia in a 2nd or subsequent remission. The results indicate that from 40–60% of patients may achieve long-term disease control. Transplantation in remission has considerably reduced deaths from infection in the immediate posttransplant period. However, a number of problems remain to be solved before bone marrow transplantation can be more widely applied as therapy for acute leukemia. Allogeneic marrow transplantation requires the availability of an HLA-matched sibling (Sec 9.58). As family size has tended to decrease, so has the proportion of patients for whom a match is available because there is only 1 chance in 4 that any sibling will be appropriate. Studies are under way to determine whether minor degrees of HLA mismatches or better immunosuppression will allow the use of donors other than HLA-matched siblings.

Although the risk of early death from infection has been decreased, the complications of graft versus host disease (Sec 9.19) and interstitial pneumonitis remain serious post-transplant problems which may be fatal. Improvements in the regimens preparing the patients for transplantation and the subsequent immunosuppressive treatment may decrease the incidence of these 2 complications.

Leukemic relapse is another problem limiting the proportion of patients achieving long-term disease control. Total body irradiation in association with various chemotherapy regimens is used to eradicate residual leukemic cells and to destroy the patient's immunocompetence and thus allow acceptance for the donor marrow engraftment. Patients with graft versus host disease have a lesser likelihood of relapse; therefore, paradoxically, reducing the incidence and severity of graft versus host disease may increase the likelihood of relapse.

The future of bone marrow transplantation as a therapeutic modality for acute leukemia is uncertain. With improved techniques marrow transplantation may have wider application as it becomes possible to use mismatched bone marrow. On the other hand, as chemotherapy regimens improve, treatment results may become better for patients at high risk for treatment failure than the results of bone marrow transplantation.

Johnson FL, et al: A comparison of marrow transplantation with chemotherapy for children with acute lymphoblastic leukemia in second or subsequent remission. N Engl J Med 305:845, 1981.

Thomas ED, et al: One hundred patients with acute leukemia treated by chemotherapy, total body irradiation and allogeneic marrow transplantation. Blood 49:511, 1977.

LYMPHOMA

Lymphoma is the third most common cancer in children in the United States; it affects 13.2/million children/yr. This rate is similar for white and black children. Two broad categories are recognized: Hodgkin disease and non-Hodgkin lymphoma. The clinical manifestations, treatment, and prognosis of each are so different from those of the other that they will be considered separately. Also see Sec 9.1 and 14.79 for related discussion of the lymphatic and immune systems.

15.6 HODGKIN DISEASE

Incidence. This tumor rarely occurs before the age of 5 yr. The rate thereafter increases steadily to a peak level at 15–34 yr of age. A 2nd peak occurs after the age of 50 yr. The bimodal frequency curve has suggested that there may be 2 forms of Hodgkin disease. The condition is almost twice as common in boys as in girls. No definitive causal factors are known, but reports of occurrence in marriage partners and among groups having close contact have suggested a virus of low virulence and infectivity. Hodgkin disease appears to have an increased frequency with the prolonged administration of hydantoin drugs known to produce lymphadenopathy.

Pathology. There are 4 histologic types of Hodgkin disease, each with special clinical features and implications for prognosis. The central histologic feature in all 4 types is the Reed-Sternberg cell, shown in Fig 15–5.

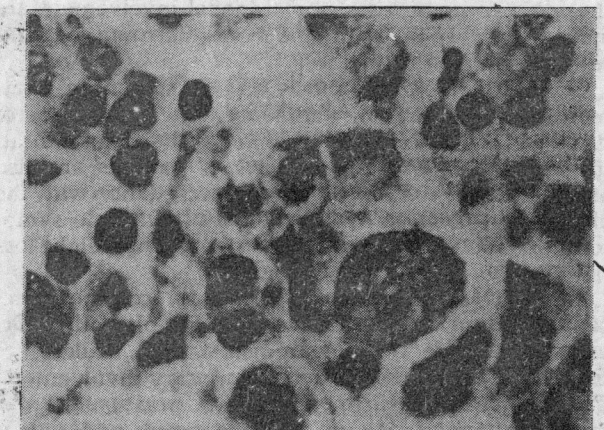

Figure 15–5 A Reed-Sternberg cell, which contains 2 nuclei, each with a prominent nucleolus and distinct nuclear membrane. The cytoplasm of this cell is relatively abundant. Other cells present are lymphocytes, plasma cells, and tissue mononuclear cells. This appearance in a lymph node is diagnostic of Hodgkin disease.

In the *lymphocyte predominant* variety almost all of the cells appear to be mature lymphocytes or a mixture of lymphocytes and benign histiocytes, with only occasional Reed-Sternberg cells. This type affects 10–20% of patients, and generally has the least dissemination at time of diagnosis, and has the best prognosis.

The next most favorable histologic type is the *nodular sclerosing* variety, which is the most common, affecting about 50% of patients. Broad bands of collagen divide the involved lymph node into nodular cellular areas. A special cytologic feature is clear spaces surrounding "lacunar cells," which are variants of the Reed-Sternberg cell. This form occurs more frequently in the mediastinum and to a lesser degree in the abdomen.

Hodgkin disease of *mixed cellularity*, the 2nd most common form, is characterized by accumulations of lymphocytes, plasma cells, eosinophils, histiocytes, malignant reticular cells, and Reed-Sternberg cells. Foci of necrosis may be present. This form is more likely to involve extranodal areas at the time of diagnosis and after further progression and has a less favorable prognosis.

The least common and least favorable form of the disease is the *lymphocyte depletion* variety, which affects fewer than 10% of patients. Numerous bizarre malignant reticular cells are found, with Reed-Sternberg cells and relatively few lymphocytes. There may also be varying degrees of partly hyalinized fibrosis with a paucity of cells, mostly of reticular and Reed-Sternberg types.

Hodgkin disease arises in lymph nodes in almost all instances. Extranodal primary sites occur in fewer than 1% of patients. The manner of spread of Hodgkin disease indicates that areas of involvement or extension are not random. Adjacent lymph node areas are found diseased in the majority of patients. With progression, the proximity of new areas of involvement to the initially involved nodes suggests that Hodgkin disease may arise in a single nodal focus and spread along adjacent lymphoid channels. These observations have provided the base for current treatment programs. When the disease is no longer confined to lymph nodes, the more common sites of extranodal involvement are spleen, liver, lung, bone and bone marrow, gastrointestinal tract, and skin.

For determining prognosis and for planning treatment, anatomic staging should be done at the time of diagnosis (Table 15–7). In addition to the stage indicating the anatomic extent of disease, patients are also assigned to an A or B category in accordance with the absence or presence, respectively, of systemic symptoms such as night sweats, fever, or recent weight loss of more than 10% of body weight.

Clinical Manifestations. The most common presenting finding is enlarged cervical lymph nodes. Occasionally, nodes of the supraclavicular, axillary, or inguinal areas may be the site of primary involvement. The enlargement is firm, nontender, and usually discrete, involving single or multiple lymph nodes. It is generally first noted by the patient or parents. Characteristically, no regional inflammation can be found to explain the lymphadenopathy. Mediastinal lymph node enlargement is common and may produce a cough,

Table 15–7   ANN ARBOR STAGING SYSTEM FOR HODGKIN DISEASE

STAGE I	Involvement of a single lymph node region or of a single extralymphatic organ or site
STAGE II	Involvement of 2 or more lymphoid regions on the same side of the diaphragm; or localized involvement of an extralymphatic organ or site and of 1 or more lymph node regions on the same side of the diaphragm
STAGE III	Involvement of lymph node regions on both sides of the diaphragm, which may be accompanied by localized involvement of an extralymphatic organ or site or by splenic involvement
STAGE IV	Diffuse or disseminated involvement of 1 or more extralymphatic organs or tissues, with or without associated lymph node enlargement

generally nonproductive, or symptoms of tracheal or bronchial compression; or it may be found on a roentgenogram of the chest taken for an unrelated purpose.

Usually, the patient initially has few, if any, systemic manifestations. Typical symptoms would be night sweats, unexplained fever, weight loss, lethargy, easy fatigability, and anorexia. Pruritus is an unusual early complaint; alone, it does not place the patient in a B category.

Extranodal involvement is unusual at the time of diagnosis but may occur with progression of the disease. Lung involvement is represented roentgenographically by diffuse fluffy exudates, difficult to distinguish from disseminated fungal infection (Fig 15–6); fever and tachypnea are usual, and pulmonary insufficiency may develop.

Liver involvement is associated early with signs of intrahepatic biliary obstructive disease, such as increased serum levels of direct and indirect bilirubin and serum alkaline phosphatase activity. With progression, signs of hepatocellular disease may develop. Bone marrow involvement may result in neutropenia, thrombocytopenia, and anemia. Infiltration of the gastrointestinal tract may produce ulceration and bleeding. Extradural tumor masses in the spinal canal can cause progressive cord compression. A variety of immune disorders may occur, such as immunohemolytic anemia, immunothrombocytopenia, or the nephrotic syndrome.

Cellular immunity is impaired in Hodgkin disease as a consequence both of the disease and of its treatment. Affected patients are at increased risk of the infections characteristic of immunosuppressed patients. Varicella-zoster infections occur in up to one third of the patients and may become disseminated, most frequently with involvement of the lungs and with a progressive pneumonia; fungal infections, such as cryptococcosis, histoplasmosis, and candidiasis, may also become disseminated.

When treatment produces neutropenia, these patients are also susceptible to severe bacterial infections. One of the most difficult diagnostic problems is the interpretation of the significance of fever in patients with Hodgkin disease. Careful consideration must be given to the full range of infectious diseases character-

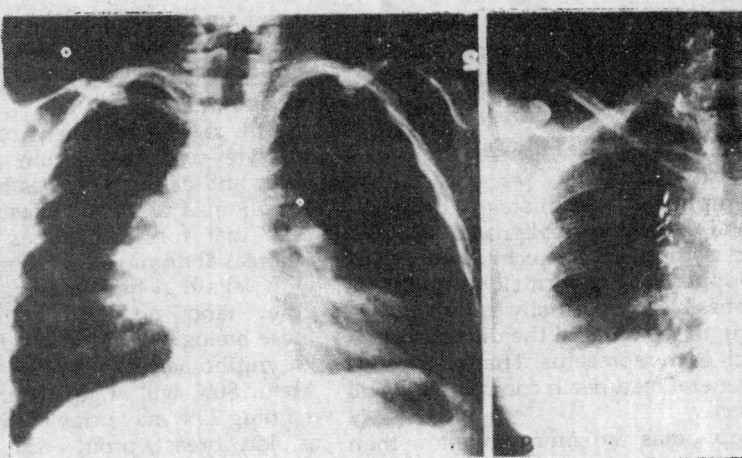

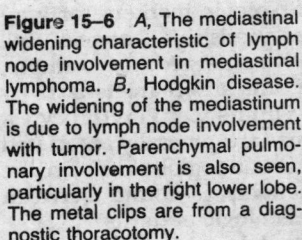

Figure 15–6 *A*, The mediastinal widening characteristic of lymph node involvement in mediastinal lymphoma. *B*, Hodgkin disease. The widening of the mediastinum is due to lymph node involvement with tumor. Parenchymal pulmonary involvement is also seen, particularly in the right lower lobe. The metal clips are from a diagnostic thoracotomy.

istic of immunosuppressed patients before fever is ascribed to the disease itself.

Diagnosis. Hodgkin disease should be suspected in the patient with persistent unexplained lymphadenopathy. The disease is more common in older children and adolescents, past the time when infectious cervical lymphadenopathy is common. If a careful history and physical examination find no evidence that an underlying inflammatory process is responsible for the enlarged nodes and if the lymphadenopathy is persistent, then a biopsy is warranted. Before biopsy of a cervical node, a chest roentgenogram should explore the possibility of mediastinal involvement. The blood counts are generally not helpful; characteristic changes in the white blood cell count include a neutrophilic leukocytosis, lymphopenia and sometimes eosinophilia, and monocytosis. Anemia and thrombopenia occur only in the patient with systemic manifestations and disseminated disease. The erythrocyte sedimentation rate may be increased, and in some patients the serum copper level is elevated, nonspecifically.

When the diagnosis is made, staging should be completed in order to establish the extent of disease. Most patients first present evidence of lymph node enlargement above the diaphragm. Liver function tests are unreliable indicators of hepatic disease, and the size of the spleen correlates poorly with splenic involvement. Lymphangiograms are generally accurate in indicating lymph node involvement below the level of the 2nd lumbar vertebra, but above that level involved lymph nodes may not be filled with the contrast material. Accordingly, for most patients a staging laparotomy is indicated to determine with certainty the presence or absence of infradiaphragmatic disease. At laparotomy the spleen is removed, a liver biopsy is obtained, and samples are taken of nodes from all accessible areas. Bone marrow biopsies are done at the same time to determine possible marrow involvement. In about one third of affected children the stage of disease assigned from clinical findings will be revised when the anatomic findings are known. The physician must determine before the laparotomy is done whether a possible change will affect the design of the treatment regimen for the patient. If so, then laparotomy is indicated; if not, the treatment should proceed without it.

Treatment. Both radiation therapy and chemotherapy are highly effective in the treatment of Hodgkin disease. Many patients have a good chance of long-term disease control or cure. Control of local disease can be obtained with radiotherapy in doses of 3500–4000 rads. Combination chemotherapy with vincristine, nitrogen mustard procarbazine, and prednisone can produce long periods free of disease for patients with advanced Hodgkin disease. Combining irradiation with chemotherapy will achieve long-term disease-free intervals in a greater proportion of patients. Questions still to be answered are whether combination chemotherapy should be used alone in patients with limited disease initially, what extent of irradiation field is optimal for limited disease, and what radiation dose is required in programs with combination chemotherapy. This knowledge is needed to determine the minimal necessary treatment plans that will be effective but reduce to a minimum the long-term complications of therapy.

Prognosis. With current treatment more than 90% of patients with Hodgkin disease initially achieve a complete clinical remission. The likelihood of prolonged remission or cure is related primarily to the stage at diagnosis. Most patients with disease in Stages I and II have remissions which last 5–10 yr. More than 50% of the patients with Stages III and IV disease also achieve 5 yr remissions.

The long survivals of these patients have created increasing concern about the complications of treatment. With the combination of radiation therapy and chemotherapy the complications depend on the site being irradiated. With irradiation of upper body node areas, there may be restriction of lung capacity, cardiac involvement, and late hypothyroidism. Esophageal stenosis and transverse myelitis are also reported. Irradiation of abdominal nodes may affect fertility in women. In the younger child growth of the vertebral column can be affected.

One–2% of patients who have had splenectomy as part of the staging laparotomy may develop the syndrome of overwhelming sepsis with *S. pneumoniae* or *H. influenzae*. They must be treated promptly with penicillin at the onset of any febrile episode. Pneumococcal vaccines may reduce the frequency of this complication. A 2nd malignancy, most frequently acute myeloblastic or lymphoblastic leukemia, may occur, usually 4–6 yr after the diagnosis of Hodgkin disease. The true risk of this development is unknown.

15.7   NON-HODGKIN LYMPHOMA

"Non-Hodgkin lymphoma" designates a heterogeneous group of solid lymphoid malignancies which have no definitive classification. As techniques evolve for identifying subpopulations of normal lymphocytes, it should become possible to reclassify non-Hodgkin lymphomas according to the stage in the differentiation of lymphocytes which each represents. These lymphoid malignancies have general features in common and will be discussed together.

Non-Hodgkin lymphomas are more common than Hodgkin disease, especially in the younger child. There is no characteristic age distribution; boys are more frequently affected than girls in a ratio of about 3:1. Both congenital and acquired immunodeficiencies predispose to their development. Children with infantile X-linked agammaglobulinemia or severe combined immunodeficiency have about a 5% incidence of malignancy, usually lymphoma. The risk for children with Wiskott-Aldrich syndrome and ataxia-telangiectasia is about 10%. The incidence of lymphomas is increased also in immunosuppressed patients after renal transplantation.

Pathology. The classification of the non-Hodgkin lymphomas is under continual revision. Table 15–8 provides a working classification developed by an international panel of experts. In addition to considering histology and architecture, it relates the appearance of the tumor to the clinical features by subdividing them into low, intermediate, and high grade lymphomas. About one third of children with non-Hodgkin lymphoma will have the diffuse large cell or large cell immunoblastic form, another third the lymphoblastic

Table 15–8 A WORKING FORMULATION OF NON-HODGKIN LYMPHOMAS FOR CLINICAL USE

Low Grade
Malignant lymphoma, small lymphocytic
Malignant lymphoma, follicular, predominantly small cleaved cell
Malignant lymphoma, follicular, mixed small cleaved and large cell

Intermediate Grade
Malignant lymphoma, follicular, predominantly large cell
Malignant lymphoma, diffuse, small cleaved cell
Malignant lymphoma, diffuse, mixed small and large cell
Malignant lymphoma, diffuse, large cell

High Grade
Malignant lymphoma, large cell, immunoblastic
Malignant lymphoma, lymphoblastic
Malignant lymphoma, small noncleaved cell

Miscellaneous
Composite malignant lymphoma
Mycosis fungoides
Extramedullary plasmacytoma
Unclassifiable
Other

form, and the remaining third the small noncleaved cell form which includes both Burkitt and non-Burkitt types. Any other form of non-Hodgkin lymphoma in children is most unusual.

With the development of biologic markers for lymphocyte subtypes certain relationships between cell types and clinical features have emerged: for example, lymphomas of the mediastinum are characterized by cells that form E-rosettes with sheep erythrocytes, whereas abdominal lymphomas are generally associated with cells that have surface immunoglobulins. On the other hand, no clear relationship is found between these biologic markers and histologic patterns.

Lymphoma may arise in nodal or extranodal areas. About 80% will arise within lymphatic tissue; the remaining 20% may originate in such extralymphatic sites as skin, breast, orbit, parotid, ovary, and bone. Lymphomas in the gastrointestinal tract arise from lymphatic structures within that system.

The spread of non-Hodgkin lymphoma is not orderly like that of Hodgkin disease; there is a tendency both for early hematogenous dissemination and for lymphatic spread. One fourth to one third of affected patients ultimately develop a leukemic transformation. Central nervous system involvement like that of acute lymphocytic leukemia also occurs in about one third of patients.

A staging system in common use for this disease is based on that developed for Hodgkin disease; the biologic characteristics of these 2 tumors are so dissimilar, however, that staging provides little useful information. Non-Hodgkin lymphoma is not commonly confined to a single node region or extranodal site at the time of diagnosis; accordingly, treatment plans for most patients must be designed for disseminated disease.

There is a form of lymphoma in American patients which resembles the Burkitt lymphoma of African children. Histologic criteria include a uniform population of undifferentiated cells with an abundance of mitotic figures, cells with discrete narrow rims of amphophilic cytoplasm, and round to oval nuclei with only slight irregularity of the nuclear membrane. The cells carry surface immunoglobulins and are derived from B lymphocytes, as in the African form of Burkitt lymphoma. Unlike the African form, however, the American lymphoma does not have the nearly universal association with the Epstein-Barr virus.

Clinical Manifestations. The clinical features of lymphoma depend upon the site of primary tumor and the extent of local and distant disease. The tumor commonly presents in the head and neck region as a painless, unexplained swelling of cervical or supraclavicular lymph nodes. The growth may be rapid, significant increases occurring within 1–2 wk. The nodes are generally nontender and firm, discrete in the early phases of growth, but often confluent later. Other areas of nodes, such as axilla or ileocecal region, may also be primary sites of tumor.

Lymphoma of the chest generally arises in the anterior mediastinum, and the presenting feature may be progressive dyspnea due to compression of trachea and bronchi. Obstruction of the superior vena cava may occur. Dyspnea may result also from a pleural effusion, which may contain lymphoma cells.

Abdominal lymphoma arises most frequently in the ileocecal region, possibly as an abdominal mass or with evidences of intestinal obstruction. Lymphoma of the bowel wall may serve as a lead point for intussusception.

Lymphoma of bone produces local or diffuse bone pain and usually represents dissemination from some other primary site.

Along with findings related to the local tumor, there may be manifestations of systemic dissemination. Central nervous system involvement may present signs of increased intracranial pressure and involvement of cranial nerves, especially of the 7th nerve. Bone marrow infiltration may result in anemia, thrombocytopenia, and neutropenia. Fever, weakness, fatigue, and weight loss may occur.

Diagnosis. The diagnosis is to be suspected in patients with painless enlargement of lymph nodes or with signs suggesting tumor in the anterior mediastinum or abdomen. Before biopsy of available tumor is done for definitive diagnosis, bone marrow, blood, and cerebrospinal fluid or pleural or ascitic fluid, when present, should be examined for tumor cells. Roentgenographic skeletal survey and radioisotopic bone scan may indicate localized areas of bone involvement. Whenever possible, a study of the cells for surface markers should be made in order to establish the type of lymphoma.

Treatment. After biopsy, surgery has no role except for the possible excision of localized lymphoma of bowel. Radiation therapy is effective in treatment of the few patients who have localized lymph node involvement. Almost all patients require chemotherapy because of the systemic nature of this tumor and its propensity for hematogenous dissemination. Most regimens involve the use of agents effective also against acute lymphoblastic leukemia, such as prednisone, cyclophosphamide, doxorubicin, vincristine, methotrexate, and 6-mercaptopurine, in varying combinations. When large anterior mediastinal masses compromise respiration, prompt irradiation and administration of prednisone are needed. A definitive role for irradiation in treatment of areas of bulky tumor in other sites is not established.

Lymphoma generally responds quite promptly to chemotherapy with rapid lysis of cells. Metabolic complications such as hyperuricemia, hyperphosphatemia, and hypocalcemia may occur. Therapy should include, therefore, the administration of allopurinol to reduce uric acid production, the maintenance of a large alkaline urine flow, and careful attention to electrolyte balance to avoid uric acid nephropathy.

Prognosis. With current treatment somewhat more than half of the children with lymphoma can expect long-term disease-free control. Mediastinal primary tumor and bulky abdominal lymphoma have the most unfavorable prognosis.

15.8 HISTIOCYTOSIS

See Sec 26.5.

A group of diseases characterized by a pathologic increase in cells of the monocyte/macrophage line have been traditionally referred to as histiocytoses or reticuloendothelioses. There are several clinically definable subgroups. Their nature is not known, nor are there precise methods by which they can be distinguished. Careful attention to the clinical features and histologic characteristics permits sufficient definition to guide treatment and determine prognosis.

Histiocytosis X

The term *histiocytosis* X or reticuloendothelioses encompasses 3 illnesses once thought to be distinct, but now believed to be expressions of the same fundamental pathologic process. These are *Hand-Schüller-Christian disease, Letterer-Siwe disease,* and *eosinophilic granuloma of bone.* They are discussed in Sec 26.5.

Other Histiocytoses

Familial Histiocytosis. A condition clinically and histologically identical to histiocytosis of the sporadic form has been reported in monozygotic twins and in nontwin siblings with both X-linked recessive and autosomal recessive patterns of inheritance. The relationship between familial and sporadic forms is unknown, and they are not clinically different.

Familial Histiocytic Dermatoarthritis. This familial condition is characterized by a papulonodular eruption, symmetric destructive arthritis, and ocular lesions, which are histologically histiocytic. It appears during childhood or adolescence, usually as cutaneous nodules around the head and in the hands and feet. Stiffness of the distal joints develops and, later, uveitis, cataracts, and glaucoma. Inheritance may follow an autosomal dominant pattern.

Hemophagocytic Reticulosis (Lymphohistiocytosis). This familial disease of the macrophage/monocyte system has distinctive clinical features. The pattern of inheritance is autosomal recessive, the usual age of onset is under 2 yr, and the condition is usually fatal within months. The onset is frequently acute, with a protracted illness associated with fever, anemia, leukopenia, thrombocytopenia, hepatosplenomegaly, pneumonitis, and meningitis. Initial diagnostic considerations almost always focus upon some forms of infection. As it proves impossible, however, to find a specific agent and as this severe illness fails to resolve, hemophagocytic reticulosis must be considered. If another child in the family has been involved, the diagnosis can be promptly established.

The characteristic pathologic finding is the infiltration of many organs by histiocytes and lymphocytes. Sites for biopsy must be selected with care because of the thrombocytopenia. A bone marrow aspirate may show the increased numbers of histiocytes and the erythrophagocytosis which are so characteristic of this condition. Limited experience suggests that such chemotherapeutic agents as vinblastine, prednisone, methotrexate, and cyclophosphamide may produce favorable responses.

Sinus Histiocytosis. In this benign form of histiocytosis the clinical manifestations are massive lymphadenopathy, particularly of the cervical region, fever, and moderate leukocytosis. Mediastinal lymph nodes may also be massively enlarged, but there is minimal, if any, enlargement of the liver and spleen. The characteristic histologic pattern in these lymph nodes involves dilatation of the subcapsular and medullary sinuses with benign-appearing macrophages frequently containing phagocytosed lymphocytes. This accumulation of macrophages may progress to total effacement of the lymph node architecture. In the bone marrow aspirate or biopsy also there will generally be an increased number of macrophages. Most patients have an onset in the 1st decade of life; the condition affects boys and girls equally.

The disease resembles an atypical inflammatory response, but no etiologic agent has been defined. Reversible alterations in cellular immunity have been reported, but the relationship of these to the fundamental process is unknown. The clinical course may run for months with gradual resolution of the lymphadenopathy. No therapy is indicated.

Histiocytosis in Congenital Rubella. In some patients congenital rubella is associated with dysgammaglobulinemia (increased IgM and decreased IgG and IgA) and with a severe histiocytic reaction replacing normal lymph node architecture with histiocytes. Affected patients have failure to thrive, hepatosplenomegaly, and lymphadenopathy. This form of histiocytosis may be the reaction to a persistent viral infection in the presence of altered immunity induced by the congenital infection.

MISCELLANEOUS CAUSES OF LYMPHADENOPATHY

Generalized lymphadenopathy and hepatosplenomegaly may occur with administration of *phenytoin* (Dilantin). The reaction may occur within weeks of beginning treatment. On biopsy the lymph nodes demonstrate lymphoid and macrophage hyperplasia with irregular hyperplasia of the follicles. Recovery follows discontinuance of the drug.

Benign giant lymphoid hyperplasia in the hilar nodes may be associated with hypergammaglobulinemia and alterations in cellular immunity. The affected individual may be entirely asymptomatic, even with massive hilar nodes demonstrated on chest roentgenogram. Numerous lymphoid structures with massive germinal centers are found in the nodes. The lymphoid follicles are surrounded by cuffs of small lymphocytes; there may be many plasma cells. Upon removal of the massive nodes the altered immune responses return to normal.

Benign *lymphoid hyperplasia of the colon* appears to be a variant response of lymphoid tissue to undetermined stimuli. It is most common in infants under the age of 2 yr and is often discovered when a roentgenographic examination is made of the colon because of rectal bleeding; the diagnostic feature is the uniform distribution of small, umbilicated, polypoid lesions over some or all of the colon and sometimes involving small intestine or stomach. When the condition involves the small intestine, it may be associated with hypogammaglobulinemia and with enlarged tonsils and spleen. This benign condition may be confused with familial polyposis.

Generalized lymphadenopathy and hepatosplenomegaly have been described in a small group of children, usually 1 mo–2 yr of age, with variable manifestations of thrombocytopenia and immunohemolytic anemia. The chronic course is associated with intermittent fever and apparent susceptibility to infections. There are variable alterations of immunoglobulins, and in some patients there may be evidence of chronic cytomegalovirus infection. The sizes of liver, spleen, and lymph nodes may vary considerably during the illness. A Coombs test–positive hemolytic anemia may be found. It is presumed that these children have an underlying immune deficiency state.

NEOPLASMS OF NERVOUS TISSUES

Tumors of the central nervous system are discussed in Sec 21.18. Tumors of the sympathetic nervous system arise from the primitive neural crest cells that form the adrenal medulla and sympathetic nervous system. In children these tumors are represented almost exclusively by neuroblastoma.

15.9   NEUROBLASTOMA

This tumor occurs at an annual rate of about 1/100,000 children under the age of 15 yr. It is slightly more common in white than black children. Lesions designated as neuroblastoma in situ have been found at autopsy with an incidence between 1 in 200 and 1 in 1000 in infants under 3 mo of age. These observations have suggested that neuroblastoma may be a relatively common tumor undergoing spontaneous involution in most infants; other studies indicate that neuroblastoma nodules are present in the adrenal gland during fetal development, with peak numbers and size found at 20 wk of gestational age. These nodules regress, and their presence in some infants in the early wk of life most likely represents the late stages of this involution rather than neoplasms in situ.

Neuroblastoma is a tumor of young children: 25% of patients have been identified by 1 yr of age, 40% by 2 yr of age, and 90% before the age of 10 yr. Male children are slightly more frequently affected than female, in a ratio of 1.2:1. There has been no association of neuroblastoma with congenital anomalies, but a few instances of familial neuroblastoma have been reported. In studies of the neuroblastoma tumor cells abnormalities of chromosome 1 have most frequently been found.

Pathology. There can be considerable variability in the degree of cell differentiation found in neuroblastoma. Most tumors consist of primitive neuroblastoma cells with little evidence of differentiation. In some tumors there are variable admixtures of cells with larger amounts of cytoplasm, cytoplasmic processes, rosettes with central fibrillar material, and mature ganglion cells (Fig 15–7). Electron microscopy reveals distinctive features, with peripheral dendritic processes containing longitudinally oriented microtubules and small, spher-

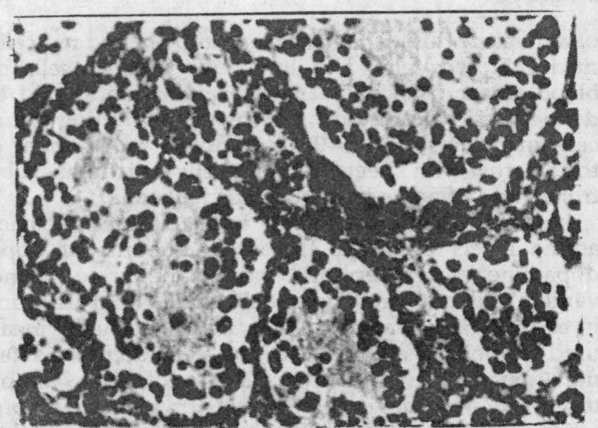

Figure 15–7 The diagnostic criteria of neuroblastoma: poorly formed compartments of cells with relatively uniform, round, dark nuclei, which surround an acellular, fibrillar central area.

ical, membrane-bound granules with electron-dense cores, which represent cytoplasmic accumulation of catecholamines. During the course of treatment serial biopsy specimens may contain increasing proportions of mature ganglion cells, and "maturation" of the tumor to a ganglioneuroma may take place at some sites.

This tumor may arise in any site where neural crest cells are present. About 50% of the tumors arise in the abdomen, about 25% in the adrenal gland. The thorax is the initial site in 15–20% of patients, less frequent sites being the cervical region, nares, liver, or an intracranial site. In some children the discovery of widely disseminated tumor makes definition of the initial site impossible.

Neuroblastoma may extend by local invasion of surrounding tissue or via the lymphatics to regional lymph nodes. There may also be hematogenous spread, most frequently with involvement of liver, bone marrow, and skeleton. Intracranial involvement of the dura can result in signs of increasing intracranial pressure.

The staging system in most general use is the following: Stage I indicates a tumor confined to the organ or structure of origin. Stage II designates tumor extending in continuity beyond the origin but not crossing the midline of the body. Stage III tumors have extended beyond the midline, and bilateral involvement of regional lymph nodes may be found. With Stage IV there is metastasis to remote areas. Some evidence suggests that a special designation (Stage IV-S) should be considered for patients who would otherwise have Stage I or II disease but who have remote involvement confined to liver, skin, or bone marrow. This special designation reflects the relatively good prognosis in this situation. Almost all of these patients are under the age of 6 mo. A new proposal for staging this tumor which is likely to become generally accepted in the coming years is shown in Table 15–9. Disseminated disease is present in 70% of children over the age of 1 yr. Forty–50% of children under the age of 1 yr have distant metastases.

Clinical Manifestations. The initial clinical features depend on the site of origin of the tumor, the degree of dissemination, and the age of the child. The primary tumor is most frequently in the abdomen. The most common finding, therefore, especially in the very young, is abdominal swelling associated with an abdominal mass, which is generally firm, irregular, and nontender. With enlargement the mass tends to cross the midline. Because the primary tumor arises frequently in the adrenal gland, the mass is usually in the upper abdomen. With metastasis to the liver there will be hepatic enlargement. Hemorrhage into the enlarging tumor is common; therefore, the patient may have pallor reflecting the resulting anemia. Bone involvement can produce pain and tenderness. In superficial bones, such as in the skull, tumor masses may be seen. Involvement of bone marrow can stop marrow production and produce pancytopenia; affected patients will have pallor, petechiae, and ecchymoses. Tumor masses may produce skin nodules, particularly in the younger infant. Intracranial metastases to dura or bones may cause increasing intracranial pressure, with irritability, pain, and vomiting. Fever may be a feature of either localized or disseminated tumor. Lethargy and anorexia are features of advanced disease.

An asymptomatic intrathoracic tumor may be found on a roentgenogram obtained for another purpose. On the other hand, a growing tumor mass may produce dyspnea and stridor. A tumor in the neck may present as a primary mass or with evidence of cervical lymph node metastasis. Cervical and mediastinal neuroblastomas may have Horner syndrome associated on the side of the tumor and, occasionally, heterochromia. Neuroblastoma arising along the vertebral column may have an extension into the spinal canal with spinal cord compression; this serious complication requires immediate treatment to prevent irreversible cord damage. Prompt treatment with chemotherapy or additional radiation therapy is frequently sufficient, and surgical decompression of the spinal canal can be avoided. Chronic diarrhea may occasionally be an early manifestation of neuroblastoma. Neuroblastoma may be congenital, usually presenting an abdominal tumor. Mothers of affected infants may have sweating, headache, and hypertension as effects of the increased catecholamines produced by the fetus. A myoclonic encephalopathy may rarely occur with neuroblastoma, associated primarily with such movement disorders as ataxia, myoclonus, or nystagmus. Initial findings with olfactory

Table 15–9 NEUROBLASTOMA STAGING SYSTEM

STAGE A	Complete gross resection of primary tumor, with or without microscopic residual; intracavitary lymph nodes, not adherent to and removed with primary,* histologically free of tumor; if primary in abdomen or pelvis, liver histologically free of tumor
STAGE B	Grossly unresected primary tumor; nodes and liver same as Stage A
STAGE C	Complete or incomplete resection of primary; intracavitary nodes not adherent to primary histologically positive for tumor; liver as in Stage A
STAGE D	Any dissemination of disease beyond intracavitary nodes, e.g., extracavitary nodes, liver, skin, bone marrow, bone

*Nodes adherent to or within tumor resection may be positive for tumor without upstaging patient to C.

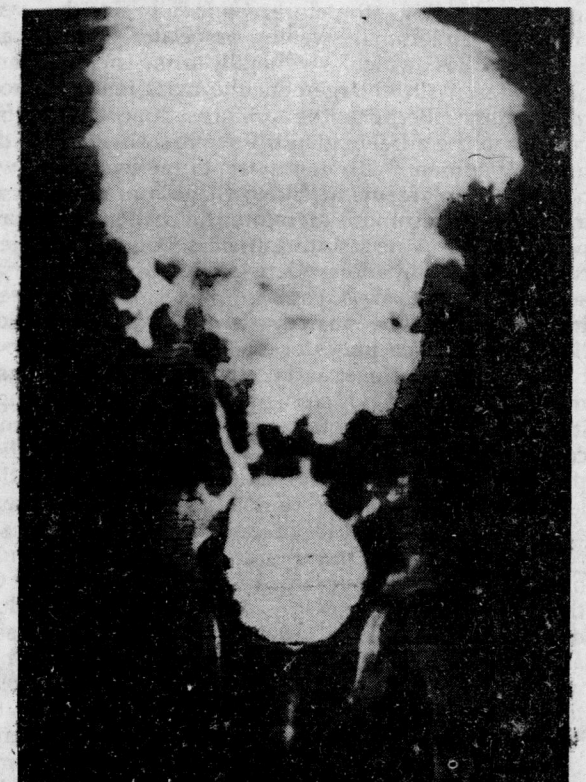

Figure 15–8 The intravenous pyelogram of a patient with a neuroblastoma arising in the right adrenal gland. The kidney is shown as displaced by the tumor mass downward and to the right.

neuroblastoma (esthesioneuroblastoma) are usually recurrent epistaxis or unilateral nasal obstruction. Local extension may lead to headaches and exophthalmos. The orbits are frequent sites of metastasis of neuroblastomas primary in other regions; proptosis, periorbital swelling, and ecchymosis may result.

Diagnostic Studies. Initial studies are determined by the site of origin and the evidence of dissemination. For adrenal tumors the intravenous pyelogram usually shows a kidney displaced by the tumor (Fig 15–8). Tumors in the thoracic region will be seen in the posterior mediastinum on roentgenograms of the chest. Widening of a vertebral foramen may be found if a paraspinal tumor has an intraspinal extension.

After the tumor has been identified at the primary site, it is necessary to assess its extension. Skeletal metastases can be revealed both by radioisotopic bone scans and by roentgenographic skeletal surveys. Radioisotopic scans of liver and spleen will demonstrate hepatic metastases. Ultrasound examination of the abdomen or pelvis may detect and measure primary tumor masses not displacing kidneys.

The associated anemia may be microcytic and hypochromic, reflecting chronic blood loss into the tumor, or normocytic if intratumor bleeding is more recent. Mechanical hemolysis within the tumor or associated with disseminated intravascular coagulation may cause fragmentation of red blood cells. Invasion of marrow by the tumor can cause pancytopenia and such features

of a myelophthisic anemia as teardrop-shaped red cells, nucleated red cells, and immature myeloid cells on blood smear. A bone marrow examination should be done for all patients and may reveal infiltrating tumor cells in clumps (Fig 15–9) or complete replacement of the marrow with sheets of tumor cells indistinguishable from those of acute lymphoblastic leukemia.

A specific diagnostic feature is the elevated catecholamine levels in urine. Increased amounts of dopa, dopamine, norepinephrine, normetanephrine, homovanillic acid, and vanillylmandelic acid (VMA) are found in about 90% of patients. The substance usually measured is vanillylmandelic acid, the most accurate determination requiring a 24-hr collection of urine. Simple tests have been devised (spot tests), which are helpful when positive but are often insensitive, giving false-negative results. Increased levels of carcinoembryonic antigen in plasma and of alpha-fetoprotein in serum occur, particularly with disseminated disease.

Final diagnosis depends upon the histologic characteristics of tumor obtained at excisional or diagnostic biopsy. The above studies to demonstrate the site of primary tumor and the degree of dissemination should be done before any surgery. The surgeon must know the extent of disease to determine whether complete removal of the primary tumor should be attempted. For some patients with widely disseminated disease, a limited diagnostic biopsy of a superficial lesion or bone marrow aspiration or biopsy will be appropriate.

Treatment. For localized tumor complete surgical resection gives the best chance for cure. For unresectable regional disease the surgeon should establish the degree and nature of the local extension for staging purposes. Biopsies should be obtained of lymph nodes draining the tumor area, and for tumors primary in the abdomen liver biopsies should be examined for microscopic involvement. For cases in which metastatic disease has already occurred, the value of an attempt at resection of the primary tumor has not been established. For patients with disseminated disease who have shown a complete clinical response to chemotherapy, attempts have been made later to resect the primary

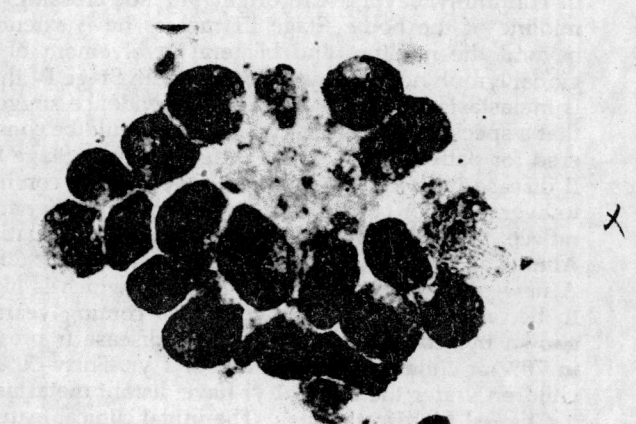

Figure 15–9 Neuroblastoma cells aspirated from the bone marrow. Clumps of cells often contain 3 or more cells without evidence of rosette formation. Rosettes of cells surrounding an inner mass of fibrillary material are characteristic of neuroblastoma.

tumor; the value of this "2nd look" also has not been established.

Most neuroblastomas are radiosensitive; irradiation may be used for local symptomatic relief of disseminated tumor or for reduction of tumor masses.

Because disseminated disease is common at the time of diagnosis of this tumor, chemotherapy is the mainstay of treatment. Responses have been demonstrated to vincristine, cyclophosphamide, doxorubicin, cis-platin, and the podophyllotoxins. A treatment regimen incorporating cyclophosphamide and doxorubicin can produce a complete response in more than 50% of children with disseminated neuroblastoma. The combination of the epipodophyllotoxin VM-26 and cis-platin has also been proved to be effective.

Prognosis. The 3 yr survival rate for all children with neuroblastoma is about 23%; after 3 yr deaths become rare. In patients under 1 yr of age at the time of diagnosis, the survival rate is about 50%, from 1–2 yr of age about 25%, and over 2 yr 15–20%.

The influence of the stage is related to the effect of age, younger children tending to have more limited disease at time of diagnosis. The 2 yr survival of children with neuroblastoma according to stage is reported to be Stage I, 84%; Stage II, 66%; Stage III, 33%; and Stage IV, 5%. The 2 yr survival for Stage IV-S (almost exclusively infants under 12 mo of age) is 84%. A better prognosis is associated with tumors arising in the thorax and cervical regions, with greater degrees of cellular differentiation, with female sex, and with the syndrome of opsomyoclonus. Laboratory indications of a favorable response to treatment are decreases in the levels of urinary catecholamine excretion and in the plasma levels of carcinoembryonic antigen.

PHEOCHROMOCYTOMA

Pheochromocytoma is a tumor of the sympathetic nervous system, rare in children and more benign than neuroblastoma. This metabolically active tumor is discussed in Sec 18.28.

NEOPLASMS OF KIDNEY

Kidney tumors occur at a rate of 7.8/million children under the age of 15 yr and with equal frequency in white and black races. In children Wilms tumor accounts for almost all renal neoplasms.

15.10 WILMS TUMOR

The diagnosis is made at a median age of 3 yr and before 5 yr in 80% of patients. The tumor is unusual in the 2nd decade of life but has occurred occasionally even in adults. It occurs with equal frequency in boys and girls.

An important feature of Wilms tumor is its association with congenital anomalies in as many as 13% of patients. The most common associations are genitourinary anomalies (4.4–7%), hemihypertrophy (2–3%), and sporadic aniridia (1–2%). Parents with hemihypertrophy have had children with Wilms tumor, and the tumor has occurred in siblings of children with hemihypertrophy. Less frequently, the neoplasm may occur with the syndrome of pseudohermaphroditism and nephropathy, with Beckwith-Wiedemann syndrome (macroglossia, gigantism, and umbilical hernia), with Klippel-Trenaunay syndrome (hemangiomas and lower extremity hypertrophy), and with a translocation involving B and C group chromosomes. In patients with Wilms tumor physical examination should include a careful search for congenital anomalies; the family history should carefully explore the possibility of related congenital anomalies in other family members. The aniridia–Wilms tumor syndrome is associated with interstitial deletion of the short arm of chromosome 11; a familial occurrence of the chromosomal abnormality with the syndrome has been described.

Pathology. Wilms tumor contains small undifferentiated blastemic cells, cells differentiating into abortive tubular or glomerular structures, and sarcomatous elements characterized by striated muscle cells. The mix of cells can vary considerably depending on the area of tumor sampled. Several histologic classification schemes are based on the proportions of different cellular elements (Fig 15–10).

The tumor is bilateral at the time of diagnosis in from 5–13% of cases. It metastasizes most frequently to the lung (80% of cases). Regional extension of the tumor may occur as it breaks through the renal capsule or involves regional lymph nodes. About 20% of patients with metastasis have involvement of the liver. Rare sites of metastases are bone marrow and the central nervous system.

The staging system most frequently used is that of the National Wilms Tumor Study Group. Stage I tumor is limited to the kidney and completely resected. Stage II tumor extends beyond the kidney but is completely resected. Stage III indicates residual nonhematogenous extension of tumor confined to the abdomen. Stage IV means hematogenous metastases, most frequently to

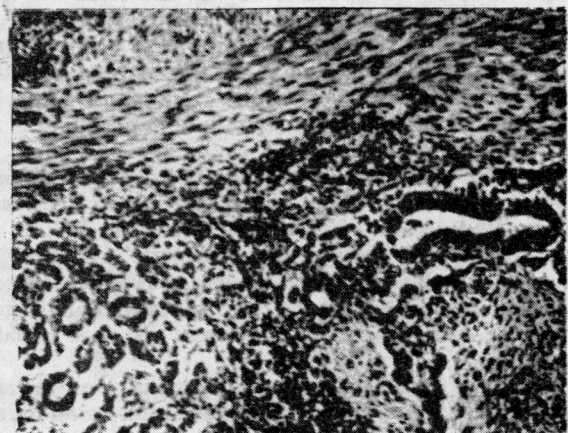

Figure 15–10 The histologic features of Wilms tumor. The epithelial component is represented by the round oval tumor tubules; an elongated tumor tubule is also present. The mesodermal component is represented by the band of aligned nuclei across the photomicrograph.

the lung. Stage V is used for bilateral renal involvement, either at time of diagnosis or later.

Clinical Manifestations. The most frequent sign of Wilms tumor is an abdominal mass; it is present in 95% of cases and is the usual reason for suspecting the diagnosis. The mass may be asymptomatic and found only on routine examination. About half of affected children have additional symptoms of abdominal pain; there may be vomiting or fever. Masses vary greatly in size at the time of discovery; half of them are 5–10 cm in diameter; one third will be larger. The mass is generally smooth and firm and rarely crosses the midline. If there are metastases in the liver, it may be enlarged and nodular. Patients with bilateral tumors have an earlier onset of disease (average age of 15 mo) and a greater frequency of associated congenital anomalies.

Hypertension occurs in 30–60% of cases. It may be sufficiently severe and prolonged to produce congestive cardiac failure. The hypertension results from increased renin levels caused by renal ischemia, usually from pressure by the tumor on the renal artery. Arteriovenous fistulas within the tumor may also lead to congestive heart failure.

Certain rare paraneoplastic syndromes may be associated with Wilms tumor. The neoplasm may produce erythropoietin, leading to polycythemia. Cushing syndrome may be caused by the secretion of ACTH; symptomatic hypoglycemia has been reported.

Diagnosis. This diagnosis must be suspected in the young child with an abdominal mass. Microscopic or gross hematuria, reported in from 10–25% of patients, may be the only indication of renal tumor.

The most important diagnostic study is an intravenous pyelogram, which will demonstrate an intrarenal mass in about 80% of patients (Fig 15–11). The remaining patients may present nondiagnostic findings, such as failure of excretion of dye. About 5% of tumors show mineralization. The intravenous pyelogram is incorrectly interpreted in about 5–10% of cases. The major problems in differential diagnosis are hydronephrosis, renal cysts, mesoblastic nephroma, or other malignancies, principally neuroblastoma but also renal cell carcinoma, lymphangial sarcoma, and fibrosarcoma. In difficult cases angiography, computed axial tomography, and ultrasonography may help to establish the nature of an abdominal mass. Arteriography may be particularly helpful in determining whether there is an otherwise undetectable tumor in the other kidney.

Pulmonary metastases will be evident on roentgenograms in about 19% of patients at the time of diagnosis. Radionuclide scans of liver and spleen are helpful in detecting hepatic metastases. Bone involvement is so rare that roentgenographic skeletal surveys and bone scans are not useful, nor is bone marrow examination necessary preoperatively. Metastases to bone usually cause pain.

Increased levels of alpha-fetoprotein are usually found but have no diagnostic significance, being found also with several other abdominal tumors. Mucoproteins have been reported in the serum or urine of some patients with Wilms tumor but generally only with advanced disease.

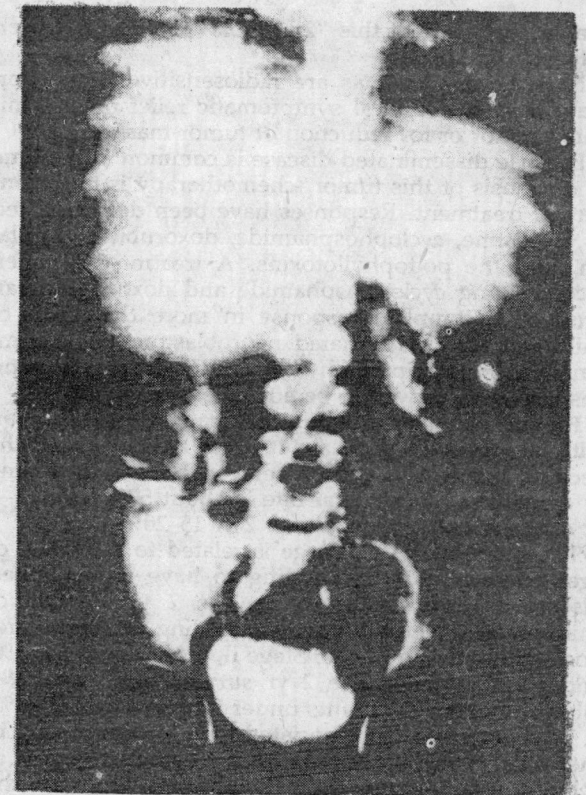

Figure 15–11 The intravenous pyelogram of a patient with a right Wilms tumor. The collecting system of the right kidney is displaced downward by the tumor mass in the upper pole of the kidney. The pelvis and caliceal system are distorted by this intrarenal tumor.

Treatment. The usual immediate treatment is surgical removal of the kidney containing the tumor, even if pulmonary metastases are present. At the time of operation careful inspection of the other kidney should be made to exclude the possibility of bilateral tumor and of the liver to discover possible metastases. Dissection of retroperitoneal lymph nodes should be made in a search for regional metastases. The surgeon should look for evidence of penetration of the capsule by the tumor and for the possibility of involvement of the renal vein. The specimen removed should be delivered intact to the pathologist so that valid staging can guide subsequent treatment.

Wilms tumor is sensitive to irradiation and to chemotherapy. There is no indication that the results are improved by preoperative use of these or by postoperative irradiation to the bed of the removed kidney.

For patients with Stage I tumor a regimen employing vincristine and actinomycin D is recommended. For patients found to have Stage II or III disease the same regimen should be accompanied by irradiation either to the renal bed (Stage II) or to the whole abdomen (Stage III). Choice of irradiation ports must be based on the surgical findings. With Stage IV disease the irradiation ports should also include the involved lung fields.

Doxorubicin (Adriamycin) is also effective for Wilms tumor but carries the serious side effect of myocardial toxicity. Its role in extending disease-free survival in patients with extensive disease is under evaluation.

For patients with bilateral Wilms tumor the surgeon must evaluate the possibilities of wedge resection for the less involved kidney. Irradiation of the kidney containing residual tumor must be done with care to avoid nephritis. In some cases successful resections of hepatic or pulmonary metastases can be done.

Prognosis. Several factors influence prognosis. Patients under 2 yr of age at time of diagnosis have a higher response rate than older children. Sex, the side affected, and the presence of associated congenital defects do not influence prognosis. However, the stage of disease is important. With rare exceptions, 2 yr of disease-free survival indicates cure. About 90% of patients with Stage I disease under 2 yr of age will survive, as will about 80% of patients with Stage I disease over 2 yr of age or patients with Stage II or III disease of any age. It is difficult to evaluate the prognosis for patients with Stage IV disease or bilateral disease at the time of diagnosis because they are so few; some of them, however, achieve 2 yr of disease-free survival. Any recurrence of disease during treatment carries a bad prognosis.

The prognosis depends also on the histologic character of the tumor. The greater the degree of epithelial differentiation, the better the prognosis. On the other hand, the finding of sarcomatous histology or anaplastic features is associated with a worse prognosis. The tumors are also more likely to be associated with bone metastasis.

OTHER RENAL NEOPLASMS

Neonatal Renal Tumor. The characteristic tumor of the infant kidney is the congenital mesoblastic nephroma (fetal renal hamartoma). The histologic feature is a preponderance of interlacing bundles of spindle cells resembling fibroblasts and smooth muscle cells. Variable cellularity and pleomorphism occur, and mitotic figures may be common. Treatment is nephrectomy alone, without chemotherapy or irradiation. Recurrences are rare.

Renal Cell Carcinoma. This tumor is infrequent in childhood and particularly rare during the 1st decade. Initial findings are an abdominal mass and hematuria. The intravenous pyelogram is the most useful means of demonstrating the intrarenal tumor. The microscopic appearance and clinical course are similar to those found in adults with this neoplasm.

15.11 SOFT TISSUE SARCOMAS

Soft tissue sarcomas have an annual incidence of 8.4/million white children under the age of 15 yr and about half that incidence in black children. Rhabdomyosarcoma accounts for more than half of these tumors.

RHABDOMYOSARCOMA

Epidemiology. Rhabdomyosarcoma has a peak incidence at 4 yr of age and again at 16-18 yr. The 2nd peak is due primarily to tumors of the genitourinary system. Forty-50% of cases occur before the age of 5 yr. Males predominate in a ratio of 1.4:1 and are highest in tumors of the genitourinary tract and lowest in tumors of the head and neck. Rhabdomyosarcoma occurs more often than expected in siblings, and among young adult relatives of affected children there is a high frequency of other cancers, especially of the breast in females.

Pathology. The vast majority of rhabdomyosarcomas in children and adolescents are thought to be derived from embryonic tissue, either from immature prospective muscular tissue or from undifferentiated mesenchymal tissue which has the potential for aberrant differentiation of muscle fibers. The tumor may occur at any site of embryonal development of muscle cells.

There are 4 histologic subtypes: the *embryonal* accounts for about 60% of all forms; the *botryoid* type (also called *sarcoma botryoides*), a variant of the embryonal form in which the tumor cells are found with an edematous stroma, accounts for 6% of the total and is commonly seen in the vagina, uterus, bladder, nasopharynx, and middle ear; the *alveolar* type comprises about 20%; and the *pleomorphic* subtype represents about 1% of these tumors. Histologic differentiation may be difficult; some sarcomas remain unclassified.

Rhabdomyosarcoma most frequently arises in the head and neck area, where it accounts for 25% of cases; the next most frequent sites are the extremities and the genitourinary system, each representing about 20% of the total. Less common sites of origin, ranging from 5-10% in frequency, are the trunk, orbit, intrathoracic area, and retroperitoneum. Metastatic disease involves regional lymph nodes and hematogenous dissemination to bone, bone marrow, and lung. Involvement of the myocardium can be found in 33% of fatal cases.

The most commonly used staging system is that of the Intergroup Rhabdomyosarcoma Study. Stage I represents localized disease completely resected. Substage IA designates tumor confined to the muscle or organ of origin, and IB, infiltration beyond this structure without involvement of regional nodes. Stage II represents grossly resected lesions: IIA describes grossly resected tumor with microscopic residual disease; IIB describes regional disease completely resected, with regional node involvement or with extension of the tumor into an adjacent organ; and IIC describes gross resection of regional disease and involved nodes, with evidence of microscopic residual tumor. Stage III is designated if there has been incomplete resection or only biopsy, with gross residual disease. Stage IV describes distant metastatic disease at the time of diagnosis. Most patients have evidence of disease extension at the time of diagnosis, only about 20% being amenable to complete resection and the majority having grossly unresectable disease or distant metastases.

Clinical Manifestations. The usual presenting feature is a mass, which may be painful. Associated features depend upon the site of origin. Nasopharyngeal tumor may be associated with nasal congestion, mouth breathing, epistaxis, and difficulty with swallowing and chewing. Regional extension into the cranium may produce cranial nerve paralysis, blindness, and signs of increasing intracranial pressure, with headache and vomiting. When the tumor develops in the face or cheek, there may be swelling, pain, trismus, and, as extension occurs, paralysis of cranial nerves. In the neck region the original finding may be progressive swelling, with neurologic features following progressive regional extension. In the orbit there may be proptosis, periorbital edema, ptosis, change in visual acuity, and local pain. When the tumor arises in the middle ear, the early signs are usually pain, loss of hearing, chronic otorrhea, or a tumor mass in the ear canal; extensions of the tumor produce cranial nerve paralysis and signs of an intracranial mass on the involved side. With tumor of the larynx there may be an unremitting croupy cough, progressive stridor, and respiratory distress. Most of these signs and symptoms can also be associated with more common problems of the head and neck area, particularly those associated with infection; accordingly, the clinician must be alert to the possibility that unusually prolonged or severe problems in this area may represent complications of a tumor.

Rhabdomyosarcoma of the trunk or extremities usually presents as a mass. Not uncommonly, this tumor is first noticed after some trauma to the region and for a time may be regarded as a hematoma. When the tumor shows little change in size, or even grows, at a time when a hematoma should be subsiding, the true diagnosis should be suspected. Tumor of the genitourinary tract may produce hematuria, obstruction of the lower urinary tract, recurrent urinary tract infections, incontinence, or a mass detectable by abdominal or rectal examination. Involvement of the paratesticular tissues usually presents a rapidly growing, painful mass in the scrotum. Vaginal rhabdomyosarcoma may present a grapelike mass of tumor tissue bulging through the vaginal orifice and may cause symptoms relating to the urinary tract or even to the large bowel. Vaginal bleeding or obstruction of the urethra or the rectum may occur. Similar findings may occur when the tumor arises in the uterus.

With tumors in any location there may be early dissemination, and the presenting findings can be bone pain or the respiratory distress of pulmonary metastases. Extensive bone involvement may produce symptomatic hypercalcemia and consequent renal disease. In patients with disseminated tumor it is sometimes difficult to identify the primary lesion, which might be in the middle ear or be such a small mass on an extremity as to be thought of no consequence.

Diagnosis. The early diagnosis of rhabdomyosarcoma requires that an alert physician exercise the keenest clinical judgment when the patient is first seen. The diagnosis should be made as soon as possible, particularly for tumors in the head and neck area, where regional extension can quickly involve vital structures. In our experience the median delay between the onset of signs and symptoms and biopsy is 2 mo.

Diagnostic procedures are determined in large degree by the area of involvement. In the head and neck area, roentgenograms and computed tomographic scans should be examined for evidences of the tumor mass and for indications of bony erosion. For abdominal tumors, intravenous pyelography, computed tomographic scans, and ultrasound examinations can help to delineate the site and size of the mass. Cystourethrograms are useful for tumors in the bladder region. Barium studies of the gastrointestinal tract are only rarely of value. Arteriography will only occasionally provide useful information. Evidence of metastatic disease should be sought in roentgenograms and computed tomographic scans of lungs as well as in roentgenograms and radionuclide scans of the skeleton and an examination of bone marrow. These studies should be evaluated before any surgical procedure so that the extent of proposed surgery can be defined. The most essential element of the diagnostic workup is the examination of tumor tissue, which may involve special stains and electron microscopy. The usual differential diagnostic problems are other small-cell sarcomas, such as Ewing sarcoma or neuroblastoma. The characteristics of rhabdomyosarcoma are shown in Fig 15–12.

Treatment. In only about 20% of the patients can the tumor be completely removed. In some locations removal is impractical because of the proximity of vital structures or the resulting disfigurement. The initial surgical procedure must at times be limited to a diagnostic biopsy.

Radiation therapy can produce regression of tumor at doses of around 3000–4000 rads. Larger doses, from 5000–6000 rads, are necessary for complete tumor destruction. The location of the tumor and the long-range consequences of radiation in this dose may limit this form of treatment. Chemotherapy with dactinomycin, cyclophosphamide, vincristine, and doxorubicin (Adriamycin), alone or in combination, has produced regression of this tumor. Each agent alone is effective in from 25–50% of patients, but current treatment regimens involve 3–4 of these drugs in combination.

The treatment program for each patient must be designed according to the location and stage of the tumor. In Stage I complete local excision is followed by chemotherapy to reduce the likelihood of subsequent metastatic disease. For Stages II and III the attempt at complete surgical removal must be followed by a regimen involving local irradiation and systemic chemotherapy. At times it is advisable to give a course of irradiation and chemotherapy before any attempt at surgical resection in an effort to shrink the tumor to a point at which it can be removed without a severely mutilating procedure. The treatment of disseminated rhabdomyosarcoma rests primarily on chemotherapy, with surgery and radiotherapy used in the management of complications caused by local tumor masses.

Prognosis. This is influenced primarily by site of origin and by stage of disease at time of diagnosis. Eighty–90% of patients with resectable tumor have a tumor-free survival. About two thirds of patients with regional tumor, incompletely resected, also achieve long-term disease-free survival. For patients with disseminated disease, only an occasional patient responds to chemotherapy with long-term control. The prognosis

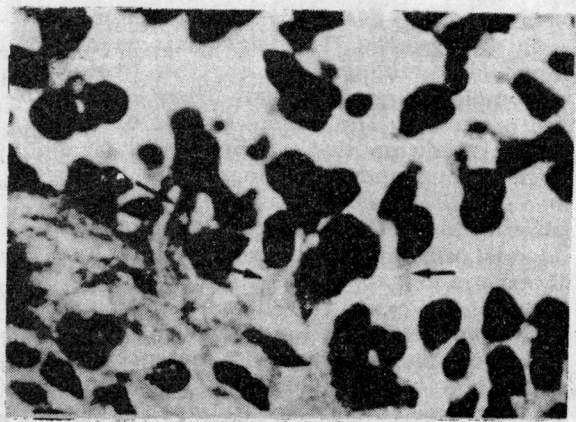

Figure 15–12 The typical histologic features of alveolar rhabdomyosarcoma. Arrows point to cytoplasmic attachments of the rhabdomyeloblasts to a connective tissue septum.

is better for tumors arising in the orbit or in the genitourinary tract. Older children have a worse prognosis; they have a greater frequency of lesions of the extremities and greater likelihood of disseminated disease at the time of diagnosis. Tumors of the alveolar form, histologically, are more likely to be disseminated early and widely.

15.12 OTHER SARCOMAS

Fibrosarcoma. This unusual tumor accounts for fewer than 10% of soft tissue sarcomas. It is particularly uncommon in the 1st decade of life. Males predominate about 2:1 in reported series.

The histologic appearance of fibrosarcoma must be carefully distinguished from that of the benign fibrous tumors of childhood. The malignant neoplasm is composed of interweaving bundles of spindle-shaped cells with varying amounts of cytoplasm. The nuclei are thin and pointed. With more differentiation the cellular growth pattern has a herringbone appearance with nuclei arranged in parallel rows. Multinucleated bizarre tumor cells may occur in the anaplastic varieties. The most common site of origin is the lower extremities, other sites being upper extremities, trunk, and head and neck region. Metastatic disease occurs in about 10% of patients. Sites of metastasis are lung and bone.

The presenting feature is a mass at the site of origin, which is generally painless and may be present for weeks or months before diagnosis. The tumors have variable rates of growth. Diagnosis is made by biopsy and careful microscopic examination of tissue.

The treatment is surgical excision, with wide margins required because of the tendency of this tumor to infiltrate locally. The major problem in management is local recurrence, which in some cases necessitates amputation of the involved extremity. Irradiation and chemotherapy with current modalities have little to offer, though there are reports of tumor regression with combination chemotherapy. For most patients long-term disease-free survival can be obtained by surgical

removal of the tumor. Careful follow-up must be done in order to detect local recurrence as early as possible.

Synovial Sarcoma. This tumor accounts for about 5% of soft tissue sarcomas in children. It is particularly uncommon during the 1st decade of life, but is rather evenly distributed from the 2nd–5th decades. Males predominate in a ratio of about 3:2.

The tumor is made up of spindle cells admixed with plump epithelioid cells characteristic of mesenchymal differentiation into synovial membranes. The degree of admixture of these 2 elements allows for classification into poorly and well-differentiated forms. Ninety-five % of these tumors arise on the extremities, 70% occurring on the legs. In only 12% of patients does the tumor appear to arise from anatomic synovium. Metastases involve the lungs predominantly but may also appear in regional lymph nodes.

This tumor is slow growing, making its presence known predominantly by a palpable mass, with 60% of patients experiencing pain or tenderness in the area. The diagnosis of this tumor depends on its histologic appearance after excisional biopsy. The only effective method of treatment is wide local excision. Response to radiation therapy or combination chemotherapy is unpredictable; for most patients these adjuvant forms of therapy are ineffective. Because of the possibility of local recurrence, patients must be carefully followed even after an apparently complete resection of tumor.

Alveolar Soft Part Sarcoma. This tumor accounts for only about 1% of soft tissue sarcomas, occurring in both children and adults. The tumor has an organoid pattern characterized by small rounded groups of cells within a fibrovascular framework. Individual cells are rounded and contain well-defined granules in the cytoplasm. Both light and electron microscopy suggest that these cells are derived from paraganglia present in the muscles throughout the body. The usual site of this tumor is the musculature of the extremities or trunk, but it may occur also in the retroperitoneal area and in the head and neck region. Metastases are hematogenous and can involve lung, bone, and brain. Lymph node metastases are uncommon.

The presenting feature is a slowly growing mass, which may be painful and tender. Diagnosis necessitates a biopsy for histologic examination. Effective treatment involves complete surgical excision, but local recurrences are common, with eventual widespread metastatic disease. Limited experience does not yet permit evaluation of the role of local radiation therapy after excision; chemotherapy with regimens similar to those for rhabdomyosarcoma has limited usefulness.

Hemangiosarcoma. This tumor is also known as *malignant hemangioendothelioma*. It is extremely rare. So few cases have been reported that it is impossible to draw conclusions about age and sex distribution. It occurs during the 1st 2 decades and seems to be evenly distributed between boys and girls. The characteristic histologic features are anastomosing capillaries lined by neoplastic endothelial cells. The cells appear within the reticulin sheaf of the vessels, and individual cells are not encircled by reticulin fibers. The tumor may arise anywhere in the body and is frequently associated with bone. Metastasis is hematogenous, most frequently to lungs but also to bone and brain. Regional lymph nodes may be involved. This tumor presents as a growing mass, and diagnosis must be made by histologic examination. Effective treatment involves complete excision. There may be temporary regression of the tumor with chemotherapy regimens similar to those for rhabdomyosarcoma. Irradiation may have some value in local control.

Hemangiopericytoma. This is a rare malignancy of the capillary pericyte of Zimmerman. It is seen more commonly in the 2nd decade of life than in younger children. Sex distribution seems to be equal. Histologically, the tumor is composed of small spindle cells, with prominent vessels lined by a single layer of normal-appearing endothelial cells. The tumor cells tend to be arranged in clusters or whorls and are outside the vessel. Clusters of these cells may bulge into and deform the vascular channels. Metastases are blood borne, primarily to lung, liver, and bone.

The tumor presents clinically as a growing mass or as local pain in involved bone. Diagnosis depends on histologic examination. Effective treatment involves complete surgical excision. Where this is impractical, a chemotherapeutic regimen similar to that for rhabdomyosarcoma may be temporarily effective, and local irradiation may provide temporary control.

Liposarcoma. Another rare soft tissue sarcoma of children, this neoplasm is characterized by an abortive differentiation of cells into lipocytes. It occurs during both decades of childhood and seems to have an even sex distribution. It may arise anywhere that fat tissue is found but occurs most frequently on the extremities. Metastases are blood borne. The presenting clinical feature is a mass, usually slowly growing. The tumor may be firm or rubbery in consistency. Associated pain or tenderness is unusual. Diagnosis depends on histologic examination. Effective treatment is wide local excision with close observation for local recurrences, which may occur late. Radiation therapy may be useful for local control, and chemotherapy with a regimen similar to that for rhabdomyosarcoma has produced regression of tumor.

Leiomyosarcoma. This tumor of smooth muscle occurs during both decades of childhood; the sex distribution appears even. The tumor is composed of spindle cells with blunt-ended nuclei, which sometimes tend to be oval with prominent nuclei. The cells are arranged in intertwining bundles or whorls with variable degrees of cellularity. The distinction from benign leiomyoma is based on the degree of cellular atypicality and the frequency of mitotic figures. The tumor may arise in many organs, including prostate, bladder, lung, stomach, and small bowel. It also may appear in the head and neck area, trunk, or extremities. Metastases occur primarily to liver and lung; regional lymph nodes may also be involved.

The initial clinical features depend on the site of origin. Gastrointestinal tumors may produce bleeding or signs of intestinal obstruction. Tumors in the lung may cause respiratory distress; those of the bladder or prostate may be associated with hematuria or with bladder neck obstruction and urine retention. A mass may be the initial clinical feature for tumors in organs

of the abdomen or elsewhere. The tumor masses are generally slow growing. The diagnosis is established by excisional biopsy if possible. Effective treatment involves complete surgical excision. There is a likelihood of local recurrence. The tumors tend to be radioresistant; there is little reported experience with chemotherapy. The recommended treatment would be a drug regimen similar to that for rhabdomyosarcoma.

Malignant Mesenchymoma. This tumor is of mixed mesodermal origin. It can occur during both decades of childhood and may also be seen as a congenital tumor. It occurs more frequently in boys than in girls. The tumor is composed of malignant cells differentiating into 2 or more unrelated forms of mesenchymal tissue other than fibrosarcoma. There may be the appearance of well differentiated bone or cartilage. The most common site of origin is the trunk or extremities, but it can also arise from pleura, gut, or retroperitoneal tissue or in the head and neck area. Metastasis can involve liver, lung, and skeleton; there may also be regional node involvement. The initial clinical feature is almost always a slowly growing mass. The diagnosis must be established by excisional biopsy. Treatment is complete surgical removal. The roles of radiation and chemotherapy have not been established. Recommended treatment for incomplete removal would be like that for rhabdomyosarcoma.

GENERAL CONSIDERATIONS

As the above discussion of soft tissue sarcomas indicates, the usual problem facing the clinician is a patient with a growing tumor mass. Few clinical features distinguish 1 sarcoma from another. The vascular sarcomas have an obvious appearance if they are superficial, but there are otherwise no distinguishing features. Rhabdomyosarcoma is more common in younger children, and fibrosarcomas occur more often during the 2nd decade, but age is not definitive for the individual patient. For many of these tumors the chance for cure rests on complete surgical excision; accordingly, the diagnosis must be established as early as possible. If a thorough search for metastatic disease finds none, then an attempt at resection of the tumor is appropriate. Preoperative chemotherapy and irradiation may be useful in patients with rhabdomyosarcoma to reduce the size of a tumor to the point of complete resectability. Histologic evaluation should include a complete range of histochemical and, as appropriate, electron microscopic examinations. Perhaps for no other group of tumors is it so important to have the careful review of tissues by an experienced pathologist, both for definition of the specific type of tumor and for an assessment of its malignant or benign nature.

NEOPLASMS OF BONE

Bone tumors have an annual incidence of 5.6/million white children and 4.8/million black children. Osteosarcoma is the most common malignant bone tumor; it is twice as common in white children as Ewing tumor.

Ewing tumor is almost completely absent in the black race. Rare bone tumors include chondrosarcomas and fibrosarcomas.

15.13 OSTEOSARCOMA

The median age of onset of osteosarcoma is 15 yr; two thirds of patients are between the ages of 10–20 yr. The incidence is identical in Blacks and Whites. During the 1st 13 yr of life boys and girls have the same incidence of osteosarcoma, but older boys have an increasing rate whereas girls reach a plateau. The distributions as to age and sex are consistent with a proposal that these tumors are related to the level of cellular activity in bone. Osteosarcoma occurs most frequently in long bones at the points of greatest growth and reconstruction, the metaphyseal ends, during periods of most active growth; the continuing increase in frequency in boys over girls follows a pattern consistent with their growth characteristics.

There is an excessive incidence of osteosarcoma of the femur in children with bilateral retinoblastoma, amounting to about 1% of survivors living into the 2nd decade of life. Accordingly, the gene associated with retinoblastoma may predispose to tumors in sites besides the retina. Certain diseases of bone, some known to be genetically determined, may also predispose to bone cancer in childhood. These conditions are multiple osteochondromatosis (Ollier disease), which also may be found with hemangiomas (Maffucci syndrome) and multiple hereditary exostoses, and osteogenesis imperfecta. Familial cases of osteosarcoma occur occasionally. Other tumors seen with increased frequency in family members with osteosarcoma are adrenocortical carcinoma, rhabdomyosarcoma, and brain tumors. Ionizing radiation in large doses is related to the development of osteosarcoma, with a latency period ranging from 4–21 yr.

Pathology. This tumor may have osteosarcomatous, chondrosarcomatous, and fibrosarcomatous differentiation within a single lesion. Different patterns may be seen in different sections of the same tumor, and osteoblastic, fibroblastic, or chondroblastic elements may predominate. A characteristic section is shown in Fig 15–13. The tumor most frequently arises in long bones, occasionally in flat bones of the trunk or cranial vault. The femur is most commonly affected, with tibia and humerus, respectively, being the next most common sites. The tumors of the long bones usually involve the metaphyseal region. The lung is the most frequent site of metastasis, and of those patients who die, 90% succumb to pulmonary insufficiency caused by metastatic tumor. Metastasis to other bones may occur, but generally after the development of pulmonary metastases. Regional lymph nodes are rarely involved. The classic osteosarcoma arises within the shaft of the medullary canal and may break through the cortex of the bone of origin to form a soft tissue mass which can achieve considerable size. The tumor may also extend along the medullary cavity.

Two important variants of osteosarcoma must be distinguished. *Parosteal osteosarcoma* is extramedullary

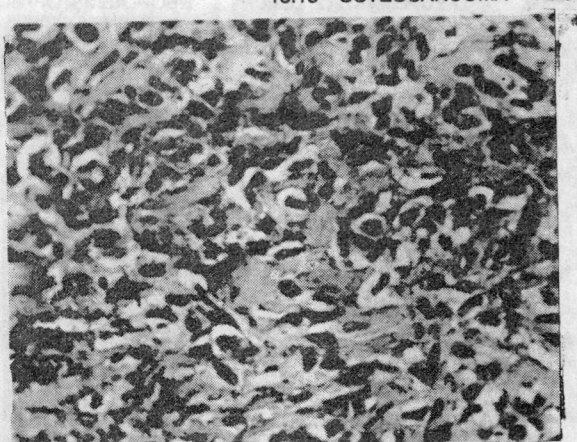

Figure 15–13 The diagnostic histologic features of osteosarcoma. The nuclei are of various sizes, shapes, and chromatin densities; most have a dark chromatin appearance. The cells are intimately involved with the background amorphous material, which is osteoid.

and attached by a broad base to the underlying bone, which is usually the lower femoral shaft. This form of the tumor tends to occur at a slightly older age and more frequently in females. The characteristic histologic appearance is as a heavily ossified lesion with areas of proliferating fibroblasts. Bands of well-formed osteoid material and bone are scattered throughout, and there may be some focal anaplastic spindle cell components. Cartilaginous participation is usually limited. *Periosteal osteosarcoma* is rare; like osteosarcoma it occurs most frequently during the 2nd decade of life with a slight male predominance. The tumor is limited to the periphery of the cortex; it most frequently involves the upper tibia but may also occur on the femur or humerus. This tumor usually contains lobulated islands of malignant cartilage, and there is little tendency to invade surrounding skeletal muscle. The osteogenic component consists of fine lacelike osteoid with absence of trabeculae of mature osteoid or bone. Clusters of malignant spindle cells are interspersed. Both of these variants of osteosarcoma metastasize less frequently in lung and other bones.

Osteosarcoma may rarely appear simultaneously at many sites, with a predominantly osteoblastic pattern (*multifocal sclerosive osteosarcoma*).

Clinical Manifestations. The most frequent initial finding is pain at the site of the tumor. Subsequently, limitation of motion may develop and a palpable or visible tumor. With involvement of the bones of the legs there may be limping or alterations of gait. Later manifestations are tenderness and local erythema and hyperthermia. With pulmonary metastases there may be progressive dyspnea, and pneumothorax may occur.

Diagnosis. Persistently unexplained bone pain, particularly when associated with a palpable mass, requires roentgenographic examination of that bone. A typical appearance of osteosarcoma is shown in Fig 15–14. These bone changes should initiate a search for metastatic disease. Roentgenographic examination of the lungs, including computed tomographic scanning, is essential. Typical pulmonary metastasis in osteosar-

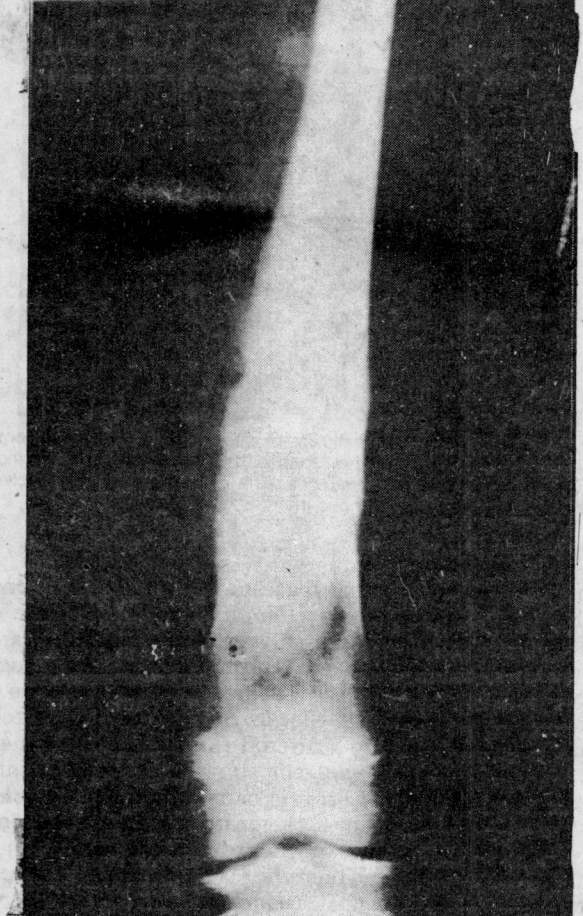

Figure 15–14 Osteosarcoma of the distal portion of the femur. The tumor has broken through the cortex; calcification of the tumor is seen in the surrounding soft tissues.

coma is shown in Fig 15–15. A roentgenographic skeletal survey should search for other possible bone lesions. The radionuclide bone scan will show increased uptake in the area of the tumor and in other skeletal areas where there are metastases. The bone scans may also reveal areas of intracortical spread of the tumor, a finding which is important in planning surgical intervention. Other laboratory studies are of less value. The serum alkaline phosphatase level may be increased, most likely because of osteoblastic activity in the area of the tumor. Confirmation of the diagnosis must be made by open biopsy of the lesion and histologic examination.

Treatment. For the patient with no evident metastatic disease the recommended treatment is amputation of the affected extremity or wide local excision of a flat bone where feasible. A transmedullary resection of the extremity, where possible, will provide the best base for a prosthesis. Samples of the medullary cavity of the residual stump must be examined as frozen sections at the time of surgery to detect any residual tumor.

A retrospective analysis of the results of amputation

found a 5 yr survival of 17%. Patients who had not survived had usually developed pulmonary metastases within 2 yr of surgery. It was thought likely that pulmonary micrometastases had been present at the time of diagnosis though not then demonstrable by roentgenograms of the chest. Accordingly, several regimens of chemotherapy adjunctive to surgery have been developed. Active drugs are methotrexate, doxorubicin (Adriamycin), cis-platin, and cyclophosphamide. Methotrexate is given in large doses followed by citrovorum factor rescue. Most regimens involve 1 or more of these drugs. Current reports indicate that about 50% of patients can achieve long-term disease-free survival if pulmonary metastases are not evident at the time of diagnosis.

Attempts have been made to preserve the involved extremity through preoperative chemotherapy followed by resection of the involved bone and a prosthetic bone replacement. Selecting this approach requires careful comparison of the functional characteristics of a likely prosthesis following amputation and those of a preserved limb after attempted bone replacement. This procedure seems most attractive for the upper extremity, where the hand of the involved arm may be preserved.

In some patients with pulmonary metastasis, resection may be considered. If the metastases are solitary or few and in the periphery of the lung, and particularly if metastatic disease appears late in the course of treatment, resection may be followed by long-term disease-free survival.

A most important consideration for patients with osteosarcoma is the careful rehabilitation which must follow the amputation. This should include not only the careful fitting of a prosthesis but also the psychologic support essential to a period of adjustment. These patients are most often adolescents, who must adjust

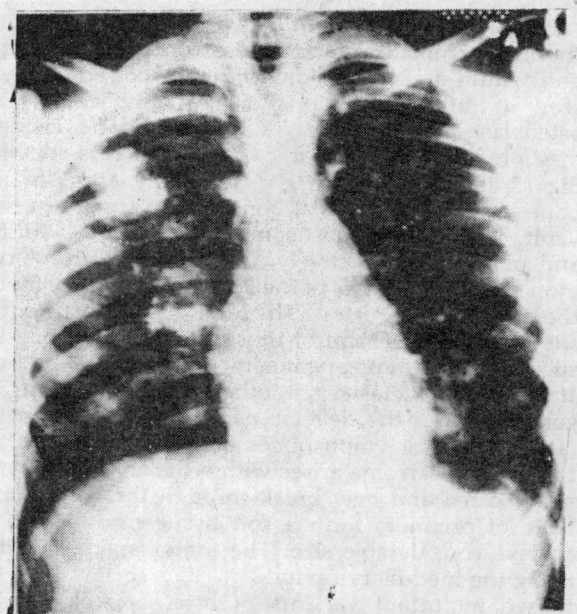

Figure 15–15 Multiple metastatic nodules of osteosarcoma.

to a major alteration of their body at the same time that they face other critical psychologic issues.

Prognosis. Patients with the periosteal or parosteal forms of osteosarcoma have a lower frequency of pulmonary metastasis and a better prognosis. Greater survival is also seen in females. Histologic predominance of chondroplastic or massive osteoid appearance conveys a somewhat better prognosis than do other histologic appearances, but within any tumor there is great variability from site to site.

15.14 EWING SARCOMA

Ewing sarcoma is also seen most frequently during the 2nd decade of life at a time of greatest bone growth. The incidence in boys and girls is identical until the age of about 15 yr, when the rate for girls decreases. The tumor is virtually absent in Blacks, both in Africa and in the United States. Ewing sarcoma has a familial pattern and has not been reported to occur with other familial tumors or syndromes. There is no indication that it is radiation induced.

Pathology. This tumor is composed of neoplastic cells with clear cytoplasma and ill-defined cytoplasmic borders (Fig 15–16). The cell nuclei are singular and markedly irregular in size and shape. Broad connective tissue bands divide the tumor into irregular lobules or sheets of neoplastic cells. The presence of glycogen, as indicated by the periodic acid–Schiff reaction, helps differentiate this tumor of small round cells from metastatic neuroblastoma. The cell of origin for this tumor is uncertain.

The tumor may arise either in long bones of the extremities or in flat bones of the head and trunk. The most commonly involved bone of the trunk is the pelvis, and of long bones, the femur. Extraskeletal neoplasms histologically resembling Ewing sarcoma have been described, most frequently arising in the soft tissues of

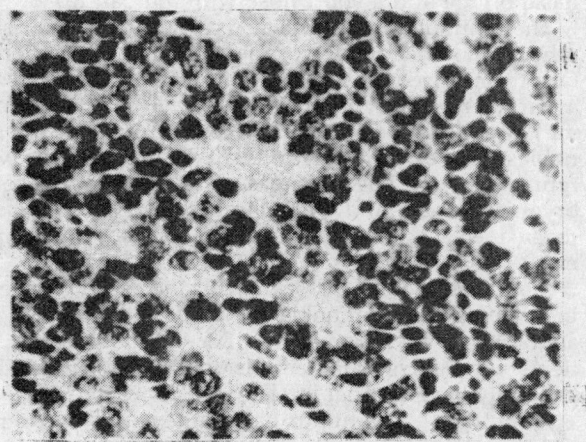

Figure 15–16 Characteristic features of Ewing sarcoma. The cells are uniform, with primitive round to oval nuclei, ill-defined cytoplasmic borders, nuclear crowding, and, in some areas, Ewing rosettes. The rosettes consist of an amorphous material which sometimes contains tumor nuclei in various stages of degeneration.

the lower extremity and paravertebral regions. Their relationship to Ewing sarcoma of bone is uncertain. Metastatic disease most frequently involves lungs and bone, occasionally the central nervous system.

Clinical Manifestations. The consistent symptom is pain at the site of tumor, usually with some swelling in the area. The site may be tender and the patient febrile. The typical roentgenographic features are shown in Fig 15–17. The usual finding is that of a bone lesion with surrounding soft tissue mass. The roentgenographic features may be indistinguishable from those of osteomyelitis.

Diagnosis. This may be suspected from clinical history and roentgenographic features; it must be confirmed by surgical biopsy. The usual problem for differential diagnosis is distinguishing the tumor from an infection of bone. The clinical features and the roentgenographic picture may not be helpful unless pulmonary metastatic disease is present. Histologically, this tumor may be difficult to distinguish from neuroblastoma or rhabdomyosarcoma metastatic to bone. A positive periodic acid–Schiff reaction will eliminate neuroblastoma from consideration. A careful search must be made for a possible primary tumor. The usual age of onset of this tumor differs from that of neuroblastoma or rhabdomyosarcoma.

The patient should have initial tomograms of lungs, a roentgenographic skeletal survey, and a radioisotopic bone scan to detect metastatic disease. If there are symptoms referable to the central nervous system, a brain scan or computed axial tomography is indicated.

Treatment. Localized Ewing sarcoma of bone is treated with a combination of high-dose irradiation and chemotherapy, but the roles of both these treatment forms remain to be established. The tumoricidal dose of radiation ranges from 5000–7000 rads. Treatment ports should give adequate coverage to the tumor with normal tissue spared as much as possible. Studies are under way evaluating the effectiveness of lower doses of irradiation in combination with chemotherapy.

Disease clinically localized at the time of diagnosis develops with high frequency into systemic disease, even if the local tumor is controlled by irradiation. All patients should, therefore, receive chemotherapy. Active agents are vincristine, cyclophosphamide, dactinomycin, and doxorubicin (Adriamycin). A 4-drug regimen combining these agents gives the longest disease-free period after initiation of therapy. Other chemotherapeutic regimens in combination with radiation therapy are under current evaluation.

Prognosis. The results of current intensive treatment regimens have not been completely evaluated. About half of patients so treated can achieve long-term disease-free survival. With intensive chemotherapy, however, there may be late appearance of metastatic disease, usually in other bones or in the central nervous system. A long period of follow-up is necessary, therefore, for accurate assessment of treatment.

Metastatic disease at the time of diagnosis indicates a poor prognosis. Tumors in the pelvis carry the least favorable prognosis, and tumors of the humerus or femur are less favored than those arising distal to the knee or elbow. Fever at the time of diagnosis is an

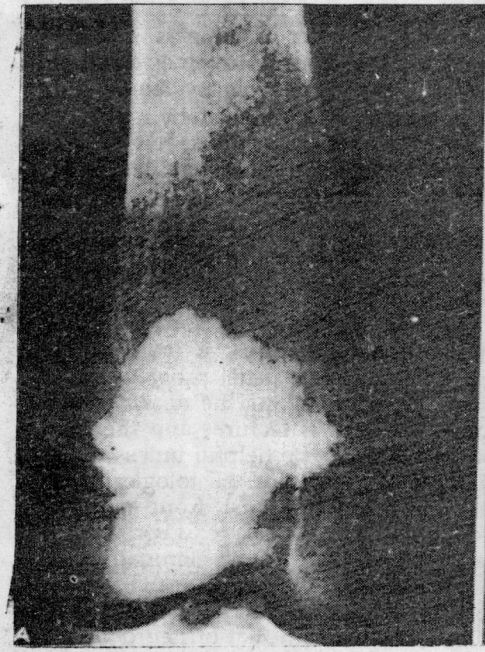
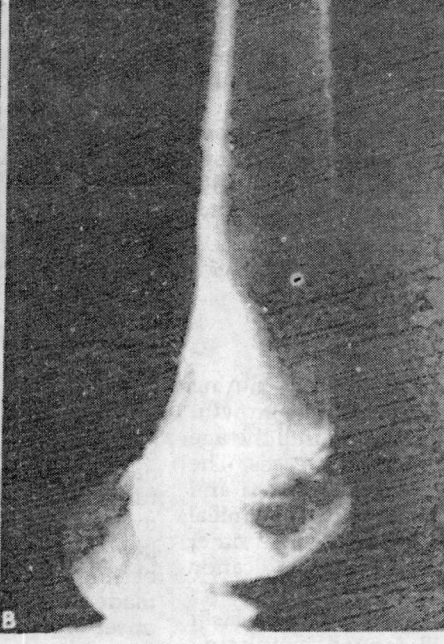

Figure 15–17 Anterior and lateral views of the distal femur of a patient with Ewing sarcoma. The lateral view shows the destruction of cortex, with growth of tumor into the surrounding soft tissues. With time, progressive calcification of periosteum lifted away from the bone may lead to a typical "sunburst" appearance.

unfavorable sign. Females respond to treatment with longer periods of disease-free survival than do males.

15.15 CHONDROSARCOMA

This tumor of bone is rare in children and is usually seen during the 2nd decade. It occurs with equal frequency in boys and girls. It is associated with Ollier disease and Maffucci syndrome. Exposure to ionizing radiation is an etiologic factor in some patients.

The histology is that of malignant formation of cartilage. The tumor may arise in any bone but is most frequent in the pelvis. It occurs in flat bones of the trunk as well as in long bones of the extremities. It can metastasize to lung and bone, but the usual form of spread is local extension to contiguous normal tissues, with recurrence following surgical removal.

The clinical features are local pain and tumor mass. Diagnosis can be suspected from the roentgenogram of the area; it must be confirmed by biopsy. These tumors must be examined histologically with great care since osteosarcoma can have a large chondrosarcomatous component. The prognosis for these 2 tumors is quite different in terms of the likelihood of metastatic disease. Treatment is surgical removal of the tumor or amputation if an extremity is involved. Chondrosarcoma is relatively radioresistant. Because of its rarity the effectiveness of chemotherapy has not been adequately evaluated.

15.16 RETINOBLASTOMA

See also Sec 25.13.

This tumor has an annual incidence of 3.4/million children, similar for black and white children. The average age at time of diagnosis is 8 mo for bilateral tumors, 26 mo for unilateral tumors. Boys and girls are equally represented in both forms.

About 30% of patients with retinoblastoma have bilateral involvement; they have a dominantly inherited predisposition to retinoblastoma. About 10–20% of patients with unilateral disease also have the genetic predisposition. The retinoblastoma gene is thought to be on the long arm of chromosome 13 because bilateral retinoblastoma is seen in patients who have deletion of or within the long arm of this chromosome. More than 50% of the children with this 13 q− chromosome syndrome will develop retinoblastoma. The syndrome also includes growth delay, mental retardation, and a characteristic facies consisting of a broad, prominent nasal bridge and a short nose with a broad tip.

The retinoblastoma gene also carries increased risk of other tumors; about 1% of the survivors of the hereditary form of retinoblastoma will develop osteosarcoma at an average age of around 10 yr. The osteosarcoma may occur in an area irradiated for treatment for retinoblastoma or at a nonirradiated site. Patients with retinoblastoma have increased levels of carcinoembryonic antigen, and, with the hereditary form, abnormally increased levels can be found also in asymptomatic family members.

Mental retardation is seen with increased frequency in patients with retinoblastoma, possibly due to the abnormality of chromosome 13. Retinoblastoma patients who have retained vision, and their families, generally have normal intelligence.

Pathology.   The tumor usually develops in the posterior portion of the retina. It consists of small, closely packed, round, malignant cells with scanty cytoplasm. Occasionally, rosette formation occurs, which is thought to be an abortive attempt at formation of rods and cones.

The tumors may grow in an exophytic or endophytic manner. Endophytic growth is more common. The endophytic tumors arise from the inner nuclear, nerve fiber, or ganglion cell layer of the retina. They have a whitish appearance with vessels overlying the surface. The exophytic type comes from the external nuclear layer and may present the appearance of a solid retinal detachment. Intraocular extension into the vitreous may occur with the endophytic type, and there may be metastatic seeding through the subretinal space or through the vitreous. Extraocular extension may occur.

The tumor may also extend by infiltration through the lamina cribrosa directly into the substance of the optic nerve and into the subarachnoid space surrounding the optic nerve. With extension to the choroid layer there may be infiltration of the veins in that area with distant hematogenous metastasis, primarily to bone and bone marrow. Direct extension through the optic nerve may lead to central nervous system invasion. Tumor cells may appear in the spinal fluid.

Stage I indicates tumor confined to the retina. Stage II tumor remains confined to the globe. With Stage III there is regional extraocular extension of the tumor, either beyond the cut end of the optic nerve at enucleation or into the orbital contents. With Stage IV there are distant metastases, either by extension into the brain or by hematogenous dissemination to bone or bone marrow.

Clinical Manifestations. It usually presents with leukokoria, an asymptomatic patient being discovered to have a yellowish-white reflex in the pupil indicative of the tumor behind the lens. Other presenting findings can be development of a squint in the affected eye, or, with more advanced tumor, complaints of poor vision, pain, pupillary irregularity, or hyphema. With far advanced tumor there may be proptosis, signs of increasing intracranial pressure, or bone pain associated with metastatic disease.

More than 80% of patients with the hereditary bilateral form have tumors involving both eyes at the time of diagnosis. Delay in involvement of the 2nd eye rarely exceeds 18 mo. The usual appearance of the eye at diagnosis is shown in Fig 25–2.

Diagnosis. The finding of leukokoria must be followed by a careful funduscopic examination, which may necessitate anesthesia. Concurrent fluorescein angiography, computed tomographic scanning, and ultrasonography of the globe will provide additional information. In about 75% of patients a roentgenogram will show mineralization within the globe. Other causes of leukokoria include retinal detachment, persistent hyperplastic primary vitreous, nematode endophthalmitis (usually visceral larva migrans), bacterial panendophthalmitis, cataract, coloboma of the choroid, and the retinopathy of prematurity. These conditions can be distinguished by an experienced ophthalmologist.

Additional studies should include a roentgenographic skeletal survey, with particular emphasis on films of the face and skull. Radionuclide scans of bone and brain should be done as well as examination of the bone marrow and cerebrospinal fluid for tumor cells. Increased levels of plasma carcinoembryonic antigen and alpha-fetoprotein are frequently found at the time of diagnosis, which decrease to normal levels after removal of the tumor. Their subsequent rise may indicate recurrence of tumor.

Treatment. The treatment of choice for unilateral tumor is enucleation, including at least 10 mm of the optic nerve. If the tumor is entirely contained within the retina (Stage I), this should be adequate for tumor control. If Stage II tumor is found, with vitreous seeding, extension to the optic nerve head, or choroidal involvement, a regimen of chemotherapy with vincristine and cyclophosphamide should be given for 1 yr because of the risk of dissemination. For Stage III tumor radiotherapy to the orbit and skull should be added, and weekly intrathecal administrations of methotrexate for 6 wk are recommended. If distant metastases are found at the time of diagnosis, an appropriate program of radiotherapy and chemotherapy should be designed.

For patients with bilateral disease, generally the more severely affected eye is removed for histologic confirmation of diagnosis and for staging. The tumor in the remaining eye may be controlled by appropriate combinations of radiotherapy, cryotherapy, or light coagulation. For these patients every effort is made to preserve sight. Radiation therapy may cause the development of cataract, which can be treated surgically.

Following enucleation an ocular prosthesis should be fitted, usually about 6 wk after the surgical procedure. With the growth of the child new prostheses must be fitted periodically to assure adequate growth of the orbital bones.

Prognosis. The overall survival rate for patients with retinoblastoma is about 85%. Deaths are caused by intracranial spread or metastatic disease. Patients with Stage I or II disease have a greater than 90% likelihood of survival, and with Stage III disease 70% can survive. Most series report few or no survivors among patients with Stage IV disease. For patients with bilateral disease the long-term prognosis must take into account the risk of subsequent osteogenic sarcoma.

Parents and patients should have genetic counseling. As more patients survive this tumor, the incidence of bilateral cases can be expected to increase. The frequency of retinoblastoma in Holland doubled from 1930–1960, bilaterally affected patients increasing from 19–36%. Each of the children of patients with bilateral retinoblastoma has a 50% risk of being similarly affected. Of patients with unilateral tumor, the risk for their children of having retinoblastoma is 4–5%. If uninvolved parents have a child with retinoblastoma, the risk for a later-born sibling is about 4–6%.

15.17 GASTROINTESTINAL NEOPLASMS

Cancer of the gastrointestinal tract is unusual in children, but an awareness of certain tumors is important for their early diagnosis.

Salivary Gland Tumors. Most lesions causing enlargement of the salivary glands result from such benign causes as inflammation or the formation of mucoceles. Most tumors involving the salivary glands are benign, such as hemangiomas, hamartomas, or the mixed tumor of salivary glands (pleomorphic adenoma).

Mixed tumors are rare during the 1st decade of life; they are occasionally seen during the 2nd decade, evenly distributed between boys and girls. The gland most usually involved is the parotid, and the most frequent presenting manifestation is a mass in that area. The mass is usually hard, movable, and nontender. Facial nerve paralysis may occur. Treatment is excision of the tumor mass. The prognosis for control of the disease is excellent, though occasional recurrences may necessitate a 2nd surgical procedure.

The mucoepidermoid carcinoma is the malignant tumor of salivary glands; it is found primarily during the 2nd decade of life in children. It presents most frequently in the parotid gland, usually as a hard, nontender mass. Metastases to regional lymph nodes are unusual, the tumor most frequently remaining confined within the gland of origin. Treatment is excision, and the prognosis is excellent, though local recurrences may necessitate a 2nd surgical procedure.

Nasopharyngeal Carcinoma (Lymphoepithelioma). This tumor occurs in the nasopharynx, usually during the 2nd decade of life; it may occasionally be seen in the younger child. The sex distribution is even. This tumor is a carcinoma of the epithelium of the nasopharynx.

The most frequent early finding is cervical lymphadenopathy, usually unilateral and frequently tender. Additional early symptoms and signs are trismus, epistaxis, sore throat, and difficulty in swallowing. There may be weight loss due to dysphagia.

On careful examination, it is possible to find the primary tumor somewhere in the nasopharynx in the majority of affected children and establish the diagnosis by biopsy of it. At times, however, the diagnosis is made through a lymph node biopsy in which the metastatic tumor is identified; it is then necessary to find the primary site by multiple biopsies of the posterior nasopharynx of the involved side. Extension occurs locally to the base of the skull and to the soft tissues surrounding the nasopharynx. Regional lymph node metastases are frequent, and there may be hematogenous spread to bone and lung.

The primary therapy is irradiation to the involved areas of the nasopharynx. Experience with chemotherapy is limited; cyclophosphamide, vincristine, and doxorubicin (Adriamycin) have been shown to have some effect. The prognosis for local control by irradiation is good. More than half of the patients should have no recurrence; late metastases to lung or bone may occur, however, and long-term follow-up is necessary.

Carcinoma of the Stomach. This form of gastrointestinal cancer has been rarely reported in children. The clinical manifestations are similar to those in adults, such as weight loss, vomiting, abdominal pain, hematemesis, a palpable upper abdominal mass, and, occasionally, perforation with peritonitis. Metastases can be found in the liver, abdominal lymph nodes, and peritoneal serosal surface. The histologic pattern is usually that of a mucinous adenocarcinoma. Resection should be done, if possible, and if metastatic disease is present,

chemotherapy with 5-fluorouracil, the nitrosoureas, or doxorubicin (Adriamycin) can be attempted. The prognosis is extremely poor.

Pancreatic Carcinoma. This tumor is extremely rare. The usual site of origin is the head of the pancreas, and the initial clinical findings are those of upper abdominal mass, weight loss, and pain. Obstruction to the common bile duct may lead to obstructive jaundice. There can be regional extension and metastasis within the abdominal cavity. Hematogenous metastasis can spread to the liver and lung. Surgical resection should be attempted, but in most reported cases the tumor has extended beyond the pancreas at the time of diagnosis. The prognosis is poor.

Carcinoma of the Colon. This unusual tumor of childhood almost never occurs before the 2nd decade of life. It is most frequently a mucinous adenocarcinoma and can arise in any segment of the large bowel. Predisposing conditions are familial multiple polyposis, ulcerative colitis, regional enteritis, and the Peutz-Jeghers syndrome.

The tumor is rarely confined to the mucosa at the time of diagnosis; it has usually extended through the serosa with involvement of the regional lymph nodes. Other metastasis can occur within the abdominal cavity, and there may be hematogenous dissemination to the liver. Late involvement of bone and bone marrow may occur.

Affected patients may present bloody stools or melena. Abdominal pain, which may be colicky, anorexia, and weight loss are common. An abdominal mass can be found, and there may be liver enlargement due to metastases. The clinical findings are usually suggestive of large bowel cancer, and the diagnosis can be confirmed by barium enema. Ultrasound examination and computed tomographic scanning may give further information concerning the extent of the disease, and radionuclide scans of liver and spleen will help detect hepatic metastasis.

Surgical removal of the tumor should be attempted, but complete resection is not usually possible. Chemotherapy with 5-fluorouracil, vincristine, the nitrosoureas, doxorubicin (Adriamycin), and methotrexate have been used, but temporary response can be expected in only about one third of the patients. The prognosis is poor.

15.18 NEOPLASMS OF THE LIVER

Malignant tumors of the liver occur with an annual frequency of 2/million children from the ages of 1–15 yr. Two kinds of primary liver cancer occur in children: hepatoblastoma and hepatocellular carcinoma (hepatoma). These vary in histology and some aspects of epidemiology, but the clinical features and approaches to treatment are quite similar.

Epidemiology. Hepatoblastoma is the more common; it is seen almost exclusively in children under the age of 3 yr, with half of the patients being 18 mo of age or younger. Boys predominate in a ratio of 1.5:1. For hepatocellular carcinoma there are 2 age peaks of onset, the 1st below the age of 4 yr and the 2nd from 12–15 yr. This tumor predominates in boys by a ratio of 1.3:1.

The congenital defects associated with hepatic malignancy are similar to those that occur in patients with Wilms tumor and adrenocortical neoplasm, such as congenital hemihypertrophy and extensive hemangiomas. Hepatic tumor and Wilms tumor have occurred in the same patient, a phenomenon which indicates that similar mechanisms may be involved in the predisposition to all 3 neoplasms. Both hepatoblastoma and hepatocellular carcinoma have been reported in siblings. Patients with the chronic form of hereditary tyrosinemia who survive beyond the age of 2 yr have about a 40% risk of developing hepatocellular carcinoma. Hepatocellular carcinoma has also occurred in patients with the cirrhosis of congenital bile duct atresia or that of neonatal hepatitis. Patients with de Toni-Fanconi syndrome and von Gierke disease have developed liver tumors.

Pathology. Hepatoblastoma may consist entirely of cells with an epithelial appearance, or there may be an admixture of mesenchymal components. Typically, the epithelial components consist of thin cords or plates of cells. These cords are surrounded by sinusoidal vessels and separated by fibrous septa. Gland-like structures may be seen. The individual cells are poorly differentiated and may resemble embryonal hepatic cells. In the mixed type of tumor, mesenchymal components also may be seen, and it is not uncommon to find areas of primitive osteoid tissue. Foci of extramedullary erythropoiesis are usual.

The hepatocellular carcinoma consists of well-differentiated large polygonal cells with a highly eosinophilic cytoplasm. The cells form hepatic cordlike structures surrounded by sinusoidal vessels. There may be nodules of cholangioma composed of sclerosing adenocarcinoma. Extramedullary erythropoiesis is found in foci throughout the tumor.

In both forms of hepatic cancer the right lobe is more frequently involved than the left. In about half of patients, however, the tumor involves both lobes or is multicentric. The most frequent site of metastasis is the lungs; local extension within the abdomen is also common. Less often, the central nervous system may be the site of metastasis. Unusual metastatic sites are lymph nodes, bone, or bone marrow. The only useful criteria for prognosis are whether the tumor is resectable and whether there are distant metastases.

Clinical Manifestations. The most frequent finding is an upper abdominal mass with abdominal enlargement. Pain is present in only 15–20% of patients at the time of diagnosis; anorexia and weight loss occur in the same frequency. Even less common initial complaints are vomiting and jaundice. Rarely, there may be virilization in affected boys due to production of gonadotropin by the tumor.

Diagnosis. The major diagnostic problem is the differentiation of hepatic enlargement due to primary tumor from that caused by other diseases, benign or malignant. A careful search should be made for another primary site of tumor, most frequently neuroblastoma. Infantile hemangioendotheliomas and cavernous hemangiomas can enlarge the liver, and a careful survey for other hemangiomas should be made. Metabolic storage diseases may also simulate hepatic tumor.

Laboratory studies of liver function are most often normal. Bilirubin levels are increased in about 20% of patients, and about the same proportion may have abnormally increased values for SGOT, SGPT, and alkaline phosphatase activities. Most patients will have increased serum levels of alpha-fetoprotein and increased urinary excretion of cystathionine.

The roentgenogram of the abdomen will demonstrate hepatic enlargement; in about 30% of patients calcification will be seen within the tumor. There is usually no displacement of the kidneys on intravenous pyelography, but large hepatic tumors occasionally displace the right kidney downward. In about 10% of patients pulmonary metastases are present at the time of diagnosis. Angiography is particularly valuable in distinguishing liver tumors from hemangiomas and can also provide the surgeon with an indication of the blood supply of a tumor. Radionuclide scan of the liver will indicate tumor as will ultrasound and computed tomography of the abdomen. Final diagnosis depends upon histologic examination.

Treatment. The only effective treatment is complete surgical resection. In only about one third of patients are the size and location of the tumor at the time of diagnosis such that complete excision can be attempted. The tumor is relatively radioresistant; there are as yet no effective chemotherapeutic regimens, though various combinations of vincristine, 5-fluorouracil, dactinomycin, cyclophosphamide, the nitrosoureas, and doxorubicin (Adriamycin) have been tested.

Prognosis. The prognosis for patients with hepatic tumors is poor. Overall survival rate in hepatoblastoma is 35% and in hepatocellular carcinoma, only 13%. The survivors are represented entirely by patients who have had complete surgical excision of the tumor. Less than complete excision is always associated with local recurrence and eventually with distant metastasis and death.

15.19 GONADAL AND GERM CELL NEOPLASMS

Epidemiology. Gonadal and germ cell tumors are uncommon in children, occurring at a rate of 2.2/million white children and approximately the same for black children. Most reports indicate a female preponderance, but the significance of this is difficult to assess because most series deal with either testicular or ovarian tumors. The age incidence for both ovarian and testicular tumors peaks below the age of 2 yr, with a 2nd increase in rate beginning after the age of 6 for ovarian tumors and after the age of 14 for testicular tumors. Gonadal dysgenesis is the consistent underlying clinical feature of patients who develop gonadoblastoma (Sec 18.37).

Pathology. The germ cell tumors are an interrelated group of malignancies expressing the multipotential characteristics of differentiation of the cells from which they arise. The tumors may express differentiation of extraembryonic tissues (choriocarcinoma or yolk sac carcinoma) or intraembryonic tissues (teratoma). Primitive tumors without evidence of differentiation are

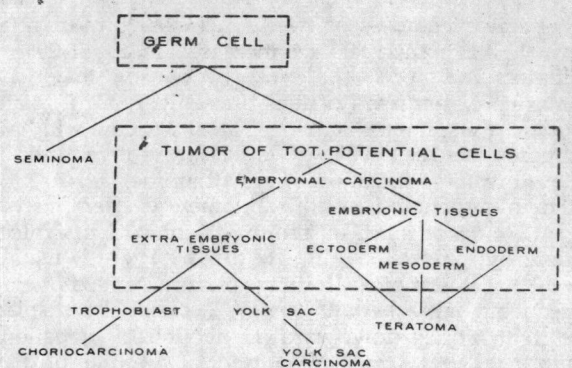

Figure 15–18   A concept of tumors of germ cell origin. (From Pierce GB, Abell MR: Pathol Annu 5:27, 1970.)

called embryonal carcinoma. These relationships are expressed graphically in Fig 15–18. That mixtures of the different cell types may be present in the same tumor confirms their interrelationship.

Germ cell tumors occur most commonly in the gonads but may infrequently appear in such sites as the retroperitoneum, mediastinum, sacrococcygeum, or central nervous system. These tumors in extragonadal sites are thought to represent aberrancies in the migration of germ cells from the yolk sac into the developing fetus.

The least differentiated of these tumors is *embryonal carcinoma*. The histologic pattern may consist of sheets of closely packed cells, of an adenocarcinomatous appearance with irregular glandular spaces, or of a mesodermal picture with an arrangement of cell types suggesting embryonal muscle or adipose tissue.

Differentiation may occur in the direction of extraembryonic tissues, resulting in *choriocarcinoma* or *yolk sac carcinoma*. Choriocarcinoma is recognized as a component of both gonadal and extragonadal germ cell neoplasms. It is encountered after puberty in the testicle but may be seen in the ovary both before and after puberty. It is uncommon as the predominant pattern of the tumor. There is frequently hemorrhagic necrosis, which may be an important clue to the presence of choriocarcinoma in a tumor of germ cell origin. There are masses of cytotrophoblast overlain by caps of syncytiotrophoblastic giant cells. The yolk sac carcinoma (endodermal sinus tumor) has histologic features resembling the endodermal sinuses of the placenta.

A pattern of differentiation predominantly in the direction of embryonic tissues leads to *teratomas* or *teratocarcinomas*, which must have elements of all 3 germ layers. The malignant component of a teratocarcinoma is usually an embryonal carcinoma.

Seminoma is considered to be a related tumor but occurs almost exclusively during the 2nd decade of life and later. The tissue is cellular, with histologically clear cells aggregated in lobules and separated by a fibrous stroma.

These tumors metastasize to regional lymph nodes, with hematogenous dissemination to lung and bone. Just as the primary tumor may contain a mixture of histologic elements, the metastatic disease is generally also mixed, but occasionally a representation purely of

1 cell type or another may be found. Metastasis from ovarian tumors may also be found within the peritoneal cavity, both by implantation and by regional extension.

Clinical Manifestations.   During the 1st yr of life, the usual initial sign of a testicular tumor is a mass in the scrotum, sometimes found at birth. Delays in diagnosis arise when the mass is initially considered a hydrocele. The tumors are usually not painful at first, nor are there signs of inflammation. An initial finding of metastatic disease is uncommon.

In the older boy a gradual swelling of the involved testicle is usually noted over some wk, and pain and tenderness are found in more than half of cases. Clinical complications of metastasis to retroperitoneal lymph nodes or to lungs may be the initial findings in some patients. Gynecomastia may occur as an effect of chorionic gonadotropin. In a few patients the early clinical findings may be those of disseminated cancer, such as weight loss, anorexia, and lethargy.

With ovarian tumors the most common initial symptoms are pain, nausea, and vomiting. Some patients have no symptoms, an abdominal mass or abdominal fullness being noted incidentally. An acute onset of abdominal pain may occur in patients who have ovarian torsion; in such patients, the findings may simulate an inflammatory process, such as appendicitis. Germ cell tumors of the ovary seldom make their initial appearance through signs of metastatic disease.

Sacrococcygeal teratoma or *teratocarcinoma* is usually detected during infancy and frequently at the time of birth. The most common finding is a mass in the area of the sacrum and buttocks. About 25% of these tumors contain a malignant component, but initial metastatic disease is uncommon. Additional symptoms and signs result if the growing mass causes obstruction of the rectum or urinary tract. Associated clinical features are congenital anomalies involving the lower vertebrae, genitourinary system, and anorectum.

Initial clinical features of patients with germ cell tumors arising in other extragonadal sites depend on the location of the primary tumor. In the abdomen, tumors will usually present as growing masses. In the chest there may be respiratory symptoms. In the head and neck area, findings will depend upon the impairment of function caused in surrounding tissues.

Diagnosis.   The chief diagnostic aid is careful examination. Testicular tumors are solid, opaque to transillumination, and usually painless; they must be distinguished from scrotal hernia or hydrocele. Abdominal pain, nausea, and vomiting in a girl must be carefully evaluated; and their acute onset must always raise the possibility of ovarian tumor. Ultrasound and computed axial tomographic examination of the abdomen may help further define the size and position of any mass felt.

A sacrococcygeal tumor in early infancy should immediately suggest teratoma. Other masses found in the same area include meningoceles, chordomas, duplications of the rectum, neurogenic tumors, lipoma, rhabdomyosarcoma, and hemangioma. At times, masses in the area may be confused with perirectal abscess, but absence of other signs of inflammation should exclude that possibility. Germ cell tumors in other extragonadal sites cannot in most cases be identified until excision or biopsy has been done and the histologic character established.

All patients with suspected germ cell tumors should have roentgenograms of the chest and radionuclide scans of bone to detect any metastatic disease. Ultrasound and computed tomographic examination of the abdomen in boys with testicular tumors may be of value in demonstrating retroperitoneal lymph node metastasis. Levels of alpha-fetoprotein may be increased, but this finding is not specific. Some patients have increased chorionic gonadotropin levels, even when later examination of tissue does not indicate a major component of choriocarcinoma. The levels of these 2 biologic markers prior to treatment may be useful in subsequent evaluation of the effectiveness of therapy.

Treatment. Therapy depends primarily upon prompt recognition and surgical removal of the tumor. Even when no definable metastatic disease is found, malignant germ cell tumors should subsequently receive combination chemotherapy because it is likely that inapparent dissemination has already occurred. Optimal chemotherapy is still uncertain; regimens using vincristine, cyclophosphamide, cis-platin, bleomycin, and dactinomycin are most commonly used. For germ cell tumors of the testicle the value of routine laparotomy to assess retroperitoneal lymph nodes for metastatic disease and the role of routine radiation therapy to retroperitoneal node areas require further study.

Prognosis. The main determinant of prognosis is the extent of disease at the time of diagnosis. It is important, therefore, that germ cell tumors be suspected as early as possible. It is difficult to assess results of treatment because only a small number of patients have been treated in any consistent manner; treatment should be planned, however, with the assumption that early intervention and adjuvant chemotherapy provide reasonable expectation for long-term disease-free survival.

OTHER GONADAL TUMORS

Other tumors of the gonads are also uncommon in children. *Sertoli tumors* are usually benign and arise from sustentacular cells originating from the primitive gonadal mesenchyme. Malignant tumors of this origin are found almost exclusively in adults but occur rarely in boys. The initial sign is usually an enlarging, firm, testicular mass. Occasionally, endocrine activity can occur, with sexual precocity or gynecomastia. The tumor is most likely to occur during the 1st yr or 2 of life but may be encountered through the 2nd decade. In patients exhibiting effects of endocrine activity, urinary excretion of 17-ketosteroids will be increased. Treatment is removal of the tumor. Because malignancy is rare, no further therapy is to be recommended other than careful follow-up.

Seminoma of the testicle is also rare in children. It appears as a firm tumor of the testis and characteristically metastasizes to retroperitoneal lymph nodes. This tumor is radiosensitive; accordingly, radiation therapy is important in the treatment of metastatic disease.

Almost half of ovarian tumors are caused by benign *ovarian cysts.* These cysts may be found incidentally at laparotomy for other purposes or on physical examination of an otherwise well child. Occasionally, torsion of the involved ovary can cause abdominal pain, nausea, and vomiting, with the picture of an acute abdomen. Other ovarian tumors are quite uncommon. The *granulosa–theca cell* tumor is usually associated with a mass in the lower abdomen and precocious puberty. Removal of the tumor alleviates the endocrine abnormality. Only rarely do these tumors manifest malignant potential by recurrence or dissemination. *Cystadenocarcinomas* of the ovary are even more uncommon and cannot be differentiated by clinical manifestations from other ovarian malignant tumors. *Dysgerminomas* of the ovary are composed of primitive germ cells and histologically resemble testicular seminomas. They are radiosensitive and respond to chemotherapy as do seminomas. Most dysgerminomas are confined to the ovary at the time of surgery, and the likelihood of long-term disease-free survival for such patients is excellent. *Hemangiomas* may involve the ovary (Sec 24.7). Occasionally, ovarian enlargement will be the initial manifestation of *lymphoma.*

Gonadoblastomas are found exclusively in patients with gonadal dysgenesis. Eighty per cent of affected patients are phenotypic females, usually with evidences of virilization. The others are phenotypic males, usually with such abnormalities as cryptorchidism, hypospadias, or female internal or secondary sex organs. The gonadoblastoma is regarded as cancer in situ from which germinomas may develop. The tumor may be bilateral; it presents as a growing mass with the added features of virilization in some female patients. Histologic examination shows an intimate mixture of germ cells and elements resembling immature granulosa or Sertoli cells, with or without Leydig cells or lutein-type cells. The tumor should be removed.

15.20 MISCELLANEOUS CARCINOMAS

CARCINOMA OF THE THYROID

Thyroid cancer is discussed in Sec 18.16. Its relationship to irradiation of the head and neck in children is of particular importance. Medullary carcinoma of the thyroid may occur sporadically or in a familial pattern. In its familial form, it is associated with Marfan-like habitus, pheochromocytoma, hyperparathyroidism, and mucosal neuromas. Its familial character and its association with other endocrine tumors (multiple endocrine neoplasia) are of particular importance.

CARCINOMA OF THE ADRENAL GLAND

Adrenocortical carcinoma is quite rare. It may occur at any age during childhood, but more often during the 1st few yr. The tumor may be associated with hemangiomas of the skin, hemihypertrophy, urinary tract anomalies, and astrocytomas. There is a predominance of girls among patients with this tumor. The usual presenting symptoms are secondary to the endocrine function of the cancer. Affected children present signs of adrenal hyperfunction (Sec 18.24), which may include Cushing syndrome (Sec 18.25), virilization (Sec 18.24), feminization (Sec 18.27), or a combination of these.

ADENOCARCINOMA OF THE VAGINA AND CERVIX

This tumor, once extremely rare, has become more common as the result of exposure in utero to diethylstilbestrol given to the mothers of affected patients during pregnancy (Sec 19.5).

CARCINOMA OF THE BREAST

Unilateral or bilateral enlargement of the breast is almost never a cause to consider cancer in children. Prepubertal enlargement is almost always related to growth of normal glandular tissue, due either to an excessively sensitive end organ or to an inappropriately early production of stimulatory hormones. By 1972 there had been reported fewer than 25 acceptable examples of carcinoma of the breast in patients under 20 yr old. The tumors tended to be fairly well differentiated and slow growing; most were localized in the breast, though axillary metastases have occasionally been found. The tumors have been circumscribed, firm, and painless in contrast to the softer, more diffuse, and generalized involvement of the breast in glandular hypertrophy. A biopsy is essential before surgery is undertaken. With removal the prognosis has been reported excellent, though local recurrences may arise.

CANCER OF THE SKIN

Cancer of the skin is rare in children (Sec 24.32). *Malignant melanoma* may occur during the 1st 2 decades of life with clinical behavior much like that in adults. It usually appears as a rapidly growing, easily traumatized, ulcerated lesion which is darkly pigmented or has changed in color. It may be found on any part of the body. Because malignant melanoma is rare in children, an excisional diagnostic biopsy is initially indicated. If malignancy is found, then wide local resection is indicated, which may necessitate skin grafting. Regional lymph nodes should be carefully examined; if they are enlarged, then a lymph node dissection also should be done. For patients with disseminated disease, temporary clinical responses may be obtained with chemotherapy.

Two conditions predispose to the development of skin cancer in children. *Xeroderma pigmentosum* is an autosomal recessive condition in which there is a defective DNA repair mechanism. When the affected person is exposed to sunlight, the ultraviolet radiation produces breaks in DNA, which provide an opportunity for mutant malignant growth. The skin because of its exposure, is the organ of primary involvement. Multiple skin cancers appear in the exposed areas, particularly on the head, arms, and legs. Surgical resection of the tumors is necessary, and affected children must be protected as much as possible from sunlight. The *nevoid basal cell carcinoma syndrome* (basal cell nevus syndrome) is discussed in Sec 24.32.

MISCELLANEOUS BENIGN TUMORS

A variety of benign tumors in infants and children present problems in differential diagnosis; many will also require treatment. Some can be life threatening though histologically benign.

15.21   BENIGN TUMORS AND TUMOR-LIKE PROCESSES IN BONE

A number of benign processes in bone must be recognized by the clinician and distinguished from malignant tumors in order to avoid tragic consequences of overtreatment. Some of them may be reactions to trauma, but the putative trauma usually cannot be identified. Others appear to be hamartomas, or true overgrowths of normal tissue in situ. Still other lesions, less well understood, are considered to be benign neoplasia, with perhaps the potential for malignancy.

Osteoid osteoma is an uncommon lesion which occurs most often in adolescent boys; it usually involves femur or tibia, much less frequently the spine, humerus, or phalanges. The cardinal clinical feature is pain, dull at first and accentuated by weight-bearing, typically more severe at night, and relieved by aspirin. After weeks or months of increasing pain there may be localized tenderness, but signs of inflammation are unusual. The roentgenogram is diagnostic, disclosing a sharply demarcated radiolucent nidus of osteoid tissue surrounded by sclerotic bone. There may be calcification of the osteoid within the nidus. The sclerotic response is more marked when the lesion is cortical, less when medullary or subperiosteal. Treatment is surgical. The nidus must be completely removed to prevent recurrence.

Osteoblastoma is the name commonly given by some investigators to a number of processes thought to be closely related (ossifying fibroma, osteogenic fibroma, osteoid fibroma, fibrous osteoma, and giant osteoid osteoma). The features of pain and distribution of lesions are those of osteoid osteoma, except that osteoblastoma appears more likely to cause nerve root pain as a consequence of spinal involvement. The roentgenographic appearance is of an expanding translucent lesion of bone, though it may contain flecks of calcification and have some sclerotic bone about it. Extension into soft tissues with formation of a mass is not uncommon. Roentgenographic differentiation from osteosarcoma or aneurysmal bone cyst may be difficult; it may be particularly difficult to distinguish an osteoblastoma from an aneurysmal bone cyst when the spine is involved. Histologic features are sometimes suggestive of true neoplasm. Treatment is curettage following histologic verification of the diagnosis.

Subperiosteal cortical defects are eccentric in location and presumably arise from the periosteum to erode the cortex from without rather than from within. They have been estimated to occur in as many as 53% of boys and 31% of girls, most commonly from 4–8 yr of age. They are found always in the metaphyses of cylindrical bones, usually of the lower extremities. The roentgenographic picture is characteristic. They are asymptomatic and heal spontaneously. Their recognition is important lest they be mistaken for malignant lesions.

Nonosteogenic fibroma occurs most commonly in late childhood and early adolescence and may be related to a subperiosteal cortical defect. Its true incidence is unknown, with about half of all cases being found incidentally when roentgenograms are made for other purposes. There are often no symptoms, but chronic bone pain may occur. A pathologic fracture may be the 1st sign. The ends of the shafts of the long bones of the lower extremity are most commonly involved. The roentgenographic picture of a rarefied scalloped lesion is so characteristic that biopsy for histologic confirmation may not be required. Treatment is often not required, spontaneous cure being expected after months or years. Curettage or other interventions may be required for weakened or fractured bones.

Osteoma represents a local overgrowth of osseous tissue occurring only in membranous bone. It is most common in adults and may produce no symptoms unless the local tumor interferes with function because of location in the orbit, in the sinuses, on the hard palate, or in the mandible. Tumors of stable size need no treatment unless they interfere with function. They may be associated with colonic polyps.

Osteochondromas (cartilaginous exostoses) are the solitary lesions corresponding to those of osteochondromatosis (hereditary multiple exostoses, Sec 23.17). They occur in any bone formed in cartilage, most often near the cartilaginous ends of femur or tibia at the knee. Growth appears in childhood or early adolescence and ceases with closure of the neighboring epiphysis, at which time calcification of its cartilaginous cap occurs. A mass may be present or pain if there is a fracture. The roentgenographic features are characteristic; some lesions are pediculated, others sessile. Reactivation of growth occurs spontaneously on rare occasions, sometimes after a fracture; such lesions should be considered malignant until proved otherwise by excision biopsy. Lesions should be removed prophylactically when possible, particularly if there are symptoms.

Enchondromas are the solitary lesions corresponding to those of *multiple enchondromatosis* (Ollier disease, Sec 23.17). They are less common than osteochondromas and are most likely to involve metacarpals and phalanges or their counterparts in the foot. Enchondromas appear as deforming masses or become apparent when they induce pathologic fractures. Roentgenograms show circumscribed areas of rarefied bone with thinning and often bulging of the cortex and stippled calcification. Lesions in the hands or feet are benign; those in the large long bones, in any diaphysis, or in membra-

nous bone have malignant potential and may be difficult to separate histologically from malignant lesions. Treatment is curettage of clearly benign lesions or wide excision of doubtful ones.

Chondroblastoma is a rare tumor seen usually in boys from the ages of 10–20 yr. It appears in the epiphyses and particularly in the femoral epiphysis and the head of the humerus. The 1st symptom is likely to be dull pain; a roentgenogram discloses a rounded or oval tumor with sharp outline, sometimes scalloped, often with islands of calcification. The histologic picture is generally characteristic but may be confused with that of a malignant lesion. Treatment has generally been curettage. Recurrences are known, however, and the malignant potential of this tumor is not yet fully assessed. Wide resection, therefore, may be indicated.

Chondromyxoid fibroma may be closely related to chondroblastoma. Differences may depend on the site of the lesion, this tumor preferring the metaphyses of long bones. It may appear at any age but usually is found in adolescents or young adults. The usual symptom is mild pain; tenderness is common, and there may be expansion of bone, a mass, or a fracture. The roentgenographic appearance includes an area of rarefaction with scalloped borders and occasional speckled calcification; the lesion is frequently septate. Histologic examination discloses the fibromyxomatous nature of the tumor; chondroblasts are found at the periphery and must not be mistaken in a shallow biopsy for chondrosarcoma. The prognosis is generally good, but the tumor has malignant potential and should be completely resected if possible.

Giant cell tumors of bone constitute a heterogeneous group of conditions historically linked only by the fact that a characteristic response of bone to injury, infection, or neoplasm includes the development of multinucleated giant cells (osteoclasts). An *osteoclastoma* is a rare tumor in children. It occurs in long bones after closure of the epiphyses and almost always before the age of 40 yr, giving a characteristic roentgenographic picture. Destruction of bone is extensive, with little reaction at the periphery. Septa may be seen within the tumor, which represent remnants of the trabeculae. Aneurysmal bone cysts may be associated. The symptoms are generally those of pain or pathologic fracture. The tumor has malignant potential and should be completely excised.

Giant cell reactions distinct from osteoclastoma may occur in the skull, jaws, and vertebrae. They are probably the result of trauma or infection and have been called *giant cell reparative granulomas*. Those of the jaw may present as an *epulis*. In *cherubism* a process indistinguishable pathologically from giant cell reparative granuloma involves the jaws of young children, appearing usually from 3–5 yr of age and leading to enlarged mandibles with a characteristic facies. The condition is familial, probably an autosomal dominant trait.

Angioma of bone may be primary and solitary or part of a more extensive hemangiomatous diathesis. The spine is particularly likely to be involved, and destruction and collapse of vertebrae may first call attention to the tumor. The roentgenographic picture may be diagnostic, showing a pseudotrabeculated, cystic lesion or a "sunburst" appearance in the calvarium. Management may require radiation as surgery is hazardous because of bleeding.

Angioma of bone may be related to *disappearing bone disease* (massive osteolysis), a rare condition in which there is slow resorption of a bone or a group of bones over a period of years. Almost any bones may be involved but most commonly the clavicle. The condition may follow trauma in older children or adolescents. The histologic process usually appears hemangiomatous, sometimes lymphangiomatous. No treatment is known. The process usually stabilizes after the partial or complete disappearance of an involved bone or group of bones. Death may result.

Aneurysmal bone cyst is an incompletely understood process in bone which may represent a congenital lesion or hypervascular organization of the results of hemorrhage following trauma. Adolescents and young adults are most often affected; the spine is involved in about 25% of cases. The roentgenographic picture is the result of the erosion of the bony cortex from within and of the stimulation of subperiosteal new bone formation, which leads to an expansile, cystic lesion. Lesions of extraosseous origin may erode bone from without. The characteristic symptoms are pain, possibly due to the elevation of periosteum, or signs or symptoms associated with vertebral involvement. Treatment is curettage, excision, or, in some cases, irradiation. Aneurysmal bone cyst may arise from or be associated with an underlying lesion, such as chondroblastoma or osteosarcoma.

Solitary (unicameral) cysts fall somewhere between dysplasias and true tumors. These common lesions begin close to the epiphysis and appear to migrate toward the diaphysis with growth of bone. The cavity is uni- or multilocular and contains fluid or blood. The origin of the cysts is unknown; they have been attributed to traumatic hematomas. Symptoms may be absent or scant; the cysts may first declare themselves as pathologic fractures. The roentgenographic appearance consists of an area of rarefaction, often pseudoloculated, which does not cross the epiphyseal line. These lesions may resolve spontaneously. Those in the upper extremity sometimes need no therapy; those of the lower extremity are at greater risk of fracture and should usually be treated with curettage or excision.

15.22   HEMANGIOMA

This tumor is among the most common neoplasms found in infants and children. Most occur in the skin and do not achieve great size (Sec 24.7).

In a few children, large, rapidly growing hemangiomas can produce serious or life-threatening complications or grotesque deformity, especially in the area of the head and neck or on an extremity. Most such hemangiomas become evident before the age of 6 mo. They are evenly distributed between boys and girls. Their natural history is unpredictable. Usually there is rapid growth during the 1st 2 yr of life, followed by slow regression. Histologically, *hemangioendotheliomas*

present multiple dilated vascular spaces separated by varying amounts of interstitial connective tissue. The vascular channels are well formed and interlined by plump endothelial cells that are cytologically benign. *Cavernous hemangiomas* have widely dilated nonseptate vascular spaces lined by flat endothelial cells and supported by fibrous tissue. These vascular lumina sometimes contain partially organized thrombi.

Hemangiomas in the head and neck area can be unsightly and progressively distort normal structures. They generally appear first as a raised erythematous nodule which with growth becomes violaceous and irregular; surface ulceration may become extensive. Growth of these tumors may produce airway obstruction, pressure necrosis of surrounding structures, difficult feeding, and obstruction of the ear canal. They may become secondarily infected through the ulceration of overlying skin. If arteriovenous communications of sufficient size develop, congestive cardiac failure may ensue.

Treatment of large tumors by resection is frequently difficult because of extensive involvement, and complete removal may be impossible. Growth and deformity may involve vital structures, making even partial resection difficult. In some patients the administration of prednisone may suppress growth of the tumor, and regression may occur. Stopping the prednisone therapy may be followed by regrowth of tumor.

Hemangioma of the liver most frequently becomes evident before the age of 6 mo. Histologically, hemangioendothelioma is much more common than are cavernous hemangiomas. The initial symptoms may be jaundice, vomiting, or diarrhea or in some infants increases in abdominal size without symptoms. The hemangioma is sometimes found when routine examination discloses an enlarged liver. Arteriovenous fistulas may lead to congestive cardiac failure. Roentgenograms of the abdomen show an enlarged liver and occasionally calcification in the tumor. Radionuclide and computed tomographic scans of liver and spleen will show the defect in hepatic tissue; hepatic angiograms will show an abnormal vascular pattern. Initial treatment with prednisone is recommended. If hemangioma of the liver is confined to a single lobe, surgical resection may be possible.

In some patients with large cavernous hemangiomas, hemolysis and intralesional clotting may produce thrombocytopenia and hypofibrinogenemia with clinical symptoms. The anemia is not easily corrected by transfusion because of the ongoing red cell destruction, and a hemorrhagic diathesis may be impossible to correct by the transfusion of platelets and plasma clotting factors (Sec 14.66).

15.23   LYMPHANGIOMA
(Cystic Hygroma)

Lymphangiomas are found in the head and neck region in about 75% of cases. Like hemangiomas they appear early in life, with almost all evident by the age of 3 yr. The embryonic origin of lymphangiomas is uncertain; it is not known whether they are malformations, benign neoplasms, or hamartomas. They may present as unilocular or multicystic masses with thin, often transparent walls. The contents of these cysts are straw colored. Histologically, there is a flat lining of the cystic areas 1–2 cell layers thick with varying amounts of intervening fibrous stroma.

On physical examination the mass is compressible and feels cystic. The tumors are not tender or painful. There may be some thinning of the overlying skin. There is no erythema unless the lesion becomes infected. With growth of the tumor there may be progressive distortion of surrounding tissues. In some patients the tongue may become involved and enlarged. On roentgenograms of the chest, intrathoracic extensions may be found in some patients. With such extension tracheal compression or involvement of the mouth and pharynx may cause respiratory difficulty. Unlike hemangiomas, these tumors do not regress spontaneously; in most patients treatment is necessary. Surgical excision most frequently requires a radical neck dissection. The earlier the tumor is removed, the better the chance for complete resection. Delay in treatment may permit involvement of vital structures, making the subsequent surgery more difficult. With successful removal the long-term prognosis is excellent; there is no recurrence in most patients.

15.24 THYMOMA

Thymoma is a rare tumor in children, seen equally in boys and girls. There are 3 histologic patterns: the lymphoepithelial is most common and presents an intermingling of lymphocytes with diffuse proliferation of epithelial cells; the epithelial pattern has sheets, cords, and nests of plump neoplastic epithelial cells; and the spindle cell tumor shows sheets, cords, and interlacing trabeculae of fusiform cells with pale cytoplasm. The normal thymic tissue is usually adjacent to the neoplasm and separated from it by a dense fibrous capsule.

This anterior mediastinal tumor may be found in an asymptomatic person on routine chest roentgenogram. With growth of the tumor there may be progressive compression of surrounding tissues with the development of cough, dyspnea, dysphagia, and even superior vena cava compression with suffusion of the head and neck. In children it is unusual for thymoma to present as myasthenia gravis.

Untreated, this tumor grows progressively and may infiltrate local tissue. Spread beyond the thorax is rare. Treatment is surgical.

15.25 SPLENIC CYSTS

Splenic cysts can produce an enlarged spleen which may suggest a malignant neoplasm (Sec 14.77).

Acknowledgments. Gratitude is expressed to Drs. Tom Coburn, Warren Johnson, Charles Pratt, and Ann Hayes and to Ms. Pam Taylor for providing the illustrative material in this chapter.

This work was supported by USPH Research Project Grant CA15956; CORE Grant CA 21765, and Leukemia Program Project Grant CA 20180 from the National Cancer Institute and by ALSAC.

ALVIN M. MAUER

15.26 TUMORS OF THE HEART

Tumors of the heart are rare in infancy and childhood. Approximately three fourths of all cardiac tumors presenting in childhood are benign. The clinical manifestations are variable but depend principally upon the location of the tumor and, to a lesser extent, upon the histologic type of tumor encountered.

Almost 50% of all reported primary tumors are benign myxomas, which generally develop in intracavitary locations. The majority are located in the left atrium, consist of a pedunculated mass which attaches to the atrial septum and protrudes into the chamber, and cause intermittent obstruction and a clinical picture consistent with mitral stenosis. The tumor may be suspected in the presence of fainting spells, a changing character to the murmur, or evidence of systemic embolization. Treatment consists of surgical excision, which must include all of the base of the tumor to prevent recurrence. Other benign tumors include myxomas or papillomas, which are attached to valve leaflets and often present in the newborn period; fibromas and lipomas, which develop in the wall of a chamber, usually the left ventricle; and rhabdomyomas, which may be familial and present as space-occupying lesions originating in the ventricular septum. Rhabdomyomas may be associated with cerebral lesions of tuberous sclerosis and adenomas of the sebaceous glands. Rarely, congenital mesotheliomas may involve the atrioventricular node and cause abnormalities of electrical conduction, including complete heart block.

Primary malignant tumors of the heart in childhood are almost exclusively sarcomas. They are usually located in the atrial septum, right atrial wall, or root of the pulmonary artery. These tumors may present as early as 3 days of age and more frequently involve the right side of the heart. The tumor may extend either into the adjacent chamber or into the pericardial cavity. Thus, the clinical presentation may be either that of obstruction to blood flow or that of pericardial disease, including effusion or tamponade.

Finally, the heart may be involved in the metastatic dissemination of a noncardiac malignant tumor, either leukemia or malignant lymphoma.

THOMAS A. RIEMENSCHNEIDER

General

Carins NU, Clark GM, Smith SD, et al: Adaptation of siblings to childhood malignancy. J Pediatr 95:484, 1979.
Failkow PJ: Clonal and stem cell origin of blood cell neoplasms. *In*: LoBue J, et al (eds): Contemporary Hematology/Oncology, Vol 1. Plenum Publishing Corporation, 1980, p 1.
Fraumeni JF Jr (ed): Persons at High Risk of Cancer: An Approach to Cancer Etiology and Control. New York, Academic Press, 1975.
Miller RW: Childhood cancer and congenital defects. A study of US death certificates during the period 1960–1966. Pediatr Res 3:389, 1969.
Miller RW, Delager NA: US childhood cancer deaths by cell type, 1960–1968. J Pediatr 85:664, 1974.
Young JL Jr, Miller RW: Incidence of malignant tumors in US children. J Pediatr 86:254, 1975.

Acute Lymphocytic Leukemia

Bowman WP, Melvin S, Mauer AM: Cell markers in lymphomas and leukemias. Adv Intern Med 25:391, 1980.
George SL, Aur RJA, Mauer A, et al: A reappraisal of the results of stopping therapy in childhood leukemia. N Engl J Med 300:269, 1979.

Mauer AM: Therapy of acute lymphoblastic leukemia in childhood. Blood 56:1, 1980.

Sallan SE, Ritz J, Pesanda J, et al: Cell surface antigens: Prognostic implications in childhood acute lymphocytic leukemia. Blood 55:395, 1980.

Simone JV: Prognostic factors in childhood acute lymphocytic leukemia. Adv Biosci 14:27, 1973.

Acute Myelocytic Leukemia

Choi SI, Simone JV: Acute nonlymphocytic leukemia in 171 children. Med Pediatr Oncol 2:119, 1976.

Fialkow PJ, Singer JW, Adamson JW, et al: Acute nonlymphocytic leukemia. N Engl J Med 301:1, 1979.

Chronic Myelocytic Leukemia

Brodeur GM, Dow LW, Williams DL: Cytogenetic features of juvenile chronic myelogenous leukemia. Blood 53:812, 1979.

Fialkow PJ, Denman AM, Jacobson RJ, et al: Chronic myelocytic leukemia. J Clin Invest 62:815, 1978.

Randall DL, et al: Familial myeloproliferative disease. Am J Dis Child 110:479, 1965.

Smith KL, Johnson W: Classification of chronic myelocytic leukemia in children. Cancer 34:670, 1974.

Hodgkin Disease

American Cancer Society (a collaborative study): Survival and complications of radiotherapy following involved and extended field therapy for Hodgkin's disease, stages I and II. Cancer 38:288, 1976.

Borum K: Increased frequency of acute myeloid leukemia complicating Hodgkin's disease: A review. Cancer 46:1247, 1980.

Chaim WC, et al: Involved field radiation therapy for early stage Hodgkin's disease in children. Cancer 37:1625, 1976.

DeVita VT, Serpick AA, Carbone P: Combination chemotherapy in the treatment of advanced Hodgkin's disease. Ann Intern Med 73:881, 1970.

Filler RM, et al: Experience with clinical and operative staging of Hodgkin's disease in children. J Pediatr Surg 10:321, 1975.

Jaffe N, Paed D, Bishop YMM: The serum iron level, hematocrit, sedimentation rate, and leukocyte alkaline phosphatase level in pediatric patients with Hodgkin's disease. Cancer 26:332, 1970.

Jenkin MB, Freedman M, McClure P, et al: Hodgkin's disease in children: Treatment with low dose radiation and MOPP without staging laparotomy. Cancer 44:80, 1979.

Kaplan HS: Role of intensive radiotherapy in the management of Hodgkin's disease. Cancer 19:356, 1966.

Newell GR, Rawlings W: Evidence for environmental factors in the etiology of Hodgkin's disease. J Chron Dis 25:261, 1972.

O'Carroll DI, McKenna RW, Brunning RD: Bone marrow manifestations of Hodgkin's disease. Cancer 38:1717, 1976.

Rapoport A, Cole P, Mason J: Correlates of survival after initiation of chemotherapy in 142 cases of Hodgkin's disease. Cancer 24:377, 1969.

Rosenberg SA, Kaplan HS: Evidence for an orderly progression in the spread of Hodgkin's disease. Cancer Res 26:1225, 1966.

Schimpff S, et al: Varicella-zoster infection in patients with cancer. Ann Intern Med 76:241, 1972.

Schnitzer B, et al: Hodgkin's disease in children. Cancer 31:560, 1973.

Smith KL, et al: Concurrent chemotherapy and radiation therapy in the treatment of childhood and adolescent Hodgkin's disease. Cancer 33:38, 1974.

Young RC, et al: Delayed hypersensitivity in Hodgkin's disease. Am J Med 52:63, 1972.

Non-Hodgkin Lymphoma

Banks PM, et al: American Burkitt's lymphoma: A clinicopathologic study of 30 cases. Am J Med 58:322, 1975.

Bernard A, Boumsell L, Bayle C, et al: Subsets of malignant lymphomas in children related to the cell phenotype. Blood 54:1058, 1979.

Frizzera F, Rosai J, Dehner LP, et al: Lymphoreticular disorders in primary immunodeficiencies: New findings based on an up-to-date histologic classification of 35 cases. Cancer 46:692, 1980.

Jaffe ES, et al: Heterogeneity of immunologic markers and surface morphology in childhood lymphoblastic lymphoma. Blood 48:213, 1976.

Mann RB, et al: Non-endemic Burkitt's lymphoma. N Engl J Med 295:685, 1976.

Murphy SB, Frizzera G, Evans AE: A study of childhood non-Hodgkin's lymphoma. Cancer 36:2121, 1975.

Schey WL, et al: Lymphosarcoma in children. Am J Roentgenol Radium Ther Nucl Med 117:59, 1973.

Familial Histiocytosis

Falletta JM, et al: A fatal X-linked recessive reticuloendothelial syndrome with hyperglobulinemia. J Pediatr 83:549, 1973.

Juberg RC, Kloepfer W, Oberman HA: Genetic determination of acute disseminated histiocytosis X (Letterer-Siwe syndrome). Pediatrics 45:753, 1970.

Miller DR: Familial reticuloendotheliosis: Concurrence of disease of five siblings. Pediatrics 38:986, 1966.

Omenn GS: Familial reticuloendotheliosis with eosinophilia. N Engl J Med 273:427, 1965.

Familial Histiocytic Dermatoarthritis

Zayid I, Farraj S: Familial histiocytic dermatoarthritis. Am J Med 54:793, 1973.

Hemophagocytic Reticulosis

Berard CW, et al: Disseminated histiocytosis associated with atypical lymphoid cells (lymphohistiocytosis). Cancer 19:1429, 1966.

Fullerton P, et al: Hemophagocytic reticulosis. Cancer 36:441, 1975.

Nelson P, et al: Generalized lymphohistiocytic infiltration. Pediatrics 27:931, 1961.

Sinus Histiocytosis

Becroft DMO, et al: Benign sinus histiocytosis with massive lymphadenopathy: Transient immunological defects in a child with mediastinal involvement. J Clin Pathol 26:463, 1973.

Rosai J, Dorfman RF: Sinus histiocytosis with massive lymphadenopathy. Arch Pathol 87:63, 1969.

Histiocytosis in Congenital Rubella

Claman HN, et al: Histiocytic reaction in dysgammaglobulinemia and congenital rubella. Pediatrics 46:89, 1970.

Miscellaneous Lymphadenopathies

Bajoghli M: Generalized lymphadenopathy and hepatosplenomegaly induced by diphenylhydantoin. Pediatrics 28:943, 1961.

Ballow M, et al: Benign giant lymphoid hyperplasia of the mediastinum with associated abnormalities of the immune system. J Pediatr 84:418, 1974.

Canale BC, Smith CH: Chronic lymphadenopathy simulating malignant lymphoma. J Pediatr 70:891, 1967.

Sympathetic Nervous System Tumors

deLorimier AA, et al: Neuroblastoma in childhood. Am J Dis Child 118:441, 1969.

Evans AE, et al: A proposed staging for children with neuroblastoma. Cancer 27:374, 1971.

Turkel SB, Itabashi HH: The natural history of neuroblastic cells in the fetal adrenal gland. Am J Pathol 76:225, 1974.

Wilson LMK, Draper GJ: Neuroblastoma, its natural history and prognosis: A study of 487 cases. Br Med J 3:301, 1974.

Neuroblastoma

Coldman AJ, Fryer CJH, Elwood JM, et al: Neuroblastoma: Influence of age at diagnosis, stage, tumor site, and sex on prognosis. Cancer 46:1896, 1980.

Green AA, Hayes FA, Hustu HO: Sequential cyclophosphamide and Adriamycin for induction of complete remissions in children with disseminated neuroblastoma. Cancer 48:2310, 1981.

LaBrosse EH, Com-Nougue C, Zucker JM, et al: Urinary excretion of 3-methoxy-4-hydroxymandelic acid and 3-methoxy-4-hydroxyphenylacetic acid by 288 patients with neuroblastoma and related neural crest tumors. Cancer Res 40:1995, 1980.

Smith EI, Krous HF, Tunell WP, et al: The impact of chemotherapy and radiation therapy on secondary operations for neuroblastoma. Ann Surg 191:561, 1980.

Renal Tumors

Beckwith JB, Palmer NF: Histopathology and prognosis of Wilms tumor. Cancer 41:1937, 1978.

Bolande RP: Congenital and infantile neoplasia of the kidney. Lancet 2:1497, 1974.

Bond JF: Bilateral Wilms' tumour. Lancet 2:482, 1975.

Favara BE, et al: Renal tumors in the neonatal period. Cancer 22:845, 1968.

Green DM, Jaffe N: The role of chemotherapy in the treatment of Wilms tumor. Cancer 44:52, 1979.

Lemerle J, et al: Wilms' tumor: Natural history and prognostic factors. Cancer 37:2557, 1976.

Medical Research Council's Working Party on Embryonal Tumours in Childhood, Morris Jones PH (ed): Management of nephroblastoma in childhood. Arch Dis Child 53:112, 1978.

Palma LD, et al: Childhood renal carcinoma. Cancer 26:1321, 1970.

Pendergrass TW: Congenital anomalies in children with Wilms' tumor. Cancer 37:403, 1976.

Pratt-Thomas HR, et al: Carcinoma of the kidney in a 15-year old boy. Cancer 31:719, 1973.

Riccardi VM, Sujansky E, Smith AC, et al: Chromosomal imbalance in the aniridia–Wilms tumor association: 11p interstitial deletion. Pediatrics 61:604, 1978.

Soft Tissue Sarcomas

Botting AJ, et al: Smooth muscle tumors in children. Cancer 18:711, 1965.

Exelby PR, et al: Soft-tissue fibrosarcoma in children. J Pediatr Surg 8:415, 1973.

Furey JG, et al: Alveolar soft-part sarcoma. J Bone Joint Surg (Am) 51-A:185, 1969.

Gerner RE, Moore GE: Synovial sarcoma. Ann Surg 181:22, 1975.

Kauffman SL, Stout AP: Malignant hemangioendothelioma in infants and children. Cancer 14:1186, 1961.

Kumar PAN, et al: Combined therapy to prevent complete pelvic exenteration for rhabdomyosarcoma of the vagina or uterus. Cancer 37:118, 1976.

Maurer HM, Moon T, Donaldson M, et al: The intergroup rhabdomyosarcoma study. Cancer 40:2015, 1977.

Mayer CMH, et al: Malignant mesenchymoma in infants. Am J Dis Child 128:847, 1974.

Miller RW, Dalager NA: Fatal rhabdomyosarcoma among children in the United States, 1960–1969. Cancer 34:1897, 1974.

Nelfeld JP, Maurer HM, Godwin D, et al: Prognostic variables in pediatric rhabdomyosarcoma before and after multi-modal therapy. J Pediatr Surg 14:699, 1979.

Ortega JA, et al: Chemotherapy of malignant hemangiopericytoma of childhood. Cancer 27:730, 1971.

Pratt CB, Smith JW, Woerner S, et al: Factors leading to delay in the diagnosis and affecting survival of children with head and neck rhabdomyosarcoma. Pediatrics 61:30, 1978.

Raney RB, Gehan EA, Maurer HM, et al: Evaluation of intensified chemotherapy in children with advanced rhabdomyosarcoma (clinical Groups III and IV). Cancer Clinical Trials, Spring, 1979.

Schuller DE, Lawrence TL, Newton WA Jr: Childhood rhabdomyosarcoma of the head and neck. Arch Otolaryngol 105:689, 1979.

Tefft M, Fernandez C, Donaldson M, et al: Incidence of meningeal involvement by rhabdomyosarcoma of the head and neck in children. Cancer 42:253, 1978.

Unni KK, et al: Hemangioma, hemangiopericytoma, and hemangioendothelioma (angiosarcoma) of bone. Cancer 27:1403, 1971.

Bone Tumors

Burgers JMV, Breuer DK, Van Dobbenburgh OA, et al: Role of metastatectomy without chemotherapy in the management of osteosarcoma in children. Cancer 45:1664, 1980.

Glaubiger DL, Makuch R, Schwarz J, et al: Determination of prognostic factors and their influence on therapeutic results in patients with Ewing sarcoma. Cancer 45:2213, 1980.

Herson J, Sutow WW, Elder K, et al: Adjuvant chemotherapy in non-metastatic osteosarcoma: A Southwest Oncology Group Study. Med Pediatr Oncol 8:343, 1980.

Jaffe N, et al: Adjuvant methotrexate and citrovorum-factor treatment of osteogenic sarcoma. N Engl J Med 291:994, 1974.

Kumar APM, et al: Transmedullary amputation and resection of metastases in combined therapy of osteosarcoma. J Pediatr Surg 12:427, 1977.

Marcove RC, et al: Osteogenic sarcoma under the age of twenty-one. J Bone Joint Surg 52A:411, 1970.

Mehta Y, Hendrickson FR: CNS involvement in Ewing's sarcoma. Cancer 33:859, 1973.

Miller RW: Etiology of childhood bone cancer: Epidemiologic observations. Recent Results Cancer Res 54:51, 1976.

Rosen G, et al: Disease-free survival in children with Ewing's sarcoma treated with radiation therapy and adjuvant four-drug sequential chemotherapy. Cancer 33:384, 1974.

Rosen G, et al: Chemotherapy, en bloc resection, and prosthetic bone replacement in the treatment of osteogenic sarcoma. Cancer 37:1, 1976.

Scranton PE Jr, et al: Prognostic factors in osteosarcoma. Cancer 36:2179, 1975.

Sinkovics JG, et al: Chondrosarcoma. J Med 1:15, 1970.

Tepper J, Glaubiger D, Lichter A, et al: Local control of Ewing sarcoma of bone with radiotherapy and combination chemotherapy. Cancer 46:1969, 1980.

Unni KK, et al: Periosteal osteogenic sarcoma. Cancer 37:2476, 1976.

Retinoblastoma

Eldridge R, et al: Superior intelligence in sighted retinoblastoma patients and their families. J Med Genet 9:331, 1972.

Francke U, Kung F: Sporadic bilateral retinoblastoma and 13q– chromosomal deletion. Med Pediatr Oncol 2:379, 1976.

Freeman CR, Esseltine DL, Whitehead VM, et al: Retinoblastoma: The case for radiotherapy and for adjuvant chemotherapy. Cancer 46:1913, 1980.

Lennox EL, et al: Retinoblastoma: A study of natural history and prognosis of 268 cases. Br Med J 3:282, 1975.

Michelson JB, et al: Fetal antigens in retinoblastoma. Cancer 37:719, 1976.

Gastrointestinal Tumors

Krolls SO, et al: Salivary gland lesions in children—a survey of 430 cases. Cancer 30:459, 1972.

Pick T, et al: Lymphoepithelioma in childhood. J Pediatr 84:96, 1974.

Pratt CB, et al: Colorectal carcinoma in adolescents; implications regarding etiology. Cancer 40:2464, 1977.

Siegel SE, et al: Carcinoma of the stomach in childhood. Cancer 38:1781, 1976.

Taxy JB: Adenocarcinoma of the pancreas in childhood. Cancer 37:1508, 1976.

Liver Tumors

Exelby PR, et al: Liver tumors in children in the particular reference to hepatoblastoma and hepatocellular carcinoma: American Academy of Pediatrics Surgical Section Survey 1974. J Pediatr Surg 10:329, 1975.

Fraumeni JF Jr, et al: Primary carcinoma of the liver in childhood: An epidemiologic study. J Natl Cancer Inst 40:1087, 1968.

Holton CP, et al: A multiple chemotherapeutic approach to management of hepatoblastoma. Cancer 35:1083, 1975.

Ito J, Johnson WW: Hepatoblastoma and hepatoma in infancy and childhood. Arch Pathol 87:259, 1969.

Moss AA, et al: Angiographic appearance of benign and malignant hepatic tumors in infants and children. Am J Roentgenol 113:61, 1971.

Smith JB, O'Neill RT: Alpha-fetoprotein: Occurrence in germinal cell and liver malignancies. Am J Med 51:767, 1971.

Sorsdahl OA, Gay BB: Roentgenologic features of a primary carcinoma of the liver in infants and children. Am J Roentgenol 100:117, 1967.

Weinberg AG, et al: The occurrence of hepatoma in the chronic form of hereditary tyrosinemia. J Pediatr 88:434, 1976.

Gonadal and Germ Cell Tumors

Brodeur GM, Howarth CB, Pratt CB, et al: Malignant germ cell tumors in 57 children and adolescents. Cancer 48:1890, 1981.

Dehner LP: Intrarenal teratoma occurring in infancy: Report of a case with discussion of extragonadal germ cell tumors in infancy. J Pediatr Res 8:369, 1973.

Ein SH, et al: Cystic and solid ovarian tumors in children: A 44-year review. J Pediatr Surg 5:148, 1970.

Ein SH, Adeyemi SD, Mancer K: Benign sacrococcygeal teratomas in infants and children. Ann Surg 191:382, 1980.

Fraumeni JF Jr, et al: Teratomas in children: Epidemiologic features. J Natl Cancer Inst 51:1425, 1973.

Ise T, et al: Management of malignant testicular tumors in children. Cancer 37:1539, 1976.

Mahour GH, et al: Sacrococcygeal teratoma: A 33-year experience. J Pediatr 19:183, 1975.

Scully RE: Gonadoblastoma—a review of 74 cases. Cancer 25:1340, 1970.

Towne BH, et al: Ovarian cysts and tumors in infancy and childhood. J Pediatr Surg 10:311, 1975.

Weitzner S: Sertoli cell tumor of testis in childhood. Am J Dis Child 128:541, 1974.

Miscellaneous Carcinomas

Forsman PJ, Jenkins ME: Medullary carcinoma of the thyroid with Marfan-like body habitus. Pediatrics 52:188, 1973.

Frohman LA: Irradiation and thyroid carcinoma: Legacy and controversy. J Chron Dis 29:609, 1976.

Herbst AL, Scully RE: Adenocarcinoma of the vagina in adolescence. Cancer 25:745, 1970.

Leape LL, et al: Total thyroidectomy for occult familial medullary carcinoma of the thyroid in children. J Pediatr Surg 11:831, 1976.

Lerman RI, et al: Malignant melanoma of childhood. Cancer 25:436, 1970.

Oberman HA, Stephens PJ: Carcinoma of the breast in childhood. Cancer 30:470, 1972.

Stewart DR, et al: Carcinoma of the adrenal gland in children. J Pediatr Surg 9:59, 1974.

Benign Tumors and Tumor-Like Lesions of Bone

Aegerter E, Kirkpatrick JA: Orthopedic Diseases. Ed 4. Philadelphia, WB Saunders, 1975.

Hemangiomas

Brown SH Jr, Heerhout RC, Fonkalsrud EW: Prednisone therapy in the management of large hemangiomas in infants and children. Surgery 71:168, 1972.

Cooper WH, Martin JF: Hemangioma of the liver with thrombocytopenia. Am J Roentgenol Radium Ther Nucl Med 88:751, 1962.

Dehner LP, Ishak KG: Vascular tumors of the liver in infants and children. Arch Pathol 92:101, 1971.

Propp RP, Scharfman WB: Hemangioma-thrombocytopenia syndrome associated with microangiopathic hemolytic anemia. Blood 28:623, 1966.

Tawes RL Jr, Nelson JA, Hyde GA: Hepatic hemangioma: Successful resection in a neonate. Surgery 70:782, 1971.

Thatcher LG, Clatanoff DV, Stiehm ER: Splenic hemangioma with thrombocytopenia and afibrinogenemia. J Pediatr 73:345, 1968.

Touloukian RJ: Hepatic hemangioendothelioma during infancy: Pathology, diagnosis and treatment with prednisone. Pediatrics 45:71, 1970.

Williams OK, et al: Giant hemangioendothelioma with thrombocytopenia and hypofibrinogenemia. Am J Roentgenol Radium Ther Nucl Med 106:204, 1969.

Lymphangiomas

Doberneck RC: Diagnosis and treatment of solitary mass in the neck. Am Surg 40:181, 1974.

Saijo M, Munro IR, Mancer K: Lymphangioma. A long term follow-up study. Plast Reconstr Surg 56:642, 1975.

Thymomas

Fonkalsrud EW, Herrmann C Jr, Mulder DG: Thymectomy for myasthenia gravis in children. J Pediatr Surg 5:157, 1970.

LeGolvan DP, Abell MR: Thymomas. Cancer 39:2142, 1977.

Zanca P, et al: True congenital mediastinal thymic cyst. Pediatrics 36:615, 1965.

Splenic Cyst

Griscom NT, et al: Huge splenic cyst in a newborn: Comparison with 10 cases in later childhood and adolescence. Am J Roentgenol 129:889, 1977.

Pearson HA, Touloukian RJ, Spencer RP: The binary spleen: A radioisotopic scan sign of splenic pseudocyst. J Pediatr 77:216, 1970.

Tumors of the Heart

Fine G: Primary tumors of the pericardium and heart. Cardiovasc Clin 5:208, 1973.

Longino LA, Meeker IA Jr: Primary cardiac tumors in infancy. J Pediatr 43:724, 1953.

Whorton CM: Primary malignant tumors of the heart. Report of a case. Cancer 2:245, 1949.

THE URINARY SYSTEM 16

THE KIDNEY

16.1 Renal Anatomy

The kidneys, ureters, and bladder are retroperitoneal structures. The kidneys are at the level of the 1st–4th lumbar vertebrae, at or slightly above the level of the umbilicus; they can usually be palpated in the neonate. Each kidney has 8–12 pyramid-shaped lobes. The external surface of the fetal kidney is lobulated; the lobulations gradually disappear with age. The base of each lobe forms the kidney surface; the apex is the papilla, which enters the urine collecting system at a minor calyx. Each lobe consists of 2 principal zones: the cortex, or outer zone, where the glomeruli and the proximal and distal convoluted tubules are located; and the medulla, or deeper zone, where the vasa recta, descending and ascending limbs of the loop of Henle, and collecting ducts are located. These structures are arranged in a fanlike distribution and funnel toward the papilla, where the urine is delivered through the ducts of Bellini, the terminal fusion of many collecting ducts, into a minor calyx. The minor calyces are subdivisions of the superior and inferior major calyces that unite to form the renal pelvis, from which urine drains into the ureter and is transported by active peristalsis to the bladder.

Blood Supply. Each kidney receives about 10% of the cardiac output; in relation to weight, this is the greatest blood flow of any organ.

The renal or main artery of each kidney arises from the aorta; occasionally, a kidney has more than 1 such artery. The principal branches are the interlobar arteries; they pass dorsally and ventrally between the lobes to the renal pelvis. At the junction of cortex and medulla the interlobar arteries divide to form the arcuate arteries, which pass between the cortex and medulla parallel to the surface of the kidney. From these arteries the interlobular arteries enter the cortex and run perpendicular to the kidney surface (Fig 16–1). The interlobular arteries branch to form the afferent arterioles, each of which supplies a glomerulus—a spherical network of capillary loops surrounded by a Bowman capsule. Other interlobular arteries pass directly to the superficial cortex to provide much of its blood supply.

About 50 μ before the afferent arteriole enters the glomerulus, the muscle cells of the media assume the appearance of secretory cells; they contain granular deposits of renin. These cells, situated at the vascular pole of the glomerulus, constitute the *juxtaglomerular apparatus.* Just beyond the point at which the arteriole enters a Bowman capsule, it subdivides into several branches which in turn branch into a network of glomerular capillary loops. These reunite to form the *efferent arteriole,* which emerges at the vascular pole, where the renal tubule, returning to the cortex, makes tangential contact with the afferent arteriole of its own glomerulus. The tubular epithelial cells become narrower here; this portion of the tubule is known as the *macula densa.*

The blood supply to cortical nephrons differs from that to the nephrons at the junction of the cortex and medulla (the so-called *juxtamedullary nephrons*) (Fig 16–2); in the latter the diameter of the efferent arteriole is slightly larger than that of the afferent arteriole, whereas the reverse is true in the arterioles of cortical nephrons. The efferent arterioles of the outer and mid-cortical nephrons divide into an anastomosing network of capillaries that surround proximal and distal convoluted tubules and the cortical portions of the loop of Henle and the collecting duct. For subcapsular or outer cortical nephrons these peritubular capillaries arise from the efferent arteriole of the associated glomerulus; for nephrons that are deeper in the cortex, there is free communication with the peritubular capillary network from the efferent arterioles of other nephrons. The walls of the peritubular capillaries are extremely thin and are

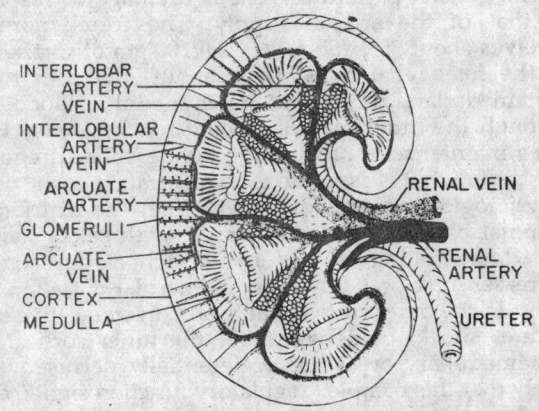

Figure 16–1 Gross morphology of the renal circulation. (From Pitts RF: Physiology of the Kidney and Body Fluids. Ed. 3. Chicago, Year Book Medical Publishers, 1974. Used by permission.)

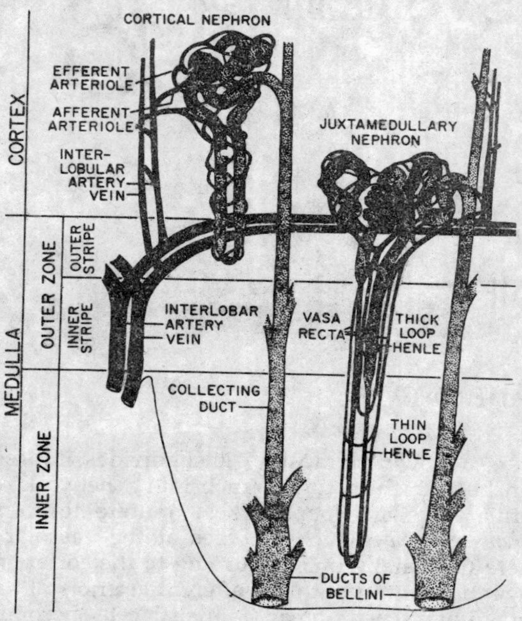

Figure 16–2 Comparison of the blood supplies of cortical and juxtamedullary nephrons. (From Pitts RF: Physiology of the Kidney and Body Fluids. Ed. 3. Chicago, Year Book Medical Publishers, 1974. Used by permission.)

in very close proximity to the basement membrane surrounding each tubule. The cortical capillaries finally merge to form the interlobular veins.

The efferent arterioles of the inner cortical and juxtamedullary nephrons provide a peritubular capillary network for the proximal and distal convoluted tubules and the loops of Henle and collecting ducts in the area. The efferent arterioles of the juxtamedullary nephrons also supply the vasa recta, which are recurrent arterial loops that parallel the loops of Henle as they descend through the medulla to the papilla. The vasa recta turn upward at the bend of the loop to the juxtamedullary region to enter an interlobular or arcuate vein. The vasa recta function as countercurrent exchangers in the process of urine concentration (Sec 16.2).

The general pattern of venous drainage corresponds to that of the arterial supply. The cortex normally receives about 75% (about 400 ml/100 gm of cortex/min) of the total renal blood flow; about 20% goes to the juxtamedullary cortex and outer medulla. Blood flow through the inner medulla, being much slower, facilitates maintenance of the high solute concentration in this region that is essential to concentration of the urine. Physiologic or pathologic factors alter the distribution of renal blood flow. For example, with saline loading or administration of a diuretic such as furosemide, increases in blood flow and glomerular filtration rate occur in the outer cortical nephrons. In congestive heart failure, shock, or dehydration, the inner cortical and juxtamedullary areas are preferentially perfused. It is likely that this complex regulatory function significantly involves the autonomic nervous system, humoral factors such as antidiuretic hormone and angiotensin, and prostaglandins.

The Nephron.   The functioning unit in the formation of urine is the nephron; there are about 1 million of them in each kidney; their anatomic and functional components are discussed below. The nephrons having glomeruli in the zone adjacent to the medulla (juxtamedullary nephrons) differ from the more superficial nephrons in that their loops of Henle extend deep into the medulla; they also have a different role in regulation of salt and water excretion. The ratio of cortical to juxtamedullary glomeruli is about 7:1.

The Glomerulus.   The glomerulus (average diameter, 150–200 μ) is the filtering apparatus of the nephron; the formation of urine is initiated there. The number of glomeruli in the adult is present in a fetus of 2–2.5 kg. Each glomerulus consists of an intricate, spherical, convoluted, capillary network arising from the afferent arteriole after it enters Bowman capsule. The walls of the capillaries of this network form a membrane across which the process of filtration occurs. The walls of the glomerular capillaries have 3 layers (Fig 16–3): (1) The *endothelium* is thin and attenuated and is traversed by multiple fenestrae, with a polyanionic glycoprotein surface coat covering the endothelial plasma membranes (Fig 16–4). (2) The *glomerular basement membrane* (GBM) is an uninterrupted, highly convoluted membrane about 1200 Å thick having a central electron dense layer (the lamina densa) and 2 relatively electron lucent layers: the lamina rara interna, which is subendothelial in location, and the lamina rara externa, which is subepithelial. (3) The *epithelium* consists of relatively large cells with extensive cytoplasmic projections; these subdivide into foot processes which interdigitate with one another and are in direct contact with the GBM. Between the foot processes are the filtration slits, which are about 240 Å in diameter. Covering the epithelial cells and filling the spaces between the foot processes is a carbohydrate rich polyanionic glycoprotein cell coat up to 800 Å in thickness, with a negative charge derived primarily from the carboxyl groups of sialic acid. The fixed negative charge conferred by the endothelial and epithelial cell coats influences the ease with which charged macromolecules traverse the glomerular capillary wall, restricting access of negatively charged molecules to the urinary space and facilitating the transit of those with positive charges (Fig 16–5).

In addition to the endothelial and epithelial cells in contact with the glomerular basement membrane, there are the mesangial cells. These cells lie deep in the central or stalk region of the glomerulus and are separated from the capillary lumina by overlying endothelial cells. The mesangial cells and the intercellular material between them (the mesangial matrix) constitute the mesangium. Macromolecules (such as immune complexes) which circulate through the glomerular capillaries may enter the mesangium through the interface between the endothelial and mesangial cells and migrate via intercellular channels toward the juxtaglomerular region, where they are disposed of by as yet poorly understood mechanisms. Macromolecules may also be phagocytosed by the mesangial cells or by infiltrating phagocytes. The mesangium thus appears to act as a component of the reticuloendothelial system for the glomerular circulation, trapping and disposing of some substances of large molecular weight. The

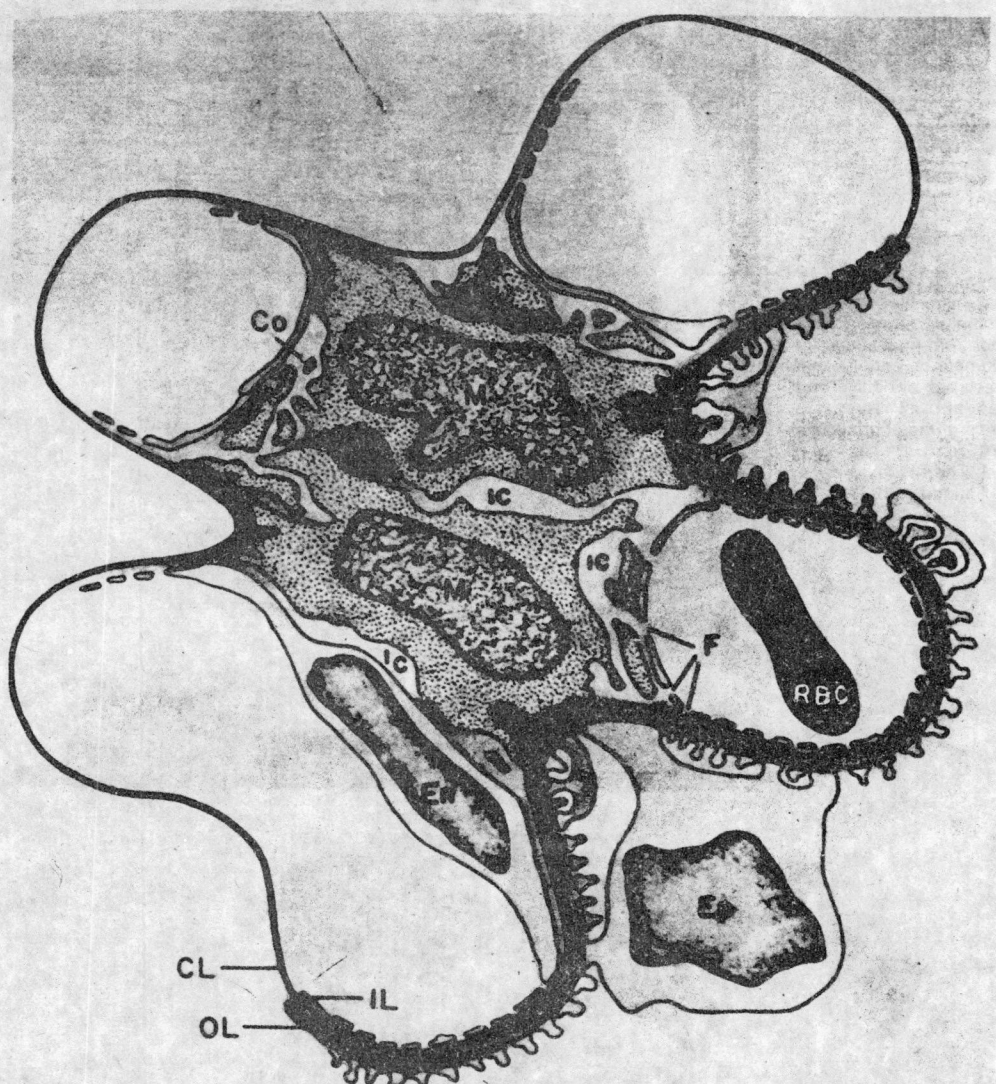

Figure 16–3 Glomerular lobule with its mesangial region. Abbreviations: CL, central layer (lamina densa) of the basement membrane of the capillary loop; OL and IL, outer and inner layers, respectively, of the basement membrane (lamina rara externa and interna); Ep, epithelial cell with foot processes; En, endothelial cell; F, fenestrae or gaps in endothelium; RBC, red blood cell; M, mesangial cell and matrix (Ma); IC, intercapillary mesangial channels. (From Orloff J, Berliner R [eds]: Handbook of Physiology, Sec 8, 1973, p 19.)

mesangial region is an important site of injury in some diseases affecting the glomerulus, responding sometimes in nonspecific ways (as with cellular and matrix proliferation), at other times with more specific or even pathognomonic changes (e.g., intercapillary nodule formation in diabetic glomerulosclerosis).

Bowman capsule surrounds the glomerulus. Its basement membrane is continuous with the basement membrane of the proximal convoluted tubule and is lined on its inner aspect by the parietal epithelial cells. The tubular portion of the nephron begins at an orifice in the capsule usually situated opposite the vascular pole.

The Tubules. Distal to the glomerulus the nephron becomes a tubule. Various segments are characterized by their location, histologic appearance, and distinct physiologic functions; they are the proximal convoluted tubule, the loop of Henle, the distal tubule, and the collecting duct. The collecting duct is not embryologically a part of the nephron, but it is a structural and functional part. Throughout their length the tubules are enveloped by a continuous basement membrane that joins the basement membrane of Bowman capsule. The tubular basement membrane provides an uninterrupted framework for the tubular epithelium.

The *proximal convoluted tubule* is situated in the cortex; it has the widest diameter of the tubular segments. Its epithelium is cuboidal and 1 cell deep; the spherical nuclei are situated at the basal surface of the cell. The spaces between cells are difficult to define by electron microscopy, but they play an important role as channels

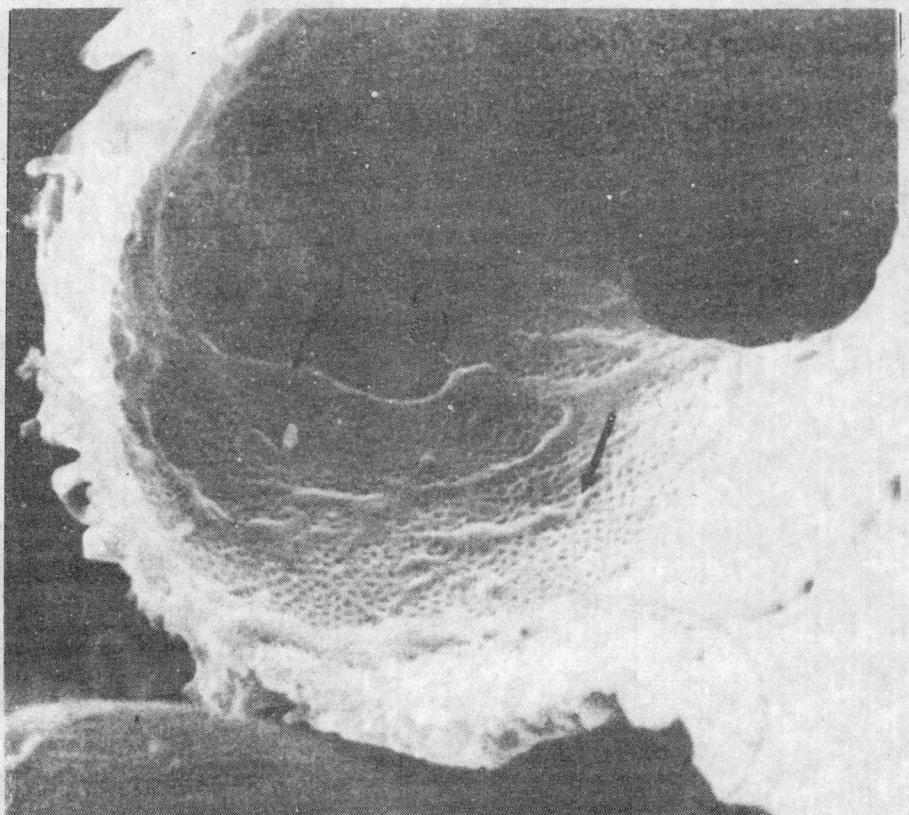

Figure 16–4 Scanning electron micrograph demonstrating the appearance of the endothelial surface of a glomerular capillary from the kidney of a normal rat. Numerous endothelial pores, or fenestrae, are evident. The ridgelike structures (arrows) represent localized thickenings of the endothelial cells. (×21,400.) (From Brenner BM, Rector FC Jr [eds]: The Kidney. Ed 2. Philadelphia, WB Saunders, 1981.)

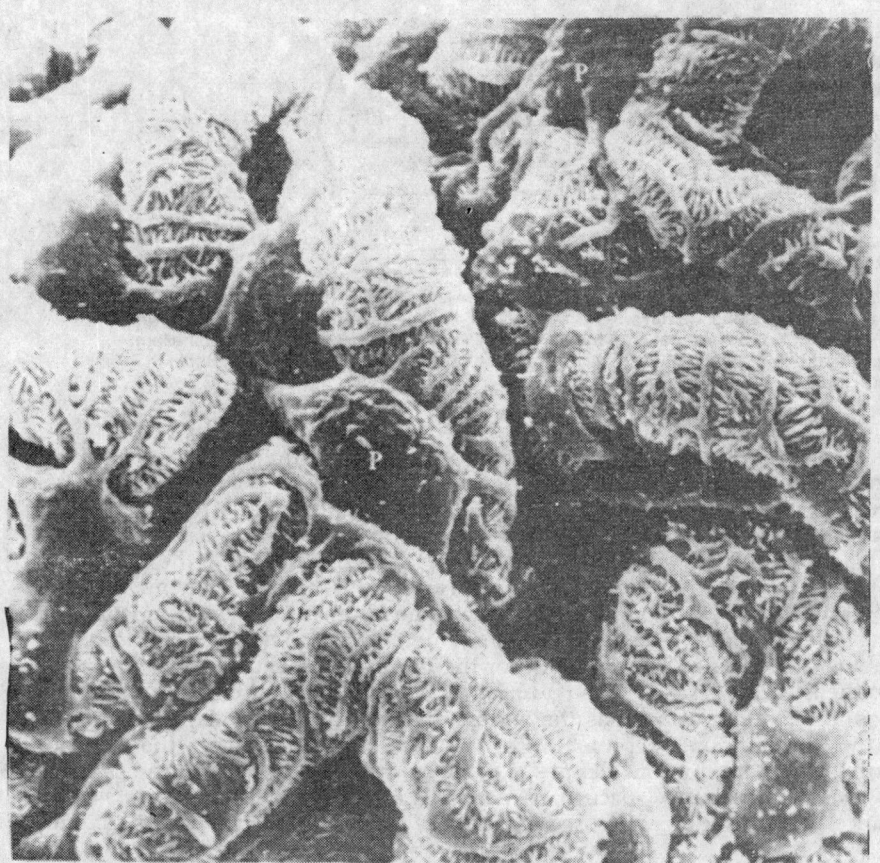

Figure 16–5 Scanning electron micrograph of a glomerulus from the kidney of a normal rat. The visceral epithelial cells, or podocytes (P), extend multiple processes outward from the main cell body to wrap around individual capillary loops. Immediately adjacent pedicels, or foot processes, arise from different podocytes. (×4800.) (From Brenner BM, Rector FC Jr [eds]: The Kidney. Ed 2. Philadelphia, WB Saunders, 1981.)

through which solutes and water reabsorbed from the lumen by the cells pass to the peritubular capillaries. An abundant luminal brush border increases the reabsorptive surface of the cells, and there is a tight junction between each of the cells at their luminal aspect. This junction is relatively impermeable to solute or water, but it is likely that back diffusion of reabsorbed solute and water into the tubular lumen occurs via these intercellular junctions. Mitochondria are numerous in the cells of the proximal tubule and occupy principally the basal two thirds of the cell; the basal surface of each tubular cell (basal plasma membrane) has numerous infoldings which bring it close to the mitochondria. The peritubular capillaries are immediately next to the basement membrane. The proximal tubular cells transport or reabsorb large quantities of water and solute from the tubular lumen. They also participate in the process of tubular secretion, by which substances derived from the circulation or synthesized within the cells are added to the luminal fluid.

The *loop of Henle* is a continuation of the proximal convoluted tubule. Its length varies according to the location of its glomerulus within the cortex. Nephrons with glomeruli situated in the outer two thirds of the cortex have short or even absent loops; those with glomeruli in the inner third have longer loops which extend toward the tips of the papillae.

After descending into the medulla, the loop turns abruptly back on itself to ascend toward the cortex, where it becomes the distal tubule. The epithelium of the descending limb of the medullary loop is flat and squamous, and the tubular diameter is considerably less than that of the proximal convoluted tubule. This section is called the thin segment of the loop of Henle; it may be confined to the descending portion or may form the bend of the loop and continue for a variable distance up the ascending segment limb. The luminal surfaces of the cells of the thin segment have short, widely spaced microvilli, and their cytoplasm has only infrequent mitochondria. The ascending limb (the thick segment) of the loop has a thicker epithelium, and the nuclei are situated in the luminal half of the cell. Numerous rod shaped mitochondria occupy the basal half of these cells; short microvilli arise from the luminal cell surface. The cleftlike infoldings of the basal plasma membrane of the cells bring it into intimate contact with the mitochondria.

The *distal tubule* continues from the ascending limb of the loop of Henle. The initial portion, the pars recta, continues in a straight course toward its glomerulus.

As the distal tubule passes its glomerulus of origin, it makes contact with the afferent arteriole; this part of the tubule is the macula densa. Thereafter, the distal tubule becomes convoluted; the cells are cuboidal and have a dense, coarsely granular cytoplasm containing numerous mitochondria. The cell nucleus is apical rather than basal. The luminal surface of the cells has numerous short microvilli that are coarser and less abundant than the brush border projections of the cells of the proximal tubule.

The *collecting duct* is formed by the junction of 2 or more terminal segments of distal convoluted tubules and receives additional branches in its course to the medullary papilla. It has a simple cuboidal epithelium. This is the final segment of the nephron; it joins one of the ducts of Bellini, through which urine from collecting ducts is discharged into a minor calyx at the papillary tip.

The Interstitium. The interstitial space and the number of cells increase as the papilla is approached. The space itself is filled with a flocculent material of low electron density. Several types of interstitial cells are recognized: Type I cells are the most numerous; they resemble fibroblasts. Type II cells have some characteristics of mononuclear cells and may have phagocytic activity. Type III, the pericyte, is found adjacent to the vasa recta.

By electron microscopy Type I cells are seen to contain many lipid bodies and an abundant granulated endoplasmic reticulum. The renal medulla is a site of prostaglandin synthesis; it is likely that these lipid droplets contain renal prostaglandin PGE_2 and $PGF_{2\alpha}$ precursors.

Nerve Supply. The kidney has rich adrenergic and cholinergic innervation. The nerve fibers course mainly along the blood vessels, i.e., along the interlobar, arcuate, and interlobular arteries and afferent arterioles. Some fibers innervate the juxtamedullary efferent arterioles that give rise to the vasa recta. The nerves play a role in regulating renal blood flow, intrarenal distribution of blood, and glomerular filtration rate. Stimulation of renal sympathetic nerves causes reduction in cortical blood flow and leads to reduction in urinary excretion of sodium. Sympathetic blocking agents induce renal vasodilatation and mild natriuresis.

Barger AC, Herd JA: Renal vascular anatomy and distribution of blood flow. In: Orloff A, Berliner W (eds): Handbook of Physiology. Section 8, Renal Physiology. Washington DC, American Physiological Society, 1973.
Latta H: Ultrastructure of the glomerulus and juxtaglomerular apparatus. Ibid.
Michael AF, Keane WF, Raij L, et al: The glomerular mesangium. Kidney Int 17:141, 1980.

16.2 Renal Physiology

GLOMERULAR FILTRATION

Formation of urine begins in the glomerulus with the formation of an ultrafiltrate of plasma by filtration across the glomerular basement membrane. The ease with which any given molecule traverses this membrane is determined principally by its molecular weight; the shape and electrical charge are modifying factors, the passage of negatively charged macromolecules being restricted to a greater degree than that of positively charged or neutral molecules of the same size and shape. Normally, molecules with molecular weight over 70,000 are not filtered in appreciable amounts; the permeability of the membrane increases as molecular weight falls. Inulin, a fructose polymer with a mean molecular weight of 5000, is completely filterable, as are smaller molecules, the concentration of which in the ultrafiltrate is thus virtually the same as in plasma. The barrier to filtration of substances of larger molecular weight is remarkably efficient. For example, the concentration of protein in the filtrate is less than 2 mg/dl, whereas the concentration within the capillary lumen is approximately 7000 mg/dl. Most evidence favors the basement membrane as the principal filtration barrier of the glomerulus, but the final barrier for substances of low molecular weight may be located at the filtration slits between the epithelial foot processes.

Glomerular Filtration Rate. The volume of the filtrate formed per unit of time (usually expressed in ml/min) is the glomerular filtration rate (GFR). About 20% of the total renal plasma flow is filtered; this is called the filtration fraction. After about 1 yr of age the GFR is approximately 70 ± 5 (1 S.D.) ml/min/M^2 or 100 l/M^2/24 hr. The latter volume in a healthy child will contain about 850 gm of salt, 100 gm of glucose, and 5 gm of calcium.

The physiologic determinants of the rate of glomerular ultrafiltration are as follows:

The *transcapillary hydraulic pressure* is the difference between the intracapillary hydraulic pressure and that within Bowman space. The former is probably constant throughout the glomerular capillary network at about 40% of the mean aortic pressure; the latter is about 10–12 mm Hg. The net hydraulic pressure favoring ultrafiltration is thus about 35 mm Hg.

The *transcapillary oncotic pressure* is created by proteins and other colloids within the capillary lumen; it opposes the hydraulic pressure that favors ultrafiltration. Since the filtrate is essentially protein free, the intracapillary protein concentration rises progressively along the capillary network; the magnitude of this increase is of the order of 3 gm/dl and corresponds to a rise in colloid osmotic pressure of from 20 mm Hg at the afferent entrance to about 35 mm Hg at the efferent outflow. The net ultrafiltration pressure, i.e., the transcapillary difference between the hydraulic and oncotic pressures, thus falls from approximately 15 mm Hg to 0 at the efferent end. At this point filtration ceases and filtration pressure equilibrium is said to exist.

An increase in *glomerular plasma flow rate* results in a situation in which the luminal colloid osmotic pressure remains less than the hydraulic pressure throughout the glomerular transit; the filtration pressure equilibrium is thus not reached, and there is a net increase in the rate of ultrafiltration.

The *ultrafiltration coefficient* is the product of the water permeability of the glomerular basement membrane and the surface area available for filtration. Values of approximately 0.08 ml/sec/mm Hg in mammals have been obtained in experimental studies. As long as the coefficient remains high enough to allow filtration-pressure equilibrium to develop, further increases in the coefficient will not lead to an increase in filtration rate. Similarly, a modest decrease in the ultrafiltration coefficient is unlikely to lead to significant reduction in the filtration rate, though extensive reduction in the coefficient or of its determinants could reduce the rate.

Since the protein concentration in the afferent end of the glomerular capillary network determines the intra-

capillary oncotic pressure, the filtration rate should vary reciprocally with the concentration; i.e., a fall in oncotic pressure opposing ultrafiltration should lead to an increase in the net ultrafiltration pressure. This mechanism, however, is complicated because the ultrafiltration coefficient is affected by the afferent protein concentration; the coefficient is reduced when the afferent protein concentration is reduced. This change blunts the increment in the GFR which would otherwise result from reduced intraluminal osmotic pressure.

TUBULAR REABSORPTION AND SECRETION

Reabsorption. Only a fraction of the fluid and solute filtered at the glomerulus is excreted in the urine; during the passage of the ultrafiltrate through the tubule, a large percentage of it is reabsorbed and returned to the plasma. This process prevents excessive loss of filtered water, electrolytes, and other solutes necessary for life. The kidney regulates both the plasma concentration and total body content of these substances by modifying, in response to differing circumstances, their rates of reabsorption and thus the amounts excreted. The renal tubular cells are also able to secrete a variety of molecules into the luminal fluid (see below).

Tubular reabsorption or secretion can be passive (i.e., in relation to an electrochemical gradient, like the chloride ion, or to an osmotic gradient, like water or urea), or active (i.e., by a mechanism that requires expenditure of energy to transport a substance against an electrochemical or concentration gradient). Energy for the active transport of many substances, notably sodium and potassium, is derived from the cleavage of adenosine triphosphate under the influence of sodium or potassium adenosine triphosphatase.

Active tubular reabsorption is mediated by a number of mechanisms, each of which is involved in the transport of a limited number of specific compounds. For example, reabsorption of amino acids involves at least 5 different mechanisms, 1 for each of the following groups: (1) neutral amino acids; (2) cystine, lysine, arginine, and ornithine; (3) imino acids and glycine; (4) dicarboxylic acids; and (5) beta amino acids. There is often competition for a transport site. For example, when the concentration of a given substance increases in the tubular fluid, it may reduce, by competitive inhibition, reabsorption of other substances transported by the same system. Capacity for active transport is limited, and the amount of solute, expressed in mg/min, which can be reabsorbed or secreted varies for different substances. This maximal tubular reabsorptive or secretory rate is known as the tubular maximum or *Tm*. Solutes with a Tm for reabsorption include glucose, sulfate, phosphate, amino acids, lactate, malate, acetoacetate, vitamin C, and β-hydroxybutyrate. When the Tm of a compound has been reached, an increment in reabsorption will not occur if the filtered amount increases; the amount filtered in excess of the Tm is excreted.

Secretion. In addition to the mechanisms with an absolute limit in reabsorptive capacity, 2 secretory mechanisms are known to have this characteristic: 1 serves a heterogeneous group of compounds of which many are carboxylic or sulfonic acids (e.g., *p*-aminohippurate, penicillin, a variety of glucuronides and sulfuric acid esters, acetylated sulfonamides, and urologic contrast media such as Diodrast); the other serves organic bases such as guanidine, choline, hexamethonium, and histamine. When the plasma concentration of a substance exceeds the level at which the specific tubular mechanism for its secretion is functioning at full capacity, additional excretion of that substance in the urine, if any, must take place by means of glomerular filtration. The existence of only 2 Tm-limited secretory mechanisms stands in marked contrast to the large number of independent specific Tm-limited reabsorptive mechanisms. Furthermore, their specificity is less than that of transport mechanisms for reabsorption.

Role of the Kidney in Water and Electrolyte Excretion and Acid-Base Balance.   See Sec 5.7.

Role of the Kidney in Regulation of Blood Pressure. See Sec 13.85.

THE CONCEPT OF RENAL CLEARANCE OF PLASMA SOLUTES

The renal clearance of a solute represents that volume of plasma which, if it were completely cleared of the solute, would provide the amount of that solute appearing in the urine within a specified time; clearance is usually expressed as ml/min. Accordingly, if the plasma concentration of a solute is p mg/ml and x mg are excreted/min, the volume of plasma which is totally cleared of this solute is $\dfrac{x \text{ mg/min}}{p \text{ mg/ml}} = \dfrac{x}{p}$ ml/min. This volume per unit time represents the renal clearance of that particular solute and is expressed:

$$\text{Clearance (ml/min)} = \frac{UV}{P}$$

where U = urinary concentration of solute (mg/ml)
V = urinary flow rate (ml/min)
P = plasma concentration of solute (mg/ml)

Measurement of Glomerular Filtration Rate (GFR). If the molecular weight of a solute is sufficiently low for it to be freely filtered through the glomerular basement membrane, and if it is neither reabsorbed nor secreted by the tubules, the amount excreted in the urine (UV) equals the amount filtered (GFR × P), or GFR × P = UV. Thus GFR = $\dfrac{UV}{P}$; i.e., the rate of clearance of such a solute is the same as the GFR. Substances having a rate of clearance $\dfrac{UV}{P}$ that may be used as a measurement of the GFR include inulin (a fructose polymer with a molecular weight of about 5000), other polyfructosans, iothalamate, EDTA, cyanocobalamin (vitamin B_{12}), and mannitol. Measurement of the inulin clearance during constant infusion of it is generally considered the most accurate means of determining the GFR (Sec 16.3).

Measurement of creatinine clearance over a 12 or 24 hr period using endogenously produced creatinine provides an approximate measurement of GFR. The concentration of endogenous creatinine in plasma is low unless the GFR is reduced by more than 50% and the presence of nonspecific chromogens which are detected by techniques commonly used to determine creatinine concentration makes measurement of plasma creatinine levels imprecise. Measurement of endogenous creatinine clearance is easily done, however, and has been widely used clinically as an index of the GFR.

Measurement of Renal Plasma Flow (RPF). Substances that are almost completely removed from the blood and excreted during 1 passage through the kidney are used for measuring renal plasma flow (RPF). The most commonly used method is measurement of para-aminohippurate (PAH) clearance during constant infusion; 85–90% of the PAH is cleared during a single passage. A single injection method based on the rate of decrease in plasma concentration of PAH is easier to carry out and is useful to provide approximate values. The renal blood flow (RBF) can be calculated from the renal plasma flow using the formula:

$$RBF = \frac{RPF}{100 - \text{hematocrit (\%)}}$$

RED BLOOD CELL PRODUCTION

The mediator of the erythropoietic response to anemia or hypoxia is *erythropoietin*, a glycoprotein hormone elaborated by the kidney in response to reduced oxygen tension. In the bone marrow this hormone acts on erythropoietin-sensitive stem cells, transforming them into hemoglobin-synthesizing pronormoblasts. Control of red blood cell production seems to involve a feedback system between the kidney and bone marrow, mediated in 1 direction by red cell–bound oxygen and in the other by erythropoietin. Red blood cell production is influenced by factors other than erythropoietin, as evidenced by the slow constant rate of erythropoiesis in patients who have received a blood transfusion or who are anephric. An inappropriately high rate of erythropoietin secretion leading to polycythemia occurs in a small percentage of patients with renal neoplasms, cystic renal disease, and hydronephrosis.

PROSTAGLANDINS

The kidney both synthesizes and metabolizes prostaglandins. The medullary interstitial and collecting duct cells are the most active sites of synthesis; the cortex contains enzymes which are largely responsible for degradation. Arachidonic acid, the common precursor, is converted (by various prostaglandin cyclooxygenase enzymes collectively called prostaglandin synthetase) to prostaglandin endoperoxides and then to such prostaglandins as PGE_2 (the principal renal prostaglandin), $PGF_{2\alpha}$, PGD_2, and possibly also to PGI_2 (prostacyclin) and thromboxane A_2. Indomethacin inhibits the converting enzymes.

The relationship between renal prostaglandin synthesis and the renin-angiotensin system is complex: angiotensin II stimulates the production and release of PGE_2 and $PGF_{2\alpha}$; on the other hand, PGE_2 increases and $PGF_{2\alpha}$ decreases the production of renin, and indomethacin inhibits renin secretion.

Both PGE_2 and $PGF_{2\alpha}$ are natriuretic in man if given in large doses, probably because of renal vasodilation. There is, however, no convincing evidence that renal prostaglandin and sodium excretion are interrelated.

In response to ischemia and vasoconstriction renal PGE_2 and $PGF_{2\alpha}$ production increases. PGE_2 has a vasodilatory effect and thus attenuates the effect of severe ischemia on the kidney; prostaglandins are probably not responsible, however, for autoregulation of renal blood flow.

The role of renal prostaglandins in hypertension is uncertain, but data suggest that they are involved either primarily or secondarily in many types of hypertension by virtue of their role as vasodilators and natriuretic substances and as actuators or inhibitors of the renin-angiotensin system.

PGE_1 and PGE_2 appear to stimulate erythropoietin production and release from the kidney and to have a direct erythropoietic action on the marrow.

Finally, prostaglandins of the E series have a major influence on renal water excretion, inhibiting vasopressin-stimulated water reabsorption by interfering with the production by vasopressin of its intracellular mediator, cyclic AMP. Indomethacin counteracts this effect by reducing the medullary content of prostaglandins and, thus, potentiates the hydro-osmolar effect of vasopressin; it has been found useful in the treatment of nephrogenic diabetes insipidus.

Renal enzymes that metabolize prostaglandins probably protect against the potent vasodilator and diuretic effects of prostaglandins synthesized elsewhere in the body.

DEVELOPMENTAL ASPECTS OF RENAL FUNCTION

Urine formation begins from the 9th–11th wk of fetal life. The role of the fetal kidney in maintaining homeostasis during subsequent gestation is speculative, although experimental studies in a variety of mammals indicate that it is able to dilute and acidify urine, to absorb phosphate, and to transport organic materials. The placenta is able to meet the excretory needs of the fetus; in the neonate with bilateral renal agenesis, for example, the composition of the body tissues does not differ from normal. Fetal renal blood flow and glomerular filtration rate are low, but within the 1st few days of extrauterine life they undergo a dramatic increase. During the 1st yr of life there is a more gradual increase in these functions, and by 1 yr of age, expressed in relation to weight or surface area, the values are comparable to those of adults. It is clearly inappropriate to

assess renal function at birth or in early infancy by the same standards used for children or adults. In early infancy, however, the kidney is ideally suited to meet the homeostatic requirements.

The dramatic increases in GFR and renal blood flow that occur after birth are principally due to a decrease in renal arteriolar vascular resistance and an increase in the fraction of the cardiac output directed to the kidneys. Circulation in the medullary and juxtamedullary nephrons develops more rapidly than in the outer cortical nephrons. Postnatal growth of the kidney is principally accounted for by increase in tubular mass. The formation of new glomeruli ceases at a fetal weight of approximately 2100–2500 gm.

Values for GFR, determined by inulin clearance, and for effective renal plasma flow, determined by para-aminohippurate clearance, at different stages during the 1st several yr of life are shown in Table 16–1.

The fraction of the renal plasma flow that is filtered is higher in infants (0.32–0.34) than in adults (0.18–0.20). Despite the low GFR value when expressed per unit of surface area, glomerular function is relatively more mature than tubular function. This differential is called *glomerular/tubular imbalance*. It results in a lower fractional reabsorption of many filtered solutes in the proximal tubule than is the case in later life and probably accounts for the fact that infants excrete a higher percentage of glucose, phosphate, and amino acids than do older children and adults. The threshold for HCO_3^- absorption is also lower in the 1st 6 mo (19–21 mEq/l). The ratio of glomerular surface area to proximal tubular volume at birth is high relative to adult values and falls rapidly during the 1st yr.

Ninety-three per cent of normal neonates void within 24 hr after birth and 99% within 48 hr. The mean value of maximal urine osmolality in the newborn period is 600–700 mOsm/kg H_2O. This low value does not reflect an inability of the immature kidney to concentrate urine but is an evidence of the small amount of dietary protein that is metabolized and excreted as urea. If the infant receives a high urea or protein intake several wk after birth, the maximal urine osmolality approximates that of the adult (1200 mOsm/kg H_2O). After the 1st 48 hr of life the urine excretion of a normal infant is 3–4 ml/kg/hr.

The capacity of the infant's kidney to dilute urine is qualitatively the same as the adult's and indicates adequate ability to deliver sodium and chloride to the

Table 16–1 GLOMERULAR FILTRATION RATE (GFR) AND EFFECTIVE RENAL PLASMA FLOW (ERPF) DURING THE FIRST THREE YEARS OF LIFE

AGE	GFR (ML/MIN/M²)	ERPF (ML/MIN/M²)
Newborn–3 days	10–20	30–50
1–2 wk	20–35	70–90
2–4 mo	35–45	135
6–12 mo	45–60	200–245
1–3 yr	60–75	310–380

Adapted from McCrory WW: Developmental Nephrology; Cambridge, Harvard University Press, 1972; and from Guignard JP, Torrado A, Da Cunha O, et al: J Pediatr 87:268, 1975.

diluting segment of the nephron. Following a water load, however, the absolute rate of urine flow is considerably less than in the mature state, a feature that may make the infant more vulnerable to sudden increases in intake of fluid.

The capacity of the neonate's kidney to conserve sodium is good; and the ability to adapt to changes in sodium intake during infancy is considerable, though less than in adults. Since the medullary region is relatively more developed than the cortical zone, the infant is better able to withstand the stress of deprivation of sodium and water than of their excessive intake.

For the 1st several days of life, the infant cannot excrete a strongly acid urine, but by the 2nd wk this capacity is comparable to that of the adult. Unlike older children, infants during their 1st yr secrete a greater proportion of H^+ as titratable acid than as ammonium.

Brenner BM, Bohrer MP, Baylis C, et al: Determinants of glomerular permselectivity: Insights derived from observations in vivo. Kidney Int 12:229, 1977.

Brenner BM, Hostetter TH, Humer HD: Molecular basis of proteinuria of glomerular origin. N Engl J Med 298:826, 1978.

Brenner BM, Humes HD: Mechanics of glomerular ultrafiltration. N Engl J Med 297:148, 1977.

Dunn MJ, Hood VL: Prostaglandins and the kidney. Am J Physiol 233:169, 1977.

Edelmann CM Jr: Pediatric nephrology. Pediatrics 51:854, 1973.

Farquhar MG: The primary glomerular filtration barrier—basement membrane or epithelial slits? Kidney Int 8:197, 1975.

Fried W: Erythropoietin. Arch Intern Med 131:929, 1973.

Lum GM, Aisenbrey GA, Dunn MJ, et al: In vivo effects of indomethacin to potentiate the renal medullary cyclic AMP response to vasopressin. J Clin Invest 59:8, 1977.

McCrory WW: Developmental Nephrology. Cambridge, Harvard University Press, 1972.

Moore ES, Glavez MB: Delayed micturition in the newborn period. J Pediatr 80:867, 1972.

Orloff J, Berliner RW (eds): Handbook of Physiology, Section 8, Renal Physiology. Washington, DC, American Physiological Society, 1973.

Pitts RF: Physiology of the Kidney and Body Fluids. Ed 3. Chicago, Year Book Medical Publishers, 1974.

Venkatachalam MA, Rennke HG: The structural and molecular basis of glomerular filtration. Circ Res 43:3, 1978.

16.3 DIAGNOSTIC ASSESSMENT OF STRUCTURE AND FUNCTION

A variety of techniques are used to evaluate the structure and function of the kidneys and other components of the urinary system. Experience and judgment are required not only in choosing the studies to be carried out but also in synthesizing and interpreting accumulated data. The skills required are those of clinician, physiologist, immunologist, pathologist, geneticist, and radiologist. Few of the presenting manifestations of renal disease in childhood are specific, but many should alert the physician to consider the possibility of a problem affecting the urinary tract and to undertake appropriate studies.

History. Important areas to be explored include:

1. Family history of renal disease, deafness, hypertension, renal calculi, structural developmental anomalies of the urinary tract, and existence in family members of syndromes known to have associated abnormalities of the urinary system.

2. Abnormalities or changes in the pattern of micturition, such as increased urinary frequency, nocturnal or daytime enuresis, increased or decreased urine volume, urgency, dribbling, poor urinary stream, and dysuria.

3. Presence of tea-colored or reddish urine suggesting hematuria or of a foul-smelling urine suggesting infection.

4. Exposure to nephrotoxic agents or potentially nephrotoxic drugs.

5. Facial or generalized edema, or both.

6. Symptoms suggestive of chronic renal failure, such as fatigue, anorexia, nausea, failure to thrive, growth arrest, bone pain, paresthesias, or tetany.

7. History of headache, irritability, seizures, visual disturbance, or facial palsy suggesting hypertension.

8. History of midline abdominal pain or flank pain suggesting renal swelling, bladder infection, obstruction, or calculus.

Physical Examination. The principal physical findings which help in assessing the presence and severity of renal disease include growth retardation, rickets, pallor or sallow complexion, tachypnea, dehydration, edema with or without ascites, hypertension, signs of circulatory congestion, enlargement of the kidneys, flank or suprapubic tenderness, distention of the bladder, abnormalities of external genitalia, single umbilical artery in a newborn infant, physical features of syndromes known to include abnormalities of the urinary tract, and evidence of systemic disease commonly associated with renal manifestations, such as anaphylactoid purpura, systemic lupus erythematosus, or chronic bacteremia.

DIAGNOSTIC EVALUATION OF URINE AND ITS FORMATION

Collection of Urine Specimen. With patience and ingenuity it is usually not difficult to obtain a urine specimen from even the smallest infant. A plastic urine collection bag, the edges of which adhere to the skin around the genitalia, can be used. The perineum and genitalia should be cleansed with soap and water and rinsed thoroughly so that the urine is free of contaminating debris. The collector should be removed as soon as the urine is voided to reduce the likelihood of fecal contamination. Children 2 yr of age or older will usually void on request, and a midstream specimen can be easily collected. In boys the foreskin should be retracted, if possible, and the glans cleansed, particularly if the urine is collected for culture. When accurately timed clearance studies are needed in infants or in children who cannot cooperate, an indwelling flexible urethral catheter of appropriate size with extra holes cut in it may be used. The techniques for collecting urine for culture, including suprapubic aspiration from the bladder in infants, are described in Sec 16.43.

Urinalysis should be performed within several hr of obtaining the specimen. For routine urinalysis the specimen should be kept at room temperature; refrigeration may cause precipitation of phosphates or urates and make microscopic examination difficult.

The *color* should be noted. Urine is normally pale

yellow or amber. If the urine is almost colorless, it is probably very dilute with a low specific gravity; however, when there is osmotic diuresis (e.g., in diabetes mellitus), the urine may be very pale yet have a high specific gravity due to the presence of a dissolved solute, in this instance, glucose. The urine may be pink or reddish because of urates, red blood cells, free hemoglobin (blood or free hemoglobin may also create a brown or tea color), myoglobin, or, rarely, porphyrins. It may have a pink color following ingestion of beets, blackberries, and vegetable dyes used in coloring foods, candies, and soft drinks. Phenolphthalein, a constituent of some laxatives, may color the urine pink or red; conjugated bilirubin, orange-red. Indigo blue, an oxidation product of indican, may cause a blue, nonwater-soluble discoloration of the diaper; the urine is not colored blue when voided; staining of the diaper develops after several hr.

The *odor* of the urine should be noted. An acetone scent indicates ketonuria. In maple syrup urine disease the urine has an odor resembling that of maple syrup. A fecal odor suggests infection with coliform bacteria as does the odor of ammonia from the diaper.

The *osmolality* or *specific gravity* should be measured. Determination of osmolality following a period of dehydration is the best means of estimating the ability to concentrate urine. After 2 mo of age normal infants and children can concentrate urine to over 900 mOsm/kg H_2O following an overnight fast. The urinary specific gravity gives similar information concerning concentrating ability and can be measured with a simple hydrometer or with a refractometer;* the latter requires only a drop of urine.

In general, there is a direct relation between urinary osmolality and specific gravity; when, however, the urine contains glucose, protein, or a compound such as urographic contrast medium, the specific gravity may be elevated to a greater extent than the osmolality as these molecules have a relatively large molecular weight and contribute only slightly to the osmolality.

Screening tests for glucose, ketones, blood, and protein should be done. The simplest way to screen for these substances is to use appropriate dipsticks.† It should be noted that the dipstick test for glucose is specific for glucose. A copper sulfate solution or Clinitest‡ tablet may be used to detect other reducing substances, such as galactose, which are not identified by the glucose oxidase test. The dipstick test§ for proteinuria is sensitive and will reliably detect protein at a concentration of 20 mg/dl or more; the test is more sensitive for detection of albumin than of other urinary proteins. A nitrite dipstick¶ is also available for detection of bacterial infection; for the test to be positive both a significant number of bacteria and sufficient

incubation time in the bladder are required. The ideal specimen of urine for testing is the 1st one voided on arising in the morning. The test may be particularly useful to detect recurrences of documented infection when used by the patient's parent in the home (Sec 16.43).

The temperature of freshly voided urine is related to oral and rectal temperatures; measurement of urinary temperature is a simple way to differentiate real from factitious fever.

For microscopic examination of the urinary sediment, 10–12 ml of urine is centrifuged in a clean centrifuge tube at 100–150 g (800–1000 rpm in the standard laboratory centrifuge) for 5 min. The supernatant is discarded to 0.5 ml in which the sediment is resuspended by brisk agitation. Several drops of the sediment are placed on a clean glass slide; a coverslip may or may not be used.

The sediment should be examined for red and white blood cells, epithelial cells, casts (red cell, white cell, mixed, granular, heme-granular, hyaline), crystals (cystine, uric acid, calcium oxaiate, triple phosphate, sulfonamide), bacteria, protozoa, and yeasts. No precise figures can be set for the number of red or white cells per high power microscopic field which should be accepted as normal because the urine concentration and the thickness of the sediment drop vary. Generally, more than 5 red or white blood cells per high power field ($\times 250$) is considered abnormal. The possibility of contamination of urine by cells from a vaginal discharge should be considered. Hyaline and granular casts or long cylindrical casts with cells attached to their outer aspect may occasionally be seen in normal urine.

The finding of tubular casts is of particular importance since they must originate in the kidney. The matrix of casts is formed of Tamm-Horsfall glycoprotein which originates in the cytoplasm of cells of the ascending limb of the loop of Henle. Their presence, in association with an excessive number of red or white blood cells, is evidence in favor of a renal disorder as distinct from one in the lower urinary tract.

PROTEINURIA

Excessive urinary protein excretion (proteinuria) may be *glomerular*, due to a defect in the filtration barrier which permits proteins of molecular weight 60,000–500,000 (principally albumin and globulin) to appear in the urine; *tubular*, due to failure of absorption of normally filtered low molecular weight proteins (1500–40,000), such as hormones, enzymes, peptides, and immunoproteins; or *overflow*, due to an excess production of proteins which surpasses the tubular reabsorptive capacity (e.g., Bence Jones proteinuria, fibrin split products). Proteins may also arise from various tissues, such as the kidney itself (e.g., Tamm-Horsfall glycoprotein), or from other organs, often as a result of tissue death or injury (e.g., SGOT, myoglobin).

Among many methods for measuring the amount of protein in the urine, the simplest are:

(1) Urine dipstick (Albustix), in which the test paper is impregnated with tetrabromophenol blue buffered to an acid pH. The color of the strip is yellow in the

---

*Total Solids Meter, American Optical Corporation, Buffalo, N.Y.

†Labstick Reagent Strips, Ames Company, Elkhart, Ind.

‡Clinitest Reagent Tablets, Ames Company, Elkhart, Ind. These contain the same essential ingredients as in Benedict solution: copper sulfate, caustic soda, sodium carbonate, and citric acid. A tablet plus 5 drops of urine and 10 drops of water will produce a blue, green-yellow, or orange-red precipitate, depending on the amount of reducing sugar present.

§Albustix Reagent Strips, Ames Company, Elkhart, Ind.

¶N-Labstix, Ames Company, Elkhart, Ind.

absence of protein, but color changes within 10 sec to a shade of green which depends on the concentration of protein present.

(2) The sulfosalicylic acid method, in which 0.5 ml of 3% sulfosalicylic acid is added to an equal volume of urine. If protein is present, the urine develops a degree of turbidity that is directly related to the protein concentration. For precise quantitation of protein concentration a spectrophotometric sulfosalicylic acid method, the biuret technique, and the Lowry technique using the Folin phenol reagent are available (see Cipriani and Looney and Walsh references).

The ratio of the clearance of albumin, as determined by a single radial gel diffusion immunochemical method, to creatinine clearance is advocated by some as an index of the severity of proteinuria and can be determined from single samples of urine and blood. Normal values are less than 0.1; 0.1–1.0, 1–10, and greater than 10 indicate mild, moderate, and marked proteinuria, respectively.

If benzalkonium, used to wash the genitalia, contaminates the urine specimen, a falsely positive dipstick test for protein may result.

In normal infants and children the concentration of protein in urine is less than 20 mg/dl, usually less than 5 mg/dl. The volume of urine depends on fluid intake and on the concentrating ability of the kidney; accordingly, when a given quantity of protein is excreted per unit time, the urine protein concentration will vary with the dilution of the urine. For this reason, if proteinuria in excess of 20–30 mg/dl is detected, the *total* quantity of protein excreted over a timed period should be measured. A 24 hr period is usually selected; the normal value for infants and children is less than 150 mg/24 hr; the majority excrete less than 50 mg/24 hr. The term *proteinuria* should apply only when the total daily excretion of protein exceeds 150 mg.

In urine from normal resting subjects about 70% of the protein has the electrophoretic mobility of globulins; urinary globulins are in general smaller than plasma globulins, and up to half of them are not present in the plasma. They probably originate in the kidney, urinary tract, or seminal glands. The rest of the urine protein has the mobility of albumin and is probably identical to plasma albumin. The *Tamm-Horsfall glycoprotein* is formed in the kidney and is a principal constituent of the matrix of urinary casts. With exercise, excretion of plasma proteins increases to the extent that they constitute about 85% of the proteins in urine.

In most disorders with increased proteinuria, albumin accounts for 60–90% of the protein, particularly in the nephrotic syndrome and other glomerular disorders. In tubular disorders, such as the Fanconi syndrome, proteinuria of 500–1000 mg/24 hr may occur, but it differs from that of glomerular disease in that low molecular weight proteins (1500–40,000) predominate. Hyperglobulinemia is found in some disorders, e.g., chronic active hepatitis, and may lead to increased urinary excretion of globulin.

With the use of sensitive immunologic techniques many of the proteins present in normal plasma can be detected in urine from normal persons and from patients with proteinuria. These proteins include transferrin, ceruloplasmin, IgG, IgA, α2 macroglobulin, a variety of other plasma globulins, and, as mentioned earlier, albumin. From a practical viewpoint, however, it is seldom helpful to determine which particular proteins are present. Immunologic or electrophoretic studies of urinary proteins are of little diagnostic value except in distinguishing tubular from glomerular proteinuria; in the former, globulins predominate, whereas albumin is the principal protein excreted in glomerular diseases.

Depending on the type and severity of injury to the glomerular basement membrane, there is a difference in the molecular weight of the proteins that are filtered and excreted. For example, in the minimal-lesion nephrotic syndrome, preferential excretion of plasma proteins of low molecular weight such as transferrin is found. In contrast, when there is more serious damage, the glomerular basement membrane loses its capacity to restrict the filtration of proteins of high molecular weights and more large proteins appear in the urine. The differential clearance of proteins depending on their weight is called "selectivity." A clearance selectivity test has some usefulness in assessing the severity of glomerular basement membrane injury, but the total amount of protein excreted bears no relation to the selectivity. In practice, the ratio of the clearance of IgG (molecular weight 160,000 daltons) to that of transferrin (88,000) or albumin (69,000) is used as an index of protein selectivity. A value of less than 0.1 (10%) represents highly selective proteinuria such as is seen in the minimal change nephrotic syndrome.

In assessing proteinuria it is important to establish whether it is *persistent* (i.e., present every day over at least several wk, throughout the day and independent of changes in posture) or *transient*. Transient proteinuria occurs after exercise, in fixed reproducible orthostatic proteinuria (postural proteinuria, see below), in acute febrile illnesses, after administration of epinephrine, following plasma or blood transfusions, in skin diseases, and in extensive burns.

When proteinuria is persistent, serial determinations of the 24 hr excretion may be a useful guide to progress of the disorder or to response to treatment. Quantitative excretion of protein must be evaluated in relation to other measures of renal function. For example, in a disorder with progressive glomerular destruction, a decrease in total excretion of protein may result from a lesser amount of protein being filtered because of reduction in the number of functioning glomeruli; such a reduction in excretion of protein could not be regarded as a sign of improvement.

Patients with persistent proteinuria may be separated arbitrarily into 3 groups, based on the amount of protein excreted in 24 hr: 150–500 mg = mild proteinuria; 500–2000 mg = moderate; and over 2000 mg = marked. Marked proteinuria is usually a sign of glomerular disease, but it may also be seen in congestive heart failure or constrictive pericarditis. Mild to moderate proteinuria is seen in some glomerular disorders, such as acute poststreptococcal glomerulonephritis, recurrent macroscopic hematuria, and hereditary nephritis with deafness (Alport disease).

Proteinuria may be absent or mild in many important renal diseases. These include polycystic kidney disease, nephronophthisis, analgesic nephropathy, hypercalcemic and hypokalemic nephropathy, most congenital renal anomalies, obstructive uropathy, nephrolithiasis, and pyelonephritis.

Tubular proteinuria is usually mild, and the proteins are of low molecular weight. Conditions include congenital metabolic disorders in which the proximal tubule is affected (e.g., cystinosis), chronic heavy metal poisoning, chronic pyelonephritis, analgesic nephropathy, acute intrinsic renal failure, interstitial nephritis, Balkan nephropathy, and renal transplantation. Appearance of specific low molecular weight proteins (1500–40,000) in the urine is suggestive of tubular damage; these include lysozyme, an enzyme derived from leukocytes and normally absorbed in the proximal tubule, β_2-microglobulin (MW 11,800) derived from the light chain of the HLA histocompatibility antigen, and N-acetyl glucosaminidase and β-glucuronidase.

Orthostatic (Postural) Proteinuria. In most normal persons the quantity of protein excreted in urine per unit of time is 5–15 times greater in the upright than in the recumbent position; the protein concentration in the upright position is, however, not above 30 mg/dl, and the total daily excretion of protein is less than 150 mg. In some persons the protein concentration in urine formed in the upright position is considerably higher and may reach 150–1200 mg/dl. Proteinuria which is present in the upright position but absent in the recumbent is called orthostatic or postural proteinuria. Orthostatic proteinuria may be present over a prolonged period (5–10 yr), in which case it is referred to as fixed and reproducible orthostatic proteinuria.

Although orthostatic proteinuria is seen in some forms of renal disease, most children with this pattern are healthy, and there is no underlying renal pathology. The sex incidence is equal, and the usual period of detection is the 2nd decade, when proteinuria is discovered incidentally on routine urinalysis. In at least 50% of patients the condition is still present 10 yr or so after detection. Currently available data indicate that postural proteinuria is a normal variant without increased risk for the development of other forms of renal disease or hypertension.

A simple test can confirm the diagnosis of orthostatic proteinuria.* Collection of a 24 hr specimen for total protein measurement can be done before the postural test.† With the information gained from these determinations and a routine urinalysis, it is possible to be confident of the diagnosis and to reassure the patient and the parents about the prognosis. The routine urinalysis shows a variable protein concentration and no other abnormal findings; the urine formed while the child is recumbent has a protein concentration of 2–25 mg/dl, and the protein concentration in the urine formed while the child is in the upright position is 75–1500 mg/dl; the total 24 hr urinary excretion of protein seldom exceeds 1000 mg.

HEMATURIA

It is difficult to quantify the number of red blood cells that are present in normal urine; usually there are fewer than 5 per high power field ($\times 250$) in the sediment of a 10 ml centrifuged fresh specimen; arbitrarily, hematuria is present when this number is exceeded. When hematuria is of clinical importance, many times this number of RBCs are usually seen. Attempts have been made to quantify the numbers of red cells, white cells, and tubular casts passed during a given time. A 12 hr Addis count has been widely used for this purpose, but this test is not reliable in the evaluation of renal disorders in children; a properly done urinalysis provides the necessary information concerning cellular elements and casts excreted.

The terms gross or macroscopic hematuria are used when the urine has a reddish or brown color due to the presence of red blood cells; free hemoglobin resulting from hemolysis of excreted RBCs may also be present. Hematuria may also be suspected when the urine has a greenish brown color. Bright red urine, with or without clots, suggests an extrarenal or lower urinary tract source of bleeding, whereas a renal source is more likely when the urine is brown or tea colored. Free hemoglobin, which may spill into the urine following acute intravascular hemolysis, may color the urine reddish brown; more commonly, free hemoglobin arises from lysis of red blood cells already present in the urine. The indicator strip on the Labstix dipstick is a sensitive test for hemoglobin, either free or contained in erythrocytes. The term microscopic hematuria is used when the color of the urine is normal and hematuria is detected only by microscopic examination or dipstick.

Hematuria, especially if only microscopic, does not necessarily represent a disorder of the kidney or urinary tract. Microscopic hematuria may occur following strenuous exercise and with a variety of intercurrent unrelated conditions, such as viral or bacterial respiratory infections, other febrile disorders, and gastroenteritis with dehydration. Urine may also be contaminated by

---

*The test is done in the morning. The night before the test the child voids at bedtime, and this specimen is discarded. One glass of water is given. Upon waking in the morning, the child voids immediately, preferably before getting out of bed or while sitting on the side of the bed. This specimen is labeled "recumbent specimen." A large glass of water or fruit juice is given and the child stands in a lordotic position for 20–30 min. Then the child voids again, and the specimen is saved in a separate container labeled "upright specimen." A comparison of the protein concentration in these 2 consecutive specimens is then made. The uncomfortableness of the upright, arched position may be alleviated by permitting the child to rest his or her head on a wall and by permitting some freedom in movement.

†The time to start the collection is not fixed; any convenient 24 hr period may be used. Beginning, for example at 8 A.M., the child voids and the specimen is discarded. All urine voided after this time up to and including the specimen voided at 8 A.M. the following day is saved. This completes the collection. The specimens may all be placed in the same bottle and should be refrigerated.

Table 16–2 CAUSES OF HEMATURIA IN CHILDREN

Acute and chronic forms of acquired glomerular injury; e.g., acute poststreptococcal glomerulonephritis, hemolytic-uremic syndrome, membranoproliferative glomerulonephritis, recurrent macroscopic hematuria with mesangial IgA and IgG deposition (Berger disease)

Hereditary or familial renal disorders; e.g., hereditary nephritis with deafness, familial benign recurrent hematuria, polycystic kidney disease

Systemic disorders with vasculitis which may affect the kidney; e.g., systemic lupus erythematosus, anaphylactoid purpura, polyarteritis

Disorders of the renal vasculature; e.g., renal vein or artery thrombosis, hemolytic-uremic syndrome, renal vascular malformation, arteriovenous fistula

Neoplasm; e.g., Wilms tumor

Trauma

Developmental anomalies, e.g., obstructive uropathy causing hydronephrosis (minor renal trauma may cause gross hematuria in patients with structural renal anomalies)

Bacterial or viral infection of the urinary tract

Nephrolithiasis

Systemic bacterial infection; e.g., bacterial endocarditis, shunt nephritis

Miscellaneous; e.g., sickle cell disease or trait, urethral meatal ulcer, malignant hypertension, coagulation disturbances, hematuria following strenuous exercise, drug- or chemical-induced hematuria (e.g., hemorrhagic cystitis due to cyclophosphamide), foreign body in lower urinary tract, schistosomiasis, hypercalciuria

---

red blood cells from the external genitalia, e.g., a urethral meatal ulcer or menstrual blood.

If proteinuria is also present, the hematuria is usually clinically important and probably has a renal source. If casts are present, the source of the hematuria must be the kidney. The association of both proteinuria and tubular casts with hematuria is evidence that the hematuria is most likely the result of a glomerular disorder, and in such circumstances extensive radiologic and urologic examination of the lower urinary tract is unnecessary.

The absence of hematuria does not exclude a number of important renal disorders including, for example, the minimal lesion nephrotic syndrome, nephronophthisis, and many of the developmental renal anomalies.

Microscopic examination of the sediment, apart from the search for casts, may be additionally helpful in elucidating the cause of hematuria. Numerous bacteria and pus cells indicate acute infection; certain crystals, such as those of cystine or a sulfonamide, suggest injury by stone formation in the collecting system.

In evaluating hematuria, there is often a tendency to focus on the bladder as the source of the bleeding, and in many hospitals children with hematuria undergo cystoscopic examination. In most instances this is unnecessary. The cause and site of origin can usually be ascertained by the history and clinical findings and by microscopic examination of the urine sediment, quantitation of proteinuria, and, if necessary, radiologic study of the urinary tract. Multisystem disorders such as systemic lupus erythematosus and anaphylactoid purpura which may cause renal damage and hematuria should be excluded by appropriate studies. In some patients with hematuria of renal origin a biopsy may be indicated to establish the diagnosis.

Table 16–2 lists some of the causes of hematuria in children.

ABILITY TO CONCENTRATE URINE

After a 12 hr period of fluid restriction the normal child can concentrate urine to 900 mOsm/l (specific gravity 1.024) or more. The mean value for children 2 yr of age or older is approximately 1100 mOsm/l (range 870–1300 mOsm/kg H_2O). The normal values are less well defined in infants, but, in general, beyond the age of 2 mo infants should be able to concentrate urine to a value of 900 mOsm/l or more after fluid deprivation; from 1 wk–2 mo of age an osmolality of 700 or more can be expected. Fluid restriction must be carried out with very close supervision in infants or in patients in whom substantial inability to concentrate the urine may be present. When impaired ability to concentrate urine is suspected, there is a simple test of urinary concentrating ability.* Care should be taken to avoid dehydration, contraction of extracellular fluid volume, and weight loss as a consequence of fluid deprivation during the test. The synthetic vasopressin analogue DDAVP (1-deamino-8-D-arginine vasopressin) is increasingly used as a means of testing the urine concentrating ability. It is given intranasally (10 µg in infants, 20 µg in children) at 7:30 A.M.; the 8:30 urine is discarded, and the osmolality is measured on a specimen collected during the next several hr. Normal values for children and infants are over 975 mOsm/kg and 475 mOsm/kg H_2O, respectively. These results are comparable to those obtained with prolonged fluid restriction. For testing infants, the fluid intake should be restricted to about 50% of the usual amount for the 2 meals following DDAVP administration, but restriction is not necessary in older children.

The ability of the kidney to form a concentrated urine is impaired in a number of renal disorders. For example, in chronic renal failure, as the glomerular filtration rate declines, so does the ability to dilute and to concentrate the urine; the maximal urine concentration, even after fluid restriction, may not exceed that of plasma by more than 150 mOsm/l. In disorders in which the renal medulla or interstitium is damaged, e.g, obstructive uropathy with hydronephrosis, pyelonephritis, or nephronophthisis, the maximal urine concentration is often below the normal range. Chronic hypokalemia, acute or chronic hypercalcemia, sickle cell disease, and nephrocalcinosis due to distal renal tubular acidosis may be associated with an impaired urinary concentrating ability. If a major defect in concentrating ability is suspected, e.g., in nephrogenic diabetes insipidus, an overnight test should not be done; the study may be done during the daytime under close observation, with frequent measurement of weight and vital signs, but it is probably wiser to test urine concentrating ability with the DDAVP test in situations in which gross polyuria is present than to use a water deprivation test.

---

*The child is given a normal diet; nothing is given by mouth after lunch except dry supper until the test is completed. The child voids before going to bed; this urine is not saved. The 1st morning specimen is obtained and the time of collection noted; the minimal amount of urine required is 2 ml, but more than 5 ml is preferable. The specimen should not be refrigerated; it should be sent in a sealed container to the laboratory for measurement of osmolality.

Renal Excretion of Acid. In most instances it is unnecessary to test the capacity of the kidney to acidify urine and excrete hydrogen ions by administration of an acid load. In children with impairment of renal acidifying capacity, metabolic acidosis is usually present, and the urine pH, titratable acidity, and ammonium excretion can be determined; in patients with an impaired ability to excrete hydrogen ions an imposed acid load has risk.

In a state of metabolic acidosis the otherwise normal child should excrete a urine of pH 5.0–5.5 or less, with titratable acid and ammonium values of approximately 30 and 42 μEq/min/M^2, respectively. During the 1st yr of life the titratable acid excretion is approximately 20% higher and the ammonium excretion approximately 20% lower than these values.

For an oral ammonium chloride loading test, the dose is about 5 g/M^2; the intent is to lower the plasma bicarbonate level 3–5 mEq/l to about 18 mEq/l. This test should not be done if the child is already acidotic (plasma bicarbonate concentration of 18 mEq/l or less). Plasma HCO_3^- and H^+ concentrations and pCO_2 are obtained 3–5 hr after giving the ammonium chloride; 2 consecutive urine collections under oil (each of 60 min duration) are obtained. A urine pH under 5.5 and the values for titratable acid and ammonium indicated above should be attained in a normal child. In cases of systemic metabolic acidosis these data should be obtained without need to give ammonium chloride; the risk of inducing more severe acidosis is not warranted.

URINARY EXCRETION OF AMINO ACIDS, ELECTROLYTES, AND OTHER METABOLITES

Paper chromatographic techniques can be used to detect excessive excretion of *amino acids* (Scriver and Rosenberg). The nitroprusside test* can be used to detect excretion of cystine.

Excretion of *calcium* may need to be determined in patients with nephrolithiasis who may have hypercalciuria, hyperparathyroidism, or inadequately controlled distal renal tubular acidosis. Normal urine calcium values are under 5 mg/kg/24 hr (usually < 2 mg/kg) while receiving a calcium intake of less than 500 mg/24 hr.

When the *sodium* intake is restricted, e.g., below 20 mEq/M^2/24 hr, the kidney can reduce excretion of it to less than 10 mEq/l. Excessive urinary loss of sodium during restricted intake may indicate inadequate secretion of adrenal mineralocorticoids or impaired renal ability to conserve sodium, as in chronic renal failure, obstructive uropathy, nephronophthisis, and pseudohypoaldosteronism. The normal kidney adapts readily to changes in intake of sodium and can excrete up to 250 mEq/M^2/24 hr, even more if the dietary intake is chronically above this level.

In health the excretion of *potassium* also is responsive to a wide range of intake, e.g., from 20–250 mEq/M^2/24 hr. Excretion in excess of intake occurs during metabolic acidosis, contraction of extracellular volume, diuretic therapy, hyperadrenalism, and corticosteroid therapy.

Determination of the amount of *chloride* excreted may help to identify the cause of metabolic alkalosis. When it is secondary to contraction of the intravascular volume, the urine chloride concentration is usually < 10 mEq/l, and correction by administration of isotonic saline is indicated. Urinary concentration of sodium is usually also very low (< 10 mEq/l) in the presence of intravascular volume contraction. In acute renal insufficiency of prerenal origin similarly low levels of sodium and chloride excretion are found; this finding may be helpful in diagnosis.

Urinary excretion of *oxalate* is elevated in oxalosis, an inherited metabolic disorder of which nephrolithiasis is one of the manifestations, and in a variety of conditions with secondary hyperoxaluria. Normal values of urinary oxalate excretion are < 40 mg/24 hr.

CLEARANCE AND REABSORPTION STUDIES

Glomerular Filtration Rate (GFR). The normal glomerular filtration rate in children over 1 yr of age is 70 ± 5 (1 S.D.) ml/min/M^2. This is the value obtained during infusion of inulin* or iothalamate ^{125}I.† (See Sec 16.2.) Single injection techniques using inulin, iothalamate ^{125}I, or ^{51}Cr EDTA permit reasonably accurate measurement of the GFR without need for constant infusion techniques in children. Single injection techniques are not reliable when the patient is edematous or when the GFR is markedly reduced. More frequently in clinical practice clearance of endogenous creatinine measured over a 6–24 hr period is used to determine the GFR. This long period of measurement tends to minimize errors introduced by incomplete collection, inaccurate timing, and possible incomplete emptying of the bladder. Values obtained with this method are usually 10–15% lower than with inulin. Because of difficulty in the accurate measurement of plasma creatinine, especially at concentrations under 1 mg/dl, there is considerable variation in the GFR based on endogenous creatinine clearance measurement. The method for measuring the endogenous creatinine clearance is: (1) collect a 12 or 24 hr urine specimen (discarding the 1st and including the last specimen of the timed collection period), (2) measure the total creatinine excreted during the period, (3) obtain a plasma creatinine value during the period of urine collection, and (4) calculate the GFR as follows:

$$GFR = \frac{\text{creatinine excreted (mg/min)}}{\text{plasma creatinine (mg/min)}} = \text{ml/min}$$

---

*Nitroprusside test reagents: 5% sodium cyanide, fresh saturated solution of sodium nitroprusside. Procedure: to 1–2 ml of urine add an equal volume of 5% sodium cyanide; wait 10 min. Add 3–4 drops of saturated sodium nitroprusside solution. A positive test is indicated by a dark magenta color.

*Inulin 10 per cent, Arnar Stone Laboratories, 601 E. Kensington Road, Mt. Prospect, Ill.

†Glofil, Abbott Laboratories Ltd., P.O. Box 68, Abbott Park, North Chicago, Ill.

Since the method using the rate of clearance of endogenous creatinine is, at best, an approximation of the GFR, when accuracy is required, the clearance of another substance such as inulin or iothalamate should be determined.

The serum creatinine concentration itself gives a rough guide to the GFR. In children under 2 yr of age the normal value is less than 0.4 mg/dl; from 2 yr to onset of puberty it is under 0.6 mg/dl; from onset of puberty to maturity it is less than 1.0 mg/dl, except for some normal muscular subjects in whom it may be up to 1.2 mg/dl. The blood urea nitrogen value may also be used as a rough index of the GFR, but it is influenced by factors other than the GFR; the normal value in infants and children is less than 15 mg/dl.

Renal Plasma Flow. See Sec 16.2.

Phosphate Clearance. Other than creatinine or inulin clearance, the phosphate clearance (C_p) is most commonly measured. The C_p is influenced principally by parathyroid hormone. The normal value is less than 8.0 ml/min/M^2. Values in excess of this may indicate an impaired ability of the proximal tubule to reabsorb phosphate or hyperparathyroidism. Values less than 2.0 ml/min occur with severely restricted phosphorus intake and in hypoparathyroidism.

The tubular reabsorption of solutes, such as phosphate, which are almost completely filtered at the glomerulus and of which concentrations in the plasma are virtually identical to those in the glomerular filtrate, can be calculated in several ways. Using phosphate as an example, the % of the phosphate filtered that is reabsorbed by the tubules—the % of tubular reabsorption of phosphate, or TRP—is determined in the following way:

(1) GFR (ml/min) can be measured by clearance of endogenous creatinine or of inulin or iothalamate ^{125}I.
(2) Filtered phosphate (mg/min) = GFR (ml/min) $\times$ plasma phosphate concentration (mg/ml).
(3) Excreted phosphate is measured for a given time interval.
(4) The % TRP, defined as the percentage of the filtered phosphate which is reabsorbed (reabsorbed phosphate = filtered phosphate − excreted phosphate),

$$= \frac{\text{reabsorbed phosphate}}{\text{filtered phosphate}} \times \frac{100}{1}$$

Normal values for TRP are >85%. Lower values occur in hyperparathyroidism (primary or secondary) and in disorders of the proximal tubule when there is a disorder in the transport mechanism for phosphate reabsorption.

Renal Biopsy. Renal biopsy often enables precise diagnosis and evaluation of severity of an illness and also facilitates decisions concerning treatment.

Percutaneous renal biopsy should be done only when it is suspected that the abnormality is not confined to a localized area of the kidney. Renal biopsy is of most help in conditions that affect the glomeruli principally, such as those that have a reduced glomerular filtration rate, hematuria, and proteinuria. A biopsy may also be helpful diagnostically in acute renal failure and in evaluating the status of a transplanted kidney. Sequential

Table 16–3 CLINICAL SITUATIONS IN WHICH RENAL BIOPSY IS OFTEN INDICATED

Persistent or recurrent hematuria of unknown cause
Atypical or severe acute glomerulonephritis
Rapidly progressive glomerulonephritis
Nephrotic syndrome resistant to corticosteroids
Nephrotic syndrome with features not typical of the minimal change type
Persistent asymptomatic proteinuria
Suspected familial or hereditary nephritis
Acute intrinsic renal failure of unknown cause
Chronic renal failure of unknown cause
Evaluation of renal involvement in systemic disease, e.g., anaphylactoid purpura, systemic lupus erythematosus
Evaluation of renal allograft
Monitoring course of glomerular disease in response to treatment

biopsies may be used to monitor the course of a disorder and response to treatment.

Biopsy should be performed only after complete evaluation by appropriate clinical, biochemical, immunologic, bacteriologic, and radiologic studies. It should be performed by an experienced physician who has facilities and personnel to prepare the renal tissue for light and electron microscopic and immunopathologic examination. In infants under 6 mo of age an open rather than a percutaneous biopsy is safer. Table 16–3 lists clinical situations in which a renal biopsy is often indicated.

UROLOGIC INVESTIGATIONS

See Sec 16.62 and 16.63.

SCREENING PROGRAMS FOR DETECTION OF URINARY TRACT DISORDERS IN PRESCHOOL AND SCHOOL AGE CHILDREN

Routine urine screening programs for children have generally been based on a dipslide method to detect urinary tract infection and on dipstick tests to detect hematuria, proteinuria, and glucosuria. Approximately 1% of girls and 0.04% of boys will be found to have previously unrecognized urinary tract infections, but a great deal more must be learned about the natural history of asymptomatic bacteriuria in children before routine screening for its detection can be recommended. The majority of children with hematuria and proteinuria detected by screening have no renal disease or, at most, self-limited conditions. Most investigators who have participated in these studies have concluded that the effort expended in detecting abnormalities of the urinary tract by means of screening programs has not warranted the cost, nor has it been convincingly shown that a positive or useful outcome accrues to the recipients of urinary screening. It is now felt that the overall effectiveness of urinary screening with early inclusion of roentgenographic or urologic investigations in children with positive tests is doubtful. On the other hand, there is evidence that when renal scarring results from urinary infection and associated vesicoureteral reflux, most of the scars have developed by 5 yr of age and it is uncommon for new scars or progressive damage to occur. These findings suggest that screening for bacteriuria well before school age has a potential role in the prevention of renal disease.

A more rational approach for the detection of kidney disease is one directed at the individual child whose medical history, symptoms, and signs warrant the use of more extensive studies to exclude disorders of the urinary tract.

KEITH N. DRUMMOND

Arbus GS: Urinary screening program to detect renal disease in preschool and kindergarten children. Can Med Assoc J 116:1141, 1977.

Aronson AS, Svenningsen NW: DDAVP test for estimation of renal concentrating capacity in infants and children. Arch Dis Child 49:654, 1974.

Barratt TM, Crawford R: Lysozyme excretion as a measure of renal tubular dysfunction in children. Clin Sci 39:457, 1970.

Barratt TM, McLaine PN, Soothill JF: Albumin excretion as a measure of glomerular dysfunction in children. Arch Dis Child 45:496, 1970.

Boylan JB, Van Liew JB (eds): Symposium on proteinuria and renal protein catabolism. Kidney Int 16:247, 1979.

Chantler C, Barratt TM: Estimation of glomerular filtration rate from the plasma clearance of Cr⁵¹ EDTA. Arch Dis Child 47:613, 1972.

Cipriani A, Brophy DA: Method for detecting cerebrospinal fluid protein by photoelectric colorimeter. J Lab Clin Med 28:1269, 1943.

Cohen ML, Smith FG Jr, Mindell RS, et al: A simple, reliable method of measuring glomerular filtration rate using single, low dose sodium iothalamate I¹³¹. Pediatrics 43:407, 1969.

Dodge WF, West EF, Smith EH, et al: Proteinuria and hematuria in school children. Epidemiology and early natural history. J Pediatr 88:327, 1976.

Edelmann CM Jr, Barnett HL, Stark H, et al: A standardized test of renal concentrating capacity in infants and children. Am J Dis Child 114:639, 1967.

Edelmann CM Jr, Boichis H, Rodriguez-Soriano J, et al: The renal response of children to acute ammonium chloride acidosis. Pediatr Res 1:452, 1967.

Forbes PA, Drummond KN: Urine screening programs in schools. Can Med Assoc J 109:979, 1973.

Harries JD, Mildenberger RR, Malowany AS, et al: A computerized cumulative integral method for the precise measurement of the glomerular filtration rate. Proc Soc Exp Biol Med 140:1148, 1972.

Looney JM, Walsh AI: The determination of spinal fluid protein with the photoelectric colorimeter. J Biol Chem 127:117, 1939.

Lowry OH, Rosebrough NJ, Farr AL, et al: Protein measurement with the Folin phenol reagent. J Biol Chem 193:254, 1951.

Manuel Y, Revillard JP, Betuel H (eds): Proteins in Normal and Pathologic Urine. Baltimore, University Park Press, 1970.

Peterson PA, Evrin PE, Berggard I: Differentiation of glomerular, tubular, and normal proteinuria: Determinations of urinary excretion of β₂-microglobulin, albumin, and total protein. J Clin Invest 48:1189, 1969.

Robinson RE, Glenn WG: Fixed and reproducible orthostatic proteinuria. IV. Urinary albumin excretion by healthy human subjects in the recumbent and upright postures. J Lab Clin Med 64:717, 1964.

Scriver CR, Rosenberg LE: Amino Acid Metabolism and Its Disorders. Philadelphia, WB Saunders, 1973.

16.4 DIAGNOSTIC IMAGING OF THE URINARY SYSTEM IN INFANTS AND CHILDREN

Radiographic imaging and image-amplified fluorography remain the primary diagnostic methods of imaging of the urinary tract, but dramatic refinements in ultrasonography and in computed axial tomography and advances in radionuclide imaging and function studies call for a fresh approach to investigation of the urinary system.

To be able to select and carry out the appropriate procedures, the radiologist should know the clinical history and be informed about pertinent physical and laboratory findings. Since the number of centers which are equipped with the complete array of modern imaging modalities for children is limited, choices may differ as to the primary imaging method.

Each diagnostic procedure has weaknesses. The pediatric radiologist should choose the least invasive and most informative method to provide baseline information with minimal exposure to ionizing radiation and the least physical and psychologic trauma to the child. Ideally, a single method should suffice, but in practice a combination of different procedures is often necessary to establish an accurate diagnosis. Until recently the primary diagnostic examination in pediatric uroradiology was urography. Voiding cystourethrography, image intensified fluorography for dynamics of the upper and lower tract, angiography, radionuclide scanning, pressure studies, ultrasonography, and computed tomography serve to complement urography in various disease states. In a number of conditions there has been increasing use of ultrasonography as the most informative and least invasive primary diagnostic tool and at times as the only necessary preoperative investigation (e.g., in case of multicystic kidney). Ultrasonography increasingly replaces an invasive baseline study in a critically ill infant (e.g., in acute renal failure). Table 16–4 lists the suggested primary imaging technique for various conditions affecting the urinary tract in children.

Table 16–4   INDICATIONS FOR DIAGNOSTIC IMAGING OF THE URINARY TRACT

INDICATION	SUGGESTED PRIMARY METHOD
Urinary tract infection	Urography
Pyelonephritis (acute)	Ultrasound
Acute renal shutdown	Ultrasound
Sepsis (newborn)	Ultrasound
Abdominal mass	Ultrasound
Bilateral flank mass	Ultrasound
Unilateral flank mass	Ultrasound
Suspected infravesical obstruction—neonate	Retrograde voiding cystourethrogram
Bilateral pneumothorax—newborn	Ultrasound
Renal insufficiency	Ultrasound
"Anuria"	Ultrasound
Failure to thrive	Ultrasound
Screening for polycystic kidney disease	Ultrasound
Abdominal pain unexplained, recurrent	Ultrasound
Abdominal trauma	Urography
Hypertension	Urography
Congenital abnormalities known to be associated with urinary tract abnormalities	Urography
Ambiguous genitalia	Urography
Enuresis (selected)	Urography
Lower urinary tract signs and symptoms	Urography
Suspected neurogenic abnormality	Urography
Prospective kidney donor for renal transplant	Urography
Patients with renal transplant	Ultrasound
Kidney localization before biopsy	Ultrasound

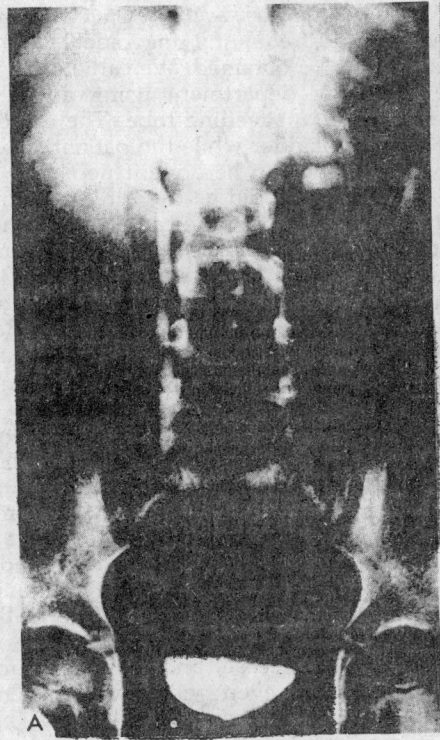

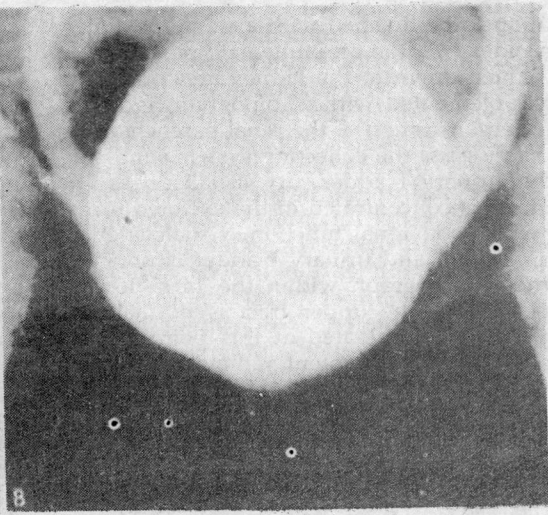

Figure 16–6 Normal kidneys and collecting systems in a 4½ yr old (A), in whom significant bilateral reflux is shown by excretory method (B).

Excretory urography (urography, intravenous pyelography [IVP]) remains the most commonly used primary imaging modality for the urinary tract in children. It consists of serial radiography using ionizing radiation subsequent to intravenous injection of an organic triiodo compound such as meglumine diatrizoate.* Urography displays the morphology of the renal parenchyma, collecting systems, and urinary bladder in relation to other retroperitoneal and intraperitoneal organs (Fig 16–6A). It also gives a crude assessment of renal function. Mobility of the kidneys, motility of the collecting systems, and function of the urinary bladder can be studied using fluoroscopy and/or fluorographic recording.

Adequate preparation of the patient prior to urography, e.g., with a cleansing enema, permits better visualization with the least number of radiographs. A preliminary radiograph is examined before the injection of any contrast medium. Presently used contrast media are hypertonic, are eliminated by glomerular filtration, and cause an osmotic diuresis. The dose is 1.5–3.0 ml/kg in infants weighing less than 5 kg and 1.5–2.0 ml/kg in children, with a maximum of 50 ml for a single bolus injection. Only superficial veins should be used for administration of contrast media. A nonionic water-soluble contrast medium (metrizamide), of low toxicity and osmolality, is in use for urography in some centers.

Contraindications to urography include dehydration and shock. In renal failure, providing the patient is well hydrated, much useful information can be obtained

with urography. Occasionally, a 2nd injection has to be given or an infusion urogram done.

Serious reactions to contrast media are extremely uncommon in children, but resuscitation facilities must be available in every radiographic room. Minor reactions such as urticaria, nausea, vomiting, or flushing do not contraindicate repeated study.

An *inferior venacavogram* may be obtained as part of a urographic study and may be helpful in investigation of a child for abdominal mass. Successful injection of a foot vein is required. Abdominal radiographs taken during the injection may display the inferior vena cava and useful conclusions be drawn.

Total body opacification occurs during and after injection, while the contrast medium is mainly in the vascular compartment. Highly vascular organs or lesions are distinguishable from avascular or less vascular structures. This phenomenon may be of diagnostic value.

Various phases of the excretory urogram are recognized. The *nephrogram* (renal parenchymal visualization) permits the study of renal size and contour and evaluation of the renal parenchyma. Since perirenal fat is absent or scarce in the young patient, a radiograph with nephrogram is mandatory for the evaluation of the homogeneity of the parenchyma, measurement of renal size, and appreciation of renal contour. In the 1st few yr of life the nephrogram is adequate within the 1st 10 min of intravenous injection of the contrast medium, and a 6 or 10 min postinjection abdominal radiograph may display the renal parenchyma, the collecting systems, and the urinary bladder, permitting

*Reno-M-60, Squibb.

the examination to be finished with a single postinjection film. In older children an immediate postinjection radiograph, coned down to the kidney area only, and sometimes supplemented with a tomogram, is necessary for best demonstration of the renal parenchyma.

In the *excretory phase* the collecting systems and subsequently the urinary bladder are visualized as the contrast medium is concentrated in the excreted urine. In children with good renal function, visualization of the collecting system and urinary bladder is obtained with 1 overhead radiograph within the 1st 5–10 min after the injection. If the upper tract is normal, the examination may be terminated at this point. If any abnormality is found, subsequent radiographic exposures are planned by viewing each radiograph and focusing on the areas of interest in order to improve detail and decrease radiation exposure.

The kidneys are immature organs in the newborn and premature infant. Hence radiologic visualization is different in this group of patients. Excretion and concentration of contrast medium are delayed and diminished in comparison with older children. These factors should be taken into account when planning urography in this age group.

Urinary tract infection is the most common indication for urography, which is still the most informative primary imaging procedure. Baseline urography is done several wk after completion of treatment of the 1st infection. If renal damage (which is present in about 15% of cases) or secondary evidence of vesicoureteric reflux is found, a micturition cystourethrogram is also obtained, with fluorographic recording. The micturition cystourethrogram displays the morphology and contractility of the urinary bladder, and, with proper positioning, the bladder neck and urethra are well seen.

Micturition (voiding) cystourethrography (MCU, VCU) can be done by the excretory method provided there is a good concentration of the contrast medium in the urinary bladder. Although sometimes more time consuming, it is always less traumatic and more physiologic than retrograde cystourethrography (Fig 16–6B).

Retrograde (catheter) voiding cystourethrography is widely practiced and frequently unavoidable if adequate information is to be obtained. We catheterize the patient in the radiology department using a No. 5 or No. 8 premature infant feeding tube. The catheter is kept in the urinary bladder while the patient is voiding so that repeated filling can be done if necessary (Fig 16–7). A Foley catheter should be used in exceptional situations only. The position of the catheter and the early filling of the bladder should be observed by fluoroscopy. An emergency retrograde cystourethrogram is done when infravesical obstruction is suspected in a baby boy. The observation of the detrusor contraction during voiding is useful; the appearance of the male urethra during different phases of filling may vary from virtually normal to grossly abnormal in appearance.

Vesicoureteric reflux is as a rule an intermittent phenomenon. Some type of fluorographic record (fluoroscopist's observation, 100 mm spot filming, videotape recording, or a combination of these) is mandatory for diagnosis of and for recording the extent of vesicoureteric reflux. The use of random overhead radiographs to record findings on voiding cystourethrography should be abandoned; major abnormalities may be missed with such a method. Reflux may alter in intensity and extent, cease, and reappear during straining and micturition, even with a well distended bladder and forceful micturition (Fig 16–8).

The *grading* of reflux should be done at the time of maximum filling of the collection system during voiding. Contractility of the renal pelvis, ureteric peristalsis, and the speed of emptying of the refluxing collecting systems are other important parameters to look for and document. Whatever grading system is used by the radiologist, the description of the severity of the reflux should be clear to the clinician. The maximal ureteric dilatation should be stated in millimeters.

Radiologic follow-up examinations in clinically well supervised patients with chronic medical or postsurgical renal abnormality should be sufficiently separated in time, and minimal radiographic exposures should be

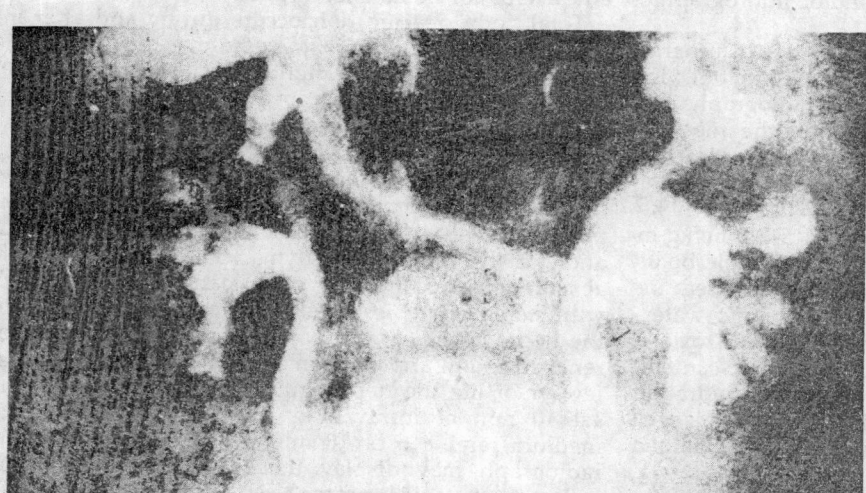

Figure 16–7 Maximum degree of reflux, as shown during fluorography during retrograde cystourethrogram; reflux from the bladder to the kidneys is evident, with dilatation of the pelvicalyceal system.

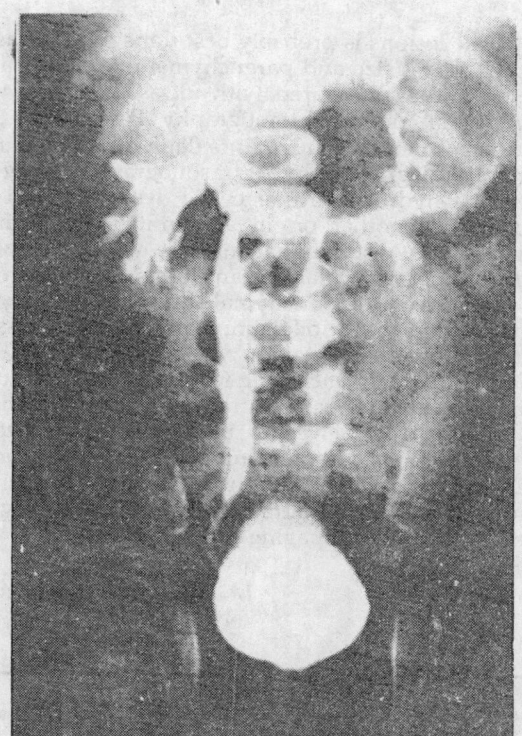

Figure 16–8 At 35 min after intravenous injection of contrast medium, while the patient is straining, vesicoureteric reflux to the inferior pole division of a duplicated system is well shown.

injury to the renal pedicle is suspected. In such cases an aortogram is done as a 1st step to exclude or demonstrate trauma to the renal artery. A renal angiogram is useful in selected cases of *hypertension*. In children with an abdominal mass, angiography is sometimes necessary for differentiation of the renal, suprarenal, or hepatic origin of the mass.

Radionuclide imaging is inferior to urography, ultrasonography, and computed tomography for delineation of morphology. Radiation dose (total, thyroid, and gonadal) is usually higher than with urography. As a physiologic *function test* radionuclide imaging has advantages, but those aspects are beyond the scope of this chapter. In some centers vesicoureteric reflux is successfully investigated by radionuclide imaging. We prefer fluorographic observation before, during, and after micturition for evaluation of reflux since, as previously mentioned, vesicoureteric reflux is usually an intermittent phenomenon.

Computed tomography (CT scan) is selectively used as a complementary imaging technique for urinary system abnormalities. This examination involves additional ionizing radiation and usually additional intravenous injection of a contrast medium; accordingly, in nonmalignant conditions it is uncommonly indicated in children. There does not currently appear to be any place for computed tomography as a primary or baseline imaging modality.

In the newborn and young or emaciated patient, computed tomography for diagnosing urinary system

used. When maximal improvement and/or renal growth are documented, urographic follow-up is no longer indicated. Since the kidneys grow during childhood, compensatory renal growth in patients with renal disorders should be documented at puberty or thereafter for future reference. Subsequently, laboratory tests and blood pressure recordings may be all that are required; there is usually no indication for consecutive follow-up radiographic studies.

Retrograde urethrography is rarely indicated in children. Post-traumatic, iatrogenic, and inflammatory strictures are uncommon in our experience. This examination is done by injecting water-soluble contrast medium under fluoroscopic control using spot film or 100 mm film recording. It is a very painful examination; adequate analgesia is necessary.

Retrograde pyelography gives additional information occasionally in preoperative workup of a patient. When required for diagnosis, it should be done under fluoroscopic control after introduction of the ureteric catheter.

Aortography and renal angiography have become much less frequently used in the diagnostic workup of childhood urinary system abnormalities. Percutaneous catheterization of femoral artery or vein can be done even in small infants. For this special examination sedation or occasionally general anesthesia may be required. During and subsequent to high pressure bolus injection, rapid sequence serial roentgenographs are exposed (Fig 16–9). Angiography is indicated in *renal trauma* when

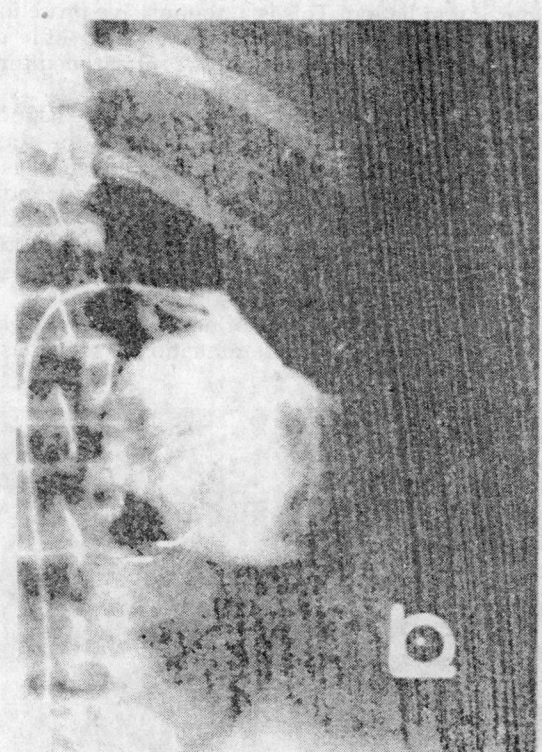

Figure 16–9 Selective renal angiogram. Multiloculated cystic mass is confirmed in the superior pole of the left kidney in a hypertensive 15 yr old boy. Duplication was excluded with an aortogram.

pathology should not be done. Motion artifacts may interfere with accurate interpretation in the older child. Scanners with less than 3 sec exposure time produce superior images. Gastrointestinal tract preparation, using contrast medium to opacify the gut and drugs to decrease motility, and intravenous injection of urographic contrast media are frequently needed to achieve satisfactory visualization of the kidneys and retroperitoneal structures. Sedation of the uncooperative child may be necessary.

In children with neoplastic conditions that involve or potentially invade the urinary system, retroperitoneal space, pelvic organ, and/or perirectal and perivesical spaces, computed tomography should definitely be part of the preoperative and/or pretreatment workup. The anatomic display with this modality is incomparably easier to understand for all physicians involved in the management of the patient than any other imaging method. With serial examinations the results of surgery, radiation, and/or chemotherapy can be assessed. Recurrences and metastases are presently best recognized with this modality, although there is no way at present to differentiate between scar tissue, inflammatory tissue, or neoplastic tissue.

Ultrasonography (echography) of the urinary system has become an increasingly important imaging modality since 1973 (gray scale ultrasonography, real time ultrasonography). Rapid technical developments have led to the potential of great diagnostic accuracy in detecting morphologic abnormalities. Present-day ultrasonography equals or surpasses imaging modalities necessitating ionizing radiation. This is a noninvasive procedure, and diagnostic images can be obtained with little discomfort to the patient. Injection of contrast medium is avoided and sedation rarely necessary.

The frequency of sound waves used for diagnosis varies from 1–10 MHz. The attenuation of the sound waves in the tissues depends on the frequency used; 2.2–7.5 MHz transducers are generally used, depending on the size of the patient and the depth and size of the organ to be examined. Ultrasonography has become the initial diagnostic imaging modality of choice in numerous conditions (Table 16–4).

Sonographic differentiation of normal renal morphology is possible today. The differentiation of solid masses from cystic lesions is probably best done with ultrasonography. Renal size and parenchymal thickness can be more accurately measured with ultrasound than with urography or computed tomography (Fig 16–10).

In newborn and young infants flank masses are most accurately diagnosed by ultrasonographic imaging. Congenital hydronephrosis, cystic dysplasia, and nephromegaly of other origin are entities that can be differentiated. A suprarenal mass is detectable earlier by ultrasonography than by any other method in the very young. Minor parenchymal abnormalities, calyceal distortion, and minor dilatations are not yet accessible to ultrasonographic imaging.

The pelvic organs including female internal genitalia, the urinary bladder, and intrapelvic anatomic abnormalities lend themselves to ultrasound examination, and, if necessary, complementary CT scanning can be done. In the diagnosis of intrascrotal abnormalities, including neoplasms, ultrasonography is already accepted as a superior imaging modality.

M. BERNADETTE NOGRADY

Ash JM, Gilday DL: Renal nuclear imaging and analysis in pediatric patients. Urol Clin North Am 7:201, 1980.

Brun B, Egeblad M: Metrizamide in pediatric urography. Ann Radiol (Paris) 22:198, 1979. Quoted in Yearbook of Urology. Chicago, Year Book Medical Publishers, 1980, p 61.

Bushong SC, Glaze D, Glaze S, Singleton E: Radiation dose to children from x-ray and radioisotope examinations. Health Physics 35:720, 1978.

Fellows KG: The uses and abuses of abdominal and peripheral arteriography in children. Radiol Clin North Am 10:349, 1972.

Freeman LM, Raymond C, Koutulidis C: Renal imaging in pediatrics. In: James AE Jr, Wagner HN Jr, Cooke RE (eds): Pediatric Nuclear Medicine. Philadelphia, WB Saunders, 1974, p 308.

Heller JO, Schneider M: Pediatric Ultrasound. Chicago, Year Book Medical Publishers, 1980.

Nogrady MB, Dunbar JS: Delayed concentration and prolonged excretion of urographic contrast medium in the first month of life. Am J Roentgenol 104:289, 1968.

Nogrady MB, Dunbar JS, Rousseau O: The technique of roentgen investigation of the urinary tract in infants and children. Prog Med Radiol 3:3, 1970.

Standen JR, Nogrady MB, Dunbar JS, et al: Osmotic effects of methylglucamine diatrizoate (Renografin 60) in intravenous urography in infants. Am J Roentgenol 93:473, 1965.

Sumner TE: Pediatric ultrasonography. In: Ultrasound in Urology. Baltimore, Williams and Wilkins, 1979, p 275.

Teele RL: Ultrasonography of the genito-urinary tract in childhood. Radiol Clin North Am 15:109, 1976.

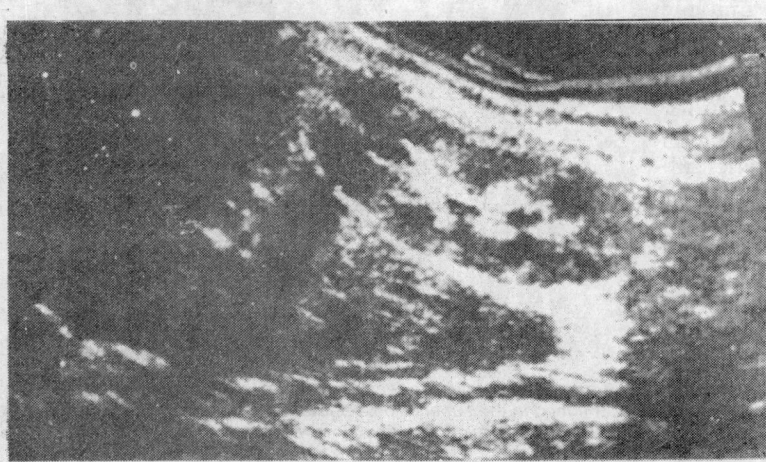

Figure 16–10 Swollen kidney demonstrated by ultrasound in a 4 yr old girl in severe renal failure prior to biopsy.

16.5 Diseases of the Glomerulus

It is clinically useful and, in most instances, theoretically sound to consider renal disease from the standpoint of the primary site of injury or of disturbed physiology, which may be the nephron (glomerulus, proximal tubule, distal tubule), the interstitial tissue, or the renal vasculature. The various parts of the nephron are closely related, however, and dependent upon the integrity of the renal blood supply and interstitium; a disturbance in or pathologic insult to 1 of the components is often reflected in altered structure or function in others. In this section disorders are discussed that affect primarily the glomerulus. It is essential to consider the etiology and pathogenesis of the injury, the types of histopathologic change that may be present, the spectrum of clinical and laboratory manifestations, the role of host factors, and the natural history of each of the currently recognized disorders. Failure to use an integrated approach is responsible for much confusion about glomerular disease.

16.6 ETIOLOGY AND PATHOGENESIS OF GLOMERULAR INJURY

In most forms of glomerular injury one cannot specify precisely the molecular basis for structural or functional changes, but a general grouping of etiologic factors is possible.

Hereditary or familial factors play a role in many forms of glomerular disease; in some there are also interstitial parenchymal and tubular lesions. A list of the heritable conditions in which there are renal manifestations comprises about 50 distinct entities. These are listed in Table 16–8 in Sec 16.30. Not all are described completely since many are rare or are manifest only in adulthood.

Immunologic Factors. A number of different types of immunologic glomerular injury are recognized. The most common results from deposition of *antigen-antibody* complexes in the glomerulus; these complexes bind complement which is believed to be the principal mediator of injury. During circulation through the glomeruli, complexes may be sequestered in the mesangium, localize in a subendothelial position within the glomerular basement membrane itself, or penetrate the glomerular basement membrane and become trapped on its epithelial aspect. Neither the antigen nor the antibody in the complex bears any immunologic relation to glomerular constituents. In immune complex injury electron microscopy finds characteristic discrete deposits or lumps in mesangial, subendothelial, or epimembranous sites. On immunofluorescence microscopy a similar granular or nodular pattern is seen, and antibody molecules such as IgG, IgM, or IgA and complement components such as C3, C4, and C2 are often identifiable within these deposits. The specific antigen against which the immunoglobulin is directed may sometimes be identified.

The pattern of tissue response depends on the site of deposition and on the number of complexes deposited. If they localize principally in the mesangium, the re-

sponse may be minimal, or a mesangiopathic change consisting of proliferation of mesangial cells and matrix may occur, which may extend between the endothelial cells and the basement membrane and compromise the filtering function of the capillary loops. When the complexes localize principally in the subendothelial or subepithelial region, the response tends to be a diffuse glomerulitis, sometimes with epithelial crescent formation. The presence of fibrin in Bowman space, presumably leaked through damaged glomerular basement membrane, is crucial for crescent development. In case of chronic deposition of complexes in the subepithelial region, the inflammatory and proliferative responses tend to be less prominent, and the glomerular basement membrane gradually becomes thickened as the complexes are incorporated into new basement membrane formed on the epithelial aspect; this results in the condition known as membranous glomerulopathy.

The mechanisms responsible for the differential distribution of immune complex deposition within the glomerulus are largely unknown; the size of the complex appears, however, to be 1 of the principal determinants. Small complexes tend to penetrate the capillary loop, undergo aggregation, and accumulate along the capillary wall beneath the epithelial cells, whereas intermediate size complexes do not penetrate the basement membrane so readily but enter the mesangium. Complexes may also localize at sites other than the glomeruli, e.g., in the tubular basement membranes, peritubular capillary walls and interstitium, and may initiate a form of interstitial nephritis.

In some diseases with immune complex deposition the amount of available antigen is limited; e.g., a bacterial antigen may be eliminated by host defense mechanisms or by specific treatment. In such conditions glomerular deposition of complexes is limited, and damage may be mild or of short duration, as in acute poststreptococcal glomerulonephritis or the nephritis of serum sickness.

When there is an unlimited or persistent source of antigen, the host continues to produce antibody to it, and chronic formation of antigen-antibody complexes results; deposition of complexes in the glomeruli continues, and progressive glomerular damage may occur, as in untreated systemic lupus erythematosus.

Many techniques exist for detecting immune complexes in the circulation. The complexes can often be found in glomerular disorders in which complex deposition is believed to be of pathogenetic importance, but the correlation is inconsistent and of limited value in diagnosis or in furthering our understanding of these disorders.

An increasing number of specific endogenous (e.g., DNA, neoplastic, and thyroglobulin) and exogenous (e.g., bacterial, viral, fungal, and parasitic) antigens have been identified within glomerular immune complexes, but in most patients with presumed immune complex glomerulopathy there is no clue as to the nature and identity of the postulated antigen.

It has recently been proposed that glomerular injury may follow in situ immune complex formation, free circulating antibody reacting with antigen already localized within the glomerulus to form insoluble immune complexes at the local site. The antigen could be a normal glomerular constituent or an exogenous one that has become fixed or trapped within the glomerulus. This mechanism may be operative in subepithelial complex formation (e.g., membranous glomerulopathy), whereas circulating preformed immune complexes are more likely to deposit in subendothelial and mesangial sites.

That immunofluorescent microscopy finds immune reactants such as antibodies and complement within the glomerulus does not necessarily signify an immunologic pathogenesis since passive and nonspecific trapping of a variety of macromolecules, including fibrin, C3, IgM, and IgG, may occur at sites of glomerular damage of nonimmunologic origin.

A 2nd type of immunologic injury is due to the formation of *host antibodies to glomerular basement membrane* antigens; these antibodies can be detected in serum in some cases. They are deposited in a linear, uninterrupted pattern along the endothelial aspect of the glomerular basement membrane. Complement is fixed at the site of this antigen-antibody reaction. The linear pattern of antibody and complement deposition contrasts with the nodular pattern of immune complex deposition described above. Possible explanations for development of antibodies to one's own glomerular antigens are as follows: (1) an alteration in glomerular antigenic structure, possibly as the result of injury, renders the glomerular antigens foreign to the host's antibody-producing cells; (2) glomerular antigens previously confined to the glomeruli, without access to antibody-producing sites, may be released into the circulation and stimulate antibody production; (3) antibodies may be produced to foreign protein, such as a viral or bacterial antigen, and may cross-react with glomerular antigens; and (4) nonrenal host antigens may be released following injury, and antibodies produced to them may cross-react with glomerular constituents that have similar antigenic determinants. Whatever the mechanism, the development of host antibodies to glomerular basement membrane antigens is operative in fewer than 10% of human immunologic renal diseases. Included are Goodpasture syndrome, some cases of rapidly progressive glomerulonephritis, and some of chronic glomerulonephritis; all are rare in children.

A 3rd type of immunologic renal injury involves activation of the *alternative complement pathway* by a mechanism independent of the relationship of immunoglobulin molecules to antigens. Either exogenous or endogenous factors activate the complement system at the 3rd component, bypassing C1, C4, and C2. The final sequence of complement activation leading to release of biologically active compounds is the same as in the classic system involving C1, C4, and C2, but the participation of an antigen-antibody reaction is not needed to initiate the sequence of complement activation after C3. This mechanism operates in membranoproliferative glomerulonephritis and may, in addition to complex deposition, be of importance in acute poststreptococcal glomerulonephritis and in the nephritis of

systemic lupus erythematosus. C3 nephritic factor (C3NeF) is detectable in sera of some patients with glomerular disease due to alternative complement pathway activation. C3NeF is an IgG autoantibody to the labile C3 convertase C3b,Bb. By binding to it, C3NeF stabilizes this enzyme and retards its decay, thus promoting C3 cleavage via the alternative pathway.

A 4th type of immunologic injury involves *mesangial deposition of IgA aggregates,* often in association with IgG and, less frequently, with complement components. The pathogenesis is not understood. Although the IgA deposits are found diffusely in the mesangial regions of most glomeruli, the histopathologic response tends to be focal and segmental. This condition is often associated with recurrent episodes of gross hematuria (Berger disease) and with the nephritis of anaphylactoid purpura.

In most recognized forms of immunologic glomerular injury the complement system participates in production of damage (1) by contributing to the inflammatory reaction through immune adherence to leukocytes and by chemotaxis, (2) by damage to biologic membranes, and (3) by enhancement of blood coagulation. The pathways by which the complement system is activated are the *classic pathway,* in which antibody molecules aggregated in relation to specific antigens interact with the C1q subunit of C1, triggering the assembly and activation of the subsequent complement components; and the *alternative pathway,* in which C1, C2, and C4 are bypassed and C3 is activated by a C3 activator enzyme derived from a serum protein called C3 proactivator. The plasma protein *properdin* is involved in activation of the alternative pathway.

Congenital absence of specific components of the complement system may be associated with glomerulonephritis. Complement deficiencies in which this association is recognized include those of C1r, C1s inhibitor, C4, C2, and C7. The mechanism by which complement deficiencies lead to glomerular damage is unknown. Two possibilities have been suggested: (1) that complement deficiency leads to an increased incidence of infection, with more immune complex formation; and (2) that complement normally plays a role in solubilizing complexes once they are formed, a deficit in complement activity retarding this dissolution.

In end-stage kidney disease, regardless of cause, deposition of immunoglobulins (primarily IgM) and components of the classic and alternative pathways is common. The deposition is focal and segmental and is limited to hyalinizing glomeruli. Properdin is found in some of these sclerosing segments. The immune deposition in focal glomerulosclerosis or in end stage kidney disease is more likely the consequence than the cause of glomerular changes. The role of cell-mediated immunity in glomerular injury is uncertain.

Metabolic or Toxic Factors. Most known nephrotoxic drugs or chemicals cause damage principally to renal tubules or interstitial tissue; glomerular damage is usually a secondary reaction. Certain drugs, such as trimethadione, however, may selectively damage the glomeruli and cause increased permeability of the glomerular basement membrane to protein; this may also occur in chronic mercury poisoning. Drugs can also serve as haptens and lead to the development of an immune complex type of glomerulopathy, as is sometimes seen with penicillamine therapy. In diabetes mellitus evidence suggests that there is a change in the carbohydrate composition of the glomerular basement membrane; an increase in mesangial tissue and thickening of the basement membrane develop early, before there is any clinical or laboratory evidence of renal disease. It has been proposed that the minimal lesion form of the nephrotic syndrome is due to a chemical or metabolic disorder of the glomerulus.

Coagulation Disturbances. The hypothesis that disturbances in coagulation or in the fibrinolytic system may play a pathogenetic role in glomerular disorders is supported by the findings of fibrin or its derivatives at the site of glomerular injury, the detection of fibrin degradation products in serum and urine, and the modification by anticoagulation of the course of some glomerular diseases. It is not established, however, that fibrin deposition is an initial or important event in human glomerular damage. Some investigators doubt that the coagulation disturbance is critical to the initial insult but think that it does participate in progressive glomerular damage. Conditions in which glomerular fibrin deposition is common include anaphylactoid purpura and lupus glomerulonephritis. Fibrin deposition in Bowman space is an important factor in the development of epithelial crescents.

Other Factors. Few causes of glomerular injury can be considered isolated factors. For example, immune complex deposition involves complement activation which may enhance blood coagulation locally; this in turn may accentuate glomerular damage. Similarly, in diabetes mellitus, which is primarily a disorder of carbohydrate metabolism, there is evidence of immunoglobulin deposition along the glomerular basement membrane in about 50% of patients. It is likely that this is a secondary event and not of pathogenetic importance. It is a good example of how interrelated and complex the factors are that may lead to glomerular injury. Furthermore, there is evidence that increased permeability of the glomerular basement membrane to protein, a common consequence of glomerular injury, may itself induce alterations in the metabolic activities of the glomerulus, with additional effects on glomerular function, structure, or both.

Glomerular damage, often manifested as the nephrotic syndrome, may be related to a variety of neoplasms. In some instances an immune complex system involving tumor antigens seems to be operative. In the case of lymphoproliferative neoplasms there is little evidence for this form of injury. In some developing countries glomerular diseases, which often present clinically as the nephrotic syndrome, are relatively common; immune complex formation involving parasitic antigens is suspected in some of these disorders.

The causes of many forms of glomerular injury remain unknown. In children the most common disorders in this category include the minimal lesion form of the nephrotic syndrome, benign recurrent hematuria, and the hemolytic-uremic syndrome.

16.7 HISTOPATHOLOGY OF GLOMERULAR DISEASE

The range of possible clinical, laboratory, and pathologic responses to glomerular injury is limited.

In assessing the pathologic changes in glomeruli by light microscopy, the following points should be considered:

1. Are there any abnormal findings?
2. Do the lesions affect all glomeruli (diffuse) or fewer than half of the glomeruli (focal)?
3. Does the lesion affect the entire glomerulus (global), or is it confined to limited areas of it (segmental)?
4. Does the lesion appear recent (acute) or longstanding (chronic)?
5. Is there abnormal lobulation of the glomeruli?
6. Is there evidence of segmental hyalinosis or sclerosis of parts of the glomerular tuft?
7. Is there cellular proliferation? If so, which cells are involved (mesangial, endothelial, or epithelial)? Has proliferation of parietal epithelial cells led to epithelial crescent formation? If crescents are present, what percentage of the glomeruli is affected? Are the crescents fibrous or cellular?
8. Are patent capillary loops reduced in number?
9. Is there an increase in mesangial matrix?
10. Is there an infiltrate of polymorphonuclear leukocytes to indicate inflammation?
11. Is there necrosis of any part of the glomerulus?
12. Are the glomerular basement membranes thickened? If so, is the thickening uniform or localized? Is it due to proliferation of the mesangial tissue that has extended between the endothelial cells and the glomerular basement membrane proper, or is it due to deposition of material, such as immune complexes, within the glomerular basement membrane or along its epithelial or endothelial aspect? Are the endothelial cells themselves swollen, with or without the formation of subendothelial space?
13. Is Bowman capsule thickened? Are there adhesions between the glomerular tuft and Bowman capsule?
14. Are the lesions minimal, moderate, or severe?
15. Are the interstitial tissue and the blood vessels involved? Are these changes secondary to or independent of the glomerular lesion? Is there periglomerular fibrosis, tubular atrophy or dilatation, interstitial scarring, or inflammation? Are foam cells present in the interstitium?

A description of the pathologic changes is achieved with this evaluation. It is then possible to assess the severity of the lesions and to decide whether they are likely to be self-limited, progressive, or amenable to therapy; it is also often possible to identify specific disease entities.

Immunopathologic studies and electron microscopic examination provide further essential data. Renal biopsy should not be undertaken unless these studies are available.

Classification of the major glomerular diseases is not yet satisfactory since in most instances causative factors are unknown and since the wide variety of insults and pathogenetic mechanisms generate a distinctly limited number of pathologic and clinical responses. A suitable classification should take account of histopathologic, immunopathologic, and electron microscopic findings; the presence of absence of systemic disease; the presumed pathogenetic mechanism and etiology; and the clinical features.

16.8 CLINICAL MANIFESTATIONS OF GLOMERULAR DISEASE

The clinical conditions resulting from glomerular disorders are determined not only by the type of injury, its extent, its severity, and its rate of progression but by host determinants, some of which are unknown, and by factors such as age, state of nutrition, amount of proteinuria, and the intake and excretion of fluid and electrolytes.

The major clinical patterns resulting from glomerular injury are listed in Table 16–5. It should be emphasized that they are not mutually exclusive and that, with time, one may supersede another.

16.9 LABORATORY DATA OF GLOMERULAR DISEASE

Apart from laboratory tests which may help in the diagnosis of a specific disease, 3 areas of laboratory investigation are particularly helpful in the assessment of glomerular involvement: (1) Measurement of glomerular filtration rate; values below normal are reflected in elevation of the blood urea nitrogen and serum creatinine concentrations. When the glomerular filtration rate falls below 25% of normal, the concentrations of serum phosphate and uric acid may also be above normal. (2) Measurement of protein excretion; a common response of the glomerulus to a wide variety of injuries is increased permeability of the glomerular basement membrane to macromolecules, which are normally excluded from the filtrate. This leads to excretion of an increased amount of protein in the urine. Values over 150 mg/24 hr are abnormal unless the child has orthostatic proteinuria. (3) Examination of the urine sediment; an abnormal number of red blood cells is a common finding in many forms of glomerular injury; polymorphonuclear leukocytes may also be present. These cells may arise from renal lesions at sites other than the glomerulus or from bleeding or inflammation in the ureters and lower urinary tract; their renal source is signified by the presence of casts. Red or white blood cells or both may be embedded in the matrix of the cast, or the cast may be hyaline or granular. In most instances the presence of casts reflects not only a renal but a glomerular origin of the abnormal sediment.

Couser WG, Salant DJ: In situ immune complex formation and glomerular injury. Kidney Int 17:1, 1980.
Daha MR, Austen KF, Fearon DT: Heterogeneity, polypeptide chain composition, and antigenic reactivity of C3 nephritic factor. J Immunol 120:1389, 1978.
Habib R, Levy M: Contribution of immunofluorescent microscopy to classification of glomerular diseases. In: Kincaid-Smith P, d'Apice AJF, Atkins RC (eds): Progress in Glomerulonephritis. New York, John Wiley and Sons, 1979.

Kim Y, Friend PS, Dresner IG, et al: Inherited deficiency of the second component of complement (C2) with membranoproliferative glomerulonephritis. Am J Med 62:765, 1977.
O'Regan S, Smith M, Drummond KN: Antigens in human immune complex nephritis. Clin Nephrol 6:417, 1976.
Velosa J, Miller K, Michael AF: Immunopathology of the end-stage kidney. Immunoglobulin and complement component deposition in nonimmune disease. Am J Pathol 84:149, 1976.
Wilson CB, Brenner BM, Stein JH, et al (eds): Immunologic mechanisms of renal disease. Contemporary Issues in Nephrology, Vol 3. New York, Edinburgh, and London, Churchill, 1979.

16.10 THE NEPHROTIC SYNDROME

The nephrotic syndrome may be a manifestation of a number of different clinical entities which share an abnormal increase in permeability of the glomerular basement membrane to protein, with marked proteinuria. Clinical features include generalized *edema, hypoproteinemia* (with serum albumin levels usually below 2 gm/dl), *hyperlipidemia* (with serum cholesterol levels above 220 mg/dl), and marked *proteinuria* (2 gm/M^2/24 hr or more). Proteinuria is the essential feature of the syndrome. In children with the nephrotic syndrome the kidney usually appears to be the only or principal organ involved; this may be termed a *primary* nephrotic

Table 16–5 CLINICAL PATTERNS OF GLOMERULAR DISEASE

Nephrotic syndrome	Generalized edema, proteinuria in excess of 2 gm/M^2/24 hr, reduced serum protein concentration, elevated serum cholesterol, transient microscopic hematuria and hypertension infrequently
Acute glomerulonephritis	Hematuria, red blood cell casts, oliguria, hypertension, mild edema, circulatory congestion, azotemia
Mixed nephritic-nephrotic picture	A combination of glomerulonephritic and nephrotic features
Acute renal failure	Anuria or severe oliguria, with fluid, acid-base, and electrolyte disturbances; hypertension, circulatory congestion, and edema may be present
Chronic renal insufficiency or failure	Growth retardation, lethargy, neurologic manifestations, anemia, azotemia, metabolic acidosis, hyperphosphatemia, hypocalcemia, renal osteodystrophy, polyuria, and polydipsia
Recurrent or persistent hematuria	Episodic gross hematuria with intermittent or persistent microscopic hematuria; moderate proteinuria may be present during episodes of hematuria
Asymptomatic proteinuria	Persistent proteinuria in an otherwise apparently healthy child
Rapidly progressive glomerulonephritis	Initial presentation with a mixed nephritic-nephrotic picture; progressive course to renal insufficiency within 6 wk to several mo

syndrome. The nephrotic syndrome may develop also during the course of a systemic disease; here it is considered *secondary*. The distinction between *primary* and *secondary* is blurred since even when the clinical and pathologic changes appear related only to the kidney, unrecognized systemic factors are usually operative.

The *primary* group includes (1) the *minimal change nephrotic syndrome* (MCNS), nephrotic syndrome with *diffuse mesangial proliferation*, and *nephrotic syndrome with focal glomerulosclerosis* (some consider these to be separate entities, but it seems more likely that they are variants of the same process; MCNS is by far the most common condition causing the nephrotic syndrome in children); and (2) a group of disorders characterized by *diffuse glomerular lesions*, including *membranoproliferative glomerulonephritis* (MPGN) types I and II, *membranous glomerulopathy*, and *idiopathic crescentic glomerulonephritis* with antiglomerular basement membrane antibodies. (Each is readily recognized by characteristic histopathologic and immunopathologic glomerular findings, and all appear to result from 1 or another of a variety of forms of immunologic renal injury.)

Secondary forms of the nephrotic syndrome develop during the course of a diverse group of unrelated diseases, including diabetes mellitus, Alport disease, systemic lupus erythematosus, syphilis, malaria, anaphylactoid purpura, amyloidosis, lymphoproliferative neoplasia, poststreptococcal glomerulonephritis, and systemic infections such as subacute bacterial endocarditis or infected atrioventricular shunt. In some of these, immunopathogenetic mechanisms identical to those operative in the *diffuse glomerular lesion* group of primary nephrotic syndrome can be identified; in others the mechanism of glomerular basement membrane injury is unknown. The most evident clinical features are frequently not those of the nephrotic syndrome.

Some authors separate the nephrotic syndrome in infancy into a 3rd group. Two principal forms are the *Finnish type* and *diffuse mesangial sclerosis*; rarely, other disorders may cause the nephrotic syndrome in the 1st yr of life.

Proteinuria. The excessive excretion of protein results from increased glomerular filtration of protein due to increased permeability of the glomerular basement membrane. Generally, plasma proteins of low molecular weight, such as albumin, IgG, and transferrin, are excreted more readily than are proteins of larger molecular weight, such as lipoproteins. This relative clearance of plasma proteins in inverse relation to their size or molecular weight reflects the *selectivity* of proteinuria.

Hypoproteinemia. The reduction in serum concentration of proteins, particularly those of low molecular weight, is primarily a consequence of the loss of protein in the urine. There is some reabsorption of filtered protein, with increased protein catabolism in tubular cells and a paradoxic increase in the serum concentration of some proteins of larger molecular weight, particularly of α_2-globulins; the plasma lipoproteins are in this fraction. Accordingly, the protein loss as a consequence of increased glomerular permeability to protein is only partly accounted for by the amount finally excreted in the urine. The plasma calcium concentration may be low as a consequence of the reduced albumin level, since about half of the plasma calcium is bound to albumin; the concentration of ionized calcium, however, remains normal.

Edema. Though edema is almost always present at some time during the course and is the sign that dominates the clinical pattern, it is the most variable of the cardinal features of the nephrotic syndrome. It is a secondary manifestation that is influenced by a number of factors other than hypoproteinemia, such as fluid and salt intake. The mechanism of its formation is complex; some of the factors are: (1) *Reduction in plasma colloid osmotic pressure* consequent to the decreased concentration of serum albumin; this is responsible for a shift of extracellular fluid from the intravascular to the interstitial compartment with edema formation and reduction in intravascular volume. (2) *Marked reduction in urinary excretion of sodium* due to an increase in tubular reabsorption. The mechanisms responsible for the enhanced sodium reabsorption are not completely understood but are principally the result of reduced intravascular volume and lowered colloid osmotic pressure. There is increased excretion of renin and elevated aldosterone secretion. (3) *Retention of water.* Reduction of plasma colloid osmotic pressure and retention of all ingested sodium would not in themselves be sufficient for the development of manifest edema in the nephrotic syndrome. In order for edema to develop, there must be a retention of water. If the concentration of electrolytes in body fluids is to remain isotonic despite retention of virtually all ingested sodium chloride, water must be conserved (for each 140 mEq of sodium retained, 1 liter of water). Normal tonicity is maintained through the secretion of antidiuretic hormone, which leads to reabsorption of water in the distal tubules and collecting ducts and the formation of a hypertonic or concentrated urine. This may be the principal explanation for water retention in most nephrotic children, as suggested by the observation that when sodium intake is markedly reduced, it is not essential to restrict the intake of water since the ability to excrete water is not usually impaired significantly. Other reasons for water retention may exist since a small percentage of nephrotic children continue to retain water even when their sodium intake is nil. Retention may result from inappropriate release of an antidiuretic hormone in response to contraction of the intravascular volume. It is also possible that a net increase in sodium reabsorption in the proximal tubule, together with passive reabsorption of water along an osmotic gradient in this segment, reduces the volume of filtrate delivered to the ascending limb of the loop of Henle and to the distal convoluted tubules for formation of dilute urine. In such a situation, ingestion of excess water could lead to fluid retention and progressive decrease in serum sodium level and plasma osmolality.

In nephrotic patients the retention of salt and water, which may be considered a physiologic response to reduced plasma oncotic pressure and hypertonicity, does not correct the contracted intravascular volume since the retained fluid escapes into the interstitial space and the patient becomes more edematous in direct relation to the amount of ingested sodium and water.

Hyperlipidemia. Most of the lipid fractions normally found in plasma are elevated in the nephrotic syndrome. There is a variable inverse relation between the degree of hyperlipidemia and the reduction in plasma albumin. A possible explanation for the elevated plasma concentration of lipoproteins is their relatively high molecular weight and consequent negligible loss in the urine in comparison with that of albumin. Since lipoproteins play a role in lipid transport, their increase in plasma may also influence lipid levels.

Albrink MJ, Hald PM, Man EB, et al: The displacement of serum water by the lipids of hyperlipidemic serum. A new method for the rapid determination of serum water. J Clin Invest 34:1483, 1955.

Bader PI, Grove J, Trygstad CW, et al: Familial nephrotic syndrome. Am J Med 56:34, 1974.

Cameron JD, White RHR: Selectivity of proteinuria in children with the nephrotic syndrome. Lancet 1:463, 1965.

Churg J, Habib R, White RHR: Pathology of the nephrotic syndrome in children. A report for the international study of kidney disease in children. Lancet 1:1299, 1970.

Habib R, Kleinknecht C: The primary nephrotic syndrome of childhood: Classification and clinicopathologic study of 406 cases. In: Sommers SC (ed): Pathology Annual, 1971. New York, Appleton-Century-Crofts, 1971.

Habib R, Levy M, Gubler M-C: Clinicopathologic correlations in the nephrotic syndrome. Pediatrician 8:325, 1979.

Michael AF, McLean RH, Roy LP, et al: Immunologic aspects of the nephrotic syndrome. Kidney Int 3:105, 1973.

16.11 MINIMUM CHANGE NEPHROTIC SYNDROME (MCNS)

(Nephrosis, Lipoid Nephrosis, Idiopathic Nephrotic Syndrome)

This condition accounts for over 75% of cases of nephrotic syndrome in childhood. It is characterized by responsiveness to corticosteroid therapy, by absence of significant glomerular lesions on light microscopy, with diffuse podocyte fusion on electron microscopy, by absence of glomerular immune globulin or complement deposition, and by highly selective proteinuria.

Etiology. This is unknown. Familial or genetic factors are found in a minority of cases. HLA antigen B12 is said to be more common than in the general population.

Incidence. The incidence of new cases from birth to 16 yr of age is about 2/100,000 children/yr in North America and is twice as high in boys as in girls. Adults with MCNS do not show this sex difference. In most cases the onset occurs from 2–7 yr; it is uncommon under 1 yr but may rarely occur at several mo of age. In adults MCNS accounts for fewer than 20% of patients with nephrotic syndrome.

Pathology and Pathogenesis. Kidney changes are absent or minimal in the biopsies of most patients near the time of onset, hence the designation minimal change nephrotic syndrome. There may be a slight increase in mesangial matrix or mild mesangial hypercellularity. These changes tend to become more pronounced as the duration of proteinuria increases; later biopsies in patients who have frequent relapses or who are resistant to therapy may show development of focal sclerotic lesions which may be either global or segmental. Tubular casts containing protein, lipid vacuoles,

and protein reabsorption droplets in proximal tubular cells and focal interstitial fibrosis may be seen. Electron microscopy reveals diffuse fusion of epithelial foot processes and hyperactivity of mesangial areas. Immunopathologic studies show absence of glomerular immune globulin and complement deposits, although occasional focal deposits of IgM and C3 may be present in the mesangial zone, near the vascular pole, or in sites where segmental sclerosis has occurred.

The cause of the increased glomerular protein leak is unknown. If an immune mechanism is operative, it is unlikely to be 1 of the types currently recognized as causing glomerular injury. A defect in lymphocyte function has been postulated.

Clinical Manifestations. The usual presenting manifestation is edema, developing over the course of several wk, sometimes with a history of transient edema during the preceding months. Sometimes the initial episode and, not uncommonly, relapses appear to be precipitated by viral upper respiratory infections. Lethargy, anorexia, weight gain of 15–20% due to accumulation of edema fluid, and decreased urine volume with increased urine concentration occur.

The patient usually does not appear seriously ill; the most striking feature is generalized edema, often with ascites and pleural effusion. The edema fluid accumulates in dependent sites; after a night's sleep the face and eyelids or sacral region may be edematous, whereas during the day swelling of the legs and abdomen is more prominent. The blood pressure is usually normal or slightly decreased; in 5–10% of cases it is elevated. An increase in susceptibility to bacterial infection is related to hypogammaglobulinemia, loss of C3 proactivator (Factor B) in urine, leading to impaired opsonization of bacteria, and reduced defense mechanisms consequent upon corticosteroid therapy. Peritonitis or septicemia, due to *Streptococcus pneumoniae, Hemophilus influenzae,* or coliform organisms, and cellulitis are not uncommon. Venous or arterial thrombosis is an infrequent but potentially serious complication, secondary to a hypercoagulable state. Hypovolemic shock may follow rapid diuresis induced by aggressive diuretic therapy in a patient whose intravascular volume is already contracted. Abdominal pain and a general malaise may result from hypovolemia and are more common than outright shock.

Untreated patients tend to have a prolonged course characterized by recurrent episodes; in some instances remission may occur spontaneously or after an intercurrent illness such as measles.

Laboratory Data. The characteristic findings are proteinuria in excess of 2 gm/M^2/24 hr, accompanied by a reduction of total plasma proteins, with the albumin level under 2.5 gm/dl; elevation of α_2-globulins; and hyperlipidemia. Hematuria is present in under 10% of cases and is microscopic and transient; oval fat bodies (tubular cells containing lipid) and hyaline casts are seen in the sediment. Proteinuria is highly selective, with relatively greater clearance of proteins of low than of high molecular weight. Anemia is absent; hemoglobin and hematocrit may even be elevated because of hemoconcentration. The white blood cell count is normal or mildly elevated. The erythrocyte sedimentation rate is elevated, and at times there is a mild azotemia, which is usually prerenal in origin as reduced intravascular volume or decreased urine flow leads to a reduced clearance of urea. If the child is well hydrated and hypovolemia insignificant, the glomerular filtration rate is usually normal. The serum level of C3 is normal. The serum sodium concentration is often decreased to 130–135 mEq/l. This may reflect a reduced ability to excrete free water and thus signifies a true dilution of body fluids; it is partly accounted for, however, by hyperlipidemia leading to a spurious hyponatremia.

Diagnosis is based on the typical clinical and laboratory features and the usual responsiveness to corticosteroid therapy. In addition, severe or persistent hypertension, gross or persistent hematuria, significant or persistent azotemia, and depression of serum C3 are absent. Renal biopsy is not indicated in the majority of patients; it should be reserved for patients with atypical features which suggest that the nephrotic syndrome is not of the minimal change type. These features include age below 1 yr or over 10 yr, antecedent proteinuria of long duration, gross hematuria, persistent azotemia, hypertension, poorly selective proteinuria, evidence of a systemic disease known to cause the nephrotic syndrome, depression of C3 level, or failure to respond to a 4 wk course of corticosteroids.

The **differential diagnosis** includes other glomerulopathies which may cause the nephrotic syndrome. These are:

Idiopathic membranous glomerulopathy, which may present identical clinical findings, except that the usual age of onset exceeds 10 yr and the response to corticosteroids is poor. Proteinuria is less selective, and renal biopsy shows thickening of the glomerular basement membrane due to deposits on the epithelial aspect which contain IgG with or without C3.

Membranoproliferative glomerulonephritis, Types I and II, in which hematuria, proteinuria, and azotemia (i.e., features suggesting a nephritic component) are usually present. Serum complement levels may be depressed. Renal biopsy shows glomerular lobulation and mesangial proliferation. The onset frequently occurs beyond 10 yr of age.

Idiopathic proliferative glomerulonephritis with epithelial crescents, which is manifested by impressive nephritic as well as nephrotic features but usually normal serum complement levels. More than 1 specific etiologic entity is included under this heading.

Membranous glomerulopathy associated with systemic disorders such as lupus erythematosus, malaria, or syphilis which is distinguished by the specific features of the respective systemic disease. A nephritic component is often present.

Glomerulonephritis of anaphylactoid purpura, which is a proliferative lesion involving primarily the mesangium, often with epithelial crescent formation. The features of the underlying disease may or may not be present at the time of the nephrotic episode. A nephritic component is common.

Drug- or toxin-induced nephrotic syndrome, secondary, for example, to trimethadione therapy, ingestion of mercury, or exposure to poison oak. The clinical and pathologic features may be indistinguishable from those of MCNS; diagnosis may be made by eliciting a history of exposure.

Focal glomerulosclerosis, which is probably part of the spectrum of MCNS but is less responsive to therapy and has a poorer prognosis. Affected patients tend to have microscopic hematuria more frequently and a less highly selective proteinuria than those with uncomplicated MCNS. The diagnosis rests on the characteristic renal biopsy changes. *Diffuse mesangial proliferation* is probably another variant of MCNS and is associated with a higher incidence of resistance to corticosteroid therapy.

Acute poststreptococcal glomerulonephritis which may occasionally present clinically as the nephrotic syndrome; the distinguishing features are discussed in Sec 16.17.

The nephrotic syndrome in the 1st yr of life, which includes a group of different disorders, is described later.

Treatment. The goal is reduction in excretion of urinary protein to a normal quantity. To this end corticosteroids should be given in sufficient dosage for an appropriate length of time. The most frequently used, least expensive, and safest drug is prednisone in a dosage of 2 mg/kg (60 mg/M^2)/24 hr, in 3–4 divided doses, up to a maximum of 80 mg/24 hr. There is no advantage to a larger dose. Treatment is continued until urinary excretion of protein has returned to and remained normal for 10–14 days. The dose is then tapered to discontinuation over a period of 3–4 days. In over 90% of patients protein excretion returns to normal within 4 wk; the mean response time is around 10 days. If a favorable response is not obtained after 1 mo of daily treatment, the likelihood of later response to continued therapy is slight. Of those whose protein excretion returns to normal on corticosteroid treatment, only 10% will do so in the 2nd mo of daily therapy; the response rate after 2 mo is virtually nil. For this reason patients with MCNS are considered steroid resistant if protein excretion has not returned to normal after 1 or, at most, 2 mo of treatment. Lack of response after 1 mo of daily steroid treatment at an adequate dose is an indication for re-evaluation or change of therapy. If the diagnosis was made on the basis of clinical and laboratory features alone, a renal biopsy should be done at this point to establish the precise diagnosis. Of the different glomerular diseases which may cause an idiopathic type of the nephrotic syndrome in childhood, only the MCNS should be treated with corticosteroids.

About 30% of children who respond to corticosteroid therapy will not have relapses, but most will have at least 1 or 2. If a tendency to relapse is demonstrated, particularly if the relapse occurs within several mo to 1 yr after discontinuance of treatment, an interrupted schedule of administration of prednisone should be given after repetition of a daily course as outlined above. A safe and effective interrupted schedule consists of prednisone in a dosage of 60 mg/M^2 on alternate days in a single dose, i.e., every 48 hr, administered in the morning soon after arising. This schedule should be continued for 6–12 mo, which reduces the number of relapses to about a third of that which would otherwise occur. There remain about 20% of children with the syndrome who relapse either during the alternate-day schedule or within several wk after it is discontinued. These are referred to as *steroid-dependent patients*.

They may be treated again with daily administration of prednisone, followed as before by an interrupted schedule. Once the patient who is steroid-dependent or who has frequent relapses is in remission for a period of 1–2 mo on alternate-day therapy, an attempt can be made gradually to lower the dosage of prednisone to a level which will keep the patient in remission; a dose as low as 0.5–1 mg/kg every 48 hr may be achievable in some of the children. Many patients, however, will require a dose of 2 mg/kg (60 mg/M^2) or even higher on alternate days to stay in remission. This regimen, even at the higher dosage level, is well tolerated without significant toxicity in the majority of patients despite therapy prolonged over many mo.

If the side effects of prolonged steroid therapy pose a threat to the child's growth and general health, it is possible to reduce the relapse rate by using an oral alkylating agent, such as cyclophosphamide. The dose is 1–2.5 mg/kg/24 hr for a period of 6 wk–3 mo. Prednisone should be given in addition, as outlined above, and continued on an alternate-day basis until administration of cyclophosphamide is discontinued. The shorter course appears to have less potential for inducing subsequent sterility, but the relapse rate is higher than with the longer course. Because of the potential risk of sterility as well as side effects such as hemorrhagic cystitis and alopecia, it is recommended that cyclophosphamide be used only in carefully selected patients and under the direct supervision of a pediatric nephrologist. There is an increased mortality from chickenpox in children who are receiving cyclophosphamide, and great care must be taken to avoid exposure of patients receiving this drug. Oral chlorambucil, 0.15–0.4 mg/kg/24 hr, is also used to induce prolonged remission in frequently relapsing MCNS.

Initiation of daily treatment with prednisone for either the 1st attack or a relapse is best delayed for 1 wk or so because (1) spontaneous remission may occur, particularly if the episode has been precipitated by an intercurrent illness; (2) latent bacterial infection, especially active or inactive tuberculosis or unrecognized urinary tract infection, which could spread or reactivate during corticosteroid treatment, must be excluded or treated before steroids are given; (3) excessive edema and ascites may make the child uncomfortable, anorexic, and unable to move about, and the skin may break down and become infected. If excessive edema can be reduced by diuretics prior to prednisone therapy, the patient's overall condition will probably be better during therapy with prednisone. For this purpose a combination of oral hydrochlorothiazide, 2 mg/kg/24 hr (maximum 100 mg), and spironolactone, 3 mg/kg/24 hr (maximum 200 mg), each given in 2–3 divided doses, may be used for induction of a gradual diuresis. Furosemide, 0.5–2.0 mg/kg per dose, orally or intravenously, may also be given every 12 hr; this potent diuretic should be used with caution in nephrotic patients since intravascular volume may already be contracted and a sudden diuresis may induce shock. Intravenous infusion of salt-poor albumin in a dose of 1 gm/kg over a 2 hr period, followed by intravenous administration of furosemide, may be useful in patients with severe hypoalbuminemia and refractory edema; care should be taken to avoid circulatory congestion, which may be induced by sudden expansion of the intravascular volume due to the elevation of intravascular osmotic pressure by the administered albumin. Because intensive diuretic therapy carries the danger of contraction of the vascular volume, thrombosis, electrolyte disturbances, and shock, it should be undertaken with caution and preferably in the hospital.

There is a marked tendency to retain sodium in the nephrotic state, and this is accentuated by steroid therapy. Accordingly, the dietary intake of salt should be restricted; an intake of 17 mEq/24 hr (1 gm of sodium chloride) is recommended as long as there is evident edema and proteinuria. Water intake should be limited only if there is progressive accumulation of edema despite dietary restriction of sodium or if there is an impaired ability to excrete a normal intake of water, leading to hyponatremia (a serum sodium concentration of 130 mEq/l or less). Physical activity during an attack of the nephrotic syndrome should be as desired and tolerated by the child. Enforced bed rest contributes more to prolonging the disability than to the patient's well being in virtually all disorders of the kidney and urinary tract. Apart from restriction of salt intake, a full nutritious diet rich in protein is recommended. Total caloric intake may have to be restricted if excessive appetite and obesity develop as a consequence of corticosteroid therapy. Daily oral penicillin is recommended by some nephrologists for prophylaxis against pneumococcal infections.

Prognosis. The prognosis for ultimate recovery is good. Although relapses are common and there is always the danger of an unpredictable event such as septicemia, peritonitis, or shock, most children with this condition will respond to treatment and can look forward to a healthy future. For those who have numerous relapses or who cannot be controlled adequately with steroid therapy alone, alkylating agents such as cyclophosphamide or chlorambucil provide the possibility of prolonged remission. The activity of the disease tends to lessen after adolescence. In a few instances the nephrotic syndrome may, after satisfactory responses, become steroid resistant, sometimes with progression to glomerular sclerosis and renal insufficiency over the course of several yr. Pregnancy in patients who are in remission does not increase the likelihood of a relapse.

In some patients the response to corticosteroids is partial, with reductions in proteinuria only to levels of 1–2 gm/24 hr; such patients may lose the clinical features of the nephrotic syndrome but are at increased risk for relapse. Some gradually reduce the protein excretion further, to normal levels, over a period of months. In such patients an expectant approach without overly agressive therapy is warranted; the long term outlook is fairly good, and few progress to chronic renal failure. The best approach is an alternate-day prednisone regimen sustained over a period of months.

Callis L, Nieto J, Vila A, et al: Chlorambucil treatment in minimal lesion nephrotic syndrome: A reappraisal of its gonadal toxicity. J Pediatr 97:653, 1980.
Cameron JS: The problem of focal segmental glomerulosclerosis. In: Kincaid-

Smith P, d'Apice AJF, Atkins RC (eds): Progress in Glomerulonephrosis. New York, John Wiley and Sons, 1979.

Chiu J, Drummond KN: Long-term follow-up of cyclophosphamide therapy in frequent relapsing minimal lesion nephrotic syndrome. J Pediatr 84:825, 1974.

Drummond KN, Kaplan BS: Glomerular disorders. In: Conn HF (ed): Current Therapy 1977. Philadelphia, WB Saunders, 1977.

Drummond KN, Michael AF, Good RA, et al: The nephrotic syndrome of childhood: Immunologic, clinical and pathologic correlations. J Clin Invest 45:620, 1966.

Etteldorf JN, West CD, Pitcock JA, et al: Gonadal function, testicular histology, and meiosis following cyclophosphamide therapy in patients with nephrotic syndrome. J Pediatr 88:206, 1976.

Gur A, Adefuin PY, Siegel NJ, et al: A study of the renal handling of water in lipoid nephrosis. Pediatr Res 10:197, 1976.

Habib R, Levy M, Gubler M-C: Clinicopathologic correlations in the nephrotic syndrome. Pediatrician 8:325, 1979.

Heymann W, Makker SP, Post RS: The preponderance of males in the idiopathic nephrotic syndrome of childhood. Pediatrics 50:814, 1972.

Lentz RD, Bergstein J, Steffes MW, et al: Postpubertal evaluation of gonadal function following cyclophosphamide therapy before and during puberty. J Pediatr 91:385, 1977.

McLean RH, Forsgren A, Bjorketen B, et al: Decreased serum factor B concentration associated with decreased opsonization of Escherichia coli in the idiopathic nephrotic syndrome. Pediatr Res 11:910, 1977.

Murphy WM, Jukkola AF, Roy S III: Nephrotic syndrome with mesangial cell proliferation in children—a distinct entity? Am J Clin Pathol 72:1, 1979.

Rothenberg MB, Heymann W: The incidence of the nephrotic syndrome in children. Pediatrics 19:446, 1957.

Seigel NJ, Goldberg B, Krassner LS, et al: Long-term follow-up of children with steroid-responsive nephrotic syndrome. J Pediatr 81:251, 1972.

Shigeko OL, Joy Y, Thachuck MT, et al: Plasminogen and antithrombin III deficiencies in the childhood nephrotic syndrome associated with plasminogenuria and antithrombinuria. J Pediatr 96:390, 1980.

Stuart MJ, Spitzer RE, Nelson DA, et al: Nephrotic syndrome: Increased platelet prostaglandin endoperoxide formation, hyperaggregability, and reduced platelet life span. Reversal following remission. Pediatr Res 14:1078, 1980.

Waldherr R, Gubler MC, Levy M, et al: The significance of pure diffuse mesangial proliferation in idiopathic nephrotic syndrome. Clin Nephrol 10:5, 1978.

Williams SA, Makker SP, Ingelfinger JR, et al: Long-term evaluation of chlorambucil plus prednisone in the idiopathic nephrotic syndrome of childhood. N Engl J Med 302:929, 1980.

16.12 NEPHROTIC SYNDROME WITH FOCAL GLOMERULOSCLEROSIS OR WITH DIFFUSE MESANGIAL PROLIFERATION

There is controversy about the relation of MCNS both to focal glomerulosclerosis (FGS) and to diffuse mesangial proliferation (DMP). Some consider that their histopathologic differences identify separate entities; we consider them to be within the spectrum of manifestations of idiopathic nephrotic syndrome of childhood. It is, however, important to distinguish patients with FGS or DMP from the typical child with MCNS since in each of the former the response to therapy and the prognosis are worse than in MCNS. Initially, the lesions of FGS are focal and segmental and tend to affect principally the glomeruli deep in the juxtamedullary zone. On light microscopy unaffected glomeruli may appear normal, but electron microscopic study shows the diffuse fusion of podocytes characteristic of MCNS. The lesions of FGS may also be superimposed on those of DMP, a histopathologic variant in which there is mesangial cell and matrix proliferation affecting all glomeruli, along with diffuse podocyte fusion. There is no evidence of an immune pathogenesis in either FGS or DMP, though IgM, C3, and fibrin-related antigens may be found in areas of segmental sclerosis. It is believed that these proteins are passively trapped in areas of local mesangial dysfunction. The histopathologic lesions of FGS and of DMP are neither specific nor pathognomonic of any disorder. FGS may, for example, be seen in the glomerulopathies of Alport disease, heroin addiction, or amyloidosis, and DMP may be seen in the resolving phase of acute poststreptococcal glomerulonephritis. Whatever the relation of FGS and DMP to MCNS may be, certain clinical and laboratory features distinguish them from typical MCNS. Proteinuria is nonselective in about 75% of cases and about 50% have microscopic hematuria. Of particular importance is the fact that although the clinical onset is the same as in other children with nephrotic syndrome, the incidence of resistance to corticosteroid therapy is increased, as high as 50% in some series, and the risk of renal failure due to progressive diffuse glomerulosclerosis may be as high as 50% in patients with FGS. Both may occur as early as 6 mo following onset of the nephrotic syndrome, but the mean interval is about 6 yr.

The finding of either FGS or DMP on biopsy should not preclude an active approach to therapy, and affected children should be treated with prednisone initially as in MCNS; if resistance is encountered, an oral alkylating agent should be tried for up to 3 mo in combination with an alternate-day regimen of prednisone. In our experience about one third of these patients ultimately enter complete remission, although some may subsequently experience frequent relapses or become steroid dependent. The prognosis is worse if FGS appears early rather than late in the patient's course or if it is superimposed on DMP. Recurrences of the nephrotic syndrome and FGS have been reported in patients who have received kidney transplants for terminal renal failure, but this phenomenon should not contraindicate transplantation since significant numbers of patients have satisfactory results.

16.13 MEMBRANOUS GLOMERULOPATHY
(Membranous Glomerulonephritis, Epi- or Extramembranous Glomerulopathy)

Membranous glomerulopathy accounts for about 5% of cases of the nephrotic syndrome in children. It is more common in late childhood; about 20% of patients with onset of nephrosis after the age of 15 have this condition.

Pathology. The characteristic pathologic change is uniform thickening of the glomerular basement membrane without evidence of inflammation or significant increase in mesangial tissue. The thickening begins with deposition of immune complexes on the epithelial aspect of the membrane, detectable by light and electron microscopic and immunopathologic techniques. The immune complexes appear as discrete nodular masses or bumps that project from the epithelial surface of the membrane which extends in a spiked or sawtoothed pattern between the complexes. As the disease progresses, the deposits are incorporated into the membrane, which becomes progressively thicker. Over a period of years gradual sclerosis of the glomeruli may occur. Immunopathologic studies demonstrate that the membranous deposits consistently contain IgG, whereas C3 is present in only a third of patients. In about two thirds the condition appears to be idiopathic; there are no associated extrarenal or systemic conditions. It is essential, however, to investigate for systemic conditions since treatment of such underlying disorders may lead to resolution of the glomerulopathy. Such conditions include congenital or acquired syphilis, D-penicillamine therapy, systemic lupus erythematosus, autoimmune thyroiditis, malaria, and sickle cell hemoglobinopathy. Some series of patients with apparent idiopathic disease have had increased incidences of hepatitis B surface antigenemia. Renal lesions other than membranous glomerulopathy may occur in some of these conditions.

Clinical Manifestations and Laboratory Data. The onset is gradual, and the clinical pattern and laboratory data are quite similar to those of the minimal lesion nephrotic syndrome. In some cases the proteinuria is not marked, and clinical manifestations may be absent. The serum complement level is usually normal; there is poorly selective proteinuria; and the urine sediment may contain hyaline casts and a few red blood cells.

Diagnosis and Treatment. Membranous glomerulopathy should be considered in nephrotic patients beyond the usual age range for MCNS and in patients with failure to respond to 1 mo of corticosteroid therapy. Systemic conditions known to be associated with membranous glomerulopathy must be excluded since their successful treatment may lead to healing of the renal lesions. In the idiopathic form there is evidence that a course of alternate-day prednisone prolonged over a period of months to several yr is beneficial. Therapy with azathioprine or alkylating agents is not indicated. Spontaneous remission occurs in about 30% of patients; 10% develop chronic renal failure within a decade.

A controlled study of short-term prednisone treatment in adults with membranous nephropathy: Collaborative study of the adult idiopathic nephrotic syndrome. N Engl J Med 301:1301, 1979.
Habib R, Kleinknecht C, Gubler MC: Extramembranous glomerulonephritis in children: Report of 50 cases. J Pediatr 82:754, 1973.
Kleinknecht C, Levy M, Peix A, et al: Membranous glomerulonephritis and hepatitis B surface antigen in children. J Pediatr 95:946, 1979.
Kleinknecht C, Levy M, Gagnadoux M-F, et al: Membranous glomerulonephritis with extra-renal disorders in children. Medicine 58:3, 1979.

16.14 MEMBRANOPROLIFERATIVE GLOMERULONEPHRITIS (MPGN)
(Mesangiocapillary Glomerulonephritis)

MPGN is a chronic diffuse form of proliferative glomerulonephritis with characteristic histopathologic, immunologic, and electron microscopic features. The renal changes may appear in several unrelated systemic clinical conditions (e.g., lipodystrophy, α_1-antitrypsin deficiency, congenital absence of the C2 component of the complement system), but MPGN usually presents as a primary renal disease, of which there are 2 well recognized variants, Types I and II. The 2 types are indistinguishable clinically. Their renal manifestations include the nephrotic syndrome, acute nephritis, a nephritic-nephrotic picture, asymptomatic proteinuria, rapidly progressive (crescentic) glomerulonephritis, chronic renal failure, or recurrent episodes of gross hematuria. Hypertension and azotemia are common. Although the specific etiology is not known, the renal damage is mediated by immunologic mechanisms involving either the classic pathway of complement activation with immune complex deposition (Type I), or alternative pathway activation, often with detectable serum C3 nephritic factor (Type II). Girls are affected more often than boys; the usual age of onset is adolescence or young adulthood. The 2 types are differentiated on the basis of histopathologic, electron microscopic, and immunologic findings. The histologic features of the 2 types overlap considerably. In each the glomeruli are enlarged and there is diffuse, fairly uniform proliferation of mesangial cells with thickening of the capillary walls. There may be a marked increase in mesangial matrix, with a tendency to glomerular lobulation. Epithelial crescent formation is often present. Glomerular neutrophil infiltration may be seen early in the course.

In Type I subendothelial deposits and interposition of mesangial matrix between the endothelial layer and the basement membrane lead to thickening of the capillary walls, creating a double contour or tramtrack appearance. In Type II thickening of the capillary wall results from a dense refractile material within the basement membrane itself, giving the basement membrane a ribbon-like appearance. Strongly electron-dense deposits are seen in the mid-portion of the basement membrane by electron microscopy, which replace and widen the lamina densa. Similar deposits are seen in the mesangium, in Bowman capsule, and in tubular basement membranes. Type II MPGN is sometimes referred to as dense deposit disease or MPGN with dense intramembranous deposits. Some authors also distinguish a Type III, with contiguous subepithelial and subendothial deposits, disruption of the basement membrane, and layering of the lamina densa.

Immunopathologic studies show several different patterns in Type I, the most common being granular deposits containing IgG, IgM, C3, C1q, and C4 along the peripheral loops, with variable mesangial fluorescence. Mesangial properdin and C3 deposition is evident in many Type I patients. By contrast, in Type II the principal finding is intense staining for C3 in round nodular deposits within the mesangium and only faint, if any, staining of the intramembranous deposits; properdin deposition is not common in Type II.

The serum complement profile in Type I shows depression of C1q and C4 and a variable decrease in C3 suggestive of classic pathway activation, whereas in Type II there is persistent depression of C3 consistent with alternative pathway activation, and C1q and C4 levels are normal; C3 nephritic factor is more frequently detected than in Type I.

Type I is 2–3 times as common as Type II; Type II may develop in patients with lipodystrophy. Type II has a greater tendency to recur in a transplanted kidney.

In the idiopathic form girls are affected more often than boys, and the usual age of onset is adolescence or young adulthood. About a third of patients with MPGN present with a nephrotic syndrome, although this accounts for under 10% of children with the nephrotic syndrome; a third have an acute nephritic-nephrotic picture, and the rest may have episodic gross hematuria, asymptomatic proteinuria, or chronic progressive renal failure. Proteinuria is nonselective. Hypertension and reduced GFR are present in about a third of patients. About 10% develop renal failure within 2 yr, and the long-term prognosis must be guarded since about half will progress to chronic renal failure in 10 yr. There is no consensus about the value of treatment in MPGN. Alternate-day high dose prednisone, dipyridamole, anticoagulants, and antimetabolic drugs have been used. Our experience suggests that the rate of progression can be slowed and improvement induced with a regimen combining azathioprine and alternate-day prednisone if it is begun early in the acute stage of illness and maintained for a period of several yr. In patients with end-stage renal failure transplantation is a worthwhile option; although transmission of the lesions to the allograft may occur, this may not be accompanied by significant clinical manifestations.

Chapman SJ, Cameron JS, Chantler C, et al: Treatment of mesangiocapillary glomerulonephritis in children with combined immunosuppression and anticoagulation. Arch Dis Child 55:446, 1980.

Dobrin RS, Hoyer JR, Nevins TE, et al: The association of familial liver disease, subepidermal immunoproteins, and membranoproliferative glomerulonephritis. J Pediatr 90:901, 1977.

Habib R, Levy M: Membranoproliferative glomerulonephritis. In: Hamburger J, Crosnier J, Grunfeld JP, et al: Nephrology. New York, John Wiley and Sons, 1979.

Lamb V, Tisher CC, McCoy RC, et al: Membranoproliferative glomerulonephritis with dense intramembranous alterations. A clinicopathologic study. Lab Invest 36:607, 1977.

Levy M, Gubler MC, Habib R: New concepts in membranoproliferative glomerulonephritis. In: Kincaid-Smith P, d'Apice AJF, Atkins RC (eds): Progress in Glomerulonephritis. New York, John Wiley and Sons, 1979.

McEnery PT, McAdams AJ, West CD: Membranoproliferative glomerulonephritis: Improved survival with alternate day prednisone therapy. Clin Nephrol 13:17, 1980.

Ooi YM, Vallota EH, West CD: Classical complement pathway activation in membranoproliferative glomerulonephritis. Kidney Int 9:46, 1976.

16.15 THE NEPHROTIC SYNDROME IN THE FIRST YEAR OF LIFE

The nephrotic syndrome in infancy requires separate consideration, mainly to identify the congenital form but also to emphasize the association of the syndrome with congenital syphilis. In approximately 5% of patients with the *minimal change nephrotic syndrome* and in 5–10% of those with *focal glomerulosclerosis*, the onset occurs in the 1st yr of life, usually after 6 mo of age but sometimes earlier. Treatment for MCNS at this age is the same as for other age groups.

Finnish Type of Congenital Nephrotic Syndrome (Infantile Microcystic Disease). This autosomal recessive condition is seen most frequently in the Scandinavian countries. Proteinuria is usually present from birth but may not be manifest for several mo. It is highly selective initially but becomes less selective and increases in amount; tubular proteinuria is added. Commonly associated features include toxemia of pregnancy, an enlarged placenta, and prematurity. The pathognomonic lesion is cystic dilatation of the proximal tubules. This change is not present in all cases; in some it is not present at birth but develops subsequently. The pathogenesis is unknown; there is no evidence of an immune mechanism. Antenatal diagnosis in patients at risk is possible by detection of an elevation in α-fetoprotein concentration in amniotic fluid. α-Fetoprotein has a molecular weight of approximately 70,000; its appearance in amniotic fluid is probably a manifestation of proteinuria in utero. In pregnancies at risk for this disease screening by amniocentesis for α-fetoprotein should be done from the 15th–20th wk. Causes of an elevated value other than infantile microcystic disease should, of course, be considered. The α-fetoprotein level may also be elevated in maternal plasma, but false negative values occur; accordingly, plasma screening may be of use in population studies, but it is not reliable in pregnancies known to be at risk. No treatment is known to be effective. Measures such as restriction of sodium intake and the provision of a nutritious diet may help to maintain the general state of health. The disease is usually fatal within the 1st 2 yr. Some success has been reported with renal transplantation.

Membranous Nephropathy of Congenital Syphilis. The onset of the nephrotic syndrome occurs within the 1st 6 mo, and other stigmata of congenital syphilis are usually present. The pathologic change is a membranous nephropathy; immunopathologic studies reveal nodular deposits containing IgG with or without C3. The pathogenetic basis is immune complex deposition; the antigen is a component of *Treponema pallidum*. Complete recovery from the nephrotic syndrome and resolution of the renal lesion usually occur in response to antisyphilitic therapy. A proliferative form of glomerulonephritis and interstitial nephritis has also been described in congenital syphilis.

Miscellaneous Conditions. Rarely, other conditions may be associated with or cause the nephrotic syndrome in infancy. These include diffuse mesangial sclerosis, idiopathic membranous glomerulopathy, mercury poisoning, congenital toxoplasmosis, nail-patella syndrome, congenital rubella, systemic lupus erythematosus, abnormal genitalia, nephroblastoma with or without pseudohermaphroditism, the hemolytic-uremic syndrome, and Alport disease.

Habib R, Bois E: Hétérogénéité des syndromes néphrotiques à début précoce du nourisson (syndrome néphrotique "infantile"). Helv Pediatr Acta 28:91, 1973.

Hallman N, Norio R, Kouvalainen K: Main features of the congenital nephrotic syndrome. Acta Paediatr Scand (Suppl) 172:75, 1976.

Hoyer JR, Kjellstrand CM, Simmons RL, et al: Successful renal transplantation in 3 children with congenital nephrotic syndrome. Lancet 1:1410, 1973.

Huttunen NF, Vehaskari M, Viikari M, et al: Proteinuria in congenital nephrotic syndrome of the Finnish type. Clin Nephrol 13:12, 1980.

Kaplan BS, Bureau MA, Drummond KN: The nephrotic syndrome in the first year of life: Is a pathologic classification possible? J Pediatr 85:615, 1974.

Kaplan BS, Drummond KN: The nephrotic syndrome in infancy. In: Hamburger J, Cosnier J, Grunefield J-P (eds): Nephrology. New York, John Wiley & Sons, 1979.

Milunsky A, Alpert E, Frigoletto FD, et al: Prenatal diagnosis of the congenital nephrotic syndrome. Pediatrics 59:770, 1977.

OTHER CONDITIONS IN WHICH THE NEPHROTIC SYNDROME MAY OCCUR

Malignant Lymphomas and Other Neoplasms. Renal manifestations associated with malignant neoplasms are much less common in children than in adults. In reticuloendothelial malignancies such as Hodgkin disease the features may be similar to the MCNS, whereas with other tumors a proliferative glomerulonephritis may be seen. Glomerulopathy with proteinuria is not rare in patients with Wilms tumor. Renal manifestations may antedate clinical evidence of the neoplasm; successful treatment of the neoplasm may lead to resolution of the glomerulopathy.

The Nephropathies of Malaria and Other Tropical Parasitic Diseases. The association of parasitic infestations with glomerular disease leading to the nephrotic syndrome has become increasingly recognized in developing countries. In some instances an immune complex type of injury involves parasitic antigens; in others the pathogenesis is less well understood. An acute transient immune complex glomerulopathy with nephritic rather than nephrotic features may occur in *P. falciparum* infection; recovery is the rule. Glomerulonephritis with the nephrotic syndrome has been described in patients with the hepatosplenic (*S. mansoni*) form of schistosomiasis. *P. malariae*, responsible for quartan malaria, is associated with childhood nephrotic syndrome in Africa. The peak age of incidence is 5 yr. Proteinuria is nonselective and hematuria uncommon. The condition is not responsive to corticosteroid or antimetabolic drugs, and despite adequate antimalarial treatment an unremitting course with progression to renal failure in 3–5 yr is the usual outcome. Only a small proportion of children with *P. malariae* infestation develop a nephropathy.

Miscellaneous. The nephrotic syndrome may also develop during the course of other primary renal diseases or in systemic disorders which may affect the kidney. Included are acute poststreptococcal glomerulonephritis, systemic lupus erythematosus, anaphylactoid purpura, diabetes mellitus, familial Mediterranean fever, and chronic bacteremia such as may occur with an infected atrioventricular shunt.

Andrade ZA, Rocha H: Schistosomal glomerulopathy. Kidney Int 16:23, 1979.
Boonpucknavig V, Sitprija V: Renal disease in acute *Plasmodium falciparum* infection in man. Kidney Int 16:44, 1979.
Eagen JW, Lewis EJ: Glomerulopathies of neoplasia. Kidney Int 11:297, 1977.
Hendrickse RG, Adeniyi A: Quartan malarial nephrotic syndrome in children. Kidney Int 16:64, 1979.
Moorthy AV, Zimmerman SW, Burkholder PM: Nephrotic syndrome in Hodgkin's disease. Evidence for pathogenesis alternative to immune complex deposition. Am J Med 61:471, 1976.

BENIGN PERSISTENT ASYMPTOMATIC PROTEINURIA

Although persistent proteinuria is usually a sign of potentially serious glomerular disease, this finding may occasionally be present over a prolonged period without evidence of clinical or pathologic progression to renal insufficiency or of the nephrotic syndrome. It is likely that proteinuria in such situations is the consequence of a variety of unrelated conditions. Renal biopsy studies have in some instances revealed minor ultrastructural abnormalities, such as slight focal thickening or splitting of the glomerular basement membrane, localized areas of increased electron density, and partial

fusion of the epithelial foot processes. Immunopathologic studies are negative. The proteinuria does not respond to corticosteroid therapy. Although the prognosis is generally favorable, some patients have been observed to develop hypertension and increasing proteinuria over a period of 3–5 yr, suggesting that the course is not always benign.

McLaine PN, Drummond KN: Benign persistent asymptomatic proteinuria in childhood. Pediatrics 46:548, 1970.
Urizar, RE, Tinglof BO, Smith FG Jr, et al: Persistent asymptomatic proteinuria in children. Am J Clin Pathol 62:461, 1974.

16.16 ACUTE GLOMERULONEPHRITIS

General Considerations. The category of acute glomerulonephritis includes a number of distinct entities. In some the glomerulus is affected as the primary event; in others renal involvement is only 1 manifestation of a systemic disorder. The clinical, laboratory, or pathologic abnormalities of the various acute glomerulonephritides may range from minimal to severe. Features include oliguria, in which the urine volume may be less than 180 ml/M^2/24 hr, the amount required for excretion of the minimal possible solute load; edema, which may be slight and is seldom as marked as in the nephrotic syndrome; **hypertension and circulatory congestion**, which are common to most forms of acute glomerulonephritis; **hematuria**, which may be grossly evident by brownish red to tea-colored urine or may be detected only microscopically, the sediment characteristically containing red blood cells, pus cells, and mixed, granular, and red blood cell casts; **proteinuria**, which varies from a modest elevation of 30–100 mg/dl to "nephrotic" levels of 1000 mg/dl or more; and findings consequent to a reduction in glomerular filtration rate, including **azotemia** and elevation of serum creatinine, phosphorus, and uric acid. The serum calcium may be depressed due to the hyperphosphatemia. The cause of the hypertension is not well understood, but retention of sodium and water appears to be of primary importance. Circulatory congestion may be manifested by pulmonary edema and other features of cardiac overload, such as hepatomegaly, distention of the external jugular veins, and gallop rhythm.

There may be a mild normochromic *anemia*. Electrolyte and acid-base disturbances include *hyperkalemia* from reduced urinary excretion of potassium in the face of continued potassium intake and tissue catabolism; *hyponatremia* from continued water intake during reduced output of urine; and *metabolic acidosis*, particularly if oliguria is severe. Acidosis may worsen hyperkalemia.

The pathologic changes depend, to a large extent, on the specific disease entity and will be discussed under the respective disorders; features common to most forms include polymorphonuclear leukocyte infiltration, cellular proliferation of 1 or more of the glomerular cell types (endothelial, mesangial, parietal, or epithelial), increased glomerular size, mesangial edema or increase of mesangial matrix (usually a fine fibrillar type), and reduction in the number of open capillary loops. In addition, there may be focal infiltration of mononuclear or polymorphonuclear leukocytes in the interstitial areas.

16.17 ACUTE POSTSTREPTOCOCCAL GLOMERULONEPHRITIS

This acute, specific, self-limited glomerulonephritis follows pharyngeal or cutaneous infection with a nephritogenic strain of group A beta-hemolytic streptococci. It is the most common form of acute glomerulonephritis, though its incidence has fallen dramatically in recent years.

Etiology and Epidemiology. The precipitating event is a streptococcal infection of the upper respiratory tract or the skin. The clinical pattern of the nephritis is the same following infection at either of these sites, but there are a number of important differences, including the types of streptococci involved, epidemiology, age, sex, seasonal incidence, the latent period between infection and onset of nephritis, and the antibody response to the infection. Only certain serotypes of group A beta-hemolytic streptococci, characterized by either their M or T antigens, cause acute poststreptococcal glomerulonephritis. The nephritogenic strains are listed in Table 16–6. The most common pharyngeal and skin streptococci are M types 12 and 49, respectively. Some of the nephritogenic strains of streptococci that infect the skin are difficult to type on the basis of their M protein antigen but are typable on the basis of T antigen agglutination. Of these strains, those with the T-14 antigen are the most common.

Acute glomerulonephritis associated with streptococcal pharyngeal infection is more common in temperate or cold climates, has a peak seasonal incidence in winter and spring, affects mainly children of early school age, and follows onset of the streptococcal infection by 9–11 days. The ratio of boys to girls is about 2:1, despite the lack of a sex difference in the incidences of streptococcal pharyngitis and impetigo. By contrast, acute glomerulonephritis associated with streptococcal infection of the skin is more common in hot or tropical climates, with a seasonal peak in late summer and early fall; preschool children are most frequently affected, the sex incidence is equal, and the latent period between onset of skin infection and onset of nephritis is 3 wk or longer. The

attack rate of nephritis in patients with either pharyngitis or impetigo is 10–15%. Multiple cases tend to occur in families, often within several wk of one another; 2nd attacks are rare.

Serum antibodies (anti-NADase) to streptococcal nicotinamide adenine dinucleotidase, alternatively designated streptococcal diphosphopyridine nucleotidase (DPNase), and, to a slightly lesser extent, to streptococcal deoxyribonuclease B (anti-DNase B) and streptolysin O (ASO) are usually present in nephritis after pharyngitis. In nephritis following impetigo a vigorous anti-DNase B or antihyaluronidase response is seen, but the ASO and anti-NADase responses are irregular or weak. Accordingly, there appears to be an advantage to using the anti-NADase (anti-DPNase) test in acute glomerulonephritis following streptococcal pharyngitis and a definite superiority to using the anti-DNase B test in nephritis induced by skin infection.

Pathogenesis and Pathology. It has been postulated since early in this century that immune mechanisms are important in the development of acute poststreptococcal glomerulonephritis. Several observations support this concept: (1) the characteristic latent period between streptococcal infection and the development of nephritis; (2) the depression of serum complement activity; (3) the finding of immune reactants at the site of glomerular injury; and (4) similarity of the immunopathologic and electron microscopic findings in acute poststreptococcal glomerulonephritis to those in immunologically induced renal disease in animals.

Acute poststreptococcal glomerulonephritis has been thought to be analogous to the serum sickness nephritis seen in human beings or in animals following injection of a foreign protein, such as horse antitetanus serum. Several perplexing problems remain unexplained, however. These include (1) the difficulty in identifying a specific streptococcal antigen at the site of the IgG and C3 deposits in the kidney; (2) the finding by immunopathologic techniques of C3 more frequently than IgG in glomerular deposits; and (3) the complement profile. The marked depression of C3 and terminal components of complement with relative sparing of C1, C4, and C2 and with a distinct decrease of properdin in the serum and its deposition in the glomeruli suggests operation of the alternative pathway of complement activation. It is probable that both the classic and the alternative pathways of complement activation are operative, as is believed to be the case in the nephritis of systemic lupus erythematosus and in Type I membranoproliferative glomerulonephritis.

The pathologic changes are confined largely to the glomeruli, in which initially infiltration with polymorphonuclear leukocytes, proliferation of endothelial and mesangial cells, increase in fibrillar mesangial matrix, and, infrequently, epithelial crescent formation take place. The glomeruli appear hypercellular and swollen, and the number of open capillary loops is reduced. Electron microscopic or ultrathin light microscopic studies demonstrate discrete nodular deposits along the epithelial aspect of the glomerular basement membrane, within the mesangium, and in a subendothelial position. Polymorphonuclear leukocytes are often seen adjacent to these deposits. Within 2–3 wk of onset most

Table 16–6 STREPTOCOCCAL M SEROTYPES ASSOCIATED WITH ACUTE NEPHRITIS

	SEROTYPE	
	Pharyngitis	*Pyoderma*
Most common and best-confirmed	12	49
Less frequent but good evidence for association	1, 3, 4	2, 55, 57
Probable or possible association	6, 25, 49	31, 52, 56

Based on Wannamaker LW: N Engl J Med 282:23, 1970.

of these changes begin to resolve; the abnormalities of the mesangial matrix are the last to return to normal. Microscopic lesions are usually not detectable after 2 mo from onset. Acute tubular and interstitial changes consist of interruptions in the tubular basement membrane, arteritis, and occasional interstitial inflammatory foci.

Clinical Manifestations and Course. Although the clinical pattern varies greatly in the degree of severity and in the extent of the various manifestations from a very mild to an extremely critical disorder, in most instances the clinical pattern and course are fairly characteristic. In many instances a history of pharyngitis or impetigo can be elicited. The onset is usually abrupt; the earliest symptoms are dark-colored urine, mild periorbital edema, decreased urinary output, flank or midline abdominal pain, irritability, general malaise, and a low-grade fever. Acute hypertension may cause headache, vomiting, somnolence, and other central nervous system manifestations, including seizures. Extensive retinal changes due to hypertensive encephalopathy are absent; if found, they should direct attention to the possibility of a more chronic problem. Symptoms related to circulatory congestion or overload, compounded by hypertension, may also be manifest: dyspnea, tachypnea, and a tender, enlarged liver. Less commonly, the 1st features of acute poststreptococcal glomerulonephritis may be seizures due to hypertensive encephalopathy or pulmonary edema and circulating congestion with cardiac decompensation. These may direct attention away from the correct diagnosis, particularly if abnormalities in urine color or sediment are minimal or absent. Infrequently, the clinical and laboratory features may be those of the nephrotic syndrome; the history of preceding pharyngeal or skin infection and the presence of hypertension, circulatory overload, and the characteristic laboratory data should clarify the diagnosis. Urinalyses or determinations of serum C3 concentrations of schoolmates and members of the patient's family show that an appreciable number of apparently healthy individuals have abnormalities in the urine and reduced C3 levels, suggesting that acute poststreptococcal glomerulonephritis may occur in a subclinical form among individuals infected with nephritogenic types of streptococci.

The acute phase usually lasts from 4–10 days. Subsequently, urine output increases, edema subsides, and blood urea nitrogen and creatinine concentrations return to normal. In a few patients elevated blood pressure and mild azotemia may persist for up to 2 wk after the urine volume returns to normal. Gross hematuria seldom persists beyond the 1st wk but microscopic hematuria and casts may persist for 1–2 mo. An increase in hematuria may occur with exercise or with an unrelated intercurrent illness during this period. Within 3 wk of onset most children have returned to their usual state of general health and experience no further problems related to this illness.

Laboratory Data. A mild normochromic anemia is found, due largely to hemodilution, along with mild leukocytosis (with a polymorphonuclear shift to the left), increased erythrocyte sedimentation rate, elevated blood urea nitrogen and serum creatinine levels, sero-

logic evidence of preceding streptococcal infection, reduction in serum C3 level, and a decrease in concentration of serum properdin. Serum complement remains low for about 10 days and returns to normal within 4–5 wk. In about 5–10% of cases the C3 level is not reduced at any time.

The *urine* is usually light to reddish brown; the sediment contains varying numbers of red and white blood cells and a mixture of casts (mostly red cell and granular). The urinary excretion of protein is usually under 1 gm/24 hr, with a protein concentration of 30–100 mg/dl. Urine volume is reduced during the 1st 3–5 days and may remain low for up to 10 days; infrequently, the child is anuric. Electrolyte and acid-base disturbances may occur, particularly in patients with anuria or oliguria; these include hyponatremia due to fluid overload in the face of reduced urinary output, hyperkalemia with levels from 5.5–9.0 mEq/l, and metabolic acidosis. *Electrocardiographic changes* may result from hyperkalemia (Sec 13.3) and should be sought in each patient since they reflect potentially serious changes in the electrical activity of the heart and may warrant immediate medical intervention.

Roentgenograms of the chest may show interstitial pulmonary edema, more pronounced in the hilar regions; with excessive circulatory overload, cardiomegaly and frank pulmonary edema are evident. *Cultures* from the pharynx or skin lesions should be obtained; if the patient has received effective antibacterial therapy, group A beta-hemolytic streptococci may not be recovered.

Diagnosis. The clinical features of acute poststreptococcal glomerulonephritis may be atypical in a small percentage of patients, but the correct diagnosis is readily made in most instances. A renal biopsy is not usually indicated unless there are atypical features such as persistently depressed or initially normal C3 level, heavy proteinuria in the nephrotic range, or persistence of clinical and/or laboratory abnormalities beyond 4 wk. Accuracy in the diagnosis of this and other glomerular disorders is important because of differences in prognosis and treatment.

The differential diagnosis includes most of the conditions which may cause hematuria, edema, hypertension, or oliguria. To be considered are the hemolytic-uremic syndrome, membranoproliferative glomerulonephritis, nephritis associated with such systemic disorders as systemic lupus erythematosus and anaphylactoid purpura, focal glomerulonephritis with recurrent hematuria, acute exacerbation of chronic glomerulonephritis, malignant hypertension, diffuse crescentic glomerulonephritis, hereditary nephritis, renal trauma, acute renal tubular injury, acute interstitial nephritis, and acute hemorrhagic cystitis. These conditions can usually be excluded without difficulty through their own characteristic clinical and laboratory features. Occasionally, the correct diagnosis can be established only by examination of renal tissue obtained by biopsy. An acute glomerulonephritis may follow other acute infections, including *Streptococcus pneumoniae*, *N. meningitidis*, *Staphylococcus pyogenes*; *Mycoplasma pneumoniae*, and infectious mononucleosis.

Prevention. Whether early antibiotic treatment of

nephritogenic streptococcal infections of the skin will prevent glomerulonephritis has not been established; it is generally considered, however, to be about 50% effective in the case of pharyngeal infections. Members of the patient's family should have appropriate bacterial cultures, and those with streptococcal infections should be treated with penicillin or erythromycin. Systemic treatment is superior to local therapy of streptococcal pyoderma. In institutional epidemics of nephritogenic streptococcal infection, early antibiotic treatment can limit the spread of nephritogenic strains.

Treatment. Since the course of the acute phase is variable and the severity not predictable, the child suspected of having acute glomerulonephritis should be hospitalized and carefully assessed. The major life-threatening problems encountered during the initial 1–2 wk are due to *acute renal insufficiency*, resulting in fluid, electrolyte, and acid-base abnormalities, and *acute hypertension*, which may cause hypertensive encephalopathy or, when compounded by severe oliguria or anuria, may lead to circulatory congestion and pulmonary edema. Present evidence does not indicate that primary myocardial failure is the cause of the circulatory congestion, which appears more likely a consequence of salt and water retention and of hypertension.

The treatment of *acute renal insufficiency* consists of the following measures: (1) Fluid restriction to an amount equal to insensible water loss (about 400 ml/M^2/24 hr) plus urinary output. (2) Provision of an adequate number of calories, at least 400/M^2/24 hr, in the form of carbohydrates to minimize endogenous tissue catabolism. If the patient is vomiting or is otherwise unable to be fed orally, fluid and carbohydrate requirements should be met by intravenous administration of 10–20% glucose in water. (Since 20% glucose solution may irritate small veins and lead to occlusion, a large vein or a cutdown may be needed.) (3) Correction of metabolic acidosis by parenteral administration of sodium bicarbonate and of other existing electrolyte and fluid disturbances by appropriate means (see Chapter 5).

Hyperkalemia can profoundly affect cardiac depolarization and may be a threat to life. The serum potassium level should be determined immediately, and a baseline electrocardiogram should be obtained. Potassium intake should be eliminated until it is certain that urinary output is adequate and hyperkalemia not present. If there is evidence of cardiac effects of hyperkalemia, immediate measures should be taken to reduce the concentration of serum potassium. Calcium gluconate should be administered intravenously under electrocardiographic monitoring over a period of 15–30 min in an amount to provide 10–15 mg/kg of elemental calcium (1 gm of calcium gluconate contains 93 mg of calcium). Correction of metabolic acidosis with sodium bicarbonate also serves to reduce hyperkalemia. Care should be taken, however, not to administer excessive amounts of sodium, particularly when circulatory congestion and edema are present. It may be necessary to repeat the administration of calcium gluconate if serious electrocardiographic changes persist during the time required to reduce the hyperkalemia. If the electrocardiographic changes are serious, crystalline insulin, 0.1 unit/kg, may

be given intravenously, and the same dose may be given subcutaneously some time after a glucose infusion has been started, to enhance the effect of glucose in reducing the serum potassium concentration. Blood glucose values should be monitored for the hypoglycemic effect of insulin.

An ion exchange resin (e.g., Kayexalate*) may be given orally or rectally to help remove excess potassium. For rectal use 10–25 gm of the resin is suspended in 50–100 ml of 5% glucose, retained for 30–60 min, and then evacuated with isotonic saline. This resin tends to cause constipation; care should be taken to avoid fecal impaction.

Infrequently, serious hyperkalemia persists and is life-threatening. When this is the case, peritoneal dialysis with a potassium-free fluid is effective in removing potassium. When severe acidosis, circulatory congestion, and hyperkalemia are present, this may be the best way to re-establish normal electrolyte, acid-base, and fluid balance. Hemodialysis is also effective but seldom required.

Hyponatremia is a consequence of continued intake or administration of hypotonic fluids during severe oliguria or anuria. Restriction of fluids alone is usually enough to permit the serum sodium level to return to normal. If, however, the concentration is less than 120 mEq/l and central nervous system signs of water intoxication occur, 3% sodium chloride solution should be administered intravenously over 15–60 min in an amount calculated to effect a half-correction of the serum sodium concentration. Furosemide, given intravenously in a dose of 1–2 mg/kg, may also be of value; the sodium content of the urine delivered is usually 70 mEq/l or less.

Acute hypertension must be anticipated, and, to identify it early, blood pressure determinations should be taken at intervals of 4–6 hr (see Sec 13.85). Judgment is required concerning the level of blood pressure at which treatment is necessary. With evidence of hypertensive encephalopathy, such as drowsiness, headache, coma, or seizures with signs of circulatory congestion and pulmonary edema, or with diastolic blood pressure over 95 mm Hg, treatment is definitely indicated. In an acute hypertensive emergency such as encephalopathy with seizures, the drug of choice is diazoxide, 5–10 mg/kg, given intravenously and as rapidly as possible. Intravenous methyldopa, 5–15 mg/kg/dose, may also be used; it is given over a 20–60 min period. Labetalol, a new agent with β and α blocking activity, also appears promising for the management of severe hypertension. It is given intravenously, 0.1 mg/kg/min, a 50 mg ampule being diluted in 125 ml of 5% glucose in water. Onset of action occurs within 30 min, and a gradual reduction in blood pressure can be achieved with little risk of sudden hypotension. Sodium nitroprusside can also be given intravenously, 0.5–1 µg/kg/min, but close monitoring is essential to avoid a precipitous fall in blood pressure. An amount of 50 mg is dissolved in 500 ml of 5% glucose in water and carefully protected from light. In less urgent situations the most frequently used and effective drugs are hydralazine, 0.1–0.5 mg/

---

*Winthrop Laboratories, 90 Park Av., New York, N.Y.

kg, and reserpine, 0.07 mg/kg (maximum dose = 2 mg); they are given together intramuscularly. The combination may be repeated if the blood pressure does not fall within 2–3 hr. More than 2 injections of reserpine are not recommended, but hydralazine, if effective, may be continued as necessary and may be given either intramuscularly or intravenously over a 5–10 min period. Oral methyldopa, 20–40 mg/kg/24 hr in 4 divided doses, or a combination of hydrochlorothiazide, 2 mg/kg/24 hr, and hydralazine, 2–4 mg/kg/24 hr in 3 divided doses, can be instituted after parenteral therapy has reduced the blood pressure to levels considered safe (diastolic pressure <90 mm Hg; systolic pressure <120). With concomitant hypertension and circulatory congestion, a potent diuretic such as furosemide, 1–2 mg/kg/dose given by intravenous or intramuscular injection, can relieve the circulatory congestion and the hypertension; it may also be effective in correcting hyperkalemia and hyponatremia.

Circulatory congestion may pose a serious problem because of pulmonary edema and cardiac decompensation. An early roentgenogram of the chest should be taken to assess the heart size and extent of pulmonary edema. Treatment consists of restricting the intake of sodium and fluid, reducing hypertension, administering parenteral diuretics such as furosemide, and, in refractory and progressive cases, phlebotomy or dialysis to reduce intravascular volume.

The *diet* should be based on the stage and severity of the illness. In the acute, oliguric, edematous, hypertensive phase, restriction in intake of sodium, potassium, protein, and fluids is necessary; most of the calories should be provided in the form of carbohydrate and fat. This period usually lasts less than 1 wk; subsequent dietary restriction is usually unnecessary.

If the child feels well and is not at risk, there is no advantage to enforced bed rest; ambulation with return to normal activities should be encouraged as the general condition permits. Increased physical activity may lead to an increase in abnormal urinary constituents, including hematuria, but this is of no consequence insofar as the healing of the renal lesion is concerned.

When there is evidence of an active pharyngeal or cutaneous streptococcal infection or the initial bacterial cultures have grown group A beta-hemolytic streptococci, an appropriate antibiotic should be prescribed.

It is essential to emphasize the great variability in the acute phase of poststreptococcal glomerulonephritis. The above descriptions pertain mainly to moderately severe to severe forms, which are relatively common. In many instances, however, the clinical manifestations are mild and require only careful monitoring of blood pressure and fluid intake and, initially, sharp reduction in intake of potassium. Even with a mild onset the patient should be hospitalized for close observation during the early days as severe manifestations may develop precipitously and need prompt threatment.

Prognosis. The long-term prognosis for acute poststreptococcal glomerulonephritis in children is excellent; complete recovery occurs in nearly all children who survive the acute stage. Some nephrologists consider that widespread glomerular sclerosis and renal failure may develop many yr after apparent recovery, but the

evidence is questionable. Mortality in the acute phase is the result of disturbances which in virtually all instances are readily amenable to appropriate medical treatment. Exacerbations during the healing phase (i.e., within the 1st 2 mo following onset) are uncommon, are usually precipitated by an intercurrent acute respiratory illness, are manifested principally by hematuria, and are self-limited. Second attacks of acute poststreptococcal glomerulonephritis are rare but may occur following infection with a different nephritogenic strain of streptococcus.

Brogden RN, Hell RC, Speight TM, et al.: Labetalol: A review of its pharmacology and therapeutic use in hypertension. Drugs 15:251, 1978.
Drummond KN, Kaplan BS: Glomerular disorders. *In*: Conn HF (ed): Current Therapy 1977. Philadelphia, WB Saunders, 1977, p 532.
Fish AJ, Herdman RC, Michael AF, et al.: Epidemic acute glomerulonephritis associated with type 49 streptococcal pyoderma. Am J Med 48:28, 1970.
Jennings RB, Earle DP: Post-streptococcal glomerulonephritis: Histopathologic and clinical studies of the acute, subsiding acute and early chronic latent phases. J Clin Invest 40:1525, 1961.
Michael AF Jr, Drummond KN, Good RA, et al: Acute poststreptococcal glomerulonephritis: Immune deposit disease. J Clin Invest 45:237, 1966.
Pruitt AW, Boles A: Diuretic effect of furosemide in acute glomerulonephritis. J Pediatr 89:306, 1976.
Rammelkamp CH Jr, Weaver RS: Acute glomerulonephritis. J Clin Invest 32:345, 1953.
Travis LB, Dodge WF, Beathard GA, et al: Acute glomerulonephritis in children. A review of the natural history with emphasis on prognosis. Clin Nephrol 1:169, 1973.
Wannamaker LW: Differences between streptococcal infections of the throat and of the skin. N Engl J Med 282:23, 78, 1970.

16.18 IDIOPATHIC RECURRENT MACROSCOPIC HEMATURIA
(IgA Nephropathy, Berger Disease, Focal Proliferative Glomerulitis, Benign Recurrent Hematuria)

This heading probably includes several unrelated disorders characterized by recurrent episodes of gross hematuria, with or without intervening persistent microscopic hematuria, and by absence of systemic disease and other known glomerular or nonglomerular causes of hematuria; focal segmental mesangial proliferation is the usual pathologic change. The etiology is unknown, but episodes of gross hematuria are often precipitated by nonspecific viral respiratory infections or febrile episodes, less frequently by strenuous exercise.

The condition occurs at any age, even in infancy; in most instances the onset occurs after the age of 2 yr. Boys are affected about twice as often as girls; familial cases are reported.

Pathology and Pathogenesis. In about a third of cases only minimal glomerular changes are present; but the most characteristic lesion is focal, segmental, mesangial, cellular, and matrix proliferation of mild severity involving a variable proportion of glomeruli, usually fewer than half. More extensive and severe changes may occur. These include diffuse proliferative glomerulonephritis with focal crescent formation, focal areas of glomerulosclerosis, and synechiae between glomerular tufts and Bowman capsule. In about a third of patients studied there is mesangial deposition of IgA, C3, and properdin (Fig 16–11); deposits of IgG, IgM,

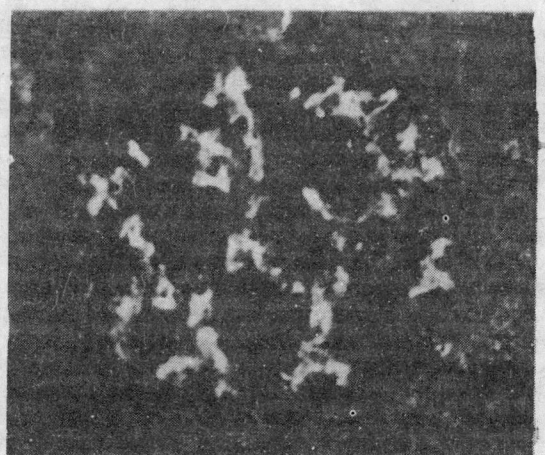

Figure 16–11 Immunopathologic preparation from a 14 yr old patient with recurrent macroscopic hematuria and focal glomerulonephritis (Berger disease); tissue is stained for human IgA. Note diffuse mesangial fluorescence. This pattern of fluorescence was seen in each glomerulus in the biopsy, even though the histopathologic changes were confined to only some segments of some glomeruli (focal segmental glomerulitis or focal glomerulonephritis). (×250.)

and fibrin-related antigens are present in about 50% of those with IgA deposits. The IgA does not contain secretory piece. The absence of C1q and C4 suggests activity of the alternative pathway, as does the demonstration of properdin deposits in some patients. The deposits are usually glomerular and mesangial in location; in some cases they involve the capillary loops and the walls of contiguous arterioles. IgA deposits may be found in small blood vessel walls of the superficial dermis. Electron microscopy reveals mesangial and, in some cases, subendothelial, intramembranous, or subepithelial deposits. Although light microscopic changes may be only focal and segmental, if IgA deposits are present, they tend to involve all glomeruli, even those without apparent histopathologic changes. Sequential biopsies over a period of years, during which the patient has repeated episodes of gross hematuria, show no distinct change or progression in most instances; in a minority, especially if there is persistent proteinuria between episodes of hematuria, there is progressive glomerular destruction with resultant chronic or end-stage renal disease. For unexplained reasons a higher percentage of patients in Europe than in North America with this clinical entity are found to have IgA deposits.

Clinical Manifestations, Course, and Prognosis. Most episodes of gross hematuria are preceded within 1–3 days by mild upper respiratory infections or febrile episodes, less often by strenuous exercise. The onset of hematuria is usually abrupt and unaccompanied by other symptoms. Some patients complain of lethargy or malaise or of abdominal, flank, or lower back pain. Hypertension, oliguria, and edema are not usually seen in children; patients presenting with the nephrotic syndrome or acute renal insufficiency have been described. Episodes of gross hematuria usually last 2–4 days; microscopic hematuria is usually present between the episodes and may occur many times over a period of 5–10 yr. The condition clears spontaneously within 5 yr

in about 50% of patients, and the prognosis is generally good, especially in children. A progressive course leading to renal insufficiency or sustained hypertension occurs in about 15% of children, principally in those who have persistent proteinuria between the episodes of hematuria. These complications are twice as common in adults. Mesangial IgA deposits have been noted in renal allografts in some of these patients.

Laboratory Data. During an attack the urine is red or tea colored. The presence of red blood cell casts indicates a renal source of the bleeding. The urinary excretion of protein is moderately elevated during episodes of gross hematuria but seldom exceeds 1.5 gm/24 hr. In most patients the proteinuria disappears as the hematuria subsides. There is no depression of serum C3 levels or of other components of complement, no evidence of group A beta-hemolytic streptococcal infection, and none of a generalized or systemic disease, such as systemic lupus erythematosus. A minority of patients have a transient decrease in glomerular filtration rate during episodes. The serum IgA level is elevated in 50% of cases, and the presence of circulating immune complexes containing IgA has been described during acute episodes.

Diagnosis and Differential Diagnosis. A renal biopsy should be performed in patients in whom this diagnosis is suspected, particularly if there is persistent proteinuria. In addition to confirming the diagnosis and providing prognostic information, it enables exclusion of other more serious and potentially treatable diseases. Conditions which must be considered include many of the causes of hematuria in children listed in Table 16–2, such as membranoproliferative glomerulonephritis, hereditary nephritis with deafness, benign familial hematuria, and chronic glomerulonephritis, each of which can be reactivated by intercurrent illness leading to episodic gross hematuria. It is essential to exclude nonglomerular causes of hematuria, such as renal tumor, hydronephrosis, trauma, calculus, polycystic kidney disease, or other congenital structural or vascular anomalies of the urinary tract. If the diagnosis is in question, particularly if red blood cell casts are not observed, an intravenous urogram should be obtained to exclude such conditions. Acute hemorrhagic cystitis of bacterial or viral etiology may occur with gross hematuria and abdominal discomfort, with or without other symptoms of urinary tract infection. Extensive and unnecessary urologic evaluations, including cytoscopy, are carried out all too frequently because of lack of awareness of this entity. Mesangial IgA deposits are seen also in other conditions, including anaphylactoid purpura; indeed, some authors consider Berger disease and anaphylactoid purpura to be related in pathogenesis. Similar deposits may be seen in systemic lupus erythematosus, in cirrhosis of the liver, and, rarely, in patients with minimal change nephrotic syndrome.

Treatment. No specific treatment for the renal lesion exists. Reassurance should be given since the attacks of gross hematuria are self-limited and the course is benign in the majority of patients. Bed rest is not indicated, but if the child does not feel well, he or she may wish to restrict activity for several days. Even if the number of episodes of gross hematuria could be reduced by avoiding exercise, the long-term prognosis would probably not be affected; the patient should be encouraged to lead a completely normal life.

Berger J: IgA glomerular deposits in renal disease. Transplant Proc 1:939, 1969.
Gervais M, Drummond KN: L'hématurie récidivante chez l'enfant. Union Med Can 99:1234, 1970.
Levy M, Beaufils H, Gubler MC et al: Idiopathic recurrent macroscopic hematuria and mesangial IgA-IgG deposits in children (Berger's disease). Clin Nephrol 1:63, 1973.
Nakamoto Y, Asano Y, Dohi K, et al: Primary IgA glomerulonephritis and Schönlein-Henoch purpura nephritis: Clinicopathological and immunohistological characteristics. Quart J Med 47:495, 1978.
Vernier RL, Resnick JS, Mauer SM: Recurrent hematuria and focal glomerulonephritis. Kidney Int 7:224, 1975.
Woodroffe AJ, Gormly AA, McKenzie PE, et al: Immunologic studies in IgA nephropathy. Kidney Int 18:366, 1980.

16.19 GLOMERULONEPHRITIS WITH SEPTICEMIA, INFECTED SHUNTS FOR HYDROCEPHALUS, OR SUBACUTE BACTERIAL ENDOCARDITIS

A proliferative glomerulonephritis may develop in the course of a variety of acute or chronic systemic bacterial infections. These include coagulase-positive staphylococcal osteomyelitis, ventriculoatrial shunts infected with coagulase-negative staphylococci, subacute bacterial endocarditis due to a variety of organisms, and chronic suppuration. The pathologic features range from focal segmental mesangial proliferative glomerulonephritis to diffuse proliferative glomerulonephritis with crescents, segmental necrosis, and interstitial mononuclear cell infiltration. A picture resembling membranoproliferative glomerulonephritis may be seen. The lesions may be acute and active or may become chronic, with focal or diffuse scarring. Mesangial, subendothelial, or membranous deposits may be seen on electron microscopy. Immunopathologic study reveals nodular deposits of IgG and C3, with or without IgM, IgA, or fibrin.

A pathogenesis involving immune complexes of antibody of the IgG or IgM type and antigens of the infecting organism is postulated. Specific bacterial antigens have been identified within the complexes in a number of these conditions.

The clinical presentation is usually that of a mixed nephritic-nephrotic type with hematuria, red cell casts, proteinuria, azotemia, and hypertension. In infants with infected shunts, the initial manifestation is that of the nephrotic syndrome in 50% of cases, whereas in patients with subacute bacterial endocarditis, hematuria and proteinuria occur usually without leading to a full-blown nephrotic syndrome. In virtually all patients, clinical evidence of bacteremia or sepsis, such as fever and hepatosplenomegaly, precedes the renal manifestations. A positive blood culture can usually be obtained, but the urine culture is frequently negative. There are findings of normochromic anemia and leukocytosis, and the serum levels of C3 and early components of the complement system are depressed. Immune complex nephritis should be suspected in patients

with chronic bacterial infection who develop abnormal urinary sediment, proteinuria, azotemia, and/or hypertension. The diagnosis is supported by reduction in serum complement levels; renal biopsy can establish the diagnosis and provide valuable information regarding its severity and prognosis.

Treatment consists of antibiotic therapy for the infecting organism; in most cases of infected shunts for hydrocephalus, the shunt should be removed. The prognosis varies with the nature of the underlying disease. If the infection can be controlled, the renal lesions tend to become inactive; uncommonly, progressive glomerular destruction leads to chronic renal failure.

Black JA, Challacombe DN, Ockenden BG: Nephrotic syndrome associated with bacteraemia after shunt operations for hydrocephalus. Lancet 2:921, 1965.
Gutman RA, Striker GE, Gilliland BC, et al: The immune complex glomerulonephritis of bacterial endocarditis. Medicine 51:1, 1972.
Levy RL, Hong R: The immune nature of subacute bacterial endocarditis (SBE) nephritis. Am J Med 54:645, 1973.
O'Regan S, Kaplan BS, Drummond KN: Antigens in human immune complex nephritis. Clin Nephrol 6:417, 1976.

16.20 NEPHRITIS IN SYSTEMIC LUPUS ERYTHEMATOSUS

See Sec 9.62 for a general discussion of systemic lupus erythematosus. Renal involvement is present in most pediatric patients with systemic lupus; its severity, however, may vary from changes detectable only by electron microscopic and immunopathologic studies of biopsied tissue associated with no clinical or laboratory evidence of disease to florid disease with severe clinical renal manifestations.

Pathology and Pathogenesis. The glomerulus is the principal site of injury. Five forms of renal involvement are recognized, but it is reasonable to consider them as a continuum since they overlap, with the possibility of transition from 1 form to another. The presence or absence of nephritis and the form that it will take are usually established early in the disease. The 5 forms are:

Mesangial Lupus Nephritis. The renal findings by light microscopy are usually normal or show only mesangial widening, associated at times with mild hypercellularity. By immunopathologic study IgG and C3 deposits are usually seen in the mesangial regions, IgA and IgM less frequently. These changes are present whether or not mesangial changes are detectable by light microscopy. By electron microscopy electron dense deposits are seen mainly in mesangial sites but occasionally in association with the glomerular basement membrane. It is likely that all of the forms of lupus nephritis begin with these mesangial changes. Hematuria and proteinuria are usually absent at this stage and urinalysis is normal; transition to focal proliferative, diffuse proliferative, membranous, or interstitial forms may occur.

Focal Proliferative Lupus Nephritis (Lupus Glomerulitis). Lesions are confined to some glomeruli and to only some lobules or segments of the affected glomeruli. Characteristically present are mesangial hypercellularity with increased mesangial matrix, reduction in patent capillary loops in affected segments, mild polymorphonuclear infiltration, localized thickening of peripheral capillary basement membranes, and, less commonly, some nuclear fragmentation. A mild periglomerulitis may be present. Electron microscopic findings include dense mesangial deposits, with occasional subendothelial or intramembranous deposits in regions where a proliferative reaction is present. Immunopathologic study reveals focal mesangial deposits of IgG and C3 and occasionally of fibrin, IgM, IgA, or properdin. Subendothelial and epimembranous deposits are also seen. These lesions tend not to progress, and a benign renal course generally follows if adequate therapy is provided.

Diffuse Proliferative Lupus Nephritis. This is the most active and serious form of renal injury and constitutes about 30% of cases of lupus nephritis in children. All glomeruli are involved. Characteristic histopathologic features are a marked increase in the mesangial matrix, with obliteration of capillary lumens, necrosis of glomerular lobules, nuclear fragmentation, localized thickening of glomerular basement membranes that creates the so-called wire-loop appearance, and infiltration with neutrophils. There may be epithelial crescent formation, interstitial edema, local interstitial perivascular inflammation and plasma cell infiltration, and necrotizing renal vasculitis. Electron microscopy reveals extensive mesangial and subendothelial deposits with marked increase in mesangial matrix. The subendothelial deposits along the glomerular basement membrane correspond to areas of wire-loop change seen by light microscopy. Heavy deposition of IgG, C3, and fibrin is widely distributed in the glomerulus, often in a lumpy, lobular pattern; IgM, IgA, and properdin may also be seen, as well as DNA and other nuclear antigens. Untreated, this form progresses rapidly to glomerular destruction with renal failure, severe hypertension, and death within months. Transition from diffuse proliferative to membranous lupus nephritis has been observed during immunosuppressive treatment.

Membranous Lupus Nephritis. This is the least common form of lupus nephritis in children, seen in about 10% of cases. It is a chronic, indolent process with little cellular proliferation but with diffuse thickening of the basement membranes. The thickening is the result of epimembranous deposits similar to those of idiopathic membranous nephropathy. In comparison with the diffuse proliferative form there is less subendothelial and mesangial deposition. The deposits contain IgG, C3, and fibrin; IgM, IgA, and DNA may also be present. This form of lupus nephritis progresses slowly and responds slowly, if at all, to treatment.

Interstitial Lupus Nephritis. In this form focal and diffuse infiltration of inflammatory cells in the interstitium, interstitial fibrosis, and tubular damage are found. Glomerular changes of 1 or another of the abovementioned forms may be present. Immune complexes containing IgG and C3 are seen along the tubular basement membranes, bound to peritubular capillaries, and within the interstitium.

In each of the forms described above glomerular sclerosis may develop.

Evidence is good that the renal lesions principally involve deposition of immune complexes. A number of distinct immune complex systems have been identified. Antibodies to nuclear constituents, such as native and single-stranded DNA, cytoplasmic constituents, clotting factors, gamma globulins, red blood cell antigens, platelets, and various tissue antigens are detectable in the serum of patients with active systemic lupus. The formation of DNA/anti-DNA immune complexes which bind complement, with the subsequent deposition of these complexes in the glomerulus, is one of the principal mechanisms of glomerular injury. Differences between the types of lupus nephritis may reflect differences in the immune complex system involved. Activation of the alternative complement pathway may also occur. There is evidence also that glomeruli have a strong capacity to bind DNA, which raises the possibility that free DNA may be trapped in the glomeruli and that in situ complex formation may occur.

Clinical Manifestations and Course. Renal disease in systemic lupus is one of the major causes of morbidity and mortality; thus, it is critical to establish whether it is present. Furthermore, since each of the forms of lupus nephritis has a different natural history and requires a different therapy, the particular type of nephritis should be established by renal biopsy. Urinalysis may be normal in the face of important progressive pathologic changes found on renal biopsy.

In **focal proliferative lupus nephritis** there may be microscopic hematuria with red blood cell casts and mild proteinuria. Hypertension, edema, and azotemia are uncommon. Usually the renal lesions do not progress, and treatment should be aimed primarily at control of the nonrenal manifestations.

In **diffuse proliferative lupus nephritis** the renal manifestations are a major clinical problem. Hypertension, edema, azotemia, microscopic or gross hematuria, and moderate or massive proteinuria are usually present (i.e., there is a mixed nephritic-nephrotic picture). If untreated, this form of lupus nephritis progresses in several mo to renal failure. In children aggressive treatment is effective (see below).

The nephrotic syndrome is the principal manifestation of **membranous lupus nephritis.** Microscopic hematuria, hypertension, and mild azotemia may also be present. The course is usually chronic, with slow progression to renal insufficiency or gradual response to treatment over a period of months to several yr.

Laboratory Data. Hematuria with red blood cell casts, pyuria, proteinuria, and azotemia are the principal laboratory manifestations. If the nephrotic syndrome is present, hypoproteinemia, particularly hypoalbuminemia, is also present. In patients with active lupus nephritis the level of serum complement, particularly C3, is low, and the titer of antinuclear antibodies, especially anti-DNA antibodies, is elevated. With treatment, these tend to return to normal levels. Normal levels of C4 and of antibodies to double-stranded DNA are reasonably good indicators of satisfactory control.

Differential Diagnosis. Other forms of renal disease may occur in patients with systemic lupus; specifically, it is essential to exclude urinary tract infection, since this may not be clinically apparent and may cause progressive renal destruction or sepsis while being masked by corticosteroid therapy. Iatrogenic urinary abnormalities may also occur; e.g., cyclophosphamide or azathioprine may produce cystitis or mucosal ulceration of the urinary tract.

The diagnosis and differential diagnosis of systemic lupus are considered in Sec 9.62. Similar findings in renal biopsy may be seen in anaphylactoid purpura, subacute bacterial endocarditis, nephritis associated with infected ventriculoatrial shunts, and other causes of membranous glomerulonephritis. What appears to be idiopathic membranous glomerulopathy may precede the full development of overt systemic lupus by 1–3 yr. In mixed connective tissue disease renal involvement is uncommon, and the serum complement level is usually normal or increased, but some patients have been reported to have an immune complex type of glomerulonephritis. Various medications can cause lupus with its renal manifestations. Discontinuation of exposure to the offending agent usually resolves the problem.

Prevention. No means of prevention of lupus nephritis is known. Likelihood of reactivation or exacerbation of systemic lupus can be reduced by avoiding exposure to ultraviolet irradiation, e.g., sunlight. Sudden changes in medication, such as rapid reduction in corticosteroid dosage or withdrawal of azathioprine, should be avoided since they can reactivate lupus nephritis, and recontrol may subsequently be difficult to achieve.

Treatment. The treatment of *focal proliferative nephritis* ordinarily requires only the usual course of prednisone (1–2 mg/kg/24 hr) for treatment of the underlying disease. An alternate-day regimen should be introduced as soon as feasible, usually after 4–6 wk of daily therapy. Close attention should be paid to urinary and biopsy findings to determine whether progression is occurring.

For *diffuse proliferative lupus nephritis* active treatment of the renal lesion itself must be undertaken. Doses of prednisone adequate to control nonrenal manifestations are often inadequate; doses of 2–3 mg/kg/24 hr should be given for 1–2 mo in conjunction with azathioprine in a dose of 3–4 mg/kg/24 hr. The course should be monitored by the usual laboratory and clinical evaluations and by sequential renal biopsies. Attention should be paid to the possible development of steroid-induced hypertension and edema; restriction of salt intake to 1–2 gm/24 hr should be instituted, and antihypertensive and/or diuretic therapy may be needed. Gradual introduction of an alternate-day regimen of prednisone therapy by reducing the dosage by 5–10 mg at weekly intervals on alternate days while maintaining the initial dose on the other days should be started after several mo of daily therapy. During the initial treatment period prednisone is given in 3 doses daily; later, a single daily dose is evolved. Daily azathioprine treatment should be continued indefinitely; gradual reduction to a maintenance dose of 2 mg/kg/24 hr may be attempted after satisfactory control has been achieved. Cyclophosphamide can be used instead of or, in some refractory cases, in addition to azathioprine.

The treatment of *membranous lupus nephritis* is controversial. Less aggressive treatment is indicated than for diffuse proliferative lupus glomerulonephritis. Long-term azathioprine and alternate-day prednisone therapy reduce the protein excretion and lessen the renal insufficiency in some patients.

Therapy should be directed toward normalizing the results of urinalysis and renal function tests and maintaining serum complement levels and antinuclear antibody titers at normal levels. It is important to be alert for the possible development of bacterial or fungal infections; the capacity of patients with lupus to resist infection has been impaired both by the underlying disease and by immunosuppressive drugs.

Prognosis. Lupus nephritis has a good prognosis if adequate treatment is given early. Improvement is most dramatic in the diffuse proliferative form, least in the membranous type. An overall 10 yr survival rate should, with optimal care, be at least 85%.

Agnello V, Koffler D, Kunkel HG: Immune complex systems in the nephritis of systemic lupus erythematosus. Kidney Int 3:90, 1973.
Baldwin DS, Gluck MC, Lowenstein J, et al.: Lupus nephritis: Clinical course as related to morphologic forms and their transitions. Am J Med 62:12, 1977.
Brentjens JR, Sepulveda M, Baliah T, et al: Interstitial immune complex nephritis in patients with systemic lupus erythematosus. Kidney Int 7:342, 1975.
Fish AJ, Blau EB, Westberg NG, et al: Systemic lupus erythematosus within the first two decades of life. Am J Med 62:99, 1977.
Kallen RJ, Lee S-K, Aronson AJ, et al: Idiopathic membranous glomerulopathy preceding the emergence of systemic lupus erythematosus in two children. J Pediatr 90:72, 1977.
Woolf A, Croher B, Osofsky SE, et al: Nephritis in children and young adults with systemic lupus erythematosus and normal urinary sediment. Pediatrics 64:678, 1979.

16.21 THE NEPHRITIS OF SCHÖNLEIN-HENOCH SYNDROME
(Anaphylactoid Purpura)

See also Sec 9.65.

About 40% of children with Schönlein-Henoch syndrome have evidence of renal involvement; serious kidney disease affects a much smaller proportion.

Pathology and Pathogenesis. On light microscopy the principal lesion is a proliferative change affecting endothelial and mesangial cells. These changes may be minor (focal and segmental glomerulitis), or there may be diffuse mesangial proliferation affecting all glomeruli. Considerable variation among glomeruli in severity of the lesion is not uncommon. Epithelial crescent formation results from the proliferation of parietal epithelial cells, affecting a percentage of glomeruli which varies among patients, with severity which ranges from limited foci of epithelial cell proliferation to fully developed circumferential crescents. Renal pathologic changes range, then, from minimal focal segmental mesangial proliferation to severe diffuse proliferative glomerulonephritis with extensive crescent formation. Interstitial inflammatory changes are not uncommon; their severity is related to that of the glomerular lesions. Immunopathologic studies regularly show IgA deposition, principally in the mesangium but occasionally in some of the capillary loops. C3 is detected in similar locations in about 75% of patients; IgG and IgM deposits are also common. Early components of the classic complement pathway, C1q and C4, are not found, but properdin is occasionally present. These findings suggest activation of the alternative complement pathway. Fibrin deposition is seen in about two thirds of patients, sometimes in a mesangial locus but especially within epithelial crescents. By electron microscopy finely granular electron dense deposits are regularly seen within the mesangium and occasionally in relation to the glomerular basement membrane in a subendothelial, intramembranous, or epimembranous location.

The pathogenesis of the Schönlein-Henoch syndrome is not well understood. Plasma IgA levels tend to be elevated during the acute phase, and circulating IgA and IgG immune complexes have been detected. The role of alternative pathway activation, possibly by IgA-containing immune complexes, is uncertain. The regular finding of fibrin within sites of crescent formation as well as in the dermis around areas of vasculitis suggests involvement of the coagulation system, possibly secondary to immunologic events.

Clinical Manifestations and Course. In most children the clinical features of the nephritis are overshadowed by the skin, joint, and gastrointestinal manifestations. In those with renal involvement the spectrum of findings is broad and includes, in decreasing order of frequency, microscopic hematuria, episodic gross hematuria, mild proteinuria, nephrotic syndrome, a mixed acute nephritic-nephrotic picture, and progressive renal failure, which is seen in about 5% of untreated patients.

The renal manifestations are usually seen within 1 mo of onset of the syndrome; in a minority of patients serious renal manifestations may appear late when other features are subsiding, even as late as several mo after other signs have disappeared. Nephritis may also first appear in association with recurrences of the purpura.

There is good correlation between early histopathologic findings and clinical features of renal disease. Patients with minimal or focal changes do not have significant clinical findings, whereas those with diffuse proliferative glomerulonephritis have more serious manifestations and severity increasing in direct relation to the percentage of glomeruli with epithelial crescent formation. Those with crescents in more than 50% of glomeruli often have the nephrotic syndrome, and both acute and chronic renal failure are seen more commonly in those with extensive crescent formation.

In most instances the nephritis is self-limited, becoming inactive within 6 mo of onset and leaving no clinically important residual renal damage. Minor abnormalities in the urine sediment may persist longer, but they do not usually signify progressive renal damage. Patients at risk for development of progressive renal failure should be identified as early as possible in order that treatment can be instituted.

Laboratory data are not diagnostic. The serum C3 level is normal, the properdin level decreased in 50% of cases within the 1st mo. About half show elevations in plasma IgA and IgM levels, which return to normal within several mo. Tests for antinuclear antibodies and rheu-matoid factor are negative. Findings indicative of renal involvement include gross or microscopic hematuria, proteinuria, and elevation of the blood urea nitrogen and creatinine levels. Typical findings of acute nephritis or the nephrotic syndrome may be present. Proteinuria is poorly selective.

Diagnosis and Differential Diagnosis. The characteristic rash, with or without typical areas of soft tissue swelling, provides the strongest evidence for the diagnosis of Schönlein-Henoch syndrome. It is accompanied in most patients by gastrointestinal and joint manifestations and in about 50% by evidence of renal involvement. The full-blown syndrome is distinctive, diagnosis resting primarily on clinical rather than on laboratory features. An identical but less extensive rash may occasionally be seen in both *systemic lupus erythematosus* and *acute poststreptococcal glomerulonephritis* with renal manifestations, but other typical clinical and laboratory features help differentiate them. In the hemolytic-uremic syndrome, purpura is secondary to thrombocytopenia, but the lesions are less discrete than in Schönlein-Henoch syndrome, and a microangiopathic hemolytic anemia and other features aid in diagnosis. The nephropathy of Schönlein-Henoch syndrome must be differentiated from other causes of focal segmental nephritis, such as subacute bacterial endocarditis, systemic lupus erythematosus, and Berger disease or from forms of diffuse proliferative glomerulonephritis, with or without crescents, such as membranoproliferative glomerulonephritis, acute poststreptococcal glomerulonephritis, and idiopathic crescentic glomerulonephritis.

Patients who develop nephropathy after other features of Schönlein-Henoch syndrome have subsided may present a difficult diagnostic problem since it may be hard to ascertain whether the renal disorder is a consequence of this condition. Patients with Schönlein-Henoch syndrome should be followed for at least 3 mo to exclude the late development of nephritis. In difficult cases a skin biopsy at a site of fresh purpura may help in establishing the diagnosis since it will reveal the characteristic leukocytoclastic vasculitis, with deposits of IgA and fibrin in the dermal vessels and surrounding connective tissue. In certain patients renal biopsy may not only clarify the diagnosis but also provide important information about the severity and extent of nephritis which may be crucial in deciding whether or not to initiate therapy. Renal biopsy is indicated in patients with proteinuria in excess of 1 gm/day, a nephrotic or nephritic syndrome, or evidence of renal insufficiency. We prefer to do the biopsy without waiting to see whether these findings resolve spontaneously.

Treatment. In most cases of Schönlein-Henoch syndrome the nephropathy is self-limited and not serious. Serious manifestations should be treated in the usual way, with supervision of the fluid and electrolyte status when there is renal failure, control of hypertension, and salt restriction in cases with the nephrotic syndrome. Patients with the major renal manifestations outlined above should be referred to a pediatric nephrologist for assessment of the need for renal biopsy and specific therapy for the nephritis. The value of cytotoxic drugs in Schönlein-Henoch syndrome has not been established by controlled studies, but we consider that they have an important place in patients with severe renal manifestations, particularly if treatment is instituted early. For patients with proteinuria in excess of 1 gm/day, the nephrotic syndrome, or nephritis with renal failure who have biopsy evidence of diffuse proliferative glomerulonephritis, we currently use azathioprine, 3–4 mg/kg/24 hr for 6–12 mo, in combination with prednisone, 2 mg/kg/24 hr up to a maximum of 60 mg/24 hr. The prednisone is given daily for 3–4 wk and then on alternate days in the morning for the duration of the azathioprine therapy. Some nephrologists use dipyridamole and anticoagulant therapy in addition for severely affected patients. Long-term follow-up is recommended for all patients who have major renal manifestations since renal failure or the development of hypertension may occur as late as 5–10 yr after the acute episode. Renal transplantation has been successful in patients with terminal renal failure following Schönlein-Henoch syndrome.

Prognosis. In the majority of cases the prognosis for the nephritis of Schönlein-Henoch syndrome is very good. Of 350 reported cases of nephritis, only 5% have developed end-stage renal failure. Seventy-five per cent of those with microscopic hematuria or transient mild proteinuria recover completely within 2 yr. Persistent active renal disease and end-stage renal failure are confined largely to patients with diffuse proliferative glomerulonephritis and epithelial crescent formation affecting over 50% of glomeruli and who have presented a nephrotic or nephritic-nephrotic syndrome within the 1st 3 mo of illness. On the other hand, about 40% of patients with these more serious features have normal renal function 5 yr after onset, even without therapy. We find that the treatment in appropriately selected cases improves this prognosis significantly.

Allen DM, Diamond LK, Howell DA: Anaphylactoid purpura in children (Schönlein-Henoch syndrome). Am J Dis Child 99:833, 1960.

Barratt TM, Drummond KN: Schönlein-Henoch syndrome or anaphylactoid purpura. In: Kelly VC (ed): Brennemann-Kelly Practice of Pediatrics. Hagerstown, Md., Harper and Row, 1980.

Counahan R, Winterborn MW, White RHR, et al: Prognosis of Henoch-Schönlein nephritis in children. Br Med J 2:11, 1977.

Levinsky RJ, Barratt TM: IgA immune complexes in Henoch-Schönlein purpura. Lancet 2:1100, 1979.

Levy M, Broyer M, Arran A, et al: Anaphylactoid purpura nephritis in childhood: natural history and immunopathology. In: Hamburger J, Crosnier J, Maxwell MH (eds): Advances in Nephrology. Chicago, Year Book Medical Publishers, 1976, p 183.

Levy M, Broyer M, Habib R: Pathology and immunopathology of Schönlein-Henoch glomerulonephritis. In: Kincaid-Smith P, d'Apice AJF, Atkins RC (eds): Progress in Glomerulonephritis. New York, John Wiley and Sons, 1979.

16.22 HEMOLYTIC-UREMIC SYNDROME

The hemolytic-uremic syndrome is an acute disorder characterized by renal failure with or without oligoanuria, microangiopathic hemolytic anemia, and thrombocytopenia. These features usually appear several days to 2 wk after a prodromal illness, which is commonly a gastroenteritis with diarrhea and less commonly an upper respiratory tract infection.

Etiology. The specific etiology is unknown, although inciting or precipitating events have been recognized in some patients, particularly in the case of small epidemics. These include infections due to agents such as coxsackievirus, arbovirus, echovirus, *Shigella*, *Salmonella, Streptococcus pneumoniae*, group A beta-hemolytic streptococcus, and *Mycoplasma*. Other precipitating factors include pregnancy, oral contraceptives, longstanding hypertension, and x-irradiation to the kidneys. Familial factors are evident in some cases. Circulating endotoxin has been proposed as an important pathogenetic factor, but there is no conclusive evidence as to its role. It is clear that while agents or events have been recognized as possible etiologic factors in some patients, in the majority there is no clue which points to a specific cause.

Epidemiology. The syndrome has been recognized mainly in Caucasians. The mean age of onset varies with geography, mainly under 1 yr in infants in the Southern Hemisphere and 2–4 yr of age in children in the Northern Hemisphere. Eighty per cent of affected children are under 4 yr; older children and adults may be affected. Argentina, California, South Africa, and the Netherlands have been considered endemic areas, but the syndrome has a worldwide distribution. Males and females are affected equally.

Pathology and Pathogenesis. Early pathologic reports suggested that renal cortical necrosis was a principal finding, but subsequent studies have shown other characteristic changes. Three overlapping groups may be recognized. Over 50% of children with hemolytic-uremic syndrome have a **microangiopathy** affecting the glomeruli and arterioles. Swelling of endothelial cells and separation of these cells from the glomerular basement membrane occur with formation of a subendothelial space in which accumulates an electron-lucent, fluffy, amorphous material containing fibrin and lipid and platelet and red blood cell fragments (Fig 16–12). The basement membrane itself is unaltered. Epithelial foot process fusion is present. The capillary lumen is narrowed or occluded, and there may be fibrin microthrombi. The mesangial matrix has a fibrillar and somewhat foamy appearance, but there is no increase in mesangial cells. A variable number of glomeruli are affected, and some glomeruli or parts of glomeruli may be normal. A similar change involving endothelial swelling and widening of the subendothelial space with consequent luminal narrowing affects a variable number of arterioles. Immunofluorescent studies may show occasional IgM or C3 deposits; the principal finding is fibrin deposition within the capillary walls and lumina and in the mesangium. Arteriolar fibrin deposition may also be seen, principally in subendothelial or intramural position. These histopathologic changes, very characteristic of the hemolytic-uremic syndrome, are sometimes referred to as *thrombotic microangiopathy*. Six mo–1 yr after onset follow-up biopsies show a variable number of sclerotic glomeruli. This histopathologic variant is most commonly seen in infants under 2 yr of age, a high percentage of whom have had a gastroenteritic prodrome and have acute renal failure, proteinuria, and gross hematuria. Severe intractable hypertension is not a prominent feature. Most patients make a complete recovery, though about 15% have some resid-

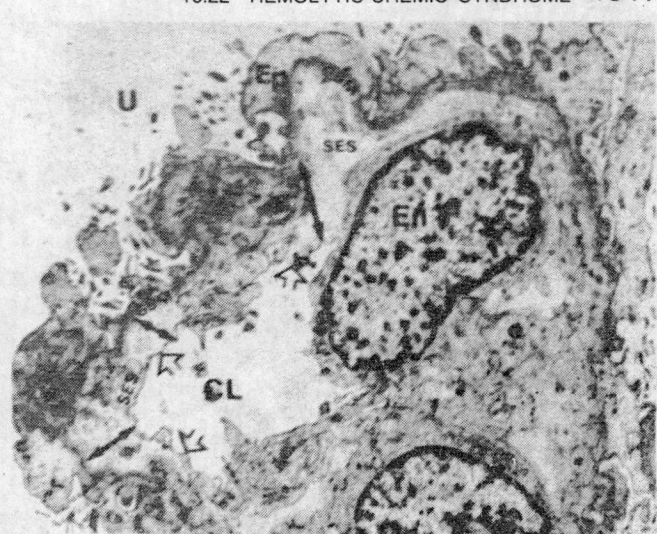

Figure 16–12 Electron micrograph illustrating uncomplicated glomerular microangiopathy in a patient with the hemolytic-uremic syndrome. C = narrowed capillary lumen. En = swollen endothelial cell. Ep = epithelial cells with fused foot processes. U = urinary space. SES = the newly formed subendothelial space; the double-headed arrows indicate its variable width, expanding from the glomerular basement membrane (GBM) to the membrana fenestrata (light arrows). (× 7500.)

ual renal symptoms such as microscopic hematuria, mild proteinuria, hypertension, or reduced renal function.

The 2nd variant has predominantly **arterial involvement** affecting mainly the interlobular arteries. Intimal edema and proliferation, necrosis of the vessel wall, and a lamellar, onion-skin appearance may be seen. Narrowing of the lumen and occlusion by thrombi occur. The glomeruli may show the changes of thrombotic microangiopathy described above, but more often the glomerular changes are ischemic in type, with diffuse wrinkling and some splitting of the basement membranes. Fibrin deposition is not prominent in this group. This variant tends to affect children over 3 yr of age and is the type seen in older children and adults; there is less often a diarrheal prodrome or severe oligoanuria, but severe hypertension is common and may be difficult to control. The prognosis for this group is worse than for the 1st group; a significant number progress to end-stage renal failure.

The 3rd variant has patchy or diffuse **cortical necrosis,** which is more common in infants and is associated with a high incidence of severe oligoanuria. Prognosis depends on the extent of the areas of necrosis.

It is not clear whether these histopathologic patterns are simply age-related variants of a single underlying disease or represent different clinical entities.

It is generally agreed that the central event in pathogenesis is damage to the vascular endothelium, probably as a consequence of 1 of many possible noxious stimuli, such as infectious agents, endotoxin, drugs, hypertension, immune complexes, and x-irradiation. The altered endothelial barrier, irregular lumen, and exposed underlying basement membrane lead to local coagulation, with fibrin strand formation in the lumina and capillary walls; platelets and red blood cells are damaged during passage through this altered capillary and arteriolar network and are subsequently trapped in the spleen. Selective platelet consumption is the only consistent coagulation abnormality, the reduction of the platelet half-life from 9.5 to around 1.5 days resulting in a variable degree of thrombocytopenia. The surviving

platelets discharge their serotonin, and platelet exhaustion can be detected as reduced aggregability of the surviving platelets to collagen, ADP, and epinephrine.

Immunologic factors do not appear to play an important role in most patients. Absence of a plasma factor which enhances formation of endothelial cell prostacyclin (an endogenous inhibitor of platelet aggregation), and an abnormality in red blood cell membrane phospholipid content suggestive of lipid peroxidation have been postulated; this could contribute to hemolysis in the face of oxidant stress.

The hemolytic anemia is Coombs-negative; there are no enzymatic defects in the red blood cells, which are fragmented, irregular, and anisocytotic. Burr cells and helmet cells are also seen (Fig 16–13). Convulsions may be secondary to hypertension or to the metabolic complications of acute renal failure as well as to microangiopathic changes within the central nervous system. Hypertension is often associated with markedly elevated plasma renin activity.

Familial forms of the syndrome are recognized. In some, genetic factors appear operative; both dominant and recessive patterns of autosomal inheritance are described. A familial pattern in which the syndrome affects infants of the same age is associated with a very poor prognosis. In other families children of several ages may be affected simultaneously; here environmental factors are probably operative, and the prognosis is good.

Clinical Manifestations and Course. The onset is acute, with extreme pallor, bruising or purpura, irritability, lethargy, and decreased urinary output. It usually follows within several days to 2 wk an episode of gastroenteritis, an acute "flu"-like illness, or an upper respiratory infection; some patients have severe colitis, associated sometimes with localized gangrene of bowel due to microangiopathic vascular occlusions.

The child is anorectic, irritable, and pale. Hypertension, edema, splenomegaly, purpura or petechiae, mild jaundice, seizures, and signs of circulatory congestion such as hepatomegaly, pulmonary edema, cardiomegaly, tachycardia, gallop rhythm, and venous distention

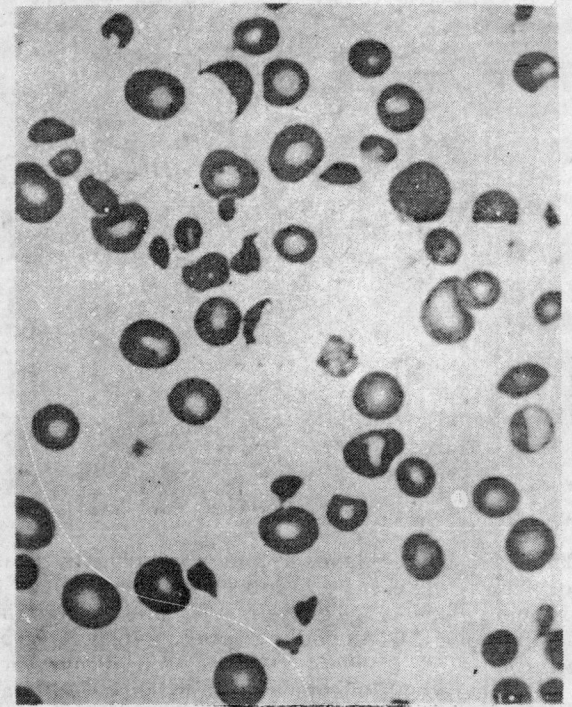

Figure 16–13   Red blood cell smear showing fragmented, anisocytotic, and helmet-shaped cells. (× 1000.)

may develop. The urine may appear dark yellow or brownish red. In mild cases the acute phase lasts 1–2 wk, followed by gradual improvement for 1–2 mo. In severe cases oligoanuria may last several wk or longer, with recovery of renal function still possible. The course is progressive in some patients, in whom chronic renal disease, hypertension, or end-stage renal disease may develop. Occasionally, renal failure follows a temporary clinical remission. Episodes of the syndrome have been reported to recur over periods of many yr.

Laboratory Data.   A severe hemolytic anemia with hemoglobin levels of 5–7 gm/dl is common. The red cells have the features of fragmentation hemolysis: anisocytosis and fragmented, helmet-shaped, and burr cells (Fig 16–13). The reticulocyte count is elevated. The platelet count may initially be normal but within the 1st wk almost always falls to a level below 100,000/mm³; the level may become supranormal later. There is no consistent change in the white blood cell count or differential, but counts of 15,000–20,000/mm³ with a predominance of polymorphonuclear leukocytes are not uncommon. The serum cholesterol, triglyceride, and phospholipid concentrations are elevated, and the serum albumin level is often decreased. The serum C3 is usually normal, but total hemolytic complement may be decreased early in the course. The serum sodium level is usually normal unless there has been fluid overload. Azotemia and the electrolyte and acid-base disturbances of acute renal failure may develop; an unexplained significant hypokalemia is sometimes seen, which is a paradoxical finding in patients with acute renal failure and hemolysis. Uric acid concentration and

serum LDH activity are high. The urine sediment reflects active glomerular damage; microscopic or gross hematuria and red blood cell or granular casts, usually with proteinuria, are present.

Diagnosis and Differential Diagnosis.   The triad of severe microangiopathic hemolytic anemia, nephropathy, and thrombocytopenia of sudden onset following an acute illness in a previously healthy child permits a diagnosis of the hemolytic-uremic syndrome. Renal biopsy may show the characteristic arteriolar or glomerular endothelial and subendothelial changes, indicate the extent and severity of the nephropathy, and exclude other disorders which must be considered in the differential diagnosis. Inciting or predisposing factors such as longstanding hypertension, oral contraceptive use, or pregnancy are not present in children, although familial or hereditary factors are recognized in a small minority of cases.

Other forms of acute hemolytic anemia, such as those of immune pathogenesis or those due to an intrinsic red cell enzyme defect, may initially resemble the hemolytic-uremic syndrome and cause dark urine and minor abnormalities in the urinary sediment. Thrombocytopenia, nephropathy, and hemolytic anemia may occur in active systemic lupus erythematosus. The anemia in this disease is not usually microangiopathic, however, and is often Coombs positive. Patients with systemic lupus erythematosus are also usually older, and other manifestations of the disease are commonly present. (See Sec 16.40 for differentiation of other glomerular or interstitial disorders leading to acute renal failure.)

Treatment.   Generally, therapeutic measures should address the complications of renal failure and the hematologic manifestations. The most frequently encountered renal problems are oligoanuria, electrolyte disorders, acidosis, hypertension, and fluid overload. Their treatment is discussed in Sec 16.17 and 16.40. If anemia is severe (hemoglobin concentration 5 gm/dl or less), transfusion with fresh, washed, packed red blood cells will be necessary, but because of hypertension and circulatory congestion the added load of a blood transfusion may be disastrous if caution is not exercised. The transfusion should be given slowly, and the hemoglobin concentration should not be raised above 7–8 gm/dl. Early and repeated peritoneal dialysis in severe cases has reduced mortality. Hemodialysis may be valuable if severe renal failure persists. Either form of dialysis should be combined with early institution of a high quality diet given either by nasogastric tube or intravenously. Transfusions with fresh frozen plasma or exchange transfusion with plasma appears to benefit some patients. Anticoagulation drugs, antiplatelet agents, corticosteroids, immunosuppressive agents, and fibrinolytic drugs are not of benefit and are not recommended. Bleeding from thrombocytopenia may require platelet transfusions. The goal of therapy is to provide adequate time for spontaneous recovery of renal function and resolution of the microangiopathy. If terminal renal failure develops, consideration must be given to institution of chronic dialysis with a view to eventual renal transplantation.

Prognosis.   The prognosis has improved dramatically in recent years; as many as 90% of patients now survive the acute phase. Unfortunately, the prognosis is poor in familial cases in which the onset of the syndrome occurs more than 1 yr apart in siblings. In these the case fatality rate is about 70%; the overall rate for patients with recurrent episodes is 30%. Recurrences have also been described after renal transplantation. The long-term prognosis varies from 1 series to another but in most is not unfavorable. Hypertension, proteinuria, and mild azotemia, the main sequelae, persist in about 15% of patients, and about 10% develop end-stage renal disease. The prognosis is worse in children over 4 yr of age and in adults, probably because of an increased incidence of the form which predominantly affects the renal arteries.

de Chadarevian J-P, Kaplan BS: The hemolytic uremic syndrome of childhood. In: Rosenberg H, Bolande R (eds): Perspectives in Pediatric Pathology. Vol 4. Chicago, Year Book Medical Publishers, 1978.

Habib R, Levy M, Gagnadoux M-F, et al: Prognosis of the hemolytic uremic syndrome in children. In: Advances in Nephrology, Vol 11. Year Book Medical Publishers, 1982, pp 99–128.

Kaplan BS, Chesney RW, Drummond KN: Hemolytic uremic syndrome in families. N Engl J Med 292:1090, 1975.

Kaplan BS, Drummond KN: The hemolytic uremic syndrome is a syndrome. N Engl J Med 298:964, 1978.

Kaplan BS, Fong JSC: Reduced platelet aggregation in hemolytic-uremic syndrome. Thromb Haemostasis 43:154, 1980.

Levy M, Gagnadoux M-F, Habib R: Pathology of hemolytic-uremic syndrome in children. In: Remuzzi G, Mecca G, de Gaetano G (eds): Hemostasis, Prostaglandins, and Renal Disease. New York, Raven Press, 1980.

Remuzzi G, Misiani R, Marchesi D, et al: Treatment of the hemolytic uremic syndrome with plasma. Clin Nephrol 12:279, 1979.

Thoenes W, John HD: Endotheliotropic (hemolytic) nephroangiopathy and its various manifestation forms (thrombotic microangiopathy, primary malignant nephrosclerosis, hemolytic-uremic syndrome). Klin Wochenschr 58:173, 1980.

Upadhyaya K, Barwick K, Fishaut M, et al: The importance of nonrenal involvement in hemolytic-uremic syndrome. Pediatrics 65:115, 1980.

DIFFUSE CRESCENTIC GLOMERULONEPHRITIS
(Endo- and Extracapillary Proliferative Glomerulonephritis, Rapidly Progressive Glomerulonephritis)

This clinicopathologic entity includes a group of unrelated disorders characterized pathologically by involvement of a majority of glomeruli in extensive epithelial crescent formation leading to obliteration of Bowman space, with changes within the glomerular tuft that depend on the nature of the underlying disease. Clinically, there is a nephritic-nephrotic picture, with oliguria, azotemia, and progression to renal failure over a period of a few wk to several mo in the majority of cases. Immunofluorescence microscopy usually reveals fibrin deposition between the proliferating cells of the epithelial crescent and either discrete deposits containing complement components and IgG, suggestive of immune complex injury, or linear deposition of IgG along the glomerular basement membrane, indicating deposition of antibodies to it.

The condition is *primary* or idiopathic when no systemic disorder is detected, secondary when it occurs in conjunction with a recognized systemic disease.

Patients with acute poststreptococcal glomerulonephritis, membranoproliferative glomerulonephritis, antibodies to glomerular basement membrane but without pulmonary hemorrhage, and circulating immune complexes are included in the primary group.

The secondary group includes patients with Goodpasture disease, Schönlein-Henoch nephritis, polyarteritis nodosa, Wegener granulomatosis, mixed cryoglobulinemia, systemic lupus erythematosus, and chronic systemic infection such as subacute bacterial endocarditis.

It is important to recognize crescentic nephritis as early as possible because, regardless of its cause, the potential for progression to end-stage renal disease is high; if therapy is available for an underlying condition, it should be initiated as soon as possible. Current therapies include a combination of corticosteroids and cytotoxic drugs such as azathioprine or cyclophosphamide, anticoagulants, dipyridamole, and plasmapheresis.

McKenzie PE, Taylor AE, Woodroffe AJ, et al: Plasmapheresis in glomerulonephritis. Clin Nephr 12:97, 1979.

16.23 Tubular Disorders

Disorders of renal tubular function include a variety of conditions in which 1 or more specific tubular functions are impaired without overall decrease in renal function or reduction in glomerular filtration rate. Many of these disorders are hereditary and involve (1) a primary defect in a transport mechanism for reabsorption of 1 or more specific solutes from the glomerular filtrate, e.g., cystinuria and renal glycosuria; (2) inability of the tubular cell to respond to normal hormonal stimuli, e.g., pseudohypoparathyroidism and nephrogenic diabetes insipidus; or (3) inability to develop or maintain the electrical or chemical gradients that permit certain specific physiologic tubular functions to be performed, e.g., distal renal tubular acidosis.

Some tubular disorders are secondary or acquired; such tubular dysfunction might occur (1) during the course of a systemic disease, usually metabolic in nature, in which deposition of a metabolic product in the tubules, e.g., cystine crystals in cystinosis, occurs or a circulating metabolite has a toxic effect on the tubule, e.g., fructose-1-phosphate in hereditary fructose intolerance; or (2) as a consequence of an exogenous drug or toxin, e.g., distal renal tubular acidosis from amphotericin B or generalized proximal tubular dysfunction from lead poisoning.

In some conditions, though only tubular function may be affected initially, subsequent interstitial or glomerular damage leads to reduction in glomerular filtration rate; e.g., nephrocalcinosis and interstitial scarring may develop in distal renal acidosis and lead to chronic renal failure; or cystine stones may form in cystinuria and result in obstructive renal damage and increased susceptibility to pyelonephritis.

Hereditary conditions in which tubular dysfunction is present either as a primary or secondary event are listed in Table 16–8 in Sec 16.30.

16.24 RENAL TUBULAR ACIDOSIS

Renal tubular acidosis (RTA) is a clinical syndrome of sustained metabolic acidosis with hyperchloremia and a normal anion gap without significant reduction in the glomerular filtration rate. It results from impaired ability of the kidney to maintain plasma HCO_3^- levels within the normal range because of defective acidification of urine or impaired reabsorption of bicarbonate. The urine pH is inappropriately high in relation to the metabolic acidosis; excretion of titratable acid and ammonia is reduced. Two physiologically distinct and some intermediate forms of RTA are recognized; the principal forms are distal RTA (type I, classic type) and proximal RTA (type II).

Table 16–7 lists causes of distal and proximal RTA; it includes hereditary disorders and many of the exogenous toxins or drugs that cause impaired tubular function. Many of the agents that cause proximal RTA may also be responsible for the Fanconi syndrome (Sec 16.25; see also Sec 23.28).

Etiology.   Both distal and proximal RTA occur as

Table 16–7 CAUSES OF RENAL TUBULAR ACIDOSIS

DISTAL TYPE	PROXIMAL TYPE
Primary	*Primary*
Sporadic, with infantile or later onset	Sporadic, with infantile or later onset
Hereditary, with infantile or later onset	Hereditary, with infantile or later onset
Hereditary, associated with nerve deafness	
*Secondary**	*Secondary†*
Amphotericin B	Cystinosis
Hyperimmunoglobulinemia	Galactosemia
Renal transplantation	Heavy metals (lead, cadmium)
Medullary nephrocalcinosis due to hypercalcemia, hyperparathyroidism, vitamin D intoxication, and so on	Hereditary fructose intolerance
	Primary or secondary hyperparathyroidism
Toluene sniffing	Hyperimmunoglobulinemia
Ehlers-Danlos syndrome	Vitamin D deficiency rickets
Obstructive uropathy	Wilson disease
Lithium salts	Lowe syndrome
	Tyrosinosis
	Outdated tetracycline
	Leigh syndrome
	Renal vascular accidents in the newborn period

*Distal renal tubular acidosis has been reported rarely in other conditions; most are listed in the references.

†Many of these disorders are expressed as the Fanconi syndrome of proximal renal tubular dysfunction and are thus associated with generalized aminoaciduria, glycosuria, hyperkaliuria, uricosuria, hypercalciuria, and phosphaturia, in addition to bicarbonaturia.

primary abnormalities in urine acidification and as secondary disorders consequent to systemic disease or intoxication. *Primary distal RTA* may be inherited in an autosomal recessive manner, particularly in the form expressed in childhood, or in an autosomal dominant manner, in which expression is delayed until adulthood, and the incidence is higher in women. Usually, however, the disorder is sporadic and without evidence of hereditary factors.

Proximal RTA also occurs as a primary defect, especially in male infants, but it is more commonly secondary to systemic disorders or toxins and is usually associated with other features of impaired proximal tubular transport.

Pathology.   In *distal RTA,* no specific pathologic lesion has been recognized. Nephrocalcinosis usually develops, particularly in the renal medulla, if adequate control of the acidosis is not achieved. Tubular degeneration and interstitial fibrosis may result from the nephrocalcinosis and from repeated episodes of hypokalemia that often complicate the course. Nephrocalcinosis and nephrolithiasis may predispose to urinary tract infection and to pyelonephritic changes.

In *primary proximal RTA* no specific lesion has been described. Proximal tubular dilatation and the "swan neck deformity" are seen in some children with proximal RTA and other features of impaired proximal tubular transport. In cystinosis, in which proximal RTA and other features of the Fanconi syndrome are present, cystine crystals are present within the interstitium, and tubular damage and interstitial scarring occur; giant cell transformations of the visceral epithelial cells of the glomerulus may occur. Nephrocalcinosis is rarely seen in proximal RTA.

Pathophysiology.   In *distal RTA* the functional defect is an inability to maintain in the distal tubule and collecting duct a steep enough H^+ gradient to permit, by excretion of titratable acid and ammonium chloride, regeneration of the HCO_3^- essential for buffering nonvolatile acids formed in normal metabolic activity. Consequently, the plasma HCO_3 level remains below normal. The fixed acids are excreted as sodium salts, and a net sodium deficit results, to which the physiologic response is secondary hyperaldosteronism. This accentuates reabsorption of sodium and chloride and loss of potassium, especially in the distal tubule; the result is a negative potassium balance, with hypokalemia. The decreased plasma HCO_3^- concentration is accompanied by a corresponding elevation in chloride concentration. Bone buffers, particularly calcium carbonate, modify the severity of the systemic acidosis, but, as a consequence, excessive amounts of calcium salts appear in the urine. Because of the relatively high urine pH and the low urinary excretion of citrate consequent to the systemic acidosis, the calcium salts precipitate in the urine and are deposited as nephrocalcinosis or -lithiasis. The ensuing interstitial medullary damage may interfere with the normal countercurrent multiplier and exchange systems by which the kidney concentrates urine. This situation is aggravated by tubular and interstitial damage caused by episodic or sustained hypokalemia. The result is impaired concentrating ability and polyuria. A fall in glomerular filtration rate sometimes develops; in concert with the bone changes induced by systemic acidosis, this may lead to osteomalacia or rickets.

In most patients with distal RTA the amount of HCO_3^- lost in the urine is less than 3% of the filtered load. This persistent slight bicarbonaturia and the inability to maintain a sufficient lumen-to-plasma H^+ gradient result in inability to reduce urine pH below 6.0 even in the face of severe acidosis. Some children also have a significant reduction in the capacity to reabsorb HCO_3^-, and bicarbonaturia may equal 5–10% of the amount filtered; in this situation HCO_3^- loss may be quantitatively more important in the pathogenesis of acidosis than impaired excretion of acid.

In *proximal RTA* the defect is reduced proximal tubular reabsorption of HCO_3^- due to a decreased Tm HCO_3^-; at normal plasma HCO_3^- levels, over 15% of filtered HCO_3^- is spilled into the urine. Bicarbonaturia also occurs when mild acidosis is present (HCO_3^- levels of 16–22 mEq/l). Below this level sufficient H^+ can be secreted by the proximal tubule to permit reabsorption of most of the filtered HCO_3^-. At this point bicarbonaturia ceases and, since distal tubular function is intact, generation of a normal H^+ gradient with a urine pH under 5.5 occurs, with normal net acid excretion as titratable acid and ammonium chloride. Proximal RTA usually occurs as part of a more complex abnormality in the proximal tubules known as the Fanconi syndrome, which is discussed later.

Potassium loss in proximal RTA, whether or not it is associated with the Fanconi syndrome, results in part from impaired proximal tubular K^+ reabsorption. In addition, the increased amount of HCO_3^- reaching the distal tubule enhances passive K^+ secretion into the lumen at this site. Morever, raising the serum HCO_3^- level by alkali therapy further increases the amount of HCO_3^- reaching the distal tubule and augments K^+ secretion. By contrast, in distal RTA, proximal HCO_3^- reabsorption is usually normal at physiologic levels of plasma HCO_3^- and a significant increment in K^+ loss consequent to therapy is not observed. In fact, many patients with distal RTA do not require potassium supplements to maintain normal serum K^+ levels, provided sustained correction of the metabolic acidosis is achieved. The hypokalemia in either proximal or distal RTA may have profound physiologic consequences. These include impairment in urine concentrating ability, muscle paralysis, and predisposition to tetany during correction of acidosis.

Hypercalciuria and resultant hypocalcemia may also occur in proximal RTA, and secondary hyperparathyroidism induced by the hypocalcemia may magnify the defects in proximal tubular transport. Correction of hypocalcemia may be important to the therapy of proximal RTA in decreasing the secretion of parathyroid hormone.

Incomplete or partial forms of RTA have been described in adults. Such patients are clinically well but, when stressed by ammonium chloride loading, do not develop an appropriately acid urine and may become acidotic. It is not established whether these patients represent examples of the heterozygote state of distal RTA.

Hyperchloremic acidosis occurs in patients with congenital or acquired deficiency in secretion of aldosterone; the pathogenesis is poorly understood. There is evidence that a proximal type of RTA reversible by mineralocorticoid administration is present in some of these patients.

Clinical Manifestations and Course. The clinical features of renal tubular acidosis reflect the associated electrolyte and fluid disturbances and, in the case of proximal RTA, abnormalities due to other defects of proximal tubular function, of which RTA may be but 1 manifestation. In systemic or toxic conditions that may cause either proximal or distal RTA the features of the underlying disorder may overshadow those due only to RTA.

The age at onset of RTA is variable. In infants with the inherited form of *distal RTA* the acidifying defect is usually present at birth, but the correct diagnosis is often not made until months or years later. Failure to thrive and polyuria may date from early infancy. Some patients with what appears to be distal RTA in infancy apparently recover spontaneously, but most do not, and alkali therapy is required throughout life. In some patients with inherited distal RTA the onset is delayed until the 3rd–4th decade. Some have nerve deafness, and a few have heterochromia iridis.

Primary proximal RTA, unassociated with the Fanconi syndrome of proximal tubular dysfunction, is more common in boys. The clinical onset occurs usually in the 1st 18 mo; growth failure and vomiting in early infancy are characteristic. In many patients the defect in HCO_3^- reabsorption is temporary; after a number of months therapy can be stopped without relapse.

In children RTA is characterized by growth failure and tachypnea due to hyperchloremic metabolic acidosis, with thirst, polyuria, and osteomalacia. Dehydration, vomiting, episodic fever, nephrolithiasis secondary to hypercalciuria, muscle weakness or paralysis due to hypokalemia, and episodes of severe, life-threatening acidemia, sometimes triggered by an intercurrent illness, are also seen. Tetany, muscle cramps, and even seizures during correction of acidosis may be prominent features in patients with hypocalcemia or hypokalemia. Recurrent urinary infections may be a problem when nephrolithiasis is present.

Correction of acidosis by alkali therapy with or without K^+ supplementation leads to dramatic improvement in the clinical condition, and normal growth resumes. If muscle weakness and polyuria secondary to hypokalemia are present, these are also ameliorated. In patients with distal RTA it is not uncommon for impaired ability to concentrate urine to persist because of permanent damage by nephrocalcinosis and episodes of hypokalemia.

Laboratory Data. The cardinal features of *distal RTA* are sustained metabolic acidosis with hypocarbia and hyperchloremia, with an inappropriately alkaline urine (pH 6.0 or higher). Infrequently, the urine pH may be as low as 5.5. Decreased serum pH may also be present. Hypokalemia, excessive excretion of potassium in the urine, hypercalciuria (over 4 mg/kg/24 hr), and hypocalcemia may be present. In the face of this sustained metabolic acidosis, the net acid excretion (urinary titratable acid, plus ammonia, minus bicarbonate) is decreased. Aminoaciduria, phosphaturia, and glucosuria are absent. The plasma level at which bicarbonate spills into the urine is usually normal (23–25 mEq/l), but some patients with distal RTA have a reduced HCO_3^- threshold. The ability to concentrate urine is often impaired; maximal values of 300–500 mOsm/l after overnight fasting are the rule. Roentgenograms may reveal medullary nephrocalcinosis and decreased bone density. Determination of the difference between the blood and urine pCO_2 following $NaHCO_3$ loading has been used as a means of differentiating patients with distal RTA from normal subjects. Normal values are above 32 mm Hg, whereas in patients with distal RTA the values range from 0–12 mm Hg.

Also in *proximal RTA*, systemic acidosis with hyperchloremia occurs. In contrast to distal RTA the urine may be acid if the plasma HCO_3^- level is sufficiently low for complete reabsorption of HCO_3^-. The urine pH will be above 6.0 because of bicarbonaturia when plasma levels are above the HCO_3^- threshold (usually 17–20 mEq/l in these patients); the pH will be appropriately acid with a normal net acid excretion when the plasma HCO_3^- level is below the threshold value. Urinary loss of K^+ is excessive and tends to increase as the plasma HCO_3^- level rises. Impaired ability to concentrate urine is a less prominent feature than in distal RTA; it may, however, occur because of tubular damage in some of the disorders with which proximal RTA may be associated and because of hypokalemia. If proximal RTA is associated with the Fanconi syndrome, laboratory features of this condition will also be present (see below).

Diagnosis and Differential Diagnosis. The diagnosis of *distal RTA* can be established by the finding of an inappropriately alkaline urine (pH >6.0) with a sustained metabolic acidosis without evidence of significantly reduced renal function, i.e., without significant elevation of blood urea nitrogen or serum creatinine. Associated clinical and laboratory features, as described earlier, are usually present. In most instances it is not necessary to perform an ammonium chloride loading test to determine maximal urine acidification; acidosis is already present, and the procedure has some risk under these circumstances.

The diagnosis of *proximal RTA* depends on the finding of both a sustained metabolic acidosis and a lowered tubular threshold for HCO_3^-. The urine pH may be appropriately acid (pH <5.5) when the plasma HCO_3^- is very low, but an alkaline urine (pH >6.0) is found when the plasma HCO_3^- is above the patient's threshold value, yet still in a range below the normal level at which bicarbonaturia appears (24–26 mEq/l). This may be verified by measurement of the HCO_3^- threshold by sodium bicarbonate infusion or by giving sufficient alkali orally to maintain the serum HCO_3^- level at 20–22 mEq/l, at which level, despite mild metabolic acidosis, the urine pH is inappropriately alkaline and net acid excretion is reduced. Other characteristic laboratory and clinical findings may provide supportive evidence.

In addition to establishing the diagnosis of either proximal or distal RTA or 1 of their variants, it is necessary to determine whether any of the known predisposing causes of RTA, as listed in Table 16–7, are present. Appropriate historic, clinical, and laboratory features of each of these conditions should be sought.

Specific conditions which may cause some of the clinical and laboratory features of RTA include severe diarrhea, small bowel fistula, ingestion of acidifying salts or of the carbonic anhydrase inhibitor acetazolamide, saline infusion, ureterosigmoidostomy, diabetes insipidus, respiratory alkalosis, lactic acidosis, acidosis of prematurity, chronic renal failure, and other disorders of metabolism that lead to metabolic acidosis.

Prevention. Except in well-documented kindreds in which genetic counseling may be of value, primary inherited RTA cannot be prevented. In many of the conditions known to be associated with RTA of either proximal or distal type, avoidance of toxic doses of drugs or awareness of the possibility that RTA may develop can permit either prevention or early diagnosis.

Treatment. In both distal and proximal RTA the central goal of therapy is to provide sufficient alkali to maintain the plasma HCO_3^- level within the normal range and to correct associated electrolyte disorders, notably hypokalemia. In distal RTA this usually requires administration of sodium bicarbonate ($NaHCO_3$), 1–3 mEq/kg/24 hr in 4 divided doses. The amount required in proximal RTA is much higher, usually 5–15 mEq/kg/24 hr, and more frequent administration may be required. The amount of potassium required is variable; an initial supplement of 2 mEq/kg/24 hr as potassium chloride should be given, but children with proximal RTA may require 4–10 mEq/kg/24 hr to maintain the serum K^+ within the normal range. Alkali may also be given in the form of sodium and potassium citrates, as Scholl solution (140 gm citric acid and 90 gm hydrated crystalline salt of sodium citrate in 1 liter of water) or as Polycitra,* either of which is slightly more palatable than sodium bicarbonate or potassium chloride. A mixture of 10% each of sodium and potassium citrate in a sweet syrup provides 1 mEq/ml each of Na^+ and K^+ and the equivalent of 2 mEq of HCO_3^-/ml.

Oral therapy will not suffice in an acutely ill, severely acidotic, dehydrated child. A reasonable solution for intravenous administration consists of sodium bicarbonate in a concentration of 60–100 mEq/l with potassium chloride in a concentration of 40–60 mEq/l. The amount given should be calculated to correct the base deficit, i.e., to raise the plasma HCO_3^- level to normal over a period of 12–24 hr. If the plasma H^+ concentration is elevated (i.e., the pH is decreased), more HCO_3^- than calculated to raise the plasma level to normal will be necessary. Care should be taken to avoid tetany, muscle cramps, and seizures, which are likely to develop if the acidosis is corrected too rapidly, especially if hypocalcemia, hypokalemia, or both are present. Administration of calcium gluconate in a dose calculated to give about 15 mg/kg of calcium over 1–2 hr via a separate intravenous route may be used to prevent or treat hypocalcemia. Water intake as high as 2–5 l/M²/24 hr may be necessary because of impaired ability to concentrate urine.

It is important to establish whether RTA is temporary or permanent and to exclude or treat any underlying

---

*Polycitra, Willen Drug Company, Baltimore, Md.

cause. Continuous administration of alkali and potassium supplements and careful surveillance over a lifetime may be required, with periodic evaluation of plasma electrolyte and acid-base status; urinary calcium excretion may also be a useful guide since hypercalciuria ceases when good control is achieved. The usual vitamin supplements are necessary.

Prognosis. The prognosis of primary distal RTA is excellent if therapy is begun early and the serum HCO_3^- level and other electrolytes are maintained within the normal range. If the diagnosis is not made until renal damage secondary to hypokalemia or nephrocalcinosis has developed, some residual functional damage may persist. Even under these circumstances proper therapy may permit normal life expectancy. A small percentage of infants with primary distal RTA recover spontaneously and require no further therapy. The prognosis in children with primary proximal RTA is less well established, but some appear to recover spontaneously over a period of 4–12 mo. Control of the acid-base and electrolyte status is not as easy in proximal RTA, and return to completely normal growth and health is less common.

In both proximal and distal RTA the presence of an underlying systemic or toxic condition is of fundamental importance in the ultimate prognosis.

Brenes LG, Brenes JN, Hernandez MM: Familial proximal renal tubular acidosis: A distinct clinical entity. Am J Med 63:244, 1977.
Halperin ML: Pathogenesis of type I (distal) renal tubular acidosis: Re-evaluation of the diagnostic criteria. Ann R Coll Phys Surg Can 7:103, 1974.
Hutcheon RA, Kaplan BS, Drummond KN: Distal renal tubular acidosis in children with chronic hydronephrosis. J Pediatr 89:372, 1976.
Nance WE, Sweeney A: Evidence for autosomal recessive inheritance of the syndrome of renal tubular acidosis with deafness. Birth Defects 7:70, 1971.
Perez GO, Oster JR, Vaamond CA: Incomplete syndrome of renal tubular acidosis induced by lithium carbonate. J Lab Clin Med 80:386, 1975.
Sebastian A, Morris RC Jr: Renal tubular acidosis. Clin Nephrol 7:216, 1977.
Stanbury JB, Wyngaarden JB, Frederickson DS: The Metabolic Basis of Inherited Disease. Ed 4. New York, McGraw-Hill, 1978.
Stark H, Geiger R: Renal tubular dysfunction following vascular accidents of the kidneys in the newborn period. J Pediatr 83:933, 1973.

16.25 FANCONI SYNDROME

The principal features of this syndrome are osteomalacia or rickets, growth retardation, proximal renal tubular acidosis with bicarbonaturia, glycosuria without hyperglycemia, phosphaturia with hypophosphatemia, generalized aminoaciduria in the absence of elevated plasma levels of amino acids, tubular proteinuria, ketonuria, excessive urinary excretion of sodium and potassium, hypokalemia, hypouricemia, variable hypercalciuria, and an impaired ability to concentrate the urine which may lead to polyuria. In patients with cystinosis, a glomerular lesion may develop and possibly proteinuria in excess of 1 g/24 hr. In this situation the protein excreted by glomeruli is the same as in other forms of glomerular injury. These findings vary in severity from patient to patient but have a common pathogenesis: a complex proximal tubular dysfunction. Depending on which transport mechanisms are principally affected, different substances appear in urine because of failure of reabsorption from the tubular lumen.

See also Sec 23.28 (Fanconi syndrome) and Sec 8.5 and 23.29 (cystinosis).

16.26 NEPHROGENIC DIABETES INSIPIDUS

In this congenital hereditary disorder the kidneys do not respond to antidiuretic hormone (vasopressin) Consequently, the urine volume is high, and its concentration is persistently hypotonic. (See also Sec 5.15.) The term nephrogenic distinguishes this condition from diabetes insipidus, which results from insufficient antidiuretic hormone production and in which the kidney is able to concentrate urine when vasopressin is administered.

In North America most affected patients are descended from Ulster Scots who reached Nova Scotia on the ship Hopewell in 1761. Clusters of affected patients are found in areas of New England and the Maritime Provinces.

Etiology. Nephrogenic diabetes insipidus occurs principally in males, probably with X-linked recessive inheritance; the degree varies in heterozygous females.

Pathology and Pathophysiology. The condition is clearly of renal origin; the neurohypophyseal system by which vasopressin is released in response to increased plasma tonicity is intact. There is no evidence that an abnormal type of vasopressin is released or that the hormone is inactivated. Unresponsiveness of the distal tubule and collecting duct to vasopressin is believed to be the primary defect. No consistent renal pathologic changes have been demonstrated; the disorder is probably due to an enzymatic or biochemical abnormality in renal tubular function.

Vasopressin normally increases the permeability of the distal tubule and collecting duct to water and thus allows passive diffusion of luminal water into the hypertonic medullary interstitium. This increase in permeability to water is mediated by cyclic adenosine-3',5'-monophosphate (3'5'-AMP). Production of this cyclic nucleotide from adenosine triphosphate (ATP) is catalyzed by adenyl cyclase in the distal tubule and collecting duct cells under the stimulus of vasopressin. In nephrogenic diabetes insipidus there is apparently failure to bind vasopressin at some receptor site or defective adenyl cyclase activity. Prostaglandins of the E series inhibit the vasopressin stimulation of adenyl cyclase and thus inhibit water reabsorption. Inhibition of prostaglandin synthetase by agents such as indomethacin leads to an increased capacity to form concentrated urine in patients with nephrogenic diabetes insipidus.

Permeability of the distal tubule and collecting ducts to water is reduced, and its diffusion from the lumen into the hypertonic interstitium is restricted. Since sodium and chloride transport from the ascending limb of Henle loop and distal tubule is intact, the urine is hypotonic to plasma regardless of the body's need to conserve water. When the capacity to concentrate the urine is thus impaired and maximal urine osmolality is

80–150 mOsm/kg H_2O, a greater urine volume is required to excrete a given solute load than would be the case if the urine osmolality were high, e.g., 800–1200 mOsm/kg H_2O. At the lower range of urine concentration, e.g., 100 mOsm/l, the volume of urine in which 1 mOsm is excreted is 10 ml, whereas at a urine concentration of 1000 mOsm/l the volume of urine is only 1 ml/mOsm. Thus the solute load is of great importance in determining the requisite volume of urine in a patient with an impaired ability to concentrate the urine. If the fluid intake needed to produce the required volume of urine is not provided, plasma solute concentration (e.g., sodium, chloride, and urea concentrations) will rise. Furthermore, given inadequate fluid intake in the face of a high obligatory water loss, the patient's total body water decreases and dehydration results. This may lead to a fall in glomerular filtration rate causing a decreased flow rate through the nephron. In some patients with nephrogenic diabetes insipidus this appears to give adequate time for some degree of urine concentration, and urine osmolality may be slightly higher than plasma in this circumstance.

Clinical Manifestations and Course. Nephrogenic diabetes insipidus is present at birth, though the diagnosis is frequently not made for several mo. Frequent urination of a large volume of dilute urine, extreme thirst, repeated episodes of dehydration, and failure to thrive are the common initial manifestations. Loss of skin turgor, constipation, vomiting, unexplained fever, and even convulsions may occur. Growth retardation results from inadequate food intake because of uncontrolled polydipsia and from general poor health because of dehydration and hypernatremia. These features may impair mental and motor development; the severity of retardation is least when the diagnosis is made and therapy begun early. Children old enough to express their needs have an insatiable thirst. Because of the large urinary volume, which may reach 6–10 l/M^2/24 hr, there may be dilatation of the renal collecting system and ureters and of the bladder.

Diagnosis and Differential Diagnosis. The clinical and laboratory features described above lead to the suspicion of nephrogenic diabetes insipidus. The initial clue is often repeated episodes of unexplained fever. A family history of a similar disorder in males provides supportive evidence.

The failure of the adequately hydrated subject to increase urine osmolality in response to administration of vasopressin differentiates nephrogenic diabetes insipidus from diabetes insipidus due to inadequacy of the posterior pituitary. Nephrogenic diabetes insipidus may be suspected when there is persistently hypotonic urine (specific gravity, 1.002–1.006; osmolality, 80–120/mOsm/kg H_2O) in the face of clinical dehydration or an elevated serum sodium concentration or osmolality. The serum chloride concentration is often elevated during periods of dehydration and sometimes the sweat chloride concentration as well. Hyperuricemia may occur in adults with nephrogenic diabetes insipidus.

Hyposthenuria and failure of the kidney to respond normally to vasopressin may be seen in other conditions; these, however, usually have characteristic features which should preclude errors in diagnosis. They include hypercalcemia, hypokalemia, distal renal tubular acidosis with nephrocalcinosis, cystinosis, obstructive uropathy, sickle cell nephropathy, nephronophthisis, uremia, the diuretic phase of recovery from acute renal tubular injury, amyloidosis, and administration of lithium salts. In patients with *psychogenic polydipsia* a poor response to vasopressin may be manifest; this is transient, however, and a normal response can be elicited after several wk of a normal fluid intake. Polyuria due to diabetes mellitus should be excluded.

Prevention. No means of prevention is known, but genetic counseling may be of value. Mothers and half of the sisters of affected males are carriers of the gene; the risk is 1 in 2 that their male children will be affected and their female children will be carriers. A decreased ability to concentrate the urine has been described in women presumed to be carriers, but overt clinical manifestations are mild or absent.

Treatment. The cornerstone of therapy is the provision of sufficient intake of water to prevent dehydration and to maintain serum osmolality, as expressed by the serum sodium concentration, within normal limits. The fluid intake required may reach 6–10 l/M^2/24 hr. Proper nutrition and caloric intake must also be maintained.

An obligatory urine volume of 8–12 ml is required to excrete each mOsm of solute; accordingly, fluid requirements can be reduced if solute load is decreased. Such a decrease requires a greater than usual proportion of dietary calories in the form of carbohydrate and fat, which are metabolized to carbon dioxide and water and do not contribute to the solute load. The intake of protein, salt, and foods containing phosphorus should be reduced.

Hydrochlorothiazide and other diuretics which lead to a negative sodium balance when used in combination with a reduced sodium intake have an important role in therapy. They lead to a reduction in urinary volume and to a modest increase in urinary concentration. The action of these saluretic drugs in this disease is not fully understood. The response results in part from the state of sodium depletion they induce, which in turn leads to reabsorption of a greater than normal proportion of filtered sodium and water in the proximal tubule. This alone reduces urine volume; in addition, less filtrate is delivered to the ascending limb of Henle loop and the distal tubule, where urine dilution occurs. A trial of hydrochlorothiazide in a dose of 0.5–1.5 mg/kg/24 hr in combination with a sodium intake of less than 1 mEq/kg/24 hr is warranted; reduction of urinary volume of 40–50% may be achieved. Hydrochlorothiazide may produce hypokalemia, and potassium supplements of 2–4 mEq/kg/24 hr may be required. Addition of indomethacin, 1–2 mg/kg/24 hr, has been very effective in some patients. Chlorpropamide is not useful in nephrogenic diabetes insipidus.

Prognosis. With early diagnosis and maintenance of adequate therapy, prognosis for life and for normal development is good. The problem of ensuring adequate hydration will be lifelong.

Blachar Y, Zakik Z, Shemesh M, et al.: The effect of inhibition of prostaglandin synthesis on free water and osmolar clearances in patients with hereditary nephrogenic diabetes insipidus. Int J Pediatr Nephrol 1:48, 1980.

Bode HH, Crawford JD: Nephrogenic diabetes insipidus in North America—the Hopewell hypothesis. N Engl J Med 280:750, 1969.

McConnell RF Jr, Lorentz WB Jr, Berger M, et al: The mechanism of urinary concentration in nephrogenic diabetes insipidus. Pediatr Res 11:33, 1977.

ten Bensel RW, Peters ER: Progressive hydronephrosis, hydroureter, and dilatation of the bladder in siblings with congenital nephrogenic diabetes insipidus. J Pediatr 77:439, 1970.

Ziegler EE, Fomon SJ: Fluid intake, renal solute load and water balance in infancy. J Pediatr 78:561, 1971.

16.27 RENAL GLYCOSURIA
(Renal Glucosuria)

With this hereditary defect in tubular glucose transport, glucose is excreted in the urine even though the blood glucose level is normal. Glucosuria resulting from impaired glucose reabsorption may also occur in the Fanconi syndrome, but the term renal glycosuria denotes the tubular abnormality in which only glucose transport is affected. The amount of glucose excreted is variable and in children may range from 1–30 gm/24 hr. The degree of glycosuria is generally independent of the diet, though the amount of glucose excreted may increase if excessive carbohydrate is ingested. Usually, all urine specimens contain glucose. The urinary loss of glucose has little effect on blood glucose concentration, and the glucose tolerance curve is either normal or flat. There is no generalized defect in glucose metabolism.

Renal glycosuria is usually detected in the 2nd decade, though it is probably present from birth. It is benign and symptomless, except that ketosis and dehydration may develop during periods of low dietary intake or during pregnancy and especially with vomiting or diarrhea. There is no association with diabetes mellitus. Renal glycosuria may be diagnosed by the consistent finding of glucosuria in conjunction with normal or slightly low concentrations of blood glucose; other features of abnormal glucose metabolism are absent. Disorders in which other sugars or reducing substances appear in the urine should be excluded by appropriate chemical tests; these include pentosuria, fructosuria, galactosuria, sucrosuria, and maltosuria.

The phenotypic expression of renal glycosuria may result from a number of different mutations. One classification proposes 2 principal forms: types A and B. In type A the defect in glucose reabsorption is diffuse, involving all nephrons, with uniformly reduced glucose Tm. In type B a variable glycosuria occurs over a range of blood sugar concentrations, but the overall glucose Tm is normal; distinct groups of nephrons appear to differ in their capacity to reabsorb glucose. Both types have been described in the same family.

In some families the condition is inherited as an autosomal dominant character; in others an autosomal recessive mode is probable.

16.28 CYSTINURIA

This defect of amino acid transport affects cells of the renal tubules and gastrointestinal tract. See also Sec 8.5 and 23.29. The transport defect involves a group of amino acids: cystine, lysine, arginine, ornithine, and cysteine-homocysteine mixed disulfide. The clinical problem arises from the cystine, which is the least soluble of the group and precipitates in the urine to form calculi. Both sexes are affected, but problems tend to be more serious in the male, possibly because of the differences in urinary tract anatomy which result in a greater likelihood of urethral obstruction by calculi. There are 2 types: type I is completely recessive (the heterozygote has a normal pattern of amino acid excretion); type II is incompletely recessive (the heterozygote has increased excretion of cystine and lysine without stone formation).

Although the transport defect is present from birth, the peak age at diagnosis is the 2nd–3rd decade. The usual presentation is that of ureteral colic or obstruction. The latter may lead to urinary infection and reduced renal function. Cystine stones form in acid urine, as do uric acid stones, but, unlike the latter, they are radiopaque. They tend to form in a staghorn pattern and to be recurrent. The simplest diagnostic test is microscopic examination of the urine for the hexagonal, flat cystine crystals. The urine cyanide nitroprusside test is positive; a positive test also is obtained in homocystinuria and acetonuria. Amino acid chromatography is of value in detecting cystine and the other amino acids that are excreted in excessive amounts.

Treatment is based on attempts to increase cystine solubility by keeping the urine dilute and alkaline and by reducing the amount of cystine excretion. At pH 7.5, approximately 300 mg/l of cystine will be in solution. Increasing the urine volume reduces cystine concentration and the likelihood of precipitation. Many cystinuric subjects excrete up to 1 gm/24 hr of cystine and require a urine output of 3–4 l to reduce the likelihood of stone formation. It is important to maintain dilution of the urine during the night as well as during the day; several glasses of water should be taken on retiring. Cystine solubility is highest at a urine pH above 7.5, and alkalinizing agents, such as sodium citrate or bicarbonate, should be given to maintain urine pH at or above this level.

D-Penicillamine leads to production of a mixed disulfide of cysteine-penicillamine which is 50 times as soluble as cystine; its use may lead to a reduction in excretion of free cystine. In patients with recurrent stone formation not controlled by dilution of urine and alkalinization, D-penicillamine may be effective in dissolving stones and in diminishing the threat of progressive renal damage. Undesirable side effects of this drug include allergic reactions and renal damage; it should be used with caution only for patients who fail to respond to conservative therapy.

If recurrent stone formation and urinary tract infection can be avoided, progressive renal damage is unlikely and the prognosis reasonably good.

Crawhall JC, Watts RWE: Cystinuria. Am J Med 45:736, 1968.

Watts RWE: Metabolic causes of renal stone formation. Postgrad Med J Vol 53, Suppl 1, Sec 1, p 7.

16.29 TUBULAR DISORDERS DUE TO ELECTROLYTE DISTURBANCES

The 2 principal electrolyte disturbances that lead to abnormal tubular function are hypercalcemia and hypokalemia.

Hypercalcemia is responsible for impaired sodium transport from the ascending limb of Henle loop and thus causes a disturbance in the medullary countercurrent multiplier system. The renal medulla is less hypertonic than normal; this results in an impaired ability to concentrate the urine. Hypercalcemia may also lead to reduced permeability to water in the distal tubule and collecting duct. The clinical consequences of these disturbances are polyuria and polydipsia. Hypercalcemia may lead also to the development of *nephrocalcinosis*, particularly in the medulla, where interstitial scarring results in destruction of nephrons and reduction in the glomerular filtration rate. It is important to know that significant nephrocalcinosis with impaired renal function may occur with no roentgenographic evidence of calcium deposition in the kidneys.

The causes of hypercalcemia are numerous and are discussed elsewhere. To avoid potentially serious renal consequences of hypercalcemia, therapy should aim at reduction of the serum calcium level to normal as soon as possible.

Potassium depletion leading to hypokalemia is also responsible for impairment of urine concentration. The degree of impairment varies with the duration and severity of the potassium deficit. As in the case of hypercalcemia, reduced concentrating ability is probably due to reduced tubular permeability to water or interference with the countercurrent multiplier and exchange systems.

Structural changes are undoubtedly important in the pathogenesis of the functional changes observed. They consist of vacuolar lesions in the proximal and, sometimes, distal tubules, lamination of the tubular basement membranes, swelling of tubular mitochondria, and increased interstitial collagen in both cortex and medulla. If potassium depletion is not corrected, the nephropathy is progressive, with interstitial nephritis and development of renal insufficiency.

Cremer W, Bock KD: Symptoms and course of chronic hypokalemic nephropathy in man. Clin Nephrol 7:112, 1977.

Other Disorders of Renal Tubular Transport

Besides renal tubular acidosis and nephrogenic diabetes insipidus, there are many other specific disorders of tubular transport affecting a variety of solutes, such as amino acids, sugars, phosphate, calcium, sodium, and potassium. Many are hereditary. Some of these conditions are listed in Tabl 16–7; some are described in Chapter 8.

Scriver CR, Chesney RW, McInnes RR: Genetic aspects of renal tubular transport: Diversity and topology of carriers. Kidney Int 9:149, 1976.

Tubular Damage by Toxins and Drugs

A variety of agents selectively damage the tubules. Tubular necrosis leading to acute renal failure or disturbances in specific areas of tubular function may result. (See Sec 16.53.)

16.30   Hereditary or Familial Diseases

The number of genetically determined conditions known to involve the kidney or urinary tract currently approaches 50. Little is known about the pathogenesis of these conditions, and attempts at pathologic classification leave much to be desired. A proposed grouping of these disorders is given in Table 16–8. The list is incomplete. A discussion of some of the entities follows; some are discussed elsewhere:

Bergsma D (ed): Conference on genetic and cellular bases of congenital renal dysfunction. Birth Defects 6:1, 1970.

Fitch N: Heterogeneity of bilateral renal agenesis. Can Med Assoc J 116:381, 1977.

Frimpter GW: Aminoacidurias due to inherited disorders of metabolism. N Engl J Med 289:835, 895, 1973.

Scriver CR, Chesney RW, McInnes RR: Genetic aspects of renal tubular transport: Diversity and topology of carriers. Kidney Int 9:149, 1976.

Senior B: Familial renal-retinal dystrophy. Am J Dis Child 125:442, 1973.

16.31   HEREDITARY NEPHRITIS WITH DEAFNESS AND OCULAR ABNORMALITIES
(Alport Syndrome)

This hereditary disease is characterized by progressive renal failure of variable severity (usually more severe in males), high-frequency sensorineural deafness, and ocular abnormalities. The disease has a wide geographic distribution and occurs in patients of various ethnic and racial backgrounds. It is the most common of the heritable renal diseases.

Pathology and Pathogenesis.   Glomerular and interstitial lesions develop simultaneously. By light microscopy the early changes may be minimal, consisting of focal and segmental areas of glomerular basement thickening and irregularity, with increased mesangial matrix and cell number. Adhesions to Bowman capsule and occasional epithelial cell proliferation may occur. Dif-

Table 16–8 HEREDITARY CONDITIONS IN WHICH RENAL MANIFESTATIONS ARE USUALLY PRESENT*

1. CONDITIONS IN WHICH ANY OF THE FOLLOWING ARE PRINCIPAL
   MANIFESTATIONS: REDUCED GLOMERULAR FILTRATION RATE, HEMATURIA,
   PROTEINURIA, HYPERTENSION
   Hereditary nephritis with deafness (Alport syndrome)
   Benign familial hematuria
   Nephronophthisis (medullary cystic disease, familial juvenile
     nephronophthisis)
   Childhood (autosomal recessive) type polycystic kidney disease
     with portal dysplasia
   Adult (autosomal dominant) type polycystic kidney disease
   Congenital nephrotic syndrome (Finnish type)
   Familial nephrotic syndrome of the minimal lesion type
   Diffuse mesangial sclerosis of infancy
   Familial renal-retinal dystrophy
   Familial hemolytic-uremic syndrome
   Hereditary thrombocytopenia, deafness, and renal disease

2. DISORDERS IN WHICH A RENAL TUBULAR DEFECT IS OF PRINCIPAL
   IMPORTANCE
   Renal tubular acidosis
   Nephrogenic diabetes insipidus
   Pseudohypoparathyroidism
   Renal glycosuria
   Hypophosphatemic rickets (familial vitamin D–resistant rickets with
     hypophosphatemia)
   Familial iminoglycinuria
   Idiopathic Fanconi syndrome with proximal tubular dysfunction
   Familial hyperglycinuria
   Essential pentosuria
   Hartnup disease
   Liddle syndrome (pseudohyperaldosteronism)
   Pseudohypoaldosteronism
   Cystinuria

3. SYSTEMIC METABOLIC DISORDERS WHICH MAY LEAD TO RENAL DAMAGE
   Cystinosis
   Fabry disease (ceramide trihexosidase deficiency)
   Oxalosis
   Lipodystrophy
   Familial Mediterranean fever with amyloidosis
   Wilson disease
   Glycogen storage disease
   Gout
   Diabetes mellitus
   Tyrosinemia
   Galactosemia
   Xanthinuria
   Hereditary fructose intolerance
   Dihydroxyadeninuria

4. MULTISYSTEM DISORDERS OR SYNDROMES
   Laurence-Moon-Biedl syndrome
   Fanconi syndrome of multiple congenital anomalies and aplastic
     anemia

   Lowe syndrome (oculocerebrorenal syndrome)
   DiGeorge syndrome
   Zellweger syndrome (cerebrohepatorenal syndrome)
   Tuberous sclerosis
   Nail-patella syndrome (hereditary onycho-osteodysplasia)
   Prune-belly syndrome (triad syndrome)
   Oral-facial-digital syndrome
   Meckel syndrome (dysencephalia splanchnocystica syndrome)
   Dandy-Walker malformation of the brain
   Autosomal trisomy syndromes D and E
   Von Hippel–Lindau disease
   Jeune asphyxiating thoracic dystrophy
   Syndrome of hamartomas, nephroblastomatosis, fetal gigantism,
     and hypoglycemia
   Thymic alymphoplasia
   Russell-Silver dwarfism
   Beckwith-Wiedemann syndrome
   Ehlers-Danlos syndrome
   Cockayne syndrome
   Branchio-otorenal dysplasia
   Cerebro-oculofacioskeletal syndrome
   Familial dysautonomia

5. DEVELOPMENTAL STRUCTURAL ABNORMALITIES AND TUMORS OF THE URI-
   NARY TRACT (*hereditary factors are not operative in most renal
   tumors and developmental structural abnormalities of the urinary
   tract*)
   Nephroblastomatosis
   Hypernephroma
   Renal sarcoma
   Unilateral hydronephrosis
   Congenital megaloureter
   Congenital renal and ear abnormalities
   Familial renal agenesis or hypoplasia (bilateral or unilateral)
   Familial renal dysplasia
   Crossed fused renal ectopia
   Familial renal dysplasia with blindness
   Childhood (autosomal recessive) type polycystic kidney disease
     with portal dysplasia
   Adult (autosomal dominant) type polycystic kidney disease
   Leopard syndrome (multiple lentigenes)
   Hemihypertrophy with nephroblastomatosis or Wilms tumor
   Nonobstructive vesicoureteral reflux with renal scarring

6. MISCELLANEOUS
   Familial urolithiasis, with or without hypercalciuria
   Familial vitamin D–dependent rickets (impaired renal 1-hydroxyla-
     tion of 25-hydroxycholecalciferol)
   Sickle cell anemia
   Hyperuricemia, renal insufficency, ataxia, and deafness
   Hereditary deficiency of 1 of the complement components (C1r, C1s
     inhibitor, C4, C7, C2) with glomerulonephritis

*The renal manifestations of the conditions listed in this table are diverse. Included are disorders expressed in a variety of unrelated ways, such as defects in tubular transport, aminoaciduria, structural developmental abnormalities, and diseases of the glomerular basement membrane. In some the renal problem is secondary or of little clinical consequence; in others it is the chief cause of morbidity and/or mortality.

fuse thickening of the glomerular basement membrane ensues, with progressive glomerular sclerosis. Immunopathologic studies show no immunoglobulin or complement deposition. Findings on electron microscopy, though not pathognomonic, are very characteristic. The change is diffuse, affecting most glomerular basement membranes. Initially, there are irregular areas of attenuation and thickening. Where the glomerular basement membrane is thickened, the lamina densa may be split or lamellated, and there are electron-lucent rarefied areas containing round dense granules or particles. The tubular basement membrane may be similarly affected.

Abnormalities in the interstitial tissue include periglomerular fibrosis, a general increase in fibrous tissue, tubular atrophy, and focal mononuclear cell infiltration. Interstitial foam cells are seen in about a third of patients, mainly at the corticomedullary junction. This finding was once considered specific for Alport syndrome but occurs also in other renal disorders.

As the lesions progress, the kidney shrinks, and an end-stage chronic glomerulonephritis results.

Clinical Manifestations and Course. The mean age of onset of renal disease is 6 yr, but it has been noted as early as the 1st few mo of life. Hematuria is the most common manifestation; initially it is microscopic, but episodes of gross hematuria occur, sometimes in relation to exercise or respiratory infection. Red blood cell or granular casts are present. Proteinuria may be absent or mild early in the course, but with time 75% of cases have some degree of proteinuria. The 24 hr protein excretion exceeds 1 gm in 25% of cases and may be associated with a nephrotic syndrome. At onset the glomerular filtration rate is usually normal but with progressive renal damage azotemia, hypertension, and other features of chronic renal failure supervene. The nephrotic syndrome is uncommon but may occur even in young children. In most kindreds the course in affected males is more serious than in affected females; terminal uremia tends to develop in the 2nd–3rd decade of life. In some families, however, girls are as seriously affected as boys.

About half the patients have sensorineural high-frequency deafness, which usually has its onset in the 1st decade and is more severe in males; the severity is roughly related to that of the nephropathy. The hearing loss is usually progressive; it may be asymmetric or even unilateral. In some kindreds deafness is not a feature. There may be severe renal disease without deafness and deafness without renal involvement. Deafness may not be evident clinically; formal audiometry may be necessary.

Ocular abnormalities occur in about 10% of patients; the most frequent are cataracts and myopia; lenticonus, keratoconus, nystagmus, and microspherophakia also occur. A characteristic symmetrical perimacular retinal granulation may be seen, without visual disturbances; this finding is more common in males and is usually associated with anterior lenticonus.

Variants of Alport syndrome have been described in which hereditary deafness and progressive nephritis are associated with macrothrombocytopathia (giant size platelets), thrombocytopenia, or both. Bruising and bleeding occur in early childhood; renal and hearing defects appear later.

Genetic Aspects. The most likely mode of inheritance is an autosomal dominant pattern with variable penetrance. Half the sons and half the daughters of either affected parent receive the mutant gene. There may, however, be reduced penetrance, and there is less likelihood that boys who receive the gene from their father will develop the disease. By contrast, penetrance is complete in sons of affected females, whose children of each sex are at equal risk of inheriting the disorder.

Laboratory Data. Initially, microscopic hematuria with red cell casts is usual; proteinuria is present in about 75% of patients, and pyuria is relatively infrequent. Serum complement level is normal. With progression of the renal disease the serum creatinine and blood urea nitrogen values increase, and other changes of chronic renal failure become evident.

Diagnosis and Differential Diagnosis. The association of progressive hereditary renal disease, deafness, ocular abnormalities, and characteristic changes on renal biopsy suggest the diagnosis of Alport syndrome. A pattern of autosomal dominant inheritance, more serious disease in male family members, and deafness even in relatives without nephritis provides strong supportive evidence. An audiogram, urinalysis, and appropriate blood studies should be obtained for each available family member. Other forms of hereditary or familial renal disease having microscopic hematuria should be considered. Of these, benign familial hematuria is important to exclude since its prognosis is excellent; deafness and progressive renal failure do not occur in this condition. The condition of recurrent macroscopic hematuria with or without mesangial IgA deposits should be excluded. Renal biopsy can be of crucial diagnostic importance, especially if immunopathologic and electron microscopic studies are done.

Prevention. Genetic counseling for affected adults may reduce the number of affected children.

Treatment. There is no specific therapy. Standard therapeutic measures for renal insufficiency and its complications should be used when specific problems arise. Dialysis or renal transplantation should be carried out when advanced renal failure supervenes.

Prognosis. The rate of progression of the renal disease tends to be typical for each kindred. In general, 50% of affected males will develop terminal renal failure before the age of 30, often before 20 yr. The remainder progress more slowly, but most eventually have seriously compromised renal function. In most females the disorder is less severe, and in many kindreds females have a nearly normal life expectancy despite persistent microscopic hematuria. The prognosis has been improved by dialysis and renal transplantation.

Eckstein JD, Filip DJ, Watts JC: Hereditary thrombocytopenia, deafness, and renal disease. Ann Intern Med 82:639, 1975.

Ferguson AC, Rance CP: Hereditary nephropathy with nerve deafness (Alport's syndrome). Am J Dis Child 124:84, 1972.

Grunfeld J-P, Bois EP, Hinglais N: Progressive and nonprogressive hereditary chronic nephritis. Kidney Int 4:216, 1973.

Gubler MC, Levy M, Broyer M, et al: Alport's syndrome: A report of 58 cases and a review of the literature. Am J Med 70:493, 1981.

Kohaut EC, Singer DB, Nevels BK, et al: The specificity of split renal membranes in hereditary nephritis. Arch Pathol Lab Med 100:475, 1976.

Penin D, Jungers P, Grunfeld JP, et al: Perimacular changes in Alport's syndrome. Clin Nephrol 13:163, 1980.

Preus M, Fraser FC: Genetics of hereditary nephropathy with deafness (Alport's disease). Clin Genet 2:331, 1971.

16.32 BENIGN FAMILIAL HEMATURIA

Benign familial hematuria is characterized by persistent microscopic hematuria of glomerular origin with episodic macroscopic hematuria that is often precipitated by an intercurrent acute respiratory illness. Inheritance is usually autosomal dominant. Males and females are affected equally. Proteinuria is absent except during episodes of gross hematuria. There are no other characteristic abnormalities and no progression to renal insufficiency. Findings on histopathologic examination are normal, though red blood cells may be seen in Bowman space. Electron microscopy shows localized areas of thinning of the glomerular capillary basement membrane.

It is important in diagnosis of this condition to exclude other potentially more serious diseases. In particular, hereditary nephritis with deafness (Alport syndrome) must be ruled out. Recurrent macroscopic hematuria with focal glomerulonephritis should be considered; this nonfamilial condition can be identified by renal biopsy.

The other causes of hematuria listed in Table 16–2 should also be considered and can be differentiated by their own clinical, laboratory, or histopathologic features. Benign familial hematuria can be confidently diagnosed only after prolonged observation to exclude other serious disorders. An overly aggressive series of investigations, however, should be avoided. The findings of casts in the urinary sediment will establish the renal origin of the hematuria. An intravenous pyelogram and measurements of the 24 hr urinary excretion of protein and of blood urea nitrogen and serum creatinine concentrations should be obtained. Renal biopsy helps to distinguish this condition from other familial forms of glomerular disease. Urinalyses of family members and careful family histories regarding episodic hematuria, serious renal disease, deafness, or ocular abnormalities will help to establish the diagnosis. No treatment is needed and the prognosis is good.

Marks MI, Drummond KN: Benign familial hematuria. Pediatrics 44:590, 1969.
Rogers PW, Kurtzman NA, Bunn SM Jr, et al: Familial benign essential hematuria. Arch Intern Med 131:257, 1973.

16.33 NEPHRONOPHTHISIS
(Medullary Cystic Disease, Familial Juvenile Nephronophthisis)

Nephronophthisis is a hereditary progressive renal disease characterized pathologically by tubular atrophy, interstitial fibrosis, glomerular sclerosis, and medullary cysts and clinically by anemia, impaired urinary concentrating ability, and renal loss of sodium. Ocular abnormalities are often associated. It is likely that this description includes more than 1 disease entity or variant.

Etiology and Epidemiology. The cause is unknown, but hereditary factors are of importance in many instances.

This disease is not common, but it has been diagnosed with increasing frequency. There is wide geographic and ethnic distribution.

Pathology and Pathophysiology. Both glomeruli and interstitial tissue are involved, with progressive interstitial scarring, tubular atrophy with thickening of the tubular basement membranes, and periglomerular fibrosis. Medullary cysts are present in about two thirds of patients who die in terminal uremia; they vary from microscopic size to 3–4 cm in diameter, involve the distal tubule and collecting duct, and are lined with flattened epithelium. The cysts may not be present initially but may develop as the disease progresses. Foci of chronic inflammatory cells may be present in the interstitium. Most glomeruli show progressive sclerosis and hyalinization.

The structural changes in the medullary interstitium account for the reduced ability to concentrate urine.

Impaired retention of sodium results from the osmotic load imposed on surviving nephrons and from the cortical and interstitial fibrosis, which interferes with normal tubular function. Progressive loss of functioning tubular and interstitial tissue may result in reduced erythropoietin production and lead to anemia; another result is decreased production of 1,25-dihydroxycholecalciferol, with reduction in the plasma calcium level and development of marked secondary hyperparathyroidism and renal osteodystrophy.

Clinical Manifestations and Course. A spectrum of clinical manifestations probably reflects differences in the stage and severity of the illness, the likelihood that more than 1 specific disease entity is included under this designation, and differences that exist between kindreds in the expression of a single genetic disorder.

Typically, the clinical onset appears from 5–20 yr of age. The initial features are polyuria, thirst, and anemia. The urine is dilute, the sediment is normal, and proteinuria is usually absent. Hypertension and edema are not present until late in the course. Initially, azotemia is mild, with levels of blood urea nitrogen of 20–40 mg/dl. An inability of the kidneys to conserve sodium is common, and, to maintain balance, some children require a large dietary intake of salt. Urinary excretion of calcium may also be high; hypocalcemia with episodes of clinical tetany may occur. Severe hyperparathyroid bone disease and renal osteodystrophy are common. Progression to renal insufficiency over a period of 5–10 yr is the usual course. In some families associated abnormalities may be present; ocular lesions such as retinitis pigmentosa, cataracts, macular degeneration, myopia, and nystagmus are the most common.

Genetic Features. In most families an autosomal recessive mode of inheritance is likely; histories of consanguinity are recorded. In some kindreds, particularly those with onset in adulthood, an autosomal dominant mode has been shown. Sporadic cases also occur and probably represent mutations or the clinical expression of rare recessive genes in homozygous persons.

Laboratory Data. There are no specific laboratory changes. Normochromic anemia is a prominent finding. Unless uremia is advanced, urinary excretion of sodium and calcium is excessive; the serum calcium level is usually low in relation to the degree of phosphate elevation. Marked secondary hyperparathyroidism with attendant osseous changes is not uncommon. Urinalysis is unremarkable except for the low specific gravity. Intravenous urography usually shows poor functioning and slightly small kidneys; the medullary cysts are seldom detected radiographically.

Diagnosis. In the recessively transmitted form a positive family history is usually not obtained, except for the possibility of consanguinity. The constellation of polyuria, thirst, renal salt wasting, hyposthenuria, normal urinary sediment, severe anemia, and absence of edema and hypertension, with or without ocular abnormalities, suggests the diagnosis.

Other causes of polyuria and hyposthenuria include the nephropathies resulting from hypercalcemia or hypokalemia, obstructive uropathy, and chronic pyelonephritis. Renal biopsy may not provide a specific diagnosis since medullary cysts are not always present or may be missed on a random biopsy. The other characteristic morphologic changes may, however, provide strong support for the diagnosis.

Prevention. No means of prevention is known, but genetic counseling, especially for those with the autosomal dominant form, may reduce the number of affected offspring.

Treatment. There is no specific treatment. Care should be taken to provide an adequate fluid and salt intake, particularly during periods of intercurrent illness when the child may not take appropriate amounts voluntarily. As the disease progresses, the amount of renal salt loss decreases and hypertension may develop. The anemia may require occasional transfusions with freshly washed, packed red blood cells. Aggressive treatment of renal osteodystrophy with vitamin D analogues and adequate supplementation of calcium are required. Apart from these measures, standard methods of treating uremia should be used. Dialysis and renal transplantation have definite roles in terminally affected patients.

Prognosis. In most patients a relentless downhill course to terminal uremia takes place over a period of 3–10 yr; in some kindreds a slower progressive course is followed.

Boichis H, Passwell J, David R, et al: Congenital hepatic fibrosis and nephronophthisis. Q J Med 42:221, 1973.
Gardner KD, Evans HP: The nephronophthisis–cystic renal medulla complex. In: Hamburger J, Crosnier J, Grunfeld JP (eds): Nephrology. New York, John Wiley & Sons, 1979.
Makker SP, Grupe WE, Perrin E, et al: Identical progression of juvenile hereditary nephronophthisis in monozygotic twins. J Pediatr 82:773, 1973.
Steele BT, Lirenman DS, Beattie GW: Nephronophthisis. Am J Med 68:531, 1980.

16.34   THE NAIL-PATELLA SYNDROME
(Hereditary Onycho-osteodysplasia)

This disorder is characterized by (1) multiple osseous abnormalities, including absence or hypoplasia of the patellae, hypoplasia of the proximal radial heads, iliac horns, and talipes equinovarus deformities of the feet; (2) flexion contractures of a variety of joints, especially of the elbows; (3) hypoplasia, absence, ridging, or flatness of the nails, especially those of the thumb and index fingers; (4) ocular abnormalities such as ptosis of the upper eyelids, abnormal pigmention of the iris, glaucoma, microcornea, and strabismus; and (5) renal disease. The condition is transmitted as an autosomal dominant trait closely linked to the ABO blood group locus.

The most common initial manifestation of renal involvement is proteinuria; it is present in about 50% of patients. A mild urinary concentrating defect or microscopic hematuria may also be present initially. The majority of patients with these manifestations of renal involvement have no associated morbidity; however, in about 20% of them slow progression to renal failure occurs within 5–25 yr, during which the only manifestation may be asymptomatic proteinuria. The nephrotic syndrome is an infrequent complication. Duplication of the urinary collecting system has been observed.

The histopathologic changes consist of focal, glomerular basement membrane thickening and an increase in mesangial matrix. The tubules of the sclerosed glomeruli become atrophic. Electron microscopic findings are probably pathognomonic and consist of lucent areas within irregularly thickened glomerular basement membranes; within the lucent areas are fibrils with the characteristic periodicity of collagen.

No specific treatment for the renal disorder is known.

Bennett WM, Musgrave JE, Campbell RA, et al: The nephropathy of the nail-patella syndrome. Am J Med 54:304, 1973.
Hoyer JR, Michael AF, Vernier RL: Renal disease in nail-patella syndrome: Clinical and morphologic studies. Kidney Int 2:231, 1972.

16.35   LIPODYSTROPHY

See also Sec 24.17.

This condition is characterized by atrophy of subcutaneous fat with variable association of other findings, such as increased height, enlarged genitalia, skin pigmentation, hirsutism, hepatomegaly, central nervous system disturbances, abnormal glucose tolerance curve or insulin-resistant diabetes mellitus, hyperlipidemia, and, in about 25% of affected persons, progressive renal disease. Both partial and total forms of lipodystrophy are described on the basis of the distribution of atrophy of subcutaneous fat. The total form displays a higher incidence of the associated abnormalities, but renal disease occurs with equal frequency in both forms. An absolute distinction between the total and partial forms of lipodystrophy appears unwarranted since there is considerable overlap in many of the features. Most cases are sporadic, but there are instances of familial involvement.

The renal pathology is indistinguishable from membranoproliferative glomerulonephritis, Type II. A high level of C3 nephritic factor is present in the serum, and the serum C3 level is low.

Evidence of renal involvement usually appears within several yr of onset of lipodystrophy. Proteinuria is found with or without microscopic hematuria; the nephrotic syndrome may develop; and progressive decrease in renal function leading to terminal uremia within a period of several yr occurs in at least half of those with renal involvement. Hypertension is a prominent feature.

There is no specific treatment for lipodystrophy or for its renal manifestations. Successful renal transplantation has been reported in a patient with terminal uremia.

Bennett WM, Bardana EJ, Wuepper K, et al: Partial lipodystrophy, C3 nephritic factor and clinically inapparent mesangiocapillary glomerulonephritis. Am J Med 62:757, 1977.
Eisinger AJ, Shortland JR, Moorhead PJ: Renal disease in partial lipodystrophy. Q J Med 41:343, 1972.

Habib R, Levy M, Gubler MC, et al: Lipodystrophie partielle, hypocomplémentémie et glomerulonéphrite. Arch Franç Pediatr 34:CXCVII, 1977.

FAMILIAL NEPHROTIC SYNDROME

In occasional families in which more than 1 member has minimal change nephrotic syndrome, it has not been established whether hereditary or environmental influences are operative. The features of the disorder are typical, including responsiveness to corticosteroid therapy.

A nephrotic syndrome may also develop during the course of several clearly hereditary disorders, including congenital nephrotic syndrome of the Finnish type, Alport syndrome, and the nail-patella syndrome. These are discussed elsewhere.

16.36 SICKLE CELL ANEMIA AND THE KIDNEY

The principal renal manifestations are gross or microscopic hematuria and impaired ability to concentrate urine; less common are the nephrotic syndrome, papillary necrosis, and progressive renal insufficiency. Hematuria is said to be more common in affected males than in females and in adults than in children; its source is usually the left kidney.

A spectrum of pathologic changes, many of which are probably nonspecific, has been described. Characteristically, the glomeruli are enlarged with dilatation of capillary loops. Glomerular sclerosis develops later, and tubular atrophy and dilatation are seen. Papillary necrosis and interstitial fibrosis have been observed.

Impaired ability to concentrate urine is an early and common functional change. This finding is not the result of the anemia per se; the defect is present in patients with the sickle cell trait who are not anemic. To some extent it is temporarily reversible by transfusion with normal blood cells. That this defect worsens with time and becomes no longer reversible by transfusion suggests that permanent structural changes supervene. The basis for the concentrating defect is not known; a likely factor is the tendency of sickling to increase in a hypertonic medium. Since the medulla is hypertonic relative to plasma, red cells in the vasa recta have a tendency to sickle. This could reduce medullary blood flow and impair the normal functioning of the countercurrent multiplier system. Episodes of painless gross hematuria or periods of microscopic hematuria occur at some time in about 20% of patients with SS, SA, or SC hemoglobinopathy. The hematuria is not yet explained but is probably related to congestion and dilatation of papillary vessels, to submucosal hemorrhage, and, uncommonly, to frank papillary necrosis. Some patients have an incomplete form of distal renal tubular acidosis.

Both renal failure and the nephrotic syndrome have been reported in conjunction with sickle cell anemia, but the association is rare in children. Since, however, renal function does deteriorate with age, some patients under adequate therapy who live longer can be expected eventually to develop chronic renal failure.

Alleyne GAO, Van Eps LWS, Addae SK, et al: The kidney in sickle cell anemia. Kidney Int 7:371, 1975.

16.37 OXALOSIS

See also Sec 8.8.

Oxalosis is a rare hereditary disorder in glyoxalate metabolism, in which hyperoxaluria, calcium oxalate nephrolithiasis, widespread extrarenal deposition of calcium oxalate crystals, and progressive renal failure leading to death, usually before adulthood, occur. Transmission is autosomal recessive. Two types of primary oxalosis have been characterized.

Secondary hyperoxaluria may occur in patients with ileal dysfunction. A genetic predisposition to the formation of calcium oxalate renal calculi has also been demonstrated in patients with no evidence of abnormal glyoxalate metabolism; hyperoxaluria is not present in these patients.

In most patients with oxalosis, symptoms from renal calculi occur in the 1st decade. Progressive renal failure resulting from calcium oxalate deposition and recurrent episodes of nephrolithiasis follow, and death from uremia usually occurs before or during the 3rd decade.

The diagnosis of oxalosis should be considered in patients with recurrent and progressive nephrolithiasis beginning in the 1st decade. Calcium oxalate calculi are radiopaque. The most consistent and diagnostic laboratory finding is an increased urinary excretion of oxalate in the absence of excess oxalate ingestion or pyridoxine deficiency. Normal children excrete less than 40 mg of oxalate/24 hr; in primary hyperoxaluria the amount excreted usually exceeds 200 mg/24 hr. As renal failure progresses, the amount of oxalate excreted decreases.

There is no specific treatment. Pharmacologic doses of pyridoxine, up to 1 gm/24 hr, may reduce oxalate excretion in about one third of cases, but this may not alter the prognosis. A copious intake of water in order to dilute the urine may reduce the likelihood of forming calculi.

In view of the extensive extrarenal deposition of calcium oxalate crystals and the likelihood of recurrent calculi in a transplanted kidney, renal transplantation does not appear to be indicated.

Boquist L, Lindquist B, Ostberg Y, et al: Primary oxalosis. Am J Med 54:673, 1973.

HEREDITARY DISORDERS WITH RENAL CYSTS

Cortical and medullary renal cysts are relatively common in genetically determined renal disorders. Renal cysts may also occur in developmental abnormalities which are not genetically determined, and they may sometimes develop even in previously normal nephrons. A discussion of 2 heritable conditions in which renal cysts are a prominent feature follows. A more complete list of these disorders, both hereditary and nonhereditary, is given in Table 16–9.

16.38   CHILDHOOD-TYPE POLYCYSTIC KIDNEYS

(Autosomal Recessive Polycystic Kidney Disease, Congenital Hepatic Fibrosis with Renal Cysts)

This autosomal recessive disorder affects the kidneys and liver. Its clinical and pathologic features are largely age related; renal abnormalities are predominant in early infancy, and problems related to the liver assume greater importance in later childhood. In a given pedigree the pattern of disease (predominantly renal, hepatic, or intermediate) and the age of presentation are relatively constant among affected members. It has been suggested that differences in pattern among various age groups reflect different genetic entities; however, since the lesions at different ages are qualitatively identical though quantitatively different, it seems more reasonable to consider this as a single disease with a spectrum of age-related manifestations.

Table 16–9 CONDITIONS IN WHICH RENAL CYSTS MAY BE PRESENT

Hereditary
Childhood (autosomal recessive) type polycystic kidneys with portal dysplasia
Adult (autosomal dominant) type polycystic kidneys
Nephronophthisis
Congenital nephrotic syndrome of the Finnish type
Genetic disorders in which renal cysts may occur:*
  Tuberous sclerosis†
  Laurence-Moon-Biedl syndrome‡
  Oral-facial-digital syndrome
  Meckel syndrome (dysencephalia splanchnocystica syndrome)
  Dandy-Walker malformation of the brain
  Zellweger syndrome (cerebrohepatorenal syndrome)
  Autosomal trisomy syndromes C, D, and E
  Von Hippel–Lindau disease
  Jeune asphyxiating thoracic dystrophy
Nonhereditary
Cystic kidneys with lower urinary tract obstruction
Multilocular renal cysts
Medullary sponge kidney§
Renal dysplasia with cysts (multicystic kidney, multicystic dysplasia)¶
Simple renal cyst**

*Renal cysts in these conditions are sometimes of no clinical importance.
†Angiomyolipomatous malformation is more common than cysts.
‡Glomerular sclerosis and interstitial fibrosis are prominent features.
§Rare in childhood; calculi in cysts are common; rare familial cases reported.
¶Often unilateral; lower urinary tract abnormalities present in 50% of cases.
**Uncommon in childhood; not bilateral; usually an incidental finding at autopsy.

Pathology and Pathogenesis.   In the newborn period, the kidneys are grossly enlarged and have a diffusely spongy appearance due to innumerable, radially arranged, fusiform cysts. The renal pelves, ureters, bladder, and urethra are normal. On microscopic examination the cysts are lined by hyperplastic, cuboidal, or low columnar epithelium. Glomeruli and remaining interstitial tissue are normal. The cysts represent dilated distal tubules and collecting ducts; there is continuity between the lumina of tubules and cysts. In affected infants about 90% of tubules are involved. In older children the kidneys are less enlarged, the cortex is not extensively involved, and there are more intervening areas of normal parenchyma. When clinical manifestations are not apparent until adolescence or later, only 10–20% of nephrons may be affected, and the principal finding is dilatation of medullary collecting ducts. At this age the renal lesion is usually of no clinical importance; radiologic examination shows good renal function with tubular ectasia. In the liver are seen proliferation, infolding, and dilatation of portal bile ducts and ductules with a variable degree of fine periportal and subcapsular fibrosis; all portal triads are involved, and the changes are distributed uniformly throughout the liver. Hepatic lesions are not severe in young infants; affected older children have progressive extensive periportal fibrosis that often leads to portal hypertension with esophageal varices and splenomegaly in the 2nd decade.

Pancreatic cysts of no clinical importance are occasionally present. The pathogenesis of the renal and hepatic lesions is unknown. The clinical presentation bears a close relationship to the predominant underlying pathologic change.

Clinical Manifestations and Course.   Affected neonates often have a history of oligohydramnios and dystocia, and they may have the so-called Potter facies. The abdomen is distended, and the enlarged kidneys are readily palpable. There may be anuria or oliguria, respiratory distress, and gross or microscopic hematuria. Hypertension is common. Roentgenographic studies show enlarged flank masses on the plain abdominal film and markedly decreased function by intravenous urography. Contrast medium may be concentrated in collecting ducts and tubules; calyces may be blunted or distorted. In most instances, however, insufficient contrast medium is concentrated in the collecting system to permit its adequate visualization, even though some appears in the bladder. Death from progressive renal failure may occur within a period of weeks to months. Pyloric stenosis occurs with greater than normal frequency. Older infants and children have fewer renal and more hepatic problems; in affected adolescents the presenting problem is likely to be the result of portal hypertension, and renal medullary tubular dilatation with or without blunted calyces is found incidentally on intravenous urography. The clinical patterns manifested from infancy to maturity are determined principally by the degree of renal involvement, as enlargement of the kidneys, variable degrees of chronic or progressive renal insufficiency, hypertension, and intermittent hematuria.

Diagnosis. The differential diagnosis in the young infant includes other causes of kidney enlargement, abdominal mass, and renal failure; these are Wilms tumor, neuroblastoma, bilateral hydronephrosis, multicystic renal dysplasia, and bilateral renal vein thrombosis. Medullary sponge kidney, a benign condition rarely seen in childhood, may require differentiation in an older child whose urogram shows medullary cysts with calyceal distortion. Other hereditary conditions in which renal cysts may occur should be considered; most present their own particular diagnostic features. The diagnosis in older children may be more difficult to establish; the association of hepatosplenomegaly and portal hypertension should suggest the possibility of childhood polycystic kidney disease, and an intravenous urogram should be obtained. In some instances biopsy of the liver may be helpful. A positive family history, particularly of a similarly affected sibling, is strong evidence for the disease.

Laboratory Data. There may be variable hematuria with minimal proteinuria as well as azotemia and other nonspecific features of chronic renal failure in the later stages. Roentgenographic and liver biopsy findings, as discussed earlier, may help in establishing the diagnosis.

Treatment. There is no specific treatment. Early death from renal failure or respiratory difficulties is not uncommon in infants. Control of hypertension is important in older children with decreased renal function; standard treatment of chronic renal failure may be used, and dialysis and renal transplantation can be considered. Surgical measures may be necessary to relieve portal hypertension in cases of recurrent esophageal bleeding.

Prognosis. When clinical manifestations are apparent in early infancy, the course may be rapidly fatal; but a prolonged course may also be followed even in infancy. In older children the renal failure develops more slowly or not at all; if esophageal varices and portal hypertension can be treated successfully, the outlook is reasonably good. A sibling has a 1 in 4 risk of being affected.

16.39 ADULT-TYPE POLYCYSTIC KIDNEYS
(Autosomal Dominant Polycystic Kidney Disease)

This is an autosomal dominant disorder with a high degree of penetrance; the clinical manifestations usually have their onset in the 2nd–3rd decade but may present in early infancy or throughout childhood. In contrast to the autosomal recessive form, the autosomal dominant form presents cysts that are larger and irregular in size and cause marked distortion of the renal outline and calyces. Collecting ducts are the principal segment affected; other segments of the nephron may be involved. The cysts are lined with flattened epithelium and increase in size with age; therefore renal enlargement is progressive. Focal cystic formation in the liver, of no clinical consequence, is present in about a third of patients; aneurysms of cerebral arteries occur in about 10% of patients. Coarctation of the aorta and cardiac abnormalities such as endocardial sclerosis are sometimes associated. In affected children the condition is usually asymptomatic, but episodic hematuria, hypertension, renal enlargement, and even progressive renal failure have been observed. The differential diagnosis includes multiple simple cysts, which are irregularly distributed and are separated by zones of uninvolved parenchyma.

There is no specific treatment for the course of progressive renal failure with hypertension; major clinical problems usually do not occur before the 4th or 5th decade.

Bernstein J: Infantile polycystic disease. In: Hamburger J, Crosnier J, Grunfeld J-P (eds): Nephrology. New York, John Wiley and Sons, 1979.
Blythe H, Ockenden BG: Polycystic disease of the kidneys and liver presenting in childhood. J Med Genet 8:257, 1971.
Kaplan BS, Rabin I, Nogrady MB, et al: Autosomal dominant polycystic renal disease in children. J Pediatr 90:782, 1977.
Lieberman E, Salinas-Madrigal L, Gwinn JL, et al: Infantile polycystic disease of the kidneys and liver. Medicine 50:277, 1971.
Murray-Lyon IM, Ockenden BG, Williams R: Congenital hepatic fibrosis—is it a single clinical entity? Gastroenterology 64:653, 1973.

Renal Failure

16.40 ACUTE RENAL FAILURE
(Acute Uremia)

Acute renal failure is a complex syndrome resulting from an acute reduction in or cessation of renal function and is characterized by anuria or oliguria (less than 180 ml/M^2/24 hr of urine), electrolyte and acid-base disturbances (notably hyperkalemia and metabolic acidosis), and impaired excretion of substances such as creatinine, urea, and phosphate. Reduction in urine volume, however, is not an essential feature of acute renal failure, and the other features can be present despite a urine output in excess of 350 ml/M^2/24 hr; this condition is known as acute nonoliguric renal failure.

Etiology. Acute renal failure can be *prerenal*, *intrinsic*, or *postrenal*, depending on where the principal disturbance lies. Major causes of acute renal failure are listed in Table 16–10, and those common in infancy are listed in Table 16–13. The most common causes in childhood are renal hypoperfusion leading to prerenal failure, hemolytic-uremic syndrome, glomerulonephritis and interstitial nephritis, congenital developmental anomalies of the kidney and urinary tract, septicemia, tubular damage, and cardiopulmonary bypass surgery for congenital heart disease.

Pathogenesis and Pathophysiology. **Acute prerenal failure** results from renal hypoperfusion and is often readily reversible when the cause of the hypoperfusion is corrected. It accounts for about 40% of acute renal

Table 16–10 PRINCIPAL CAUSES OF ACUTE RENAL FAILURE IN CHILDREN

TYPE OF ACUTE RENAL FAILURE	CAUSE OR CLINICAL CONDITION
Prerenal (renal hypoperfusion)	Hypovolemia, dehydration, hemorrhage, burns, shock, septicemia, nephrotic syndrome, 3rd space losses (e.g., ileus, peritonitis), reduced cardiac output, congestive heart failure
Intrinsic	
Vascular disorders	Hemolytic-uremic syndrome, renal arterial or venous thrombosis, malignant hypertension, disseminated intravascular coagulation
Septicemia	E. coli, Bacteroides, clostridia, acute pyelonephritis (especially if associated with calculi or obstruction)
Tubular damage	Anoxia, shock, drugs, diethylene glycol, mercury, carbon tetrachloride
Tubular obstruction	Uric acid nephropathy, sulfonamides, xanthine crystals
Postoperative	Cardiopulmonary bypass surgery for congenital heart disease
Interstitial nephritis	Systemic or renal infection, sulfonamides, diphenylhydantoin, penicillin analogues, cephalosporins, etc.
Glomerulonephritis	Acute poststreptococcal glomerulonephritis, diffuse crescentic glomerulonephritis
Developmental structural anomalies of the kidney	Renal dysplasia
Acute insult superimposed on underlying chronic renal disease	Gastroenteritis with vomiting and diarrhea leading to fluid and electrolyte loss; acute exacerbation of a chronic glomerular disease
Miscellaneous	Lymphomatous infiltration of the kidneys in acute leukemia
Postrenal (obstructive)	
Obstructive uropathy	Calculi, stomal closure, blood clots, developmental structural abnormalities such as posterior urethral valves or pelviureteric junction obstruction; superimposed infection may precipitate acute obstruction in these conditions

failure in children. The oliguria and the retention of products normally excreted results from *reduction in effective plasma volume* (e.g., due to shock or dehydration) or from *decreased cardiac output* (e.g., in congestive heart failure). The renal response is a predictable physiologic adaptation to these stimuli. The urine sodium concentration is very low, usually under 10 mEq/l; the urine urea and creatinine concentrations and the osmolality are high. Normal renal function and increased urine output usually return shortly after correction of the renal hypoperfusion, but prolonged contraction of intravascular volume may lead to intrinsic renal failure which does not respond to restoration of volume or cardiac output; this sequence has been reported to be as high as 50% in some series.

In **acute intrinsic renal failure,** when the principal site of injury is the renal tubule, the urine concentration of sodium is often 50–90 mEq/l; when glomerular injury predominates and tubular function is intact, a urine sodium concentration less than 20 mEq/l may be expected. The urine volume is usually low, but a nonoliguric form of acute renal failure may sometimes develop following burns, trauma, or exposure to nephrotoxins. The cause of oliguria in acute intrinsic renal failure has been the subject of much discussion. With severe glomerular damage, reduction of the filtration rate may be assumed. In conditions in which tubular or interstitial changes are present, it is reasonable to distinguish between pathogenetic factors which initiate and those which maintain the state of renal failure. Vascular events, notably ischemia and afferent arteriolar constriction, are important in the initiation of acute renal failure and also play a role in its maintenance. After acute renal failure has been established, renal blood flow may return to normal levels without improvement in renal function. Intratubular obstruction by swollen or sloughed tubular cells, casts, and other debris is probably important in maintaining the state of renal failure. Reflux of filtered luminal fluid across damaged tubular epithelium and reduced permeability of the glomerular basement membrane are probably not significant factors. Tubular cell necrosis, with or without damage to the tubular basement membrane, is often cited as an important feature of acute intrinsic renal failure, but it is present in under 20% of cases. In classic acute intrinsic renal failure resulting from tubular damage, the course may be divided into 3 stages: anuric or oliguric, diuretic, and convalescent; the management of these stages differs. In children this sequence often is not clear cut.

Acute postrenal failure results from obstruction of urine flow at some point in the pelvicalyceal collecting system or in the ureters. Causes of obstruction include renal calculi, crystal formation during sulfonamide therapy, and trauma responsible for blood clots.

Hyperkalemia develops in acute renal failure because of decreased renal excretion of potassium and cellular release of potassium as a result of trauma, hemolysis, infection, or hypoxia. In the metabolic acidosis which often accompanies acute renal failure an increased plasma K^+ concentration results from an intracellular shift of H^+ in exchange for K^+. The cardiotoxic effects of hyperkalemia result from a decreased ratio of intracellular to extracellular K^+.

Sodium and water overload during reduced excretion of urine may lead to interstitial and pulmonary edema, pleural effusion, hypertension, and circulatory congestion. Hyponatremia in acute renal failure is the result of dilution of body fluids as a consequence of excessive intake of water relative to that of sodium.

Metabolic acidosis, with or without increased plasma H^+ concentration (acidemia), is common in acute renal failure and reflects impaired ability of the kidney to eliminate acid as well as increased catabolic production of acid.

The *blood pressure* may be normal, reduced, or elevated depending on the underlying cause of acute renal failure. *Acute hypertension* may result in hypertensive encephalopathy or aggravate circulatory congestion. It is common in acute poststreptococcal glomerulonephritis and may occur in other conditions, such as the hemolytic-uremic syndrome, burns, and acute obstructive nephropathy.

Blood urea nitrogen, plasma creatinine, and uric acid concentrations are elevated because of reduced excretion. *Anemia, thrombocytopenia, leukocytosis, impaired carbohydrate tolerance,* and *hyperlipidemia* may also occur in acute renal failure.

Clinical Manifestations. The clinical pattern of acute renal failure is often overshadowed by manifestations of the precipitating cause. For example, the patient may be in shock as a result of endotoxemia, severely dehydrated with gastroenteritis, jaundiced with carbon tetrachloride poisoning, or subject to seizures due to the hypertensive encephalopathy of acute glomerulonephritis. Initially, attention must be paid to the possible presence of each of the following precipitating or associated findings: shock, trauma, hemolysis, sepsis, dehydration, intoxication, hemorrhage, hypertension, cardiac arrhythmia secondary to hyperkalemia, circulatory congestion, metabolic acidosis, congestive heart failure, pelvicalyceal or ureteral obstruction, and underlying chronic renal disease.

The clinical features related more specifically to acute renal failure include decreased urinary output (oliguria to anuria), edema, drowsiness, the cardiac arrhythmia of hyperkalemia, circulatory congestion, and tachypnea as a result of metabolic acidosis. Seizures may be due to hyponatremia or hypocalcemia. If the underlying disorder can be treated successfully, recovery of renal function is often surprisingly complete, even following severe oliguria lasting several days to several wk. In acute renal failure of acute poststreptococcal glomerulonephritis, complete recovery is the rule provided the electrolyte and acid-base disturbances, circulatory congestion, and hypertensive complications are managed satisfactorily.

Laboratory Data. The usual abnormalities include hyperkalemia; hyponatremia; metabolic acidosis; elevation of serum concentrations of urea, phosphate, uric acid, and creatinine; and hypocalcemia. The urine may contain red blood cells, protein, casts, and tubular cells, but it is usually normal in prerenal failure. The urinary concentration of sodium is generally low (<20 mEq/l)

in prerenal acute failure and in failure due to glomerular disease and elevated (50–90 mEq/l) in tubular disorders. Indices useful in distinguishing among the 3 types of acute renal failure are given in Table 16–11. Electrocardiographic changes may reflect hyperkalemia. Roentgenographic studies may reveal cardiomegaly, pulmonary congestion, radiopaque calculi, and shrunken or enlarged kidneys. Radionuclide studies may be used to assess blood flow and to determine whether renal necrosis or ureteral obstruction is present. In nonoliguric acute intrinsic renal failure the urine sodium concentration is usually lower and the osmolality higher than in acute oliguric intrinsic renal failure.

Treatment. It is essential to ascertain immediately which of the 3 principal types of acute renal failure is present since therapy differs for each. The following investigations are recommended for initial evaluation: (1) history and general clinical assessment, including blood pressure, weight, and evaluation of state of hydration; (2) examination of urine obtained by catheterization for volume, routine urinalysis, electrolyte content, osmolality, pH, culture, and indices listed in Table 16–11 (time of collection is noted also); (3) examination of blood for Na^+, Cl^-, K^+, calcium, phosphorus, pH, pCO_2, HCO_3^-, urea nitrogen, creatinine, uric acid, and hemoglobin; a white blood cell and platelet count; a blood smear for fragmented erythrocytes; and a blood culture; (4) electrocardiography; and (5) roentgenogram of the chest and abdomen (to detect renal calculi and estimate kidney size).

A decision must be made about the urgency of restoring the circulating blood volume to normal as opposed to the need for peritoneal or hemodialysis, the main indications for which are severe hyperkalemia or circulatory overload. Central venous pressure measurement may help to assess the contribution of cardiac function and circulating volume to the renal failure. If the patient is dehydrated or in shock, measures to reestablish intravascular volume and to rehydrate should be carried out immediately. If sepsis is suspected, appropriate antibiotics should be given as soon as blood and urine cultures have been obtained.

If the patient is well hydrated and not in shock, or if circulatory congestion is present, a diuretic such as furosemide (1–2 mg/kg intravenously) should be used. If intrinsic renal damage is potentially reversible, furo-

Table 16-11 INDICES IN RENAL FAILURE

TYPES OF ACUTE RENAL FAILURE	U_{OSM}	U_{OSM}/P_{OSM}	U_{REA}/P_{UREA}	U_{Cr}/P_{Cr}	U_{Na}	RFI	FRACTIONAL Na EXCRETION
Prerenal	>500	>1.3	>8	>40	<20	<1	<1
Intrinsic	<350	<1.1	<8	<20	>50	>1	>1
Obstructive	<350	<1.1	<8	<20	>50	>1	>1

U = urine.
P = plasma.
UREA = urea nitrogen.
Cr = creatinine.

RFI = renal failure index = $\dfrac{U_{Na\,(mEq/l)}}{U_{Cr}/P_{Cr}}$

Fractional Na excretion = $\dfrac{U_{Na}/P_{Na}}{U_{Cr}/P_{Cr}}$

semide may induce a temporary diuresis; in irreversible acute renal failure an increase in urinary output rarely occurs. If circulatory congestion is not present, mannitol (0.2–0.4 gm/kg intravenously) can be given for the same purpose. Mannitol and furosemide may also help to prevent the development of oliguric acute intrinsic failure or to convert it to the nonoliguric form, which is easier to treat and has a better prognosis. Serial specimens of urine should be examined for volume, proteinuria, and electrolyte loss. Less urgent blood studies are measurements of antistreptolysin O titer, C3 level, and total serum protein concentration. Intravenous urography may be indicated if anuria persists after the patient is out of shock or when circulatory congestion is no longer present; a radionuclide study may be useful. These studies may help assess renal size and perfusion and exclude obstruction. Retrograde contrast studies may also be necessary to exclude obstruction and define the anatomy of the urinary tract. Ultrasound examination is of great value in excluding obstruction. Renal biopsy may be indicated to establish the nature and severity of the renal damage but only when there is no coagulation disturbance.

The indications for each of the above studies must be considered carefully for each patient; not all are required in each case, and in some they may pose undue risk or expense.

Hyperkalemia and Hyponatremia. See Sec 16.17, Treatment.

Shock and Dehydration. Correction of hypovolemia is urgent, whatever its cause. Twenty ml/kg (about 450 ml/M²) of plasma or lactated Ringer solution can be infused rapidly as initial replacement over 15–45 min; the patient must be carefully monitored, and continuous measurement of central venous pressure may be required. The patient is then reassessed. If the acute renal failure is the result of prerenal failure, an increase in urine output may be anticipated. Fluids are required for replacement of remaining electrolyte deficits and of ongoing losses and for normal maintenance. If an increase in urine output does not follow correction of volume depletion, a test dose of 20% mannitol (0.2 gm/kg intravenously), can be given over a 20–30 min period, with or without furosemide (1 mg/kg intravenously). Mannitol should not be given to a patient in cardiac failure, nor furosemide to one who is hypovolemic. Mannitol and furosemide may induce diuresis in reversible intrinsic renal failure.

Metabolic Acidosis. General measures include correction of the catabolic state by treatment of shock, infection, and hypoxia and by provision of an adequate caloric intake. At least 300 calories/M²/24 hr given as carbohydrate or fat is required to minimize endogenous catabolism. During the oliguric or anuric phase 10–30% glucose may be given intravenously. With improving renal function high quality proteins may gradually be introduced. There is evidence that provision of essential amino acids and glucose intravenously may speed recovery. Specific measures for correction of metabolic acidosis are discussed in Sec 5.32.

Fluid, Electrolyte, and Caloric Requirements. A meticulous balance sheet of intake and output of all fluids and electrolytes should be kept. This should include losses by vomiting or gastric suction as well as urinary losses and oral as well as intravenous intake. Maintenance fluids should include replacement of insensible water loss (300–400 ml/M²/24 hr); they can be given intravenously as 10–30% dextrose. Such a concentration of glucose will irritate small veins, and it may be necessary to use a cut-down or a large vein. The fluid can be given orally if the patient tolerates it. Oral feeding of carbohydrate (as hard candy) and fat can be used to increase the caloric intake. The usual vitamin requirements should be met. Unless the patient is voiding or has a definite sodium deficit, it is unnecessary to give sodium; excess sodium will increase edema and aggravate circulatory congestion and hypertension.

The use of an indwelling urethral catheter to collect specimens of urine should be avoided.

Hypertension. (See Sec 16.17, Treatment.)

Infection. Since bacterial infection accounts for about a third of deaths in acute renal failure, it should be anticipated, promptly diagnosed by appropriate cultures, and promptly treated. Prophylactic use of antibiotics is not indicated. Unexplained persistent hyperkalemia may be caused by infection. During renal failure dosages of antibiotics should be adjusted if their primary route of excretion is the kidney. Such adjustment is particularly important in the case of potentially toxic drugs, e.g., the aminoglycosides.

Dialysis. The indications for peritoneal dialysis or hemodialysis in patients with acute renal failure are (1) severe metabolic acidosis or acidemia which cannot be safely corrected with NaHCO₃; (2) failure of the previously discussed measures to reduce serum potassium concentrations to a safe range; and (3) circulatory congestion, pulmonary edema, and severe fluid overload that are threatening survival. Table 16–12 lists indications for dialysis in patients with acute renal failure as well as in those with chronic renal failure or with intoxication by endogenous or exogenous toxins. Contraindications to peritoneal dialysis include recent abdominal or diaphragmatic surgery, a diaphragmatic defect, or an open abdominal wound. Age is not a contraindication; successful dialysis can be carried out in newborn infants.

The peritoneum is a semipermeable membrane that

Table 16–12 INDICATIONS FOR DIALYSIS

Acute renal failure
  BUN >100 mg/dl
  Uncontrollable hyperkalemia
  Intractable severe metabolic acidosis or acidemia which cannot safely be corrected with NaHCO₃
  Severe hypo- or hypernatremia
  Fluid overload with circulatory congestion and pulmonary edema
Chronic renal failure with severe symptoms or any of first 5 entries above, or pending institution of hemodialysis or transplantation
Other indications:
  Intractable lactic acidosis
  Inborn errors of metabolism with organic acidemia or hyperammonemia
  Hyperuricemia
  Intoxication with dialyzable toxins, e.g., barbiturates, glutethimide, methylprylon, amphetamines, methanol,* acetylsalicylate*

*Hemodialysis is more effective than peritoneal dialysis.

allows diffusion of water and solutes along concentration gradients. The relative peritoneal clearance rates of endogenous solutes in decreasing order are as follows: urea, K, Cl, Na, creatinine, PO_4, uric acid, HCO_3, Ca, and Mg. Maximum peritoneal clearance of urea in children is achieved with a dialysate exchange rate of 50 ml/kg/hr using solutions warmed to 37° C.

See other sources (Day and White; Gault) for selection of dialysis solutions and for details of the technique of peritoneal dialysis.

Most children with acute renal failure can be satisfactorily treated using the measures outlined above, with or without peritoneal dialysis. If there is a hypercatabolic state or if a prolonged period of renal failure is anticipated, consideration should be given to early use of hemodialysis, which will permit easier management of fluid and electrolyte problems and better nutrition.

Diuretic or Recovery Phase. During recovery from acute renal failure the patient may undergo a period of diuresis. When severe glomerular disease is improving, though the urine volume may be high, the tubules are usually able to exhibit homeostatic functions, and excessive losses of fluid and electrolytes do not occur. In this situation the diuresis represents excretion of excess fluid and electrolytes accumulated during the oliguric phase. When, on the other hand, acute renal failure is the consequence of tubular damage, an excessive diuresis may occur as tubular function begins to return. Regenerating tubular epithelium may be unable to respond to the stimuli that normally regulate excretion of electrolytes and water, and serious urinary losses of them may occur. During this time, adequate measurement and replacement of fluids and electrolytes should be maintained; at some stage during the diuretic phase, a test to determine whether normal tubular function has returned can be made by reduction of the quantities administered.

Prognosis. The prognosis in acute renal failure depends largely on the nature and severity of the precipitating event and on promptness and adequacy of management. The mortality rate in children is under 20%, much lower than in adults. Sepsis, respiratory and cardiac failure, and brain damage are the main causes of death. The ultimate level of renal function depends on the type and severity of the renal damage. Although clinical recovery is apparently complete in many patients with acute intrinsic failure, about half of them have residual renal dysfunction, such as impaired urine concentrating ability or reduced glomerular filtration. In many instances the residual problems may be of little or no clinical consequence. Patients with nonoliguric acute renal failure have fewer complications, have shorter periods of azotemia, require dialysis less frequently, and have lower mortality than those with oliguric acute renal failure.

Day RE, White RHR: Peritoneal dialysis in children. Arch Dis Child 52:56, 1977.
Feldman W, Baliah T, Drummond KN: Intermittent peritoneal dialysis in the management of chronic renal failure in children. Am J Dis Child 116:30, 1968.
Gault MH: Peritoneal dialysis solutions. Can Med Assoc J 108:325, 1972.

16.41 ACUTE RENAL FAILURE IN INFANCY

Approximately 70% of instances of renal failure in the 1st yr of life occur in the 1st wk. The symptoms may not be characteristic of renal failure; rather, they are apt to consist of poor feeding, vomiting, lethargy, and pallor. By far the most common sign of possible renal failure is oliguria (normal urine volume after the 1st 48 hr of life is 3–4 ml/kg/24 hr). Congenital structural anomalies of the kidneys and urinary tract and asphyxia account for approximately 80% of cases of renal failure in the 1st mo of life. Shock, dehydration, sepsis, pyelonephritis, urate nephropathy, or renal vascular disorders account for most of the remaining cases in early infancy. Nonrenal congenital anomalies will be found in over half of the infants.

Causes of acute renal failure in infancy are listed in Table 16–13.

Anderson RJ, Linas SL, Berns AS, et al: Nonoliguric acute renal failure. N Engl J Med 296:1134, 1977.
Cameron JS, Brown C: The investigation and management of acute uremia. In: Hamburger J, Crosnier J, Grunfeld J-P (eds): Nephrology. New York, John Wiley and Sons, 1979.
Chesney RW, Kaplan BS, Freedom RM, et al: Acute renal failure: An important complication of cardiac surgery in infants. J Pediatr 87:381, 1975.
Counahan R, Cameron JS, Ogg CS, et al: Presentation, management, complications, and outcome of acute renal failure in childhood: Five years experience. Br Med J 1:599, 1971.
Dauber IM, Krauss AN, Symchych PS, et al: Renal failure following perinatal anoxia. J Pediatr 88:851, 1976.
Griffin NK, McElnea J, Barratt TM: Acute renal failure in early life. Arch Dis Child 51:459, 1976.
Guignard J-P, Torrado A, Mazouni SM, et al: Renal function in respiratory distress syndrome. J Pediatr 88:845, 1976.
Matthew OP, Jones AS, James E, et al: Neonatal renal failure: Usefulness of diagnostic indices. Pediatrics 65:57, 1980.
Reimold EW, Don TD, Worthen HG: Renal failure during the first year of life. Pediatrics 69:987, 1977.
Rigden S, Barratt TM, et al: Acute renal failure following cardiopulmonary bypass surgery. Arch Dis Child 57:425, 1982.
Schrier RW: Acute renal failure. Kidney Int 15:205, 1979.
Schrier RW, Gardenswartz MJ, Burke TJ: Insuffisance rénale aiguë: Pathogénie, diagnostic et traitement. In: Hamburger J, Crosnier J, Funck-Bretano JL (eds): Actualités néphrologiques de l'Hôpital Necker, 1980. Paris, Flammarion Medecine Sciences, 1980.
Tiller DJ, Mudge GH: Pharmacologic agents used in the management of acute renal failure. Kidney Int 18:700, 1980.
Wilson DM, Turner DR, Cameron JS, et al: Value of renal biopsy in acute intrinsic renal failure. Br Med J 2:459, 1976.

Table 16–13 CAUSES OF ACUTE RENAL FAILURE IN INFANCY

Renovascular accident
   Renal vein thrombosis
   Renal artery thrombosis
Perinatal anoxia
Respiratory distress syndrome
Hemorrhage (maternal antepartum hemorrhage, neonatal hemorrhage)
Septicemia and disseminated intravascular coagulation
Acute pyelonephritis
Hemolytic-uremic syndrome
Congenital obstructive structural abnormality
Renal agenesis
Cardiopulmonary bypass surgery for congenital heart disease

16.42 CHRONIC RENAL FAILURE
(Chronic Uremia)

Chronic renal failure is a complex of clinical, chemical, and metabolic disturbances that result from chronic reduction in renal function, of which the essential feature is a decreased glomerular filtration rate. Clinical problems are usually not evident until the GFR is below 20 ml/min/M²; in preadolescent children with GFR at this level the blood urea nitrogen is usually above 40 mg/dl and the serum creatinine is over 1.6 mg/dl. The normal GFR in children over 1 yr of age is 70 ± 5 (1 S.D.) ml/M²/min.

Etiology. The causes of chronic renal failure in children are diseases of the glomeruli (40%); developmental abnormalities of the kidneys and urinary tract, with or without obstruction (20%); hereditary renal diseases (15%); pyelonephritis with reflux nephropathy (15%); and a miscellaneous group (10%), including vascular disorders of the kidney, hemolytic-uremic syndrome, papillary or cortical necrosis, etc.

Congenital anomalies of the kidney and urinary tract tend to produce signs of chronic renal failure before the age of 5 yr, whereas glomerular and hereditary renal diseases usually lead to its development from 5–15 yr of age. The principal congenital renal and urinary tract abnormalities leading to chronic renal failure are renal hypoplasia, with or without dysplasia, and bilateral severe vesicoureteral reflux, with or without obstruction of the lower tract. Urinary tract abnormalities are about 3 times as common in males as in females. The glomerular disorders leading most frequently to chronic renal failure are membranoproliferative glomerulonephritis, focal and segmental glomerulosclerosis with the nephrotic syndrome, and glomerulopathy in such systemic diseases as anaphylactoid purpura. The hereditary renal disorders which most commonly lead to chronic renal failure in children are nephronophthisis, Alport syndrome, autosomal recessive polycystic renal disease, the renal lesion of Laurence-Moon-Biedl syndrome, cystinosis, oxalosis, and the congenital nephrotic syndrome.

Pathology. The pathologic changes depend on the type of underlying renal disease; these are discussed elsewhere.

Pathophysiology. The GFR may be reduced to about 25% of normal before clinical signs and symptoms appear, and prolonged survival is possible even when the GFR is reduced to about 5% of normal. As destruction proceeds, each surviving nephron responds in an orderly, predictable manner to the increasing requirements for maintaining homeostasis. For solutes which are filtered and partially reabsorbed, there must be a progressive decrease in the fraction of the filtered load which is reabsorbed. For example, when the GFR is normal, only 0.5% or less of filtered sodium is excreted; in contrast, the surviving nephrons of a patient with a GFR of 5 ml/M²/min excrete 20–30% of filtered sodium.

The mechanisms by which modification in tubular function is mediated are not completely understood. The mediator of the increased fractional excretion rate of phosphate is parathyroid hormone. With each decrement in GFR a minimal increment in plasma phosphate concentration leads to a reciprocal decrease in plasma concentration of ionized calcium. This, in turn, induces an increased secretion of parathyroid hormone that returns calcium and phosphate plasma concentrations toward normal by reducing the rate of tubular reabsorption of phosphate and increasing reabsorption of calcium.

These adaptive changes of surviving nephrons permit a remarkably good balance between intake and excretion of water, solutes, and electrolytes. Eventually, the balance becomes precarious, and a further increase in intake may not be accompanied by an equivalent increment in excretion. Fluid, solute, and electrolytes may then accumulate. Moreover, the ability to concentrate the urine to an osmolality much above that of the plasma and to conserve sodium decreases as renal failure progresses. Under these circumstances a *sudden* restriction in intake of fluid or electrolytes may not be followed by a suitable reduction in the excretory rate, with the result that volume contraction may occur. With a *gradual* stepwise reduction in intake of sodium, the surviving nephrons are able to reduce excretion of it to an amount equivalent to the dietary intake. Prolonged administration of diuretics in chronic renal failure may lead to salt depletion and volume contraction.

Excretion of potassium in chronic renal failure is remarkably efficient, and adequate balance between intake and output is usually maintained. Acute K⁺ loads, however, may result in hyperkalemia, as may also such acute catabolic events as bacterial infections or hemolysis; acute metabolic acidosis may accentuate hyperkalemia. Hypokalemia may reflect an inadequate intake of potassium or an excessive loss induced by continuous diuretic therapy.

A sustained metabolic acidosis is usual in chronic renal failure when the GFR is decreased to 15 ml/min/M² or less. The acidosis results from several factors; the principal one is reduction of ammonium excretion to about 50% of normal. There is also impaired excretion of endogenous or dietary acid metabolites because of reduction in the GFR. In order for excretion of acid and regeneration of HCO_3^- to occur, it is necessary for the acid salt to be filtered so that reclamation of $NaHCO_3$ by physiologic tubular mechanisms can take place. Titratable acid may be normal or slightly decreased.

An appropriately acid urine with a pH less than 5.5 is usual in chronic renal failure, even though net urinary acid excretion is less than normal. Rarely, there may be impaired HCO_3^- reabsorption. Since a progressively more acidotic state does not usually develop, some buffering mechanisms must maintain the plasma pH at a level compatible with life, with bone salts, notably calcium bicarbonate, appearing to play a vital role as buffers in this regard. The plasma HCO_3^- usually stabilizes at 18–20 mEq/l.

Profound changes in calcium and phosphorus homeostasis occur in chronic renal failure. As noted above, systemic acidosis leads to leaching of bone salts to be used as buffers. Secondary hyperparathyroidism also results in excessive reabsorption of bone. Calcium absorption from the small intestine is decreased, principally as the result of marked reduction in renal production of 1,25(OH)$_2$-cholecalciferol, which normally stimulates gut calcium absorption. This contributes to the secondary hyperparathyroidism.

This complex disturbance in calcium, phosphorus, and bone metabolism is expressed principally as growth arrest or retardation, hypocalcemia, hyperphosphatemia, and hyperparathyroid bone disease. The bony changes are referred to as **renal osteodystrophy** (Sec 23.32).

A moderate to severe **normochromic anemia** is common; its causes include depression of erythropoiesis by uremic toxins, decreased erythropoietin production, shortened red blood cell survival time, blood loss, and defective utilization of iron.

Abnormalities in the coagulation system include decreased platelet adhesiveness, reduced activation of platelet factor 3, and prolongation of the bleeding time.

The causes of **delayed growth and sexual maturation** are poorly understood; renal osteodystrophy, chronic acidosis, inadequate caloric intake, chronic anemia, sodium loss, and recurrent infections may all be factors, as may inhibitors of somatomedin action.

Neurologic manifestations may appear as renal failure advances. These include impaired ability to concentrate, neuromuscular irritability, cramps, seizures, and vomiting. The pathogenesis of these alterations is believed to be related to accumulation of uremic toxins such as guanidinosuccinic acid, phenolic compounds, methyl guanidine, and other metabolites such as urea and uric acid. Parathyroid hormone is probably a major uremic toxin; its level is markedly elevated in chronic renal failure. It is believed to be partly responsible for the nervous system disturbances, pruritus, skin lesions, anemia, and sexual dysfunction which may occur. Disturbances in water and electrolyte balance and altered calcium ion concentration may also play a role. Sudden reduction in the concentrations of some of these compounds following hemodialysis may precipitate confusion and seizures in uremic patients. Severe hypertension may be a factor in uremic encephalopathy.

Peripheral sensory and motor neuropathy may develop in longstanding cases; demyelination of the distal peripheral nerves has been observed.

The kidney normally has a role in degradation of the hormone *gastrin;* in uremic or anephric patients, elevated plasma gastrin levels may lead to gastric hypersecretion and peptic ulceration.

The principal **disturbance in carbohydrate metabolism** is an elevation in peak blood glucose level following an oral glucose load and a delayed return to the fasting level, probably due to peripheral antagonism to the action of insulin. Decreased catabolism of glucagon also occurs in uremia and contributes to hyperglycemia.

Progressive reduction in the glomerular filtration rate leads to depression of both cellular and humoral immunity.

Clinical Manifestations and Course. The discussion here will be confined to the features of chronic renal failure; manifestations of the underlying disease must also be taken into account in management of the patient.

The onset is usually gradual; initial complaints, often vague or nonspecific, include lassitude, fatigue, headache, anorexia, and nausea. More specific symptoms are polyuria, nocturia, polydipsia, mild facial puffiness, bone or joint pain, growth retardation, dryness or itchiness of the skin, muscle cramps, paresthesias, and signs of sensory or motor neuropathy.

As chronic renal failure advances, there may be vomiting, diarrhea (sometimes bloody), confusion, easy bruising, edema, and a declining volume of urine. Hypertension, acidosis, fluid retention, and anemia may produce symptoms of cardiac failure and circulatory congestion (tachypnea, shortness of breath, and tenderness of the liver and abdomen). Headache is common; seizures may occur.

Physical findings vary with the severity or stage: pallor and a sallow, brownish complexion; growth retardation; muscle weakness and wasting; edema; dry or bruised skin with scratch marks from pruritus; systolic and diastolic hypertension; signs of circulatory overload (such as pulmonary edema, tachycardia, tachypnea, jugulovenous distention, cardiomegaly, gallop rhythm and an ejection systolic murmur); bony deformity with or without tenderness resulting from renal osteodystrophy; characteristic uremic breath; coated tongue; signs of neuropathy, such as loss of deep tendon reflexes, of sensation, or of muscular strength; and uremic retinopathy with exudates, vascular narrowing, and possibly hemorrhages.

The course depends principally on the nature of the underlying disease, which may lead to progressive, inexorable nephron destruction over a relatively short period (several mo–1 yr) or may cause a stable reduction in renal function which does not progress and may be compatible with an indefinite period of relatively good health. When chronic renal failure develops in infancy, impairment of growth will be much more profound than when it occurs in a previously healthy teenager; the medical management is also more difficult in the younger child.

Laboratory Data. The essential features are a reduction in GFR as shown by decreased inulin, iothalamate, or creatinine clearance and elevation of the blood urea nitrogen and serum creatinine concentrations. The extent of reduction in GFR is the major determinant of the severity of other abnormal changes such as hyperphosphatemia, hypocalcemia, hyperuricemia, metabolic acidosis, hyperkalemia, hypoproteinemia, normochromic anemia, reduced platelet-adhesiveness, prolonged bleeding time, and isosthenuria. Depending on the cause of chronic renal failure, there may be renal salt wasting, proteinuria, and/or an abnormal urinary sediment.

Roentgenographic examination of the chest may show cardiomegaly, aortic dilatation, left ventricular hypertrophy, pulmonary edema, and pleural effusion. Renal osteodystrophy (Sec 23.32) is most pronounced at areas of rapid growth (upper humerus, knees, wrists, and lateral aspect of the clavicle). The changes include demineralization, coarsened trabeculation, patchy erosion, thinning or loss of cortex owing to secondary hyperparathyroidism, rickets or osteomalacia, osteitis fibrosa, retarded bone age, foci of osteosclerosis, and, in advanced cases, actual bone deformity, particularly at sites of weight-bearing such as at the hips and knees.

Subperiosteal erosion of the edges of the distal phalanges of the index and middle fingers are indicators of hyperparathyroidism in uremia.

Diagnosis and Differential Diagnosis. It is essential, if possible, to establish the nature of the underlying disease leading to chronic renal failure. Conditions that may aggravate chronic renal insufficiency include congestive heart failure; uncontrolled hypertension; hypovolemia resulting from gastrointestinal or urinary losses related to diuretic therapy or impaired ability to conserve fluid and electrolytes in the face of inadequate intake; infection of the urinary tract; obstruction by calculi, stomal closure, or uric acid nephropathy; disturbances in plasma electrolytes (e.g., hypercalcemia or hypokalemia) which impair renal function; and nephrotoxicity of drugs or other exogenous agents (discussed elsewhere in this chapter).

Prevention. With early diagnosis and proper therapy, a high proportion of children with chronic renal failure need never reach the stage of advanced renal insufficiency that requires hemodialysis and renal transplantation to prolong life. To this end the following must be considered: proper antibacterial agents for treatment of urinary tract infection; avoidance or cessation of use of nephrotoxic drugs; use of corticosteroid or cytotoxic drugs in specific glomerular diseases; prevention and treatment of nephrocalcinosis or urolithiasis in renal tubular acidosis, hyperuricemia, and cystinuria; diagnosis and treatment of obstructive uropathy; and control of hypertension.

Treatment. Management of chronic renal failure demands not only an understanding of the complex physiologic disturbances and skills in diagnosis and treatment but also an awareness of the tremendous impact that chronic progressive renal disease has on the patient and the family. Nurse, social worker, dietitian, teacher, and psychiatrist can help to provide the assistance and guidance that may be needed to deal effectively with these problems. Specific treatments for individual conditions which may lead to chronic renal failure are discussed elsewhere. The following features are applicable to most patients regardless of the underlying disorder:

Provision of the caloric and nutritional requirements of the child with chronic renal failure is a major problem. When there is severe impairment of renal function, the child's appetite is poor, nausea and other gastrointestinal complaints are common, and constraints on the dietary intake of fluid, phosphorus, electrolytes, and nitrogen are imposed by the kidney's impaired excretory ability. Phosphorus is the principal substance which must be restricted; its retention is one of the crucial factors in the pathogenesis of renal osteodystrophy. Decreasing the dietary intake of phosphorus requires restriction of milk and other sources of protein though these are important for good nutrition. When the GFR falls to 15 ml/min/M² or less, the serum phosphorus level usually begins to rise, and restriction of dietary phosphorus to 200–500 mg/24 hr and the administration of oral aluminum hydroxide gel* (1 or 2 tablets

or the equivalent in liquid form with each meal) may be necessary to keep the plasma phosphorus level below 6 mg/dl. When the blood urea nitrogen level is above 70–80 mg/dl, the child's appetite for nitrogen-containing foods often declines. Consequently, the diet often is a compromise between what the child will eat and what is optimal in light of the altered pathophysiology. An attempt should be made to supply an adequate caloric intake for growth and to give high quality protein such as that in eggs or calves' liver.

Restriction of milk to decrease phosphorus intake results in reduction of calcium intake. A calcium supplement of approximately 1 gm of calcium/24 hr should be given as a calcium salt in a syrup.* Supplementation with vitamin D or 1 of its analogues is also necessary, the usual requirement being 2000–25,000 units of vitamin D (calciferol)/24 hr. This should be introduced gradually to avoid hypercalcemia. Dihydrotachysterol in a dose of 0.05–0.15 mg/24 hr may be used instead of vitamin D. Some prefer to use 1α-OH-cholecalciferol (30–100 μg/kg/24 hr) or 1,25(OH)₂-cholecalciferol. A normal intake of other vitamins and minerals should be assured.

Sodium, Potassium, Water, and Acid-Base Balance. In the absence of salt wasting, edema, or an abnormal plasma concentration of sodium it is usually not necessary to modify the intake of sodium or water. In general, the thirst mechanism regulates intake of water satisfactorily, and the child's usual intake of salt should be permitted. Vigorous restriction of sodium, particularly during continuous diuretic therapy, can cause extracellular volume contraction and a further decline in GFR. In nephronophthisis excessive obligatory urinary excretion of salt is common so that the intake must be compensatorily high, sometimes 15–20 gm/24 hr.

When edema is present, it is necessary to restrict the intake of sodium, even to as low as 15–20 mEq/24 hr. A low plasma concentration of albumin may contribute to salt and water retention. Congestive cardiac failure due to longstanding hypertension, fluid overload, and anemia can accentuate fluid retention; control of hypertension, diuretic therapy, transfusion with washed, packed red blood cells, and digitalization may be indicated.

In advanced *uremia* the ability to dilute urine may be impaired, and hyponatremia may develop from excessive intake of water. Refractory edema with or without hyponatremia can develop despite restriction of sodium and fluid intake. In such circumstances the use of furosemide either orally or intravenously in a dose of 1–2 mg/kg/24 hr may be helpful; *this drug is potentially ototoxic.* Peritoneal dialysis and hemodialysis are effective in removing edema fluid if other measures fail; they are particularly helpful with circulatory congestion and congestive cardiac failure.

The capacity to excrete potassium remains remarkably adequate, even when renal function is severely reduced. Unless the urinary volume is decreased to the extent that fluid is retained or unless the plasma potas-

---

*Aluminum hydroxide–dimethylpolysiloxane compound tablets (Amphojel 65), Wyeth International, PO Box 8616, Philadelphia, Pa. 19101.

*Calcium Sandoz Syrup, now marketed as Neo-Calgucon Syrup, Dorsey Laboratories, Division of Sandoz Inc., Lincoln, Neb. 68501.

sium is above 7.0 mEq/l with accompanying electrocardiographic changes of hyperkalemia, it is generally not necessary to reduce the intake of potassium. Chronic hyperkalemia can usually be tolerated in chronic renal failure; sudden elevations in the concentration of plasma K^+, however, may result in life-threatening hyperkalemia.

Long-term diuretic or antihypertensive therapy with furosemide or hydrochlorothiazide can cause potassium depletion and chronic hypokalemia. Hypokalemia may also contribute to digitalis toxicity; nausea and vomiting in such a situation may be mistaken for symptoms of chronic renal failure.

Sodium bicarbonate or citrate, in a dose to supply the equivalent of 1–3 mEq/kg/24 hr of bicarbonate and given in 3–4 divided doses, may be used to treat *metabolic acidosis*. It is not desirable to attempt complete correction of the plasma base deficit; a plasma bicarbonate level of 18–20 mEq/l is acceptable when the GFR is 15 ml/min/M^2 or less. Severe metabolic acidosis may require dialysis. Reduction of plasma potassium concentration during dialysis may aggravate digitalis toxicity, and rapid correction of acidosis may precipitate tetany in a hypocalcemic patient.

Hypertension, Cardiac Failure, and Circulatory Congestion. An attempt should be made to maintain the *blood pressure* within the normal range, but at times an elevation of 10–15 mm Hg in diastolic pressure may have to be accepted. Conservative measures using standard antihypertensive agents with or without sodium restriction, depending on whether there is edema, are usually successful. Hydrochlorothiazide in combination with hydralazine should be used as initial therapy; propranolol is also a useful drug in combination with hydrochlorothiazide and/or hydralazine. Other antihypertensive drugs include captopril, prazosin, labetalol, and minoxidil. Strict restriction of sodium may be necessary in oliguric hypertensive patients. (See also discussions of acute renal failure and acute nephritis.)

Emergency treatment of hypertensive crises with encephalopathy, pulmonary edema, or cardiac failure consists of the administration of diazoxide, labetalol, hydralazine, or methyldopa intravenously (as outlined in the section on acute poststreptococcal glomerulonephritis) and parenteral administration of furosemide.

Cardiac failure requires skillful balancing of several types of therapy, including (1) reduction of blood pressure to normal; (2) increasing the hemoglobin concentration to 8–9 gm slowly by small transfusions of washed, packed red blood cells; (3) decreasing circulatory congestion by restriction of salt and fluids and the use of diuretics such as furosemide; and (4) judicious use of digoxin. Since digoxin is excreted largely by the kidney, the dose must be reduced in chronic renal failure. The digitalizing dose should be about half the usual amount; the maintenance dose is reduced to about one quarter and should be given at extended intervals, such as every 2nd or 3rd day. Digitalis is not dialyzable, and care must be taken to avoid digitalis toxicity. When cardiac failure becomes life threatening and is not amenable to conservative measures, consideration must be given to peritoneal dialysis or hemodialysis.

Circulatory congestion is best treated by rigid restriction of intake of sodium and fluids and by oral or parenteral administration of furosemide. Hypertension, cardiac decompensation, and circulatory congestion are interrelated, as are the measures used in their treatment. Improvement achieved in 1 of these circulatory problems by a single intervention is often accompanied by improvement in the others.

Renal Osteodystrophy. The principal measures for prevention and treatment are restriction of dietary phosphorus; administration of aluminum hydroxide gel to bind phosphorus in the intestine; provision of supplemental calcium; provision of vitamin D, dihydrotachysterol, 1α-OH-cholecalciferol, or 1,25$(OH)_2$-cholecalciferol; control of metabolic acidosis; and provision of a nutritious diet (Sec 23.32).

Radical measures such as parathyroidectomy to treat hyperparathyroid bone disease are seldom required. If the plasma phosphorus is elevated, calcium supplementation and vitamin D should be used judiciously so that a gradual elevation of plasma calcium to normal is achieved. Hypercalcemia and metastatic calcification should be considered potential complications when vitamin D and calcium supplements are given to uremic patients.

Anemia. It is unwise to attempt to keep the hemoglobin at normal levels by transfusions. If the level falls below 6 gm/dl, the danger of cardiac decompensation makes it reasonable to give small (20–75 ml) transfusions of fresh packed, washed red blood cells to raise the hemoglobin to 7–8 gm/dl. Caution should be exercised to avoid circulatory overload during the transfusion; it is sometimes necessary to withdraw an equivalent volume of blood from the patient.

A normal intake of dietary iron should be assured to avoid iron deficiency. Erythropoiesis may be improved by treatment of infections, by proper nutrition, and by regular dialysis.

Drug Dosage in Chronic Renal Failure. If the dosage of drugs excreted by the kidneys is not reduced or the intervals between administrations of them lengthened during impaired renal function, retention of them or their metabolites may result in high blood and tissue concentrations that may have deleterious effects. Should the drug be potentially nephrotoxic, the risk of increasing the degree of renal insufficiency is extremely serious. The complex question of drug dosage cannot be completely covered here. Table 16–14 lists drugs used in children that are excreted principally by the kidney; the dosages and the intervals of their administration must be modified in chronic renal failure. Table 16–15 lists drugs the dosage of which does not need to be modified in children with renal failure. Methods for determining drug dosage in relation to renal failure are to measure the rate of disappearance from the plasma following a single dose and thus establish the half-life of the drug or to determine the plasma concentration in order to know whether a safe and therapeutic level is present. For most drugs, however, this is not practicable, and modification in dosage is based on an "educated guess" which takes into account the degree of renal failure, the extent to which the drug is normally

Table 16–14 DRUGS THAT REQUIRE MODIFIED DOSAGE IN CHILDREN WITH RENAL FAILURE

Antibacterial and antifungal drugs

Aminoglycosides
 Amikacin
 Amphotericin B*
 Gentamicin*
 Kanamycin*
 Tobramycin

Antituberculous drugs
 Aminosalicylic acid†
 Ethambutol
 Isoniazid
 Streptomycin

Cephalosporins
 Cephalexin
 Cephalothin*
 Colistimethate*
 5-Fluorocytosine
 Lincomycin
 Nitrofurantoin†

Penicillins*
 Amoxicillin
 Ampicillin
 Penicillin G

Miscellaneous
 Pentamidine
 Polymyxin B*
 Sulfonamides*
 Tetracycline
 Vancomycin

Sedative, anticonvulsant, and analgesic drugs

Acetaminophen†
Aspirin
Phenobarbital
Phenothiazines
Phenylbutazone*†
Primidone
Trimethadione*

Antihypertensive, cardiovascular, and diuretic drugs

Acetazolamide†
Digitoxin
Digoxin
Ethacrynic acid†
Guanethidine
Mercurials*†
Methyldopa
Quinidine
Spironolactone†
Thiazides†
Triamterene†

Miscellaneous drugs

Allopurinol*
Aminocaproic acid†
Azathioprine
Chlorpropamide†
Gold salts*†
Insulin
Lithium salts
6-Mercaptopurine
Methotrexate
Penicillamine*
Propylthiouracil

*Potentially nephrotoxic.
†Should be avoided or used with great care when the GFR is below 15 ml/M²/24 hr.

Table 16–15 DRUGS NOT REQUIRING MODIFIED DOSAGE IN CHILDREN WITH RENAL FAILURE

Antibacterial drugs

Chloramphenicol
Clindamycin
Cloxacillin
Erythromycin
Oxacillin
Rifampin

Antihypertensive and cardiovascular drugs

Beta blockers
Clonidine
Diazoxide
Furosemide
Hydralazine
Lidocaine
Minoxidil

Miscellaneous drugs

Codeine
Corticosteroids
Heparin
Indomethacin
Morphine
Pentobarbital
Phenothiazines
Theophylline
Tricyclic antidepressants
Tubocurarine
Warfarin

excreted by the kidney, the potential toxicity of the drug if elevated levels are inadvertently reached, and clinical observations that suggest drug toxicity.

The modification of gentamicin dosage in chronic renal failure can be cited as an example since this drug is used frequently and is potentially both ototoxic and nephrotoxic. The risk depends on the total dose of gentamicin and on whether there is simultaneous administration of a diuretic such as furosemide. In normal individuals the half-life of gentamicin is 2 hr; peak serum levels are obtained sooner with intravenous than with intramuscular injection, and the volume of distribution is equivalent to that of the extracellular fluid (about 15% of the body weight); an unknown amount is bound to serum proteins. Gentamicin is cleared by glomerular filtration, and little is reabsorbed or secreted in the tubule. The therapeutic range is 2.5–

10 µg/ml in the serum. Ototoxicity is associated with high peak serum levels: in excess of 20 µg/ml 5 min after intravenous injection, or sustained serum levels above 10 µg/ml. The half-life of gentamicin in uremia may be as long as 48 hr. Nomograms have been developed to calculate gentamicin doses in uremia, but they are less helpful than direct measurement of serum levels. The principles that should govern gentamicin usage in patients with renal failure are as follows: (1) use the normal loading dose; (2) the peak serum concentration of the drug should be measured 5 min after the drug has been infused; (3) if the level is not satisfactory, the dose can be adjusted as shown in Table 16–16; and (4) gentamicin is cleared by peritoneal dialysis and hemodialysis, and the dose may have to be adjusted in patients who are being dialyzed.

Peritoneal dialysis, hemodialysis, and renal transplantation are effective forms of therapy for children with advanced renal failure. The indications for them have changed dramatically in recent years; it is inevitable that they will continue to change in response to advances in technology, availability of dialysis and transplantation facilities, and developments in transplantation biology. End-stage renal failure requiring dialysis or transplantation develops in 2–3.5 children/million population/yr. In children the problems encountered differ from those of adults and involve psycho-

Table 16–16 MODIFICATION OF GENTAMICIN ADMINISTRATION IN RENAL FAILURE

DEGREE OF RENAL FAILURE	NORMAL	MILD	MODERATE	SEVERE
Glomerular filtration rate (ml/min)	Normal	50–80	10–50	<10
Maintenance dose intervals	q 8 hr	q 8–12 hr	q 12–24 hr	q 48 hr

social and emotional development, physical growth, and technical difficulties related to the comparably smaller size of the child.

The decision to begin chronic dialysis or to perform transplantation should be made after careful consideration of the total constellation of problems presented by the child and the family. Ideally, decisions concerning these procedures should be made in consultation with a pediatric nephrologist and carried out in a center with all the necessary laboratory facilities and qualified allied professional personnel. Dialysis and transplantation should be considered when the conservative measures detailed above are no longer effective. The principal indicators of need for consideration are growth arrest; severe renal osteodystrophy; cardiovascular, circulatory, fluid, and acid-base disturbances; malnutrition and inadequate caloric intake; and inability to carry out the normal activities essential for emotional well-being and development. Indications for institution of dialysis include plasma creatinine levels over 10 mg/dl in older children, or over 4–5 mg/dl in children under 2 yr old. Clinical indications, however, supersede laboratory values, and it is wise to initiate dialysis before complications of uremia develop.

Hemodialysis in children is usually a means of sustaining the patient in preparation for renal transplantation and not generally recommended as definitive treatment, but it is being used in hospital or at home by several centers for long-term management of some children with chronic renal failure, and ambulatory peritoneal dialysis in the home is being increasingly widely used. Technical improvements permit hemodialysis to be done even in infants. Acute complications of hemodialysis include hypotension, muscle cramps, nausea, headache, and hypertension; long-term complications are anemia, neurologic effects, pericarditis, growth retardation, osteodystrophy, and potentially severe psychosocial problems. Dialysis does not adequately ameliorate the delays in growth and sexual development associated with chronic renal failure. Catch-up growth is seldom seen.

Renal transplantation must now be regarded as the preferred form of treatment for many children with chronic renal failure. Many are returned to satisfactory health by this procedure. A remarkable surge in emotional and intellectual development is not uncommon in patients previously managed conservatively or by dialysis. Patients whose weight is over 10 kg may be considered for transplantation.

The original kidney disease may recur in the transplanted kidney, but often there are few important clinical consequences, and the graft may survive and function adequately for a prolonged period. Possible recurrence of the disease in the graft does not contribute an important contraindication to renal transplantation in most instances. Five yr survivals following living donor and cadaver donor grafts should now be over 85% and 75%, respectively. Many children have had successful 2nd renal transplants after failure of the 1st graft. Complications of transplantation include hyperacute, acute, or chronic rejections, growth retardation, infections, hypertension, and psychologic problems. The quality of life of patients with well-functioning grafts may, however, be excellent.

Prognosis. The prognosis for children with chronic renal failure has improved dramatically; few children need die of uremia at this time. In a significant proportion of affected children, however, the physical and emotional goal of complete rehabilitation is still not achieved.

Anderson RJ, Gambertoglio JG, Schrier RW: Clinical Use of Drugs in Renal Failure. Springfield, Ill., Charles C Thomas, 1976.
Bennett WM, Muther RS, Parker RA, et al: Drug therapy in renal failure: Dosing guidelines for adults. Ann Int Med 93:62, 1980.
Bricker NS: On the meaning of the intact nephron hypothesis. Am J Med 46:1, 1969.
Bricker NS, Fine LG: The trade-off hypothesis. Current status. Kidney Int 13:S-5, 1978.
Bricker NS, Fine LG, Kaplan M, et al: "Magnification phenomenon" in chronic renal disease. N Engl J Med 299:1287, 1978.
Byron PR, Mallick NP, Taylor G: Immune potential in human uraemia. 1. Relationship of glomerular filtration rate to depression of immune potential. J Clin Pathol 29:765, 1976.
Chantler C, Carter JE, Bewick M, et al: 10 years' experience with regular hemodialysis and renal transplantation. Arch Dis Child 55:435, 1980.
Cleigh JS: Drug administration in renal failure. Am J Med 62:555, 1977.
Danovitch GM, Bourgoignie J, Bricker NS: Reversibility of the "salt-losing" tendency of chronic renal failure. N Engl J Med 296:14, 1977.
DeFronzo RA, Andres R, Edgar P, et al: Carbohydrate metabolism in uremia: A review. Medicine 52:469, 1973.
Holliday MA: Calorie deficiency in children with uremia: Effect upon growth. Pediatrics 50:590, 1972.
Lloyd-Mostyn RH, Lord IJ: Ototoxicity of intravenous furosemide. Lancet 2:1156, 1971.
Massry SG, Goldstein DA: The search for uremic toxin(s) "X"; X-PTH. Clin Nephrol 11:181, 1979.
Mauer SM, Shideman JR, Buselmeier TJ, et al: Long term hemodialysis in the neonatal period. Am J Dis Child 125:369, 1973.
Potter DE, Holliday MA, Piel CF, et al: Treatment of end stage renal disease in children—a 15 yr experience. Kidney Int 18:103, 1980.
Rubin AL, Stenzel KH, Reidenberg MM: Symposium on drug action and metabolism in renal failure. Am J Med 62:459, 1977.
Slatopolsky E, Bricker NS: The role of phosphorus restriction in the prevention of secondary hyperparathyroidism in chronic renal failure. Kidney Int 4:141, 1973.

16.43 Infection of the Urinary Tract

Though it might be useful to classify bacterial infections of the urinary tract on the basis of the areas involved, e.g., the bladder (cystitis) or the kidney (pyelonephritis), it is usually impossible in children to establish whether infection is confined to upper, lower, or both areas of the tract.

In the early 1960's 2 observations led to concern that infections of the urinary tract constituted a major unrecognized health hazard: the discovery of clinically unrecognized chronic pyelonephritis in 2–20% of un-

selected autopsies and the detection of asymptomatic bacteriuria in about 6% of adult women and in 1–2% of apparently healthy female children. These 2 observations were interpreted as causally related and led to unnecessarily aggressive medical, urologic, and radiologic approaches to the diagnosis and treatment of urinary tract infection in children in an attempt to prevent a presumed gradual but relentless development of renal insufficiency.

The past 2 decades have altered the perspective; it is

now assumed that only very few children who have a urinary tract infection have a serious, potentially permanent or life-threatening problem and that surgical procedures are probably indicated for only a relatively small number of them, i.e., those who have repeated infections associated with *gross structural abnormalities of the urinary tract which are amenable to surgical correction.*

Etiology. The susceptibility of the urinary tract to infection by organisms which are not ordinarily pathogenic is poorly understood. The bacteria are predominantly coliform bacilli. *E. coli* is the most common species; *Proteus* accounts for about 30% of infections in boys but only 10–15% in girls. Anaerobic and CO_2-dependent organisms are increasingly recognized. Other organisms usually considered not pathogenic such as *Staphylococcus epidermidis* may also be responsible. The bacterial source is generally the patient's fecal flora. Congenital structural anomalies of the urinary tract, particularly those that obstruct the flow of urine, predispose to urinary tract infection. Other predisposing factors are foreign bodies, indwelling urethral catheters, nephrolithiasis, and, possibly, constipation. Most urinary tract infections, however, are not related to a primary structural or functional abnormality. On the other hand, some anatomic or functional abnormalities, such as thickening of the bladder wall, vesicoureteral reflux, or an abnormal voiding pattern, are apt to be sequelae of infection. The consistently higher incidence in girls beyond infancy may result from the short female urethra; the usual route of infection is an ascending one from external genitalia. There is no substantial evidence that poor perineal hygiene predisposes girls to urinary infection. In infants urinary tract infection is hematogenous.

Incidence. In girls this is 10 times that in boys except in infancy, when the ratio is about equal. In infancy congenital structural anomalies of the urinary tract probably account in part for the higher incidence in boys. Screening programs in apparently healthy schoolchildren show that at any given time from 1–2% of girls have an active urinary tract infection which is usually asymptomatic. About 5% or more have at least 1 such infection prior to maturity.

Pathogenesis and Pathology. There is little understanding of the factors which enable bacteria to establish a foothold and initiate an actual infection. It is possible that unrecognized host factors enhance bacterial colonization in some children and not in others.

In acute uncomplicated infection the principal inflammatory changes are usually confined to the bladder (cystitis), where they may be responsible for urinary urgency and frequency. Rarely, hemorrhage into inflamed areas may lead to passage of bloody urine.

Recurrent infection of the bladder may cause inflammatory changes which distort the normal anatomic relationships of the ureter as it traverses the bladder wall, leading to incompetence of the vesicoureteral valve. This may permit reflux of urine into the ureter, especially during voiding, with subsequent ureteral dilatation and access of organisms to the upper tract. Infection of the kidney—pyelitis or pyelonephritis—may then develop. Infection of renal parenchyma may also be introduced hematogenously; this is a more common route in infants in association with septicemia. Inflammation causes irritability and spasm of smooth muscle and is responsible for urinary urgency and frequency. Infection of the renal medulla may interfere with the mechanisms for concentration of urine and result in polyuria.

Infection of the upper collecting system and kidney is much less common than that of the lower urinary tract and is usually acquired via the collecting system. Acute and chronic inflammatory changes in the pelvis and medulla develop. Calyceal blunting results from parenchymal infection, principally in patients with reflux of infected urine to the kidney. Intrarenal reflux (i.e., the extension of vesicoureteral reflux from the calyces into the collecting ducts and nephrons) appears to be the route by which organisms are directly introduced into the kidney. Scarring and loss of renal tissue result. These changes are asymmetrical. If there are recurrent or chronic episodes of renal infection, the kidney contracts. Foci of acute and chronic inflammatory cells are seen in the interstitium, and with time there is an increase in fibrous tissue. In acute fulminating pyelonephritis the kidney is swollen and edematous, and there is a diffuse interstitial infiltrate of polymorphonuclear cells. The development of parenchymal scars in association with reflux appears to occur principally in children under 5 yr of age.

Clinical Manifestations and Course. A large proportion of children with active urinary tract infection are essentially asymptomatic; when there are complaints, they may or may not be related to the urinary system.

Urgency, frequency, dysuria, dribbling, nocturnal enuresis or daytime incontinence in a previously dry child, and foul-smelling urine are common presenting complaints. Fever, irritability, abdominal pain, loss of appetite or vomiting, inflammation of the mucous membrane of the external genitalia, and hematuria are not uncommon. Infants may have unexplained jaundice or lethargy or appear septic. High fever, chills, flank pain, and leukocytosis suggest *acute pyelonephritis*. Examination may reveal an enlarged, very tender kidney, and acute renal failure may be a presenting feature.

If untreated, the clinical features often subside within several wk; the infection, however, can persist, and clinical recurrences are common. In the absence of structural abnormalities or marked vesicoureteral reflux, recurrent or chronic infections over a period of years do not usually result in serious renal or ureteral damage.

Laboratory Data. The diagnosis of urinary tract infection rests primarily on the detection of bacteriuria. Numerous leukocytes may also be found; white cell casts suggest the diagnosis of pyelonephritis.

Urine Collection. The external genitalia may harbor bacteria, feces, vaginal secretions containing pus and epithelial cells, and, in uncircumcised males, debris under the foreskin; accordingly, a randomly voided urine often contains bacteria, cells, and other material not present in bladder urine. To avoid contamination, it is important that the external genitalia be cleansed and, whenever possible, a midstream specimen obtained. This is desirable in collection of urine for routine urinalysis but essential when the urine is to be cultured. Sterile cotton balls soaked in a nonirritating antiseptic solution such as aqueous benzalkonium chloride 1:1000 may be used to cleanse the genitalia. With sterile precautions the labia should be separated and the vulva wiped gently from front to back with 3–4 separate antiseptic-soaked cotton balls. The antiseptic solution should be rinsed off with sterile water. In boys the foreskin should be retracted and the glans and prepuce thoroughly cleansed and then rinsed. The genitalia should then be dried with sterile absorbent gauze or cotton. The child is then asked to void into a sterile container, from which urine for culture and urinalysis can be taken. In infants a sterile urine collection bag may be attached to the penis or vulva following cleansing; it is important that frequent checks be made to determine when voiding has occurred and to avoid fecal contamination. The mother can be of help in this task.

Despite the most diligent attempts some contamination of the urine commonly occurs; it is essential that the specimen obtained for quantitative bacterial culture be plated immediately or in less than half an hour. If this is not possible, the specimen should be refrigerated at 4° C to inhibit multiplication of contaminating bacteria which could lead to a falsely positive culture. The specimen for culture can be kept at this temperature for 24 hr and then plated without danger of spurious results.

When it is not feasible to obtain a clean voided urine specimen, urine may be obtained under sterile conditions by urethral catheterization or by direct aspiration of the bladder. The latter technique has been used extensively in infants because the bladder is not as low in the pelvis as it is later and because it is more difficult to obtain noncontaminated voided specimens. The technique is simple and should be done after the baby has not voided for 1–2 hr to ensure that the bladder contains urine. Unless the bladder is palpable, the procedure should be deferred. The infant is placed on a flat, firm surface. An assistant should stand opposite the operator and immobilize the infant by grasping the lower thorax in 1 hand and the thighs and hips with the other. A 10 ml syringe is used with a 22 gauge, 38 mm (1.5 in) long needle. The skin is cleansed with an antiseptic solution, and the needle is inserted in the midline 1–2 cm above the symphysis pubis; the angle of the syringe is slightly downward, 10–20° from perpendicular. A steady motion is used as the needle is inserted until a change in resistance is felt as the bladder is entered. Gentle suction is then applied to aspirate the urine specimen. The procedure should be done quite rapidly before spontaneous voiding stimulated by the procedure occurs. Aspiration should be limited to 1 attempt. Though this technique is widely used and is generally safe, it is not entirely without risk; bladder hemorrhage and perforations of other intra-abdominal structures have occurred. Normal bladder urine is sterile.

Urinalysis. Infected urine often has a strong coliform odor. The urine may be faintly clouded, because of the presence of numerous pus cells, or it may have a reddish color if blood is present. The protein concentration is usually less than 100 mg/dl. Alkaline urine suggests the presence of such organisms as *Proteus* species, which split urea and thus lead to the formation of ammonia.

Microscopic examination of the urinary sediment after centrifugation usually shows numerous pus cells and, less frequently, red blood cells. An active urinary tract infection can be present without pus cells in the urine; conversely, the presence of pus cells does not necessarily indicate urinary tract infection. For example, pyuria may occur during a febrile illness or with dehydration, and numerous pus cells are often seen in the urine in acute poststreptococcal glomerulonephritis. Innumerable bacteria per high power field are commonly seen in the unstained urine specimen; this finding correlates well with urine bacterial colony counts over 100,000/ml and may, in the absence of bacteriologic culture data, permit a tentative diagnosis of urinary tract infection.

Bacteriologic Studies. The importance is stressed of obtaining a suitable specimen of urine and culturing it immediately or refrigerating it for later culture. Measurement of the number of bacterial colonies in a known volume of urine is of value in differentiating between infection and bacterial contamination of cleanly voided specimens. Infected urine usually contains over 100,000 colonies/ml, contaminated urine under 10,000. When there is urinary tract infection, a single organism is normally found, whereas it is not uncommon to find 2 or more different species in contaminated urine.

When the results of a single colony count are equivocal (e.g., the number of colonies is between 10,000–100,000/ml), the study should be repeated. Falsely positive colony counts may be due to a variety of causes, which include bacterial contamination from the external genitalia, delay between urine collection and plating, or keeping the urine at a temperature that permits contaminating bacteria to multiply. Falsely low colony counts in the presence of infection may occur when the urine is dilute or very acid, when the specimen is contaminated with the cleansing antiseptic, or when the patient is receiving antibacterial therapy. Also, when the infection is chronic or indolent, the colony count may be less than 100,000/ml. When the child is voiding frequently, bacterial multiplication in the bladder is limited; for this reason the 1st morning specimen voided is most suitable for colony count.

Use of an agar-coated slide that can be dipped in the freshly voided urine has gained wide acceptance. It is particularly useful in the pediatrician's office. The number of bacterial colonies on the dip slide after incubation for 24 hr can be estimated by comparison with standard charts; the results correlate closely with colony counts performed in the laboratory. When there is a significant count, a culture of the organism can be taken from the dip slide for identification and for antibiotic sensitivity studies. This technique also has value in screening programs for urinary tract infection and in monitoring patients with recurrent infection. Another simple test that may be used to detect bacterial infection and to monitor relapses or recurrences is a plastic dipstick* containing 3 reagent pads: 1 for immediate recognition

---

*Microstix, Ames Company, Division of Miles Laboratories, Inc., Elkhart, Ind.

of nitrite in the urine; a 2nd for quantitating the gram-negative bacterial count; and a 3rd for quantitating both gram-negative and gram-positive bacterial counts. This test yields only 1.6% falsely positive results and detects approximately 90% of positive cultures. (See also Sec 16.3.)

Various means have been used to differentiate upper from lower urinary tract infection (pyelonephritis from cystitis). Though symptomatology may be of some help, the most reliable basis is a satisfactory roentgenographic study. Elevation in antibody titer to the infecting organism is said to be more common in pyelonephritis than in cystitis, as is the finding of antibody-coated bacteria in the urine, but these tests are of limited value in children. A blood culture should be obtained in all infants with suspected urinary tract infection since pyelonephritis is often associated with septicemia in the newborn period and in older children suspected of having acute pyelonephritis.

Roentgenographic Examination. For details of the technique for roentgenographic assessment of the urinary tract, see Sec 16.4 and 16.62.

It is essential to assess the anatomic integrity of the urinary tract, to identify any structural or functional abnormalities, and to detect renal parenchymal damage because these findings have an important bearing on the treatment, recurrence rate, and ultimate prognosis of urinary tract infections. In the majority of cases roentgenographic study should be deferred until 1–2 mo after infection has been successfully treated since minor abnormalities, including mild vesicoureteral reflux, may be temporary manifestations of the acute inflammatory reaction. In about 15% of children who have roentgenographic examination after their 1st recognized urinary tract infection, important urinary tract abnormalities are detected. These include congenital anomalies of the kidney, obstructive lesions at any level of the urinary tract, renal parenchymal scarring, and significant vesicoureteral reflux with ureteral dilatation. It is uncommon that new renal scars develop beyond 5 yr of age, even with recurrent or persistent infection. Of the remaining children about 35% have less serious abnormalities, such as irregularity or thickening of the bladder wall, an abnormal or intermittent voiding pattern with or without postvoiding residuum, or minimal vesicoureteral reflux. Many of these minor abnormalities result from the acute inflammation and resolve over a period of months if the urine remains uninfected. About 50% of patients with minor abnormalities will have recurrences after adequate courses of treatment, whereas fewer than 10% of children with entirely normal roentgenographic studies have recurrences.

In the newborn infant marked hydronephrosis with dilatation of the ureters and vesicoureteral reflux may occur as a consequence of acute urinary infection. This may resolve spontaneously and without surgical intervention when the infection is brought under control. As mentioned earlier, pyelonephritis in the neonate is often associated with septicemia; follow-up roentgenographic studies 6 mo–several yr later may reveal a significant incidence of renal parenchymal scarring, vesicoureteral reflux, and generalized renal atrophy.

In **acute bacterial pyelonephritis** the affected kidney is swollen, and on intravenous urography there is decreased concentration of contrast medium. Normal patterns are usually found within 1–2 mo if appropriate antibacterial therapy is initiated promptly.

Renal Function Studies. In most children with urinary tract infection there are no changes in renal function unless pyelonephritis is present. In *acute pyelonephritis* there may be mild elevation of the blood urea nitrogen and serum creatinine concentrations; these usually return to normal with treatment. The most consistent early finding in *chronic pyelonephritis* is an impaired ability to concentrate the urine, due to damage to the renal medulla; progressive interstitial scarring and nephron destruction may occur. The glomerular filtration rate is reduced, and there is persistent elevation of the blood urea nitrogen and serum creatinine, as well as other findings of chronic renal failure. In some instances, as a consequence of tubular dysfunction, there may be impaired ability to conserve sodium. Progression to chronic renal failure is uncommon in children with acute or chronic urinary tract infection unless important anatomic structural changes such as obstruction or extensive vesicoureteral reflux are present.

Diagnosis and Differential Diagnosis. The diagnosis rests on the detection of bacteria in the urine but, as noted above, there are numerous pitfalls. Roentgenographic findings may provide supplementary evidence. Since congenital anomalies of the urinary tract predispose to urinary tract infection, which can lead to abnormal roentgenographic patterns, it may be difficult to know the genesis of some of the abnormal findings. Renal vascular accidents in infancy may impair later kidney growth and lead to irregular anatomic development; these changes may be difficult to distinguish from those of chronic pyelonephritis. In the former, ureteral dilatation and reflux are usually absent.

Prevention. In patients with recurrent urinary tract infections it may be necessary to give antibacterial drugs in an attempt to prevent or to decrease the number of recurrences. This is particularly important if there is evidence of structural abnormalities with urinary stasis or reflux, or if recurrent infections have already caused significant damage to the kidneys or collecting system. (See Treatment of Recurrent Infections, below.)

Treatment. *Acute Uncomplicated Infections.* The organisms most commonly involved in acute uncomplicated urinary tract infection are strains of *Escherichia coli;* an excellent therapeutic response is usually obtained with a short-acting sulfonamide such as sulfisoxazole in a dose of 100–125 mg/kg/24 hr in 4 divided doses. Two wk is an adequate treatment period; there is no reduction in the recurrence rate when treatment is continued for a longer time. Amoxicillin, 50 mg/kg/24 hr, may also be used for initial treatment, but it has no advantage over sulfonamides. The clinical condition usually improves within several days. A follow-up urine culture should be obtained 1–2 wk after therapy is completed. Cephadroxil, 40–60 mg/kg/24 hr orally, cefaclor, 40 mg/kg/24 hr orally, or cefamandole, 100 mg/kg/24 hr intravenously or intramuscularly, is very useful, particularly if pyelonephritis is suspected.

In acutely ill children a parenteral route may be

necessary. If there is no response to intravenously administered sulfisoxazole or ampicillin, if the patient's condition is serious or deteriorating, or if infection with less common organisms such as *Pseudomonas aeruginosa*, *Klebsiella-Enterobacter*, or *Proteus* is present, the choice of an antibiotic will depend on bacterial sensitivity studies; alternatively, a potent broad-spectrum antibiotic active against gram-negative organisms may be used empirically. In this situation gentamicin, 1.0–1.5 mg/kg/24 hr, may be used. Attention must be paid to possible ototoxic and nephrotoxic effects of any of the antibiotics chosen, particularly when renal function is impaired and a potentially toxic blood concentration of the drug may be reached if usual doses are given. Cefamandole intravenously is a useful drug in this situation since it has neither ototoxic nor nephrotoxic effects. Penicillin G may be effective in *Proteus mirabilis* infections; erythromycin, 30–75 mg/kg/24 hr, with sodium bicarbonate to alkalinize the urine, is effective in certain gram-negative infections, such as *Pseudomonas*; nitrofurantoin, 5–7 mg/kg/24 hr, is also a valuable drug, particularly in infections due to *Klebsiella-Enterobacter*. The combination of sulfamethoxazole and trimethoprim (co-trimoxazole) is an effective medication for the treatment of a wide spectrum of infections due to gram-negative organisms, including *E. coli*, *Proteus*, and *Klebsiella-Enterobacter*; it is not effective against *Pseudomonas aeruginosa*. The dosage is 20 mg/kg/24 hr of sulfamethoxazole (4 mg/kg/24 hr of trimethoprim), given in 2 divided doses. *Staphylococcus epidermidis* may also cause acute pyelonephritis, cystitis, or both; this organism is often resistant to penicillin; bacterial sensitivity studies should be obtained.

Recurrent Infections. There is a tendency for urinary tract infection to recur even in the absence of major anatomic abnormalities; moreover, recurrences are often asymptomatic. Studies of the serotype of the infecting organisms indicate that, in the majority of instances, recurrent infections are due to different organisms rather than to recrudescences of partially treated infection. It is thus essential to secure follow-up cultures of urine every 1–4 mo for a sufficient time, usually 1–2 yr, even when the patient appears well. The choice of antibacterial therapy for recurrences depends on bacterial sensitivity studies; medication should be given for 2–4 wk. If recurrences are frequent, prolonged therapy for periods up to several yr may be considered; such a regimen can significantly reduce the number of infections. For this type of prophylactic therapy nitrofurantoin, methenamine mandelate, or sulfisoxazole is usually safe and effective. The combination of sulfamethoxazole and trimethoprim is also useful. The dosage of drug required to prevent infection in patients with a demonstrated tendency to recurrence is about half that recommended for the treatment of active infections; the medication may be effective if given only once a day at bedtime. Potentially toxic antibiotics should be avoided unless clearly warranted by the patient's condition.

Abnormal Bladder Function with Intermittent, Prolonged Voiding. This condition is seen almost exclusively in girls with recurrent urinary tract infection. It is characterized by daytime incontinence or dribbling and an abnormal voiding pattern demonstrable by cystourethrography. The bladder contracts irregularly, voiding is prolonged, and emptying may be incomplete. Involvement of the upper tract and kidneys is uncommon, although minor degrees of vesicoureteral reflux occur. Long-term prophylactic antibacterial treatment as discussed previously is indicated, and regular voiding at approximately 2 hr intervals during the daytime should be encouraged; the latter may be of considerable help in overcoming urinary incontinence. Urologic procedures such as ureteral reimplantation, meatotomy, and urethral dilatation have no beneficial effect on the course of this problem. This type of abnormal voiding is most common from 3–10 yr of age; improvement is often noted after puberty.

Vesicoureteral Reflux (Sec 16.63). The treatment of ureteral reflux associated with urinary tract infection remains an unresolved problem. Minor degrees of reflux are seen in about 25% of children with acute urinary tract infection and usually resolve with control of the infection. Urinary infections in general and vesicoureteral reflux in particular are less common in black girls than in white girls. A familial incidence of vesicoureteral reflux is sometimes seen, probably inherited as an autosomal dominant. The patient should be observed for at least 1 yr on conservative medical management with prophylactic antibacterial therapy and regular urine cultures. Surgical therapy should be considered only if there is the coincidence of reflux and obstruction or if there is continued urinary infection with reflux in spite of well supervised antibacterial therapy. Renal scarring alone is not an indication for ureteric reimplantation. Results of long-term conservative therapy, including prophylactic antibacterial drugs, regular complete voiding, double micturition at bedtime, and correction of constipation, indicate that resolution of vesicoureteral reflux and normal kidney growth can be achieved in the majority of cases.

The fact that most renal scars associated with reflux are present at the time of initial diagnosis and few develop after the age of 5 yr suggests that in young children with urinary tract infection, careful examination for vesicoureteral reflux should be made. If it is detected, the urinary tract must be kept free from infection for a prolonged period in the hope that renal scarring can be avoided or minimized. Segmental corticopapillary scarring probably results from urinary infection with reflux in early childhood and is an important cause of renal hypertension in children; since hypertension usually does not appear for 8–10 yr, the need for long-term follow-up with regular monitoring of the blood pressure is emphasized.

Meatal Stenosis (Sec 16.60). Many children have been subjected to a variety of surgical procedures, such as meatotomy, urethrotomy, or urethral dilatation, on the assumption that urethral obstruction contributed to the development of urinary tract infection. It is clear that true meatal stenosis is *very uncommon* in children with urinary tract infection, that surgical procedures on the urethra do not affect the infection recurrence rate, and that operations of any sort for correction of presumed narrowing or stenosis of the bladder neck, urethra, or meatus are rarely indicated in children with urinary tract infection.

Renal Parenchymal Involvement (Pyelonephritis)

(Sec. 16.43).   Acute bacterial pyelonephritis is a serious condition and should be treated with appropriate antibiotics for at least 2 wk. Cefamandole, gentamicin, and ampicillin are useful drugs for this purpose and can be given parenterally. Loss of renal tissue, distortion and clubbing of the calyceal system, and irregularity of the outline of the kidney indicate that the condition is chronic or recurrent. Significant vesicoureteral reflux is commonly associated. If recurrent infections occur, long-term prophylactic therapy as outlined should be given. Attention should be directed to possible deterioration in renal function and to the development of hypertension. Roentgenographic reassessment every 1–3 yr may be indicated to determine whether the condition is progressive or stable.

With evidence of *upper tract and renal involvement*, it is important that, in addition to control of the urinary tract infection, other aspects of renal function such as urine concentrating ability, blood urea nitrogen, and serum creatinine be assessed periodically and that attention be paid to the possible development of hypertension, acid-base disturbances, growth failure, and other complications of chronic renal insufficiency.

Symptomatic treatment for dysuria may be needed during the acute infection. A urinary analgesic such as phenazopyridine HCl, 10 mg/kg/24 hr orally in 3–4 divided doses, may be helpful for acute dysuria; diluting the urine by increasing the fluid intake may also reduce dysuria. Fever may be treated with acetylsalicylic acid.

Neurogenic Bladder.   Urinary infection can present a serious problem in a child with neurogenic bladder. Infection should be treated with appropriate antibacterial drugs and a program initiated which will permit regular complete emptying of the bladder. Intermittent self-catheterization every 6–8 hr, sometimes in combination with drugs to facilitate bladder contraction and emptying, has proved of value in eliminating infection and permitting the children to be continent.

Prognosis.   The prognosis for uncomplicated urinary tract infection is excellent if adequate therapy is instituted for the acute infection and if recurrences are promptly recognized and treated. The long-term prognosis is less favorable for patients with significant structural abnormalities complicated by infection and for patients with renal parenchymal damage. Here the underlying abnormality or the damage already present at the time of the 1st diagnosed urinary tract infection may not be amenable to medical or surgical therapy, even though further deterioration in renal function from the urinary tract infection per se can usually be prevented. The late development of hypertension occurs in some patients with segmental scarring of the kidney due to pyelonephritis and reflux nephropathy.

Cardiff-Oxford Bacteriuria Study Group: Sequelae of covert bacteriuria in school-girls: A four-year follow-up study. Lancet 1:889, 1978.
Cohen, M: Urinary tract infections in children. I. Females aged 2 through 14, first two infections. Pediatrics 50:271, 1972.
Drummond, KN, Forbes PA: Bacterial infections of the urinary tract (female children). In: Conn HF (ed): Current Therapy 1973. Philadelphia, WB Saunders, 1973.

Forbes PA, Drummond KN: Trimethoprim-sulfamethoxazole in recurrent urinary tract infection in children. J Infect Dis 128:S626, 1973.
Forbes PA, Drummond KN, Nogrady MB: Initial urinary tract infections. J Pediatr 75:187, 1969.
Forbes PA, Drummond KN, Nogrady MB: Meatotomy in girls with meatal stenosis and urinary tract infections. J Pediatr 75:937, 1969.
Gillenwater JY, Gleason CH. Lohr JA, et al: Home urine cultures by the dip-strip method: Results in 289 cultures. Pediatrics 58:508, 1976.
Guignard JP. Pathogénès et prévention de la néphropathie de reflux. Helv Paediatr Acta 35:205, 1980.
Hodson J, Kincaid-Smith P (eds): Reflux Nephropathy. Masson Publishing USA Inc, 1979.
Kunin CM, Halmagyi NE: Urinary tract infections in schoolchildren. II. Characterization of invading organisms. N Engl J Med 266:1297, 1962.
Kunin CM, Zacha E, Paquin AJ: Urinary tract infections in schoolchildren. Prevalence of bacteriuria and associated urologic findings. N Engl J Med 266:1287, 1962.
Nelson JD, Peters PC: Suprapubic aspiration of urine in premature and term infants. Pediatrics 36:132, 1965.
Pais VM, Retik AB: Reversible hydronephrosis in the neonate with urinary sepsis. N Engl J Med 292:465, 1975.
Pryles CV, Eliot CR: Pyuria and bacteriuria in infants and children. Am J Dis Child 110:628, 1965.
Ransley PG, Risdon RA: Reflux and renal scarring. Br J Radiol Suppl 14:1, 1978.
Saccharow L, Pryles CV: Further experience with the use of percutaneous suprapubic aspiration of the urinary bladder: Bacteriologic studies in 654 infants and children. Pediatrics 43:1018, 1969.
Smellie JM, Normand ICS, Katz G: Children with urinary infection: A comparison of those with and without vesicoureteral reflux. Kidney Int 20:717, 1981.
Tamminen TE, Kapric EA: The relation of the shape of renal papillae and of collecting duct opening to intrarenal reflux. Br J Urol 49:343, 1977.

TUBERCULOSIS OF THE URINARY TRACT

Tuberculosis of any part of the urinary or genital tract in children usually results from a generalized tuberculous infection (Sec 10.52). Hematogenous seeding begins in the glomerulus, spreads down the tubule, and invades the medulla. A tuberculoma forms, and caseous material containing mycobacteria spills into the calyx to involve adjacent areas of the renal pelvis, ureter, and bladder. Symptoms depend on the sites of involvement. There may be fever, emaciation, flank tenderness, dysuria, frequency, or hematuria. Persistent sterile pyuria suggests renal tuberculosis. Roentgenographic findings may be suggestive and include calcification of tuberculous lesions, calyceal cavities, stenosis of the excretory tract with dilatation above the stenosis, and contraction of the bladder. Multiple sites of involvement are typical. Tubercle bacilli must be differentiated from smegma bacilli and must be identified by culture. Treatment is that of progressive pulmonary tuberculosis, Rarely, surgical removal of an affected kidney may be indicated.

16.44   ACUTE NONBACTERIAL CYSTITIS
(Acute Hemorrhagic Cystitis)

Acute hemorrhagic cystitis of viral etiology is a self-limited, benign disease seen most often in school age males. Adenovirus types 11 and 21 have been recovered from the urine of some patients and are likely causative agents. The symptoms are those of acute cystitis of bacterial origin. The most common initial complaint is sudden onset of gross hematuria. Microscopic examination of the urine reveals numerous red and white blood cells; the usual duration of symptoms and hematuria is about 4 days. Urine culture for bacteria is negative. Treatment is not required except for relief of dysuria when it is severe (see Treatment of Dysuria in Sec 16.43).

Acute hemorrhagic cystitis may also occur in patients who are receiving **cyclophosphamide.** Chemical irritation of the bladder mucosa by cyclophosphamide excreted in the urine is potentially a serious problem since the lesion may respond slowly to termination of cyclophosphamide therapy, and fibrosis of the bladder and neoplastic transformation are possible long-term complications. Patients receiving cyclophosphamide should be given a high fluid intake to dilute the cyclophospha-

mide in the urine; regular urinalyses should be carried out to detect hematuria or pyuria that may signal the beginning of bladder irritation; the drug should be discontinued if there is evidence of cystitis.

Mufson MA, Bleshe RB, Horrigan TJ, et al: Cause of acute hemorrhagic cystitis in children. Am J Dis Child 126:605, 1973.
Numazaki Y, Kumasaka T, Yano N, et al: Further study on acute hemorrhagic cystitis due to adenovirus Type II. N Engl J Med 289:344, 1973.

16.45 Developmental Abnormalities of the Kidney and Urinary Collecting System

About 10% of people have developmental abnormalities of the kidney and urinary tract. Some are of no clinical significance; others pose problems to the patient's health and survival. Collectively, they account for about 45% of cases of chronic renal failure in childhood; they often have a hereditary basis and are frequently associated with abnormalities in other organ systems. The prognosis is often worsened by failure to recognize the anomaly at an early age.

A satisfactory classification of the abnormalities is not yet possible because little is known of their pathogenesis and because similar pathologic changes may be seen in conditions that are almost certainly unrelated. One classification which takes into account both clinical and pathologic features is presented in Table 16–17. Many of these conditions are hereditary, but in terms of the number of patients affected, there is no evidence of genetic influence in the majority.

A number of developmental abnormalities may be present in a given patient; for example, renal dysplasia may be accompanied by renal cyst formation and obstructive uropathy. A discussion of some of these developmental abnormalities follows. Some of the syndromes are discussed in other chapters.

RENAL AGENESIS AND HYPOPLASIA

Renal agenesis may be unilateral or bilateral; it may be sporadic or hereditary or occur as an isolated entity or a problem associated with other unrelated disorders. Ultrasound studies can detect renal agenesis at about 34 wk gestation. Any pathogenetic distinction between unilateral and bilateral agenesis may be uncertain since monoamniotic twins have been reported of whom 1 twin had unilateral and the other bilateral renal agenesis.

Unilateral renal agenesis occurs in about 1 of 1000 live births. The single kidney may be completely normal and without associated abnormalities. Affected children may have a normal life expectancy without morbidity; it has been suggested, however, that the risk of urinary infection and calculus formation is higher than in patients with 2 normal kidneys. In some instances the single kidney is abnormally formed, and there may be associated abnormalities of its collecting system; extrarenal congenital abnormalities are relatively more common in patients with unilateral renal agenesis. These include the following anomalies: cardiac (ventricular septal defect), nervous system (meningomyelocele), gastrointestinal (strictures, esophageal atresia, tracheoesophageal fistula, imperforate anus), skeletal (vertebral, limb, digital, long bone, rib), and genital (ipsilateral unicornate uterus, absence of fallopian tube, absent or hypoplastic testes). Abnormalities in shape and position of the ipsilateral ear pinna may also be associated.

The normal solitary kidney increases in size by compensatory hypertrophy after birth so that by the time the child is several yr of age its volume may approach twice normal. Inadvertent surgical removal of a solitary kidney following trauma has been reported. Most nephrologists consider that biopsy of a solitary kidney is contraindicated.

Bilateral renal agenesis (**Potter syndrome**) occurs in about 1 in 4000 births. Seventy-five per cent of those affected are males. Oligohydramnios, amnion nodosum, prematurity, small size for gestational age, and breech presentation are common. Extrarenal abnormalities are usual and include characteristic facies (wide-set eyes, parrot-beak nose, pliable low-set ears, receding chin); spade-like hands; dry, wrinkled skin; pulmonary hypoplasia or dysplasia; limb abnormalities; ovoid adrenal glands; and lower urinary tract or genital abnormalities.

The abnormal facies, though characteristic, is not specific for bilateral renal agenesis. It has been suggested that the oligohydramnios resulting from absent urine formation in utero is important in the pathogenesis of some of the extrarenal anomalies, particularly pulmonary hypoplasia. Spontaneous pneumothorax or pneumomediastinum is common in patients with renal agenesis. Conversely, approximately 20% of newborn infants with spontaneous pneumothorax have some form of renal anomaly; nephrologic examination is warranted in such infants.

About 40% of affected infants are stillborn. The liveborn usually die within several wk of age from renal failure or pulmonary problems.

Table 16–17 DEVELOPMENTAL STRUCTURAL ABNORMALITIES

Abnormalities in the amount of renal tissue
Unilateral or bilateral agenesis
Hypoplasia
Supernumerary kidneys

Abnormalities in renal location or shape
Ectopia
Fusion (horseshoe kidney)

Abnormalities in renal differentiation
Dysplasia, with or without cysts
Polycystic renal disease
Congenital renal neoplasms (nephroblastomatosis, Wilms tumor)

Renal and urinary tract abnormalities in multisystem disorders or syndromes*
Laurence-Moon-Biedl syndrome
Fanconi syndrome of multiple congenital anomalies and aplastic anemia
DiGeorge syndrome
Zellweger syndrome
Tuberous sclerosis
Prune-belly syndrome
Oral-facial-digital syndrome
Branchio-otorenal dysplasia
Cerebro-oculofacioskeletal syndrome
Meckel syndrome
Dandy-Walker malformation of the brain
Turner syndrome
Autosomal trisomy syndromes D and E
Von Hippel–Lindau disease
Jeune asphyxiating thoracic dystrophy
Thymic alymphoplasia
Russell-Silver dwarfism
Syndrome of renal hamartomas, nephroblastomatosis, and fetal gigantism
Beckwith-Wiedemann syndrome
Congenital renal and ear abnormalities
Familial renal dysplasia with blindness
Cat-eye syndrome
Ehlers-Danlos syndrome
Rubinstein-Taybi syndrome
Cockayne syndrome
Syndromes with abnormalities of the urinary tract, müllerian ducts, ears, and distal extremities
Neurofibromatosis
Familial dysautonomia
Hereditary osteolysis with nephropathy
"VATER" association
Nail-patella syndrome
Pseudohermaphroditism, glomerulopathy, and Wilms tumor

Abnormalities of the collecting system, bladder, and/or urethra
Hydronephrosis due to pelviureteric obstruction
Hydroureter and megaureter
Vesicoureteral reflux
Ureterocele
Duplication of the kidney and collecting system
Ectopic ureteral insertion
Epispadias and bladder exstrophy
Hypospadias
Posterior urethral valve
Other anomalies of the urethra

*In many of these conditions the renal lesion is asymptomatic and is an incidental finding; in others it causes severe impairment of renal function. The most common types of renal anomalies in these conditions are (1) gross or microscopic cysts beneath the capsule and along the columns of Bertin and (2) cystic dysplasia of the kidney. Other types of anomalies may also occur.

Renal hypoplasia is a rare anomaly in which the number of renal lobules is reduced to 5 or fewer and the number of calyces is correspondingly low. The kidney weighs only a fraction of normal, but normal nephron differentiation has occurred. The renal artery is also small. In most cases both kidneys are involved. Usually there are no associated abnormalities in the urinary collecting system.

In bilateral hypoplasia the total mass of functioning renal tissue is inadequate to sustain normal growth and development, and renal failure with growth arrest ensues. Clinical recognition may occur as early as several wk of age and as late as the 2nd decade. Unilateral hypoplasia may present no clinical problems.

Other more common causes of reduced kidney size which should be differentiated from renal hypoplasia include renal dysplasia, atrophy as a result of reflux or pyelonephritis, and a renal vascular insult, such as thrombosis of the renal vein in infancy.

Segmental Hypoplasia (Ask-Upmark Kidney). The importance of this condition is its common association with severe hypertension, which develops from 8–15 yr of age, usually in the absence of any reduction in glomerular filtration rate. This was once considered a developmental anomaly, but the current consensus is that the renal lesion is a consequence of urinary tract infection with vesicoureteral and intrarenal reflux in early childhood. Renal scarring occurs particularly at the superior and inferior poles, with cessation of normal renal growth in these regions. Three quarters of the patients are girls. Both kidneys may be involved, and affected kidneys are usually smaller than normal. Intravenous urography shows depression of the external contour over affected segments, with dilatation or clubbing of the underlying calyx or calyces and thinning of the intervening parenchyma. Vesicoureteral reflux is commonly associated. Histologically, there is sharp demarcation of the involved segments from the spared adjacent areas. Arteries in the affected areas are thick walled and tortuous; tubules are atrophic and sometimes filled with colloid casts resembling thyroid tissue. Marked hyperreninemia has been detected in hypertensive patients.

Terms applied to this condition have included reflux nephropathy, segmental hypoplasia, Ask-Upmark kidney, and chronic atrophic pyelonephritis. Habib suggests, pending further information on pathogenesis, that the descriptive title *renal segmental corticopapillary scarring* be used.

SUPERNUMERARY KIDNEY

This rare abnormality consists of an extra mass of renal tissue, usually smaller than a normal kidney; it has no connection with the normal kidney and usually lies caudal to it. Ureteral drainage into the normal ureter of the same side is common, but the insertion of the ureter may be ectopic (e.g., into the vagina). The clinical problem is usually that of urinary tract infection. When the infection cannot be controlled medically, surgical removal of the extra kidney may sometimes be necessary.

RENAL ECTOPIA

This is a congenital malposition of 1 or both kidneys. The ectopic kidneys may be displaced but normally lateralized, or there may be crossed ectopia, in which case lateralization is not normal, and the ureter from the ectopic kidney crosses the midline before draining into the bladder. The most common site of the unilateral ectopic kidney is the pelvis; the renal mass is often small or dysplastic, with associated abnormalities in arterial supply and in ureteral origin or insertion. In crossed ectopia, the ectopic kidney is usually caudal to and fused with the normal kidney. Crossed fused renal ectopia is found in about 1 in 7500 births, has occurred in identical twins, and is said to be more common in males than females.

Renal ectopia often causes no clinical problem, except that the ectopic kidney may be more subject to infection; if the site of ureteral insertion is into the vagina, there may be a persistent vaginal discharge of urine.

HORSESHOE KIDNEY

This is the most common form of renal fusion; the kidneys are joined inferiorly by an isthmus of renal parenchyma which passes anterior to the aorta and to the inferior vena cava. Some caudal displacement of the fused kidney is common. In this sense the horseshoe kidney could be considered as a form of bilateral renal ectopia with fusion. Usually the nephrons in the parenchyma of the isthmus drain into 1 or 2 calyces which, in turn, drain into the pelvis of 1 of the kidneys. The pelves of each half of the horseshoe kidney and their ureters arise more anteriorly than normal. In children, the condition is usually asymptomatic; there is, however, an increased incidence of urinary infection, and the kidney may be more susceptible to trauma. Adults rather commonly have episodes of abdominal pain which may be consequent to obstruction of the ureters as they angulate in passing over the isthmus. Horseshoe kidney is seen in children with Turner syndrome, in whom intravenous urography should be done routinely since renal anomalies are common.

RENAL DYSPLASIA

This developmental defect in differentiation of nephrogenic tissue may be partial or total and involve either or both kidneys. Dysplastic tissue in the kidney may include any of the following: mesenchymal stroma, dilated ducts lined by tall columnar epithelium, smooth muscle, cartilage, bone, immature ductules, primitive glomeruli, and abundant fibrous tissue. Cysts are common in dysplastic kidneys and may be a prominent feature on gross examination. This admixture of various embryonic elements may alter the organ's shape so that it bears no resemblance to a kidney. The dysplastic kidney may be abnormally small; however, if cysts are present, the total renal mass may be several times normal size. **Unilateral renal dysplasia with cysts** (also called *unilateral multicystic kidney*) is the most common cystic renal disorder in infants and children and the most common cause of a unilateral abdominal mass in the newborn.

Table 16–18 CONDITIONS IN WHICH THERE IS BILATERAL RENAL ENLARGEMENT IN INFANCY

Bilateral cystic renal dysplasia
Autosomal recessive (infantile type) polycystic kidney disease
Autosomal dominant (adult type) polycystic kidney disease
Bilateral renal vein or artery thrombosis
Bilateral hydronephrosis owing to obstruction at the ureteropelvic junction
Maternal diabetes mellitus
Beckwith-Wiedemann syndrome
Syndrome of nephroblastomatosis, renal hamartomas, and fetal gigantism
Bilateral Wilms tumor
Bilateral mesoblastic nephroma
Nephroblastomatosis (familial or nonfamilial forms)
Tuberous sclerosis with renal angiomyolipomas and/or polycystic kidneys
Conditions with infiltration or accumulation of substances not normally stored in the kidney, e.g., glycogen storage disease type I and acute leukemia

About 90% of patients with renal dysplasia have other anomalies of the urinary tract; most common is absence, atresia, or obstruction of the ureter. Abnormalities of the lower tract such as posterior urethral valves or bladder anomalies are sometimes seen, especially when renal dysplasia is bilateral. There is no evidence of hereditary or familial factors in the majority of cases and no sex predilection. Renal dysplasia occurs in some of the multisystem disorders listed in Tables 16–8 and 16–17; a number of these are hereditary.

The clinical problem of renal dysplasia is renal failure in patients with bilateral dysplasia, likely to be present in the newborn period. Affected infants often have the extrarenal features associated with bilateral renal agenesis; abdominal mass, which may be unilateral or bilateral in infants with cystic renal dysplasia; obstructive uropathy at any point along the course of the collecting system; hypertension; or urinary infection.

BILATERAL RENAL ENLARGEMENT IN THE NEWBORN INFANT

A number of conditions may cause bilateral nephromegaly in the newborn infant and must be considered when enlarged kidneys are found on abdominal examination. Some may not, strictly speaking, be considered as developmental anomalies, but since they develop during the course of gestation, they are included in Table 16–18, which lists these disorders.

DUPLICATIONS OF THE KIDNEY AND COLLECTING SYSTEM

Duplications of varying degrees, involving the kidney and collecting system, with or without ectopy, fusion, or malrotation, are the most common developmental abnormality of the kidney, affecting about 10% of the population. They are discussed in Sec 16.58.

Arant BS, Sotelo-Avila C, Bernstein J: Segmental "hypoplasia" of the kidney (Ask-Upmark). J Pediatr 95:931, 1979.
Bashour BN, Balfe JW: Urinary tract anomalies in neonates with spontaneous pneumothorax and/or pneumomediastinum. Pediatrics 59:1048, 1977.

Emanuel B, Nachman R, Aronson N, et al: Congenital solitary kidney. Am J Dis Child 127:17, 1974.

Fitch N: Heterogeneity of bilateral renal agenesis. Can Med Assoc J 116:381, 1977.

Gilbert E, Opitz J: Renal involvement in genetic-hereditary malformation syndromes. In: Hamburger J, Crosnier J, Grunfeld J-P (eds): Nephrology. New York, John Wiley & Sons, 1979.

Habib R: Pathology of renal segmental corticopapillary scarring in children with hypertension: The concept of segmental hypoplasia. In Hodson J, Kincaid-Smith P (eds): Reflux Nephropathy. Masson Publishing USA Inc, 1979.

Kissane JM: Congenital malformations. In: Hamburger J, Crosnier J, Grunfeld J-P (eds): Nephrology. New York, John Wiley and Sons, 1979.

Mauer SM, Dobrin RS, Vernier RL: Unilateral and bilateral renal agenesis in monoamniotic twins. J Pediatr 84:236, 1974.

Perlman M, Goldberg GM, Bar-Ziv J, et al: Renal hamartomas and nephroblastomatosis in fetal gigantism. A familial syndrome. J Pediatr 83:414, 1973.

Pinsky L: A community of human malformation syndromes involving the müllerian ducts, distal extremities, urinary tract, and ears. Teratology 9:65, 1974.

Straub E, Spranger J: Etiology and pathogenesis of the prune belly syndrome. Kidney Int 20:695, 1981.

INTERMITTENT HYDRONEPHROSIS INDUCED BY OVERHYDRATION

Some children with recurrent episodes of abdominal pain have an intermittent form of hydronephrosis which occurs and is detectable only following excessive fluid intake. This condition is usually difficult to diagnose because the complaints may be nonspecific; the pain is usually in the flank or abdomen. To establish the diagnosis, it is important to carry out intravenous urography during an attack of pain while the patient is being overhydrated by either the oral or intravenous route.

CONGENITAL MALFORMATIONS OF THE URINARY COLLECTING SYSTEM, BLADDER, AND URETHRA

A heterogeneous group of malformations is included under this heading; they are about 3 times more common in males than in females, are often associated with anatomic or functional obstruction to urine flow, and are clinically important because they account for a significant proportion of cases of chronic renal failure in childhood; they are not infrequently associated with renal and extrarenal congenital abnormalities; they predispose to recurrent infection and urolithiasis of the urinary tract; and the prognosis often depends on early diagnosis and appropriate surgical therapy.

Some anomalies are hereditary, but most occur sporadically. Suspicion should be directed to the existence of 1 of these anomalies if there is a history of oligohydramnios and if there are such physical findings as abnormal external genitalia, unusually shaped or positioned external ears, anorectal anomalies, spina bifida, a single umbilical artery, or spontaneous pneumothorax in the neonatal period. In children with features of the multisystem disorders or syndromes listed in Tables 16–8 and 16–17, the possibility of these associated urinary tract anomalies should also be considered. Since many of these disorders require urologic evaluation and correction, they are discussed in Sec 16.57.

KEITH N. DRUMMOND

16.46   Miscellaneous Conditions

16.47   UROLITHIASIS
(Renal Calculus)

Renal calculi are much less common in children than in adults and are more common in boys than girls. They sometimes signal an important underlying disorder needing specific therapy. Calculi are endemic in some developing countries, but the incidence has declined in these regions as the standard of living rises. The principal causes of nephrolithiasis in children are urinary infection, idiopathic, hypercalciuria, cystinuria, and a heterogeneous group of metabolic disorders.

Calculi in patients with urinary tract infection are most common in children under 5 yr of age and are associated with infections caused by urea-splitting organisms, particularly *Proteus* species. *Pseudomonas aeruginosa* and some strains of Enterobacteriaceae and Micrococcaceae may also split urea. Urease produced by the bacteria converts urea to ammonia, which favors calculus formation by increasing the alkalinity of the urine. The stones consist principally of magnesium ammonium phosphate (struvite), with calcium phosphate sometimes admixed. The upper collecting system is the usual site of calculus formation, with the left side affected more than the right. In a third of cases there is an underlying congenital structural abnormality lead-

ing to urinary stasis. The treatment is removal of the calculus, sterilization of the urine with appropriate antibacterial therapy, and correction of any anatomic abnormality. The prognosis is good and the recurrence rate low if the calculi can be removed.

Calculi in *idiopathic nephrolithiasis* usually consist of calcium oxalate; there is no evidence of excessive excretion of any urinary crystalloid. A genetic predisposition exists to the formation of calcium oxalate stones, besides that in patients with hyperoxaluria; it is probably polygenic, with males at greater risk and with a peak age of onset at 10–15 yr.

Hypercalciuria may result from a variety of causes. Increased intestinal absorption of calcium and hyperparathyroidism are seen in some patients. Hypercalciuria also occurs in uncontrolled distal renal tubular acidosis, with hypercortisonism or with corticosteroid therapy, during total parenteral alimentation, in hypercalcemia, and during immobilization for major fractures or extensive bone lesions. It may also be idiopathic. Normal values for urinary calcium excretion in children are less than 4 mg/kg/24 hr. In some of the conditions in which hypercalciuria is seen there may also be *nephrocalcinosis*, a condition in which there is radiologically demonstrable calcium deposition within the kidney parenchyma itself, usually in the medulla.

Metabolic conditions account for less than 10% of

urolithiasis in children and include cystinuria, hyperoxaluria (primary or secondary), dihydroxyadeninuria, xanthinuria, and orotic aciduria.

Ammonium acid urate bladder stones are not rare in the Far East, Thailand, and Turkey, and in endemic areas bladder stones consisting of magnesium ammonium phosphate result from *Schistosoma haematobium* infestation with subsequent bacterial urinary tract infection.

The signs and symptoms of renal calculi include colicky abdominal or flank pain, hematuria, repeated urinary infections, passing of the calculus, and, uncommonly, urethral obstruction. When an underlying disorder (e.g., renal tubular acidosis or chronic renal failure due to oxalosis) is present, clinical manifestations of the basic disorder may also be observed.

Evaluation for nephrolithiasis should include family history; an examination of the urine for red blood cells and for crystals, which may provide a clue to the diagnosis; urine culture; simultaneous determination of urine pH and serum bicarbonate concentration to exclude renal tubular acidosis; determination of blood levels of calcium, phosphorus, alkaline phosphatase, and uric acid; chromatographic examination of urine for amino acids; nitroprusside test for cystine; 24 hr urine determination of calcium and oxalic acid excretion; roentgenogram of the abdomen for stones; and chemical analysis of any stones passed.

Treatment. A high intake of fluids should be assured throughout each 24 hr period in order to reduce the concentration of precipitable crystalloids. If there is acute renal colic, an analgesic should be given. Surgical intervention is infrequently warranted during an acute episode; given time, the calculus usually will either pass or be dissolved. Calculi may remain lodged at the ureterovesical junction for several days or longer and yet ultimately pass spontaneously without urologic intervention. Urinary infection, when present, should be treated with appropriate antibacterial therapy. Surgical removal is indicated in the case of calculous disease due to urinary infection with organisms such as *Proteus* species, particularly if the stone is lodged in the upper collecting system.

Specific measures include correction of major anatomic obstructive lesions; antibacterial therapy when calculi are associated with urinary infection; reduction of calcium intake and administration of hydrochlorothiazide in idiopathic hypercalciuria (oral cellulose phosphate, 5 gm 2–3 times daily, is effective in adults with this disorder); and specific treatment of recognizable causes of nephrolithiasis such as renal tubular acidosis, cystinuria, and dihydroxyadeninuria.

Uric Acid Nephropathy and Lithiasis. Uric acid is the end product of purine metabolism in man. Four inborn errors of metabolism are known to lead to excess uric acid production, but most urate-containing stones in children have other causes. Urate stones do occur in the *Lesch-Nyhan syndrome* and in glucose-6-phosphatase deficiency at adolescence or in early adult life. Ammonium acid urate stones were once common in Europe and North America but have now virtually disappeared with improvements in the standard of living; they are, however, still endemic in the Far East, Thailand, Tur-

key, and India. They appear in sterile acid urine in children whose diet contains principally whole grain cereals, oxalate-rich vegetables, and little animal protein.

The principal cause of uric acid nephropathy in western countries is the *breakdown of large amounts of nucleoprotein* as a consequence of treatment for various reticuloendothelial malignancies, sarcomas, and acute leukemias. If allopurinol therapy is not given before treatment of such malignant conditions, increases in plasma uric acid levels to as high as 25–40 mg/dl may occur, with urate and uric acid deposition in the renal collecting ducts and pelvis. Anuria may result. Uric acid excretion may also rise and uric acid nephropathy result in patients with hemolytic crises due to thalassemia. Urate stones are radiolucent; simple help in diagnosis comes with finding numerous urate crystals in the urine sediment; also, the ratio of uric acid to creatinine in a random urine specimen is greater than 1.0. Treatment involves allopurinol, furosemide, high fluid intake to initiate a diuresis, and alkalinization of the urine with $NaHCO_3$. The prognosis of the uric acid nephropathy is excellent if this therapy is used. Prophylactic treatment with allopurinol is advised in patients about to undergo chemotherapy for childhood malignancies in order to prevent untoward elevation of the plasma uric acid level.

2,8-Dihydroxyadeninuria results from a complete deficiency of the enzyme adenine phosphoribosyltransferase, with precipitation of dihydroxyadenine crystals or stone. These radiolucent stones have been confused with urate stones in the past because of lack of specificity in analytic techniques. Sometimes these stones are admixed with uric acid. The enzyme defect can be detected in lysed red blood cells. Patients may have calculi in early childhood. Treatment with allopurinol is successful.

Treatment with allopurinol may lead to so great an increase in excretion of xanthine and hypoxanthine that xanthine crystals will form. Treatment is diuresis and alkalinization of urine.

Barkrop D (ed): Renal calculi. Section I. In: Paediatric Implications for Some Adult Disorders. London, Fellowship of Postgraduate Medicine, 1977.

Coe FL, Canterbury JM, Firpo JJ, et al.: Evidence for secondary hyperparathyroidism in idiopathic hypercalciuria. J Clin Invest 52:134, 1973.

Kelton J, Kelley WN, Holmes EW: A rapid method for the diagnosis of acute uric acid nephropathy. Arch Int Med 138:612, 1978.

Simmonds HA: 2,8-Dihydroxyadeninuria—or when is a uric acid stone not a uric acid stone? Clin Nephrol 12:195, 1979.

Williams HE: Nephrolithiasis. N Engl J Med 280:33, 1974.

16.48 RENAL VASCULAR DISORDERS

Renal venous thrombosis occurs in 2 unrelated and distinct situations in childhood: in infants as an acute, potentially catastrophic event and in children with the nephrotic syndrome as an associated and often unrecognized event.

16.49 RENAL VENOUS THROMBOSIS IN INFANTS

Etiology. Renal venous thrombosis usually occurs in high-risk infants with dehydration, shock, septicemia, severe pyelonephritis, congenital renal anomaly, asphyxia, or cyanotic congenital heart disease, or it may follow angiography for congenital heart lesions. Infrequently, there is no recognized predisposing cause. Maternal diabetes mellitus has been considered a predisposing cause; this association is now rarely seen.

Ninety per cent of patients are under 1 yr of age, and 75% are less than 1 mo. In the 1st yr of life boys are affected more frequently than girls (1.5:1); this is even more pronounced in the 1st mo, reflecting male vulnerability to precipitating or contributory disorders.

Pathology and Pathophysiology. Morbid anatomy depends on the extent and duration of venous thrombosis. The kidney may be enlarged, red, tense, and friable. The thrombus may be undergoing organization and may obstruct the main renal vein and its branches and extend into the inferior vena cava. In approximately 50% of patients thrombosis is bilateral. Thrombi are found in other organs in about 50% at postmortem examination. On microscopic examination microthrombi are found in the kidney, and there are infarcted and necrotic areas, interstitial edema, and hemorrhage. Calcification of the kidney and adrenal gland may occur in infants who survive.

The pathogenesis of renal venous thrombosis is related to sludging associated with polycythemia or to venous stasis produced by hypovolemia associated with dehydration, shock, infection, and/or hypernatremia. Infection of the renal parenchyma may be a factor in initiation of the thrombosis. Thrombocytopenia and extrarenal thrombi suggest that the renal thrombosis may be associated with disseminated intravascular coagulation. The thrombus usually starts in a small vein, such as an arcuate or interlobular one, and then spreads to the cortex or medulla or along the interlobar vein to the renal vein. The inferior vena cava or adrenal veins may also be affected.

Clinical Manifestations. The typical presenting pattern is the sudden deterioration of the infant's clinical condition, associated with hematuria, oliguria, and a flank mass. Fever, diarrhea, vomiting, and shock are common; edema and hypertension are usually absent. Manifestations of the predisposing condition are usually evident.

Laboratory Data. Anemia, leukocytosis, thrombocytopenia, moderate azotemia, and metabolic acidosis may be present. Roentgenographic examination reveals an enlarged kidney with poor or no excretion of dye during intravenous urography. Inferior vena cavagrams may demonstrate thrombosis of 1 or both renal veins and possibly of the inferior vena cava. Ultrasonography and radionuclide studies may provide valuable diagnostic information.

Differential Diagnosis. The differential diagnosis includes other conditions in which any of the following are present in a seriously ill infant: a flank mass, oliguria or anuria, hematuria, and a unilateral nonfunctioning kidney. Conditions to be considered include renal cortical or papillary necrosis, acute tubular necrosis, unilateral cystic kidney, renal arterial thrombosis, renal trauma with perirenal hemorrhage, acute obstructive uropathy, nephroblastoma, nephroblastomatosis, and neuroblastoma.

Prevention. There is no specific means of preventing renal venous thrombosis; correction of the underlying or predisposing illness may be presumed to diminish the likelihood of its development. Of special importance is the avoidance of dehydration in a seriously ill infant.

Treatment. The most important aspect is correction or management of the underlying disorder. Bacteriologic culture of the blood, urine, and cerebrospinal fluid should be obtained if septicemia is suspected, and appropriate antibacterial treatment should be instituted. Rehydration and measures to correct shock are essential. The value of heparin in renal venous thrombosis is controversial since the above supportive measures may suffice. If there is thrombocytopenia or if other features suggest widespread intravascular coagulation, the patient may be heparinized with the intent to maintain the clotting time longer than 20 min. In the past the diagnosis of renal venous thrombosis was an indication for immediate nephrectomy; results with conservative treatment, however, justify a nonsurgical approach except when there is bilateral involvement or associated inferior vena cava thrombosis. In these circumstances a thrombectomy is indicated as soon as the patient's condition permits. Angiography or intravenous urography should be obtained only when the patient is adequately hydrated and not in shock.

Prognosis. The prognosis depends to a large extent on the severity of the underlying condition and on whether the thrombosis is bilateral. If the patient's general condition and underlying problem can be managed satisfactorily for several days, there is reasonable possibility of survival. Recovery of renal function on the affected side is then not uncommon; this is a compelling reason to avoid nephrectomy if at all possible. Subsequent roentgenographic studies may reveal a poorly functioning small kidney or a normal kidney. Renal calcification may also be seen. Hypertension is an occasional late complication, and renal tubular dysfunction has been reported following recovery from renal venous thrombosis in infancy.

Arneil GC, MacDonald AM, Murphy AV, et al: Renal venous thrombosis. Clin Nephrol 1:119, 1973.
Renfield ML, Kraybill EN: Consumptive coagulopathy with renal vein thrombosis. J Pediatr 82:1054, 1973.

16.50 RENAL VENOUS THROMBOSIS AND THE NEPHROTIC SYNDROME

An association between the nephrotic syndrome and renal venous thrombosis has been recognized since 1840, but only in recent years has it been established that the nephrotic syndrome is a cause rather than a consequence of the thrombosis. Renal venous thrombosis has been reported in approximately a third of adult patients with the nephrotic syndrome; the incidence in children is much lower.

Pathology and Pathogenesis. In some patients the thrombosis is bilateral or involves the inferior vena cava; thrombi may occur also at extrarenal sites. The affected kidney initially is enlarged, tense, and congested; subsequently, fibrosis may lead to renal contraction. A number of different causes may account for renal venous thrombosis in patients with the nephrotic syndrome. Specific pathologic features of the underlying renal disease are detectable in the kidney with the thrombosed renal vein as well as in the uninvolved contralateral kidney. These conditions include the congenital nephrotic syndrome, membranous nephropathy, minimal lesion nephrotic syndrome, lupus nephritis, and membranoproliferative glomerulonephritis. The pathologic lesions related to renal venous thrombosis include interstitial edema and congestion, foci of polymorphonuclear and round cell infiltration, interstitial fibrosis, tubular atrophy, margination of polymorphonuclear leukocytes in capillary lumina, and glomerular capillary loop ectasia with stasis of blood and microthrombi.

The pathogenesis of renal venous thrombosis and of thrombi in many other organs of patients with the nephrotic syndrome can be better understood in the context of the abnormalities of coagulation found in nephrotic patients, with or without thromboses. These include elevated plasma levels of fibrinogen, factors V, VII, VIII, and X, thrombocytosis, accelerated thromboplastin generation, urinary loss of antithrombin III, and activation of the Hageman factor. Since thromboses have occurred in patients not treated with corticosteroid or diuretic therapy, it appears that there is no relationship to administration of these agents; rather, it appears that the pathogenesis is related to a hypercoagulable state; hyperlipidemia and volume contraction may be additional predisposing factors.

Clinical Manifestations and Course. Renal venous thrombosis may be clinically silent in a nephrotic patient. Flank pain with renal tenderness, gross hematuria, worsening of the clinical state, and deterioration in renal function occur in some patients. Hypertension occasionally develops in a previously normotensive patient. With bilateral thrombosis or inferior vena cava thrombosis the morbidity is increased. The ultimate course depends largely on the nature of the underlying disorder.

Laboratory Data. There are no specific laboratory manifestations of renal venous thrombosis. Microscopic or gross hematuria may develop, and the urinary excretion of protein may increase. Roentgenographic or radionuclide studies reveal an enlarged kidney with less function than the uninvolved kidney has. Inferior vena cavagram may reveal thrombosis of the inferior vena cava or a clot extending into its lumen from the affected vein. Renal biopsy may confirm the diagnosis and give information concerning the underlying glomerular pathology.

Prevention. Appropriate treatment of the nephrotic syndrome, resulting in reducing the excretion of protein to normal and in reducing the frequency of relapse,

may be expected to decrease the incidence of renal venous thrombosis. Avoidance of hypovolemia by treatment with albumin infusions when indicated, hydration, and the judicious use of diuretics only when necessary may also help prevent renal venous thrombosis.

Treatment. Anticoagulation with heparin is the accepted initial treatment; it is followed by long-term use of oral anticoagulants. Some nephrologists advocate thrombectomy in addition to anticoagulation; this is particularly important when there is bilateral involvement or involvement of the inferior vena cava. There is no reason to discontinue any concurrent therapy for the nephrotic syndrome, but aggressive diuretic therapy should be avoided.

Prognosis. The prognosis of treated unilateral renal venous thrombosis is good, particularly if measures to treat the nephrotic syndrome itself are successful. With bilateral or inferior vena caval involvement the prognosis is serious, though early diagnosis, surgical intervention, and anticoagulation therapy increase the survival rate. The long-term prognosis is influenced by the nature of the primary renal disease.

Kaplan BS, Chesney RW, Drummond KN: The nephrotic syndrome and renal vein thrombosis. Am J Dis Child 132:367, 1978.
Kendall AG, Lohman RC, Dossetor JB: Nephrotic syndrome: A hypercoagulable state. Arch Intern Med 127:1021, 1971.
Llach F, Papper S, Massry SG: The clinical spectrum of renal vein thrombosis: Acute and chronic. Am J Med 69:819, 1980.
Shigeko OL, Tkachuck JY, Hasegawa DK, et al: Plasminogen and antithrombin III deficiencies in the childhood nephrotic syndrome associated with plasminogenuria and antithrombinuria. J Pediatr 96:390, 1980.
Stuart MJ, Spitzer RE, Nelson DA, et al: Nephrotic syndrome: Increased platelet prostaglandin endoperoxide formation, hyperaggregability, and reduced platelet life span. Reversal following remission. Pediatr Res 14:1078, 1980.

16.51 RENOVASCULAR HYPERTENSION AND RENAL ARTERIAL DISORDERS

See also Sec 13.85.

Renovascular hypertension (RVHT) occurs when a lesion or compression of the renal artery or 1 of its branches results in reduced blood flow to all or part of the ipsilateral kidney. Localized renal scarring or other disruptive or space-occupying processes which may distort and compromise the renal blood supply, even to a very limited volume of the parenchyma, may also cause RVHT. The pathogenesis of the hypertension involves activation of the renin-angiotensin system. RVHT is responsible for 10–15% of cases of severe hypertension in childhood. Table 16–19 lists the principal causes.

Fibromuscular dysplasia of the renal artery and its branches is the most common cause of the arterial narrowing leading to RVHT in children. This is a hyperplastic disruptive process involving the tunica media, leading to stenosis of the lumen. In 40% of cases the lesions affect both kidneys. Arterial stenosis may be associated with a poststenotic dilatation or aneurysm, and a beaded appearance on renal angiography is characteristic. The affected kidney may be smaller

Table 16–19 CAUSES OF RENOVASCULAR HYPERTENSION IN CHILDHOOD

Unilateral or bilateral segmental corticopapillary scarring (segmental hypoplasia)

Fibromuscular dysplasia of renal artery

Renal artery thrombosis secondary to umbilical artery catheterization, closure of patent ductus arteriosus, post-traumatic, etc.

Neurofibromatosis with renal arterial stenosis

Congenital isolated renal artery stenosis

Renal artery stenosis secondary to lesions affecting the abdominal aorta, e.g., Takayasu disease, Marfan syndrome, coarctation

Aneurysm of renal artery

Intrarenal arteriovenous fistula—congenital, traumatic

External compression or displacement of the renal artery, e.g., Wilms tumor, neurinoma

Polyarteritis affecting renal artery

Stenosis of renal artery in Williams syndrome (hypercalcemia with supravalvular aortic or pulmonary artery stenosis, elfin facies)

Renal arterial stenosis following transplantation

Congenital developmental renal anomalies with associated renal arterial abnormalities, e.g., narrowing

---

than normal. Girls are affected more frequently than boys.

Unilateral or bilateral *renal parenchymal scarring* (segmental hypoplasia), possibly a late consequence of vesicoureteral and intrarenal reflux, is an important cause of RVHT.

Thrombosis of the renal artery is an important cause of RVHT in early infancy. This may result from a high indwelling umbilical artery catheter, sepsis, or a thrombus dislodged following closure of a patent ductus arteriosus. Hypertension may be defined in premature and term infants as systolic and diastolic blood pressures at or above 80/50 and 90/60 mm Hg, respectively. Signs of hypertension in infants include respiratory distress, congestive heart failure, and neurologic signs (sometimes secondary to intracranial hemorrhage). With renal artery thrombosis the kidney may be enlarged, proteinuria and hematuria are present, the plasma renin level is elevated, and the blood urea nitrogen and creatinine levels are raised. If the hypertension is severe, prompt treatment with diuretics, hydralazine, and propranolol (0.5–2 mg/kg, intravenously) is warranted. The long-term prognosis is usually good, and it is possible to discontinue all medications in 3–6 mo.

In *neurofibromatosis* hyperplasia of the media and intima may lead to renal artery stenosis, usually in the proximal 1 cm of the renal artery. By contrast, the lesions of the fibromuscular dysplasia tend to affect more distal regions of the artery. Other possible causes of RVHT in neurofibromatosis include aneurysm of the renal artery, compression of the renal pedicle by neurinoma, and pheochromocytoma. Males are affected more often than females.

RVHT can also result from a *congenital or acquired abnormality of the arterial supply to a segment of a kidney.*

Clinical Manifestations. These relate to the hypertension itself and to the underlying cause when there is one (see Table 16–19). When the hypertension is mild, there may be no symptoms. More often, however, headaches, irritability, and, at times, visual disturbances occur. In extreme cases there may be encephalop-

athy and seizures. Congestive heart failure and respiratory distress may be the presenting signs of hypertension in infancy.

Laboratory Data. In patients with suspected RVHT intravenous urography is the 1st and often most useful study since it may indicate the likelihood of RVHT, extent of the problem (unilateral or bilateral), and nature of the lesion. Asymmetry of renal size is a clue; the fully grown left kidney is normally about 0.5 cm longer than the right. If the left is smaller than the right by more than 1 cm or the right smaller by more than 1.5 cm, the difference should be considered significant. Delayed appearance of the contrast medium may reflect reduced blood supply to the affected side, as may hyperconcentration of the media or delay in washout with a diuretic such as furosemide. A segmental abnormality or scar may be identified. Radionuclide renography is valuable for dynamic studies of renal perfusion and glomerular filtration rate. Renal arteriography can delineate the site, type, and extent of renal arterial disease. Selective study of individual segments of the kidney may be indicated.

Investigation of the renin-angiotensin system is indicated in suspected RVHT. The peripheral plasma renin activity (PRA) may be elevated, providing an initial clue, but peripheral values may be normal even when RVHT is present. Renal vein PRA is more helpful, and selective segmental studies from individual renal lobes are often rewarding. In over 90% of cases the ratio of PRA on the affected side to that on the unaffected side is 1.5:1 or higher.

Treatment. Selection of therapy is influenced by the nature of the problem. Conservative management using antihypertensive medication should be tried initially; a combination of propranolol, hydralazine, and hydrochlotothiazide is often effective. Captopril alone or in combination with other antihypertensive drugs is very useful. If there is unequivocal localized arterial disease or isolated segmental disease and if there are supportive data from PRA studies, reconstructive vascular surgery or resection of the affected segment may be indicated. Nephrectomy is seldom indicated and, in any event, should not be done unless it has been demonstrated that conservative treatment has failed to control the blood pressure satisfactorily. Bilateral involvement drastically reduces the likelihood of success by surgical treatment. (See discussion of hypertension in Sec 13.85.)

Prognosis. This varies with the type of lesion, the degree of damage to the contralateral kidney, and the presence or absence of diffuse vascular changes. Generally, with early diagnosis and optimal medical and/or surgical management the outlook is good.

Adelman RD, Merten D, Vogel J, et al: Nonsurgical management of renovascular hypertension in the neonate. Pediatrics 62:71, 1978.

Korobkin M, Perloff DL, Palubinskas AJ: Renal arteriography in the evaluation of unexplained hypertension in children and adolescents. J Pediatr 88:388, 1976.

Magilavy DB, Petty RE, Cassidy JT, et al: A syndrome of childhood polyarteritis. J Pediatr 91:25, 1977.

Makker SP, Moorthy B: Fibromuscular dysplasia of renal arteries. An important cause of renovascular hypertension in children. J Pediatr 95:340, 1979.

Plumer LB, Kaplan GW, Mendoza SA: Hypertension in infants—a complication of umbilical arterial catheterization. J Pediatr 89:302, 1976.

16.52 ENURESIS

See also Sec 2.50.

Enuresis, or involuntary emptying of the bladder beyond the age when bladder control should have been established, may be nocturnal or diurnal; the former is more common. A distinction should also be made between *primary enuresis*, in which the child has never been reliably dry, and *secondary* enuresis, which is the development of enuresis in a child who has achieved bladder control for a period of 1 yr or more. Primary enuresis is more common and is much less often associated with an underlying organic problem. Nocturnal enuresis is present in about 10% of otherwise normal 5 yr old children and in about 1% of normal children at 15 yr. It is slightly more common in boys, in lower socioeconomic classes, and in 1st-born children. There is a fairly prominent family tendency. Primary nocturnal enuresis has no organic basis in the great majority of cases and is due to delayed maturation of bladder control or to emotional factors. Separation from the family, death of a parent, and birth of a sibling are examples of events which may precipitate nocturnal enuresis in a previously continent child.

Organic disorders that may cause nocturnal enuresis include urinary tract infection, increased urinary volume in diabetes mellitus, diabetes insipidus, obstructive uropathy, chronic renal failure, other conditions in which the ability to concentrate urine is impaired, and nocturnal epilepsy. Urinary tract infection is the most common organic cause by far; 15% of girls with urinary infection, whether symptomatic or not, have enuresis.

The initial examination of the child should include an evaluation of possible psychogenic factors, a complete physical examination, routine urinalysis, urine culture, and measurement of the urine specific gravity after an overnight fast. If there is reason to suspect an underlying organic disorder, appropriate blood and urine studies should be carried out, including intravenous urography. These studies are warranted only in a minority of patients with nocturnal enuresis. A more extensive evaluation is indicated in children with secondary enuresis, especially in those over 10 yr of age, than in those with primary nocturnal enuresis.

A number of forms of therapy for nocturnal enuresis not associated with organic disease have been used. The point to emphasize is that the condition is benign and self-limited, and steps should be taken to eliminate the emotional impact of the problem on the child. Reassurance, support, and avoidance of overinvestigation or overtreatment are indicated. There should be no shame or guilt associated with enuresis—it seems that the more the child wishes to be dry the more likely is failure; a matter-of-fact attitude toward success or failure should be adopted.

Appropriate techniques for motivating, encouraging, and helping enuretic children are given in Sec 2.50.

Burke EC, Stickler GB: Enuresis—Is it being overtreated? Mayo Clin Proc 55:118, 1980.
Foxx RM, Azrin NH: Dry pants: A rapid method of toilet training in children. Behav Res Ther 11:435, 1973.

Imipramine for enuresis. Med Lett Drugs Ther 16:22, 1974.
Marshall S, Marshall HH, Lyon RP: Enuresis: An analysis of various therapeutic approaches. Pediatrics 52:813, 1973.

16.53 TOXIC NEPHROPATHY

A wide variety of compounds may damage the kidney. Often the damage is transient and reversible if exposure to the noxious agent is discontinued. Potentiation of a toxic effect of 1 drug may occur with administration of a 2nd drug (e.g., gentamicin and cephalothin). Table 16–20 lists the most common nephrotoxins grouped according to the principal site of injury or the clinical pattern they induce (see References for an exhaustive list of agents potentially damaging to the kidney). In addition, Table 16–14, which lists drugs for which dosages should be modified in children with reduced renal function, and Table 16–7, which lists the causes of renal tubular acidosis, should be consulted. Drug-induced renal diseases probably represent the most common of the toxic nephropathies at this time. Given the frequency with which exposure to drugs occurs, the frequency of nephrotoxic reactions is low, and lower in children than in adults exposed to the same drugs. Two types of pathogenetic mechanisms are involved: (1) a direct toxic reaction which is largely dose dependent, e.g., the reactions caused by aminoglycosides, cephalosporins, and polymyxin B and E; and (2) an allergic or hypersensitivity reaction, which may involve immune complex deposition, anti–basement membrane antibodies, or cell-mediated injury. Cell-mediated or other immunopathologic types of injury are considered to be operative in many patients, but it is uncommon to find good evidence for them. Most of the drug-induced nephropathies are self-limited and respond without further treatment when administration of the offending drug is discontinued. Patients with acute allergic interstitial nephritis may be improved by corticosteroid therapy.

Penicillins, Cephalosporins, and Rifampin. Acute interstitial nephritis is the most common type of reaction and is presumed to be allergic. Penicillin and its analogues are the foremost offenders. Nephrotoxicity may occur after only 1 dose of these drugs but typically occurs in a patient receiving a prolonged course for a serious infection. There may be recurrence exposure to the same or a closely related drug. Reactions have been reported more often with methicillin than with other penicillins; cephalothin and cephaloridine are the most nephrotoxic of the cephalosporins.

Aminoglycoside Antibiotics. All of the aminoglycosides are potentially nephrotoxic, streptomycin and neomycin being the least and most nephrotoxic, respectively. Gentamicin is the most common offender in children, possibly because of its frequent use. When it occurs, toxicity develops after 7–10 days of therapy; the usual problem is nonoliguric acute renal failure. Tubular damage may be manifested as proximal tubular dysfunction (Fanconi syndrome), proteinuria, and lysozymuria. Volume depletion induced by furosemide diuresis, pre-existing renal disease, or simultaneous administration of cephalothin will increase the neph-

Table 16–20 NEPHROTOXIC COMPOUNDS*

Nephrotic syndrome
Gold salts
Mercurial diuretics
Miscellaneous compounds containing mercury
Paramethadione
Penicillamine
Perchlorate
Probenecid
Tolbutamide
Trimethadione

Nephrogenic diabetes insipidus
Amphotericin B
Demeclocycline
Lithium carbonate
Methoxyflurane
Propoxyphene

Fanconi syndrome
Cadmium
Gentamicin
Lead
Lysol
Mercury
Nitrobenzene
Outdated tetracycline
Salicylate
Uranium

Renal tubular acidosis
Lithium salts
Toluene sniffing

Interstitial nephritis with or without papillary necrosis
Amidopyrine
p-Aminosalicylate
Bunamiodyl (papillary necrosis only)
Penicillins (especially methicillin)
Phenacetin
Phenylbutazone
Salicylate
Sulfonamides

Renal vasculitis with or without glomerular capillary involvement
Hydralazine
Isoniazid
Sulfonamides
Any of the numerous other drugs that may cause a hypersensitivity reaction

Nephrocalcinosis or nephrolithiasis
Allopurinol
Ethylene glycol
Methoxyflurane
Vitamin D

Miscellaneous renal manifestations including proteinuria, hematuria, oliguria, tubular necrosis, and renal failure
Arsenic
Bacitracin
Cadmium
Carbon tetrachloride
Cephaloridine
Cephalothin
Colistin
Copper
Ethylene glycol
Gentamicin
Gold salts
Indomethacin
Iron
Kanamycin
Mercury salts
Neomycin
Pentamidine
Poisonous mushrooms
Polymyxin B
Streptomycin
Sulfonamides
Tetrachlorethylene
Vancomycin
Viomycin

*The agents are grouped according to the principal site of injury or manifestation. (Dr. Sean O'Regan assisted in the preparation of this table.)

---

rotoxic potential of gentamicin. Recovery usually occurs within 1 wk following cessation of drug administration.

Amphotericin B. Nephrotoxicity relates to the total dose; irreversible damage occurs in 50% of patients receiving over 5 gm total. Amphotericin B may cause decreased glomerular filtration rate and renal blood flow, renal tubular acidosis, and increased clearance of potassium and uric acid. Associated reactions include abnormal urine sediment, azotemia, acidosis, and hypokalemia. Functional changes appear early; histologic changes occur later and include nephrocalcinosis and glomerular and tubular lesions with degenerative changes in tubular cells. The renal failure may be reversible after decreasing or discontinuing therapy.

Cyclophosphamide. Hyponatremia associated with cyclophosphamide therapy appears to be caused by damage to the distal nephron, with inability to excrete a normal water load.

Diuretics. Furosemide and thiazides may cause acute allergic interstitial nephritis, possibly on the basis of hypersensitivity. Improvement of renal function has occurred after discontinuation of therapy. Furosemide may potentiate the nephrotoxic and ototoxic effects of gentamicin.

Vitamin D. Large doses of vitamin D cause hypercalcemia and nephrocalcinosis. Adverse reactions include polydipsia and polyuria, with impaired ability to concentrate the urine.

Appel GB, Neu HC: The nephrotoxicity of antimicrobial agents. N Engl J Med 296:663, 722, 784, 1977.
Kovnat P, Labovitz E, Levison S: Antibiotics and the kidney. Med Clin North Am 57:1045, 1973.
Schreiner GE: Toxic nephropathy due to drugs, solvents and metals. Progr Biochem Pharmacol 7:248, 1972.

16.54 INTERSTITIAL NEPHRITIS (Interstitial Renal Inflammation)

This heading includes a number of different conditions which lead to nonsuppurative inflammation of the renal interstitial tissue and may be either acute or chronic. Many causes (Table 16–21) are recognized; the principal ones are drugs and systemic infection. In children acute interstitial nephritis may occur also in association with iridocyclitis, inflammatory bowel disease, or chronic active hepatitis. In the *acute* form there is diffuse infiltration of the interstitium by mononuclear

Table 16-21 CAUSES OF INTERSTITIAL NEPHRITIS

Acute interstitial nephritis
  Drugs: sulfonamides, penicillin and its analogues, cephalosporins, furosemide, thiazide diuretics, diphenylhydantoin, phenylbutazone, rifampin, phenindione, allopurinol
  Infection: toxoplasmosis, leptospirosis, infectious mononucleosis, diphtheria, syphilis, measles, typhoid fever, subacute bacterial endocarditis
  Connective tissue diseases: systemic lupus erythematosus, Sjögren syndrome
  Miscellaneous: sarcoidosis, inflammatory bowel disease, acute glomerulonephritis, iridocyclitis, renal allograft rejection, minimal change nephrotic syndrome, hypergammaglobulinemia
Chronic interstitial nephritis*
  Radiation nephritis
  Prolonged hypokalemia
  Hypercalcemia with nephrocalcinosis
  Analgesic abuse
  Uric acid nephropathy in gout
  Balkan nephropathy
  Heavy metal exposure
  Cystinosis
  Reflux nephropathy
  Sickle cell disease

*Chronic interstitial fibrosis may be a more accurate term for the changes seen in some of these conditions.

cells, lymphocytes, plasma cells, eosinophils, and occasional neutrophils. Patchy tubular cell damage and interstitial edema may be present. Immunopathologic studies occasionally show granular IgG deposits around the tubular basement membrane and in the interstitium; antibodies to tubular basement membrane may be deposited in a linear pattern. Clinically, there is acute onset of oliguria with a variable degree of renal insufficiency, gross hematuria, proteinuria, eosinophilia, eosinophils in the urine, and bilateral kidney enlargement; evidence of proximal tubular dysfunction (Fanconi syndrome) may be present. Systemic signs may also be present and include nausea, fever, chills, rash, arthralgias, lumbar pain, and jaundice. The condition is usually self-limited and recovery spontaneous; dramatic response to corticosteroids has been seen in some patients with acute allergic interstitial nephritis. Treatment of a defined predisposing condition, e.g., leptospirosis, or withdrawal of a precipitating agent, e.g., methicillin, is indicated. Progression to chronic renal failure may rarely occur. Renal biopsy may be required to establish the diagnosis.

Chronic interstitial nephritis is associated with tubular atrophy, interstitial fibrosis, and, occasionally, papillary necrosis. Chronic renal failure, inability to concentrate the urine, salt wasting, and hypertension may be present.

KEITH N. DRUMMOND

Appel GB: A decade of penicillin related acute interstitial nephritis—more questions than answers. Clin Nephrol 13:151, 1980.
Cremer W, Bock KD: Symptoms and course of chronic hypokalemic nephropathy in man. Clin Nephrol 7:112, 1977.
Heptinstall RH: Interstitial nephritis. A brief review. Am J Pathol 83:214, 1976.
Levy M, Guesry P, Loirat C, et al: Immunologically mediated tubulo-interstitial nephritis in children. Contr Nephol 16:132, 1979.
Van Ypersele de Strihou C: Acute oliguric interstitial nephritis. Kidney Int 16:751, 1979.
Woodroffe AJ, Row PG, Meadows R, et al: Nephritis in infectious mononucleosis. Q J Med 43:451, 1974.

16.55 GENERAL CONSIDERATIONS OF OBSTRUCTIVE LESIONS OF THE URINARY TRACT

See Sec 16.57 for details of individual lesions.

Children with obstructive uropathy are usually first seen and evaluated by their primary physician and frequently require careful follow-up for many yr after surgical therapy.

Etiology. Both congenital and acquired defects can cause obstructive uropathy; the manifestations may be acute or chronic. Boys are affected more commonly than girls. Malformation of the urinary tract must be suspected in patients with other congenital defects, such as the prune-belly syndrome, the VATER* constellation of anomalies, chromosomal abnormalities (XO, Down syndrome, trisomies 13 and 18), and in patients with apparently isolated defects including congenital heart disease, an absent or deformed pinna, preauricular pits, hypospadias, sacral agenesis, and anorectal malformations. The causes and sites of urinary obstruction are listed in Table 16-22.

Pathology. The pathologic changes depend on the nature of the underlying defect, the site of obstruction (e.g., dilatation of the pelvicalyceal system with pelviureteric obstruction or dilatation of the entire urinary tract with obstruction by posterior urethral valves), the duration of obstruction, and complications such as infection or urinary calculi. Histologically, there may be dilated atrophic or hypertrophied tubules, interstitial nephritis, interstitial fibrosis, peritubular and periglomerular fibrosis, dilatation of Bowman space, and glomerular obsolescence.

Pathophysiology. Experimental studies have revealed reduction in glomerular filtration and underperfusion of distal nephrons in acute obstruction. In chronic obstruction there is increased glomerular filtration in the residual nephrons but an overall reduction in the glomerular filtration rate.

The pathophysiology of acute or chronic renal failure with obstructive uropathy is described in detail in Sec 16.40 and 16.42. It is important to stress, however, that many clinical features and metabolic consequences of obstructive uropathy are caused not only by the reduced glomerular filtration rate but also by damage to the distal nephron. Polyuria in chronic obstructive uropathy is the result of increased delivery of filtrate per nephron and inability of the damaged collecting tubules to concentrate the urine. Similarly, metabolic acidosis is caused not only by decreased excretion of acid secondary to reduction in GFR but also by an impaired ability of the distal nephron to secrete hydrogen ions. Thus, hyperchloremic metabolic acidosis with an inappro-

*Quan L, Smith DW: The VATER association. Vertebral defects, Anal atresia, T-E fistula with esophageal atresia, Radial and Renal dysplasia: A spectrum of associated defects. J Pediatr 82:104, 1973.

Table 16–22 CAUSES OF OBSTRUCTIVE UROPATHY

SITE OF OBSTRUCTION/CAUSE

Any site in the urinary tract
  Calculi
  Trauma causing interruption or distortion of tract for urine flow
  Blood clots
  Fungus balls
Tubule
  Uric acid crystals
  Polycystic kidneys
Renal pelvis
  Wilms tumor
  Ectopic kidney
  Tuberculosis
  Obstruction at ureteropelvic junction by fibrous bands, aberrant
    vessel, stenosis
Ureter
  Retroperitoneal disease
    Tumor
    Retroperitoneal fibrosis
    Hemangioma
    Retroperitoneal hemorrhage, abscess, urinoma
    Lymphocele
  Congenital
    Stricture
    Ureterocele
    Retrocaval ureter
    Ectopic kidney
    Diverticulum
    Adynamic segment
  Miscellaneous
    Ureteral valve
    Mesenteric cyst
    Peritonitis
    Abdominal tumors
Bladder
  Foreign body
  Hydrocolpos, hematocolpos
  Neurogenic bladder
  Chronic constipation
Urethra
  Valves
  Diverticulum
  Phimosis
  Meatal stenosis (males)
  Stricture (acquired or congenital)
  Foreign body
  Meatal atresia
  Hypospadias, epispadias
  Ectopic ureter

Adapted from Howards SS, Wright FS, In: Brenner BM, and Rector
FC (eds): The Kidney. Philadelphia, WB Saunders, 1976, p 1297.

priately high urine pH can occur in patients with only
mild or moderate reduction in the GFR.

Clinical Manifestations and Course. The clinical
features depend on whether the obstruction is acute or
chronic, partial or complete, and on whether there are
complications, such as infection. A history of oligohydramnios and occasionally of polyhydramnios during
the pregnancy may be obtained for infants with severe
obstructive uropathy. Acute obstruction usually presents with pain or strangury, and, if due to calculi,
with hematuria. The type of pain depends on the site
of obstruction and can be abdominal, in the costovertebral angle, along the ureters, or over the suprapubic
area; it can also radiate to the testicle or the inguinal
region. Hypertension can occur in patients with acute
obstruction. Polyuria due to inability to concentrate the

urine may result from acute bilateral partial obstruction.
The manifestations of *chronic obstruction* include polydipsia, polyuria, anemia, failure to thrive, chronic irritability, unexplained febrile episodes due to urinary
infection, frequent voiding, a weak urinary stream in
some and a forceful stream in other patients, and
daytime and nocturnal enuresis. Examination of the
abdomen may reveal a full bladder, an enlarged kidney,
or both. The course is often one of gradual reduction
in renal function. Inability to conserve sodium may be
a feature of chronic obstruction in infancy, and this
may lead to salt wasting and hyponatremia.

Postoperatively, after relief of obstruction a period of
increased urine output may last for days to weeks and
can be complicated by dehydration and by loss of
electrolytes. Another postoperative phenomenon is
transient but often severe hypertension, apparently due
to manipulation of the ureters or kidneys.

Laboratory Data. The laboratory data are those of
either acute or chronic renal failure. Azotemia, hyperkalemia, and metabolic acidosis are found in *acute
obstructive uropathy* if the obstruction is bilateral or if the
contralateral kidney is abnormal. In *chronic obstructive
uropathy*, the abnormalities include anemia, azotemia,
hypocalcemia, hyperphosphatemia, and a hyperchloremic metabolic acidosis. Urine concentrating ability is
impaired, and urine osmolality of 300 mOsm/kg H_2O is
not uncommon after 12 hr of water deprivation. Roentgenograms of bones may reveal evidence of hyperparathyroidism, osteoporosis, rickets, or sclerosis. Intravenous urography may identify the site of obstruction
and show reduced function and delayed excretion of
the contrast media. A voiding cystourethrogram can
help to demonstrate posterior urethral valves or vesicoureteral reflux. Ultrasound and radionuclide studies
can help to determine the presence of obstructive uropathy and to locate the site of obstruction.

Treatment. Though the treatment is usually surgical
correction or diversion of the urinary flow to bypass
the obstruction, the medical complications must be
treated as outlined in Sec 16.40 and 16.42. Furthermore,
children with ileal conduits or cutaneous ureterostomies
require psychologic support and counseling, especially
when they reach adolescence. Severe congenital chronic
hydronephrosis must be corrected before 1 yr of age if
there is to be a lasting improvement in renal function.

Prognosis. This depends on many factors, including
the degree of irreversible renal damage, the presence
of renal dysplasia, the age at which the diagnosis is
made, the type of obstruction, and the severity of
complications. Hypertension, renal osteodystrophy,
and urinary tract infection can adversely affect the
prognosis if not treated adequately.

BERNARD KAPLAN

Bensman A, Baudon JJ, Jablonski JP, et al: Uropathies diagnosed in the neonatal
  period: Symptomatology and course. Acta Pediatr Scand 69:449, 1980.
Hutcheon RA, Kaplan BS, Drummond KN: Distal renal tubular acidosis in children
  with chronic hydronephrosis. J Pediatr 89:372, 1976.
Mayor G, Genton N, Torrado A, et al: Renal function in obstructive nephropathy:
  Long-term effect of reconstructive surgery. Pediatrics 56:740, 1975.
Wilson DR: Pathophysiology of obstructive uropathy. Kidney Int 18:281, 1980.

16.56 MYOGLOBINURIA WITH RHABDOMYOLYSIS

There is confusion concerning the relation of myoglobinuria and hemoglobinuria to acute renal failure. Current evidence indicates that neither myoglobin nor hemoglobin is nephrotoxic but that under certain circumstances (e.g., severe dehydration, acidosis, or shock) the appearance of either of these substances in the circulation and urine may be associated with tubular injury and acute renal failure. The nephrotoxic agent released during injury or death of muscle (rhabdomyolysis) is probably not myoglobin but some other constituent such as tissue thromboplastin which may have a direct toxic effect on the renal tubules, induce hypotension, and trigger the coagulation system. Rhabdomyolysis with myoglobinuria, shock, and acute renal failure has been reported in patients with malignant hyperthermia, after muscle trauma or intense exercise, with heat stroke, with polymyositis, after intravenous administration of amphetamine, with different forms of muscular dystrophy (particularly after undergoing general anesthesia), in association with severe hypernatremia, in certain viral illnesses, and in hereditary disorders of muscle metabolism (such as lack of muscle phosphorylase, phosphofructokinase, or carnitine palmityl transferase). The presence of myoglobinuria, pigmented tubular casts, and an elevation in plasma creatine phosphokinase levels in a patient with acute renal failure suggests the diagnosis. There is no specific treatment, and general measures for treatment of acute renal failure are followed.

Bank WJ, DiMauro S, Bonilla E, et al: A disorder of muscle lipid metabolism and myoglobinuria. N Engl J Med 292:443, 1975.
Herman J, Nadler HL: Recurrent myoglobinuria and muscle carnitine palmityl transferase deficiency. J Pediatr 91:247, 1977.
Opas LM, Adler R, Robinson R, et al: Rhabdomyolysis with severe hypernatremia. J Pediatr 90:713, 1977.

DIABETIC NEPHROPATHY

Also see Sec 17.1.
Renal functional changes in diabetes mellitus occur long before there is clinical evidence of diabetic nephropathy. Initially, there is an unexplained elevation of glomerular filtration rate, and the filtration fraction is high. The glomerular size and glomerular filtering surface are increased. Within 1–2 yr there is an increased thickness in the glomerular basement membrane and mesangial deposition of basement membrane–like material.

Proteinuria is the most common clinical feature of diabetic nephropathy, and decreased renal function is uncommon in patients who do not have proteinuria. Proteinuria appears within 2 decades of onset in juvenile diabetes mellitus in many patients. The proteinuria is of glomerular origin; the quantity is usually under 2 gm/24 hr. The interval between onset of proteinuria and appearance of azotemia varies considerably, but the time from appearance of azotemia (defined as blood urea nitrogen 30 mg/dl or more) to end-stage renal disease seldom exceeds 2 yr. Patients with proteinuria are more likely to be hypertensive than those without proteinuria.

Diabetic nephropathy is the principal cause of death in patients whose onset of diabetes occurs in childhood. The need for management of these renal problems will usually arise in early and mid-adulthood and may, therefore, not be of concern to the pediatrician, but it is important to be aware of the serious renal problems which these children will ultimately have to face. Proteinuria, hypertension, and moderate azotemia occur in some diabetic children by their mid and late teens. At present there is no effective treatment to slow or change the course of diabetic nephropathy.

KEITH N. DRUMMOND

Knowles HC Jr: Magnitude of the renal failure problem in diabetic patients. Kidney Int (Suppl) 6(No 4): S2, 1974.
Shapiro FL, Kjellstrand CM, Goetz FC (guest eds): End-stage diabetic nephropathy. Kidney Int (Suppl) 6(No 4), 1974.
Viberti GC: Early functional and morphological changes in diabetic nephropathy. Clin Nephrol 12:47, 1979.

16.57 THE GENITOURINARY SYSTEM

16.58 ANOMALIES OF THE URINARY COLLECTING SYSTEM

The shape and form of the pyelocalyceal system may be altered by congenital malformation, obstruction, or infection. Calyceal diverticula and hydrocalycosis are focal areas of dilatation associated with congenital or acquired infundibular obstruction, occasionally including obstruction of the lower urinary tract from posterior urethral valves. Secondary infection and a stone or stones can develop within the cavity. At times, surgical repair is necessary. Differentiation of acquired abnormalities from congenital megacalycosis (generalized nonobstructive calyceal dilatation) is essential because surgery for the latter anomaly is of no benefit.

Complete duplication of the collecting system occurs when multiple ureteral buds originate from the mesonephric duct. Incomplete duplication ("Y" ureter) results from early division of the developing ureter.

Incompletely duplicated systems are usually asymptomatic except that stasis from to-and-fro passage of urine between the limbs (ureteroureteral reflux) may dispose to infection, with loin pain or discomfort. Total duplication is often an incidental finding, but it may be associated with an ectopic ureteral orifice, a ureterocele (involving the upper pole ureter), or vesicoureteral reflux (generally into the lower pole ureter). Duplication is more common in girls and more often unilateral. The ureteral orifice for the upper pole of a duplex collecting system is typically located more medial in the genitourinary tract than the orifice for the lower pole and can terminate inside or outside the urinary tract. The ectopic segment is generally dilated and associated with obstruction and dysplasia of the associated renal segment. Abnormality of the lower pole segment is usually associated with vesicoureteral reflux because the intravesical ureter is too short. This reflux may regress, but more often reflux associated with total duplication persists, often with parenchymal hypoplasia. Surgical correction generally has a favorable outcome.

Ectopic ureteral orifices terminate along the path of migration of the developing mesonephric duct or into structures of mesonephric origin, for example, at the vesical neck in both girls and boys or in the prostatic urethra, seminal vesicle, vas deferens, or ejaculatory duct in boys. Ectopic orifices in males are always suprasphincteric and do not produce incontinence. With infection of these segments, however, dysuria, asymptomatic pyuria, urinary infection, and recurrent epididymitis are possible, depending on the site of the orifice. Physical examination may disclose a rectal mass or an enlarged seminal vesicle. In boys ectopic ureters most often represent a single and dilated collecting system with a dysplastic renal unit, and total nephroureterectomy is indicated. In girls ectopic ureteral orifices can enter the vestibule, the urethra, or the vagina, and, less commonly, the uterus. When these ectopic orifices are extrasphincteric in location, continuous urinary dribbling occurs independent of voiding and can mimic vaginal discharge. Careful review of the intravenous urography with attention to calyceal asymmetry will usually reveal the duplication; the upper pole segment is often diminutive and poorly visualized. Physical examination may reveal wetness or a flow of urine in the vestibule provided the involved renal segment has sufficient function (Fig 16–14). Obstruction, infection, and renal dysplasia make preservation of the duplicated renal segment seldom worthwhile; the usual treatment is partial nephrectomy with ureterectomy. Ureteral reimplantations or other conservative procedures are occasionally possible.

Obstruction at the ureteropelvic junction is the most common cause of hydronephrosis in childhood. It is often the result of a congenitally abnormal zone of muscle function that interferes with propagation of ureteropelvic peristalsis; urinary stasis, pelvic dilatation, and further secondary mechanical obstruction result. Other causes of ureteropelvic junction obstruction include true stenosis, kinks, bands, adhesions, and aberrant renal vessels. Vesicoureteral reflux may also cause pelvic dilatation; accordingly, a voiding cystourethrogram should usually be included in the evaluation of apparent obstruction at the ureteropelvic junction.

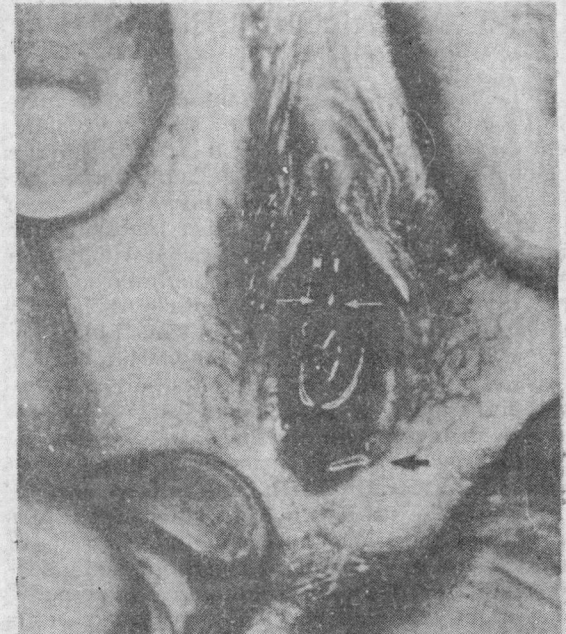

Figure 16–14   Ectopic ureter in perineum. Upper arrows (white) point to ectopic ureteral orifice between urethra and vagina; lower arrow (black) indicates perineal wetness.

The common symptoms of obstruction at the ureteropelvic junction in infancy are vomiting, sepsis, failure to thrive, and a palpable abdominal mass. Older children will often have vague gastrointestinal complaints, recurrent colicky or flank pain, and gross or microscopic hematuria after minimal trauma; at times, episodes of renal pain occur only after a large fluid intake (acute, intermittent hydronephrosis). Intravenous urography is usually diagnostic; with severe hydronephrosis the involved collecting system appears lucent during the earliest phase of the study, initially surrounded by crescents of opacification representing renal parenchyma stretched around dilated calyces; opacification within the collecting system follows (Fig 16–15). Delayed films (up to 24 hr) may be necessary to define the nature and extent of the obstruction. When the visualization is poor, ultrasonography may provide confirmatory evidence of hydronephrosis.

Transillumination with a fiberoptic light source in a darkened room may demonstrate a reddish glow of the hydronephrotic or multicystic kidney. Most hydronephroses and up to two thirds of multicystic kidneys transilluminate easily (Fig 16–16).

Surgical repair aims at creation of a dependent, funnel-shaped, ureteropelvic junction of sufficient caliber to allow adequate drainage of urine into the ureter, with sufficient reduction of renal pelvic size to improve the efficiency of emptying. Since the potential for recovery and growth of damaged parenchyma is excellent in infants, every effort should be made to preserve the kidney. In 20–40% of cases some degree of contralateral hydronephrosis is also present or may appear after correction of the 1st obstruction. Mild contralateral obstruction will often remain stable or even improve. Periodic postoperative intravenous urography is essen-

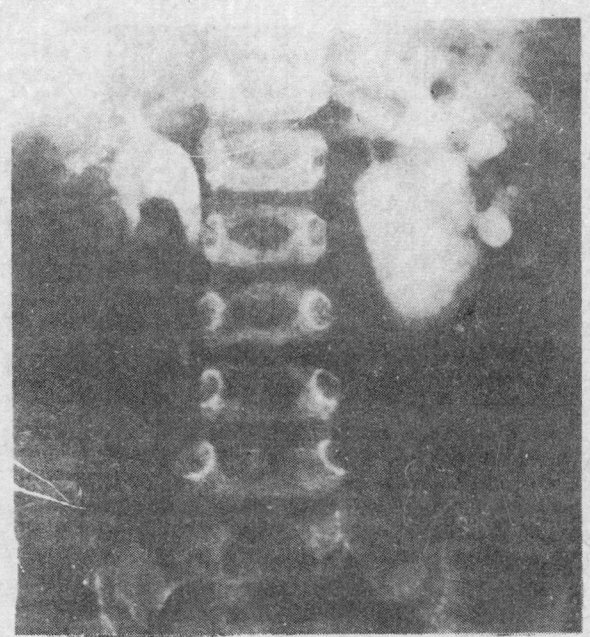

Figure 16–15 Ureteropelvic junction obstruction. Left ureteropelvic junction obstruction and hydronephrosis; right kidney is normal.

tial in following the status of both the operated and the contralateral kidney. Many yr may be required for final assessment.

Retrocaval ureter (circumcaval ureter) is an uncommon cause of upper urinary obstruction, the ureter passing medially behind and around the vena cava. It usually occurs on the right side when persistence of the ventral infrarenal subcardinal venous system traps the ureter behind it. Most retrocaval ureters are asymptomatic and are rarely found in childhood. Presenting symptoms are those of upper urinary tract obstruction and/or infection. Diagnosis is usually possible by intravenous urography; retrograde pyelography may be useful but carries risk of infection. The usual treatment is

division of the ureter and reanastomosis anterior to the vena cava.

Megaureter, or a wide or dilated ureter, may occur without distal ureteral obstruction (idiopathic), with juxtavesical ureteral obstruction (primary obstructed), or with vesicoureteral reflux; at times the obstruction is acquired as the result of extrinsic causes (e.g., pelvic masses) or iatrogenic factors. The diagnosis of megaureter is usually made on intravenous urography or voiding cystourethrography performed during investigation of urinary infection, hematuria, or abdominal pain. The dilatation of the ureter is typically more severe in its distal portion, with variable hydronephrotic changes in the upper urinary system. Because of the potential for progressive dilatation, infection, and renal deterioration, obstructive megaureter must be differentiated from the idiopathic; the former should be corrected surgically, usually by resection of the obstructing segment and by distal ureteral tapering and reimplantation. The documentation of obstruction is best made by means of percutaneous intrapelvic perfusion pressure and flow studies; fluoroscopic studies after retrograde instillation of contrast material into the ureter may also be helpful. Idiopathic megaureter (Fig 16–17) is more apt to be found in older children; it does not involve the pyelocalyceal system and requires no treatment unless recurrent infection is a problem. Treatment of megaureter secondary to vesicoureteral reflux will be considered later. The result of surgical repair of megaureter is generally good but depends upon the extent of pre-existing renal and ureteral damage.

Ureterocele is a congenital cystic ballooning of the distal portion of a ureter into the bladder; it is the result of an obstructed ureteral orifice. Ureteroceles may be simple (arising from a single ureter with a trigonal orifice) or ectopic (arising from a ureter with an ectopic orifice in the urethra). Ureteroceles are 4–6 times more common in girls than in boys and are bilateral in about 10% of cases.

Simple ureteroceles are associated with a single collecting system, are generally small, and are frequently asymptomatic; they are less often diagnosed in early

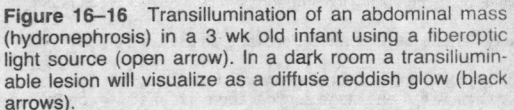

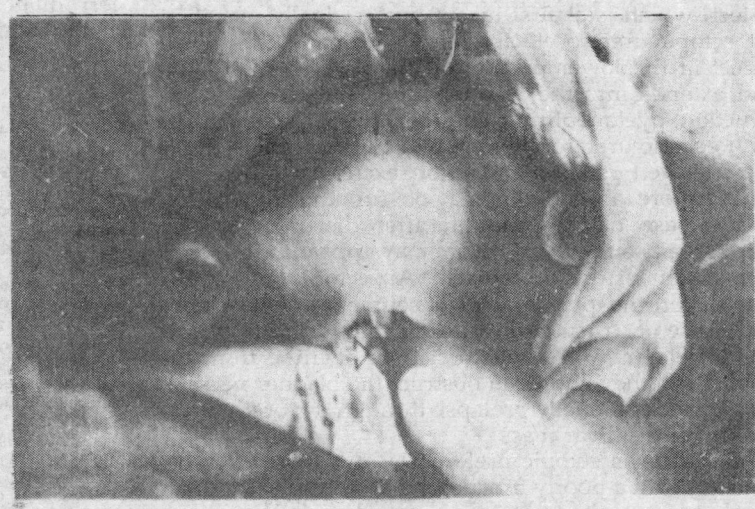

Figure 16–16 Transillumination of an abdominal mass (hydronephrosis) in a 3 wk old infant using a fiberoptic light source (open arrow). In a dark room a transilluminable lesion will visualize as a diffuse reddish glow (black arrows).

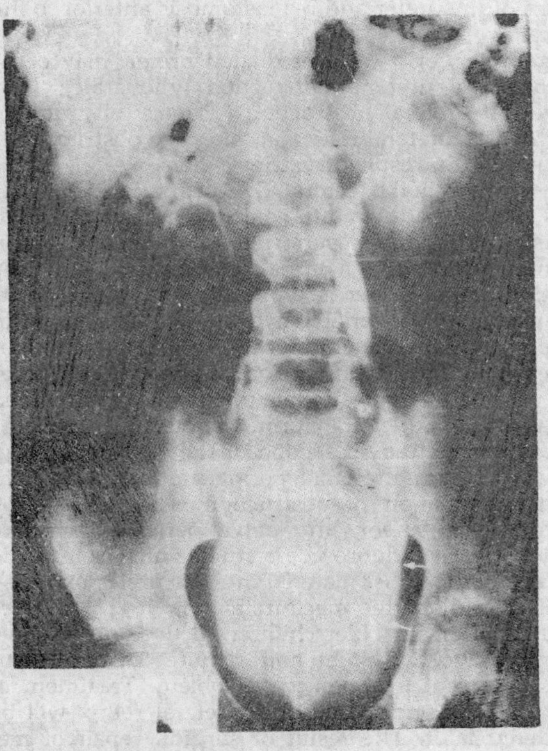

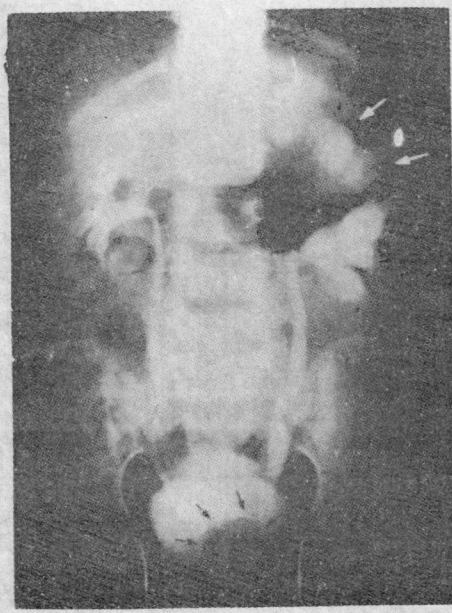

Figure 16–18 Ectopic ureterocele. Duplicated left kidney and collecting system: lucent filling defect of ureterocele in bladder (dark arrows); obstructed, hydronephrotic upper pole collecting system (white arrows).

Figure 16–17 Idiopathic megaureter: 14 yr old boy with fusiform distal ureteral dilation (arrows); also note mild upper ureteral dilation and minimal calycectasis. The right kidney and ureter are normal.

childhood than ectopic ureteroceles, which are almost always associated with the upper segment of a duplicated collecting system. Because of their size and location, the ectopic ureterocele is most often manifest early in life, with evidence of urinary infection or obstruction and, especially in infants, with septicemia and azotemia.

The simple ureterocele appears in the bladder on intravenous urography as a sharply defined, oval filling defect, which is at first lucent but gradually opacifies. An ectopic ureterocele appears as a broad-based filling defect in the lower portion of the bladder (Fig 16–18) and extends into the bladder neck. The effects of obstruction, pyelonephritis, and renal dysplasia associated with ectopic ureterocele may make it impossible to see the involved renal segment on excretory urography. Furthermore, a cystogram may obscure the filling defect at the base of the bladder; after distention of the bladder, a pseudodiverticulum may appear as the result of eversion of the ureterocele. An ectopic ureterocele may distort the ipsilateral lower segment ureteral orifice and cause obstruction of or reflux into it. Large ectopic ureteroceles may also obstruct flow of urine from the opposite kidney and even obstruct the bladder neck. In girls they occasionally prolapse through the urethra and present as a vulvar mass.

Inasmuch as ectopic ureteroceles are most often associated with a poorly functioning and dysplastic upper renal segment, the treatment is usually partial nephrec-

tomy and distal ureterectomy and at times ureterocelectomy. On occasion, the upper pole of the kidney can be saved and its ureter reimplanted into the bladder or anastomosed to the renal pelvis of the lower pole.

Simple ureteroceles are often small, cause no demonstrable obstruction, and require no treatment. Stones may form as a result of urinary stasis and/or infection in untreated simple ureteroceles, usually in the adult years; transurethral meatotomy and stone removal are then the simplest treatment. Treatment in childhood is reserved for larger lesions and those with pelvicalyceal dilatation. Transurethral resection may create reflux; simple meatotomy is less likely to do so. If reflux results, reimplantation of the ureter may be required. With a very dilated lower ureter, ureteral reconstruction and reimplantation is the best initial management.

Eklof O, Lohr G, Ringertz H, et al: Ectopic ureterocele in the male infant. Acta Radiologica Diagnosis 19:145, 1978.
Gray WS, Skandalakis JE: Embryology for Surgeons. Philadelphia, WB Saunders, 1972.
Hidai H, Kohdaira T, Terashima K, et al: Retrocaval ureter in children. Eur Urol 4:127, 1978.
Johnston JH: Megacalycosis: A burnt-out obstruction? J Urol 110:344, 1973.
Kroovand RL, Perlmutter AD: A one-stage surgical approach to ectopic ureterocele. J Urol 122:367, 1979.
Lockhart J, Singer A, Glenn JF: Congenital megaureter. J Urol 122:310, 1979.
Mann CM Jr, Ellis DG: Ureteropelvic junction obstruction. In: Holden TM, Ashcraft KW (eds): Pediatric Surgery. Philadelphia, WB Saunders, 1980.
Marshall FF, Jeffs RD, Smolev JK: Neonatal bilateral ureteropelvic junction obstruction. J Urol 123:107, 1980.
Michigan S, Whitton PK, Walsh PC: Forgotten kidney: Asynchronous bilateral ureteropelvic junction obstruction. Urology 12:565, 1978.
Perlmutter AD, Retik AB, Bauer SB: Anomalies of the upper urinary tract. In: Harrison JH, Gittes RF, Perlmutter AD, et al (eds): Campbell's Urology. Ed 4. Philadelphia, WB Saunders, 1979.

Retik AD: Ectopic ureter and ureterocele. *In:* Harrison JH, Gittes RF, Perlmutter AD, et al (eds): Campbell's Urology. Ed 4. Philadelphia, WB Saunders, 1979.

Smith P, Dunn M: Duplication of the upper urinary tract. Ann Roy Coll Surg 61:281, 1979.

Sullivan M, Halpern L, Hodges CV: Extravesical ureteral ectopia. Urology 11:577, 1978.

Williams DI: The natural history of reflux—a review. Urol Int 26:350, 1971.

16.59 ANOMALIES OF THE BLADDER AND URETHRA

During the 5th–7th wk of gestation the urorectal (cloacal) septum divides the terminal hindgut (cloaca) into an anterior urogenital sinus (ventral cloaca) and a posterior rectal canal (dorsal cloaca). The urogenital sinus lengthens during the 6th wk, and the more proximal portion dilates to form the urinary bladder; that portion closest to the umbilicus becomes the urachus, which usually becomes obliterated with continued development. The lower portion of the urogenital sinus produces the upper portion of the urethra. The developing ureteral buds and the terminal portions of the wolffian (mesonephric) ducts are absorbed into the urogenital sinus, where they create separate openings for the ureters and wolffian ducts (ejaculatory ducts) in the male; the wolffian ducts are vestigial in the female. Further development of the urogenital sinus in the male contributes to the major portion of the urethra and forms the prostate and in the female, to the vestibule, distal urethra, and lower vagina.

Urachal anomalies are rare and twice as common in boys as in girls. In infants they occur as a persistently patent urachus or as a persistent umbilical sinus and in older children as diverticula of the bladder dome, umbilical sinus, or urachal cyst. A patent urachus is not uncommon with the prune-belly syndrome or with obstruction of the lower urinary tract. Urachal cysts are formed when both ends of the urachal tract become closed without obliteration of the lumen; this may produce a lower abdominal mass, sometimes with abscess formation. Intraperitoneal rupture can occur, or an abscess may drain into the bladder. External umbilical sinuses may have a purulent discharge. Urachal lesions are correctable by surgery.

Exstrophy of the bladder with epispadias is the most common of a spectrum of related anomalies of the lower urinary and genital tracts; it occurs in 1:30,000–40,000 live births, is more common in males, and is not familial. In the exstrophic anomalies an abnormally large cloacal membrane prevents mesodermal ingrowth and midline fusion between the endodermal and ectodermal layers, dislocating the primordial tissues. Rupture of the membrane leads to deficiency in development of the anterior abdominal wall, pubis, bladder, and urethra. Since the paired primordia of the phallus remain apart, the clitoris and occasionally the penis fail to fuse in the midline.

The form of exstrophy depends upon the size and stage of development of the cloacal membrane at the time of rupture. Usually, the bladder is everted and its mucosa exposed, the rectus muscles diverge and are inserted into widely separated pubic bones, and the

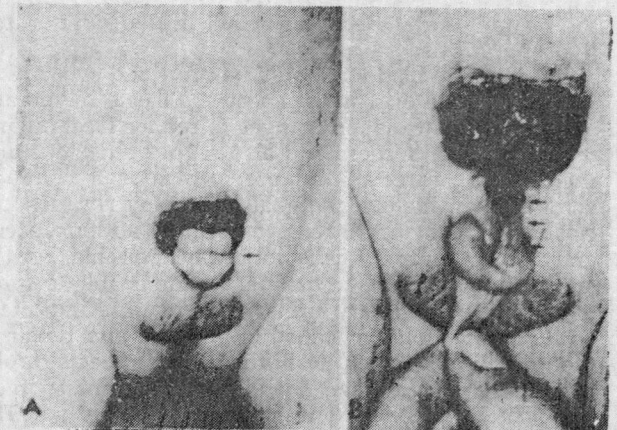

Figure 16–19 Exstrophy of the bladder. *A,* Male infant with exstrophy; epispadias of penis with dorsal chordee (arrow). *B,* Dorsal view of the short broad epispadias; arrows indicate open urethral strip on dorsum of penis.

umbilicus is located at the top edge of the exstrophy, giving the upper abdomen an overdeveloped appearance (Fig 16–19). The perineum is flattened, and the anus is more anterior than usual. The bony pelvic ring is open anteriorly, and the femoral heads are externally rotated; the child has a waddling gait but no other orthopedic deformity. Umbilical and inguinal hernias are common but often not apparent at birth. Unrelated anomalies occur in other systems, but there is no pattern to their occurrence.

In males the epispadic penis is broad, short, and spadelike with dorsal chordee and an open urethral strip on the dorsum of the penis (Fig 16–20). In females the clitoris is bifid or double; the labia are widely separated, and the vagina is located more anteriorly than usual.

The affected infant should be examined by a pediatrician and by a urologist familiar with exstrophy. Findings on intravenous urography are usually normal at first, but ureteral dilatation may follow inflammation of

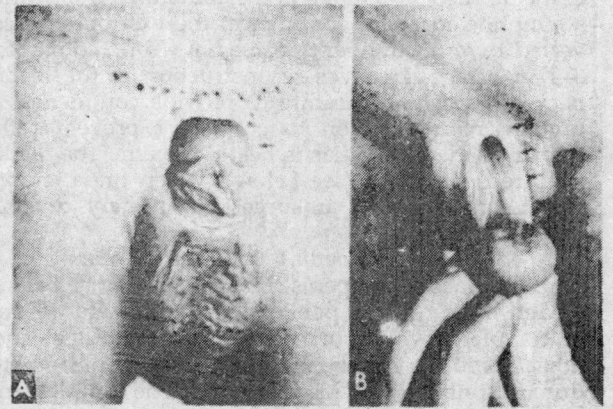

Figure 16–20 Complete epispadias. *A,* Male with short spade-shaped penis with dorsal chordee (arrow). Marks on abdomen are preoperative for repair. *B,* Epispadias; dorsal urethral gutter extending into incompetent bladder neck (arrows).

the bladder surface and can result in hydroureter and hydronephrosis.

The exposed bladder should be protected by strips of Vaseline gauze or a moist sheet of Silastic membrane and by frequent diaper changes to reduce local inflammation and tenderness and also reduce tenesmus and the chance of rectal prolapse, which is a common complication. Ideally, the goal of therapy is functional closure of the defect to achieve normal bladder capacity and urinary control; this is not always possible. For the small, fibrotic, platelike bladder not amenable to functional closure, primary urinary diversion is indicated, with simultaneous or staged cystectomy and repair of the anterior abdominal wall; the genital defects can be corrected at a later date. The surgery for urinary diversion can be postponed until the 2nd or 3rd yr. The current choice for external urinary diversion is a nonrefluxing ureterosigmoid cutaneous diversion (sigmoid colon conduit); for internal diversion, ureterosigmoid anastomosis. The antirefluxing sigmoid conduit appears not to have many of the late complications of uretero-ileal-cutaneous diversion (ileal conduit). Internal urinary diversion (ureterosigmoidostomy) is an excellent alternative to external urinary diversion and avoids the psychologic trauma associated with an external appliance. The procedure is contraindicated in patients with diminished renal function, dilated ureters, or a weak anal sphincter.

Complications of ureterosigmoidostomy include hyperchloremic acidosis, hypokalemia, recurrent pyelonephritis, and growth impairment. Supplementary potassium and sodium citrate or bicarbonate can reduce the likelihood of chronic metabolic acidosis. Frequent emptying of the bowel on a timed schedule is also important to minimize acidosis and postrenal azotemia. Failure of ureterosigmoidostomy will require cutaneous diversion. Continued follow-up is essential for children with any type of urinary diversion.

In patients for whom functional bladder closure seems possible, achievement of continence requires several stages of difficult repair; complications and failure are common. The bladder should be closed shortly after birth; the 1st operation is limited to closure of the detrusor and repair of the abdominal wall without attempting to attain continence; the exstrophy is converted to an incontinent epispadias. The 2nd stage, at 3–4 yr of age, involves reconstruction of the bladder neck and posterior urethra to provide continence and ureteral reimplantation to correct or prevent reflux. Repair of the epispadias is best done after the bladder neck reconstruction (see below). When the attempt at functional closure is unsuccessful, urinary diversion becomes necessary.

In boys with epispadias the urethra opens on the dorsal surface of the penis. Epispadias may be balanitic (a cleft in the glans), penile (glans and shaft affected), or complete (with short penis, dorsal chordee, and a dorsal urethral gutter extending into an incompetent urinary sphincter and bladder neck). The complete form of epispadias is the most common; it often accompanies exstrophy. Repair of complete epispadias, including that remaining after treatment of exstrophy, involves cosmetic and functional reconstruction of the penis and urethra. Incontinence may require repair of the underdeveloped bladder neck and posterior urethra–sphincter areas; an artificial urinary sphincter may be implanted.

Girls with epispadias have a bifid clitoris and a short wide urethra, often with incontinence due to involvement of the bladder neck. The condition is sometimes diagnosed only when careful genital examination is made of the incontinent girl. Monsplasty and clitoral approximation are indicated unless the defect is very minor; correction of incontinence is required.

Cloacal exstrophy is the most complex and severe of the exstrophic anomalies and is often associated with other anomalies. Here, perforation of the cloacal membrane before complete descent of the urorectal septum allows eversion of the hindgut between the bladder plates. Many affected infants do not survive the neonatal period; those who do survive require a thorough evaluation, especially of the urogenital, nervous, and cardiovascular systems. Initial management involves treatment of excessive fluid losses from the short intestinal tract. Immediate surgical intervention is not generally necessary, but separate urinary and fecal diversions should be established at an appropriate time, and genital abnormalities should be corrected. Sex assignment should be assessed in the neonatal period since the double penis of the male with cloacal exstrophy is usually diminutive and inadequate.

Diverticulum of the bladder in children is usually a developmental anomaly but occasionally associated with urinary obstruction or with neurogenic bladder. The diverticulum is a herniation of the bladder mucosa through a muscular defect in the wall of the bladder, most often near or at the ureteral hiatus. Discovery is commonly made during roentgenographic investigation of urinary tract infection or of a voiding problem. A periureteral diverticulum may produce vesicoureteral reflux or, when large, ureteral obstruction. Large diverticula which drain poorly contain residual urine and should be removed; ureteral reimplantation may be necessary.

Duplication of the urethra is an uncommon anomaly that appears in a variety of forms. The duplication is usually sagittal; rare horizontal duplications are typically associated with penile duplication. In boys with sagittal urethral duplication the true urethra is most often in its normal position, with the orifice of the accessory urethra usually situated in an epispadic location along the dorsal glans or penile shaft. The accessory urethra tends to create a dorsal chordee. It can end blindly under the pubis or extend all the way into the neck of the bladder; if the accessory urethra exits the bladder outside the sphincter mechanism, the boy will be incontinent through this accessory channel. Rarely, the true urethra terminates in an anal or perianal (hypospadic) location with a hypoplastic accessory channel more dorsal in the penile shaft.

In girls the accessory urethra may penetrate the clitoris. As in the male, side-by-side (horizontal) urethral duplications may be associated with duplications of the bladder, vagina, or clitoris.

Some accessory urethras cause no symptoms. Surgical repair is required when there is incontinence, chordee, or local infection or when the true urethra is ectopic in the perineum.

Posterior urethral valves consist of hyperplastic folds of tissue located in the posterior urethra just below the verumontanum; they are the most common cause of lower urinary obstruction in male neonates, infants, and young boys. Their embryogenesis is poorly understood. Clinical presentation is variable and often insidious; the effects may be disastrous. The most important diagnostic clues in the neonate or young infant are a distended bladder and a weak, dribbling urinary stream. When the obstruction has been severe during fetal development, there may be oligohydramnios and failure to thrive, with sepsis, anemia, and renal failure. Toddlers may have dysuria, hematuria, urinary infection, or azotemia. Older children who have had lesser degrees of obstruction are generally identified because of diurnal dribbling and sometimes infection; hydroureter and hydronephrosis are less common. Infants with posterior urethral valves or other lower urinary tract obstruction should have urethral catheter drainage for a few days, preferably using an infant feeding tube. Voiding cystourethrography is diagnostic; it shows a dilated and elongated posterior urethra, a trabeculated bladder, and often the valvular folds (Fig 16–21). Vesicoureteral reflux may be present. In infants in whom renal function permits visualization, intravenous urography usually shows extensive hydronephrosis and hydroureter; at times, the findings are nearly normal.

Definitive treatment is usually the transurethral destruction of the valvular leaflets. Relief of obstruction may be followed by diuresis, which must be anticipated, recognized promptly, and treated appropriately. Rarely, critically ill or septic infants may require temporary cutaneous vesicostomy or supravesical drainage, such as loop cutaneous ureterostomy, with treatment of the valves and urinary tract reconstruction postponed. The prognosis depends upon the severity of renal damage and dysplasia at the time of diagnosis. Careful postoperative medical management now allows many infants

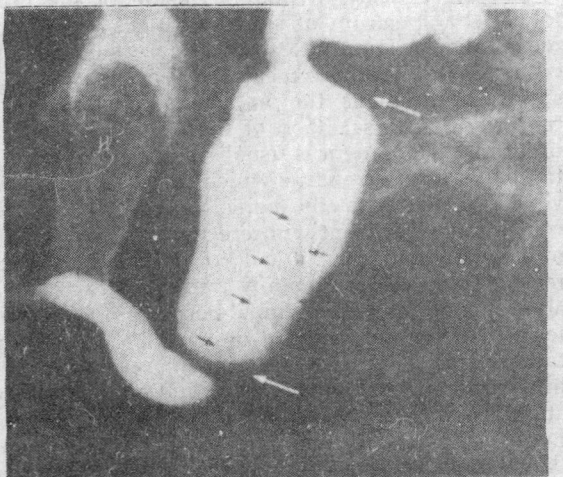

Figure 16–21 Oblique cystogram showing posterior urethral valves. Elongated prostatic urethra (white arrows) from obstruction; valve leaflets (dark arrows).

with severe chronic renal insufficiency to survive to an age when they become candidates for renal transplantation.

Congenital urethral diverticula and anterior urethral valves are similar, uncommon lesions. Most anterior valves do not appear to exist as isolated lesions but rather as the obstructing distal lip (rim) of a small urethral diverticulum, often initially unrecognized.

In prepubertal girls urethral diverticula are very rare. In boys most diverticula are a manifestation of abnormal development of the corpus spongiosum; they may be saccular or fusiform. Megalourethra, a diffuse enlargement of the entire anterior urethra, is a related lesion. Diverticula located in the deep bulbous urethra arise from anomalous openings of the bulbourethral (Cowper) gland ducts.

The age at diagnosis of anterior urethral valves depends on the severity of obstruction. Diagnosis is suggested by a weak urinary stream and ballooning of the proximal urethra during voiding. Saccular diverticula can similarly produce urinary obstruction by the flaplike action of the distal lip. When severe, the obstruction is associated with urinary stasis, infection, and postvoiding dribbling; upper urinary tract damage can result. A ventral penile or perineal mass may be felt. Fusiform diverticula, idiopathic megalourethra, and megalourethra associated with the prune-belly syndrome may appear as a dorsally curved or redundant, flabby penis, with ventral urethral ballooning during voiding; there is no obstructive component.

Voiding cystourethrography defines the nature and extent of the anomaly; excretory urography will assess the effects on the upper urinary tract. Anterior urethral valves or obstructing diverticula are managed by transurethral resection of the obstructing flap or rim. Large diverticula may require open excision and repair.

The **prune-belly syndrome** (triad [Eagle-Barrett] syndrome) occurs in 1/30,000–40,000 live births, almost invariably in males; it has a wide spectrum of severity and of clinical presentation. Typically, there is deficiency of the abdominal musculature, nonobstructive dilatation and dysplasia of the urinary tract, and cryptorchidism. Many affected infants are stillborn or die early in the neonatal period from pulmonary hypoplasia or ventilation problems related to the muscular deficiencies. Others with lesser manifestations of the syndrome may remain undetected until roentgenographic investigation for other reasons reveals the characteristic abnormalities of the urinary tract: elongated and dilated ureters with ineffective peristalsis, a bladder of large capacity, and frequently a urachal diverticulum which empties poorly. The posterior urethra is dilated, and the prostate may be hypoplastic or absent. The corpus spongiosum and the tissues of the anterior urethra may be deficient, with resultant megalourethra. Rarely, urethral stenosis or atresia will be associated with a patent urachus. The kidneys are variably dysmorphic, the testes almost invariably intra-abdominal. Associated malformations may involve the skeletal and cardiovascular symptoms or the gastrointestinal tract (with malrotation).

Early treatment is symptomatic. The dilatation of the urinary tract may be striking, but the hydronephrosis is of low pressure; unless infection develops which cannot be cleared readily, no surgery is necessary. For some children who have demonstrable anatomic obstruction or acquire intractable infection, temporary cutaneous vesicostomy or a more proximal urinary diversion will decompress the urinary tract and, with appropriate antibacterial therapy, will control the urinary infection. In selected instances, other corrective surgery may improve bladder and ureteral function.

Chisolm TC: Exstrophy of the urinary bladder. In: Holder TM, Ashcraft KW (eds): Pediatric Surgery. Philadelphia, WB Saunders, 1980.
Duckett JW Jr: Anomalies of the urethra. In: Harrison JH, Gittes RF, Perlmutter AD, et al (eds): Campbell's Urology. Ed 4. Philadelphia, WB Saunders, 1979.
Duckett JW Jr: Prune-belly syndrome. In: Holder TM, Ashcraft KW (eds): Pediatric Surgery. Philadelphia, WB Saunders, 1980.
Griffith GL, Mulcahy JJ, McRoberts WJ: Umbilical anomalies. South Med J 72:981, 1979.
Jeffs RD: Exstrophy. In: Harrison JH, Gittes RF, Perlmutter AD, et al (eds): Campbell's Urology. Ed 4. Philadelphia, WB Saunders, 1979.
Johnston JH: Epispadias. In: Harrison JH, Gittes RF, Perlmutter AD, et al (eds): Campbell's Urology. Ed 4. Philadelphia, WB Saunders, 1979.
Lebowitz RL, Colodny AH, Crissey M: Neonatal hydronephrosis caused by vesical diverticula. Urology 13:335, 1979.
Muecke EC: The role for the cloacal membrane in exstrophy: The first successful experimental study. J Urol 92:659, 1964.
Muecke EC: Exstrophy, epispadias and other anomalies of the bladder. In: Harrison JH, Gittes RF, Perlmutter AD, et al (eds): Campbell's Urology. Ed 4. Philadelphia, WB Saunders, 1979.
Perlmutter AD: Urachal disorders. In: Harrison JH, Gittes RF, Perlmutter AD, et al (eds): Campbell's Urology. Ed 4. Philadelphia, WB Saunders, 1979.
Sahney S, Perlmutter AD, Fleischmann LE, et al: The importance of supportive medical management in infants with posterior urethral valves. Presented at Section on Urology, American Academy of Pediatrics, November, 1976.
Shapiro SR, Lebowitz R, Colodny AH: Fate of 90 children with ileal conduit urinary diversion a decade later: Analysis of complications, pyelography, renal function, and bacteriology. J Urol 114:289, 1975.
Silverman FN, Huang N: Congenital absence of the abdominal muscle associated with malformation of the genitourinary and alimentary tracts: Report of cases and a review of literature. Am J Dis Child 80:91, 1950.
Smith ED: Malformations of the bladder and urethra and hypospadias. In: Holder TM, Ashcraft KW (eds): Pediatric Surgery. Philadelphia, WB Saunders, 1980.
Sohrabi A, Bellis JA, Durig JC, et al: Duplication of male urethra. Urol 12:704, 1978.
Williams DI: Prune-belly syndrome. In: Harrison JH, Gittes RF, Perlmutter AD, et al (eds): Campbell's Urology. Ed 4. Philadelphia, WB Saunders, 1979.

16.60 ANOMALIES OF THE MALE EXTERNAL GENITALIA

EMBRYOLOGY

The genital tubercle develops cephalad to the cloacal membrane; paired genital folds develop, flanking its ventral surface, and paired genital swellings develop laterally. In response to androgen secreted by the fetal testis the genital tubercle enlarges and extends outward to form the penis. The genital folds fuse in the midline to enclose the urethra, and the genital swellings migrate inferiorly and fuse to form the scrotum. During the 3rd mo of development the prepuce develops from tissue at the base of the glans penis, grows over the dorsal penis to surround the glans, and fuses ventrally to form the frenulum.

In the female the genital tubercle grows less, forming the clitoris. There is no fusion of the genital folds or genital swellings, which become the labia minora and labia majora, respectively.

The gonads develop from mesenchyme of the paired genital ridges, to which germ cells migrate from the yolk sac. Differentiation of the gonads into testis or ovary depends on chromosomal sex and on the presence or absence of testosterone. The sex ducts differentiate from the paired wolffian or müllerian ducts in accordance with genetic sex. In the male each wolffian duct forms an epididymis, vas deferens, seminal vesicle, and ejaculatory duct; the müllerian system regresses. In the female the müllerian ducts contribute to formation of the fallopian tubes, uterus, and proximal vagina; the wolffian ducts regress.

ANOMALIES OF THE PENIS

Agenesis of the penis is rare and is due to failure of the genital tubercle to develop. The urethral opening is usually located near the anus; the condition is frequently associated with anorectal anomalies and renal dysplasia. The condition is best managed by surgical conversion to female status in early infancy.

Micropenis is also unusual; the penis is diminutive but anatomically normal, with a urethral meatus at the tip of the glans. Micropenis has a variety of associations (microphallus, Prader-Willi syndrome, anencephalia, apituitarism, Kallmann syndrome, various forms of dwarfism, etc.). It is due to failure of the testis or pituitary to provide adequate hormonal stimulation during the final 2 trimesters of pregnancy or to failure of the genital tubercle to respond to this stimulus. Endocrine evaluation will identify those children who may respond to endocrine therapy, but some are undiagnosed until puberty, when anticipated genital growth fails to occur. If at an early age studies show end-organ unresponsiveness, or if the stretched penile length is less than 2.0 cm in the newborn (2 or more standard deviations below the normal mean) and there is associated gonadal dysgenesis, sex reassignment should be considered.

Hypospadias is the most common anomaly of the penis; it affects 1–3.3/1000 live births and is the result of failure or delay in midline fusion of the urethral folds. The spectrum of severity ranges from minimal meatal displacement to extreme degrees of genital ambiguity. The urethral meatus opens on the ventral surface of the penis; the prepuce is deficient ventrally, presenting a dorsal hood or flap. The distal failure of urethral development is usually associated with a ventral band of fibrous tissue which causes some degree of ventral curvature of the penis (chordee). Chordee becomes more apparent with erection; when it is severe, intercourse may be difficult or impossible. Urethral meatal stenosis is commonly present; other associated abnormalities include inguinal hernia and undescended testes. With mild degrees of hypospadias associated urinary tract anomalies are uncommon and usually of little consequence; pyelographic and endoscopic evaluation is unnecessary. With the more severe degrees of hypospadias and genital ambiguity, a vaginal remnant (large utriculus masculinus) may enter the prostatic urethra and lead to lower urinary tract infections.

In assessment of the severity of hypospadias it is useful to describe the position of the urethral meatus (glandular, coronal, distal penile, and so on) and the location and degree of chordee (glandular, midshaft, mild, moderate, severe, and so on). These are important in planning management. An embarrassment due to more severe degrees of hypospadias is the need to sit to void. In evaluating hypospadias, chordee is often overlooked or its severity underestimated. The extent of chordee is revealed by compression of the corpora cavernosa in the perineum; the penile shaft will become engorged and with additional compression at the base of the penis may mimic erection (Fig 16–22).

The treatment for hypospadias with chordee consists of straightening the curved penis and establishing a more distal meatus. Most surgeons agree that reconstruction should not be attempted during infancy but should be completed prior to school age. Some hold that for psychologic reasons the best time for elective surgery on the genitalia is during the 4th yr. For most children with hypospadias distal to the penoscrotal angle, 1-stage repairs consisting of release of chordee and urethroplasty using preputial skin provide excellent functional and cosmetic results. Hypospadias may occur without chordee or severe chordee without hypospadias. The management is modified appropriately in each case.

Penoscrotal transposition associated with hypospadias may result in a scrotum that partially or completely surrounds the penis. Surgical repositioning of the scrotum, with release of any chordee, will improve the cosmetic appearance and function of the genitalia.

Phimosis is a narrowness (congenital or acquired) of the opening of the prepuce that prevents its being drawn back over the glans penis. In the newborn male infant the preputial space is incompletely developed, and the prepuce is adherent to the glans and not easily retracted. With normal development and physiologic erections these adhesions gradually disappear, the opening at the prepuce widens, and the prepuce becomes freely retractile by the age of 3 yr. After this time a prepuce that cannot be retracted or has a tight ring may be identified as phimotic. Attempts at forcible retraction of the prepuce in the neonate or infant should be avoided as they tend to tear the prepuce, with scarring that may cause persistent phimosis. Phimosis may also result from infection or trauma.

Paraphimosis is incarceration of the glans penis by a phimotic prepuce which has retracted behind it; local pain and swelling may be intense. Reduction is sought by firm pressure against the glans with countertraction on the prepuce. If this is unsuccessful, immediate incision of the constricting band, or circumcision, is indicated.

Circumcision in infancy is generally done for social or religious reasons. The major medical indications for circumcision are persistent phimosis or balanoposthitis, but these are not problems of infancy. If circumcision of the newborn infant is to be done, a careful prior inspection of the penis should be made for conditions such as epispadias, hypospadias, isolated chordee, or anomalous investment of penile skin. If any of these are present, circumcision should be avoided because the prepuce will be needed for reconstructive surgery.

Urethral **meatal stenosis** is the result of perimeatal inflammation or ulceration after circumcision, usually

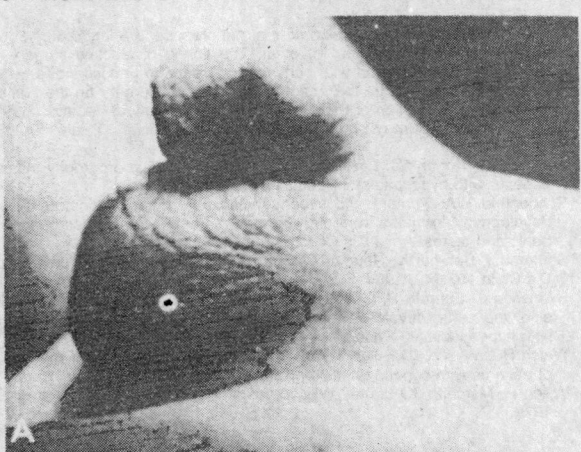
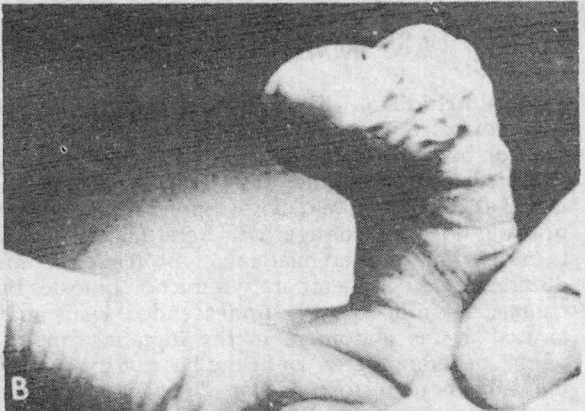

Figure 16–22 Hypospadias. *A*, Appearance of penis and dorsal hooded prepuce. *B*, Compression of corpora cavernosa to engorge penile shaft, simulate erection, and demonstrate presence of chordee.

secondary to diaper dermatitis. Meatitis is treated by frequent diaper changes, exposure of the penis to air, and local cleansing in an attempt to reduce the effects of inflammation and irritation (Sec 24.26). Meatal stenosis may be asymptomatic or cause dysuria, terminal hematuria, or urinary spotting. The urinary stream is needle-like and often dorsally deflected. The diagnosis of meatal stenosis cannot be made solely on the appearance of the meatus; a narrow-looking meatal orifice may widen adequately during voiding. The appearance of the urinary stream is the important diagnostic criterion.

Meatal stenosis almost never produces serious urinary obstruction. Urologic investigations are necessary only with other indications. Symptomatic meatal stenosis can usually be corrected as an office procedure, with local anesthesia and light sedation as needed.

Allen JS, Summers JL: Meatal stenosis in children. J Urol 112:526, 1974.

Bauer SB, Bull MJ, Retik AB: Hypospadias: A familial study. J Urol 121:474, 1979.

Gibbons MB: Why circumcise. Pediatr Nursing 5:9, 1979.

Grimes DA: Routine circumcision of the newborn infant: A reappraisal. Am J Obstet Gynecol 130:125, 1978.

Hunter RH: Notes on the development of the prepuce. J Anat 70:68, 1935.

Kelalis PP, Bunge R, Barker M, et al: The timing of elective surgery on the genitalia in male children with particular reference to undescended testes and hypospadias. Report by the Action Committee on Surgery on the Genitalia of Male Children, Section of Urology, American Academy of Pediatrics, 1974.

Lisa L, Hanah J, Cerney M, et al: Agenesis of the penis. J Pediatr Surg 7:442, 1972.

Lutzker CG, Kogan SJ, Levitt SB: Is routine intravenous urography indicated in patients with hypospadias? Pediatrics 59:630, 1977.

Schoenfeld WA: Primary and secondary sexual characteristics; study of their development in males from birth through maturity, with biometric study of the penis and testes. Am J Dis Child 65:535, 1943.

Shulman J, Ben-hur N, Neuman Z: Surgical complications of circumcision. Am J Dis Child 107:149, 1964.

Svensson J, Eneroth P, Gustafsson J, et al: Metabolism of androstenedione in skin and serum levels of gonadotropins and androgens in prepubertal boys with hypospadias. J Endocrinol 76:399, 1978.

Walsh PC, Wilson JD, Allen TD, et al: Clinical and endocrinological evaluations of patients with congenital microphallus. J Urol 120:90, 1978.

Wilkin P, Metcalfe JO, Lahey WH: Hypospadias: A review. Can J Surg 22:532, 1979.

16.61   ANOMALIES OF THE TESTIS

Cryptorchidism.   Descent of the testes into the scrotum normally occurs during the 8th mo of fetal life. One or both testes are undescended in about 30% of low birth weight infants, in 3–4% of term infants, and in 0.3–0.7% of 1 yr old boys. Spontaneous descent is unusual after 1 yr of age. Unilateral failure of descent is more common than bilateral; cryptorchidism must be differentiated from temporary retraction of testes by the cremasteric muscles. An undescended testis may be located in the abdomen, in the inguinal canal, perineum, or femoral area, or at the base of the penis over the pubic bone (ectopic testis). The causes of testicular maldescent appear to be multiple and may be related to testicular failure, to deficient gonadotropic stimulation, to mechanical obstruction, or to an ectopic attachment of the gubernaculum.

Evaluation of undescended testes requires examination in a warm relaxed environment. If retractile testes are suspected, repeated examinations may be needed. When the testis is in the inguinal canal, it may often be trapped by sliding the fingers from the internal inguinal ring toward the neck of the scrotum. Examination in the squatting position may aid in locating a highly placed testis. Retractile testes require no treatment.

The undescended testis is likely to be smaller than its normally descended mate, is more susceptible to development of malignancy, and is a poor sperm producer. There frequently are associated abnormalities of the corresponding mesonephric derivatives and, in up to 90%, an associated inguinal hernia. Associated anomalies of the urinary system are uncommon; accordingly, routine pyelography in cases of simple undescended testis does not seem warranted. The higher the position of the undescended testis, the greater will be the abnormality of the testis, the likelihood of associated ductal structures, and the likelihood of anomalies in other systems.

Torsion of the undescended testicle is an uncommon event that may be confused with incarcerated inguinal hernia. Both conditions produce a tender, nonreducible inguinal mass requiring prompt surgical consultation and often exploration. The prognosis for future function of the testis is poor, usually because of delays in diagnosis and treatment. The cause of spermatic cord torsion in the undescended testicle is poorly understood. In patients with bilateral cryptorchidism, unilateral torsion warrants prompt elective contralateral orchiopexy.

In 3–5% of surgical explorations for unilateral cryptorchidism no testis is found. The cause may be failure of the testis to develop from its primordial tissue or a loss of its blood supply during fetal life or early infancy. When the vas deferens is also absent, the ipsilateral ureter and kidney are sometimes absent.

Bilateral congenital absence of the testes (anorchism) is rare; its occurrence in a male with normal phallus implies that an embryologic disaster followed early sexual differentiation. In order to detect bilateral anorchism and avoid unnecessary exploratory surgery, children with bilateral cryptorchidism should have measurements of urinary gonadotropin levels and of serum testosterone levels before and after administration of human chorionic gonadotropin (hCG). With bilateral agenesis, levels of urinary gonadotropins are elevated, and serum testosterone levels are low and unresponsive to challenge with gonadotropin; under such circumstances, surgical exploration is not required to confirm anorchism. Therapy with testosterone at puberty will produce masculinization and prevent a eunuchoid appearance. In children with cryptorchidism who have normal levels of urinary gonadotropins and appropriate increases in testosterone levels after hCG challenge, surgical exploration is indicated. The role of treatment by hCG for cryptorchidism is unclear; its administration may differentiate between maldescended and potentially retractile testes, but it is usually not effective in securing or maintaining descent of the former. In selected cases, a course of such therapy (1000 units hCG intramuscularly 3 times weekly for 3 wk) can be tried; if testicular descent does not occur, orchiopexy should be performed. Orchiopexy should include correction of the associated hernia.

When an abdominal testis is too high to be brought into the scrotum and appears worthy of salvage, orchiopexy may be done in 2 stages, or a 1-stage procedure may be done which involves mobilization of the testis and the vas deferens and its blood supply, with microsurgical relocation of the spermatic vessels to the inferior epigastric vessels. These procedures are followed by testicular atrophy in a substantial number of cases.

Malignant change, usually seminoma, occurs in undescended testes at least 14 times more frequently than in scrotal testes, but it is uncommon. Testicular tumors account for about 1% of malignancies in males; 5–12% of testicular tumors occur in undescended testicles. These tumors do not occur before puberty. Orchiopexy does not appear to change the risk of tumor but does make the testis accessible to examination. There is also a higher than normal frequency of malignancy in the contralateral descended testis; this suggests that the end-organ defect of unilateral cryptorchidism may be bilateral. This assumption is supported by the fact that about a third of adults who have had an orchiopexy in childhood for a unilateral undescended testis are oligospermic.

Cosmetic results after orchiopexy are generally good,

but whether fertility is apt to be improved is undetermined. Histologic studies have shown that irreversible and progressive changes in the germinal epithelium of the undescended testis can first be seen at 2–3 yr of age. In view of these degenerative changes and the infrequency of spontaneous descent after 1 yr of age, elective orchiopexy should be performed during the 2nd–3rd yr of life—earlier than has been recommended in the past. Simple orchiopexy for the undescended but palpable testis can usually be performed without the need for overnight hospitalization.

Torsion of the spermatic cord (including the testis) is the most common intrascrotal disorder in children and must be differentiated from torsion of testicular appendage and from epididymitis. Torsion may be inside or outside the tunica vaginalis which surrounds the testis. Intravaginal torsion (torsion of the testis) is the most common form and is due to absence of the posterior attachments of the testis within the tunica vaginalis which normally prevent the testis from twisting. Such torsion has its peak incidence in early adolescence. Affected children typically have sudden onset of scrotal pain, nausea, and vomiting; occasionally attacks are intermittent. Early examination reveals a swollen, tender, elevated testis and a variable degree of scrotal edema. The epididymis is usually anterior. Progressive scrotal edema and the development of a hydrocele may obscure intrascrotal anatomy and make differentiation from epididymitis difficult.

Extravaginal torsion (torsion of the entire spermatic cord and scrotal contents at the external inguinal ring) is found only in neonates, in whom it has often had an antenatal onset. Extravaginal torsion may be related to lack of fixation of the testis and its membranes to the scrotum. Extravaginal torsion characteristically presents a smooth, firm, painless mass in a discolored scrotum. At surgery the testis is usually found to be infarcted, but torsion should be reduced and the testis biopsied; orchiopexy should be performed unless the testis is necrotic. Prophylactic contralateral testicular fixation is usually advisable to prevent contralateral torsion.

Torsion of a testicular or epididymal appendage occurs most often in the preadolescent boy; it produces less severe symptoms than torsion of the testis. In the early phases the twisted appendage may be palpable as a tender nodule at the upper, outer aspect of the testis (Fig 16–23); if it is infarcted, the upper outer scrotal skin may be bluish in color (blue dot sign).

Epididymitis (Sec 16.67) is unusual in prepubertal children; it is likely to present as a swollen tender epididymis in its normal anatomic position, superior and posterior to the testis. Most cases are idiopathic; the etiology may be gonorrheal or tuberculous or related to reflux of urine, infected or sterile, into the ejaculatory ducts. Epididymitis is frequently accompanied by evidence of urinary infection. The prognosis in boys with epididymitis appears more favorable than in adults; subsequent testicular atrophy is rare.

Whenever acute scrotal pain of undetermined origin is associated with swelling of intrascrotal contents, prompt consultation with an experienced surgeon is indicated. Only when the diagnosis of epididymitis or of torsion of an appendage is unmistakable is nonop-

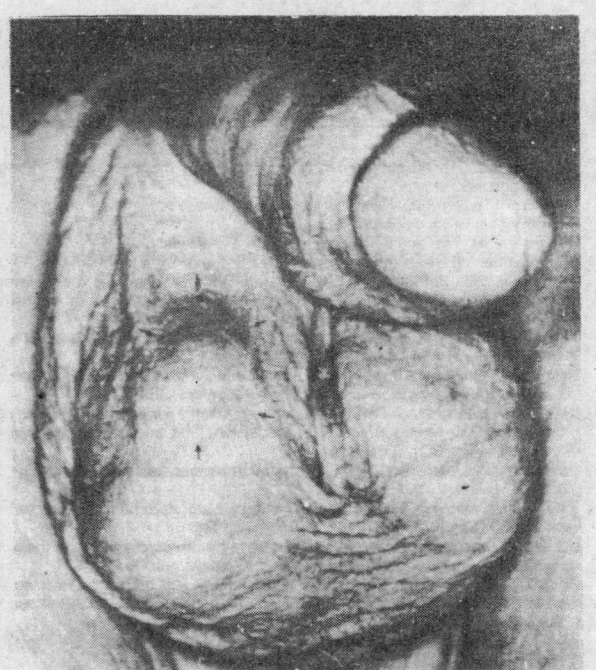

Figure 16–23 Torsion of appendix testis: note swollen nodule above testes (arrows). The "blue dot sign" is not evident here.

erative management appropriate; even then, surgical removal of an infarcted appendage may hasten recovery. When torsion of the cord has occurred, surgical exploration within 6–8 hr of the onset of symptoms will generally permit salvage of the testis. A necrotic testis should be removed. Because the anomaly of fixation that allows torsion to occur is bilateral in about 80% of instances and contralateral torsion occurs later in up to 30% of cases, fixation of the contralateral testis should be done at the time of initial surgery.

Hydrocele of the tunica vaginalis in infants is the result of failure of obliteration of the processus vaginalis. Segmental closure of the processus vaginalis may produce a hydrocele of the spermatic cord. In infancy or childhood patency of the processus vaginalis allows the hydrocele to communicate with the peritoneal cavity; communicating hydroceles will fluctuate in size and tend to be soft and small after a period of sleep. The distended hydrocele can be readily transilluminated. It usually resolves after spontaneous closure of the processus. Hydroceles that persist after 1 yr of age and those associated with demonstrable inguinal hernia at any age require surgical correction. Infection, trauma, and torsion may produce acute reactive hydroceles; these resolve with resolution of the primary problem.

Varicocele, the abnormal dilatation of the pampiniform plexus of spermatic veins, is the result of incompetent valves in the internal spermatic venous system and occurs almost always on the left side. In adults large varicoceles are often associated with subnormal fertility, but little is known about the desirability or need for repair of these lesions in childhood. Correction of a large lesion may prevent impairment of fertility, especially if the left testis is smaller and softer than the right. Surgical correction is made by high ligation of the internal spermatic vein.

Dresner ML: Torsed appendage: Diagnosis and management; blue dot sign. Urology 1:63, 1973.

Gislason T, Noronha RFX, Gregory JG: Acute epididymitis in boys. A 5-year retrospective study. J Urol 124:533, 1980.

Johnston JH: The acute scrotum in childhood. Practitioner 223:306, 1979.

Kiesewetter WB: Hernias and hydroceles. Pediatr Clin North Am 6:1129, 1959.

Kroovand RL, Perlmutter AD: Congenital anomalies of the vas deferens and epididymis. In: Kogan SG, Hafez ESE (eds): Clinics in Andrology, Pediatric Andrology. The Hague, Martines Nijhoff, 1981.

Levitt SB, Kogan SJ, Engel RM, et al: The impalpable testes: A rational approach to management. J Urol 120:515, 1978.

Lipshultz LD, Snyder PJ, Greenspan C: Testicular function following orchidopexy for unilaterally undescended testicles. N Engl J Med 295:15, 1976.

Mengel W, Heinz HA, et al: Studies on cryptorchidism: A comparison of histological findings in the germinative epithelium before and after the second year of life. J Pediatr Surg 9:445, 1974.

Mowad JJ, Konvolinka CW: Torsion of undescended testes. Urology 12:567, 1978.

Noe HN, Patterson TH: Screening urography in asymptomatic cryptorchid patients. J Urol 119:669, 1978.

Oster J: Varicocele in children and adolescents: An investigation of the incidence among Danish school children. Scand J Urol Nephrol 5:27, 1971.

Scorer CG, Farrington GH: Congenital anomalies of the testis. In: Harrison JH, Gittes RF, Perlmutter AD, et al (eds): Campbell's Urology. Ed 4. Philadelphia, WB Saunders, 1979.

Whitesel JA: Intrauterine and newborn torsion of spermatic cord. J Urol 106:786, 1971.

Williams CB, Litvak AS, McRoberts JW: Epididymitis in infancy. J Urol 121:125, 1979.

Wyllie GG: The diagnosis of undescended testes. M J Aust 1:639, 1978.

16.62 INFECTION OF THE URINARY TRACT

See also Sec 16.43.

Children with proven urinary infection or symptoms suggestive of infection should be examined by voiding cystourethrography and intravenous pyelography to identify those with anomalies of the urinary tract or with vesicoureteral reflux who may be at particular risk for renal damage.

To avoid confusion by findings associated only with active infection (e.g., transitory vesicoureteral reflux, ureteral atony, edema of the bladder mucosa) uroradiographic studies should be delayed until a few wk after acute infection and its effects have subsided unless the patient is seriously ill and/or is responding poorly to treatment.

A *voiding cystourethrogram* is best performed under fluoroscopic control to observe the timing and degree of vesicoureteral reflux, the nature of ureteral peristalsis, the urethral anatomy in boys, and the completeness of bladder emptying. Residual bladder urine is measured at the time of catheterization and a sample obtained for culture and sensitivity. Measurements of residual urine obtained by catheterization before or after voiding cystourethrography may be inaccurate as urine drains from the ureter after reflux or as the child, because of anxiety or embarrassment, may be unable to void completely. When a urethral abnormality is suspected in a child unable to void because of modesty or fear, expression cystourethrography under anesthesia offers an alternative means of examination; but it is less physiologic than voiding studies, and up to 35% of cases of vesicoureteral reflux may be missed. Grading the severity of reflux (Fig 16–24) is useful as a guide to therapy and prognosis. Both the American and International classifications are presented.

Intravenous urography can be obtained on the same day as voiding cystourethrography after all refluxed contrast material has left the upper collecting system. The use of voiding films made during intravenous pyelography should not be relied upon to give accurate information regarding reflux or the completeness of bladder emptying.

When vesicoureteral reflux is present, intravenous

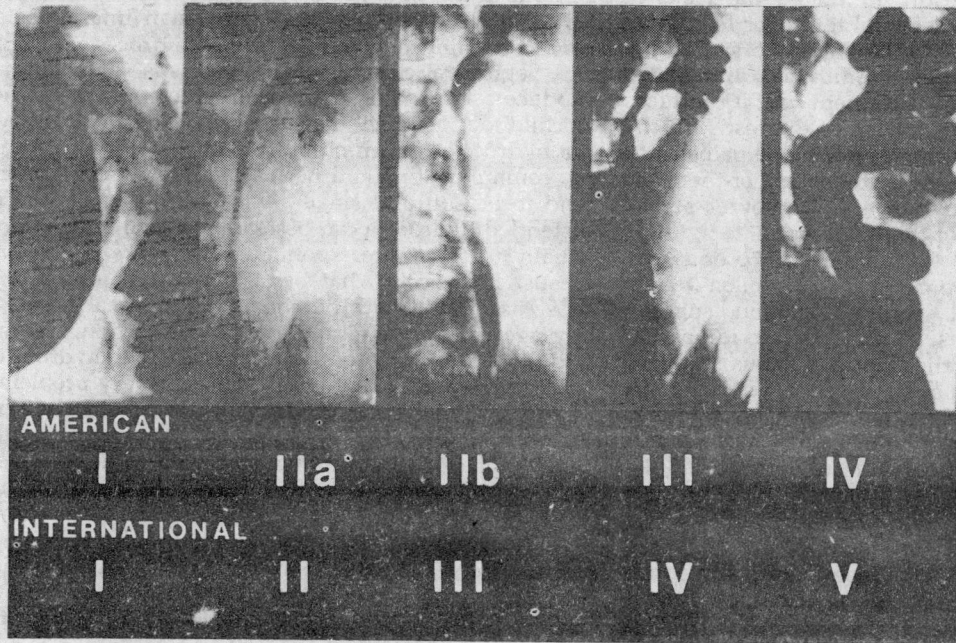

AMERICAN

I   IIa   IIb   III   IV

INTERNATIONAL

I   II   III   IV   V

Figure 16–24 Grades of vesicoureteral reflux. Both the American and International classifications of vesicoureteral reflux are presented (the latter in parentheses). The maximal observed reflux is classified Grade I (I)—lower ureteral filling only; Grade IIa (II)—ureteral and pelvicalyceal filling, without other changes (dilation); Grade IIb (III)—ureteral and pelvicalyceal filling with *mild* dilation of the renal pelvis and with *mild* calyceal blunting without clubbing, with maintenance of papillary impressions in the *majority* of calyces, and with no ureteral tortuosity; Grade III (IV)—ureteral and pelvicalyceal filling with *moderate* dilation and/or tortuosity of the ureter and *moderate* dilation of the renal pelvis and calyces, with *significant blunting* of the majority of the calyceal fornices and *loss* of papillary impressions in the *majority* of the calyces; Grade IV (V)—*gross* dilation and tortuosity of the ureter, renal pelvis, and calyces.

pyelography reveals focal renal scarring (segmental pyelonephritis) in up to 40% of instances. The scarring is usually polar or bipolar and may appear as deformed, elongated calyces with overlying wedge-shaped parenchymal defects. Focal scarring may be more subtle and, when limited to the medial parenchyma of the upper pole of the kidney, is easily overlooked. Ureterectasis, pyelectasis, and longitudinal mucosal striae in the ureter and renal pelvis all result from intermittent distention and are additional clues to reflux.

The use of *radionuclide imaging* in evaluation of children with urinary infection and vesicoureteral reflux greatly reduces radiation exposure and is excellent for periodic reassessment; poor image resolution, however, makes it unsuitable for initial evaluation. When renal damage is present, baseline and periodic renal function studies should be obtained.

The role of *cystoscopy* in evaluation of children with urinary infection is changing; it is now used less frequently than in the past. Cystoscopy provides information about the trigone, ureteral orifices, and submucosal ureteral tunnels that is important in assessing the prognosis for children with the higher grades of reflux. In children with symptoms of severe chronic cystitis, cystoscopy is helpful in evaluating the inflammatory changes. Cystoscopy is usually unnecessary in children who have occasional uncomplicated urinary infections, normal findings on urography, or minimal (grade I) reflux; these children generally have normal trigonal anatomy and bladder mucosa. Calibration of the urethra in girls at the time of cystoscopy rarely defines significant outlet obstruction. The value of urethral dilation or internal urethrotomy in girls is now questioned; evidence indicates that these procedures offer no protection against further infections. At the time of cystoscopy in girls, vaginoscopy and bimanual rectal examination should be done to disclose or exclude other anomalies or inflammations.

Acute cystitis may be bacterial or nonbacterial and presents symptoms of dysuria, frequency, urgency, and lower abdominal or suprapubic pain but few systemic symptoms. (See Sec 16.43 and 16.44.)

Allen RP, Burrows EH: Micturition cysto-urethrography in the investigation of the urinary tract diseases in children. Arch Dis Child 39:95, 1964.

Filly R, Friedland GW, Govan DE, et al: Development and progression of clubbing and scarring in children with recurrent urinary tract infections. Radiology 113:145, 1974.

Goodall J: Bacteria and renal tract pathology in children. Practitioner 221:248, 1978.

Govan DE: Investigation and management of urinary tract infections in female children. Urol Clin North Am 1:397, 1974.

Helin I, Okmian L: Hemorrhagic cystitis complicating cyclophosphamide treatment in children. Acta Paediatr Scand 62:497, 1973.

Hodson CJ: Formation of renal scars with special reference to reflux nephropathy. Contr Nephrol 16:83, 1979.

Johnson DK, Kroovand RL, Perlmutter AD: The changing role of cystoscopy in the pediatric patient. J Urol 123:232, 1980.

Kaplan GW, King LR: Cystitis cystica in childhood. J Urol 103:657, 1970.

McCarthy JM, Pryles CV: Clean voided and catheter neonatal urine specimens: Bacteriology in the male and female neonate. Am J Dis Child 106:473, 1963.

Merrick MV, Utley WS, Wild R: A comparison of two techniques of detecting vesico-ureteric reflux. Br J Urol 50:792, 1979.

Mufson MA, Zollar LM, Mankad VN, et al: Adenovirus infection in acute hemorrhagic cystitis. Am J Dis Child 121:281, 1971.

Nasrallah PF, Anway JJ, King LR, et al: Quantitative nuclear cystogram. Urology 12:654, 1978.

Ransley PG, Risdon RA: The pathogenesis of reflux nephropathy. Contr Nephrol 16:90, 1979.

Smellie JM, Hodson CJ, Edwards D, et al: Clinical and radiological features of urinary infection in childhood. Br Med J 2:1222, 1964.

Walther PC, Kaplan TW: Cystoscopy in children: Indications for its use in common urologic problems. J Urol 122:712, 1979.

Wenzl JE, Greene LF, Harris LE: Eosinophilic cystitis. J Pediatr 64:746, 1964.

16.63 VESICOURETERAL REFLUX

Vesicoureteral reflux may be primary or secondary; primary reflux, a developmental anomaly, is more common. Reflux occurs when there is inadequate intravesical submucosal tunnel (valve mechanism) or defective attachment of the ureter to the trigone. The degree of deficiency varies: a marginally developed intravesical submucosal tunnel may allow reflux only when infection and edema impair effective valvular function; with more severe deformities reflux can be continuous and severe. Secondary or acquired reflux can result from injury to the ureteral orifice (e.g., during surgical procedure or by an intravesical foreign body), or it may be produced by a persistent increase in intravesical pressure resulting from severe bladder outflow obstruction.

In the majority of instances primary reflux is mild and associated with a normal pyelocalyceal system and ureter; more severe grades are associated with significant ureteral and renal pelvic dilatation and a high likelihood of renal scarring. Pelviureteral fullness with reflux, even on intravenous urography, may appear more severe in infancy than in later childhood because of the greater compliance of the young infant's urinary tract. After spontaneous cessation or surgical correction of reflux, the findings on urography should gradually improve, though some radiographic ureteral widening or columning may be permanent.

The combination of reflux and infection can produce segmental renal scarring (reflux nephropathy); children under 5 yr of age appear to be especially vulnerable. With recurrent or persistent infection the scarring may progress or may appear in kidneys which were normal at the initial examination. Segmental intrarenal reflux (reflux into the renal parenchyma) has been associated with the development and progression of renal scarring involving these same areas; it is still unclear whether concurrent infection is essential to production of this focal parenchymal damage.

Treatment. The majority of children with reflux respond to nonoperative management. Effective antibacterial treatment minimizes the likelihood of recurrent infections and progressive renal damage. Renal growth arrest, progressive scarring, and increasing hydronephrosis do not follow mild or moderate reflux in the absence of infection or obstruction. Periodic urinalyses and urine cultures should be done. Roentgenographic or radionuclide re-evaluation is conducted at intervals of 6–24 mo, depending on the severity of the reflux and the age of the child. The older child and those with mild degrees of reflux require less frequent study. In infants and in any patients with severe reflux or pre-existing parenchymal scars, renal damage may occur rapidly, and the 1st follow-up roentgenographic studies should be made after 4–6 mo of therapy in these children.

Spontaneous remission of reflux is more common in children under 5 yr of age and may be anticipated in 30–60% overall. Resolution is less likely in those with more severe degrees of reflux and in those with deficient ureteral valvular mechanisms. There is no substantial tendency for persistent reflux to cease spontaneously at puberty.

Some indications for the operative correction of reflux remain controversial, but most urologists agree that persistent severe reflux, progressive renal scarring, renal growth arrest, absence of the submucosal ureteral tunnel, an anomalous or ectopic ureteral orifice, breakthrough infections while on appropriate antibacterial regimens, and poor compliance of patients or parents with a nonoperative program are indications for surgical procedures to correct reflux. In patients in whom reflux persists after physical growth is complete, antireflux surgery should be considered.

After apparently successful surgery, follow-up intravenous urography annually is justified for 2–3 yr to determine whether any late ureteral obstruction or progressive renal deterioration has occurred. Focal parenchymal scarring can progress for up to 2 yr after elimination of infection, whether or not surgery has been performed, although renal growth will often resume at a normal or accelerated rate. Most children who have had appropriate surgical repair will have no further reflux; they may have episodes of bacteriuria or cystitis, but pyelonephritis is unusual.

Atwell JD, Vijay MR: Renal growth following reimplantation of the ureters for reflux. Br J Urol 50:367, 1978.
Dwoskin JY, Perlmutter AD: Vesicoureteral reflux in children: A computerized review. J Urol 109:888, 1973.
Hodson CJ, Maling TMJ, McManamon PJ, et al: The pathogenesis of reflux nephropathy (chronic atrophic pyelonephritis). Br J Radiol Suppl 13, 1975.
Merrell RW, Mowad JJ: Increased physical growth after successful antireflux operation. J Urol 122:523, 1979.
Perlmutter AD, Kroovand RL: Vesicoureteral reflux. In Ravitch M, et al (eds): Pediatric Surgery. Ed 3. Chicago, Year Book Medical Publishers, 1979.
Ransley PG: Vesicoureteral reflux: Continuing surgical dilemma. Urology 12:246, 1978.
Rolleston GL, Maling TMJ, Hodson CJ: Intrarenal reflux and the scarred kidney. Arch Dis Child 49:531, 1974.
Rolleston GL, Shannon FT, Utley WLF: Relationship of infantile vesicoureteric reflux to renal damage. Br Med J 1:460, 1970.
Wallace DMA, Rothwell DC, Williams DI: The long-term follow-up of surgically treated vesicoureteric reflux. Br J Urol 50:479, 1978.
Williams DI: The natural history of reflux—a review. Urol Int 26:350, 1971.
Willscher MK, Bauer SB, Zammuto PJ, et al: Renal growth and urinary infection following antireflux surgery in infants and children. J Urol 115:722, 1976.

16.64 RENAL AND PERIRENAL INFECTIONS

Renal carbuncle or abscess may be acquired by the hematogenous route (e.g., with *Staphylococcus aureus* metastatic from another site) or by ascending infections secondary to severe vesicoureteral reflux (usually with gram-negative organisms). Initial symptoms tend to be vague and nonlocalizing, followed by gradual evolution of fever, flank pain, and mass. On intravenous urography the renal mass may resemble a neoplasm. Small abscesses heal with antibiotic treatment alone; large abscesses may require surgical drainage in addition to appropriate antibiotic therapy. Nephrectomy is usually not required except when there is xanthogranulomatous pyelonephritis (see below).

Pyonephrosis or purulent hydronephrosis can occasionally be managed successfully by surgical drainage and antibiotic therapy with subsequent repair of the obstructing lesion; nephrectomy is indicated when there is widespread destruction of renal parenchyma.

Perinephric abscess follows rupture of a renal carbuncle or of pyonephrosis into the tissue around the kidney; findings include diffuse swelling, erythema and edema of the flank, and progressive toxicity. On intravenous urography the psoas shadow is obliterated and the involved kidney and ureter are displaced. Irritation of the psoas muscle is often reflected by a limp or by fixed flexion of the hip. Treatment consists of surgical drainage and administration of an appropriate antibiotic.

Xanthogranulomatous pyelonephritis is a chronic, diffuse renal disorder characterized by yellow nodules containing plasma cells and xanthine cells. It occurs infrequently in children with longstanding, untreated, or inadequately treated febrile infections involving the kidney. Underlying obstructive and/or calculous disease is often present. Differentiation from renal neoplasm can be difficult. Nephrectomy generally provides both diagnosis and cure as the lesion is usually unilateral.

OTHER INFECTIONS AND INFLAMMATIONS OF THE URINARY TRACT

Fungal infections of the urinary tract are becoming more common, in part because of prolonged or inappropriate broad-spectrum antibiotic therapy, especially in association with indwelling catheters. Urinary fungal infections are generally confined to the collecting and drainage portions of the urinary tract; when they are part of a generalized systemic fungal infection, the patient is generally severely and chronically debilitated (Sec 10.100–10.106). Instillations of amphotericin B or nystatin into the urinary tract will usually cure localized infections of the collecting system or bladder.

Cobb OE: Carbuncle of the kidney. Br J Urol 38:262, 1966.
Fahr K, Opperman HC, Scharer K, et al: Xanthogranulomatous pyelonephritis in childhood. Pediatr Radiol 8:10, 1979.
Jimenez JF, Pacios AL, Llamazares G, et al: Treatment of pyonephrosis: A comparative study. J Urol 120:287, 1978.
Laval KU, Lutzeyer W: Paranephric abscess: A changing concept. Eur Urol 5:81, 1979.
Malek RS, Elder JS: Xanthogranulomatous pyelonephritis: A critical analysis of 26 cases and of the literature. J Urol 119:589, 1978.
Timmons JW, Perlmutter AD: Renal abscess: A changing concept. J Urol 115:299, 1976.
Wise GJ, Wainstein S, Goldberg P, et al: Candidal cystitis: Management by continuous bladder irrigation with amphotericin B. JAMA 224:1636, 1973.

16.65 ANTERIOR URETHRITIS

In preadolescent boys anterior urethritis is a nonspecific infection evidenced by a postvoiding bloody discharge or by spotty urethral bleeding between voidings; often there is terminal dysuria or pain in the glans penis. Cultures for bacteria, *Ureaplasma*, and *Chlamydia* are usually negative. On urethroscopy fibrinous or granular inflammation can be seen in the bulbar urethra. The course of the condition is generally protracted but self-limited; treatment is generally unsatisfactory. Administration of tetracycline or 1 of its analogues appears at times to control the inflammation and is occasionally followed by resolution of symptoms and bleeding. The use of tetracycline must be limited to children in whom the permanent dentition is complete. The disorder is often persistent or recurrent and occasionally results in urethral stricture; long-term observation is necessary. If on initial study voiding cystography outlines a normal urethra, cystoscopic examination is best omitted to avoid increasing the likelihood of stricture formation.

Urethral inflammation and hematuria may also follow injury by foreign objects introduced into the urethra during masturbation or self-exploration. Treatment is symptomatic unless the urethra has been torn. Treatment of urethral injury is discussed in Sec 16.71. Treatment of gonorrhea is discussed in Sec 10.26.

Williams DI, Mikhael BR: Urethritis in male children. Proc R Soc Med 64:133, 1971.

16.66 PROSTATITIS

Acute staphylococcal abscess of the prostate has been reported in neonates; the swelling can cause urinary retention. The cystic prostatic mass is readily palpable by rectal examination. Treatment consists of antibiotic therapy and surgical drainage through the perineum.

Prostatitis is rare in prepubertal boys but not unusual in adolescents. It may be caused by gonococci as well as by other organisms. In adolescents, as in adults, acute prostatitis may be evidenced by fever, vesical irritability (burning, frequency, urgency, nocturia), a weak urinary stream, cloudy urine, purulent urethral discharge, and perineal or low back pain. The enlarged and tender prostate can be identified on rectal examination. Treatment consists of culture-specific antibiotics or erythromycin, oleandomycin, or trimethoprim-sulfamethoxazole when an organism is not recovered. (For treatment of gonorrhea, see Sec 10.26.) Warm baths and anticholinergic medications may help in the relief of symptoms. Prostatic massage is contraindicated during the acute phase because it can lead to septicemia. If symptoms of prostatitis recur, an anatomic cause should be sought.

Chronic bacterial prostatitis is unusual in childhood and adolescence but may follow repeated episodes of acute prostatitis. Symptoms of vesical irritability and perineal or low back pain may be relieved by prostatic massage, sitz baths, and appropriate long-term antibiotic therapy. Psychosomatic or psychosexual symptoms may mimic those of chronic prostatitis; the evidence for prostatitis should be confirmed by appropriate bacteriologic studies before that diagnosis is accepted.

Mann S: Prostatic abscess in the newborn. Arch Dis Child 35:396, 1960.
Mears EM Jr, Stamey TE: The diagnosis and management of bacterial prostatitis. Br J Urol 44:175, 1972.

16.67 EPIDIDYMITIS

Epididymitis is far less common in prepubertal or adolescent boys than torsion of the testis or of a testicular appendage. Epididymitis may be associated with urinary infection or with an ectopic ureter emptying into the vas deferens or seminal vesicle, or it may be a primary infection of bacterial or viral origin (e.g., mumps or coxsackievirus). Treatment is symptomatic, with rest, elevation of the scrotum, sitz baths, analgesics, and antibiotics when indicated. During the acute phase local cooling is preferable to heat for relief of pain and swelling. Sterility is unusual after unilateral disease but can follow severe bilateral involvement.

Doolittle KH, Smith JP, Saylor ML: Epididymitis in the prepubertal boy. J Urol 96:364, 1966.
Gislason T, Noronha RFX, Gregory JG: Acute epididymitis in boys: 5-year retrospective study. J Urol 124:533, 1980.
Williams CB, Litvak AS, McRoberts JW: Epididymitis in infancy. J Urol 121:125, 1979.

Orchitis may be infectious or post-traumatic; mumps orchitis rarely occurs prior to puberty but is relatively common thereafter and is usually, but not always, associated with parotitis (Sec 10.77).

Lyon RP, Bruyn HB: Treatment of mumps epididymitis. JAMA 196:736, 1966.
Riggs S, Sanford JP: Viral orchitis. N Engl J Med 266:990, 1962.

16.68 INFLAMMATION OF THE EXTERNAL GENITALIA

Inflammation of the glans penis (**balanitis**) or the prepuce (**posthitis**) or both (**balanoposthitis**) is common in infants and is usually the result of irritation from wet diapers or poor genital hygiene. Mild cases of balanoposthitis will respond to local cleansing and topical antibiotic preparations; more severe cases may require systemic antibiotic therapy. When phimosis is associated, a relaxing incision in the phimotic prepuce speeds healing; circumcision can be performed at a later date. *Candida albicans* may also produce inflammation of the prepuce and causes a foul-smelling, sticky preputial discharge. Local cleansing and a topical nystatin preparation are effective in treatment; occasionally, circumcision is required.

Inflammation and swelling of the scrotal skin are usually caused by bacterial or fungal infections or by trauma. Skin infections are usually treatable by appropriate topical preparations; when severe, systemic antibiotic therapy is indicated. Swelling alone may be associated with Schönlein-Henoch purpura, urinary extravasation, torsion of the testis, or epididymitis, or it may be congenital or idiopathic. Neonatal scrotal edema (congenital) is of uncertain etiology and resolves spontaneously. *Idiopathic scrotal edema* is a condition of early childhood. It appears rapidly, is usually unilateral, and is unaccompanied by pain or other symptoms. The involved scrotum becomes swollen, firm, and pink. Spontaneous resolution usually occurs within 24–48 hr. The lack of local or systemic symptoms, with the findings of palpable, normal, nontender testis and epididymis, rules out torsion or epididymitis.

Inflammation of the vulva in the preadolescent girl is common and is usually limited to the vestibule; unlike vaginitis, it does not extend proximal to the hymenal ring. Mild vulvar irritation is usually asymptomatic and does not require treatment, but severe vulvitis may mimic symptoms of urinary infection. When the inflammation is symptomatic, local hygiene and sitz baths are usually curative. Occasionally, topical application of an estrogen cream for 4–5 days helps resolution.

Gonococcal vulvovaginitis is discussed in Sec 10.26.

Adhesions of the labia minora (synechiae) are acquired lesions of the prepubertal girl. The adhesions probably follow local inflammation. They are thin, translucent, epithelial bridges. The condition is usually asymptomatic. Occasionally, when the length of fusion is extensive, trapping of urine behind the membrane results in vulvar irritation, postvoiding dribbling, or bacteriuria. Unless the synechiae are quite tenuous, forcible disruption as an office procedure can be quite painful and should be avoided. The application of topical estrogen cream for 1–2 wk will generally result in spontaneous lysis, and the residual adhesions can then be gently separated. Rarely, dense adhesions will require surgical division.

Argemi J, Valls A, Casanova-Bellido M, et al: Candida infections. Paediatrician 8:35, 1979.

Emans SJH, Goldstein DP: Pediatric and Adolescent Gynecology. Boston, Little, Brown, 1977.

Farrell MK, Billmire ME, Shamroy JA, et al: Prepubertal gonorrhea: A multidisciplinary approach. Pediatrics 67:151, 1981.

Glenn JF: Labial fusion and urinary infection. J Urol 87:485, 1962.

Johnston JH: The testicles and the scrotum. In: Williams DI (ed): Pediatric Urology. New York, Appleton-Century-Crofts, 1970.

Lang WR: Premenarchal vaginitis. Obstet Gynecol 13:723, 1959.

Nicholas JL, Morgan A, Zachary RB: Idiopathic edema of scrotum in young boys. Surgery 67:847, 1970.

Smith DR: Disorders of the penis and male urethra. In: Smith DR (ed): General Urology. Ed 8. Los Altos, Calif., Lange Medical Publications, 1975.

Sparks JP: Torsion of the testis in adolescents and young adults: Some comments on clinical expressions and management. Clin Pediatr 11:484, 1972.

Ster J: Further fate of the foreskin: Incidence of preputial adhesions, phimosis, and smegma among Danish schoolboys. Arch Dis Child 43:200, 1968.

Tomeh MO, Wilfert CM: Venereal diseases of infants and children at Duke University Medical Center. NC Med J 34:109, 1973.

Williams BH, Cramm CJ Jr: Adhesions of the labia minora: Treatment with topical estrogenic ointment. South Med J 50:573, 1957.

16.69 DISTURBANCES OF MICTURITION

Abnormal patterns of urinary frequency, incontinence, retention, or abnormal or difficult voiding are indications for urologic consultation. Evaluation of children with voiding dysfunction should be adapted to the type and severity of symptoms and requires a thorough history, a physical examination that includes watching or hearing the child void, and urinalysis, including culture and antibiotic sensitivity studies as indicated. Knowledge of the normal stages in acquisition of urinary control is helpful in identifying those children whose abnormal voiding pattern is simply a delay in maturation.

Children with urinary infection, residual urine, a poor urinary stream, or daytime wetting should have additional studies. Intravenous urography and voiding cystourethrography provide basic structural and functional information about the urinary tract. Cystometrography may demonstrate an uninhibited small bladder; urethral pressure profile studies or electromyographic tracings of urethral sphincter activity may reveal a lack of coordination between detrusor and external sphincter functions. Cystoscopy occasionally reveals unsuspected inflammatory changes as a cause of voiding symptoms, especially when there has been prolonged bacteriuria or a history of recurrent urinary infections.

Enuresis is inappropriate or involuntary voiding at any age when urinary control should be achieved. Nocturnal wetting occurs in approximately 20% of 4 yr olds, with 14–16% of persistent enuretics ceasing to wet each year thereafter. Nocturnal enuresis may be primary (child has never been dry) or secondary (wetting follows a dry period usually after an identifiable stress). Nocturnal enuresis may be due to a maturational lag in the development of the central nervous system, to stress factors during the developmental period from 2–4 yr, to genetic factors, to psychologic factors, or, uncommonly, to organic factors. A careful, systematic evaluation of the enuretic child, avoiding unnecessary manipulation, is essential. In the absence of other indications, a full urologic evaluation is usually unnecessary, especially when the physical and neurologic examinations are normal and the child has a normal voiding pattern, complete bladder emptying, and normal urine specific gravity and microscopic urinalysis. Treatment for nocturnal enuresis is discussed in Sec 2.50 and 16.52, and in references listed below.

Kass EJ, Diokno AC, Montealegre A: Enuresis: Principles of management and results of treatment. J Urol 121:794, 1979.

Perlmutter AD: Enuresis. In: Harrison JH, Gittes RF, Perlmutter AD, et al (eds): Campbell's Urology. Ed 4. Philadelphia, WB Saunders, 1979.

16.70 NEUROGENIC BLADDER DYSFUNCTION

Normal bladder function is complex, involving the storage of urine at low pressure with continence, periodic complete emptying at appropriate intervals, and the ability to initiate or postpone voiding voluntarily. In patients with myelomeningocele, sacral agenesis, or trauma to or degenerative disease of the central nervous system or spinal cord, the bladder may become enlarged and unable to empty or it may have diminished functional capacity due to uninhibited contractions or lack of sphincter resistance. In either case, urinary incontinence results. Infection may be followed by vesicoureteral reflux, hydronephrosis, and functional renal deterioration; these can be avoided by appropriate management. Pharmacologic agents will often increase the functional capacity of the bladder and control incontinence by inhibiting detrusor contractions and enhancing the tone of the bladder outlet. Many affected children benefit from intermittent catheterization or self-catheterization, periodically emptying the bladder to achieve socially acceptable urinary control. Those children with adequate bladder capacity who remain incontinent in spite of appropriate neuropharmacologic manipulation and/or intermittent catheterization may achieve urinary continence and control of bladder emptying after a surgical procedure which reconstructs the bladder outlet or after placement of an artificial, inflatable urinary sphincter.

Allen TD: The non-neurogenic bladder. J Urol 117:232, 1977.

Bruskewitz R, Raz S, Smith RB, et al: AMS 742 sphincter: UCLA experience. J Urol 124:812, 1980.

Colodny A: Artificial urinary sphincter. In: Holder TM, Ashcraft KW (eds): Pediatric Surgery. Philadelphia, WB Saunders, 1980.

Dorfman LE, Bailey J, Smith JP: Subclinical neurogenic bladder in children. J Urol 101:48, 1969.

Galdston R, Perlmutter AD: The urinary manifestations of anxiety in childhood. Pediatrics 52:818, 1973.

Gonzalez R, Dewolf WC: The artificial bladder sphincter AS-721 for the treatment of incontinence in patients with neurogenic bladder. J Urol 121:71, 1979.

Hannigan KF: Teaching intermittent self-catheterization to young children with myelodysplasia. Dev Med Child Neurol 21:365, 1979.

Hardy DA, Melick WF, Gregory JG, et al: Intermittent catheterization in children. Urology 5:206, 1975.

Hilwa N, Perlmutter AD: The role of adjunctive drug therapy for intermittent catheterization and self-catheterization in children with vesical dysfunction. J Urol 119:551, 1978.

Hinman F, Bauman FW: Vesical and ureteral damage from voiding dysfunction in boys without neurogenic or obstructive disease. J Urol 109:727, 1973.

Kass EJ, McHugh T, Diokno AC: Intermittent catheterization in children less than 6 years old. J Urol 121:792, 1979.

Kroovand RL, Perlmutter AD: Neurogenic bladder. In: Holder TM, Ashcraft KW (eds): Pediatric Surgery. Philadelphia, WB Saunders, 1980.

Martin DC, Datta NS, Schweitz B: The occult neurological bladder. J Urol 105:733, 1971.

Mulcahy JJ, James HE: Management of neurogenic bladder in infancy and childhood. Urology 13:235, 1979.

16.71 TRAUMA

Up to 7% of all trauma to children involves injuries to the genitourinary system. Genitourinary trauma may be accidental, intentional, or iatrogenic, blunt or penetrating, direct or indirect. Genital trauma can be a sign of child abuse. External evidence of trauma and gross or microscopic hematuria usually alert the physician to the possibility of urologic injury, but the absence of these signs does not exclude genitourinary trauma.

Many children with genitourinary injuries also have other serious injuries. As many as 40% of pediatric renal injuries are accompanied by cerebral, spinal cord, bone, pulmonary, and intraperitoneal injuries as well as damage to other genitourinary organs. Despite these multiple injuries children tend to recover with fewer sequelae than do adults. In evaluating the child with multiple serious injuries, an orderly multidisciplinary approach is essential. Maintenance of an adequate airway and pulmonary function, control of hemorrhage, restoration of blood volume, and control of shock have the highest priority.

After appropriate resuscitation and stabilization, children suspected of having injury to the kidneys, bladder, or urethra should have retrograde cystourethrography and infusion excretory urography with "delayed films" and tomography. Children with fracture of the bony pelvis or with symptoms suggestive of urethral injury should have retrograde urethrography with soluble contrast material. If this study demonstrates urethral rupture, attempts at passage of a catheter may be ill-advised as this may convert partial transection of the urethra into a complete disruption. In 90% of urologic injuries these studies are diagnostic. When the need appears urgent, uroradiographic evaluation may be performed during resuscitation and stabilization, but it should not interfere with lifesaving efforts of higher priority.

Renal Injuries. In infants and children the kidneys have proportionately greater size and a less sturdy fatty and fascial envelope than in adults, and they are less protected because of greater flexibility of the overlying lower ribs. Accordingly, the kidneys of infants and children are more prone to injury than those of adults. The large size and relative noncompressibility of such renal abnormalities as hydronephrosis, renal ectopia, or tumor make such abnormal kidneys especially vulnerable to injury. Most renal injuries in children are produced by blunt trauma from falls, athletic injuries, and auto accidents. Renal injuries are more common in boys and have 2 peaks of age incidence: from 5–7 yr and during adolescence.

Most renal injuries in children are minor and can be managed nonoperatively. Management includes analgesia, general medical support, serial urinalyses, hematocrit measurements, repeated gentle abdominal examinations to detect any expanding or changing masses, and strict bed rest until microhematuria resolves. Stabilization usually occurs within 48 hr.

For major renal injuries, in which the kidneys are not visualized by intravenous urography or there are possibilities of severe parenchymal disruption, of extensive urinary extravasation, or of an expanding mass, arteriography should be performed to define more precisely the nature of the injury.

Immediate surgical intervention is required for major vascular injuries or for uncontrolled bleeding. The treatment of deep parenchymal lacerations, complete renal fractures, and tears of the collecting system is controversial. Certain of these injuries will stabilize and resolve with nonoperative management; in those that do not, delayed (2–5 days) surgery generally provides better conditions for a more limited debridement, repair, or partial nephrectomy than can be accomplished in the initial phase. Serial pyelograms, renal scans, and computed tomography of the kidney are of value in the nonoperative management of blunt renal trauma.

Ureteral Injuries. Because of the small size of the ureters and their protected position, ureteral injuries from blunt trauma are unusual, but hyperextension of the spinal column, penetrating trauma, or endoscopic manipulation can injure them. Not infrequently, ureteral injuries are initially asymptomatic or overshadowed by other injuries, only to present later as an abdominal mass, flank pain, fever, or urinary fistula. Infusion pyelography with delayed films is usually diagnostic.

Most ureteral injuries will require prompt surgical repair. For patients in poor condition or with multiple injuries preliminary temporary urinary diversion (nephrostomy) may be advisable, with definitive repair later. Whether the ureter is repaired primarily or after a period of temporary diversion, the prognosis is good.

Bladder Injuries. In infants and children the bladder is an abdominal rather than a pelvic organ. It is especially vulnerable when full to rupture from blunt trauma, penetrating wounds of the lower abdomen, and pelvic fractures. Spontaneous rupture of a normal bladder is unusual. Small extraperitoneal tears of the bladder may be treated by urethral catheter drainage, but most ruptures require exploration, debridement, primary repair, and temporary suprapubic drainage, especially when the tear is intraperitoneal.

Injuries of the Anterior Urethra. The anterior urethra in boys may be injured by blunt or penetrating wounds. A gently performed retrograde urethrogram, using a soluble contrast material, should define the extent and location of the urethral injury. Small or incomplete urethral tears can be simply managed with catheter drainage for 7–10 days; more extensive injuries require evacuation of periurethral hematoma, debridement, primary repair (if possible), and longer term urinary diversion.

Injuries of the prostatomembranous urethra in boys may result from pelvic trauma, with or without fracture. The clinical manifestations are bloody urethral spotting, urinary retention, and a fluctuant pelvic mass on rectal examination. Infusion urography will usually demonstrate upward displacement of a distended bladder, and a gently performed retrograde urethrogram confirms the disruption. Forcible attempts at catheterization may totally disrupt an incompletely separated urethra and are ill-advised.

Total disruption of the prostatic urethra from the membranous urethra is most simply and safely managed initially by insertion of a suprapubic bladder tube, with repair of the urethra delayed for 6 mo or more; on the other hand, some urologists recommend an early attempt at primary realignment of the severed urethra whenever possible.

Injuries to the External Genitalia. Injuries may be accidental, intentional, or iatrogenic and are often frightening to the child; examination and treatment should be gentle and usually done under general anesthesia, at which time diagnosis and treatment can be combined.

Male External Genitalia. The penis and scrotum may be injured during breech delivery, at circumcision, at play, by zippers and falling toilet seats, or by winding hair or other foreign objects around the penis, sometimes placed intentionally for erotic purposes or in an effort to improve urinary control.

The testis, epididymis, and spermatic cord are so mobile that severe injury from blunt or penetrating trauma is relatively uncommon. Because of its relatively exposed and fixed position, the undescended or ectopic testis is more vulnerable to trauma than is its scrotal counterpart. When a traumatic hematocele accompanies testicular injury, the capsule of the testicle has been ruptured; in such a case surgical exploration and primary testicular repair are indicated.

The penis and scrotum have a rich vascular supply and heal well after debridement and primary repair. Skin grafting is necessary after total avulsion of penile skin; temporary placement of the testes into the thighs

and secondary scrotal reconstruction may be required for extensive scrotal injuries.

Female External Genitalia. Blunt and penetrating injuries to the external genitalia of girls are usually the result of straddle or crush injuries or of sexual assault. Uterine, vaginal, and bladder injuries may complicate therapeutic abortions in teenage girls. Profuse bleeding may follow even minor labial, urethral, or vaginal injuries and generally obscures the distorted tissues. Proper examination and treatment often require general anesthesia; the rectal area should also be examined for injury.

Urethral injuries in girls are uncommon but may accompany pelvic fracture or penetrating injuries to the perineum. Such injuries may be treated by repair of any torn and bleeding urethral edges; catheter drainage may be required for a few days. Hematomas in the labia will resorb spontaneously; lacerations should be repaired.

Urethral prolapse in girls is often confused with vaginal bleeding or neoplasm. The prolapsed urethral mucosa appears as a granular red mass in the perineum, entrapped distal to the urethral meatus. A central opening in the mass distinguishes it from a prolapse of an ectopic ureterocele and from sarcoma botryoides. Despite its appearance symptoms are usually absent or minimal, though spotty bleeding can occur. Resection of the prolapsed mucosa is curative; recurrence is unusual.

Priapism (sustained nonerotic erection) is rare in children but may occur in a variety of conditions, especially in sickle cell disease, in leukemia, and in association with perineal trauma. Resolution can be spontaneous; treatment is recommended for priapism persisting longer than 24–36 hours. In sickle cell disease rapid hypertransfusion with packed red cells may be effective, and in leukemia chemotherapy combined with local radiation is the treatment of choice. Persistent post-traumatic priapism requires prompt surgical drainage of the injured area and creation of a vascular shunt between the corpora cavernosa and corpus spongiosum to produce detumescence. Impotence often follows prolonged post-traumatic priapism; it is less common after priapism associated with sickle cell disease.

R. LAWRENCE KROOVAND
ALAN D. PERLMUTTER

Baron M, Leiter E: The management of priapism in sickle cell anemia. J Urol 119:610, 1978.

Bulfin MJ: A new problem in adolescent gynecology. South Med J 72:967, 1979.

Buxton RA: Rupture of the urethra in a female child with a fractured pelvis: A case report. Injury 9:209, 1978.

Cromie WJ: Genitourinary injuries in the neonate. Clin Pediatr 18:292, 1979.

Ellerstein NS: Sexual abuse of boys. Am J Dis Child 134:255, 1980.

Emond AM, Holman R, Hayes RJ, et al: Priapism and impotence in homozygous sickle cell disease. Arch Int Med 140:1434, 1980.

Glassberg KI, Kassner EG, Haller JO, et al: The radiographic approach to injuries of the prostatomembranous urethra in children. J Urol 122:678, 1979.

LaBerge I, Homsey YL, Dadour G, et al: Avulsion of ureter by blunt trauma. Urology 13:172, 1979.

Leal J, Walker D, Egan EA: Idiopathic priapism in the newborn. J Urol 120:376, 1978.

Persky L: Childhood urethral trauma. Urology 11:603, 1978.

Seeler RA: Intensive transfusion therapy for priapism in boys with sickle cell anemia. J Urol 110:360, 1973.

Uson AC, Lattimer JK: Genitourinary tract injuries. In: Ravitch MM, Welch KJ, Benson CD, et al (eds): Pediatric Surgery. Chicago, Year Book Medical Publishers, 1979.

METABOLIC DISORDERS 17

17.1 DIABETES MELLITUS

Diabetes mellitus, a disturbance of energy metabolism, is due to a deficiency of insulin or of its action and is characterized by altered homeostasis of carbohydrate, protein, and fat. It is the most common endocrine/metabolic disorder of childhood that has important consequences on physical and emotional development. Its impact on the quality of life, and on morbidity and mortality, stems mainly from the complications that affect small and large blood vessels and result in retinopathy, nephropathy, neuropathy, ischemic heart disease, and obstruction of large vessels. Especially during the past decade, fresh insights have evolved concerning the synthesis, secretion, and actions of insulin as well as more precise understanding of the pathophysiology of the disease, of its acute and chronic clinical features, of its genetic and other etiologic factors, and of rational approaches to its treatment.

Epidemiology. Surveys in the United States indicate that the prevalence of diabetes among school age children is about 1.9/1000. The frequency, however, is highly correlated with increasing age; available data indicate a range of about 1 case/1430 children at 5 yr of age to 1 case/360 children at 16 yr. Data on prevalence in relation to racial or ethnic backgrounds are incomplete. Among American Blacks the occurrence of insulin-dependent diabetes has been estimated to be 20–30% of that in American Caucasians, although there are reports as high as two thirds. These observations have genetic implications (see below). The annual incidence increases at the rate of about 16 new cases/100,000 of the childhood population. Males and females appear to be almost equally affected; there is no apparent correlation with socioeconomic status. Peaks of presentation occur in 2 age groups: at 5–7 yr of age and at the time of puberty. The 1st peak corresponds to the time of increased exposure to infectious agents coincident with the beginning of school, the latter, to the pubertal growth spurt induced by gonadal steroids, which may antagonize insulin action, and to the emotional stresses accompanying puberty. These possible cause-and-effect relationships remain to be proved. The prevalence and incidence of insulin-dependent diabetes in childhood in the United States are similar to those reported in Great Britain, Sweden, and Australia.

Seasonal and long term cyclic variations have been noted in the incidence of insulin-dependent diabetes mellitus. Newly recognized cases appear to occur with greater frequency in the autumn and winter months in both the Northern and Southern Hemispheres. Children under 6 yr of age appear to have an exaggerated seasonal variation. In some instances the long term cycle has appeared to parallel the incidence of mumps when allowance was made for a 4 yr time lag. There is also an increased incidence of diabetes in children with congenital rubella. These associations with viral infections suggest a potential role for viruses as direct or indirect triggering mechanisms in the etiology of diabetes.

Classification. It has become increasingly apparent that diabetes mellitus is not a single entity but rather a heterogeneous group of disorders in which there are distinct genetic patterns as well as other etiologic and pathophysiologic mechanisms that lead to impairment of glucose tolerance. The National Diabetes Data Group has proposed a classification of diabetes and other categories of glucose intolerance based on contemporary knowledge; this classification has been endorsed and accepted by various diabetes associations throughout the world as well as by pediatric investigators (Table 17–1). Three major forms of diabetes and several forms of carbohydrate intolerance have been identified:

Type I Diabetes (Juvenile-Onset Diabetes). This con-

Table 17–1 SUMMARY OF CLASSIFICATION OF DIABETES MELLITUS IN CHILDREN AND ADOLESCENTS*

CLASSIFICATION	CRITERIA
Diabetes mellitus	
1. Insulin-dependent (IDDM, Type I)	Typical manifestations: glucosuria, ketonuria, random plasma glucose (PG) >200 mg/dl
2. Non-insulin-dependent (NIDDM, Type II)	FPG >140 mg/dl and 2 hr value >200 mg/dl during OGTT on more than 1 occasion and in absence of precipitating factors
3. Other types	Type I or II criteria in association with certain genetic syndromes, drugs, cystic fibrosis, and other disorders (see text)
Impaired glucose tolerance (IGT)	FPG <140 mg/dl with 2 hr value >140 mg/dl during OGTT
Gestational diabetes (GDM)	2 or more of following abnormalities during OGTT: FPG >105 mg/dl; 1 hr, >190 mg/dl; 2 hr, >165 mg/dl; 3 hr, >145 mg/dl
Statistical risk classes	
1. Previous abnormality of glucose tolerance	Normal OGTT following a previous abnormal OGTT, spontaneous hyperglycemia or gestational diabetes
2. Potential abnormality of glucose tolerance	Genetic propensity (e.g., identical nondiabetic twin of a diabetic mate); islet-cell antibodies

*Proposed by National Diabetes Data Group.

Abbreviations: PG = Plasma glucose.
FPG = Fasting plasma glucose.
OGTT = Oral glucose tolerance test.

dition is characterized by severe insulinopenia and dependence on exogenous insulin to prevent ketosis and to preserve life; it is therefore also termed **insulin-dependent diabetes mellitus (IDDM)**. There may, on occasion, be preketotic, non-insulin-dependent phases in the natural history of the disease. Although the onset occurs predominantly in childhood, it may come at any age. Hence, such terms as juvenile diabetes, ketosis-prone diabetes, and brittle diabetes should be abandoned in favor of Type I or IDDM. Type I diabetes is clearly distinct by virtue of its association with certain HLA antigens (histocompatibility loci antigens), autoimmunity, and the presence of circulating antibodies to cytoplasmic and cell-surface components of islet cells. With few exceptions, diabetes in children is insulin dependent and fits the Type I category.

Type II Diabetes. Persons in this subclass (formerly known as adult-onset diabetes, maturity-onset diabetes [MOD], or stable diabetes) are not insulin dependent and only infrequently develop ketosis; some may use insulin for correction of symptomatic hyperglycemia, and ketosis may develop in some during severe infections or other stress.

Serum concentration of insulin may be normal or moderately depressed, but it is usually elevated. In the majority of instances the onset of non-insulin-dependent diabetes mellitus occurs after age 40, but it may occur at any age. It is rare in childhood, when it may be manifested as abnormal glucose tolerance, usually in obese individuals; there is adequate secretion of insulin but resistance to it. Weight reduction is indicated in these children. Abnormal carbohydrate tolerance may also occur in children who have a strong family history of Type II diabetes in a pattern suggestive of dominant inheritance; this pattern of diabetes has been termed **MODY** (maturity-onset diabetes of the young) and may require treatment with insulin. Of importance is that there is no association in this type of diabetes with HLA antigens, autoimmunity, and/or islet-cell antibodies.

Secondary Diabetes. This subclass contains a variety of types of diabetes, for some of which the etiologic relationship is known. Examples include diabetes secondary to exocrine pancreatic diseases, such as cystic fibrosis; endocrine other than pancreatic diseases, e.g., Cushing syndrome; and ingestion of certain drugs or poisons, e.g., the rodenticide Vacor. Certain genetic syndromes, including those with abnormalities of the insulin receptor, also are included in this category. There are no associations with HLA antigens, autoimmunity, or islet cell antibodies among the entities in this subdivision.

TYPE I DIABETES MELLITUS
(Insulin-Dependent Diabetes [IDD]; Juvenile-Onset Diabetes)

Etiology and Pathogenesis. The basic cause of the initial clinical findings in this predominant form of diabetes in childhood is the sharply diminished secre-

tion of insulin. Although basal insulin concentrations in plasma may be normal in newly diagnosed patients, insulin production in response to a variety of potent secretagogues is blunted and usually disappears over a period of months to years, rarely exceeding 5 yr. The greater the residual insulin secreting capacity, as assessed by measurements employing C-peptide, the easier it is to maintain metabolic control with relatively small doses of exogenous insulin.

The mechanisms that lead to failure of pancreatic beta-cell function are incompletely understood; in some predisposed individuals they may be related to an autoimmune destruction of pancreatic islets. Type I diabetes has long been known to have an increased prevalence among persons with such disorders as Addison disease, Hashimoto thyroiditis, and pernicious anemia, in which autoimmune mechanisms are known to be pathogenic (Sec 17.3). These conditions, as well as insulin-dependent Type I diabetes mellitus, are now known to be associated with an increased frequency of certain *histocompatibility antigens*, in particular HLA-B8, HLA-BW15, -DW3, and -DW4. The HLA system is the major histocompatibility complex; it is located on chromosome number 6 and consists of a cluster of genes that code transplantation antigens and play a central role in immune responses.

Increased susceptibility to a number of diseases has been related to 1 or more of the identified HLA antigens. The inheritance of HLA-B8 or -BW15 antigens appears to confer a 2–3-fold increased risk for developing Type I diabetes. When both B8 and BW15 are inherited, the relative risk for developing diabetes is 7–10-fold. A rare genetic type of properdin factor B (BfF1) that is closely linked to the HLA system on chromosome 6 is found in more than 20% of Type I diabetics but in only 2% of healthy subjects; thus there is a relative risk factor of 15 for those who inherit this genetic marker. The association of B8 with diabetes may be secondary to its linkage disequilibrium with the antigen DW3, whereas the association of BW15 may be secondary to its linkage disequilibrium with CW3; specificities in the D region appear to be the more frequent associations with Type I diabetes. Because there appear to be substantial differences in certain immune responses and possibly in the complication rates among those with B8-associated disease in contrast to those with BW15, and because B8 and BW15 are additive in conferring risk for developing diabetes, it has been suggested that there is genetic heterogeneity within Type I, insulin-dependent diabetes mellitus.

These observations and speculations provide a rational framework for the long-assumed association of Type I diabetes with genetic factors on the bases of the increased incidence in some families, of the concordance rates in monozygotic twins, and of ethnic and racial differences in prevalence. For example, Type I diabetes among American Blacks is associated with the same HLA genes as it is in American Caucasians. Because the ratios of the prevalence of these genes and of Type I diabetes in the American Black and Caucasian populations (about 0.2–0.3:1) are quite similar, it has been argued that the disease may be transmitted by autosomal dominant inheritance. On the other hand, a more complex 3-allele genetic model that exhibits the features of both dominant and recessive inheritance also fits the available data. It would thus appear that there should be lower recurrence risks to relatives of Black, as compared to those of Caucasian, diabetics. From multiple family pedigrees and HLA typing data, it can be safely predicted that in Caucasians the recurrence risks to siblings are approximately 6% if the proband is under 10 yr of age and 3% if older at the time of diagnosis; the risk to offspring is 2–5%. In American Blacks these risks are only one half to two thirds of those in Caucasians.

Factors other than pure inheritance are also involved in evoking clinical diabetes. For example, the concordance among identical twins of whom 1 has insulin-dependent diabetes is only 50%, suggesting the participation of environmental triggering factors. Such a triggering factor might be a viral infection. In animals a number of viruses can cause a diabetic syndrome, the appearance and severity of which depend on the genetic strain and immune competence of the species of animal tested. In man, epidemics of mumps, rubella, and coxsackie virus infections have been associated with subsequent increases in the incidence of Type I diabetes; the acute onset of diabetes mellitus, presumably induced by coxsackievirus B4, has been described. Certain viruses may be pancreatropic and initiate an inflammatory response in the islets (insulinitis). Observed pathologic changes are characterized by lymphocytic infiltration around the islets of Langerhans. Later, the islets become progressively hyalinized and scarred, a process suggesting an ongoing inflammatory response, possibly autoimmune in nature.

In support of an autoimmune basis for Type I diabetes, a high prevalence of circulating antibodies directed against the cytoplasmic components of islet cells and against the cell-surface components of insulin-producing beta cells has been observed. These antibodies are present in over 75% of patients examined at the clinical onset of disease and prior to insulin treatment; they are, therefore, not insulin antibodies of the kind found universally in insulin-treated diabetics. The islet-cell surface antibodies, in the presence of complement, are cytotoxic for beta cells in vitro. Similarly, T lymphocytes from diabetics have been shown to be cytotoxic to human insulinoma cells in culture. These findings suggest that Type I diabetes, akin to other autoimmune diseases such as Hashimoto thyroiditis, is a disease of "autoaggression," in which autoantibodies in cooperation with complement, T cells, or other factors induce toxic reactions in their target cell, the insulin-producing islet cell. Thus, the inheritance of certain genes intimately associated with the HLA system on chromosome 6 appears to confer a predisposition for autoimmune disease, including diabetes, when triggered by an appropriate stimulus, such as a virus. It should be understood, however, that some insulin-dependent diabetic patients have none of the frequently associated HLA antigens.

Pathophysiology. The progressive destruction of beta cells leads to progressive deficiency of insulin. Insulin is the major anabolic hormone. Its normal secretion in response to feeding is exquisitely modulated by neural, hormonal, and substrate-related mechanisms to permit controlled disposition of ingested foodstuff as energy for immediate or future use; mobilization of energy during the fasted state depends on low plasma levels of insulin. Thus, in normal metabolism there are regular swings between the postprandial high-insulin anabolic state and the fasted low-insulin catabolic state that affect 3 major tissues (liver, muscle, and adipose— Table 17–2). Type I diabetes mellitus, as it evolves, becomes a permanent low-insulin catabolic state in which feeding will not reverse but rather exaggerate these catabolic processes.

Although insulin deficiency is the primary defect, several secondary changes that involve the stress hormones (epinephrine, cortisol, growth hormone, and glucagon) accelerate and exaggerate the rate and magnitude of metabolic decompensation. Increased plasma concentrations of these counterregulatory hormones magnify metabolic derangements by further impairing insulin secretion (epinephrine), by antagonizing its action (epinephrine, cortisol, growth hormone), and by promoting glycogenolysis, gluconeogenesis, lipolysis, and ketogenesis while decreasing glucose utilization and renal clearance. All of these secondary changes are restored to normal by adequate insulin therapy. There may, however, be selective suppression of some of the counterregulatory hormones. For example, the suppression of glucagon, growth hormone, and splanchnic blood flow by the hormone somatostatin ameliorates the hyperglycemia of diabetes, slows the rate of progression to ketoacidosis, and facilitates metabolic control; somatostatin is not available for noninvestigative use.

Table 17–2 INFLUENCE OF FEEDING (HIGH INSULIN) OR OF FASTING (LOW INSULIN) ON SOME METABOLIC PROCESSES IN LIVER, MUSCLE, AND ADIPOSE TISSUE

Insulin is considered to be the major factor governing these metabolic processes. Diabetes mellitus may be viewed as a permanent low-insulin state that, untreated, results in exaggerated fasting.

	HIGH INSULIN (POSTPRANDIAL STATE)	LOW INSULIN (FASTED STATE)
Liver:	Glucose uptake	Glucose production
	Glycogen synthesis	Glycogenolysis
	Absence of gluconeogenesis	Gluconeogenesis
	Lipogenesis	Absence of lipogenesis
	Absence of ketogenesis	Ketogenesis
Muscle:	Glucose uptake	Absence of glucose uptake
	Glucose oxidation	Fatty acid and ketone oxidation
	Glycogen synthesis	Glycogenolysis
	Protein synthesis	Proteolysis and amino acid release
Adipose tissue:	Glucose uptake	Absence of glucose uptake
	Lipid synthesis	Lipolysis and fatty acid release
	Triglyceride uptake	Absence of triglyceride uptake

Insulin deficiency, in concert with the excessive plasma concentrations of epinephrine, cortisol, growth hormone, and glucagon, results in unrestrained production of glucose and impairment of its utilization; hence hyperglycemia and an increase in osmolality develop. Glucosuria occurs when the renal threshold of approximately 160 mg/dl is exceeded; the resultant osmotic diuresis produces polyuria, dehydration, and compensatory polydipsia. Plasma osmolality can be calculated by the following formula:

$$\text{Serum osmolality in mOsm/kg} = \text{Serum [Na}^+ \text{ (mEq/l)}$$
$$\text{plus K}^+ \text{ (mEq/l)]} \times 2 \text{ plus } \frac{\text{glucose mg/dl)}}{18}$$

Hyperosmolality is commonly encountered and is almost universally present during episodes of ketoacidosis. It contributes to the symptomatology, in particular to cerebral obtundation during ketoacidosis, and has important implications for therapy.

The combination of insulin deficiency and elevated plasma values of the counterregulatory hormones is also responsible for accelerated lipolysis and impaired lipid synthesis, with resulting increased plasma concentrations of total lipids, cholesterol, triglycerides, and free fatty acids. The hormonal interplay of insulin deficiency and glucagon excess shunts the free fatty acids into ketone formation; the rate of formation of these ketone bodies, principally beta-hydroxybutyrate and acetoacetate, exceeds the capacity for peripheral utilization and for renal excretion. Accumulation of these ketoacids results in metabolic acidosis and in compensatory rapid deep breathing in an attempt to excrete excess CO_2 (Kussmaul respiration). Acetone, formed by nonenzymatic conversion of acetoacetate, is responsible for the characteristic fruity odor of the breath. Ketones are excreted in the urine in association with cations and thus further increase losses of water and electrolytes (Table 17–3 and Sec 5.27). With progressive dehydration, acidosis, hyperosmolality, and diminished cerebral oxygen utilization, consciousness becomes impaired, the patient ultimately becoming comatose. Thus, insulin deficiency produces a profound catabolic state—an exaggerated starvation—in which all of the initial clinical features can be explained on the basis of known alterations in intermediary metabolism.

Table 17–3 FLUID AND ELECTROLYTE MAINTENANCE REQUIREMENTS AND ESTIMATED LOSSES IN DIABETIC KETOACIDOSIS

	Approximate Daily Maintenance Requirements*	Approximate Accumulated Losses†
Water	2000 ml/M²	100 ml/kg (range 60–100 ml/kg)
Sodium	45 mEq/M²	6 mEq/kg (range 5–13 mEq/kg)
Potassium	35 mEq/M²	5 mEq/kg (range 4–6 mEq/kg)
Chloride	30 mEq/M²	4 mEq/kg (range 3–9 mEq/kg)
Phosphate	10 mEq/M²	3 mEq/kg (range 2–5 mEq/kg)

*Maintenance is expressed in surface area to permit uniformity because fluid requirements change as weight increases. Also see Sec 5.27.

†Losses are expressed per unit of body weight since the losses remain relatively constant in relation to total body weight.

The severity and duration of the symptoms are a reflection of the extent of insulinopenia.

Clinical Manifestations. Most diabetic children present initially with a history of polyuria, polydipsia, polyphagia, and weight loss. The duration of these symptoms varies, but it is often less than 1 mo. A clue to the existence of polyuria may be the onset of enuresis in a previously toilet-trained child. An insidious onset with lethargy, weakness, and weight loss is also quite common. The loss of weight in spite of an increased dietary intake is readily explicable by the following illustration:

The average healthy 10 yr old child has a daily caloric intake of 2000 or more calories, of which approximately 50% are derived from carbohydrate. With the development of diabetes, daily losses of water and glucose may be as much as 5 l and 250 gm, respectively. Despite the child's compensatory increased intake of food and water, the calories cannot be utilized, and increasing catabolism and weight loss ensue.

Pyogenic skin infections are not common presenting complaints; monilial vaginitis is occasionally observed in teenage girls.

Ketoacidosis is responsible for the initial presentation of many diabetic children. The early manifestations may be relatively mild and consist of vomiting, dehydration, hyperglycemia, ketonemia, glucosuria, and ketonuria. In the more prolonged and severe cases the child is comatose; air hunger is manifested by Kussmaul respiration, and there is an odor of acetone in the breath. Leukocytosis and abdominal rigidity and/or pain that may mimic appendicitis are common; there may also be an associated elevation of serum amylase, but this does not necessarily indicate pancreatitis. It should not be assumed that these findings are evidence of a surgical emergency prior to a period of appropriate fluid, electrolyte, and insulin therapy to correct the acidosis; the abdominal manifestations frequently disappear after several hr of such treatment.

Nonketotic hyperosmolar coma is a syndrome characterized by severe hyperglycemia (blood glucose greater than 600 mg/dl); absence of or only very slight ketosis; nonketotic acidosis; severe dehydration; depressed sensorium or frank coma; and various neurologic signs that may include grand mal seizures, hyperthermia, hemiparesis, and positive Babinski signs. Respiration is usually shallow, but coexistent metabolic (lactic) acidosis may be manifested by Kussmaul breathing. Serum osmolarity is commonly 350 mOsm/kg or higher. This condition usually occurs in middle-aged or elderly individuals who have "mild" diabetes; among them mortality rates have been as high as 40–70%, possibly in part because of delays in recognition and in institution of appropriate therapy. In children this condition is infrequent; among reported cases there has been a high incidence of existing neurologic damage. The profound hyperglycemia may develop over a period of days, and, initially, the obligatory osmotic polyuria and dehydration may be partially compensated by increasing fluid intake. With progression, thirst becomes impaired, possibly because of alteration of the hypothalamic thirst center by hyperosmolarity and possibly in some instances because of a pre-existing defect in the hypothalamic osmoregulating mechanism.

The low production of ketones is attributed mainly to the hyperosmolarity which in vitro blunts the lipolytic effect of epinephrine and the antilipolytic effect of insulin; blunting of lipolysis by the therapeutic use of beta-adrenergic blockers may contribute to the syndrome. Depression of consciousness is closely correlated with the degree of hyperosmolarity in this condition as well as in diabetic ketoacidosis; hemoconcentration may also predispose to cerebral arterial and venous thromboses.

Treatment is directed at repletion of the vascular volume deficit and correction of the hyperosmolar state (also see management of ketoacidosis). One half isotonic saline (0.45% NaCl) is administered at a rate estimated to replace 50% of the volume deficit in the 1st 12 hr and the remainder over the ensuing 24 hr. When the blood glucose concentration approaches 300 mg/dl, the hydrating fluid should be changed to 5% dextrose in water. Approximately 20 mEq/l of potassium chloride should be added to each of these fluids to prevent hypokalemia. Serum potassium and plasma glucose concentrations should be monitored at 2 hr intervals for the 1st 12 hr and at 4 hr intervals for the next 24 hr to permit appropriate adjustments of administered potassium and insulin.

Insulin can be given by continuous intravenous infusion beginning with the 2nd hr of fluid therapy. Inasmuch as blood glucose may decrease dramatically with fluid therapy alone, the intravenous loading dose should be 0.05 U/kg of regular (fast-acting) insulin followed by 0.05 U/kg/hr of the same insulin, rather than 0.1 U/kg/hr as advocated for diabetic ketoacidosis. During the recovery period, therapy with insulin and diet and monitoring of the patient are as described for patients recovering from diabetic ketoacidosis (See Table 17–4 and related text).

Diagnosis. Children in whom the diagnosis of diabetes mellitus must be considered may, for practical purposes, be divided into 3 general categories: (1) those who have a history suggestive of diabetes, especially polyuria and failure to gain or a loss of weight in spite of a voracious appetite; (2) those who have a transient or persistent glucosuria; and (3) those who have clinical manifestations of metabolic acidosis with or without stupor or coma. *In all instances the diagnosis of diabetes mellitus is dependent on the demonstration of glucosuria, with or without ketonuria, in association with otherwise unexplained hyperglycemia.* In such instances the glucose tolerance test is not needed to support the diagnosis.

Renal glucosuria is a manifestation in a variety of conditions in addition to its isolated occurrence as a congenital disorder (Sec 16.27); these include the Fan-

Table 17–4 FLUID AND ELECTROLYTE LOSSES BASED ON ASSUMED 10% DEHYDRATION WITH RECOMMENDED REPLACEMENTS IN A CHILD WITH DIABETIC KETOACIDOSIS WHO WEIGHS 30 KG (SURFACE AREA 1.0 M²)

REPLACEMENT FLUIDS

	APPROXIMATE ACCUMULATED LOSSES WITH 10% DEHYDRATION	APPROXIMATE REQUIREMENTS FOR DAILY MAINTENANCE	TOTAL	WORKING TOTAL
Water (ml)	3000	2000	5000	5000
Sodium (mEq)	180	50	230	250
Potassium (mEq)	150	40	190	200
Chloride (mEq)	120	30	150	150
Phosphate (mEq)	90	10	100	100

REPLACEMENT SCHEDULE

APPROXIMATE DURATION	FLUIDS (ML)	SODIUM (MEQ)	CHLORIDE (MEQ)	POTASSIUM (MEQ)	PHOSPHATE (MEQ)
1st hr	500 0.9% NaCl	75	75	—	—
2nd hr	500 0.45% NaCl	35	45	10*	—
3rd–5th hr	1000 0.45% NaCl	75	75	40†	40
6th–8th hr	1000 0.45% NaCl	75	75	40†	40
9th–30th hr	2000 G5W‡	—	40	80§	40
	5000 ml	260 mEq	310 mEq	170 mEq	120 mEq

Note: All replacement values should be halved if dehydration is estimated to be 5%. Maintenance requirements remain the same.
*Potassium chloride.
†Potassium phosphate.
‡G5W = 5% glucose in water.
§aa Potassium chloride and potassium phosphate.

ADDITIONAL GUIDELINES

A diabetic flow-sheet with laboratory data appropriately recorded must be maintained in the patient's chart.

Insulin therapy by continuous low-dose intravenous method: Priming dose—0.1 unit/kg regular insulin IV. Continuous IV infusion—0.1 unit/kg/hr regular insulin beginning with 2nd hr.

Directions for making insulin infusion: Add 30 units regular insulin to 300 ml of physiologic saline. Flush 50 ml through the tubing to saturate insulin binding sites. For 30 kg patient, infuse at rate of 30 ml/hr. When the blood glucose concentration approaches 300 mg/dl, discontinue the insulin infusion and start insulin therapy by subcutaneous injections of 0.25 U/kg at 6 hr intervals.

Bicarbonate therapy: For pH >7.20, no therapy necessary. For pH 7.10–7.20, 40 mEq/M² of bicarbonate over 2 hr; then re-evaluate. For pH <7.10, 80 mEq/M² of bicarbonate over 2 hr; then re-evaluate. New diabetics <2 yr of age with diabetic ketoacidosis and 10% dehydration, or any diabetic with pH <7.00, should be managed in an intensive care unit.

coni renal syndrome, severe lead intoxication with associated renal tubular damage, and ingestion of certain drugs (e.g., phlorizin). When vomiting, diarrhea, and/or inadequate intake of food are complicating factors in any of these conditions, starvation ketosis may ensue and simulate diabetic ketoacidosis. The absence of hyperglycemia eliminates the possibility of diabetes. It is also important to recognize that not all urinary sugar is glucose, and infrequently galactosemia, pentosuria, and the fructosurias will require consideration as diagnostic possibilities.

The discovery of glucosuria, with or without a mild degree of hyperglycemia, during a hospital admission for trauma or infection or even during the associated emotional upheaval may, but usually does not, herald the existence of diabetes; in most of these instances the glucosuria remits during recovery. Inasmuch as this circumstance may indicate a limited capacity for insulin secretion, which is unmasked by elevated plasma concentrations of the stress hormones, these patients should be rechecked at a later date for the possibility of hyperglycemia and/or clinical features of diabetes mellitus.

Diabetic ketoacidosis must be differentiated from acidosis and/or coma from other causes; these include hypoglycemia, uremia, gastroenteritis with metabolic acidosis, lactic acidosis, salicylate intoxication, encephalitis, and other intracranial lesions. Diabetic ketoacidosis can be said to exist when there is hyperglycemia (glucose ≥300 mg/dl), ketonemia (ketones strongly positive at greater than 1:2 dilution of serum), acidosis (pH <7.30 and bicarbonate less than 15 mEq/l), glycosuria, and ketonuria in addition to the clinical features described. Precipitating factors, even for the initial presentation, include stress such as trauma, infections, vomiting, and psychologic disturbances. Recurrent episodes of ketoacidosis in established diabetics often represent deliberate errors in recommended insulin dosage or unusual stress responses that indicate psychologic disturbances and, at times, pleas to be removed from a home environment perceived to be stressful or intolerable.

Screening procedures, such as postprandial determinations of blood glucose or oral glucose tolerance tests, have yielded low detection rates in children, even among those considered at risk, such as siblings of diabetic children.

Treatment. The management of insulin-dependent diabetes mellitus may be divided into 3 phases: that of ketoacidosis; the postacidotic or transition period for establishment of metabolic control; and the continuing phase of guidance of the diabetic child and his or her family. Each of these phases has separate goals, although in practice they merge into a continuum.

Ketoacidosis. The immediate aims of therapy are expansion of intravascular volume, correction of deficits in fluid, electrolyte, and acid-base status, and initiation of insulin therapy to correct intermediary metabolism. Treatment should be instituted as soon as the clinical diagnosis is confirmed by the presence of hyperglycemia and ketonemia. Determinations of blood pH and electrolytes should also be obtained; an ECG is useful to provide a rapid reference for the existence of hyper-

kalemia. If sepsis is suspected as a possible precipitating factor, a blood culture should be obtained and the urine examined for the presence of bacteria and leukocytes. A flow sheet to record chronologically the rate and composition of fluid input, urine output, amount of insulin administered, and the acid-base and electrolyte values of the blood is most useful. Catheterization of the bladder is not recommended in children; if considered necessary, bag collection or condom drainage permits an assessment of urinary output.

FLUID AND ELECTROLYTE THERAPY (Sec 5.15).   The expansion of reduced intravascular volume and correction of depleted fluid and electrolyte stores are most important in the treatment of diabetic ketoacidosis. It must be stressed, however, that exogenous insulin is essential to arrest further metabolic decompensation and restore intermediary metabolism.

Dehydration is commonly of the order of 10%; initial fluid therapy can be based on this estimate, with subsequent adjustments to be related to clinical and laboratory data. The initial hydrating fluid should be isotonic saline (0.9%); in children under 10 yr of age, it may be a 0.45% solution. Because of the hyperglycemia, hyperosmolarity is universal in diabetic ketoacidosis; thus, even 0.9% saline is hypotonic relative to the patient's serum osmolality. A gradual decline in osmolality is desirable as too rapid a decline contributes to cerebral edema, 1 of the major complications of therapy in children. For the same reason the rate of fluid replacement is adjusted to provide only 50% of the calculated deficit within the initial 8 hr; the remaining 50% is administered during the next 20–30 hr. Administration of glucose (5% solution in water) is initiated when blood glucose concentration approaches 300 mg/dl (Table 17–4).

Administration of potassium (K^+) should be started early. Total body potassium may be considerably depleted during acidosis, even when the serum potassium concentration is normal or elevated. Whereas potassium moves from intra- to extracellular sites during acidosis, the reverse occurs with alkalosis, particularly when exogenous insulin and endogenous and/or exogenous glucose are available in the circulation. This shift of potassium back to the intracellular compartment may result in hypokalemia, a problem more common than hyperkalemia. Hence, after the initial fluid replacement of approximately 20 ml/kg of isotonic saline (0.9%) has been provided, potassium should be added to subsequent infusates if urinary output is adequate; serum potassium concentration should then be monitored periodically. An ECG provides a rapid assessment of serum potassium concentration; T waves are peaked in hyperkalemia and are low and associated with U waves in hypokalemia (Sec 13.3). Because the total potassium deficit cannot be replaced within the initial 24 hr of treatment, potassium supplementation should be continued as long as fluids are administered intravenously (Table 17–4).

It is almost inevitable that the patient will receive an excess of chloride, which may aggravate acidosis; the extent of acidosis, however, can be reduced by substitution of phosphate, which is also significantly depleted in diabetic ketoacidosis. Moreover, phosphate in conjunction with glycolysis is essential for the formation of 2,3-diphosphoglycerate (2,3-DPG), which governs the oxygen dissociation curve. During deficiency of 2,3-DPG, the oxygen dissociation curve is shifted to the left, i.e., more oxygen is retained by hemoglobin and less is available to tissues, a situation that predisposes to lactic acidosis. Acidosis per se tends to shift the oxygen dissociation curve toward the right (Bohr effect) and thus partially "compensates" for 2,3-DPG deficiency. As acidosis resulting from the accumulation of ketones is corrected by the provision of insulin, with or without administration of bicarbonate, the effects of 2,3-DPG deficiency may no longer be "compensated" and the release of oxygen to tissues may again be impaired. Exogenous phosphate, by contributing to the formation of 2,3-DPG, permits the oxygen dissociation curve to shift to the right and thus facilitates release of oxygen to tissues and aids in the correction of acidosis. Furthermore, resistance to insulin action is associated with hypophosphatemia. Hence, we recommend the administration of potassium phosphate as outlined in Table 17–4. Since excessive use of phosphate may result in hypocalcemia, serum calcium should be measured periodically. Symptomatic hypocalcemia should be corrected with calcium gluconate.

ALKALI THERAPY. With provision of fluids, electrolytes, glucose, and insulin, metabolic acidosis is usually corrected through the interruption of ketogenesis, the metabolism of ketones to bicarbonate, and the generation of bicarbonate by the distal renal tubule. Concerns over the therapeutic administration of bicarbonate center on 4 issues: (1) Alkalosis, by shifting the oxygen dissociation curve to the left, may diminish the release of oxygen to tissues and hence predipose to lactic acidosis. (2) Alkalosis accelerates the entry of potassium into cells and hence may produce hypokalemia. (3) Provision of bicarbonate according to the calculated base deficit overcorrects and may result in alkalosis. (4) Perhaps most important, bicarbonate may lead to worsening of cerebral acidosis while the plasma pH is being restored to normal because HCO_3^- combines with H^+ and dissociates to CO_2 and H_2O. Whereas bicarbonate passes the blood-brain barrier slowly, CO_2 diffuses freely, thereby exacerbating cerebral acidosis and possibly cerebral depression. On the other hand, severe acidosis, with a blood pH of 7.1 or less, diminishes respiratory minute volume, may produce hypotension by means of peripheral vasodilation, impairs myocardial function, and may be a factor in insulin resistance. For these reasons, administration of bicarbonate is recommended only when the pH is 7.2 or below (Table 17–4). At pH 7.1–7.2, 40 mEq of HCO_3^-/M^2, and below pH 7.1, 80 mEq of HCO_3^-/M^2, should be infused over a period of 2 hr; acid-base status should then be re-evaluated prior to further alkali therapy. Bicarbonate should not be given by bolus infusion as it may precipitate cardiac arrhythmias.

INSULIN THERAPY. Several regimens of insulin therapy during ketoacidosis are in current use; each is effective in experienced hands provided that care is taken to avoid hypoglycemia.

The traditional approach has been the administration of insulin by repeated intramuscular or subcutaneous bolus injections; a portion of the initial dose is usually injected intravenously. One such regimen based on body weight is outlined in Table 17–5; if plasma ketones are only moderately elevated, the recommended doses may be half of those listed. Administrations are repeated every 2–4 hr, and blood glucose values and acid-base status are monitored. When the concentration of blood glucose has fallen to approximately 300 mg/dl, subsequent insulin therapy at a dose of 0.25–0.5 U/kg may be given subcutaneously every 6–8 hr while maintaining an infusion of 5% glucose in water with potassium added (Table 17–4) until the child can tolerate solid food. Sips of clear liquid, broth, or carbonated beverages may be given during this interval.

When food intake is tolerated, half of the total insulin dose of the previous day is administered subcutaneously in an intermediate-acting form (NPH or lente; Table 17–6). Blood glucose should be measured before each meal; a value greater than 250 mg/dl is an indication for an additional subcutaneous injection of regular (short-acting) insulin (0.25 U/kg). After 1–2 days of this regimen the total daily dose of insulin may be given by combining two thirds of the intermediate and one third of the short-acting forms as a single injection before breakfast. Alternatively, two thirds of the total daily dose of insulin may be given in the morning before breakfast and one third in the evening before dinner; each injection combines intermediate and short-acting insulin in a ratio of 2:1. The choice between the single or twice-daily regimens depends on the degree of metabolic control achieved. The aim is to minimize glycosuria and hyperglycemia without precipitating hypoglycemia.

Table 17–5 INTERMITTENT OR "TRADITIONAL" INSULIN REGIMEN FOR DIABETIC KETOACIDOSIS

BLOOD GLUCOSE	TOTAL INSULIN DOSE	INTRAVENOUS DOSE	INTRAMUSCULAR OR SUBCUTANEOUS DOSE	FREQUENCY
>900 mg/dl	2 units/kg	1 unit/kg	1 unit/kg	Every 2–4 hr
>600–900 mg/dl	1 unit/kg	½ unit/kg	½ unit/kg	Every 2–4 hr
>300–600 mg/dl	½ unit/kg	¼ unit/kg	¼ unit/kg	Every 2–4 hr

These doses may be halved if serum ketones are only modestly elevated.

When blood glucose approaches 300 mg/dl, the intravenous infusion for fluid and electrolyte replacement should contain 5% glucose (see Table 17–4 for rate of administration). Continue subcutaneous injections of insulin at 0.25 U/kg every 6 hr and monitor blood glucose concentration at the same time. If blood glucose concentration rises, increase the next insulin dose by 50%; if glucose concentration falls, decrease the next insulin dose by 50%. Continue this insulin regimen for 24 hr after oral fluid and food intake is established. (See text for subsequent management.)

Table 17–6 SOME COMMON TYPES OF AVAILABLE INSULIN

	DURATION OF ACTION IN HOURS		
PRODUCT	Onset	Peak Effect	Approximate Duration
Rapid onset—short duration			
Regular*	1/2	2–4	6–8
Quick†	1/2	2–4	6–8
Actrapid‡	1/2	2–4	6–8
Semilente*	1/2	2–4	10–12
Semitard‡	1/2	2–4	12–16
Intermediate onset and duration			
NPH*	2	4–12	24
NPH†	2	4–12	24
Lente* (70% ultra, 30% semi lente)	2	8–10	24
Mixtard† (70% NPH, 30% quick)	1/2	4–8	24
Monotard‡	2	4–12	24
Lentard‡	2	4–12	24
Delayed onset—long duration			
Protamine zinc insulin* (PZI)	4–8	14–20	24–36
Ultra lente*	4–8	14–20	36
Ultratard‡	8–10	10–30	36

*Eli Lilly Co.
†Nordisk Insulin.
‡Novo Lab. Inc.
All 3 manufacturers distribute in the United States and Europe. Different brand names may prevail in some countries. Highly purified pork, beef, or beef-pork preparations are available.

The *continuous low-dose intravenous infusion method,* in which a priming dose of 0.1 U/kg of regular insulin is followed by a constant infusion of 0.1 U/kg/hr, is outlined in Table 17–4. This method is effective, simple, and physiologically sound and has gained wide acceptance as the preferred method for administering insulin during diabetic ketoacidosis. It provides a constant steady concentration of insulin in plasma that approximates the peak attained in normal individuals during an oral glucose tolerance test. Presumably, the same steady concentration is attained at the cellular level and permits a steady metabolic response without the fluctuations that must occur with intermittent injections of insulin. Concern that the insulin may adhere to glass and tubing has proved to be unfounded, and effective delivery of insulin can be provided without the use of albumin or gelatin added to the infusate. Moreover, insulin infusion can be provided by gravity drip without the use of a special pump although such a pump may be helpful. We recommend infusion of the insulin into a vein other than the one used for fluid and electrolyte therapy so that adjustments in the dosage of each can be made independently. After the amount of insulin for the initial 6–8 hr has been calculated, this quantity is added to a 250 or 500 ml bottle of 0.5% saline (see Table 17–4 for specific instructions).

As with the traditional approach, when the blood glucose concentration approaches 300 mg/dl, the ongoing potassium requirement is added to 5% glucose in water (Table 17–4), and the rate of insulin infusion is reduced to 0.05 U/kg/hr. Alternatively, the continuous insulin infusion may be discontinued, and insulin may be given subcutaneously in bolus injections at a dose of 0.25–0.5 U/kg every 6–8 hr while maintaining the glucose infusion until the child can fully tolerate food. Subsequent insulin therapy, using a combination of intermediate and short-acting insulin, is as described above. With this regimen, intermediate-acting insulin is usually begun within 24–36 hr after commencing therapy for ketoacidosis.

Ketonemia and ketonuria may persist despite clinical improvement. The nitroprusside reaction that is routinely used to measure "ketones" reacts with acetoacetate and weakly with acetone but not with beta-hydroxybutyrate. The usual ratio of beta-hydroxybutyrate to acetoacetate is approximately 3:1, but it is commonly as much as 8:1 or more in diabetic ketoacidosis. With correction of acidosis, beta-hydroxybutyrate dissociates to acetoacetate, which is identified by the nitroprusside reaction. Hence, persistence of ketonuria for a day or more may not reliably reflect the clinical improvement and should not be interpreted as an index of poor therapeutic response.

Postacidotic Phase or Transition Period for Establishment of Metabolic Control. Diabetic ketoacidosis is usually corrected within 36–48 hr by the foregoing therapeutic regimen. At this time food and fluids are usually tolerated orally, and insulin can be given by subcutaneous injection. The aims during the postacidotic phase are treatment of any recognized precipitating cause such as an infection; stabilization of metabolic control by adjustments of insulin dosage; institution of an appropriate nutritional pattern for the child; and education of the parents and patient in the principles of diabetic management. These include techniques of insulin injection, monitoring of urine or blood glucose, an understanding of nutritional requirements, recognition of hypoglycemia (insulin shock) and its management, and adjustments of insulin dosage during minor illnesses and for regularly planned exercise. This education is best carried out by the coordinated participation of physician, dietitian, and nurse educator who have had special training in diabetes. For newly diagnosed patients this phase commonly lasts 7–10 days; less time may be required for stabilization and re-education of previously diagnosed patients. Ongoing education and adjustment of insulin dosage are continued after discharge from hospital through outpatient visits; during this phase, gradual reductions in insulin dosage are frequently required, and the patients should be so advised (see Residual Beta Cell Function, below). Details and rationale of insulin and dietary therapy as well as other aspects of long term management are provided in the following section.

Ongoing Management. The immediate goals in the management of children with Type I diabetes are the provision of adequate nutrition and exogenous insulin in a manner that prevents polydipsia and polyuria, including nocturia; avoids ketoacidosis and severe hypoglycemia; and permits normal growth and development with an active life pattern. These goals are achievable by most patients and their parents if they come to understand the principles of the pathophysiology and management of this disease. Ongoing supervision by the physician is essential and should be provided in a manner that avoids undue anxiety and psychologic dependence on the part of the child or parents or a sense of guilt on the part of the parents.

Evidence is emerging that the long term complications of diabetes are related to the degree of metabolic control; therefore, one should aim for as nearly normal metabolism as possible. The achievement of completely normal metabolism, however, is not possible by the standard pattern of treatment that consists of 1–2 daily injections of insulin and attention to nutritional intake and exercise. In highly motivated adolescents, however, near-normal metabolism can now be achieved in 1 of 2 ways: (1) Monitoring of blood glucose values at home with appropriate adjustments of insulin dosage 2–3 times a day and close attention to nutritional intake can be effective. (2) The continuous subcutaneous insulin infusion by a pump worn externally which can be programmed to provide a basal rate of delivery with meal-related increments is also an extremely effective means for selected patients (See Future Directions at end of this section). For the majority of pediatric patients, however, these newer approaches are not available or applicable, and management consists primarily of guidance in respect to insulin dosage, nutritional intake, and exercise.

INSULIN REGIMENS. The diurnal pattern of insulin concentration in the plasma of normal persons is characterized by a basal level on which are superimposed secretory episodes that coincide with intake of food. Each rise in plasma insulin concentration during feeding is synchronous with, and proportional to, the rise in blood glucose. Plasma insulin concentrations, however, do not reflect total insulin secretion. Because insulin is secreted into the portal circulation, its 1st target organ is the liver, the key organ governing the initial disposal of a glucose load (Table 17–2).

Currently available insulins are listed in Table 17–6. They are classified as short-acting, intermediate-acting, and long-acting types; each is available in a concentration of 100 units/ml (U-100); higher (but not lower) concentrations are available for the unusual patient who has high resistance to insulin. Refinements in manufacture are now responsible for insulins with distinctly less contamination than formerly by such other pancreatic hormones as proinsulin, glucagon, pancreatic polypeptide, and some somatostatin. Antibodies to these and other contaminants have been demonstrated in the sera of insulin-treated diabetics. It is unclear whether the new and more highly purified insulins facilitate metabolic control, but they probably do result in fewer local and systemic allergic reactions, including lipoatrophy and lipohypertrophy. The currently available insulins are extracted from beef and pork pancreases and are marketed separately or as a mixture of the 2 insulins. Human insulin, synthesized in bacteria via recombinant DNA technology, has undergone some preliminary testing and should be available for therapy in the future.

Because exogenous insulins are injected subcutaneously rather than directly into the portal vein, their rate of absorption may be variable; and because the dose injected is determined empirically, it lacks the precision of endogenously supplied insulin. Hence, it should be

apparent that a single injection of intermediate-acting insulin cannot duplicate the pattern of normal insulin secretion, and periods of excessive plasma insulin that may produce hypoglycemia and/or periods of inadequate insulin that permit hyperglycemia are virtually inevitable. Even with injections of regular fast-acting insulin prior to each meal, normalization of blood glucose values is not entirely achieved, although the degree of control is clearly improved. Hence, the regimen of insulin administration selected for the diabetic child must represent a compromise designed to achieve as nearly normal intermediary metabolism as will permit normal growth and development and avoid frequent hypoglycemic reactions and the consequences of unrestrained hyperglycemia.

At the onset of diabetes, or after recovery from ketoacidosis, the total daily dose of insulin is about 0.5–1.0 U/kg. Long-acting insulins are not often used in children. In most instances 1 of the intermediate insulins is employed, but, because of its delayed action, a fast acting (regular) insulin is usually combined with it. With the *single daily dose regimen* on the latter basis, approximately two thirds of the total dose is an intermediate-acting insulin (NPH, lente, etc.), and the remainder is regular insulin; the injection is given 30 min before breakfast. The 2 insulins should always be drawn into the syringe in the same sequence so that the residual insulin in the "dead space" is always the same type; thus, greater stability of the patient can be assured once a therapeutic dose is established. Disposable syringes with fine needles, minimal dead space, and easy-to-read calibration for use with U-100 insulin are available. For small children syringes calibrated to a maximum of 50 units are also available; in some European countries diluted insulins are marketed.

In order to avoid hypoglycemia, the *single daily dose regimen* combining intermediate and short-acting insulin is initially calculated on the basis of a total daily dose of 0.5 unit/kg. Step increases or decreases of 10% can then be made daily during the initial phase in hospital until the desired degree of control is achieved. The initial phase of recovery of metabolic equilibrium is characterized by a period of replenishment of body stores of glycogen, protein, and fat that were depleted during the evolution of diabetes. Hence, insulin requirements for the 1st few days may on occasion be found to be even greater than 1 unit/kg/day. Adjustments in the dose of insulin are made in relation to the pattern of blood glucose values and/or of the excretion of glucose. If the predominant glucosuria occurs in late morning, then the quick-acting form of insulin is increased by 10%. If the predominant glucosuria occurs in late afternoon or evening, then the intermediate-acting insulin is increased by 10%. Should hypoglycemic reactions occur in mid-morning to noon, the quick-acting form of insulin is reduced by 10%, and, if hypoglycemia occurs in late afternoon or evening, the intermediate-acting insulin is decreased by 10%. In anticipation of increased exercise at home the daily dose of insulin should be decreased by 10% at the time of discharge from the initial hospitalization.

Although many children can be managed with a single daily injection of insulin, some will achieve better control with 2 *daily injections*. When there is persistent nocturia associated with excessive fasting hyperglycemia and morning glucosuria in response to a single daily injection of insulin, consideration should be given to dividing the total daily dose into 2 injections. In this plan two thirds of the daily total dose is given before breakfast and one third before the evening meal; each injection consists of intermediate and short-acting insulins in proportions of 2:1 to 3:1. For example, assuming a total daily dose of 1 unit/kg for a 30 kg child, 14 units of NPH or lente combined with 6 units of regular insulin would be given before breakfast, and 6 units of NPH or lente with 4 units of regular insulin before the evening meal. As with the single daily dose regimen, stepwise increases or decreases, each consisting of 10%, should be made to minimize hypoglycemic reactions and undue hyperglycemia (see above paragraph for guidelines).

Two daily injections of insulin are especially applicable and tend to result in smoother metabolic control with fewer hypoglycemic reactions and less uncontrolled hyperglycemia when the evening meal is the major one (see under Nutritional Management); this approach is more effective also for infants and children under 5 yr of age, in whom intake of food and extent of activity are not always predictable and for adolescents, especially during the pubertal growth spurt. With explanation of the rationale, compliance with this twice-daily regimen by patients and parents has been remarkably good. When compliance is not good, we attempt to avoid an attitude of rigidity, particularly with adolescents in whom there is evidence that 2 daily injections may not always result in better metabolic control than the 1 daily injection. The physician must in all instances attempt to determine what may be in the best interest of the patient. For children who insist on only 1 daily injection of insulin, we comply by adjusting the daily dose according to carefully kept records of blood and/or urinary glucose values until the best possible degree of metabolic control is achieved. In this way, it is hoped that confidence in the patient-family-physician relationship is maintained and that a sense of guilt in patient and/or family is avoided.

The technique for injection of insulin should be taught to the parents and to the patient when he or she is ready for it. Injections are given vertical to the plane of the tissue, rotating sites on arms, thighs, buttocks, and abdomen in a regular sequence. An appropriate rotation helps to ensure adequate absorption of insulin, prevent fibrosis, and minimize lipodystrophic changes. Indeed, with this rotation and the availability of the purer, single peak insulins, lipoatrophy and lipohypertrophy are now quite unusual. If children find that injection in the abdominal wall is difficult or painful, this site may be omitted. Depending on the physical and psychologic maturity of the child, those over the age of 10–12 yr should be encouraged to administer their own insulin and to monitor their own responses to it. The assumption of responsibility for self-monitoring will be a gradual process in which the parents and child all participate. Once the child has assumed total responsibility, the parents must resist a tendency to overprotection. Guidelines for adjusting the dose of

insulin have been outlined above, and those for adjusting the dose of insulin with exercise, infection, and "brittle" diabetes are provided in greater detail in the following section. It should be stressed, however, that the adolescent growth spurt is regularly associated with an increase in insulin requirements, which may be lower when puberty is completed.

Hypersensitivity to insulin is uncommon in children. Local skin reactions are characterized by erythema or urticaria, with burning, itching, and tenderness within hours or less after an injection. These reactions usually resolve spontaneously over a period of days; antihistamines may be used if necessary. Generalized reactions with severe urticaria or angioedema are extremely rare and may also spontaneously resolve, but a change in the type of insulin is usually indicated, e.g., from a mixed beef-pork preparation to a pure pork preparation. Desensitization may also be necessary, as may a course of systemic corticosteroid therapy for 1–2 wk. Rarely, insulin resistance develops in response to a local tissue enzyme which destroys injected insulin; some of these patients have benefited from the addition of a protease enzyme inhibitor to the insulin solution; others have required chronic intravenous infusion and are best managed in a hospital with a specialized diabetes unit.

After several mo of insulin therapy nearly all patients will have acquired antibodies to insulin. In the majority, they do not interfere with the metabolic response. They may, however, promote instability by creating a reservoir of insulin that may be released at unpredictable times. Rarely, children with antibodies develop true resistance to insulin and require more than 2 units of insulin/kg/24 hr. A change to a preparation of pure pork or pure beef insulin usually resolves this problem; in some instances a period of corticosteroid therapy or a course of desensitization may be necessary. Antibodies causing allergy are usually of the IgE class; IgA and IgM antibodies may be responsible for resistance to insulin.

NUTRITIONAL MANAGEMENT. Because the word diet may connote restriction and denial and impose a source of anxiety and rebellion on the part of parent and/or patient, we tend to avoid its use and categorize our instructional discussion under such terms as "nutritional requirements" and "meal plans." Actually, there are no special nutritional requirements for the diabetic child other than those for optimal growth and development. Inasmuch, however, as the capacity to secrete insulin in response to the intake of food is negligible in the diabetic child, and since the dose of insulin is predicated on caloric intake, regularity of the eating pattern for the determined insulin regimen becomes paramount. In outlining nutritional requirements for the child on the basis of age, sex, weight, and activity, food preferences including any based on cultural and ethnic backgrounds must be considered. Although general guidelines are usually applicable, individualization for each child should be programmed.

Total recommended caloric intake is based on size or surface area and can be obtained from standard tables. The caloric mixture should comprise approximately 55% carbohydrate, 30% fat, and 15% protein. In general, we recommend that approximately 70% of the carbohydrate content be derived from complex carbohydrates such as starch and that intake of sucrose and highly refined sugars be avoided. Complex carbohydrates require prolonged digestion and absorption so that plasma glucose rises slowly, whereas glucose in refined sugars including those in carbonated beverages is rapidly absorbed and causes wide swings in the metabolic pattern; carbonated beverages should therefore be of the sugar-free variety. In the United States the ban on saccharin as an artificial sweetener has been removed pending further evidence of its toxic or teratogenic effect. Although in children there is concern about the potential cumulative effect, available data do not support an association of moderate amounts with bladder cancer. Sorbitol and xylitol should not be used as artificial sweeteners; they are products of the polyol pathway and are implicated in some of the complications of diabetes.

The intake of fat is adjusted so that the polyunsaturated/saturated (P/S) ratio is increased to about 1.2:1.0, in contrast to the estimated American average of 0.3:1.0. Dietary fats derived from animal sources are therefore reduced and are replaced by polyunsaturated fats from vegetable sources. Substituting margarine for butter, vegetable oil for animal oils in cooking, and lean cuts of beef, veal, chicken, turkey, and fish for such fatty meats as ham, bacon, and fatty ground beef achieves the proper ratio. The intake of cholesterol is also reduced by these measures and by limiting the number of egg yolks consumed. There is ample evidence that these simple measures reduce serum LDL cholesterol, a predisposing factor to atherosclerotic disease.

The total daily caloric intake may be divided to provide 20% at breakfast, 20% at lunch, and 30% at dinner, leaving 10% for each of the mid-morning, mid-afternoon, and evening snacks, if they are desired. In older children, the mid-morning snack may be omitted and its caloric equivalent added to the lunch. Special brochures and pamphlets describing the exchanges and sample meal plans for children are usually available from regional diabetes associations; their use should be encouraged as part of the educational process. Meal plans are often based on groups of food exchanges; within each of the exchange lists of the foods that are principal sources of carbohydrates, proteins, and fats, respectively, there is a wide variety of foods that can be substituted or exchanged. For practical purposes there are few restrictions so that each child may select a diet based on personal taste or preferences with the help of the physician and/or dietitian. Emphasis should be placed on regularity of food intake and on the constancy of carbohydrate intake. Occasional excesses for birthdays and other parties are permissible and are tolerated so as not to foster rebellion and stealth in obtaining desired food. Similarly, cakes, doughnuts, and even candies are permissible on special occasions as long as the food exchange value and carbohydrate context are adjusted in the meal plan. Adjustments in meal planning must be made for anticipated vigorous exercise (see below). Above all, adjustments must constantly be made to meet the needs as well as the desires of each child.

MONITORING. Success in the daily management of the diabetic child can be measured to a considerable extent by the competence acquired by the family, and subsequently by the child, in assuming responsibility for day-to-day "diabetic care." Their initial and ongoing instruction in conjunction with their supervised experience can lead to a sense of confidence in making intermittent adjustments in insulin dosage for dietary deviations, unusual physical activity, and even, for some, minor intercurrent illnesses as well as for otherwise unexplained repeated hypoglycemic reactions and excessive glucosuria. Within limits such acceptance of responsibility should make them independent of the physician for their ordinary care. Independence is good provided that there is ongoing interested supervision and shared responsibility by the physician with the family and with the child.

Self-monitoring is essential to such a plan and necessitates a regimen that includes measurements of urinary glucose and at times of ketones, the keeping of a standardized record of the results and of the corresponding data of dietary deviations, unusual physical activity, hypoglycemic reactions, intercurrent illness, the daily dose of insulin, and other items of possible relevance. Many of these records are patently unreliable for a number of reasons. There may be self-delusion, reliance on memory with charting just prior to the visit to the physician, attempts to please the physician and avoid rebuke, as well as reluctance to perform some aspects of the urinary tests. In spite of these problems, asking patients to keep records does appear to be justified. Initially, following dismissal from the hospital, the parent is apt to be particularly attentive to a prescribed regimen. It is after some months of satisfactory experience that parents tend to become less attentive to detail. When the physician apparently accepts the contrived report, the parent or the child may come to find increasing reasons for nonconformance. When the physician mistrusts the report, he may think it justifiable to make evaluations of his own selection (see below). Should his data be counter to those in the parent's or child's report, he then can attempt to clarify the situation with them in such a manner as not to undermine their mutual confidence. Such situations test the physician's skill in the management of patients with persistent but not confining illness.

The daily tests for glucosuria are appropriately scheduled to be performed just prior to each of the 3 major meals and at the time of the evening snack. This timing is designed to secure an estimate of the effect of the prescribed insulin 3–4 hr after each meal. The preciseness of this estimate is increased if the child voids a half hour or so prior to the test voiding; the initial specimen is discarded. When reliable measurements consistently indicate 2% or more glucose in the urine for a given portion of the day, the appropriate dose of the short- or intermediate-acting insulin should be increased by 10%. Conversely, when urine is consistently free of glucose for any portion of the day, the insulin dose may need to be reduced by 10% if hypoglycemic reactions ensue or the blood glucose concentration, as determined by the glucose oxidase strip, is 60 mg/dl or less. In the absence of symptomatic hypoglycemia and of documented low blood glucose concentrations, absence of glucosuria does not warrant a reduction in insulin dosage; such patients are manifesting desirable metabolic control. Consistent patterns of excessive glucosuria at fixed times in the morning or afternoon are indications for appropriate increases in the morning and/or evening doses and at times for a change to another type of insulin. When more precise adjustments are deemed necessary, the physician may request a fractional 24 hr collection of urine. The urine should be collected in three fractions: 8:00 AM to 2:00 PM; 2:00 PM to 8:00 PM; and 8:00 PM to 8:00 AM. Assessment of volume and semiquantitative or quantitative glucose values in each sample permits a rational basis for adjusting the respective doses of the rapid- and intermediate-acting insulins.

Measurement of glycosylated hemoglobin (glycohemoglobin or HbA_{1c}) in blood provides a reliable index of long term control. Glycohemoglobin (HbA_{1c}) represents the fraction of hemoglobin to which glucose has been nonenzymatically attached in the bloodstream. The formation of HbA_{1c} is a slow reaction that is dependent on the prevailing concentration of blood glucose; it continues irreversibly throughout the red blood cell's life span of approximately 120 days. The higher the blood glucose concentration and the longer the red blood cell's exposure to it, the higher will be the fraction of HbA_{1c}, which is expressed as a percentage of total hemoglobin. Since a blood sample at any given time contains a mixture of red blood cells of varying ages, exposed for varying times to varying blood glucose concentrations, an HbA_{1c} measurement reflects the average blood glucose concentration of the preceding 2–3 mo. The fraction of HbA_{1c} is not influenced by an isolated episode of hyperglycemia. As an index of long term compliance and of metabolic control as well as of the patient's compliance with an insulin regimen, a measurement of HbA_{1c} is superior to measurements of glycosuria or of a single blood glucose determination. Periodic measurements of HbA_{1c} may also help to resolve questions relating the degree of metabolic control to subsequent development of complications. Although values of HbA_{1c} may vary according to the method used for its measurement, in normal individuals the HbA_{1c} fraction is usually less than 7%; in diabetics, values of 6–9% represent very good metabolic control, values of 9–12%, fair control, and values above 12%, poor control.

In highly motivated adolescents or young adults who become sufficiently knowledgeable about diabetes, self-monitoring of blood glucose before and 2 hr after each meal permits appropriate adjustment of insulin dosage based on blood glucose concentrations. The blood glucose measurement is performed with a glucose oxidase strip such as Dextrostix in conjunction with a reflectance meter, or with a Chemstrip, on which blood glucose concentration can be read directly. A small portable device that automates capillary blood letting in a relatively painless fashion is now commercially available (Autolet). Although this method of monitoring clearly permits the achievement of near-normal metabolic control, it remains to be seen whether it is practical in children; the required discipline may preclude this possibility.

EXERCISE. Exercise is an integral component of

growth and development. No form of exercise, including competitive sports of any kind, should be forbidden to the diabetic child, who should not be made to feel different or restricted. Examples of diabetics who have excelled in national or international sports are not rare. A major complication of exercise in diabetics is hypoglycemic reaction during or within hours after exercise. If hypoglycemia does not occur with exercise, adjustments in diet or insulin are not necessary, and glucoregulation is likely to be improved through the increased utilization of glucose by muscles. The major contributing factor to hypoglycemia with exercise is an increased rate of absorption of insulin from its injection site. Regular exercise also improves glucoregulation by increasing insulin receptors.

In anticipation of vigorous exercise 1 additional carbohydrate exchange may be taken prior to the exercise, and glucose in the form of orange juice, carbonated beverage, or candy should be available during and after exercise. With experience and trial and error each child and parent, guided by the physician, should develop an appropriate regimen for regularly planned exercise that is frequently associated with hypoglycemia; in such instances, the preceding dose of insulin may be reduced by about 10% on the day of the scheduled exercise.

RESIDUAL BETA CELL FUNCTION (SO-CALLED HONEYMOON PERIOD). After the initial stabilization some 75% of newly diagnosed diabetic children will require a progressive reduction in their daily dose of insulin from approximately 1 unit/kg–0.5 unit/kg or less. Recurrent hypoglycemia is the manifestation that prompts a reduction in the insulin dose. A minority of children can even maintain normoglycemia for a time without any administered insulin; this complete remission occurs in only 2% of diabetics or fewer, but even in these patients glucose tolerance tests will demonstrate abnormal carbohydrate metabolism. The duration of this "honeymoon" phase is variable; it commonly lasts several wk or mo but may last as long as 1–2 yr. Recent investigations clearly demonstrate that residual insulin secretion, measured as C-peptide, is present during this remission period and to some extent in virtually all diabetic children in the initial year of their disease; in approximately 20% there will be some C-peptide response even after 5 yr. Stable, well controlled subjects have higher C-peptide secretion than nonstable subjects, and the required dose of insulin is inversely correlated to the basal or the stimulated C-peptide response.

It is not completely clear why this residual insulin secretion is inadequate to prevent the evolution of diabetes including ketoacidosis, but the reasons presumably relate to stress-provoked secretion of catecholamines that inhibit still further the insulin secretory capacity of the pancreatic beta cells. In any event, the clinical remission phase is limited; with isolated exceptions, insulin-dependent diabetes inevitably recurs. Although opinion varies, it is our policy to maintain insulin treatment unless a daily dose of 0.1 unit/kg still causes hypoglycemia, in which case we discontinue insulin treatment and periodically test the patient for the re-emergence of glycosuria. The physician may decide to discontinue insulin treatment completely if it appears to be in the patient's best interests to do so.

The patient and family, however, should not be led to believe that the disease is "cured" and should continue to examine the child's urine for glucose.

Hypoglycemic Reactions (Insulin Shock). Virtually all diabetic children experience a hypoglycemic reaction at some time during the course of their disease. Hypoglycemia occurs suddenly or over minutes, in contrast to diabetic ketoacidosis which develops over hours or days. The symptoms and signs are those due to an outpouring of catecholamines, which include pallor, sweating, apprehension, trembling, and tachycardia, and those due to cerebral glucopenia, which include hunger, drowsiness, mental confusion, seizures, and coma. Mood and personality changes plus some abnormal physical patterns may be characteristic for an individual and provide an early clue to the more pronounced reaction. There is some evidence that these symptoms may occur with a sudden drop in blood glucose to levels that do not meet the criteria for hypoglycemia (less than 60 mg/dl) in healthy subjects.

The occurrence of hypoglycemia in a diabetic child indicates too much insulin relative to food intake and energy expenditure. Common causes include the evolution of the "honeymoon" phase (see above) after the initial diagnosis, deliberate or accidental errors in insulin dosage, inadequate caloric intake, and strenuous and sustained physical activity in the absence of increased caloric intake.

The most important factors in the management of hypoglycemia are an understanding by patient and family of the symptoms and signs of the reaction, especially of the patient's individual pattern, and the avoidance of known precipitating factors. For the acute attack a carbohydrate-containing snack or drink such as orange juice or a sugar-containing carbonated beverage or candy (equivalent to 5–10 gm of glucose) should be taken. Patients, parents, and teachers should also be instructed in the administration of glucagon; 0.5 mg given intramuscularly is particularly useful when the patient is losing consciousness or is vomiting. If exercise has been the precipitating factor, the patient should be instructed as a preventive measure to take additional calories prior to exercise. If hypoglycemic attacks persist subsequently under similar circumstances, a reduction in the morning dose of insulin by 10% for that day is indicated. The avoidance of severe hypoglycemic episodes should be a major objective of treatment; they have been implicated in ultimately provoking epileptic seizures, and there is an increased frequency of abnormal EEG changes in diabetics.

The Somogyi Phenomenon and "Brittle Diabetes." Hypoglycemic episodes, which may be mild and manifest as late nocturnal or early morning sweating, night terrors, and headaches alternating rapidly, within 4–6 hr, with ketosis, hyperglycemia, ketonuria, and excessive glucosuria, should suggest the possibility of the Somogyi phenomenon. This syndrome has been aptly described as "hypoglycemia begetting hyperglycemia" and is believed to be due to an outpouring of counterregulatory hormones in response to insulin-induced hypoglycemia. The coexistence of this brittle form of diabetes with daily doses of more than 2 units/kg of insulin suggests the presence of this phenomenon and

the need to reduce the dose of insulin. The term brittle diabetes implies that control of blood glucose fluctuates widely and rapidly despite frequent upward adjustments of the dose of insulin. The Somogyi phenomenon may be the most common cause of instability or "brittleness" in diabetic children. Early morning elevations of blood glucose concentration following recognized or unrecognized nocturnal hypoglycemia appear to be due mainly to waning of biologically available insulin and not to plasma increases in counterregulatory hormones. Therein lies the dilemma; increases in the dose of insulin may exacerbate the nocturnal hypoglycemic episodes without improving metabolic control. When this syndrome is suspected, the dose of intermediate insulin should be decreased by about 10%, and further reductions should be made at intervals of 3 days; abrupt larger reductions may precipitate ketoacidosis.

In other patients with brittle diabetes better control is often achieved by a change from 1 to 2 daily injections of insulin and/or by a change from beef-pork mixtures to pure pork or pure beef insulins, which may circumvent problems with antibodies that bind insulin. Attention should also be directed to psychologic problems within or without the home that may be bases for deliberate errors in insulin and/or nutritional intake.

Psychologic Aspects. Diabetes in a child affects the lifstyle and interpersonal relationships of the entire family. Feelings of anxiety and guilt are common in parents. Similar feelings, coupled with denial and rejection, are equally common in children, particularly during the rebellious teenage years. No specific personality disorder or psychopathology is characteristic of diabetes; similar feelings are observed in families with other chronic disorders.

In diabetics these feelings find expression in nonadherence to instructions regarding nutritional and insulin therapy and in noncompliance with self-monitoring. Deliberate overdosage with insulin resulting in hypoglycemia, omission of insulin, or excesses in nutritional intake resulting in ketoacidosis may be pleas for psychologic help or manipulative events to escape an environment perceived as undesirable or intolerable; occasionally, they may be manifestations of suicidal intent. Frequent admissions to hospital for ketoacidosis or hypoglycemia should arouse suspicion of underlying emotional conflict. Overprotection on the part of parents is common and often is not in the best interest of the patient. Feelings of being different and/or of being alone are common and may be justified in view of the restrictive schedules imposed by testing of urine, administration of insulin, and nutritional limitations. Furthermore, publicity regarding the likelihood of developing complications and of decreased life span in Type I diabetes must foster anxiety. Unfortunately, misinformation abounds regarding the risks of development of diabetes in siblings or in offspring and of pregnancy in young diabetic women. In turn, even appropriate information often causes further anxiety.

Many, but not all, of these problems can be averted through continued empathic counseling based on correct information and attempts to build attitudes of normality in the patient as a productive and potentially reproductive member of society. Recognizing the potential impact of these problems, peer discussion groups have been organized in many locales; feelings of isolation and frustration tend to be lessened by the sharing of common problems. Summer camps for diabetic children afford an excellent opportunity for learning and sharing under expert supervision. Education regarding the pathophysiology of diabetes, insulin dose and technique of administration, nutrition, exercise, and hypoglycemic reactions can be reinforced by medical and paramedical personnel. The presence of numerous peers with similar problems affords new insights for the diabetic child.

The physician managing a child or adolescent with diabetes should be aware of his pivotal role as counselor and advisor and should anticipate the common emotional problems of his patient. When emotional problems are clearly responsible for poor compliance with the medical regimen, referral for psychologic help is indicated. Such help is often available in pediatric centers where psychologists form part of the management team for diabetic children.

Management During Infections.   Systemic and local infections are no more common in diabetic children than in nondiabetic ones. During intercurrent illnesses, either infectious or traumatic, diabetic children nearly always will require additional insulin, especially during prolonged serious episodes that necessitate inactivity. In the latter situations, when glucosuria is excessive, a good working rule is to add 10–20% of the total daily dose as regular (short-acting) insulin prior to each meal. Subsequent increases or decreases should then be based on careful monitoring of urinary and plasma glucose values.

Patients who are vomiting should nevertheless take some insulin; approximately 50% of the daily dose is a general rule, followed by careful monitoring of urinary or blood glucose and subsequent adjustments of the dose of insulin as indicated. If vomiting continues and the patient cannot tolerate clear liquids, admission to hospital and consideration of intravenous therapy with glucose, electrolytes, and insulin are warranted.

Management During Surgery.   The objectives are the prevention of hypoglycemia during anesthesia, of severe loss of fluids, and of diabetic acidosis. The regimens described below are generally applicable, but vigilance and individual adjustments for each patient are necessary to achieve these goals.

When surgery is elective, the patient should be admitted to hospital 24 hr prior to surgery; during this time the usual nutritional requirements and insulin dose are provided. Supplemental regular insulin may be given to achieve better control of blood glucose when the need is demonstrated. On the morning of surgery an infusion of 5% glucose in 0.45% saline solution plus 20 mEq/l of potassium chloride is begun; initially 1 unit of regular insulin is added to the infusate for each 4 gm of administered glucose. The rate of infusion should provide maintenance fluid requirements plus estimated losses during surgery. The blood glucose concentration should be monitored at periodic intervals before, during, and after surgery; concentrations of approximately 120–150 mg/dl should be the goal; this can be achieved by varying the rate of infusion of the glucose and electrolyte mixture or the amount of insulin added. This regimen may be discontinued when the patient is awake and capable of taking food and fluid orally. Prior to reinstitution of the patient's usual diet, regular insulin may be administered at a dose of 0.25 unit/kg at 6 hr intervals; appropriate adjustments in the dose are based on blood or urinary concentrations of glucose.

An equally effective plan that is particuarly useful for surgery of short duration is as follows: on the morning of surgery administer one half of the usual morning dose of insulin subcutaneously and initiate intravenous infusion of the electrolyte and glucose solution described in the preceding paragraph, but do not include insulin in it. After surgery regular insulin in a dose of 0.25 unit/kg is administered subcutaneously; subsequent doses at 6 hr intervals are adjusted on the basis of blood glucose concentrations until the patient is ready for his or her usual dietary pattern.

For emergency surgery an intravenous infusion is initiated that provides 5–10% glucose in 0.45% saline solution, 20 mEq/l of potassium chloride, and 1 unit of regular insulin for each 2–4 gm of glucose. Blood glucose concentration should be maintained at approximately 120–150 mg/dl. When possible, rehydration and metabolic balance should precede the surgery. After surgery the regimen described above can be instituted.

For minor surgery under local anesthesia the usual insulin and dietary regimens can be maintained. If there should be extensive vomiting, the losses can usually be compensated with glucose solution administered intravenously.

Neurovascular and Other Complications: Relation to Glycemic Control.   It has become apparent that the increasingly prolonged survival of the diabetic child, due principally to insulin therapy, is associated with an increasing prevalence of complications that affect the microcirculation of the eye (retinopathy), the kidney (nephropathy), and the nerves (neuropathy) as well as the large vessels (atherosclerosis) and the lens (cataracts). Recent statistics indicate that retinopathy is present in 45–60% of insulin-dependent diabetics after 20 yr of known disease and in 20% after 10 yr; lens opacities are present in at least 5% of those under 19 yr of age. Diabetic nephropathy is also common; it is present in about 40% after 25 yr of insulin-dependent diabetes when the onset was in childhood; this complication may account for about 50% of deaths in long term, insulin-dependent diabetics.

After extensive debate, many now consider that clinical experience and experimental data strongly suggest an association between glycemic control and the later development of complications. In addition, studies implicate some possible biochemical pathways that might be responsible for these complications. For example, the process of glycosylation of erythrocytic hemoglobin, which is directly proportional to the blood glucose concentration, also involves other serum and tissue proteins; it has been implicated in basement membrane thickening in the glomeruli. There is evidence that activation of the polyol pathway and disturbances in myoinositol metabolism are related, respectively, to cataracts and to neuropathy. In humans, typical lesions of diabetic nephropathy develop in normal kidneys within several yr after they have been transplanted to diabetics with chronic renal failure; it would appear that it is the diabetic environment and not the genetic background that predisposes to these renal changes. Similarly, renal lesions that mimic those of human diabetes develop in animals rendered diabetic, and these changes tend to regress following cure of the diabetes by islet transplantation.

Other complications that have been described in diabetic children include *dwarfism associated with a glycogen-laden enlarged liver (Mauriac syndrome), osteopenia, and a syndrome of limited joint mobility associated with tight, waxy skin, growth impairment, and maturational delay.* The Mauriac syndrome is clearly related to underinsulinization; it is now rare because of the availability of the longer acting insulins. The syndrome of limited joint mobility is frequently associated with the early development of diabetic microvascular complications, such as retinopathy and nephropathy, which may appear before the age of 18 yr. None of these complications has been demonstrated in a nondiabetic identical twin, even after 20 yr of recognized diabetes in his or her insulin-dependent twin. Genetic predisposition to the development of diabetic vascular complications does, however, play a role.

Despite the hard evidence in experimental animals and suggestive evidence in human diabetics, a possible relationship of the degree of glycemic control to these complications in humans remains moot because none of the available modes of treatment has resulted in sufficiently normal metabolic control to provide an adequate study group. Nevertheless, there does appear to be a relationship. Consequently, as long as reduction of these late complications remains a possibility, physicians have the responsibility to maintain as nearly normal metabolism as is compatible with the physical and psychologic limits of each diabetic child. Despite the potential for developing complications, survival for 40 yr and more is feasible; the goal should be to make these years increasingly free of debilitating diabetic-related disease.

Long-Term Outcome. Type I diabetes mellitus is not a benign disease. In 1 study on the long term outcome of 45 children under 12 yr of age at the time of diagnosis, there were 7 deaths within 10–25 yr of diagnosis: 3 were directly attributable to diabetes, and 2 were due to suicide; 3 patients attempted suicide unsuccessfully. Visual, renal, neuropathic, and other complications were relatively frequent. Furthermore, although diabetic children eventually attain a height within the normal adult range, puberty may be considerably delayed, and the final height may be less than the genetic potential. From studies in identical twins it is apparent that, despite apparently satisfactory control, the diabetic twin manifests delayed puberty and a substantial reduction in height with a mean difference of 5 cm when onset of disease occurs before puberty. These observations indicate that our conventional criteria for judging control are inadequate, that adequate control of insulin-dependent diabetes is almost never achieved by presently available means, and that the resolution of these problems should be viewed as a matter of urgency.

The recent introduction of portable devices that can be programmed to provide continuous subcutaneous infusion of insulin with meal-related pulses is 1 approach to the resolution of these long term problems. In selected individuals, nearly normal patterns of blood glucose and other indices of metabolic control including HbA_{1c} have been maintained for over 1 yr. This approach, however, is presently limited to clinical investigational studies.

17.2 IMPAIRED GLUCOSE TOLERANCE AND TYPE II NON-INSULIN-DEPENDENT DIABETES

In the classification of diabetes mellitus and other clinical impairments of glucose tolerance proposed by the National Diabetes Data Group (Table 17–1) the term *"impaired glucose tolerance"* is used to characterize individuals who have a plasma glucose concentration in excess of 140 mg/dl 2 hr after initiation of the standard oral glucose tolerance test but who do not have symptoms of diabetes or fasting hyperglycemia. The indication for an oral glucose tolerance test may be the discovery of isolated or intermittent glucosuria or the occurrence of hyperglycemia during a stressful illness or during corticosteroid therapy. Individuals considered at risk for abnormal glucose metabolism should also be tested; these include obese children, those who have symptoms suggestive of reactive postprandial hypoglycemia, and close relatives of known diabetics. An oral glucose tolerance test is *not indicated* in a child who has characteristic diabetic symptoms and a random blood glucose value in excess of 200 mg/dl.

The term impaired glucose tolerance is suggested as a replacement for such terms as asymptomatic diabetes, chemical diabetes, subclinical diabetes, borderline diabetes, or latent diabetes in order to avoid the stigma associated with the term diabetes mellitus, which may influence the choice of vocation, eligibility for health or life insurance, and self image. Furthermore, although impaired glucose tolerance represents a biochemical intermediate between normal glucose metabolism and that of diabetes, experience has shown that few children with impaired glucose tolerance go on to develop diabetes; estimates range from 0–10%. There is disagreement whether the degree of glucose intolerance is useful as a prognostic index of the likelihood of progression, but there is evidence that among the few who do progress, the insulin response during glucose tolerance testing is severely impaired. In the majority of children with impaired glucose tolerance, particularly the obese, insulin responses during oral glucose tolerance tests are higher than is the mean of age-adjusted controls; it appears that these individuals have some resistance to the effects of insulin rather than an inability to secrete it.

In normal children the glucose response during an oral glucose tolerance test is similar at all ages. In contrast, plasma insulin responses during the test increase progressively within the age span of about 3–15 yr so that interpretation of them requires comparison with age-adjusted criteria.

The performance of the glucose tolerance test should be standardized according to currently accepted criteria. These include at least 3 days of a well-balanced diet containing approximately 50% of calories from carbohydrates; fasting from midnight until the time of the test in the morning; and a dose of glucose for the test of 1.75 gm/kg but not in excess of 75 gm. Plasma samples are obtained prior to ingestion of the glucose and at 1, 2, and 3 hr thereafter. The arbitrarily designated response to the test that identifies "impaired glucose tolerance" is a fasting plasma glucose value <140 mg/dl and a value at 2 hr >140 mg/dl. The determination of serum insulin responses during the glucose tolerance test is not necessary in reaching a diagnosis; the magnitude of the response, however, may have prognostic value.

In children with impaired glucose tolerance but without fasting hyperglycemia, repeated oral glucose tolerance tests are not recommended. Investigations in such children indicate that the degree of impaired glucose tolerance tends to remain stable or may actually decrease over a period of years, even in patients with subnormal insulin responses. Consequently, apart from reduction in weight for the obese child, no therapy is indicated. In particular, the use of oral hypoglycemic agents should be restricted for investigational studies. If fasting hyperglycemia and/or characteristic symptoms of diabetes should develop, the affected children will have the characteristics of non-insulin-dependent diabetes (Type II), previously known as adult-onset diabetes (Table 17–1 and brief description in text under Classification).

17.3 DISEASES ASSOCIATED WITH DIABETES

Cystic Fibrosis. Because of improvements in the medical care of children with cystic fibrosis, many survive to the late teen and early adult years. In addition to the primary insufficiency of pancreatic exocrine function, there is an increasing incidence of pancreatic endocrine dysfunction manifested as glucose intolerance that progresses occasionally to overt diabetes mellitus. When hyperglycemia develops, the accompanying metabolic derangements are usually mild, and, if insulin therapy becomes necessary, relatively low doses usually suffice for adequate management. Ketoacidosis is uncommon but may occur with progressive deterioration of islet cell function. Treatment with insulin is as outlined for Type I diabetes, but dietary management may be limited by the constraints of the primary disturbance.

Autoimmune Diseases. *Chronic lymphocytic thyroiditis* (Hashimoto thyroiditis) is frequently associated with Type I diabetes in children. As many as 1 in 5 insulin-dependent diabetics may have thyroid antibodies in their serum; the prevalence is 2–20 times greater than that observed in control populations. Only a small proportion of these diabetics, however, develop clinical hypothyroidism; the interval between diagnosis of diabetes and of thyroid disease averages about 5 yr. Periodic palpation of the thyroid gland is indicated in all diabetic children; if the gland feels firm and/or enlarged, serum measurements of thyroid antibodies and thyroid stimulating hormone (TSH) should be obtained. A TSH level of greater than 10 microU/ml indicates existing or incipient thyroid dysfunction that warrants replacement with thyroid hormone. Deceleration in the rate of growth may also be due to thyroid failure and is, in itself, a reason for securing serum measurements of thyroxine and TSH concentrations.

When diabetes and thyroid disease coexist, the possibility of **adrenal insufficiency** should also be considered. It may be heralded by decreasing insulin requirements, increasing pigmentation of the skin and buccal mucosa, salt craving, weakness, asthenia and postural hypotension, or even frank addisonian crisis as evidence of primary adrenal failure. This syndrome is most unusual in the 1st decade of life, but it may become apparent in the 2nd decade or later.

Circulating antibodies to gastric parietal cells and to intrinsic factor are 2–3 times more common in patients with Type I diabetes than in control subjects. There are good correlations of antibodies to gastric parietal cells with atrophic gastritis and of antibodies to intrinsic factor with malabsorption of vitamin B_{12}. Although the possibility of megaloblastic anemia should be considered in children with Type I diabetes, its occurrence is rare.

A variant of the *multiple endocrine deficiency syndrome* is characterized by Type I diabetes, idiopathic intestinal mucosal atrophy with associated inflammation and severe malabsorption, IgA deficiency, and circulating antibodies to multiple endocrine organs including the thyroid, adrenal, pancreas, parathyroid, and gonads. In addition, nondiabetic family members have an increased frequency of vitiligo, Graves disease, and multiple sclerosis, low complement levels, and a high frequency of antibodies to endocrine tissues.

That Type I diabetes may itself be an autoimmune disease has been discussed above.

17.4 GENETIC SYNDROMES ASSOCIATED WITH DIABETES MELLITUS

A number of rare genetic syndromes associated with insulin-dependent diabetes mellitus or with carbohydrate intolerance have been described. These syndromes represent a broad spectrum of diseases ranging from premature cellular aging, as in the Werner and Cockayne syndromes, to excessive obesity associated with hyperinsulinism, resistance to insulin action, and carbohydrate intolerance as in the Prader-Willi syndrome. Some of these syndromes are characterized by primary disturbances in the insulin receptor or in antibodies to the insulin receptor without any impairment in insulin secretion. Although rare, these syndromes provide unique models to study the multiple causes of disturbed carbohydrate metabolism from defective insulin secretion or from defective insulin action at the cell receptor or postreceptor step. (A description of some of these syndromes may be found in the report of the National Diabetes Data Group; Diabetes 28:1039, 1979.)

17.5 TRANSIENT DIABETES MELLITUS OF NEWBORN

Onset of persistent insulin-dependent diabetes before the age of 6 mo is most unusual. The syndrome of transient diabetes mellitus in the newborn infant has its onset in the 1st weeks of life and persists only several wk to mo before spontaneous resolution. It occurs most often in infants who are small for gestational age and is characterized by hyperglycemia and pronounced glycosuria resulting in severe dehydration and at times metabolic acidosis, but with only minimal or no ketonemia or ketonuria. Insulin responses to glucose or tolbutamide are low to absent; basal plasma insulin concentrations, however, are normal. After spontaneous recovery the insulin responses to these same stimuli are brisk and normal. Occurrence of the syndrome in consecutive siblings has been reported. Permanent diabetes is apparently not known to have developed in any affected infant who has recovered from the transient syndrome. This syndrome should be distinguished from severe hyperglycemia which may occur in hypertonic dehydration; this occurs usually in infants beyond the newborn period, who respond promptly to rehydration with a minimal requirement for insulin.

Administration of insulin is mandatory during the active phase of this syndrome. One–2 units/kg/24 hr of an intermediate-acting insulin in 2 divided doses usually results in dramatic improvement and accelerated growth and gain in weight. Attempts at gradually reducing the dose of insulin may be made as soon as recurrent hypoglycemia becomes manifest or after 2 mo of age. The parents should be assured of the transient nature of the disease and the excellent prognosis.

FUTURE DIRECTIONS

Several avenues of research are being followed to elucidate the etiology of Type I diabetes, find a "cure," improve methods of insulin delivery, and reduce long term complications. The association of certain HLA types and their relation to viral and autoimmune diseases may provide leads for unmasking the primary cause of insulin-dependent diabetes mellitus and determine directions for attempts to prevent its appearance in genetically predisposed individuals. Transplantation of whole pancreas has been performed, but success has been severely limited by problems of rejection and by leakage of pancreatic enzymes. Transplantation of iso-lated pancreatic islets obviates the problems associated with pancreatic enzymes; culture of islets prior to their transplantation has demonstrated some success in overcoming the problems of rejection between and within species of diabetic animals. Development of portable insulin delivery systems that may be computer-controlled and that could provide insulin in a more physiologic manner shows increasing promise. Of these devices, those depending on continuous monitoring of blood glucose with computer-controlled insulin delivery (closed loop) are too cumbersome for long term use; success with such devices must await the development of an implantable glucose sensor. The portable devices that provide preprogrammed continuous subcutaneous insulin delivery at 2 rates, constant basal and meal-related increments (open loop), can be adjusted for individual needs and have been used by some patients for periods exceeding 1 yr; blood glucose, serum lipids, hormonal profiles, and glycosylated hemoglobin are maintained within normal ranges.

Human insulin can now be synthesized by recombinant DNA technology; it has been tested in preliminary trials and is likely to be available for therapy in the future. Inhibitors of certain enzymes that are believed to participate in the development of diabetic complications are also undergoing clinical trials. These advances justify some optimism toward solving the problems of diabetes mellitus.

MARK A. SPERLING

Epidemiology, Etiology, Pathophysiology, and Classification

Cahill GF, McDevitt HO: Insulin-dependent diabetes mellitus: The initial lesion. N Engl J Med 304:1454, 1981.
Craighead JE: Current views on the etiology of insulin-dependent diabetes mellitus. N Engl J Med 299:1439, 1978.
Dobersen MJ, Scharff JE, Ginsberg-Fellner F, et al: Cytotoxic autoantibodies to beta cells in the serum of patients with insulin-dependent diabetes mellitus. N Engl J Med 303:1493, 1980.
Fajans SS, Cloutier MC, Crowther RL: Clinical and etiologic heterogeneity of idiopathic diabetes mellitus. Diabetes 27:1112, 1978.
Fleegler FM, Rogers KD, Drash AL, et al: Age, sex and season of onset of juvenile diabetes in different geographic areas. Pediatrics 63:374, 1979.
Gamble DR: An epidemiological study of childhood diabetes affecting two or more siblings. Diabetologia 19:341, 1980.
Huang SW, MacLaren NK: Insulin-dependent diabetes: A disease of autoaggression. Science 192:64, 1976.
Irvine WF, McCallu CF, Campbell CJ, et al: Pancreatic islet-cell antibodies in diabetes mellitus correlated with the duration and type of diabetes, coexistent autoimmune disease and HLA type. Diabetes 26:138, 1977.
Karam JH, Lewitt PE, Young CW, et al: Insulinopenic diabetes after rodenticide (Vacor) ingestion: A unique model of acquired diabetes in man. Diabetes 29:971, 1980.
Kyllo DF, Nuttall FQ: Prevalence of diabetes mellitus in school-aged children in Minnesota. Diabetes 27:57, 1978.
LaPorte RE, Fishbein HA, Drash AL, et al: The incidence of insulin dependent diabetes mellitus in Allegheny County, Pennsylvania (1965–1976). Diabetes 30:279, 1981.
National Diabetes Data Group: Classification and diagnosis of diabetes mellitus and other categories of glucose intolerance. Diabetes 28:1039, 1979.
Neufeld M, MacLaren NK, Riley NF, et al: Islet cell and other organ-specific antibodies in US Caucasians and Blacks with insulin-dependent diabetes mellitus. Diabetes 29:589, 1980.
Rayfield EJ, Seto Y: Viruses and the pathogenesis of diabetes mellitus. Diabetes 26:1126, 1978.
Rosenbloom AL, Kohrman A, Sperling M: Classification and diagnosis of diabetes mellitus in children and adolescents. J Pediatr 98:320, 1981.
Yoon JW, Austin M, Onodera T, et al: Virus-induced diabetes mellitus: Isolation of a virus from the pancreas of a child with diabetic ketoacidosis. N Engl J Med 300:1173, 1979.

Genetics

Cudworth AG, Gorsuch AN, Woif E, et al: A new look at HLA genetics with particular reference to type I diabetes. Lancet 2:389, 1979.

Pyke DA: Diabetes: The genetic connections. Diabetologia 17:333, 1979.

Raum D, Stein R, Alper CA, et al: Genetic marker for insulin-dependent diabetes mellitus. Lancet 1:1208, 1979.

Rotter JI, Hodge SE: Racial differences in juvenile-type diabetes are consistent with more than one mode of inheritance. Diabetes 29:115, 1980.

Rotter JI, Rimoin DL: Heterogeneity in diabetes mellitus—update 1978. Diabetes 27:599, 1978.

Diabetic Ketoacidosis

Duck SC, Weldon VV, Pagliara AS, et al: Cerebral edema complicating therapy for ketoacidosis. Diabetes 25:111, 1976.

Hammeke M, Bear R, Lee R, et al: Hyperchloremic metabolic acidosis in diabetes mellitus. Diabetes 27:16, 1978.

Heber D, Molitch M, Sperling MA: Low-dose continuous insulin therapy for diabetic ketoacidosis: Prospective comparison with "conventional" insulin therapy. Arch Intern Med 137:1377, 1977.

Kanter Y, Gerson JR, Bessman AN: 2,3-Diphosphoglycerate, nucleotide phosphate, and organic and inorganic phosphate levels during the early phases of diabetic ketoacidosis. Diabetes 26:429, 1977.

Kaye R: Diabetic ketoacidosis—the bicarbonate controversy. J Pediatr 87:156, 1975.

Keller U, Berger W: Prevention of hypophosphatemia by phosphate infusion during treatment of diabetic ketoacidosis and hyperosmolar coma. Diabetes 29:87, 1980.

Kreisberg RA: Diabetic ketoacidosis: New concepts and trends in pathogenesis and treatment. Ann Intern Med 88:681, 1978.

Podolsky S: Hyperosmolar nonketotic coma in the elderly diabetic. Med Clin North Am 62:815, 1978.

Rubin HM, Kramer R, Drash A: Hyperosmolality complicating diabetes mellitus in childhood. J Pediatr 74:177, 1969.

Schade DS, Eaton RP: The temporal relationship between endogenously secreted stress hormones and metabolic decompensation in diabetic man. J Clin Endocrinol Metab 50:131, 1980.

Waldhausl W, Kleinberger G, Korn A, et al: Severe hyperglycemia: Effects of rehydration on endocrine derangements and blood glucose concentration. Diabetes 28:577, 1979.

Management of Type I Diabetes in Children

American Diabetes Association: Principles of nutrition and dietary recommendations for individuals with diabetes mellitus: 1979. Diabetes 28:1027, 1979.

Editorial: A plethora of insulins. Diabetes Care 3:638, 1980.

Felig P, Wahren J: Fuel homeostasis in exercise. N Engl J Med 293:1078, 1975.

Forman BJ, Goldstein PS, Genel M: Management of juvenile diabetes mellitus: Usefulness of 24-hour fractional quantitative urine glucose. Pediatrics 53:257, 1974.

Gabbay KH, Hasty K, Breslow JL, et al: Glycosylated hemoglobin and long-term blood glucose control in diabetes mellitus. J Clin Endocrinol Metab 44:859, 1977.

Gale EAM, Kurtz AB, Tattersall RB: In search of the Somogyi effect. Lancet 2:279, 1980.

Goldstein DE, Walker B, Rawlings SS, et al: Hemoglobin A₁c levels in children and adolescents with diabetes mellitus. Diabetes Care 3:503, 1980.

Isenberg PL, Barnett DM: Psychological problems in diabetes mellitus. Med Clin North Am 49:1125, 1965.

Rosenbloom AL, Giordano BP: Chronic overtreatment with insulin in children and adolescents. Am J Dis Child 131:881, 1977.

Saccharin and bladder cancer. Lancet 1:855, 1980.

Santiago JV, Clarke WL, Shah SD, et al: Epinephrine, norepinephrine, glucagon, and growth hormone release in association with physiological decrements in the plasma glucose concentration in normal and diabetic man. J Clin Endocrinol Metab 51:877, 1980.

Sonksen PH, Judd SL, Lowy D: Home-monitoring of blood-glucose: Method for improving diabetic control. Lancet 1:729, 1978.

Sperling MA: Insulin biosynthesis and C-peptide. Am J Dis Child 134:1119, 1980.

Tamborlane WV, Sherwin RS, Genel M, et al: Reduction to normal of plasma glucose in juvenile diabetes by subcutaneous administration of insulin with a portable infusion pump. N Engl J Med 300:573, 1979.

Werther GA, Jenkins PA, Turner RC, et al: Twenty-four-hour metabolic profiles in diabetic children receiving insulin injections once or twice daily. Br Med J 281:414, 1980.

Witters LA, Ohman JL, Weir GC, et al: Insulin antibodies in the pathogenesis of insulin allergy and resistance. Am J Med 63:703, 1977.

Long Term Outcome of Childhood Diabetes: Relation of Control to Development of Complications

Diabetes Data: U.S. Department of Health, Education and Welfare. Publication No. 78:1468 (NIH), compiled 1977.

Gabbay KH: The sorbitol pathway and complications of diabetes. N Engl J Med 288:831, 1973.

Karam JH, Rosenthal M, O'Donnell JJ, et al: Discordance of diabetic microangiopathy in identical twins. Diabetes 25:24, 1976.

MacGregor M: Juvenile diabetics growing up. Lancet 1:944, 1977.

Mauer SM, Barbosa J, Vernier R, et al: Development of diabetic vascular lesions in normal kidneys transplanted into patients with diabetes mellitus. N Engl J Med 295:916, 1976.

Pax-Guevara AT, Hsu TH, White P: Juvenile diabetes after forty years. Diabetes 24:559, 1976.

Rosenbloom AL, Lezotte DC, Weber FT, et al: Diminution of bone mass in childhood diabetes. Diabetes 26:1052, 1977.

Rosenbloom AL, Silverstein JH, Lezotte DC, et al: Limited joint mobility in childhood diabetes mellitus indicates increased risk for microvascular disease. N Engl J Med 305:191, 1981.

Skyler JS: Complications of diabetes mellitus: Relationship to metabolic dysfunction. Diabetes Care 2:499, 1979.

Tattersall, RB, Pyke DA: Growth in diabetic children: Studies in identical twins. Lancet 2:1105, 1973.

White NW, Waltman SR, Krupin T, et al: Reversal of neuropathic and gastrointestinal complications related to diabetes mellitus in adolescents with improved metabolic control. J Pediatr 99:41, 1981.

Diseases and Syndromes Associated with Diabetes

Flier JS, Kahn CR, Roth J: Receptors, antireceptor antibodies and mechanisms of insulin resistance. N Engl J Med 300:413, 1979.

Lippe BM, Sperling MA, Dooley RR: Pancreatic alpha and beta cell functions in cystic fibrosis. J Pediatr 90:751, 1977.

Maccuish AC, Irvine WJ: Autoimmunological aspects of diabetes mellitus. Clin Endocrinol Metab 4:435, 1975.

National Diabetes Data Group: Classification and diagnosis of diabetes mellitus and other categories of glucose intolerance. Diabetes 28:1039, 1979.

Pollett RJ, Levey GS: Principles of membrane receptor physiology and their application to clinical medicine. Ann Intern Med 92:663, 1980.

Transient Diabetes of the Newborn

Blethen SL, White NH, Santiago JV, et al: Plasma somatomedins, endogenous insulin secretion, and growth in transient neonatal diabetes mellitus. J Clin Endocrinol Metab 52:144, 1981.

Pagliara AS, Karl IE, Kipnis DB: Transient neonatal diabetes: Delayed maturation of the pancreatic beta cell. J Pediatr 82:97, 1973.

Schiff D, Colle E, Stern L: Metabolic and growth patterns in transient neonatal diabetes. N Engl J Med 267:119, 1972.

Future Directions

Lacy PE, Davie JM, Finke EH: Prolongation of islet xenograft survival without continuous immunosuppression. Science 209:283, 1980.

Santiago JV, Clemens AH, Clarke WL, et al: Closed-loop and open-loop devices for blood glucose control in normal and diabetic subjects. Diabetes 28:71, 1979.

Skyler JS, Raptis R: Symposium in biosynthetic human insulin. Diabetes Care 4:139, 1981.

Tamborlane WV, Hintz RL, Bergman M, et al: Insulin-infusion-pump treatment of diabetes: Influence of improved metabolic control on plasma somatomedin levels. N Engl J Med 305:303, 1981.

17.6 HYPOGLYCEMIA

Hypoglycemia is a state in which there is an abnormally low level of blood glucose, the principal and physiologically most important circulating hexose. The normal fasting blood glucose level is lower in infants than in children. Hypoglycemia is especially common in the newly born, affecting 4/1000 live-born fullterm infants and 16/1000 premature infants. It may occur immediately (within 30 min) after birth, as in infants of diabetic mothers; or it may be delayed (24–48 hr), as in infants who are small for gestational age, in the smaller of discordant twins, and in those infants whose mothers have had hypertensive disease of pregnancy. Hypoglycemia in the neonate may be asymptomatic, mild, and transient, or severe, persistent, and intractable to usual modes of treatment.

The precise definition of hypoglycemia in the newborn period is still unsettled, but it is generally agreed that if 2 determinations of glucose level in plasma fall below 35 mg/dl in the fullterm infant or below 25 mg/dl in the premature infant, such findings are definitely pathologic. After 72 hr of age the plasma glucose level is normally over 45 mg/dl, and in older infants and children fasting levels below 50 mg/dl may be considered hypoglycemic.

The diagnosis and management of hypoglycemia in the newborn are discussed in Sec 7.57.

Physiologic Considerations. Glucose may be derived directly from dietary intake by intestinal absorption, by conversion of other hexoses after absorption (galactose, fructose), by hydrolysis of polyglucose units (maltose, starch, glycogen), or by combinations of these processes (lactose, sucrose). Glucose can also be derived from dietary or endogenous amino acids, but there is no *net* synthesis of glucose from exogenous or endogenous lipids.

Fig 17–1 depicts some of the pathways of glucose metabolism. Although free glucose may passively diffuse through most cell membranes, insulin is required for glucose to enter adipose and muscle cells. It is usually taken up from the lumen of the intestinal tract by the mucosal cells, from the lumen of the renal tubules by their epithelial cells, or from the bloodstream by various parenchymal cells using an active process requiring energy. The phosphorylation of glucose requires ATP and either hexokinase(s) or glucokinase. Within the cells, the glucose-6-phosphate may be metabolized or may be hydrolyzed in intestinal, renal tubular, or liver cells to glucose, which is then free to diffuse out of the cells again. The main routes of metabolism are as follows: (1) The Embden-Meyerhof pathway of anaerobic glycolysis converts the 6-carbon glucose to 3-carbon acids (pyruvic and lactic) with a small release of energy. (2) The pentose-phosphate shunt, initiated by the enzyme glucose-6-phosphate dehydrogenase, yields ribose among other sugars or joins the Embden-Meyerhof scheme at the level of glyceraldehyde-3-phosphate. The reduction of NADP along this pathway is important for a variety of oxido-reductive processes, such as for lipid synthesis and for the maintenance of glutathione in the reduced form. (3)

Glucose is also converted to glucose-1-phosphate, which is in equilibrium with galactose-1-phosphate. Glycogen is the form in which glucose units are stored, mainly in the liver, and is in equilibrium with circulating glucose via the pathways depicted.

The ultimate product of glycolysis is pyruvic acid. After the addition of carbon dioxide or after oxidation to acetyl coenzyme A, it enters the citric acid cycle (tricarboxylic acid or Krebs cycle). Acetyl coenzyme A can also be used in the synthesis of fatty acids, cholesterol, and steroid hormones or in the formation of ketone bodies (acetone, acetoacetic acid, and beta-hydroxybutyric acid). The enzymes of the citric acid cycle are found in the mitochondria within the cells where most of the energy resident in glucose is released and captured in the form of ATP. It is in the citric acid cycle that many amino acids are in equilibrium with glucose. By transamination or oxidation, glutamic acid is converted to alpha-ketoglutaric acid, aspartic acid to oxaloacetic acid, and alanine to pyruvic acid.

The process of gluconeogenesis involves overcoming the thermodynamically unfavorable reaction which changes pyruvic acid to phosphoenolpyruvic acid as illustrated in Fig 17–1, by the transfer of pyruvic acid from the cytosol to the mitochondrion. Once within the mitochondrion, pyruvic acid is converted to either oxaloacetic acid or malic acid, both of which can then diffuse out into the cytosol, where they are in equilibrium with each other. Once in the cytosol, oxaloacetic acid is converted to phosphoenolpyruvic acid by phosphoenol-pyruvate carboxykinase, one of the key rate-limiting enzymes in the gluconeogenic pathway.

Many of the enzyme systems involved in the metabolism of glucose are under hormonal control. The mechanisms and sites of action of the various hormones have been the subject of intensive investigation. Insulin is known to increase the activity of glucokinase in liver and of glycogen synthase in muscle and liver and to suppress key enzymes of gluconeogenesis in liver. In contrast, glucagon and epinephrine act via specific membrane receptors to stimulate the adenyl cyclase system, thereby producing 3',5'-cyclic AMP and initiating a complex series of integrated reactions. In particular, glycogen degradation by activation of the phosphorylase cascade and glucose synthesis via gluconeogenetic mechanisms are stimulated. The enzymatic sites of action of growth hormone, corticotropin, and glucocorticoids, all of which produce hyperglycemia, are activated through similar mechanisms. One of the effects of glucocorticoids is to promote gluconeogenesis via amino acids. The interaction of hormones and of neural control on enzymatic processes and the availability of substrates in the liver are essential to the mature, fine control of glucose homeostasis. Blood glucose concentration is then dependent upon gastrointestinal or hepatic production of glucose to meet the requirements of nervous tissue and blood elements. A low blood glucose level may reflect diminished hepatic production or increased peripheral tissue uptake or some combination of both.

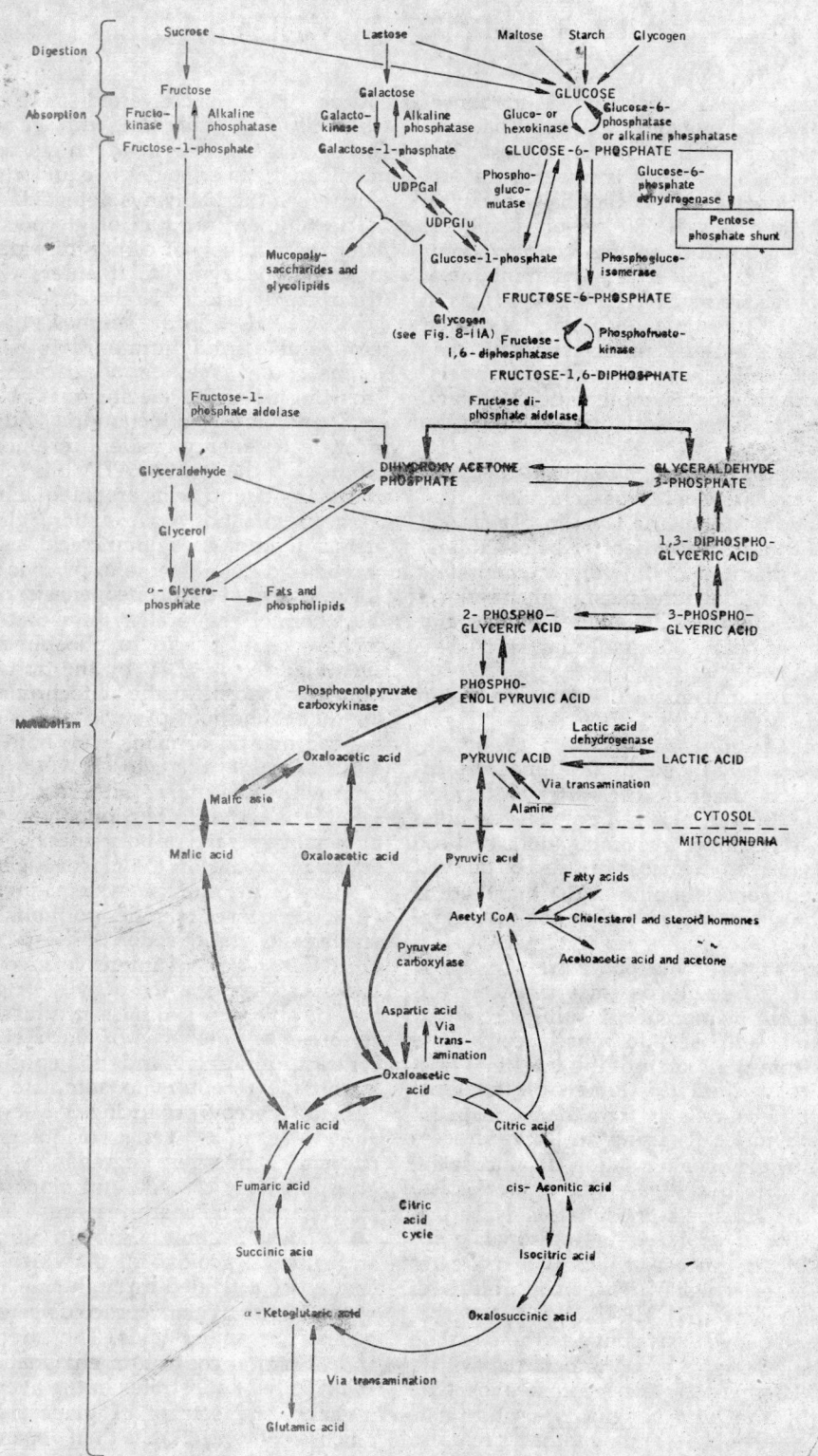

Figure 17–1 The metabolism of glucose. The compounds of the Embden-Meyerhof pathway are indicated in capital letters. The pathway for gluconeogenesis is indicated by heavy arrows.

Table 17-7 CLASSIFICATION OF HYPOGLYCEMIAS

A. With hyperinsulinism
 1. Islet (beta)-cell tumors
 2. Beta-cell adenomatosis
 3. Nesidioblastosis
 4. Beta-cell hyperplasia
  a. In association with hypopituitarism
  b. Infant of diabetic mother
  c. Infant with erythroblastosis fetalis
  d. Beckwith syndrome
  e. Leprechaunism
  f. Etiology unknown
 5. Teratoma containing pancreatic tissue
 6. Functional beta-cell secretory defect
B. With hepatic enzyme deficiencies
 1. Glucose-6-phosphatase
 2. Amylo-1,6-glucosidase
 3. Phosphorylase system
 4. Glycogen synthase
 5. Fructose-1-phosphate aldolase
 6. Fructose-1,6-diphosphatase
 7. Pyruvate carboxylase
 8. Phosphoenolpyruvate carboxykinase deficiency
 9. Galactose-1-phosphate uridyl transferase
 10. Branched chain amino acid abnormalities
C. With endocrine deficiencies
 1. Pituitary
  a. Isolated growth hormone deficiency
  b. Isolated ACTH deficiency
  c. Panhypopituitarism
   (1) With hypoinsulinism
   (2) With hyperinsulinism
 2. Adrenal
  a. Addison disease
  b. Congenital adrenal hypoplasia
  c. Congenital adrenal hyperplasia
  d. Familial glucocorticoid deficiency
  e. Adrenal medullary unresponsiveness
 3. Glucagon deficiency
D. Ketotic hypoglycemia
E. Due to drugs and toxins
 1. Ethyl alcohol
 2. Salicylates
 3. Sulfonylureas
 4. Propranolol
 5. Jamaican vomiting sickness
F. Other
 1. Hepatic damage
  a. Reye syndrome
  b. Leukemia
 2. Malabsorption
 3. Renal glycosuria
 4. Malnutrition
  a. Kwashiorkor
  b. Low phenylalanine diet
 5. Extrapancreatic neoplasms

Hypoglycemia in the neonate may be caused by many of the conditions listed above as well as by other less well delineated factors (Sec 7.57).

CAUSES OF HYPOGLYCEMIA

There are numerous loci where aberrations of control of glucose metabolism can lead to hypoglycemia. Defects in the control mechanisms may involve inborn errors of metabolism, alterations of endocrine balance, or exogenous drugs and toxins (Table 17–7). Since hypoglycemia may result from a wide variety of factors, and since rational treatment and prognosis depend upon the nature of the disorder, it is essential to determine its cause.

17.7 HYPERINSULINISM

When blood glucose falls to hypoglycemic levels, a concomitant fall of insulin to unmeasurable levels occurs in patients with normal homeostasis. Levels of insulin greater than 10 µU/ml in the presence of hypoglycemia are abnormal; in some infants even lower levels of insulin may be inappropriate for the degree of hypoglycemia and indicate autonomous secretion of insulin. A majority of patients with the condition previously called *idiopathic hypoglycemia of infancy* are now known to have hyperinsulinism.

Many children with hyperinsulinism exhibit marked sensitivity to administration of L-leucine with a fall of glucose to hypoglycemic levels. In normal children leucine produces only a small rise in the level of insulin in blood and a concomitant decrease of approximately 10 mg/dl in the level of glucose. Leucine stimulates beta cell secretory activity directly. Patients with islet cell adenoma, islet cell hyperplasia, or nesidioblastosis usually, but not always, exhibit an exaggerated response to leucine. Many of the children diagnosed as having *leucine-sensitive hypoglycemia* in the past probably had nesidioblastosis rather than a discrete diagnostic entity related to leucine.

Islet Cell Adenoma. Functioning beta cell adenoma of the pancreas is a rare lesion now reported in over 80 children. In most instances onset of symptoms has occurred after 4 yr of age, but in approximately one third hypoglycemia was manifested during the neonatal period. Symptoms may be severe and unremitting or may be mild and intermittent. The adenoma is usually solitary but may be multiple or associated with adenomatosis. Four cell types, including beta (insulin), alpha (glucagon), delta (somatostatin), and pp (pancreatic polypeptide), have been identified in varying proportions in islet adenomas. Plasma insulin levels are usually disproportionately elevated relative to glucose levels and indicate autonomous secretion. In adults approximately 10% of beta cell tumors are malignant, but in children malignancy is rarer.

Nesidioblastosis. Hyperinsulinism occurs more frequently in the absence of a discrete islet cell adenoma. It is believed that the pancreatic duct cell is the primordial cell of the pancreas from which the duct and acinar and islet cells arise when appropriately stimulated (hence the term nesidioblast, meaning "islet builder"). It has been suggested that nesidioblastosis results from inappropriate control of early development of the endocrine pancreas, but the cause is not known.

The histologic findings consist of diffuse proliferation of islet cells throughout the pancreas. These cells vary in size and are found budding from pancreatic duct epithelium. All 4 islet cell types are involved in the process; disorganization as well as proliferation characterizes the condition. These cells may be scattered singly or in small clusters throughout the pancreas and occur in association with islets which are normal or which have increased cell numbers. A 5-fold increase in total endocrine area is found. The various islet cell types can be detected by electron microscopy or by immunocytochemistry. Approximately 50–60% of cells are beta cells; the remainder are cells which secrete glucagon, somatostatin, or pancreatic polypeptide.

The hypoglycemia most often begins in the 1st weeks or months of life and is usually severe and intractable. Other infants may be asymptomatic or only mildly irritable with similar degrees of hypoglycemia. Insulin levels may be only slightly increased in serum, beta cell proliferation may not be increased, and pancreatic insulin content may not be elevated. In such patients, deficiency of glucagon and/or somatostatin secretory cells results in alteration of pancreatic hormone balance and may explain the hypoglycemia. Differentiation of this condition from islet cell adenoma is usually not possible without pathologic examination of the pancreas.

That nesidioblastosis has been reported in siblings in 6 families suggests a recessive mode of inheritance. The condition has been seen in association with multiple endocrine adenomatosis, an autosomal dominant condition. Heterogeneity of nesidioblastosis seems likely.

Hyperinsulinism in Association with Panhypopituitarism. In this entity hypoglycemia usually has its onset during the 1st days of life. In spite of deficiencies of growth hormone, ACTH, and TSH, serum insulin levels are inappropriately elevated for the level of glucose. Hyperplasia of the beta cells occurs in some patients. The hypopituitarism appears to be hypothalamic in origin, but the cause for the hyperinsulinism is obscure. In newborn males with hypoglycemia, microphallus provides an important clinical clue to the syndrome.

Newborn Infants of Diabetic and Prediabetic Mothers. Hypoglycemia is common but may not be symptomatic (Sec 7.56).

Other Hypoglycemias. In newborn infants with moderate or severe *erythroblastosis fetalis* clinical manifestations of hypoglycemia and blood glucose levels under 30 mg/dl occur with some frequency. Hyperplasia of the pancreatic islets has been observed in many infants dying with this disorder; it is not as marked as that which occurs in infants of diabetic mothers, and eosinophilic infiltrations are usually not present. The insulin content of the pancreas is increased as are insulin levels in blood and urine. The stimulus which leads to the hyperplasia of the islet cells is not known. The condition is ordinarily transitory, but hypoglycemia has been reported in 2 siblings at 7 and 25 mo of age, presumably as a late sequel of severe erythroblastosis fetalis.

The use of blood containing acid citrate dextrose (ACD) for exchange transfusion of affected infants may lead to a hypoglycemic response which is delayed for 2–3 hr after completion of the transfusion. The high level of glucose in ACD blood corrects any initial hypoglycemia but causes an increased secretion of insulin which may provoke a precipitous fall of blood glucose. Careful monitoring of glucose levels should continue beyond the period of exchange transfusion.

Hyperplasia of the pancreatic islets has also been observed in *Beckwith syndrome* (Sec 7.57).

Hypoglycemia associated with a marked increase in the size and number of islets has been observed in *leprechaunism (Donohue syndrome)*. A defect in insulin receptors has been found.

Teratomas, especially mediastinal and sacrococcygeal, frequently contain pancreatic tissue. Asymptomatic hypoglycemia and an increased level of insulin were detected in a 5 yr old boy with a mediastinal teratoma. This type of hypoglycemia may occur more often than heretofore suspected.

Most infants with hyperinsulinism do not come to surgery; it is not firmly established, therefore, that increased numbers of beta cells are invariably present in these patients. A deranged homeostatic mechanism leading to increased responsiveness of the islet cells remains a possible cause of hypoglycemia. It is even possible that *functional hyperinsulinism* is a primary defect leading to increased numbers of beta cells.

The most common form of hyperinsulinemic hypoglycemia is that associated with treatment of known Type I, insulin-dependent diabetes mellitus.

17.8 HEPATIC ENZYME DEFICIENCIES

Glycogenoses. *Deficiency of glucose-6-phosphatase* leads to severe hypoglycemia in the fasting state and 4–6 hr after meals. In the liver, this is the most important enzyme involved in the release of glucose whether derived from glycogenolysis or via gluconeogenesis. Its deficiency leads to accumulation of glycogen and fat and to hepatomegaly (Sec 8.21). After even a short period of fasting, rather than yielding a normal release of glucose, the glycogen is metabolized via the Embden-Meyerhof pathway with release of pyruvic and lactic acids (Fig 17–1). As a consequence, the hypoglycemia is associated with metabolic acidosis. Patients may have levels of glucose as low as 10 mg/dl and of lactate as high as 200 mg/dl.

Affected children are not, as a rule, mentally retarded or excessively prone to convulsions even at these low concentrations of glucose. It is believed that their brains adapt to the utilization of ketones, amino acids, and/or lactate and pyruvate.

When there is *deficiency of debranching enzyme (amylo-1,6-glucosidase)*, glycogen can be degraded only up to branch points in the molecule. The decreased production of glucose from the liver leads to hypoglycemia, but this is largely compensated for by increased gluconeogenesis. Marked hepatomegaly and growth failure are common; spontaneous improvement occurs at puberty.

Children with, *deficiency of the phosphorylase system* manifest hepatomegaly, mild muscular weakness, growth retardation, and mild hypoglycemia. Glycogen is slightly increased in liver (10% compared with normal <5%) and in muscle (1.5% compared with normal <1%). Considerable degradation of glycogen is possible since injection of glucagon may result in an appropriate rise in the level of blood glucose. All other hepatic enzymatic defects resulting in hypoglycemia are inherited in autosomal recessive fashion; this "defect" may be inherited as an X-linked trait. Heterozygous females may manifest enlargement of the liver in childhood. The signs and symptoms of this disorder disappear at puberty.

In the very rare instances of *deficiency of glycogen synthase*, only small amounts of glycogen can be synthesized in the liver. In this disorder severe hypoglycemia occurs after an overnight fast.

Hereditary Fructose Intolerance. The ingestion of fructose leads to abnormally elevated blood levels of fructose (fructosemia) in 2 conditions: *benign fructosemia*, also known as fructosuria, is an asymptomatic disorder resulting from a deficiency of fructokinase; *hereditary fructose intolerance* is a serious disorder of infancy and an easily treated cause of hypoglycemia (Sec 8.19).

The clinical symptoms of hypoglycemia in hereditary fructose intolerance are associated with other systemic manifestations. Affected infants do not exhibit symptoms until fructose or sucrose is added to the diet. The infant then becomes anorexic, vomits, and fails to thrive. Hypoglycemic manifestations include drowsiness during feeding, excessive sweating, pallor, rolling of the eyes, twitching, and convulsions. Jaundice and hepatosplenomegaly develop and may be the presenting manifestations. Renal tubular involvement may result in glycosuria, aminoaciduria, proteinuria, and acidosis. A low blood glucose concentration may be masked by elevated levels of fructose unless the measurement is made by a specific enzymatic method, such as the glucose oxidase method. If not recognized and treated, the disorder may be fatal. The development of an aversion to fruits and other fructose containing foods or to sucrose results in the spontaneous amelioration of symptoms and may account for survival into childhood before recognition of the disorder. The hepatomegaly may persist for many yr but liver function returns to normal.

This genetic disorder is transmitted in an autosomal recessive manner. The primary defect is a structural mutation of 1 of the 2 isozymes of aldolase, the so-called liver type. This enzyme normally reacts with both fructose-1-phosphate and fructose-1,6-diphosphate. The muscle type of aldolase which remains in the liver reacts more readily with the diphosphate than the monophosphate; accordingly, the accumulation is primarily of fructose-1-phosphate.

The mechanism of the hypoglycemia is not known. It has been suggested that accumulation of fructose-1-phosphate may inhibit hepatic enzymes involved in the release of glucose.

Fructose-1,6-Diphosphatase Deficiency. Hypoglycemia, acidosis, and hepatomegaly are the characteristic hallmarks of this disorder; these findings are also typical of Type I glycogen storage disease (glucose-6-phosphatase deficiency). Fasting hypoglycemia may be severe or moderate and frequently has its onset in the newborn period. Episodes of dyspnea, tachypnea, and hypotonia may occur, and there is progressive hepatomegaly. Increased plasma levels of lactate, pyruvate, free fatty acids, ketones, alanine, and uric acid are present. Reported pedigrees have been of Dutch, German, and Italian ancestry; the error is inherited as an autosomal recessive trait.

Administration of glucagon results in a hyperglycemic response in the fed state but not in the fasting

state. Glucose, galactose, maltose, and lactose can be utilized, or stored as glycogen and then metabolized since the glycogenolytic pathway is intact. However, with periods of fasting and depletion of glycogen stores, the gluconeogenic precursors, including alanine, lactate, pyruvate, and glycerol, cannot be converted to glucose. In patients with complete enzymatic deficiency, oral administration of fructose, glycerol, or alanine induces profound hypoglycemia. In several patients with partial deficiency of the enzymatic defect, improved tolerance to these precursors appears to have occurred following oral administration of folic acid.

Pyruvate Carboxylase Deficiency. Severe hypoglycemia with lactic acidosis has been reported in a neonate with deficiency of 1 of the 2 enzymatic activities of pyruvate carboxylase normally found in liver. The defective activity involved the low Km (high substrate affinity) component, and the infant was responsive to thiamine. It is not known how thiamine enhanced disposal of pyruvate and corrected lactic acidosis.

Mild hypoglycemia has been noted in some patients with *Leigh syndrome (subacute necrotizing encephalomyelopathy)*, a disorder also presumably due to a defect in pyruvate carboxylase. This enzyme has been found markedly reduced late in the course of Leigh syndrome, but it is unlikely that the lack of a normal amount is in itself a cause of the disorder (Sec 8.20).

Alanine, lactate, and pyruvate equilibrate with one another and are all elevated when there is deficiency of pyruvate carboxylase (Fig 17–1).

Phosphoenolpyruvate Carboxykinase Deficiency. Severe, persistent neonatal hypoglycemia has been reported in association with an absence of the extramitochondrial form of hepatic phosphoenolpyruvate carboxykinase, a key gluconeogenic enzyme. Similarities to other enzymatic defects of gluconeogenesis include lactic acidosis and hepatomegaly with fatty infiltration.

Galactosemia. In the event that this defect is not discovered by routine neonatal metabolic screening, hypoglycemia may occur in the presence of weight loss, jaundice, and evidence of hepatocellular dysfunction following milk ingestion. The absence of galactose-1-phosphate uridyl transferase results in diverse toxic effects due to galactose-1-phosphate or galactitol accumulation. (See also Sec 8.19.) Specific enzymatic methods are necessary to identify hypoglucosemia and galactose excretion. Removal of all galactose from the diet prevents mental retardation, cataracts, and renal and hepatic dysfunction.

Branched Chain Amino Acid Defects. Fasting hypoglycemia in patients with maple syrup urine disease appears to be related to a defect in gluconeogenesis from amino acids (Sec 8.7). A related defect involving hydroxymethylglutaryl–coenzyme A lyase has resulted in severe hypoglycemia and organic acidosis in the newborn.

17.9 ENDOCRINE DEFICIENCIES

Cortisol and growth hormone are 2 of the principal hormones antagonistic to insulin and are necessary to maintain glucose homeostasis. Symptomatic hypoglycemia, especially after fasting, occurs in 10–20% of patients with *isolated deficiency of growth hormone* or with *panhypopituitarism*. Prolonged and profound hypoglycemia in the neonatal period may be the 1st clue to severe hypopituitarism. The hypoglycemia appears to result from an inadequate supply of endogenous gluconeogenic substrates. For example, concentrations of amino acids 2–4 hr after a meal are markedly reduced. The hepatic gluconeogenic enzyme system is normal. When there is deficiency of both ACTH and growth hormone, replacement therapy with both cortisol and growth hormone is necessary to restore carbohydrate metabolism to normal. "Ketotic" hypoglycemia has been described in patients with isolated deficiency of ACTH or of growth hormone.

Children with failure to thrive or *maternal deprivation syndrome* may first be seen with an episode of seizure or coma resulting from severe hypoglycemia. Deficiencies of ACTH, growth hormone, or both have been incriminated, but they probably only aggravate the effects of the already deficient gluconeogenic substrates present in these patients.

Fasting hypoglycemia is a frequent concomitant of *Addison disease* but is an uncommon presenting manifestation. In *congenital virilizing adrenal hyperplasia*, hypoglycemia has been noted only rarely. By contrast, hypoglycemia is frequently the presenting manifestation in the newborn with *congenital adrenal hypoplasia* and in children with *familial glucocorticoid insufficiency* (Sec 18.22). The increased pigmentation which is almost invariably associated with the latter disorder is an important diagnostic clue.

Patients with hypopituitarism generally have decreased insulin release, but a subgroup of patients has been identified who have *hyperinsulinism* in association with deficiencies of growth hormone, ACTH, and TSH (Sec 18.2).

Adrenal medullary unresponsiveness has been thought to be the cause of hypoglycemia in some children. Evidence indicates that failure to increase levels of epinephrine in response to hypoglycemia is a concomitant of ketotic hypoglycemia.

Glucagon deficiency has been found in a newborn with severe, persistent neonatal hypoglycemia. Insulin secretion was normal, while glucagon did not rise in response to intravenous alanine. The infant responded remarkably to exogenous glucagon administration. This disorder may be autosomal recessive.

17.10   KETOTIC HYPOGLYCEMIA

Ketotic hypoglycemia is the most common cause of hypoglycemia in childhood, accounting for more than 50% of cases. Onset usually occurs from 18 mo–5 yr of age with spontaneous remission by 9–10 yr. Boys are affected twice as often as girls, and low birth weight is a common characteristic of affected children. The attacks are episodic, most apt to occur in the morning, and frequently associated with ketonuria. Episodes seem to be related to periods of illness, vomiting, or deprivation of food. Otherwise, affected children are in good health but tend to be small and thin. Hypogly-

cemic episodes respond promptly to administration of glucose.

Between attacks, carbohydrate tolerance tests give normal results. Hypoglycemia can be precipitated by a prolonged fasting (18–24 hr) or by a low calorie, high fat, low carbohydrate (ketogenic) diet. Ketonuria frequently occurs under these conditions but is not a specific finding since it may occur in normal children during fasting; moreover, unlike adults, about 20% of normal children have blood glucose levels below 40 mg/dl after a 24 hr fast. Children with ketotic hypoglycemia usually do not respond to administration of glucagon with appropriate rises in blood glucose during either spontaneous or induced episodes of hypoglycemia; by contrast, 1 study found 49 of 52 normal children to have a >10 mg/dl rise in glucose following administration of glucagon after a 24 hr fast. Failure to respond to glucagon reflects depletion of hepatic glycogen, but it may also be noted occasionally in fasted normal children and is not diagnostic. Between hypoglycemic episodes the normal response to glucagon indicates normal hepatic glycogenolysis. During hypoglycemic episodes or during prolonged fasting, levels of insulin are appropriately low for the level of glucose. Insulin levels are normal after overnight fasting or after glucose tolerance tests made between attacks.

The precise mechanism of ketotic hypoglycemia is unsettled. The underlying defect is probably present at birth but does not become manifest until the child is stressed with caloric deprivation. Some believe this entity represents 1 end of a spectrum of variability, related to the large relative mass of glucose-requiring tissues (e.g., brain) in the young. Physiologic observations are compatible with the hypothesis that persistent oxidation of glucose occurs with an accelerated adaptation to starvation in which there is a failure of gluconeogenesis, in some circumstances due to deficient substrate. Concentrations of plasma alanine may be abnormally low in these children under basal and fasting conditions; infusions of alanine restore the hypoglycemic blood glucose level to normal without altering concentrations of pyruvate or lactate. The cause for the hypoalaninemia in some of these patients is unknown. Patients with deficiency of pituitary or adrenocortical hormones are also deficient in the same substrate; it is not surprising, therefore, that "ketotic" hypoglycemia has been reported in these conditions. Patients with ketotic hypoglycemia may also have increased excretion of the keto derivatives of branched chain amino acids in urine (Sec 8.7).

Children with an inability to increase their plasma levels of epinephrine (*adrenal medullary hyporesponsiveness*) when they are subjected to hypoglycemia have ketotic hypoglycemia. In normal persons during hypoglycemic episodes excretion of epinephrine in the urine and levels in plasma are increased 5–20-fold above euglycemic levels. In children with ketotic hypoglycemia, both urinary excretion and rises in plasma levels of epinephrine are deficient when hypoglycemia is induced either by insulin or by a ketogenic diet. The cause for this effect is not known, nor is it settled whether it is specific for ketotic hypoglycemia or a primary or secondary effect. Many affected children also exhibit a subnormal response of endogenous cortisol level to hypoglycemia. Adrenomedullary and adrenocortical hyporesponsiveness are independent of each other, and it has been suggested that the primary defect may be in the hypothalamus or in delayed maturation of adrenal medullary synthesis of epinephrine.

17.11 DRUGS AND TOXINS

Ingestion of ethyl alcohol precipitates hypoglycemia in normal adults after a fast of 2–3 days, but in persons in whom the gluconeogenic reserve is decreased, the hypoglycemic potential of alcohol is revealed after only 12 hr or so of fasting. The hypoglycemia is not mediated by an increase in insulin secretion and is not responsive to glucagon administration. It has been shown that ethanol itself, and not congeners or denaturants, is responsible for the hypoglycemia; the effect results from suppression of hepatic gluconeogenesis and reduction of hepatic glucose output secondary to changes in the oxidoreductive state associated with the metabolism of ethanol.

Young children are unusually susceptible to alcohol and may develop profound, disabling, and even lethal hypoglycemic coma within 1 hr of drinking a leftover cocktail. There are many reports of children developing hypoglycemia following ingestion of alcoholic beverages or substances containing alcohol; in 1 case the hypoglycemia was induced in a 6 mo old febrile infant by sponging with alcohol. Convulsions are common, and deaths have occurred. The prevalence of this cause of hypoglycemia is much greater than the number of reported cases indicates. Immediate intravenous administration of glucose corrects the condition; relapse is uncommon, and continued administration of glucose is rarely necessary. Hypoglycemia has not been found in infants receiving transplacental ethanol from mothers treated for premature labor, presumably because of the immaturity of the alcohol dehydrogenase system in the fetal liver.

Salicylates and related compounds such as acetaminophen may cause hypoglycemia. This effect does not appear to be mediated through increased release of insulin; these drugs may interfere with enzyme systems involved in glucose homeostasis.

Therapy with sulfonylureas during the last trimester of pregnancy has resulted in life-threatening hypoglycemia in newborn infants within hours of birth. Chlorpropamide, acetohexamide, and tolbutamide have all been incriminated. Sulfonylureas cross the placenta and stimulate secretion of insulin from fetal islets. Intravenous glucose may be required continuously for as long as 4 days. Exchange transfusion has also been effective in treatment.

Propranolol, a beta-adrenergic blocking agent, has caused hypoglycemia in children who have been fasted in preparation for surgery or who have been on diminished oral intakes because of illness. In such instances, tachycardia and sweating may not be manifest because of the effect of the drug.

Jamaican vomiting sickness results from ingestion of "bush tea" made from unripe fruits of the ackee, which is grown in Jamaica. This disorder is characterized by severe vomiting, prostration, drowsiness, convulsions, hypoglycemia, and coma, with blood glucose levels as low as 10 mg/dl. The mortality rate is high, death occurring within 24 hr. There are severe hepatic changes including depletion of liver glycogen and fatty degeneration. The agent responsible is the plant toxin hypoglycin A, an unusual amino acid, the chemical structure of which is α-aminomethylenecyclopropylpropionic acid. Hypoglycin A is a specific inhibitor of isovaleryl CoA dehydrogenase and leads to increased concentrations of isovaleric acid with some features of isovaleric acidemia (Sec 8.7). Accumulation of branched pentanoic acids may account for the fact that some patients with the illness fail to respond even to massive infusions of glucose.

17.12 OTHER CAUSES OF HYPOGLYCEMIA

Hepatic Damage. Severe hepatic damage may disturb the metabolism of carbohydrates sufficiently to produce hypoglycemia. Hepatotoxic agents such as phosphorus, halogenated hydrocarbons (carbon tetrachloride), and hydrazine may be responsible for hypoglycemia. Extensive infiltration of the liver by neoplastic cells, fibrous tissue, granulomas, or fat may also lead to hypoglycemia, as may acute and chronic infectious hepatitis in the terminal stages. The mechanisms are not completely understood, but the hypoglycemia probably results from failure to store glycogen, impaired release of glucose into the bloodstream, and decreased net synthesis of glucose from amino acids.

Reye syndrome is characterized by encephalopathy and fatty degeneration of the viscera; blood glucose levels below 25–30 mg/dl are common in younger children. Serum insulin levels are normal, and blood glucose levels are not increased by administration of glucagon. The hypoglycemia appears to be secondary to decreased hepatic glucose production; it is easily managed by infusion of glucose, but such treatment appears to have little influence on the outcome (Sec 11.95).

On rare occasions hypoglycemia occurs in patients with *leukemia*. The cause is not known; it has been suggested that reduced levels of glucose-6-phosphatase in the liver infiltrated by leukemia may play a role.

Impaired Intestinal Absorption of Glucose. Unlike most adults, children and especially infants may exhibit lowering of the blood glucose level when carbohydrate is withheld for 24–48 hr. Fasting is rarely, however, by itself a cause of clinical hypoglycemia; it may be a precipitating factor when other defects that may cause hypoglycemia are present. This may be the case when the level of blood glucose is lowered by impaired intestinal absorption accompanying chronic diarrhea, celiac disease, or the edematous phase of the nephrotic syndrome. Several specific defects in the intestinal absorption of sugars (Sec 11.45), such as of glucose and galactose, of sucrose and isomaltose, and of lactose, are characterized by diarrhea, but they do not lead to significant hypoglycemia. Delayed absorption of glucose occurs in hypothyroidism but is rarely of sufficient magnitude to lead to hypoglycemia.

Renal Glycosuria. Glycosuria due to defective tubular reabsorption of glucose occurs in a variety of clinical entities. It occurs as an isolated hereditary condition, in combination with glycinuria, in the de Toni–Fanconi syndrome, and in some patients with lead poisoning. It is rare that any of these conditions leads to hypoglycemia.

Other. Mild hypoglycemia is a complication of *kwashiorkor*, in which it may be secondary to impaired gluconeogenesis.

Hypoglycemia has occurred in *phenylketonuric* children when dietary restriction of phenylalanine has been too severe during the course of treatment. In these instances general malnutrition is probably the principal factor causing the hypoglycemia.

Hypoglycemia has been observed repeatedly in association with some *extrapancreatic tumors*. The tumors are usually large mesodermal neoplasms (sarcomas) arising in the abdominal or thoracic cavity. The majority of reported patients have been adults; the phenomenon has been observed in children with Wilms tumor and infants with congenital neuroblastoma. Hypoglycemia due to tumor is probably underdiagnosed since fasting blood glucose levels are not determined routinely in children with tumors; its mechanism is unsettled.

Though the residuum of instances in which no cause for hypoglycemia can be established has decreased markedly in recent yr, new pathogenetic causes continue to be discovered. A defect in glycerol metabolism has been found to account for hypoglycemia and ketonuria in a young child. Other reports of unique and bizarre symptom complexes with hypoglycemia suggest that much remains to be learned concerning glucose homeostasis.

17.13 CLINICAL MANIFESTATIONS OF HYPOGLYCEMIA

There is no constant relationship between blood glucose levels and the development or severity of symptoms of hypoglycemia in different patients or even in the same patient at different times. The rate of fall of blood glucose is important; a rapid fall is especially likely to produce symptoms. Even at extremely low blood levels of glucose, children manifest great variability in their responses. Some become conditioned to repeated hypoglycemic episodes or to hypoglycemia of long duration so that they have few or no symptoms, especially children with Type I glycogenosis (von Gierke disease).

The symptoms of hypoglycemia are derived chiefly from disturbances of the central nervous system. Neural tissue has little stored carbohydrate and, unlike other tissues, cannot utilize sugars other than glucose; it is therefore dependent upon a continuous and adequate supply of blood glucose to maintain its normal functions. There is evidence that neural tissue can utilize ketones or amino acid as sources of energy as is thought to be the case in children with prolonged hypoglycemia who are asymptomatic.

Hypoglycemic symptoms are protean but often produce more or less characteristic patterns in individual patients. Sweating, pallor, fatigue, hunger, tachycardia, and nervousness occur as a result of excessive secretion of epinephrine in response to the hypoglycemia. Central nervous system dysfunction is manifested by headache, irritability, negativism, alterations in behavior, drowsiness, mental confusion, psychotic behavior, seizures, and coma.

In newborn and young infants recognition and evaluation of symptoms may be difficult. Convulsions are often the 1st recognized manifestation, but irritability, poor feeding, lethargy, excessive drowsiness, eye-rolling, sweating, and twitching are more common symptoms. Even with very low glucose levels, hypoglycemic symptoms may be absent in the neonate. Young infants with hypoglycemia may manifest cardiomegaly and even heart failure, which remit promptly with elevation of the blood level of glucose.

17.14 DIAGNOSIS OF HYPOGLYCEMIA

Two distinct problems are posed: (1) the detection of hypoglycemia and (2) the determination of its cause. Many children in whom clinical manifestations on 1 or more occasions suggest hypoglycemia can be demonstrated to be hypoglycemic only under specific conditions. In others, hypoglycemia is readily demonstrated by blood glucose determinations. Once hypoglycemia is established, it is essential to determine the cause. There is no routine approach for the study of patients with manifestations of hypoglycemia; individualization in the choice of diagnostic procedures is essential.

The information garnered from the history and physical examination should be evaluated before undertaking exhaustive tests of carbohydrate function. Since many of the causes for hypoglycemia are genetically determined, a family history of other affected persons or of consanguinity may be pertinent. The initial episode of hypoglycemia caused by ingestion of alcohol or other toxins can usually be identified by the history. The infant with galactosemia usually has other clinical manifestations to suggest the diagnosis before hypoglycemia is suspected. A history of aversion to fruits and sweets and the occurrence of gastrointestinal manifestations, as well as those of hypoglycemia, following ingestion of foods containing fructose should suggest hereditary fructose intolerance. Aggravation of hypoglycemic symptoms by meals rich in protein suggests leucine sensitivity and hyperinsulinism.

Hepatomegaly should alert one to the hepatic causes of hypoglycemia. Growth failure directs attention to pituitary hypofunction, whereas manifestations of Addison disease lead to consideration of adrenal hypofunction. The association of large tumors in the thoracic or abdominal cavity with hypoglycemia should suggest appropriate studies. The presence of acidosis points to a deficiency of 1 of the hepatic enzymes.

Hypoglycemic episodes which follow periods of undereating or of vomiting and which have their onset after 1–2 yr of age are suggestive of ketotic hypoglycemia. Once the acute episode is over, all the usual tolerance tests are normal and it generally requires a period of prolonged fasting (18–24 hr) to provoke hypoglycemia.

One of the most difficult differentials is to distinguish the child with a functioning islet cell tumor. Levels of insulin in other conditions may not be clearly elevated. In the presence of abnormally low glucose levels, however, plasma insulin should normally be suppressed; levels as low as 7–15 μU/ml associated with very low levels of plasma beta-hydroxybutyrate, therefore, may be indicative of hyperinsulinism. The leucine and tolbutamide tests are useful for detecting states of insulin hypersecretion, and once it is established, trial therapy with diazoxide may be useful for treatment as well as diagnosis. Most patients with functioning beta cell tumors will not respond to diazoxide, and laparotomy is then usually necessary to establish the diagnosis. Somatostatin infusion should suppress insulin, glucagon, and growth hormone secretion. It may be beneficial acutely and during surgery.

Laboratory Data. The most important period of observation is the time of a spontaneous hypoglycemic episode. Ideally, blood should be obtained then for plasma glucose, beta-hydroxybutyrate, and specific amino acids as well as for hormones (insulin, glucagon, and growth hormone). An aliquot of plasma should be frozen for additional studies to be determined by the patient's future course. Examination of the initial urine for substrates and catecholamines may also be important. However, tests for the evaluation of carbohydrate metabolism (Table 17–8) are usually performed after an overnight fast except in young infants, for whom a 6 hr period is adequate. Occasionally, shorter periods of fasting are indicated if the hypoglycemia is severe. When the expected response of a given test is a lowering of the blood glucose level, the fasting glucose level should be 50 mg/dl or higher to permit a sufficient differential in glucose levels for comparative purposes. The patient should be in reasonably good nutritional state and free of fever when a test is performed.

Appropriate analytic methods should be used to determine the concentration of glucose. Glucose is measured specifically when glucose oxidase or certain other enzymatic methods are used, whereas methods depending upon reduction are not specific for glucose. Values for serum or plasma levels of glucose are approximately 15% higher than those obtained when whole blood is utilized.

A number of tests have evolved for the study of the patient with hypoglycemia. Some are of little value and others of importance only in the delineation of specific disorders. The appropriate use of these tests is based on a knowledge of carbohydrate metabolism and the purposes for which the tests were designed. Precise diagnosis of some hypoglycemic conditions requires measurements of lactate, ketones, growth hormone, or cortisol or assay of specific enzyme activities.

Levels of insulin should be measured in all hypoglycemic patients. The fasting level is rarely above 10 μU/ml. A level above 10 μU/ml in plasma with a blood glucose under 50 mg/dl is abnormal and suggests hyperinsulinism.

The *glucagon tolerance test* is a useful procedure to study the ability of the liver to release glucose into the circulation from stored glycogen. (The *epinephrine tolerance test* has been replaced by the safer glucagon test.) Normally, a rise of blood glucose of 25–50 mg/dl should occur within 15–45 minutes. Failure of an adequate response may be due to depletion of liver glycogen by starvation or hepatic disease. It may be necessary to test the patient in both the fed and fasting state. For example, in glucose-6-phosphatase deficiency there is

Table 17–8 TOLERANCE TESTS FOR THE EVALUATION OF CARBOHYDRATE METABOLISM

COMPOUND	ROUTE		TIME TO OBTAIN SAMPLES (MINUTES)	CRITICAL MEASUREMENTS
L-Alanine	Oral	500 mg/kg	0,30,60,90	Glucose and lactate
	IV	250 mg/kg (as 10% solution in sterile pyrogen-free water)	0,10,20,30,45,60,90	
Glucose	Oral	1.75 gm/kg	0,30,60,90,120, 180,240,300	Glucose and insulin
	IV	0.5 gm/kg (as 10 to 20% solution over 4 min period)	0,5,10,20,30,40, 50,60	
Galactose	Oral	1.75 gm/kg	0,30,60,90,120	Glucose and lactate
Glycerol	Oral	1 gm/kg	0,10,20,30,45,60,90,120	Glucose and lactate
Fructose	Oral	0.5 gm/kg	0,30,45,60,90	Glucose, phosphate and lactate
	IV	0.25 gm/kg (as 10% solution over 4 min period)	0,10,20,30,45,60,90,120	
L-Leucine	Oral	150 mg/kg (as 2% solution or slurry)	0,15,30,45,60,90,120	Glucose and insulin
	IV	75 mg/kg (as 2% solution in 0.45% NaCl)	0,10,20,30,45,60,90	
Glucagon	IM	30 μg/kg (1 mg maximum)	0,15,30,45,60,90,120	Glucose and lactate
Tolbutamide	IV	20 mg/kg (1 gm maximum) (over 1 min period)	0,5,10,20,30,45, 60,90,120	Glucose and insulin

IV = intravenous; IM = intramuscular.

no rise in glucose level following administration of glucagon in either the fasting or fed state, whereas in debrancher deficiency the response is normal postprandially but not after fasting. Children with ketotic hypoglycemia exhibit an inadequate response to glucagon during the hypoglycemic episode or after a 24 hr fast but respond normally between attacks.

The *galactose tolerance test* should not be used for the diagnosis of galactosemia since it may be toxic to the nervous system and may induce severe hypoglycemia; direct assay of uridyl transferase activity is the appropriate diagnostic method. Infusion of galactose provokes a rise in the level of lactate in patients with glucose-6-phosphatase deficiency but not with other conditions.

The *fructose tolerance test* is primarily of use in the detection of hereditary fructose intolerance and of fructose-1,6-diphosphatase deficiency. Administration of fructose to patients results in a decrease of blood glucose to hypoglycemic levels and a rise in the level of blood fructose. In addition, the level of serum inorganic phosphorus is decreased, the concentration of lactic acid is increased, and the insulin level remains unchanged. For this test the blood glucose level must be measured by the glucose oxidase method since the total concentration of reducing sugar remains relatively constant.

The *leucine tolerance test* is used to determine whether this amino acid provokes an exaggerated release of insulin. It is helpful in unmasking hypersecretory states (see above). Normal children exhibit a small but significant rise in concentration of insulin in blood and a decrease of approximately 10 mg/dl in concentration of glucose. In some pathologic states a marked rise in level of insulin is accompanied by a profound fall in level of glucose, as in leucine-sensitive hypoglycemia. In other conditions, such as obesity, a marked rise in the level of insulin is associated with only a normal decline in level of blood glucose.

The *tolbutamide tolerance test* measures the ability of the pancreas to release insulin as determined by the degree and duration of the hypoglycemic response. In normal children the blood glucose level falls about 20–40% within 20–30 min and returns to normal within 60–90 min. In hypoglycemic patients there is an exaggerated response in the increase of insulin level and in the decrease of glucose level. The increase in level of insulin in response to tolbutamide is quite rapid and can be easily missed if blood levels are not obtained early. Infants with hyperinsulinism of any etiology may exhibit a profound and prolonged response to tolbutamide.

The *alanine tolerance test* is useful for evaluating gluconeogenesis. In normal individuals administration of L-alanine results in an increase in blood levels of glucose if the patient has been suitably fasted and hepatic glycogen stores are depleted. Patients with deficiency of fructose-1,6-diphosphatase do not exhibit a rise in blood glucose; instead, the already elevated level of lactate is increased further.

The *glycerol tolerance test* may be utilized for the same purpose as alanine.

17.15 TREATMENT OF HYPOGLYCEMIA

During a hypoglycemic attack the child should under no circumstances be left unattended. The immediate symptoms may be relieved by the administration of glucose, but it should be kept in mind that hypoglycemia of either the organic or functional type may be only temporarily abated by the administration of glucose and may rebound to hypoglycemic levels as the release of additional insulin is evoked. In such situations frequent feedings of small amounts of carbohydrates are advisable until the patient is stabilized. When the cause of the hypoglycemia is established, treatment should be related to it.

For some conditions glucagon in a dose of 1 mg intramuscularly is usually effective in terminating a hypoglycemic episode. This form of therapy is a useful emergency measure which parents can be trained to utilize in the home. It is *not* effective in the glycogenoses, in other hepatic disease, or in ketotic hypoglycemia. Even when it is effective, it should be followed by the oral administration of sugar in some readily absorbable form acceptable to the child.

Patients with ketotic hypoglycemia do well with a program of frequent feedings (4–5 meals a day) of a diet high in protein and carbohydrate. During periods of illness and fasting, high carbohydrate liquids should be offered at frequent intervals. Patients with deficiencies of specific hepatic enzymes may require special dietary management to remove offending foodstuffs. Children with pituitary or adrenocortical insufficiency require replacement therapy with the appropriate hormones.

The most difficult patients to manage have been those with hyperinsulinism. Diazoxide, a nondiuretic benzothiodiazine, has proved to be an effective agent in controlling hypoglycemia in some of these patients. The drug acts primarily by suppressing insulin release. The usual dose is 10 mg/kg/24 hr given orally in 2 divided doses; the dose range has been 5–20 mg/kg/24 hr. The most common side effect is hypertrichosis, particularly of the back, extremities, and face. Once the drug is discontinued, the hypertrichosis disappears. The majority of children with hyperinsulinism of any etiology other than adenoma, the infants of diabetic mothers, and those with erythroblastosis fetalis ordinarily respond satisfactorily. Failure to respond suggests a functioning adenoma, though there have been occasional patients with proven adenomas who have responded quite satisfactorily to diazoxide. On the other hand, some patients with beta cell hyperplasia or nesidioblastosis have failed to respond. Patients who fail to respond to treatment with diazoxide should be explored for an adenoma. If none is found, a subtotal pancreatectomy will often be helpful in reducing the frequency and severity of hypoglycemic attacks. In the event of recurrence of hypoglycemia after pancreatectomy, another course of diazoxide is indicated since the drug may then be effective. The occasional refractory patient may require corticosteroids, repeated attempts at surgical control, or even streptozotocin, a potent diabetogenic antibiotic used primarily to treat carcinoma of the pancreatic islet cells.

A significant number of patients with hyperinsulinism exhibit spontaneous remissions. The hypoglycemic episodes become less frequent and fasting glucose levels gradually rise. Diazoxide may be discontinued and the patient remains asymptomatic. Some such patients still exhibit leucine sensitivity. Patients with ketotic hypoglycemia characteristically experience remission by 10 yr of age.

Brain damage is a frequent concomitant of hypoglycemia. The earlier in life the onset and the more protracted and profound its course, the more likely is brain damage a sequel. It is usually manifested by mental retardation, learning and behavior problems, ataxia, and/or seizures. The electroencephalogram is usually abnormal during hypoglycemic episodes and may remain abnormal between seizures. Even after hypoglycemia is in remission, abnormal EEG tracings and seizures may persist; such normoglycemic seizures require treatment with anticonvulsant agents. Psychologic guidance of the hypoglycemic child and his or her family is of paramount importance.

ANGELO M. DIGEORGE
ROBERT SCHWARTZ

Aynsley-Green A, Polak JM, Bloom SR, et al: Nesidioblastosis of the pancreas: Definition of the syndrome and management of the severe neonatal hyperinsulinemic hypoglycemia. Arch Dis Child 56:496, 1981.

Baker L, Kaye R, Root AW, et al: Diazoxide treatment of idiopathic hypoglycemia of infancy. J Pediatr 71:494, 1967.

Balsam MJ, Baker L, Bishop HC, et al: Beta cell adenoma in a child with hypoglycemia controlled with diazoxide. J Pediatr 80:788, 1972.

Bishop AE, Polak JM, Chesa PG, et al: Decrease of pancreatic somatostatin in neonatal nesidioblastosis. Diabetes 30:122, 1981.

Bord C, Ravazzola M, Pollack A, et al: Neonatal islet cell adenoma: A distinct type of islet cell tumor? Diabetes Care 5:122, 1982.

Breitweser JA, Meyer RA, Sperling MA, et al: Cardiac septal hypertrophy in hyperinsulinemic infants. J Pediatr 96:535, 1980.

Brunette M, Delvin E, Hazel B, et al: Thiamine-responsive lactic acidosis in a patient with deficient low-Km pyruvate carboxylase activity in liver. Pediatrics 50:702, 1972.

Chaussain JL: Glycemic response to 24 hour fast in normal children and children with ketotic hypoglycemia. J Pediatr 82:438, 1973.

Christensen NJ: Hypoadrenalinemia during insulin hypoglycemia in children with ketotic hypoglycemia. J Clin Endocrinol Metab 38:107, 1974.

Colle E, Ulstrom RA: Ketotic hypoglycemia. J Pediatr 64:632, 1964.

Collipp PJ: Hypoglycemia and leukemia. Pediatrics 46:788, 1970.

Combs JT, Grunt JA, Brandt IK: New syndrome of neonatal hypoglycemia: Association with visceromegaly, macroglossia, microcephaly and abnormal umbilicus. N Engl J Med 275:236, 1966.

Cornblath M, Schwartz R: Disorders of Carbohydrate Metabolism in Infancy. Ed 2. Philadelphia, WB Saunders, 1976.

Dahlquist G, Genta J, Hagenfeldt L, et al: Ketotic hypoglycemia in childhood. A clinical trial of several unifying etiological hypotheses. Acta Pediatr Scand 68:649, 1979.

Dahms BB, Landing BH, Blaskovics M, et al: Nesidioblastosis and other islet cell abnormalities in hyperinsulinemic hypoglycemia of childhood. Human Pathol 11:641, 1980.

DiGeorge AM, Auerbach VH, Mabry CC: Leucine-induced hypoglycemia. III. The blood glucose depressant action of leucine in normal individuals. J Pediatr 63:295, 1963.

Ehrlich RM, Martin JM: Tolbutamide tolerance test and plasma-insulin response in children with idiopathic hypoglycemia. J Pediatr 71:485, 1967.

Falorni A, Fracassini F, Mass-Benedetti F, et al: Glucose metabolism, plasma insulin, and growth hormone secretion in newborn infants with erythroblastosis

fetalis compared with normal newborns and those born to diabetic mothers. Pediatrics 49:682, 1972.

Glasgow AM, Cotton RB, Dhiensiri K: Reye syndrome. 3. The hypoglycemia. Am J Dis Child 125:809, 1973.

Goodall McC, Cragan M, Sidbury J: Decreased epinephrine excretion in idiopathic hypoglycemia. Am J Dis Child 123:569, 1972.

Grover WD, Auerbach VH, Patel MS: Biochemical studies and therapy in subacute necrotizing encephalomyelopathy (Leigh's syndrome). J Pediatr 81:39, 1972.

Haymond MW, Karl IE, Feigin RD, et al: Hypoglycemia and maple syrup urine disease: Defective gluconeogenesis. Pediatr Res 7:500, 1973.

Hirsch JH, Loo S, Evans N, et al: Hypoglycemia of infancy and nesidioblastosis. N Engl J Med 296:1323, 1977.

Honicky RE, dePapp EW: Mediastinal teratoma with endocrine function. Am J Dis Child 126:650, 1973.

Hopwood NJ, Forsman PJ, Kenny FM, et al: Hypoglycemia in hypopituitary children. Am J Dis Child 129:918, 1975.

Johnson JD, Hansen RC, Albritton WL, et al: Hypoplasia of the anterior pituitary and neonatal hypoglycemia. J Pediatr 82:634, 1973.

Kerr DS, Stevens MCG, Picon DIM: Estimation of Fasting Glucose Flux in Malnourished and Hypoglycemic Children by Constant Infusion of U-13c Glucose. Argonne, Ill., Second International Conference on Stable Isotopes, October, 1975.

Kirkland J, Ben-Menachem Y, Akhtar M, et al: Islet cell tumor in a neonate: Diagnosis by selective angiography and histologic findings. Pediatrics 61:790, 1978.

Koffler H, Schubert WK, Hug G: Sporadic hypoglycemia: Abnormal epinephrine response to the ketogenic diet or to insulin. J Pediatr 78:448, 1971.

Kühl C, Anderson GE, Hertel J, et al: Metabolic events in infants of diabetic mothers during the first 24 hours after birth. I. Changes in plasma glucose, insulin and glucagon. Acta Paediatr Scand 71:19, 1982.

Levin B, Snodgrass GJAI, Oberholzer VG, et al: Fructosaemia. Observations on seven cases. Am J Med 45:826, 1948.

Loridan L, Sadeghi-Nejad A, Senior B: Hypersecretion of insulin after the administration of L-leucine to obese children. J Pediatr 78:53, 1971.

Loutfi AH, Mehrez I, Shahbender S, et al: Hypoglycaemia with Wilms' tumour. Arch Dis Child 39:197, 1964.

McBride JT, McBride MC, Viles PH: Hypoglycemia associated with propranolol. Pediatrics 51:1085, 1973.

Odievre M, Gentil C, Gautier M, et al: Hereditary fructose intolerance in childhood. Am J Dis Child 132:605, 1978.

Pagliara AS, Karl IE, Haymond M, et al: Hypoglycemia in infants and childhood. J Pediatr 82:365, 1973.

Pagliara AS, Karl IE, Keating JP, et al: Hepatic fructose-1,6-diphosphate deficiency. A cause of lactic acidosis and hypoglycemia in infancy. J Clin Invest 51:2115, 1972.

Rallison ML, Meikle AW, Zigrang WD: Hypoglycemia and lactic acidosis associated with fructose-1,6-diphosphate deficiency. J Pediatr 94:933, 1979.

Roe TF, Kogut MD: Idiopathic leucine-sensitive hypoglycemia syndrome: Insulin and glucagon responses and effects of diazoxide. Pediatr Res 16:1, 1982.

Schutgens RBH, Heymans H, Ketal A, et al: Lethal hypoglycemia in a child with a deficiency of 3-hydroxy-3 methylglutaryl-coenzyme A lyase. J Pediatr 94:89, 1979.

Schutt-Aine JC, Drash AL, Kenny FM: Possible relationship between spontaneous hypoglycemia and "maternal deprivation syndrome." J Pediatr 82:809, 1973.

Schwartz JF, Zwiren GT: Islet cell adenomatosis and adenoma in an infant. J Pediatr 79:232, 1971.

Schwartz SS, Rich BH, Lucky AW, et al: Familial nesidioblastosis: Severe neonatal hypoglycemia in two families. J Pediatr 95:44, 1979.

Seltzer HS: Drug-induced hypoglycemia. A review based on 473 cases. Diabetes 21:955, 1972.

Shapiro M, Sincha A, Rosenmann E, et al: Hypoglycemia associated with neonatal neuroblastoma and abnormal responses of serum glucose and free fatty acids to epinephrine injection. Israel J Med Sci 2:705, 1966.

Stanley CA, Baker L: Hyperinsulinism in infancy: Diagnosis by demonstration of abnormal response to fasting hypoglycemia. Pediatrics 57:702, 1976.

Tanaka K, Isselbacher KJ, Shih V: Isovaleric and α-methylbutyric acidemias induced by hypoglycin A: Mechanism of Jamaican vomiting sickness. Science 175:69, 1972.

Tietze HU, Zurbrugg RP, Zuppinger KA, et al: Occurrence of impaired cortisol regulation in children with hypoglycemia associated with adrenal medullary hyporesponsiveness. J Clin Endocrinol Metab 34:948, 1972.

Van Obberghen-Schilling EE, Rechler MM, Romanus JA, et al: Receptors for insulin-like growth factor I are defective in fibroblasts cultured from a patient with leprechaunism. J Clin Invest 68:1356, 1981.

Vidnes J, Sovik O: Gluconeogenesis in infancy and childhood. III. Deficiency of the extramitochondrial form of hepatic phosphoenolpyruvate carboxykinase in a case of persistent neonatal hypoglycemia. Acta Pediatr Scand 65:307, 1976.

Vidnes J, Oyasaeter S: Glucagon deficiency causing severe neonatal hypoglycemia in a patient with normal insulin secretion. Pediatr Res 11:943, 1977.

Yakovac WC, Baker L, Hummeler K: Beta cell nesidioblastosis in idiopathic hypoglycemia of infancy. J Pediatr 79:226, 1971.

18 THE ENDOCRINE SYSTEM

18.1 DISORDERS OF THE HYPOTHALAMUS AND PITUITARY GLAND

The hypothalamus and pituitary gland consist of 7 or more functional units working in concert to maintain endocrine homeostasis. Certain conditions formerly classified as pituitary have a hypothalamic origin, and advances in isolation and synthesis of hypothalamic hormones have permitted more precise delineation of many endocrinologic conditions. Techniques can help differentiate between hypopituitary and hypothalamic aberrations, and new therapeutic approaches are in sight.

The pituitary gland is attached by a stalk to the median eminence of the brain and consists of a posterior lobe (neurohypophysis) and an anterior lobe. The differing connections of each lobe to the hypothalamus reflect their different embryologic origins. The posterior lobe is derived from the infundibulum of the diencephalon; it has direct neural connections via a large tract of fibers with neurons in the supraoptic and paraventricular nuclei of the anterior hypothalamus. The anterior lobe develops from ectoderm of the stomadeum (Rathke pouch) and is controlled by hypothalamic secretions. The endings of some hypothalamic nerve fibers liberate neurohormones into the capillaries of the median eminence, from which they are carried by portal vessels to the pituitary gland. Accordingly, the median eminence is the final common pathway of all releasing factors. Fetal rests of the original connection of the Rathke pouch with the primitive oral cavity may persist in postnatal life; tumors developing from such rests, known as craniopharyngiomas, are the most common tumors arising in this region during childhood.

Function. *Anterior Lobe.* The anterior pituitary has at least 6 different types of secretory cells, which synthesize and secrete a variety of protein hormones. These hormones act either on other endocrine glands or directly on certain body cells to affect almost every organ. The pituitary gland itself is under the control of hypothalamic secretions, each of which regulates specific pituitary cells. Hypothalamic secretions are of 2 types: releasing hormones, which release pituitary hormones, and inhibitory hormones, which inhibit such secretion. Pituitary hormones which lack feedback control from the product of a target gland (growth hormone, prolactin, and melanocyte-stimulating hormone) require hypothalamic inhibitors and stimulators for their control. Only stimulators are known for corticotropin, thyrotropin, luteinizing hormone, and follicle-stimulating hormone; inhibition is effected by target gland hormones (corticosteroids, thyroxine, and sex steroids).

Growth hormone (hGH) is a protein with 191 amino acids; its gene is located on chromosome 17. Growth hormone is closely related to chorionic somatomammotropin (85% homology) and more distantly related to prolactin (26% homology). Unlike other pituitary hormones, it is relatively species-specific; only primate growth hormone is effective in man. Growth hormone currently used to treat hGH-deficient children is obtained from human pituitaries collected at autopsy. Recently hGH has been prepared by recombinant DNA technology; it is currently undergoing clinical trials. The hypothalamic growth hormone–releasing factor (GRF) has been isolated. The somatotropin release–inhibiting factor (SRIF) is a tetradecapeptide, *somatostatin*. It is widely distributed in the central nervous system outside of the hypothalamus and is found also in pancreatic islet cells and in endocrine cells of the gastrointestinal tract; evidence suggests that somatostatin is a secretory product of neurons and acts as a neurotransmitter or neuromodulator in these sites. In the hypothalamus, however, somatostatin has a physiologic role in direct regulation of growth hormone release.

Deficiency of growth hormone results in dwarfism and an excess in gigantism or acromegaly. It appears that growth hormone stimulates skeletal growth through production of intermediary hormones named somatomedins (formerly known as sulfation factor). Several somatomedins have been purified, including somatomedin-A, somatomedin-C, insulin-like growth factors (IGF) I and II, and others. Somatomedins are peptides with molecular weights about one third that of growth hormone and appear to be synthesized in liver and kidney. They circulate in plasma bound to carrier proteins and are believed to mediate the effects of growth hormone on cartilage and other skeletal tissues; their effects on other tissues remain undefined. How many somatomedins exist, their structures, the manner in which they are formed, and their physiologic roles remain to be determined. Defects in this class of potent insulin-like substances account for some types of growth disorders; pure somatomedins might prove to be potent therapeutic agents. Growth hormone–deficient children have low levels of somatomedins, which return to normal during treatment with hGH.

Levels of growth hormone in normal children may be quite low for much of the day. Hence, provocative tests are employed for clinical evaluation of pituitary growth hormone reserves. Both insulin-induced hypoglycemia and intravenous infusion of arginine evoke prompt rises in serum GH in normal patients. A single oral dose of L-dopa (500 mg) is a reliable stimulus of growth hormone secretion, circumventing the need for intravenous infusion or the risk of hypoglycemia. L-

Dopa crosses the blood-brain barrier and probably increases hypothalamic levels of dopamine, which stimulate secretion of growth hormone–releasing hormone and, in turn, of growth hormone. This test is the preferred initial test to evaluate growth hormone secretory reserve. If the results are abnormal, provocative tests with insulin and/or arginine are indicated. After 3–6 mo of age, a cycle develops in GH levels, with sharp rises during deep sleep. A single normal growth hormone level 45–90 min after onset of sleep is strong indication that growth hormone deficiency is not present, whereas a low level requires provocative tests. A short period of exercise strenuous enough to make the patient breathless is also a potent stimulator of growth hormone secretion and can be used as a screening test to rule out growth hormone deficiency.

Human *prolactin* is composed of 199 amino acid residues; its gene is located on chromosome 6. The only established role for prolactin is the initiation and maintenance of lactation. Stimulation of the nipple is a potent stimulus to prolactin secretion. Mean serum levels in children and in fasting adults of both sexes are about 5–20 ng/ml. Elevated levels occur in full term neonates and during pregnancy. Extremely high levels of prolactin occur in amniotic fluid, where concentrations are 10–100 times the levels in maternal or fetal serum. The major source of amniotic prolactin appears to be the decidua.

Prolactin is controlled primarily by prolactin-inhibiting factor (PIF). There is evidence that a prolactin-releasing factor (PRF) exists, but neither PIF nor PRF has been isolated or characterized. Chlorpromazine increases and L-dopa decreases serum prolactin, presumably by altering catecholamine levels in the hypothalamus, with resultant decrease or increase in prolactin-inhibiting factor. Thyrotropin-releasing factor also increases prolactin levels, but it acts directly on the pituitary gland. These drugs are useful in the functional evaluation of prolactin secretion in man and allow the differentiation of pituitary defects from hypothalamic defects.

Prolactin is pathologically elevated with section of the pituitary stalk, in certain pituitary tumors, and in a variety of hypothalamic disorders. Elevated levels of both TSH and prolactin occur in primary hypothyroidism. Absence of an increase in prolactin following administration of thyrotropin-releasing factor (TRH) is the hallmark of primary pituitary disease.

Thyrotropin (TSH) is a glycoprotein with a molecular weight of about 26,000. TSH increases iodine uptake, iodide clearance from the plasma, iodotyrosine and iodothyronine formation, thyroglobulin proteolysis, and release of thyroxine and triiodothyronine from the thyroid. Deficiency results in inactivity and atrophy of the thyroid, and excess results in hypertrophy and hyperplasia. A sensitive radioimmunoassay for TSH in serum aids in the study of clinical problems.

The releasing factor (TRH) for TSH was the 1st hypothalamic hormone to be isolated, characterized, and synthesized; it is a tripeptide ([pyro] Glu-His-Pro-NH$_2$). Thyroxine and triiodothyronine inhibit TSH secretion by blocking the action of TRF upon the pituitary cell. Surprisingly, TRH also stimulates the release of prolactin, in males as well as in females. Synthetic TRH is available for clinical studies and is useful for testing pituitary reserves of TSH and prolactin. Through such studies it is possible to discriminate between the hypothalamic and pituitary origins of many disorders.

Adrenocorticotropin (ACTH) is a single unbranched glycoprotein chain of 39 amino acids; it acts primarily on the adrenal cortex. ACTH is derived from a prohormone which also yields the 91 amino acids of β-lipotropin (β-LPH). ACTH produces changes in adrenal structure, chemical composition, and enzymatic activity and stimulates the release of cortical steroid hormones. Corticotropin-releasing factor was the 1st hypothalamic hormone to be identified, but only recently has a 41-residue peptide been isolated and synthesized which stimulates secretion of corticotropin and β-endorphin. Radioimmunoassays exist for ACTH in plasma.

Melanocyte-stimulating hormone (MSH) consists of 2 separate peptides. One, α-MSH, contains 13 amino acids identical to the 1st 13 amino acids of ACTH but has no corticotropic activity. The 2nd peptide, β-MSH, consists of 22 amino acids and shares a sequence in common with both α-MSH and ACTH. Human β-MSH is not a natural pituitary peptide but an artifact formed by degradation of β-lipotropin during extraction. Plasma levels of ACTH correlate well with β-MSH activity when the steroid feedback mechanism is interfered with, as in Addison disease and in Cushing disease. It appears that ACTH is the principal pigmentary hormone in humans and that MSH has extrapigmentary effects on the brain.

β-Lipotropin (β-LPH) is a 91-residue polypeptide isolated from the pituitary in several species. It is a prohormone; its cleavage results in neurotropic peptides with morphinomimetic activity. Fragment 61–65 is α-endorphin; fragment 61–77 is γ-endorphin; and fragment 61–91 is β-endorphin. β-LPH is stored in the same secretory granules as ACTH, and they are secreted together. Most of the β-MSH activity in human plasma and pituitary is due to β-LPH. Plasma levels of β-endorphin are elevated in endocrine disorders associated with increased ACTH and β-lipotropin production. The fetus at term has high β-endorphin and lipotropin levels.

Gonadotropic hormones include 2 specific glycoproteins: luteinizing hormone (LH) and follicle-stimulating hormone (FSH). Each has an α subunit and a β subunit. The α subunits of these 2 hormones and of TSH are very similar; specificity of hormone action resides in the β subunit, which is different for each of these 3 hormones. Receptors for FSH on the ovarian granulosa cells and on the testicular Sertoli cells mediate FSH stimulation of follicular development in the ovary and of gametogenesis in the testis. On binding to specific receptors on ovarian theca cells and testicular Leydig cells, LH promotes luteinization of the ovary and Leydig cell function of the testis. Both LH and FSH activate adenyl cyclase. Highly specific and sensitive radioimmunoassays for FSH and LH are available. Both hormones are measurable in the plasma of prepubertal children.

Hypothalamic control of gonadotropic hormones has long been known, and separate releasing hormones for

FSH and LH were once anticipated. Luteinizing hormone–releasing hormone (LRH), a decapeptide, has been isolated and synthesized. Since it leads to the release of both LH and FSH, it is now proposed that there may be only 1 gonadotropin-releasing hormone. Use of LRH for clinical studies is giving new insights into dysfunctions of the hypothalamic-pituitary-gonadal axis. Thus far, LRH has not proved as effective as TRF in differentiating between hypothalamic and pituitary disorders.

Posterior Lobe. The posterior lobe of the pituitary is part of a functional unit known as the neurohypophysis, which consists of (1) the neurons of the supraoptic and paraventricular nuclei of the hypothalamus; (2) their axons, which form the pituitary stalk; and (3) their terminals, either in the median eminence or in the posterior lobe.

The neurohypophysis is the source of *arginine vasopressin* (AVP), the antidiuretic hormone, and of *oxytocin;* both are octapeptides, differing in only 2 amino acids. These hormones are produced by a process of neurosecretion in the hypothalamic nuclei. The neurons of the supraoptic and paraventricular nuclei also synthesize specific *neurophysins* during the biosynthesis of vasopressin and oxytocin. These are transported to nerve terminals in the posterior pituitary, where they are released together with oxytocin or vasopressin. Radioimmunoassays of the neurophysins provide a direct index of vasopressin and oxytocin levels in plasma. The concentration of arginine vasopressin in umbilical cord plasma appears to be a sensitive indicator of fetal stress.

Vasopressin has a short half-life and responds very quickly to changes in hydration. It changes the permeability of the cell membrane via cyclic AMP. Vasopressin and oxytocin are thought to be synthesized in separate and specific cells. A synthetic analogue, deamino-8-D-arginine vasopressin is resistant to peptidases and has a prolonged half-life. Small amounts administered intranasally are effective in therapy of patients with diabetes insipidus.

18.2 HYPOPITUITARISM

Here we shall discuss only those hypopituitary states associated with deficiency of growth hormone (Table 18–1). Affected children have usually been referred to as pituitary dwarfs, a designation best avoided. Isolated deficiencies of thyrotropin, corticotropin, and gonadotropin are discussed later.

Etiology. *Congenital Defects.* Aplasia or hypoplasia of the pituitary is rare. Developmental abnormalities of the pituitary are associated with such defects as anencephaly, holoprosencephaly (cyclopia, cebocephaly, orbital hypotelorism), and septo-optic dysplasia. Recently, in 6 neonates absence of the pituitary gland has been reported associated with hypothalamic hamartoblastoma, imperforate anus, postaxial polydactyly, and other congenital defects. The cause is unknown; chromosomes have been normal; no familial cases have occurred. Hypoplasia of the pituitary with anencephaly has long been known, but recent obser-

Table 18–1 ETIOLOGIC CLASSIFICATION OF HYPOPITUITARISM

Aplasia or hypoplasia of pituitary
  Developmental defects
    Anencephaly
    Holoprosencephaly (cyclopia, cebocephaly, orbital hypotelorism)
    Midfacial anomalies (hypertelorism, etc.)
    Basal encephalocele
    Septo-optic dysplasia (de Morsier syndrome)
    Cleft lip and palate
    Solitary maxillary central incisor
    Hall-Pallister syndrome (hypothalamic hamartoblastoma, imperforate anus, polydactyly)
    Rieger syndrome
    Fanconi syndrome
  Idiopathic (usually hypothalamic deficiency)
    Sporadic
    Autosomal recessive
    Autosomal dominant
    Polygenic
    X-linked associated with hypogammaglobulinemia
Destructive lesions
  Trauma
    Perinatal (trauma, anoxia, hemorrhagic infarction)
    Basal skull fractures
    Child abuse
  Infiltrative lesions
    Tumors
      Histocytosis X
      Craniopharyngioma
      Hypothalamic tumors
      Germinoma
      Optic glioma
      Pituitary adenomas
    Sarcoidosis
    Hemochromatosis
    Tuberculosis
    Toxoplasmosis
  Irradiation (CNS, eyes, middle ears)
  Autoimmune hypophysitis
  Surgery
    Removal of pharyngeal pituitary
    Surgery for craniopharyngioma and other tumors
  Vascular
    Infarctions (e.g., hemoglobinopathy)
    Aneurysm
Functional deficiency
  Psychosocial deprivation
  Anorexia nervosa

vations reveal a large residuum of normal pituitary function and suggest that hypoplasia may be secondary to the hypothalamic defect. With hypothalamic-releasing hormones it is possible to determine whether defects in pituitary function reside in the pituitary or in the hypothalamus. Many of these conditions are lethal early in life, but partial defects may occur in siblings. A child has been reported with isolated deficiency of growth hormone and mild hypotelorism who had 2 siblings with holoprosencephaly with hypopituitarism. Deficiency of growth hormone occurs in 4% of all patients with *cleft lip* or *cleft palate* and in 32% of those who have short stature. Midfacial anomalies or the presence of a *solitary maxillary central incisor* will indicate high likelihood of growth hormone deficiency.

Septo-optic dysplasia (de Morsier syndrome) should be suspected in visually impaired children of short stature. Hypoplasia of the optic nerves and absence of the septum pellucidum characterize this sporadic developmental defect. The fundus exhibits hypoplastic discs with typical double rims and sparse retinal vessels. Computed tomography usually reveals absence of the septum pellucidum and inferior pointing of the antero-inferior margins and flattening of the roofs of the frontal horns. The hormonal deficiency may involve growth hormone alone or panhypopituitarism, including diabetes insipidus. The defect in this condition is believed to reside in the hypothalamus.

Aplasia of the pituitary without abnormalities of the brain or skull is very rare, but affected infants are being increasingly recognized because hypoglycemia occurs early and there is microphallus in males. Some have had evidence of the neonatal hepatitis syndrome, but the relationship of hypopituitarism is obscure. The condition has been reported in siblings of both sexes, and consanguinity has been noted in 2 families; autosomal recessive inheritance is suggested. Studies in some children have placed the defect in the hypothalamus. This may be a heterogeneous group of disorders.

Hypogammaglobulinemia has been associated with isolated growth hormone deficiency in 1 family as an X-linked trait. The relationship between the 2 disorders is not clear.

Destructive Lesions. Any lesion which damages the anterior pituitary or hypothalamus may cause cessation of growth. Since such lesions are not selective, multiple hormonal deficiencies are usually observed. The most common lesion responsible for this condition is the craniopharyngioma; central nervous system germinoma and other hypothalamic tumors, tuberculosis, sarcoidosis, toxoplasmosis, and aneurysms may also cause hypothalamic-hypophyseal destruction. These lesions are frequently associated with roentgenographic changes in the skull. Diabetes insipidus is a well-known complication of histiocytosis, but deficiency of growth hormone and other pituitary hormones may occur in almost half of affected children. Enlargement of the sella or deformation or destruction of the clinoid processes usually indicates a tumor. Intrasellar or suprasellar calcifications usually indicate a craniopharyngioma. Trauma, including child abuse, traction at delivery, anoxia, and hemorrhagic infarction may also damage the pituitary, its stalk, or the hypothalamus.

Irradiation for tumors of the central nervous system, eyes, and middle ears and cranial irradiation in acute leukemia may cause hypothalamic-pituitary damage. Deficiency of growth hormone is the most common defect, but deficiencies of TSH, ACTH, and gonadotropins may also occur. The latent period may be long between irradiation and onset of clinical manifestations.

Idiopathic Hypopituitarism. More than half of patients with hypopituitarism have no demonstrable lesion of the pituitary or hypothalamus, and the cause is not known. The disorder is 3 times as common in males as in females. Increased incidences in breech birth, forceps delivery, and intrapartum maternal bleeding suggest that birth trauma and anoxia may be pathogenic factors. It is increasingly apparent that the functional defect occurs more frequently in the hypothalamus than in the pituitary.

Approximately half of children with growth hormone deficiency also have deficiencies of other pituitary hormones. The multiple deficiencies may be manifest in infancy, or there may be progressive development of the various deficiencies; for example, a child with initially only GH deficiency may eventually exhibit deficiencies of TSH and ACTH. Hypopituitarism is usually sporadic, but affected siblings are not uncommon.

In the other half of children with idiopathic hypopituitarism, growth hormone deficiency occurs as an isolated defect and is often familial. Autosomal recessive inheritance is most common, but autosomal dominant inheritance has also been noted. It has been suggested that interaction of a polygenic susceptibility with environmental agents (birth trauma) may explain many of the familial cases. Puberty may be markedly delayed, but it does occur spontaneously.

Clinical Manifestations. *In Patients Without Demonstrable Lesion of the Pituitary.* The hypopituitary child is usually of normal size and weight at birth. The retardation of growth has a variable onset; in about half of affected children the retardation of growth is noticed by 1 yr of age. In others there may be regular but slow growth in height, with the increments always below those of coevals, or periods of lack of growth may alternate with short spurts of growth. Delayed closure of the epiphyses permits growth beyond the age when normal persons cease to grow.

Infants with congenital defects of the pituitary or hypothalamus usually present such neonatal emergencies as apnea, cyanosis, or severe hypoglycemia. Microphallus in the male is an important diagnostic clue. Deficiency of growth hormone is accompanied by hypoadrenalism and hypothyroidism, and clinical manifestations of hypopituitarism evolve more rapidly than in the usual hypopituitary child.

The head is round and the face short and broad. The frontal bone is prominent and the bridge of the nose depressed and saddle-shaped. The nose is small, and the nasolabial folds are well developed. The eyes are somewhat bulging. The mandible and the chin are underdeveloped and infantile, and the teeth, which erupt late, are frequently crowded. The neck is short and the larynx small. The voice is high-pitched and remains high after puberty. The extremities are well proportioned, the hands and feet being small. The genitalia are usually underdeveloped for the child's age, and sexual maturation may be delayed or absent. Facial, axillary, and pubic hair is usually absent; the hair of the scalp is fine. Symptomatic hypoglycemia, usually after fasting, occurs in 10–15% of children with panhypopituitarism as well as with isolated growth hormone deficiency. Intelligence is usually normal. Affected children may become shy and retiring as they grow older.

In Patients with Demonstrable Lesions of the Pituitary. The child is normal initially, and manifestations similar to those seen in idiopathic pituitary growth failure gradually appear and progress. When complete or almost complete destruction of the pituitary gland occurs, severe manifestations of pituitary insufficiency are present. Atrophy of the adrenal cortex, thyroid, and gonads results in loss of weight, asthenia, sensitivity to cold, mental torpor, and absence of sweating. Sexual maturation fails to take place or regresses if already present. Thus, there may be atrophy of the gonads and genital tract with amenorrhea and loss of pubic and axillary hair. There is a tendency to hypoglycemia and coma. Growth ceases. Diabetes insipidus may be present early but tends to improve spontaneously with progressive destruction of the anterior pituitary.

If the lesion is an expanding tumor, symptoms such as headache, vomiting, visual disturbances, pathologic sleep, decreased school performance, seizures, polyuria, and growth failure may be present. Although growth failure frequently antedates the neurologic signs and symptoms, especially in patients with craniopharyngiomas, symptoms of hormonal deficit account for only 10% of presenting complaints. In other patients the neurologic manifestations may precede the endocrinologic, or evidence of pituitary insufficiency may first appear after surgical intervention. In children with craniopharyngiomas visual field defects, optic atrophy, papilledema, and cranial nerve palsy are common.

Laboratory Data. The diagnosis of growth hormone deficiency rests upon demonstration of absent or subnormal reserve of pituitary GH. Random serum levels of growth hormone over 10 ng/ml exclude growth hormone deficiency, but lower levels must be studied further. Exercise is a benign and physiologic stimulus to growth hormone release; in most normal children elevated levels of growth hormone will be found after 20 min of strenuous exercise. Levels of growth hormone are also elevated 45–90 min after onset of sleep. If only low levels are found under these conditions, provocative tests for growth hormone release are required to verify a deficiency and to identify those children who will not respond to treatment with growth hormone. The usual provocative agents are L-dopa, insulin-arginine, and glucagon, and tests with each may be required. Finding levels below 5 ng/ml after 2 provocative tests establishes the diagnosis of growth hormone deficiency. Great care must be taken in the administration of insulin to patients with hypopituitarism because of their decreased ability to overcome hypoglycemia. At greatest risk are thin children under 5 yr of age, particularly if they exhibit low levels of glucose when fasting. Levels of somatomedin-C are increasingly utilized as indicators of growth hormone deficiency. Diagnostic use of measurements of somatomedin-C requires comparison with age- and sex-matched controls. In normal children levels gradually increase from birth to peak levels at puberty with peak levels 2 yr earlier in girls than in boys. Boys with constitutional growth delay have lower levels than age-matched controls. In growth hormone–deficient children levels are very low but rise significantly within 16–28 hr of hGH administration in the majority of patients.

Decreased growth hormone responses may also occur in children with primary hypothyroidism or with emotional deprivation, but in these conditions correction of the underlying disorder restores growth hormone levels to normal.

Once deficiency of GH is established, it is necessary to examine the functions of the remainder of the pituitary-hypothalamic axis. When there is deficiency of thyrotropin, serum levels of thyroxine and TSH are low. A normal rise in TSH and prolactin following stimulation with thyrotropin-releasing hormone places the defect in the hypothalamus, whereas absence of response localizes the defect in the pituitary. In most patients with idiopathic multiple anterior pituitary hormone deficiency, normal responses to TRH indicate that the deficiency is primary in the hypothalamus and secondary in the pituitary. An elevated random level of plasma prolactin in the hypopituitary patient is also strong evidence that there is a defect in the hypothalamus rather than in the pituitary. Some children with craniopharyngioma have elevated levels of prolactin before surgery, whereas after surgery they have prolactin deficiency due to pituitary damage.

Decreased urinary corticosteroid and plasma cortisol levels indicate deficiency of corticotropin. Insulin-induced hypoglycemia provokes a rise in cortisol levels by stimulating ACTH release; measurements of cortisol levels, therefore, during the provocative test for growth hormone with insulin provide information concerning corticotropin reserve. The response to metyrapone also may indicate corticotropin production. Serum FSH and LH levels may be decreased even below the ordinarily low prepubertal levels. Gonadotropin deficiency cannot be excluded, however, until after the child has gone through puberty. Antidiuretic hormone deficiency may be established by appropriate studies.

Roentgenographic Examination. The long bones are slender and poor in minerals, the centers of ossification appear late, and the epiphyseal clefts remain open. The fontanels may remain open beyond the 2nd yr and intersutural wormian bones may be found. The sella turcica may be abnormally small, but a normal sellar volume does not exclude the diagnosis. Roentgenograms of the skull are most helpful when there is a destructive or space-occupying lesion causing hypopituitarism. A history of nausea, vomiting, loss of vision, headache, or increase in circumference of the head suggests increased intracranial pressure. Enlargement of the sella, especially ballooning with erosion and calcifications within or above the sella, may be detected. Computed tomography, radionuclide scans, or carotid angiograms may be required for diagnosis and localization.

Differential Diagnosis. The causes of growth disorders are legion; only those which most closely mimic hypopituitarism are considered here.

Children with *Laron syndrome* have all the clinical findings of those with idiopathic hypopituitarism, but plasma levels of growth hormone are elevated whereas those of somatomedin are low. There is no response to administration of hGH. The primary defect appears to be cellular unresponsiveness to growth hormone. In many families an autosomal recessive mode of inheritance is suggested, but sporadic cases have been noted.

Decreased serum somatomedin levels also occur in β-thalassemia, presumably secondary to hemosiderosis of the liver and other organs.

Primary hypothyroidism is usually easily distinguished on clinical grounds. Responses to growth hormone provocative tests may be subnormal, however, and enlargement of the sella may be present. Elevated levels of TSH clearly establish the diagnosis, and these secondary changes disappear following treatment with thyroid hormone.

Turner syndrome must always be considered in short

girls. When this is associated with the usual characteristic congenital deformities, the diagnosis is not difficult, but in other instances there may be few characteristic findings other than shortness of stature. Chromosomal analysis is necessary to establish the diagnosis.

Emotional deprivation is an important cause of retardation of growth and mimics hypopituitarism. The condition is known as psychosocial dwarfism, deprivation dwarfism, or reversible hyposomatotropism. The mechanisms whereby sensory and emotional deprivation interferes with growth are not fully understood. Functional hypopituitarism is indicated by low levels of somatomedin, by inadequate responses of growth hormone to provocative stimuli, by decreased pituitary responses to metyrapone stimulation, and perhaps by delayed puberty. Appropriate history and careful observations reveal disturbed mother-child or family relations and provide clues to diagnosis. Proof may be difficult to establish because the adults responsible often hide from professionals the true situation in the family and the children rarely divulge their plight. Emotionally deprived children frequently have perverted or voracious appetites, enuresis, encopresis, insomnia, crying spasms, and sudden tantrums. They may be excessively passive or aggressive and are borderline or dull-normal in intelligence. When child-rearing practices are altered or when the child is removed from the domicile of abuse, the rate of growth improves significantly. During this period of catch-up growth, separation of the cranial sutures and other evidence of pseudotumor cerebri may occur; these should not be mistaken for signs of a mass lesion.

In *primordial dwarfism* the growth retardation begins during intrauterine life, is present at birth, and is frequently associated with other minor or major defects. This is a heterogeneous group with diverse causative factors. Growth hormone levels are normal. *African pygmies* in the rain forests of Equatorial Africa resemble patients with deficiency of growth hormone but have normal levels of growth hormone and do not respond to administration of hGH. Recent studies indicate that pygmies have a deficiency of a potent insulin-like growth factor (IGF-I), which may be identical to somatomedin C.

The *Silver-Russell syndrome* is characterized by short stature, frontal bossing, small triangular facies, sparse subcutaneous tissue, shortened and incurved 5th fingers, and, in many cases, asymmetry. Affected children have low birth weights for gestational age. Growth hormone levels are usually normal, but 5 affected patients have had growth hormone deficiencies, 1 due to a craniopharyngioma and 4 idiopathic.

The growth problem most frequently encountered by the pediatrician is the apparently normal child who is below the 3rd percentile in height but who has a normal growth velocity. When skeletal maturation is below the chronologic age but is consistent with height age, the condition is referred to as *constitutional delay in growth*. In such children growth potential is adequate; puberty and adult height will be achieved later than average. If skeletal maturation is consistent with chronologic age, the condition is known as *genetic short stature*. Other

family members with short stature will be commonly found, and the growth potential is limited. Growth hormone studies in these 2 groups of children are normal.

Prognosis. Prognosis for life depends upon the causative factor. In the absence of an anatomic lesion the affected person may reach old age.

Prognosis of ultimate height is difficult since continued growth is possible long after the usual age of adolescence because open epiphyses persist. Sexual maturation may also take place 10–20 yr later than in normal persons. Catchup growth is frequently observed in children who have had surgical treatment of craniopharyngiomas or other tumors in the hypothalamic area. Surprisingly, growth may occur even in the absence of demonstrable hGH. Growth appears to be dependent on somatomedin since its plasma levels are normal. The stimulus for somatomedin production in these patients is unknown.

Treatment. In patients with demonstrable organic lesions treatment should be directed to the underlying disease process. Evaluation of pituitary function is indicated after surgery and/or irradiation.

Replacement of the essential hormonal deficiencies is possible. Administration of growth hormone has been successful in increasing the growth velocity of at least 80% of growth hormone–deficient children, whereas it has failed to alter growth rates in most other conditions of deficient growth. A variety of dosage regimens have been used. The standard and effective dose is 2 IU by intramuscular injection 3 times a week, but 2.5 IU of hGH weekly appears just as effective during the 1st yr of therapy. Maximal growth response occurs during the 1st yr of treatment; the rate may reach twice that expected for chronologic age, whereas, by the 3rd yr of treatment, it averages less than 1.5 times that expected for age. Although almost half the treated patients develop antibodies to human growth hormone, this rarely accounts for diminished effectiveness of the hormone. Younger children appear to respond better than older.

The hormone is now available in adequate amounts to treat most children with hypopituitarism; 1 human pituitary yields about 5 mg of growth hormone. hGH prepared by recombinant DNA technology should also soon be available.

Therapy with hydrocortisone is indicated if hypoglycemia or proven adrenal insufficiency is present and with thyroid hormone when there is secondary hypothyroidism. The doses of these hormones should be kept in the physiologic range. For infants with microphallus 1 or 2 3-mo courses of monthly intramuscular injections of 25 mg of testosterone enanthate may bring the penis to normal size without inordinate effect on osseous maturation.

18.3 DIABETES INSIPIDUS
(Arginine Vasopressin Deficiency)

Diabetes insipidus is characterized by polyuria and polydipsia and results from lack of the antidiuretic hormone, arginine vasopressin. Destruction of the supraoptic and paraventricular nuclei or division of the supraoptic-hypophyseal tract above the median eminence results in permanent diabetes insipidus. Transection of the tract below the median eminence or removal of just the posterior lobe may result in transitory polyuria, but in this case arginine vasopressin released into the median eminence prevents occurrence of diabetes insipidus. Vasopressin acts directly on the distal tubules and collecting ducts of the kidney to facilitate reabsorption of water. Vasopressin deficiency may be total or partial with varying degrees of polydipsia and polyuria.

Etiology. Any lesion which damages the neurohypophyseal unit may result in diabetes insipidus. Tumors of the suprasellar and chiasmatic regions, particularly craniopharygiomas (Fig 18–1) and optic gliomas, are common causes; the symptoms of increased intracranial pressure may accompany those of diabetes insipidus or may follow years later. Approximately 25–50% of patients with histiocytosis have diabetes insipidus as a consequence of histiocytic infiltration of the hypothalamus and pituitary. Deficiency of growth hormone is found in most patients with reticuloendothelioses who manifest diabetes insipidus. Encephalitis, sarcoidosis, tuberculosis, actinomycosis, and leukemia are occasional causes. Injuries to the head, especially basal skull fractures, may produce diabetes insipidus immediately or after a delay of several mo. Operative procedures near the pituitary or hypothalamus may result in transitory or permanent diabetes insipidus.

In a minority of instances diabetes insipidus is hereditary. Autosomal dominant and X-linked recessive forms occur; affected males with either type are indistinguishable. In the genetic forms of the disorder there is marked reduction in neurosecretory cells of the supraoptic and paraventricular nuclei. In the Brattleboro strain of rat, diabetes insipidus is transmitted as an autosomal recessive trait; the neurosecretory cells are normal or hypertrophied; thus, the basic defect is in the synthesis of the peptide hormone.

Diabetes insipidus also occurs as part of a rare syndrome in which it is associated with diabetes mellitus, optic atrophy, and sensorineural deafness (*Wolfram syndrome*). The order of appearance of the various components varies. Pathologic studies suggest that a systemic degenerative process involves the optic nerve, supraoptic and paraventricular nuclei, and 8th cranial nerve. Incomplete forms of the syndrome may occur in patients or in their siblings; an autosomal recessive mode of inheritance is likely.

Diabetes insipidus is increasingly recognized in the newborn infant. It has been reported following asphyxia, intraventricular hemorrhage, intravascular coagulopathy, *Listeria monocytogenes* sepsis, and group B beta-hemolytic streptococcal meningitis.

In many instances no specific cause can be found; some of these may represent genetic forms of the disease. Since diabetes insipidus may be the 1st recognizable sign of an intracranial tumor and may antedate neurologic signs by years, periodic re-evaluation is required for a long time.

Clinical Manifestations. Polydipsia and polyuria are the outstanding symptoms of diabetes insipidus. In families with the hereditary disorder the polyuria is noted in early infancy. The infant cries excessively and will not be satisfied with additional milk but is quieted with water. Hyperthermia, rapid loss of weight, and collapse are common in infancy. Vomiting, constipation, and growth failure may be observed. Dehydration in early infancy may result in brain damage and mental impairment. In the familial forms of vasopressin deficiency there is wide variability in manifestations. Severity tends to increase with age, some affected members being asymptomatic until adolescence. Many affected families accept polydipsia and polyuria as a family habit and do not seek medical attention or may even prefer the symptoms to injections of vasopressin.

In a child who has acquired bladder control, enuresis

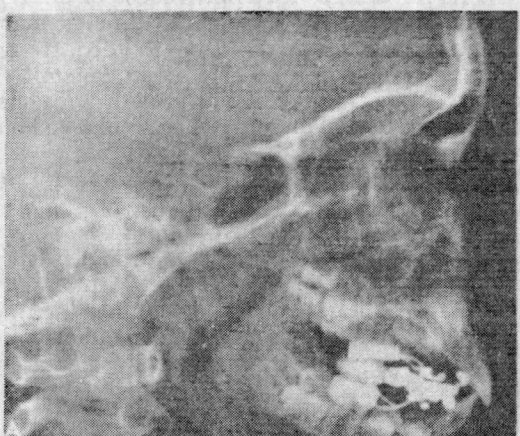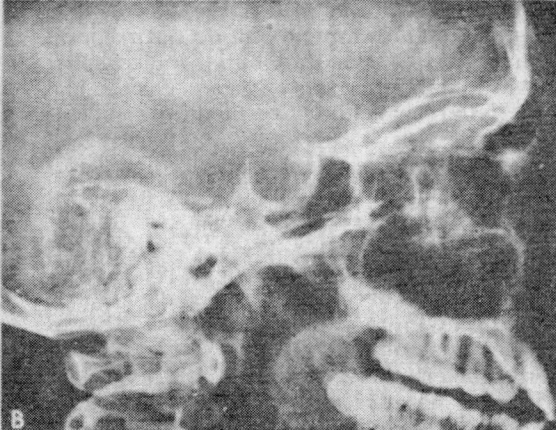

Figure 18–1 *A*, Roentgenograph of skull of 9 yr old boy with polydipsia, polyuria, nocturia, and enuresis. Urine specific gravity was 1.016 after water deprivation. Growth was normal, and the sella turcica was considered roentgenographically to be at upper limit of normal, but was probably enlarged. Over the ensuing 6 mo the symptoms of diabetes insipidus abated. *B*, The patient returned at 14 yr of age because of growth failure and delay in sexual maturation. Studies revealed a deficiency of growth hormone, gonadotropins, corticotropin, and thyrotropin. Note enlargement and thinning of the sella turcica but absence of intrasellar or suprasellar calcification. Neurologic and ophthalmologic examinations were normal. There was exacerbation of diabetes insipidus with administration of hydrocortisone and thyroxine. At surgery a large craniopharyngioma was found.

may be the 1st symptom. The excessive thirst is disturbing and interferes with play, learning, and sleep. Children with diabetes insipidus do not perspire; their skin is dry and pale. Anorexia is common; there is a preference for carbohydrates.

Other signs and symptoms depend on the primary lesion; for example, patients with tumors in the region of the hypothalamus may have disturbance of growth, progressive cachexia or obesity, hyperpyrexia, sleep disturbance, sexual precocity, or emotional disorders. Lesions initially causing diabetes insipidus may eventually destroy the anterior pituitary; in such instances the diabetes insipidus tends to become milder or disappear completely.

Laboratory Data. The daily volume of urine may be 4–10 or more liters. The urine is pale or colorless; the specific gravity varies from 1.001–1.005, with a corresponding osmolality of 50–200 mOsm/kg water. During periods of severe dehydration the specific gravity may rise to 1.010 and the osmolality to 300. Other renal function studies are normal. Serum osmolality is normal with adequate hydration. During water deprivation tests patients must be closely observed to prevent surreptitious intake of water on the one hand and to avoid severe and rapid development of dehydration on the other. In patients with severe deficiency a 3 hr period of dehydration leads to elevation of plasma osmolality, while urine osmolality characteristically remains below plasma levels. Administration of exogenous DDAVP or vasopressin quickly raises urine osmolality. When the polyuria is mild and the deficiency incomplete, urine osmolality may exceed that of plasma and the response to vasopressin is attenuated.

A highly sensitive radioimmunoassay for vasopressin may eventually replace water deprivation tests. Plasma levels consistently below 0.5 pg/ml indicate severe neurogenic diabetes insipidus. Vasopressin levels that are subnormal for the concomitant hyperosmolality indicate partial neurogenic diabetes insipidus. The assay is particularly useful in distinguishing partial diabetes insipidus from primary polydipsia.

Roentgenograms of the skull may reveal evidence of an intracranial tumor such as calcifications, enlargement of the sella turcica, erosion of the clinoid processes, or increased width of the suture lines. Roentgenograms of the skull or other bones in patients with the reticuloendothelioses may reveal areas of rarefaction. Computed tomography of the brain is indicated.

Differential Diagnosis. Polydipsia, polyuria, and impaired concentration are common in patients with hypercalcemia or potassium deficiency. In the young male infant nephrogenic diabetes insipidus must be differentiated from congenital or inherited types of vasopressin deficiency; failure of response to exogenous vasopressin (Pitressin) is a critical differential criterion.

Compulsive water drinking (*psychogenic polydipsia*) is rare but may easily be confused with diabetes insipidus. Affected persons are usually able to produce a concentrated urine when fluids are withheld. Occasionally, however, diagnosis is difficult because prolonged polydipsia lowers the maximal urinary concentrations achievable following dehydration or even following infusion of hypertonic saline solution. As a rule, a urine osmolality greater after dehydration than after administration of vasopressin alone indicates the ability to secrete vasopressin. On the other hand, if administration of vasopressin produces a urinary osmolality substantially higher than dehydration alone, vasopressin secretion is deficient. This rule seems to apply no matter how low or high urinary concentration may be.

Defects in urinary concentrations also occur in a variety of chronic renal disorders. Familial nephronophthisis, in particular, can mimic diabetes insipidus. Elevated plasma levels of urea and creatinine, anemia, and isotonic rather than hypotonic urine are characteristics of primary renal disease.

A familial syndrome is characterized by *intermittent polyuria, seizures,* and *hyperphosphatemia.* Three of 4 children of a nonconsanguineous marriage had intermittent attacks of profound polyuria (up to 3500 ml/12 hr), massive phosphaturia (up to 500 mg/8 hr), and hypocalcemic tetany. Serum levels of inorganic phosphorus ranged from 12–19 mg/dl. Investigations failed to reveal any renal or endocrine disorder. Between attacks the patients were quite normal.

Prognosis. With the diagnosis of diabetes insipidus the underlying process must be determined. Diabetes insipidus itself rarely threatens life, but it may signify a serious underlying condition. It may be only transitory following trauma or surgical intervention in the region of the hypothalamus or pituitary. In some patients with reticuloendothelioses spontaneous remission occurs, whereas in others diabetes insipidus may be the only residuum long after remission of the primary condition. Amelioration of clinical diabetes insipidus may herald the development of anterior pituitary insufficiency. The prognosis of patients with brain tumors depends upon the site of the lesion and upon the type of neoplastic cell. Occasionally, disturbances of the thirst center accompany diabetes insipidus and seriously complicate the management of problems of water balance.

Treatment. The causative factor deserves 1st consideration in the treatment. Patients with uncomplicated diabetes insipidus may go untreated for years with only the inconvenience of polyuria and polydipsia so long as they have an intact thirst mechanism and are allowed free access to water. Of the effective preparations available for symptomatic treatment the best known is Pitressin tannate in oil, a long-acting preparation which provides relief for 24–72 hr when 0.5–1.0 ml is administered. The dose must be individualized for each patient and should not be repeated until symptoms recur. Since Pitressin tannate is suspended in a viscous oil, careful attention must be given to resuspension by warming under a hot water faucet and shaking vigorously before injecting. Intramuscular injections should be made deep with a 1-inch 20- to 22-gauge needle. Pitressin may also be administered as snuff or nose drops intranasally, or synthetic lysine-8-vasopressin may be administered as a liquid nasal spray; these forms are less satisfactory because they require frequent administration and cause local irritation.

A highly effective agent for the treatment of vasopressin-sensitive diabetes insipidus, 1-desamino-8-D-arginine vasopressin (DDAVP, or desmopressin acetate), is administered intranasally in a dose of 2.5–20 µg

(0.025–0.2 ml) once or twice daily. This vasopressin analogue has the advantage of ease of administration, long duration of action (about 12 hr), and low pressor activity; it is replacing Pitressin preparations as treatment of choice.

Many patients respond satisfactorily to oral administration of chlorpropamide. Though this agent has no antidiuretic effect itself, it potentiates the action of suboptimal amounts of vasopressin. In responsive patients an effect is noted within 24–48 hr. Hypoglycemia is a frequent side effect of treatment, particularly in children with anterior pituitary insufficiency, but a decrease in the dose usually averts this problem. An initial dose of 20 mg/kg/24 hr in 2 divided doses should be reduced to the minimal effective level.

Chlorpropamide is especially useful in those patients who also have hypodipsia from associated involvement of the thirst center since it appears to restore drinking behavior to normal besides controlling the diabetes insipidus.

Great care must be taken with patients with diabetes insipidus who are comatose, undergoing surgery, or receiving intravenous fluids for any reason. Patients receiving Pitressin or chlorpropamide are at considerable risk of the clinical manifestations of hypersecretion of vasopressin (see below) unless the total fluid allotment is kept low; serum sodium concentration must be monitored twice daily.

In children under 2 yr of age, and especially in the newborn, one should avoid the use of Pitressin and particularly of Pitressin tannate in oil. Young children can frequently be managed by low solute feedings, by frequent water between feedings, and, when necessary, by short-acting intranasal Pitressin.

NEPHROGENIC DIABETES INSIPIDUS
(Vasopressin-Insensitive Diabetes Insipidus)

This disorder closely mimics vasopressin deficiency, but levels of the hormone in plasma and urine are normal. Affected patients show no antidiuresis even with large doses of vasopressin, and renal medullary production or release of cyclic AMP is deficient. Administration of vasopressin does result in increased cortisol levels, indicating that at least 1 extrarenal effect of vasopressin is intact and that the end-organ resistance is probably limited to the kidney. The disorder occurs primarily in males as an X-linked dominant trait. Heterozygous females are usually asymptomatic but may exhibit a variable defect in concentration, which is probably explained by the Lyon hypothesis of sex-chromosome inactivation.

For further discussion see Sec 16.26.

18.4 INAPPROPRIATE SECRETION OF ANTIDIURETIC HORMONE
(Hypersecretion of Vasopressin)

The syndrome of inappropriate secretion of antidiuretic hormone (ISADH) is now recognized as one of the most common aberrations of arginine vasopressin (AVP) secretion. In this condition plasma levels of AVP are inappropriately high for the concurrent osmolality of the blood and are not suppressed by further dilution of body fluids.

Etiology.   The syndrome is being recognized in an increasing number of clinical conditions, particularly those involving the central nervous system, including meningitis, encephalitis, brain tumor and abscesses, subarachnoid hemorrhage, Guillain-Barré syndrome, and head trauma. Pneumonia, tuberculosis, acute intermittent porphyria, cystic fibrosis, perinatal asphyxia, use of positive pressure respirators, and certain drugs such as vincristine and vinblastine also produce the syndrome. The mechanism of the disturbed regulation of vasopressin in these conditions is not fully understood, but in many instances it is clear that there is direct involvement of the hypothalamus. The syndrome has been observed in patients with Ewing sarcoma; malignant tumors of the pancreas, duodenum, or thymus; and particularly oat cell carcinoma of the lung. In these instances the tumor presumably synthesizes and secretes vasopressin, the syndrome disappearing when the tumor is removed. In rare instances no cause for the syndrome has been found.

The syndrome has also occurred during chlorpropamide therapy for diabetes mellitus, presumably because this drug potentiates vasopressin. Patients with diabetes insipidus treated with Pitressin or chlorpropamide readily develop the syndrome during periods of excessive ingestion of fluids or during intravenous fluid therapy.

Clinical Manifestations.   The syndrome is probably most often latent and asymptomatic and forms the basis for the long known observation that serum sodium levels may be unexpectedly low in conditions such as pneumonia, tuberculosis, and meningitis. Careful attention to fluid replacement in patients with conditions known to be associated with the syndrome may prevent the development of symptoms.

The clinical manifestations are attributable to hypotonicity of body fluids and are those of water intoxication. If the serum sodium is not below 120 mEq/l, there may be no symptoms. Early, there is loss of appetite followed by nausea and sometimes vomiting. Irritability and personality changes, including hostility and confusion, may occur. When the serum sodium falls below 110 mEq/l, neurologic abnormalities and/or stupor are common, and convulsive seizures may also occur. Skin turgor and blood pressure are normal, and there is no evidence of dehydration.

Serum sodium and chloride concentrations are low, whereas serum bicarbonate usually remains normal. Despite low serum sodium there is continued renal excretion of sodium. The serum is hypo-osmolar, but the urine is less than maximally dilute and its osmolality greater than appropriate for the tonicity of the serum. Renal and adrenal functions are normal.

Treatment.   Successful treatment of the underlying disorder (meningitis, pneumonia) is followed by spontaneous remission. Immediate management of the hyponatremia consists simply of *restriction of fluids*. Sodium should be made available to replace the sodium loss; hypertonic saline solution is usually of little benefit, however, since even large sodium loads are excreted in the urine. In instances of severe water intoxication, with convulsions or coma, administration of hypertonic saline solution will increase osmolality and control the central nervous system manifestations. In such emergencies administration of furosemide with 300 ml/M² of 1.5% sodium chloride will cause both a rise in sodium levels and a diuresis. Demeclocycline interferes with the action of AVP on the renal tubule. Experience in adults with ISADH indicates that this agent may be useful, but its role in the treatment of children is not established.

18.5 HYPERPITUITARISM

Hypersecretion of pituitary hormones is an expected finding in conditions in which deficiency of a target organ gives decreased hormonal feedback, as in primary hypogonadism or hypoadrenalism. In primary hypothyroidism pituitary hyperfunction and hyperplasia can enlarge and erode the sella and on rare occasions increase intracranial pressure. Such changes are not to be confused with primary pituitary tumors; they disappear when the underlying thyroid condition is treated.

Primary hypersecretion of pituitary hormones is usually associated with a suspected or proven neoplasm of the pituitary; it is rare in childhood. The principal hormone-secreting tumors are eosinophilic adenoma (growth hormone), basophilic adenoma (ACTH), and chromophobe adenoma (prolactin). There is mounting evidence that these tumors may in some instances be secondary to primary defects in the hypothalamus, with stimulation of the pituitary by hypothalamic releasing factors. Any pituitary tumor may cause pituitary insufficiency by compression of pituitary tissue.

PITUITARY GIGANTISM AND ACROMEGALY

In young persons with open epiphyses, overproduction of growth hormone results in gigantism; in persons with closed epiphyses, acromegaly results. Often some acromegalic features are seen with gigantism, even in children and adolescents; after closure of the epiphyses, the acromegalic features become more prominent.

Etiology. Pituitary gigantism is rare. The cause is most often an eosinophilic adenoma, but gigantism has been observed in a 2.5 yr old boy with a hypothalamic tumor. Two boys with McCune-Albright syndrome and accelerated growth have had functioning pituitary tumors; levels of growth hormone were markedly elevated and were not suppressed by a glucose tolerance test. Because of the rarity of eosinophilic adenoma few children with this tumor have had evaluation of pituitary function by currently available techniques. Tumors in many adults with acromegaly as well as in a 5 yr old child have responded with changes in growth hormone levels to administration of provocative or suppressive agents. These data suggest that in some patients gigantism and acromegaly may begin as a hypothalamic disturbance, resulting in hypertrophy and hyperplasia and, ultimately, in tumors of somatotropic cells.

Clinical Manifestations. In most of the recorded cases the abnormal growth became evident at puberty, but the condition has been established as early as 5 yr of age. Giants may grow to a height of 8 ft or more. Acromegaly consists chiefly in enlargement of the distal parts of the body, but manifestations of abnormal growth actually involve all portions. The circumference of the skull increases, the nose becomes broad, and the tongue is often enlarged, with coarsening of the facial features. The mandible grows excessively, and the teeth become separated. The fingers and toes grow chiefly in thickness. There may be dorsal kyphosis. Fatigue and lassitude are early symptoms. Delayed sexual maturation or hypogonadism may occur. Signs of increased intracranial pressure appear later; visual loss may be demonstrable only on careful examination of visual fields.

Laboratory Data. Growth hormone levels are elevated and may occasionally reach 400 ng/ml. Random fluctuations are common, with no increase in secretion during deep sleep. There is usually no suppression of growth hormone levels by the hyperglycemia of a glucose tolerance test. There may be no response, normal responses, or paradoxical responses to various other stimuli. For example, L-dopa may paradoxically decrease growth hormone levels. Surprisingly, administration of TRF results in increased growth hormone levels in some acromegalics and in a 5 yr old giant resulted in a 3-fold increase in levels of growth hormone. Somatomedin C levels are consistently elevated in acromegaly, levels in 1 study ranging from 2.6–21.7 U/ml in contrast to normal levels of 0.31–1.4 U/ml. Detailed evaluation of each child is indicated because the results of such studies not only increase insight into pathologic mechanisms but also provide clues to therapeutic management.

Adenomas may compromise other anterior pituitary function through growth or cystic degeneration. Secretion of gonadotropins, TSH, and/or ACTH may be impaired. Prolactin levels may be elevated; and in 1 instance a tumor was shown to secrete prolactin and growth hormone.

Roentgenograms of the skull may reveal enlargement of the sella turcica and of the paranasal sinuses. Tufting of the phalanges and increased heel pad thickness are common. Osseous maturation is normal.

Differential Diagnosis. In the differential diagnosis hereditary tall stature must be considered; in this condition there is usually abnormal height in 1 or both parents or in close relatives. Such tall persons are well proportioned and free of signs of increased intracranial pressure. Excessive growth during preadolescence in obese children is a temporary state; though such children may become tall, they do not attain the height of giants. Children with precocious puberty are often unusually tall but do not develop into giants since their epiphyses close early and growth ceases prematurely. Patients with tall stature associated with untreated thyrotoxicosis, hypogonadism, or Marfan syndrome are easily distinguished clinically and have normal levels of growth hormone. Gigantism and increased growth hormone levels may occur in some patients with lipodystrophy, but absence of subcutaneous fat is a characteristic finding; there is increasing evidence for disordered hypothalamic function in this condition. Cerebral gigantism, which is far more common than pituitary gigantism, can usually be differentiated on clinical grounds (see below).

Treatment.   Treatment is difficult and controversial. If there is evidence of increased intracranial pressure, surgical intervention is indicated. In the absence of ocular symptoms such as choked discs and constricted visual fields, irradiation, either conventional or with high energy proton beams, may be an effective form of therapy. Bromocriptine, a dopamine agonist, has been effective in managing a 9 yr old boy in whom surgery and irradiation were not successful.

CEREBRAL GIGANTISM

This disorder, like pituitary gigantism, is characterized by rapid growth; growth hormone levels in the serum are not elevated, however, and evidence suggests a cerebral defect for the pathogenetic mechanism. Birth weight and length are above the 90th percentile in most affected infants, and macrocrania may be noted. Growth is rapid, and by 1 yr of age all affected infants are over the 97th percentile in height. Accelerated growth continues for the 1st 4–5 yr, and then a normal rate is observed. Puberty usually occurs at the normal time but may occur slightly early. The hands and feet are large, with thickened subcutaneous tissue. The head is large and dolichocephalic, the jaw prominent; there is hypertelorism, and the eyes have an antimongoloid slant. Clumsiness and awkward gait are characteristic, and affected children have great difficulty in sports, in learning to ride a bicycle, and in other tasks requiring coordination. Mental retardation is almost always associated; it may vary considerably in degree but is not progressive. (See Fig 18–2.)

Roentgenograms reveal a large skull, a high orbital roof, a sella of normal size but slightly posterior inclination, and an increased interorbital distance. Osseous maturation is compatible with the patient's height. Growth hormone levels are normal, and 17-ketosteroids are only slightly increased. Abnormal electroencephalograms are common; other studies will frequently reveal a dilated ventricular system.

The cause of the disorder is unknown; nor is it clear whether all patients with this syndrome have the same defect. This syndrome may be caused by a hypothalamic defect, but none has been demonstrated. Familial cases have been reported. Affected patients may be at increased risk of development of malignancies such as Wilms tumor and hepatic carcinoma.

PROLACTINOMA

Prolactin-secreting pituitary adenomas are the most common tumor of the pituitary in adults but have been only recently recognized in children. Headache is a common presenting finding. Decreased growth rate, delayed puberty, secondary amenorrhea, galactorrhea, and gynecomastia are other manifestations. Primary amenorrhea may be a presenting manifestation on occasion. Prolactin levels are markedly elevated (as high as 5000 ng/ml) and are not increased by TRH stimulation. Some of the tumors are large and invasive but

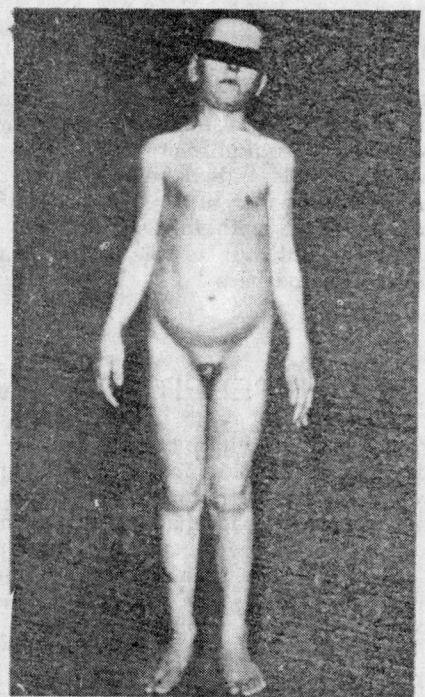

Figure 18–2   Cerebral gigantism in an 8 yr old boy. Height age was 12 yr; bone age, 12 yr; IQ, 60; abnormal electroencephalogram. Note prominence of forehead and jaw and the large hands and feet. Sexual development was consistent with chronologic age. Hormone studies were normal. Adult height was 208 cm (6 ft, 10 in); normal sexual development. He wears size 18 shoes.

may be circumscribed. The sella may be enlarged; high-resolution computed tomography may reveal an intersellar mass. Treatment consists of surgical excision and/or radiotherapy.

18.6   PRECOCIOUS PUBERTY

Physiology of Puberty.   The hypothalamus, pituitary, and gonads are active and interacting for years before appearance of the secondary sex characteristics associated with puberty. Levels of FSH and LH are low but measurable throughout childhood and rise slowly during the prepubertal years. An active hypothalamic-pituitary-gonadal interaction prior to puberty is demonstrated by the fact that patients with Turner syndrome or with anorchia have levels of gonadotropins higher than those of normal children of the same age. The prepubertal gonad is capable of responding to stimulation; administration of human chorionic gonadotropin to prepubertal boys results in marked increases in testosterone levels. Factors which influence the onset of puberty are being unraveled, but the details remain obscure. Prior to puberty very small amounts of gonadal steroids are able to suppress the hypothalamus and pituitary. With the onset of puberty the hypothalamic "gonadostat" becomes progressively less sensitive to the suppressive effects of sex steroids on gonadotropin secretion. Consequently LH and FSH levels increase and stimulate the gonad, and a new homeostatic level is achieved (gonadarche). This decrease in hypothalamic sensitivity is thought to be important to the onset of puberty. In girls at puberty, a sharp rise in FSH production precedes the increase in plasma estradiol; in boys LH production rises prior to the sharp increase in testosterone. Plasma levels of bioactive LH increase more during puberty than those of immunoreactive LH; thus, qualitative as well as quantitative changes occur in LH. FSH and LH act synergistically to promote changes in the gonad at puberty.

Other evidence suggests that neither pituitary nor gonadal maturation is involved in the initiation of puberty; for example, pulsed administration of luteinizing hormone–releasing hormone (LRH) can induce puberty in the infantile monkey. The factors which activate the dormant hypothalamic mechanism are unknown. It appears that a neuronal oscillator discharging at approximately hourly intervals causes a discharge of LRH and in turn LH. Pulsatile discharge of LH is of considerable significance in onset of puberty and in reproductive physiology.

A 2nd critical event occurs in middle or late adolescence, at least in girls, in whom cyclicity and ovulation occur. A positive feedback mechanism develops whereby rising levels of estrogen in midcycle cause a distinct increase (rather than decrease) of LH. Prior to midadolescence this ability of estrogen to release LH is not found. Other changes known to occur at the onset of puberty include an increase in LH release during sleep and increased ability of the pituitary to release LH in response to LRH administration.

Adrenal cortical androgens also play a role in pubertal maturation (adrenarche). Levels of dehydroepiandrosterone (DHA) and its sulfate (DHAS) begin to rise before the earliest physical changes of puberty. This increase occurs before those of gonadotropins, testosterone, or estradiol at about 6 yr of age; the rise is more rapid in girls than in boys. DHAS is the most abundant adrenal C-19 steroid in blood, but its function is unknown. It has been postulated that an adrenal androgen-stimulating factor other than ACTH initiates adrenarche, but direct evidence is lacking.

Age of onset of puberty is variable and more closely correlated with osseous maturation than with chronologic age. In girls the breast bud is usually the 1st sign of puberty (10–11 yr) and the interval to menarche is usually 2–2.5 yr but may be as long as 6 yr. In the United States about 95% of girls have at least 1 sign of puberty by 12 yr, and the mean age of menarche is about 12½ yr. Peak height velocity always precedes menarche and is attained about 2 yr earlier in girls than in boys. There are, however, wide variations in the sequence of changes involving growth spurt, breast, pubic hair, and genital development.

Genetic and environmental factors also affect onset of puberty. The drop in menarchal age in the past century is probably due to better nutrition and improved general health. Black girls are significantly more advanced in development of secondary sex characteristics than white girls. Ballet dancers, gymnasts, swimmers, runners, and other girl athletes in whom leanness

and strenuous physical activity have coexisted from early childhood frequently exhibit a marked delay in puberty and/or menarche. This observation supports the thesis that there may be a relation between weight and body composition and pubertal maturation.

In boys, growth of the testes is the 1st sign of puberty (prepubertal testicular volume is 2–4 cc). This is followed by pigmentation and thinning of the scrotum and growth of the penis. Pubic hair then appears. Appearance of axillary hair usually marks the midpoint of puberty. In boys, unlike girls, acceleration of growth begins after puberty is well under way and is maximal from 14–16 yr of age; growth may continue well beyond 18 yr of age.

Precocious puberty is difficult to define because of the marked variation in the age at which puberty begins normally. Onset of puberty before 8.5 yr of age in girls and 10 yr in boys may be considered precocious, but these are arbitrary guidelines.

Precocious pubertal development may be classified as true precocious puberty or precocious pseudopuberty. True precocious puberty is always isosexual and indicates not only precocity of the secondary sexual characteristics but also an increase in the size and activity of the gonads. In precocious pseudopuberty some of the secondary sex characteristics appear, but the gonads do not mature and there is no activation of normal pituitary-hypothalamic-gonadal interplay. In this latter group the sex characteristics may be isosexual or heterosexual and will be discussed later. (See Sec 18.23, 18.30, and 18.34.)

18.7 TRUE PRECOCIOUS PUBERTY

PRECOCIOUS PUBERTY WITHOUT OTHER PATHOLOGIC FINDINGS (CONSTITUTIONAL)

In about 80–90% of girls and about 50% of boys with precocious puberty no causative factor can be found. Presumably the normal hypothalamic mechanism which initiates puberty is precociously activated. In many affected children there are electroencephalographic abnormalities, suggesting a primary cerebral abnormality. The condition occurs far more frequently in girls and is usually sporadic. In males the disorder may be familial; the usual pattern of transmission is as a sex-limited autosomal dominant trait transmitted only by affected males to half their sons.

Clinical Manifestations. The clinical course is extremely variable. Affected children may complete sexual maturation rapidly or slowly; manifestations may remain stationary or even regress, only to resume development later. Sexual development may begin at any age. In girls the 1st sign is development of the breasts; pubic hair may appear simultaneously but more often appears later. Development of the external genitalia, the appearance of axillary hair, and the onset of menstruation follow. The early menstrual cycles may be more irregular than with normal puberty. Menarche has been observed within the 1st yr of life. The initial cycles are usually anovulatory, but pregnancy has been reported as early as 5.5 yr of age (Fig 18–3).

In boys enlargement of the penis and testes, appear-

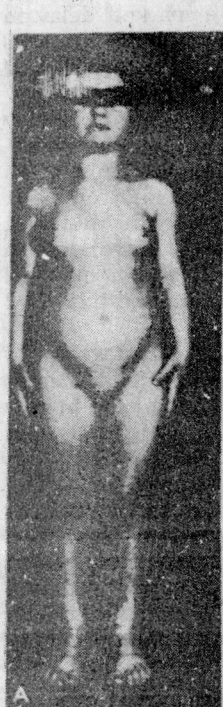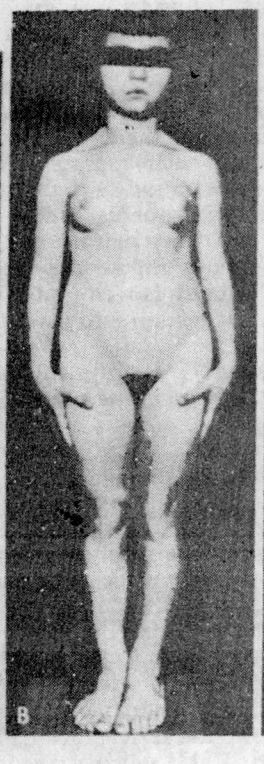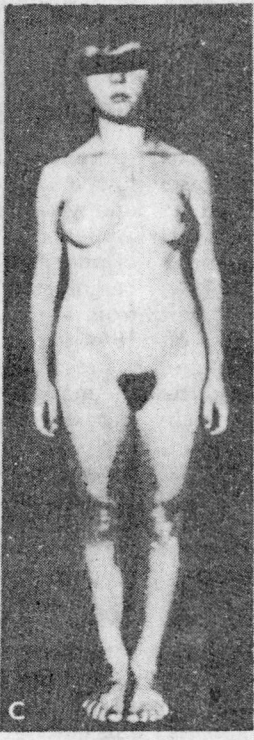

Figure 18–3 Idiopathic precocious puberty. Patient at *(A)* 3¹¹/₁₂, *(B)* at 5⁸/₁₂, and *(C)* at 8½ yr of age. Breast development and vaginal bleeding began at 2½ yr of age. Osseous age was 7½ yr at 3¹¹/₁₂ and 14 yr at 8 yr of age. Repeated estrogen assays have varied between 12–132 mouse units. Urinary gonadotropins were not demonstrable until the child was 5 yr of age. 17-Ketosteroids varied between 1.6–2.1 mg/24 hr during the 1st 5 yr of life. Intelligence and dental age are normal for chronologic age. Growth was completed at 10 yr; ultimate height was 14 cm (56 in).

ance of pubic hair, acne, and frequent erections occur. The voice deepens, and linear growth is accelerated. Spermatogenesis has been observed as early as 5–6 yr of age, and nocturnal emissions may occur. Testicular biopsies have shown all elements of the testes to be stimulated. If the precocity is complete, various degrees of spermatogenesis are present; even if it is incomplete, the interstitial cells are present (Fig 18–4).

In both girls and boys height, weight, and osseous maturation are advanced. The increased rate of ossification results in early closure of epiphyses so that ultimate stature is less than it would have been otherwise. Approximately one third of patients do not achieve a height of 152 cm (5 ft) as adults. Dental age and mental development are usually compatible with chronologic age.

Laboratory Data. Levels of plasma FSH and LH may be elevated for the age of the patient. In as many as 50% of patients, however, there is overlap with levels in normal children of the same age. Serial determinations often reveal that elevated and normal levels alternate. Measurements of gonadotropin excretion in timed collections of urine, either for 3 hr or overnight, provide more accurate and sensitive tests of gonadotropin function in children. Markedly elevated LH levels should suggest the presence of a human chorionic gonadotropin (hCG) secreting tumor since most assays for LH cross-react with hCG.

Plasma testosterone (in boys) and estradiol (in girls) are usually elevated to levels consistent with the stage of puberty and osseous maturation. Like normal pubertal girls, girls with idiopathic precocious puberty may have wide fluctuations of levels of estrogens.

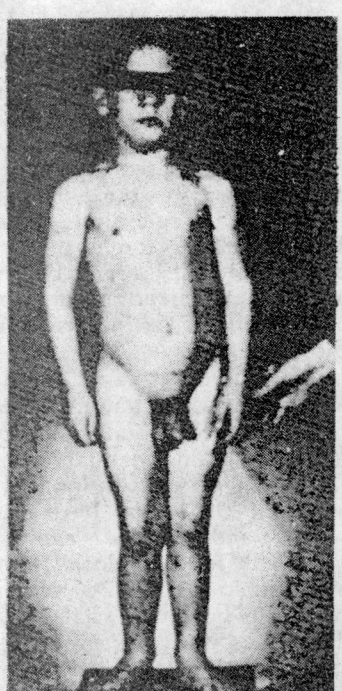

Figure 18–4 Precocious puberty without a demonstrable lesion in a 3.5 yr old boy. Height age was 5 yr and bone age, 8 yr. Urinary gonadotropins were demonstrable; 17-ketosteroids, 1.9 mg/24 hr. Note well developed testes; testicular biopsy revealed Leydig cells and well developed tubules with adult spermatogonia. At 5 yr of age the boy had a height age of 10 yr and osseous maturation of 14 yr. Growth ceased at 9 yr; ultimate stature was 148.6 cm (58.5 in). He had no neurologic abnormalities and was bright-normal in intelligence and well-adjusted emotionally.

Table 18-2 CONDITIONS CAUSING PRECOCIOUS PUBERTY

True precocious puberty
  Central nervous system lesions
    Brain tumor, hypothalamic hamartoma, craniopharyngioma,
      germinoma, pineal tumor, neurofibromatosis, postencephalitis
      scar, tuberous sclerosis, hydrocephalus
  McCune-Albright syndrome
  Prolonged primary hypothyroidism
  Gonadotropin-secreting tumor
    Hepatoblastoma, hepatoma
    Chorionepithelioma
    Polyembryoma
    Posterior mediastinum in association with Klinefelter syndrome
  Therapy of virilizing adrenal hyperplasia
  Idiopathic (constitutional, functional)
    Sporadic
    Familial
      Male limited autosomal dominant
      Isolated elevation of LH
  Administration of gonadotropins
Precocious pseudopuberty
  Females
    Isosexual (feminization)
      Ovarian tumors
        Granulosa–theca cell tumor
        Teratoma, chorionepithelioma
        Sex cord tumor with annular tubules (associated with Peutz-
          Jeghers syndrome)
        Autonomous functional cyst of ovary
        McCune-Albright syndrome
      Adrenocortical tumor
      Exogenous estrogen
    Heterosexual (virilization)
      Congenital adrenal hyperplasia
      Adrenocortical tumor
        Testosterone-secreting tumor
      Androblastoma (arrhenoblastoma)
      Androgen-producing teratoma
      Exogenous androgen
  Males
    Isosexual (masculinization)
      Congenital adrenal hyperplasia
      Adrenocortical tumor
      Leydig cell hyperplasia
      Leydig cell tumor
      Teratoma (containing adenocortical tissue)
      Exogenous androgen
    Heterosexual (feminization)
      Adrenocortical tumor
      Exogenous estrogen
      Sertoli cell tumor
      Sex cord tumor with annular tubules (associated with Peutz-
        Jeghers syndrome)
Partial precocious puberty
  Premature adrenarche (pubarche)
  Premature thelarche

Urinary 17-ketosteroids may be normal or only slightly elevated. Osseous maturation is advanced and consistent with the stage of pubertal development. Electroencephalographic abnormalities may be present.

Differential Diagnosis. In girls, lesions of the central nervous system, tumors of the ovaries, feminizing adrenocortical tumors, McCune-Albright syndrome, and exogenous sources of estrogens must be considered in the differential diagnosis. A carefully obtained history, a complete physical examination, and appropriate laboratory studies usually resolve the diagnosis. Examination by ultrasonography may be indicated to outline the ovaries. Computed tomography of the brain is helpful in ruling out tumors. Early, true precocious puberty may be impossible to differentiate from premature thelarche when breast development is the only manifestation. Plasma gonadotropin levels may be normal or only slightly elevated. A period of follow-up may be necessary to establish the diagnosis.

In boys, cerebral lesions, adrenogenital syndrome, Leydig cell tumor, and gonadotropin-producing hepatoma must be considered diagnostic possibilities. In the *adrenogenital syndrome* the testes are small relative to the degree of sexual maturation. A *Leydig cell tumor* can usually be detected on physical examination, and a *hepatoma* usually causes hepatomegaly.

When there is no evidence of a cerebral lesion, even on computed tomography, the child must be carefully and repeatedly observed for several yr before the possibility of an intracranial lesion can be excluded.

Treatment. Treatment consists essentially of psychologic management of patient and family. A detailed explanation to the parents with the reassurance of the harmlessness of the condition is imperative. They should also be told that the precocious manifestations will persist but that by the age of 10–14 yr the child will not be different from other children. Such children should also be guarded against abuses that could result in pregnancy. The few data available indicate that these patients have a normal reproductive span and that menopause takes place within the usual time.

Medroxyprogesterone acetate (Provera) has been used to treat children with precocious puberty; it results in cessation of menses and regression of breast development in girls and will depress testosterone levels in boys. On the other hand, growth and skeletal maturation usually continue unabated with common side effects, including suppression of the pituitary-adrenal axis, cushingoid manifestations, and alterations of testicular histology. These considerations markedly limit the usefulness of this agent. Danazol, an ethinyl analogue, has antigonadotropic but also androgenic activity; its usefulness is limited. Cyproterone acetate, an antiandrogen, has not been used in the United States; it seems to offer little advantage over medroxyprogesterone acetate.

A new but still investigative approach to treatment consists of daily subcutaneous administration of an analogue of luteinizing hormone–releasing hormone (LRH) that is more potent and has a longer duration of action than native LRH. To maintain sustained release of gonadotropin, pituitary gonadotropic cells require intermittent periods of absence of stimulation by LRH. Intermittent administration of a long-acting LRH suppresses pulsatile discharges of gonadotropins. Short term studies indicate that the effect is reversible when the agent is discontinued. Long term studies are under way to evaluate the usefulness of the agent in the management of true precocious puberty.

PRECOCIOUS PUBERTY WITH POLYOSTOTIC FIBROUS DYSPLASIA AND ABNORMAL PIGMENTATION
(McCune-Albright Syndrome)

When fibrous dysplasia of the skeletal system is associated with patchy cutaneous pigmentation and endocrine dysfunction, the association is referred to as McCune-Albright syndrome. The most common endocrine disturbance is sexual precocity, but hyperthyroidism or Cushing syndrome may also occur. The condition affects many more girls than boys. For many years the disorder was presumed to originate in the hypothalamus, but data now suggest that endocrine disorders in this syndrome may result from autonomous hyperfunction of the peripheral target glands. For example, it is now established that the hyperthyroidism in this condition is not hypothalamic in origin since TSH is suppressed. The hyperthyroidism differs from Graves disease in that the goiters tend to be multinodular and there is an equal distribution between males and females. In the instances of associated Cushing syndrome the lesions were bilateral nodular adrenocortical hyperplasia; in 1 case the plasma levels of ACTH were low. Studies of the sexual precocity in some girls found suppressed levels of FSH and LH and markedly elevated plasma levels of estradiol and estrone; functioning ovarian cysts were found, and surgical excision resulted in return to normal of the levels of estrogen. It is still uncertain whether hypothalamic dysfunction may have initiated the sequence of events leading to autonomous ovarian, adrenal, or pituitary lesions (Fig 18–5).

The average age of menarche in affected girls is about 3 yr, but vaginal bleeding has occurred as early as 4 mo of age and secondary sex characteristics at 6 mo. The Cushing syndrome has occurred in early infancy, antedating the sexual precocity. The onset of hyperthyroidism occurs in most instances from 3–12 yr, though it has occurred as early as 9 mo. Gigantism and acromegaly may occur with or without precocious puberty. In 2 boys, markedly elevated levels of growth hormone

were not suppressed during a glucose tolerance test; a functioning pituitary chromophobe adenoma was found in 1, an eosinophilic adenoma in the other.

In view of these findings, it cannot be assumed that the precocity is central in origin; accordingly, all patients must be thoroughly investigated. Elevated FSH and LH levels will suggest a hypothalamic etiology, but suppressed levels point to a functional ovarian lesion that may require surgical intervention. Cushing syndrome requires adrenalectomy; hyperthyroidism is treated as in any other patient with Graves disease. Prognosis is favorable for longevity, but deformities may result from the bony lesions and repeated pathologic fractures. The osseous lesions become static in adult life.

PRECOCIOUS PUBERTY RESULTING FROM ORGANIC BRAIN LESIONS

Etiology. A wide variety of lesions of the central nervous system have been associated with sexual precocity. How these lesions activate the hypothalamic mechanisms which initiate puberty is not known, but they all involve the hypothalamus by scarring, invasion, or pressure. Among the more common lesions are pinealomas, optic gliomas, suprasellar teratomas, neurofibromas, astrocytomas, and ependymomas. Hypothalamic hamartomas (benign nodules composed of nerve cells and attached to both the maxillary bodies and tuber cinereum) are often associated with precocious puberty. Evidence suggests that their autonomous function may release luteinizing hormone–releasing hormone into vessels which communicate with the pituitary portal blood system. Rarely, intracranial tumors cause precocious puberty in boys by secreting human chorionic gonadotropin (hCG), which stimulates

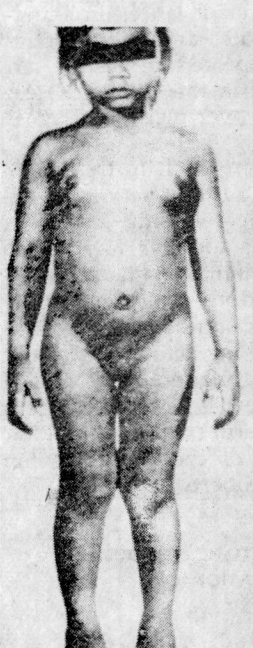
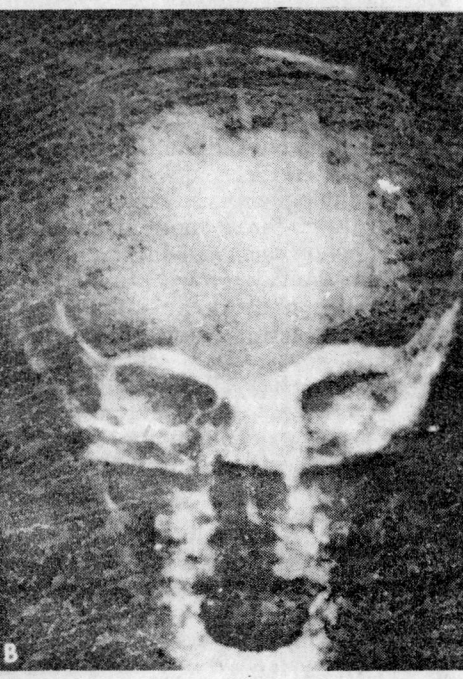

Figure 18–5 Precocious puberty associated with polyostotic fibrous dysplasia (McCune-Albright syndrome) in a girl 4.5 yr of age; at this time her height age and osseous age were normal. Menarche occurred at 4 yr. A, Note bilateral breast development, hyperpigmented spots on abdomen, and prominence on left side of face. B, Roentgenograms revealed fibrous dysplasia in the distal end of the left ulna and the thickening of the bones about the left orbit and the maxillary portion of the frontal bones shown here.

the Leydig cells of the testes. An intracranial hCG-secreting germinoma found in a prepubertal girl did not cause precocious puberty because FSH was not present. Postencephalitic scars, tuberculous meningoencephalitis, hydrocephalus, and tuberous sclerosis have all, on occasion, been etiologic factors (Fig 18–6).

Some of these tumors grow slowly and produce no signs other than precocious puberty. Accordingly, a child who is considered initially to have precocious puberty without a lesion may eventually exhibit signs of increased intracranial pressure and be found to have a tumor. Other hypothalamic signs or symptoms such as diabetes insipidus, hypernatremia secondary to impaired osmoregulation of ADH secretion, hyperthermia, obesity, cachexia, and unnatural crying or laughing may suggest the possibility of an intracranial lesion. A history of convulsions, retarded mental development, or other neurologic signs should also suggest a lesion of the central nervous system.

Clinical Manifestations. An intracranial tumor is the cause of precocious puberty in about 40% of boys and 10% of girls; the diagnosis of idiopathic precocious puberty can be made with less confidence in boys, therefore, than in girls. The precocity is always isosexual, and the endocrine pattern and laboratory findings are the same as those found in children without demonstrable organic lesions.

Roentgenographic examination of the skull, electroencephalographic studies, and brain scans are essential to adequate examination. Computed tomography (CT scan) is indicated in all boys with true precocious puberty when no specific cause can be found. Whenever neurologic manifestations suggest a space-taking lesion, CT scan, cerebral angiography, pneumoenceph-

alography, or ventriculography may be required to localize the lesion. Gelastic (laughing) seizures in a child with precocious puberty suggest a hypothalamic tumor.

Treatment. Therapy depends on the nature and location of the lesion. Surgical decompression followed by roentgen therapy is usually indicated when removal of the tumor is not possible.

SYNDROME OF PRECOCIOUS PUBERTY AND HYPOTHYROIDISM

In children with untreated hypothyroidism, onset of puberty is usually delayed until epiphyseal maturation has reached 12–13 yr of age. Precocious puberty in a child with untreated hypothyroidism and a prepubertal bone age presents, therefore, a striking appearance and an unexpected association. There have been only several dozen reported instances, but the phenomenon appears to be not uncommon. Among 54 carefully studied children with primary hypothyroidism, half had varying degrees of isosexual development in advance of their osseous maturation.

All affected patients had severe hypothyroidism of long duration with the usual manifestations including retardation of growth and of osseous maturation. The causes of the hypothyroidism include lymphocytic thyroiditis, thyroidectomy, and overtreatment with antithyroid drugs.

A preponderance of the reported instances involved girls, probably reflecting the higher incidence of hypothyroidism in females. A significant number have also had Down syndrome; this observation probably relates to the delay in recognition of hypothyroidism in chil-

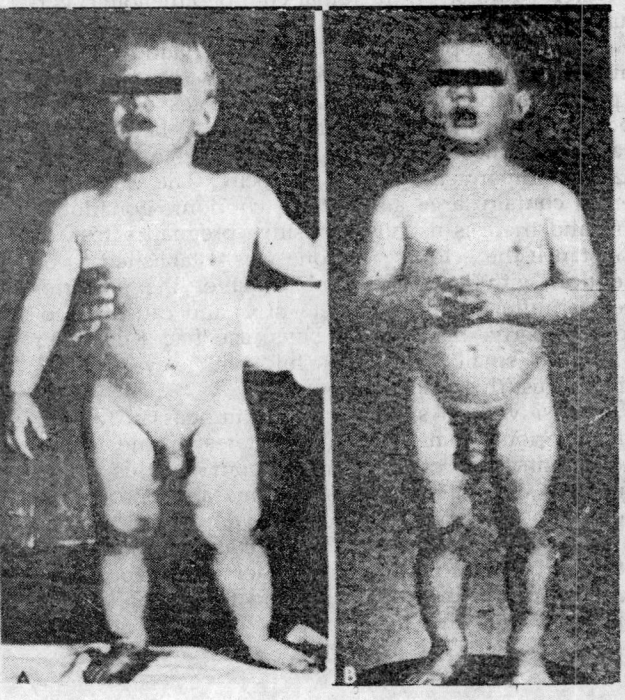

Figure 18–6 Precocious puberty with central nervous system lesion. Photographs at (A) 1.5 and (B) 2.5 yr of age. Accelerated growth, muscular development, osseous maturation, and testicular development were consistent with the degree of secondary sexual maturation. Urinary gonadotropins were repeatedly negative, 17-ketosteroids usually 2–3 mg/24 hr. In early infancy he began having frequent spells of rapid, purposeless motion; later in life he had episodes of uncontrollable laughing with ocular movements. At 7 yr he exhibited emotional lability, aggressive behavior, and destructive tendencies. Although a hypothalamic disorder has been suspected, repeated studies have failed to reveal a space-taking lesion.

dren with Down syndrome. Sexual maturation usually includes breast development in girls and testicular enlargement in boys. Adrenarchal changes of puberty are mild as reflected in sparse or absent pubic and axillary hair. Menstrual bleeding is a common feature, even in girls with minimal breast development. Enlargement of the sella turcica, galactorrhea, excessive pigmentation, and papilledema were present in some. In all instances treatment with thyroid hormone resulted in regression of sexual precocity.

Plasma levels of TSH are markedly elevated. LH, FSH, and prolactin levels are also elevated for reasons as yet unknown. Presumably, thyrotropin-releasing factor is markedly elevated, but in normal individuals it does not cause release of LH and FSH. Whatever the derangement, hypothalamic-pituitary regulating mechanisms rapidly return to normal upon treatment with thyroid hormone.

GONADOTROPIN-SECRETING TUMORS

Hepatic Tumors. Nine instances of isosexual precocious puberty associated with hepatoblastoma or hepatoma have been recorded. All have involved males, the age of onset varying from 8 mo–7 yr. An enlarged liver or mass in the upper quadrant should suggest the diagnosis. Testicular histology reveals interstitial cell hyperplasia and absence of spermatogenesis. The tumor cells produce an ectopic gonadotropin which stimulates precocious maturation of the testes. In 1 instance the gonadotropin was proved to be identical with human chorionic gonadotropin. Plasma levels of alpha-fetoprotein may also be elevated. These 2 biochemical markers are useful for following the effects of therapy. Treatment for these tumors is the same as that for other carcinomas of the liver. All recorded patients with this condition survived less than 1 yr.

Other Tumors. Intracranial chorioepithelioma, germinoma, and other unidentified intracranial tumors may secrete ectopic human chorionic gonadotropin and cause sexual precocity. Choriocarcinoma has also been reported to arise in the ovaries and testes; sexual precocity may be produced by stimulation of the contralateral gonad. These tumors are highly malignant; cachexia may accompany the sexual precocity. The urine and serum contain large amounts of chorionic gonadotropin, and there is usually a positive pregnancy test. In 1 instance the ectopic hormone was established to be identical with hCG. Polyembryoma of the posterior mediastinum may also secrete hCG and cause precocious puberty. Six affected boys also had Klinefelter syndrome; small testes in a child with elevated hCG will suggest this association.

A sensitive and specific radioimmunoassay for human chorionic gonadotropin facilitates diagnosis and the identification of the gonadotropin. By this assay, one third of patients with seminoma and one half of those with embryonal carcinoma have hCG production. In adults it is one of the more common hormones ectopically produced by nontrophoblastic neoplasms. No systematic studies of childhood tumors have been conducted thus far.

PRECOCIOUS PSEUDOPUBERTY

The adrenal causes of pseudopuberty are discussed in Sec 18.24 (adrenogenital syndrome) and in Sec 18.34 and 18.41 (gonads).

18.8 INCOMPLETE (PARTIAL) PRECOCIOUS DEVELOPMENT

Isolated manifestations of precocity without development of other signs of puberty are not unusual; development of the breasts and growth of sexual hair are the 2 most common.

Precocious Thelarche (Simple Development of Breasts). Precocious development of breasts may occur without any other pubertal changes. It most often appears during the 1st yr of life and in about one third of affected infants is present at birth and persists. Breast development in the neonatal period may regress and reappear. The enlargement may involve only 1 breast or 1 breast more than the other. The breast development regresses within 2 yr in 50% of infants; it may persist unchanged 5 yr or longer. Premature thelarche is usually benign; it may be familial in some instances. Growth and osseous maturation are normal; menarche occurs at the normal time. The usual tests for urinary estrogens are negative, and there is no cornification of vaginal epithelium, but plasma levels of estradiol may occasionally be increased. Plasma levels of gonadotropins and prolactin are normal. It is thought that the condition is caused by secretion of small amounts of estrogens by the ovaries, perhaps intermittently. Since enlargement of breasts may be the 1st sign of pseudoprecocious or of true puberty, a prolonged period of observation is indicated in all instances. (See Fig 18–7.)

Premature Adrenarche (Simple Development of Sexual Hair). The appearance of sexual hair at an early age without any other evidence of maturation has been termed *premature adrenarche*. It occurs much more frequently in girls than in boys. Hair appears first on the labia majora, then in the pubic region, and finally in the axilla. Affected children are taller than average, and osseous age is generally 1–4 yr in advance of chronologic age. Urinary 17-ketosteroids and plasma testosterone levels may be slightly increased beyond values normal for age. On the other hand, serum levels of dehydroepiandrosterone sulfate and of other C-19 adrenal steroids are significantly elevated and may be 10 times normal. Gonadotropin levels are usually normal. When this disorder occurs in children with cerebral damage, as it often does, they are usually small for chronologic age and osseous maturation is not advanced. (See Fig 18–8.)

This condition appears to result from premature activation of the adrenal cortex, with secretion of adrenal androgens before the pituitary gonadotropic mechanism becomes activated. The reason for the relatively frequent association of the disorder with cerebral damage is not known. Premature adrenarche must be differentiated from early true precocious puberty, adrenal

18.9 MEDICATIONAL PRECOCITY

A variety of medicaments can induce the appearance of secondary sexual characteristics which may be confused with precocious puberty. A careful history to explore the possibility of accidental exposure to or ingestion of sex hormones is of paramount importance. Precocious pseudopuberty has occurred in both boys and girls from the accidental ingestion of estrogens (including contraceptive pills) and from the administration of anabolic steroids. Contamination of foodstuffs and of vitamin tablets by sex hormones has been reported to cause precocious pseudopuberty. Estrogens in cosmetics may be absorbed through the skin. Exogenous estrogens may produce an intense, dark brown color in the areola of the breasts which is not usually seen in endogenous types of precocity. The precocious changes disappear after cessation of administration of the exogenous hormones.

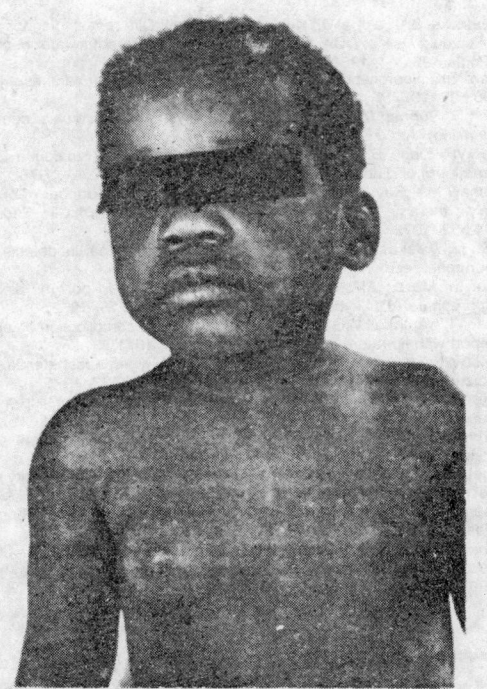

Figure 18–7 Premature thelarche. Simple hypertrophy of the breasts in a 23 mo old girl. No demonstrable urinary estrogens or gonadotropin. Normal genitalia and growth. The disparity in size of the breasts is a common finding in this condition as well as in normal puberty.

cortical tumors, and adrenal hyperplasia. Measurement of plasma androgens, including $17\text{-}\alpha\text{-}$hydroxyprogesterone, testosterone, and androstenedione, may be necessary to rule out mild cases of congenital adrenal hyperplasia. Parents should then be assured that this condition is a harmless variation of development.

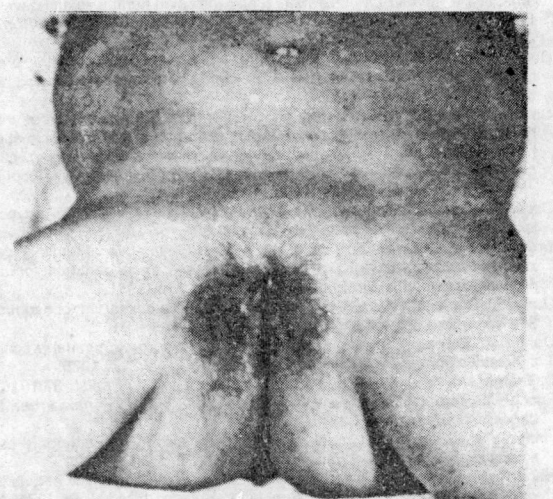

Figure 18–8 Premature adrenarche (pubarche). Isolated development of sexual hair in a 6 yr old girl with cerebral palsy. Urinary 17-ketosteroids varied between 1.5–3.4 mg/24 hr.

General

Grumbach MM, Grave GD, Mayer FF (eds): The Control of the Onset of Puberty. New York, Wiley, 1974.
Williams RH: Textbook of Endocrinology. Ed 6. Philadelphia, WB Saunders, 1981.

Hypopituitarism

Asa SL, Bilbao JM, Kovacs K, et al: Lymphocytic hypophysitis of pregnancy resulting in hypopituitarism: A distinct clinicopathologic entity. Ann Intern Med 95:166, 1981.
Bala RM, Lopatka J, Leung A, et al: Serum immunoreactive somatomedin levels in normal adults, pregnant women at term, children at various ages, and children with constitutionally delayed growth. J Clin Endocrinol Metab 52:508, 1981.
Brooke CGD, Sanders MD, Hoare RD: Septo-optic dysplasia. Br Med J 2:811, 1973.
Draznin M, Steeling MW, Johanson AJ: Silver-Russell syndrome and craniopharyngioma. J Pediatr 96:887, 1970.
Ellyin F, Khatir AH, Singh SP: Hypothalamic-pituitary functions in patients with transsphenoidal encephalocele and midfacial anomalies. J Clin Endocrinol Metab 51:854, 1980.
Fleisher TA, White RM, Broder S, et al: X-linked hypogammaglobulinemia and isolated growth hormone deficiency. N Engl J Med 302:1429, 1980.
Frasier SD: A review of growth hormone stimulation tests in children. Pediatrics 53:929, 1974.
Frasier SD, Aceto T Jr, Hayles AB, et al: Collaborative study of the effects of human growth hormone in growth hormone deficiency. IV. Treatment with low doses of human hormone based on body weight. J Clin Endocrinol Metab 44:22, 1977.
Golde DW, Bersch N, Kaplan SA, et al: Peripheral unresponsiveness to human growth hormone in Laron dwarfism. N Engl J Med 303:1156, 1980.
Hall JG, Pallister PD, Carren SK, et al: Congenital hypothalamic hamartoblastoma, hypopituitarism, imperforate anus, and postaxial polydactyly—a new syndrome? Part 1: Clinical, causal and pathogenetic considerations. Am J Med Genet 7:47, 1980.
Herman SP, Baggenstoss AM, Clothier MD: Liver dysfunction and histologic abnormalities in neonatal hypopituitarism. J Pediatr 87:892, 1975.
Holdaway IM, Rees LH, Landon J: Circulating corticotropin levels in severe hypopituitarism and in the neonate. Lancet 2:1170, 1973.
Jacobs LS, Sneid DS, Garland JT, et al: Receptor-active growth hormone in Laron dwarfism. J Clin Endocrinol Metab 42:403, 1976.
Johanson AJ, Morris GL: A single growth hormone determination to rule out growth hormone deficiency. Pediatrics 59:467, 1977.
Johnson JD, et al: Hypoplasia of the anterior pituitary and neonatal hypoglycemia. J Pediatr 82:634, 1973.
Kaplan SL, Grumbach MM, Triesen HG, et al: Thyrotropin-releasing factor (TRF) effect on secretion of human pituitary prolactin and thyrotropin in children and in idiopathic hypopituitary dwarfism: Further evidence for hypophysiotropic hormone deficiencies. J Clin Endocrinol Metab 35:825, 1972.
Klachko DM, Winder N, Burns TW, et al: Traumatic hypopituitarism occurring before puberty: Survival 35 years untreated. J Clin Endocrinol Metab 28:1768, 1968.
Kleinmann RE, Kazarian EL, Raptopoulos V, et al: Primary empty sella and Rieger's anomaly of the anterior chamber of the eye. N Engl J Med 304:90, 1981.

LaFranchi SH, Lippe BM, Kaplan SA: Hypoglycemia during testing for growth hormone deficiency. J Pediatr 90:244, 1977.

Laron Z, Saul R: Penis and testicular size in patients with growth hormone insufficiency. Acta Endocrinol 63:625, 1970.

Latorre H, Kenney FM, Lahey ME, et al: Short stature and growth hormone deficiency in histiocytosis X. J Pediatr 85:813, 1974.

Lovinger RD, Kaplan SL, Grumbach MM: Congenital hypopituitarism associated with neonatal hypoglycemia and microphallus: Four cases secondary to hypothalamic hormone deficiencies. J Pediatr 87:1171, 1975.

Marks LJ, Bergeson PS: The Silver-Russell syndrome, a case with sexual ambiguity, and a review of the literature. Am J Dis Child 131:447, 1977.

Merimee TJ, Rimoin DL, Cavalli-Sforza LL: Metabolic studies in the African pygmy. J Clin Invest 51:395, 1972.

Merimee TJ, Zapf J, Froesch ER: Dwarfism in the pygmy. An isolated deficiency of insulin-like growth factor I. N Engl J Med 305:965, 1981.

Miller WL, Kaplan SL, Grumbach MM: Child abuse as a cause of post-traumatic hypopituitarism. N Engl J Med 302:724, 1980.

Money J: The syndrome of abuse dwarfism (psychosocial) or reversible hyposomatotropism. Am J Dis Child 131:508, 1977.

O'Dwyer JA, Newton TH, Hoyt WF: Radiologic features of septo-optic dysplasia (deMorsier syndrome). Am J Neuroradiol 1:443, 1980.

Richards GE, et al: Delayed onset of hypopituitarism: Sequelae of therapeutic irradiation of the central nervous system, eye and middle ear tumors. J Pediatr 89:553, 1976.

Rona RJ, Tanner JM: Aetiology of idiopathic growth hormone deficiency in England and Wales. Arch Dis Child 52:197, 1977.

Rosenbloom AL, Riley WJ, Silverstein JH, et al: Low dose single weekly injections of growth hormone? Response during first year of therapy of hypopituitarism. Pediatrics 66:272, 1980.

Rudman D, Davis GT, Priest JH. et al: Prevalence of growth hormone deficiency in children with cleft lip or palate. J Pediatr 93:378, 1978.

Shalet SM, Beardwell CG, Morris Jones PH, et al: Growth hormone deficiency after treatment of acute leukemia in children. Arch Dis Child 51:489, 1976.

Shalet SM, Beardwell CG, Twomey JA, et al: Endocrine function following the treatment of acute leukemia in childhood. J Pediatr 90:920, 1977.

Sklar CA, Grumbach MM, Kaplan SL, Conte FA: Hormonal and metabolic abnormalities associated with central nervous system germinoma in children and adolescents and effect of therapy: Report of 10 patients. J Clin Endocrinol Metab 52:9, 1981.

Tanner JM, Lejarraga H, Cameron N: The natural history of the Silver-Russell syndrome: A longitudinal study of thirty-nine cases. Pediatr Res 9:611, 1975.

Thomasett MJ, Conte FA, Kaplan SL, Grumbach MM: Endocrine and neurologic outcome in childhood craniopharyngioma: Review of effect of treatment in 42 patients. J Pediatr 97:728, 1980.

Hyperpituitarism

AvRuskin TW, Sau K, Tang S, et al: Childhood acromegaly: Successful therapy with conventional radiation and effects of chlorpromazine on growth hormone and prolactin secretin. J Clin Endocrinol Metab 37:380, 1973.

Clemmons DR, Van Wyk JJ, Ridgway EC, et al: Evaluation of acromegaly by radioimmunoassay of somatomedin-C. N Engl J Med 301:1138, 1979.

Costin G, Fefferman RA, Kogut MD: Hypothalamic gigantism. J Pediatr 83:419, 1973.

Guyda H, Robert F, Colle E, et al: Histologic, ultrastructural and hormonal characterization of a pituitary tumor secreting both HGH and prolactin. J Clin Endocrinol Metab 36:531, 1973.

Lightner ES, Winter JSD: Treatment of juvenile acromegaly with bromocriptine. J Pediatr 98:494, 1981.

Lucas C: Diagnostic and developmental aspects of prolactin adenomas in children. Arch Fr Pediatr 37:79, 1980.

Musa BU, Paulsen CA, Conway MJ: Pituitary gigantism. Am J Med 52:399, 1972.

Rappaport EB, Ulstrom RA, Gorlin RJ, et al: Solitary maxillary central incisor and short stature. J Pediatr 91:924, 1977.

Sadeghi-Nejad A, Wolfsdorf JI, Biller BJ, et al: Hyperprolactinemia causing primary amenorrhea. J Pediatr 99:802, 1981.

Sotos JF, Cutler EA: Cerebral gigantism. Am J Dis Child 131:625, 1977.

Spence JH, Trias EP, Raiti S: Acromegaly in a 9½ year old boy. Am J Dis Child 123:504, 1972.

Diabetes Insipidus

Adams JM, Kenny JD, Rudolph AJ: Central diabetes insipidus following intraventricular hemorrhage. J Pediatr 88:292, 1976.

Bartter FC, Schwartz WB: The syndrome of inappropriate secretion of antidiuretic hormone. Am J Med 42:790, 1967.

Bode HH, Harley BM, Crawford JD: Restoration of normal drinking behavior by chlorpropamide in patients with hypodipsia and diabetes insipidus. Am J Med 51:304, 1971.

Braverman LE, Mancini JP, McGoldrick DM: Hereditary idiopathic diabetes insipidus. A case report with autopsy findings. Ann Intern Med 63:503, 1965.

Coggins CH, Leaf A: Diabetes insipidus. Am J Med 42:807, 1967.

Crigler JF: Commentary: On the use of Pitressin in infants with neurogenic diabetes insipidus. J Pediatr 88:295, 1976.

Friedman AL, Segar WE: Antidiuretic hormone excess. J Pediatr 94:521, 1979.

Hays RM: Antidiuretic hormone. N Engl J Med 295:659, 1976.

Hendricks SA, Lippe B, Kaplan SA, et al: Differential diagnosis of diabetes insipidus: Use of DDAVP to terminate the seven-hour water deprivation test. J Pediatr 98:244, 1981.

Khare SK: Neurohypophyseal dysfunction following perinatal asphyxia. J Pediatr 90:628, 1977.

Kohn B, Norman ME, Feldman H, et al: Hysterical polydipsia (compulsive water drinking) Am J Dis Child 130:210, 1976.

Lee WP, Lippe B, LaFranchi SH, et al: Vasopressin analogue DDAVP in the treatment of diabetes insipidus. Am J Dis Child 130:166, 1976.

Linshaw MA, Sey M, DiGeorge AM, et al: A potential danger of oral chlorpropamide therapy: Impaired excretion of a water load. J Clin Endocrinol Metab 34:562, 1972.

Miller M, Dalakos T, Moses AM, et al: Recognition of partial defects in antidiuretic hormone secretion. Ann Intern Med 73:721, 1970.

Miller M, Moses AM: Urinary antidiuretic hormone in polyuric disorders and in appropriate ADH syndrome. Ann Intern Med 77:715, 1972,

Miller VI, Campbell WG Jr: Diabetes insipidus as complication of leukemia: Case report with literature review. Cancer 28:666, 1971.

Muller WL, Meyer WJ, Bartter FC: Intermittent hyperphosphatemia, polyuria, and seizures—a new familial syndrome. J Pediatr 86:233, 1975.

Rallison ML, Tyler FH: Treatment of diabetes insipidus in children with lysine-8-vasopressin. J Pediatr 70:122, 1967.

Richman RA, Post EM, Notman DD, et al: Simplifying the diagnosis of diabetes insipidus in children. Am J Dis Child 135:839, 1981.

Robertson GL, Bhoopalam N, Zelkowitz LJ: Vincristine neurotoxicity and abnormal secretion of antidiuretic hormone. Arch Intern Med 132:717, 1973.

Rosenbloom AL: Chlorpropamide in diabetes insipidus in childhood. Curr Ther Res 13:671, 1971.

Zerbe RL, Robertson GL: A comparison of plasma vasopressin with a standard direct test in the differential diagnosis of polyuria. N Engl J Med 305:1539, 1981.

Precocious Puberty

Aarskog D, Tveteraas E: McCune-Albright syndrome following adrenalectomy for Cushing's syndrome in infancy. J Pediatr 73:89, 1968.

August GP, Hung W, Mayes DM: Plasma androgens in premature pubarche: Value of 17-α-hydroxyprogesterone in differentiation from congenital adrenal hyperplasia. J Pediatr 87:246, 1975.

Barnes ND, Hayles AB, Ryan RJ: Sexual maturation in juvenile hypothyroidism. Mayo Clin Proc 48:849, 1973.

Beas F, Zurbrugg RP, Leibow SG, et al: Familial male sexual precocity: Report of the eleventh kindred found, with observations on blood group linkage and urinary C_{19}-steroid excretion. J Clin Endocrinol Metab 22:1095, 1962.

Bidlingmair F, Butenandt O, Knorr D: Plasma gonadotropins and estrogens in girls with precocious puberty. Pediatr Res 17:91, 1977.

Braunstein GD, Boidson WE, Glass A, et al: In vivo and in vitro production of human chorionic gonadotropin and alpha-fetoprotein by a virilizing hepatoblastoma. J Clin Endocrinol Metab 35:857, 1972.

Braunstein GD, Vaitukaitis JL, Carbone PP, et al: Ectopic production of human chorionic gonadotropin by neoplasms. Ann Intern Med 78:39, 1973.

Bruton OC, Martz DC, Gerard ES: Precocious puberty due to secreting chorionepithelioma (teratoma) of the brain. J Pediatr 59:719, 1961.

Bullough VL: Age at menarche: A misunderstanding. Science 213:365, 1981.

Clements JA, Reyes FI, Winter JSD, et al: Studies on human sexual development. IV. Fetal pituitary and serum, and amniotic fluid concentrations of prolactin. J Clin Endocrinol Metab 44:408, 1977.

Comite F, Cutler GB Jr, River J, et al: Short-term treatment of idiopathic precocious puberty with a long-acting analogue of luteinizing hormone–releasing hormone. N Engl J Med 305:1546, 1981.

Conte FA, Grumbach MM, Kaplan SL, Reiter EO: Correlation of luteinizing hormone–releasing factor–induced luteinizing hormone and follicle-stimulating hormone release from infancy to 19 years with the changing pattern of gonadotropin secretion in agonadal patients: Relation to the restraint of puberty. J Clin Endocrinol Metab 50:163, 1980.

Costin G, Kershnar AK, Kogut MD, et al: Prolactin activity in juvenile hypothyroidism and precocious puberty. Pediatrics 50:881, 1972.

Crowley WF Jr, Comite F, Vale W, et al: Therapeutic use of pituitary desensitization with a long-acting LHRH agonist: A potential new treatment for idiopathic precocious puberty. Clin Endocrinol Metab 52:370, 1981.

Curi JFJ, Vanucci RC, Grossman H, et al: Elevated serum gonadotropins in Silver's syndrome. Am J Dis Child 114:658, 1967.

Danon M, Robboy SJ, Sully R, et al: Cushing syndrome, sexual precocity and polyostotic fibrous dysplasia in infancy. J Pediatr 87:817, 1975.

DiGeorge AM: Albright syndrome: Is it coming of age? J Pediatr 87:1018, 1975.

Frisch RE, Wyshak G, Vincent L: Delayed menarche and amenorrhea in ballet dancers. N Engl J Med 303:17, 1980.

Harlan WR, Grillo GP, Cornoni-Huntley J, Leaverton PE: Secondary sex characteristics of boys 12–17 years of age. J Pediatr 95:293, 1979.

Harlan WR, Harlan EA, Grillo GP: Secondary sex characteristics of girls 12 to 17 years of age: The US Health Examination Survey. J Pediatr 96:1074, 1980.

Hertz R: Accidental ingestion of estrogens by children. Pediatrics 21:203, 1958.

Hung W, Milhorat TH, Nelson KB, et al: Sexual precocity as the only sign of a brain tumor in a 9-year-old boy. Am J Dis Child 121:524, 1971.

Jenner MR, Kelch KP, Kaplan SL, et al: Plasma estradiol in prepubertal children, pubertal females, and in precocious puberty, premature thelarche, hypogonadism, and in a child with a feminizing ovarian tumor. J Clin Endocrinol 34:521, 1972.

Judge DM, Kulin HE, Page R, et al: Hypothalamic hamartoma and luteinizing-hormone release in precocious puberty. N Engl J Med 296:7, 1977.

Korth-Schotz S, Levin LS, New MI: Dehydroepiandrosterone sulfate (DS) levels, a rapid test for abnormal adrenal androgen secretion. J Clin Endocrinol Metab 42:1005, 1976.

Kulin HE, Reiter EO: Gonadotropins during childhood and adolescence: A review. Pediatrics 51:260, 1973.

Kulin HE, Santner SJ: Timed urinary gonadotropin measurements in normal infants, children, and adults, and in patients with disorders of sexual maturation. J Pediatr 90:760, 1977.

Lee PA, Xenakis T, Winer J, et al: Puberty in girls: Correlation of serum levels of gonadotropins, prolactin, androgens, estrogens, and progestins with physical changes. J Clin Endocrinol Metab 42:775, 1976.

Lightner ES, Penny R, Frasier SD: Growth hormone excess and sexual precocity in polyostotic fibrous dysplasia (McCune-Albright syndrome): Evidence for abnormal hypothalamic function. J Pediatr 87:922, 1975.

Lightner ES, Penny R, Frasier SD: Pituitary adenoma in McCune-Albright syndrome: Follow-up information. J Pediatr 89:159, 1976.

Lucky AW, Rich BH, Rosenfield RL, et al: LH bioactivity increases more than immunoactivity during puberty. J Pediatr 97:205, 1980.

Mills JL, Stolley PD, Davies J, Moshang T Jr: Premature thelarche. Natural history and etiologic investigation. Am J Dis Child 135:743, 1981.

Penny R, Goldstein IP, Frasier SD: Overnight gonadotropin excretion in normal females. J Clin Endocrinol Metab 44:780, 1977.

Rieter EO, Fuldauer VG, Root AW: Secretion of the adrenal androgen dehydroepiandrosterone sulfate, during normal infancy, childhood and adolescence in sick infants, and in children with endocrinologic abnormalities. J Pediatr 90:766, 1977.

Romshe CA, Sotos JF: Intracranial human chorionic gonadotropin–secreting tumor with precocious puberty. J Pediatr 86:250, 1975.

Rosenfeld RG, Reitz RE, King AB, Hintz RL: Familial precocious puberty associated with isolated elevation of luteinizing hormone. N Engl J Med 303:859, 1980.

Sigurjonsdottir TJ, Hayles AB: Precocious puberty. A report of 96 cases. Am J Dis Child 115:309, 1968.

Wohltmann H, Mathur RS, Williamson HO, et al: Sexual precocity in a female infant due to feminizing adrenal carcinoma. J Clin Endocrinol Metab 50:186, 1980.

Zachmann M, Illig R: Precocious puberty after surgery for craniopharyngioma. J Pediatr 95:86, 1979.

18.10 DISORDERS OF THE THYROID GLAND

The main function of the thyroid gland is to synthesize thyroxine (T_4) and 3,5,3'-triiodothyronine (T_3). The only known physiologic role of iodine is effecting the synthesis of these hormones; the estimated requirement is 75–150 μg/day. The daily intake in North America varies from 240 to more than 700 μg. Whatever the chemical form ingested, iodine eventually reaches the thyroid gland as iodide. Thyroid tissue has an avidity for iodine and is able to trap (with a gradient of 100–1), transport, and concentrate it in the follicular lumen for synthesis of thyroid hormone.

Before trapped iodide can react with tyrosine, it must be oxidized; this reaction is catalyzed by thyroidal peroxidase. The thyroid cells also elaborate a specific thyroprotein, a globulin with approximately 120 tyrosine units. After iodination of tyrosine to form monoiodotyrosine and diiodotyrosine, 2 molecules of diiodotyrosine couple to form 1 molecule of thyroxine, or 1 molecule of diiodotyrosine and 1 of monoiodotyrosine combine to form triiodothyronine. It is uncertain whether a coupling enzyme exists. Once formed, hormones are stored as thyroglobulin in the lumen of the follicle (colloid) until ready to be delivered to the body cells. Thyroglobulin (Tg) is a large globular glycoprotein with a molecular weight of about 660,000 and under normal conditions is detectable in the blood of most individuals at nanogram levels. T_4 and T_3 are liberated from thyroglobulin by activation of proteases and peptidases.

The metabolic potency of T_3 is 3–4 times that of T_4. Only 20% of circulating T_3 is secreted by the thyroid; the remainder is produced by deiodination of T_4 in the liver, kidney, and other peripheral tissues by thyroxine-5'-deiodinase. T_3 carries out most of the physiologic actions of the thyroid hormones. T_4 is more abundant, but it binds weakly to nuclear receptors, and most of its physiologic effects occur via conversion to T_3. Reliable methods now measure the level of T_3 directly in blood; its concentration is 1/50 that of T_4. The thyroid hormones increase oxygen consumption, stimulate protein synthesis, influence growth and differentiation, and affect carbohydrate, lipid, and vitamin metabolism.

The free hormones enter cells, bind to cytosol receptors specific for T_3 or T_4, and are transported to the mitochondria or the nucleus where they participate in activating transcription.

The circulating thyroid hormones (T_4 and T_3) are firmly bound to thyroxine-binding proteins, of which the major one is thyroxine-binding globulin (TBG); less important are thyroxine-binding prealbumin (TBPA) and albumin. The concentration or binding capacity of TBG is altered in many clinical circumstances; its status must be considered in the interpretation of T_4 or T_3 levels.

The thyroid is regulated by thyroid-stimulating hormone (TSH), a glycoprotein produced and secreted by the anterior pituitary. This hormone activates adenylate cyclase in the thyroid gland to effect release of thyroid hormones. TSH is composed of 2 noncovalently bound subunits (chains): an alpha (hTSH-α) and a beta subunit (hTSH-β). The free subunits as well as TSH can be measured in blood by specific radioimmunoassays. TSH synthesis and release are stimulated by thyroid-releasing hormone (TRH), which is synthesized in the hypothalamus and secreted into the pituitary. TRH is a simple tripeptide which is available for clinical use. In states of decreased production of thyroid hormone, TSH and presumably TRH are increased. An excess of TRH or of TSH results in hypertrophy and hyperplasia of thyroid cells, increased trapping of iodine, and increased synthesis of thyroid hormones. Exogenous thyroid hormone or increased thyroid hormone synthesis inhibits TSH production.

Further control of the level of circulating thyroid hormones occurs in the periphery. In many nonthyroidal illnesses extrathyroidal production of T_3 decreases; factors which inhibit thyroxine-5'-deiodinase include fasting, chronic malnutrition, acute illness, and certain drugs. Levels of T_3 may be significantly decreased while levels of T_4 and TSH remain normal. Presumably, the decreased levels of T_3 result in decreased rates of oxygen production, of substrate utilization, and of other catabolic processes.

18.11 THYROID HORMONE STUDIES

SERUM THYROID HORMONES

Of the methods which have been utilized to measure T_4 and T_3 most have been made obsolete by the radioimmunoassay (RIA) method. Measurements of T_3 (3,5,3'-triiodothyronine) are valuable in the diagnosis of thyroid disorders, particularly in hyperthyroidism. A metabolically inert form of T_3, reverse T_3 (3,3',5'-triiodothyronine), is also present in sera; both T_3 and rT_3 are measurable by radioimmunoassay. Normal levels of T_4, T_3, and rT_3 vary with age; therefore age must be considered in interpreting results, particulately in the neonate (see below).

Thyroglobulin (Tg) is present in measurable amounts in the circulation of normal subjects but is absent in the sera of congenitally athyrotic infants. Its production appears to be controlled by TSH. Elevated levels of Tg are found in patients with differentiated carcinoma of the thyroid, where it serves as a useful marker in their post-treatment follow-up.

Thyrotropin (TSH) is readily measured by radioimmunoassay (RIA) and is 1 of the most sensitive tests for the detection of primary hypothyroidism. After the neonatal period, normal levels are below 7 μU/ml. TSH secretion can be stimulated by intravenous administration (7 μg/kg) of thyrotropin-releasing hormone (TRH). In normal subjects TRH administration increases baseline levels of TSH within 30 min. In hyperthyroidism there is no rise in serum levels of TSH in response to TRH because the elevated levels of thyroid hormones block the effect of TRH on the pituitary. On the other hand, in patients with even very mild degrees of thyroid failure, administration of TRH results in an exaggerated TSH response. Patients with pituitary or hypothalamic failure have low basal levels of TSH; a normal response to TRH localizes the defect in the hypothalamus.

FETAL AND NEWBORN THYROID

The fetal thyroid develops by 10–12 wk of gestation and is able to concentrate iodine and to synthesize iodothyronines. At the same time the fetal pituitary develops; it contains TSH, but the fetal hypothalamic-pituitary-thyroid system develops independently of maternal influence. T_4, T_3, and TSH do not cross the mammalian placenta. Fetal serum T_4 increases progressively from midgestation to approximately 11.5 μg/dl at term. Fetal levels of T_3 are below measurable levels before 30 wk and then gradually rise to about 50 ng/dl at term. Reverse T_3 levels, however, are very high in the fetus (250 ng/dl at 30 wk) and fall to 150 ng/dl at term. Serum levels of TSH peak in the fetus at 20–24 wk to about 15 μU/ml and then gradually decrease to 10 μU/ml at term.

NEWBORN THYROID

At birth there is an acute release of TSH; peak serum concentrations reach 70 μU/ml in 30 min in full term infants. A rapid decline occurs in the ensuing 24 hr and a more gradual decline within the next 2 days to below 10 μU/ml. The acute increase in TSH produces a dramatic rise in levels of T_3 to approximately 300 ng/dl in about 4 hr. This T_3 seems largely derived from increased peripheral conversion of T_4 to T_3. T_3 levels then decline during the 1st wk of life to levels under 200 ng/ml. rT_3 levels are maintained for the 2 wk of life (200 ng/dl) and fall by 4 wk to around 50 ng/dl.

Serum Thyroxine-Binding Globulin (TBG). The thyroid hormones are transported in plasma bound to TBG. Estimation of TBG levels is occasionally necessary because TBG is increased or decreased in a variety of clinical situations, with effects on the level of thyroxine. TBG binds about 70% of T_4 and 50% of T_3. TBG levels increase in pregnancy and in the newborn period. Estrogens (oral contraceptives), perphenazine, heroin, and clofibrate also raise TBG levels; androgens, anabolic steroids, glucocorticoids, and L-asparaginase decrease them. These effects are the results of modulation of hepatic synthesis of TBG. Phenytoin (diphenylhydantoin) is the most common cause of drug-induced abnormality of thyroid function tests. Phenytoin, an inducer of hepatic enzymes, stimulates hepatic degradation of T_4 and accelerates transport of T_4 into tissues. Phenobarbital has a similar effect. Some drugs, particularly phenytoin, also inhibit binding of T_4 and T_3 to TBG. Decreased or increased levels of TBG also occur as genetic traits (see below).

A variety of methods measure TBG or TBG-binding capacity. Most commonly used are the many variations of the resin triiodothyronine uptake test, RT_3U, a screening test with which to interpret T_4 results; it should never be used as an autonomous test of thyroid function. The product of the serum T_4 concentration and T_3 uptake (thyroxine-resin T_3 index or T_4-RT_3U index) correlates closely with free T_4 concentration in serum. This index increases in hyperthyroidism, decreases in hypothyroidism, and is normal in euthyroid patients with abnormalities in the concentration of TBG. It is important to know that normal values vary among laboratories since T_4 levels and T_3 uptakes are often determined by a variety of kit methods and the index is calculated and expressed differently in different laboratories. A radioimmunoassay method to measure TBG is available.

In Vivo Radionuclide Studies. Markedly improved direct tests of thyroid function have made radioiodine uptake studies less useful. The iodine-trapping or concentrating mechanism of the thyroid can be evaluated by the radioactive isotope ^{123}I (half-life 13 hr). Present technology allows doses of radioiodine that are only a fraction of those formerly used (0.1–0.5 μCi). Technetium (^{99m}Tc) is a particularly useful radioisotope for children since, in contrast to iodine, it is trapped but not organified by the thyroid and has a half-life of only 6 hr. Thyroid scanning may be indicated to detect ectopic thyroid tissue, to evaluate thyroid nodules, and to assess presence of thyroid tissue in questions of thyroid agenesis. These studies should be performed with ^{99m}Tc as pertechnetate since it has the advantages of lower radiation exposure and high quality scintigrams. Use of ^{131}I in children should be limited to those with known thyroid cancer.

DEFECTS OF THYROXINE-BINDING GLOBULIN

Abnormalities in the level of TBG are not associated with clinical disease and do not require treatment. They are discussed here because aberrations of TBG levels may be sources of confusion in the diagnosis of hypo- or hyperthyroidism.

TBG deficiency occurs as an X-linked dominant disorder. Affected males are euthyroid. TBG is absent or low, T_4 is low, and levels of RT_3U are high. Heterozygous females have intermediate levels of TBG, low normal levels of T_4 and high normal levels of RT_3U. Homozygous females have not been reported, but an affected 45,X female is known. Absence of TBG from the cord blood of affected males indicates that it does not cross the placenta. A rare instance of total deficiency of TBG in a normal woman established that TBG is not necessary for normal pregnancy.

Congenital deficiency of TBG is being detected through screening programs for neonatal hypothyroidism. It occurs in 1/14,000 neonates. Levels of T_4 in affected infants are usually as low as with congenital hypothyroidism; in contrast to hypothyroidism, however, serum levels of TSH are not elevated. The diagnosis is confirmed by finding low levels of TBG by radioimmunoassay.

There appears to be also an autosomal dominant form of the disorder in which deficiency of TBG is partial.

Elevated TBG also occurs as an X-linked dominant disorder. Affected patients are euthyroid. The nature of the regulatory genetic defect is unknown. TBG and T_4 levels are elevated, and RT_3U levels are low.

Levels of TSH and free T_4 are normal in euthyroid patients with either deficiency or excess of TBG. A study of relatives in the family is usually necessary to establish the genetic origin of the aberrant level of TBG.

Table 18–3 ETIOLOGIC CLASSIFICATION OF HYPOTHYROIDISM

Deficiency of TRF
  Isolated
  Multiple hypothalamic deficiencies (e.g., idiopathic hypopituitarism)
Deficiency of TSH
  Isolated
  Multiple pituitary deficiencies (e.g., craniopharyngioma)
Deficiency of thyroid hormone
  Aplasia, hypoplasia or ectopia of thyroid
    Developmental defects (thyroid dysgenesis)
    Maternal radioiodine
    Maternal autoimmune disease?
  Defective synthesis of thyroid hormone (goitrous hypothyroidism)
    Iodide-trapping defect
    Iodide-organification defects
      Absent peroxidase
      Defective binding of peroxidase
      Inactive bound peroxidase
      Pendred syndrome
    Iodotyrosine coupling defect
    Iodotyrosine deiodination defect
    Thyroglobulin synthesis defect
  Iodine deficiency (endemic cretinism)
  Damage to thyroid gland
    Autoimmune disease (lymphocytic thyroiditis)
    Cystinosis
  Maternal ingestion of medications (neonatal goiter)
    Iodides
    Propylthiouracil, methimazole
  Iatrogenic
    Thyroidectomy
    Drugs (iodides, lithium, cobalt, propylthiouracil, methimazole, para-aminosalicylic acid)
    Neck irradiation (e.g., for Hodgkin disease)
End-organ defect
  TSH unresponsiveness
    Defective TSH receptor
    Defective TSH receptor–adenylate cyclase system
    Maternal TSH-binding inhibitor
  Thyroid hormone unresponsiveness
    Autosomal recessive
    Autosomal dominant

18.12 HYPOTHYROIDISM

Hypothyroidism results from deficient production of thyroid hormone (Table 18–3). The disorder may be manifest very early in life. When symptoms appear after a period of apparently normal thyroid function, the disorder may either be truly "acquired" or only appear so as a result of 1 of a variety of congenital defects in which the manifestation of the deficiency is delayed. The term "cretinism" is often used synonymously with congenital hypothyroidism but should be avoided.

CONGENITAL HYPOTHYROIDISM

All the congenital causes of hypothyroidism, whether sporadic or familial, goitrous or nongoitrous, will be discussed together. In many of these conditions the deficiency of thyroid hormone is severe, and symptoms develop in the early weeks of life. In others, lesser degrees of deficiency occur, and manifestations may be delayed for months or years.

Etiology. *Aplasia and Hypoplasia.* Developmental defects of the thyroid gland are the most common causes of congenital hypothyroidism. Neonatal screening programs find an incidence of approximately 1/3500–4000 white infants and 1/30,000 black infants. Radionuclide scans find no thyroid in about one third of affected infants, whereas rudiments of thyroid tissue may be found in the others when sensitive scanning techniques are used. The thyroid rudiment is frequently found in an ectopic location anywhere from the base of the tongue to the normal position in the neck. Functional abnormalities may occur in 1–2% of newborn infants and are most common in premature infants. Little is known of the factors which interfere with normal migration and development of the thyroid gland. The disorder is usually sporadic, but familial cases have been described. Twice as many females as males are affected. Congenital hypothyroidism has been seen confined to 1 of monozygotic twins; this observation suggests that a deleterious factor operated during intrauterine life; occasionally, the onset of hypothyroidism in the 2nd twin is delayed. In 1 instance of identical twins hypothyroidism associated with an inadequate thyroid in the normal position was diagnosed at 4 mo of age; in the 2nd twin an ectopic thyroid did not lose adequate function until about 4–6 yr of age. The disorder has been noted occasionally in siblings; that both males and females have been affected suggests recessive inheritance in some instances.

Lingual thyroid represents extreme failure of migration of the thyroid gland; the ectopic tissue may provide adequate amounts of thyroid hormone for many yr, or may fail in early childhood. Hypothyroidism usually follows surgical removal of a lingual thyroid from a euthyroid patient since most such patient have no other thyroid tissue. Lingual thyroid has been associated with thyroglossal duct cysts and with a family history of other thyroid disorders. In 1 family, 2 siblings had lingual thyroids, and a 3rd sibling had hypoplasia of 1 lobe of a normally situated thyroid.

Several patients with developmental thyroid defects, including siblings, have been reported whose mothers had thyroid antibodies; in a study of 104 infants with congenital hypothyroidism, however, only 1 had detectable antithyroid microsomal antibodies. Deficiency of fetal TSH has also been proposed as a possible cause of defective thyroid development. Possible deficiencies in early fetal life cannot be excluded, but TSH is always elevated postnatally.

Radioiodine. Administration of radioiodine during pregnancy for treatment of cancer of the thyroid or of hyperthyroidism has been reported to damage the fetal thyroid. In most instances of hypothyroidism resulting from this cause, pregnancy was not suspected at the time of administration of ^{131}I. Whenever radioiodine is administered to a woman of child-bearing age, a pregnancy test must be made before a therapeutic dose of ^{131}I is given. The fetal thyroid gland is capable of trapping iodine by 70–75 days. In 1 instance, ^{131}I was administered to the mother at 14 wk of gestation for treatment of thyroid carcinoma; the athyreotic infant had a tracheal stricture at the site of the thyroid, T_4 and T_3 were undetectable in cord serum, and TSH was markedly elevated (340 μU/ml). This is clear evidence that fetal hypothyroidism occurs and that maternal thyroid hormones do not cross the placenta in significant amounts late in pregnancy. Administration of radioactive iodine to lactating women is also contraindicated since it is readily excreted in milk.

Thyrotropin Deficiency. Deficiency of TSH and hypothyroidism may occur in any of the conditions associated with developmental defects of the pituitary or hypothalamus or in children with idiopathic hypopituitarism (Sec 18.2). More often in these conditions the deficiency of TSH is secondary to a deficiency of thyrotropin-releasing factor (hypothalamic hypothyroidism). With administration of TRH an increase of TSH indicates a primary hypothalamic defect. TSH-deficient hypothyroidism is found in 1/110,000 infants screened for neonatal hypothyroidism.

Isolated deficiency of TSH is rare and has been reported only about 20 times, mostly in adults. It has been reported in association with pseudohypoparathyroidism (Sec 18.19). Isolated TSH deficiency might also be primary or secondary to TRH deficiency.

Thyrotropin Unresponsiveness. Congenital nongoitrous hypothyroidism has been reported in 2 boys of 2 consanguineous matings who had elevated levels of biologically active TSH and normal ^{131}I uptake. Absence of response to thyrotropin was shown in vivo and in metabolism of thyroid tissue in vitro.

Thyroid Hormone Unresponsiveness. An increasing number of patients are being found who are resistant to thyroid hormones. Most have a goiter and clearly elevated levels of T_4, T_3, free T_4, and free T_3. These findings have often led to the erroneous diagnosis of Graves disease although the patients are clinically euthyroid. TSH levels are normal or elevated and inappropriate for the levels of T_4 and T_3. Abnormally large doses of T_3 are required to suppress the levels of TSH. The resistance to thyroid hormone appears to vary among different tissues and is believed to be due to a defect in the nuclear receptor. Both autosomal recessive and autosomal dominant modes of inheritance have been described, suggesting heterogeneity of the disorder. Usually no treatment is necessary.

Defective Synthesis of Thyroxine. Congenital hypothyroidism may be due to a variety of defects in the biosynthesis of thyroid hormone. The presence of a goiter is the hallmark of these defects, and the condition is termed goitrous hypothyroidism or goitrous cretinism. Goitrous hypothyroidism is detected in 1/30,000–50,000 live births in neonatal screening programs. It is genetically determined and in most instances transmitted in an autosomal recessive manner. The following defects have been identified:

IODIDE-TRAPPING DEFECT. Of the 14 instances of this defect which have been reported, 8 were from Japan. A goiter is present, but in contrast to all the other defects the uptake of radioiodine is low. The salivary glands and stomach also lack ability to concentrate iodide. The biochemical defect is unknown, but deficiency of iodide permease is a possibility. Goiter and hypothyroidism usually occur in the 1st few mo of life; in Japan, however, goiter and hypothyroidism often occur after 10 yr of age, perhaps because of the very high iodine content (often 19 mg/day) of the Japanese diet.

IODIDE ORGANIFICATION DEFECT. After iodide is trapped by the thyroid, it is rapidly oxidized by H_2O_2 and thyroid peroxidase and is incorporated into tyrosine. In this defect, iodide is not organified and may be rapidly discharged from the thyroid by administration of perchlorate. Three different organification defects have now been characterized:

1. Complete absence of peroxidase activity in a severe form of goitrous hypothyroidism.

2. Failure of a prosthetic hematin group to bind to thyroidal apoperoxidase in euthyroid goitrous patients.

3. Inactive peroxidase due to an abnormality in its bound state.

Deficient organification also occurs in Pendred syndrome, but peroxidase activity is normal and the biochemical defect unknown.

COUPLING DEFECT. After iodine is incorporated into tyrosine in thyroglobulin to form iodotyrosine, an intramolecular rearrangement occurs, leading to coupling of iodotyrosines to form diiodothyronines. Because this reaction is complex, heterogeneity of defects is likely, but little is known of the biochemical aberrations involved. It has been proposed that errors may involve defects in coupling enzymes or an abnormality in steric configuration.

DEIODINASE DEFECT. Free monoiodotyrosine and diiodotyrosine are normally deiodinated within the thyroid or in peripheral tissues by a deiodinase. The iodine thus liberated is then reutilized in synthesis of hormone. Patients with iodotyrosine-dehalogenase deficiency have large amounts of monoiodotyrosine and diiodotyrosine in blood and in urine. The constant loss of iodine from the thyroid into the urine leads to hormone deficiency and goiter.

DEFECT OF THYROGLOBULIN SYNTHESIS. Patients with this disorder release from the thyroid into the bloodstream iodinated proteins or polypeptides which are calorigenically inactive. Because thyroglobulin synthesis is complex, this category almost certainly has diverse etiologies.

In some patients with genetic absence of thyroglobulin synthesis there is iodination of inappropriate proteins, mainly albumin, and very little thyroxine biosynthesis. There is a high production rate of iodohistidines which are not deiodinated but are excreted in urine and may serve as a clue to detection of defective thyroglobulin synthesis. Some reported cases of defects of "coupling" or of abnormal iodinated compounds in serum and thyroid have probably been the result of defects in thyroglobulin synthesis.

Clinical Manifestations. Congenital hypothyroidism is twice as common in girls as in boys. Prior to neonatal screening programs congenital hypothyroidism was rarely recognized in the newborn since the signs and symptoms are usually not sufficiently developed. It can be suspected and the diagnosis established during the early weeks of life if the initial but less characteristic manifestations are recognized. Hypothyroid infants may be significantly heavier at birth than normal newborn infants, but there is little diagnostic value to this observation. Unexplained or unusual prolongation of physiologic icterus, due to delayed maturation of glucuronide conjugation, may be the earliest sign. Feeding difficulties, especially sluggishness, lack of interest, somnolence, and choking spells during nursing, are often present during the 1st mo of life. Respiratory difficulties, due in part to the large tongue, include apneic episodes, noisy respirations, and nasal obstruction. Typical respiratory distress syndrome may also occur. Affected infants cry little, sleep much, have poor appetites, and are generally sluggish. There may be constipation which does not usually respond to treatment. The abdomen is large, and an umbilical hernia is usually present. The temperature is subnormal, often below 35° C (95° F), and the skin, particularly of the extremities, may be cold and mottled. Edema of the genitals and extremities may be present. The pulse is slow; heart murmurs and cardiomegaly are common. Anemia is often present and is refractory to treatment with hematinics. Since symptoms appear gradually, the diagnosis is often delayed.

These manifestations progress; retardation of physical and mental development becomes greater during the following months, and by 3–6 mo of age the clinical picture is fully developed. (See Fig 18–9.) When there is only a partial deficiency of thyroid hormone, the symptoms may be milder, the syndrome incomplete, and the onset delayed. Although breast milk contains significant amounts of thyroid hormones, particularly T_3, it is inadequate to protect the breast-fed infant with congenital hypothyroidism.

The child is stunted in growth, the extremities being short, whereas head size is normal or even increased. The anterior and posterior fontanels are widely open; observation of this sign at birth may serve as an initial clue for early recognition of congenital hypothyroidism. Only 3% of normal newborn infants have a posterior fontanel larger than 0.5 cm. The eyes appear far apart, and the bridge of the broad nose is depressed. The palpebral fissures are narrow and the eyelids swollen. The mouth is kept open, and the thick and broad tongue protrudes from it. Dentition is delayed. The neck is short and thick, and there may be deposits of fat above the clavicles and between the neck and shoulders. The hands are broad and the fingers short. The skin is dry

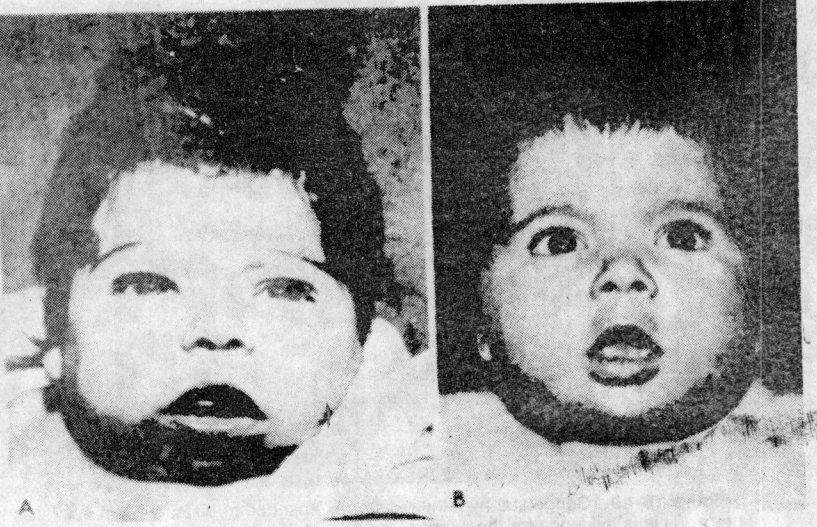

Figure 18–9 Congenital hypothyroidism in an infant 6 mo of age. The infant fed poorly in the neonatal period and was constipated. She had a persistent nasal discharge and a large tongue, was very lethargic, and had no social smile and no head control. *A,* Note puffy face, dull expression, hirsute forehead. Negligible uptake of radioiodine. Osseous development was that of newborn. *B,* Four mo after treatment. Note decreased puffiness of face, decreased hirsutism of forehead, and alert appearance.

and scaly, and there is little perspiration. Myxedema manifests itself, particularly in the skin of the eyelids, of the back of the hands, and of the external genitalia. Carotenemia may cause a yellow discoloration of the skin, but the scleras remain white. The scalp is thickened, and the hair is coarse, brittle, and scanty. The hairline reaches far down on the forehead, which usually appears wrinkled, especially when the infant cries.

Development is usually retarded. Hypothyroid infants appear lethargic and are late in sitting and standing. The voice is hoarse, and they do not learn to talk. The degree of physical and mental retardation increases with age. Sexual maturation may be delayed or not take place at all or may occur precociously. (Sec 18.7).

The muscles are usually hypotonic, but in rare instances generalized muscular hypertrophy occurs (*Kocher-Debré-Sémélaigne syndrome*). Affected children may have an athletic appearance due to pseudohypertrophy, particularly in the calf muscles. Its pathogenesis is unknown; nonspecific histochemical and ultrastructural changes seen on muscle biopsy return to normal with treatment. Boys are more prone to develop the syndrome, which has been observed in siblings born to a consanguineous mating. Affected patients have hypothyroidism of longer duration and severity.

Laboratory Data. Serum levels of T_4 and T_3 are low or borderline. If the defect is primarily in the thyroid, levels of TSH in serum exceed 20 μU/ml and are commonly above 100 μU/ml. Most newborn screening programs measure levels of T_4, but the diagnosis is confirmed by assay of TSH, which should always be measured to confirm a diagnosis of primary hypothyroidism at any age. Euthyroid patients with low levels of TBG caused by genetic deficiencies or medications will have low levels of T_4 but will have normal levels of TSH. Hypothyroid patients with low levels of TSH may have pituitary or hypothalamic defects and require study with TRH stimulation. With all these assays, special care must be given to the normal range of values for the age of the patient, particularly in the newborn period.

Retardation of osseous development can be shown roentgenographically at birth in about 60% of congenitally hypothyroid infants and indicates some deprivation of thyroid hormone during intrauterine life. For example, the distal femoral epiphysis, normally present at birth, is often absent. In untreated patients the discrepancy between chronologic age and osseous development increases. The epiphyses often have multiple foci of ossification (epiphyseal dysgenesis); deformity ("beaking") of the 12th thoracic or 1st or 2nd lumbar vertebra is common. (See Fig 18–10.) Roentgenograms of the skull show large fontanelles and wide sutures; intersutural bones (wormian bones) are common. The sella turcica is often enlarged and round; in rare instances there may be erosion and thinning. Delays in formation of dental buds and in eruption of teeth may occur. Cardiac enlargement or pericardial effusion may be present.

Levels of growth hormone and responses to provocative stimuli may be abnormally low in primary hypothyroidism but return to normal after treatment with thyroid.

Technetium scanning may be indicated to determine whether there is any thyroid tissue. Patients with goitrous hypothyroidism may require extensive evaluation, including radioiodine studies, perchlorate discharge tests, kinetic studies, chromatography, and studies of thyroid tissue if the biochemical nature of the defect is to be determined.

The electrocardiogram may show low voltage P and T waves with diminished amplitude of QRS complexes. The electroencephalogram frequently shows low voltage. In children over 2 yr of age the serum cholesterol level is usually elevated.

Differential Diagnosis. With the careful plotting on growth charts of lengths and heights of all infants and children, deceleration of growth velocity frequently

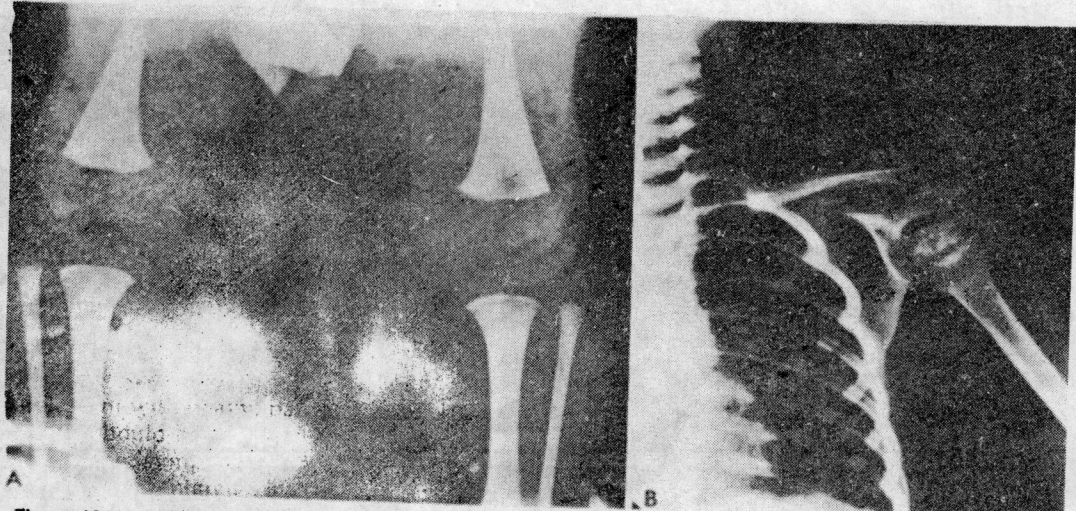

Figure 18–10 Congenital hypothyroidism. *A*, Absence of distal femoral epiphysis in a 3 mo old infant who was born at term. This is evidence for the onset of the hypothyroid state during fetal life. *B*, Epiphyseal dysgenesis in the head of the humerus in a 9 yr old girl who had been inadequately treated with thyroid.

provides the 1st clue to the diagnosis. Once it has been considered, confirmation is not difficult since direct tests of thyroid function are generally available and reliable. Familiarity with those conditions which alter test results, such as alterations in TBG, is essential.

Prognosis. Without treatment, affected infants may die of respiratory obstruction or intercurrent infections, and those who live may become mentally deficient dwarfs. Treatment with thyroid hormone results in normal linear growth, osseous maturation, and sexual development. Mental development, however, is much less predictable. Thyroid hormone is critical for normal cerebral development in the early postnatal months. Hence, the diagnosis must be made early in life and effective treatment initiated promptly in order to minimize irreversible brain damage. In general, the more profound the deprivation of the thyroid hormone in the early of life, the poorer the prognosis for mental development. With the advent of neonatal screening programs for detection of congenital hypothyroidism, the prognosis for affected infants has improved dramatically. Infants detected before the appearance of clinical manifestations with adequate treatment begun in the 1st mo of life have normal IQs at 3–4 yr. The prognosis is guarded for infants who manifest clinical signs of hypothyroidism in the 1st few wk of life and in whom scans show no evidence of thyroid remnant.

There is no conclusive evidence that treatment of the pregnant woman with huge doses of thyroid hormone to enhance transplacental transfer of protective levels of hormone to the hypothyroid fetus is effective. When clinical evidence of hypothyroidism is delayed in onset, the outlook for normal mental development is much better; children who acquire hypothyroidism after 2 yr of age and are treated appropriately have a good prognosis for mental development.

Treatment. Whatever the cause of hypothyroidism, replacement therapy with thyroid hormone is indicated and effective. Sodium-L-thyroxine given orally is the drug of choice. It has been estimated that normally 30–50% of circulating thyroxine undergoes peripheral deiodination to become triiodothyronine, most circulat-

ing T_3 being derived from T_4 rather than directly from the thyroid gland. Hence, treatment with sodium-L-thyroxine provides both T_4 and T_3. In infants the dose is 6–8 μg/kg. Older children appear to require about 4 μg/kg and may be treated initially with 100–150 μg/24 hr; only rarely is more than 200 μg/24 hr required.

Levels of both T_4 and TSH should be monitored and maintained within the normal range. It was formerly thought that when thyroxine was used for replacement therapy, levels of T_4 should be maintained slightly elevated to compensate for the deficiency of T_3, but it is known now that normal levels of T_4 ensure normal levels of T_3. In older children, after catch-up growth is complete, the growth rate provides an excellent index of adequacy of therapy. Parents should be forewarned of changes in behavior and activity expected with therapy, and special attention must be given to any developmental or neurologic deficits.

JUVENILE HYPOTHYROIDISM
(Acquired Hypothyroidism)

The development of hypothyroidism in a child who was previously euthyroid may be due to a wide variety of defects. A congenitally hypoplastic thyroid gland may furnish amounts of hormone sufficient for the 1st few yr, but the deficiency may become manifest when rapid growth of the body increases demands on the gland. Accordingly, any or all of the etiologic causes of congenital hypothyroidism must be considered. Clinical manifestations of congenital defects may develop as if they were acquired lesions.

Complete or subtotal thyroidectomy for thyrotoxicosis or cancer may result in hypothyroidism, as may removal of an anomalous thyroid when it constitutes the sole source of thyroid hormone. For example, a thyroid ectopically placed at the base of the tongue (lingual thyroid) is often the only thyroid tissue, or the entire thyroid gland may consist of a midline nodule and be mistaken for a thyroglossal duct cyst.

In nephropathic *cystinosis* accumulation of intracellu-

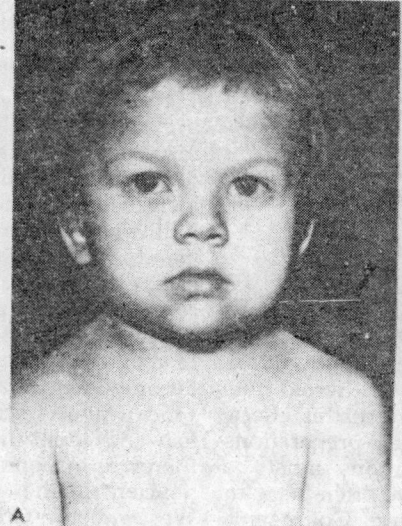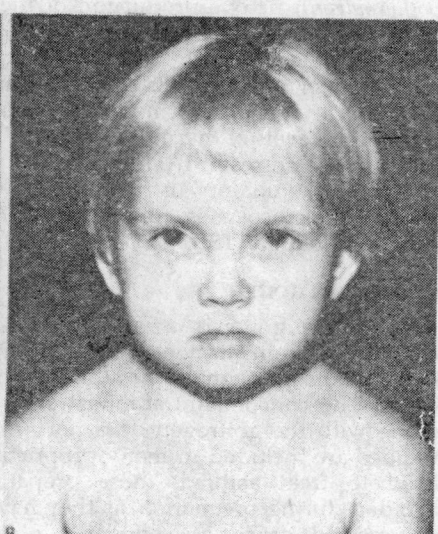

Figure 18–11 Acquired hypothyroidism in a girl 6 yr of age. She was treated with a wide variety of hematinics for refractory anemia for 3 yr. She had almost complete cessation of growth, constipation, and sluggishness of 3 yr duration. Height age was 3 yr; bone age, 4 yr. She had a sallow complexion and immature facies with a poorly developed nasal bridge. *A*, Serum cholesterol, 501 mg/dl; radioiodine uptake, 7% at 24 hr; PBI, 2.8 μg/dl. *B*, After therapy for 18 mo. Note nasal development, increased luster and decreased pigmentation of hair, and maturation of face. Height age was 5.5 yr; bone age, 7 yr. There was decided improvement in her general condition. Menarche occurred at 14 yr. Ultimate height was 61 in (155 cm). She graduated from high school. She was well controlled with 200 μg of sodium-L-thyroxine daily.

lar cystine results in impaired thyroid function with eventual destruction of the gland. Hypothyroidism may be overt, but compensated forms are more frequent and periodic assessment of TSH levels is indicated.

Irradiation to the area of the thyroid which occurs incidentally to the treatment of Hodgkin disease and other malignancies or prior to bone marrow transplantation results in thyroid dysfunction in approximately one third of children and adolescents. These are other groups of patients requiring periodic assessment of TSH.

Hypothyroidism associated with a goiter may be caused occasionally by chronic infectious processes or by the protracted ingestion of medications such as iodides or cobalt. Acquired hypothyroidism, however, most often results from *lymphocytic thyroiditis*, which may or may not be associated with a goiter. (See Sec 18.13.)

The clinical manifestations depend upon the age of the child at onset and upon the extent of dysfunction. The later in life hypothyroidism is acquired, the less will be the impairment of growth and development. Nevertheless, myxedematous changes of the skin, constipation, sleepiness, and a mental decline may be manifested at any age. Cessation or retardation of growth in a child whose growth has previously been normal should always alert one to the possibility of hypothyroidism (Fig 18–11). Obese children are frequently, but usually erroneously, considered to have hypothyroidism. Most obese children are tall and have warm moist skin, a ruddy complexion, and normal thyroid function.

Diagnostic studies and treatment are the same as described for congenital hypothyroidism.

18.13 GOITER

A goiter is an enlargement of the thyroid gland. Persons with enlarged thyroids may have normal function of the gland (*euthyroidism*), thyroid deficiency (*hypothyroidism*), or overproduction of the hormones (*hyperthyroidism*). Goiter may be congenital or acquired, endemic or sporadic.

The goiter often results from increased secretion of pituitary thyrotropic hormone in response to decreased circulating levels of thyroid hormones. Thyroid enlargement may also result from infiltrative processes which may be inflammatory or neoplastic. Goiter in patients with thyrotoxicosis is caused by thyroid-stimulating immunoglobulin (TSI).

CONGENITAL GOITER

Congenital goiter is usually sporadic and may result from the administration of antithyroid drugs and/or iodides during pregnancy for the treatment of thyrotoxicosis. The concomitant administration of thyroid hormone with the goitrogen does not prevent this effect. Iodides are included in many proprietary preparations used to treat asthma; these preparations must be avoided during pregnancy, as they have often been an unexpected cause of congenital goiter. Goitrogenic

drugs and iodides cross the placenta and at high doses may interfere with synthesis of thyroid hormone, resulting in goiter and hypothyroidism in the fetus. Even when the infant is clinically euthyroid, there may be retardation of osseous maturation, low levels of T_4, and elevated levels of TSH. Since these effects can occur when the mother takes only 100–200 mg of propylthiouracil/day, all such infants should be carefully examined. Administration of thyroid hormone to affected infants may be indicated to treat clinical hypothyroidism, to hasten the disappearance of the goiter, and to prevent brain damage. Since the condition is rarely permanent, thyroid hormone may be safely discontinued after several mo.

Enlargement of the thyroid at birth may occasionally be sufficient to cause respiratory distress which interferes with nursing and may even cause death. The head may be maintained in extreme hyperextension. When respiratory obstruction is severe, partial thyroidectomy rather than tracheostomy is indicated (Fig 18–12).

Goiter is almost always present in the congenitally hyperthyroid infant. These goiters are usually not large; the infant manifests clinical symptoms of hyperthyroidism, and the mother often has a history of Graves disease (Sec 18.15).

When no causative factor is identifiable, a defect in synthesis of thyroid hormone must be suspected. One in 30,000–50,000 live births is found in neonatal screening programs to have such a defect. Study of this group of infants is complex. If the infant is hypothyroid, it is advisable to treat immediately with thyroid hormone and to postpone more detailed studies for later in life. Since these defects are transmitted by recessive genes, precise diagnosis is important for sound counseling.

Iodine deficiency as a cause of congenital goiters has become rare but persists in isolated endemic areas (see below). More important is the recent recognition that severe iodine deficiency early in pregnancy may cause neurologic damage during fetal development even in the absence of goiter.

When the "goiter" is lobulated, asymmetric, firm, or large to an unusual degree, a teratoma within or in the vicinity of the thyroid must be considered in the differential diagnosis (Sec 15.19).

ENDEMIC GOITER AND CRETINISM

The association between deficiency of iodine and the prevalence of goiter and/or cretinism has been recognized for over half a century. If there is a moderate deficiency of iodine, the demand can be satisfied by increased efficiency in synthesis of thyroid hormone. Iodine liberated in the tissues is returned rapidly to the gland, which resynthesizes the hormone at a higher rate than normal. This increased activity is achieved by compensatory hypertrophy and hyperplasia, which satisfy the demands of the tissues for thyroid hormone. In geographic areas where deficiency of iodine is severe, decompensation and hypothyroidism may result.

Sea water is rich in iodine, and the iodine content of fish and shellfish is also high. Endemic goiter is rare therefore in populations living along the sea. Iodine is deficient in the water and native foods in the Pacific West and the Great Lakes areas of the United States.

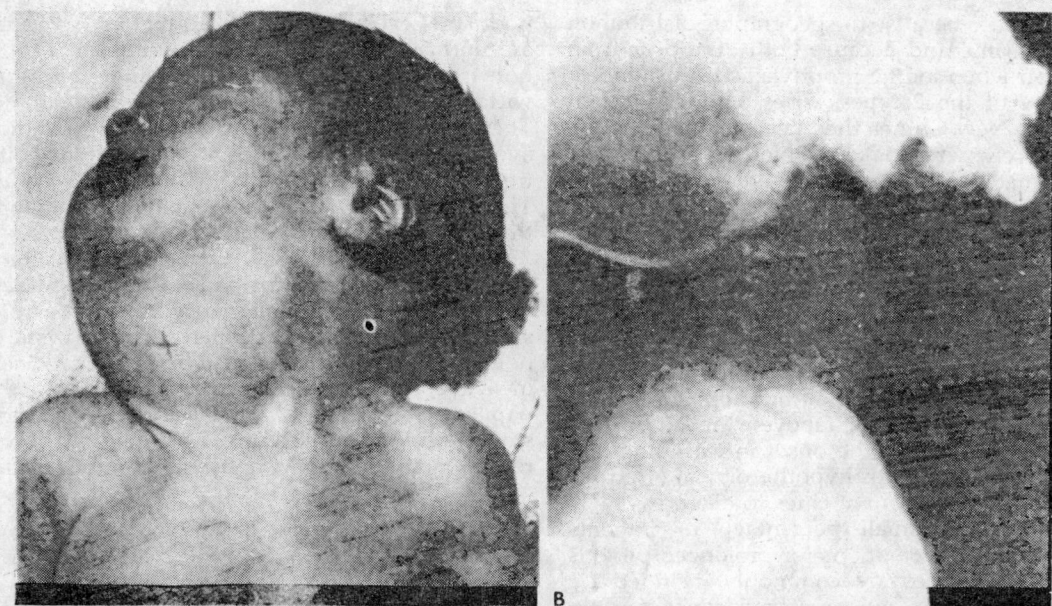

Figure 18–12 Congenital goiter in infancy. *A*, Large congenital goiter in an infant born to a mother with thyrotoxicosis who had been treated with iodides and methimazole during pregnancy. *B*, A 6 wk old infant with increasing respiratory distress and cervical mass since birth. Operation revealed a large goiter which almost completely encircled the trachea. Note anterior deviation and posterior compression of the trachea. Partial thyroidectomy completely relieved the symptoms. No cause for goiter was found. It is apparent why a tracheostomy is not adequate treatment for these infants.

Deficiency of dietary iodine is even greater in certain Alpine valleys, the Himalayas, the Andes, the Congo, and the Highlands of New Guinea. In areas such as in the United States, where iodine is provided in foods from other areas and in iodized salt, endemic goiter has disappeared. Iodized salt in the United States contains potassium iodide (100 μg/gm) and provides excellent prophylaxis. Further iodine intake in the United States is contributed by iodates used in baking, iodine-containing coloring agents, and iodine-containing disinfectants used in the dairy industry. It has been shown in New Guinea that a single intramuscular injection of 4 ml of iodinated poppy seed oil provides prophylactic effects lasting more than 4 yr.

Clinical Manifestations. If the deficiency of iodine is mild, the enlargement of the thyroid does not become noticeable except when there is an increased demand for the hormone during periods of rapid growth, as in adolescence and during pregnancy. In regions of moderate iodine deficiency, goiter may be observed in school children. It may disappear with maturity and reappear during pregnancy or lactation. Iodine-deficient goiters are more common in girls than in boys. Where iodine deficiency is severe, as in the hyperendemic Highlands of New Guinea, nearly half the population have large goiters, and endemic cretinism is common.

Serum thyroxine levels are often low in endemic goiter, though clinical hypothyroidism is rare. This is true in New Guinea, the Congo, the Himalayas, and South America. Despite low serum levels of thyroid hormone, serum TSH concentrations are often only moderately increased. In such patients circulating levels of T_3 are elevated. Moreover, T_3 levels are also elevated in those patients with normal T_4 levels, indicating a preferential secretion of T_3 by the thyroid in this disease.

Endemic cretinism has been recognized for centuries and only in geographic association with endemic goiter. On the other hand, endemic goiter may occur in the absence of endemic cretinism. For many yr there was great confusion concerning the pathogenesis of endemic cretinism. It is now recognized that the confusion was caused by including in the term "endemic cretinism" 2 very different but overlapping syndromes.

The "nervous" syndrome is characterized by ataxia, spasticity, deaf-mutism, and mental retardation. These "cretins" may be normal in stature and may have little or no impairment of thyroid function. Recent evidence from New Guinea strongly suggests that in the "nervous" type a deficiency of iodine throughout fetal life has damaged the developing nervous system quite apart from its role in the synthesis of thyroid hormone, the damage occurring in the 1st trimester of pregnancy even before the fetal thyroid has developed.

The "myxedematous" syndrome is characterized by marked delays in growth and sexual development and by mental retardation and myxedema. Neurologic examination is normal, and perceptive deafness is absent. In these patients the iodine deficiency occurred in late fetal life and postnatally. About 25% of the "myxedematous" type have goiters, but enlargement of the gland is minimal. Serum thyroid hormone levels are low, and TSH levels are markedly elevated. Thyroid scans are normal and preclude thyroid dysgenesis. There is marked delay in osseous maturation, which indicates that hypothyroidism appears around birth or during the 1st months of life. It is hypothesized that iodine deficiency in conjunction with an unknown toxic factor (goitrogen in food?) may alter thyroid function during fetal and neonatal life.

The term "endemic cretinism" continues to be used

for both syndromes because the geographic distribution of both is the same and because both disappear from the population when iodine prophylaxis is introduced. The frequency of the 2 types varies among different populations; in New Guinea the "nervous" type occurs almost exclusively, whereas in the Northeastern Congo the "myxedematous" type predominates.

SPORADIC GOITER

Sporadic goiter is a descriptive term which encompasses goiters developing from a variety of etiologic factors; patients are usually euthyroid but may be hypothyroid. The most common cause of sporadic goiter is lymphocytic thyroiditis (below). Intrinsic biochemical defects in the synthesis of thyroid hormone are almost always associated with goiter (above); the occurrence of the disorder in siblings, the onset in early life, and the possible association with hypothyroidism (goitrous hypothyroidism) are important clues to diagnosis.

Iodide Goiter. A small percentage of patients treated with iodide preparations for prolonged periods develop goiters. Iodides are commonly included for their expectorant effect in cough medicines and in proprietary mixtures for asthma. The goiter is firm and diffusely enlarged, and in some instances hypothyroidism may develop. In normal subjects acute administration of large doses of iodine inhibits the organification of iodine and the synthesis of thyroid hormone (Wolff-Chaikoff effect). This effect is short-lived and does not lead to hypothyroidism. When iodide administration continues, an autoregulatory mechanism in normal persons limits iodine trapping and thus permits the level of iodide in the thyroid to fall and organification to proceed normally. In patients with iodide-induced goiter this escape does not occur because of an underlying abnormality of biosynthesis of thyroid hormone. Subjects most susceptible to the development of iodide goiter are those with lymphocytic thyroiditis or with a subclinical inborn error in thyroid hormone synthesis as well as those who have been treated with radioactive iodine for thyrotoxicosis.

Lithium carbonate also causes goiters; it is currently widely used as a psychotropic drug. Lithium competes with iodide; the mechanism producing the goiter and/or hypothyroidism is similar to that described above for iodide goiter. Lithium and iodide also act synergistically to produce goiter; their combined use should be avoided.

Prolonged administration of para-aminosalicylic acid or cobalt and externally applied resorcinol have caused goiter. Discontinuation of contact with the causative agent results in regression of the goiter.

Simple Goiter (Colloid Goiter). About one third of children with euthyroid nontoxic goiters have simple goiters, a condition of unknown etiology not associated with hypothyroidism or hyperthyroidism and not caused by inflammation or neoplasia. The condition predominates in girls and has a peak incidence before and during the pubertal years. Histologic examination of the thyroid either is normal or reveals variable follicular size, dense colloid, and flattened epithelium. The goiter may be small or large. It is firm in consistency in half the patients and is occasionally asymmetric or nodular. Levels of TSH are normal or low; scintiscans are normal; thyroid antibodies are absent. Differentiation from lymphocytic thyroiditis may not be possible without a biopsy, but biopsy is ordinarily not indicated. Therapy with thyroid hormone may be indicated to avoid progression to a large multinodular goiter. Untreated patients should be re-evaluated periodically. This condition must be differentiated from lymphocytic thyroiditis (below).

Adenomatous Goiter. Rarely, a firm goiter with a lobulated surface and palpable solitary nodules is encountered. Because malignancy cannot be ruled out, surgical exploration is indicated. Areas of cystic change, hemorrhage, and fibrosis may be present. Follicles vary in size; epithelium is flat or cuboidal, and there may be papillary infoldings. A fetal pattern characterized by small follicles and absent colloid may also occur. Full replacement therapy with thyroid hormone is indicated.

PENDRED SYNDROME
(Goiter and Congenital Deafness)

This syndrome of congenital deafness and goiter is transmitted in an autosomal recessive fashion and is not to be confused with the deaf-mutism seen in endemic cretinism or with the minor impairment of hearing which may be found in severely hypothyroid persons. The hearing loss is usually severe and present at birth, although it may not be recognized until later. It is most pronounced in the higher frequencies, is of the perceptive type, and exhibits recruitment. The goiter generally appears at puberty or later but may be present in early childhood; it may be barely detectable or pronounced. Initially, the goiter is soft and diffuse; it tends to become nodular in adult life. Most affected persons are clinically euthyroid, but hypothyroidism may ensue even during childhood. Affected persons are otherwise normal.

Administration of perchlorate causes a significant discharge of iodide from the thyroid gland, indicating a defect in organification. The biochemical defect is not known. There does not appear to be a deficiency in iodide peroxidase or iodotyrosine synthesis or any defect in binding to apoenzyme. Lifelong substitution treatment with thyroid hormone is indicated to prevent development or progression of the goiter.

INTRATRACHEAL GOITER

One of the many ectopic locations of thyroid tissue is within the trachea. The intraluminal thyroid lies beneath the tracheal mucosa and is frequently continuous with the normally situated extratracheal thyroid. The thyroid tissue is susceptible to goitrous enlargement, which involves the normally situated as well as the ectopic thyroid. When there is obstruction of the airway associated with a goiter, it must be ascertained whether the obstruction is extratracheal or endotracheal. If obstructive manifestations are mild, administration of sodium-L-thyroxine (100–200 μg/24 hr) will usually cause the goiter to decrease in size. When symptoms are severe, surgical removal of the endotracheal goiter is indicated.

18.14 THYROIDITIS

LYMPHOCYTIC THYROIDITIS
(Hashimoto Thyroiditis; Autoimmune Thyroiditis)

Lymphocytic thyroiditis is the most common cause of thyroid disease in children and adolescents and accounts for many of the enlarged thyroids formerly designated "adolescent" goiter. It is also the most common cause of juvenile hypothyroidism, with or without goiter. Its incidence may be as high as 1% in schoolchildren.

Etiology. An autoimmune mechanism defines the disorder. There is a genetic predisposition to the development of thyroid autoantibodies, but the basic stimulus or immunologic defect is not known. The condition is characterized histologically by lymphocytic infiltration of the thyroid. Early in the course of the disease there may be only hyperplasia; this is followed by infiltration of lymphocytes and plasma cells between the follicles and by atrophy of the follicles. Lymphoid follicle formation with germinal centers is almost always present; the degree of atrophy and of fibrosis of the follicles varies from mild to moderate.

Clinical Manifestations. The disorder is 4–7 times more frequent in girls than in boys. It may occur during the 1st 3 yr of life but becomes sharply more common after 6 yr of age and reaches a peak incidence during adolescence. The goiter may appear insidiously and vary in size from slight to marked. In the majority of children the thyroid is diffusely enlarged, firm, and nontender. In about a third of the patients the gland is lobular and may seem to be nodular. Most of the affected children are clinically euthyroid and asymptomatic; some may have symptoms of pressure in the neck. Some children have clinical signs of hypothyroidism, while others who appear clinically euthyroid have laboratory evidence of hypothyroidism. A few children have manifestations suggestive of hyperthyroidism, such as nervousness, irritability, increased sweating, or hyperactivity, but results of laboratory studies are not those of hyperthyroidism. Occasionally, the disorder may coexist with Graves disease. Ophthalmopathy may occur in lymphocytic thyroiditis in the absence of Graves disease.

The clinical course is variable. The goiter may become smaller or disappear spontaneously, or it may persist unchanged for years while the patient remains euthyroid. A significant percentage of patients who are euthyroid initially exhibit hypothyroidism gradually within months or years; thyroiditis is the cause of most instances of nongoitrous juvenile hypothyroidism. Lymphocytic thyroiditis may also occur without symptoms, and in many children complete recovery occurs spontaneously.

Familial clusters of lymphocytic thyroiditis are common; the incidence in siblings and/or parents of affected children may be as high as 25%. The concurrence within families of cases of lymphocytic thyroiditis, "idiopathic" hypothyroidism, and Graves disease provides cogent evidence for a basic relationship among these 3 conditions. The disorder has been found associated with many of the other autoimmune disorders more often than expected by chance alone. The association of Addison disease with insulin-dependent diabetes mellitus and/or autoimmune thyroid disease is known as *Schmidt syndrome* or *type II polyglandular autoimmune disease*. Autoimmune thyroid disease also tends to be associated with pernicious anemia, vitiligo, and/or alopecia. Thyroid microsomal antibodies are found in approximately 20% of Caucasian and 4% of black children with diabetes mellitus. Autoimmune thyroid disease has an increased incidence in children with congenital rubella. Lymphocytic thyroiditis is also associated with certain chromosomal aberrations, particularly Turner syndrome and Down syndrome. The pathogenetic mechanisms for these associations is not known.

Since thyroid antibodies cross the placenta, it has been suspected that they may cause fetal thyroid damage and congenital cretinism. Autoimmunity is not, however, a frequent cause of congenital hypothyroidism.

Laboratory Data. The definitive diagnosis can be established by biopsy of the thyroid, but this procedure is rarely indicated for clinical purposes alone. Thyroid function tests are usually normal, though the level of TSH may be slightly or even moderately elevated in some euthyroid individuals. With progressive thyroid failure a decrease in the levels of T_4 is followed by a decrease in levels of T_3 with progressive increases in levels of TSH. The fact that many patients with lymphocytic thyroiditis do not have elevated levels of TSH indicates that the goiter may be caused by the lymphocytic infiltrations. In 50% of patients thyroid scans reveal irregular and patchy distribution of the radioisotope, and in about 60% or more the administration of perchlorate results in a greater than 10% discharge of iodide from the thyroid gland. The majority of patients with lymphocytic thyroiditis have serum antibody titers to thyroid microsomal antigens, whereas the tanned red blood cell hemagglutination test for thyroid antibodies is positive in fewer than 50%. When both tests are used, approximately 95% of patients with thyroid autoimmunity will be detected. In general, levels in children are lower than those in adults with lymphocytic thyroiditis, and repeated measurements are indicated in questionable instances since titers may increase later in the course of the disease.

Antithyroid antibodies may be found also in almost half the siblings of affected patients and in a significant percentage of the mothers of children with Down syndrome or Turner syndrome without demonstrable thyroid disease. They are also found in a significant number of children with diabetes mellitus and with a variety of other autoimmune disorders.

Differential Diagnosis. It is not possible to distinguish lymphocytic thyroiditis from simple goiter (above) on clinical grounds alone. The signs and symptoms are usually identical. The finding of a positive antibody titer clearly points to lymphocytic thyroiditis whereas a negative titer does not rule it out. An elevated level of TSH points to lymphocytic thyroiditis since patients with simple goiter have normal levels.

Treatment. If there is evidence of hypothyroidism, replacement treatment with sodium-L-thyroxine (100–200 µg daily) is indicated. The goiter slowly decreases in size, but antibody levels remain unchanged. Since the disease may be self-limited in some instances, the need for continued therapy requires periodic re-evaluation. Untreated patients should also be periodically checked.

OTHER CAUSES OF THYROIDITIS

Specific conditions such as tuberculosis, sarcoidosis, mumps, and cat scratch disease are rare causes of thyroiditis.

Acute suppurative thyroiditis is infrequent; it is usually preceded by a respiratory infection or is secondary to trauma. Abscess formation may occur. Recurrent episodes and/or the detection of a mixed bacterial flora suggest that the infection arises from a thyroglossal duct remnant. Exquisite tenderness of the gland, swelling, erythema, dysphagia, and limitation of head motion are characteristic findings. Systemic manifestations are often but not invariably absent. Scintigrams of the thyroid often reveal decreased uptake in the affected areas. Thyroid function is usually normal, but thyrotoxicosis due to escape of thyroid hormone has been encountered in a child with suppurative thyroiditis resulting from *Aspergillus*. When suppuration occurs, incision and drainage and administration of antibiotics are indicated.

18.15   HYPERTHYROIDISM

Hyperthyroidism results from excessive secretion of thyroid hormone and, with few exceptions, is due to diffuse toxic goiter (Graves disease) during childhood. Other rare causes of hyperthyroidism which have been observed in children include toxic uninodular goiter (Plummer disease), hyperfunctioning thyroid carcinoma, thyrotoxicosis factitia, and acute suppurative thyroiditis. Hyperthyroidism is common in patients with McCune-Albright syndrome; suppression of plasma TSH indicates that the hyperthyroidism is not hypothalamic in origin. Hyperthyroidism due to excess thyrotropin secretion is rare and in most instances is caused by a TSH-secreting pituitary tumor. One child with thyrotoxicosis and elevated levels of TSH has been reported; since no pituitary tumor was found, disordered hypothalamic-pituitary homeostasis was suggested as the cause. In infants born to mothers with Graves disease hyperthyroidism may occur as a transitory phenomenon or as classic Graves disease during the neonatal period. Choriocarcinoma, hydatidiform mole, and struma ovarii have caused hyperthyroidism in adults but have not as yet been recognized as causes in children.

GRAVES DISEASE

Etiology. There is evidence that immune factors participate in the pathogenesis of Graves disease and may be essential to its initiation. Enlargement of the thymus, splenomegaly, lymphadenopathy, infiltration of the thyroid gland and of retro-ocular tissues with lymphocytes and plasma cells, and peripheral lymphocytosis are common findings in Graves disease.

Patients with this condition produce an immunoglobulin which binds to the receptor for TSH and on such binding stimulates the process which normally is set in motion by TSH. This sequence leads to thyroid autonomy and hyperthyroidism. Graves disease is the only disease known to be caused by an antibody which stimulates endocrine cells. A variety of antibodies may be demonstrated, including long-acting thyroid stimulator (LATS), LATS protector, and thyroid-stimulating antibody (TSAb) or thyroid-stimulating immunoglobulin (TSI). The levels of these antibodies correlate poorly with exophthalmos, and they are probably not responsible for the ophthalmopathy. Evidence is increasing that cell-mediated immunity is distorted in this disorder; some believe the primary defect resides there. There is an association between HLA-B8 and thyrotoxicosis which is believed to represent linkage between HLA-B8 and a gene controlling the immune response to thyroid antigen.

Other evidence for an autoimmune basis for Graves disease is its coexistence with lymphocytic thyroiditis in the same gland. Like lymphocytic thyroiditis, Graves disease is often associated with other autoimmune disorders such as pernicious anemia, idiopathic adrenal insufficiency, myasthenia gravis, and insulin-dependent diabetes mellitus. Antimicrosomal thyroid autoantibodies and other autoantibodies are frequently found in patients with Graves disease as well as in other members of their families.

Clinical Manifestations. About 5% of all patients with hyperthyroidism are under 15 yr of age; the peak incidence occurs during adolescence. The disease is being increasingly recognized in early infancy apart from the transitory condition which occurs in infants of thyrotoxic mothers (see below); Graves disease has had its onset between 6 wk–2 yr of age in children born to mothers without a history of hyperthyroidism. The incidence is about 5 times higher in girls than in boys.

The clinical course is highly variable but is in general not so fulminant as in many adults. Symptoms develop gradually; the usual interval between onset and diagnosis is 6–12 mo. The earliest signs in children may be emotional disturbances accompanied by motor hyperactivity. They become irritable and excitable and cry easily. Their schoolwork suffers, and their restlessness, which may resemble that of chorea, causes conflicts. Tremor of the fingers can be noticed if the arm is extended. There may be a voracious appetite combined with loss of or no increase in weight. The thyroid is enlarged, palpable, and visible, and bruits may be audible over it. Exophthalmos is noticeable in the majority of patients but is rarely severe. *Graefe sign* (lagging of the upper eyelid as the eye looks downward), *Moebius sign* (impairment of convergence), and *Stellwag sign* (retraction of the upper eyelid and infrequent blinking) may be present. The skin is smooth and flushed, with excessive sweating. Muscular weakness is uncommon but may be so severe as to result in falling spells. Tachycardia, palpitation, dyspnea, and cardiac enlargement and insufficiency cause discomfort and may endanger the patient's life. Atrial fibrillation is a rare complication. Mitral regurgitation, probably resulting from papillary muscle dysfunction, is the cause of the apical systolic murmur present in some patients. The systolic blood pressure and the pulse pressure are increased. Children with hyperthyroidism are usually tall; their osseous development is advanced for their age, but sexual maturation is not altered.

Thyroid "crisis" or "storm" is a form of hyperthyroidism manifested by an acute onset, hyperthermia, and severe tachycardia and restlessness. There may be rapid progression to delirium, coma, and death. "Apathetic" or "masked" hyperthyroidism is another variety of hyperthyroidism characterized by extreme listlessness, apathy, and cachexia. A combination of both forms may also occur. These symptom complexes are rare in children.

Laboratory Data. Levels of both T_4 and T_3 are usually increased, and TSH is suppressed to unmeasurable levels. Radionuclide is rapidly and diffusely concentrated in the enlarged thyroid. In some patients the level of T_4 may be normal and only the level of T_3 elevated, a situation which is termed T_3 *toxicosis*. After treatment of hyperthyroidism the level of T_4 may be low even though the patient is clinically euthyroid. In such patients T_3 levels may be normal. More extensive investigation is rarely necessary if the clinical manifestations are characteristic. For borderline cases evaluation of the response to TRH may be necessary. Elevated levels of thyroid-stimulating immunoglobulin may be found in most patients with newly diagnosed Graves disease; levels appear to correlate with activity of the disorder. Serum levels of thyroglobulin are also increased and remain constant during treatment with antithyroid drugs. A return to normal of thyroglobulin and disappearance of thyroid-stimulating immunoglobulins predict remission of the Graves disease. Antithyroid antibodies are found in most children with Graves disease but are not helpful in predicting remission. Very young children with Graves disease often have advanced skeletal maturation and craniostenosis.

Differential Diagnosis. Diagnosis is rarely difficult once it has been considered. Functional nodules producing hyperthyroidism (Plummer disease) tend to secrete T_3 preferentially and can be detected on radionuclide scanning. Patients with lymphocytic thyroiditis may, on occasion, present manifestations of hyperthyroidism and must be differentiated by appropriate laboratory studies. The clinical pattern of pheochromocytoma may resemble hyperthyroidism, but the elevation of blood pressure is greater, the level of thyroid hormones is within the normal range, and that of catecholamines is elevated. Patients with thyroid hormone unresponsiveness have a goiter and elevated levels of T_4 and T_3. Many patients with this disorder have been erroneously treated for hyperthyroidism, but their normal or elevated levels of TSH should suggest the correct diagnosis.

Treatment. There is no consensus as to the preferred method of treatment. Some prefer subtotal thyroidectomy; others, including ourselves, elect a trial of medical therapy before considering surgery. Most pediatric endocrinologists and radiotherapists avoid the use of radioactive iodine to treat children except for the exceptional patient in whom medical treatment is not feasible and operation is contraindicated or refused.

The recommended antithyroid drugs are propylthiouracil and methimazole (Tapazole). These compounds inhibit incorporation of trapped inorganic iodide into organic compounds and extrathyroidal conversion of T_4 to T_3; recent evidence suggests that they may also inhibit synthesis of thyroid autoantibodies. Toxic reactions occur with about equal frequency with both drugs. The initial dose of propylthiouracil is 100–150 mg, 3 times daily, and that of methimazole is 10–15 mg, 3 times daily. Subsequently, the dose is increased or decreased as indicated. Smaller initial doses should be used in early childhood. Overdosage can lead to a hypothyroid state. Clinical response becomes apparent in 2–3 wk, and adequate control in 1–3 mo. The dose of the medication is then reduced to the minimal level that will maintain the child in a euthyroid state. Careful surveillance is required. Serum levels of T_4 and T_3 should be maintained in the normal range. Rising of serum levels of TSH above 10 μU/ml indicates overtreatment, which will lead to increased size of the goiter.

Drug therapy may be continued for 6 yr or longer since there appears to be a remission rate of about 25% every 2 yr. If a relapse occurs, it will usually appear within 3 mo and almost always within 6 mo after therapy has been discontinued. Therapy may be resumed in case of a relapse. Patients over 13 yr of age, boys, and those with small goiters and modestly elevated T_3 levels appear to have earlier remissions.

The most common toxic reactions are urticarial rashes, leukopenia, fever, arthritis, or arthralgia. In most instances these reactions are transitory even with continued use of the drug. More serious reactions such as agranulocytosis, hepatitis, or a lupus-like syndrome are uncommon. These reactions have been noted with both propylthiouracil and methimazole with about the same incidence, but changing from 1 drug to the other may avert the undesirable effect. A cutaneous vasculitis consisting of intermittent purpuric lesions has been reported in a few children treated with propylthiouracil. It is probably best to treat unusually hypersensitive patients by thyroidectomy.

A beta-adrenergic blocking agent such as propranolol is a useful supplement in the management of the severely toxic patient. Thyroid hormones potentiate the actions of catecholamines, which are manifest as tachycardia, tremor, excessive sweating, lid lag, and stare. These symptoms abate with the use of propranolol, which does not, however, alter thyroid function or exophthalmos.

Operation is indicated when adequate cooperation for medical management is not possible or when adequate trial of medical management has failed to result in permanent remission. Subtotal thyroidectomy, a rather safe procedure, is performed only after the patient has been brought to a euthyroid state. This may be accomplished with propylthiouracil or methimazole over 2–3 mo. After a euthyroid state has been attained, 5 drops of a saturated solution of potassium iodide/day are added to the regimen for 2 wk before operation in order to decrease the vascularity of the gland. Complications of surgical treatment are rare and include hypoparathyroidism (transient or permanent) and paralysis of the vocal cords. The incidence of residual or recurrent hyperthyroidism or of hypothyroidism depends upon the extent of the surgery. With extensive thyroidectomy the incidence of recurrence may be low, but that of hypothyroidism may exceed 50%.

The ophthalmopathy remits gradually and usually independently of the hyperthyroidism.

CONGENITAL HYPERTHYROIDISM

When hyperthyroidism has its onset in the newborn period, the condition is usually transitory, remitting within 3 mo. Infants with transient hyperthyroidism have thyroid-stimulating immunoglobulin (TSI) in their circulation, and their mothers have a history of active or recently active Graves disease. Remission of the condition is paralleled by disappearance of TSI in the infant. The condition is caused by transplacental passage of TSI or other maternal factors as yet unidentified. High levels of TSI in the mother during pregnancy are a good predictor of neonatal thyrotoxicosis. Unlike Graves disease at every other age, the transitory variety affects males as often as females. Occasionally, the condition does not remit but persists for several yr or longer. These patients appear to have typical Graves disease and frequently have impressive family histories of Graves disease. In some infants TSI transfer from the mother appears to blend with autonomous Graves disease of infantile onset.

The clinical course is variable. Many of the infants are premature; the majority, but not all, have goiters. The infant is extremely restless, irritable, and hyperactive and appears anxious and unusually alert. The eyes are widely opened and appear exophthalmic. There may be extreme tachycardia and tachypnea, and the temperature is elevated. In severely affected infants there is progression of symptoms; weight loss occurs despite a ravenous appetite, hepatomegaly increases, and jaundice may become manifest. Cardiac decompensation is common. The condition usually resolves in 6–12 wk, but the infant may die if therapy is not instituted promptly. The serum level of T_4 is markedly elevated. Advanced bone age, frontal bossing, and cranial synostosis are common, especially in those infants with persistent clinical manifestations of hyperthyroidism. Prognosis for intellectual development is guarded for infants with craniostenosis.

Treatment consists of administration of Lugol solution (1 drop every 8 hr) and propylthiouracil (10 mg every 8 hr). If the thyrotoxic state is severe, parenteral fluid therapy, digitalization, and propranolol (2 mg/kg/24 hr given in 3 divided doses) may be indicated. When propranolol is used during pregnancy to treat thyrotoxicosis, it crosses the placenta and may cause respiratory depression in the newborn infant.

18.16 CARCINOMA OF THE THYROID

Carcinoma of the thyroid is rare in children. The ultimate cause is unknown, but about 80% of 227 patients were found to have had irradiation during infancy to the neck and adjacent areas for such benign conditions as "enlarged" thymus, hypertrophied tonsils and adenoids, hemangiomas, nevi, acne, eczema, tinea capitis, and "cervical adenitis." Irradiation for thymic enlargement in infancy has been found to carry a 4% risk of thyroid carcinoma and an approximately 30% risk of thyroid nodularity. In a study of 735 adults with a history of radiation therapy to the head and neck for benign conditions during childhood, 159 were found to have palpable nodules. Of 49 patients operated upon because of growth of the nodule despite suppression therapy with thyroxine, 11 were found to have carcinoma. The interval between irradiation and discovery of a tumor has been as long as 35 yr. Exposure to radioactive fallout containing isotopes of iodine (especially ^{131}I) appears to be a greater risk factor in the child than in the adult. All persons with a history of head or neck irradiation should have careful examination of the thyroid at least every 2 yr for an indefinite period.

Girls are affected twice as often as boys. The average age at diagnosis is 9 yr, but the onset may be as early as the 1st yr of life. A painless nodule in the thyroid or in the neck is the usual 1st evidence of disease. Cervical lymph node involvement is usually present at the time of the initial diagnosis and is often bilateral. Any unexplained cervical lymph node enlargement requires examination of the thyroid, which will occasionally have a primary tumor too small to be felt, the diagnosis being made on biopsy. The lungs are the most common site of metastases beyond the neck. There may be no clinical manifestations referable to them; roentgenographically, they appear as diffuse miliary or nodular infiltrations, principally in the basal portions. They may be mistaken for tuberculosis, histoplasmosis, or sarcoidosis. Other sites of metastases include the mediastinum, long bones, skull, and axilla. On rare occasions the carcinoma may be functional and produce symptoms of hyperthyroidism.

Histologically, the carcinomas are usually papillary, follicular, or mixed differentiated tumors. There is no evidence that the natural history of irradiation-induced thyroid cancer differs from that of papillary or follicular thyroid cancer occurring "spontaneously." The neoplasm frequently grows slowly and may even remain dormant for years; undifferentiated neoplasms, however, may have a rapidly fatal course. The case fatality rate is approximately 20%; death usually occurs in the 1st postoperative yr.

A thyroid scan should be performed whenever a thyroid nodule is found. ^{123}Iodine or ^{99m}technetium pertechnetate is the preferred scanning agent. Most malignant lesions show decreased concentration of radioisotope (are "cold"), but some cold lesions are benign. Serum levels of thyroglobulin (Tg) are often elevated and return to normal after surgical removal of differentiated tumors; this test also permits early detection of metastases. The thyroglobulin levels do not correlate with any histologic characteristics or with malignancy or benignity of thyroid tumors.

The treatment of proven carcinoma of the thyroid is controversial. Some recommend thyroidectomy (hemithyroidectomy with removal of the isthmus if the disease is unilateral), resection of any enlarged cervical nodes, and postoperative roentgen therapy. Others recommend total thyroidectomy and regional resection of lymph nodes even though there is no evidence of involvement of them. Unresectable tumors should be removed as fully as possible along with any normal thyroid tissue in preparation for the possible use of radioiodine. Radioiodine should be used only when the lesion cannot be completely removed surgically and when the cancerous tissue is capable of concentrating therapeutic doses. Regression of extensive pulmonary metastases has been observed to follow the use of radioiodine. Doxorubicin appears to offer benefit for some patients with progressive and refractory metastatic disease.

After surgery all patients should be treated with sodium-L-thyroxine in doses sufficient to suppress TSH. Periodic determinations of serum levels of Tg provide an excellent marker for recurrence in patients taking T_4 and are supplanting routine radionuclide scans.

SOLITARY THYROID NODULE

Solitary nodules of the thyroid are uncommon in children. In the past it was estimated that as many as half were carcinoma, but more recent studies indicate a much lower incidence of malignancy, perhaps because of decreasing exposure of children to irradiation. Children exposed to irradiation have a high incidence of benign adenoma as well as of carcinoma of the thyroid.

Benign disorders which may present as solitary thyroid nodules include benign adenomas (follicular, embryonal, Hurthle cell), lymphocytic thyroiditis, thyroglossal duct cyst, ectopically located normal thyroid tissue, a single median thyroid, agenesis of 1 of the lateral thyroid lobes with hypertrophy of the contralateral lobe, thyroid cysts, and abscess. Sudden appearance of or rapidly enlarging thyroid mass may indicate hemorrhage into a benign adenoma. In most instances the child is euthyroid and thyroid function studies are normal. A ^{99m}Tc scan is usually indicated. Ultrasonography is particularly useful in detecting cystic lesions. When lymphocytic thyroiditis is the cause of the nodule, T_4 may be low, TSH may be elevated, and thyroid antibodies are usually present. The scan may reveal a motheaten appearance. Rarely, lymphocytic thyroiditis may be associated with carcinoma of the thyroid.

Some nodules are "cold" on ^{99m}Tc scan, as is the case for carcinoma, but other lesions, such as developmental defects of the thyroid, are usually "hot." In questionable cases one may use suppressive therapy with 0.2–0.3 mg daily of sodium-L-thyroxine. Cold nodules that continue to grow over 4–6 mo or that do not reduce in size by 50% in 1 yr should be surgically explored. Surgery without delay is indicated when the nodule is hard or has grown rapidly, when there is evidence of tracheal or vocal cord involvement, or when there is enlargement of adjacent lymph nodes.

Very rarely, thyroid nodules may be functional, producing hyperthyroidism (Plummer disease). The uptake of radionuclide is concentrated in the nodule ("hot" nodule), and thyroid function studies indicate that the nodule is functioning autonomously. Such nodules are almost always benign. They may secrete T_3 preferen-

tially; hence, T_4 levels may be normal, whereas T_3 levels are elevated (T_3 toxicosis).

A suppressible functioning nodule in a euthyroid child has been reported only once.

MEDULLARY CARCINOMA

This familial (usually autosomal dominant) carcinoma of the thyroid arises from the parafollicular cells (C cells) of the thyroid and accounts for about 10% of thyroid malignancies. The tumor is pleomorphic, with sheets of spindle or small cells with eosinophilic granular cytoplasm. Amyloid is invariably deposited in the stroma, and calcification is common. The most common symptom is goiter or a palpable thyroid nodule. In about a third of patients roentgenograms reveal dense, conglomerate, homogeneous calcification in the thyroid. Metastases to regional lymph nodes and to liver are common, and these too may calcify. Death may result, but long survivals are not uncommon.

These tumors arise from the cells which secrete calcitonin; accordingly, circulating levels of calcitonin are consistently elevated. Normal levels of calcitonin, either basal or after calcium infusion, usually do not exceed 0.5 ng/ml as measured by a sensitive radioimmunoassay method, whereas levels in patients with tumors are commonly 25–50 ng/ml. Measurement of calcitonin levels in subjects at risk can uncover occult tumors; tumors too small to be found by palpation or by scanning have been detected as early as 2 yr of age. These tumors elaborate other specific biochemical markers, particularly histaminase and dopa decarboxylase. In addition, elevated levels of prostaglandins, serotonin, and ACTH have been detected in tumors and in serum of some patients and have accounted for the diarrhea or for the Cushing syndrome, both of which are occasionally associated. Monitoring the levels of calcitonin and/or histaminase is useful for detecting metastatic lesions and for following the course of disease after operation.

Treatment consists of total thyroidectomy since the tumor is usually present in both lobes. Diagnosis of medullary thyroid carcinoma should always lead one to search for other associated tumors, pheochromocytoma in particular.

Multiple Endocrine Neoplasia, Type II (MEN). In some families medullary carcinoma of the thyroid is associated with pheochromocytoma and parathyroid hyperplasia. This association is also known as Sipple syndrome or multiple endocrine adenomatosis (MEA). Penetrance for the various components of the syndrome is high. When pheochromocytomas are found, they are frequently bilateral and may be multiple. The parathyroid glands may reveal only hypercellularity or may manifest chief-cell hyperplasia. Hypercalcemia may be present. The hyperparathyroidism is probably the result of the same genetic defect responsible for the thyroid carcinoma and for the pheochromocytoma; it does not seem to be secondary to the elevated calcitonin level since elevated levels of parathormone have been found in patients with normal levels of calcitonin. A primary defect of the neural crest can account for all the findings in the syndrome.

Mucosal Neuroma Syndrome. Some patients with medullary carcinoma and pheochromocytoma exhibit mucosal neuromas and skeletal anomalies. They represent a distinct subgroup of the MEN syndrome, also referred to as MEN IIa or IIb or MEN III. The neuromas most often occur on the tongue, buccal mucosa, lips, and conjunctivae. Peripheral neurofibromas and café au lait patches may be present, and intestinal ganglioneuromatosis is common. The patients may be tall, with arachnodactyly, and present a Marfan-like appearance. Scoliosis, pectus excavatum, pes cavus, and muscular hypotonia are common. The eyelids may be thickened, the lips patulous, the jaw prognathic.

The diffuse ganglioneuromatosis of the submucosal and myenteric plexuses may involve the esophagus as well as the small and large intestines. Diarrhea or constipation or both may begin in infancy or childhood and precede the endocrine manifestations by many yr.

Thyroidectomy has been recommended for children with increased calcitonin levels even if the thyroid is normal to palpation and on radionuclide scan. Infants born to an affected parent have a 50% risk of being affected and must be carefully evaluated for evidence of the syndrome in early infancy.

General

Williams RH (ed): Textbook of Endocrinology. Ed 6. Philadelphia, WB Saunders, 1981.

Hypothyroidism

Abassi V, Steinour TA: Successful diagnosis of congenital hypothyroidism in four breast-fed neonates. J Pediatr 97:259, 1980.
Anderson HJ: Studies of hypothyroidism in children. Acta Pediatr 50 (Suppl 125), 1961.
Burrow GN, Dussault JH (eds): Neonatal Thyroid Screening. New York, Raven Press, 1980.
Burt L, Kulin HE: Head circumference in children with short stature secondary to primary hypothyroidism. Pediatrics 59:628, 1977.
Codaocioni JL, Cargyon P, Miche-Bechet M, et al: Congenital hypothyroidism associated with thyrotropin unresponsiveness and thyroid cell membrane alterations. J Clin Endocrinol Metab 50:932, 1980.
Dussault JH, Letarte J, Guyda H, et al: Thyroid function in neonatal hypothyroidism. J Pediatr 89:541, 1976.
Dussault JH, Letarte J, Guyda H, et al: Serum thyroid hormone and TSH concentrations in newborn infants with congenital absence of thyroxine-binding globulin. J Pediatr 90:264, 1977.
Dussault JH, Letarte J, Guyda H, et al: Lack of influence of thyroid antibodies on thyroid function in the newborn infant and on a mass screening program for congenital hypothyroidism. J Pediatr 96:385, 1980.
Effects of neonatal screening for hypothyroidism: Prevention of mental retardation by treatment before clinical manifestations. Congenital Hypothyroidism Collaborative. Lancet 1:1095, 1981.
Fisher DA, Klein AH: Thyroid development and disorders of thyroid function in the newborn. N Engl J Med 304:702, 1981.
Greig WR, Hendersen AS, Boyle JA, et al: Thyroid dysgenesis in two pairs of monozygotic twins and a mother and child. J Clin Endocrinol Metab 26:1309, 1966.
Kaplan MM, Swartz SL, Larsen PR: Partial peripheral resistance to thyroid hormone. Am J Med 70:1115, 1981.
Klein AH, Foley TP Jr, Larsen PR, et al: Neonatal thyroid function in congenital hypothyroidism. J Pediatr 89:545, 1976.
Letarte J, Guyda H, Dussault JH, Glorieux J: Lack of protective effect of breastfeeding in congenital hypothyroidism: Report of 12 cases. Pediatrics 65:703, 1980.
Little G, Meador CK, Cunningham R, et al: "Cryptothyroidism." The major cause of sporadic "athyreotic" cretinism. J Clin Endocrinol Metab 25:1529, 1965.
Matsura N, Yamada Y, Nohara Y, et al: Familial neonatal transient hypothyroidism due to maternal TSH-binding inhibitor immunoglobulins. N Engl J Med 303:738, 1980.
Miyai K, Azukizawa M, Komahara Y: Familial isolated thyrotropin deficiency with cretinism. N Engl J Med 285:1043, 1971.
Moncrief MW, McArthur RG: Hypothyroidism in one of monozygotic twins. Postgrad Med J 44:423, 1968.
Najjar SS: Muscular hypertrophy in hypothyroid children. The Kocher-Debré-Sémélaigne syndrome. J Pediatr 85:236, 1974.
Neinas FW, Groman CA, Devine KD, et al: Lingual thyroid. Clinical characteristics of 15 cases. Ann Intern Med 79:205, 1973.

Refetoff S, DeGroot LJ, Barsano CP: Defective thyroid hormone feedback regulation in the syndrome of peripheral resistance to thyroid hormone. J Clin Endocrinol Metab 51:41, 1980.
Rezvani I, DiGeorge AM: Reassessment of the daily dose of oral thyroxine for replacement therapy in hypothyroid children. J Pediatr 90:291, 1977.
Rezvani I, DiGeorge AM, Cote ML: Primary hypothyroidism in cystinosis. J Pediatr 91:340, 1973.
Smith DW, Klein AM, Henderson JR, et al: Congenital hypothyroidism—signs and symptoms in the newborn period. J Pediatr 87:958, 1975.
Smith DW, Popich G: Large fontanels in congenital hypothyroidism: A potential clue toward earlier recognition. J Pediatr 80:753, 1972.
Staffer SS, Hamburger JI: Inadvertent ^{131}I therapy for hypothyroidism in the first trimester of pregnancy. J Nucl Med 17:146, 1976.
VanHerle AJ, Vassart G, Dumont JE: Control of thyroglobulin synthesis and secretion. N Engl J Med 301:239, 307, 1979.

Goitrous Cretinism

Burrow GN, Spaulding SW, Alexander NM, et al: Normal peroxidase activity in Pendred's syndrome. J Clin Endocrinol Metab 36:522, 1973.
Gattereau A, Bernard B, Bellabarba D, et al: Congenital goiter in four euthyroid siblings with glandular and circulating iodoproteins and defective iodothyronine synthesis. J Clin Endocrinol Metab 37:118, 1973.
Goslings BM, et al: Hypothyroidism in an area of endemic goiter and cretinism in central Java, Indonesia. J Clin Endocrinol Metab 44:481, 1977.
Illum P, Kiaer HW, Hvidberg-Hansen J, et al: Fifteen cases of Pendred's syndrome. Congenital deafness and sporadic goiter. Arch Otolaryngol 96:297, 1972.
Lissitzky S, et al: Congenital goiter with impaired thyroglobulin synthesis. J Clin Endocrinol Metab 36:17, 1973.
Riesco G, Bernal J, Sanchez-Franco F: Thyroglobulin defect in a human congenital goiter. J Clin Endocrinol Metab 38:33, 1974.
Saito K, Yamamoto K, Yoshida S, et al: Goitrous hypothyroidism due to iodide-trapping defect. J Clin Endocrinol Metab 53:1267, 1981.
Savoie JC, Massin JP, Savoie F: Studies of mono- and diiodohistidine. II. Congenital goitrous hypothyroidism with thyroglobulin defect and iodohistidine-rich iodoalbumin production. J Clin Invest 52:116, 1973.
Stanbury JB: Familial goiter. In Stanbury JB, Wyngaarden JB, Fredrickson DS (eds): The Metabolic Basis of Inherited Disease. Ed 3. New York, McGraw-Hill, 1972.
Valenta LJ, Bode H, Vickery AL, et al: Lack of thyroid peroxidase activity as a cause of congenital goitrous hypothyroidism. J Clin Endocrinol Metab 36:830, 1972.

Goiter

Delange F, Ermans AM, Vis HL, et al: Endemic cretinism in Idjwi Island (Kivu Lake, Republic of the Congo). J Clin Endocrinol Metab 34:1059, 1972.
Galina MP, Avnet NL, Fanhorn A: Iodides during pregnancy. An apparent cause of neonatal death. N Engl J Med 267:1124, 1962.
Martin MM, Renato RD: Iodide goiter with hypothyroidism in two newborn infants. J Pediatr 61:94, 1962.
Patel YC, Pharoah POD, Hornabrook RW, et al: Serum triiodothyronine, thyroxine and thyroid-stimulating hormone in endemic goiter: A comparison of goitrous and non-goitrous subjects in New Guinea. J Clin Endocrinol Metab 7:783, 1973.
Pharoah POD, Buttfield IH, Hetzel BS: Neurological damage to the foetus resulting from severe iodine deficiency during pregnancy. Lancet 1:308, 1971.
Ramalingaswami V: Endemic goiter in Southeast Asia. New clothes on an old body. Ann Intern Med 78:277, 1973.
Randolph J, Grunt JA, Vawter GF: The medical and surgical aspects of intratracheal goiter. N Engl J Med 268:457, 1963.

Hyperthyroidism

Amrheim JA, Kenny FM, Ross D: Granulocytopenia, lupus-like syndrome, and other complications of propylthiouracil therapy. J Pediatr 76:54, 1970.
Cheron RG, Kaplan MM, Larsen PR, et al: Neonatal thyroid function after propylthiouracil therapy for maternal Graves' disease. N Engl J Med 304:525, 1981.
Collen RJ, Landaw EM, Kaplan SA, Lippe BM: Remission rates of children and adolescents with thyrotoxicosis treated with antithyroid drugs. Pediatrics 65:550, 1980.
Daneman D, Howard NJ: Neonatal thyrotoxicosis: Intellectual impairment and craniosynostosis in later years. J Pediatr 97:257, 1980.
Darby CP: Three episodes of spontaneous thyroid storm occurring in a nine year-old child. Pediatrics 30:927, 1962.
Hayles AB: Problems of childhood Graves' disease. Mayo Clin Proc 47:850, 1972.
Hollingsworth DR, Mabry CC: Congenital Graves disease. Am J Dis Child 130:148, 1976.
Hulazun JF, Anst CS, Lukens JN: Thyrotoxicosis associated with Aspergillus thyroiditis in chronic granulomatosis disease. J Pediatr 80:106, 1972.
Kogut MD, Kaplan SA, Collipp PJ, et al: Treatment of hyperthyroidism in children. N Engl J Med 272:217, 1965.

Lightner ES, Allen HD, Laughlin G: Neonatal hyperthyroidism and heart failure. Am J Dis Child 131:68, 1977.

McGregor AM, Peterson MM, McLachlan SM et al: Carbimazole and the autoimmune response in Graves' disease. N Engl J Med 303:302, 1980.

Mihailovic V, Feller MS, Kourides IA, Utiger RD: Hyperthyroidism due to excess thyrotropin secretion: Follow-up studies. J Clin Endocrinol Metab 50:1135, 1980.

Perry LW, Hung W: Atrial fibrillation and hyperthyroidism in a 14-year-old boy. J Pediatr 79:668, 1971.

Pompa BH, Cloutier MD, Hayles AB: Thyroid nodule producing T_3 toxicosis in a child. Mayo Clin Proc 48:273, 1973.

Reynolds JL, Woody HB: Thyrotoxic mitral regurgitation. Am J Dis Child 122:544, 1971.

Riggs W Jr, Wilroy RS Jr, Etteldorf JN: Neonatal hyperthyroidism with accelerated skeletal maturation, craniosynostosis, and brachydactyly. Radiology 105:621, 1972.

Samuel S, Gilman S, Maurer HS, et al: Hyperthyroidism in an infant with McCune-Albright syndrome: Report of a case with myeloid dysplasia. J Pediatr 80:275, 1972.

Smith CS, Howard NJ: Propranolol in treatment of neonatal thyrotoxicosis. J Pediatr 83:1046, 1973.

Vasily DB, Tyler SB: Propylthiouracil-induced cutaneous vasculitis. JAMA 243:458, 1980.

Wilroy RS Jr, Etteldorf JN: Familial hypothyroidism including two siblings with neonatal Graves' disease. J Pediatr 78:625, 1971.

Zakarija M, McKenzie JM, Banovic K: Clinical significance of assay of thyroid-stimulating antibody in Graves' disease. Ann Intern Med 93:28, 1980.

Lymphocytic Thyroiditis

Doniach D, Nilsson LR, Roitt IM: Autoimmune thyroiditis in children and adolescents. Acta Pediatr 54:260, 1965.

Greenberg AH, Czernichow P, Hung W, et al: Juvenile chronic lymphocytic thyroiditis: Clinical, laboratory and histologic correlations. J Clin Endocrinol Metab 30:293, 1970.

Goldsmith RE, McAdams AJ, Larsen PR, et al: Familial autoimmune thyroiditis: Maternal-fetal relationship and the role of generalized autoimmunity. J Clin Endocrinol Metab 37:265, 1973.

Humbert JR, Gotlin RW, Hotetter G, et al: Lymphocytic (auto-immune, Hashimoto's) thyroiditis. Arch Dis Child 43:80, 1968.

Hung W, Chandra R, August GP, et al: Clinical, laboratory and histologic observations in euthyroid children and adolescents with goiters. J Pediatr 82:10, 1973.

Leboeuf G, Bongiovanni AM: Thyroiditis in childhood. Adv Pediatr 13:183, 1964.

Loeb PB, Drash AL, Kenny FM: Prevalence of low titer and "negative" antithyroglobulin antibodies in biopsy-proven juvenile Hashimoto's thyroiditis. J Pediatr 82:17, 1973.

Monteleone JA, Danis RK, Tung KSK, et al: Differentiation of chronic lymphocytic thyroiditis and simple goiter in pediatrics. J Pediatr 83:381, 1973.

Rallison ML, Dobyns BM, Keating FR, et al: Occurrence and natural history of chronic lymphocytic thyroiditis in childhood. J Pediatr 86:675, 1975.

Riley WJ, Maclaren NK, Lezotte DC, et al: Thyroid autoimmunity in insulin-dependent diabetes mellitus. The case for routine screening. J Pediatr 98:350, 1981.

Winter J, Eberlein WR, Bongiovanni AM: The relationship of juvenile hypothyroidism to chronic lymphocytic thyroiditis. J Pediatr 69:709, 1966.

Ziring PR, et al: Chronic lymphocytic thyroiditis: Identification of rubella virus antigen in the thyroid of a child with congenital rubella. J Pediatr 90:419, 1977.

Carcinoma of the Thyroid

Ashcroft NW, Van Herle AJ: The comparative value of serum thyroglobulin measurements and iodine I^{131} total body scans in the follow-up of patients treated with differentiated thyroid cancer. Am J Med 71:806, 1981.

Black EG, Cassoni A, Gimlette TMD, et al: Serum thyroglobulin in thyroid cancer. Lancet 2:443, 1981.

Carney JA, Go VLW, Sizemore GW, et al: Alimentary tract ganglioneuromatosis. A major component of the syndrome of multiple endocrine neoplasia, type 2b. N Engl J Med 295:1287, 1976.

Fisher DA: Thyroid nodules in children and their management. J Pediatr 89:866, 1976.

Forsman PJ, Jenkins ME: Medullary carcinoma of the thyroid with Marfan-like body habitus. Pediatrics 52:188, 1973.

Green DM, Brecher ML, Yakar D, et al: Thyroid function in pediatric patients after neck irradiation for Hodgkin disease. Med Pediatr Oncol 8:127, 1980.

Gutjahr P, Spranger J: Thyroidectomy in Type IIb multiple-endocrine-neoplasia syndrome. Lancet 1:1149, 1977.

Hempelmann LH, Hall WJ, Phillips M, et al: Neoplasma in persons treated with x-rays in infancy: Fourth survey in 20 years. J Natl Cancer Inst 55:519, 1975.

Keiser HR, Beaven MA, Doppham J, et al: Sipple's syndrome: Medullary thyroid carcinoma, pheochromocytoma and parathyroid disease. Ann Intern Med 78:561, 1973.

Kirkland RT, Kirkland JL, Rosenberg HS, et al: Solitary thyroid nodules in 30 children and report of a child with a thyroid abscess. Pediatrics 51:85, 1973.

Levin DL, Perlia C, Tashjian AH: Medullary carcinoma of the thyroid gland: The complete syndrome in a child. Pediatrics 52:192, 1973.

Pilch BZ, Kahn R, Ketcham AS, et al: Thyroid cancer after radioactive iodine diagnostic procedures in childhood. Pediatrics 51:898, 1973.

Razack MS, Sako K, Shimaoka K, et al: Radiation-associated thyroid carcinoma. J Surg Oncol 14:287, 1980.

Refetoff S, Harrison J, Karanifilski BT, et al: Continuing occurrence of thyroid carcinoma after irradiation to the neck in infancy and childhood. N Engl J Med 292:171, 1975.

Rosenbloom AL: Functioning solitary nodule of the thyroid in a child. J Pediatr 82:491, 1973.

Scott MD, Crawford JD: Solitary thyroid nodules in childhood: Is the incidence of thyroid carcinoma declining? Pediatrics 58:521, 1976.

Stjernholm MR, Freudenborrg JC, Mooney HS, et al: Medullary carcinoma of the thyroid before age 2 years. J Clin Endocrinol Metab 51:252, 1980.

Sussman L, Librik L, Clayton GW: Hyperthyroidism attributable to a hyperfunctioning thyroid carcinoma. J Pediatr 72:208, 1968.

18.17 DISORDERS OF THE PARATHYROID GLANDS

Parathyroid hormone (PTH), vitamin D, and calcitonin are the principal regulators of calcium homeostasis.

Parathyroid Hormone. PTH is an 84 amino acid chain (9500 dalton), but its biologic activity resides in the 1st 34 residues. In the parathyroid gland a proparathyroid hormone (90 amino acid chain) and a pre-pro-PTH (115 amino acid chain) are synthesized. Pre-pro-PTH is converted to pro-PTH in the endoplasmic reticulum and pro-PTH to PTH in the Golgi apparatus. PTH (1–84) is the major secretory product of the gland, but it is rapidly cleaved, probably in the liver and kidney, into smaller COOH-terminal and NH_2-terminal fragments. The 1–34 amino-terminal fragment possesses biologic activity but is poorly immunoreactive. Discrepancies in the results of radioimmunoassays (iPTH) are due in part to the fact that various assays for PTH have differing specificities for species of PTH in serum or plasma which vary in immunologic activities. It is now generally agreed that carboxy-terminal fragments represent 80% of circulating iPTH. Although these fragments are biologically inactive, there is a good correlation of their quantity with hyperparathyroidism.

When serum levels of calcium fall, secretion of PTH increases, and PTH mobilizes calcium by direct enhancement of bone resorption; this effect requires normal levels of 1,25-dihydroxycholecalciferol (1,25-$[OH]_2$-D_3). PTH also decreases renal excretion of calcium, but this effect plays a relatively minor role in restoration of normocalcemia. The effects of PTH on bone and kidney are mediated through binding to specific receptors on the membranes of target cells and subsequent activation of the adenylate cyclase system. Cyclic AMP, in turn, binds to specific intracellular receptor proteins which mediate the hormone effect. The most important action of PTH is to increase absorption of calcium from the intestine. This effect is achieved indirectly by activation of $l\alpha$-hydroxylase activity, with ensuing increase in the synthesis of 1,25-$(OH)_2$-D_3 (Fig 18–13); 1,25-$(OH)_2$-D_3 induces synthesis of calcium-binding protein in the intestinal mucosa, with resultant increased absorption of calicum.

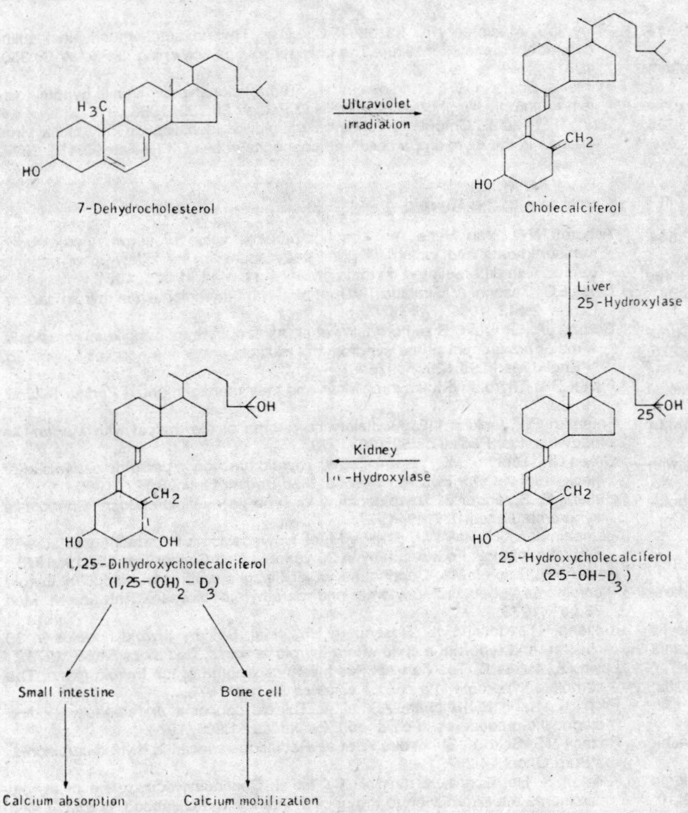

Figure 18–13   Scheme of 1.25·(OH)$_2$-D$_3$ synthesis.

Vitamin D. The mode of action of vitamin D at the molecular level and its relationship to PTH have remained elusive until recently. Its native form, cholecalciferol (vitamin D$_3$), is formed in the skin from a precursor by the action of ultraviolet light; cholecalciferol is hydroxylated primarily in the liver to 25-hydroxycholecalciferol (25-OH-D$_3$ or calcitriol) (Fig 18–13). This is the major circulating compound with vitamin D activity (approximately 20–50 ng/dl), but it must be further hydroxylated to form the physiologically active compound 1,25-dihydroxycholecalciferol (1,25-(OH)$_2$-D$_3$ or calcitriol). Hydroxylation of the 1α position occurs exclusively in the kidneys and is regulated by levels of PTH rather than by a direct effect of calcium in blood. Evidence suggests that decreased levels of phosphate also result in increased synthesis of 1,25-(OH)$_2$-D$_3$ even in the absence of the parathyroids.

Circulating levels of 1,25-(OH)$_2$-D$_3$ are about 1/250th those of 25-OH-D$_3$. This "vitamin" has all the characteristics of a sterol hormone. It localizes in the nuclei of target cells, primarily in intestine and bone. It binds initially to a cytosol receptor, is transported to nuclear chromatin, and induces synthesis of specific mRNA which codes for specific functional proteins. The calcium-binding protein in the mucosal cells of the intestine is regulated in this fashion by 1,25-(OH)$_2$-D$_3$. Though we now have new insights into clinical disorders involving calcium, parathyroids, and rachitic conditions, the full story of vitamin D is yet to be unfolded. Synthetic 1α-hydroxycholecalciferol is equipotent with 1,25-(OH)$_2$-D$_3$ (calcitriol) to which it is presumably converted in the body; both are available for therapy.

Calcitonin. Calcitonin, discovered in 1961, is a polypeptide of 32 amino acids. In birds, amphibians, and teleost fish calcitonin is synthesized in a discrete structure, the ultimobranchial gland. In mammals this gland has become incorporated into the thyroid gland as the parafollicular or C-cells. Although calcitonin was discovered through its hypocalcemic effect, patients with medullary carcinoma of the thyroid, a tumor arising from the parafollicular cells, usually have normal plasma levels of calcium in spite of markedly increased levels of calcitonin.

The physiologic role of calcitonin remains uncertain. Its action appears to be independent of PTH and of vitamin D. Its main biologic effect appears to be the inhibition of bone resorption by decreasing the number and activity of bone-resorbing osteoclasts. This action of calcitonin is the rationale behind its use in treatment of Paget disease. Calcitonin is synthesized also in other organs, such as the gastrointestinal tract, pancreas, brain, and pituitary. In these organs calcitonin is believed to behave as a neurotransmitter to impose a local inhibitory effect on cell function.

18.18 HYPOPARATHYROIDISM

Etiology (see Table 18–4). The normal level of PTH in cord blood is low; it doubles by the 6th day to reach a level nearly that of normal infants and children. Hypocalcemia is common from 12–72 hr of life, especially in premature infants, in infants with asphyxia at birth, and in infants of diabetic mothers (*early neonatal*

Table 18–4 ETIOLOGIC CLASSIFICATION OF HYPOCALCEMIA

Parathyroid hormone (PTH) deficiency
  Transient hypofunction
    Early neonatal hypocalcemia
    Late neonatal hypocalcemia
    Maternal hyperparathyroidism
    Other
  Congenital aplasia or hypoplasia of parathyroids
    With thymic and other III–IV arch defects (DiGeorge syndrome)
    With Zellweger syndrome
    With chromosomal abnormalities (especially 22p−)
    With congenital hypothyroidism due to maternal [131]I
    With maternal diabetes mellitus or alcoholism
    Isolated defects
  Familial hypoparathyroidism
    X-linked
    Autosomal dominant
  Idiopathic hypoparathyroidism
    Autoimmune hypoparathyroiditis
      Isolated
      Associated with other autoimmune disorders and/or mucocutaneous candidiasis
    Congenital hypoplasia
  Surgical removal or damage to parathyroids
  Hemosiderosis (thalassemia major)
  Ineffective parathyroid hormone (pseudoidiopathic hypoparathyroidism)
  Parathyroid hormone unresponsiveness
    Defect in generation of cyclic AMP (Type I pseudohypoparathyroidism)
    Defect in reception of cyclic AMP signal (Type II pseudohypoparathyroidism)
Calcitonin excess?—medullary carcinoma of thyroid
Vitamin D deficiency
  Inadequate irradiation (clothing, housing, smog, climate)
  Dietary deficiency
  Malabsorption
    Deficiency of bile salts (liver disease)
    Deficiency of calcium-binding protein (gluten-sensitive enteropathy)
    Intestinal bypass operations
  Depletion (bile fistulas)
  Altered metabolism (chronic therapy with phenytoin [diphenylhydantoin] and/or phenobarbital)
  Impaired synthesis of 25-(OH)-D_3 (severe hepatic disease)
  Impaired synthesis of 1,25-$(OH)_2$-D_3
    Renal failure
    Renal tubular disease?
    Genetic deficiency of 1α-hydroxylase (vitamin D–dependent rickets, Type I)
    Hypoparathyroidism
  End-organ resistance to 1,25-$(OH)_2$-D_3 (vitamin D–dependent rickets, Type II)
    With alopecia
    Without alopecia
Magnesium deficiency
  Familial hypomagnesemia
  Other malabsorption syndromes
Inorganic phosphate excess
  Poisoning
  Initial therapy of leukemia

hypocalcemia). (See also Sec 7.54). After the 2nd–3rd day and during the 1st wk of life, the type of feeding is also a determinant of the level of serum calcium (*late neonatal hypocalcemia*). The role played by the parathyroids in these hypocalcemic infants remains to be clarified though functional immaturity of the parathyroids has often been invoked as pathogenetic. In a group of infants with *transient idiopathic hypocalcemia* (1–8 wk of age) serum levels of parathormone were significantly lower than in normal infants. It is possible that the functional immaturity is a manifestation of a delay in development of the enzymes which convert glandular PTH to secreted PTH; other mechanisms are possible.

Transient hypocalcemia also occurs in infants born to *mothers with hyperparathyroidism*. It appears that the hypocalcemia in such infants results from suppression of the fetal parathyroids by exposure to elevated levels of calcium in maternal serum. Tetany usually develops within 3 wk but may be delayed 1 mo or more; hypocalcemia may persist for weeks or months. When the cause of hypocalcemia in young infants is unknown, their mothers should have measurements of calcium, phosphorus, and parathyroid hormone.

Aplasia of the parathyroid glands is often associated with other developmental defects arising from the 3rd and 4th pharyngeal pouches (*DiGeorge syndrome*) (see Fig 18–14 and Sec 9.11). The most common associations are aplasia of the thymus and congenital heart defects (especially those involving the aorta, such as truncus arteriosus and interruption of the aortic arch). Absences of the isthmus of the thyroid and of the parafollicular cells have been noted. Micrognathia, cleft lip and/or palate, and abnormalities of the ears are occasional external clues. The disorder is usually sporadic, but autosomal dominant and autosomal recessive inheritance have been reported. In other instances deletions of the short arm of chromosome 22 have been associated. The syndrome has occurred in infants of diabetic mothers and in association with the fetal alcohol syndrome. Accordingly, evidence suggests a heterogeneous etiology for congenital aplasia of the parathyroids. Incomplete forms of the syndrome (*hypoplasia of the parathyroids*) occur more often than the complete syndrome. Tetany may have a delayed onset, and the manifestations of thymic deficiency may be attenuated.

Affected patients would not be expected to have circulating antiparathyroid antibodies or to have other associated autoimmune disorders. Roentgenograms of the chest for visualization of the thymus should be routinely obtained in the study of infants with tetany. Administration of ^{131}I during pregnancy has resulted in hypoparathyroidism as well as in hypothyroidism.

Familial Congenital Hypoparathyroidism. In 2 large pedigrees this disorder appears to be transmitted by an X-linked recessive gene. Onset of afebrile seizures characteristically occurs from 2 wk–6 mo of age. Familial hypoparathyroidism that has been observed also in both sexes in successive generations suggests autosomal dominant inheritance. The age of onset ranges from infancy to young adulthood. The nature of the defect is not known for either type, and there are no associated congenital defects. Hypocalcemia, hyperphosphatemia,

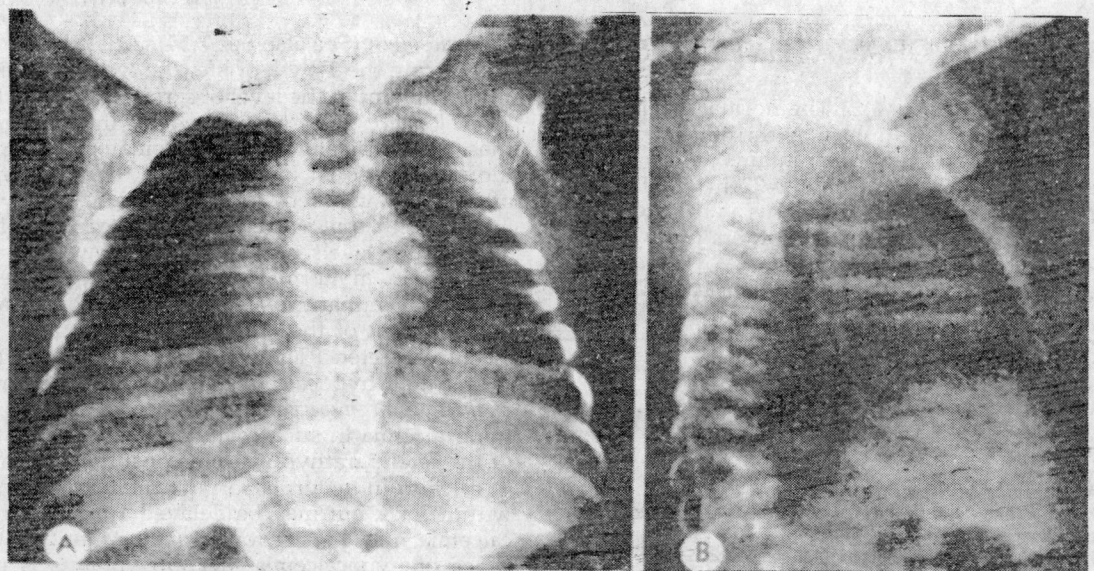

Figure 18–14   Congenital absence of parathyroid glands. Roentgenograms of chest exposed at 6 days of age reveal no evidence of thymus. *A,* The mediastinum is narrow; *B,* the substernal area is radiolucent. (Kirkpatrick, DiGeorge: Am. J Roentgenol 103:32, 1968.)

low levels of immunoreactive PTH, and absence of parathyroid antibodies occur in both types.

Removal or damage of the parathyroid glands may complicate thyroidectomy *(surgical hypoparathyroidism).* Hypoparathyroidism has developed even when the parathyroid glands have been identified and left undisturbed at the time of operation. This, presumably, is the result of interference with the blood supply or of postoperative edema and fibrosis. Symptoms of tetany may occur abruptly postoperatively and be temporary or permanent. In some instances symptoms develop insidiously and go undetected until months after thyroidectomy. Occasionally, the 1st evidence of surgical hypoparathryoidism may be the development of cataracts. All patients subjected to thyroidectomy should have the status of parathyroid function carefully monitored.

Hemosiderosis may produce hypoparathyroidism through progressive deposition of iron pigment in the parathyroid glands.

Idiopathic Hypoparathyroidism. This term is a carryover from the time when the etiology of most instances of acquired hypoparathyroidism was unknown. It is now clear that the majority of children in whom hypoparathyroidism has an onset after the 1st few yr of life have an autoimmune condition. A much smaller percentage of children have the incomplete form of the DiGeorge syndrome or the autosomal dominant type of familial hypoparathyroidism. The term "idiopathic" should be reserved for the small residuum of children with hypoparathyroidism for which no etiologic mechanism can be defined.

Autoimmune Hypoparathyroidism. An autoimmune mechanism for hypoparathyroidism is strongly suggested by the finding of parathyroid antibodies and by the frequent association with other autoimmune disorders and/or organ-specific antibodies. Autoimmune hypoparathyroidism occurs most often in association with Addison disease and chronic mucocutaneous candidiasis. The association of at least 2 of these 3 conditions has been tentatively classified as *polyglandular autoimmune disease, type I.* One third of patients with this syndrome have all 3 components; two thirds have only 2 of 3 conditions. The candidiasis almost always precedes the other disorders (70% under 5 yr of age); the hypoparathyroidism (90% after 3 yr of age) usually occurs before the Addison disease (90% after 6 yr of age). In addition, a variety of other disorders occur at variable times; these include alopecia areata or totalis, malabsorption disorder, pernicious anemia, gonadal failure, chronic active hepatitis, autoimmune thyroid disease, and vitiligo. These associations may occur in 10–25% of patients; insulin-independent diabetes and IgA deficiency are much less frequent concomitants.

Affected siblings may have the same or different constellations of disorders (e.g., hypoparathyroidism and Addison disease). No HLA type has been found in excess in these patients. There is a slight predominance of affected females (4–3), but the disorder is thought to have an autosomal recessive mode of inheritance.

Siblings have been observed with nephrosis, nerve deafness, and hypoparathyroidism, a constellation also likely to have an autoimmune basis.

Pseudoidiopathic hypoparathyroidism designates the hypoparathyroidism found in a young adult who had the onset of tetany at 8 yr of age, with all the laboratory findings of idiopathic hypoparathyroidism. He had a normal response to administration of PTH. His serum contained normal to high levels of immunoreactive parathyroid hormone by several assay systems. This patient's endogenous parathyroid hormone appeared to lack biologic effect, possibly because of a defect in conversion of proparathyroid hormone to parathyroid hormone in the gland or a defect in peripheral activation of a secreted, precursor form of PTH.

Clinical Manifestations. There is a spectrum of parathyroid deficiencies with clinical manifestations varying from no symptoms to those of complete and longstanding deficiency. Mild deficiency may be revealed only by appropriate laboratory studies. Muscular pain and cramps are early manifestations; they progress to numbness, stiffness, and tingling of the hands and feet. There may be only positive Chvostek and/or Trousseau signs or laryngeal and carpopedal spasms. Convulsions with loss of consciousness may occur at intervals of days, weeks, or months. These may begin with abdominal pain, followed by tonic rigidity, retraction of the head, and cyanosis. Hypoparathyroidism is frequently mistaken for epilepsy. Headache, vomiting, increased intracranial pressure, and papilledema may be associated with convulsions and may suggest a brain tumor.

The teeth erupt late and irregularly. Enamel formation is irregular, and the teeth may be unusually soft. The skin may be dry and scaly, and the nails of the fingers and toes may have horizontal lines. Manifestations of a wide variety of other disorders which are not direct consequences of parathyroid hormone deficiency may also be seen. Mucocutaneous candidiasis, when present, antedates the development of hypoparathyroidism; the monilia infection most often involves the nails, the oral mucosa, the angles of the mouth, and, less often, the skin.

Cataracts in patients with longstanding untreated disease are a direct consequence of hypoparathyroidism; other ocular disorders such as keratoconjunctivitis may also occur. Manifestations of Addison disease, lymphocytic thyroiditis, pernicious anemia, alopecia areata or totalis, hepatitis, and primary gonadal insufficiency may also be associated with those of hypoparathyroidism.

Permanent physical and mental deterioration occurs if initiation of treatment is long delayed.

Laboratory Data. The serum calcium level is low (5–7 mg/dl) and the phosphorus elevated (7–12 mg/dl). The serum phosphatase level is normal or low. The level of magnesium is normal but should always be checked in hypocalcemic patients (see below). Serum levels of PTH and of $1,25\text{-}(OH)_2\text{-}D_3$ are low, even in the presence of hypocalcemia. Roentgenograms of the bones occasionally reveal an increased density limited to the metaphyses, suggestive of heavy metal poisoning, or an increased density of the lamina dura. Roentgenograms or computed tomography of the skull may reveal calcifications in the basal ganglia. There is a prolongation of the Q-T interval on the electrocardiogram, which disappears when the hypocalcemia is corrected. The electroencephalogram usually reveals widespread slow activity; the tracing returns to normal after the serum calcium has been within the normal range for a few wk unless irreversible brain damage has occurred or unless the parathyroid insufficiency is associated with epilepsy. When hypoparathyroidism occurs concurrently with Addison disease, the serum level of calcium may be normal, but hypocalcemia

appears after effective treatment of the adrenal insufficiency.

Treatment. Emergency treatment for tetany consists in intravenous injections of 5–10 ml of a 10% solution of calcium gluconate at the rate of 0.5–1 ml/min. Initially, either vitamin D_2 or dihydrotachysterol should also be administered. Dihydrotachysterol acts more rapidly and is more rapidly inactivated in the body than vitamin D_2. These attributes are advantageous in the early stages of treatment, especially when hypercalcemia may occur from excessive therapy. The usual doses of vitamin D_2 are 0.1–0.5 mg/24 hr in infants and young children and 0.5–1.0 mg/24 hr in older children. One mg of vitamin D_2 or vitamin D_3 has a biologic activity of 40,000 IU. It is now possible to treat hypoparathyroidism with the acute metabolite of vitamin D, 1,25-dihydroxycholecalciferol (calcitriol). Minute doses (0.03–0.08 U/kg/24 hr—1–2 μg/24 hr) are very effective, but this agent has not yet been approved for treatment of hypoparathyroidism. Foods with a high phosphorus content, such as milk, eggs, and cheese, should be reduced in the diet.

Maintenance therapy consists of oral administration of vitamin D_2 in daily doses of 50,000–150,000 IU (1.25–3.75 mg) or 2000 IU/kg/24 hr (50 μg/kg/24 hr). Serum levels of $1,25\text{-}(OH)_2\text{-}D_3$ return to the low normal range with these doses. The main advantage of vitamin D_2 is its low cost. During the period of stabilization some patients require supplemental calcium, which can be given orally in the form of calcium gluconate or calcium lactate (3–9 gm/24 hr).

Treatment with $1,25\text{-}(OH)_2\text{-}D_3$ has the advantages of rapid onset of effect (1–4 days) and short half-life (9 days), permitting rapid reversal of hypercalcemia after discontinuation in the event of overdosage. Its cost is approximately 20 times that of vitamin D_2; its use should be considered only for patients who may be otherwise difficult to control.

Clinical evaluation of the patient and frequent determinations of the serum calcium level are indicated in the early stages of treatment in order to determine the dosage requirements of vitamin D_2 and of calcium. Maintenance treatment must be continued indefinitely. If vitamin D_2 therapy is discontinued, the serum calcium level may remain normal for months; hence, a permanent remission cannot be assumed until there has been an adequate period of observation. If hypercalcemia occurs, vitamin D_2 should be discontinued and resumed at a lower dose after the serum calcium level has returned to normal. In cases of long standing, repair of cerebral and dental changes is not likely. Pigmentation, lowering of the blood pressure, or weight loss may indicate adrenal insufficiency, which requires specific treatment.

Differential Diagnosis. *Magnesium deficiency* must be considered in patients with unexplained hypocalcemia. Concentrations of magnesium in serum below 1.0 mg/dl (0.8 mEq/l) are usually abnormal. *Familial hypomagnesemia* with secondary hypocalcemia has been reported in 18 patients, most of whom developed tetany and seizures from 2–4 wk of age. Administration of calcium is ineffective, but administration of magnesium promptly corrects both calcium and magnesium levels.

Oral supplements of magnesium, 0.5–0.75 mmole/kg/24 hr, are necessary to maintain levels of magnesium in the normal range. The low levels of magnesium result from a specific defect in intestinal absorption. The disorder has been most frequently diagnosed in boys, but it is thought to be caused by an autosomal recessive gene. (See also Sec 7.54.)

Hypomagnesemia also occurs in malabsorption syndromes and has been noted in granulomatous colitis. Patients with autoimmune hypoparathyroidism may have concurrent steatorrhea and low magnesium levels.

It is not clear how low levels of magnesium lead to hypocalcemia. There is no evidence for decreased absorption or for excessive renal loss of calcium. Synthesis of 1,25-dihydroxycholecalciferol and its localization in the intestine occur normally in the magnesium-depleted chick. On the other hand, both low and elevated levels of PTH have been reported in patients with primary magnesium deficiency. The skeleton appears to be unresponsive to PTH during magnesium depletion.

Poisoning with inorganic phosphate leads to hypocalcemia and tetany. Infants poisoned with large doses of inorganic phosphates, either as laxatives or as sodium phosphate enemas, have had sudden onset of tetany, with serum calcium levels below 5 mg/dl and markedly elevated levels of phosphate. Symptoms are quickly relieved by intravenous administration of calcium. The mechanism of the hypocalcemia is not clear.

Hypocalcemia may occur early in the course of treatment of *acute lymphoblastic leukemia*. It is usually associated with hyperphosphatemia (resulting from destruction of lymphoblasts), which is probably the primary cause of hypocalcemia.

18.19 PSEUDOHYPOPARATHY-ROIDISM
(Albright Syndrome; Hereditary Osteodystrophy)

In this syndrome, in contrast to the situation in idiopathic hypoparathyroidism, the parathyroid glands are normal or hyperplastic histologically, and they can synthesize and secrete parathyroid hormone. Serum levels of immunoreactive PTH are elevated even when the patient is hypocalcemic. The disorder is caused by a genetic defect in receptor tissues, particularly of the kidney and skeleton. Neither endogenous nor administered parathyroid hormone raises serum levels of calcium or lowers levels of phosphorus. Serum levels of 1,25-dihydroxycholecalciferol are low.

In the majority of patients (*pseudohypoparathyroidism, Type I*), an infusion of parathyroid extract evokes an inadequate increase in levels of cAMP in plasma and urine. Some patients with Type I PHP have decreased activity of a guanine nucleotide-binding protein (G unit) in erythrocytes and cultured fibroblasts that is required for stimulation of adenylate cyclase by hormonal signals from membrane receptors. A generalized deficiency of this coupling may account for associated endocrine disorders involving cyclic AMP activation such as hypothyroidism.

In a 2nd condition (*pseudohypoparathyroidism, Type II*) PTH normally activates intracellular cyclic AMP, the urinary excretion of which is elevated both in the basal state and after stimulation. It has been suggested that the defect here lies in an inability of the target cells to respond to the intracellular cyclic AMP signal.

In addition to clinical and chemical findings similar to those of idiopathic hypoparathyroidism, patients have a short, stocky build and a round face. Growth failure may be striking. There is brachydactylia; the 1st, 4th, and 5th metacarpals are most often involved, and the 1st and 5th metatarsals are also often affected. As a result, the index finger may be longer than the middle finger. There may be other skeletal abnormalities such as short and wide phalanges, bowing, exostoses, thickening of the calvaria, and general demineralization of the bones. These patients frequently have calcium deposits and metaplastic bone formation subcutaneously. Mental retardation is common as are calcifications of the basal ganglia and lenticular cataracts.

In some patients with pseudohypoparathyroidism, the resistance to PTH appears to be limited to the kidneys, the bones being normally responsive to the elevated levels of circulating hormone. As a result, in addition to the skeletal changes described above, these patients exhibit subperiosteal resorption, osteitis fibrosa, and, in children, widening and irregularity of the epiphyseal plates. The condition has been termed *pseudohypohyperthyroidism* by some, but *pseudohypoparathyroidism with osteitis fibrosa* appears to be a less confusing designation.

Some patients have the usual anatomic stigmata of pseudohypoparathyroidism but normal serum calcium and phosphorus levels. Their condition has been called pseudopseudohypoparathyroidism. Transition from the normocalcemic to the hypocalcemic form has been observed, however, and some families have normocalcemic and hypocalcemic forms in different members. The disorder has been regarded as X-linked dominant, but females appear to be more severely affected than males; a family exhibiting both the normocalcemic and hypocalcemic forms of the syndrome as well as male-to-male transmission has been reported. Heterogeneity of the Type I condition is known; in 1 family without the classic skeletal features, levels of N protein were normal.

Other endocrine disorders which may be associated with pseudohypoparathyroidism include hypothyroidism (with low or elevated TSH), partial resistance to the urine-concentrating effect of ADH, and perhaps resistance to the metabolic effects of glucagon and gonadotropins. Since each of these abnormalities can be related to deficient synthesis of cyclic AMP, it appears that the defect in some patients is not limited to PTH receptor but may be a more generalized one. The occasional finding of prolactin deficiency in pseudohypoparathyroidism cannot be explained on this basis since its secretion is not controlled primarily by cyclic AMP.

Diagnosis rests on the demonstration that no increase in urinary phosphate and cyclic AMP occurs after slow intravenous infusion (15 min) of 150 U of bovine parathyroid extract (8 U/kg in infants). This test can also be used to reveal latent pseudohypoparathyroidism in persons at genetic risk who have no other signs of the condition. Failure of the level of serum calcium to rise after 3 days' administration of intramuscular parathyroid hormone (200 U/24 hr) also indicates resistance to the hormone.

Treatment is the same as for hypoparathyroidism.

18.20 HYPERPARATHYROIDISM

Excessive production of parathyroid hormone may result from a primary defect of the parathyroid glands such as an adenoma or idiopathic hyperplasia (*primary hyperparathyroidism*).

More often, the increased production of parathyroid hormone is compensatory, usually aimed at correcting hypocalcemic states of diverse origins (*secondary hyperparathyroidism*). In vitamin D–deficient rickets and in the malabsorption syndromes intestinal absorption of calcium is deficient, but hypocalcemia and tetany may be averted by increased activity of the parathyroid glands. In chronic renal disease, hyperphosphatemia and the consequent hypocalcemia result in compensatory hyperparathyroidism with marked increases in serum levels of parathyroid hormone. In some instances, if stimulation of the parathyroids has been sufficiently intense and protracted, the glands may continue to secrete increased levels of PTH for months or years after renal transplantation, with resulting hypercalcemia (Table 18–5). This situation, where there may be some autonomy of the parathyroids, has been called *tertiary hyperparathyroidism*.

Primary hyperparathyroidism is uncommon in chil-

Table 18–5 CAUSES OF HYPERCALCEMIA

Parathyroid hormone (PTH) excess
  Primary hyperparathyroidism
    Sporadic—adenoma
    Familial
      Clear cell hyperplasia of infancy (recessive)
      Chief cell hyperplasia (dominant) with familial hypocalciuric
        hypercalcemia
      Adenoma-hyperplasia (dominant)
      Multiple endocrine neoplasia I (dominant)
      Multiple endocrine neoplasia II (dominant)
  Tertiary hyperparathyroidism—postrenal transplantation
  Malignancies
    Leukemia, lymphoma
    Rhabdomyosarcoma, neuroblastoma, bone tumors
  Transient neonatal hyperparathyroidism—maternal
    hypoparathyroidism
Without PTH excess
  Idiopathic hypercalcemia of infancy (Williams syndrome)
  Familial hypocalciuric hypercalcemia
  Vitamin D excess
  Hypervitaminosis A
  Thyrotoxicosis
  Hypophosphatasia
  Prolonged immobilization
  Subcutaneous fat necrosis
  Leukemia
  Metaphyseal chondrodysplasia (Jansen type)
  Sarcoidosis

---

dren and is usually due to a single *adenoma*. Symptoms generally begin after 10 yr of age.

There have been many kindreds with 3 or more members with hyperparathyroidism. In such instances of *familial hyperparathyroidism* most affected members are adults, but children have been involved in about a third of the pedigrees. Some affected patients in these families are asymptomatic and are revealed only by careful study. In some kindreds, in addition to parathyroid tumors, there is a high frequency of peptic ulcer with islet cell tumors (Zollinger-Ellison syndrome) and prolactin-secreting pituitary adenomas; this constellation is known as multiple endocrine neoplasia, type I (MEN I). In other families there is an association with medullary carcinoma of the thyroid and pheochromocytoma; this syndrome is known as multiple endocrine neoplasia, type II (MEN II) (see Sec 18.16). In familial hyperparathyroidism the adenomas are apt to be multiple, and in some patients the parathyroid may reveal only hyperplasia. Inheritance is autosomal dominant, with a high degree of penetrance.

Another form of familial hyperparathyroidism consists of *clear-cell hyperplasia of the parathyroids in infancy*. The condition has its onset in the early weeks of life and may have a rapidly fatal course if diagnosis is delayed. Its occurrence in siblings and with parental consanguinity in some families suggests autosomal recessive inheritance. In 1 kindred the disorder displayed autosomal dominant transmission and involved adults, children, and a newborn infant with chief-cell hyperplasia. At least 4 instances of neonatal primary hyperparathyroidism have occurred in families with familial hypocalciuric hypercalcemia. The mechanism of this association is unknown.

Ectopic PTH production has been suggested as an explanation for the hypercalcemia which occurs with various nonendocrine tumors in adults, including those arising in lung, kidney, cervix, ovary, parotid gland, and reticulum cell sarcoma, but ectopic hyperparathyroidism has not been proved. Hypercalcemia and hypophosphatemia are the usual diagnostic clues. Hypercalcemia without hypophosphatemia frequently occurs in other malignancies, especially carcinoma of the breast. The cause for hypercalcemia in these patients is not known.

Transient neonatal hyperparathyroidism has occurred in a few infants born to mothers with hypoparathyroidism (idiopathic or surgical) or with pseudohypoparathyroidism. In each instance the maternal disorder had been undiagnosed or inadequately treated during pregnancy. The cause of the condition is chronic intrauterine exposure to hypocalcemia with resultant hyperplasia of the fetal parathyroid glands. In the newborn, manifestations involve the bones primarily, and healing occurs between 4–7 mo.

Clinical Manifestations. At all ages the clinical manifestations of hypercalcemia of any cause include muscular weakness, anorexia, nausea, vomiting, constipation, polydipsia, polyuria, loss of weight, and fever. Calcium may be deposited in the renal parenchyma (nephrocalcinosis), with progressively diminished renal function. Renal calculi (noted in 12 of 46 children with adenoma) may produce renal colic and hematuria. Osseous changes may produce pain in the back or extremities, disturbances of gait, deformities, fractures, and tumors. Height may decrease from compression of vertebrae; the patient may become bedridden.

Abdominal pain is occasionally prominent and may be associated with acute pancreatitis. Parathyroid crisis may occur, manifested by serum calcium levels greater than 15 mg/dl and progressive oliguria, azotemia, stupor, and coma. In infants failure to thrive, poor feeding, and hypotonia are common. Mental retardation, convulsions, and blindness may occur as sequelae.

Laboratory Data. The serum calcium is elevated; 39 of 45 children with adenomas had levels over 12 mg/dl. The hypercalcemia is more severe in infants with parathyroid hyperplasia; concentrations from 15–20 mg/dl are common, and values as high as 30 mg/dl have been reported. Ionic (ultrafiltrable) calcium levels are often elevated even when serum calcium is borderline or only slightly elevated. The serum phosphorus level is reduced to about 3 mg/dl or less, and the level of serum magnesium is low. The urine may have a low and fixed specific gravity, and serum levels of nonprotein nitrogen and uric acid may be elevated. In patients with adenomas who have skeletal involvement serum phosphatase is elevated, whereas in infants with hyperplasia the levels of alkaline phosphatase may be normal even when there is extensive involvement of bone.

Serum levels of parathyroid hormone (PTH), as measured by carboxyterminal antisera, are elevated, especially in relation to the level of calcium. Results may vary markedly from 1 laboratory to another, depending on the antibody used. Assays of thyroid venous blood for PTH are preferred because intact hormone is assayed before fragmentation occurs in the periphery. Calcitonin levels are normal. Acute hypercalcemia can stimulate calcitonin release, but with prolonged hypercalcemia, hypercalcitoninemia does not occur.

The most consistent and characteristic roentgenographic findings are resorption of subperiosteal bone, best seen along the margins of the phalanges of the hands. In the skull there may be gross trabeculation or a granular appearance resulting from focal rarefaction; the lamina dura may be absent. In more advanced disease there may be generalized rarefaction, cysts, tumors, fractures, and deformities. Roentgenograms of the abdomen may reveal renal calculi or nephrocalcinosis. In infants with parathyroid hyperplasia, cupping and fraying at the ends of the long bones and ribs may suggest rickets, and severe demineralization and pathologic fractures are common.

Differential Diagnosis. *Hypercalcemia* of any origin results in a similar clinical pattern; other causes must be differentiated from hyperparathyroidism. A low serum phosphorus level with hypercalcemia is characteristic of primary hyperparathyroidism; elevated levels of PTH are also diagnostic. Pharmacologic doses of corticosteroids lower the serum calcium level to normal in patients with hypercalcemia from other causes but generally do not affect the calcium level in patients with hyperparathyroidism. Administration of corticosteroids may be useful in differential diagnosis.

Vitamin D intoxication can be excluded by history, by a normal level of serum phosphorus, and by roentgenographic evidence of increased bone density. *Idiopathic hypercalcemia* of infancy may be easily confused with hyperparathyroidism; however, the serum phosphorus level is normal or slightly elevated and the increased bone density of idiopathic hypercalcemia contrasts strikingly with the rarefaction of primary hyperparathyroidism. Affected infants may have an elfin face, supravalvular aortic stenosis or other cardiac defects, mental retardation, and other abnormalities (*Williams syndrome*). Hypercalcemia may also occur in infants with *subcutaneous fat necrosis*. PTH and vitamin D metabolite levels are normal; the cause for this condition is unknown. *Hypophosphatasia*, especially when severe, is frequently associated with mild to moderate hypercalcemia. The serum phosphorus level is normal; alkaline phosphatase activity is depressed. Roentgenograms of the bones may reveal disappearance of the zone of provisional calcification and lack of calcification of the metaphyseal bone. (See Table 18–5.)

Prolonged immobilization may lead to hypercalcemia and occasionally to decreased renal function, hypertension, and encephalopathy. Hypercalcemia has been associated also with leukemia, lymphoma, neuroblastoma, rhabdomyosarcoma, and bone tumors in children; elevated serum levels of PTH have been demonstrated in some of these patients. Hypercalcemia occurs in 30–50% of children with *sarcoidosis*. Levels of iPTH are suppressed and levels of $1,25\text{-}(OH)_2\text{-}D_3$ elevated. These findings in an anephric patient with sarcoidosis suggest that the $1,25\text{-}(OH)_2\text{-}D_3$ is produced in tissues other than kidney and possibly in the granuloma. Therapy with prednisone lowers serum levels of $1,25\text{-}(OH)_2\text{-}D_3$ to normal and corrects the hypercalcemia. Elevated serum calcium levels have also been observed in patients with *hypervitaminosis A*, in *thyrotoxicosis*, and in malignant disease with *osseous metastases*. Administration of *thiazide diuretics* to hypoparathyroid patients treated with vitamin D can lead to hypercalcemia.

Familial hypocalciuric hypercalcemia, a disorder with autosomal dominant transmission, occurs in children and adults; it may also be asymptomatic. The clinical course is mild, the usual renal problems of hyperparathyroidism are absent, and no other endocrine disorders are associated. Parathyroid hyperplasia is often found, but PTH levels are rarely elevated, and subtotal parathyroidectomy does not correct the hypercalcemia. The rate of urinary excretion of calcium is one third that in primary hyperparathyroidism. The basic defect in the condition is unknown; the insensitivity of the kidneys and parathyroid glands to hypercalcemia suggests a generalized insensitivity to calcium ion. Screening of family members is worthwhile; affected persons aware of the diagnosis can avoid inappropriate parathyroid surgery. No treatment is necessary for the condition.

Hypercalcemia in patients with *familial pheochromocytoma* is usually due to hyperparathyroidism. However, the reported return to normal of the calcium level in a 12 yr old boy after removal of a pheochromocytoma suggests that the tumor itself may have produced a calcium-affecting factor.

Treatment. Surgical exploration is indicated in all instances. All glands should be carefully inspected; if an adenoma is discovered, it should be removed. If there is only generalized hyperplasia, total parathyroidectomy appears indicated to avoid recurrence of the hypercalcemia. Nests of ectopic parathyroid cells in adipose tissue of the neck or mediastinum may also become hyperplastic and may lead to recurrent hyperparathyroidism *(parathyromatosis)*. The patient should be carefully observed postoperatively for the development of hypocalcemia and tetany; intravenous administration of calcium gluconate may be required for a few days. The serum calcium level then gradually returns to normal, and, under ordinary circumstances, a diet high in calcium and phosphorus needs to be maintained for only several mo after operation.

Arteriography and selective venous sampling with radioimmunoassay of PTH have been used successfully for preoperative localization and for differentiation of a single adenoma from hyperplasia in adults. These procedures are particularly advisable before re-exploration in cases of persistent or recurrent hyperparathyroidism.

Prognosis. The prognosis is good if the disease is recognized early and there is appropriate surgical treatment. When extensive osseous lesions are present, deformities may be permanent; with renal disease the prognosis is less hopeful. A search for other affected family members is indicated.

Arnaud CD: Parathyroid hormone: Coming of age in clinical medicine. Am J Med 55:577, 1973.

Aurbach GH, Mallette LE, Patten BM, et al: Hyperparathyroidism: Recent studies. Ann Intern Med 79:566, 1973.

Barakat AY, D'Albora JB, Martin MM, et al: Familial nephrosis, nerve deafness and hypoparathyroidism. J Pediatr 91:61, 1977.

Bergman L, Hagberg S: Primary hyperparathyroidism in a child investigated by determination of ultrafiltrable calcium. Am J Dis Child 123:174, 1972.

Berliner BC, Shenker IR, Weinstock MS: Hypercalcemia associated with hypertension due to prolonged immobilization. (An unusual complication of extensive burns.) Pediatrics 49:92, 1972.

Blizzard RM, Chee D, Davis W: The incidence of parathyroid and other antibodies in the sera of patients with idiopathic hypoparathyroidism. Clin Exp Immunol 1:119, 1966.

Bronsky D, Kiamko RT, Moncado R, et al: Intrauterine hyperparathyroidism secondary to maternal hypoparathyroidism. Pediatrics 42:606, 1968.

Chesney RW, Hamstra AJ, DeLuca HF, et al: Elevated serum 1,25-dihydroxyvitamin D concentrations in the hypercalcemia of sarcoidosis: Correction by glucocorticoid therapy. J Pediatr 98:919, 1981.

Daum F, Rosen JF, Boley SJ: Parathyroid adenoma, parathyroid crisis and acute pancreatitis in an adolescent. J Pediatr 83:275, 1973.

Davis RF, Eichner JM, Bleyer WA, et al: Hypocalcemia, hyperphosphatemia, and dehydration following a single hypertonic phosphate enema. J Pediatr 90:484, 1977.

Deftos LJ, Powell D, Parthemore JG, et al: Secretion of calcitonin in hypocalcemic states in man. J Clin Invest 52:3109, 1973.

DiGeorge AM: Congenital absence of the thymus and its immunologic consequences, concurrence with congenital hypoparathyroidism. In: Bergsma D, Good RA (eds): Birth Defects. Original Article Series, No 1, Vol IV. New York, The National Foundation, 1968.

Drezner M, Neelon FA, Lebovitz HE: Pseudohypoparathyroidism Type II. A possible defect in the reception of the cyclic AMP signal. N Engl J Med 289:1056, 1973.

Fairney A, Jackson D, Clayton BE: Measurement of serum parathyroid hormone, with particular reference to some infants with hypocalcemia. Arch Dis Child 48:419, 1973.

Fartel Z, Brickman AS, Kaslow HR, et al: Defect of receptor-cyclase coupling protein in pseudohypoparathyroidism. N Engl J Med 303:237, 1980.

Fisher G, Skillern PG: Hypercalcemia due to hypervitaminosis A. JAMA 227:1413, 1974.

Glass EJ, Barr DGD: Transient neonatal hyperparathyroidism secondary to maternal pseudohypoparathyroidism. Arch Dis Child 56:555, 1981.

Goldbloom RM, Gillis DA, Prasad M: Hereditary parathyroid hyperplasia: A surgical emergency of early infancy. Pediatrics 49:514, 1972.

Hutchinson RJ, Shapiro SA, Raney RB: Elevated parathyroid hormone levels in association with rhabdomyosarcoma. J Pediatr 92:780, 1978.

Jacobsen BB, Terslev E, Lund B, Sorensen OH: Neonatal hypocalcemia associated with maternal hyperparathyroidism. Arch Dis Child 53:308, 1978.

Kind HP, Handysides A, Kook SW, et al: Vitamin D therapy in hypoparathyroidism and pseudohypoparathyroidism: Weight-related doses for initiation of therapy and maintenance therapy. J Pediatr 91:1006, 1977.

Kooh SW, Fraser D, DeLuca HF, et al: Treatment of hypoparathyroidism and pseudohypoparathyroidism with metabolites of vitamin D: Evidence for impaired conversion of 25-hydroxyvitamin D to 1α,25-dihydroxyvitamin D. N Engl J Med 293:840, 1975.

Levitt M, Gessert C, Finberg L: Inorganic phosphate (laxative) poisoning resulting in tetany in an infant. J Pediatr 82:479, 1973.

Lund B, Sorensen OH, Lund B, et al: Vitamin D metabolism in hypoparathyroidism. J Clin Endocrinol Metab 51:606, 1980.

Martin KJ, Hruska KA, Freitag JJ et al: The peripheral metabolism of parathyroid hormone. N Engl J Med 301:1092, 1979.

Marx SJ, Attie MF, Spiegel AM, et al: An association between neonatal severe primary hyperparathyroidism and familial hypocalciuric hypercalcemia in three kindreds. N Engl J Med 306:257, 1982.

Marx SJ, Spiegel AM, Levine MA, et al: Familial hypocalciuric hypercalcemia. The relation to primary parathyroid hyperplasia. N Engl J Med 307:426, 1982.

Neufeld M, Blizzard RM: Polyglandular autoimmune disease. In: Pinchera A, Doniach D, Fenzi GF, Baschieri L (eds): Autoimmune Aspects of Endocrine Disorders. New York, Academic Press, 1980.

Nusynowitz ML, Klein MH: Pseudoidiopathic hypoparathyroidism. Hypoparathyroidism with ineffective parathyroid hormone. Am J Med 55:677, 1973.

Öberg K, Wälinder O, Boström H, et al: Peptide hormone markers in screening for endocrine tumors in multiple endocrine adenomatosis Type I. Am J Med 73:619, 1982.

Olambiwonnu NO, Ebbin AJ, Frasier DS: Primary hypoparathyroidism associated with ring chromosome 18. J Pediatr 80:833, 1972.

Parfitt AM: Thiazide-induced hypercalcemia in vitamin D-treated hypoparathyroidism. Ann Intern Med 77:557, 1972.

Patterson CR, Gunn A: Familial benign hypercalcemia. Lancet 2:61, 1981.

Reddick RL, Costa JC, Marx SJ: Parathyroid hyperplasia and parathyromatosis. Lancet 1:549, 1977.

Reddy CR, et al: Studies on mechanisms of hypocalcemia of magnesium depletion. J Clin Invest 52:3000, 1973.

Roof BS, Carpenter B, Fink DJ, et al: Some thoughts on the nature of ectopic parathyroid hormones. Am J Med 50:686, 1971.

Root A, Gruskin A, Reber RM: Serum concentrations of parathyroid hormone in infants, children and adolescents. J Pediatr 85:329, 1974.

Shapiro MS, Bernheim J, Gutman A, et al: Multiple abnormalities of anterior pituitary hormone secretion in association with pseudohypoparathyroidism. J Clin Endocrinol Metab 51:483, 1980.

Stanbury SW: Azotaemic renal osteodystrophy. Clin Endocrinol Metab 1:267, 1972.

Stromme JH, Steen-Johnson J, Harnaes K, et al: Familial hypomagnesemia—a follow-up examination of three patients after 9 to 12 years of treatment. Pediatr Res 15:1134, 1981.

Swinton NW, Clerkin EP, Flint LD: Hypercalcemia and familial pheochromocytoma. Correction after adrenalectomy. Ann Intern Med 76:455, 1972.

Veldhuis JD, Kulin HE, Demers LM, Lambert PW: Infantile hypercalcemia with subcutaneous fat necrosis: Endocrine studies. J Pediatr 95:460, 1979.

Weinberg AG, Stone RT: Autosomal dominant inheritance in Albright's hereditary osteodystrophy. J Pediatr 79:997, 1971.

Whyte MP, Weldon VV: Idiopathic hypoparathyroidism presenting with seizures during infancy: X-linked recessive inheritance in a large Missouri kindred. J Pediatr 99:608, 1981.

18.21 DISORDERS OF THE ADRENAL GLANDS

The adrenal gland is composed of 2 endocrine systems, the medullary and the cortical systems. Mesodermal cells contribute to the development of the adrenal cortex, the gonads, and the liver; these 3 tissues are active in steroid metabolism in the fetus. Adrenals and gonads have in common certain enzymes involved in steroid synthesis, and an inborn defect in 1 tissue may also involve the other.

At about the 7th wk of gestation the primordium of the adrenal cortex is invaded by sympathetic neural elements. About 1 wk later these cells begin to differentiate into the chromaffin cells capable of synthesizing and storing catecholamines; the methyl transferase which converts norepinephrine to epinephrine develops later.

In a fetus of 2 mo the adrenals are larger than the kidneys, but from the 4th mo the kidneys grow rapidly, becoming about twice as large as the adrenals by the end of the 6th mo. In the fullterm infant the adrenal gland is one third the size of the kidney, and the combined weight of both glands is 7–9 gm.

The adrenal cortex in the fetus and the newborn infant has 2 histologically distinct components: an outer portion, the true cortex, and a more central portion, the "fetal cortex." At birth the "fetal" cortex makes up about 80% of the gland. Within a few days it begins to involute, undergoing a 50% reduction by 2 wk of age and disappearing completely by about 6 mo of age.

The true cortex consists of 3 zones. In the zona glomerulosa, situated beneath the capsule, there is an alveolar arrangement of the cells; in the broader zona fasciculata the columns of cells are radially arranged; in the zona reticularis the cells form a network next to the medulla.

Fetoplacental Unit. Fetal adrenal does not possess the 3β-hydroxysteroid dehydrogenase necessary to form progesterone; it utilizes placental pregnenolone to synthesize cortisol, aldosterone, and particularly dehydroepiandrosterone sulfate (DHAS). The placenta in turn utilizes the fetal DHAS to produce estrone and estriol. Estriol is the major estrogen found in maternal urine in pregnancy, especially in the late stages. In instances of fetal adrenal hypoplasia, maternal urinary estriol levels are markedly reduced.

Adrenal Cortex. The adrenal cortex secretes various steroid compounds essential to life. The known compounds can be divided into several general categories:

Glucocorticoids. These steroids have a 21-carbon structure and are also referred to as 17-hydroxycorticosteroids or simply as corticosteroids. The principal one is cortisol, which is also known as compound F or hydrocortisone. Cortisone (compound E) is a metabolite of cortisol. Glucocorticoids are produced by the zona fasciculata and zona reticularis.

Glucocorticoids affect the metabolism of most tissues. They attach to specific intracellular receptor proteins which then bind to the cell nucleus to influence RNA and protein synthesis. In many tissues glucocorticoids have a catabolic effect, resulting in increased degradation of protein; primarily affected are muscles and skin and connective, adipose, and lymphoid tissues. On the other hand, glucocorticoids are anabolic in the liver, where they stimulate a number of enzymes, increase protein and glycogen content, and enhance its capacity for gluconeogenesis. Patients with cortisol excess (e.g., Cushing syndrome) have increased glucose production, whereas those with deficiency of cortisol (Addison disease) have decreased gluconeogenesis, with hypoglycemia. Insulin and androgens have effects antagonistic to glucocorticoids. Some actions of catecholamines and of glucagon are facilitated by glucocorticoids.

The 17-hydroxycorticosteroids are excreted in urine; cortisol itself is also excreted in urine in amounts less than 1% of the adrenal production. Urinary levels of 17-hydroxycorticosteroids and cortisol, when expressed respectively as mg or μg/gm of creatinine, are comparable in children and adults and are useful indices of adrenocortical function. Plasma cortisol may be measured by a variety of techniques; methods using competitive protein-binding and radioimmunoassay are replacing all others. Levels of cortisol in plasma vary with the time of day; after the 1st few yr of life a circadian rhythm follows that of corticotropin.

A radioimmunoassay for ACTH is capable of measuring levels as low as 10 pg/ml in plasma. A test for pituitary reserve of ACTH is also available. Metyrapone, which inhibits 11β-hydroxylation by the adrenal, is administered. The effect of this drug is decreased secretion of cortisol, with increased secretion of 11-deoxycortisol. This latter compound can be measured directly or indirectly, either in urine or in plasma. When there is deficiency of corticotropin, levels of 11-deoxycortisol fail to rise.

Many synthetic analogues of cortisone and hydrocortisone are available. Derivatives with an additional double bond in ring A are known as prednisone and prednisolone. They are 3–4 times as potent in anti-inflammatory and carbohydrate activity as the natural steroids but have less effect on salt and water retention. Halogenated derivatives have different effects; 9α-fluorohydrocortisone is approximately 15 times as active as hydrocortisone in anti-inflammatory activity but is more than 20 times as active in salt and water retention. Betamethasone and dexamethasone are approximately 25 times as potent as cortisol and have little effect on the retention of water and electrolytes. These analogues are usually used in pharmacologic doses for their anti-inflammatory or immunosuppressive properties.

Aldosterone. A potent mineralocorticoid, aldosterone is the 18-aldehyde of corticosterone and is produced primarily in the zona glomerulosa. Its secretion is regulated by activation of the renin-angiotensin system. Renin is a proteolytic enzyme which acts upon renin substrate to yield the inactive decapeptide, angiotensin I. A converting enzyme in the lungs rapidly changes angiotensin I to the biologically active octapeptide, angiotensin II. Angiotensin II is a pressor agent 50 times more potent than norepinephrine. One of its main functions is to act directly on the adrenal cortex to stimulate the secretion of aldosterone.

In good health and on a normal dietary intake, ACTH plays a minor role in regulation of aldosterone secretion, but under some conditions, as in anephric man, it may have a more significant effect. On the other hand, potassium may be of equal importance to the renin-angiotensin system in the regulation of aldosterone secretion. In studies of aldosterone secretion, dietary potassium and sodium must be rigidly controlled. Aldosterone and renin activity in plasma can be measured by radioimmunoassay.

Sodium deprivation is a potent stimulus to secretion of aldosterone. Changes in intake of sodium result in small changes in blood volume, arterial pressure, and renal blood flow. These changes are sensitively monitored by the juxtaglomerular cells on the renal afferent arterioles, which form the receptor site or volume receptor. Activation of the juxtaglomerular apparatus results in increased output of angiotensin II followed by increased secretion of aldosterone.

The principal action of aldosterone is the maintenance of electrolyte equilibrium, which in turn contributes to the stabilization of blood volume and blood pressure. Aldosterone controls sodium reabsorption (and hence water reabsorption) in the distal tubule of the kidney.

Androgens. Dehydroepiandrosterone and androstenedione are produced mainly by the zona reticularis but also by the zona fasciculata. These hormones are capable of increasing retention of nitrogen, potassium, phosphorus, and sulfate. They promote growth and have androgenic effects which are most conspicuous when adrenal hyperplasia or adrenal tumors induce precocious growth and development of secondary male sex characteristics. There is evidence that the adrenal androgens are partly responsible for the development of axillary and pubic hair in the female.

Dehydroepiandrosterone sulfate (DHAS) is the most abundant of the C19 steroids in blood and serves as a precursor for dehydroepiandrosterone. The function of these hormones is not fully understood. Levels of DHAS rise prior to the other hormonal changes of puberty, but the fact that boys and girls have equal levels indicates that DHAS does not have significant virilizing or feminizing actions. Levels of DHAS are undetectable in hypopituitarism, low in Addison disease, and elevated in untreated congenital adrenal hyperplasia, in precocious adrenarche, and in sick premature and full term infants. Levels do not change with insulin-induced hypoglycemia or with administration of hCG or LH-RH but do rise with ACTH stimulation.

Metabolites of adrenal androgens appear in the urine as 17-ketosteroids. Their measurement is a crude index of the production of adrenal androgens in the female. In the male approximately one third of the urinary 17-ketosteroids can be attributed to testicular and two thirds to adrenal androgens. In children under 8–10 yr of age the urinary excretion of these substances is small, but a constant increase is seen throughout adolescence until adult levels are reached. Increased production of adrenal androgens is usually reflected in increased secretion of urinary 17-ketosteroids.

Adrenal Medulla. The principal hormones of the adrenal medulla are the physiologically active catecholamines: dopamine, norepinephrine, and epinephrine. The sequence of their biosynthetic reactions is depicted in Fig 18–15. Catecholamine synthesis occurs also in the brain, in sympathetic nerve endings, and in chromaffin tissue outside the adrenal medulla. Metabolites of catecholamines are excreted in the urine. The principal ones are 3-methoxy-4-hydroxymandelic acid (VMA), metanephrine, and normetanephrine. Measurement of VMA in urine has been the usual method for detection of functioning tumors of the adrenal medulla;

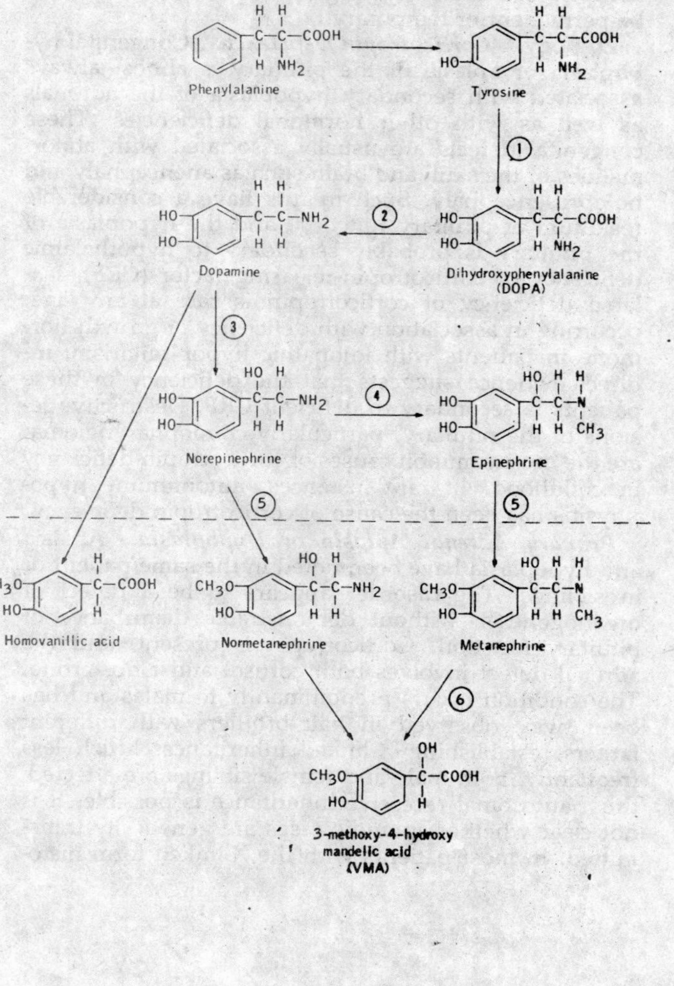

Figure 18–15 Biosynthesis (above dashed line) and metabolism (below dashed line) of the catecholamines: norepinephrine and epinephrine.

1. Tyrosine hydroxylase
2. Dopa decarboxylase
3. Dopamine-β-hydroxylase
4. Phenylethanolamine-*N*-methyltransferase
5. Catechol-o-methyltransferase
6. Monoamine oxidase

new methods now measure levels of catecholamines directly.

The proportions of epinephrine and norepinephrine in the adrenal vary with age. In early fetal stages there is practically no epinephrine, and even at birth norepinephrine is predominant. In adults norepinephrine makes up only 10–30% of the pressor amines in the medulla. Both epinephrine and norepinephrine raise the mean arterial blood pressure, norepinephrine without changing the cardiac output. By increasing peripheral vascular resistance, it increases systolic and diastolic blood pressures with only a slight reduction in the pulse rate. Epinephrine increases the pulse rate and, by decreasing the peripheral vascular resistance, decreases the diastolic pressure. The hyperglycemic and calorigenic effects of norepinephrine are much less pronounced than those of epinephrine.

18.22 ADRENOCORTICAL INSUFFICIENCY

Deficient production of cortisol and/or aldosterone may result from a wide variety of congenital or acquired lesions of the hypothalamus, pituitary, or adrenal cortex (Table 18–6). Depending upon the pathologic lesions, symptoms may be severe or mild, become manifest abruptly or insidiously, begin in infancy or later, and be permanent or temporary.

Etiology. *Corticotropin Deficiency.* Congenital hypoplasia or aplasia of the pituitary is almost always associated with secondary hypoplasia of the adrenals as well as with other hormonal deficiencies. These congenital defects are usually associated with abnormalities of the skull and brain such as anencephaly and holoprosencephaly. Such infants have a considerable residuum of pituitary function, and the hypoplasia of the pituitary is probably secondary to hypothalamic deficiency of corticotropin-releasing factor (CRF). Isolated deficiency of corticotropin is rare at any age, occurring in association with deficiency of growth hormone in patients with idiopathic hypopituitarism; indirect evidence suggests that the deficiency in these patients is secondary to deficient CRF. Destructive lesions of the pituitary, particularly craniopharyngioma, are the most common causes of corticotropin deficiency in childhood. In rare instances, autoimmune hypophysitis has been the cause of corticotropin deficiency.

Primary Adrenal Aplasia or Hypoplasia. Aplasia and hypoplasia have been noted in the same patient or in siblings. The disorder appears to be a defect of organogenesis, without demonstrable disturbance of pituitary function. Corticotropin is present, and the adrenal defect involves both cortisol and aldosterone. The condition occurs predominantly in males and has been twice observed in half brothers with different fathers, establishing X-linked inheritance. Much less frequently, both male and female siblings are affected; thus, autosomal recessive inheritance is possible. It is not clear whether sporadic cases are genetically transmitted. In most patients with the X-linked form histologic examination of hypoplastic adrenal cortex reveals disorganization and cytomegaly, findings not present in the adrenals from corticotropin-deficient infants.

Most boys with the X-linked disorder do not spontaneously undergo puberty because of deficiency of gonadotropins. The mechanism is not clear; either failure of adrenal androgens to activate hypothalamic-pituitary secretion of gonadotropins or primary congen-

Table 18–6 ETIOLOGIC CLASSIFICATION OF ADRENOCORTICAL HYPOFUNCTION

Corticotropin-releasing factor deficiency
  Hypothalamic defects (e.g., anencephaly, holoprosencephaly, septo-optic dysplasia)
  Destructive lesions (e.g., tumor, trauma)
  Idiopathic (e.g., idiopathic hypopituitarism)
Corticotropin deficiency
  Pituitary hypoplasia or aplasia
  Destructive lesions of pituitary (e.g., craniopharyngioma, trauma)
  Autoimmune hypophysitis
Primary adrenal hypoplasia or aplasia
  X-linked
  With glycerol kinase deficiency
  Autosomal recessive
  Sporadic?
Familial glucocorticoid deficiency
  With autonomic dysfunction
  Without autonomic dysfunction
Inborn defects of steroidogenesis
  Congenital adrenal hyperplasia
    Lipoid adrenal hyperplasia (desmolase defect)
      Severe
      Mild
    3β-Hydroxysteroid dehydrogenase deficiency
      Severe
      Mild
    21-Hydroxylase deficiency
      Classic
        Salt-loser
        Non-salt-loser
      Variants
        Late onset
        Cryptic
  Isolated defects of aldosterone synthesis
    Corticosterone methyl oxidase I
    Corticosterone methyl oxidase II
Aldosterone unresponsiveness—pseudohypoaldosteronism
Destructive lesions of adrenal cortex
  Granulomatous lesions (e.g., tuberculosis)
  Autoimmune adrenalitis (idiopathic Addison disease)
    Isolated
    Associated with hypoparathyroidism and/or mucocutaneous candidiasis (Type I autoimmune polyglandular syndrome)
    Associated with autoimmune thyroid disease and insulin-requiring diabetes (Type II autoimmune polyglandular syndrome)
  Adrenoleukodystrophy and adrenomyeloneuropathy
  X-linked Addison disease
  Neonatal hemorrhage
  Acute infection (Waterhouse-Friderichsen syndrome)
  Lysosomal acid lipase deficiency (Wolman syndrome)
Iatrogenic
  Abrupt cessation of exogenous corticosteroids or corticotropin
  Removal of functioning adrenal tumor
  Adrenalectomy for Cushing disease
  Drugs
    Aminoglutethimide
    Mitotane (o,p'-DDD)
    Metyrapone
Fetal adrenal suppression—maternal hypercortisolism
  Endogenous
  Therapeutic

ital gonadotropin deficiency may be possible. Cryptorchidism is occasionally associated, but the testes respond normally to hCG stimulation.

Siblings with X-linked adrenal hypoplasia from 2 families have been described with coexisting glycerol kinase deficiency. The reason for this concordance is unknown.

Familial Glucocorticoid Deficiency. This form of chronic adrenal insufficiency is characterized by isolated deficiency of glucocorticoids and elevated levels of corticotropin in association with normal aldosterone production. As a consequence, the salt-losing manifestations of most other forms of adrenal insufficiency do not occur. Instead, patients present primarily with hypoglycemia, seizures, and pigmentation. The disorder affects both sexes equally and appears to be inherited in an autosomal recessive manner. Histologically, there is marked adrenocortical atrophy with relative sparing of the zona glomerulosa. It has been suggested that the unresponsiveness of the adrenal cortex may be due to failure of membrane attachment or to failure of activation of adenyl cyclase by corticotropin, but evidence suggests that the adrenocortical defect may result from a degenerative process. The syndrome may be heterogeneous. Most patients exhibit achalasia of the cardia, deficient tear production, and other autonomic dysfunction. The relationship of these manifestations to the adrenal disorder is not clear.

Inborn Defects of Steroidogenesis. The most common causes of adrenocortical insufficiency in infancy are the salt-losing forms of congenital adrenal hyperplasia (Sec 18.24). About half the infants with the 21-hydroxylase defect, all infants with lipoid adrenal hyperplasia, and most infants with deficiency of 3β-hydroxysteroid dehydrogenase manifest salt-losing symptoms in the newborn period. In these defects there is a deficiency in the synthesis of both cortisol and aldosterone.

Isolated Deficiency of Aldosterone. This rare disorder is due to a defect in either of 2 mixed-function oxidases, corticosterone methyl oxidase, type I or type II (CMO I or CMO II) (see Fig 18–16). Levels of aldosterone and its metabolites are relatively or absolutely low, and levels of plasma renin activity are markedly elevated. In CMO II deficiency levels of 18-hydroxycorticosterone are greatly increased; levels of 17-ketosteroids, cortisol, and pregnanetriol are normal. There is no unusual pigmentation, and clinical manifestations consist primarily of hyponatremia, hyperkalemia, metabolic acidosis in the neonate, failure to thrive in infancy, or retardation of growth during childhood. Some adaptation or compensation occurs, the salt-losing manifestations improving with increasing age. The biosynthetic defect persists, however, and can be demonstrated in adults. The type II defect has been detected in 8 families of Iranian Jews, in a large North American pedigree, and in other siblings; its inheritance is autosomal recessive. Specific diagnosis depends on measurement of the ratio of 18-hydroxycorticosterone to aldosterone in plasma and/or urine. Treatment consists of administration of enough salt and/or mineralocorticoid to return plasma renin activity to normal.

Pseudohypoaldosteronism. About a dozen infants have been described with a salt-losing syndrome despite normal adrenocortical and renal function. Secretion and urinary excretion rates of aldosterone are elevated and remain so after salt supplementation. Administration of DOCA or aldosterone does not correct the urinary sodium loss. Elevated renin activity in plasma indicates that the hyperaldosteronism is secondary to hyperactivity of the renin-angiotensin system. No response occurs to high doses of 9-α-fluorocortisol; evidence suggests a defect in mineralocorticoid receptors. Besides distal renal tubules, the defect may involve salivary and sweat glands and colonic mucosal cells.

Destructive Lesions of Adrenal Cortex. In older children 1 of the more common causes of adrenal insufficiency is a destructive lesion of the adrenal gland; the condition is referred to as *Addison disease*. Tuberculosis was once the most frequent cause of Addison disease but no longer. Histoplasmosis, coccidioidomycosis, torulosis, mycosis fungoides, amyloidosis, and metastatic malignancies have been identified as causative agents in adults but not in children, in whom in most instances "idiopathic atrophy" is noted. The adrenal glands may be so small that they are not visible at autopsy, and only remnants of tissue are found in microscopic sections. Usually, however, the medulla is not destroyed, and there is lymphocytic infiltration in the area of the former cortex and in the medulla. About half of affected patients have antibodies against adrenal tissue, a finding which suggests that the adrenocortical insufficiency results from an *autoimmune adrenalitis*.

Patients with idiopathic Addison disease are exceptionally prone to a variety of other conditions known or believed to be autoimmune in origin. In individuals and families with associated hypoparathyroidism and chronic mucocutaneous moniliasis, there is a high association of alopecia, malabsorption, pernicious anemia, gonadal failure, chronic active hepatitis, and vitiligo. The candidiasis and hypoparathyroidism almost always antedate the Addison disease. These patients do not have any HLA predominance. Another group of patients with Addison disease have a conspicuous association with autoimmune thyroid disease and insulin-dependent diabetes, with a predominance of HLA-B8 (A1). The genetics are not clear; heterogeneity in affected families is common. Selective IgA deficiency and defective suppressor T-cell function have been noted in some patients, but the underlying defect is not known.

Adrenoleukodystrophy. This rare X-linked recessive adrenal disorder is also known as *melanodermic leukodystrophy* or *sudanophilic leukodystrophy*. Symptoms usually begin from 3–12 yr of age. Central nervous system manifestations dominate the clinical course and consist of behavioral changes, disturbance of gait, dysarthria, dysphagia, and loss of vision. Eventually seizures, spastic quadriparesis, and decorticate posturing occur. Approximately a third of patients exhibit signs and symptoms of adrenal insufficiency, usually after 4 yr of age. These develop insidiously and may antedate or appear concomitantly with the neurologic manifestations. Reduced adrenal cortical reserve may be demonstrable even in children without clinical manifestations of the disorder. *Adrenomyeloneuropathy* is a milder form of the disorder occurring later in life.

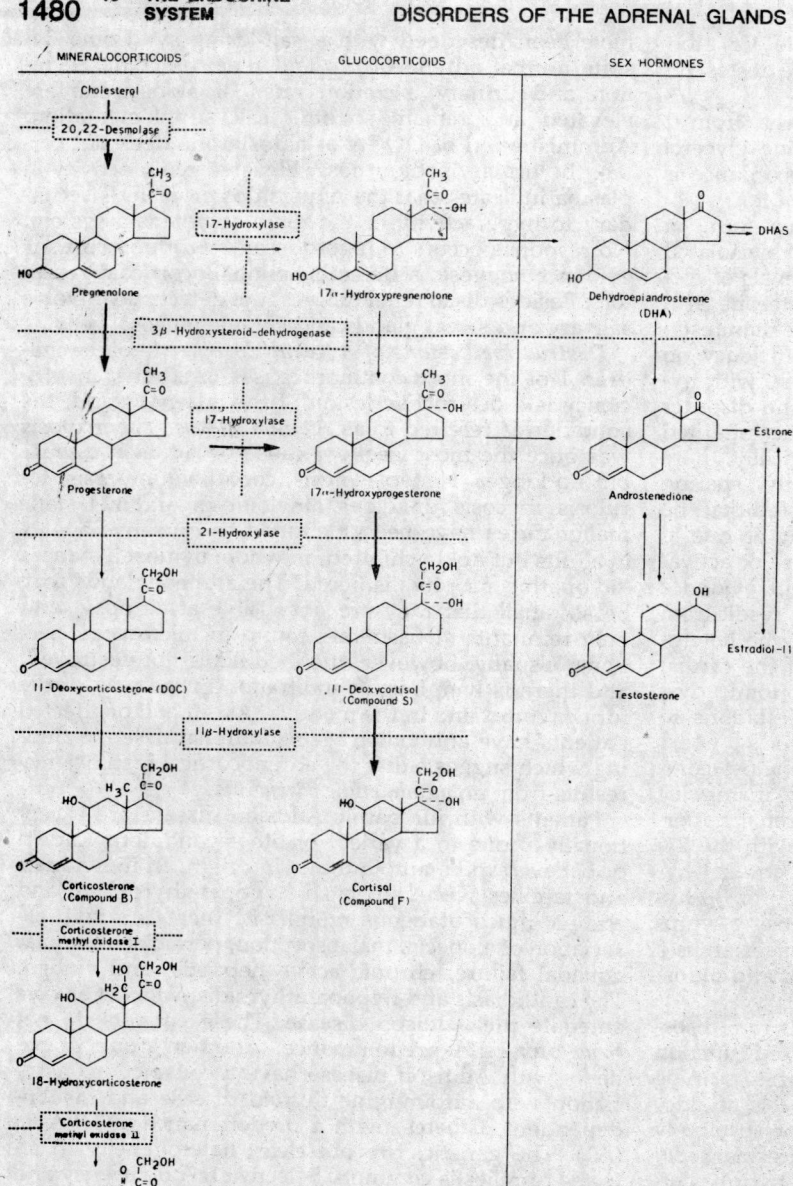

MINERALOCORTICOIDS   GLUCOCORTICOIDS   SEX HORMONES

Figure 18–16 The synthesis of cortisol and aldosterone are shown to the left of the vertical line. The heavy arrows indicate the principal pathway of cortisol synthesis. The enzymatic defects that cause virilizing adrenal hyperplasia and the defects in aldosterone synthesis are shown by horizontal dotted lines. Vertical dotted lines show the defect in 17-hydroxylation. To the right of the solid vertical line are the predominant adrenal androgens that lead to peripheral conversion to testosterone.

Patients with this disorder are unable to oxidate very long chain fatty acids. Increased levels of saturated very long chain fatty acids, particularly hexicosanoic acid (C 26), have been demonstrated in plasma, adrenal cortex, and cerebral white matter and in cultured fibroblasts from skin and amniotic fluid. Heterozygous females from families with affected children can be identified, and prenatal diagnosis has been successfully accomplished.

Hemorrhage into Adrenal Glands. This may occur in the neonatal period as a consequence of difficult labor or of asphyxia. The hemorrhage may be sufficiently extensive to result in death from exsanguination or from hypoadrenalism. Often the hemorrhage is asymptomatic initially and is identified by later calcification of the adrenal. On rare occasions, gradual impairment in function resulting from progressive fibrosis or cystic changes may culminate in adrenocortical insufficiency in infancy or childhood.

Waterhouse-Friderichsen Syndrome. This characteristic state of shock resulting from bacterial infection is usually associated with hemorrhage into the adrenal glands. The syndrome has been recognized most often in patients with fulminating meningococcemia, but it also occurs with septicemia caused by other organisms. The various lesions, including the adrenal hemorrhage, have been attributed to a generalized Shwartzman reaction. The circulatory collapse has been attributed to impaired adrenocortical function, but in most patients blood levels of corticoids are appropriately elevated. On the other hand, in some children with hemorrhagic adrenals, serum levels of corticoids have been undetectable. It appears that the circulatory collapse results in most instances from severe toxemia, but it may be aggravated by adrenal insufficiency.

Abrupt cessation of administration of corticotropin or a corticosteroid may result in adrenal insufficiency. Symptoms are most likely to occur after these substances have been given in large doses for a long time to patients who are subsequently subjected to stressful situations such as severe infections or surgical procedures. Administration of these substances results in impaired pituitary or adrenocortical function, and these effects may sometimes persist for a long time after treatment is discontinued.

Clinical Manifestations. The age of onset of symptoms and the clinical manifestations depend upon the specific etiologic factor involved. In patients with adrenal hypoplasia, defects in steroidogenesis, or pseudohypoaldosteronism, symptoms and signs begin shortly after birth and are those of salt loss. Failure to thrive, vomiting, lethargy, anorexia, and dehydration occur; circulatory collapse may be fatal.

In older children with Addison disease the onset is usually more gradual and characterized by muscular weakness, lassitude, anorexia, loss of weight, general wasting, and low blood pressure. Abdominal pain may simulate an acute abdominal process, and there may be an intense craving for salt. If the condition is not recognized and treated, *adrenal crisis* may supervene. The patient suddenly becomes cyanotic, the skin cold, and the pulse weak and rapid. The blood pressure falls, and respirations are rapid and labored. In the absence of immediate and intensive therapy, the course is rapidly fatal. In patients with inadequately treated chronic adrenal insufficiency, crises may be precipitated by infection, trauma, excessive fatigue, or drugs such as morphine, barbiturates, laxatives, thyroid hormone, or insulin.

Increased pigmentation of the skin should always alert the clinician to the possibility of adrenocortical insufficiency. This manifestation occurs in those conditions in which there are deficiency of cortisol and excessive secretion of corticotropin, as in primary adrenal hypoplasia, familial glucocorticoid deficiency, and Addison disease. Pigmentation may be first apparent on the face and hands and is most intense around the genitalia, umbilicus, axillae, nipples, and joints. Scars and freckles may be especially pigmented. Areas of depigmentation may be interspersed with dark areas. The exposed areas of the skin are the most intensely affected, and failure of a suntan to disappear may be the 1st clue to the condition. In the buccal mucosa the pigmentation is usually bluish brown.

The presenting manifestations may be those of hypoglycemia, particularly in the neonate with congenital adrenal hypoplasia. Patients with adrenocortical insufficiency are deficient in gluconeogenic substrates; the hypoglycemia may be associated with ketosis, therefore, and confused with ketotic hypoglycemia. (See Sec 17.10.)

In young children with familial glucocorticoid deficiency, salt-losing manifestations do not occur, and the symptoms are primarily increased pigmentation and hypoglycemia. Symptoms may begin shortly after birth and almost always by 5 yr of age. Many affected children have had other treatment for seizures before the hypoglycemic cause was recognized.

In patients with deficiency of corticotropin, pigmentation does not occur. Hypoglycemia may be manifest, but salt-losing is uncommon, presumably because of residual ability of the adrenal to secrete aldosterone.

In those conditions known to have a genetic basis it is important to evaluate fully the adrenocortical function of siblings.

Laboratory Data. When salt-losing manifestations are present, the levels of sodium and chloride in the serum are usually low and that of potassium elevated, with increased plasma renin activity. Urinary excretions of sodium and chloride are increased and that of potassium decreased. The nonprotein nitrogen level in plasma is elevated if there is dehydration. Hypoglycemia may be striking or become manifest only after prolonged fasting. The blood eosinophils may be increased in number. When hemorrhage, adrenal cysts, or tuberculosis have been causative factors, roentgenograms of the abdomen may reveal calcifications in the area of the adrenals. Ultrasonography and computed tomography may also be helpful. A small and narrow roentgenographic shadow of the heart reflects hypovolemia (Fig 18–17). Electrocardiographic changes reflect potassium levels. The electroencephalogram may show a greatly decreased content or absence of low-voltage, fast-frequency waves.

The most definitive test is measurement of urinary or

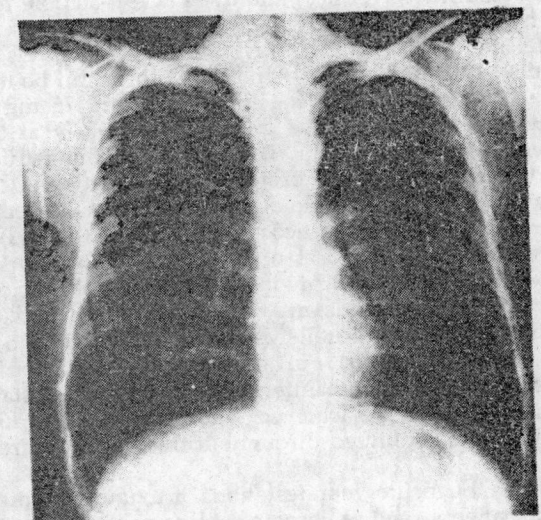

Figure 18–17 Addison disease in a 10 yr old boy. On admission he was dehydrated; there was bronzing of the skin and hypotension. Note the microcardia characteristic of untreated Addison disease. Hypoparathyroidism developed subsequently. One sibling died of Addison disease and another developed mucocutaneous candidiasis, hypoparathyroidism, and ovarian failure.

plasma levels of corticosteroids before and after administration of corticotropin. Resting levels of corticosteroids are low, and no increase occurs after administration of corticotropin. Occasionally, normal resting levels which do not increase after administration of corticotropin indicate an absence of adrenocortical reserve. A low initial level followed by a significant response to corticotropin may indicate adrenal insufficiency secondary to endogenous insufficiency of corticotropin. When corticotropin deficiency is suspected (as in hypothalamic and pituitary disorders), residual reserve of pituitary corticotropin can be evaluated by using metyrapone (q.v.). Patients with corticotropin deficiency show little response to this test. The ideal test is to measure plasma cortisol and corticotropin simultaneously.

Measurement of plasma levels of 17-hydroxyprogesterone is necessary in infants suspected of congenital adrenal hyperplasia. Aldosterone secretion is low in salt-losing congenital adrenal hyperplasia, in adrenal hypoplasia, and in Addison disease, but its measurement is rarely needed for diagnosis. Measurement of aldosterone is necessary in infants suspected of isolated defects of aldosterone synthesis (in whom it is low) and in those suspected of pseudohypoaldosteronism (in whom it is usually elevated). In patients with familial glucocorticoid deficiency aldosterone levels are normal and rise appropriately to salt deprivation.

Treatment. Treatment for acute adrenal insufficiency or for crises must be immediate and vigorous. If the cause of adrenal insufficiency has not been established, a blood sample should be obtained prior to therapy for determination of levels of cortisol, 17-hydroxyprogesterone, and adrenal androgens. Intravenous administration of 5% glucose in 0.9% saline solution should be given to correct the hypoglycemia and the sodium loss. Concomitantly, a water-soluble form of hydrocortisone, such as hydrocortisone hemisuccinate, should be given intravenously. High levels are achieved instantaneously, and large doses can be used safely. As much as 25 mg for infants and 75 mg for older children should be given intravenously at 6-hr intervals for the 1st 24 hr. These doses may be reduced during the next 24 hr if progress is satisfactory. A salt-retaining hormone should be added to maintain electrolyte balance; desoxycorticosterone acetate (DOCA) in oil may be used in doses of 1–5 mg/24 hr intramuscularly. After the 1st 48 hr, if oral intake is satisfactory, the intravenous fluids may be discontinued and the corticosteroid given orally as cortisol in doses of 5–20 mg at 8-hr intervals. Further reduction can then be accomplished until maintenance levels and a stable clinical situation are achieved. The daily administration of DOCA is continued throughout this period of treatment.

Once the acute manifestations are under control, most patients require chronic replacement therapy for their deficiencies of aldosterone and cortisol. The cortisol may be given orally in daily doses of 10 mg for infants to 40 mg for adolescents; the daily dose should be divided and administered at breakfast and in the evening. During situations of stress, such as periods of infection or operative procedures, the dose of hydrocortisone should be increased. The daily injections of

DOCA can be replaced by monthly injections of a long-acting preparation, desoxycorticosterone pivalate, which may be given intramuscularly every 3–4 wk; or DOCA may be replaced by fluorohydrocortisone, which is administered orally in doses of 0.05–0.1 mg/24 hr. Measurements of serum electrolyte levels and plasma renin activity are useful in monitoring adequacy of mineralocorticoid replacement.

Overdosage with DOCA or fluorohydrocortisone results in hypertension and may lead to cardiac enlargement and edema because of excessive retention of sodium chloride and water; excessive loss of potassium may produce weakness or paralysis.

Patients with primary corticotropin deficiency or with familial glucocorticoid deficiency do not require a salt-retaining hormone since their ability to secrete aldosterone is intact. On the other hand, patients with primary defects in aldosterone synthesis do not require cortisol; a salt-retaining hormone may be required, but in milder forms the addition of salt to the diet is adequate to maintain homeostasis. In patients with pseudohypoaldosteronism administration of DOCA does not correct the urinary sodium loss; therapy must consist of supplementation with sodium chloride. The disorder is self-limited and treatment may be discontinued after 1–2 yr. In newborn infants with adrenal hemorrhage vitamins K and C and transfusions with whole blood may be indicated.

Patients with Addison disease must be closely observed for the development of other endocrine disorders. Appropriate counseling is indicated for disorders known to have a genetic basis.

18.23 ADRENOCORTICAL HYPERFUNCTION

Four syndromes are attributable to hyperadrenocorticism: the *adrenogenital syndrome, Cushing syndrome, hyperaldosteronism,* and *feminization* (Table 18–7).

18.24 ADRENOGENITAL SYNDROME

CONGENITAL ADRENAL HYPERPLASIA

Pathogenesis. When the adrenogenital syndrome is associated with congenital adrenal hyperplasia, it is caused by an inborn defect in the biosynthesis of adrenal corticoids. Five different enzymatic defects are known (Fig 18–16); virilization is associated with some, not with others. The deficiency of cortisol results in increased secretion of corticotropin, which in turn leads to adrenocortical hyperplasia and overproduction of intermediary metabolites. Each defect is inherited as an autosomal recessive trait, and each exhibits severe and mild forms, presumably because of allelic variants. The incidence of the condition varies among populations; in the United States it is on the order of 1/15,000 births. The Yupik Eskimos have an incidence of 1/500 live births of the salt-losing form of the disease.

Deficiency of 21-Hydroxylase. This defect accounts

Table 18–7 ETIOLOGIC CLASSIFICATION OF ADRENOCORTICAL HYPERFUNCTION

Excess androgen (adrenogenital syndrome)
  Congenital adrenal hyperplasia
    21-Hydroxylase defect
    11β-Hydroxylase defect
    3β-Hydroxysteroid dehydrogenase defect (females)
  Tumor
    Carcinoma
  Adenoma—isolated testosterone secretion
Excess cortisol (Cushing syndrome)
  Bilateral adrenal hyperplasia
    Pituitary corticotropin-producing tumor
    Adrenocortical nodular dysplasia
    Adrenocortical nodular hyperplasia
    Extra-adrenal corticotropin-producing tumor
    Exogenous corticotropin
  Tumor
    Carcinoma
    Benign adenoma
Excess mineralocorticoid (hypertensive hypokalemic syndrome)
  Primary hyperaldosteronism
    Adrenal hyperplasia
      Glucocorticoid suppressible
      Nonsuppressible
    Tumor
      Adenoma
      Carcinoma
  Desoxycorticosterone excess
    Adrenal hyperplasia
      11β-Hydroxylase defect
      17-Hydroxylase defect
    Tumor—carcinoma
Excess estrogen (adrenal feminization syndrome)—tumor
  Carcinoma
  Adenoma
Mixed hypercorticism—tumor

for 95% of affected patients. The gene is on the short arm of chromosome 6 and is closely linked to the locus for HLA-B. In the classic form of the disease, approximately half of the patients have salt-losing manifestations and half are "non-salt losers." Variants include a late onset form and a cryptic form. Since these variants are also HLA-B linked, they are best explained on the basis of allelic variability of the enzyme. Each defect is genetically specific; if 1 form occurs in a family, subsequently affected infants will almost always have the same form. However, genetic compounds are known and both the classic and cryptic forms have been reported in the same family.

Genetic linkage disequilibrium between the 21-hydroxylase deficiency allele and specific HLA-B locus antigens as well as specific HLA-A, HLA-B, and DR antigen combinations has been reported.

Deficiency of 11β-Hydroxylase. This is the second most frequent defect causing this syndrome. In Israel, among Jews of North African origin, this defect is the most common cause of congenital adrenal hyperplasia. Of the reported cases, most have been adults or children several yr old, and little is known of their steroid production early in life. Clinical and laboratory findings have been somewhat heterogeneous, but the plasma and urine characteristically contain large amounts of 11-desoxycortisol (compound S), the immediate precursor of cortisol. Excessive production and urinary excretion of desoxycorticosterone (DOC) also occur. The elevated

levels of DOC prevent salt-losing symptoms in spite of decreased aldosterone secretion and account for the hypertension which is characteristic of this enzymatic defect. In 1 young infant studied there appeared to be a defect in conversion of compound S to cortisol but not in conversion of DOC to corticosterone. (See Fig 18–16.) The study suggests that there may be 2 11β-hydroxylating systems, at least in infancy. As in the case for deficiency of 21-hydroxylase, females have ambiguous genitalia and males are virilized. A mild form of the disorder has been detected in normotensive women with normal genitalia who have hirsutism, acne, and menstrual irregularities.

Deficiency of 3β-Hydroxysteroid Dehydrogenase (3β-HSD). This has been reported in only 14 patients. Deficiency of both cortisol and aldosterone occurs with this defect. Salt wasting is usual, but incomplete defects without salt losing have been reported. Girls are only slightly virilized at birth; boys are usually incompletely virilized, with hypospadias. Patients with partial enzymatic defects may have normal genitalia. The enzyme is required for biosynthesis of testicular hormones; its absence in fetal testes explains the incomplete virilization of males.

Lipoid Adrenal Hyperplasia. This has been reported in 17 patients. Failure of conversion of cholesterol into pregnenolone is due to absence of 1 of the 3 enzymes needed for this conversion, presumably 20,22-desmolase. There is marked accumulation of lipids and cholesterol in the adrenal cortex, with failure of synthesis of any adrenal steroids. The same enzymatic defect is present in the testis, preventing synthesis of testicular hormones. As a consequence, males are phenotypically female and females exhibit no genital abnormality. Salt-losing manifestations are usual, and most patients have died in early infancy. Because urinary 17-ketosteroid levels are not elevated in this form of adrenal hyperplasia, affected infants are apt to be confused with those with adrenal hypoplasia.

17-Hydroxylase Deficiency. This defect has been described in 14 adults. There is deficiency of cortisol synthesis, the major adrenal corticosteroid being corticosterone (Fig 18–16). Increased production of deoxycorticosterone leads to hypokalemic alkalosis and hypertension. Urinary 17-ketosteroids and estrogens are absent; as a consequence, affected females exhibit no secondary sexual characteristics and amenorrhea is common. In the affected genotypic male the fetal testis is also involved, and the genitalia may be ambiguous, with hypospadias, cryptorchidism, and a rudimentary vagina, or they may be completely female in form, with inguinal testes. This defect must be considered in the differential diagnosis of male pseudohermaphroditism or of testicular feminization. Affected females must be considered in the differential diagnosis of primary hypogonadism (See Sec 18.46.)

Clinical Manifestations. The majority of patients with congenital adrenal hyperplasia have the defect in 21-hydroxylation and exhibit the classic form of the disease. About 50% of affected patients have the compensated variant of the disorder without salt losing.

Patients Without Salt Losing. In the *male* the main clinical manifestations are those of premature isosexual

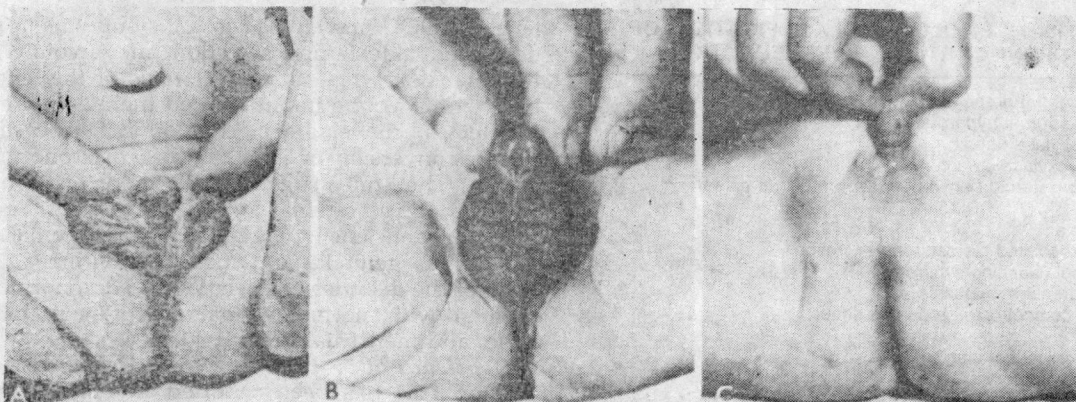

Figure 18–18   Three female pseudohermaphrodites with untreated congenital adrenal hyperplasia. All were erroneously assigned male sex at birth, and each had normal female sex-chromosome complement. Infants A and B were salt-losers and were diagnosed in early infancy. Infant C was referred at 1 yr of age because of bilateral cryptorchidism. Note completely penile urethra; such complete degrees of masculinization in females with adrenal hyperplasia are not extremely rare; most such infants are salt-losers.

development. The infant usually appears normal at birth, but signs of sexual and somatic precocity may appear within the 1st 6 mo of life or develop more gradually, becoming evident at 4–5 yr of age or later. Enlargement of the penis, scrotum, and prostate, appearance of pubic hair, and development of acne and a deep voice are noted. Muscles are well developed, and bone age is advanced for chronologic age. Premature closure of the epiphyses causes growth to stop relatively early, and adult stature is stunted.

The testes are normal in size so that they appear relatively small in contrast to the enlarged penis. Occasionally, ectopic adrenocortical cells in the testes of patients with adrenal hyperplasia become hyperplastic just as the adrenal glands do, producing enlargement of the testes. Spermatogenesis does not take place. Mental development is usually normal, but the abnormal physical development may result in behavioral problems.

In the *female* congenital adrenal hyperplasia results in female pseudohermaphroditism (Fig 18–18 and 18–19). Since the disorder of steroidogenesis begins early in fetal life, there is almost always evidence of some degree of masculinization at birth. It is manifested by enlargement of the clitoris and varying degrees of labial fusion. The vagina has a common opening with the urethra (urogenital sinus). The clitoris may be so enlarged that it resembles a penis, and, since the urethra opens below

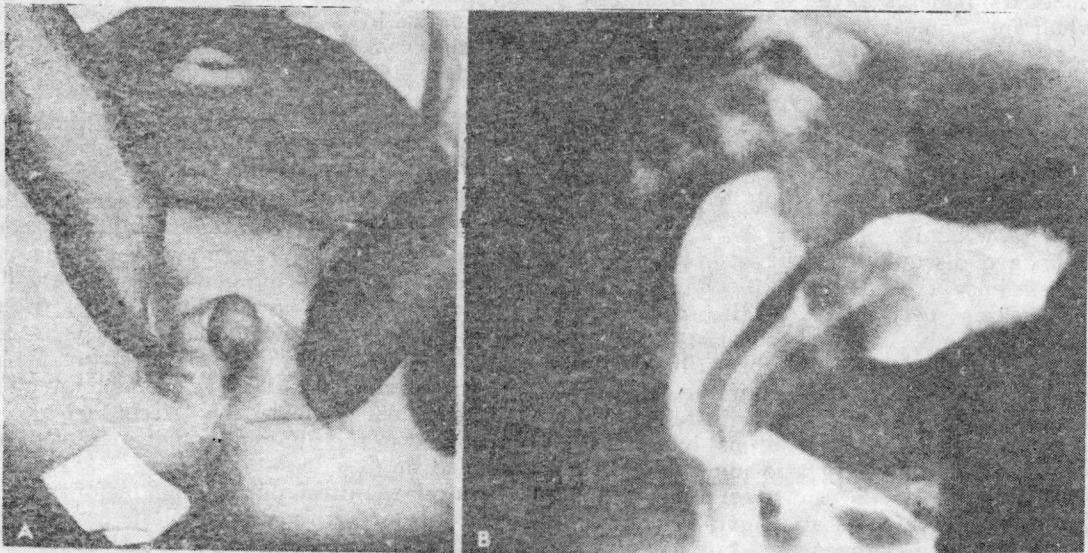

Figure 18–19   Female hermaphroditism. A, One wk old infant with clitoral enlargement and labial fusion. Normal excretion of 17-ketosteroids and normal female karyotype. B, Contrast medium injected into the urogenital sinus visualized the vagina with indentation of the cervix as well as the urinary bladder. The mother had received progesterone during the 1st trimester of pregnancy; this agent is a rare cause of masculinization of the female fetus.

this organ, a mistaken diagnosis of hypospadias and cryptorchidism is often made. Occasionally, the urogenital sinus extends to the tip of the phallus, and the genitalia resemble those of a cryptorchid male. The severity of the virilization is in general greater in infants who are salt-losers than in those who are not. The internal genital organs are those of a normal female (Fig 18-20).

After birth the masculinization progresses. Pubic and axillary hair develops prematurely, acne appears, and the voice assumes a masculine quality. Affected girls are tall for their age, and ossification is advanced; they show good muscular development and, in general, have the body build of a boy. Although the internal genitalia are female, breast development and menstruation do not occur unless the excessive production of androgens is suppressed by adequate threatment.

A number of such virilized female pseudohermaphrodites whose condition was not diagnosed until adult life have been erroneously reared as males. These patients have behaved in every way as males, including having sexual intercourse; some have had satisfactory marriages.

With the *11-hydroxylase defect* salt-losing manifestations do not occur. Most patients are hypertensive, but several have been normotensive or have had intermittent hypertension only. The disorder has been diagnosed only rarely early in life, but 2 affected infants did not have hypertension during the 1st yr of life. A 1 yr old with this defect presented with gynecomastia. Virilization occurs in all patients and is as severe as with the 21-hydroxylase defect.

Patients with Salt Losing. In patients with salt-losing variant, symptoms begin shortly after birth, with failure to regain birth weight, progressive weight loss, and dehydration. Vomiting is prominent, with ano-

rexia. Disturbances in cardiac rate and rhythm may occur, with cyanosis and dyspnea. Without treatment, collapse and death usually occur within a few wk.

In females virilization of the external genitalia in an infant with the above manifestations directs attention to the correct diagnosis. In the male, on the other hand, the genitalia appear normal, and clinical manifestations are apt to be confused with those of pyloric stenosis, intestinal obstruction, heart disease, cow milk intolerance, or other causes of failure to thrive. As a consequence, the diagnosis is established more frequently in females than in males though the disorder affects both sexes equally.

Familial homogeneity of defect is usually observed for the salt-losing and non-salt-losing forms. Under conditions of stress or sodium deprivation, salt losing may be provoked in compensated patients.

Patients with the *3β-hydroxysteroid dehydrogenase* defect are usually salt losers but less virilized. Enlargement of the clitoris may be mild and escape detection. Labial fusion is usually present; a female with normal genitalia has been reported. In the male varying degrees of hypospadias may occur, with or without bifid scrotum and/or cryptorchidism.

Patients with Variant Forms. In variant forms of late onset, symptoms of androgen excess do not appear until late childhood or during puberty. Patients with the *cryptic variant* have no clinical evidence of androgen excess even as adults and appear to be normally fertile; they have been detected through biochemical studies of unaffected parents of children with classic virilizing adrenal hyperplasia. Affected persons appear to be genetic compounds who have inherited 1 gene for classic (severe) 21-hydroxylase deficiency and 1 gene for a less severe (cryptic) 21-hydroxylase deficiency (21-OH^{CAH}/21-OH^{CRYPTIC}). Why they are asymptomatic even

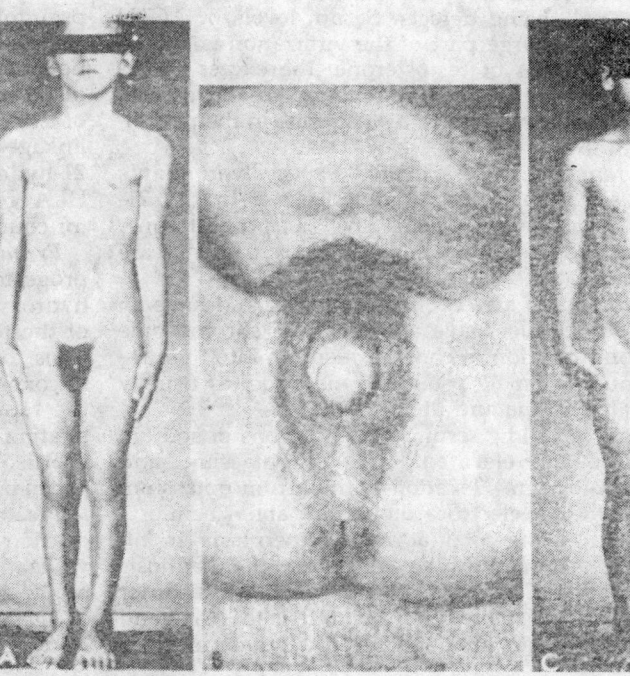
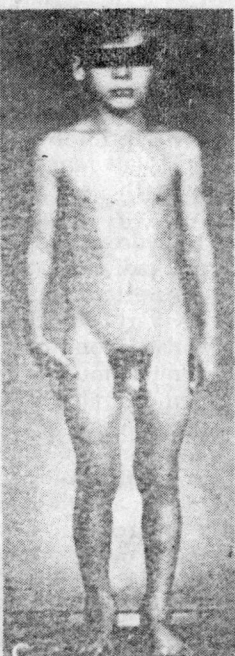

Figure 18-20 *A*, A 6 yr old girl with congenital virilizing adrenal hyperplasia. Height age, 8.5 yr; bone age, 13 yr; urinary 17-ketosteroids, 50 mg/24 hr. *B*, Note clitoral enlargement and labial fusion. *C*, Five yr old brother of girl in *A* was not considered abnormal by parents. Height age, 8 yr; bone age, 12.5 yr; urinary 17-ketosteroids, 36 mg/24 hr.

when baseline levels of 17-hydroxyprogesterone are elevated is not clear. Like the classic form, the late onset and cryptic variants of 21-hydroxylase deficiency are HLA linked.

Laboratory Data. These 3 enzymatic defects are characterized by levels of urinary 17-ketosteroids higher than normal for the age of the patient. Because of the normally somewhat elevated 17-ketosteroid levels during the 1st few days of life (up to 2.5 mg/24 hr), there may be difficulty in diagnosis at this time, and repeated determinations may be indicated. After this time up to 5 yr of age, normal excretion of 17-ketosteroids is below 0.5 mg/24 hr. Examination of the urine for the dominant steroids permits identification of the enzymatic defect. In the 21-hydroxylase defect 17-hydroxyprogesterone and pregnanetriol predominate. With the 11-hydroxylase defect increased excretion of compounds S and DOC is characteristic, whereas pregnanetriol is only moderately increased. Steroids with the Δ^5-3β-OH configuration characterize the 3-hydroxysteroid dehydrogenase defect. In this defect pregnanetriol levels are low initially, but after a few mo may rise as a consequence of hepatic 3β-hydroxysteroid dehydrogenase activity. Radioimmunoassay now permits measurement of levels in plasma of many of the steroids involved in congenital adrenal hyperplasia; accordingly, 24 hr urine collections are now often unnecessary. Plasma levels of 17-hydroxyprogesterone (17-OHP) are especially helpful in diagnosis of 21-hydroxylase deficiency and in monitoring adequacy of treatment. Levels of 17-OHP are normally high during the 1st few days of life and may overlap levels in affected patients, but by the 3rd day levels in normal infants fall and those in affected infants rise to clearly diagnostic levels.

Blood levels of cortisol and urinary excretion of its metabolites are usually normal in the compensated variant of 21-hydroxylase deficiency but do not increase further upon stimulation with ACTH. Cortisol is usually low in the salt-losing defects. Serum levels of ACTH are increased. A large part of the virilization is caused by increased levels of testosterone; the excess 17-hydroxyprogesterone is partially diverted to androstenedione, which is converted to testosterone in the periphery (Fig 18–16).

Plasma renin activity is elevated, especially in infants with the salt-losing form of the disease. In the 21-hydroxylase deficiency, plasma levels of progesterone, 17-hydroxyprogesterone, and 21-deoxycortisol are markedly elevated.

Affected females are chromatin positive and have an XX karyotype; males have a normal XY chromosome constitution. Injection of contrast medium into the urogenital sinus of female pseudohermaphrodites usually demonstrates vagina and uterus.

Salt-losers have low serum concentrations of sodium and chloride and elevated levels of potassium and nonprotein nitrogen. Elevation of the serum potassium level may produce electrocardiographic abnormalities.

Diagnosis. Congenital adrenal hyperplasia in an infant or child should always alert one to the diagnosis in later siblings. The salt-losing form of the disorder must be suspected in any infant who fails to thrive and especially in female infants with ambiguous external genitalia. When virilization occurs postnatally, in either male or female, a virilizing adrenocortical tumor must be considered in the differential diagnosis.

An adrenal tumor may be palpable or suggested on pyelography by displacement of the adjacent kidney. Urinary 17-ketosteroid excretion is elevated with congenital hyperplasia and with cortical tumors, but very high values favor the diagnosis of neoplasm. High levels of urinary pregnanetriol are highly suggestive of adrenal hyperplasia. A therapeutic test with a corticosteroid is a reliable differential procedure; administration of hydrocortisone quickly reduces excretion of urinary 17-ketosteroids to normal levels in patients with congenital adrenal hyperplasia but does not do so in those with a virilizing tumor. Corticosteroids, by inhibiting secretion of corticotropin, reduce the excessive stimulation of the adrenals in patients with hyperplasia, whereas adrenocortical tumors are not subject to pituitary regulation.

In males with virilization an interstitial cell tumor of the testis and true precocious puberty must also be considered in differential diagnosis. In true precocious puberty, gonadotropins may be elevated. The urinary 17-ketosteroid level is never above normal adult values; pregnanetriol is not found in the urine; 17-hydroxyprogesterone levels in plasma are normal; the testes are usually well developed; and interstitial cells may be seen in biopsy specimens.

Females with this condition must be differentiated from those with other causes for ambiguity of the external genitalia. Only in this condition are urinary 17-ketosteroids and plasma 17-hydroxyprogesterone levels elevated. Males with 3β-hydroxysteroid dehydrogenase defect may be confused with female pseudohermaphrodites because they lack normal virilization of the external genitalia. These male patients are 46,XY and do not have elevated urinary pregnanetriol levels; they are thus easily differentiated from the 46,XX female pseudohermaphrodite.

Detection of the heterozygous carrier is often, but not always, possible by measuring the rates of increase of 1α-hydroxyprogesterone after intravenous infusion of ACTH. With the recent documentation of genetic linkage between congenital adrenal hyperplasia due to 21-hydroxylase deficiency and HLA, it appears that HLA genotyping of families provides a reliable basis for counseling.

Prenatal Diagnosis. Concentrations of 17-hydroxyprogesterone in amniotic fluids of fetuses with 21-hydroxylase deficiency are clearly elevated. HLA typing of the fetus is also possible. These studies give a firm basis to prenatal diagnosis of the most common form of congenital adrenal hyperplasia. Prenatal diagnosis of the 11β-hydroxylase defect has been made by demonstrating increased concentrations of tetrahydro-11-deoxycortisol in maternal urine and in amniotic fluid during pregnancy.

Treatment. Hydrocortisone inhibits excessive production of adrenal androgens and stems the progressive virilization. The maintenance dose may be administered orally as follows: 10–15 mg/24 hr to children under 5 yr of age; 15–20 mg/24 hr to children from 5–12; and 20–30 mg/24 hr after 12 yr of age. These daily doses should be divided into 2 or 3 administrations. Such amounts suppress excessive secretion of androgens without producing undesirable effects. Analogues of hydrocortisone or cortisone are effective in suppressing adrenal androgens but do not provide complete physiologic replacement; they are therefore contraindicated in the treatment of adrenal hyperplasia. Serial determinations of the urinary levels of 17-ketosteroids and pregnanetriol are helpful but not essential guides to dosage. Concentrations in plasma of 17-hydroxyprogesterone or of androstenedione at 9 A.M. reflect adrenal suppression reliably and may indicate inadequate control earlier than urinary studies. The goal is to maintain the level of 17-hydroxyprogesterone below 200 ng/dl. Measurements of growth, bone age, and plasma renin activity also give important indications of adequacy of treatment.

Patients who have disturbances of electrolyte regulation ("salt losers") and elevated plasma renin activity must receive a high salt intake and mineralocorticoid therapy in addition to hydrocortisone. Dehydrated infants may require 4–8 gm of sodium chloride for adequate replacement therapy during the 1st 24 hr. DOCA, 2–4 mg, should be given daily by intramuscular injection. The blood pressure should be carefully monitored since excessive mineralocorticoid can cause hypertension. Once control has been achieved, maintenance therapy is instituted with fluorohydrocortisone, in once daily doses of 0.10–0.15 mg; the dose should be sufficient to reduce plasma renin activity to normal. This medication is continued indefinitely in salt-losers. Non-salt-losers also may manifest elevated plasma renin activity and require a mineralocorticoid. With this regimen additional sodium chloride is usually not required, but patients are given free access to salt.

The administration of hydrocortisone must be continued indefinitely in *all* patients. Increased doses are indicated during periods of stress such as infection or surgery or during periods of decreased salt intake for both salt-losers and non-salt-losers, including those with the 11-hydroxylase defect, since they all have defective adrenal reserve.

The enlarged clitoris of female infants usually requires surgical correction; a good age for this elective surgery is 6–12 mo. Recession of the clitoris is preferred, rather than its removal; the clitoris is freed and repositioned beneath the pubis with preservation of the glans, corporal components, and all neural and vascular elements. Parents should be reassured that it has been established that complete sexual gratification, including orgasm, can be achieved. The menarche occurs at the appropriate age in most girls who have been well controlled. In others there may be significant delay, and it is not exceptional for adolescents past 16 not to have begun menstruating. The delay in menarche is probably related to suboptimal control.

Non-salt-losers, particularly males, are frequently not diagnosed until 3–7 yr of age, at which time osseous maturation may be 5 yr or more in advance of chronologic age. Institution of treatment slows growth and osseous maturation to more nearly normal rates in some children; in others, especially if the bone age is 12 yr or more, spontaneous puberty may occur, therapy with hydrocortisone having suppressed production of adrenal androgens and permitted release of pituitary gonadotropins if the appropriate level of hypothalamic maturation is present.

Males who have had inadequate corticosteroid therapy may develop bilateral testicular tumors, which may or may not regress with increased dosage. The tumors are thought to arise from hilar cells or from adrenal rest tissue.

Adenomatous changes may also occur in the adrenal glands, which are then incompletely suppressible.

VIRILIZING ADRENOCORTICAL TUMORS

Tumors of the adrenal cortex may result in masculinization in girls and pseudoprecocious puberty in boys. Hypertension is common, and manifestations of Cushing syndrome may accompany virilization since these tumors frequently secrete excessive cortisol and mineralocorticoids in addition to androgens.

In males the symptoms are usually the same as those occurring with non-salt-losing congenital adrenal hyperplasia. It is virtually impossible to differentiate the 2 conditions on clinical grounds. *In females* virilizing tumors of the adrenal cause masculinization of a previously normal female, whereas congenital hyperplasia is almost always associated with genital abnormalities at birth. In late onset congenital adrenal hyperplasia, virilization may have its onset during childhood; an adrenal adenoma is known to have caused intrauterine clitoral enlargement and mild labial fusion.

Tumors of the adrenal (with or without Cushing syndrome) may be associated with hemihypertrophy, usually during the 1st few yr of life. These tumors are also associated with Beckwith syndrome and other congenital defects, particularly genitourinary tract and central nervous system abnormalities and hamartomatous defects.

Urinary 17-ketosteroid levels are usually increased, occasionally only modestly but more often markedly, and may exceed 100 mg/24 hr. Some adrenal adenomas secrete testosterone without significant amounts of adrenal androgens. Assay of testosterone production is essential to the investigation of virilized patients. Selective venous sampling may be indicated to localize small tumors. Roentgenographic studies may reveal calcification in the tumor or displacement of a kidney. Ultrasonography and computed tomography are indicated.

The treatment is surgical; a transperitoneal approach is usually recommended. Some of these neoplasms are highly malignant and metastasize widely, but cure with regression of the masculinizing features may follow removal of less malignant encapsulated tumors.

A neoplasm of 1 adrenal may produce atrophy of the other as excessive production of cortical hormones by the tumor suppresses stimulation of the normal gland by ACTH. Consequently, adrenal insufficiency may follow surgical removal of the tumor. This situation can be avoided by giving 100 mg of hydrocortisone daily, starting on the day of operation and continuing for 3–4 days postoperatively. It may also be necessary to give corticotropin concurrently with cortisol to reactivate the atrophied gland. Adequate quantities of water, sodium chloride, and glucose must also be provided. On rare occasions the tumors are bilateral, and in at least 5 instances the contralateral adrenal was absent; in such instances replacement therapy must be continued indefinitely.

The recurrence rate of these tumors may be as high as 90%; tumors weighing less than 50 gm have a much better prognosis than tumors greater than 200 gm. Urinary excretion of 17-ketosteroids returns to normal postoperatively if removal of the tumor is complete. Adrenal androgen levels should be measured at monthly intervals to detect recurrences early. Intensive therapy with mitotane (o,p'-DDD), an isomer of DDD, is indicated for inoperable tumors and for recurrences. This agent can induce regression of metastases and of abnormal steroid excretion through suppression of hormonal production in the tumor; it has not produced cures. In at least 8 patients a 2nd primary tumor has developed, the central nervous system being the most frequent site.

18.25 CUSHING SYNDROME

Cushing syndrome, a characteristic pattern of obesity in association with hypertension, is the result of maintenance of abnormally high blood levels of hydrocortisone due to hyperfunction of the adrenal cortex.

Etiology. In infants Cushing syndrome is most often caused by a *functioning adrenocortical tumor,* usually a malignant carcinoma but occasionally a benign adenoma. Over 50% of cortical tumors occur in children 3 yr of age or younger and 85% in children 7 or under. Patients with cortical tumors often exhibit a mixed form of hypercorticism due to overproduction of such other steroids as androgens, estrogens, and aldosterone.

Primary adrenocortical nodular dysplasia is being increasingly recognized as another cause of Cushing syndrome in infants. This condition is characterized by micro- or macronodules with extreme internodular atrophy.

In *adrenocortical nodular hyperplasia* the glands show hyperplasia between the nodules; this condition is the cause of Cushing syndrome in children with the McCune-Albright syndrome. There are only 2 reports of an *ACTH-producing pituitary tumor* in an infant with Cushing syndrome.

In children over 7 yr of age the etiology is usually *bilateral adrenal hyperplasia* (Cushing disease). When Harvey Cushing described this entity in 1932, he attributed it to a basophilic adenoma of the pituitary, but such tumors are rarely demonstrable in children. On the other hand, covert pituitary adenomas (microadenomas) are present in most instances of Cushing disease, and resection of these tumors results in correction of the hypercorticalism. In some children the pituitary tumors become overt after adrenalectomy (*Nelson syndrome);* these consist principally of chromophobe cells and produce increased levels of β-lipotropin and β-endorphin as well as of ACTH.

Bilateral hyperplasia of the adrenals may also result from *ectopic production of ACTH* or of material with ACTH-like activity. In adults a variety of tumors have caused this form of Cushing syndrome, in particular thymoma and bronchogenic carcinoma. Cushing syndrome has been associated with an islet cell tumor of the pancreas in a 2 yr old boy, with neuroblastoma or ganglioneuroblastoma in several children, with a hemangiopericytoma arising from the cerebral tentorium in a 7 yr old boy, and in 2 children with Wilms tumors.

Prolonged exogenous administration of corticotropin or hydrocortisone or its analogues results in a clinical pattern identical to the spontaneous disorder and is frequently referred to as *cushingoid syndrome.*

Clinical Manifestations. Symptoms may begin in the neonatal period and have been recognized in infants under 1 yr of age on at least 35 occasions. Early in life girls outnumber boys 3–1, and adrenocortical tumors (carcinoma, adenoma, and nodular hyperplasia) are the usual causative lesions. The disorder appears to be more severe and the clinical findings more flagrant than later in life. The face is rounded, with cheeks prominent and flushed (moon facies). The chin is doubled, there is a buffalo hump, and generalized obesity is common. Signs of abnormal masculinization, due to the androgen production of tumors, occur frequently; accordingly, there may be hypertrichosis on the face and trunk, pubic hair, acne, deepening of the voice, and, in girls, enlargement of the clitoris. Growth is impaired, length falling below the 3rd percentile; when significant virilization is present, growth may be normal or even accelerated. Hypertension is common and may lead to heart failure. There is increased susceptibility to infection, which may lead to fatal sepsis. Infants with Cushing syndrome, despite a robust appearance, are generally very fragile. Occasionally, the condition may be associated with hemihypertrophy or other congenital defects.

In older children bilateral hyperplasia of the adrenals is the most common lesion, and the sex incidence is equal. In addition to obesity, short stature is a common presenting feature. Gradual onset of obesity and deceleration or cessation of growth may be the only early manifestations. Purplish striae on the hips, abdomen, and thighs are common. Pubertal development may be delayed, or amenorrhea may occur in girls past menarche. Weakness, headache, deterioration in schoolwork, and emotional lability may be prominent. Hypertension is usual. Renal stones have occurred both in older children and in infants.

Laboratory Data. Polycythemia, lymphopenia, and eosinopenia are common. The glucose tolerance test may be diabetic despite elevated levels of insulin. Levels of serum electrolytes are usually normal, but potassium may be decreased.

Corticosteroid levels in blood and urine are usually elevated, but these may fluctuate widely from day to day, and repeated determinations may be required to establish the diagnosis. Quantitation of free cortisol in 24-hr collections of urine is particularly useful; normal adult values are 15–65 μg/24 hr. In most patients with Cushing syndrome, the normal diurnal rhythm in levels of plasma cortisol is abolished; measurements of the levels at 8 A.M. and 8 P.M. may be useful except in children under 3 yr of age, in whom the circadian rhythm is not always established. Urinary 17-ketosteroids may be increased, particularly in virilized patients; very high levels usually indicate adrenal carcinoma.

Special studies are frequently necessary to establish

the definitive diagnosis or to differentiate hyperplasia from tumor. Multiple tests may be necessary, particularly in children with adrenal hyperplasia who have only moderate symptoms. The dexamethasone suppression test may be helpful. Administration of 0.5 mg of dexamethasone every 6 hr for 2 days suppresses urinary excretion of corticosteroids in normal adults but not in patients with Cushing syndrome. The same test with a larger dose, 2 mg every 6 hr for 2 days, results in suppression in patients with Cushing disease due to bilateral adrenal hyperplasia but not in those with adrenocortical tumors. The test has given both false-positive and false-negative results. An appropriate dose of dexamethasone for children is 5 µg/kg every 6 hr. On the 2nd day 17-hydroxycorticoid excretion falls below 1 mg/gm/24 hr of creatinine in normal children. The reliability of the dexamethasone test is improved when free cortisol excretion is measured.

Osseous maturation is usually moderately retarded but may be normal; in virilized children the bone age is apt to be advanced. Osteoporosis is common and is most evident in roentgenograms of the spine. Pathologic fractures may be noted. Sellar tomography is indicated, though the pituitary sella is usually normal. The growth hormone response to hypoglycemia may be impaired but usually returns to normal when the hypercortisolism is corrected. Diminution of muscle mass and increased deposition of adipose tissue may be noted in roentgenograms of the extremities. The thymic shadow is absent because involution occurs due to excessive cortisol. Adrenal tumors occasionally have calcifications and frequently displace the kidney on the affected side. Computed tomography is helpful in diagnosis and localization of tumors.

Differential Diagnosis. Cushing syndrome is frequently suspected in children with obesity, particularly when striae and hypertension are present. Differential diagnosis is complicated by the fact that elevated urinary concentrations of corticosteroids are frequently secondary to obesity itself. Children with simple obesity are usually tall, whereas those with Cushing syndrome are short or decelerating in growth rate. The excretion of urinary corticoids is rapidly suppressed by oral administration of low doses of dexamethasone in persons with uncomplicated obesity.

Treatment. If the lesion is benign cortical adenoma, unilateral adrenalectomy is indicated. Such adenomas are occasionally bilateral, and the treatment of choice is subtotal adrenalectomy. In either instance an excellent therapeutic result is achieved by removal of the tumor. Adrenocortical carcinomas, on the other hand, frequently metastasize, especially to the liver and lungs, and the prognosis may be unfavorable in spite of removal of the primary lesion. Rarely, the tumors are bilateral and require total adrenalectomy. It is often impossible to differentiate benign and malignant tumors by histologic appearance alone.

The management of bilateral adrenal hyperplasia (Cushing disease) is still unsettled. Total adrenalectomy has been recommended, but current treatment is increasingly directed at the pituitary. Irradiation of the pituitary appears to induce remission in children, though not in adults; it is being increasingly advocated

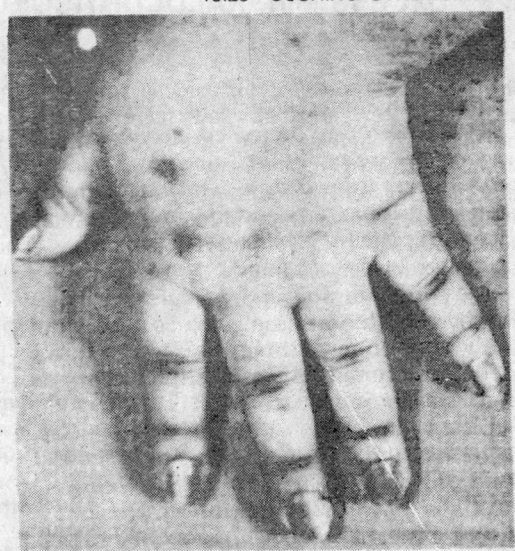

Figure 18–21 Pigmentation of skin in a 12 yr old girl with postadrenalectomy pituitary tumor. Note pigmentation of nails and skin folds. Adrenalectomy was performed for Cushing syndrome due to bilateral adrenal hyperplasia, when the girl was 10 yr of age. Pigmentation, headaches, and enlargement of the sella turcica developed 1 yr after adrenalectomy.

as the initial treatment of choice. When a pituitary tumor can be demonstrated, surgical resection should be considered. Cyproheptadine, a serotonin antagonist, administered over a 3–6 mo period has been reported to induce remissions in 50% of adult patients with Cushing disease, but further experience is required with this agent in children.

After subtotal adrenalectomy, the remaining adrenal tissue frequently undergoes hyperplasia, and symptoms recur. In some patients after adrenalectomy, enlargement of the sella occurs and chromophobe adenomas appear, even with adequate replacement therapy with cortisol. Slight increase in pigmentation may occur after adrenalectomy (Fig 18–21) and is of no clinical import, but intense melanosis is generally a harbinger of a pituitary tumor (Nelson syndrome). Large doses of hydrocortisone pre- and postoperatively have been recommended to avert possibly too rapid withdrawal of endogenous cortisol. Cyproheptadine appears effective in reducing ACTH levels and in ameliorating clinical symptoms in some patients with Nelson syndrome.

Management of patients undergoing adrenalectomy requires adequate pre- and postoperative replacement therapy with a corticosteroid. Tumors which produce corticosteroids usually lead to atrophy of the normal adrenal tissue, and replacement with both cortisol and corticotropin may be required. Patients with adrenal hyperplasia must be carefully watched after adrenalectomy for the development of pituitary tumor. Periodic examination of the pituitary fossa and of the ocular system is indicated. Postoperative complications have included sepsis, pancreatitis, thrombosis, poor wound healing, and sudden collapse, particularly in infants with Cushing syndrome. Substantial catch-up growth occurs, but adult height is often compromised.

18.26 EXCESS MINERALOCORTICOID SECRETION

The principal mineralocorticoid secreted by the adrenal is aldosterone. Increased secretion may result from a primary defect of the adrenal (primary hyperaldosteronism) or from factors which activate the renin-angiotensin system (secondary hyperaldosteronism). Patients with primary hyperaldosteronism usually have hypertension or hypokalemia; those with secondary hyperaldosteronism do not.

Desoxycorticosterone is a precursor of aldosterone, with only about one thirtieth the sodium-retaining potency of aldosterone (see Fig 18–16). Overproduction of desoxycorticosterone occurs with 2 distinct defects of adrenal steroidogenesis: the 1st defect involves 11-hydroxylation, which also leads to androgen excess and presents clinically as the hypertensive form of the adrenogenital syndrome (see above); the 2nd involves 17-hydroxylation, producing hypogonadism in the female and male pseudohermaphroditism in the male since the synthesis of androgens and estrogens as well as of adrenal steroids is impaired.

Etiology. Primary hyperaldosteronism is rare in children, occurring most often in the 3rd and 4th decades of life; aldosterone-producing adenomas account for 50–90% of cases in adults. Children reported to have aldosterone-secreting adenomas have ranged in age from 3–16 yr; all have been girls. In other children hyperaldosteronism is associated with bilateral hyperplasia of the zona glomerulosa. A subgroup of these children respond to treatment with glucocorticoids (glucocorticoid-suppressible hyperaldosteronism). This variant should be especially considered in children. Glucocorticoid-suppressible hyperaldosteronism has been reported in 5 kindreds; an autosomal dominant mode of transmission has been established. When the diagnosis is established in a proband, family members at risk should be investigated for this easily treated cause of hypertension.

Clinical Manifestations. Some affected children have had no symptoms, the diagnosis being established after incidental discovery of moderate hypertension. Others have had severe hypertension (up to 240/150 mm Hg), with headache, dizziness, and visual disturbances. Chronic hypokalemia may lead to "clear cell nephrosis," polyuria, nocturia, enuresis, and polydipsia. Muscle weakness and discomfort, tetany, intermittent paralysis, fatigue, and growth failure have been noted.

Laboratory Studies. Hypertension, hypokalemia, and suppressed plasma renin activity are the hallmarks of hyperaldosteronism. The serum pH, carbon dioxide content, and sodium concentrations may be elevated and the serum chloride and magnesium levels decreased. Serum levels of calcium are normal, even in children who manifest tetany. The urine is neutral or alkaline. Plasma and urine levels of aldosterone are increased and plasma levels of renin persistently low.

Differential Diagnosis. After establishing the diagnosis of primary aldosteronism, it is necessary to determine the etiology. All children should have a therapeutic trial with dexamethasone before invasive studies are

performed. Daily administration of 1–2 mg/24 hr results in marked suppression of aldosterone and disappearance of hypertension in those patients with the glucocorticoid-suppressible variant of hyperaldosteronism. If there is no response to dexamethasone, computed tomography (CT scan) may be helpful in visualizing an adrenal adenoma, but the tumors are often quite small and there is little experience with this diagnostic study in this condition. If CT scans are normal, adrenal vein catheterization is indicated. High concentrations of aldosterone are found in only 1 adrenal vein when an adenoma is present and in both when bilateral hyperplasia is the cause. If adrenal vein catheterization is not successful, exploratory laparotomy may be required to establish the diagnosis.

Hyperaldosteronism occurs in many other conditions in which it is a normal homeostatic response. In such secondary hyperaldosteronism, serum renin activity is high or rises with a low salt diet, whereas in primary hyperaldosteronism the renin-angiotensin system is suppressed. Increased aldosterone secretion occurs in edematous disorders with reduced effective volume, such as nephrotic syndrome, congestive cardiac failure, and cirrhosis of the liver. Increased secretion of aldosterone also occurs in conditions in which compromise of renal perfusion results in increased secretion of renin, such as in stenosis of the renal artery. Wilms tumor and juxtaglomerular cell tumors may also secrete renin and cause secondary hyperaldosteronism.

In pseudohypoaldosteronism the increased levels of aldosterone are due to a defect in mineralocorticoid receptors, with ensuing activation of the renin-angiotensin system.

Bartter syndrome is also characterized by hypokalemic alkalosis, hypochloremia, and hyperaldosteronism. The blood pressure is normal, however, and secretion of renin is increased. Growth failure is the usual presenting complaint. Renal biopsy reveals hyperplasia of the juxtaglomerular apparatus. Urinary excretion of prostaglandin $F_{1\alpha}$ has been demonstrated, and it has been suggested that this mediates the hyperreninemia. Drugs which reduce prostaglandin levels, such as indomethacin, correct the aldosterone, renin, and prostaglandin abnormalities but do not completely correct the hypokalemia.

Treatment. Glucocorticoid-suppressible hyperaldosteronism is managed by daily administration of dexamethasone. Bilateral adrenal hyperplasia which does not respond to this therapy requires bilateral adrenalectomy; the results are excellent, but adrenal replacement therapy is required. Removal of an aldosterone-secreting adenoma results in a cure.

Treatment of secondary hyperaldosteronism is directed to the specific causative disorder.

18.27 FEMINIZING ADRENAL TUMORS

Adrenocortical tumors have been associated in 9 boys with excessive production of estrogens and heterosexual precocious puberty. Gynecomastia was the initial manifestation, appearing from 6 mo–7 yr of age. Growth and development were otherwise normal, or concomitant virilization was sometimes evidenced by acne, deep voice, phallic enlargement, and advanced osseous maturation. The testes were not enlarged. Hypertension is common in affected adults but has not been observed in children. Levels of estrogens in plasma and urine are markedly elevated, and urinary 17-ketosteroids may be abnormally high. Tumors may be either carcinomas or benign adenomas and may be calcified on roentgenography. Gynecomastia regresses after removal of the tumor, and hormone values return to normal.

Estrogen-secreting adrenocortical tumors have been reported in 11 girls ranging in age from 6 mo–10 yr. The majority of the tumors were adenomas, some of which also elaborated androgens (with virilization) and/or mineralocorticoids (with hypertension). In addition to elevated plasma and urinary levels of estrogens, there were usually elevated levels of 17-ketosteroids in urine and of DHAS in plasma. Plasma gonadotropin levels were suppressed.

Intravenous pyelography, ultrasonography, and/or computed tomography may localize the tumor, and venacavagraphic examination may detect vascular invasion and identify a carcinoma.

18.28 EXCESSIVE SECRETION OF CATECHOLAMINES

PHEOCHROMOCYTOMA

The pheochromocytoma, a catecholamine-secreting tumor, arises from the chromaffin cells. The most common site of origin is the adrenal medulla; tumors may develop, however, anywhere along the abdominal sympathetic chain and are particularly apt to be located near the aorta at the level of the inferior mesenteric artery or at its bifurcation. They also appear in the periadrenal area, the urinary bladder or ureteral walls, the thoracic cavity, and the cervical region. Fewer than 5% of reported instances have occurred in children. Tumors vary from about 1–10 cm in diameter; they are found more often on the right side than on the left. In 20% of affected children the adrenal tumors are bilateral, and in 30% tumors are found in both the adrenal and extra-adrenal areas or only in an extra-adrenal area.

Pheochromocytoma is frequently inherited as an autosomal dominant trait. In affected families the ages of patients at the time of diagnosis have varied from the 1st–5th decade of life; more than half the patients have had multiple tumors.

Pheochromocytoma is frequently associated with other syndromes or tumors. Approximately 5% of patients with pheochromocytoma have neurofibromatosis. Sporadic as well as familial instances of pheochromocytoma have been noted in patients with von Hippel-Lindau disease. Kinships have been reported in which some affected members also have asymptomatic islet cell adenomas and some with pheochromocytoma are asymptomatic despite elevated urinary concentrations of catecholamines.

Pheochromocytoma also may coexist with medullary carcinoma of the thyroid; this association is known as *Sipple syndrome*. Of patients with these 2 tumors, some also have parathyroid disease (*multiple endocrine neoplasia, type II*); others have *mucosal neuromas* (*multiple endocrine neoplasia, type IIb or type III*). Mucosal neuromas appear early in life and affect primarily the tongue and lips; they may also affect the gingival, buccal, or conjunctival mucosa. *Ganglioneuromatosis* of the alimentary tract is often a major component of the syndrome, leading to constipation or diarrhea before other manifestations appear.

These syndromes are all inherited in an autosomal dominant fashion, with highly variable expression.

Clinical Manifestations. These result from excessive secretion of epinephrine and norepinephrine; the clinical picture varies with quantitative variations in their secretion. All patients have hypertension at some time. The hypertension is usually sustained, but it may often be *paroxysmal*. Paroxysms should particularly suggest pheochromocytoma as a diagnostic possibility. When there are paroxysms of hypertension, the attacks are usually infrequent at first but become more frequent and eventually give way to a continuous hypertensive state. Between attacks of hypertension the patient may be free of symptoms. During attacks the patient complains of headache and palpitation, and pallor, vomiting, and sweating also occur. Convulsions and other manifestations of hypertensive encephalopathy may occur. In severe cases precordial pains radiate into the arms, and pulmonary edema and cardiac and hepatic enlargement may develop. The child has a good appetite but because of hypermetabolism does not gain weight, and severe cachexia may develop. Polyuria and polydipsia can be sufficiently severe to suggest diabetes insipidus. Growth failure may be striking. The blood pressure may range from 180–260 systolic and 120–210 diastolic, and the heart may be enlarged. Ophthalmoscopic examination may reveal papilledema, hemorrhages, exudate, and arterial constriction.

Laboratory Data. The urine contains protein, a few casts, and occasionally glucose. Gross hematuria suggests that the tumor is in the bladder wall. Polycythemia is occasionally noted.

The most direct and specific test is the demonstration of increased basal plasma levels or excretion of catecholamines. Pheochromocytomas produce both norepinephrine and epinephrine; norepinephrine in plasma is derived, however, from both the adrenal gland and adrenergic nerve endings, whereas epinephrine is derived primarily from the adrenal. In affected children the predominant catecholamine is norepinephrine, and total urinary catecholamine excretion usually exceeds 300 µg/24 hr. The concentrations of catecholamines in urine are directly related to those in the tumor. Urinary excretion of VMA (3-methoxy-4-hydroxymandelic acid), the major metabolite of epinephrine and norepinephrine, and of metanephrine (Fig 18–15) is also increased. Measurement of plasma catecholamines in the resting, supine state (by radioenzymatic assay) may replace urinary studies. Excretion of catecholamine metabolites may be similar in children with neuroblastoma and with pheochromocytoma, but levels are usually higher with pheochromocytoma. Daily urinary excretion of these compounds by normal children increases with age, and vanilla-containing foods and fruits can produce falsely elevated levels of VMA. Certain drugs interfere with fluorometric determinations of catecholamines.

Plasma renin levels may be elevated secondary to reduced renal cortical blood flow.

Differential Diagnosis. The various causes of hypertension in children must be considered, such as renal or renovascular disease, coarctation of the aorta, acrodynia, thallium intoxication, hyperthyroidism, Cushing syndrome, congenital adrenal hyperplasia, and essential hypertension. A nonfunctioning kidney may result from compression of a ureter or of a renal artery by a pheochromocytoma. Paroxysmal hypertension may be associated with familial dysautonomia. Urinary excretion of VMA is low in familial dysautonomia because of a defect in release rather than in synthesis of catecholamines. Cerebral disorders, diabetes insipidus, diabetes mellitus, and hyperthyroidism must also be considered in the differential diagnosis. Hypertension in patients with neurofibromatosis may be caused by renal vascular involvement as well as by concurrent pheochromocytoma.

Neuroblastoma, ganglioneuroblastoma, and ganglioneuroma frequently produce catecholamines. Secreting neurogenic tumors commonly produce hypertension, excessive sweating, flushing, pallor, rash, polyuria, and polydipsia. Diarrhea may also be associated with these tumors, particularly with ganglioneuroma, and may at times be sufficiently persistent to suggest the "celiac syndrome."

Management. Localization of the tumor is often difficult; only rarely can it be discovered by palpation. Pyelography may locate the tumor, or a tumor blush may be detected by angiography. With the advent of body computed tomography, venous catheterization with sampling of blood at different levels for catecholamine determinations is now only rarely necessary to localize the tumor. A new radiopharmaceutical agent, [131]meta-iodobenzylguanidine, offers hope for more reliable localization of pheochromocytomas. Since these tumors are often multiple, especially in children, a thorough transabdominal exploration of all the usual sites offers the best chance of finding all of them. Removal of the tumor(s) results in cure. Although these tumors often appear malignant histologically, only rarely has malignancy been unequivocally established, as demonstrated by the metastasis to lymph nodes of hormonally active chromaffin cells. The operation is not without danger because an extreme rise of blood pressure may result from massive discharge of hormone during operative manipulation. Shock from a precipitous drop of blood pressure during operation or within the 1st 48 hr postoperatively is also a danger. These risks can be lessened by alpha- and beta-adrenergic blockade preoperatively, by careful monitoring during surgery, and by continuous postoperative surveillance. The urinary excretion of catecholamines should be determined after operation as a measure of the completeness of the surgical removal. Prolonged follow-up is indicated since functioning tumors at other sites may become manifest many yr after the initial operation.

Examination of relatives of affected patients may reveal other persons harboring unsuspected tumors. In 1 family with 10 affected individuals the highest blood pressures and urinary concentrations of catecholamines were found in the children, whereas some of the affected adults were normotensive and had only moderately elevated urinary concentration of catecholamines and VMA.

OTHER CATECHOLAMINE-SECRETING NEURAL TUMORS

Excessive elaboration of catecholamines is not exclusive to pheochromocytomas but frequently occurs with other neurogenic tumors (neuroblastoma, ganglioneuroblastoma, and, less frequently, ganglioneuroma). Consequently, many of the systemic manifestations characteristic of pheochromocytoma may be seen in patients with other tumors of neural origin. Hypertension, excessive sweating, flushing, pallor, rash, polyuria, and polydipsia are the most common findings. *Chronic diarrhea* occurs with other manifestations or may be the only symptom. It occurs in approximately 8% of patients with these tumors but only rarely in patients with pheochromocytoma. The diarrhea is voluminous, may result in severe electrolyte depletion, and is intractable to treatment; it ceases abruptly with removal of the tumor. Diarrhea is more apt to occur in association with ganglioneuroma and ganglioneuroblastoma, but it may occur with neuroblastoma. Increased levels of *vasoactive intestinal peptide* (VIP) are present in the tumor and/or plasma. This peptide is a potent stimulator of water and electrolyte secretion and stimulates adenylate cyclase production in the mucosa of the small intestine.

Benign adrenal cortical hyperplasia with Cushing disease has been observed in children with these neural tumors; the secretion of an ACTH-like hormone by the tumor is a likely but not proven explanation. An 18 mo old girl has been reported to have a ganglioneuroblastoma as well as an adrenocortical adenoma in each adrenal.

Many patients with these tumors have increased excretion of dopa, dopamine, norepinephrine, normetanephrine, homovanillic acid, and vanillylmandelic acid (VMA). Patients with pheochromocytoma usually excrete only epinephrine, norepinephrine, their methoxy analogues, and VMA (Fig 18–15). Elevated excretion of homovanillic acid generally indicates malignant pheochromocytoma or other malignant neural tumors, but it has been noted also with benign phenochromocytoma. Biochemical differentiation between neuroblastomas, ganglioneuroblastomas, and benign ganglioneuromas is not possible. Serial determinations of VMA and catecholamines, and particularly of norepinephrine and dopamine, help in detecting recurrences and in assessing the effectiveness of therapy in the postoperative evaluation of children whose VMA levels were elevated prior to treatment. Excretion of these compounds returns to normal if the tumor is completely removed.

Screening tests for VMA excretion may detect neuroblastoma. Negative tests do not exclude the tumor since only about 80% are associated with increased urinary excretion of VMA; false-positive tests also occur.

18.29 CALCIFICATION WITHIN THE ADRENAL

Calcification within the adrenal glands may occur in a wide variety of situations, some serious and others of no obvious consequence. Adrenal calcifications are often detected as incidental findings in roentgeno-graphic studies of the abdomen in infants and children. One may elicit a history of anoxia or trauma at birth. Hemorrhage into the adrenal at or immediately after birth is probably the common factor which leads to subsequent calcification. Though it is advisable to assess the adrenocortical reserve of such patients, there is rarely any functional disorder.

Neuroblastomas, ganglioneuromas, cortical carcinomas, pheochromocytomas, and cysts of the adrenal gland may each be responsible for calcifications, particularly if hemorrhage has occurred within the tumor. Calcification in such lesions is almost always unilateral.

The most common infection associated with calcifications within the adrenal is tuberculosis, and the patient usually has the clinical manifestations of Addison disease. Calcifications may also develop in the adrenal glands of children who recover from the Waterhouse-Friderichsen syndrome; such patients are usually asymptomatic.

Infants with *Wolman syndrome*, a rare lipid disorder due to deficiency of lysosomal acid lipase, have extensive bilateral calcifications of the adrenal glands. The clinical manifestations include hepatosplenomegaly, gastrointestinal symptoms, and failure to thrive; rapid clinical deterioration and death by 3–4 mo of age are the usual course. The lipids stored in the affected tissues are cholesteryl esters and triglycerides. Deposition of lipids is especially heavy in the adrenal, but the cause of the calcifications is not known. The disorder is recessively transmitted. Prenatal diagnosis is possible through study of cultured fibroblasts obtained by amniocentesis. Late in pregnancy the calcified adrenals may be detected roentgenographically. It is probable that patients who have been reported to have had adrenal calcifications with Niemann-Pick disease have had this form of xanthomatosis.

General

Baxter JD, Forsham PH: Tissue effects of glucocorticoids. Am J Med 53:573, 1972.
Franks RC: Urinary 17-hydroxycorticosteroid and cortisol excretion in childhood. J Clin Endocrinol Metab 36:702, 1973.
Johannisson E: The foetal adrenal cortex in the human. Its ultrastructure at different stages of development and in different functional states. Acta Endocrinol Suppl 130, 1968.
Lee PL, Plotnick LP, Kowarski A, et al (eds): Treatment of Congenital Adrenal Hyperplasia: A Quarter of a Century Later. Baltimore, University Park Press, 1977.
Tyler FH, West CD: Laboratory evaluation of disorders of the adrenal cortex. Am J Med 53:664, 1972.
Villee DB: The development of steroidogenesis. Am J Med 53:533, 1972.

Adrenal Cortical Insufficiency

Allgrove J, Clayden GS, Grant DB, et al: Familial glucocorticoid deficiency with achalasia of the cardia and deficient tear production. Lancet 1:1284, 1978.
Arulananthan K, Dwyer JM, Genel M: Evidence for defective immunoregulation in the syndrome of familial candidiasis endocrinopathy. N Engl J Med 300:165, 1979.
Blizzard RM, Kyle M: Studies of the adrenal antigens and antibodies in Addison's disease. J Clin Invest 42:1653, 1963.
Boyd JF, McDonald AM: Adrenal cortical hypoplasia in siblings. Arch Dis Child 35:561, 1960.
Camacho AM, Kowarski A, Migeon CJ, et al: Congenital adrenal hyperplasia due to a deficiency of one of the enzymes in the biosynthesis of pregnenolone. J Clin Endocrinol 28:153, 1968.
Cathelineau G, Brerault J, Fiet J, et al: Adrenocortical 11β-hydroxylation defect in adult women with postmenarchial onset of symptoms. J Clin Endocrinol Metab 51:287, 1980.
Hay ID: Pubertal failure in congenital adrenocortical hypoplasia. Lancet 2:1035, 1977.
Hintz RL, Menking M, Sotos JF: Familial holoprosencephaly with endocrine dysgenesis. J Pediatr 72:81, 1968.
Honour JW, Dillon MJ, Shackleton CHL: Analysis of steroids in urine for differentiation of pseudohypoaldosteronism and aldosterone biosynthetic defect. J Clin Endocrinol Metab 54:325, 1982.
Kelch RP, Kaplan SL, Biglieri EG, et al: Hereditary adrenocortical unresponsiveness to adrenocorticotropic hormone. J Pediatr 81:726, 1972.
Kenny FM, Reynolds JW, Green OC: Partial 3β-hydroxysteroid dehydrogenase (3β-HSD) deficiency in a family with congenital adrenal hyperplasia: Evidence for increasing 3β-HSD activity with age. Pediatrics 48:256, 1971.
Kirkland RT, Kirkland JL, Johnson CM, et al: Congenital lipoid adrenal hyperplasia in an eight-year-old phenotypic female. J Clin Endocrinol Metab 36:488, 1973.
Kreines K, DeVaux WD: Neonatal adrenal insufficiency associated with maternal Cushing syndrome. Pediatrics 47:516, 1971.
Migeon CJ, Kenny FM, Hung W, et al: Study of adrenal function in children with meningitis. Pediatrics 40:163, 1967.
Mittelstaedt CA, Volberg FM, Merten DF, et al: Sonographic diagnosis of neonatal adrenal hemorrhage. Radiology 131:453, 1979.
Moser HW, Moser AB, Kawamura N, et al: Adrenoleukodystrophy: Studies of the phenotype, genetics and biochemistry. Johns Hopkins Med J 147:217, 1980.
Moser HW, Moser AB, Powers JM, et al: The prenatal diagnosis of adrenoleukodystrophy. Demonstration of increased hexacosanic acid levels in cultured amniocytes and fetal gland. Pediatr Res 16:171, 1982.
Moshang T, Rosenfield RL, Bongiovanni AM, et al: Familial glucocorticoid insufficiency. J Pediatr 82:821, 1973.
Rosenfeld RL, Rich BH, Wolfsdorf JI, et al: Pubertal presentation of congenital Δ⁵-3β-hydroxysteroid dehydrogenase deficiency. J Clin Endocrinol Metab 51:345, 1980.
Rosler A, Rabinowitz D, Theodor R, et al: The nature of the defect in a salt-wasting disorder in Jews of Iran. J Clin Endocrinol Metab 44:279, 1977.
Savage MO, Jefferson IG, Dillon MJ, et al: Pseudohypoaldosteronism: Severe salt wasting in infancy caused by generalized mineralocorticoid unresponsiveness. J Pediatr 101:239, 1982.
Sperling MA, Wolfsen AR, Fisher DA: Congenital adrenal hypoplasia: An isolated defect of organogenesis. J Pediatr 82:444, 1973.
Ulick S, Eberlein WR, Blitfeld AR, et al: Evidence for an aldosterone biosynthetic defect in congenital adrenal hyperplasia. J Clin Endocrinol Metab 51:1346, 1980.
Veldhuis JD, Kulin HE, Santen RJ, et al: Inborn error in the terminal steps of aldosterone biosynthesis. Corticosterone methyl oxidase Type II deficiency in a North American pedigree. N Engl J Med 303:117, 1980.
Zachman M, Illig R, Prader A: Gonadotropin deficiency and cryptorchidism in three prepubertal brothers with congenital adrenal hypoplasia. J Pediatr 97:255, 1980.

Adrenal Cortical Hyperfunction

Aronin N, Krieger DT: Sustained remission of Nelson's syndrome after stopping cyproheptadine treatment. N Engl J Med 302:453, 1980.
Bergstrand CG, Nilsson KO: Treatment of Cushing's disease in children. Acta Paediatr Scand 71:1, 1982.
Bhettay E, Bonnier F: Pure estrogen-secreting feminizing adrenocortical adenoma. Arch Dis Child 52:241, 1977.
Bongiovanni AM: Disorders of adrenocortical steroid biogenesis. The adrenogenital syndrome associated with congenital adrenal hyperplasia. In: Stanbury JB, Wyngaarden JB, Fredrickson DS (eds): The Metabolic Basis of Inherited Disease. Ed 3. New York, McGraw-Hill, 1972.
Bricaire H, et al: A new male pseudohermaphroditism associated with hypertension due to a block of a 17α-hydroxylation. J Clin Endocrinol Metab 35:67, 1972.
Brook CGD, Bambach M, Zachmann M, et al: Familial congenital adrenal hyperplasia. Helv Paediatr Acta 28:277, 1973.
Burr IM, Sullivan J, Graham T, et al: A testosterone-secreting tumour of the adrenal producing virilization in a female infant. Lancet 2:643, 1973.
Dahms WT, Gray G, Vrana M, et al: Adrenocortical adenoma and ganglioneuroblastoma in a child. Am J Dis Child 125:608, 1973.
Duck SC: Acceptable linear growth in congenital adrenal hyperplasia. J Pediatr 97:93, 1980.
Fraumeni JF Jr, Miller RW: Adrenocortical neoplasms with hemihypertrophy, brain tumors, and other disorders. J Pediatr 70:129, 1967.
Gabrilove JL, Sharma DC, Wotiz HH, et al: Feminizing adrenocortical tumors in the male. A review of 52 cases including a case report. Medicine 44:37, 1965.

Ganguly A, Bergstein J, Grim CE, et al: Childhood primary aldosteronism due to an adrenal adenoma: Preoperative localization by adrenal vein catheterization. Pediatrics 65:605, 1980.

Ganguly A, Grim CE, Bergstein J, et al: Genetic and pathophysiologic studies of a new kindred with glucocorticoid-supressible hyperaldosteronism manifest in three generations. J Clin Endocrinol Metab 53:1040, 1981.

Grim CE, McBryde AC, Glenn JF, et al: Childhood primary aldosteronism with bilateral adrenocortical hyperplasia. Plasma renin activity as an aid to diagnosis. J Pediatr 71:377, 1967.

Grim CE, Weinberg MH: Familial, dexamethasone-suppressible, normokalemic hyperaldosteronism. Pediatrics 65:597, 1980.

Gullner HG, Cerletti C, Bartter FC, et al: Prostacycline overproduction in Bartter's syndrome. Lancet 2:767, 1979.

Haicken BN, Schulman NH, Schneider KM: Adrenocortical carcinoma and congenital hemihypertrophy. J Pediatr 33:284, 1973.

Hodgkinson DJ, Telander RL, Sheps SG, et al: Extra-adrenal intrathoracic functioning paraganglioma (pheochromocytoma) in childhood. Mayo Clin Proc 55:271, 1980.

Howard CP, Takahashi H, Hayles AB: Feminizing adrenal adenoma in a boy. Case report and literature review. Mayo Clin Proc 52:354, 1977.

Jennings AS, Liddle TW, Orth DN: Results of treating childhood Cushing's disease with pituitary irradiation. N Engl J Med 297:957, 1977.

Jones HW, Verkauf BS: Congenital adrenal hyperplasia: Age at menarche and related events at puberty. Am J Obstet Gynecol 109:292, 1971.

Kenny FM, Hashaida Y, Askari A, et al: Virilizing tumors of the adrenal cortex. Am J Dis Child 115:445, 1968.

Kershnar AK, Borut D, Kogut MD, et al: Studies on a phenotypic female with 17-α-hydroxylase deficiency. J Pediatr 89:395, 1976.

Kirkland RT, Kirkland JL, Keenan BS, et al: Bilateral testicular tumors in congenital hyperplasia. J Clin Endocrinol Metab 44:369, 1977.

Klecker RL, Roth JB: Visceral neurofibromatosis and hypertension in childhood. Pediatrics 53:417, 1974.

Levine LS, Dupont B, Lorenzen F, et al: Genetic and hormonal characterization of cryptic 21-hydroxylase deficiency. J Clin Endocrinol Metab 53:1193, 1981.

Levy SR, Val Wynne C Jr, Lorentz WB Jr: Cushing's syndrome in infancy secondary to pituitary adenoma. Am J Dis Child 136:605, 1982.

Lorenzen F, Pan S, New MI, et al: Hormonal phenotype and HLA-genotype in families of patients with congenital adrenal hyperplasia (21-hydroxylase deficiency). Pediatr Res 13:1356, 1979.

Loridan L, Senior B: Cushing's syndrome in infancy. J Pediatr 75:349, 1969.

McArthur RG, Bahn RC, Hayles AB: Primary adrenocortical nodular dysplasia as a cause of Cushing's syndrome in infants and children. Mayo Clin Proc 57:58, 1982.

McArthur RG, Bloutier MD, Hayles AB, et al: Cushing's disease in children. Findings in 13 cases. Mayo Clin Proc 47:379, 1972.

McArthur RG, Hayles AB, Salassa RM: Childhood Cushing disease: Results of bilateral adrenalectomy. J Pediatr 95:214, 1979.

Modlinger RS, Nicolis GL, Krakoff LR, et al: Some observations on the pathogenesis of Bartter's syndrome. N Engl J Med 289:1022, 1973.

Mosier HD Jr, Smith FG, Schultz MA: Failure of catch-up growth after Cushing's syndrome in childhood. Am J Dis Child 124:251, 1972.

Pollack MS, Levine LS, O'Neill GJ, et al: HLA linkage and B14, DR1, BfS haplotype association with the genes for late onset and cryptic 21-hydroxylase deficiency. Am J Hum Genet 33:540, 1981.

Pombo M, Alvez F, Varela-Cives R, et al: Ectopic production of ACTH by Wilms' tumor. Hormone Res 16:160, 1982.

Raiti S, Grant DB, Williams DI, et al: Cushing's syndrome in childhood: Postoperative management. Arch Dis Child 47:597, 1972.

Rosler A, Leiberman E, Rosenmann A, et al: Prenatal diagnosis of 11β-hydroxylase deficiency congenital adrenal hyperplasia. J Clin Endocrinol Metab 49:546, 1979.

Snaith AH: A case of feminizing adrenal tumor in a girl. J Clin Endocrinol Metab 18:318, 1958.

Solomon JL, Schoen EJ: Juvenile Cushing syndrome manifested primarily by growth failure. Am J Dis Child 130:200, 1976.

Streetan DHP, Faas FH, Elders MJ, et al: Hypercortisolism in childhood: Shortcomings of conventional diagnostic criteria. Pediatrics 56:797, 1975.

Sultan C, Descomps B, Garandeau P, et al: Pubertal gynecomastia due to an estrogen-producing adrenal adenoma. J Pediatr 95:744, 1979.

Tyrell JB, Wiener-Kronish J, Lorenzi M, et al: Cushing's disease: Growth hormone response to hypoglycemia after correction of hypercortisolism. J Clin Endocrinol Metab 44:218, 1977.

Zachmann M, Vollmin JA, New MI, et al: Congenital adrenal hyperplasia due to deficiency of 11β-hydroxylation of 17α-hydroxylated steroids. J Clin Endocrinol Metab 33:501, 1971.

Zancan L, Zacchello F, Mantero F: Indomethacin for Bartter's syndrome. Lancet 2:1334, 1976.

Pheochromocytoma and Other Neural Tumors

Gitlow SE, Bertani LM, Greenwood SM, et al: Benign pheochromocytoma associated with elevated excretion of homovanillic acid. J Pediatr 81:1112, 1972.

Keiser HR, Beauen MA, Doppman J, et al: Sipple's syndrome: Medullary thyroid carcinoma, pheochromocytoma, and parathyroid disease. Ann Intern Med 78:561, 1973.

Kogut MD, Kaplan SA: Systemic manifestations of neurogenic tumors. J Pediatr 60:697, 1962.

Mitchell CH, et al: Intractable watery diarrhea, ganglioneuroblastoma, and vasoactive intestinal peptide. J Pediatr 89:593, 1976.

Phillips AF, McMurty RJ, Taubman J: Malignant pheochromocytoma in childhood. Am J Dis Child 130:1252, 1976.

Schimke RN, Hartman WH, Prout TE, et al: Syndrome of bilateral pheochromocytoma, medullary thyroid carcinoma and multiple neuromas. A possible regulatory defect in the differentiation of chromaffin tissue. N Engl J Med 279:1, 1968.

Sisson JC, Frager MS, Valk TW, et al: Scintigraphic localization of pheochromocytoma. N Engl J Med 305:12, 1981.

Smith AA, Dancis J: Catecholamine release in familial dysautonomia. N Engl J Med 277:61, 1967.

Stackpole RH, Melicow MM, Uson AC: Pheochromocytoma in children. Report of 9 cases and review of the first 100 published cases with follow-up studies. J Pediatr 63:315, 1963.

Voorhess ML: Urinary catecholamine excretion by healthy children. I. Daily excretion of dopamine, norepinephrine, epinephrine and 3-methoxy-4-hydroxymandelic acid. Pediatrics 39:252, 1967.

Voorhess ML: Neuroblastoma-pheochromocytoma: Products and pathogenesis. Ann NY Acad Sci 230:187, 1974.

Wise KS, Gibson JA: Von Hippel—Lindau's disease and pheochromocytoma. Br Med J 1:441, 1971.

Adrenal Calcification

Crocker AC, Vawter GF, Neuhauser EBO, et al: Wolman's disease: Three new patients with recently described lipidosis. Pediatrics 35:627, 1965.

Hill EE, Williams JA: Massive adrenal haemorrhage in the newborn. Arch Dis Child 34:178, 1959.

Jarvis JL, Seaman WB: Idiopathic adrenal calcification in infants and children. Am J Roentgenol 82:510, 1959.

Stevenson J, MacGregor AM, Connelly P: Calcification of the adrenal glands in young children. A report of three cases with a review of the literature. Arch Dis Child 36:316, 1961.

18.30   DISORDERS OF THE GONADS

Maturation in Boys. The main hormonal product of the testis is testosterone. It is produced in the Leydig cells, which have many enzymes in common with cells of the adrenal cortex. Defects have now been described for each of the steps in biosynthesis of testosterone (see Fig 18–25). Because testosterone is important to normal virilization of the XY fetus, each of these defects has produced some degree of male pseudohermaphroditism. Defects in synthesis of testosterone become more clearly evident at puberty when normal masculinization fails to occur. These defects are all genetic and almost surely all autosomal recessive.

Within specific target cells, testosterone is converted by 5α-reductase to dihydrotestosterone, another potent androgen (see Fig 18–25). There appears to be differential binding of these 2 androgens in different cells, with differences in functional activity. In the male fetus at the critical time of masculinization (8–12 wk) these 2 androgens appear to have distinct and separate functions. Patients with deficiency of 5α-reductase clearly demonstrate that testosterone is necessary for wolffian differentiation, whereas dihydrotestosterone is necessary for masculinization of the external genitalia. Evidence from these same patients suggests that growth of facial hair and prostate may also be dependent upon dihydrotestosterone.

In prepubertal boys and girls the plasma levels of testosterone are at the same low levels. The level of testosterone rises sharply in boys during puberty, particularly in stage 3 (generally after 12 yr of age). The size of the testis increases slightly from 6–12 yr of age, before testosterone levels rise; thereafter, growth of the testis is markedly accelerated. Pubic hair growth, acne, voice change, and axillary hair growth correlate with the rising levels of testosterone. Estradiol and adrenal androgens also increase during puberty. In the early stages of puberty a nocturnal rise of plasma testosterone occurs 40–80 min after onset of sleep because of a slightly earlier sharp rise in the level of LH.

The ability of prepubertal testis to secrete testosterone can be assessed by administration of chorionic gonadotropin (hCG), which stimulates the testis in a manner analogous to luteinizing hormone (LH). After administration of hCG for 1–3 days, levels of testosterone rise in all stages of puberty; after administration for 2–6 wk, adult levels of plasma testosterone are achieved.

Progressive maturation of the testis occurs under the influence of gradually rising levels of gonadotropins. The normally low levels of FSH and LH begin to rise slowly around the age of 6–8 yr; there is slight growth of the testis during this period. A sharper rise in the levels of FSH and LH occurs at the onset of puberty. Plasma levels of FSH increase only to midpuberty, whereas plasma levels of LH continue to rise until about 17 yr of age. The somatic changes of puberty and the rising levels of testosterone correlate best with the levels of LH.

The hormonal changes described above are initiated by maturation of the hypothalamus, a process still poorly understood. The key physiologic change at puberty is a decreasing sensitivity of the hypothalamus to the negative feedback effects of the sex steroids. This change is presumably associated with increasing synthesis and release of gonadotropin-releasing factor(s). Increasing sensitivity of the pituitary to luteinizing hormone–releasing hormone (LRH) also occurs. Administration of LRH to the prepubertal child results in a smaller release of LH than occurs when LRH is administered during puberty. Thus, puberty and gonadal maturation are associated with stepwise maturation, first in the hypothalamus, then in the pituitary, and lastly in the gonad.

Clinical patterns of pubertal changes vary widely. In 95% of boys enlargement of the genitalia begins between 9½–13½ yr, reaching maturity from 13–17 yr. In a small minority of normal boys puberty begins after 15 yr of age. In 50% of boys pubic hair is present by 11 yr of age, and by 13–17½ yr it is equivalent in amount to that of normal adult females. In some boys pubertal development is completed in less than 2 yr, whereas in others it may take longer than 4½ yr. The adolescent growth spurt occurs later in boys than in girls at corresponding levels of sexual maturation; for example, the peak velocity of change in height is not attained in boys until the genitalia are well developed, whereas in girls the growth rate is usually at its maximum when the nipple and areola have developed but before there is any other significant breast development.

Maturation in Girls. The most important estrogens produced by the ovary are estradiol-17β (E_2) and estrone (E_1); estriol is a metabolic product of these 2, and all 3 estrogens may be found in the urine of mature females. Estrogens also arise from androgens, both in the adrenal and in the testis; the pathway for this conversion is shown in Fig 18–22. (This conversion explains why in certain types of male pseudohermaphroditism feminization occurs at puberty; in 17β-hydroxysteroid dehydrogenase deficiency, for example, the enzymatic block results in markedly increased secretion of androstenedione, which is converted in the peripheral tissues to estradiol and estrone; these estrogens, in addition to that directly secreted by the testis, result in normal breast development in XY hermaphrodites with testes.) The ovary also synthesizes progesterone, a progestational steroid; adrenal cortex and testis also synthesize progesterone as a precursor for other adrenal and testicular hormones.

Plasma levels of estradiol increase slowly but steadily with advancing sexual maturation and correlate well with clinical evaluation of pubertal development, skeletal age, and rising levels of FSH. Levels of LH do not rise until secondary sexual characteristics are well de-

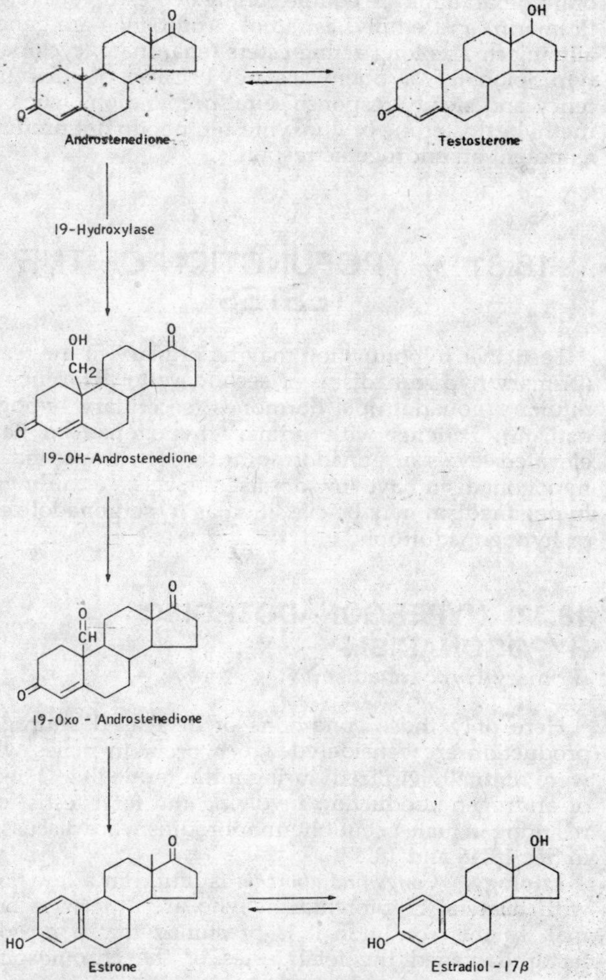

Figure 18–22 Conversion of androgens to estrogens.

veloped. Estrogens, like androgens, inhibit secretion of both LH and FSH (negative feedback). It now appears, however, that in females estrogens also provoke the surge of LH secretion which occurs in the midmenstrual cycle. The capacity for this positive feedback is another maturational milestone of puberty. The average age at menarche in American girls is 12½–13 yr, but the range of normal is wide, and 1–2% of normal girls have not menstruated by 16 yr of age. Menarche generally correlates closely with skeletal age.

Diagnostic Aids. Rapid advances in understanding the hypothalamic-pituitary-gonadal interactions involved with puberty and in the clinical diagnosis of aberrations of pubertal development have been made possible by markedly improved assays for FSH, LH, testosterone, and estradiol. These can be measured in small amounts of blood, and the burdensome collection of 24-hr specimens of urine for hormone assays has become less necessary. With LRH it is now also possible to differentiate between primary pituitary and hypothalamic defects in hypogonadotropic patients.

Therapeutic Aids. Naturally occurring estrogens administered orally are rapidly destroyed by gastrointestinal and liver enzymes; accordingly, they are usually given as conjugates or esters. The most widely used oral preparations are equine conjugated estrogens (e.g., Premarin) and ethinyl estradiol. Androgens are generally injected as long acting esters (enanthate, cyclopentylpropionate, or phenylacetate) because of their potency and steady response. Oral preparations, such as methyltestosterone or fluoxymesterone, do not produce as potent an androgenic response.

18.31 HYPOFUNCTION OF THE TESTES

Testicular hypofunction may be primary in the testis (primary hypogonadism) or secondary to deficiency of pituitary gonadotropic hormones (secondary hypogonadism). Patients with primary hypogonadism have elevated levels of gonadotropin; those with secondary hypogonadism have low or absent levels. Accordingly, hypogonadism may be classified as hypergonadotropic or hypogonadotropic.

18.32 HYPERGONADOTROPIC HYPOGONADISM
(Primary Hypogonadism)

Here only those conditions of decreased androgen production are considered which occur in males who were normally virilized during intrauterine life. Defects of androgen production involving the fetal testis and resulting in male pseudohermaphroditism are discussed in Sec 18.46 and 18.47.

Etiology. *Congenital anorchia* is found in a few boys with bilateral cryptorchidism who are otherwise normal. In this condition it is presumed that a noxious factor damaged the fetal testes of the chromosomal

male some time after sexual differentiation had taken place. When testicular function fails before the 7th–14th wk of fetal life, normal male somatic differentiation does not take place and an intersex results.

A syndrome of *rudimentary testes* has been described in which the testes are exceedingly small; it appears to be inherited as an autosomal or X-linked recessive trait. The etiology is unknown. *Atrophy* of the testes may follow damage to the vascular supply as a result of unskillful manipulation of the testes during surgical procedures for correction of cryptorchidism or as a result of bilateral torsion of the testes. *Acute orchitis* in pubertal or adult males with mumps may also damage the testes; usually, only the reproductive function of the testes is impaired. The routine immunization of all prepubertal males with mumps vaccine should prevent this complication.

The immunosuppressive drug *cyclophosphamide* can cause testicular damage in prepubertal boys, with elevated levels of FSH and LH and excessive responses to LRH. After puberty, oligo- and azoospermia may be present. Gonadal damage appears dose related prepubertally; smaller doses for shorter periods appear to spare gonadal function. Safe regimens of treatment are not yet defined, but it appears that a course of up to 3 mg/kg/24 hr for 8 wk is reasonably safe. Pubertal boys treated with MOPP combination chemotherapy frequently develop gynecomastia several yr later; levels of FSH and LH are elevated, and testicular biopsy reveals germinal aplasia. Most young boys treated with combination therapy for acute lymphoblastic leukemia have intact Leydig cell function and undergo normal pubertal development.

In *germinal cell aplasia (Del Castillo syndrome)* sexual maturation occurs normally, Leydig cells are normal, and testosterone secretion is normal. The testes are small, however, and the seminiferous tubules are small and devoid of germ cells. Azoospermia and infertility are the rule. The disorder has affected brothers, but the mode of transmission is not clear. FSH levels are elevated, LH levels normal. These findings support the current hypothesis that the germ cells produce a specific inhibitor of FSH.

The term hypogonadism has been widely used to describe aspects of children with a variety of syndromes of multiple malformations. It often refers simply to cryptorchidism, a small phallus, or a scrotal anomaly. For many of these syndromes little is known concerning the function of the testes; hyper- or hypogonadotropic hypogonadism has been proved in some instances.

Varying degrees of hypogonadism also occur in a significant percentage of patients with chromosomal aberrations such as Klinefelter syndrome or the XY Turner phenotype (see below).

Clinical Manifestations. The clinical manifestations of hypogonadism are noted only at puberty or subsequently. Secondary sex characters fail to develop. Facial, pubic, and axillary hair is scant or absent; there is neither acne nor regression of scalp hair, and the voice remains high pitched. The penis and scrotum remain infantile and may be almost obscured by pubic fat; the testes are small or absent. Fat accumulates in the region of the hips and buttocks and sometimes also in the breasts and on the abdomen. The epiphyses close late in life; therefore, extremities are long. The span is several inches longer than the height, and the measurement from the symphysis pubis to the soles of the feet is much greater than from the symphysis pubis to the vertex. This clinical state is also known as *eunuchism*, and the proportions of the body are described as "eunuchoid."

Diagnosis. Levels of serum FSH and, to a lesser extent, of LH are elevated above age-specific normal values. These elevated levels indicate that even in the prepubertal child there is an active hypothalamic-gonadal feedback relationship. After the age of 11 yr levels of FSH and LH rise significantly, reaching the postmenopausal range. Plasma testosterone levels are ordinarily low in normal prepubertal children, rising during puberty to attain adult levels. During puberty these levels correlate better with testicular size and stage of sexual maturation than with age. In patients with primary hypogonadism, testosterone levels remain low at all ages, and there is no rise following administration of human chorionic gonadotropin (hCG), whereas in normal males at any stage of development hCG produces a significant rise in plasma testosterone.

XY TURNER PHENOTYPE
(Noonan Syndrome)

The term "male Turner syndrome" has been applied to phenotypic males who have certain anomalies which also occur in females with Turner syndrome. These boys have normal karyotypes. Moreover, this syndrome also occurs in girls with normal karyotypes. Affected patients, both boys and girls, have been given various designations, including Turner phenotype with normal chromosomes, XY Turner phenotype (males), XX Turner phenotype (females), Ullrich-Turner syndrome, Ullrich syndrome, familial Turner phenotype, pseudo-Turner syndrome, male Turner syndrome, and Noonan syndrome.

The most common abnormalities are short stature, webbing of the neck, pectus carinatum or pectus excavatum, cubitum valgum, congenital heart disease, and a characteristic facies. Hypertelorism, epicanthus, an antimongoloid palpebral slant, ptosis, micrognathia, and ear abnormalities are common. Other abnormalities such as clinodactyly, hernias, and vertebral anomalies occur less frequently. The phenotype differs from true Turner syndrome in the following respects: (1) Mental retardation is much more common. (2) The cardiac defect is most often pulmonary valvular stenosis or atrial septal defect, whereas coarctation of the aorta is rare; the reverse is seen in true Turner syndrome. (3) Gonadal defects vary from severe deficiency to apparently normal sexual development. Males frequently have cryptorchidism and small testes; they may be hypogonadal or normal. Puberty may be normal or arrive late or never.

The cause is not known. Chromosomes appear normal. The disorder is usually sporadic, but affected siblings of the same and different sexes have been reported, with concordance noted in probably monozygotic twins. Partial expression of the syndrome is often present in 1st degree relatives. Male-to-male transmission has been reported, suggesting an autosomal dominant gene with variable expressivity.

KLINEFELTER SYNDROME

Etiology. Approximately 1/750 newborn males has a 47,XXY chromosome complement. Accordingly, Klinefelter syndrome is slightly more common than Down syndrome. The incidence approximates 1% among the mentally retarded, clustering among patients with IQs above 50 and among children admitted to psychiatric hospitals or referred to psychiatric clinics. The chromosomal aberration may result from meiotic nondisjunction of an X chromosome during parental gametogenesis or from mitotic nondisjunction in the zygote. Increased maternal age predisposes to meiotic nondisjunction and to this syndrome, but in most instances maternal age is not advanced.

The 47,XXY complement is the most common chromosomal pattern in persons with Klinefelter syndrome; some have mosaic patterns: 46,XY/47,XXY; 46,XY/48,XXYY; 45,X/46,XY/47,XXY; or 46,XX/47,XXY. Rarely, occurrence of more than 2 X chromosomes may result in Klinefelter variants: 48,XXXY; 49,XXXYY; 49,XXXXY; 50,XXXXYY; 47,XXY/48,XXXY; 47,XXY/49,XXXXY; or 48,XXYY karyotypes. It is noteworthy than even with as many as 4 X chromosomes, the Y chromosome determines a male phenotype.

Clinical Manifestations. The diagnosis is rarely made prior to puberty because of the paucity or subtleness of clinical manifestations in childhood. Since behavioral or psychiatric disorders may often be apparent long before defects in sexual development, the condition should be considered in all boys with mental retardation as well as in children with psychosocial, learning, or school adjustment problems. Affected children may be anxious, immature, excessively shy, or aggressive; they may engage in antisocial acts. Problems often first become apparent after the child begins school. The patients tend to be tall, slim, and underweight and to have relatively long legs; but body habitus can vary markedly. The testes tend to be small for age, but this sign may become substantially apparent only after puberty, when normal testicular growth fails to occur. The phallus tends to be smaller than average, and cryptorchidism and/or hypospadias may occur in a few patients.

Pubertal development may be delayed. Some degree of androgen deficiency is usually noted, though some patients may undergo almost normal masculinization. About 40% of adults have gynecomastia; they have sparser facial hair, most shaving less than daily. Azoospermia and infertility are usual, though rare instances of fertility are known. Height tends to be increased. There is an increased frequency of antisocial behavior and delinquency. There is also an increased incidence of pulmonary disease, varicose veins, and cancer of the breast.

In a prospective study a group of children with 47,XXY karyotypes identified at birth exhibited relatively mild deviations from normal during the 1st 5 yr of life. None had major physical, intellectual, or emotional disabilities; some were inactive, with poorly organized motor function and mild delay in language acquistion. Whether more serious impairments will develop later in these children is unknown.

In adults with *XY/XXY mosaicism* the features of Klinefelter syndrome are decreased in severity and frequency. Little is known of children with mosaicism, but they may have a better prognosis for virilization, fertility, and psychosocial adjustment. The *XXYY male* phenotype is not distinctively different from that of the XXY patient except that XXYY adults tend to be taller than the average XXY patient.

Klinefelter Variants. When the number of X chromosomes exceeds 2, the clinical manifestations, including the mental retardation and the impairment of virilization, are more severe. The rare *49,XXXXY variant* is sufficiently distinctive to be detected in childhood. Affected patients are severely retarded, and many have large malformed ears, a short neck, and a typical facies with wide-set eyes which have a mild mongoloid slant; epicanthus, strabismus, a wide, flat upturned nose, and a large open mouth may also be present. The testes are small and may be undescended, the scrotum is hypoplastic, and the penis is very small. Defects suggestive of Down syndrome (such as short incurved terminal 5th phalanges, single palmar creases, and hypotonia) and other skeletal abnormalities (including defects in the carrying angle of the elbows and restricted supination) are common. The most frequent radiographic abnormalities are radioulnar synostosis or dislocation, elongated radius, pseudoepiphyses, scoliosis or kyphosis, coxa valga, and retarded osseous age. Most patients with such extensive changes have a 49,XXXXY chromosome karyotype; the following mosaic patterns have also been observed: 48,XXXY/49,XXXXY; 48,XXXY/49,XXXXY/50,XXXXXY; and 48,XXXY/49,XXXXY/50XXXXYY (Fig 18–23).

Laboratory Data. Buccal smears should be examined in all patients suspected of Klinefelter syndrome, particularly those attending child guidance, psychiatric, and mental retardation clinics; the number of X chromosomes can be deduced from the number of sex-chromatin bodies. All chromatin-positive boys should have complete study of chromosomes so that mosaics such as XY/XXY and patients with the XXYY constitution may be identified.

Gonadotropin levels are usually elevated by the time of puberty, but they may be normal, depending upon the amount of testicular androgen produced. Plasma testosterone levels in men with Klinefelter syndrome are low or low normal.

Testicular biopsy before puberty may reveal only a deficiency or absence of germinal cells. After puberty the seminiferous tubular membranes are hyalinized, and there is adenomatous clumping of Leydig cells. Azoospermia is characteristic; only rarely is spermatogenesis sufficient to permit fertility.

Treatment. Replacement therapy with long-acting testosterone preparation should begin at 11–12 yr of age. The cyclopentylpropionate ester may be used in a starting dose of 50 mg injected intramuscularly every 3 wk with 50 mg increments every 6–9 mo until a maintenance dose for adults (250 mg every 3 wk) is achieved.

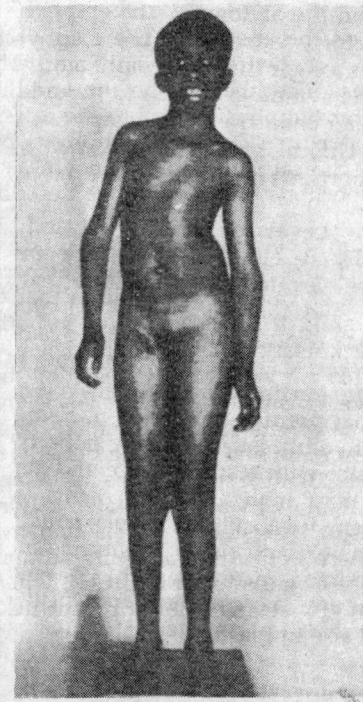

Figure 18–23 A 12 yr old boy with 48,XXXY/49,XXXXY mosaicism, who has prognathism, epicanthal folds, scoliosis, very small testes, severe mental retardation, clinodactyly, and radioulnar synostoses.

For older boys larger initial doses and increments can achieve more rapid virilization.

XX MALES

Approximately 50 males with 46,XX chromosome constitution have been identified. They have a male phenotype, small testes, a small phallus, and no evidence of ovarian or müllerian duct tissue; they appear, therefore, to be distinct from the XX true hermaphrodite (below). They are suspected of having occult Y chromosomal material; all patients examined thus far have been H-Y antigen positive. This disorder resembles Klinefelter syndrome, but stature is greater in the latter. The histologic features of the testes are essentially the same in the 2 conditions. Only about 20% of reported patients have been prepubertal, the condition usually coming to medical attention in adult life because of hypogonadism or gynecomastia. About 50% of those detected as children have had hypospadias and/or chordee. Hypergonadotropic hypogonadism occurs secondary to testicular failure.

The same explanations have been proposed for these findings as for 46,XX true hermaphroditism. The 1st possibility is undetected mosaicism; indeed, in some otherwise XX males who appear not to have mosaicism, it has been theorized that male-determining genes have been translocated from Y chromosomes to X chromosomes or autosomes. Male-determining genes are located on the pericentric region of the short arm of the Y chromosome and would not be expected to show fluorescence with quinacrine. Studies of the Xg blood group in some families have suggested such X-Y interchanges. Finally, autosomal inheritance of a male-determining gene has been proposed; the finding of this rare syndrome in 2nd cousins suggests such a gene effect. The disorder may be heterogeneous.

XYY MALES

The 47,XYY male does not have hypogonadism; his condition is discussed here for easy comparison with the XXY and the XX male syndromes.

Approximately 1/1000 newborn males have an XYY chromosome pattern. Thus far, in a small number of children detected at birth as part of routine screening programs and followed prospectively, no abnormal physical, intellectual, or behavioral characteristics have been detected except for a tendency to tall stature. When this disorder was first discovered in adults, studies of XYY individuals in mental or penal institutions created a stereotype of affected individuals as having deviant behavior marked by physical aggressiveness and violence. It now appears that the rate at which XYY males are found in mental or penal settings may be as high as 20 times the rate at which they are born, but studies not biased by behavioral ascertainment do not show deviant behavior to be a prominent feature. Recent studies indicate that adults with this karyotype may be relatively impulsive, antisocial, and apt to break the law, but they are not especially aggressive.

The XYY adult has few phenotypic manifestations. He tends to be tall and to have severe nodulocystic acne. Dermatoglyphics do not differ significantly from XY males. In affected persons genital abnormalities have been noted, but cryptic mosaicism, such as X/XYY, is a possibility in these instances. Prolonged P-R intervals on electrocardiography and radioulnar synostosis appear to occur more often than in the general population. No clear-cut endocrine abnormalities have been found. It is not certain why XYY individuals are more apt to be found in mental or penal institutions though it is possible that an abnormality of neural development due to the XYY genotype favors deviant behavior in some persons. The nature and extent of such an association are yet to be determined. This condition poses a serious dilemma for counseling of parents of infants or children discovered to have this sex chromosome complement. The risks for behavioral disability may not be trivial; neither do they appear as dire as earlier thought.

18.33 HYPOGONADOTROPIC HYPOGONADISM
(Secondary Hypogonadism)

In hypogonadotropic hypogonadism there is deficiency of follicle-stimulating hormone (FSH) and/or of luteinizing hormone (LH). The primary defect may lie in the anterior pituitary or in the hypothalamus as a deficiency of gonadotropin-releasing hormone (LRH). The testes are normal but remain in the prepubertal state because stimulation by gonadotropins is lacking.

The classification of these disorders is in active evolution.

Etiology. *Hypopituitarism.* Patients with deficiency of growth hormone frequently have associated deficiency of 1 or more of the other pituitary hormones. The most frequently associated deficiency is that of gonadotropin. In patients with organic lesions in or near the pituitary (e.g., craniopharyngiomas), the gonadotropin deficiency is pituitary in origin. On the other hand, in many patients with "idiopathic" or "familial" hypopituitarism, it now appears that the defect lies in the hypothalamus; administration of LRH to these patients indicates that the pituitary is capable of response. In some patients in whom the rise of FSH and LH in response to acute administration of LRH has been impaired or absent, more intensive stimulation produced a response. These findings suggest that the pituitary cells responsible for gonadotropin production can release hormone into the circulation if appropriately stimulated.

Isolated Deficiency of Gonadotropin. When deficiency of gonadotropin occurs as an isolated deficiency, the defect usually involves the hypothalamus rather than the pituitary. Persons with *Kallmann syndrome* (hypogonadotropic hypogonadism with anosmia) fail to develop sexually or exhibit only minimal development at puberty. Inability to smell is present from early childhood, but it is usually not discovered except on direct questioning. Both FSH and LH remain at prepubertal levels in adult life. Agenesis of the olfactory lobes of the brain accounts for the anosmia. No histologic lesion has been defined, but a hypothalamic defect is the cause for the gonadotropin deficiency inasmuch as administration of LRH to affected patients produces increases in FSH and LH.

Other somatic defects observed in some patients with Kallmann syndrome include cryptorchidism, choanal abnormalities, and renal abnormalities. Familial occurrences have suggested X-linked transmission, but male-to-male transmission has been observed, and an autosomal dominant defect is now thought likely. The expression is variable; some kindreds contain anosmic individuals without, as well as others with, hypogonadism; other kindreds contain individuals with only harelip or cleft palate or with only hypogonadism or anosmia. The incidence of hyposmia in affected families is not known; more males than females have been recognized with the syndrome. Genetic heterogeneity is possible. Spermatogenesis can be induced by treatment with human menopausal gonadotropins (hMG).

Isolated deficiency of LH has been observed in patients with the *fertile eunuch syndrome.* Failure of the Leydig cells to mature at puberty is accompanied by delayed pubertal development. The testes may be normal in size, however, and spermatogenesis may occur. A good response to administration of chorionic gonadotropin reveals the presence of normal Leydig cell precursors. Serum and urine FSH concentrations are normal, whereas those of LH are undetectable or low. An increase in LH levels follows administration of LRH, indicating a hypothalamic defect. Fertility has occasionally been noted, but evidence suggests that testicular androgen is necessary for completely normal spermatogenesis. This rare syndrome has been observed in brothers and in association with Kallmann syndrome.

Biologically inactive LH has been demonstrated in 1 hypogonadal male born of a consanguineous union who had immunologically active LH of normal molecular weight. The defect may reside in the primary structure of the molecule.

Other Syndromes. Some syndromes of hypogonadism with gonadotropin deficiency have not yet been evaluated by up-to-date techniques, and the sites of their defects are unknown. In the recessively inherited *Laurence-Moon-Biedl syndrome* hypogonadism occurs in both males and females, but its incidence is unknown. On occasion, the hypogonadism is primary, but there is usually hypothalamic-pituitary dysfunction. Several syndromes of ataxia and hypogonadotropic hypogonadism appear to have distinctive genetic origins. Ichthyosis and male hypogonadism has been described in several families. In 10 males in 4 generations of 1 kindred, hypogonadotropic hypogonadism and ichthyosis were associated with anosmia and mild mental retardation. In the *multiple lentigines syndrome*, an autosomal dominant disorder, delayed puberty occurs in about 25% of affected patients. An 18 yr old male with this syndrome and delayed puberty had deficiency of FSH and LH and anosmia, suggesting a hypothalamic defect. The *Prader-Willi syndrome* presents variable hypogonadotropic hypogonadism as well as hypergonadotropic hypogonadism. We have observed hypogonadotropic hypogonadism in *Carpenter syndrome* and in *Lowe syndrome.*

Diagnosis. Physiologic delay of puberty is extremely difficult to differentiate from hypogonadotropic hypogonadism since in both conditions gonadotropin levels remain low after the usual age of puberty. The diagnosis should always be considered if puberty is delayed beyond 16–17 yr of age. The detection of other pituitary deficits, the discovery of anosmia by careful questioning, and the history of hypogonadism in other family members are important clues. Plasma levels of LH and of testosterone during sleep may identify boys with delayed puberty who are on the verge of spontaneous puberty inasmuch as augmentation of LH secretion during sleep has its onset in early puberty. In hypogonadotropic hypogonadism there is no sleep-associated rise in LH secretion. Though they may have blunted gonadotropin responses to LRH during the prepubertal years, most children (76–90%) with isolated growth hormone deficiency undergo normal puberty. Accordingly, the response to LRH is not a reliable prepubertal indicator of gonadotropin status in children with isolated growth hormone deficiency. In the hypopituitary patient absent or delayed adrenarche, as compared with bone age, usually indicates gonadotropin deficiency. Children with ACTH deficiency are also usually deficient in gonadotropins.

Treatment. Administration of chorionic gonadotropin induces satisfactory development of secondary sex characters by stimulating the Leydig cells. The recommended dose is 4000–5000 IU 3 times weekly for 6 wk. After discontinuation of therapy a period of observation for evidence of regression is necessary to establish the diagnosis. If puberty regresses, the patient probably has hypogonadotropic hypogonadism, whereas if puberty continues, the patient has had physiologic delay of maturation. Several such courses may be necessary to exclude the diagnosis of physiologic delayed adolescence. When the diagnosis of secondary hypogonadism is established, maintenance therapy with androgen is initiated.

18.34 PSEUDOPRECOCITY RESULTING FROM TUMORS OF THE TESTES

Functional tumors of the testis are rare causes of sexual pseudoprecocity. Such tumors arise from the Leydig cells, which are sparse before puberty. Tumors derived from them are more common in the adult; about 50 cases in children have been reported, including 1 member in each of 2 pairs of identical twins. Leydig cell tumors are usually benign.

The clinical manifestations are those of puberty in the male; onset occurs usually from 4–6 yr of age. Gynecomastia has occurred in 5 patients. The tumor of the testis can usually be readily felt; the contralateral unaffected testis is normal in size for the age of the patient.

Urinary 17-ketosteroids are only slightly or moderately increased, but testosterone levels are markedly elevated. FSH and LH levels are suppressed. Treatment consists of surgical removal of the affected testis. Progression of virilization ceases, and partial reversal of the signs of precocity may occur.

There are few other causes of testicular enlargement to be considered in the differential diagnosis. Leydig cell hyperplasia of unknown etiology has been reported as the cause of early onset and rapidly progressive sexual precocity in 2 young brothers. Enlargement of the testes, hyperplasia of the Leydig cells, elevation of testosterone levels, and low serum levels of immunoreactive and bioactive gonadotropins characterize the syndrome. Rarely, in untreated congenital adrenal hyperplasia, the testes will contain ectopic adrenal cortical cells, which give rise to bilateral testicular enlargement; treatment with corticosteroids suppresses adrenocortical activity, and they return to normal size. Occasionally, boys with inadequately treated congenital adrenal hyperplasia develop bilateral testicular tumors which are not suppressed by corticosteroids; these are thought to arise from hilar cells or adrenal rest tissue. In boys with unilateral cryptorchidism, the contralateral testis is about 25% larger than normal for age. The enlargement of the testes which occurs in boys with true precocious puberty is bilateral and symmetrical.

The association of marked enlargement of the testes (macro-orchidism) with mental retardation occurs in the *fragile X syndrome,* in which, after puberty, the testicular size reaches 30–40 ml. The penis is normal in size, and there is no evidence of precocious puberty. Hormonal studies and testicular histology are normal. Many of those patients with macro-orchidism have a fragile site at the terminus of the long arm of the X chromosome (Xq 27 fra). The relationship between chromosomal abnormality and clinical disorder is not understood, but the fragile X serves as a useful marker to study affected families. The identification of affected boys is important to genetic counseling in families where macro-orchidism is associated with X-linked mental retardation.

18.35 GYNECOMASTIA

Gynecomastia, or the occurrence of mammary tissue in the male, is a common condition. It occurs in most newborn males as a result of stimulation by maternal hormones. The effect disappears in a few wk.

During pubertal development approximately two thirds of boys develop varying degrees of subareolar hyperplasia of the breasts. *Physiologic pubertal gynecomastia* may involve only 1 breast, and it is not unusual for both breasts to enlarge at disproportionate rates or at different times. Tenderness of the breast is common but transitory. Spontaneous regression may occur within a few mo; it rarely persists longer than 2 yr. Mean concentrations of FSH, LH, prolactin, testosterone, estrone, and estradiol are the same as in boys without gynecomastia. When, however, levels are correlated with stage of puberty, a decreased ratio of testosterone to estradiol is found in boys with gynecomastia. Treatment usually consists of reassurance of the boy and his family of the physiologic and transient nature of the phenomenon. Surgical removal of the breast is rarely indicated; when enlargement is striking and persistent and causes serious emotional disturbance to the patient, removal may be justified. *Pubertal macromastia* designates female breast development (to Tanner stages 3–5) in boys which does not abate spontaneously. Histology is that of chronic idiopathic gynecomastia. Plasma levels of gonadotropins, prolactin, sex steroids, and steroid binding globulins are normal. In several kindreds gynecomastia has occurred in many males without apparent endocrinopathy. Such *familial gynecomastia* is probably inherited as a male-limited autosomal dominant trait.

In young children with gynecomastia an exogenous source of estrogens must be sought. Either accidental or therapeutic exposure to small amounts of estrogens by inhalation, percutaneous absorption, or ingestion may cause gynecomastia. Increased pigmentation of the nipple and areola should suggest this cause. Gynecomastia may also be caused by exogenously administered androgens.

A number of other pathologic conditions may cause gynecomastia. It has been noted in a 1 yr old child with the 11β-hydroxylase–deficient form of congenital virilizing adrenal hyperplasia, probably due to excessive adrenal production of estrogens. It may be associated with Leydig cell tumors of the testis or with feminizing tumors of the adrenal. A young boy with the *Peutz-Jeghers syndrome* and gynecomastia had a *sex-cord tumor with annular tubules* of the testes. Gynecomastia occurs in Klinefelter syndrome and with other types of testicular failure (hypergonadotropic states). It is a common finding in certain types of male pseudohermaphroditism, particularly in Reifenstein syndrome, in the testicular feminization syndrome, and in patients with the 17β-hydroxysteroid dehydrogenase defect. When gynecomastia is associated with galactorrhea, a prolactinoma

should be considered. In adults gynecomastia occurs with liver cirrhosis, with digitalis therapy for congestive heart failure, with bronchogenic carcinoma, with administration of various nonsteroidal therapeutic agents, and with heavy marijuana smoking. Ketoconazole, a new antifungal drug, causes gynecomastia by direct inhibition of testosterone synthesis.

18.36 HYPOFUNCTION OF THE OVARIES

Hypofunction of the ovaries may be due to congenital failure of development or to postnatal destruction (primary or hypergonadotropic hypogonadism) or to lack of stimulation by the pituitary (secondary or hypogonadotropic hypogonadism). Many chronic diseases may result in the latter type.

18.37 HYPERGONADOTROPIC HYPOGONADISM
(Primary Hypogonadism)

Diagnosis of hypergonadotropic hypogonadism prior to puberty is possible. Except in the case of Turner syndrome, most of the affected patients have no prepubertal clinical manifestations.

TURNER SYNDROME
(Gonadal Dysgenesis)

In 1938 Turner described a syndrome consisting of sexual infantilism, webbed neck, and cubitum valgum in adult females. It was found that such women have elevated levels of urinary gonadotropins and that the gonads consist of rudimentary elongated streaks containing no germinal elements but consisting of whorls of connective tissue suggestive of ovarian stroma.

Pathogenesis. In 1959 it was demonstrated that patients with Turner syndrome have a single X chromosome; they have a 45,X chromosome constitution. The X chromosome is more often maternal than paternal, but in contrast to Klinefelter syndrome, the occurrence of Turner syndrome is not influenced by maternal age. Most cases probably arise from nondisjunction or anaphase lag in the zygote. A large prospective study found a seasonal pattern, two thirds of births with nondisjunction occurring between May and October.

The 45,X disorder occurs in about 1/3000 live born females and is much less common than Klinefelter syndrome. It appears that over 95% of all 45,X conceptions are aborted; 5–10% of all abortuses are 45,X. Mosaicism (46,XX/45,X) among patients with Turner syndrome is 25%, a proportion higher than with any other aneuploid state, whereas the mosaic Turner constitution is rare among the abortuses; these findings indicate preferential survival for mosaic forms.

Other types of mosaics, such as isochromosome for

the long arm, deletion of the short arm, and rings of the X chromosome, are less common.

Primordial germ cells are found in the gonadal ridges of aborted 45,X fetuses up to 3 mo of gestation but disappear thereafter. In the normal fetus the number of germ cells declines rapidly at about 5 mo of gestation and then decreases at a slower rate after birth. In the 45,X patient this normal process may be hastened and exaggerated. The streak gonads usually consist of only connective tissue; rarely, a few germ cells may be found to explain partial sexual maturation.

Clinical Manifestations. In the past the diagnosis was generally first suspected in childhood or at puberty when sexual maturation failed to occur. It is now clear that most 45,X patients are recognizable at birth because a characteristic edema of the dorsum of the hands and feet and loose skin folds at the nape are present. Significantly low birth weight and short stature are common. Clinical manifestations in childhood include webbing of the neck, a low posterior hairline, small mandible, prominent ears, epicanthic folds, high arched palate, a broad chest presenting the illusion of widely spaced nipples, cubitum valgum, and hyperconvex fingernails. Stature is almost always below the 3rd percentile; an adult height of more than 147 cm (58 in) is rare. With increasing age, pigmented nevi become more prominent. At the expected age sexual maturation fails to occur.

Associated defects are common. Coarctation of the aorta is the most frequent cardiovascular lesion, but hypertension of unknown etiology and other congenital heart defects may occur. A dissecting aortic aneurysm is a rare complication. Approximately half the patients have abnormal urograms, horseshoe kidney and malrotation being the most common anomalies. Hearing and cognitive problems are more common than in the general population.

Goiter should suggest lymphocytic thyroiditis; abdominal pain, tenesmus, or bloody diarrhea may represent inflammatory bowel disease; and recurrent gastrointestinal bleeding may indicate gastrointestinal telangiectasia. Patients with Turner syndrome have a higher than expected incidence of these conditions.

In the 45,X/46,XX *mosaic* the abnormalities are attenuated and fewer. The affected newborn usually has no recognizable findings. Webbing of the neck, coarctation of the aorta, and edema of hands and feet are infrequent. Short stature is almost as frequent as in the 45,X patient and may be the only manifestation (Fig 18–24).

Sexual maturation fails to occur in both the 45,X and 45,X/46,XX patients; occasional patients with some degree of breast development or even menstruation are likely to be 45,X/46,XX mosaics. Fertility has been reported in occasional 45,X patients in whom mosaicism was not detected in the tissues examined.

Laboratory Data. Chromosomal analysis should be done in all suspected patients. The sex-chromatin pattern is usually negative, but patients with 45,X/46,XX mosaicism or with abnormal X chromosomes could be overlooked. Unusually large sex-chromatin bodies are seen in patients with isochromosomes of the X chromosome; smaller than normal sex-chromatin bodies suggest a deletion in 1 of the X chromosomes.

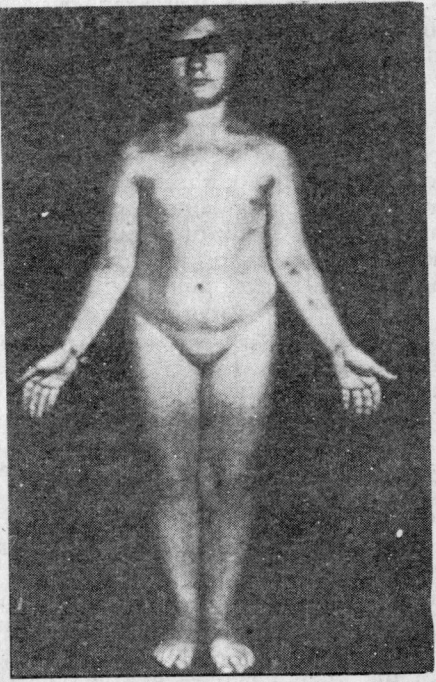

Figure 18–24 Turner syndrome in a 15 yr old girl exhibiting failure of sexual maturation, short stature, cubitus valgus, and a goiter. There is no webbing of the neck. Karyotype revealed 45,X/46,XX chromosome complement, and urinary gonadotropin was over 96 mouse units/24 hr. T_4 was 2.2 µg/dl. Biopsy of the thyroid revealed lymphocytic thyroiditis.

Plasma levels of gonadotropins, particularly of FSH, are usually elevated above those of age-matched controls, even in infancy. In prepubertal children occasional levels of FSH may not be clearly abnormal because of the overlap with the range of normal values. After 10 yr of age plasma levels are markedly elevated and approximate menopausal levels. At puberty the pulsatile release of FSH and LH probably accounts for day-to-day variability in plasma levels. Urinary gonadotropins are clearly elevated after 10–12 yr of age but are less helpful in prepubertal children. Urinary excretion of estrogens and plasma levels of estradiol are very low. Growth hormone secretion in response to provocative stimuli is normal.

Roentgenographic studies may reveal cardiovascular or renal abnormalities. The most common skeletal abnormalities are shortening of the 4th metatarsal and metacarpal bones, epiphyseal dysgenesis in the joints of the knee and elbow, inadequate osseous mineralization, scoliosis, and spina bifida occulta.

A high percentage of patients and other family members have significant titers of antithyroid antibodies. Mild chemical diabetes is present in about one third of patients.

Treatment. Replacement therapy with estrogens to initiate and sustain sexual maturation may be deferred until age 13–15 yr in order to avoid early closure of the epiphyses. An oral estrogen is administered daily for 6 mo or until menstrual bleeding occurs. Thereafter, cyclic estrogen-progestogen therapy may be given in the form of 1 of the · sequential contraceptive regimens.

Diethylstilbestrol is contraindicated since it is suspected of provoking endometrial carcinoma in these patients.

XX GONADAL DYSGENESIS

Some phenotypically normal females have gonadal lesions identical to those in 45,X patients but without somatic features of Turner syndrome; their condition is termed "pure gonadal dysgenesis." Some with a 46,XY karyotype are also designated as having the Swyer syndrome, which is discussed below, with male pseudohermaphroditism. Here we discuss only those with the XX chromosome constitution. These 2 conditions are quite distinct entities; in no instance have XX and XY gonadal dysgenesis been reported in the same family.

The disorder is rarely recognized in children because the external genitalia are normal, no other abnormalities are visible, and growth is normal. At pubertal age sexual maturation fails to take place. Plasma gonadotropin levels are elevated. Delay of epiphyseal fusion results in a eunuchoid habitus.

Affected siblings, parental consanguinity, and failure to uncover mosaicism (even in the streak gonads) all point to autosomal recessive inheritance. It appears that autosomal genes have an important role in the differentiation of normal ovaries. In 5 families XX gonadal dysgenesis has been associated with sensorineural deafness; therefore there may be distinct genetic forms of this disorder. Tumors of the gonads have not been reported in these patients. Treatment consists of replacement therapy with estrogens.

MIXED GONADAL DYSGENESIS

Patients with this condition may be considered as part of a spectrum between 45,X females and 46,XY males. All patients are chromatin negative, the majority being 45,X/46,XY mosaics, with varying proportions of each cell line in different individuals. In instances where only XY or X cell lines have been found it is suspected that mosaicism may have gone undetected. The cytogenetic defect probably occurs early in embryogenesis.

The phenotype is rather characteristic and can be related to the mixture of X and XY cell lines. The presence of some cells with a Y chromosome always results in some virilization; on occasion, the phenotype may be male, but in most instances the genitalia are ambiguous, with a unilateral testis. A vagina and an infantile uterus are present, and there are usually bilateral fallopian tubes though there may be only 1. A streak gonad is usually present on the side contralateral to the testis. The streak gonad differs somewhat from that in Turner syndrome; in addition to wavy connective tissue there are often tubular or cord-like structures, occasional clumps of granulosa cells, and frequently mesonephric or hilus cells. Somatic signs of Turner syndrome are commonly present.

Puberty occurs at the normal time, with virilization; growth of the phallus may be striking. Adult height is greater than in Turner syndrome, particularly if none of the stigmata of Turner syndrome are present. A delay in maturation of the fetal testis might explain the discrepancy between failure of complete genital masculinization during fetal life, with persistence of müllerian ducts, and normal Leydig cell function at puberty.

Gonadal tumors, particularly gonadoblastomas, are reported to have increased frequency in patients with mixed gonadal dysgenesis. Analysis of cases with tumors reveals that these patients are often less virilized at birth, are more apt to have normal stature, undergo little or no virilization at puberty, and are the only ones with breast development. In addition, most of them have a 46,XX karyotype and fewer stigmata of Turner syndrome. These observations suggest that many of the reports of patients with mixed gonadal dysgenesis and tumor are more akin to pure 46,XY gonadal dysgenesis; the true incidence of tumors in patients with mixed gonadal dysgenesis may not be so high as formerly thought.

XX TURNER PHENOTYPE
(Noonan Syndrome)

Girls with a phenotype resembling that of Turner syndrome but with normal sex chromosomes constitute a separate entity which is described above, with XY Turner phenotype (Sec 18.31).

OTHER OVARIAN DEFECTS

An increasing number of other young women with no chromosomal abnormality are being found to have "streak" gonads which may contain only occasional germ cells, if any. Gonadotropins are increased. *Cytotoxic drugs* and exposure of the ovaries to radiation for the treatment of malignancy are increasingly frequent causes of ovarian failure. A study of young women with Hodgkin disease found that combination chemotherapy and pelvic irradiation may be more deleterious than either therapy alone. Teenagers are more apt than older women to retain or have recovery of ovarian function after either irradiation or combined chemotherapy; normal pregnancies have occurred after such treatment. Further experience is required to determine the long range effects of current treatment regimens on ovarian function.

Autoimmune ovarian disease occurs predominantly in association with Addison disease. Affected girls may not develop sexually, or secondary amenorrhea may occur in young women. The ovaries may have lymphocytic infiltration or appear simply as streaks. The majority of affected patients have circulating steroid cell antibodies.

Galactosemia may cause ovarian failure, with primary or secondary amenorrhea the presenting clinical manifestation. Elevated levels of FSH and LH, even early in life, reflect early ovarian failure. Antiovarian antibodies are not found. Ovarian failure may begin during intrauterine life since it has occurred even in girls treated with a galactose-free diet from birth. Women known to be heterozygous for galactosemia should follow a galactose-free diet during pregnancy.

Ataxia-telangiectasia may be associated with ovarian hypoplasia and elevated gonadotropins; the cause is not known, but it appears to be an integral part of the syndrome.

18.38   HYPOGONADOTROPIC HYPOGONADISM
(Secondary Hypogonadism)

Hypofunction of the ovaries can result from failure to secrete normal levels of gonadotropins. The defect may lie in the anterior pituitary, but as in the male, there is increasing evidence for a hypothalamic defect in many such hypogonadal females.

Etiology. *Hypopituitarism.* Destructive lesions in or near the pituitary almost always result in impaired secretion of gonadotropins as well as of other pituitary hormones. In patients with idiopathic hypopituitarism, however, the defect is most often found in the hypothalamus. In these patients administration of LRH results in increased plasma levels of FSH and LH, and administration of TRH provokes a rise in plasma level of TSH, establishing the integrity of the pituitary gland.

Isolated Deficiency of Gonadotropins. This heterogeneous group of disorders is only now being sorted out with the help of LRH. Isolated pituitary deficiency of FSH has been documented, but in most patients the pituitary is normal, the defect residing in the hypothalamus.

Several sporadic instances of anosmia with hypogonadotropic hypogonadism have been reported. Anosmic hypogonadal females have also been reported in kindreds with Kallmann syndrome, but hypogonadism more frequently affects the males in these families.

Some autosomal recessive disorders such as the Laurence-Moon-Biedl, multiple lentigines, and Carpenter syndromes also appear in some instances to include gonadotropic hormone deficiency.

Diagnosis. The diagnosis is not difficult in patients with other deficiencies of pituitary tropic hormones. On the other hand, it is difficult to differentiate isolated hypogonadotropic hypogonadism from physiologic delay of puberty. Repeated measurements of FSH and LH, particularly during sleep, may reveal rising levels which herald the onset of puberty.

18.39   POLYCYSTIC OVARIES
(Stein-Leventhal Syndrome)

This syndrome is characterized by amenorrhea, hirsutism, obesity, and sterility. Enlarged ovaries are covered by a condensation of collagen resembling a "thickened capsule." Beneath this layer the ovaries are studded with atretic follicles. This disorder accounts for many more instances of virilism than do ovarian tumors. The disorder commonly begins at puberty or shortly thereafter; it should be considered in adolescent girls with menstrual irregularities and hirsutism. In married women the most frequent complaint is infertility; anovulation is the sine qua non of diagnosis. The enlarged ovaries can often be felt on combined rectal and abdominal palpation.

The cause of the disorder is unsettled. Deficiency of secretion of FSH and abnormal follicular maturation are thought to be central to pathogenesis. Basal levels of LH in plasma are moderately elevated during the follicular phase of the cycle; levels of FSH are consistently depressed. That the elevated level of LH can be suppressed by estradiol indicates a normal negative feedback mechanism. The secretion of estradiol is decreased, whereas rates of production of testosterone and androstenedione are significantly elevated. The increase in ovarian androgens is presumed to result from the elevated levels of LH.

Late onset congenital virilizing adrenal hyperplasia may mimic polycystic ovarian disease. Basal levels of 17-hydroxyprogesterone may be normal, and an ACTH stimulation test may be required to reveal the defect.

Bilateral wedge resections of the ovaries result in normal ovulatory menstrual cycles in 70–80% of patients, in some way relieving the suppression of FSH and restoring normal follicular maturation. Success of this therapy is often of short duration; accordingly, surgery may be deferred until the patient wishes to become pregnant. For young girls therapy with clomiphene citrate is probably preferable.

18.40   SEX CHROMOSOME ABNORMALITIES WITHOUT GONADAL DEFECTS

Some sex chromosomal abnormalities have been uncovered which are not associated with defects in the gonads. These are of concern to the pediatrician primarily because mental retardation may be associated.

XXX Females. The 47,XXX chromosomal constitution is the most frequent X chromosomal abnormality in females, occurring in almost 1/1000 live born females. Affected infants are not usually recognized but frequently have minor anomalies, particularly clinodactyly, epicanthal folds, and wide-set eyes. As with 47,XYY males, little is known of the natural history of this condition since large numbers of affected persons have only recently been discovered in screening studies of the newborn. Ascertainment of XXX females has been biased, most patients having been found in studies of the mentally retarded in institutions. Affected adult women have been found, however, who are completely normal, even in respect to fertility. Among 9 triple-X girls identified at birth, only 1 was clearly retarded at 1 yr of age. Further follow-up of such patients is required to determine the full spectrum of the syndrome.

XXXX and XXXXX Females. About 17 females with 4 X and 6 with 5 X chromosomes have been described. All have been mentally retarded except for 1 of the 48,XXXX girls. Commonly associated defects are epicanthal folds, hypertelorism, clinodactyly, simian crease, radioulnar synostosis, and congenital heart disease.

18.41   PSEUDOPRECOCITY DUE TO LESIONS OF THE OVARY

Most of the functioning lesions of the ovary in children are neoplasms. The majority synthesize estrogens; a few synthesize androgens. Infrequently, a lesion produces both estrogens and androgens, or the same lesion may produce estrogenic manifestations in 1 patient and androgenic in another; for example, the rare androblastoma of the ovary has caused isosexual precocity in some girls, masculinization in others. (See also Sec 15.19.)

18.42 ESTROGENIC LESIONS OF THE OVARY

These lesions cause isosexual precocious sexual development but account for only a small percentage of all instances of precocity.

GRANULOSA-THECA CELL TUMOR

In childhood the most common neoplasm of the ovary with estrogenic manifestations is the granulosa-theca cell tumor. These tumors have varying proportions of granulosa and theca cells; in childhood the granulosa cell is dominant, and only very rare tumors consist almost completely of theca cells (thecoma). Though their morphology varies, these tumors produce similar clinical manifestations through their synthesis of estrogen.

Clinical Manifestations. The tumor has been observed in a newborn infant, but clinical manifestations usually do not appear until after 2 yr of age. The breasts become enlarged, rounded, and firm and the nipples prominent. The external genitalia resemble those of a normal girl at puberty, and the uterus is enlarged. A white vaginal discharge is followed by irregular or cyclic menstruation. Ovulation, however, does not occur; the sexual development is of the pseudoprecocious variety. Pubic hair is usually absent unless there is mild virilization.

A mass is readily palpable in the lower portion of the abdomen in most patients by the time sexual precocity is evident. The tumor may be small, however, and escape detection even on careful rectal and abdominal examination.

Association of these tumors with ascites and hydrothorax has been observed in children and is more likely with the thecoma. Such manifestations, known as *Meigs syndrome*, should not be confused with metastases and the primary tumor mistakenly considered inoperable.

Plasma estradiol levels are markedly elevated; a 9 yr old girl with a granulosa cell tumor had a level of 413 pg/dl, whereas levels in fully mature women or in children with idiopathic precocious puberty are under 100 pg/dl. Usually, urinary estrogens are also markedly elevated, whereas both plasma and urinary levels of gonadotropins are suppressed. Urinary 17-ketosteroids are normal or only slightly elevated and of little value in diagnosis. Osseous development is moderately advanced.

The tumor should be removed as soon as the diagnosis is established. The mortality rate in adults with these tumors is 7% at 10 yr; prognosis in children appears better, but data are limited. Vaginal bleeding immediately after removal of the tumor is common. Signs of precocious puberty abate and may disappear within a few mo after operation. The secretion of estrogens returns to normal.

In at least 1 instance of functioning granulosa cell tumor *Peutz-Jeghers syndrome* has been associated. The most common ovarian tumor occurring with the *Peutz-Jeghers syndrome* is a distinctive *sex cord tumor with annular tubules*, but evidence suggests that this tumor arises from granulosa cells.

FOLLICULAR CYST

Ovarian cysts are common in childhood, but most are nonfunctioning and hence not feminizing. Ovarian cysts are common also in children with constitutional sexual precocity, in whom the cyst is a secondary event; it is not the cause of sexual precocity, and its removal does not alter the course of sexual precocity. In rare instances, on the other hand, removal of a follicular cyst has resulted in regression of clinical signs of sexual precocity. Such functional cysts are being increasingly recognized through the use of sensitive hormone assays and have been found in children with McCune-Albright syndrome and in other cases of precocious puberty. Clinical manifestations are those of true precocious puberty. Since these cysts function autonomously, gonadotropins are suppressed and estradiol levels markedly elevated, though they may fluctuate widely and even return spontaneously to normal. Stimulation of these children with luteinizing hormone–releasing factor (LRH) results in a prepubertal type of response rather than the pubertal type response expected in true precocious puberty. Ultrasonography may detect the cyst, or it may be palpable on rectal examination. If the condition does not show evidence of remission, surgery is indicated since it is not possible to differentiate the lesion from a functioning ovarian tumor.

18.43 ANDROGENIC LESIONS OF THE OVARY

Virilizing ovarian tumors are rare at all ages but particularly so in prepubertal girls. The *androblastoma (arrhenoblastoma)* has been reported as early as 4 yr of age, but fewer than 2 dozen cases have been reported under 16 yr of age. Other androgen-secreting tumors include lipoid cell tumors and such benign ovarian lesions as ovarian hyperthecosis. The clinical features are the same as for virilizing adrenal tumors and include acne, hirsutism, and clitoral enlargement. These conditions must be given consideration in adolescent girls with hirsutism and secondary amenorrhea. Urinary 17-ketosteroids may be normal or only slightly elevated, but plasma levels of testosterone are usually elevated, and levels of LH are suppressed. In order to differentiate these lesions from adrenal tumors, dexamethasone suppression and chorionic gonadotropin stimulation studies may be necessary. Even such studies, however, may not differentiate among them, and selective venography and venous blood sampling or exploratory laparotomy may be indicated.

Patients with *ovarian thecosis* usually have elevated plasma levels of LH as well as of testosterone, and they may exhibit excessive response to LRH. Wedge resection of the ovary may be beneficial.

18.44   HERMAPHRODITISM
(Intersexuality)

Hermaphroditism in man implies a discrepancy between the morphology of the gonads and of the external genitalia. Many chromosomal aberrations resulting in ambiguity of the external genitalia have been discussed

**Table 18–8   ETIOLOGIC CLASSIFICATION OF
· HERMAPHRODITISM**

Female pseudohermaphroditism
  Androgen exposure
    Fetal source
      Congenital adrenal hyperplasia
        21-Hydroxylase deficiency
        11β-Hydroxylase deficiency
        3β-Hydroxysteroid dehydrogenase deficiency
      Adrenal tumor?
    Maternal source
      Virilizing tumor
        Ovary
        Adrenal
      Androgenic drugs
      Progestational drugs
  Undetermined origin
    Usually associated with other defects (skeleton, urinary and
      gastrointestinal tracts)
Male pseudohermaphroditism
  Defect in testicular differentiation
    Deletion short arm of Y chromosome
    XY pure gonadal dysgenesis (Swyer syndrome)
    XY gonadal agenesis syndrome
    XY antigen deficiency with camptomelic dysplasia
  Defect in testicular hormones
    Leydig cell aplasia—abnormality of hCG-LH receptor?
    Inborn errors of testosterone synthesis
      Cholesterol 20α,22-hydroxylase and/or 20,22-desmolase
        deficiency
      3β-Hydroxysteroid dehydrogenase deficiency
      17α-Hydroxylase deficiency
      17,20-Desmolase deficiency
      17β-Hydroxysteroid dehydrogenase deficiency
    Defect in antimüllerian hormone action (uterine hernia
      syndrome)
      Defective synthesis
      Defective response
  Defect in androgen action
    Defect in conversion of testosterone to dihydrotestosterone—5α-
      reductase deficiency
    Testicular feminization syndrome
      Cytosol receptor defect
      Post-receptor defect
    Incomplete testicular feminization
    Reifenstein syndrome (Lubs, Gilbert-Dryfus, Rosewater
      syndromes)
      Decreased cytoplasmic receptor
      Normal cytoplasmic receptor
  Undetermined—male pseudohermaphroditism
    With aniridia
    With Wilms tumor
    With nephrosis or nephritis
True hermaphroditism
  XX
  XY
  XX/XY chimeras
  Familial

earlier in this section. Here we discuss those conditions of aberrant sexual differentiation imposed on the XX or XY genotype (female and male pseudohermaphrodites). (See Table 18–8.) An increasing number of such conditions are now understood through advances in the understanding of normal sexual differentiation. The category known as true hermaphroditism, with few exceptions, is still a poorly understood heterogeneous group of disorders.

Embryonic Sexual Differentiation. In normal differentiation, the final form of all sexual structures is consistent with normal sex chromosomes (either XX or XY). A 46,XX complement of chromosomes is necessary for the development of normal ovaries. Both the long and the short arms of X chromosomes bear genes for normal ovarian development. An autosomal gene also appears to play a role in normal ovarian organogenesis (see XX gonadal dysgenesis, above). A deletion affecting the short arm of the X chromosome produces the typical somatic anomalies of Turner syndrome. Development of the male phenotype is more complex. Testicular differentiation is controlled by the Y chromosome. With few exceptions the finding of testes indicates presence of a Y chromosome; the exceptions (XX males and XX true hermaphrodites) usually have translocations of male-determining genes onto paternal X chromosomes or autosomes. Male-determining genes are on the short arm of the Y chromosome, deletion of which produces a female phenotype with streaked gonads.

The Y chromosome determines the male sex by causing the initially indifferent gonad to differentiate as a testis, beginning around the 5th–6th wk of intrauterine life. The H-Y antigen, a cell-surface component, is required for testicular differentiation. In its absence even patients with normal XY chromosomes fail to virilize and exhibit sex reversal. The structural gene for H-Y antigen is now believed to be autosomal but controlled by genes on the X and Y chromosomes. It appears that the H-Y gene is the primary male-determining gene. If it is present, the male phenotype develops even if many X chromosomes are present. A serologic assay for H-Y antigen can detect the effect of genes of the Y chromosome even when the Y chromosome cannot be found in the karyotype. In the XX fetus the female phenotype develops simply because there are no male-determining genes or H-Y antigen. The original bipotential gonad in the H-Y negative fetus develops into an ovary but not until about the 12th wk.

In the male fetus, once the indifferent gonad has differentiated into a testis, it begins to produce hormones, and masculinization of the fetus begins at about 8 wk. During this period of masculinization (8–12 wk) the fetal testis secretes 2 hormones. The 1st of these is testosterone, as shown indirectly by correlation with cytodifferentiation of the Leydig cells and directly by measurement of testosterone concentration of fetal testes and plasma. Secretion of testosterone during this critical period of differentiation probably occurs in response to placental chorionic gonadotropin (hCG). It appears that testosterone initiates virilization of the wolffian duct into the epididymis, vas deferens, and seminal vesicle. Testosterone is also converted by a 5α-reductase to an active metabolite, dihydrotestosterone, which causes virilization of the urogenital sinus and the external genitalia. A functional androgen receptor, controlled by an X-linked gene, is required for testosterone to give a masculine phenotype to XY individuals. When there is a defect in the synthesis of testosterone, normal masculinization may not occur, even when the testis has H-Y antigen and there are normal androgen receptors. The pathway for testosterone biosynthesis is given in Fig 18–25, which also indicates the various biosynthetic defects.

The 2nd hormone produced by the fetal testis is the müllerian duct inhibiting factor (MIF); it is a glycoprotein of high molecular weight produced by the Sertoli cells. Though it has its effect only during a short critical period, it is produced from shortly after testicular differentiation until the perinatal period. MIF causes the müllerian ducts to regress; in its absence they persist. It is clear, therefore, that the female phenotype develops independently of the gonads. Normal female differentiation requires that there be no H-Y antigen, no testosterone, and no anti-müllerian hormone; maleness is imposed upon a basically female potential by the hormones of the fetal testis. Defects are now known at each of these steps.

18.45 FEMALE PSEUDOHERMAPHRODITISM

In the female pseudohermaphrodite the genotype is XX and the gonads are ovaries, but the external genitalia are virilized. Since there is no anti-müllerian hormone, uterus, tubes, and ovaries develop. The mechanisms involved in normal female differentiation are considerably less complex than those required for male differentiation, and the varieties and causes of female pseudohermaphroditism are fewer. Most instances result from exposure of the female fetus to excessive androgens during intrauterine life; and the changes consist principally of virilization of the external genitalia (clitoral hypertrophy and labioscrotal fusion).

Congenital Adrenal Hyperplasia. This is by far the most common cause of the condition. Females with the 21-hydroxylase and 11-hydroxylase defects are the most highly virilized, though minimal virilization also occurs with the 3β-hydroxysteroid dehydrogenase defect. Salt-losers tend to have greater degrees of virilization than non-salt-losers. The masculinization may be so intense as to result in a complete penile urethra and may mimic a male with cryptorchidism.

Masculinizing Maternal Tumors. In 13 instances the female fetus has been virilized during fetal life by a maternal androgen-producing tumor. In 1 instance the lesion was a benign adrenal adenoma, but all others were ovarian tumors, particularly androblastomas, luteomas, and Krukenberg tumors. Maternal virilization may be manifested by enlargement of the clitoris, acne, deepening of the voice, decreased lactation, hirsutism, and elevated levels of androgens. In the infant there is enlargement of the clitoris of varying degrees, often with labial fusion. Mothers of children with unexplained female pseudohermaphroditism should have measurements of their own levels of plasma testosterone.

Administration of Androgenic Drugs to Women During Pregnancy. Testosterone and 17-methyltestosterone have been reported to cause female pseudohermaphroditism in some instances. The greatest number of cases, however, have resulted from the use of certain progestational compounds for the treatment of threatened abortion. In recent yr most of these progestins have been replaced by nonvirilizing ones.

Infants with female pseudohermaphroditism have been reported for whom no masculinizing agent could be identified. In such instances the disorder is usually associated with other congenital defects, particularly of the urinary and gastrointestinal tracts. No etiologic factors are known.

18.46 MALE PSEUDOHERMAPHRODITISM

In the male pseudohermaphrodite the genotype is XY, but the external genitalia are incompletely virilized, ambiguous, or completely female. When gonads can be found, they are invariably testes; their development may range from rudimentary to normal. Because the process of normal virilization in the fetus is so complex, it is not surprising that there are many varieties of male hermaphroditism.

DEFECTS IN TESTICULAR DIFFERENTIATION

The 1st step in male differentiation is conversion of the indifferent gonad to a testis. If in the XY fetus there is a deletion of the *short arm of the Y chromosome* and/or deletion of the male-determining genes, male differentiation does not occur. The phenotype is female; müllerian ducts are well developed, but gonads consist of undifferentiated streaks. By contrast, even extreme deletions of the *long arm of the Y chromosome* (Yq−) have been found in normally developed and fertile males. In other syndromes in which the testes fail to differentiate, Y chromosomes are morphologically normal.

Camptomelic dysplasia, a form of short-limbed dysplasia, is probably inherited as an autosomal trait (Sec 23.17). Many of the affected phenotypic females have an XY karyotype and exhibit sex reversal. Uterus and fallopian tubes are present. The gonads appear grossly to be ovaries; histologically, some resemble dysgenetic testicular tissue, and others more closely resemble the ovaries of the newborn. H-Y antigen was absent in 3 cases examined. It is postulated that the mutation causing camptomelic dysplasia may also prevent the production of H-Y antigen or prevent its association with the cell surface; hence, normal testicular differentiation may not occur.

XY Pure Gonadal Dysgenesis (Swyer Syndrome). The designation "pure" distinguishes this from forms of gonadal dysgenesis which are of chromosomal origin and associated with somatic anomalies. Affected patients have a female phenotype, including vagina, uterus, and fallopian tubes, but at pubertal age breast development and primary amenorrhea fail to occur. The gonads consist of almost totally undifferentiated streaks despite the presence of a cytogenetically normal Y chromosome. Although H-Y antigen is demonstrable in most patients, it is postulated that the embryonic gonad has failed to respond to the H-Y antigen for reasons not known. In patients who are H-Y negative it has been suggested that a gene on the short arm of the X chromosome which regulates production of H-Y antigen is mutated. In either case the primitive gonad fails to differentiate and cannot accomplish any testicular function, including suppression of müllerian ducts. There may be hilar cells in the gonad capable of producing some androgens; accordingly, some virilization, such as clitoral enlargement, may occur at the age of puberty. Growth is normal; there are no associated defects. The streak gonads may undergo neoplastic changes, such as gonadoblastomas and dysgerminomas, and even earlier than in the testicular feminization syndrome. The gonads should, therefore be removed shortly after ascertainment, irrespective of age.

Pure gonadal dysgenesis also occurs in XX individuals (Sec 18.37).

XY Gonadal Agenesis Syndrome (Embryonic Testicular Regression Syndrome). In this rare syndrome the external genitalia are slightly ambiguous but more nearly female. Hypoplasia of the labia, some degree of labioscrotal fusion, a small clitoris-like phallus, and a perineal urethral opening are present. No uterus, no gonadal tissue, and usually no vagina can be found. At the age of puberty no sexual development occurs, and gonadotropins are elevated. Most patients have been reared as females. In this condition it is presumed that testicular tissue was active long enough during fetal life to inhibit müllerian duct development but that its Leydig cell function was minimal.

In several patients with XY gonadal agenesis in whom no gonads could be found on exploration, significant rises in testosterone followed stimulation with human chorionic gonadotropin, indicating Leydig cell function somewhere. Siblings with the disorder are known.

In *bilateral anorchia* testes are absent, but the male phenotype is complete; it is presumed that tissue with fetal testicular function was active during the critical period of genital differentiation but that sometime later it was damaged. Bilateral anorchia in identical twins and unilateral anorchia both in identical twins and in siblings suggest a genetic predisposition. Coexistence of anorchia and the gonadal agenesis syndrome in a sibship is evidence for embryonic testicular regression in affected children and for a relationship between the disorders.

DEFECTS IN TESTICULAR HORMONES

Five genetic defects have been delineated in the enzymatic synthesis of testosterone by fetal testis, and a defect in Leydig cell differentiation has been described. These defects produce male pseudohermaphroditism through inadequate masculinization of the XY fetus (Fig 18–25). Since levels of testosterone are normally low prior to puberty, a chorionic gonadotropin stimulation test must be used in children to assess the ability of the testes to synthesize testosterone.

Leydig Cell Aplasia. Two patients with this defect

were phenotypic female adults with a shallow vagina, absent uterus, and bilateral inguinal testes. One prepubertal child had genital ambiguity. Unlike patients with testicular feminization, they had no breast development. Pubic hair was sparse or normal; levels of testosterone were low and did not rise after stimulation with chorionic gonadotropin. Low levels of precursors to testosterone synthesis ruled out a defect in synthesis of testosterone. Plasma LH was elevated, but FSH was normal. No Leydig cells were present in the testes.

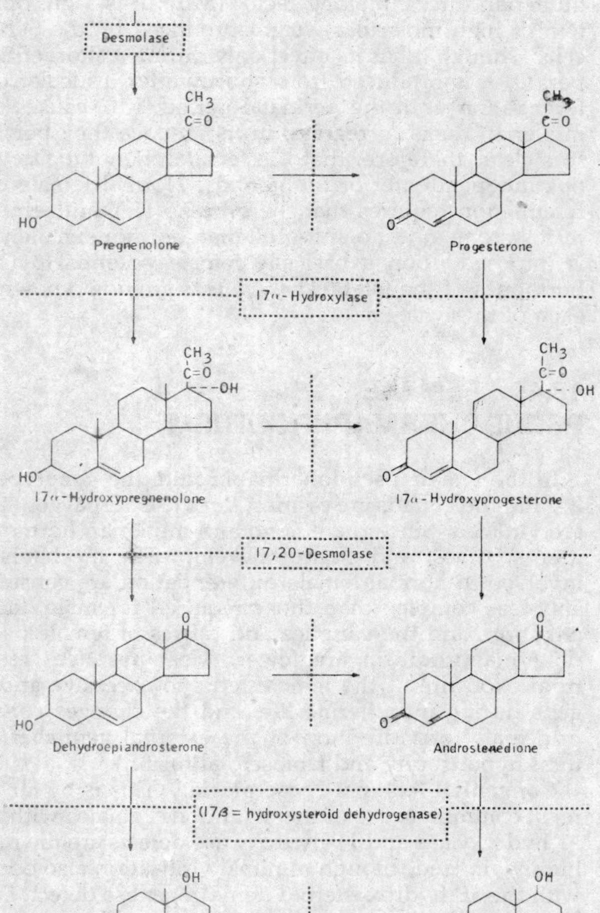

Figure 18–25 Biosynthesis of androgens. Dotted lines indicate enzymatic defects associated with male pseudohermaphroditism. Vertical dotted line indicates defect in 3β-hydroxysteroid dehydrogenase.

Selective agenesis of the Leydig cells could explain all these findings. It is possible that Leydig cells failed to differentiate because of a lack of receptors that permit a response to chorionic gonadotropin. Absence of müllerian ducts indicates that the fetal testis produced antimüllerian hormone. Parents of 1 patient were 1st cousins; thus, autosomal recessive inheritance is suggested.

20,22-Desmolase Deficiency. This enzyme is required early in the biosynthetic pathway for both hydrocortisone and testosterone. Deficiency is also known as lipoid adrenal hyperplasia (Sec 18.24). The fetal testis cannot synthesize testosterone, and affected XY patients are considered normal females until salt-losing symptoms intervene. In at least 1 instance a partial defect has resulted in a partially masculinized male with ambiguous genitalia and delayed onset of salt loss.

3β-Hydroxysteroid Dehydrogenase Deficiency. Males with this form of congenital adrenal hyperplasia (Sec 18.24) have varying degrees of hypospadias, with or without bifid scrotum and cryptorchidism. Affected infants usually develop salt-losing manifestations shortly after birth; incomplete defects have been reported, and in a pubertal boy the defect seemed to be complete in the adrenal but only partial in the testis.

Deficiency of 17-Hydroxylase. Males with this defect have ambiguous genitalia, with hypospadias, cryptorchidism, and a rudimentary vagina. The phallus may be so small as to suggest a female phenotype, and several patients were reared to adult life as females. Because of the overproduction of DOC and corticosterone, hypertension and hypokalemic alkalosis are characteristic, but in less severely affected males the blood pressure may be normal in early life. With failure of adrenal and testicular synthesis of androgens, puberty does not occur and the patient remains eunuchoid. Absence of müllerian duct remnants indicates that fetal production of müllerian-inhibiting substance is normal. The diagnosis can be suspected after puberty if low levels of 17-ketosteroids, of 21-hydroxycorticoids, and of plasma androgens are found. To establish the diagnosis before puberty, it is necessary to determine secretion rates of DOC, corticosterone, cortisol, and compound S. This defect follows autosomal recessive inheritance.

Deficiency of Steroid 17,20-Desmolase. In 2 1st cousins and a maternal "aunt" in 1 family and in 2 siblings in another family, ambiguous external genitalia and XY constitutions have been associated with deficiency of the enzyme which cleaves the side chain of 17-hydroxypregnenolone and 17-hydroxyprogesterone (Fig 18–25). As a consequence, levels of both of these precursors as well as of pregnenolone and progesterone are elevated. Since plasma androgens are normally low in the prepubertal period, they are of no help in diagnosis in the basal state. The enzymatic defect also involves the adrenal since ACTH administration fails to increase adrenal androgens but results in exaggerated rise in progestogens even after castration. The inguinal testes in these patients revealed no specific abnormalities. There were no müllerian structures. The functional defect was probably incomplete since with total absence of testosterone one would expect complete feminization. This diagnosis can be investigated in male pseudohermaphrodites with histologically normal testes by measuring plasma levels of progestogens and androgens following stimulation with hCG and ACTH. Both X-linked and autosomal recessive inheritance are possible; only XY subjects have been reported thus far.

Deficiency of 17β-Hydroxysteroid Dehydrogenase. A defect in testicular 17β-hydroxysteroid dehydrogenase has been identified as a cause of pseudohermaphroditism in a few XY patients. Affected persons were completely feminized and reared as females until, at puberty, virilization and primary amenorrhea occurred and, in some patients, gynecomastia. A shallow vagina is present, but no cervix or uterus. The defect in testosterone synthesis results in low plasma levels of testosterone and in marked accumulation of its precursor androstenedione (Fig 18–25). The testis also produces estrone at increased rates. The testicular tubules are small, with a fibrotic lamina propria, and spermatogenesis is arrested at early stages. Marked Leydig cell hyperplasia is present. The defect has been detected only in adults. In prepubertal children the disorder would be easily confused with the testicular feminization syndrome, but it could be suspected if there were no rise in testosterone following administration of human chorionic gonadotropin. Consanguinity of parents in 1 family suggests autosomal recessive transmission. Removal of the defective testis prevents or halts virilization. Replacement therapy with estrogens is indicated.

Uterine Hernia Syndrome. In this disorder fetal testosterone production is normal and affected males completely virilized. There is, however, a deficiency of testicular müllerian duct inhibiting factor (MIF), with persistence of müllerian ducts. These are usually detected when surgical correction of an inguinal hernia in an otherwise normal male discloses uterus and uterine tubes. The degree of müllerian development is variable and may be asymmetrical. Testicular function, including spermatogenesis, may be normal. The disorder may result from a biosynthetic defect or from end-organ unresponsiveness to anti-müllerian hormone. At least 6 sibships have been reported, each with several affected males; these suggest recessive inheritance, either X-linked or autosomal. Treatment consists of removal of as much of the müllerian structures as possible without damage to testis, epididymis, or vas deferens. About 10% of affected patients have developed testicular tumors after puberty.

DEFECTS IN ANDROGEN ACTION

In the following group of disorders it has now been established that fetal synthesis of testosterone is normal, and defective virilization results from inherited abnormalities in androgen action.

5α-Reductase Deficiency. In this disorder decreased production of dihydrotestosterone in utero results in severe ambiguity of the external genitalia of the affected male fetus. Biosynthesis and peripheral action of testosterone are normal.

Affected boys have a small phallus, bifid scrotum, urogenital sinus with perineal hypospadias, and a blind vaginal pouch. Testes are in the inguinal canals or labial-scrotal folds and are normal histologically. There are no müllerian structures; the vas deferens, epididymis, and seminal vesicles are present. At puberty, masculinization occurs normally; the phallus enlarges, the testes descend and grow normally, and spermatogenesis occurs. There is no gynecomastia. Beard growth is scanty, acne is absent, the prostate is small, and recession of the temporal hair line fails to occur.

These findings are consistent with studies in animals which show virilization of the wolffian duct to be due to the action of testosterone itself, whereas masculinization of the urogenital sinus and external genitalia depends on the action of dihydrotestosterone during the critical period of fetal masculinization. Growth of facial hair and of the prostate also appears to be dihydrotestosterone dependent. The disorder is inherited as an autosomal recessive but is limited to males; normal homozygous females with normal fertility indicate that in females dihydrotestosterone has no role in sexual differentiation or in ovarian function later in life. In 23 interrelated families in the Dominican Republic, although many of the 38 affected males had been reared as females, most assumed a male gender role coincident with masculinization at puberty. It appears that exposures to testosterone in utero, neonatally, and at puberty contribute to the formation of male gender identity.

Testicular Feminization Syndrome. This is 1 of the more common and most extreme examples of failure of virilization. These XY patients appear female at birth and are invariably reared accordingly. The external genitalia are female; the vagina ends blindly in a pouch, and the uterus is absent. The gonads are testes which consist largely of seminiferous tubules. They are usually intra-abdominal but may descend into the inguinal canal. At puberty there is normal development of breasts and the habitus is female, but menstruation does not occur and sexual hair is often absent. Psychosexual orientation of such persons is entirely female.

The testes of affected adult patients produce normal male levels of testosterone. Affected patients are able to convert testosterone to 5α-dihydrotestosterone. The absence of androgenic effects is due to a striking resistance to the action of endogenous or exogenous testosterone at the peripheral cellular level. Evidence suggests that there are clinically identical but genetically distinct variants: in some the cytosol receptor for dihydrotestosterone may be absent or structurally abnormal (thermolabile); in others the receptor is normal and the defect presumed to be postreceptor. Failure of normal male differentiation during fetal life reflects the defective response to testicular androgens at that time.

In adults amenorrhea is the usual presenting symptom. Prepubertal children with this disorder are often detected when inguinal masses prove to be testes or when a testis is unexpectedly found during herniorrhaphy in a phenotypic female. Examination of a buccal smear is indicated for any female with an inguinal hernia; 1–2% will prove to have this syndrome.

The disorder follows X-linked recessive inheritance, the gene being transmitted by female carriers. About half of all XY offspring are affected, while half of the daughters are carriers. In prepubertal children the condition must be differentiated from other types of XY male pseudohermaphroditism in which there is complete feminization. These include XY pure gonadal dysgenesis (Swyer syndrome), true agonadism, Leydig-cell aplasia, and the testicular 17-ketosteroid reductase defect.

Affected patients should always be reared as females. The testes should be removed since there is about a 4% incidence of tumors by the age of 25 yr and about 33% by the age of 50 yr. Some recommend not removing the testes until after completion of secondary sexual development, but a testicular tumor has been found in an affected 18 mo old infant. To relieve parental anxiety and to avoid adverse effects on psychosexual orientation of the child, we recommend that the testes be removed as soon as they are discovered. Replacement therapy with estrogens is then indicated at the age of puberty.

Incomplete Testicular Feminization. In this disorder patients exhibit some degree of masculinization and at birth may have enlargement of the phallus and labioscrotal fusion. The vagina ends blindly, and the uterus is absent. Testes are present in the inguinal canal or in the labioscrotal folds. At puberty, breast development occurs as well as axillary and pubic hair. These patients have lesser degrees of insensitivity to androgen than those with the complete syndrome; the androgen receptor may have low responsiveness or be structurally abnormal. In a family studied by the author the pattern of inheritance is compatible with X-linkage; the "complete" and "incomplete" forms have not been reported in the same family.

Reifenstein Syndrome. This type of male pseudohermaphroditism is caused by decreased end-organ responsiveness rather than decreased androgen production. It is best described as *partial androgen insensitivity*. In childhood the disorder presents severe perineal hypospadias and small testes, which may be found in the scrotal sac or may be cryptorchid. The phallus is usually normal in size and affected patients are usually considered male. After puberty there is inadequate masculinization. There is lack of facial hair and voice change. Female escutcheon, azoospermia, and infertility are usual. Within affected families the severity ranges from a mild defect (microphallus and bifid scrotum) to the severe abnormality described above. Three other syndromes of defective virilization (described by Lubs, by Gilbert-Dreyfus, and by Rosewater and their coworkers) may represent the variable manifestations of the same defect as in Reifenstein syndrome.

In adults plasma levels of testosterone and of dihydrotestosterone are normal or elevated. Levels of LH, and often of FSH, are also elevated. Androgen receptor studies in skin fibroblasts reveal low or normal androgen-binding capacity. There appear to be 2 variants of the syndrome, as in the case of testicular feminization. The cause of the insensitivity to androgen in patients with normal dihydrotestosterone binding is not known. Inheritance is believed to be X-linked recessive.

UNDETERMINED CAUSES

Other XY male pseudohermaphrodites display much variability of the external and internal genitalia and varying degrees of phallic and müllerian development. Testes may be histologically normal or rudimentary, or there may only be 1. Some reported cases may belong to 1 of the above-described categories, without having been studied by newer techniques. Some ambiguity of genitalia is associated with a wide variety of chromosomal aberrations, which must always be considered in the differential, the most common being the 45,X/46,XY syndrome (Sec 18.37). It may be necessary to examine several tissues in order to establish mosaicism. Other complex genetic syndromes, many resulting from single gene mutations, are associated with varying degrees of ambiguity of the genitalia, particularly in the male. These entities must be identified on the basis of the associated extragenital malformations.

PSEUDOHERMAPHRODITISM AND WILMS TUMOR

Some XY male pseudohermaphrodites are at increased risk of Wilms tumor, usually in the 1st 2–3 yr of life. Such children often also develop nephritis and/or nephrosis which may rapidly progress to renal failure. Hermaphroditism in these instances is of unknown cause; it is not due to any of the mechanisms discussed above.

Male infants with *sporadic aniridia* also often have cryptorchidism and/or hypospadias as well as mental retardation. In at least 5 instances a gonadoblastoma has arisen in the presumably dysgenetic testis. Most patients with this syndrome have deletions of the short arm of chromosome 11 (11p−), usually involving the 11p 12–13 bands. Wilms tumor occurs in about half of all children with this chromosome abnormality.

18.47 TRUE HERMAPHRODITISM

In true hermaphroditism both ovarian and testicular tissue are present, either in the same or in opposite gonads. The clinical features may include any of those described for the other types of hermaphroditism. The phenotype may be male or female; usually, the external genitalia are ambiguous.

Examination of the chromosomes of 19 true hermaphrodites found 50% to be XX, 20% to be XY, and 30% to be mosaics. The most common mosaic conditions have been 45,X/46,XY; 46,XX/47,XXY; and 45,XX/46,XY. To establish mosaicism may require study of many different tissues; its possibility can never be completely eliminated. On the other hand, some instances of XX true hermaphroditism have been very intensively investigated, with no evidence found of a Y chromosome. In such patients the portion of the Y chromosome containing the male-determining genes may have been translocated to the X chromosome or to an autosome. In a few cases cytologic evidence for such translocations has been presented; and a number of XX true hermaphrodites with no cytologic evidence of translocation have been found to have H-Y antigen, indicating the activity of Y-linked or Y-autosome translocations. The situation is comparable to that which occurs in XX males (see above).

Patients with XX/XY mosaicism are of special interest and are the best understood of patients with true hermaphroditism. Of 12 reported cases, 9 were derived from more than 1 zygote; that is, they were chimeras (chi 46,XX/46,XY). Chimerism has usually been established by blood group studies. The presence of both paternal alleles for some blood groups and of both maternal alleles for other blood groups is clear evidence for it. A variety of mechanisms are possible. In 1 instance study of chromosome heteromorphisms established that 2 different spermatozoa had fertilized an ovum and its 2nd meiotic division polar body, with subsequent fusion of the 2 zygotes.

Diagnosis and Management. The diagnosis of hermaphroditism depends upon a thorough review of the numerous mechanisms which may lead to the condition. Screening tests (examination of sex chromatin or fluorescence of the Y chromosome) must always be supplemented by complete chromosomal analysis. It is important in conditions in which mosaicism is a possibility to establish the chromosomal constitution of tissues other than blood, such as skin or any tissues removed at biopsy or exploration.

For all XX patients a detailed search for the source of virilization should be undertaken. Studies of adrenal hormones, 17-ketosteroids, pregnanetriol, and 17-dehydroxyprogesterone are needed to exclude the common varieties of adrenogenital syndrome. Urethrovaginography or endoscopic examination is indicated to establish whether vagina and/or cervix may exist in patients with ambiguous external genitalia.

For XY patients it is necessary to determine whether testicular production of androgen is normal. In the prepubertal child determination requires stimulation of the testes with hCG. It may be necessary to verify the ability to convert testosterone to dihydrotestosterone and the ability of fibroblasts to bind androgen. Precise diagnosis is essential to genetic counseling since genes both on autosomes and on the X chromosome are known to cause hermaphroditism. Many XY hermaphrodites are at high risk of gonadal neoplasia; it is important to identify them and to remove the gonads promptly.

Many male pseudohermaphrodites, like boys with hypopituitarism, have a small penis (*microphallus*). A course of 3 monthly intramuscular injections of testosterone (25–50 mg testosterone enanthate) may assist differential diagnosis as well as treatment. The phallus will respond in patients with defects in testosterone synthesis or with hypopituitarism but not in those with complete androgen insensitivity. Such a course of treatment must precede any plan for surgical reconstruction of XY males as anatomic females.

The assignment of sex of rearing should be settled as early in life as possible. The decision is based largely on the possibilities for correction of the ambiguous genitalia and not on the chromosomal constitution. Female pseudohermaphrodites should almost always be reared as females even when highly virilized. Male pseudohermaphrodites who are totally or significantly feminized should also be reared as females. It is more feasible to reconstruct the external genitalia to create a functional female, particularly when a vagina is already present, than to create a functional male phallus. The management of the potential psychologic upheaval that such problems can generate in patient and/or family is of paramount importance and requires physicians with sensitivity and with training and experience in this field. Once the appropriate sex of rearing has been established, parents should be left with no ambiguity in their minds as to the sex of the child.

In some mammals the female exposed to androgens prenatally or in early postnatal life will exhibit aberrant sexual behavior in adult life. Girls who have undergone fetal masculinization from congenital adrenal hyperplasia or from maternal progestin therapy have no such problems in sexual identity, though during childhood they may appear to prefer male playmates and activities to girl playmates and feminine play with dolls in mothering roles.

ANGELO M. DiGEORGE

General

Simpson JL: Disorders of Sexual Differentiation: Etiology and Clinical Delineation. New York, Academic Press, 1976.
Williams RH: Textbook of Endocrinology. Ed 6. Philadelphia, WB Saunders, 1981.

Hypofunction of Testes

Borgaonkar DS, Mules E, Char F: Do the 48 XXYY males have a characteristic phenotype? Clin Genet 1:272, 1970.
Bowen P, et al: Hereditary male pseudohermaphroditism with hypogonadism, hypospadias, and gynecomastia (Reifenstein's syndrome). Arch Intern Med 62:252, 1965.
Caldwell PD, Smith DW: The XXY (Klinefelter's) syndrome in childhood: Detection and treatment. J Pediatr 80:250, 1972.
Chaussain JL, Lemerle J, Roger M, et al: Klinefelter syndrome, tumor and sexual precocity. J Pediatr 97:607, 1980.
Court Brown MW: Males with an XYY sex chromosome complement. Review article. J Med Genet 5:341, 1968.
Dekaban AS, Parks JS, Ross GT: Laurence-Moon syndrome: Evaluation of endocrinological function and phenotypic concordance and report of cases. Med Ann District Columbia 41:687, 1972.
DeLaChapelle A, Hortling H: Cytogenetical and clinical observations in male hypogonadism. Acta Endocrinol 44:165, 1963.
DeLaChapelle A, Schroder J, Murros J, et al: Two XX males in one family and additional observations bearing on the etiology of XX males. Clin Genet 11:91, 1977.
Ewer RW: Familial monotropic pituitary gonadotropin insufficiency. J Clin Endocrinol 28:783, 1968.
Faiman C, Hoffman DL, Ryan RJ, et al: The "fertile eunuch" syndrome: Demonstration of isolated luteinizing hormone deficiency by radioimmunoassay technique. Mayo Clin Proc 43:661, 1968.
Haseltine FP, Genel M, Crawford JD, Breg WR: HY antigen negative patients with testicular tissue and 46, XY karyotype. Hum Genet 57:265, 1981.
Hook EB: Behavioral implications of the human XYY genotype. Science 179:139, 1973.
Karpouzas J, Papaioannov AC: Noonan syndrome in twins. J Pediatr 85:84, 1974.
Kasdan R, Nankin HR, Troen P, et al: Paternal transmission of maleness in XX human beings. N Engl J Med 288:539, 1973.
Kirkland RT, Bongiovanni AM, Cornfeld D, et al: Gonadotropin responses to luteinizing releasing factor in boys treated with cyclophosphamide for nephrotic syndrome. J Pediatr 89:941, 1976.
Leonard MF, Land G, Ruddle FH, et al: Early development of children with abnormalities of the sex chromosomes: A prospective study. Pediatrics 54:208, 1974.
Levy EP, Pashasyan H, Fraser FC, et al: XX and XY Turner phenotypes in a family. Am J Dis Child 120:36, 1970.
Lieblich JM, Rogol AD, White BJ, et al: Syndrome of anosmia with hypogonadotropic hypogonadism (Kallmann syndrome). Clinical and laboratory studies in 23 cases. Am J Med 73:506, 1982.

Marynick SP, Nisula BC, Pita JC Jr, Loriaux DL: Persistent pubertal macromastia. J Clin Endocrinol Metab 50:128, 1980.
Meisner LF, Inhorn SL: Normal male development with Y chromosome long arm deletion (Yq –). J Med Genet 9:373, 1972.
Melman A, Leiter E, Perez JM, et al: The influence of neonatal orchiopexy upon the testis in persistent müllerian duct syndrome. J Urol 125:856, 1981.
Money J, Franzke A, Borgaonkar DS: XYY syndrome, stigmatization, social class, and aggression. South Med J 68:1536, 1975.
Naftolin F, Harris GW: Effect of purified luteinizing hormone–releasing factor on normal and hypogonadotropic anosmic men. Nature (Lond) 232:496, 1971.
Najjar SS, Takla RJ, Nassar VH: The syndrome of rudimentary testes: Occurrence in five siblings. J Pediatr 84:119, 1974.
Neuhauser G, Opitz JM: Autosomal recessive syndrome of cerebellar ataxia and hypogonadotropic hypogonadism. Clin Genet 7:426, 1975.
Noonan JA: Hypertelorism with Turner phenotype. A new syndrome with associated congenital heart disease. Am J Dis Child 116:373, 1968.
Nora JJ, Torres FG, Sinha AK, et al: Characteristic cardiovascular anomalies of XO Turner syndrome, XX and XY phenotype and XO/XX Turner mosaic. Am J Cardiol 25:639, 1970.
Pescia G, Jotterand M: Possible evidence of X/Y interchange in an XX male. Lancet 1:550, 1977.
Philip J, Lundsteen C, Owen D, et al: The frequency of chromosome aberrations in tall men with special reference to 47,XYY and 47,XXY. Am J Hum Genet 28:404, 1976.
Reinfrank RF, Nicholl FL: Hypogonadotropic hypogonadism in the Laurence-Moon syndrome. J Clin Endocrinol 24:48, 1964.
Roe TF, Alfi OS: Ambiguous genitalia in XY male children: Report of two infants. Pediatrics 60:55, 1977.
Roth JC, Kelch RP, Kaplan SE, et al: FSH and LH response to luteinizing hormone–releasing factor in prepubertal and pubertal children, adult males and patients with hypogonadotropic and hypergonadotropic hypogonadism. J Clin Endocrinol Metab 35:926, 1972.
Salbenblatt JA, Bender BG, Puck MH, et al: Development of eight pubertal males with 47,XXY karyotype. Clin Genet 20:141, 1981.
Santen RJ, Paulsen CA: Hypogonadotropic eunuchoidism. I. Clinical study of the mode of inheritance. J Clin Endocrinol Metab 36:47, 1973.
Saunder SE, Corley KP, Hopwood NJ, Kelch RP: Subnormal gonadotropin responses for gonadotropin-releasing hormone persist into puberty in children with isolated growth hormone deficiency. J Clin Endocrinol Metab 53:1186, 1981.
Seyler LE, Arulananthan K, O'Connor CF: Hypergonadotropic-hypogonadism in the Prader-Labhart-Willi syndrome. J Pediatr 94:435, 1979.
Shalet SM, Hann IM, Lendon M, et al: Testicular function after combination chemotherapy in childhood for acute lymphoblastic leukaemia. Arch Dis Child 56:275, 1981.
Sherins RJ, Olweny CLM, Ziegler JL: Gynecomastia and gonadal dysfunction in adolescent boys treated with combination chemotherapy for Hodgkin's disease. N Engl J Med 299:12, 1978.
Shilsky RL, Lewis BJ, Sherins RJ, Young RC: Gonadal dysfunction in patients receiving chemotherapy for cancer. Ann Intern Med 93:109, 1980.
Sparkes RS, Simpson RW, Paulsen CA: Familial hypogonadotropic hypogonadism with anosmia. Arch Intern Med 121:534, 1968.
Swanson SL, Santen RJ, Smith DW: Multiple lentigenes syndrome: New findings of hypogonadotrophism, hyposmia, and unilateral renal agenesis. J Pediatr 78:1037, 1971.
Tennes K, Puck M, Orfanakis D, et al: The early childhood development of 17 boys with sex chromosome anomalies: A prospective study. Pediatrics 59:574, 1977.
Tolis G, Lewis W, Verdy M, et al: Anterior pituitary function in the Prader-Labhart-Willi (PLW) syndrome. J Clin Endocrinol Metab 39:1061, 1974.
Valentine GH, McClelland MA, Sergovich FR: The growth and development of four XYY infants. Pediatrics 48:853, 1971.
Volpe R, Metzler WS, Johnston MW: Familial hypogonadotropic eunuchoidism with cerebellar ataxia. J Clin Endocrinol Metab 23:107, 1963.
Wachtel SS, Koo GC, Greg WR, et al: Serologic detection of a Y-linked gene in XX males and XX true hermaphrodites. N Engl J Med 295:750, 1976.
Wieland RC, Folk RI, Taylor JN, et al: Studies of male hypogonadism. I. Androgen metabolism in a male with gynecomastia and galactorrhea. J Clin Endocrinol Metab 27:763, 1967.
Williams C, Wieland AG, Zorn EM, et al: Effect of synthetic gonadotropin-releasing hormone (GnRH) in a patient with the "fertile eunuch" syndrome. J Clin Endocrinol Metab 41:176, 1975.
Winter JSD, Faiman C: Serum gonadotropin concentrations in agonadal children and adults. J Clin Endocrinol Metab 35:561, 1972.
Witkin HA, Mednick SA, Schulsinger F, et al: Criminality in XYY and XXY men. Science 193:547, 1976.
Zarate A, Kastin AJ, Soria J, et al: Effect of synthetic luteinizing hormone–releasing hormone (LH-RH) in two brothers with hypogonadotropic hypogonadism and anosmia. J Clin Endocrinol Metab 36:612, 1973.

Tumors of the Testes

Canty JM, Seaglia HE, Medina M, et al: Inherited congenital normofunctional testicular hyperplasia and mental deficiency. Hum Genet 33:23, 1975.
Engel FL, et al: Clinical, morphological and biochemical studies on a malignant testicular tumor. J Clin Endocrinol Metab 24:528, 1964.

Martin MM, Canary JJ, Balsamo PA: Virilizing tumor of the testis in one twin. J Clin Endocrinol Metab 22:345, 1962.

Nisula BC, Loriaux DL, Sherins RJ, et al: Benign bilateral testicular enlargement. J Clin Endocrinol Metab 38:440, 1974.

Savard K, et al: Clinical, morphological and biochemical studies of a virilizing tumor of the testis. J Clin Invest 39:534, 1960.

Schedewie HK, Reiter EO, Teitins IZ et al: Testicular Leydig cell hyperplasia as a cause of familial sexual precocity. J Clin Endocrinol Metab 52:271, 1981.

Turner G, Daniel A, Frost M: X-linked mental retardation, macro-orchidism, and the Xq 27 fragile site. J Pediatr 96:837, 1980.

Turner WR, Derrick FC, Wohltmann W: Leydig cell tumor in identical twin. Urology 7:194, 1976.

Gynecomastia

August GP, Chandra R, Hung W: Prepubertal male gynecomastia. J Pediatr 80:259, 1972.

Goldfine I, Rosenfeld RL, Landau KL: Hyperleydigism: A cause of severe pubertal gynecomastia. J Clin Endocrinol Metab 32:751, 1971.

Green M: Gynecomastia and pseudoprecocious puberty following diethylstilbestrol exposure. Am J Dis Child 95:637, 1958.

Laron Z: Breast development induced by methandrostenolone (Dianabol). J Clin Endocrinol Metab 22:450, 1962.

Lee PA: The relationship of concentrations of serum hormones to pubertal gynecomastia. J Pediatr 86:212, 1975.

Maclaren NK, Migeon CJ, Raiti S: Gynecomastia with congenital virilizing adrenal hyperplasia (11β-hydroxylase deficiency). J Pediatr 86:579, 1975.

Nydick M, Bustos J, Dale JH Jr, et al: Gynecomastia in adolescent boys. JAMA 178:449, 1961.

Van Meter QL, Gareis FJ, Hayes JW, et al: Galactorrhea in a 12-year old boy with a chromophobe adenoma. J Pediatr 90:756, 1977.

Wallach EE, Garcia C: Familial gynecomastia without hypogonadism: A report of three cases in one family. J Clin Endocrinol Metab 22:1201, 1962.

Hypofunction of the Ovaries

Arulanantham K, Kramer MS, Gryboski J: The association of inflammatory bowel disease and X chromosomal abnormality. Pediatrics 66:63, 1980.

Carneiro IJ, Vorhees ML, Schlegel RJ, et al: XX/XO mosaicism in nine preadolescent girls with short stature as presenting complaint. Pediatrics 38:972, 1966.

Chang RJ, Davidson BJ, Carlson HE, et al: Hypogonadotropic hypogonadism associated with retinitis pigmentosa in a female sibship: Evidence for gonadotropin deficiency. J Clin Endocrinol Metab 53:1179, 1981.

Collins E: The illusion of widely spaced nipples in the Noonan and Turner syndromes. J Pediatr 83:557, 1973.

Davidoff F, Federman DD: Mixed gonadal dysgenesis. Pediatrics 52:725, 1973.

Eller E, Frankenberg W, Puck M, et al: Prognosis in newborn infants with X chromosomal abnormalities. Pediatrics 47:681, 1971.

Friedrich U, Nielsen J: Chromosome studies in 5,049 consecutive newborn children. Clin Genet 4:333, 1973.

Hecht F, MacFarlane JP: Mosaicism in Turner's syndrome reflects the lethality of XO. Lancet 2:1197, 1969.

Horning SJ, Hoppe RT, Kaplan HS, et al: Female reproductive potential after treatment for Hodgkin's disease. N Engl J Med 304:1377, 1981.

Kaufman FR, Kogut MD, Donnell GH, et al: Hypergonadotropic hypogonadism in female patients with galactosemia. N Engl J Med 304:994, 1981.

Lemli L, Smith DW: The XO syndrome: A study of the differentiated phenotype in 25 patients. J Pediatr 63:577, 1963.

Lindsten J: The Nature and Origin of X Chromosome Aberrations in Turner's Syndrome. A Cytogenetical and Clinical Study of 57 Patients. Stockholm, Almqvist-Wiksells, 1963.

Polychronakos C, Letarte K, Collu R, Ducharme JR: Carbohydrate intolerance in children and adolescents with Turner syndrome. J Pediatr 96:1009, 1980.

Spitz IM, et al: Isolated gonadotropin deficiency: A heterogeneous syndrome. N Engl J Med 290:10, 1974.

Tagatz G, Fialkow PJ, Smith D, et al: Hypogonadotropic hypogonadism associated with anosmia in the female. N Engl J Med 282:1326, 1970.

Warne GL, Fairley KF, Hobbs JB, et al: Cyclophosphamide-induced ovarian failure. N Engl J Med 29:1159, 1973.

Tumors of the Ovary

Ammann AJ, Kaufman S, Gilbert A: Virilizing ovarian tumor in a 2½-year-old girl. J Pediatr 70:782, 1967.

Campbell PE, Danks DM: Pseudoprecocity in an infant due to a luteoma of the ovary. Arch Dis Child 38:519, 1963.

Eberlein WR, Bongiovanni AM, Jones IT, et al: Ovarian tumors and cysts associated with sexual precocity. J Pediatr 57:484, 1960.

Faber HK: Meigs' syndrome with thecomas of both ovaries in a 4-year-old girl. J Pediatr 61:769, 1962.

Lack EE, Perez-Atayde AR, Murthy AS, et al: Granulosa theca cell tumors in premenarchal girls: A clinical and pathologic study of ten cases. Cancer 48:1846, 1981.

Tucci JR, Zäh W, Kalderon AE: Endocrine studies in arrhenoblastoma responsive to dexamethasone, ACTH and human chorionic gonadotropin. Am J Med 55:681, 1973.

Hermaphroditism

Amrhein JA, Jones Klingensmith G, Walsh PC, et al: Partial androgen insensitivity. The Reifenstein syndrome revisited. N Engl J Med 297:350, 1977.

Armendares S, Buentello L, Frenk S: Two male sibs with uterus and fallopian tubes. A rare, probably inherited disorder. Clin Genet 4:291, 1973.

Bell RJM: Fetal virilization due to maternal Krukenberg tumor. Lancet 1:1162, 1977.

Benirschke K, Naftolin G, Gittes R, et al: True hermaphroditism and chimerism. Am J Obstet Gynec 113:449, 1971.

Bernstein R, Koo GC, Wachtel SS: Abnormality of the X chromosome in human 46,XY female siblings with dysgenetic ovaries. Science 207:768, 1980.

Berthezene F, Forest MG, Grimaud JA, et al: Leydig-cell agenesis. A cause of male pseudohermaphroditism. N Engl J Med 295:696, 1976.

Bond JV: Wilms' tumor, hypospadias, and cryptorchidism in twins. Arch Dis Child 52:243, 1977.

Bongiovanni AM, DiGeorge AM, Grumbach MM: Masculinization of the female infant associated with estrogenic therapy alone during gestation: Four cases. J Clin Endocrinol Metab 19:1004, 1959.

Book JA, Eilon B, Halbrecht I, et al: Isochromosome Y (46,X,I, (Yq)) and female phenotype. Clin Genet 4:410, 1973.

Bricaire H, et al: A new male pseudohermaphroditism associated with hypertension due to a block of 17α-hydroxylation. J Clin Endocrinol Metab 35:67, 1972.

Bricarelle FD, Fraccaro M, Lindsten J, et al: Sex-reversed XY females with camptomelic dysplasia are H-Y negative. Hum Genet 47:12, 1981.

Brook CGB, Wagner H, et al: Familial occurrence of persistent müllerian structures in otherwise normal males. Br Med J 1:771, 1973.

Brown DM, Markland C, Dehner LP: Leydig cell hypoplasia: A cause of male pseudohermaphroditism. J Clin Endocrinol Metab 46:1, 1978.

Bullock LP, Bardin W: Androgen receptors in testicular feminization. J Clin Endocrinol Metab 35:935, 1972.

Burstein S, Grumbach MM, Kaplan SL: Early determination of androgen-responsiveness is important in the management of microphallus. Lancet 2:983, 1979.

Corey MJ, Miller JR, MacLean JR, et al: A case of XX/XY mosaicism. Am J Hum Genet 19:389, 1967.

Dewald G, Haymond MW, Spurbeck JL, Moore SB: Origin of chi 46,XX/46,XY chimerism in a true hermaphrodite. Science 207:321, 1980.

Fitzgerald PH, Donald RA, Kirk RL: A true hermaphrodite dispermic chimera with 46,XX and 46,XY karyotypes. Clin Genet 15:89, 1979.

Forest MG, Lecornu M, DePeretti E: Familial male pseudohermaphroditism due to 17,20-desmolase deficiency. I. In vivo endocrine studies. J Clin Endocrinol Metab 50:826, 1980.

Givens JR, Wiser WL, Summitt RL, et al: Familial male pseudohermaphroditism without gynecomastia due to deficient testicular 17-ketosteroid reductase activity. N Engl J Med 291:938, 1974.

Goebelsmann U, et al: Male pseudohermaphroditism due to testicular 17β-hydroxysteroid dehydrogenase deficiency. J Clin Endocrinol Metab 36:867, 1973.

Griffin JE, Wilson JD: The syndromes of androgen resistance. N Engl J Med 302:198, 1980.

Hall JG, Morgan A, Blizzard RM: Familial congenital anorchia. In: Bergsma D (ed): Genetic Forms of Hypogohadism. Birth Defects, Original Article Series 2(4):115, 1975.

Haymond MW, Weldon VV: Female pseudohermaphroditism secondary to a maternal virilizing tumor. J Pediatr 82:682, 1973.

Imperato-McGinley J, Peterson RE: Male pseudohermaphroditism: The complexities of male phenotypic development. Am J Med 61:261, 1976.

Imperato-McGinley J, Peterson RE, Gautier T, Sturla E: Androgens and the evolution of male gender identity among male pseudohermaphrodites with 5α-reductase deficiency. N Engl J Med 300:1233, 1979.

Josso N, Briard ML: Embryonic testicular regression syndrome: Variable phenotypic expression in siblings. J Pediatr 97:200, 1980.

Jost A: A new look at the mechanisms controlling sex differentiation in mammals. Johns Hopkins Med J 130:38, 1972.

Keenan BS, Kirkland JL, Kirkand RT, et al: Male pseudohermaphroditism with partial androgen insensitivity. Pediatrics 59:224, 1977.

Kershnar AK, Borut D, Kogut MD, et al: Studies in a phenotypic female with 17α-hydroxylase deficiency. J Pediatr 89:395, 1976.

Kirkland RT, Kirkland JL, Johnson CM, et al: Congenital lipoid adrenal hyperplasia in an eight-year-old phenotypic female. J Clin Endocrinol Metab 36:488, 1973.

Manuel M, Katayama KP, Jones HW Jr: Age of occurrence of gonadal tumors in intersex patients with a Y chromosome. Am J Obstet Gynecol 124:293, 1976.

Medina M, Chavez B, Perez-Palacios G: Defective androgen action at the cellular level in the androgen resistance syndromes. I. Differences between the complete and incomplete testicular feminization syndromes. J Clin Endocrinol Metab 53:1243, 1981.

Meisner LF, Inhorn SL: Normal male development with chromosome long arm deletion (Yq−). J Med Genet 9:373, 1972.

Meyer WJ III, Migeon BR, Migeon CJ: Locus on human X chromosome for dihydrotestosterone receptor and androgen insensitivity. Proc Natl Acad Sci 72:1469, 1975.

New MI: Male pseudohermaphroditism due to 17α-hydroxylase deficiency. J Clin Invest 49:1930, 1970.

Opitz JM, Simpson JL, Sarto GE, et al: Pseudovaginal perineoscrotal hypo-spadias. Clin Genet 31:1, 1971.

Pergament E, Heimler A, Shah P: Testicular feminization and inguinal hernia. Lancet 2:740, 1973.

Peterson RE, Imperato-McGinley K, Gautier T, et al: Male pseudohermaphroditism due to steroid 5α-reductase deficiency. Am J Med 62:170, 1977.

Pittaway DE, Anderson RN, Givens JR: Deficient 17β-hydroxysteroid oxireductase activity in testes from a male pseudohermaphrodite. J Clin Endocrinol Metab 43:457, 1976.

Reyes FI, Winter JJD, Faiman C: Studies on human sexual development. I. Fetal gonadal and adrenal sex steroids. J Clin Endocrinol Metab 37:74, 1973.

Rivarola MC, Bergada C, Cullen M: HCG stimulation test in prepubertal boys with cryptorchidism, in bilateral anorchia and in male pseudohermaphroditism. J Clin Endocrinol Metab 31:526, 1970.

Rosenberg HS, Clayton GW, Hsu TC: Familial true hermaphroditism. J Clin Endocrinol Metab 23:203, 1963.

Saenger P, Levine LS, Wachtel SS, et al: Presence of H-Y antigen and testis in 46,XX true hermaphroditism, evidence for Y chromosomal function. J Clin Endocrinol Metab 43:1243, 1976.

Sarto GE, Opitz JM: The XY gonadal agenesis syndrome. J Med Genet 10:288, 1973.

Schneider G, Genel M, Bongiovanni AM, et al: Persistent testicular $\triangle^5$-isomerase-3β-hydroxysteroid dihydrogenase ($\triangle^5$-3β-HSD) deficiency in the $\triangle^5$-3β-HSD form of congenital hyperplasia. J Clin Invest 55:681, 1975.

Schwartz M, Imperato-McGinley J, Paterson RE, et al: Male pseudohermaphro-ditism secondary to an abnormality in Leydig cell differentiation. J Clin Endo-crinol Metab 53:123, 1981.

Shanfield I, Young RB, Hume DM: True hermaphroditism with XX/XY mosaicism: Report of a case. J Pediatr 83:471, 1973.

Siiteri PK, Wilson JD: Testosterone formation and metabolism during male sexual differentiation in the human embryo. J Clin Endocrinol Metab 38:113, 1974.

Silvers WK, Wachtel SS: H/Y antigen behavior and function. Science 195:956, 1977.

Spear GS, Hyde TP, Gruppo RA, et al: Pseudohermaphroditism, glomeruloneph-ritis with the nephrotic syndrome, and Wilms' tumor in infancy. J Pediatr 79:677, 1971.

Stallings MW, Rose AH, Auman GL, et al: Persistent müllerian structures in a male neonate. Pediatrics 57:568, 1976.

Tourniaire J, et al: Male pseudohermaphroditism with hypertension due to a 17α-hydroxylation deficiency. Clin Endocrinol 5:53, 1976.

Turleau C, de Grouchy J, Dufier JL, et al: Aniridia, male pseudohermaphroditism, gonadoblastoma, mental retardation, and del 11 p13. Hum Genet 57:300, 1981.

Wachtel SS, Koo GC, Greg WR, et al: Serologic detection of a Y-linked gene in XX males and XX true hermaphrodites. N Engl J Med 295:750, 1976.

Walsh P, Madden JD, Harrdo MJ, et al: Familial incomplete male pseudoher-maphroditism, type 2. Decreased dihydrotestosterone formation in pseudova-ginal perineoscrotal hypospadias. N Engl J Med 291:944, 1974.

Wilkins L, Jones HW Jr, Holman G, et al: Masculinization of the female fetus associated with administration of oral and intramuscular progestins during gestation; non-adrenal female pseudohermaphroditism. J Clin Endocrinol Metab 18:559, 1958.

Winter JSD, Faiman C, Reyes FL: Sex steroid production by the human fetus: Its role in morphogenesis and control by gonadotropins. In: Blandau RJ, Bergsma D (eds): Morphogenesis and Malformation of the Genital System. Birth Defects: Original Article Series 13(2):41, 1977.

Wu RH, Boyer RM, Knight R, et al: Endocrine studies in a phenotypic girl with XY gonadal agenesis. J Clin Endocrinol Metab 43:506, 1976.

Zachmann M, Vollmin JA, Hamilton W: Steroid 17,20-desmolase deficiency. A new cause of male pseudohermaphroditism. Clin Endocrinol 1:369, 1972.

PEDIATRIC GYNECOLOGY AND ADOLESCENT ISSUES 19

PEDIATRIC GYNECOLOGY

See also Sec 2.13, 2.61, and 18.6.

Pediatric gynecology has long been neglected in the training of young physicians. Some of the problems are uncommon and require special attention. Others reflect new common concerns of our society related to increased sexual awareness and activity, sex education, and sexual abuse. Adolescents lead the nation in rate of rise of venereal diseases, particularly gonorrhea. Similarly, the birth rate continues to increase among teenagers.

Although there are approximately 40 million adolescents in the United States, they represent only 17% of visits to pediatricians' offices, and the average adolescent sees a doctor one third to one half as often as does a child under 4 yr of age. However, a number of so-called "adult" health problems may be present during adolescence in preclinical form, e.g., hypertension, hypercholesterolemia, and carcinoma in situ of the cervix. In addition, a variety of health problems may be related to the rapid growth and maturation which characterize puberty, such as scoliosis, slipped capital femoral epiphysis, Osgood-Schlatter disease, goiter, and acne. Surveys have revealed that the incidence of undiagnosed problems may be as high as 20%.

Violence, in the forms of accidents (Sec 5.43), homicides, or suicides (Sec 2.54), accounts for 70% of all deaths in this age group; neoplasms, 7%; and infectious disease or diseases of a congenital nature, 7%. Among the neoplasms, testicular tumors and tumors of bone and lymphatics are most prevalent. Rubella, rubeola, and infectious mononucleosis have their peak occurrence among adolescents. Chemical dependency (alcohol and drugs) and increased consumption of cigarettes continue to be major problems in the teenage population.

19.1 EXAMINATION OF THE GENITALIA

The examination of the genitalia should be part of a complete gynecologic assessment of children, which includes a general history and physical examination, assessment of growth and development, evaluation of sexual maturation (Sec 2.61), and the pelvic examination. An understanding of the child's stage of psychologic and cognitive development as well as the emotional state is critical to a sensitive and appropriate relationship during the examination and subsequently. A toddler being examined after traumatic sexual abuse may be fearful of pain when placed in an uncomfortable position but not cognizant of any sexual connotation of the examination. Evaluation of an adolescent girl requires appropriate concern for her sexual consciousness and feelings of privacy.

Position. The pelvic examination in the young child is best performed in that position most comfortable for both the physician and child. The classic lithotomy position used for adolescents and adults is not well received by most youngsters It is strange and often invokes fear in young children, requiring restraint by parents or assistants. The modified frog leg position with hips flexed and feet on the table is better received, but some advocate the Sims or the knee-chest position. In the latter position the abdomen faces the table and weight is supported on bent knees kept comfortably separated, 15–20 cm (6–8 in) apart, with the child's head resting on her hands and turned to 1 side. This allows good eye contact with physician, parent, or assistant and assists in overcoming anxiety and fear. It also permits a good view of the labia, hymen, vagina, and sometimes cervix without instrumentation.

When either the lithotomy or frog leg position is utilized, relaxation, comfort, and diminishing anxiety are critical for a successful examination. For adolescents, the lithotomy position is essential, especially if instrumentation is to be performed. Adequate draping and explanation are imperative. Many authorities recommend examining adolescents without the mother's presence. However, although privacy is critical for adolescents, especially when their sexual activities are being discussed, the presence of mother or friend may be extremely comforting to these young girls. Their preferences should be discussed with them and honored, including topics to be discussed as well as the method and extent of examination. A female assistant should be present with a male physician, not just for medical-legal protection but for important support to the adolescent girl. Some children of any age are best examined without the mother in attendance; these decisions are best made by a physician familiar with past parent-child interactions.

Specimens. Specimens for microscopic examination, wet preps, Pap smears, estrogen effect, and culture can be obtained using simple equipment. Vaginal secretions can be secured with a small, soft plastic eye dropper with light suction. A "butterfly" needle from which the needle has been removed from the tubing becomes an effective aspirating device by inserting the very small, soft plastic tube through essentially any hymenal opening. Insertion of 1–2 ml of sterile saline may facilitate aspiration. A dry cotton swab should not be used for these procedures, as the twisting motion necessary to insert such a swab into the prepubertal, dry vagina with its thin, noncornified epithelium may be very painful. A swab moistened with saline may be useful for obtaining cultures.

Instrumentation. A number of good instruments are available for vaginoscopy in prepubertal girls and virginal adolescents. For most purposes adequate illumination of the external genitalia and vagina can be obtained with an ordinary otoscope head without a speculum, although this will not be sufficient for a more detailed examination and visualization of the cervix, etc. The Cameron-Miller or Huffman-Huber fiberoptic vaginoscopes are expensive but easy to use with young children. They utilize cylindrically designed specula of varying lengths which are easy to insert and facilitate good visualization. Simple and less costly variants of these instruments are veterinary otoscope specula which come in lengths up to 7 cm and diameters up to 7 mm and fit on traditional Welch-Allyn otoscopes.

For older but virginal girls a Huffman-Graves virginal bivalved speculum is useful as it has been designed for the adolescent vagina which is almost of adult length but very narrow. Metal specula should be adequately warmed and lubricated with water and inserted on a 45 degree angle using a gentle rotary movement.

The Mini-Examination in Young Children. *Inspection* is one of the most useful components of the genital examination in young children. Adequate illumination, comfortable positioning, and cooperation are essential.

Superficial palpation of the labia and vagina is best done by depressing the perineum on either side of the labia with both thumbs or by gently pulling the labia apart. In the knee-chest position little manipulation may be required; simply holding the buttocks apart pressing laterally and slightly upward will provide good visualization.

Bi-manual examination is usually not possible and often, when it is possible, is not indicated. An alternative abbreviated examination placing the little or index finger in the rectum and palpating the abdomen with the other hand can provide considerable information regarding the identification of the uterus, masses, or hard foreign bodies in the vagina. The adnexa of young girls and early adolescents are very difficult to palpate.

19.2   DEVELOPMENTAL ABNORMALITIES PRESENTING IN THE NEWBORN PERIOD

The newborn infant must be carefully examined to determine the *morphology of the external genitalia.* Virilization of the female fetus in utero may lead to development of ambiguous genitalia (Sec 18.24), with varying degrees of masculinization. The most common etiology is congenital adrenal hyperplasia with virilization ranging from an enlarged clitoris to a distinct phallus (Sec 18.24). Chromosomal dysgenesis and several developmental hormonal defects may lead to varying degrees of discrepancy between the external and internal genitalia. Early recognition of ambiguous genitalia and etiologic diagnosis is important for treatment and for determination of sexual identity, which will govern parental child-rearing attitudes.

Imperforate hymen is generally not identified until menarche when the patient may present with amenorrhea, abdominal pain, and lower abdominal swelling with or without a bulging introitus. Occasionally it may

be identified in the newborn period by a bulging of the introitus due to the accumulation of vaginal secretions from the newborn's estrogenized vagina; the volume of secretions is generally small and may contain blood as the result of endometrial sloughing in response to withdrawal of maternal estrogens. Excision of the membrane is the treatment of choice; vaginal or biologic defects are rarely associated.

Congenital absence of vagina associated with normal labia is usually overlooked in the newborn period. In the 1st several mo of life many infant girls develop *adhesions of the labia* from recurrent or continuous irritation and inflammation (labial agglutination). Although this may suggest absence of the vagina, it is distinguished by a markedly translucent midline raphe at the site of adhesion. Local estrogen cream followed by good hygiene and elimination of irritation will reverse the adhesion. This may become a recurrent problem which resolves itself at puberty with the onset of endogenous estrogen stimulation. Rarely, urinary retention and infection occur, requiring immediate separation of the labia. If absolutely necessary, this can be accomplished using a well lubricated probe or cotton swab, followed by application of estrogen creams to maintain the separation.

19.3   INFECTIONS AND SKIN DISORDERS OF THE GENITALIA

Vulvovaginitis is the most common gynecologic problem of children and adolescents. It has numerous infectious and noninfectious etiologies. A variety of infectious agents are seen in both pre- and postmenarchal girls. The physiologic state of the vagina is the most important determinant of pathologic and nonpathologic vaginal flora.

Physiology of Vagina. At birth, the vagina, having been stimulated in utero by maternal estrogens, is hypertrophied with numerous layers of glycogen-containing stratified squamous epithelium. The pH is 5.5–7.0. This normal physiologic state results in the thick milky-white discharge seen during the 1st 3 wk of life which rapidly diminishes as estrogen stimulation ceases. From about 3 wk of age to immediately preceding menarche, the vaginal mucosa is atrophic, lacks glycogen, and has a neutral to alkaline pH (ranging from 6.5–7.4); it is an excellent culture medium for bacteria.

The anatomy of the prepubertal vagina lying close to the anus, lacking the pubic hair and thickened labial fat pads of the older girl, in conjunction with frequent poor hygiene, leads to repeated bouts of vulvovaginitis.

History and Physical Examination. Complaints will vary with the age of the child. The young child may rub and scratch the genitals and cry with voiding or defecation; the older child will describe itching and pain. Vaginal discharge is variable, and frequently it is not the 1st sign of vaginitis. There should be specific inquiries about foreign bodies which are commonly missed etiologic agents. Even the older girl may have a retained tampon or other paper product used as a substitute for a sanitary napkin. Contact irritants in-

Table 19-1 COMMON SKIN DISORDERS AFFECTING THE GENITALIA

	AGE	SYMPTOMS/INVOLVED AREA	APPEARANCE	MANAGEMENT
Seborrhea	Common <3 mo, may occur at any age	In folds of diaper area between labia minora and labia majora; pruritic, frequent secondary infection; often seborrhea elsewhere	Elevated red lesions with yellow, greasy scales	Hydrocortisone cream 1%; treat secondary infection
Psoriasis	Any age	Usually associated with disease elsewhere, pruritic	Variable sized, sharply demarcated, erythematous plaques with silvery scale on flat surface	Hydrocortisone cream 1%; Burow soaks if acute and exudative
Atopic dermatis	Any age	Common on surface areas in contact with offending agent; severe pruritus and secondary infection	Erythema; vesicles may be excoriated and exudative	Remove offending agent (clothes, diapers, perfumes); hydrocortisone cream 1%; Burow soaks if exudative; treat secondary infection
Lichen sclerosis	Any age; generally improves at puberty	Vulva and labia; chronic, severe pruritus	White parchment appearance of vulva, fissuring, easily traumatized	Hydrocortisone cream 1%; testosterone petrolatum 2% if severe

clude soaps, perfumes, feminine hygiene sprays, and clothing. The common use of synthetic fabrics and tight clothing such as leotards has added significantly to this problem. Antibiotics used for several wk preceding the onset of vaginal symptoms may alter vaginal flora, allowing colonization by organisms such as *Cantlida* which are more commonly seen in postmenarchal women. A family history of diabetes mellitus, of pinworms or other parasites, or of skin problems such as eczema, atopic dermatitis, psoriasis, or seborrhea may be important. This group of skin problems may accompany, aggravate, or trigger vulvovaginitis.

Clinical Manifestations. Disorders may affect primarily the skin and vulva or be the result of a true vulvovaginitis, and there is considerable overlap in the etiologies within these 2 categories. Table 19-1 reviews the most common skin disorders affecting the external genitalia; the effects are often only a component of a generalized skin disorder. Secondary infection in the perineal area of young children may result from contamination with urine and stool, making the diagnosis and therapy more difficult. Table 19-2 presents the most common viral and parasitic infestations of the perineum; these affect primarily the skin of the external

genitalia. Herpes simplex infection may have serious systemic manifestations and present a major risk to an infant born to an infected female. It has become 1 of the most prevalent venereal diseases among adolescents and adults. Table 19-3 summarizes the most common causes of vulvovaginitis.

Venereal diseases, primarily gonococcal infections (Sec 10.26), are seen with increasing frequency in the adolescent age group as a result of increased sexual activity. In girls, gonococcal infection is generally associated with intense redness and swelling of the vulva, a tender cervix, and a thick purulent discharge. Smear usually reveals gram-negative intracellular diplococci. Upper genital tract infection (pelvic inflammatory disease [PID]) is rare in prepubertal girls but is seen in adolescents and should be considered in the differential diagnosis of abdominal pain in these young girls. Other organisms, primarily *Chlamydia* and more rarely tuberculosis, actinomycosis, and ameba, are also associated with pelvic inflammatory disease. Gonorrheal infection should also be considered in the differential diagnosis of a vaginal discharge in prepubertal girls. It may occur as a result of sexual activity, sexual abuse, or occasionally close physical contact with an infected adult.

Table 19-2 COMMON INFECTIONS OR INFESTATIONS OF VULVA

AGENT	MENARCHAL Pre-	Post-	SOURCE	SYMPTOMS	DIAGNOSIS	MANAGEMENT
Herpes—herpes simplex virus type 2 primarily	±	+ +	Maternal contamination; venereal	Pruritus; small vesicles on erythematous base; ulcerations; may have systemic symptoms: fever, lymphadenopathy; dysuria	Inspection; scraping—multinucleated giant cells seen with Wright stain	No satisfactory therapy; sitz baths; local anesthetic; light therapy
Pediculosis pubis—*Phthirus pubis*, "crab lice"	–	+	Venereal or close contact	Pruritus	Inspection; lice; eggs (nits) attached to hair follicle	Gamma benzene hexachloride 1%
Molluscum contagiosum—DNA virus of poxvirus group	±	+	Veneral or close contact	Pruritus—autoinoculation from lesions elsewhere; may be secondarily infected	2–4 mm flesh-colored papules with central umbilication containing a "cheesy" plug	Spontaneous regression; curetted or cauterized
Scabies—mite, *Sarcoptes scabiei*	+	+	Close physical contact	Pruritic, present in other family members or sexual partners; small erythematous papules with wavy burrows	Scrapings or skin biopsy to visualize mite	Wash clothing and bedding; gamma benzene hexachloride 1%; crotamiton (Eurax)
Condylomata acuminata—papova-papilloma virus	±	+	Close physical contact or venereal	Dry, warty lesions on skin of labia, perineum, and vestibule associated with irritating vaginal discharge	Inspection	Podophyllin (20%) in tincture of benzoin at 2–4 wk intervals (not in pregnancy or young child); freezing; cauterization

Table 19-3   ETIOLOGY OF VULVOVAGINITIS

AGENT	MENARCHAL PRE	MENARCHAL POST	SOURCE	SYMPTOMS	DIAGNOSIS	MANAGEMENT
Nonspecific—Hemophilus vaginalis (Corynebacterium vaginale)	±	+	Normal flora potentially pathogenic; venereal	Few symptoms; gray-white, thick discharge; fishy odor	Wet prep—"clue cells" epithelial cells with organisms adherent to surface; culture-chocolate agar gram-negative bacilli	Vaginal sulfonamides, bid; metronidazole, 250 mg tid × 1 wk, PO; treat asymptomatic male consort
Trichomonas—flagellated parasite	±	+	Maternal colonization in newborn; venereal—male asymptomatic	Asymptomatic to severe; profuse watery, frothy, yellow-green discharge	Wet prep—flagellated organisms	Metronidazole, 250 mg tid × 1 wk, PO or 2 gms in single dose (contraindicated in pregnancy); use local—clotrimazole, 100 mg vaginal suppositories qd × 7 days; treat asymptomatic male consort
Candida—Candida albicans	±	+ +	Secondary—diabetes, antibiotics, skin disease, oral contraceptives, obesity; not venereal	Pruritic, thick cheesy discharge; red, edematous vulva	KOH prep—spores and hyphae; culture—Nickerson agar	Sitz baths; mycostatin—child, cream applied to vulva, adolescent, suppositories 1 bid × 14 days; hydrocortisone cream for severe symptoms and erythema; oral mycostatin if recurrent; gentian violet, 1% aqueous preparation, 3 ×/wk for 2 wk when above fails
Pinworms—Enterobius vermicularis	+ +	±	Poor hygiene; spread from anus	Pruritic, erythema	Scotch tape test to visualize ova	Mebendazole (Vermox), 1 tab, PO
Foreign body	+ +	+	Foreign body, tampon	Foul-smelling discharge; secondary bacterial infection	Examination, rectal x-ray for opaque foreign body	Removal; good hygiene

Syphilis is uncommon (Sec 10.55) but must be investigated in sexually promiscuous adolescents, rape victims, and sexually abused young girls.

19.4 Neoplasms

Accurate statistics regarding gynecologic neoplasms in infancy and childhood are not available. All types are rare, and only individual case reports or small series have been reported. No consolidated reporting has been instituted, except for diethylstilbestrol (DES)-exposed females. Therefore, routine gynecologic examination of otherwise normal young girls and adolescents for detection of neoplasm prior to menstruation and established sexual activity is not medically indicated or cost effective. Pelvic examination should be limited to those presenting with unusual genital lesions, abnormal genital bleeding, vaginal discharge, tissue protruding from the vagina, unexplained abdominal swelling, or abnormalities of growth.

The most common gynecologic neoplasms of children are of ovarian origin and generally present as an abdominal mass. These are highly malignant, and vigorous investigation with tissue diagnosis is necessary to plan treatment and to preserve ovarian function. Rarely, the vagina and vulva may be the sites of benign or malignant lesions in childhood. Benign lesions include mesonephric duct cysts, paraurethral cysts, and simple inclusion cysts. The most common malignant lesions of the vagina is the clear cell adenocarcinoma associated with diethylstilbestrol exposure in utero. (See also Chapter 15.)

19.5 DES-EXPOSED FEMALES

From 1940–1960's, in an attempt to prevent fetal wastage a number of women were treated with diethylstilbestrol (DES) during pregnancy. The association between DES and clear cell adenocarcinoma was first identified in 1971 when a statistically significant association was described between this therapy and the occurrence of vaginal adenosis and subsequent malignancy in offspring of these women in a retrospective epidemiologic survey. Subsequently the Food and Drug Administration recommended that DES not be used in pregnancy, a centralized registry was established, and a large cooperative study of adenosis was carried out.

The incidence of adenosis (the presence of mucinous columnar cells and/or metaplastic squamous cells with or without mucinous droplets in vaginal scrapings) varies from 20–90% depending on the following variables: (1) whether the term adenosis is defined to include cervical as well as vaginal abnormalities; (2) time of DES exposure in utero (more frequent if given prior to 18th wk); (3) length and dose of exposure; (4) age of index case; and (5) method of selection of exposed subjects (lowest rates in those identified by retrospective review of medical records and highest in self-referred women). Although women exposed to DES in utero are at greater risk for vaginal adenosis and development of clear cell adenocarcinoma, they are not at increased risk for invasive squamous cell carcinomas; the increase of squamous cell dysplasia appears to be the result of healing and aging.

Appropriate management of women exposed to DES in utero starts with a complete history, including evaluation of prenatal records. A pelvic examination of all exposed women should be performed by age 14 yr or after menses by an experienced gynecologist. This should include meticulous inspection and palpation of the entire vagina, cytologic samples from the vagina and cervix, iodine staining (½ strength Lugol solution) of the vagina, and colposcopy and direct biopsy of any suspicious lesions. Subsequently, similar examinations should be performed every 1–2 yr unless an abnormality is found. Treatment of clear cell adenocarcinoma is radical with vaginectomy, hysterectomy, and lymphadenectomy. Survival rates are 80% overall and 90% in those identified with Stage I disease. Ovarian function is generally preserved. New therapies combining surgery, radiation, and chemotherapy are being evaluated, but clear advantages have not yet been demonstrated.

It is suspected that these women may have increased rates of miscarriage, premature births, infertility, and menstrual irregularities. In males exposed to DES in utero there appears to be a greater incidence of hypoplastic testes, epididymal cysts, testicular capsular induration, and alterations in sperm production, but no increased risk for neoplasms has been demonstrated.

19.6 PREPUBERTAL VAGINAL BLEEDING

A number of conditions in young girls are associated with vaginal bleeding, including estrogen withdrawal in the newborn, severe vulvovaginitis, foreign bodies, and genital neoplasms. Several others deserve special comment.

Traumatic lesions are common in young girls associated with physical activity such as fence or straddle injuries. Sexual abuse is discussed in Sec 2.67. If not extensive, simple tears of the vagina and vulva heal readily without scarring and require only supportive and symptomatic treatment including cold compresses, local anesthetics, and antibiotic creams for superficial infections. If bleeding is persistent or trauma is known to be more extensive with or without visible signs, a complete vaginal examination must be performed, under anesthesia if necessary. Puncture or other penetrating wounds are of particular concern as rectal perforation and urethral or bladder injuries are possible; if suspected, appropriate investigation is required.

Urethral prolapse may occur in prepubertal girls because adequate supporting tissue of the distal urethra is in part dependent on estrogen stimulation. It is seen most commonly with extreme straining leading to increased intra-abdominal pressure as may occur in temper tantrums, but it may occur spontaneously. Irritation and excoriation with bleeding of the friable mucosa may be mistaken for vaginal bleeding. Usually the prolapse is self-limited and repair is rarely necessary. The diagnosis may be made by passing a urinary catheter into the bladder. Associated urologic anomalies or complications are rare.

Precocious puberty results in true menstrual bleeding although at an unexpectedly early age. Problems associated with early menarche are discussed in Sec 18.7 and 18.42.

Sarcoma botryoides (Sec 15.11) arises from the upper vagina and cervix and generally presents with a bloody vaginal discharge. This is a highly malignant lesion and survival is rare. Any diagnosis of vaginal polyps in the young child should suggest sarcoma botryoides which must be specifically ruled out. Radical surgery of vagina, cervix, and uterus may be required. Radiation and chemotherapy are being evaluated.

I. BRUCE GORDON

Bibbo M, Gill WB, et al: Follow-up study of male and female offspring of DES exposed mothers. Obstet Gynecol 49:1, 1977.

Billmire ME, Farrell MK, et al: A simplified procedure for pediatric vaginal examination. Use of veterinary otoscope specula. Pediatrics 65:823, 1980.

Cowell CA (ed): Symposium on Pediatric and Adolescent Gynecology. Pediatr Clin North Am 28:245, 1981.

Emans SJ, Goldstein DP: Pediatric and Adolescent Gynecology. Boston, Little, Brown and Co, 1977.

Emans SJ, Goldstein DP: The gynecologic examination of the pre-pubertal child with vulvovaginitis. Pediatrics 65:758, 1980.

Eschenbach DA: Epidemiology and diagnosis of acute pelvic inflammatory disease. Obstet Gynecol 55 Suppl:142, 1980.

Hammerschlag MR, Alpert S, et al: Microbiology of the vagina in children: Normal and potentially pathogenic organisms. Pediatrics 62:57, 1978.

Herbst AL: Clear cell adenocarcinoma and the current status of DES-exposed females. Cancer 48 (Suppl):484, 1981.

Herbst AL, Hubby MM, et al: A comparison of pregnancy experience in DES-exposed and DES-unexposed daughters. J Reprod Med 24:62, 1980.

Herbst AL, Scully RE, et al: Complications of prenatal therapy with diethylstilbestrol. Pediatrics 62:1151, 1978.

Jacobs AH (ed): Symposium on Pediatric Dermatology. Pediatr Clin North Am 25:189, 1978.

Robboy SJ, et al: Dysplasia and cytologic findings in 4589 young women enrolled in diethyl-adenosis (DESAD) project. Am J Obstet Gynecol 140:579, 1981.

Shafer MB, et al: Acute salpingitis in the adolescent female. J Pediatr 100:339, 1982.

Singleton AF: Vaginal discharge in children and adolescents. Clin Pediatr 19:799, 1980.

19.7 DISORDERS OF MENSTRUATION

19.8 Menometrorrhagia

Excessive menstrual bleeding is one of the few gynecologic emergencies of adolescence. Bleeding may be severe enough to cause hypovolemia and anemia and is always frightening to the young adolescent. Diagnosis and therapy must be accomplished expeditiously while reassurance is given to the worried patient and her family.

Painless Bleeding

Dysfunctional uterine bleeding or excessive menstrual bleeding is most often secondary to the anovulatory cycles which normally occur in the 1st 2 yr postmenarche. In the absence of ovulation, the effect of estrogen on the endometrium is unopposed by progesterone; the continued endometrial proliferation results in eventual massive shedding. The continued estrogen effect also serves to inhibit the LH surge responsible for ovulation, thus perpetuating the problem. FSH levels are usually higher than LH around the time of menarche. Basal body temperature determinations will reveal absence of ovulation.

Treatment is necessary only when significant bleeding continues; it is directed at correcting the estrogen-progesterone imbalance, as well as providing the hemostatic effect of exogenous estrogens. The immediate administration of 25 mg Enovid orally has the advantage of causing rapid cessation of bleeding, typically within 2 hr, although the patient may become nauseated. The dose is then tapered by 5 mg daily until a daily dose of 5 mg is reached. The patient is kept on this dose (1 tablet) daily for the duration of a 21-day cycle, calculating the cycle from the day treatment began. If bleeding should recur at any point in the tapering cycle, the previous day's dose is resumed and tapering not resumed until bleeding stops. A normal menstrual period should begin 1–2 day after the last pill is taken. On the 5th day of bleeding a 3 mo course of oral contraceptive therapy should be initiated (with a preparation containing 50 μg of estrogen and 1 mg of progestin) utilizing the same cycling used for contraceptive purposes. If the patient is sexually active, she may be continued on oral contraceptives, being cognizant of the increased risk of post-pill amenorrhea in those adolescents who had anovulatory cycles prior to initiation of oral contraceptive therapy. An alternative to the initial high dose Enovid therapy is oral administration of Ortho-Novum (2 mg) or Enovid-E (2.5 mg) every 4 hr until the bleeding slows or stops, after which it is given twice daily until the dispenser is finished. In the rare patient whose bleeding cannot be brought under control by 1 of these approaches, an endometrial curettage may be indicated. Although this procedure is frequently undertaken in adult women with menometrorrhagia, the rarity of endometrial pathology (such as carcinoma) and the usual effectiveness of hormonal therapy in the adolescent markedly limit its indications.

Far less frequently, excessive vaginal bleeding in the adolescent may be associated with a bleeding diathesis such as *von Willebrand disease* (Sec 14.58). This condition should be suspected when there is excessive bleeding at the onset of the 1st menstrual period and a prolonged bleeding time. Although the pathophysiology of bleeding is different, the same approach to management as for dysfunctional uterine bleeding is effective; therapy may be required for the entire premenopausal life of the patient. *Ingestion of aspirin* in therapeutic doses within 14 days of menses may also produce excessive menstrual flow. *Thrombocytopenia* resulting from toxins, marrow infiltration, hypersplenism, or the idiopathic variety (ITP) may be complicated by menometrorrhagia, but it is rarely the presenting symptom. Treatment as described for dysfunctional uterine bleeding is effective in combination with platelet transfusions for those whose bleeding is secondary to thrombocytopenia or to thrombopathies.

A common *hormonal cause* of excessive vaginal bleeding in the adolescent is the improper use of oral contraceptives agents. Some who harbor the mistaken belief that the pills are to be used only when intercourse is experienced or others who interrupt a cycle before its completion may experience this symptom. A history of intermittent ingestion may not be readily volunteered, out of embarrassment or the desire to protect a friend whose pills were shared. Hypothyroidism (Sec 18.12), if acquired after menarche, is often associated with excessive menstrual bleeding as well as increased frequency of menses. Occasionally, menometrorrhagia may be the 1st sign. Rarely, hyperthyroidism, adrenal dysfunction, diabetes mellitus, and estrogen-secreting ovarian tumors may be associated with this symptom.

Painful Bleeding

Approximately 15% of pregnancies in the 15–19 yr age group terminate in *spontaneous abortion*. Therefore, in any adolescent with heavy, painful vaginal bleeding, this diagnosis should be considered. History of unprotected intercourse, symptoms of pregnancy, and physical evidence of an enlarged uterus are suggestive of abortion. A serum β-subunit HCG will remain positive for 10–15 days although urine pregnancy tests may become negative from 5–8 days after abortion. Dilation

and curettage is often necessary to stop the bleeding and ensure complete evacuation of the uterine contents.

Ectopic pregnancy may rarely present with excessive vaginal bleeding, although typically it is associated with amenorrhea. Unilateral adnexal tenderness or mass should suggest this diagnosis, which demands immediate surgical intervention.

Lacerations of the genital tract induced by 1st or forceful intercourse or trauma must always be considered in the adolescent with painful, heavy vaginal bleeding. The circumstances of the injury may be embarrassing or frightening for her, requiring a gentle and caring approach. Involvement of the gynecologist is necessary as examination can be coupled with suturing and resolution of the bleeding.

For *toxic shock syndrome* see Sec 10.24.

For *sexually transmitted disease*, see appropriate section in Chapter 10.

19.9   Dysmenorrhea

Painful menstrual cramps are experienced by nearly two thirds of postmenarchal teenagers in the United States; more than 10% of this group suffer sufficiently to miss school, making dysmenorrhea the leading cause of short-term school absenteeism in female adolescents. Dysmenorrhea may be primary or secondary, the former being the more common. Secondary dysmenorrhea results from an underlying structural abnormality of the cervix or uterus, a foreign body such as an intrauterine device (IUD), or a disease entity such as endometriosis or endometritis. Primary dysmenorrhea refers to painful menstrual cramps without any associated abnormality. Although dysmenorrhea was long thought to be a psychosomatic symptom, research has now implicated prostaglandins $F_{2\alpha}$ and E_2 in its pathogenesis. These substances, produced in the endometrium, are capable of smooth muscle stimulation. Their concentration is higher in women suffering from dysmenorrhea than in controls, and their suppression by agents which inhibit prostaglandin synthetase is associated with alleviation of cramps. Dysmenorrhea may be successfully treated by the use of oral contraceptives to inhibit ovulation and its resultant progesterone sensitization of the myometrium to the effects of prostaglandins. This approach is advisable for adolescents who are also in need of contraception. An alternative is the administration of pharmacologic agents which inhibit prostaglandins such as aspirin (500 mg, 4 times daily for 3 days prior to the expected menstrual period) or, for those with irregular menses, naproxen sodium (275 mg every 6 hr on the 1st day of menstruation).

19.10   Amenorrhea

Absence of menses is a common concern among adolescents. Amenorrhea may be primary (never menstruated) or secondary (missed 4 or more menstrual periods). The range of normal for menarche is broad (from 10.5–16 yr) with a mean age of 12.5 yr and is influenced by familial pattern, ethnic origin, body weight, nutrition, and presence of chronic illness or blindness. Accordingly, a diagnosis of primary amenorrhea is usually not entertained until the otherwise normal appearing adolescent is over 16 yr, has not menstruated within 4 yr of onset of secondary sex characteristics, or is more than 1 yr older than her mother was at menarche.

Primary Amenorrhea

This may result from a number of chromosomal, endocrinologic, or structural defects. In order to determine its etiology, it is helpful to classify the condition according to associated findings. Primary amenorrhea in the absence of other signs of pubertal development may be associated with chronic illness, such as inflammatory bowel disease or cyanotic congenital heart disease; gonadal dysgenesis associated with chromosomal anomalies (Sec 18.30); hypogonadotropic hypogonadism (Sec 18.33); and ovarian failure secondary to earlier therapy with irradiation or cyclophosphamide. Central nervous system tumors, most commonly a craniopharyngioma (Sec 21.18); hyperthyroidism (Sec 18.15); and anorexia nervosa (Sec 2.50) may also present in this manner.

Primary amenorrhea in the presence of signs of pubertal development is usually due to a structural abnormality of the genitalia. *Imperforate hymen* associated with recurrent abdominal pain is the most frequent of these and, as it progresses, is frequently accompanied by a midline lower abdominal mass (the blood-filled vagina, "hematocolpos"). Diagnosis is made by inspection of the introitus, revealing a bulging hymen with bluish discoloration. Primary amenorrhea may also be due to *cervical stenosis;* the external examination will be normal, but the blood-filled uterus (hematometrium) will be apparent at bimanual examination. History and pregnancy test will distinguish this condition from the rare occurrence of pregnancy prior to menarche. Even less common is *agenesis of the cervix* or *uterus,* which may accompany anomalies of the urinary tract or sacral agenesis. Diagnosis is suspected on physical examination and confirmed by ultrasonography. In all of these cases the presence of intact ovarian function will result in normal gonadotropin levels. The presence of high FSH and LH in the patient with some signs of pubertal development, particularly those which are androgen, rather than estrogen, dependent, should suggest the diagnosis of gonadal dysgenesis with mosaicism, a condition diagnosed by obtaining chromosomal analysis (Sec 6.11). Another reason for performing a karyotype is the rare possibility of testicular feminization in an XY individual with normal gonadotropin levels (Sec 18.46). Disorders associated with primary amenorrhea in the absence of signs of pubertal development may also present in those with some signs of puberty.

Primary amenorrhea in the presence of signs of virilization such as clitoromegaly, hirsutism, or excessive acne suggests adrenal tumors (Sec 18.27), congenital adrenal hyperplasia (Sec 18.24), or rare virilizing ovarian tumor such as a Sertoli-Leydig cell or lipoid cell tumor. Hermaphroditism, gonadal dysgenesis, or incomplete testicular feminization may also present in this way.

Secondary Amenorrhea

This is defined as cessation of menses for 4 mo or more in an individual with previously regular monthly menstrual periods. Pregnancy is suggested by a history of sexual activity, nausea, breast tenderness, pigmentation of nipples and linea alba, cyanosis and softening of the cervix, and an enlarged uterus. Confirmation with a β-subunit human chorionic gonadotropin analysis of a blood sample is the most sensitive and specific of tests now available. Phenothiazines, propranolol, oral contraceptives, and heroin have also been shown to cause amenorrhea, either by interference with hypothalamic monoamine synthesis or by affecting gonadotropin production. Psychogenic factors such as the stress of going away to camp or school have been implicated in the etiology of certain cases of secondary amenorrhea. It is often difficult to separate these from nutritional factors as weight loss is a common confounding variable in many of these cases, e.g., anorexia nervosa.

Endocrinopathies involving pituitary, thyroid, or adrenal glands, similar to those discussed above in connection with primary amenorrhea, may also be responsible for secondary amenorrhea if acquired after menarche. Ovarian tumors, which are feminizing or masculinizing, should also be considered in the differential diagnosis of secondary amenorrhea.

Polycystic ovary syndrome (Stein-Leventhal) previously thought to be limited to obese, hirsute, infertile older women has more recently been identified with increasing frequency in young, otherwise normal-appearing adolescents with secondary amenorrhea or oligomenorrhea. Typically, FSH is normal with elevated LH levels (more than twice that of FSH), and histologically thickened tunica albuginea and ovarian cysts are observed. The elevated LH levels may stimulate excessive estrogen production by the ovaries and cause the histologic findings as well as amenorrhea. (See also Sec 18.39.)

When the cause of amenorrhea cannot be established by history, physical examination, lateral skull roentgenogram, and hormonal and chromosomal studies, ultrasonography may be helpful in confirming the presence and size of uterus and ovaries and of tumor and cysts. Also, ovarian biopsy in conjunction with laparoscopy is often helpful in diagnosing amenorrhea; Anteby et, using laparoscopy as the initial procedure, made the diagnosis in 14 of 37 cases of primary and 38 of 87 cases of secondary amenorrhea.

Diagnosis of the etiology of amenorrhea may permit initiation of specific therapy. However, when the underlying cause may not lend itself to remediation, consideration should then be given to establishing regular pseudo-menses in order to allow the adolescent to feel like her peers. If a vaginal smear is positive for estrogen effect, regular cycling can be accomplished using medroxyprogesterone in a dose of 10 mg orally, on days 17–21 of the cycle.

19.11 THE BREAST

Breast development is the obvious sign of female puberty (Sec 2.14). Accordingly, it is more often the focus of attention than are the other pubertal manifestations, and *asymmetric* growth or development of the breasts during puberty is a common cause of anxiety. In most instances, wearing a padded bra is sufficient, and completion of development will equalize the discrepancy. Rarely, however, the asymmetry is so marked as to cause severe self-consciousness and interfere with normal peer relations. In such cases, consideration should be given to corrective surgery. Both augmentation and reduction mammoplasty are possible, but should not be done prior to completion of breast growth, that is, before sex maturity rating 5 is reached.

Presence of a *mass* is another common problem usually discovered in the process of breast self-examination. The majority of these masses are cysts or benign fibroadenomas. A cyst will vary in size over the course of the menstrual cycle so that the patient should be re-examined 2 wk after the initial examination. Persistence of the tumor or its enlargement over several menstrual cycles is an indication for surgical consultation. Aspiration is generally attempted under local anesthesia and may be diagnostically and therapeutically conclusive. If fluid is not obtained, an excisional biopsy is performed. The incision should be circumareolar to prevent a disfiguring scar. In a series of biopsies performed on adolescents with breast masses at Montefiore Hospital, 71 were found to be fibroadenomas, 2 cystosarcoma phylloides, and 11 abscesses. Carcinoma of the breast in the adolescent is sufficiently rare and the risks of mammography sufficiently serious to preclude its use in this age group.

Multiple small lumps in the breast suggest *fibrocystic disease*. Because these patients may be more prone to develop other forms of breast disease, they should be taught careful self-examination. Combination oral contraceptives may be beneficial in such patients and should be considered if birth control is indicated.

Discharge from the nipple is less common than either masses or asymmetry and in this age group is due to nipple manipulation, oral contraceptives or other medications, and pregnancy. Rarely, it is encountered in association with amenorrhea (Chiari-Frommel, Forbes-Albright, Del Castillo syndromes), a pituitary neoplasm, infection, or breast neoplasm. Benign conditions are associated with a milky or sticky and thick discharge, infection with a purulent one, and intraductal papilloma and cancer with serous, serosanguineous, or bloody discharge. Elevation of serum prolactin may be found in the amenorrhea-galactorrhea syndromes; may be associated with the use of certain antihypertensives, oral contraceptives, and tranquilizers; or may occur secondary to a pituitary neoplasm. Infection in the non-breast-feeding adolescent is rare.

19.12 PREGNANCY PREVENTION

There were 1 million pregnancies among adolescents in 1978, and 600,000 of those resulted in live births. By 13 yr of age, 10% of females in the United States have experienced intercourse, and 33% of sexually active females become pregnant before 19 yr of age. In addition, one third to one half of rape victims are adolescents, who are thereby placed at risk for pregnancy. The emotional, physical, educational, and economic toll of pregnancy in this age group makes knowledge of preventive techniques imperative. While delaying intercourse may be the best advice, it is unrealistic; pediatricians should thus be able to counsel the sexually active teenager about contraception. It is appropriate and necessary to inquire about sexual activity in all females who have entered puberty and to do so giving assurance of confidentiality.

The discovery of unprotected intercourse is an indication for discussion of contraception. However, first it is important to explore with the young patient her feelings about the risk of pregnancy as well as her perception about the reasons she has not yet become pregnant. Many teenagers feel invulnerable to the risk of pregnancy; others desire pregnancy, and some are convinced that they are sterile because past intercourse did not result in pregnancy. These issues must be raised and accurate information provided in order to motivate adolescents to accept and continue to use contraception properly. The method of contraception should then be individualized to the needs of each adolescent.

Barrier Methods

Condom. There are no major side effects, but the effectiveness of the condom in preventing pregnancy is low, with 15 pregnancies occurring/100 adult woman years. There may also be lack of acceptance because of perceived or actual decrease in sensitivity for the male partner. The main advantages are low price, availability without prescription, little need for advanced planning, and effectiveness in preventing transmission of venereal diseases. In a 1979 study 23% of 15–19 yr old females reported condom use by their partner.

Diaphragm. This acts by preventing access of sperm to the cervix while placing spermicidal jelly in a position to be effective. Aside from rare instances of contact vaginitis caused by the latex or powder, the diaphragm has no associated side effects. It is effective in only 85% of women who use it properly over a 1 yr period of time. In 1 study of adolescents who were highly motivated to avoid pregnancy, however, diaphragm use was associated with only 2 pregnancies/100 woman years. Adolescents may object to the messiness of the jelly or to the fact that diaphragm insertion may interrupt the spontaneity of sex, or they may express discomfort about touching their genitalia. The college health service at Stanford University reports that this method is currently used by 21% of sexually active women students, while only 3.5% of 15–19 yr olds studied by Zelnik and Kantner chose this method.

A diaphragm must be fitted individually. Once fitted, the same diaphragm may be used for 3 yr unless extreme weight gain or loss or pregnancy occurs. After the proper diaphragm is selected, it is important that the teenager be given instruction and ample opportunity to insert and remove it before leaving the office.

Cervical Cap. Currently under evaluation, this is a rubber cap which, after proper fitting, remains affixed to the cervix by suction for 1–3 days of an intermenstrual period.

Chemical Methods. A variety of agents containing the spermicide nonoxynol have been developed and are available as foams, jellies, or effervescent vaginal suppositories which must be inserted shortly before intercourse and repeated prior to each subsequent ejaculation. Side effects are minimal, consisting of only contact dermatitis; but effectiveness is only about 85%. However, nonoxynol is gonococcidal and spirocheticidal.

Gossypol. Developed and widely used in China, this cottonseed derivative results in temporary male infertility; it is not approved for use in the United States. Lack of data on long-term effects should preclude its use in adolescents at this time.

Combination Methods. Combination of condom by the male and spermicidal foam by the female is extremely effective, resulting in a pregnancy rate of only 2% in studies of adult couples. In addition, it is effective in preventing transmission of venereal disease.

Hormonal Methods

Available preparations consist of either an estrogenic substance in combination with a progestin or a progestin alone. The mechanism of action of the estrogen-progestin combination is to prevent the surge of luteinizing hormone and, as a result, to inhibit ovulation. While the progestin alone may also prevent ovulation, it does not reliably do so. However, it does effect fallopian tube transport and composition of cervical mucus.

Combination Oral Contraceptives. Commonly referred to as "the pill," these are available containing either 80, 50, or 35 μg of the estrogenic substance, typically either mestranol or ethinyl estradiol. Thrombophlebitis, hepatic adenomas, myocardial infarction, and carbohydrate intolerance are some of the more serious associated complications. Other side effects, such as hypertension, are not clearly related to either the estrogen or progestin alone. A beneficial increase in high density lipoproteins also occurs in adolescent users.

The long term consequences of use of oral contraceptives beginning in adolescence are still unknown; however, concern over long term effects of these agents has led to utilization of smaller amounts of estrogen. Estrogen use has the potential for limiting pubertal growth. A period of anovulation and amenorrhea twice that observed for adult women, lasting as long as 18 mo following discontinuation of pill use by adolescents, has been another concern. There is evidence, however, that ovulation will return but that underweight teenagers or those with oligomenorrhea prior to initiation of pill use are at greater risk for post-pill amenorrhea. The pill remains the most reliable contraceptive method available, with a pregnancy rate in the range of 0.8%. With the use of the 35 μg preparation there may be a higher incidence of breakthrough bleeding leading to noncompliance.

All-Progestin Contraceptives. For the adolescent in whom use of estrogen is potentially deleterious (e.g., those with liver disease, replaced cardiac valves, or hypercoagulable states), an all-progestin, so-called "mini-pill" is available. It is less reliable in inhibiting ovulation and is associated with a 2.4% pregnancy rate. The necessity to take the pill daily, plus the higher incidence of associated amenorrhea or, conversely, increased bleeding, frequently limits its acceptance by some adolescents.

An injectable progestin, medroxyprogesterone (Depo-Provera), is a highly effective agent for birth control. The fact that this substance need be administered only once every 3 mo and is completely reversible in its anovulatory action, coupled with the cessation of menses coterminous with its use, makes this a particularly attractive contraceptive for adolescents who have difficulty with compliance or for retarded teenagers. It is not available for use as a contraceptive in the United States because of concern over its apparent association with breast tumors in experimental animals.

Postcoital Contraception. Unprotected intercourse at mid-cycle carries a pregnancy risk of 2–30%. This risk may be reduced or eliminated within 72 hr after unprotected intercourse by either hormonal or mechanical methods. The so-called "morning after" pill, DES (diethylstilbestrol), is a nonsteroidal synthetic estrogen which is administered in an oral dose of 25 mg twice daily for 5 days, beginning within 72 hr of intercourse. It reduces the risk of pregnancy to about 4%. The potential teratogenic effect of DES in producing genital anomalies and malignancies makes it necessary to consider therapeutic abortion if pregnancy occurs in a DES-treated female. Alternatively, ethinyl estradiol, in a dose of 2.5 mg twice daily for 5 days, is being used, but its safety has not been established.

Intrauterine Device (IUD). IUD's are small, flexible, plastic objects introduced into the uterine cavity through the cervix. They differ in size, shape, and the presence or absence of pharmacologically active substances (such as copper or progesterone). The mechanism of action of the IUD is uncertain, but they are effective in preventing pregnancy in 97–99% of women. Expulsion rates in adolescent nulliparas are comparable to those of parous women. Women who become pregnant with an IUD in place are at greater risk for having an ectopic pregnancy; the risk is greatest in those having a progesterone-containing IUD.

Additional problems associated with IUD use are increased menstrual bleeding (less a factor with the newer smaller IUD's such as Copper-7); increased dysmenorrhea (which may, however, be decreased by use of progesterone-containing devices); and increased risk of infection. There is a higher incidence of salpingitis when women using an IUD are compared retrospectively to women hospitalized for other reasons.

The insertion of a copper-7 intrauterine device provides long-term contraception as well as emergency protection.

OTHER ADOLESCENT ISSUES

19.13 SUBSTANCE ABUSE DURING ADOLESCENCE

Epidemiology. Substance abuse is not a new adolescent phenomenon; an outbreak of ether inhalation by teenagers was reported in the latter half of the 19th century in Ireland. However, the types of drugs abused and the resulting medical and psychosocial consequences continue to change. During the decade of the 1970's, a heroin epidemic in the United States claimed many adolescent victims. From a peak of 58% of heroin users among a drug-using population identified in a juvenile detention facility in New York City in 1970, the proportion fell to 4% by 1977, corresponding to a nationwide decrease in hepatitis and overdose deaths. However, there has been a concurrent increase in abuse of a variety of other substances by adolescents since 1970.

Marijuana and alcohol are currently the most common psychoactive agents used by teenagers with estimates varying from 50–90% with an approximately equal frequency in both sexes. It has been reported that 6% of high school seniors use alcohol daily. Stimulant use has remained fairly constant, with cocaine gaining ascendency in the latter half of the 70's. Phencyclidine (PCP) is now considered the 3rd most popular drug of abuse in the United States. Another pattern that has emerged is the poly-drug user, the youngster who will ingest whatever drug is available, typically in combination with others.

Etiology. A number of factors contribute to the initial decision to use a substance of abuse such as the desire to explore the limits of emotionality; the need to try on new "adult" roles; the wish to expand one's consciousness; availability, coupled with peer pressures; and a desire to escape. Continued use of a drug after the 1st experience usually indicates a more serious problem. Drug use is more prevalent among depressed teenagers. Similarly, the seriousness of the problem may be inferred from the type of drug used, the circumstances and frequency of its use, the premorbid setting, and the adolescent's functional status (Table 19–4). In general, use of opiates, hard liquor, or sedatives or any drug by injection should be viewed as high-risk behavior. Substance abuse on a weekday, particularly before or instead of school, is more serious than that which occurs only on weekends. The use of any drug when the teenager is alone and/or depressed suggests a more significant problem than its occurrence in a group context. In addition, the adolescent who uses a psychoactive substance in conjunction with operating a motor vehicle or the one whose school attendance and/or grades have fallen off is in need of immediate counseling for his or her own protection.

Pathophysiology. The process of physical growth and development which characterizes puberty may be adversely affected by the use of drugs. In adolescent females who utilized heroin, for example, one third have secondary amenorrhea, even in the absence of associated weight loss. It is postulated that the higher incidence of menstrual abnormalities noted in the adolescent heroin users is the result of the greater vulnerability of the hypothalamic-pituitary-ovarian axis in the maturing individual. Another possible contributing factor relates to the effect of certain psychoactive drugs on sleep stages; the release of gonadotropins in stage 4 sleep in the early adolescent may be inhibited by substances such as amphetamines which interfere with that sleep stage. Deriving calories largely from ethanol during the peak of pubertal growth spurt deprives the body of protein necessary for growth of muscles. Malnutrition, although rarely observed among adolescent drug users, may also interfere with establishing normal menstrual cycles.

The metabolism of certain drugs prescribed for adolescents may be affected by coincident abuse of drugs and alcohol (Table 19–5). Induction of hepatic smooth endoplasmic reticulum by barbiturate or alcohol may result in accelerated metabolism and hence excretion of those substances requiring glucuronidation, such as estrogen-containing oral contraceptives. The adolescent relying on this method of birth control may, in fact, be vulnerable to pregnancy if she is abusing either of these substances. Conversely, those on "the pill" are at a greater risk of intoxication from alcohol as estrogens decrease the rate of ethanol metabolism. The potentiating interaction of alcohol and barbiturates must also be taken into consideration when prescribing anticonvul-

Table 19–4 ASSESSING THE SERIOUSNESS OF ADOLESCENT DRUG ABUSE

	0	+1	+2
Age	>15	<15	
Sex	Male	Female	
Family history of drug abuse		+	
Setting of drug use	In group		Alone
Affect before drug use	Happy		Sad
School performance	Good/improving	Always poor	Recently poor
Use before driving			×
History of accidents			×
Time of week	Weekend	Weekdays	
Time of day		After school	Before school
Type of drug	Marijuana, beer, wine	Hallucinogens, amphetamines	Whiskey, opiates, cocaine, barbiturates

Total score: 0–3 less worrisome; 3–8 serious; 8–18 very serious.

Table 19–5 INTERACTIONS BETWEEN ALCOHOL AND PRESCRIPTION DRUGS

ADDITIVE (REDUCE DOSE)	CROSS-TOLERANT (NEED HIGHER DOSE)	ANTAGONISTIC (ANTABUSE-LIKE EFFECT)
Salicylates	Chloroform	Metronidazole
Acetaminophen	Fluorinated anesthetics	Isoniazid
Antihypertensives	Ether	Chloramphenicol
Anticoagulants (acute intoxication)	Anticoagulants (chronic intoxication)	Griseofulvin
Antihistamines		Cefamandole
Barbiturates		
Benzodiazepines	Phenytoin	Moxalactum
Phenothiazines		
Propoxyphene		

sant medications. A more immediate and dramatic interaction occurs when metronidazole is ingested by an alcohol-abusing adolescent because of the antagonistic effect of alcohol on acetaldehyde.

Psychosocial Sequelae. Youth may engage in robbery, burglary, drug-dealing, or prostitution for the purpose of acquiring the money necessary to buy drugs or alcohol. Regular use of any drug will eventually diminish ability to function in school, to hold a job, or to operate a motor vehicle. An "amotivational" syndrome has been described in chronic marijuana users who lose interest in age-appropriate behavior.

Opiates

Heroin and methadone are the opiates most subject to abuse by adolescents because of greater availability. Heroin, derived from the opium poppy *Papaver somniferum*, is a bitter crystalline powder which produces euphoria and analgesia. It is hydrolyzed to morphine, which undergoes hepatic conjugation with glucuronic acid before being excreted, usually within 24 hr of administration. It can be detected by thin layer chromatography up to 48 hr following administration.

The route of administration influences the timing of onset of action. When the drug is inhaled ("snorting"), it will require almost 30 min until the desired effect is achieved. By the subcutaneous route ("skinpopping"), the effect is achieved within minutes; and when injected intravenously ("mainlining"), it has an almost instantaneous effect. A larger dose can be administered by the intravenous route. Tolerance is first developed to the euphoric effect, whereas it is rare for an individual to become tolerant to the inhibitory effect on smooth muscle, typically manifested by constipation or miosis.

Clinical Manifestations. The pharmacologic effects of heroin, or its adulterants, combined with the conditions and route of administration are responsible for the manifestations in major organ systems.

The cerebral effect is manifested by the sought-after euphoria, diminution in pain, and sleep-like EEG pattern. Coma, depressed respiration, miosis, and tachycardia are characteristically found, while seizures and increased intracranial pressure may complicate overdosages. An effect on the hypothalamus is suggested by the lowering of body temperature. In addition, the lack of sterile technique in the injection process is responsible for the occurrence of multiple cerebral microabscesses, usually caused by *Staphylococcus aureus*.

Transverse myelitis of the thoracic segments has been reported in patients resuming heroin use after a period of abstinence, suggesting a possible hypersensitivity reaction. Rarely, Guillain-Barré syndrome and toxic amblyopia, the latter presumably due to the quinine additive, are found in heroin addicts. Brachial and lumbosacral plexitis and poly- and mononeuropathies, the latter manifested by ankle or wrist drop, are the more common peripheral neurologic findings.

Acute *rhabdomyolysis* with myoglobinuria may occur in association with intravenous injection of heroin and is manifested by generalized muscle tenderness, edema, and marked weakness of extremities. Necrotizing fasciitis is a rare complication after subfascial injections of heroin. Another rare complication is contractures of the fingers resulting from infection and scarring medial to the proximal interphalangeal joint secondary to injection into the small veins of the hand, such injections necessitated by sclerosis of the larger veins or used to avoid detection by authorities.

Vasodilation is a major cardiovascular manifestation related to the method of administration of the drug. Lack of antisepsis with parenteral administration is responsible for the occurrence of endocarditis with a high incidence of infection with coagulase-positive *Staphylococcus aureus*, involvement of the tricuspid valve, and high mortality. Rare complications of parenteral heroin administration include arteriovenous fistula, arterial and venous thrombosis, embolism, necrotizing arteritis, and mycotic aneurysm.

Respiratory depression is caused by heroin's effect on the central nervous system and is characterized by alveolar underventilation with a fall of arterial oxygen tension and saturation. In addition, particles of cotton fibers or nonsoluble adulterants inadvertently injected with the heroin are responsible for granulomatosis and pulmonary fibrosis which may result in pulmonary hypertension and decrease in lung volume and in diffusing capacity. Pulmonary edema is common in the *overdose syndrome* and may occur in association with intranasal as well as parenteral administration. Although it is invariably found in those who die of heroin overdose, it may occur as an incidental roentgenologic finding in an otherwise asymptomatic adolescent. Pulmonary infections have not been a prominent finding in adolescent heroin users.

The most common dermatologic lesions are the so-called "tracks," the hypertrophic linear scars which follow the course of large veins. Smaller, discrete peripheral scars, resembling healed insect bites, may be easily overlooked. In the adolescent who injects heroin subcutaneously, fat necrosis, lipodystrophy, and atrophy over portions of extremities may be found. Attempts at concealment of these stigmata may include amateur tattoos in unusual sites. Abscesses secondary to unsterile techniques of drug administration are commonly found.

The mechanism for the reported loss of libido is unknown. The female heroin user may resort to prostitution to support the habit, adding the risk of venereal disease and pregnancy to other sequelae.

Urinary retention may result from increased tone of the detrusor muscles, and constipation may result from the drug's ability to decrease smooth muscle propulsive contractions and to increase anal sphincter tone. The practice of swallowing the cotton used as a filter for heroin solutions or a condom or balloon filled with heroin to escape detection may result in intestinal obstruction or sudden, often fatal, overdosage if the container opens.

Hepatic enzymes are frequently elevated in heroin users, and the majority have serologic evidence suggesting viral infection with hepatitis B. Elements of chronic-aggressive hepatitis on biopsy and persistence of enzyme elevations suggest a poor prognosis in some patients.

Elevations in IgM are consistently noted in parenteral heroin users, while IgA elevations are reported in those who inhale the drug. Abnormal serologic reactions are also common, including false-positive VDRL and latex fixation tests. Depression of lymphocyte response to stimulation by mitogens in culture has also been demonstrated. The significance of these findings is confused by the high incidence of viral hepatitis.

After a period of 8 hr or more without heroin, the addicted individual will undergo over a course of 24–36 hr a series of physiologic disturbances referred to collectively as "withdrawal" or the *abstinence syndrome.* The earliest sign is yawning, followed by lacrimation, mydriasis, insomnia, and "gooseflesh," cramping of the voluntary musculature, hyperactive bowel sounds and diarrhea, tachycardia, and systolic hypertension. The occurrence of grand mal seizures is rare in adolescent addicts. A short course of diazepam is effective and safe for heroin detoxification in our experience. An oral dose of 10 mg every 6 hr for 3 days is recommended for those with mild withdrawal (no evidence of gastrointestinal hypermotility or change in vital signs) within 24 hr of last dose of heroin or prophylactically for those known to be addicted. For moderate withdrawal (evidence of gastrointestinal effect or change in vital signs), treatment is begun with the intramuscular administration of 2 doses of 10 mg of diazepam given 4 hr apart followed by the oral regimen. For severe withdrawal, 10 mg of diazepam is administered intramuscularly every 4 hr for a 24-hr period followed by oral administration. Insomnia is not eliminated by this regimen, but hypnotics should not be administered as they are ineffective and may lead to a new addiction.

An alternative to diazepam is methadone. This synthetic opiate is effective by the oral route and is pharmacologically similar to heroin with the exception of its lack of euphoric effect. An initial oral dose of 10 mg is administered and repeated every 6 hr, not to exceed 40 mg daily, if withdrawal symptoms reappear or do not abate. On the 2nd day, the same dose is administered; thereafter, the daily dose is reduced by 20%. Treatment should not extend beyond 21 days as only licensed methadone maintenance programs are authorized for prolonged administration. Neither the safety nor the dosage of methadone has been established for the pediatric age group.

The *overdose syndrome* is an acute reaction following administration of heroin. It is the leading cause of death among drug users. The rapidity of onset, eosinophilia after recovery, and the fact that it occurs only in those who have used the drug previously suggest an allergic mechanism. The clinical signs include stupor or coma, miotic pupils (unless severe anoxia has occurred), respiratory depression, cyanosis, and pulmonary edema. The differential diagnosis includes central nervous system trauma, diabetic coma, hepatic (and other) encephalopathy, Reye syndrome, as well as overdose of alcohol, barbiturates, PCP, and other agents, including methadone. Diagnosis of opiate toxicity is facilitated by intravenous administration of the opiate antagonist naloxone, 0.01 mg/kg (a vial of 0.4 mg usually suffices for an adolescent), which will cause dilatation of pupils constricted by an opiate; diagnosis is confirmed by the finding of morphine in the blood. Treatment consists of maintaining adequate oxygenation and continued administration of naloxone every 5 min as necessary to improve and maintain adequate ventilation. Naloxone may have to be continued for 24 hr if methadone, rather than shorter-acting heroin, was taken.

Hallucinogens

A number of naturally occurring and synthetic substances have been used by adolescents for their hallucinogenic properties. Some which enjoyed popularity in the past, such as LSD, have been shunned by the current generation for others which are equally dangerous, such as PCP. Marijuana is the most popular, although phencyclidine use is increasing.

Phencyclidine (PCP, sternyl, angel dust, "hog," "peace pill," "sheets") is an arylcyclohexalamine. Part of its popularity relates to its ease of synthesis in home laboratories, with a minimum of expense; however, this may result in contamination by a toxic byproduct which causes cramps, diarrhea, and hematemesis. The drug is thought to potentiate adrenergic effects by inhibiting neuronal re-uptake of catecholamines. PCP is available as a tablet, liquid, or powder which may be used alone or sprinkled on cigarettes ("joints"). The powders and tablets generally contain 2–6 mg of PCP, while "joints" average 1 mg PCP for every 150 mg of tobacco leaves, or approximately 30–50 mg per joint.

Symptoms are dose related with euphoria, nystagmus, ataxia, and emotional lability occurring with doses of 1–5 mg within 2–3 min after smoking and lasting for hours. Hallucinations may involve bizarre distortions of body image which often precipitate panic. In the range of 5–15 mg a toxic psychosis may occur in association with disorientation, hypersalivation, and abusive language lasting for more than 1 hr after consumption. Above 15 mg the patient usually becomes comatose within 30 to 60 min after oral administration, with alternating periods of wakefulness, dystonic posturing, muscular rigidity, or myoclonic jerks. Hypotension, generalized seizures, and cardiac arrhythmias commonly occur with plasma concentrations from 40–200 μg/dl. Death from hypertension, hypotension, hypothermia, seizures, and trauma occurring during psychotic delirium is reported. The coma of PCP may be distinguished from that of the opiates by the absence of respiratory depression; the presence of muscle rigidity, hyperreflexia, and nystagmus; and lack of response to naloxone. PCP psychosis may be difficult to distinguish from schizophrenia. In the absence of history of use, analysis of urine must be depended upon.

Management of the PCP-intoxicated patient includes placement in a darkened, quiet room on a floor pad, safe from injury. Diazepam, in a dose of 10–20 mg orally or 10 mg intramuscularly every 4 hr, may be helpful if the patient is agitated and not comatose. Ammonium chloride, 500 mg every 6 hr, may be given orally or by nasogastric tube to maintain urinary pH at 5.5–6, which enhances urinary clearance of PCP. Supportive therapy of the comatose patient is indicated with particular attention to hydration, which may be compromised by PCP-induced diuresis.

Marijuana and **alcohol** are presently the most popular drugs of abuse among adolescents. In contrast with most other drugs discussed, these agents are abused as frequently by the well-adjusted as by the alienated youth in our society. However, there is a high correlation between marijuana use and incidence of drunkenness in 7th–12th graders, and drinking and marijuana smoking have similar psychosocial correlates such as poor school performance, lower expectations for academic achievement, generally deviant behavior, greater value placed on independence than academic achievement, and less compatibility between parents and friends.

These substances also share some similar psychopharmacologic qualities in that both decrease short term memory, reaction time, and fine coordination and produce "mental clouding," as assessed by the Smith and Beecher questionnaire; testing has shown 300 mg of cannabis to be equivalent to about 70 gm of alcohol. Alcohol use is generally legal for those over 18–21 yr, whereas in many states the use of marijuana by anyone constitutes a criminal act punishable by incarceration. In the remaining states possession of small amounts (from 1–3.5 oz) constitutes a civil offense punishable by a fine, and only larger amounts involve criminal penalties.

Marijuana (THC, "pot," "hash," "grass") is synthesized from the resin of the *Cannabis sativa* plant, which flourishes in temperate and hot, dry climates. The tetrahydrocannabinol (THC) fraction of the resin is responsible for its hallucinogenic properties and has been synthesized (delta-9-THC). THC is rapidly absorbed by the nasal or oral routes, producing a peak of subjective effect at 10 min and 1 hr, respectively. Marijuana is generally consumed as a "reefer" or "joint," made by rolling the crushed plant material in paper. Although there is much variation in content, each marijuana cigarette contains approximately 1 gm of marijuana or 20 mg of delta-9-THC.

Clinical manifestations: In addition to the "desired" effects of elation and euphoria, marijuana may cause impairment of short-term memory, poor performance of divided attention tasks such as those involved in driving, loss of critical judgment, and distortion of time perception. Visual hallucinations and perceived body distortions occur rarely, but there may be "flashbacks" or recall of frightening hallucinations experienced under marijuana's influence which occur usually during stress or with fever.

Temperature may be lowered. Tachycardia is apparent within 20 min of smoking marijuana and is followed by transient systolic and diastolic hypertension ½ hr later, which disappears by 3 hr. Tachypnea is observed only in the chronic user. In placebo-controlled studies of experienced users smoking marijuana caused hypercapnic ventilation and a decrease in forced expired volume, maximal mid-expiratory flow rate, airway conductance, and diffusing capacity. Reduction in bronchospasm has also been demonstrated. Both delta-9-THC and marijuana (smoking a single "joint") cause a significant fall in intraocular pressure, lasting up to 5 hr in normals as well as in subjects with glaucoma.

Dose-related suppression of plasma testosterone and spermatogenesis as a result of smoking marijuana for a minimum of 4 days/wk for 6 mo was demonstrated by Kolodny, prompting concern over the potential deleterious effect of smoking marijuana before completion of pubertal growth and development. Smoking marijuana for 1 week also increases glucose intolerance. There is an antiemetic effect of oral THC or smoked marijuana, often followed by appetite stimulation, which is the basis of the drug's use in patients receiving cancer chemotherapy. Although the possibility of teratogenicity and carcinogenesis has been raised because of findings in lower animals, there is no evidence for such effects in humans. Nor is there proof of physiologic dependency.

Alcohol use among adolescents has increased over the past decade and poses a threat to the normal functioning of the teenager as well as to the lives of those potentially jeopardized by drunken drivers. The usual progression is from beer to wine to hard liquor; 4 oz of hard liquor (86 proof alcohol) consumed on an empty stomach will produce a plasma level of approximately 65 mg/dl in an adult male and 80 mg/dl in a premenstrual female. The legal definition of intoxication in the United States is a blood level of 200 mg/dl (0.2%).

Pathophysiology: Alcohol is ethyl alcohol or ethanol (C_2H_5OH), a substance which is rapidly absorbed from the stomach, transported to the liver, and metabolized by 1 of 2 pathways. The primary pathway involves removal of 2 hydrogen atoms to form acetaldehyde, a reaction catalyzed by alcohol dehydrogenase through reduction of a cofactor NAD. The removed hydrogen atoms supply energy (7.1 calories/gm of alcohol) and contribute to the synthesis of excess triglycerides, a phenomenon which is responsible for producing a fatty liver, even in those who are well nourished. Engorgement of hepatocytes with fat causes necrosis, triggering an inflammatory process, so-called alcoholic hepatitis, which is followed by fibrosis, the hallmark of cirrhosis. Early hepatic involvement may result in elevations in gamma glutamyl transpeptidase and serum glutamic pyruvic transaminase; cirrhosis has been reported in native American adolescents. The 2nd metabolic pathway which is utilized at high serum alcohol levels involves the microsomal system of the liver in which the cofactor is reduced NADPH. The net effect of activation of this pathway is to decrease metabolism of drugs which share this system and to allow for their accumulation and hence enhance their effect, e.g., drinking alcohol and ingesting tranquilizers results in potentiation of each and greater toxicity (Table 19–5).

Clinical manifestations: Alcohol acts primarily as a central nervous system depressant. It produces euphoria, grogginess, talkativeness, and impaired short-term memory, and it increases the pain threshold and the time needed to brake a car under simulated driving conditions. Alcohol's ability to produce vasodilation and hypothermia is also centrally mediated. At very elevated serum levels, respiratory depression occurs. Its inhibitory effect on release of antidiuretic hormone by the posterior pituitary is responsible for its well-known diuretic effect.

The most common gastrointestinal complication of alcohol use is acute erosive gastritis, which is manifested by epigastric pain, anorexia, vomiting, and guaiac-positive stools. Less commonly, vomiting and mid-abdominal pain may be caused by acute alcoholic pancreatitis; diagnosis is confirmed by the finding of an elevated serum amylase and lipase.

Physiologic dependence upon alcohol may develop in the adolescent who uses it on a daily basis over a period of weeks. In such individuals, alcohol deprivation may precipitate a *withdrawal syndrome* whose manifestations in adolescents are generally mild, occurring within 8 hr of the last dose of alcohol and lasting no longer than 48 hr in the untreated patient. Anxiety, tremor, insomnia, and irritability are common symptoms. Only rarely are severe reactions found in older adolescents who have been drinking steadily for 1 yr or more; these consist of auditory or visual hallucinations, hyperthermia, delirium, and seizures occurring 48 hr or more after the last drink. Treatment of the alcohol withdrawal or abstinence syndrome is based on utilization of drugs which are cross-tolerant with alcohol but which have a longer duration of action such as benzodiazepine derivatives, of which chlordiazepoxide (Librium) is the most popular. The usual regimen consists of an initial oral dose of 25 mg every 6 hr. If a satisfactory effect is not achieved, the dose is repeated at 2-hr intervals. Once symptomatic relief is obtained, the dose is tapered by 25 mg daily.

The *alcohol overdose syndrome* should be suspected in any teenager who appears disoriented, lethargic, or comatose. While the distinctive aroma of alcohol may assist in diagnosis, confirmation by analysis of blood is recommended. At levels above 200 mg/dl the adolescent is at risk, and levels above 500 mg/dl are usually associated with a fatal outcome (LD_{50}). There is high correlation between results obtained by serum and by breath analysis (r—0.956) so that the latter method may also be used. The usual mechanism of death is respiratory depression so that artificial ventilatory support must be provided until the liver can eliminate sufficient amounts of alcohol from the body. In the nonalcoholic it generally takes 20 hr to reduce the blood level of alcohol from 400 mg/dl to zero. Dialysis should be considered when the blood level is higher than 400 mg/dl. When the level of depression appears excessive for the reported blood level, head trauma or ingestion of other drugs should be considered.

Sniffing of **volatile substances** such as airplane glue enjoyed wide popularity among young adolescents from the inner cities in the late 1950's and 1960's. Although hepatic and renal abnormalities did not occur in this group, others who inhaled cleaning fluid (Carbona) containing 1,1,1,trichloroethane and trichloroethylene experienced the sudden onset of vomiting, abdominal pain, and jaundice. Severe hepatotoxicity, often complicated by oliguria, or anuria, and elevated blood urea nitrogen levels also occurred with such cleaning fluid inhalations. Many heroin-using adolescents claim to have begun their drug use with glue-sniffing. Sniffing of toluene-containing substances such as paints, lacquer thinners, and various household glues has also been associated with renal tubular acidosis; glues containing n-hexane have caused polyneuropathies.

Gasoline sniffing is popular among rural adolescents and American Indian youths and may cause ataxia, nausea, and loss of consciousness. Euphoria followed by violent excitement and then coma may result from prolonged or rapid inhalation. The long-term effects of chronic exposure include irreversible encephalopathy and bone marrow aplasia (from benzene) and lead encephalopathy when tetraethyl lead is added.

Inhalation of aerosol products, such as hair sprays, deodorants, frypan lubricants, and cocktail glass chillants has also become popular. This method of dispensation involves pressurizers, fluorocarbon propellants known as Freons, which have been implicated as the cause of cardiac sensitization to epinephrine resulting in arrhythmias and death in those who inhale it.

A variety of volatile nitrites such as amyl nitrite, butyl nitrite, and related compounds marketed as room deodorizers are used as euphoriants, enhancers of musical appreciation, and aphrodisiacs among older adolescents and adults. They may result in headaches, syncope, and lightheadedness; in profound hypotension and cutaneous flushing followed by vasoconstriction and tachycardia; in transiently inverted T waves and depressed S-T segments in ECG; and in methemoglobinemia, increased bronchial irritation, and increased intraocular pressure. Their potential for producing carcinogenic nitrosamines has not been evaluated.

Cocaine is the most expensive of the inhalants. The alkaloid extracted from the leaves of the South American *Erythroxylon coca* is supplied as the hydrochloride salt in crystalline form. It is rapidly absorbed from the nasal mucosa, detoxified by the liver, and excreted in the urine as benzoyl ecgonine. Its half-life is slightly more than 1 hr, yet social custom often dictates its repeated administration every 15 min. The perceived effect of "snorting" cocaine may be influenced by some of the many diluents now being added to or actually substituted for the drug, e.g., heroin, amphetamines, PCP, or fillers such as mannitol or quinine. Cocaine causes euphoria, increased motor activity, decreased fatigability, and, occasionally, paranoid ideation. Its sympathomimetic properties are responsible for tachycardia, hypertension, and hyperthermia. The chronic user may develop tolerance to these physiologic effects and psychologic dependence may occur. Withdrawal symptoms upon its discontinuation have not, however, been reported.

19.14 LEGAL ISSUES IN ADOLESCENT CARE

In the United States the right of a minor to consent to treatment without parental knowledge is governed by various state laws. In all states, however, self-consent is granted when there is suspicion of a venereal disease. Since such disease is often asymptomatic, this provision in the various public health codes is often interpreted as enabling the physician to perform a pelvic examination on any sexually active adolescent solely upon her own consent. In many states, adolescents may consent to receive care for drug abuse or mental health problems. The minor's right to contraceptives has not been reviewed by the Supreme Court, although the minor's right to privacy has been upheld and the majority of states now permit the provision of contraceptives to teenagers upon their own consent. The right to obtain an abortion without parental consent or over parental objections is unsettled.

With the exception of Delaware, which has an age limit of 17 yr, all other states require that an individual be 18 yr of age in order to consent to blood donation. Organ donation by a consenting minor generally requires parental consent as well as a court order to ensure that there is no adult alternative donor, that the transplant is absolutely necessary in order to save the life of the recipient, and that the adolescent will not suffer physically or psychologically as a result of the procedure.

In addition, minors are exempt from the requirement of parental consent for medical treatment under the following circumstances: (1) Emancipated minors—those who live away from home, are no longer subject to parental control, are economically self-supporting, are married, or are members of the military. (2) Emergencies. In a medical emergency a minor may be treated without consent of parents if, in the physician's judgement, the delay resulting from attempts to contact them would jeopardize the life or health of the minor. (3)

The Mature Minor Rule. An emerging trend in the law is the recognition that many minors are sufficiently mature to understand the nature of their illness and the potential risks and benefits of proposed therapy and, therefore, should receive such treatment upon their own consent. In these cases the physician should document that the adolescent has acted in a responsible manner.

IRIS F. LITT

Pregnancy and Contraception

Eleven Million Teenagers: What Can Be Done About the Epidemic of Adolescent Pregnancies in the United States. Planned Parenthood Federation of America, Inc., 1976.
Hatcher RA, Stewart GK, Stewart F, et al: Contraceptive Technology, 1980–1981. Ed 10. New York, Irvington Publishers Inc., 1980.
Sorenson RC: Adolescent Sexuality in Contemporary America. New York, World, 1973.
Zelnik M, Kantner JF: Sexual activity. Contraceptive use and pregnancy among metropolitan-area teenagers: 1971–1979. Fam Planning Perspect 12:230, 1980.

Substance Abuse

Burns RS, Lerner SE: Perspectives: Acute phencyclidine intoxication. Clin Toxicol 9:477, 1976.
Donovan JE, Jessor R: Adolescent problem drinking. Psychosocial correlates in a national sample study. J Studies Alcohol 39:1506, 1978.
Garriott J, Petty CS: Death from inhalant abuse: Toxicological and pathological evaluation in 34 cases. Clin Toxicol 16:305, 1980.
Jessor R, Chase JA, Donovan JE: Psychosocial correlates of marijuana use and problem drinking in a national sample of adolescents. Am J Publ Health 70:604, 1980.
Kolodny RC, Masters WH, Kolodner RM, et al: Depression of plasma testosterone after chronic intensive marijuana use. N Engl J Med 290:872, 1974.
Lieber CS: The metabolism of alcohol. Sci Am 234:25, 1976.
Litt IF, Cohen MI: The drug using adolescent as a pediatric patient. J Pediatr 77:195, 1970.
Louria DB, Hensle T, Rose J: The major medical complications of heroin addiction. Ann Intern Med 67:1, 1967.
Mayer J, Filstead WJ: The adolescent alcohol involvement scale. J Studies Alcohol 40:291, 1979.
Sigell LT, Kapp FT, Fusaro GA, et al: Popping and snorting volatile nitrites: A current fad for getting high. Am J Psychiatry 135:1216, 1978.

Legal Issues

Holder AR: Legal Issues in Pediatrics and Adolescent Medicine. New York, John Wiley & Sons, 1977.

SEXUAL MISUSE

See also Sec 2.67.

Sexual misuse, which always existed, is now being identified and addressed more often. It includes child molestation, incest, and rape. Physician understanding, sensitivity, appropriate inquiry, treatment, and adequate follow-up are critical to maintaining the well-being of the misused child. Victims of child molestation have a median age of 11 yr, but molestation has often involved preschool girls. Young boys as well as girls are subject to sexual misuse. Family members, including close relatives, neighbors, and friends account for 30–50% of all incidents. Very few children are molested by strangers. Adolescent victims account for over 30% of reported cases of rape, with a large percentage sustaining significant genital injury. Incest often starts before adolescence and may continue throughout this period with associated severe psychologic disturbances.

Rape should be viewed as more than physical assault, although this is what usually brings the victim to the physician's attention. The "rape trauma syndrome" as described by Burgess and Holmstrom includes 2 phases of psychologic adaptation: (1) the acute phase of disorganization, and (2) the long term phase of reorganization. This is particularly relevant when dealing with adolescent rape victims. Sensitivity to the patient's feelings and needs should be maintained while meeting the medical-legal requirements, which include (1) detailed history of the event, (2) physical examination with emphasis on trauma and visible signs of rape, and (3) laboratory data to confirm rape, such as the presence of sperm.

Treatment for rape victims includes (1) repair of trauma, (2) prophylactic treatment for venereal disease and appropriate related diagnostic tests, (3) pregnancy prophylaxis with diethylstilbestrol in postmenarchal girls at risk for pregnancy, and (4) appropriate counseling for emotional problems and pregnancy if it occurs.

I. BRUCE GORDON

Burgess AW, Holmstrom LL: Rape trauma syndrome. Am J Psychiatry 131:981, 1974.

CONVULSIVE DISORDERS 20

20.1 ALTERED STATES OF CONSCIOUSNESS

Consciousness can be defined as the state of awareness, including responsiveness to stimulation, and ability to recall past events. When alterations in consciousness occur in a child, the physician who first sees the patient will need to judge the severity of the condition, its acuteness, any immediate threat to life, and the possibility of the condition's worsening in the near future. History should be elicited regarding possible trauma, accident, acute or chronic illness, and use of drugs. Evidence of head trauma, shock, crush injuries, seizures, hypoglycemia, "stroke," and infection will be of major concern. Following whatever immediate intervention is indicated, more detailed neurologic examination, further history, and additional therapy can be considered. Changes in condition must be carefully recorded and decisions made concerning what facilities will be needed for further care.

The above steps in care are often provided by a single physician; intensive care of a serious problem is less likely to be his or her sole responsibility. Facilities and resources needed may be sophisticated, or the size and age of the patient may call for special instrumentation. Consultation with other physicians may be essential, and results of laboratory tests may indicate modification of an initial therapeutic program.

Altered awareness will be harder to assess if the child is known to have a developmental disability or if the prior states of health and function are not known. Parents or caretakers can often help define a child's prior abilities and what alterations of speech or affect have occurred.

Children may need evaluation while awake or drowsy, in light or deep sleep, or in stupor or coma. The depth of natural sleep can be assessed with electroencephalographic (EEG) findings. Assessment of deep normal sleep may be difficult in a child who may also be in the postictal phase of a recent seizure, have a history of recent head injury, or have a past history of diabetic acidosis. Altered states of consciousness may require exquisite judgment as to how to avoid doing either too little or too much.

The assessment of the comatose child is discussed in Sec 21.6.

The most common cause of sudden transient loss of consciousness is a convulsive disorder due to a disturbance of the central nervous system. Less frequent are syncopal attacks, which are presumed to be circulatory in origin, and breath-holding episodes; these may be difficult to distinguish from convulsions. Syncopal episodes are more likely to be preceded by anxiety and excitement. Clonic movements can occur in both syncopal attacks and breath-holding episodes. An accurate history, the occurrence of postictal sleep, and the EEG help distinguish among these.

20.2 CONVULSIVE DISORDERS

Convulsive phenomena are common in children and occur with a wide variety of disorders of the central nervous system. Seizures may be classified according to (1) their cause or pathogenesis (Table 20–1), (2) their clinical manifestations (Table 20–2), or (3) their electroencephalographic patterns.

Incidence. Consideration of the relative incidence of the various causative factors at different ages is frequently helpful in arriving at a correct diagnosis and in evaluating prognosis.

Convulsions are far more common during the 1st 2 yr than at any other period of life. Intracranial birth injuries, including the effects of anoxia and hemorrhage and congenital defects of the brain, are the most frequent causes of convulsions in very young infants. In the later part of infancy and in early childhood acute infections (extracranial and intracranial) are the most frequent causes. Far less frequent causes in infants are tetany, idiopathic epilepsy, hypoglycemia, brain tumors, renal insufficiency, poisoning, asphyxia, spontaneous intracranial hemorrhage and thrombosis, postnatal trauma, and others listed in Table 20–1.

By midchildhood acute extracranial infections have become an infrequent cause of convulsions, and idiopathic epilepsy, first appearing as an important cause of convulsions about the 3rd yr of life, becomes the most common factor. Other causes after infancy are congenital defects of the brain, residual cerebral damage from earlier trauma, infection, lead poisoning, brain tumors, acute or chronic glomerulonephritis, certain degenerative diseases of the brain, and drug ingestion.

20.3 Acute or Nonrecurrent Convulsions

Convulsions in the Newborn Infant. A clinical seizure at any age is associated with a paroxysmal burst of electrical activity within the central nervous system. In the newborn infant the electrical activity of the cerebral hemispheres is underdeveloped; subcortical rhythms are present. Mass myoclonic movements have been reported to occur in utero, but the tonic and clonic movements that characterize grand mal seizures are rarely apparent during the 1st several wk of life. The low incidence of grand mal seizures reported during

Table 20–1 ETIOLOGIC CLASSIFICATION OF CONVULSIVE DISORDERS

I. **Acute or nonrecurrent forms**
   "Febrile convulsions" (e.g., at onset of acute extracranial infections or in association with high environmental temperatures)
   Intracranial infections (e.g., acute meningitis, encephalitis, sinus thrombophlebitis, cerebral abscess, malaria, typhus fever)
   Intracranial hemorrhage (e.g., from birth or other trauma, hemorrhagic disease, rupture of defective vessels, sickle cell disease)
   Toxic:
   1. Convulsant drugs (e.g., aminophylline, antihistamines, camphor, propoxyphene, pentylenetetrazol, phenothiazine, hexachlorophene, corticosteroids, strychnine, and thujone)
   2. Tetanus
   3. Lead encephalopathy
   4. Shigellosis, salmonellosis
   Anoxic (e.g., sudden severe asphyxia, inhalation anesthesia)
   Metabolic or nutritional (e.g., acute hypocalcemia and hypomagnesemic tetany, hyponatremia and hypernatremia, alkalosis, therapeutic hypoglycemia, pyridoxine deficiency, phenylketonuria, copper deficiency [Menkes], maple syrup urine disease, hyperammonemia, argininuria, argininosuccinic aciduria, hyperlysinemia, tyrosinemia, glycinemia)
   Organic acidurias (propionic, lactic, green acyl dehydrogenase deficiency)
   Acute cerebral edema (e.g., in acute glomerulonephritis or allergic edema of the brain)
   Brain tumor
   Miscellaneous (porphyria, systemic lupus erythematosus)
II. **Chronic or recurrent forms**
   Epilepsy:
   1. Idiopathic (primary, cryptogenic, essential or genuine epilepsy)
      a. Hereditary or genetic type
      b. Nongenetic or acquired idiopathic type (?)
   2. Organic (secondary or symptomatic epilepsy—with residual brain damage from previous focal or diffuse injuries)
      a. Post-traumatic (e.g., from direct laceration of brain tissue)
      b. Posthemorrhagic (e.g., from injury at birth or later, from hemorrhagic diseases, pachymeningitis, rupture of miliary aneurysm)
      c. Postanoxic (e.g., from severe asphyxia neonatorum)
      d. Postinfectious (e.g., following encephalitis, meningitis, sinus thrombophlebitis, or abscess)
      e. Post-toxic (e.g., kernicterus, encephalopathy following lead, arsenic, or other chronic poisoning)
      f. Degenerative (e.g., "idiopathic atrophy," cerebromacular degeneration, encephalitis periaxialis diffusa, intracranial neurofibromatosis, incontinentia pigmenti)
      g. Congenital (e.g., cerebral aplasia, porencephaly, tuberous sclerosis, hydrocephalus, vascular anomalies such as the Sturge-Weber type, and arteriovenous aneurysms)
      h. Parasitic brain disease (cysticercosis, toxoplasmosis, syphilis)
      i. Posthypoglycemic injury
   3. Sensory (reading, touch, light, sound, music, self-induced)
   Epilepsy-simulating states:
   1. Narcolepsy and cataplexy
   2. Hysteria ("psychogenic epilepsy")
   Tetany:
   1. Hypocalcemic (e.g., idiopathic, postoperative, neonatal, vitamin D deficiency, deficient intestinal absorption)
   2. Of alkalosis (e.g., vomiting, administration of bicarbonate, hyperventilation)
   Hypoglycemic states:
   1. Hyperinsulinism (e.g., tumor or hyperplasia of islets of Langerhans)
   2. Hypopituitarism (e.g., deficiency of adrenocorticotropic, thyrotropic, and growth hormones)
   3. Adrenocortical insufficiency
   4. Hepatic disorders (e.g., von Gierke disease)
   5. Miscellaneous (e.g., leucine-induced, idiopathic ketotic)
   Uremia
   "Cerebral" allergy
   Cardiovascular dysfunction or syncopal attacks (e.g., simple fainting attacks, Stokes-Adams syndrome, hyperactive carotid sinus reflex)
   Migraine

Table 20–2 CLINICAL CLASSIFICATION OF "EPILEPTIC" SEIZURES*

I. Partial seizures (seizures beginning locally)
   A. Partial seizures with elementary symptomatology, generally without impairment of consciousness
      1. With motor symptoms (includes jacksonian seizures)
      2. With special sensory or somatosensory symptoms
      3. With autonomic symptoms
      4. Compound forms (partial complex seizures without loss of consciousness)†
   B. Partial seizures with complex symptomatology (temporal lobe or psychomotor seizures), generally with impaired consciousness
      1. With impairment of consciousness only
      2. With cognitive symptomatology
      3. With affective symptomatology
      4. With psychosensory symptomatology
      5. With psychomotor symptomatology (automatisms)
      6. Compound forms (descriptions vary with the patient—"psychomotor seizures")†
   C. Partial seizures secondarily generalized
II. Generalized seizures (bilaterally symmetrical, without local onset)
   A. Absences (petit mal)†
   B. Bilateral massive epileptic myoclonus (Lennox-Gastaut)†
   C. Infantile spasms (infantile myoclonic seizures)†
   D. Clonic seizures
   E. Tonic seizures
   F. Tonic-clonic seizures (grand mal)†
   G. Atonic seizures
   H. Akinetic seizures†
III. Unilateral seizures (or predominantly unilateral)
IV. Epileptic seizures as yet unclassified (because of incomplete data)

*Abstracted from the International Classification proposal by Gastaut (1970).

†These are the types most often recognized in infants and children; older patients can often describe their experiences more fully, making more precise classification possible.

the neonatal period probably reflects both the immaturity of the cerebral cortex and lack of uniformity in recognizing or classifying seizures or their equivalents. The electroencephalogram, though not so informative as later in infancy and childhood and technically difficult to obtain, may be the only objective means of detecting seizures in some instances.

After an episode of acute anoxia, a convulsion in the newborn may take the form of a tonic spasm preceded by a few clonic jerks. The electroencephalogram becomes flattened. Focal seizures may be associated with irregular jerky movements and nystagmus or with staring, pallor, and hypotonia. Paroxysmal bursts of multiple spike and slow wave discharges may appear on the electroencephalogram. In some instances the respiration becomes slow and irregular, with periods of apnea and a feeble cry. The neck becomes rigid, the pupils dilate, and the infant drools. Alteration of the electroencephalogram may also occur in association with slight movements of the fingers, toes, or eyelids, with a change in color, or with chewing.

The occurrence of a seizure suggests a cerebral insult and calls for examination of possible causative factors, particularly those which can be altered favorably. The maternal use of drugs should be considered. Disorders of amino acid metabolism should be sought or excluded through chromatographic examination of urine or serum. A clinical trial of pyridoxine or examination of the urine for maple syrup urine disease may be lifesaving. (See Sec 8.7.) Convulsions are rarely the only manifestation of a bacterial infection, but this possibility cannot be excluded by clinical examination alone.

The prognosis for the newborn infant who has a seizure is best if the episode is early in onset, of brief duration, and associated with no other disease state. Tremors occurring during the 1st day of life seem to have the best prognosis if the child's subsequent neonatal course is entirely normal. If the heart rate is consistently slow or if symptoms of any kind persist for more than 72 hr, the risk of later motor and/or mental impairment is high.

Treatment and management of the newborn infant with seizures primarily involve adequate supportive care. This includes prevention of shock, maintenance of an adequate airway, and sedation appropriate to the infant's needs. Diazepam and phenobarbital are the most widely used anticonvulsive agents.

Acute Convulsions in Infants and Children. Any of the types of acute convulsive attacks in children may occur as a transient manifestation of acute disease involving the brain, but generalized tonic and clonic convulsions similar to the grand mal attack of epilepsy are by far the most common. Practically all seizures resulting from extracranial disorders are of this type.

Febrile convulsions occurred in slightly more than 3% of the 54,000 infants examined in the National Collaborative Perinatal Project, a significant number of whom were known to have had prior neurologic deficits or developmental delays. Most febrile convulsions occur after the 1st 6 mo of life but within the 1st 2–3 yr. The incidence decreases up to 6–8 yr after which such seizures are rare. Males are more often affected than females, and there appears to be an increased susceptibility in some families.

Diagnosis. In the latter part of infancy and in the 1st few yr of childhood most convulsions merely represent an initial symptom of an acute benign febrile illness. The affected child should, however, be examined for the possibility of some other cause. Such disorders as tetany, lead encephalopathy, intracranial injury, hemorrhage or tumor, poisoning with a convulsant drug, hypoglycemia, asphyxia, cerebral sinus thrombosis (associated with cyanotic congenital heart disease or cachexia), acute nephritis, and epilepsy should be considered.

A carefully taken history should record any previous attacks; immediately preceding symptoms such as hyperirritability, fever, muscular cramps, headache, vomiting, or dizziness; any possibilities of dietary deficiency, poisoning of any kind, cranial injury, or hemorrhagic tendency; exposure to infection; or familial predisposition to seizures.

Thorough physical examination and neurologic appraisal are essential, with special attention to features which may point to specific causes for seizures. For example, depigmented areas resembling a white mountain ash leaf or the lesions of adenoma sebaceum suggest the diagnosis of tuberous sclerosis. Other dermatologic findings which may be helpful include port wine hemangiomas of the face and adjacent areas (Sturge-Weber), irregular hyperpigmented areas or subcutaneous nodules (neurofibromatosis), bronzed skin (Addison disease), linear nevus, eczematoid areas (un-

treated PKU), or butterfly rash of the nose and cheeks (systemic lupus erythematosus). Inspection of the eyegrounds may give the 1st clue to the nature of the primary illness by revealing an optic neuritis or choking of the discs. These may occur in the presence of an expanding intracranial lesion (tumor, cyst, hemorrhage, or abscess), acute hydrocephalus, or severe encephalitis. Such examination may also reveal the presence of retinal hemorrhages, suggesting intracranial bleeding from trauma or a blood dyscrasia. Albuminuric retinitis may furnish the 1st clue to the presence of subacute or chronic nephritis. There may be slight choking of the optic discs in acute nephritis with arterial hypertension. Chorioretinitis is suggestive of toxoplasmosis but is not diagnostic of it. The reddish areas of degeneration in the macular region in cerebromacular degenerative disease and the choroidal tubercles of miliary tuberculosis are highly characteristic.

Determinations of serum calcium, blood sugar, and urea nitrogen levels will aid in the diagnosis of hypocalcemic tetany, hypoglycemia, and acute nephritis, respectively. Coexisting hypertension, proteinuria, and cylindruria are evidences of nephritis. Roentgenograms may show the "lead line" of lead poisoning in the long bones, multiple recent or healed fractures in instances of child abuse, or thinning of the skull and separation of the sutures in the presence of an expanding intracranial lesion. Examination of the urine for coproporphyrin and for type III uroporphyrin (Sec 8.43) may reveal evidence of lead intoxication or of acute intermittent porphyria.

If the primary disease is infectious, it is necessary to determine whether the infection is extracranial (febrile or prefebrile convulsions) or intracranial, and if the latter, whether it is meningitis, encephalitis, abscess, or sinus thrombophlebitis. Certain other infectious diseases, such as typhus, shigellosis, salmonellosis, and malaria, may occasionally cause convulsions; in some instances convulsions reflect disturbances of water and electrolyte balance (Sec 5.30), or tetanus (Sec 10.40).

Treatment. For the control of "febrile" convulsions, which occasionally occur at the onset of acute extracranial infections, reduction of the elevated body temperature usually suffices.

If the convulsion is prolonged or if the child has a 2nd convulsion before recovering fully from the 1st, more vigorous anticonvulsant treatment is indicated. Appropriate treatment for shock and for the primary condition must, of course, be provided.

Seizures secondary to electrolyte disturbances require special therapy (Sec 5.30). In young infants, after other causes for seizures have been excluded, a clinical trial of pyridoxine may be indicated.

Prognosis. In 1980 a panel of experts convened by the National Institutes of Health reached a "consensus" that in view of the benign nature of most febrile seizures there is no need for medication, but that anticonvulsant prophylaxis might be considered (1) if the neurologic examination is abnormal, (2) if a seizure is prolonged (greater than 15 min) or focal or associated with transient or permanent neurologic defect, or (3) if there is a family history of nonfebrile seizures. After a single febrile seizure the family can be reassured that the probability of chronic epilepsy is not great. Recurrence of febrile seizures increases the probability of later spontaneous nonfebrile convulsions. There is a relatively high probability that idiopathic epilepsy will develop in children who have more than 5 febrile convulsions in a 12 mo period, single seizures which last for more than 1 hr, or persistent electroencephalographic abnormalities. (Note that the electroencephalogram of a child who has had a febrile convulsion may be abnormal as long as 1 wk afterward.) About 25% of epileptic children have a history of febrile seizure. For children with febrile seizures who had been judged to be normal prior to the 1st seizure, data from the National Collaborative Perinatal Project found no association of seizures with intelligence when these children were compared with unaffected siblings.

Opinions differ sharply as to the advisability of daily anticonvulsant medication for the child who has had 1 or more febrile convulsions. Some recommend that daily anticonvulsant therapy be maintained for 2–4 yr after a single seizure and others that continuing therapy be withheld until after the 1st afebrile seizure. The reasons given for daily treatment are (1) that a significant number of young adults who develop psychomotor seizures have a history of "febrile" convulsions, and (2) that data of Lennox suggest that febrile seizures do not recur if a serum level of phenobarbital higher than 15 µg/ml is maintained. Intermittent administration of phenobarbital is ineffective in preventing recurrences. Arguments against continuous prophylactic therapy are (1) that 3–5% of all children would be treated for at least 2 yr if such a program were carried out, and (2) that the administration of full therapeutic amounts of phenobarbital is needed to maintain the level of 15 µg/ml. The long term effects of administration of other anticonvulsant medications such as diazepam (Valium) or valproic acid (Depakene) are not fully known.

Our opinion is that daily anticonvulsant therapy as usually prescribed does not seem to reduce the number or duration of febrile convulsions and that as long as convulsions are felt to be febrile seizures, such therapy is not indicated. If convulsions recur with little or no evidence of infection or if the electroencephalogram is significantly abnormal 2 wk or more after the last seizure, a trial of daily anticonvulsant therapy may be indicated. The usual EEG itself has not been proved to be a reliable predictor of the development of epilepsy under these circumstances.

An infant or young child who has had 1 or more febrile seizures is entitled to more prompt antipyretic measures (such as aspirin or tepid sponging) and *anti-infectious* therapy than might otherwise seem indicated. Some physicians give phenobarbital prophylactically to such infants during febrile episodes. If anti-infectious or anticonvulsant therapy is prescribed, the physician must observe the child closely for the possibility that a serious infection such as meningitis may be masked. The value of routine examination of cerebrospinal fluid in instances of febrile seizures is questionable. The physician must consider the need for this or for other laboratory tests in the context of the individual patient.

Chronic or Recurrent Convulsions

20.4 EPILEPSY

The terms *epilepsy* and *recurrent convulsive disorder* can be used interchangeably. These terms designate various symptom complexes characterized by recurrent, paroxysmal attacks of unconsciousness or impaired consciousness, usually with a succession of tonic or clonic muscular spasms or other abnormal behavior. If a cause of seizures cannot be found, the patient may be said to have *idiopathic* or *cryptogenic epilepsy;* if a cerebral abnormality is demonstrable, *organic* or *symptomatic epilepsy.*

Because many persons, from prejudice or ignorance, feel that persons with epilepsy will somehow fail to make adequate social adjustments, some physicians are reluctant to use the term "epilepsy" in discussing the problem with parents. Its use, even with gentle and dispassionate explanation of its meaning, may be immediately alarming to parents or patient, but letting an affected family know the term and how it applies to them is part of educating the family toward living more comfortably with a chronic illness. The ability and desire of families to acquire information about a chronic illness vary along with the rate at which information can be assimilated. Too much information on a single visit is undesirable. Orientation should be an evolving process, especially during the early period of medical supervision.

Idiopathic Epilepsy. Although in the majority of instances the cause of recurrent seizures cannot be established, is seems probable that specific genetic defects in cerebral metabolism are responsible in many children.

Electroencephalographic tracings, particularly during sleep, show generalized abnormalities in 90% of children with idiopathic seizures. Often there are focal electrical abnormalities on the electroencephalogram which are seen to migrate from 1 area to another in serial examinations and are rarely associated with anatomic defects. Lennox pointed out that electroencephalographic abnormalities (cerebral dysrhythmias) are more likely to be found in parents and siblings of affected children than in the population at large. The abnormality most frequently found in otherwise unaffected relatives is the spike-wave discharge.

Organic Epilepsies. A variety of genetically determined conditions (Table 20–1) have seizures associated. Some have anatomic (e.g., congenital ectodermoses) or biochemical (e.g., phenylketonuria) abnormalities. In addition, convulsions may occur after cerebral damage acquired in the prenatal, natal, or postnatal period. Such children frequently display motor handicaps of central nervous system origin (cerebral palsy) and mental retardation, and these almost always have electroencephalographic abnormalities.

The recognition of genetically determined conditions is important. (1) Cerebral damage in younger siblings of affected patients may be prevented by prompt therapy (e.g., leucine-induced hypoglycemia, phenylketonuria, kernicterus). (2) Indefinite signs and symptoms in siblings may be more readily recognized (e.g., tuberous sclerosis, cerebromacular degeneration, neurofibromatosis). (3) Identification of an organic cause of the seizures is important prognostically; in general, control of such seizures is less satisfactory and social adjustment of the child less adequate than with idiopathic seizures.

Clinical Manifestations. *Tonic-Clonic (Grand Mal) Seizures.* Grand mal seizures are generalized convulsions, usually with tonic and clonic phases of the muscular spasms. Fewer than a third of epileptic children can give a definite description of an aura preceding their seizures. In some instances a preliminary, localized spasm or twitching of muscles may precede a generalized seizure. This is often referred to as a "motor aura" or warning. Vague prodromal symptoms or signs, such as irritability, intestinal disturbances, headache, and mental dullness, may forewarn patients or their parents of impending motor seizures. The period intervening is usually short but may be hours or even 1–2 days.

The onset of the typical seizure is abrupt, and the tonic spasm may occur simultaneously with loss of consciousness. The patient, if sitting or standing, falls to the ground. The face suddenly becomes pale, the pupils dilate, the corneas become insensitive to touch, the eyeballs roll upward or to 1 side, the face is distorted, the glottis is closed, the head may be thrown backward or to 1 side, the abdominal and chest muscles are held rigidly, and the limbs contract irregularly or stiffen out. As the air is forced out of the lungs through the glottis by sudden contraction of the diaphragm and the intercostal muscles, a short, startling cry may be heard. The tongue may be severely bitten as a result of the rapid contraction of the jaw muscles. Micturition and, less frequently, defecation may follow the sudden forceful contraction of the abdominal muscles. As the tonic phase of the seizure continues, facial pallor is quickly followed by suffusion and this, in turn, by cyanosis, occasionally severe, due to absence of effective respiratory movements. At the end of this phase, which usually lasts not more than 20–40 sec, the clonic phase sets in with variable duration. Generalized motor seizures tend to be predominantly tonic during infancy, though the clonic feature is always present to some degree.

Patients may awaken from their postconvulsive sleep with a severe, generalized headache and in a state of confusion and may go about in a semidazed or stuporous state in which they may perform more or less automatic acts without being able to recollect what they have experienced. These postparoxysmal or postictal reactions presumably represent malfunction of neurons which have not yet recovered from the effects of the seizure. Sometimes prolonged automatism, transient paresis, or, more rarely, hemiplegia or other paralystic manifestations of focal injury or hemorrhage occur. Grand mal seizures may occur at night (*nocturnal epilepsy*) without the patient's being aware of them. A bitten tongue or lip, headache, blood on the pillow, or a bed wet with urine may be the only clue.

So-called secondary symptomatology, which includes chiefly such personality traits as egocentricity, shallowness, religiosity, and chronic negativism and is considered by some to be characteristic of epilepsy, is much less prominent in children than in adults. Such personality traits usually represent a response to long exposure to psychogenically injurious attitudes of other people toward the disability. These traits are not to be attributed to the disease itself or confused with the transient behavior disturbances of psychomotor attacks. Similar personality disturbances develop frequently for the same general reasons in children with other chronic handicapping conditions.

Petit Mal Absences. These seizures consist of a transient loss of consciousness. There may be such additional minor manifestations as an upward rolling of the eyes, moving of the lids, drooping or rhythmic nodding of the head, or slight quivering of the trunk and limb muscles. Clinical evidence of petit mal rarely appears before 3 yr of age and frequently disappears by puberty. Girls are more often affected than boys. Intellectual development is rarely impaired in children who have only simple, staring, petit mal seizures. Attacks of this type last less than 30 sec and are commonly described by lay observers as "dizzy spells," "absences," "lapses," or "fainting turns." The patient rarely falls but usually drops articles he or she may have in hand or mouth. For example, a child engaged in an activity such as writing or reading will suddenly discontinue it and then resume it at the end of the seizure, often unaware of having had a convulsion. Such seizures vary in frequency from 1–2/mo to several hundred/day. Hyperventilation or exposure to blinking lights may evoke typical episodes. Individual petit mal seizures may, in rare instances, become progressively prolonged and gradually resemble a mild form of grand mal. Prolonged episodes of confusion, inappropriate action, and loss of ability to speak or understand (*petit mal status*) are rare and can be distinguished from psychomotor seizures only by electroencephalographic findings during the attack.

Psychomotor Seizures. Psychomotor seizures are the most difficult to recognize and among the more difficult to control. They consist in purposeful but inappropriate motor acts which are repetitive and often complicated. Frequently a slight aura in a young child is manifested in a shrill cry or an attempt to run for help. The seizure itself often consists of a gradual loss of postural tone. For example, the child may extend an arm and make a slow half-turn to 1 side while falling slowly to the ground. There are often vasomotor changes, such as circumoral pallor. After a 1–5 min episode of unconsciousness the child may resume normal activity. The child is often drowsy or sleeps for a short time after the spell. There are usually no tonic or clonic movements. Fugue states or episodes of confusion, which may resemble petit mal, are rarely found in children. The electroencephalogram, except at the time of psychomotor seizure, is often normal.

Focal Partial Seizures. These seizures may be sensory or motor (*jacksonian epilepsy*) depending upon the location of the focal area of abnormal neuronal discharge. Focal seizures may occasionally occur in the absence of organic lesions. Localized sensory attacks, which may give a variety of symptoms, are rare in children. Unilateral motor or jacksonian attacks, though not infrequently preceded by à brief tonic phase, are typically clonic, indicating their origin in the motor cortex. The muscles most frequently involved in jacksonian seizures are those most specialized for voluntary movements, as in the hand, face, and tongue, less often those of the foot and trunk.

As might be expected from the relation of the areas of representation of the various muscle groups in the precentral gyrus, a focal motor seizure beginning in 1 member spreads or extends to others according to a fixed pattern, e.g., from thumb to fingers, to wrists, to arm, to face, and then to the leg on the same side ("jacksonian march"). When such an attack is of brief duration and remains localized to 1 area, consciousness may not be disturbed. When its spread is extensive and rapid, however, consciousness is lost, and a generalized convulsion follows, indistinguishable from a typical grand mal seizure.

Infantile Myoclonic Seizures. The convulsive seizure has also been called "infantile spasm," "lightning major," and "jackknife epilepsy." Unlike true petit mal seizures, these episodes occur before 2 yr of age and involve more than 1 group of muscles. The most common type of mass myoclonus is a sudden dropping of the head and flexion of the arms. The attack may be repeated several hundred times a day. The electroencephalographic changes consist of random high-voltage slow waves and spikes (*hypsarrhythmia*) and suggest a diffuse, disorganized state. It is 1 of the most characteristic encephalographic patterns and probably represents the response of the immature brain to a profound disturbance.

Infants with myoclonic seizures may be placed in 1 of 2 groups in accordance with age and developmental ability at the time of onset. If the developmental level has never been normal or if seizures occur before 4 mo of age, a congenital cerebral defect (Table 20–1) or other organic cause is likely. If the infant appeared to progress normally until 6 mo or more of age before the hypsarrhythmia was detected, an unrecognized encephalitis or an underlying defect in cerebral metabolism may be responsible. In either case, significant developmental retardation is to be expected; only about 10% of the infants in the 2nd group retain intellectual ability within the normal range. Often the children in the 2nd group have good motor ability but poor adaptive and language abilities for their chronologic age. Infantile myoclonic seizures usually disappear spontaneously before the 4th yr of life; other seizures may occur subsequently. The evaluation of treatment, such as with corticotropin, is difficult.

A therapeutic trial with corticotropin, a corticosteroid, or pyridoxine is indicated. Such therapy, when started early, has sometimes appeared to produce improvement in the clinical status and in the electroencephalographic pattern, but interpretation is speculative since spontaneous improvement occasionally occurs.

Myoclonic and Akinetic Seizures. Myoclonic jerks or involuntary muscular contractions may occur in conjunction with other manifestations of epilepsy, including loss of consciousness, or they may occur alone. A single group of muscles is usually affected. A normal electroencephalogram may accompany myoclonic jerks involving 1 side or extremity; the origin of such seizures is presumed to be subcortical.

An akinetic seizure is associated with a sudden generalized loss of postural tone. These seizures in young children may resemble infantile myoclonic seizures and are sometimes called motor petit mal, jackknife, or akinetic seizures. The electroencephalogram usually reveals a spike and wave pattern at fewer than 3/sec (*petit mal variant*).

Minor motor seizures are often a sign of degenerative disease or other central nervous system disorders and may be difficult to control.

Nocturnal Seizures. The true incidence of seizures during sleep is unknown. Night terrors and sleep walking (somnambulism) most commonly occur during the deep sleep that occurs 1–2 hr after retiring. Later, during the rapid eye movement (REM) phase of sleep, brief myoclonic movements or motions associated with dreaming occur. The EEGs of children who are dreaming during REM sleep show low-voltage fast activity and lack sleep spindles.

A specific form of benign nocturnal seizures has been described. The episodes consist of somatosensory aura, brief hemifacial movements, and sometimes self-limited generalized tonic and clonic movements. The typical EEG has unilateral or bilateral foci of spikes in midtemporal or rolandic centrotemporal areas. These seizures appear in the 1st decade and disappear in the 2nd. Whether this type of seizure can be controlled by currently available anticonvulsant drugs or seizures prevented from recurring in later life is uncertain.

Self-Induced Seizures. It is possible for some children to induce petit mal or grand mal seizures by overbreathing, by watching a blinking light, or by some other form of learned behavior. Self-induced seizures should be distinguished clinically from other types of convulsions because drug therapy alone is usually unsatisfactory. After a child has learned to draw attention in this manner, it is difficult to alter this behavior. Complex family problems probably underlie this kind of behavior. Behavioral modification therapy has been successful in some instances.

20.5 DIAGNOSIS

Electroencephalography. The electroencephalogram (EEG) records spontaneous electrical activity in the scalp; the recorded compound harmonic waves represent various cortical and subcortical events. The record may be made while the subject is awake, asleep, or hyperventilating or during spontaneous or induced seizures.

The EEG has been most useful in the recognition and classification of seizure disorders, though virtually any metabolic or disease state may affect it. Responses of the EEG to controlled auditory, visual, and other stimuli (evoked potentials) have expanded its usefulness.

The technique is noninvasive and requires minimal cooperation. Placement of scalp electrodes by the so-called 10–20 system allows the electrodes to be placed in the same relative locations from subject to subject and (more important) from hemisphere to hemisphere. Three types of rhythms have been described in the normal human adult. The most common, the alpha rhythm, consists of regular sinusoidal waves, which occur at frequencies of 8–12/sec, with a voltage of 20–60 microvolts. The 2nd most common is the beta rhythm, most prominent in the frontal cortex, with lower amplitude and a frequency of 13–32/sec. The least common is the gamma rhythm, which arises from the frontal lobes and consists of a more rapid rate, 33–55/sec, with waves of extremely low voltage. Slower waves

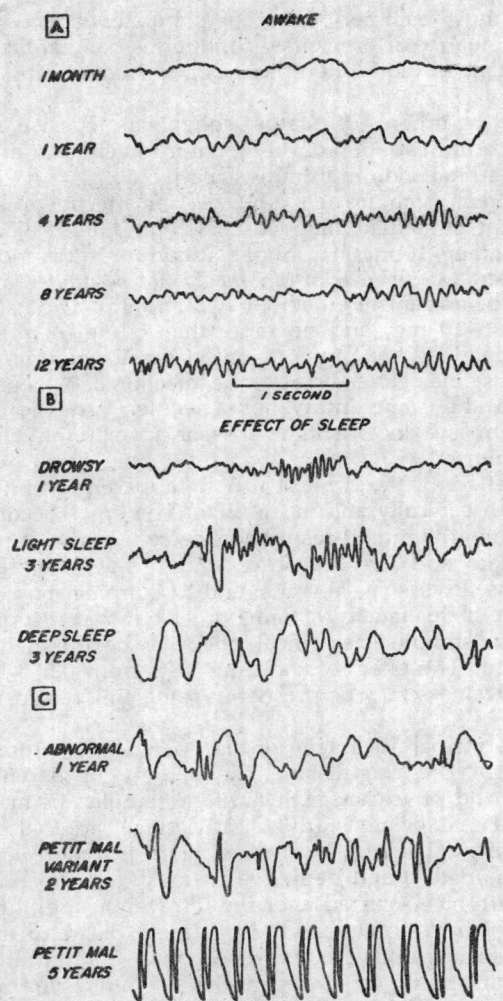

Figure 20–1 Electroencephalograms of infants and children. A, Tracings from comparable areas of the scalp illustrating variations with age of electrical activity in the motor cortex; all were secured during a quiet phase just before sleep. B, The effects of sleep, variations of patterns in normal children; compare with tracings in A and C. C, Abnormal waves.

(theta, 4–7/sec, and delta, 1–4/sec) are not present in normal adults during the waking state.

The interpretation of EEGs of infants and children is more difficult than it is for those of adults because slow rhythms (3–8/sec) are normal in children (Fig 20–1). Cortical rhythm is poorly developed in the newborn infant. With normal maturation, random 3–7/sec waves appear and some faster low voltage activity. Gradually, the basic rhythm becomes more regular; by 6 yr of age the pattern is made up principally of 5–7/sec waves, and by 10 yr alpha waves, 8–12/sec, predominate. During childhood 14 and 16/sec positive spikes (ctenoids) are commonly found in presumably healthy subjects. During adolescence some slow wave activity, 4–8/sec, is not uncommon and may be incorrectly interpreted if adult standards are used.

Sleep (without the use of a hypnotic), hyperventilation for 2 min, pentylenetetrazol (Metrazol), artificially induced fever, vasopressin (Pitressin), and flickering light bring out latent abnormalities in the EEG and may on occasion produce a seizure. Sleep and hyperventilation are most frequently used in cooperative subjects.

When there is clinical evidence of a convulsive disorder, an EEG should almost always be obtained. Findings of spike-wave or other characteristic patterns may give valuable guidance to long-term management.

ABNORMAL WAVES. Lack of stability of the central nervous system is associated with electroencephalographic abnormalities. If a cell membrane is damaged, the increased permeability alters membrane function (excessive depolarization). In humans, repair of the leak (repolarization) probably depends upon a chemical reaction involving "high energy" phosphate compounds, which quickly re-establish the gradients of potassium and sodium across the cell wall. If excessive release of energy from a damaged or leaking cell occurs, neighboring cells become involved, and alterations in many cells and their connections may take place. The ensuing disorderly transmission of information from 1 cell to another is presumed to be a major cause of seizures. Kindling, an elaboration of a convulsive response to an original minimal or subconvulsive stimulus, may be a key phenomenon in the pathophysiology of recurrent convulsive disorders.

Most patients with frequent *grand mal seizures* have definite abnormalities in their EEGs in the intervals between seizures. These consist of random spike discharges or diffuse high-voltage slow waves, or of a pattern not consistent with chronologic age. An EEG obtained during a grand mal seizure shows multiple high-voltage spike discharges. After the seizure there are asymmetries between the 2 hemispheres and diffuse slowing.

Patients with seizures other than grand mal have a variety of abnormalities. The most easily recognized is that of *infantile myoclonic seizures*: a high voltage, 1–2/sec, spike and wave pattern called hypsarrhythmia (hyps = high and lofty). The EEG appears completely disorganized. During *petit mal attacks* there is characteristically a 3/sec spike and wave pattern.

Persistent asymmetry between opposite sides may be significant, especially if the electrical activity shows phase reversal of slow waves. Shifting foci are more common in children than in adults and indicate a functional disturbance rather than an anatomic lesion.

Absence of electrical activity over an area suggests a large lesion such as a subdural collection of fluid or an abscess. Serial EEGs of children with hydrocephalus show a disturbance of function as the process progresses.

After cerebral insults such as trauma, encephalitis, cerebral thrombosis, and prolonged seizures, electrical activity may be slow for a time and may be roughly correlated with the child's clinical course. Metabolic disorders, such as hypoglycemia, hyperthyroidism, and adrenal insufficiency, alter cortical activity.

Short bursts of various types of cerebral dysrhythmia may occur between clinical seizures (subclinical or larval seizures) as single wave and spike formations or short series of spikes similar to those in grand mal seizures. These subclinical bursts may, at times, predict the onset of clinical seizures.

Computer analysis of the clinical EEG will probably permit more sophisticated and precise interpretation.

Roentgenography. A roentgenographic examination of the skull is an essential element of the diagnostic appraisal; it seeks such abnormalities as intracranial calcifications, erosion of the base, or increased densities, which may indicate reasons for seizures. A hammered-silver pattern of the cranium is so common that in isolation it has no significance. Computed (CT scan) tomography is an excellent method for detecting cerebral lesions responsible for recurrent seizures and establishing both their location and nature. Alterations in CT scans due to transitory vascular phenomena are commonly seen for 1 wk after a prolonged seizure. These must be distinguished from significant anatomic changes by repeating the test or by studies using contrast media. Indications for CT scans are findings which suggest the possibility of space-occupying or vascular lesions. The suggestion of some that all individuals receiving anticonvulsant medication should have regular or routine CT scans has only rarely produced any significant finding.

Other Studies. Decisions about the need for laboratory examinations should be based on leads obtained from medical history, physical examination, and clinical course. Examination of the cerebrospinal fluid need not be routine, but it may provide useful information when diagnostic considerations include lead poisoning, certain instances of mental deterioration, or encephalitis.

When hypoglycemia (Sec 17.6), nephritis (Sec 16.16), lead poisoning (Sec 28.15), and tetany (Sec 10.40) are considered possible causes of convulsions, appropriate diagnostic steps are indicated.

20.6 TREATMENT OF RECURRENT CONVULSIONS

Management of the Individual Seizure. Little should be done for a patient having an isolated seizure other than protecting him or her from bodily injury. This necessitates constant supervision in severe cases. At the beginning of a major seizure, clothing about the neck should be loosened. The patient should then be turned to 1 side so that pooled secretions are not aspirated. The patient should be observed for changes in color; administration of oxygen is indicated during prolonged convulsions. Any injury to the tongue or other tissues of the oral cavity during a convulsion is most apt to occur at the onset. Since subsequent injury is not very likely and because additional damage often results from crude interventions, the family should be counseled against placing a stick or other object between the teeth.

Status Epilepticus. If a series of grand mal convulsions occurs before the patient has fully recovered, the prolonged seizure is termed status epilepticus. The intervals between individual convulsions may be so short that the seizures are virtually continuous. During status epilepticus the muscular contractions may appear to be 1 sided or to shift from 1 group of muscles to another. This does not represent a true focal (jacksonian) seizure.

The most common cause of status epilepticus is discontinuance of previously continuous daily anticonvulsant medication; often this has occurred within less than 2 wk.

Drug treatment of status epilepticus consists of prompt administration of diazepam intravenously or of phenobarbital sodium intramuscularly.

Diazepam (Valium, see Table 29–1) is effective in the treatment of status epilepticus. Each ampule of diazepam contains 10 mg in 2 ml of solution for intravenous administration. The solution *should not be diluted* and should be administered slowly (0.5 ml/min). The usual dose is 5–10 mg, and no more than 3 mg (6 ml) is recommended. We prefer to inject small amounts of isotonic saline before and after the injection of diazepam through the same intravenous needle. Extravasated diazepam is a local irritant; loss of an extremity has been reported.

The effect of the drug is usually apparent within 1 min both clinically and in the EEG. The limbs become hypotonic, the rate of respiration decreases, the pupils first dilate and later constrict, and nystagmus often develops. Excessive salivation and hiccupping may occur. The child usually remains quiet but will respond to painful stimuli. The corneal reflex may be diminished or absent. The effect of the drug lasts from 0.5–3 hr, but drowsiness may be present in some children for as long as 18 hr.

The principal advantage of diazepam is the prompt control of the convulsion. The anxiety of parents, nurses, and physicians, which often complicates management, is alleviated early. Disadvantages are that the underlying cause may be masked (e.g., infection, lead encephalopathy) and definitive therapy delayed. Sudden death has occurred after the intravenous administration of barbiturates for the treatment of grand mal status but has not yet been reported in children after the administration of diazepam. Its side effects are not fully known. Tolerance tends to occur after 3 or 4 intravenous administrations of diazepam so that increasing amounts must be administered to regain the initial effect.

In a hospital setting, where the treatment of seizures is often an adjunct to management of another disorder, prompt administration of diazepam is often desirable. Children may have acute convulsive disorders for many reasons, and the place and circumstance will influence management. The physician must guard against promiscuous use of either diazepam or phenobarbital.

The dose of phenobarbital for intramuscular injection averages 60 mg at 6 mo of age to 120 mg at 2–3 yr or 5–6 mg/kg; the maximum single dose is 200 mg. If the convulsion is not controlled within 15 min, the initial dose should be repeated; if the convulsion has been partially controlled by this time, half the initial dose should be given. Subsequent administrations may be necessary. The rhythmic contraction of 1 group of muscles after a severe convulsion does not require additional therapy. Sedative therapy should be limited to a single agent. If the convulsions are not controlled by a total dose of phenobarbital of 15 mg/kg within 60 min, the possibility of some organic lesion such as encephalitis, metabolic disturbance, or vascular accident should be considered. The administration of a small dose of phenobarbital (under 2–3 mg/kg) to a child in status should be avoided; it is likely to be inadequate and subsequent control may then be difficult.

The dangers of intravenously administered barbiturates and of inhalation anesthesia are similar to those of anesthetizing an excited child. Such procedures are rarely necessary; when they are indicated, there should be an experienced anesthesiologist in attendance. Laryngeal spasm and sudden death may occur if treatment is too vigorous.

Administration of oxygen is indicated during prolonged convulsions, and administration of 5% glucose in 0.45% saline solution intravenously may shorten the recovery time.

A quiet and calm atmosphere, reassurance, and avoidance of unnecessary annoyance to the patient are important factors in general management, especially during the recovery phase.

Continuous Therapy of the Epileptic Child. The aims of treatment are to reduce the number of seizures, to encourage the child to function at a level commensurate with his or her natural endowment, and to promote acceptance at home and in the community in accordance with capabilities. The responsibilities of the physician include diagnostic and therapeutic services for the child, information and counsel for the parents, and guidance to the community and the school. The success of the physician in each arena will often affect both the child's adjustment and the number of seizures. Factors limiting success include duration and severity of symptoms, the kind of seizures, genetic factors, complicating cerebral lesions, and capacity of patient and family to cooperate. Patients or families who have been unduly frightened by laboratory studies, by folk tales, or by reading poorly selected medical information will require additional special attention and explanations. Usually, however, the medical management of an idiopathic convulsive disorder is relatively easy after the diagnosis has been established.

Orientation of the Child. The attitude of the child toward his or her disease generally reflects that of the parents. It is usually desirable for the child to be present during conferences with the parents. Even if the medical terms are puzzling, the child will sense the philosophy of the physician, which, if it combines realism with optimism, can produce long-term benefits. Parents are often poorly equipped to explain chronic illness to a child. Giving parents and child chances to ask questions in each other's presence can resolve many doubts and fears. Attempts to disguise the existence of seizures are unwise and often harmful.

The questions of the child are apt to be related to activity in school, sports, and the like or to the duration of therapy. Most children are pleased to find that their participation in regular activity is encouraged. Customary restrictions against riding a horse alone or swimming except when attended by a responsible adult are readily accepted. Participation in competitive sports, in which injury to the child or others is possible, must be decided on an individual basis. Seizures during athletic activities are rare in otherwise well controlled children.

The issue of driving an automobile presents special problems for an adolescent with a seizure disorder, the family, and the physician. The decision should be individualized and take into account the degree of control on regular medication, monitoring of blood levels, state law, and the social and behavioral adjustment of the youth, including acceptance of reasonable constraints on driving activity and the like.

The duration of therapy cannot be predicted. It is preferable to maintain medication for a long time even if the dose of the drug is small. A workable rule is to continue medication until annual EEGs are consistently normal. It is difficult for both child and parents if therapy must be resumed because seizures recur.

It is usually best to leave discussion about discontinuation of medication until the child has been without seizures for 1 yr. Early in the course of treatment it is enough for children to know that they may not always have to take medication. Later, if they can lead an otherwise normal life, they will be willing to accept this minor inconvenience.

After the diagnosis of an idiopathic convulsive disorder has been made, return visits to the physician every 2–4 wk may be helpful. Additional questions, the possibility of additional history, information about environmental factors, physical findings, and drug toxicity may be dealt with appropriately at these times.

Orientation of the Adolescent. The behavioral changes during adolescence of patients with convulsive disorders are similar to those of unaffected children, but they are more likely to be brought to the attention of the physician. Unexplained tearfulness, hostility, clumsiness, inattention (particularly in school), forgetfulness, increased sibling rivalry, antiauthoritarianism, and overreaction (by adult standards) to petty annoyance are often part of normal adolescent behavior; but in patients with convulsive disorders they may be attributed to medication or to the disease. If the physician has previously discussed the increasing need for independence during adolescence, reassurance offered after development of symptoms is more likely to be successful. It may be helpful to have the child's teachers and a psychologist work together toward finding a realistic educational program.

The child with epilepsy wants to be "normal," to be

independent, to be accepted and admired by peers, and to achieve status symbols which are sometimes unrealistic. To achieve these goals, the adolescent with a convulsive disorder may test the fantasy that there is nothing wrong and refuse or forget to take medication. If a seizure occurs, this "forgetfulness," personality changes (depression), and recurrent seizures may lead to unnecessary hospitalization and unjustified diagnostic procedures which may further delay the development of independence and self-sufficiency. In some instances 1 or both parents may be reluctant to give up control of the child. The patient who has had little opportunity to exercise judgment in activities of daily life is likely to use the handicap as a shield.

Orientation of the Parents. Among the pertinent questions asked of physicians by parents after the diagnosis of epilepsy has been established are these: Will punishment of the child cause a seizure? What of the child's future? Is mental development likely to be retarded by the disease? Will mental deterioration occur? Will life be shortened by it? Should the child attend school? Should he or she marry and have children? As the physician helps the family to understand the general problem, the following points are fundamental:

1. The seizure is a symptom. Unless it is associated with clinical evidence of shock (peripheral vascular collapse), it will rarely produce irreversible damage to the central nervous system.

2. If the child gains excessive attention by having seizures, control by medication alone is likely to be difficult.

3. In most instances, avoidance of emphasis on the number or recurrence of seizures is helpful.

4. Restoration of confidence, in both the parents and the child, is important. The adults need to feel that they are competent and capable persons who can meet their responsibilities appropriately.

5. If the child receives medication in the proper amount, therapy should in no way influence mental ability or personality or cause drug addiction.

6. It is best to rear the child in accordance with the family's standards of reward or punishment. To modify them only because of seizures will lead to behavioral difficulties.

7. The patient needs access to activities in which he or she can compete successfully.

With some parents it is prudent for the physician to say in effect to the parents, "You give the medication and handle the child in a normal fashion, and let me be concerned with the spells." As members of the family become more mature in their attitudes, they will become more receptive to consideration of any important underlying difficulties such as previously unrecognized mental retardation, behavioral difficulties, inappropriate placement in school, or intrafamily conflicts.

Orientation of the Community. If educational facilities appropriate to the child's needs are available, he or she should attend school close to home and participate in activities to which he or she is naturally inclined. It is the duty of the physician, the nurse, and the social worker who are acquainted with the problem to do everything possible to improve the attitude of the public toward the epileptic patient and the disease. Nearly every intelligent epileptic child sooner or later encounters attitudes of pity and oversolicitousness or of disgust and horror. These are likely to be a source of constant anxiety unless supports enable the child to acquire an adequate philosophy for coping.

Drugs. Since the introduction of bromides for the treatment of epilepsy in 1858, drug therapy has been the choice and usually the only form of treatment. The tendency to rely upon medication alone was encouraged by the introduction of phenobarbital in 1912. Diet therapy came into use later when it was discovered that fasting, the ketogenic diet, and reduction of water intake all tended to prevent epileptic seizures. Since 1938, when Merritt and Putnam showed that phenytoin (diphenylhydantoin [Dilantin]) was effective in the treatment of some patients not controlled by phenobarbital, reliance mainly upon drug therapy has again increased.

The successful management of the epileptic child requires finding the most appropriate anticonvulsant drug or combination of drugs as well as the most appropriate dosages (Table 20–3). If control of seizures proves to be difficult, determinations of drug levels in the serum are essential. Unless these are readily available on a timely basis, a drug which might have been useful in a different dose or with proper compliance may have to be abandoned. When the administration of more than 1 drug is necessary, the serum levels are less predictable (usually lower) than when either one is given alone.

Valproic Acid (Depakene). The advent of dipropyl acetic acid has led to a change in the traditional patterns of prescribing barbiturates, hydantoins, and ethosuximide. The administration of valproic acid in amounts sufficient to sustain serum levels at about 100 μg/dl is often adequate for control of seizures in infancy and childhood. The starting dose in children is 15 mg/kg/24 hr. The dose may be increased in steps of 5 mg/kg/24 hr until a clinical effect is seen. Increases beyond 30 mg/kg/24 hr, if required, probably should be monitored by timely serum levels. A range of 50–100 μg/dl is usually appropriate. The presumed action of this drug is to increase the content of GABA (gamma aminobutyric acid) in the brain by inhibition of the enzyme GABA transaminase. The drug does not cause sedation if used alone. Side effects include nausea and temporary loss of small amounts of hair. These are said to be minor complaints which do not interfere with the continued administration of the drug. Clinical trials suggest that valproic acid may become the drug of choice for treatment of both grand mal and petit mal epilepsy. It has been less successful in controlling temporal lobe (psychomotor) seizures and those associated with hypsarrhythmia. If valproic acid is used in association with other medication, the amounts of other drugs can often be decreased. In many instances children receiving valproic acid seem brighter and more alert. It is suggested that children receiving this drug should have periodic studies of liver function and should have blood studies for possible thrombocytopenia prior to surgery.

Phenobarbital. If tolerance to valproic acid occurs or if there are other contraindications to its administration, phenobarbital in tablet form is the drug of choice for prolonged use in the usual patient with grand mal epilepsy. Its virtues are its relative effectiveness, its comparative harmlessness with prolonged administra-

---

Table 20–3 SUGGESTED SCHEDULE FOR A THERAPEUTIC PROGRAM IN EPILEPSY

Unless there is a specific contraindication, the administration of phenobarbital, 3–5 mg/kg/24 hr in 2 or 3 divided doses, is the treatment of choice for every child with grand mal (tonic-clonic seizures, psychomotor seizures [partial seizures with complex symptomatology also called or including "temporal lobe seizures"]), petit mal absences, infantile myoclonic seizures (infantile spasms), or mixed seizures.

Example: 20 kg (44 lb) × 3 mg/kg = 60 mg daily; 1 30 mg tablet on arising and bedtime.

Note: (1) If circumstances demand, a "loading dose" of phenobarbital of 60 mg/kg (maximum 180 mg) may be given. (2) Periodic monitoring of serum levels of phenobarbital is essential. Levels between 15–30 μg/ml (depending upon laboratory) are usually sufficient. (3) See alternative (below) for petit mal.

Grand mal (tonic-clonic) seizures—If seizures persist despite appropriate drug levels, attention should be given to improvement of environmental factors, to ascertaining that the best possible diagnosis has been reached, and to evaluating any changes in symptoms or side effects of medication. If phenobarbital in amounts sufficient to give serum levels consistently in the therapeutic range (with 2 or more determinations each wk) does not produce side effects, add valproic acid (Depakene), 15 mg/kg/24 hr, increasing by 5–10 mg/kg/24 hr at 1 wk intervals. Use measurement of serum levels to establish levels in the expected therapeutic range. If control of seizure is attained, move toward control by a single drug. Valproic acid (Depakene) is relatively new and more expensive and requires more careful studies for possible hepatic and other damage (see drug section). Drowsiness, ataxia, and loss of spontaneity are rarely associated with valproic acid.

Petit mal absences—An alternative to phenobarbital is the administration of valproic acid (Depakene), alone or in addition to phenobarbital. The petit mal absences associated with bursts of 3/sec spike wave discharges on the EEG often respond dramatically to valproic acid alone (see text). Slight gastric distress (transitory), expense, the size and number of capsules or amount of liquid required, and uncertainty as to side effects of a relatively new agent have limited the exclusive use of valproic acid.

Administration of ethosuximide (Zarontin) or trimethadione (Tridione) is rarely necessary.

Psychomotor (partial seizures with and without loss of consciousness ["temporal lobe"]).—It is generally preferable to undertake a trial of phenobarbital (as above) unless the evidence is convincing that the patient has this type of seizure alone. The choice between primidone (Mysoline) and carbamazepine (Tegretol) must be based upon clinical trial. Primidone has fewer systemic side effects, is less expensive, and after initial transient drowsiness usually has no detectable effect on mental abilities. Those individuals whose seizures have been difficult to control often respond well to carbamazepine without significant side effects. Carbamazepine depresses white blood cell counts and is potentially associated with other side effects; accordingly, careful observation is essential, and monitoring of serum levels is advisable.

Infantile myoclonic seizures (infantile spasms)—For infantile myoclonic seizures of recent origin (under 1 mo) the administration, in relatively large amounts, of corticotropin (ACTH) is suggested (40 units daily for 2 wk, then 80 units every other day for not less than 3 mo). This is combined with phenobarbital, 3 mg/kg/24 hr. The EEG is monitored for correlation with clinical progress; and regular measurements of serum levels of phenobarbital are needed.

Lennox syndrome (massive myoclonus)—If the administration of phenobarbital (as above) is not successful, valproic acid (Depakene) administered with the cautions given above is preferred. Start with 15 mg/kg/24 hr and increase at 1 wk intervals by 5–10 mg/kg/24 hr. The serum level should be monitored, with a goal of 50–100 μg/ml. Usually, 2 doses daily are sufficient. Other possible choices of medications are diazepam (Valium), clonazepam (Clonopin), chlordiazepoxide (Librium), primidone (Mysoline), phenytoin (Dilantin), ethosuximide (Zarontin), acetazolamide (Diamox), and phensuximide (Milontin) alone or in combination with phenobarbital or mephobarbital (Mebaral).

---

tion, its ease of administration, and its low cost. Doses range from 8 mg (1/8 grain) 1–3 times daily for an infant up to 100 mg (1½ grains) 1–3 times daily for an older child. On the basis of weight, an initial dose of 3 mg/kg/24 hr in 2 divided doses can be given, with gradual increases to the required maintenance dose. More than 6 mg/kg/24 hr may result in drowsiness. Concentrations of phenobarbital and other anticonvulsant medications in serum and other tissues can be measured accurately through gas-liquid or high pressure chromatography. Serum levels of 15–35 μg/ml are within the therapeutic range. Serum levels of phenobarbital often reach 30–60 μg/ml without apparent alteration of mental or motor functions. Because lack of compliance (failure of the child to receive prescribed amounts of medication) is a common cause of poor seizure control, determination of serum levels on 1 or more occasions is highly desirable. Otherwise, less effective or more expensive drugs may be substituted prematurely.

Two wk after initiation of daily therapeutic dosage of phenobarbital, the level in serum reaches a value which tends to remain constant. This stable state can be identified through serum specimens obtained just prior to the administration of a morning dose and 3 hr later. A significant variation between the concentrations in the 2 specimens is strong evidence that the administration of the drug has been irregular.

Occasionally a child will have an idiosyncrasy to phenobarbital. A maculopapular eruption on the skin and mucous membranes, excessive drowsiness, and fever may be signs of sensitivity or overdosage. These soon disappear without permanent harm if the dose is reduced or if the drug is withdrawn. Rarely, and particularly in the case of petit mal, a patient appears to be made worse by phenobarbital and has petit mal variants or psychomotor attacks. In such cases phenytoin may be added to the regimen. Rarely, it is necessary to discontinue phenobarbital, always gradually, and to substitute another drug. Mephobarbital (Mebaral) is of value in some cases. The dose is approximately double that recommended for phenobarbital.

Phenytoin. The only drugs that rival the barbiturates in the control of grand mal seizures are certain hydantoin compounds. Phenytoin (diphenylhydantoin [Dilantin]) is administered to older children in capsules and to younger ones in tablet form crushed in a little food or fruit juice. Doses range from 25 mg (½ tablet) 1 or 2 times daily in infants to as much as 100 mg once or twice daily in older children. The drug may also be prescribed in an initial dose of 3 mg/kg/24 hr in 2 doses, with gradual increases to the required maintenance dose. More than 8 mg/kg/24 hr may result in toxic manifestations. The chief advantage of hydantoin compounds over the barbiturates is that they act as efficient anticonvulsants without producing excessive drowsiness. Whenever grand mal seizures are not adequately controlled by phenobarbital alone in nondepressing doses, a hydantoin drug should be tried. Replacement should be made gradually, however, since sudden changes may result in increased convulsive reactivity. The therapeutic range of serum levels of phenytoin is usually 15–30 μg/ml. Somewhat lower levels may be satisfactory.

Painless, nonhemorrhagic hypertrophy of the gums usually follows the administration of phenytoin. It usually requires no special treatment other than good dental hygiene. If it becomes unattractive cosmetically, another drug should be substituted.

Ataxia and drowsiness may occur if the initial dose is too large, if the dose is increased too rapidly, or if the total daily dose exceeds about 8 mg/kg/24 hr. Serious toxic reactions, such as nausea or vomiting, erythema, or a morbilliform eruption, and nervous manifestations such as tremor of the hands, ataxia, diplopia with nystagmus, paralytic manifestations, and mild psychoses are relatively uncommon and disappear after reduction of the dose, usually to about two thirds of its former level. *Phenytoin (Dilantin) should not be administered to infants and young children in the form of a suspension because most parents are not able to administer the small dose accurately.*

Chemical and roentgenographic evidences of rickets (Sec 23.23) have been associated with the administration of phenytoin. In our experience correction of dietary factors and reduction of the level in the serum to the currently accepted therapeutic range have been associated with prompt improvement. Most reported instances have occurred among patients in institutions who had received medication for long periods of time. Adequacy of nutrition is difficult to assess in these settings; nutritional factors and the relatively high dosage schedules employed probably account for most cases. These emphasize the need for periodic review of dietary habits, recent weight gain and loss, and other evidences of mental and physical growth. In institutions, children unable to make their needs known may require especially careful medical supervision.

Trimethadione (Tridione). Tridione (3,5,5-trimethyl-oxazolidine-2,4-dione) is an effective drug for the treatment of petit mal epilepsy in doses of 0.3 gm (5 grains) 1–4 times daily. The drug may also be prescribed on the basis of weight, with an initial dose of 25 mg/kg/24 hr in 2–4 doses, which may be gradually increased if necessary to 80 mg/kg/24 hr. Tridione is now rarely used. It is occasionally needed for children who have petit mal seizures refractory to valproic acid and ethosuximide. Tridione may increase frequency of grand mal attacks if they coexist; the additional administration of a barbiturate or hydantoin will be indicated. Excessive doses or prolonged use of Tridione may result in photophobia, hemeralopia (day blindness), drowsiness, nausea, skin eruptions, or nephrosis. Such manifestations tend to disappear after withdrawal of the drug. Fatal aplastic anemia has been reported in patients receiving Tridione; when it is given for more than a short time, periodic blood cell counts should be obtained and the drug discontinued if any abnormality is found.

Ethosuximide (Zarontin). Zarontin is useful in the treatment of petit mal seizures if the administration of valproic acid (Depakene) is contraindicated, and is probably more useful than Tridione. Side effects reported to follow the administration of Zarontin usually disappear if the amount of medication is decreased. These effects include nausea, dizziness, drowsiness, rash, and hiccups; they are unlikely to return if the drug is administered at a lower dose, which is then increased gradually to a maintenance level lower than the one not tolerated. The occurrence of a blood dyscrasia following the administration of Zarontin is unusual. White blood cell and differential counts should be obtained before starting therapy, after 1 mo, and then every 3–6 mo. Routine examination of the urine at these times is also desirable.

Because many children with petit mal seizures can be controlled by valproic acid or phenobarbital alone, the administration of Zarontin is suggested only when necessary in addition to phenobarbital or Mebaral. Occasionally, a child with more than 1 type of convulsion may have an increased number of seizures after Zarontin has been administered.

The recommended starting dose is 1 capsule (250 mg) daily for 1 wk. If necessary, the daily number of capsules is increased by 1 each wk, until a total of 6 capsules daily is reached (2 capsules, 3 times daily). The drug may also be prescribed by weight, 20–40 mg/kg/24 hr. Serum levels of 40–120 µg/ml are often required. If the administration of the capsule is impractical in young children, the drug may be given in the form of syrup (250 mg/4 ml).

Primidone (Mysoline). Mysoline (5-phenyl-5-ethyl-hexahydropyrimidine-4:6-dione) is used in the treatment of grand mal and psychomotor seizures. It may be used alone or with other drugs and does not depress hematopoietic activity. The chief side effects, drowsiness, ataxia, and dermatitis, can be minimized by starting with small amounts (125 mg) at bedtime and by increasing the dose slowly at 7–10 day intervals to a maximum dose of 250 mg, 3 times daily. In patients receiving both Mysoline and phenobarbital the serum will contain both primidone and a breakdown product, phenylethylmalonic acid (PEMA), but the control of seizures seems to depend chiefly upon the phenobarbital.

Diazepam (Valium) (Table 29–1). The use of diazepam for the treatment of chronic convulsive disorders is under study. Some children respond favorably, particularly those with petit mal who have been refractory to Zarontin and other agents. The dose is 1–10 mg 3 times a day as tolerated. In many instances tolerance occurs after 3–14 days of therapy. If the dosage is further increased, side effects may occur, such as drowsiness, ataxia, and slurred speech.

Children who have seizures associated with degenerative disease of the central nervous system often tolerate diazepam well. The dosage must be adjusted individually. The oral administration of diazepam with phenobarbital and phenytoin is a useful combination in some instances.

Carbamazepine (Tegretol). Tegretol (200 mg tablets only) has been widely used for relief of pain, primarily for trigeminal neuralgia. This drug may also help to control seizures (particularly of the psychomotor type). Common side effects include dizziness, drowsiness, nausea, vomiting, and ataxia. Serious side effects reported in adults may reflect the severity of the conditions for which it has been prescribed. The starting dose of 100 mg (half a tablet) 2–3 times daily, with or without other medications, can be increased to 400 mg

(2 tablets) 2–3 times daily in adolescence. Maintenance of serum levels of 3–10 µg/ml is usually associated with control of seizures. If the administration of the drug is successful, the principal advantage is the lack of sedation.

The Ketogenic Diet. Fasting causes cessation of grand mal seizures in a majority of epileptic children, the effect usually manifesting itself shortly after ketosis has appeared on the 3rd day. A strongly ketogenic diet has a comparable anticonvulsive effect once ketosis has developed. Stringent restriction of fluid intake, even when the diet is nonketogenic, results in cessation of grand mal seizures in most of those patients who respond favorably to fasting or to the ketogenic diet. Establishment of a negative water balance, by restricting the intake or increasing the output, intensifies the anticonvulsive effects of the ketogenic regimen. Administration of alkaline salts in sufficient amount to neutralize the acidogenic effect of fasting or of the ketogenic diet abolishes the anticonvulsive action, whereas administration of inorganic acids or acid-forming salts intensifies such action. The ketogenic diet has been used for both grand mal and petit mal epilepsy.

The use of the ketogenic diet is limited because of the difficulties of consistent adherence to a restricted dietary intake and because of the possibility of attendant emotional disturbances. It may be helpful as adjunctive therapy for children who have frequent seizures which are not controlled by moderate doses of 1 or more of the anticonvulsant drugs. Both child and family must be able to accept the dietary regimen without emotional conflict. Because of these difficulties the diet is no longer widely used. The use of medium chain triglycerides has been suggested.

Prognosis. The prognosis of a convulsive disorder depends upon any coexisting mental retardation, physical handicaps, or possible organic disease and upon the adequacy of medical and social management. The results of therapy are generally not satisfactory in infants and young children with infantile myoclonic seizures.

A tendency to repeated seizures, with or without apparent organic cause, is found in some families, but the risk of occurrence of a convulsive disorder in siblings or in offspring of affected persons cannot be assessed accurately. It may be helpful for parents to know that residual effects of a convulsion are rare and that children with convulsions who had parents with convulsive disorders have been better adjusted and had fewer seizures than those whose parents had not had seizures.

A severe prolonged seizure of 1 hr or more may deplete stores of glucose, interfere with oxygenation, and cause secondary cerebral changes, but there is reason to believe that the usual convulsive episode does not cause irreversible damage. Permanent hemiplegia following a convulsion is probably more often the result of a vascular accident which occurred before the seizure than to injury during it. In such instances recurrent convulsions are likely to be more difficult to control than those of idiopathic epilepsy.

Grand mal seizures tend to become more numerous unless the course is modified by therapy. On the other hand, some patients with unquestioned diagnoses of idiopathic grand mal epilepsy appear to have spontaneous cessation of seizures after adequate treatment. Epileptic patients who are otherwise normal seldom die or sustain serious injuries as a result of their disorder.

It is generally stated that 80% or more of children with epilepsy can expect to lead useful lives, but continuing changes in treatment, management, and facilities available to children and their families make inferences from longitudinal studies unreliable. A 25 yr study reported by Harrison and Taylor (1976) found that among 200 epileptic children residual handicap was minimal in two thirds, but many of these had educational difficulties and reduced employability, with a need for special education 7 times greater than in the population at large. The remaining one third were profoundly affected (death, institutional care, or unemployability and dependence on family). The cost of seizure disorders to the community is high, both in the use of human and medical resources and in the mental anguish and hardship imposed on patients, parents, and relatives.

20.7 DISORDERS SIMULATING EPILEPSY
(Including Epileptic Equivalents)

Narcolepsy. Narcolepsy is characterized by diurnal attacks of irrepressible sleep, usually precipitated by sudden emotional changes. It is rare in children and is said to be more frequent in boys than in girls. Six categories of narcolepsy have been described: toxic-infective, e.g., postencephalitic; circulatory; post-traumatic; endocrine; neoplastic; and psychopathologic.

The attacks resemble those of epilepsy in their brevity, in their abruptness of onset, and in their paroxysmal and involuntary nature. The overpowering sleep of narcolepsy may come on suddenly while the patient is engaged in some activity such as talking, walking, or driving. Activity ceases and the patient falls "in a heap." The "sleep" is usually shallow, and the patient is easily aroused. The disturbance apparently has no relation to the physiologic need for sleep. Regular nocturnal sleep is normal. The patient exhibits mental alertness rather than somnolence after arousal.

The disorder tends to be chronic, but spontaneous improvement and cure are more common than in epilepsy. The administration of amphetamines has generally proved effective. Dosage for a child should be the minimum amount which will produce the desired effect.

Abdominal Epilepsy. Otherwise unexplained recurrent episodes of abdominal pain, nausea, and vomiting have on occasion been considered to be a manifestation of epilepsy. Some epileptic children with psychomotor or grand mal seizures do have abdominal pain just prior to the onset of a convulsion, but abdominal pain as the only overt manifestation of epilepsy must, if it does occur, be extremely rare. Recurrent abdominal pain associated with headache, but without nausea or vomiting, has also been attributed to migraine (see below). If abdominal epilepsy is to be accepted as a diagnosis, the criteria for making it should be quite restrictive, probably as follows: recurrent episodes of abdominal pain, with or without headache but without twitching or convulsive movements; somnolence as a postictal manifestation; an abnormal electroencephalogram; and relief from the attacks of abdominal pain with anticonvulsive therapy.

Breath-Holding. See Sec 2.55. These spells, common in early childhood, are sometimes associated with tonic and clonic movements.

Hysterical Fits. These can superficially resemble true epileptic seizures, but are fairly easily distinguished. There is usually a typical neurotic background. Between attacks the patient may exhibit motor or sensory disturbances which do not follow the true neural patterns, and the gag reflex may be absent. Dilation of the pupils and pallor of the skin and mucous membranes rarely accompany an attack. Loss of consciousness is superficial and variable. Sphincter control is not lost, and bodily injury from the seizure does not occur. Crying, moaning, and disconnected talk throughout the attack, which may last half an hour or longer, are common. Hysterical patients, like other neurotic children with behavior problems, commonly have some abnormalities in the electroencephalogram. The treatment of hysterical seizures is that of the underlying psychologic disorder.

Syncope. Syncopal attacks of various types due chiefly to transient cerebral anemia are frequently complicated by slight tonic and clonic convulsive reactions of short duration confined mostly to the face and arms. The most common form in early life is the *simple fainting spell*, which is brought on reflexly in certain children by simple procedures such as removal of a sliver or insertion of a needle into the skin or by a sudden fright while in a standing or sitting posture. The susceptibility to fainting appears to be related to a defect in reflex regulation of the vascular system, which permits sudden relaxation of the visceral venous system with bradycardia and a fall in blood pressure. Placing the patient in a horizontal position or with the head tilted downward at a 45° angle will tend to shorten the period of unconsciousness. When it is necessary to subject a child known to faint easily to some painful test or treatment, it is advisable to have him or her lie on a table during the procedure. Vigorous crying before and during such a procedure as taking a blood sample tends to prevent fainting. In an older child active gripping of some object and voluntary contraction of the abdominal muscles have the same effect. It is not uncommon for persons with undoubted seizure disorders of cerebral origin to faint during emotional upsets.

Over 25% of "normal" young adults and probably many adolescents can produce loss of consciousness by hyperventilating in the upright position and then straining voluntarily against a closed glottis. At this time both EEG and ECG show changes. The clinical effects can be prevented by the administration of atropine or (in some instances) of a beta-adrenergic blocker. The fainting episodes usually happen while the person is standing in a warm, stuffy atmosphere or is suffering pain or an emotional upset. They rarely occur in supine persons. Just before the episode, affected persons may experience muscle weakness, tremor, nausea, a sinking feeling in the abdomen, sweating, and lightheadedness. After the faint these symptoms may continue briefly as consciousness is regained, whereas after a seizure of central nervous system origin, the description of the state of feeling is usually markedly altered.

In the *Stokes-Adams syndrome*, which occurs in heart block (Sec 13.69), a short convulsive reaction often accompanies the syncopal attack. The seizure appears within 10–20 sec after the onset of asystole. Similar syncopal attacks have been reported in patients as a result of *paroxysmal tachycardia*, and attacks occur fairly frequently after muscular effort in young children with certain congenital anomalies of the heart, such as the tetralogy of Fallot.

A *hyperactive carotid sinus reflex* manifests itself by episodes of unconsciousness with or without brief tonic and clonic convulsive attacks. This condition is extremely rare. Pressure over the carotid sinuses in the anterior cervical region causes a slowing or temporary arrest of the pulse in persons subject to attacks. Associated with the asystole are symptoms of faintness, weakness, loss of consciousness, and finally the convulsive reaction.

Apneic Episodes During Swimming. These episodes, especially in competitive events, have, in rare instances, been responsible for sudden loss of consciousness and at times for clonic movements. Such attacks presumably have been observed most frequently in adolescent boys and more often in association with the breast stroke than with other forms of swimming. Even expert underwater swimmers can, by forced hyperventilation before submerging, so deplete the body of carbon dioxide that hypoxia may produce unconsciousness before the respiratory center initiates a breath, or perhaps an overwhelming desire to attain a competitive goal may dominate the urge to breathe. When respiration cannot be restarted by prompt artificial respiration, it is presumed that ventricular fibrillation has occurred.

Migraine (Hemicrania) (Sec 21.14). In its paroxysmal nature, its chronicity, and its genetic features, migraine has long been regarded as akin in some respects to epilepsy. The 2 frequently occur in the same family. Occasionally, attacks of migraine are replaced by typical epileptic seizures. The use of the designation "sensory epilepsy" for migraine is inappropriate; the visual seizures of true epilepsy are much shorter in duration than the visual symptoms in migraine and are bilateral.

HENRY W. BAIRD

Baird HW, John ER, Ahn H, et al: Neurometric evaluation of epileptic children who do well and poorly in school. Electroencephalography Clin Neurophysiol 48:683, 1980.
Costeff AH: Reported seizures in early childhood: A 14-year follow-up. Dev Med Child Neurol 24:472, 1982.

Ellenberg JH, Nelson KB: Febrile seizures and later intellectual performance. Arch Neurol 35:17, 1978.

Ellenberg JH, Nelson KB: Birth weight and gestational age in children with cerebral palsy or seizure disorders. Am J Dis Child 133:1044, 1979.

Febrile convulsions: A suitable case for treatment. Lancet 72:680, 1980.

Freeman JM: Febrile seizures: A consensus of their significance, evaluation, and treatment. Pediatrics 66:1009, 1976.

Glaser GH: Kindling. Dev Med Child Neurol 25:137, 1983.

Kurokawa T, Goya N, Fukuyama Y, et al: West syndrome and Lennox-Gastaut syndrome: A survey of natural history. Pediatrics 65:81, 1980.

Lacy JR, Penry JK: Infantile Spasms. New York, Raven Press, 1976.

Lindsay J, Ounsted C, Richards P: Long-term outcome in children with temporal lobe seizures. I: Social outcome and childhood factors. Dev Med Child Neurol 21:285, 1979.

O'Donohoe NV: Epilepsies of Childhood. London, Butterworths, 1979.

Pedley TA: The pathophysiology of focal epilepsy: Neurophysiological considerations. Ann Neurol 3:2, 1978.

Penry JK, Daly DD: Advances in Neurology, Vol 11: Complex Partial Seizures and Their Treatment. New York, Raven Press, 1975.

Purpura DP: Dendritic differentiation in human cerebral cortex. Normal and aberrant developmental patterns. In: Advances in Neurology, Vol 12. New York, Raven Press, 1975, p 91.

Sillanpää M: The significance of motor handicap in the prognosis of childhood epilepsy. Dev Med Child Neurol 17:52, 1975.

Singer WD, Rabe EF, Haller JS: The effect of ACTH therapy upon infantile spasms. J Pediatr 96:485, 1980.

Ware S, Millward-Sadler GH: Acute liver disease associated with sodium valproate. Lancet 2:1110, 1980.

21 THE NERVOUS SYSTEM

EVALUATION OF THE CHILD WITH NEUROLOGIC DISEASE

21.1 HISTORY—THE SYMPTOMATOLOGY OF NEUROLOGIC DISORDERS

The neurologic evaluation should include a thorough pediatric history, with special attention to the evolution of the illness, which may provide important clues regarding the category of neurologic disorder. A static disability dating from early infancy suggests a congenital malformation or a lesion acquired in the perinatal period, but even in static brain lesions new symptoms emerge as the brain matures since the expression of a disorder of a particular function cannot become apparent until the age at which that function normally appears. Steady progression of disability with loss of previously acquired functions is seen in degenerative brain diseases, such as chronic encephalitis, uncompensated hydrocephalus, and brain tumors. Arrest of development generally precedes loss of function in progressive brain disease in infancy. Sudden disability followed by gradual improvement is characteristic of cerebral vascular diseases. Episodes of exacerbation followed by partial remission are seen most commonly in the demyelinating diseases. Histories of deterioration in school performance, loss of interest, irritability, and emotional lability are common in children with cerebral dysfunction.

Unsteadiness of gait, limping, stumbling, clumsiness, floppiness, tightness of muscles, and loss of skill in handwriting are all symptoms of motor dysfunction, but the history should never be relied upon for localization of motor disorders. This is accomplished only by neurologic examination.

Because children rarely complain of sensory deficits, these often go unnoticed until quite severe. Absence of visual following, random searching eye movements, and a tendency to look directly at bright lights without evidence of discomfort suggest severe visual defects in the infant. In the older child loss of visual acuity manifests itself by a tendency to walk into objects and to hold objects close to the eyes for inspection. Unilateral visual loss is usually asymptomatic even in the school-age child until formal testing of vision is carried out. A lack of response to sounds suggests severe hearing loss in the young child but is easily confused with the inattention of the retarded or autistic child. Partial hearing loss may express itself only as absence of speech or delay in its development, which may also be presenting complaints in retardation or autism. Repeated injuries of which the child fails to complain suggest loss of pain sensation.

The history is especially important in the diagnosis of paroxysmal disorders of the nervous system, such as seizures, syncope, and paroxysmal vertigo. When such attacks occur at infrequent intervals, decisions regarding diagnostic studies or therapy may have to depend on historical data alone. The events that precede an attack may provide clues. Anxiety, excitement, pain, or crying may commonly precede syncopal attacks but only rarely seizures. Exposure to unusual sensory stimuli such as flickering lights (e.g., television) may precipitate seizures. The older child who has seizures may describe a warning sensation or aura. The state of the patient during an attack should be ascertained as completely as possible. Was he or she unconscious, in a state of confusion, or lucid? Were there convulsive movements? If so, were they lateralized? Was there incontinence of urine or feces? Was recovery rapid, or was there a period of sleep or drowsiness? In infancy and early childhood manifestations of seizures may be so slight as not to be mentioned by parents unless specific inquiry is made. This is especially true of infantile myoclonic seizures; the momentary flexion of head, trunk, and arm is often dismissed as a normal startle response or as colic.

Vertigo, the sensation that the environment is turning or tilting, is easily misinterpreted in the young child who is unable to describe this sensation. The outward manifestations of an attack include unsteadiness, vomiting, fright, and unwillingness to move the head, which may be kept rigidly in 1 position. The child with vertigo remains lucid throughout the attack, in contrast to the child with epilepsy.

The correct diagnosis of headache is largely dependent on a careful history, which should ascertain time of occurrence of head pain, localization, quality (throbbing, dull, sharp, pressing, or bandlike), and associated symptoms such as nausea, vomiting, or visual disturbance. Headache that occurs principally after the child arises from bed and is associated with vomiting and drowsiness should suggest the possibility of increased intracranial pressure.

21.2 THE NEUROLOGIC EXAMINATION

A careful neurologic examination is essential for the correct localization of neurologic illness; it is a challenging task in the potentially uncooperative young child. The confidence of the child is secured by being gentle and informal and by making the procedure interesting to the patient. Uncomfortable tests, such as the funduscopic examination and sensory testing, should be postponed to the last portion of the examination. Much can be learned by observing the child playing, walking, or running. A portion of the examination can be carried out with the child sitting comfortably and securely on the mother's lap. Examination of the newborn infant, the child with psychiatric disorder, and the comatose patient presents special problems. The usual neurologic examination should record the following observations.

ASSESSMENT OF THE CHILD'S MENTAL STATUS AND BEHAVIOR

Important aspects of behavior are the child's ability to relate to others, level of activity, distractibility, attention span, and mood. The ability and/or willingness to cooperate with the examination and the appropriateness of responses to various situations provide important clues.

Speech functions are divided into expressive speech (talking) and receptive speech (understanding). Their evaluation is discussed in Sec 2.78. Isolated disorders of central speech mechanisms are referred to as *aphasias*. Several types of aphasia can be distinguished. In *expressive (Broca) aphasia* the patient is unable to speak, or speech is sparse and labored in telegraphic style. Understanding of verbal commands is preserved. In *receptive (Wernicke) aphasia* there is loss of comprehension of speech. The patient speaks fluently but with little content and may use empty words such as "that thing," circumlocutions, or made-up words (neologisms). The ability to repeat verbatim is impaired in both types of aphasia. In *global asphasia* both receptive and expressive speech are affected. Aphasia usually implies a lesion in the dominant temporal lobe. It must be distinguished from speech disorders secondary to hearing loss and from dysarthria, a speech defect resulting from dysfunction of muscles of articulation.

Ability to read is tested by use of graded reading paragraphs. An isolated inability to read in a child of otherwise normal intellectual functions is referred to as *dyslexia*. The neurologic examination should include an assessment of writing, drawing, and copying of shapes. For example, the drawing of a man tests the ability to control a pencil, to produce recognizable shapes, and to arrange shapes in space in proper proportions. As a rough approximation, a 4 yr old child should be able to draw a figure with 4 recognizable parts, a 5 yr old with 8 recognizable features. Ability to draw shapes can also be tested by having the child copy geometric figures, such as circle and cross (3 yr), square (4 yr), and triangle and diamond (5 yr). In a child with otherwise normal motor functions and with good ability to recognize shapes inability to draw objects is referred to as *apraxia*. This type of defect is associated with lesions of a parietal lobe. It also occurs as a transient maturational lag in early school-age children with learning disabilities.

Handedness should be noted. Normally, clear preference for 1 hand in writing, eating, and reaching is established by the age of 3 yr. Delayed development of handedness is found in children with mental slowness and learning disorders. Right-handed children have left cerebral dominance for speech, but the dominant hemisphere cannot be predicted for left-handed children, more than 50% of whom also have speech localization in the left hemisphere. Memory can be tested by giving the child a list of 4 or 5 object words to be recalled 5 min later. Testing of arithmetic ability such as counting, addition, and subtraction is helpful in the assessment of children with possible mental slowness, in whom the understanding of abstract mathematical concepts tends to be especially poor. Formal psychologic testing is often helpful.

MOTOR EXAMINATION

The motor examination requires an understanding of the organization of the motor system (Fig 21–1). Voluntary movements depend on intact neural pathways, including at least 2 motor neurons, upper and lower. The axons of the upper motor neurons, whose cells of origin are in the motor cortex, form the *pyramidal tract*, which passes via the internal capsule and brain stem to the spinal cord. The pyramidal tract fibers cross to the opposite side in the lower medulla and synapse on anterior horn cells in the spinal cord. The anterior horn cells (lower motor neurons) send their axons via peripheral nerves to muscle. Each lower motor neuron innervates a group of muscle fibers, up to several hundred in some of the large muscles of the extremities. A lower motor neuron and the group of muscle fibers it innervates are known as a *motor unit*. The basic motor pathway (Fig 21–1) is influenced by a number of other centers, which as a group are known as the *extrapyramidal motor system*. These include the basal ganglia and the cerebellum. The functions of the extrapyramidal motor system include the control of repetitive motor acts and the coordination of movements. In general, lesions of the upper motor neuron or of the extrapyramidal motor system interfere with voluntary motor activities without interrupting involuntary and reflex motor functions. In many instances such lesions result in enhancement of involuntary and reflex motor activity through release from central inhibitory influences. Lesions of the lower motor neuron lead to loss of both voluntary and involuntary motor activities. In addition, the denervation of muscle leads to atrophy and to spontaneous activity (*fibrillation*) of individual muscle fibers. Fibrillations are visible only in the tongue, where they appear as worm-like movements. Coarse, irregular twitches, due to simultaneous contraction of entire motor units (*fasciculations*), are seen primarily in diseases involving the anterior horn cells.

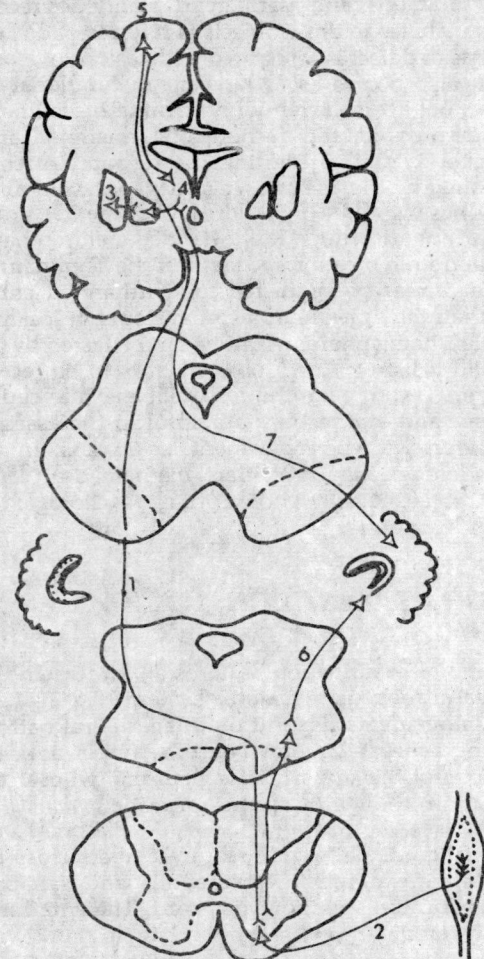

Figure 21-1 Schematic representation of the more important motor pathways. 1 = Upper motor neuron; 2 = Lower motor neuron; 3 = Basal ganglia, which send efferent fibers to the thalamus (4), which in turn influences the motor cortex (5). 6 = Descending fibers from cerebellum influencing motor neuron activity in spinal cord. 7 = Ascending fibers from cerebellum, which act on motor cortex via the thalamus.

It is usually possible to localize a motor lesion in upper or lower motor neurons or in the extrapyramidal motor system by the following simple clinical tests:

Assessment of Muscle Strength.   Strength is tested informally in the younger child. Ability to stand up from the supine position tests back, hip, and proximal leg muscles. Walking on tiptoes and on heels tests the gastrocnemius-soleus and the tibialis anterior, respectively. Shoulder muscles are tested by supporting and/or lifting the child with the examiner's hands in the child's axillae. Intercostal muscles can be assessed by observing spontaneous respirations and by asking the child to blow out a match. In the older child strength is tested separately in individual muscle groups and is graded on a 0–5 scale as follows:

0 = no movement
1 = movement with gravity eliminated
2 = full range against gravity

3 = movement against slight resistance
4 = movement against moderate resistance
5 = normal strength

Muscular weakness occurs with lesions of upper or lower motor neurons but is usually absent in extrapyramidal disorders. Upper motor neuron lesions produce weakness, especially in the extensor muscles of the upper limbs and in the flexors of the legs. Diseases of the peripheral nerve result in distal weakness; most muscle diseases affect proximal muscles.

Assessment of Muscle Bulk.   Atrophy of muscle is marked in lower motor neuron lesions, less striking in diseases of upper motor neurons. Fasciculations should always be looked for in atrophic muscles since their presence tends to localize the lesion in the anterior horn cells. Both upper and lower motor neuron lesions interfere with growth of the affected extremity. Excessive muscle bulk or muscular hypertrophy is usually due to increased muscular activity. It occurs normally in athletes and abnormally in muscle diseases with myotonia and in the adrenogenital syndrome. Pseudohypertrophy refers to enlargement of muscles that are weak. It is usually due to infiltration of muscle with fat, such as occurs in muscular dystrophy, or to distention of muscle by an abnormal substance, e.g., glycogen in type II glycogenosis (Pompe disease).

Assessment of Muscle Tone.   This is estimated by the resistance to passive movement of an extremity. It ranges from atonia and hypotonia to severe rigidity. Diminished muscle tone occurs in lower motor neuron diseases and in some extrapyramidal disorders, especially those of the cerebellum. *Rigidity* is an increase in resistance throughout passive movement of a joint; it occurs in disorders of the basal ganglia. It must be distinguished from *spasticity*, or increased resistance to passive movement which gives way suddenly (*clasp-knife effect*). Spasticity is a sign of upper motor neuron disease.

Tests of Fine Motor Coordination.   Impairment of skilled movements is found in disorders of upper motor neurons and in cerebellar diseases. It can be assessed informally by watching the child manipulate toys, control a pencil, or put on clothing. A more formal test consists of rapid alternating supination and pronation of the hands. Irregular and slow performance of this test is seen in children with cerebellar disease, but care must be exercised in interpretation since the adult level of performance is not reached until the midteens. Incoordination of gait (ataxia) is also characteristic of cerebellar lesions. In diseases of a cerebellar hemisphere the patient tends to reel to the side of the lesion. When cerebellar involvement is diffuse or confined to the midline vermis, the child may stagger to either side. Mild degrees of ataxia can be brought out by having the child walk a line with heel to toe or hop on 1 foot.

Involuntary Movements.   These occur principally in diseases of basal ganglia and of the cerebellum. They are usually absent during complete relaxation, especially during sleep; they are brought out by attempts to maintain a given posture or to carry out a skilled motor act. *Tremor* is defined as a rapid, regular, repetitive involuntary movement, usually of the distal extremities. A fine tremor of the outstretched hands is seen in

Table 21-1 DISEASES OF THE NEUROMUSCULAR SYSTEM

	UPPER MOTOR NEURON	BASAL GANGLIA	CEREBELLUM	ANTERIOR HORN CELLS	PERIPHERAL NERVE	MUSCLE
Strength	Decreased	Normal	Normal	Decreased	Decreased	Decreased
Muscle tone	Spasticity (usually)	Hypotonia or rigidity	Hypotonia	Hypotonia	Hypotonia	Normal or hypotonia
Coordination	Decreased	Decreased	Decreased	Normal	Normal	Normal
Involuntary movements	None	Chorea, athetosis, or dystonia	Intention tremor	Fasciculations	None	None
Tendon reflexes	Hyperactive	Normal	Decreased	Absent or decreased	Absent or decreased	Decreased
Babinski sign	Present	Absent	Absent	Absent	Absent	Absent
Sensory deficit	Usually present	Absent	Absent	Absent	Present	Absent

anxiety and in thyrotoxicosis. A similar, somewhat coarser tremor occurs as a benign hereditary trait. A more proximal tremor of the outstretched arms and wrists (wing-beating tremor) is seen in Wilson disease. Tremor that becomes more marked on approach to the target is known as intention tremor; it is a sign of cerebellar disorder. It can be observed in the young child reaching for a toy. In the older child it is brought out by the finger-to-nose test, in which the child touches the examiner's finger and his or her own nose alternately.

Three characteristic disorders of movement—chorea, athetosis, and dystonia—are seen in diseases of the basal ganglia:

Chorea consists of irregular jerking and writhing movements, often in proximal muscles such as the tongue, face, neck, and shoulder. These may be quite violent and may cause the child to fling the arms or suddenly to drop a held object. Gait is irregular, with sudden lurching to the side; walking may be impossible when chorea is severe. Mild chorea is to be distinguished from tic, which is a stereotyped sudden movement, always involving the same muscle group. Tic can be voluntarily inhibited by the patient for a short period of time.

Athetosis is a slow writhing movement, often more marked in the distal extremities, consisting of alternating supination-pronation and flexion-extension of the limbs.

Dystonia is a tendency toward hyperextension of joints, brought out especially when the patient tries to walk. Typically, there is plantar flexion of the feet, hyperextension of the legs, extension and pronation of arms, arching of the back, and extension and rotation of the neck.

All abnormal extrapyramidal movements are accentuated during emotional stress and disappear during sleep. Failure to appreciate these features may lead to the erroneous impression that there is a psychiatric disorder.

Examination of Reflexes. The tendon reflexes are elicited by stretching of a tendon, usually by a quick tap with a reflex hammer. They provide evidence of the intactness of a particular reflex arc which includes sensory nerve endings in tendon, sensory nerve fibers, spinal cord, motor neuron, and muscle. The tendon reflexes are decreased or absent in disorders of peripheral nerves or muscle and in diseases that affect the

spinal cord or brain stem at the level of the reflex arc. The intactness of specific segments of the neuraxis can be assessed as follows:

Central Segment	Related Reflex
pons	Jaw jerk
C5–6	Biceps jerk
C5–6	Supinator jerk
C6,7,8	Triceps jerk
L3–4	Knee jerk
S1–2	Ankle jerk

A tense or anxious patient may have difficulty relaxing sufficiently for demonstration of the tendon reflexes. Distraction of the patient by having him or her squeeze hands together may produce the necessary relaxation. Hyperactivity of tendon reflexes, especially when associated with clonus, is a sign of upper motor neuron disease.

Several superficial reflexes are elicited by stroking the skin. The plantar reflex is produced by a firm stroke against the lateral aspect of the sole, moving from the heel forward. A normal response consists of flexion of the toes. The abnormal response or Babinski sign consists of extension of the great toe, often associated with fanning of the other toes. Beyond the age of 2 yr it indicates pyramidal tract dysfunction. Abdominal reflexes consist of contraction of the abdominal muscles following stroking of the overlying skin. Their absence suggests either a lesion of the spinal cord segment that is stimulated (T10–L1) or a central motor lesion. The cremasteric reflex consists of ascent of the testis upon stroking the skin of the medial thigh; it is absent in lesions involving the L1–2 segment. The anal reflex, elicited by stroking the perianal skin, assesses the lower sacral segments.

Table 21–1 summarizes the clinical abnormalities in various categories of neuromuscular disease.

SENSORY EXAMINATION

This is necessarily limited in the infant and young child. Response to pain can be tested by observation of withdrawal and of emotional reaction to pinprick. This maneuver tests intactness of peripheral pain fibers and of pain pathways up to the level of the thalamus. In the evaluation of unilateral sensory impairment it has to be remembered that near the midline there is an overlap of innervation from the 2 sides. A sensory defect which ends abruptly at the midline is due to hysteria or malingering rather than to neurologic disease. Function of the posterior columns in the spinal cord is tested by asking the child to identify direction of passive movement of a joint (*position sense*) and by response to the vibration of a tuning fork placed on a bony prominence such as the lateral malleolus. Intactness of the sensory cortex is determined by a number of sensory discrimination tests, such as identification of objects placed into the hand (*stereognosis*), ability to recognize numbers drawn onto the skin (*graphesthesia*), or responses to simultaneous stimulation of 2 points (*2-point discrimination*) and to bilateral simultaneous stimulation.

EXAMINATION OF CRANIAL NERVES AND THEIR CENTRAL CONNECTIONS

The cranial nerves innervate the eye muscles, facial muscles, and muscles of deglutition, and they carry somatosensory fibers from the face and fibers from the special sensory organs. In testing muscles innervated by cranial nerves, the same principles apply as in the examination of motor function in the extremities: motor abnormalities in muscles supplied by cranial nerves may be due to lower motor neuron, upper motor neuron, or extrapyramidal disorders.

Cranial Nerve I (Olfactory Nerve). Ability to identify odors such as peppermint or coffee is determined for each nostril separately. Chronic rhinitis is the most common cause of *anosmia*.

Cranial Nerve II (Optic Nerve). *Vision* is frequently affected in children with neurologic disease. In the toddler rough assessment of acuity is possible through observation of the response to a small object, such as a bread crumb. The Snellen picture charts may be used for preschool children. The young child is normally myopic; 20/20 vision is reached at age 6 yr. Gross evaluation of visual fields is possible as soon as the infant is able to fixate and to follow visually. A test object such as a reflex hammer or a red block is gradually moved into the field of vision. The child fixes on the object as soon as it is seen. In the older child, visual fields are tested by confrontation: the child closes 1 eye and fixes with the other on the nose of the examiner who confronts the child. The examiner gradually moves 1 finger or another test object into the field of vision, and the child reports when it is first seen. Formal perimetry is possible by school age. The course of visual pathways from the different retinal areas is indicated schematically in Fig 21–2.

Homonymous hemianopsia, in which the defect involves the temporal field of 1 eye and the nasal fields of the opposite eye, is seen in lesions of the optic radiations or of the visual cortex. The cerebral lesion is opposite the side of the field defect. A homonymous upper quadrant defect indicates a lesion in the temporal lobe white matter, through which the optic radiation fibers from the inferior portion of the retina pass on their way to the visual cortex.

Bitemporal hemianopsia implies a lesion in the region

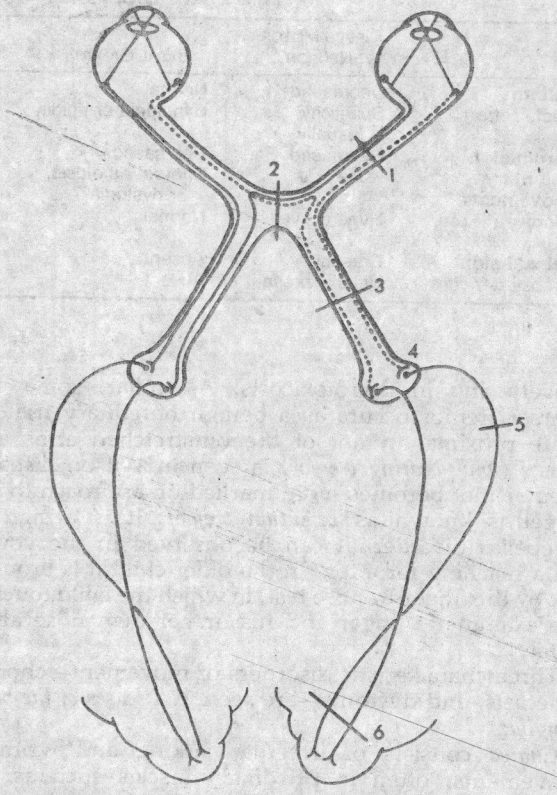

Figure 21–2 Schematic representation of visual pathways. 1 = Optic nerve. Lesion in this location causes unilateral visual loss. 2 = Optic chiasm. Lesion results in bitemporal hemianopsia because it interrupts fibers to the nasal half of both retinas. 3 = Optic tract. Lesion causes homonymous hemianopsia by interrupting temporal fibers on the same side and nasal fibers on the opposite side. 4 = Lateral geniculate body. 5 = Optic radiation. Fibers are widely separated and partial lesions are common. The fibers from the lower part of the retina pass in the white matter beneath the temporal cortex; thus homonymous upper quadrant anopsia in temporal lobe lesions is frequent. 6 = Visual cortex. Lesions may cause partial or complete homonymous hemianopsia.

of the optic chiasm, most often in children with craniopharyngioma.

Funduscopic examination is always included in a complete neurologic examination. A pale optic nerve head with sparsity of capillary vessels on the disc indicates optic atrophy. In papilledema the optic disc is hyperemic, the optic cup is obliterated, and the disc may protrude forward into the vitreous. The retinal veins are distended, and venous pulsations are absent. Hemorrhage may be present on the disc or adjacent to it. The appearance of papilledema may be indistinguishable from inflammation of the optic disc or papillitis. In papilledema, however, visual acuity tends to be preserved until late, whereas it is lost early in papillitis.

Cranial Nerve III. This nerve carries the pupilloconstrictor fibers and innervates all the extraocular muscles except the lateral rectus and superior oblique. Pupillary asymmetry at rest may be due to unilateral visual loss, a midbrain lesion, 3rd nerve palsy, or a lesion of cervical sympathetic nerves (Horner syndrome, Sec 21.28). Slight but definite asymmetry of pupillary size is not uncommon, however, in normal children. In unilateral visual loss the pupil on the affected side is dilated and the pupillary reflex diminished or absent when the affected eye is exposed to light; the pupil constricts normally, however, when the opposite (seeing) eye is stimulated (consensual light reflex). In lesions of the 3rd nerve or of its cells of origin in the upper midbrain the pupil of the affected side is dilated, and both direct and consensual light reflexes are lost. Third nerve palsy causes deviation of the eye down and out as a result of unopposed action of the superior oblique and the lateral rectus; there also is ptosis due to paralysis of the voluntary portion of the levator palpebrae.

Cranial Nerve IV. This nerve innervates the superior oblique muscle only. An isolated palsy, which is rare, causes inability to turn the affected eye downward when it is in the adducted position.

Cranial Nerve VI. Palsy of the 6th nerve results in inability to abduct the eye on the affected side. The lesion has to be distinguished from convergent strabismus. In strabismus, eye movements generally are full when each eye is tested alone; the abnormality is evident only when both eyes are open. Patching of the good eye for a time may be necessary before the child becomes able to abduct the squinting eye.

Abnormalities of Eye Movements Secondary to Supranuclear Lesions. Brain stem lesions may result in abnormalities of eye movements because of disruption of the fibers connecting the various oculomotor nuclei. In *internuclear ophthalmoplegia* the patient is unable to adduct either eye during visual following movements, but adduction during convergence is usually preserved. In *skew deviation*, 1 eye is elevated with respect to the other in all directions of gaze. Lesions of the upper brain stem in the pineal region cause paralysis of upward gaze. Paralysis of conjugate lateral gaze may be due to a lesion in the pons on the same side, but more commonly it is caused by a cortical lesion involving the gaze centers in the frontal or the occipital cortex on the opposite side. With cortical lesions, only voluntary eye movements are affected. Reflex eye turning, such as may be induced by vestibular stimulation, is preserved.

Lesions involving cerebellar and vestibular pathways produce rhythmic jerking of the eyes (*nystagmus*). Most forms of nystagmus have a slow and a fast component. In nystagmus due to dysfunction of the cerebellum or of cerebellar connections in the brain stem the nystagmus becomes more marked when the eyes are deviated laterally; the slow component is always toward the midline. This type of nystagmus is seen in intoxication with certain drugs such as phenytoin and the barbiturates. It may also occur with structural lesions of the cerebellum or brain stem, and it is often present in children with cerebellar tumors. The nystagmus tends to be coarser and of greater amplitude when the eye is deviated to the side of the tumor.

Nystagmus due to cerebellar or brain stem disorders has to be distinguished from nystagmus caused by labyrinthine dysfunction and from congenital nystagmus. Labyrinthine nystagmus often varies with head position, tends to have a rotary component, is most obvious at rest when the patient is not fixing on any object, and is associated with vertigo and nausea. It occurs acutely following trauma to or inflammation of the labyrinth (labyrinthitis). Congenital nystagmus is pendular at rest, with irregular jerking when the eyes are deviated to the sides. It is usually associated with poor visual acuity and is thought to be due to failure of development of visual fixation in infancy.

Cranial Nerve V. The trigeminal nerve conveys sensation, including touch and pain, from the entire face except for a small area at the angle of the mandible. Its upper (ophthalmic) division is tested by the corneal reflex. The 5th nerve also has a motor component which innervates the muscles of mastication. Unilateral paralysis causes deviation of the jaw to the side of the lesion. The intactness of the segmental arc involving the muscles of mastication is tested by means of the jaw jerk. A brisk jaw jerk or jaw clonus implies a bilateral upper motor neuron lesion.

Cranial Nerve VII. The facial nerve is frequently affected in childhood as a result of congenital anomalies, birth injury, inflammation (Bell palsy), and tumor. It innervates all the facial muscles except the levator palpebrae. Mild weakness is made evident by asking the child to show the teeth; it can be detected in the infant by watching facial movements during crying. The palpebral fissure is larger on the side of the weakness. In addition to motor fibers, the facial nerve carries parasympathetic fibers to the lacrimal and salivary glands and a sensory branch which transmits taste sensation from the anterior two thirds of the tongue. Lacrimation, salivation, and taste are affected only in lesions of the proximal portion of the nerve in its course through the facial canal in the temporal bone. Taste is tested by placing salt or sugar on the outstretched tip of the tongue by means of a cotton applicator and having the patient indicate by head nods which taste sensation is felt. Peripheral facial nerve weakness has to be distinguished from weakness due to a central (corticobulbar) lesion. In weakness of facial muscles due to a central nervous system lesion the upper face is less severely affected, and the patient continues to be able to wrinkle the forehead. There is often associated weakness of arm, hand, and leg on the same side.

Cranial Nerve VIII. This consists of auditory and vestibular divisions. Hearing can be tested grossly in the young child by observing the response to the noise made by rubbing the fingers together or by crinkling a piece of paper and in the older child by asking for identification of whispered words. Formal audiometry is indicated in any child suspected of hearing or speech disorder since partial deafness, especially for high tones, is easily missed by gross clinical testing. Vestibular dysfunction is rare in childhood but should be suspected in a child with episodic vertigo, staggering, and vomiting, especially when there is associated labyrinthine nystagmus. It can be confirmed by caloric testing with cold water, which normally produces deviation of the eyes to the side of stimulation. A more comfortable test consists of rotation of the child while being held upright under the arms of the examiner. If vestibular functions are intact, ocular deviation toward the direction of rotation will occur.

Cranial Nerves IX and X. Dysfunction of these

nerves produces difficulty in swallowing and in phonation. Palatal paralysis can be observed by inspection
of the soft palate and uvula when the patient says "ah."
The gag reflex is diminished or absent. Secretions pool
in the oropharynx, and the patient drools excessively.
With unilateral lesions the voice is nasal or hoarse;
bilateral lesions cause aphonia and stridor.

Cranial Nerve XI (Spinal Accessory).   This nerve
innervates the sternocleidomastoid and trapezius muscles. Paralysis causes weakness in head rotation toward
the opposite side and in elevation of the shoulder on
the affected side.

Cranial Nerve XII (Hypoglossal).   Lesions of this
nerve produce paralysis of tongue movements and
atrophy and fibrillations of the tongue. In unilateral
involvement the tongue is deviated to the side of the
lesion on attempted protrusion.

Lesions of the 9th, 10th, and 12th cranial nerves have
to be distinguished from impairment of swallowing,
phonation, and tongue movement resulting from bilateral central nervous system (corticobulbar) disorders.
The latter lesions, known collectively as *pseudobulbar
palsy*, are manifested by difficulty in swallowing, slurred
speech, and impaired control of emotional expression,
with inappropriate laughing and crying, and by brisk
reflex responses involving the bulbar muscles, including
a brisk gag reflex. This type of deficit is common in
children with spastic cerebral palsy.

EXAMINATION OF THE CRANIUM

The neurologic examination includes measurement of
head circumference and inspection of the skull for
symmetry and shape. Abnormalities of shape, especially those associated with palpable bony ridges, suggest craniosynostosis. Auscultation over the skull or
over the eyes may reveal a cranial bruit. This is a normal
finding up to about age 6 yr. In the older child it
suggests the possibility of a cerebral vascular malformation or of increased intracranial pressure. Percussion
of the skull gives a sound resembling that of a cracked
pot (*Macewen sign*) when the cranial structures are
separated because of increased intracranial pressure.

EXAMINATION OF THE AUTONOMIC
NERVOUS SYSTEM

A limited number of clinical tests can be used to
assess intactness of the autonomic nervous system.
These consist of measurement of blood pressure and of
body temperature, including diurnal variations. Absence of sweating can be shown by painting a portion
of the skin involved with iodine and covering it with
starch powder, which fails to turn dark blue in areas of
anhidrosis. Parasympathetic function is tested by the
Mecholyl test: a 2% solution of methacholine (Mecholyl)
is instilled into 1 conjunctival sac. This produces constriction of the pupil in patients with parasympathetic
disorders such as familial dysautonomia. Disorders of
the parasympathetic innervation of the bladder result
in urinary retention and incomplete emptying. The
cystometrogram helps to evaluate partial lesions.

21.3 NEUROLOGIC EXAMINATION
OF THE INFANT

At birth human neurologic function is largely at a
subcortical (brain stem and spinal cord) level. Cortical
functions cannot be tested reliably, and even major
cerebral defects may go unnoticed. Accordingly, extreme caution is indicated in giving a prognosis as to
future intellectual function from neurologic findings in
the neonatal period. Measurement of head size can at
times give indirect evidence of major cerebral defect. A
head circumference more than 3 standard deviations
below the normal for gestational age suggests a defect
in brain growth that will usually be permanent. Major
malformations of the cerebrum can sometimes be detected by transillumination of the skull with a bright
flashlight equipped with a soft rubber cuff or with a
specially constructed (commercially available) high-in-
tensity transilluminator. A totally darkened room is
essential. A light beam applied to the occiput can be
seen shining through the globes of the eyes in infants
with hydranencephaly. Less marked transillumination
is seen with subdural effusions or extreme hydrocephalus. A localized area of increased transillumination,
usually unilateral, is found in porencephaly. During
the 1st yr of life intracranial pressure can be assessed
clinically by palpation of the anterior fontanelle. Normally the fontanelle of the sitting infant is soft and
slightly depressed. The fontanelle is tense and bulging
in the infant with increased intracranial pressure; it is
sunken with dehydration or with destructive brain
lesions which lead to low intracranial pressure. Chronic
increase in intracranial pressure is manifested by abnormal head enlargement.

Reflexes.   Many reflex patterns mediated by brain
stem and spinal cord mechanisms are found in the
newborn infant and during the 1st months of postnatal
life. The responses are stereotyped; they are normally
present but may be less brisk in the sleepy or recently
fed infant. Absence of reflex responses indicates general
depression of central or peripheral motor functions;
asymmetric responses suggest focal motor lesions,
either peripheral or central. As the infant matures, the
neonatal reflexes disappear in a predictable order as
voluntary motor functions supersede them. Abnormal
persistence of these reflexes is seen in infants with
general developmental lag or with central motor lesions;
ages of appearance and disappearance of certain of the
reflexes are shown in Table 21–2.

The *Moro reflex* (Fig 21–3) is elicited by placing the
infant supine upon the examining table, the head supported by the examiner's hand. The support is withdrawn suddenly, and the head is allowed to fall backward for 10–15 degrees. The reflex consists of extension
of the trunk and extension and abduction followed by
flexion and adduction of the arms, with less regular
participation of the legs. The *stepping reflex* consists of
movements of walking which are elicited when the
infant is held upright and inclined forward with soles
of feet touching a flat surface. The *placing reflex* occurs
when the infant is held erect and the dorsum of 1 foot
is drawn along the under edge of a table top. The
response consists of flexion followed by extension of
the leg that is stimulated.

Table 21-2 REFLEXES OF NEONATES

REFLEX	AGE AT WHICH REFLEX USUALLY APPEARS	AGE AT WHICH REFLEX IS NORMALLY NO LONGER OBTAINABLE
Moro	Birth	3 mo
Stepping	Birth	6 wk
Placing	Birth	6 wk
Sucking and rooting	Birth	4 mo awake 7 mo asleep
Palmar grasp	Birth	6 mo
Plantar grasp	Birth	10 mo
Adductor spread of knee jerk	Birth	7 mo
Tonic neck	2 mo	6 mo
Neck righting	4–6 mo	24 mo
Landau	3 mo	24 mo
Parachute reaction	9 mo	Persists

Several *postural reflexes* can be easily observed in the infant. The *tonic neck reflex* (Fig 21–3), which is elicited by rapidly turning the head of the supine infant to 1 side, consists of extension of the arm and leg on the side to which the face is turned and flexion of the limbs on the opposite side (fencing posture). Tonic neck patterns are normally prominent in the 2–4 mo old infant. Their persistence past the age of 6–9 mo occurs with central motor lesions, especially in infants with spastic cerebral palsy. The *neck righting reflex* consists of rotation of the trunk in the direction in which the head of the supine infant is turned. It is absent or decreased in infants with spasticity. The *Landau reflex* is demonstrated by supporting the infant in the prone position with the examiner's hand beneath the abdomen. A normal response consists of extension of head, trunk, and hips. Flexion of trunk and hips occurs when the examiner flexes the head. The *parachute reflex* consists of extension of arms, hands, and fingers when the infant, suspended in prone position, is suddenly allowed to fall for a short distance onto a soft pad.

The *sucking reflex* is initiated by stroking the lips. Stroking of the cheek produces the *rooting reflex*, which consists of turning the mouth toward the stimulus. *Grasp reflexes* are elicited by light pressure on the palms or on the soles of the feet. *Tendon reflexes* are generally present in the normal neonate; only the knee jerk may be easily obtainable. Brisk tendon jerks may be normal, and there may be adductor spread of the knee jerk and unsustained ankle clonus. Spontaneous clonus of arms, legs, and feet is seen in infants with cerebral disorders. Absence of tendon reflexes suggests a neuromuscular disorder, such as Werdnig-Hoffmann disease. The *Babinski sign* is not helpful in infancy since either flexion or extension of toes may normally be obtained.

Assessment of Motor Functions. This includes careful observation of spontaneous activity, which should be symmetrical. Consistent fisting of hands with adduction of thumbs is abnormal and suggests a central motor lesion. Maintained opisthotonus is evidence of severe spasticity; it is rarely seen in neonatal meningitis except in the terminal stage but is common in kernicterus and may be seen in other conditions, including congenital toxoplasmosis, maple syrup urine disease, and poisoning, e.g., with the phenothiazines and strychnine. *Scissoring* of legs as a result of increased

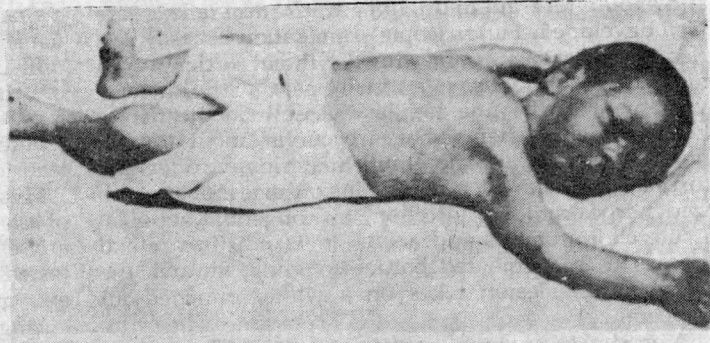

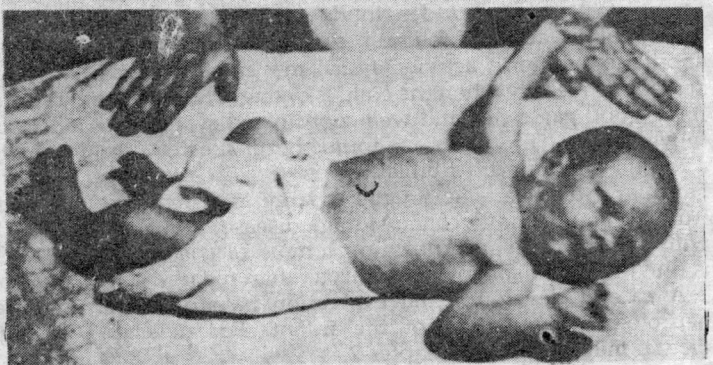

Figure 21-3 Upper photograph shows a spontaneous tonic neck reflex. Lower photograph shows the Moro reflex.

tone in adductors of the hips is a sign of spasticity. *Diminished muscle tone* is seen in infants with diffuse cerebral dysfunction and in peripheral neuromuscular diseases. Hypotonic infants tend to lie in the frog-leg position, with arms abducted at the shoulders. There is head lag and absence of contraction of shoulder muscles (absent traction response) when the supine infant is pulled to the sitting position. Rapid *tremors* of the limbs (jitteriness) are seen in infants with metabolic disturbances such as hypoglycemia or hypocalcemia but may occur without obvious cause. They must be distinguished from the slower and often focal intermittent clonic movements characteristic of seizure activity in infancy.

The quality of the *infant's cry* can be of diagnostic help. The cry is high-pitched in the infant with increased intracranial pressure, hoarse in cretinism, feeble in the infant with Werdnig-Hoffmann disease, and catlike in the cri-du-chat syndrome.

Examination of the Cranial Nerves. In the neonate the presence of vision is indicated by blinking in response to a bright light. Visual following can usually be demonstrated in the normal fullterm infant. It is one of the few signs of cerebral cortical function in the immediate neonatal period. A light or the examiner's face, moved slowly 9–12 in from the child's eyes, is an adequate stimulus. Visual following movements of the infant are irregular and poorly sustained. The eyes tend to move conjugately, but intermittent disconjugate eye movements may occur normally. The presence of full lateral eye movements can be ascertained by rotation of the infant's head, which results in deviation of the eyes to the side opposite the rotation. The pupils of the newborn infant should be approximately equal in size and should respond to bright light. Corneal reflexes are well developed. Funduscopic examination is easily carried out in a dark room with the infant sucking on a nipple. The optic disc is normally pale, with underdevelopment of the fine capillary vessels on the nervehead. Preretinal hemorrhages occur in about 10% of normal neonates. Chorioretinitis may signify congenital toxoplasmosis, cytomegalic inclusion disease, generalized herpes simplex infection, or congenital syphilis. Acute chorioretinitis appears as gray, indistinct retinal masses with pigmented borders. After a few wk the center of the lesion takes on a white, punched-out appearance.

A gross assessment of hearing is possible. The normal infant startles to a sudden loud noise. Responses to more subtle auditory stimuli consist of changes in spontaneous motor activity. Facial movements are assessed most easily when the child is crying. The neonate has a good gag reflex and well-coordinated swallowing movements. The tongue should be inspected. An atrophic tongue with fibrillations is seen in Werdnig-Hoffmann disease. The tongue is large and may protrude in cretinism, glycogen storage disease, and Beckwith syndrome. The protruding tongue of trisomy 21 is due more to a shallow oropharynx than to large size.

A careful developmental evaluation is part of the neurologic examination of the infant. For developmental milestones see Chapter 2.

21.4 NEUROLOGIC EVALUATION OF THE CHILD WITH PSYCHIATRIC DISEASE

Older children and adolescents with psychiatric disorders may have symptoms and signs mimicking neurologic disease. Problems in differential diagnosis arise especially in *hysteria*. The history is helpful since the hysterical patient has often had a variety of previous symptoms. Fairly characteristic ones include a sensation of compression of the throat (*globus hystericus*) and recurrent abdominal pain without associated positive physical findings. The patient tends to relate symptoms and disabilities in a matter-of-fact, detached manner, an emotional state referred to as *"la belle indifférence."* Common manifestations easily confused with neurologic dysfunction include hysterical blindness, spasm of convergence, gait disturbance, paralysis, sensory loss, seizures, and urinary retention.

Hysterical blindness can usually be distinguished from true visual loss by the absence of funduscopic findings and by preservation of pupillary constriction to light and of opticokinetic nystagmus. Differentiation from cortical blindness, such as may occur transiently after head injury or cerebral angiography, may be difficult. Hysterical visual field defects tend to be concentric, with general constriction of the fields in both eyes. Characteristically, the absolute size of the visual fields on a screen remains the same no matter at what distance from the screen the field is tested. Demonstration of this type of *"tunnel vision"* is very helpful since it cannot be explained on the basis of any organic lesion.

Spasm of convergence tends to be of sudden onset, usually during some traumatic experience such as a difficult school examination. The child complains of blurring vision or double vision, and on examination it is noted that the eyes are disconjugate, both in the adducted position. Reassurance and suggestion usually lead to rapid improvement.

Hysterical gait disturbances usually occur in the form of *astasia abasia*, an inability to stand or to walk without any evidence of neurologic deficit when the patient is tested in the lying position. The gait is bizarre, with extreme lurching to the sides, requiring exquisite balancing acts to prevent a fall. It has to be distinguished from cerebellar ataxia, in which the patient walks on a wide base and has great difficulty maintaining balance.

Hysterical paralysis is distinguished from true paralysis by presence of normal muscle tone, normal tendon reflexes, and negative Babinski signs. *Hoover sign* is helpful in unilateral paralysis involving the legs. The examiner places a hand under the heel of the paralyzed leg and then asks the patient to raise the normal leg against resistance. In hysteria forceful raising of the normal leg leads to downward pressure of the "paralyzed" leg against the examiner's hand; no such pressure occurs in true paralysis.

When sensory loss is unilateral, hysterical loss ends exactly at the midline, whereas loss due to an organic lesion is restored about 2.5 cm short of the midline because of overlapping innervation of the midline areas. Anesthesia in glove and stocking distribution is commonly hysterical. In sensory neuropathy the transition from abnormal to normal is more gradual. A useful maneuver is to test repeatedly, each time shifting the point at which testing is begun. As one starts higher, the boundary of the hysterical sensory loss also moves upward. Occasionally, the child with hysteria can be persuaded to report touches felt as "yes" and ones supposedly not felt as "no" during testing with eyes closed. The anesthetic side may shift from left to right or vice versa when the patient is moved from supine to prone. The *Japanese illusion* may be used to bring out left-right confusion in unilateral anesthesia. The patient is asked to cross arms, oppose the palms, and clasp fingers. The clasped hands are then rotated inward and the arms extended. This maneuver makes it very difficult for the patient to tell right fingers from left.

Hysterical seizures may be difficult to distinguish from epilepsy unless evaluated by an experienced observer. The seizure activity tends to be bizarre, often with rhythmic thrusting and writhing of the trunk. Tongue-biting, apnea, and incontinence are absent. The eyes tend to be held forcibly closed.

Hysterical urinary retention may have to be distinguished from bladder paralysis secondary to spinal cord lesions. The cystometrogram is normal when urinary retention is due to hysteria.

21.5 SPECIAL DIAGNOSTIC PROCEDURES

Lumbar Puncture. This procedure provides much valuable information when it is carefully performed. It is contraindicated in patients with increased intracranial pressure caused by a space-occupying lesion and in the presence of an untreated clotting defect. The puncture should not be done through an area of infected skin. If possible, the child should be kept from struggling during the tap; local procaine infiltration is helpful, even in the infant. The young child should be allowed to suck on a pacifier; sedation may be necessary in later childhood, but barbiturates should be avoided since the stimulus of pain after barbiturate administration often leads to wild and unreasoning behavior. The puncture is made in the lateral recumbent position except in the neonate, for whom the sitting position may be preferable. The neck and back are held flexed by an attendant. Careful cleansing of the skin is essential; drapes are unnecessary. The needle should not be inserted above the L2–3 interspace; L3–4 is the preferred site. A sharp needle with stylet should be used. Omission of the stylet may increase the chance of carrying a fragment of skin into the spinal canal, with formation of a spinal epidermoid tumor. The needle is advanced slowly, exactly in the midline, the tip of the needle pointed slightly cephalad. In the small child it often is not possible to feel the change in resistance that occurs as the dura is penetrated and the subarachnoid space is

entered. It therefore is necessary to remove the stylet repeatedly during advance of the needle until the cerebrospinal fluid drips out. A bloody tap usually occurs when the needle is advanced too far.

Cerebrospinal fluid pressure should be measured whenever it is possible to obtain relaxation. The pressure measurement is most accurate when legs and neck are extended prior to the reading. The normal opening pressure ranges from 60–160 mm of water.

The color of the fluid should be compared with that of distilled water against a white background. After the neonatal period *xanthochromia*—a yellow tint—is always abnormal. It may be due to elevation of spinal fluid protein or to accumulation of bilirubin. The latter usually implies recent subarachnoid hemorrhage, but it may also be seen in the absence of central nervous system lesions in patients with hyperbilirubinemia. Fluid that contains more than about 100 leukocytes/mm^3 appears cloudy. Bloody fluid may be due to a traumatic tap or a recent subarachnoid hemorrhage. To discover the origin of the blood, the fluid should be centrifuged and the supernatant inspected; in subarachnoid hemorrhage the supernatant is xanthochromic, and equal amounts of blood are present in successive fractional specimens of fluid. In a bloody tap the supernatant is clear or only faintly yellow, and the amount of blood decreases in successive tubes.

Normally, the spinal fluid contains no red blood cells and at most 5 leukocytes/mm^3 except in the newborn infant, in whom up to 500 red cells and up to 15 leukocytes, including granulocytes, may be insignificant. Later in childhood, predominance of granulocytes most often indicates bacterial infection but is occasionally seen during the early phase of acute viral meningitis. Elevation in numbers of lymphocytes is seen in a large variety of illnesses in which meningeal irritation and inflammation are factors.

The protein content of lumbar spinal fluid in childhood normally ranges from 10–30 mg/dl except in the 1st weeks of infancy, when values up to 100 mg/dl are accepted as normal. By the age of 3 mo the protein should be below 30 mg/dl. Elevation in protein is usually due to increased permeability of meningeal vessels and occasionally to obstruction of spinal fluid circulation, with decrease in resorption of protein. Elevations in the concentration of protein are seen in many neurologic disorders, including brain and spinal cord tumors, degenerative brain diseases, and inflammatory diseases of the central nervous system and of peripheral nerves.

Elevation in spinal fluid globulins is detected by immunoelectrophoresis. Normally about 30% of the protein in spinal fluid is represented by globulins, 6–8% by gamma globulins. When electrophoresis is not available, the colloidal gold curve may be used as a general measure; a "1st zone" colloidal gold curve implies elevation in globulins. An increased gamma globulin or a 1st zone colloidal gold curve content in the absence of general elevation in spinal fluid protein is of considerable diagnostic value. This finding is associated with only a few illnesses, which include multiple sclerosis, subacute sclerosing panencephalitis, neurosyphilis, and postinfectious encephalomyelitis. Measurement of measles antibody titer in spinal fluid is an important diagnostic aid in subacute sclerosing panencephalitis.

The glucose concentration of spinal fluid is normally about 50% that of blood. The ratio between spinal fluid and blood glucose values rather than the absolute value of the former is of importance. A low ratio is seen in bacterial meningitis, fungal meningitis, meningeal tumor, and, rarely, in aseptic meningitis.

Spinal fluid should always be cultured for bacteria and, when indicated, for fungi, acid-fast bacilli, and viruses. When meningitis is suspected, the fluid is centrifuged and a Gram-stained smear of the sediment examined. An excellent method of spinal fluid preparation for morphologic examination is to add a drop of liquid albumin to an aliquot of spinal fluid and spin the mixture in a cytocentrifuge. The sediment is dried and then stained with Wright stain. Histiocytes and tumor cells as well as normal leukocytes can be readily identified.

Subdural Tap.   This procedure is helpful to rule out subdural effusion in infancy. Indications for its performance may include unexplained excessive head growth, a bulging anterior fontanelle, and positive transillumination of the skull. The scalp hair must be shaved and strict aseptic precautions observed. The head is firmly held by an attendant. A blunt, short-beveled #20 needle with a stylet is used. The needle is introduced into the lateral angle of the fontanelle or into the coronal suture, *at least 2 cm lateral to the midline;* it is advanced perpendicular to the scalp surface. A popping sensation usually occurs when the dura is penetrated. The needle should be advanced slowly, never more than 1.5 cm from the scalp surface, and the stylet should be removed repeatedly to determine whether a fluid-filled space has been reached. If intracranial pressure is not elevated; it is advisable to hold the head in a somewhat dependent position during the tap so that flow is aided by gravity. Care has to be taken to avoid to and fro movements of the needle, which could lead to laceration of the meninges or cerebral cortex.

Subdural fluid is xanthochromic, bloody, or reddish brown in color, depending on the age of the effusion and the amount of admixed blood. The protein content is always elevated, usually above 100 mg/dl. At times, a fairly copious amount of clear fluid with low protein content is obtained. This is subarachnoid fluid, the presence of which is usually of no pathologic significance. In general, the protein content of subarachnoid fluid obtained over the convexities is about twice that obtained from a lumbar tap.

Subdural fluid should be removed slowly, with no more than 15 ml taken from 1 side in any 1 tap. Rapid removal of large quantities may cause shock or intracranial hemorrhage from sudden shift of the intracranial structures. The opposite side should always be tapped when subdural fluid is found; subdural effusions in infancy are bilateral in 80% of cases. After the tap a pressure dressing is applied and the infant placed in a semi-erect position in an infant seat to diminish the chance of prolonged leakage from the puncture site.

Ventricular Taps.   These taps should not be performed by the pediatrician except in cases of life-threatening increase in intracranial pressure when a neurosurgeon is not immediately available. The needle is introduced as for a subdural tap but is inclined slightly forward, toward the nasion. The needle is advanced until ventricular fluid is obtained, usually fewer than 4 cm from the surface when intracranial pressure is elevated because of ventricular obstruction. The procedure carries the risk of intracerebral or ventricular hemorrhage, and it always leads to some damage to cerebral cortex.

Electroencephalography. Electroencephalography (EEG) records the electrical activity of the cerebral cortex. Normally, fairly regular wave forms predominate. They are classified according to their frequency as delta (1–3/sec), theta (4–7/sec), alpha (8–12/sec), or beta waves (13–20/sec). During maturation the waves gradually become more regular and increase in frequency. Theta and delta waves are normally seen during waking periods in the infant and young child. By the age of 10 yr the normal background rhythm in the waking state consists largely of alpha and beta activity. Slower waves are normal during sleep. Spike discharges, which may replace or be superimposed on the basic brain waves, indicate a lowered seizure threshold and are an important confirmatory sign in the child with a suspected seizure disorder. Metabolic and inflammatory diseases of cerebral cortex tend to be associated with generalized high voltage slow wave (delta) activity. Focal structural lesions of cerebral cortex, such as brain abscesses or brain tumors, cause localized slow wave activity.

Electromyography.   Electromyography is useful in the differential diagnosis of neuromuscular disease. A needle is inserted into the muscle to record the electrical activity. Normal muscle is electrically silent at rest. Spontaneous discharges of single muscle fibers at rest (*fibrillation potentials*) indicate denervation. During normal muscular contraction, groups of muscle fibers in a motor unit are activated in unison and generate a *motor unit potential.* Decrease in size of motor unit potentials is seen in primary diseases of muscle. In diseases of peripheral nerves the motor units are decreased in number, but they often are of abnormally large size as a result of collateral innervation of denervated muscle fibers. Measurements of velocity of nerve conduction are helpful in the confirmation of peripheral nerve disorders. Maximum velocity is decreased in inflammatory and metabolic diseases of peripheral nerves, especially when the myelin sheaths of the nerve fibers are affected.

Muscle Biopsy.   This is frequently necessary to establish the diagnosis of a specific neuromuscular disease. Both histochemical and electronmicroscopic examination of the biopsy tissue may be needed.

Neuroroentgenography.   *Skull roentgenograms* are valuable to identify intracranial calcifications, craniosynostosis, skull fractures, or bony defects. They may also provide information regarding intracranial pressure. Elevated pressure in the child causes separation of the cranial sutures; if it is longstanding, the posterior clinoid processes are eroded, the sella turcica may be flattened and enlarged, and the convolutional impressions on the inner table of the skull are accentuated and have a "beaten-silver" appearance. This pattern of the skull is not by itself necessarily evidence of increased intracranial pressure or of any abnormality.

Computed tomography (CT scan) is a noninvasive technique for demonstration of intracranial structures. The method detects small variations in tissue density by computerized assembly of information from multiple tomographic sections through the head. Brain tissue is clearly distinguishable from cerebrospinal fluid–filled spaces; the technique is therefore well suited for the demonstration of ventricular size, displacements of the ventricular system by mass lesions, and subdural collections of fluid. Edematous brain, as in the area of an infarct or contusion, has lower density than normal brain. Cerebral hemorrhages, calcifications, and some solid tumors are detectable as areas of high density. The resolution of the method is increased if the study is repeated after intravenous infusion of a radiopaque contrast material. Such infusion results in increased density in areas of heightened vascularity such as vascular malformations, the capsule surrounding a brain abscess, and vascular tumors.

Computed tomography now is the primary method for the study of space-occupying intracranial lesions. It has largely replaced *pneumoencephalography* and *ventriculography*. These 2 techniques, in which the ventricular system and the subarachnoid spaces are outlined by displacement of CSF with air or with oxygen, are still used occasionally, especially for diagnosis of lesions in the brain stem and in the parasellar region.

Cerebral *angiography* remains the definitive test for the study of cerebral vascular disorders, including arteriovenous malformations, arterial occlusions, and venous thrombosis. In the child, the procedure is carried out most easily and safely via an arterial catheter introduced into 1 of the femoral arteries.

Radionuclide brain scan is of value for detection of certain local brain lesions. A radioactive material, usually ^{99m}technetium, is injected intravenously, and radioactivity over the skull is counted after a fixed time interval. The test material tends to accumulate in areas of brain where the blood-brain barrier is defective, especially in tumors and around brain abscesses. Positive uptakes are also seen with encephalitis and with subdural hematoma. Cerebral infarcts due to vascular occlusion often result in positive brain scans starting about 1 wk after infarction; reversion to normal occurs in 3–4 wk.

Two-dimensional (B mode) *ultrasound scanning* of the head can safely and rapidly evaluate ventricular size and detect intracranial hemorrhages or masses in infants with open anterior fontanelles.

Myelography is important in the diagnosis of mass lesions situated in or encroaching upon the spinal cord. Either iophendylate (Pantopaque) or air is used as contrast material. The injection is made through a lumbar spinal needle when possible. Pantopaque myelography carries some small definite risk of meningeal reaction to the injected material, which may result in incapacitating and occasionally fatal arachnoiditis.

Babcock DS, Han BK, LeQuesne GW: B-mode gray scale ultrasound of the head in the newborn and young infant. Am J Roentgenol 134:457, 1980.

Bachman DS, Hodges FJ III, Freeman JM: Computerized axial tomography in neurologic disorders of children. Pediatrics 59:352, 1977.

Brazelton TB, Scholl ML, Robey JS: Visual responses in the newborn. Pediatrics 37:284, 1966.

Denny-Brown D: Handbook of Neurological Examination and Case Recording. Cambridge, Harvard University Press, 1965.

Dodge PR, Porter P: Demonstration of intracranial pathology by transillumination. Arch Neurol 5:594, 1961.

Fois A: Clinical Electroencephalography in Epilepsy and Related Conditions in Childhood. Springfield Ill., Charles C Thomas, 1963.

Harwood-Nash D, Fitz CR: Neuroradiology in Infants and Children. St. Louis, CV Mosby, 1976.

Hurley PJ, Wagner HN: Diagnostic value of brain scanning in children. JAMA 221:877, 1972.

Lorber J, Granger RG: Cerebral cavities following ventricular puncture in infants. Clin Radiol 14:98, 1963.

Norris F: The EMG: A Guide and Atlas for Practical Electromyography. New York, Grune & Stratton, 1963.

Paine RS, Oppe TE: Neurologic Examinations of Children. Clinics in Developmental Medicine, Vol 20–21. London, William Heinemann, Ltd., 1966.

Shaywitz BA: Epidermoid spinal cord tumors and previous lumbar puncture. J Pediatr 80:638, 1972.

Widell S: On the cerebrospinal fluid in normal children and in patients with acute abacterial meningo-encephalitis. Acta Pediatr Suppl 115, 1958.

21.6 THE COMATOSE CHILD

Clinical Assessment. Evaluation of the comatose child must provide certain critical information as soon as possible: Is circulation adequate? Is the airway patent, with sufficient respiratory exchange? Is intracranial pressure elevated, and, if so, is the elevation great enough to be life-threatening? Is there a focal neurologic deficit which might indicate a localized, surgically remediable brain lesion? Is the coma likely to be due to remediable metabolic disease?

The *vital signs*—pulse, respiration, and blood pressure—evaluate circulation and airway and may give clues to the diagnosis. The pulse is often slow and blood pressure elevated when intracranial pressure is high. Hyperventilation is usually the result of metabolic acidosis, but it may also occur in respiratory alkalosis because of abnormal stimulation of the medullary respiratory center (e.g., in salicylate poisoning, hepatic coma, or Reye syndrome). Periodic breathing and irregular (ataxic) breathing are signs of medullary dysfunction; they often precede complete apnea.

The *pupillary reactions* should be assessed when the patient is first seen and at frequent intervals thereafter. Unilateral dilatation with decrease in the light reflex is usually secondary to 3rd nerve damage by tentorial herniation of the brain (Fig 21–4). It is often an indication for emergency medical or surgical measures to reduce intracranial pressure. A dilated pupil may also be due to eye trauma, or it may be a transient postictal finding following a grand mal seizure. Bilateral fixed dilated pupils often, but not invariably, imply irreversible brain stem damage when present for more than 5 min. The pupils may be unreactive in hypothermia and in reversible coma resulting from poisoning by sedative or atropine-like drugs. Dilated, unreactive pupils may

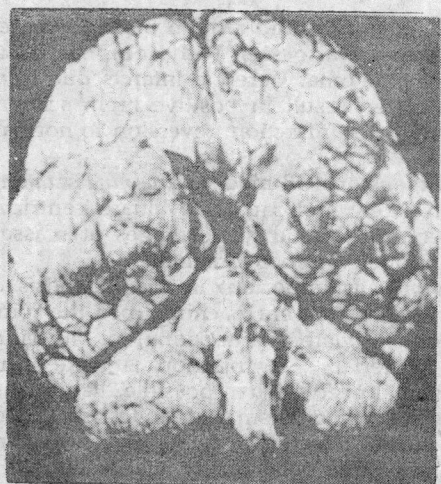

Figure 21–4 Tentorial herniation secondary to diffuse cerebral edema. The arrow points to the portion of temporal lobe that has herniated through the tentorium. A groove, produced by the tentorial edge, is clearly visible. The 3rd nerve is just below and medial to the area of herniation.

also be due to previous local instillation of mydriatics. Pinpoint pupils are seen in poisoning with opiates, during barbiturate coma, and with pontine lesions.

Eye movements in comatose patients are tested by the *doll's head maneuver*. The head is quickly rotated to 1 side, then to the other. The eyes show conjugate deviation to the side opposite the direction of head rotation. Absence of this response in a comatose patient implies dysfunction of brain stem or of oculomotor nerves. Deviation of the eye down and laterally is frequently seen in association with pupillary dilatation in 3rd nerve dysfunction due to tentorial herniation. Sixth nerve palsy is usually due to increased intracranial pressure; it does not carry as ominous a prognosis as does 3rd nerve dysfunction.

Funduscopic examination should be carried out to determine whether papilledema is present. Mydriatics should not be used since they interfere with pupillary reactions, which are invaluable for the clinical assessment of the comatose patient. The absence of papilledema does not rule out increased intracranial pressure of recent onset since papilledema takes 24–48 hr to develop. Distention of retinal veins and absence of venous pulsations are early signs of elevated intracranial tension. Preretinal hemorrhages are usually the result of subarachnoid or subdural bleeding.

Assessment of motor functions includes observations of spontaneous activity, posture, and response to noxious stimuli. In deep coma, primitive postural reflex patterns emerge as cortical control over motor functions is lost. In *"decorticate posturing"* the arms are flexed on the chest, hands are fisted, and legs extended. This position is seen in severe, diffuse dysfunction of the cerebral cortex. *"Decerebrate posturing"* is characterized by rigid extension and pronation of arms and extension of legs, often in response to painful stimulation. It is a sign of dysfunction at the level of the midbrain. When decerebrate posturing is unilateral, it is often caused by

tentorial herniation, in which case there may be associated contralateral paralysis of the 3rd nerve.

Hemiplegia can be diagnosed even in the deeply comatose patient. The paretic leg lies in external rotation. It moves less than the opposite leg, both spontaneously and in response to pain. The paretic extremity drops more limply when it is picked up and allowed to fall.

Grading of the *stage of coma* is helpful in charting the course of the patient:

Stage I—stupor. The patient can be roused for brief periods, during which he may be able to make simple verbal and voluntary motor responses. Stupor may alternate with *delirium*, which is a state of mental confusion and motor excitement.

Stage II—light coma. The patient cannot be roused, even with painful stimuli. He may moan and make semipurposeful avoidance movements.

Stage III—deep coma. Painful stimuli now fail to produce a response, or they lead to extension and pronation of arms (decerebrate posturing).

Stage IV—patient is flaccid and apneic. All brain stem functions are lost. Some spinal reflexes may be preserved. The use of artificial ventilation has made it possible to maintain circulation after all brain function is irreversibly lost. The term *brain death* has been applied to this state. The criteria for brain death are as follows: (1) absence of all cerebral function, including pupillary responses, spontaneous respiratory efforts, and all but local spinal reflexes for a period of at least 24 hr; (2) total absence of brain waves on at least 2 EEG recordings obtained 24 hr apart; (3) certainty that absence of brain functions is secondary to conditions other than drug intoxication or hypothermia. Termination of resuscitative efforts is justified when each of these 3 conditions has been appropriately determined to be present.

Differential Diagnosis. Information gained during the examination will usually make it possible to place the patient into 1 of 4 categories, depending on whether intracranial pressure is elevated and on whether there are focal neurologic signs. Table 21–3 provides the likely diagnostic possibilities in each category.

Laboratory studies which may be needed include blood sugar, serum electrolytes, blood gases, BUN, liver function tests, and toxicologic screening. Examination of CSF is usually necessary to rule out bacterial meningitis. Lumbar puncture carries a risk of tentorial herniation in the patient with increased intracranial pressure, especially when a focal brain lesion is present. Neurosurgical consultation should be obtained prior to spinal tap in a child with increased intracranial pressure and focal neurologic signs. Diagnosis of the comatose child with focal signs usually requires computed tomography.

Management. The comatose child requires meticulous attention to respiratory status. The child should not be placed flat on his/her back but rather should be kept on his/her side or in a semiprone position to minimize the danger of aspiration of saliva or of vomitus. Frequent suctioning of secretions is essential. The comatose patient should never be left unattended.

Moderately severe hypoxia may not be clinically evident; therefore, repeated determinations of blood gases

Table 21-3 DIFFERENTIAL DIAGNOSIS OF COMA

No Focal Signs		Focal Signs	
Normal CSF Pressure	*Increased CSF Pressure*	*Normal CSF Pressure*	*Increased CSF Pressure*
Most metabolic encephalopathies	Some metabolic encephalopathies (lead poisoning, water intoxication, Reye syndrome, severe anoxia)	Vascular disease (cerebral artery occlusion)	Trauma (subdural, epidural or intracerebral hemorrhage, cerebral contusion)
Drug intoxication			Brain tumor
CNS infection (meningitis, encephalitis)	CNS infection (meningitis, encephalitis)	CNS infection (encephalitis)	CNS infection (brain abscess, subdural empyema, encephalitis)
Trauma (concussion)	Trauma (subdural hemorrhage in infants, subarachnoid hemorrhage)	Trauma (cerebral contusion)	
Epilepsy (postictal state)	Brain tumor (midline tumors) Hydrocephalus	Epilepsy (postictal state with Todd paralysis)	Vascular disease (arteriovenous malformation)

are necessary. Hyperventilation may also occur and lead to respiratory alkalosis. It is important to remember that the electrolyte changes in respiratory alkalosis can best be distinguished from those of metabolic acidosis only by measurement of pH.

Intravenous fluid therapy in the comatose child must be carefully monitored by repeated determinations of serum electrolytes. The most common mistake is overhydration, which may result in water intoxication; frequently, the child in coma is unable to cope with what would be a moderate water load at other times. This inability is thought to be the result of dysfunction of the hypothalamus, with inappropriate secretion of antidiuretic hormone (ADH). The patient with inappropriate ADH secretion excretes scant quantities of concentrated urine in the face of hypervolemia and hyponatremia. Attention to urine output alone may give the erroneous impression that the child is dehydrated. Fatal cerebral edema may result if administration of hypotonic solutions is continued. The treatment of inappropriate ADH secretion is simple; it consists only of fluid restriction until serum electrolytes and osmolality return to normal (Sec 5.30).

Prompt therapeutic intervention may be lifesaving in the comatose patient with marked increase in intracranial pressure, especially when evidence of tentorial herniation is present. When increased intracranial pressure is due to hydrocephalus or to ventricular obstruction by tumor, it is relieved most quickly and effectively by ventricular tap. Several medical measures can reduce the increased intracranial pressure caused by brain swelling. Controlled hyperventilation rapidly lowers intracranial pressure through constriction of cerebral vessels. Osmotic diuretics also are useful in emergencies; they lead to decrease in brain volume and to lowering in pressure within minutes of the start of infusion. Mannitol (1–2 gm/kg) and urea (0.5–1 gm/kg) administered rapidly by vein are most effective. An

indwelling urinary catheter is needed to prevent overdistention of the bladder by the induced diuresis. The effect of these agents is transient, rarely lasting over 6 hr. Their effectiveness decreases markedly on repeated use. High doses of synthetic corticosteroids are useful for more prolonged control of cerebral edema. Dexamethasone, 0.2–0.4 mg/kg intravenously, followed by 0.1–0.2 mg/kg intramuscularly every 6 hr, is commonly employed. A therapeutic response is usually seen within 6 hr. Stools must be checked for occult blood, and serum electrolytes must be carefully monitored while the child is receiving steroids. The above measures should not replace or delay definitive therapy for the underlying disease when it is available. In the management of severe cerebral edema such as occurs in major head injury and in Reye syndrome, continuous monitoring of intracranial pressure by means of intraventricular catheters or devices implanted in the subdural or subarachnoid spaces is useful.

Adequate nutritional intake must be assured when coma is prolonged. Nasogastric or nasojejunal feeding should be initiated as soon as the acute phase of the illness has subsided. The usual hospital diet mixed in a food blender makes an excellent feeding mixture, which is often tolerated better than many artificial formulas.

Guidelines for the determination of death. Report of the Medical Consultants on the Diagnosis of Death to the President's Commission for the Study of Ethical Problems in Medicine and Biomedical and Behavioral Research. JAMA 246:2184, 1981.
Goldberg M: Hyponatremia and the inappropriate secretion of antidiuretic hormone. Am J Med 35:293, 1963.
Mickell JJ, Reigel DH, Cook DR, et al: Intracranial pressure: Monitoring and normalization therapy in children. Pediatrics 59:606, 1977.
Plum F, Posner JB: The Diagnosis of Stupor and Coma. Ed 2. Philadelphia, FA Davis Co, 1972.

21.7 DISEASES OF THE NERVOUS SYSTEM

STATIC AND DEVELOPMENTAL LESIONS

Most neurologic disabilities in childhood result from congenital malformations or from brain damage in the perinatal period and are usually nonprogressive. Understanding of their etiology is often incomplete, and any classification is at best only partly satisfactory. The following classification is based on presumed time of onset of the defect, on the structures involved, and on etiology when known.

I. *Developmental defects of the nervous system (congenital malformations)*
   A. *Defects of closure of the neural tube*
   Anencephaly
   Encephalocele
   Myelomeningocele and the
       Arnold-Chiari malformation
   Spina bifida occulta
   Dermal sinus
   Neurenteric cyst
   B. *Defects in the differentiation and growth of the cerebral hemispheres*
   Chromosomal defects (see other
       sections)
   Morphologic syndromes with
       mental retardation (see Chapter 6)
   Holoprosencephaly (arhinencephaly)
   Agenesis of corpus callosum
   Porencephaly and hydranencephaly
   Lissencephaly
   Polymicrogyria
   Microcephaly
   Megalencephaly
   C. *Defects in development of cerebrospinal fluid circulation (congenital hydrocephalus)*
   Aqueductal stenosis
   The Dandy-Walker malformation
   "Communicating" hydrocephalus
   D. *Developmental defects of brain stem*
   Moebius syndrome
   Spasmus nutans
II. *Perinatally acquired cerebral lesions*
   A. *Intrauterine and neonatal infections of the nervous system*
   Congenital syphilis
   Congenital toxoplasmosis
   Cytomegalic inclusion disease
   Neonatal herpesvirus infection
   Other viral encephalitides
   Neonatal bacterial meningitis
   B. *Perinatal anoxic encephalopathy*
   C. *Cerebral trauma incident to birth*
   Intraventricular hemorrhage (not necessarily traumatic, see also Sec 7.49)
   Intracerebral hemorrhage and cerebral
       contusion

Subarachnoid hemorrhage
Subdural hemorrhage
   D. *Neonatal metabolic encephalopathies*
   Bilirubin encephalopathy (kernicterus)
   Hypoglycemic encephalopathy
   The aminoacidurias
   Cretinism

21.8 DEFECTS OF CLOSURE OF THE NEURAL TUBE

(See Sec 6.29 for recurrence risks and prenatal diagnosis.)

These developmental anomalies are best understood in the context of normal formative stages of the nervous system as indicated in Fig 21–5. In the human the 1st evidence of development of neural tissue occurs at about 20 days' gestation, at which time a distinct depression, the neural groove, appears in the dorsal ectoderm of the embryo (Fig 21–5A). This groove quickly deepens, and its 2 margins become apposed and fuse. This fusion forms the neural tube; it begins near the center of the embryo and progresses cephalad and caudad. By about 23 days' gestation the neural tube is complete, except for an opening at each end, the anterior and posterior neuropores (Fig 21–5B). Failure of closure of the anterior neuropore causes anencephaly and encephalocele; a closure defect of the posterior neuropore leads to spina bifida and meningomyelocele. The term *rachischisis* is sometimes used for very widespread spinal closure defects involving most or all of the dorsal, lumbar, and sacral regions.

Anencephaly. Anencephaly is evident immediately at birth; the membranous skull is absent, as well as the cerebral hemispheres. Brain stem and basal nuclei may be well formed and are visible at the base of the skull. Affected infants are stillborn or die within a few days.

Encephalocele. Encephalocele consists of a herniation of brain and meninges through a defect in the skull, resulting in a sac-like structure. When the defect contains only meninges it is referred to as a *cranial meningocele*. About 75% of encephaloceles occur in the occipital area; the remainder are parietal, frontal, or nasopharyngeal.

Encephalocele is usually obvious at birth as a midline skull defect through which a large pedunculated or sessile mass protrudes. Nasopharyngeal encephaloceles, however, may have no externally visible anomaly. The child may present with nasal airway obstruction or with cleft palate; the nasal passages contain a smooth, round mass projecting downward, which must be differentiated from nasal polyp. A frontal encephalocele may extend into the orbit and produce proptosis of 1 eye.

The differentiation of encephalocele from cranial meningocele is made by palpation and transillumination of the mass and by computed tomography. The latter shows associated hydrocephalus in approximately two thirds of infants with encephalocele.

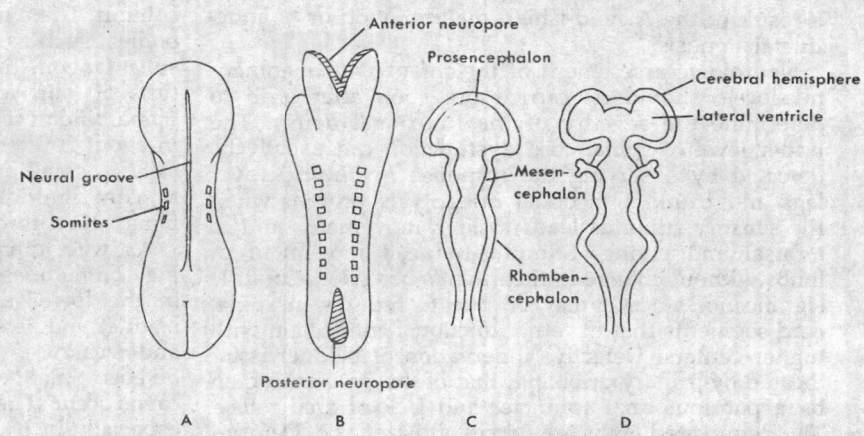

Figure 21–5 Early developmental stages of the human central nervous system. *A,* Dorsal view of embryo at 20 days of age. The future nervous system is indicated by a midline depression, the neural groove. *B,* 23 days' gestational age. The neural groove has closed dorsally, except for openings at either end (the anterior and posterior neuropores), to form the neural tube. *C,* Cephalic portion of the embryo, 28 days. The cerebral hemispheres are represented by a single midline structure, the prosencephalon. *D,* 36 days' gestational age. Paired lateral ventricles and cerebral hemispheres are formed. The outlines of the ventricular system, including the 3rd ventricle, aqueduct of Sylvius, and 4th ventricle, are discernible.

Therapy of encephalocele consists of surgical repair of the defect unless a major associated malformation of the brain is severe enough to preclude the possibility of meaningful survival. The associated hydrocephalus frequently requires a shunt operation. The prognosis is good in cranial meningocele, with normal intellectual and motor function in 60% of affected infants; it is guarded in occipital encephalocele, with only about a 10% chance of normal intelligence.

Spina Bifida with Meningomyelocele. This is a midline defect of skin, vertebral arches, and neural tube, usually in the lumbosacral region. It is 1 of the most common developmental anomalies of the nervous system; the incidence ranges from 0.2–0.4/1000 births in different population groups; the highest incidence is reported in the Welsh and Irish. Little is known about the etiology of meningomyelocele, though it appears to be linked with anencephaly. A woman who has had a child with either anencephaly or meningomyelocele has an increased risk of either in subsequent pregnancies (see *Anencephaly* above). Each defect has been observed

following administration of aminopterin during the 1st mo of pregnancy.

Meningomyelocele is evident at birth as a skin defect over the back, bordered laterally by bony prominences of the unfused neural arches of the vertebrae. The defect is usually covered by a transparent membrane which may have neural tissue attached to its inner surface. Cerebrospinal fluid leaks from this membrane initially, but soon after birth drying of the membrane tends to decrease its permeability. As cerebrospinal fluid accumulates, the membrane begins to bulge, and it may eventually form a large sac unless surgical closure of the defect is carried out. In almost all cases meningomyelocele is associated with the *Arnold-Chiari malformation* (Fig 21–6), which consists of maldevelopment and downward displacement into the cervical spinal canal of parts of the cerebellum, 4th ventricle, and medulla oblongata. Other developmental anomalies of neural tissue, including aqueductal stenosis and arrest of migration of cerebral neurons, may coexist. Hydrocephalus develops in about 90% of affected children as

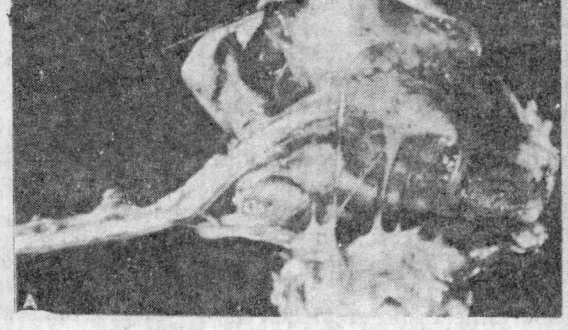
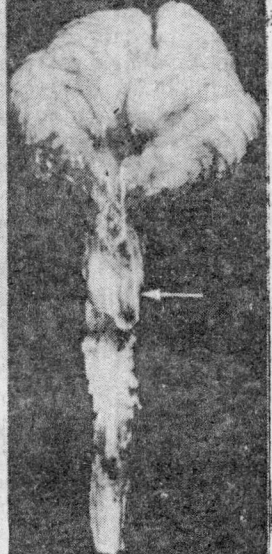

Figure 21–6 Meningomyelocele and Arnold-Chiari malformation. *A,* Characteristic deformity of the spinal cord. The normally formed thoracic spinal cord (left side of figure) gradually becomes flattened; the lumbar cord is represented by a platelike structure which is firmly adherent to the surrounding skin. The lumbar spinal nerves can be seen to emerge from the malformed neural plate. *B,* Arnold-Chiari malformation, same case. The medulla oblongata and 4th ventricle (arrow) show marked downward displacement. The malformed cerebellum is visible above.

a result of the Arnold-Chiari malformation or of aqueductal stenosis.

Neurologic assessment of the infant with meningomyelocele should be carried out soon after birth to determine the severity of the functional defect. The upper level of spinal cord dysfunction can usually be detected by observing the response to pinprick over legs and trunk. Functional integrity is present when the sensory stimulus leads to limb movements and to arousal and crying. Stimulus-induced movement of limbs without change in the infant's behavior is of little significance since it may be due to reflexes in spinal cord segments that have no functional connection with higher centers. Defective innervation of bladder is indicated by urinary dribbling, that of the perianal region by a patulous anal sphincter and lack of anal reflex. The denervated limbs are flaccid and areflexic. Deformities such as talipes equinovarus and dislocated hips are often present. The Arnold-Chiari malformation may lead to medullary and lower cranial nerve dysfunction, including difficulty in swallowing, stridor, and atrophy of tongue.

Optimal therapy of meningomyelocele consists of prompt surgical closure of the skin defect, preferably within 48 hr after birth, to prevent meningeal infection. Wide excision of the membranous covering is contraindicated since the membrane may contain functioning neural tissue. After closure of the defect the infant must be carefully observed for development of hydrocephalus, which is treated surgically when indicated. Urinary retention can be managed by repeated catheterizations, done by the caretakers in infants and young children, in older children by the patients themselves. Orthopedic procedures are sometimes helpful to correct the hip and foot deformities but should be considered only when the child has some chance of useful function of his lower extremities. An organized plan for management by a specialized multidisciplinary clinical group is essential.

The prognosis depends on the extent of the motor deficit present at birth, on involvement of bladder innervation, and on the presence of associated cerebral anomalies. For the infant with total paralysis of legs and urinary bladder the outlook is poor even with optimal medical care; most such infants die during early childhood from complications of therapy for hydrocephalus or from chronic renal failure. The remainder are severely restricted by their motor disability, and 50% are mentally retarded. Advanced hydrocephalus at birth also carries a poor prognosis. Children with lesser degrees of involvement may lead successful lives, especially those with spina bifida and meningocele without evidence of neurologic deficit at birth. In the severely affected infant the decision to carry out operative procedures or to allow the disorder to take its natural course presents serious ethical problems. Unoperated, over 90% of affected infants die in their 1st yr.

Spina Bifida Occulta. This consists of a defect of the vertebral arch with failure of posterior fusion of the vertebral laminae and often with absence of the spinous processes. The anomaly is most common at L5 and S1 levels, but it may affect any portion of the vertebral column. There may be associated anomalies of vertebral bodies, such as hemivertebrae. The overlying skin and subcutaneous tissues may be normal or show abnormal tufts of hair, telangiectasia, or subcutaneous lipoma. Spina bifida occulta is an isolated, insignificant finding in about 20% of all spines examined roentgenographically. A small percentage of affected infants have functionally significant developmental defects of the underlying spinal cord and spinal roots.

As with meningomyelocele, the neurologic deficit may be manifested as motor and sensory disturbances in the lower extremities and/or disturbances of the bladder and bowel sphincters. Unilateral foot deformity and weakness of foot muscles are the most common defects. Smallness of the foot, trophic ulcers, and pes cavus occur. These may be associated with sensory loss, especially in L5 and S1 distribution. Bladder sphincter disturbance is seen in about 25% of infants with neurologic involvement and leads to urinary incontinence, dribbling, and recurrent urinary infections. It is usually associated with weakness of the anal sphincters and with sensory impairment in the perineal region. The neurologic impairments may gradually worsen, especially during adolescent growth.

The differential diagnosis includes spinal cord tumor, poliomyelitis, developmental defects of the spine such as diastematomyelia, and foot deformities. Diagnostic studies should be limited to roentgenograms of the spine unless there is progressive neurologic impairment. In that case myelography, either with iophendylate (Pantopaque) or with air is performed to rule out associated surgically remediable defects. Lipoma is especially common; it has been found on surgical exploration in about 40% of children with neurologic impairment associated with spina bifida occulta; a dermoid cyst has been present in about 5%. If these tumors can be removed without damage to neural structures, they should be.

Diastematomyelia. Diastematomyelia is a fissure or cleft of the spinal cord, usually in the lumbar region. The cleft is often transfixed by a bony or fibrous septum which prevents the normal ascent of the spinal cord in the vertebral canal as the child grows. Tethering of the spinal cord in the vertebral canal may lead to progressive neurologic deficit. Progressive flaccid paraparesis, weakness of 1 leg, or bladder dysfunction may occur. Frequently, associated anomalies include spina bifida with meningomyelocele, spina bifida occulta, dermal sinus, and hemivertebrae. Cutaneous hemangioma, lipoma, or a tuft of hair may overlie the site of the spinal defect.

The diagnosis can often be made by roentgenographic demonstration of a bony spicule in the spinal canal. Myelography further delineates the abnormality. Surgical exploration and resection of the abnormal bone and fibrous tissue is indicated when the lesion is discovered in infancy or in early childhood.

Dermal Sinus. Dermal sinus is a small midline closure defect which is of importance primarily because the sinus may be a route of entry of bacteria into the subarachnoid space and thus lead to recurrent meningitis. It is usually located in the lumbosacral area but may occur at any level of the spine or in the midline of the cranium. Its point of origin on the skin is visible as a dimple, often surrounded by a tuft of hair or by a small hemangioma. The low sacral defects known as *pilonidal dimples or sinuses* usually end blindly without communication with the subarachnoid space and are therefore rarely significant. Sinus tracts above that level should be surgically explored and closed.

Neurenteric Cyst.   These rare lesions arise from incorporation of entodermal tissue into developing neural tissue of the early embryo. They consist of epithelium-lined tracts and cysts which protrude into the spinal canal. They are most common in the thoracic and lower cervical regions. Neurologic dysfunction results from compression of the spinal cord by the cystic mass.

The symptoms and signs are those of spinal cord tumor or of infection of the subarachnoid space (sometimes recurrent or chronic meningitis). The diagnosis can occasionally be suspected from examination of an anterior view of the spine, which may show a rounded, midline defect in 1 of the vertebral bodies through which the neurenteric tract gains entry to the spinal canal. In other cases these lesions have been entirely intraspinal without any associated bony defect. The diagnosis then depends on myelography and on pathologic examination of tissue removed at surgery. Therapy consists of surgical excision of the cyst.

Alter M: Anencephalus, hydrocephalus and spina bifida. Epidemiology with special reference to a survey in Charleston, S.C. Arch Neurol 7:411, 1962.

Holcomb GW Jr, Matson DD: Thoracic neurenteric cyst. Surgery 35:115, 1954.

Ingraham FD: Spina Bifida and Cranium Bifidum. Papers reprinted from the New England Journal of Medicine with addition of a comprehensive bibliography. Boston, Massachusetts Medical Society, 1944.

Laurence KM: The recurrence risk in spina bifida cystica and anencephaly. Develop Med Child Neurol Suppl 13, 1967, p 75.

Lorber J: Results of treatment of myelomeningocele. Develop Med Child Neurol 13:279, 1971.

Matson DD: Neurosurgery of Infancy and Childhood. Springfield, Ill., Charles C Thomas, 1969.

Matson DD, Jerva MJ: Recurrent meningitis associated with lumbosacral dermal sinus tracts. J Neurosurg 25:288, 1966.

Sheptak PR, Susen AF: Diastematomyelia. Am J Dis Child 113:210, 1967.

Sieben RL, Hamida MB, Shulman K: Multiple cranial nerve deficits associated with the Arnold-Chiari malformation. Neurology 21:673, 1971.

Swinyard CA: The Child with Spina Bifida. New York, Association for the Aid of Crippled Children, 1971.

Thiersch JB: Therapeutic abortions with a folic acid antagonist, 4-amino-pteroyl-glutamic acid administered by the oral route. Am J Obstet Gynecol 63:1298, 1952.

21.9   DEFECTS IN THE DIFFERENTIATION AND GROWTH OF THE CEREBRAL HEMISPHERES

The future cerebrum makes its appearance as a recognizable structure in the human embryo at about 28 days' gestation, when the anterior end of the neural tube shows a globular expansion, *the prosencephalon* (Fig 21–5C). Over the next several days the prosencephalon cleaves into 2 lateral expansions which represent the beginnings of the cerebral hemispheres and of the lateral ventricles (Fig 21–5D). The walls of the ventricles at this stage are formed by a germinal layer of actively dividing neuroblasts. Newly formed neuroblasts migrate away from the ventricular wall toward the surface of the primitive cerebral hemisphere, where their accumulation leads to formation of the cerebral cortex. The 1st arrivals form the lower cortical layers, and later arrivals migrate past them to form the upper layers. Differentiation of neuroblasts leads to formation of neurons and of glial cells. Migrating neuroblasts tend to maintain contact with the ventricular lumen through cellular extensions which steadily increase in length and which eventually make up the axons of the subcortical white matter. Axons crossing from 1 hemisphere to the other in the future corpus callosum first appear during the 3rd mo of gestation; the formation of the corpus callosum is complete by the 5th mo. About then, the surface of the cerebral cortex begins to show indentations which are progressively elaborated during the last trimester until at term major cerebral sulci and gyri are clearly delineated.

The brain of the term infant contains the full adult complement of neurons, but its weight is only about one third that of the adult. The postnatal increase in weight is the result of myelination of subcortical white matter, of elaboration of neuronal processes, both dendrites and axons, and of increase in glial cells (Fig 21–7).

Generally, abnormal influences occurring prior to the 6th mo of gestation tend to affect development of the gross structure of the brain and to diminish total neuronal number. Pathologic influences in the perinatal period tend to have more subtle effects, such as retardation of myelination and decrease in elaboration of dendrites. Loss of brain substance due to destructive lesions may occur in the late fetal and early infancy periods, either alone or in combination with developmental defects.

Holoprosencephaly.   Holoprosencephaly is an early developmental defect of brain in which there is failure to form paired cerebral hemispheres. The cerebrum is made up of an unpaired sphere, and the lateral ventricles are represented by a single midline cavity. Usually there is associated *arrhinencephaly*—absence of olfactory bulbs and tracts, cleft lip, and microphthalmia or cyclopia. Occasionally, holoprosencephaly occurs with trisomy 13–15; in other instances the etiology is unknown. Severe mental and motor defects are usually present; affected children rarely survive past infancy.

Agenesis of the Corpus Callosum.   In this developmental anomaly the major fiber tracts that connect the 2 cerebral hemispheres are absent. Rarely, partial agenesis of the corpus callosum is transmitted by X-linked recessive inheritance; most cases are of unknown etiology. *Two clinical syndromes are recognized:* (1) The patient has normal intellectual and motor functions, and the malformation manifests itself only as an inability to transfer information from 1 cerebral hemisphere to the other. For example, the patient, if right-handed, may have difficulty in naming objects placed in the left hand since this requires transfer of information from right sensory cortex to the speech areas in the left cerebral hemisphere. (2) More commonly, the condition is associated with other developmental defects of the cerebrum, including failure of migration of neurons and hydrocephalus; affected children present in infancy with seizures, developmental retardation, abnormal head enlargement, and, often, hypertelorism. The diagnosis is made by computed tomography.

Porencephaly. Porencephaly is a defect in the cerebral mantle resulting in a cyst-like expansion of the lateral ventricle, which may extend up to the pia-arachnoid membrane.

Porencephaly is occasionally due to a primary defect in development of the cerebral mantle, in which case it tends to be bilateral, with replacement of the temporoparietal areas by fluid-filled spaces; affected infants have severe amentia. More commonly, porencephaly is unilateral and is secondary to local damage of the cerebrum during the later fetal or early infantile period. Vascular occlusion, encephalitis, and needle puncture of the brain have been implicated as possible etiologic factors.

Depending on the location of the porencephaly, the child may have spastic hemiparesis, hemisensory defects, or homonymous hemianopsia. The skull may expand laterally and be thinner on the side of the porencephaly, apparently as a result of fluid waves set up in the porencephalic cavity by pulsations of the choroid plexus.

Transillumination of the skull is of great value in the diagnosis of porencephaly and should always be performed in infants with unexplained hemiparesis. The differential diagnosis includes chronic subdural effusion, in which skull transillumination is also positive. The differentiation can be made by subdural tap and by computed tomography. Shunt surgery may be indicated in the rare instance when porencephaly is asso-

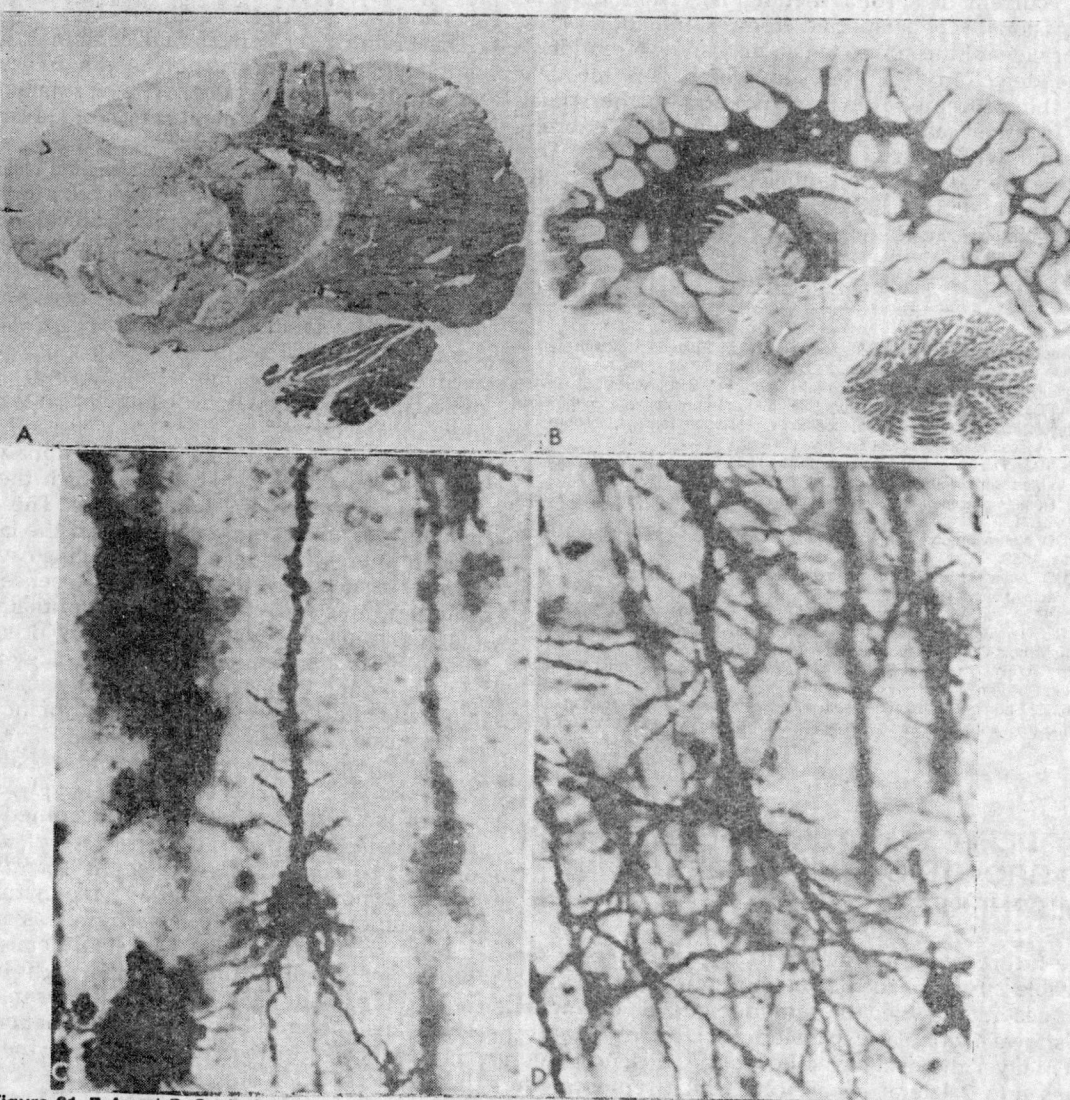

Figure 21–7 *A* and *B,* Sagittal sections of brain stained with myelin stain. *A,* The brain of a newborn shows little myelin in the subcortical white matter. *B,* The brain of a 9 mo old shows extensive myelination, especially in the primary visual, somatosensory, and motor areas. *C* and *D,* Single cortical pyramidal neurons stained by the Golgi method to show dendritic development. *C* is from frontal cortex of a newborn, *D* from the same area in a 4 yr old child, showing marked increase in length and complexity of dendritic branching. (× 100.)

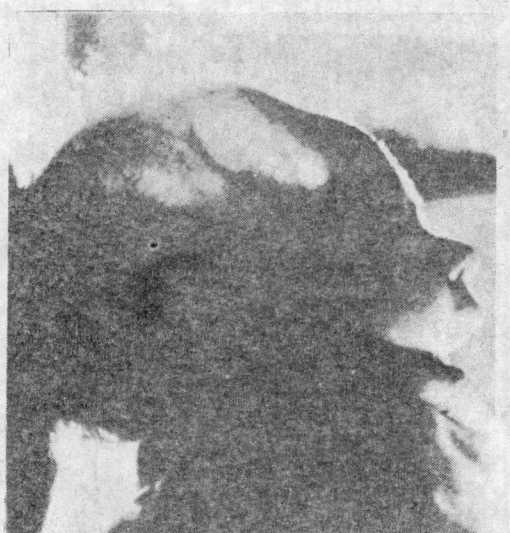

Figure 21–8 Hydranencephaly shown by transillumination.

ciated with abnormal enlargement of the head and with progressive motor deficit.

Hydranencephaly. Hydranencephaly is defined as congenital absence of the cerebral hemispheres. The cerebrum is replaced by a large, fluid-filled cavity. The brain stem and basal ganglia are well formed, and rudiments of frontal and occipital cortex may be present. The etiology is unknown. Failure of development of the cerebral arteries and destruction of brain by severe intrauterine infection have been suggested as possible etiologic factors.

The hydranencephalic infant may look remarkably normal at birth. Head size is normal or slightly enlarged. All the normal neonatal reflex patterns may be present. The infant does not have visual following, however, and there is failure of further voluntary motor and intellectual development. Seizures may occur. The diagnosis is suggested by total transillumination of the skull (Fig 21–8). A similar clinical picture may be seen in advanced congenital hydrocephalus and with extensive bilateral subdural effusions. The diagnosis should be confirmed by cerebral angiography, which shows absence of the major cerebral vessels. Most of the affected infants die within 1 yr, but survival past 3 yr has been reported.

Lissencephaly. In this defect in migration of cerebral neurons, cortical gyri fail to develop. The surface of the cerebral hemispheres is smooth; microscopic examination shows absence of the normal cortical cell layers and persistence of groups of neurons in the subcortical white matter. The clinical picture is that of severe mental retardation. The diagnosis can be made by computed tomography.

Polymicrogyria. Polymicrogyria is another defect in neuronal migration; a great excess of poorly developed cerebral gyri is formed. The abnormality has been associated with intrauterine cytomegaloviral infection, but in most cases the etiology is obscure. Severe mental retardation is always present. The diagnosis is made at autopsy.

Microcephaly. This is a defect in the growth of the brain as a whole, resulting from developmental abnormalities and destructive processes affecting the brain during the fetal and early infancy periods. Head size is more than 3 standard deviations below the normal mean. The more important known causes are listed in Table 21–4.

The microcephalic brain always shows a decrease in weight, which may be as low as 25% of normal. The number and complexity of cortical gyri may be diminished. The frontal lobes are most severely stunted; the cerebellum is often disproportionately large. In microcephaly due to perinatal or postnatal disorders there may be neuronal loss and gliosis in the cerebral cortex.

The most severe microcephaly tends to occur in the recessively inherited form. Affected children have marked backward sloping of the forehead and disproportionately large ears. Motor development is often remarkably good, but mental retardation becomes progressively more evident and is often profound.

The various conditions listed in Table 21–4 have to be considered in the differential diagnosis of the microcephalic infant or child. A backward-sloping forehead, large ears, or a history of parental consanguinity suggests the diagnosis of hereditary microcephaly. The possibility that microcephaly may be due to maternal phenylketonuria should always be pursued by appropriate examination of the mother's urine. Skull roentgenograms, lumbar puncture, and serologic tests are useful in the diagnosis of microcephaly secondary to intrauterine infection. Diffuse cerebral calcifications are frequently found in congenital toxoplasmosis; periventricular calcifications are more prevalent in cytomegaloviral disease (Fig 21–9). The fetal alcohol syndrome has to be considered in a microcephalic child whose mother has a history of alcoholism.

Microcephaly must be distinguished from small head size

Table 21–4   CAUSES OF MICROCEPHALY

DEFECTS IN BRAIN DEVELOPMENT	INTRAUTERINE INFECTIONS	PERINATAL AND POSTNATAL DISORDERS
Hereditary (recessive) microcephaly	Congenital rubella	Intrauterine or neonatal anoxia
Mongolism and other autosomal trisomy syndromes	Cytomegaloviral infection	Severe malnutrition in early infancy
Fetal ionizing radiation exposure	Congenital toxoplasmosis	Neonatal herpes virus infection
Maternal phenylketonuria	Congenital syphilis	
Seckel dwarfism		
Cornelia de Lange syndrome		
Rubinstein-Taybi syndrome		
Smith-Lemli-Opitz syndrome		
Fetal alcohol syndrome		

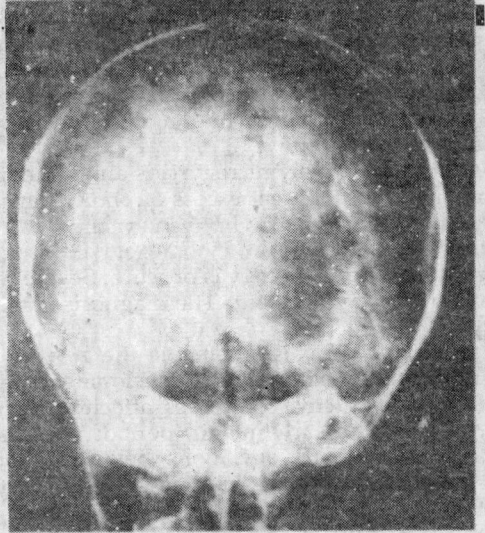
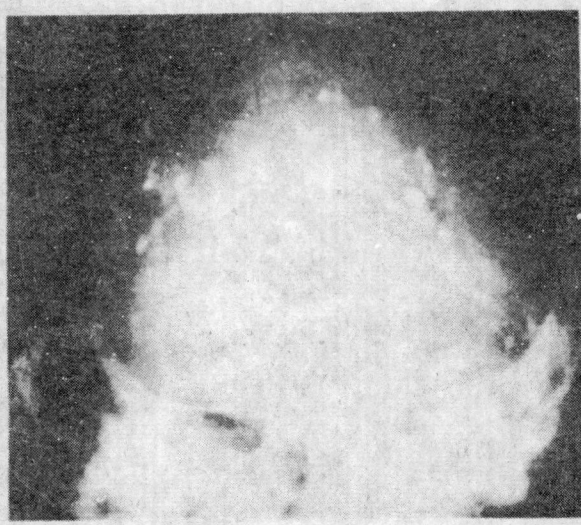

A   B

Figure 21–9 *A*, Periventricular calcification and hydrocephalus following cytomegalic inclusion disease in the newborn. *B*, Diffuse intracerebral calcifications following congenital toxoplasmosis.

secondary to synostosis of sagittal and coronal sutures. In craniosynostosis a palpable ridge is present in the region of the prematurely closed suture, and there is evidence of increased intracranial pressure, including papilledema and increase in convolutional markings on skull radiographs.

None of the forms of microcephaly are treatable, but accurate diagnosis is important for genetic counseling, some disorders being hereditary, others clearly sporadic.

Megalencephaly. In this rare developmental defect excessive growth of brain occurs during infancy and is responsible for abnormally rapid enlargement of the head. Brains weighing up to 2800 gm have been reported, the excessive weight usually due to overgrowth of glial cells rather than of neurons. Similar excessive growth of brain may occur in Hurler syndrome, in Tay-Sachs disease, and in metachromatic leukodystrophy, but the cause of megalencephaly is often unknown. Affected infants usually have considerable developmental delay. Signs of increased intracranial pressure are absent. Differentiation from hydrocephalus is made by computed tomography. The prognosis is guarded; severe mental deficiency is common.

Baron J, et al: The incidence of cytomegaloviruses, herpes simplex, rubella and toxoplasma antibodies in microcephalic, mentally retarded and normocephalic children. Pediatrics 44:932, 1969.

Bishop K, Connolly JM, Carter CH, et al: Holoprosencephaly. J Pediatr 65:406, 1964.

DeMyer W: Megalencephaly in children. Clinical syndromes, genetic patterns, and differential diagnosis from other causes of megalocephaly. Neurology 22:634, 1972.

Freeman JM, Gold AP: Porencephaly simulating subdural hematoma in childhood. Am J Dis Child 107:327, 1964.

Haberland C, Brunngraber E: Micropolygyria: A histopathological and biochemical study. J Ment Defic Res 16:1, 1972.

Hamby WB, Krauss RF, Beswick WF: Hydranencephaly: Clinical diagnosis. Presentation of seven cases. Pediatrics 6:371, 1950.

Hansen, H: Epidemiological considerations on maternal hyperphenylalaninemia. Am J Ment Defic 75:22, 1970.

Jones KL, Smith DW: Recognition of the fetal alcohol syndrome in early infancy. Lancet 2:999, 1973.

Koch FP, Doyle PJ: Agenesis of the corpus callosum. Report of eight cases in infancy. J Pediatr 50:345, 1957.

Lorber J, Granger RG: Cerebral cavities following ventricular puncture in infants. Clin Radiol 14:98, 1963.

Menkes JH, Philippart M, Clark DB: Hereditary partial agenesis of corpus callosum. Arch Neurol 11:198, 1964.

Murphy DP, Shirlock ME, Doll EA: Microcephaly following maternal pelvic irradiation for interruption of pregnancy. Am J Roentgenol 48:356, 1942.

Osburn BI, Silverstein AM, Prendergast RA, et al: Experimental viral-induced congenital encephalopathies. I. Pathology of hydranencephaly and porencephaly caused by bluetongue vaccine virus. Lab Invest 25:197, 1971.

Penrose LS: Microcephaly. Folia Hered Pathol 5:79, 1956.

Yakovlev PI, Wadsworth RC: Schizencephalies. A study of congenital clefts in the cerebral mantle; Clefts with fused lips. J Neuropathol Exp Neurol 5:169, 1946.

Yu JS, O'Halloran MT: Children of mothers with phenylketonuria. Lancet 1:210, 1970.

21.10 HYDROCEPHALUS

Definition. The term "hydrocephalus" is applied to any condition in which enlargement of the ventricular system occurs as a result of an imbalance between production and absorption of cerebrospinal fluid (CSF). CSF pressure is usually elevated in progressive hydrocephalus, but occasionally it may be normal or nearly so.

Pathophysiology and Etiology. CSF production depends largely on the active transport of ions, especially sodium, across the specialized epithelial membrane of the choroid plexus into the ventricular cavities. Water follows passively to re-establish osmotic equilibrium; the result is the passage of fluid into the cerebral ventricles. This fluid circulates via the aqueduct of Sylvius and the 4th ventricle and gains access to the subarachnoid spaces through the foramina of Luschka and Magendie. It is reabsorbed into the venous circulation from the subarachnoid spaces over the brain, to

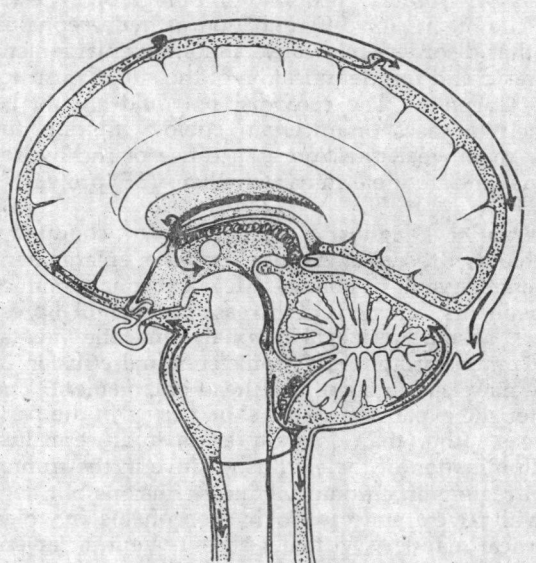

Figure 21–10 Schematic representation of CSF circulation.

some extent from those over the spinal cord, and from the ependymal lining of the ventricles. The circulation of CSF is shown schematically in Fig 21–10.

Hydrocephalus is almost always due to interference with the circulation and absorption of CSF. Rarely, it is due to overproduction of fluid. Excessive fluid production is best documented in papilloma of the choroid plexus, a tumor which actively secretes CSF.

Two anatomic types of hydrocephalus are distinguished: (1) In *obstructive hydrocephalus* there is interference with circulation of CSF within the ventricular system itself. As a result ventricular fluid cannot gain rcady access to the subarachnoid spaces. Enlargement of the ventricular system occurs proximal to the site of obstruction. (2) In *communicating hydrocephalus* CSF pathways inside the ventricular system are open and ventricular fluid is able to move freely into the spinal subarachnoid space. Interference with absorption of CSF is due either to occlusion of the subarachnoid cisterns around the brain stem or to obliteration of subarachnoid spaces over the convexities of the brain. The entire ventricular system becomes uniformly dis-

tended. A number of congenital and acquired conditions may lead to hydrocephalus (Table 21–5).

Obstructive Hydrocephalus. This is due most commonly to *congenital aqueductal stenosis.* The aqueduct of Sylvius is narrowed or is replaced by multiple small channels or "forks" which end blindly (Fig 21–11). In a small number of cases aqueductal stenosis is transmitted as an X-linked recessive trait. It may also be a residuum of inflammation in the periaqueductal region. Experimental evidence in several animal species implicates fetal viral infection, especially mumps, as an etiologic factor. Occasionally, obstructive hydrocephalus is due to compression of the aqueduct by an extrinsic lesion posterior to the brain stem, such as congenital aneurysm of the vein of Galen or subdural hematoma in the posterior fossa. The latter occurs as a birth injury; the bleeding is secondary to traumatic rupture of veins bridging from the surface of the cerebellum to the transverse sinuses. The diagnosis of posterior fossa subdural hematoma has to be considered in infants who develop hydrocephalus during the 1st postnatal weeks, especially when there is a history of difficult birth. The *Dandy-Walker malformation* is a congenital defect of midline cerebellar structures in which hydrocephalus is caused by atresia of the foramina of Luschka and Magendie. When obstructive hydrocephalus is acquired postnatally, it is often due to brain tumors which compress or extend into the ventricular system. Aqueductal stenosis also may be of postnatal onset and may not become manifest until late in childhood or adolescence.

Communicating Hydrocephalus. Often of unknown etiology, this occurs in the *Arnold-Chiari malformation* where it is due to obstruction of subarachnoid pathways around the brain stem by downward displacement of the medulla oblongata and cerebellum. Communicating hydrocephalus may follow bacterial meningitis, toxoplasmosis, cytomegaloviral infection, and subarachnoid

Table 21–5 CAUSES OF HYDROCEPHALUS

OBSTRUCTIVE HYDROCEPHALUS	COMMUNICATING HYDROCEPHALUS

Aqueductal stenosis
  Congenital
  Acquired (postinfectious)
Midline brain tumors
Vein of Galen malformation
Posterior fossa subdural
  hematoma
Dandy-Walker malformation
	Arnold-Chiari malformation
	Postinfectious (meningitis,
	  toxoplasmosis, cytomegaloviral
	  infection)
	Secondary to subarachnoid
	  hemorrhage
	Secondary to excessive production
	  of CSF (papilloma of choroid
	  plexus)
	Diseases of connective tissue
	  (Hurler syndrome, achondroplasia)
	Vitamin A intoxication

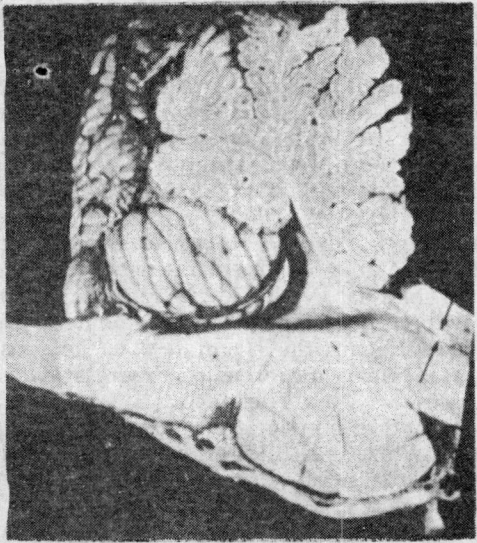

Figure 21–11 Congenital stenosis of aqueduct of Sylvius (arrows). Despite severe obstructive hydrocephalus, patient lived to 6th decade as a self-supporting person.

hemorrhage as a result of obliteration of subarachnoid spaces by fibrous tissue reaction to meningeal inflammation or to hemorrhage. Hydrocephalus may complicate *Hurler syndrome* because of fibrous tissue proliferation in the subarachnoid spaces. In *achondroplasia* hydrocephalus is probably due to underdevelopment of the occipital skull, an abnormally small posterior fossa interfering with circulation of CSF in the subarachnoid spaces at the base of the brain. *Vitamin A intoxication* is a rare cause of communicating hydrocephalus; the mechanism is unknown.

Incidence. The incidence of congenital hydrocephalus varies in different populations, especially hydrocephalus associated with meningomyelocele, the incidence of which varies from about 4.0/1000 births in some parts of Wales and of Northern Ireland to about 0.2/1000 in Japan. The incidence of all other forms of hydrocephalus is nearly 1/1000. Aqueductal stenosis is found in about one third of all hydrocephalic children.

Clinical Manifestations. Signs and symptoms of hydrocephalus depend on the time of onset and on the severity of the imbalance between CSF production and resorptive capacity. Abnormal enlargement of the head is an invariable feature of congenital hydrocephalus and of hydrocephalus with onset in infancy. In the most severe cases of congenital hydrocephalus massive enlargement of the head during the fetal period precludes normal delivery of the infant. In milder forms the head is of normal size at birth but then grows at an excessive rate. Serial measurements of head circumference are essential for early diagnosis and for assessment of rate of progression. The skull is distended in all directions but especially in the frontal area. Occipital expansion is seen in the Dandy-Walker malformation as a result of massive dilatation of the 4th ventricle, which can be demonstrated by occipital transillumination of the skull. Infants with rapidly progressive hydrocephalus have a large, bulging anterior fontanelle and palpable separation of cranial sutures. Apparently normal fontanelle tension, however, does not rule out the diagnosis. Separation of the cranial sutures leads to a resonant note on percussion of the skull (Macewen or "cracked-pot" sign). The scalp veins are often prominent and the scalp skin is thin and shiny. The cry becomes high-pitched as intracranial pressure rises. In severe infantile hydrocephalus the eyes are often deviated downward ("setting-sun" sign). Optic atrophy, resulting from compression of the optic nerve and chiasm, occurs in chronic, untreated cases.

When the onset of hydrocephalus is late in childhood, there may be no appreciable enlargement of the head. Instead, the child has evidence of increased intracranial pressure with chronic papilledema. Combined spasticity and ataxia affecting the legs more than the arms are common, as is urinary incontinence. Progressive decline in mental activity occurs. Higher cortical functions such as judgment and reasoning tend to be affected disproportionately, while speech, often preserved, results in rather characteristic empty chatter. There is poor correlation between degree of hydrocephalus and intellectual dysfunction. Some children with hugely dilated ventricular systems and thin cerebral mantles have normal intelligence.

Laboratory Studies. Computed tomography is a reliable, safe means for differentiation of hydrocephalus from other disorders that cause abnormal enlargement of the head and for identification of the site of obstruction to CSF flow. The cerebrospinal fluid should be examined in cases of uncertain etiology to rule out chronic meningeal infection as a cause of the hydrocephalus and to determine whether CSF protein is elevated.

Differential Diagnosis. A number of conditions other than hydrocephalus cause abnormal enlargement of the cranial vault in infancy. Megalencephaly mimics hydrocephalus, but signs of increased intracranial pressure are absent in megalencephaly and the mental defect is more profound. Chronic subdural effusion in infancy may lead to significant head enlargement. The characteristic expansion of the skull occurs in the parietal areas rather than frontally as in hydrocephalus. Transillumination of the skull is positive in the fronto-parietal regions in chronic subdural effusions but negative in all but extreme cases of hydrocephalus, in which the cortical mantle is virtually absent. Ventricular enlargement follows cerebral atrophy in degenerative and metabolic brain diseases, in which head size is normal or small.

The possibility that hydrocephalus may be secondary to midline brain tumor always has to be considered. Cerebellar, pineal region, and 3rd ventricular tumors are likely to produce head enlargement in the absence of focal neurologic signs. Brain tumor has to be considered especially when enlargement of the head is very rapid in a previously normal infant and when papilledema is present. An underlying cerebral neoplasm can be ruled out by computed tomography with infusion of radiopaque contrast material.

Therapy. The treatment of hydrocephalus has improved in recent yr but continues to present many formidable problems. Ideally, the goal is to re-establish equilibrium between CSF production and resorption. Acetazolamide in a dose of 40–75 mg/kg/24 hr diminishes CSF production by about one third and is occasionally effective in mild, slowly progressive hydrocephalus. In most cases, however, shunt operations provide the best available treatment for progressive hydrocephalus.

In obstructive hydrocephalus the site of obstruction can sometimes be bypassed. The Torkildsen operation bypasses aqueductal stenosis with a plastic tube that connects 1 lateral ventricle with the cisterna magna and the spinal subarachnoid spaces; the operation is not successful in infants since these spaces are as yet poorly developed. At present, the most widely used and successful treatments depend on shunting of the excess fluid into some extracranial body compartment. Ventriculoperitoneal shunts are most commonly used. A 1-way valve that closes when ventricular fluid pressure falls below a fixed value is inserted into the tubing to prevent complete drainage of CSF and collapse of the cerebral ventricles. Complications with this type of shunt include bacterial colonization of the shunt (especially with *Staphylococcus albus*), kinking, plugging, or separation of the shunt tubing, and subdural hematoma due to low intracranial pressure. Shunt infection may cause recurrent episodes of septicemia and ventriculitis. In either case, cure of the infection usually requires removal of the shunt in addition to antibiotic therapy. Plugging of the shunt tubing is especially apt to occur when CSF protein is elevated. Growth of the head, neck, and chest necessitates repeated shunt revisions during early childhood. Ventriculoatrial shunts, which deliver ventricular fluid from a lateral ventricle to the right atrium, are used less commonly now because of higher rates of infection and the complications of pulmonary embolism, superior vena caval occlusion, and nephritis.

Careful initial evaluation is essential to determine whether a shunt operation is needed or spontaneous arrest of hydrocephalus has occurred. In general, a shunt is not indicated in hydrocephalic infants whose head growth has become arrested or is progressing at or below the normal rate. Repeated lumbar punctures rather than shunt surgery appear to be the initial treatment of choice when acute hydrocephalus occurs after subarachnoid hemorrhage or bacterial meningitis.

When a successful shunt has been established, it usually has to be maintained for the life of the patient. Such a child needs careful medical supervision for early detection of evidences of shunt malfunction. Acute shunt failure in the older child causes rapidly progressive increase in intracranial pressure, with headache, vomiting, and stupor, progressing to coma and death unless shunt revision is performed promptly. Chronic shunt malfunction may result in school failure, lethargy, and deterioration of gait. Serial computed tomography is useful for detection of early shunt failure.

Prognosis. The prognosis of infantile hydrocephalus has been significantly but not dramatically improved by introduction of shunt operations. Untreated, 50–60% of infants with hydrocephalus succumb to the disorder itself or to intercurrent illnesses. About 40% of survivors are of near-normal intelligence. With good neurosurgical and medical management about 70% can be expected to live beyond infancy; of these, about 40% will have normal intellect, and about 60% will have significant intellectual and motor handicaps. The prognosis of infants with both hydrocephalus and meningomyelocele is considerably worse.

Ameli NO: Arrest of development and Dandy-Walker malformation. Brain 89:459, 1966.
Drachman DA, Richardson EP: Aqueductal narrowing, congenital and acquired. Arch Neurol 5:552, 1961.
Foltz EL, Shurtleff DB: Five-year comparative study of hydrocephalus in children with and without operation (113 cases). J Neurosurg 20:1064, 1963.
Gilles F, Shillito J: Infantile hydrocephalus: Retrocerebellar subdural hematoma. J Pediatr 76:529, 1970.
Goldstein GW, et al: Transient hydrocephalus in premature infants: Treatment by lumbar punctures. Lancet 1:512, 1976.
Hagberg B, Naglo AS: The conservative management of infantile hydrocephalus. Acta Paediatr Scand 61:165, 1972.
Hagberg B, Sjorgen I: The chronic brain syndrome of infantile hydrocephalus. Am J Dis Child 112:189, 1966.
Hart MN, Malamud N, Ellis WG: The Dandy-Walker syndrome: A clinical-pathological study of 28 cases. Neurology 22:771, 1972.
Huttenlocher PR: Treatment of hydrocephalus with acetazolamide. Results in 15 cases. J Pediatr 66:1023, 1965.
Ignelzi RJ, Kirsch WM: Follow-up analysis of ventriculoperitoneal and ventriculoatrial shunts for hydrocephalus. J Neurosurg 42:679, 1975.
Johnson RT, Johnson KP: Hydrocephalus following viral infection: The pathology of aqueductal stenosis developing after experimental mumps virus infection. J Neuropathol Exp Neurol 27:591, 1968.
Laurence KM, Coates S: The natural history of hydrocephalus. Detailed analysis of 182 unoperated cases. Arch Dis Child 37:345, 1962.
Milhorat TH: Hydrocephalus and the Cerebrospinal Fluid. Baltimore, Williams & Wilkins, 1972.
Noonan JA, Ehmke DA: Complications of ventriculovenous shunts for control of hydrocephalus. Report of three cases with thromboemboli to the lungs. N Engl J Med 269:70, 1963.
Ransohoff J, Shulman K, Fishman RA: Hydrocephalus. A review of etiology and treatment. J Pediatr 56:399, 1960.
Russell DS: Observations on the pathology of hydrocephalus. Special Report No 265. Medical Research Council London, His Majesty's Stationery Office, 1949.
Scarff JE: Treatment of hydrocephalus: An historical and critical review of methods and results. J Neurol Neurosurg Psychiat 26:1, 1963.
Schick RW, Matson DD: What is arrested hydrocephalus? J Pediatr 58:791, 1961.
Stauffer UG: "Shunt nephritis": Diffuse glomerulonephritis complicating ventriculoatrial shunts. Develop Med Child Neurol 22(Suppl):161, 1970.
Woodard WK, Miller LJ, Legant O: Acute and chronic hypervitaminosis A in a 4 month old infant. J Pediatr 59:260, 1961.
Yashon D: Prognosis of infantile hydrocephalus, past and present. J Neurosurg 20:105, 1963.

21.11 DEFECTS IN DEVELOPMENT OF THE BRAIN STEM

Moebius Syndrome. In this syndrome, also known as congenital nuclear aplasia, there is absence or maldevelopment of cranial nerve nuclei and of their nerves. The 7th nerves are affected most frequently, but most of the cranial nerves may be involved. The most severely affected children have ptosis, complete ophthalmoplegia, inability to close the eyes, facial immobility, and difficulty with chewing and swallowing. Congenital anomalies often associated include absence of pectoralis muscles and clubfoot deformities. The expressionless face and constant drooling may give the erroneous impression of mental defect. When lid closure is defective, it is important to protect the corneas by use of artificial tears and by taping the eyelids at night. Familial cases have been reported.

Spasmus Nutans. This disorder of eye movements is peculiar to infancy and is usually first noted from the ages of 4–12 mo. It consists of intermittent rapid pendular nystagmoid movements, often confined to 1 eye, and, when bilateral, almost always more prominent on 1 side. About 80% of infants have intermittent head nodding. The etiology is unknown. Insufficient lighting and relative absence of visual stimuli for the infant to fix on have been implicated as possible etiologic factors without convincing evidence. Spontaneous improvement always occurs.

Spasmus nutans has to be distinguished from searching nystagmus due to decreased visual acuity and from hereditary congenital nystagmus. In congenital nystagmus the abnormal movement of the eyes is bilaterally symmetrical, with pendular movements when the eyes are at rest giving way to jerk nystagmus on attempted lateral gaze.

Becker-Christensen F, Lund HT: A family wtih Möbius syndrome. J Pediatr 84:115, 1974.
Hoefnagel D, Biery B: Spasmus nutans. Develop Med Child Neurol 10:32, 1968.
Van Allen MW, Blodi FC: Neurologic aspects of the Moebius syndrome. Neurology 10:249, 1960.

21.12 PERINATALLY ACQUIRED CEREBRAL LESIONS

Damage to the central nervous system in the perinatal period is a major cause of intellectual handicap and of nonprogressive motor disorders. In part, this is related to the unusual stresses to the infant incident to birth, in part to the peculiar susceptibility of the immature central nervous system to injury by a variety of agents. Cerebral anoxia, traumatic injury to brain, infection, hyperbilirubinemia, hypoglycemia, hypothyroidism, and the inborn errors of amino acid metabolism are important causes of brain damage in the infant. The reaction of the immature brain to these agents differs markedly from that of the mature central nervous system.

Cerebral anoxia in the infant, contrary to that in the older child or adult, frequently causes selective damage to subcortical structures rather than to cortical neurons; this is especially the case in the premature infant, in whom the subcortical white matter is particularly vulnerable. The resulting brain lesion, periventricular leukomalacia, is frequently demonstrated at autopsy of premature infants who have had repeated anoxic episodes. The basal ganglia are also susceptible to anoxic damage in the neonate. Pathologically, one finds loss of neurons in basal ganglia and abnormal deposition of myelin to replace them, giving with myelin stains a marbled appearance, "status marmoratus," to the basal ganglia.

Meningeal infection results in cerebritis and cerebral vasculitis much more frequently in the neonate than in the older child, and these account for brain damage in the majority of survivors. Infections with rubella, cytomegalovirus, herpesvirus, coxsackievirus, and toxoplasma are more likely to involve brain in the fetus and neonate than in the older person. The reaction in the nervous system is usually one of widespread necrosis of tissue.

Elevation in the blood level of unconjugated bilirubin above 15–20 mg/dl causes damage in selected structures of the neonatal brain, especially the basal ganglia and cranial nerve nuclei in the lower brain stem, including those of the 8th nerve (Sec 7.44). The most prominent acute, pathologic change is yellow staining of the affected nuclei *(kernicterus)* due to deposition of bilirubin in the damaged tissues. The chronic lesion consists of loss of nerve cells, gliosis, and defective myelination.

Severe neonatal *hypoglycemia* (Sec 7.57) may cause diffuse necrosis of cortical neurons and damage to cerebellum. However, these lesions are uncommon, and it is generally assumed that the immature brain is less sensitive to damage by hypoglycemia than is the mature one.

A number of *metabolic diseases* lead to cerebral dysfunction by interference with the normal developmental events in postnatal brain; these include congenital hypothyroidism (cretinism) and the large group of inborn errors of amino acid metabolism, of which phenylketonuria is the most common. Myelination of subcortical white matter and the elaboration of dendrites and of synaptic connections between nerve cells are the 2 most important developmental events in postnatal brain (Fig 21–7). They are most likely to be disturbed in the metabolic encephalopathies of the infant. Defective myelination has been well demonstrated in phenylketonuria and in maple syrup urine disease. In cretinism both the elaboration of cortical dendrites and myelination appear to be inhibited.

A major problem in care of the newborn is the paucity of early clinical evidences of CNS lesions in many infants damaged in the perinatal period. The infant may initially appear to improve, with cerebral dysfunction becoming manifest only as he or she matures. Intellectual handicaps ranging from severe mental defect to mild learning disabilities are common sequelae of neonatal brain damage. In some damaged infants motor deficits predominate, and there may be relative preservation of intellectual functions. (See Cerebral Palsy below.) Others may develop seizures, sometimes 1 yr or more after the initial insult. Since the mental and motor manifestations of cerebral damage may not appear until much later, it often is difficult to ascribe them with certainty to specific events; accordingly the causes of static cerebral lesions in many children are unknown or conjectural.

Anderson JM, Milner RDG, Stritch SJ: Effects of neonatal hypoglycemia on the nervous system: A pathological study. J Neurol Neurosurg Psychiat 30:295, 1967.
Banker BQ, Larroche JC: Periventricular leukomalacia of infancy: A form of neonatal anoxic encephalopathy. Arch Neurol 7:386, 1962.
Berman PH, Banker BQ: Neonatal meningitis. A clinical and pathological study of 29 cases. Pediatrics 38:6, 1966.
Diamond I, et al: Kernicterus: Revised concepts of pathogenesis and management. Pediatrics 38:539, 1966.
Eayres JT, Horn G: The development of cerebral cortex in hypothyroid and starved rats. Anat Rec 121:53, 1955.
Norman RM: État marbré of the corpus striatum following birth injury. J Neurol Neurosurg Psychiat 10:12, 1947.
Prensky AL, Carr S, Moser HW: Development of myelin in inherited disorders of amino acid metabolism. Arch Neurol 19:552, 1968.
Rosman NP, et al: The effect of thyroid deficiency on myelination of brain. Neurology 22:99, 1972.
Towbin A: Central nervous system damage in the human fetus and newborn infant. Am J Dis Child 119:529, 1970.

21.13 CEREBRAL PALSY (Little Disease)

Cerebral palsy is defined as any nonprogressive central motor deficit dating to events in the prenatal or perinatal periods. It is 1 of the most common crippling conditions of childhood; almost 300,000 children are affected in the United States alone. It is not a specific disease but a group of disorders of varied causes.

Etiology. The relationship of cerebral palsy to neonatal anoxia was first established by Little in 1843. Recent studies find that more than one third of children with cerebral palsy weighed less than 2500 gm at birth. The most likely etiologic event in these infants is cerebral anoxia, often complicated by intraventricular and subependymal hemorrhages (Sec 7.23); mechanical trauma to the brain at birth is also a cause, especially in those with spastic hemiplegia. Congenital malformations of brain and cerebral vascular occlusions during fetal life appear to account for a smaller percentage. Kernicterus, an important cause of cerebral palsy prior to the introduction of exchange transfusion for neonatal hyperbilirubinemia, is now relatively uncommon.

Pathology. The most severely disabled children are apt to have widespread cerebral atrophy, often with cavity formation in subcortical white matter. Atrophy of basal ganglia is found when rigidity and extrapyramidal movement disorders were present during life. With hemiplegia, atrophy and gliosis of the opposite cerebral hemisphere often occur, usually confined to the areas supplied by the middle cerebral artery and probably due to arterial occlusion. Porencephaly occurs in some cases. In milder forms of cerebral palsy the brain may appear grossly normal but is often reduced in weight. The sparseness of subcortical white matter suggests that some nerve fibers may have been destroyed by the initial cerebral insult.

Clinical Manifestations. Clinical classification of patients with cerebral palsy is based on the nature of the observed motor deficit. The following classification is useful: (1) *Spastic cerebral palsy* (quadriplegia, paraplegia, hemiplegia, monoplegia); (2) *extrapyramidal cerebral palsy* (choreoathetosis, dystonia); (3) *atonic cerebral palsy* (atonic diplegia, congenital cerebellar ataxia); and (4) *mixed types*.

Spastic Cerebral Palsy. This is the most common type of palsy. Early manifestations are those of reflex hyperexcitability and abnormal persistence of neonatal reflexes. Hyperactivity of the grasp reflex leads to tight fisting of the hands. Tonic neck reflexes are often obligatory and may continue to be present long after the normal age of disappearance. Vertical suspension of the infant leads to extensor postures (arching of the back and rigid extension and adduction and internal rotation of the legs). When hip adduction is marked, it leads to crossing (scissoring) of the legs. The severely spastic infant may have arching of the back and scissoring even at rest. Tendon reflexes are brisk, often with sustained ankle clonus. A positive Babinski sign is helpful in the diagnosis after the age of 2 yr. Spasticity and rigidity become more evident as the child matures and often lead to abnormal postures of limbs and to contractures. Heel cord contractures, limitation in abduction and external rotation of the hips, and limitation in extension and supination of the forearms are common. Pseudobulbar palsy is present when spasticity is bilateral; it accounts for the swallowing difficulties and excessive drooling of these children.

In *spastic quadriplegia* all 4 limbs are involved. There is usually associated mental defect. Pseudobulbar palsy is prominent, and convulsions are common. *Diplegia* refers to a motor deficit that affects all 4 limbs but is much more severe in the lower extremities than in the upper ones. The involvement of hands may be minimal, expressing itself only in clumsiness in grasping and, later in life, in awkwardness of hand movements. Evidence of pseudobulbar palsy may be absent or lim-

ited to a brisk jaw jerk. Intelligence is often normal or borderline, but apraxias are common and may lead to difficulties in learning to draw and to form letters. More than 50% of children with diplegia had low birth weights.

In *spastic paraplegia*, a rare form of cerebral palsy, only the lower extremities are affected. The possibility of a spinal cord lesion must always be carefully considered in the child who has spasticity confined to the legs.

Spastic hemiplegia accounts for about one third of children with cerebral palsy. There is often homonymous hemianopsia and a hemisensory deficit on the side of the hemiplegia. The posture of the affected arm is quite characteristic: maintained flexion and pronation of the forearm and flexion of the wrist. The gait of these children is characterized by limping, often with circumduction of the affected leg. The intellectual level depends largely on whether the brain lesion is confined to 1 hemisphere. Convulsions early in life decrease the likelihood of normal intellectual development.

Monoplegia, spastic weakness confined to 1 limb, is rare. Careful examination will usually disclose an asymmetric diplegia or hemiplegia with 1 limb more severely affected than the other.

Extrapyramidal Cerebral Palsy. This is manifest as hypotonia in early infancy and by choreoathetoid movements and dystonia later in childhood. Identification is unusual until after the age of 6 mo; abnormal posturing of hands when the infant attempts to reach for an object is an early sign. When choreoathetosis is associated with deafness, it is almost always the result of kernicterus. The combination of motor handicap and absence of speech function caused by deafness may give an erroneous impression of severe mental retardation; intellectual capacity can be surmised only after prolonged study.

Atonic Diplegia. Atonic diplegia is a diagnostic term designating hypotonia and motor disability due to central nervous system damage. Severe mental defect is usual. The tendon reflexes are easily obtainable and may be quite brisk, in contrast to the pattern in hypotonia due to peripheral neuromuscular diseases. Some degree of spasticity in later childhood is common.

Congenital Cerebellar Ataxia. In this rare form of cerebral palsy hypotonia and hypoactive tendon reflexes are present in infancy. Usually by the 2nd yr intention tremor and gait ataxia are present. Nystagmus is uncommon. There may be an associated mental defect, usually mild.

Differential Diagnosis. *Spastic cerebral palsy* has to be distinguished from the leukodystrophies. In doubtful cases a spinal tap may provide helpful diagnostic information; spinal fluid protein is almost always elevated in the leukodystrophies but not in cerebral palsy. The possibility that spastic weakness may be due to hydrocephalus or to subdural effusion should be considered whenever head size is large or when signs of increased intracranial pressure are present. Rarely, a slowly growing tumor of a cerebral hemisphere may be confused with the hemiplegic form of cerebral palsy. In brain tumor the disability is always progressive, and signs of increased intracranial pressure are usually present.

Spinal cord lesions, including birth injuries to the cervical cord, tumors, and congenital malformations, should be considered when spasticity and weakness are limited to the muscle groups below the neck. Spastic diplegia is sometimes confused with muscular dystrophy; heel cord contractures and weakness of legs occur in both. Spasticity, however, is absent in muscular dystrophy, and the tendon reflexes are normal or reduced. In doubtful and early cases measurement of serum enzymes is helpful, especially of creatine phosphokinase, which is always increased in Duchenne muscular dystrophy. *Atonic diplegia* must be distinguished from neuromuscular diseases of infancy, including Werdnig-Hoffmann disease and benign congenital hypotonia. The presence of mental defect and the preservation of tendon reflexes in atonic diplegia usually make clinical differentiation possible. *Congenital cerebellar ataxia* must be differentiated from a number of slowly progressive cerebellar degenerations. Early in the course the distinction from ataxia-telangiectasia may be especially difficult; children with this illness are often diagnosed as having cerebral palsy. The presence of more than 1 child with motor deficit in the same family should always suggest a disease other than cerebral palsy; there is no "familial cerebral palsy."

Prognosis. The outlook for the child with cerebral palsy depends largely on the severity of any associated intellectual handicaps. Good adjustment can be made to fairly severe motor deficits as long as intellectual capacity is good. The response of the family to the situation and the availability of adequate educational and therapeutic facilities are of great importance.

Treatment and Prevention. Treatment of the child with cerebral palsy consists of ensuring the fullest physical and social development possible. This is discussed in general terms in Sec 2.80. In specific terms, treatment consists of early application of stretching exercises to prevent contractures, orthopedic appliances and surgical procedures to improve mobility, and special educational techniques to compensate for motor and intellectual defects insofar as possible.

The prevention of cerebral palsy constitutes a great challenge to the pediatrician. Much has been accomplished in the prevention of kernicterus through therapy of neonatal hyperbilirubinemia. Meticulous care of low birth weight infants may reduce the number of children with spastic diplegia. Careful attention to the respiratory status of the infant and prompt therapy of apneic episodes appear to be especially important.

Crothers B, Paine R: The Natural History of Cerebral Palsy. Cambridge, Harvard University Press, 1959.

Ford FR: Cerebral birth injuries and their results. Medicine 5:121, 1926.

McDonald AD: The aetiology of spastic diplegia. A synthesis of epidemiological and pathological evidence. Dev Med Child Neurol 6:277, 1964.

Mitchell RG: The prevention of cerebral palsy. Dev Med Child Neurol 13:137, 1971.

Myers RE: Atrophic cortical sclerosis with status marmoratus in the perinatally damaged monkey. Neurology 19:1177, 1969.

Plum P: Aetiology of athetosis with special reference to neonatal asphyxia, idiopathic icterus and ABO-incompatibility. Arch Dis Child 40:376, 1965.

Towbin A: The Pathology of Cerebral Palsy. Springfield, Ill., Charles C Thomas, 1960.

Twitchell TE: The neurological examination in infantile cerebral palsy. Dev Med Child Neurol 5:271, 1963.

21.14　HEADACHE AND VERTIGO

Recurrent head pain is a common, frequently benign symptom late in childhood and in adolescence; in the young child it is unusual and more often indicative of serious underlying disease. Headache may stem from any of the pain-sensitive structures of the head, including all the tissues covering the cranium, the intracranial blood vessels, the cranial nerves that carry sensory fibers (V, IX, X), the upper cervical nerves, and the meninges near the base of the brain. The brain itself, the calvarium, and the meninges overlying the cerebral hemispheres are insensitive to pain.

The following is a useful classification of the various types of headache.

1. *Vascular headache*
   Migraine
   Headache secondary to fever
   Hypertensive headache
2. *Headache related to epilepsy*
3. *Headache secondary to changes in intracranial pressure*
   Brain tumor headache
   Low CSF pressure headache
4. *Tension headache*
5. *Headache related to psychiatric disease*
6. *Headache due to eye strain*
7. *Nasal sinus pain*

Migraine. This is a common cause of vascular headache in a child.

Pathogenesis. Migraine is incompletely understood. The aura preceding the onset of head pain is thought to be due to abnormal constriction of intracranial arteries, with localized transient ischemia of cerebral tissue. The headache itself is secondary to vasodilatation of cranial vessels, especially those of the scalp. Pain fibers in the vessel walls are stimulated by the abnormal vascular distention and pulsations.

Clinical Manifestations. Over two thirds of affected patients have a positive family history; a dominant pattern of inheritance is suggested in many families. The onset usually occurs late in childhood or in early adolescence. In some instances there is a history of repeated vomiting in infancy, suggesting that the attacks may start at a time when the child is unable to verbalize his symptoms. Classically, an attack of migraine is preceded by an aura, which often consists of transient visual disturbance but which may include a variety of other fleeting neurologic disabilities. The visual aura consists of scintillating scotomas and of zigzag lines (*"fortification phenomena"*) which move slowly across the visual field. Less commonly, the aura consists of diplopia due to oculomotor nerve palsy (ophthalmoplegic migraine) or of transient ataxia, vertigo, hemisensory loss, hemiparesis, or aphasia. Within minutes or at most a few hours the aura is followed by throbbing unilateral head pain and by nausea and vomiting. Sleep usually terminates an attack. The frequency of attacks varies greatly even in the same patient; stress appears to increase the number of attacks. Partial forms, in which there is no aura, and atypical attacks with bilateral head pain and without vomiting are probably considerably more common than is the classic migraine described above.

Differential Diagnosis. The diagnosis of migraine can usually be made from the history in combination with the absence of any positive findings on careful funduscopic, physical, and neurologic examination. Fever may produce a similar throbbing head pain secondary to peripheral vasodilatation and increased cerebral blood flow. Hypertension should always be ruled out. Congenital cerebrovascular malformations are a rare cause of vascular headache. They usually produce an audible cranial bruit over the head or eyes. Headache due to increased intracranial pressure must be ruled out.

Laboratory Studies. These are of little value. Occasionally, it may be necessary to obtain skull roentgenograms, a brain scan, and an electroencephalogram to supplement the clinical evaluation. More extensive evaluations, such as cerebral angiography, should be avoided.

Treatment. Therapy is often only partially satisfactory. Vasoconstrictors such as ergotamine and caffeine taken at the very onset of symptoms may abort an attack; a combination of these 2 agents (Cafergot) is widely used. The dosage in a child over age 10 yr is 1 tablet at the 1st sign of an attack, repeated twice at 30 min intervals if necessary. Simple analgesics, such as aspirin, may be as effective and should be tried first. Maintenance therapy with phenobarbital or with propranolol sometimes prevents attacks but is justifiable only if attacks are frequent and incapacitating. Reassurance that the child has a benign condition is often more helpful than drugs. Potentially dangerous medications such as methysergide and narcotics are to be strictly avoided.

Headache as a Symptom in Epilepsy. Headache may occur as part of the aura preceding a grand mal seizure or as a postictal event. In autonomic seizures headache may be a striking part of the attack itself. Other autonomic disturbances, such as pallor, tachycardia, or pupillary dilatation, are easily overlooked. The concept that headache may be the only manifestation of a seizure is difficult to prove. Finding an abnormal electroencephalogram in a child with recurrent head pain is of little help since abnormal EEG records are common in children with classic migraine, especially at the time of attack.

Headache Secondary to Changes in Intracranial Pressure. This head pain is probably the result of stretching and deformation of cerebral vessels and of meninges. The headache of increased intracranial pressure often occurs following changes in position of the head, such as after arising from sleep. Morning headache in a child should always arouse the suspicion of brain tumor. There may be associated vomiting, often with minimal nausea, followed by a feeling of well-being. The location of head pain is a good localizing sign in brain tumor. Headache due to posterior fossa tumor is almost always occipital.

Low pressure headache is usually due to a persistent CSF leak after spinal tap. It may also be seen after traumatic meningeal tears with CSF fistula. The pain appears almost immediately on assumption of the upright position and is relieved by lying down. This type of headache is best treated by bed rest, preferably in the prone position.

Tension Headache. This is thought to be due to persistent contraction of neck and temporalis muscles, leading to localized ischemia of these structures. It is often described as a dull, steady pain, increasing as the day advances, and relieved after sleep. In its classic form it is rarely seen prior to adolescence.

Headache Related to Psychiatric Disease. Headache is a rather common symptom of depression in childhood. This type of headache is described as continuously present, whereas organic head pain is almost always intermittent. The facial expression of the depressed child with headache bespeaks suffering. Speech may be reduced to a whisper. Poor appetite, constipation, and insomnia are frequently associated. Failure to recognize this syndrome often leads to extensive and potentially harmful diagnostic studies.

Eye Strain. Eye strain is often blamed for headache, and glasses are prescribed for relief, but there is little evidence of such an association. Occasionally, prolonged reading by a child with a refractive error may lead to tension headache.

BENIGN PAROXYSMAL VERTIGO IN CHILDHOOD

This syndrome has its onset in young children, usually from 1–4 yr of age. It is thought to be secondary to a disturbance in vestibular function. During a typical attack the child suddenly becomes unsteady on his or her feet, appears frightened, and may clutch at a parent. The older child may be able to describe a rotational experience. There is no alteration of consciousness, and after a few minutes the child returns to his or her former state. The condition is self-limited, tending to subside within 2–3 yr. Benign paroxysmal vertigo is often misdiagnosed as epilepsy, and anticonvulsant drugs are prescribed unnecessarily. Preservation of normal alertness during the attack is the most important differential point from epilepsy.

Cold water caloric tests may show diminished or absent vestibular response in 1 or both ears. Audiograms and electroencephalograms are normal. A trial of dimenhydrinate (Dramamine) is indicated for frequent attacks.

Golden GS, French JH: Basilar artery migraine in children. Pediatrics 56:722, 1975
Graham JH, et al: Fibrotic disorders associated with methysergide therapy for headache. N Engl J Med 274:360, 1966.
Holguin J, Fenichel G: Migraine. J Pediatr 70:290, 1967.
Koenigsberger MR, Chutorian AM, Gold AP, et al: Benign paroxysmal vertigo of childhood. Neurology 20:1108, 1970.
Ludvigsson J. Propranolol used in prophylaxis of migraine in children. Acta Neurol Scand 50:109, 1974.
Malmquist CP: Depressions in childhood and adolescence. N Engl J Med 284:955, 1971.
Pearce J: Migraine. Springfield, Ill., Charles C Thomas, 1969.
Waters WF: Headache and the eye. Lancet 2:1, 1970.
Wolff HG: Headache and Other Head Pain. New York, Oxford University Press, 1963.

21.15 THE NEUROCUTANEOUS SYNDROMES

These syndromes, also known as phakomatoses and ectodermal dysplasias, include congenital lesions of the skin and of the central nervous system, often in association with ocular and visceral abnormalities. Several clearly distinct syndromes are recognized.

TUBEROUS SCLEROSIS
(Bourneville Disease)

See Sec 24.11.

This disorder, a major cause of mental defect and of intractable convulsions, is inherited as a dominant trait, with wide variation in expression. About 50% of cases appear to be new mutations. The fully developed disease involves numerous organs, including brain, skin, eyes, kidneys, heart, bones, and lungs.

The characteristic cerebral lesions are sclerotic patches (tubers) scattered throughout the cortical gray matter. They consist of collections of astrocytes, neurons, and bizarre giant cells without the cellular organization characteristic of normal cerebral cortex. In addition, glial nodules occur in a periventricular distribution. These lesions, present at birth, gradually enlarge and become calcified. Periventricular tumors consisting of giant astrocytes and blood vessels may form large masses, obstructing the foramina of Monro.

Convulsions are the most common clinical sign of brain involvement and occur in more than 90% of patients. Myoclonic seizures may occur during the 1st yr of life; grand mal and psychomotor seizures predominate later. Mental defect, varying from mild to severe, is present in 60–70% of patients. Behavior disorders, especially hyperactivity and destructiveness, are common. Focal neurologic signs such as hemiparesis are rare except in patients with periventricular giant cell astrocytoma, in which case headache and papilledema related to ventricular obstruction are usually also found.

Adenoma sebaceum is the most characteristic skin lesion of tuberous sclerosis. It consists of small bright red or brownish nodules in a butterfly distribution on the nose and cheeks. Histologically, these lesions consist of a mixture of fibrous tissue and blood vessels. They usually appear from 2–5 yr of age and, by late childhood, are found in more than 80% of patients. *Hypopigmented macules* on the skin of arms, legs, and trunk are usually present from birth; they may be oval or irregular in outline and a few mm to several cm in diameter. These skin lesions in an infant with infantile spasms strongly suggest the diagnosis of tuberous sclerosis. Other skin manifestations include slightly raised, indurated areas of skin, usually over the back (*shagreen patches*), and gingival and periungual fibromas.

Benign tumors made up of a mixture of fibrous tissue, fat, blood vessels, and smooth muscle, often partly cystic, are found in numerous organs, especially kidneys, heart, liver, spleen, and lungs. The renal tumors are present in about 80% of patients and may cause renal failure by compression of the ureters or renal

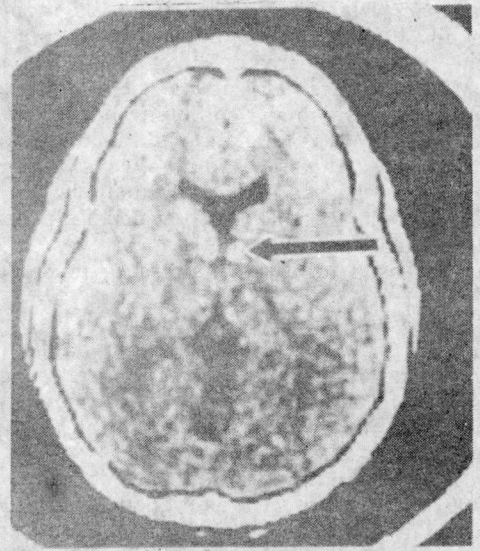

Figure 21–12 Computed tomogram (CT scan) of a 9 yr old girl with hypopigmented skin macules, mental retardation, and history of infantile myoclonic seizures. Two very dense, calcified lesions are seen in a periventricular location, typical of tuberous sclerosis.

pelvis. Rhabdomyoma of the heart is an uncommon but important complication of tuberous sclerosis, manifested clinically by progressive cardiac failure, arrhythmias, or sudden death. Small tumor nodules and cystic malformations throughout the lungs may lead to recurrent pneumothorax. About 50% of patients have retinal lesions, visible on funduscopic examination as white or yellow raised areas, often near the edge of the optic disc. These are malformations in the nerve fiber layer of the retina, consisting primarily of glial fibers and malformed retinal neuroglial cells. Such lesions usually do not impair vision.

The *diagnosis* of tuberous sclerosis is based on clinical findings. Demonstration of characteristic calcifications on skull roentgenograms and computed tomography is confirmatory (Fig 21–12). Roentgenograms of long bones may disclose areas of sclerosis and of rarefaction, especially in metacarpal and metatarsal bones.

The *prognosis* is extremely variable. Patients with mild involvement may have full, productive lives. Institutional care is required for those with severe mental deficiency. Early death may be due to status epilepticus, brain tumor, renal failure, or tumor of the heart.

Proper *management* includes treatment of seizures and assessment of intellectual function as a guide to an appropriate educational program. Methylphenidate (Ritalin) or dextroamphetamine may be helpful for control of hyperactivity in young children with tuberous sclerosis. Surgical excision of tumors is indicated only if they are symptomatic. Genetic counseling is essential. Both parents should be carefully examined for stigmata, including those of skin, retina, and brain (roentgenogram or CT scan of head). Evidence of tuberous sclerosis in 1 parent suggests a 50% likelihood of occurrence in subsequent children; a new mutation can be assumed if both parents are free of stigmata.

NEUROFIBROMATOSIS
(von Recklinghausen Disease)

See also Sec 24.10.

Neurofibromatosis is transmitted as an autosomal dominant trait, but new mutations are common and have been estimated to account for about 50% of cases. Manifestations are extremely varied. The skin is involved in the great majority of patients. *Café-au-lait spots*, irregularly shaped areas of increased skin pigmentation, are a hallmark of the disease (Fig 21–13). A few such spots are commonly found in otherwise normal persons, but the presence of more than 6 that are greater than 1.5 cm in diameter is pathognomonic of neurofibromatosis. In addition, there tends to be freckling, especially in the axillae, and general hyperpigmentation of skin.

Cutaneous and subcutaneous neurofibromas commonly make their appearance in late childhood or in adolescence. These are thought to arise from the Schwann cells of peripheral nerves. The cutaneous tumors tend to form multiple soft pedunculated masses (*molluscum fibrosum*); the subcutaneous ones are usually felt as soft nodules attached to the larger peripheral nerves. Less common are plexiform neuromas, which are large infiltrative tumors; they cause considerable disfigurement, usually involving the face or 1 extremity. Sarcomatous degeneration of 1 or more neurofibromas occurs in about 10% of patients; it is rare in childhood.

Neurofibromas on cranial or spinal nerve roots may lead to a variety of neurologic symptoms. Tumor of the 8th nerve (acoustic neuroma) causes tinnitus, nerve deafness, loss of corneal reflex, vertigo, ataxia, and signs of increased intracranial pressure. Neurofibroma involving a spinal root may be manifested as an extramedullary spinal cord tumor. There is also increased incidence of other types of neural tumors, such as glioma of the optic nerve and optic chiasm, meningioma, and pheochromocytoma.

A large variety of congenital malformations have been associated, including congenital bowing and pseudarthrosis of the tibia, cysts of long bones, overgrowth of bone and of soft tissue, scoliosis, megalencephaly, and malformation of the greater wing of the sphenoid bone (with pulsating exophthalmos). Mild impairment of intellectual function is common, but severe mental defect rarely occurs. Convulsions occur in about 5% of patients. Life expectancy is near normal; the increased incidence of neural tumors and sarcomas is the principal risk.

The diagnosis of neurofibromatosis is based on the physical findings. Confirmation by biopsy of a subcutaneous nodule may be necessary if cutaneous manifestations are lacking. A careful family history and examination of immediate family members are essential in determining whether the disease occurs as a dominant trait or whether the propositus represents a new mutation. The family should be advised that any offspring of a patient with neurofibromatosis has a 50% chance of inheriting the disorder. Therapy is limited to excision of tumors which produce pain or impairment in function and of rapidly growing masses suspected of malignant transformation.

STURGE-WEBER DISEASE
(Encephalotrigeminal Angiomatosis)

Sturge-Weber disease occurs sporadically without known hereditary factors. The basic lesion is a congenital capillary hemangioma which involves skin of the face and cervical area, mucous membranes, meninges, and choroid, usually unilaterally. The skin angioma (*"nevus flammeus"* or *"port wine stain"*) is in the trigeminal distribution, most commonly in the ophthalmic division, but it may extend more widely over cervical segments. In the meninges the malformation often is confined to the pial vessels in the occipitoparietal areas. Sluggish flow of blood in malformed pial vessels leads to anoxic injury in underlying cerebral cortex. The clinical manifestations of cortical damage include convulsions, mental defect, and hemiparesis or hemianopsia on the side opposite that of the lesion. Subarachnoid hemorrhage rarely occurs. Calcifications in the damaged cortical layers may become visible roentgenographically even in infancy and nearly always by late childhood (Fig 21–14). They are often curvilinear and double contoured ("railroad track pattern") and are pathognomonic in a child with facial nevus. Angioma in the choroid may lead to buphthalmos in infancy or to glaucoma in childhood.

Management of the child with Sturge-Weber disease is determined by clinical manifestations: e.g., anticonvulsant drugs for seizures, physiotherapy for paretic limbs, and periodic eye examination for early detection

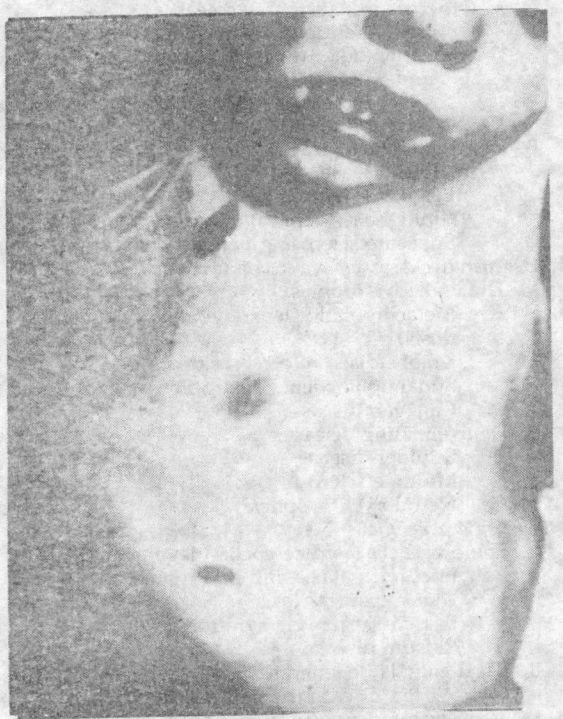

Figure 21–13 Café-au-lait spots in neurofibromatosis.

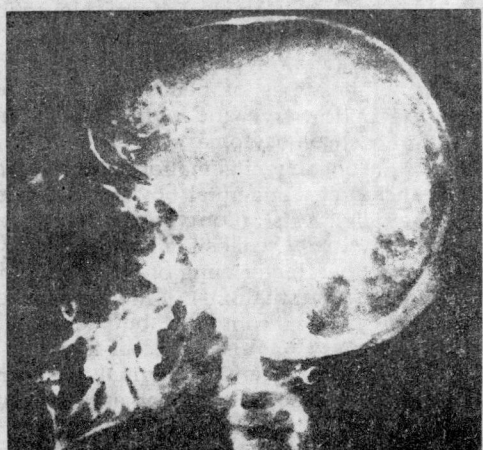

Figure 21–14 Extensive calcification of cerebral cortex in Sturge-Weber disease.

of glaucoma. Local resection of the cerebral cortical lesion may be indicated when severe convulsions are refractory to medication. A covering cream may be used on the face for cosmetic purposes.

VON HIPPEL–LINDAU DISEASE

This disorder is often included among the neurocutaneous disorders although the skin is not involved. Retinal angiomas are associated with hemangioblastoma of the cerebellum and less frequently with such other tumors as hemangioma of spinal cord, hypernephroma, and cystadenomas of visceral organs. Dominant inheritance has occurred in several families. Symptoms include visual loss and evidences of cerebellar and spinal cord dysfunction; these do not usually appear until adolescence or later.

Alexander GL, Norman RM: The Sturge-Weber Syndrome. Bristol, John Wright and Sons, 1960.
Cooper JR: Brain tumors in hereditary multiple system hamartomatosis (tuberous sclerosis). J Neurosurg 34:194, 1971.
Crowe FW, Schull WJ, Neel JV: Multiple Neurofibromatosis. Springfield, Ill., Charles C Thomas, 1956.
Fienman NL, Yakovac WC: Neurofibromatosis in childhood. J Pediatr 76:339, 1970.
Gold AG, Freeman JM: Depigmented nevi: The earliest sign of tuberous sclerosis. Pediatrics 35:1003, 1965.
Gomez MR (ed): Tuberous Sclerosis. New York, Raven Press, 1979.
Hurwitz S, Braverman IM: White spots in tuberous sclerosis. J Pediatr 77:587, 1970.
Peterman AF, et al: Encephalotrigeminal angiomatosis (Sturge-Weber disease). Clinical study of 35 cases. JAMA 167:2169, 1958.
Pitt MJ, Mosher JF, Ederken J: Abnormal periosteum and bone in neurofibromatosis. Radiology 103:143, 1972.

21.16 DEGENERATIVE BRAIN DISEASES

The outstanding characteristic of these illnesses is progressive loss of previously acquired intellectual, mo-

tor, and sensory functions. Most of them are genetically autosomal recessive; specific enzymatic defects have been demonstrated in some. Identification of carriers (heterozygotes) and intrauterine diagnosis are now possible by enzymatic assays in several of the disorders. Some cerebral degenerations, however, cannot be specifically categorized. Effective therapy is lacking for most of them.

Classification usually divides the disorders into those which principally affect cerebral gray matter and those which affect the white matter. Subdivisions are based, at least in part, on the functional systems involved (e.g., the basal ganglia and the spinocerebellar system). Dementia and seizures are the predominant early manifestations in the gray matter diseases, whereas deterioration in motor function, manifested by spasticity, hypotonia, or ataxia, is the early sign of degenerations involving the white matter. Eventually, the entire nervous system tends to become affected in both varieties, and, in general, the end-stage clinical picture of all the disorders is similar: the child becomes helpless, with loss of all intellectual and voluntary motor functions.

The following is a useful classification:
I. *Degenerations of cerebral gray matter*
  A. Neuronal storage diseases
    1. Ganglioside storage diseases
      Tay-Sachs disease
      Generalized gangliosidosis
    2. Storage diseases with accumulation of sphingolipids other than ganglioside
      Infantile Gaucher disease
      Niemann-Pick disease
      Farber disease (lipogranulomatosis)
    3. Other neuronal storage diseases
      Late infantile and juvenile cerebromacular degeneration (Bielschowsky, Spielmeyer-Vogt, and Batten)
      Glycogen storage disease of heart, muscle, and central nervous system (Pompe disease)
  B. Degenerations of gray matter without neuronal storage
    Alper disease
    Leigh disease
    Kinky-hair (Menkes) disease
    Subacute sclerosing panencephalitis (SSPE)
II. *Degenerative disorders of cerebral white matter*
  A. The leukodystrophies
    Metachromatic leukodystrophy (sulfatide lipidosis)
    Krabbe disease (cerebroside lipidosis)
    Sudanophilic leukodystrophies
    Canavan disease
  B. Demyelinating diseases
    Schilder disease
    Multiple sclerosis
    Neuromyelitis optica
III. *System degenerations*
  A. Spinocerebellar and cerebellar degenerations
    Friedreich ataxia and its variants
    Ataxia-telangiectasia
    Bassen-Kornzweig syndrome
    Refsum disease
  B. Basal ganglia degenerations
    Wilson disease (hepatolenticular degeneration)
    Dystonia musculorum deformans
    Huntington chorea

Table 21–6 SPHINGOLIPIDS WHICH ARE THE MAJOR STORAGE MATERIALS IN THE LIPID STORAGE DISEASES

DISEASE	STORAGE COMPOUND
Niemann-Pick disease	Ceramide-p-choline (sphingomyelin)
Infantile Gaucher disease	Ceramide-glucose (glucocerebroside)
Generalized gangliosidosis Juvenile GM, gangliosidosis	Ceramide-glucose-galactose-acetylgalactosamine-galactose (GM₁)* | Sialic acid
Tay-Sachs disease Sandhoff disease	Ceramide-glucose-galactose-acetylgalactosamine (GM₂) | Sialic acid

*GM, also is the major ganglioside found in normal human brain.

21.17 DEGENERATIONS OF CEREBRAL GRAY MATTER

Neuronal Storage Diseases

These diseases are characterized by accumulation of lipid substances in cerebral neurons. In most instances the stored material is a sphingolipid, in some, a ganglioside. The sphingolipids are normal components of all cell membranes. The simplest sphingolipids are made up of the base, sphingosine, and a fatty acid. The resulting compound is referred to as ceramide. In the more complex sphingolipids a variety of side chains are added to the ceramide molecule. Several compounds of ceramide are of particular importance in neuronal lipid storage disease (see Table 21–6). Gangliosides are complex sphingolipids, which are normally present in high concentration in neurons; their function is unknown. Neuronal lipid storage is due to deficiency of specific enzymes which normally degrade the sphingolipids. In general, the substrate of the defective enzyme is stored in the cells.

The terminology of Svennerholm is generally used to classify the gangliosides. In this system the letter G refers to ganglioside; M, D, or T refers to the number of sialic acid groups (mono-, di-, or trisialic acid), and the subscript (1, 2, or 3) refers to the number of hexosides in the molecule. Tetrahexosides are assigned the number 1, trihexosides, the number 2, dihexosides, the number 3.

Ganglioside Storage Diseases

See also Sec 8.29 and 8.30.

At least 5 illnesses in this category are recognized; they can be differentiated on the basis of clinical findings, age of onset, and specific enzyme assays. Each of them is transmitted on an autosomal recessive basis. Their salient features are summarized in Table 21–7. The enzymatic defect in each disorder affects all body cells, but functional derangement appears to be limited to the central nervous system in all except generalized gangliosidosis, in which visceral and osseous lesions are associated with cerebral degeneration. In each disorder specific diagnosis is possible by assay of the affected enzyme in white blood cells. Heterozygous carriers of the trait can be identified on the basis of partial deficiency of the enzyme. Intrauterine diagnosis can be established by enzyme assay of cultured amniotic fluid cells.

Tay-Sachs Disease. Infantile cerebromacular degeneration is by far the most common of the gangliosidoses. It is most frequently found in children of Eastern European Jewish (Ashkenazi) ancestry; the incidence of the carrier state among Ashkenazi Jews is estimated to be 2.7%, about 10 times higher than in other population groups. The clinical findings are quite characteristic. At 2–6 mo of age a previously well infant becomes apathetic and loses interest in his or her surroundings. There is progressive loss of acquired motor functions and of visual ability. An exaggerated startle response to noise (hyperacusis) is an early sign. Progressive

Table 21–7 GANGLIOSIDE STORAGE DISEASES

DISEASE	ENZYME DEFECT	AGE AT ONSET	CHARACTERISTIC PHYSICAL FEATURES
Tay-Sachs disease (GM₂ gangliosidosis, type 1)	Absence of hexosaminidase A	3–6 mo	Hyperacusis, dementia, seizures, cherry-red spot of macula, blindness, macrocephaly
Sandhoff disease (GM₂ gangliosidosis, type 2)	Absence of hexosaminidase A and B	3–6 mo	Same as Tay-Sachs disease
Juvenile GM₂ gangliosidosis (GM₂ gangliosidosis, type 3)	Partial deficiency of hexosaminidase A	2–6 yr	Dementia, ataxia, spasticity, seizures
Generalized gangliosidosis (GM₁ gangliosidosis, type 1)	Absence of β-galactosidase A, B and C	In utero or early infancy	Hepatosplenomegaly, Hurler-like features and bone changes, failure of intellectual and motor development
Juvenile GM₁ gangliosidosis (GM₁ gangliosidosis, type 2)	Absence of β-galactosidase B and C	6 mo–3 yr	Spasticity, ataxia, dementia

spasticity with hyperreflexia and decerebrate posturing, feeding difficulties, and emaciation occur in the late stages of the illness, and the head may become abnormally large. Grand mal, tonic, or myoclonic seizures are seen. The most characteristic feature is the cherry-red spot of the macula, a bright red area in the region of the fovea surrounded by a grayish-white rim (Fig 21–15). The latter is due to lipid accumulation in the surrounding retinal ganglion cells. The cherry-red spot may also occur in Niemann-Pick and Sandhoff diseases (Table 21–7).

Routine laboratory examinations are not helpful in the diagnosis. The cerebrospinal fluid protein is usually normal, but there may be an increase in cerebrospinal fluid enzymes, including lactic dehydrogenase and glutamic oxaloacetic transaminase. The basic defect is virtual absence of the enzyme hexosaminidase A from all body tissues. Measurement of this enzyme in serum, amniotic fluid cells, or white cells has become the definitive diagnostic measure. Deficiency of hexosaminidase A results in marked accumulation of GM_2 ganglioside in all neurons, including those in the peripheral autonomic nervous system. GM_2 gangliosides, which normally make up only 1–3% of total brain gangliosides, account for more than 90% in patients with Tay-Sachs disease. The accumulation of ganglioside is visible by light microscopy as marked ballooning of neurons. By electron microscopy the ganglioside is seen as discrete intracellular concretions with a characteristic lamellar structure. Neuronal degeneration and gliosis are marked in infants who survive for several years.

There is no therapy for Tay-Sachs disease. Death usually occurs prior to the age of 4 yr. Heterozygous carriers in populations known to be at risk can be identified by serum assay of hexosaminidase A. Diagnostic amniocentesis should be offered when both parents are known to be heterozygotes. It should be carried out at about 18 wk gestation, in time for safe therapeutic abortion of an affected fetus, if desired.

Other Ganglioside Storage Diseases. See Table 21–7.

Late Infantile and Juvenile Cerebromacular Degenerations

See also Sec 8.41.

These disorders are the 2nd most common group of degenerative disorders of the cerebral gray matter. Onset occurs from 1–3 yr of age in the late infantile form (*Bielschowsky syndrome*) and usually from 5–7 yr in the more common juvenile variety (*Spielmeyer-Vogt* or *Batten* disease). As yet, it is unknown whether the 2 represent variants of the same illness or different genetic defects. Transmission of both occurs on an autosomal recessive basis.

Pathologically, neurons are distended with material that has the staining characteristics of lipofuscin. Electron microscopy shows curvilinear and lattice-like neuronal cytoplasmic inclusions. Neuronal involvement includes cells in the anterior horn of the spinal cord and in the peripheral autonomic ganglia. Lipofuscin-like material also accumulates in other organs, especially in the thyroid gland and in sweat glands. The storage material in brain is a retinoyl complex.

The illness often starts with progressive loss of vision. Ophthalmologic changes vary among affected families; they may consist of retinitis pigmentosa, pigmentary degeneration of the macular region, or simple optic atrophy. The electroencephalogram may be abnormal, with diffuse spike-wave activity, long before the onset of neurologic deterioration. Grand mal or myoclonic seizures and symptoms of dementia may appear 1–3 yr after onset of visual loss. The child becomes hyperactive and irritable. Speech deteriorates, often with a peculiar stammering, slurring, and repetition of words. Cerebellar ataxia, tremor, rigidity, spastic paralysis, and complete dementia appear late. Progression is slow; the later the onset, the slower the course. Some patients survive into adolescence or early adult years.

The diagnosis should be suspected in a child with progressive visual loss, seizures, and mental deterioration. Ganglioside storage disease may present identical clinical findings but can be ruled out by assay of

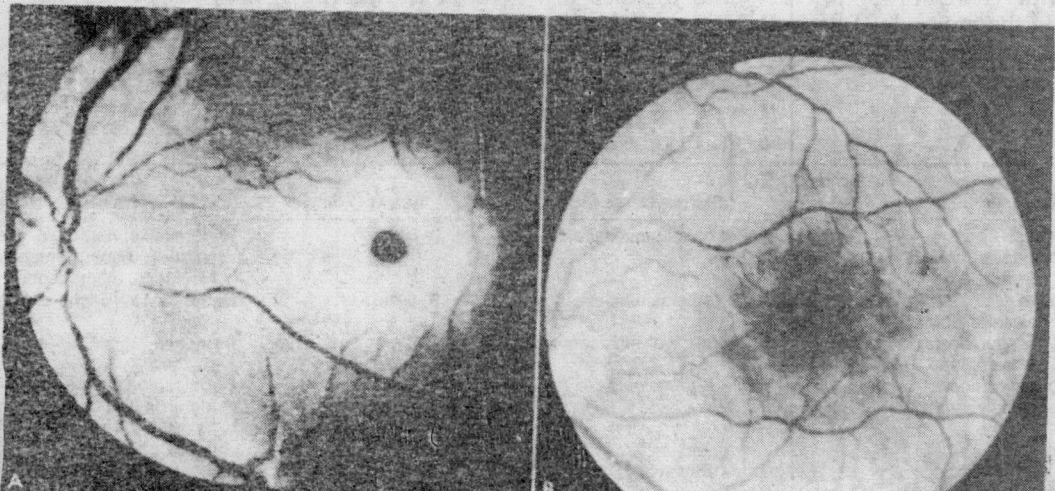

Figure 21–15 *A*, cherry-red spot of the macula in Tay-Sachs disease. *B*, Normal macula for comparison.

hexosaminidases and beta-galactosidases in white cells. Electron microscopic examination of muscle or of sweat glands may show electron-dense bodies similar to those found in neurons.

Aronson SM, Volk BW (eds): Cerebral sphingolipidoses. A Symposium on Tay-Sachs Disease and Allied Disorders. New York, Academic Press, 1962.

Carpenter S, Karpati G, Andermann F: Specific involvement of muscle, nerve and skin in late infantile and juvenile amaurotic idiocy. Neurology 22:170, 1972.

Fawcett JS, et al: On the natural history of late infantile cerebromacular degeneration. Neurology 16:1130, 1966.

Jervis GA: Juvenile amaurotic idiocy. J Dis Child 97:663, 1959.

Landing BH, Silverman FN, et al: Familial neurovisceral lipidosis. Am J Dis Child 108:503, 1964.

Milunsky A, Littlefield JW, et al: Prenatal genetic diagnosis. N Engl J Med 283:1370, 1441, 1498, 1970.

O'Brien JS, et al: Generalized gangliosidosis. Am J Dis Child 109:338, 1965.

O'Brien JS, Okada S, et al: Tay-Sachs disease. Detection of heterozygotes and homozygotes by serum hexosaminidase assay. N Engl J Med 283:15, 1970.

Wolfe LS, et al: Identification of retinoyl complexes as the autofluorescent compound of the neuronal storage material in Batten's disease. Science 195:1360, 1977.

Zeman W, Dyken P: Neuronal ceroid-lipo-fuscinosis (Batten's disease): Relationship to amaurotic family idiocy. Pediatrics 44:570, 1969.

Degeneration of Gray Matter Without Neuronal Storage

Poliodystrophy (Alpers Disease). A heterogeneous group of degenerations of cerebral cortex with onset in infancy or early childhood is referred to as poliodystrophy or as Alper disease. Pathologic changes in brain are nonspecific in all of these cases; widespread neuronal loss and gliosis occur in cerebral cortex and in cerebellum. The most prominent symptoms are recurrent seizures and dementia. Involvement of siblings may suggest recessive inheritance, but several ill-defined metabolic errors may be included in this category. Some cases have lactic acidosis, probably secondary to deficiency of an enzyme in the pyruvate dehydrogenase complex. Others have progressive hepatic cirrhosis. Treatment with corticosteroids or with a ketogenic diet may produce transient clinical improvement in patients with poliodystrophy who have lactic acidosis.

Leigh Disease. *Subacute necrotizing encephalomyelopathy* is a metabolic brain disease which leads to widespread cerebral damage, especially in the brain stem. It is autosomal recessive.

Pathologic changes include degeneration of neural structures and capillary proliferation in a characteristic distribution surrounding the 3rd ventricle, the aqueduct of Sylvius, and the 4th ventricle. The lesions are strikingly similar to those of thiamine deficiency (Wernicke) encephalopathy. Leigh disease may be related to an inborn error in thiamine metabolism. (See Sec 8.20.)

Onset usually occurs in infancy; it may be subacute, with vomiting, weight loss, weakness, seizures, and stupor, or the course may be more chronic, with developmental arrest, loss of vision, and dementia. Nystagmus and extraocular palsies are common. Both spastic weakness due to upper motor neuron degeneration and flaccidity due to spinal cord and peripheral nerve involvement are seen. Irregular respirations, periodic hyperventilation, and sudden apnea are late manifestations. The course is often one of exacerbations and remissions, a feature which may aid in differentiation from other cerebral degenerations; time of survival may be a few wk or many yr. Therapy with massive doses of thiamine has given inconclusive results.

Kinky Hair Disease. *Menkes syndrome* is a sex-linked recessive abnormality in copper metabolism in which severe cerebral degeneration and arterial changes lead to death in infancy.

Pathologic changes include widespread cerebral degeneration with loss of cerebral cortical neurons; gliosis and cysts replace the most severely damaged areas. Extensive vascular changes include fragmentation of the elastica and intimal thickening. The basic defect appears to consist of excessive binding of copper to certain tissues, including fibroblasts and intestinal mucosa. The defect in the intestinal mucosa may account for the observed decrease in absorption and serum level of copper, which accounts for diminished synthesis of ceruloplasmin. (See Sec 8.28.)

Inadequate gain in weight and hypothermia are manifest from birth, with unusual susceptibility to sepsis. The scalp hair is initially normal but rapidly becomes sparse and brittle. Microscopically the shaft has a twisted appearance (pili torti). Seborrheic dermatitis is common. Developmental retardation becomes evident within the 1st few mo of life, and myoclonic seizures may occur. Death usually occurs within the 1st yr.

Laboratory studies are necessary for definitive diagnosis. Roentgenograms of long bones show changes resembling those of scurvy. Serum copper and ceruloplasmin levels are low. Parenteral copper therapy does not seem to prevent cerebral damage, even when begun in early infancy.

Subacute Sclerosing Panencephalitis (SSPE). (See also Sec 10.67.) This disease, though of viral etiology, is included among the cerebral degenerative disorders because of its chronic course and absence of clinical evidences of infection. The incidence varies with geographic area from 1–4/million; a high incidence is reported in the southeastern United States.

Pathologic changes in brain include perivascular lymphocytic infiltrates, intranuclear viral inclusions in neurons and glial cells, widespread loss of cortical neurons, and gliosis. Measles virus has been grown from cerebral tissue. It is thought that the disease is caused by entry of measles virus into the brain during acute measles infection or (10 times less frequently) following immunization with live measles vaccine, with subsequent chronic intracellular propagation. Cerebral degeneration becomes apparent at an average of 7 yr after primary infection.

Clinical manifestations appear from 2–21 yr of age, with peak incidence from 8–14 yr. The 1st signs are those of progressive decline in higher cerebral functions (especially school failure), subtle personality changes, and emotional lability. Generalized myoclonic jerks, at regular intervals of several sec, are characteristic. Barely noticeable at first, they eventually become so severe that ambulation is hampered. Grand mal seizures also may occur. In the late stages the child becomes demented and is bedridden with generalized rigidity.

Changes in the cerebrospinal fluid include elevated gamma globulin levels, a 1st-zone colloidal gold curve, and a measurable antibody titer against measles virus. CSF protein concentration and cell count are often normal. The titer of measles antibody in serum is usually above 1:128 by the complement-fixation method. The electroencephalographic pattern is fairly characteristic, consisting of regularly repeated bursts of generalized high-voltage slow wave complexes.

The disease is usually fatal within 2 yr of onset, but rare instances of prolonged spontaneous remission have been reported.

Blackwood W, Buxton PH, Cummings JN et al: Diffuse cerebral degeneration of infancy (Alper's disease). Arch Dis Child 38:193, 1963.
Danks DM, et al: Menkes' kinky hair syndrome. An inherited defect in copper absorption with widespread effects. Pediatrics 50:188, 1972.
Detels R, et al: Further epidemiologic studies of subacute sclerosing panencephalitis. Lancet 2:11, 1973.
Falk RE, et al: Ketonic diet in the management of pyruvate dehydrogenase deficiency. Pediatrics 58:713, 1976.
Goka TJ, et al: Menkes' disease: A biochemical abnormality in cultured human fibroblasts. Proc Natl Acad Sci USA 73:604, 1976.
Katz M, et al: Subacute sclerosing panencephalitis: Isolation of a virus encephalitogenic for ferrets. J Infect Dis 121:188, 1970.
Pincus JH: Subacute necrotizing encephalomyelopathy (Leigh's disease): A consideration of clinical features and etiology. Dev Med Child Neurol 14:87, 1972.
Sever JL, Zeman W (eds): Measles virus and subacute sclerosing panencephalitis. Neurology 18 (pt 2):1, 1968.
Shapira Y, et al: Familial poliodystrophy, mitochondrial myopathy and lactate acidemia. Neurology 25:614, 1975.

21.18   DEGENERATIVE DISORDERS OF CEREBRAL WHITE MATTER

In most of these diseases there is faulty formation or excessive breakdown of myelin, a major component of cerebral white matter, which consists of proteolipid membranes wrapped around axons in concentric layers. Myelination markedly increases the speed and efficiency of conduction of nerve impulses; it is essential for normal function of the mammalian nervous system. In the human, myelination of axons in subcortical white matter is largely postnatal with maximal formation occurring within the 1st yr of life. Accordingly, diseases in which there is faulty formation of central myelin tend to have their onset during infancy; they present clinically as arrest of motor development or as progressive disturbances of gait, weakness, spasticity, and ataxia.

Two groups of degenerative diseases involve cerebral white matter. In one, the *leukodystrophies*, enzymatic defects in myelin lipid metabolism lead to excessive tissue deposition of a normal component of myelin lipids or of breakdown products of myelin. The clinical disorders include *metachromatic leukodystrophy* and *Krabbe disease*. In the 2nd group, the *demyelinating diseases*, degeneration of previously normal myelin is caused by an unknown exogenous factor. *Multiple sclerosis*, *neuromyelitis optica*, and *Schilder disease* belong in this group.

The Leukodystrophies

See also Sec 8.35 and 8.36.

Metachromatic Leukodystrophy.   *Sulfatide lipidosis* is the most common leukodystrophy in childhood. It is autosomal recessive.

The basic defect in metachromatic leukodystrophy is deficiency of aryl sulfatase A in brain and other tissues. This enzyme normally splits the sulfate group from ceramide-galactose-sulfate or sulfatide, a normal component of myelin lipids. Sulfatide accumulates in white matter and can be identified on light microscopy by metachromatic (reddish-brown) staining with toluidine blue. Similar deposits are found in peripheral nerves. There is diffuse demyelination of white matter tracts throughout the nervous system, most extensive in tracts which myelinate late.

Clinical manifestations usually appear at about 1 yr of age, but onset may occur later in childhood. Initially there is a disturbance in gait, and the child may be unable to learn to run or to walk up stairs. Spasticity of limbs, hyperreflexia, and extensor plantar responses are noted early. Though most of the tendon reflexes are brisk, the ankle jerks may be diminished or absent because of involvement of peripheral nerves. Flaccid weakness and atrophy of distal muscles, especially in the lower extremities, occur when peripheral nerve involvement is severe. Eventually the child becomes demented and bedridden. Death usually occurs before the age of 10 yr.

Definitive diagnosis depends on finding absent or significantly reduced activity of aryl sulfatase A in 1 or more body tissues. Renal tubular cells from urinary sediment, white blood cells, or cultured fibroblasts are suitable for this analysis. A screening test, rapid but unreliable, involves the demonstration of metachromatic material in urinary sediment stained with toluidine blue. Dysfunction of the gallbladder, resulting from storage of sulfatide in its wall, leads to failure of filling on oral cholecystography. Conduction velocity in peripheral motor and sensory nerves is decreased. The concentration of protein in CSF is usually increased, the elevation aiding the differentiation of leukodystrophy from the much larger group of nonprogressive motor deficits classified as cerebral palsy. Differentiation is of considerable importance for genetic counseling and for prognosis. Intrauterine diagnosis of metachromatic leukodystrophy is possible by measurement of aryl sulfatase A in cultured cells from the amniotic fluid; the test should be offered to prospective parents who are both known to be carriers of the abnormal gene.

Krabbe Disease.   *Cerebroside lipidosis*, or *globoid leukodystrophy*, is autosomal recessive. The pathologic changes in brain consist of diffuse lack of myelin in white matter and an accumulation of peculiar multinucleated giant cells (globoid cells). The white matter contains an increased ratio of cerebroside (ceramide galactose) to sulfatide (ceramide-galactose-sulfate) but usually no absolute increase in the quantity of cerebroside. These changes are thought to be secondary to a deficiency of galactocerebrosidase activity.

The illness becomes evident in early infancy with progressive rigidity, hyperreflexia, and swallowing difficulties and with failure of normal motor and intellectual development. Peripheral nerve involvement may lead to hypotonia; death usually occurs within 2 yr. The diagnosis is established by assay of galactocerebrosidase in peripheral white blood cells. Spinal fluid protein is elevated, and the velocity of peripheral nerve conduction is slowed. Intrauterine diagnosis is possible by enzymatic assay of cultured amniotic fluid cells.

Several other forms of leukodystrophy are as yet incompletely defined and usually are diagnosable only by postmortem examination of the brain:

Canavan Disease (Spongy Degeneration of the Cerebral White Matter). This condition is autosomal recessive. The characteristic pathologic change is diffuse vacuolization in the deep cortical layers and in subcortical white matter, apparently secondary to excessive accumulation of water in glial cells and in myelin. Clinical manifestations appear in early infancy with poor head control, blindness, optic atrophy, rigidity, hyperreflexia, and progressive macrocephaly. The last may suggest hydrocephalus or subdural effusion. The ventricular system, however, is normal in size or only mildly dilated. Death occurs within 5 yr.

The Sudanophilic Leukodystrophies. These derive their name from the accumulation in white matter of breakdown products of myelin, especially neutral fats, which stain positively with Sudan stains.

Adrenoleukodystrophy, the most common disorder in this group, is X-linked recessive. Onset occurs toward the end of the 1st decade, with progressive spasticity and dementia and later the increased pigmentation of skin and other evidence of Addison disease. The metabolic defect is as yet unknown. Hexacosanoate (C26 fatty acid) is increased in brain, adrenal glands, muscle, cultured fibroblasts, and plasma. Measurement of this fatty acid in plasma is used for diagnosis and for carrier identification. In some cases spinal cord and peripheral nerves are predominantly involved (adrenomyeloneuropathy).

Pelizaeus-Merzbacher disease is also X-linked recessive. The onset occurs in infancy, with nystagmus and head nodding, followed by progressive ataxia, spasticity, and choreoathetosis. Progression is slow, with survival into adulthood. Clinical differentiation from cerebral palsy may be difficult.

Austin J: Studies in globoid (Krabbe) leukodystrophy. Arch Neurol 9:207, 1963.

Austin J, et al: Metachromatic leukodystrophy. Arch Neurol 18:225, 1968.

Banker BQ, Robertson JT, Victor M: Spongy degeneration of the central nervous system in infancy. Neurology 14:981, 1964.

Griffin JW, Goren E, Schaumberg H, et al: Adrenomyeloneuropathy: A probable variant of adrenoleukodystrophy. Neurology 27:1107, 1977.

Leroy JG, et al: Infantile metachromatic leukodystrophy. Confirmation of a prenatal diagnosis. N Engl J Med 288:1365, 1973.

Moser HW, et al: Adrenoleukodystrophy: Increased plasma content of saturated very long chain fatty acids. Neurology 31:1241, 1981.

Norman RM, et al: Pelizaeus-Merzbacher disease: A form of sudanophilic leucodystrophy. J Neurol Neurosurg Psychiat 29:521, 1966.

Percy AK, Brady RO: Metachromatic leukodystrophy: Diagnosis with sample of venous blood. Science 161:594, 1968.

Schaumberg HH, et al: Adrenoleukodystrophy. A clinical and pathological study of 17 cases. Arch Neurol 33:577, 1975.

Suzuki Y, Suzuki K: Krabbe's globoid cell leukodystrophy: Deficiency of galacto-cerebrosidase in serum, leukocytes, and fibroblasts. Science 171:73, 1971.

The Demyelinating Diseases

These illnesses, which include *Schilder disease, multiple sclerosis,* and *neuromyelitis optica,* occur sporadically without known genetic factors. It is not clear whether they are separate entities or different manifestations of the same pathologic process. Transitional forms have been described. In all 3 there is breakdown of myelin in the central nervous system without involvement of the myelin of the peripheral nerves. A perivascular lymphocytic inflammatory reaction is present in the areas of demyelination, suggesting the possibility of an autoimmune disorder or of a viral infection; definite evidence for either possibility is lacking.

Schilder Disease. *Diffuse sclerosis* may occur at any age but is most common in late childhood. Conclusive diagnosis is usually possible only at autopsy; there is diffuse demyelination of central white matter with relative sparing of subcortical U fibers. Lipid breakdown products of myelin accumulate in the areas of demyelination. The pathologic picture resembles that of the sudanophilic leukodystrophies. Neurologic findings are extremely varied. Cortical blindness, optic neuritis, spastic hemiplegia, paraparesis, cortical deafness, aphasia, and seizures have been described in the early phase. Late manifestations include dementia and coma. Occasionally, there are signs of increased intracranial pressure, with papilledema secondary to cerebral swelling. The course may be acute, death occurring within a few wk of onset, or the illness may be protracted over months or years. Rarely, there is partial remission or a relapsing course. The cerebrospinal fluid may be normal or show an increase in protein and lymphocytes. The differential diagnosis includes brain tumor, viral encephalitis, subacute sclerosing panencephalitis (SSPE), and the leukodystrophies.

Multiple Sclerosis. *Disseminated sclerosis* is a chronic cerebral disorder characterized by remissions and exacerbations and by multifocal lesions. The disease is uncommon in childhood; in about 1% of cases the onset occurs before 15 yr of age. The changes in the brain consist of scattered foci of demyelination in cerebral white matter, often in a perivenous distribution with associated perivascular lymphocytic infiltrates. Lesions may occur also in brain stem and spinal cord.

In order of frequency, the most common presenting signs in childhood or adolescence are cerebellar ataxia, spastic weakness (often asymmetric), optic neuritis, and diplopia. The optic neuritis tends to be retrobulbar. Loss of vision occurs without funduscopic changes at first. Temporal pallor of the optic discs indicative of optic atrophy develops over weeks or months. The onset may be acute or subacute over several wk. Recovery from acute episodes may initially be complete or nearly so, but after repeated attacks the patient is left with fixed neurologic deficits, often including spastic paralysis and ataxia. Intellectual functions are preserved until late. The clinical diagnosis is based on (1) the finding of multiple neurologic deficits which cannot be due to a single anatomic lesion and (2) the relapsing course. A definite clinical diagnosis cannot be established at the time of the 1st attack. Differentiation from hysteria may be difficult initially, especially when visual disturbance occurs without objective eye findings. The spinal fluid may be normal or show an increase in gamma globulin which is responsible for a positive 1st-zone colloidal gold curve. A pleocytosis up to 100 lymphocytes/mm³ may occur during acute exacerbations.

Treatment of acute exacerbations of multiple sclerosis with short courses of ACTH has a slight but statistically significant beneficial effect. ACTH gel is given intramuscularly, 40–80 units/24 hr for 2 wk; the dose is then tapered and discontinued over the subsequent week. Physiotherapy can help patients with spastic weakness. Careful bladder care and therapy of urinary tract infections are essential when spinal cord involvement results in bladder dysfunction. The prognosis is guarded but not hopeless; exacerbations may be infrequent with symptom-free intervals of many yr.

Neuromyelitis Optica. *Devic disease* probably is a variant of multiple sclerosis in which demyelination occurs in the optic nerves and in the spinal cord. The only reason for separation from multiple sclerosis is that there may be a single attack without later exacerbations. A relapsing course with eventual involvement of other white matter tracts is also possible. The illness starts acutely, usually with eye pain followed by loss of vision, which may affect 1 or both eyes. Funduscopic examination may reveal swelling and hyperemia of the optic disc, distended retinal veins, and peripapillary hemorrhages; in some instances the fundi initially appear normal. The onset of spinal cord involvement is also acute, at times with fever, back pain, and nuchal rigidity. It usually follows the visual loss by several days but may precede it. A level of sensory involvement on the trunk can be demonstrated, usually in the thoracic area. Initially the legs are weak, flaccid, and areflexic, and the plantar responses are absent or flexor. The bladder is distended. After a few days the involved extremities become spastic, the tendon reflexes hyperactive, with clonus at the ankles and a positive Babinski sign.

The spinal fluid may be normal or show pleocytosis; polymorphonuclear cells may be present initially. Myelography may be necessary to rule out acute compression of the cord, especially by spinal epidural abscess. This study is usually normal in neuromyelitis optica, but partial obstruction at the level of the cord lesion may reflect edema of the spinal cord. Dexamethasone in high doses for a period 5–7 days during the acute illness may help prevent pressure necrosis of the edematous segment of the cord. The prognosis for return of vision is good, but some degree of persistent paraparesis and bladder dysfunction can be expected.

Gall JC Jr, et al: Multiple sclerosis in children: Clinical study of 40 cases with onset in childhood. Pediatrics 21:703, 1958.

Kennedy C, Carter S: Relationships of optic neuritis to multiple sclerosis in children. Pediatrics 28:377, 1961.

Low NL, Carter S: Multiple sclerosis in children. Pediatrics 18:24, 1956.

Rose AS, et al: Cooperative study in the evaluation of therapy in multiple sclerosis: ACTH vs. placebo—final report. Neurology 20, May, 1970 (Suppl).

Salguero LF, Itsabashi JH, Gutierrez NB: Childhood multiple sclerosis with psychotic manifestations. J Neurol Neurosurg Psychiat 32:572, 1969.

Suzuki K, Grover WD: Ultrastructural and biochemical studies of Schilder's disease. J Neuropathol Exp Neurol 29:392, 1970.

Walsh FB: Neuromyelitis optica. An anatomical-pathological study of one case. Clinical studies of three additional cases. Bull Johns Hopkins Hosp 56:183, 1935.

21.19   DEGENERATIVE DISEASES OF THE CEREBELLUM AND BASAL GANGLIA

In this category are included a number of illnesses in which spinocerebellar pathways or basal ganglia are selectively involved in degenerative processes. Most are genetically determined; in a few the metabolic error has been defined, but the etiology of the majority is unknown. See also Sec 8.28.

The Spinocerebellar Degenerations

Friedreich Ataxia. This term is applied to a heterogeneous group of disorders which have in common onset in late childhood or adolescence of progressive cerebellar and spinal cord dysfunction. As new knowledge has accumulated, several disorders such as ataxia-telangiectasia and the Bassen-Kornzweig syndrome have been clearly separated from Friedreich ataxia. It is likely that there will be further subdivision as underlying metabolic disturbances are defined. In most families so-called Friedreich ataxia displays autosomal recessive transmission. A few families with similar abnormalities, but usually somewhat later in onset, have dominant inheritance.

Pathologic changes include degeneration of spinocerebellar, posterior column, and corticospinal tracts. In addition, necrosis and degeneration of cardiac muscle fibers are often present.

The clinical history is that of a progressive gait disturbance, followed by incoordination of the upper limbs. Initially, associated skeletal deformities, including a highly arched foot (pes cavus) (Fig 21–16), hammer toes, and scoliosis, may attract more attention than the neurologic disabilities. Occasionally, the child presents in cardiac failure, with cardiomegaly and arrhythmias. Clinical signs of cerebellar disorder include gait ataxia,

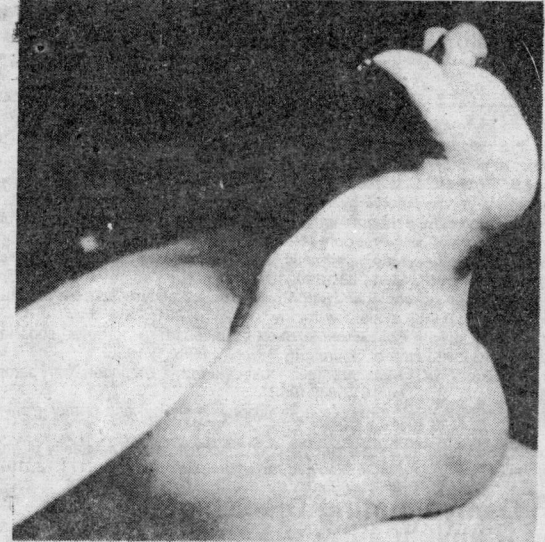

Figure 21–16 Pes cavus in a 12 yr old child with Friedreich ataxia.

dysarthria, intention tremor, and, less commonly, nystagmus. In addition, affected patients usually have evidence of corticospinal tract dysfunction and peripheral neuropathy. The former leads to a positive Babinski sign, the latter to loss of tendon reflexes and to distal weakness and muscle atrophy. The combination of ataxia, Babinski sign, and absent ankle jerks is almost pathognomonic. Sensory loss occurs, especially in the feet, with position and vibration senses most severely affected.

Several related syndromes cannot be clearly separated from Friedreich ataxia. Hyperreflexia and spasticity, rather than areflexia and muscle atrophy, are seen in some families. Some patients have onset of areflexic ataxia and pes cavus in infancy, with very slow progression consistent with a normal life span. This condition (known as the *Roussy-Lévy syndrome*) is dominantly inherited.

Diagnosis is almost totally dependent on the clinical findings. Laboratory examinations are negative, except for electrocardiographic changes suggestive of myocarditis and in some instances slowing of nerve conduction velocity due to peripheral neuropathy. Mild elevation in blood lactate and pyruvate, apparently secondary to decreased oxidation of pyruvate, has been reported. There is no effective treatment. Extensive orthopedic procedures, especially those requiring prolonged confinement to bed, should be avoided. The disease tends to be relentlessly progressive; the gait ataxia usually precludes independent walking by early adult years. Death in childhood is almost always due to myocardial failure.

Ataxia-Telangiectasia. In this complex disorder a specific immunologic dysfunction is associated with progressive cerebellar degeneration, telangiectasis of bulbar conjunctiva and skin, and an increased likelihood of malignancy. The disease is autosomal recessive. Affected children have immunologic deficits, including a decrease in delayed hypersensitivity which suggests early thymic dysfunction. It is not known how the immunologic disorder and the cerebellar degeneration are related. Pathologic changes in the nervous system tend to be limited to degeneration in the cerebellum and spinocerebellar tracts.

The *neurologic manifestations* usually begin in infancy. Affected children walk late, always with an ataxic gait. Late in childhood progressive dysarthria, nystagmus, intention tremor, and choreoathetosis appear. Tendon reflexes are diminished or absent. A peculiar abnormality of eye movements is characteristic, the child being unable to move the eyes on command, whereas involuntary movements are retained. The *skin changes*, usually evident by 5 yr of age, consist of telangiectases over the bulbar conjunctiva (Fig 21–17), along the nasolabial folds, over the external ears, and along flexor creases of the extremities. Clinical evidences of *immunologic deficiency* are variable: some children have severe recurrent sinus, ear, and pulmonary infections from early childhood; some never suffer from increased susceptibility to infection. Tonsillar tissue is diminished or absent; there are usually no palpable lymph nodes. The illness runs a slowly progressive course. The neurologic

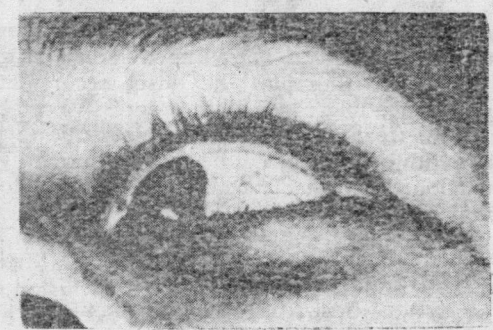

Figure 21–17 Ataxia-telangiectasia. Arterial telangiectasis on bulbar conjunctiva.

deficits often lead to scoliosis in late childhood; by early adolescence independent ambulation becomes impossible. Mild dementia is seen during the late stages of the illness. Death usually occurs in adolescence or in early adulthood as a result of pulmonary failure, infection, or malignancy. The incidence of several tumors is increased (especially lymphomas and brain tumors).

Laboratory findings include, in varying combinations, a decrease or absence of serum IgA and IgE, a decrease in the number of circulating small lymphocytes, and decrease or absence of delayed hypersensitivity reactions to intradermal injection of mumps or *Candida* antigens. The skin sensitization reaction to dinitrochlorobenzene is usually absent. These tests help differentiate the condition from Friedreich ataxia and from the ataxic form of cerebral palsy, which are easily confused with ataxia-telangiectasia during the early stages. Further, a positive Babinski sign is found in Friedreich ataxia but not in ataxia-telangiectasia. Friedreich ataxia tends to be of later onset and lacks the eye movement abnormalities seen in ataxia-telangiectasia.

Therapy is limited to the prompt treatment of the associated infections; replacement therapy with gamma globulin does not appear to be helpful. See also Sec 9.17.

Abetalipoproteinemia (Acanthocytosis, Bassen-Kornzweig Syndrome) (Sec 8.26). In this rare, recessively inherited disease malabsorption of fat and abetalipoproteinemia are associated with progressive cerebellar ataxia and pigmentary degeneration of the retina. Onset occurs in infancy with manifestations of intestinal malabsorption. Slowly progressive ataxia appears later in childhood; retinal degeneration becomes evident during adolescence. The clinical pattern may resemble that of Friedreich ataxia, including the Babinski sign, distal sensory loss, areflexia, scoliosis, and pes cavus.

Low density lipoproteins are absent or markedly reduced in serum; carotene, vitamin A, and cholesterol levels are also low, the last below 60 mg/dl. Lipid droplets (triglycerides) can be seen in intestinal mucosal cells obtained by peroral biopsy. The red blood cells have multiple spiny projections, a feature which accounts for the term acanthocytosis as well as for the low sedimentation rate. The basic defect is unknown. Therapy at present is limited to supplementary administration of the fat-soluble vitamins.

Refsum Syndrome. Refsum syndrome, another rare form of hereditary ataxia, has a known metabolic defect and an effective therapy. The onset occurs late in childhood or in adolescence, with progressive cerebellar ataxia, distal weakness and sensory loss due to polyneuritis, retinitis pigmentosa, deafness, and ichthyosis. The metabolic abnormality consists of inability to oxidize phytanic acid (3,7,11,15-tetramethylhexadecanoic acid), which accumulates in serum and in body tissues. The CSF protein is elevated. Therapy with a diet low in foods containing phytanic acid (i.e., exclusion of all green vegetables) has resulted in improvement in the neurologic deficit (Sec 8.40).

Myoclonic Encephalopathy of Childhood. *Kinsbourne syndrome* is a rare neurologic disorder of unknown etiology which has its onset from 1–3 yr of age. It is characterized by irregular, rapid jerking movements of limbs and trunk (myoclonus) and by similar chaotic, irregular jerking of the eyes (opsoclonus). In addition, gait ataxia, intention tremor, and nystagmus are present. Some cases have been associated with occult neuroblastoma, with removal of the tumor bringing striking improvement in the neurologic state. In children without tumor and in those with inoperable neoplasms, therapy with ACTH may induce remissions.

Blass JP: Low activities of the pyruvate and oxoglutarate dehydrogenase complexes in five patients with Friedreich's ataxia. N Engl J Med 295:62, 1976.

Boder E, Sedgwick RP: Ataxia-telangiectasia: Familial syndrome of progressive cerebellar ataxia, oculocutaneous telangiectasia, and frequent pulmonary infection. Pediatrics 21:526, 1958.

Boyer SH, Chisolm AW, McKusick VA: Cardiac aspects of Friedreich's ataxia. Circulation 25:493, 1962.

Critchley EMR: The genetic basis of hereditary ataxias. J Roy Coll Physicians Lond 4:88, 1969.

Greenfield JC: The Spino-Cerebellar Degenerations. Springfield, Ill., Charles C Thomas, 1954.

Herbert PN, Gotto AM, Fredrickson DS: Familial lipoprotein deficiency. In Stanbury JB, Wyngaarden JB, Fredrickson DS (eds): The Metabolic Basis of Inherited Disease. Ed 4. New York, McGraw-Hill, 1978.

Herndon JH Jr, Steinberg D, Uhlendorf BW: Refsum's disease: Defective oxidation of phytanic acid in tissue cultures derived from homozygotes and heterozygotes. N Engl J Med 281:1034, 1969.

Kinsbourne M: Myoclonic encephalopathy of infants. J Neurol Neurosurg Psychiat 25:271, 1962.

McFarlin DE, Strober W, Waldman TA: Ataxia-telangiectasia. Medicine 51:281, 1972.

Moe PG, Nellhaus G: Infantile polymyoclonus-opsoclonus syndrome and neural crest tumors. Neurology 20:756, 1970.

21.20   Degenerations of the Basal Ganglia

Wilson Disease. *Hepatolenticular degeneration* is a recessively inherited disorder of copper metabolism which leads to injury of liver and of basal ganglia. Changes in the brain include cavitation, gliosis, and neuronal degeneration in basal ganglia, most severe in the putamen. Similar changes may occur in the cerebral cortex, especially in the frontal lobes. The pathogenesis is not completely understood, but a defect in the synthesis of the copper-carrying protein, ceruloplasmin, explains many of the findings. Decreased protein-binding of serum copper appears to lead to increased leakage of copper into the tissues. Copper poisoning is a plausible explanation for the damage to the liver, basal ganglia, and renal tubules. (See also Sec 8.28 and 11.98.)

Clinical Manifestations. Clinical onset may occur as subacute or chronic hepatic failure in early childhood. Neurologic abnormalities generally do not appear until later in childhood or in adolescence, but they may precede clinical evidence of liver disease. The diagnosis of Wilson disease should be considered in any child past 8 yr of age who develops a motor disorder or unexplained mental changes. A peculiar flapping tremor of the shoulders and wrists (*wing-beating tremor*) is characteristic but not always present. Instead, there may be dysarthria, choreoathetoid movements, or rigidity. Dysfunction of the bulbar musculature tends to occur early and leads to an immobile grinning facial expression, drooling, and dysarthria. Rarely, there is spasticity, hemiparesis, or a positive Babinski sign. Wilson disease may present with mental changes in the absence of any other neurologic changes. Emotional lability, progressive school failure, and frank psychotic states may occur. The most important physical finding is the *Kayser-Fleischer ring* of the cornea, a greenish yellow rim near the limbus, often most evident superiorly and inferiorly. It is due to deposition of copper in Descemet membrane and is seen only in Wilson disease and in exogenous copper poisoning. It is usually visible; if not, it will show up on slit lamp examination.

Laboratory Data. The diagnosis is confirmed by measurement of serum ceruloplasmin (the copper-carrying protein) and urinary copper excretion. A serum ceruloplasmin level under 50% of normal suggests the diagnosis, but a normal value does not rule it out. Urine copper values are usually above 200 μg/24 hr, as they may also be in hepatic cirrhosis from other causes. Increase in excretion after administration of penicillamine is a helpful diagnostic test in doubtful cases. Serum copper concentrations tend to be lower than normal because of deficiency of the fraction bound to ceruloplasmin. Other laboratory findings include generalized aminoaciduria, low serum concentration of uric acid, and glycosuria (all due to renal tubular damage) and usually chemical evidence of liver disease.

Prognosis. The prognosis of untreated Wilson disease is poor, with a fatal outcome normally by 5 yr after onset. Early treatment, directed at removal of excessive copper stores from tissues, has greatly improved the outlook.

Therapy. Various chelating agents have been used; penicillamine, 1–2 gm/24 hr by mouth, is most effective. Allergic reactions, including fever, rash, and leukopenia, unfortunately are common. Penicillamine is a pyridoxine antimetabolite, and supplemental pyridoxine should be given during long-term therapy. A diet low in copper is a valuable adjunct to penicillamine therapy. Foods to be avoided include liver, shellfish, nuts, and chocolate.

Dystonia Musculorum Deformans (Torsion Dystonia). Dystonia occurs in a number of static and progressive brain diseases. The static disorders are perinatal brain injuries and postencephalitic syndromes; the progressive ones include Wilson disease, Huntington disease, and several other rare degenerative brain disorders.

The term *dystonia musculorum deformans* (torsion dystonia) is applied to a clinical entity characterized by dystonia as an isolated, genetically determined abnormality. Inheritance may be dominant or recessive, the latter especially among East European (Ashkenazi) Jews. The pathogenesis is obscure, and there are no consistent pathologic lesions in the brain. A biochemical rather than structural lesion of the basal ganglia appears to be responsible. Torsion dystonia has its onset during childhood or early adolescence in the recessive group, usually somewhat later in families with dominant inheritance. Progression tends to be rapid, with grotesque distortion of limbs (Fig 21–18) and incapacitation within a few yr of onset. Intelligence is preserved, and there is no evidence of disorder of the pyramidal motor system. Wilson disease should be ruled out by appropriate laboratory tests. There are no other helpful laboratory studies. A few patients with torsion dystonia

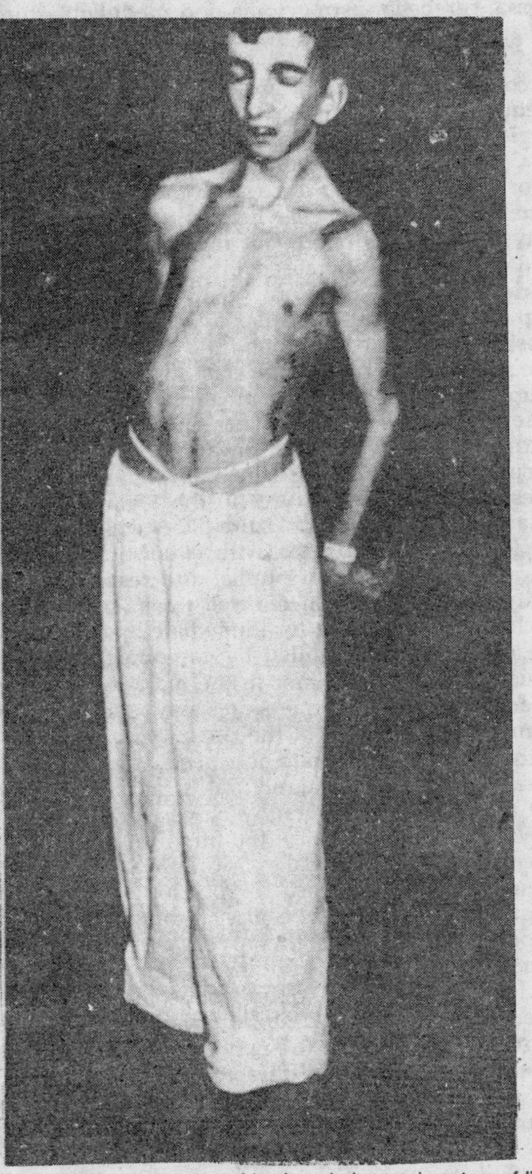

Figure 21–18 Hyperextension of back and abnormal posture of limbs in a patient with dystonia.

have responded to therapy with L-dopa; trihexyphenidyl and carbamazepine have occasionally been helpful. Stereotactic thalamotomy produces dramatic but often transient improvement.

Huntington Disease. Huntington disease is a dominantly inherited degeneration of the basal ganglia, especially of the caudate nucleus, manifested clinically by dementia, choreiform movements, and irregular, dancing gait. Onset usually occurs in middle age but may occur in childhood, with learning disorders, seizures, and rigidity or with chorea. In the latter instance it must be differentiated from Sydenham chorea, from Wilson disease, and from a dominantly inherited *benign chorea* which does not lead to dementia or to marked incapacitation. Usually, the diagnosis of Huntington chorea in childhood is possible only if a parent has the fully developed disease. L-Dopa may cause chorea in an asymptomatic person who is a carrier of the gene for Huntington chorea; this test is unreliable for early diagnosis. At present, there is no effective therapy. Genetic counseling is important.

Byers RK, Dodge JA: Huntington's chorea in children. Neurology 17:587, 1967.
Chun RWM, et al: Benign familial chorea with onset in childhood. JAMA 225:1603, 1973.
Denny-Brown D: Hepatolenticular degeneration (Wilson's disease). N Engl J Med 270:1149, 1964.
Eldridge R (ed): Torsion dystonias (dystonia musculorum deformans). Neurology 20(pt 2):1, 1970.
Goldstein NP, et al: Wilson's disease (hepato-lenticular degeneration). Treatment with penicillamine and changes in hepatic trapping of radioactive copper. Arch Neurol 24:391, 1971.
Klawans HL, Paulson GW, Ringel SP, et al: Use of L-dopa in the detection of presymptomatic Huntington's chorea. N Engl J Med 286:1332, 1972.
Markham CH, Knox JW: Observations on Huntington's chorea in childhood. J Pediatr 67:46, 1965.
Oliver J, Dewhurst K: Childhood and adolescent forms of Huntington's chorea. J Neurol Neurosurg Psychiat 32:455, 1969.
O'Reilly S: Problems in Wilson's disease. Neurology 17:137, 1967.
Pincus JH, and Chutorian A: Familial benign chorea with intention tremor: A clinical entity. J Pediatr 70:724, 1967.
Sternlieb I, Scheinberg IH: Prevention of Wilson's disease in asymptomatic patients. N Engl J Med 278:352, 1968.
Tu J, et al: DL-Penicillamine as a cause of optic axial neuritis. JAMA 185:83, 1963.
Walshe JM: The physiology of copper in man and its relation to Wilson's disease. Brain 90:149, 1967.

21.21 NEOPLASMS OF THE BRAIN

General Considerations. After leukemias, brain tumors are the most common type of neoplasms in children. Incidence is highest during the 2nd half of the 1st decade, but they may occur at any age, including early infancy. The incidences of the various cerebral neoplasms and their locations differ greatly from those observed in adults. Tumors of the cerebellum are most common and account for about 40% of the total. Tumors in other posterior fossa structures, including the brain stem and the 4th ventricle, make up about 15%. Suprasellar lesions, which include craniopharyngiomas, optic pathway gliomas, and gliomas of the hypothalamus, are also relatively common and account for another 15%. Tumors of the cerebral hemispheres, the ventricles, and the meninges account for the remainder. In about 80% of neoplasms in children the basic cell is glial. The remainder are craniopharyngiomas, teratomas, hemangiomas, sarcomas, and meningiomas. Metastatic tumors of the brain are rare in childhood.

Most brain tumors occur sporadically and are of unknown cause; several, including teratomas and craniopharyngiomas, result from congenital malformations. An increased incidence of certain intracranial neoplasms is seen in the neurocutaneous syndromes. Irradiation of the brain increases the incidence of cerebral sarcomas.

Clinical Manifestations. The clinical manifestations in childhood are largely those of increased intracranial pressure because the majority of the tumors are in the posterior fossa and midline, where a mass lesion will obstruct CSF circulation. An important exception is the brain stem glioma, which, despite a midline location, rarely leads to increased intracranial pressure.

The manifestations of increased intracranial pressure vary somewhat with age. In infancy there is abnormal enlargement of the head. (Brain tumor should always be considered in the differential diagnosis of hydrocephalus.) Later in childhood marked expansion of the skull is no longer possible, and the increased intracranial pressure produces symptoms by compression of brain, meninges, and cerebral vessels. Headache is a common early symptom, characteristically occurring shortly after the child arises from bed or following changes in head position at other times of day. As pressure rises, headache becomes more severe and prolonged, but it is rarely continuous. The site of the pain has some localizing value; it tends to be suboccipital with posterior fossa tumors and on the side of the lesion in tumors of the cerebral hemisphere. Vomiting is common. It eventually becomes projectile and is characteristically unaccompanied by nausea. It is due to compression of the medulla and is therefore most severe in tumors of the posterior fossa. Drowsiness and stupor are rather late signs and are most likely due to pressure on the midbrain. Compression of vagal nuclei in the medulla leads to slowing of the pulse. Blood pressure is frequently elevated. Papilledema is often present but less likely in early infancy. Several intracranial structures are especially susceptible to damage by increased intracranial pressure. Sixth nerve palsies are common, with blurring of vision and diplopia; damage to optic nerves causes diminished visual acuity and may lead to total blindness. Important shifts of brain substance may also occur; inferior portions of cerebellum, i.e., the inferior vermis and the cerebellar tonsils, may herniate downward through the foramen magnum, producing the syndrome of *tonsillar herniation*. This is especially apt to occur with posterior fossa tumors. It is manifested by neck stiffness and often by a head tilt toward the side of herniation. Respirations become irregular and may suddenly cease because the respiratory centers in the medulla are compromised. Forceful neck flexion must be carefully avoided since it may lead to further compression of the medulla and sudden respiratory arrest. Supratentorial lesions, especially the laterally located ones, may lead to *tentorial herniation*.

The diagnostic study and management of brain tumor present many problems which fall outside the scope of pediatrics. The pediatrician needs to be thoroughly familiar with the presenting symptoms and signs, however, since he or she is likely to be the first to evaluate the child. The differential diagnosis includes some common and benign syndromes, even school phobia. The pediatrician also has a role in the pre- and postoperative care of children with brain tumors, especially those with suprasellar tumors which may lead to severe disorders of fluid and electrolyte balance. Perhaps the most important role will be to provide support and comfort to parents during the course of a very trying illness.

INFRATENTORIAL NEOPLASMS

Four types of neoplasm are common in the posterior fossa: cerebellar astrocytoma and medulloblastoma are of approximately equal incidence and account for about 65% of the tumors in this location; brain stem gliomas account for about 20% and ependymomas of the 4th ventricle for about 10%. Acoustic neuromas and meningiomas in this area are rare in childhood.

Cerebellar Astrocytoma. This is usually a cystic tumor which tends to arise near the midline but often extends into 1 cerebellar hemisphere. It may occur at any time in childhood, but incidence is highest from 2–8 yr. Signs of increased intracranial pressure occur early and may be the only changes; more commonly, signs of unilateral cerebellar dysfunction are superimposed, including hypotonia and intention tremor on the side of the lesion and nystagmus which is of greater amplitude when the child attempts to look toward the side of the tumor. Gait ataxia may be present, often with a tendency to veer toward 1 side. Somnolence occurs eventually because the brain stem is compressed. Pressure on vital structures in the brain stem appears to account for peculiar seizure-like states characterized by loss of consciousness with extensor rigidity, neck retraction, dilatation of pupils, and respiratory irregularity which have been referred to as "cerebellar fits"; such attacks are cause for immediate investigation.

Early diagnosis is aided by computed tomography, which localizes the tumor in the majority of instances. Roentgenograms of the skull may show lateralized thinning and bulging of the occipital bone on the side of the lesion in addition to nonspecific signs of increased intracranial pressure. Rarely, calcifications are visible in the tumor. Ventriculography or vertebral angiography may be needed to localize the tumor in doubtful cases. Therapy requires surgical excision. Expert surgical management results in close to 90% long-term survivals; most of these appear to be cures, though late recurrence is possible. Radiation therapy is used only when a tumor is recurrent or is not completely resectable.

Medulloblastoma. Medulloblastoma is a midline cerebellar tumor made up of undifferentiated small round cells. It grows extremely rapidly, has a tendency to seed along the entire cerebrospinal axis, and is 1 of the few brain tumors that may metastasize to extraneural tissues. Incidence peaks from 2–6 yr, with boys affected about twice as frequently as girls. It is not possible to differentiate this tumor reliably from cere-

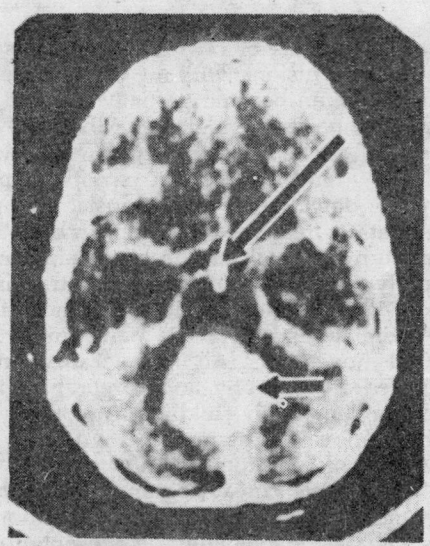

Figure 21–19 Computed tomogram (CT scan) after intravenous infusion of radiopaque material in a 4 yr old girl with morning vomiting, cachexia, and irritability but without positive findings on neurologic or funduscopic examination. A large tumor mass is shown in midline cerebellum (short arrow). A smaller, metastatic lesion is seen in the suprasellar cistern (long arrow). The temporal horns of the lateral ventricles are enlarged because the 4th ventricle is obstructed by the cerebellar tumor, which proved to be a medulloblastoma.

bellar astrocytoma on the basis of history or clinical examination, though the tumor is particularly likely to be found in a boy who has a history of rapidly progressive signs of increased intracranial pressure. There is often gait ataxia without lateralizing signs. Roentgenograms of the skull show evidence of increased intracranial pressure but no focal abnormalities. The tumor can usually be localized by computed tomography (Fig 21–19).

Therapy consists of surgical excision of accessible tumor followed by focal radiation to the posterior fossa and low dose radiation to the entire neuraxis. After completion of a course of radiation, chemotherapy may be advisable. A simple and well-tolerated regimen consists of weekly intravenous injections alternately of vincristine and cyclophosphamides, continued for 12–18 mo. The prognosis of medulloblastoma is hopeless with surgical therapy alone but improves somewhat with the use of combined treatment. A 20–30% cure rate has been achieved with surgery plus radiation. The effects of the addition of chemotherapy are not yet known. The outlook is hopeful if the child has no evidence of recurrence 18 mo after initial surgery.

Ependymoma. Ependymoma in the posterior fossa arises from the ependymal lining of the floor of the 4th ventricle. Upward extension into the ventricle causes early obstruction to CSF flow. The symptoms and signs are those of increased intracranial pressure. Cranial nerve palsies and positive Babinski signs may be present because of infiltration of the brain stem. These tumors may calcify, and the diagnosis can occasionally be made by visualization of calcification in the area of the 4th ventricle on a lateral roentgenogram of the skull. Surgical excision of accessible tumor often results in transient improvement, but surgical removal is rarely

possible. Postoperative radiation therapy is given to the posterior fossa. There are few long-term survivors.

Glioma of the Brain Stem. Pontine glioma has its peak incidence from 6–8 yr of age. The clinical history and physical findings are almost pathognomonic. They consist of progressive appearance of multiple bilateral cranial nerve palsies in combination with pyramidal tract signs (hyperreflexia and Babinski sign) and ataxia. Usually, there is no evidence of increased intracranial pressure. All the cranial nerves may be affected, with 6th and 7th nerve palsies being most common. The diagnosis is established by computed tomography, which shows enlargement of the pons and posterior displacement of the 4th ventricle and aqueduct of Sylvius.

The tumors cannot be removed surgically; therapy consists of local radiation. Most patients die within 18 mo of diagnosis; a few long-term survivors have been reported.

SUPRATENTORIAL NEOPLASMS

Craniopharyngioma. Craniopharyngioma is the most common tumor of the sellar and suprasellar regions in childhood. Its special pediatric interest is due to the numerous problems in management which arise from hypothalamic and pituitary dysfunctions. The tumor arises from squamous epithelial cell rests of the embryonic Rathke pouch. It often has a large cystic component; the growth features are those of a benign neoplasm.

Symptoms may appear at any time during childhood and adolescence and include (1) growth failure, (2) progressive visual loss, and (3) symptoms of increased intracranial pressure. These may occur singly or in any combination. The diagnosis should be considered whenever there is an arrest of linear growth after a period of normal gain in height. Other endocrine abnormalities are rare initially. Diabetes insipidus occurs *preoperatively* in fewer than 10%. Puberty is delayed. The visual impairment classically consists of bitemporal hemianopsia but may consist of asymmetric field defects, unilateral blindness, or bilateral decrease in visual acuity. Funduscopic examination reveals optic atrophy or papilledema. Roentgenograms of the skull show calcifications in a supra- or intrasellar location in about 80% of craniopharyngiomas that present during childhood (Fig 21–20). The sella turcica may be ballooned or distorted. Bone age is often retarded.

The location of the craniopharyngioma makes therapy a formidable problem. Cure by complete surgical removal requires both unusual surgical skill and meticulous postoperative care. Therapy with cortisone is initiated on the day prior to operation, at a dosage of about 40 mg/M²/24 hr, and is continued for at least 2 wk postoperatively. Supplementary hydrocortisone is given intravenously during the operation. Postoperatively, fluid intake is carefully matched to output; diabetes insipidus occurs almost invariably and must be controlled by replacement therapy. A marked decrease in urine output often occurs on the 2nd or 3rd postoperative day because of inappropriate release of antidi-

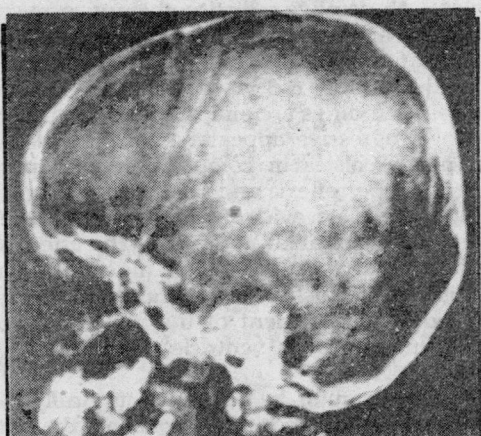

Figure 21–20 Craniopharyngioma in a boy 8 yr of age. Note fluffy suprasellar calcification, enlarged sella turcica, digital markings of skull, and early sutural separation.

uretic hormone. It is essential that fluids be restricted during this period to prevent water intoxication and cerebral edema. Serum electrolytes must also be carefully monitored and imbalances corrected. Occasionally, there is persistent hypernatremia due to damage to the hypothalamic thirst-regulating mechanism. A satisfactory result can be achieved in approximately 60% of patients. Aspiration of the tumor cyst followed by radiation of the tumor has been proposed as an alternative method of therapy.

Gliomas of the Optic Pathways.   These occur with increased frequency in patients with neurofibromatosis. They present with unilateral or bilateral visual loss. Extension of the tumor into the orbit may cause proptosis. Evidences of hypothalamic dysfunction and of increased intracranial pressure appear late. Surgical cure can be achieved when the tumor is confined to 1 optic nerve; those involving the optic chiasm are inoperable. These lesions progress very slowly, however, and survival without treatment may be as long as 20 yr. Radiation therapy has been advocated.

Hypothalamic Gliomas.   These occur mainly in infants, in whom they produce a very characteristic syndrome of emaciation, *the diencephalic syndrome of infancy*. Tumors of the hypothalamus occurring later in childhood usually present as precocious puberty in children who tend to be excessively large for age. They may have increased intracranial pressure due to extension of the tumor into the 3rd ventricle and visual loss due to involvement of the optic chiasm. Various types of tumor are seen, including hamartomas, gliomas, ectopic pinealomas, and teratomas.

TUMORS OF THE CEREBRAL HEMISPHERES

In childhood, tumors of the cerebral hemispheres include astrocytoma, oligodendroglioma, ependymoma, glioblastoma, and sarcoma. The symptoms and signs depend on the location of the tumor and its growth characteristics. Low-grade hemispheral tumors such as astrocytomas or oligodendrogliomas may initially cause convulsions without other abnormalities. These lesions often become partially calcified, a possibility warranting roentgenograms of the skull as part of the study of a child with seizures. As the tumors enlarge, they tend to produce spastic hemiparesis, hemisensory defects, or hemianopsia. Symptoms of increased intracranial pressure appear late. The more malignant tumors, such as the glioblastomas, present with rapidly progressive increase in intracranial pressure and with focal neurologic signs, including hemiparesis, hemianopsia, aphasia, and unilateral choreoathetoid movements. Accurate localization is made by computed tomography and cerebral angiography. Hemispheric tumors in childhood are rarely curable, but partial removal of the more benign types may lead to many years of symptom-free life.

Neoplasms in the Pineal Region.   These are uncommon in childhood, but they deserve mention in view of their characteristic clinical presentation. Early compression of the upper midbrain produces pupillary dilatation with diminution in the light reflex (*Parinaud syndrome*) and paralysis of upward gaze. Hydrocephalus is due to obstruction of the posterior 3rd ventricle and the aqueduct. The lesions cannot be removed surgically, but palliation can be achieved by a shunt operation followed by radiation.

Developmental tumors (*epidermoids, dermoids*, and *teratomas*) may occur in the pineal region and elsewhere along the midline. Epidermoids contain only stratified squamous epithelium; dermoids are made up of all skin structures, including hair and sebaceous glands; teratomas contain mesodermal and endodermal tissues as well. Occasionally, teratomas may be diagnosable roentgenographically by the visualization of bones or of teeth in the tumor. These developmental tumors may form large cysts filled with sebaceous secretions and desquamated skin. Depending on location, complete surgical removal may be possible.

Papillomas of the Choroid Plexus.   Papillomas are most common prior to 3 yr of age. They usually arise from choroid plexus of a lateral ventricle. Focal neurologic signs are rare. Increased production of CSF and obstruction to CSF flow by the tumor mass lead to early hydrocephalus. This tumor needs to be considered in the differential diagnosis of any child with hydrocephalus of obscure etiology. Diagnosis is usually apparent by computed tomography. Complete surgical removal is possible and leads to cure of the associated hydrocephalus.

PSEUDOTUMOR CEREBRI

As the name implies, this condition produces symptoms and signs which mimic those of brain tumor. The increased intracranial pressure is caused by diffuse cerebral edema.

Pseudotumor cerebri may occur as a complication of hypoparathyroidism; galactosemia; corticosteroid therapy, especially while the dose is being tapered off or after it has been discontinued; tetracycline therapy; or high doses of vitamin A. The majority of cases are of obscure etiology; obese adolescent girls are especially apt to acquire this condition.

The clinical presentation includes headache, morning vomiting, papilledema, and sometimes a 6th nerve palsy. Somnolence may occur but is rarely marked. Signs of focal neurologic disease are absent. A child with this combination of symptoms and signs usually requires special neuroroentgenographic studies, such as computed tomography, to rule out a focal mass lesion. The diagnosis of pseudotumor cerebri should be suspected in a child with increased intracranial pressure in whom neither a mass lesion nor enlargement of the ventricular system is found. The lateral ventricles may be reduced in size because of compression by the edematous brain. The CSF is normal except for a low protein content in some instances.

The elevation in intracranial pressure may persist for several mo, but it always subsides eventually. The chief danger is damage to optic nerves from chronic compression. No treatment is needed in mild cases. Patients with severe increase in pressure may be helped by repeated removal of CSF via lumbar puncture. Adrenocortical steroid therapy is very effective, but relapse may occur when therapy is discontinued. Weight reduction is indicated if the child is obese.

Banna M, et al: Craniopharyngioma in children. J Pediatr 83:781, 1973.
Bray PF, Carter S, Taveras JM: Brain stem tumors in children. Neurology 8:1, 1958.
Chutorian AM, et al: Optic gliomas in children. Neurology 14:83, 1964.
Farwell JR, Dohrmann GJ, Flannery JT: Central nervous system tumors in children. Cancer 40:3123, 1977.
Gareis FJ, Johnson JA: Inanition in infants associated with diencephalic neoplasms. Am J Dis Child 102:349, 1965.
Greer M: Benign intracranial hypertension. Neurology 12:472, 1962; 14:469, 1964; 15:382, 1965.
Kramer S: The value of radiation therapy for pituitary and parapituitary tumors. Can Med Assn J 99:1120, 1968.
Lassman LP, et al: Sensitivity of intracranial gliomas to vincristine sulfate. Lancet 1:296, 1965.
Lysak WR, Svien JH: Long-term follow-up on patients with diagnosis of pseudotumor cerebri. J Neurosurg 25:284, 1966.
Matson DD: Neurosurgery of Infancy and Childhood. Springfield, Ill., Charles C Thomas, 1969.
Matson DD, Crigler JF Jr: Radical treatment of craniopharyngioma. Ann Surg 152:699, 1960.
McFarland DR, et al: Medulloblastoma—a review of prognosis and survival. Br J Radiol 42:198, 1969.
Rose A, Matson DD: Benign intracranial hypertension in children. Pediatrics 39:227, 1967.
Wilson CB: Medulloblastoma. Current views regarding the tumor and its treatment. Oncology 24:273, 1970.

21.22 INTRACRANIAL MASS LESIONS SECONDARY TO INFECTION

Pyogenic infections may lead to abscess formation within the brain or to effusions or purulent exudates in subdural or epidural spaces. In each of these conditions intracranial pressure is increased by a local mass effect. When signs of infection are absent, differentiation from other conditions which cause increased intracranial pressure may be difficult.

BRAIN ABSCESS

Children with cyanotic congenital heart disease are at increased risk of development of pyogenic abscess of the brain. This peculiar susceptibility appears to be due to the fact that a right to left shunt eliminates the normal filtering of venous blood by the capillary bed of the lungs. In addition, the hypoxic brain appears to be an especially good culture medium for the anaerobic bacteria that are usually found in such lesions. Somewhat fewer than half of brain abscesses in childhood represent spread from foci of infection in other locations. Some occur by intracranial extension of infection from mastoids, paranasal sinuses, and skull; these were much more common prior to the widespread use of antibiotics. Occasionally brain abscess is metastatic from lung abscess, empyema, or endocarditis. Rarely, it is a complication of bacterial meningitis or of a penetrating injury to the skull. Some affected children have no history of any major preceding infection. The organisms found in brain abscess include microaerophilic or anaerobic streptococci, *Staphylococcus aureus*, pneumococcus, *Proteus*, and *Hemophilus influenzae* and *aphrophilus*.

Clinical signs of infection may be absent throughout the course of the illness. When present, they usually consist of low-grade fever and stiffness of the neck. Neurologic signs depend on the location of the abscess. Focal seizures and hemiparesis occur with abscess of a cerebral hemisphere. Temporal lobe abscess, which may complicate mastoiditis, causes aphasia if the dominant side is involved. Cerebellar abscess, also usually secondary to mastoiditis, results in ataxia and nystagmus.

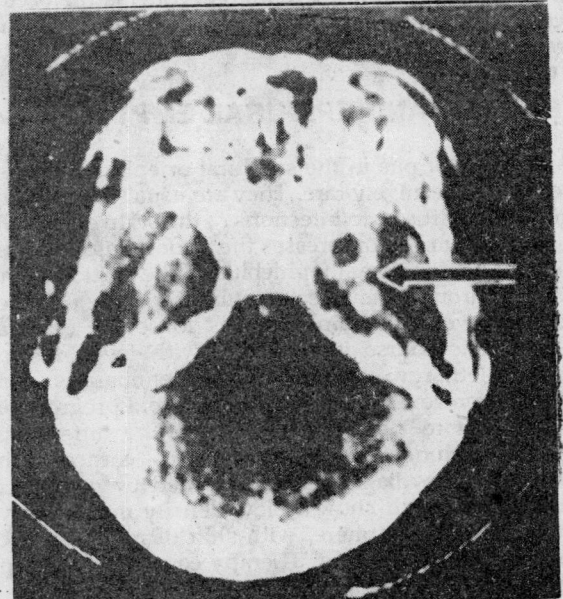

Figure 21–21 Two ring-shaped lesions in the right temporal lobe (arrow) in a computed tomogram obtained after intravenous injection of radiopaque material. The patient, an 11 yr old boy, had a history of frontal and sphenoid sinusitis and headache. The appearance of the lesions is typical of brain abscess. Resolution occurred following long-term antibiotic therapy.

Evidence of increased intracranial pressure is almost always present. Headache, vomiting, irritability, and drowsiness may be the presenting symptoms, and papilledema is usually present. The course is usually subacute over a period of weeks. Untreated, the child eventually becomes comatose. Death results from rupture of the abscess with overwhelming meningitis or from tentorial or cerebellar herniation.

Leukocytosis and elevated sedimentation rate may or may not be present. Computed tomography (Fig 21–21), radionuclide brain scan, and electroencephalography are useful initial laboratory tools. The radionuclide scan is almost always positive; it may show a ring-shaped area of increased uptake corresponding to the capsule of the abscess. In supratentorial abscesses the EEG shows a prominent slow-wave focus in the area of the lesion. CSF is of limited diagnostic help, and lumbar puncture should be avoided when intracranial pressure is high. The CSF is sterile unless the abscess has ruptured. The protein content is usually elevated, and white blood cells may be increased, with lymphocytes predominating. A roentgenogram of the chest is essential to look for a suppurative lesion of the lungs.

As soon as a tentative diagnosis of brain abscess is made, broad spectrum intravenous antibiotic therapy should be initiated and maintained for at least 6 wk. Use of osmotic diuretics, such as mannitol, will be important when intracranial pressure is elevated. Surgical drainage of the abscess is performed when there is a large collection of purulent material, and may be an emergency procedure in the comatose child with markedly increased intracranial pressure. Excision of the abscess, including its capsule, is advocated by some neurosurgeons. The most common sequel is the occurrence of seizures, for which continuous anticonvulsant therapy is usually needed.

SUBDURAL AND EPIDURAL EMPYEMA

Collections of pus in the subdural or epidural spaces have become relatively rare. They are usually secondary to frontal sinusitis or to infections of the scalp and skull. The purulent mass compresses the underlying brain. In addition, there is thrombophlebitis of the cortical veins that pass through the infected subdural space; interference with venous drainage leads to severe cerebral swelling. The course is subacute, with fever, severe headache, lethargy, convulsions, and hemiparesis. Papilledema is present, and there may be rapid progression to coma and to tentorial herniation. The differential diagnosis includes brain abscess and cortical vein thrombosis. The diagnosis is confirmed by computed tomography, which shows a low-density mass overlying a cerebral hemisphere, with shift of midline structures to the opposite side. Therapy consists of prompt surgical drainage and appropriate antibiotic therapy.

SUBDURAL EFFUSION COMPLICATING MENINGITIS

This disorder is thought to be peculiar to infancy. Incidence peaks from 4–6 mo of age; it is rarely recognized beyond 1 yr. Subdural effusion may be associated with any of the bacterial meningitides but occurs most often following *Hemophilus influenzae* meningitis. It seems probable that there are small collections of fluid in the subdural spaces in most persons with meningitis, the great majority of which are insignificant and resorb spontaneously. The incidence of large collections which require therapy is much smaller and probably less than has been thought to be the case.

The pathogenesis of subdural fluid collections with meningitis is incompletely understood. The arachnoid membrane in the infant is a poor barrier to the spread of infection into the subdural space. Early in the course of meningitis subdural fluid is often purulent and bacteria may be grown from it. After the infection has been controlled, several mechanisms appear to act to maintain and enlarge the fluid collection. As the subdural space becomes expanded, there may be rupture of small bridging veins; hemorrhage into the space is suggested by the fact that the fluid is frequently bloody. Transudation of fluid from inflamed capillary vessels may also be important; the protein content of subdural fluid is that of a transudate of plasma. The formation of large collections of fluid is aided by the distensibility of the skull of the infant. Longstanding effusions lead to the formation of vascular membranes, which become especially well developed along the outer wall of the subdural space. These membranes are friable, and capillary bleeding may occur from their surface.

It is difficult to identify symptoms that are clearly related to postmeningitic subdural effusions. Convulsions, vomiting, irritability, and persistent drowsiness are also seen in infants with meningitis not complicated by effusion. Physical findings in infants with subdural effusions include persistent fever, a bulging anterior fontanelle, and abnormal head enlargement. The diagnosis is confirmed by transillumination of the skull and by computed tomography. The effusions are bilateral in over two-thirds of cases. Treatment is directed toward prevention of large fluid collections, which may damage the brain by compression. It is not necessary to tap small collections which are not associated with increased intracranial pressure. Too many taps may actually worsen the problem by causing bleeding into the subdural spaces. Small collections subside spontaneously. In infants with bulging fontanelle or abnormal head enlargement, subdural taps are repeated every 24–48 hr, always bilaterally if fluid collections have been demonstrated on both sides. If large quantities of high-protein or bloody fluid continue to accumulate after 2 wk of repeated tapping, the subdural spaces should be surgically drained via bilateral burr holes. Surgical excision of subdural membranes has been advocated, but it has not been proved effective.

Berg B, Franklin G, Cuneo R, et al: Nonsurgical cure of brain abscess: Early diagnosis and follow-up with computerized tomography. Ann Neurol 3:474, 1978.

Farmer TW, Wise GR: Subdural empyema in infants, children and adults. Neurology 23:254, 1973.

Gitlin D: Pathogenesis of subdural collections of fluid. Pediatrics 16:345, 1955.

Hitchcock E, Andreadis A: Subdural empyema: A review of 29 cases. J Neurol Neurosurg Psychiat 27:422, 1964.

Liske E, Weikers NJ: Changing aspects of brain abscess. Neurology 14:294, 1964.

Matson DD, Salam M: Brain abscess in congenital heart disease. Pediatrics 27:772, 1961.

McKay RJ Jr, Ingraham FS, Matson DD: Subdural fluid complicating bacterial meningitis. JAMA 152:387, 1953.

Raimondi AJ, Matsumo S, Miller RA: Brain abscess in children with congenital heart disease. J Neurosurg 23:588, 1965.

Tefft M, Matson DD, Neuhauser EBD: Brain abscess in children. Radiologic methods for early recognition. Am J Roentgenol 98:675, 1966.

21.23 ACUTE TOXIC ENCEPHALOPATHY AND REYE SYNDROME

The label acute toxic encephalopathy has been applied to a clinical syndrome in which acute depression in state of consciousness occurs without apparent cause. The history is that of a previously well child who lapses into stupor and coma, often with associated convulsions. The cerebrospinal fluid may be under increased pressure but is otherwise normal.

In 1963 Reye et al reported abnormal liver function and pathologic changes in the liver and other visceral organs in a group of children with "acute toxic encephalopathy." Since then hepatic dysfunction has been found in a majority of children who fall within the diagnostic category. A rather distinct, easily recognizable clinical syndrome is referred to as *Reye syndrome*.

Pathology and Pathophysiology. The pathologic changes in Reye syndrome consist of marked fatty infiltration of liver cells in the form of small lipid droplets and similar but less intense fatty infiltration in the proximal tubules of the kidneys, in myocardium, and in other visceral organs. Electron microscopy of the liver shows evidence of mitochondrial damage. Biochemical study of biopsy of liver tissue has shown decreased activity of 2 mitochondrial enzymes of the Krebs urea cycle, ornithine transcarbamylase and carbamylphosphate synthetase. Inflammatory changes are lacking. The brain is markedly edematous, and there may be widespread neuronal necrosis, often in a distribution suggestive of anoxic damage.

Little is known about the pathogenesis of this syndrome. The pathologic findings suggest the action of a mitochondrial or general cellular poison, but none has been identified to date. The neurologic dysfunction may be in part secondary to ammonia intoxication and to fatty acidemia. Exogenous toxins such as acetylsalicylic acid have been implicated as possible etiologic factors. Epidemiologic and clinical data suggest a relationship to preceding viral infection.

Incidence. Reye syndrome is emerging as 1 of the more common causes of death in childhood. Small epidemics have occurred at the time of influenza outbreaks, and a few instances of simultaneous involvement of more than 1 child in a family have been reported.

Clinical Manifestations. The clinical history is remarkably uniform. The illness may occur at any age from infancy to adolescence. It almost always follows an acute viral infection, which has been identified as influenza type B in a large proportion of cases and as influenza A, chickenpox, or adenovirus infection in a smaller number. The child appears to be recovering from the initial disease but then has recurrent vomiting which may last for 24–48 hr. Toward the end of this period stupor and delirium supervene. The child rapidly lapses into coma and may have convulsions. There are no focal neurologic signs but general hyperreflexia and a positive Babinski sign. Hyperventilation is characteristic. Decerebrate rigidity and dilation of pupils occur in the most severely affected children, as does evidence of increased intracranial pressure, including papilledema. Terminally, signs of tentorial herniation of the brain supervene, with appearance of 3rd nerve palsy, followed by respiratory arrest. Clinical evidence of liver disease is limited to mild hepatomegaly. There is no jaundice. Survivors recover rapidly, often within 2–3 days. Residual disability is uncommon except in infants under 1 yr of age.

Laboratory data show evidence of hepatic dysfunction. SGOT and LDH are markedly elevated, and the liver-dependent blood clotting factors such as prothrombin are diminished. Serum bilirubin is normal or only mildly elevated. Early in the course blood ammonia is always increased. Elevation in blood level of several short chain fatty acids, including propionic, butyric, isobutyric, isovaleric, and octanoic, has been described, as well as elevated blood levels of lactate and several amino acids, including alanine, glutamine, lysine, and α-amino-N-butyrate. Hypoglycemia is common in young children. Mild evidence of renal dysfunction, including elevation in blood urea nitrogen and generalized aminoaciduria, occurs inconstantly. Respiratory alkalosis is common. The leukocyte count may reach 40,000/mm³, with predominance of granulocytes.

Differential Diagnosis. The differential diagnosis includes a number of toxic and metabolic disorders, including drug poisoning (especially with salicylates), hypoglycemic encephalopathy, hepatic coma due to acute hepatitis, and acute water intoxication. When convulsions occur early, the possibility of anoxic brain damage secondary to a seizure has to be considered. Sudden obstruction to CSF flow by an intraventricular tumor may cause a similar clinical picture, as may the occasional case of encephalitis without spinal fluid pleocytosis. Chemical evidence of hepatic dysfunction, including ammonia intoxication, is of great value for the rapid differentiation of Reye syndrome from most other severe, acute encephalopathies. Acute hepatitis can usually be excluded by the absence of jaundice. The liver tends to be small and nonpalpable in the rare cases of fulminant anicteric hepatitis.

Treatment. Therapy consists of supportive measures, including administration of 10% glucose and electrolyte solution by vein. Overhydration must be avoided since it may exacerbate cerebral edema. Anticonvulsant drugs are indicated when seizures occur. Care should be taken not to administer drugs such as acetylsalicylic acid or phenothiazines which may exacerbate the cerebral and hepatic dysfunctions. Strict attention to respiratory status is important. Assisted ventilation is indicated in the severely affected child. Curarization may be necessary if the patient's respiratory efforts preclude adequate ventilation. Control of cerebral edema is essential since death is usually the result of diminished cerebral perfusion secondary to increased intracranial pressure. Continuous pressure monitoring, either by a pressure transducer placed in the epidural or subdural space or by an intraventricular catheter, is a useful aid to management of the critically ill child since a major objective of management is to keep intracranial pressure below life-threatening levels, i.e., below 50% of mean arterial pressure. Osmotic agents such as 20% mannitol are frequently effective. Mannitol is given as repeated, rapid intravenous infusions, the amount being determined by the response of the intracranial pressure. The total dose should not be over 2 gm/kg/6 hr; larger amounts may lead to a hyperosmolar state. Repeated removal of small amounts (1 ml or less) of ventricular fluid, controlled hyperventilation, and curarization may also be used to maintain intracranial pressure below life-threatening levels. Exchange blood transfusion has been reported to result in decreased intracranial pressure, lessening of depth of coma, and improvement in the electroencephalogram. It also corrects blood clotting abnormalities, but it is uncertain that it diminishes the mortality or incidence of neurologic sequelae.

The mortality of Reye syndrome, which varied from 40–80% in series reported prior to 1972, has decreased to 10–20% in centers where an intensive therapeutic program is employed. It is not clear whether this decrease in mortality is due to intensive treatment or to increased diagnosis of previously unidentified mild cases with inherently good prognosis.

Berman W, et al: The effects of exchange transfusion on intracranial pressure in patients with Reye's syndrome. J Pediatr 87:887, 1975.

DeVivo DC: Reye syndrome: A metabolic response to an acute mitochondrial insult? Neurology 28:105, 1978.

Huttenlocher PR, Trauner DA: Reye's syndrome in infancy. Pediatrics 62:84, 1978.

Kindt GW, et al: Intracranial pressure in Reye's syndrome: Monitoring and control. JAMA 231:822, 1975.

Lyon G, Dodge PR, Adams RD: The acute encephalopathies of obscure origin in infants and children. Brain 84:680, 1961.

Partin JC, Schubert WK, Partin JS: Mitochondrial ultrastructure in Reye's syndrome (encephalopathy and fatty degeneration of the viscera). N Engl J Med 285:1339, 1971.

Pollack JD (ed): Reye's Syndrome. New York, Grune & Stratton, 1975.

Reye RDC, Morgan G, Baral J: Encephalopathy and fatty degeneration of the viscera. Lancet 2:749, 1963.

Trauner DA, Nyhan WL, Sweetman L: Short-chain organic acidemia and Reye's syndrome. Neurology 25:296, 1975.

21.24   CEREBRAL VASCULAR DISEASES

This group of illnesses is characterized by the precipitous onset of signs and symptoms of neurologic dysfunction. They fall into 2 categories: *intracranial hemorrhage* and *vascular occlusion*.

INTRACRANIAL HEMORRHAGE

(See also Sec 7.23.)

Spontaneous intracranial hemorrhage in childhood usually results from the rupture of a congenital vascular lesion such as an arteriovenous malformation or an arterial aneurysm. Hemorrhage from a vascular malformation or an aneurysm has to be differentiated from intracranial bleeding secondary to blood coagulation defects and from traumatic hemorrhage. Intracranial bleeding occurs occasionally in hemophilia and in idiopathic thrombocytopenia and may be a terminal event in leukemia. Traumatic hemorrhage may be especially difficult to distinguish in the small child with no history of head trauma.

Arteriovenous Malformations (Fistulas). These may occur in any part of the brain; they consist of large arterial feeding vessels, a mass of dilated communicating channels, and large draining veins that carry arterialized blood. The larger malformations may produce symptoms in infancy without hemorrhage. This is especially true of malformations involving the posterior cerebral artery and the great vein of Galen; the arteriovenous shunt may be so large as to cause congestive heart failure and polycythemia. Enormous saccular dilatation of the vein of Galen may also lead to hydrocephalus in infancy by obstruction of the aqueduct of Sylvius. The majority of arteriovenous malformations, however, are clinically silent for a number of years, then suddenly cause symptoms when rupture of 1 of the communicating vessels leads to subarachnoid and intracerebral hemorrhage.

Sudden severe headache, drowsiness, and nuchal rigidity due to subarachnoid hemorrhage and focal neurologic signs from damage of brain tissue at the site of the hemorrhage are the most common presenting signs. Detection of an intracranial bruit is a helpful confirmatory sign, especially after the age of 4 or 5 yr. With massive intracranial bleeding the child rapidly lapses into coma. Funduscopic examination may show retinal and preretinal hemorrhages. Occasionally, there are repeated episodes of headache and focal convulsions, which probably represent recurrent minor episodes of bleeding.

The diagnosis is confirmed by bloody or xanthochromic cerebrospinal fluid. Cerebral angiography is essential for determination of the exact location and extent of the lesion. Arteriovenous malformations superficially located in the cerebral cortex may be amenable to complete surgical excision. Embolization of the abnormal vessels is the preferred method of treatment in large or deeply situated malformations. Ligation of feeding arteries alone is usually of limited effectiveness.

Intracranial Arterial Aneurysms. The most common aneurysms are due to *congenital malformations* in the media of arterial walls at points of bifurcation (berry aneurysm). The incidence is increased in patients with coarctation of the aorta and with polycystic disease of the kidney. The most common sites are the anterior communicating and anterior cerebral arteries and the terminal branching of the internal carotid artery. Occasionally, aneurysms form at sites of damage to cerebral arteries by infection (*mycotic aneurysms*).

Intracranial arterial aneurysms are rarely diagnosed in childhood. Though the defect is almost always congenital, it is not apt to be manifested until early adult years. Symptoms are mainly those of subarachnoid and intracerebral hemorrhage following rupture. The typical history involves a previously well child who suddenly develops excruciating headache and then lapses into stupor and coma. Nuchal rigidity and preretinal hemorrhage are signs of subarachnoid bleeding. Third nerve palsy is common after rupture of an aneurysm of the carotid artery, hemiparesis after rupture of a middle cerebral artery aneurysm. The CSF is bloody and xanthochromic and is under increased pressure. Cerebral angiography is needed for definitive diagnosis. Surgical ligation or clipping of the aneurysm is indicated if it is possible. The mortality of unoperated ruptured aneurysms is about 50%. Bleeding may recur many yr later in survivors.

CEREBRAL VASCULAR OCCLUSIONS

Occlusive cerebral vascular disorders include arterial occlusions, either thrombotic or embolic, and venous occlusions, which are due to thrombosis or thrombophlebitis in cerebral veins.

Arterial Occlusions (Acute Infantile Hemiplegia). Occlusion of cerebral arteries is uncommon in childhood; it has its peak incidence from 1–3 yr of age. It is due to thrombosis or embolism in a major cerebral artery, usually the internal carotid or middle cerebral. Thrombosis in the extracranial (cervical) portion of the internal carotid artery may be caused by localized vasculitis from spread of tonsillar infection or cervical adenitis or by local trauma, especially from a pencil point or other sharp object pushed into the region of the tonsillar fossa. The cause is less often evident in occlusions of the intracranial vessels. Local arteritis, atherosclerosis, and fibromuscular hyperplasia of the vessel wall have been implicated, often without proof. Thrombocytosis has been associated, but its relationship to the thrombosis is uncertain. Systemic illnesses which may be complicated by arterial occlusions in childhood include sickle cell disease, lupus erythematosus, polyarteritis nodosa, and cyanotic heart disease. Infants under 2 yr of age with cyanotic congenital heart disease who have both polycythemia and iron deficiency are especially prone to cerebral arterial occlusion. The possibility of cerebral embolus has to be considered in the older child with congenital heart disease.

The clinical manifestations of cerebral vascular occlusion in childhood resemble those of stroke in the adult. In the child there is often a preceding acute febrile illness. The child may be found to be hemiparetic on awakening from sleep. In other instances weakness is progressive over a period of hours. The child may remain lucid; aphasia is common when the dominant hemisphere is affected. Convulsions, either focal or generalized, frequently occur during the acute phase. There are no signs of increased intracranial pressure, and the CSF remains normal. The diagnosis may be confirmed by cerebral angiography if it is performed early. Recanalization of the occluded vessel occurs rapidly, and arteriography a few wk after the onset may show a normal vascular system.

The differential diagnosis of cerebral arterial occlusion includes postictal (Todd) paralysis when the acute illness is complicated by convulsions. Encephalitis has to be considered but can usually be ruled out if the child remains fairly alert and if there are no inflammatory changes in the CSF.

Therapy is limited to treatment of definable underlying conditions such as infection. The prognosis for recovery of speech is good, but almost always there is some residual hemiparesis. Spasticity tends to develop over a period of weeks or months. Recurrent seizures are common, especially following acute hemiplegia in infancy. Many children are left with mild intellectual impairment and behavioral abnormalities.

Venous Occlusions. Thrombosis of cerebral veins occurs principally as a complication of severe dehydration or as an extension of local infection. Several clinical syndromes depend on the site of the venous occlusion.

Sagittal Sinus Thrombosis. This may be a complication of severe dehydration, especially in the infant with diarrhea. Obstruction of the sinus leads to cerebral swelling, which produces signs of increased intracranial pressure, including stupor, coma, and bulging anterior fontanelle. When thrombosis extends into the cortical veins, there may be widespread hemorrhagic infarction of the brain. Seizures and quadriparesis may occur. The clinical diagnosis can rarely be made with certainty. The clinical picture may mimic encephalitis and various metabolic encephalopathies, especially water intoxication in the dehydrated infant who has been rehydrated too rapidly.

Lateral Sinus Thrombosis. This complication of neglected otitis media and mastoiditis has become rare. Obstruction to the sinus results from septic thrombophlebitis. There may be chills and fever, or the onset may be insidious with signs of increased intracranial pressure. Focal neurologic signs are usually absent.

Cavernous Sinus Thrombosis. This follows infection of the face, orbit, or nasal sinuses which spreads via anastomoses from the facial vein to the ophthalmic veins, which drain directly into the cavernous sinus. Pyogenic infections of the nose are a common source. Onset occurs with high fever, drowsiness, and proptosis of the eye on the affected side. Within hours or at most 1–2 days the veins of the lid become distended and chemosis develops. There is paralysis of 1 or more of the ocular muscles. On funduscopic examination disc margins are blurred and retinal veins engorged. Untreated, the thrombophlebitis spreads to the other side via the circular sinus, and fatal intracranial extension usually follows.

The *diagnosis* of cerebral venous thrombosis is based to a large extent on the clinical findings. CSF examination is of little help. CSF pressure is usually elevated; the fluid may be bloody, and it may show white cells and an elevated protein content. Cerebral angiography is of value in localizing the site of obstruction.

Treatment. Therapy of cerebral vein thrombosis consists of appropriate antibiotic therapy if thrombosis is secondary to infection. Localized collections of pus should be drained surgically. Life-threatening increases in intracranial pressure may be treated with mannitol or dexamethasone. Anticoagulant therapy is not indicated; it may worsen hemorrhage into infarcted brain.

Brown P: Septic cavernous thrombosis. Bull Johns Hopkins Hosp 109:68, 1961.

Gold AP, Ransohoff J, Carter S: Vein of Galen malformation. Acta Neurol Scand 8 (Suppl) 1964.

Greer M: Benign intracranial hypertension. 1. Mastoiditis and lateral sinus obstruction. Neurology 12:472, 1962.

Isler W: Acute Hemiplegias and Hemisyndromes in Childhood. Clinics in Developmental Medicine, Nos 41/42. Philadelphia, JB Lippincott, 1971.

Levine OR, Jameson AG, Nelhaus G, et al: Cardiac complications of cerebral arteriovenous fistula in infancy. Pediatrics 30:563, 1962.

Matson DD: Intracranial arterial aneurysms in childhood. J Neurosurg 23:578, 1965.

Pool JL, Potts DG: Aneurysms and Arteriovenous Anomalies of the Brain: Diagnosis and Treatment. New York, Paul B Hoeber, 1965.

Solomon GE, et al: Natural history of acute hemiplegia of childhood. Brain 93:107, 1970.

Tyler HR, Clark DB: Incidence of neurological complications in congenital heart disease. Arch Neurol Psychiat 77:17, 1957.

21.25   HEAD INJURY

Craniocerebral trauma is a major cause of serious disability and death in childhood. About 200,000 children each year are admitted to United States hospitals for observation and treatment following head injury. A much larger number are managed at home. The decision as to whether a potentially life-threatening head injury requires hospitalization is frequently difficult.

MINOR HEAD TRAUMA

Normally a closed head injury can be assumed to be insignificant when the initial blow to the head is not followed by unconsciousness; the child can usually be followed at home without special diagnostic study. Dizziness, nausea, occasional vomiting, and headache may be seen during the 1st 24–48 hr after minor head trauma. They are not cause for alarm unless they are accompanied by marked or progressive lethargy. But even after apparently mild head trauma the parents should be instructed to make certain at least once during the 1st night that the child is rousable and that there has not been a significant drop in heart rate (to 60 or below) since intracranial hemorrhage, especially into the subdural space, occasionally follows apparently trivial head trauma.

CONCUSSION

This is defined as a head injury which is immediately followed by a period of unconsciousness. Concussion is not associated with obvious pathologic changes in brain; it is assumed to be due to disturbance in function of the brain stem caused by sudden jarring. After a concussion the patient may have loss of memory for events that preceded the injury (retrograde amnesia) or for occurrences after the injury (antegrade amnesia). In general, the duration of unconsciousness and the extent of retrograde amnesia correlate well with the severity of injury. Retrograde amnesia diminishes during recovery but never disappears completely.

Concussion implies a significant blow to the head, with sufficient distortion of intracranial structures to make severance of intracranial vessels a possibility. After a concussion the child should be carefully observed for delayed signs of intracranial hemorrhage. A baseline neurologic examination should include a check for pupillary size and reaction to light, funduscopic examination, and assessment of reflexes for symmetry and for the Babinski sign. In the infant, tension of the fontanelle should be assessed and the head size measured. It is advisable to obtain roentgenograms of the skull for skull fractures. Not every child with concussion or even skull fracture needs to be treated in the hospital. Close observation at home may be sufficient if the initial evaluation finds no neurologic abnormality, if the child has regained normal alertness, and if the parents are reliable and responsible.

SKULL FRACTURE

The roentgenographic demonstration of a skull fracture provides important information regarding the site of injury but does not necessarily indicate serious brain injury. The possibility of intracranial hemorrhage must, of course, be assessed. A fracture that crosses the groove for the middle meningeal artery suggests the possibility of epidural hemorrhage. Occipital skull fracture may be associated with posterior fossa hemorrhage (see below). Basal skull fractures may lead to leakage of CSF into the middle ear with bulging of the tympanic membrane and to otorrhea if the tympanic membrane is ruptured. Rhinorrhea due to escape of CSF from the nose occurs with fractures through the cribriform plate. Basal skull fractures may lead to meningitis by spread of organisms from the nose or ear. Prophylactic use of 1 of the penicillins is justifiable for basal skull fracture with rhinorrhea or otorrhea. Linear fractures require no specific therapy. Depressed fractures should be elevated surgically unless depression is minimal. Occasionally, surgical closure of dural defects is necessary to control CSF leakage.

Skull fractures in infancy may lead to progressively enlarging defects of the skull (spreading fractures) over a period of months or years because the meninges are trapped in the fracture line. Large leptomeningeal cysts may form and need surgical resection.

SEVERE HEAD INJURY

This should be assumed when a child fails to awaken within some minutes after an accident. Structural damage to brain has to be expected in such a patient. This may take the form of contusion or bruising of brain, usually either at the site of the blow (coup) or opposite the site (contracoup). Actual laceration of brain tissue and meninges may occur, often with intracerebral, subarachnoid, or subdural hemorrhage. Intracranial pressure may increase rapidly as a result both of hemorrhage and of edema of injured tissue.

The acute management of the child with severe head injury is demanding. Generally, the child is comatose. The 1st priorities are that the patient have adequate blood pressure, that the airway be patent, and that respirations be well maintained. Movement of the patient should be avoided until it is clear that there are no other serious injuries such as fractures of the spine or of other major bones. Prompt neurologic assessment should be carried out as summarized above for the comatose patient. This is repeated at frequent intervals until the patient's condition is stable. Neuroroentgenographic studies and/or neurosurgical intervention may be indicated when coma progressively deepens or when signs of tentorial herniation appear. The medical management of the child who remains comatose following severe head injury is that of coma from any cause. Management of cerebral edema complicating head injury includes use of dexamethasone, intravenous mannitol, and controlled ventilation as indicated. Continuous monitoring of intracranial pressure (via an intraventricular catheter or a pressure transducer inserted into the epidural or subdural space) is a valuable aid to management of critically ill children with head injury.

POST-TRAUMATIC SYNDROMES

The brain of the child shows remarkable capacity for recovery from acute injury. Good functional recoveries have been reported in children comatose for over 2 mo. Post-traumatic epilepsy occurs in about 10% of survivors from severe head injury and usually has its onset within 1 yr. The most common residuals are minor changes in behavior and in learning. Headache and dizziness are rather common. Hydrocephalus may follow subarachnoid hemorrhage.

EPIDURAL HEMORRHAGE

This is usually secondary to severance of the middle meningeal artery, most often as a result of a fracture that crosses the artery's groove in the skull. Fracture is less likely in the infant or small child with epidural hemorrhage, in whom bleeding is frequently venous from dural veins. The patient with epidural hemorrhage characteristically awakens from a concussion and after a brief lucid interval lapses into coma again. Signs of tentorial herniation rapidly follow unless therapy is promptly instituted. If the initial injury is severe enough to cause cerebral contusion, the lucid interval is absent and coma progressively deepens. Prompt surgical evacuation of blood from the epidural space is lifesaving.

When epidural hemorrhage is venous in origin, the course is less rapid and is clinically indistinguishable from that of subdural hematoma. Hemorrhage into the epidural space of the posterior fossa may follow trauma to the occiput, with or without fracture. The bleeding originates in the lateral sinus or tributary veins. The child becomes progressively drowsy after a lucid interval. Vomiting and irregular respirations occur early because the brain stem is compressed. Hydrocephalus may follow compression of the aqueduct and 4th ventricle; this lesion is a possibility in infants who develop hydrocephalus following traumatic deliveries.

21.26 SUBDURAL HEMATOMA

Subdural hematoma may be acute or chronic. The latter is most common in infants, in whom it presents special problems.

Acute Subdural Hematoma. This is almost always associated with meningeal tears and with contusion and hemorrhage in the underlying brain. The affected child with severe head trauma remains in deep coma and has evidence of progressively increasing intracranial pressure. Prognosis is guarded even when the collection of blood is removed promptly because there is usually severe injury to the brain.

Chronic Subdural Hematoma. In the child, as in the infant, there is gradual leakage of blood from torn frontal or parietal cortical veins which traverse the subdural space in their course to the sagittal sinus. The initial injury may be minor, often a concussion from which the child appears at first to recover. Within days or sometimes weeks signs of increased intracranial pressure develop, including headache, vomiting, drowsiness, unsteadiness of gait, and 6th nerve palsy. Hemiparesis and convulsions may occur. Papilledema is usually present. The initial injury may have been forgotten, and the 1st consideration may be of brain tumor. Coma and signs of tentorial herniation develop in neglected cases. The diagnosis is made by computed tomography, which shows a low-density mass between the inner table of the skull and the surface of the brain, with displacement of the ventricular system. Radionuclide brain scan may show increased uptake in the area of the hematoma. The EEG may show lower amplitude on the affected side, but this finding is not reliable. Surgical evacuation of the chronic subdural hematoma in the older child usually results in cure.

Chronic Subdural Hematoma in the Infant. This occurs with maximum incidence from 2–6 mo of age. About 25% of affected infants have a history of birth trauma, and about an equal number have a history of postnatal head injury. There may be no clear history of trauma even when there are distinct evidences of such injuries as fractures of long bones, ribs, and skull. (See Sec 2.67.) The evolution of chronic subdural hematoma in infancy is as follows: the initial clot liquefies, and water moves into the subdural space to maintain osmotic equilibrium. Repeated small hemorrhages occur from rupture of bridging veins, which are put under stress as the subdural space enlarges. The infant's skull expands in response to increasing intracranial pressure. Very large collections of fluid may form. The fluid is initially bloody; it gradually clears and becomes straw-colored, with a high protein content. Chronic subdural effusions become encapsulated by vascular inner and outer membranes. The outer membrane may become quite thick and occasionally calcifies.

Presenting symptoms include vomiting, failure to gain weight, unexplained fever, irritability, drowsiness, and convulsions. Focal neurologic signs are rare; rather, one finds signs of increased intracranial pressure, including a bulging fontanelle and mild head enlargement. Biparietal prominence of the skull is characteristic, in contrast to hydrocephalus, in which the

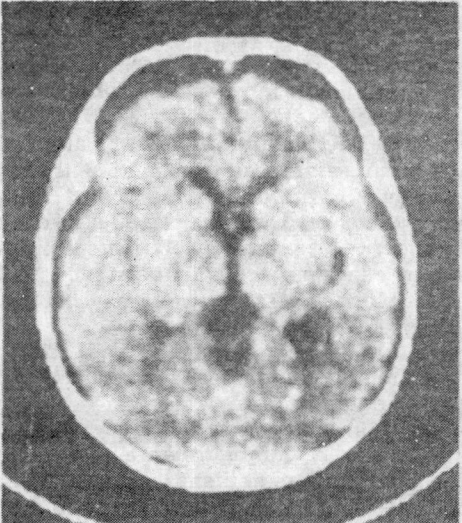

Figure 21–22 Computed tomogram (CT scan) of a 7 mo old boy with a history of lethargy and vomiting and with bilateral retinal hemorrhages on funduscopic examination. Bilateral fluid collections are seen between the inner table of the skull and the brain surface, typical of chronic subdural hematoma.

prominence tends to be frontal. Transillumination of the skull is increased after liquefaction of the initial hematoma has occurred. Retinal hemorrhages are found in more than 50% of infants.

The diagnosis is made by subdural tap and by computed tomography (Fig 21–22). Initially, therapy consists of repeated subdural taps, but surgical drainage is frequently required. Shunting of the subdural fluid to the peritoneal cavity or right atrium may be indicated if other measures fail. The prognosis depends on the severity of cerebral damage which occurred at the time of the initial trauma and on the size and duration of the subdural effusion at the time therapy was initiated. The outcome is satisfactory in about 60% of patients. Mental defects, convulsions, and quadriparesis are the most common residuals.

Collins W, Pucci G: Peritoneal drainage of subdural hematomas in infants. J Pediatr 58:682, 1961.
DeVivo DC, Dodge PR: The critically ill child: Diagnosis and management of head injury. Pediatrics 48:129, 1971.
Ingraham FD, Matson DD: Subdural hematoma in infancy. J Pediatr 24:1, 1944.
Mealey J Jr: Pediatric Head Injuries. Springfield, Ill., Charles C Thomas, 1968.
Richardson F: Some effects of severe head injury. A follow-up study of children and adolescents after protracted coma. Dev Med Child Neurol 5:471, 1963.
Shulman K, Ransohoff J: Subdural hematoma in children. The fate of children with retained membranes. J Neurosurg 18:175, 1961.
Taveras TM, Ransohoff J: Leptomeningeal cysts of the brain following trauma with erosions of the skull: A study of 7 cases treated by surgery. J Neurosurg 10:233, 1953.
Till K: Subdural hematoma and effusion in infancy. Br Med J 3:400, 1968.

21.27   DISEASES OF THE SPINAL CORD

General Considerations.   Diseases of the spinal cord are uncommon in childhood, but their prompt recog-

nition is urgent since early diagnosis and treatment may avoid permanent paraplegia and incontinence.

Compression of the spinal cord results in a variety of characteristic symptoms and signs, which vary with the location of the spinal lesion. These include localized back tenderness, pain and immobility, scoliosis, and bladder dysfunction, manifested initially as frequency and urgency and later as distention and incontinence. The most common motor manifestation is a disturbance of gait, initially a limp, which may progress to paraplegia. Lesions involving the cervical cord may produce a quadriparesis, usually with muscle atrophy, areflexia, and hypotonia in the upper limbs and hyperreflexia and spasticity in the legs. In general, flaccid weakness and areflexia are found at the level of the lesion, with spasticity below that level. In acute lesions, however, the paralysis is flaccid throughout because of spinal "shock." A sensory level on the trunk identified by pinprick and touch is indicative of spinal cord disease and establishes the approximate site of the lesion. Often the actual lesion is several segments above the upper extent of sensory impairment.

NEOPLASMS OF THE SPINAL CORD

When spinal cord dysfunction evolves in a subacute or chronic manner, it is most often due to a neoplasm. Gliomas, including astrocytomas and ependymomas, are the most common types. Neuroblastoma is next in frequency; it is the most likely cause of spinal cord compression in the infant. In lymphoma the spinal cord may be compressed by tumor masses in the epidural space. Spinal neurofibroma may be associated with generalized neurofibromatosis. Various developmental lesions, including teratoma, lipoma, and neurenteric cysts, account for most of the remaining spinal cord tumors in childhood. Spinal cord compression occurs occasionally with chronic hemolytic anemia as a result of extramedullary hematopoiesis in the extradural space.

Careful neurologic examination of the child with unexplained limp or bladder dysfunction is essential for early diagnosis of spinal tumors. Roentgenograms of the spine may be helpful; with slowly growing tumors, the spinal canal is widened in the area of the lesion and there is bony erosion, especially of the pedicles. Defects of neural arches are found in developmental tumors. The lumbar spinal fluid is xanthochromic and high in protein content when there is obstruction of the spinal subarachnoid space at a higher level. Myelography is needed to define the level and extent of the tumor and to determine whether it is extrinsic or intrinsic to the cord.

Intrinsic spinal cord tumors may be difficult to distinguish from *syringomyelia*, a condition of unknown cause producing cavitation in the cord, usually in the cervical area. Atrophy of hand muscles and loss of pain sensation in the upper limbs are the most common clinical findings.

Prompt surgical exploration is indicated in most types of spinal cord tumor. Local irradiation manages cord compression due to lymphoma.

ACUTE SPINAL CORD LESIONS

Spinal Cord Trauma. Spinal cord trauma in childhood most often is the result of breech deliveries, automobile accidents, and diving injuries. It is usually associated with fracture or dislocation of vertebrae. Dislocations are especially common at the C1–2 level with fractures of the odontoid process, at the lower cervical level, and at T12–L1. Complete cord transection at the upper cervical level leads to rapid death from respiratory paralysis. Less severe injury at this level causes quadriparesis and often respiratory embarrassment requiring assisted ventilation. It is very important to avoid movement of such a patient; when absolutely necessary, movement must be accomplished en bloc. If possible, the patient should be kept supine on a firm support. Gentle neck traction is helpful during transportation of the patient with cervical spine injury. Complete loss of function below the level of the lesion lasting over 24 hr is almost always permanent. Surgical exploration of the damaged area, to have any chance of success, must be carried out within the 1st few hr.

Atlantoaxial (C1–2) Dislocation. This may occur without a clear history of trauma, especially in patients with congenital malformations of the spine or with metabolic bone diseases such as the chondrodystrophies. Flexion of the neck causes compression of the cervical cord in such patients. There is a history of progressive weakness and gait disturbance. Spastic paresis of arms and legs occurs without dysfunction of cranial nerves. The lesion must be differentiated from spastic cerebral palsy and from the leukodystrophies and demyelinating diseases. Therapy consists of reduction of the dislocation by neck traction followed by immobilization of the neck.

Spinal Epidural Abscess. This is a localized accumulation of pus in the spinal epidural space, usually posterior to the cord in the thoracic area. It may be acute, usually staphylococcal in origin, or subacute, from extension of tuberculous osteomyelitis of the spine. Exquisite pain and percussion tenderness are present over the abscess, and the spine is held rigidly extended. Signs of spinal cord dysfunction, including paraparesis, loss of bladder and bowel control, and a sensory level on the trunk, evolve rapidly. Systemic evidence of infection may be absent. The diagnosis is occasionally made at lumbar puncture when pus under pressure is obtained before the dura is penetrated. Myelography may be necessary to define spinal cord compression. Spinal epidural abscess represents a neurosurgical emergency; prompt drainage may prevent permanent paraplegia.

Vascular Anomalies of the Spinal Cord. These include arteriovenous malformations, venous angiomas, and telangiectasia. These lesions may cause sudden spinal cord dysfunction if rupture of an abnormal blood vessel leads to hemorrhage into the spinal cord or into the spinal subarachnoid space. Nuchal rigidity occurs when subarachnoid hemorrhage is massive. Recurrent, acute exacerbations and partial remissions are characteristic. The cerebrospinal fluid may be bloody or the protein content elevated. Myelography is usually diagnostic, showing tortuous, dilated vascular channels. At times, the vascular anomaly may be suspected from the presence of a port wine stain (nevus flammeus) covering the skin in a segmental distribution corresponding to the level of the vascular malformation. Surgical removal of vascular anomalies of the spinal cord is not often successful.

Transverse Myelopathy. Often misdesignated transverse myelitis, transverse myelopathy is a syndrome in which segmental spinal cord dysfunction appears rapidly, usually within hours, without evidence of a compressive lesion or of hemorrhage. In some instances the disorder is secondary to demyelinating disease. In others segmental necrosis of the cord probably is a result of vascular occlusion. Occlusion of the anterior spinal artery is likely when posterior column functions (position and vibration senses) are spared. The onset of transverse myelopathy may follow a mild febrile illness or be sudden in a previously healthy child. Back pain at the site of the lesion is usually present but is much less severe than in spinal epidural abscess. This is followed by paraparesis, a sensory level, and inability to void. The CSF is usually normal, but there may be mild elevation in protein content and in cell count. Myelography may be needed to rule out compressive lesions. Corticosteroid therapy has produced equivocal results. Partial recovery of function is usual.

CHRONIC CARE OF THE PARAPLEGIC CHILD

Children who survive acute spinal cord diseases are frequently left with paraplegia and bladder dysfunction. The paraplegia is initially flaccid, but spasticity develops gradually, often with appearance of painful flexor spasms. These are especially common in paraplegics with decubitus ulcers due to stimulation of pain fibers in the areas of skin breakdown which activates flexor reflexes in the severed spinal cord segments. Frequent turning, use of an air mattress, and physiotherapy may prevent both decubitus ulcers and flexor spasms. The urinary bladder of the acutely paraplegic patient is atonic and becomes massively distended unless catheter drainage is instituted. Chronically, the bladder may become spastic with frequent partial reflex emptying. Chronic urinary tract infection from inadequate drainage and calciuria from immobility lead to renal and bladder calculi (Sec 2.80).

Alexander E Jr, Masland R, Harris C: Anterior dislocation of first cervical vertebra simulating cerebral birth injury in infancy. Am J Dis Child 85:151, 1953.

Matson DD: Neurosurgery of Infancy and Childhood. Springfield, Ill., Charles C Thomas, 1969.

Paine RS, Byers RK: Transverse myelopathy in childhood. Am J Dis Child 85:151, 1953.

Rand RW, Rand CW: Intraspinal Tumors of Childhood. Springfield, Ill., Charles C Thomas, 1960.

Rowland LP, Shapiro JH, Jacobson HG: Neurological syndromes associated with congenital absence of the odontoid process. Arch Neurol Psychiat 80:286, 1958.

Tarlov IM: Spinal cord injuries—early treatment. Surg Clin North Am 35:2, 1955.

21.28 DISORDERS OF THE AUTONOMIC NERVOUS SYSTEM

The autonomic nervous system provides neural control over a large variety of vegetative functions such as heart rate, blood pressure, temperature regulation, micturition, and intestinal motility. Its 2 large divisions are sympathetic and parasympathetic; their actions are often but not always antagonistic. The highest level of integration of autonomic functions occurs in the hypothalamus; from there central parasympathetic and sympathetic pathways descend to the brain stem and spinal cord.

Parasympathetic nerve fibers leave the central nervous system via the cranial nerves and the sacral spinal nerves. These fibers synapse in peripherally located parasympathetic ganglia, whence the peripheral fibers are in turn distributed to the visceral organs as follows:

Nerves in which parasympathetic fibers travel	Organ innervated
Cranial III	Sphincter of pupil
VII	Submaxillary and sublingual glands
IX	Parotid gland
X	esophagus, bronchi, lungs, heart, stomach, pancreas, small intestine, proximal colon
Sacral ($S_2 - S_4$)	Distal colon, rectum, bladder, external genitalia

Stimulation of parasympathetic nerves releases acetylcholine at the nerve terminals. The actions of this system can be explained entirely in terms of pharmacologic effects of acetylcholine and can be reproduced by administration of such parasympathomimetic drugs as methacholine (Mecholyl) and pilocarpine and blocked by atropine and atropine-like drugs. Parasympathetic effects include constriction of the pupils, salivation, bronchial constriction, slowing of the heart rate, gastric secretion of hydrochloric acid, stimulation of peristalsis, and micturition.

Sympathetic nerve fibers leave the central nervous system only at the spinal level and travel with the thoracic and upper 2 lumbar spinal nerves. They synapse in peripheral sympathetic ganglia and are distributed to the visceral organs and to blood vessels, hair follicles, sweat glands, and adrenal medulla. Stimulation of the sympathetic nervous system releases norepinephrine at most of the peripheral nerve endings; exceptions are the sweat glands, where the neurohumoral substance is acetylcholine, and the adrenal medulla, where it is epinephrine. Many of the effects of sympathetic nervous system stimulation can be reproduced by administration of norepinephrine or of such sympathomimetic drugs as amphetamine and ephedrine and blocked by adrenergic blocking agents. Effects of sympathetic nervous system stimulation include pupillary dilatation, constriction of blood vessels, acceleration of heart rate, sweating, piloerection, and bronchodilatation.

Autonomic nervous system functions are disturbed in a large number of systemic and neurologic illnesses.

In the following disorders abnormalities of the autonomic nervous system are particularly prominent:

1. *Developmental defects*
   Familial dysautonomia (Riley-Day syndrome)
   Hirschsprung disease
2. *Tumors*
   Neuroblastoma
   Ganglioneuroma
   Pheochromocytoma
   Hypothalamic tumor—the diencephalic syndrome of infancy
3. *Poisonings*
   Atropinism
   Botulism
4. *Injuries to autonomic nerves*
   Horner syndrome
   Adie syndrome
5. *Inflammatory disorders of autonomic nerves*
   Autonomic neuropathy
   Postinfectious polyneuritis (Guillain-Barré syndrome)
6. *"Psychosomatic" disorders*
   Cushing-Rokitansky ulcer
   Curling ulcer

FAMILIAL DYSAUTONOMIA

The *Riley-Day syndrome* is a genetically determined disturbance in autonomic and peripheral sensory functions; inheritance is autosomal recessive. It is most common in Ashkenazi Jews, among whom the frequency of the carrier state is estimated at about 1%.

Neuropathologic findings are sparse and are confined to the peripheral sensory system. The taste buds (fungiform papillae) of the tongue are absent or decreased in number. The peripheral nerves have a deficit in the number of small unmyelinated fibers, which normally carry pain, temperature, and taste sensations, and of the large myelinated fibers, which carry afferent impulses from muscle spindles. These abnormalities are not always present, and the autonomic nervous system usually has no demonstrable pathologic changes. Disturbed autonomic function is reflected in metabolic abnormalities: the plasma of about 25% of affected children shows no dopamine-beta-hydroxylase, the enzyme which catalyzes the conversion of dopamine to norepinephrine; vanillylmandelic acid (VMA), an excretion product of norepinephrine, is usually diminished in the urine of patients; and homovanillic acid (HVA), a metabolite of dopamine, is increased in urine and in CSF.

Clinical manifestations are prominent in infancy. Swallowing movements are poorly coordinated and therefore lead to gagging, vomiting, and aspiration. Excessive bronchial secretions and repeated aspiration contribute to recurrent bouts of pulmonary infection with eventual chronic pulmonary failure. Evidences of autonomic disturbances include excessive salivation and sweating, decrease or absence of tear formation, marked blotching of the skin during excitement, urinary incontinence, labile hypertension and orthostatic hypotension, and defective temperature regulation with periodic fevers. Clinical manifestations of peripheral sensory dysfunction consist of absence of taste sensation, diminished or absent pain sense leading to repeated skin trauma and to asymptomatic fractures, and absence of corneal sensation. The latter, together with the defect in tear formation, increases the susceptibility to corneal ulceration. Tendon reflexes are diminished or absent, probably as a result of defective formation of afferent fibers of muscle spindles. The central nervous system is usually affected; the manifestations include mental defect, dysarthria, clumsiness, and emotional lability.

Laboratory Data. Roentgenograms of the chest show atelectasis and pulmonary infiltrates similar to the changes in cystic fibrosis. The Mecholyl test for denervation hypersensitivity of the pupil (a fresh 2% solution of Mecholyl instilled into 1 conjunctival sac, the other eye serving as a control) is positive: constriction of the pupil appears within 10 min. There is no response to the histamine skin test (0.05 ml of a 1:1000 solution of histamine injected intradermally), which is normally characterized by a red flare and pain at the injection site. Urinary VMA is decreased; HVA is increased. Slow intravenous infusion of norepinephrine produces an exaggerated pressor response. The hypotensive response to infusion of Mecholyl is increased.

The **differential diagnosis** of familial dysautonomia includes other causes of "failure to thrive" in infancy, chronic pulmonary diseases in childhood, congenital universal indifference to pain, and congenital sensory neuropathy.

Treatment is directed toward control of recurrent respiratory infections, prevention of corneal ulceration by use of artificial tears, and protection from injuries related to lack of pain sensation. Bethanecol (Urecholine) has been used to increase tear formation.

The **prognosis** for the child with familial dysautonomia is poor. A majority die prior to adulthood, usually from chronic pulmonary failure.

DIENCEPHALIC SYNDROME OF INFANCY

This cause of failure to thrive is usually due to glioma of the anterior hypothalamus, but the same syndrome may also occur with inflammatory or destructive lesions in this region. Affected infants have endocrine and central autonomic disturbances secondary to hypothalamic dysfunction. The most striking clinical findings are extreme emaciation in spite of apparently adequate food intake and a hypermetabolic state with overactivity and "hyperalertness." The autonomic disturbances consist of excessive sweating, easy flushing of the skin, tachycardia, and vomiting. Evidences of endocrine abnormality include increased linear growth, advanced bone age, and excessive size of hands and feet. Late in the course the infants develop enlargement of the head, optic atrophy, and searching nystagmus secondary to visual loss. The syndrome may appear at any time from 3 mo–4 yr of age.

Soft tissue roentgenograms of the extremities show complete absence of the normal subcutaneous fat shadow. There may be fasting hypoglycemia. The CSF protein level is increased if there is an underlying hypothalamic tumor. The neoplasm is usually demon-strable by computed tomography. Therapy is generally unsatisfactory: long remissions have been induced by radiation therapy.

INJURY TO AUTONOMIC NERVES

Horner Syndrome. This refers to a lesion of the cervical sympathetic nerve fibers; it is usually unilateral. These fibers are especially prone to injury because of their long intra- and extracranial course. Central sympathetic neurons descend in the lateral medulla and spinal cord to the upper thoracic spinal level. Preganglionic cervical sympathetic fibers then leave the spinal cord in the upper thoracic ventral spinal roots and pass upward in the paravertebral sympathetic chain; the majority of fibers synapse in the superior cervical ganglion and then follow the course of the common carotid artery in the neck. Sudomotor and vasomotor fibers travel in close relation to the external carotid artery to be distributed to the skin over the face; fibers innervating the pupil and the upper eyelid (oculosympathetic fibers) follow the internal carotid and ophthalmic arteries to the orbit. The Horner syndrome may follow lesions at any of these anatomic levels, i.e., at the medulla oblongata, cervical or upper thoracic spinal cord, posterior mediastinum, or neck. A partial syndrome in which only the oculosympathetic fibers are affected occurs with lesions near the internal carotid artery or in the orbit.

The clinical manifestations of the Horner syndrome consist of ptosis due to weakness of the levator palpebrae muscle, meiosis due to dysfunction of pupillodilator fibers, and absence of sweating over the ipsilateral face. In congenital Horner syndrome there is heterochromia iridis as a result of failure in pigmentation of the iris on the affected side.

Pharmacologic tests are of some help in differentiating Horner syndrome caused by a central nervous system lesion from that caused by a peripheral sympathetic lesion. Instillation of a 4% solution of cocaine into the conjunctival sac normally produces dilatation of the pupil by potentiation of the effect of locally released norepinephrine. This response is absent in the Horner syndrome associated with a peripheral sympathetic lesion, whereas it is preserved in a lesion involving central sympathetic pathways. Instillation of a 1:1000 solution of epinephrine normally produces no pupillary reaction but will result in dilatation of the pupil in Horner syndrome caused by a peripheral sympathetic lesion. The results of these tests may be equivocal when the Horner syndrome is incomplete. A search for tumor or other compressive lesion is indicated in any patient who develops Horner syndrome. This should include careful palpation of the neck and of the supraclavicular areas and roentgenograms of the chest and the cervical spine. Horner syndrome per se does not produce significant disability and requires no therapy.

Adie Syndrome. Adie syndrome is a disorder of the parasympathetic innervation of the iris of unknown etiology; it usually first appears in young adults but may occasionally occur in childhood. The affected pupil is large and reacts little or not at all to light but will often react slowly to accommodation. Patients with Adie pupil often have hyporeflexia, especially absence of the knee jerk. Occasionally, there is associated anhidrosis over the trunk. The Adie pupil is hypersensitive to parasympathomimetic agents, and instillation of 2% Mecholyl into the conjunctival sac produces brisk contraction. The Adie syndrome is an essentially benign condition, needing no therapy; its prompt recognition may avert unnecessary studies.

INFLAMMATORY DISORDERS OF AUTONOMIC NERVES

The peripheral autonomic nervous system is occasionally involved in inflammatory diseases of nerve. In postinfectious polyneuritis (Guillain-Barré syndrome), autonomic dysfunction may represent a clinically significant complication. Evidences of autonomic disturbance include postural hypotension, hypertension, unexplained tachycardia, sweating, and urinary retention. Urinary excretion of VMA may be increased.

A few cases of *acute autonomic neuropathy* have been reported. Such patients have acute onset of diminished pupillary reaction to light, dryness of mouth, hypohidrosis, urinary retention, and vomiting. Recovery is gradual over a period of weeks or months. The condition must be distinguished from atropinism and from botulism.

AUTONOMIC STIMULATION LEADING TO VISCERAL LESIONS

It has long been known that lesions of the central nervous system may induce visceral abnormalities through stimulation of central autonomic pathways. A striking example is the *Cushing-Rokitansky ulcer* of the stomach or duodenum which occurs in children with posterior fossa tumor, often a few days after surgical resection of the neoplasm. Gastric ulceration in these children is probably due to abnormal stimulation of vagal (parasympathetic) nuclei in the medulla, which leads to increased gastric hydrochloric acid secretion. Stress may lead to overactivity of hypothalamic parasympathetic centers with the same result of gastric and duodenal ulceration and hemorrhage. This complication has been observed with special frequency in patients suffering from extensive burns (*Curling ulcer*).

It has been suggested that less specific stresses of life may be causative factors in the formation of gastric and duodenal ulcers as well as in the etiology of a number of other disorders such as ulcerative colitis, asthma, and essential hypertension. However, proof of cause-effect relationships has been inconclusive. (See also Sec 2.49.)

PETER R. HUTTENLOCHER

Aguayo A, Nair P, Bray G: Peripheral nerve abnormalities in the Riley-Day syndrome. Arch Neurol 24:106, 1971.

Axelrod FB: Treatment of familial dysautonomia with bethanecol (Urecholine). J Pediatr 81:573, 1972.

Dancis J, Smith AA: Familial dysautonomia. N Engl J Med 274:207, 1966.

Esterly N, Cantoline SJ, Alter BP, et al: Pupillotonia, hyporeflexia and segmental hypohidrosis: Autonomic dysfunction in a child. J Pediatr 73:852, 1968.

Loggie JMH, Van Maanen EF: The autonomic nervous system and some aspects of the use of autonomic drugs in children. J Pediatr 81:205, 432, 1972.

Mitchell PL, Meilman E: The mechanism of hypertension in the Guillain-Barré syndrome. Am J Med 42:986, 1967.

Poznanski AK, Manson G: Radiographic appearance of the soft tissues in the diencephalic syndrome of infancy. Radiology 81:101, 1963.

Riley CM, Moore RH: Familial dysautonomia differentiated from related disorders. Pediatrics 37:435, 1966.

Russell A: A diencephalic syndrome of emaciation in infancy and childhood. Arch Dis Child 26:274, 1951.

Sauer C, Levinsohn MW: Horner's syndrome in childhood. Neurology 26:216, 1976.

Smith AA, Dancis J: Catecholamine release in familial dysautonomia. N Engl J Med 277:61, 1967.

Thomashefsky AJ, Horowitz SJ, Feingold MH: Acute autonomic neuropathy. Neurology 22:251, 1972.

Weinshilboum RM, Axelrod J: Reduced plasma dopamine-hydroxylase activity in familial dysautonomia. N Engl J Med 285:938, 1971.

NEUROMUSCULAR DISEASES 22

22.1 CLASSIFICATION OF NEUROMUSCULAR DISORDERS

Disorders of the peripheral motor and sensory systems are known collectively as the neuromuscular diseases. These illnesses involve 1 or more of the structures concerned with the segmental spinal reflex arc: the anterior horn cells, motor nerve fibers, neuromuscular junction, muscle, and sensory nerve fibers from muscle and tendons (Fig 22–1). Interference with this reflex arc leads to depression of tendon reflexes, which is characteristic of all neuromuscular diseases. In addition, weakness and muscle atrophy usually are present.

The following is a useful classification of the more common disorders:

1. *Anterior horn cell diseases*
    Werdnig-Hoffmann disease
    Poliomyelitis (Sec 10.84)
    Other viral infections (Sec 10.78)
2. *Polyneuropathies*
    Postinfectious polyneuritis (Guillain-Barré syndrome)
    Diphtheritic polyneuritis (Sec 10.23)
    Toxic neuropathies (heavy metal poisoning, Sec 28.12 and 28.15), drug-induced neuropathies, metabolic diseases with polyneuropathy (Table 22–2)
    Hypertrophic interstitial neuritis (Dejerine-Sottas disease)
    Charcot-Marie-Tooth disease (peroneal muscular atrophy)
    Congenital sensory neuropathy
    Congenital indifference to pain
3. *Mononeuropathies*
    Congenital ptosis
    Oculomotor nerve palsy (Tolosa-Hunt syndrome)
    Sixth nerve palsy (Duane syndrome)
    Facial palsy (Bell palsy)
    Erb palsy (Sec 7.25)
    Peroneal palsy
    Sciatic nerve injury
4. *Diseases of the neuromuscular junction*
    Myasthenia gravis
    Botulism (Sec 10.43 and 28.2)
5. *Diseases of muscle*
    Inflammatory diseases of muscle
        Polymyositis
        Myositis ossificans
    Endocrine myopathies
        Hyperthyroid myopathy
        Hypothyroid myopathy
        Corticosteroid myopathy
    Congenital defects of muscle
        Absence of muscle
        Congenital torticollis
        Congenital myopathies (central core disease and nemaline myopathy)
    Myotonia
        Myotonia congenita (Thomsen disease)
    Periodic paralyses
        Hyperkalemic form (adynamia episodica herediaria)
        Hypokalemic form
        Paroxysmal myoglobinuria
        McArdle disease (Sec 8.21)
    The muscular dystrophies
        Pseudohypertrophic form (Duchenne)
        Congenital muscular dystrophy
        Facioscapulohumeral form
        Limb-girdle form
        Ocular myopathy
        Myotonic dystrophy

22.2 ANTERIOR HORN CELL DISEASES

The anterior horn cells are selectively affected in poliomyelitis and occasionally by infection with other viruses, including coxsackieviruses and echoviruses. Inherited degeneration of the anterior horn cells occurs primarily in infancy.

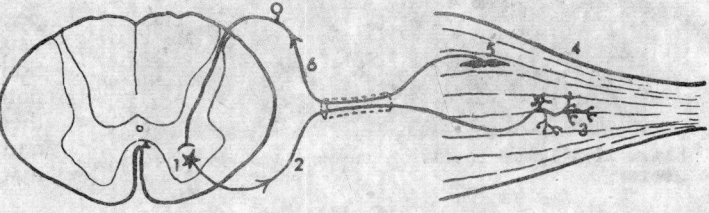

Figure 22–1 Schematic representation of the structures that make up the neuromuscular system. 1 = anterior horn cell; 2 = motor nerve fiber; 3 = motor end-plate on muscle; 4 = muscle; 5 = sensory receptor in muscle (muscle spindle); 6 = sensory nerve fiber.

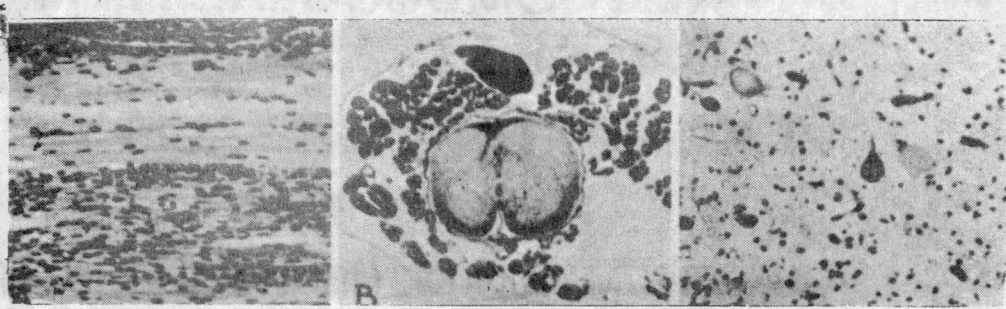

Figure 22–2 Werdnig-Hoffmann disease. *A*, Fascicular atrophy of muscle. *B*, Pallor of ventral roots. *C*, Degenerating motor neurons.

Infantile Spinal Muscular Atrophy. *Werdnig-Hoffmann disease* is transmitted as a recessive trait. The primary pathologic change is atrophy of anterior horn cells in the spinal cord and of motor nuclei in the brain stem (Fig 22–2), with secondary atrophy of motor nerve roots and of muscle.

Onset occurs prior to the age of 2 yr and often in utero. Rare instances of similar illness with onset later in childhood have been described. Early manifestations are weakness and hypotonia of the proximal and distal limb and intercostal and bulbar muscles. The legs tend to lie in a frog-leg position, with hips abducted and knees flexed (Fig 22–3). The diaphragms are relatively

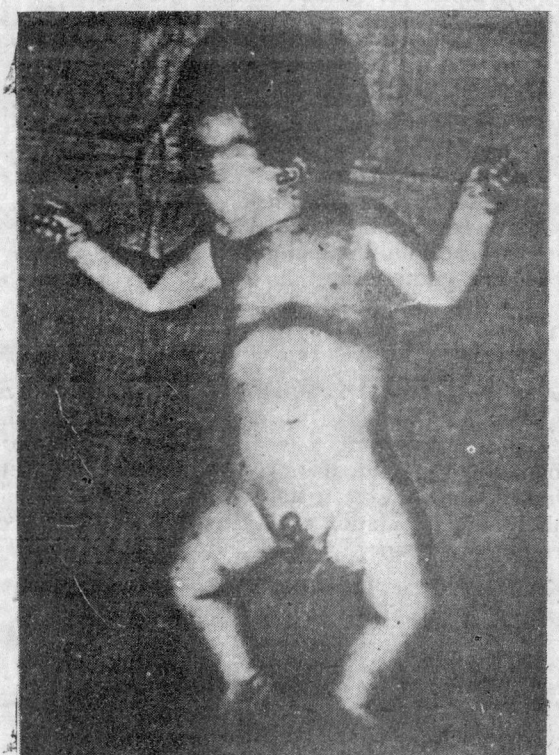

Figure 22–3 Typical posture of the infant with Werdnig-Hoffmann disease.

spared; diaphragmatic function in the presence of weakness of the intercostal muscles results in characteristic paradoxic breathing, with inward movement of the chest on inspiration. Extraocular muscles are unaffected. Fibrillations usually are visible in the tongue. Tendon reflexes are almost always absent. Mental development is normal, and the bright look of these infants provides striking contrast to their lack of motor activity. Initially, the infants tend to be obese. In the late stages swallowing becomes impossible. Death results from respiratory failure and from aspiration of food. Infants with onset in utero usually die prior to the age of 2 yr. Those with later onset may survive for some years, occasionally to adulthood.

The *diagnosis* of Werdnig-Hoffmann disease is based largely on the clinical findings. Electromyography often shows evidence of denervation of muscle, including fibrillation potentials and fasciculations. In biopsied muscle, groups of cells are seen in varying states of degeneration; each group represents cells innervated by a single motor neuron. Spinal fluid, nerve conduction measurements, and serum enzyme activities are within normal ranges.

The *differential diagnosis* of Werdnig-Hoffmann disease includes a large number of less common conditions in which hypotonia and weakness occur in infancy. The term "floppy infant" is used for this group of disorders (Table 22–1).

Disorders of the central nervous system presenting with hypotonia can usually be differentiated from the peripheral neuromuscular diseases by decreased alertness and visual responsiveness and by the preservation of tendon reflexes. Special studies, including examination of CSF, nerve conduction velocity measurements, serum enzyme determinations, and muscle biopsy, may be needed to distinguish Werdnig-Hoffmann disease from disorders of peripheral nerves or of muscle. A small number of hypotonic infants cannot be placed into the classification of Table 22–1. These infants appear normally alert. Tendon reflexes are depressed but usually not completely absent. Laboratory investigations, including muscle biopsy, are unrevealing. Hypotonia and weakness gradually improve in most of these infants. Such labels as *benign congenital hypotonia* and *amyotonia congenita* have been used; it is unlikely that this group represents a single entity.

Table 22-1 DISEASES INCLUDED IN THE DIAGNOSTIC TERM "FLOPPY INFANT" AND CHARACTERIZED BY PERSISTENT HYPOTONIA

CENTRAL NERVOUS SYSTEM DISORDERS	SPINAL CORD DISEASES	DISEASES OF PERIPHERAL NERVE	DISEASES OF THE NEUROMUSCULAR JUNCTION	MUSCLE DISEASES
Atonic diplegia	Spinal cord trauma	Polyneuritis (Guillain-Barré syndrome)	Myasthenia gravis	Congenital muscular dystrophy
Congenital cerebellar ataxia	Werdnig-Hoffmann disease	Familial dysautonomia	Infantile botulism	Myotonic dystrophy
Kernicterus		Congenital sensory neuropathy		Glycogen storage disease of muscle and heart (Pompe)
Chromosomal defects				
Oculocerebrorenal syndrome (Lowe)				Central core disease
Cerebral lipidoses				Nemaline myopathy
Prader-Willi syndrome				Mitochondrial myopathies

Brandt S: Werdnig-Hoffmann's Infantile Progressive Muscular Atrophy. Copenhagen, Ejnar Munksgaard, 1950.

Byers RK, Banker BQ: Infantile muscular atrophy. Arch Neurol 4:140, 1961.

Chambers R, MacDermot V: Polyneuritis as a cause of "amyotonia congenita." Lancet 1:397, 1957.

Dubowitz V: The Floppy Infant. London, William Heinemann, 1969.

Eden AN: Guillain-Barré syndrome in a 6 month old infant. Am J Dis Child 102:224, 1961.

Garvie JM, Woolf AL: Kugelberg-Welander syndrome (hereditary spinal muscular atrophy). Br Med J 1:1458, 1966.

Paine RS: The future of the "floppy infant." A follow-up study of 133 patients. Dev Med Child Neurol 5:115, 1963.

Pickett J, Berg B, Chaplin E, et al: Syndrome of botulism in infancy: Clinical and electrophysiological study. N Engl J Med 295:770, 1976.

Rabe EF: The hypotonic infant. J Pediatr 64:422, 1964.

Walton JN: Amyotonia congenita. A follow-up study. Lancet 1:1023, 1956.

22.3 POLYNEUROPATHIES

Involvement of multiple peripheral nerves is found in many systemic diseases, intoxications, and infections. In addition, there are a number of genetically determined illnesses in which degeneration of peripheral nerves is the primary abnormality. The more common causes of polyneuropathy are listed in Table 22-2.

The *clinical manifestations of polyneuropathy* include weakness, muscular atrophy, loss of tendon reflexes, and sensory impairment. The distal limbs—feet and hands—are affected first, and there is gradual proximal progression as the disorder becomes more severe. Motor fibers are more severely affected than sensory ones in some polyneuropathies, including lead poisoning, the Guillain-Barré syndrome, and Charcot-Marie-Tooth disease. Gait disturbance with foot drop is an early manifestation in these illnesses. Fairly selective damage to sensory fibers occurs in diabetes mellitus and in some of the genetically determined neuropathies. All types of sensation, including pain, touch, temperature, position, and vibration sense, are impaired, often in a "stocking and glove" distribution. Injured sensory nerve endings may become abnormally sensitive to stimulation, and innocuous stimuli may be interpreted as being painful (hyperpathia), while tingling or "pins and needles" sensations may occur in the absence of stimulation. Loss of sensory and autonomic innervation results in trophic changes in skin and nails and occasionally in loss of toes and fingers. Remarkable recovery from polyneuritis may follow removal of the offending agent because of the capacity of peripheral nerves, in contrast to central neural pathways, to regenerate after injury.

The *pathologic changes* in some peripheral neuropathies consist of patchy loss of the myelin sheath of the nerve fibers (segmental demyelination); in other instances, degeneration of the axons appears to be the primary process. In chronic neuropathies there is often considerable fibrous tissue reaction which may result in palpable enlargement of the affected nerves.

Measurement of nerve conduction velocity is the most helpful diagnostic aid. Decrease in conduction velocity is seen exclusively in disorders of peripheral nerves and is especially striking when demyelination is a prominent pathologic feature. Biopsy of the sural nerve may also be useful in confirming the diagnosis except in predominantly motor neuropathies, in which this sensory nerve may be spared. Neither of these measures, however, provides information regarding the specific cause of the neuropathy. The recognizable toxic and metabolic causes listed in Table 22-2 must, when possible, be identified by toxicologic and other special tests. A careful family history and examination of family members are important for the diagnosis of the genetically determined polyneuropathies. Included in this group are hypertrophic interstitial neuritis, Charcot-Marie-Tooth disease (peroneal muscular atrophy), and several forms of sensory neuropathy.

Guillain-Barré Syndrome (Postinfectious or Idiopathic Polyneuritis). This acute or subacute disease affects nerve roots and peripheral nerves in a diffuse

Table 22-2 THE MORE COMMON POLYNEUROPATHIES

POISONING	DRUG TOXICITY	INFECTIONS	METABOLIC DISORDERS	DEGENERATIVE DISEASES
Lead	Vincristine	Diphtheria	Diabetes mellitus	Hypertrophic interstitial neuritis
Mercury	Isoniazid	Guillain-Barré syndrome	Uremia	Charcot-Marie-Tooth disease
Thallium	Nitrofuran	Leprosy	Porphyria	Congenital sensory neuropathy
Arsenic			Thiamine deficiency	Metachromatic leukodystrophy
			Vitamin B_{12} deficiency	Krabbe disease
			Refsum disease	Leigh disease
				Spinocerebellar degeneration

manner. The disorder occurs sporadically at any age from early infancy. It usually follows viral infections; occasional cases occur after immunizations. A variety of viral illnesses, including infectious mononucleosis, mumps, measles, echovirus, coxsackievirus, and influenza viral infections, have been observed prior to the development of Guillain-Barré syndrome. The viral illness, however, has usually run its course by the time the neurologic symptoms appear, and there is no evidence for viral invasion of the nervous system. About 2.5% of cases occur in patients with immune disorders, including lupus erythematosus and rheumatoid arthritis.

Sensitization of lymphocytes to a protein component of myelin has been found in Guillain-Barré syndrome and is likely to be of etiologic importance. Migration of sensitized lymphocytes into peripheral nerves appears to be the earliest pathologic change; myelin breakdown follows. The disease can be reproduced in animals by sensitization to the basic protein of myelin derived from peripheral nerves.

Clinical manifestations appear within about 2 wk after the onset of a viral illness in about two thirds of cases. The remainder have no evidence of prior illness. Pain suggestive of nerve root irritation and paresthesias in the legs and feet are early symptoms; sensory loss is rarely demonstrable. Cranial nerve involvement occurs in over 75% of cases; facial weakness is the most common, may be unilateral, may precede other neurologic findings, and may initially be indistinguishable from Bell palsy. Muscle weakness evolves over a period of 3–21 days, often starting in the legs and spreading to the arms and to the muscles of respiration. The weakness is both proximal and distal and tends to be symmetric. Tendon reflexes are lost, but plantar responses usually remain normal. Muscle tone is diminished. Occasionally, autonomic nerves are involved, in which case there may be urinary retention, postural hypotension, or hypertension. Drowsiness, mental changes, papilledema, and Babinski signs indicative of concurrent involvement of the central nervous system are observed in a small proportion of affected children.

The *diagnosis* is made largely from the clinical manifestations. Spinal fluid changes may be confirmatory; the protein concentration becomes elevated in about 75% of cases, but this finding may not appear until 1–2 wk after the onset of clinical manifestations. CSF protein often remains elevated for several mo, even after clinical improvement is clearly evident. Typically, there are no cells in the CSF, but up to 10 lymphocytes/mm³ have been observed. Nerve conduction is slow in both motor and sensory nerves.

The *differential diagnosis* includes poliomyelitis, polymyositis, spinal cord tumors, transverse myelopathy, and, in the young child, acute cerebellar ataxia. In poliomyelitis, weakness is less symmetric, and there is an increase in white cells, primarily lymphocytes, in the CSF and usually a normal protein content. In polymyositis the CSF is normal, but serum enzymes such as creatine phosphokinase and aldolase are usually elevated as is the erythrocyte sedimentation rate. Spinal cord tumors and transverse myelopathy may initially cause flaccid weakness and areflexia, but these rapidly give way to spasticity, hyperreflexia, and positive Babinski signs. A level of sensory loss on the trunk and the early and severe involvement of bladder and rectal sphincter functions also aid in the differentiation of spinal cord lesions from Guillain-Barré syndrome. Cerebellar ataxia presents a problem of differentiation in the young child when formal testing of strength is not possible and when gait ataxia may be confused with leg weakness.

Respiratory insufficiency secondary to paralysis of intercostal muscles is the most serious complication of the Guillain-Barré syndrome. Patients should be closely observed by serial measurements of vital capacity. Blood gas determinations are necessary if confusion, drowsiness, or tachypnea appears. Tracheal intubation and assisted ventilation should be performed before there is advanced respiratory failure. Recovery has occurred after more than 8 mo of complete ventilatory support. With good supportive treatment, more than 90% of children with Guillain-Barré syndrome recover. Complications of tracheostomy and of respiratory therapy, pneumonia, and cardiac arrhythmia account for the occasional fatal outcome. Recovery is usually complete in children, but it tends to be slow, over a period of up to 2 yr. Physiotherapy may be helpful during the recovery period. Rarely, there is a relapsing course with multiple attacks or a chronic progressive course. Therapy with corticosteroid hormones is probably ineffective in acute cases but may improve the outcome in the chronic form of the disease.

Hypertrophic Interstitial Neuritis (Dejerine-Sottas Disease). This is an uncommon, recessively inherited disease that has its onset in late infancy or early childhood. Motor development may be slow from the start. Later in childhood there is progressive gait disturbance, with foot drop and ataxia caused by loss of position sense. Associated findings include pes cavus and scoliosis. Eventually, but rarely during childhood, the peripheral nerves become palpably enlarged. The disease is slowly progressive and permits a normal life span. The CSF protein content is usually elevated, a finding of some value in differentiation from most other chronic neuropathies and from diseases of muscle.

Charcot-Marie-Tooth Disease. *Peroneal muscular atrophy* is a motor neuropathy that disproportionately affects the nerves to the legs. Inheritance is usually on a dominant basis. Onset occurs during late childhood or adolescence, with pes cavus, foot drop, and peroneal myatrophy. The distal wasting of the legs gives the characteristic "stork leg" appearance. Foot drop leads to a high "steppage" gait. The intrinsic hand muscles are affected eventually. Mild distal sensory impairment may be present. Progression is slow, and the disease rarely becomes severe enough to preclude ambulation. The CSF is normal.

Congenital Sensory Neuropathy. This recessively inherited abnormality is usually noted in late infancy when the child fails to respond to painful stimuli to the hands or feet. These children tend to bite and otherwise injure their fingers. Ulceration and progressive loss of digits are common. All sensory modalities are affected, with distal limbs involved more severely than proximal. Anhidrosis may be present and may be manifest by recurrent fever. Associated abnormalities include mental retardation, deafness, and retinitis pigmentosa. The differential diagnosis includes hereditary ectodermal dysplasia, Lesch-Nyhan syndrome (Sec 8.24), infantile autism, the Riley-Day syndrome (Sec 21.28), and congenital indifference to pain.

Congenital Indifference to Pain. In this rare syndrome absence of appropriate responses to painful stimuli is found as an isolated abnormality. Failure to appreciate pain leads to repeated minor skin trauma and to burns. Acute surgical abdominal disorders and fractures may go undetected for a long time. Other sensory functions are intact. In some patients the condition has been associated with anhidrosis and mental defect. The cause of congenital indifference to pain is unknown. The condition is distinguished from congenital sensory neuropathy by the universal absence of pain sensation and by the preservation of touch, position, vibration, and temperature senses.

Asbury AK, Arnason BG, Adams RD: The inflammatory lesion in idiopathic polyneuritis. Its role in pathogenesis. Medicine 48:173, 1969.

Baxter DW, Olszewski J: Congenital universal indifference to pain. Brain 83:381, 1960.

Byers RK, Taft LT: Chronic multiple peripheral neuropathy in childhood. Pediatrics 20:517, 1957.

Colan RV, Snead OC, Or SJ, et al: Steroid-responsive polyneuropathy with subacute onset in childhood. J Pediatr 97:374, 1980.

Dyck PJ, Lambert EH: Lower motor and primary sensory neuron diseases with peroneal muscular atrophy. 1. Neurologic, genetic and electrophysiologic findings in hereditary polyneuropathies. Arch Neurol 18:603, 1968.

Gamstorp I: Encephalo-myelo-radiculo-neuropathy: Involvement of the CNS in children with Guillain-Barré-Strohl syndrome. Dev Med Child Neurol 16:654, 1974.

Haymaker W, Kernohan JW: The Landry-Guillain-Barré syndrome. Medicine 28:59, 1949.

Hughes RAC, Newsom-Davis JM, Perkin GD, et al: Controlled trial of prednisolone in acute polyneuropathy. Lancet 2:750, 1978.

Linarelli LG, Prichard JW: Congenital sensory neuropathy. Am J Dis Child 119:513, 1970.

Pinsky L, DiGeorge AM: Congenital familial sensory neuropathy with anhidrosis. J Pediatr 68:1, 1966.

Wiederholt WC, Mulder CW, Lambert EH: The Landry-Guillain-Barré-Strohl syndrome or polyradiculo-neuropathy: Historical review, report on 97 patients, and present concepts. Proc Staff Meetings Mayo Clinic 39:427, 1964.

22.4 MONONEUROPATHIES

Defects involving single peripheral nerves may be congenital or secondary to inflammation, trauma, or injection of irritant materials.

Congenital Ptosis. Congenital ptosis is probably secondary to faulty innervation of the levator palpebrae muscle. It is often transmitted by dominant inheritance. Drooping of 1 or both eyelids is noted in the neonatal period and persists throughout life. The ptosis is rarely complete. Occasionally, movements of the jaw will elevate the ptotic eyelid. This finding ("jaw winking" or Marcus Gunn phenomenon) is due to innervation of the levator palpebrae with an admixture of 3rd and 5th cranial nerve fibers.

Congenital ptosis has to be differentiated from myasthenia gravis, brain stem lesions, and ocular myopathy. Surgical correction for cosmetic reasons is indicated when the defect is severe.

Tolosa-Hunt Syndrome. *Oculomotor nerve palsy* consists of painful, unilateral paralysis of 1 or more oculomotor nerves (usually the 3rd) of unknown etiology. The onset is acute, with retroorbital pain and diplopia, and usually with ptosis and mydriasis on the affected side. Gradual improvement always occurs, but there may be repeated attacks. Distinction from ophthalmoplegic migraine may be difficult. Aneurysm of the internal carotid artery and parasellar neoplasms have to be excluded by appropriate studies; carotid angiography is usually required. A rapid response to corticosteroids is said to be characteristic.

Sixth Nerve Palsy. This may occur as an isolated congenital anomaly. There is inability to abduct the eye on the affected side. The abducens muscle may be replaced by a fibrous band that also prevents full adduction of the eye. Attempted adduction leads to retraction of the globe (Duane syndrome). The differentiation of congenital 6th nerve palsy from convergent strabismus may be difficult. In strabismus, however, the squinting eye will move fully after a period of patching.

Seventh (Facial) Nerve Palsy. This may be congenital or acquired.

Congenital Facial Nerve Palsy. The palsy is often partial; selective weakness of muscles innervated by the mandibular branch results in paralysis of the lower lip and the angle of the mouth. The unopposed action of the opposite lower facial muscles pulls the mouth toward the normal side (Fig 22–4). The cosmetic defect tends to be quite mild; other anomalies may be associated.

Bell Palsy. Bell palsy refers to 7th nerve paralysis of sudden onset and usually of obscure etiology. Otitis media and herpes zoster of the geniculate ganglion have been implicated in some instances. The facial weakness appears over a few hr, occasionally with associated pain in the ear on the affected side. The face is pulled toward the normal side; the nasolabial fold on the affected side is flattened, and the child is unable to close the eye. Attempted closure leads to upward deviation of the eye (Bell sign). Loss of taste may occur over the anterior two thirds of the tongue, and there may be hyperacusis due to involvement of the nerve to the stapedius muscle. Occasionally, recurrent attacks of 7th nerve weakness of obscure etiology are associated with edema of the lips (*Melkersson syndrome*).

The *differential diagnosis* includes tumor of the brain stem or temporal bone, demyelinating disease, basal skull fracture, otitis media, and mastoiditis. Therapy consists of protection of the cornea on the affected side by taping the eye in a closed position or by instillation of artificial tears into the conjunctival sac. ACTH and corticosteroids have been used to reduce inflammatory swelling of the facial nerve; there is some evidence of benefit. The incidence of permanent residual weakness is 10–20%.

Trauma to Peripheral Nerves. Trauma occurs rather frequently at birth (Erb palsy, Sec 7.25). Later in infancy or childhood peripheral nerves may be injured by pressure such as may occur from an improperly applied cast or restraint or from failure to position the limbs properly in a comatose child. The *peroneal nerve* is most frequently affected, damage leading to foot drop and to

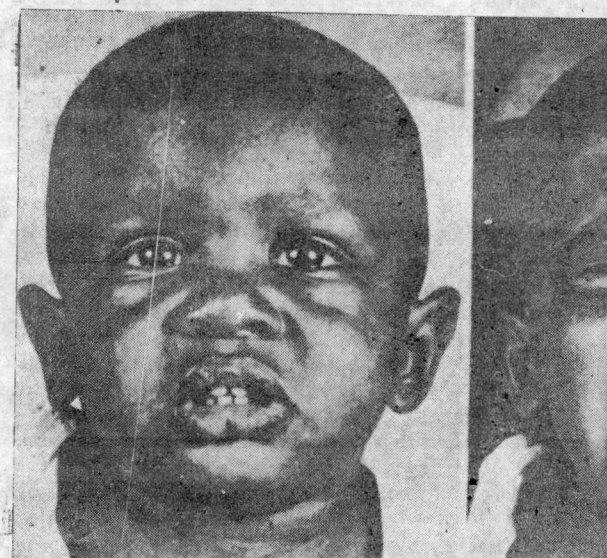

Figure 22–4 Congenital paralysis of left inferior angle of mouth. *A*, At rest, face is symmetrical. *B*, During crying the left labial angle does not depress, and *right* facial palsy may be misdiagnosed.

sensory impairment over the lateral aspect of the leg and dorsum of the foot. *Radial nerve* injury causes wrist drop. Paralysis of intrinsic hand muscles with claw-hand deformity is characteristic of *ulnar nerve* palsy.

Sciatic nerve injury by faulty intramuscular injection in the buttock is an important cause of mononeuropathy in early childhood. When such injury is severe, there is paralysis of knee flexion and of all movements below the knee as well as anesthesia over the foot and over the lateral aspect of the lower leg.

Pressure neuropathies are usually self-terminating if the nerve is protected from repeated compression. Lacerations of peripheral nerves require surgical suture of the severed nerve ends. Surgical lysis of adhesions has been recommended for postinjection injuries of the sciatic nerve when there is no improvement 3 mo after the injury. Permanent sciatic nerve damage in early childhood results in considerable disability, including arrest of growth of the affected limb.

Adour KK, et al: Prednisone treatment for idiopathic facial paralysis (Bell's palsy). N Engl J Med 287:1268, 1972.
Gilles FH, French JH: Postinjection sciatic nerve palsies in infants and children. J Pediatr 58:195, 1961.
Hoefnagel D, Penry JK: Partial facial paralysis in young children. N Engl J Med 262:1126, 1963.
Lloyd AVC, Jewitt DE, Still JDL: Facial paralysis in children with hypertension. Arch Dis Child 41:292, 1966.
McHugh HE, Sowden KA, Levitt MN: Facial paralysis and muscle agenesis in the newborn. Arch Otolaryngol 89:157, 1969.
Manning JJ, Adour KK: Facial paralysis in children. Pediatrics 49:102, 1972.
Paine RS: Facial paralysis in children. Pediatrics 19:303, 1957.
Pape KE, Pickering D: Asymmetric crying facies and other congenital anomalies. J Pediatr 81:21, 1972.
Terrence CF, Samaha FJ: The Tolosa-Hunt syndrome (painful ophthalmoplegia) in children. Dev Med Child Neurol 15:506, 1973.

22.5 DISEASES OF THE NEUROMUSCULAR JUNCTION

There are several disorders in which muscular weakness is caused by a defect in neuromuscular transmission. Normal transmission of the nerve impulse to muscle involves 3 steps: (1) release of acetylcholine at terminal nerve endings; (2) action of acetylcholine at receptor sites in the muscle membrane, leading to depolarization of this membrane; and (3) removal of excess released acetylcholine through hydrolysis by the enzyme cholinesterase. Blockade of neuromuscular transmission may result from interference with any of these steps.

Several toxins, such as those of botulinus and of the tick, act by preventing step 1. Step 2 is blocked by curare. The lesion in myasthenia gravis appears to lie at the muscle receptor sites. Step 3 is prevented by inhibitors of acetylcholinesterase, which include certain organic phosphate insecticides (Sec 28.16) and drugs such as neostigmine. Poisoning by these substances leads to excessive accumulation of acetylcholine in the synaptic cleft and to paralysis by persistent depolarization of the muscle membrane (depolarized block).

Myasthenia Gravis. Myasthenia gravis is uncommon in childhood, but prompt recognition and proper therapy may be lifesaving. The disorder appears to be secondary to an autoimmune reaction directed against acetylcholine receptors in muscle. Both circulating antibodies and a lymphocyte-mediated immune response to acetylcholine receptors have been identified. Myasthenia can be passively transferred from affected patients to mice by repeated injection of immunoglobulin fractions derived from the patient's serum. Other immunologic disorders may coexist, in particular, thymic hyperplasia, thymoma, and lupus erythematosus. Three myasthenic syndromes occur in childhood: *transient neonatal myasthenia gravis, persistent neonatal myasthenia gravis,* and *juvenile myasthenia gravis.*

Transient Neonatal Myasthenia Gravis. This is seen only in infants whose mothers have myasthenia. The disease in the mother may be mild or unrecognized. The infant is weak and hypotonic, with poor suck, feeble respiratory effort, and ptosis. Untreated, these infants may die within hours or days or may gradually improve. Recovery occurs within 2–4 wk.

Persistent Neonatal Myasthenia Gravis. In the neonatal period, symptoms are identical to those of the transient form, but there is no indication of myasthenia in the mother. More than 1 sibling may be affected. The disease persists throughout life. The eyelids and extraocular muscles tend to be most severely affected.

Juvenile Myasthenia Gravis. Onset usually occurs after the age of 10 yr; girls are affected 6 times as often as boys. Ptosis and double vision due to weakness of extraocular muscles are the most common initial symptoms. Neck, facial, bulbar, and intercostal muscles are also frequently affected. Paralysis of virtually all muscles occurs in the most severe form. A striking feature of the weakness is its amelioration after rest and its exacerbation on repetitive movement. Sudden, life-threatening exacerbations known as *myasthenic crises* may occur during intercurrent infections or during stresses such as minor surgical procedures.

The diagnosis is based on the characteristic distribution of weakness and on the demonstration of progressive weakness after repetitive or sustained muscular contractions. The latter can often be brought out by having the patient maintain upward gaze, which leads to progressively increasing ptosis. The diagnosis is confirmed by the response to anticholinesterase drugs. Edrophonium chloride (Tensilon), 0.2 mg/kg intravenously, or neostigmine, 0.04 mg/kg intramuscularly, may be used. Increase in strength after intravenous edrophonium chloride is almost immediate but lasts for less than 5 min. A more prolonged response is obtained with neostigmine. Atropine sulfate, 0.01 mg/kg, should be readily available during the neostigmine test and should be given if the patient develops signs of excessive parasympathetic stimulation, such as abdominal cramps, salivation, or bradycardia. Electrical testing of neuromuscular transmission is a helpful adjunct to diagnosis; there is progressive decrease in muscle response on repetitive stimulation of nerve at low rates. The possible presence of thymoma should be explored.

Anticholinesterase drugs are effective therapeutic agents. Pyridostigmine bromide (Mestinon) is the least toxic. The beginning dose is about 30 mg orally every 4 hr in the older child and 5 mg every 4 hr for the infant. Neostigmine (Prostigmin) or ambenonium chloride (Mytelase) may be used instead of or in addition to pyridostigmine. The dosage of the anticholinesterase drug is gradually increased until the weakness is controlled or until symptoms of parasympathetic stimulation occur such as lacrimation, salivation, vomiting, diarrhea, abdominal cramps, or bradycardia. Further increase in dosage may be dangerous and may actually exacerbate weakness because of excessive accumulation of acetylcholine at the neuromuscular junction (see above). At times it may be difficult to be certain whether increase in weakness is due to worsening of the myasthenia or to overdosage of anticholinesterase drugs. The edrophonium test is helpful in the differentiation; edrophonium will improve myasthenic symptoms but will transiently increase weakness due to excess of anticholinesterase drugs. The parents of a child with myasthenia gravis should be warned of the possibility of sudden exacerbation at times of stress and of the need for immediate medical attention in such an event.

If possible, the therapy of severe myasthenia should be supervised by physicians with wide experience in the management of this disease. Intermittent assisted ventilation and tracheostomy may be needed. Thymectomy or corticosteroid therapy may be indicated in intractable, severe myasthenia.

The prognosis of myasthenia gravis in childhood is somewhat better than in later life. With optimal therapy most children can lead near-normal lives. Complete remissions occur in about 25% of affected children.

Appel SH, Almon RR, Levy N: Acetylcholine receptor antibodies in myasthenia gravis. N Engl J Med 293:760, 1975.
Brunner NG, Namba T, Grob D: Corticosteroids in management of severe generalized myasthenia gravis. Neurology 22:603, 1972.
Mackay RI: Congenital myasthenia gravis. Arch Dis Child 26:289, 1951.
Millichap JG, Dodge PR: Diagnosis and treatment of myasthenia gravis in infancy, childhood and adolescence. Neurology 10:1007, 1960.
Richman DP, Patrick J, Arnason BGW: Cellular immunity in myasthenia gravis. N Engl J Med 294:694, 1976.
Snead OC, Benton JW, Dwyer D, et al: Juvenile myasthenia gravis. Neurology 30:732, 1980.
Teng P, Osserman KE: Studies in myasthenia gravis: Neonatal and juvenile types. A report of 21 and a review of 188 cases. J Mt Sinai Hosp (NY) 23:711, 1956.
Toyka KV, et al: Myasthenia gravis: Passive transfer from man to mouse. Science 190:397, 1975.

22.6 DISEASES OF MUSCLE

Skeletal muscle is affected in a large number of degenerative, metabolic, and inflammatory disorders. Degeneration of muscle fibers occurs in most of these, and, in the chronic state, there is often replacement of muscle by fibrous connective tissue and fat. Proximal muscles tend to be affected more severely than distal ones and lower extremities more than the upper ones. Affected children often have a waddling gait, are unable to run, and have difficulty climbing stairs and standing up from the sitting position. The tendon reflexes are usually depressed in proportion to the degree of weakness. There are no sensory abnormalities.

Measurement of serum enzyme activity, especially that of creatine phosphokinase (CPK), is often a helpful laboratory test in the differential diagnosis of muscle disease. The enzyme, which catalyzes the reaction, phosphocreatine + ADP → creatine + ATP, is present primarily in brain and muscle tissues. Excessive leakage of the enzyme into the extracellular spaces and into blood occurs in several diffuse muscle diseases, especially in the muscular dystrophies. Serum lactic dehydrogenase and glutamic-oxaloacetic transaminase are also often elevated in muscle disease, but the wide distribution of these enzymes in other tissues, including liver, makes these tests less specific. A muscle biopsy is usually needed for the definitive diagnosis of muscle disease.

Inflammatory Diseases of Muscle. Inflammation of muscle occurs in a number of infectious illnesses, especially in trichinosis (Sec 10.123), toxoplasmosis, and coxsackievirus infections. It also is a component of the collagen diseases (Sec 9.58), including dermatomyositis, lupus erythematosus, polyarteritis nodosa, and rheumatoid arthritis.

Polymyositis. Diffuse inflammation of muscles, as an isolated abnormality of unknown cause, is known as polymyositis. It presents progressive, principally proximal, muscular weakness and pain. The neck muscles are frequently affected, and the child may have difficulty lifting the head or supporting it in the upright position. Laboratory evidence of inflammation includes elevation of sedimentation rate and of the leukocyte count, but their absence does not rule out the diagnosis. The serum enzymes are usually elevated. Muscle biopsy shows degeneration and attempted regeneration of muscle fibers and lymphocytic infiltration. Differentiation from muscular dystrophy or dermatomyositis may be difficult. Polymyositis may represent a forme fruste of dermatomyositis, but the histologic appearance of muscle differs somewhat in the 2 conditions. Vasculitis is prominent in dermatomyositis but usually absent in polymyositis. The prognosis is somewhat better in polymyositis. Therapy with a corticosteroid frequently leads to remission, but relapse may occur following withdrawal of the drug.

Myositis Ossificans Progressiva. This is a rare progressive disease of connective tissue and muscle of unknown etiology. It has been described in siblings, including identical twins, and in successive generations. An autosomal dominant pattern of inheritance with variable expression has been suggested. Boys are more commonly affected than girls at a ratio of 2–3:1.

Pathologic changes depend on the age of the lesions. During the early stages localized areas of edema and inflammatory cell infiltrates are found in muscle and tendons. Later, granulation tissue replaces the areas of inflammation and, eventually, sheets of cartilage and of bone are laid down in involved areas.

About 75% of affected children have congenital malformations, most commonly microdactyly and ankylosis of phalanges of the great toes; there may also be small thumbs, polydactyly, incurving of digits, webbing of toes, deformity of the ears, deafness, and absence of teeth. The same anomalies may occur in relatives who do not develop the progressive connective tissue and muscle lesions. Age of onset of these lesions varies from birth to late childhood. A typical lesion evolves through 3 stages: (1) a localized, often hot and tender doughy swelling of soft tissue may follow mild local trauma; (2) after a few days evidences of inflammation subside, and the affected area becomes indurated; and (3) the lesion becomes ossified. New lesions appear periodically, especially in the cervical and dorsal regions. Torticollis, due to lesions in the sternocleidomastoid, may be the initial feature. Eventually, there is widespread ossification of tendons and fascia. The spine and the joints of the extremities become ankylosed (Fig 22–5). The masseter and mandibular joints are likely to be affected, and difficulty in chewing results. Spicules of bone may be extruded through the skin. Severe incapacitation and death from respiratory failure often occur in the early adult years; cases of survival to old age have been reported. The incidence of osteosarcoma is increased.

The process may at times remain localized to 1 area, usually following trauma to soft tissue (*myositis ossificans circumscripta*). Widespread calcification of muscle also

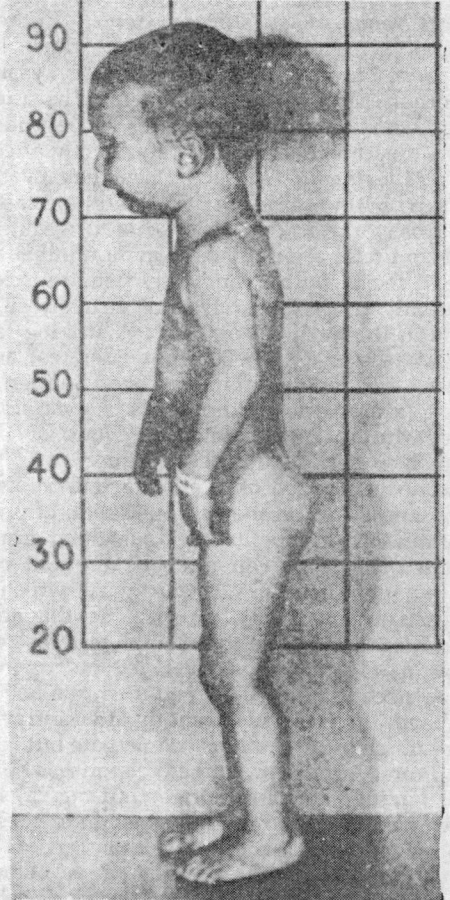

Figure 22–5 Myositis ossificans progressiva. No roentgenographically demonstrable calcification, but typical histologic changes. Note posture and rigidity of neck and back.

may occur in chronic polymyositis and dermatomyositis.

Laboratory studies are of little help in the diagnosis. Serum calcium, phosphate, and alkaline phosphatase values are normal as are those of creatine phosphokinase and the other serum enzymes. Analysis of the bone in the soft tissues has shown no difference from normal bone.

Therapy is unsatisfactory; corticosteroids and ACTH have been reported to decrease the rate of progression in a few cases. It is doubtful that they have an effect on the eventual outcome.

Endocrine Myopathies. Muscular weakness occurs in some endocrine disorders.

Hyperthyroid Myopathy. This is an uncommon complication of thyrotoxicosis. Ptosis, bifacial weakness, and proximal weakness of limb muscles are manifestations. Some of the usual signs of hyperthyroidism may be masked by the weakness; tachycardia, excessive sweating, and enlargement of the thyroid gland, however, are manifest. The tendon reflexes remain brisk, in contrast to those in most other forms of myopathy. The weakness disappears slowly after correction of the hyperthyroid state.

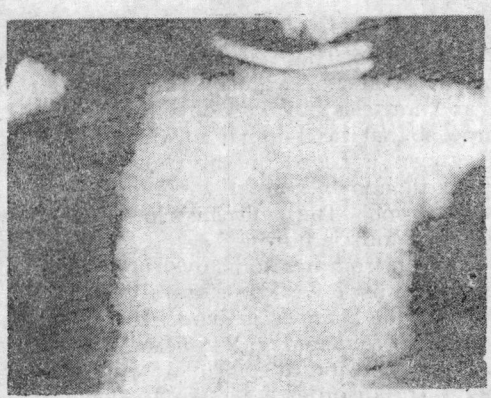

Figure 22–6 Congenital absence of left pectoral muscle. Note absence of anterior axillary fold and low placement of nipple.

Hypothyroidism. Hypothyroidism in the infant is associated with weakness and hypotonia. In the older child with myxedema, weakness, slowness of muscular contraction and relaxation, and, at times, muscular hypertrophy (Debré-Sémélaigne syndrome) are present. The combination of weakness and hypertrophy may suggest the diagnosis of muscular dystrophy.

Corticosteroid Myopathy. This may complicate Cushing disease but occurs more commonly during therapy with high doses of synthetic steroids. Weakness is most marked in hip girdle muscles, leading to a waddling gait and to difficulty in standing and in climbing stairs. Knee jerks are depressed. Muscle wasting may be marked. Myopathic changes seen in muscle tissue are usually mild, even when weakness is profound. Recovery after discontinuance of steroid therapy is slow, requiring months.

Hyperparathyroidism. Hyperparathyroidism leads to weakness and hyporeflexia, which appear to be secondary to hypercalcemia; they are readily reversed after correction of the metabolic abnormality by parathyroidectomy (Sec 18.20).

Congenital Defects of Muscle. *Congenital Absence of Muscle.* Failure of muscle development may be widespread, leading to immobility of multiple joints or arthrogryposis multiplex congenita (Sec 23.18). More commonly, congenital absence is limited to 1 muscle. Absence of the sternal head of the pectoralis major is a common anomaly (Fig 22–6), occasionally with syndactyly on the same side (see Poland Syndrome, Sec 6.32). Absence of the pectoral muscle is found with increased frequency in children with muscular dystrophy. Congenital absence of abdominal muscles is often associated with anomalies of the urinary tract (Sec 16.57).

Congenital Torticollis. Torticollis or *wryneck* is due to shortening or contracture of the sternocleidomastoid muscle on 1 side. The head is tilted toward the side of the contracture, and the chin is turned toward the opposite side (Fig 22–7). Considerable resistance is encountered in attempts to correct the deviation. A firm mass may be palpable in the involved muscle. The cause is unclear; birth trauma has long been incriminated, but torticollis has been observed at cesarean section, suggesting a prenatal cause in some cases.

The differential diagnosis of congenital torticollis in-

cludes head tilt secondary to malformation of the cervical spine, such as occurs in the Klippel-Feil anomaly, and fracture or dislocation of cervical vertebrae. Roentgenograms of the cervical spine should be obtained to rule these out. In the older child, head tilt may also occur secondary to strabismus, dystonia, posterior fossa or cervical cord tumor, myositis ossificans, cervical adenitis, or hiatus hernia. Most infants with congenital torticollis improve with simple muscle-stretching exercises. Persistent torticollis leads to asymmetric development of the face and skull (Fig 22–7) and may require surgical section of the affected muscle for a good cosmetic outcome.

Congenital Myopathies. This group includes several rare inherited disorders in which weakness and hypotonia are present from infancy. (See the "floppy infant," Table 22–1.) The correct diagnosis of these disorders is important from a prognostic standpoint. In general, the outlook for a normal life span and useful existence is good, in contrast to that of the hypotonic infant with Werdnig-Hoffmann disease or with congenital muscular dystrophy. Identification of the congenital myopathies is made by study of biopsied skeletal muscle.

CENTRAL CORE DISEASE. The center of each muscle fiber stains abnormally but homogeneously. Electron microscopy shows a decrease of mitochondria and of sarcoplastic reticulum in the central portion of the affected fibers.

NEMALINE MYOPATHY. Nemaline myopathy derives its name from the presence of threadlike structures within muscle cells. Electron microscopy indicates that these are the result of abnormalities of the Z bands of myofibrils.

Mitochondrial Myopathies. Several myopathies have been described in which alteration of muscle mitochondria is the most prominent pathologic finding.

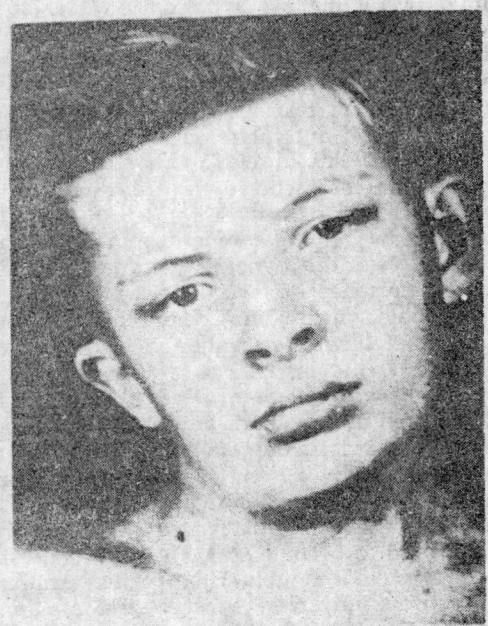

Figure 22–7 Congenital torticollis, untreated until the age of 12 yr. Note wryneck and asymmetry of face.

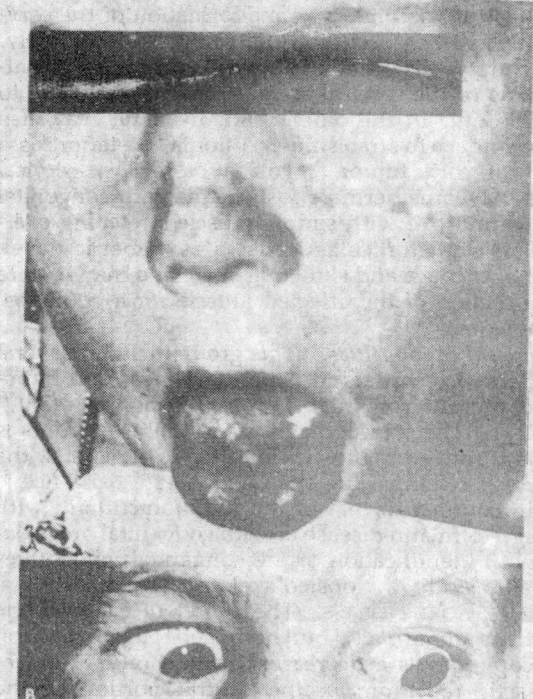

Figure 22–8 *A,* Myotonia following tap of the right tongue with a reflex hammer. *B,* Myotonia of the eyelid in a child with the hyperkalemic form of familial periodic paralysis. The lid remains retracted when the child is asked to look down.

Mitochondria may be extremely numerous, increased in size, or both. Weakness and hypotonia may be present from infancy and may become episodic later in childhood.

Myotonia. Myotonia is a symptom of a variety of muscle diseases, including myotonic dystrophy, the hyperkalemic form of familial periodic paralysis, and glycogen storage disease of muscle. It is defined as abnormal slowness in relaxation of muscle following voluntary or induced muscular contraction. Clinically, it is manifest by inability to relax the hand grip and by visible maintained contraction following direct stimulation of a muscle by sharp tap (Fig 22–8A). The latter is demonstrated by tapping a superficial muscle group such as the tongue or the thenar eminence with a reflex hammer. The presence of myotonia is confirmed by electromyography, which shows persistence of muscle action potentials following relaxation of voluntary contraction (myotonic discharges).

Myotonia Congenita (Thomsen Disease). In this disorder, transmitted by dominant inheritance, myotonia occurs as an isolated finding. It may be manifest in infancy as slow swallowing and gagging due to failure of normal relaxation of oropharyngeal muscles or, later in childhood, as inability to release a firm hand grip. The muscles tend to become stiff when the child first attempts to carry out a motion. This stiffness gradually subsides when the movement is repeated a few times. For example, an affected child may have difficulty initiating the act of walking. The 1st few steps tend to

be slow and awkward. After a few sec the gait becomes normal, or nearly so. These symptoms are worse during emotional upset and on exposure to cold. Strength is normal, and muscles are well developed, often unusually large, so that the child has an athletic appearance.

The diagnosis is based on the clinical and electromyographic demonstration of myotonia. Serum enzymes are normal. The only histologic alteration is hypertrophy of muscle fibers.

Differentiation from myotonic dystrophy is based on the absence of muscle weakness or atrophy and on the lack of dystrophic changes in biopsied muscle tissue. Therapy with procainamide or quinidine sulfate lessens the myotonia and is indicated when there is functional impairment. The disorder is benign and may improve with age.

The Periodic Paralyses. In this group of illnesses weakness is intermittent, with complete or nearly complete recovery of strength between attacks. The group includes also muscle phosphorylase deficiency (McArdle disease, Sec 8.21).

Hyperkalemic Periodic Paralysis. *Adynamia episodica hereditaria or paramyotonia* is transmitted as a dominant trait, with more severe expression in the male. Onset occurs during early childhood and sometimes in infancy. Rest after strong exertion appears to precipitate paralytic episodes. Weakness develops rapidly and lasts up to a few hr. Legs are most severely affected; respiration is usually spared. Myotonia is common and may persist between attacks. It tends to be most marked in the eyelids, with lid lag on downward gaze (Fig 22–8B).

During the attack the serum concentration of potassium is often elevated, but repeated measurements in several episodes may be needed to demonstrate it. An oral potassium load of 2–3 gm may be used to precipitate an attack but should be given only with monitoring of the ECG. Acetazolamide prevents recurrent paralysis. Severely affected patients eventually develop mild persistent weakness and dystrophic changes in muscle.

Hypokalemic Periodic Paralysis. *Familial periodic paralysis* also is transmitted in a dominant manner, with symptoms more severe in males. In contrast to the hyperkalemic form, 1st attacks usually occur in late childhood or early adolescence. Large carbohydrate meals or rest after exertion may precipitate paralysis. Typically, the patient awakens paralyzed on the morning after a day of heavy exercise capped by a large evening meal. During the attack the limbs are flaccid and areflexic. Respiration may be affected. Cardiac arrhythmias may include ventricular premature beats and ventricular tachycardia. An attack may last longer than 24 hr. Serum potassium levels are usually low, 2–3 mEq/l, during the paralytic phase. The basic defect is unknown. Patients with repeated severe attacks develop fixed weakness and dystrophic changes in muscle. Therapy during an attack consists of oral potassium chloride, beginning with a dose of 2–3 gm. Acetazolamide reduces the frequency of attacks.

Paroxysmal Myoglobinuria (Idiopathic Myoglobinuria). Idiopathic myoglobinurias are a heterogeneous group of entities in which attacks of paralysis with myoglobinuria occur spontaneously or following strenuous exercise. Dominant and X-linked inheritance have been reported. Affected muscles, often of the calf and thigh, become painful and swollen during an attack. The urine becomes dark red or brown. The myoglobinuria may cause renal tubular necrosis, with death from renal failure.

The diagnosis is confirmed by demonstration of myoglobin in urine. A positive benzidine test in urine free of red cells suggests the presence of myoglobin, especially when a concomitant serum sample is clear (free of hemoglobin). Definite differentiation from hemoglobin is made on spectrophotometry. Paroxysmal myoglobinuria must be distinguished from McArdle disease (Sec 8.21) and from the myoglobinuria which may occur in a normal person following severe unaccustomed exertion or crushing injury of muscle. Myoglobinuria after heavy exertion occurs occasionally in pseudohypertrophic (Duchenne) muscular dystrophy.

Treatment consists of bed rest, assisted ventilation when necessary, and hydration to minimize the danger of renal injury.

The Muscular Dystrophies. The muscular dystrophies are a group of familial disorders in which degeneration of muscle fibers occurs. Classification is based on age of onset, rate of progression, distribution of muscular involvement, and mode of inheritance.

Pseudohypertrophic Muscular Dystrophy. The *childhood* or *Duchenne* form of muscular dystrophy is the most common of this group of muscle diseases; the incidence is about 0.14/1000 children. Its classic form occurs only in boys, with a history of X-linked inheritance in about 50% of propositi. The remainder appear to represent new mutations. The diagnosis is rarely made prior to the age of 3 yr. A history of slow motor development with late onset of sitting, walking, and running is usually obtained, however, indicating a

much earlier onset. Waddling gait, difficulty in climbing stairs, and hypertrophy of calf muscles are the common presenting findings. Occasionally, muscles other than the calf, including deltoid, brachioradialis, or tongue, are increased in bulk. Early in the disease the hypertrophied muscles have considerable strength, but later the enlarged muscles are often weak (pseudohypertrophy) since much of the increased bulk is due to fatty infiltration. The hypertrophic calf muscles are stronger than the anterior leg muscles; accordingly, toe walking and contracture of the heel cords are common. Weakness of pelvic girdle muscles results in characteristic waddling, lordotic gait, and difficulty in arising from the floor. The child with moderately severe muscular dystrophy demonstrates Gowers sign: in getting up from the floor he first rolls to the prone position, kneels, and then raises himself to standing by pushing with his hands against shins, knees, and thighs (Fig 22–9). Weakness of shoulder girdle muscles can be brought out by lifting the child by means of hands placed under the axillae. He will slip through the hands rather than support himself by adducting the arms. Eventually the child becomes unable to lift his arms above his head. Profound muscle atrophy occurs in late stages. Ambulation usually becomes impossible by the age of 12 yr, and death occurs prior to 20 yr in 75% of patients. The majority of patients have cardiomyopathy; it is occasionally the cause of sudden death. Instances of X-linked pseudohypertrophic muscular dystrophy occur with onset in late childhood and prolonged survival (Becker muscular dystrophy). The mean IQ of children with Duchenne muscular dystrophy is 80; 25% have frank mental defect.

The *differential diagnosis* of Duchenne muscular dystrophy includes the late infantile form of Werdnig-Hoffmann disease and such diseases of muscle as the

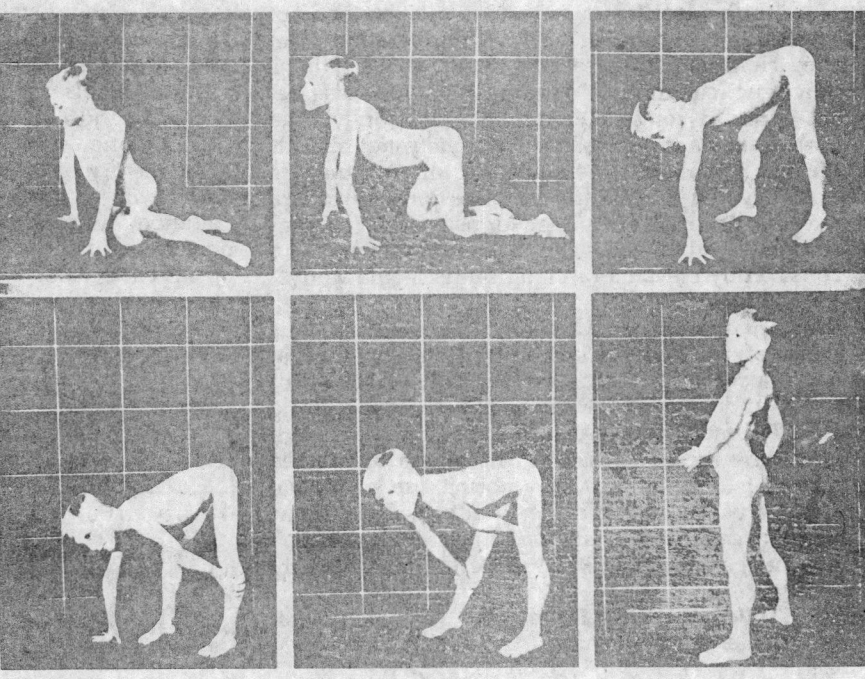

Figure 22–9 A child 7 yr of age with pseudohypertrophic muscular dystrophy, showing characteristic manner of rising from the floor (Gowers sign). The last picture shows the standing position with the severe lordosis.

endocrine myopathies, glycogen storage disease of muscle, and polymyositis. Occasionally, the presence of heel cord contractures and of toe walking suggests cerebral palsy, but the spasticity and hyperreflexia of cerebral palsy are absent in muscular dystrophy.

The *diagnosis* of Duchenne muscular dystrophy is confirmed by measurement of serum enzymes, by electromyography, and by muscle biopsy. The serum enzymes, especially CPK, often are increased to more than 10 times normal, even in infancy prior to onset of clinical weakness. Electromyographic changes consist primarily of decreases in amplitude and duration of motor unit potentials. Histologic changes in muscle include degeneration of muscle fibers, with variation in fiber size and central nuclei and replacement of muscle fibers by fat and connective tissue. The diagnosis can be established at birth by measurement of CPK levels; intrauterine diagnosis is not yet possible. Identification of female carriers of the disease cannot be achieved with certainty, but mild to moderate elevations of serum CPK are found in 60–80% of known carriers; this finding is more likely during childhood than in later life.

There is no effective treatment for muscular dystrophy. The children should be kept active and ambulatory as long as possible. Strenuous exercise is to be avoided since it may hasten the breakdown of muscle fibers. Occasionally, surgical lengthening of heel cords may improve ambulation, but prolonged bed rest after orthopedic procedures may hasten muscle atrophy. Genetic counseling is an important aspect of management. With X-linked inheritance, male siblings of an affected child have a 50% chance of being afflicted; the sisters have a 50% chance of being carriers.

Congenital Muscular Dystrophy. This autosomal recessive disorder is characterized by hypotonia and weakness in infancy and should be considered in the differential diagnosis of the "floppy infant" (Table 22–1). The onset occurs in utero. Occasionally, profound muscle atrophy, contractures, and limitation of joint movements are present at birth. Differentiation from Werdnig-Hoffmann disease is difficult. Fasciculations of the tongue, common in Werdnig-Hoffmann disease, do not occur in congenital muscular dystrophy. The tendon reflexes are depressed but usually not absent. Muscles of respiration, including the diaphragm, are affected. Severely ill infants die of respiratory failure prior to the age of 1 yr; milder forms may have compatibility with prolonged survival. Serum enzymes are not consistently elevated, although muscle shows dystrophic changes.

Facioscapulohumeral Muscular Dystrophy. This mild form of dystrophy has autosomal dominant transmission. Onset usually occurs in the 2nd decade, with weakness and atrophy of facial and shoulder girdle muscles. The face is expressionless; forceful eye closure and whistling are not possible. The illness progresses slowly and is compatible with a normal life span. The diagnosis is based on the clinical findings and pattern of inheritance. Biopsy of affected muscles shows dystrophic changes. Serum CPK may be normal or mildly elevated.

Limb-Girdle Muscular Dystrophy. This heterogeneous disorder is characterized by slowly progressive muscular dystrophy, usually autosomal recessive. Onset may occur in late childhood, adolescence, or adulthood. The pelvic girdle muscles are most commonly affected.

Ocular Myopathy. This dystrophic process affects principally the extraocular muscles. Onset occurs usually during childhood or adolescence, with progressive ptosis and limitation of eye movements; occasionally, weakness extends to facial and neck muscles. There is no clear inheritance pattern. This disorder must be differentiated from myasthenia gravis and from cranial nerve palsies due to brain stem tumor.

A progressive ophthalmoplegia beginning in childhood or adolescence is associated with atypical pigmentary degeneration of the retina and heart block (*Kearns-Sayre syndrome*). Progressive ataxia, nerve deafness, growth retardation, and delayed sexual maturation are common. Changes in muscle consist of large subsarcolemmal collections of abnormal mitochondria. There is no evidence that the syndrome is genetic in origin. Sudden death is due to the cardiac conduction defect and may be prevented by use of a cardiac pacemaker.

Myotonic Dystrophy. Myotonic dystrophy has usually been thought to have its onset in adulthood but the onset begins in infancy or childhood with considerable frequency. Its transmission is autosomal dominant. When the onset occurs in childhood, the mother is apt to have the disorder also; thus it seems that a factor in the intrauterine environment influences the severity of expression. Hypotonia and poor sucking ability may be present at birth. Developmental delay is noted later in infancy as is mental retardation. In early childhood muscle weakness and atrophy are found principally in the facial, jaw, and temporalis muscles; bilateral ptosis is common. Myotonia may be demonstrated by percussion of muscle, by electromyography, or by the child's inability to relax a hand grip (see Myotonia Congenita). Weakness and atrophy of limb muscles, often distal in distribution, become evident in later childhood and adolescence. Cataracts, baldness, and testicular atrophy are characteristic of the adult form of the disease.

The diagnosis is based on the demonstration of myotonia along with characteristic distribution of weakness, history of dominant inheritance, and findings of dystrophic changes in muscle. The prognosis of the childhood form of the disease must be guarded. Mental defect is usually present, and the muscle weakness is apt to be a major handicap by early adulthood. Treatment with procainamide or quinidine is indicated if the myotonia leads to functional impairment.

PETER R. HUTTENLOCHER

Berenberg RA, Pellock JM, DiMauro S, et al: "Ophthalmoplegia plus" or Kearns-Sayre syndrome? Ann Neurol 1:37, 1977.
Byers RK, Bergman AB, Jospeh MC: Steroid myopathy. Pediatrics 29:26, 1962.
Dodge PR, Gamstorp I, Byers RK, et al: Myotonic dystrophy in infancy and childhood. Pediatrics 35:3, 1965.
Dowben RM, Vawter GF, et al: Polymyositis and other diseases resembling muscular dystrophy. Arch Intern Med 115:584, 1965.

Dubowitz V: Intellectual impairment in muscular dystrophy. Arch Dis Child 40:296, 1965.

Dubowitz V: Muscle Disorders in Childhood. Philadelphia, WB Saunders, 1978.

Engel WK, et al: Central core disease—an investigation of a rare muscle cell abnormality. Brain 84:167, 1961.

Favara BE, Vawter GF, et al: Familial paroxysmal rhabdomyolysis in children. Am J Med 42:196, 1967.

Frame B, et al: Myopathy in primary hyperparathyroidism. Ann Intern Med 68:1022, 1968.

Gonatas NK, Shy GM, Godfrey EH: Nemaline myopathy: The origin of nemaline structures. N Engl J Med 274:535, 1966.

Harper PS, Dyken PR: Early-onset dystrophia myotonica. Evidence supporting a maternal environmental factor. Lancet 1:53, 1972.

Illingworth RS: Myositis ossificans progressiva (Munchmeyer disease). Arch Dis Child 46:264, 1971.

Jackson CE, Strehler DA: Limb-girdle muscular dystrophy: Clinical manifestations and detection of preclinical disease. Pediatrics 41:495, 1968.

Layzer RB, Lovelace RE, Rowland LP: Hyperkalemic periodic paralysis. Arch Neurol 16:455, 1967.

Levitt LP, Rose LI, Dawson DM: Hypokalemic periodic paralysis with arrhythmia. N Engl J Med 286:253, 1972.

McArdle B: Familial periodic paralysis. Br Med Bull 12:226, 1956.

Najjar SS, Nachman HS: Kocher-Debré-Sémélaigne syndrome: Hypothyroidism with muscular "hypertrophy." J Pediatr 66:901, 1965.

Pearson CM: The periodic paralyses: Differential features and pathological observations in permanent myopathic weakness. Brain 87:391, 1964.

Ramsey I: Thyrotoxic muscle disease. Postgrad Med J 44:385, 1968.

Resnick JS, Engel WK, Griggs RC, et al: Acetazolamide prophylaxis in hypokalemic periodic paralysis. N Engl J Med 278:582, 1968.

Shy GM, Gonatas NK, Perez M: Two childhood myopathies with abnormal mitochondria. 1. Megaconial myopathy. 2. Pleoconial myopathy. Brain 89:133, 1966.

Smith HL, Amick LD, Johnson WW: Detection of subclinical and carrier states in Duchenne muscular dystrophy. J Pediatr 69:67, 1966.

Thompson CE: Polymyositis in children. Clin Pediatr 7:24, 1968.

Vignos PJ Jr, Bowling GF, Watkins MP: Polymyositis. Effect of corticosteroids on final results. Arch Intern Med 114:263, 1964.

Walton J: Disorders of Voluntary Muscle. Ed 3. Edinburgh, Churchill, Livingstone, 1974.

Zellweger H, Afifi A, McCormick WF, et al: Severe congenital muscular dystrophy. J Dis Child 114:591, 1967.

Zundel WS, Tyler FH: The muscular dystrophies. N Engl J Med 273:537, 1965.

23.1 ORTHOPEDIC PROBLEMS

In this section, musculoskeletal problems will be presented by anatomic region and according to the frequency with which they are encountered. The problems commonly faced by pediatricians are grouped by age. Neoplasms of bone are discussed in Sec 15.13 to 15.15; infections of bone in Sec 10.14.

23.2 THE FEET AND TOES

The Infant

The foot of the normal infant at birth is proportionately longer and thinner than that of the older child, and the joints of the ankle and foot are very supple. The foot can be dorsiflexed so that the top of the foot touches the tibia anteriorly, plantar flexed so that the dorsum of the forefoot is parallel with the tibia, and inverted or everted in the hindpart 45°. The forefoot should be flexible enough to be moved into 45° of adduction or abduction.

The feet of a newborn infant may appear to be in abnormal positions, but if the feet can be moved through the range of motion described above, there is no need for concern. Such "positional" foot configurations resolve spontaneously.

In-toeing. This condition is common in newborn infants. It may be due to inturning of the forepart of the foot (i.e., metatarsus varus, see below) or inturning of the entire foot (i.e., medial tibial torsion). Both conditions are aggravated by sleeping face down or crawling with the feet and toes turned inward. With standing and walking, in-toeing in which the entire foot turns inward diminishes. In general, if the amount of in-toeing is greater than 45° at 3 mo, 30° at 9 mo, or 20° at 1 yr, orthopedic evaluation should be considered.

Treatment usually employs some method of holding the feet turned outward during sleeping hours. This can be achieved in a number of ways, from simply pinning or sewing the pajama legs together to sewing each half of a wristwatch strap to the backs of soft shoes. The most commonly used device is a bar as long as the pelvis is wide attached to shoes. Six–12 mo of treatment is usually satisfactory. Children over 1.5 yr of age often will not tolerate the restrictions of the nighttime footwear and are best left alone until after about the age of 3, when they may again use a night brace.

Out-toeing. Out-toeing may slightly delay walking since standing with the feet externally rotated is unstable. It is usually the entire leg that points outward rather than just the foot. Correction of out-toeing is usually spontaneous but is hastened by exercises. The child's thighs are grasped above the knee, rotated medially, and held at maximum medial rotation for a count of 5. This is repeated 5 times at each diaper change. In addition, the legs of the pajamas can be sewn or pinned together to prevent sleeping in the "frog position."

Metatarsus Varus (Metatarsus Adductus). In the normal foot a line along the middle of the heel should run through the 2nd toe (see Fig 23–1). Many infants are born with the front part of the foot turned inward. If the foot becomes fixed in such a position, proper fit of shoes may be a lifelong problem.

If the forefoot can be abducted past the midline but less than 30° beyond, exercises provided by the parents at each diaper change are usually sufficient treatment. Stretching can be done by holding the heel in neutral position with the thumb and index finger of 1 hand while moving the forefoot into abduction with the other hand, where it is held for a count of 5, repeated 5 times. Parents need encouragement to be moderately vigorous with the exercises. Since pushing on the great toe can create hallux valgus, the pressure should be over the 1st metatarsal head. If the forepart of the foot cannot be moved beyond the neutral point, the infant should be referred for orthopedic care. The feet are stretched by manipulation and held with casts, a procedure that is repeated at approximately weekly intervals. Casting is usually followed by the use of outflare shoes until the child is walking.

Clubfoot. The term clubfoot is used for a number of congenital anomalies of the foot. The most common (about 95% of clubfeet) is an equinovarus deformity. This deformity has 3 elements: the ankle is in equinus; the subtalar joint is in varus; and the mid and foreparts of the foot are in varus. If this form of clubfoot is not treated, further stiffening occurs in the abnormal position, with secondary changes in osseous development.

Early treatment is critical and should be started within the 1st hours after birth since the joints of the foot are maximally flexible at that time. The feet are manipulated to the position of maximum correction and held there by casts or adhesive taping. Manipulation and casting are repeated every few days for 1–2 wk and then at 1–2 wk intervals. In the past, emphasis was given to manipulation and casting for the entire course of therapy, and operative treatment was viewed as a mark of failure. Manipulation against very thickened ligaments, however, leads to distortion of the cartilaginous anlage of the bones with permanent damage. If manipulation becomes ineffective, surgical release of the Achilles

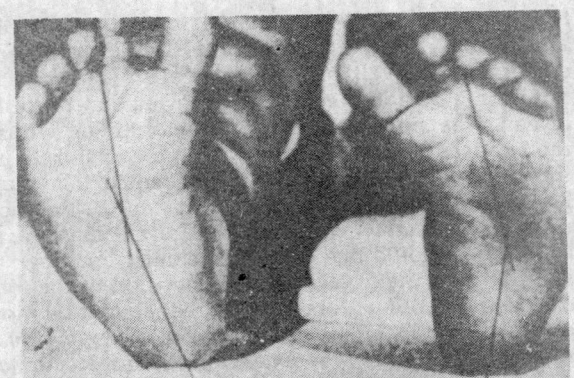

Figure 23–1 Metatarsus varus: A line bisecting the hindpart of the foot should pass through the 2nd toe or between the 2nd and 3rd toes.

Though this condition is of concern to parents, it does not result in functional problems and resolves spontaneously with weight bearing. Adhesive tape or a Band-Aid wrapped under the 1st toe, over the 2nd, and under the 3rd may relieve anxiety in some parents.

Extra Toes. These may make it difficult to fit shoes and should be removed. They are often associated with a partial or complete extra metatarsal, usually the major offender in problems with shoes. Since segments of the metatarsals may not be sufficiently ossified to be recognized by roentgenograms in the neonate, resection should be delayed until about 1 yr of age when they are visible. There will be ample time for healing before the child is walking a great deal.

Syndactyly of the Toes. This condition is rarely a problem except cosmetically; separation of such toes is usually unnecessary.

tendon, capsules of the ankle, subtalar joints, medial ligaments, and joint capsules is required. The age at which surgery is necessary may be as early as 2–3 mo. Parents should be advised early that surgery is often necessary.

By the 1st yr of life a treated clubfoot may look relatively normal. However, the lateral part of the foot will always have excess soft tissue and the calf of that leg will be thinner. Because this disorder tends to recur, orthopedic care is necessary throughout childhood.

Other forms of clubfoot, such as calcaneovalgus, usually present less difficult problems; the principles of treatment are the same.

Vertical Talus (Congenital Rocker-Bottom Foot). This condition is characterized by malposition of the navicular on the neck of the talus. The ankle is held in marked equinus and the forefoot in dorsiflexion; thus the foot has a rocker-bottom shape. Palpation of the sole of the foot reveals a hard mass, the head of the talus. A patient with vertical talus should be referred to the orthopedic surgeon immediately.

Overlapping Toes. Most commonly the 2nd toe is displaced dorsally while the 3rd toe touches the 1st.

The Toddler

The normal foot of the toddler is somewhat chubby and wider than that of the older child. The fat pad on the medial aspect creates a fullness so that the foot appears flat. When the child first stands and walks, the foot may be everted; eversion is accentuated if the child stands with the legs externally rotated. Such an appearance should not be of concern. Only after the child has attained a stable standing and walking pattern does the pediatrician need to be concerned about the configuration of the foot.

Flat Foot. With weight bearing, some children's feet appear flat because of a loss of the longitudinal arch. If the feet are otherwise normal, particularly the hind and foreparts of the feet, they need no treatment. In other children the feet collapse with weight bearing and display valgus of the hindfoot, or eversion, and pronation of the forefoot (Fig 23–2). This collapse may be due to ligamentous laxity, muscular weakness, or a tight Achilles tendon. Valgus of less than 10° need not be treated. In more severe instances the bones of the

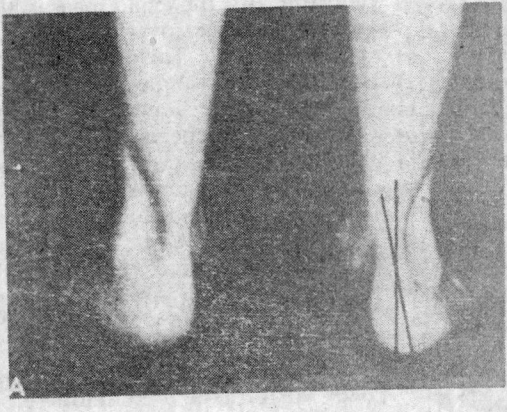
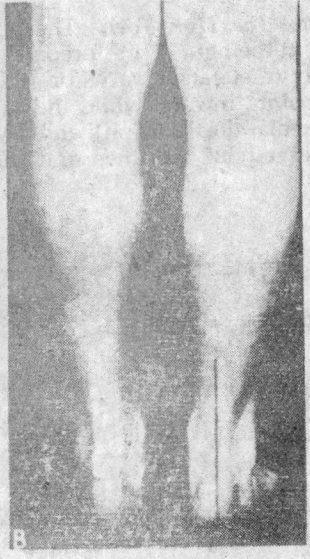

Figure 23–2 A, The heel in valgus; B, normal heel.

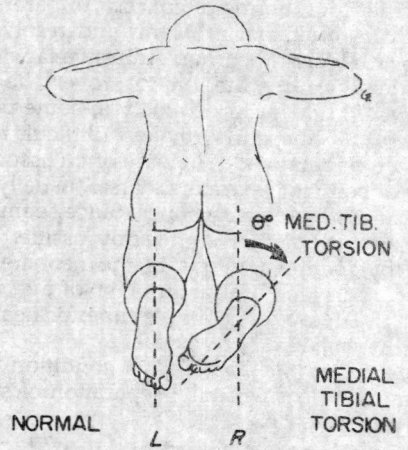

Figure 23–3 With the patient lying prone and the knees flexed 90°, the position of the foot is examined for medial tibial torsion. The left foot is normal; the right foot is in medial torsion.

foot will adapt to the abnormal position, with a "flat-foot" configuration becoming permanent and sometimes with painful feet in adulthood.

The goal of treatment is to maintain the foot in as near normal shape as possible during growth so that the bones will develop normally. Because the underlying ligamentous laxity and muscular weakness remain unaltered, when maturity is reached, the feet may be flat but the bones relatively normal. Treatment may consist of exercises to strengthen the muscles or stretch the heel cord. Because they require active effort by the child, treatment is usually fruitless. If the condition is mild, the foot may be supported by an arch pad (usually 3/16–1/4 inch thick) glued into the shoe and a medial heel wedge (usually 1/8 inch thick). In the severe form a molded plastic insert ("UCB insert," University of California–Berkeley insert) designed to hold the foot in a neutral position can be worn inside the shoe. Occasionally, corrective surgery may be needed. The so-called "Thomas Heel" adds nothing to the treatment of flat feet.

In-toeing (Pigeon Toe, Ding Toe). There are 3 common reasons for in-toeing: (1) the forepart of the foot is turned medially (metatarsus varus or adductus); (2) the entire foot points inward while the knee points straight ahead (medial tibial torsion); and (3) the entire leg turns in so that both the knee and the foot are

facing medially (medial femoral torsion or increased anteversion of the hips). The child should be observed standing and walking with shoes on and barefoot, noting the position of the knees in relation to the line of gait. The simplest method of determining which of the 3 causes is responsible for the in-toed gait is to have the child lie prone with the knees bent to 90° (see Fig 23–3). This gives a good view of the sole of the foot to disclose metatarsus varus. A line drawn along the sole of the foot should line up with a similar line down the length of the thigh; any inward deviation of the foot is due to medial tibial torsion. The feet should be moved outward (Fig 23–4) to demonstrate the degree of *medial* rotation of the femora in extension. Both feet should be moved simultaneously so that the pelvis stays in a neutral position. Similarly, the feet may be moved inward in order to measure the *lateral* rotation of the femora in extension. The femora normally rotate 45 ° in each direction; excessive medial rotation with a concomitant decrease in lateral rotation is called medial femoral torsion or increased anteversion.

Metatarsus varus of more than 10° which cannot be readily brought to the midline may cause problems with the proper fit of shoes and should be evaluated by an orthopedic surgeon. Otherwise, the condition can be ignored.

The problems of in-toeing from **medial tibial torsion** are more cosmetic than functional. In later childhood and adulthood, in-toeing from medial tibial torsion, even 20–30°, does not impair function and may even enhance it in athletics. Some children trip over their own feet, but this tendency vanishes by the age of 4 or 5 yr, even if there has been no change in rotation. Rarely, in later years, medial tibial torsion of greater than 20° may be a functional problem.

Medial femoral torsion (increased anteversion of the hips) usually becomes apparent to parents after the child reaches 2 yr of age. They frequently report that the children trip over their own feet, a problem that generally disappears spontaneously after the age of 4–5 yr. Only in extreme circumstances does this condition lead to any decrease in function; it is mainly a cosmetic concern. As the child passes the age of 10, parents usually learn to overlook the condition. Treatment is rarely required. The only realistic treatment for an axial deformity of a single long bone is surgical and requires division of the bone and realignment and fixation so that the bone heals in the new position. If needed, surgery can be performed as late as the age of 10. The longer the decision is delayed, the less likely it is that the parents or the child will want such treatment.

Out-toeing. When children start to walk, they often do so with their feet laterally rotated. Almost invariably this rotation will correct itself and deserves attention only if it persists beyond the age of 1–1.5 yr, with lateral rotation at the thighs.

Toewalking. A child who walks on tiptoes usually does so for 1 of 3 common reasons. The 1st is *habit*, which may be treated by having the parents encourage the child to walk heel/toe and indulge in exercises or game playing with the child walking on the heels. The 2nd is *cerebral palsy* with mild spasticity. Toewalking combined with limited abduction of the hips may provide the clue for this diagnosis in its milder form. The

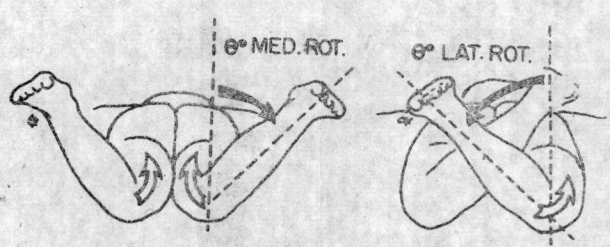

Figure 23–4 With the patient lying prone and the knees flexed 90°, the femurs are examined for their range of motion at the hips in extension.

3rd is *congenital tight heelcords*. With the knees in extension the normal foot should be capable of dorsiflexion to 20° above a right angle. If this cannot be attained, stretching exercises with assistance by the parents can be of help. Surgical lengthening of the tendon may be necessary if a 6 wk trial of immobilization in a plaster cast is unsuccessful.

Shoes. Shoes serve 2 purposes for the normal child: to protect the feet from sharp objects on the ground or floor and to keep the feet warm. They are not required to learn to walk. "Orthopedic shoes" (a term coined by the manufacturer) are of no benefit to a normal child and are potentially harmful by being too stiff. For the youngster learning to walk, shoes should be soft so that the child can sense the contours of the ground. They should not have a heel which can catch on objects. High shoes are not needed for the support of a normal foot but may prevent a child from kicking them off. There is nothing inappropriate about the use of sneakers for a child with a normal foot. A new shoe should be long enough to allow for growth (a distance about the width of the child's thumb from the end of the big toe to the end of the shoe measured while the child stands). The shoe should be wide enough at the metatarsal heads so that when the child stands, a pinch of leather can be squeezed between the fingers.

The Older Child and Adolescent

The Painful Foot. A child or adolescent, especially if obese or undergoing a growth spurt, may complain of pain in the feet, particularly after vigorous activity, and should be referred to an orthopedist for evaluation. If the pain is secondary to *pronated feet*, treatment by exercises and footpads will often suffice. Occasionally, *flexible flat feet* that are painful may require surgical realignment of the tendons or bones.

Pain may also result from a *coalition between the tarsal bones*. Before the age of 10 yr coalition may be composed of cartilage or fibrous tissue not easily recognized on a roentgenogram, but the altered joint motion will lead to a painful subtalar joint with spasm of the peroneal muscles. Sharp medial motion of the hindfoot by the examiner will produce not only pain but a reactive spasm of the peroneal muscles. Prior to the age of 11 or 12 such a coalition may be excised. Older children usually require a triple arthrodesis to relieve the pain.

Pain may be caused by *osteochondritis dissecans of the talus*, a condition of unknown etiology. A small segment of the bone just under the articular cartilage becomes avascular. Occasionally, the fragment breaks free into the joint and requires surgical removal. Other causes of painful foot in the adolescent are *juvenile rheumatoid arthritis*, which may present monarticular disease in the foot; *infection*; *Kohler disease*, avascular necrosis of the tarsal navicular; *Freiberg disease*, avascular necrosis of the head of the metatarsals, commonly the 2nd; and *stress fractures* of metatarsals.

Cavus Foot. Whereas the flat foot is commonly brought to the pediatrician's attention by the parents, its opposite, the high arched foot, is rarely noted but is far more significant and should immediately alert one

to the possibility of a neurologic condition, such as spinal dysrhaphia or Charcot-Marie-Tooth disease.

Toe Conditions in the Adolescent. *Hallux valgus* may be seen in the adolescent, commonly with a family history and with girls more frequently affected than boys. Once the deformity begins, the forces created by growing bones generally make matters worse. Nonoperative treatments such as spacers between the 1st and 2nd toes and wider shoes are not usually successful in the adolescent; surgical correction may be necessary. This condition may reflect faulty development of the bones as in pseudo- or pseudopseudohypoparathyroidism.

Overlapping or Underlapping Fifth Toe. Such anomalies are very common. Underlapping of the 5th toe beneath the 4th is not a functional problem, but if wearing shoes causes pain, surgical correction may be necessary. In overlapping 5th toe, if the joint capsule and the extensor tendons become so tight that the fit of shoes is difficult, surgical correction is indicated.

Macrodactyly (Enlargement of One Toe). This may be associated with vascular anomalies or neurofibromatosis. Surgical fusion of the epiphyses at the appropriate age may ultimately result in normal length, but the diameter of the toe is not so easily controlled. When fitting of a shoe becomes a problem, amputation of all or part of the toe may be needed.

23.3 THE HIP

Congenital Dysplasia of the Hip. This lesion results from abnormal development of 1 or all of the components of the hip joint: the acetabulum, the femoral head, and the surrounding capsule and soft tissues. The head of the femur may be dislocated and may or may not be relocatable in the acetabulum. Alternatively, the hip joint may be so lax that the femoral head in the acetabulum is dislocatable and spontaneously relocates. In subluxation the capsule is lax enough that the femoral head may be partially displaced from its position within the acetabulum but cannot be dislocated. In acetabular dysplasia the femoral head is well seated and the capsule sufficiently tight that there is no subluxation, but the angle of the acetabulum faces laterally to such an extent that dislocation may occur later in childhood.

The etiology of congenital dysplasia of the hip is clearly multifactorial. There are genetic factors. Girls are more commonly affected than boys. It may be associated with other abnormalities such as clubfeet and arthrogryposis or with a breech delivery, in which case uterine position or the trauma of delivery may be important factors. Abnormal laxity of the surrounding capsule and the ligaments may reflect hormonal changes in the mother.

Diagnosis. The hips should be examined in every newborn child and re-examined at every routine follow-up visit during the 1st yr of life. With the infant supine the examiner should inspect the contours of the lower extremities. While asymmetric folds may be seen in normal children, extra skin folds on the medial aspect of 1 thigh suggest that the femur has been dislocated proximally. *With the legs extended, the perineum should not* *be readily visible.* If it is, one should suspect bilateral dislocation, a condition likely to be missed when 1 hip is compared to the other.

The thighs are flexed, then abducted fully. In the neonate each thigh should abduct to almost 90°. Abduction less than 60–70° indicates an abnormality. The stability of the hip joint should also be evaluated to see whether the femoral head can be displaced from the acetabulum and then replaced. During this motion the examiner may get the sensation of the head "clunking" out of the acetabulum and over its posterior margin. Stability is determined in the following manner (Fig 23–5*A* and *B*): both the tibia and the femur are held in the palm of the hand so that any clicking sensations in the knees will not be confused with those in the hip. The long finger of the examiner is placed over the greater trochanter; the thumb is placed medially and just distal to the position of the long finger. The thighs are held in midabduction. The femoral head is then pulled out of the acetabulum by lateral pressure of the thumb and by rocking the knee medially with the knuckle of the index finger (Barlow test). If the femoral head can be displaced out of the acetabulum and over its posterior rim, the reverse maneuver is performed by pressing the long finger on the greater trochanter and rocking the knee laterally in order to replace the femoral head into the acetabulum (Ortolani maneuver).

If the femoral head can be felt to move laterally without coming out of the joint, the hip is classified as *subluxable.* If the head can be totally displaced out of the joint and replaced, it is classified as *dislocatable/relocatable.* The head may be found in the dislocated position and be relocatable but so unstable that dislocation immediately occurs again. This would be classified *dislocated/relocatable.* In the newborn period there are few dislocated hips which cannot be relocated, except in arthrogryposis. After the 1st weeks of life, however, an unstable hip may become fixed in the dislocated position. The adductor muscles and tendons will shorten so that limitation of abduction is even more obvious. At this point it is probable that the femoral head cannot be relocated by the Ortolani maneuver.

As the hip joint is moved through abduction, the examiner may feel the sensation of a high-pitched "click." This is not the same as the "clunk" which is felt as the femoral head is being displaced over the posterior acetabular margin and dropped either behind the acetabulum or back into it. The cause of the "click" is unknown. It usually disappears in the 1st weeks of life and is by itself of no significance.

Roentgenographic examination of the newborn's hips may be difficult to interpret because of the large ratio of cartilage to bone and absence of an ossified head. An anteroposterior roentgenogram will usually reveal lateral and superior displacement of the femoral head from the shallow acetabulum, which may be appreciated better after drawing certain lines in relation to the acetabula (Fig 23–6). In the 1st few days of life dislocation may be seen on an anteroposterior roentgenogram of the pelvis and hips made with the femora abducted 45° and rotated medially (von Rosen maneuver).

Treatment. Therapy of the dysplastic hip depends on the age of the child at the time of diagnosis and the

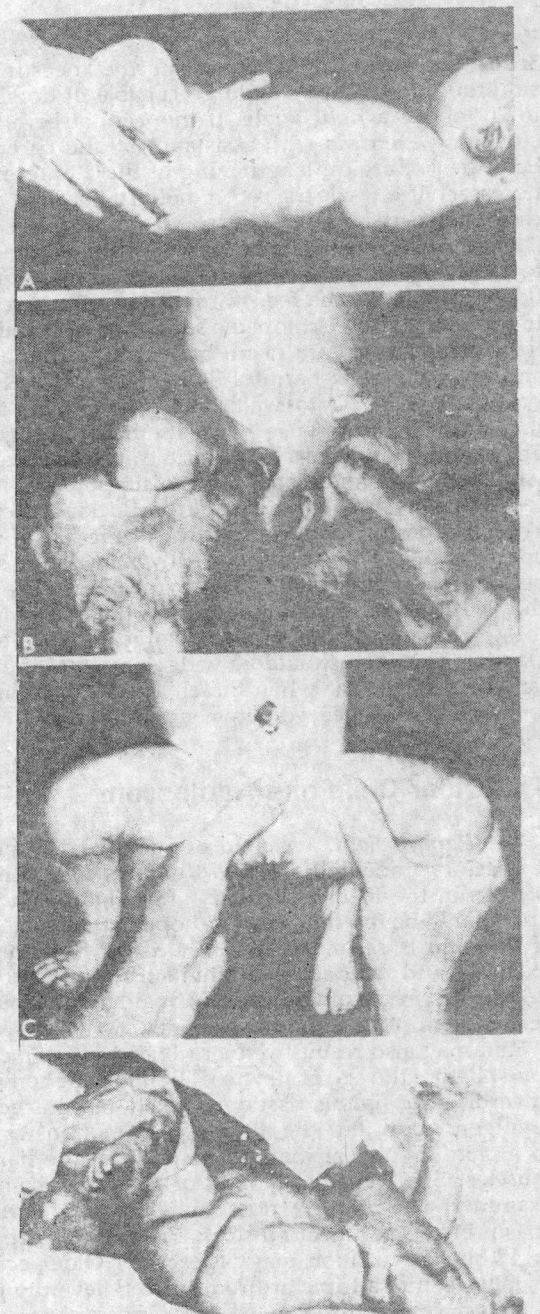

Figure 23–5 *A,* The newborn child is laid on its back with the hips and knees flexed, and the middle finger of each hand is placed over each greater trochanter. *B,* The thumb of each hand is applied to the inner side of the thigh opposite the lesser trochanter. *C,* In a doubtful case the pelvis may be steadied between a thumb over the pubis and fingers under the sacrum while the hip is tested with the other hand. *D,* Limitation of abduction is an early sign of congenital dislocation of the hip. Note restriction in abduction of right leg.

age of the abnormality on clinical examination. In a neonate with subluxation (i.e., femoral head and acetabulum are normal but the capsule is lax) the goal of treatment is to hold the legs in abduction until the capsule tightens, about 6 wk. This can be accomplished

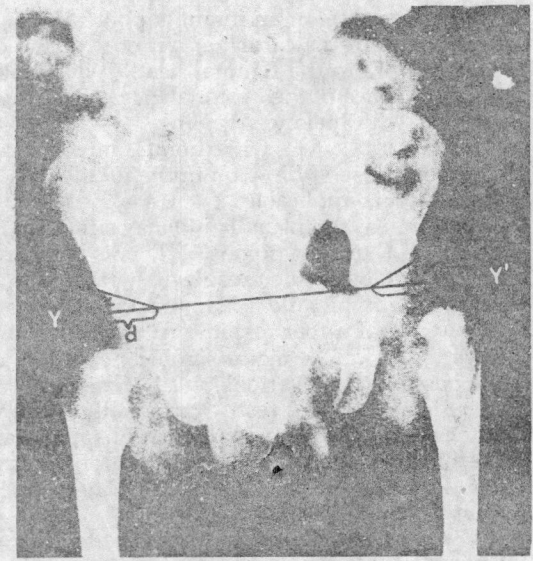
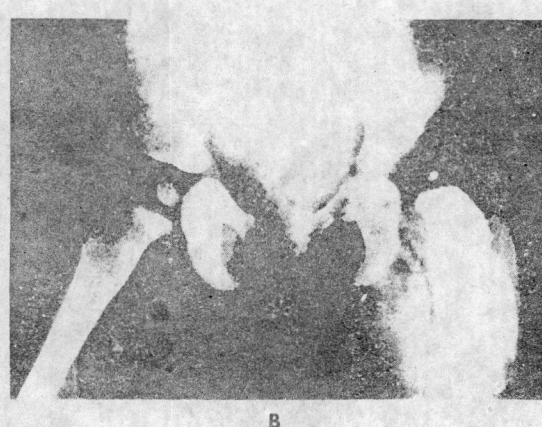

Figure 23–6 *A*, The Hilgenreiner method for identification of dysplasia of the hip prior to ossification of the capital femoral epiphysis. α' is greater than α, indicating greater obliquity of the acetabular roof. *d'* is greater than *d*, indicating lateral displacement of the femur *h* is greater than *h'*, indicating cephalic displacement of the femur. These relations indicate dysplasia of the patient's left hip. *B*, Congenital dislocation of left hip. The bony roof of the left acetabulum is quite oblique and there is the beginning of a false acetabulum above its most lateral aspect. The left femur is displaced laterally and superiorly. The left femoral capital epiphyseal center is smaller than the right.

with a rigid device, such as a von Rosen splint or an Ilfeld brace, or one that allows some mobility, such as a Frejka pillow or Pavlik harness. The simple use of multiple diapers is not advised because adductor muscles of the thigh usually overpower soggy diapers and abduction is not maintained.

For the hip which is dislocatable and relocatable, a more reliable form of fixation is preferable, especially one which is not removed by the mother at each diaper change (e.g., Pavlik stirrups or von Rosen splint). In the child whose hip is very unstable, a more fixed form of holding device, a plaster spica, may be required for a few mo before switching to a splint.

Children older than 2–3 mo with dislocated and unrelocatable hips require traction in order to stretch the tight muscles around the hip, and an adductor tenotomy may be required in order to relocate the femoral head. Under no circumstances should the hips be forcefully relocated without preceding traction because of the increased risk of avascular necrosis of the femoral head. When traction has stretched the tissues sufficiently to allow the hip to be placed easily into the acetabulum, the dislocation is reduced under general anesthesia and held in a spica cast with the hips abducted about 45–60°. The cast is changed approximately every 6 wk to allow for the child's growth; immobilization is continued for a time equal to the age of the child at the time of diagnosis but not longer than 6 mo. Thereafter, a splinting device may be needed to maintain the hips in abduction until the acetabulum has developed satisfactorily. Occasionally, in spite of traction and an adductor tenotomy, the femoral head cannot be reduced. Under such circumstances open reduction may be performed.

In a child whose dislocation of the hip has not been discovered until after 18 mo of age, open reduction with a simultaneous osteotomy of the pelvis to create a better roof over the femoral head (Salter innominate osteotomy) is usually the most satisfactory form of therapy.

In **acetabular dysplasia** the acetabulum itself may be inadequately developed so that it faces more laterally than is normal; further maldevelopment may lead to a dislocation of the hip. The diagnosis of acetabular dysplasia is made on a roentgenogram taken because of limited hip abduction; the acetabular angle will be high, and the contour of the bony acetabulum will not be concave. The very young child may be treated by any device that holds the hip in abduction, usually for 3–6 mo. For a child over 18 mo of age, surgery may be required to provide better coverage for the femoral head and prevent dislocation.

In **congenital coxa vara** the neck of the femur makes less than the expected 135° angle with the shaft of the femur. It is not usually encountered under 2–3 yr of age, and the etiology is not known. The physical findings may simulate a dislocated hip because the shaft of the femur is located proximally relative to the normal side. On the other hand, the motion of the hip will be virtually normal, and there will be no laxity of the femoral head within the acetabulum. If this condition is left untreated, the varus deformity usually worsens. Treatment is osteotomy of the proximal femur to increase the femoral neck/shaft angle.

The Painful Hip. The causes of painful hip in a child and its evalution vary considerably from age to age.

THE INFANT. The most likely cause of a painful hip joint in an infant is a **bacterial infection** (Sec 10.52).

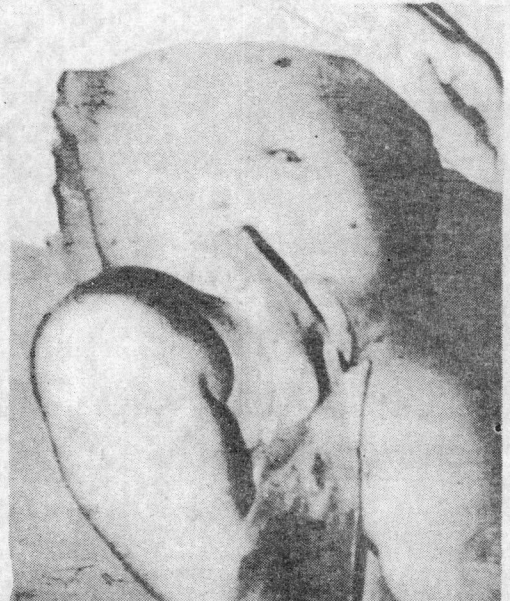

Figure 23–7 An infant with a bacterial infection of the hip holds the joint flexed, abducted, and laterally rotated.

This infection may be a direct bloodborne contamination of the hip joint or may be secondary to extension of osteomyelitis of the neck of the femur into the hip joint. The capacity of the hip joint to hold an increased volume of fluid is maximal when the hip is held in about 20° of flexion, abduction, and lateral rotation (see Fig 23–7). Any attempt to move the thigh from this position will cause distress.

A roentgenogram of the infant's hip often reveals lateral displacement of the femoral head and of the fat adjacent to the capsule due to fluid accumulation. Aspiration of the hip joint will confirm the diagnosis and permit appropriate bacteriologic study. A needle of at least 18 gauge caliber is necessary for extraction of the thick pus. This procedure requires considerable expertise. General anesthesia is often helpful; fluoroscopic control should be used.

A septic hip joint should be treated immediately. The joint must be opened and the pus removed, with liberal irrigation and subsequent closed tube drainage. Antibiotics should be chosen initially with the knowledge that infecting agents commonly include *H. influenzae* and salmonella as well as *Staphylococcus aureus*.

The prognosis in an infant is poor. Not only is there destruction of the cartilage, but obstruction of the vascular supply to the femoral head, which passes across the joint space of the hip, may occur, causing avascular necrosis with lifelong crippling.

THE TODDLER. As with infants, infection is the most common cause of hip pain in the toddler, and the same discussion is applicable.

Children as young as 18 mo may suffer from **transient synovitis** ("toxic synovitis"). This is a disorder of unknown etiology which results in a painful hip and gives all the signs of mild inflammation. The episode may follow a viral upper respiratory tract infection by a few days to 2 wk. The major significance of the disorder is the possibility of overlooking a bacterial infection. Treatment is usually bed rest. Occasionally, the pain may be sufficiently severe to require in-hospital traction with the hip in flexion. The sedimentation rate can be elevated; however, the alpha$_2$-globulin is rarely greater than 1.0 mg/dl.

Other causes of painful hip in the toddler are *juvenile rheumatoid arthritis* and *leukemia* (in which monarticular pain is the 1st sign in 5% of cases).

THE 2 TO 10 YEAR OLD. In the child of 4 yr and older, infection is much less common, but it results in severe damage to the joint if the diagnosis is delayed. It must always be suspected and excluded, but transient synovitis and Legg-Perthes disease are more common causes of painful hip.

Legg-Calvé-Perthes disease is an avascular necrosis of the femoral head. Boys are affected more often than girls. The common age range is 5–9 yr, but children 2–11 may be affected.

At the onset of the avascular event the hip is painful and the symptoms indistinguishable from transient synovitis; a roentgenogram of the hips may show bulging of the capsule but will often be normal. If there has been disuse of the leg, the metaphysis may be more lucent than the epiphyseal center. A radioisotope bone scan (in anteroposterior and in frog leg lateral) may show decreased uptake in the femoral head (see Fig 23–8). Subsequently, in the repair process there is revascularization of the femoral head. As new bone is laid down upon the dead trabecular bone, resorption of the dead areas begins. At this point a roentgenogram will show increased density in the femoral head where new bone has been added. A subarticular fracture line may be seen anterolaterally, and there will be gradual distortion of the femoral head (Fig 23–9). Healing occurs over 2–3 yr. While the repair proceeds, marked distor-

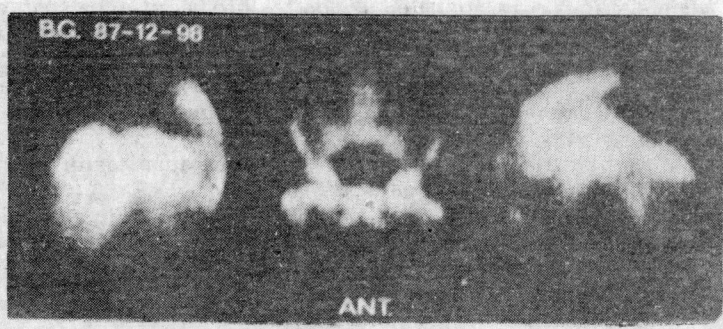

B.G. 87-12-98

ANT.

Figure 23–8 Legg-Calvé-Perthes disease. The radionuclide scan of the pelvis and hips reveals an area of decreased uptake in the head of the right femur. This is best seen in the isolated image on the right and can be compared with the normal left hip.

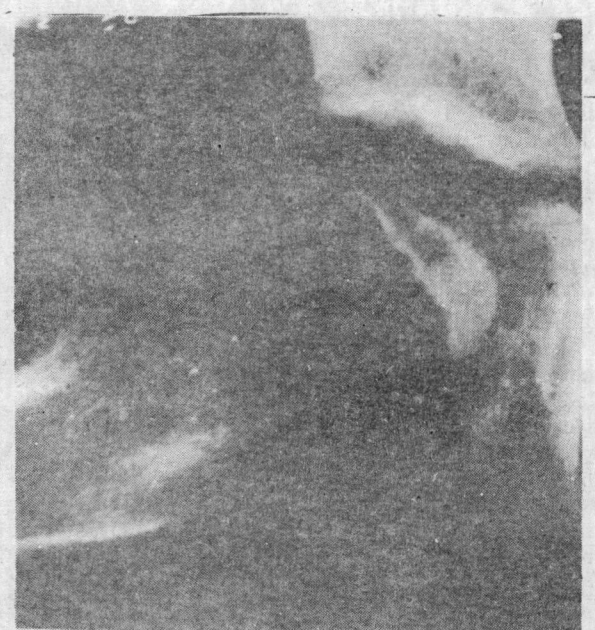

Figure 23–9 Legg-Calvé-Perthes disease. The lateral radiograph of the right hip reveals the epiphyseal line to be irregularly widened. The femoral capital epiphyseal center is flattened; there is a lucent defect in the anterior aspect of the center. Relative to the femoral neck, the secondary center is opaque.

tion of the femoral head and neck can lead to an imperfect joint.

The goal of *treatment* of Legg-Perthes disease is to retain the normal spherical shape of the femoral head. In the past this was attempted by efforts to relieve the hip of weight bearing: by bed rest (up to several yr) or a variety of braces which kept the affected limb off the ground. Many children have been successfully treated by these methods, but the proportion of patients who were left with distorted femoral heads was high. Current therapy allows the child to continue weight bearing but with the femur in an abducted position so that the head is well contained by the acetabulum. This decreases focal areas of increased load and minimizes distortion. Weight bearing in abduction may be accomplished by Petrie casts (long leg casts with the legs held in abduction and medial rotation by a bar between the 2 casts) or by braces which hold the legs in the same position. Surgical procedures have been developed to keep the femoral head abducted in relation to the acetabulum, either by varus osteotomy of the proximal femur or by Salter innominate osteotomy, which orients the acetabulum anterolaterally to cover the femoral head.

Tuberculosis of the Hip. The hip is the joint most often affected by tuberculosis. The disease may begin in the synovial membrane but usually starts as an infection in the femoral epiphysis or greater trochanteric apophysis with subsequent breakthrough into the joint. Also see Sec 10.52.

The 1st symptom is usually an intermittent slight limp, occurring when the patient first gets out of bed and after exercise. It may disappear for days or weeks at a time. Pain may be present at this stage or develop later and is usually referred to the knee or the medial aspect of the thigh. As destruction of the joint proceeds, the thigh is flexed and adducted, and rotation which initially was lateral becomes medial. Swelling about the hip increases and, if an abscess forms, pus may discharge anteriorly or be disseminated in other directions. Absorption of the head and neck of the femur may take place without evidence of suppuration.

Distinction must be made between Legg-Perthes disease and tuberculous infections on the hip. In the former, roentgenographic changes do not extend beyond the femoral capital epiphysis and metaphysis and the femoral capital epiphyseal center is relatively dense, not lucent. In the latter the acetabulum may also be affected. The 2 conditions may be indistinguishable in the early stage, and the clinical course and tuberculin reaction must be relied upon to differentiate them. The insidious onset of a tuberculous hip infection serves to distinguish it from rheumatic fever and acute arthritis.

Systemic isoniazid and ethambutol are indicated for 18 mo to treat tuberculosis of the hip and *tuberculous arthritis* of other joints (Table 10–32). Intra-articular administration of drugs is not indicated. No controlled studies support bed rest immobilization, but it is recommended.

THE ADOLESCENT. Among adolescents, infection of the hip is rare. More common causes of hip pain are slipped capital femoral epiphysis and traumatic avulsion of a muscle from its insertion.

In **slipped capital femoral epiphysis** the upper femoral epiphysis slips posteromedially off the metaphysis. This disorder occurs often in obese boys and can be bilateral. The slip may occur gradually or suddenly. Gradual slip may give symptoms and signs like those of synovitis; often the diagnosis is delayed because the pain is referred to the medial aspect of the knee. Abduction and internal rotation are limited. Acute slip usually follows trauma, with pain, limited motion, and inability to walk.

The goal of *treatment* is to prevent further slipping. Threaded pins or screws may be inserted along the neck of the femur and across the epiphyseal cartilage. Occasionally, the slip may be so severe that there is marked limitation of medial rotation and flexion. In this situation the fixation of the epiphysis is accompanied by an osteotomy of the upper femur to regain the lost motions. Reduction of a slipped epiphysis may be successful but carries a very high risk of avascular necrosis.

Avulsion of muscles results when an adolescent does physical exertion more appropriate for an adult and pulls the origin or insertion of a muscle from its bony anchorage. The apophysis usually pulls free with the muscle. The sartorius can be pulled off the anterior superior iliac spine, the rectus femoris can be pulled off the anterior inferior spine, the iliopsoas from the lesser trochanter, or the hamstring muscles from the ischial tuberosity. If the apophysis to which the muscle is attached is not ossified, the diagnosis by roentgenogram is more difficult. Suspicion of these possibilities and individually stressing these 4 muscles provide the clues for this diagnosis. The rectus femoris can be stressed by passive flexion of the knee with the hip extended, the psoas by medially rotating the thigh with the hip and knee fixed 90°, the hamstrings by flexing the hip with the knee extended, and the sartorius by placing the foot of the affected limb on top of the opposite knee and then resisting the patient's effort to flex the affected hip.

23.4   THE KNEE

Knee problems are not common in infants and young children, but the knee is a common site for disorders in the preadolescent and adolescent. Pain in the hip may be referred to the knee, and *an examination of the hip should be part of any examination of the knee joint*. The knee is also a common site of monarticular juvenile rheumatoid arthritis; since this may be preceded by trauma, diagnostic confusion is common.

Popliteal Cysts.   Characteristically, these are found posteriorly at the origin of the medial head of the gastrocnemius or the semitendinosus muscle. True Baker cysts (posterior herniations of the knee joint) are rare in childhood, but the term Baker cyst is commonly applied to popliteal cysts. Reasons to excise these benign lesions include pain, limitation of motion, cosmetic concern, increasing size, or worry by parents who cannot be assured. They may recur.

Discoid Meniscus.   This is a congenital disorder of the semilunar cartilage of the knee joint, almost invariably of the lateral side. Instead of being semilunar in configuration, the meniscus is disclike and may be cystic. Characteristically, it causes a popping sensation, and the child or parents may notice a small mass that protrudes laterally at the knee joint. It is frequently bilateral. The treatment consists of excision of the meniscus to prevent later degenerative arthritis of the knee.

Osgood-Schlatter Disease.   This is a disease of the anterior tibial tubercle. The apophysis onto which the infrapatellar ligament of the quadriceps is attached is not well anchored so that excessive activity involving the quadriceps results in pain and swelling in the region. The anterior tibial tubercle becomes prominent and is tender to direct pressure. Any activity which stresses the quadriceps will reproduce this pain.

The goal of treatment is to decrease the stress at the tubercle. Often a period of 4–8 wk of restriction from strenuous physical activity, especially activities requiring deep knee bending, is sufficient. If the pain is not satisfactorily controlled in this manner, a cast may be required to rest the knee, a situation that is particularly difficult if the condition is bilateral. The problem ceases when the apophysis fuses to the metaphysis, but there may be several yr of annoying pain. The bump at the anterior tubercle often alarms parents. Rarely, in the older adolescent excision of a residual ossicle deep to the ligament is needed to bring relief.

Osteochondritis Dissecans.   In this condition of unknown etiology a small fragment of the bone underlying the articular cartilage of the knee becomes avascular. It characteristically occurs on the lateral aspect of the medial condyle of the femur but may occur anywhere over the distal femoral surface. Treatment is generally symptomatic. Application of a cast for as little as 6 wk may suffice, though the roentgenographic defect may persist for several yr. Occasionally, the fragment and its adjacent articular cartilage break off and float freely in the knee joint. The fragment is either excised or repositioned and held in place with bone pegs or nails. The prognosis for patients under 17 yr is good, for those over 17 only fair.

Dislocating Patella.   The patella may dislocate laterally because of loose ligamentous structures (as seen in the child with Down syndrome) or a laterally inserted infrapatellar ligament. If the dislocation recurs, surgical reconstruction of the attachments of the patella may be needed. Sometimes a child's knee dislocates and then pops back prior to clinical examination. In such cases the knee should be examined in full extension and the patella pushed laterally as far as possible. The child who has a dislocating patella will have an involuntary contraction of the quadriceps to resist this maneuver, whereas the child with a normal knee will not.

Chondromalacia of the Patella.   This is a condition of 1 or both patellae characterized by pain within the knee whenever the leg is actively used with the knee flexed, as in going up or down stairs. There may be a sensation of buckling or giving way. Its cause is unknown, but it is often aggravated by poor mechanics of the patella sliding on the femur. It is most common in teenage girls. Examination of the knee in a child with chondromalacia rarely shows any effusion, which is common in adults. With the knee in full extension, downward pressure on the patella, impacting it against the femur, is very painful. This is exaggerated if the patient is asked to stress the quadriceps during the maneuver. Tenderness along the medial border of the articular margin of the patella is common.

Reassurance that the child is not suffering from juvenile rheumatoid arthritis or bone malignancy is often adequate treatment for the mild case. The next order of treatment is an exercise program aimed at strengthening the medial portion of the quadriceps muscle to realign the patella's motion on the femur, often with the administration of aspirin. These exercises should be done with the knee in extension. Occasionally, surgery is required to realign the patella or to excise areas of softened cartilage and drill the underlying cortical bone to allow the ingrowth of fibrocartilage.

23.5   THE LEG

Bowing of the Tibia.   In the newborn, anterior or anterolateral bowing, as seen in neurofibromatosis, is often preliminary to fracture and ultimate nonunion (pseudoarthrosis), sometimes requiring amputation. It is important that affected infants have bone grafting procedures done early before the tibia breaks. Posterior bowing of the tibia is not associated with this sequence of events and may gradually remodel spontaneously.

Bowleg.   Infants generally have bowing of the legs. By 12–18 mo of age the legs have straightened and progressed to mild knock knee; they will gradually assume their ultimate configuration by 6–7 yr of age

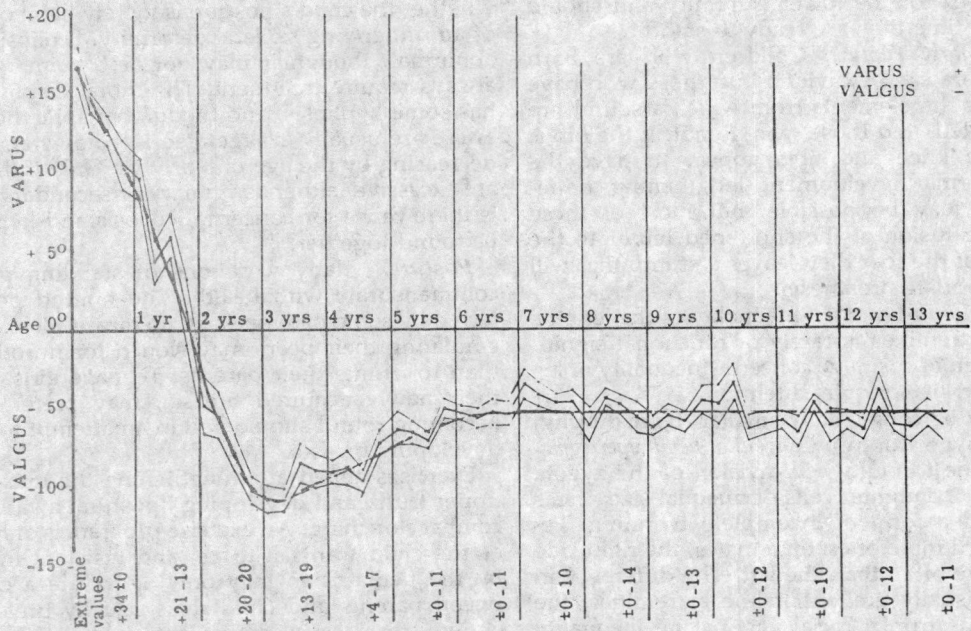

Figure 23–10 Development of the tibiofemoral angle during growth. (Salenius P, Vankka E: J Bone Joint Surg 57A:259, 1975.)

(Fig 23–10). If the bowing is outside the range shown in the graph, roentgenographic examination, with the child standing if possible, is required. In the absence of evidence for rickets of nutritional or of renal origin, the roentgenogram can be used to assess future change. Increasing bowing of the legs should be referred for evaluation.

Blount Disease (Tibia Vara). Of unknown etiology, this is a disorder of growth of the medial part of the proximal tibial epiphysis. Roentgenograms show irregularity of the medial aspect of the tibial metaphysis adjacent to the epiphysis, with distortion of the adjacent epiphyseal center (Fig 23–11). The bowing begins as a sharp angulation at the metaphysis. Treatment is usually osteotomy of the proximal tibia and fibula, which may have to be repeated 1 or more times.

Knock Knees (Genu Valgum). This deformity can be assessed by measuring the distance between the medial malleoli of the ankles when the medial parts of the distal thighs are touching. Progressive knock knees after the age of 6 yr should be evaluated for an underlying abnormality and the need for surgical correction. There is no evidence that shoe wedges alter this abnormality or are needed to "protect" the feet from pronation.

"Growing Pains." Pain in the shins is common from the ages of 3–6 yr, especially at night after the child has gone to bed. The etiology is unknown but may involve edema of the muscle bodies within the tight fascial sheaths following a day of vigorous activity. Reassurance, the application of local heat, massage, and aspirin are usually adequate treatment. If the pain is severe and frequent, quinine sulfate given at suppertime can alleviate the problem.

Congenital Anomalies. Part or all of 1 of the bones of the lower extremity may be absent. Affected children

should be cared for in centers where such deformities are frequently treated. Many of these children are best treated by appropriate removal of nonfunctional parts; rather than spending years in hospitals, they can then become fully active in prostheses. Small children readily

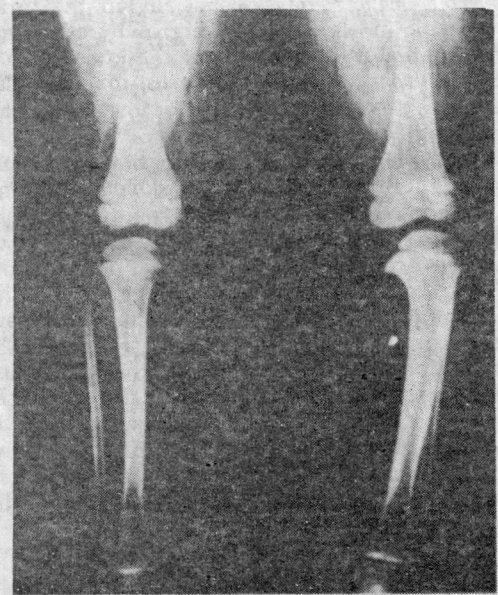

Figure 23–11 Blount disease. The medial aspect of the proximal end of the left tibia is irregular and "beaked." There is also minimal involvement of medial aspects of the proximal tibial epiphyseal center. As a consequence of the proximal tibial deformity, there was abnormal weight bearing, which in turn was responsible for the thickening shown in the medial cortex of the left tibia. The right tibia is normal.

accept prostheses for the lower extremity and should be fitted by the time they are ready to stand.

Congenital Short Femur. Children who are born with short femora can be divided into those who have a sound hip (or the elements from which a sound hip can be constructed) and those who do not. If the hip is sound and the knee and tibia appear to have the potential for normal development, lengthening the femur surgically may be possible, but most of these children require fusion of the shortened femur to the tibia. Removal of the foot then leaves a stump that will accept an appropriate prosthesis.

Inequality of Limb Length. Inequality of the lengths of the upper extremities is rarely of functional significance and seldom of cosmetic concern. Inequality of leg length, however, may require attention.

One side may be congenitally smaller (hemiatrophy) or larger (hemihypertrophy). *Congenital hemihypertrophy* is most likely due to faulty cell division of the zygote which results in 2 daughter cells of unequal size; it has been considered a form of incomplete twinning. Females are affected more often than males, the right side of the body more often than the left. The difference in the 2 sides is usually greatest in the extremities, the genitalia, and the trunk. Facial and palatal inequality may also be present. Paired internal organs are sometimes of unequal size. The bones of the larger size are longer and thicker than their counterparts and may differ in osseous maturation. Other malformations may be associated, such as aniridia, polydactyly, hypospadias, cryptorchidism, nevi, and hemangiomas. There is an association with Wilms tumor and adrenal and hepatic neoplasms. Hemihypertrophy may be a feature of Beckwith-Wiedemann syndrome, in which the same neoplasms have been encountered.

Arteriovenous malformations, especially in the groin, may also result in significant overgrowth of a limb. Chronic inflammatory lesions about the knee, such as longstanding *juvenile rheumatoid arthritis*, may stimulate growth, as may *fractures*, particularly those adjacent to epiphyseal cartilage plates.

A treatment plan begins with estimation of the ultimate limb length discrepancy at skeletal maturity through periodic (usually yearly) roentgenographic measurements of the extremities, together with an evaluation of the bone age in the left hand and wrist. Differences expected to be less than 2 cm at maturity usually do not need treatment. Anticipated greater differences can be treated by making the short leg longer or the long leg shorter. Usually the longer limb is shortened by surgically scraping away the epiphyseal cartilage at the appropriate end of the bone or by putting staples across it. The short leg continues growing and catches up with the long one. Shoe lifts are usually used until the child reaches the age for the definitive operation.

23.6 THE SPINE

The spinal problems most frequently encountered by the pediatrician are questions by parents about children's poor posture. The problem is to determine whether the child's posture is merely habit or the result of an underlying skeletal deformity. Scoliosis is always abnormal, though it may not be a primary defect or always require treatment. The thoracic spine normally has some kyphosis, and the lumbar spine has lordosis. These are usually exaggerated in youngsters, gradually decreasing by the age of 8 or 9 yr. Only if these curves are excessive, either as primary or secondary problems, is there cause for concern. Scoliosis and kyphosis may be found together.

Posture. Many variations of standing posture are commensurate with health. The ramrod posture preferred by some patients is by no means ideal. Teenagers emulating their peers may slouch for no other reason than to irritate their parents. Teenage girls, shy about their newly acquired breasts, may prefer to slump, becoming round shouldered in an attempt to hide their developing breasts.

Exercises aimed at strengthening the muscles of the upper trunk and developing "postural awareness" can combat slouching. An exercise program is only as useful as the child wants it to be, and insistent intervention by the pediatrician may only aggravate a conflict between parents and child. It is usually preferable and enough to reassure the parents that slouched posture does not lead to structural changes and that when the children are older and want to sit or stand differently, they will be able to do so.

Scoliosis. Side-to-side curves of the spine can be nonstructural or structural. Nonstructural curves have no axial rotation and show no residual deformity on bending as seen by roentgenograms. They are secondary to causes such as posture, short leg, muscle spasm, or, rarely, hysteria. Structural curves may be congenital in origin or secondary to metabolic problems, such as idiopathic juvenile osteoporosis or the Prader-Willi syndrome, or they may be secondary to neuromuscular abnormality. Scoliosis is most commonly idiopathic. Idiopathic scoliosis is rarely seen within the 1st yr of life ("infantile idiopathic") in North America, and uncommonly from 1–10 yr of age ("juvenile idiopathic"); it usually has its onset after 10 yr ("adolescent idiopathic").

The *etiology* of idiopathic scoliosis is multifactorial, with an autosomal dominant genetic component with incomplete penetrance. Girls are much more commonly affected than boys. All members of the family should be carefully examined for scoliosis if 1 is found with the disorder. Patients with scoliosis should be warned to pay special attention to their offspring as they approach their teens.

Congenital scoliosis due to absence of a part of the spine or a fusion of several segments of the spine is often associated with congenital anomalies of other organ systems within the same segmental level, particularly of the genitourinary tract and heart. One third of children with congenital scoliosis have abnormalities on intravenous urography.

Structural curves can be separated from nonstructural curves on clinical examination by their associated spinal rotation. As the spine bends from side to side in scoliosis, there is an associated axial rotation. The bodies of the vertebral segments rotate toward the convex-

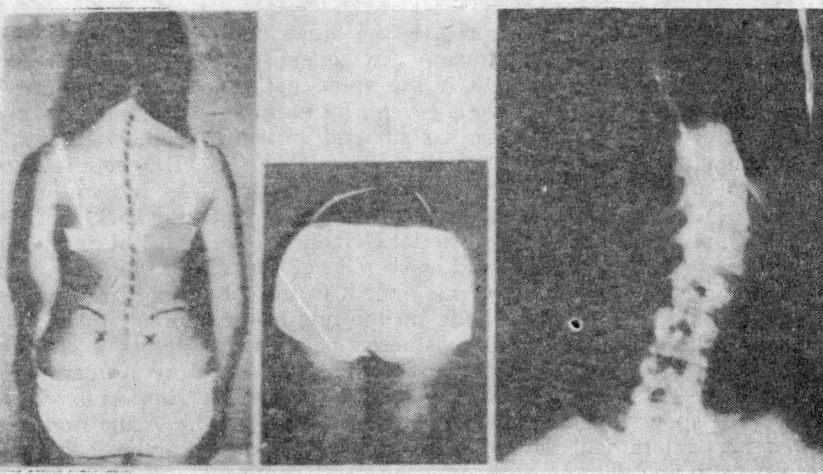

Figure 23–12 Scoliosis. The spine rotates as it curves, with the spinous processes moving toward the concavity. The severe curve of 46° seen by roentgenogram on the right is only partly recognizable when the patient stands upright. However, examination with the child's spine flexed shows the rotation on the right that indicates a structural scoliosis.

ity and the spinous processes toward the concavity of the curve. Rotation of the spine is most readily appreciated if the patient is asked to bend forward with the arms hanging freely. In this position any prominence of 1 side of the rib cage is seen easily (more commonly on the right; see Fig 23–12). In the lumbar region only the short transverse processes protrude to push the paraspinous muscles posteriorly; therefore rotation is not as prominent. Patients who have rotational components to their curves should have a roentgenogram of the entire spine, anteroposterior, erect, preferably on a single film showing the full extent of the vertebral column from the chin to the anterior superior iliac spines.

The rotary component of scoliosis is its serious aspect. As the rotation of the thorax progresses, there is less room for the heart and lungs; pulmonary restriction may ultimately shorten the lifespan of the individual. In addition, curves of the lumbar region can be a source of significant pain in adult life.

The goal of *therapy* is to keep the curve from increasing so that when growth ceases, the curve will be less than 40° (by the Cobb method). This gives a reasonable expectation that progression thereafter will not present problems, whereas curves over 40° can increase after growth stops. For small curves (less than 10–15°) treatment is usually not required. Curves from 20–40° in growing children can usually be managed with a brace; the brace is worn 23 out of 24 hr a day throughout the period of growth. Curves over 40° are generally managed by spinal fusion (most commonly posterior) and the insertion of metal rod (Harrington rod) to obtain correction and to help hold the curve during the time required for the fusion to become solid. Some children must have their spines fused anteriorly. There has been concern that fusion before growth ceases will prevent that segment of the spine from growing. Fusion does prevent growth, but a spine with a marked curve is short anyway. A short straight spine is more desirable than a short crooked spine, particularly in congenital scoliosis in which lack of segmentation on 1 side of the spine will lead to an ever-progressing curve that must be fused as soon as it is recognized, even as early as a few mo of age.

Kyphosis. Excessive thoracic kyphosis may be congenital or acquired. Congenital kyphosis is secondary to a lack of segmentation of the vertebral bodies anteriorly or to a lack of formation of 1 or more vertebral bodies. Generally, this requires surgical fusion; delay can lead to paraplegia.

Acquired kyphosis is a condition of unknown etiology. The child stands with an increased roundback in the thoracic region. There may be pain. Usually, there is a compensatory increase in lumbar lordosis.

The examiner should have the child bend forward as far as possible, allowing the arms to dangle freely. The spine is observed from the side. There should be a smooth curve going from the neck to the buttocks with no sharp angulation (Fig 23–13). Normal lumbar lordosis should completely correct either to flat or to slight kyphosis. Any suspicion of abnormality is an indication for a standing lateral roentgenogram of the thoracolumbar spine. The thoracic kyphosis should not measure more than 40°; irregularity of the apophyseal growing areas of the vertebral bodies may be apparent (Scheuermann disease).

Excessive kyphosis may increase after the end of growth and become a major problem in later life if there is osteoporosis.

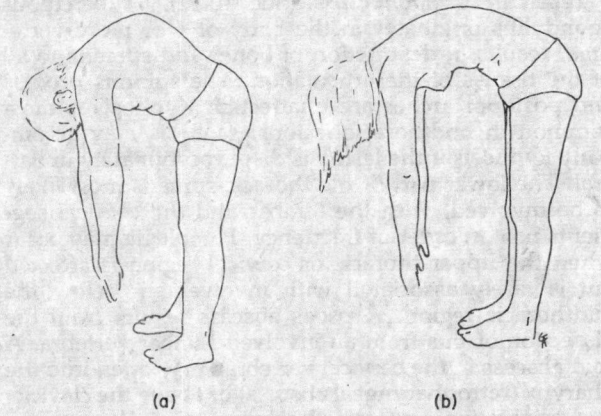

(a)   (b)

Figure 23–13 Note the sharp break in contour in the child with abnormal kyphosis *(a)* compared with the contour in the normal child *(b)*.

The goal of treatment is to reduce the thoracic kyphosis to less than 40°. Reduction can generally be achieved with brace treatment if the spine has not completed growth. If the curve is severe, for example, in excess of 60°, or if the spine has stopped growing, fusion may be required.

Spondylolysis and Spondylolisthesis. In these conditions of unknown etiology there is a discontinuity in the pars interarticularis of the posterior elements of the spine between the superior and inferior facet joints. The discontinuity (*spondylolysis*) may result in the forward slipping of 1 vertebral body on the one below, creating a lesion called spondylolisthesis. This occurs most frequently between L5 and the sacrum but may occur between L4, L5, and even higher. A congenital variety of spondylolisthesis associated with an elongated pars interarticularis and defective facets allows forward slipping without a break in the pars. Trauma, especially stress in hyperextension, may cause a fracture in the pars interarticularis. Genetic factors are prominent.

Spondylolisthesis is usually associated with low back pain. The propensity to slip forward is exaggerated during the growth spurt, and the forward slip can be so severe that the vertebral body can fall off the one below. Irritation of the L5 and S1 roots is common and results in limitation in straight leg raising with hamstringing spasm. The diagnosis of spondylolisthesis can be made from a standing lateral roentgenogram of the lumbosacral spine. Diagnosis of spondylolysis requires oblique roentgenograms of the lumbosacral spine to show the defective pars interarticularis. When roentgenograms are inconclusive, tomography or radionuclide bone scan may be helpful.

Treatment is directed at relieving pain and preventing further slipping. Excessive lumbar lordosis will increase the mechanical sheer forces leading to slipping; therefore exercises to reduce lumbar lordosis may relieve pain. Activities associated with hyperextension of the lumbar spine should be avoided. Braces may be helpful, or surgery may be required to relieve pain. Even if pain is under control, patients should be monitored for roentgenographic evidence of progressive slipping of the vertebrae. For progressive slipping, spinal fusion is necessary.

Tuberculous Spondylitis (Sec 10.52). Tuberculous spondylitis originates in the body of 1 or more vertebrae, results in destruction of bone, and spreads to all of the tissues of the articulation. The spinous process and posterior arches are unaffected. Kyphosis is most common in midthoracic lesions; scoliosis may accompany kyphosis if the lesion is disproportionately unilateral. The lower part of the thoracic spine is most likely to be involved, with the lumbar and the cervical segments next in order of frequency. Paraplegia may occur when the upper thoracic or cervical region is affected but is rarely associated with involvement below the midthoracic region. A psoas abscess results from the dissection of pus from an involved lumbar vertebra. A cold abscess in the cervical vertebrae may open into the pharynx (retropharyngeal abscess) or above the clavicle; one originating opposite the lower cervical or upper thoracic vertebrae may rupture into the pleura or penetrate to the scapula, but often it gravitates and points above Poupart ligament.

Symptoms are insidious in onset. Persistent or intermittent pain may occur over the distribution of the spinal nerves arising adjacent to the affected vertebrae. This pain is increased by pressure on the head but not by pressure over the lesions. Muscular rigidity splints the back, and the child assumes a position that reduces weight on the diseased spine and prevents jarring. He or she may avoid bending to reach an object on the floor, may walk stiffly or carefully on the toes, or may prefer to lie on the abdomen and to rest frequently across a chair or over a parent's lap. With cervical involvement the child may hold the head stiffly or support it with a hand.

Acute nontuberculous osteomyelitis of the vertebrae can be distinguished by its greater toxicity, leukocytosis, and fever. Roentgenographic abnormalities are usually well established in a tuberculous lesion of the vertebrae when symptoms first become manifest, whereas they are not likely to be demonstrable during the 1st days of acute pyogenic osteomyelitis.

With *treatment* the reparative process may not begin for 1–3 yr, but recovery with ankylosis and little or no deformity can be expected in the majority of well-treated cases. Paraplegia may resolve completely. Traditional therapy consisted of holding the patient in continuous extension on a Bradford frame or in a plaster body jacket until there was no evidence of active infection. Immobilization has not been shown, however, to improve the results of antibiotic treatment of tuberculosis of the thoracic or lumbar vertebrae. In paraplegic patients or those with extensive bone destruction and necrosis, surgical debridement and bone grafting, with 18 mo of systemic administration of isoniazid and ethambutol (Table 10–32), have produced the best results. A 3rd drug may be indicated in areas of the world where resistant organisms are prevalent. When surgical facilities and skills are not available, ambulatory 2-drug antibiotic treatment alone may be effective but is associated with increased morbidity (scoliosis).

Back Pain in Children. Back pain in children is frequently a sign of a significant underlying disorder. Roentgenographic examination should be made in order to identify Scheuermann disease, spondylolisthesis, evidence of infection in the vertebral bodies, or narrowing of the disc space that might indicate an adjacent bony infection ("discitis"). Lesions such as osteoid osteoma and infection may be the cause of considerable pain and yet be very difficult to locate by roentgenography; children with persistent back pain and no roentgenographic abnormalities should have a radionuclide bone scan.

Sacral Agenesis. This abnormality has a high incidence in infants of diabetic mothers. There is an absence of 1 or more lumbar vertebral segments, the iliac wings are not anchored to any bone structure, and the femora and tibias are usually short. There are marked flexion contractures and webbing of the skin between the leg and the thigh. The feet are usually abnormal. Renal anomalies are frequently associated.

For this devastating anomaly rehabilitation usually requires amputation of the lower extremities at the knees or hips, with prosthetic replacement. The absence of connection between the ilia and the lumbar vertebrae presents difficulties with spinal curvature.

23.7 THE NECK

Congenital Torticollis. It should be possible to turn the head of a newborn infant 90° in both directions, but limitation of motion of the neck may not become apparent until 1 wk of age. The inability to achieve this range of motion should suggest congenital torticollis, a condition in which the sternocleidomastoid muscle on 1 side is shortened. In early infancy the muscle may contain a firm mass in its midportion, but this is not evident after 2–3 mo. If this condition goes untreated, the muscle becomes fibrotic and shortened, the head and face become asymmetric, and there will be permanent limitation of motion in the neck. The etiology of this condition is unknown. See also Sec 22.6.

The treatment initially is exercise to stretch the involved sternocleidomastoid muscle. This requires turning the face toward the affected muscle but tilting it in the opposite direction and extending the neck. For example, if the right sternocleidomastoid muscle is affected, the chin should be turned to the right, the left ear brought down toward the left shoulder, and the neck extended. This position should be held for a count of 5 and repeated 10 times, twice daily. This exercise requires 1 person to hold the thorax and shoulders and another to hold the infant's head with a hand on each side. It is best done with the infant's head extended over the end of a table (Fig 23–14). The exercise requires very explicit instruction to the parents. In addition, the crib should be placed so that the child who turns the head in the wrong direction sees less interesting objects. Similarly, the way in which the parents feed and play with the child can be used to encourage turning the head in the proper direction. If exercises do not give full correction, surgical release of the sternocleidomastoid muscle will be necessary.

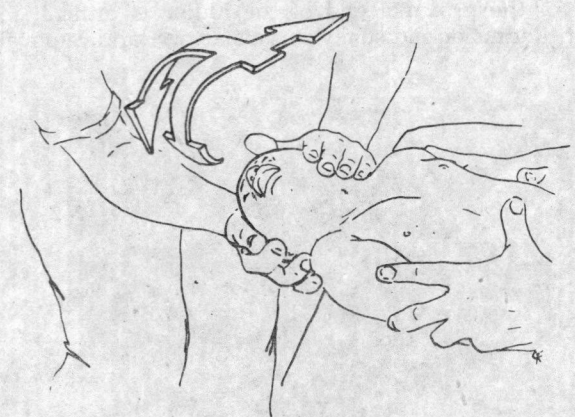

Figure 23–14 Exercises to stretch out a tight-sternocleidomastoideus muscle in congenital torticollis. The motion is a combination of rotation toward the affected (right) side, tilting away from the affected side, and extension of the neck.

Spastic Torticollis. After mild trauma or a tonsillar infection a child may complain of pain in the neck and hold the neck to 1 side in a fixed position. Such behavior immediately suggests a rotary subluxation of the atlantoaxial joint. If there is no roentgenographic evidence of subluxation, treatment with a soft collar (which can be readily made from a rolled towel pinned or taped in place), application of local heat, and the use of aspirin are usually sufficient. Occasionally, cervical traction is required. Mild or persistent cervical pain should suggest the possibility of juvenile rheumatoid arthritis. Intraspinal tumors can also cause torticollis.

Klippel-Feil Disorder. This congenital dysgenesis consists of failure of segmentation of the cervical spine and is often associated with congenital anomalies of other skeletal parts of the same segment, such as Sprengel deformity. Generally, no treatment is required for the cervical spine itself.

23.8 DEFORMITIES OF THE STERNUM

Fissure of the sternum is the term used when the halves of the sternum remain separated. *Pigeon breast* is prominence of the sternum and the cartilaginous parts of the ribs, with lateral depressions of the thorax. A short sternum is a common manifestation of trisomy 18.

Pectus excavatum (Sec 12.102), or indentation of the lower half of the sternum, may be rachitic in origin or the result of chronic obstruction to respiration. In most instances, however, the condition is congenital. The manubrium is at the normal level, but the inferior parts are depressed, the xiphoid approaching the vertebral bodies. The deformity can have adverse psychologic effects on the child. Surgical improvement may be attempted for cosmetic reasons if the deformity is severe or if compression causes pulmonary embarrassment.

23.9 THE UPPER EXTREMITIES

Sprengel Deformity. In this congenital condition the scapula fails to descend completely from its embryonic position in the neck to its usual thoracic location. It may be unilateral or bilateral. There may be a fibrous, cartilaginous, or osseous connection between the scapula and the spine (an omovertebral connection). The scapula is smaller than usual, and abduction of the arm may be limited. There is webbing of the neck, which is often exaggerated by a short neck resulting from associated congenital anomalies of the cervical spine (Klippel-Feil disorder). There may be associated abnormalities of the kidneys and decreased hearing acuity. Treatment is directed at releasing the omovertebral connection to allow greater motion. Removal of the upper segment of the scapula and repositioning the scapula inferiorly improve the appearance.

Congenital Amputations of the Upper Extremity. Congenital amputations more commonly involve the upper extremity than the lower. They may involve only parts of fingers or may extend to the loss of an entire arm and represent intrauterine destruction of limbs that were originally normally formed. Children with con-

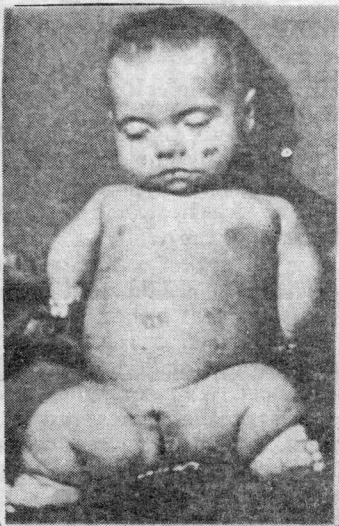

Figure 23–15 Partial phocomelia in an infant 11 mo of age, picture taken at autopsy.

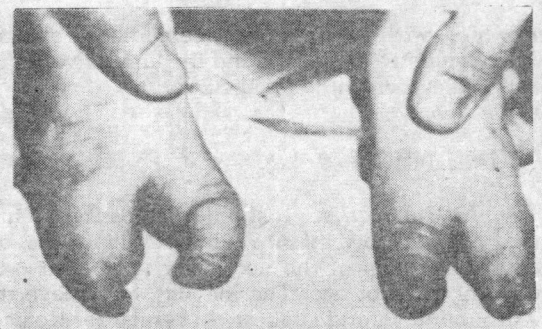

Figure 23–17 Split feet (lobster claws) in a child whose mother, maternal aunt, and maternal grandfather had similar malformations.

genital amputations of the upper extremities should be seen in specialized facilities as soon as possible. An appropriate prosthesis can be used after the child is able to sit. The 1st prosthesis is usually nothing more than a paddle to allow 2-handed functions. When a child is 1.5–2 yr of age, an active terminal device can be fitted. If prosthetic management is not started early, children develop 1-handed patterns which are virtually impossible to break. Cosmetic prostheses with actively operated hands are not available for children under about 5 yr of age and are very expensive. In the absence of sensory feedback children frequently abuse such structures (e.g., use a hand as a hammer); accordingly, most physicians are reluctant to prescribe expensive and delicate prosthetic devices.

Deformities of the Extremities. Severe deformities of the extremities are often associated with other malformations incompatible with life. Surviving children with extensive defects of the limbs were rare until the epidemic resulting from maternal ingestion of thalidomide. Limb defects due to primary inhibition of development or growth are called *reduction malformations* and frequently have terminal fingers or nails, indicating that no true amputation has occurred.

Amelia means absence of limbs. *Hemimelia* refers to defects of the distal parts of the extremities, such as absence of forearm and hand or lower leg and foot. *Phocomelia* signifies a great reduction in size of the proximal parts of the limb, resulting in an approach of distal parts toward the trunk (Fig 23–15). In complete phocomelia the hand or foot seems to spring directly from the trunk. *Acheiria* and *apodia* are terms for absence of the hand or foot; *adactyly* for absence of digits (Fig 23–16); and *aphalangia* for absence of phalanges.

Split hand and *split foot* are deep clefts in the anterior part of the hand or foot (Fig 23–17), the foot appearing split where the 2nd or 3rd toe should be. Fingers and toes may have various degrees of syndactyly (Fig 23–18). *Brachydactyly*, abnormal shortness of fingers or toes resulting from lack of or reduction in size of the phalanx or metacarpal bone, may be genetically determined. It may also be seen in pseudohypoparathyroidism, pseudopseudohypoparathyroidism, and Turner syndrome. *Clinodactyly*, incurving of the little finger, may be inherited as a dominant trait and is often seen in Down syndrome. *Camptodactyly*, permanently flexed fingers, can be transmitted as a dominant trait; it also occurs in trisomies D and E. *Macrodactyly* is a hypertrophy of 1 or several fingers and toes and may be a manifestation of neurofibromatosis.

Congenitally Dislocated Radial Head. This dislocation of the proximal end of the radius is difficult to treat. Reduction is usually unsatisfactory, and removal

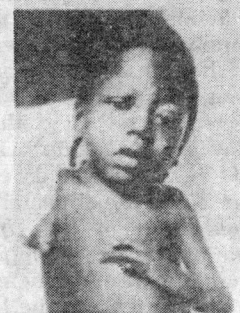

Figure 23–16 Phocomelia and partial adactyly in a girl 3.5 yr of age.

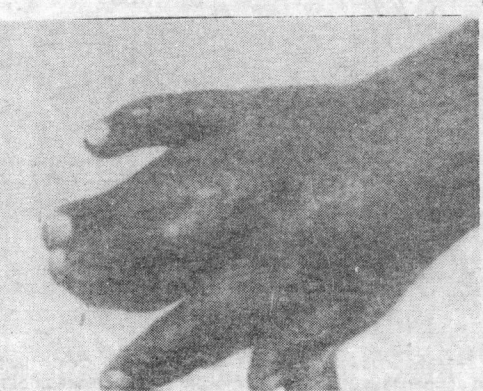

Figure 23–18 Syndactyly.

of the head of the radius before the end of growth leads to shortening of the radius with radial deviation of the hand and consequent dysfunction of the wrist. After the child has attained full growth, the radial head may be removed if it is a cosmetic problem.

Congenital Radioulnar Synostosis. Fusion at birth of the proximal end of the radius and ulna results in an inability to pronate and supinate the forearm. Since attempts to divide this synostosis to allow motion have almost always failed, surgical treatment is directed at correcting extremes of position in order to leave the forearm in a useful neutral position.

Absence of the Radius or Ulna ("Club Hand"). Congenital absence of the radius or ulna is rare. In the former, which is more common, the soft tissues of the radial side of the arm act as a tension band, drawing the hand radially so that the wrist is pulled off the end of the ulna. Treatment is directed at stretching out the soft tissues during infancy, followed by surgical release and positioning the wrist on the ulna. Retention of this new position is a major problem; a number of operations may be required during the growing period to keep the hand appropriately placed. Radial anomalies of the hand, wrist, and forearm may be associated with congenital cardiac disease and certain blood dyscrasias (Sec 14.4).

Pulled Elbow (Traumatic Subluxation of the Radial Head, Nursemaid's Elbow). This very common condition occurs in children from 1–4 yr of age. The child refuses to move the arm and holds it slightly flexed at the elbow and pronated at the forearm. The cause of this disorder is sudden forceful longitudinal traction upon the arm, which may happen when a parent tries to drag a reluctant child by the arm or the child trips while being held by the arm. The sudden traction carries the head of the radius slightly distally and may partially tear the annular ligament at its attachment on the radius. When the traction is released, the annular ligament becomes impacted between the radius and the capitellum. Roentgenographic examination will not demonstrate the abnormality.

The condition is treated simply by supinating the arm fully, as may, on occasion, unwittingly be done when positioning the forearm for a lateral roentgenogram. If a finger is held over the proximal radius as the arm is supinated, a click may be felt. Following reduction, the child may not move the arm immediately, but over the next 20–30 min spontaneous motion is usually noted. No postreduction fixation is needed unless the condition has recurred, in which case a collar-and-cuff sling is used. The parents should be alerted to the cause of the disorder to prevent recurrence.

Osteochondrosis of the Elbow. Children may suffer from osteochondrosis of the capitellum, the trochlea, or both. The etiology is unknown and is presumed to be analogous to osteochondritis dissecans of the knee. Trauma may play a role, especially in youngsters trying to emulate professional baseball pitchers. Treatment is usually supportive, but if fragments of the articular cartilage drop free into the joint, they must be surgically removed.

Polydactyly. Extra digits in the hand are most commonly seen at either the 5th finger or the thumb. These are frequently nothing more than skin tabs and can be readily removed. If they contain any bony element, it is preferable to delay their removal until the child is older than 9 mo, when there is more ossification of the cartilaginous anlage and a better assessment can be made of the amount of bone that must be removed.

Syndactyly. Syndactyly of the fingers (Fig 23–18) generally requires surgical treatment. Because of the varied lengths of the metacarpals and phalanges in the different fingers, the joints of 2 adjacent and fused fingers do not line up side by side; their flexion and extension are therefore limited. If syndactyly is allowed to persist, there will be bony deformities at the joint with significant loss of function.

Tuberculous Dactylitis. Dactylitis occurs most frequently in early childhood and involves 1 or more of the phalanges, the metacarpal bones, or the corresponding bones of the feet. The medullary canal of the involved bone becomes caseous; the cortex, thinned and expanded; and the periosteum, thickened. The entire digit develops a spindle-shaped, hard, red swelling as the soft tissues are affected. The process is comparatively painless, but it lasts many mo and may leave a permanent deformity. The differential diagnosis involves chiefly the dactylitis of congenital syphilis, which is more often multiple and symmetric. Dactylitis may also occur in sickle cell anemia and in coccidioidomycosis. The involved region should be put at rest with a splint or cast; surgical drainage is indicated if an abscess develops.

23.10 THE HEAD

Craniosynostosis. Premature closure of 1 or more sutures of the skull results in deformity of the head and, depending on which suture is involved, may cause damage to the brain and the eyes.

Congenital craniosynostoses originate in embryonic life for unknown reasons and may be associated with other skeletal defects. In other instances craniostenoses may be postnatal and associated with rickets, hypophosphatasia, and idiopathic hypercalcemia and may follow shunt procedures for hydrocephalus.

In the normal newborn infant the bones of the cranium are separated, but soon after birth the definitive sutures are established. The edges of the flat bones are separated by fibrous tissue in which growth takes place perpendicular to the line of the suture. Premature closure of a suture results in failure of growth of the vault at right angles to the involved suture and compensatory growth in regions where the sutures are patent.

When the *sagittal sutures* close prematurely, the head becomes long and narrow (scaphocephaly) and a bony ridge often marks the obliterated sutures. Males are affected more often than females. Ocular or neurologic abnormalities are rarely related to the abnormality of the suture.

Closure of the *coronal suture* results in severe deformity of the head (oxycephaly, acrocephaly) and in deformity of the face and orbits. The roof of the orbit is depressed, exophthalmos develops, and there may be strabismus, nystagmus, papilledema, optic atrophy, and loss of vision. The complications are more severe when both coronal sutures are obliterated or when other sutures are involved. Other malformations such as cardiac anomalies, choanal atresia, or defects of the elbow and knee joints may be associated. Syndactyly is the most commonly associated anomaly. A familial form of closure of the coronal sutures associated with hemolytic jaundice has been reported.

Acrocephalosyndactyly (Apert syndrome) consists of deformity of the skull secondary to closure of the coronal sutures and syndactyly of the hands and sometimes of the feet. It is thought to follow autosomal dominant transmission. Acrocephalopolysyndactyly (Carpenter syndrome) has certain similarities to the Apert syndrome and to the Laurence-Moon-Biedl syndrome. Besides acrocephaly, there is a peculiar facies, brachysyndactyly of the fingers, preaxial polydactyly and syndactyly of the toes, hypogenitalism, obesity, and mental retardation. Transmission is autosomal recessive. Craniofacial dysostosis (Crouzon disease) is characterized by acrocephaly, a beak-shaped nose, hypoplastic maxilla, short upper and protruding lower lips, hypertelorism, exophthalmos, and external strabismus. In clover-leaf skull syndrome (Kleeblattschädel) the severely deformed skull has a trilobed configuration as seen on a frontal roentgenogram. It is due to premature synostosis of some cranial sutures and is associated with marked hydrocephalus. The skull bulges toward the vertex and the temporal regions. It is often associated with skeletal dysplasias.

Oxycephaly or acrocephaly must be distinguished from a familial form of high skull in which premature closure of the sutures does not take place. In microcephaly the head is small, the vault is symmetric, and the sutures are patent; there is failure of the brain to grow. In craniosynostosis, roentgenograms of the skull reveal abnormality in shape depending on the suture or sutures involved. The involved suture may be obliterated or marked by a thin lucent line, but there is frequently thickening of bone along the suture and bony bridging.

Closure of the sagittal suture is rarely associated with complications except for the cosmetic problem of a long narrow head. In other congenital forms of craniosynostosis compression of the brain or cranial nerves may require surgical *treatment*. When the lesion is one which may result in significant cerebral or visual damage, surgical intervention in early infancy may lessen or avoid such damage. Surgical treatment consists of linear craniectomy along the prematurely closed suture. Since there is rapid growth of the brain during the 1st 6 mo of life, surgery will be most effective when performed soon after birth. Secondary closure of 1 or more of the cranial sutures occurs months after birth and only rarely requires surgical treatment. In Crouzon and Apert syndromes, maxillary advancement, a complex surgical technique, may be of value.

Lacunar Skull. This cranial anomaly is characterized by defects in the vault in the form of shadow depressions or deep cavitations extending to the outer surface and occurring mainly in the frontal or parietal regions. The thinned areas of bone are lined by dura and bordered by regions of osseous tissue. The outer surface of the skull is smooth. The roentgenographic appearance is diagnostic and shows diminution in the thickness of the bones of the skull and variations in their density as irregular areas of rarefaction, or lacunae, separated by ridges of increased density (Fig 23–19). Differentiation should be made from the generalized "hammered silver" or "digital impression" appearance of the bones of the skull, which is observed sometimes without apparent explanation or, in other instances, in association with increased intracranial pressure, particularly in later childhood.

Lacunar skull is found roentgenographically in approximately half the infants with meningocele or myelomeningocele. When the latter is associated with the lacunar skull, progressive hydrocephalus is a frequent complication. As the cranium enlarges, the bony ridges become thin and the lacunae disappear.

Parietal Foramina. These are irregularly shaped congenital defects of varying size and well-defined margins symmetrically placed on each side of the posterior third of the sagittal suture. They are palpable but frequently discovered only roentgenographically. They may be transmitted through several generations or occur sporadically in otherwise normal persons. They must be distinguished from defects of the skull associated with meningoencephalocele or from defects caused by reticuloendotheliosis, infection, multiple myeloma, or metastases. Parietal foramina cause no discomfort, and no treatment is indicated.

Basilar Impression (Occipitalization of the Atlas; Platybasia). This condition may be primary or secondary. In primary basilar impression there is encroachment upon the cervical vertebral canal and posterior cranial fossa. The 1st and 2nd occipital segments and the 1st and 2nd cervical vertebrae may be fused into a bony mass. This anomaly is similar to the Klippel-Feil syndrome except that the latter involves the cervical segments below the 2nd. Secondary basilar impression occurs when the cranial bones are so softened by disease that they no longer support the weight of the

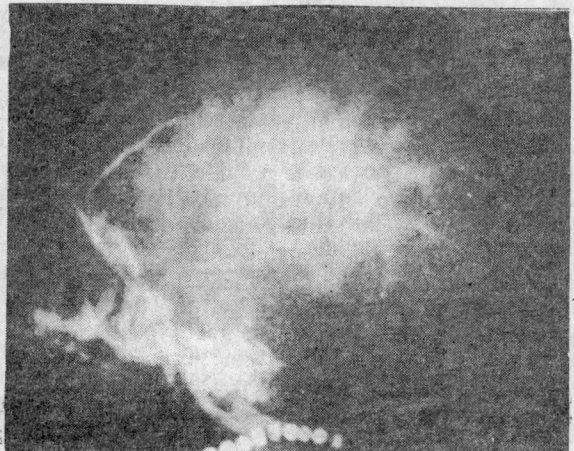

Figure 23–19 Lacunar skull. Multiple areas of decreased density in the frontal and parietal bones are delineated by thick bony ridges. The external surface of the cranial bones is smooth. The patient had a lumbar meningocele.

head. It may occur in rickets (osteomalacia). The cranial vertex approaches the occiput, encroaching upon the posterior cranial fossa. Flattening of the base of the skull (platybasia or an increased basal angle) is at times associated with basilar impression.

In either primary or secondary basilar impression, upward displacement of the odontoid process occurs which narrows the foramen magnum. Kinking of the medulla over the odontoid process may produce pressure upon the spinal cord. Localized thickening of the dura at the craniovertebral junction is frequently associated and contributes to constriction of the brain stem. This constriction may, in some instances, be relieved by surgery.

Ocular Hypertelorism. This condition consists of an abnormally large distance between the eyes and apparent broadening of the root of the nose; it is a nonspecific sign and not a disease entity. The diagnosis is made by determining the distance between the pupils rather than by inspection alone. It is often associated with mental deficiency or with other congenital defects. Mild forms occur in otherwise normal children. The lesser wings of the sphenoid bone are overdeveloped, the greater wings relatively small. Hypertelorism can be transmitted through several generations. Epicanthal folds may result in an appearance resembling hypertelorism, but with normal intrapupillary distance. Hypertelorism may be a sign of an ethmoid encephalocele.

23.11 TRAUMA

Epiphyseal Fractures. Fractures of an epiphysis can be innocuous or disastrous. In a growing bone the area of least resistance to stress is the junction between the metaphysis of the bone and the cartilaginous epiphyseal plate. If a bone breaks at this junction and is repositioned accurately, the rapid turnover of bone at this site allows for healing in 2–4 wk. Alternatively, a blow along the axis of a long bone which crushes the cartilaginous cells or injures the blood supply to them may destroy the epiphyseal cartilage plate, with subsequent loss of growth. If fractures at approximately right angles across the epiphyseal cartilage plate are not repositioned exactly, bone from the metaphysis will bridge to the epiphysis and there will be marked distortion of subsequent bony growth.

Harris-Salter Type I fractures (Fig 23–20) are not easily recognized on roentgenograms since there is no discontinuity in the outline of the bone. They are suspected only from the nature of the injury and from the swelling seen clinically or roentgenographically. "Ankle sprains" in young children are likely to involve Harris-Salter I epiphyseal fractures of the distal fibula.

Stress Fractures. Children, especially adolescents, engaging in intense physical activity after a period of decreased activity (such as football training after a summer's layoff) may develop pains in the region of the proximal tibia or at the junction of the distal three quarters of the femur. These represent fractures through an area of remodeling where the body is trying to improve the structure of the bone (Sec 23.13). Roentgenograms may show an area of reactive bone healing in the periosteum, often mistaken for a malignant tumor. Treatment is to refrain from such activity. Crutches may be needed.

Avulsion Injuries. Avulsions of the origins of muscles about the hip are common (Sec 23.3). These may also be seen at the insertion of the peroneus brevis on the 5th metatarsal of the foot.

23.12 SPORTS PARTICIPATION

The past decade has seen a marked increase in organized sports activities for adolescents and preadolescents and the inclusion of girls in many of them. This rapid growth has been accompanied by problems and controversies, including whether this age group's physical activities should be organized or spontaneous, individual or team-oriented.

Advocates of organized sports believe that the availability of adult supervision reduces risks of bodily trauma. Trained coaches teach better techniques of play, which reduce injuries. Risk of injury is inherently less in children since the energy of collision (proportional

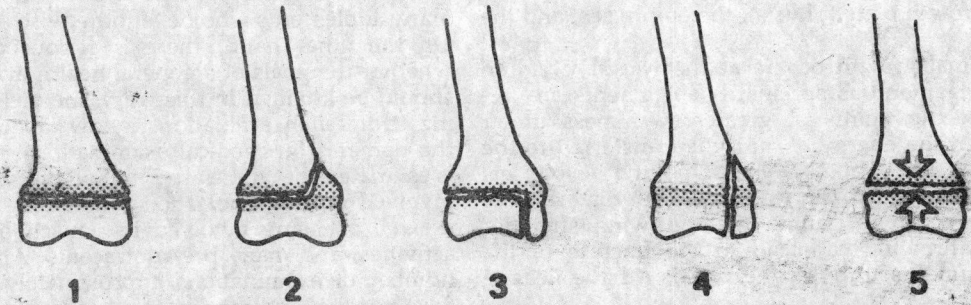

1   2   3   4   5

Figure 23-20 Salter-Harris classification of epiphyseal fractures. (1) The epiphysis separates from the metaphysis. The germinal cells remain with the epiphysis, usually uninjured. Healing is rapid and growth seldom arrested. (2) Similar to type 1, except that a small piece of metaphysis breaks free to remain with the epiphysis. Healing is rapid and growth is usually normal. Types 1 and 2 are the most common. (3) Separation passes a variable distance along the growth plate, then enters the joint. Accurate reduction of the intra-articular fracture is necessary to prevent lateral traumatic arthritis. Open reduction may be needed. Growth disturbances are not usually a problem. (4) The fracture extends from the joint, across the growth plate, and into the metaphysis. This usually requires open reduction to prevent unilateral growth arrest and traumatic arthritis from malposition. (5) This is a crushing injury which leads to death of the germinal cells of the epiphyseal cartilage and arrest of growth. This type is rare.

to the mass and the square of the velocity) is smaller in children than in adults. Data show, for example, that football injuries in organized leagues of preadolescents are less frequent or serious than in college leagues.

Opponents argue, however, that poor leadership frequently leads growing children into physical activity more appropriate for adults. Injuries will increase in frequency as the number of participants and exposure time are increased, and recurrent minor trauma may ultimately exact a major toll upon the growing skeleton.

Advocates believe that children gain self-confidence and enjoyment from learning to play well under organized coaching. They also find organized sports desirable as outlets for children's energies which might otherwise be spent in unwholesome activities. The substantial involvement of girls in organized sports can help eliminate some sex discrimination in expectation of gender roles. Opponents see the dangers of poor leadership, which can overemphasize and overvalue winning rather than sportsmanship, and undue emphasis on the trappings of the sport (in the form of uniforms and cheerleaders, for example) which can distort values and judgment as to what is good, desirable, and fair in play. "Not making the team" can represent serious emotional trauma for a child. The manner in which funds are allocated to the cost of equipment and transportation can easily be recognized in some communities as reflecting socially discriminatory decision making. Some of the organizations which promote certain sports have been blatantly sexist.

Advocates of team sports believe that they contribute to socialization in preparation for adult activities that involve "team efforts" and that teams may also provide good training for leadership, with players other than "stars" able to participate within the framework of the whole team. Critics of emphasis on teams point to the importance of individual sport to adult lives. They are concerned also that the "team mentality" decreases self-reliance in thought and action.

23.13 SPORTS INJURIES PECULIAR TO CHILDREN

The skeleton that is still growing has special areas of susceptibility to injury not found in adults; these include the growth plate (physis), the epiphyses, and the apophyses.

Longitudinal growth occurs at the *physis*. Children can suffer ligamentous sprains, but ligaments are frequently not the points of greatest weakness under stress. When the energy of injury is transferred to the bone, it may break at its weakest point, the physeal cartilage. Such a break can lead to growth disturbances (Sec 23.11). Chronic trauma to a growing shoulder caused by throwing can lead to the fracture of the proximal humerus through the physis ("Little League shoulder").

The *epiphysis*, in addition to the end of the bone and its articular cartilage, contains a layer of physeal cartilage (indistinguishable from the cells of the physis). The epiphysis is responsible for growth in diameter of the bone ends and for the sculpturing of the joint. The articular cartilage has beneath it a layer of physeal cells (like those of the growth plate) which are supported by the bony center in the epiphysis. Repeated excessive axial loading compresses these cells against the underlying bony support, causing not only temporary injury but also alteration of the joint configuration and lifelong arthritis, e.g., injury to the distal humerus (known as "Little League elbow") (Sec 23.9). Osteochondritis dissecans, which characteristically afflicts the knee, may be secondary to trauma (Sec 23.4).

Major tendons attach to bones at *apophyses* via an interfacing layer of physeal cartilage. Tendons which insert on the bones through apophyseal cartilaginous plates are prone to avulsion. This occurs most commonly around the hip, involving muscles which originate in the pelvis (Sec 23.3). Osgood-Schlatter disease is a chronic partial avulsion of the infrapatellar ligament of the quadriceps from the anterior tibial tubercle (Sec 23.4).

Stress Fractures. Stress fractures are not limited to children, but children's growing bones are especially susceptible. Cortical bone under unusual stress responds by seeking a structurally stronger form. Osteoclastic activity dissolves some bone, which is replaced with concentric lamellae. At the point where the bone substance has been weakened temporarily by osteoclasts (a process which may take several wk) the bone may fracture under stress. Stress fractures are typically noted after a few wk of vigorous physical activity which has followed a prolonged rest (for example, during the 1st weeks of spring training after a winter layoff). These are most commonly seen in tibia, distal fibula, and metatarsals (See also Sec 23.11).

Excessive lumbar extension, such as back walk-overs in young gymnasts, may lead to stress fracture of the pars interarticularis of the lumbar spine (spondylolysis) (See also Sec 23.6).

23.14 PREVENTION OF SPORTS INJURIES

Pre-participation Medical Evaluation. Physical examination prior to participation in organized sports is frequently mandated, either to exclude children susceptible to injury or to counsel children and assign them to physically appropriate activities. Such pre-participation examinations provide a medical evaluation for many adolescents who never otherwise see a physician. On the other hand, there is serious question as to whether the goals of a general health evaluation can or should be attained in this way. The yield of abnormalities from such evaluations is low (about 1%), though the demand for medical examinations is enormous. It is estimated that there are 7 million high school children involved in interscholastic sports in the United States, as well as many involved in nonschool-related sport activities, and many pre-adolescents. Among the large number of examinations approximately 15% result in false-positive findings; these cause unnecessary anguish and considerable cost for the consultations required to determine that the affected children can participate. Some sports physicians have advised that children with lax ligaments should avoid contact sports or that they should be put on pre-participation training, but no substantial data indicate that these measures decrease the rate of injuries.

If pre-participation evaluation is to be done, the goals of the evaluation should be clear. If it is a yearly routine examination, then a complete physical examination can be done. If the goal is a matter simply of pre-sports evaluation, the aim is to find conditions which might interfere with the ability of the child to participate in a specific sport, be made worse by the sport, or indicate an increased susceptibility to injury.

The medical history is the primary source of significant findings, especially in respect to head injury, syncope with exercise, and recurrent sprains. Examination of the eyes, ears, nose, and throat, auscultation of the lungs, or eliciting deep tendon reflexes, for example, are of little value. Blood pressure should be measured. This is especially important for primarily isometric activities, such as weight-lifting, in which marked increases in pressure will occur. Assessment of sex maturity ratings (Tanner) has been advocated so that later-maturing children can be counseled to avoid collision sports; on the other hand, no data yet show that this advice decreases rates of injury. Estimation of joint laxity, either for individual joints or overall, is advocated by some, but awaits evaluation. Urine or blood analyses have not proved to be useful to these evaluations.

Education for Sports Participation. The child, parents, and coaches should understand the necessity for pre-season conditioning and for proper stretching and warming-up exercises prior to practice or competitive events. Such practices as achieving rapid weight loss to enter a lower wrestling weight category should be discouraged. Considerable effort may need to be expended in assessment of the appropriateness of the sport activities engaged in. An over-enthusiastic coach may push children to excessively vigorous activity or to undue prolongation of an activity. In muscle-strengthening exercises children should be encouraged to work with less weight and increased frequency; the converse can be harmful. Some parents feel that certain practices, rule changes, or use of protective equipment designed to limit injuries are to protect "sissy kids." When this feeling leads to laxity on the part of officials (who may be the parents thenselves), failure to enforce the rules may place the children in jeopardy. Education about these and other issues may require that the physician observe the sports program and talk with students, parents, and coaches.

Physicians may be in a strategic position to influence community attitudes toward sports. In an educational role the physician should be concerned with emotional as well as physical stress.

Protective Equipment. Advances have been made in protective equipment for children involved in sports of violence; use of this protective equipment can sometimes be overdone, however, in the desire to emulate the adult model. Cleats on football boots, for example, lead to a higher incidence of ankle injuries; the longer the cleats, the higher the accident rate. Playing in running shoes may appear less professional but can be safer. Equipment manufacturers have not always provided equipment of appropriate size for pre-adolescents. It is sometimes difficult to find the child inside the protective layer of padding; a child so equipped cannot move with good coordination.

Rule Changes. Organizations responsible for some sports have tried to alter the rules to make the games safer for children (for example, a rule limits pitching in Little League baseball to 6 innings/wk to minimize the likelihood of "Little League elbow"). Benefits of such rules can be undone by lack of awareness on the part of parents who allow the child to practice pitching at home considerably in excess of the rules. Prohibiting "spearing" and cross-body blocking in football and base-sliding in baseball has helped diminish injuries. Physicians who monitor such games should encourage vigorous enforcement of these rules.

Clinical. Injuries may be minimized by paying early attention to any child complaining of pain; minor microtrauma can be identified and/or stopped before disaster strikes.

INFECTIONS OF BONES AND JOINTS

See Sec 10.14 and 10.15.

HUGH G. WATTS
JOHN KIRKPATRICK, JR.

Currarine G: Normal variants in congenital anomalies in the region of the obelion. Am J Roentgenol 127:487, 1976.

D'Angielis JA, Fisher RL, Ozonoff MB, et al: 99m Tc-polyphosphate bone imaging in Legg-Perthes disease. Radiology 115:407, 1975.

Fraumani JF, Geiser GG, Manning MD: Wilms' tumor and congenital hemihypertrophy: Report of five new cases in review of literature. Pediatrics 40:886, 1967.

Garrick JG, Smith NJ: Preparticipation sports assessment. Pediatrics 66:803, 1980.

Hemple DJ, Harris LE, Svien HJ, et al: Craniosynostosis involving the sagittal suture only. Guilt by association? J Pediatr 58:342, 1961.

Ianaconne G, Guerlini G: So-called clover-leaf skull syndrome: Report of three cases with discussion of its relationships with thanatophoric dwarfism and the craniosynostosis. Pediatr Radiol 2:157, 1974.

Micheli LJ: Sports injuries in children and adolescents. *In:* Straus R (ed): Sports Medicine and Physiology. Philadelphia, WB Saunders, 1979, pp 268–303.

Passarge E, Lenz W: Syndrome of caudal regression in infants of diabetic mothers. Pediatrics 37:672, 1966.

Rang M: Children's Fractures. Philadelphia, JB Lippincott, 1974.

Riseborough EG, Herndon JH: Scoliosis and Other Deformities of the Axial Skeleton, Boston, Little, Brown, 1975.

Smith DW: Recognizable Patterns of Human Malformation. Ed 2. Philadelphia, WB Saunders, 1977.

Tachdjian MO: Pediatric Orthopedics. Philadelphia, WB Saunders, 1972.

Warkany J: Congenital Malformations, Notes and Comments. Chicago, Year Book Medical Publishers, 1971.

23.15   GENETIC SKELETAL DYSPLASIAS

Developmental defects affecting the skeleton, while individually rare, contribute a major portion of the burden of short stature and skeletal deformity at all ages. They include dysplasias (disorders of growth), dysostoses (malformations of the bone), idiopathic osteolyses (pathologic resorption of bone), chromosomal aberrations with skeletal malformations, and metabolic disorders affecting the skeleton.

Nomenclature. The term "dwarfism" has been replaced by "dysplasia." The nomenclature of the genetic dysplasias reflects clinical, genetic, and/or roentgenographic features. A name will describe the skeletal segment involved or some other feature of the disorder. Some disorders are eponymous. Disorders with short stature are divided into short-trunk and short-limb conditions; the latter are divided into rhizomelic (shortening involving mainly the proximal segment of the limbs), mesomelic (shortening of the middle segments), and acromelic (shortening of the distal segments). In acromesomelic dysplasia both middle and distal segments are involved. Other names of skeletal dysplasias describe unique roentgenographic features (e.g., chondrodysplasia punctata) or the pattern of involvement of skeletal elements (e.g., epiphyseal, metaphyseal, or diaphyseal). With primary involvement of skull the prefix cranio- may be used; with significant involvement of the spine, spondylo- may be used.

Diagnosis and Assessment. The majority of congenital skeletal dysplasias show disproportionate lengths of limbs and trunk. Usually, it is the limbs which are relatively short, even in conditions such as spondyloepiphyseal dysplasia congenita and metatropic dysplasia, in which, as the child grows, disproportion becomes manifestly greater in the shortened trunk than in the limbs. When the disproportion between limbs and trunk is not obvious, the disproportionately large head size may suggest dysplasia (e.g., with achondroplasia or hypochondroplasia). Associated abnormalities aid in diagnosis. Cleft palate occurs with high frequency in Kniest dysplasia, in spondyloepiphyseal dysplasia (SED) congenita, and in Stickler arthro-ophthalmopathy; polydactyly is often associated with chondroectodermal dysplasia (Ellis–van Creveld), asphyxiating thoracic dysplasia, and other short rib–polydactyly syndromes.

In infants with the short rib–polydactyly syndromes, thanatophoric dysplasia, and lethal perinatal osteogenesis imperfecta, respiratory distress due to a short, small thorax is largely responsible for neonatal death.

Skeletal dysplasias vary in the ages at which they become apparent. When patients present beyond the newborn period, the most frequent reason for referral is disproportionate short stature, due either to relatively short limbs or to a short trunk, with kyphosis or scoliosis. Asymmetric growth of the limbs also occurs, as in chondrodysplasia punctata (Conradi-Hünermann), hemimelic epiphyseal dysplasia (Trevor), and multiple cartilaginous exostoses. Symptoms may arise from decreased density of the skeleton, as in osteogenesis imperfecta syndromes, or from increased density

with hematologic or neurologic complications, as in hyperostotic skeletal dysplasias.

Whatever the presentation, the approach to these disorders of skeletal development is the same. Prenatal, perinatal, and postnatal growth history should be reviewed and the family history taken. Physical examination should assess the symmetry and proportions of the patient, with a search for associated skeletal or extraskeletal malformations. Measurements should include height, length of upper segment (US) and lower segment (LS), span, head circumference, and chest circumference; these measurements should be made periodically and plotted on appropriate growth charts. Specific growth charts exist for patients with achondroplastic dysplasia or with other diagnoses. The upper segment/lower segment (US/LS) ratio and span/length ratio may aid in diagnosis. For example, a high US/LS ratio is characteristic of short-limb dysplasias (in which also span is usually less than height), whereas a decrease in US/LS ratio is found in short-trunk conditions, such as spondyloepiphyseal dysplasia.

Roentgenographic studies are required for the diagnostic differentiation of skeletal dysplasias; serial examinations are necessary for delineation of some conditions and for assessment of complications specific to each dysplasia.

At the 1st consultation a full series of skeletal views is usually required for liveborn or stillborn infants and for children of any age. These views include anteroposterior (AP), lateral, and Towne views of the skull, AP and lateral views of the spine, and AP views of the pelvis and extremities, with separate views of hands and feet. Lateral views of the foot are particularly helpful in identifying punctate calcification of the calcaneus and in detecting absence or hypoplasia of calcaneus and talus in the epiphyseal dysplasias.

In certain disorders radiologic features are diagnostic; others may require serial studies or the review of films by physicians with special experience in these conditions. In several countries registries of skeletal dysplasias exist for this purpose.

Pathologic Studies. Specific histologic or ultrastructural changes are found in many dysplasias, especially in the lethal neonatal disorders. When affected infants die, autopsy should be obtained whenever possible, with specimens preserved of costochondral junction and of growth plates of iliac crest and of long bones such as femur, tibia, or fibula.

The best diagnostic study during life is biopsy of a rib or of the iliac crest. A trephine biopsy of the iliac crest is suitable. Appropriate studies may differentiate closely related conditions, but some dysplasias show only nonspecific histopathologic changes; in such cases pathologic examination is useful in excluding other diagnoses.

Biochemical Studies. Patients with severe congenital hypophosphatasia have markedly low serum alkaline phosphatase activities and elevated urinary levels of phosphorylethanolamine, and bone and liver isoenzymes of alkaline phosphatase can be studied in cul-

Table 23-1 SKELETAL DYSPLASIAS WITH ASSOCIATED IMMUNE DEFICIENCY

	McKusick No.*
Metaphyseal chondrodysplasia McKusick type	25025
Metaphyseal chondrodysplasia with thymolymphopenia	20090
Metaphyseal dysplasia with severe combined immunodeficiency (adenosine deaminase deficiency)	24275
Metaphyseal dysplasia with pancreatic insufficiency and neutropenia (Shwachman)	26040†
Metaphyseal dysplasia with short ribs, neutropenia, and pancreatic insufficiency	26040†

*McKusick VA: Mendelian Inheritance in Man, 1978.
†Probably 2 distinct syndromes.

tured fibroblasts. Patients with lysosomal storage disease have deficiencies of specific lysosomal enzymes in serum, blood leukocytes, or cultured skin fibroblasts. On the other hand, the underlying biochemical defect in most cases of skeletal dysplasia is unknown. Biochemical research is active; the birth of an affected infant warrants prompt consultation with research workers in this field.

Certain skeletal dysplasias are characterized by disordered immune (Table 23–1), renal (Table 23–2), neurologic, cardiovascular, ophthalmologic, or hearing and speech functions (Table 23–3). These complications should be sought at the time of diagnosis and with periodic screening throughout life.

Management. Effective management requires (1) precise diagnosis, (2) prompt recognition of specific skeletal and nonskeletal complications, (3) appropriate orthopedic and rehabilitative care, (4) emotional support and psychosocial counseling, and (5) genetic counseling. There is no specific cure for any of these conditions. Use of growth hormone is not indicated for short stature due to skeletal dysplasia. Use of androgenic hormones has given no evidence of sustained growth and no gains which outweigh their potentially serious side effects.

Orthopedic management aims at maximizing mobility and correcting deformity; if deformities in the lower limbs are left uncorrected beyond puberty, early onset of osteoarthritis may lead to mechanically unsound joints. Early recognition of spinal deformity and its early treatment with bracing or minimal surgical intervention may reduce morbidity (from scoliosis, etc.) in adult life.

The need for educational and emotional support and

Table 23-2 SKELETAL DYSPLASIAS FREQUENTLY ASSOCIATED WITH RENAL COMPLICATIONS

	McKusick No.*
Lethal to newborn	
Short rib–polydactyly syndrome I (Saldino-Noonan)	26353
Short rib–polydactyly syndrome II (Majewski)	26352
Usually nonlethal	
Asphyxiating thoracic dysplasia	20850
Acrodysplasia with retinitis pigmentosa and nephropathy (Saldino-Mainzer)	26692

*McKusick VA: Mendelian Inheritance in Man, 1978.

Table 23-3 SKELETAL DYSPLASIAS ASSOCIATED WITH HEARING IMPAIRMENT

	McKusick No.*
Predominantly sensorineural	
Congenital	
Spondyloepiphyseal dysplasia congenita	18390
Kniest dysplasia	18655
Diastrophic dysplasia	22260
Otopalatodigital syndrome	31130
Stickler syndrome	10830
Due to progressive 8th nerve encroachment	
Osteopetrosis	16660
Craniodiaphyseal dysplasia	21830
Craniometaphyseal dysplasia	12300 and 21840
Endosteal hyperostosis (van Buchem)	23910
Sclerosteosis	26950
Hyperphosphatasia	23900
Frontometaphyseal dysplasia	13674
Predominantly conductive	
Achondroplasia†	10080
Hypochondroplasia‡	14600
Osteogenesis imperfecta (A.D.)	16620
Metaphyseal dysplasia and mental retardation	25042

*McKusick VA: Mendelian Inheritance in Man, 1978.
†Recurrent and chronic serous otitis media.
‡Infrequent.

counseling is often intense and chronic. Several lay organizations (see references) may help to provide emotional support and an environment in which short persons can learn together to adjust to a world of taller people.

23.16 DEFECTS OF THE GROWTH OF TUBULAR BONES AND/OR SPINE

ACHONDROPLASIA

Achondroplasia is the most common genetic skeletal dysplasia; it is inherited as an autosomal dominant trait (Fig 23–21). About 80% of cases represent new mutations. Achondroplasia occurs in about 1 in 25,000 births. Its pathogenesis is unknown. Disordered growth seems to involve mainly a reduced rate of qualitatively normal enchondral bone formation, with marked disturbance in craniofacial growth.

Clinical Manifestations. Rhizomelic shortening of the limbs can be recognized at birth, when most achondroplastic infants will already have large head size, frontal bossing, depression of the nasal bridge, and short stature. The limbs are covered with fatty folds of skin in infancy and early childhood. The hands are short and broad, with an appearance resembling a trident consisting of the thumb, the 2nd and 3rd digits, and the 4th and 5th digits, a wedge-shaped gap separating the 3rd and 4th fingers. The trident appearance is usually lost in late childhood or adolescence, the hand remaining short and broad. The elbows may be limited in extension and pronation. A lumbar gibbus is common in infancy, but after the 1st yr this almost always disappears, being replaced frequently by a

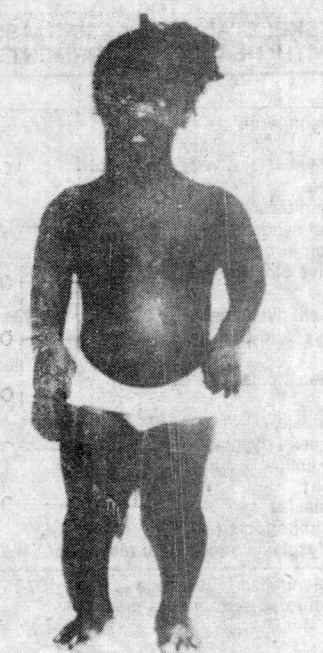

Figure 23–21 Achondroplasia demonstrating predominantly proximal (rhizomelic) limb shortening.

straight back, invariably with a prominent lumbar lordosis.

Achondroplastic infants are often hypotonic with delayed motor development. Normal neuromuscular tone is usually gained by 2–3 yr of age. Joint laxity, particularly in the interphalangeal joints, may persist throughout childhood. In the absence of hydrocephalus, mental and motor development are usually normal.

The head is large throughout life, with prominent frontal bossing, hypoplasia of the maxilla, and relative mandibular prognathism. The mean head circumference in achondroplasia follows a growth curve above the 97th percentile for normal individuals. Specific growth curves for achondroplasia have been developed, which are particularly valuable in monitoring the rapid growth in head size in infancy since hydrocephalus may complicate achondroplasia.

Dental malocclusion with anterior open bite is common and should be managed by an orthodontist familiar with the problem of achondroplasia. High frequencies of recurrent otitis media and chronic serous otitis media are found in children and lead to a high incidence of conductive hearing loss in adults.

Roentgenographic Manifestations. Roentgenograms show a short pelvis with broad iliac wings, horizontal acetabular roofs, and narrow, deep sacrosciatic notches. The vertebral interpedicular distance diminishes from L1–L5, in contrast to the normal caudal widening; this is a distinctive feature of achondroplasia though it may not be apparent in the newborn. The disc spaces are increased at the expense of the vertebral bodies, and the spinal canal is narrowed. There may be anterior tonguing and wedging of a lower thoracic or upper lumbar vertebra. There is posterior scalloping of the lumbar vertebrae; the pedicles appear short on lateral view. The base of the skull is shortened, and the foramen magnum is small and irregular. The cranium is large relative to the face, with frontal prominence and maxillary hypoplasia. The long bones are decreased in length, particularly in proximal limb segments, and appear rather wide and squat. The metaphyses have some flaring and may appear V-shaped (circumflex sign). The femoral neck may be radiolucent in infancy, and there is relative overgrowth of the fibulae. The short tubular bones of the hands and feet are shorter and wider than normal; the shortening is greatest in the phalanges. The chest has a decreased anteroposterior diameter, with anterior cupping of the ribs.

Management. Achondroplasia may be complicated by hydrocephalus (see above and Sec 21.10), which results from obstruction at the foramen magnum and by lumbar cord and nerve root compression syndromes, dental malocclusion, hearing impairment from repeated otitis media, and strabismus (resulting from craniofacial dysmorphism). Bowing of the legs and persistent kyphosis may also require attention. Besides the prompt recognition and appropriate treatment of these problems, management during childhood will mainly be concerned with the social and psychologic effects of severe short stature and unusual appearance and with genetic counseling. Prompt and appropriate therapy is particularly necessary for each episode of acute otitis media. Hydrocephalus is not common but must be recognized as early as possible. There is some evidence that physiotherapy and bracing during childhood can ameliorate the complications of prolonged infantile kyphosis or of the severe lordosis which may aggravate lumbar stenosis in adult life. Fibular epiphysiodesis is currently being evaluated for some children with severe progressive bowing of the legs. Osteotomies may be indicated during adolescence or later.

Prognosis. Except for the rare patient with hydrocephalus or with severe complications of cervical or lumbar spinal cord compression, the life span in achondroplasia is normal. The mean adult height in achondroplasia is about 131.5 cm (51.8 in) in men and 125 cm (49.2 in) in women.

HYPOCHONDROPLASIA

This form of short-limbed (rhizomelic) short stature is usually recognized from 2–3 yr of age. It appears to be distinct from achondroplasia, but there is wide variability in severity and much overlap in appearance with persons with achondroplasia. Morphologic studies of chondro-osseous tissue show qualitatively normal chondro-osseous transformation. Achondroplasia and hypochondroplasia appear to be allelic autosomal dominant disorders.

Clinical Manifestations. Hypochondroplasia is not usually recognized at birth. Head size is commonly within the normal range but may fall between the normal range and the range for achondroplasia. Usually, the nasal bridge is not depressed, nor is the mandible unusually prominent. Affected persons appear rather stocky and muscular. The hands and feet are short and broad but not trident, and the legs are usually straight, but mild genu varum may develop.

There may be a mild lumbar lordosis, pelvic tilt, and mild limitation of extension at the elbows, features which are always prominent in achondroplasia.

Roentgenographic Findings. These resemble those in achondroplasia but may be very mild. Features include prominent deltoid tubercles, relatively short ulnae with prominent radial styloids, relatively long fibulae, and narrowing or constancy of the interpedicular distance between L1–L5.

Complications. A small number of patients with hypochondroplasia and mental retardation have been reported. Whether this is a chance finding is not known.

Management. Hypochondroplasia causes little morbidity apart from short stature. The condition may require orthopedic management of problems such as leg bowing or lumbar spinal cord claudication.

THANATOPHORIC DYSPLASIA

Thanatophoric dysplasia is probably the most frequent lethal congenital skeletal dysplasia. Most cases have been sporadic. An instance of familial occurrence of thanatophoric dysplasia with clover-leaf skull deformity (Kleeblattschädel) has been reported.

Infants with thanatophoric dysplasia are shorter at birth than those with achondroplasia. They have a prominent forehead and depressed nasal bridge, with bulging eyes (Fig 23–22). The limbs are extremely short and held extended from the body. The chest is small and pear shaped. Affected infants are hypotonic and lack primitive reflexes. Roentgenograms show marked rhizomelic shortening of the long bones, with metaphyseal flaring, marginal spicules, and cupping. The changes in lumbar vertebrae are characteristic: inverted-U-shaped appearance in the anteroposterior view and marked flattening of vertebrae, with a notch-like defect in the central portion of the body, in the lateral view. The pelvis resembles that of achondroplasia, with short,

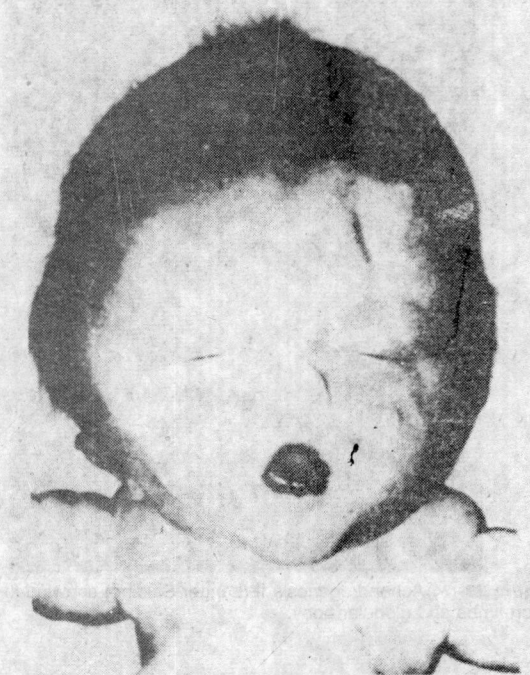

Figure 23–23 Cloverleaf skull deformity in association with thanatophoric dysplasia.

flat acetabula and small sacrosciatic notches, but spicules of bone protrude from both acetabula and ischia. The cranium is large, with a constricted base and a small foramen magnum. Clover-leaf skull deformity is found in some babies with thanatophoric dysplasia, all of whom have had hydrocephalus at autopsy (Fig 23–23).

ACHONDROGENESIS I (PARENTI-FRACCARO) AND ACHONDROGENESIS II (LANGER-SALDINO)

These rare autosomal recessive conditions are both lethal. They have clinical features in common and are distinguished by roentgenographic findings. Infants with achondrogenesis I have heads which appear large relative to the trunk, and the skull is extremely soft, with multiple small bone islands palpable in a membranous calvarium. The neck is very short, and the arms are extremely short and stubby. The thorax is small and barrel shaped rather than pear shaped. Roentgenograms show no ossification in any vertebral body, although ossification of the pedicles and neural arches is present down to the mid-sacrum. The ribs are thin and may contain multiple fractures; there are usually no fractures of the long bones. The femora appear short and square with prominent bony projections at the border of the metaphyses.

Infants with achondrogenesis II (Fig 23–24) have severe short limb stature, but the head is more proportionate to the body. The neck is short and hidden in skin folds; the trunk is short, with abdomen distended. The roentgenographic features differ from those of achondrogenesis I or of thanatophoric dysplasia. The skull is poorly mineralized but not so defective as in

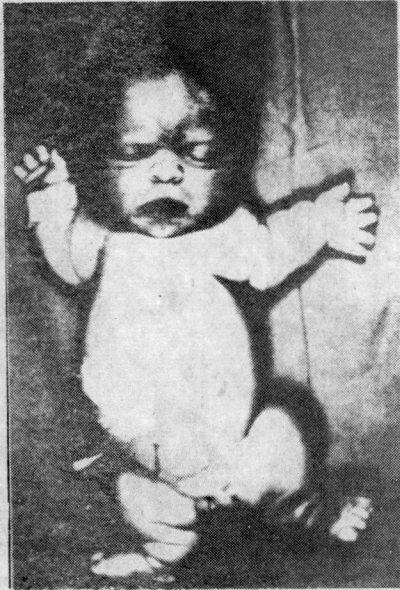

Figure 23–22 Thanatophoric dysplasia with short limbs, large head, prominent forehead, and depressed nasal bridge.

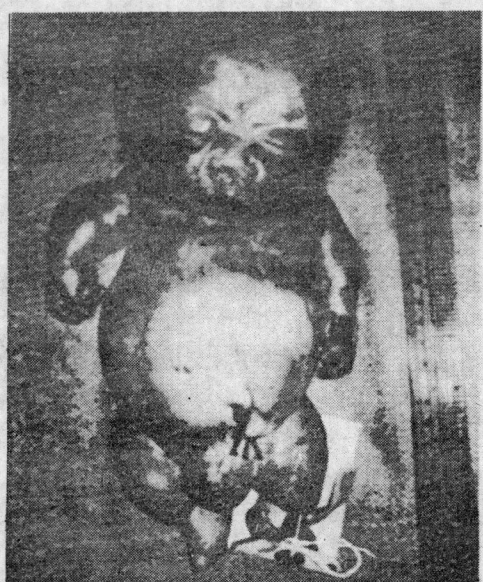

Figure 23–24 Achondrogenesis II (Langer-Saldino) showing extremely short limbs and globular body.

achondrogenesis I. The ribs are short but relatively normal in diameter. There is often lack of ossification of the vertebral bodies, but some infants show some ossification of the lower thoracic and upper lumbar vertebral centers. The ilia are small, with concave medial and inferior margins; ossification of the ischium and pubis is usually absent. The long bones are very short with metaphyseal flaring, spicules of ossification at both lateral and medial borders of the growth plate, and marked cupping.

SHORT RIB–POLYDACTYLY (SRP) SYNDROMES

SRP syndromes include lethal newborn skeletal dysplasias (Fig 23–25), SRP I (Saldino-Noonan) and SRP II (Majewski), and usually nonlethal disorders, asphyxiating thoracic dysplasia (ATD) and chondroectodermal dysplasia (Ellis–van Creveld). All are inherited as autosomal recessive conditions. They have in common respiratory distress due to pulmonary hypoplasia within a narrow dysplastic thorax with extremely short ribs. Polydactyly is almost always found in patients with SRP I, SRP II, and chondroectodermal dysplasia, but not as often in those with ATD.

SRP I (Saldino-Noonan) is characterized by relatively high frequencies of cloacal abnormalities (anal atresia, urogenital sinus) and of postaxial polydactyly, whereas *SRP II* (Majewski) has high frequencies of associated cleft upper lip or palate, multiple internal anomalies including hypoplastic epiglottis, cardiovascular defects, and pre- as well as postaxial polydactyly. Roentgenographically, both show extremely short horizontal ribs. The pelvis is small and hypoplastic in SRP I, with an irregular acetabular margin, whereas in SRP II the pelvis is normal. In some cases of SRP I long bones are hypoplastic, with poor corticomedullary demarcation; other cases have longitudinal spurs at the margins of the metaphyses, with a convex central metaphysis. In

SRP II long bones appear relatively normal apart from disproportionately short tibiae.

In the newborn it may be difficult to distinguish between *asphyxiating thoracic dysplasia* and *chondroectodermal dysplasia*. Both have short limbs and polydactyly and respiratory distress due to thoracic dysplasia. There is considerable clinical and roentgenographic variability in both. Roentgenograms may show short, horizontally oriented ribs and short pelvic bones with marked spurlike projections at the medial and lateral margins of the acetabula. Many patients survive the newborn period. Respiratory symptoms decrease with age.

In *asphyxiating thoracic dysplasia*, polydactyly may be absent or limited to the hands. Cardiac defects are uncommon. Many surviving patients develop a progressive renal disease which has glomerular, cystic, and interstitial elements.

Patients with *chondroectodermal dysplasia* often have congenital cardiac anomalies (usually atrial septal defects) and ectodermal abnormalities including hypoplastic nails, natal teeth, multiple frenula of the upper lip, cleft lip and palate, and epispadias.

Short ribs are found with other dysplasias besides the SRP syndromes (e.g., in thanatophoric dysplasia, sometimes in spondyloepiphyseal dysplasia congenita, in chondrodysplasia punctata, and in a syndrome of metaphyseal dysplasia associated with neutropenia), but polydactyly is associated with none of these conditions.

The respiratory distress of infants with SRP I and SRP II is not remediable. Some infants with asphyxiating thoracic dysplasia or severe chondroectodermal dys-

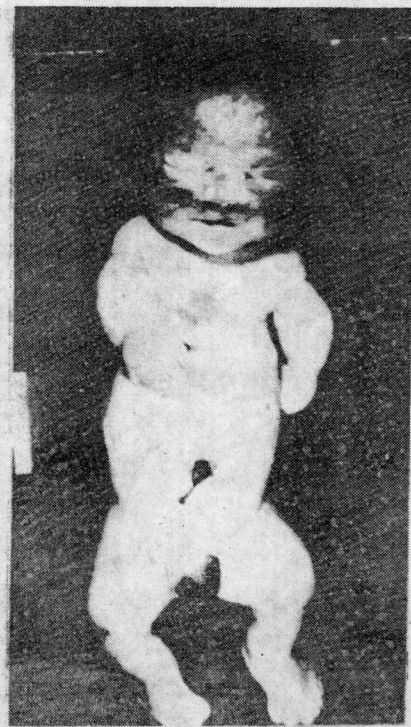

Figure 23–25 Short-rib polydactyly I (Saldino-Noonan) showing small thorax, postaxial hexadactyly in the fingers, and both pre- and postaxial heptadactyly of the feet.

plasia who have severe respiratory distress will show spontaneous improvement in respiratory function. In asphyxiating thoracic dysplasia, surgical enlargement of the thoracic cage with prolonged respirator management has permitted survival beyond the newborn period. Survivors have a high incidence of chronic renal failure.

CAMPOMELIC DYSPLASIAS

Campomelic dysplasia is characterized by short-limbed short stature, with bowing or bending of the long bones, particularly in the lower limbs; pretibial skin dimples at the site of the bowing; and associated anomalies. It is inherited as an autosomal recessive trait. The majority of reported cases are phenotypic females, some of whom have 46,XY karyotypes. Cases with intersex have been reported. The relationship between sex reversal and the skeletal dysplasia is not yet explained.

The classic finding in campomelic dysplasia is that the long bones are long and slender and usually bent at their midpoint. Cutaneous dimples may overlie the points of maximum curvature in tibia or fibula. Severe respiratory distress usually leads to early death, presumably due to small thoracic cage, narrow larynx, and hypoplasia of tracheal rings. Many other congenital abnormalities have been associated.

Roentgenograms show an enlarged dolichocephalic skull with narrow shallow orbits. The ribs usually number 11 and are often narrow. The cervical vertebral bodies may be hypoplastic and the lumbar interpedicular distance increased. The pelvis is usually tall, narrow, and hypoplastic.

Campomelia (bent limbs) is observed in the campomelic dysplasias, in osteogenesis imperfecta (at least 4 varieties), and in hypophosphatasia (dominant and recessive varieties). Bowing or angulation of the limbs is found also with other skeletal dysplasias and malformations.

CHONDRODYSPLASIA PUNCTATA
(Punctate Epiphyseal Dysplasia)

Chondrodysplasia punctata comprises several dysplasias in which roentgenograms of the epiphyses, periarticular tissues, and growth plate zones show stippled calcification. At least 3 defined genetic skeletal dysplasias showing this finding have been referred to as Conradi disease, chondrodystrophia calcificans congenita, punctate epiphyseal dysplasia, stippled epiphyses, or other names. These defined syndromes include a severe autosomal recessive rhizomelic form, an autosomal dominant form (Conradi-Hünermann), and a milder X-linked form. Laryngomalacia with stippling of the laryngeal cartilages occurs in some patients, who may have significant respiratory distress with upper airway obstruction during inspiration.

EPIPHYSEAL DYSPLASIAS

These are characterized by flattened, fragmented, or irregular epiphyses. The earliest feature may be delay in the development of certain epiphyses. The epiphyseal dysplasias can be broadly divided into those with spinal involvement (the spondyloepiphyseal dysplasias) and those without spinal involvement (the multiple epiphyseal or polyepiphyseal dysplasias). Many patients cannot be precisely classified.

Spondyloepiphyseal Dysplasias. These are characterized by flattening and irregularity of the vertebrae, with delay in ossification of the vertebral bodies. These changes are not pathognomonic of spondyloepiphyseal dysplasia (SED) since vertebral irregularity, including an increased incidence of Schmorl nodes, also occurs in adults with multiple epiphyseal dysplasias. Accurate diagnosis can be made only from serial roentgenographic assessments of the vertebrae at various ages. In some spondyloepiphyseal dysplasias (SED), skeletal dysplasia is evident at birth (SED congenita); in others, short stature develops during infancy or childhood (SED tarda). SED congenita has autosomal dominant inheritance with variable expressivity; SED tarda appears in both X-linked recessive and autosomal dominant forms.

Newborn infants with *SED congenita* have rhizomelic shortening of the limbs, but these appear long relative to the trunk. Hands and feet are of normal size so that the fingers appear excessively long. Club feet are common. The head is also normal in size, but the neck is extremely short with limited flexion. Odontoid hypoplasia is common and may lead to atlanto-occipital dislocation with cervical cord and root compression. Exaggerated dorsal kyphosis contributes to a broad barrel chest, and scoliosis commonly develops during adolescence. Marked lumbar lordosis, often with genu valgum or varum, leads to a waddling gait. Cleft palate is common. Over 50% of patients have severe myopia predisposing to retinal degeneration and detachment.

Roentgenographically, SED congenita is characterized by platyspondyly and epiphyseal dysplasia. In the newborn, ossification of the epiphyseal centers is retarded, especially at the ankles, knees, and hips. Epiphyseal ossification centers ultimately appear but are irregular, fragmented, and flattened. The proximal femoral epiphysis is severely affected; severe coxa vara results. The long bones appear shortened, especially the humerus and femur, but the hands are normal or show only minor abnormalities. In childhood the vertebrae are ovoid but later become flat and irregular with narrowed disc spaces. Odontoid hypoplasia may be found with subluxation of C1 on C2.

Some patients with SED congenita later show other features or have a relatively mild disorder, suggesting genetic heterogeneity.

Short stature in *SED tarda* (X-linked recessive type) is recognized from 5–10 yr of age, when spinal growth appears to be slowed and the shoulders assume a humped appearance. Mild to severe kyphoscoliosis may develop, and US/LS ratio is reduced. As adults, affected men have mild short stature, with short trunk, large chest capacity, and relatively normal limb length. The hands, head, and feet appear normal. During late childhood or adolescence vague back pain may occur; in early adulthood painful osteoarthritis with limited mobility of the back and hips is usually present. Symptoms may also affect the shoulder and, less commonly, the knees and ankles.

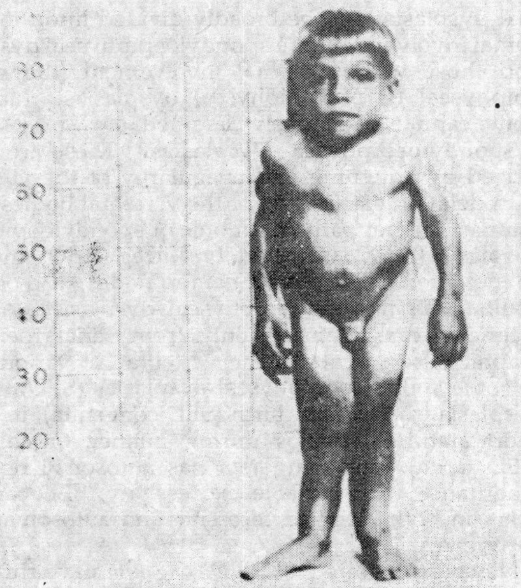

Figure 23–26 Spondylometepiphyseal dysplasia showing predominant shortening of the trunk characteristic of the spondylodysplasias.

Roentgenograms in SED tarda reveal diagnostic changes in the lumbar vertebrae by childhood or adolescence. Vertebral bodies show generalized mild flattening, with a hump-shaped build-up of bones in the central and posterior portions of the superior and inferior plates. No bone is visible in the areas of the ring epiphyses. Disc spaces appear narrowed and may appear to be calcified, but the calcification is part of the vertebral body itself. Premature disc degeneration occurs, and osteospondylotic changes develop in early childhood. The acetabula are deep and the femoral neck short. Mild dysplastic changes are seen in all large joints, especially the hips.

Differential Diagnosis. A dominantly inherited form of SED tarda has variable onset of manifestations after infancy, with distinctive roentgenographic features. Several conditions having metaphyseal as well as epiphyseal changes are called spondyloepimetaphyseal dysplasia or spondylometepiphyseal dysplasia, depending on the relative severity of metaphyseal or epiphyseal lesions (Fig. 23–26). *Stickler syndrome* (hereditary arthro-ophthalmopathy) is characterized by tall stature, myopia, and premature osteoarthritis. In the *Schwartz-Jampel* syndrome (myotonic chondrodysplasia) myotonia is associated with skeletal abnormalities. *Kniest dysplasia* is described below. Heterogeneity is marked among the spondyloepiphyseal dysplasias, many patients being unclassifiable.

Kniest Dysplasia. In this autosomal dominant condition there is a marked delay in epiphyseal ossification at the hips, short-trunk short stature, progressive kyphoscoliosis, and progressive joint limitation. The joint deformity and limitation are most marked at the knee and the small joints of the hands. The face is round and flat. Myopia and cleft palate are common. Roentgenographic features include coronal clefts in the ver-

tebrae, hypoplastic iliac bones with wide and irregular acetabular margins, dysplastic femoral heads which are very delayed in appearance, and short, thin tubular bones with flared metaphyses. Epiphyseal ossification is irregular and punctate, and with age a peculiar stippling occurs at the epiphyses and adjacent metaphyses.

Kniest syndrome must be differentiated from *Weissenbacher-Zweymuller syndrome*, an autosomal recessive condition characterized by only mild short stature and by improvement in the clinical and roentgenographic findings with age, and from *Rolland-Desbuquois syndrome*, an autosomal recessive condition having many features in common with Kniest dysplasia but showing more severe vertebral segmentation defects.

DIASTROPHIC DYSPLASIA

In this autosomal recessive disorder the dysplastic changes occur in auricular, tracheal, articular, and ligamentous tissues as well as chondro-osseous tissues. Affected persons have short-limb (rhizomelic) short stature, severe club feet, joint contractures, and deformity of the hands with a proximally placed hypermobile (hitchhiker) thumb (Fig 23–27). In about 85% of cases the pinnae of the ears become acutely inflamed and swollen during the 1st 2–5 wk of life and remain thickened, firm, and irregular (cauliflower ear). With time, the ear lesions calcify and may ossify. The palate is broad and high arched; cleft palate occurs in about 25% of cases. Laryngomalacia may lead to respiratory distress. Midline frontal hemangiomas are common.

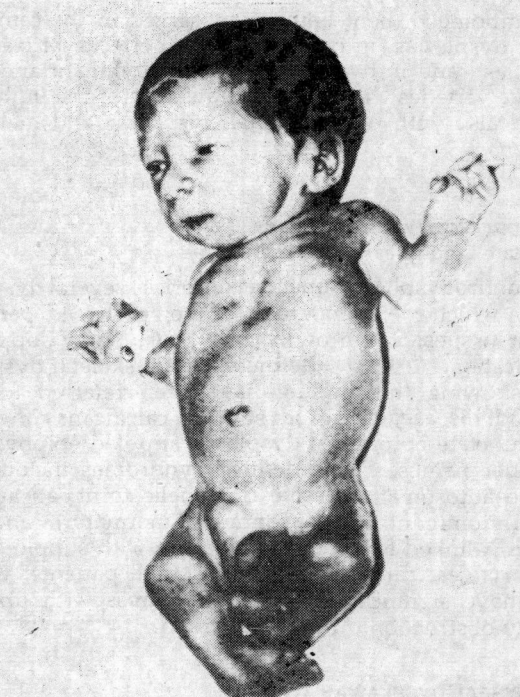

Figure 23–27 Diastrophic dysplasia showing fixed deformities of the knees and elbows, and "hitch-hiker" thumbs (and halluces).

The hips are normal at birth, but hip and knee dislocations frequently develop on weight bearing. Both stiff joints and loose joints may occur in the same patient, with subluxations and dislocations as well as contractures. Progressive scoliosis may develop during the 1st yr of life. Kyphosis of the spine may begin at adolescence and lead to respiratory difficulty in adults. The head and skull are normal. Some patients with milder features of diastrophic dysplasia have been termed "diastrophic variant."

Roentgenographic manifestations include hypoplasia of the epiphyses and flaring of the metaphyses in long tubular bones, carpal bone irregularities (including extra carpal bones), and twisted or fused metatarsals with equinovarus deformity. Caudal narrowing of the spinal canal may be present, and the cervical spine may be kyphotic, with C2–C3 dislocation. Metacarpals and phalanges are short and wide, and the 1st metacarpal is oval or triangular in shape and set low on the carpus.

METATROPIC DYSPLASIA

Metatropic dysplasia is characterized by short extremities, bulbous enlargement of the joints, joint limitation, and progressive and ultimately severe kyphoscoliosis. It is probably genetically heterogeneous, with both dominant and recessive autosomal varieties. At birth, affected children have a short-limbed appearance, but kyphoscoliosis develops rapidly, and a short-trunk appearance supervenes. The kyphosis may produce neurologic complications from acute angulation of the spinal cord. Some patients have a peculiar tail-like skin fold over the sacrum. Some patients die in infancy.

Roentgenographic findings at birth include extreme platyspondyly with tongue-like flattening of vertebrae and relatively large intervertebral spaces. The long bones are short, with irregularly expanded metaphyses resembling barbells. Epiphyses are deformed, flattened and irregular, and delayed in ossification. The tubular bones of the hands are short and broad with irregular epiphyses and metaphyses. Carpal ossification is delayed. The ribs are short, with flared and cupped costochondral junctions. Marked flaring of the iliac crests produces a "battle-axe" (halberd) appearance.

The kyphoscoliosis has generally been resistant to bracing or surgical treatment. Electrical stimulation to the sacrospinalis muscles with bracing has been reported to limit progression of kyphoscoliosis.

MESOMELIC DYSPLASIAS

This heterogeneous group of skeletal dysplasias is characterized predominantly by shortening in the mesomelic segments of the limbs (Fig 23–28). Modes of inheritance vary. Five syndromes manifest at birth are clearly delineated: The Nievergelt, Langer, Robinow, Rheinhardt, and Werner mesomelic dysplasias. The most common mesomelic dysplasia, dyschondrosteosis, is not manifest until late childhood. A number of other conditions with mesomelia, short stature, and other congenital abnormalities do not fit into these categories.

Dyschondrosteosis (Léri-Weill syndrome) results in mild mesomelic short stature with Madelung deformity at the wrist. Inheritance is autosomal dominant, with

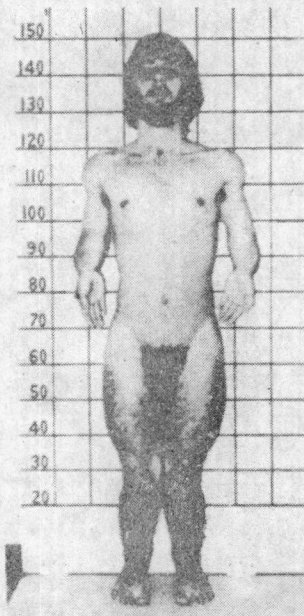

Figure 23–28 Mesomelic dysplasia with predominantly middle (mesomelic) limb shortening.

variable penetrance and expression. The bones of the forearm and leg are disproportionately shortened and appear wide. Hypoplasia and dorsal dislocation of the distal ends of the ulnae result in bilateral Madelung deformity. The carpal bones are wedged into a small triangular space between the deformed distal radius and ulna. The tibia and fibula appear widened. In some family members of normal stature the diagnosis is made solely on the basis of Madelung deformity.

Robinow mesomelic dysplasia is an autosomal dominant condition recognized by the flat facial profile, mesomelic shortening, and high frequency of genital hypoplasia. The distal ulna is hypoplastic; in some cases there is radial head dislocation. Prominent forehead, hypoplastic mandible and hypertelorism, and down-slanting palpebral fissures with a short, flat nose are characteristic. Genital hypoplasia may occur, with or without cryptorchidism. The nails are commonly hypoplastic.

Acromesomelic dysplasias include several distinct skeletal dysplasias characterized by disproportionate shortening, predominantly affecting the forearms, hands, feet, and legs, which can be recognized at birth or within the 1st months of life (Fig 23–29). In these the face and head are usually normal and the trunk only slightly shortened. The epiphyses and metaphyses of the long bones are unaffected.

CLEIDOCRANIAL DYSPLASIA

The disorder is characterized by varying degrees of hypoplasia of membranous bones. Inheritance is autosomal dominant, with variable expressivity. Hypoplasia of the anterior ends of the clavicles and sacral rami and delayed closure of the anterior fontanelle with multiple wormian bones are characteristic. The hypoplasia of the clavicles leads to abnormally low positioning of the

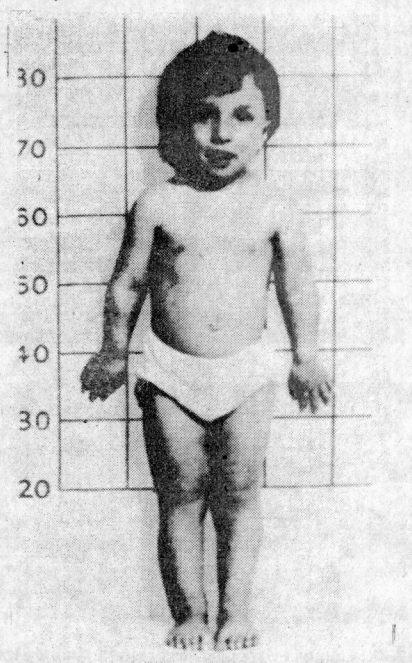

Figure 23–29 Peripheral dysostosis with disproportionate (acromelic) shortening of the fingers.

shoulders, which can commonly be apposed anteriorly. Frontal bossing, joint hyperlaxity leading to genu valgum, and dental anomalies are common. The primary dentition appears late and is frequently incomplete. The secondary dentition is similarly delayed and frequently malaligned, malformed, or hypoplastic. Proportionate short stature may occur.

Roentgenographically, there are variable degrees of hypoplasia of clavicles and scapulae and marked delay in ossification of the pubis and ischiopubic segments, with widening of the symphysis pubis.

LARSEN SYNDROME

This is a genetically heterogeneous group of disorders characterized by marked hyperlaxity and multiple dislocations, especially of the hips, knees, and elbows. Skin hyperlaxity and dermatorrhexis are not features. Autosomal dominant and, rarely, autosomal recessive transmissions occur. Affected patients characteristically have a prominent forehead, low nasal bridge, hypertelorism with a flattened face, disproportionate short stature, and, in about 50% of cases, cleft uvula and/or palate.

Roentgenographically, joint dislocations with secondary epiphyseal deformities are seen. Supernumerary carpal and tarsal ossification centers develop, and the 1st–4th metacarpals are short and broad. There may be premature fusion of the epiphysis and shaft of the 1st distal phalanx.

Larsen syndrome must be distinguished from Ehlers-Danlos syndrome, types III (benign hypermobility) and VII (arthrochalasis multiplex congenita), in which associated skeletal abnormalities and craniofacial dispro-

portion are not present. Multiple joint dislocations occur also in the otopalatodigital syndrome.

OTOPALATODIGITAL SYNDROME

This disorder is characterized by a distinct facies, abnormalities of the hands and feet, proportionate short stature, and, sometimes, mental retardation. Inheritance is X-linked dominant, with complete expression in males and milder features in carrier females. The facies has prominent supraorbital ridges, with a broad nasal root, flattening of the midface, and a small jaw. The thumbs and distal segments of the other fingers are short and broad. Dislocation of the radial heads and/or hips may be present. Midline cleft palate and conductive deafness are commonly associated.

METAPHYSEAL DYSPLASIAS

The metaphyseal dysplasias (formerly called metaphyseal dysostoses) are a heterogeneous group of disorders predominantly involving the metaphyses, with relatively normal epiphyses and spine. They should always be considered in the differential diagnosis of vitamin D–resistant rickets. Four principal types are the Jansen type (autosomal dominant), the Schmid type (autosomal dominant), the Spahr type (autosomal recessive), and the McKusick type (autosomal recessive), which is also called cartilage-hair hypoplasia.

The *Jansen type* produces the most severe short stature (adult height about 125 cm) and can be recognized in the newborn period or early infancy by the predominantly rhizomelic short stature, severe bowing of the legs, and mandibular hypoplasia. Joints are large, with contractures, and since the legs are more severely affected than the arms, the arms appear to hang down around the knees. Roentgenographically, all metaphyses, including those of hands and feet, are severely involved, appearing markedly enlarged, wide, irregular, and cystic. Epiphyses and spine appear relatively normal. The long bones are broad and short, and bowing is evident. Deafness has been associated with hyperostosis of the calvarium. Serum calcium levels are elevated in some patients. Serum alkaline phosphatase activity is slightly elevated. New mutations account for most cases.

The *Schmid type* of metaphyseal dysplasia is characterized by mild to moderate short stature (adult height 130–160 cm), bowing of the legs, and a waddling gait. It is usually recognized when the infant commences walking. Enlarged wrists and flaring of the rib cage are usually present. Roentgenographically, the metaphyseal changes are much less severe than those of the Jansen type. The metaphyses are flared and irregular and may be fragmented, with radiolucent streaks. Changes are most prominent in the hips, shoulders, knees, ankles, and wrists. In contrast to the McKusick variety, involvement of the femoral neck may be quite severe and result in marked coxa vara. This disorder has been frequently confused with vitamin D–resistant rickets, but calcium and phosphorus metabolism appears to be normal.

In the *McKusick type* of metaphyseal dysplasia (cartilage-hair hypoplasia) severe growth deficiency of postnatal onset, bowing deformities of the limbs, and particularly short, broad hands with loose joints are characteristic. Affected individuals also have an ectodermal dysplasia manifested by fine, light, sparse hair and a light complexion. Increased susceptibility to severe varicella infection in some patients reflects a deficiency in cellular immunity. Serum immunoglobulins have been reported to be normal. Aganglionic megacolon may be associated.

Roentgenographically, cartilage-hair hypoplasia is characterized by multiple metaphyseal lesions in the long and short tubular bones, with normal skull, spine, and epiphyses. Lesions especially involve the knees, and, in contrast to the Schmid type, the proximal femoral metaphyses are very mildly involved. The affected metaphyses are wide and irregular with sclerotic radiolucent cystic areas and linear streaks. The fibula is long relative to the tibia, producing an unstable ankle joint. Genu valgum is prominent. The ribs are short, with anterior cupping.

The *combination of metaphyseal abnormalities and immune deficiency* is found in at least 3 other autosomal recessive syndromes: (1) the Shwachman syndrome, in which skeletal lesions are associated with pancreatic exocrine insufficiency and chronic neutropenia; (2) metaphyseal chondrodysplasia–thymic alymphopenia syndrome; and (3) immunodeficiency due to adenosine deaminase deficiency, in which growth failure with metaphyseal irregularities and flaring of the ribs may occur.

SPONDYLOMETAPHYSEAL DYSPLASIAS

In these conditions abnormalities primarily involve the vertebrae and metaphyses.

Spondylometaphyseal dysplasia (SMD) Kozlowski is an autosomal dominant condition. Growth retardation is not usually apparent until 1–2 yr of age, when short-trunk short stature and waddling gait develop, with mild pectus carinatum, kyphoscoliosis, and precocious osteoarthritis in some patients. Affected children frequently have limb pains which are aggravated by exercise and relieved by rest; these may be misdiagnosed as "growing pains." Skeletal roentgenograms show generalized metaphyseal irregularities in the tubular bones, with normal or small and irregular epiphyses and platyspondyly. On anteroposterior view the vertebral bodies appear flat and broad, with prominent articular facets and spinal processes contributing to an "open staircase" appearance.

Spondylometaphyseal dysplasias other than the Kozlowski type have been described, some with other modes of inheritance.

PSEUDOACHONDROPLASIA

The pseudoachondroplasias are a group of disorders producing short-limb short stature with moderately severe reduction of trunk height and normal face. Both dominant and autosomal recessive forms have been described. Growth retardation is usually not apparent until 2–3 yr of age, with considerable variability in its severity. In some patients shortening is predominantly rhizomelic, in others predominantly mesomelic.

There is an exaggerated lumbar lordosis. Hypolaxity

of the joint in the periphery may lead to valgus or varus deformities at the knees. Deformities of the legs lead to a waddling gait. The hands and feet are short and broad, ligamentous laxity permitting telescoping of the fingers similar to that seen in cartilage-hair hypoplasia. Dislocations may be troublesome, particularly at the knees. Contractures may also occur at the hips and knees, and there may be limitation of extension at the elbow. Ulnar deviation at the wrist is characteristic. The major complication is precocious osteoarthritis.

Roentgenographically, the epiphyses and metaphyses of the tubular bones are involved, with platyspondyly and irregularity of the vertebrae. The vertebrae have irregular end-plates; anterior tonguing of the vertebral bodies is common.

DYGGVE-MELCHIOR-CLAUSEN SYNDROME

This rare dysplasia is characterized by short-trunk short stature with a barrel chest, accentuated lumbar lordosis, restricted joint mobility, and a waddling gait. Inheritance is autosomal recessive. In some sibships mental retardation has been associated. Roentgenographically, this is a spondyloepiphyseal dysplasia showing flat anteriorly beaked vertebral bodies, a fine lace-like ossification above the iliac crest, and irregular small carpal and metacarpal bones.

TRICHORHINOPHALANGEAL (TRP) SYNDROME

This is characterized by mild disproportionate short stature involving deformities of the fingers with a typical facies including sparse hair, pear-shaped nose, and medial accentuation of the eyebrows. Inheritance is autosomal dominant. The main roentgenographic features are numerous phalangeal cone-shaped epiphyses of the hands (PhCSEH), often associated with brachymetacarpism and brachymetatarsism. Legg-Perthes–like changes may occasionally occur in the hips.

OSTEOCHONDRODYSPLASIAS WITH ANARCHIC DEVELOPMENT OF CARTILAGINOUS OR FIBROUS TISSUE

These form a group of disorders in which development of abnormally placed cartilage or fibrous elements leads to skeletal deformity during growth, with relative hyperplasia or hypoplasia of skeletal elements. Two subgroups can be distinguished according to whether the anarchic proliferation involves cartilage or fibrous tissue: those involving cartilage include dysplasia epiphysealis hemimelica, multiple cartilaginous exostoses, Langer-Giedion syndrome (multiple cartilaginous exostoses–peripheral dysplasia), multiple enchondromatosis (Ollier), enchondromatosis with hemangioma (Maffucci), and metachondromatosis. Those involving fibrous tissue include fibrous dysplasia (Jaffe-Lichtenstein), fibrous dysplasia with skin pigmentation and precocious puberty (McCune-Albright), cherubism, and neurofibromatosis. The latter group is discussed elsewhere.

Abnormally situated growths of osteocartilaginous tissue may be localized to the epiphyses, the metaphyses, or the diaphyses of the long bones. Dysplasia epiphysealis hemimelica or tarsomegaly affects the skeleton of only 1 portion of the lower extremity. Cartilage may develop within bone (i.e., as an enchondroma) or on the surface of bone, commonly at the edge of the metaphyses (i.e., as exostosis or enchondroma).

In **dysplasia epiphysealis hemimelica (Trevor disease)** there is asymmetric overgrowth of the epiphyses, tarsal centers, and, rarely, carpal centers. All cases have been sporadic, with a male predominance noted. Because there may be involvement of an entire epiphysis rather than half, the term "unilateral epiphyseal dysplasia" has been suggested as an alternative name for this disease.

This condition is usually recognized in the 1st years of life because of foot or knee deformity, a limp, or a painful gait. Usually, there is a medial or lateral firm swelling at the knee or tibiotarsal joint with minimal loss of length in the involved leg. Roentgenographically, fragmentation and excessive growth of the involved epiphysis are seen, which commonly involves only 1 part of the epiphysis. Simultaneous involvement of several epiphyses is common, especially of foot and knee. The talus, distal femoral, and distal tibial epiphyses are the most common sites of disease. Lesions of the upper extremities are rare.

Multiple cartilaginous exostoses (MCE) are bony projections found near the ends of the tubular bones and ribs, the vertebral bodies, the scapulae, and the iliac crest. Roentgenographically, these tumors appear to originate at the borders of metaphyses and sometimes along the shafts (diaphyses) of the long bones. They are distinct from enchondromata (chondromata), which arise within the metaphyses and sometimes the diaphyses and which appear to be expanding within the metaphyses into the epiphyses. Inheritance is autosomal dominant with high penetrance but widely variable expression. It is generally believed that the pathogenesis involves proliferation of normal cartilage at the borders of the metaphyses, along the diaphyses, or alongside the cartilaginous borders of the vertebrae and scapulae. Because regular endochondral ossification occurs within these cartilaginous tumors, the center of the tumor becomes ossified. The medullary cavity of this central ossified area may communicate with the marrow space of the shaft of the affected bone.

The tumors may undergo rapid growth during infancy but are rarely detected roentgenographically prior to 3 yr of age, when they appear as bony projections from the affected bones, with a normal pattern of ossification. Exostoses at the ends of the long bones point away from the epiphyses. Involvement of metacarpals and phalanges frequently occurs, but the exostoses are small and rarely deform the fingers. Exostoses of the shaft of the humerus characteristically occur at the junction of the upper and middle thirds on the medial surface. The exostoses are not only unsightly but disturbing to the growth of long bones, producing deformation and sometimes compression of nerves and blood vessels. Severe deformity of the distal ulna is often associated with an asymmetric growth disturbance, dislocation of the radial head, and ulnar deviation of the hand. Involvement of the lower limbs may lead to coxa valga, genu valgum, or obliquity of the distal tibial epiphyses and limb length discrepancy. Final

adult height tends to be in the normal range, but mild skeletal disproportion may occur since limb involvement (often asymmetric) is much greater than spinal involvement. Malignant degeneration may occur, but rarely, if ever, in childhood.

Surgical treatment is indicated for cosmetically deforming lesions or those producing neurovascular complications. Wherever possible, surgery should be delayed until the end of growth because of the high chance of regression of the lesions.

Multiple cartilaginous exostoses–peripheral dysplasia (Langer-Giedion syndrome) is characterized by predominantly acromelic or acromesomelic short stature of postnatal onset, facial appearance similar to that in the trichorhinophalangeal syndrome (see above), mild microcephaly of postnatal onset, and multiple cartilaginous exostoses. All reported cases have been sporadic. The characteristic facies includes large, poorly developed, laterally protruding ears, sparse scalp hair with thick eyebrows, a large bulbous nose with a thick prominent septum, a simple prominent elongated philtrum, and a relatively recessed chin. Redundant or loose skin folds and hyperextensibility of skin and ligaments in infancy may lead to confusion with the Ehlers-Danlos syndrome.

Roentgenographically, 2 types of lesions are apparent: (1) multiple exostoses with all the possibilities for skeletal deformity produced by MCE alone, and (2) abnormalities in metacarpal and proximal phalanges consisting of cone-shaped epiphyses (see TRP syndrome), widening with lack of normal funnelization, and a hook-like, often asymmetric, projection of the metaphyses.

Enchondromata arise within bone, usually within areas of endochondral ossification. Single enchondromata of bone are not uncommon and may be incidentally detected. They may, on the other hand, produce local pain due to intramedullary expansion. *Multiple enchondromata* (Ollier disease) have widespread involvement of the skeleton, involving the hands; they are detected because of bone pain or deformity. All cases have been sporadic. Roentgenographically, the lesions may be detectable in early infancy as clear, homogeneous, oval lesions with axes parallel to the longitudinal axis of the bone.

Patients present because of growth disturbance, which may be asymmetric, leading to limp, or because of swelling of the fingers and toes in infancy. The tumors may produce visible or palpable swelling, particularly in the hands or the growing ends of the long bones; they are somewhat elastic and may limit mobility of neighboring joints. Phalangeal chondromas may lead to severe deformation of the fingers.

The effect of enchondromas on growth is usually much more serious than that of exostoses, and the prognosis is more serious than in MCE. Asymmetric growth disturbance is more severe. Involvement of distal ulna and radius may produce a severe deformation at the wrist leading to ulnar deviation of the hand. Malignant change is uncommon in childhood but has a high frequency in adults. Pain and rapid growth in size and/or radiologic evidence of endosteal erosion may indicate malignant change.

Surgical intervention is indicated for lesions causing local symptoms or growth plate deformation leading to marked limb asymmetry. Radionuclide scanning may be useful in investigating large enchondromata at risk of malignant change.

In **enchondromatosis with hemangiomatosis (Maffucci syndrome)** multiple enchondromata and hemangiomata of bone and overlying skin develop during childhood. The majority of affected persons are normal at birth; the lesions develop during infancy. All reported cases have been sporadic. The cutaneous lesions are usually cavernous or capillary hemangiomas, with or without lymphangiomas. Their distribution in skin appears to be independent of skeletal lesions; they may be found also in mucous membranes and intra-abdominal viscera. The skeletal lesions are typical enchondromata, involving metaphyses throughout the body; in some cases unilateral deformity predominates.

Maffucci syndrome produces a severe, cosmetically unsightly and often painful deformation of the skeleton. Neither the hemangiomata nor the enchondromata are amenable to surgical intervention except for palliation. The lesions lead to short stature, or if predominantly unilateral, to leg length discrepancy and scoliosis. The most serious complication is the development of malignancy, which has a higher incidence than malignant change in MCE. Chondrosarcomatous transformation of 1 or more enchondromata may occur; sarcomatous degeneration of hemangiomas and lymphangiomas has been reported.

Metachondromatosis is an exceedingly rare condition in which typical multiple cartilaginous exostoses and multiple enchondromata are found in the same patient. Inheritance is autosomal dominant. Affected patients are normal at birth; in infancy they acquire lesions in digits and long bones. Short stature may occur, although the majority of patients have normal stature.

23.17 ABNORMALITIES OF DENSITY OR MODELING OF THE SKELETON

This group of genetic skeletal dysplasias includes heritable conditions associated with osteoporosis (diminished or fragile bone), osteopetrosis, and hyperostosis or hyperplasia of bone producing abnormal modeling of the skull, long bones, or axial skeleton.

INHERITED OSTEOPOROSES

Osteopenia (insufficiency of bone) is a roentgenographic feature of many inherited or acquired disorders of childhood; it results from reduced production or increased breakdown of bone, or both. Osteoporosis (the clinical syndrome resulting from osteopenia) is characterized by susceptibility to fractures and particularly to crush fractures of vertebrae. Osteogenesis imperfecta is the most prevalent of the osteoporosis syndromes.

The term "osteogenesis imperfecta" (OI) was adopted by Vrolik in 1840 to explain a syndrome of osteoporosis, fractures, and skeletal deformities. Some of the affected die in the newborn period with extreme fragility of bone and numerous fractures (osteogenesis imperfecta congenita); others manifest bone fragility in life and live a normal life span (osteogenesis imperfecta tarda). The condition was once thought to be due to a single autosomal dominant gene, but it appears that at least 4 genetic syndromes account for variability in osteogenesis imperfecta. Serum alkaline phosphatase activity is elevated in all forms.

Osteogenesis Imperfecta Type I (OI Type I). This is characterized by osteoporosis and excessive bone fragility, with distinctly blue sclerae and presenile conductive hearing loss in adolescents and adults. Inheritance is autosomal dominant. This most common variety of osteogenesis imperfecta has an incidence of about 1:30,000 live births.

The sclerae in affected patients are generally of a deep blue-black hue. Fractures result from minimal trauma, but not all accidental trauma produces fractures. About 10% of affected infants have fractures at birth but generally only a few. Occurrence of neonatal fractures does not predict more deformity, more handicap, or a greater number of fractures than in other patients who have their 1st fractures after 1 yr of age. Deformities of the limbs in OI type I are largely the result of fractures, but bowing, particularly of the lower limbs, is common. Other deformities such as genu valgum and flat feet with metatarsus varus are common. About 20% of affected adults have progressive kyphoscoliosis which may be severe. Kyphosis alone is common in older adults but rarely seen in children. There is usually excessive hyperlaxity of ligaments, particularly at the small joints of the hands, feet, and knees, but this feature is less marked in adults. There is usually mild short stature, with body proportions depending on the relative involvement of limbs or spine. During adolescence there is a marked spontaneous reduction in the frequency of fractures.

Hearing impairment affects about 35% of patients; it is rare, however, before the end of the 1st decade.

Hereditary opalescent dentin (dentinogenesis imperfecta) is observed in some families with this trait. It produces distinctively yellow (or sometimes grayish-blue) transparent teeth, which are frequently prematurely eroded or broken. These teeth have short roots, with constricted coronoradicular junctions. Opalescent dentin may distinguish 2 hereditary types of osteogenesis imperfecta: OI type IA with normal teeth and OI type IB with opalescent dentin.

Roentgenographic studies in OI type I show generalized osteopenia, evidence of previous fractures, and normal callus formation at the site of recent fractures. Deformities are usually the result of angulation at the site of previous fractures, but bowing of the femora and tibia and fibula occurs as well as deformity in the bones of the feet, particularly metatarsus varus. Severe osteoporosis of the spine with codfish vertebrae is occasionally seen; kyphoscoliosis is not usually observed in childhood.

Osteogenesis Imperfecta Type II (OI Type II). This lethal syndrome is characterized by low birth weight

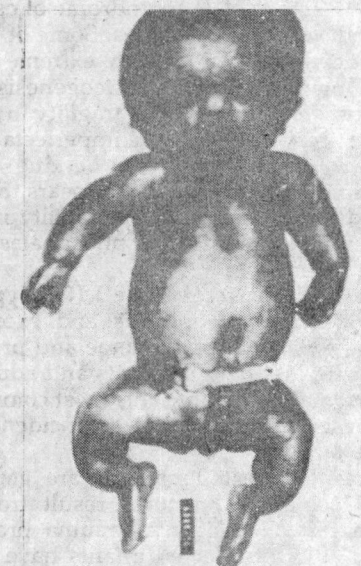

Figure 23–30 Osteogenesis imperfecta (OI) type II (lethal crumpled bone variety) with broad thighs and angulation deformities of the limbs.

and length and typical roentgenographic findings of crumpled long bones and beaded ribs. Autosomal recessive inheritance is probable. The condition affects about 1 infant in 60,000 live births.

Approximately 50% are stillborn, and the remainder die soon after birth, of respiratory insufficiency due to a defective thoracic cage. The skull is soft, with multiple palpable bone islands. The face may show beaking of the nose and apparent hypotelorism, and the limbs are extremely short, bent, and deformed. The thighs are broad and fixed at right angles to the trunk (Fig 23–30). The skin is thin and fragile and may be torn during delivery.

Roentgenograms show multiple fractures of the ribs and a crumpled (accordion-like) appearance of the long bones (especially the femora), with diffuse osteopenia in the face and skull and multiple bone islands in the vault.

Osteogenesis Imperfecta Type III (OI Type III). This syndrome of osteogenesis imperfecta is characteristically manifested in the newborn or young infant by severe bone fragility and multiple fractures, which lead to progressive skeletal deformity (Fig 23–31). The sclerae may be blue at birth and become less blue with age. Inheritance is autosomal recessive; clinical variability suggests genetic heterogeneity.

Very few patients with OI type III reach adult life. Infants generally have normal birth weight and often normal birth length, but the latter may be reduced by deformities of the lower limbs. Fractures are present in the majority of cases at birth and occur frequently during childhood. Kyphoscoliosis develops during childhood and progresses into adolescence. Final stature is very short. Hearing impairment has not been reported in children with this syndrome. A considerable proportion of patients succumb to cardiorespiratory complications in infancy or childhood.

Skeletal roentgenograms in OI type III show generalized osteopenia with multiple fractures, without the beading of the ribs or crumpling of long bones seen in OI type II. Osteopenia appears to be progressive, with platyspondyly and codfish vertebrae. The skull shows osteopenia and multiple wormian bones.

Osteogenesis Imperfecta Type IV (OI Type IV). This syndrome is characterized by osteoporosis leading to bone fragility without other features of classic OI type I. Inheritance is autosomal dominant. The sclerae in OI type IV may be bluish at birth but become less blue as the patient matures. Hearing impairment has not been observed; on the other hand, opalescent dentin has been observed in some families, suggesting heterogeneity within this group.

Patients with OI type IV have variable ages of onset of fractures, ranging from birth to adult life, and variable deformity of long bones and spine. Significant bowing of the lower limbs at birth may be the only feature of this syndrome, and progressive deformity of the long bones and spine has been reported without fractures. In several patients bowing has lessened with age. Like those with OI type I, patients with OI type IV show spontaneous improvement with puberty, few fractures showing up in adolescents and adults. Most patients, however, have short stature. Roentgenographically, there is generalized osteopenia. Multiple fractures may be observed at birth and occur throughout life, but these patients have less osteopenia and fewer fractures than infants with recessive varieties of osteogenesis imperfecta.

Management of Osteogenesis Imperfecta. For OI type II, no therapeutic intervention will be effective. For other forms of OI careful nursing of the newborn on a firm mattress or pillows may prevent excessive

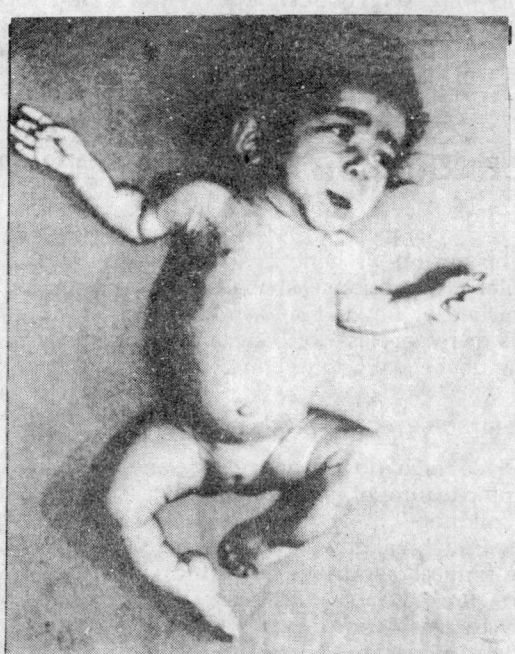

Figure 23–31 OI type III showing less shortening of limbs but angulation deformities of legs.

fractures. Beyond the newborn period the mainstay of management is an aggressive orthopedic regimen aimed at prompt splinting of fractures, correction of deformities arising from fractures, and correction of deformities arising from the progressive bowing or bending of the skeleton. Therapeutic regimens including supplements of calcium or fluoride, of vitamin C, or of magnesium oxide have shown no clear benefit. Calcitonin therapy has been reported to increase skeletal mass and decrease the frequency of fractures in some patients, but its use is investigative at present. Genetic counseling for affected families should aim at primary prevention. Reliable antenatal diagnosis is not available for osteogenesis imperfecta, but some severely affected fetuses with OI type II may be recognized prenatally through a combination of ultrasound and roentgenographic studies.

Osteoporosis with Pseudogliomatous Blindness. This rare autosomal recessive syndrome is characterized by generalized osteoporosis leading to fractures and deformities of long bones and spine. Ocular pseudogliomata, which may be mistaken for retinoblastoma, develop in infancy. Mild mental retardation has been observed in several of those affected but may be unrelated.

OSTEOPETROSIS, PYKNODYSOSTOSIS, AND DYSOSTEOSCLEROSIS

These conditions are characterized by generalized increase in skeletal density. Individually, they are distinguished by their mode of inheritance, age of onset, and pattern of skeletal involvement. Several forms of osteopetrosis have been described with overlapping spectra of clinical and roentgenographic features. A form with manifestations in the newborn and a progressive course leading to death at an early age is called *osteopetrosis with precocious manifestations*. A usually milder disorder with delayed manifestations is known as *osteopetrosis tarda* or *Albers-Schönberg disease*.

Osteopetrosis with Precocious Manifestations. The precocious form of osteopetrosis is most frequently discovered during the 1st months of life; it may appear as failure to thrive, malignant hypocalcemia, anemia with thrombocytopenia, or severe, perhaps overwhelming infection. Inheritance is generally autosomal recessive, but some cases may show autosomal dominant inheritance.

Rarely, fractures lead to medical attention. Hyperostosis may crowd the marrow cavity, with anemia and extramedullary hematopoiesis, hepatosplenomegaly, and thrombocytopenia. Anemia appears to result not from inadequate erythropoiesis but from excessive hemolysis. A defect in macrophage killing of bacteria may account for recurrent and sometimes overwhelming infection. Bony encroachment on the optic foramina may lead to optic atrophy and blindness, in some cases detectable at birth. Hypocalcemia is not uncommon, and serum phosphorus may be low. Serum alkaline phosphatase activity is elevated. Roentgenographically, the diagnostic findings are a generalized increase in bone density, with defective metaphyseal modeling and a "bone in bone" appearance most marked in the

vertebral bodies. Diffuse hyperostosis leads to loss of demarcation between the cortex and the medullary cavity. Irregular condensation of bone at the metaphyses may produce the appearance of parallel plates of dense bone at the ends of the long bones. The base of the skull is dense, with normal to increased density of the vault and markedly increased density in the orbital margins.

Treatment is aimed at decreasing or arresting progressive hyperostosis, correcting anemia and thrombocytopenia, and treating infections promptly and vigorously; a regimen of oral cellulose phosphate, prednisone, and low calcium diet has been reported effective in some but not all patients. The prednisone arrests the progress of anemia. Neurosurgical unroofing of the optic foramina has been tried in some patients, but results are difficult to interpret. Bone marrow transplantation with appropriately HLA-matched donor marrow has been reported to be curative in several patients, but the long-term success of this treatment remains to be learned. Generally, the prognosis for survival is poor, and death in the 1st few mo or yr from anemia, bleeding, or overwhelming infection is not uncommon.

Osteopetrosis Tarda (Albers-Schönberg Disease). This condition is found in childhood, adolescence, or young adult life because of fractures (about 10% of patients), mild craniofacial disproportion, mild anemia, complications arising from neurologic involvement, or osteitis with osteonecrosis (usually of the mandible). Increased bone density may be discovered incidentally on a roentgenographic study made for some other problem. Most cases appear to represent autosomal dominant inheritance, a few autosomal recessive.

Skeletal roentgenograms show generalized increase in density of cortical bone, with a club-shaped appearance of the long bones due to defective metaphyseal modeling. Over 50% of patients have longitudinal and transverse dense striations at the ends of the long bones. The vertebrae show alternating lucent and dense bands. The base of the skull is dense and thickened, but face and vault are less affected.

Management should be directed at recognition and treatment of complications, with frequent testing of visual fields and acuity and periodic roentgenograms of the optic foramina. Transfusion may be required for anemia, and splenectomy may be useful in some patients.

Pyknodysostosis. This autosomal recessive disorder is characterized by postnatal onset of short-limbed short stature and generalized hyperostosis. A disproportionately large skull, with frontal and occipital bossing and wide anterior fontanelle, may bring the patient to attention. The hands and feet are short and broad, and the nails may be deformed and brittle. The sclerae are often blue; this evidence combined with a tendency to fractures may lead to confusion with osteogenesis imperfecta.

Roentgenographically, there is a generalized increase in bone density without metaphyseal striation. The distal phalanges are characteristically hypoplastic or aplastic. The skull has wide sutures and wormian bones, the face a small mandible with an obtuse mandibular angle.

Dysosteosclerosis. This rare autosomal recessive disorder is characterized by generalized increase in bone density and short stature of postnatal onset. Dysosteosclerosis differs from osteopetrosis and pyknodysostosis in showing platyspondyly with superior and inferior irregularity of vertebral ossification. Developmental defects of the teeth are common, with delayed eruption of primary dentition, severe hypodontia, and early loss of the teeth. Secondary dentition may fail to erupt. Other complications (fractures, visual and hearing loss, and recurrent infections of mandible and paranasal sinuses) are similar to those of osteopetrosis.

OSTEOPOIKILOSIS, OSTEOPATHIA STRIATA, AND MELORHEOSTOSIS

These 3 conditions are usually asymptomatic and encountered incidentally through roentgenographic studies. Some patients have several types of lesions.

In *osteopoikilosis*, numerous small osteodense round or oval foci are seen in the skeleton, most commonly in the epiphyses and carpal and tarsal centers. Joint pain is associated in about 20% of cases, and skin lesions occur in some patients. The latter are slightly elevated whitish-yellow fibrocollagenous infiltrations (dermatofibrosis lenticularis disseminata). The incidence of keloid formation is increased. Inheritance is autosomal dominant.

In *osteopathia striata*, linear regular bands of increased density radiate from the metaphyses throughout the skeleton, with a fan-like array in the iliac wings. Inheritance is possibly autosomal dominant. The lesions should be differentiated from those of osteopetrosis, which are associated with modeling defects and transverse bands of osteodensity at the metaphyses. Osteopathia occurs with focal dermal hypoplasia (Goltz syndrome), in which linear lesions of dermal hypoplasia with herniation of the adipose tissue are associated with skeletal defects (hypoplasia or aplasia of limbs or syndactyly).

In *melorheostosis*, irregular linear osteodense lesions are seen along the axes of the tubular bones in single or multiple areas of the skeleton. No hereditary basis has been established. The osteodense lesions have been likened to wax flowing down the side of a candle. Since the pattern of lesions may follow the sensory sclerotomes, it has been suggested that melorheostosis may result from lesions of the sensory nerve supply to skeletal elements. The lesions may be associated with shortening of certain bones, with contractures of the joints or palmar and plantar fasciae, and with intermittently painful swelling of joints.

CRANIOTUBULAR REMODELING DISORDERS

A distinction has been drawn between craniotubular dysplasias, e.g., craniodiaphyseal dysplasia, in which modeling abnormalities are present, and craniotubular hyperostoses, e.g., endosteal hyperostosis (van Buchem), in which deformity is due to overgrowth of osseous tissue rather than to defective bone modeling. This distinction may be arbitrary since these disorders must be the resultant of bone resorption and bone deposition, albeit with different patterns of skeletal involvement. In all of them there is generally minimal involvement of the spine, as compared to osteopetrosis, pyknodysostosis, and dysosteosclerosis.

In diaphyseal dysplasia (Camurati-Engelmann), craniodiaphyseal dysplasia, the craniometaphyseal dysplasias, frontometaphyseal dysplasia, and pachydermoperiostosis, sclerosis in the region of optic foramina may lead to visual impairment, papilledema, and optic atrophy. Sclerosis of internal acoustic foramina and the middle ear may lead to conductive or sensorineural hearing loss. Encroachment on the facial nerve foramina may lead to facial paresis and encroachment on the foramen magnum to long tract signs, hyperreflexia, weakness, and even sudden death or paraplegia.

Diaphyseal Dysplasia (Camurati-Engelmann). This rare disorder is also known as progressive hereditary diaphyseal dysplasia. Significant neuromuscular involvement is associated. Inheritance is autosomal dominant, with variable penetrance and expression. Signs, symptoms, and severity vary among affected individuals within the same family. Symptoms usually begin from 4–10 yr of age but have occurred as early as 3 mo of age and as late as the 6th decade. Failure to thrive or gain weight, easy tiring, and abnormal gait are common presenting symptoms. Increasing leg pain may occur. The gait is waddling, with reduced muscle mass and poor muscle tone. Flexion contractures may develop at the elbows and knees. Bowleg or knock-knee may be seen; the feet may be flat and pronated. Deep tendon reflexes may be hypoactive or hyperactive, occasionally with ankle clonus. Lumbar lordosis and scoliosis may occur, with back pain. Symptoms and signs of encroachment on cranial nerves may be present.

The roentgenographic features include symmetric fusiform enlargement of the diaphyses of the long bones, with normal epiphyses and metaphyses. Diaphyseal cortex is enlarged by accretion of mottled endosteal and periosteal new bone. The lesions are often first noted in the centers of long bones, with gradual involvement of adjacent proximal and distal bone. The skull may show sclerosis of frontal areas and base. Blood chemical findings are characteristically normal. Muscle has been reported to show loss of individual muscle fibers with replacement by adipose tissue, atrophic muscle fibers, and slightly pyknotic sarcolemmal cell nuclei, with hyalinization and decreased prominence of cross-striations.

Management should aim for maximal mobility of the patient. Orthopedic correction of deformity of the lower limbs by appropriate osteotomy may help. A symptomatic response to low dose corticosteroid therapy has been reported.

Craniodiaphyseal Dysplasia. This rare disorder is characterized by massive hyperostosis and sclerosis of the skull and facial bones, with hyperostosis and defective modeling of the shafts of the tubular bones. Inheritance is autosomal recessive. The early symptoms may be respiratory difficulty due to narrowing of the nasal passages. Flattening of the nasal root may be noted at birth, and symptoms may occur as early as 3 mo of age. Progressive hyperostosis of the cranial and facial bones usually leads to prominence of nasal and adjacent maxillary bones by 1–2 yr of age. Symptoms and signs produced by encroachment on cranial foramina are marked. Affected patients are often of normal to tall stature. Serum alkaline phosphatase activity is markedly decreased.

Roentgenograms show massive hyperostosis of the cranial bones, which develops rapidly during infancy and completely obscures structural detail. The spine, ribs, clavicles, and scapulae appear hypermineralized but normal in shape. The metaphyses of the long bones show loss of normal funnelization and tubulation, which causes the long bones to appear broad and undermodeled.

At present, no medical or surgical treatment can prevent progressive hyperostosis and sclerosis or their complications. Special attention should be given to amelioration of hearing and visual impairment and to psychosocial and genetic counseling.

Endosteal Hyperostosis and Sclerosteosis. These form a group of disorders characterized by marked accretion of osseous tissue at the endosteal (inner) surface of bone leading to narrowing of the medullary canal or obliteration of the medullary space.

A rare, dominantly inherited variety of *endosteal hyperostosis* (Worth type) is frequently associated with torus palatinus. A recessively inherited variety (van Buchem) is characterized by progressive mandibular enlargement from childhood; in adult life signs and symptoms result from sclerotic encroachment on optic and acoustic foramina. Serum alkaline phosphatase activity is markedly elevated. Roentgenographically, there is marked thickening of the skull, from base to vault, and increased density of the mandible after puberty. Cortices of tubular bones show increased density, with narrowing of the marrow cavity.

Sclerosteosis, an autosomal recessive trait, is clinically and roentgenographically almost indistinguishable from van Buchem disease, of which it may be a variant. It is differentiated by a high incidence of hyperostosis in nasal and facial bones, which produces a broad, flat nasal bridge and hypertelorism, and by minor hand malformations consisting of cutaneous syndactyly, radial deviation of the 2nd and 3rd fingers, and absent or hypoplastic nails.

Tubular Stenosis (Caffey-Kenny). This autosomal dominant syndrome is characterized by narrowing of the medullary canal. Features include delayed closure of the anterior fontanelle, tetanic seizures secondary to hypocalcemia, and myopia. Roentgenographically, the medullary cavity is reduced, often markedly, with normal or increased cortical thickness. The diploic space may be absent.

Frontometaphyseal Dysplasia. This X-linked dominant condition produces a clinically striking facial appearance, with a pronounced supraorbital ridge resulting from a torus-like bony overgrowth of the supraorbital ridges of the frontal bones. Changes are more severe in males. Affected patients show hirsutism, conductive deafness, and wasting of the muscles of arms and legs and particularly of the hypothenar and interosseous muscles of the hands. A prominent supraorbital ridge extends across the entire frontal bone and is associated with poor development of frontal and other paranasal sinuses and with mandibular hypoplasia. The metaphyses of all the long and short tubular bones are undermodeled.

Craniometaphyseal Dysplasias. These conditions manifest severe progressive cranial hyperostosis and undermodeling of the metaphyses. Both autosomal dominant and recessive transmissions have been reported. The time of onset of symptoms and signs shows wide variability in families with dominant inheritance; some cases are recognized in infancy. Clinically, both dominant and recessively inherited forms show progressive facial dysmorphology, with broad osseous prominence of the nasal root extending across the zygoma. Difficulty in breathing due to encroachment on the nasal passages may be recognized in early infancy. The severity of sclerotic encroachment on cranial foramina is variable.

The essential roentgenographic features are hyperostosis of the skull; of the nasal and maxillary bones, extending bilaterally across the zygoma, with failure of pneumatization of the paranasal sinuses and mastoids; and of the mandible. The long bones show flaring and decreased density of the metaphyses (Ehrlenmeyer flask deformity). Hyperostosis and sclerosis of the mandible are less severe than in craniodiaphyseal dysplasia.

OSTEODYSPLASTY
(Melnick-Needles)

This disorder or group of disorders is characterized by "abnormally shaped" bones. The majority of familial cases have shown autosomal dominant inheritance. An autosomal recessive variant is reported. The age at diagnosis is variable, and affected children are usually first evaluated because of an abnormal gait, with bowing of the extremities, occasionally because of dislocation of hips or delayed closure of the anterior fontanelle. On the whole, these patients do not have short stature, and psychomotor development and adult height are normal. Facial appearance is somewhat typical, with slight exophthalmos, protruding cheeks, a high, narrow forehead, prominent orbital rims, micrognathia, and malaligned teeth. The lower thorax is narrow. Distal segments of the thumbs are incurved.

Roentgenographically, there is uneven thickening of the cortex of the long bones, in which irregular contours and multiple constrictions produce a wavy border. The diaphyses are slightly curved and show metaphyseal modeling defects.

Coxa valga and dislocation of the hips are common. The ribs are wavy in appearance. The supra-acetabular iliac wings appear narrowed.

HYPERPHOSPHATASEMIA WITH OSTEOECTASIA

In this group of patients, progressive skeletal deformation is associated with marked elevation of alkaline phosphatase activity. Inheritance is autosomal recessive. The disease usually has its onset by 2–3 yr, when painful deformity developing in the extremities leads to abnormal gait and sometimes fractures. Clinical findings resemble those of Paget disease in adults but are more generalized and symmetric. Short stature results.

The skull is large, and roentgenographically the diploë is widened, with loss of normal calvarial structure. Bony texture is variable, with dense areas (showing a teased cotton-wool appearance) interspersed with radiolucent areas and general demineralization. Long bones appear cylindrical, with loss of metaphyseal modeling, and contain pseudocysts showing a dense bony halo. (See also Sec 23.27.)

INFANTILE CORTICAL HYPEROSTOSIS
(Caffey Disease)

This condition of unknown cause must be differentiated from hyperphosphatasemia with osteoectasia (see above). The disorder is usually recognized in the 1st 3 mo of life. The course is febrile with marked swelling of soft tissues over the face and jaws and progressive cortical thickening of long bones and flat bones. Alkaline phosphatase activity is usually mildly increased. The condition has exacerbations and remissions with spontaneous regression after several yr. Corticosteroids can relieve symptoms during exacerbations.

HYPOPHOSPHATASIA

A number of hypophosphatasias exist, with overlapping phenotypes but differing modes of inheritance. All show bowing deformities of the skeleton and reduced or absent serum alkaline phosphatase activity due to total absence of the bone-liver isoenzyme. Serum and urine levels of phosphorylethanolamine are elevated. (See also Sec 23.25.)

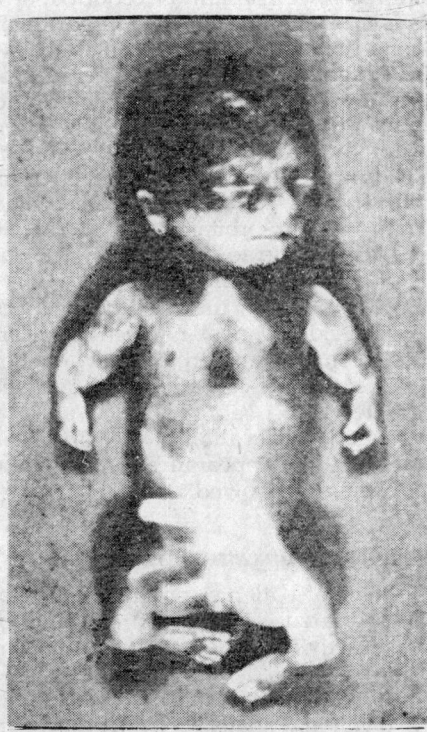

Figure 23–32 Congenital lethal hypophosphatasia showing short limbs with angulation deformities. The roentgenographic picture is quite distinctive and different from OI type II (see text).

Congenital lethal hypophosphatasia is a severe, autosomal recessive form usually leading to neonatal death (Fig. 23–32). It is characterized by a moth-eaten appearance at the ends of the long bones and by severe deficiency of ossification throughout the skeleton, with marked shortening of the long bones. Prenatal diagnosis is possible through enzymatic examination of cultured fibroblasts.

Hypophosphatasia tarda is a mild disease, with both dominant and recessive inheritance. Bowing of the legs with variable statural shortening may be observed. The activity of the bone-liver isoenzyme of alkaline phosphatase is reduced in serum. Rare patients with identical clinical and roentgenographic findings will have normal serum alkaline phosphatase activities. Their disease has been labeled pseudohypophosphatasia.

DAVID O. SILLENCE

General

Akeson WH, Bornstein P, Glimcher MJ: American Academy of Orthopaedic Surgeons Symposium on Heritable Disorders of Connective Tissue. St. Louis, CV Mosby, 1982.
Beighton P: Inherited Disorders of the Skeleton. Edinburgh, Churchill Livingstone, 1978.
Maroteaux P: Bone Disease of Children. Philadelphia, JB Lippincott, 1979.
McKusick VA: Heritable Disorders of Connective Tissues. St. Louis, CV Mosby, 1978.
McKusick VA: Mendelian Inheritance in Man. Ed 5. Baltimore, The Johns Hopkins Press, 1978.
Rimoin DL (ed): International nomenclature of constitutional disease of bone with bibliography. Birth Defects 14(6B)39, 1978.
Rimoin DL (ed): Skeletal dysplasias. Clin Orthop 114:2, 1976.
Rimoin DL, Horton WA: Short stature, Parts I and II. J Pediatr 92:523, 93:697, 1978.
Silence DO, Lachman R, Rimoin DL: Neonatal dwarfism. Pediatr Clin North Am 25:453, 1978.

Radiology

Lachman R: Radiology of pediatric syndromes. Curr Probl Pediatr 9(4):52, 1979.
Spranger JW, Langer LO, Wiedemann HR: Bone Dysplasias. An Atlas of Constitutional Disorders of Skeletal Development. Philadelphia, WB Saunders, 1974.

Chondro-osseous Morphology and Biochemical Investigation

Sillence DO, Horton WA, Rimoin DL: Morphologic studies in skeletal dysplasias. Am J Pathol 96:813, 1979.
Stanescu V, Stanescu R, Maroteaux P: Morphological and biochemical studies of epiphyseal cartilage in dyschondroplasias. Arch Franc Pediatr 34, Suppl 3:1, 1977.
Teitelbaum SL, Bullough PG: The pathophysiology of bone and joint disease. Am J Pathol 96:283, 1979.
Temtamy SA, McKusick VA: The genetics of hand malformations. Birth Defects, Original Article Series 14(3), 1978.
Yang SS, Heidelberger KP, Brough AJ, et al: Lethal short-limbed chondrodysplasia in early infancy. Perspect Pediatr Pathol 3:1, 1976.

Management

Amstutz HC, Sakai DN (eds): Equalization of leg length. Clin Orthop Rel Research 136:2, 1978.
Coccia PF, Krivit W, Cervenka J, et al: Successful bone-marrow transplantation for infantile malignant osteopetrosis. N Engl J Med 302:701, 1980.
Goldberg MJ: Orthopedic aspects of bone dysplasias. Orthop Clin North Am 7:445, 1976.
Horton WA, Rotter JI, Rimoin DL, et al: Standard growth curves for achondroplasia. J Pediatr 93:435, 1978.
Kopits SE: Orthopedic complications of dwarfism. Clin Orthop Rel Research 114:153, 1979.

Nonprofessional Organizations of and for Patients with Skeletal Short Stature

American Brittle Bone Society, National Headquarters, Suite LL-3, Cherry Hill Plaza, 1415 East Marlton Pike, Cherry Hill, N.J. 08034.

Human Growth Foundation, 11740 East 5th Street, Tulsa, Okla. 74128.
Little People of America, Inc., Box 126, Owatonna, Minn. 55060.
Osteogenesis Imperfecta Foundation, Inc., 632 Center Street, Van Wert, Ohio
45891.

23.18 Mucopolysaccharidoses

The mucopolysaccharidoses are a group of heritable syndromes resulting from defects in the degradation of certain complex carbohydrates, the mucopolysaccharides (glycosaminoglycans), normally present in connective tissues. Patients who have these diseases show widespread deformity of many organs and tissues as a result of accumulation of incompletely degraded mucopolysaccharides in lysosomes.

The mucopolysaccharides are heteropolysaccharides, most of which contain repeating disaccharide units of N-acetylglucosamine or N-acetylgalactosamine and glucuronic acid or iduronic acid and ester sulfate groups. Hyaluronic acid contains no ester sulfate, and keratan sulfate contains galactose instead of uronic acid. Heparan and heparan sulfate also have sulfate linked to the amino group of glucosamine. The sulfated mucopolysaccharides (chondroitin 4-sulfate, chondroitin 6-sulfate, heparan sulfate, heparin, and keratan sulfate) are covalently linked to proteins through a linkage region to form macromolecules, which may be parts of larger aggregates in tissues.

Normally, the mucopolysaccharides are degraded by endoglycosidases as well as exoglycosidases and sulfatases. These lysosomal hydrolases, together with proteases, lead to the stepwise degradation of the macromolecules within lysosomes. Genetic mutations which lead to loss of enzymatic activity of specific hydrolases will impair degradation and result in the accumulation of the undegraded mucopolysaccharide residue in lysosomes. The distended lysosomes distort cell architecture throughout tissues and organs and interfere with cell function. With incomplete degradation, urinary excretion of partially degraded mucopolysaccharides results.

The mucopolysaccharidoses are inherited as autosomal recessive diseases with the exception of the Hunter syndrome, which is an X-linked recessive disease. Table 23–4 lists the various mucopolysaccharidoses and their genetics, products accumulated, and enzymatic deficiencies. The gene defects in other variants, including those classified as mucolipidoses, have not as yet been defined. The gene frequencies of these diseases are not precisely known, though, taken together, they appear to be among the more common of the rare genetic diseases.

Hurler Syndrome (Mucopolysaccharidosis IH). Hurler syndrome has been the prototype of these diseases. The facies of a typical patient is illustrated in Fig 23–33. There is a marked retardation of growth and enlargement of the skull. The thick lips are usually separated, revealing an enlarged tongue, widely separated, peglike teeth, and hypertrophic gums. Hypertelorism is present, and the bridge of the nose is depressed under a prominent forehead covered by characteristic coarse hair. The ears are low set. The chest is enlarged with flaring of the ribs. A gibbus is usually present which, like the other signs, becomes more prominent with age. The strikingly abnormal extremities show contractures of the hips, knees, elbows, and fingers. The hands are broad. The liver and usually the spleen are markedly enlarged. Diastasis recti and umbilical and inguinal hernias are characteristic. The skin is thickened; hirsutism is common. Corneal clouding is a constant characteristic, as is progressive deafness. Respiratory infection as a result of nasal obstruction is common. Heart disease results from distortion of the valves and thickening of the walls of the coronary arteries. On post mortem examination all of the valves are affected, usually the mitral valve most severely. Neurologic findings are sometimes difficult to distinguish from the effects on connective tissues; mental retardation, however, is severe and progressive.

Roentgenographic changes (Fig 23–34 and 23–35) are characteristic and show thickening of the skull, marked deformity of the sella turcica, broad spatulate ribs, ovoid

Table 23–4 SUMMARY OF ENZYMATIC DEFECTS IN MUCOPOLYSACCHARIDOSES

Name	Genetics	Accumulated Product	Enzyme Deficiency
Mucopolysaccharidosis IH (Hurler)	Autosomal recessive	Heparan sulfate, dermatan sulfate	α-L-Iduronidase (EC 3.2.1.76)
Mucopolysaccharidosis IS (Scheie)	Autosomal recessive	Heparan sulfate, dermatan sulfate	α-L-Iduronidase (EC 3.2.1.76)
Mucopolysaccharidosis II (Hunter)	X-linked recessive	Heparan sulfate, dermatan sulfate	L-Iduronosulfate sulfatase
Mucopolysaccharidosis IIIA (Sanfilippo A)	Autosomal recessive	Heparan sulfate	Sulfamidase (EC 3.10.1.1)
Mucopolysaccharidosis IIIB (Sanfilippo B)	Autosomal recessive	Heparan sulfate	α-N-Acetylglucosaminidase (EC 3.2.1.50)
Mucopolysaccharidosis IV (Morquio)	Autosomal recessive	Keratan sulfate, chondroitin sulfate	N-Acetylgalactosamine 6-SO$_4$ sulfatase (EC 3.1.6.4)
Mucopolysaccharidosis IVB (Morquio-like)	Autosomal recessive	Keratan sulfate	β-Galactosidase (3.2.1.23)
Mucopolysaccharidosis VI (Maroteaux-Lamy)	Autosomal recessive	Dermatan sulfate	N-Acetylgalactosamine 4-SO$_4$ sulfatase Arylsulfatase B (EC 3.1.6.1)
Mucopolysaccharidosis VII (β-glucuronidase deficiency)	Autosomal recessive	Dermatan sulfate, heparan sulfate, chondroitin sulfate	β-Glucuronidase (EC 3.2.1.31)
Mucopolysaccharidosis VIII	Autosomal recessive	Heparan sulfate, keratan sulfate	N-Acetylglucosamine 6-SO$_4$ sulfatase

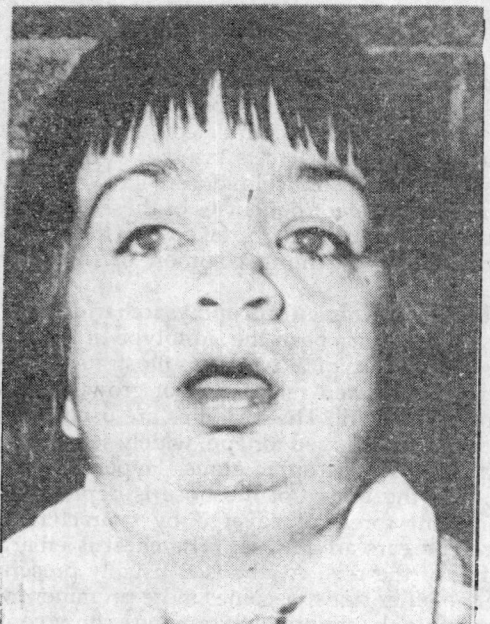

Figure 23–33 Typical appearance of a patient with Hurler syndrome.

beaked vertebrae, and broad heavy bones of the hand. There is no specific treatment and patients usually survive only to 12–14 yr of age.

Scheie Syndrome (Mucopolysaccharidosis IS). The

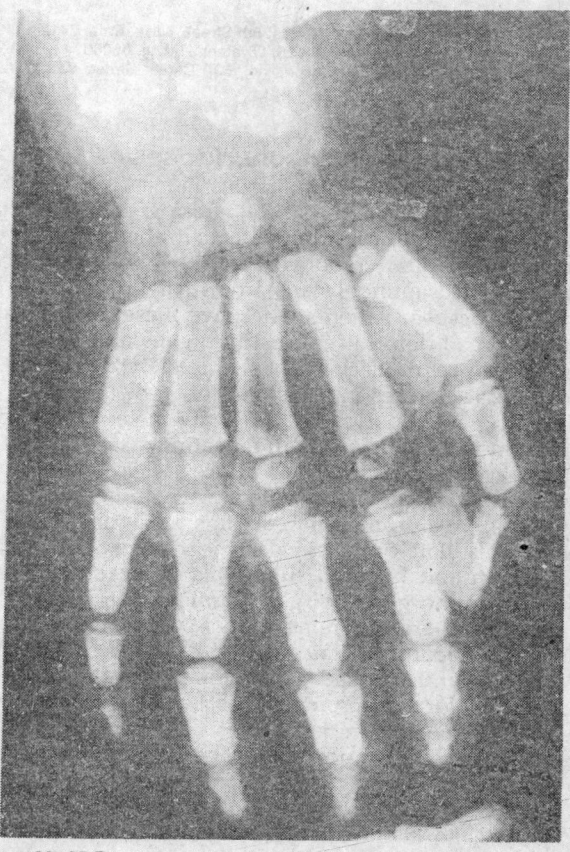

Figure 23–35 Roentgenogram of hand of patient with Hurler syndrome.

physical findings are milder than in Hurler syndrome. Most characteristic are corneal opacities, some dwarfing, and contractures. Patients with Scheie disease may show little or no mental retardation and survive to adulthood.

Hunter Syndrome (Mucopolysaccharidosis II). Patients with this condition resemble those with Hurler syndrome but have less severe somatic and neurologic changes. Corneal opacities usually do not occur. In some patients characteristic nodules are present in the skin, primarily over the scapular region extending to the axilla. Roentgenographic findings are like those of Hurler disease, but vertebral changes are less severe. Two varieties of Hunter syndrome affect the same enzyme but differ in severity of clinical manifestations. Some patients with this syndrome survive to adulthood.

Sanfilippo Syndromes (Mucopolysaccharidoses IIIA and B). Two different Sanfilippo syndromes have been distinguished on the basis of enzymatic defects; they are clinically indistinguishable. In general, patients with the Sanfilippo syndromes show less severe somatic changes than do those with the Hurler syndrome; growth is not restricted. Severe neurologic changes, however, are present, including seizures, athetosis, and marked mental retardation. Corneal clouding and cardiac involvement do not usually occur. Roentgenographic changes are much less severe than those of Hurler syndrome. Death usually occurs by 10–14 yr of age.

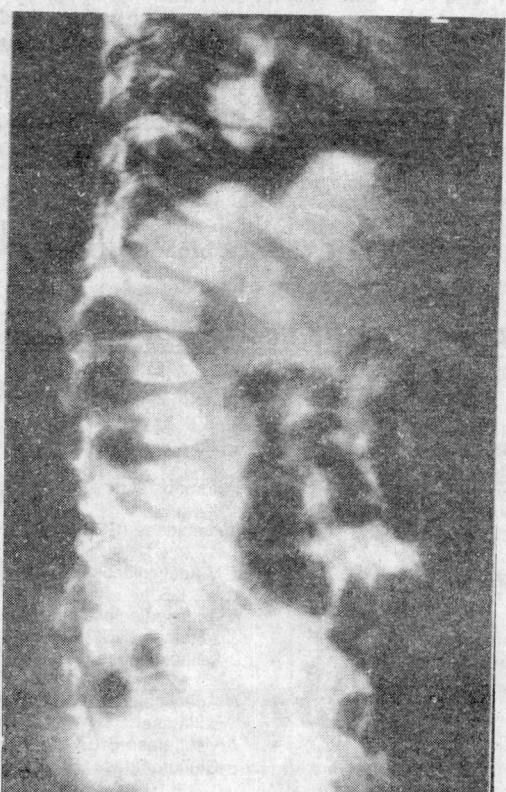

Figure 23–34 Lateral spine roentgenogram of patient with Hurler syndrome.

Morquio Syndrome (Mucopolysaccharidosis IV). Morquio (or Morquio-Brailsford) syndrome is 1 of the larger group of spondyloepiphyseal dysplasias. In Morquio syndrome, skeletal changes and disturbances of linear growth are most prominent. Characteristic are platyspondyly, knock knees, widespread changes in epiphyses, and generalized osteoporosis. There is marked shortening of the trunk, with deformities of the extremities and chest. The spinal curvature, together with rib deformities, results in a typical barrel chest with pigeon breast and short neck. The characteristic facial appearance shows prominent maxillae, broad mouth, short nose, and widely spaced teeth with defective enamel. Corneal opacities and hepatosplenomegaly occur in some patients. Neurologic complications result in deformity of the spine, but mental retardation is absent. Cardiac complications have been reported to result from deformity of the chest. A variant demonstrating β-galactosidase deficiency has recently been reported.

Maroteaux-Lamy Syndrome (Mucopolysaccharidosis VI). This syndrome, sometimes referred to as polydystrophic dysplasia (dwarfism), is characterized by severe somatic changes including short stature, lumbar kyphosis, protrusion of the sternum, and contractures. Hepatosplenomegaly and corneal clouding are present, but mental retardation is much less prominent than in Hurler syndrome. Hydrocephalus has been associated.

β-Glucuronidase Deficiency (Mucopolysaccharidosis VII). This rare syndrome shows clinical and roentgenographic features similar to those of the other mucopolysaccharidoses. Hepatosplenomegaly, corneal clouding, and gibbus of the spine occur. Developmental retardation has been reported, but sufficient follow-up is not available to evaluate the eventual course and the extent of mental retardation.

Mucopolysaccharidosis VIII. Recently, several patients have been described with the Morquio phenotype who also show mental retardation. As indicated in Table 23-4, these have been shown to have a distinct enzyme defect.

Differential Diagnosis. The suspicion of mucopolysaccharidoses usually results from the characteristic history of clinical and roentgenographic findings. The presence of elevated urinary mucopolysaccharides and their qualitative identification are confirmatory and also aid in the identification of specific syndromes indicated in Table 23-4. The individual syndromes are identified by specific enzyme assays of cultured fibroblasts and leukocytes. Heterozygote determination has been accomplished in some cases. There is no effective treatment other than supportive management of individual complications.

Genetic Counseling. Accurate diagnosis is important to permit genetic counseling in general and more particularly prenatal diagnosis in subsequent pregnancies, which should be possible in all affected fetuses.

ALBERT DORFMAN*

Dorfman A, Matalon R: The mucopolysaccharidoses (a review). Proc Natl Acad Sci USA 73:630, 1976.
McKusick VA: The mucopolysaccharidoses. In Heritable Disorders of Connective Tissue. Ed. 4. St Louis, CV Mosby, 1972.
McKusick VA, Neufeld EF, Kelly TE: The mucopolysaccharide storage diseases. In Stanbury JB, Wyngaarden JB, Fredrickson JS (eds): The Metabolic Basis of Inherited Disease. Ed 4. New York, McGraw-Hill, 1978.
Spranger J: The systemic mucopolysaccharidoses. In: Frick P, von Harnack GA, Muller AF, et al (eds): Ergebnisse der Inneren Medizin und Kinderheilkunde. Berlin, Springer-Verlag, 1972.

*Deceased.

23.19 METABOLIC BONE DISEASE

The bone lesions which can result from a number of metabolic disorders are in most instances classified as forms of rickets not resulting from dietary deficiency. Certain other bone conditions are more difficult to classify.

23.20 Rickets

Rickets may be defined as inadequate mineralization of osteoid tissue in the growing animal. Remodeling of bone continues, with resorption and new formation of matrix (osteoid). In mature animals, failure of mineralization results in osteomalacia. In both rickets and osteomalacia excess osteoid tissue is formed. Osteoporosis is the result of demineralization with the calcifying process intact; it should not be confused with rickets.

Most of the body calcium is found in the skeleton, along with phosphate and magnesium. It exists mostly in the form of crystalline hydroxyapatite, which is in equilibrium with the ionized calcium and phosphate of the extracellular fluids. The level of ionized calcium in extracellular fluids is held relatively constant by several homeostatic mechanisms. Details are discussed in Sec 3.6 and 18.21. Features of non-nutritional rickets are discussed in this section. Nutritional rickets and rickets resulting from malabsorption are discussed in Sec 3.28 and 11.45.

Table 23-5 lists various types of rickets and some conditions resembling rickets; it is modified from the classification proposed by Harrison and Harrison and shows the expected laboratory findings in serum and urine and the mode of genetic transmission where applicable.

In Type I rickets there is a deficiency of 1,25-dihydroxy-vitamin D_3 (1,25-$(OH)_2$-D_3), which may result from a variety of causes. Secondary hyperparathyroidism occurs as a result of calcium malabsorption. In Type II rickets the primary problem appears to be phosphate deficiency, which usually results from failure of normal resorption of phosphate by the renal tubule. Secondary hyperparathyroidism is not usually found with Type II

Table 23–5   CLINICAL VARIANTS OF RICKETS AND RELATED CONDITIONS

TYPE	SERUM CALCIUM LEVEL	SERUM PHOSPHORUS LEVEL	ALKALINE PHOSPHATASE ACTIVITY	URINE CONCENTRATION, AMINO ACIDS	GENETICS
I. Deficiency of 1,25-(OH)$_2$-D$_3$					
1. Lack of vitamin D					
a. Lack of exposure to sunlight	N or L	L	E	E	
b. Dietary deficiency of vitamin D	N or L	L	E	E	
c. Congenital	N or L	L	E	E	
2. Malabsorption of vitamin D	N or L	L	E	E	
3. Hepatic disease	N or L	L	E	E	
4. Anticonvulsive drugs	N or L	L	E	E	
5. Renal osteodystrophy	N or L	E	E	V	
6. Vitamin D–dependent Type I	L	N or L	E	E	AR
II. Primary phosphate deficiency					
(No secondary hyperparathyroidism)					
1. Genetic primary hypophosphatemia	N	L	E	N	XD
2. Fanconi syndromes					
a. Cystinosis	N	L	E	E	AR
b. Tyrosinosis	N	L	E	E	AR
c. Lowe syndrome	N	L	E	E	XR
d. Acquired	N	L	E	E	
3. Renal tubular acidosis	N	L	E	N	
4. Oncogenic hypophosphatemia	N	L	E	N	
5. Phosphate deficiency or malabsorption					
a. Parenteral hyperalimentation	N	L	E	N	
b. Low phosphate intake	N	L	E	N	
III. End-organ resistance to 1,25-(OH)$_2$-D$_3$					
1. Vitamin D–dependent Type II					
(several variants)	L	L or N	E	E	
IV. Related conditions resembling rickets					
1. Hypophosphatasia	N	N	L	Phosphoethano-lamine elevated	AR
2. Metaphyseal dysostosis					
a. Jansen type	E	N	E	N	AD
b. Schmid type	N	N	N	N	AD

N = normal; L = low; E = elevated; V = variable; X = X-linked; A = autosomal; D = dominant; R = recessive.

rickets. Both in primary (genetic) hypophosphatemia and in oncogenous hypophosphatemia there is evidence of an associated disorder of vitamin D metabolism; moreover, deficiency of 1,25-(OH)$_2$-D$_3$ may develop in some cases of Type II rickets as a complication of renal tubular injury. Type III rickets is incompletely understood; the primary abnormality appears to be end-organ resistance to 1,25-(OH)$_2$-D$_3$.

Metabolism.   A knowledge of vitamin D metabolism is essential for understanding rickets (Fig 23–36). Vitamin D$_3$ (cholecalciferol) is synthesized in the skin through ultraviolet radiation of 7-dehydrocholesterol. The reaction is apparently nonenzymatic. Vitamin D$_3$ is also effectively absorbed from the gastrointestinal tract with the help of bile salts. Vitamin D$_2$ (ergocalciferol), produced by irradiation of ergosterol, is also efficiently absorbed from the intestine. After absorption, vitamin D is transported with chylomicra through the lymphatics and bloodstream to the liver (Fig 23–37). Vitamin D in blood is bound to an alpha globulin of approximately 52,000 molecular weight. In the liver vitamin D$_3$ (Fig 23–38) is hydroxylated at carbon 25 to 25-hydroxyvitamin D$_3$ (25-OH-D$_3$). The reaction is microsomal, requires molecular oxygen, NADPH, and magnesium ions, and is controlled to some extent by feedback regulation. The 25-OH-D$_3$ subsequently appears in the plasma bound to alpha globulin, 1 molecule of 25-OH-D$_3$ to 1 of protein. The usual level is approximately 30

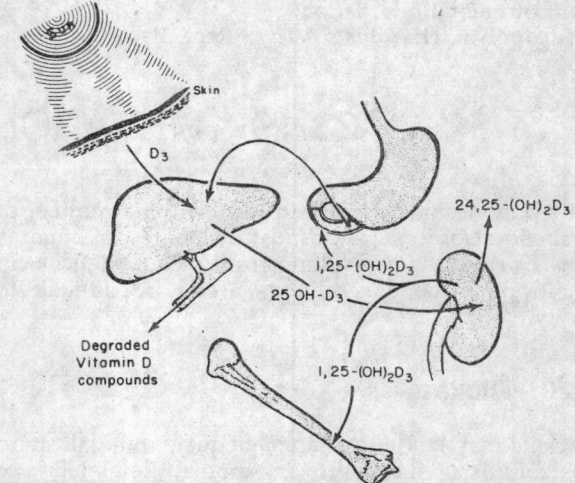

Figure 23–36 Vitamin D pathways. D$_3$ = vitamin D$_3$ (cholecalciferol); 25-OH-D$_3$ = 25-hydroxycholecalciferol; 1,25-(OH)$_2$-D$_3$ = 1,25-dihydroxycholecalciferol; 24,25-(OH)$_2$-D$_3$ = 24,25-dihydroxycholecalciferol. Arrows toward the liver and kidney indicate sites of hydroxylation. Arrows from these organs indicate sites of action. Note that 24,25-(OH)$_2$-D$_3$ has no significant effect on bone or gut. (Also see Fig 23–37.)

ng/ml. Heavy ingestion of vitamin D can raise the level considerably. Vitamin D$_2$, after ingestion, follows the same metabolic pathway.

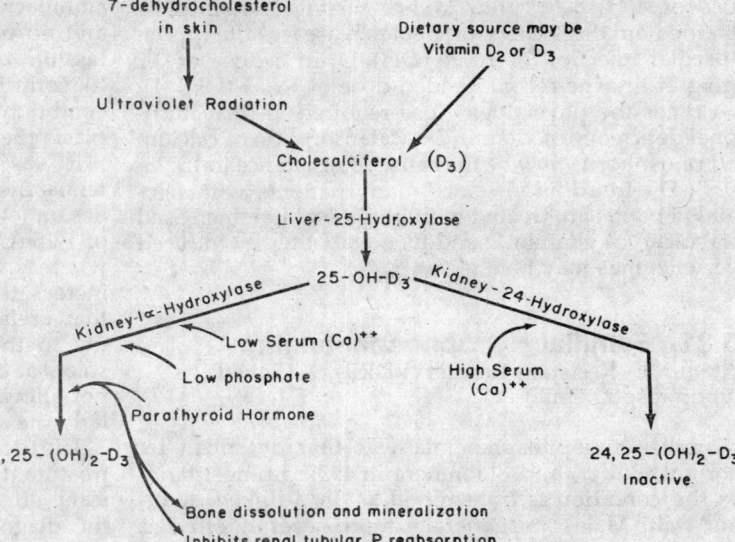

Figure 23–37 The metabolic pathway of vitamin D, indicating its conversion to the hormone 1,25-$(OH)_2$-D_3 and the inactive degraded compound 24,25-$(OH)_2$-D_3. Vitamin D_2 (ergosterol) appears to go through similar hydroxylations.

In the kidney 25-OH-D_3 undergoes further hydroxylation. If the serum calcium is low, the mitochondrial enzyme 25-OH-D_3-1α-hydroxylase produces hydroxylation at carbon 1, forming 1α,25-$(OH)_2$-D_3. The reaction requires NADPH, which reduces ferredoxin reductase (a flavoprotein); this in turn reduces renal ferredoxin (an iron-sulfur protein). Renal ferredoxin then reduces 25-OH-D_3-1α-hydroxylase (a cytochrome P450), which is specific for 25-OH-D_3, producing 1α-25-$(OH)_2$-D_3. This last compound is the metabolically active form of vitamin D. Synthesis of 1α,25-$(OH)_2$-D_3 is tightly regulated by feedback mechanisms involving plasma calcium and phosphorus levels.

If calcium levels are elevated, the mitochondrial mixed function mono-oxygenase enzyme 25-OH-D_3-24-hydroxylase produces hydroxylation at carbon 24, yielding 24,25-$(OH)_2$-D_3, an inactive compound. If calcium levels are normal, both 1α,25-$(OH)_2$-D_3 and 24,25-$(OH)_2$-D_3 are produced. In effect, vitamin D is a prohormone ultimately converted to a hormone, 1α,25-$(OH)_2$-D_3, with intestine and bone as target organs; the hormone rapidly induces absorption of calcium by action on the brush borders of intestinal epithelial cells. The functional hormone, 1α,25-$(OH)_2$-D_3, requires no further conversion. It is 10 times more active than cholecalciferol and 4 times more active than 25-OH-D_3.

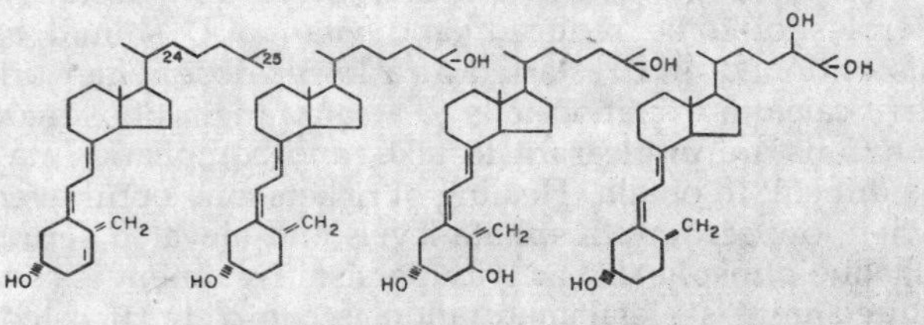

In addition to stimulating calcium absorption, 1α,25-$(OH)_2$-D_3 also enhances intestinal absorption of phosphate. Low serum levels of phosphate also stimulate production of 1α,25-$(OH)_2$-D_3 by the kidney. It is postulated that high phosphate levels may stimulate synthesis of 24,25-$(OH)_2$-D_3. Parathyroid hormone not only stimulates the formation of 1α,25-$(OH)_2$-D_3 by the kidney but also enhances the response of bone to 1α,25-$(OH)_2$-D_3.

The major route of excretion of vitamin D and its metabolites is through the liver into the bowel, probably after sulfation or glucuronidation. Compounds hydroxylated at carbon 24 are very rapidly metabolized and excreted.

Normal serum levels for 1α,25-$(OH)_2$-D_3 are about 36 pg/ml as measured by radioreceptor ligand assay. The level of 25-OH-D_3 can also be measured by radioligand assay or by high pressure liquid chromatography. It is expected that serum measurements of D_3, 25-OH-D_3, and 1α,25-$(OH)_2$-D_3 will become generally available through centralized laboratories.

Hepatic Diseases Associated with Rickets. Rickets can occur in children with hepatic disease. It is found in about 60% of cases of congenital atresia of the extrahepatic biliary ducts, probably due to vitamin D malabsorption resulting from absence of bile salts in the intestine. Rickets occurs in about 50% of cases of neonatal hepatitis, presumably because of inadequate 25-hydroxylation of cholecalciferol; in this condition cholestasis and parenchymal injury can also lead to diminished bile salt concentration in the intestine. In hepatic rickets reduced levels of serum 25-OH-D_3 are found, with hypocalcemia and roentgenographic evidence of rickets. Elevations of serum alkaline phosphatase activity may reflect liver disease as well as rickets.

Rickets associated with hepatic disease can be treated with 25-OH-D_3 in a dose of 50 μg/24 hr; healing occurs in about 30 days. Rickets associated with neonatal hepatitis will respond to vitamin D given orally in a

Figure 23–38 The four compounds are vitamin D_3 (cholecalciferol) and the principal hydroxylation compounds to which it is converted. The numbering system for the carbon atoms of cholecalciferol is also indicated.

dose of 4000–8000 units/24 hr. Healing can also be obtained in the rickets of hepatic disease after intramuscular injection of $1\alpha,25\text{-}(OH)_2\text{-}D_3$ in a dose of 0.2 μg/kg/24 hr. The recommended dose of $1\alpha,25\text{-}(OH)_2\text{-}D_3$ is 4 times the physiologic dose required to treat nutritional deficiency of vitamin D. Malabsorption of calcium and phosphorus may be the cause of resistance to $1\alpha,25\text{-}(OH)_2\text{-}D_3$. In addition, since many patients with neonatal hepatitis are treated with phenobarbital, increased catabolism of vitamin D and its metabolites by induced liver enzymes may be a factor.

23.21 Familial Hypophosphatemia
(Vitamin D–Resistant Rickets (VDRR), X-Linked Hypophosphatemia)

Familial hypophosphatemia was first described by Albright, Butler, and Bloomberg in 1937. In most families the condition is transmitted as an X-linked dominant trait. Males are generally more severely affected than heterozygous females, though some females have the characteristic bone abnormalities. Other females manifest hypophosphatemia with minimal or no bone changes. There are some families in which the disease appears to be transmitted as an autosomal recessive trait, and there is 1 report of a family with autosomal dominant transmission. A number of presumably sporadic cases have been identified.

Children with this disease appear normal at birth, and growth appears to be normal during the 1st 6 mo of life, after which growth retardation occurs. Characteristically, genu varum or genu valgum develops with weight bearing, along with coxa vara and medial tibial torsion. A waddling gait often results. In contrast to vitamin D–deficient rickets, there is minimal involvement of the bones of the chest and head. Enlargement of the costochondral junctions is not seen; Harrison grooves do not develop, and deformities of the vertebrae are rare. Significant functional deformities of the pelvis also do not occur. Most patients have short stature, adult height ranging from 130–160 cm. In contrast to vitamin D–deficient rickets, muscle strength is not impaired.

The teeth are often abnormal, with large pulp chambers, and enamel hypoplasia is sometimes found. Dental eruption may be delayed. There is increased incidence of periapical infections.

Roentgenographic findings include fraying, widening, and cupping of metaphyseal ends of long bones, including the proximal and distal tibia and the distal femur, radius, and ulna. Changes in the wrist may improve with time, but ankle and knee abnormalities persist.

At birth serum phosphate levels are normal. After approximately 6 mo phosphate levels fall below 4 mg/dl, and after infancy alkaline phosphatase activity is elevated while serum calcium levels are normal. The maintenance of normal phosphate levels during the 1st few mo may be related to the low glomerular filtration rate found in infants. The basic abnormality appears to be a defect in the renal tubular reabsorption of phosphate, probably in the proximal renal tubule. Pathologic aminoaciduria does not occur. There is no glycosuria, and no pathologic loss of bicarbonate, sodium, or potassium occurs. Hyperparathyroidism does not appear to contribute significantly to the pathogenesis. The condition must be differentiated from metaphyseal dysplasia (Sec 23.17).

It was once believed that in familial hypophosphatemia there was no defect in vitamin D metabolism. Serum levels of $25\text{-}OH\text{-}D_3$ are normal, but serum levels of $1,25\text{-}(OH)_2\text{-}D_3$ appear to be in the low normal range, whereas low serum phosphate levels should result in increased levels of $1,25\text{-}(OH)_2\text{-}D_3$. It has been postulated that a relative deficiency of this compound may contribute to the pathogenesis. Moreover, treatment aimed solely at correction of low serum phosphate levels does not alleviate all manifestations of the disease, particularly the short stature.

The doses of vitamin D usually employed in the treatment of vitamin D–deficient rickets have no significant effect upon familial hypophosphatemic rickets, the diagnosis of vitamin D–resistant rickets being in some cases first considered only after rickets thought to be nutritional has failed to respond to the usual therapy.

The earliest treatment for familial hypophosphatemic rickets was the administration of massive doses of vitamin D, ranging from 50,000–150,000 units/24 hr. Healing of rickets could be obtained, but there was significant risk of hypercalcemia, with nephrocalcinosis and renal injury. In most patients, despite healing of the rickets, understature was not prevented.

Dihydrotachysterol produced by irradiation of ergosterol can be used in place of vitamin D. Dihydrotachysterol, like cholecalciferol, needs hepatic 25-hydroxylation for activation, but 1α-hydroxylation is not required. Dihydrotachysterol is more rapidly inactivated than vitamin D and thus has less cumulative toxicity. The dose required is 0.5–1.0 mg/24 hr. Careful monitoring is necessary in order to avoid hypercalcemia and renal injury.

Oral administration of heavy doses of phosphate was later introduced to therapy. Approximately 0.5–1.5 gm/24 hr is required for a young child and 1.5–2.0 gm/24 hr for older children. Phosphate can be given as Joulie solution (dibasic sodium phosphate 136 gm/l and phosphoric acid 58.8 gm/l), 1 ml of which contains 30.4 mg of inorganic phosphorus. Potassium phosphate can also be used. In addition to phosphate, dihydrotachysterol in a dose of 0.02 mg/kg/24 hr or vitamin D 2000 units/kg/24 hr should be given. If the urinary calcium excretion exceeds 4 mg/kg/24 hr, the dose of dihydrotachysterol should be reduced, and vitamin D should be discontinued and restarted at a lower dose when urinary calcium excretion falls to a safe range. Phosphate solutions are unpleasant to take, and compliance may be difficult to obtain. Healing of rickets may occur even when low serum phosphate levels and elevated serum alkaline phosphatase activity persist. Treatment is continued until skeletal maturation is complete. If osteomalacia develops after cessation of growth, reinstitution of therapy may be required.

With early diagnosis and good compliance, deformities can be minimized, but the patients remain short.

Osteotomies may be required to correct deformities. It is generally preferable to defer osteotomy until growth has been completed. It is recommended that administration of vitamin D or dihydrotachysterol be suspended for about 1 mo before surgery in order to avoid hypercalcemia from immobilization. Medication can be resumed when the patient begins using crutches.

Recent observations indicate that 1,25-(OH)$_2$-D$_3$ may replace vitamin D or dihydrotachysterol in treatment. The relatively low serum levels of 1,25-(OH)$_2$-D$_3$ in familial hypophosphatemic rickets suggest that a defect in 1-hydroxylation coexists with defective renal tubular absorption of phosphate. The dose of 1,25-(OH)$_2$-D$_3$ used has ranged from 1–3 µg/24 hr, generally supplemented by oral phosphate. Increased gastrointestinal absorption of phosphate produces a positive phosphate balance, serum phosphate levels rise, and a fall in plasma levels of parathyroid hormone has been noted. Rickets heals, and the rate of growth increases. It is not yet clear whether this increased rate of growth will be sustained or whether the ultimate height attained will exceed that attained with other modes of treatment.

23.22 Vitamin D–Dependent Rickets
(Pseudovitamin D Deficiency, Hypocalcemic Vitamin D–Resistant Rickets)

Vitamin D–dependent rickets was first described by Prader in 1961. In affected children rickets develops despite ingestion of normally adequate amounts of vitamin D. The disease usually becomes apparent from 3–12 mo of age, but some patients have onset of symptoms in later childhood. Both serum calcium and serum phosphate levels are low, and serum alkaline phosphatase activity is elevated. Generalized aminoaciduria and increased urinary excretion of cyclic AMP result from secondary hyperparathyroidism. Roentgenograms show progressive rickets. Serum levels of 1α,25-(OH)$_2$-D$_3$ are low despite normal or elevated levels of 25-OH-D$_3$. That the physiologic abnormalities can be corrected by administration of physiologic amounts of 1α,25-(OH)$_2$-D$_3$ indicates a deficiency in the 25-OH-D$_3$-1α-hydroxylase enzyme system of the kidney.

Vitamin D–dependent rickets is transmitted as an autosomal recessive trait. Treatment with vitamin D in a dose of 10,000–50,000 units/24 hr will generally correct the rickets, the dose required varying from patient to patient. Care must be taken to avoid hypercalcemia. Treatment with 1α,25-(OH)$_2$-D$_3$ in a dose of 0.5–1.0 µg/24 hr will also result in healing in most patients; some patients require 1.5–2.0 µg/24 hr.

Occasionally, patients with vitamin D–dependent rickets require very high doses of 1α,25-(OH)$_2$-D$_3$ or do not heal at all with this medication. In these cases, serum levels of 1α,25-(OH)$_2$-D$_3$ are normal, and there appears to be end-organ resistance to 1α,25-(OH)$_2$-D$_3$, the postulated end-organ not yet defined. This condition has been called vitamin D–dependent rickets Type II; its genetic transmission is uncertain. Some patients have alopecia.

23.23 Rickets Associated with Anticonvulsant Drug Therapy
(Toxic Hepatic Hydroxylation)

Rickets may develop in children being treated with anticonvulsant drugs despite apparently adequate vitamin D intake. This is more likely in patients taking combinations of drugs, phenobarbital and phenytoin having been the drugs primarily implicated, with some evidence of a similar effect from primidone. Affected patients have low serum levels of 25-OH-D$_3$. Both phenobarbital and phenytoin can induce liver enzymes of the cytochrome 450 system of mixed oxidases, producing accelerated degradation of vitamin D and its excretion into bile as inactive glucuronides. Phenobarbital and phenytoin appear also to inhibit directly the intestinal absorption of calcium. Many of the affected children may have been relatively deprived of sunlight.

Serum levels of calcium and phosphorus should be determined periodically in patients receiving these anticonvulsant agents. Serum alkaline phosphatase levels may be elevated because of drug ingestion itself. A daily dose of 500–1000 units of vitamin D added to normal requirements will prevent or correct this type of rickets. Also effective is 25-OH-D$_3$ in a dose of 50–100 µg/24 hr.

23.24 Oncogenous Rickets
(Primary Hypophosphatemic Rickets Associated with Tumor)

Rickets is occasionally associated with tumors of mesenchymal origin. The original report by Prader concerned association with a bone tumor; after excision of the tumor, the rickets healed. Tumors associated with oncogenous rickets have included nonossifying fibromas, giant cell tumors of bone, histiocytomas, pericytomas, and fibroangiomas. Also associated have been the epidermal nevus syndrome and neurofibromatosis. The tumors may be difficult to locate; they have been found in bone, rectoabdominal sheath, nasal antrum, pharyngeal wall, and skin. Most of the tumors associated with this condition have been benign.

Hypophosphatemia is present. Some patients have glycinemia and glycinuria. There is evidence that these tumors secrete an agent which inhibits renal tubular reabsorption of phosphate. It has also been suggested that some tumors may elaborate a substance which inhibits normal vitamin D metabolism. Recent studies of a few cases indicate that the serum levels of 25-OH-D$_3$ are normal and the levels of 1α,25-(OH)$_2$-D$_3$ low, suggesting inhibition of 25-OH-D$_3$-1α-hydroxylase. In patients with acquired hypophosphatemic rickets, the possibility of oncogenous rickets should be considered and search made for a tumor. Excision of the tumor results in a rapid rise of serum phosphate and healing of the rickets. In a few cases studied, low serum levels of 1α,25-(OH)$_2$-D$_3$ have returned to normal after removal of the tumor. If the tumor cannot be removed, treatment with 1α,25-(OH)$_2$-D$_3$ and oral phosphate can be considered.

23.25   Hypophosphatasia

Hypophosphatasia is characterized by low serum alkaline phosphatase activity. There is wide variation in the severity of the disease. Some cases are evident at birth; in a few the roentgenographic diagnosis has been made in utero. In severe cases the skull is soft at birth, with lack of calcification of frontal, parietal, and occipital bones, only the base of the skull being calcified. The long bones show incomplete ossification in the metaphyseal areas with bowing. There may be abnormalities of the thoracic cage with fractures. Severely affected infants are usually stillborn or die early in infancy. (See also Sec 23.17.)

In moderately severe cases cranial sutures may be wide, with bulging of the anterior fontanelle. The ribs may be short, with a rosary resembling that of rickets. Skeletal deformities are present, with irregular metaphyseal mineralization; cutaneous dimples may be present. Hypotonia is usual. Hypercalcemia and hypercalcemic nephrocalcinosis may develop. Failure to thrive is common; about half of affected children die in infancy.

In mild cases skeletal deformities may be present. Bone pain may develop and occasional fractures occur. Some of the roentgenographic changes resemble those of rickets, with poor mineralization of the primary spongiosa and growth plates. The metaphyseal abnormalities in hypophosphatasia are sharply defined, with irregular ossification, punched-out areas, and cupping deformities in the metaphyseal regions. Loss of deciduous teeth occurs prematurely.

Hypophosphatasia is transmitted as an autosomal recessive trait. There is increased urinary excretion of phosphoethanolamine, which is not restricted to hypophosphatasia. Heterozygotes may have mildly increased urinary excretion of phosphoethanolamine and slight reduction of serum alkaline phosphatase activity. The diagnosis can be made by determination of serum calcium and phosphorus levels and alkaline phosphatase activity. There is no definitive therapy.

23.26   Idiopathic Hypercalcemia

Many cases of idiopathic hypercalcemia occurred in the United Kingdom following World War II, when milk was fortified with vitamin D to a concentration of 1800 units/quart. Given their other sources of vitamin D, some infants were receiving as much as 3500 units/day. That only a very small percentage of the exposed infants developed hypercalcemia suggests a defective degradative mechanism as the cause of the condition. Affected infants had hypercalcemia with normal serum phosphate levels. Failure to thrive and loss of renal function occurred. Roentgenograms showed osteosclerosis with development of dense bone in the metaphyseal areas. When fortification of milk was reduced to 400 units of vitamin D/quart in Britain, idiopathic hypercalcemia in infants became very rare. Treatment consisted of a diet low in vitamin D and calcium.

Williams syndrome (elfin facies syndrome) is sometimes confused with idiopathic hypercalcemia. The characteristic facies of Williams syndrome includes small mandible, prominent maxilla, and a sharp upturned nose. The upper lip is prominent, and malocclusion is common. Feeding problems and failure to thrive are common during the 1st yr of life. Mild mental retardation is found. Many affected patients have supravalvular aortic stenosis; some have mild stenosis of peripheral pulmonary arteries, hypoplasia of the aorta, or atrial or ventricular septal defects. Some patients develop nephrocalcinosis with impaired renal function. Extracellular calcification and sclerosis of the base of the skull, the long bones, and the vertebrae are found. At the time of diagnosis serum calcium and phosphorus levels are normal.

The clinical features strongly suggest that Williams syndrome has an intrauterine onset. There is no evidence of excessive vitamin D intake by mothers or children. The disease appears to be sporadic. It has been hypothesized that a placental abnormality increasing fetal serum calcium levels may be responsible for the condition. A transient abnormality of vitamin D metabolism has also been suggested to explain the condition.

23.27   Hyperphosphatasia

In primary hyperphosphatasia the serum alkaline phosphatase activity is markedly elevated. The enzyme appears to be of osseous origin. The condition generally becomes evident during the 1st yr of life with growth deficiency. There is marked proliferation of osteoid in the subperiosteal areas of bone. The periosteum becomes separated from the cortex of bone. The long bones become osteopenic, and fractures may occur as a result of minimal trauma. Deformities may develop, with thickening of diaphyses and bowing, and there may be bone pain. Pectus carinatum may be present; kyphoscoliosis may develop, and the ribs may be frayed. The cranium is thickened and may be deformed. Serum calcium and phosphorus levels are normal. Serum acid phosphatase activity may be elevated with increased urinary excretion of leucine amino acid peptidase. This rare disease is presumably transmitted as an autosomal recessive trait. (See also Sec 23.17.)

IRA M. ROSENTHAL

Chen JC, Bartter FC: Hypophosphatemic rickets, effect of 1α,25-dihydroxy vitamin D₃ on growth and mineral metabolism. Pediatrics 64:488, 1979.

DeLuca, HF: Vitamin D metabolism and function. Arch Int Med 138:836, 1978.

DeLuca HF, Anast CS: Pediatric Disease in Relation to Calcium. New York, Elsevier, 1980.

Fraser D, Kooh SW, Kind HP, et al: Pathogenesis of hereditary vitamin D–dependent rickets. N Engl J Med 289:817, 1973.

Harrison HH, Harrison HC: Disorders of Calcium and Phosphate Metabolism in Childhood and Adolescence. Philadelphia, WB Saunders, 1979.

Heubi JE, Tsang RC, Steicher JJ, et al: 1α,25-Dihydroxy vitamin D₃ in childhood hepatic osteodystrophy. J Pediatr 94:97, 1979.

Parker MS, Klein I, Haussler MF, et al: Tumor-induced osteomalacia. JAMA 245:492, 1981.

Sockalosky J, Ulstrom R, DeLuca HF, et al: Vitamin D–resistant rickets; end-organ unresponsiveness to 1,25(OH)₂D₃. J Pediatr 96:701, 1980.

23.28 Fanconi Syndrome
(Rickets Associated with Multiple Defects of the Proximal Renal Tubule; de Toni-Debré-Fanconi Syndrome)

Generalized aminoaciduria, renal glycosuria, and phosphaturia resulting in hypophosphatemia characterize Fanconi syndrome. Associated but inconstant renal tubular abnormalities include excessive bicarbonaturia leading to metabolic acidosis, hyperkaliuria leading to hypokalemia, sodium wasting, uricosuria, proteinuria, and hyposthenuria. Clinical hallmarks are linear growth failure and rickets resistant to doses of vitamin D that are ordinarily adequate for treatment of nutritional deficiency (1000–2000 units/day).

Etiology. Fanconi syndrome occurs with genetically transmitted inborn errors of metabolism (cystinosis, fructose intolerance, galactosemia, glycogenosis, Lowe syndrome, tyrosinemia, and Wilson disease) and with some acquired diseases, including exposure to environmental toxins, e.g., heavy metals (Cd, Pb, Hg) or outdated tetracycline. Most commonly, it is idiopathic, and its occurrence in this form may be sporadic or inherited as a mendelian dominant or recessive trait, including X-linked recessive. The following description of the primary idiopathic form is representative of the syndrome in general.

Pathogenesis. Clinical and experimental studies point to an abnormality in some final common pathway for normal membrane transport in the proximal renal tubules. It is not clear whether the defect is structural (in the membrane itself) or biochemical (involving energy production). A spontaneously occurring Fanconi syndrome which mimics the human disorder occurs in the basenji breed of dogs. In this animal excessive urinary losses of amino acids, sugar, and phosphate result from decreased proximal renal tubular reabsorption of the glomerular filtrate. Also, loss of bicarbonate in the urine leads to proximal renal tubular acidosis (Sec 16.24). Renal potassium wasting results from excessive urinary losses of bicarbonate and glucose. Urinary sodium losses are obligatory because of the large excretion of urinary anions. Serum calcium level is normal to low; urinary calcium levels vary. A urinary concentrating defect is often present but unexplained.

Rickets can result from the combined effects of metabolic acidosis and hypophosphatemia or from hypophosphatemia alone. Simple calcium deficiency does not appear to play a role in the bone disease. Vitamin D resistance may be due to impaired conversion of vitamin D to its active metabolites in the presence of metabolic acidosis.

Microscopic findings are nonspecific. Renal tubules may show dilatation, variation in size and shape, swelling of epithelial cells, and atrophy. Foci of interstitial fibrosis are common. Enlarged mitochondria may be seen on electron microscopy. Typically, glomerular architecture is preserved until late in the disease.

Clinical Manifestation. Primary Fanconi syndrome may occur at any age and may persist for many yr. Symptoms typically appear in the 1st 6 mo of life, when vomiting, polydipsia, polyuria, and constipation are noted. Episodes of weakness, fever with dehydration, and metabolic acidosis may also occur. Failure to thrive is often pronounced, especially in linear growth.

Roentgenographic signs of rickets or osteopenia may appear despite a history of adequate vitamin D intake and the absence of glomerular insufficiency, indicating a renal tubular cause.

Laboratory Data. Usually, a hyperchloremic metabolic acidosis is noted, with normal "anion gap" (Sec 5.12), hypokalemia, hypophosphatemia, and hypouricemia. Fractional excretion of phosphate is elevated. Alkaline phosphatase activity is elevated if rickets is present. Glycosuria occurs at normal serum glucose concentrations. There is generalized nonspecific aminoaciduria. Urinary pH is inappropriately elevated, with low levels of urinary ammonia and titratable acid. When the glomerular filtration rate falls late in the course of the disease, there may be a "paradoxical" improvement in the levels of serum electrolytes and an amelioration of aminoaciduria, glycosuria, and phosphaturia.

Diagnosis. There is no definitive diagnostic test for idiopathic Fanconi syndrome. Aminoaciduria, diminished tubular reabsorption of phosphate, and elevated alkaline phosphatase activities accompany other forms of rickets. In a child with stunted growth and rickets refractory to ordinary doses of vitamin D the finding of renal glycosuria indicates multiple tubular dysfunction. Metabolic acidosis and hypokalemia are corroborative. Fluid deprivation to test urinary concentrating ability is risky in the face of obligatory hyposthenuria, and glucose loading may cause profound symptomatic hypokalemia by shifting potassium into cells.

Treatment. The Fanconi syndrome represents a rather uniform response of renal tubules to various insults, but the clinical and biochemical expressions vary from patient to patient; accordingly, treatment is not uniform. For patients with secondary Fanconi syndrome, underlying causes should be sought. In those with primary Fanconi syndrome, symptomatic therapy can restore mineral and electrolyte balance, prolong survival, and often permit a normal life. Rickets can be corrected and skeletal deformities prevented, but fully normal growth rates are rarely achieved.

Rickets or osteopenia will respond to large doses of vitamin D. The usual starting dose is 5000 units/24 hr, which should be increased gradually to a maximal dose of 2000–4000 units/kg/24 hr. Most patients require at least 25,000 units to heal rickets. Dihydrotachysterol may be substituted for vitamin D at a starting dose of 0.05–0.1 mg/24 hr (1 mg is equivalent to 120,000 units of vitamin D). Serum calcium levels must be followed closely (weekly at first, then monthly) to avoid hypercalcemia from vitamin D overdose. Hypophosphatemia can be treated by oral supplementation with 1–3 gm of neutral phosphate/24 hr given in 4–5 equally spaced doses through the waking hours. If abdominal pain or diarrhea ensues, therapy should be temporarily discontinued and then reinstituted at a lower dose. Phosphate should not be given without concomitant vitamin D lest it cause or aggravate hypocalcemia.

Correction of metabolic acidosis due to excessive bicarbonaturia may require large amounts of alkali. From 2–15 mEq/kg/24 hr of alkali may be needed, as sodium bicarbonate solution (1 mEq of Na = 1 ml), Shohl solution (140 gm citric acid, 90 gm sodium citrate qs to 1 l with water; 1 mEq of Na = 1 ml) or Polycitra (5 ml = 550 mg potassium citrate, 500 mg sodium citrate, 334 mg citric acid; 2 mEq of base = 1 ml). Doses should be adjusted to raise serum bicarbonate only to near normal levels (18–20 mEq/l). Attempts to normalize serum bicarbonate may exaggerate urinary bicarbonate loss as a result of extracellular fluid volume expansion with excessive sodium loads. Alkali is administered in 3–4 divided doses/day, and, if Polycitra is not used, extra potassium should be given as either potassium triplex or potassium chloride at a starting dose of 2–3 mEq/kg/24 hr. Extra salt and water should be provided to counter excessive losses, especially in warm weather.

Bovee KC, Joyce T, Reynolds R, et al: The Fanconi syndrome in basenji dogs—a new model for renal transport defects. Science 201:1179, 1978.
Brodehl J: The Fanconi syndrome. In: Edelmann CM, Jr (ed): Pediatric Kidney Disease. Boston, Little, Brown, 1978.

23.29 Cystinosis
(Lignac Syndrome; Fanconi Syndrome with Cystinosis)

Cystinosis presents the clinical and laboratory features of Fanconi syndrome with the additional distinctive finding of abnormal accumulation of cystine in various tissues (see also Sec 23.28).

Pathogenesis. The cause is unknown. Cystine accumulates in lysosomes, where it cannot be maintained in reduced form. It is not clear whether there is failure in lysosomal release or in degradation of this amino acid. No specific enzyme defect has yet been identified. Tissue levels of cystine do not correlate with degree of renal tubular dysfunction; accordingly, a simple toxic effect of cystine on tubules is not the cause of Fanconi syndrome in cystinosis.

Cystine is deposited in the reticuloendothelial system, especially in spleen, liver, lymph nodes, and bone marrow. Deposits occur in renal tubular cells, cornea, and conjunctiva. Cystine also accumulates in peripheral blood leukocytes and fibroblasts. Early renal changes are similar to those of primary Fanconi syndrome; the characteristic "swan neck" lesion consists of atrophy and shortening of the proximal tubule just beneath the glomerulus. Birefringent cystine crystals may be seen in interstitial tissue; they are sometimes recognizable only on electron microscopy. Cystine crystals are rarely noted in tubular cells. With advancing renal failure, the kidneys become shrunken and contracted, with glomerular sclerosis and interstitial fibrosis.

Clinical Manifestations. There are 3 clinical patterns. Patients with the infantile or nephropathic form present Fanconi syndrome at 3–6 mo of age. A generalized aminoaciduria is found without predominance of cystine. Glomerular filtration rate falls progressively, and chronic renal failure develops within the 1st decade. Severe growth failure and hypothyroidism accompany this state. Distinctive clinical features include blond hair and fair complexion, due to a defect in melanin synthesis, and photophobia secondary to deposit of cystine crystals in the conjunctivae. The adolescent or intermediate form is characterized by mild renal involvement, with onset in the 2nd decade and slow progression. The adult type of cystinosis (benign) causes no renal disease. Cystine crystals may be found in the cornea, bone marrow, and leukocytes.

Laboratory Data. Other than the deposition of cystine crystals, laboratory abnormalities are similar to those described for the Fanconi syndrome. Tubular proteinuria characterizes the early phase of nephropathic cystinosis, but glomerular proteinuria supervenes as renal failure ensues.

Diagnosis. In the asymptomatic newborn infant from an affected family the diagnosis of cystinosis can be made by measuring the cystine content of leukocytes or fibroblasts, which will be 80–100 times normal. Later, granular and circinate irregularities in the peripheral pigmentation of the retina may be noted. Cystine crystals may be detected in the bone marrow, lymph nodes, conjunctiva, and rectal mucosa. Slit lamp examination will show crystals in the cornea. Prenatal diagnosis can be made by finding an increased concentration of cystine in amniotic fluid cells. Cystinosis must not be confused with cystinuria, which is an inborn error of specific amino acid transport, with neither cystine deposition nor Fanconi syndrome.

Treatment. No specific treatment is as yet available that reduces tissue levels of cystine or reverses the abnormalities of renal function. Symptomatic therapy is similar to that for primary Fanconi syndrome.

For patients with end-stage renal failure, hemodialysis and renal transplantation are recommended. Hemodialysis does not lower tissue cystine levels. Cystine will accumulate in the transplanted kidney, but it does not produce Fanconi syndrome; this finding suggests either that the cystine is stored in a different location or that the cause of renal dysfunction is not cystine per se.

States B, Blazer B, Harris D, et al: Prenatal diagnosis of cystinosis. J Pediatr 87:558, 1975.

23.30 Rickets Associated with Renal Tubular Acidosis
(Lightwood Syndrome; Infantile or Transient Distal Renal Tubular Acidosis)

This disorder is characterized by a hyperchloremic metabolic acidosis due to an inability to form an adequately acid urine; hypercalciuria and hyperkaliuria are frequently associated. (See Sec 5.12.) Affected children often develop growth retardation and rickets or osteopenia and pathologic fractures.

Pathogenesis. If hypercalciuria leads to transient hypocalcemia, secondary hyperparathyroidism will develop and cause diminished tubular reabsorption of phosphate, resulting in turn in hypophosphatemia. These disturbances cause rickets, especially if there is concomitant impairment in the conversion of vitamin D to its active metabolite $1,25\text{-}(OH)_2\text{-}D_3$ (Sec 23.22).

Treatment. The metabolic abnormalities leading to bone disease can usually be reversed by alkali therapy. Doses vary with the child's age, expected growth rate, and glomerular filtration rate. A starting dose of 2 mEq/kg/24 hr given in 2–3 divided doses is appropriate, but up to 10–15 mEq/kg/24 hr may be necessary to restore a normal linear growth pattern.

Rodriguez–Soriano J: Renal tubular acidosis. *In*: Edelmann, CM Jr (ed): Pediatric Kidney Disease. Boston, Little, Brown, 1978.

23.31 Oculocerebrorenal Dystrophy
(Lowe Syndrome)

This rare disorder is transmitted as an X-linked recessive trait. In addition to Fanconi syndrome, organic aciduria, decreased production of urinary ammonia, and occasionally heavy proteinuria occur. Distinctive clinical features include congenital cataracts, glaucoma, and buphthalmos that lead to severe visual impairment. Severe hypotonia and hyporeflexia appear in the 1st yr. Mental retardation is severe and often progressive. Rickets, marked osteopenia, and pathologic fracture may develop as a result of metabolic acidosis and phosphate depletion.

Pathogenesis. The pathogenesis is not known. Pathologic studies have shown splitting of the glomerular basement membranes, with marked variation in their thickness. These changes may not be confined to the kidney.

Clinical Features. Early in life the eye findings and mental retardation predominate; the Fanconi syndrome becomes clinically apparent later. If the patient survives childhood, the Fanconi syndrome may resolve spontaneously, only to be supplanted by chronic renal failure. There is no specific therapy. Treatment is supportive, as in primary Fanconi syndrome.

Abbassi V, Lowe CU, Calcagno PL: Oculo-cerebro-renal syndrome. A review. Am J Dis Child 15:145, 1968.

23.32 Renal Osteodystrophy

The term renal osteodystrophy designates the alterations in skeletal growth and remodeling which occur in children with chronic renal disease because of abnormalities in mineral and bone metabolism. These abnormalities include malabsorption of calcium, hyperfunction of the parathyroid glands, cutaneous vascular and visceral calcification, and impairment in the renal production of biologically active vitamin D. Renal osteodystrophy can occur with tubular dysfunction while glomerular filtration remains intact (Sec 23.32 and 16.2) but more commonly follows progressive loss of nephrons, with glomerular insufficiency and uremia.

The condition was formerly called renal (uremic) rickets or renal dwarfism because severe linear growth failure was associated with rickets-like roentgenographic changes. These findings were first thought to be due primarily to mineralization defect resulting from vitamin D deficiency, but recent studies of immuno-parathyroid physiology and bone histology indicate that secondary hyperparathyroidism is an equally important contributor to the clinical and roentgenographic findings in uremic osteodystrophy. Since hemodialysis and kidney transplantation have become available to children, the major complication of chronic renal failure in childhood has become renal osteodystrophy.

Pathogenesis. The pathogenesis is complex. The bony abnormalities do not respond to physiologic doses of vitamin D adequate to treat simple vitamin D deficiency. This vitamin D resistance leads to a malabsorption of calcium and phosphate and, through unknown mechanisms, to defective mineralization of osteoid (osteomalacia). The fact that the kidney is the site of final synthesis of the major vitamin D metabolites may explain the vitamin D resistance.

Secondary hyperparathyroidism occurs as the glomerular filtration falls; serum phosphate levels rise and lead to hypocalcemia and release of parathyroid hormone (PTH). At some critical renal threshold, e. g., when glomerular filtration rate falls to approximately 25–30% of normal, the phosphaturic renal response to elevated PTH is lost, and compensatory hyperparathyroidism supervenes in an attempt to restore serum calcium to normal. The consequences are roentgenographic and histologic evidence of exaggerated osteoclast-mediated resorption of bone (osteitis fibrosa). Also, endosteal fibrosis, increased bone turnover, and replacement of regularly textured lamellar bone with disorganized and structurally deficient woven bone are seen. Chronic metabolic acidosis probably contributes to the bony changes by increasing calcium resorption and impairing conversion of vitamin D to its biologically active forms.

The pathology varies. On biopsy, trabecular bone may show predominant osteomalacia, predominant osteitis fibrosa, or, most commonly, a mixed pattern. The mineralization defect can be demonstrated by giving the patient tetracycline prior to biopsy; this fluorescent antibiotic is deposited at the mineralization front.

Roentgenographic abnormalities at the epiphyseal growth plate may occasionally resemble those of nutritional rickets but are often quite distinct; histologically, they reflect osteitis fibrosa rather than rickets. The growth plate is not actually increased in longitudinal width but appears to be because of the formation of a bar of metaphyseal fibrosis with dysplastic trabeculae. The concomitant defect in mineralization leads to a failure in modeling, with persistence of cartilage, an expanded epiphyseal diameter, and frequent overriding of the lateral border of the metaphysis.

Clinical Manifestations. The younger the child at onset of chronic renal failure and the longer the duration of renal failure, the greater the incidence and severity of osteodystrophy. In children with congenital diseases of the kidney, which predominate under the age of 5 yr, the interval between onset of disease and end-stage renal failure is longer than it is in the glomerulonephritides, which occur later in childhood. In children with congenital nephropathies, bone disease is accelerated because it occurs at a time of maximal growth and bone modeling and remodeling.

The earliest sign of renal osteodystrophy is usually growth failure, to which metabolic acidosis, protein-calorie malnutrition, hormonal disorders, and trace mineral deficiencies associated with chronic renal failure may contribute. Growth failure may occur with no roentgenographic skeletal abnormalities. With advancing (untreated) disease, additional clinical manifestations appear, including muscle weakness, bone pain, bone deformities, slipped epiphyses, metaphyseal fractures, metastatic calcification, and pruritus. Genu varum, frontal bossing, and dental abnormalities are particularly evident in young children. Tetany is rare (despite hypocalcemia) because of the combined protective effects of metabolic acidosis and hyperparathyroidism.

Laboratory Data. There may be mild hypocalcemia, but the Ca × P product is usually elevated by increased levels of serum phosphorus. Elevated alkaline phosphatase activity reflects increased bone turnover but is not as reliable a sign in children as in adults.

In roentgenograms of the hands and wrists subperiosteal erosions of the middle and distal phalanges are considered by some to be sensitive early indicators of osteitis fibrosa. Erosions may also occur in the distal clavicle and on inner aspects of the distal femur and proximal tibia. Findings on percutaneous bone biopsy (which is not yet widely done) might give still earlier indications, but elevated serum levels of PTH will generally give the earliest indication of bone disease and may be found when glomerular filtration rates are reduced to as little as 40–50 ml/min/1.73 M^2. The degree of elevation of PTH correlates with roentgenographic and histologic evidence of osteitis fibrosa, but the degree of histologic osteomalacia does not correlate well with chemical abnormalities in serum or with roentgenographic evidence of rickets, osteopenia, or coarsening of trabeculae.

Treatment. Renal osteodystrophy can usually be successfully managed by (1) controlling hyperphosphatemia, (2) supplying adequate oral calcium intake, and (3) providing extra vitamin D. Treatment should begin early since growth failure in infancy can greatly influence the attainment of ultimate stature. An unresolved question is whether therapy should be initiated before definite roentgenographic or biochemical abnormalities appear.

Hyperphosphatemia should be controlled with oral administration of phosphate binders. Aluminum hydroxide or aluminum carbonate gel can be given at a starting dose of 20–30 mg/kg/24 hr and the dose adjusted to keep the serum phosphorus between 4–5 mg/dl. The dose may have to be increased when vitamin D is given. Calcium supplementation in the form of calcium carbonate should be added to the diet to provide 1–1.5 gm of elemental calcium/day. We prefer calcium carbonate because, of the available calcium preparations, it contains the highest percentage of elemental

calcium. Strict control of acidosis should be achieved with administration of sodium bicarbonate. Starting doses are usually 1–2 mEq/kg/24 hr (see Sec 23.28 for specific agents).

Some form of vitamin D appears necessary for successful treatment of uremic osteodystrophy. Large doses of ordinary vitamin D may produce improvement of bone lesions and partial suppression of hyperparathyroidism. Starting doses are from 5000–10,000 units/24 hr, but the dose may need to be increased to as high as 100,000–200,000 units/24 hr. The therapeutic to toxic ratio is narrow; hypercalcemia is frequently encountered and may be persistent because of the long half-life of the agent in patients with chronic renal failure. In recent years dihydrotachysterol (DHT) has been favored over vitamin D because it has a shorter half-life. Moreover, it has the theoretical benefit of requiring only hepatic 25-hydroxylation and not renal 1-hydroxylation to become active. Starting doses are 0.1–0.2 mg/24 hr. With either form of treatment, doses are adjusted to normalize levels of serum calcium and to heal roentgenographic abnormalities. Doses can be lowered once these goals are achieved. Frequent measurements of serum calcium and phosphorus are required, weekly at first, then monthly. Striking therapeutic effects have been reported for 1,25-(OH)$_2$-D$_3$ and 25-(OH)-D$_3$ in the healing of bone lesions of osteodystrophy; these agents are as yet investigational but appear to hold promise for the future.

Hemodialysis may either ameliorate or exacerbate bone disease; the effect cannot be predicted. Unrecognized or untreated hypercalcemia may accelerate renal insufficiency or foster metastatic calcification of the tympanic membranes, cornea, conjunctiva, skin, and vascular tree. When hypercalcemia is found, administration of vitamin D must be suspended until the serum calcium level is normal; therapy can then be reinstituted at a lower dose.

Parathyroidectomy is indicated in carefully selected patients with severe secondary hyperparathyroidism refractory to medical therapy. Indications include severe bone pain, mental aberrations, severe pruritus, fractures, chronic hypercalcemia, and, less commonly, metastatic calcification. In all cases marked elevation of serum PTH levels should be proved prior to surgery.

MICHAEL E. NORMAN

Avioli LV, Teitelbaum SL: Renal osteodystrophy. In: Edelmann CM (ed): Pediatric Kidney Disease. Boston, Little, Brown, 1978.
Chesney RW, Moorthy AV, Jax DK, et al: Increased linear growth after long-term oral 1,25(OH)$_2$D therapy in childhood renal osteodystrophy. N Engl J Med 298:238, 1978.
DeLuca HF: The vitamin D hormonal system: Implications for bone diseases. Hosp Pract 15:57, 1980.
Dent CE, Harper CM, Philpot GR: The treatment of renal-glomerular osteodystrophy. Q J Med 30:1, 1961.
Norman ME, Mazur AT, Borden S, et al: Early diagnosis of juvenile renal osteodystrophy. J Pediatr 97:226, 1980.

24.1 MORPHOLOGY OF THE SKIN

The Epidermis. The mature epidermis, a stratified epithelial tissue, is constantly renewed by mitotic division of the cells of the basal layer. In addition to the squamous cells or keratinocytes, the epidermis contains melanocytes, the pigment-forming cells, and Langerhans cells, dendritic cells of the mononuclear phagocyte system.

The renewal of the surface cells of the epidermis is a continuous process that normally proceeds in an orderly fashion as the cells of the basal cell layer move upward to the stratum corneum. The transit time of the epidermal cell is relatively fixed; the total life span is approximately 28 days. In hyperproliferative diseases the movement of the cells is more rapid so that the newly arrived epidermal cells in the stratum corneum, being immature, form a defective barrier junction of the skin and allow increased permeability.

Epidermal melanocytes are derived from the neural crest and migrate to the skin during embryonic life. They reside in the interfollicular epidermis and in the hair follicles and multiply by mitosis to repopulate the epidermis. Melanocytes are responsible for skin color; melanosomes containing melanin are ingested by the keratinocytes, and the melanin is shed with the stratum corneum cells.

The Langerhans cells have a dendritic form and, in that respect, resemble melanocytes, but rather than melanosomes, they contain a specific organelle, the Birbeck granule. These cells appear to be of mesenchymal origin and participate in immune reactions in the skin, playing an active role in antigen presentation and processing.

The Dermis. The dermis, or corium, forms a tough, pliable, fibrous supporting structure between the epidermis and the subcutaneous fat. It is composed of collagen and elastic and reticular fibers embedded in an amorphous ground substance and contains blood vessels, lymphatics, neural structures, eccrine and apocrine sweat glands, hair follicles, sebaceous glands, and smooth muscle. Morphologically, the dermis can be divided into 2 layers, the superficial papillary layer that interdigitates with the rete ridges of the epidermis and the deeper reticular layer that lies beneath the papillary dermis. The papillary layer is less dense and more cellular, whereas the reticular layer appears more compact because of the coarse network of interlaced collagen and elastic fibers.

The predominant cell is a spindle-shaped fibroblast that is responsible for the synthesis of collagen, elastic fibers, and mucopolysaccharides. Phagocytic histiocytes, mast cells, and motile leukocytes are also present.

The gelatinous ground substance serves as a supporting medium for the fibrillar and cellular components as well as a storage place for a substantial portion of body water. Nutrients are supplied to both epidermis and dermis via the dermal blood vessels.

The Subcutaneous Tissue. Panniculus, or subcutaneous tissue, is composed of fat cells, which form and store lipid, and of fibrous septa that divide it into lobules and anchor it to the underlying fascia and periosteum. Blood vessels and nerves are also present in this layer, which serves as a storage depot for lipid, an insulator to conserve body heat, and a protective cushion against trauma.

The appendageal structures are derived from aggregates of epidermal cells that become specialized during early embryonic development. Small buds, called the primary epithelial germs, appear during the 3rd fetal mo and give rise to hair follicles, sebaceous and apocrine glands, and the attachment bulges for the arrector pili muscles. Eccrine sweat glands are derived from separate epidermal downgrowths that arise during the 2nd fetal mo and are completely formed by the 5th mo. Formation of nails is initiated during the 3rd intrauterine mo.

The hair follicle is the most prominent structure in the pilary complex, which includes the sebaceous gland, the arrector pili muscle, and in certain areas such as the axillae, an apocrine gland. Hair follicles are distributed throughout the skin except in the palms, soles, lips, and glans penis; if destroyed, they cannot regenerate. Individual follicles extend from the surface of the epidermis to the deep dermis, where the matrix cells with the dermal papilla form a bulbous hair root. The growing hair consists of a bulb and a matrix from which the keratinized hair shaft is generated; the shaft is composed of an inner medulla, a cortex, and an outer cuticular layer.

Human hair growth is cyclical, with alternate periods of growth (anagen) and rest (telogen). The length of the anagen phase varies from months to years. At birth, all hairs are in the anagen phase. Subsequent generative activity lacks synchrony so that an overall random pattern of growth and shedding prevails. Scalp hair usually grows about 0.35 mm/24 hr.

The sebaceous glands occur in all areas except the palms, soles, and dorsa of the feet, but they are most numerous on the face, upper chest, and back. Their ducts open into the hair follicles except on the lips, prepuce, and labia minora, where they emerge directly onto the mucosal surface. These holocrine glands are saccular structures that are often branched and lobulated and consist of a proliferative basal layer of small flat cells peripheral to the central mass of lipidized cells. The latter cells disintegrate as they move toward the duct and form the lipid secretion known as sebum that is composed of cellular debris, triglycerides, phospholipids, and cholesterol esters.

Sebaceous glands are dependent upon hormonal stimulation and are activated by the increasing androgenic activity at puberty. Fetal sebaceous glands are stimulated by maternal androgens, and their lipid secretion together with desquamated stratum corneum cells comprise the vernix caseosa.

The apocrine glands are located in the axillae, areolae, perianal and genital areas, and the periumbilical region. These large, coiled, tubular structures continuously secrete an odorless milky fluid which is discharged in response to adrenergic stimuli, usually the result of emotional stress. Bacterial decomposition of apocrine sweat accounts for the unpleasant odor associated with perspiration.

Apocrine glands remain dormant until puberty, when they enlarge and secretion begins through increasing androgenic activity. The secretory coil of the gland consists of a single layer of cells enclosed by a layer of contractile myoepithelial cells. The duct is lined with a double layer of cuboidal cells and opens into the pilosebaceous complex. Although apocrine glands do not function in thermoregulation, they are involved in certain disease processes.

Eccrine sweat glands are distributed over the entire body surface including the palms and soles, where they are most abundant. Those on the hairy skin respond to thermal stimuli and serve to regulate the body temperature by delivering water to the skin surface for evaporation; in contrast, sweat glands on the palms and soles respond mainly to psychogenic stimuli.

Each eccrine gland is composed of a secretory coil, which is located in the reticular dermis or subcutaneous fat, and a secretory duct, which opens onto the skin surface. The sweat pores can be identified on the epidermal ridges of the palm and fingers with a magnifying lens, but they are not readily visualized elsewhere.

Two types of cells compose the single-layered secretory coil: small dark cells and large clear cells; these rest on a layer of contractile myoepithelial cells and a basement membrane. The glands are supplied by sympathetic nerve fibers, but the pharmacologic mediator of sweating is acetylcholine rather than epinephrine. The composition of sweat varies with the rate of sweating but is always hypotonic in normal children.

Nails are specialized epidermal structures that form convex, translucent plates on the distal dorsal surfaces of the fingers and toes. The nail plate, which is derived from a metabolically active matrix of multiplying cells situated beneath the posterior nail fold, grows forward at the rate of approximately 0.1 mm/24 hr. The nail plate is bounded by the lateral and posterior nail folds; a thin eponychium, the cuticle, protrudes from the posterior fold over a crescent-shaped white area called the lunula. The pink color above it reflects the underlying vascular bed.

24.2   EXAMINATION OF THE PATIENT

Though many skin disorders are easily recognized by simple inspection, a painstaking history and physical examination are often necessary for accurate assessment. In all instances the entire body surface, the mucous membranes, the hair, and nails should be thoroughly examined under adequate illumination. The color, turgor, texture, temperature, and moisture of the skin and the growth, texture, caliber, and luster of the hair and nails should be noted. Skin lesions should be palpated as well as inspected and should be classified on the bases of morphology, size, color, texture, firmness, configuration, location, and distribution. One must also decide whether the changes are those of the primary lesion itself or whether the clinical pattern has been altered by a secondary factor such as infection, trauma, or therapy.

Primary lesions are classified as macules, papules, nodules, tumors, vesicles, bullae, pustules, wheals, and cysts. A *macular* lesion represents an alteration in skin color but cannot be felt. *Papules* are palpable solid lesions smaller than 1 cm, whereas *nodules* are larger in circumference. *Tumors* are usually larger than nodules and vary considerably in mobility and consistency. *Vesicles* are raised, fluid-filled lesions less than 0.5 cm in diameter; when larger, they are called *bullae*. *Pustules* contain purulent material. *Wheals* are flat-topped, palpable lesions of variable size and configuration that represent dermal collections of edema fluid. *Cysts* are circumscribed, thick-walled lesions that are located deep in the skin, are covered by a normal epidermis, and contain fluid or semisolid material. Aggregations of any of the primary lesions may be referred to as *plaques*.

Secondary lesions include scales, ulcers, excoriations, fissures, crusts, and scars. *Scales* are composed of compressed layers of stratum corneum cells that are retained on the skin surface. *Ulcers* are excavations of necrotic or traumatized tissue. Ulcerated lesions inflicted by scratching are often linear or angular in configuration and are called *excoriations*. *Fissures* are caused by splitting or cracking; they usually occur in diseased skin. *Crusts* consist of matted, retained accumulations of blood, serum, pus, and epithelial debris on the surface of a weeping lesion. *Scars* are end-stage lesions that can be thin, depressed and atrophic, raised and hypertrophic, or flat and pliable; they are composed of fibrous connective tissue.

If the diagnosis is not clear after a thorough examination as indicated above, 1 or more of several diagnostic procedures may be indicated. In addition to those discussed below, others are identified in appropriate subsections. These include scrapings of scabies lesions and smears and cultures of vesicles and pustules for detection of bacteria.

Biopsy of skin by an excision is rarely required for diagnostic purposes in children. A *punch biopsy* is a simple and relatively painless procedure and usually provides adequate tissue for examination. A fresh but well-developed lesion should be selected for removal. Xylocaine, 1 or 2%, with or without epinephrine should be injected intradermally with a 25-gauge needle following cleansing of the site. A punch, 3 or 4 mm in diameter, is pressed firmly against the skin and rotated until it sinks to the proper depth. All 3 layers (epidermis, dermis, and subcutis) should be contained in the plug. The plug should be gently lifted with forceps or extracted with a needle and separated from the underlying tissue with an iris scissors. Bleeding abates with firm pressure; suturing is optional. The biopsy specimen should be placed in 10% formalin for appropriate processing.

The **Wood lamp** transmits ultraviolet light mainly in a wave length of 3650 A. The examination, which is performed in a darkened room, is useful mainly in certain superficial fungus infections of the scalp. Blue-green fluorescence is detectable at the base of each infected hair shaft in ectothrix and in some endothrix infections. Scales and crusts may appear pale yellow, but this observation is not evidence of a fungus infection. Dermatophyte lesions of the skin (tinea corporis) do not fluoresce; the macules of tinea versicolor, however, do have a golden fluorescence under the Wood lamp.

Discrete areas of altered pigment can also be visualized more clearly by use of a Wood lamp, particularly if the pigmentary change is epidermal. Hyperpigmented lesions appear darker and hypopigmented lesions lighter than the surrounding skin.

The **KOH preparation** provides a rapid and reliable method for the detection of fungal elements of both yeasts and dermatophytes. Scaly lesions should be scraped at the active border for optimal recovery of mycelia and spores. Vesicles should be unroofed, and the blister top should be clipped and placed on a slide for examination. In tinea capitis, infected hairs must be plucked from the follicle; scales from the scalp usually will not contain mycelia. A few drops of 10% potassium hydroxide are added to the specimen, which is then gently heated over an alcohol lamp until it begins to bubble. The preparation is examined under low-intensity light for fungal elements.

A **Tzanck smear** is useful in the diagnosis of some viral infections (herpes simplex, varicella, herpes zoster, and eczema herpeticum) as well as for detection of acantholytic cells in pemphigus. An intact, fresh blister should be ruptured and drained of fluid. The base of the blister is then vigorously scraped with a dull-edged instrument; the material is smeared on a clear glass slide and air-dried. Staining with Giemsa stain is preferable, but Wright stain is acceptable. Balloon cells and multinucleated giant cells are diagnostic of herpesvirus infection; acantholytic epidermal cells are characteristic of pemphigus.

Immunofluorescent studies of skin can be used to detect tissue-fixed antibodies to skin components; characteristic staining patterns under the fluorescent microscope are specific for certain skin disorders. Serum can be used for identification of circulating antibodies. Skin biopsies for direct immunofluorescent preparations should be obtained from involved sites except in those diseases for which paralesional skin or uninvolved skin is required. A punch biopsy is obtained, and the tissue is placed in a special transport medium or *immediately* frozen in liquid nitrogen for transport or storage. Thin cryostat sections of the specimen are incubated with fluorescein-conjugated goat or rabbit antihuman globulin or complement.

Serum of patients can be examined by indirect immunofluorescent techniques in which a section of normal human skin, guinea pig lip, or monkey esophagus is used as a substrate. A substrate is incubated with fresh or thawed frozen serum and then with fluorescein-conjugated antihuman globulin. If the serum contains antibody to epithelial components, the immunoglobulin can be identified by its specific staining pattern as seen on fluorescent microscopy. By serial dilutions, the titer of circulating antibody can be estimated.

DISEASES OF THE SKIN

24.3 TRANSIENT LESIONS OF THE NEONATE

Minor evanescent lesions of the newborn infant, particularly when florid, may cause undue concern. Most of the entities described in this section are relatively common, benign, and transient; they do not require therapy.

Sebaceous Hyperplasia. Minute profuse yellow-white papules are frequently found on the forehead, nose, upper lip, and cheeks of the term infant; they represent hyperplastic sebaceous glands. These tiny papules gradually diminish in size and disappear entirely within the 1st few wk of life.

Milia. The milium is a superficial epidermal inclusion cyst that contains laminated keratinized material. The lesion is a firm papule, 1–2 mm in diameter and pearly, opalescent white in color. Milia may occur at any age but in the neonate are most frequently scattered over the face and gingivae and on the midline of the palate, where they are called *Epstein pearls*. Milia exfoliate spontaneously in most infants and may be ignored; those that appear in scars or sites of trauma in older children may be gently unroofed and "shelled out" with a fine-gauge needle.

Sucking Blisters. Solitary or scattered superficial bullae on the upper limbs and lips of infants at birth are presumed to be induced by vigorous sucking on the affected part in utero. Common sites are the radial aspect of the forearm, the thumb, the index finger, and the central portion of the upper lip. These bullae resolve rapidly without sequelae.

Cutis Marmorata. When the newborn infant is exposed to low environmental temperatures, an evanescent, lacy, reticulated red or blue cutaneous vascular pattern appears over most of the body surface. This vascular change represents an accentuated physiologic vasomotor response that disappears with increasing age, although it is sometimes discernible even in older children. Persistent and pronounced cutis marmorata occurs in the Cornelia de Lange, Down, and trisomy 18 syndromes. Cutis marmorata telangiectasia congenita (Sec 24.7) is clinically similar, but the lesions are more intense and are persistent.

Harlequin Color Change. The so-called harlequin color change in the immediate newborn period is a rare but dramatic vascular event that occurs more commonly in infants of low birth weight. It probably reflects an imbalance in the autonomic vascular regulatory mechanism. When the infant is placed on his or her side, the body is bisected longitudinally into a pale upper half and a deep red dependent half. The color change is transient, lasting only a few minutes, and occasionally affects only a portion of the trunk or face. The pattern may be reversed by changing the infant's position. Muscular activity will cause generalized flushing and obliterate the color differential. Multiple episodes may occur but are not indicative of other or permanent autonomic imbalance.

Salmon Patch (Macular Hemangioma, Nevus Simplex). Salmon patches are small, pale pink, ill-defined, flat vascular lesions that occur most commonly on the glabella, eyelids, upper lip, and nuchal area of 30–50% of normal newborn infants. These lesions, which represent localized plaques of vascular ectasia, persist for several mo and may become more visible during crying or changes in environmental temperature. The lesions on the face eventually fade and disappear completely, but those on the posterior neck and occipital area persist in a number of infants. When they become covered with hair, they are not noticeable. The facial lesions should not be confused with nevus flammeus, which is a permanent lesion.

Mongolian Spots. These are blue or slate-gray macular lesions with variably defined margins; they occur most commonly in the presacral area but may be found over the posterior thighs, legs, backs, and shoulders. They may be solitary or multiple and often involve large areas. More than 80% of black, oriental, and East Indian infants have these lesions, whereas the incidence in white infants is less than 10%. The peculiar hue of these lesions is due to the dermal location of melanin-containing melanocytes which are presumed to have been arrested in their migration from neural crest to epidermis. Mongolian spots usually fade during the 1st few yr of life, but they may persist. Widespread multiple lesions, particularly those in unusual sites, are unlikely to disappear.

Erythema Toxicum. This benign, self-limited, evanescent eruption occurs in approximately 50% of full-term infants; preterm infants are affected less commonly. The lesions are firm, yellow-white, 1–2 mm papules or pustules localized in a patch of erythema (Fig 24–1, p. xxxiv). At times, splotchy erythema is the only manifestation. Lesions may be sparse or numerous and clustered in several sites or widely dispersed over much of the body surface. Palms and soles are virtually always spared. Peak incidence occurs in the 2nd day of life, but new lesions may erupt during the 1st few days.

The pustules are below the stratum corneum or in the epidermis; there is a dense infiltrate of eosinophils in the upper portion of the pilosebaceous follicle which can be demonstrated in Wright-stained smears of the intralesional contents. Cultures are always sterile.

The cause of erythema toxicum is unknown. The lesions can mimic pyoderma, candidiasis, transient neonatal pustular melanosis, and miliaria but may be differentiated by the characteristic infiltrate of eosinophils and the absence of organisms on a stained smear. The course is brief, and no therapy is required.

Transient Neonatal Pustular Melanosis. Pustular melanosis, which appears more often in black than in white infants, is a transient, benign, self-limited dermatosis of unknown cause that is characterized by 3 types of lesions: (1) superficial, small pustules; (2) ruptured pustules with a collarette of fine scale, at times with a central hyperpigmented macule; and (3) hyperpigmented macules (Fig 24–2). The lesions are present at birth, and 1 or all types of lesions may be found in a profuse or sparse distribution. The pustules represent the early phase of each lesion, the macules, the late phase. Sites of predilection are the anterior neck, forehead, lower back, and shins, although the scalp, trunk, limbs, and soles may be affected.

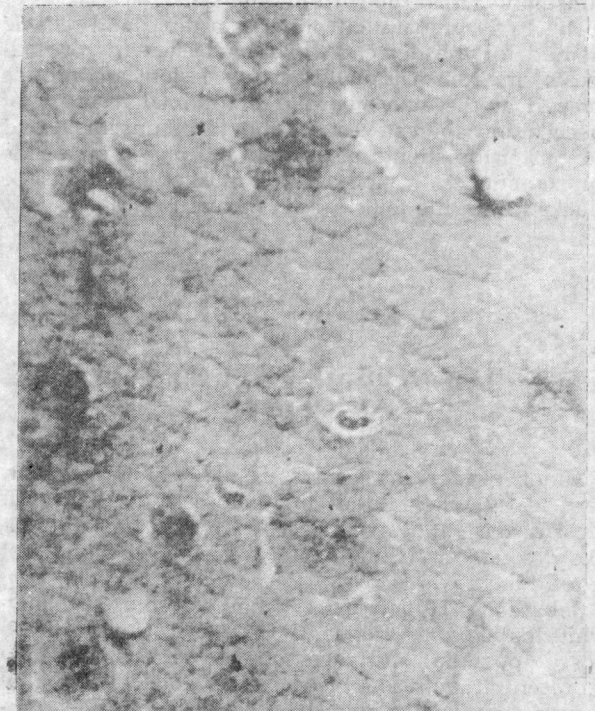

Figure 24–2 Transient neonatal pustular melanosis showing pustules, rings of scales, and hyperpigmented macules.

In biopsies of tissue during the active phase, an intracorneal or subcorneal pustule filled with polymorphonuclear leukocytes, debris, and an occasional eosinophil is demonstrable. The macules are characterized only by increased melanization of epidermal cells. Cultures of pustules can be used to distinguish the lesions from those of erythema toxicum and pyoderma since they do not contain bacteria or dense aggregates of eosinophils.

The pustular phase rarely lasts more than 2–3 days; hyperpigmented macules may persist for as long as 3 mo. No therapy is required.

24.4 DEVELOPMENTAL DEFECTS

24.5 CUTANEOUS DEFECTS

Skin Dimples. Deep dimpling over bony prominences and in the sacral area, at times associated with pits and creases, may occur in normal children as well as in association with some dysmorphologic syndromes, such as those of congenital rubella, deletion of the long arm of chromosome 18, Bloom, and the cerebrohepatorenal syndromes.

Redundant Skin. Loose folds of skin must be differentiated from cutis laxa, a congenital defect of elastic tissue. Redundant skin over the posterior neck is common in the Turner and Down syndromes; more generalized folds of the skin occur in infants with trisomy 18, with combined immunodeficiency disease, and with short-limbed dwarfism.

Amniotic Constriction Bands. Partial or complete constriction bands that produce defects in extremities and digits are found occasionally in otherwise normal infants. They are thought to result from intrauterine rupture of amnion with formation of fibrous strands which encircle the fetal parts and cause permanent depression of the underlying tissue. Rarely, amputation of 1 or more digits may result. Constriction bands on the limbs may be removed by plastic procedures.

Preauricular Sinuses and Pits. Pits and sinus tracts anterior to the pinna may be the result of imperfect fusion of the tubercles of the 1st 2 branchial arches, from which the tragus and pinna are derived. These anomalies may be unilateral or bilateral, at times associated with other anomalies of the ears and face. When the tracts become chronically infected, retention cysts may form and drain intermittently; such lesions may require excision.

Accessory Tragi. Multiple or single, unilateral or bilateral, sessile or pedunculated skin tags may occur in the preauricular area or on the neck anterior to the sternocleidomastoid muscle. They may occur as an isolated defect or in syndromes that include anomalies of the ears and face. Surgical excision is appropriate.

Branchial Cleft and Thyroglossal Cysts and Sinuses. Cysts and sinuses in the neck may be formed along the course of the 1st and 2nd branchial clefts as a result of improper closure during embryonic life. The lesions may be unilateral or bilateral and may open onto the cutaneous surface or drain into the pharynx. Secondary infection is an indication for systemic antibiotic therapy. These anomalies may be inherited as autosomal dominant traits.

Thyroglossal cysts and fistulas are similar defects located in or near the midline of the neck; they may extend to the base of the tongue. Occasionally these cysts contain aberrant thyroid tissue as well as the usual mucinous material. Surgical excision is the appropriate treatment, but care must be taken to preserve thyroid tissue (Sec 18.16).

Supernumerary Nipples. Solitary or multiple accessory nipples may occur in a unilateral or bilateral distribution along a line from the midaxilla to the inguinal area. The accessory nipples may or may not have areolae and may be mistaken for congenital nevi. They may be excised for cosmetic reasons. Rarely, they undergo malignant change.

Aplasia Cutis Congenita (Congenital Absence of Skin). Developmental absence of skin is most frequently noted on the scalp as multiple or solitary, noninflammatory, well demarcated, oval or circular 1–2 cm ulcers. The majority occur at the vertex just lateral to the midline, but similar defects may also occur on the face, trunk, and limbs, where they are often symmetrical. The depth of the ulcer is variable; it may involve only the epidermis and upper dermis, or it may extend to the deep dermis, subcutaneous tissue, and, rarely, to the periosteum, skull, and dura. Occasionally the defects are covered by a tough membrane and simulate a bulla. In some instances, multiple family members have been afflicted; both autosomal recessive and dominant patterns of inheritance have been observed.

The major complications are massive hemorrhage, secondary local infection, and meningitis. Associated developmental defects are rare; they include cleft lip and palate, vascular malformations, congenital heart disease, limb anomalies, and defects of the central nervous system. Cutis aplasia of the scalp is commonly associated with trisomy 13 syndrome; congenital localized defects of skin, generalized recurrent blisters of skin and mucous membranes, and nail defects inherited as an autosomal dominant trait are known as Bart syndrome.

If the defect is small, recovery is uneventful with gradual epithelialization and formation of a hairless atrophic scar over a period of several mo (Fig 24–3). Small bony defects usually close spontaneously during the 1st yr of life. Large or multiple defects may require excision and primary closure, if feasible, or rotation of a flap to fill the defect. In some instances, punch graft transplants of hair have been successful.

Bitemporal aplasia cutis congenita, also called ectodermal dysplasia of the face, is a rare defect that has been observed mostly in Puerto Rican children. The children have a peculiar facies with widow's peak, frontal bossing, atrophic depressed defects of the temporal skin, upward slanting eyebrows, absence of or multiple rows of eyelashes, and a prominent chin with a median ridge. The pattern of inheritance is not established, but the defect may be an autosomal recessive trait in some instances.

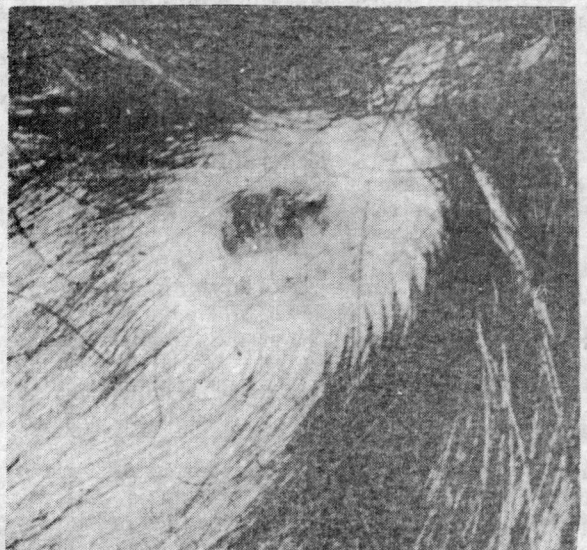

Figure 24–3 Healing solitary lesion of aplasia cutis.

Focal Dermal Hypoplasia (Goltz Syndrome). This is a rare congenital mesoectodermal disorder characterized by herniations of fat through thinned, partially deficient dermis that are responsible for multiple soft, tan-colored papillomas. Other types of skin changes include linear cribriform atrophic lesions, reticulated hypopigmentation and hyperpigmentation, telangiectasia, congenital absence of skin, angiofibromas presenting as verrucous excrescences, and papillomas of the lips, tongue, circumoral region, vulva, anus, and the inguinal, axillary and periumbilical areas. Partial alopecia, sweating disorders, and dystrophic nails are additional less common ectodermal anomalies.

The most frequent skeletal defects include syndactyly, clinodactyly and polydactyly, and scoliosis and other spinal anomalies. Ocular abnormalities are legion, but the most common are colobomas, strabismus, nystagmus, and microphthalmia. Small stature, dental defects, soft tissue anomalies, and peculiar dermatoglyphic patterns are also common. Mental deficiency occurs occasionally.

This familial disorder occurs principally in girls. It has been postulated that an X-linked dominant gene, lethal in males, or an autosomal dominant sex-limited mode of inheritance may account for the sex distribution. This disorder is often confused with incontinentia pigmenti since it shares a sex predilection for females and has some similar skin manifestations and mesodermal anomalies. The cutaneous lesions may also superficially resemble epidermal nevi. Treatment should be directed at amelioration of specific anomalies; genetic counseling is advisable.

Congenital Dyskeratosis (Zinsser-Engman-Cole Syndrome). This is a rare familial syndrome that affects only males and is probably inherited in an X-linked fashion. The onset occurs during childhood; nail dystrophy is the usual initial manifestation. The nails become ridged and atrophic, and there is considerable loss of the nail plate. The skin changes resemble a poikiloderma with reticulated gray-brown pigmentation, atrophy, and telangiectasia, especially on the neck, face, and chest. Hyperhidrosis and hyperkeratosis of the palms and soles, acrocyanosis, and occasional bullae on the hands and feet are also characteristic. Blepharitis, ectropion, and excessive tearing due to atresia of the lacrimal ducts are occasional manifestations. Vesiculobullous lesions may occur on the oral mucous membranes and result in ulceration, formation of epithelial tags, atrophic changes of the tongue, and premalignant oral leukokeratosis. Similar changes have been noted in the urethral and anal mucosa. The scalp hair, eyebrows, and lashes may become sparse. Hypoplastic anemia, at times of the Fanconi variety, is a common complication; immune deficiency has been noted.

The differential diagnosis includes the ectodermal dysplasias, pachyonychia congenita, poikilodermas, epidermolysis bullosa, keratoderma of the palms and soles, and lichen sclerosus et atrophicus. The abnormalities noted in skin biopsies are those of poikiloderma. Congenital dyskeratosis is progressive and may be complicated by squamous cell carcinoma of the mouth and/or anus as well as by the potentially lethal hematologic abnormalities.

Cutis Verticis Gyrata. This bizarre alteration of the scalp, which is more common in males, may be present at birth or during adolescence. The scalp is characterized by convoluted elevated folds, 1–2 cm in thickness, usually in the fronto-occipital axis. Unlike the lax skin of other disorders, the convolutions cannot be flattened by traction.

Primary cutis gyrata is often associated with mental retardation, cataracts, abnormal size and shape of the head, seizures, and spasticity. Secondary cutis gyrata may be due to chronic inflammatory diseases, tumors, nevi, acromegaly, and pachydermoperiostosis, a syndrome characterized by hypertrophy of the skin and bones.

24.6 ECTODERMAL DYSPLASIAS

The term ectodermal dysplasia has been used to designate a group of disorders characterized by a constellation of defects involving the teeth, skin, and appendageal structures, including hair, nails, and eccrine and sebaceous glands. In addition to alterations in various ectodermal structures, disturbances in tissue derived from other embryologic layers are not uncommon. Many of the following syndromes have overlapping features and are distinguished by the presence or absence of a single defect:

Hypohidrotic (Anhidrotic) Ectodermal Dysplasia. This syndrome is manifested by a triad of defects: hypohidrosis, anomalous dentition, and hypotrichosis. It is usually inherited as an X-linked recessive trait, with full expression only in males; however, in some families an autosomal recessive mode of inheritance permits full expression in both sexes.

Affected children unable to sweat may experience episodes of high fever when they are in a warm environment and be mistakenly considered to have fever of unknown origin. The typical facies is characterized by

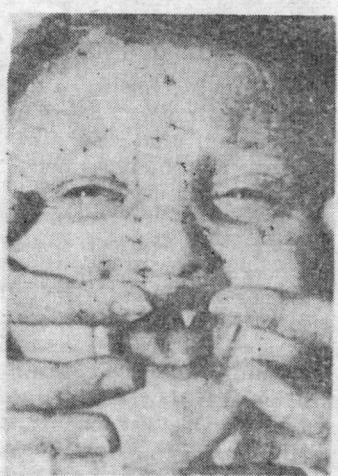

Figure 24–4 Hypohidrotic ectodermal dysplasia is characterized by pointed ears, wispy hair, periorbital hyperpigmentation, midfacial hypoplasia, and pegged teeth.

frontal bossing, malar hypoplasia, a flattened nasal bridge and recessed columella, thick, everted lips, wrinkled, hyperpigmented periorbital skin, and prominent, low set ears (Fig 24–4). The skin over the entire body is thin, dry, and hypopigmented, often with a prominent venous pattern. The hair is sparse, unruly, and lightly pigmented, and eyebrows and lashes are sparse or absent. Anodontia or hypodontia with widely spaced, peg-shaped teeth is a consistent feature (Fig 24–4). Less commonly, stenotic lacrimal puncta, corneal dysplasia, cataracts, gonadal abnormalities, and conductive hearing loss have been observed. The incidence of atopic diseases in these children is relatively high.

The sweating deficit is a reflection of hypoplasia or absence of the eccrine glands; this may be confirmed by skin biopsy. The palmar skin is an appropriate site for biopsy. Reduction or absence of sweating can be documented by pilocarpine iontophoresis or by topical application of o-phthalaldehyde to the palmar skin. Sweat pores are not visible in the palmar ridges in affected children and are decreased in number in carrier females. Diminished lacrimation and atrophic rhinitis are due to maldevelopment of the secretory glands. These glands are also deficient in the tracheobronchial mucosa, the esophagus, and the duodenum; recurrent pulmonary infections, hoarseness, and dysphonia are the clinical manifestations.

Children with hypohidrotic ectodermal dysplasia must be protected from exposure to high ambient temperatures. Early dental evaluation is necessary so that prostheses can be provided for cosmetic reasons and for adequate nutrition. The use of artificial tears will prevent damage to the cornea in patients with defective lacrimation. Alopecia may necessitate the wearing of a wig to improve the appearance.

Hidrotic Ectodermal Dysplasia (Clouston Type). Dystrophic, hypoplastic, or absent nails, sparse hair, and hyperkeratosis of the palms and soles are the salient features of this autosomal dominant disorder. The dentition is usually normal although small teeth and ram-

pant caries are occasionally associated. Sweating is always normal. Absence of eyebrows and lashes and hyperpigmentation over the knees, elbows, and knuckles have been noted in some affected individuals.

EEC Syndrome. Ectrodactyly, ectodermal dysplasia, and cleft lip and palate compose the EEC syndrome, which is probably inherited as an autosomal dominant trait of low penetrance and variable expressivity. The ectodermal dysplasia consists of a thin, dry, poorly pigmented integument, light-colored, wispy, sparse scalp hair and eyebrows, and absence of lashes. Decreased numbers of hair follicles and sebaceous glands have been demonstrated by biopsy.

Associated defects include anomalies of the hands and feet, nail hypoplasia, granulomatous perlèche frequently complicated by candidiasis, defective dentition, ocular abnormalities such as blepharophimosis, atretic or absent lacrimal puncta, strabismus, and abnormalities of the urinary tract.

Rapp-Hodgkin ectodermal dysplasia is inherited as an autosomal dominant trait and consists of hypohidrosis with reduced numbers of sweat pores, sparse, fine hair, dysplastic nails, oral clefts, variable growth deficiency, and hypospadias.

Robinson-type ectodermal dysplasia, an autosomal dominant disorder, combines sensorineural deafness, nail dystrophy, and peg-shaped teeth with partial anodontia.

24.7 VASCULAR LESIONS

Developmental vascular anomalies may occur as isolated defects or as part of a syndrome. Hemangiomas (vascular nevi) are the most common vascular defects and, with rare exception, occur sporadically and without a genetic basis. Cutaneous hemangiomas are superficial in approximately 65% of instances, subcutaneous in 15%, and mixed in about 20%. The terms *capillary* and *cavernous* distinguish the histologic patterns. Capillary hemangiomas are composed of dilated capillaries with or without endothelial proliferation, whereas cavernous hemangiomas consist of large, blood-filled cavities that have a compressed single-layered endothelial lining.

Nevus Flammeus (Port Wine Nevus, Flat Hemangioma). Port wine nevi are always present at birth; they consist of mature dilated capillaries and represent a permanent developmental defect. The lesions are macular, sharply circumscribed, pink to purple in color (or occasionally black in deeply pigmented infants), and tremendously varied in size, occasionally involving up to one half of the body surface (Fig 24–5). The posterior surface of the neck is a common site, and in this area the nevus is known as Unna nevus. The face is also a site of predilection; distribution is often unilateral, and the mucous membranes can be involved. With maturation, the port wine nevus may become slightly raised and pebbly in consistency; alternatively, the paler lesions may fade until almost imperceptible.

True nevus flammeus should be distinguished from the common salmon patch of the neonate, which is, in contrast, a relatively transient lesion. When the nevus

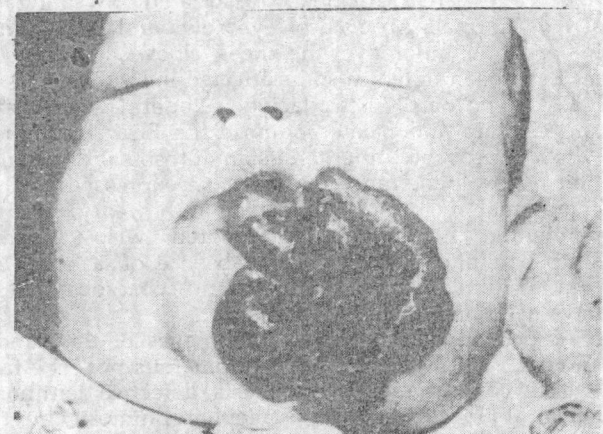

Figure 24-5 Large mixed capillary and cavernous hemangioma with central crusted ulcer.

is localized to the trigeminal area of the face, the diagnosis of *Sturge-Weber syndrome* (seizures, hemiparesis contralateral to the facial lesion, and ipsilateral intracranial calcification) must be considered. Associated glaucoma or other ocular defects may cause irreparable damage if not diagnosed and treated immediately. Rarely, Sturge-Weber syndrome occurs in association with a bilateral facial lesion or with a nevus flammeus elsewhere on the body surface. Nevus flammeus also occurs as a component of Klippel-Trenaunay-Weber syndrome and with moderate frequency in other syndromes, which include the Rubinstein-Taybi, Cobb (spinal arteriovenous malformation and nevus flammeus), Wiedemann-Beckwith, and trisomy 13 syndromes.

Several types of therapy including cryosurgery, excision and grafting, laser beam treatments, and tattooing have been utilized in the management of this defect. The disguise provided by makeup (e.g., Covermark), which is compounded to match the patient's normal facial skin, provides the most dependable means of therapy.

Capillary Hemangioma (Strawberry Nevus). So-called strawberry hemangiomas are bright red, protuberant, compressible, sharply demarcated lesions that may occur on any area of the body. Although sometimes present at birth, more often they appear within the 1st 2 mo heralded by an erythematous mark or by an area of pallor, which subsequently develops a fine telangiectatic pattern prior to the phase of expansion. Girls are affected more often than boys. Favored sites are the face, scalp, back, and anterior chest; lesions may be solitary or multiple.

Most strawberry hemangiomas undergo a phase of rapid expansion followed by a stationary period and finally by spontaneous involution. Regression may be anticipated when the lesion develops blanched or pale gray areas which are indicative of fibrosis. The course of a particular lesion is unpredictable; however, in general, approximately 60% of these lesions have involuted by age 5 yr, and 90-95% by age 9 yr. Spontaneous involution cannot be correlated with size or site

of involvement, but lip lesions seem to persist most often. Complications include ulceration, secondary infection, and, rarely, hemorrhage.

In the usual patient who has no serious complications or extensive overgrowth that results in tissue destruction and severe disfigurement, a course of expectant observation should be followed. Since almost all of these lesions resolve spontaneously, interference is rarely indicated and may, in fact, cause further harm. Parents require repeated reassurance and support. After spontaneous resolution, approximately 10% of patients are left with small cosmetic defects such as puckering or discoloration of skin. These defects can be eliminated or minimized by judicious plastic repair if it is desired.

In the rare instance that intervention is required, excision may be advisable; the extent of scarring anticipated should influence the final decision. Radiation can be hazardous and should be considered only in life-threatening situations, such as the Kasabach-Merritt syndrome. Application of solid carbon dioxide is rarely effective and may produce scarring. Elastic bandages may reduce the amount of tissue distortion resulting from rapid growth, but they are appropriate only in selected patients with large hemangiomas.

Cavernous Hemangiomas. These are more deeply situated than strawberry hemangiomas and, hence, appear more diffuse and ill-defined. The lesions are cystic, firm, or compressible, and the overlying skin may appear normal in color or have a bluish hue. Mixed hemangiomas consist of a cavernous component with a superimposed strawberry nevus (Fig 24-5).

Cavernous hemangiomas progress from a growth phase to a stationary phase to a period of involution. These lesions are as likely to regress as strawberry hemangiomas, and the outcome cannot be predicted from size or site of involvement. A course of expectant observation should be followed in most instances. If involvement of underlying structures is suspected, appropriate radiologic studies should be performed for elucidation. Rarely, these lesions impinge on vital structures, interfere with functions such as vision or feeding, cause grotesque disfigurement because of rapid growth, or are associated with life-threatening complications such as thrombocytopenia and hemorrhage (see Kasabach-Merritt syndrome below). If it becomes necessary to intervene, a course of prednisone (2-4 mg/kg/24 hr) has proved effective in some infants. Termination of growth and sometimes regression may be evident after approximately 4 wk of therapy. When a response is obtained the dosage should be decreased gradually. Alternate day corticosteroid therapy has also been administered with success.

Cavernous hemangiomas are associated with macrocephaly and pseudopapilledema in a rare autosomal dominant syndrome and occur with variable frequency in I cell disease and in Gorham disease (cavernous hemangiomas and disappearing bones).

Kasabach-Merritt syndrome is a combination of a rapidly enlarging hemangioma and thrombocytopenia; it is usually clinically evident during early infancy, but occasionally the onset is later. The hemangiomas are often present at birth and characteristically are solitary and large, although multiple and small hemangiomas have also been associated with thrombocytopenia. The vascular lesions are usually cutaneous and are only rarely located in viscera. The associated platelet defect may lead to precipitous hemorrhage accompanied by ecchymoses, petechiae, and a rapid increase in size of the hemangioma. Severe anemia may ensue. The platelet count is depressed, but the bone marrow contains increased numbers of normal or immature megakaryocytes. The thrombocytopenia has been attributed to sequestration or increased destruction of platelets within the hemangioma. Hypofibrinogenemia and decreased levels of consumable clotting factors are relatively common (Sec 14.60).

Disseminated Hemangiomatosis. This is a serious condition in which multiple hemangiomas are widely distributed cutaneously and internally; on the skin there are usually numerous small, red or purple papular hemangiomas, but infrequently they may be sparse or absent. The internal hemangiomas may involve any of the viscera; the liver, gastrointestinal tract, central nervous system, and lung are the more common sites. The disorder is often fatal because of high-output cardiac failure, obstruction of the respiratory tract, and/or compression of central neural tissue. In a few instances systemic corticosteroid therapy alone or in combination with surgery and/or irradiation has apparently been lifesaving. Rarely, there are myriads of cutaneous hemangiomas in the absence of visceral involvement; spontaneous regression of the lesions is a possibility in such instances.

Multiple hemangiomas may also occur in several rare syndromes such as macrocephaly combined with pseudopapilledema or lipomas.

Blue Rubber Bleb Nevus. This syndrome consists of multiple cavernous hemangiomas of the skin, mucous membranes, and gastrointestinal tract. Typical lesions are blue-purple in color and rubbery in consistency; they vary in size from a few mm to a few cm in diameter. At times they are painful or tender. The lesions, which are also rarely located in liver, spleen, and central nervous system in addition to the skin, do not involute spontaneously. Recurrent gastrointestinal hemorrhage may lead to severe anemia. Palliation by excision of involved bowel is the only remedial measure.

Maffucci Syndrome. The association of cavernous hemangiomas, phlebectasias, lymphangiomas, and lymphangiectasias with nodular echondromas in the metaphyseal or diaphyseal portion of long bones is known as the Maffucci syndrome. Onset occurs during childhood. Pigmentary changes reflecting diminution or excess of melanin have been associated.

Klippel-Trenaunay-Weber Syndrome. A macular vascular nevus (port-wine nevus) in combination with bony and soft tissue hypertrophy and venous varicosities constitutes the triad of defects of this nonheritable disorder. The anomaly may be confined to a single limb or involve more than one as well as portions of the trunk or face (Fig 24-6). Enlargement of the soft tissues may be gradual and may involve the entire extremity, a portion of it, or selected digits. In addition to venous varicosities, arteriovenous fistulas can develop, and bruits are audible in the affected part. This disorder can

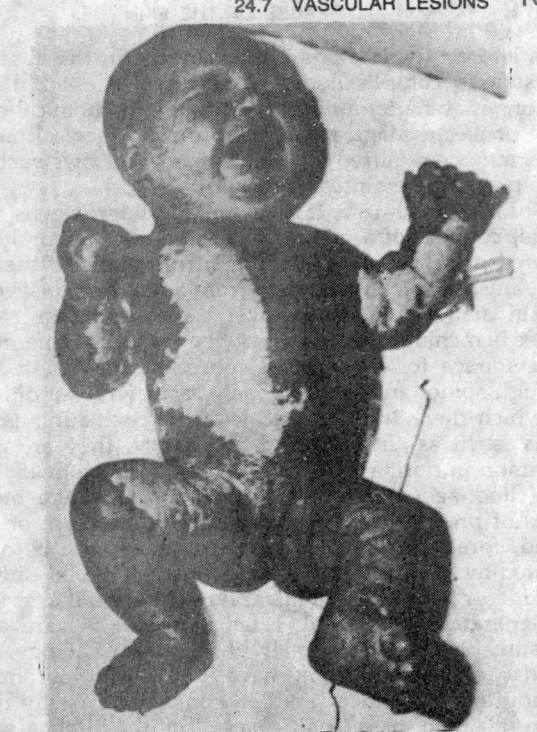

Figure 24–6 Widespread nevus flammeus in an infant with Klippel-Trenaunay-Weber syndrome.

be confused with Maffucci syndrome or, if the surface hemangioma is minimal, with Milroy disease. Thrombophlebitis, dislocations of joints, gangrene of the affected extremity, congestive heart failure, hematuria secondary to urinary tract hemangiomas, rectal bleeding from lesions of the gastrointestinal tract, pulmonary lesions, and malformations of the lymphatic vessels are infrequent complications. Arteriograms and venograms may delineate the extent of the anomaly, but surgical correction or palliation is often difficult. The indications for radiologic studies of viscera and bones are best determined by clinical evaluation.

Hereditary Hemorrhagic Telangiectasia. Also known as *Osler-Weber-Rendu disease*, this familial disorder is inherited as an autosomal dominant trait. Affected children may experience recurrent epistaxis prior to detection of the characteristic skin and mucous membrane lesions. The mucocutaneous lesions, which usually develop at puberty, are 1–4 mm, sharply demarcated, red to purple macules, papules, or spider-like projections, each of which is composed of a tightly woven mat of tortuous telangiectatic vessels. The nasal mucosa, lips, and tongue are usually involved; less commonly, cutaneous lesions occur on the face, ears, palms, and nail beds. Vascular ectasias may also arise in the conjunctivae, larynx, pharynx, gastrointestinal tract, bladder, vagina, bronchi, brain, and liver.

Massive hemorrhage is the most serious complication and may result in severe anemia. Bleeding may occur from the nose, mouth, gastrointestinal tract, genitourinary tract, and lungs. Persons with hereditary hemorrhagic telangiectasia have normal levels of clotting factors and an intact clotting mechanism. In the absence of serious complications, life span is normal. Local lesions may be temporarily ablated with chemical cautery or electrocoagulation. More drastic surgical measures may be required for lesions in critical sites such as the lung or gastrointestinal tract.

Spider Angiomas. The vascular spider (nevus araneus) consists of a central feeder artery with multiple dilated radiating vessels and a surrounding erythematous flush. Lesions may vary from a few mm to several cm in diameter. Pressure over the central vessel will cause blanching; pulsations may be visible in larger nevi as evidence for the arterial source of the lesion. Although spider angiomas are associated with conditions in which there are increased levels of circulating estrogens, such as cirrhosis and pregnancy, they are also common in normal children, occurring in up to 15% of preschool-age children and 45% of school-age ones. Sites of predilection in children are the dorsum of the hand, forearm, face, and ears. Angiomas can be obliterated by application of liquid nitrogen or solid carbon dioxide or by electrocoagulation of the central artery.

Generalized Essential Telangiectasia. A rare and presumably nevoid anomaly of unknown etiology, essential telangiectasia may have its onset in childhood or adulthood. Mild expression consists of patchy retiform telangiectases, particularly on the limbs, with occasional progression to involve large areas of the body surface. The condition must be distinguished from the secondary telangiectasia of connective tissue diseases, xeroderma pigmentosum, poikiloderma, and ataxia-telangiectasia. There is no treatment; however, patients can be reassured that their health will not be affected by the cutaneous disorder.

Unilateral Nevoid Telangiectasia. This unusual entity is characterized by the appearance of telangiectasia in a unilateral distribution, particularly in females at onset of menses or during pregnancy. The appearance of these lesions usually is coincident with elevated levels of circulating estrogens, whatever the cause. When initiated by pregnancy, the telangiectasia may fade or disappear postpartum.

Cutis Marmorata Telangiectatica Congenita (Congenital Generalized Phlebectasia). This benign vascular anomaly represents dilatation of superficial capillaries and veins and is apparent at birth. Involved areas of skin have a reticulated pattern of a red or purple hue which resembles physiologic cutis marmorata but is more pronounced and relatively unvarying (Fig 24–7, p. xxxiv). The lesions may be restricted to a single limb and a portion of the trunk or may be more widespread. The lesions become more pronounced during changes in environmental temperature, physical activity, or crying. In some instances, the underlying subcutaneous tissue is underdeveloped, and ulceration may occur within the reticulated bands. Flat capillary nevi may also be associated. Rarely, defective growth of bone and soft tissue and other congenital abnormalities may be associated. No specific therapy is indicated; the expected course is one of gradual steady improvement, with partial or complete resolution during adolescence.

Ataxia-Telangiectasia (Sec 6.32 and 21.17). This disorder, also known as Louis-Bar syndrome, is transmitted as an autosomal recessive trait. Onset during infancy or early childhood is heralded by a disturbance in gait with subsequent development of choreoathetosis, aberrant ocular movements, nystagmus, drooling, a peculiar stooped posture, and a dull facies. The ataxia is progressive, suggestive of a vestibular defect. Mental deficiency occurs in about half the children, and seizures may coexist. The characteristic telangiectasia develops at about 3 yr of age, first on the bulbar conjunctivae and later on the nasal bridge, malar areas, external ears, hard palate, upper anterior chest, and antecubital and popliteal fossae. Additional cutaneous stigmata include café-au-lait spots, premature graying of the hair, and sclerodermatous changes.

Angiokeratomas. Several forms of angiokeratomas have been described, but some of them do not occur during childhood or adolescence. *Angiokeratoma of Mibelli*, which is probably transmitted in an autosomal dominant pattern, is characterized by 1–8 mm red, purple, or black scaly, verrucous, occasionally crusted papules and nodules that appear on the dorsum of the fingers and toes and on the knees and the elbows. Less commonly, palms, soles, and ears may be affected. In many patients, onset has followed frostbite or chilblains. These nodules bleed freely following injury and may involute in response to trauma or may be effectively eradicated by cryotherapy or fulguration. *Angiokeratoma circumscriptum* is a rare solitary lesion that presents as a small plaque of papules, usually during adolescence. The lower limb is the site of predilection. Excision is the treatment of choice.

Angiokeratoma corporis diffusum (Fabry disease) (Sec 8.32), an inborn error of glycolipid metabolism, is an X-linked recessive disorder fully penetrant in males and of variable penetrance in carrier females. The skin lesions have their onset prior to puberty and occur in profusion over the genitalia, hips, buttocks, and thighs and in the umbilical and inguinal regions. They consist of 0.1–3.0 mm red to blue-black papules which may have a hyperkeratotic surface. Telangiectasias are seen in mucosa and in the conjunctivae. On light microscopy these angiokeratomas appear as blood-filled, dilated, endothelial-lined vascular spaces. Granular lipid deposits that stain with Sudan black and periodic acid–Schiff reagent are demonstrable in dermal macrophages, fibrocytes, and endothelial cells.

Additional clinical features include recurrent episodes of fever and agonizing limb pain, cyanosis and flushing of the acral areas, paresthesias of the hands and feet, corneal opacities detectable by slit-lamp examination, and hypohidrosis. Renal and cardiac failure secondary to involvement of those organs are the usual causes of death. The biochemical defect is a deficiency of the lysosomal enzyme α-galactosidase, which results in accumulation of ceramide trihexoside in the tissues and in massive excretion of it in the urine.

Similar cutaneous lesions have also been described in another lysosomal enzyme disorder, α-L-fucosidase deficiency (Sec 8.20).

Nevus Anemicus. Although nevus anemicus is present at birth, it may not be detectable until early childhood. The nevus consists of solitary or multiple, sharply delineated, pale macules; the lesions are most often on the trunk but may also appear on the neck or limbs. The lesions may simulate hypopigmented plaques of vitiligo, leukoderma, or nevoid pigmentary defects, but they can be readily distinguished by the response to firm stroking. Stroking will evoke an erythematous line and flare in hypopigmented nevi, but the skin of a nevus anemicus fails to redden. Although the cutaneous vasculature appears normal histologically, the blood vessels within the pale area do not respond to injection of vasodilators. It has been postulated that the persistent pallor may represent a sustained localized adrenergic vasoconstriction.

LYMPHANGIOMAS

See Sec 15.23.

24.8 CUTANEOUS NEVI

The term *nevus* often causes semantic confusion because the precise definition of the word has been blurred by common usage. In this section it is used to designate skin lesions that histologically are characterized by collections of well-differentiated cell types normally found in the skin. Not all nevi, however, are discussed in this section; the most notable exceptions are vascular nevi (hemangiomas), which are described in the preceding section.

Acquired Pigmented Nevi. Common pigmented nevi or moles are also termed *nevus cell nevi* to distinguish them from the pigmented lesions arising from mature melanocytes. Nevus cells are closely related to melanocytes and may be derived from a common stem cell (*nevoblast*). An alternative theory is that nevus cells are of dual origin with superficially located cells arising from melanocytes (*melanocytic nevus*) and that the cells in the deeper layers arise from Schwann cells (*neuroid nevus*).

Nevus cell nevi have a well-defined life history. Early lesions are usually junctional in type. Although some nevi remain junctional throughout life, most become compound or intradermal and change morphologically as well as histologically. Classification of nevi as junctional, compound, or dermal is determined by the exact location of the nevus cells in the skin.

Junctional nevi may be present at birth but most often appear in early childhood or during adolescence. The lesions appear in varying shades of brown; they are relatively small, discrete, flat, and variable in shape. They may appear anywhere on the body; those on the palms, soles, and genitalia usually remain junctional throughout life. The melanized nevus cells are cuboidal or epithelioid in configuration and occur in nests on the epidermal side of the basement membrane.

With maturation *compound and intradermal nevi* may become raised, dome-shaped, verrucous, or pedunculated. Slightly elevated lesions are usually compound, i.e., the nevus cells inhabit both the epidermis and the dermis. Distinctly elevated lesions are usually intradermal. The amount of melanin in a lesion may vary greatly, or there may be none.

Acquired pigmented nevi are benign lesions and need be removed only to improve appearance or to avoid chronic irritation and infection if they are subject to repeated trauma. A very small percentage of nevi undergo malignant transformation; there is no way, however, to determine which are potentially dangerous, and random excision is neither feasible nor rational. Suspicious changes such as rapid increase in size, development of satellite lesions, itching, or pain are indications for excision and histologic evaluation. Most of these changes will be due to irritation, infection, or maturation; color change and gradual increase in size and elevation normally occur during adolescence and should not be cause for concern. Nevertheless, if there is doubt about the benignity of a nevus, excision is a safe and simple outpatient procedure that may be justified to allay anxiety.

Congenital giant pigmented nevus (giant hairy nevus) (Fig 24–8) is not generally regarded as heritable though multiple cases within a few families have been recorded. Sites of predilection are the lower trunk, upper back and shoulders, chest, and proximal limbs. The lesions may be flat, elevated, verrucous, or nodular; they may appear in various shades of brown, blue, or black; and they may develop numerous coarse hairs or remain hairless and leathery in texture. The size may vary tremendously, and a large area of the body surface is often involved; numerous smaller pigmented nevi may be scattered elsewhere, and there may also be café-au-lait spots, lipomas, and fibromas. The lesions, if significantly disfiguring, may cause severe emotional problems.

The histologic features are usually those of an ordinary junctional, compound, or intradermal nevus and may differ in biopsy specimens obtained from several sites. Less commonly, the histologic pattern is that of a neural nevus, blue nevus, or spindle and epithelioid cell nevus.

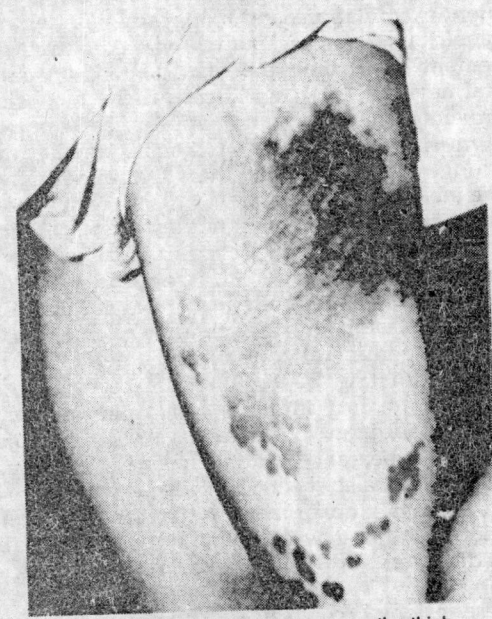

Figure 24–8   Giant hair nevus on the thigh.

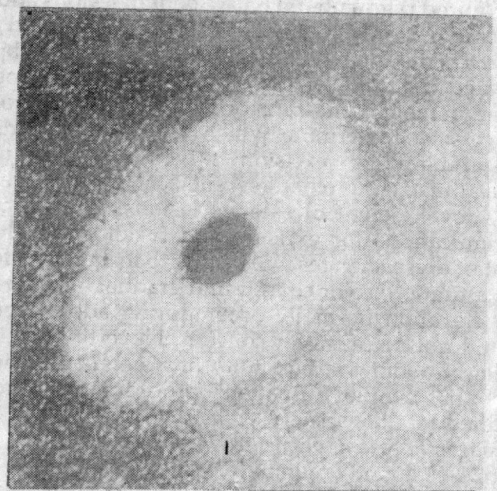

Figure 24–9 Well-developed halo nevus.

Giant congenital pigmented nevi are of special significance for 2 reasons: (1) the association of leptomeningeal melanocytosis and (2) the predisposition for development of malignant melanoma. Leptomeningeal involvement may cause hydrocephalus, seizures, retardation, and motor deficits and may result in melanoma. Malignancy can be identified by careful cytologic examination of the cerebrospinal fluid for melanin-containing cells. Most of these patients succumb despite palliative measures. The incidence of cutaneous malignant melanoma varies from 1–30% in reported series; the true incidence is unknown, but it is estimated to be approximately 10%. Early total excision and grafting is the treatment of choice. Extensive spotty involvement of peripheral skin with small nevi often limits the use of the patient's skin for grafting. If excision is delayed, frequent examinations and biopsy of enlarging nodules or suspicious areas are mandatory. Although there is agreement concerning the management of giant congenital nevi (larger than 2.0 cm), there is considerable controversy concerning the appropriate approach to medium-sized (1.5–2.0 cm) and small (smaller than 1.5 cm) congenital nevi. While there are no definitive data on the incidence of melanomas arising in these lesions, it is now the prevailing, but not universal, opinion that these nevi should be excised during infancy or childhood.

Halo Nevus (Leukoderma Acquisitum Centrifugum). Occasionally, the common pigmented nevus develops a peripheral zone of depigmentation up to 5 mm in width (Fig 24–9). In tissue biopsy there is a dense inflammatory infiltrate of lymphocytes and histiocytes in addition to the nevus cells. The pale halo reflects disappearance of the melanocytes. This phenomenon has also been associated with blue nevi, neurofibromas, and primary and secondary malignant melanoma. Patients with certain organ-specific autoimmune disorders and vitiligo have an increased incidence of halo nevi.

These lesions occur primarily in children and young adults; development of the halo may coincide with puberty or pregnancy. Frequently, several pigmented nevi will develop halos simultaneously. Subsequent disappearance of the central nevus is the usual outcome, and the depigmented area may or may not be repigmented. Excision and histopathologic examination of the lesion is indicated only when the nature of the central lesion is in question.

Spindle and epithelioid cell nevus (Spitz nevus) is commonly referred to as a *juvenile melanoma*; however, since it is always benign, the anxiety-provoking term melanoma should be avoided. Spindle and epithelioid cell nevi are pink to red, smooth, dome-shaped, firm, hairless nodules, which appear suddenly, grow rapidly, and are most often situated on the face, shoulder, or upper limb. They achieve a maximal size of about 1.5 cm. Visually similar lesions include pyogenic granuloma, hemangioma, nevus cell nevus, and basal cell carcinoma, but histologically these entities are distinguishable. The spindle and epithelioid cell nevus, a variant of the compound nevus, presents epidermal changes, vascular ectasias, and dermal and epidermal collections of pleomorphic, fusiform, and polygonal nevus cells, giant cells, and multinucleated giant cells. Although the histologic pattern may appear ominous to the inexperienced observer, the benign nature of the lesion permits conservative excision with little likelihood of reappearance or spread.

Zosteriform lentiginous nevus is a unilateral, linear, band-like lesion composed of multiple small brown or black macules on the face, trunk, or limbs. The lesions may be present at birth or develop during childhood; they represent collections of melanin-containing nevus cells at the tips of the dermal papillae.

Nevus spilus (speckled lentiginous nevus) is a flat, pigmented lesion with interspersed, darker brown, speckled macules. The lesions may be quite large and can resemble café-au-lait spots or junctional nevi. They are benign and need not be excised.

Nevus of Ota is a permanent, blue-gray, macular, facial stain caused by aggregates of melanocytes in the dermis. The macular nevi resemble mongolian spots in color and occur unilaterally in the areas supplied by the 1st and 2nd divisions of the trigeminal nerve. Although usually present at birth, they may arise during the 1st or 2nd decade of life. Patchy involvement of the sclera and other ocular tissues and of the nasal and buccal mucosa occurs in some patients. Nevus of Ota is more common in females and in oriental and black patients.

Nevus of Ito is localized to the shoulder, supraclavicular area, lateral neck, and upper arm. It can also be regarded as a persistent mongolian spot. The only available treatment is masking with cosmetics.

Blue nevi are solitary lesions that may be present at birth or develop during childhood, most frequently on the face, neck, arms, buttocks, hands, and feet; they are more common in females. Typical lesions are smooth, dome-shaped, hairless, blue or black nodules that rarely exceed 1 cm in diameter. Microscopically, they are characterized by groups of intensely pigmented, spindle-shaped melanocytes in the dermis and around appendicular structures.

Cellular blue nevi, which differ somewhat histologically, are larger and occur most frequently on the buttocks and in the sacrococcygeal area. They have a low but definite incidence of malignant transformation, and hence excision is the treatment of choice.

Achromic nevi (nevus depigmentosus) are usually present at birth; they are localized macular hypopigmented patches or streaks, often with bizarre, irregular borders. They resemble hypomelanosis of Ito clinically except that they are smaller, more localized, and often unilateral. They appear to represent a focal defect in melanin production.

Epidermal nevi may be visible at birth or may develop within the 1st months of years of life. They affect both sexes equally and only very rarely occur in more than 1 family member. Initially the epidermal nevus may appear as a discolored, slightly scaly patch that, with maturation, becomes more thickened, verrucous, and hyperpigmented. There are several morphologic types that include pigmented papillomas, often in a linear distribution; unilateral hyperkeratotic streaks (nevus unius lateris) involving a limb and perhaps a portion of the trunk; velvety hyperpigmented plaques; and feathered, whorled, or marbled hyperkeratotic lesions in localized plaques (Fig 24–10) or over extensive areas of the body. An inflammatory linear verrucous form which is markedly pruritic and may become eczematized is another variant.

The histologic pattern evolves as the lesion matures; but epidermal hyperplasia of some degree is apparent in all stages of development. One or another dermal appendage may predominate in a particular lesion. The diagnosis can be confirmed by biopsy. These nevi must be distinguished from lichen striatus, lymphangioma circumscriptum, shagreen patch of tuberous sclerosis, congenital hairy nevi, and nevus sebaceus (Jadassohn). Keratolytic agents such as vitamin A acid or salicylic acid may be moderately effective in reducing scaling and controlling pruritus, but definitive treatment requires full-thickness excision; recurrence is usual if more superficial removal is attempted. Alternatively, the nevus may be left intact.

With some frequency, epidermal nevi are associated with abnormalities of other organs; this combination has been designated as the *epidermal nevus syndrome*. The additional defects include localized soft tissue hy-

pertrophy, hemangiomas, pigmentary changes, skeletal anomalies of various sorts, ocular defects, and neurologic abnormalities such as developmental delay, seizures, motor deficits, and cerebrovascular malformations. Associated malignancies such as Wilms tumor and astrocytoma, although rare, are being reported with increasing frequency.

Nevus sebaceus (Jadassohn) is a relatively small, sharply demarcated, oval or linear, yellow-orange, elevated plaque that is usually devoid of hair and occurs on the head and neck of infants. Although characterized histologically by an abundance of sebaceous glands, all elements of the skin are represented. With maturity, the lesions become verrucous and studded with large rubbery nodules. The changing clinical appearance reflects the histologic pattern, which is characterized by a variable degree of hyperkeratosis, hyperplasia of the epidermis, malformed hair follicles, and often a profusion of sebaceous and apocrine glands. During adolescence or adulthood, these nevi are frequently complicated by secondary malignancies and benign adnexal tumors, most commonly basal cell carcinoma or syringocystadenoma papilliferum. The diagnosis can be established by biopsy; the treatment of choice is total excision prior to adolescence. Sebaceous nevi associated with central nervous system, skeletal, and ocular defects probably represent variants of the epidermal nevus syndrome.

Comedone nevi (nevus comedonicus) consist of linear plaques simulating comedones; they may be present at birth or appear during childhood. The horny plugs represent keratinous debris within dilated, malformed pilosebaceous follicles. The lesions are most often unilateral and may develop at any site. They appear to be a harmless developmental anomaly not associated with other congenital malformations. There is no effective treatment except full thickness excision; palliation of larger lesions may be achieved by regular applications of a vitamin A acid preparation.

Connective tissue nevus may occur as a solitary defect or may be a manifestation of an associated disorder. These nevi may occur at any site but are most common on the trunk. They are skin colored, ivory, or yellow plaques, 2–15 cm in diameter, composed of multiple tiny papules or grouped nodules which are frequently difficult to appreciate visually because of the subtle color changes. The plaques have a rubbery or cobblestone consistency on palpation. Biopsy findings are variable and include increased amounts of dermal elastic tissue or a predominance of thickened collagen bundles. Similar lesions occurring with tuberous sclerosis are called shagreen patches.

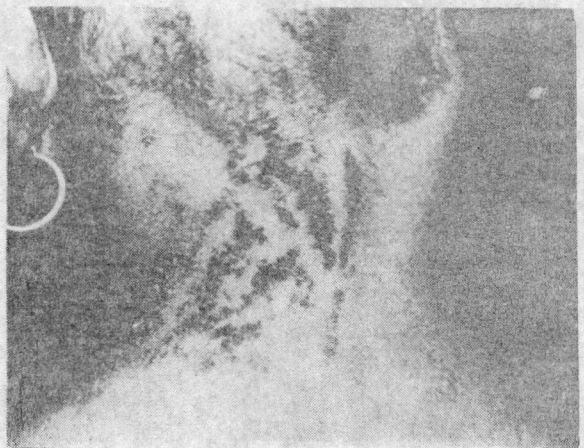

Figure 24–10 Verrucous streaky epidermal nevus on the neck.

24.9 DISORDERS OF PIGMENT

Alterations in skin color may be generalized or localized and may result from a variety of defects ranging from absence of melanocytes and defective melanization of melanosomes to overproduction of melanin and increased numbers of melanocytic cells. Some of these aberrations are induced by hormones (hyperpigmentation of Addison disease); others represent focal developmental defects (white spots of tuberous sclerosis); still others may be nonspecific and the result of cutaneous inflammation (postinflammatory hypopigmentation or hyperpigmentation).

24.10 HYPERPIGMENTED LESIONS

Ephelides or **freckles** are light or dark brown macules that occur in sun-exposed areas, such as the face, upper back, arms, and hands. They are induced by exposure to sun, particularly during the summer months, and may fade or disappear during the winter. They are more common in fairhaired individuals, appear first during the preschool years, and are probably genetically determined. Histologically, they are marked by increased melanin pigment in the epidermal basal layer with no increase in the number of melanocytes. Actually the freckle contains fewer but larger melanocytes than the surrounding paler skin.

Lentigines, often mistaken for freckles or pigmented nevi, are small (1–3 cm), round, dark brown macules that can appear anywhere on the body, are unrelated to sun exposure, and remain permanently. They differ from other hyperpigmented macules histologically in that they have elongated, club-shaped, epidermal rete ridges with increased numbers of melanocytes and dense epidermal deposits of melanin. The lesions are benign and, when few, may be viewed as a normal occurrence. Some juvenile lentigines may be precursors of nevus cell nevi (pigmented moles). The *multiple lentigines syndrome (leopard syndrome)* is an autosomal dominant entity consisting of a generalized distribution of lentigines in association with profound sensorineural deafness and other anomalies that include retarded growth, hypertelorism, cardiac defects such as pulmonic stenosis, and abnormalities of the genitalia.

The Peutz-Jeghers syndrome (see also Sec 6.32) is characterized by melanotic macules on the lips and mucous membranes and by polyposis of the small intestine. It is inherited as an autosomal dominant trait. Onset is noted during early childhood when pigmented macules appear on the lips, buccal mucosa, and gingivae and occasionally on the nose, hands, and feet. Polyposis usually involves the small intestine but may also occur in the stomach and large intestine. Episodic abdominal pain, melena, and intussusception are frequent complications. Although malignant degeneration has been reported, the risk of malignancy is small, and a normal life span is usual in affected individuals. Peutz-Jeghers syndrome must be differentiated from other syndromes associated with multiple lentigines, from ordinary freckling, and from Gardner syndrome and Cronkhite-Canada syndrome, a disorder characterized by gastrointestinal polyposis, alopecia, onychodystrophy, and skin pigmentation.

Café-au-lait spots are uniformly hyperpigmented, sharply demarcated, macular lesions, the hues of which vary depending on the normal depth of pigmentation of the individual: they are tan or light brown in white individuals and may be dark brown in black children. Café-au-lait spots vary tremendously in size and may be quite large, covering a significant portion of the trunk or limb. Generally, the borders are smooth, but some have an exceedingly irregular border. These lesions are characterized by increased numbers of melanocytes and melanin in the epidermis but lack the clubbed rete ridges that typify lentigines. One to 3 café-au-lait spots are common in normal children. They may be present at birth or develop during childhood.

Large, often unilateral café-au-lait spots with irregular borders are characteristic of patients with *McCune-Albright syndrome* (see Sec 18.5 and 23.15), a disorder that includes polyostotic bone dysplasia, precocious puberty, and multiple endocrine dysfunctions. The macular hyperpigmentation may be present at birth or develop late in childhood; if segmentally localized, it suggests an embryonic developmental defect.

Neurofibromatosis (von Recklinghausen disease). The café-au-lait spot is the most familiar cutaneous hallmark of this autosomal dominant neurocutaneous syndrome; it is present in up to 90% of affected children. Since these lesions occur in normal children and in association with certain other disorders, 6 lesions, each >1.5 cm in its largest diameter, are considered diagnostic of neurofibromatosis. The lesions may not be present at birth; therefore, a definitive diagnosis during the early years of life may not be possible unless other evidence of the disease is present. Axillary freckling (Crowe sign) and speckled hyperpigmentation on the upper chest, groin, and perineal skin are also common manifestations of neurofibromatosis.

Neurofibromas rarely develop before late childhood or adolescence and may occur anywhere, including the oral mucous membranes and tongue. These lesions are soft, skin-colored, sessile or pedunculated nodules (Fig 24–11) that may grow to considerable size and occasionally undergo sarcomatous change. Subcutaneous nodules may also occur along the course of nerve trunks.

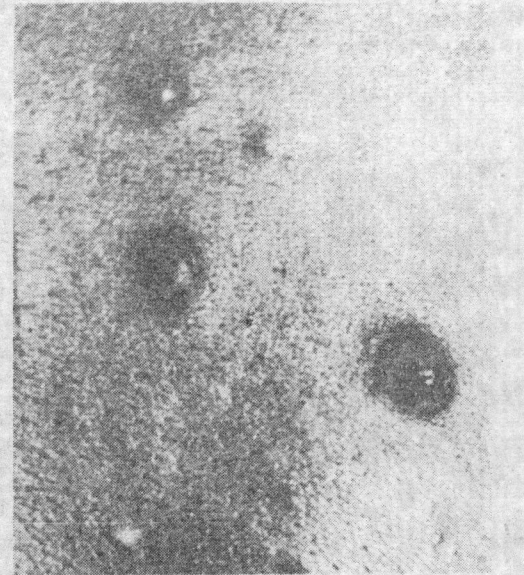

Figure 24–11 Multiple sessile neurofibromas.

Deforming plexiform neuromas are another cutaneous feature. The histologic changes of these lesions are diagnostic.

Neurofibromatosis also affects the musculoskeletal system, eye, gastrointestinal tract, vascular system, and central nervous system (Sec 21.15). There is also an increased incidence of pheochromocytomas and central nervous system neoplasms in these patients.

Incontinentia pigmenti (Bloch-Sulzberger disease) is a rare, heritable, multisystem disorder that is thought to be transmitted as an X-linked dominant trait, lethal in males. The paucity of affected males and the high frequency of spontaneous abortions in carrier females lend credence to this supposition.

The cutaneous manifestations can be divided into 3 phases, which are not present in all affected individuals: (1) the 1st phase is present at birth or is evident shortly thereafter and consists of erythematous, linear streaks and plaques of vesicles which are most pronounced on the limbs (Fig 24–12A). The lesions may be confused with those of herpes simplex, bullous impetigo, or mastocytosis, but the linear configuration is unique, and smears of vesicle fluid prepared with Wright stain demonstrate masses of eosinophils. Peripheral eosinophilia up to 65% is common but disappears after 4–5 mo of age. (2) The vesicular phase is followed by an intermediate verrucous stage, which may persist up to approximately 6 mo of age. These lesions eventually involute, at times leaving atrophic or depigmented areas. (3) The final pigmentary stage is variable in time of onset; it may overlap the earlier phases and even be evident at birth or, more commonly, within the 1st few wk of life; sites of involvement are not necessarily those of the preceding vesicular and warty lesions. The pigment is distributed in macular whorls, reticulated patches, flecks, splashes, and linear streaks and, once present, persists throughout childhood (Fig 24–12B).

Histologically, an early vesicular lesion is character-ized by epidermal edema and an interepidermal vesicle filled with eosinophils. Epidermal hyperplasia, hyperkeratosis, and papillomatosis are characteristic of the 2nd phase. The end-stage pigmentary lesion typically shows vacuolar degeneration of the epidermal basal cells and melanin in melanophages of the upper dermis. The name of the disease is derived from the latter histologic feature.

Although the skin lesions may constitute the only manifestation, approximately 80% of affected children have other defects. Alopecia, which may be scarring and patchy or diffuse, occurs in up to 40% of patients; dental anomalies, present in over half the children, consist of late dentition, conical teeth, and partial anodontia. Central nervous system manifestations, including developmental retardation, seizures, microcephaly, spasticity, and paralysis, are found in about a third of affected children; ocular anomalies resulting in severe impairment of vision or blindness occur in over 15% of children. Less common abnormalities include dystrophy of nails and skeletal defects. The choice of investigative studies and the plan of management depend on the occurrence of particular noncutaneous abnormalities since skin lesions are benign and often become less evident during adulthood. The high incidence of major anomalies associated with this disease is a strong reason for genetic counseling.

Postinflammatory Pigmentary Changes. Either hyperpigmentation or hypopigmentation can occur as a result of cutaneous inflammation. Alteration in pigmentation usually follows a severe inflammatory reaction but may result from mild dermatitis. Dark-skinned children are more likely to show these changes than fair-skinned ones. Although altered pigmentation may persist for weeks to months, patients can be reassured that these lesions are usually temporary. These changes must be distinguished from nevoid lesions and diseases manifested by pigmentary alterations such as vitiligo.

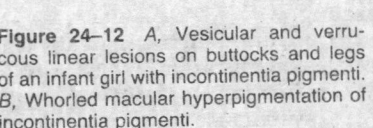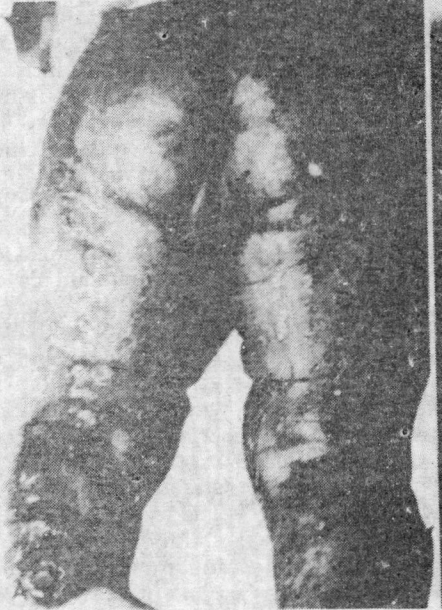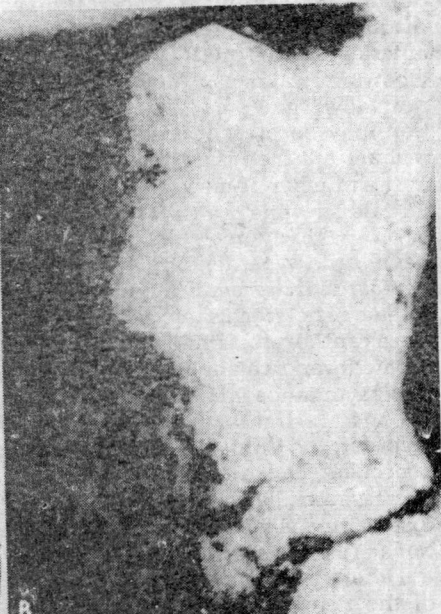

Figure 24–12 *A,* Vesicular and verrucous linear lesions on buttocks and legs of an infant girl with incontinentia pigmenti. *B,* Whorled macular hyperpigmentation of incontinentia pigmenti.

24.11 HYPOPIGMENTED LESIONS

Albinism. Several types of oculocutaneous albinism have been defined, each of which is inherited in an autosomal recessive fashion. The various forms of albinism may be distinguished by clinical manifestations, morphology of the melanosomes, and the hair bulb incubation test which determines whether tyrosinase is present. The well-defined types of oculocutaneous albinism are as follows:

Tyrosinase-negative albinism is characterized by lack of visible pigment in hair, skin, and eyes that results in photophobia, nystagmus, defective visual acuity, white hair, and white skin. The irides are blue-gray in oblique light and pink in reflected light.

Tyrosinase-positive albinism may resemble the above pattern except that the hair may be straw colored or light brown. With aging, the irides may accumulate some brown pigment and hence some improvement in visual acuity. The skin color is cream or pink.

In *tyrosinase-variable albinism* (yellow mutant) the infant has white hair, pink skin, and gray eyes at birth but develops bright yellow hair, light tanning of skin on sun exposure, and some pigment in the iris. Photophobia and nystagmus are present but mild.

The *Hermansky-Pudlak syndrome* is tyrosinase-negative albinism with platelet defects and a hemorrhagic diathesis.

The *Cross-McKusick-Breen* syndrome consists of tyrosinase-positive albinism with microphthalmia, retardation, spasticity, and athetosis.

Because of the absence of normal protection by adequate amounts of epidermal melanin, persons with albinism are predisposed to develop actinic keratoses and cutaneous carcinoma secondary to skin damage by ultraviolet light. Protection with a broad-spectrum sunscreen preparation (Sec 24.32) should be provided during exposure to sunlight.

Partial Albinism (Piebaldism). This autosomal dominant disorder is characterized by amelanotic plaques; they occur most frequently on the forehead, anterior scalp (producing a white forelock), thorax, elbows, and knees. Though sharply demarcated from normally pigmented skin, islands of normal pigmentation may be present within the amelanotic areas. The plaques are the result of localized absence or reduction in the number of melanocytes; the defect is permanent. Piebaldism must be differentiated from vitiligo, which is progressive and is not usually congenital; achromic nevus; and Waardenburg syndrome.

Waardenburg syndrome is characterized by a white forelock, heterochromic irides, broad nasal root, dystopia canthorum, congenital deafness, defects in fundus pigment, and cutaneous hypopigmentation; it is inherited as an autosomal dominant trait.

Chédiak-Higashi syndrome is an autosomal recessive disorder; the diffuse dilution in pigmentation results in a peculiar bluish hue of skin and hair, photophobia, decreased ocular pigmentation, and nystagmus. Hepatosplenomegaly and increased susceptibility to infections are also features (Sec 9.31 and 14.49).

Tuberous sclerosis (Sec 21.15), as is the case in many of the neurocutaneous syndromes, is a multisystem disorder affecting primarily tissues derived from ectoderm but also involving organs of mesodermal and endodermal origin. It is inherited as an autosomal dominant trait of variable penetrance and expressivity. In addition to multiple cutaneous stigmata, it is characterized by mental retardation, epilepsy, cerebral calcification, tuberous nodules of the cortex and subependymal area, retinal phakomas, rhabdomyomas of the heart, renal cysts and tumors, and cysts of bone and lung.

The most reliable early cutaneous sign is the *white leaf macule*, which is present but not always easily detectable at birth. At least 80% of patients have these lesions, which may be identified by examination with the Wood lamp. The white macules are sharply demarcated, pale, 0.5–3 cm lesions that often assume the shape of a mountain ash leaflet. Single or multiple lesions are most often found on the trunk (Fig 24–13A) but also occur on the face and limbs. Small, confetti-like, hypopigmented macules are also present in some instances. Hypopigmentation reflects inadequate melanization of the melanosomes of the pigment-generating cells.

Adenoma sebaceum is the most commonly recognized cutaneous marker of tuberous sclerosis; the lesions appear on the face during mid to late childhood or adolescence in approximately 80% of patients. These pink or flesh-colored papulonodular growths may erupt in profusion on the cheeks, nose, forehead, and chin but often spare the upper lip (Fig 24–13B). The term adenoma sebaceum is a misnomer since these growths are angiofibromas rather than tumors of the sebaceous glands. Similar fibromatous nodules may be scattered on the forehead, trunk, and limbs. Large, skin-colored, raised or flat collagenous plaques with an orange peel or cobblestone texture (*shagreen patches*) occur with some frequency in the lumbosacral area. At puberty, distinctive, clove-like, periungual fibromas (Fig 24–13C) appear on the fingers and toes of some children; gingival fibromas may also occur, unassociated with the administration of anticonvulsant medications. Café-au-lait spots occur with increased frequency but are not as numerous as in neurofibromatosis.

The cutaneous markers of this disorder are incontrovertible evidence for tuberous sclerosis and should be sought in any child with suggestive central nervous system manifestations. Appreciation of the significance of white leaf macules with seizures and retardation can provide a focus for the diagnostic evaluation and permit effective genetic counseling.

Hypomelanosis of Ito (incontinentia pigmenti achromians) is a congenital skin disorder, which affects children of both sexes, is frequently associated with defects in several organ systems, and should be regarded as a neurocutaneous syndrome. The role of genetic transmission has not been established. The skin lesions consist of bizarre, patterned, hypopigmented macules arranged in sharply demarcated whorls, streaks, and patches over the body surface (Fig 24–14). The hypopigmentation remains unchanged throughout childhood but is said to fade during adulthood. Neither inflammatory nor vesicular lesions precede the development of the pigmentary changes as in incontinentia

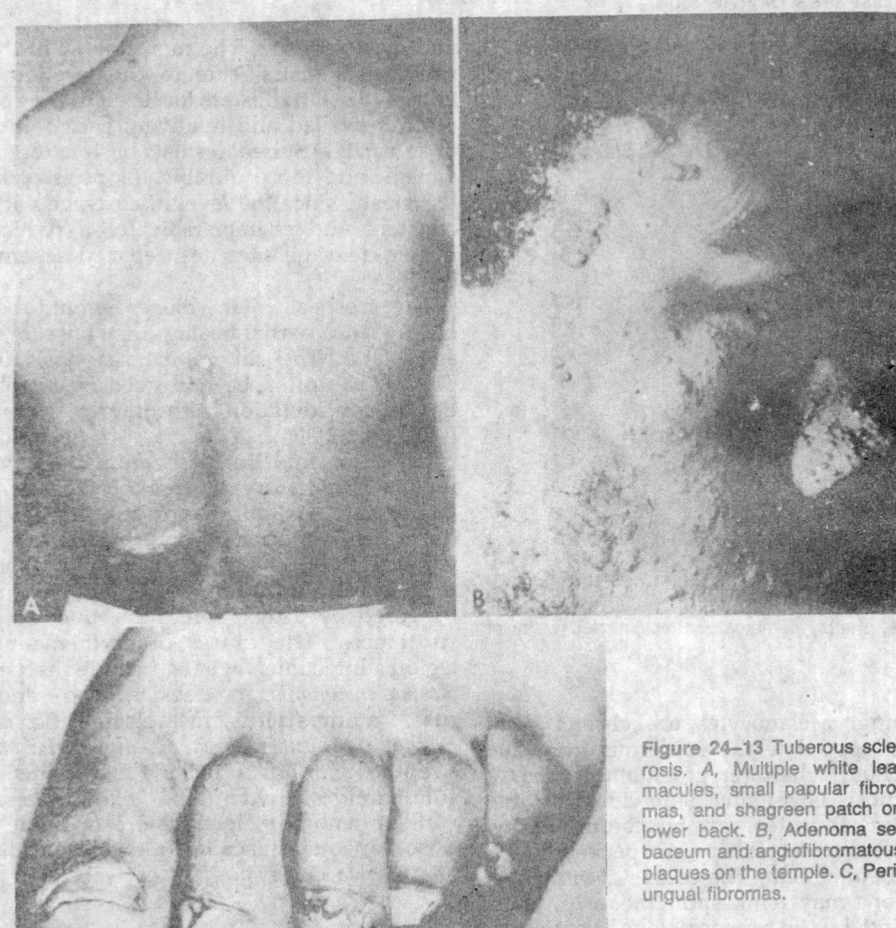

Figure 24–13 Tuberous sclerosis. *A*, Multiple white leaf macules, small papular fibromas, and shagreen patch on lower back. *B*, Adenoma sebaceum and angiofibromatous plaques on the temple. *C*, Periungual fibromas.

pigmenti. Histologic changes in affected skin are nonspecific and consist of decreased numbers of melanocytes detectable on DOPA stains and of incomplete melanization of melanosomes demonstrable by electron microscopy. Commonly associated abnormalities include seizures, developmental retardation, scoliosis, limb asymmetry, and ophthalmologic defects. Children with this pigmentary anomaly should have constant medical supervision.

Vitiligo is an acquired pigmentary defect that may occur at any age in persons of any skin color. The lesions are depigmented macules, sharply circumscribed, often with a hyperpigmented border; they vary in size and shape. Preferred sites are the face, particularly around the eyes or mouth (Fig 24–15), the genitalia, hands and feet, elbows, knees, and upper chest. When the scalp or brow is affected, the hair may also lose its pigment.

Although no clear-cut pattern of genetic transmission has been established, vitiligo is known to occur with increased frequency in some families. It is also more prevalent in patients with hyperthyroidism, adrenal insufficiency, pernicious anemia, and diabetes mellitus; some patients have detectable circulating antibodies to thyroid, adrenal, and other tissues.

The cause is unknown, but trauma appears to play a role in induction of the lesions. An autoimmune mechanism has been suggested; however, direct evidence to

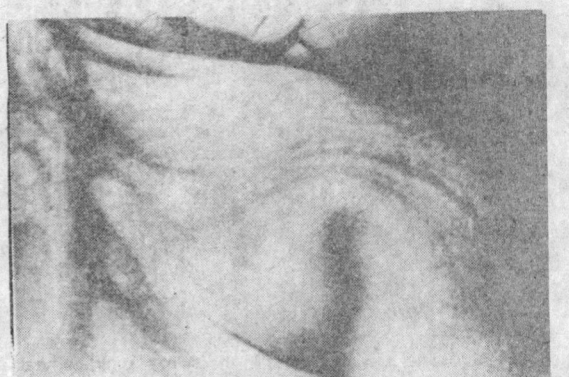

Figure 24–14 Marbled hypopigmented streaks of hypomelanosis of Ito.

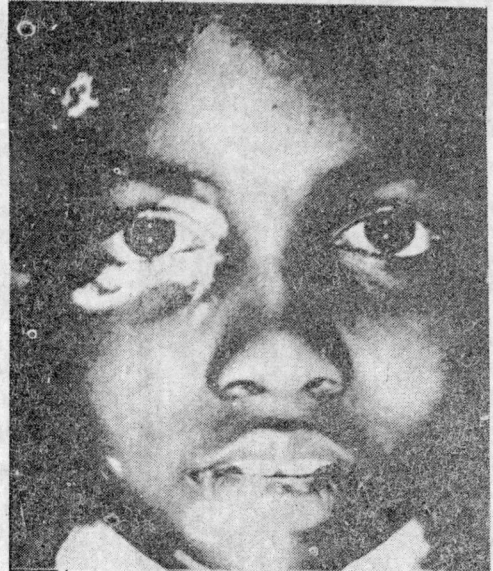

Figure 24–15 Multiple, sharply demarcated, depigmented areas of vitiligo.

support it is lacking. Melanocytes are absent from involved sites and repopulate the epidermis from the hair follicle epithelium when repigmentation occurs. Although the diagnosis is usually made clinically, the disappearance of melanocytes can be confirmed by DOPA stains or electron microscopy of specimens obtained from depigmented skin. The course of vitiligo is variable; some lesions may remit spontaneously while others are developing, but on rare occasions relentlessly progressive depigmentation occurs. Treatment is difficult and usually involves administration of oral or topical psoralen compounds (8-methoxypsoralen or Trisoralen) in conjunction with exposure to sunlight or an ultraviolet light source several times weekly. Repigmentation may be partial or complete, but many mo of therapy may be required and should be carefully monitored by physicians experienced in the use of photosensitizing drugs. Small lesions may be camouflaged by application of a specially prepared makeup (Covermark). Because of the absence of melanin, vitiliginous skin will burn readily on sun exposure and should be protected at all times by the use of an appropriate sunscreen agent.

24.12 VESICOBULLOUS DISORDERS

Many diseases are characterized by vesicobullous lesions; they vary considerably in etiology, in age of occurrence, and in the pattern of the lesion. Some of them (e.g., varicella) are discussed in other chapters; some are described in other sections of this chapter since the vesicobullous lesions represent only a transient stage of the disease (e.g., incontinentia pigmenti

and mastocytosis). The morphology of the blister often provides a visual clue to the location of the lesion within the skin. Blisters localized to the epidermal layers are thin-walled and relatively flaccid and tend to rupture easily. Subepidermal blisters are tense, thick-walled, and more durable. Biopsies of blisters can be diagnostic since the level of cleavage within the skin is constant and characteristic for a particular disorder. Blister cleavage sites are depicted schematically in Fig 24–16.

The freshest intact blister should be selected for biopsy since partial healing may obscure the true cleavage plane. The differential diagnosis of the disease process can often be narrowed by histologic examination in consideration with other diagnostic procedures (see Table 24–1).

Erythema multiforme is an acute, sometimes recurrent, inflammatory disease of the skin and mucous membranes. It occurs at any age, but it is more common during childhood and more frequent in males than in females. The pathogenesis is unknown, but the disorder is generally regarded as a hypersensitivity reaction triggered by drugs, infections, and exposure to toxic substances. The causes of erythema multiforme are legion. Infectious agents include herpesvirus, *Mycoplasma pneumoniae*, coxsackie-, echo-, and influenza viruses, mumps virus, histoplasma, *Coccidioides immitis*, *S. typhi*, *M. tuberculosis*, *C. diphtheriae*, and hemolytic streptococci. Drugs include penicillins, tetracyclines, sulfonamides, hydantoins, barbiturates, phenylbutazone, phenolphthalein, chlorpropamide, and aspirin. Miscellaneous causes include collagen diseases, malignancies, vaccines (polio, BCG, vaccinia), radiation ther-

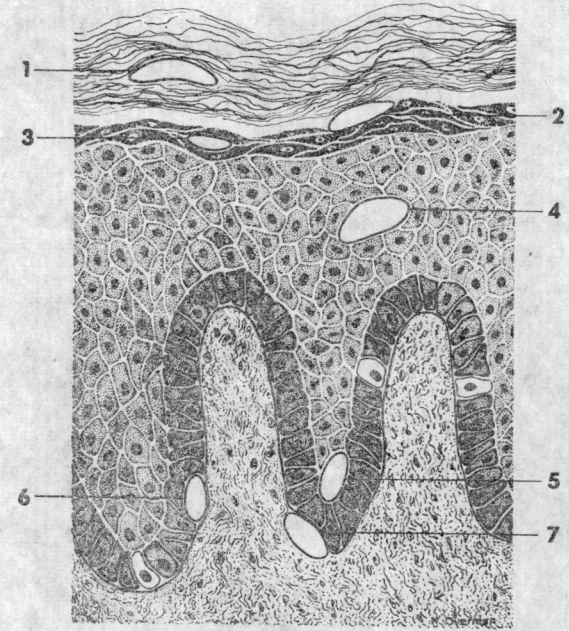

Figure 24–16 Blister cleavage sites in the skin: (1) intracorneal, (2) subcorneal, (3) granular layer, (4) intraepidermal, (5) suprabasal, (6) junctional (between basal cell membrane and basement membrane), and (7) subepidermal.

Table 24–1 SITES OF BLISTER FORMATION AND DIAGNOSTIC STUDIES FOR THE VESICOBULLOUS DISORDERS

DISORDER	BLISTER CLEAVAGE SITE	CUTANEOUS DIAGNOSTIC STUDIES
Acrodermatitis enteropathica	IE	—
Bullous impetigo	GL	Smear, culture
Bullous pemphigoid	SE (junctional)	Direct and indirect immunofluorescent studies
Candidiasis	SC	KOH preparation, culture
Chronic bullous dermatosis of childhood	SE	Direct immunofluorescent studies
Dermatitis herpetiformis	SE	Direct immunofluorescent studies
Dermatophytosis	IE	KOH preparation, culture
Dyshidrotic eczema	IE	—
Epidermolysis bullosa simplex	IE	—
hands and feet	IE	—
letalis	SE (junctional)	—
recessive dystrophic	SE	—
dominant dystrophic	SE	—
Epidermolytic hyperkeratosis	IE	—
Erythema multiforme	SE	—
Erythema toxicum	SC, IE	Smear for eosinophils
Incontinentia pigmenti	IE	Smear for eosinophils
Insect bites	SE	—
Mastocytosis	SE	Smear for mast cells
Miliaria crystallina	IC	—
Pachyonychia congenita	IE	—
Pemphigus foliaceus	GL	Direct and indirect immunofluorescent studies; Tzanck smear
Pemphigus vulgaris	SB	Direct and indirect immunofluorescent studies; Tzanck smear
Pseudomonas infection	IE, SE	Smear, culture
Scabies	IE	Scraping
Staphylococcal scalded skin syndrome	GL	Frozen section biopsy
Syphilis	SE	Darkfield preparation
Toxic epidermal necrolysis (Lyell)	SE	Frozen section biopsy
Transient neonatal pustular melanosis	SC, IE	Smear for cells
Viral blisters	IE	Tzanck smear for herpesvirus infections

GL, granular layer; IC, intracorneal; IE, intraepidermal; SB, suprabasal; SC, subcorneal; SE, subepidermal

apy, plant allergens, and 9-bromofluorine. There are several forms of the disease. In *erythema multiforme simplex,* the most common type, the diverse morphology of the skin lesions is the prominent manifestation. In *bullous erythema multiforme,* the mouth is often affected and the skin lesions are characteristically bullous. The *Stevens-Johnson syndrome* is a serious systemic disorder in which at least 2 mucous membranes as well as skin are involved (Sec 9.74).

The cutaneous lesions of erythema multiforme are usually symmetrical, appear in crops, and show a predilection for the extensor surfaces of the hands, arms, feet, legs, palms, and soles. The lesions vary considerably in extent and severity and may involve the entire body except the scalp. Lesions may be macular, papular, nodular, or urticarial. Vesicobullous lesions arise centrally within pre-existent lesions; urticarial lesions may fuse to form annular polycyclic plaques of bizarre outline. Intradermal hemorrhage is common and may be florid or may consist only of petechiae. Iris or target lesions, pathognomonic for erythema multiforme, are formed by urticarial lesions that have dusky centers and develop successively darker rings that may blister when the reaction is intense. Oral lesions occur in 25% of patients and consist of erythematous macules surmounted by vesicobullae that rapidly form painful necrotic ulcers, often with a pseudomembranous surface.

Skin lesions appear in crops for up to 3 wk and heal with hypo- or hyperpigmentation but without scarring. Pruritus is minimal to absent. The differential diagnosis includes bullous pemphigoid, pemphigus, urticaria, viral infections, Reiter disease, Behçet disease, allergic vasculitis, and periarteritis nodosa.

The diagnosis can usually be made from the clinical features, particularly when iris lesions are apparent. When the diagnosis is uncertain, a skin biopsy should be performed. The histologic changes vary with the severity of the lesions. There is intraepidermal edema with vesicular alteration in the epidermal basal layer and necrosis of individual epidermal cells. The dermis is edematous, with lymphocytic infiltration around the vessels and at the dermal-epidermal junction. When the changes are severe, red blood cells may be extravasated into the dermis, subepidermal bullae may form, and the epidermis may become necrotic. Eosinophils and neutrophils are sparse.

Treatment is local and symptomatic. Oral lesions should be cleaned with mouthwashes and glycerin swabs. Topical anesthetics (Benadryl, dyclonine, and viscous Xylocaine) may provide relief from pain, particularly when applied prior to eating. Denuded skin lesions can be cleansed with a Betadine-water solution. Patients with recurrent erythema multiforme may experience rapid relief following early systemic therapy with a corticosteroid or occasionally with a topical steroid preparation.

Toxic epidermal necrolysis (Lyell disease) appears to

be a hypersensitivity phenomenon triggered by many of the same factors responsible for erythema multiforme: drugs, infections, vaccination, radiotherapy, and malignancies. It may represent the most devastating form of erythema multiforme; widespread epidermal necrosis rapidly follows blister formation at the dermal-epidermal junction.

The prodrome consists of fever, malaise, and localized skin tenderness and erythema. Flaccid bullae develop, desquamate rapidly, and peel in large sheets. Nikolsky sign (denudation of the skin with gentle pressure) is positive but only in the areas of blistering. Conjunctivitis and oral lesions are common and may mimic those of Stevens-Johnson syndrome. The course may be relentlessly progressive, complicated by severe dehydration, electrolyte imbalance, shock, and secondary localized infection and septicemia.

The differential diagnosis includes the staphylococcal scalded skin syndrome, in which the blister cleavage plane is intraepidermal; pemphigus; and the Stevens-Johnson syndrome. Appreciation of the specific etiologic factor is crucial, particularly when the disorder is drug-induced. Management is similar to that for severe burns: strict isolation, appropriately calculated fluid and electrolyte therapy, and daily cultures. Systemic antibiotic therapy is indicated when secondary infection is evident or suspected. Skin care consists of cleansing with isotonic saline or Betadine and applications of Silvadene. The case fatality rate is approximately 25%.

Epidermolysis Bullosa. The diseases categorized under this general term are a heterogeneous group of congenital, hereditary blistering disorders in which the lesions are produced by mechanical trauma. They differ in severity and prognosis, clinical and histologic features, and inheritance patterns. In each, the basic defect is unknown, although increased skin content of collagenase is present in the more severe forms. Five major types are readily distinguishable; 2 of these are scarring disorders. Since mechanical trauma and high environmental temperatures are provocative factors in all of the types, affected children should be protected to the extent warranted by the severity of their disease. Parents usually become quite knowledgeable about what their child will tolerate. Metal closures on clothing, tape of any kind, rough or tight clothing, and sharp-edged toys should be avoided. Hot baths may also initiate new lesions. Large blisters may be drained by puncturing, but the blister tops should be left intact to protect the underlying skin. Management must be individualized to permit maximum safe participation in childhood activities. Genetic counseling should be offered to families of affected children; therefore, early diagnosis of the type of the disease is critical.

Epidermolysis bullosa simplex is a nonscarring, autosomal dominant disorder. Blisters can usually be induced at birth or during the neonatal period. The bullae are intraepidermal and result from disintegration of the basal cells. These lesions may be mistaken for cutis aplasia. Sites of predilection are the hands, feet, elbows, knees, legs, and scalp; intraoral lesions are minimal, and nails may become dystrophic and may be shed but usually regrow. The infants are usually vigorous. Secondary infection is the only serious compli-

cation. The propensity to blister decreases with age, and the long-term prognosis is good.

Epidermolysis bullosa of hands and feet (Weber-Cockayne type) is also an autosomal dominant disorder. This nonscarring variant begins some time after the 1st yr of life. Bullae are usually restricted to the hands and feet, including the palms and soles; rarely, they occur elsewhere. The intraepidermal blisters involve the cells of the suprabasal and granular layers, which may be dyskeratotic with clumped tonofilaments. The disorder is only mildly incapacitating.

Epidermolysis bullosa letalis, although basically a nonscarring condition, is life-threatening, and the complications are such that serious morbidity and disfigurement can be predicted. The infant is usually blistered at birth or develops lesions during the neonatal period, particularly on the perioral area, scalp, legs, diaper area, and thorax. Large, moist, erosive plaques may provide a portal of entry for bacteria, and septicemia is a frequent cause of death. Healing is delayed, and vegetating granulomas may persist for a long time. Mucous membrane lesions are mild. Defective dentition with early loss of teeth due to rampant caries is characteristic. In contrast to other variants of epidermolysis bullosa, sparing of the hands and feet is striking, with the exception of the nail plates; these are dystrophic or permanently lost. Growth retardation and recalcitrant anemia are almost invariable. A subepidermal blister is found on light microscopic examination, and electron microscopy demonstrates a cleavage plane between the plasma membranes of the basal cells and the basement membrane.

Therapy is supportive; an adequate caloric diet and iron should be provided. Infections should be treated promptly with antibiotics. Transfusions of packed red blood cells may be required at times as supplementary therapy. In addition to infection, cachexia and circulatory failure are common causes of death. Occasionally in mildly affected individuals, the disorder is compatible with a restricted but relatively normal life.

Dominant dystrophic epidermolysis bullosa appears to occur sporadically in many instances, although an autosomal dominant mode of transmission has been documented in several generations of some families. Blisters may be present at birth and are often limited to the hands, feet, and sacrum. The lesions heal promptly with the formation of soft, wrinkled scars, milia, and alterations in pigmentation. The general health is unimpaired, and in many instances the blistering process is rather mild, causing little restriction of activity and unimpaired growth and development. Mucous membrane involvement tends to be minimal, but nail loss is common. The blister is subepidermal with separation beneath the basement membrane.

Recessive dystrophic epidermolysis bullosa is probably the most incapacitating form of the disorder. Extensive erosions and blister formation may occur at birth and seriously impede the care and feeding of the infant. Mucous membrane lesions are common and may cause severe nutritional deprivation, even in older children, whose growth may be retarded. During childhood, esophageal erosions and strictures, scarring of the buccal mucosa, flexion contractures of joints secondary to

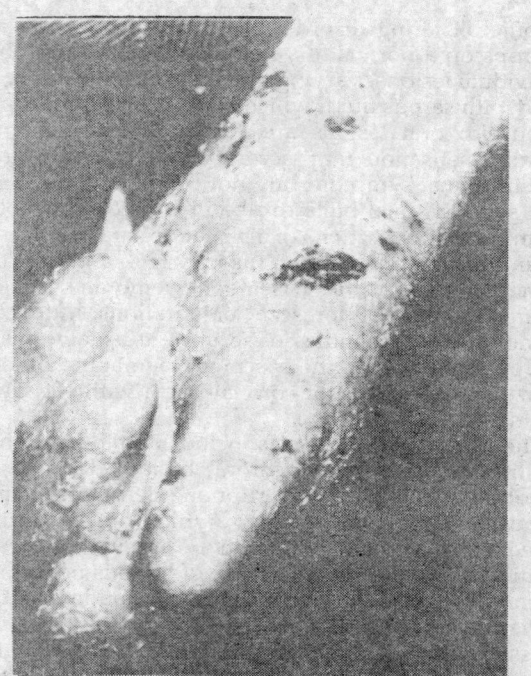

Figure 24–17 Mitten-hand deformity of recessive dystrophic epidermolysis bullosa.

scarring of the integument, and the development of the characteristic mitten deformity of the hands and feet due to digital fusion (Fig 24–17) significantly limit the quality of life. The subepidermal bullae are located beneath the basement membrane, and absence of anchoring fibrils can be confirmed by electron microscopy.

Although the skin becomes less sensitive to trauma with aging, the progressive and permanent deformities complicate management tremendously, and the overall prognosis is poor. Systemic corticosteroid therapy may reduce esophageal scarring in some patients who, nevertheless, may require a semiliquid diet. In infants, severe oropharyngeal involvement may necessitate the use of special feeding devices. Continuous iron therapy for anemia, intermittent antibiotic therapy for secondary infections, and periodic plastic procedures for release of digits may reduce morbidity.

Acrodermatitis enteropathica is a rare, autosomal recessive disorder of zinc deficiency that appears to be somewhat more common in girls. The onset is insidious, occurring usually during the 1st yr of life. Initial symptoms often are noted following weaning from breast milk to cow milk. The cutaneous eruption consists of vesicobullous and eczematous skin lesions symmetrically distributed in the perioral, acral, and perineal areas as well as on the cheeks, knees, and elbows. Initially these lesions are intensely erythematous and erosive, but with chronicity they become dry, hyperkeratotic, and psoriasiform in appearance (Fig 24–18A and B). The hair often has a peculiar reddish tint, and alopecia of some degree is characteristic. Ocular manifestations include photophobia, conjunctivitis, blepharitis, and corneal dystrophy, which is detectable by slit-

lamp examination. Associated manifestations include chronic diarrhea, stomatitis, glossitis, paronychia, nail dystrophy, growth retardation, personality changes, intercurrent bacterial infections, and superinfection with *Candida albicans*. The course without treatment is chronic and intermittent but often relentlessly progressive, terminating in severe marasmus and death. When the disease is less severe, only growth retardation and delayed development may be apparent.

The diagnosis is established by the constellation of clinical findings and low concentrations of plasma zinc and alkaline phosphatase, a zinc-dependent enzyme. Histopathologic changes in the skin are nonspecific, as they are in the gastrointestinal tract, except that a cytoplasmic inclusion body has been noted in the Paneth cells. The basic metabolic defect in the disease appears to relate to intestinal absorption of zinc. A possible deficiency in amount or function of a zinc-binding ligand has been suggested as a pathogenetic factor.

For many yr, acrodermatitis enteropathica was treated empirically, but often successfully, with diiodohydroxyquin and breast milk; the possibility, however, of serious untoward effects of the drug, particularly optic atrophy, was a hazard. Oral therapy with zinc compounds has now replaced diiodohydroxyquin as the treatment of choice. Optimal doses are in the range of 50 mg of zinc sulfate, acetate, or gluconate daily for infants and up to 150 mg daily for children; plasma zinc levels, however, should be monitored to individualize the dosage. Zinc therapy rapidly abolishes the manifestations of the disease. A few patients with

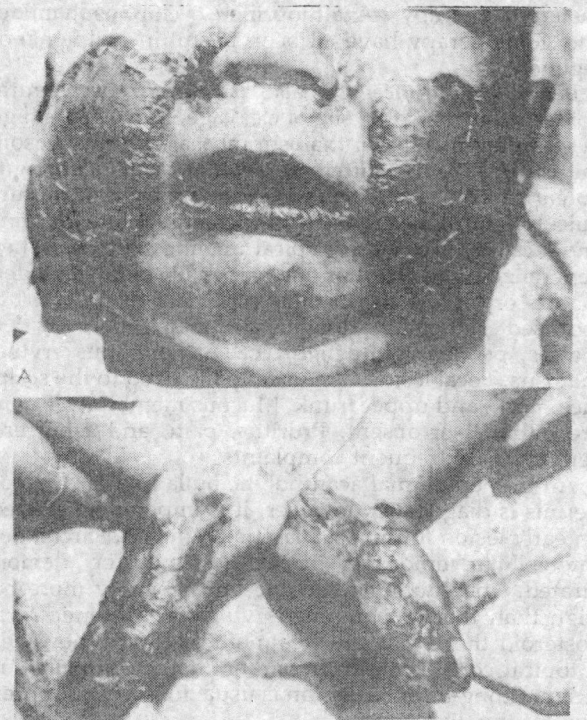

Figure 24–18 *A,* Psoriasiform facial lesions of acrodermatitis enteropathica. *B,* Similar lesions on the feet with secondary nail dystrophy.

acrodermatitis enteropathica but without hypozincemia have also been shown to recover on pharmacologic doses of zinc. In addition, a syndrome resembling acrodermatitis enteropathica has been observed in individuals of all ages receiving total parenteral nutrition without supplemental zinc.

Pemphigus occurs during childhood as pemphigus vulgaris or as pemphigus foliaceus.

Pemphigus vulgaris is usually first manifested as painful oral ulcers, which may be the only evidence of the disease for weeks or months. Subsequently, large, flaccid bullae emerge on nonerythematous skin, most commonly on the head and trunk. The lesions rupture and enlarge peripherally, producing painful, raw, denuded areas that have little tendency to heal. Malodorous verrucous and granulomatous lesions may develop at the sites of ruptured bullae. Nikolsky sign, the avulsion of epidermis on gentle pressure, is always positive.

Histologically, the lesion is a suprabasal (intraepidermal) blister containing loose, acantholytic epidermal cells. IgG antibody to epidermal intercellular substance produces a characteristic pattern on direct immunofluorescent preparations. Circulating serum antibody to the epidermal intercellular substance usually correlates with the clinical course; hence serial determinations may have predictive value.

The disease can be confused with erythema multiforme, bullous pemphigoid, Stevens-Johnson syndrome, and toxic epidermal necrolysis. Since the course may be rapidly progressive leading to debility, malnutrition, and death, prompt diagnosis is essential. The disease is best controlled initially with systemic corticosteroid therapy. Azathioprine, cyclophosphamide, and gold therapy have all been useful in maintenance regimens.

Pemphigus foliaceus is also characterized by intraepidermal blisters; the site of cleavage, however, is high in the epidermis rather than suprabasal. For this reason, the clinical picture differs somewhat from pemphigus vulgaris in that the blisters are very superficial, rupture quickly, and may be missed on examination. Crusting and scaling are more typical manifestations. When generalized, the eruption may resemble exfoliative dermatitis or any of the chronic blistering disorders, but localized erythematous plaques simulate seborrheic dermatitis, psoriasis, impetigo, eczema, or lupus erythematosus. Focal lesions are usually localized to the scalp, face, neck, and upper trunk. Mucous membrane lesions are minimal or absent. Pruritus, pain, and a burning sensation are frequent complaints.

An intraepidermal acantholytic bulla high in the epidermis is diagnostic; however, it is imperative to select an early lesion for biopsy. Tissue-bound and circulating intercellular epidermal antibodies may be demonstrated. The course is variable but generally more benign than that of pemphigus vulgaris. Systemic corticosteroid therapy is the treatment of choice; however, a topical corticosteroid preparation is occasionally sufficient. Long-term remission is usual following suppression of the disease.

Bullous pemphigoid rarely occurs in children, but it must be considered in the differential diagnosis of any chronic blistering disorder. Typically the blisters arise in crops on a normal, erythematous, or urticarial base. Individual lesions, varying greatly in size, are tense and filled with serous fluid, which may become hemorrhagic or turbid; oral lesions are common. Pruritus and a burning sensation may accompany the eruption, but constitutional symptoms are not prominent.

A subepidermal bulla can be identified by histologic examination. In sections of a blister or paralesional skin, a band of immunoglobulin (usually IgG) and C3 can be demonstrated in the basement membrane zone by means of immunofluorescent preparations. Indirect immunofluorescent studies of serum are usually positive for IgG antibodies to the basement membrane zone; the titers, however, do not correlate well with the clinical course.

The differential diagnosis includes bullous erythema multiforme, pemphigus, chronic bullous dermatosis of childhood, bullous drug eruption, dermatitis herpetiformis, and bullous impetigo, which can be differentiated by histologic examination, immunofluorescent studies, and cultures. The cause of bullous pemphigoid is unknown, and the course is chronic and intermittent. Nevertheless, the disease can be successfully suppressed with systemic corticosteroid therapy alone or in combination with azathioprine, and ultimately it usually remits permanently. Local skin care consists of compresses and a drying lotion.

Dermatitis herpetiformis is characterized by grouped, small, tense, erythematous, pruritic papules and vesicles. The eruption tends to be symmetrically distributed; the sites of predilection are the knees, elbows, shoulders, buttocks, and scalp; mucous membranes are usually spared. When pruritus is severe, excoriations may be the only visible sign.

The cause is unknown; however, an association with celiac sprue (gluten-sensitive enteropathy) is found with some frequency (Sec 11.45). Subepidermal blisters are found on skin biopsy, and IgA can be detected in the dermal papillae of paralesional skin by direct immunofluorescent studies. The frequent demonstration of circulating immune complexes and autoimmune antibodies in these patients as well as the association with certain HLA types suggests an immunodeficiency mechanism.

Dermatitis herpetiformis may mimic other chronic blistering diseases and may also resemble scabies, papular urticaria, insect bites, contact dermatitis, and papular eczema. The most effective treatment is administration of oral sulfapyridine or dapsone. These drugs afford immediate relief from the intense pruritus, but must be used with caution because of the hazards of serious side effects. Local antipruritic measures may also be useful. The enteropathy will respond to a gluten-free diet, but skin lesions respond extremely slowly to dietary therapy.

Chronic bullous dermatosis of childhood (linear IgA dermatosis) is a disease of the 1st decade of life with a peak incidence during the preschool years. The eruption consists of multiple large, tense bullae filled with clear or hemorrhagic fluid that emerge from a normal or erythematous base. Areas of predilection are the trunk, genitalia, and legs, as well as the face, scalp,

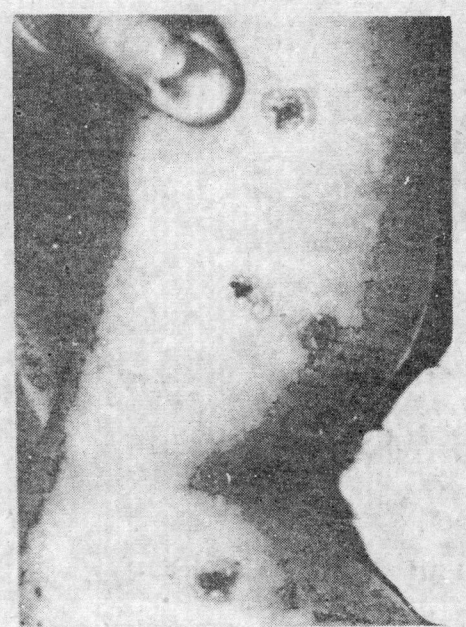

Figure 24—19 Rosette-like blisters around a central crust typical of chronic bullous dermatosis of childhood.

and dorsum of the feet. In the smaller lesions sausage-shaped bullae may be arranged in an annular or rosette-like fashion around a central crust (Fig 24–19). Erythematous plaques with gyrate margins bordered by intact bullae may develop over larger areas. Pruritus may be absent or very intense.

The cause of the eruption is unknown. Histologic examination discloses a subepidermal bulla infiltrated with a mixture of inflammatory cells. Direct immunofluorescent studies demonstrate linear deposition of IgA and sometimes C3 at the dermal-epidermal junction. Indirect immunofluorescent studies are sometimes positive for circulating antibodies. These studies serve to differentiate this eruption from pemphigus, bullous pemphigoid, dermatitis herpetiformis, and erythema multiforme, with which it may be confused. Gram stain and culture will exclude the diagnosis of bullous impetigo. The lack of bullous formation in response to trauma differentiates epidermolysis bullosa.

Many children respond favorably to oral sulfapyridine or dapsone. During therapy with sulfapyridine, attention should be paid to urinary output and alkalinization of the urine to avoid crystal formation and deposition within the renal parenchyma. Hematologic and biochemical studies must be obtained at regular intervals during treatment with either drug to avoid serious side effects. Children who do not respond to either of these drugs may benefit from oral therapy with a corticosteroid. The usual course is 2–4 yr; there are no long-term sequelae.

24.13   ECZEMA

Eczema is a generic term used to designate a particular type of reaction pattern in the skin. Acute eczematous lesions are characterized by erythema, weeping, oozing, and the formation of microvesicles within the epidermis. Chronic lesions are generally thickened, dry, and scaly with coarse skin markings (lichenification) and altered pigmentation. Many types of eczema occur in children, of which the most common is atopic dermatitis (Sec 9.50); however, seborrheic dermatitis, allergic and primary irritant contact dermatitis, nummular eczema, and dyshidrosis are also relatively common childhood eczemas. Pyoderma may become eczematized from scratching as may insect bites, papular urticaria, dermatophytosis, and a variety of dermatoses. Once the diagnosis of eczema has been established, it is important to classify the eruption more specifically for proper management. Pertinent historical data will often provide the clue. In some instances the subsequent course and character of the eruption permit classification. Histologic changes are relatively nonspecific, but all types of eczematous dermatitis are characterized by intraepidermal edema known as spongiosis.

Contact dermatitis can be subdivided into primary irritant eczema, resulting from nonspecific injury to the skin, and allergic contact dermatitis, in which the mechanism is known to be a delayed hypersensitivity reaction. Of the 2, primary irritant dermatitis is more frequent in children, particularly during the early years of life.

Primary irritant contact dermatitis can result from prolonged or repetitive contact with a variety of substances that include saliva, citrus juices, bubble bath, detergents, abrasive materials, strong soaps, and proprietary medications. Saliva is probably one of the most common offenders; it may cause dermatitis on the face and in the neck folds of the drooling infant or retarded child. The older child who habitually licks his lips because of dryness may develop a striking, sharply demarcated perioral rash (Fig 24–20). Among the exogenous irritants, citrus juices, proprietary medications, and bubble bath preparations are relatively common; bubble bath dermatitis is a cause of severe pruritus. Excessive accumulation of sweat and moisture as a result of wearing occlusive shoes may also be responsible for irritant dermatitis.

Clinically, primary irritant contact dermatitis may be indistinguishable from atopic dermatitis or allergic contact dermatitis. A detailed history and consideration of the sites of involvement, age of the child, and contactants will usually provide clues to the etiology. The propensity to develop irritant dermatitis varies considerably among children, and some may respond to minimal injury in this fashion. In general, all primary irritant contact dermatitis will clear after removal of the stimulus and temporary treatment with a topical corticosteroid preparation. Education of patient and parents as to the causes of contact dermatitis is crucial to successful therapy.

Diaper dermatitis can be regarded as the prototype of primary irritant contact dermatitis. As a reaction to friction, maceration, and prolonged contact with urine and feces, retained soaps, and topical preparations, the skin of the diaper area may become erythematous and scaly, often with papulovesicular or bullous lesions, fissures, and erosions. The eruption can be patchy or confluent, but the genitocrural folds are often spared.

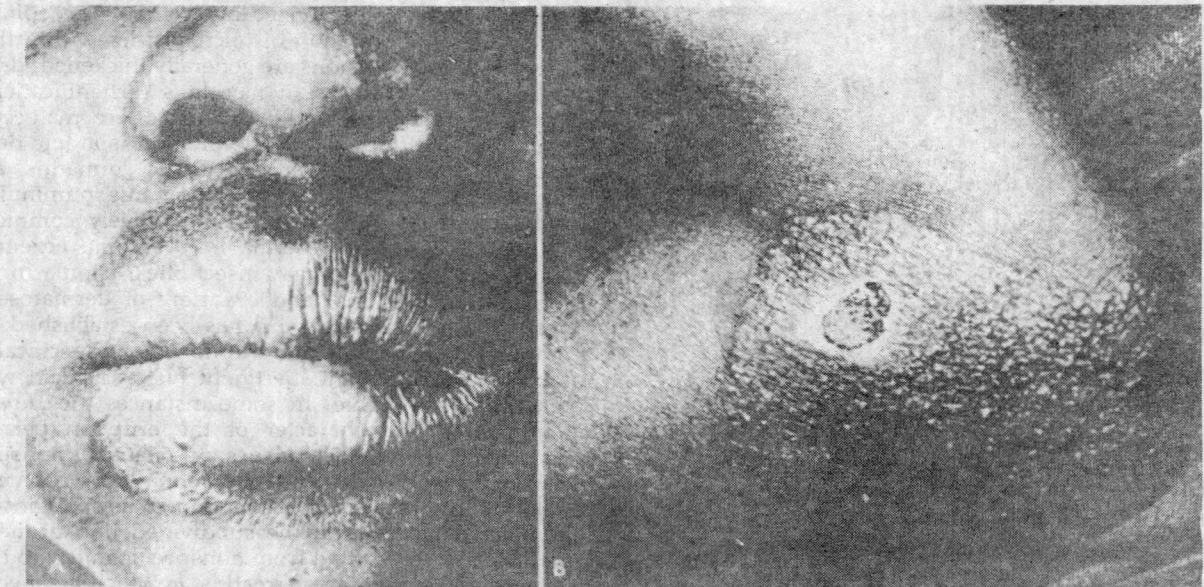

Figure 24–20 *A*, Primary irritant perioral contact dermatitis from lip-licking. *B*, Allergic contact dermatitis in Merthiolate spray. Note the sharp angular border of vesicular eruption.

Chronic hypertrophic, flat-topped papules and infiltrative nodules may simulate syphilitic lesions. Secondary infection with bacteria and yeasts is common; discomfort may be marked because of intense inflammation. Such conditions as allergic contact dermatitis, seborrheic dermatitis, candidiasis, atopic dermatitis, and rare disorders such as histiocytosis X and acrodermatitis enteropathica should be considered when the eruption is persistent or recalcitrant to simple therapeutic measures.

Diaper dermatitis will often respond to simple measures; however, some infants seem predisposed to diaper dermatitis, and management of them may be difficult. The damaging effects of prolonged contact with feces and ammoniacal urine can be obviated by frequent changing of diapers and meticulous washing of the genitalia with warm water without irritating soaps. Occlusive plastic pants which accentuate maceration should not be used; disposable diapers are a practical substitute. Frequent applications of a bland protective topical agent (petrolatum or zinc oxide paste) following thorough gentle cleansing may suffice to prevent dermatitis.

When the above measures are not sufficient to promote healing, a light application of 0.5–1% topical hydrocortisone ointment after each diaper change for a limited time is often effective. Prior to initiation of such therapy the possibility of candidal infection should be excluded by a KOH preparation or culture. For infants requiring additional protection, zinc oxide paste can be applied after the steroid as a thick covering. Secondary complications can result from prolonged use of corticosteroids, especially the fluorinated ones.

Allergic contact dermatitis is a T cell–mediated hypersensitivity reaction that is provoked by application of an antigen to the skin surface. The antigen penetrates the skin, where it is conjugated with a cutaneous protein, and the hapten-protein complex is transported to the regional lymph nodes. A primary immunologic response occurs locally in the nodes and becomes generalized, presumably because of dissemination of sensitized T cells. Sensitization requires several days and, when followed by a fresh antigenic challenge, becomes manifest as allergic contact dermatitis. Generalized distribution may occur if substantial quantities of antigen find their way into the circulation. Once sensitization has occurred, each new antigenic challenge may provoke an inflammatory reaction within 8–12 hr; sensitization to a particular antigen usually persists for many yr.

Acute allergic contact dermatitis is an erythematous, intensely pruritic, eczematous dermatitis, which, if severe, may be edematous and vesicobullous. Chronic contact dermatitis has the features of a longstanding eczema: lichenification, scaling, fissuring, and pigmentary change. The distribution of the eruption often provides a clue to the diagnosis. Volatile sensitizers usually affect exposed areas such as face and arms. Jewelry, topical agents, shoes, clothing, and plants cause dermatitis at points of contact.

Rhus dermatitis (poison ivy or poison oak) is often vesicobullous and may be distinguished by linear streaks of vesicles where the plant leaves have brushed against the skin. Contrary to popular opinion, fluid from ruptured vesicles does not spread the eruption; however, antigen retained on the skin, under the fingernails, and on clothing will initiate new plaques of dermatitis if not removed by washing. Antigen may also be carried by animals on their fur.

Nickel dermatitis usually develops from contact with jewelry or metal closures on clothing and is seen most frequently on the ear lobes, e.g., when nickel-containing posts rather than nonmetallic materials or stainless steel are used to keep a pierced tract open. Some children are quite exquisitely sensitive to nickel, and even the traces found in gold jewelry may provoke an eruption.

Shoe dermatitis typically affects the dorsum of the feet and toes, sparing the interdigital spaces; it is usually symmetric. Allergic contact dermatitis, in contrast to irritant dermatitis, rarely involves the palms and soles. Common allergens are the antioxidants and accelerators in shoe rubber and the chromium salts in tanned leather or shoe dyes. These substances are often leached out by excessive sweating.

Wearing apparel contains a number of sensitizers, including dyes, mordants, fabric finishers, fibers, resins, and cleaning solutions. Dye may be poorly fixed to clothing and leached out with sweating, as are the partially cured formaldehyde resins. The elastic in garments is also a frequent cause of clothing dermatitis.

Topical medications and cosmetics may be unsuspected as allergens, particularly if the medication is being used for a pre-existing dermatitis. The most common offenders are neomycin, Merthiolate (Fig 24–20B), topical antihistamines (e.g, Caladryl), anesthetics (e.g., Nupercaine and Surfacaine), preservatives (e.g., parabens), and ethylenediamine, a stabilizer present in many medications (e.g., Mycolog cream). All types of cosmetics can cause facial dermatitis; involvement of the eyelids is characteristic for nail polish sensitivity.

Contact dermatitis can be confused with other types of eczema, dermatophytosis, and vesicobullous diseases. Patch testing may clarify the situation but should be performed only by an experienced person. The essential principle in treatment is elimination of contact with the allergen. Acute dermatitis responds to cool compresses and a corticosteroid cream applied several times daily. Chronic dermatitis often requires a more potent fluorinated steroid ointment with protective covering at night. An oral antihistamine may be used for its sedative effect. Massive bullous acute reactions such as those of poison ivy are best treated by a short course of therapy with an oral corticosteroid. If secondary infection has occurred, an appropriate systemic antibiotic should be prescribed. Desensitization therapy is rarely indicated.

Nummular eczema is unusual in children and unrelated to other types of eczema. The eczematous plaques are more or less coin-shaped. Common sites are the extensor surfaces of the extremities (Fig 24–21), the buttocks, and the shoulders. The plaques are relatively discrete, boggy, vesicular, severely pruritic, and exudative; when chronic, they often become thickened and lichenified. The cause is unknown. Most frequently, these lesions are mistaken for tinea corporis, but the plaques of nummular eczema are distinguished by the lack of a raised, sharply circumscribed border, and they often weep or bleed when scraped. A KOH study can be helpful in differentiation. Secondary infection is a frequent complication. Control of pruritus is usually achieved with a fluorinated corticosteroid preparation with or without occlusion with a polyethylene wrap. Sedation with an antihistamine is helpful, particularly at night. Antibiotics are indicated for secondary infection.

Pityriasis alba occurs mainly in children; the lesions

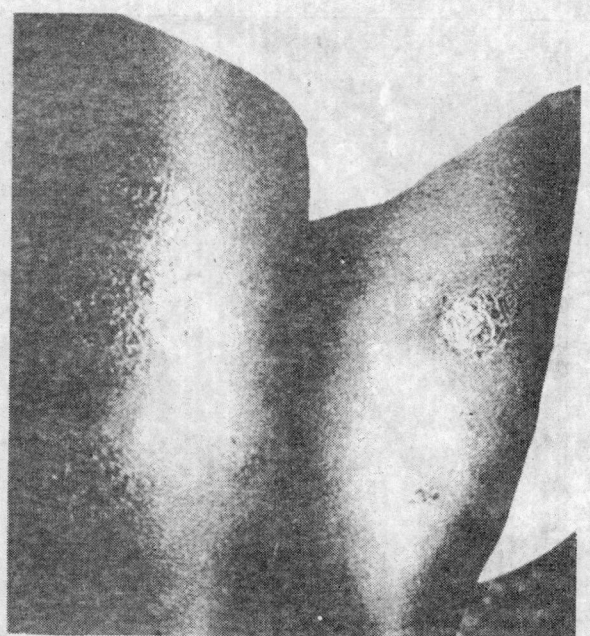

Figure 24–21 Multiple hyperpigmented scaly plaques of nummular eczema.

are hypopigmented, round or oval, macular or slightly elevated patches with fine adherent scales (Fig 24–22, p. xxxiv). They may be mildly erythematous, and, although relatively well defined, they lack a sharply marginated border. Lesions occur on the face, neck, upper trunk, and proximal arms. Itching is minimal or absent.

The etiology is unknown, but the eruption appears to be exacerbated by dryness and is often regarded as a mild form of eczema. Pityriasis alba is frequently misdiagnosed as tinea versicolor or tinea corporis, each of which can be readily excluded by performing a KOH examination of surface scales. The lesions wax and wane but eventually disappear spontaneously. Application of a lubricant may ameliorate the condition; if pruritus is troublesome, a 1% hydrocortisone topical preparation applied 3–4 times daily may be more effective. Return of normal pigmentation requires weeks to months.

Lichen simplex chronicus is characterized by a chronic pruritic, eczematous, circumscribed, solitary plaque that is usually lichenified and hyperpigmented. The most common sites are the posterior neck, dorsum of the feet, wrists, and ankles. Trauma from rubbing and scratching accounts for persistence of the plaque, although the initiating event may be a transient irritating lesion such as an insect bite. Pruritus must be controlled to permit healing. A topical fluorinated corticosteroid preparation should be applied at frequent intervals throughout the day; a covering to prevent scratching is usually necessary.

Dyshidrotic eczema (dyshidrosis, pompholyx) is a recurrent, sometimes seasonal, blistering disorder of the hands and feet; it occurs in all age groups but is uncommon in infancy. The pathogenesis is not known;

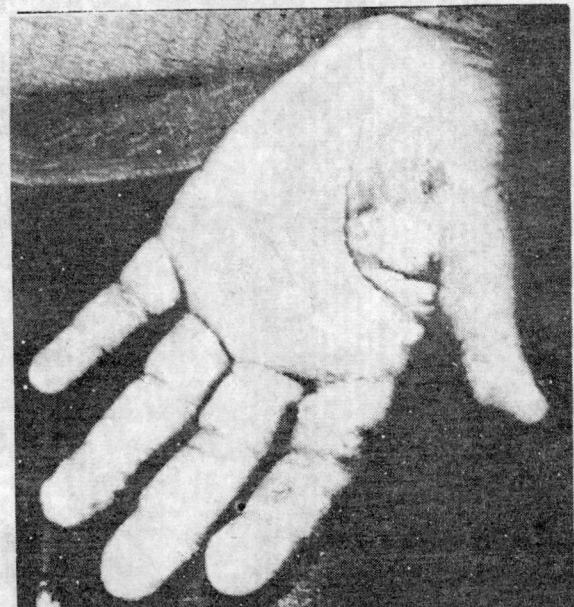

Figure 24—23 Vesicular palmar lesions of dyshidrotic eczema that have become secondarily infected.

there does not appear to be a genetic factor, although an increased incidence of atopy has been recorded in patients and their relatives.

The disease is characterized by recurrent crops of intensely pruritic, small vesicles on the hands and feet. Sites of predilection are the palms, soles, and lateral aspects of the fingers and toes. Primary lesions are noninflammatory and filled with clear fluid, which, unlike sweat, has a physiologic pH and contains protein. Larger vesicobullae may occur, and maceration and secondary infection are frequent because of scratching (Fig 24—23). The chronic phase is characterized by thickened, fissured plaques that may cause considerable discomfort. Hyperhidrosis is common in many patients, but the association may be fortuituous.

The diagnosis is made clinically. The disorder may be confused with allergic contact dermatitis, which usually affects the dorsal rather than the volar surfaces, and with dermatophytosis, which can be distinguished by a KOH preparation of the roof of a vesicle and by appropriate cultures.

Dyshidrotic eczema responds to wet dressings, followed by a topical corticosteroid preparation during the acute phase. Control of the chronic stage is difficult; lubricants containing mild keratolytic agents in conjunction with a potent topical fluorinated corticosteroid preparation and occlusion with a polyethylene wrap may be indicated. Secondary bacterial infection should be treated systemically with an appropriate antibiotic. Patients should be told to expect recurrence and should protect their hands and feet from the damaging effects of excessive sweating, chemicals, harsh soaps, and adverse weather.

Seborrheic dermatitis is a chronic inflammatory disease that occurs at all ages; in the pediatric age group it is most common during infancy and adolescence. The cause is unknown, as is the role of the sebaceous gland.

In infancy the disorder may begin within the 1st mo of life and be most troublesome during the 1st yr. Diffuse or focal scaling and crusting of the scalp, sometimes called *cradle cap*, may be the initial and at times the only manifestation. A dry, scaly, erythematous papular dermatitis, which is usually nonpruritic, may involve the face, neck, retroauricular areas, axillae, and diaper area. The dermatitis may be patchy and focal or may spread to involve almost the entire body (Fig 24—24). Postinflammatory pigmentary changes are common, particularly in black infants. When the scaling becomes pronounced, the condition may resemble psoriasis and at times can be distinguished only with difficulty. The possibility of coexistent atopic dermatitis must be considered when there is an acute weeping dermatitis with pruritus. An intractable seborrheic-like dermatitis, sometimes called *Leiner disease*, may reflect a functional disorder of the 5th component of complement. A seborrheic-like pattern may also result from cutaneous histiocytic infiltrates in infants with histiocytosis X.

During childhood and adolescence, seborrheic dermatitis is more localized and may be confined to the scalp and intertriginous areas. There may also be marginal blepharitis and involvement of the external auditory canal. Scalp changes may vary from diffuse, branny scaling to focal areas of thick, yellow crusts with underlying erythema. Loss of hair is not uncommon, and pruritus may be absent to marked. When the dermatitis is severe, erythema and scaling may occur at the frontal hairline, at the medial aspects of the eyebrows, and in the nasolabial and retroauricular folds. Red, scaly plaques may appear in the axillae, inguinal region, gluteal cleft, and umbilicus. On the extremities seborrheic plaques may be more eczematous and less erythematous and demarcated.

Seborrheic dermatitis is a condition that is reactivated in some patients by stressful situations, poor hygiene, and excessive perspiration. The differential diagnosis includes psoriasis, atopic dermatitis, dermatophytosis, and candidiasis. Secondary bacterial infections and superimposed candidiasis are not uncommon.

Scalp lesions should be controlled with an antisebor-

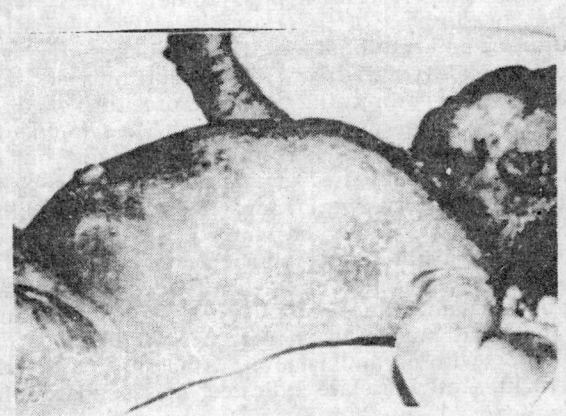

Figure 24—24 Widespread seborrheic dermatitis in an infant.

rheic shampoo, which may be used daily if necessary. Inflamed lesions will usually respond promptly to a topical corticosteroid preparation, 2–4 times daily. A 3% sulfur ointment in a washable base is an alternative means of therapy. Wet compresses should be applied to the moist or fissured lesions prior to application of the steroid ointment. Many patients require the continued use of an antiseborrheic shampoo for control. Response to therapy is usually rapid unless there are complicating factors or the diagnosis is in error.

24.14 PHOTOSENSITIVITY

Photosensitivity denotes a qualitatively or quantitatively abnormal cutaneous reaction to sunlight or, less commonly, to artificial light. The adverse effects of sunlight are due principally to wavelengths of light ranging from 250–800 nm, a range which includes both ultraviolet and visible light. Host factors play an important role, particularly natural skin pigmentation, since melanin serves to reflect, absorb, and scatter light.

Acute sunburn reaction is the most common light-induced effect seen in children; it is caused mainly by rays in the 290–320 nm band. Erythema appears 6–12 hr after initial exposure and reaches a peak in 24 hr when intense redness, exquisite tenderness, pain, edema, and blistering may occur. Additional effects of sun exposure include increase in thickness of the stratum corneum and increased formation and melanization of melanosomes, resulting in deepening of the skin color (tanning). Acute severe sunburn should be managed with cool tap water compresses and shake lotions and, if necessary, a mild oral analgesic. Topical corticosteroids, judiciously chosen, may diminish inflammation and pain. Proprietary preparations containing topical anesthetics are relatively ineffective and potentially hazardous because of their propensity to cause contact dermatitis. A bland emollient is effective in the desquamative phase.

Although the long-term sequelae of chronic and intense sun exposure are not often seen in children, pediatricians should advise patients regarding the harmful effects and irreversible skin damage that results from unduly prolonged sun exposure. Premature aging, senile elastosis, actinic keratoses, squamous and basal cell carcinomas, and probably melanomas all occur with greater frequency in sun-damaged skin. Adequate protection is readily provided by a wide variety of sunscreen agents.

Phototoxicity and Photoallergy. *Exogenous photosensitizers* in combination with a particular wavelength of light will cause dermatitis which can be classified as a phototoxic or a photoallergic reaction.

Phototoxic reactions occur in all individuals who accumulate adequate amounts of a photosensitizing drug or chemical within the skin. The eruption is confined to light-exposed areas and often resembles an exaggerated sunburn, but it may be urticarial or bullous, and it results in hyperpigmentation.

Photoallergic reactions, in contrast, occur only in a small percentage of persons exposed to photosensitizers and light and require a time interval for sensitization to take place. A photoallergic dermatitis is a T cell–mediated delayed hypersensitivity reaction in which the drug, acting as a hapten, combines with a skin protein to form the antigenic substance. Photoallergic reactions vary in morphology and may occur on partially covered as well as on light-exposed skin. Some of the important classes of drugs and chemicals responsible for photosensitivity reactions are listed in Table 24–2.

Although photodermatitis due to drugs or chemicals may be diagnosed by photopatch testing, facilities for this diagnostic procedure are not widely available. A high index of suspicion coupled with an appreciation of the distribution pattern of the eruption (sparing of eyelids, areas beneath the nose and chin, wrists, and antecubital fossae) and a history of application or ingestion of a known photosensitizing agent are all that is required to make a diagnosis. Discontinuation of the offending medication or avoidance of sun exposure, oral administration of an antihistamine, and application of a topical corticosteroid preparation to alleviate pruritus are appropriate therapeutic measures. Severe reactions may necessitate systemic corticosteroid therapy for a brief time.

The porphyrias are acquired or inborn abnormalities of specific enzymes in the heme biosynthetic pathway; they are quite diverse in their clinical manifestations

Table 24–2 CUTANEOUS REACTIONS TO SUNLIGHT

Sunburn
Photo-induced drug eruptions
  Systemic drugs include tetracyclines (Declomycin), psoralens, chlorothiazides, sulfonamides, barbiturates, griseofulvin, phenothiazines
  Topical agents include coal tar derivatives, furocoumarins (plants), psoralens, halogenated salicylanilides (soaps), perfume oils (e.g., oil of bergamot)
Genetic disorders with photosensitivity
  Xeroderma pigmentosum
  Bloom syndrome
  Cockayne syndrome
  Rothmund-Thomson syndrome
Disorders involving immune mechanisms
  Lupus erythematosus
  Dermatomyositis
  Scleroderma
  Solar urticaria
  Polymorphous light eruptions (?)
Inborn errors of metabolism
  Porphyrias
  Hartnup disease
Infectious diseases associated with photosensitivity
  Recurrent herpes simplex infection
  Lymphogranuloma venereum
  Viral exanthems (accentuated photodistribution)
Skin diseases exacerbated or precipitated by light
  Lichen planus
  Darier disease
  Granuloma annulare
  Psoriasis
  Erythema multiforme
  Sarcoid
  Atopic dermatitis
Deficient protection due to lack of pigment
  Vitiligo
  Oculocutaneous albinism
  Partial albinism
  Phenylketonuria
  Chédiak-Higashi syndrome

(Sec 8.43). Two in particular occur in children and have photosensitivity as a consistent feature. Signs and symptoms may be negligible during the winter, when sun exposure is minimal.

Congenital erythropoietic porphyria (Gunther) is a rare autosomal recessive disorder. Affected persons are exquisitely sensitive to light, which may induce repeated severe bullous eruptions that result in mutilating scars. Hyperpigmentation, hyperkeratosis, vesiculation, and fragility of skin in light-exposed areas are a consequence of permanent skin damage. Hirsutism, red urine, erythrodontia, hemolytic anemia, splenomegaly, and increased amounts of uroporphyrin I in urine, plasma, and erythrocytes and coproporphyrin I in feces are additional characteristic manifestations.

Erythropoietic protoporphyria is inherited as an autosomal dominant trait; photosensitivity becomes apparent in early childhood and is manifested by pain, pruritus, and a sensation of burning within half an hour of sun exposure, followed by erythema, edema, urticaria, vesicles, and, rarely, bullae on light-exposed areas. Nail changes consist of opacification of the nail plate, onycholysis, pain, and tenderness. Mild systemic symptoms of malaise, chills, and fever may accompany the acute skin reaction. Recurrent sun exposure produces a chronic eczematous dermatitis with thickened, lichenified skin, especially over the finger joints, and persistent violaceous erythema, ulcers, and pitted or vermicular atrophic scars on the face and rims of the ears. Protoporphyrin is elevated in the red blood cells, plasma, and feces.

The *porphyrias* may be confused with other diseases characterized by photosensitivity. Biopsies of affected skin from patients with porphyria have demonstrated deposits of an amorphous material histochemically identifiable as a lipomucopolysaccharide-protein complex in the papillary dermis and around the blood vessels.

The wavelengths of light mainly responsible for eliciting cutaneous reactions in porphyria are in the region of 400 nm. Window glass, which transmits wavelengths greater than 320 nm but absorbs light or shorter wavelengths, is not protective. Patients must avoid direct sunlight, wear protective clothing, and use a sunscreen agent that effectively blocks wavelengths in the region of 400 nm. The administration of β-carotene (Solatene) quenches the fluorescence of the porphyrin molecule by imparting a yellow color to the skin; it effectively reduces the photosensitivity in patients with protoporphyria.

Colloid milium is a rare childhood disorder that occurs on the face and dorsum of the hands as a profuse eruption of ivory to yellow, firm, tiny, grouped papules. Although the translucent quality of the lesions suggests vesiculation, no fluid is obtained by puncture. The eruption is asymptomatic and usually remits spontaneously after puberty.

Polymorphous light eruption includes a wide spectrum of cutaneous lesions clearly attributable to photosensitivity, which have not been accounted for by ingestion of drugs, use of topical medications, or known systemic diseases (see Table 24–2). The pathogenesis is obscure, but immune mechanisms have been implicated. The skin manifestations include erythematous plaques, urticaria, vesicles, bullae, papules, and eczematous dermatitis and are usually limited to sun-exposed areas. For some unknown reason, incidence peaks in spring and early summer, prior to the time when ultraviolet radiation is at a maximum. The greatest difficulty lies with light in the sunburn spectrum (290–320 nm), although patients with solar urticaria may have difficulty with the entire spectrum of ultraviolet light. Testing for light sensitivity with a monochromator is usually positive.

Patients must be instructed to avoid prolonged exposure during peak hours of sunlight. Appropriately selected sunscreens can afford excellent protection (Sec 24.14). Pruritus may be alleviated by administration of an oral antihistamine and by applications of a mild corticosteroid preparation.

Children who have lesions clinically indistinguishable from other polymorphous light eruptions but who do not have a positive response to photo-testing with ultraviolet light are said to have *summer prurigo*. They must be protected from sunlight by an appropriate sunscreen agent.

Hydroa vacciniforme and **hydroa aestivale** are characterized by a vesicobullous eruption on portions of the body exposed to sunlight; the pathogenetic mechanism is unknown. Peak incidence occurs during the spring and summer months, a feature that is responsible for the designation of the milder form of the disease, hydroa aestivale, in which scarring does not result. It is possible that these disorders are subtypes of polymorphous light eruption. Itching and burning precede the eruption of lesions, which occur in crops in a symmetrical arrangement over the nose, cheeks, ears, lips, dorsum of the hands, and forearms. Severe lesions resemble the vesicles of smallpox; they become ulcerated and crusted and heal as deep pitted scars. The disorder occurs with greater frequency in boys; it begins in early childhood and may remit at puberty. It must be distinguished from erythropoietic protoporphyria. Therapy with a topical corticosteroid preparation is effective in the inflammatory phase of the eruption. Protective sunscreens are mandatory for affected children.

Cockayne syndrome is inherited as an autosomal recessive trait and is characterized by photosensitivity, loss of adipose tissue, dwarfism, mental retardation, and thin, atrophic, hyperpigmented skin, particularly over the face. The ears are large and protuberant, the nose pinched, the teeth carious, the hands and feet cool and sometimes cyanotic. An unsteady gait with tremor, limitation of joint mobility, partial deafness, cataracts, retinal pigmentary abnormalities, optic atrophy, decreased sweating and tearing, and premature graying of the hair are additional features. The syndrome is distinguished from progeria (Sec 26.4) by photosensitivity and the ocular abnormalities.

Rothmund-Thomson syndrome is also known as poikiloderma congenitale because of the striking skin changes; it is thought to be inherited as an autosomal recessive trait, although a preponderance of affected females has been reported. Skin changes are noted in infancy as early as the 3rd mo. Plaques of erythema and edema appear on the cheeks, buttocks, hands, and feet and are gradually replaced by reticulated, atrophic, hyperpigmented, telangiectatic plaques., Exposure to the sun may provoke formation of bullae. Short stature, small hands and feet, sparse eyebrows and eyelashes, sparse, prematurely gray hair or alopecia, dystrophic nails, defective dentition, bony defects, hypogenitalism, and mental retardation are additional common features. Cataracts are common and become apparent from 2–7 yr of age.

Hartnup disease (Sec 8.6) is a rare inborn error of metabolism inherited in an autosomal recessive fashion; renal aminoaciduria is associated with a photo-induced, pellagra-like eruption. Approximately 20% of affected patients are mentally retarded and others evidence emotional instability and episodic cerebellar ataxia. The initial cutaneous manifestations are detectable during the early months of life when an eczematous, occasionally vesicobullous, eruption is noted on the face and on the extremities in a glove and stocking pattern. Hyperpigmentation and hyperkeratosis may supervene and are intensified by further exposure to sunlight. Episodic flares may be precipitated by febrile illness, sun exposure, emotional stress, and poor nutrition. Administration of nicotinamide and protection from sunlight are the most effective therapeutic measures and result in improvement of both the cutaneous and neurologic manifestations.

Bloom syndrome is inherited in an autosomal recessive fashion and is characterized by erythema and telangiectasia in a butterfly distribution on the face, photosensitivity, and dwarfism of prenatal onset. The facial erythema develops during infancy following exposure to sunlight. A bullous eruption may appear on the lips and telangiectatic erythema on the hands and forearms. Café-au-lait spots, ichthyosis, acanthosis nigricans, and hypertrichosis are less constant cutaneous manifestations. Defective dentition, prominent ears, pilonidal cysts, sacral dimples, syndactyly, polydactyly, clinodactyly of the 5th fingers, shortened lower extremities, and club feet are additional inconstant features. Mentation is normal. Chromosomal breaks and rearrangements are commonly observed, and affected children have an unusual tendency to develop lymphoreticular malignancies.

Xeroderma pigmentosum is a rare genetic disorder, inherited as an autosomal recessive trait, in which the skin changes are first noted during infancy or early childhood. Affected children, who are unable to repair DNA damaged by ultraviolet light, are sensitive to light in the wavelength range of 280–310 nm (UVB) and develop extensive solar changes in exposed skin. Sun-exposed areas such as the face, neck, hands, and arms are most severely involved, but lesions may occur at other sites including the scalp. The skin lesions consist of erythema, scaling, bullae, crusting, ephelides, telangiectasia, keratoses, basal and squamous cell carcinomas, and malignant melanomas. Ocular manifestations include photophobia, lacrimation, blepharitis, symblepharon, keratitis, corneal opacities, tumors of the lids, and possible eventual blindness. The association of xeroderma pigmentosum with microcephaly, mental retardation, dwarfism, and hypogonadism is known as *De Sanctis-Cacchione syndrome.*

This disease is a serious, mutilating disorder, and the life span is often quite brief. Affected families should have genetic counseling. Amniocentesis and possible interruption of pregnancy can be offered inasmuch as the defect is detectable in cells cultured from amniotic fluid. Affected children should be protected from sun exposure; opaque broad-spectrum sunscreens should be employed even for mildly affected children. Early detection and removal of malignancies is mandatory. Grafting of skin from non-light-exposed areas may be helpful, as is the use of topical antimitotic agents such as 5-fluorouracil.

24.15 DISEASES OF THE EPIDERMIS

Psoriasis, a common, chronic skin disorder among adults, is first evident in approximately one third of affected individuals within the 1st 2 decades of life. When the onset occurs during childhood, about 50% have a positive family history of the disease, and girls are more frequently affected. The mode of transmission is unknown; a multifactorial type of inheritance has been proposed. The pathogenesis is also unknown; epidermal turnover time, however, is distinctly accelerated compared with that of normal epidermis.

The lesions consist of erythematous papules which coalesce to form plaques with sharply demarcated, irregular borders. If they are unaltered by treatment, a thick silvery or yellow-white scale develops; removal of it may result in pinpoint bleeding (Auspitz sign). The Koebner, or isomorphic, response in which new lesions appear at sites of trauma is a valuable diagnostic feature. Lesions may occur anywhere, but preferred sites are the scalp, knees (Fig 24–25A), elbows, umbilicus, and genitalia. Scalp lesions may be confused with seborrheic dermatitis or tinea capitis. Small, raindrop-like lesions on the face are moderately common. Nail involvement, a valuable diagnostic sign, is characterized by pitting of the nail plate (Fig 24–25B), detachment of the plate (onycholysis), and accumulation of subungual debris.

Age is an important factor in determining the clinical pattern. Psoriasis is rare in the neonate but may be severe and recalcitrant and pose a diagnostic problem. The initial lesions may involve the diaper area and mimic seborrheic dermatitis, eczematous diaper dermatitis, or candidiasis. Biopsy and/or prolonged observation may be required for definitive diagnosis. Other rare forms include psoriatic erythroderma, localized or generalized pustular psoriasis, and linear psoriasis. In severe forms of the disease, hospitalization may be required.

Guttate psoriasis, a variant that occurs predominantly in children, is characterized by an explosive eruption of profuse, small, oval or round lesions that morphologically are identical to the larger plaques of psoriasis (Fig 24–25C). Sites of predilection are the trunk, face, and proximal portions of the limbs. The onset frequently follows a recent streptococcal respiratory infection; a culture of the throat and serologic titers should be obtained. Guttate psoriasis has also been observed

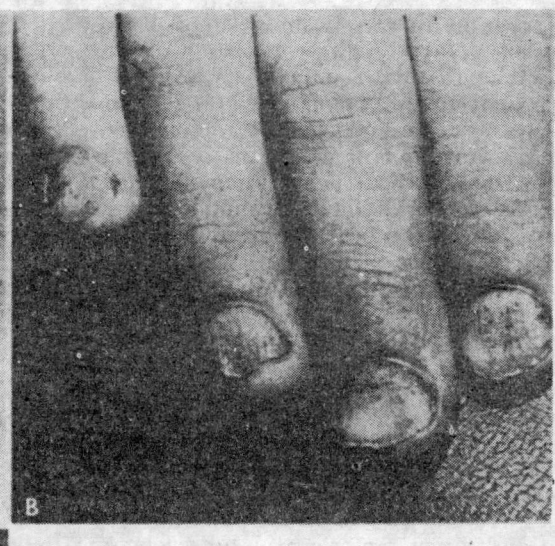

Figure 24–25 A, Chronic psoriatic plaques on the knee. B, Psoriatic nail changes of pitting and dystrophy. C, Guttate psoriasis in widespread distribution over the trunk.

following viral infections, sunburn, and withdrawal from systemic corticosteroid therapy. The lesions may be confused with viral exanthems and guttate parapsoriasis (see below).

When the diagnosis is in question, a biopsy of skin may provide supportive evidence. In a typical psoriatic lesion, the stratum corneum is thickened and parakeratotic, and the epidermis is hyperplastic with irregular elongation of the rete ridges, thinning of the suprapapillary epidermis, and microabscesses. The dermis contains a proliferative vascular network and an infiltrate of inflammatory cells.

The therapeutic approach varies with the age of the child, type of psoriasis, sites of involvement, and extent of disease. Therapy is mainly palliative and should not be overly aggressive. Physical and chemical trauma to the skin should be avoided insofar as possible (see Koebner response, above).

Tar preparations may be used in the form of an emulsion added to the daily bath, gel preparations, or ointments such as crude coal tar (1–5%) and liquor carbonis detergens (5–15%) in petrolatum alone or in conjunction with ultraviolet light or natural sunlight (Sec 24.14). Occasionally, sunlight has an adverse rather than a beneficial effect, and the use of tar preparations may have to be decreased during the summer to avoid phototoxic reactions. Salicylic acid ointment (1–3%) may provide an alternative for removal of scale, but extensive application may result in toxicity, particularly in small children. Topical corticosteroid preparations are extremely effective, but they must be used with caution; fluorinated compounds produce cutaneous atrophy if applied excessively or if occluded with polyethylene film for prolonged periods of time. The least potent effective preparation should be applied 3–4 times daily. For scalp lesions, applications of a phenol and saline solution (Baker P & S) followed by a tar shampoo are effective in the removal of scales. A corticosteroid in a lotion or gel base may be applied when the scaling is diminished. Rarely, the more severe forms of psoriasis may require systemic therapy; such management should be under the direction of an experienced physician. The use of psoralens and ultraviolet light (PUVA) is effective in severe psoriasis in adults, but the safety of this therapy has not been established for children. Psoriasis in infants and acute guttate psoriasis may flare with vigorous treatment and should be managed conservatively. Nail lesions are usually recalcitrant to therapy.

Guttate parapsoriasis (pityriasis lichenoides chronica), an uncommon chronic skin disorder, may occur at any age but most frequently affects older children. The etiology is not known. The eruption can be polymorphous in appearance, but typical lesions are small (1–5 mm), superficial, erythematous papules covered by a fine, white scale. Occasional lesions may become infiltrated, vesicular, hemorrhagic, and crusted and may be followed by a transient alteration of pigmentation. There is a predilection for involvement of the trunk, but all body sites may be affected except the nails and mucous membranes. An individual lesion may persist for 2–6 wk, but exacerbations and remissions of the disease persist for months to years.

Despite the prolonged course, guttate parapsoriasis is benign and unassociated with systemic manifestations. The lesions may be asymptomatic or cause minimal pruritus. The diagnosis is entirely clinical. Differential diagnosis includes guttate psoriasis, pityriasis rosea, drug eruptions, secondary syphilis, viral exanthems, lichen planus, and, occasionally, Mucha-Habermann disease. Since the pathologic changes are specific in some of these disorders, a skin biopsy may be indicated to exclude them. The chronicity of guttate parapsoriasis helps to exclude pityriasis rosea, viral exanthems, and some drug eruptions.

No effective treatment has been established. Some patients show remarkable improvement during times of intense sun exposure. Topical corticosteroid-tar preparations and ultraviolet light have been employed with variable success. A lubricant to remove excessive scaling may be all that is necessary if the patient is asymptomatic. Parents may be reassured that the child will remain well.

Keratosis pilaris, a moderately common papular eruption, may vary in extent from sparse lesions over the extensor aspects of the limbs to involvement of most of the body surface. The lesions may resemble gooseflesh; they are noninflammatory, scaly, follicular papules that do not coalesce. Because the lesions are associated with and accentuated by dry skin, they are often more prominent during the winter months; they also occur with greater frequency in association with atopic dermatitis and are most common during childhood and early adulthood. They tend to subside during the 3rd decade of life. Mild or localized eruptions respond to lubrication with a bland emollient; more pronounced or widespread lesions require regular applications of a 10–20% urea cream or a vitamin A acid preparation.

Lichen spinulosus, an uncommon disorder, occurs principally in children and more frequently in boys. The cause is unknown. The lesions consist of sharply circumscribed irregular plaques of spiny, keratinous projections which protrude from the orifices of the pilosebaceous canals (Fig 24–26). Plaques may occur anywhere on the body and are often distributed symmetrically on the trunk, elbows, knees, and extensor surfaces of the limbs. Although sometimes erythematous, the lesions are usually skin-colored. They are readily palpable and represent keratotic follicular plugs.

Lichen spinulosus is easily differentiated from keratosis pilaris since the latter lesions are never grouped to form plaques. More commonly, it is confused with papular eczema.

Treatment is usually unnecessary. For patients who regard the eruption as a cosmetic defect, keratolytic agents such as salicylic acid ointment (3–7%), urea-containing lubricants (10–20%), and vitamin A acid preparations often are effective in flattening the projections. The plaques usually disappear spontaneously after several mo or yr.

Pityriasis rosea, a benign, common eruption, occurs most frequently in children and young adults. Although a prodrome of fever, malaise, arthralgia, and pharyngitis may precede the eruption, children rarely complain of such symptoms. A *herald patch*, a solitary, round or oval lesion that may occur anywhere on the body and is often but not always identifiable by its large size, usually precedes the generalized eruption. When present, the herald lesions vary from 1–10 cm in diameter, are annular in configuration, and have a raised border with fine, adherent scales. Approximately 5–10 days following appearance of the herald patch, a widespread, symmetrical eruption becomes evident involving mainly the trunk and proximal limbs (Fig 24–27). When the disease is extensive, the face, scalp, and distal limbs may be involved, or, in the inverse form of pityriasis

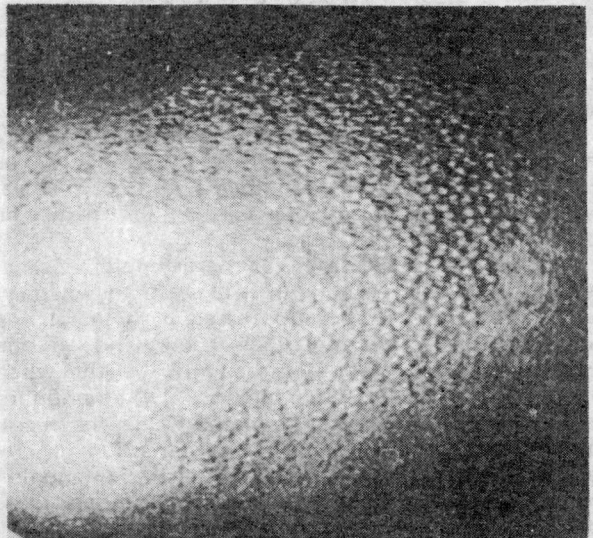

Figure 24–26 Sharply circumscribed plaque of follicular papules characteristic of lichen spinulosus.

Figure 24–27 Ovoid, maculopapular lesions of pityriasis rosea. Note distribution along skin lines and herald patch on the chest.

rosea, only those sites may be affected. Lesions may appear in crops over a period of several days. Typical lesions are oval or round, less than 1 cm in diameter, slightly raised, and pink to brown in color. The developed lesion is covered by a fine scale which gives the skin a crinkly appearance; some lesions clear centrally, producing a collarette of scale which is attached only at the periphery. Papular, vesicular, urticarial, and large, annular lesions are unusual variants. The eruption is usually distributed so that the long axis of each lesion is aligned with the cutaneous cleavage lines, a feature that creates the so-called "Christmas tree" pattern on the back. Actually, conformation to skin lines is often more discernible in the anterior and posterior axillary folds and in the supraclavicular areas. Duration of the eruption varies from 2–12 wk. The lesions may be asymptomatic or mildly to severely pruritic. The cause of pityriasis rosea is unknown; a viral etiologic agent has been sought but not identified.

The diagnosis is entirely clinical. The herald patch may be mistaken for tinea corporis, a pitfall which can be avoided if a KOH preparation is obtained. The generalized eruption resembles a number of other diseases; of these, secondary syphilis is the most important. Drug eruptions, viral exanthems, guttate psoriasis, parapsoriasis, and eczematous dermatitides can also be confused with pityriasis rosea.

Treatment is unnecessary for the asymptomatic patient. If scaling is prominent, a bland emollient may suffice. Pruritus may be suppressed by a lubricating lotion containing menthol (0.25–0.50%) and an oral antihistamine for sedation, particularly at night, when itching may be troublesome. Occasionally, a nonfluorinated topical corticosteroid preparation may be necessary to alleviate pruritus. After the eruption has resolved, postinflammatory hypo- or hyperpigmentation may be pronounced, particularly in black patients; these changes will disappear during subsequent weeks.

Pityriasis rubra pilaris, a rare chronic dermatosis, often has an insidious onset with diffuse scaling and erythema of the scalp, indistinguishable from seborrheic dermatitis, and with thick hyperkeratosis of the palms and soles. The characteristic primary lesion is a firm, dome-shaped, tiny, acuminate papule, which is pink to red in color and has a central keratotic plug pierced by a vellus hair. Masses of these papules coalesce to form large, erythematous, sharply demarcated plaques, within which islands of normal skin can be distinguished, creating a bizarre effect. Typical papules on the dorsum of the proximal phalanges are readily palpated and have been compared to the surface of a nutmeg grater. Gray plaques or papules resembling lichen planus may be found in the oral cavity. Dystrophic changes in the nails may occur and mimic those of psoriasis. In advanced stages, marked hyperkeratosis of the scalp and face cause alopecia and ectropion. Differential diagnosis includes ichthyosis, seborrheic dermatitis, keratoderma of the palms and soles, and psoriasis.

The etiology is unknown. A genetic form of pityriasis rubra pilaris with autosomal dominant transmission has been said to account for most of the cases in childhood; nevertheless, the majority of reported cases seem to be sporadic. Attempts to link the disease with a defect in vitamin A metabolism have not been definitive. Skin biopsy may aid in differentiating this condition from psoriasis and seborrheic dermatitis, which it resembles most closely.

Numerous therapeutic regimens have been recommended and are difficult to evaluate since the disease has a capricious course with exacerbations and remissions. Oral and topical vitamin A preparations have been used extensively; such therapy may be reasonable for patients who repeatedly demonstrate decreased levels of serum vitamin A. When vitamin A is administered orally, the child should be observed carefully for signs of toxicity. In childhood the prognosis for eventual resolution is relatively good.

Darier disease (keratosis follicularis) is a rare genetic disorder inherited as an autosomal dominant trait. Onset occurs usually during late childhood. Typical lesions are small, firm, skin-colored papules which are not always follicular in location. Eventually, the lesions acquire yellow, malodorous crusts; coalesce to form large, gray-brown, vegetative plaques; and usually involve the face, neck, shoulders, chest, back, and limb flexures in a symmetrical distribution. Papules, fissures, crusts, and ulcers may appear on the mucous membranes of the lips, tongue, buccal mucosa, pharynx, larynx, and vulva. Hyperkeratosis of the palms and soles and nail dystrophy with subungual hyperkeratosis are variable features. Severe pruritus, secondary infection, offensive odor, and aggravation of the dermatosis on exposure to sunlight are annoying features.

Darier disease is most likely to be confused with seborrheic dermatitis or juvenile flat warts. Histologic changes are diagnostic; hyperkeratosis, intraepidermal separation with formation of suprabasal clefts, and dyskeratotic epidermal cells are characteristic features.

Therapy is nonspecific. Some patients have responded to large oral doses of vitamin A or to topical vitamin A acid, with or without occlusive dressings. Secondary infection may require local cleansing and

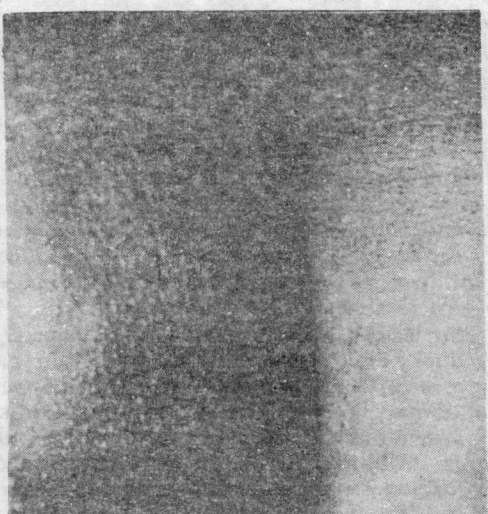

Figurre 24–28 Tiny flat-topped papules of lichen nitidus on the arm and trunk. Note the Koebner response on the arm (papules in a line of scratch).

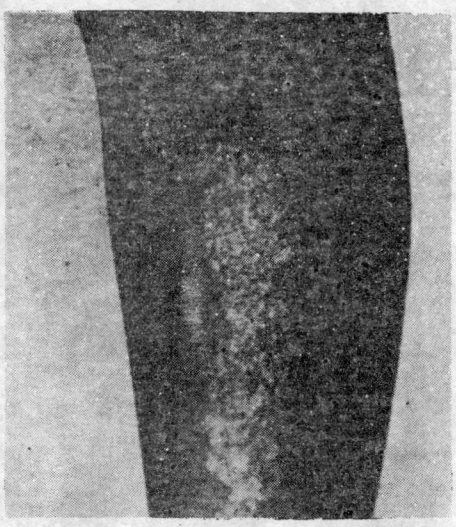

Figure 24–29 Multiple linear plaques and streaks of lichen striatus.

systemically administered antibiotics. Affected individuals usually suffer more during the summer months.

Lichen nitidus is a chronic, benign, papular eruption characterized by minute (1–2 mm), flat-topped, shiny, firm papules of uniform size which are most often skin-colored but may be pink or red and, in black individuals, are usually hypopigmented. Sites of predilection are the genitalia, abdomen, chest, forearms, wrists, and inner aspects of the thighs. The lesions may be sparse or numerous and form large plaques; careful examination will usually disclose linear papules in a line of scratch (Koebner phenomenon), a valuable clue to the diagnosis since it occurs in only a few diseases (Fig 24–28).

Lichen nitidus occurs in all age groups. The cause is unknown. Patients are usually asymptomatic and constitutionally well. The lesions may be confused with and rarely coexist with those of lichen planus. Widespread keratosis pilaris also can be confused with lichen nitidus, but the follicular localization of the papules and the absence of the Koebner phenomenon in keratosis pilaris will distinguish them. Verruca plana (flat warts), if small and uniform in size, may occasionally resemble lichen nitidus. Although the diagnosis can be made clinically, a biopsy is occasionally indicated. Histopathologically, the lichen nitidus papule consists of sharply circumscribed nests of lymphocytes and histiocytes in the upper dermis enclosed by claw-like epidermal rete ridges. The course of lichen nitidus is months to years, but the lesions eventually involute completely. There is no effective therapy.

Lichen striatus, a benign, self-limited eruption, consists of a continuous or discontinuous linear band of papules in a zosteriform distribution. The primary lesion is a flat-topped red to violaceous papule covered with a fine scale. Aggregates of these papules form multiple bands or plaques (Fig 24–29). In black patients the lesions may be hypopigmented.

The etiology and explanation for the linear distribution are unknown. The eruption evolves over a period of days or weeks in an otherwise healthy child, remains stationary for weeks to months, and finally remits without sequelae. Symptoms are usually absent; some children complain of itching. Nail dystrophy may occur if the eruption involves the posterior nail fold and matrix.

Lichen striatus is rarely confused with other disorders. The initial plaque may resemble papular eczema or lichen nitidus until the linear configuration becomes apparent. Linear lichen planus and linear psoriasis are often associated with typical individual lesions elsewhere on the body. Linear epidermal nevi are permanent lesions that often become more hyperkeratotic and hyperpigmented than those of lichen striatus. A lubricating lotion containing menthol and phenol or a mild corticosteroid preparation provides sufficient relief when pruritus is a problem.

Lichen planus is a rare disorder in the young child and uncommon in the older one. The primary lesion is a violaceous, sharply demarcated, polygonal papule with fine lines or thin white scales on the surface; papules may coalesce to form large plaques. The papules are intensely pruritic, and additional ones are often induced by scratching (Koebner phenomenon) so that lines of them are often detectable (Fig 24–30). Sites of predilection are the flexor surfaces of the wrists, the forearms, and inner aspects of the thighs. Characteristic lesions of the mucous membrane consist of pinhead-sized, white papules that coalesce to form reticulated and lacy patterns on the oral mucosa and sometimes on the lips and tongue.

There are several subtypes of the disease. Acute eruptive lichen planus is probably the most common form in children. The lesions erupt in an explosive fashion, much like a viral exanthem, and spread to involve most of the body surface. Hypertrophic, linear, bullous, atrophic, annular, follicular, erosive, and ulcerative forms of lichen planus may also occur. Nail

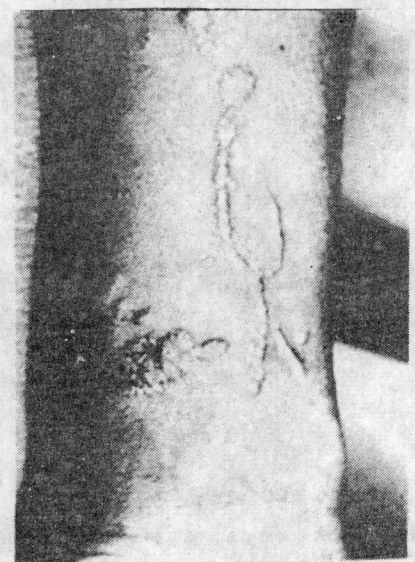

cells with retained nuclei) which is responsible for the linear ridge of the lesion, an invariable clinical feature.

The disease is slowly progressive but relatively asymptomatic. Lesions are sometimes responsive to applications of liquid nitrogen or may be surgically excised, a procedure which may not be feasible.

Papular acrodermatitis of childhood (Gianotti-Crosti syndrome) is a distinctive eruption associated with malaise and low-grade fever but few other constitutional symptoms. The incidence peaks in early childhood. Occurrences are usually sporadic, but epidemics have been recorded.

The skin lesion is a monomorphous, usually nonpruritic, dusky or coppery red, flat-topped, firm papule ranging in size from 1–5 mm. The papules appear in crops and may become profuse but remain discrete forming a symmetrical eruption on the face, buttocks, and limbs including the palms and soles. Lines of papules (Koebner phenomenon) may be noted on the extremities. The trunk is relatively spared, as are the scalp and mucous membranes. Generalized lymphadenopathy and hepatomegaly constitute the only other abnormal physical findings. The eruption resolves spontaneously in about 3 wk. Lymphadenopathy and hepatomegaly may persist for several mo.

The disorder represents a primary natural infection with hepatitis B virus and is, therefore, associated with hepatitis B surface antigenemia. Subtyping of the HB_sAg in most instances has demonstrated the determinant *ayw*. Elevation of serum transaminase and alkaline phosphatase values without concomitant hyperbilirubinemia is usual, and histologic changes of viral hepatitis are demonstrable on liver biopsy. Skin biopsy is characterized by a perivascular mononuclear cell infiltrate and capillary endothelial swelling.

Generally the disease is benign and self-limited and does not recur. The hepatitis usually resolves in 2–3 mo but, occasionally, may progress to chronic hepatitis with persistent antigenemia and elevated transaminase activity. The surface antibody of the hepatitis B virus is not detected during the phase of dermatitis appearing approximately 6–12 mo later in patients who become HB_sAg negative.

The eruption can be confused with viral exanthems, lichen planus, erythema multiforme and histiocytosis X, and Henoch-Schönlein purpura. The term papulovesicular acrolocated syndrome has been devised for those eruptions of unknown or presumed viral etiology which mimic papular acrodermatitis of childhood.

24.16 ICHTHYOSIS

The ichthyosiform dermatoses are a group of inherited keratinizing disorders characterized by visible scaling in distinctive patterns of distribution. They are usually distinguishable on the basis of inheritance patterns, clinical features, associated defects, and histologic changes. Since some of these conditions cause disfigurement and considerable mental anguish, early diagnosis is helpful in order to predict probable course and prognosis and to provide supportive management for the patient and family.

Figure 24–30 Violaceous polygonal papules of lichen planus. Note the striking Koebner response.

involvement may occur in the chronic forms but is rarely evident in children (see Twenty Nail Dystrophy, Sec 24.22). The disorder may persist for months to years; the acute eruptive form is most likely to involute permanently. Frequently, intense hyperpigmentation persists for a long time following resolution of lesions. The pathology of lichen planus is quite specific, and a biopsy is indicated if the diagnosis is unclear.

Treatment is directed at alleviation of the intense pruritus as well as amelioration of the skin lesions. Oral antihistamines and/or tranquilizers are often helpful. The skin lesions respond best to regular applications of a topical corticosteroid preparation. Rarely, systemic corticosteroid therapy is necessary to gain control of widespread, intractable lesions.

Porokeratosis is a rare, chronic, progressive disease that is inherited as an autosomal dominant trait. Several forms have been delineated: solitary plaques, linear porokeratosis, hyperkeratotic lesions of the palms and soles, disseminated eruptive lesions, and superficial actinic porokeratosis. The last form, probably induced by excessive sun exposure, occurs more commonly in adult females. Other types of porokeratosis are more common in males and begin during childhood. Sites of predilection are the limbs, face, neck, and genitalia. The primary lesion is a small, keratotic papule that enlarges peripherally so that the center becomes depressed, the edge forming an elevated wall or collar. The configuration of the plaque may be round, oval, or gyrate; its elevated border is split by a thin groove from which minute cornified projections protrude. The enclosed central area is yellow, gray, or tan, sclerotic, smooth, and dry, whereas the hyperkeratotic border is a darker gray, brown, or black.

The differential diagnosis includes warts, epidermal nevi, lichen planus, granuloma annulare, and elastosis perforans serpiginosa. A skin biopsy will disclose the characteristic cornoid lamella (plug of stratum corneum

Harlequin fetus is a very rare keratinizing disorder that is inherited as an autosomal recessive trait. Affected infants are extremely grotesque. Markedly thickened, ridged, and cracked skin forms horny plates over the entire body, disfiguring the facial features and constricting the digits. Severe ectropion and chemosis obscure the orbits; the nose and ears are flattened, and the lips are everted and gaping. Nails and hair may be absent. Joint mobility is restricted, and the hands and feet appear fixed and ischemic. The infants have respiratory difficulty and suck poorly. Most succumb within the 1st wk of life; few live beyond 6 wk. The prognosis is hopeless, and all that can be offered is genetic counseling.

The **collodion baby** is covered at birth by a thick, taut membrane resembling oiled parchment or collodion, which is subsequently shed. The condition is usually a primary manifestation of 1 of the ichthyoses, most often of the lamellar variety. Infrequently an affected infant has normal skin after the membrane is shed. There is ectropion, flattening of the ears and nose, and fixation of the lips in an O-shaped configuration (Fig 24–31). Hair may be absent or may perforate the horny covering. The membrane cracks with initial respiratory efforts and, shortly after birth, begins to desquamate in large sheets. Complete shedding may take several wk, and occasionally a new membrane may form in localized areas.

The nursery course may be complicated by cutaneous infection with yeasts and bacteria. Since the outcome is uncertain, accurate prognostic information is impossible in respect to the subsequent development of ichthyosis. Maintenance in a high-humidity environment and application of nonocclusive lubricants may facilitate shedding of the membrane.

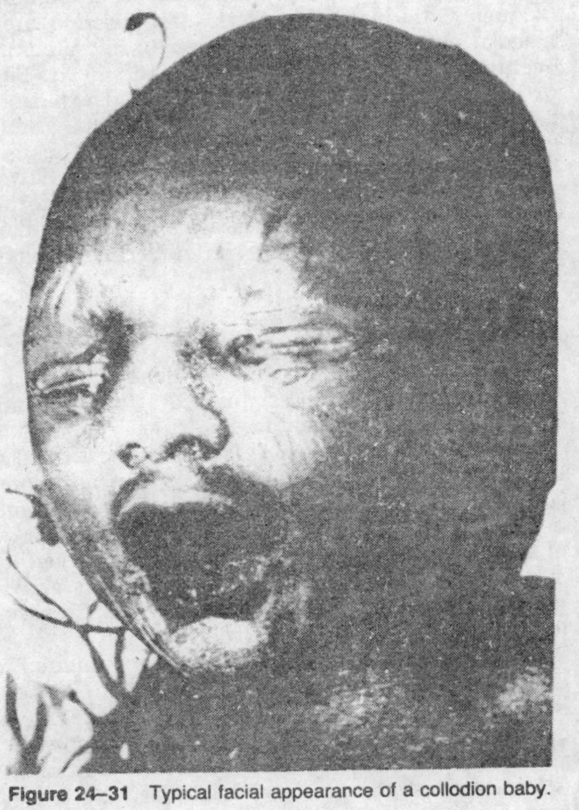

Ichthyosis vulgaris, the most common type of ichthyosis, is transmitted as an autosomal dominant trait. Onset occurs sometime after the 1st yr of life. Scaling is most prominent on the extensor aspects of the extremities and back. The flexures are spared, and the abdomen and face are relatively uninvolved. Accentuated markings and creases are apparent on palms and soles. Atopy is relatively common.

The histologic changes differ from those of other types of ichthyosis in that the hyperkeratosis is associated with a decreased or absent granular layer. Epidermal transit time is normal. Scaling is most pronounced during the winter months and may abate completely during warm weather. The condition may improve and even disappear with age. Scaling may be diminished by use of a bath oil and daily applications of an emollient or a urea-containing lubricant.

X-linked ichthyosis is limited to males and is usually present at birth. Scaling is most pronounced on the scalp, neck, sides of the face, anterior trunk, and limbs. The face, palms, and soles are usually spared. Although the distribution pattern of scaling differs somewhat from that of ichthyosis vulgaris, a skin biopsy may be required to distinguish the 2 conditions. Histologic changes in X-linked ichthyosis include hyperkeratosis of the stratum corneum, a well-developed granular layer, a hyperplastic epidermis, and a mononuclear, perivascular dermal infiltrate. Epidermal transit time is normal.

The inherited biochemical defect in X-linked ichthyosis is a deficiency of the enzyme steroid sulfatase. This defect can be demonstrated in the fibroblasts of affected males. Carrier mothers demonstrate a placental steroid sulfatase deficiency reflected by low urinary and serum estriol values, prolonged labors, and insensitivity of the uterus to oxytocin and prostaglandins. In addition, microsomal arylsulfatase C is absent from the placenta and the epidermis of affected boys. The role these enzymes play in the keratinization process is as yet unknown; therefore, the mechanism by which ichthyosis is produced has not been elucidated. The gene for steroid sulfatase is located on the short arm of the X chromosome and is closely linked with the Xg^2 blood group locus.

Deep corneal opacities that do not interfere with vision develop during late childhood or adolescence and are a useful marker for the disease since they may also be present in carrier females. Although the disease does not represent a serious keratinizing defect, affected boys are usually embarrassed by the disfigurement and request treatment. Hydration by bathing with bath oil and daily application of emollients and a urea-containing lubricant are usually effective. Citric or lactic acid (5%) in an emollient base is an alternative form of topical therapy.

Lamellar ichthyosis, an autosomal recessive disorder, is always evident at birth; the neonate may have a "collodion membrane." Universal erythema is characteristic in infancy and may persist during childhood; it

Figure 24–31 Typical facial appearance of a collodion baby.

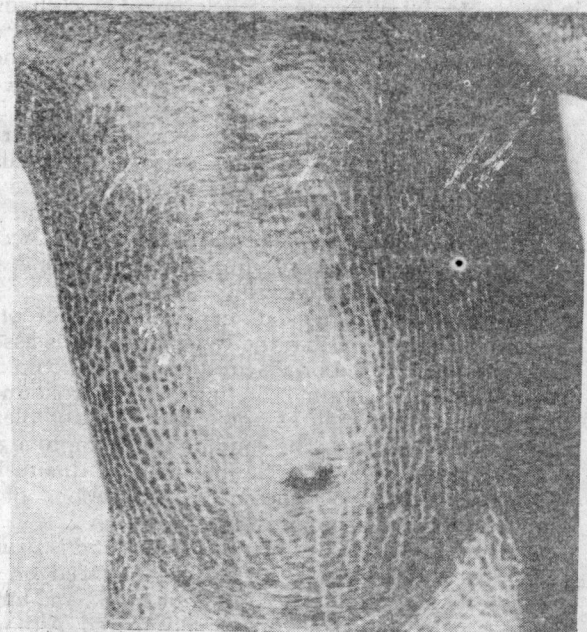

Figure 24–32 Generalized scaling of lamellar ichthyosis. Note involvement of axillary areas.

accounts for the obsolete designation, **congenital ichthyosiform erythroderma**. Scaling is often pronounced and involves the entire body surface including flexures and palms and soles (Fig 24–32). Pruritus may be severe, and it responds only minimally to antipruritic measures. Ectropion of variable degree is usually present.

Skin biopsy demonstrates hyperkeratosis, a well-developed granular layer, epidermal hyperplasia, and a mononuclear, perivascular dermal infiltrate. Epidermal transit time is significantly decreased. Growth of hair may be curtailed, and affected children may suffer in hot weather because of an inability to sweat freely through plugged sweat ducts. The unattractive appearance of the child and the malodor from bacterial colonization of macerated scales may create serious psychologic problems.

Effective measures include prolonged baths with bath oil to remove excessive scales. The restriction of bathing, on the erroneous premise that accentuation of dryness will occur, only promotes malodor and accumulation of keratinous debris and contributes to pruritus and discomfort. A high-humidity environment in winter and air conditioning in summer will lessen discomfort. Generous and frequent applications of emollients as well as keratolytic agents such as lactic or citric acid (5%), urea (10–20%), and vitamin A acid (0.1% cream) may lessen the scaling to some extent. Ectropion requires ophthalmologic care and, at times, plastic procedures. Genetic counseling should be provided.

Epidermolytic hyperkeratosis (bullous congenital ichthyosiform erythroderma), an autosomal dominant keratinizing disorder, is characterized by onset at birth, generalized erythroderma, and severe hyperkeratosis

with accentuation in the flexural areas. The scales are small, hard, and verrucous and differ from those of other forms of ichthyosis. Recurrent bullae, which are characteristic during childhood and are usually localized to the lower limbs, may be widespread in the neonate and cause diagnostic confusion with other blistering disorders. Secondary infection, usually with β-hemolytic streptococci, is common and requires appropriate antibiotic therapy.

The histologic pattern in this disorder is pathognomonic and consists of hyperkeratosis and vacuolization of the cells of the granular layer and mid-epidermis with abnormally large clumped keratohyaline granules. Epidermal transit time is decreased. Localized forms of the disease may resemble epidermal nevi (ichthyosis hystrix) or keratoderma of the palms and soles but share the distinctive histologic changes of epidermolytic hyperkeratosis.

Effective therapeutic agents are the same as those recommended for lamellar ichthyosis. Genetic counseling should be provided.

Ichthyosis linearis circumflexa, a rare autosomal recessive disorder, is characterized by migratory hyperkeratotic lesions, hyperkeratosis of the flexures, and hyperhidrosis of the palms and soles. The skin is diffusely red and scaly at birth. Superimposed serpiginous scaly plaques, bordered by a distinctive double-edged scale, appear at various sites on the trunk and limbs. This type of ichthyosis is characteristic of patients with the Netherton syndrome (see below).

Erythrokeratoderma variabilis is characterized by 2 types of lesions: sharply demarcated hyperkeratotic plaques with bizarre borders, and discrete areas of macular erythema which disappear or migrate but may eventually become hyperkeratotic and fixed. Sites of predilection are the face, buttocks, and extensor surfaces of the limbs. The palms and soles may be thickened, but hair, teeth, and nails are normal. The disorder is inherited as an autosomal dominant trait. Histologic changes include lamination of the stratum corneum, focal parakeratosis, papillomatosis, and irregular hyperplasia of the epidermis. The epidermal transit time is normal.

ICHTHYOSIS SYNDROMES

Several syndromes that include ichthyosis as a constant feature have been established as distinct entities. Each of them is relatively rare.

Sjögren-Larssen syndrome (see also Sec 25.4), an autosomal recessive disorder, has 3 major and constant components: ichthyosis of the lamellar type, mental deficiency, and spastic diplegia. A degenerative defect of retinal pigment epithelium has been detected in 20–30% of affected individuals; it is evident as early as 2 yr. Some patients may walk with the aid of braces, but most are confined to a wheelchair.

Rud syndrome, as described, consists of mental retardation, epilepsy, ichthyosis (type uncertain), and sexual infantilism. Associated defects of the skeleton, eyes, dentition, and hearing have also been reported. The authenticity of this syndrome has been questioned.

Netherton syndrome is characterized by ichthyosis (usually ichthyosis linearis circumflexa but occasionally the lamellar type), trichorrhexis invaginata, and other hair shaft anomalies and atopic diatheses. The ichthyosis is present at birth. Scalp hair is sparse and fractures easily; eyebrows, eyelashes, and body hair are also abnormal. The most frequent allergic manifestations are urticaria, angioedema, and asthma. Some affected children are mentally retarded. Although the disease is believed to be inherited in an autosomal recessive fashion, a preponderance of females has been reported.

Refsum syndrome (see also Sec 8.40), a multi-system disorder, is inherited as an autosomal recessive trait and becomes symptomatic during the 1st or 2nd decade of life. The ichthyosis is relatively mild and not clinically distinctive. Chronic polyneuritis with progressive paralysis and ataxia, atypical retinitis pigmentosa, anosmia, deafness, body abnormalities, and electrocardiographic changes are the most characteristic features. Affected patients have a deficiency of the enzyme alpha-decarboxylase and cannot degrade phytic acid, a constituent of chlorophyll, that accumulates in the serum and tissues. Dietary avoidance of chlorophyll-containing foods is all that is available therapeutically.

Chondrodysplasia punctata (see also Sec 23.16) includes several genetically heterogeneous disorders. Two major types have been distinguished: *Conradi-Hunermann syndrome*, inherited as an autosomal dominant trait, and *rhizomelic dwarfism*, transmitted as an autosomal recessive trait. Approximately 25% of patients with each type of chondrodysplasia have a distinctive ichthyosiform eruption at birth. Thick, yellow, tightly adherent keratinized plaques are distributed in a whorled pattern over the entire body, which may be intensely erythematous. The histologic changes include hyperkeratosis that penetrates to the depths of the hair follicles. The eruption disappears completely during the 1st few wk of life and may be superseded by a follicular atrophoderma. Patchy alopecia may be associated. Additional features include cataracts with or without optic atrophy, an abnormal facies with saddle nose and hypertelorism, and cardiovascular and central nervous system abnormalities. The pathognomonic defect, which also disappears with age, is stippled epiphyses in the cartilaginous skeleton. Other bony abnormalities consist of shortened femora and humeri, flexion contractures of joints, dysplasia of the hips, and asymmetrical deformities of the limbs. Severely affected patients may die in infancy.

A number of other rare syndromes with ichthyosis as a consistent feature include the following: *ichthyosis with defective hair having a banded pattern under polarized light and a low sulfur content, and mental and growth retardation; ichthyosis with atrophy, mental retardation, dwarfism, and generalized aminoaciduria; and ichthyosis with mental retardation, dwarfism, and renal impairment.*

Keratoderma of palms and soles (keratosis palmaris et plantaris) is due to excessive accumulation of stratum corneum and may occur as a manifestation of a focal or generalized congenital hereditary skin disorder or may result from such chronic skin diseases as psoriasis, eczema, or pityriasis rubra pilaris.

Although strict classification is difficult, the hereditary types of keratoderma may be categorized as follows:

Diffuse hyperkeratosis of palms and soles (tylosis) is an autosomal dominant disorder characterized by sharply demarcated areas of scaling. Striate and punctate forms have also been described.

Localized epidermolytic hyperkeratosis of palms and soles is an autosomal dominant defect with characteristic histologic changes.

Mal de Meleda is a rare, progressive autosomal recessive condition characterized by erythema and thick scales on palms, soles, and dorsal surfaces of the limbs, hyperhidrosis, EEG abnormalities, and mental retardation.

Keratoma hereditaria mutilans (progressive dystrophic hyperkeratosis) is a progressive autosomal dominant disease with honeycombed hyperkeratosis of palms and soles, starfish-like linear and annular keratoses on the dorsum of the hands and feet, and ainhum-like constriction of the digits that at times leads to autoamputation. This disorder may be associated with scarring, alopecia, and deafness.

Papillon-Lefèvre syndrome is an autosomal recessive erythematous hyperkeratosis of palms and soles characterized by periodontal inflammation and early shedding of teeth, nail dystrophy, and ectopic calcification of the dura.

Keratoderma of palms and soles also occurs in association with corneal dystrophy and with carcinoma of the esophagus as an autosomal dominant trait and as a feature of pachyonychia congenita, ichthyosis, ectodermal dysplasia, dyskeratosis congenita, and tyrosinemia as well as of several other conditions.

Patients with hyperhidrosis may develop macerated plaques that become secondarily infected and malodorous. Morbidity is lessened if the hyperkeratosis can be controlled; however, treatment is difficult, and only mild palliation is achieved with applications of lubricants, keratolytic agents (urea, salicylic acid, lactic acid), and vitamin A acid. Excision and split-skin grafting have been successful in patients with extreme hyperkeratosis and painful fissuring that cause chronic disability.

Acanthosis nigricans is a symmetrical dermatosis characterized by papillary hypertrophy and hyperpigmentation, which give the skin a velvety appearance and texture. The neck, axillae, genitalia, groin, umbilicus, and inner aspects of the thighs, elbows, and knees are most often affected. Mucous membranes are occasionally involved as are the palms and soles. Four types of acanthosis nigricans have been delineated:

Benign acanthosis nigricans, usually inherited as an autosomal dominant trait, is present at birth or may develop during childhood. The lesions may resemble widespread epidermal nevi.

Pseudoacanthosis nigricans is common in obese, dark-complexioned individuals and may be related to exogenous factors such as friction or to various endocrine disorders. This type may be induced by administration of diethylstilbestrol and nicotinic acid. Pseudoacanthosis nigricans is often reversible.

Syndromal acanthosis nigricans occurs as a feature of a number of disorders including the Seip-Lawrence, Bloom, and Rud syndromes.

Malignant acanthosis nigricans is only rarely observed

during childhood and occurs mainly in association with adenocarcinoma of the gastrointestinal tract, breast, and lung.

Pachyonychia congenita is a heritable disorder transmitted as an autosomal dominant trait with variable expressivity. The salient features include keratoderma of the palms and soles, follicular hyperkeratosis, hyperhidrosis, oral leukokeratosis, and nail dystrophy. Less common findings include epidermal cysts, corneal dystrophy, natal teeth, and abnormalities of the hair. The nail dystrophy is the most striking feature and may be present at birth or develop early in life. The nails are thickened and tubular, projecting upward at the free edge to form a conical roof over a mass of subungual keratotic debris. Repeated paronychial inflammation may result in shedding of the nails.

Treatment is relatively ineffective, although keratolytic agents may be of some benefit. The oral leukokeratosis should be evaluated periodically since malignant change may occur as early as the 2nd decade of life.

Essential fatty acid deficiency may be responsible for generalized, scaly dermatitis that resembles congenital ichthyosis. The eruption has also been observed in patients sustained on fat-free diets or fat-free parenteral alimentation and is caused by a deficiency of linoleic and arachidonic acids. Additional manifestations of essential fatty acid deficiency include alopecia, thrombocytopenia, increased susceptibility to bacterial infections, and failure to thrive. Daily application of sunflower seed oil, which contains linoleic acid, may ameliorate the clinical and biochemical manifestations, but it does not readily replenish tissue stores of linoleic acid. This condition should be distinguished from ichthyosis since it is amenable to therapy.

24.17   DISEASES OF THE DERMIS

Granuloma annulare is a common dermatosis that occurs predominantly in children; it can be polymorphous in its presentation. Typical lesions begin as erythematous, firm, flat-topped papulonodules; they gradually enlarge to form ring-shaped plaques with a normal, slightly atrophic or discolored central area (Fig 24–33) that varies in size up to several cm. Lesions occur most frequently on the dorsum of the hands and feet and on the scalp, trunk, arms, and legs. *Annular lesions* are often mistaken for tinea corporis because of the elevated advancing border; they differ in that they are almost never scaly. *Papular lesions*, another variant, may simulate rheumatoid nodules, particularly when grouped on the fingers and elbows. The generalized papular form is rare in children. *Subcutaneous granuloma annulare*, a less common form, may appear on the palms, soles, scalp, and limbs, particularly in the pretibial area. These lesions are firm, usually nontender, skin-colored nodules. They may be confused with other nodular and cystic lesions; identification of typical annular lesions elsewhere on the body will resolve the diagnostic dilemma.

Occasionally a biopsy is required for identification. Histologic changes are sufficiently characteristic to con-

Figure 24–33 Annular lesion with a raised papular border and depressed center characteristic of granuloma annulare.

firm the diagnosis. The lesions consist of a granuloma with a central area of necrotic collagen, mucin deposition, and a peripheral palisading infiltrate of lymphocytes, histiocytes, and foreign body giant cells. The pattern resembles that of necrobiosis lipoidica and rheumatoid nodule, but subtle histologic differences usually permit differentiation. The cause of granuloma annulare is unknown, and affected children are usually healthy. The eruption persists for months to years, but eventual spontaneous resolution without residual change is usual. Application of a potent topical corticosteroid preparation or intralesional injections of corticosteroid may hasten involution.

Lichen sclerosus et atrophicus, a dermatosis of unknown etiology, occurs rarely in children. Initial lesions consist of ivory-colored, shiny, indurated papules, often with violaceous halos that coalesce to form irregular atrophic plaques of variable size, in the margins of which hemorrhagic bullae may occur. Sites of predilection are the anogenital skin, buttocks, upper back, chest, forearms, and face. In boys, the prepuce and glans penis are involved most often. In girls, extensive involvement of the anogenital area may produce a sclerotic, atrophic plaque of hourglass configuration. Severe itching and burning are common.

Lichen sclerosus et atrophicus in children is most frequently confused with focal scleroderma (morphea). Biopsy is diagnostic, demonstrating hyperkeratosis, atrophy of the epidermis, edema and degeneration of the basal cell layer, homogenization of the collagen fibers, and edema of the upper dermis. The lesions may involute spontaneously and, in children, resolve without residua. Resolution has coincided with menarche. In therapy, the topical corticosteroid creams, local injection of corticosteroid, and topical progesterone have been most effective; none has been invariably curative; the risks of side effects must be weighed against the benefits of therapy.

Macular atrophies (anetoderma) may occur in the absence of inflammation (primary macular atrophy) or as a sequel of an inflammatory process (secondary macular atrophy). Lesions vary from 0.5–1 cm in diameter and, if inflammatory, may initially be erythematous but subsequently become thinned, wrinkled, and blue-white in color or hypopigmented. Often the lesions protrude as small outpouchings which, on palpation, may be readily indented into the subcutaneous tissue because of the dermal atrophy. Secondary macular atrophy may follow cutaneous lesions of lupus erythematosus, sarcoidosis, and certain other dermatoses.

All types of macular atrophy show loss of elastic tissue on histopathologic examination, a change which is not recognizable unless special stains are used. These lesions occasionally resemble morphea, lichen sclerosus et atrophicus, or end-stage lesions of chronic bullous dermatoses.

Necrobiosis lipoidica is rare in children and usually occurs in association with diabetes mellitus. The lesions begin as erythematous papules and evolve into irregularly shaped, yellow, sclerotic plaques with central telangiectasia and a violaceous border. Scaling, crusting, and ulceration are frequent. Preferred sites are the pretibial areas, but plaques may occur on the arms, trunk, and scalp. Histologically, necrosis of collagen, a granulomatous infiltrate, deposition of lipid, and proliferation of the small dermal vessels are evident. Necrobiosis must be differentiated clinically from xanthomas, morphea, and pretibial myxedema. The lesions persist in spite of good control of the diabetes but may improve minimally after local injection of a corticosteroid.

Keloid is a sharply demarcated benign growth of connective tissue in the dermis; it is composed of whorled and interlaced hyalinized collagen fibers. The lesions are firm, raised, pink, and rubbery; they may be tender or extremely pruritic. Sites of predilection are the face, ears, sternum, and extremities. Keloids are usually induced by trauma and commonly follow ear piercing, burns and scalds, and surgical procedures. Certain individuals, especially Blacks, seem predisposed to keloid formation. Keloids may enlarge to form grotesque excrescences with numerous claw-like projections, and, on the ear lobe, where they tend to be round, may hang in a pendulous fashion.

Keloids must be differentiated from hypertrophic scars, which differ histologically. Young keloids may diminish in size if injected intralesionally at 2 wk intervals with triamcinolone suspension (10 mg/ml). At times a more concentrated suspension is required. Large or old keloids may require surgical excision to be followed by intralesional injections of corticosteroid. The risk of recurrence at the same site argues against surgical excision alone.

Striae distensae are thinned, depressed, erythematous bands of atrophic skin which, with time, become silvery, opalescent, and smooth in consistency. They occur most frequently in areas that have been subject to distention, such as the lower back, buttocks, thighs, breasts, abdomen, and shoulders. The most frequent causes are rapid growth, as in adolescent males, pregnancy, obesity, Cushing disease, or prolonged corticosteroid therapy. The lesions result from rupture, retraction, and disintegration of the dermal elastic fibers.

Scleredema (scleredema adultorum, scleredema of Buschke) occurs in children as well as in adults. The onset is sudden with brawny edema of the face and neck that spreads rapidly to involve the thorax and arms but usually spares the abdomen, hands, and feet. The face acquires a waxy, mask-like appearance; the involved areas feel indurated and woody and are nonpitting. The overlying skin cannot be wrinkled, but it is normal in color and there are no atrophic changes. Systemic involvement, which is uncommon, is marked by thickening of the tongue, dysarthria, dysphagia, restriction of eye movements, and pleural, pericardial, and peritoneal effusions. Electrocardiographic changes may also be observed.

Though the disease often follows an infection such as tonsillitis, influenza, or scarlet fever after an interval of days or weeks, the cause remains obscure. Onset may be heralded by a prodrome of fever, arthralgia, myalgia, and malaise. Laboratory data are not helpful. Skin biopsy demonstrates an increase in dermal thickness due to swelling and homogenization of the collagen bundles, which are separated by large interfibrous spaces. Increased amounts of mucopolysaccharides in the dermis can be identifed by special stains.

The active phase of the disease persists for 2–8 wk; spontaneous and complete resolution usually occurs in 6 mo–2 yr. Recurrent attacks are unusual. The disorder must be differentiated from scleroderma, myxedema, trichinosis, dermatomyositis, and other conditions causing widespread edema. There is no specific therapy.

Lipoid proteinosis, an autosomal recessive disorder, may be initially noted in early infancy as hoarseness. Skin lesions appear during childhood and consist of yellowish papules and nodules which may coalesce to form plaques on the face, forearms, neck, genitalia, dorsum of the fingers, and scalp, where they result in patchy alopecia. Similar deposits are found on the lips, tongue, fauces, uvula, epiglottis, and vocal cords. Translucent nodules along the margins of the eyelids are the most characteristic clinical manifestation. Hypertrophic, hyperkeratotic nodules occur at sites of friction such as the elbows and knees; the palms may be diffusely thickened. The distinctive histologic pattern includes extreme dilatation of the dermal blood vessels and infiltration of the dermis with extracellular hyaline material, which is also deposited in the vessel walls. Calcification of the hippocampal gyri, identifiable roentgenographically, is pathognomonic, although it is not invariably present. The biochemical defect is unknown; the infiltrates appear to contain both lipid and mucopolysaccharide substances. There is no specific treatment.

Cutis laxa (dermatomegaly, generalized elastolysis) is a congenital heritable disorder that occurs in 2 forms: 1 as an autosomal recessive trait, the other as an autosomal dominant trait. When the apparent onset occurs during childhood or adulthood, usually after a febrile illness or a course of drug therapy, the disorder is designated as acquired cutis laxa; such clinical expression may, however, represent the variable expressivity of the congenital types.

In each form of cutis laxa, the skin hangs in pendulous folds. Characteristic facial features include an aged appearance, a hooked nose with everted nostrils, a

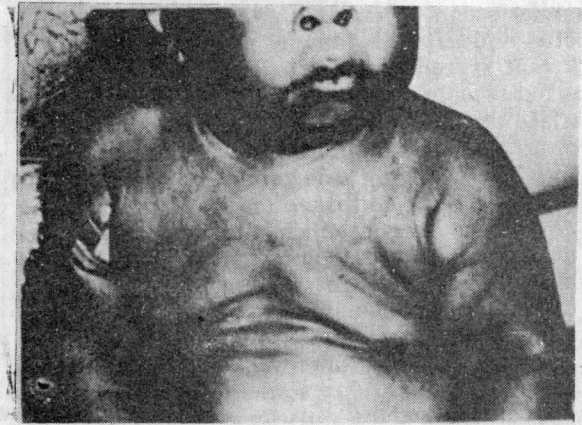

Figure 24–34 Pendulous folds of skin of an infant with cutis laxa. Note the long upper lip and upturned nose.

short columella, a long upper lip, and everted lower eyelids. The skin is lax elsewhere on the body and may resemble an ill-fitting suit (Fig 24–34). Hyperelasticity and hypermobility of the joints are not present as they are in the Ehlers-Danlos syndrome. Tensile strength of the skin is normal. Many infants have a hoarse cry, probably due to laxity of the vocal cords.

The dominant form of cutis laxa is essentially benign and mainly of cosmetic significance; a few affected individuals have had mild cardiovascular or pulmonary manifestations. In contrast, those with the recessive form of the disease are prone to severe complications such as multiple hernias, diaphragmatic atony, diverticula of the gastrointestinal and genitourinary tracts, and cardiopulmonary disease with emphysema, peripheral pulmonary artery stenosis, and aortic dilatation; they often have a shortened life span. Skeletal anomalies, growth retardation, and developmental delay have also been noted.

Histologically, elastic tissue is reduced throughout the dermis with fragmentation, distention, and clumping of the elastic fibers. Plastic procedures may be helpful in ameliorating the cutaneous defect.

Ehlers-Danlos syndrome, a genetically heterogeneous connective tissue disorder, has been differentiated into 8 distinct clinical forms:

I. *Gravis type*—autosomal dominant. Skin hyperelasticity and fragility, easy bruising, generalized and severe joint hypermobility, preterm birth.

II. *Mitis type*—autosomal dominant. Mild skin and joint manifestations, the latter limited to hands and feet.

III. *Benign, hypermobile type*—autosomal dominant. Generalized severe joint hypermobility and minimal skin manifestations.

IV. *Ecchymotic (Sack) type*—autosomal dominant. Joint hypermobility limited to digits, skin hyperextensibility minimal, severe bruisability with prominent venous network, extensive ecchymoses from trauma, high incidence of keloids and contractures, rupture of bowel and great vessels common. Absence of type III collagen.

V. *X-linked-type*. Limited joint hypermobility, extensive hyperelasticity, moderate bruising, fragility, and scarring. Lysyl oxidase deficiency.

VI. *Ocular type*—autosomal recessive. Ocular abnormalities (fragile cornea, sclera, deformed cornea), joint hyperextensibility, skin hyperelasticity, fragile bones. Lysyl hydroxylase deficiency.

VII. *Arthrochalasis multiplex congenita*—autosomal recessive. Short stature, marked joint hyperextensibility and dislocation, moderate hyperelasticity and bruisability of skin. Procollagen peptidase deficiency.

VIII. *Periodontitis type*—autosomal dominant. Mild skin hyperelasticity, joint hypermobility and bruisability, moderate cutaneous fragility, and severe periodontitis leading to premature loss of teeth and alveolar bone.

Ehlers-Danlos syndrome has been confused with cutis laxa, but the features of the 2 disorders differ considerably. The skin in Ehlers-Danlos syndrome is hyperextensible and snaps back into place when stretched. Because of its marked fragility, minor trauma results in ecchymoses, bleeding, and poor healing with atrophic cigarette-paper scars, which are most prominent on the forehead and lower legs and over pressure points. Surgical procedures are fraught with risk; dehiscence of wounds is common. Additional cutaneous manifestations include molluscoid pseudotumors over pressure points, small, subcutaneous, lipid-containing cysts that often calcify, and redundant skin on the palms and soles. Joint hypermobility with skeletal deformity, ocular defects, and ruptures of the bowel, great vessels, and lung are the major complications. Hernias and gastrointestinal diverticula may also occur.

All types of Ehlers-Danlos syndrome have been attributed to a defect of collagen, each presumably the reflection of a distinct biochemical defect.

Pseudoxanthoma elasticum is a rare, heritable, generalized disorder of elastic tissue which involves the skin, eyes, cardiovascular system, and gastrointestinal tract. Four distinct forms of the disease have been described; 2 of them are transmitted in an autosomal dominant fashion, 2 as an autosomal recessive trait.

Onset of skin manifestations occurs often during childhood; however, the changes produced by early lesions are subtle and may not be recognized. The characteristic cutaneous lesions are asymptomatic; 1–3 mm yellow papules are arranged in a linear or reticulated pattern or in confluent plaques. Preferred sites are the neck, axillary and inguinal folds, umbilicus, and antecubital and popliteal fossae. As the lesions become more pronounced, the skin acquires a velvety texture and droops in lax, inelastic folds. Mucous membrane lesions of the lips, buccal cavity, rectum, and vagina may also occur. Additional manifestations include visual disturbances, angioid streaks and other chorioretinal changes, intermittent claudication, cerebral and coronary occlusion, hypertension, and hemorrhage from the gastrointestinal tract and uterus.

The 4 forms of the disorder can be distinguished by pedigree data and the clinical patterns. Most of the features described above occur in each of the 2 autosomal dominant forms of the disease; they differ principally in the incidence of vascular and ophthalmologic complications. Patients with the type 1 disorder tend to have extensive disease with numerous complications, whereas those with type 2 have a less prominent macular skin eruption and low incidences of vascular involvement and of debilitating ophthalmologic disease. Patients with the recessive type 1 form have the classic flexural skin changes, but vascular changes are minimal, and the degenerative retinopathy is localized. In the recessive type 2 form there is elastic tissue degeneration of the entire integument, in contrast to the flexural accentuation in the other forms of the disease, and systemic involvement does not occur.

The basic defect is unknown, but the pathologic and clinical manifestations are related to deposition of calcium and to degenerative changes in the elastic fibers of the skin and blood vessels. Because of the serious nature of the systemic complications, even suggestive skin changes are an indication for skin biopsy. There is no effective therapy.

Elastosis perforans serpiginosa is an unusual skin disorder in which 1–3 mm, skin-colored, keratotic, firm papules tend to cluster in arcuate and annular patterns on the posterolateral neck and limbs and occasionally on the face and trunk. Onset usually occurs during childhood or adolescence. The etiology is unknown, but of particular interest is the frequent coexistence of this disorder with other ones such as osteogenesis imperfecta, Marfan syndrome, pseudoxanthoma elasticum, Ehlers-Danlos syndrome, Rothmund-Thomson syndrome, and Down syndrome.

Proliferation, thickening, and branching of dermal elastic fibers which perforate the epidermis and stimulate a reactive epidermal hyperplasia and inflammatory response are diagnostic. Differential diagnosis includes tinea corporis, granuloma annulare, lichen planus, creeping eruption, and porokeratosis of Mibelli. Treatment is ineffective; however, the lesions are asymptomatic and disappear spontaneously.

Xanthomas. (Sec 8.42.)

Farber disease (lipogranulomatosis). (Sec 8.37.)

The **mucopolysaccharidoses (MPS)** are distinguished by differences in clinical and genetic patterns and specific enzymatic defects (Sec 23.18). In several of these disorders, thick, inelastic, rough skin, particularly on the extremities, and generalized hirsutism are characteristic but nonspecific features. Telangiectasias on the face, forearms, trunk, and legs have been noted in the Scheie and Morquio syndromes. In some patients with Hunter syndrome, distinctive lesions have been noted; they are skin- to ivory-colored papulonodules that aggregate to form plaques on the upper trunk, arms, and thighs. They are firm and have a corrugated surface texture. Onset of these unusual lesions occurs during the 1st decade, and spontaneous disappearance has been noted.

Biopsies of affected skin and nodular lesions demonstrate thickening of the dermis with swelling and separation of the collagen bundles and deposition of metachromatic material. The epidermal cells may be vacuolated, and large mononuclear "gargoyle" cells, which also contain metachromatic material, may be identified in the upper dermis.

Mastocytosis encompasses a spectrum of disorders that range from solitary cutaneous nodules to diffuse infiltration of skin associated with involvement of other organs. All the disorders are characterized by aggregates of tissue mast cells in the dermis; the local and systemic manifestations of the disease are due to release of histamine and heparin from mast cell granules. Biopsy of involved skin is diagnostic provided special stains such as Giemsa or toluidine blue are employed to identify the infiltrates of mast cells.

Affected children may have intense pruritus. Systemic signs of histamine release, such as episodic flushing, tachycardia, respiratory distress, headache, colic, diarrhea, hypotension, and syncope, occur most frequently in the more severe types of mastocytosis. Flushing can be precipitated by excessively hot baths, by vigorous rubbing of the skin, and by certain drugs such as codeine, aspirin, morphine, atropine, and polymyxin B. Avoidance of these triggering factors will reduce discomfort considerably. For those patients who are symptomatic, oral antihistamines, particularly cyproheptadine, may be palliative.

The cause is unknown, and most cases are sporadic; however, in rare instances, other family members have been affected.

Mastocytomas are solitary lesions that constitute approximately 10% of childhood cases of mastocytosis. Lesions may be present at birth or arise during early infancy; they can occur at any site, although the wrist, neck, and trunk are sites of predilection. Initially the lesions may present as recurrent, evanescent wheals or bullae; however, in time, an infiltrated, rubbery, pink, yellow, or tan plaque develops at the site of whealing or blistering (Fig 24–35A). The surface acquires a pebbly, orange-peel–like texture, and hyperpigmentation may become prominent. Stroking or trauma to the nodule may result in urtication (Darier sign); rarely, systemic signs of histamine release become apparent. The differential diagnosis includes recurrent bullous impetigo, nevi, and juvenile xanthogranuloma. Mastocytomas usually involute spontaneously during early childhood; troublesome lesions can be excised and do not recur. Only rarely do multiple cutaneous lesions develop.

Urticaria pigmentosa is the most common form of mastocytosis and occurs primarily in infants and children; onset occurs before the 2nd yr. Lesions may be present at birth but more often erupt in crops over a period of several mo. In some cases, early lesions are bullous or urticarial and fade repeatedly only to recur at the same site until they become fixed and hyperpigmented; in others, the initial lesions are hyperpigmented. Vesiculation usually abates by age 2 yr. Individual lesions range in size from a few mm to several cm and may be macular, papular, or nodular; in color they range from yellow-tan to chocolate brown and often have ill-defined borders (Fig 24–35B). Larger nodular lesions, like mastocytomas, may have a characteristic orange-peel texture (Fig 24–35C).

Lesions may be sparse or numerous and are often symmetrically distributed. Palms, soles, and face are sometimes spared, as are the mucous membranes. The rapid appearance of erythema and whealing in response to vigorous stroking of a lesion (Darier sign) can usually be elicited; dermographism of intervening normal skin is also common. Urticaria pigmentosa can be confused with drug eruptions, postinflammatory pigmentary change, juvenile xanthogranuloma, pigmented nevi, ephelides, xanthomas, chronic urticaria, insect bites, and bullous impetigo.

The prognosis is good; spontaneous involution occurs

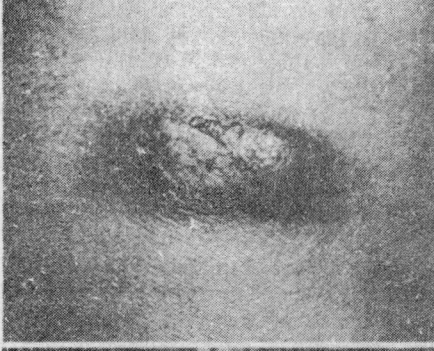

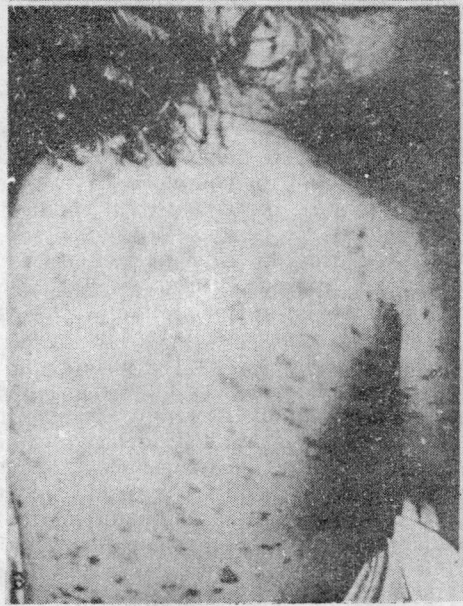

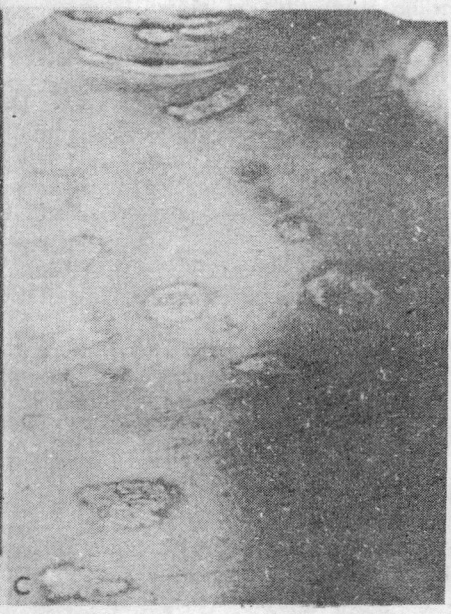

Figure 24–35 *A,* Solitary mastocytoma which is partially blistered. *B,* Hyperpigmented papular lesions of urticaria pigmentosa, some of which exhibit a surrounding flare. *C,* Infiltrated plaques of urticaria pigmentosa.

in about 50% of patients by puberty. Another 25% of them will have partial resolution of lesions by adulthood.

Diffuse mastocytosis is characterized by diffuse involvement of the skin rather than discrete hyperpigmented lesions. Rarely, there are no discernible skin changes, but usually the skin appears thickened and pink to yellow in color; it may also have a doughy feel and rough texture. Surface changes are accentuated in the flexural areas. Recurrent bullae, intractable pruritus, and flushing attacks are common, as is systemic involvement.

Systemic mastocytosis occurs in approximately 5–10% of patients with mastocytosis. Bone lesions may be silent but are detectable radiologically as osteoporotic or osteosclerotic areas, principally in the axial skeleton. Gastrointestinal tract involvement may be manifested clinically by diarrhea and steatorrhea. Mucosal infiltrates may be detectable by barium studies or by small bowel biopsy. Peptic ulcers are also a complication. Hepatosplenomegaly due to mast cell infiltrates and fibrosis as well as mast cell proliferation in lymph nodes, kidneys, periadrenal fat, bone marrow, and peripheral blood have been described. The prognosis is guarded.

The need for laboratory studies is determined by the symptoms and physical findings. Urinary excretion of free histamine and its metabolites is increased. Coagulation abnormalities are rare.

Epidermal inclusion cysts are sharply circumscribed, firm, freely movable, skin-colored nodules, often with a central dimple or dilated pore. They form most frequently on the face, neck, or trunk and may periodically become inflamed and secondarily infected. The wall of the cyst is composed of stratified epithelium that surrounds a mass of layered keratinized material which may have a cheesy consistency. Epidermal cysts may be confused with dermatofibromas, branchial cleft cysts, and small lipomas. Excision of the cysts with removal of the entire sac and its contents is the appropriate procedure.

24.18 DISORDERS OF SUBCUTANEOUS TISSUE

Diseases involving the subcutis are usually characterized histologically by necrosis or inflammation of the subcutaneous tissue; each of them may occur either as a primary event or as a secondary response to a variety of stimuli or disease processes. Unfortunately, these disorders are not all separable on the basis of the histologic changes; the histologic pattern may merely reflect the stage of the lesion at biopsy. The clinician must rely principally on the appearance and distribution of the lesions, the associated symptoms, and his or her appreciation of the exogenous provocative factors as diagnostic criteria.

Lipogranulomatosis subcutanea (Rothmann-Makai syndrome) is a type of panniculitis that occurs mainly in children, most frequently on the legs but occasionally on the arms and trunk. Typically, nodules appear singly or a few at a time and are unaccompanied by fever or other constitutional symptoms. The nodules are 0.5–3 cm in diameter, tender, firm, and elastic; they may be skin-colored or hyperemic, and only rarely do they rupture and discharge liquefied material. The duration of an individual lesion is several wk, but new ones appear over a period of 6–12 mo; the disease is usually self-limited.

Histologic findings vary with the stage of the lesion. In the acute stage, necrotic foci are surrounded by polymorphonuclear leukocytes. Subsequent granuloma formation with phagocytosis of fat by histiocytes is finally superseded by a fibrotic stage with homogenization of connective tissue fibers. Lipogranulomatosis subcutanea must be differentiated from Weber-Christian panniculitis, nodular vasculitis, erythema nodosum, and erythema induratum. There is no known effective treatment.

Weber-Christian panniculitis. (Sec 9.77.)

Corticosteroid atrophy. The injection of a corticosteroid intradermally can produce deep atrophy accompanied by surface pigmentary changes and telangiectasia. These changes occur approximately 2 wk after injection and may last for months. The deltoid area is most susceptible to this complication, but lesions also occur on the buttocks and thighs.

Postcorticosteroid panniculitis has been observed in children who have received corticosteroids orally for relatively short periods of time. Within 1–2 wk after discontinuation of the drug, multiple nodules appear on the face, trunk, and arms. Lesions range in size from 0.5–4.0 cm; they are erythematous or skin-colored and may be pruritic. The mechanism of the inflammatory reaction in the fat is unknown. Treatment is unnecessary as the lesions remit spontaneously without scarring.

Cold panniculitis may result in localized lesions in infants after prolonged cold exposure, especially on the cheeks, or after prolonged application of a cold object such as an ice cube, ice bag, or Popsicle to any area of the skin. Erythematous, indurated lesions arise within hours of exposure, persist for 2–3 wk, and heal without residua. The pathogenic mechanism may be similar to that of subcutaneous fat necrosis. Familiarity with this reaction will permit the physician to elicit pertinent information since avoidance of a biopsy may be desirable, particularly when the cheeks are involved.

Lipodystrophy. Several rare conditions are associated with loss of fatty tissue in a partial or generalized distribution.

Partial lipodystrophy occurs more commonly in females, often with onset during the 1st decade. There is gradual symmetrical loss of subcutaneous tissue over the face, upper trunk, and arms, resulting in a cadaverous facies and marked disproportion between the upper and lower halves of the body. Loss of adipose tissue is not preceded by an inflammatory phase, and histologic examination reveals only absence of subcutaneous fat. Some of these patients have had associated renal disease, disordered glucose metabolism, or abnormal serum lipid profiles. The etiology of the disorder is not understood, and there is no effective treatment.

Congenital generalized lipodystrophy (Seip-Lawrence syndrome) is a progressive multisystem disorder inherited as an autosomal recessive trait. The earliest manifestation is generalized loss of subcutaneous and visceral fat; it may be evident at birth or occur during early infancy. Associated cutaneous changes include prominent superficial veins, hirsutism, and skin pigmentation with acanthosis nigricans. Accelerated skeletal and muscle growth and advanced bone age are seen. Abnormalities of carbohydrate homeostasis, insulin production, and growth hormone appear to be age-dependent. Hyperlipidemia, hyperinsulinism, and insulin-resistant nonketotic diabetes mellitus develop gradually and are reflected by increasing hepatomegaly due to fatty infiltration and cirrhosis. Although serum concentrations of growth hormone may be normal, responses of it to stimuli may be disturbed. Hypothalamic releasing factors not ordinarily detectable in plasma have been identified in these patients and suggest a lack of hypothalamic regulation. There is no treatment.

Sclerema neonatorum is an uncommon disorder of adipose tissue that occurs primarily in preterm, sick, or debilitated infants. There is abrupt onset of a diffuse and generalized hardening of the skin, which becomes stony in consistency, cold, and nonpitting. Joint mobility may be compromised, and the face assumes a mask-like expression because of the inflexibility of the integument.

Sclerematous change is nonspecific and virtually always associated with serious illness such as sepsis, gastroenteritis, pneumonia, or multiple congenital anomalies. The outcome is dependent upon the response to treatment of the underlying disorder; however, the appearance of sclerema in a sick infant should be regarded as an ominous prognostic sign. When recovery is imminent, sclerema tends to disappear rapidly.

The histologic changes in sclerema are minimal, consisting only of edema and thickening of the connective tissue septa. Early and extensive subcutaneous fat necrosis may resemble sclerema; however, the evolution of the process usually permits differentiation. Edema of the newborn is localized to dependent parts, pits easily with pressure, and should not be confused with sclerema.

Scleroderma. (Sec 9.72.)

Subcutaneous fat necrosis is an inflammatory disorder of adipose tissue that occurs in the newborn infant. Sites of predilection are the buttocks, thighs, back, upper arms, and face. Lesions may be focal or extensive and may be preceded by a brawny edema of the affected skin. Typical well-developed lesions are firm, irregular nodules that may be skin colored or have a red or violaceous hue (Fig 24–36, p. xxxiv). They appear to be tender during the acute phase.

Uncomplicated lesions involute spontaneously within weeks to months, usually without scarring or atrophy. Occasionally, calcium deposition may occur within areas of fat necrosis and at times may result in rupture and drainage of liquid material. Rarely, constitutional symptoms such as hypotonia, poor feeding, vomiting, and fever are complications. Hypercalcemia and hyperlipemia have also been associated.

Fat necrosis in the infant has been attributed to birth trauma, asphyxia, overexposure to cold, and prolonged hypothermia; however, provocative factors are historically absent in many of the affected infants. Susceptibility has been attributed to differences in the composition of the subcutaneous tissue of the young infant as compared to that of older infants and children. Clinical studies have demonstrated a high melting point and an altered ratio of saturated to unsaturated fatty acids. Nevertheless, the etiology and pathogenesis are poorly understood.

Subcutaneous fat necrosis can be confused with sclerema neonatorum, panniculitis, or hematoma. Histologic changes are diagnostic and consist of thickening of the fibrous septa, increased vascularity, crystal deposition within the fat cells, and a granulomatous cellular infiltrate composed of lymphocytes, histiocytes, foreign body giant cells, and fibroblasts. Lipid-stained frozen sections are required to demonstrate the crystals, which are dissolved by fixatives. Since the lesions are self-limited, therapy is not required. Careful needle aspiration of fluctuant lesions may prevent rupture and subsequent scarring; the possibility of introducing infection, however, must be considered.

24.19 DISEASES OF THE SWEAT GLANDS

Miliaria, or *prickly heat,* as it is known to the layman, results from retention of sweat in ducts and pores of the eccrine sweat glands when they are occluded by keratinous plugs. Retrograde pressure may result in rupture of the duct and leakage of sweat into the dermis, where an inflammatory response is evoked. The eruption is most often induced by hot, humid weather, but it may also be caused by high fever. Infants who are kept too warmly dressed indoors may develop this eruption even in wintertime.

In *miliaria crystallina* the lesions are very superficial and noninflammatory. The tiny clear vesicles rupture readily with gentle pressure. They can erupt suddenly and occur in profusion over large areas of the body surface (Fig 24–37). The clarity of the fluid, the extreme superficiality of the vesicles, and the absence of inflammation permit differentiation from other blistering disorders. This type of miliaria occurs most frequently in newborn infants and in older patients with hyperpyrexia. *Miliaria rubra* is a less superficial eruption and is characterized by papulovesicles with intense erythema.

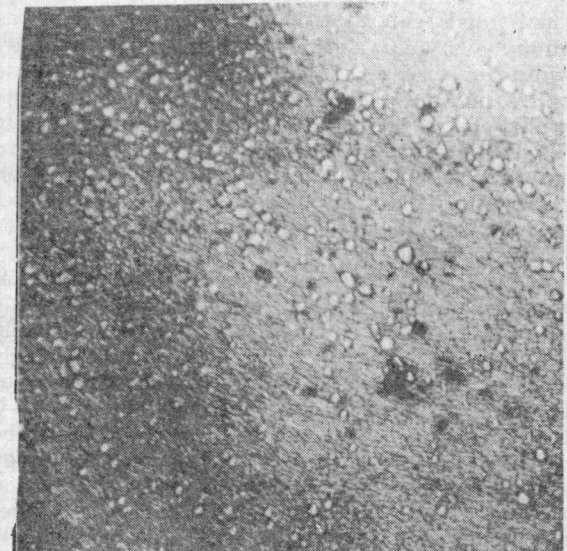

Figure 24–37 Superficial clear vesicles of miliaria crystallina in a patient with hyperpyrexia and lymphoma.

The lesions are usually localized to sites of occlusion or to flexural areas where the skin may become macerated and eroded. This lesion may be confused with or superimposed on other diaper area eruptions including candidiasis and folliculitis. *Pustular miliaria,* unusual in children, is often a consequence of sweat retention associated with an underlying dermatitis.

All forms of miliaria respond dramatically to cooling the patient by regulation of environmental temperatures and removal of excessive clothing and, in patients with fever, to administration of antipyretics. Topical agents are usually ineffective and may exacerbate the eruption. A cool bath is often helpful in alleviating pruritus.

Hidradenitis suppurativa, an inflammatory suppurative disease of the apocrine glands, is a chronic, indolent disorder which involves the axillae and genitocrural area and, rarely, the scalp and mammary and umbilical skin. Onset usually occurs during puberty or early adulthood. The disease is probably initiated by plugging of apocrine gland ducts with keratinous debris. Progressive dilatation below the obstruction leads to rupture of the duct and inflammation and often to secondary bacterial infection. Healing is by fibrosis and scarring. Clinically these patients have solitary or multiple painful, erythematous nodules, deep abscesses, and contracted scars, sharply confined to areas of skin containing apocrine glands. When the disease is severe and chronic, sinus tracts, ulcers, and fistulas develop.

Early lesions are often mistaken for infected epidermal cysts or for furuncles (abscesses of the hair follicles), but the sharp localization to particular areas of the body should suggest hidradenitis.

Systemic antibiotics chosen on the basis of bacterial culture and sensitivity tests should be administered in the acute phase even though such therapy is not always effective. Warm compresses will encourage spontaneous rupture of abscesses; those which are "pointing" should be incised and drained. The addition of a limited course of prednisone (40–60 mg/24 hr) to the regimen of patients who respond poorly to antibiotics may decrease fibrosis and scarring. Axillary shaving and the use of deodorants should be avoided. Ultimately, surgical measures are required for control or cure. Solitary lesions can be excised and closed by primary intention, and sinus tracts and fistulas should be exteriorized and excised. Extensive involvement may require removal of all diseased tissue and placement of skin grafts. Surgical management should not be withheld in the mistaken belief that such an approach is radical.

24.20 DISORDERS OF HAIR

Disorders of hair in infants and children may result from intrinsic disturbances of hair growth; they may be due to structural anomalies of the hair shafts, or they may reflect an underlying biochemical or metabolic defect. Excessive and abnormal hair growth is referred to as hypertrichosis or hirsutism. Deficient hair growth is known as hypotrichosis, and hair loss, which may be partial or complete, is termed alopecia. Alopecia may be classified as nonscarring or scarring; the latter type is rare in children and, if present, is most often due to prolonged or untreated inflammatory conditions such as pyoderma or tinea capitis.

HYPERTRICHOSIS

Hypertrichosis is rare in children and may be localized or generalized, permanent or transient. Localized hypertrichosis is most often due to a heritable condition or to a nevoid defect. Generalized hypertrichosis has a multiplicity of causes; some of them are listed in Table 24–3.

HYPOTRICHOSIS AND ALOPECIA

Some of the disorders associated with hypotrichosis and alopecia are listed in Table 24–4. True alopecia is only rarely congenital; it is more often related to infec-

Table 24–3 CAUSES OF AND CONDITIONS ASSOCIATED WITH HYPERTRICHOSIS

1. *Intrinsic factors*
   Racial and familial forms such as hairy ears, hairy elbows, intraphalangeal hair or generalized hirsutism
2. *Extrinsic factors*
   Local trauma or casts
   Drugs
   Diazoxide, Dilantin, corticosteroids, corticotropin, androgens, anabolic agents, hexachlorobenzene
3. *Hamartomas or nevi*
   Congenital hairy nevus, nevus pilosus, Becker nevus
4. *Endocrine disorders*
   Virilizing ovarian tumors, Cushing syndrome, acromegaly, congenital adrenal hyperplasia, adrenal tumors, gonadal dysgenesis, male pseudohermaphroditism, nonendocrine hormone–secreting tumors
5. *Congenital abnormalities*
   Hypertrichosis lanuginosa, mucopolysaccharidoses, leprechaunism, congenital generalized lipodystrophy, Cornelia de Lange syndrome, craniofacial dysostosis, trisomy 18, Rubinstein-Taybi syndrome, Bloom syndrome, congenital hemihypertrophy

Table 24–4 DISORDERS ASSOCIATED WITH ALOPECIA AND HYPOTRICHOSIS

1. Congenital universal alopecia, atrichia with papular lesions
2. Localized congenital alopecia: aplasia cutis, alopecia triangularis
3. Ectodermal dysplasias
4. Heritable syndromes: Marie Unna hypotrichosis, Cockayne, progeria, Rothmund-Thomson, dyskeratosis congenita, Seckel, cartilage-hair hypoplasia, Conradi, trichorhinophalangeal, pachyonychia congenita, Hallermann-Streiff, Treacher Collins, popliteal web, oculodentodigital, oral-facial-digital, incontinentia pigmenti, focal dermal hypoplasia, keratosis follicularis spinulosa decalvans
5. Metabolic defects: homocystinuria, acrodermatitis enteropathica
6. Hamartomas of the scalp and the hair follicles

tions, an inflammatory dermatosis, drug ingestion, or mechanical factors. Hair loss as well as alterations in texture and quality occur in association with some of the endocrinopathies that involve the ovary, thyroid, parathyroid, adrenal, and pituitary glands. Bacterial, viral, and fungal infections of the scalp may also cause focal or diffuse hair loss. Metabolic disturbances, such as protein deprivation, celiac disease, hypervitaminosis A, and hypozincemia associated with acrodermatitis enteropathica, are additional causes. Any inflammatory condition of the scalp, such as atopic dermatitis and seborrheic dermatitis, if severe enough, may result in partial alopecia. In all these disorders, hair growth will return to normal if the underlying condition is treated successfully unless there has been permanent damage to the hair follicle.

Telogen effluvium, or loss of scalp hair because of premature conversion of growing hairs to the resting phase, accounts for the loss of hair by infants during the 1st few mo of life, for postpartum loss, and for that lost 2–4 mo after an acute febrile illness. Telogen effluvium may also occur after discontinuation of oral contraceptives. There is no inflammatory reaction; the hair follicles remain intact, and telogen bulbs can be demonstrated microscopically on shed hairs. Since more than 50% of the scalp hair is rarely lost, alopecia is usually not severe; the sudden loss of large amounts of hair with brushing, combing, and washing of hair, however, can generate considerable anxiety. Parents should be reassured that normal hair growth will return shortly and alopecia will not be permanent.

Traction alopecia (marginal or traumatic alopecia) that results in follicular damage may be caused by tight braiding or "ponytails," headbands, rubber bands, curlers, and rollers (Fig 24–38A). Associated folliculitis in the parietal areas, if severe, may cause scarring. The alopecia is usually reversible; children and parents must be encouraged to avoid these devices and, if necessary, alter the hair style. Otherwise, irreparable damage to hair follicles may occur.

Toxic alopecia is a side effect of radiation and certain drugs. Cancer chemotherapeutic agents, such as antimetabolites, alkylating agents, and mitotic inhibitors, inhibit synthesis of hair in growing (anagen) follicles. Hairs become dystrophic, and the hair shaft breaks at the narrowed segment. Loss is diffuse, rapid (1–3 wk after treatment), and temporary; regrowth occurs when administration of the drug(s) is discontinued. Thallium, heparin, and the coumarins induce shedding of the hair

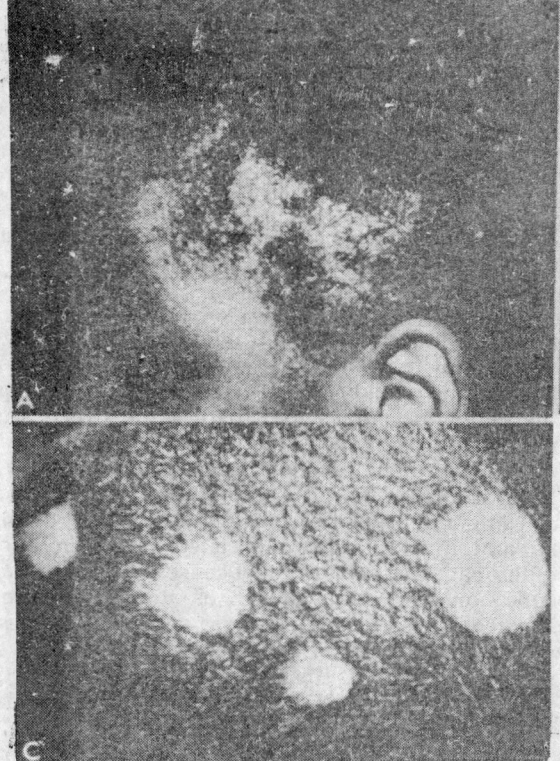
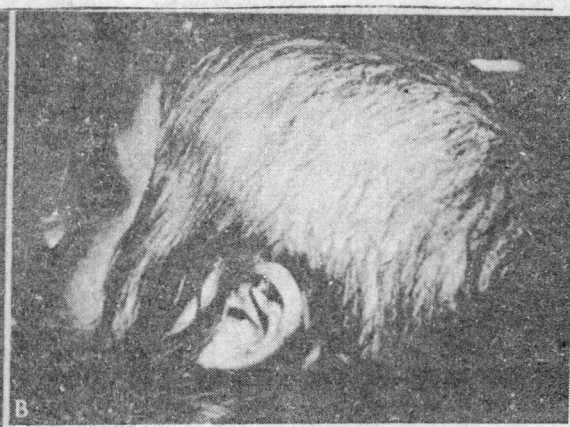

Figure 24–38 *A*, Marginal alopecia due to traction. *B*, Partial alopecia with bizarre pattern typical of trichotillomania. *C*, Multiple areas of total alopecia characteristic of alopecia areata. The scalp is normal.

by converting it from the growing (anagen) to the resting (telogen) phase. Hair loss is diffuse and temporary.

Trichotillomania, or compulsive pulling, twisting, and breaking of hair, is responsible for irregular areas of incomplete hair loss. These are most often located on the crown and in the occipital and parietal areas of the scalp (Fig 24–38*B*), but occasionally eyebrows, eyelashes, and body hair are traumatized. Some plaques of alopecia may have a linear outline. The hairs remaining within the areas of loss are of varying lengths and are typically blunt-tipped because of breakage. The scalp is normal in appearance.

The diagnosis of trichotillomania is often difficult and may require biopsy confirmation. Histologic changes include coexistent normal and damaged follicles, parafollicular hemorrhages, atrophy of some follicles, and catagen transformation of hair. Tinea capitis and alopecia areata must be considered in the differential diagnosis. Parents will often acknowledge that the child frequently plucks or twists the hair. Amelioration of the condition requires the patient's cooperation. Denial on the part of both patient and parents complicates management, and occasionally psychiatric counseling is required. Long-term repeated trauma may result in irreversible damage and permanent alopecia.

Alopecia areata is an idiopathic disorder characterized by rapid and complete loss of hair in round or oval patches on the scalp (Fig 24–38*C*) as well as on other body sites. In *alopecia totalis* all the scalp hair is lost; in *alopecia universalis* body as well as scalp hair is non-

existent. Peripheral spread and confluence of plaques of alopecia areata often result in bizarre patterns. At the margin of active plaques, the hairs can often be extracted with gentle traction and, on examination, demonstrate an attenuated or catagen bulb at the termination of a tapered, poorly pigmented shaft. The skin within the plaques of hair loss is normal in appearance. In patients with severe alopecia, dystrophy of the nails is relatively common.

Although the cause of alopecia areata is unknown, a perifollicular infiltrate of inflammatory round cells is seen in biopsy specimens from affected areas. Emotional factors and stress have been suggested as triggering factors, but supportive evidence is tenuous. A family history of alopecia areata is obtainable in about 20% of patients. The infrequent but striking association with autoimmune diseases, such as Hashimoto thyroiditis, Addison disease, pernicious anemia, collagen diseases, and vitiligo, has suggested an autoimmune pathogenetic mechanism. Some patients have detectable circulating antibodies to thyroglobulin, parietal cells, and adrenal gland. An increased incidence of alopecia areata has also been reported in patients with Down syndrome.

The differential diagnosis includes tinea capitis, seborrheic dermatitis, trichotillomania, traumatic alopecia, and lupus erythematosus. The course is unpredictable since spontaneous resolution is usual, but recurrences are common. In general, onset at a young age and extensive or prolonged hair loss are poor prognostic signs. Alopecia universalis and totalis as well as *ophiasis*, a type of alopecia areata in which hair loss is circumferential, are less likely to resolve permanently.

Treatment is difficult to evaluate since the course is erratic and unpredictable. The use of high-potency topical, fluorinated corticosteroids with occlusion at night is thought to be minimally effective in some patients. Intradermal injections of steroid may also stimulate hair growth locally, but this mode of treatment is impractical in young children or in those with extensive hair loss. Systemic corticosteroid therapy has, on occasion, been associated with good results; however, the permanence of cure is questionable, and the side effects are a serious deterrent. In general, parents and patients can be reassured that spontaneous remission will usually occur. New hair growth may initially be of finer caliber and lighter color, but replacement by normal terminal hair can be expected.

24.21 STRUCTURAL DEFECTS OF HAIR

Structural defects of the hair shaft can be congenital or acquired. Some reflect a known biochemical aberration; others are of unknown cause; and 1, at least, appears to be related to damaging grooming practices. All the defects can be demonstrated by microscopic examination of wet-mount preparations of affected hairs. Scanning and transmission electron microscopy has contributed greatly to an understanding of the structural abnormalities.

Trichorrhexis nodosa is the most common of the structural defects. Clinically, the defect appears as a node or swelling on the hair shaft. Microscopically, it has the appearance of 2 interlocking brushes. The defect is due to a fracture of the hair shaft with derangement of the cells in the cortex. Weakness at the nodal points accounts for the fragility of the shaft, resulting in broken stubs and partial alopecia. Trichorrhexis nodosa has been noted as a congenital defect in some families and has also been observed in some infants with argininosuccinic aciduria.

Acquired trichorrhexis nodosa, the most common cause of hair breakage, occurs in 2 forms. *Proximal defects* are found most frequently in black children, whose complaint is not of alopecia but of the failure of their hair to grow. The hair is short, often in brush-stroke patches; easy breakage is demonstrated by gentle traction on the hair shafts. A history of other affected family members may be obtained. The problem is thought to be caused by a combination of genetic predisposition and the cumulative mechanical trauma of rough combing and brushing, hair straightening procedures, and "permanents." The longitudinal splits, knots, and nodal defects can be demonstrated in wet-mounts. The patient must be cautioned to avoid damaging grooming techniques. A soft, natural-bristle brush and a wide-toothed comb should be used. The condition is self-limited with resolution in 2–4 yr if the patient avoids damaging practices.

Distal trichorrhexis nodosa is seen more frequently in white and oriental children; it also is traumatic in origin. The distal portions of the hair shafts are thinned, ragged, and faded and may have white specks (sometimes mistaken for nits) along the shaft. Wet-mounts reveal the paint-brush defect and the sites of excessive fragility and breakage. Avoidance of diverse insults, including saltwater soaking and traumatic grooming, as well as regular trimming of affected ends and the use of cream rinses to lessen tangling will ameliorate the condition.

Monilethrix, a rare defect of the hair shaft, is inherited as an autosomal dominant trait. The hair appears dry, lusterless, and brittle, and it fractures spontaneously or with mild trauma. Eyebrows, lashes, and body and sexual hair as well as scalp hair may be affected. Keratosis pilaris is always present, and, less commonly, there are other ectodermal defects. Microscopically, a distinctive, regular beading pattern of the hair shafts is evident; the narrowed internodal portions of the shaft lack a medulla and are the sites of fracture. The etiology is unknown, and treatment is ineffective. Spontaneous improvement at puberty has been noted in some children.

Trichorrhexis invaginata (bamboo hair) is a distinguishing feature of the Netherton syndrome. Dry, fragile hair without apparent growth is characteristic. The nodal defects of the shaft have the appearance of a ball and socket joint in which the distal portion has been invaginated into the cup-like proximal portion. The abnormality is thought to result from a transient defect in keratinization. The defects may be identified in body hair as well as scalp hair and seem to decrease in frequency as the child matures. Hair growth may improve significantly at puberty.

Trichoschisis applies to a defect that has the appearance of a clean fracture perpendicular to the hair shaft. Under the light microscope, the hair resembles a flat ribbon and folds back on itself at intervals along the hair shaft. On scanning electron microscopy, near absence of the cuticular hair cells can be demonstrated along with ridging and fluting of the shaft. A zebra-striped pattern of alternating bright and dark bands is characteristic on polarizing microscopy.

Trichoschisis occurs in association with diminished hair sulfur content. Affected children have brittle hair as well as variable intellectual impairment, short stature, ichthyosis, and defects of the teeth, nails, and eyes. It has been suggested that this constellation of findings is inherited as an autosomal recessive trait, and the term trichothiodystrophy has been proposed as a general designation for children with some or all of these features.

Pili torti is a structural defect in which the hair shaft is grooved and flattened at irregular intervals and twisted on its axis in varying degrees. Minor twists that occur in normal hair should not be misconstrued as pili torti. Pili torti is usually first recognized at about 2–3 yr of age, when the hair acquires a striking spangled appearance and increased fragility. The hair is often ash-blond in color.

Both autosomal dominant and recessive forms have been described; most cases, however, are sporadic. Pili torti has, on occasion, been associated with sensorineural hearing loss, mental retardation, and ectodermal defects of the hair and teeth. It has also been observed in patients with Menkes syndrome.

Pili annulati, ringed hair, is characterized by hair

shafts banded with bright rings when viewed in reflected light. The bands are caused by reflection of light from focal aggregates of abnormal air-filled cavities within the hair shafts. The hair is not fragile. The defect may be familial or sporadic.

Pseudo-pili annulati is a variant of normal blond hair; an optical effect caused by the refraction and reflection of light from the flattened and twisted shaft creates the phenomenon of banding.

Wooly hair disease. In this disease a peculiarly tight, curly, abnormal hair has been noted at birth. Three types have been recognized: (1) an autosomal dominant form in which other ectodermal structures and hair color are normal; (2) an autosomal recessive type in which the scalp hair has a bleached appearance and body hair is short and pale; and (3) wooly hair nevus, a sporadic form in which only a portion of the scalp hair is involved.

24.22   DISEASES OF THE NAILS

Nail abnormalities in children are often puzzling; they may be a manifestation of generalized skin disease or of systemic disease. They may also be due to trauma, localized bacterial and fungal infections, or skin diseases involving the nail fold. Diseases that cause nail changes include psoriasis, Reiter disease, Norwegian scabies, lichen planus, lichen striatus, Darier disease, alopecia areata, hypoparathyroidism, and acrodermatitis enteropathica. Nail anomalies are also common in certain congenital disorders (Table 24–5).

Anonychia is absence of the nail plate, usually the result of a congenital disorder or trauma. *Koilonychia* is flattening and concavity of the nail plate with loss of normal contour. *Macronychia* is an abnormally large nail, *micronychia*, an unusually small one. *Leukonychia* is a white opacity of the nail plate that may involve the entire plate or may be punctate or striate; the nail plate, however, remains smooth and undamaged. Leukonychia can be traumatic or may be a benign hereditary defect. *Onychogryphosis* is an acquired defect characterized by a thickened, overgrown, distorted nail plate. *Onycholysis* indicates separation of the nail plate from the nail bed. Common causes are trauma, psoriasis, fungal infection (distal onycholysis), contact dermatitis, and drug-induced phototoxicity. *Beau lines* are transverse grooves in the nail plate that represent an inability of the nail matrix to produce a nail plate of normal thickness. Usually, Beau lines are indicative of periodic

Table 24–5   CONGENITAL DISEASES WITH NAIL DEFECTS

Large nails: Pachyonychia congenita, Rubinstein-Taybi syndrome, hemihypertrophy

Small or absent nails: Syndromes: the ectodermal dysplasias, nail-patella, dyskeratosis congenita, focal dermal hypoplasia, cartilage-hair hypoplasia, Ellis–van Creveld, Larsen, epidermolysis bullosa, incontinentia pigmenti, Rothmund-Thomson, Turner, popliteal web, trisomy 13, trisomy 18, Apert, Gorlin-Pindborg, long arm 21 deletion, otopalatodigital, fetal alcohol, and elfin facies

trauma or episodic shutdown of the nail matrix secondary to a systemic disease.

Pigmentation of an entire nail plate or linear bands of pigmentation are common in black individuals. The pigment is produced by melanocytes in the nail matrix and nail bed and is of no consequence. Pigmentation may also be due to nevus cells in the nail matrix (junctional nevus). Extension or alteration in pigment in the latter lesion should be evaluated by biopsy because of the possibility of malignant change.

Paronychial inflammation is often responsible for dystrophies of the nail plate which are due to damage of the nail matrix; the lesions include bacterial infections, candidiasis, eczema, psoriasis, and lichen striatus. Tumors in the paronychial area include pyogenic granulomas, mucous cysts, and junctional nevi. Periungual fibromas that appear during late childhood should suggest a diagnosis of tuberous sclerosis.

Twenty nail dystrophy, a recently described entity, is a disease of children characterized by longitudinal ridging, fragility, distal notching, and opalescent discoloration of all the nails. The onset is insidious; there are no associated skin or systemic diseases and no other ectodermal defects. It has been suggested that the disorder is due to lichen planus, but the nail dystrophy is never associated with typical skin lesions of lichen planus. The disorder must be differentiated from fungal infections, psoriasis, nail changes of alopecia areata, and nail dystrophy secondary to eczema. Eczema and fungal infections rarely produce changes of all the nails simultaneously. The disorder is self-limited and eventually remits; treatment is ineffective.

24.23   DISEASES OF THE MUCOUS MEMBRANES

The mucous membranes may be involved in developmental disorders, infections, acute and chronic skin diseases, genodermatoses, and benign and malignant tumors. A few of the more common diseases specific to mucous membranes are discussed below.

Fordyce disease is characterized by multiple, yellow-white papules which may be located on the mucosa of the lips and the buccal surface. They are aberrant sebaceous glands and may be found in otherwise normal individuals. They are asymptomatic and require no therapy.

Geographic tongue, or glossitis areata migrans, is seen most often in children and young adults. The lesions consist of sharply demarcated, irregular, smooth red plaques, often with elevated, gray margins. The erythematous areas are due to loss of the normal papillae other than the fungiform ones. The cause is unknown. Symptoms of mild burning or irritation are occasionally bothersome. Onset is rapid, and individual lesions may persist for months. These lesions should not be confused with mucous patches of secondary syphilis. No therapy other than reassurance is necessary.

Cheilitis, or inflammation of the lips and angles of

the mouth (angular cheilitis), may be due to a variety of causes. In children it is commonly due to dryness, chapping, and constant lip-licking; excessive salivation and drooling, particularly in children with neurologic deficits, may also cause chronic irritation. The lesions of oral thrush may occasionally extend to the angles of the mouth. Protection can be provided by frequent applications of a bland ointment such as petrolatum. Candidiasis should be treated with an appropriate antifungal agent and contact dermatitis of the perioral skin with a topical corticosteroid preparation with a lubricant for protection.

Lip pits and fistulas are usually located symmetrically in the vermilion of the lower lip; they represent the mucosa-lined sinus tracts from underlying minor salivary glands. They may occasionally exude a mucous secretion and should be excised for cosmetic reasons.

Mucoceles, or mucous retention cysts, usually form as a result of trauma to the lips or buccal mucosa. Severance of the duct of a mucous gland leads to retention of mucous secretion within the interrupted duct lumen and subsequent cystic dilatation. Lesions are common on the lips, tongue, palate, and buccal mucosa. Those on the floor of the mouth are known as *ranulas* when the submaxillary or sublingual salivary ducts are involved. Fluctuations in size are usual, and the lesions may disappear temporarily after traumatic rupture. Mucoceles must be excised to prevent recurrence.

Aphthous stomatitis (canker sores), recurrent painful ulcers of the oral mucous membranes, is a common condition in which several factors probably play a role. Solitary or multiple lesions occur on the labial, buccal, and lingual mucosa as well as on the sublingual, palatal, and gingival mucosa. Initial lesions are erythematous and indurated papules that erode rapidly to form sharply circumscribed, necrotic ulcers with a gray fibrinous exudate and an erythematous halo. The lesions heal spontaneously in 10–14 days. A more severe form of this disorder in which there are larger, more debilitating lesions is called *periadenitis aphthae.*

Aphthous stomatitis is often cyclical in occurrence. It has been attributed to a variety of causes that include food hypersensitivity, allergic or toxic drug reactions, infectious agents, endocrine factors, emotional stress, and trauma. Immunologic studies have demonstrated lymphocytotoxicity for oral epithelial cells, suggesting a cell-mediated pathogenesis. It is a common misconception that aphthous stomatitis is a manifestation of herpes simplex. Recurrent herpes infections remain localized to the lips and rarely cross the mucocutaneous junction; involvement of the oral mucosa occurs only in primary infections.

Treatment of aphthous stomatitis is extremely difficult and palliative at best. Relief of pain, particularly before eating, may be achieved by use of a topical anesthetic such as viscous Xylocaine or an oral rinse with 1 teaspoonful of elixir of Benadryl. A topical corticosteroid in a mucosal adhering agent (0.1% triamcinolone in Orabase) may be helpful if applied 2–3 times daily. Alternatively, Orabase emollient of Gelusil used as a rinse may provide some relief.

24.24 VASCULITIS

Cutaneous vasculitis can occur as a variable feature of a large number of disorders including connective tissue diseases, infections, and hypersensitivity reactions. Although the morphology of the skin lesions may vary considerably in these diseases, palpable purpura can be regarded as pathognomonic of vasculitis, reflecting the intense inflammatory process in the dermal vessels (Sec 9.64).

Mucha-Habermann disease (pityriasis lichenoides et varioliformis acuta), which can occur at any age, is sometimes classified as a form of parapsoriasis but is, in fact, a type of vasculitis. The eruption is polymorphous; small, red-brown, scaly papules and varicelliform vesicles appear in crops and evolve as papulonecrotic, crusted, hemorrhagic lesions that heal as pitted scars. The anterior trunk and proximal limbs are preferred sites; the palms, soles, and mucous membranes are spared. There are no constitutional signs, and mild itching is often the only symptom.

The disease must be differentiated from varicella, other viral exanthems, papular urticaria, drug eruptions, and other vasculitides. The protracted episodic course of weeks to months (or even years) serves to exclude some of these disorders. The histologic changes are lymphocytic vasculitis, invasion of the epidermis by lymphocytes and erythrocytes, edema, necrosis, and vesicle formation. Cultures of intact lesions are always negative. The general health is unimpaired, and the process eventually resolves spontaneously. There is no effective treatment other than reassurance of the patient.

24.25 CUTANEOUS BACTERIAL INFECTIONS

Impetigo contagiosa, a superficial form of pyoderma, occurs most commonly in children and is most prevalent during the hot, humid summer months. The infection is characterized by erythematous macules that very rapidly evolve into thin-walled vesicles and pustules (Fig 24–39A). The vesicopustular stage is also brief, and, following rupture, sticky, heaped-up, honey-colored crusts are formed (Fig 24–39B). Removal of crusts leaves a moist, red base over which a fresh exudate quickly accumulates. The lesions often spread peripherally and clear centrally to form circinate plaques and gyrate patterns. The infection may be spread to other parts of the body by the fingers, clothing, and towels. The sites usually involved are exposed areas such as the face, neck, and limbs, but lesions may develop anywhere on the body. Insect bites, scabies, cutaneous injuries, and preceding dermatitis serve as portals of entry for the organism, which does not penetrate intact skin. Regional lymphadenopathy is frequently associated.

Impetigo is usually initiated by infection with group A β-hemolytic streptococci, which are present on normal skin. Subsequently, superinfection with staphylo-

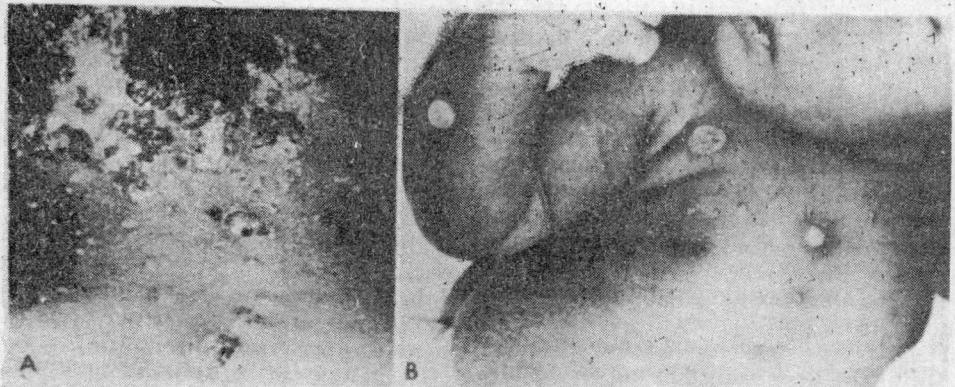

Figure 24–39 *A,* Multiple crusted and oozing lesions of streptococcal impetigo. *B,* Multiple tense and flaccid blisters of bullous impetigo on the trunk and arm of an infant.

cocci, usually of nasal origin, can occur. Thus, streptococci alone or in combination with staphylococci can be isolated from impetiginous lesions. In later stages of the infection, staphylococci may be the only agent isolated by usual means although streptococci are present. Historically, these variable results of culture have led to the belief that staphylococci were initiators of impetigo and could occur alone in this disease. These older concepts have been challenged by the new data.

The strains of streptococci that colonize the skin and cause impetigo are different from the strains that are usually responsible for pharyngeal infection. Although skin strains elaborate streptolysin, hyaluronidase, and DNase B, ASO and antihyluronidase titers are not consistently elevated; anti-DNase B titers are more frequently elevated. The total differential and white blood cell counts and erythrocyte sedimentation rate are usually normal.

Type specificity and virulence of streptococci are associated with their M protein, and only certain types are known to be associated with the development of poststreptococcal acute glomerulonephritis. The incidence of nephritis as a complication of streptococcal impetigo varies considerably in epidemiologic studies and is higher in areas where cutaneous infection is endemic (Sec 16.17).

Impetigo is an indolent but self-limited disease. It should, however, be treated to decrease morbidity and prevent spread to other children. Local measures should include improvement of personal hygiene, compresses with Burow solution applied 4 times a day to remove crusts, and washing with an antibacterial soap. Systemic antibiotic therapy will result in more rapid recovery; penicillin is the drug of choice. Intramuscular benzathine penicillin is the most efficacious preparation when inadequate compliance with oral therapy can be expected. Oral erythromycin is a suitable alternative for penicillin-allergic patients. Topical antibiotics such as bacitracin or neosporin are less effective in eradicating the organisms. Although the staphylococci are often penicillin-resistant, in most instances penicillin will eradicate the infection, a fact that further supports the presumed secondary role of the staphylococcus in impetigo contagiosa. Early treatment of impetigo caused by nephritogenic strains of streptococci does not appear to lessen the occurrence of acute glomerulonephritis.

Ecthyma resembles impetigo in onset and appearance but gradually evolves into a deeper, more chronic infection. The initial lesion is a vesicle or vesicopustule with an erythematous base that erodes through the epidermis into the dermis to form an ulcer with elevated margins. The ulcer becomes obscured by a dry, heaped-up, tightly adherent crust that contributes to the persistence of the infection and to scar formation. Lesions vary in size and may be as large as 4 cm. Sites of predilection are the legs, where trauma probably plays a major role. Pruritic lesions such as insect bites, scabies, or pediculosis, which are subject to frequent scratching, act as a focus for the infection.

The causative agent is usually a β-hemolytic streptococcus; the lesions are infectious and may be spread by autoinoculation. Crusts should be softened by frequent warm compresses and then removed with an antibacterial soap or hydrogen peroxide. Systemic antibiotic therapy, as for impetigo, is indicated.

Blistering distal dactylitis is a β-hemolytic streptococcal infection of the fingertips. The superficial bullae are located over the volar fat pad on the distal portion of the fingers or thumb. If left untreated, they may continue to enlarge and extend to the paronychial area. Polymorphonuclear leukocytes and chains of gram-positive cocci are demonstrable in the purulent exudate obtained from the blister. The infection responds to incision and drainage and a 10-day course of systemic penicillin or erythromycin.

Bullous impetigo is a localized skin infection that is sometimes regarded as a form of the staphylococcal scalded skin syndrome because it is also caused by group 2 phage types of *Staphylococcus aureus*. It is mainly an infection of infants and children. Typical bullae arise on normal skin or have a narrow, erythematous halo; they are filled with a clear, pale to dark yellow fluid which may become turbid if the bullae remain intact. The blisters are relatively superficial and rupture easily, leaving a moist denuded base that is rapidly covered with a thin crust. The skin adjacent to the blister is firmly attached to the underlying layers. The lesions occasionally become widespread, particularly in young infants, but they rarely have systemic manifestations.

The differential diagnosis in the neonate includes epidermolysis bullosa, bullous mastocytosis, herpetic infections, and early scalded skin syndrome. In older children, erythema multiforme, chronic bullous dermatosis of childhood, pemphigus, and pemphigoid must be considered, particularly if the lesions fail to respond to therapy. Examination of smears of blister fluid will disclose polymorphonuclear leukocytes and clusters of gram-positive cocci. Cultures of fluid from an intact blister should yield the causative agent; when the patient appears ill, blood cultures should be obtained. Bullae will rupture and dry rapidly with frequent application of wet compresses followed by gentle cleansing. Localized lesions can be treated with a topical antibiotic such as Polysporin, 3–4 times daily. Patients with widespread lesions and small infants should receive a 5–7 day course of oral therapy with a penicillinase-resistant penicillin. Cephalexin or erythromycin may be substituted in the case of the penicillin-allergic patient.

Staphylococcal scalded skin syndrome (Ritter disease) is, almost without exception, a disease of infants and children under 10 yr of age. In most instances it appears to be caused by a group 2 phage type *Staphylococcus aureus* although, rarely, group 1 phage types have been isolated. The clinical manifestations are due to the elaboration of an exotoxin (exfoliatin) by the infecting strain of bacteria. This extracellular toxin is distinct from other staphylococcal toxins. The toxin has reproduced the disease in both animal models and human volunteers.

The onset of the rash may be preceded by a prodrome of malaise, fever, and irritability associated with exquisite tenderness of the skin, or the appearance of generalized erythema may be abrupt without preceding symptoms. Initially, the eruption is macular and involves the face, neck, axilla, and groin; rapid extension is usual, and the brightly erythematous skin may acquire a wrinkled appearance due to the formation of ill-defined flaccid bullae filled with clear fluid. At this stage, areas of epidermis may separate in response to gentle stroking (the characteristic Nikolsky sign). Facial edema and perioral crusting are usual and result in a typically lugubrious facies. As large sheets of epidermis peel away, moist, glistening, denuded areas become apparent, initially in the flexures and subsequently over much of the body surface (Fig 24–40, p. xxxiv). These areas dry quickly and heal by postinflammatory desquamation, which begins within 2–3 days. Additional variable findings include pharyngitis, conjunctivitis, and superficial erosions of the oral mucous membranes. Although some patients appear desperately ill, many are reasonably comfortable except for the marked skin tenderness. Once the desquamative phase has started, healing proceeds at a rapid rate and is complete in 10–14 days.

A presumed abortive form of the disease (resembling *scarlet fever*) is less dramatic in presentation. The facial appearance is similar to that of the classic scalded skin syndrome, but the generalized scarlatiniform eruption, which may be accentuated in the flexural areas, never progresses to blister formation. In these patients Nikolsky sign may be negative.

It is important to recognize that the portal of entry for the toxin-producing staphylococcus may be a preceding impetiginous skin eruption, conjunctivitis, gastroenteritis, or pharyngitis. Cultures, therefore, should be obtained from all suspected sites of infection and from the blood, although septicemia is a rare complication. Intact bullae are consistently sterile, unlike those of bullous impetigo; the organism, however, may be cultured from other cutaneous sites.

In staphylococcal scalded skin syndrome the site of blister cleavage is the granular layer, the feature that accounts for the rapid healing of denuded areas of skin. Scattered acantholytic cells are evident in the cleft-like bullae; mild edema and vascular ectasia are present in the dermis, but the absence of inflammatory infiltrate is striking. Ultrastructural studies have consistently demonstrated separation of the 2 halves of the desmosome without preceding cytolysis or demonstrable removal of the cellular surface.

The differential diagnosis varies with the presentation and age of the child. Incipient scalded skin syndrome in infants may be mistaken for bullous impetigo, epidermolysis bullosa, epidermolytic hyperkeratosis, a type of ichthyosis, or boric acid poisoning. Florid lesions of the scalded skin syndrome in older children may mimic erythema multiforme, toxic epidermal necrolysis of the drug-induced type (Lyell disease), pemphigus, and other blistering disorders. Toxic epidermal necrolysis can often be distinguished by a history of drug ingestion, absence of severe skin tenderness, a positive Nikolsky sign only at the site of erythema, absence of perioral crusting, and a deeper blister cleavage plane. A frozen biopsy specimen of exfoliated epidermis provides a rapid means to distinguish the scalded skin syndrome from toxic epidermal necrolysis since the entire thickness of epidermis will be exfoliated only in the latter. The scarlatiniform variety of scalded skin syndrome is most frequently mistaken for streptococcal scarlet fever, but it lacks the palatal enanthem, strawberry tongue, and perioral pallor of scarlet fever. Drug eruptions and other hypersensitivity reactions must also be considered in the differential diagnosis.

Systemic therapy, either orally or parenterally, with one of the semisynthetic penicillinase-resistant penicillins should be prescribed since the staphylococci are usually penicillin-resistant. Corticosteroid therapy is not indicated and may be hazardous. The skin should be gently moistened and cleansed with Burow solution, isotonic saline, or 0.25% silver nitrate compresses. During the desquamative phase, applications of a bland nonocclusive emollient will provide lubrication and decrease itching. Topical antibiotics are unnecessary. Recovery is usually rapid, but occasionally complicating factors such as excessive fluid loss, electrolyte imbalance, faulty temperature regulation, pneumonia, septicemia, and cellulitis cause increased morbidity. The skin lesions, if uncomplicated, should heal without scarring.

Folliculitis is a superficial infection of the hair follicle which is most often caused by *Staphylococcus aureus*. The lesions are typically small, dome-shaped pustules with an erythematous base; they are located at the mouth of the pilosebaceous canals. Hair growth is unimpaired. Favored sites include the scalp, extremities, and perioral and paranasal areas. Poor hygiene, maceration, and drainage from wounds and abscesses can be provocative factors. Folliculitis can also occur as a result of tar therapy or occlusive wraps; the moist environment encourages bacterial proliferation.

The causative organism can be identified by Gram stain and culture of the pus. Treatment includes frequent cleansing; the use of an antibacterial soap may be helpful. Local antibiotic therapy is usually all that is required. In chronic recurrent folliculitis, daily application of a benzoyl peroxide lotion or gel may facilitate resolution.

Furuncles and **carbuncles** are follicular lesions that may originate from a preceding folliculitis or may arise initially as a deep-seated, tender, erythematous nodule. Although lesions are initially indurated, central necrosis and suppuration follow and lead to rupture and discharge of a central core of necrotic tissue. Pain may be intense if the lesion is situated in an area where the skin is relatively fixed such as in the external auditory canal or over the nasal cartilages. Sites of predilection are the face, neck, buttocks, and axillae. Confluent furuncles with multiple drainage points are termed carbuncles. Furuncles may become chronic and recurrent, particularly in obese individuals and in those with poor hygiene and hyperhidrosis.

Patients with furuncles usually have no constitutional symptoms, whereas carbuncles may be accompanied by fever, leukocytosis, and bacteremia. The causative agent is almost always *Staphylococcus aureus* though, rarely, other bacteria or fungi may be responsible. For this reason, Gram stain and culture of the pus are indicated.

Initial treatment should consist of frequent applications of hot, moist compresses to encourage localization and drainage. Large lesions may be drained by a small incision or by repeated needle aspirations but should not be tampered with until fluctuant. Lesions in the paranasal area should not be incised because of the danger of extension to the cavernous sinus. Carbuncles and large or multiple furuncles should be treated with systemic antibiotics. Since penicillinase-producing staphylococci are frequently involved, 1 of the penicillinase-resistant penicillins, e.g., cloxacillin orally or oxacillin parenterally, should be used. The penicillin-allergic patient can be treated with 1 of the cephalosporins.

Treatment of chronic furunculosis is often difficult. Attention to personal hygiene, the use of an antibacterial soap, and frequent hand washing may be beneficial.

Pitted keratolysis arises in chronically moist and macerated skin and is most often attributable to the wearing of occlusive footgear or to frequent swimming. The lesions consist of plaques of irregularly shaped, superficial erosions of the horny layer which produce crateriform defects on the soles. Occasionally they become secondarily infected. Although usually mild and asymptomatic, the lesions may be quite painful.

The etiologic agent is thought to be a species of keratinophilic diphtheroid. A KOH preparation of scrapings from the lesion demonstrates filamentous coccobacilli. Of the various therapeutic agents that have been tried, 20% formalin solution in Aquaphor applied topically and avoidance of maceration have been the most effective measures.

Erythrasma is a benign chronic superficial infection of the skin in adolescents, particularly obese ones, and occurs more commonly in warmer climates. It is caused by the filamentous diphtheroid, *Corynebacterium minutissimum*. The most frequently affected sites are moist intertriginous areas such as the groin, axillae, and toe webs. Sharply demarcated, brownish-red, slightly scaly macular patches are characteristic of the disease. Mild pruritus is the only constant symptom.

The diagnosis is readily made by examination with a Wood lamp; the lesions fluoresce to a brilliant coral-red color under ultraviolet light. The gram-positive pleomorphic coccobacilli can be cultured on routine laboratory media.

Erythrasma can be differentiated from dermatophyte infections and from tinea versicolor by the Wood lamp examination. A 10–14 day course of orally administered erythromycin is usually curative. Recurrence may be inhibited by frequent cleansing with an antibacterial soap.

Tuberculosis of the skin. Primary cutaneous tuberculosis is rare in the United States but occurs with the greatest frequency in infants and children. Primary lesions result when *Mycobacterium tuberculosis* is inoculated at a site of injury on the skin or mucous membranes. Sites of predilection are the chin, lips, nose, limbs, and genitalia. The initial lesion, referred to as a *tuberculous chancre,* develops 2–3 wk after introduction of the organism into the damaged tissue. A red-brown papule gradually enlarges and ulcerates, forming an indolent, firm, sharply demarcated ulcer. Some lesions acquire a crust resembling impetigo, and others become heaped-up and verrucous at the margins. Regional adenopathy with or without lymphangitis appears at approximately 3–4 wk.

The primary lesion is a tuberculoid granuloma with caseation necrosis. *M. tuberculosis* is demonstrable in the skin lesion and local lymph nodes. Clinically, the lesions can resemble syphilitic chancres or deep fungal infections. Spontaneous healing coincides with acquisition of immunity, at which time the skin lesions and infected nodes may become calcified. Antituberculous therapy is indicated (Sec 10.52).

Miliary tuberculosis may rarely be manifested cutaneously. The skin lesions result from bloodstream invasion by massive numbers of mycobacteria. The eruption consists of symmetrically distributed, erythematous papules that ulcerate and crust and may become purpuric. Subcutaneous gummatous nodules are often associated. Tubercle bacilli are readily identified in an active lesion. A fulminant course should be anticipated, and aggressive antituberculous therapy is indicated.

Lupus vulgaris is, fortunately, relatively rare today and represents reinfection tuberculosis in children with immunity induced by previous infection. Infection follows traumatic cutaneous inoculation of mycobacteria or the drainage of a tuberculous lymph node. Typical lesions consist of tiny red papules that evolve into small nodules. When examined by diascopy, these lesions are discerned as sharply marginated, yellow-brown macules. Relentless progression occurs by peripheral spread and coalescence of nodules to form irregular plaques of varying sizes, often with central spontaneous healing. These lesions usually ulcerate and cause extreme disfigurement with eventual formation of atrophic and hypertrophic scars.

Lupus vulgaris occurs most frequently on the head and neck, but no site is exempt. Lesions involving the nasal, buccal, and conjunctival mucosa may cause extensive facial deformity. Chronicity is characteristic, and persistence of plaques for many yr is not uncommon. The histopathologic changes are those of a tuberculoid granuloma without caseation; organisms are extremely difficult to demonstrate. Small lesions of lupus vulgaris can be excised; the administration of antituberculous drugs will usually halt further spread and induce involution.

Scrofuloderma is caused by infection of the skin from caseous tuberculous cervical lymph nodes. The infection is initiated in the larynx and is believed to be caused most often by the ingestion of milk containing *M. tuberculosis*. The lymph nodes become enlarged and fluctuant, stretching the overlying skin, which may slough, forming ulcerations and multiple draining sinuses. Healing results in cord-like cicatrices.

Caseous tubercles can be demonstrated in the deep dermis and subcutaneous tissue. Tubercle bacilli are readily identified.

Scrofuloderma may occasionally resemble actinomycosis, sporotrichosis, or pyogenic lymphadenitis. The course is predictably indolent, but constitutional symptoms are typically absent. Antituberculous therapy is usually effective.

Tuberculids represent a variety of noninfectious cutaneous lesions and have been ascribed to hypersensitivity to the tubercle bacillus. The most commonly observed reaction pattern is the *papulonecrotic tuberculid*; lesions appear in crops of symmetrically distributed, sterile papules that undergo central ulceration and eventually heal, leaving sharply delineated, circular, depressed scars. Preferred sites are the extensor aspects of the limbs and the dorsum of the hand and foot. Histologically, nonspecific inflammation, tubercles, and minimal caseation coexist with an obliterative vasculitis of the deep dermis. The duration of the eruption is variable, but disappearance usually follows eradication of the primary infection.

Lichen scrofulosorum, another form of tuberculid, is characterized by grouped, pinhead-sized, pink or red papules which form large plaques, mainly on the trunk. Clinically and histologically, the eruption can simulate sarcoidosis; in such instances hypersensitivity to tuberculin is supportive evidence of tuberculous disease. Healing occurs without scarring.

Atypical mycobacterial infection (swimming pool granuloma) may be responsible for cutaneous lesions in children; *M. marinum*, an organism found in saltwater fish and in swimming pools, is responsible for most of the infections. Swimming pool granulomas are usually initiated by traumatic abrasion of the skin, which serves as a portal of entry for the organism; the knees and elbows are most often affected. Approximately 3 wk after inoculation with the organism, single or multilple reddish papules develop and enlarge slowly to form violaceous nodules. Occasionally the lesions break down and become covered with adherent brown crusts.

Systemic signs and symptoms, including regional lymphadenopathy, are absent.

M. marinum granulomas may mimic sporotrichosis or pyoderma. A biopsy specimen of a fully developed lesion will demonstrate a granulomatous infiltrate with tuberculoid architecture and caseation necrosis; intracellular organisms can be identified within the histiocytes with appropriate stains. Cultures of material obtained from the granuloma must be incubated at 30–33°C since *M. marinum* does not grow at 37°C. This organism is a photochromogen; therefore, colonies will change color (white to yellow) on exposure to daylight.

There is no specific treatment since these organisms are resistant to antituberculous drugs. Minocycline hydrochloride has been effective in some instances. Surgical excision may be curative for small lesions; however, recurrences are not uncommon. Spontaneous healing can be expected within a period of several yr.

24.26 CUTANEOUS FUNGAL INFECTIONS

Tinea versicolor is a rather common, innocuous, chronic fungus infection caused by the dimorphic yeast *Pityrosporon orbiculare (Malassezia furfur)*. The lesions vary widely in color; in white individuals they are typically reddish-brown, whereas in Blacks they may be either hypo- or hyperpigmented. The characteristic macules, which are covered with a fine scale, often begin in a perifollicular location, enlarge, and merge to form confluent patches, most commonly on the neck, upper chest, back, and upper arms (Fig 24–41A). Facial lesions are not unusual in the adolescent, and occasionally lesions are observed on the forearms, the dorsum of the hands, and the pubis. There may be little or no pruritus. Involved areas do not tan following sun exposure.

P. orbiculare exists as part of the normal flora, predominantly in the yeast form, but proliferation of filamentous forms occurs in the disease state. Predisposing factors include excessive sweating, high plasma cortisol levels, debilitating diseases, and genetically determined susceptibility. The disease is most prevalent in adolescents and young adults.

Examination with a Wood lamp will disclose a deep gold fluorescence. A KOH preparation of scrapings is diagnostic, demonstrating groups of thick-walled spores and myriads of short, thick, angular hyphae (Fig 24–41B).

Tinea versicolor must be distinguished from dermatophyte infections and scaling disorders such as seborrheic dermatitis and pityriasis alba. Nonscaling pigmentary disorders such as postinflammatory pigmentary change may be mimicked if the patient has removed the scales by scrubbing.

Many therapeutic agents can be used to treat this disease successfully; however, it must be appreciated that the causative agent is a normal human saprophyte, and the disorder will recur in predisposed individuals. Appropriate therapy may include one of the following:

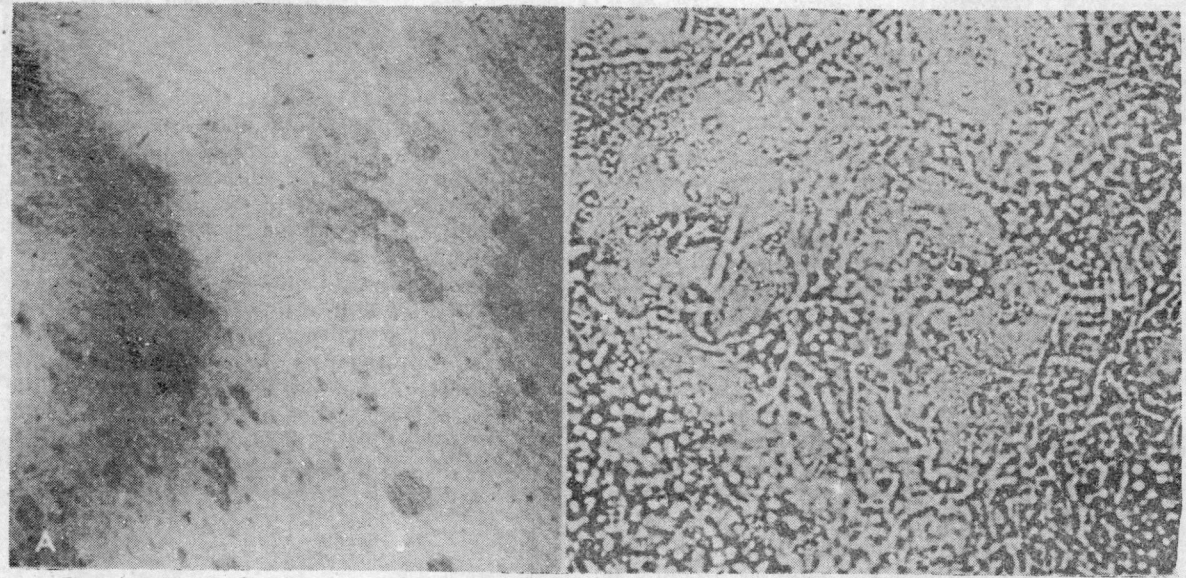

Figure 24–41 *A,* Hyperpigmented, sharply demarcated macules of varying sizes on the upper trunk characteristic of tinea versicolor. *B,* KOH preparation of *Pityrosporon orbiculare* demonstrating short, thick hyphae and clusters of spores.

a selenium sulfide suspension applied for 4 consecutive evenings and repeated the following week; 25% sodium hyposulfite solution or 25% sodium thiosulfate lotion applied twice daily for 2–4 wk; lotions, ointments, or creams containing 3–6% salicylic acid twice daily for 2–4 wk; haloprogin, miconazole, or clotrimazole twice daily for 2–4 wk. The latter antifungal agents are relatively expensive. Recurrent episodes continue to respond promptly to the above agents.

24.27 THE DERMATOPHYTOSES

The **dermatophytoses (ringworm)** are caused by a group of closely related filamentous fungi with a propensity for invading the stratum corneum, hair, and nails. The 3 principal genera responsible for dermatophyte infections are *Trichophyton, Microsporum,* and *Epidermophyton.* The *Trichophyton* species cause lesions of all keratinized tissue, including skin, nails, and hair; the *Microsporum* species principally invade the hair, and the *Epidermophyton* species, the intertriginous skin. The dermatophytic infections are designated by the word tinea followed by the Latin word for the anatomic site of involvement. The dermatophytes are also classified according to source and natural habitat. Fungi acquired from the soil are called *geophilic,* those from animals, *zoophilic;* dermatophytes acquired from humans are referred to as *anthropophilic. Epidermophyton* infections are transmitted only by humans, but various species of *Trichophyton* and *Microsporum* can be acquired from both human and nonhuman sources.

Anthropophilic dermatophytes apparently elicit a delayed-type hypersensitivity response in the infected host, although some dermatophytes, most notably the zoophilic species, tend to elicit a more severe, suppurative inflammation in humans. Some degree of resistance to reinfection apparently is acquired by most infected persons and may be associated with a positive delayed hypersensitivity response. Although humoral immunity to dermatophytes can be detected by serologic techniques, no relationship between circulating antibody and resistance to infection has been demonstrated.

Occasionally a secondary skin eruption referred to as a dermatophytid or "id" reaction appears in sensitized individuals and has been attributed to circulating fungal antigens derived from the primary infection. The eruption occurs most frequently on the fingers, hands, and arms and is characterized by grouped papules, vesicles, and occasionally sterile pustules. Symmetrical urticarial lesions and a more generalized maculopapular eruption can also occur. Id reactions are most often associated with tinea pedis but also occur with tinea capitis and, in the latter instance, most often appear as scattered papulovesicular follicular lesions on the trunk.

The important diagnostic procedures for the various dermatophyte diseases include examination with a Wood lamp of infected hairs, microscopic examination of potassium hydroxide (KOH) preparations of infected material, and cultural identification of the etiologic agent. Hairs infected with common *Microsporum* species fluoresce to a bright blue-green color; most *Trichophyton*-infected hairs do not fluoresce.

Tinea capitis is a dermatophyte infection of the scalp most often caused by the species *Microsporum audouini, Microsporum canis,* or *Trichophyton tonsurans* and much less commonly by other microsporum and trichophyton species. In microsporum and some trichophyton infections, the spores are distributed in a sheath-like fashion around the hair shaft (ectothrix infection), whereas *T. tonsurans* produces an infection within the hair shaft. The clinical presentation of tinea capitis varies with the infecting organism. The pattern produced by *M. audouini* is characterized initially by a small papule at the base of a hair follicle. The infection spreads peripherally, forming an erythematous and scaly circular plaque within which the infected hairs become brittle and broken. Multiple, confluent patches of alopecia develop, and the patient may complain of severe pruritus. Although *M. audouini* infection was formerly the most common type of scalp ringworm, this organism is no longer ubiquitous. Endothrix infections such as those caused by *T. tonsurans* create a pattern known as "black-dot ringworm"; it is characterized initially by multiple, small, circular patches with only a few hairs involved; they are broken off close to the hair follicle and create a polka-dot appearance. This organism also may produce a chronic and more diffuse alopecia (Fig 24–42A). A severe inflammatory response will produce elevated, boggy granulomatous masses (*kerions*); they are often studded with sterile pustules (Fig 24–42B). Permanent scarring and alopecia may result. *Favus*, a form of tinea capitis that is rare in the United States, is caused by the fungus *Trichophyton schoenleini*; it is characterized by development of scaly, erythematous patches with yellow, honeycomb-like crust and a dull green fluorescence under the Wood lamp.

M. audouini and *T. tonsurans* are anthropophilic species acquired most often by contact with infected hairs and epithelial cells that are on such surfaces as theater seats, hats, and combs. Dermatophyte spores may also be airborne within the immediate environment, and high carriage rates have been demonstrated in noninfected schoolmates. *Microsporum canis* is a zoophilic species whose preferred hosts are cats and dogs; children acquire it from them.

In microsporum-infected lesions a characteristic bright green fluorescence is seen at the base of each hair on examination with the Wood lamp, whereas lesions caused by *T. tonsurans* fail to fluoresce. Microscopic examination of a KOH preparation of infected hair from the active border of a lesion discloses tiny spores surrounding the hair shaft in microsporum infections and chains of spores within the hair shaft in *T. tonsurans* infections. Fungal elements are not seen on scales. A specific etiologic diagnosis of tinea capitis may be obtained by planting infected hairs on Sabouraud medium or Mycosel agar; such identification may require 2 wk or more.

Tinea capitis can be confused with seborrheic dermatitis, psoriasis, alopecia areata, trichotillomania, and certain dystrophic hair disorders. When inflammation is pronounced, as in kerion, primary or secondary bacterial infection must also be considered. In adolescents, the patchy, motheaten type of alopecia associated with secondary syphilis may resemble tinea capitis.

Oral administration of griseofulvin microcrystalline (10 mg/kg/24 hr) is recommended for all forms of tinea capitis. Treatment may be necessary for 4–8 wk and should be terminated only after examination by the Wood lamp or KOH preparation is negative. Adverse reactions to griseofulvin include gastrointestinal disturbances, headache, rare blood dyscrasias, and hepatotoxicity. Although the possible carcinogenicity of this antibiotic is unconfirmed, use of it should be reserved for indicated diseases.

Topical therapy alone is ineffective; it may be an important adjunct since it may decrease the shedding of spores. For this purpose vigorous shampooing with antiseborrheic preparations and/or application of mild keratolytic agents may be used. It is not necessary to shave the scalp.

Tinea corporis, or dermatophytic infection of the skin of the face, trunk, and extremities, can be caused by most of the dermatophyte species although *Trichophyton rubrum* and *Trichophyton mentagrophytes* are the most prevalent etiologic organisms. In children, infections with *Microsporum canis* are also frequent. The most typical clinical lesion begins as a dry, mildly erythematous, elevated, scaly papule or plaque and spreads centrifugally as it clears centrally to form the characteristic annular lesion responsible for the designation "ringworm" (Fig 24–43). At times plaques with advancing borders may spread over large areas. Grouped pustules are another variant. Although most lesions clear spontaneously within several mo, some may become chronic. Central clearing does not always occur, and differences in host response may result in tremendous variability in the clinical apparance, e.g., granu-

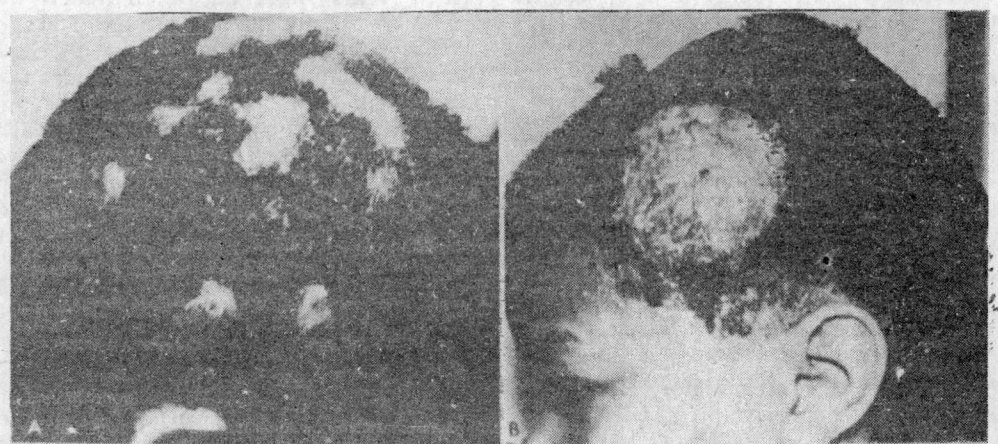

Figure 24–42 *A*, Patchy alopecia associated with tinea capitis. *B*, Elevated, boggy granuloma with multiple pustules (kerion) due to inflammatory tinea capitis.

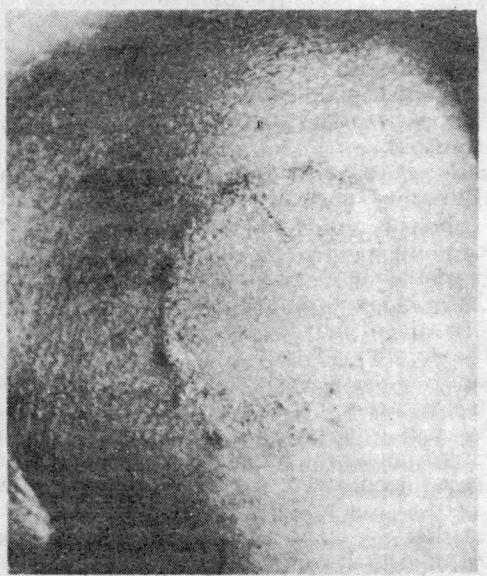

Figure 21—43 Circinate lesion of tinea corporis on the shoulder. Note the active papular border, scaling, and relative clearing centrally.

lomatous lesions and the kerion-like lesions referred to as tinea profunda.

Tinea corporis can be acquired by direct contact with infected persons or by contact with infected scales or hairs deposited on environmental surfaces. *M. canis* infections are usually acquired from infected pets. Not infrequently, a single dermatophyte lesion is responsible for dissemination.

Many skin lesions, both infectious and noninfectious, must be differentiated from the lesions of tinea corporis. Those most frequently confused are granuloma annulare, nummular eczema, pityriasis rosea, psoriasis, seborrheic dermatitis, and tinea versicolor. Microscopic examination of KOH wet mount preparations or cultures should always be obtained when fungal infection is considered.

Tinea corporis will usually respond to treatment with 1 of the topical antifungal agents (haloprogin, tolnaftate, miconazole, clotrimazole) twice daily for 2–4 wk. In usually severe or extensive disease, a course of therapy with oral griseofulvin microcrystalline may be required for several wk.

Tinea cruris, or dermatophyte infection of the groin, occurs most often in adolescent males and is usually caused by the anthropophilic species, *Epidermophyton floccosum* or *Trichophyton rubrum,* but occasionally by the zoophilic species *Trichophyton mentagrophytes.* The initial lesion is a small, raised, scaly, erythematous patch on the inner aspect of the thigh which spreads peripherally, often developing multiple tiny vesicles at the advancing margin. It eventually forms bilateral, irregular, sharply bordered patches with hyperpigmented, scaly centers. In some instances, particularly in infections of *T. mentagrophytes,* the inflammatory reaction is more severe, and the infection may spread beyond the crural region. Pruritus may be severe initially but abates as the inflammatory reaction subsides. Bacterial super-

infection may alter the clinical appearance, and erythrasma or candidiasis may coexist with the dermatophytosis. Tinea cruris is more prevalent in obese persons and in those who perspire excessively and wear tight-fitting clothing.

The diagnosis is confirmed by culture and by demonstrating septate hyphae on a KOH preparation of epidermal scrapings. Tinea cruris must be differentiated from intertrigo, allergic contact dermatitis, candidiasis, and erythrasma. Bacterial superinfection must be excluded when there is a severe inflammatory reaction.

The patient should be advised to use a bland absorbent powder and to wear loose cotton underwear. Topical therapy with clotrimazole or miconazole is recommended for severe infection, especially since these agents are effective in mixed candidal-dermatophyte infections. Pure dermatophyte infection may also be treated with haloprogin or tolnaftate.

Tinea pedis (athlete's foot), a dermatophyte infection of the toe webs and soles of the feet, is uncommon in young children but occurs with some frequency in preadolescent and adolescent males. The usual etiologic agents are *Trichophyton rubrum, Trichophyton mentagrophytes,* and *Epidermophyton floccosum.* Most commonly the toe webs in the 3rd and 4th interdigital spaces and the subdigital crevice are fissured with maceration and peeling of the surrounding skin. Severe tenderness, itching, and a persistent, foul odor are characteristic. These lesions may become chronic, but they can usually be treated effectively. Less commonly, a chronic, diffuse hyperkeratosis of the sole of the foot occurs with only mild erythema. This type of infection is more refractory to treatment and tends to recur.

An inflammatory, vesicular type of reaction may occur with *T. mentagrophytes* infection; this type is most common in young children. These lesions involve any area of the foot, including the dorsal surface, and are usually circumscribed. The initial papules progress to vesicles and bullae which may become pustular (Fig 24–44). A number of factors, such as occlusive footwear and warm, humid weather, predispose to infection. The disease may be transmitted in shower facilities and swimming pool areas. Despite its severity, the infection tends to resolve spontaneously.

Tinea pedis must be differentiated from simple maceration and peeling of the interdigital spaces, which is common in children. Infection with *Candida albicans* and with a variety of bacterial organisms may cause confusion or may coexist with primary tinea pedis. Contact dermatitis, dyshidrotic eczema, and atopic dermatitis also simulate tinea pedis. Fungal mycelia can be demonstrated by microscopic examination of a KOH preparation and/or by culture; the 4th toe web provides a high yield of infected scales; a blister top can also be utilized.

Simple measures such as avoidance of occlusive footwear, careful drying between the toes after bathing, and the use of an absorbent antifungal powder such as zinc undecylenate may suffice for milder infections. Topical therapy with clotrimazole or miconazole is curative in most instances; each of these agents is also effective against candidal infection. Haloprogin and tolnaftate can be used in uncomplicated dermatophyte

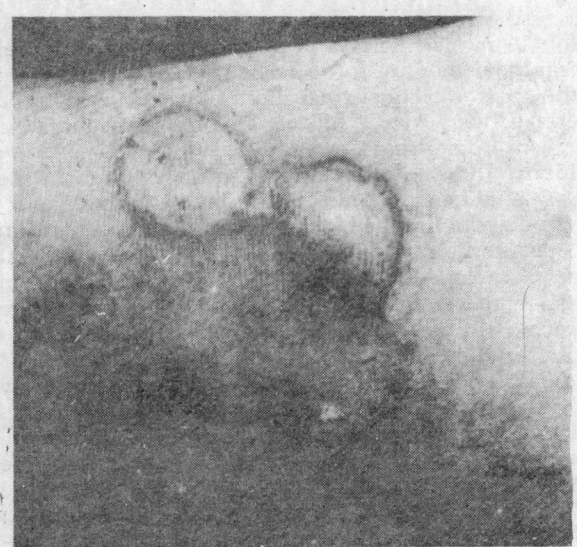

Figure 24—44   Multiple inflammatory bullae of tinea pedis.

infections. Several wk of therapy may be necessary, and low-grade, chronic infections, particularly those caused by *Trichophyton rubrum*, may be refractory. In such patients, oral griseofulvin therapy may effect a cure. Response may be only temporary, however, since infection may recur.

Tinea unguium is a dermatophyte infection of the nail plate; it occurs most often in patients with tinea pedis, but it may occur as a primary infection. It can be caused by a number of dermatophytes, of which *Trichophyton rubrum* and *Trichophyton mentagrophytes* are the most common. The most superficial form of tinea unguium is often due to *T. mentagrophytes*; it is manifested by irregular, single, or multiple white patches on the surface of the nail unassociated with paronychial inflammation or deep infection. *T. rubrum* generally causes a more invasive, subungual infection that is initiated at the lateral distal margins of the nail and often preceded by mild paronychia. The middle and ventral layers of the nail plate, and perhaps the nail bed, are the sites of infection. The nail initially develops a yellowish discoloration and slowly becomes thickened, brittle, and loosened from the nail bed. In advanced infection the nail may turn dark brown to black and may crack or break off.

Tinea unguium must be differentiated from a variety of dystrophic nail disorders. Changes due to trauma, psoriasis, lichen planus, and eczema can all be confused with tinea unguium. Nails infected with *Candida albicans* have several distinguishing features, most prominently the presence of pronounced paronychial swelling. Thin shavings taken from the infected nail, preferably from the deeper areas, should be examined microscopically with KOH and cultured. Repeated attempts may be required to demonstrate the fungus.

Therapy of tinea unguium is frequently disappointing. Prolonged therapy with griseofulvin and the application of topical fungistatic agents to the nail bed may be effective in some instances. Griseofulvin ther-

apy may be required for more than 1 yr and should be reserved for especially severe disease in patients who are motivated to obtain a cure.

Tinea nigra palmaris is a rare but distinctive superficial fungal infection that occurs principally in children and adolescents. It is caused by the dimorphic fungus *Cladosporium wernecki*, which imparts a gray-black color to the affected palm. The characteristic lesion is a well-defined hyperpigmented macule; scaling and erythema are rare, and the lesions are asymptomatic. Tinea nigra is often mistaken for a junctional nevus, melanoma, or staining of the skin by contactants. A KOH preparation of scrapings will permit identification of the fungal hyphae; the organism can also be grown on Sabouraud agar. Treatment with Whitfield ointment, undecylenic acid ointment, or tincture of iodine is most successful.

24.28   CANDIDAL INFECTIONS
(Candidiasis)

The dimorphic yeasts of the genus *Candida* are ubiquitous in the environment, but *Candida albicans* is the one that usually causes candidiasis in children. This yeast is not a member of the normal skin flora, but it is a frequent transient on skin and may colonize the human alimentary tract and the vagina as a saprophytic organism. Certain environmental conditions, notably elevated temperature and humidity, are associated with an increased frequency of isolation of *C. albicans* from the skin. Many bacterial species inhibit the growth of *C. albicans*, and alteration of normal flora by the use of antibiotics may promote overgrowth of the yeast.

Candidal infections in infants and children may be acute or chronic and localized or generalized; widespread lesions may occur in the newborn infant, in children with an immunodeficiency or with a serious disease of any etiology, and in patients with the multiple endocrinopathy syndrome (Sec 9.18). In such instances, species other than *C. albicans* may also be important etiologic agents. In addition to the mucocutaneous lesions, candidiasis may occur as a granulomatous process (candidal granuloma).

Oral candidiasis (thrush). (Sec. 7.42 and 11.13.)

Vaginal candidiasis. (Sec. 19.3.) *Candida albicans* is an inhabitant of the adult female vagina in at least 5% of women, and vaginal candidiasis is not uncommon in adolescent girls. A number of factors can predispose to this infection, including antibiotic therapy, corticosteroid therapy, diabetes mellitus, pregnancy, and the use of oral contraceptives. The infection is manifested by cheesy white plaques on an erythematous vaginal mucosa and by a thick white-yellow discharge. The disease may be relatively mild by or it may be accompanied by pronounced inflammation and scaling of the external genitalia and surrounding skin with progression to vesiculation and ulceration. Patients often complain of severe itching and burning in the vaginal area. The infection may be eradicated by insertion of nystatin vaginal tablets or suppositories twice daily for 2 wk. If this regimen is ineffective, the addition of oral nystatin tablets, 1–2 tablets 3 times daily, may eliminate or decrease the candidal population in the gastrointestinal tract.

Congenital generalized candidiasis is an infrequent intrauterine infection which may include the umbilical cord and fetal adnexa. The viscera and oropharynx are rarely involved. The infection is thought to occur by the transplacental route or via the placental membranes from an infected vagina. The skin lesions are widespread and profuse and consist of scaling, erythema, moist erosions, and scattered vesicopustules on an erythematous base. They affect the entire body, including the palms and soles. Yellow-white, flat nodules, a few mm in diameter, may be discernible on the surface of the umbilical cord and fetal adnexa. The diagnosis can be made by culture or by KOH preparation of material obtained from an active lesion. Generalized application of an anticandidal agent (nystatin, amphotericin B, miconazole, or clotrimazole) 4 times daily will effect a cure unless there is visceral involvement. Infants with disseminated candidiasis usually do not survive.

Candidal diaper dermatitis is a ubiquitous problem in infants and, although relatively benign, is often frustrating to manage because of its tendency to recur. Predisposed infants usually carry *C. albicans* in their intestinal tract, and the warm, moist, occluded skin of the diaper area provides optimal environment for its growth. Usually a seborrheic, atopic, or primary irritant contact dermatitis provides a portal of entry for the yeast.

Candidal diaper dermatitis is an intensely erythematous, confluent plaque with a scalloped border and a sharply demarcated edge. It is formed by the confluence of numerous papules and vesicopustules; satellite pustules, those which stud the contiguous skin, are a hallmark of localized candidal infections. Usually the perirectal skin, inguinal folds, perineum, and lower abdomen are involved (Fig 24–45, p. xxxiv). In males the entire scrotum and penis may be involved with an erosive balanitis of the perimeatal skin; in females the lesions may be found on the vaginal mucosa as well as on the labia. In some infants the process is generalized, with erythematous lesions distant from the diaper area; in some instances it may represent a fungal id (hypersensitivity) reaction.

The differential diagnosis includes other eruptions of the diaper area which may coexist with candidal infection. For this reason, it is important to establish a diagnosis by a KOH preparation or culture.

Treatment consists of applications of an anticandidal agent (nystatin, amphotericin B, miconazole, clotrimazole) with each diaper change or 4 times daily. Ointments are better tolerated than creams; lotions and creams may cause a burning sensation when applied to irritated skin, and powder may cake and cause erosion from friction during movement. The combination of a corticosteroid and antifungal agent is justified if inflammation is severe but may confuse the situation if the diagnosis is not firmly established. Protection of the diaper area by an application of thick zinc oxide paste overlying the anticandidal preparation may be helpful; the paste is more easily removed with mineral oil than with soap and water. Fungal id reactions will gradually abate with successful treatment of the diaper dermatitis or may be treated with a mild corticosteroid preparation. When recurrences of diaper candidiasis are frequent, it may be helpful to prescribe a course of oral anticandidal therapy to decrease the yeast population in the gastrointestinal tract. Some infants seem to be receptive hosts for *C. albicans* and may reacquire the organism from a colonized adult.

Intertriginous candidiasis occurs most often in the axillae and the groin, under the breasts, under overhanging abdominal fat folds, in the umbilicus, and in the gluteal cleft. Typical lesions are large, confluent areas of moist, denuded, erythematous skin with an irregular, macerated, scaly border. Satellite lesions are characteristic and consist of small vesicles or pustules on an erythematous base. With time, intertriginous candidal lesions may become lichenified, dry, scaly plaques. The lesions develop on skin subjected to irritation and maceration. Candidal superinfection is more prone to occur under conditions which lead to excessive perspiration, especially in obese children and in those with underlying disorders, such as diabetes mellitus.

A similar condition, interdigital candidiasis, commonly occurs in individuals whose hands are constantly immersed in water; fissures occur between the fingers and have red, denuded centers, with an overhanging, white epithelial fringe. Similar lesions between the toes may be secondary to occlusive footgear. Treatment is the same as for other candidal infections.

Perianal candidiasis. The perianal skin is erythematous, excoriated, and pruritic; it is aggravated by occlusive, moist underclothing, poor hygiene, anal fissures, and pinworms and may become superinfected with *C. albicans*, especially in children who are receiving oral antibiotic or corticosteroid medication. The involved skin becomes denuded and macerated, and the lesions are identical to those of candidal intertrigo or candidal diaper rash. Application of a topical antifungal agent in conjunction with improved hygiene is usually effective. Underlying disorders such as pinworm infection must also be treated.

Candidal paronychia and onychia are characterized by tender, erythematous swellings at the base of the nails (posterior nail fold) that occasionally discharge purulent material. If the lesion becomes chronic, the nail is secondarily invaded and becomes brittle and thickened, initially in the proximal portion but subsequently over the entire nail plate. The nail may develop a brownish discoloration and prominent transverse ridges or grooves, or it may be completely destroyed. Associated infection with *Pseudomonas* imparts a green color to the nail plate, particularly at the lateral margins.

This type of onychia is more common on the fingers, particularly in thumb-sucking children and in those whose hands are frequently immersed in water. The candidal paronychia is often mistaken for a dermatophyte infection, which is rare in children and has different clinical characteristics. It may also be confused with bacterial paronychia. *C. albicans* can usually be cultured from the posterior nail fold and can often be identified on a KOH preparation of nail scrapings or a Gram stain of exudate. Effective management necessitates keeping the finger as dry as possible and applying nystatin, amphotericin B, miconazole, or clotrimazole 3 times daily for weeks to months, until the nail plate grows out normally.

Candidal granuloma is a rare response to an invasive candidal infection of skin. Clinically the lesions appear as crusted, verrucous plaques and horn-like projections on the scalp, face, and distal limbs. Affected patients may have single or multiple defects in immune mechanisms and are often refractory to topical therapy. When antifungal agents prove ineffective, a systemic anticandidal agent may be required for palliation or eradication of the infection.

24.29 CUTANEOUS VIRAL INFECTIONS

Warts (verrucae) of all types are caused by DNA viruses in the papova group; those which infect humans are not readily transmissible to animals. Warts can affect the skin and the mucous membranes, including the larynx (laryngeal papillomas). Histologically, the various types of verrucae differ in minor ways, but the basic changes consist of hyperplasia of the epidermal cells and vacuolization of the spinous keratinocytes, which may contain basophilic intranuclear inclusions (viral particles). Parakeratosis (retained stratum corneum cell nuclei), papillomatosis, and eosinophilic cytoplasmic inclusions thought to represent altered keratohyalin are additional variable histologic changes.

The incidence of all types of warts is highest in children and adolescents. The warts are probably transferred by direct contact, although transmission by contaminated fomites is possible. Incubation periods range from 1–8 mo. Once acquired, warts are spread by autoinoculation. Antibodies do occur in response to infection but appear to have little protective effect.

Common warts (verruca vulgaris) occur most frequently on the fingers, dorsum of the hands, paronychial areas, face, knees, and elbows. They are well-circumscribed papules with a roughened, keratotic, irregular surface. When the surface is pared away, multiple black dots representing thrombosed dermal capillary loops are often visible. Periungual warts are less sharply circumscribed and often painful and may spread beneath the nail plate separating it from the nail bed.

Filiform warts are frequently located on the face or neck; the lesion is a single projection of several mm which has a sharply circumscribed base. The digitate wart is a related morphologic type of verruca that is often found on the scalp and neck. It has multiple projections from a sessile base.

Plantar warts, although essentially similar to the common wart, are usually flush with the surface of the sole because of the constant pressure from weight bearing. Similar lesions (palmar) can also occur on the palms. They are sharply demarcated, often with a ring of thick callus. Sometimes the surface keratotic material must be removed before the boundaries of the wart can be appreciated; in contrast to calluses, warts obliterate normal skin markings. Several contiguous warts may fuse to form a large plaque, the so-called mosaic wart. Plantar warts may be exceeding painful.

Juvenile flat warts (verruca plana) are slightly elevated, minimally hyperkeratotic papules that usually remain less than 3 mm in size and vary in color from pink to brown. They may occur in profusion on the face, arms, dorsum of the hands, and knees. The distribution of multiple lesions along a line of scratch is a helpful diagnostic feature. Lesions may be disseminated in the beard area by shaving and from the hairline onto the scalp by combing the hair.

Condylomata acuminata (mucous membrane warts) are moist, fleshy, papillomatous lesions that occur on the perianal mucosa (Fig 24–46), the labia, vaginal introitus, and perineal raphe and on the shaft, corona, and glans penis. Occasionally, they may obstruct the urethral meatus or the vaginal introitus. Because they are located in intertriginous areas, they may become moist and friable. When untreated, condylomata proliferate and become confluent, at times forming large cauliflower-like masses. Condylomata acuminata can be transmitted by sexual contact and are often referred to as veneral warts. Lesions can also occur on the lips, gingivae, and tongue.

Differential Diagnosis. Common warts are most often confused with molluscum contagiosum. Plantar and palmar warts may be difficult to distinguish from punctate keratoses, corns, and calluses. Juvenile flat warts mimic lichen planus, lichen nitidus, adenoma sebaceum, syringomas, milia, and acne papules. Condylomata acuminata may resemble condylomata lata of secondary syphilis.

Treatment. A variety of therapeutic measures are effective in the treatment of warts. More than 50% of warts will disappear spontaneously within 2 yr, but failure to treat incurs the risk of spread to other sites. Warts are epidermal lesions and usually do not produce scarring unless they are surgically managed or treated in an overly aggressive fashion. Hyperkeratotic lesions (common, plantar, and palmar warts) are more responsive to therapy if the excess keratotic debris is gently pared with a scalpel only until thrombosed capillaries are apparent; further paring will induce bleeding.

Common warts can be destroyed by light electrodesiccation and curettage or by applications of liquid nitro-

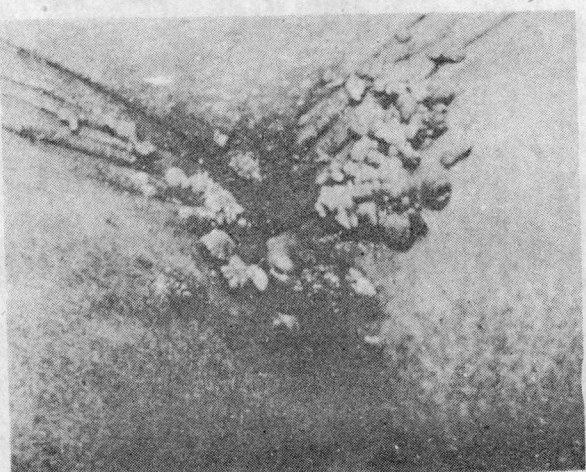

Figure 24–46 Condylomata acuminata in the perianal area of a toddler.

gen or cantharidin. Daily applications of 10–17% lactic acid and 10–17% salicylic acid in flexible collodion is a slow but painless method of removal. Filiform, digitate, and periungual warts respond best to liquid nitrogen. Plantar and palmar warts may be treated with cantharidin, liquid nitrogen, salicylic and lactic acids in collodion, or 40% salicylic acid plasters. After prolonged soaking keratotic debris can be removed by an emery board or pumice stone. Condylomata respond best to weekly applications of 25% podophyllin in tincture of benzoin; the medication should be left on the warts for 4–6 hr and then removed by bathing. Condylomata localized to keratinized sites (e.g., buttocks) may not respond to podophyllin. Resistant lesions can usually be eradicated by weekly freezing with liquid nitrogen. With all types of therapy, extreme care should be taken to protect the surrounding normal skin from irritation.

Molluscum contagiosum is a common cutaneous viral infection. It is caused by a DNA virus, the largest member of the poxvirus group and the largest true virus that infects man. The disease is acquired by direct contact with an infected person or from fomites and is spread by autoinoculation. The incubation period is estimated to be 2–8 wk.

The lesions are discrete, pearly, skin-colored, dome-shaped papules varying in size from 1–5 mm; typically they have central umbilication from which a plug of cheesy material can be expressed (Fig 24–47). The papules may occur anywhere on the body, but the face, eyelids, neck, axillae, and thighs are sites of predilection. They may be found in clusters on the genitalia or in the groin of adolescents and may be associated with other veneral diseases in sexually active individuals. Mucosal lesions are rarely evident. Eczematous dermatitis infrequently obscures the molluscum papules.

Although biopsy is not indicated, an appreciation of the histologic pattern of the lesions is helpful diagnostically. The molluscum papule consists of a lobulated

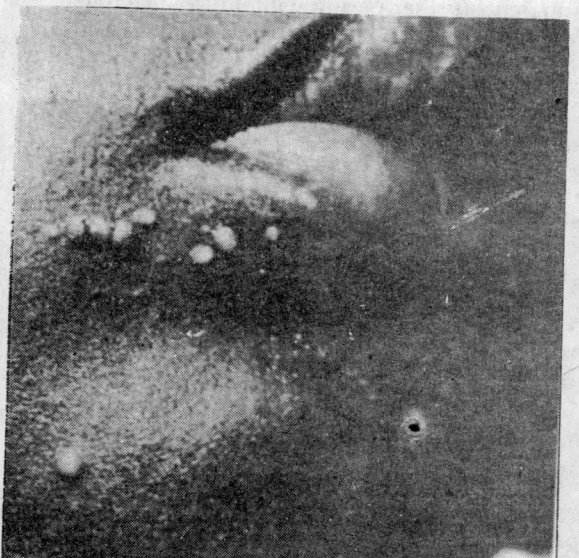

Figure 24–47 Grouped papules of molluscum contagiosum on the face.

adhesive mass of virus-infected epidermal cells which degenerate gradually as they move upward from basal layer to stratum corneum. The eosinophilic viral inclusions become more prominent as the cells reach the surface and pack the cytoplasm. The central plug of material which represents these virus-laden cells (molluscum bodies) may be shelled out from a lesion (see below) and examined under the microscope with 10% KOH or with Wright or Giemsa stain. The rounded, cup-shaped mass of homogeneous cells, often with identifiable lobules, is diagnostic for molluscum contagiosum and distinguishes it from warts that are likely to cause confusion in the differential diagnosis.

Molluscum contagiosum is a self-limited disease, but lesions can persist for months to years, can be spread to distant sites, and may be transmitted to others. It is therefore advisable to eradicate the lesions in all infected children. It is mandatory to treat children who also have atopic dermatitis or an immunodeficiency since the infection may spread rapidly in them and produce hundreds of lesions. The papules can be destroyed by expressing the plug with a needle, a sharp curette, a comedo extractor, or a curved forceps; the base of the lesion can be touched with iodine. Brief application of liquid nitrogen to each lesion is also very effective. Cantharidin 0.9% may be applied without occlusion and frequently causes enough inflammation to facilitate spontaneous extrusion of the plug. Similarly, daily applications of a 10% benzoyl peroxide gel may result in adequate surface peeling and spontaneous extrusion of the molluscum bodies. Molluscum is an epidermal disease and should not be overtreated so that scarring results.

24.30   INSECT BITES AND PARASITIC INFESTATIONS

INSECT BITES

Insect bites are a common affliction of children and usually pose no problem in diagnosis. Occasionally, however, the patient is unaware of the source of the lesions or denies being bitten; in these instances, precise interpretation of the eruption may be difficult. Insect bites may occur as solitary, multiple, or profuse lesions but, when numerous, are usually grouped because of the tendency of a single insect to inflict several bites in a localized area.

The type of reaction that occurs depends on the species of insect and the age group and reactivity of the human host. Infants often display no reaction, young children manifest only a delayed hypersensitivity reaction, and older children experience both an immediate and a delayed reaction. By adolescence or adulthood, the delayed component of the insect bite reaction is lost, and the host responds only with an immediate reaction, which is characterized by an evanescent, erythematous wheal. Usually there is a visible central punctum, but the punctum may disappear as the lesion ages, and, if edema is marked, the wheal may be surmounted by a tiny vesicle. Bullous lesions are produced by certain beetles as a result of the action of cantharidin, and hemorrhagic lesions may be caused by a variety of insects including beetles and spiders. Delayed hypersensitivity reactions to insect bites are characterized by firm persistent papules which may become hyperpigmented and are often excoriated and crusted. Pruritus may be mild or severe, transient or persistent. The reaction is a response to introduction of insect toxins and antigens into the tissues of the host. Severe hypersensitivity reactions that occur as a result of certain types of bites and stings are discussed in Chapters 10 and 28.

Acute local reactions may be ameliorated by cool water compresses followed by application of a soothing shake lotion such as calamine, to which 0.25% menthol and 0.5% phenol can be added. Topical corticosteroids can also be helpful for control of pruritus. If lesions are extensive and extremely pruritic, an oral antihistamine may provide some relief. Topical antihistamines are potent sensitizers and have no role in the treatment of insect bite reactions or other skin diseases. Insect repellents containing diethyltoluamide or ethyl hexanediol may afford moderate protection against mosquitoes, fleas, flies, chiggers, and ticks but are relatively ineffective against wasps, bees, and spiders.

Papular urticaria is a persistent, annoying eruption which occurs principally in the 1st decade of life and appears to represent a delayed hypersensitivity reaction to the bites of insects, the most common of which are species of fleas and mites, bedbugs, gnats, mosquitoes, and animal lice. The disorder is most prevalent during the warmer months.

Typical lesions are firm, hyperpigmented, intensely pruritic, discrete papules which cluster mainly on the trunk and extensor surfaces of the extremities (Fig 24–48). The initial and acute lesion may be an urticarial wheal that in turn is replaced by a papule. When new lesions are acquired, quiescent papules may flare and become erythematous and edematous. A central punctum is visible initially; however, when the lesions become severely excoriated, central crusting or a secondary pyoderma can obscure the typical morphologic aspects.

It is important to identify the etiologic agent. The nature of the eruption may not be suspected because older family members are usually not afflicted. When it is appreciated that papular urticaria represents a delayed hypersensitivity reaction to insect bites and that this phenomenon is age related, the sparing of others in the household becomes explicable.

Papular urticaria can be confused with papular exanthems, varicella, and scabies. The histologic changes are relatively nonspecific; they consist of dermal edema and a mixed inflammatory perivascular infiltrate. At times, however, the dermal cellular infiltrate is so dense that a lymphoma or foreign body reaction may be suspected.

Treatment is directed at alleviation of pruritus by oral antihistamines, cool compresses, soothing lotions, and topical corticosteroid creams or lotions for the more annoying lesions. A concerted effort should be made to identify the etiologic agent: pets should be carefully inspected; crawl spaces, eaves, and other sites of the

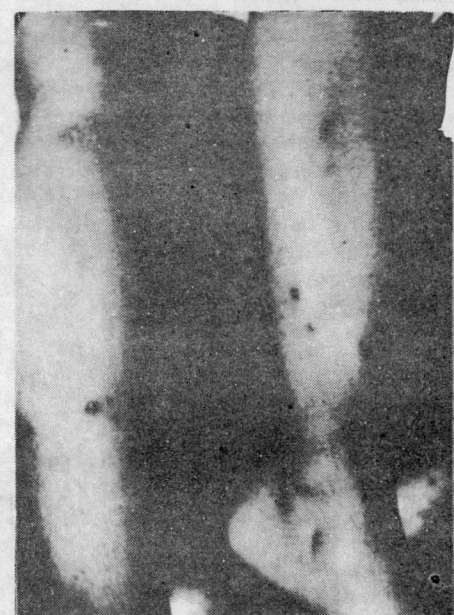

Figure 24–48   Hyperpigmented papulonodular lesions, some of which are grouped, characteristic of papular urticaria.

house and/or outbuildings frequented by animals and birds should be decontaminated since insects such as fleas can survive for many mo without feeding; baseboard crevices, mattresses, rugs, furniture, and animal sleeping quarters should also be sprayed with an insecticide.

PARASITIC INFESTATIONS

Scabies is caused by the itch mite *Sarcoptes scabiei* var. *hominis*. The recent worldwide epidemic has resulted in an increased incidence of the disease in all age groups.

The intensely pruritic eruption consists of wheals, papules, vesicles, threadlike burrows, and a superimposed eczematous dermatitis. In older children and adolescents the clinical pattern is similar to that in adults; preferred sites are the interdigital spaces, wrists, elbows, ankles, buttocks, umbilicus, groin, genitalia, areolae, and axillae (Fig 24–49A). The head, neck, palms and soles are generally spared. In infants, bullae and pustules are relatively common; burrows are absent, and the palms, soles (Fig 24–49B), face, and scalp are often affected. Red-brown nodules, most often located in the axillae and groin and on the genitalia, constitute a less common variant. All the lesions are extremely pruritic, particularly at night; scratching inevitably results in eczematization, excoriation, and secondary pyoderma, which may mask the true nature of the disorder.

Scabies is transmitted by direct contact with infected persons and only rarely by contaminated fomites since the mite dies within 2–3 days. The adult female mite measures approximately 0.4 mm in length and has 4 sets of legs and a hemispherical body marked by transverse corrugations and brown spines and bristles on the dorsal surface. The male mite is approximately half

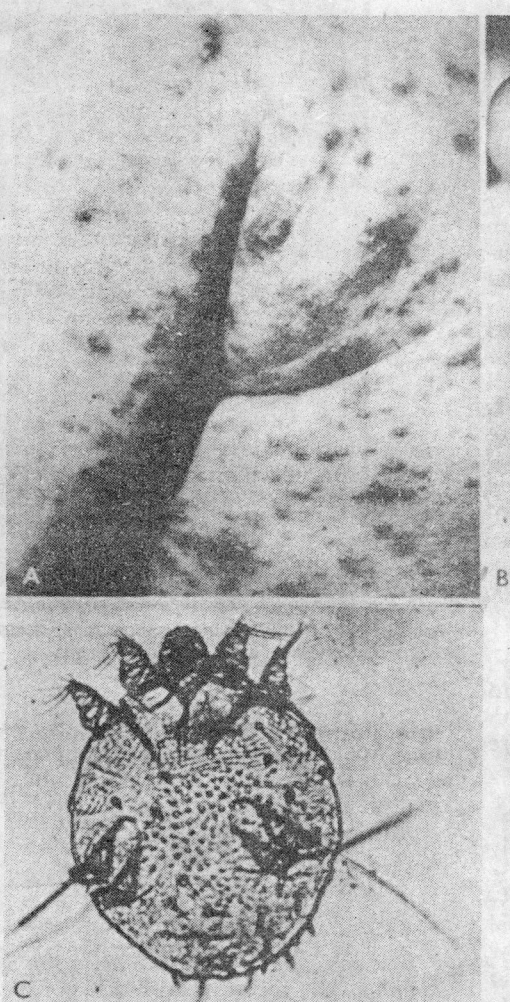

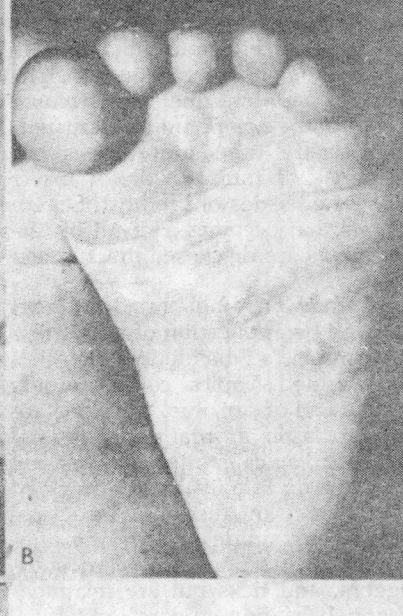

Figure 24–49 *A*, Eczematous dermatitis, papules, and nodules of human scabies. *B*, Vesiculopustular lesions of scabies on the soles of an infant. *C*, Human scabies mite obtained from scraping.

her size and is similar in configuration. After fertilization on the cutaneous surface, the gravid female burrows into the stratum corneum and gradually extends this tract as she deposits 1–3 oval eggs daily and numerous brown fecal pellets (scybala). When egg-laying is completed in 4–5 wk she dies within the burrow. The eggs hatch in 3 to 5 days, releasing larvae which grow and molt into nymphs on the skin surface. Maturity is achieved in about 2–3 wk. Mating occurs, and the gravid female invades the skin to complete the life cycle.

Diagnosis is made by microscopic identification of mites (Fig 24–49C), ova, and scybala in epithelial debris. Scrapings are most often positive when obtained from burrows, eczematous lesions, or fresh papules. The most reliable method is application of a drop of mineral oil on the selected lesion, vigorous scraping of it with a dull-edged instrument, and transfer of the oil and scrapings to a glass slide. The mite can be detected microscopically by its movement.

The differential diagnosis depends on the types of lesions present. Burrows are virtually pathognomonic for human scabies. Papulovesicular lesions are confused with papular urticaria, canine scabies, chickenpox, viral exanthems, drug eruptions, dermatitis herpetiformis, and folliculitis. Eczematous lesions may mimic atopic dermatitis and seborrheic dermatitis, and the less common bullous disorders of childhood may be suspected in the infant with predominantly bullous lesions. Nodular scabies is frequently misdiagnosed as urticaria pigmentosa, histiocytosis X, and insect bite granuloma.

Treatment by application of 1% gamma benzene hexachloride cream or lotion to the entire body from the neck down, with particular attention to intensely involved areas, is effective. The medication is left on the skin for 8–12 hr, and if necessary it may be reapplied in 1 wk for another 8–12 hr period. The vulnerability of small infants to percutaneous absorption of this potentially neurotoxic substance should dictate extreme caution in prescribing it for them. A shorter application time (6–8 hr) is less hazardous for infants under 1 yr of age. For infants less than 6 mo, as well as older individuals, alternative therapy includes 10% crotamiton cream or lotion applied twice during a 48 hr period or a 6% sulfur ointment applied for 24 hr and repeated in 1 wk. Pruritus, which is due to hypersensitivity to mite antigens, may persist for a number of days and may be alleviated by a topical corticosteroid preparation. Nodules are extremely resistant to treatment and may not respond for several mo. Persistent pruritus may not reflect inadequate treatment since the hypersensitivity reaction to the mite may outlast the presence of live parasites. The entire family should be carefully examined and all affected members treated appropriately. A latent period of approximately 1 mo follows infestation so that itching may be absent and lesions relatively inapparent in family members who are asymptomatic carriers. Clothing, bed linens, and towels should be throughly laundered.

Norwegian scabies, a variant of human scabies, is highly contagious and occurs mainly in institutions among mentally and physically debilitated patients. Affected individuals are infested by myriads of mites which inhabit the crusts and exfoliating scales of the skin and scalp lesions in this form of the disease. The nails may become thickened and dystrophic and are densely populated by mites. Management is extremely difficult; it requires scrupulous isolation measures and repeated but careful applications of antiscabetic preparations.

Canine scabies is caused by *Sarcoptes scabiei* var. *canis*, the dog mite that is associated with mange. The eruption in the human, which is most frequently acquired by cuddling an infested puppy, consists of tiny papules, vesicles, wheals, and excoriated eczematous plaques. Burrows are not present since the mite infrequently inhabits human stratum corneum. The rash is pruritic and has a predilection for the arms, chest, and abdomen, the usual sites of contact. Onset is sudden and usually follows exposure by 1–10 days, possibly resulting from development of a hypersensitivity reaction to mite antigens. Recovery of mites or ova from scrapings of human skin is rare. The disease is self-limited in humans, but removal and/or treatment of the infested animal is necessary. Symptomatic therapy for itching is helpful. In the rare instances that mites are demonstrated in scrapings from the affected child, they can be eradicated by the same measures applicable to human scabies.

Pediculosis: Three types of lice are obligate parasites of the human host: pubic or crab lice (*Phthirus pubis*), head lice (*Pediculus humanus capitis*), and body lice (*Pediculus humanus corporis*). Only the body louse is a vector for pathogens of human disease (typhus, trench fever, relapsing fever). Body and head lice are related and have similar physical characteristics; they are about 2–4 mm in length, whereas pubic lice have a striking crablike anatomy and are only 1–2 mm in length. Female lice live for approximately 1 mo and deposit up to 10 eggs daily on the human host. Ova hatch in 1 wk and require another wk to mature. Both nymphs and adult lice feed on human blood, injecting their salivary juices into the host and depositing their fecal matter on the skin.

Pediculosis pubis is usually encountered in adolescents, though small children may acquire pubic lice, e.g., on the eyelashes by close contact with an infested individual. Patients experience moderate to severe pruritus and may develop a secondary pyoderma from scratching. Maculae caeruleae (blue spots) may appear in the pubic area and on the abdomen and thighs; they are thought to represent altered blood pigments or excretion from the salivary gland of the louse. Oval, translucent nits, which are firmly attached to the hair shafts, may be visible to the naked eye or may be readily identified by a hand lens or by microscopic examination (Fig 24–50). Adult lice are occasionally detected.

Since the pubic louse may occasionally wander or be transferred to other sites on fomites, terminal hair on the trunk, thighs, axillary region, beard area, and eyelashes should be examined for nits. The patient also should be checked for manifestations of other venereal diseases. Infestation may be effectively treated by application of 1% gamma benzene hexachloride cream or lotion; it should be massaged into affected areas and permitted to remain for 24 hr. Alternatively, the shampoo is lathered for 4 min and removed by thorough rinsing. Retreatment may be required in 8–9 days. Nits can be removed with a fine-toothed comb. Infestation of eyelashes is eradicated by 0.25% physostigmine ophthalmic ointment applied twice daily for 8 days. Pubic lice survive for only a short time when separated from the host; nevertheless, clothing, towels, and bed linens may be contaminated with nit-bearing hairs and should be thoroughly laundered or dry-cleaned.

Pediculosis corporis is rare in children except under conditions of poor hygiene since the parasite is transmitted mainly on contaminated clothing or bedding. The lesions consist of papules, wheals, excoriations, secondary eczematization, and pyoderma; itching is intense in all stages. Lice are found on the skin only when they are feeding; at other times they inhabit the seams of clothing, which are also a repository for nits. Therapy consists of improved hygiene and laundering or boiling all infested clothing and bedding. Gamma

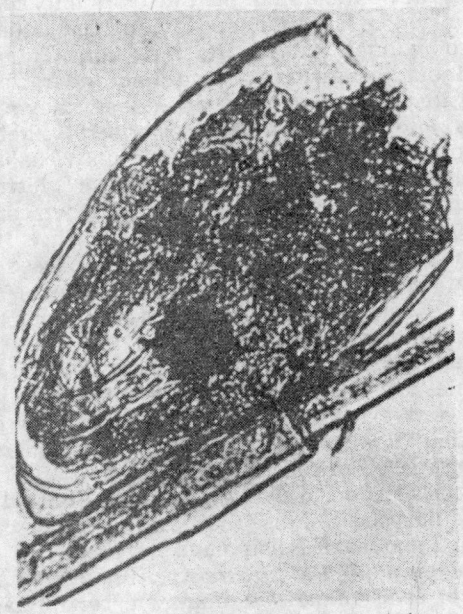

Figure 24–50 Intact nit on a human hair.

benzene hexachloride can be used to eradicate nits on body hair.

Pediculosis capitis is responsible for intense pruritus, and the infestation may be complicated by secondary pyoderma and lymphadenopathy. Pediculi are not always visible, but nits are detectable on the hairs, most commonly in the occipital region and above the ears. Dermatitis may also be noted on the neck and pinnae. Head lice can be transmitted on infested clothing, combs, brushes, and furniture or by direct human contact. Shampooing with 1% gamma benzene hexachloride for 4 min. is effective; treatment may be repeated in 24 hr. Nits can be removed with a fine-toothed comb or, if tenacious, by a 1:1 vinegar-water rinse followed by vigorous combing. Clothing and bed linens should be laundered in very hot water or dry-cleaned; brushes and combs should be discarded or thoroughly cleaned in boiling water.

Creeping eruption. (Sec. 10.122.)

24.31   ACNE

Acne vulgaris is often regarded as a physiologic event since it occurs most universally during adolescence and frequently persists into adulthood. It is a self-limited inflammatory process of the pilosebaceous unit and is somewhat more common in males. Occurrence for girls peaks between 14–17 yr of age and for boys between 16–19 yr of age. Genetic factors probably play some role, but no clear-cut patterns of transmission are evident.

Pathology. The lesions of acne vulgaris develop in sebaceous follicles; these appendicular structures have a large, multilobular sebaceous gland and a wide follicular canal containing a rudimentary hair. The primary histologic alteration appears to be abnormal keratinization of the epithelium in the duct with impaction of the keratinized cells within the lumen. The initial lesions are comedones, which are impactions of lamellated keratinous material containing lipid and bacteria. Two types are recognized: open comedones, known as blackheads, and closed comedones, termed whiteheads. A patulous pilosebaceous orifice permits visualization of the plug (open comedo), the surface of which is darkened by the accumulation of melanin. Open comedones are presumed to be mature lesions since they less commonly become inflammatory. The closed comedo has only a pinpoint opening and represents a follicular sac filled with densely aggregated keratinous material, lipids, and bacteria.

Inflammatory papules and nodules develop from comedones in which the follicular epithelium has ruptured and extruded the follicular contents into the subjacent dermis, where a neutrophilic inflammatory response is produced. Suppuration and an occasional giant cell reaction to the keratin and hair are the cause of nodulocystic lesions; these are not true cysts but liquefied masses of inflammatory debris.

Etiology and Pathogenesis. Although the direct cause of acne vulgaris is unknown, certain aspects of the pathogenesis are understood. A functionally mature sebaceous gland is fundamental to the disease process. At puberty, the sebaceous gland enlarges and sebum production increases in response to the increased activities of testicular, ovarian, and adrenal androgens. Usually, but not invariably, sebum production is greater in adolescents with extensive acne. Studies of testosterone metabolism in acne skin have implicated a local tissue abnormality as a possible mechanism in the pathogenesis.

Freshly formed sebum consists of a mixture of lipids with a predominance of triglycerides. Normal follicular bacteria convert sebum triglycerides to free fatty acids, and those of medium chain length (C8–C14) may be 1 of the minor provocative factors in initiating an inflammatory reaction. There is also evidence that free fatty acids may stimulate formation of comedones.

The sebaceous follicles are colonized by organisms of 3 types: an anaerobic diphtheroid, *Propionibacterium acnes (Corynebacterium acnes)*; coagulase-negative *Staphylococcus epidermidis*; and a dimorphic yeast, *Pityrosporon ovale.* Each of these organisms possesses lipolytic enzymes; however, *P. acnes* appears to be largely responsible for the formation of free fatty acids. It is probable that bacterial proteases, hyaluronidases, and chemotactic factors play a significant role in eliciting an inflammatory reaction.

Clinical Manifestations. Acne vulgaris is characterized by 4 basic types of lesions: open and closed comedones, papules, pustules, and nodulocystic lesions. The last may be firm and indolent, resembling true cysts, or fluctuant or draining, resembling furuncles. Pitted, atrophic or hypertrophic scars may be interspersed, depending on the severity and chronicity of the process. One or more types of lesions may predominate whether acne is mild or severe. Lesions may be confined to the face or may also involve the chest, upper back, and deltoid areas. A predominance of lesions on the forehead, particularly closed comedones, is often attributable to prolonged use of greasy hair preparations (pomade acne). Marked involvement on the trunk is most often seen in males. The diagnosis is rarely difficult, although flat warts, folliculitis, and other types of acne may be confused with acne vulgaris.

Treatment. There is no evidence that early treatment will prevent the emergence of acne lesions; however, acne can be controlled and severe scarring prevented by judicious therapy maintained until the disease process has spontaneously abated.

It is important to establish rapport with the adolescent patient and to explain the basic pathogenetic events in clear simple language. Parents should be included in discussions since their misconceptions about acne may lead to needless harassment of the afflicted adolescent.

GENERAL MEASURES. Diet plays *no* significant role in the pathogenesis of the usual case of acne. There is little evidence that ingestion of particular foods can trigger acne flares. When a patient is convinced that certain dietary items exacerbate acne, it is permissible to omit those foods; it is unnecessary, however, to impose unwarranted restrictions on most teenagers. A balanced diet should be encouraged for reasons of general health.

Climate appears to influence acne in that improvement frequently occurs during the summer months, and flares are more common during the wintertime. Remission during summer may be a direct effect of increased exposure to ultraviolet light or may relate, in part, to the relative absence of stress. Emotional tension and fatigue seem to exacerbate acne in many individuals.

Additional factors which should be discussed are cleansing, cosmetics, hair preparations, and facial manipulation. Although cleansing removes surface lipid and renders the skin less oily in appearance, there is no evidence that surface lipid is harmful in acne. Only minimal drying and peeling are achieved by cleansing; repetitive cleansing can be harmful since it irritates and chaps the skin. Greasy cosmetic and hair preparations must be discontinued as they will exacerbate pre-existing acne and cause further plugging of follicular pores. Manipulation and squeezing of facial lesions will serve only to rupture intact lesions and provoke localized inflammatory reactions.

TOPICAL THERAPY. Cleansing agents that contain keratolytic agents, such as sulfur and salicylic acid, may exert a mild drying and peeling effect and are acceptable if tolerated. Cleansers containing abrasives probably provide little additional help and may be excessively drying and irritating. There is no evidence that preparations containing alcohol or hexachlorophene decrease acne since surface bacteria are not involved in the pathogenesis.

Topical lotions, creams, and gels containing sulfur, salicylic acid, and resorcinol may be added to a cleanser for additional mild keratolytic effect. Tinted preparations intended to replace cosmetics often mismatch normal skin color and highlight rather than mask the lesions.

The most effective topical preparations, particularly for comedones and papulopustular acne, include the benzoyl peroxide gels and vitamin A acid. Benzoyl peroxide is an organic peroxide and oxidizing agent that dries and peels the skin and suppresses growth of *P. acnes*. Preparations are available in concentration of 5% and 10% (e.g., Desquam-X, Benzagel, PanOxyl) and may be applied as a thin film once or twice daily as tolerated. Water-based gels are less irritating than alcohol-based gels for patients with sensitive skin. Vitamin A acid (Retin-A) affects keratinization in the sebaceous follicle by increasing turnover of epidermal cells and by decreasing the cohesiveness of the squamous cells; it thus aids in elimination of the keratinous plug. Some erythema and peeling may be expected, and pustular flares due to rupture of microcomedones are common. Vitamin A acid may be applied once daily, a half hour after washing, in the form best tolerated (0.025% gel; 0.01% gel; 0.1% cream; 0.05% cream, in decreasing order of potency). Increased sensitivity to sunlight may occur, and a sunscreen should be provided until partial tanning has occurred.

Topical antibiotics in a vehicle appropriate for use in patients with acne are now commercially available. These products contain either clindamycin (Cleocin-T) or erythromycin (Staticin) and may be applied once or twice daily. While not as effective as orally administered antibiotics, they serve as a useful therapeutic adjunct.

All topical preparations require several wk for a demonstrable positive effect. They may be used alone or together in selected patients, e.g., benzoyl peroxide gel in the morning and vitamin A acid at night.

SYSTEMIC THERAPY. Certain antibiotics, especially tetracycline and erythromycin, have been used in the treatment of papulopustular and nodulocystic acne. These drugs appear to act by suppressing the normal follicular flora, mainly *P. acnes*, and by decreasing the inflammatory reaction. For most patients, initiation of therapy with 1 gm daily for 2–4 wk and gradual decrease in dosage to a maintenance dose of 250–500 mg daily will be effective. The drugs should always be administered in combination with topical therapy. Patients should be instructed to take the drug between meals and should be forewarned of such side effects as secondary candidal vaginitis and transient nausea. Tetracycline is contraindicated in pregnant adolescents.

Estrogen therapy is appropriate only for young women with premenstrual flares of acne; it is sometimes effective in such circumstances. The hazards of side effects must be considered. Diuretics, oral vitamin A, and staphylococcal vaccines are ineffective therapy for acne and should not be used.

PHYSICAL THERAPY. Ultraviolet light, cryotherapy, and radiation therapy may be included under this heading. Ultraviolet light appears to be beneficial in some patients who tan easily, possibly because of the peeling effect of tanning. It is best provided by natural sunlight. Periodic applications of CO_2 snow or slush for a peeling effect may be therapeutic for some patients. Radiation therapy is contraindicated.

SURGICAL THERAPY. Extraction of open and closed comedones, needle aspiration of nodulocystic lesions, and injection of corticosteroid into acne cysts are additional helpful measures in selected patients. Planing of the skin by dermabrasion to minimize scarring is indicated only after the active process is quiescent. Not all patients, however, will be improved by dermabrasion, and some risks accompany it.

Steroid acne. Pubertal and postpubertal patients who are receiving systemic corticosteroid therapy or potent topical steroids are predisposed to steroid-induced acne, a monomorphous folliculitis that occurs on the face, neck, chest (Fig 24–51A), shoulders, upper back, arms, and, rarely, the scalp. Onset follows the initiation of steroid therapy by 2 wk. The lesions are small, erythematous papules or pustules that may erupt in profusion and are all in the same stage of development. Comedones may occur subsequently, but nodulocystic lesions and scarring are rare. Pruritus is occasional. The steroid appears to induce focal degeneration of the follicular epithelium with a localized neutrophilic inflammatory response. Although steroid acne is relatively refractory if there is continued use of the drug, the eruption may respond to use of vitamin A acid and a benzoyl peroxide gel.

Endogenous steroid (androgen) production may produce acne in children with congenital adrenal hyperplasia, including the cryptic form, of which severe acne in adolescence may be the only clinical manifestation. Studies of adrenal function are indicated in appropriate patients (Sec 18.24).

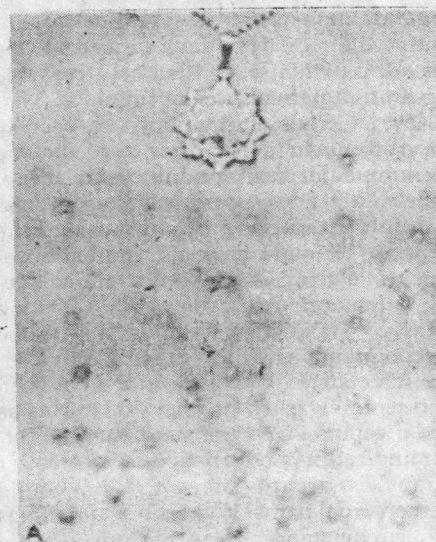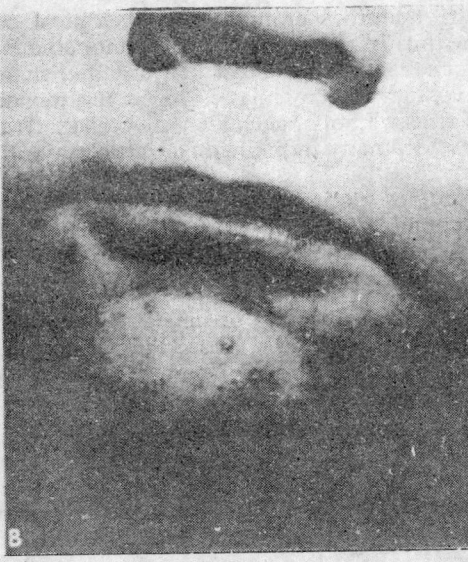

Figure 24–51 *A*, Monomorphous papular eruption of steroid acne. *B*, Acne in a male infant.

Halogen acne may be induced by administration of medications containing iodides or bromides or, rarely, by ingestion of massive amounts of vitamin-mineral preparations or iodine-containing "health foods" such as kelp. The lesions are often very inflammatory. Discontinuation of the provocative agent and appropriate topical preparations will usually achieve reasonable therapeutic results.

Infantile acne. Acne vulgaris may occur in infants, principally in males; it has been attributed to a hypersensitive end-organ response to hormones, but the etiology is unknown. Onset may occur within the 1st mo of life, and lesions are confined to the face (Fig 24–51*B*). Papules, pustules, and open and closed comedones are usual, but only occasionally do nodulocystic lesions develop; pitted scarring is rare. The course may be relatively brief, or the lesions may persist for many mo. Rarely, an unusual exposure to an occlusive ointment, a halogenated compound, or a topical fluorinated corticosteroid may cause the acneiform eruption, and appropriate history should be sought. The use of a mild acne lotion or a benzoyl peroxide gel will usually clear the eruption within a few wk. Often there is a history of severe acne in 1 or both parents, and the child may be predisposed to more severe acne in adolescence.

Tropical acne. A severe form of acne occurs in tropical climates and is believed to be due to the intense heat and humidity. Lesions occur mainly on the back, chest, and buttocks, with a predominance of suppurating nodulocystic lesions. Secondary infection with *S. aureus* may be a complication. The eruption is refractory to acne therapy if the environmental factors are not eliminated.

Acne conglobata, a rare disorder, is a chronic, progressive inflammatory disease that occurs mainly in adult males but may begin during adolescence. Papules, pustules, nodules, cysts, abscesses, sinus tracts, and severe scarring are characteristic. The face is relatively spared, but, in addition to the back and chest, the buttocks, abdomen, arms, and thighs may be involved.

Constitutional symptoms and anemia may accompany the inflammatory process. Acne conglobata has been related to hidradenitis suppurativa and may occur coincidentally. Routine acne therapy is generally ineffective. Systemic therapy with a corticosteroid or sulfones may be required to suppress the intense inflammatory activity. A course of isoretenoin (Accutare) may prove to be the most effective form of therapy.

24.32   TUMORS OF THE SKIN

Also see Sec 15.20.

Pyogenic granuloma (telangiectatic granuloma) is a small, red, moist, sessile or pedunculated growth that often has a discernible epithelial collarette (Fig 24–52). The surface of the lesion may be weeping and crusted, or it may be completely epithelialized. Pyogenic granulomas initially grow rapidly and bleed easily when traumatized since they are composed of exuberant granulation tissue. They are relatively common in children, particularly on the face, arms, and hands. Generally they arise at sites of injury, but often a history of previous trauma cannot be elicited. Clinically, they resemble and often are indistinguishable from small hemangiomas.

Microscopically, the lesions consist of a dense proliferation of capillaries and fibroblastic stroma. Masses of polymorphonuclear leukocytes which infiltrate the stroma account for the designation pyogenic granuloma. Although benign, these lesions are a nuisance since they bleed easily when traumatized and may recur if incompletely removed. Small lesions may regress after cauterization with silver nitrate; larger lesions require excision and electrodesiccation of the base of the granuloma.

Infantile digital fibromatoses are benign but destructive tumors identifiable as firm, smooth, erythematous or skin-colored nodules on the dorsal or lateral surfaces

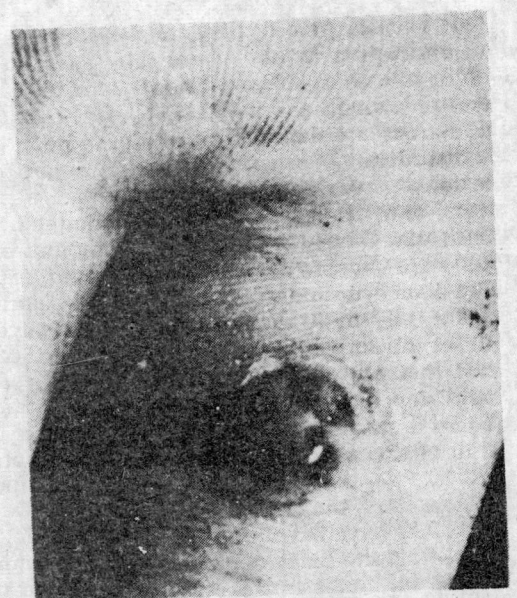

Figure 24–52 Pyogenic granuloma with a moist surface and epithelial collarette at the base.

of the distal phalanges of the fingers and toes. More than 80% of these tumors have been reported in infants less than 1 yr of age. Lesions may be solitary or multiple. Generally, they are asymptomatic, but flexion deformity of the digits may occur.

Clinically, the lesions resemble fibromas, leiomyomas, angiofibromas, and mucous cysts. The diagnosis is confirmed by finding characteristic pyroninophilic intracellular inclusion bodies within the proliferating fibroblasts on biopsy. A viral etiology has been postulated. Local recurrence following simple excision of this tumor has been described in 60% of reported patients. Since the tumor does not metastasize and occasionally may regress spontaneously, a course of expectant observation is advised. If functional impairment or flexion deformity of the digit becomes apparent, prompt surgical intervention with full excision of the tumor is indicated.

Dermatofibromas (histiocytomas) are benign dermal tumors which rarely exceed 1 cm and arise most frequently on the limbs. They may be nodular, flat, or pedunculated and are usually firm and well circumscribed but occasionally feel soft on palpation. The overlying skin is usually hyperpigmented. The differential diagnosis includes sclerosing hemangioma, epidermal inclusion cyst, juvenile xanthogranuloma, hypertrophic scar, and neurofibroma. Dermatofibromas may be excised or left intact according to patient preference. They represent collections of histiocytes, fibroblasts, and small capillaries in the dermis.

The association of multiple small, papular, skin-colored fibromas with osteopoikilosis is called *dermatofibrosis lenticularis disseminata* (Buschke-Ollendorff syndrome).

Basal cell epithelioma (basal cell carcinoma) is rare in children in the absence of a predisposing condition such as basal cell nevus syndrome, xeroderma pigmen-

tosum, nevus sebaceus of Jadassohn, or preceding exposure to irradiation. Nevertheless, it has been reported as isolated lesions in children as young as 7 yr of age. Sites of predilection are the face, scalp, and upper back; the lesions are yellow to pink, smooth, crusted or verrucous papulonodules which enlarge slowly and may bleed occasionally or become chronically irritated. The differential diagnosis includes pyogenic granuloma, nevus cell nevus, epidermal inclusion cyst, closed comedo, dermatofibroma, and the various appendicular tumors. Simple excision is usually curative, although occasional recurrences have been reported.

Basal cell nevus syndrome includes a wide spectrum of defects involving the skin, eyes, central nervous system, bones, and endocrine system. The typical facies of this autosomal dominant syndrome is characterized by temporoparietal bossing, prominent supraorbital ridges, a broad nasal root, ocular hypertelorism or dystopia canthorum, and prognathism. Appearing in early childhood, the basal cell carcinomas erupt in crops and vary in size, color, and number, mimicking numerous other types of skin lesions. Sites of predilection are the periorbital skin, nose, malar areas, and upper lip, but the lesions can develop on the trunk and limbs and are not restricted to sun-exposed areas. Ulceration, bleeding, and crusting occur with considerable destruction of surrounding tissue if the lesions are not removed. Small milia, epidermal cysts, pigmented lesions, hirsutism, and palmar and plantar pits are additional cutaneous findings.

Cysts in the maxilla and mandible occur in 65–75% of these patients. These cysts may result in maldevelopment of the teeth and also cause pain, fever, swelling of the jaw, facial deformity, bone erosion, pathologic fractures, and suppurating sinus tracts. Osseous defects such as anomalous rib development, spina bifida, kyphoscoliosis, and brachymetacarpalism occur in two thirds of patients and ocular abnormalities including cataracts, coloboma, strabismus, and blindness in approximately one third. Neurologic manifestations include calcification of the falx, seizures, mental retardation, partial agenesis of the corpus callosum, hydrocephalus, and nerve deafness. There is increased incidence of medulloblastoma.

The management of these patients requires participation of various specialists according to individual clinical problems. Genetic counseling is also indicated.

Syringomas are benign adnexal tumors which are inherited in an autosomal dominant fashion but are more frequent in females. They develop during childhood or adolescence. The tumors are soft, small, skin-colored, red, or brown papules which erupt in profusion on the face, particularly in the periorbital regions, and on the neck, upper chest, lower abdomen, and pubic area. Syringomas are derived from the sweat gland ducts and are readily distinguishable from other adnexal tumors by their histologic pattern. They are of cosmetic significance only. Sparse lesions may be excised, but they are often too numerous to remove.

Trichoepitheliomas (epithelioma adenoides cysticum) are benign nevoid tumors derived from the hair follicles and are inherited as an autosomal dominant trait. They occur on the face in a symmetrical distribu-

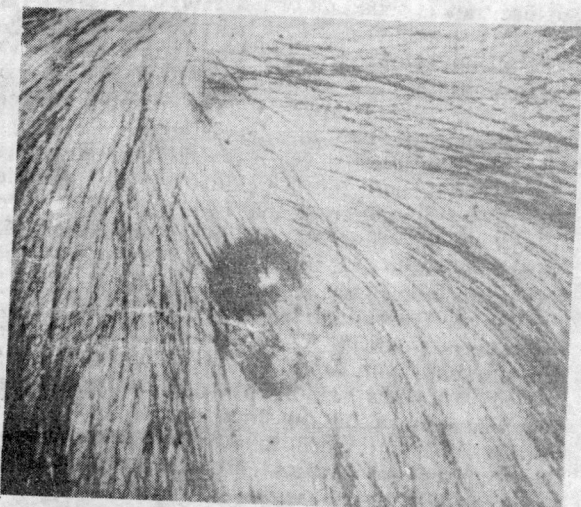

Figure 24–53 Multiple papulonodular juvenile xanthogranulomas on the scalp.

tion but may also appear on the scalp, ears, neck, upper trunk, arms, and thighs. Trichoepitheliomas arise during childhood and adolescence as firm, pink, yellow, or skin-colored papules which enlarge gradually, reaching a final size of 0.5–2 cm. They may be distinguished from other adnexal tumors, basal cell epitheliomas, syringomas, and adenoma sebaceum by biopsy. Surgical excision is the only available therapy.

Lipomas are benign collections of fatty tissue, which appear on the trunk, neck, and proximal limbs. They are soft, compressible, lobulated growths which form skin-colored masses that are usually subcutaneous in location. They attain a maximum size and thereafter persist indefinitely. Occasionally, multiple lesions may occur, particularly in association with neurofibromatosis. At times, atrophy, calcification, liquefaction, or xanthomatous change may complicate their course. They represent a cosmetic defect and may be surgically excised or subjected to biopsy if diagnosis is in doubt.

Juvenile xanthogranulomas (nevoxanthoendothelioma) may be present at birth or develop within the 1st several mo of life. The lesions are firm, dome-shaped, yellow, pink, or orange papules or nodules, varying in size from a few mm to approximately 4 cm in diameter. Rarely, they are macular, annular, or reticulated. Sites of predilection are the scalp (Fig 24–53), face, and upper trunk, where they may erupt in profusion or remain as solitary lesions. Affected infants are otherwise normal, and blood lipid values are never elevated, as they are with xanthomas of hyperlipoproteinemic disorders.

The lesions may resemble papulonodular urticaria pigmentosa, dermatofibromas, or xanthomas of hyperlipoproteinemia. Biopsy is helpful diagnostically; mature lesions are characterized by a dermal infiltrate of lipid-laden histiocytes, admixed inflammatory cells, and Touton giant cells (multinucleated vacuolated cells with a wreath of nuclei and a peripheral rim of foamy cytoplasm) that are pathognomonic for xanthogranuloma. Lipid deposits may be demonstrated by special stains. There is no need to remove these lesions since virtually all of them regress spontaneously during the 1st few yr.

Rare instances of similar lesions in the lung, testes, and pericardium have been reported. More commonly, juvenile xanthogranulomas occur in the ocular tissues, presenting as infiltrates in the orbit, iris, episclera, or ciliary body or as glaucoma, hyphema, uveitis, heterochromia iridum, iritis, or sudden proptosis (see Chapter 25).

Mucosal neuroma syndrome (Sipple syndrome) is inherited as an autosomal dominant trait and is easily recognized during the 1st few wk of life by characteristic physical features. An asthenic or Marfanoid habitus is accompanied by scoliosis, pectus excavatum, pes cavus, and muscular hypotonia. There are thick, patulous lips and soft tissue prognathism simulating acromegaly. Multiple mucosal neuromas or neurofibromas appear as pink, pedunculated, or sessile nodules on the anterior third of the tongue, at the commissures of the lips, and on the buccal mucosa and palpebral conjunctiva. A variety of ophthalmologic defects and intestinal ganglioneuromatosis with recurrent diarrhea are additional common findings.

Of major concern in these patients is the high incidence of medullary thyroid carcinoma associated with high calcitonin levels, pheochromocytoma, and hyperparathyroidism, probably a compensatory response to the high levels of circulating calcitonin. Rarely, these patients are mistakenly diagnosed as having neurofibromatosis. Periodic screening tests for the associated malignant tumors are mandatory.

24.33 PRINCIPLES OF THERAPY

Dermatologic therapy is a mixture of art and science in which the nuances often determine the success of management. Competent skin care requires a specific diagnosis and knowledge of the natural course of the disease as well as an appreciation of primary versus secondary lesions. If the diagnosis is uncertain, it is better to err on the side of less rather than more aggressive treatment. Even when the diagnosis is clear, an acute dermatitis may require gentle and bland therapy initially.

In the use of topical medication, consideration of vehicle is as important as the specific therapeutic agent. Acute weeping lesions respond best to wet compresses, followed by lotions, aerosols, or creams. When the skin is dry, thickened, and scaly, an ointment base is more effective. Gels and solutions are most useful for the scalp and other hairy areas. The site of involvement is of considerable importance since the most desirable vehicle may not be cosmetically or functionally appropriate, e.g., ointment on the face or hands. Patient preference should also play a significant role in choice of vehicle since compliance is poor if the medication is not acceptable to the patient.

Therapy should be kept as simple as possible, and specific written instructions as to frequency and duration of application should be provided. Drug combinations in a single vehicle may exacerbate a dermatitis and cause diagnostic confusion. The physician should become familiar with 1 or 2 preparations in each category and learn to use them appropriately. The careless prescribing of nonspecific proprietary medications that often contain sensitizing agents is not to be condoned. Certain preparations such as topical antihistamines and anesthetics are never indicated in good dermatologic practice.

Wet dressings will alleviate pruritus, burning, and stinging sensations; they are indicated for any acutely inflamed moist or oozing dermatitis. Although a variety of astringent and antiseptic substances may be added to the solution, tap water compresses are just as effective.

Open wet dressings cool and dry the skin by evaporation and cleanse by removal of crusts and exudates that cause further irritation if permitted to remain. The solution should be cool or tepid and consist of tap water, isotonic saline, or aluminum acetate (Burow solution) in a 1:20 or 1:40 dilution. Potassium permanganate is messy and offers no advantage. Boric acid can be toxic if absorbed and should *never* be used for compresses. Dressings of multiple layers of Kerlix, gauze, or soft cotton material should be saturated with the solution and remoistened as often as necessary. Compresses should be applied for 10–20 min at least every 4 hr and continued as necessary, usually for 24–48 hr.

Closed wet dressings are indicated for abscesses and cellulitis. The solution should be warm, and the dressings should be covered with plastic to prevent evaporation. Closed wet dressings, if prolonged, cause maceration because they prevent evaporation and heat loss.

Bath oils, colloids, soaps. *Bath oil* may be added to the bath or to compressing solutions when the skin is dry. These preparations, which are highly dispersible and have surfactant activity, may be obtained scented or unscented for the allergic patient. Bath oils leave a fine film of oil on the skin for lubrication; parents should be cautioned that the child and tub will be slippery. Alpha Keri oil, Lubath, and Domol are examples of commercial preparations. Bath oils containing tar (Balnetar, Zetar) can be prescribed for psoriasis.

Colloids such as starch powder or Aveeno are soothing and antipruritic for some patients when added to the bath water. Oilated Aveeno contains mineral oil and lanolin derivatives to provide lubrication if the skin is dry.

Ordinary toilet *soaps* may be irritating and drying if patients have dry skin or dermatitis. Examples of soaps that are usually not harmful to skin are Dove, Lowila, Aveeno, Neutrogena, Basis, Alpha Keri, Lubriderm, and Oilatum. When skin is acutely inflamed, avoidance of soap is advised.

Lubricants, such as lotions, creams, and ointments, can be used as emollients for dry skin and as vehicles for topical agents such as corticosteroids and keratolytics. In general, ointments are the most effective emollients. Numerous commercial preparations are available in addition to standard U.S.P. items, such as petrolatum, cold cream, stearin-lanolin cream, and hydrophilic ointment. Some patients do not tolerate ointments on their skin, and some may be sensitized to 1 of the components of the lubricant; some preservatives of creams, most commonly parabens, are known sensitizers.

Useful lubricating lotions include Lubriderm, Keri lotion, Nutraderm, and Nivea. Creams include Eucerin, Neutrogena, Nutraderm, and Lubriderm. Aquaphor is a cosmetically acceptable alternative to petrolatum. These preparations can be applied several times a day if necessary for lubrication. Maximal effect is achieved when they are applied *immediately* following a bath or shower.

Shampoos. Special shampoos containing sulfur, salicylic acid, antiseptics, and selenium sulfide (Selsun, Exsel) are useful for conditions in which there is scaling of the scalp. Most shampoos also contain surfactants and detergents. Shampoos with sulfur and/or salicylic acid include Ionil, Sebulex, Fostex, and Vansek. Those with only antiseptic agents include Zincon, Danex, and Head and Shoulders. Tar-containing shampoos such as T-gel, Ionil-T, Sebutone, and Polytar are useful for psoriasis and severe seborrheic dermatitis. In general, they can be used as frequently as necessary to control scaling, but use must be limited to avoid irritation. Patients should be instructed to leave the lathered shampoo in contact with the scalp for 5–10 min.

Shake lotions are useful antipruritic agents; they consist of a suspension of powder in a liquid vehicle. A water-dispersible oil may be added for lubrication. Calamine lotion is acceptable but tends to cake on the skin. A prototype lotion is zinc oxide 20 gm, talc 20 gm, glycerine 20 gm, Alpha Keri 5 gm, and water to make 120 gm. These preparations can be used effectively in combination with wet dressings for exudative dermatitis. Cooling occurs as the lotion evaporates and moisture is absorbed by the powder deposited on the skin.

Powders are hygroscopic and serve as effective absorptive agents in areas of excessive moisture. They are most useful in the intertriginous areas and between the toes, where maceration and abrasion may result from friction on movement. Coarse powders may cake; therefore they should be of fine particle size and inert unless medication has been incorporated in the formulation. Cornstarch may be a growth medium for *Candida* and should not be used. Zeasorb is a bland, finely milled, general purpose powder that can be applied to any area of the body.

Pastes contain a fine powder in an ointment vehicle and are not often prescribed in current dermatologic therapy; in certain situations, however, they can be used effectively to protect vulnerable or damaged skin. For example, a stiff zinc oxide paste is bland and inert and can be applied to the diaper area to avert irritant diaper dermatitis. Zinc paste should be applied in a thick layer completely obscuring the skin and is more easily removed with mineral oil than with soap and water.

Keratolytic agents. *Urea*-containing agents are hydrophilic; they hydrate the stratum corneum and make the skin more pliable. In addition, because urea dissolves hydrogen bonds and epidermal keratin, it is effective in treatment of scaling disorders. A concentration of 10–25% is available in several commercial lotions and creams (Carmol, Carmol 10, Nutraplus, Uhramide, Aquacare HP), which can be applied once or twice daily as tolerated.

Salicylic acid is an effective keratolytic agent and can be incorporated into a variety of vehicles in concentrations up to 6% to be applied 2–3 times daily. Salicylic acid preparations should not be used in the treatment of small infants or on large surface areas and denuded skin; percutaneous absorption may result in salicylism.

The α-hydroxy acids, particularly *lactic acid* and *citric acid*, can be incorporated in an ointment vehicle such as petrolatum or Aquaphor in concentrations up to 5%. These preparations are useful for the treatment of keratinizing disorders and may be applied once or twice daily. Some patients complain of burning; in this event, the frequency of application should be decreased.

Tar compounds. Coal tars are obtained from bituminous coal, shales, petrolatum, and woods. They are antipruritic and astringent and appear to promote normal keratinization. They are particularly useful for chronic eczema and psoriasis, and their efficacy may be increased if the affected area is exposed to ultraviolet light. However, the tar should be removed prior to exposure to light; otherwise a phototoxic dermatitis may ensue. Tars *should not be used* in acute inflammatory lesions.

Tars may be incorporated into shampoos, bath oils, lotions, and ointments. A useful preparation for pediatric patients is liquor carbonis detergens (LCD) 2–5% in a cream or ointment vehicle. The newer tar gels (Psorigel and Estargel), are relatively pleasant cosmetic preparations which cause minimum staining of skin and fabrics. Tars can also be incorporated into a vehicle with a topical corticosteroid. The frequency of application varies from 1–3 times daily according to tolerance.

Antifungal agents are now available as powders, lotions, creams, and ointments for the treatment of dermatophyte and yeast infections. Nystatin and amphotericin B (Fungizone) are specific for *Candida* and are ineffective in other fungal disorders. Tolnaftate (Tinactin) is effective against the dermatophytes and somewhat effective in the treatment of tinea versicolor. The spectrum for haloprogin (Halotex) includes the dermatophytes, *Pityrosporon orbiculare* and *Candida albicans*. The newest agents, miconazole (Micatin) and clotrimazole (Lotimin), have a spectrum similar to haloprogin. They should be applied 2–3 times a day for most fungal infections. All these agents have a low sensitizing potential; however, additives such as preservatives and stabilizers in the vehicles may cause allergic contact dermatitis. Whitfield ointment (6% benzoic acid and 3% salicylic acid) is a potent keratolytic agent that has also been used for the treatment of dermatophyte infections. Irritant reactions are common.

Topical antibiotics have been used to treat local cutaneous infections for many yr; recently their efficacy has been questioned. Ointments are the preferable vehicle, and combinations with other topical agents, such as corticosteroids, are in general inadvisable. Whenever possible, the etiologic agent should be identified and treated specifically. Antibiotics in wide use as systemic preparations should be avoided because of the risk of sensitization. The sensitizing potential of certain other antibiotics (e.g., neomycin, Furacin) should be kept in mind. Polysporin and bacitracin are probably the 2 most useful preparations for pyoderma; Silvadene cream is effective in the treatment of patients with large denuded areas of skin.

Topical corticosteroids are potent antiinflammatory agents and effective antipruritic agents. Successful therapeutic results have been achieved in a wide variety of skin conditions. In general, corticosteroids fall into 2 classes: nonfluorinated preparations such as hydrocortisone (Hytone) and desonide (Tridesilon); and fluorinated compounds including triamcinolone (Kenalog, Aristocort), flurandrenolone (Cordran), fluocinolone (Synalar), betamethasone (Valisone, Benisone, Flurobate), and flumethasone (Locorten). The nonfluorinated steroids are of lesser potency but also cause fewer local and systemic side effects, whereas fluorinated steroids are potentially more harmful, particularly with long-term use. Other fluorinated compounds, e.g., fluocinonide (Lidex) and halcinonide (Halog), are extremely potent and should be prescribed with care. Some of these compounds are formulated in several strengths.

Virtually all of the corticosteroids can be obtained in a variety of vehicles, including creams, ointments, solutions, gels, and aerosols. Absorption is enhanced by an ointment or gel vehicle; however, the selection of the vehicle should be based on the type of disorder and site of involvement. Frequency of application should be determined by the potency of the preparation and the severity of the eruption. In general, the application of a *thin film* 2–4 times daily will suffice. Adverse local effects include cutaneous atrophy, striae, telangiectasia, hypopigmentation, and increased hair growth.

Percutaneous absorption of corticosteroids can be enhanced up to 100-fold by the use of occlusive pliable plastic wraps (Handi-Wrap, Saran Wrap). The steroid is applied in a thin film and tightly covered with a strip of plastic which is taped to the skin. Baggies may be used for the feet and disposable plastic gloves for the hands. Occlusion should be carried out for no more than 8–10 hr since prolonged occlusion may produce undesirable side effects such as pyoderma, folliculitis, miliaria, and malodor from maceration and bacterial overgrowth. This procedure is appropriate in chronic recalcitrant disorders such as lichen simplex chronicus, dyshidrotic eczema, and psoriasis. The possibility of systemic absorption and adrenal suppression must be considered if large areas are occluded. Fluorinated corticosteroids with or without occlusion are seldom indicated in infancy.

In selected circumstances, corticosteroids may be administered by intralesional injection for acne cysts, keloids, psoriatic plaques, and persistent insect bite reactions. This method of administration should be used only by physicians experienced in dermatologic therapeutic techniques.

Sunscreens are of 2 general types: those which reflect all wavelengths of the ultraviolet and visible spectrums, such as zinc oxide and titanium dioxide; and a heterogeneous group of chemicals that selectively absorb energy of various wavelengths within the ultraviolet spectrum. Some sunscreens permit tanning without burning; others prevent both. In addition to the spectrum of light which is blocked, other factors to be considered include cosmetic acceptance, sensitizing potential, retention on skin while swimming or sweating, required frequency of application, and cost. Effective opaque total barrier agents are A-Fil, zinc oxide ointment, and RVPaque. Para-aminobenzoic acid-ethanol (Pabanol, PreSun) and cinnamate-benzophenone combinations (Maxafil, Solbar, Uval) effectively prevent transmission of UVB and at least some UVA wavelengths. PABA-esters (Eclipse, Pabafilm, Sundown) afford partial protection. Lip protectants that absorb in the UVB range (Sunstick, RVPaba lipstick, Uval Sun 'N Wind Stick) are also available for patients with photo-induced lip disorders such as recurrent herpesvirus infections. Sunscreens are now designated by sun protection factor (SPF) values ranging from 2 (minimal protection) to 15 (maximal protection) and are so labeled on the container. Examples of sunscreens offering maximal protection are Supershade 15 and Total Eclipse. The efficacy of these agents depends on careful attention to instructions for use. PABA-containing sunscreens should be applied at least ½ hr prior to sun exposure to permit penetration of the epidermis. Most patients with photosensitivity eruptions will require protection by agents that absorb UVB wavelengths; patients with porphyria, phototoxic eruptions, and some types of solar urticaria require agents with a broader spectrum of prevention.

NANCY B. ESTERLY

General

Arndt KA: Manual of Dermatologic Therapeutics. Ed 2. Boston, Little, Brown, 1978.
Cunliff WJ, Cutterill JA: The Acnes. London, WB Saunders, 1975.
Hurwitz S: Clinical Pediatric Dermatology. Philadelphia, WB Saunders, 1981.
Moschella SL, Pillsbury DM, Hurley HM: Dermatology. Vols I and II. Philadelphia, WB Saunders, 1975.
Solomon LM, Esterly NB, Loeffel ED: Adolescent Dermatology. Philadelphia, WB Saunders, 1978.
Weston WL: Practical Pediatric Dermatology. Boston, Little, Brown, 1979.

Specific Diseases

Altman J, Perry HO: The variations of course of lichen planus. Arch Dermatol 84:179, 1961.
Bean SF: Bullous scabies. JAMA 230:878, 1974.
Beckett IH, Jacobs AH: Recurring digital fibrous tumors of childhood. Pediatrics 59:401, 1977.

Beighton P: The dominant and recessive forms of cutis laxa. J Med Genet 9:216, 1972.
Brown SH Jr, Neerhout RC, Founkalsrud FW: Prednisone therapy in the management of large hemangiomas in infants and children. Surgery 71:168, 1972.
Burgoon CF Jr, Graham JH, McCaffree DL: Mast cell disease. A cutaneous variant with multisystem involvement. Arch Dermatol 98:590, 1968.
Carney RG Jr: Incontinentia pigmenti. A world statistical analysis. Arch Dermatol 112:535, 1976.
Chalhub EG: Neurocutaneous syndromes in children. Pediatr Clin North Am 23:499, 1976.
Dajani AS, Ferrieri P, Wannamaker LW: Natural history of impetigo. II. Etiologic agents and bacterial interactions. J Clin Invest 51:2863, 1972.
Elias PM, Fritsch P, Epstein J: Staphylococcal scalded skin syndrome. Arch Dermatol 113:207, 1977.
Epstein EH Jr, Oren ME: Popsicle panniculitis. N Engl J Med 282:966, 1970.
Esterly NB, Furey NL, Kirschner BS, et al: Chronic bullous dermatosis of childhood. Arch Dermatol 113:42, 1977.
Ferrieri P, Dajani AS, Wannamaker LW, et al: Natural history of impetigo. I. Site sequence of acquisition and familial patterns of spread of cutaneous streptococci. J Clin Invest 51:2851, 1972.
Flanagan BP, Helwig EB: Cutaneous lymphangioma. Arch Dermatol 113:24, 1977.
Fost NC, Esterly NB: Successful treatment of juvenile hemangiomas with prednisone. J Pediatr 72:351, 1968.
Friedman Z, Schochat SJ, Maisela MJ, et al: Correction of essential fatty acid deficiency in newborn infants by cutaneous application of sunflower seed oil. Pediatrics 58:650, 1976.
Gianotti F: Papular acrodermatitis of childhood and other papulo-vesicular acro-located syndromes. Br J Dermatol 100:49, 1979.
Hawthorne HC Jr, Nelson JS, Giangiacomo Z: Blanching subcutaneous nodules in neonatal neuroblastoma. J Pediatr 77:297, 1970.
Hazelrigg DE, Duncan C, Jarrett M: Twenty-nail dystrophy of childhood. Arch Dermatol 113:73, 1977.
Holder KR, Pilchard WA: Diffuse neonatal hemangiomatosis. Pediatrics 46:411, 1971.
Jacobs AH, Walton RG: The incidence of birthmarks in the neonate. Pediatrics 58:281, 1976.
Jobsis AC, DeGrout WP, Tigges AJ, et al.: X-linked ichthyosis and X-linked placental sulfatase deficiency: A disease entity. Am J Pathol 99:279, 1980.
Kaplan EN: The risk of malignancy in large congenital nevi. Plast Reconstr Surg 53:421, 1974.
King LE Jr: Darier's disease: Genetic and isolated forms. Arch Dermatol 110:657, 1974.
Kopf AN, Bart RS, Hennessey P: Congenital nevocytic nevi and malignant melanomas. J Am Acad Dermatol 1:123, 1979.
Krieger I, Evans GW: Acrodermatitis enteropathica without hypozincemia: Therapeutic effect of a pancreatic enzyme preparation due to a zinc-binding ligand. J Pediatr 96:32, 1980.
Laymon CW, Peterson WC: Lipogranulomatosis subcutanea (Rothmann-Makai). Arch Dermatol 90:288, 1954.
Lees MH, Stroud CE: Bone lesions of urticaria pigmentosa in childhood. Arch Dis Child 34:205, 1959.
Lynch HT, Frichot BC III, Lynch JF: Cancer control in xeroderma pigmentosum. Arch Dermatol 113:193, 1977.
Mabry CC, Hollingsworth DR, Upton GV, et al: Pituitary-hypothalamic dysfunction in generalized lipodystrophy. J Pediatr 82:625, 1973.
Mikat DM, Ackerman HR Jr, Mikat KW: Balanitis xerotica obliterans: Report of a case in an 11-year-old and review of the literature. Pediatrics 52:25, 1973.
Milstone EG, Helwig EB: Basal cell carcinoma in children. Arch Dermatol 180:523, 1973.
Mulbauer JE: Granuloma annulare. J Am Acad Derm 3:217, 1980.
Neldner KH, Hambidge KM: Zinc deficiency of acrodermatitis enteropathica. N Eng J Med 292:879, 1975.
Nyfors A, Lemholt K: Psoriasis in childhood. Br J Dermatol 92:437, 1975.
Ortega JA, Swanson VL, Landing BH, et al: Congenital dyskeratosis. Am J Dis Child 124:701, 1972.
Papa CM, Mills OH Jr, Hanshaw W: Seasonal trichorrhexis nodosa. Arch Dermatol 106:888, 1972.
Pinnell SR, Krane SM, Kenzora JR, et al: A heritable disorder of connective tissues: Hydroxylysine-deficient collagen disease. N Engl J Med 286:1013, 1972.
Pope FM: Two types of autosomal recessive pseudoxanthoma elasticum. Arch Dermatol 110:209, 1974.
Prystowsky SD, Maumenee IH, Freeman RG, et al: A cutaneous marker in the Hunter syndrome. Arch Dermatol 113:602, 1977.
Rasmussen J: Erythema multiforme: Responses to treatment with systemic corticosteroid. Br J Dermatol 95:181, 1976.
Roenigk HH, Haserick JR, Arundell FD: Poststeroid panniculitis. Arch Dermatol 90:387, 1964.
Rook A: Papular urticaria. Pediatr Clin N Am 8:817, 1961.
Rosenmann A, Shapira T, Cohen MM: Ectodactyly, ectodermal dysplasia and cleft palate (EEC syndrome). Clin Genet 9:347, 1976.
Schachner L, Young D: Pseudoxanthoma elasticum with severe cardiovascular disease in a child. Am J Dis Child 127:571, 1974.

Schmidt H, Knitker G, Thomsen K, et al: Erythropoietic protoporphyria. A clinical study based on 29 cases in 14 families. Arch Dermatol 110:58, 1974.

Schwartz MF Jr, Esterly NB, Fretzin DF, et al: Hypomelanosis of Ito (incontinentia pigmenti achromians): A neurocutaneous syndrome. J Pediatr 90:236, 1977.

Shaw JCL: Trace elements in the fetus and young infant. Am J Dis Child 133:1260, 1979.

Solomon LM: The management of congenital melanocytic nevi. Arch Dermatol 116:1017, 1980.

Solomon LM, Esterly NB: Epidermal and other congenital organoid nevi. Curr Probl Pediatr 6:1, 1975.

Tunnessen WW Jr, Neiburg PJ, Voorhess ML: Hypothyroidism and pityriasis rubra pilaris. J Pediatr 88:456, 1976.

Wanzl JE, Bugert EO Jr: The spider nevus in infancy and childhood. Pediatrics 33:227, 1964.

Watson W, Farber EM: Psoriasis in childhood. Pediatr Clin North Am 18:875, 1971.

Wilkin JK: Unilateral nevoid telangiectasia. Three new cases and the role of estrogen. Arch Dermatol 113:486, 1977.

PEDIATRIC OPHTHALMOLOGY 25

THE EYE IN INFANCY AND CHILDHOOD

25.1 GROWTH AND DEVELOPMENT

At birth the eye of the normal fullterm infant is approximately three quarters of adult size. Postnatal growth is maximal during the 1st yr, proceeds at a rapid but decelerating rate until the 3rd yr, and continues at a slower rate thereafter until puberty, after which little change occurs. Various parts of the eye have different growth rates. In general, the anterior structures of the eye are relatively large at birth and grow proportionately less thereafter than the posterior structures. This growth pattern results in a progressive change in the shape of the globe; it becomes more nearly spherical.

In the infant the *sclera* is thin and translucent, with a bluish tinge. The *cornea* is relatively large in the newborn (averaging 10 mm) and attains adult size (nearly 12 mm) by the age of 2 yr or earlier. Its curvature tends to flatten with age, with progressive change in the refractive properties of the eye. The normal cornea is perfectly clear. In infants born prematurely there may be an opalescent haze that is transient. The anterior chamber in the newborn appears shallow, and the angle structures, so important to the maintenance of normal intraocular pressure, must undergo further differentiation after birth. The *iris*, typically light blue at birth in Caucasians, undergoes progressive change of color as the pigmentation of the stroma increases in the early months and years. The pupils of the newborn infant tend to be small and are often difficult to dilate. Often remnants of the pupillary membrane are evident on ophthalmoscopic examination as cobweb-like lines crossing the pupillary aperture; these developmental features tend to disappear.

The *lens* of the newborn infant is more nearly spherical than that of the adult; its greater refractive power helps to compensate for the relative shortness of the young eye. The lens continues to grow throughout life; new fibers added to the periphery continually push older fibers toward the center of the lens. With age, the lens becomes progressively more dense and more resistant to change of shape during accommodation.

The *fundus* of the newborn eye is less pigmented than that of the adult; the choroidal vascular pattern is highly visible, and the retinal pigmentary pattern often has a fine "peppery" or mottled appearance. In addition, the macular landmarks, particularly the foveal light reflex, are less well defined and not readily apparent to ophthalmoscopic examination. The peripheral retina appears pale or grayish, and the peripheral retinal vasculature is immature, especially in the premature infant. The optic nervehead also tends to appear slightly pale, sometimes grayish. Within 4–6 mo the appearance of the fundus more nearly approximates that of the mature eye.

Superficial retinal hemorrhages may be observed in as many as 25% of newborn infants. These usually absorb promptly and only rarely leave any permanent effect. Conjunctival hemorrhages also may occur at birth and resorb spontaneously without consequence.

Remnants of the primitive hyaloid vascular system may also be seen on ophthalmoscopic examination. They appear as small tufts or worm-like structures projecting from the disc or as a fine strand traversing the vitreous; in some cases only a small dot (Mittendorf dot) remains on the posterior aspect of the lens capsule.

As a rule, the infant eye is somewhat hyperopic (farsighted), but the refractive state at any time in life depends on the net effect of many factors, the principal ones being the size of the eye, the state of the lens, and the curvature of the cornea.

Newborn infants tend to keep their eyes closed much of the time, but the normal newborn can see, will respond to changes in illumination, and can fixate points of contrast. The visual acuity in the newborn is estimated to be in the range of 20/600. One of the earliest responses to a formed visual stimulus is the infant's regard for the mother's face, evident especially during feeding. By 2 wk of age the infant shows more sustained interest in large objects, and by 8–10 wk of age the normal infant can follow an object through an arc of 180°. The acuity improves rapidly and may reach 20/30–20/20 by the age of 3 yr or earlier.

In many normal infants there may be imperfect coordination of the *eye movements* and *alignment* during the early days and weeks, but proper coordination should be achieved by age 4–6 mo, usually sooner. Persistent deviation of an eye in an infant requires evaluation.

25.2 EXAMINATION OF THE EYE

Examination of the eye should be a routine part of the periodic pediatric assessment. Screening in schools and community programs can also be effective in detecting problems early. The child should be examined by an ophthalmologist whenever a significant ocular abnormality or vision defect is noted. Ideally, every child should have a thorough ophthalmologic examination sometime in early childhood, preferably by the age of 3–4 yr; these are the crucial years for the detection and treatment of amblyopia, strabismus, high refractive errors, and certain tumors of childhood.

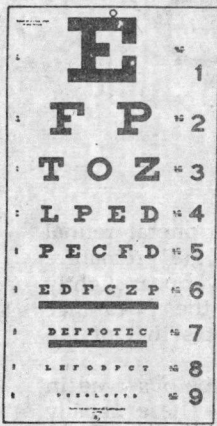 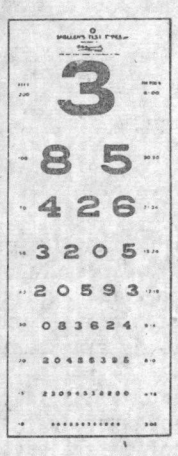 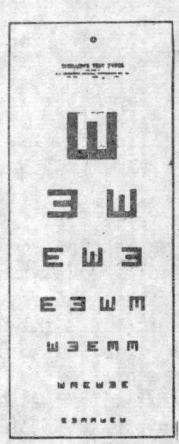 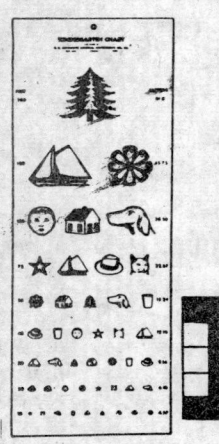

Figure 25–1 Various types of visual acuity charts. As illustrated by the Snellen E, each optotype is designed to subtend 5 min of arc, each component 1 min of arc.

Basic examination, whether done by the pediatrician or ophthalmologist, must include evaluation of visual acuity and the visual fields, assessment of the pupils, ocular motility and alignment, a general external examination, and an ophthalmoscopic examination of the media and fundi. When indicated, biomicroscopy (slit lamp examination), cycloplegic refraction, and tonometry are performed by the ophthalmologist. In some cases special diagnostic procedures, such as ultrasonic examination, fluorescein angiography, electroretinography (ERG), or visual evoked response (VER) testing, are also indicated.

Visual acuity is best measured by the standard Snellen chart (Fig 25–1), and this method should be used as early as the child's ability to name, copy, or match letters or numbers will allow. The "E" chart, consisting of rows of the letter E in various sizes and directions, can also be used; children are asked to indicate the direction of the selected E by pointing their hand or fingers (or a matching cardboard E) up, down, right, or left. For the very young child or the retarded, shy, or frightened child, a calibrated picture test can be used. In infants and toddlers, in the very retarded, and in the psychiatrically disturbed youngster, vision can be estimated by the response to balls and familiar objects of various sizes, recording the distance at which the response is elicited. Optokinetic nystagmus, the response to a sequence of moving targets ("railroad" nystagmus), can also be used to assess vision; this can be calibrated by various sized targets (stripes or dots) or a rotating drum at specified distances. The visual evoked response (VER), an electrophysiologic method of evaluating the cerebral response to light and special visual stimuli, such as a changing checkerboard pattern, can also be used to study visual function in selected cases.

Subnormal vision in 1 or both eyes warrants further evaluation.

Visual field assessment, like visual acuity testing, must be geared to the child's age and abilities. Formal visual field examination (perimetry and scotometry) can often be accomplished in the school age child. Often, however, the examiner must rely on confrontation techniques and finger counting in quadrants of the visual field. In many children only testing by attraction can be accomplished; the examiner observes the child's response to familiar objects brought into each of the 4 quadrants of the visual field of each eye in turn. The child's bottle, a favorite toy, and lollipops are particularly effective attention-getting items. Even such gross methods can often detect diagnostically significant field changes such as the bitemporal hemiopsia of a chiasmal lesion or the homonymous hemianopsia of a cerebral lesion.

Color vision testing can be accomplished whenever the child is able to name or trace the test symbols; these may be either numbers or Xs, Os, and triangles. Color vision testing is not frequently necessary in young children, but parents will sometimes request it, particularly if the child seems to be slow in learning colors. Defective color vision is not uncommon in males but rare in females. Occasionally, there is achromatopsia, a total color vision defect with subnormal visual acuity, nystagmus, and photophobia. A change in color discrimination can be a sign of optic nerve or retinal disease.

The pupillary examination includes evaluation of both the direct and consensual reactions to light, the reaction on near gaze, and the response to reduced illumination, noting the size and symmetry of the pupils under all conditions. Special care must be taken to differentiate the reaction to light from the reaction to near gaze; the natural tendency of a child is to look directly at the approaching light, inducing the near gaze reflex when one is attempting to test only the reaction to light; accordingly, every effort must be made to control fixation. The swinging flashlight test is especially useful for detecting unilateral or asymmetric prechiasmatic afferent defects in children (see Marcus Gunn pupil, below).

Ocular motility is tested by having the child follow an object into the various positions of gaze. Movements of each eye individually (ductions) and of the 2 eyes together (versions, conjugate movements, and convergence) are assessed. Alignment is judged by the symmetry of the corneal light reflexes and by the response to alternate occlusion of each eye (see *cover tests for strabismus*, Sec 25.6).

External examination begins with general inspection in good illumination, noting size, shape, and symmetry of the orbits; position and movement of the lids; and the position and symmetry of the globes. Viewing the eyes and lids from above will aid in detection of orbital asymmetry, lid masses, proptosis (exophthalmos), and abnormal pulsations. Palpation too is important in detection of orbital and lid masses.

The lacrimal apparatus is assessed by looking for evidence of tear deficiency, overflow of tears (epiphora), and erythema and swelling in the region of the tear sac or gland. The sac is massaged to check for reflux when obstruction is suspected. The presence and position of the puncta are also checked.

The lids and conjunctiva are specifically examined for focal lesions, foreign bodies, and inflammatory signs; loss and maldirection of lashes are also to be noted. When necessary, the lids can be everted in the following manner: (1) instruct the patient to look down; (2) grasp the lashes of the patient's upper lid between the thumb and index finger of 1 hand; (3) place a probe, a cotton-tipped applicator, or the thumb of the other hand at the upper margin of the tarsal plate; and (4) pulling the lid down and outward, evert it over the probe, using the instrument as a fulcrum. Skill at eversion of the lid should be acquired. Foreign bodies commonly lodge in the concavity just above the lid margin and are exposed only by fully everting the lid.

The anterior segment of the eye is then evaluated with oblique focal illumination, noting luster and clarity of the cornea, depth and clarity of the anterior chamber, and features of the iris. Transillumination of the anterior segment will aid in detecting opacities and in demonstrating atrophy or hypopigmentation of the iris; these latter signs are important when ocular albinism is suspected. Fluorescein dye will also aid in the diagnosis of abrasions, ulcerations, and foreign bodies.

Biomicroscopy (slit lamp examination) provides a highly magnified view of the various structures of the eye and an optical section through the media of the eye—that is, the cornea, aqueous humor, lens, and vitreous. Lesions can be not only identified but also localized as to their depth within the eye, and the resolution is sufficient to allow detection even of individual inflammatory cells in the aqueous and vitreous. With addition of special lenses and prisms, the angle of the anterior chamber and regions of the fundus also can be examined with the slit lamp. Biomicroscopy is often crucial in trauma and in examination for iritis. It is also helpful in the diagnosis of many metabolic diseases of childhood.

Fundus examination is best done with the pupil dilated unless there are neurologic or other contraindications. Tropicamide (Mydriacyl), 0.5–1%, or phenylephrine (Neo-Synephrine), 2.5%, are recommended as mydriatics of short duration. Beginning with posterior landmarks, the disc and the macula, the 4 quadrants are systematically examined by following each of the major vessel groups to the periphery. More of the fundus can be seen if the child is directed to look up, down, right, and left. Even with care, only a limited amount of the fundus can be seen with the direct or handheld ophthalmoscope. For examination of the far periphery the indirect ophthalmoscope is used, and full dilation of the pupil is essential.

It should be noted that before an examination of the retina is made, the ophthalmoscope is used to examine the clarity of the media; with a high plus lens (+8 or +10) in place, the ophthalmoscope can also be used for examination of external lesions and foreign bodies as it provides magnification and good illumination.

Refraction is the determination of the refractive state of the eye, that is, the degree of nearsightedness, farsightedness, or astigmatism. Retinoscopy gives an objective determination of the amount of correction required and can be done at any age. In young children it is best done with cycloplegia. Subjective refinement of the refraction, involving asking the patient for preferences in the strength and axis of corrective lenses, can be accomplished in many school age children. Refraction and determination of the visual acuity with appropriate corrective lenses in place are essential steps in deciding whether or not the patient has a pathologic visual defect.

Tonometry, the measurement of intraocular pressure, is usually done by the traditional indentation method with the Schiøtz gauge or by the applanation method with the slit lamp. Alternative methods are pneumatic and electronic tonometry. When accurate measurement of the pressure is necessary in a child who cannot cooperate, it may be done with sedation or general anesthesia. A gross estimate of pressure can be made by palpating the globe with the index fingers placed side by side on the upper lid above the tarsal plate.

25.3 ABNORMALITIES OF REFRACTION AND ACCOMMODATION

If parallel rays of light come to focus on the retina with the eye in a state of rest (nonaccommodating), emmetropia exists. Such an ideal optical state is not uncommon, but more often the opposite condition, ametropia, exists. Three principal types occur: hyperopia (farsightedness), myopia (nearsightedness), and astigmatism. Approximately 80% of children are physiologically hyperopic at birth; about 5% are born myopic.

The refractive state of the eye in children is most accurately measured by cycloplegic refraction, with the use of such drugs as tropicamide (Mydriacyl), cyclopentolate hydrochloride (Cyclogyl), homatropine hydrobromide, or atropine sulfate to relax accommodation.

Hyperopia. If parallel rays of light come to focus posterior to the retina with the eye in a state of rest (nonaccommodating), hyperopia or farsightedness exists. This may result because the anteroposterior diameter of the eye is too short, because the refractive power of the cornea or lens is less than normal, or because the lens is dislocated posteriorly.

In hyperopia, accommodation is used to bring objects into focus for both far and near gaze. If the accommodative effort required is not too great, the child will have clear vision and will be comfortable for both distant and close work. In high degrees of hyperopia requiring greater accommodative effort, vision may be blurred, and the child may complain of "eye strain," headaches, or fatigue. Squinting, eye rubbing, lid inflammation, and lack of interest in reading are also frequent manifestations. There may be associated esotropia (convergent strabismus, accommodative esotropia, Sec 25.6). Convex lenses (spectacles) of sufficient strength to provide clear vision and comfort are prescribed when indicated.

Myopia. In myopia parallel rays of light come to focus anterior to the retina, possibly because the anteroposterior diameter of the eye is too long, because the refractive power of the cornea or lens is greater than normal, or because the lens is dislocated forward. The principal symptom is blurred vision for distant objects. The far point of clear vision varies inversely with the degree of myopia; as the myopia increases, the far point of clear vision comes closer. With myopia of 1 diopter, for example, the far point of clear focus is 1 meter from the eye; with myopia of 3 diopters, the far point of clear vision is only one third of a meter from the eye. Thus myopic children tend to hold objects and reading matter close, prefer to be close to the blackboard, and may be uninterested in distant activities. Frowning and squinting are common since the visual acuity is improved when the lid aperture is reduced; the effect is similar to that achieved by closing or "stopping down" the aperture of the diaphragm of a camera.

Concave lenses (spectacles or contact lenses) of appropriate strength to provide clear vision and comfort are prescribed. Yearly re-evaluation is advised; simple myopia tends to increase through adolescence. There is a hereditary tendency to myopia, and children of myopic parents should be examined at an early age. In some cases of myopia there are associated degenerative changes of the retina.

Astigmatism. In astigmatism there is a difference in the refractive power of the various meridians of the eye. Most cases are due to irregularity in the curvature of the cornea; some astigmatism is due to changes in the lens. A mild degree of astigmatism is very common and may produce no symptoms. With greater degrees there may be distortion of vision. In an effort to achieve a clearer image, the person with astigmatism will use accommodation or frown or squint to obtain a pinhole effect, as in myopia. Symptoms include "eye strain," headache, and fatigue. Eye rubbing and lid hyperemia, indifference to schoolwork, and holding reading matter close are common manifestations in childhood. Cylindric or spherocylindric lenses are used to provide optical correction when indicated. Glasses may be needed constantly or only part-time, depending on the degree of astigmatism and the severity of the attendant symptoms.

Anisometropia. When the refractive state of 1 eye is significantly different from the refractive state of the fellow eye, anisometropia exists. Uncorrected, this may lead to sensory deprivation amblyopia or "lazy eye." Early detection and correction are essential if normal visual development in both eyes is to be achieved.

Paralysis of Accommodation. The most frequent cause of paralysis of accommodation in children is the intentional or inadvertent use of cycloplegic substances, topically or systemically; included are all the anticholi-

nergic drugs and poisons as well as plants and plant substances containing naturally occurring alkaloids. Neurogenic causes of accommodative paralysis include lesions affecting the oculomotor nerve (3rd cranial nerve) in any part of its course. Differential diagnosis includes tumors, degenerative diseases, vascular lesions, and trauma. Infectious diseases also may affect accommodation; diphtheria, for example, may cause paralysis of the ciliary muscle. Rarely, inability to accommodate is due to a congenital defect of the ciliary muscle. An apparent defect in accommodation may be psychogenic in origin; it is not uncommon for a child to feign inability to read when it can be demonstrated that visual acuity and ability to focus are normal.

25.4 DISORDERS OF VISION

Amblyopia. Amblyopia is subnormal visual acuity in 1 or both eyes despite appropriate correction of any significant refractive error. In its broadest sense the term may embrace a variety of vision defects of organic or nonorganic origin; for example, organic amblyopia designates vision loss directly attributable to trauma or to an organic lesion or disease of the eye or visual pathways. The term amblyopia is preferentially used, however, in its restricted sense to denote a specific developmental disorder of visual function arising from (1) sensory stimulation deprivation or (2) abnormal binocular interaction (i.e., malalignment or strabismus). In this sense amblyopia is familiarly known as "lazy eye."

Under normal conditions the development of visual acuity proceeds rapidly in infancy and early childhood. Anything that interferes with the formation of a clear retinal image during this early developmental period can produce *sensory deprivation amblyopia*. For example, a cataract in early life can interefere with retinal stimulation during a critical developmental period to the degree that even after the cataract is successfully removed and the aphakic refractive error is corrected with appropriate glasses or a contact lens, providing a clear retinal image, the vision will be relatively poor. Similarly, uncorrected anisometropia in the young child can lead to amblyopia; in this condition the eye with the more normal refractive state and clearer retinal image is used for definitive seeing and the eye with the greater refractive error and blurred retinal image becomes amblyopic from sensory deprivation or disuse.

In children with strabismus there is a tendency to suppress or "tune out" the image of the deviating eye as a sensory adaptation to avoid diplopia. If allowed to persist untreated in the young child, such suppression can result in amblyopia.

Susceptibility to amblyopia is greatest within the 1st 2–3 yr of life and especially in the 1st mo of life, but the risk of amblyopia exists until full visual potential and stability have been achieved, generally by the age of 5–6 yr.

Amblyopia can be treated; the key to success is early detection and prompt intervention. In an infant amblyopia can often be reversed in a matter of days or weeks.

Text continued on page 1748

Table 25–1 OCULAR CHANGES IN DEVELOPMENTAL PEDIATRIC SYNDROMES

ORGANIZATION OF TABLE HEADINGS

CNS Anomalies	Demyelinating Scleroses
Craniostenosis Syndromes	Hamartomatoses/Phakomatoses
Miscellaneous Craniofacial Defects and Syndromes	Neurocutaneous Syndromes
Chromosomal Abnormalities	Special Neurobiotrophies
Disorders of Amino Acid Metabolism	Disorders of Connective Tissues, Bones, and Joints
The Mucopolysaccharidoses	Dermatologic Disorders
Sphingolipidoses	Syndromes of Multiple Developmental Abnormalities
Ceroid Lipofuscinoses	Miscellaneous Multisystem Disorders
Leukodystrophies	Congenital Infection Syndromes

GENERAL DESCRIPTION	OPHTHALMOLOGIC MANIFESTATIONS
CNS ANOMALIES	
Anencephaly See Sec 21.8	Optic nerve aplasia or hypoplasia
Holoprosencephaly See Sec 21.9	Hypotelorism; in extreme form, cyclopia; in some cases, iris coloboma
Cyclopia A single eye, usually accompanied by proboscis-like structure on forehead; often associated with holoprosencephaly; defect in development of anterior notochord and surrounding mesoderm; malformations of brain commonly include agenesis of corpus callosum, septum pellucidum, and fornix, fusion of thalami, hydrocephalus, and absence of olfactory nerves	Single eye of variable complexity; sometimes fusion of both eyes with duplication of lenses, corneas, and other structures; rosette formation in retina; optic nerve rudimentary or absent; orbit diamond shaped
Arnold-Chiari malformation See Sec 21.8	Nystagmus, usually vertical, often downbeat; ocular motor palsies with diplopia; sometimes skew deviation
Dandy-Walker syndrome See Sec 21.10	Ophthalmic manifestations of increased intracranial pressure
Septo-optic dysplasia (deMorsier syndrome) Malformation of anterior midline structures (agenesis of septum pellucidum, primitive optic ventricle, with hypoplasia of optic nerves, chiasm, and infundibulum); sometimes associated endocrine abnormalities, ranging from panhypopituitarism to selective growth hormone deficiency	Optic nerve hypoplasia, bilateral or unilateral, of varying severity; vision defects, strabismus, nystagmus; in some cases, other anomalies of eyes
CRANIOSTENOSIS SYNDROMES	
Apert syndrome (acrocephalosyndactyly) See Sec 23.10	Orbits shallow, eyes protuberant (proptosis) and widely spaced; antimongoloid slant of palpebral fissures; ocular motor abnormalities (strabismus, partial ophthalmoplegia, nystagmus); papilledema; optic atrophy; cataracts; sometimes dislocated lenses; occasionally iris and fundus colobomata
Carpenter syndrome (acrocephalopolysyndactyly) Sec Sec 23.10	Orbits shallow; lateral displacement of medial canthi; epicanthus; antimongoloid slant of palpebral fissures; optic atrophy; microcornea and corneal opacities in some cases
Crouzon syndrome (dysostosis craniofacialis) See Sec 23.10	Eyes protuberant (proptosis) and widely spaced; luxation of globe may occur; antimongoloid slant of palpebral fissures; strabismus; papilledema; optic atrophy; vision loss; cataracts in some patients
Kleeblattschädel syndrome (cloverleaf skull) See Sec 23.10	Shallow orbits with proptosis; high risk of corneal ulceration
MISCELLANEOUS CRANIOFACIAL DEFECTS AND SYNDROMES	
Frontonasal dysplasia (median cleft-face syndrome) Maldevelopment of nasal capsule; primitive brain vesicle filling space normally occupied by the nasal capsule; facial dysmorphism of varying severity; in complete form, anterior cranium bifidum occultum, median facial cleft involving nose and often upper lip, broad nasal root, hypertelorism, unilateral or bilateral clefting of alae nasi and lack of formation of nasal tip; sometimes limb anomalies	Hypertelorism (radiographic interorbital distance 2 standard deviations above normal for age); in some cases, anophthalmia, microphthalmia, epibulbar dermoids, lid colobomata, congenital cataracts
Opitz syndrome Midline defects of the craniofacial structures, heart, and genitalia occurring in males; hypertelorism particularly associated with hypospadias	Hypertelorism; antimongoloid slant of palpebral fissures; epicanthus; strabismus
Waardenburg syndrome Familial syndrome of dystopia canthorum, heterochromia, and pigmentary disturbances of hair and skin (commonly white forelock), with sensorineural deafness in most cases; prognathism common	Lateral displacement of medial canthi and inferior puncta; heterochromia iridis, total or partial; in some cases both irides completely blue (isochromia)

Table 25–1 OCULAR CHANGES IN DEVELOPMENTAL PEDIATRIC SYNDROMES (*Continued*)

GENERAL DESCRIPTION	OPHTHALMOLOGIC MANIFESTATIONS
Oculodentodigital dysplasia (Meyer-Schwickerath syndrome) Hypotelorism, microphthalmos, microcornea, dental anomalies and enamel hypoplasia, camptodactyly, syndactyly, and other skeletal defects; typical facies with thin nose, high cheek bones, small mandible; hair fine, with slow growth	Microphthalmos, microcornea, hypotelorism, persistent pupillary membrane; glaucoma
Hallermann-Streiff syndrome (dyscephalia oculomandibulofacialis) Craniofacial dysostosis giving a bird-headed appearance (brachycephaly, micrognathia, small mouth, beaked nose), in association with ectodermal dysplasia and hypotrichosis, and with dwarfism	Microphthalmos, cataract, sparse eyebrows and lashes, blue sclerae, nystagmus
Pierre Robin syndrome Micrognathia, cleft palate, and glossoptosis; in some cases cardiac and skeletal anomalies, mental retardation	Congenital glaucoma; retinal detachment; strabismus
Treacher Collins syndrome (mandibulofacial dysostosis; Franceschetti-Klein syndrome) First branchial arch defects, with malar and mandibular hypoplasia, eyelid and ear malformations, conductive deafness; mouth commonly large and fish-like	Antimongoloid slant of palpebral fissures; underdevelopment of supraorbital ridges; coloboma of lower eyelids and in some cases of iris or choroid
Goldenhar syndrome (oculo-auriculo-vertebral dysplasia) Defects of eyes and ears associated with abnormalities of vertebrae, heart, and lungs; complete or partial agenesis of external, middle, inner ear; conductive hearing defects; preauricular skin appendages; mandibular hypoplasia; hemivertebrae, supernumerary vertebrae, or fusion of vertebral bodies	Antimongoloid slant of palpebral fissures; colobomata of eyelid, upper lid more commonly involved than lower; hypoplasia or coloboma of iris; hypertelorism; sometimes microphthalmos
CHROMOSOMAL ABNORMALITIES	
Trisomy 21 (Down syndrome) See Sec 6.11	Mongoloid slant of palpebral fissures; epicanthus; dacryostenosis; blepharitis; Brushfield spots of iris; peripheral thinning of iris stroma; keratoconus and corneal hydrops; cataracts; high refractive errors; strabismus; nystagmus
Trisomy 18 (Edwards syndrome) See Sec 6.12	Ptosis; short palpebral fissures; epicanthus; hypoplastic supraorbital ridges; microphthalmia; corneal opacities; anisocoria; cataracts; fundus and disc colobomata; retinal hypopigmentation
Trisomy 13 (Patau syndrome) See Sec 6.13	Microphthalmos; anophthalmos; cyclopia in some cases; dysgenesis of anterior segment (iris hypoplasia, iris adhesions, chamber angle abnormalities); corneal opacities; congenital glaucoma; cataracts; persistent hyperplastic primary vitreous; retinal dysplasia; colobomata of iris, ciliary body, fundus; intraocular cartilage; optic nerve hypoplasia
Trisomy 9 Microcephaly; prominent forehead; prominent nose; prominent ears; fish-like mouth; micrognathia; digital hypoplasia; congenital heart disease; urinary tract anomalies; mental retardation	Antimongoloid slant of palpebral fissures; deeply set eyes; corectopia; strabismus
Trisomy 8 Dysmorphic skull; prominent forehead; dysplastic ears; high palate; micrognathia; vertebral anomalies; short stature; limited joint mobility; congenital heart disease; mental retardation	Strabismus
Syndrome 45X (Turner) (and mosaic variants) See Sec 6.22 and 18.30	Ptosis; epicanthus; blue sclerae; defective color vision; cataracts; strabismus; nystagmus
47,XXY; 48,XXXY; 49, XXXXY (Klinefelter) syndromes See Sec 6.23 and 18.32	Hypertelorism; epicanthus; Brushfield spots of iris; myopia; strabismus
Partial deletion short arm chromosome 4 (4p−) See Sec 6.18	Ptosis; hypertelorism; epicanthus; colobomata
Partial deletion short arm chromosome 5 (5p−) (cri-du-chat syndrome) See Sec 6.18	Antimongoloid slant of palpebral fissures; hypertelorism; epicanthus; strabismus
Partial deletion short arm chromosome 9 (9p−) See Sec 6.18	Mongoloid slant of palpebral fissures; epicanthus; arched brows
Partial deletion long arm chromosome 13 (13q−) Microcephaly; trigonocephaly; facial asymmetry; micrognathia; hypoplastic thumbs; syndactyly; congenital heart disease; hip dysplasia; cryptorchidism; failure to thrive; mental retardation	Ptosis; epicanthus; hypertelorism; microphthalmos; colobomata; retinoblastoma
Partial deletion long arm chromosome 18 (18q−) See Sec 6.18	Horizontal palpebral fissures; epicanthus; deeply set eyes; optic disc pallor; tapetoretinal degeneration; nystagmus

Table 25–1 OCULAR CHANGES IN DEVELOPMENTAL PEDIATRIC SYNDROMES (Continued)

GENERAL DESCRIPTION	OPHTHALMOLOGIC MANIFESTATIONS
Partial deletion long arm chromosome 21 (21q−) Microcephaly; mental retardation; growth retardation; hypertonia; skeletal malformations; micrognathia; high palate; prominent nasal bridge; pyloric stenosis; cryptorchidism	Downward slanting palpebral fissues
Partial deletion long arm chromosome 22 (22q−) Microcephaly; mental retardation; hypotonia; high palate; bifid uvula; syndactyly of toes	Ptosis; epicanthus
Extrachromosomal material (cat eye syndrome) Anal atresia; congenital cardiac and renal malformations; preauricular skin tags or pits; mild to moderate mental retardation	Antimongoloid slant of palpebral fissures; epicanthus; hypertelorism; microphthalmos; colobomata of iris, fundus, optic nerve; macular defects; pale discs; cataracts; strabismus; nystagmus

DISORDERS OF AMINO ACID METABOLISM

GENERAL DESCRIPTION	OPHTHALMOLOGIC MANIFESTATIONS
Albinism* Defect in the formation of melanin; several forms include: (1) *Oculocutaneous albinism, tyrosine negative;* generalized hypopigmentation	Iris blue or gray; generalized hypopigmentation of eye; typical pink or orange reflex; fundus bright, with increased choroidal vascular pattern; macula/fovea poorly defined (hypoplastic); photophobia; nystagmus; subnormal vision; often high refractive error
(2) *Oculocutaneous albinism, tyrosinase positive;* pigmentation may increase with age	Iris color blue, yellow, or brownish; color increasing with age; photophobia; nystagmus; subnormal vision, which may improve with age
(3) *Amish* or *yellow* mutant; generalized albinism in which a yellowish pigment is produced instead of melanin, providing some skin and hair color	Ocular signs of albinism throughout life
(4) *Hermansky-Pudlak syndrome;* tyrosine negative albinism associated with a hemorrhagic diathesis	Iris blue-gray to brown; photophobia; nystagmus; slight to moderate vision defect
(5) *Cross syndrome,* tyrosine positive; a syndrome of hypopigmentation, gingival fibromatosis, spasticity, athetoid movements, and microphthalmos	Iris blue-gray; microphthalmos; cataracts; severe vision defect; nystagmus
(6) *Ocular albinism;* pigment deficiency limited to the eye	Generalized ocular hypopigmentation; macular hypoplasia; nystagmus (in Blacks, fundus tessellated)
Alcaptonuria See Sec 8.3	Black discoloration of sclera, most noticeable at insertion of extraocular muscles
Tyrosinemia (Richner-Hanhart syndrome) See Sec 8.3	Corneal ulceration, "herpetiform"
Cystinosis See Sec 8.5	Accumulation of refractile crystals in cornea (best seen with slit lamp, but corneal haze may be detected grossly); photophobia; pigmentary retinopathy; fundi generally hypopigmented, with fine to coarse spotty pigmentation, most marked peripherally; vision usually normal to nearly normal
Homocystinemia, type I See Sec 8.4	Ectopia lentis; cataract; secondary glaucoma; peripheral cystic degeneration of retina
Sulfite oxidase deficiency See Sec 8.5	Subluxation of lens; spherophakia; strabismus
Hartnup disease See Sec 8.6	Photophobia; nystagmus; strabismus
Maple syrup urine disease See Sec 8.7	Strabismus, varying with condition of child

THE MUCOPOLYSACCHARIDOSES (MPS)

GENERAL DESCRIPTION	OPHTHALMOLOGIC MANIFESTATIONS
Hurler syndrome (MPS IH) (α-L-iduronidase deficiency) See Sec 23.18	Hypertelorism, prominent eyes; puffy lids; heavy brows; deposition of MPS and attendant cellular changes throughout most regions of eye, particularly the conjunctiva, cornea, sclera, iris, ciliary body, retina, and optic nerve; characteristic corneal clouding, clinically evident early in life, and progressing to dense milky "ground-glass" haze, often with associated photophobia; progressive retinal degeneration with pigmentary dispersion and clumping, arteriolar attenuation and disc pallor, and reduced ERG; optic atrophy; vision loss, owing principally to corneal, retinal, and optic nerve changes; hydrocephalus and cerebral changes; glaucoma in some cases
Scheie syndrome (MPS IS; α-L-iduronidase deficiency) See Sec 23.18	Progressive corneal clouding, diffuse but sometimes more dense peripherally than centrally; progressive retinal degeneration; visual symptoms, field loss and night blindness often commencing in 2nd or 3rd decade; glaucoma in some cases

*To be differentiated from these forms of albinism is the **Chédiak-Higashi syndrome**, in which the defect is in morphology of the melanosomes, not in formation of melanin. Ocular signs include hypopigmentation of iris and fundus, photophobia, nystagmus, and papilledema with lymphocytic infiltration of optic nerve.

Table 25–1   OCULAR CHANGES IN DEVELOPMENTAL PEDIATRIC SYNDROMES (Continued)

GENERAL DESCRIPTION	OPHTHALMOLOGIC MANIFESTATIONS
Hurler-Scheie Compound (MPS IH/S; α-L-Iduronidase deficiency) See Sec 23.18	Corneal clouding, diffuse and progressive; glaucoma in some cases; vision loss owing to corneal clouding or to optic nerve effects of arachnoid cysts
Hunter syndrome (MPS II; iduronosulfate sulfatase deficiency) Phenotypically similar to MPS IH; both mild and severe forms occur	Progressive retinal degeneration with pigmentary changes, arteriolar attenuation, optic atrophy, vision loss, reduced ERG; corneas macroscopically (clinically) clear, but microscopic corneal changes documented; papilledema secondary to hydrocephalus in some cases
Sanfilippo syndrome (MPS III; types A [heparan sulfate sulfatase deficiency], B [N-acetyl α-D-glucosaminidase deficiency], and C [acetyl-Co A:α-glucosaminide N-acetyl transferase deficiency]) Three biochemically different, clinically indistinguishable forms; severe mental retardation, with relatively less severe somatic manifestations than with MPS IH	Retinal changes in some patients—arteriolar narrowing; reduced ERG; corneas clinically clear but some microscopic changes reported
Morquio syndrome (MPS IV) (galactosamine-6-sulfate sulfatase deficiency in classic form; β-galactosidase deficiency reported in variants) See Sec 23.18.	Fine corneal clouding in many patients; slowly progressive; often not clinically apparent for several years
Moroteaux-Lamy syndrome (MPS VI; arylsulfatase-B deficiency) See Sec 23.18.	Diffuse corneal clouding; usually evident within 1st few yr of life; tortuosity of retinal vessels in some patients; papilledema and 6th nerve paresis in some patients with hydrocephalus
Sly syndrome (MPS VII; β-D-glucuronidase deficiency) Some diversity of phenotype; many classic features of MPS, including skeletal deformity, macrocephaly, coarse features, hepatosplenomegaly, mental retardation, cardiac and respiratory complications	Corneas clear or cloudy; corneal haze of either fine or coarse type
Di Ferrenti syndrome (MPS VIII; N-acetylglucosamine-6-sulfate sulfatase deficiency) Short stature; mild dysostosis multiplex; odontoid hypoplasia; hepatosplenomegaly; mental retardation	Not yet described
SPHINGOLIPIDOSES **Generalized gangliosidosis (GM$_1$ gangliosidosis type 1; β-galactosidase deficiency)** See Sec 8.29	Diffuse corneal clouding (MPS accumulation); macular cherry red spot of retinal ganglioside accumulation; retinal vascular tortuosity and retinal hemorrhages; optic atrophy; vision loss, nystagmus, strabismus
Juvenile GM$_1$ gangliosidosis (GM$_1$ gangliosidosis type 2; β-galactosidase deficiency) See Sec 8.29	Corneas clinically clear; histologic changes of retinal ganglioside storage without clinically obvious signs; optic atrophy and vision loss; nystagmus and strabismus
Tay-Sachs disease (GM$_2$ gangliosidosis type 1; hexosaminidase A deficiency) See Sec 8.30	Macular cherry red spot; optic atrophy (demyelination and degeneration of optic nerves, chiasm, and tracts); progressive loss of vision, owing both to ocular and to cerebral abnormalities; sequential deterioration of eye movements
Sandhoff variant (GM$_2$ gangliosidosis type 2; hexosaminidase A and B deficiency) See Sec 8.30	Macular cherry red spot; optic atrophy and progressive loss of vision; corneas clinically clear or slightly opalescent; histologic evidence of storage cytosomes in cornea
Juvenile GM$_2$ gangliosidosis (GM$_2$ gangliosidosis type 3; partial deficiency of hexosaminidase A) See Sec 8.30	Retinal pigmentary degeneration; macular changes (cherry-red spot type) in some cases; optic atrophy; blindness later in course of disease
Krabbe globoid cell leukodystrophy (galactosyl ceramide lipidosis; galactosylceramide β-galactosidase deficiency) See Sec 8.36	Cortical blindness and optic atrophy, owing to degenerative changes in brain and visual pathways; nystagmus; strabismus

Table 25-1 OCULAR CHANGES IN DEVELOPMENTAL PEDIATRIC SYNDROMES (Continued)

GENERAL DESCRIPTION	OPHTHALMOLOGIC MANIFESTATIONS
Gaucher disease (glycosyl ceramide lipidosis; glucosyl ceramide β-glucosidase deiciency) See Sec 8.33	Paralytic strabismus due to brain stem and cranial nerve involvement in neuronopathic forms; nystagmus; macular changes (grayness) in some cases; retinal hemorrhages secondary to anemia, thrombocytopenia; discrete white spots in or on retina reported in juvenile form; pingueculae (wedge-shaped conjunctival lesions) in chronic non-neuronopathic form; possibly corneal clouding
Niemann-Pick disease (sphingomyelin lipidoses; sphingomyelinase deficiency) See Sec 8.34	Macular cherry red–like spot or grayish macular haze in classic infantile neuronopathic form (type A); and in subacute neurovisceral or juvenile form (type C); corneal clouding, lens opacities in some cases (Type A); vertical gaze palsy in some patients
Fabry disease (glycosphingolipid lipidosis; α-galactosidase A deficiency) See Sec 8.32	Corneal dystrophy related to epithelial lipid deposits (radiating lines/whorls in affected males and in carrier females); aneurysmal dilatation and tortuosity of conjunctival and retinal vessels; renovascular signs of renal hypertension; papilledema; orbital and lid edema; cataracts (spoke-like posterior cortical lens opacities—anterior lens opacities in some cases)
Farber disease (ceramide lipidosis; ceramidase deficiency) See Sec 8.37	Cherry red–like spot; grayish posterior pole; retinal pigmentary mottling; granulomata in and around eye
CEROID LIPOFUSCINOSES (See also Sec 8.41 and 21.17) **Infantile (Finnish variant; unsaturated fatty acid lipidosis)** Microcephaly; marked atrophy of brain; granular inclusions; ataxia, myoclonus; profound dementia, decorticate state; onset 1–2 yr; death by 10 yr	Loss of vision
Late Infantile (Jansky-Bielschowsky) Intellectual deterioration, seizures, ataxia; inclusions of curvilinear type; onset 2–4 yr; death by 10 yr	Pigmentary retinal degeneration, in some cases, predominantly macular; ERG abnormal; optic atrophy
Juvenile (Batten-Mayou-Spielmeyer-Vogt) Intellectual deterioration, seizures, ataxia, progressive loss of motor function; mixed inclusion, including curvilinear and fingerprint types, and lipofuscin in brain; onset 5–8 yr, sometimes later; death in teens or 20's	Pigmentary retinal degeneration, resembling retinitis pigmentosa, with progressive loss of vision; in some cases predominantly macular degeneration; ERG abnormal; optic atrophy as a late manifestation
Late juvenile or adult (Kufs) Behavior disturbances and intellectual impairment; ataxia, spasticity, myoclonic seizures; mostly lipofuscin in brain; onset in childhood, adolescence, or early adult life	Vision and fundi usually normal; macular degeneration in some cases
Cherry red spot myoclonus syndrome Intention myoclonus; variable inclusions in brain; light inclusions in hepatocytes and Kupffer cells; onset in childhood; survival to adulthood	Macular cherry red spot; vision loss
LEUKODYSTROPHIES (See also Sec 8.35 and 21.18) **Metachromatic leukodystrophy (arylsulfatase A deficiency)**	Retinal degeneration resembling retinitis pigmentosa; in some cases, early macular involvement (macular grayness with accentuation of central red spot); optic atrophy; vision loss; strabismus and nystagmus
Pelizaeus-Merzbacher syndrome	"Eye-rolling" (arrhythmic eye movements) noted soon after birth, sometimes with rotary movements of the head; optic atrophy as a late manifestation
Canavan disease	Vacuolization of ganglion cell layer of retina reportedly detectable with slit lamp; retinal pigmentary changes; optic atrophy; blindness early in course; ERG normal; VER reduced; strabismus, roving eye movements, and nystagmus
DEMYELINATING SCLEROSES (See Sec 21.18) **Schilder disease (encephalitis periaxialis diffusa)**	Involvement of visual pathways, producing retrobulbar neuritis, optic atrophy, central scotomas, chiasmal syndromes, homonymous field defects; disorders of cortical gaze functions; nystagmus

Table 25–1   OCULAR CHANGES IN DEVELOPMENTAL PEDIATRIC SYNDROMES (Continued)

GENERAL DESCRIPTION	OPHTHALMOLOGIC MANIFESTATIONS
Multiple sclerosis	Retrobulbar neuritis (episodic loss of vision, typically a central scotoma, unilateral more often than bilateral, often with retrobulbar pain); other visual pathway lesions (variety of field defects); internuclear ophthalmoplegia; supranuclear gaze palsies; nystagmus; sheathing of peripheral retinal vessels in some cases
Neuromyelitis optica (Devic disease)	Optic neuritis (usually papillitis with visible disc edema), with resultant optic atrophy; other visual pathway lesions (variety of visual field defects); in some cases, extraocular muscle palsies, conjugate gaze palsies, nystagmus, pupil abnormalities
HAMARTOMATOSES/PHAKOMATOSES	
Tuberous sclerosis (Bourneville disease) See Sec 21.15 and 24.11	Retinal phakomata (glial hamartomas, ranging from small flat or slightly elevated white or yellowish lesions to large elevated refractile yellowish multinodular or cystic masses often likened to an unripe mulberry); fibroangioma of the lids; in some, papilledema or optic atrophy, vision defects, pupil or ocular motor signs related to CNS changes (tumors, hydrocephalus)
Neurofibromatosis (von Recklinghausen syndrome) See Sec 21.15 and 24.10	Plexiform neuromas of eyelids, often producing ptosis; episcleral and conjunctival neurifibromas; prominent corneal nerves; iris nodules; uveal hypercellularity; glaucoma (related to angle anomalies, uveal hypercellularity, neovascularization, or synechiae); hamartomas (phakomata) of disc and retina; fundus pigmentary changes likened to café-au-lait spots; optic gliomas and vision loss (presenting with proptosis, strabismus, nystagmus if intraorbital—with signs of increased intracranial pressure, hydrocephalus, or diencephalic syndrome when intracranial); orbital asymmetry; orbital wall defects; pulsatile exophthalmos; intraorbital neurofibromas, with proptosis
Angiomatosis of the retina and cerebellum (von Hippel–Lindau disease) See Sec 21.15	Retinal hemangioblastoma (reddish or yellowish globular mass with paired vessels coursing to and from the lesion, sometimes likened to a toy balloon in the fundus); may lead to hemorrhage, exudates, retinal detachment
Encephalofacial angiomatosis (Sturge-Weber syndrome) See Sec 21.15	Lid and conjunctival involvement of facial nevus flammeus; choroidal hemangioma; dilated and tortuous retinal vessels; glaucoma, congenital or later in infancy or childhood, (related to possible angle anomalies, vascular lesion, or hypersecretion); visual field defects associated with CNS lesions; hemianopsia in some cases
Angiomatosis of mid-brain and retina (Wyburn-Mason syndrome) Extensive vascular malformations involving principally the midbrain and eye; rare	Angiomatosis of the retina; vessels dilated and tortuous; angiomatosis affecting optic nerve and orbit
NEUROCUTANEOUS SYNDROMES	
Ataxia-telangiectasia (Louis-Bar syndrome) See Sec 21.19	Telangiectasias of bulbar conjunctivae, usually by the age of 4–6 yr; apraxic disorder of conjugate eye movements; horizontal and vertical gaze performed in halting dyssynergic fashion; difficulty in maintaining eccentric gaze; sometimes convergence defect; nystagmus
Sjögren-Larsson syndromes See also Sec 24.16 Triad of congenital ichthyosiform dermatitis, mental deficiency, and spastic paresis of the extremities; seizures and speech disorders in some cases	Chorioretinal lesions; discrete defects in retinal pigment epithelium of unknown etiology; circumscribed symmetrical lesions of varying size in and about the macula in approximately 25% of cases
Incontinentia pigmenti (Bloch-Sulzberger Syndrome) See Sec 24.10	Intraocular retrolental masses ("pseudogliomas") and membranes, apparently secondary to an underlying retinal vascular disorder characterized by aneurysmal dilatation, abnormal arteriovenous connections, and vasoproliferative changes; sometimes intraocular hemorrhage and inflammation; microphthalmos; corneal opacities; cataracts; optic atrophy
Linear nevus sebaceus of Jadassohn See also Sec 24.8 A rare and probably sporadic syndrome of neurologic and ocular abnormalities occurring in association with linear nevus sebaceus; well-demarcated plaques present from birth; epilepsy, retardation, facial paresis, and hearing defects in some cases	Coloboma of the eyelids, iris, and fundus; corectopia; epibulbar lipodermoids; orbital teratomas; proptosis; aberrant lacrimal gland; corneal vascularization; ocular motor palsies; nystagmus; defective vision

Table 25–1 OCULAR CHANGES IN DEVELOPMENTAL PEDIATRIC SYNDROMES (Continued)

GENERAL DESCRIPTION	OPHTHALMOLOGIC MANIFESTATIONS
Xerodermic idiocy of de Sanctis and Cacchione See Sec 24.14	Atrophy of eyelids; loss of cilia, ectropion, entropion, symblepharon, ankyloblepharon; drying and infection of conjunctiva; ulceration of cornea; iritis; photophobia
Klippel-Trenaunay-Weber syndrome See Sec 24.7	Conjunctival telangiectasias; choroidal hemangioma; iris coloboma; heterochromia; glaucoma; strabismus
SPECIAL NEUROBIOTROPHIES **Subacute sclerosing panencephalitis (Dawson disease; Van Bogaert disease)** See Sec 10.86	Focal retinitis (edema, hemorrhage, pigmentary changes), with chorioretinal scarring (usually macular or paramacular, usually bilateral)—may precede other neurologic manifestations; papilledema; optic atrophy; visual symptoms of retinal and optic nerve involvement; field defects of cerebral involvement; nystagmus; extraocular muscle palsies; ptosis
Subacute necrotizing encephalomyopathy (Leigh disease) See Sec 8.20 and 21.16	Abnormal eye movements (bizarre rolling eye movements, disconjugate eye movements, horizontal and vertical nystagmus, saccadic ocular movements); extraocular muscle palsies (sometimes complete external ophthalmoplegia); blepharoptosis; progressive optic atrophy and vision loss; sometimes retinal changes (diminished macular reflex); afferent and efferent pupil defects
Hepatolenticular degeneration (Wilson disease) See Sec 8.28, 11.98, and 21.20	Kayser-Fleischer ring of cornea (copper deposition in periphery of Descemet membrane, particularly in deepest zone adjacent to endothelium, seen as granules of golden, greenish, grayish, or brown hue); Sonnenblumenkatarakt ("sunflower" cataract); occasionally ocular motor abnormalities (jerky oscillations of eyes, involuntary upward deviation of eyes, or paresis of upward gaze); accommodation sometimes affected; in some cases, optic neuritis secondary to penicillamine therapy
Trichopoliodystrophy (Menkes disease; kinky hair disease) See Sec 8.28 and 21.17	Decrease in retinal ganglion cells, thinning of retinal nerve fiber layer, and partial atrophy of optic nerve; progressive vision loss; abnormal ERG; microcysts of pigment epithelium of iris
Abetalipoproteinemia (acanthocytosis; Bassen-Kornzweig disease) See Sec 8.26 and 21.19	Pigmentary retinal degeneration with progressive impairment of visual function (pigment dispersion, arteriolar attenuation, disc pallor, impaired dark adaptation); cataracts, ptosis, and ocular motor abnormalities; in some cases, progressive exotropia, paresis of medial recti, and dissociated nystagmus on lateral gaze
Heredopathia atactica polyneuritiformis (Refsum syndrome; phytanic acid α-hydrolase deficiency) See Sec 8.40, 21.19, and 24.16	Pigmentary retinal degeneration (pigmentary clumping, arteriolar attenuation, optic atrophy, progressive impairment of night vision and visual field); ERG abnormal; sometimes vitreous opacities, cataracts, cornea guttata, miosis; ophthalmoparesis; nystagmus
Familial dysautonomia (Riley-Day syndrome) See Sec 21.28	Depressed or absent corneal sensation, with corneal ulceration and scarring common; defective lacrimation; tortuosity of retinal vessels; tonic pupil in some cases; myopia and exotropia common
Congenital familial sensory neuropathy with anhidrosis (Pinsky-DiGeorge syndrome) See Sec 22.3	Defective corneal sensation, with defective lacrimation; corneal ulceration and scarring may result
DISORDERS OF CONNECTIVE TISSUES, BONES, AND JOINTS **Arachnodactyly (Marfan syndrome)** See Sec 23.18	Ectopia lentis (lens dislocation, usually upward) and iridodonesis (tremulous iris); microphakia, spherophakia; cataract; myopia; glaucoma; retinal changes: degeneration, detachment
Cutis hyperelastica (Ehlers-Danlos syndrome) See Sec 23.18 and 24.17	Epicanthus; blue sclera; keratoconus; subluxation of lens; retinal detachment
Pseudoxanthoma elasticum See Sec 24.17	Angioid streaks (breaks in Bruch membrane appearing as dark lines in the fundus radiating from the disc); tendency to retinal hemorrhage

Table 25–1 OCULAR CHANGES IN DEVELOPMENTAL PEDIATRIC SYNDROMES (*Continued*)

GENERAL DESCRIPTION	OPHTHALMOLOGIC MANIFESTATIONS
Osteogenesis imperfecta See Sec 23.17	Blue sclera; prominent eyes; in some cases, megalocornea, keratoconus, corneal opacities
Polyostotic fibrous dysplasia (McCune-Albright syndrome) See Sec 23.18	Thickening of bones of orbit
Osteopetrosis (Albers-Schönberg disease; "marble bones") See Sec 23.17	Vision loss and extraocular muscle palsies, due to bony overgrowth of cranial foramina; in some cases, retinal degeneration, optic atrophy
Chondrodystrophia calcificans congenita (Conradi syndrome) See Sec 23.16	Cataract; optic atrophy; hypertelorism
Spondyloepiphyseal dysplasia congenita See Sec 23.16	Myopia; retinal detachment; cataract; buphthalmos
Spondyloepiphyseal dysplasia variants See Sec 23.13 and 23.16	Punctate corneal dystrophy without impairment of vision
Hereditary onchyo-osteodysplasia (nail-patella syndrome) See Sec 16.34	Dark "cloverleaf" pigmentation of iris; cataract; microphakia; microcornea; keratoconus; ptosis
Progressive arthro-ophthalmopathy (Stickler syndrome) Pain and stiffness of joints with bony enlargement; kyphosis; cleft palate; Pierre Robin anomaly; deafness	Progressive myopia; retinal detachment; glaucoma
DERMATOLOGIC DISORDERS **Focal dermal hypoplasia (Goltz syndrome)** See Sec. 24.5	Nystagmus; strabismus; microphthalmos; coloboma
Hypohidrotic (anhidrotic) ectodermal dysplasia See Sec 24.6	Deficiency of tears, leading to keratopathy, photophobia; stenosis of the lacrimal puncta; cataracts; lashes and brows sparse
Dyskeratosis congenita See Sec 24.5	Bullous conjunctivitis, with minimal scarring of cornea; chronic blepharitis, loss of lashes and ectropion; keratinization of lacrimal puncta
Ichthyosis See Sec 24.16	Conjunctivitis, ectropion, and corneal erosions in lamellar and sex-linked forms; cataracts in congenital and vulgaris forms
Basal cell nevus syndrome See Sec 24.32	Prominent supraorbital ridges; hypertelorism or dystopia canthorum; cataracts; coloboma; vision defects; strabismus
Juvenile xanthogranuloma (nevoxanthoendothelioma) See Sec 24.32	Xanthogranuloma in ocular tissues, as infiltrates in orbit, iris, episclera, ciliary body; presenting signs may be proptosis, heterochromia, spontaneous hyphema, uveitis, glaucoma
Poikiloderma congenitale (Rothmund-Thomson syndrome) See Sec 24.14	Sparse eyebrows and eyelashes; cataracts (onset 2–7 yr); corneal dystrophy
Bloom syndrome See Sec 24.14	Conjunctivitis; conjunctival telangiectasias; drusen at posterior pole of fundus
SYNDROMES OF MULTIPLE DEVELOPMENTAL ABNORMALITIES **Cornelia de Lange syndrome** Microbrachycephaly, short neck, low hair line, confluent brows, long lashes, anteverted nares, micrognathism, and low set ears; physical and mental retardation; limb defects, including micromelia, phocomelia, oligodactyly, polydactyly; cardiac and urogenital anomalies	Synophrys (confluent eyebrows) and long curly eyelashes; ptosis; epicanthus; microphthalmos with eccentric pupils; corneal opacities; optic atrophy; strabismus
Fraser syndrome Cryptophthalmos with facial, genitourinary, skeletal anomalies (including lateral cleft of nostril, ear deformity, renal agenesis, hydronephrosis, hypospadias, cryptorchidism, syndactyly); cerebral defects, meningoencephalocele	Cryptophthalmos (eye hidden, fused lids—absence of palpebral fissure), sometimes with symblepharon (adhesion of lid to globe); microphthalmos in some cases; flat supraorbital ridge
Rieger syndrome Dysplasia of anterior segment of the eye associated with various dental and limb anomalies; occasionally intellectual retardation, muscular dystrophy, and myotonic distrophy	Posterior embryotoxon (prominence and anterior displacement of Schwalbe line), often with bands of iris tissue attached (Axenfeld syndrome); iris hypoplasia; glaucoma; cataracts; ectopia lentis; colobomata; micro- or megalocornea; strabismus; ptosis; optic atrophy
Peter syndrome Skeletal anomalies; developmental defects of the gastrointestinal tract and central nervous system; hydrocephalus and mental retardation	Central defect of Descemet membrane, with central corneal leukoma, shallow anterior chamber, peripheral anterior synechia; cataracts

Table 25-1 OCULAR CHANGES IN DEVELOPMENTAL PEDIATRIC SYNDROMES (Continued)

GENERAL DESCRIPTION	OPHTHALMOLOGIC MANIFESTATIONS
Lenz syndrome Microcephaly, mental retardation; short stature, digital anomalies, and dental defects	Colobomatous microphthalmos; blepharoptosis; nystagmus; strabismus
Meckel syndrome (Meckel-Gruber syndrome) Microcephaly, occipital encephalocele, or anencephaly; polycystic kidneys; polydactyly; congenital heart disease; genital abnormalities	Microphthalmos, anophthalmos, cryptophthalmos; sclerocornea; partial aniridia; cataract; retinal dysplasia; optic nerve hypoplasia
Otopalatodigital syndrome (Rubinstein-Taybi syndrome) Intellectual and growth retardation; abnormally broad thumbs and broad great toes; characteristic facies with hypoplasia of maxilla and mandible, beaked nose, posterior rotation of ears; hypertrichosis; cryptorchidism; cardiac and renal anomalies	Hypertelorism, with epicanthus, ptosis, and antimongoloid slant of palpebral fissures; cataract; colobomata; strabismus
Seckel syndrome Growth retardation, with small head circumference and characteristic face, narrow with beak-like nose ("bird head"); micrognathism and apparent prominence of maxilla; sometimes musculoskeletal and genitourinary anomalies	Hypertelorism, with antimongoloid slant of palpebral fissures, prominent eyes; strabismus
Freeman-Sheldon syndrome Syndrome characterized by mask-like face with small pursed mouth, "whistling-face"; ulnar deviation of the hand and fingers; talipes equinovarus	Deep-set eyes; epicanthus, blepharophimosis, ptosis; strabismus
Aicardi syndrome Agenesis of the corpus callosum, with cortical heterotopia; seizures; mental retardation; costovertebral anomalies	Multiple discrete chorioretinal defects of varying size; sometimes microphthalmos
Wildervanck syndrome Association of the Klippel-Feil malformation with congenital deafness and Duane syndrome	Unilateral or bilateral Duane syndrome (congenital defect in abduction with retraction of the globe on attempted adduction of the affected eye); epibulbar dermoid cysts
Falls-Kertesz syndrome Pterygium colli; later onset of lymphedema of lower extremities	Distichiasis of all 4 lids; partial ectropion of lower lids
Kartagener syndrome See Sec 13.28	Pigmentary retinal disorder; cataracts

MISCELLANEOUS MULTISYSTEM DISORDERS

GENERAL DESCRIPTION	OPHTHALMOLOGIC MANIFESTATIONS
Oculocerebrorenal syndrome (Lowe syndrome) See Sec 23.31	Congenital cataracts in affected males; fine lens opacities in carrier females; glaucoma; rarely, microphthalmos
Cerebrohepatorenal syndrome (Zellweger syndrome) Profound hypotonia, growth retardation, and failure to thrive; hepatomegaly, jaundice, hypoprothrombinemia; renal cortical cysts; characteristic facies, flat profile; accumulation of iron in various organs	Mild hypertelorism, flat supraorbital ridges, and epicanthal folds; cataracts; glaucoma (also, nonglaucomatous corneal haze); vitreous opacities; optic nerve hypoplasia; retinal pigmentary disorder (fundi generally hypopigmented, with fine to coarse spotty pigmentation, most marked peripherally)
Lawrence-Moon-Biedl syndrome See Sec 18.32	Pleomorphic pigmentary retinal degeneration (retinitis pigmentosa type, with prominent macular involvement in some cases), with progressive vision impairment
Prader-Willi syndrome A syndrome of hypotonia, hypomentia, hypogonadism, and obesity, with tendency to diabetes mellitus	Strabismus
Cockayne syndrome See Sec 24.14	Pigmentary retinal degeneration; optic atrophy; cataracts; photophobia
Werner syndrome A syndrome of premature aging; in the 2nd decade, with cessation of growth, graying of the hair, alopecia, scleroderma-like changes of the skin, atherosclerosis, and diabetes mellitus; hypogonadism; increased risk of neoplasia	Cataracts, juvenile onset; pigmentary retinal degeneration ("retinitis pigmentosa"); macular degeneration; glaucoma
Asphyxiating thoracic dysplasia (Jeune syndrome) See Sec 23.17	Pigmentary retinal degeneration, with progressive vision impairment in some cases
Alstrom disease Nerve deafness, diabetes mellitus, and obesity in childhood	Pigmentary retinal degeneration; cataracts
Renal-retinal dystrophy Interstitial nephritis	Progressive pigmentary retinal degeneration, with attenuation of arterioles, reduced ERG, optic atrophy, and loss of vision
Usher syndrome Nerve deafness; mental retardation; epilepsy	Pigmentary retinal degeneration ("retinitis pigmentosa"); cataracts
Norrie disease A syndrome of retinal malformation, mental retardation, and deafness	Retinal malformation; congenital retinal pseudoglioma; persistent hyperplastic primary vitreous, with vision loss; degenerative changes with phthisis bulbi; corneal opacities; cataracts

Table 25–1   OCULAR CHANGES IN DEVELOPMENTAL PEDIATRIC SYNDROMES (*Continued*)

GENERAL DESCRIPTION	OPHTHALMOLOGIC MANIFESTATIONS
CONGENITAL INFECTION SYNDROMES	
Congenital rubella See Sec 7.70	Sequelae both teratogenic and inflammatory; bilateral or unilateral effects; persistence of virus in the eye for months or years; microphthalmia; cataract (usually a dense pearly nuclear opacity with relatively clearer cortical rim); iris hypoplasia, atrophy, synechiae (pupils often difficult to dilate); congenital glaucoma; transient nonglaucomatous corneal clouding in the newborn; retinopathy (pigmentary mottling "salt and pepper," focal or generalized, without loss of function); acute maculopathy (submacular neovascularization) as a delayed complication later in childhood in some cases, with attendant vision impairment; optic atrophy; vision defects and ocular motor abnormalities (nystagmus, strabismus) related not only to ocular involvement but also to effects of encephalomyelitis
Congenital cytomegalovirus infection See Sec 10.75	Chorioretinitis (single or multifocal atrophic and pigmented fundus lesions, more often peripheral than macular—sometimes perivascular retinal exudates and hemorrhages); anterior uveitis, conjunctivitis, and corneal clouding; optic atrophy; optic nerve hypoplasia; coloboma; microphthalmos; vision defects with strabismus, nystagmus
Congenital toxoplasmosis See Sec 10.113	Retinochoroiditis (retinitis, with secondary choroiditis, often with exudate into vitreous in early stages, resulting in single or multifocal atrophic and pigmented scars); often large macular lesions; satellite lesions and recurrent inflammation common in later years due to persistence of organism in eye; vision loss, optic atrophy, retinal detachment, cataract, and glaucoma common; attendant ocular motor abnormalities (strabismus, nystagmus) attributed to ocular and/or CNS involvement; congenital anomalies of eye (e.g., microphthalmos)
Congenital syphilis See Sec 10.55	Perivascular infiltration by *T. pallidum*, with inflammation in the cornea, uvea, retina, and optic nerve; persistence of the organism in the eye for years; interstitial keratitis, usually appearing after age 5 or 6 yr (iridocyclitis and intense photophobia in acute phase, vascularization and corneal opacification later, with decreased vision); retinopathy ("salt and pepper" pigmentary changes, frequently with arteriolar attenuation and disc pallor); retinal periphlebitis, sometimes with vascular occlusion; exudative uveitis in some cases; phthisis may result; disc edema; optic atrophy

In an older child with longstanding amblyopia, months or years of treatment may be required.

Treatment of amblyopia involves (1) providing the clearest possible retinal image (for example, by correction of refractive error, removal of cataract), and (2) stimulation or forced use of the amblyopic eye. The latter is accomplished by occlusion therapy, often referred to as "patching"; the better eye is simply covered to force use of the amblyopic eye. Best results are achieved with complete and constant occlusion throughout the waking hours by the use of adhesive eye pads or "patches" (Opticlude, Elastoplast); occluders placed on spectacles allow peeking, and the adjustable head band type of cloth or plastic occluder is too easily removed by the child. In selected cases an opaque contact lens or a contact lens of sufficiently high power to blur the vision in the better eye is used. In certain cases cycloplegic drops are used to blur the image in the better eye. Most children and their families tolerate occlusion therapy well. In some cases the child resists therapy because of the severity of the vision defect, the cosmetic blemish of the patching, or related psychologic disturbances. The goals of treatment must be thoroughly understood and the treatment carefully supervised. Close monitoring of occlusion therapy is essential, especially in the very young, to avoid deprivation amblyopia in the occluded eye.

Amaurosis. The term amaurosis refers to partial or total loss of vision; it is usually reserved for profound impairment, blindness or near blindness. When amaurosis exists from birth, primary consideration in differential diagnosis must be given to developmental malformations, damage consequent to gestational or perinatal infection, anoxia or hypoxia, perinatal trauma, and the genetically determined diseases that can affect the eye itself or the visual pathways. In certain cases the reason for the amaurosis can be readily determined by objective ophthalmic examination; examples are severe microphthalmia, corneal opacification, dense cataracts, atrophic chorioretinal scars, macular colobomata, retinal dysplasia, and severe optic nerve hypoplasia. In some cases there is intrinsic retinal disease that may not be apparent on initial ophthalmoscopic examination; an example is Leber congenital retinal amaurosis.

In this retinal dystrophy the fundus may appear normal or near normal for some time before ophthalmoscopically appreciable signs of retinal degeneration (pigmentary deposits, arteriolar attenuation, optic pallor, etc.) develop; in such cases electroretinography is highly important in diagnosis, as the electroretinographic response in this condition will be markedly reduced or absent. In many cases of amaurosis the defect lies not in the eye or optic nerve but in the brain, requiring neurologic and sophisticated neuroradiologic evaluation. The development of computed tomography has been of great help in this area.

Amaurosis that develops in a child who once had useful vision has somewhat different implications. In the absence of obvious ocular disease (cataract, chorioretinitis, retinoblastoma, retinitis pigmentosa, etc.) consideration must be given to many neurologic and systemic disorders that can affect the visual pathways. Amaurosis of rather rapid onset may indicate an encephalopathy (such as might occur with hypertension), infectious or parainfectious processes, vasculitis, leukemia, toxins, or trauma. It may be due to acute demyelinating disease affecting the optic nerves, chiasm, or cerebrum. In some cases precipitous loss of vision is the result of increased intracranial pressure, a rapidly progressive hydrocephalus, or dysfunction of a shunt. More slowly progressive visual loss suggests tumor or neurodegenerative disease. Gliomas of the optic nerve and chiasm and craniopharyngiomas are primary diagnostic considerations in children who show progressive loss of vision with or without other neurologic signs. It is to be stressed that manifestations of impairment of vision vary with the age and abilities of the child, the mode of onset, and the laterality and severity of the deficit. The 1st clue to amaurosis in an infant may be nystagmus or strabismus, the vision defect itself passing undetected for some time. Timidity, clumsiness, or behavioral change may be the initial clues in the very young. Deterioration in school progress and indifference to school activities are common signs in the older child. School age children will often try to hide their disability and, in the case of very slowly progressive disorders, may not themselves realize the severity of the problem; some will detect and promptly report small changes in their vision.

Any evidence of loss of vision requires prompt and thorough ophthalmic evaluation. More often than not, the complete delineation of childhood amaurosis and its etiology will require extensive investigation involving neurologic evaluation, electrophysiologic tests, neuroradiologic procedures, and sometimes metabolic and genetic studies.

Nyctalopia. Nyctalopia or "night blindness" refers to vision that is defective in reduced illumination. It generally implies impairment in function of the rods, particularly in dark adaptation time and perceptual threshold. *Stationary congenital night blindness* may occur as an autosomal dominant, autosomal recessive, or X-linked recessive condition. *Progressive night blindness* usually indicates primary or secondary retinal, choroidal, or vitrioretinal degeneration. Progressive impairment of night vision may also occur in vitamin A deficiency or as the result of retinotoxic drugs such as quinine.

Diplopia. Diplopia or "double vision" is most frequently due to malalignment of the visual axes—that is, displacement or deviation of the eye. It is common in heterophoria, in heterotropia of recent onset (particularly when due to acquired nerve palsy), and in proptosis. Because in such cases occluding 1 eye relieves the diplopia, it is common for affected children to squint, to cover 1 eye with a hand, or to assume an abnormal head posture (a face turn or head tilt) to alleviate the bothersome sensation. These mannerisms in children, especially in preverbal children, are important clues to diplopia. The onset of diplopia in any child warrants prompt evaluation; it may signal the onset of a serious problem such as increased intracranial pressure, a brain tumor, an orbital mass, or myasthenia gravis.

Less commonly, diplopia is monocular, the result of dislocation of the lens or some defect in the media or macula.

Psychogenic Disturbances of Vision. Vision problems of psychogenic origin are not uncommon in school age children. Both conversion reactions and willful feigning are encountered. The usual manifestation is reduced visual acuity in 1 or both eyes. Another common manifestation is constriction of the visual field. In some cases the symptom is diplopia or polyopia.

Important clues to the diagnosis are inappropriate affect, excessive grimacing, inconsistency in performance, and suggestibility. Thorough ophthalmologic examination is essential to differentiate organic from functional visual disorders.

As a rule, affected children do well with reassurance and positive suggestion. In some cases psychiatric care is indicated. In all cases the approach must be supportive and nonpunitive.

Dyslexia. The term dyslexia is used to describe a specific reading disability that is attributable to a primary or developmental defect in the higher cortical processing of graphic symbols. It is to be differentiated from (1) reading retardation that may be secondary to other causes such as intellectual impairment, maturational delay, cultural or educational deprivation, emotional disturbances, organic brain disease, or sensory defects, and from (2) acquired word blindness (alexia) occurring as the result of a lesion in the dominant cerebral hemisphere.

Neither dyslexia nor the often associated symptoms such as letter or word reversal and so-called mirror writing are due to any defect in the eye or visual acuity per se, nor are they attributable to a defect in ocular motility or binocular alignment, but ophthalmologic evaluation of the child with a reading problem is recommended for the following reasons: (1) this assessment is of value in the differential diagnosis; (2) correction of any concurrent ocular problems such as a significant refractive error, amblyopia, or strabismus is important to ensure the best possible visual function and efficiency for the child's education; and (3) the ophthalmologist can be of help in counseling and directing the family.

The approach to treatment is remedial instruction. Treatment directed to the eyes themselves cannot be expected to correct developmental dyslexia.

25.5 ABNORMALITIES OF PUPIL AND IRIS

Aniridia. With this developmental anomaly there is almost complete absence of iris. The defect is usually accompanied by photophobia, nystagmus, and defective vision. There may be associated glaucoma, progressive corneal degenerative changes, cataracts, macular hypoplasia, and optic nerve hypoplasia. The condition may be familial (the transmission being dominant) or sporadic. Sporadic aniridia is associated with an increased incidence of Wilms tumor; periodic abdominal examination, supplemented by ultrasound examination or intravenous pyelography, is advised in all children with sporadic aniridia. (See also Sec 15.10).

Coloboma of the Iris. Coloboma is a developmental defect that may take the form of a defect in a sector of the iris, a hole in the substance of the iris, or a notch in the pupillary margin. Simple colobomata are frequently transmitted as an autosomal dominant characteristic. This defect may occur alone or in association with other anomalies. An iris coloboma may be part of an extensive coloboma involving the fundus and optic nerve as a result of malclosure of the embryonic fissure. Such defects are commonly associated with chromosomal abnormalities, particularly trisomies 13 and 18.

Heterochromia. In heterochromia the 2 irides are of different color, or a portion of an iris differs in color from the remainder. Simple heterochromia may occur as an autosomal dominant characteristic. Congenital heterochromia is also a feature of Waardenburg syndrome, an autosomal dominant condition characterized principally by lateral displacement of the inner canthi and puncta, pigmentary disturbances (usually a median white forelock and patches of depigmentation of the skin), and defective hearing. Change in the color of the iris (acquired heterochromia) may occur as the result of trauma, hemorrhage, intraocular inflammation (iridocyclitis, uveitis), intraocular tumor (especially retinoblastoma), intraocular foreign body, glaucoma, iris atrophy, or oculosympathetic palsy (Horner syndrome).

Other Iris Lesions. Discrete nodules of the iris may be seen in patients with neurofibromatosis (von Recklinghausen disease). The lesions vary from slightly elevated pigmented areas to distinct ball-like excrescences. Slit lamp examination may aid in the diagnosis of neurofibromatosis.

In leukemia there may be infiltration of the iris, sometimes with hypopyon, an accumulation of white cells in the anterior chamber which may herald relapse or involvement of the central nervous system.

The lesion of juvenile xanthogranuloma (nevoxanthoendothelioma) may occur in the eye as a yellowish fleshy mass or plaque of the iris. Spontaneous hyphema (blood in the anterior chamber), glaucoma, or a red eye with signs of uveitis may be associated. A search for the skin lesions of xanthogranuloma (see also Sec 24.31)

should be made in any infant or young child with spontaneous hyphema. In many cases the ocular lesion will respond to topical corticosteroid therapy.

Dyscoria and Corectopia. Dyscoria is abnormal shape of the pupil, and corectopia is abnormal pupillary position. They may occur together or independently as congenital anomalies. Corectopia may be associated with dislocation of the lens. Distortion and displacement of the pupil are frequently the result of trauma and are important signs of prolapse of the iris in perforating injuries of the eye; they may also be seen with tears of the iris, with segmental iridoplegia, and with synechiae (inflammatory adhesions of iris to lens or cornea).

Leukocoria. This term describes any white pupillary reflex or so-called cat's eye reflex. Primary diagnostic considerations in any child with leukocoria are cataract, persistent hyperplastic primary vitreous, retrolental fibroplasia, retinal detachment and retinoschisis, larval granulomatosis, and retinoblastoma (Fig 25–2). Also to be considered are endophthalmitis, organized vitreous hemorrhage, leukemic ophthalmopathy, exudative retinopathy (as in Coats disease), and a few rare conditions such as medulloepithelioma, massive retinal gliosis, the retinal pseudotumor of Norrie disease, the so-called pseudoglioma of the Bloch-Sulzberger syndrome, and the retinal lesions of the phakomatoses, to name just a few. A white reflex may also be seen with fundus coloboma, large atrophic chorioretinal scars, and ectopic medullation of retinal nerve fibers.

Often the diagnosis can readily be made by direct examination of the eye by ophthalmoscopy and biomicroscopy. Ultrasound and radiologic examinations are helpful. In some cases the final diagnosis rests with the pathologist.

Anisocoria. This is inequality of the pupils. As a general rule, if the inequality is more pronounced in the presence of bright focal illumination or on near gaze, the larger pupil is abnormal, whereas if the anisocoria is worse in reduced illumination, the smaller pupil is abnormal. Neurologic causes of anisocoria (parasympathetic or sympathetic lesions) must be differentiated from local causes such as synechiae (adhesions), congenital iris defects (colobomata, aniridia), and pharmacologic effects.

The Dilated Fixed Pupil. Differential diagnosis of the dilated unreactive pupil includes internal ophthalmoplegia due to a central or peripheral lesion, the Hutchinson pupil of transtentorial herniation, tonic pupil, pharmacologic blockade, and iridoplegia secondary to ocular trauma.

The most common cause of a dilated unreactive pupil is the purposeful or accidental instillation of a cyclo-

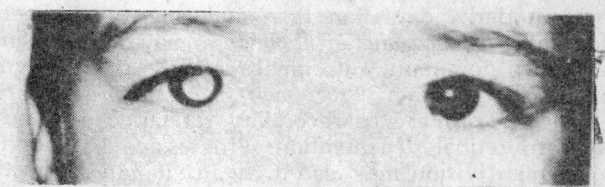

Figure 25–2 Leukocoria. White pupillary reflex in a child with retinoblastoma.

plegic agent, particularly atropine and related substances. Internal ophthalmoplegia may occur with central lesions, and in children the possibility of pinealoma must be considered. The "blown pupil" of transtentorial herniation, as occurs with subdural hematoma and increasing intracranial pressure, is usually unilateral, and usually the patient is obviously ill. The pilocarpine test can help to differentiate neurologic iridoplegia from pharmacologic blockade. In the case of neurologic iridoplegia the dilated pupil will constrict within minutes after the instillation of 1 or 2 drops of 1–2% pilocarpine; if the pupil has been dilated with atropine, the pilocarpine will have no effect. Because pilocarpine is a long-acting drug, this test is not to be used in acute situations in which pupillary signs must be carefully monitored.

Tonic Pupil. This is typically a large pupil that reacts poorly to light (the reaction may be very slow or essentially nil), reacts poorly and slowly to accommodation, and redilates in a slow, tonic manner. A distinctive feature of the tonic pupil is its sensitivity to dilute cholinergic agents, such as 0.125% pilocarpine or 2.5% methacholine (Mecholyl). The condition is usually unilateral. Its occurrence in association with decreased deep tendon reflexes in young women is referred to as Adie syndrome. It may also occur in familial dysautonomia.

Tonic pupil is usually attributed to a lesion affecting the ciliary ganglion in the orbit; the condition is sometimes referred to as ciliary ganglion iridoplegia. In most cases it is benign.

Marcus Gunn Pupil. The Marcus Gunn pupil sign indicates an asymmetric, prechiasmatic, afferent conduction defect. It is best demonstrated by the swinging flashlight test; this allows comparison of the direct and consensual pupillary responses in both eyes. With the patient fixing on a distant target (to control accommodation) a bright focal light is directed into each eye in turn, moving alternately from 1 eye to the other. In the presence of an afferent lesion, both the direct response to light in the affected eye and the consensual response in the fellow eye will be defective. Swinging the light to the better or normal eye causes both pupils to react (constrict) normally. Swinging the light back to the affected eye causes both pupils to redilate to some degree, reflecting the defective conduction. This is a very sensitive and useful test for detecting and confirming optic nerve and retinal disease.

Horner Syndrome. The principal signs of oculosympathetic paresis (Horner syndrome) are homolateral miosis, mild ptosis, and apparent enophthalmos with slight elevation of the lower lid. There may also be decrease in facial sweating, increased amplitude of accommodation, and transient decrease in intraocular pressure. If paralysis of the ocular sympathetic fibers occurs before the age of 2 yr, there may be heterochromia iridis with hypopigmentation of the iris on the affected side.

Oculosympathetic paralysis may be due to a lesion in the midbrain, brain stem, upper spinal cord, neck, middle fossa, or orbit.

Congenital oculosympathetic paresis due to birth trauma is common, though the ocular signs, particularly the anisocoria, may pass undetected for years. Acquired oculosympathetic paresis may signal the presence of mediastinal disease, including neuroblastoma.

The cocaine test is useful in the diagnosis of oculosympathetic paralysis; a normal pupil will dilate within 20–45 min after instillation of 1 or 2 drops of 4–10% cocaine while the miotic pupil of an oculosympathetic paresis will dilate poorly if at all to cocaine. In some cases there is denervation supersensitivity to dilute phenylephrine; 1 or 2 drops of a 1% solution will dilate the affected but not the normal pupil. Furthermore the instillation of 1% hydroxyamphetamine hydrobromide will dilate the pupil only if the postganglionic sympathetic neuron is intact.

25.6 DISORDERS OF EYE MOVEMENT AND ALIGNMENT

STRABISMUS
(Squint, Cast; Tropia, Phoria; Cross-Eye, Wall-Eye)

In humans the development of normal vision in each eye, the maintenance of proper alignment of the visual axes (orthophoria), and the ability to integrate the images from the 2 eyes into a single visual perception are essential to a refined sense of depth perception, or stereopsis. Any variation from normal sensorimotor development in early life may result in lifelong patterns of defective vision or abnormal ocular alignment. Early detection and treatment of strabismus in children is of primary importance; and proper assessment and management require a working knowledge of the various clinical types of strabismus, the methods of detection, and the principles of treatment.

Clinical Types of Strabismus; Classification and Terminology. The 2 principal types of deviation or malalignment of the eyes are heterophoria and heterotropia. *Heterophoria* is a latent tendency to malalignment; the eye deviates only under certain conditions (such as fatigue, illness, stress, or dissociative testing) that interfere with maintenance of normal fusion. Phorias are common and may or may not give rise to bothersome symptoms such as transient diplopia, asthenopia ("eye strain"), or headaches. When the deviation exceeds the amplitude of fusion and becomes manifest, the malalignment is termed *heterotropia* or simply tropia. The condition may be monocular or alternating, depending on the vision and fixation pattern. In *alternating strabismus* the patient uses either eye for fixation or definitive seeing while the fellow eye deviates; since each eye is being used in turn, vision develops more or less equally in both. The patient in effect learns to suppress the image in the deviating (nonfixating) eye. When only 1 eye is used (or preferred) for fixation and the fellow eye consistently deviates, the deviation may be referred to as monocular or as right or left strabismus; in this situation the child is prone to amblyopia or defective central vision in the deviating eye as the result of disuse or misuse.

Strabismus is further described according to the direction of the deviation. Convergent deviation, a crossing or turning in of the eyes, is designated by the prefix *eso-* (hence esotropia, esophoria), while a divergent deviation or turning outward of the eyes (commonly referred to as wall-eye) is designated by the prefix *exo-*. Vertical deviations are indicated by the prefixes *hyper-* and *hypo-*. These may occur singly or in various combinations; in addition, torsional or cyclovertical deviations may occur.

The etiologic classification of strabismus is complex and knowledge of the causative factors and mechanisms incomplete. Certain major types must be distinguished; these are paralytic (noncomitant), nonparalytic (comitant), accommodative, and nonaccommodative.

Paralytic strabismus is due to weakness or paralysis of 1 or more of the extraocular muscles. The deviation characteristically worsens on gaze into the field of action of the affected muscle. Hence, in the case of a right abducent paresis the eyes appear crossed on looking to the right but appear straight (orthophoric) on looking to the left. The subjective manifestation is diplopia; to avoid this bothersome sensation, the child may turn the head to compensate for the paretic muscle or may close or cover 1 eye to eliminate the double image. Such mannerisms are important clues to the presence of an extraocular muscle palsy. With few exceptions, acquired extraocular muscle palsies are ominous signs of a serious pathologic process; the development of a noncomitant strabismus may be the 1st sign of an intracranial tumor, an infectious or parainfectious process (meningitis, encephalitis, neuritis), a demyelinizing or neurodegenerative disease, myasthenia gravis, or a progressive myopathy. A notable exception is benign 6th nerve palsy (see below). Congenital paralytic strabismus is more commonly due to developmental defects of the cranial nerve nuclei or fibers, to muscle anomalies, to congenital infection syndromes, or to birth trauma.

Nonparalytic strabismus is the more common type. There is no defect in the action of the individual extraocular muscles, and the amount of deviation is constant or relatively constant in all directions of gaze. The majority of the congenital or infantile esotropias are of the nonparalytic or comitant type; this type is best treated surgically, but successful treatment must also involve treatment of any concurrent amblyopia.

Some cases of nonparalytic strabismus are due to underlying ocular or visual defects, such as may occur with cataracts, lesions of the optic nerve or macula, high refractive errors, or asymmetric refractive errors (anisometropia). When possible, the underlying ocular condition is corrected first; in selected cases surgery may then be offered to "straighten" the eyes.

A special type of nonparalytic strabismus is *accom-* *modative esotropia* (Fig 25–3). This type depends on the relationship between the accommodation and convergence reflexes. In certain individuals activation of accommodation results in overconvergence or crossing of the eyes; in some cases also the amount of crossing with near gaze is greater than that with gaze into the distance. This type of deviation most commonly appears at 2–3 yr of age, with a range of onset from approximately 6 mo–7 or 8 yr. The majority of affected children have some degree of hyperopia (farsightedness). In most cases the crossing can be controlled with glasses that correct the hyperopia; some children require the use of bifocal lenses to control fully the excessive convergence for near gaze. Some respond to topical miotics such as phospholine iodide, but these must be used with great care as they are long-acting cholinesterase inhibitors. With early treatment of accommodative esotropia good vision should be maintained in both eyes; when amblyopia occurs, it is necessary to use occlusion therapy as well as glasses. A few children with accommodative esotropia require surgery for a residual amount of crossing that cannot be controlled with glasses alone.

True strabismus must be differentiated from the false impression of deviation created by certain anatomic variations. Children with prominent epicanthal folds and broad, flat nasal bridges will often appear crosseyed when they are in fact orthophoric; this is *pseudoesotropia*. Similarly, an orthophoric child may appear to have a divergent strabismus because of an increased interpupillary distance or a slight disparity between the position of the corneal light reflex and the pupillary axis; this is *pseudoexotropia*. Various types of facial asymmetry can also contribute to the false impression of vertical malalignment of the eyes.

Methods of Testing for Strabismus.   Two relatively simple and reliable techniques for assessing the alignment of the eyes in children are the Hirschberg or corneal light reflex test and the cover, uncover, and cross-cover tests. The *Hirschberg test* involves simply observing the position of the corneal reflexes (reflections) when a small focal light is directed toward the patient's face. If the light reflex is well centered in each eye or falls symmetrically on corresponding points, such as the 3 o'clock position of the corneoscleral junction of both eyes simultaneously, the eyes are properly aligned. If the light reflex in 1 eye is well centered while the light reflex in the fellow eye falls nasally or temporally, superiorly or inferiorly, a deviation exists. The amount of prism needed to recenter the light reflex in the deviating eye gives an accurate measurement of the degree of deviation.

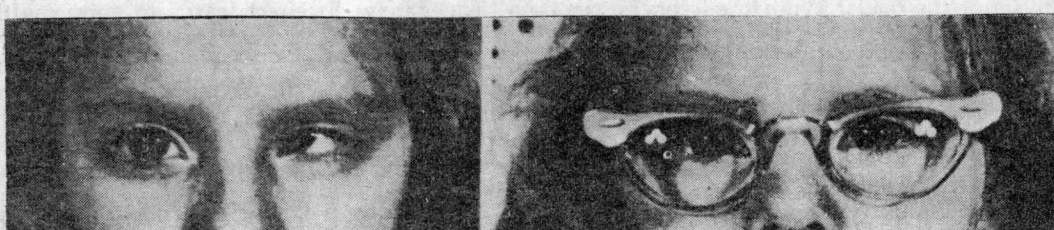

Figure 25–3   Accommodative esotropia; control of deviation with corrective lenses.

In the *cover, uncover, and cross-cover tests* the eyes are observed for compensatory or adjustive refixation movements. With the patient fixating a distant target, the examiner alternately covers each eye in turn with an occluder. If no movement of either eye occurs as the occluder is moved back and forth from 1 eye to the other, alignment is normal (orthophoria). If there is esotropia, the deviating eye will be seen to move outward as the fixating eye is occluded; if there is exotropia, the deviating eye will move inward as the fixating eye is occluded. In the case of a phoria or latent deviation it is the occluded eye that tends to deviate because of the temporary disruption of binocular fusion; the adjustive or refixation movement will be seen at the moment of uncovering. The tests should be performed both for distance and for near gaze to assure detection of any accommodative component or any abnormality of the distance-near relationship; the tests should also be done in the cardinal positions of gaze to assure detection of any incomitancy. In addition, the extraocular muscle functions of each eye should be tested individually. Simple toys, particularly those that create a gentle noise, are especially useful in attracting the attention of young children for these tests, but detailed targets such as letters, numbers, and pictures are needed to elicit accommodative deviations.

Before proceeding with the light reflex and cover testing it is advisable to take time simply to observe the child at a nonthreatening distance in quiet, pleasant surroundings while the child plays or sits comfortably with a parent, particularly when the child is very young, shy, fearful, or retarded.

Principles of Treatment. The 1st goal of treatment is to develop the best possible vision in each eye, and, if possible, equal or nearly equal vision in both eyes. Any correctable underlying defect such as a cataract must be dealt with, contributing refractive errors must be corrected with lenses, and any amblyopia must be vigorously treated with occlusion therapy.

The 2nd goal is to achieve the best possible ocular alignment, especially for the primary or forward gaze position and for the reading or eyes-down position. In many cases surgery is required. Surgical treatment is particularly important in congenital strabismus, and it should be accomplished at the earliest possible time to give the child the best possible opportunity to develop normal sensorimotor patterns. The longer the deviation persists untreated, the less chance there is for development of good or reasonably good function. Surgery is also required in some children with accommodative or partially accommodative esotropia when there is some degree of residual crossing that cannot be controlled with glasses and/or miotics. Surgical correction of a deviation is also offered in selected cases for cosmetic reasons, particularly when there is an underlying ocular defect such as an optic nerve or macular lesion or a dense amblyopia that cannot be altered. In some cases multiple surgical procedures are required for strabismus, but the majority of uncomplicated cases can be corrected with only 1 or 2 procedures.

The ultimate goal of treatment is to develop fusion and depth perception. In some cases the ophthalmologist and the patient must be satisfied with less than the ideal functional result.

OTHER DISORDERS

Duane Syndrome. This is a congenital ocular motor disorder in which there is a defect in abduction with an associated retraction of the globe on adduction. The retraction is typically accompanied by narrowing of the palpebral fissure. There may also be a defect in adduction of the affected eye, with vertical or oblique movement of the eye on attempted adduction. The condition may be unilateral or bilateral, may occur as an isolated defect or in association with other anomalies, and in some instances is familial.

A number of defects have been associated, including fibrosis or abnormal insertion of the lateral rectus, hypoplasia of cranial nerve VI, aberrant innervation of the lateral rectus by cranial nerve III, and dual innervation of the lateral rectus muscle by cranial nerves VI and III. Electrophysiologic evidence has been found for a co-contraction phenomenon or supranuclear disorder.

Moebius Syndrome. This consists of congenital facial palsy and inability to abduct the eye. The facial palsy is commonly bilateral, frequently asymmetric, and often incomplete, tending to spare the lower face and platysma. Ectropion, epiphora, and exposure keratopathy may develop. The abduction defect may be unilateral or bilateral. It is usually complete, and esotropia is common. Surgical correction of the esotropia can be done in selected cases.

There may be associated developmental defects, including ptosis, palatal and lingual palsy, hearing loss, pectoral and lingual muscle defects, micrognathia, syndactyly, supernumerary digits, or absence of hands, feet, fingers, or toes. The etiology is unknown.

Gradenigo Syndrome. This is characterized by an acquired abducens palsy with pain in the distribution of the homolateral trigeminal nerve, indicating involvement of the petrous portion of the 6th cranial nerve and the adjacent gasserian ganglion. The usual causes are otitis media or mastoiditis with inflammation extending into the petrous bone, its meninges, and the inferior petrosal sinus. Tumor is rarely the cause. Principal signs and symptoms are weakness of the lateral rectus, diplopia, ocular and facial pain, photophobia, lacrimation, and sometimes corneal hypesthesia. There may also be involvement of the 7th nerve, with facial palsy.

Benign Sixth Nerve Palsy. This is a painless acquired abducens palsy that resolves spontaneously, usually without residua. The palsy typically develops 1–3 wk after a nonspecific febrile illness or upper respiratory infection; in some cases the palsy precedes other symptoms of infection or occurs during the prodrome of an exanthem. Improvement in abduction usually begins within 3–6 wk after onset of the palsy, and recovery is usually complete within 10–12 wk. Episodes may be recurrent. The paresis is thought to be a neurotropic effect of a viral infection. Except for benign 6th nerve palsy the development of a cranial nerve palsy in a child is usually a sign of a serious pathologic process, such as intracranial tumor, increased intracranial pressure, meningitis, or demyelinating disease.

Brown Syndrome. In this syndrome elevation of the eye in the adducted position is restricted or absent.

Often, there is an associated downward deviation of the affected eye in adduction. There may be a compensatory tilt of the head. Various causes have been described. In some cases there is congenital shortening of the anterior sheath of the superior oblique tendon; in others there are fine adhesions between the sheath and the tendon. In many cases no anatomic abnormality is found. Acquired and intermittent cases have been related to inflammation or injury in the region of the trochlea of the superior oblique. Surgery is helpful in selected cases.

Parinaud Syndrome. This is the eponymic designation for a palsy of vertical gaze, isolated or in association with pupillary or nuclear oculomotor (cranial nerve III) paresis. It indicates a lesion affecting the mesencephalic tegmentum. The ophthalmic signs of midbrain disease include vertical gaze palsy, dissociation of the pupillary responses to light and to near focus, general pupillomotor paralysis, corectopia, dyscoria, accommodative disturbances, pathologic lid retraction, ptosis, extraocular muscle paresis, and convergence paralysis. In some cases there are spasms of convergence, convergent retraction nystagmus, and vertical nystagmus, particularly on attempted vertical gaze. Combinations of these signs are variously referred to as the Koerber-Salus-Elschnig syndrome or the sylvian aqueduct syndrome.

A principal cause of vertical gaze palsy and associated mesencephalic signs in children is tumor of the pineal gland or 3rd ventricle. Differential diagnosis also includes trauma and demyelinating disease. In children with hydrocephalus, impairment of vertical gaze and pathologic lid retraction are familiarly referred to as the *setting sun sign*.

Congenital Ocular Motor Apraxia. This congenital disorder of conjugate gaze is characterized by (1) a defect in voluntary horizontal gaze, (2) compensatory jerking movement of the head, and (3) retention of slow pursuit and reflexive eye movements. Additional features are absence of the fast (refixation) phase of optokinetic nystagmus and obligate contraversive deviation of the eyes on rotation of the body. Typically, the affected child is unable to look quickly to either side voluntarily in response to command or in response to an eccentrically presented object but may, however, be able to follow a slowly moving target to either side. To compensate for the defect in purposive lateral eye movements, the child jerks the head to bring the eyes into the desired position and may also blink repetitively in an attempt to change fixation.

The pathogenesis of congenital ocular motor apraxia is unknown; it may be due to delayed myelination of the ocular motor pathways. The condition tends to become less conspicuous with age. It may be associated with some clumsiness and with slowness in reading.

Nystagmus. Nystagmus, rhythmic oscillations of 1 or both eyes, may be due to abnormality in any 1 of the 3 basic mechanisms that regulate the position and movement of the eyes: the fixation mechanism, the conjugate gaze mechanism, or the vestibular system. In addition, physiologic types of nystagmus may be elicited by appropriate stimuli.

Congenital pendular nystagmus is commonly associated with ocular and visual defects; it typically occurs with albinism, aniridia, achromatopsia, congenital cataracts, congenital macular lesions, congenital optic atrophy, and high refractive errors. In some instances pendular nystagmus occurs in families as a dominant or X-linked characteristic without obvious ocular abnormalities. There may be associated rhythmic movements of the head.

Congenital jerky nystagmus is characterized by horizontal jerky oscillations with gaze preponderance; the nystagmus is coarser in 1 direction of gaze than in the other with the jerk toward the direction of gaze. There is usually a point of reversal or null point in which the nystagmus lessens and in which position vision is best; compensatory posturing, turning of the head to bring the eyes into the position of least nystagmus, is characteristic. The cause of congenital jerky nystagmus is unknown; in some instances it is familial.

Acquired nystagmus requires prompt and thorough evaluation. Worrisome pathologic types are the gaze-paretic or gaze-evoked oscillations of cerebellar, brain stem, or cerebral disease.

Nystagmus retractorius or *convergent nystagmus* is repetitive jerking of the eyes into the orbit or toward each other. It is usually seen in association with vertical gaze palsy as a feature of the Parinaud or Koerber-Salus-Elschnig syndrome of the sylvian aqueduct. While the causal condition may be neoplastic, vascular, or inflammatory, nystagmus retractorius in children suggests particularly the presence of pinealoma or hydrocephalus.

A special type of acquired nystagmus in childhood is *spasmus nutans*. In its complete form spasmus nutans is characterized by the triad of pendular nystagmus, head nodding, and torticollis. The nystagmus is characteristically very fine, very rapid, horizontal, and pendular; it is often asymmetric, sometimes unilateral. Signs usually develop within the 1st yr or 2 of life. Components of the triad may develop at varying times. The cause is unknown, but poor illumination and deprivation have been implicated. The condition is benign and self-limited, usually lasting a few mo though sometimes years. Certain insidious lesions such as optic glioma may produce a fine rapid nystagmus (asymmetric or monocular) that initially mimics spasmus nutans. Children with nystagmus warrant close follow-up.

To be differentiated from true nystagmus are certain special types of abnormal eye movements, particularly opsoclonus, ocular dysmetria, and flutter.

Opsoclonus. Opsoclonus and ataxic conjugate movements are terms which describe spontaneous, nonrhythmic, multidirectional, chaotic movements of the eyes. The eyes appear to be in agitation, with bursts of conjugate movement of varying amplitude in varying directions. Opsoclonus is most often associated with encephalitis. It may be the 1st sign of neuroblastoma.

Ocular Motor Dysmetria. This is analogous to dysmetria of the limbs. There is lack of precision in performing movements of refixation, characterized by an overshoot (or undershoot) of the eyes with several corrective to and fro oscillations on looking from 1 point to another. Ocular motor dysmetria is a sign of cerebellar or cerebellar pathway disease.

Flutter-Like Oscillations. These intermittent to and fro horizontal oscillations of the eyes may occur spontaneously or on change of fixation. They are characteristic of cerebellar disease.

25.7 ABNORMALITIES OF THE LIDS

Ptosis. Blepharoptosis exists when the upper eyelid droops below its normal level. Congenital ptosis is usually due to faulty development of the levator muscle or its innervating branch of the 3rd nerve. There may be associated involvement of the superior rectus muscle and attendant impairment in elevation of the eye. The condition may be familial, transmitted as a dominant trait. Congenital ptosis can be corrected surgically; the age at which surgery is done depends on its degree, its cosmetic and functional severity, the presence or absence of compensatory posturing, the wishes of the parents, and the discretion of the surgeon; unless the ptosis is complete, surgery is generally deferred until the child is 3–4 yr old.

Congenital ptosis occurs with a large number of syndromes. In the Marcus Gunn jaw winking syndrome of aberrant innervation, there is abnormal synkinesis of lid and jaw movements; paradoxical elevation of the ptotic lid occurs as the child sucks, chews, or cries. In the congenital fibrosis syndrome, a hereditary condition, ptosis is associated with paralysis or "fibrosis" of other extraocular muscles. Minimal ptosis occurs in the Horner syndrome (oculosympathetic palsy). In the Sturge-Weber syndrome ptosis is often secondary to hemangiomatous involvement of the upper lid, and in von Recklinghausen syndrome there may be ptosis due to plexiform neuroma of the upper lid.

Differential diagnosis of acquired ptosis in childhood includes myasthenia gravis, progressive external ophthalmoplegia, progressive intracranial lesions affecting the 3rd nerve, and inflammation or tumors affecting the levator, the orbit, or lid. Ptosis may also result from trauma. Aberrant regeneration of injured 3rd nerve fibers may produce paradoxic lid and eye movements.

Epicanthal Folds. These vertical or oblique folds of skin extend on either side of the bridge of the nose from the brow or lid area, covering the inner canthal region. They are present to some degree in most young children and become less apparent with age. The folds may be sufficiently broad to cover the medial aspect of the eye, making the eyes appear crossed (pseudoesotropia).

Epicanthal folds are a common feature of many syndromes, including chromosomal aberrations (particularly the trisomies) or disorders of single genes.

Lagophthalmos. This exists when complete closure of the lids over the globe is difficult or impossible. It may be paralytic, due to a facial palsy involving the orbicularis muscle, or spastic, as in thyrotoxicosis. It may be structural when retraction or shortening of the lids results from scarring or atrophy consequent to injury or disease; in children burns are an all too frequent cause. Infants with collodion membrane may have temporary lagophthalmos due to the restrictive effect of the membrane on the lids. Lagophthalmos may accompany proptosis or buphthalmos when the lids, although normal, cannot effectively cover the enlarged or protuberant eye. A degree of physiologic lagophthalmos may occur normally during sleep, but functional lagophthalmos in the unconscious or debilitated can be a problem.

When lagophthalmos exists, exposure of the eye may lead to drying, infection, corneal ulceration, or perforation; the result may be loss of vision, even loss of the eye. In lagophthalmos protection of the eye by means of artificial tear preparations, ophthalmic ointment, or moisture chambers is essential. Gauze pads are to be avoided as the gauze may abrade the cornea. In some cases surgical closure of the lids (tarsorrhaphy) may be necessary for long term protection of the eye.

Lid Retraction. Pathologic retraction of the lid may be myogenic or neurogenic. Myogenic retraction of the upper lid occurs in thyrotoxicosis, in which it is associated with 3 classic signs: a staring appearance (Dalrymple sign), infrequent blinking (Stellwag sign), and lag of the upper lid on downward gaze (von Graefe sign).

Neurogenic retraction of the lids may occur in conditions affecting the anterior mesencephalon. Lid retraction is a feature of the syndrome of the sylvian aqueduct. In children it is commonly a sign of hydrocephalus. It may occur with meningitis.

Paradoxical retraction of the lid is a feature of the Marcus Gunn jaw winking syndrome. Paradoxical lid retraction may also occur during recovery from a 3rd nerve palsy as a result of aberrant regeneration or misdirection of oculomotor fibers.

To be differentiated from pathologic lid retractions are simple staring and the physiologic or reflexive lid retraction ("eye popping") that occurs in infants in response to sudden reduction in illumination or as a startle reaction.

Entropion. Entropion is inversion of the lid margin, which may cause discomfort and corneal damage due to the inward turning of the lashes (trichiasis). A principal cause is scarring secondary to inflammation such as occurs in trachoma. There is also a rare congenital form. Surgical correction is effective.

Ectropion. Ectropion is eversion of the lid margin; it may lead to overflow of tears (epiphora) and subsequent maceration of the skin of the lid, to inflammation of exposed conjunctiva, or to superficial exposure keratopathy. Common causes are scarring consequent to inflammation, burns, or trauma or weakness of the orbicularis muscle due to facial palsy; these forms may be corrected surgically.

Ectropion is also seen in certain children who have faulty development of the lateral canthal ligament; this may occur in Down syndrome.

Blepharospasm. This is spastic or repetitive closure of the lids. It may be due to irritative disease of the cornea, conjunctiva, or facial nerve, to fatigue or uncorrected refractive error, or to psychogenic causes. Excessive repetitive blinking in children is a common tic, but thorough ophthalmic examination for pathologic causes such as trichiasis, keratitis, conjunctivitis, or foreign body is indicated.

Blepharitis. This inflammation of the lid margins is

characterized by erythema and crusting or scaling; the usual symptoms are irritation, burning, and itching. The condition is commonly bilateral and chronic or recurrent. There are 2 main types: staphylococcal and seborrheic. In *staphylococcal blepharitis* ulceration of the lid margin is common, the lashes tend to fall out, and there is often associated conjunctivitis and superficial keratitis. In *seborrheic blepharitis* the scales tend to be greasy, the lid margins are less red, and ulceration does not occur. The blepharitis is often of mixed type.

Thorough daily cleansing of the lid margins with a moistened cotton applicator to remove scales and crusts is essential in the treatment of both forms of blepharitis. Staphylococcal blepharitis is treated with antistaphylococcal antibiotic or sulfonamide ophthalmic ointment applied directly to the lid margins daily at bedtime. When seborrhea exists, concurrent treatment of the scalp is important; local treatment using selenium sulfide ointment is effective.*

Hordeolum. This infection of the glands of the lid may be acute or subacute; there is tender focal swelling and redness in the lid. The usual agent is *Staphylococcus aureus.*

When the meibomian glands are involved, the lesion is referred to as an *internal hordeolum;* the abscess tends to be large and may point through either the skin or conjunctival surface. When the infection involves the glands of Zeis or Moll, the abscess tends to be smaller and more superficial and points at the lid margin; it is then referred to as an *external hordeolum* or *stye.*

As with abscesses elsewhere, treatment is frequent warm compresses and, if necessary, surgical incision and drainage. In addition, topical antibiotic or sulfonamide preparations are often used. Untreated, the infection may progress to cellulitis of the lid or orbit, requiring use of systemic antibiotics. Recurrence is common, possibly by reinfection through contaminated hands. Itching due to an underlying allergy is a common contributory factor. Recurrent styes in children may also signal an immunologic defect.

Chalazion. Chalazion is granulomatous inflammation of a meibomian gland characterized by a firm, nontender nodule in the upper or lower lid. This lesion tends to be chronic and differs from internal hordeolum in the absence of acute inflammatory signs. When a chalazion is large enough to distort vision (it may cause astigmatism by exerting pressure on the globe) or to be a cosmetic blemish, excision is advised. Rarely will a chalazion subside spontaneously.

Vaccinia. Vaccinia of the lids or conjunctiva has followed accidental inoculation, with great danger of corneal involvement; dense scarring and visual loss can result.

Coloboma of the Eyelid. This cleftlike deformity may vary from a small indentation or notch of the free margin of the lid to a large defect involving almost the entire lid. If the gap is extensive, xerosis, ulceration, and corneal opacities may result from exposure. Early surgical correction of the lid defect is recommended.

---

*Selenium sulfide (Selsun) ointment is toxic to the cornea and should be used on the lid margins only with great care; its application is best done by the physician, once a week, until the condition subsides.

Other deformities frequently associated with lid colobomata include dermoid cysts or dermolipomata on the globe; often, they occur in a position corresponding to the site of the lid defect. Lid colobomata may also be associated with extensive facial malformation, as in mandibulofacial dysostosis (Franceschetti or Treacher Collins syndrome).

Tumors of the Lid. A number of lid tumors arise from surface structures (the epithelium and sebaceous glands). Nevi may appear in early childhood; most are junctional. Compound nevi tend to develop in the prepubertal years. Dermal nevi first appear at puberty. Malignant epithelial tumors (basal cell carcinoma and squamous cell carcinoma) are rare in children, but the basal cell nevus syndrome, the malignant lesions of xeroderma pigmentosum, and the skin cancers of the Rothmund-Thomson syndrome may develop in childhood. Adenoma sebaceum (vascular fibroma) of tuberous sclerosis may also occur in the lid, sometimes forming extensive masses. The small yellowish papules of juvenile xanthogranuloma may occur on the lids, with or without cutaneous lesions elsewhere; these usually appear in infancy and regress spontaneously by the age of 1–2 yr.

Of the lid tumors that arise from deeper structures (the neural, vascular, and connective tissues) hemangiomas are especially common. The majority tend to regress spontaneously, though they may show alarmingly rapid growth in infancy; usually, the best management of such hemangiomas is patient observation, allowing spontaneous regression to occur. Alternative treatment methods include surgery, radiotherapy, injection of sclerosing agents, and administration of corticosteroids. In the case of a rapidly expanding lesion that threatens to obstruct vision, corticosteroid treatment should be considered.

Nevus flammeus (port wine stain), a noninvoluting hemangioma, occurs as isolated lesions or in association with other signs of Sturge-Weber syndrome. Affected patients should be examined for glaucoma.

Lymphangiomas of the lid appear as firm masses at or soon after birth and tend to enlarge slowly during the growing years. Associated conjunctival involvement, appearing as a clear, cystic, sinuous conjunctival mass, may provide a clue to the diagnosis. In some cases there is also orbital involvement. The treatment is surgical excision.

Plexiform neuromas of the lids occur in children with von Recklinghausen disease; the presenting sign is often ptosis.

The lids may also be involved by other tumors such as retinoblastoma, neuroblastoma, and rhabdomyosarcoma of the orbit; these conditions are discussed elsewhere.

25.8 DISORDERS OF THE LACRIMAL SYSTEM

Dacryocystitis. In this inflammation of the nasolacrimal sac and duct, the usual signs are epiphora (tearing), accumulation of purulent or mucopurulent discharge in the conjunctival sac, and sometimes swelling and erythema at the site of the sac; gentle massage over the sac will often produce reflux of mucopus.

In childhood, dacryocystitis occurs most often in the newborn period (dacryocystitis neonatorum) because of developmental obstruction in the lacrimal passages; there may be epithelial remnants in the duct or membranous occlusion of the lower ostium. Rarely, there is absence of the puncta.

The condition usually runs a mild and somewhat chronic course, responding well to conservative treatment consisting of massage of the sac and instillation of antibiotic drops. If signs of obstruction persist, probing is indicated. Acute dacryocystitis, with swelling over the sac and pericystic spread, requires more aggressive treatment, including warm compresses and use of systemic antibiotics; often the condition will not improve until the sac is incised and drained. In some cases of obstruction a new opening from the tear sac to the nasal cavity must be created surgically.

Dacryoadenitis. Dacryoadenitis, or inflammation of the lacrimal gland, is uncommon in childhood. It may occur with mumps, in which case it is usually acute and bilateral, subsiding in a few days or weeks. Acute dacryoadenitis may also be seen with infectious mononucleosis in young patients. Chronic dacryoadenitis is associated with certain systemic diseases, particularly sarcoidosis, tuberculosis, and syphilis. A variety of systemic diseases may produce enlargement of the lacrimal and salivary glands (Mikulicz syndrome).

Alacrima ("Dry Eye"). Marked deficiency of tears may occur as an isolated unilateral or bilateral congenital defect or in association with other nervous system anomalies, such as aplasia of cranial nerve nuclei. It occurs congenitally in familial dysautonomia (Riley-Day syndrome) and in the anhidrotic type of ectodermal dysplasia. Deficiency of tears may also follow inflammation; it is not uncommon after Stevens-Johnson syndrome. Drying of the eye, corneal ulceration, and scarring may result. Preventive care includes the frequent instillation of an artificial tear preparation. In some cases occlusion of the lacrimal puncta is helpful. In severe cases tarsorrhaphy may be necessary to protect the cornea.

25.9 DISORDERS OF THE CONJUNCTIVA

CONJUNCTIVITIS

The conjunctiva reacts to a wide range of bacterial and viral agents, allergens, irritants, toxins, and systemic diseases. Conjunctivitis is common in childhood and may be infectious or noninfectious.

Acute purulent conjunctivitis is characterized by more or less generalized conjunctival hyperemia, edema, mucopurulent exudate, and various degrees of ocular discomfort. It is usually due to bacterial infection. The most frequent causes are staphylococci, pneumococci, *Hemophilus influenzae*, and streptococci. Conjunctival

smear and culture are helpful in differentiating specific types. These common forms of acute purulent conjunctivitis usually respond well to warm compresses and frequent topical instillation of antibiotic drops.

Ophthalmia neonatorum is acute conjunctivitis in the newborn infant. Any of the common bacterial conjunctivitides can occur in the newborn period, but emphasis in differential diagnosis must be given to recognition of gonococcal infection and inclusion blennorhea.

Ophthalmia neonatorum due to *Neisseria gonorrhoeae* usually appears from 1–3 or 4 days after birth; there is generally profuse discharge with marked edema and hyperemia of the eyelids and conjunctiva. Gonococcal infection can lead to corneal perforation and blindness. Prompt diagnosis is aided by identification of gram-negative diplococci in smears of conjunctival scrapings. Culture and fermentation tests must differentiate the gonococcus from other members of the *Neisseria* group. Systemic treatment with penicillin with the frequent topical instillation of antibiotic drops is usually effective, but the emergence of penicillinase-producing *Neisseria gonorrhoeae* in the United States makes it necessary to determine the antibiotic susceptibility in individual cases. Great care must be taken in handling infected infants to avoid spread to others.

Inclusion blennorrhea, the more common form of ophthalmia neonatorum, is due to *Chlamydia oculogenitalis*. The infant is infected by organisms in the maternal genital tract during birth. The incubation period is usually 1 wk or more. The clinical picture is commonly that of an acute purulent conjunctivitis, but the discharge and scrapings are bacteriologically sterile; the diagnostic feature is intracytoplasmic inclusion bodies. Inclusion blennorrhea and the sometimes associated pulmonary involvement can be effectively treated with erythromycin (Sec 10.63).

To be differentiated from the infectious types of ophthalmia neonatorum is the chemical conjunctivitis due to prophylactic use of silver nitrate. This usually develops 12–24 hr after instillation and lasts only 24–48 hr; no pathogen is grown on culture.

Viral conjunctivitis is generally characterized by a watery discharge. Often, there are follicular changes, pinhead-sized aggregates of lymphocytes, of the palpebral conjunctiva. Conjunctivitis due to adenovirus infection is relatively common. In some types there is corneal involvement. Sulfonamides are useful in treatment.

Conjunctivitides are commonly associated with such systemic viral infections as the childhood exanthems, particularly measles. These are self-limited.

Epidemic keratoconjunctivitis is caused by adenovirus type 8 and is transmitted by direct contact. Initially, there is a sensation of a foreign body beneath the lids with itching and burning. Edema and photophobia develop rapidly, and large oval follicles appear within the conjunctiva. Preauricular adenopathy and a pseudomembrane on the conjunctival surface occur frequently. Blurring of vision results from subepithelial corneal infiltrates; these usually disappear but have been known to reduce visual acuity permanently. Corneal complications are less common in children than in adults. Children may have associated upper respiratory infection.

Membranous and pseudomembranous conjunctivitis can be seen in a number of diseases. The classic example of membranous conjunctivitis is that of diphtheria. The membrane results when fibrin-rich exudate forms on the conjunctival surface and permeates the epithelium; the membrane is removed with difficulty and leaves raw bleeding areas. In pseudomembranous conjunctivitis the layer of fibrin-rich exudate is superficial and can be stripped with ease, leaving the surface smooth. This type occurs in a wide range of bacterial and viral infections, including staphylococcal, pneumococcal, streptococcal, or chlamydial conjunctivitis, and in epidemic keratoconjunctivitis. It is also seen in vernal conjunctivitis and in Stevens-Johnson disease.

Allergic conjunctivitis is usually accompanied by intense itching, tearing, and conjunctival edema. It is commonly seasonal. Symptomatic relief is afforded by cold compresses and decongestant drops. Topical steroids are used only under close ophthalmic supervision.

Vernal conjunctivitis is a bilateral disease that usually begins in the prepubertal years and may recur for many years. Atopy appears to play a role in its origin, but the pathogenesis is uncertain. Extreme itching and tearing are the usual complaints. Large flattened cobblestone-like papillary lesions of the palpebral conjunctiva are characteristic. A stringy exudate and a milky conjunctival pseudomembrane are frequently present. There may be small elevated lesions of the bulbar conjunctiva adjacent to the limbus (limbal form). Smear of the conjunctival exudate will show many eosinophils. Topical steroid therapy and cold compresses afford some relief.

Chemical conjunctivitis can result when an irritating substance enters the conjunctival sac. The common example is the acute but benign conjunctivitis due to silver nitrate in the newborn. Other common offenders are household cleaning substances, sprays, smoke, smog, and industrial pollutants.

Alkalis tend to linger in the conjunctival tissues and continue to inflict damage over a period of hours or days. Acids precipitate the proteins in tissues and so produce their effect immediately. In either case, prompt, thorough, and copious irrigation is crucial. Extensive tissue damage, even loss of the eye, can result, especially if the offending agent is an alkali.

OTHER CONJUNCTIVAL DISORDERS

Subconjunctival Hemorrhage. This is manifested by bright or dark red patches in the bulbar conjunctiva and may result from injury or inflammation. It may occasionally result from severe sneezing or coughing or be a manifestation of a blood dyscrasia.

Pingueculum. A pingueculum is a benign lesion, a yellowish white, slightly elevated mass on the bulbar conjunctiva, usually in the interpalpebral region. It represents elastic and hyaline degenerative change of the conjunctiva. No treatment is required except for cosmetic reasons, in which case simple excision is all that is needed.

Pterygium. A pterygium is a fleshy triangular conjunctival lesion that may encroach on the cornea. It typically occurs in the nasal interpalpebral region. The pathologic findings are similar to those of a pingueculum. Irritation such as exposure to dust and wind is thought to aggravate the lesion. Removal is suggested when the lesion encroaches far onto the cornea.

Dermoid Cyst and Dermolipoma. These benign lesions are clinically similar in appearance. They are smooth, elevated, round to oval lesions of various sizes. The color varies from yellowish white to a fleshy pink. The most frequent site is the upper outer quadrant of the globe, though they commonly occur near or straddle the limbus. The dermolipoma is composed of adipose and connective tissue. Dermoid cysts may also contain glandular tissue, hair follicles, and hair shafts. Excision for cosmetic reasons is feasible.

Nevus. A conjunctival nevus is a small, slightly elevated lesion that may vary in pigmentation from pale salmon to dark brown. It is usually benign, but careful observation for progressive growth or changes suggestive of malignancy is advised.

Symblepharon. This is a cicatricial adhesion between the conjunctiva of the lid and the globe; the lower lid is usually affected. It follows operation or injuries, especially burns from lye, acids, or molten metals. It may interfere with motion of the eyeball and cause diplopia. The band should be separated and the raw surfaces kept from uniting during healing. Grafts of oral mucous membrane may be necessary.

25.10 ABNORMALITIES OF THE CORNEA

Megalocornea. This term denotes a developmental anomaly in which the diameter of the cornea is greater than 13 mm. The condition is nonprogressive and produces no ill effects, though there is often a high refractive error.

To be differentiated from this anomaly is pathologic corneal enlargement due to glaucoma. Any progressive increase in the size of the cornea, especially when accompanied by photophobia, lacrimation, or haziness of the cornea, requires prompt ophthalmologic evaluation.

Microcornea. Microcornea or anterior microphthalmia describes an abnormally small cornea in an otherwise relatively normal eye. This may occur as a hereditary condition, the transmission being dominant more often than recessive. More commonly, a small cornea is just 1 feature of an otherwise developmentally abnormal or microphthalmic eye; associated defects include colobomata, microphakia, congenital cataract, and glaucoma.

Keratoconus. Keratoconus or conical cornea is a condition characterized by ectasia and increased curvature of the central or axial portion of the cornea. It commonly appears in adolescence and with increased frequency in Down syndrome. The etiology is obscure. There is usually considerable impairment of vision due to a high degree of astigmatism, though vision can often be improved with contact lenses. In some cases acute ectasia and corneal edema (hydrops) develop. In selected cases perforating keratoplasty (corneal transplant) is done.

Dendritic Keratitis. Infection of the eye with the virus of herpes simplex produces a characteristic lesion of the corneal epithelium referred to as a dendrite; it has a branching tree–like pattern that can be demonstrated by fluorescein staining. The acute episode is accompanied by pain, photophobia, tearing, blepharospasm, and conjunctival injection. Specific treatment is 5-iodo-2'-deoxyuridine (IDU) in the form of drops or ointment; in the early stages debridement is also helpful. In addition, a cycloplegic agent, preferably atropine sulfate, is used. Recurrent infection and deep stromal involvement may occur and can lead to corneal scarring.

It has been clearly demonstrated that topical use of corticosteroids causes exacerbation of superficial herpetic disease of the eye; eyedrops combining steroids and antibiotics, are, therefore, to be avoided in treatment of "red eye" unless there are clear-cut indications for their use and close supervision during therapy.

Corneal Ulcers. The usual signs and symptoms of corneal ulcer are focal or diffuse corneal haze, hyperemia, lid edema, pain, photophobia, tearing, and blepharospasm. Often, there is hypopyon (pus in the anterior chamber).

Corneal ulcers are cause for immediate concern and require prompt treatment. They result most frequently from traumatic lesions which become secondarily infected. Many organisms are capable of infecting the cornea. One of the most troublesome is *Pseudomonas aeruginosa;* it can rapidly destroy stromal tissue and lead to corneal perforation. *Neisseria gonorrhoeae* also is particularly damaging to the cornea. Indolent ulcers are often found to be due to fungi. In each case scrapings of the cornea must be studied in an effort to identify the causative infectious agent and to determine the best therapeutic agent. Generally, both systemic and local treatment are needed to save the eye. Perforation or scarring due to corneal ulceration is an important cause of blindness throughout the world and is estimated to be responsible for 10% of blindness in the United States.

Phlyctenules. These are small, yellowish, slightly elevated lesions usually located at the corneal limbus; they may encroach on the cornea and extend centrally. Often, there is a small corneal ulcer at the head of the advancing lesion, with a fascicle of blood vessels behind the head of the lesion. Phlyctenular keratoconjunctivitis was previously thought to be most commonly due to hypersensitivity to tuberculin proteins, but a specific cause is not really known. Staphylococcal infections also may be associated with phlyctenular changes, but the lesion is not primarily due to staphylococcal invasion. The condition usually responds to topical steroid therapy, leaving superficial stromal pannus and scarring.

Interstitial Keratitis. The term interstitial keratitis denotes inflammation of the corneal stroma. The most common cause is syphilis, interstitial keratitis being 1 of the characteristic late manifestations of congenital syphilis. The deep inflammation produces pain, photophobia, tearing, circumcorneal injection, and corneal haze. Corneal vascularization and opacities develop and generally remain as permanent stigmata of the disease.

Less frequently, interstitial keratitis is due to other infectious diseases, such as tuberculosis or leprosy.

Corneal Manifestations of Systemic Disease. Several metabolic diseases produce distinctive corneal changes in childhood. Refractile polychromatic crystals are deposited throughout the cornea in cystinosis. Corneal deposits producing various degrees of corneal haze also occur in certain of the mucopolysaccharidoses, particularly MPS IH (Hurler), MPS IS (Scheie), MPS I H/S (Hurler-Scheie compound), MPS IV (Morquio), MPS VI (Maroteaux-Lamy), and sometimes MPS VII (Sly). Corneal deposits may develop in patients with G_{M1} (generalized) gangliosidosis. In Fabry disease fine opacities radiating in a whorl or fanlike pattern occur, and corneal changes can be important in identifying the carrier state. A spray-like pattern of corneal opacities may also be seen in the Bloch-Sulzberger syndrome. In Wilson disease the distinctive corneal sign is the Kayser-Fleischer ring, a golden brown ring in the peripheral cornea due to changes in Descemet membrane.

25.11 ABNORMALITIES OF THE LENS

Cataracts. Cataract may be defined simply as any opacity of the lens. Cataracts vary considerably, however, in their morphology, etiology, and effects on vision.

Early developmental processes in the lens may lead to a number of different types of congenital cataract. Not uncommon are discrete dots or small white plaque-like opacities of the lens capsule, sometimes with involvement of the contiguous subcapsular region. Such opacities of the posterior capsule may be associated with persistent remnants of the hyaloid system, while those of the anterior capsule may be associated with persistent strands of the pupillary membrane or vascular sheath of the lens. Congenital opacities of this type are usually stable and rarely interfere with vision.

To be differentiated from capsular and capsulolenticular opacities are congenital cataracts involving the central nucleus of the lens or the developing lamellae laid down immediately around the fetal nucleus. Some are hereditary, dominant transmission being more common than recessive or sex-linked, and examination of other family members is important in the differential diagnosis of congenital cataracts. Some are the result of gestational infection, rubella being a more frequent cause of congenital cataract than syphilis or toxoplasmosis. In congenital rubella the cataract tends to be a dense, pearly, nuclear opacity surrounded by clearer cortex, often with associated ocular abnormalities such as microphthalmos, iris hypoplasia, inflammatory iris adhesions (synechiae), glaucoma, pigmentary retinopathy, and optic atrophy. In many cases congenital cataract is just 1 facet of a complex syndrome; in Lowe syndrome, for example, congenital cataract and glaucoma are associated with mental retardation, hypotonia, renal tubular dysfunction, and aminoaciduria. In this sex-linked disorder affected males tend to have a dense nuclear or total cataract readily visible at birth, whereas fine punctate cortical opacities can be detected in many carrier females.

As lens growth continues throughout life, opacities of various layers may occur as the result of disease appearing at any age. Metabolic diseases are major considerations in the differential diagnosis of cataracts. In infants with galactosemia, cataracts may form in the 1st weeks of life; opacities in the cortex create a refractive ring and an "oil droplet" appearance on ophthalmoscopic examination, best seen with the pupil well dilated. Infants and children with hypocalcemic tetany may develop cataracts; these opacities are zonular, affected lamellae often being separated by clear layers. Young persons with diabetes mellitus may develop cataracts that progress rapidly, with the formation of fine vacuoles and punctate "snowflake" opacities in the subcapsular layers occurring in a matter of hours, days or weeks. Development of the cataract may be heralded by rapid changes in the refractive state. This may occur in adolescence, rarely earlier. In Wilson disease a brilliant array of anterior capsular and subcapsular opacities arranged in a radiating pattern may develop; it is referred to as "sunflower cataract."

Certain drugs and toxins may also produce cataract at various ages. Cataract is a well documented effect of prolonged corticosteroid therapy, and it is recommended that all children being treated long term with steroids have periodic eye examinations. As a rule, steroid-induced lens opacities develop in the posterior subcapsular region. The effect on vision depends on the extent and density of the opacity. In many cases the acuity is reduced to only a minimal or moderate degree.

Trauma at any age can produce cataracts. Opacities may result either from contusion or from penetrating injury. Other physical agents such as radiation can also damage the lens and result in cataract.

Cataract may also develop secondary to a variety of intraocular processes such as retrolental fibroplasia, retinal detachment, retinitis pigmentosa, and uveitis.

A special type of lens change seen in some newborns is the so-called "cataract of prematurity." The opacities appear as clusters of tiny vacuoles in the distribution of the "Y" sutures of the lens; they can be visualized with the ophthalmoscope and are best seen with the pupil well dilated. The etiology is unclear; fortunately, in most cases the opacities disappear spontaneously, often within a few wk.

The treatment of cataracts that significantly interfere with vision involves (1) surgical removal of the lens to provide an optically clear visual axis, (2) correction of the resultant aphakic refractive error with either spectacles or contact lenses, and (3) treatment of any associated sensory deprivation amblyopia. The last may be the most demanding and difficult step in the visual rehabilitation of a child with cataract.

The prognosis depends on numerous factors, including the nature of associated ocular abnormalities (such as microphthalmia, retinal lesions, optic atrophy, nystagmus, strabismus, etc.). In addition, affected children may have cardiac, renal, skeletal, or central nervous system disorders. There is often amblyopia requiring intensive treatment. The ultimate management decisions must rest jointly with the ophthalmologist, the pediatrician, and the family.

Dislocation of the Lens (Ectopia Lentis). Dislocation or subluxation of the lens in children is usually associated with trauma, Marfan syndrome, Marchesani syndrome, or homocystinuria; displacement of the lens is also seen in aniridia, sulfite oxidase deficiency, hyperlysinemia, and Ehlers-Danlos syndrome. The abnormal position of the lens produces refractive changes with various degrees of impairment of vision. In many instances vision can be improved with corrective lenses. In selected cases surgery is performed. Complications associated with subluxation of the lens are glaucoma and retinal detachment. The external sign of dislocation is iridodonesis, a shimmering movement of the iris due to its loss of support by the lens.

25.12 DISEASE OF THE UVEAL TRACT

Uveitis (Iritis, Cyclitis, Chorioretinitis). The uveal tract, the inner vascular coat of the eye consisting of iris, ciliary body, and choroid, is subject to inflammatory involvement in a number of systemic diseases, both infectious and noninfectious, and in response to exogenous factors, including trauma and toxic agents. Inflammation may affect any 1 portion of the uveal tract preferentially or all parts together.

Iritis may occur alone or in conjunction with inflammation of the ciliary body as iridocyclitis or in association with pars planitis. Pain, photophobia, and lacrimation are the characteristic symptoms of acute anterior uveitis, but the inflammation may develop insidiously without disturbing symptoms. Signs of anterior uveitis include conjunctival hyperemia, particularly in the perilimbal region (ciliary flush), cells and protein ("flare") in the aqueous humor, inflammatory deposits on the posterior surface of the cornea (keratic precipitates or "KP"), congestion of the iris, and sometimes neovascularization of the iris. In more chronic cases there may be degenerative changes of the cornea (band keratopathy), lenticular opacities (cataract), and impairment of vision. In many cases the etiology of anterior uveitis remains obscure. Primary etiologic considerations in children are rheumatoid disease, particularly pauciarticular rheumatoid arthritis, and sarcoidosis. Iritis may also develop secondary to corneal disease, such as herpetic keratitis or a bacterial or fungal corneal ulcer, or secondary to a corneal abrasion or foreign body. Traumatic iritis and iridocyclitis are especially common in children.

Choroiditis, inflammation of the posterior portion of the uveal tract, invariably also involves the retina; when both are obviously affected, the term chorioretinitis is used (Fig 25–4). The causes of posterior uveitis are protean; the more common are toxoplasmosis, histoplasmosis, cytomegalic inclusion disease, sarcoidosis, syphilis, tuberculosis, and toxocariasis. Depending on the etiology, the inflammatory signs may be diffuse or focal. Often there is vitreous reaction as well. With many types the result is atrophic chorioretinal scarring

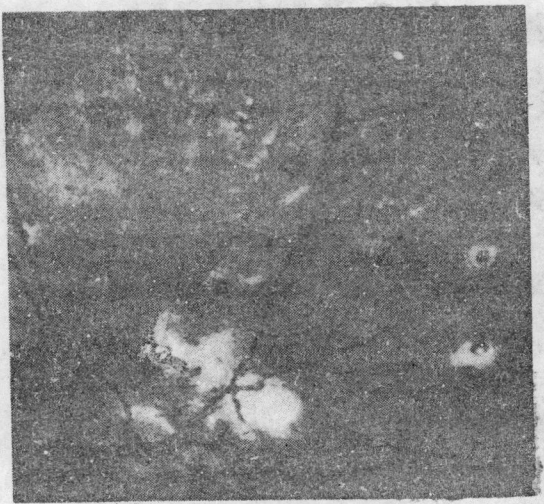

Figure 25–4 Focal atrophic and pigmented scars of chorioretinitis.

demarcated by pigmentation, often with visual impairment. Secondary complications include retinal detachment, glaucoma, or phthisis.

Panophthalmitis is inflammation involving all parts of the eye. It is frequently suppurative, most often as a result of a perforating injury or of septicemia. It produces severe pain, marked congestion of the eye, inflammation of the adjacent orbital tissues and eyelids, and loss of vision. In many cases the eye is lost despite intensive treatment of the infection and inflammation. Enucleation or evisceration of the eye may be necessary.

Sympathetic ophthalmia is a rare type of inflammatory response that affects both eyes following perforating injury of 1 eye. It may occur weeks or even months after the injury. A hypersensitivity phenomenon is the most probable cause. Loss of vision may result.

Treatment of the various forms of intraocular inflammation varies with the etiologic factors. In few cases can an identified process be treated specifically. A primary goal of treatment is prevention or reduction of the inflammatory sequelae, often with topical or systemic use of corticosteroids. Cycloplegic agents, particularly atropine, are also used to reduce inflammation and to prevent adhesion of the iris to the lens, especially in anterior uveitis.

25.13 DISORDERS OF THE RETINA AND VITREOUS

Retrolental Fibroplasia. Active modeling of the primitive retinal capillary network into more mature capillaries, arterioles, and venules proceeds from the disc to the periphery of the retina, normally reaching the ora serrata by 38–44 wk gestation. The developing vascular system of the immature retina is susceptible to pathologic changes and alterations that are referred to collectively as retrolental fibroplasia (RLF) or retinopathy of prematurity (ROP). Immaturity and periods of relative retinal hyperoxia are considered to be major factors in the development of the disorder. At greatest risk is the very small premature infant, often critically ill for days, weeks, or months after birth, who has required oxygen therapy to sustain life and neurologic function; typically today, the affected infant has had neonatal respiratory distress, periods of apnea or bradycardia, anemia, or sepsis and has received the best of modern therapy and careful monitoring. For reasons not yet determined, RLF develops in rare instances in the full term or healthy infant who has required little or no oxygen therapy.

Two major processes or phases in the development of RLF are vaso-obliteration and vasoproliferation. During periods of relative hyperoxia, endothelial damage and closure of developing retinal capillaries may occur. There may follow neovascularization and proliferation of neovascular tissue consequent to retinal ischemia and a state of relative retinal hypoxia. The precise level of oxygen and duration of exposure sufficient to produce the initial damage in the susceptible infant have yet to be determined.

In acute RLF one usually can observe an abrupt termination of the retinal vasculature, the peripheral retina appearing pale and gray to ophthalmoscopic examination (Fig 25–5A). There may be signs of a mesenchymal arteriovenous shunt in the region of the destroyed capillary bed, characterized by a distinct demarcation line with large tortuous arteries and veins arranged in fan-shaped arcades emptying into an opaque gray to white structure. Retinal neovascularization, or sometimes neovascular membranes growing into the vitreous, may also be observed. There may be retinal hemorrhages or exudates, and some degree of retinal detachment may be observed.

The active changes may continue for up to 6 mo after birth or terminate earlier. Fortunately, in many cases spontaneous regression of active proliferative RLF occurs; in others there is progressive overgrowth of vasoproliferative tissue into the vitreous, on the surface of the retina, over the ciliary body, and around the back surface of the lens, with progessive cicatrization. There may be massive detachment of the retina, shallowing of the anterior chamber, and in the final stages secondary angle closure glaucoma in a blind painful eye. All gradations from slight retinal pigmentary disorder to total organized retinal detachment may be found. A typical sign of cicatricial RLF of moderate severity is displacement or "dragging" of the disc (Fig 25–5B) and macula temporally; a common associated finding is myopia, generally of more than 6 diopters. The cause of the myopia is obscure; early refraction of premature infants is recommended.

The prevention of RLF remains a problem. The fact that hyperoxia damages immature retinal vasculature is proved, but other variables and biologic factors must be considered. Retinopathy may develop even when administration of oxygen has been carefully monitored and strictly controlled, and no absolute or "safe" level of oxygen has been determined. Currently, the biologic antioxidant tocopherol (vitamin E) is being studied as a means of protecting premature infants who are at risk for RLF; preliminary studies suggest that administration of tocopherol may decrease the incidence and the severity of RLF.

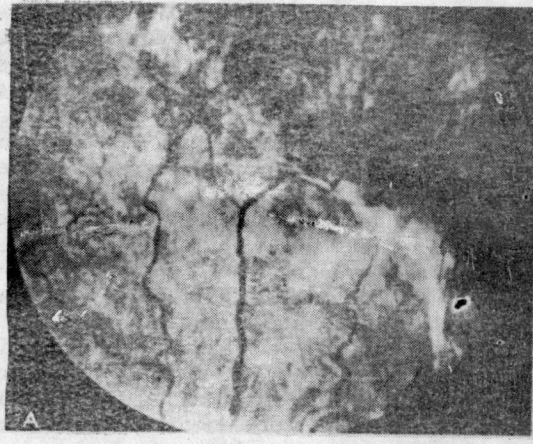
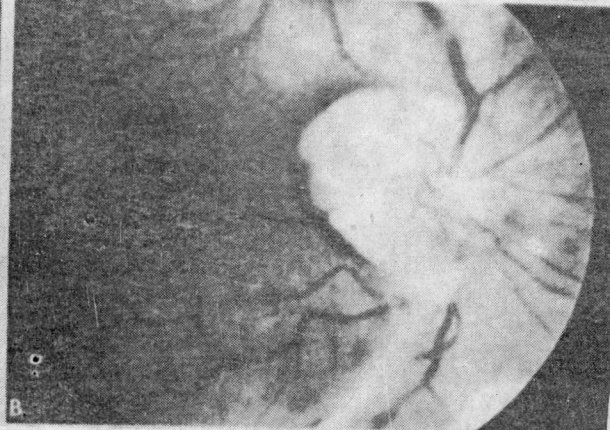

Figure 25–5 *A,* Developing retrolental fibroplasia in the temporal periphery. *B,* "Dragged disc" phenomenon in retrolental fibroplasia.

Pediatricians are truly faced with a dilemma; they must recognize the risks of retinopathy and inform parents of the risk early. It is recommended that infants born at less than 36 wk gestation or at birth weights of less than 2000 gm (4.4 lb) be examined before discharge from the nursery and periodically thereafter, depending on the findings on the initial examination.

Persistent Hyperplastic Primary Vitreous. In some persons there is persistence of the fetal hyaloid vascular system of the eye and the posterior part of the fibrovascular sheath of the lens. At times fibroblastic hyperplasia may be associated, forming a retrolental fibrous mass or opacity. The condition is referred to as persistent hyperplastic primary vitreous (PHPV). It is usually unilateral. Often, the affected eye is slightly small or microphthalmic. Complications include cataract, glaucoma, corneal opacification, intraocular hemorrhage, and retinal traction or detachment.

Surgical excision of the fibrovascular mass may be of value in preventing complications and degenerative changes, but the visual results tend to be disappointing. In some cases affected eyes may be enucleated as the differential diagnosis between the white mass of this developmental disorder and that of retinoblastoma may be difficult.

Retinoblastoma (Fig 25–6). Retinoblastoma occurs either as a nonheritable sporadic mutation involving the retinal cells or as a heritable germinal mutation transmitted as a dominant characteristic with high penetrance. Most unilateral retinoblastomas are the result of somatic mutation. All patients with bilateral retinoblastoma have either a new or inherited germinal mutation.

This malignant tumor usually appears before the age of 5 yr, most commonly in the earlier years. The most frequent 1st sign is leukocoria, a white or "cat's eye" reflex in the pupil. Another frequent sign is strabismus, secondary to impairment of vision. Some children present ocular inflammation, intraocular hemorrhage, glaucoma, or heterochromia iridis. Differential diagnosis

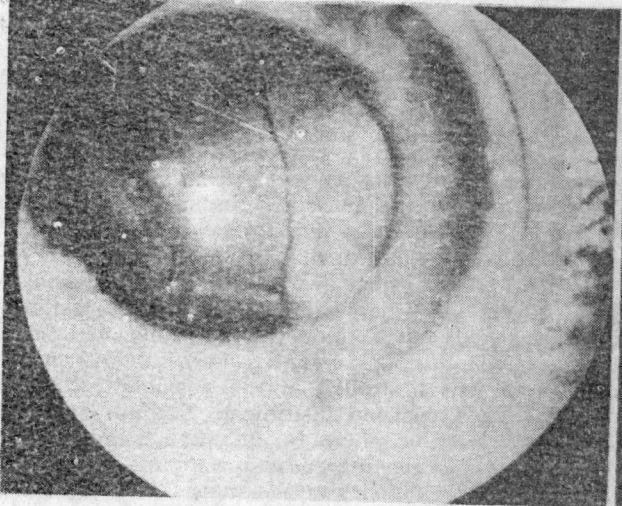
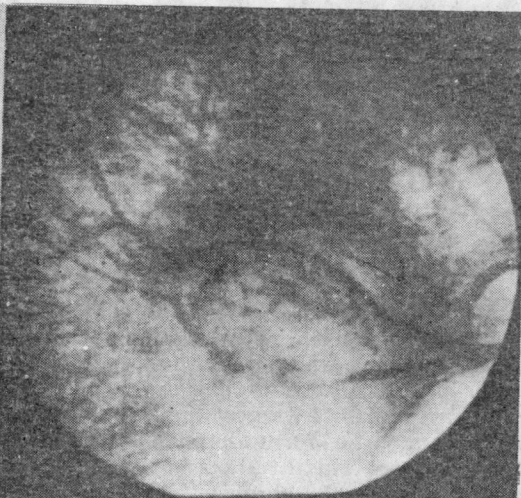

Figure 25–6 Retinoblastoma.

includes lesions such as retrolental fibroplasia, nematode endophthalmitis, persistent hyperplastic primary vitreous, and retinal dysplasia. As calcification occurs in the majority of retinoblastomas, standard orbital roentgenograms, computed tomography of the eye and orbit, and ultrasonography can be helpful in the diagnosis.

The goals of treatment are to destroy the tumor and to retain useful vision whenever possible without endangering life. The primary treatment of unilateral retinoblastoma is usually enucleation, though in selected cases alternative treatment such as cryotherapy, photocoagulation, or irradiation can be considered. In the treatment of bilateral retinoblastoma much depends on the number, size, location, and symmetry of the lesions in the 2 eyes. In some cases adjunctive chemotherapy is used.

The prognosis is uncertain. Extensive central nervous system involvement may follow, traveling along the optic nerve; or hematogenous metastasis may occur to other organs, particularly bone, liver, kidney, and the adrenal glands. Mortality is approximately 15–19%. Patients with germinal mutation (hereditary) retinoblastoma are also at increased risk for other malignancies; the most common is osteogenic sarcoma, others including rhabdomyosarcoma, leukemia, melanoma, thyroid adenosarcoma, fibrosarcoma, malignant mesenchymoma, chondrosarcoma, and angiosarcoma.

Other features of retinoblastoma and its management are discussed in Sec 15.16.

Retinitis Pigmentosa. This progressive retinal degeneration is characterized by pigmentary changes, arteriolar attenuation, usually some degree of optic atrophy, and progressive impairment of visual function. Dispersion and aggregation of the retinal pigment produce a variety of ophthalmoscopically visible changes, ranging from granularity or mottling of the retinal pigment pattern to distinctive focal pigment aggregates with the configuration of bone spicules (Fig 25–7).

Impairment of night vision or dark adaptation is often the 1st symptom. Progressive loss of peripheral vision, often in the form of an expanding ring scotoma or concentric contraction of the field, is usual. There may or may not be loss of central vision. Retinal function as measured by electroretinography (ERG) is characteristically reduced. Manifestations commonly begin in childhood. The disorder may be autosomal recessive, autosomal dominant, or sex-linked.

To be differentiated from retinitis pigmentosa are clinically similar, secondary, pigmentary retinal degenerations that occur in a wide variety of metabolic diseases, neurodegenerative processes, and multifaceted syndromes. Examples include the progressive retinal changes of the mucopolysaccharidoses (particulary the syndromes of Hurler, Hunter, Scheie, and Sanfilippo) and certain of the late-onset gangliosidoses (the syndromes of Batten-Mayou, Spielmeyer-Vogt, and Jansky-Bielschowsky), the progressive retinal degeneration that occurs in association with progressive external ophthalmoplegia (as in the Kearns-Sayre syndrome), and the retinitis pigmentosa–like changes in the Laurence-Moon-Biedl syndrome, to name just a few.

Stargardt Disease. This autosomal recessive retinal disorder is characterized by slowly progressive bilateral macular degeneration and vision impairment. It usually appears from 8–14 yr of age. The foveal reflex becomes obtunded or appears grayish, pigment spots develop in the macular area, and eventually macular depigmentation and chorioretinal atrophy occur. Macular hemorrhages also may develop. Central visual acuity is reduced, often to 20/200, but total loss of vision does not occur.

Best Vitelliform Degeneration. This macular dystrophy is characterized by a distinctive yellow or orange discoid subretinal lesion in the macula, resembling the intact yolk of a fried egg. Diagnosis is usually made from 5–15 yr of age; usually, vision is normal at this stage. The condition may be progressive; the yolk-like lesion may eventually degenerate ("scramble") and result in pigmentation, chorioretinal atrophy, and vision impairment. Inheritance is usually autosomal dominant.

In vitelliform macular degeneration the electroretinographic response is normal. The electro-oculogram, however, is abnormal in affected patients and in carriers and is therefore a useful test in diagnosis and in genetic counseling.

Cherry Red Spot. Because of the special histologic features of the macula, certain pathologic processes affecting the retina produce an ophthalmoscopically visible sign referred to as a cherry red spot, a bright to dull red spot at the center of the macula surrounded and accentuated by a grayish white or yellowish halo. The halo is the result of loss of transparency of the multilayered ganglion cell ring, due to edema or lipid accumulation or to both. The sign occurs typically in certain sphingolipidoses, principally in Tay-Sachs disease (G_{M2} type 1), in the Sandhoff variant (G_{M2} type 2), and in generalized gangliosidosis (G_{M1} type 1). Similar but less distinctive macular changes occur in some cases of metachromatic leukodystrophy (sulfatide lipidosis), in some forms of neuronopathic Niemann-Pick disease, and in certain mucolipidoses, such as Farber disease

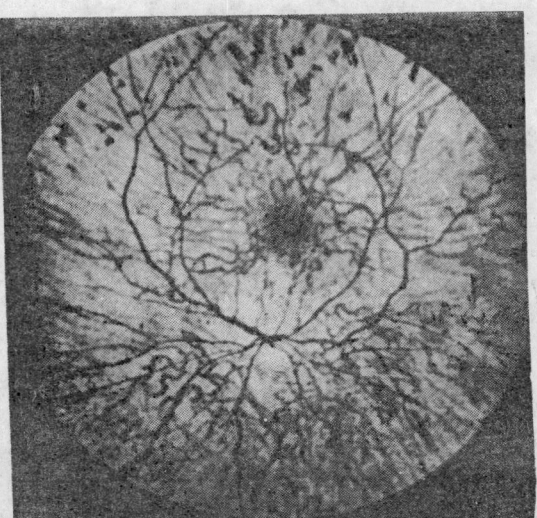

Figure 25–7   Retinitis pigmentosa.

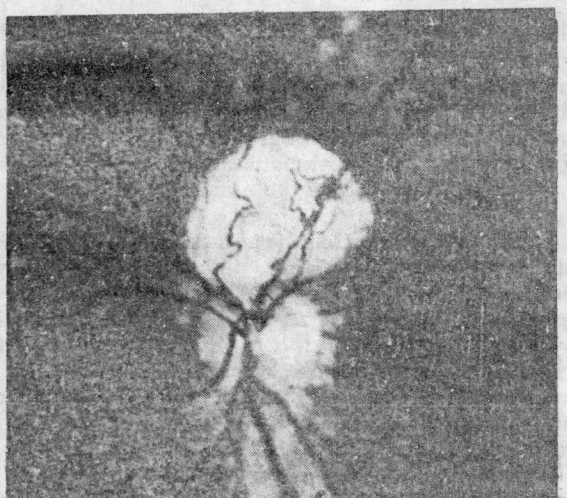

Figure 25–8 Retinal phakoma of tuberous sclerosis.

and Spranger disease. To be differentiated from the cherry red spot of neurodegenerative disease is the cherry red spot that characteristically occurs as the result of retinal ischemia secondary to vasospasm, ocular contusion, or occlusion of the central retinal artery.

Phakomata. These are the herald lesions of the hamartomatous disorders. In Bourneville disease (tuberous sclerosis) the distinctive ocular lesion is a refractile, yellowish, multinodular cystic lesion arising from the disc or retina; the appearance of this typical lesion is often likened to that of an unripe mulberry (Fig 25–8). Equally characteristic and more common in tuberous sclerosis are flatter, yellow to whitish retinal lesions, varying in size from minute dots to large lesions approaching the size of the disc. These lesions are benign astrocytic proliferations. Similar retinal phakomata occur in von Recklinghausen disease (neurofibromatosis). In von Hippel–Lindau disease (angiomatosis of the retina and cerebellum) the distinctive fundus lesion is a hemangioblastoma; this vascular lesion usually appears as a reddish globular mass with large paired arteries and veins passing to and from the lesion. In Sturge-Weber syndrome (encephalofacial angiomatosis) the fundus abnormality is a choroidal hemangioma; the hemangioma may impart a dark color to the affected area of the fundus, but the lesion is best seen with fluorescein angiography.

Retinoschisis. Congenital retinoschisis is a splitting of the retina into an inner and outer layer. This hereditary disorder is transmitted as a sex-linked recessive condition. It may be stationary or progressive. Often good vision is retained.

The most characteristic ophthalmoscopic sign is an elevation of the inner layer of the retina, most commonly in the inferotemporal quadrant of the fundus, often with round or oval holes visible in the inner layer. There are often associated cystoid macular changes. In some cases frank retinal detachment or vitreous hemorrhage occurs.

Retinal Detachment. In retinal detachment the neuroretina separates from the underlying layers. The most common cause of retinal detachment in children is trauma; there is usually a tear of the retina, with accumulation of subretinal fluid. Retinal detachment may also be associated with retinopathy of prematurity (cicatricial retrolental fibroplasia), myopia, aphakia (following cataract surgery), lattice degeneration, or congenital retinoschisis or occur secondary to inflammatory or exudative processes, such as uveitis, hypertensive renal disease, or leukemia.

The principal effect is blurring or loss of vision in the corresponding field of vision, though in some cases retinal detachment can be asymptomatic. Some patients experience a shower of floaters or flashes of light.

In most cases treatment is surgical.

Coats Disease. This is the generally accepted term for a peculiar ocular disorder characterized by exudation beneath or in the retina, often associated with telangiectasis or angiomatosis of the retina and recurrent retinal hemorrhages. The cause of this reaction remains obscure, but some vascular abnormality leading to leakage is considered to be a factor. Retinal detachment and loss of vision may result. The process is usually unilateral and occurs most commonly in male children.

Familial Exudative Vitreoretinopathy. This autosomal dominant disorder of the vitreous and retina is characterized by the presence of organized membranes in the vitreous (which often contain large blood vessels), by peripheral retinal exudation (subretinal and intraretinal), and in some cases by localized retinal detachment and recurrent vitreous hemorrhages. The ocular changes are progressive and tend to run a downhill course.

Hypertensive Retinopathy. In the early stages of hypertension there may be no observable retinal changes. Generalized constriction and irregular narrowing of the arterioles are usually the 1st signs in the fundus. Other alterations include retinal edema, flame-shaped hemorrhages, "cotton-wool patches," and papilledema (Fig 25–9). These changes are reversible if the disease process can be controlled in the early stages, but in hypertension of long standing, irreversible

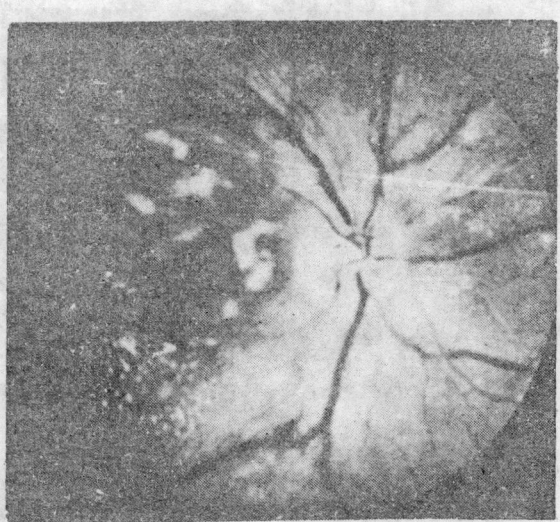

Figure 25–9 Hypertensive retinopathy.

changes may occur. Thickening of the vessel wall may produce a silver- or copper-wire appearance.

Hypertensive retinal changes in the child should alert the physician to renal disease, pheochromocytoma, collagen disease, and cardiovascular disorders, particularly coarctation of the aorta.

Renal Retinopathy. Renal and other hypertensive retinopathies are often indistinguishable; pallor of the disc and macular star formations are more commonly associated with nephritis.

Cyanosis of the Retina. This may occur with congenital heart diseases, chronic pulmonary insufficiency, or other disorders responsible for cyanosis. The retinal veins are dark, tortuous, and dilated, and the retina appears cyanotic at times, with scattered hemorrhages. The conjunctival vessels may be congested and dark.

The Retina in Subacute Bacterial Endocarditis. At some time during the course of the disease, retinopathy is present in approximately 40% of cases of subacute bacterial endocarditis; the lesions include hemorrhages, hemorrhages with white centers (Roth spots), papilledema, and, rarely, embolic occlusion of the central retinal artery.

The Retina in Blood Disorders. In primary and secondary anemias retinopathy in the form of hemorrhages and "cotton-wool patches" may occur. Vision can be affected if hemorrhage occurs in the macular area. The hemorrhages may be light and feathery or dense and preretinal. In polycythemia vera the retinal veins are dark, dilated, and tortuous. Retinal hemorrhages, retinal edema, and papilledema may be observed. In leukemia the veins are characteristically dilated, with sausage-shaped constrictions. Hemorrhages, particularly white-centered hemorrhages and exudates, are common during the severe stage.

Diabetic Retinopathy. The retinal changes of diabetes mellitus are described as simple or nonproliferative (early) or proliferative (more advanced).

Nonproliferative diabetic retinopathy is characterized by retinal microaneurysms, venous dilatation, and retinal hemorrhages and exudates. These signs may wax and wane. They are seen primarily in the posterior pole, around the disc and macula, well within the range of direct ophthalmoscopy.

Proliferative retinopathy, the more serious form, is characterized by neovascularization and proliferation of connective tissue on the retina, extending into the vitreous. The vision-threatening complications of proliferative diabetic retinopathy are retinal and vitreous hemorrhages, cicatrization, traction, and retinal detachment. Rubeosis of the iris and secondary glaucoma may develop.

Many factors may influence the course of diabetic retinitis. Recent studies indicate that a high degree of metabolic control of the diabetes may delay and even prevent microvascular changes and that the degree of control may be a more important factor than the duration of diabetes in the development of retinopathy in patients with childhood onset of diabetes. Detectable microvascular changes rarely occur in children prior to puberty; these changes can be expected in most post-pubescent patients within 15 yr unless a relatively high degree of control is maintained.

Recent advances in ocular therapy, such as retinal photocoagulation and vitrectomy, offer hope in reducing the visual morbidity in some patients with diabetes. Whether technologic advances such as insulin infusion pumps and pancreatic transplantation will be of value in the prevention of the ocular complications has yet to be determined.

Medullated Nerve Fibers. Myelination of the optic nerve fibers normally terminates at the level of the disc, but in some individuals ectopic medullation extends to nerve fibers of the retina. The condition is most commonly seen adjacent to the disc, though more peripheral areas of the retina may be involved. In most cases vision is not affected.

The characteristic ophthalmoscopic picture is a focal white patch with a feathered edge or brush-stroke appearance.

Coloboma of the Fundus. The term coloboma refers to a condition wherein a portion of a structure of the eye is lacking. The majority of colobomatous defects are due to malclosure of the embryonic fissure; these are termed "typical" colobomata and characteristically occur in the inferonasal position. Defects of similar appearance but of different etiology are referred to as atypical colobomata.

A typical fundus coloboma appears as a chorioretinal defect below the disc, exposing sclera in the inferonasal position. The defect may be extensive, engulfing the optic nerve entrance and including the ciliary body, iris, and even the lens, or it may be localized to any 1 or more portions of the fissure. In extreme cases there may be cyst formation or marked ectasia in the region of the cleft. Minimal colobomatous defects may appear as only small focal chorioretinal defects or anomalous pigmentation of the fundus. The defect may be unilateral or bilateral. The degree of visual impairment varies with the extent and position of the coloboma. Typical colobomata can be hereditary, the transmission being irregularly dominant. They may occur as isolated defects or as 1 facet of a variety of syndromes of multiple congenital anomalies.

25.14 ABNORMALITIES OF THE OPTIC NERVE

Hypoplasia of the optic nerve is a developmental deficiency of optic nerve fibers. This anomaly is associated with defects of vision and of visual fields of varying severity, ranging from blindness to normal or nearly normal vision in the affected eye. Hypoplasia may be unilateral or bilateral, and the manner of clinical presentation varies with severity and laterality of the condition. Unilateral and asymmetric hypoplasia commonly presents as a deviation (heterotropia, strabismus) of the more severely affected eye; the deviation usually develops early in life, but often the underlying visual defect is not suspected or detected until a later age. When there is bilateral hypoplasia of relatively severe degree, the defect in vision is usually appreciated early, and there is often an obvious strabismus or secondary nystagmus. Mild hypoplasia may be unrecognized for years.

Optic nerve hypoplasia may occur alone or with other developmental abnormalities, including microphthalmia, anencephaly, hydrocephalus, and encephalocele. Optic hypoplasia is a principal feature of septo-optic dysplasia of de Morsier, a developmental disorder characterized by association of anomalies of the midline structures of the brain with anomalies of the optic nerves, optic chiasm, and optic tracts; typically, there is agenesis of the septum pellucidum and malformation of the fornix, with a large chiasmatic cistern. There may be hypothalamic abnormalities and endocrine defects; growth failure is a major manifestation.

Papilledema. The term papilledema ("choked disc") can be applied to swelling of the nervehead of diverse etiologies, but it preferentially denotes the disc changes of increased intracranial pressure, including edematous blurring of the disc margins, fullness or elevation of the nervehead, partial or complete obliteration of the disc cup, capillary congestion and hyperemia of the disc, generalized engorgement of the veins, loss of spontaneous venous pulsation, nerve fiber layer hemorrhages around the disc, and peripapillary exudates. In some cases there may be edema extending into the macula, producing a fan- or star-shaped figure. In addition, there may be concentric peripapillary retinal wrinkling. Typically, the blind spot enlarges, and there may be transient obscuration of vision, lasting seconds. Visual acuity is generally preserved. Normally, when the intracranial pressure is relieved, the papilledema will resolve and the disc return to a normal or nearly normal appearance within 6–8 wk. Sustained chronic papilledema or longstanding unrelieved increased intracranial pressure may, however, lead to permanent nerve fiber damage, atrophic changes of the disc, and impairment of vision.

The sequence of events as increased intracranial pressure leads to papilledema is probably as follows: elevation of intracranial subarachnoid cerebrospinal fluid pressure, elevation of cerebrospinal fluid pressure in the sheath of the optic nerve, elevation of tissue pressure in the optic nerve, stasis of axoplasmic flow and swelling of the nerve fibers in the optic nervehead, and then secondary vascular changes and the characteristic ophthalmoscopic signs of venous stasis.

The common causes of increased intracranial pressure and choked disc in childhood are intracranial tumors and obstructive hydrocephalus, encephalopathies of various types, and "pseudotumor cerebri." Whatever the etiology, the disc signs of increased intracranial pressure in childhood may be modified by the distensibility of the young skull.

To be differentiated from true papilledema are certain structural changes of the disc ("pseudopapilledema," "pseudoneuritis," drusen, and medullated fibers) with which it may be confused.

Optic Neuritis. This term is used to describe any inflammation, demyelinization, or degeneration of the optic nerve with attendant impairment of function. The process is usually acute, with rapidly progressive loss of vision. It may be unilateral or bilateral. Pain on movement of the globe or pain on palpation of the globe may precede or accompany the onset of visual symptoms.

When the retrobulbar portion of the nerve is affected without ophthalmoscopically visible signs of inflammation at the disc, the term retrobulbar neuritis is applied. When there is ophthalmoscopically visible evidence of inflammation of the nervehead, the term papillitis or intraocular optic neuritis is used. When there is involvement of both the retina and papilla, the term optic neuroretinitis is used.

In childhood, optic neuritis rarely occurs as an isolated condition but is usually a manifestation of a neurologic or systemic disease. It may occur with bacterial meningitis or with viral infection (often accompanying encephalomyelitis following an exanthem). It may signify 1 of the many demyelinating diseases of childhood, particularly neuromyelitis optica (Devic) or Schilder disease. Alternatively, the cause may be an exogenous toxin or drug; optic neuritis may develop, for example, with lead poisoning or as a complication of long term, high dose treatment with chloramphenicol.

In most cases of acute optic neuritis there is some improvement in vision beginning within 1–4 wk after the onset, and vision may improve to normal or near normal within weeks or months. In some cases there is permanent impairment of vision. The course will vary with etiology.

Optic Atrophy. This denotes degeneration of optic nerve axons with attendant loss of function. The ophthalmoscopic signs of optic atrophy are pallor of the disc and loss of substance of the nervehead, sometimes with enlargement of the disc cup. The associated vision defect varies with the nature and site of the primary disease or lesion.

Optic atrophy is the common expression of a wide variety of congenital or acquired pathologic processes. The cause may be traumatic, inflammatory, degenerative, neoplastic, or vascular; intracranial tumors and hydrocephalus are principal causes of optic atrophy in children. In some instances optic atrophy is hereditary. Dominantly inherited infantile optic atrophy is a relatively mild heredodegenerative type that tends to progress through childhood and adolescence. Autosomal recessively inherited congenital optic atrophy is a rare condition that is evident at birth or develops at a very early age; the visual defect is usually profound. Behr optic atrophy is a hereditary type associated with hypertonia of the extremities, increased deep tendon reflexes, mild cerebellar ataxia, some degree of mental deficiency, and possibly external ophthalmoplegia; this disorder afflicts principally males from 3–11 yr of age. Leber hereditary optic atrophy occurs predominantly in males and usually appears from 18–23 yr of age; in the early stages inflammatory changes at the disc may be evident. Some forms of heredodegenerative optic atrophy are associated with sensorineural hearing loss, as may occur in some children with juvenile onset (insulin-dependent) diabetes mellitus.

Optic Glioma. The most frequent tumor of the optic nerve in childhood is optic glioma. This neuroglial tumor may develop in the intraorbital, intracanalicular, or intracranial portion of the nerve; often the chiasm is involved.

Histologically, optic glioma is a benign lesion; its deleterious effects vary with its location and growth pattern. The principal manifestations of intraorbital optic glioma are unilateral loss of vision, proptosis, and deviation of the eye; there may be optic atrophy or congestion of the optic nervehead. With chiasmal gliomas there may be a variety of defects of vision and visual fields (often bitemporal hemianopsia), increased intracranial pressure, papilledema or optic atrophy, hypothalamic dysfunction, pituitary dysfunction, and even evidence of brainstem effects such as nystagmus.

The natural clinical course of optic glioma often involves relatively slow, often self-limited progression; there may, however, be relentless progression to death.

Management of optic glioma is controversial. When the tumor is confined to the intraorbital, intracanalicular, or prechiasmal portion of the nerve, resection is often done, especially when there is unsightly proptosis with complete or nearly complete loss of vision of the affected eye. When the chiasm is involved, surgery is not advised, though surgical intervention to control secondary hydrocephalus may be necessary. Radiation is advocated by some clinicians; it may or may not alter growth of the tumor.

Optic glioma occurs with increased frequency in patients with neurofibromatosis.

25.15 DISORDERS OF OCULAR PRESSURE

Glaucoma. This term embraces a number of conditions in which there is abnormal elevation of intraocular pressure of degree sufficient to cause ocular damage and changes in vision. In infants and young children the principal signs and symptoms are tearing, photophobia, blepharospasm, corneal clouding (edema), and progressive enla. gement of the eye ("buphthalmos"). Optic nervehead cupping and visual loss may result.

Congenital glaucoma is usually due to a developmental abnormality of the angle of the anterior chamber; commonly there is residual mesodermal tissue blocking drainage through the trabecular meshwork. This primary or simple type of congenital glaucoma is inherited as a recessive condition. Congenital or infantile glaucoma may also be associated with other ocular anomalies such as aniridia, mesodermal dysgenesis of the anterior segments, and spherophakia, with certain of the hamartomatoses (neurofibromatosis, Sturge-Weber syndrome), and with a variety of syndromes such as those of Lowe and Marfan. Glaucoma in infants and children may also develop secondary to trauma, intraocular hemorrhage, inflammatory processes (uveitis), and intraocular tumor.

Treatment of congenital and infantile glaucoma is surgical; surgery should be performed as early as the child's general medical condition will allow. Procedures currently used to reduce and control ocular tension are goniotomy, goniopuncture, trabeculotomy, trabeculectomy, and, in some cases, cyclocryotherapy. Frequently, multiple surgical procedures are required. The prognosis for vision depends on normalization of intraocular pressure, and in the majority of cases surgery can lead to normal tension. Other factors, however, significantly affect prognosis. Even following an early normalization of tension, further therapy must be directed toward the correction of amblyopia and refractive errors. In some children there are also such complicating factors as cataracts, retinal disease, and abnormalities of the optic nerve.

Hypotony. This is abnormally low intraocular pressure. It may result from perforating ocular injury. It may also result from ocular inflammation (cyclitis/uveitis) that impairs aqueous secretion. Acute hypotony may be found in infants or children with moderate to severe dehydration.

25.16 ORBITAL ABNORMALITIES

Hypertelorism. This term denotes wide separation of the eyes or an increased interorbital distance, which may occur as a morphogenetic variant, a primary deformity, or a secondary phenomenon in association with developmental abnormalities, such as frontal meningocele or encephalocele or the persistence of a facial cleft. There is often associated strabismus, generally exotropia, and sometimes optic atrophy.

Hypotelorism. This term denotes narrowness of the interorbital distance, which may occur as a morphogenetic variant alone or in association with other anomalies, such as epicanthus, or secondary to a cranial dystrophy, such as scaphocephaly.

Exophthalmos. Protrusion of the eye is referred to as exophthalmos or proptosis. It may be due to shallowness of the orbits as seen in many craniofacial malformations or to increased tissue mass within the orbit as occurs with neoplastic, vascular, and inflammatory disorders. Ocular complications include exposure keratopathy, ocular motor disturbances, and optic atrophy with loss of vision.

Enophthalmos. Posterior displacement or sinking of the eye back into the orbit is referred to as enophthalmos. This may occur with fracture of the orbit or with atrophy of orbital tissue. It is also described as a feature of Horner syndrome (oculosympathetic palsy).

Orbital Cellulitis. This describes a condition involving inflammation of the tissues of the orbit, with proptosis, limitation of movement of the eye, edema of the conjunctiva (chemosis), and inflammation and swelling of the eyelids. There is often some discomfort, usually with general symptoms of toxicity, fever, and leukocytosis.

In general, orbital cellulitis may follow (1) direct infection of the orbit from a wound, (2) metastatic deposition of organisms during bacteremia, or (3) direct extension or venous spread of infection from contiguous sites such as the lids, the conjunctiva, the globe, the lacrimal gland, the nasolacrimal sac, or the paranasal sinuses. In some cases primary or metastatic tumor in the orbit can produce the clinical picture of orbital cellulitis.

By far the most common cause of orbital cellulitis in children is paranasal sinusitis, the most frequent pathogenic organisms being *Staphylococcus aureus*, group A beta-hemolytic streptococci, *Streptococcus pneumoniae*, and *Hemophilus influenzae*.

The orbital inflammatory manifestations of paranasal sinusitis can be classified in various stages depending on the location and extent of involvement. Stage 1 is swelling of the lids—the edema of impaired venous drainage or the reactive inflammation of underlying periostitis; in this stage the infection is still confined to the sinus. The 2nd stage is subperiosteal abscess, a collection of pus between the periosteum and the wall of the orbit, often with localized tenderness, displacement of the globe, and some limitation of eye movement. The 3rd stage is true orbital cellulitis, diffuse inflammation of the tissues within the orbit, with proptosis and impairment of ocular motility. The 4th stage is orbital abscess, resulting from localization of infection in the orbit or from extension of a subperiosteal abscess through the periosteum.

The potential for complications is great. Involvement of the optic nerve may result in loss of vision. Extension of infection from the orbit into the cranial cavity may occur, resulting in cavernous sinus thrombosis or meningitis or in epidural, subdural, or brain abscess.

Orbital cellulitis must be recognized promptly and treated aggressively. In most cases hospitalization and systemic antibiotic therapy are indicated. In some cases surgical intervention is necessary to drain infected sinuses or a subperiosteal or orbital abscess.

Tumors of the Orbit. A variety of tumors occur in and about the orbit in childhood. Among benign tumors, the most common are vascular lesions (principally hemangiomas) and dermoids. Among malignant neoplasms rhabdomyosarcoma, lymphosarcoma, and metastatic neuroblastoma are the most frequent. Optic gliomata and retinoblastomas that extend into the orbit also occur.

The effects of orbital tumors vary with their locations and growth patterns. The principal signs are proptosis, resistance to retroplacement of the eye, and impairment of eye movement. There may be a palpable mass. Other significant signs are ptosis, optic nervehead congestion, optic atrophy, and loss of vision. Bruit and visible pulsation of the globe are important clues to vascular lesions.

The differential diagnosis of orbital tumors is difficult; ultrasonography and computed tomography may be particularly helpful.

25.17 INJURIES TO THE EYE

About one third of all blindness in children results from trauma, usually avoidable. Injuries are caused by air rifles, arrows, darts, stones and missile-throwing toys, sticks, sharp tools, explosives, and strong chemicals. Many injuries cause acute pain, photophobia, tearing, blepharospasm, redness, or bleeding, prompting immediate consultation with a physician; unfortunately, some injuries do not produce such signs and symptoms and are often ignored.

Ecchymoses and swelling of the eyelids are common after blunt trauma. Hemorrhage into the lids and periorbital region (the so-called "black eye" or "shiner") is usually of no consequence and will absorb spontaneously, but it should prompt careful examination of the eye for deeper, more serious injury, such as intraocular hemorrhage or rupture of the globe.

Lacerations of the eyelids require careful management. Horizontal laceration of the upper lid may involve the levator, the tarsal plate, or the orbital septum. Faulty repair can result in ptosis, distortion of the lid, or herniation of orbital fat. Lacerations involving the lid margins require meticulous surgical apposition to prevent notching, eversion, or inversion of the margin or misdirection of the lashes that might lead to epiphora (tear overflow) and chronic irritation. Lacerations situated near the medial canthus may involve the punctum, canaliculi, or nasolacrimal duct and require the attention of an experienced ophthalmic surgeon. In all cases of lid laceration, examination of the globe for perforating injury is mandatory.

Superficial abrasions of the cornea usually produce pain or a foreign body sensation, sensitivity to light, tearing, redness, blepharospasm, and sometimes blurring of vision. The diagnosis is facilitated by fluorescein staining. Individually packaged sterile paper strips impregnated with fluorescein dye are available. When the strip is moistened and applied to the conjunctiva, the yellow dye diffuses in the tear film and will "stain" any epithelial defect; the stain is best seen with the aid of a blue light.

Fortunately, most superficial corneal abrasions heal promptly without complication. The injury is best treated initially by instillation of an antibiotic eye drop or ophthalmic ointment to prevent infection and application of a firm bandage (eye pad) to reduce eyelid movement and promote healing. The eye should then be examined within a day, preferably by an ophthalmologist, to determine the progress of healing and the need for further treatment (such as removal of a foreign body). In some cases there will be attendant iritis, requiring the topical use of a cycloplegic agent and/or cortical steroids.

A foreign body on or in the cornea or conjunctiva usually produces acute discomfort, lacrimation, and inflammation. Most foreign bodies can be detected by examination in good light with the aid of magnification; the direct ophthalmoscope set on a high plus lens (+10 or +12) is helpful. In many cases slit lamp examination will be necessary, especially if the particle is deep or metallic. Some conjunctival foreign bodies tend to lodge under the upper eyelid, producing the sensation of corneal foreign body as they come into contact with the globe on eyelid movement; eversion of the lid may be necessary to detect such foreign particles (Sec 25.2). If a foreign body is suspected but not found, further examination is indicated. If the history suggests injury with a high velocity particle, roentgenographic examination of the eye may be needed to explore the possibility of intraocular foreign body.

Removal of a foreign body can be facilitated by the instillation of a drop of topical anesthetic. Many foreign bodies can be removed by irrigating or by gently wiping them away with a moistened cotton-tipped applicator. Embedded foreign bodies require instrumentation and should be handled by an ophthalmologist. Removal of corneal foreign bodies may leave epithelial defects; these are treated as corneal abrasions (Sec 25.10). Metallic foreign bodies may cause rust to form in the corneal tissues; examination by an ophthalmologist a day or 2 after removal of a foreign body is recommended since a rust ring would require further treatment (curettage).

Lacerations and perforating wounds of the cornea or sclera require immediate referral to an ophthalmologist and prompt surgical repair if the eye and vision are to be saved. Emergency treatment consists of protecting the injured eye from further damage by applying a sterile bandage and a rigid eye shield. If these medical supplies are not on hand, an adequate eye shield can be fashioned from a plastic or styrofoam cup or from a piece of cardboard bent into a box or cone shape. Manipulation must be kept to a minimum, and no medication should be instilled except under the direction of an ophthalmologist.

Important clues to perforating injury of the eye are collapse of the anterior chamber, distortion and displacement of the pupil, and protrusion of dark tissue (uvea) into the wound.

Hyphema is the presence of blood in the anterior chamber of the eye. It may occur with either blunt or perforating injury. Hyphema appears as a bright or dark red fluid level between the cornea and iris or as a diffuse murkiness of the aqueous humor. The treatment of hyphema is bed rest, with the head elevated 30–45 degrees to promote settling and resorption of the blood. In some cases secondary bleeding occurs 3–5 days after the initial hemorrhage, increasing the risk of sequelae. The blood in the anterior chamber may produce elevation of intraocular pressure (glaucoma) and blood staining of the cornea. These complications may affect vision. In such cases surgical intervention (evacuation of the clot and irrigation of the anterior chamber) may be necessary.

Chemical injuries require immediate, thorough, and copious irrigation. Whereas acids do their damage on contact, caustic alkalis may continue to penetrate and damage the tissue long after the initial contact and require long term ophthalmic care. In some cases reparative surgery is necessary for resultant corneal and conjunctival scarring.

Fracture of the orbit is a common result of blunt trauma. Routine roentgenograms may fail to show the fracture; tomography is frequently necessary. Whereas any portion of the orbital rim or any wall may be involved, fracture of the floor of the orbit ("blow-out" fracture) is of special concern. The possible complications are (1) entrapment of the extraocular muscles (resulting in

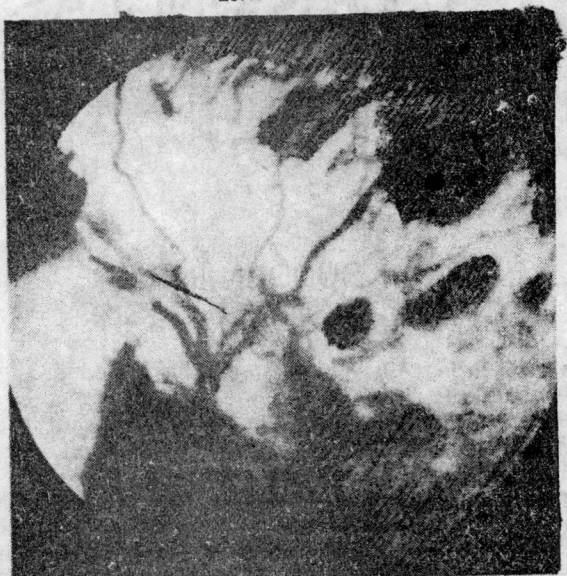

Figure 25–10 "Battered child syndrome." Retinal hemorrhages in abused child with subdural hematoma.

restriction of movement of the eye and diplopia) and (2) herniation of orbital fat or of the eye itself (resulting in enophthalmos); in such cases surgical repair is indicated.

Penetrating wounds of the orbit demand careful evaluation for possible damage to the eye, the optic nerve, or the brain. Examination should include investigation for retained foreign body. Orbital hemorrhage and infection are common with penetrating wounds of the orbit; such injuries must be treated as emergencies.

Child abuse is a major cause of injuries to the eye and orbital region. The manifestations are numerous and may play a prominent role in the recognition of this syndrome. The possibility of nonaccidental trauma must be considered in any child with ecchymosis or laceration of the lids, hemorrhage in or about the eye, cataract or dislocated lens, retinal detachment, or fracture of the orbit (Fig 25–10).

LOIS J. MARTYN

General References

Duke-Elder S (Ed): System of Ophthalmology. Vol III, Part 2: Congenital Deformities. St Louis, CV Mosby, 1963.
Francois J: Heredity in Ophthalmology. St Louis, CV Mosby, 1961.
Harley RD (ed): Pediatric Ophthalmology. Philadelphia, WB Saunders, 1974.
McKusick VA: Mendelian Inheritance in Man: Catalogue of Autosomal Dominant, Autosomal Recessive, and X-linked Phenotypes. Ed 5. Baltimore, The Johns Hopkins University Press, 1978.
Salmon MA: Developmental Defects and Syndromes. Aylesbury, England, HM&M Publishers, Ltd, 1978.
Stanbury JB, Wyngaarden JB, Fredrickson DS (eds): The Metabolic Basis of Inherited Disease. Ed 4. New York, McGraw-Hill Book Co, 1978.
Walsh FB, Hoyt WF: Clinical Neuro-Ophthalmology. Baltimore, Williams & Wilkins, 1969.

26 UNCLASSIFIED DISEASES

26.1 SUDDEN INFANT DEATH SYNDROME (SIDS)

Definition. The sudden and unexpected death of an infant, for reasons that are unclear even after an autopsy, is the most common manner of death in the 1st yr of life following the neonatal period. Its occurrence defines the *sudden infant death syndrome* (SIDS). In the typical case an apparently healthy infant of 2–3 mo of age is put to bed without suspicion that anything is out of the ordinary. Some time later the infant is found dead, and a conventional autopsy fails to reveal a cause of death. We have stated that these infants appear healthy before death, but more detailed perinatal histories and more intensive studies of cardiorespiratory and neurologic function have produced evidence that affected children have not been normal earlier. The needs to separate this tragic condition from confusion with child abuse and to supply stricken families with psychologic support have been highlighted in recent years largely through the efforts of families who have had infants die in this way.

Epidemiology. SIDS is a worldwide phenomenon; incidence rates vary from 0.3–3.0/1000 live births. Part of this variability may reflect the thoroughness with which other diagnoses are sought and accuracy of reporting. In the United States the average incidence ranges from 1.6–2.3/1000 live births, with considerable ethnic variation. The rates per 1000 live births are 0.5 among Orientals; 1.3 among Whites; 1.7 among Hispanics, 2.9 among Blacks; and 5.9 among American Indians. Incidence peaks at 2–3 mo of age; few cases occur before 2 wk or after 6 mo of age. Males are at higher risk than females. The incidence of SIDS is higher during the colder months of the year.

Since the greatest number of deaths have been reported between midnight and 9 AM, SIDS has been presumed to take place during sleep, but it is difficult to prove that SIDS actually occurs during sleep. The association of SIDS with sleep may simply reflect the larger proportion of time that infants in the susceptible age group spend in sleep. On the other hand (see below), there may be additional vulnerability to cardiorespiratory collapse during sleep.

A variety of genetic, environmental, or social factors have been associated with increased risk of SIDS, including premature births, especially with history of apnea; low birth weight for gestational age; cold weather; young unmarried mother; poor socioeconomic conditions, including crowding; maternal history of smoking, anemia, or narcotic ingestion; history of a sibling with SIDS; and history of a "near miss" or aborted episode of SIDS (i.e., an episode in which an infant ceases to breathe, develops cyanosis or pallor, and becomes unresponsive, but is successfully resuscitated). The risk of SIDS varies inversely with maternal age and directly with parity. The Apgar scores of infants with SIDS average lower than those of their surviving peers. Breast feeding does not protect. The peak incidence of SIDS (2–3 mo) coincides with normally low levels of circulating immunoglobulins, but no specific pathogens have been found.

In a family having an infant with SIDS the risk for the next or a subsequent child is about 20/1000 (2.0%) or 5–10 times the usual risk. Although the data are conflicting, recent studies do not show that twins or triplets are at higher risk for SIDS than subsequent siblings, nor is the risk higher for monozygotic than for dizygotic twins. Present evidence suggests that environmental factors (prenatal or postnatal) are important rather than genetic factors, with no evidence for any classic mendelian inheritance of susceptibility.

Pathology. Among the wide variety of findings that have been reported in infants dying of SIDS (Table 26–1), we believe that the increase in pulmonary arterial smooth muscle is the most important. This not only involves the muscular walls of the larger pulmonary arteries, but extends to smaller blood vessels close to the alveoli. The finding has been considered indirect evidence that infants with SIDS had sustained chronic hypoxia; there is as yet, however, no direct evidence of this hypoxia. Many victims of SIDS were retarded in postnatal physical growth.

Pathogenesis. Much of the present confusion about the pathogenesis of SIDS may reflect the great variability in the thoroughness with which specific abnormalities are sought post partum. Moreover, it seems likely that SIDS may have several etiologies, and several rare conditions may masquerade as SIDS. For example, prolonged sleep apnea in infancy has been associated with a space-occupying lesion (left temporal lobe astrocytoma), with a congenital CNS anomaly (absence of the corpus callosum), and with the neuromuscular dysfunction accompanying infantile botulism. Sudden death has also been caused by vascular rings, usually with antecedent evidence of upper airway obstruction.

Table 26–1 PATHOLOGIC FINDINGS IN SIDS

Increased pulmonary arterial smooth muscle
Increased right ventricular muscle mass
Increased extramedullary hematopoiesis
Retention of brown fat
Hyperplastic adrenal chromaffin tissue

Abnormal carotid body	80% hypoplastic
	20% hyperplastic

Brain stem gliosis
Intrathoracic petechiae

Infants with familial prolongation of the Q-T interval on electrocardiogram (Romano-Ward and Jervell–Lange-Nielsen syndromes) may die suddenly; on the other hand, infants with near-miss or aborted SIDS have been found to have shorter than normal Q-T intervals. When such conditions as the above are excluded, we believe that a majority of patients with SIDS share a common etiology involving an abnormality in cardiorespiratory control. Since there is no satisfactory animal model, much of the recent research in this field has focused on respiratory and cardiovascular controls in groups of infants believed to be at increased risk for SIDS, including siblings of infants with SIDS and infants with near-miss or aborted SIDS.

Respiratory Pauses. The precise role of apneic episodes (or more precisely, of respiratory pauses) in the pathogenesis of SIDS remains unclear. Prolonged apnea and cyanosis during sleep have been observed in 2 infants who subsequently died of what was presumed to be SIDS, and upper airway obstruction, with prolonged pauses in respiration and bradycardia, has been noted in infants with aborted SIDS. It is uncertain, however, whether apnea of central or of obstructive origin is more important in the genesis of SIDS. Difficulties in reconciling much of the reported data stem from arbitrary definitions of apnea and from absence of normal standards for the frequency and duration of respiration pauses. In studies of a group of normal fullterm infants during the 1st 4 mo of life, we found that the mean duration of respiratory pauses (defined as durations of expiratory phase greater than average by 2 standard deviations or more) was 5–7 sec, with some lasting as long as 13 sec. Pauses were longer and less frequent in quiet than in REM sleep in these infants. Surprisingly, we did not find pauses that were abnormal with respect either to frequency or to duration in infants with aborted SIDS; such infants have had distributions of respiratory pauses during sleep similar to those of age-matched normal fullterm infants. None of the normal or high-risk infants that we studied had any apneic episode longer than 13 sec during the 1st 4 mo of life. It has not been easy to reconcile these findings with the observations of others who have noted prolonged apneic periods (15 sec or longer) except to point out that others have included in their study populations prematurely born infants with apnea. In addition, we have seen the instantaneously recorded heart rate drop transiently to approximately 70/min in both normal and abortive SIDS infants during sleep, but there was no cyanosis or other evidence of cardiorespiratory embarrassment in either group.

Brain Stem Defect. At least 2 pieces of evidence have suggested that infants with SIDS have an abnormality in the central nervous system, presumably at the level of the brain stem: 1st, abnormalities in evoked auditory brain stem potentials have been observed in some infants with aborted SIDS; 2nd, a higher than normal resting $PaCO_2$ and a blunted ventilatory response to CO_2 have been found in a group of infants with aborted SIDS. The data with respect to ventilatory responsiveness are conflicting, other studies showing that responsiveness to CO_2 in infants with aborted SIDS is normal or increased. We believe that infants with

markedly decreased responses to CO_2, especially during sleep, belong to a separate group (failure of automatic control of ventilation or Ondine's curse) and should not be confused with SIDS.

Abnormal Upper Airway Function. UPPER AIRWAY OBSTRUCTION. The young infant is believed to be vulnerable to upper airway obstruction for anatomic and developmental reasons, including posterior displacement of the tongue and vulnerability to obstruction following flexion of the neck. It is possible also that abnormal neuromuscular control of the oropharyngeal muscle leads to airway obstruction. There is evidence that patency of the upper airway is maintained by muscles such as genioglossus, the activation of which is coordinated with excitation of respiratory muscles. Phase shifts in the contraction of these muscles could lead to upper airway obstruction. Whether this occurs in SIDS is not known.

HYPERREACTIVE AIRWAY REFLEXES. The laryngeal chemoreflex system, mediated through the superior laryngeal nerve, is capable of overriding central and peripheral respiratory drive mechanisms, and a number of studies are focusing on the maturation of this system in early life. Because the introduction of some fluids into the larynx can stimulate this reflex, presumably leading to apnea, there has been great interest in the possibility that gastroesophageal reflux with aspiration is an underlying mechanism for SIDS in some infants. With massive reflux there have been clear-cut episodes of apnea and severe bradycardia. Moreover, such episodes have ceased when feedings were thickened and the infants were kept continuously upright. On the other hand, the normal infant demonstrates gastroesophageal reflux at least up to 2 mo of age, and it is difficult, therefore, to know to what extent apneic episodes can be attributed to mild or moderate reflux.

Cardiac Abnormalities. Some have proposed that electrical instability may be present in the young heart, but there is no convincing evidence yet to indicate that cardiac arrhythmias play a role in SIDS.

Findings in Infants Who Later Died of SIDS. Several infants who subsequently died of SIDS were studied before death. One infant had a high-pitched, weaker than normal cry. Another had tachycardia, with less than normal beat-to-beat variability. Still another infant showed an increased respiratory rate and a decreased incidence of apnea. Finally, in response to auditory stimuli 1 infant showed greater than normal lability and poorer stabilization of cardiac rate.

Findings in Infants at High Risk for SIDS. SIBLINGS OF INFANTS WITH SIDS. Studies are at variance. One group of infant siblings of infants with SIDS was found to have an increased incidence and longer duration of periodic breathing in sleep than a control group, whereas other investigators found an increased respiratory rate and decreased incidence of breathing pauses in sleep among siblings of infants with SIDS; so far as frequency of long pauses (more than 10 sec) is concerned, these latter siblings could not be differentiated from normal infants. Siblings of SIDS victims also have had a faster heart rate in early infancy than control infants, with a delay in the normal decrease in heart rate with age.

INFANTS WITH NEAR-MISS OR ABORTED SIDS. In a group of 21 infants with evidence of near-miss or aborted SIDS (found to be unresponsive, cyanotic, and apneic, and having had mouth-to-mouth resuscitation) we found during the 1st 4 mo of life that they had in comparison to normal infants faster heart rates, smaller heart rate variability (both beat-to-beat and overall variability), shorter Q-T intervals even when corrected for the increased heart rate, and normal or increased ventilatory responses to elevated concentrations of inspired CO_2. In a similar group of near-miss infants others have noted an increase in the frequency and duration of respiratory pauses on exposure to gases with low oxygen tension. At present there are few data which describe the ventilatory responses to hypoxia. These may be important in the pathogenesis of SIDS, together with the levels of CO_2 and O_2 required to stimulate arousal from sleep. In another group of near-miss infants detailed neurologic examination has revealed consistent abnormalities of muscle tone, particularly shoulder hypotonia in infants under 3 mo of age.

Two studies of the respiratory control mechanisms of parents of SIDS victims have given conflicting results; in 1 there was no abnormal finding in the ventilatory response to hypoxia or to hypercapnia during wakefulness in either parent; in the other a significantly lower ventilatory response to CO_2 was found, with or without the imposition of added resistance to breathing.

The discrepancies in the result of investigations of infants at high risk for SIDS stem, we believe, from at least 2 sources: (1) differences in the techniques for measuring cardiorespiratory function in infants during sleep, some methods producing more alterations in the measured variables than others; and (2) differences in criteria for patient selection. In some small premature infants prolonged episodes of apnea may be fatal, but whether these fatalities share pathogenetic mechanisms with those of fullterm infants with SIDS is unknown. Some of the discrepancies between studies may relate to whether infants with apnea of prematurity are included.

Abnormal Autonomic Nervous System and Chemical Mediators. The increased heart rate and decreased heart rate variability, the smaller Q-T index, and the greater ventilatory response to CO_2 found in abortive SIDS infants have led us to advance the hypothesis that these infants have an abnormality in the autonomic nervous system, possibly an increase in sympathetic nervous activity. The adrenal medullary hyperplasia reported in postmortem studies of infants with SIDS supports this notion. Whether the hypothetical increase in sympathoadrenal activity is likely to be secondary to hypoxia or to some other stimulus is not known. Although the findings in several postmortem studies have led to the hypothesis that infants with SIDS have sustained chronic hypoxic insult before death, arterial oxygen desaturation has not to our knowledge been documented before death and no direct evidence of hypoxemia exists. The possible roles of such chemical mediators as catecholamines, endorphins, and serotonin in the cardiorespiratory response to hypoxia and hypercapnia and in the maturation of these responses during sleep represent important areas of research.

Diagnosis. Evidence is accumulating that some infants at risk for SIDS have physiologic handicaps before birth. In the neonatal period they may demonstrate low Apgar scores and abnormalities in control of respiration, heart rate, and temperature, and they may have postnatal growth retardation. Near-miss or aborted SIDS remains a diagnosis which can be made only by exclusion of such conditions as seizure disorders, other neurologic abnormalities, metabolic abnormalities (including hypoglycemia), cardiac anomalies and arrhythmias, vascular anomalies (especially vascular ring), massive gastroesophageal reflux, infantile botulism, and fulminant infection. In suspected cases our laboratory investigation includes (1) blood chemistries (serum glucose, Na, K, Cl, Ca, P, Mg, and BUN); (2) pH and blood gas analysis; (3) chest roentgenogram (including magnification films of the upper airways) and upper gastrointestinal study with barium swallow; (4) a 12-lead electrocardiogram (ECG) and 12–24 hr ECG monitoring for rhythm analysis; and (5) an electroencephalogram.

Home Monitoring of High-Risk Infants. As technology has improved and more parents have become informed about SIDS, pressure to monitor ventilation or heart rate has increased. The need exists to establish the normal ranges during sleep of heart rate, of heart rate variability, of respiratory rate, and of frequency and duration of respiratory pauses so that infants most likely to benefit from monitoring can be identified. Monitoring of heart rate (ECG) is at present further advanced technically than monitoring of ventilation (apnea monitor). Apnea monitors depending upon impedance may not detect complete airway obstruction as infants continue to make respiratory movements. Since serious apnea may be missed if only thoracoabdominal movements are monitored, monitoring of heart rate should also be included.

At present, it is difficult to decide whether home monitoring is necessary or desirable or how long it should go on. The abilities of members of the household to handle monitors and to make the appropriate responses to alarms and false alarms are critical factors in the decision. For the present, we believe that home monitoring programs should not be independent from research evaluating the program and its effects.

Even if, in all infants at high risk, it were possible to prevent SIDS, some cases would occur among those not recognized as being at risk. For this reason, and because, by definition, death comes swiftly and without forewarning, attention must also be given to providing psychologic and emotional support to all members of the family in cases of SIDS and to avoiding confusion with child abuse.

ROBERT B. MELLINS
GABRIEL G. HADDAD

Haddad GG, Leistner, HL, Lai TL, Mellins RB: Ventilation and ventilatory pattern during sleep in aborted sudden infant death syndrome. Pediatr Res 15:879, 1981.
Haddad GG, Mazza NM, Defendini R, Blanc WA, Driscoll JM, Epstein MAF,

Mellins RB: Congenital failure of automatic control of ventilation, gastrointestinal motility and heart rate. Medicine 57:517; 1978.
Harper RM, Leake B, Hoppenbrouwers T, Sterman MB, McGinty DJ, Hodgman J: Polygraphic studies of normal infants and infants at risk for the sudden infant death syndrome: Heart rate and heart rate variability as a function of state. Pediatr Res 12:778, 1978.
Hasselmeyer EG, Hunter JC: The sudden infant death syndrome. Obstet Gynecol Ann 4:213, 1975.
Leistner HL, Haddad GG, Epstein RA, Lai TL, Epstein MAF, Mellins RB: Heart rate and heart rate variability during sleep in aborted sudden infant death syndrome. J Pediatr 97:51, 1980.
Naeye RL, Ladis B, Drage JS: Sudden infant death syndrome: A prospective study. Am J Dis Child 130:1207, 1976.
Naeye RL: Pulmonary arterial abnormalities in the sudden infant death syndrome. N Engl J Med 289:1167, 1973.
Nelson NM: But who shall monitor the monitor. Pediatrics 4:663, 1978.
Peterson DR: Evolution of the epidemiology of sudden infant death syndrome. Epidemiol Rev 2:97, 1980.
Shannon DC, Kelly DH, O'Connel K: Abnormal regulation of ventilation in infants at risk for sudden infant death syndrome. N Engl J Med 297:747, 1977.
Steinschneider A: Prolonged apnea and the sudden infant death syndrome: Clinical and laboratory observations. Pediatrics 50:646, 1972.
Valdes-Dapena, MA: Sudden infant death syndrome: A review of the medical literature 1974–1979. Pediatrics 66:597, 1980.
Williams A, Vawter G, Reid L: Increased muscularity of the pulmonary circulation in victims of sudden infant death. Pediatrics 63:18, 1979.

26.2 THE AMYLOID DISEASES

Definition and Classification. The amyloid diseases include a number of entities of diverse etiology having in common the extracellular deposition of a proteinaceous material which displays a green birefringence when stained with Congo red and viewed under a polarizing microscope. The amyloid deposits appear homogeneous by light microscopy, but reveal 10–15 nm wide fibrils on electron microscopy. On x-ray crystallography the fibrils show a β-pleated sheet structure. Amyloid deposits compress and destroy involved tissues.

Based on the clinical features of the amyloid diseases and the nature of the major protein component of the fibrils, a tentative classification was proposed at the Third International Symposium on Amyloidosis in Portugal, 1979. As the structures of the various types of amyloid become defined, it seems likely that the widely used clinical classification will be replaced by one based on the structure of the major protein subunit, as shown in Table 26–2.

Etiology and Pathogenesis. Significant insight into the complexity of these diseases has come with recognition of their heterogeneity and the elucidation of the nature of some of the amyloid fibrils. Each type of amyloid deposit in man and in all experimental animals consists of 2 components. One of these, the P component, is common to all types of amyloid though it constitutes only about 5% of the deposits. It is derived from a 220,000 dalton serum component, a globulin which is composed of 10 identical subunits, each with a molecular weight of 22,000, and has a characteristic doughnut appearance in the electron microscope. It is closely related in structure and perhaps also in function to C-reactive protein. It is present in all types of amyloid, but its role in pathogenesis is unknown, though it seems possible that it may serve as a scaffold for the fibril deposition. The major component of all amyloid deposits, which constitutes 70–90% of the mass, is the 10–15 nm fibril which can be readily isolated by virtue of its unusual solubility properties in water. The different protein subunits of the fibrils of the several types of amyloid confer distinctive properties upon each of them. In spite of their biochemical differences, which are reflected to a slight extent in staining properties, the ultrastructural appearance of the various types of fibrils is identical.

Because the nature of the associated disorders varies with the amyloid protein subunits, it is necessary to consider the pathogenesis of the major types of amyloid individually. Abundant data implicate disordered function of the immune system in pathogenesis of amyloidosis, but we regard the data as often contradictory and far from convincing; we prefer to view all types of amyloidosis as the result primarily of the overproduction of normal or, perhaps in some instances, an unusual "amyloidogenic" protein. This overproduction is not sufficient explanation, however, since only a fraction of patients producing such proteins develop amyloid. Additional factors, perhaps contributed by the host and related to the processing of the precursor of the fibril, may also play a role. Current data support this concept only for the types of amyloid related to the L chain and AA protein.

In the AA type of amyloid the 8000 dalton AA protein, a molecule the entire primary structure of which is known, appears to be derived by proteolysis from a 12,000 dalton precursor known as SAA. SAA, a molecule of unknown function, exists in plasma complexed to other proteins, predominantly the high density lipoproteins. Subtle structural polymorphisms have been observed in the SAA and AA proteins, but these seem insufficient to account for differences in susceptibility to amyloidosis noted among different individuals. Consequently, differences in processing of the precursor or the fibril have been suggested as responsible for predisposing certain individuals to amyloidosis. Serum SAA levels are of little value in the diagnosis of amyloidosis since SAA behaves as an acute phase reactant.

AL fibrils consist of fragments of L chains; the fibrils always include the variable region and at times also part or all of the constant region. Sometimes an entire light chain has been identified. Since amyloid fibrils can be created in vitro by proteolysis of certain L chains, it seems likely that in vivo degradation of L chains is

Table 26–2 CLASSIFICATION OF THE AMYLOID DISEASES

PROPOSED	CLINICAL	PROTEIN SUBUNIT*
Light chain (AL)	Primary and myeloma-associated	AL
AA protein (AA)	Secondary	AA
Familial (AF)	Familial (many types)	AF
Endocrine (AE)	Endocrine	AE
Dermal (AD)	Localized (dermal, cutaneous)	AD
Senile (AS)	Senile	AS

*The 1st A stands for amyloid; among the 2nd letters, L = immunoglobulin light chain, F = familial, A = A protein, E = endocrine, D = dermatologic, S = senile. When the nature of the protein is known, a subscript is added (e.g., p for prealbumin, c for cardiac, t for thyrocalcitonin, etc.).

responsible for the formation of AL amyloid deposits. Because of the unexpectedly high frequency of λ-related amyloid proteins and the almost invariable association of amyloidosis with certain λ chain subclasses (especially λ VI), some light chains appear to be more "amyloidogenic" than others. Immunologically, amyloid fibrils of the AL type can react with antisera to κ or λ chains. It seems likely that proteolysis of a soluble precursor may also affect proteins like prealbumin in some of the familial forms of amyloidosis, peptide hormones in the endocrine types, and the proteins with β-pleated sheet structure in some of the other variants.

Even though proteolysis of the amyloid precursors seems to play a role in the deposition of the fibrils, once formed, they resist phagocytosis and proteolytic degradation. The body has few mechanisms to remove these deposits, a factor which may well account for the generally relentless progression of the diseases.

Incidence. Amyloidosis is a rather rare disease. With the near eradication of chronic suppurative diseases, the most common type of amyloidosis in adults has become the AL (primary) type, which is seen in association with myeloma and related plasma cell dyscrasias; these disorders are exceedingly rare among children. Among the diseases giving rise to AA (secondary) amyloidosis in children are rheumatoid arthritis, regional ileitis, and, on rare occasions, chronic suppurative disorders. Among children with juvenile rheumatoid arthritis in the United States the frequency of amyloidosis is low, whereas for unknown reasons it is more common in certain European countries. Regional ileitis is more frequently complicated by amyloidosis than ulcerative colitis. Amyloidosis is rarely associated with Hodgkin disease, renal carcinoma, or chronic suppurative conditions in children. In young adults amyloidosis is beginning to be seen with some frequency as a consequence of the suppurative and infectious complications of drug addiction. In developing countries such endemic infectious diseases as leprosy and malaria often give rise to secondary amyloidosis.

Some of the rare familial forms of amyloidosis, especially that associated with familial Mediterranean fever (most common among Sephardic Jews) and the Portuguese type, can affect children. The localized forms of amyloidosis, such as that involving the skin, are rare in children.

Clinical Manifestations. The clinical features of all types of amyloidosis stem from the infiltration of tissues by amyloid deposits, with the ultimate destruction of the affected organs. Symptoms depend upon the tissues involved; especially when the liver, kidney, or heart is affected, functional impairment may ultimately lead to death. In certain localized forms of amyloidosis, such as the cutaneous ones, the disease remains limited; otherwise it tends to be progressive, and even with control or treatment of the underlying disease significant regression is rare. An exception is seen with familial Mediterranean fever, the amyloidosis of which often improves with the administration of colchicine.

Secondary (AA) amyloidosis occurs with underlying disorders that are usually severe and of long duration; sometimes, however, amyloid deposits appear rapidly or with mild disease. In secondary amyloidosis, deposits occur predominantly in the kidneys, spleen, liver, and adrenals and rarely involve the heart, musculoskeletal, or gastrointestinal systems. Since amyloid in the kidney is deposited primarily in the glomeruli, the major manifestations are proteinuria, hyposthenuria, and hematuria; as the disease progresses, the nephrotic syndrome and ultimately renal failure make their appearance and, if left untreated, lead to death. Renal vein thrombosis is a common complication; hypertension is rare.

Hepatic and splenic enlargement may be massive but are generally asymptomatic or give rise only to abdominal discomfort since liver function usually is not significantly impaired. Tests of liver function may be only minimally altered, with increased hepatic alkaline phosphatase activity and Bromsulphalein retention, with or without increased transaminase activities.

AL amyloid is rarely seen in children whether idiopathic (primary) or associated with myeloma, macroglobulinemia, or other plasmacytic or lymphocytic neoplasms. In addition to producing the hepatic, splenic, and renal infiltrates seen in secondary amyloidosis, L chain amyloid also infiltrates the tongue, heart, skeletal muscles, subcutaneous tissues, ligaments, skin, and gastrointestinal tract. Accordingly, macroglossia, carpal tunnel syndrome, peripheral neuropathy, arrhythmias and congestive heart failure, purpura, subcutaneous infiltrates, and gastrointestinal bleeding and malabsorption may be early signs of this type of amyloidosis. A monoclonal protein is present in the serum of almost all patients whose amyloidosis is associated with myeloma; Bence Jones proteinurea is found even more often. Findings on bone marrow examination vary from a mild plasma cellular infiltrate to full-blown myeloma; at times amyloid infiltrates can be seen.

There are many familial forms of amyloidosis, each with characteristic clinical features and often with unique geographic distribution. Their variety and their rarity make clinical description of all of them impossible (see the review by Andrade et al). Probably the most common and widespread of the familial forms of amyloidosis is associated with familial Mediterranean fever (FMF) in Sephardic Jews and certain other ethnic groups of the Middle East. It is manifested as recurrent bouts of fever at irregular intervals, accompanied by abdominal, chest, or joint pains. The appearance of amyloidosis, which resembles the AA form clinically, is not related to the frequency or severity of attacks. Independent inheritance of FMF and amyloidosis is suggested by the appearance in certain individuals and families of amyloidosis as the 1st or sole clinical manifestation of the syndrome and by the absence of amyloidosis in the FMF syndrome in Armenians. FMF is inherited as an autosomal recessive trait, whereas most of the familial forms of amyloidosis are inherited in an autosomal dominant fashion. The diagnosis of FMF is based on the typical clinical features in the proper familial setting. The amyloidosis of FMF is unique in that its appearance can be delayed or prevented and the deposits made to regress by the administration of colchicine, 0.6 mg 2–3 times/day, a regimen which also aborts the febrile attacks. Since colchicine can produce

Table 26–3 COMPARISON OF THE HEREDITARY AMYLOIDOSES

PHASE	PORTUGUESE-JAPANESE FAMILIES	INDIANA-MARYLAND FAMILIES	IOWA FAMILY	FAMILIAL MEDITERRANEAN FEVER
Genetic mode of transmission	Autosomal dominant	Autosomal dominant	Autosomal dominant	Autosomal recessive
Ethnicity	Portuguese and Japanese	Swiss and German	Scotch-English-Irish	Mediterranean Jews
Age of onset (decades)	3rd–4th	4th–5th	3rd–5th	1st–2nd
Time from clinical onset to death (yr)	10–12	16–35	1–26	2–10
Neuropathy	+ + + + in lower extremities	+ + + + in upper extremities	+ + + + in lower extremities; + + in upper extremities	—
Nephropathy	—	—	+ + + +	+ + + +
Vitreous opacities	—	+ +	—	—

Adapted from Andrade et al., 1970.

chromosomal alterations and azoospermia, it should be used with caution in children and in adults in their reproductive period. To date, however, no fetal abnormalities have been attributed to the drug. Table 26–3 summarizes the salient features of 4 of the most common hereditary types. It is noteworthy that the common Portuguese and Japanese forms have prominent neuropathic components in addition to marked visceral involvement.

Diagnosis. Amyloidosis can be suspected clinically, but histologic studies with proper staining of the tissues are needed to establish the diagnosis. Ideally, biopsy is made of a clinically involved organ, but if biopsy of an affected organ is not possible (for example, if the liver is likely to bleed or rupture or if renal biopsy seems risky), rectal or gingival biopsy will yield positive results in over 90% of cases even when the rectum or gums are not obviously clinically involved. Accordingly, since it is rarely associated with complications, rectal biopsy is the procedure of 1st choice for diagnosis of amyloidosis, with the caveat that a positive rectal biopsy does not necessarily prove that renal or hepatic dysfunction is due to amyloidosis; the patients may have another associated disease. Tissues should be stained with Congo red and examined in a polarizing microscope to demonstrate the typical green birefringence. The recent elucidation of the structure of different types of amyloid subunits permits more precise classification of the deposits by immunohistochemical techniques employing appropriate specific antisera conjugated with peroxidase or fluorescein isothiocyanate. If these tests are not available, the tissues can be treated with trypsin or permanganate prior to Congo red staining. L chain amyloid is resistant to digestion, whereas AA amyloid loses its staining characteristics after such treatment. The finding of amyloid-like fibrils has recently been reported to be diagnostic of amyloidosis, but false-positive and false-negative results are common.

In the differential diagnosis other causes of nephrotic syndrome must be ruled out when renal involvement is prominent or other causes of hepatosplenomegaly when liver involvement prevails.

Treatment. With the exception of the amyloidosis associated with FMF, there is no effective treatment for amyloidosis since the material resists resorption. Treatment of the underlying disease may halt progression, however, and perhaps achieve some spontaneous resorption. In the AA protein type, eradication of a septic focus or treatment of the underlying disease may be of help. Administration of colchicine may prevent, arrest, or at times even cause regression of the amyloid deposits in FMF but has been disappointing in the other types. Use of dimethyl sulfoxide is currently under investigation. Amyloidosis associated with myeloma and primary amyloidosis are treated with chemotherapy, most often using melphalan or cyclophosphamide, in regimens similar to those used in myeloma. The renal manifestations can be managed by dialysis and, if necessary, transplantation, which has been about as effective as in other types of renal failure. Amyloid has been found to involve transplanted kidneys after periods of 5–10 yr.

Prognosis. In the absence of effective therapy the systemic forms of amyloidosis tend to be progressive and result in death in 1–5 yr, most often from renal failure or sepsis. The course can be slowed by dialysis or transplantation, but the disease cannot be arrested by any of the currently available forms of therapy.

EDWARD C. FRANKLIN*

Andrade C, Araki S, Block WD, Cohen AS, Jackson CE, Kuroiwa Y, McKusick VA, Nissim J, Sohar E, Van Allen MW: Hereditary amyloidosis. Arthritis Rheum 13:902, 1970.

Benson MD, Skinner M, Cohen S: Amyloid deposition in a renal transplant in familial Mediterranean fever. Ann Int Med 87:31, 1977.

Filipowicz-Sosnowski AM, Roztropowicz-Densiewicz K, Rosenthal CJ, Baum J: The amyloidosis of juvenile rheumatoid arthritis—comparative studies in Polish and American children. Arthritis Rheum 21:699, 1978.

Franklin EC, Zucker-Franklin D: Current concepts of amyloid. Adv Immunol 15:249, 1972.

Gafni J, Sohar E: Rectal biopsy for the diagnosis of amyloidosis. Am J Med Sci 240:332, 1960.

Glenner GG: Amyloid deposits and amyloidosis. The β-fibrilloses. N Engl J Med 302:1283, 1333, 1980.

Glenner GG, Costa PP, Freitas F (eds): Amyloid and Amyloidosis. Amsterdam, Excerpta Medica, 1980.

Kyle RA, Bayrd ED: Amyloidosis: Review of 236 cases. Medicine 54:271, 1975.

Lavie G, Zucker-Franklin D, Franklin EC: Degradation of SAA by surface associated enzymes of human blood monocytes. J Exp Med 148:1020, 1978.

Levin M, Franklin EC, Frangione B, Pras M: The amino acid sequence of the major non-immunoglobulin component of some amyloid fibrils. J Clin Invest 51:2773, 1972.

Rosenthal CJ, Franklin EC: Variation with age and disease of an amyloid A protein-related serum component. J Clin Invest 55:746, 1975.

Zemer D, Pras M, Sohar E, Gafni J: Colchicine in familial Mediterranean fever. N Engl J Med 294:170, 1976.

*Deceased.

26.3 SARCOIDOSIS

Sarcoidosis, a chronic, multisystem disease of obscure origin and variable pattern, occurs in children but is uncommon below the age of 10 yr. Weight loss, fever, abdominal pain, and anorexia are the most frequent signs and symptoms.

The *pathologic abnormalities* of sarcoidosis simulate those of chronic granulomatous diseases, especially tuberculosis. *Mycobacterium tuberculosis* has not been demonstrated in the lesions, and most patients with sarcoidosis do not have dermal reactions to tuberculin. Depression of cell-mediated hypersensitivity and of in vitro lymphocyte stimulation, which is common in adults, seems to be uncommon in children.

The *epidemiology* is obscure. Blacks are more commonly affected than Caucasians, and most patients in the United States, regardless of race, have come from rural communities in the southeastern region.

The lung is the organ most frequently affected; pulmonary involvement is variable in its extent and characteristics; the latter include parenchymal infiltrates, miliary nodules, and hilar and paratracheal lymphadenopathy (Fig 26–1). Hepatic involvement, skin lesions, and uveitis or iritis occur frequently. Uveoparotid fever may occur, with painless swelling of the parotid or salivary glands, fever, and uveitis. Cystic lesions in the bones of the hands and feet have been noted in some patients, as has disseminated sarcoidosis involving most of the viscera. Characteristic features of rare cases in infants under 1 yr of age are arthritis, skin lesions, and eye involvement. The arthritis, which can be confused with rheumatoid arthritis, produces large, painless, boggy synovial effusions of the tendon sheaths; there is little limitation of motion.

There are no specific diagnostic tests. Hyperproteinemia, hyperglobulinemia, hypercalcemia, hypercalci-

uria, and eosinophilia are common. The Kveim test, consisting of the formation of a granuloma several wk after intradermal injection of material from a sarcoid lesion, is positive in the majority of active cases; examination of biopsied tissue of affected areas is the most valuable diagnostic measure.

Because of its protean manifestations the *differential diagnosis* of sarcoidosis is extremely broad; it includes tuberculosis, the various pulmonary mycoses, and inflammatory ocular lesions such as phlyctenular conjunctivitis.

Treatment is symptomatic and supportive. Corticosteroids may suppress the acute manifestations, especially the inflammatory ocular lesions and the hypercalcemia.

The prognosis and natural history of sarcoidosis in children are uncertain. Spontaneous recovery may occur after a prolonged illness of several mo to several yr, or the condition may be very chronic, involving progressive and obstructive lung disease. Eye involvement may lead to blindness.

FLOYD W. DENNY

Gordis L: Epidemiology of Chronic Lung Diseases in Children. Chapter 3: Sarcoidosis. Baltimore, John Hopkins University Press, 1973.
James DG: Kveim revisited, reassessed. N Engl J Med 292:860, 1975.
Jasper PL, Denny FW: Sarcoidosis in children. J Pediatr 73:499, 1968.
North AF, Fink CW, Gibson WM, et al: Sarcoid arthritis in children. Am J Med 48:449, 1970.
Siltzbach LE: Sarcoidosis and mycobacteria. Am Rev Resp Dis 97:1, 1968.

26.4 PROGERIA

The Hutchinson-Gilford progeria syndrome has been reported in about 80 patients since first described in 1886. The mode of inheritance is unknown.

Children with progeria are usually considered to be normal in early infancy, but such manifestations as "scleroderma," midfacial cyanosis, and "sculptured nose" may suggest the existence of the syndrome at birth. Profound growth failure occurs during the 1st yr of life. The characteristic facies, alopecia, loss of subcutaneous fat, abnormal posture, stiffness of joints, and bone and skin changes become apparent during the 2nd yr (Fig 26–2). Motor and mental development are normal.

Features *always* present when the condition has become apparent are short stature; weight distinctly low for height; failure to complete sexual maturation; diminished subcutaneous fat; head disproportionately large for face; micrognathia; prominent scalp veins; generalized alopecia; prominent eyes; "plucked-bird appearance"; delayed and abnormal dentition; pyriform thorax; short, dystrophic clavicles; "horse-riding" stance; widebased shuffling gait; and coxa valga, thin limbs, and prominent, stiff joints.

Features *frequently* present are skin which may be thin, taut, dry, wrinkled, brown-spotted in various areas, or "sclerodermatous" over lower abdomen, prox-

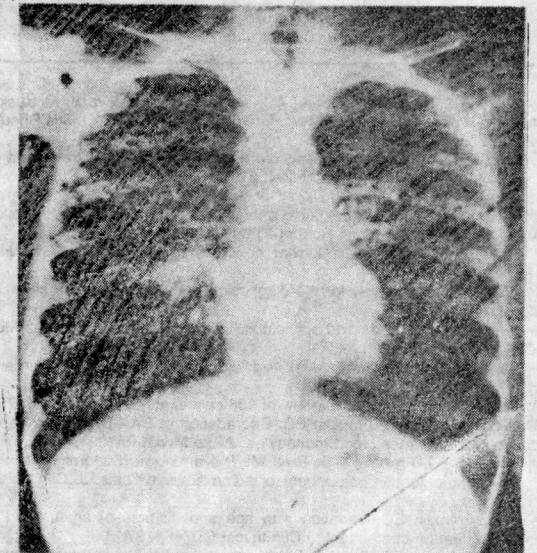

Figure 26–1 Sarcoidosis in a white girl 10 yr old. There are widely disseminated peribronchial infiltrations, multiple small nodular densities, overaeration of the lungs, and hilar adenopathy.

26.5 HISTIOCYTOSIS X

See also Sec 15.8.

Although knowledge about the group of conditions included under this designation has increased, many uncertainties remain about their nature, etiology, and therapy. Originally, 3 clinical conditions were described that shared the common histologic feature of an infiltrating histiocytosis but had widely varied clinical manifestations. *Eosinophilic granuloma* of bone usually presented as a solitary lesion in an older child. The *Hand-Schüller-Christian syndrome* characteristically seen in younger children, also termed multifocal eosinophilic granuloma, not only produced multiple bone lesions but to a variable degree affected a variety of soft tissues as well. The *Letterer-Siwe syndrome*, as originally described, usually occurred in infancy, was more rapidly progressive, and primarily affected soft tissues with minimal or no bone involvement.

These 3 clinical entities are now considered as variable expressions of the same underlying disease process. However, since the etiology is unknown and there is considerable uncertainty about the pathogenesis of the disease, the exact nature of interrelationship among these clinical patterns is unknown. It is possible that they are a heterogeneous group of conditions that have features in common because of the presence of a reactive histiocytosis.

The term "histiocytosis X" was intended to suggest a unitary hypothesis and implies that the condition is caused by a reactive histiocytosis to some unknown infecting agent X. The therapeutic regimens, on the other hand, have been designated as if to suppress a malignant proliferation of histiocytes. Others have considered the atypical histiocytic reaction to be the response of an immunodeficient host to a variety of common infecting agents. Such fundamental uncertainty about the nature of the disease process is a critical impediment to the design of clinical care programs for these patients.

Etiology.   The syndrome has been described in monozygotic twins and also in a familial pattern consistent with the inheritance of an autosomal recessive gene. Immunologic abnormalities have also been demonstrated in some of these patients; there appears to be a functional lack of suppressor T lymphocytes. This has led to the hypothesis that this condition represents an overly exuberant response of normal histiocytes to an inflammatory stimulus unimpeded by the normal regulatory activity of a specific subset of T lymphocytes.

There is no specific evidence to support the idea that the histiocytic proliferation and infiltration is neoplastic. However, the fatal outcomes, especially in infants, and the responsiveness of some patients to anticancer treatment programs suggest the need to continue consideration of malignancy as 1 of the possible causes. No epidemiologic studies suggest as yet a transmissible disease, and no microorganisms have been consistently identified. It is likely that the etiologic or predisposing factors for this condition are heterogeneous.

Pathology.   The characteristic histiocytic cells have a deeply indented nucleus and cytoplasmic structures known as Langerhans granules (Fig 26–3). These cells

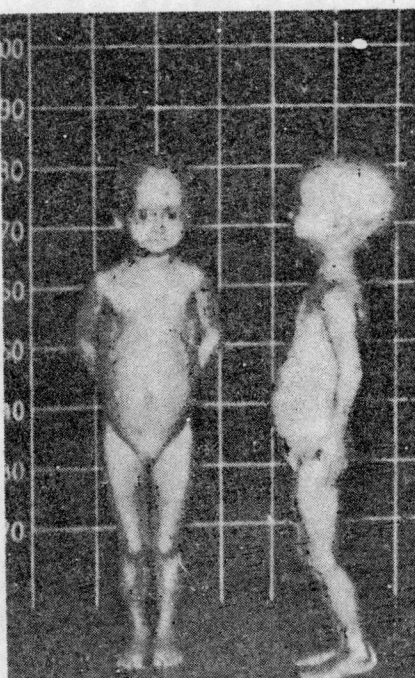

Figure 26–2 *A*, 4.5 yr old girl with height age of 1.75 yr and bone age of 4 yr. (From Wilkins, L.: Diagnosis and Treatment of Endocrine Disorders in Childhood and Adolescence. Ed 3. Springfield, Ill., Charles C Thomas, 1965.)

imal thighs, and buttocks; prominent superficial veins; loss of eyebrows and eyelashes; persistently patent anterior fontanel; "sculptured," beaked nasal tip; faint nasolabial cyanosis; thin lips; protruding ears; absence of ear lobes; thin, high-pitched voice; dystrophic nails; and progressive radiolucency of terminal phalanges.

Insulin resistance, abnormal collagen, increased metabolic rate, and variable abnormalities of serum lipids are found, but there are no demonstrable abnormalities of thyroid, parathyroid, pituitary, or adrenal function. Growth hormone responses are normal. Studies of cultured skin fibroblasts show reduced replicative life spans, increased fractions of heat-labile cellular enzymes, and increased tissue procoagulant activity.

Progeric patients ordinarily develop atherosclerosis and die of cardiac or cerebral vascular disease between 7–27 yr of age, with a median age of 13.4 yr at death. Such features associated with normal aging as cataracts, presbycusis, presbyopia, arcus senilis, osteoarthritis, or senile personality changes are not found.

FRANKLIN L. DEBUSK

DeBusk FL: The Hutchinson-Gilford progeria syndrome. J Pediatr 80:697, 1972.

Goldstein S: Studies on age-related diseases in cultured skin fibroblasts. J Invest Dermatol 73:19, 1979.

Ville DB, Nichols G Jr, Talbot NB: Metabolic studies in two boys with classical progeria. Pediatrics 43:207, 1969.

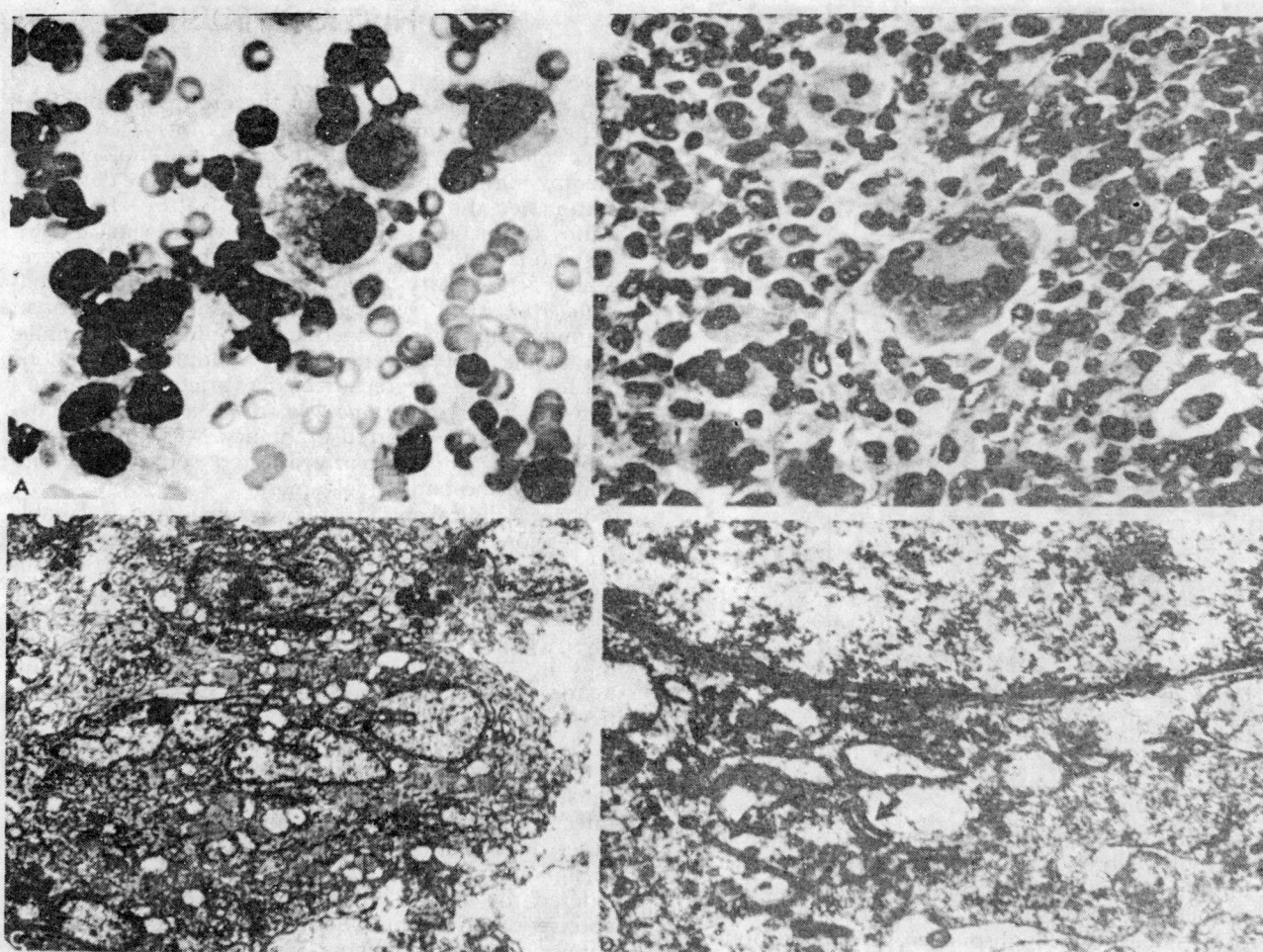

Figure 26–3 *A*, Imprint of a lymph node involved by histiocytosis X shows histiocytes with abundant pale cytoplasm and bland-appearing nuclei with characteristic grooves. (Air-dried, Wright stain, × 680). *B*, Lymph node, histiocytosis X (eosinophilic granuloma). Admixture of mononucleated and multinucleated cells; nuclei in multinucleated variants show same features as those of mononuclear cells. Note deep nuclear grooves. (B5 fixation, H and E, × 480.) *C*, Lymph node, histiocytosis X. Cytoplasm contains lipid vacuoles and lysosomes. Characteristic nuclear grooves are best appreciated at the ultrastructural level. (Uranyl acetate and lead nitrate, × 4500.) *D*, Lymph node, histiocytosis X. Langerhans or Birbeck granules (arrows) which are characteristic of the histiocytes in histiocytosis X. They are multilaminar structures with osmiphilic cores and terminal extensions. (Uranyl acetate and lead nitrate, × 19,000.) (We are grateful to Dr. Thomas Callihan for providing these illustrations.)

closely resemble the normal Langerhans cells which are widely distributed in normal skin and some reticuloendothelial organs. Although Langerhans cells may be derived from the bone marrow monocyte/macrophage cell line, recent evidence suggests the alternative possibility that they might be related to a subpopulation of thymic cells. The possibility that histiocytosis X cells are abnormal Langerhans cells derived from thymus is supported by the structural and functional abnormalities of the thymus seen in some patients. Various histologic abnormalities of the thymus have been described, including histiocytic and eosinophilic infiltration, severe lymphocyte depletion with residual atypical epithelial cells, and foci of ill-characterized abnormal cells. The functional abnormalities that may be thymus related include circulating lymphocytes spontaneously

cytotoxic to cultured human fibroblasts and the presence of antibodies to autologous erythrocytes. Some patients have decreased numbers of circulating lymphocytes characteristic of T-suppressor cells.

Accompanying these characteristic histiocytosis X cells may be variable numbers of other inflammatory and reactive cells such as eosinophils, neutrophils, and, less commonly, lymphocytes and plasma cells. The younger the patient and the more disseminated and rapidly progressive the disease, the more likely it is that the lesions will contain a greater proportion of histiocytosis X cells. With healing, the lesions are gradually replaced by fibrosis. This infiltrative process can affect tissues in any region of the body, but marrow, skin, lymph nodes, lung, liver, and meninges are the more common sites. Variable degrees of histologic and functional abnormalities of the involved normal tissue can be found, depending on the intensity of the infiltrate and the reactive inflammatory process.

Clinical Manifestations. There are 3 characteristic modes of presentation, and the clinical manifestations are determined by the extent and distribution of the lesions and the associated organ dysfunction. The older child, usually presents with only 1 or more bone lesions typical of eosinophilic granuloma. The child with bone and soft tissue involvement will have the clinical features characteristic of the Hand-Schüller-Christian syndrome. The infant and younger child usually have only soft tissue involvement and the greater degree of organ dysfunction typical of the Letterer-Siwe disease pattern.

The skeleton is the most commonly involved tissue and in the child over 5 yr of age may be the only site of involvement. The lesions may be single or multiple, are most commonly found in the skull, long bones, spine, and pelvis, and may be asymptomatic or associated with pain and local swelling. Involvement of the spine may result in collapse of the vertebral body and the roentgenographic finding of vertebra plana. In flat and long bones, the roentgenographic picture is that of an osteolytic lesion with sharp borders and no evidence of reactive new bone formation (Fig 26–4). Lesions involving weight-bearing long bones may result in pathologic fractures. The clinical course of solitary lesions is variable, and there may be resolution after several mo. Complete healing also usually follows curettage.

Skin involvement occurs in about one third of the patients at some time during their course. The usual lesion is a seborrheic dermatitis of the scalp (Fig 26–4). The lesions may spread to involve the trunk and the palms and soles. The exanthem may be petechial or hemorrhagic even in the absence of thrombocytopenia. The skin lesions, when present, are quite suggestive of this disease. Localized or disseminated *lymphadenopathy* is present in about 50% of the patients. *Hepatosplenomegaly* occurs in about 20%. The degree of liver involvement in some patients may be so severe that jaundice,

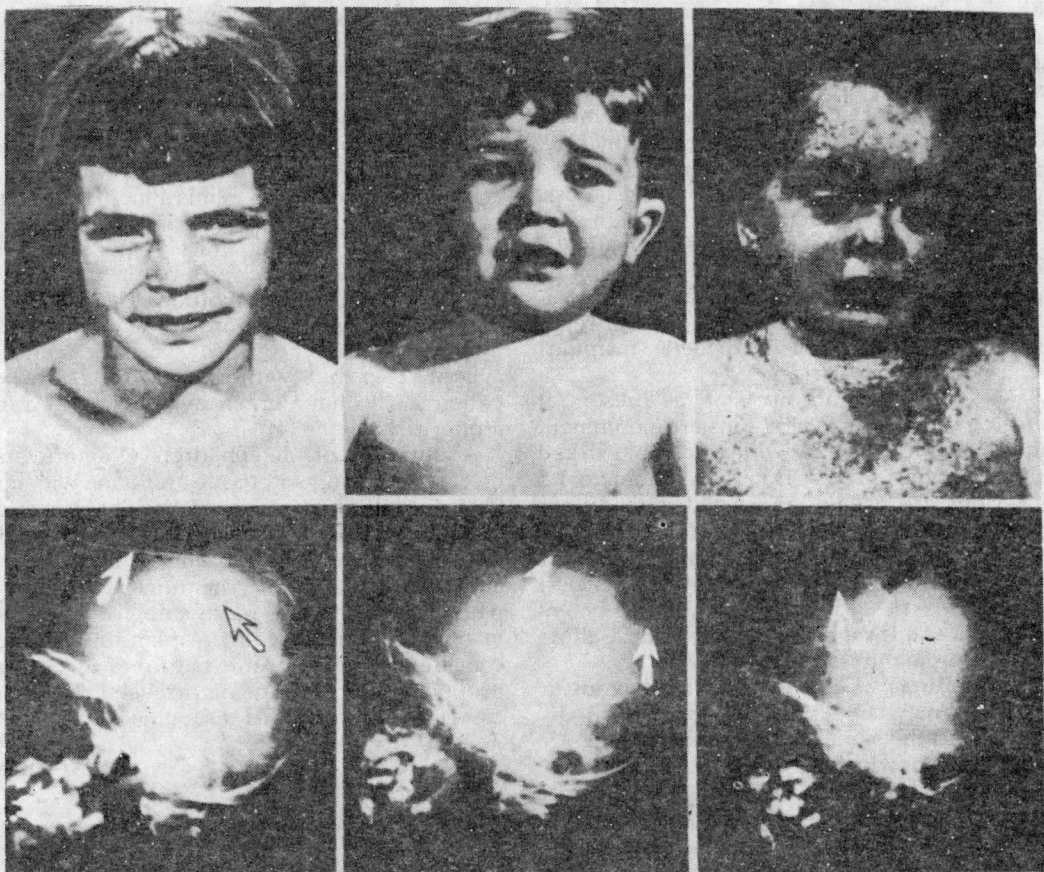

Figure 26–4 Common clinical patterns. Girl on left did not progress beyond brief involvement and isolated bone lesions which could be categorized as eosinophilic granuloma, and had good recovery. Girl in middle had several dozen bone lesions, a papular skin eruption, scalp "seborrhea," stomatitis, vaginitis, pulmonary infiltration, and diabetes insipidus. The diagnostic term Schüller-Christian syndrome is applicable here. Her disease responded well to chlorambucil therapy. Girl on right had extensive bone disease, plus a febrile course, anemia, severe skin eruption, generalized adenopathy, hepatosplenomegaly, pulmonary infiltration, and a fatal outcome in spite of antitumor chemotherapy. This patient fits the category of Letterer-Siwe syndrome.

Early biopsies of bone lesions from all 3 patients showed a similar type of histiocytic granuloma.

ascites, and laboratory evidence of liver dysfunction are present.

There are several characteristic features which may occur in the *head and neck* region. Involvement of the mandible and overlying gum tissue may leave teeth unsupported by bony matrix and result in their loss; on roentgenograms these teeth appear to be floating free. With response to therapy, there may be complete healing and reformation of normal bony support. Exophthalmos, when present, is usually bilateral and is caused by retro-orbital accumulation of granulomatous tissue. Bony destruction around the orbit may also be found. There may be chronic drainage from the ears and roentgenographic evidence of bony destruction around the involved canals. The drainage material may contain the histiocytosis X cells.

In 10–15% of the patients *pulmonary* infiltrates are found on roentgenograms. The lesions may vary from diffuse fibrosis and disseminated nodular infiltrates to diffuse cystic changes. Rarely, pneumothorax may be a complication. If the lung is severely involved, tachypnea and progressive respiratory failure may result. Symptomatic involvement of the *central nervous system* is uncommon but may be serious. Hypothalamic involvement may result in growth retardation and variable degrees of pituitary dysfunction. There may be increased intracranial pressure because of a communicating hydrocephalus. Cerebellar involvement may result in disturbances of balance and coordination and less frequently dysarthria, hyporeflexia, and weakness. There may be patchy involvement of the cerebrum with the development of seizure disorders. In some patients, the histiocytosis X cells can be demonstrated in the cerebrospinal fluid when neurologic disease is present. *Pituitary* dysfunction may be manifest in growth retardation. In addition, there may be diabetes insipidus and, rarely, a panhypopituitarism.

Histiocytosis X may on rare occasion be present at birth. In affected infants the skin lesions are a dominant feature and are characterized by widespread bluish-red maculopapules varying in size from a few mm to 1.5 cm. These lesions are usually associated with diffuse soft tissue involvement.

More severely affected patients may have systemic manifestations including fever, weight loss, malaise, irritability, and weakness. Bone marrow involvement may cause anemia and thrombocytopenia with resulting pallor and bleeding manifestations.

Laboratory Findings. *Tissue biopsy* is diagnostic. Any involved area may be helpful such as lymph node, bone, and liver, but the skin lesions, when present, are the easiest site from which to obtain the diagnosis. Smears of skin scrapings and drainage from the ear canal may be suggestive when the abnormal histiocytosis X cell is present, but these studies should not be regarded as definitive. *Blood counts* may be normal, or in patients with disseminated disease or marrow infiltration, anemia, thrombocytopenia, or even pancytopenia may occur. Monocytosis has also been described. The infiltrating abnormal histiocytes can be demonstrated on *bone marrow examination.*

Other laboratory findings may reflect the severity of specific organ involvement. Hepatic infiltration may result in intrahepatic bile duct obstruction with super-imposed parenchymal damage. Hypothalamic involvement may be associated with variable degrees of pituitary dysfunction and related laboratory abnormalities. The roentgenographic examination is particularly useful in assessing skeletal and pulmonary involvement.

Treatment. The design of appropriate therapy for histiocytosis X has been hampered by the uncertainty surrounding the nature of this condition. For patients with disseminated and progressive disease, treatment programs have incorporated a variety of cancer chemotherapeutic agents including cyclophosphamide, vinca alkaloids, prednisone, methotrexate, 6-mercaptopurine, and chlorambucil. Single agents appear to be as useful as combination chemotherapy and carry less risk of toxic side effects. Comparative studies of various regimens have not demonstrated a convincingly superior regimen. Prednisone may be useful for patients with systemic manifestations, especially fever. Response rates to therapy depend upon initial prognostic factors (see below) but are reported to be from 50–75% in various series.

For solitary bone lesions, curettage may be sufficient when indicated. Radiation therapy is usually reserved for patients with symptomatic bone disease as part of a disseminated histiocytosis X. The dose levels are limited to those necessary for response and should not exceed 1000 rads.

A small group of patients has been treated with a crude extract of calf thymus gland, with 10 of 17 patients achieving a complete remission. These results were equivalent to those expected for chemotherapy.

Prognosis. Several clinical features may be used to classify patients into 3 groups of good, intermediate, and poor risks. Patients without organ dysfunction who are over the age of 2 yr are in the good risk group. The intermediate risk group consists of patients under the age of 2 yr but without organ dysfunction. Those patients who have organ dysfunction at any age have a poor risk.

About half of the children who are survivors of disease involving soft tissue and bone will have serious, long-term disabilities. These disabilities include diabetes insipidus, skeletal abnormalities, growth failure, neurologic and intellectual deficits, hearing impairment, and chronic pulmonary insufficiency. In an occasional patient, there may be reactivation of disease after many yr of quiescence. Treatment planning should take into consideration the chronic nature of this disease and its propensity for producing irreversible organ damage associated with serious disabilities.

ALVIN M. MAUER

Groopman JE, Golde DW: The histiocytic disorders: A pathophysiologic analysis. Ann Intern Med 94:95, 1981.

Komp DM, Vietti TJ, Berry DH, et al: Combination chemotherapy in histiocytosis X. Med Pediatr Oncol 3:267, 1977.

Lahey ME: Histiocytosis X—comparison of three treatment regimens. J Pediatr 87:179, 1975.

Lahey ME: Histiocytosis X—an analysis of prognostic factors. J Pediatr 87:184, 1975.

Osband ME, Lipton JM, Lavin P, et al: Histiocytosis-X. N Engl J Med 304:146, 1981.

RADIATION INJURY 27

The possibility of untoward biologic effects of radiation is of special interest in pediatrics since these effects may be most serious in growing tissues. By judicious limitation of roentgen procedures during childhood a margin of safety for unavoidable radiation exposure later in life can be preserved.

Ionizing radiation produces injury in the same manner regardless of the type of particle or ray emitted. The variation is quantitative rather than qualitative. Absorption of energy may cause molecules in the path of the radiations to become ionized. In attaining stability these molecules may form substances which alter, temporarily or perhaps permanently, biochemical processes within the cell or its environment. These effects upon cellular structures explain the deaths of persons exposed to ionizing radiations, the death of certain cancer cells treated with roentgen rays, genetic mutations, and the production of cancer as a late effect of exposures to radiations.

Susceptibility of tissues to roentgen rays is, generally speaking, greater in the more rapidly mitosing and the more undifferentiated cells. Because of an abundance of this type of tissue in the abdomen, a patient is more likely to have radiation sickness from roentgen therapy to this region than from comparable exposure elsewhere.

Dosage Factors. Radiation absorption increases with the volume of the child's body exposed, with prolongation of exposure, or with an increase in amperage or voltage. Absorption decreases in relation to the effectiveness of filters used and with an increase in distance between the patient and the roentgen tube.

Adverse acute effects of roentgen rays are diminished when the total dose is administered in several exposures separated by sufficient time for recovery from the subclinical effects of each. Repeated exposures may produce pathologic effects not manifested until years later. Some of the chemical changes produced in cells by roentgen rays are irreversible and may lie dormant until aging, infection, hormonal alterations, or further exposure to toxic agents activates them.

The infant may be more susceptible to the effects of roentgen rays than is the adult. Moreover, even if there are no essential differences in susceptibility, the infant's longer life span provides more time for such changes to develop.

Early Effects of Irradiation. Exposure of the entire body to 100 roentgens usually produces illness in humans. A dose of about 450 roentgens will cause death in 50% of exposed persons. Higher doses can be tolerated if only a part of the body is exposed. Death results within hours to days when the entire body is exposed to the overwhelming dosage of an atomic bomb.

Symptoms of radiation sickness, which vary with the exposure, are malaise, fever, nausea, vomiting, and diarrhea. Leukopenia develops rapidly, and in more severe instances thrombocytopenia may appear within 1 wk. When the initial symptoms are not severe, they are followed by a temporary period of well-being. Epilation begins about 2 wk after the exposure. The leukopenia increases susceptibility to infection, and the low platelet count predisposes to hemorrhage. When autopsy does not reveal the cause of death, one can only assume that the radiation injury was responsible for lethal "cytochemical changes." If the patient survives for 6 wk, death is not likely from these effects of radiation.

Only a small percentage of deaths caused by an atomic explosion can be attributed to radiation effects alone; thermal and blast injuries account for most of them. Traumatic injuries do not heal effectively in persons with radiation sickness.

Clinical observation of the effects of radiation on children with genetic disease has led to a new understanding of molecular biology. Children with ataxia-telangiectasia are markedly predisposed to lymphoma and when treated for it with the usual doses of radiotherapy, sometimes suffer severe reactions. These patients have defective repair of DNA after damage by γ radiation, analogous to defective repair of DNA damage by ultraviolet light (UV) in xeroderma pigmentosum. The repair defects after γ or UV damage are enzyme-mediated and nonoverlapping. Another interaction involving genetics, neoplasia, and radiosensitivity may occur in the heritable (usually bilateral) form of retinoblastoma. For example, radiogenic tumors of the orbit occur more frequently and after a shorter latent period than in patients with nonheritable cancers given similar doses of radiotherapy.

Late Effects of Irradiation. Within the decade following the detonations of the atomic bombs in Japan there was a significant rise in the incidence of leukemia in those who were within 1500 meters of the hypocenter (the spot on the ground immediately under the center of an air burst). An increase in leukemia rates has been observed at doses as low as 20–49 rads among Hiroshima survivors of all ages. Children 10 yr of age at the time of the bombing were more susceptible to leukemogenesis than were older persons.

In Britain and in the United States, in utero exposures to diagnostic radiation have been reported to increase the relative risk of death from cancer before 10 yr of age by about 50%. No such effect was found among children exposed in utero to the atomic bomb.

Among persons exposed in utero to radiation from the Hiroshima atomic bomb (beginning at 10–19 rads) before the 18th wk of gestation, small head circumference occurred with excessive frequency. The effect increased in frequency and severity with increasing dose. Mental retardation occurred in those exposed to doses of 50 rads and above and affected the majority exposed before the 18th wk of gestation to 150 rads or more. The observations at low doses are not directly applicable to medical radiology because of the possible influence of (1) neutrons in the Hiroshima explosion and (2) interactions with nutritional deprivation and infection following the bomb explosion.

Complex chromosomal abnormalities are still found in the peripheral lymphocytes of atomic bomb survivors more than 35 yr after exposure, including those who were in utero—even in the 1st trimester—but not among persons conceived after the explosion. On the basis of animal experimentation, there is no doubt that point mutations occurred, but no effect could be demonstrated among the 75,000 1st generation offspring examined.

Small lenticular opacities of the posterior capsule of the lens have developed in 85% of those who epilated soon after the bomb explosion; the lesions are asymptomatic. Only 10 of the thousands of survivors have grade III or IV radiation-induced cataracts.

Radiation-induced premature aging has been described in animals, characterized by early senescence and death in middle age from diseases that ordinarily beset the elderly members of the species. It has not been demonstrated in humans.

Therapeutic doses of partial-body radiation may predispose to cancer. This is indicated by reports of a greater incidence of leukemia among adults treated for ankylosing spondylitis and of thyroid tumors among persons treated in early infancy for thymic enlargement. That repeated small doses of radiation to the entire body may predispose to leukemia is indicated by the increased occurrence of this disease among radiologists in the past.

Effects of exposure of parts of the body include temporary sterility, dermatitis, bone and skin tumors, and developmental defects in the teeth. Arrest in bone growth may occur in children who received cancericidal doses of roentgen rays.

Low-Level Radiation. Claims that low levels of radiation can induce cancer are based on data from persons in the area of fallout from nuclear weapons tests in Nevada in the 1950's. Increased mortality from leukemia has been reported in children in southwestern Utah and in military participants on maneuvers at the test site. The exposures were presumably low. Worries about low-dose exposures were amplified by the near melt-down at a nuclear power plant at Three Mile Island. In addition, controversial claims have been made that atomic energy workers in decades past now have increased cancer rates. The findings are not in accord with expectation based on a linear-quadratic extrapolation from effects at high or intermediate levels, as among Japanese atomic-bomb survivors. The question about low-level effects is unlikely to be solved by further epidemiologic studies because the number of exposed persons needed for study far exceeds the number available. Judgments will probably eventually have to be based on a knowledge of the fundamental biology of radiation carcinogenesis.

Preventive Measures.   Exposures to ionizing radiation should be limited to situations in which commensurate benefits are expected. The average *whole-body* exposure of the general population, based on the genetically significant dose, should not exceed 0.17 rem/yr, according to the National Council on Radiation Protection and Measurements.

It is thought that radiation changes within somatic cells are *incompletely* additive throughout life. The child of today is likely to have repeated exposures to ionizing radiations, and there is a possibility that tolerance may be dissipated. The pediatrician should limit as much as possible the exposure of patients (and self) to the emanations of roentgen ray machines and radioisotopes, but should not refrain from using them for essential diagnostic and therapeutic procedures. The patient's gonads should be shielded whenever possible. When a roentgen examination is needed, a film study should be obtained initially whenever possible. Subsequent fluoroscopic examination can be made if it is still required.

Roentgen therapy should never be used except when the indications are unmistakable or the risk justified, as, for example, in the treatment of malignant tumors. Extreme care must be exercised to avoid unnecessary damage to osseous growth centers and tooth buds.

Roentgen ray machines should be checked at least once a year for leakage that might be a hazard to personnel. The physician should wear a lead apron and gloves whenever the machine is in operation and should not expose unshielded body parts to the radiation beam.

ROBERT W. MILLER

Boice JD Jr, Fraumeni JF Jr; (eds): Radiation Carcinogenesis. Epidemiology and Biological Significance. New York, Raven Press (in press).

Bureau of Radiological Health: Gonad Shielding in Diagnostic Radiology. Washington, D.C., U.S. DHEW Publ. (FDA) 75-8024, June 1975.

Conard RA: Review of Medical Findings in a Marshallese Population Twenty-six Years after Accidental Exposure to Radioactive Fallout. National Technical Information Service, U.S. Dept. of Commerce, 5285 Port Royal Road, Springfield, Va. 22161, January 1980.

Favus MJ, Schneider AB, Stachura ME, et al: Thyroid cancer occurring as a late consequence of head-and-neck irradiation: Evaluation of 1056 patients. N Engl J Med 294:1019, 1976.

Miller RW, Boice JD Jr: Radiogenic cancer after prenatal or childhood exposure. In Upton AC, Albert RE, Burns F, Shore RF (eds): Radiation Carcinogenesis. New York, Elsevier–North Holland Inc. (in press).

Miller RW Mulvihill JJ: Small head size after atomic irradiation. Teratology 14:355, 1976.

Okada S, Hamilton HB, Egami N, et al (eds): A review of 30 years study of Hiroshima and Nagasaki atomic bomb survivors. J Radiat Res 16:1, 1975.

Strong LC: Theories of pathogenesis: Mutation and cancer. In Mulvihill JJ, Miller RW, Fraumeni JF Jr (eds): The Genetics of Human Cancer. New York, Raven Press, 1977.

United Nations Scientific Committee on Effects of Atomic Radiation 1982 Report to the General Assembly, with annexes: Ionizing Radiation: Sources and Biological Effects. New York, United Nations Publ. E. 82 IX. 8, 1982.

POISONINGS FROM FOOD, DRUGS AND CHEMICALS, POLLUTANTS, AND VENOMOUS BITES; MAMMALIAN BITES

28

28.1 FOOD POISONING

Foodborne illness resulted in a significant incidence of infant mortality in the United States until the early part of this century, but with the development of improved methods of refrigeration, pasteurization, preparation, inspection, and preservation of food, such illness has become an uncommon cause of death. However, food poisoning continues to be an important health problem; in 1977 there were 436 outbreaks of foodborne disease involving 9896 persons. Of the 157 outbreaks with confirmed etiology, the cause was bacterial in 64%, chemical in 24%, parasitic in 10%, and viral in 3%. In 73% of outbreaks the contaminated or responsible food was eaten at home (25%) or in a restaurant (48%).

Food substances may be intrinsically poisonous or contaminated with poisons. Microbial organisms may release toxins into the food (botulism), may convert a component of the food into a toxin (scombroid fish poisoning), or may have a direct effect on the intestinal tract (enterobacterial food poisoning). Organic or inorganic chemical contamination may also be toxic. Because the incidence of food poisoning remains low and pediatricians encounter few patients in their practices, cases may be misdiagnosed or go undetected. The possibility of food poisoning should be considered in individual patients as well as in clusters of patients.

28.2 BACTERIAL FOOD POISONING

STAPHYLOCOCCAL FOOD POISONING

Staphylococci are responsible for 25% of the cases of bacterial food poisoning in the United States. Those varieties of staphylococcus that cause illness are coagulase-positive organisms capable of producing enterotoxin (Sec 10.24).

Epidemiology. These organisms are ubiquitous and can be recovered from the hands and nasopharynges of 20–50% of healthy people. Contamination of everything the staphylococcal carrier touches, such as food, kitchen utensils, and dishes, is almost unavoidable. Pathogenic organisms have been recovered from the air, dust, and flies. The organisms multiply rapidly and produce enterotoxins in cooked food that is cooled slowly or is kept at room temperature. Contaminated meats and confectionary constitute the source of most outbreaks. Microbial concentrations sufficient to produce illness can be reached within several hr if conditions are favorable. A single staphylococcal strain may produce more than 1 type of enterotoxin; organisms producing type A or A and D enterotoxins are most often responsible for poisoning. Attack rates vary and have averaged 70% in a number of epidemics.

Pathogenesis. Five serologically distinct staphylococcal enterotoxins, A through E, have been identified; they do not cross-react and are not produced at ordinary refrigerator temperatures. The enterotoxins are heat stable and can withstand boiling for 30 min. Previously contaminated food rendered sterile by reheating prior to eating may still contain sufficient enterotoxin to cause food poisoning. As little as 1 mg of toxin can produce symptoms by acting on the central and autonomic nervous systems. The time interval between the ingestion of food containing enterotoxin and the onset of illness usually ranges from 3–6 hr but may be as short as 30 min.

Clinical Manifestations. Vomiting, retching, and severe abdominal cramps are the prominent symptoms. Diarrhea, fever, headache, chills, dizziness, and muscular weakness occur occasionally. Patients with underlying debilitating diseases may develop life-threatening vascular collapse. The acute symptoms usually subside within 12 hr but sometimes persist for 24–28 hr.

Treatment and Prevention. The majority of patients require no specific treatment. If vomiting is severe or persistent, a parenteral injection of antiemetic may be indicated. Infants and young children may manifest dehydration and require intravenous fluids. The prevention of staphylococcal food poisoning depends upon employment of proper hygienic techniques in food preparation and refrigeration.

SALMONELLA FOOD POISONING

Salmonellae are responsible for over 40% of cases of bacterial food poisoning in the United States. Salmonella colonization of poultry, pigs, and cattle is widespread, and there is a significant potential for the development of the carrier state in humans. Food and food products derived from domestic animals are subjected to a variety of manipulative procedures in their preparation, marketing, and distribution that increase the risk of contamination by salmonella. In the United

States the serotypes most frequently causing illness in man include *S. typhimurim, S. enteritidis, S. newport, S. heidelberg, S. infantis, S. saint-paul, S. oranienburg, S. montevideo,* and *S. derby.* Salmonella food poisoning is caused by the direct invasion of the intestinal tract (Sec 10.30).

Epidemiology. The pig is the most commonly infected farm animal and, in addition to being a specific host for *S. choleraesuis,* is also often infected with *S. typhimurium* and a wide variety of other salmonellae. It is not uncommon for 3–4% of pork sausages to be infected with salmonella. In the United States a significant number of cases of food poisoning are also associated with the eating of poultry; many incidents also result from the use of dried, liquid, or frozen egg products. In 1 study salmonellae were recovered in 35% of spray-dried egg samples, 34% of frozen dried eggs, and 15% of powdered albumin samples. Salmonellae may also infect milk, desiccated coconut, candy, shellfish, pet foods, and pets such as turtles and hamsters.

Salmonellae are readily killed by heat and are destroyed at normal baking and pasteurization temperatures. However, if cream or other materials contaminated with the organism are added after baking or if contaminated utensils are used in final preparation following cooking or baking, contamination takes place. Also, though lethal temperatures for the organism may occur at the surface, the temperature at the center of the food may remain below the lethal level.

The organisms have low virulence, and poisoning requires a heavy growth of organisms in the foodstuffs. The attack rate in epidemics is approximately 50%. Though large outbreaks, as at banquets and picnics and in school lunchrooms, are most frequently reported, smaller outbreaks involving members of single families probably account for the majority of cases.

Clinical Manifestations. Symptoms usually begin 12–18 hr after ingestion of contaminated food. Diarrhea and colicky abdominal pain are prominent but may not have their onset for up to 72 hr. Fever, chills, dizziness, headaches, meningismus, nausea, and vomiting commonly occur. The stools are watery and may contain mucus, pus, and blood, particularly in infants. The disease subsides within 24 hr in approximately 50% of patients. In young infants, immunologically compromised patients, or those with a large inoculum of a virulent strain the duration of illness may extend to 1 wk or more. On occasion, patients may develop severe dehydration, cyanosis, hypothermia, and circulatory collapse. The diagnosis depends upon the isolation of the offending organism from the stool; cultures are usually positive during the acute phase of the illness and for several wk thereafter.

Treatment. Fluid and electrolyte disturbances should be corrected by oral or parenteral hydration. Severe colicky abdominal pain may require sedation or analgesia. Antibiotics are rarely indicated; there is no evidence that they shorten the course of illness, and they may prolong the carrier state.

FOOD POISONING BY CLOSTRIDIUM BOTULINUM
(Botulism)

See Sec 10.43 for clinical manifestations and treatment. This form of food poisoning by *C. botulinum* results primarily from ingestion of the toxin produced by the organism in contaminated commercial and home-canned food. Improved commercial food processing procedures in the United States destroy the bacterial spores; therefore, almost all cases of botulism in the United States now result from contamination of home-preserved foods or importation of contaminated canned foods from other countries. Commercially processed foods frequently implicated in outbreaks of botulism are liver paste, vacuum-packed smoked fish, canned tuna, and canned soups. Contaminated food may look and taste normal or be recognized as being spoiled.

Botulism is rarely associated with food that has a pH below 4.5 because of inhibited multiplication of spores at this low pH. The spores are destroyed at temperatures of 121° C or greater, but cooking at temperatures below this level is conducive to spore germination. Freezing of foods does not necessarily prevent botulism as the organisms can produce toxin at temperatures as low as 5° C.

Infants, usually under 6 mo of age, also may develop botulism from the ingestion of spores of *Clostridium botulinum* (Sec 10.43). The enteric environment of affected infants is such that spores are capable of germinating and multiplying, producing botulinal toxin in vivo. This *infant botulism* is characterized by a history of constipation, weakness, and difficulty in sucking, swallowing, crying, or breathing. Honey has been implicated as a source of *Clostridium botulinum* organisms in a number of cases of infant botulism and therefore should not be given to infants under 1 yr of age.

FOOD POISONING BY CLOSTRIDIUM PERFRINGENS

See Sec 10.42.

Meat and poultry dishes contaminated with *C. perfringens* that are responsible for food poisoning usually have been cooked slowly at low temperatures. Ingestion of living organisms is usually necessary for the occurrence of disease, although a heat-labile, nondiffusible toxin causing diarrhea in human volunteers has been isolated from strains of *C. perfringens.* The incubation period is 8–12 hr after ingestion of contaminated food, with extremes of 1–25 hr.

FOOD POISONING DUE TO OTHER BACTERIA

Vibrio parahaemolyticus, a marine organism, is being identified with increasing frequency as a cause of food poisoning in the United States; 70% of reported cases of food poisoning in Japan are due to this organism. A majority of the outbreaks of *V. parahaemolyticus* enteritis have been caused by contaminated cooked seafood. The organism can survive temperatures from below −20° C to above 70° C. Explosive diarrhea, which is occasionally mucoid or bloody, is the prominent manifestation. Abdominal cramps, vomiting, and fever also frequently occur. Treatment consists of correction of fluid and electrolyte disturbances and symptomatic relief of abdominal pain.

Outbreaks of food poisoning have also been caused by *Bacillus cereus, Escherichia coli, Proteus, Citrobacteria, Klebsiella,* and *Enterobacter.*

28.3 NONBACTERIAL FOOD POISONING

MUSHROOM POISONING

There are approximately 3000 species of mushrooms, and at least 50 of these are toxic. In spite of the fact that there has been a significant increase in the production and consumption of mushrooms during the past decade, mushroom poisoning remains relatively uncommon in the United States because commercial mushroom farming is carefully controlled to prevent the contamination of the commercial crop by toxic varieties. Almost all cases of mushroom poisoning result from the gathering and consumption of wild mushrooms. More than 90% of mushroom fatalities in North America and Europe are due to the ingestion of members of the *Amanita* genus, particularly *Amanita pantherina* (flashbluster), *A. muscaria* (fly agaric), *A. phalloides* (death cup), *A. verna* (fool's mushroom), and *A. virosa* (destroying angel). The majority of deaths are due to *A. phalloides* and *A. verna*. Identification of the mushroom should always be attempted in cases of mushroom poisoning.

A. phalloides and *A. virosa* derive their poisonous properties mainly from amanitine, but they also contain the toxins phallia and phalloidin. The clinical manifestations of amanitine poisoning can be divided into 3 stages. In the 1st stage, occurring 6–18 hr following ingestion, the patient experiences severe crampy abdominal pain, nausea, vomiting, and diarrhea. The 2nd stage is characterized by apparent clinical improvement. However, during this 3–4 day period there may be serologic evidence of progressive hepatocellular and renal dysfunctions. In the 3rd stage the patient may develop acute hepatic or renal failure. Initial treatment involves attempts to remove unabsorbed toxin from the gastrointestinal tract; this treatment will be effective only in patients seen shortly after ingestion. Fluid replacement and correction of electrolyte imbalance is frequently necessary in the 1st stage. Hospitalization and careful monitoring of hepatic and renal function are indicated in any patient who manifests evidence of mushroom poisoning; deaths have been reported in patients within 3–6 days following premature hospital discharge. Deaths occur in 50–90% of patients with *A. phalloides* or *A. virosa* poisoning. Although some investigators have reported beneficial effects from treatment with lipoic acid, others have not been able to verify these results. Recent studies suggest that thioctic acid may be of benefit to patients who have ingested hepatotoxic mushrooms.

The toxic syndrome following the ingestion of *A. muscarina* and *A. pantherina* is due to the toxin muscarine. Clinical manifestations occur rapidly after ingestion and include abdominal pain, vomiting, excessive salivation, severe diarrhea, sweating, miosis, diplopia, twitching, muscle incoordination, convulsions, and bradycardia. In addition to supportive care, 0.02 mg/kg of atropine administered intravenously may reverse many of the muscarinic effects. Death rates of 30–50% have been reported.

SOLANINE POISONING

Solanine is a water-soluble alkaloid found in potato sprouts and in potato shoots above the ground. Potatoes that have begun to sprout have the highest concentration of solanine. Most of the alkaloid can be removed if the potatoes are peeled and boiled; however, the alkaloid remains in the potatoes if they are baked in their skins. The clinical manifestations include headache, fever, abdominal pain, vomiting, diarrhea, weakness, and depression, Fatalities are rare, most patients recovering within several days with supportive treatment.

PARALYTIC SHELLFISH POISONING

The ingestion of bivalve mollusks which have ingested toxic dinoflagellates may produce a form of food poisoning known as paralytic shellfish poisoning. The toxic dinoflagellates responsible for most poisonings in the United States are *Gonyaulax catanella* and *Gonyaulax tamarensis*. These organisms are major components of the "red tide," which may plague coastal waters. The neurotoxin produced by toxic dinoflagellates is heat and acid stable. It is thought to block the propagation of nerve and muscle action potentials by altering membrane permeability for sodium.

Symptoms may appear within 30 min following the eating of contaminated shellfish. Patients experience a burning sensation of the oral mucous membranes; paresthesias and numbness of the mouth, face, and extremities; nausea; vomiting; and diarrhea. In severe cases the patient may develop dysphagia, dysphonia, ataxia, severe muscle weakness, and, in extreme instances, respiratory paralysis. Treatment includes inducing emesis, or gastric lavage when the patient has not vomited spontaneously, and the administration of cathartics or enemas to remove unabsorbed toxin. Mechanical ventilation may be lifesaving in patients with respiratory distress. Death, which occurs in approximately 5% of patients, results from respiratory failure and myocardial complications.

SCOMBROID FISH POISONING

Scombroid fish poisoning or scombrotoxism is 1 of the most adverse reactions to fish ingestion. The toxic syndrome is characterized by flushing of the face, arms, and trunk; generalized pruritus; urticaria; angioedema; throbbing headache; tachycardia; palpitations; oral blistering or burning; abdominal cramps; and diarrhea. Bronchospasm and respiratory distress may occur in severe cases. Symptoms begin within 30–60 min following the ingestion of dark meat fish, particularly those belonging to the family Scombridae, e.g., tuna, bonito, mackerel, and albacore. Fish belonging to other families, particularly the mahimahi or dolphinfish, have also been incriminated.

Scombrotoxin consists of a mixture of thermostable substances, including histamine and saurine, which may not be destroyed by normal canning procedures. It is produced by the bacterial decarboxylation of histidine in the muscle of dead dark meat fishes which have been improperly refrigerated. *Proteus morgani*, a normal constituent of surface marine microflora of the fish, is the microorganism most commonly responsible for the bacterial decarboxylation. The spoiled fish is usually normal in appearance, odor, and taste.

The manifestations of scombroid fish poisoning, although extremely uncomfortable and temporarily disabling, are self-limited. Death is extremely rare. Treatment is symptomatic and supportive. If vomiting and diarrhea have not occurred, an emetic and cathartic should be given. Antihistamines may provide symptomatic relief.

CIGUATERA FISH POISONING

This results from eating certain tropical marine reef fish that sporadically acquire ciguatoxin. The toxin or toxins are stable to heat, cold, and drying and have as yet not been specifically identified or characterized. The affected fish acquire the toxins from the ingestion of small marine organisms such as the dinoflagellates gambier discus toxicus. Those fish most commonly involved include the lumberjack, red snapper, grouper, dolphin, and barracuda.

The symptoms of ciguatera fish poisoning occur from 2–30 hr after ingestion of toxic fish and are predominantly gastrointestinal and neurologic. They include abdominal cramps, diarrhea, vomiting, severe myalgia, a profound sense of weakness, dysesthesias and paresthesias of the perioral region and extremities, dizziness, ataxia, and visual disturbances. The neurologic symptoms may persist for many mo. Death is usually due to respiratory paralysis; however, the mortality rate is extremely low.

RUSSELL S. ASNES

Arnon SS: Infant botulism. Ann Rev Med 31:541, 1980.
Center for Disease Control: Foodborne and Waterborne Disease Outbreaks: Annual Summary 1977. Issued Aug 1979.
Cherington M: Botulism: Clinical and therapeutic observations. Rocky Mt Med J 69:55, 1972.
Hughes JM, Merson MH: Fish and shellfish poisoning. N Engl J Med 295:1117, 1976.
Kim R: Flushing syndrome due to mahimahi (scombroid fish) poisoning. Arch Dermatol 115:963, 1979.
Lawrence DN, Enriquez MB, Lumish RM, et al: Ciguatera fish poisoning in Miami. JAMA 244:254, 1980.
McCormick DJ, Aubel AJ, Gibbons RB: Nonlethal mushroom poisoning. Ann Int Med 90:332, 1979.
Paaso B, Harrison DC: A new look at an old problem: Mushroom poisoning. Am J Med 58:505, 1975.
Rieman H (ed): Foodborne Infections and Intoxications. New York, Academic Press, 1965.

CHEMICAL AND DRUG POISONING

In general, 2 distinct patterns of poisonings occur in pediatric practice. The toddler accidentally ingests an incredible array of plants, chemicals, and drugs; though the consequences are usually benign, the occasional occurrence of life-threatening ingestion requires constant vigilance and parental education. The adolescent intentionally ingests a much narrower range of agents, usually drugs, either in response to social pressure from peers or to environmental stress or as an attention-getting gesture or suicidal attempt (Sec 2.54). This section will discuss principles of management of poisonings and illustrate them with a few substances chosen for high poisoning incidence or the availability of specific antidotes that may require prompt administration. See References for complete coverage of the various poisons.

28.4   MANAGEMENT OF POISONINGS

Think of Poisoning. While the majority of cases of poisonings are obvious, some are subtle and the physician should always be alert to the possibility of poisoning as a diagnosis, especially in an unclear, confusing case.

Maintenance of Vital Signs. The maintenance of respiratory and cardiac function is of immediate importance. Respiration may be impaired by central respiratory depression (as with sedatives and opioids), excessive secretions (as with the anticholinesterase effects of organic phosphate insecticides), defective oxygen transport (as with carbon monoxide poisoning), and ineffective tissue utilization of oxygen (as with cyanide intoxication). While specific antidotes are available and useful for several of the above poisons (naloxone for opioids, atropine for anticholinesterases, and sodium nitrate and sodium thiosulfate for cyanide), nonspecific supportive respiratory care is more frequently the only therapy that can be offered and may be lifesaving.

Patency of the airway is of paramount importance. Measures to maintain its adequacy include positioning the patient in a lateral Trendelenburg or supine position with the head extended; ensuring a patent oropharyngeal or nasopharyngeal airway; suctioning as necessary; passing an endotracheal tube if the preceding are insufficient; performing a tracheostomy if endotracheal intubation is impractical or if it is anticipated that the need for intubation will be longer than 3 days; removing mucus with bronchoscopy by direct visualization; and treating or preventing atelectasis by providing physical therapy, rolling the patient periodically, and encouraging coughing. Respiratory stimulants are seldom, if ever, indicated and may cause more harm than good as a result of their side effects, which include cardiac arrhythmias and convulsions.

Hypotension is the most common serious cardiovascular complication, and its treatment is central to the patient's overall response. Whether the hypotension is related to hypovolemia or widespread vasodilation, the initial approach is expansion of the intravascular volume using a rapid-acting plasma expander. If this is insufficient, use of a pressor agent should be considered. Dopamine is recommended since it can be titrated to produce alpha-adrenergic stimulation, beta-adrenergic stimulation, or dopaminergic stimulation by increasing the rate of infusion of the drug. It has the added advantage of producing renal arteriolar vasodilation and enhancing renal blood flow; the latter may also be helpful in hastening the elimination of some poisons.

Identification of the Poison. The offending agent may be identified by a careful history, including obtaining a list of drugs kept in the home. Parents should be asked to search quickly through the house for clues. It is also occasionally rewarding for the probable containers of the ingested poisons to be brought to the physician since it is not unusual to find that the medicine in a bottle differs from the label on the bottle. A check of tablet or capsule size, shape, color, and markings may lead to an identification of the drug in question. A home visit is frequently fruitful in finding a possible agent not considered by the anxious parents or friends.

Many laboratories offer a "toxicology screen" in addition to specific assays for various agents. However, no toxicology screen is exhaustive, and the clinician should maintain a list of the drugs and chemicals that are detectable with the particular screen used. While most of the currently available methods for the identification of poisons rely on thin-layer, gas, or high pressure liquid chromatographic separation, the enormous capability of mass spectroscopy for rapid identification of poisons will substantially improve their laboratory evaluation in the future.

Quantification of the Poison. The blood concentration of a drug or toxin is rarely significant in terms of prognosis or therapy. The most important example of usefulness of an elevated plasma level is acetaminophen intoxication since in this condition the clinical picture may be benign at a time when the antidote must be given. Plasma levels of lead, salicylate, and barbiturate may also be important, but therapeutic decisions seldom rest solely on these levels.

Prevention of Continued Absorption. In an attempt to minimize the effect of an ingested poison, it is frequently feasible to remove the unabsorbed poison that remains in the stomach or to bind it to substances within the intestinal lumen so that continuing absorption from the gastrointestinal tract is minimized. Caution should be exercised in this approach and special consideration given to the comatose patient (in whom vomiting may lead to aspiration), to the patient who has ingested a strong alkali (in whom the damage to the esophagus with attempted removal may be more harmful than allowing the alkali to remain in the acidic milieu of the stomach), and possibly to the patient who has ingested a hydrocarbon (in whom aspiration may represent a greater hazard than intestinal absorption).

In the alert child the production of emesis is generally believed to be more efficacious than gastric lavage because of more complete gastric emptying and the inability of most unbroken tablets or capsules to enter even the largest available gastric tube. Emesis is most commonly induced by the administration of syrup of ipecac. An initial dose of 15 ml of syrup of ipecac should produce effective vomiting within 30 min. If this dose is ineffective, a 2nd dose of 15 ml will usually succeed. Ipecac is more effective with a full stomach, and it is important to provide several glasses of water prior to giving ipecac. Since ipecac is adsorbed onto charcoal, it is also important to withhold charcoal until after vomiting has occurred. Although apomorphine has the advantages of a more immediate onset of action (usually within 10 min) and of a parenteral mode of administration (subcutaneous), the time gained is relatively un-

important considering the fact that the poisoned patient is seldom seen within 1 hr of ingestion. Apomorphine may also cause a greater degree of respiratory depression than ipecac. Positioning of the patient is important if emesis is produced; vomiting should occur with the patient lying on the side with the head lower than the body or in a child who is kneeling with the head dependent.

In the comatose patient and possibly in the patient who has ingested a hydrocarbon (Sec 28.9), lavage may be indicated in place of induced emesis. Lavage may also be advantageous after emesis. The comatose patient can be treated most safely by providing a cuffed endotracheal tube prior to the initiation of gastric lavage.

Several important aspects of the lavage technique deserve emphasis. The lavage should be performed with the largest bore tubing available (24 French or greater in an adolescent, 8–12 French in a child) to allow removal of broken but undissolved tablets. Nasal passage of the lavage tube is usually easier in an adolescent and oral passage in a child. Lavage should be carried out with the patient on his or her right side with the head lower than the body to minimize aspiration and should be performed with copious total amounts of fluid (10–40 l) to dissolve and remove as much of the gastric contents as possible. The fluid selected for lavage is usually immaterial since most is removed; warm water is generally adequate. Occasionally, a specific antidote (such as deferoxamine) is added to the lavage fluid.

Continued absorption can often be reduced by the administration of activated charcoal, either by mouth or by gastric tube, upon completion of the lavage. A slurry containing a heaping teaspoonful of charcoal in 200 ml of water is recommended. A large array of organic molecules are nonspecifically adsorbed by charcoal and bound to it during their subsequent transit through the intestine.

The time beyond which emesis or lavage is of no value is ill defined. In many poisonings, emesis or lavage is probably of little value after 4 hr. However, exceptions to this rule occur with drugs that slow gastric emptying, such as salicylates and the tricyclic antidepressants.

Enhancement of Elimination. The duration of action of a drug is nearly always a function of the length of time it remains in contact with its receptor site and the concentration of drug at the receptor site. However, in the rare instance when a drug binds irreversibly to a receptor, the action of the drug may last long after removal of the drug from the plasma or the fluid adjacent to the receptor. Usually, the duration of drug toxicity can be lessened if the elimination of the drug can be hastened. In general, enhancement of elimination is based either on the augmentation of its normal renal elimination or on an artificial means of drug removal, including hemodialysis, peritoneal dialysis, or perfusion of blood through a charcoal or resin column.

The renal elimination of most drugs depends on adequate renal perfusion; consequently, normal hydration is important. Overhydration, however, offers little in the way of further elimination and is probably more dangerous than beneficial. A few drugs can be eliminated considerably more rapidly in an alkaline urine (salicylates and phenobarbital) or an acid urine (amphetamine and quinine). The principle involved is that the ionized drug cannot cross lipid membranes easily; the promotion, therefore, of ionization of the drug in urine, as compared with plasma, leads to trapping the ionized drug in urine, with subsequent excretion. Weak acids such as salicylates or phenobarbital have a pK_a (the pH at which half the drug is ionized) in a range (3.4–7.4) that allows significant alteration of ionization by adjusting the urinary pH to greater than 7. Amphetamine and quinine, as weak bases, are more ionized at a low pH and, therefore, more of the drug is trapped in urine that is acid relative to plasma.

Rarely, the use of hemodialysis, peritoneal dialysis, or perfusion of blood through charcoal or resin columns may be lifesaving. Factors that are associated with good dialysance include small molecular weight (less than 300), lack of significant plasma protein binding, lack of significant extravascular tissue distribution, and water solubility. A concise summary of the principles of dialysis with a review of dialyzable drugs has been published by Maher and Schreiner. Both charcoal hemoperfusion and resin hemoperfusion have considerable potential for adsorbing numerous drugs and chemicals.

Correction of the Pathophysiology. While most poisonings must be treated at a symptomatic level, the pathophysiology of some poisonings is sufficiently well understood to allow rational intervention. The diversity of potential mechanisms of toxicity precludes generalizations.

Additional Information. Since no physician can remain abreast of the toxicologic aspects of all the potential poisons ingested by the exploring child, it is important that the physician use the added help of an effective poison control center. These centers, some of which are loosely organized into a regional network, serve as repositories of the latest information on numerous poisonings.

Attention to Psychiatric Needs. The older child or adolescent who is seen because of an attempted suicide is frequently in need of significant psychiatric help even though the physiologic aspect of the poisoning may be mild. The prevention of subsequent attempts requires continuing care (Sec 2.54).

Arena JM: Poisonings, Toxicology, Symptoms, Treatments. Ed 4. Springfield Ill., Charles C Thomas, 1979.

Baselt RC, Wright JA, Cravey RH: Therapeutic and toxic concentrations of more than 100 toxicologically significant drugs in blood, plasma, or serum: A tabulation. Clin Chem 21:44, 1975.

Billets S, Carruth J, Einolf N, et al: Rapid identification of acute drug intoxications. Johns Hopkins Med J 133:148, 1973.

Dreisbach RH: Handbook of Poisoning. Ed 10. Los Altos Calif., Lange Medical Publications, 1980.

Dukes MNG: Side Effects of Drugs, Annual 4. Amsterdam, Excerpta Medica, 1980.

Goodman AG, Goodman LS, Gilman A: The Pharmacological Basis of Therapeutics. Ed 6. New York, Macmillan, 1980.

Grosselin RE, Hodge HC, Smith RP, et al: Clinical Toxicology of Commercial Products. Ed 4. Baltimore, Williams and Wilkins, 1976.

Koffler A, Bernstein M, LaSette A, et al: Fixed-bed charcoal hemoperfusion: Treatment of drug overdose. Arch Int Med 138:1691, 1978.

Maher JF: Principles of dialysis and dialysis of drugs. Am J Med 62:475, 1977.

Maher JF, Schreiner GE: The dialysis of poisons and drugs. Trans Am Soc Artif Intern Organs 14:440, 1968.

Matthew H, Lawson AAH: Treatment of Common Acute Poisonings. Ed 4. New York, Churchill Livingstone, 1979.

Rumack BH (ed): Poisindex. Englewood, Col., Micromedex Inc, 1974–1981.

Simon NM, Krumlovsky FA: The role of dialysis in the treatment of poisoning. Ration Drug Ther 5:1, 1971.

Thompson WL: Poisoning: The twentieth-century black death. In: Shoemaker WC, Thompson WL (ed): Critical Care: State of the Art, Vol 1. Fullerton Calif., Society of Critical Care Medicine, 1980.

Trafford JAP, Jones RH, Evans R, et al: Haemoperfusion with R004 Amberlite resin for treating acute poisoning. Br Med J 2:1453, 1977.

28.5   ACETAMINOPHEN

Poisoning with acetaminophen (paracetamol) is particularly important since it is increasingly chosen by adolescents and young adults as a suicidal agent. Its potentially serious hepatotoxicity is well characterized at a biochemical level, and an effective antidote to the liver disease is available but must be given very promptly after the ingestion to be effective. In contrast to the adolescent, the toddler who accidentally ingests acetaminophen rarely suffers severe consequences.

Death has been associated with the ingestion of 10 gm of acetaminophen, but much larger doses have been ingested with benign outcomes. Some individual variation in the response relates to the ability to metabolize acetaminophen to a toxic metabolite essential for the hepatotoxicity, to enhancement or protection by other drugs that induce or inhibit microsomal drug-metabolizing enzymes, to liver glutathione content, and probably to genetic factors.

Pathophysiology. A product of acetaminophen metabolism by the liver, acetimidoquinone, is probably responsible for the liver cell damage. The metabolite may cause damage by binding to intracellular proteins or nucleic acids. This metabolic pathway is a minor one with respect to the overall elimination of acetaminophen; most of the acetaminophen is conjugated with glucuronic acid or sulfate, and the nontoxic metabolites are eliminated into the urine. With usual therapeutic doses the minor toxic metabolite is conjugated with glutathione and eliminated as a mercapturic acid derivative of acetaminophen. With an overdose, however, once the liver's supply of glutathione is depleted, the toxic metabolite is available to bind to other substances within the liver with consequent liver cell damage. Successful prevention of liver damage may be related to lowering the rate of metabolism of acetaminophen to the toxic compound, providing an alternative protector to glutathione, or enhancing the supply of glutathione.

The pharmacokinetics of acetaminophen are important in understanding the time course of its toxicity. Absorption is complete and rapid after oral administration. Peak levels are usually seen at about 1–2 hr. However, the peak may be delayed if gastric emptying is delayed. Quantification of plasma acetaminophen levels should be delayed until about 4 hr after ingestion since prior to that time continued absorption may occur, producing even higher plasma levels. Since therapy should be determined primarily by plasma levels, timing is important. Once absorbed, acetaminophen is distributed into a space equivalent to 85–100% of the body weight. The half-life of acetaminophen is normally about 2.5 hr and is prolonged with hepatic dysfunction. A prolonged half-life (greater than 4 hr) has been correlated with severe hepatic cellular damage.

Clinical Manifestations. Nausea and vomiting are the most frequent symptoms associated with acetaminophen overdose for the 1st 1–2 days. Only at day 3–4 does the hepatic damage become clinically evident. Signs and symptoms of myocardial, renal, and central nervous system injury are far less frequent. The diagnosis of acetaminophen ingestion must be made by history and laboratory results since there are no pathognomonic signs or symptoms associated with even massive overdoses. It must be remembered that numerous over-the-counter preparations contain acetaminophen as an ingredient, often in substantial amounts (300–500 mg) per tablet or capsule.

Laboratory Data. A plasma level of acetaminophen greater than 300 μg/ml at 4 hr almost always correlates with hepatotoxicity and with some mortality (perhaps 20%). A plasma level of less than 150 μg/ml at 4 hr indicates minimal or absent liver damage; levels from 150–300 μg/ml at 4 hr are associated with minimal to moderate liver damage but are unlikely to be associated with mortality. Levels obtained after 4 hr can be assessed against a curve connecting the 4 hr levels cited above and levels of 100 μg/ml for severe toxicity and 50 μg/ml for minimal toxicity at 10 hr. Since it is currently believed that the initiation of specific therapy later than 10 hr after ingestion is probably of no value, levels after 10 hr may be of prognostic value but are of little therapeutic importance. A prolongation of prothrombin time is often an early sign of hepatocellular dysfunction. Serum transaminase elevations also reflect early hepatocellular damage, but hyperbilirubinemia is usually seen somewhat later. One cannot wait for abnormalities of liver function to initiate treatment.

Treatment. The prevention of continued acetaminophen absorption is the 1st step in therapy and is best accomplished by the immediate production of emesis. (Coma is seldom a problem unless other drugs have been consumed simultaneously.) Charcoal instillation into the stomach is used to bind residual acetaminophen.

Success in prevention of liver damage has been achieved by the prompt (after ingestion) intravenous administration of cysteamine (β-mercaptoethylamine), which may provide an alternative sulfhydryl compound to serve as a scavenger of the toxic metabolite that normally would bind to glutathione or may inhibit the metabolic conversion of acetaminophen to a toxic metabolite. However, cysteamine is not produced as a drug for use in humans, and it causes severe nausea, vomiting, abdominal pain, and occasional hypotension.

Methionine is probably as effective as cysteamine in humans and is commercially available in the United States as an agent approved for use in urinary tract infections. It is administered orally and causes a few side effects and no major untoward reactions. Nausea and vomiting may occasionally occur and may make administration difficult. A potential disadvantage is methionine's ability to precipitate hepatic coma in a patient in precoma due to severe liver disease. To be effective, methionine must be given early after ingestion (within 10 hr). A dose of 10 gm orally, divided into 4 doses and given over about 10 hr, has been used with success. Methionine may act as a source of cysteine, with the cysteine in turn serving to replenish the exhausted liver stores of glutathione and with the glutathione then acting as a natural protective mechanism for the liver.

Acetylcysteine offers an equipotent alternative to methionine. The suggested regimen is 140 mg/kg as an oral or intragastric loading dose, delivered as soon after ingestion as possible, followed by 70 mg/kg as a maintenance dose every 4 hr for 17 total maintenance doses. The commercially available vials of acetylcysteine, Mucomyst, contain 30 ml of a 20% solution (6 g) and can be administered in carbonated beverages or tap water. If diluted with 3 parts of water, the solution is isotonic. Intravenous acetylcysteine is also efficacious.

Hemodialysis or perfusion of blood through an adsorbent column has been ineffective in preventing subsequent hepatotoxicity.

Ameer B, Greenblatt DJ: Acetaminophen. Ann Int Med 87:202, 1977.
Gillette JR: An integrated approach to the study of chemically reactive metabolites of acetaminophen. Arch Int Med 141:375, 1981.
Goulding R: Acetaminophen poisoning. Pediatrics 52:883, 1973.
Mitchell JR, Thorgiersson SS, Potter WZ, et al: Acetaminophen-induced hepatic injury: Protective role of glutathione in man and rationale for therapy. Clin Pharmacol Ther 16:676, 1974.
Prescott LF: Treatment of severe acetaminophen poisoning with intravenous acetylcysteine. Arch Int Med 141:386, 1981.
Prescott LF, Newton RW, Swainson CP, et al: Successful treatment of severe paracetamol overdose with cysteamine. Lancet 1:588, 1974.
Rumack BH, Peterson RC, Koch GG, et al: Acetaminophen overdose. Arch Int Med 141:380, 1981.
Vale JA, Meredith TJ, Goulding R: Treatment of acetaminophen poisoning. Arch Int Med 141:394, 1981.

28.6 SALICYLATES

Salicylate intoxication accounts for a large number of accidental ingestions in young children and a moderate number of intentional ingestions in adolescents and young adults. Fatalities are infrequent, as are serious sequelae. In part, this favorable outcome may be attributable to early recognition and the application of effective therapeutic measures since delayed diagnosis and therapy can be lethal. The frequency of accidental ingestions by toddlers is related to the presence of salicylate-containing drugs in most homes and the enticing flavor of most baby aspirins. Though infrequent, the accidental ingestion of methylsalicylate is attributable to its aroma as oil of wintergreen.

While individual salicylate formulations may give rise to some unique features, such as the rapid absorption of methylsalicylate or the ready acetylation of proteins by acetylsalicylic acid, the prominent aspects of salicylate intoxication are shared by all salicylates. The acute dosage of salicylates necessary to produce serious intoxication in an otherwise healthy toddler is probably in excess of 200 mg/kg. However, individual variation is significant, and infancy, dehydration, and renal failure may enhance the severity of an otherwise safe dose.

Pathophysiology. Salicylate intoxication primarily involves the direct effects of the drug on the respiratory center of the brain and metabolic effects. Salicylates stimulate the respiratory center with a resultant increase in both depth and rate of respiration. CO_2 is eliminated and respiratory alkalosis quickly follows. This phenomenon probably occurs regardless of age and is the predominant situation in most adults with salicylism. In severely intoxicated adults and most children, this respiratory effect is rapidly balanced by a significant metabolic acidosis. The salicylate ion itself probably accounts for only a minor fraction of the acidosis. More important are the accumulation of lactate as a result of the ability of salicylates to alter the proper functioning of the Krebs cycle and the accumulation of organic acids as intermediates in this cycle. Children appear to be especially susceptible to these metabolic effects of salicylates and usually present with metabolic acidosis. The effects of salicylates on the Krebs cycle and as uncouplers of oxidation from phosphorylation are responsible for another occasional manifestation of salicylism, the hyperpyrexia associated with enhanced oxidation without conservation of the energy generated in adenosine triphosphate.

Salicylates can also cause bleeding, hypokalemia, and hypo- or hyperglycemia. The *bleeding* may be a result of local gastrointestinal irritation, altered platelet function on the basis of an inhibition of prostaglandin (and thromboxane) biosynthesis, and defective prothrombin synthesis secondary to impaired liver function. However, bleeding is rarely a clinically significant problem in acute salicylate intoxication.

Hypokalemia frequently accompanies acute salicylate intoxication. Salicylates may exert a direct effect on the renal tubular mechanism responsible for potassium excretion; they may also exert an indirect effect through their ability to produce a respiratory alkalosis. The alkalosis may produce hypokalemia both through promotion of an intracellular shift of potassium and through excessive renal loss. The hypokalemia may be associated with electrocardiographic effects (flattened T waves and depressed ST segments) and areflexia. The hypokalemia can also be responsible for a loss of concentrating ability of the renal tubule with secondary polyuria and dehydration.

Either *hyperglycemia* or *hypoglycemia* may occur. The hyperglycemia appears to be relatively unimportant at a clinical level, but the hypoglycemia can be serious. Perhaps even more important is the recently reported lowering by salicylates of brain glucose levels in young experimental animals even though blood glucose levels remained normal. The therapeutic importance of this finding was shown by the complete protection provided by glucose administration to mice given an otherwise lethal dose of salicylates. The administration of glucose also curtailed the fall in brain glucose.

The pharmacokinetics of salicylates is important in the therapeutic approach to salicylism. After ingestion the tablets of salicylate disintegrate into small pieces in the stomach and then dissolve prior to absorption. An alkaline milieu enhances dissolution of the tablets but

also retards absorption of the dissolved drug since a greater percentage of the molecules exist in the poorly absorbed ionized form.

Once absorbed, the acetyl group of aspirin is quickly removed by plasma esterases, leaving salicylate as the predominant species. Other products are absorbed as salicylates. Salicylate distributes widely in the body, entering cells as well as extracellular spaces; the distribution is, in part, a function of the relative pH of the plasma compared with other spaces (e.g., cerebrospinal fluid or cells). Should the plasma have a low pH, compared with other spaces, more salicylate will be nonionized and capable of passing across membranes and entering these other spaces.

Salicylates are eliminated from plasma as a result of several metabolic conversions occurring primarily in the liver and the simultaneous excretion of unchanged salicylate by the kidney. Since at least 2 of the hepatic enzymes responsible for its conversions are easily saturated at high levels of salicylates, the kinetics of elimination change as the plasma levels of salicylates change. While it is incorrect to speak of half-lives under these circumstances, one can view the "dose-related kinetics" as the changing of the "half-life" of a drug with changing plasma levels; higher plasma levels are correlated with longer "half-lives." Clinically, this means that it will take longer for the body to eliminate a specified percentage of the total body load at higher plasma levels than it will take to eliminate the same percentage at lower plasma levels.

A relatively small proportion of the body burden of salicylate (about 20%) is normally eliminated by the kidneys as unchanged drug by a process called "nonionic diffusion" or "ion-trapping." The salicylate is delivered to the tubular urine by both glomerular filtration and, to a lesser extent, tubular secretion. Reabsorption of the salicylate then occurs to a variable extent depending on the relationship between the urinary pH and that of the renal tubular cells and adjacent plasma. If the urine is alkaline relative to the pK_a of the salicylate (i.e., the pH at which a drug is 50% ionized), the urinary salicylate will exist primarily in an ionized form, incapable of crossing the renal tubular membranes and, therefore, unavailable for reabsorption. If, on the other hand, the urinary pH is acid relative to the pK_a of salicylates (about 3.0), then most of the salicylate will exist in a nonionized form and will be available for reabsorption. Thus, the usual small percentage of salicylates eliminated unchanged can be significantly augmented by alkalinization of the urine.

Clinical Manifestations. The signs and symptoms of salicylism are seldom diagnostic. Hyperpnea is the most frequent sign. Vomiting, confusion, lethargy, hyperpyrexia, and coma may also occur. The diagnosis of salicylate intoxication is often made by history. It should be recognized, however, that salicylates are contained in numerous over-the-counter preparations and that other toxic drugs may accompany the salicylates.

Laboratory Data. The identification of salicylates can be rapidly ascertained by simple bedside tests. A positive ferric chloride test (violet-purple color) on urine, persisting even though the urine is acidified and boiled prior to testing (in order to eliminate ketones), is good evidence that salicylates have been consumed. The test is so sensitive, however, that nontoxic quantities will produce a positive result. Phenistix can be used on urine; the presence of a brown to purple color will indicate the presence of salicylates. Since acetylsalicylic acid will not (until hydrolyzed to salicylic acid) produce a positive result with either of these 2 tests, neither is of value for the identification of aspirin vomitus or lavage fluids.

Quantification of plasma or serum salicylate concentration is of value in assessing the severity of poisoning; a rough and rapid estimate can be gained by dipping the Phenistix into plasma or serum. If there is less than 40 mg/dl of salicylate, the Phenistix will be tan. If the concentration is 40–90 mg/dl, a deeper brown to purple color will appear; a pure purple color indicates greater than 90 mg/dl. More precise quantification can be provided by several chemical assays available in most clinical chemistry laboratories. The plasma level should be interpreted as a function of time elapsed since ingestion (Fig 5–18). Severe poisoning can be anticipated if the plasma salicylate level exceeds 100 mg/dl at 6 hr, 80 mg/dl at 12 hr, or 50 mg/dl at 24 hr after ingestion.

Treatment. In an alert patient emesis should be induced to prevent continued salicylate absorption from the stomach. In a comatose patient lavage should be initiated after placement of a cuffed endotracheal tube to prevent aspiration. Charcoal may be given after emesis has been induced.

The elimination of salicylates can be dramatically enhanced by alkalinizing the urine to take advantage of the nonionic diffusion previously described. Both the decision to alkalinize the urine and the choice of an agent to produce an alkaline urine are subjects of debate. Sodium bicarbonate intravenously, acetazolamide subcutaneously, and THAM (tris-[hydroxymethyl]aminomethane) intravenously have each been advocated, and each can clearly augment the urinary excretion of salicylate. *Sodium bicarbonate* has the potential advantages of counteracting the systemic acidosis usually seen in childhood salicylate poisoning, of widespread acceptance, and of clinical familiarity. It has the disadvantages of potentially aggravating the alkalosis usually seen in adult salicylate poisoning, of requiring constant monitoring of the urinary pH to assure that enough is given to alkalinize the urine, of necessitating a considerable sodium load with the possibility of hypernatremia and fluid overload, and of failing in the most severely affected and acidotic patients. Alkalinization of the urine with bicarbonate is especially difficult, if not impossible, in the hypokalemic patient. *Acetazolamide* has the advantage of rapidly and consistently producing an alkaline urine after subcutaneous administration and the potential advantage of partially counteracting systemic alkalosis. It has the disadvantage of potentially aggravating the usual metabolic acidosis of childhood poisoning, of tending to alkalinize the cerebrospinal fluid relative to the plasma with the consequent enhancement of central nervous system salicylate concentration, and of proving deleterious to the central nervous system in an animal model. However, the deleterious effect of acetazolamide may be related to an inhibition of red cell carbonic anhydrase with attendant accumulation of carbon dioxide. This effect may be reduced by giving a smaller dose than is capable of inhibiting the red cell enzyme. A combination of bicarbonate and acetazolamide may overcome most of the disadvantages of either agent used alone. Done argues against the immediate utilization of alkalinizing agents in mildly or moderately affected patients since these patients will uniformly do well with attention to their fluid, potassium, and glucose status and since alkalinization of the urine is most difficult (with bicarbonate alone) or most hazardous (with acetazolamide) in the severely affected patients.

Rarely, it may be necessary to consider other means of removing salicylates quickly; both peritoneal dialysis (with 5% human albumin added to the dialyzing solution) and hemodialysis are effective in the rapid clearance of salicylates.

For details of fluid therapy of salicylate intoxication, see Sec 5.29.

Done AK: Aspirin overdosage: Incidence, diagnosis, and management. Pediatrics 62(Suppl):890, 1978.
Levy G: Clinical pharmacokinetics of aspirin. Pediatrics 62(Suppl):867, 1978.
Reimold EW, Worthen HG, Reilly TP Jr: Salicylate poisoning: Comparison of acetazolamide administration and alkaline diuresis in the treatment of experimental salicylate intoxication in puppies. Am J Dis Child 125:668, 1973.
Robin ED, David RP, Rees SB: Salicylate intoxication with special reference to the development of hypokalemia. Am J Med 26:869, 1969.
Smith MJH: The metabolic basis of the major symptoms in acute salicylate intoxication. Clin Toxicol 1:387, 1968.
Temple AR: Pathophysiology of aspirin overdosage toxicity, with implications for management. Pediatrics 62(Suppl):873, 1978.
Thurston JH, Pollock PG, Warren SK, et al: Reduced brain glucose with normal plasma glucose in salicylate poisoning. J Clin Invest 49:2139, 1970.

28.7 STRONG ALKALIS

The accidental ingestion of highly alkaline substances (lyes or caustics) accounts for considerable morbidity and some mortality in the toddler. The use of "childproof" containers and restriction on the concentration of strong alkalis in liquid preparations may have reduced the incidence of severe consequences of caustics, but the problem persists. An occasional older child or adult unwittingly ingests strongly alkaline tablets in the form of Clinitest tablets containing sodium hydroxide. A very small amount of a strong alkali can cause considerable local damage; a single Clinitest tablet may produce significant oral or esophageal lesions.

Pathology. The severity of the lesions produced by strong alkalis depends on the concentration of alkali that comes in contact with the skin, oral and pharyngeal mucosa, and esophagus and also on the duration of such contact. Liquid preparations (usually drain cleaners) are dangerous because of the ease with which they reach the esophagus and because of their tendency to produce circumferential damage to the esophagus. Tablets have the disadvantage of producing very high local concentrations of alkali and of becoming lodged for relatively long periods of time. The time necessary for significant damage is probably seconds to a very few minutes. Damage is usually confined to the mouth, pharynx, and esophagus since the acid milieu of the stomach offers considerable protection at that site. The caustics cause local damage to mucosa and submucosal tissue by liquefaction necrosis, which involves the saponification of fats and solubilization of proteins with thrombosis of local blood vessels and subsequent tissue necrosis.

The lesion produced may be classified like thermal burns. A 1st degree lesion is characterized by superficial damage, including hyperemia, edema, and sloughing of the mucosa only. A 2nd degree lesion involves mucosal and submucosal areas of the esophagus with exudation, ulceration, loss of mucosa, and erosion through the esophageal wall. A 3rd degree lesion includes the above as well as erosion into the mediastinal, pleural, or peritoneal spaces. In addition to the immediate direct effects of the strong alkali, there is an intense inflammatory reaction. Within several days of the acute damage the necrotic tissue is replaced by granulation tissue. Later, scar tissue may supervene with subsequent stricture formation. The strictures ultimately become quite significant as a result of nutritional deprivation and aspiration pneumonia.

Clinical Manifestations. The diagnosis of a strong alkali burn is often based on history alone. The clinical picture may include an inability to swallow, substernal or back pain, and excessive drooling. However, the existence of esophageal damage must be determined by esophagoscopy as the absence of oral or pharyngeal lesions does not prove the absence of esophageal lesions.

Treatment. Oral lesions should be washed with copious amounts of water to dilute the alkali quickly. For potential esophageal lesions it is probably best to avoid any fluids orally prior to esophagoscopy. Emesis and gastric lavage are contraindicated since the gastric acidity will usually neutralize the alkali quite effectively and both enhance the possibility of aspiration. See Sec 11.20 for diagnosis and management of esophageal lesions.

Haller JA, Andrews HG, White JJ, et al: Pathophysiology and management of acute corrosive burns of the esophagus: Results of treatment of 285 children. J Pediatr Surg 6:578, 1971.
Kirsch MM, Ritter F: Caustic ingestion and subsequent damage to the oropharyngeal and digestive passages. Ann Thorac Surg 21:74, 1976.
Leape LL, Ashcraft KW, Scarpelli DG, et al: Hazard to health—liquid lye. N Engl J Med 284:578, 1971.

28.8 BARBITURATES

Barbiturate poisoning is not common among toddlers, but it accounts for more poisoning deaths than any other category of drugs in the adolescent age group and in the adult. About 1500 deaths/yr in the United States are due to barbiturate poisoning.

The magnitude of the oral dose that should be considered dangerous is variable. In adolescents or adults an acute oral ingestion of 1 gm of any barbiturate should be viewed with concern, and 3 gm should be considered

potentially lethal. Ingestion by a toddler of about one third of the above adult values should be considered as serious or potentially lethal.

Pathophysiology. Central nervous system depression is the predominant feature of barbiturate poisoning and results in a marked inhibition of respiration at a central level. Most of the serious manifestations can be related to hypoxia secondary to central respiratory depression, including many of the cardiovascular and renal effects and probably most irreversible central nervous system effects. Though the direct central nervous system effects can be profound and devastating, they are (in the absence of secondary hypoxia) almost always reversible with elimination of the barbiturate itself. Complete reversibility has been documented even after a flat EEG.

Barbiturates may affect the cardiovascular system directly with vasodilation and fluid loss from the vascular compartment. Direct myocardial depression can also be seen. While all of the barbiturates produce about the same pathophysiologic effects, the pharmacokinetics of the individual barbiturates differ considerably, and these differences are significant in the rational management of individual intoxications.

The absorption of all of the oral barbiturate preparations is nearly complete. The rate of absorption, however, is variable, with maximum levels occurring 1–18 hr after ingestion. One cannot predict the time at which peak concentrations are likely since the rate-limiting step in absorption is probably the rate of dispersion and dissolution of the particular formulation ingested.

Absorbed barbiturates are widely distributed into most tissues of the body; the volume of distribution is about 60% of the body weight. About 50% of plasma barbiturate is protein-bound; the remainder is free and capable of equilibrating with extravascular tissues. The duration of action of the oral barbiturates is primarily a result of the hepatic metabolism for the short-acting drugs and is usually a function of both hepatic metabolism and renal elimination of the long-acting drugs. The fact that about 50% of a usual therapeutic dose of phenobarbital appears unchanged in the urine is important from a therapeutic standpoint since it is this fraction that can be increased by raising the pH of the urine. Since a much smaller proportion of the short-acting barbiturates is excreted unchanged and since the more lipid-soluble short-acting barbiturates are much more extensively reabsorbed by the renal tubules, there is less opportunity for significantly increasing the renal elimination of the short-acting barbiturates by changing the urinary pH. Furthermore, the pK_a of each of the short-acting barbiturates (pentobarbital = 8.0; secobarbital = 7.9) is higher than that of phenobarbital (7.3) so that one cannot significantly change the renal excretion by the mechanism of nonionic diffusion. The plasma half-life of phenobarbital is approximately 86 hr, while those of secobarbital and pentobarbital are considerably less (20–40 hr). Thus, the duration of toxicity is usually considerably longer after an overdose of phenobarbital, compared with that of pentobarbital or secobarbital.

Clinical Manifestations. The diagnosis of barbiturate intoxication depends largely on history and on laboratory identification of the ingested drug since the clinical symptoms and signs are similar to those of other hypnotic sedatives. However, the assessment of clinical severity is of considerable value from both a prognostic and therapeutic standpoint. The degree of central nervous system depression can be graded by the classification proposed by Matthew.

Grade I—Drowsy but responds to vocal command.
Grade II—Unconscious but responds to minimal stimuli.
Grade III—Unconscious and responds only to maximal painful stimuli.
Grade IV—Unconscious and shows no response whatever.

The standard painful stimulus is the rubbing of the sternum with a clenched fist. Pupillary signs are of little diagnostic value.

Respiratory depression can be assessed by the depth and rate of respiration and by blood gases. The absence of bowel sounds is usually associated with grade III depression and nearly always with grade IV depression. Presence of bowel sounds indicates lesser depression but also suggests that continued absorption may occur. Bullous lesions are associated with barbiturate intoxication in about 6% of cases.

Laboratory Data. Barbiturates can be identified by analyzing the gastric aspirate or plasma. However, the value of quantification of the plasma barbiturate level is the subject of continuing debate. Some place little value on the actual barbiturate level in terms of therapeutic decisions and rely nearly completely on their assessment of the clinical severity of each patient. Others believe that the plasma barbiturate level may indicate whether the degree of coma seen is due to the barbiturate or due to another drug or disease. A level of phenobarbital of 150 μg/ml has been used as a factor in the decision to initiate therapy with alkaline diuresis. Lastly, the levels of several barbiturates have been suggested as prime determinants in the decision to institute dialysis or hemoperfusion. However, the clinical status is probably more useful in this decision than is a plasma barbiturate level.

Treatment. Initial attention to the adequacy of oxygenation is imperative. The patency of the airway should be assured and assisted ventilation should be available. The management of hypotension associated with severe barbiturate intoxication is controversial. Dopamine appears to have advantages over other pressors and has been shown to be effective in animal models of phenobarbital intoxication.

Emesis should not be attempted in the comatose patient, and gastric lavage must be carefully performed after first placing a cuffed endotracheal tube. Charcoal administration is recommended at the end of the lavage.

Three approaches are effective in hastening the excretion of barbiturates to lessen the duration of coma and cardiovascular and respiratory depression: alkaline diuresis, dialysis, and hemoperfusion. Each significantly increases the clearance of the long-acting barbiturates; dialysis and hemoperfusion have also been effective in increasing the clearance of the short-acting barbiturates.

The combination of an induced osmotic diuresis and alkalinization of the urine can enhance the urinary elimination of phenobarbital and other long-acting barbiturates by entrapment of the ionized phenobarbital in the urine, with subsequent inability of the ionized phenobarbital to cross the tubular membrane and be reabsorbed. Diuresis by itself is of limited value. Alkalinization of the urine can be achieved by the administration of bicarbonate, lactate, acetazolamide, or THAM. A useful regimen in the adolescent or young adult consists of infusing a solution containing 5% dextrose, 0.45% sodium chloride, 40 mEq of sodium bicarbonate/l, and 10% mannitol at a rate of 2 l/hr for 3 hr and 500 ml/hr thereafter. Sodium and potassium must be monitored and potassium added as needed as soon as adequate urinary output is assured. It is essential to give enough alkalinizing agent to ensure an alkaline (pH = 8) urine.

If an adequate diuresis cannot be achieved or if vigorous fluid therapy is contraindicated, peritoneal dialysis is effective, especially with long-acting barbiturates. Hemodialysis is indicated in the presence of severe and persistent hypotension and is more efficient than peritoneal dialysis, both for long- and short-acting barbiturates.

Blood perfusion through charcoal columns has also been demonstrated to remove barbiturates efficiently.

There is no specific antidote for counteracting the pathophysiologic effects of barbiturate poisoning. Respiratory and central nervous system stimulants are probably more harmful than helpful in barbiturate intoxication.

Editorial: Haemoperfusion for acute intoxication with hypnotic drugs. Lancet 2:1116, 1979.
Koffler A, Bernstein M, LaSette A, et al: Fixed-bed charcoal hemoperfusion: Treatment of drug overdose. Arch Int Med 138:1691, 1978.
Maher JF, Schreiner GE: An evaluation of the effectiveness of dialysis for sedative and analgesic poisoning. In: Kerr DNS (ed): Dialysis and Renal Transplantation. Amsterdam, Excerpta Medica, 1969.
Matthew H: Acute Barbiturate Poisoning. Amsterdam, Excerpta Medica, 1971.
Shubin H, Wile MH: Shock associated with barbiturate intoxication. JAMA 215:263, 1971.
Vale JA, Rees AJ, Widdop B, et al: Use of charcoal haemoperfusion in the management of severely poisoned patients. Br Med J 1:5, 1975.

28.9 HYDROCARBONS

The ingestion of various hydrocarbons in the form of petroleum distillates (including petroleum ether, naphtha, gasoline, mineral spirits, kerosene, fuel oil, furnace oil, mineral seal oil, and turpentine) is a common problem. More than 90% of hydrocarbon ingestions (approximately 28,000/yr) occur in children under 5 yr of age, causing about 100 deaths/yr.

The severity of intoxication is a function of the amount ingested (death has occurred after as little as 15 ml) and the viscosity of the particular product. The effects of products with a very low viscosity (and a very high volatility) result primarily from aspiration occurring at the time of ingestion, with subsequent chemical irritation of the respiratory tract. Products with a higher viscosity are less frequently toxic, and the pathology is more like that of a lipoid pneumonia.

Pathology. The effects of petroleum distillates on the lungs include hyperemia, edema, hemorrhage, focal interstitial inflammation, and cellular infiltration. Edema, fibrin, polymorphonuclear leukocytes, mononuclear cells, and, occasionally, foreign body giant cells are found in the alveoli. These findings are characteristic of acute hemorrhagic edema and bronchopneumonia. Hypoxia as a consequence of the marked pulmonary pathology is the most serious aspect of the pathophysiology of hydrocarbon ingestion and chemical pneumonitis. In addition, large ingestions of petroleum distillates can produce degenerative changes in the liver, myocardium, kidney, and gastrointestinal tract.

Clinical Manifestations. (See also Sec 12.70.) The pneumonitis occurs promptly after hydrocarbon ingestion (and aspiration). Roentgenographic evidence of pneumonia often precedes clinical appearance and may be visible 15 min after the ingestion. Pneumonitis, if it occurs, usually appears roentgenographically within the 1st 24 hr following ingestion; the roentgenographic findings typically consist of fine mottled densities extending from the perihilar regions into the lung bases, often with peripheral hyperaeration. These initial findings may progress to confluent densities (consolidation or atelectasis) associated with surrounding areas of compensatory emphysema. Additional pulmonary complications are rare and include pleural effusions, pneumothorax, pneumomediastinum, and pneumatoceles. Though resolution of the roentgenographic picture may be rapid, more commonly it is slow, requiring 2–3 wk.

The diagnosis of hydrocarbon ingestion is usually obvious from the history, coupled with the odor of the petroleum distillate. However, it is important to identify the exact product ingested, both because of differing inherent toxicities based on the viscosity of the products and because of the possibility that the hydrocarbon may have served as a solvent for a more toxic ingredient, such as an insecticide. Leukocytosis and fever can occur in the absence of bacterial infection. Their presence makes it virtually impossible to rule out a bacterial superinfection in any individual case.

Treatment. The therapy for hydrocarbon ingestions is controversial. In general, emesis is contraindicated because of the risk of aspiration. Recently, emesis with ipecac syrup has been advocated by some for an alert patient and for a patient whose ingestion was so large that one fears the consequences of gastrointestinal tract absorption. Similarly, the use of lavage has been controversial. Though it is argued that lavage should be used in preference to emesis for large ingestions of hydrocarbons (greater than 30 ml), it has also been demonstrated that the incidence of aspiration with lavage is not negligible. In the comatose patient, lavage must be preceded by insertion of a cuffed endotracheal tube to prevent aspiration. In the alert patient it is probable that a properly performed lavage is not harmful. Therefore, after a large ingestion it would appear justifiable from the standpoint of risk to remove the hydrocarbon by lavage or possibly even by emesis. However, the benefits derived from removing even large amounts of hydrocarbon from the stomach are largely theoretic and poorly substantiated. A study using a baboon model has cast doubt on systemic absorption as the pathogenetic route to central nervous system toxicity and emphasized the prominent role played by the pulmonary pathology and hypoxia in the subsequent central nervous system pathology.

The instillation of olive oil to slow gastric emptying may decrease the intestinal absorption of petroleum distillates. Once the absorption has occurred, there is currently no known method of hastening elimination. Adrenocortical steroids have been advocated to reduce the inflammatory response and edema associated with the chemical pneumonitis, but controlled studies do not show a statistically significant advantage to steroid treatment. However, the question of efficacy of steroids remains inconclusively answered since these studies did not include many severely affected patients. In animal models (baboon and guinea pig) steroids do not alter the acute inflammatory response of kerosene pneumonitis and may diminish the mononuclear cell infiltration and raise the secondary bacterial infection rate. Thus, the weight of evidence is against the use of steroids in hydrocarbon pneumonitis.

There is no evidence to support the initial use of prophylactic antibiotics to reduce secondary bacterial superinfection at the onset of the pulmonary pathology. However, the usual signs of bacterial infection, including fever, leukocytosis, and pulmonary infiltration evidenced by roentgenograms, are commonly seen in hydrocarbon pneumonitis and may justify use of antibiotics.

Hypoxia is the most serious complication of hydrocarbon ingestion; careful attention to the adequacy of ventilation is imperative.

Baldachin BJ, Melmed RN: Clinical and therapeutic aspects of kerosene poisoning: A series of 200 cases. Br Med J 2:28, 1964.

Griffin JW, Daeschner CW, Collins VP, et al: Hydrocarbon pneumonitis following furniture polish ingestion: A report of fifteen cases. J Pediatr 45:13, 1954.

Marks MI, Chicoine L, Legere G, et al: Adrenocorticosteroid treatment of hydrocarbon pneumonia in children—a cooperative study. J Pediatr 81:366, 1972.

Subcommittee on Accidental Poisoning, American Academy of Pediatrics: Cooperative kerosene poisoning study: Evaluation of gastric lavage and other factors in the treatment of accidental ingestion of petroleum distillate products. Pediatrics 29:648, 1962.

Wolfsdorf J: Kerosene intoxication: An experimental approach to the etiology of the CNS manifestations in primates. J Pediatr 88:1037, 1976.

Wolfsdorf J, Kundig H: Dexamethasone in the management of kerosene pneumonia. Pediatrics 53:86, 1974.

28.10   IRON

Iron poisoning is frequent in childhood, in part related to the prevalence of iron-containing tablets in many homes and the resemblance of many iron tablets to candy. Though iron poisoning rarely results in death, prompt action by the physician may be lifesaving. An understanding of iron poisoning and its therapy is of considerable importance since it may be necessary to treat a relatively asymptomatic child.

The severity of iron poisoning is related to the amount of elemental iron ingested. Death has been reported after ingestion of as little as 900 mg of elemental iron, an amount contained in only 15 ferrous sulfate tablets. The pathophysiology is related principally to the local irritative effects of iron on the gastrointestinal mucosa and the metabolic effects produced in the liver as a result of iron deposition. Additionally, central nervous system effects are sometimes present.

Clinical Manifestations. The diagnosis of iron poisoning is usually made by history. Roentgenographic confirmation is often possible since undisintegrated iron tablets are radiopaque.

Four phases may be observed with serious iron poisoning. The 1st is due to the local irritative effects of iron on the gastrointestinal mucosa, occurs rapidly after iron ingestion, and usually subsides after 6–12 hr. The manifestations are the result of local necrosis and hemorrhage at the sites of iron contact. Nausea, vomiting, diarrhea, abdominal pain, hematemesis, and melena occur as a result. In extreme cases profound fluid and blood loss into the gastrointestinal lumen may occur and result in shock. Lethargy, coma, and seizures rarely occur during this phase. Both shock and coma during this stage are ominous signs.

A 2nd phase of deceptive quiescence follows. During both the 1st and 2nd phases of iron poisoning, the ingested iron is absorbed, passes briefly through the circulatory system, and is delivered to various organs but principally to the liver, where it accumulates within mitochondria causing profound metabolic effects. The rapidity of transport of iron into the liver makes plasma iron levels unreliable as an indicator of the severity of poisoning. Thus, while high levels (>500 μg/dl) of iron indicate a significant ingestion, low levels cannot be viewed as safe since the transient peak of plasma iron prior to hepatic deposition may have been missed. The quiescent interval may last for 12–36 hr.

The 3rd phase of iron poisoning begins 12–48 hr after ingestion and reflects the hepatic damage produced by the iron. Liver function may be abnormal, as reflected in the prothrombin time or in hypoglycemia; liver cell damage is evidenced by plasma transaminase elevations: and a metabolic acidosis may follow, attributable to an impairment of electron transport by the damaged mitochondrial membranes. The precise biochemical events culminating in hepatotoxicity are not known but may include lipid peroxidation with subsequent damage to lipid-containing cell membranes, an electron sink provided by iron with resultant shunting of electrons away from the electron transport system, or direct uncoupling of oxidative phosphorylation within mitochondria. The time course of this phase depends on the extent of liver damage produced, ranging from a few days to weeks. Most deaths occur during this 3rd phase.

A 4th phase occasionally follows, with scarring and stenosis of the pyloric area as a residuum of the local irritative action during the 1st phase. This stenosis may be symptomatic and occasionally requires surgical intervention.

A single intramuscular (or intravenous if the patient is hypotensive) administration of the specific chelator of iron, deferoxamine, in a dose of 1 gm, may be useful as a predictor of the severity of iron poisoning. If there is excess iron, beyond that bound to transferrin, the deferoxamine will chelate it, and the iron chelate of deferoxamine, feroxamine, will appear in the urine.

While deferoxamine is colorless, urine containing feroxamine will be pink or red. Absence of this color in urine formed after the delivery of deferoxamine is a sign that the overdose has been minimal.

Treatment. The therapy for iron poisoning must be initiated rapidly following ingestion to be maximally effective. The basic principle is that iron must be kept from accumulating in the hepatic mitochondria since, once there, it cannot be removed nor can the pathology be reversed.

The prevention of continued absorption is important and is aided by the slow disintegration of most iron tablets. Emesis should be induced and is to be preferred over initial lavage to remove the large iron tablets and fragments. Roentgenograms can assess removal since iron tablets are radiopaque. Emesis should be followed by gastric lavage with a solution containing 2 gm of deferoxamine/liter to remove smaller particles and precipitate or chelate residual iron in the stomach. Deferoxamine, the specific and highly tenacious chelator of iron, and feroxamine, the iron chelate of deferoxamine, are poorly absorbed from the gastrointestinal tract. Deferoxamine should chelate unabsorbed iron and aid in its removal. Deferoxamine binds iron preferentially in the ferric form, therefore, the lavage should be performed with sodium bicarbonate sufficient to maintain the pH above 5. Though bicarbonate itself will form insoluble ferrous carbonate, and phosphates (available as Fleet enemas) will form insoluble aggregates with iron, neither of these maneuvers alone is of proven efficacy.

Upon completion of the lavage an additional 10 gm of deferoxamine should be instilled into the stomach to bind any residual iron during its continued passage through the gastrointestinal tract. Though feroxamine may be absorbed to a small extent and is potentially toxic, it is less toxic than an equimolar amount of iron alone.

It is also important to prevent the excess free iron from accumulating within hepatic mitochondria and to hasten its renal elimination. Both of these goals are met, to some extent, by the parenteral administration of deferoxamine. The feroxamine formed outside cells cannot enter them and will prevent the iron from reaching its site of toxicity. Furthermore, feroxamine is eliminated into the urine and enhances urinary iron excretion.

Deferoxamine is rapidly metabolized to inactive products. Feroxamine is slowly metabolized and eliminated unchanged into the urine. As a result, it is optimal to provide the parenteral deferoxamine at frequent intervals intramuscularly or by continuous intravenous infusion. The only serious side effect is hypotension, and this has not been observed after intramuscular administration. If the intravenous administration is given at a dose of less than 15 mg/kg/hr, hypotension should not occur. The removal of iron is a function of the amount of deferoxamine given; consequently, the maximal effect can be realized by administering the maximal safe dose for a total daily dose of 360 mg/kg. In the older child or adult the maximum daily dose is 6 gm.

The duration of therapy with deferoxamine is not clearly established. As long as the urine remains pink, it can, be assumed that free iron is being removed. When normal color is seen, the deferoxamine is probably no longer removing iron and therapy should be discontinued within 24 hr. The same dose per 24 hr can be given subcutaneously, by continuous infusion, or by intermittent infusion every hr. The intramuscular administration is somewhat less efficient, and the injections should be spaced at 1–2 hr intervals to maintain plasma levels.

In renal failure feroxamine cannot be eliminated and can be toxic. It is dialyzable, however, and dialysis after the administration of deferoxamine would seem appropriate.

Covey TJ: Ferrous sulfate poisoning: A review, case summaries, and therapeutic regimen. J Pediatr 64:218, 1964.
Keberle H: The biochemistry of desferrioxamine and its relation to iron metabolism. Ann NY Acad Sci 119:758, 1964.
Propper RD, Cooper B, Rufo RR, et al: Continuous subcutaneous administration of deferoxamine in patients with iron overload. N Engl J Med 297:418, 1977.
Reissman KR, Coleman TJ, Budai BS, et al: Acute intestinal iron intoxication: I. Iron absorption, serum iron and autopsy findings. Blood 10:35, 1955.
Robotham JL, Lietman PS: Acute iron poisonings. Am J Dis Child 134:875, 1980.
Whitten CF, Brough AJ: The pathophysiology of acute iron poisoning. Clin Toxicol 4:585, 1971.
Whitten CF, Chen YC, Gibson GW: Studies in acute iron poisoning: II. Further observations on desferrioxamine in the treatment of acute experimental iron poisoning. Pediatrics 38:102, 1966.

28.11   TRICYCLIC ANTIDEPRESSANTS

The easy availability of tricyclic antidepressants to the small child resulting from their widespread use in adults has led to an increasing incidence of accidental ingestions. The 2 principal representatives of the group are amitriptyline and imipramine; others are nortriptyline (demethylated amitriptyline), desmethylimipramine (demethylated imipramine), protriptyline, and doxepin.

Fatalities are rare. However, an ingestion of as little as 9 mg/kg of imipramine has been reported fatal in a child. Since the dose of 2.5 mg/kg/24 hr is an accepted dose for the treatment of enuresis in children, the margin of safety of these drugs in children is quite small. On the other hand, the ingestion of as much as 5.4 gm has been reported without mortality in an adult.

Pathophysiology.   There may be considerable individual variation in the toxicologic response to a given dose of tricyclic antidepressants as a function of age, with children more susceptible than adults. Possible reasons for greater susceptibility to cardiotoxicity in children include less fat to allow storage of the drug in inactive sites; less protein-binding of the drug, allowing more to be free and toxic; and greater liver mass relative to body mass, providing greater capacity to produce toxic metabolites of the drug, which may also have untoward synergistic interactions with other drugs. The principal toxicologic effects of the tricyclic antidepressants are attributable to the anticholinergic properties of these drugs on the central and peripheral nervous systems. In addition, the tricyclic antidepressants or their metabolites may have a direct effect on the myocardium, reducing the force of myocardial contraction, and on the brain, leading to a diminished uptake of dopamine and serotonin with an increased effect of these endogenous neurotransmitters at their postsynaptic receptors.

Both amitriptyline and imipramine are rapidly and completely absorbed from the gastrointestinal tract. They are then widely distributed into many tissues where they are concentrated relative to the plasma, possibly on the basis of lipid solubility and tissue macromolecular binding. Plasma protein-binding is extensive. The elimination of amitriptyline and imipramine is a result of hepatic metabolism and urinary excretion of the parent drug and the metabolites. Though less effective, the metabolites may be even more toxic than the parent compounds. A very small proportion is eliminated as the unchanged drug. Neither unchanged drug nor metabolites are significantly affected by the urinary volume or pH. The volume of distribution of the drug is about 30 l/kg, and the half-life is 24 hr. However, because of individual variations, one cannot count on a specific half-life in any individual patient.

Clinical Manifestations.   The diagnosis of tricyclic antidepressant ingestion is often made by history alone. The clinical syndrome in children involves primarily the central nervous system, the peripheral autonomic nervous system, and the cardiovascular system and is attributable to the anticholinergic effects of these drugs.

The central nervous system manifestations include drowsiness or mild coma (Grade I of Matthew) alternating with agitation (especially upon stimulation), twitching or jerking, extrapyramidal rigidity, confusion, and hallucinations. Convulsions occur in the more severely affected children. The usual coma is described as coma vigil, a light coma from which the patient may be easily aroused and which is interrupted by myoclonic jerks and irritability. The peripheral autonomic nervous system manifestations include mydriasis, constipation, dry mouth, blurred vision, pyrexia, urinary retention, and absent bowel sounds. The cardiovascular signs include tachycardia in most patients. In severe cases ventricular premature contractions and conduction defects as well as hypotension may occur.

The onset of clinical disturbances occurs usually within 1 hr of ingestion, and the duration is usually less than 2 days. The physician should be alert to the possibility of recurrence of early symptoms, even in an improving patient, since such recurrences have been associated with late fatalities. Noble and Matthew have noted an absence of detectable blood levels of tricyclic antidepressant in most of their substantial series of cases in adults. The quantification of plasma levels is probably of little practical value since a relationship between severity of intoxication and plasma levels has been reported in only a very few patients. Imipramine in the gastric aspirate or urine may be identified in a qualitative manner by adding 1 ml of urine or gastric contents to 1 ml of Forest solution (25 parts of 0.2% potassium dichromate, 25 parts of 30% [by volume] sulfuric acid, 25 parts of 50% [by volume] nitric acid, and 25 parts of 20% perchloric acid). A pale olive to emerald green color indicates the presence of imipramine; a darker color occurs with greater concentrations.

Treatment. The prevention of continued absorption of tricyclic antidepressants requires a combination of emesis and the subsequent oral administration of charcoal. The charcoal may bind both the drug and its metabolic products that have been excreted into the intestine via the bile, which otherwise would be reabsorbed via the enterohepatic circulation.

It is not possible to increase the elimination of tricyclic antidepressants significantly by diuresis, dialysis, and hemoperfusion through columns since renal elimination occurs only after extensive metabolism, the drugs are highly protein-bound, and the drugs and their active metabolites are widely distributed in areas outside the vascular system. Nevertheless, hemoperfusion has been associated with prompt clinical improvement in several small series of poisoned patients. Forced diuresis may cause harm by increasing the cardiovascular work load, which is 1 of the factors contributing to severe cardiovascular toxicity.

Physostigmine is clinically effective in counteracting most of the serious consequences of tricyclic antidepressant poisoning. It enters the central nervous system and inhibits acetylcholinesterase, the enzyme responsible for the physiologic destruction of acetylcholine. It thus increases the effective levels of acetylcholine and overcomes the anticholinergic properties of these drugs. Coma is reversed by physostigmine as are at least some of the cardiovascular effects of tricyclic antidepressant drugs. The onset of action of physostigmine is rapid. A failure to respond within 10 min is an indication for a 2nd dose, but it is also highly suggestive that a tricyclic antidepressant is not solely responsible for the symptomatology. The physostigmine should be administered slowly (over 2 min) by intravenous infusion at a dose of 0.5 mg in toddlers (adult dose, 2.0 mg) and may be repeated at 5 min intervals until a total of 4 doses has been given. The duration of action of physostigmine is short compared with that of the tricyclic antidepressants, and additional doses (0.5 mg in a toddler; 2 mg in an adult) may be necessary at 1–3 hr intervals. Side effects of physostigmine include increased salivation, diarrhea, and bradycardia. If these are marked, a peripherally acting anticholinergic agent, such as propantheline bromide, may counteract the peripheral effects without diminishing the central effects of physostigmine.

The potentially serious cardiovascular effects of the tricyclic antidepressants may also respond to sodium bicarbonate, lidocaine, or propranolol. In adults a dose of 40 mEq of sodium bicarbonate intravenously has been suggested. Propranolol has also been advocated to block the prominent beta-adrenergic effects on the heart that may be involved with the inhibition of norepinephrine reuptake by tricyclic antidepressants. Lidocaine may be particularly useful in the presence of premature ventricular contractions. The use of cardiac glycosides should be avoided because of their potential for increasing the atrioventricular block produced by the tricyclic antidepressants. Norepinephrine should not be given since the inhibition of reuptake may contribute to a marked accentuation of the activity of this and other catecholamines. Monoamine oxidase inhibitors should not be given because of the potentiating effect of the tricyclic antidepressants in raising and maintaining catecholamine levels.

The lack of significant effect of tricyclic antidepressants on dopamine receptors favors the selection of dopamine as a pressor, should a pressor be necessary.

If physostigmine fails to control convulsions, diazepam is effective and is unlikely to contribute materially to respiratory depression. The barbiturates should be avoided because of their propensity to aggravate the respiratory depressive effects of the tricyclic antidepressants.

PAUL S. LIETMAN

Callaham M: Tricyclic antidepressant overdose. JACEP 8:413, 1979.
Crome P, Braithwaite RA: Relationship between clinical features of tricyclic antidepressant poisoning and plasma concentrations in children. Arch Dis Child 53:902, 1978.
Editorial: Physostigmine for tricyclic antidepressant overdosage. The Medical Letter 22:55, 1980.
Goel KM, Shanks RA: Amitriptyline and imipramine poisoning in children. Br Med J 1:261, 1974.
Noble J, Matthew H: Acute poisoning by tricyclic antidepressants: Clinical features and management of 100 patients. Clin Toxicol 2:403, 1969.
Pedersen RS: Haemoperfusion in tricyclic antidepressant poisoning. Lancet 1:154, 1980.
Robinson DS, Barker E: Tricyclic antidepressant cardiotoxicity. JAMA 236:2089, 1976.
Starkey IR, Lawson AAH: Poisoning with tricyclic and related antidepressants—A ten-year review. Quart J Med (NS) XLIX 193:33, 1980.
Young JA, Galloway WH: Treatment of severe imipramine poisoning. Arch Dis Child 46:353, 1971.

MERCURY

Mercury, both inorganic and organic, has been widely used for household, medical, agricultural, and industrial purposes and is known to cause acute and chronic poisoning. It has reversible or irreversible effects predominantly on the gastrointestinal tract and kidney in acute poisoning and on the central nervous system and skin in chronic poisoning. Because community poisoning from mercury is occurring worldwide with increasing frequency, it is essential to understand the implications and mechanisms of environmental contamination.

28.12 Acute and Chronic Mercury Poisoning

Etiology. Mercury vapor is highly toxic. Mercurous chloride, or calomel, is still used in some skin creams as an antiseptic. The mercurial diuretic chlormerodrin has also been used in roentgenographic scanning of kidney and brain. Phenylmercuric salts are used as a fungicide for seeds and in paints. Methylmercury compounds have been used extensively as fungicides, and poisonings have been reported from the ingestion of bread made from wheat treated with these compounds. Mercuric salts have wide application in industry, and contamination from these industries has led to problems of environmental pollution, notably methylmercury poisoning resulting from the ingestion of contaminated fish.

Clinical Manifestations. Exposure to high concentrations of mercury vapor may cause pulmonary irritation or bronchitis, nausea, vomiting, diarrhea, abdominal pain, and headache. Oral intake of mercury may cause stomatitis; gingivitis; esophagitis; gastroenteritis with excessive salivation; nausea, vomiting, and abdominal pain; and severe bloody diarrhea. Patients with kidney damage develop anuria, albuminuria, and uremia and frequently have a fatal outcome. Central nervous system symptoms include ataxia, slurring of speech, numbness of the hands and feet, visual and hearing impairment, and delirium.

Treatment. The emergency treatment of acute mercury poisoning consists of intravenous replacement of fluid and electrolytes to prevent peripheral vascular collapse and gastric lavage to remove the mercury in the stomach. Lavage is done first with milk and then repeated with 2–5% sodium bicarbonate.

The most effective antidote for acute mercury poisoning is BAL, British antilewisite or dimercaprol. The drug is administered intramuscularly in a 10% solution with a recommended dosage of 5 mg/kg for the 1st injection and 3 mg/kg every 4 hr for 2 days; this dose is then tapered to every 6 hr for 1 day, followed by administration every 12 hr for 7 days. BAL may be effective as protection against kidney damage from acute poisoning when given within 3 hr after ingestion of mercury. It may produce unpleasant side effects, such as nausea, vomiting, and fever, as the dose is increased. Penicillamine (N-acetyl-D,L-penicillamine) is not as effective as BAL in acute poisoning.

Symptomatic treatment is also important. Hydroxyzine and chlorpromazine may be useful for restlessness and tolazoline hydrochloride for tachycardia.

Peritoneal dialysis or hemodialysis may be indicated for acute renal failure.

Chronic mercury poisoning is generally occupational in adults and rare among children. However, acrodynia and Minamata disease are both well known as important clinical conditions in children. The central nervous system and skin are most frequently involved, and the symptoms are variable and irreversible in severe cases.

28.13 Acrodynia
(Pink Disease, Swift Disease; Feer Disease; Erythredema; Dermatopolyneuritis)

Acrodynia (the term, derived from Greek, denotes painful extremities) is principally a syndrome of chronic mercury poisoning in infants and young children consisting of many unusual symptoms which, in the well established cases, are so distinctive that there is practically no differential diagnosis. In few other conditions is extreme and persistent misery such a prominent part of the clinical picture. The condition was recognized in Australia as early as 1890 and established as a clinical entity in the British and American literature by Byfield and Bilderback in 1920.

Etiology. Most, and perhaps all, cases of acrodynia represent the clinical response to repeated contact with

or ingestion of mercury in products such as house paints, wallpapers, teething powders, vermifuges, and diaper rinses. The interval between mercury exposure and onset of symptoms may vary from 1 wk to several mo. The condition is probably the manifestation of a sensitization to mercury in the hypersensitive child.

Pathology. Pathologic findings are mainly present in the central nervous system. Degeneration and chromatolysis of the cerebral and cerebellar cortex are prominent.

Clinical Manifestations. The natural course of acrodynia is prolonged, extending from several mo to 1 yr. There are all grades of severity. The child becomes listless, no longer interested in play, restless, and irritable. Generalized inconstant rashes, which are protean, recur from time to time. Early, the tips of the fingers, toes, and nose acquire a pinkish color, and later the hands and feet become a dusky pink, with patchy areas of ischemia and cyanotic congestion. The coloring shades off at the wrists and ankles. These changes in the extremities are the most distinctive features of the syndrome and are responsible for the term pink disease. Frequently the cheeks and the tip of the nose acquire a scarlet color.

As the disease becomes established, the sweat glands are enormously dilated and enlarged, and perspiration is profuse. Secondary infection may lead to a severe pyoderma. There is desquamation of the soles and palms, which, though usually superficial, may be severe and recur during the course of the disease. The fingers and toes appear edematous; the swelling is due to hyperplasia and hyperkeratosis of the skin. An outstanding symptom is constant pruritus with excruciating pain in the hands and feet. Children will rub their hands together for hours, and older children will complain of a severe burning sensation.

The nails become dark and frequently drop off. Occasionally, gangrene of the toes and fingers develops, and trophic ulcers may result from the constant rubbing of the hands and feet. The hair tends to fall out and is often pulled out by the child.

There is photophobia without evidence of local inflammation of the eyes. The children shield their eyes or bury their faces in their pillows. The lax ligaments and hypotonia permit the children to assume unusual positions (Fig 28–1).

In extreme cases the teeth may be lost; necrosis of the jaw bones frequently follows. Initially, the gums appear normal except for a slightly deeper red color; later they become inflamed and swollen. Salivation then becomes pronounced, and the saliva often flows from the mouth in a constant stream. Anorexia is prominent, but because of the excessive perspiration large quantities of water are consumed. There may be diarrhea, and prolapse of the rectum is a frequent complication. The blood pressure and pulse rate may be increased significantly. Fever is usually not present unless there is some complication such as a urinary tract infection or bronchopneumonia.

Neurologic symptoms are an important part of the syndrome and include neuritis, mental apathy, and irritability. Early in the disease the tendon reflexes may be normal or increased, but later they disappear. There

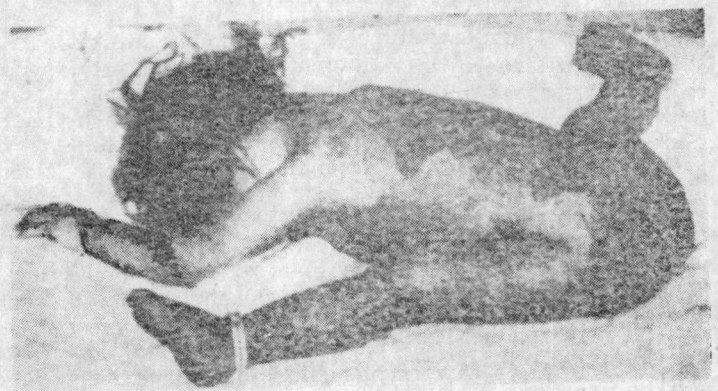

Figure 28–1 Extreme hypotonia and photophobia in an infant with acrodynia. This bizarre position may be maintained for hours.

is not a true motor paralysis, but because of the soft, flabby musculature the child has no desire to walk and is hypotonic, listless, and hypomotile. The severe pain prevents normal sleep. There is no time when a child with acrodynia appears happy or comfortable; the child does not play or smile but appears dejected and melancholic, a picture of abject misery.

Laboratory Data. There are no characteristic changes in the blood or cerebrospinal fluid. Proteinuria may occur, and a nephrotic syndrome may develop. Slit lamp examination may show a lenticular gray or red brown reflex.

Prevention. The withdrawal of mercury from various household products has led to a marked decrease in the incidence of acrodynia. However, mercurial drugs should be avoided in pediatric practice whenever possible, and the physician should be alert to other sources of mercury, especially contamination of food sources from agricultural processes and industrial waste.

Treatment. The treatment of acrodynia includes the removal of mercury, the administration of antidotes, and careful supportive measures.

BAL is effective, especially when given early in the disease, and the dose and side effects are the same as for acute poisonings (Sec 28.12). L-*Penicillamine* (N-acetyl-D,L-penicillamine) has been used successfully to treat acrodynia and has an advantage over BAL in that it can be given orally. The effective dose is 30 mg/kg daily in 2–3 divided doses for 4 wk or until symptoms improve. Side effects include fever, rashes, proteinuria, leukopenia, and thrombocytopenia.

Barbiturates, paraldehyde, hydroxyzine, or chlorpromazine may be used for irritability and pain. Nourishing foods containing proteins, minerals, and vitamins should be given. Frequently, nasogastric tube feeding is necessary for severe anorexia. Intravenous replacement of fluid and electrolytes may be required for severe dehydration. Appropriate antibiotics should be given for secondary pyogenic cutaneous and urinary infections.

28.14 Minamata Disease

Minamata disease (Fig 28–2) is a form of mercury poisoning which occurred among villagers, both adults and children, living in towns facing Minamata Bay, Kumamoto prefecture, Japan, from 1953–1966. The disease has become symbolic of the catastrophic health risks of industrial pollution (Sec 28.16).

Etiology. The causative agent of this disease is methylmercury which was released as industrial waste during the manufacture of acetaldehyde and vinyl chloride and was absorbed into the body by the ingestion of contaminated fish and shellfish. Congenital Minamata disease was produced by placental transfer of methylmercury to the fetus from the pregnant mother who had eaten contaminated fish. The fetus is more sensitive than the mother or the postnatal infant to toxic effects of methylmercury.

Pathology. Various degrees of regressive changes in the brain have been observed. Degeneration and loss of granular cells in the cortex of the cerebellum and central convolutions are prominent. In the congenital type more severe and widespread damage of the nerve cells in the cerebral and cerebellar cortices has been demonstrated.

Clinical Manifestations. The principal symptoms in the infantile form of Minamata disease include disturbance in hand coordination, gait, and speech. Masticating and swallowing difficulty and visual blurring also occur. Some patients complain of numbness and pain in the extremities, and in severe cases there are involuntary movements. Tremor, clouded consciousness,

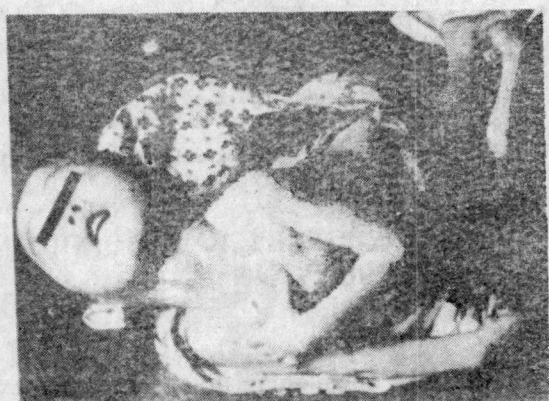

Figure 28–2 Congenital Minamata disease, showing severe hypertonicity and opisthotonos. (Courtesy of Dr. Y. Harada.)

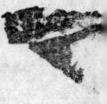

convulsions, and rigidity of the extremities are observed. Some patients have impaired hearing and constriction of the visual field. More generalized damage to the nervous system results from fetal poisoning. The principal clinical features of the congenital form include physical retardation, severe mental disturbance, delay in development, abnormal movement, or lack of smoothness in movement.

Laboratory Data. Mercury content in the hair of most patients is high, more than 20 p.p.m. Some patients have abnormal electroencephalograms and constricted visual fields. In the congenital form most patients have an abnormal pneumoencephalogram, cortical atrophy, and microcephalus. Chromosomal aberrations are not found.

Prevention. The environment should be kept free of mercury hazards. Special care should be taken with pregnant women because of the high sensitivity of fetuses to mercury. The maximum safe concentration of mercury in food is 0.3 p.p.m. of methylmercury. A level of over 40–50 p.p.m. of mercury in the hair is considered dangerous.

Treatment. In the early stages elimination of organic mercury exposure may be sufficient. Feeding of any foods suspected of contamination should be discontinued. Since transmission of mercury to infants in human milk has been proved, breast feeding should also be discontinued. BAL is effective in eliminating systemic mercury, and the dosage regimen is identical to that prescribed in acrodynia and acute poisonings. The diet should contain nourishing food rich in proteins, minerals, and vitamins. In severe cases tube feeding is necessary. Symptomatic treatment is increasingly important as time goes on. Anticonvulsive drugs are indicated for seizures. Damage is irreversible, and survivors require extensive rehabilitation, education, and long-term care.

TARO AKABANE

Amin-Zaki L, Elhassani S, Majeed MA, et al: Studies of infants postnatally exposed to methylmercury. J Pediatr 85:81, 1974.

Bilderback JB: Group of cases of unknown etiology and diagnosis. Northwest Med 19:263, 1920.

Bivings L: Acrodynia: A summary of BAL therapy reports and a case report of calomel disease. J Pediatr 34:322, 1949.

Harada Y, Moriyama H: Congenital Minamata disease. Bull Inst Constitut Med Kumamoto Univ 26:1, 1976.

Jabbtt SN: Acrodynia. In: Gellis SS, Kagan BM (eds): Current Pediatric Therapy. Ed 7. Philadelphia, WB Saunders, 1976.

Takeuchi T: Study group of Minamata disease. In: Katsuma M (ed): Minamata Disease. Japan. Kumamoto University, 1966.

Warkany J, Hubbard DM: Acrodynia and mercury. J Pediatr 42:365, 1953.

28.15 INCREASED LEAD ABSORPTION AND LEAD POISONING
(Plumbism)

Lead poisoning is a reportable chronic disease. It is most prevalent in children 1–6 yr of age who live in old, deteriorating dwellings. Most affected children have evidence of disturbed heme synthesis, but few have clear-cut symptoms. Acute encephalopathy is the most severe form of the disease. Chelation therapy substantially reduces mortality, but 50% or more of the survivors of encephalopathy treated *after* the onset of symptoms have sustained *severe* and permanent brain damage. An increased frequency of behavioral and cognitive deficits, which can impede progress in school, has been reported among some groups of children who had chronically increased lead absorption without symptoms during the preschool years. Such prognoses emphasize the need to detect and treat children with lead toxicity early. Screening tests for lead are now being incorporated more widely into Early Periodic Screening and Development Testing (EPSDT) programs.

Exposure. Food, water, and air contain small amounts of lead: the amount ingested daily in food and beverages is <100 μg Pb; in drinking water, <50 μg Pb/liter; in air, <1 μg Pb/M^3. Such usual exposures are associated with average blood lead levels (PbB)* of 10–15 μg and are without evident adverse effects on health. In adults an increase in airborne respirable lead of 1 μg Pb/M^3 increases lead in blood by 1 μg/dl.

Children may have multiple nondietary sources of exposure to lead. The powdering of paint from the surfaces of old buildings and the lead in automotive exhausts are major contributors to the lead content of surface soil and dust. While average daily diets may contain <100 μg Pb, house dust in old housing may average from 750–11,000 μg Pb/gm, and multilayered chips of old lead-pigment paints may contain 20,000–100,000 μg Pb/cm^2. Increased absorption of lead occurs among children living near lead-processing smelters or among children of workers who bring leaded dust into their homes on their work clothes. Sporadic cases of clinical plumbism have been traced to other sources of very high concentrations of lead, including (1) lead shot, fishing weights, and leaded jewelry swallowed and retained in the stomach, where the lead is dissolved and absorbed; (2) juices conveyed or stored in improperly lead-glazed earthenware; (3) lead type or toys, on which children may chew; (4) lead nipple shields; (5) "soft" drinking water stored in lead-lined cisterns; (6) lead-soldered vessels used in cooking; (7) fumes from burning casings of storage batteries; and (8) dust from sanding and burning of paint containing lead. The above exposures cause *inorganic* lead poisoning. Sniffing of leaded gasoline by older children and adolescents causes organic lead poisoning characterized by toxic encephalopathy.

Epidemiology. Factors which influence the occurrence, chronicity, and severity of lead poisoning include season, size of lead-containing particulates, residence, parental occupation, and, in the child, age, hand-to-mouth activity, and pica. PbB fluctuates seasonally, being highest in summer, when most acute symptomatic episodes occur. Absorption of lead from the intestinal tract is inversely proportional to particle size. In the United States, 90% or more of homes built and painted before 1950 contain lead paints on exposed surfaces. Many are now in a deteriorated state with

---

*See Table 28–1 for key to abbreviations used in this chapter.

powdering, flaking paint and crumbling old putty. Household dust in such homes is often rich in lead, and exterior surface soil generally has a high lead content. In young children PbB is most closely correlated with Pb on the surface of their hands and the Pb content of household dust in their homes. The usual hand-to-mouth activity found in preschool children can, if they are exposed to dust containing greater than 1000 μg Pb/gm of dust, produce PbB values falling in Groups II and III (Table 28–1). The more severe degrees of poisoning (Group IV, Table 28–1) are generally associated with repetitive ingestion (pica) of leaded paint flakes.

Metabolism. Absorption of lead from the gastrointestinal tract is affected by age, diet, and nutritional deficiencies. Although adults absorb 5–10% of dietary lead and retain little of it, young children absorb 40–50% and retain 20–25%. Spontaneous urinary excretion of lead is <50 μg/24 hr; it may be higher in acute poisoning. Studies in young growing animals have shown that diets high in fat and, especially, those low in calcium, magnesium, iron, zinc, and copper increase the absorption of lead. Diets suboptimal in calcium and iron are prevalent among children in low income groups. The total body lead burden is divided into 2 major compartments: bone, in which the amount increases with age and has a residence time of 27 yr, and soft tissues, in which the residence time is about 40 days. The lead sequestered in bone is removed from the active metabolic pool. The toxicity of lead is related to its concentration in the small, mobile, soft tissue pool.

Untoward Effects. The principal toxic effects occur in the erythroid cells of the bone marrow, the central and peripheral nervous systems, and the kidney. Abnormalities in cardiac conduction and thyroid function

have also been reported in severe cases. Lead causes partial inhibition in the synthesis of heme at several enzymatic steps (Fig 8–33). Heme synthetase and δ-aminolevulinate dehydratase (ALAD) are the enzymes most sensitive to inhibition by lead. There is a compensatory increase in the activity of the 1st enzyme in the pathway, δ-aminolevulinate synthetase. The following combination is pathognomonic for lead poisoning: increased activity of δ-aminolevulinate synthetase, decreased activity of δ-aminolevulinate dehydratase in erythrocytes, increased δ-aminolevulinic acid in plasma and urine, normal or slightly increased urinary porphobilinogen and uroporphyrin, increased urinary coproporphyrin, and increased free erythrocyte protoporphyrin (FEP). Though the porphyrin found in the circulating erythrocytes in lead poisoning and in iron deficiency is the metalloporphyrin zinc protoporphyrin, this metabolite is generally *measured* as "free" erythrocyte protoporphyrin. Bioavailability of iron and the rates of heme and globin formation are reduced. Compensatory erythroid hyperplasia and reticulocytosis result. Basophilic stippling is best seen in normoblasts in bone marrow. As the concentration of lead in blood increases above 50–60 μg/dl, hemoglobin decreases. The microcytic, hypochromic anemia of plumbism is usually indistinguishable, morphologically, from that of iron deficiency.

Severe acute lead poisoning may be responsible for the Fanconi syndrome (generalized renal aminoaciduria, mellituria, hyperphosphaturia, and hypophosphatemia) because of acute proximal renal tubular injury. The lesion is reversible. Lead nephropathy, characterized by hyperuricemia with or without gout, has been reported as a sequel of chronic plumbism in children in Australia. Acute lead encephalopathy is characterized by massive cerebral edema due primarily to a general-

Table 28–1 LABORATORY TEST RESULTS USUALLY ASSOCIATED WITH VARIOUS LEVELS OF LEAD ABSORPTION

Blood Lead (PbB) Groups*	Normal	Increased Lead Absorption		
	I	II	III	IV
Indicators of internal dose (soft tissue concentrations)				
PbB (μg/dl w.b.)	5–29	30–49	50–69	$\overline{>}70$
PbU-EDTA†	0.23 ± 0.08		>1	>2.2
Indicators of disturbed heme synthesis				
ALAD‡	1.1 + 0.37		<10–15%	<10–15%
ALAU§			>3	$\overline{>}6$
EP (μg/dl w.b.)¶	<49	50–109	110–249	$\geq$250
FEP (μg/dl rbc)**	70 ± 22	132–288	289–655	>658

*Adapted from Statement by Center for Disease Control, J Pediatr 93:709, 1978.

†Results expressed as μg Pb excreted/mg CaEDTA administered during 24 hr following a single intramuscular injection of CaEDTA in a dosage of 500 mg/M². Mean normal value for PbB is 20 μg.

‡Results vary according to method; however, for most methods when PbB >50–60 μg, then ALAD <10–15% of normal for each method, PbU-EDTA >1 and ALA-U begins to increase exponentially from 3 mg/M²/24 hr.

§ALAU results expressed as mg/M²/24 hr. Less specific screening methods give values for ALAU (1) 0.5–1.0 mg/M²/24 hr higher than values shown above. See Nordberg GF: Effects and Dose-Response Relationships of Toxic Metals. New York, Elsevier, 1976, Chapter B16.

¶Note results expressed as μg erythrocyte protoporphyrin (EP)/dl whole blood as used in many screening programs.

**Normal values based on several reports. FEP values for Groups II, III, and IV calculated from EP values on basis of 38% hematocrit. EP and FEP values are for microfluorometric methods.

Abbreviations:
ALAD = δ-aminolevulinate dehydratase in erythrocytes.
ALAU = δ-aminolevulinic acid in urine.
CaEDTA = edathamil calcium disodium.
EP = erythrocyte protoporphyrin (as μg/dl whole blood).
FEP = "free" erythrocyte protoporphyrin (as μg/dl erythrocytes).

Pb = lead.
PbB = μg Pb/dl whole blood.
PbU = μg Pb/24 hr in urine.
PbU-EDTA = chelatable lead (μg Pb excreted in urine after standard dose of CaEDTA).

ized increase in vascular permeability. Neuronal destruction also occurs. In suckling animals, but not in mature animals, slowness in learning and behavioral changes can be induced by doses of lead insufficient to produce histopathologic changes.

Clinical Manifestations.   The chronic course of unrecognized lead poisoning is characterized by recurrent symptomatic episodes which may abate spontaneously. The occurrence and severity of symptoms depend upon the episodic nature of pica and the amount of lead ingestion. The earliest symptoms are hyperirritability, anorexia, and decreased play activity. Sporadic vomiting, intermittent abdominal pain, and constipation are manifestations of lead colic. Colic may occur at blood levels of lead as low as 60 µg/dl, but children with levels of up to 250 µg may appear clinically well. Loss of recently acquired developmental skills may occur, and anemia is usually present.

The above symptoms usually, but not always, appear 4–6 wk prior to the start of acute encephalopathy, which is heralded by the sudden onset of persistent vomiting, ataxia, impairment of consciousness, coma, and seizures. Massive cerebral edema is present, though the classic signs of increased intracranial pressure may not be found. Subtle premonitory behavioral changes may not have been appreciated. Acute encephalopathy, in which blood lead concentrations almost always exceed 100 µg/dl and usually exceed 150 µg/dl, is most common during the summer months. The diagnosis can usually be made without lumbar puncture, which is very risky. If examination of the cerebrospinal fluid is considered essential for differential diagnosis, the least amount of fluid required should be obtained (several drops). In lead encephalopathy the changes in the fluid consist of mild pleocytosis and mild to moderate increase in protein, and there is increased intracranial pressure. Observation for inappropriate secretion of antidiuretic hormone, partial heart block, and profoundly impaired renal function must be maintained in the seriously ill child. Peripheral neuropathy in lead poisoning, manifested in adults principally by motor weakness in the distal muscles of the arms and legs, is rare in children.

Clinical Diagnosis.   Symptoms are subtle and nonspecific, and physical examination generally reveals little or nothing abnormal unless there is acute encephalopathy. Plumbism should be included in the differential diagnosis of anemia, seizure disorders, mental retardation, and severe behavioral disorders. Isolated seizures and self-limited episodes of vomiting during the recent past may represent episodes of plumbism, particularly if the child lives in or visits an old house, if a parent is unavailable for much of the time, and if a history of pica for any substance is obtained. Recent changes of address, recent renovations in the home, and, especially, time spent unsupervised or with babysitters and relatives should be ascertained since persistent pica is particularly associated with inadequate mothering. This information is essential in planning the details of management appropriate for each patient. Emphasis must be placed on environmental and behavioral history, environmental sampling for sources of lead, and laboratory data. Whenever an index case is found, other housemates aged 1–6 yr should also be examined.

Laboratory Diagnosis.   Because clinical diagnosis is exceedingly difficult in children prior to the occurrence of severe injury to the nervous system, early diagnosis depends on laboratory determinations. At least 2 tests are required: an indicator of the internal accumulation of lead and an indicator of adverse metabolic effect (Table 28–1). Blood lead and "free" erythrocyte protoporphyrin (FEP) can be determined in micro blood samples as well as in venous blood obtained in hematology Vacutainers containing EDTA as anticoagulant. Special precautions are needed to prevent contamination of blood and urine samples by exogenous lead. Serial tests are needed to determine trends of the blood concentrations. Iron deficiency may cause erythrocyte protoporphyrin (FEP) to be as high as 500 µg/dl of packed red blood cells when the blood lead level is normal; higher values generally indicate lead toxicity (blood lead Groups III and IV, Table 28–1) with or without iron deficiency. In Groups III and IV toxic effects of lead increase at an exponential rate. In emergencies, when these tests are not immediately available and acute lead encephalopathy is a diagnostic possibility, a strongly positive qualitative urinary coproporphyrin test, many stippled erythroblasts in bone marrow, glycosuria, and hypophosphatemia constitute presumptive evidence of plumbism. The diagnostic edathamil calcium disodium (CaEDTA) mobilization test for chelatable lead in urine *should not be used in patients with symptoms compatible with plumbism*. Radiopaque flecks in the intestinal tract indicate recent ingestion of foreign matter containing lead. Broad bands of increased density at the metaphyses of the long bones usually represent increased storage of lead in bone, but roentgenograms of long bones may be normal or equivocal in severe acute plumbism.

Short-term responses to treatment may be monitored by urinary output of lead δ-aminolevulinic acid in urine (ALAU) or δ-aminolevulinate dehydratase in erythrocytes (ALAD). FEP values, which tend to change slowly, are not predictive of chelatable lead (PbU-EDTA, Table 28–1); however, serial FEP tests are useful to monitor long-term responses to therapy and trends in lead absorption. Blood lead values or measurement of chelatable lead in urine following a standard dose of edathamil calcium disodium (CaEDTA) in an asymptomatic patient should be obtained since laws requiring the abatement of housing hazards are tied directly to the measurement of lead in the child.

Treatment.   The principal concern of therapy is prompt separation of the child from the source(s) of lead followed by timely reduction of lead hazards in his or her environment. Removal of hazards is usually the local health agency's responsibility. Children and pregnant women should remain out of the home *day and night* until the burning and sanding to remove old leaded paint are completed and the premises have been thoroughly scrubbed with high phosphate detergents 2–3 times to remove the fine particulate lead generated by the burning and sanding process. Thereafter, regular wet cleaning with high phosphate detergents for dust control should be continued, particularly in old housing areas. Play in dirt areas adjacent to such housing should also be avoided. Preschool age children should be tested periodically according to CDC and EPSDT guidelines to determine trends in lead absorption.

Most children detected in current screening programs are asymptomatic and fall into Groups II and III (Table 28–1). For those in Group II, the above measures and improved diet should suffice, and chelation therapy is probably not advisable.

Chelation therapy is advised for children in Groups III and IV, even for the asymptomatic ones. Intramuscular therapy with CaEDTA should be limited to 3–5 days at a daily dose of 1000 mg/M² in 2 divided portions, when venous PbB >50 but <90–100 µg/dl whole blood. Chelation therapy prior to the onset of symptoms may lessen the risk of cerebral injury. Oral treatment with CaEDTA is contraindicated. Oral D-penicillamine is effective only if current exposure to lead is definitely excluded. In the United States D-penicillamine is presently classed by the FDA as an investigational drug when it is used for lead poisoning. Side effects of this drug include allergic reactions, nephrotic syndrome, and bone marrow suppression, especially neutropenia.

Symptomatic plumbism (colic, seizures, acute encephalopathy) should be treated promptly with chelating agents if presumptive laboratory tests are positive. Since the onset and clinical course of encephalopathy are unpredictable, the risk of delay outweighs the risk of a few days of chelation therapy. If subsequent tests do not indicate an increased absorption of lead, treatment should be discontinued and the presumptive diagnosis should be reconsidered.

When acute encephalopathy is present and when PbB >90–100 µg/dl whole blood, a regimen of BAL and CaEDTA is recommended: the dose for BAL is 500 mg/M²/24 hr and that for CaEDTA is 1500 mg/M²/24 hr. The drugs are injected simultaneously at separate intramuscular sites in 6 divided doses each day for 5 days, after an initial priming dose of BAL only. In moderately ill children who show immediate clinical improvement after initiation of this regimen, BAL may be stopped after 3 days, and the total daily dose of CaEDTA should be reduced by one third after 72 hr. If repeated 3–5 day courses are needed, a daily dose of 1000 mg/M²/24 hr of CaEDTA is safer and adequate. If the patient becomes anuric, administration of CaEDTA, but not of BAL, should be temporarily withheld. CaEDTA is a nonmetabolizable drug that is excreted solely by the kidney. Side effects of CaEDTA include hypercalcemia, elevation of blood urea nitrogen, and renal injury. Side effects of BAL include vomiting, hypertension, and tachycardia. Side effects of each drug require careful evaluation since some of them are also features of acute lead encephalopathy. BAL may occasionally evoke intravascular hemolysis in patients with severe glucose-6-phosphate dehydrogenase deficiency.

Fluid and electrolyte management are critical in lead encephalopathy. After an initial infusion of 10% dextrose in water (and of mannitol, if necessary to decrease intracranial pressure) to establish urine flow, continuous intravenous infusion should be restricted to basal requirements and a minimal estimate of the amounts required for replacement of losses due to vomiting, dehydration, and activity associated with seizures. It is prudent to manage administration of parenteral fluids initially in the same manner in mildly symptomatic patients and in asymptomatic ones who have very high tissue levels of lead until the trend of the clinical course becomes clear. The use of enemas to remove lead from the lower bowel should never be permitted to delay treatment in symptomatic patients.

Seizures can be controlled initially with diazepam and thereafter with repeated doses of paraldehyde until the patient's state of consciousness is much improved. As the dose of paraldehyde is lowered, long-term anticonvulsant therapy with diphenylhydantoin or phenobarbital is started (see Table 29–1B and Sec 20.3 and 20.4). When lead poisoning results from ingestion of lead paint, effective long-term management requires the cooperative efforts of local health department personnel, the medical social worker, the psychologist or psychiatrist, and the pediatrician. Control of pica is particularly difficult to accomplish.

Prognosis. Sequelae are related to the degree and duration of excessive lead ingestion. Recurrence of clinical manifestations increases the chance of permanent injury. Residual brain damage may not be evident until school age. Some survivors of encephalopathy may require residential care; sequelae include seizure disorders, impaired mentation, and attentional deficit. Seizures and altered behavior tend to abate during adolescence, but intellectual deficits persist. Blindness and hemiparesis are restricted to the most severe cases of encephalopathy.

There is general agreement that PbB, if sustained during early childhood in the range of Groups III and IV, presents an unacceptable risk for long lasting but subtle injury to the nervous system even if no symptoms are ever detected. An increased frequency of learning difficulties in school has been reported among groups of children with a previous record of PbB values in Groups III and IV who had no symptoms and were never treated. There is some evidence that chelation therapy to reduce body lead burden and prompt steps to reduce further excess Pb intake may improve prognosis in asymptomatic children in Groups III and IV. Recently, in a study of over 2000 children, a dose-response relationship was shown between the frequency of behavioral and attentional problems in school and the dentin Pb content of shed deciduous teeth. Some of these children had earlier PbB values in the range of Group II (Table 28–1).

Prevention. Various federal agencies have taken steps during the past decade to reduce air Pb levels, enforce the drinking water standard for Pb, and reduce the Pb content of foods, particularly canned foods. The use of lead additives in residential paints was banned by the United States Consumer Product Safety Commission in 1977. However, a large stock of older residential housing coated with Pb paints remains in use. Until this housing is renovated or replaced, screening programs will be needed for early detection of lead toxicity in young children.

J. JULIAN CHISOLM, JR.

Baker EL Jr, Folland DS, Taylor TA, et al: Lead poisoning in children of lead workers. Home contamination with industrial dust. N Engl J Med 296:260, 1977.

Barltrop D: The prevalence of pica. Am J Dis Child 112:116, 1966.

Boeckx RL, Posti B, Coodin FJ: Gasoline sniffing and tetraethyl lead poisoning in children. Pediatrics 60:140, 1977.

Center for Disease Control: Preventing lead poisoning in young children, 1978 Statement. J Pediatr 93:709, 1978.

Chisolm JJ Jr: The use of chelating agents in the treatment of acute and chronic lead intoxication in childhood. J Pediatr 73:1, 1968.

Chisolm JJ Jr, Barrett MB, Mellits ED: Dose-effect and dose-response relationships for lead in children. J Pediatr 87:1152, 1975.

Chisolm JJ Jr, Barltrop D: Recognition and management of children with increased lead absorption. Arch Dis Child 54:249, 1979.

Emmerson BT: The clinical differentiation of lead gout from primary gout. Arthritis Rheum 11:623, 1968.

Lourie RS, Layman EM, Millican FK: Why children eat things that are not food. Children 10:143, 1963.

Needleman HL, Gunnoe C, Leviton A, et al: Deficits in psychologic and classroom performance of children with elevated dentine lead levels. N Engl J Med 300:689, 1979.

Perlstein MA, Attala R: Neurologic sequelae of plumbism in children. Clin Pediatr 5:292, 1966.

Rabinowitz MB, Wetherill GW, Kopple JD: Kinetic analysis of lead metabolism in healthy humans. J Clin Invest 58:260, 1976.

Roels HA, Buchet JP, Lauwerys RR, et al: Exposure to lead by the oral and the pulmonary routes of children living in the vicinity of a primary lead smelter. Env Res 22:81, 1980.

Rutter M: Raised lead levels and impaired cognitive/behavioural functioning: A review of the evidence. Develop Med Child Neurol 22(Suppl), 26 pp, 1980.

Sayre JW, Charney E, Vostal J, et al: House and hand dust as a potential source of childhood lead exposure. Am J Dis Child 127:167, 1974.

USEPA: Air Quality Criteria for Lead. Office of Research and Development, USEPA, EPA-600/8-77-017, Dec 1977.

28.16   CHEMICAL POLLUTANTS

As chemicals increasingly permeate our environment, there is a need to consider special exposures and vulnerability of the fetus and child. Since no federal health agency has the responsibility for this area of concern, it is up to each pediatrician to be alert for evidence of new environmental effects on child health. Alert clinical observers have discovered virtually all known human teratogens and carcinogens.

INTRAUTERINE EFFECTS

Methylmercury.   In the mid 1950s methylmercury caused the 1st epidemic of congenital cerebral palsy attributable to intrauterine exposures to a chemical pollutant (Sec 28.14). It was associated with severe, sometimes fatal, neurologic disorders in the population at large and was traced to contamination of fish by waste dumped into Minamata Bay, Japan, by a factory that made vinyl plastics. Similar episodes have occurred elsewhere in the world, among them a family affected in Alamogordo, New Mexico, and thousands of people affected in Iraq. Both occurred because grain treated prior to planting with a methylmercury-containing fungicide was mistakenly used for animal feed and baking.

Polychlorinated Biphenyls (PCBs).   In 1968 in Kyushu, Japan, there was an epidemic of chloracne, and women who were pregnant at the time gave birth to infants who were small for gestational age and had, among other findings, dark skin which cleared with time. The outbreak was traced to contamination of cooking oil by PCBs, a heat-transfer agent, through pinhole erosions in pipes during the manufacture of the oil. PCBs from factory waste have now been found in major waterways of the United States and other countries. A similar compound, polybrominated biphenyl (PBB), was accidentally mixed with animal feed in Michigan and widely distributed within the state. Animals became ill and died, but as yet no fetal effects or other overt illnesses have been found in human beings. PBBs from factory waste have also been found in catfish in the Ohio River.

Dioxin.   In 1976 a runaway reaction in a factory in Seveso, Italy, spewed a chemical cloud downwind over farms and homes. Many animals died, and 2 wk later about 40 exposed children developed chloracne. It was then learned that the chemical in the cloud was dioxin, a potent teratogen in laboratory animals. No human teratogenesis has been found among the abortuses or liveborn children of Seveso women exposed early in pregnancy. In Missouri, horse arenas and roads were sprayed with waste oil to which dioxin had been added; about 60 horses died, and foals were malformed. Transient illness, but not chloracne, occurred in 1 arena owner and her 2 children.

Cigarette Smoke.   On the average, the birth weight of infants whose mothers smoke heavily during pregnancy is 200 gm less than normal, and perinatal morbidity is increased when medical care is inadequate (Sec 7.6).

Transplacental Carcinogenesis.   The discovery that cancer of the cervix or vagina occurs in women up to 28 yr of age after intrauterine exposure to diethylstilbestrol raises the possibility that other chemicals, including pollutants, may also be transplacental carcinogens. Four children have now been reported with fetal hydantoin syndrome and neuroblastoma, suggesting that diphenylhydantoin is a transplacental carcinogen. Among other possible carcinogens is benzene, which causes leukemia after heavy occupational exposures.

LACTATIONAL EFFECTS

Because of chemical pollution, new questions are being raised about the safety of breast feeding. PCBs, PBBs, dioxin, and certain pesticides are stored in fat and are not readily cleared from the body except in the fat of breast milk. Japanese infants whose mothers were exposed postpartum to PCB-contaminated cooking oil were exposed to high levels in their mothers' milk while nursing. Elsewhere, samples of breast milk to date have rarely shown high levels of these chemicals. When unusual exposures occur, however, before advice on breast feeding is given, the milk should be tested, e.g., for dioxin in Seveso, for PBBs in Michigan, or for PCBs in upper New York State or anywhere where game fish come from PCB-polluted waters. No general recommendation against breast feeding should be made because of its many benefits. Cows' milk may also contain these chemicals, but tests are routinely made to determine that the milk sold commercially does not exceed limits set by federal regulation.

EFFECTS OF OTHER EXPOSURES

Water.   Pollution of drinking water has come from asbestos discharged into Lake Superior by a factory near Duluth, Minnesota. No effect among the populace has been detected yet, but asbestos is known to cause mesothelioma after occupational, neighborhood, or household exposures. Water that passes through serpentine rock also contains small amounts of asbestos fibers.

About 200 chemicals have been found in small amounts in various water supplies. Some are known to cause human cancer after heavy occupational exposure, but the claim that regional increases in cancer mortality rates are attributable to chemicals in the water supply is not generally accepted. Fluoride, added to water or naturally occurring, is not associated with human cancer.

Air. Major air pollutants generated by fossil fuel consumption are sulfur oxides, carbon monoxide, photochemical oxidants (especially ozone), and nitrogen oxides. The most common respiratory diseases associated with these pollutants are asthma, chronic bronchitis, and emphysema. Automotive exhausts add lead to the atmosphere and, in enclosed spaces, can cause intense pollution with carbon monoxide to which children have been especially susceptible, as in underground garages or at skating rinks where gasoline-powered vehicles were used to scrape the ice. Some industries have caused specific diseases in neighboring residential areas through air pollution with asbestos, beryllium, lead, methylmercury, or dioxin. There is an increased mortality from lung cancer among persons living in counties with arsenic-emitting smelters or petrochemical industries.

Workclothes. Illnesses in the child are at times traceable to a parent's workclothes; toxicity from lead, beryllium, and asbestos has occurred. Pediatricians, in considering the origins of noninfectious diseases, should ask about parental occupation, unusual household exposures, and neighborhood factories (mesothelioma induced by asbestos has a latent period of about 40 yr).

Food. In addition to the foregoing chemical pollutants which may enter the food chain, many other chemicals are intentionally added to food to improve appearance, taste, texture, or preservation. Evaluation of the safety of these chemicals is difficult because of problems in measuring exposures and in separating them from the effects of the myriad of variables which may confound interpretation of the observations made.

INTERACTIONS

Little is known at present about the interactions of chemicals with one another, with physical or viral agents, or with susceptibilities. Furthermore, chemicals may be activated or inactivated by metabolic processes, thus altering their disease potential. One would expect children with heritable methemoglobin reductase deficiency to be especially susceptible to the effects of nitrates or aniline dyes. Other children from the general population may be exceptionally resistant. Some chemicals photosensitize the skin as a consequence of an interaction with a physical agent, ultraviolet light. Asbestos greatly potentiates the capacity of cigarette smoke to induce lung cancer, the frequency being 92 times greater than that in people who neither smoke

nor are occupationally exposed to asbestos. Children with asbestos in their homes or neighborhoods may be especially prone to the carcinogenicity of cigarette smoking later in life. An interaction between old viruses and new chemicals may explain the increased frequency of diseases such as Reye syndrome, necrotizing enterocolitis, or the mucocutaneous lymph node syndrome.

Susceptibility to chemical pollutants varies markedly from conception through adolescence. Exposures also vary as the environment changes from that within the uterus to the nursery, home, school, neighborhood, recreational area, and, occasionally, the hospital. Greater attention must be given by pediatricians to the effects of chemical pollutants, and environmental experts must become more aware of the special biology and surroundings of the fetus and child.

ROBERT W. MILLER

Allen RW Jr, Ogden B, Bentley FL, et al: Fetal hydantoin syndrome, neuroblastoma, and hemorrhagic disease in a neonate. JAMA 244:1464, 1980.
Chisolm JJ Jr: Fouling one's own nest. Pediatrics 62:614, 1978.
Miller RW (ed): The susceptibility of the fetus and child to chemical pollutants. Pediatrics 53(Suppl):777, 1974.
Miller RW: Environmental cuases of cancer in childhood. Adv Pediatr 25:97, 1978.
Miller RW: Areawide chemical contamination: Lessons from case histories. JAMA 245:1548, 1981.
O'Brien PC, Noller KL, Robboy SF, et al: Vaginal epithelial changes in young women enrolled in the National Cooperative Diethylstilbestrol Adenosis (DESAD) Project. Obstet Gynecol 53:300, 1979.
Rogan WJ: The sources and routes of childhood chemical exposures. J Pediatr 97:861, 1980.
Rogan WJ, Bagniewska A, Damstra T: Pollutants in breast milk. N Engl J Med 302:1450, 1980.

28.17 FETAL ALCOHOL SYNDROME

High levels of alcohol ingestion during pregnancy can be damaging to embryonic and fetal development. A specific pattern of malformation identified as the fetal alcohol syndrome has been documented, and major and minor components of the syndrome are expressed in 1–2 infants/1000 live births. Both moderate and high levels of alcohol intake during early pregnancy may result in alterations in growth and morphogenesis of the fetus; the greater the intake, the more severe the signs. Ouellette prospectively evaluated the risk to offspring of heavy drinking during pregnancy and documented that infants born to heavy drinkers had twice the risk of abnormality compared with those born to abstinent or moderate drinkers; 32% of infants born to heavy drinkers demonstrated congenital anomalies, compared with 9% in the abstinent and 14% in the moderate group. The majority of affected children who are retrospectively identified have serious mental handicaps. A significant relationship exists between the severity of dysmorphogenesis and mental dysfunction.

The characteristics of the fetal alcohol syndrome include the following: (1) prenatal onset and persistence of growth deficiency for length, weight, and head circumference; (2) facial abnormalities, including short palpebral fissures, epicanthal folds, maxillary hypoplasia, micrognathia, and thin upper lip; (3) cardiac defects, primarily septal defects; (4) minor joint and limb abnormalities, including some restriction of movement and altered palmar crease patterns; and (5) delayed development and mental deficiency varying from borderline to severe. The severity of dysmorphogenesis may range from the severely affected with full manifestations of the fetal alcohol syndrome to those mildly affected with only a few manifestations.

The detrimental effects may be due to the alcohol itself or to 1 of its breakdown products. Complications of alcohol ingestion, including hypoglycemia, ketosis, and lacticacidemia, may be contributory. However, Chernoff produced a pattern of malformation in mice similar to the fetal alcohol syndrome, including prenatal growth deficiency, neural and cardiac anomalies, skeletal dysmorphogenesis, and prenatal wastage. He controlled energy, vitamin, and nutrient intake and found a dose response curve to varying ethanol intakes; high alcohol blood levels were embryolethal and lower levels caused brain malformations. There is suggestive evidence that alcohol may impair placental transfer of essential amino acids and zinc, which are necessary for protein synthesis, accounting for the intrauterine growth retardation.

The *management* of these infants may be difficult. No specific therapy, apart from the correction of hypoglycemia when it occurs, is indicated. The infants may remain hypotonic and tremulous despite sedation, and the prognosis is poor. Counseling with regard to recurrence is important. *Prevention* is achieved by restricting alcohol intake to an absolute maximum of 2 drinks/day (1$\frac{1}{3}$ oz of absolute alcohol) during pregnancy.

Alcohol withdrawal may occur when alcohol has been used to suppress premature labor. Infants may have an odor of alcohol on the breath and for 48–72 hr exhibit hyperactivity, tremors, and seizures. This period is followed by a lethargic phase before resumption of normal activity and responsiveness.

AVROY A. FANAROFF

Chernoff GG: The fetal alcohol syndrome in mice. Teratology 15:223, 1977.
Clarren SK, Alvord EC Jr, Sumi SM, et al: Brain malformations related to prenatal exposure to ethanol. J Pediatr 92:64, 1978.
Fisher SE, Atkinson M, Holzman I, et al: Selective fetal malnutrition. A new concept in the fetal alcohol syndrome (abstract). Pediatr Res 15:532, 1981.
Jones KL, Smith DH, Ulleland CN, et al: Patterns of malformation in offspring of chronic alcoholic mothers. Lancet 1:1267, 1973.
Ouellette EM, Rosett HL, Rosman P, et al: Adverse effects on offspring of maternal alcohol abuse during pregnancy. N Engl J Med 297:528, 1977.
Streissguth AP, Herman CS, Smith DW: Intelligence, behavior and dysmorphogenesis in the fetal alcoholic syndrome: A report on 20 patients. J Pediatr 92:363, 1978.

28.18   VENOM DISEASES; POISONING BY VENOMOUS SNAKES, LIZARDS, AND MARINE ANIMALS

The fear of venomous animals dates from antiquity, but the knowledge of venomous disease remains limited. As modern transportation makes remote areas of the world more accessible and interest in outdoor recreational activities expands, contact with venomous animals is likely to increase.

SNAKE BITE

Of the more than 3500 known species of snakes, only 200 that belong to the following 4 families are poisonous to man. They have in common a modified salivary gland which secretes and stores venom and maxillary fangs for conducting the venom to the victim.

The Colubridae family includes most of the world's snakes, but only the African boomslang (*Dispholidus typus*) and the vine, twig, or bird snake (*Thelotornis kirtlandi*) have been associated with human fatalities.

The Elapidae family includes many of the world's deadliest snakes. The Afro-Asian cobras, the African mambas, the Indo-Malayan kraits, and the New World coral snakes are poisonous members of this family. The elapids are particularly numerous and diverse in Australia, where all dangerous land snakes are elapids (black tiger snake, brown snake, death adder, taipan, and copperheads).

The Hydrophiodae family includes 52 different species of poisonous sea snakes that inhabit tropical waters throughout the world.

The Viperidae (true vipers) are all poisonous and inhabit Europe, Africa, and Asia; the subfamily Crotalidae (pit vipers) are common in the Americas and Southeast Asia. Many species have adapted to relatively cool climates, spending the winter in hibernation and, therefore, show seasonal variations in growth and reproduction. Species common to North America include rattlesnakes, water moccasins, and copperheads.

Epidemiology.   It has been estimated that 300,000 poisonous snake bites responsible for 30,000 to 40,000 deaths occur throughout the world each yr. The largest number of fatalities occurs in Southeast Asia; most are due to cobra bites. In the Western Hemisphere most fatalities from snake bites occur in Brazil. About 45,000 people are bitten by snakes every year in the United States, and about 20% of these are bitten by poisonous snakes; the fatalities number fewer than 20 and are usually due to bites by rattlesnakes, water moccasins, or coral snakes.

Clinical Manifestations.   *Local Effects.*   Bites by members of the Viperidae (true vipers) and Crotalidae (pit vipers) are characterized by localized pain and swelling. Necrosis of the skin with formation of bullae, ecchymoses, and discoloration soon follows. There is extensive local edema with oozing of serosanguineous fluid into the bullae and subcutaneous tissue. The bites by members of the Elapidae family vary among species. The Eastern coral snake bite causes minimal pain and tissue destruction; cobra bites are characterized by severe pain with extensive necrosis and sloughing. Bites by the Hydrophiodae are remarkable in that they are painless, fang marks are often inconspicuous, and no local reaction is observed.

Systemic Effects.   A bite by a member of the Viperidae family or the subfamily Crotalidae produces predominantly hemorrhagic symptoms. Disseminated intravascular coagulation develops rapidly and leads to subcutaneous hemorrhage, hematuria, hemoptysis, and hematemesis. Acute renal insufficiency may develop. Neurologic abnormalities are then manifest as delirium, disorientation, coma, and seizures. Death is usually secondary to intracranial hemorrhage.

The venoms of other species of poisonous snakes are neurotoxins, and death is secondary to respiratory paralysis. Cobra bites often produce drowsiness within 15 min, followed by progressive involvement of cranial nerves, including ptosis and ophthalmoplegia. Palatal and pharyngeal involvement leads to slurred speech and difficulty in handling oral secretions. Varying degrees of motor paralysis ensue as do seizures and coma. The reaction to the bite of the sea snake differs from that of the cobra bite in that the above sequence is heralded by diffuse myalgia and progressive muscular weakness. The bite of the Eastern coral snake initially produces paresthesia in the involved extremity followed rapidly by involvement of the cranial nerves, respiratory insufficiency, and death.

Treatment. Initially, one should determine whether the attacking snake is poisonous; knowledge of the species indigenous to the geographic area is helpful. Examination of the wound may be informative as bites by nonpoisonous species lack distinct fang punctures and do not cause local pain or swelling. There is also a lack of progressive symptomatology from nonpoisonous snake bites. Bites on the extremities and into adipose tissue are less dangerous than bites into highly vascularized areas such as the face.

When the victim has been bitten on an extremity, a tourniquet should be placed above the bite area, tightly enough to occlude venous and lymphatic return but loosely enough to preserve a distal pulse. The involved extremity should be immobilized, and, if possible, the patient should avoid exercise, including walking, thus lessening the spread of the venom. Applying ice directly to the wound or cooling the involved extremity may be harmful and should be avoided. Incision and suction soon after the bite can remove substantial amounts of venom from the wound. The skin should be cleaned and a single linear incision 1 cm in length and 0.5 cm in depth made through each fang mark. Suction with cups provided in commercial snake bite kits or oral suction should be continued for at least 1 hr before the tourniquet is released.

The wound should be cultured, irrigated with saline, and treated with a topical antiseptic preparation. Extensive swelling that compromises the peripheral circulation is an indication for immediate fasciotomy. Surgical debridement of vesicles and necrotic skin can often be delayed for 1 wk.

Systemic Measures. Specific therapy with antivenin (see below) should be followed by appropriate supportive therapy, which often consists of blood transfusions for bites by snakes with a strongly hematotoxic venom. Adjustment of fluid and electrolyte balance is indicated in the presence of vomiting, renal insufficiency, and shock. Systemic complications include paralysis, respiratory insufficiency, disseminated intravascular coagulation, and cardiac arrhythmias. Tetanus prophylaxis with toxoid or antitoxin is indicated if the child has not been adequately immunized, and parenteral therapy

with penicillin is indicated to prevent secondary bacterial infection. Pain is often severe and may require narcotic administration.

Nonpoisonous snake bites generally require no treatment.

Serum Therapy. Snake venom antisera or antivenins are prepared by hyperimmunization of horses against 1 or more venoms. Though the chemical composition of snake venom varies from species to species, there is enough antigenic similarity between venoms of related species to produce clinically useful polyvalent antisera. Two antivenin preparations are commercially available in the United States.* Antivenin for the treatment of bites by exotic species can usually be obtained through local zoological societies. These products can cause anaphylaxis and will cause serum sickness in 30–75% of patients, depending on the amount administered. Administration, therefore, is best performed in a hospital setting following skin testing with the normal horse serum present in the commercial antivenin kits. Severe allergic reactions have occurred after a negative test, and some patients have been safely treated even after a positive test. Some clinicians routinely give epinephrine subcutaneously or antihistamines intravenously before infusing antivenin. After bites by unidentified snakes or snakes known not to be highly poisonous, antivenin treatment should be withheld until the development of local symptoms.

GILA MONSTER

This is the only lizard poisonous to man. The 2 species inhabit the Sahuaro desert regions of Arizona and New Mexico as well as the desert regions of Mexico. Most bites occur during attempted capture or in handling captive animals. After a bite it is often difficult to remove the lizard. There is considerable injury locally, severe pain, erythema, and edema. The venom contains a potent neurotoxin. Initial systemic symptoms include nausea and vomiting and are followed rapidly by generalized weakness, cranial nerve paralysis, and respiratory insufficiency. Fatalities are uncommon. No antivenin is available. Treatment consists of local care of the wound and supportive therapy as described for snake bites.

VENOMOUS MARINE ANIMALS

Venomous fish include certain sharks, scorpion fish, stonefish, weeverfish, toadfish, catfish, and stingrays. Most of them inhabit tropical waters and are especially plentiful around coral reefs.

The clinical manifestations of poisoning are remarkably similar in all cases. There is immediate pain at the puncture sight that spreads to involve the entire extremity. The venom produces local ischemia and circumscribed cyanosis, followed by edema and erythema that may spread to involve the entire extremity. Tissue necrosis may be extensive locally and contributes to secondary bacterial infection. The wound produced by

---

*Wyeth Antivenin (Crotalidae) polyvalent: venom effective against rattlesnakes, water moccasins, and copperheads. Wyeth Antivenin (*Micrurus fulvius*): effective against North American coral snake venom.

stingrays is unique in that the laceration is several cm deep and often contains bony and epithelial fragments of the venom apparatus. Systemic manifestations include pallor, nausea, vomiting, diaphoresis, and loss of consciousness. Convulsions, paralysis, and death have been reported.

Treatment consists of the appropriate application of a tourniquet and copious irrigation of the wound to remove fragments of the venom apparatus. The only available antivenin is one for stonefish venom. Many venoms are heat labile; for this reason immersion of the involved extremity in water as hot as can be tolerated is recommended. Tetanus toxoid or antitoxin is administered except when the immune status of the patient is adequate. Broad spectrum antibiotic therapy should be prescribed to prevent superinfection. Narcotics may be required to control pain.

COELENTERATE STINGS

The venomous coelenterates include hydroids, jellyfish, sea anemones, and coral. They are equipped with tentacles that have a venom apparatus consisting of nematocysts or nettle cells. The stings vary from a mild stinging sensation produced by the smaller jellyfish to an extremely painful, almost shock-like sensation produced by the most dangerous member of the phylum (Portuguese man-of-war). The local signs include erythema and urticaria. Systemic involvement may be manifested by weakness, chills, fever, nausea, and vomiting. In extreme situations there may be respiratory failure and death.

The intensity of symptoms depends upon the length of time the tentacles remain in contact with the skin; the tentacles should therefore be removed as promptly as possible. Caution must be observed since some species of jellyfish have powerful nematocysts which may penetrate gloves and other clothing. Topical treatment consists of warm soaks with normal saline. Antihistamines and corticosteroids are indicated in the presence of extensive swelling and urticaria.

Prevention of stings is best accomplished by caution when swimming in tropical waters. Damaged tentacles, which often float in water following a storm, are capable of inflicting stings, as are jellyfish washed up on beaches and often presumed to be dead.

WILLIAM T. SPECK

Bücherl W: Venomous Animals and Their Venoms, Vols I and II. New York, Academic Press, 1968.
Halstead BW: Poisonous and Venomous Marine Animals of the World, Vols I and II. Washington DC, US Government Printing Office, 1965 and 1967.
Watt CH: Poisonous snakebite: Treatment in the United States. JAMA 240:654, 1978.

28.19 MAMMALIAN BITES: DOG, HUMAN, CAT, AND RAT

Mammalian bites are a relatively common cause of morbidity and a rare cause of mortality among children.

Bite wounds account for 1% of all emergency room visits; there are an estimated 300 reported bites/100,000 people/yr in the United States. Children are overrepresented among the population of bite victims. However, there are probably fewer than 50 bite-related deaths/yr.

Epidemiology.   Dog bites account for 50–95% of bite injuries. Children are commonly victims of dog bites, and males sustain almost 60% of them. More than 70% of dog bites to the face occur in children under 15 yr old. Most dog bites occur in summer months and in the afternoon. Fewer than 25% of bites involve stray dogs. Large breed dogs account for 50% of bite injuries.

Human bite injuries consist of self-inflicted wounds of the lips or tongue, bites into other soft tissues, and injuries to hands when they strike the tooth of another person. Rat bites are uncommon; most occur in the summer, on the extremities, and in children less than 6 yr old, usually while the child is asleep.

Clinical Manifestations.   Animal and human bites consist of scratches, lacerations, punctures, and abrasions. Dogs and humans also have the strength to produce crush injuries. Because cats have long, thin, sharp teeth, their puncture wounds are often deep. Hand wounds resulting from striking the teeth of another person are usually seen on the dorsal surface near the metacarpophalangeal joint. Such wounds may involve the joint or spread to other parts of the hand; when the hand is unclenched, folds of skin may partially cover the wound and prevent adequate drainage.

Complications.   The most feared complication of an animal bite, rabies, is now very rare in the United States (Sec 10.85). The most common complication is infection (Sec 10.49). *Pasteurella multocida* may be an important pathogen in dog bite wound infections. Streptococci and staphylococci are the most common causes of infection after human bites. Organisms cultured from cat bite wounds include *Pasteurella multocida, Staph. epidermidis, Strep. viridans,* and diphtheroids. Depending on the location and severity of the bite, cosmetic and/or functional problems may also arise. Psychologic sequelae of bite injuries are probably rare if the child receives adequate support from the family in the post-injury period. Most rat bites heal without sequelae. Rare complications are caused by *Streptobacillus moniliformis* or *Spirillum minus* (Sec 10.49 and 10.60).

Prevention.   Prevention depends upon keeping children away from animals or people who might bite them and educating children and parents about safe interaction with animals. All dogs should be leashed or confined in a fenced yard. All strays should be removed from streets by the animal warden. Rat bites can be prevented only by appropriate public health measures which clean up breeding grounds and upgrade homes to prevent infestation.

Treatment.   The management of bite injuries should include scrupulous cleansing, debridement of devitalized tissue, and care to ensure that neural and vascular structures are not injured or are repaired. Osteomyelitis must be considered in deep or crush wounds. Tetanus prophylaxis should be administered if indicated (Sec 10.40).

Cleansing should be performed by high pressure irrigation with normal saline using a large syringe connected to a large bore needle. A considerable volume of fluid should be used. Bite lacerations, except for those of the hand, seen within several hr of injury can be closed primarily after adequate irrigation and debridement. Lacerations of the face may be closed primarily up to 6–8 hr after the injury. Lacerations presenting after these time limits should be cultured and allowed to close by secondary intention. Scar revision can be done at a later date. Puncture wounds, except those of the hand, should be excised and irrigated prior to closure.

Cultures of fresh wounds and the use of prophylactic antibiotics are not indicated for most bites. Wounds that appear infected should be cultured. Penicillin or a semisynthetic penicillin is the appropriate choice of antibiotic until culture or sensitivity results are known. For patients allergic to penicillin, erythromycin or a cephalosporin may be used.

Patients presenting with uninfected or only superficially infected hand wounds may be managed as outpatients. The wound should be well irrigated, left open, and elevated. The hand should be soaked frequently and checked daily. Some authorities recommend the prophylactic use of antibiotics with coverage including penicillinase-producing staphylococci. Patients presenting with infected hand wounds—swollen, stiff, tender finger, involvement of other structures—should be admitted. The wounds should be cleaned, debrided, and left open. After cultures are taken, the patient should be started on a semisynthetic penicillin or similar antibiotic and the hand kept elevated.

Bailie WE, Stowe EC, Schmett AM: Aerobic bacterial flora or oral and nasal fluids of canines with reference to bacteria associated with bites. J Clin Microbiol 7:223, 1978.

Berzon DR: The animal bite epidemic in Baltimore, Maryland: Review and update. Am J Pub Health 63:593, 1978.

Berzon DR, DeHoff JB: Medical costs and other aspects of dog bites in Baltimore. Pub Health Reports 89:377, 1979.

Berzon DR, Farber RE, Gordon J, et al: Animal bites in a large city—a report on Baltimore, Maryland. Am J Pub Health 62:442, 1972.

Callahan ML: Treatment of common dog bites: Infection risk factors. JACEP 7:83, 1978.

Callahan ML: Prophylactic antibiotics in common dog bite wounds: A controlled study. Ann Emerg Med 9:410, 1980.

Goldstein EJC, Citron DM, Finegold SM: Dog bite wounds and infections: A prospective clinical study. Ann Emerg Med 9:508, 1980.

Goldstein EJC, Citron DM, Wield B, et al: Bacteriology of human and animal bite wounds. J Clin Microbiol 8:667, 1970.

Harris D, Imperato PJ, Oken B: Dog bites—an unrecognized epidemic. Bull NY Acad Med 50:981, 1979.

Kizer KW: Epidemiologic and clinical aspects of animal bite injuries. JACEP 8:134, 1979.

Malinowski RW, Strate RG, Perry JF, et al: The management of human bite injuries of the hand. J Trauma 19:655, 1979.

Marr JS, Beck AM, Lugo JA: An epidemiologic study of the human bite. Pub Health Reports 94:514, 1979.

Sallow W: An analysis of rat bites in Baltimore, 1948–52. Pub Health Reports 68:1239, 1953.

28.20 SPIDER BITES

The term spider is widely used to include both spiders (Order Araneae which includes tarantulas) and scorpions (Order Scorpionida). Spiders and scorpions are feared although the incidence of morbidity and mortality is very low; 27 spider bite deaths and 6 scorpion bite deaths were reported in the United States from 1960–1969.

In the United States the spiders which may cause problems include members of the *Latrodectus* genus, the most famous being *L. mactans mactans* or the black widow, and members of the *Loxosceles* genus, the most famous being *L. reclusa* or the brown recluse. Tarantulas in the United States have a venom which is not toxic to humans, and the only scorpion in the United States which can cause severe systemic reactions is *Centruroides sculpturatus*. *Hadrurus arizonensis* is a scorpion which has a venom which causes only local reactions.

Latrodectus Bites. Patients usually come into contact with the spiders outdoors in trash piles, outhouses, and stacks of old lumber. The black widow is found in the eastern United States, although there are other members of the *Latrodectus* in other parts of the country.

The bite initially produces local, mild to moderate pain. After a brief period of time, systemic symptoms occur consisting of sweating, nausea, headache, apprehension, hyperesthesias and paresthesias, muscular cramps with a rigid abdomen, and fever. The blood pressure is elevated, and there may be ECG changes. Coma may occur. The symptoms resolve over a period of hours or days.

There is a *Latrodectus* antivenin made in horses which may be given intravenously after appropriate skin tests. Cramps, headache, and nausea may be treated with intravenous calcium gluconate. Muscle relaxants such as methocarbamol may also be used. Morphine or meperidine can be used for analgesia. Tetanus prophylaxis and antibiotics may be indicated.

Loxosceles Bites. Patients usually come into contact with these spiders in abandoned houses, cellars, wood piles, and trash piles. The recluse spider is found predominantly in the central and southern United States, but other *Loxosceles* spiders are found throughout the south and west.

The venom of *Loxosceles* spiders contains enzymes which cause endothelial damage. This is followed by thrombocytopenia, decreased fibrinogen, and a prolonged partial thromboplastin time. Small vessel thrombosis accounts for skin necrosis.

The *Loxosceles* bite has local and systemic manifestations. The bite is initially painless. Two–4 hr later itching, swelling, pain, and redness occur locally. A blister may form which may be hemorrhagic. Over 3–4 days the area becomes necrotic. It then becomes mummified over the next 1–2 wk, and eventually an ulcer develops which, if larger than 1 cm, may last for weeks or months. The ulcer may become secondarily infected. Systemic reactions, while rare, are more common in children. These include fever, chills, malaise, weakness, nausea, vomiting, chest pain, petechiae, seizures, and intravascular hemolysis.

There is no antivenin for *Loxosceles* bites. It is unclear whether treatment other than supportive therapy is beneficial. Some authorities recommend excision of the bite to limit the size of the resultant ulcer; others recommend the use of steroids for treatment of the systemic reactions. Tetanus prophylaxis and antibiotics may be indicated.

Scorpion Bites. *Centruroides sculpturatus* is a nocturnal creature usually encountered in tree bark in Arizona and New Mexico. Bites are most common in May through August.

The venom contains neurotoxins, enzymes, and other substances. The bite causes local pain followed by paresthesias. Systemic reactions, which are rare, consist of difficulty in speaking and swallowing, salivation, sweating, nausea, vomiting, restlessness, and hyperreflexia. Seizures may occur in children.

Local application of ice as soon as possible is the 1st treatment. Antivenin is available for use in severe cases. Barbiturates will control seizures; paraldehyde is contraindicated. Nerve blocks should be used for pain control; morphine, meperidine, and other morphine derivatives are contraindicated.

JEROME A. PAULSON

Arnold RE: What to do about bites and stings of venomous animals. New York, Macmillan, 1973.

Auer AI, Hershey FB: Surgery for neurotic bites of the brown spider. Arch Surg 108:612, 1979.

Minton SA: Venomous arthropods. *In:* Hubbert WT, McCulloch WF, Schnurenberger PR (eds): Diseases Transmitted from Animals to Man. Ed 6. Springfield, Ill., Charles C Thomas, 1975.

Wasserman GS, Siegel C: Loxoscalism (brown recluse spider bites): A review of the literature. Clin Tox 19:353, 1979.

TABLES 29–1*A* AND *B*: DRUGS*

Table 29–1*A* SELECTED DRUGS FOR SYSTEMIC THERAPY GROUPED ALPHABETICALLY BY CATEGORY OF INDICATION FOR THEIR USE.
Individual drugs with their dosages are listed alphabetically by generic names in Table 29–1*B*, p. 1814.

ANALGESIC AGENTS
1. Narcotic analgesics
   codeine phosphate, codeine sulfate
   meperidine hydrochloride, DEMEROL hydrochloride
   morphine sulfate
   pentazocine hydrochloride, TALWIN hydrochloride
   propoxyphene hydrochloride, DARVON, ‡
2. Non-narcotic analgesics
   acetaminophen, LIQUIPRIN, TYLENOL, ‡
   acetylsalicylic acid, ASPIRIN, BUFFERIN, ‡
   sodium salicylate

ANTHELMINTIC AGENTS
1. Against *Giardia lamblia* (*Lamblia intestinalis*)
   quinacrine, ATABRINE
2. Against pinworms (*Enterobius vermicularis*), roundworms (*Ascaris lumbricoides*), and hookworms (*Necator americanus, Ancylostoma duodenale*)
   mebendazole, VERMOX
   pyrantel pamoate, ANTIMINTH
3. Against tapeworms (*Diphyllobotirium latum, Taenia saginata, Taenia solium, Hymenolepis nana*)
   niclosamide, YOMESAN
4. Against whipworms (*Trichuris trichiura*)
   mebendazole, VERMOX

ANTIALLERGIC AGENTS
1. Antihistamines
   brompheniramine maleate, DIMETANE
   carbinoxamine maleate, CLISTIN
   chlorpheniramine maleate, CHLOR-TRIMETON
   dimenhydrinate, DRAMAMINE
   diphenhydramine hydrochloride, BENADRYL
   tripelennamine hydrochloride, PYRIBENZAMINE
2. Antihistamine and antiserotonin
   cyproheptadine, PERIACTIN
3. Inhibition of immunologic reaction
   corticosteroid

ANTIASTHMA MEDICATION
1. Bronchodilators
   β-adrenergic stimulants
      bronchodilator inhalation
      epinephrine
      metaproterenol sulfate, ALUPENT, METAPREL
      terbutaline sulfate, BRETHINE, BRICANYL
   Phosphodiesterase inhibitors
      theophylline, ELIXOPHYLLIN, LUFYLLIN, SLOPHYLLIN, ‡ and many combinations
      aminophylline, SOMOPHYLLIN ‡
2. In status asthmaticus resistant to other treatment modalities
   corticosteroid, in addition to other supportive measures

3. Inhibition of mastocyte degranulation (only for prevention)
   cromolyn sodium inhalation, AARANE, INTAL Spinhaler
4. Topical corticosteroid treatment (in steroid-dependent cases)
   beclomethasone aerosol, VANCERIL Inhaler

ANTICHOLINERGIC AGENTS
atropine sulfate
propantheline, PRO-BANTHINE
scopolamine methylbromide, PAMINE

ANTICONVULSANT DRUGS
1. Treatment of partial cortical seizures with elementary symptomatology (focal motor epilepsy, focal somatosensory epilepsy, or autonomic or compound forms thereof), and generalized tonic-clonic seizures (grand mal epilepsy)
   carbamazepine,* TEGRETOL
   phenobarbital,* LUMINAL
   phenytoin,* DILANTIN
   primidone, MYSOLINE
2. Treatment of partial seizures with complex symptomatology (temporal lobe or psychomotor epilepsy)
   carbamazepine,* TEGRETOL
   phenytoin,* DILANTIN
   primidone, MYSOLINE
3. Treatment of petit mal (with 3/sec spike and wave pattern)
   clonazepam, CLONOPIN
   ethosuximide,* ZARONTIN
   phenobarbital* (to prevent secondary generalization to tonic-clonic seizures)
   trimethadione, TRIDIONE
   valproate sodium, DEPAKENE
4. Treatment of mixed seizure patterns (akinetic seizures, myoclonic seizures, petit mal variant, and combinations thereof with tonic-clonic seizures): use rational combination of drugs listed above, including, in particular, valproate sodium, DEPAKENE. At times, addition of acetazolamide, DIAMOX.
5. Treatment of status epilepticus (by parenteral route)
   diazepam,* VALIUM
   paraldehyde
   phenobarbital, LUMINAL
   phenytoin sodium, DILANTIN

ANTIEMETIC MEDICATION
chlorpromazine, THORAZINE
dimenhydrinate, DRAMAMINE
promethazine, PHENERGAN

ANTIFUNGAL AGENTS
amphotericin B, FUNGIZONE
griseofulvin, FULVICIN, GRISACTIN,‡
miconazole, MONISTAT
nystatin, MYCOSTATIN, NILSTAT

To be used in conjunction with Sec 5.47, p. 275.
Consult also the following:

DRUGS

Table 29–1A SELECTED DRUGS FOR SYSTEMIC THERAPY GROUPED ALPHABETICALLY BY CATEGORY OF INDICATION FOR THEIR USE (Continued)

DRUGS (side tab)

ANTIHYPERTENSIVE AGENTS (See Table 13–16)
1. Diuretics: see chlorothiazide, hydrochlorothiazide
2. Agents with antiadrenergic effect
   methyldopa, ALDOMET
   propranolol, INDERAL
   reserpine, SANDRIL, SERPASIL, ‡
3. Vasodilators
   hydralazine, DRALZINE, APRESOLINE
   in hypertensive emergency: diazoxide, HYPERSTAT;
   nitroprusside, NIPRIDE
   minoxidil, LONITEN
4. Against hypertension associated with catecholamine-secreting tumors
   phenoxybenzamine (α-adrenergic blockade), DI-BENZYLINE
   phentolamine (α-adrenergic blockade), REGITINE
   See Sec 18.28 on catecholamine-secreting tumors.
5. Against hypertension associated with adrenocortical hyperfunction
   See Sec 16.51 and 18.26, and Fig. 13–81 and 13–82.

ANTIMALARIAL AGENTS
1. For prevention of clinical manifestations of disease
   chloroquine diphosphate, ARALEN, RESOCHIN
   pyrimethamine, DARAPRIM
2. For treatment of malarial attack
   chloroquine diphosphate, ARALEN, RESOCHIN
   quinine sulfate or dihydrochloride, with either tetracycline or pyrimethamine and sulfadiazine
3. For "radical" cure
   primaquine diphosphate

ANTIMICROBIAL AGENTS (mechanism of action)
1. Aminoglycosides (interfere with function of ribosomes in sensitive bacteria)
   amikacin sulfate, AMIKIN
   gentamicin sulfate, GARAMYCIN
   kanamycin sulfate, KANTREX
   neomycin sulfate, MYCIFRADIN, NEOBIOTIC
   streptomycin sulfate
2. Cephalosporins (interfere with cell wall synthesis in sensitive bacteria)
   cefaclor, CECLOR
   cefadroxil, DURICEF
   cephalexin, KEFLEX
   cephaloglycin, KAFOCIN
   cephaloridine, LORIDINE
   cephalothin sodium, KEFLIN
   cephapirin, CEFADYL
   cephradine, ANSPOR, VELOSEF
3. Chloramphenicol (impairs peptide bond formation by ribosomes in sensitive bacteria)
   chloramphenicol, CHLOROMYCETIN
4. Macrolides (impair peptide bond formation by ribosomes in sensitive bacteria)
   clindamycin hydrochloride, clindamycin palmitate hydrochloride, clindamycin phosphate, CLEOCIN
   erythromycin, ILOTYCIN, ‡
   erythromycin estolate, ILOSONE
   erythromycin ethylsuccinate, ERYTHROCIN ethylsuccinate, PEDIAMYCIN
   erythromycin stearate, ERYTHROCIN stearate, ETHRIL, ‡
   lincomycin, LINCOCIN
5. Penicillins (interfere with cell wall synthesis in sensitive bacteria)
   amoxicillin, AMOXIL, LAROTID, ‡
   ampicillin sodium, OMNIPEN-N, PENBRITIN-S, ‡
   ampicillin trihydrate, OMNIPEN, PENBRITIN, ‡
   benzathine penicillin G, BICILLIN
   benzylpenicillin, penicillin G, PENTIDS, PFIZERPEN G, ‡
   carbenicillin disodium, GEOPEN
   cloxacillin sodium, TEGOPEN
   dicloxacillin sodium, DYNAPEN, PATHOCIL
   methicillin sodium, CELBENIN, STAPHCILLIN
   nafcillin sodium, NAFCIL, UNIPEN

oxacillin sodium, BACTOCILL, PROSTAPHLIN
   phenoxymethylpenicillin, penicillin V, PEN-VEE K, VEETIDS, ‡
   procaine penicillin G, DURACILLIN, WYCILLIN
   ticarcillin disodium, TICAR
6. Polypeptide antimicrobials (increase permeability of cytoplasmic membrane in sensitive bacteria)
   colistimethate sodium, COLY-MYCIN M
   colistin sulfate, COLY-MYCIN S
7. Sulfonamides (inhibit tetrahydrofolic acid synthesis in sensitive bacteria)
   sulfadiazine, SULADYNE
   sulfamethoxazole, GANTANOL
   sulfisoxazole, GANTRISIN, ‡
   trimethoprim-sulfamethoxazole, BACTRIM, SEPTRA
   trisulfapyrimidines
8. Tetracyclines (interfere with function of ribosomes in sensitive microorganisms)
   chlortetracycline, AUREOMYCIN
   demeclocycline, DECLOMYCIN
   doxycycline, VIBRAMYCIN
   methacycline, RONDOMYCIN
   minocycline, MINOCIN, VECTRIN
   oxytetracycline, TERRAMYCIN, UROBIOTIC
   tetracycline, ACHROMYCIN, TETRACYN, ‡
9. Additional antimicrobial agents used in urinary tract infections
   methenamine mandelate, MANDELAMINE, ‡
   nalidixic acid, NEGGRAM
   nitrofurantoin, FURADANTIN, MACRODANTIN, ‡

ANTIPYRETIC AGENTS
   acetaminophen, LIQUIPRIN, TEMPRA, TYLENOL, ‡
   acetylsalicylic acid, ASPIRIN, BUFFERIN, ‡
   sodium salicylate

ANTIRHEUMATIC AGENTS
   acetylsalicylic acid, ASPIRIN, BUFFERIN, ‡
   sodium salicylate
   Other nonsteroidal anti-inflammatory agents have not been conclusively evaluated in the pediatric age group. See Sec 9.59.

ANTITUBERCULOUS AGENTS
   aminosalicylate sodium, PAS, PARASAL-sodium, ‡
   ethambutol, MYAMBUTOL
   isoniazid, INH, NYDRAZID, ‡
   rifampin, RIFADIN, RIMACTANE
   streptomycin

ANTITUSSIVE AGENTS
   codeine phosphate or sulfate (addictive on long-term use)
   dextromethorphan hydrobromide, ROMILAR, component in many combinations

CALCIUM PREPARATIONS
   calcium gluconate
   calcium lactate

CARDIOACTIVE AGENTS
1. Agents with inotropic effect
   digitoxin, CRYSTODIGIN, PURODIGIN
   digoxin,* LANOXIN
   dopamine, INTROPIN
   isoproterenol, ISUPREL
2. Antiarrhythmic agents
   a. against sinus node disturbances
      sinus bradycardia
         atropine sulfate (anticholinergic effect)
      sinus tachycardia
         associated with congestive heart failure
            digoxin (inotropic effect), LANOXIN
         associated with increased sympathetic tone or induced by excess of catecholamines
            propranolol (β-adrenergic blockade), INDERAL
   b. against paroxysmal atrial tachycardia, supraventricular tachycardia, atrial flutter, or atrial fibrillation
      measures to increase vagal tone (cholinergic stimulation) (carotid massage)
         cholinesterase-inhibiting agents
            edrophonium, TENSILON

Table 29-1A SELECTED DRUGS FOR SYSTEMIC THERAPY GROUPED ALPHABETICALLY BY CATEGORY OF INDICATION FOR THEIR USE (Continued)

neostigmine methylsulfate, PROSTIGMINE
triggering of reflex vagal discharge
  phenylephrine hydrochloride, NEO-SYNEPH-
  RHINE (α-adrenergic agent, peripheral
  vasoconstrictor)
digoxin,* LANOXIN
β-adrenergic blockade
  propranolol hydrochloride, INDERAL (in association with
  digoxin, if digoxin not effective alone)
  After reversal of arrhythmia, for protection from recurrence:
  digoxin,* quinidine,* procainamide, propranolol
c. in atrioventricular conduction block
  isoproterenol IV* (β-adrenergic agonist), ISUPREL
  (ventricular pacing)
d. against paroxysmal ventricular tachycardia or tachyarrhythmia
  lidocaine hydrochloride IV,* XYLOCAINE
  procainamide hydrochloride, PRONESTYL
  .quinidine gluconate, QUINAGLUTE prn associated
  with propranolol hydrochloride, INDERAL
  phenytoin, D!LANTIN (cardioconversion)
  After reversal of arrhythmias, for protection from recurrence: quinidine,* procainamide, propranolol*
e. against digitalis-induced arrhythmia
  (correct hypokalemia, if present)
  lidocaine hydrochloride IV, XYLOCAINE
  phenytoin, DILANTIN
  propranolol,* INDERAL

CENTRAL STIMULANTS
caffeine
dextroamphetamine sulfate, DEXEDRINE, ‡
methylphenidate hydrochloride, RITALIN
pemoline, CYLERT

CHOLINERGIC AGENTS (cholinesterase inhibitors)
edrophonium chloride, TENSILON
pyridostigmine bromide, MESTINON

CORTICOSTEROIDS
for physiologic replacement
for pharmacologic effects

DIURETICS
1. osmotic diuretic
   mannitol, OSMITROL
2. saluretic agents
   with moderate effect
     chlorothiazide, DIURIL
     chlorthalidone, HYGROTON
     hydrochlorothiazide, ESIDRIX, HYDRODIURIL, ‡
     triamterene, DYRENIUM
   with rapid and accentuated effect
     ethacrynic acid, EDECRIN
     furosemide, LASIX
3. aldosterone antagonist
   spironolactone, ALDACTONE

ENURESIS (adjunct medication used in enuresis)
imipramine, TOFRANIL, W.D.D., ‡

GASTRIC ACID SECRETION INHIBITION
cimetidine, TAGAMET

HYPNOTIC AND SEDATIVE AGENTS
amobarbital, amobarbital sodium, AMYTAL
chloral hydrate, NOCTEC
pentobarbital, pentobarbital sodium, NEMBUTAL

phenobarbital, phenobarbital sodium, LUMINAL
secobarbital, secobarbital sodium, SECONAL
For selected uses, see diazepam, diphenhydramine, and "lytic cocktail" (Table 29-1B).

IRON PREPARATIONS
ferrous sulfate
iron-dextran complex, IMFERON

LAXATIVES, CATHARTICS, DEMULCENTS
bisacodyl, DULCOLAX
cascara sagrada (extract containing anthraquinones), component of
  PERI-COLACE
dioctyl sodium sulfosuccinate, COLACE, ‡
magnesium hydroxide, magnesium sulfate, milk of magnesia, components of HALEY'S M-O
mineral oil, component of AGORAL, HALEY'S M-O
phenolphthalein, PRULET, component of AGORAL
senna (extract of senna fruit), SENOKOT, X-PREP
sodium sulfate

MAGNESIUM
magnesium sulfate

MOTION SICKNESS MEDICATION (in ascending order of effective-
ness)
cyclizine, MAREZINE
dimenhydrinate, DRAMAMINE
promethazine, PHENERGAN

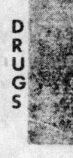

NASAL DECONGESTANTS
phenylephrine, NEO-SYNEPHRINE, component of many combinations
pseudoephedrine hydrochloride, D-FEDA, SUDAFED, component of
  many combinations

NEUROLEPTIC AGENTS
chlorpromazine hydrochloride, THORAZINE
hydroxyzine hydrochloride, or pamoate, ATARAX, VISTARIL
"lytic cocktail"
methotrimeprazine, LEVOPROME
prochlorperazine, COMPAZINE
promethazine hydrochloride, PHENERGAN
thioridazine, MELLARIL

OPIATE ANTAGONIST
naloxone hydrochloride, NARCAN

PRESSOR AGENTS
epinephrine
phenylephrine hydrochloride, NEO-SYNEPHRINE

RENAL TUBULAR SECRETION (inhibition of renal tubular secretion)
probenecid, BENEMID

URIC ACID LOWERING AGENT (inhibition of synthesis)
allopurinol, ZYLOPRIM

VASCULAR HEADACHE
1. in acute attack
   acetylsalicylic acid, ASPIRIN, BUFFERIN, ‡
   atropine sulfate
   caffeine, component in many combinations
   ergotamine tartrate, GYNERGEN, component in
     many combinations
   sedative (amobarbital, pentobarbital, secobarbital,
     phenobarbital)
2. for prevention of attacks
   cyproheptadine hydrochloride, PERIACTIN
   phenytoin, DILANTIN
   propranolol hydrochloride, INDERAL

*First-line drug; drug of choice.
‡Available also under other brand name(s).
The drug tables in several recent editions were prepared by Harry C. Shirkey, M.D.

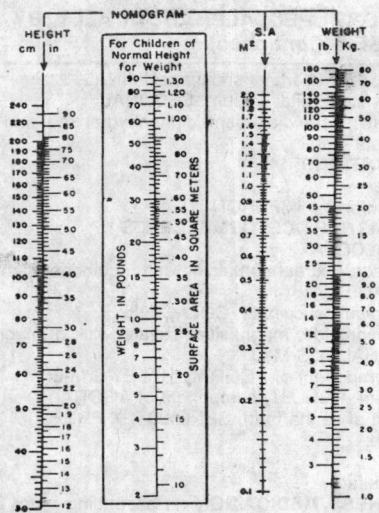

Figure 29-1 Nomogram for estimation of surface area. The surface area is indicated where a straight line which connects the height and weight levels intersects the surface area column; or the patient is roughly of average size, from the weight alone (enclosed area). (Nomogram modified from data of E. Boyd by C. D. West.)

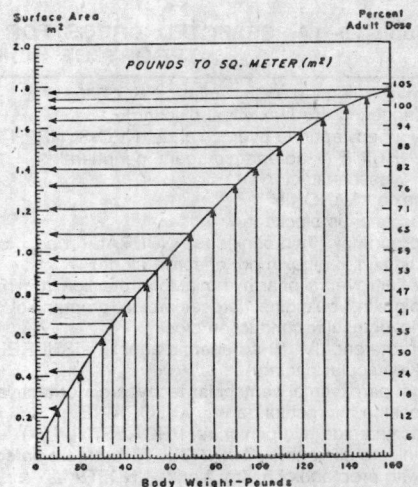

Figure 29-2 Relations between body weight in pounds, body surface area, and adult dosage. The surface area values correspond to those set forth by Crawford et al (1950). Note that the 100% adult dose is for a patient weighing about 140 lb and having a surface area of about 1.7 m². (From Talbot NB, et al: Metabolic Homeostasis—A Syllabus for Those Concerned with the Care of Patients. Cambridge, Harvard University Press, 1959.)

Table 29–1B DRUG DOSES* (Drugs Listed Alphabetically by Generic Name)

KEY:

NB	newborn (birth–end of 1st mo)
IN	infant (1–12 mo)
CH	child (1–12 yr)
AD	adult

caps	capsules
div	divided
D/W	dextrose in water
IM	intramuscular
inj	injection
IV	intravenous
PO	per os, oral
PR	per rectum
SC	subcutaneous
SL	sublingual
sol	solution
susp	suspension
tabl	tablets

†	available as generic preparation
‡	available also under other brand name(s)

g	gram
mg	milligram = 10^{-3} g
μg	microgram = 10^{-6} g
	(sometimes abbreviated "mcg")
ng	nanogram = 10^{-9} g
kg	kilogram = 10^{3} g
ml	milliliter = 10^{-3} liter ≃
	cm^{3} = cc
	(cubic centimeter)

Acetaminophen, paracetamol, APAP, NAPAP
  ℞ antipyretic, analgesic: IN, CH = PO: 30–40 mg/kg/24 hr, div, every 4–6 hr, prn
    †, LIQUIPRIN, TYLENOL, ‡; tabl, liquid preparations
  Caution: Massive overdose may cause hepatic necrosis through formation of a toxic metabolite. Lesser overdoses frequently cause reversible jaundice (Sec 28.6).

Acetazolamide, carbonic anhydrase inhibitor
  ℞ as adjunct in the treatment of convulsive disorders (ketotic effect): CH = PO: 8–30 mg/kg/24 hr, div, every 6–8 hr
    †, DIAMOX; tabl

Acetylsalicylic acid, ASA
  ℞ antipyretic, analgesic, anti-inflammatory: IN, CH = PO: 30–65 mg/kg/24 hr, div, every 4–6 hr, prn. This dosage corresponds to 27–58 mg salicylate sodium/kg/24 hr, or 20–50 mg salicylic acid/kg/24 hr.

  ℞ antirheumatic: CH = PO: 65–130 mg/kg/24 hr, div, every 4–6 hr
    †, ASPIRIN, BUFFERIN, ‡: tabl; also contained in many combination products
  Caution: Acute or chronic overdose may cause life-threatening poisoning syndrome (Sec 5.29 and 28.6).

Allopurinol, analogue of hypoxanthine; inhibitor of xanthine oxidase and thereby of the terminal steps of uric acid biosynthesis
  ℞ against hyperuricemia and urate deposition in tissues and kidneys, especially in patients receiving antineoplastic chemotherapy: CH = PO: 10 mg/kg/24 hr, div or in single daily dose. Note that allopurinol and its metabolite alloxanthine (oxypurinol) inhibit xanthine oxidase, and that reduced glomerular filtration requires lowering the dose to compensate for delayed excretion. A high urine output should be established—with a neutral or slightly alkaline urine pH—to allow for excretion of uric acid precursors.

*No attempt has been made to reproduce a comprehensive list of adverse side effects or of formulations available for the drugs listed. For these, the reader is again referred to standard textbooks of pharmacology, to the package inserts accompanying the commercial preparations of each drug, and to Physicians' Desk Reference, distributed annually in the United States by Physicians' Desk Reference, Box 210, Westwood, N.J. 07675.

Dosages listed in the Table are not specifically intended for premature and newborn infants unless so indicated.

All doses are average doses and are approximate. Variability of individual response may require alteration of dosage upward or downward. Doses based on different criteria (e.g., body weight, surface area) frequently do not correspond. Surface area may be calculated from Fig 29–1 and 29–2, p. 1814.

Doses are generally expressed as grams or milligrams per kilogram of body weight per 24 hours (g or mg/kg/24 hr), even for drugs ordinarily administered on a prn (as needed or indicated) basis.

For teratogenic effects of drugs, see Sec 6.30, package inserts, and Physicians' Desk Reference.

Because of the multiplicity of proprietary names and formulations of the drugs listed, only a few representative examples have been given of the many proprietary preparations available in most instances. We have intended no bias in selecting the proprietary names used, and make due apology to any manufacturers and distributors whose products may appear to have been slighted.

Table 29–1B DRUG DOSES (Continued)

Caution: If azathioprine or mercaptopurine, which are metabolized by xanthine oxidase, are to be given concomitantly with allopurinol, the dosage of azathioprine or mercaptopurine should be reduced substantially (to ¼–⅓ of usual dosage). ZYLOPRIM; tabl

Amikacin, antimicrobial aminoglycoside
  NB (≤2000 g and/or ≤7 days old) = IM, IV (over 20–30 min): 15 mg/kg/24 hr, div, every 12 hr
  NB (>2000 g and >7 days old), IN, CH = IM, IV (over 20–30 min): 15–22.5 mg/kg/24 hr, div, every 8 hr
    Usual duration of treatment: 7–10 days.
  AMIKIN; inj

Aminosalicylate sodium, para-aminosalicylate sodium, PAS sodium; structural analogue of para-aminobenzoic acid with weak bacteriostatic activity against *Mycobacterium tuberculosis,* used only in combination with other antituberculous agents
  ℞ as adjunct to isoniazid therapy: CH = PO: 200–300 mg/kg/24 hr, div, every 4–6 hr
  †, PAMISYL-Sodium, PARASAL-Sodium, ‡; tabl, caps
  Note: Frequent nausea, vomiting, diarrhea, abdominal pain, and poor acceptance by patients restrict the usefulness of this substance. 1 g of aminosalicylate sodium contains 4.7 mEq Na⁺.

Amobarbital, central nervous system depressant with intermediate duration of action. Tolerance to its hypnotic effect may develop on continued use. Initially, hypnotic effect lasts 3–8 hr.
  ℞ for sedation: IN, CH = PO, IM: 1–2 mg/kg/24 hr, div, every 6 hr
  ℞ for sleep: IN, CH = PO, IM: 2–3 mg/kg/dose, repeat prn after 12–24 hr
  †, AMYTAL; tabl, elixir ● amobarbital sodium, †, AMYTAL sodium; inj, caps

Amoxicillin, acid-resistant ampicillin congener
  IN, CH = PO: 20–40 mg/kg/24 hr, div, every 8 hr
  †, AMOXIL, LAROTID; ‡, caps, oral susp, pediatric drops

Amphotericin B; antifungal agent of the "polyene" type (nystatin, another example); insoluble in water, unstable below pH 4, must be given IV. Effective through binding to sterol components of the membrane of sensitive fungi, thereby altering its permeability; interference with renal function of patients seems an extension of the mode of action of this drug, demanding caution and continued monitoring during amphotericin B therapy.
  Due to potential toxicity for a variety of biologic functions amphotericin B should be used only in progressive and potentially fatal infections with fungi sensitive to it. Guidelines not available at this time for dosage in children as compared with adults.
  Use as solution of amphotericin B at concentration of 0.1 mg/ml in 5% dextrose (all other drugs, including antimicrobial agents, and electrolytes must be kept away from the colloidal suspension of amphotericin B).
  See Sec 10.105 for dose and administration. Optimal dose and duration of therapy not clearly determined.
  Available as lyophilized powder containing sodium deoxycholate as emulsifier. Colloidal suspension prepared by adding required volume of sterile water and shaking appropriately, subsequently diluted in 5% sterile dextrose in water to a final concentration of amphotericin B of 0.1 mg/ml, for slow IV administration; FUNGIZONE intravenous; inj

Ampicillin; acid-resistant penicillin congener
  NB (≤7 days old) = IV (over 15–30 min), IM: 50 mg/kg/24 hr, div, every 12 hr
    ℞ for meningitis: IV: 100 mg/kg/24 hr, div, every 4 hr
  NB (>7 days old) = IV (over 15–30 min), IM: 75 mg/kg/24 hr, div, every 8 hr
    ℞ for meningitis: IV: 200 mg/kg/24 hr, div, every 4 hr
  IN, CH = PO: 50–100 mg/kg/24 hr, div, every 6 hr
    ℞ for septicemia: IV (over 15–30 min), IM: 100–200 mg/kg/24 hr, div, every 4 hr (IV) or every 6 hr (IM)
    ℞ for meningitis: IV (over 15–30 min): 400 mg/kg/24 hr, div, every 4 hr
  ampicillin sodium, for injection, OMNIPEN-N, PENBRITIN-S, ‡; inj ● ampicillin trihydrate, †, OMNIPEN, PENBRITIN, ‡; caps, oral susp, pediatric drops

Atropine sulfate, *dl*-hyoscyamine; anticholinergic agent used mainly in premedication for anesthesia, as antiarrhythmic agent and as antispasmodic. Dosage varies according to indications and sensitivity of patients. On the average for IN, CH = SC, PO (IV): 0.01 mg/kg/dose, to be repeated prn after 2 hr until desired effect is obtained or adverse effects preclude further increase; for continued ℞: PO: 0.04 mg/kg/24 hr, div, every 6 hr, preferably with meals
  †; inj, tabl
  Caution: As for belladonna, below.

Beclomethasone diproprionate, chlorinated synthetic corticosteroid
  ℞ topical treatment to the bronchial tissues in long-term, steroid-dependent asthma. Delivered from metered-dose aerosol unit, releasing approximately 50 μg beclomethasone by activation of the dispenser unit: CH (6–12 yr): 1–2 inhalations every 6–8 hr. Effect usually apparent within 1–4 wk after beginning of steroid inhalations
  Caution: on transfer from systemic steroid therapy for asthma to inhalation therapy, adrenocortical competency of the patient must be watched and supported, if indicated, since inhalation therapy does not contribute to systemic corticosteroid supply. VANCERIL inhaler

Belladonna tincture, aqueous-alcoholic extract of belladonna leaves; anticholinergic preparation; used chiefly as antispasmodic
  Contains the equivalent of approximately 0.3 mg atropine sulfate per ml. Usual dose: 1 drop/4.5 kg (10 lbs) body weight 15–30 min before meals, 3 times per day
  Caution: Erythematous skin, persistently dilated pupils, or tachycardia are indications for discontinuing, then lowering dose. Extreme hypersensitivity may exist in patients with Down syndrome.

Bisacodyl, cathartic, structurally related to phenolphthalein
  ℞ laxative: PO: 0.3 mg/kg/dose, 6–8 hr before desired large bowel action. *Note:* tablets are enteric-coated and should be swallowed whole, with the added precaution of avoiding oral antacids or milk within at least 1 hr of ingestion.
  DULCOLAX; tabl, suppos

Brompheniramine maleate; alkylamine; antihistamine with mild anticholinergic and mild sedative effects
  ℞ antiallergic effect: CH = PO: 0.5 mg/kg/24 hr, div, every 6 hr
  †, DIMETANE; elixir, tabl, inj

See KEY to abbreviations, p. 1814; for further information about drugs, see package insert.

DRUGS

Table 29–1B DRUG DOSES (Continued)

Bronchodilator aerosols
℞ in acute asthmatic attack, provided effective inhalation is possible, e.g., in early stage of attack, or with assisted ventilation (IPPB). Effectiveness of a delivered dose depends on the microdispersion in the aerosol generated from different types of nebulizers. Onset of effect 2–5 min after inhalation of aerosol. Risk of overuse or overdosage in children is high with aerosol treatment, particularly in emergency situations. These limitations apply to all bronchodilator aerosols (epinephrine, racemic epinephrine, isoproterenol, metaproterenol, isoetharine), some of which can be dispensed from "metered" nebulization nozzles in products for use in adults.

Caffeine, CNS stimulant and vasoconstrictor of cerebral vessels
℞ against vascular headache and as an analeptic: CH = PO: 10 mg/kg/24 hr, div, prn every 4–6 hr; single dose usually 2–3 mg/kg/dose.
Note: In newborn, caffeine elimination markedly diminished compared with adult (including parturient woman) so that transplacentally acquired blood concentrations of caffeine are maintained within possibly effective range for several days after delivery. Danger of toxic manifestations by cumulation if additional caffeine administered without adjustment for this particular situation.

Calcium gluconate $[CH_2OH(CHOH)_4COO]_2Ca \cdot H_2O$
1 g equivalent to 89 mg elemental calcium or to 4.46 mEq Ca^{++}. Solution "10%" contains 100 mg/ml of calcium gluconate. This concentration equivalent to elemental calcium, 8.9 mg/ml or Ca^{++} 0.45 mEq/ml.
℞ to compensate for manifestations of hypocalcemia (tetany, seizures, myocardial insufficiency, hypoparathyroidism). Urgency and severity of clinical situation dictate dose and route of administration: IN, CH = IV (infused slowly, with monitoring of heart for bradycardia, arrest): "10%" calcium gluconate solution: 1–2 ml/kg/dose, equivalent to Ca^{++} 0.45–0.90 mEq/kg/dose, repeat prn after 6 hr. Daily dose needed might be as high as Ca^{++} 2.7 mEq/kg/24 hr.
Caution: Do not use any calcium preparation for intramuscular injection because of risk of sterile abscess formation. Extravascular leakage may cause local necrosis.
IN, CH = PO: calcium gluconate 500 mg/kg/24 hr, equivalent to elemental calcium 45 mg/kg/24 hr or Ca^{++} 2.3 mEq/kg/24 hr, div, every 4–8 hr
Note: Concomitant oral intake of phosphate exerts a major influence on the amount of calcium made available for absorption in the intestine;
†, powder, tabl

Calcium lactate $[CH_3CHOHCOO]_2Ca \cdot 5H_2O$
1 g of Ca lactate equivalent to 130 mg elemental calcium or to 6.49 mEq Ca^{++}.
IN, CH = PO: 500 mg/kg/24 hr, equivalent to elemental calcium 65 mg/kg/24 hr or Ca^{++} 3.2 mEq/kg/24 hr, div, every 4–8 hr
Note: Concomitant oral intake of phosphate exerts major influence on amount of calcium available for absorption in intestine. To ensure appropriate absorption in neonatal transient hypoparathyroidism, a calcium:phosphorus ratio of 4:1 (by weight, corresponding to 3:1 on molar basis) should be achieved in the feeding. This would require 10 g calcium lactate powder added to a daily formula containing 500 ml of whole cow milk.
†; powder, tabl

Carbamazepine, anticonvulsant agent; structurally related to tricyclic antidepressants
CH = PO: initially 10 mg/kg/24 hr, div, every 8–12 hr; to be increased progressively, if needed, to 20 mg/kg/24 hr, div, every 12 hr or as a single daily dose, if tolerated. On the basis of presently available information 25 mg/kg/24 hr should not be exceeded.
TEGRETOL; tabl

Carbenicillin disodium; semisynthetic penicillin susceptible to destruction by penicillinase
℞ for systemic use: NB = IV (over 15–30 min), IM: initial dose

100 mg/kg, followed by maintenance therapy according to the following criteria:
≤2000 g + ≤7 days old: 225 mg/kg/24 hr, div, every 8 hr
≤2000 g + >7 days old: 400 mg/kg/24 hr, div, every 6 hr
>2000 g + ≤7 days old: 300 mg/kg/24 hr, div, every 6 hr
>2000 g + >7 days old: 400 mg/kg/24 hr, div, every 6 hr
IN, CH = IV (over 15–30 min), IM: 400–600 mg/kg/24 hr, div, every 4 hr (IV) or every 6 hr (IM)
GEOPEN; inj; 1 g carbenicillin disodium contains 6.5 mEq Na^+
℞ for treatment of urinary tract infection only: CH = PO: 10–30 mg/kg/24 hr, div, every 6 hr carbenicillin indanyl sodium, GEOCILLIN; tabl

Carbinoxamine maleate, ethanolamine; antihistamine with mild anticholinergic effect and low incidence of sedation and drowsiness.
℞ antiallergic effect: IN, CH = PO: 0.6 mg/kg/24 hr, div, every 6 hr
CLISTIN; elixir, tabl; component of many combination products

Cascara sagrada aromatic fluid extract; contains anthraquinones as active ingredients
℞ laxative: IN = PO: 1–2 ml/dose; CH = PO: 2–8 ml/dose

Cephalosporins; semisynthetic derivatives of 7-aminocephalosporanic acid, structurally related to penicillins
Cefaclor; effective against some beta-lactamase–producing ampicillin-resistant strains of *H. influenzae;* absorption not affected by food intake.
℞ for treatment of otitis media and infections of the upper and lower respiratory tracts, urinary tract, skin, and soft tissues with susceptible organisms: IN, CH = PO: 20–40 mg/kg/24 hr, div, every 8 hr
CECLOR; powder for oral susp, caps
Cefadroxil; relatively resistant against beta-lactamases; absorption appears unaffected by food intake; minimal inhibitory concentrations for *E. coli, P. mirabilis, Klebsiella* species may be maintained in urine for about 20 hr after single dose.
℞ for treatment of urinary tract infections: CH = PO: 30 mg/kg/24 hr, div, every 12 hr
DURICEF; caps, powder for oral susp
Cephazolin sodium: NB = IV (over 15–30 min), IM: 40 mg/kg/24 hr, div, every 12 hr; IN, CH = IV (over 15–30 min), IM: 50–100 mg/kg/24 hr, div, every 6 hr
ANCEF, KEFZOL; inj
Cephalexin: IN, CH = PO: 25–50 mg/kg/24 hr, div, every 6 hr
KEFLEX; caps, oral susp
Cephalothin: NB = IV (over 15–30 min), IM: ≤ 7 days old: 40 mg/kg/24 hr, div, every 12 hr; > 7 days old: 60 mg/kg/24 hr, div, every 8 hr; IN, CH = IV, IM: 80–160 mg/kg/24 hr, div, every 4 hr
KEFLIN; inj
Cephapirin sodium: CH = IV, IM: 40–80 mg/kg/24 hr, div, every 6 hr
CEFADYL; inj
Cephradine: CH = PO: 50–100 mg/kg/24 hr, div, every 6 hr; IV, IM: 50–100–300 mg/kg/24 hr, div, every 6 hr
ANSPOR, VELOSEF; caps, oral susp, inj

Chloral hydrate; trichloro derivative of acetaldehyde; tolerance to its hypnotic effect may develop
℞ for sedation: IN, CH = PO: 25 mg/kg/24 hr, div, every 6–8 hr
℞ for sleep: IN, CH = PO, (PR): 20 mg/kg/dose, to be repeated prn after 12–24 hr (maximum total daily dose: 50 mg/kg/24 hr)
†, NOCTEC, SOMNOS, ‡; elixir, syrup, suppos

Chloramphenicol; derivative of dichloracetic acid combined to a structure containing a nitrobenzene ring
NB = IV (over 15–30 min), (PO):
≤ 14 days old, irrespective of weight: 25 mg/kg/24 hr, div, every 4 hr
15–30 days old and ≤2000 g: 25 mg/kg/24 hr, div, every 4 hr
15–30 days old and >2000 g: 50 mg/kg/24 hr, div, every 4 hr
IN, CH = PO: 50–100 mg/kg/24 hr, div, every 6 hr; IV (over 15–30 min): 100 mg/kg/24 hr, div, every 4 hr
Caution: Newborn infants susceptible to development of high blood levels and gray-baby syndrome on usual doses; therefore, careful

DRUGS

Table 29–1B DRUG DOSES (Continued)

monitoring (of blood levels, if available) mandatory. Dose-duration–related suppression of erythrocyte production universal; weekly hematocrit or hemoglobin and reticulocyte count mandatory. Idiosyncratic aplastic anemia occasionally occurs without warning and may be lethal. **Use only when specifically indicated.**
CHLOROMYCETIN; caps ● chloramphenicol palmitate, CHLOROMYCETIN palmitate; oral susp ● chloramphenicol sodium succinate, CHLOROMYCETIN sodium succinate; inj

Chloroquine, a 4-aminoquinoline antimalarial agent; drug of choice for the treatment of attacks of malaria caused by *P. vivax, P. ovale, P. malariae,* and susceptible strains of *P. falciparum.* Not advised for use in treatment of juvenile rheumatoid arthritis.
℞ oral treatment of uncomplicated attacks (excluding those caused by chloroquine-resistant *P. falciparum):*
Chloroquine diphosphate: CH = PO:
first day: 25 mg/kg/first 24 hr (equivalent to base: 15 mg/kg/first 24 hr), div in initial dose of 16.5 mg/kg (equivalent to base 10 mg/kg) and subsequent dose of 8.5 mg/kg (equivalent to base 5 mg/kg) 6 hr later;
second and third day: 8.5 mg/kg/24 hr (equivalent to base 5 mg/kg/24 hr), as single daily dose
℞ intramuscular treatment of severe illness (excluding malaria caused by chloroquine-resistant *P. falciparum):*
Chloroquine dihydrochloride: CH = IM: 6 mg/kg/dose (equivalent to base 5 mg/kg/dose), every 12 hr, until clinical response is obtained and treatment can be completed by the oral route
℞ clinical prophylaxis of malaria (prevention of clinical manifestations from infection with any of the *Plasmodium* species):
Chloroquine diphosphate: CH = PO: 8.5 mg/kg/dose (equivalent to base 5 mg/kg/dose) once every 7 days, beginning 2 wk before entering the malarious area and continuing for 8 wk after return. For eradication of *P. vivax* and *P. ovale,* treatment for 14 days with primaquine should be considered on leaving malarious area.
chloroquine diphosphate, ARALEN diphosphate, (RESOCHIN) diphosphate, tabl; chloroquine dihydrochloride, ARALEN dihydrochloride, inj; (1 mg chloroquine base is equivalent to 1.65 mg chloroquine diphosphate or 1.2 mg chloroquine dihydrochloride)
Caution: Irreversible retinal damage may occur with prolonged use; frequent ophthalmologic examination necessary to detect early changes. *Note:* Chloroquine does *not* cause hemolysis in individuals with G-6-PD deficiency

Chlorothiazide; saluretic, inhibiting sodium reabsorption and interfering with dilution of urine
IN, CH = PO: 20 mg/kg/24 hr, div. every 12 hr.
†. DIURIL; tabl, oral susp

Chlorpheniramine maleate; alkylamine; antihistamine with anticholinergic and mild sedative effects
℞ antiallergic effect: CH = PO: 0.35 mg/kg/24 hr, div. every 6 hr
†, CHLORTRIMETON, ‡; tabl, syrup, inj

Chlorpromazine; phenothiazine with aliphatic side chain
℞ for sedation: CH = PO: 2 mg/kg/24 hr, div, every 4–6 hr, prn; IM: 1.6 mg/kg/24 hr, div, every 6–8 hr, prn
THORAZINE; suppos; chlorpromazine hydrochloride, THORAZINE hydrochloride; tabl, syrup, inj
Caution: Overdose may produce parkinsonian syndrome. Diphenhydramine may be antidotal

Chlortetracycline; see Tetracyclines

Chlorthalidone; nonthiazide saluretic with protracted duration of action
CH = PO: 2 mg/kg/dose, as single dose; to be repeated with adjusted single dose 3 times/wk
HYGROTON; tabl

Cimetidine; H_2-receptor antagonist inhibiting gastric acid secretion

℞ for treatment of duodenal and gastric ulcers and for relief of symptoms caused by gastroesophageal reflux; compatible with concomitant treatment with oral antacids (which should be given at frequent intervals and in adequate dosage) and/or anticholinergic antispasmodics. Clinical experience in children is extremely limited, and the benefit/risk ratio should be carefully considered: PO: 20–40 mg/kg/24 hr, div and given with every meal, have been used, as well as same dosage, IV, div, every 4 hr.
TAGAMET; tabl, inj

Clindamycin; semisynthetic derivative of lincomycin
IN, CH = PO: 10–25 mg/kg/24 hr, div, every 6–8 hr (expressed in terms of the base); IV (infusion over 30–60 min), IM: 25–40 mg/kg/24 hr, div, every 6–8 hr (expressed in terms of the base)
clindamycin hydrochloride, CLEOCIN hydrochloride; caps ● clindamycin palmitate hydrochloride, CLEOCIN pediatric; oral susp ● clindamycin phosphate, CLEOCIN phosphate; inj

Clonazepam; benzodiazepine with selective anticonvulsant effect
CH = PO: start with 0.01–0.03 mg/kg/24 hr, div, every 8 hr, and progressively increase up to 0.3 mg/kg/24 hr, div, every 8 hr, if needed.
Caution: Concomitant use of clonazepam and valproate sodium may lead to petit mal status.
CLONOPIN; tabl

Cloxacillin sodium monohydrate; penicillinase-resistant penicillin
IN, CH = PO: 50–100 mg/kg/24 hr, div, every 6 hr (expressed in terms of the base)
TEGOPEN; caps, oral susp

Codeine phosphate or sulfate; narcotic analgesic
℞ as antitussive: CH = 1–1.5 mg/kg/24 hr, div, every 4 hr, prn
℞ against moderately severe pain: CH = PO: 4 mg/kg/24 hr, div, every 4–6 hr, prn; SC: 3 mg/kg/24 hr, div, every 4–6 hr, prn
†; tabl, oral susp, inj; mostly in combination with other drugs

Colistin sodium methanesulfonate, colistimethate sodium, and **colistin** sulfate, polymyxin E; polypeptide antimicrobial agent with cationic detergent activity
℞ inhibition of gastrointestinal flora, justified only in selected cases (gastroenteritis with susceptible organism): IN, CH = PO (colistin sulfate): 5–15 mg/kg/24 hr, div, every 8 hr; IM, IV (by slow infusion): 3–5 mg/kg/24 hr, div, every 8 hr
Caution against overgrowth of abnormal organisms
colistimethate sodium, COLY-MYCIN N; inj ● colistin sulfate, COLY-MYCIN S; oral susp

Corticosteroids
℞ physiologic replacement: *cortisone:* PO: 1 mg/kg/24 hr, div, every 8 hr; IM: 0.5 mg/kg/24 hr, div, every 24 hr. (*Note:* "Increased demand" under stressful situation; e.g., in children with congenital adrenogenital syndrome, receiving replacement therapy, for stressful situation which 2 mg/kg/24 hr of cortisol may be safer)
℞ use in pharmacologic doses (leukemia, lymphoma, nephrosis, rheumatic carditis, certain types of tuberculosis, immunologic reactions, and other types of autoimmune disease): adjust dosage to the specific situation.
cortisone: PO: 10 mg/kg/24 hr, div, every 6–8 hr; IM: 3–6 mg/kg/24 hr, div, every 12 hr
prednisone: PO: 2 mg/kg/24 hr, div, every 6–8 hr (or analogue in equally effective dosage; see Table)
(For continued treatment after initial response, adjust dosage, frequency of administration, and duration of treatment according to type of disease and side effects to be avoided.)
℞ in status asthmaticus refractory to other types of treatment: hydrocortisone sodium phosphate or succinate: IV: 10–20 mg/kg/24 hr, div, every 6 hr *or* 4 mg/kg/dose every 4 hr until response is obtained
℞ in endotoxic shock: hydrocortisone sodium phosphate or succinate: IV: 50 mg/kg/initial dose, followed by 50–75 mg/kg/24 hr, div, every 6 hr

DRUGS

Relative Potencies of Corticosteroids:

	ANTI-INFLAMMATORY EFFECT, GLUCONEOGENESIS	SODIUM-RETAINING EFFECT
hydrocortisone (cortisol)	1	1
cortisone	0.8	0.8
prednisolone	4	0.8
prednisone	4	0.8
methylprednisolone	5	0.5
triamcinolone	4	0
dexamethasone	25	0
desoxycorticosterone	0	100
aldosterone	0.3	3000

dexamethasone, DECADRON, GAMMACORTEN, ‡; tabl, elixir ●
dexamethasone sodium phosphate, DECADRON phosphate; inj
hydrocortisone, †, CORTEF, HYDROCORTONE, ‡; tabl, oral susp
● hydrocortisone sodium phosphate, †, HYDROCORTONE
phosphate; inj ● hydrocortisone sodium succinate, †, SOLU-
CORTEF; inj
methylprednisolone, MEDROL; tabl ● methylprednisolone sodium
succinate, SOLU-MEDROL; inj
prednisone, †, DELTASONE, METICORTEN, ‡; tabl ●
prednisolone, †, DELTA-CORTEF, METICORTELONE, ‡; tabl
triamcinolone, ARISTOCORT, KENACORT; tabl, syrup
Caution: May inhibit clinical signs of infection.

Cortisone; see Corticosteroids

Cromolyn sodium
  ℞ topical prophylaxis of bronchial asthma; not useful in the
  treatment of acute asthmatic attack since it is not a
  bronchodilator. CH (5 yr and older) = inhalation of the content
  of 1 capsule every 6 hr through the specially devised turboinhaler; 1 capsule contains 20 μg cromolyn sodium
  AARANE, INTAL; inhalation with spinhaler

Cyclizine hydrochloride; antihistamine, antiemetic, and anticholinergic
  agent
  ℞ for prevention and relief of symptoms of motion sickness: CH
  (6–10 yr) = PO: 3 mg/kg/24 hr, div, every 8 hr. The 1st dose
  should be taken about 20 min before departure.
  MAREZINE; tabl; cyclizine lactate for IM inj

Cyproheptadine hydrochloride; piperidine; serotonin and histamine
  antagonist with mild anticholinergic and mild sedative effects
  ℞ antiallergic effect: CH = PO: 0.25 mg/kg/24 hr, div, every 6 hr
  PERIACTIN; tabl, syrup

Demeclocycline; see Tetracyclines

Dexamethasone; see Corticosteroids

Dextroamphetamine sulfate; noncatecholamine sympathomimetic
  agent
  ℞ in minimal brain dysfunction: drug treatment not recommended
  below age of 3 yr or in nonstructured therapeutic situation. CH
  (above 3 yr) = PO: initiate treatment with 2.5 mg/dose given at
  onset of daytime activities and again 4–6 hr later. If needed,
  increase at weekly intervals by increments of 2.5 mg/dose and
  adjust respective size of separate doses according to response.
  Daily dose should not exceed 1 mg/kg/24 hr.
  ℞ in narcolepsy: PO: proceed for dosage as in minimal brain
  dysfunction. End points: control of symptoms, maximal dose.
  To avoid insomnia do not administer closer than 6 hr before
  bedtime. **Caution** against diversion of CNS stimulants from
  legitimate use in patient to misuse in adults.
  †, DEXEDRINE; tabl
  Caution: Severe mental depression may follow withdrawal.
  Overdose may produce extreme restlessness and psychotic
  behavior.

Dextromethorphan hydrobromide; D-isomer of a codeine analogue,
  and probably free of addictive effects
  ℞ antitussive agent: IN, CH = PO: 1 mg/kg/24 hr, div, every 6–8
  hr
  †, ROMILAR; syrup; contained in many combination products

Diazepam; benzodiazepine with anxiolytic and muscle-relaxant
  effects
  ℞ in status epilepticus: NB, IN, CH = IV (slowly, as controlled
  "push" injection): 0.3 mg/kg/dose; may be repeated 2 times after
  intervals of 5 min; give IM if impossible to give it IV (efficacy
  diminished)
  ℞ for symptomatic relief of anxiety: CH = PO: 0.2–0.3 mg/kg/24
  hr, div, every 6 hr; adjust dosage according to response
  VALIUM; tabl and VALIUM injectable
  Caution: Confusion and prolonged extreme drowsiness may follow
  overdose or concurrent ingestion of alcohol in any form.

Diazoxide, nondiuretic benzothiadiazine derivative with several
  prominent actions: (1) relaxation of smooth muscles in the
  peripheral arterioles after IV injection only; (2) hyperglycemic
  effect (beginning 1 hr after administration and lasting for
  approximately 8 hr) through inhibition of release of insulin; (3)
  retention of sodium and concomitantly of water; (4) hyperuricemic
  effect
  ℞ for emergency reduction of hypertension: CH = IV (injection
  within 30 sec of calculated amount of undiluted diazoxide solution into a peripheral vein): 5 mg/kg/dose. If 1st injection fails to
  elicit adequate response within 30 min, administer a 2nd complementary dose. Hypotensive effect usually lasts 2–12 hr. Successive injections frequently give a better response than the
  initial dose. As soon as possible, switch to oral regimen with
  alternative antihypertensive medication (Table 13–16).
  Note: Diazoxide is ineffective against hypertension due to pheochromocytoma. A concurrently administered thiazide diuretic
  (which characteristically exerts a diuretic response) may potentiate the antihypertensive, hyperglycemic, and hyperuricemic effects of diazoxide.
  Caution: hypotensive circulatory failure (responding to catecholamine such as norepinephrine), congestive heart failure (responding to plasma volume depletion by saluretic), and hyperosmolar coma in patients with diabetes mellitus (responding to
  insulin) may occur.
  HYPERSTAT; inj

Dicloxacillin sodium monohydrate; penicillinase-resistant penicillin
  IN, CH = PO: 12.5–25 mg/kg/24 hr, div, every 6 hr
  DYNAPEN; caps, oral susp

Digitoxin; cardiac glycoside with long half-life (5–9 days): main glycoside in digitalis leaf
  ℞ for digitalization: 0.5 × digitalizing dose initially, 0.25 × digitalizing dose 8 and 16 hr later. (Digitalizing dose: NB = IV, IM:
  0.035 mg/kg, div in fractions, or PO: 0.050 mg/kg, div in fractions.
  IN = IV, IM 0.050 mg/kg, div in fractions, or PO: 0.070 mg/kg,
  div in fractions
  CH = IM, PO: 0.030 mg/kg, divided into fractions as indicated
  above)
  ℞ for maintenance: begin maintenance dosage 24 hr after 1st
  fraction of digitalizing dose. NB, IN, CH = 0.1 × digitalizing
  dose, every 24 hr
  Note: Digitalizing and maintenance doses must be adjusted to
  condition of patient.
  †, CRYSTODIGIN, PURODIGIN; tabl, inj
  Caution: Fatal arrhythmia may follow overdose.

Digoxin; cardiac glycoside with rapid onset of action and half-life of
  approximately 48 hr
  ℞ for digitalization: 0.5 × digitalizing dose initially, 0.25 × digitalizing dose 8 and 16 hr later.
  (Digitalizing dose: NB = IV, IM: 0.035 mg/kg div in fractions, or
  PO: 0.050 mg/kg, div in fractions.
  IN = IV, IM 0.050 mg/kg div in fractions, or PO: 0.070 mg/kg, in
  fractions
  CH = IV, IM, PO: same doses as indicated for NB)
  ℞ for maintenance: begin maintenance dosage 24 hr after 1st
  fraction of digitalizing dose. NB = PO: 0.010 mg/kg/24 hr, div,
  every 12 hr. IN, CH = PO: 0.017 mg/kg/24 hr, div, every 12 hr
  Note: Digitalizing and maintenance doses must be adjusted to the
  condition of the patient.
  †, LANOXIN; tabl, elixir, inj
  Caution: Fatal arrhythmia may follow overdose.

See KEY to abbreviations, p. 1814; for further information about drugs, see package insert.

DRUGS

Table 29–1B DRUG DOSES (Continued)

Dimenhydrinate, chlorotheophylline salt of diphenhydramine
 ℞ for the prevention and treatment of motion sickness: CH = PO: 5 mg/kg/24 hr, div, every 6 hr
 DRAMAMINE; tabl, oral susp, suppos

Dioctyl sodium sulfosuccinate; wetting agent, emulsifier, demulcent
 ℞ as stool softener: IN, CH = PO: 5 mg/kg/24 hr, div, with meals
 †, COLACE, DOXINATE, ‡; caps, oral sol, syrup

Diphenhydramine hydrochloride; ethanolamine; antihistamine with mild anticholinergic, sedative, antiemetic and antitussive effects
 ℞ antiallergic effect; sometimes used as sedative. IN, CH = PO, IM, IV: 5 mg/kg/24 hr, div, every 6–8 hr
 †, BENADRYL; caps, elixir, inj

Dopamine, α- and β-adrenergic as well as dopaminergic agent (positive inotropic effect on heart)
 ℞ to increase cardiac output and improve organ perfusion: IV infusion (into large vein): Example: to prepare a solution containing 0.400 mg/ml, mix 100 mg dopamine HCl in 250 ml 5% D/W or appropriate electrolyte solution with pH below 7.0 (do not include bicarbonate!), and infuse at rate adjusted to response in patient, beginning with 0.002–0.005 mg/kg/min and increasing by increments of 0.005 mg/kg/min if needed up to 0.050 mg/kg/min. In case of extravasation causing peripheral ischemia, use phentolamine (REGITINE) for local infiltration.
 INTROPIN; inj

Doxycycline; see Tetracyclines

Edrophonium chloride; cholinesterase inhibitor with short duration of action
 ℞ for myasthenia in NB of myasthenic mother = IV (slowly) or IM: 0.2 mg/kg/dose. Symptoms should be relieved almost immediately. Continue cholinesterase-inhibiting treatment, if indicated, with pyridostigmine.
 ℞ for differential diagnosis of myasthenic crisis, or as adjunct treatment to carotid massage in supraventricular tachycardia: NB, IN, CH = IV: 0.05 mg/kg/dose, and watch for effect after 15–30 sec, or IM: 0.1 mg/kg/dose, and expect effect after 2–10 min
 If edrophonium test is given during "cholinergic crisis," weakness of affected muscles, including respiratory muscles, will worsen or not improve. Ventilation should be assisted, if needed, and bradycardia can be influenced by atropine. If recovery from weakness occurs, continuation of cholinesterase inhibition is indicated using inhibitors with longer duration of action, such as pyridostigmine, neostigmine, ambenonium. Their dosage must be individually titrated and adjusted.
 Manifestations of overdosage with cholinesterase-inhibiting medication: increase in muscle weakness and worsening of respiratory difficulty and dysphagia after each dose of drug; fasciculations of muscles; excessive salivation, increase in bronchial secretion; vomiting, diarrhea, pallor, sweating, bradycardia.
 TENSILON; inj
 Caution: Administration during cholinergic crisis may cause paralysis of respiratory muscles. Use only when ventilatory assistance available.

Ephedrine, phenylethylamine (direct and indirect sympathomimetic)
 ℞ for treatment of asthma in subacute stage; tolerance develops. CH = PO: 3 mg/kg/24 hr, div, every 4–6 hr. Contained in many antiasthma preparations; should be replaced with more selectively active drug
 ephedrine hydrochloride; ephedrine sulfate; caps, tabl, syrup
 Caution: Acute overdose may produce seizures and coma.

Epinephrine, catecholamine (α- and β-adrenergic agonist)
 ℞ bronchodilator (β₂ stimulatory effect), in acute asthma attack: IN, CH = SC: 0.01 mg/kg/dose, repeat prn every 20 min, 2 times
 Note: With epinephrine solution 1:1000 this corresponds to 0.01 ml/kg/dose.
 Caution: Cardiac arrhythmia and/or acute hypertension may follow overdose.

Ergotamine, adrenergic blocking agent as well as direct vasoconstrictor of vessels to the brain, and serotonin antagonist
 ℞ against acute attack of vascular headache (migraine): older child and adolescent = IM, SC (in acute attack): 0.25–0.50 mg/dose,

in single application. Minimal effective dose should be established for each patient by titration of the amount required to control headaches in that patient. Older child and adolescent = SL, PO (at 1st symptoms of attack): 1 mg/dose; if no improvement within following 30 min, repeat same dose once.
 Note: Signs of therapeutic overdosage: nausea, vomiting, diarrhea, tingling of hands and feet, weakness, muscle pain.
 ergotamine tartrate: CYNERGEN; inj, tabl ● ergotamine tartrate + caffeine: CAFERGOT, tabl, suppos ● dihydroergotamine mesylate: D.H.E.45, inj

Erythromycin; macrolide antimicrobial agent
 IN, GH = PO: 30–50 mg/kg/24 hr, div, every 6 hr; IV: 15–20 mg/kg/24 hr, div, every 6 hr
 erythromycin, †, ILOTYCIN, ‡; tabl ● erythromycin estolate, ILOSONE; tabl, oral susp ● erythromycin ethylsuccinate, PEDIAMYCIN, ‡; tabl, oral susp, drops ● erythromycin glucceptate, ILOTYCIN glucceptate IV; inj ● erythromycin lactobionate, ERYTHROCIN lactobionate iV; inj ● erythromycin stearate, ERYTHROCIN stearate, ‡; tabl

Ethacrynic acid; saluretic, inhibiting chloride and sodium reabsorption and interfering mainly with concentration of urine
 CH = PO: approximately 1 mg/kg/dose, as single daily dose. Adjust according to effect, and repeat prn on alternate days; dosage in infants and children not firmly established (PO, IV)
 EDECRIN; tabl ● ethacrynate sodium, IV, sodium EDECRIN; inj (IV only)

Ethambutol hydrochloride; antituberculous agent used concomitantly with isoniazid
 ℞ in the treatment of tuberculosis as part of multiple drug regimen. Conditions for safe use in children not firmly established. In adults: 15–25 mg/kg/24 hr, as single daily dose, for course of treatment or retreatment. *Because of rare side effects of optic neuritis and decreased visual acuity,* eye examinations are indicated before inception of treatment and at monthly intervals thereafter.
 MYAMBUTOL; tabl

Ethosuximide; anticonvulsant agent of the succinimide type
 CH = PO: 20 mg/kg/24 hr, div, every 12 hr
 ZARONTIN; caps, syrup

Furosemide; saluretic with a duration of action of about 2 hr when given IV; inhibits chloride and sodium reabsorption and interferes with concentration of urine
 IN, CH = PO: start with 2 mg/kg/dose; if needed, increase progressively to 3–6 mg/kg/dose, at intervals of 6–8 hr. IV: start with 1 mg/kg/dose; if needed, increase progressively to 6 mg/kg/dose, with an interval of at least 2 hr between doses
 LASIX; tabl, oral sol, inj

Gentamicin sulfate; antimicrobial aminoglycoside
 NB = IM, IV (over 1–2 hr). ≤ 7 days old: 5 mg/kg/24 hr, div, every 12 hr; > 7 days old: 7.5 mg/kg/24 hr, div, every 8 hr. CH = IM, IV (over 0.5–2 hr): 6–7.5 mg/kg/24 hr, div, every 8 hr
 Usual duration of treatment: 7–10 days.
 GARAMYCIN; inj
 Caution: Ototoxic; nephrotoxic, perhaps especially with concomitant administration of cephalosporins

Griseofulvin; antifungal agent
 ℞ against deep-seated mycotic infections (skin, hair, nails) with organisms of the species *Microsporum, Trichophyton, Epidermophyton:* CH = PO (microcrystalline): 10 mg/kg/24 hr for 4–6 wk (4–6 mo for fingernails, 6–12 mo for toenails)
 Note: "Ultramicrosize" form is an ultramicrocrystalline suspension for which 125 mg is biologically equivalent to 250 mg of a "microsize" preparation. The daily dose of an ultramicrosize preparation is reduced to 5 mg/kg/24 hr and offers comparable efficacy without additional advantages.
 griseofulvin, microcrystalline, †, FULVICIN-U/F, GRIFULVIN V, ‡; tabl, oral susp ● griseofulvin, ultramicrocrystalline GRIS-PEG; tabl

Hydralazine hydrochloride; phthalazine derivative; causes relaxation of vascular smooth muscles, especially of arterioles
 ℞ as antihypertensive in long-term treatment: CH = PO: initially

See KEY to abbreviations, p. 1814; for further information about drugs, see package insert.

Table 29-1B DRUG DOSES (Continued)

0.75 mg/kg/24 hr, div, every 6 hr; increase progressively until desired response or daily maximum dose of 3.5 mg/kg/24 hr is reached

℞ for emergency reduction of hypertension: IV (immediate onset of action), IM (onset of action after 15–20 min): 0.15 mg/kg/dose; repeat prn every 30–90 min up to daily dose of 1.7–3.6 mg/kg/24 hr; switch to oral administration if conditions permit

Note: Hydralazine may produce sodium retention and usually increases plasma renin activity.

Caution: May induce lupus erythematosus–like syndrome; frequency related to dosage.

†, APRESOLINE, ‡; tabl, inj

Hydrochlorothiazide; saluretic, inhibiting sodium reabsorption and interfering with dilution of urine

IN, CH = PO: 2 mg/kg/24 hr, div, every 12 hr

†, ESIDRIX, HYDRODIURIL, ‡; tabl

Hydroxyzine hydrochloride; neuroleptic agent of the piperazine type, with sedative and antihistamine effects

℞ for sedation and/or antihistamine effect: CH = PO: 2 mg/kg/24 hr, div, every 6–8 hr, prn

ATARAX: tabl, syrup; VISTARIL I.M.: inj (IM) ● hydroxyzine pamoate, VISTARIL; caps, oral susp

Imipramine hydrochloride; tricyclic antidepressant

℞ against enuresis, as adjunct therapy to proper medical and educational approach, after age 4 yr: CH (after age 4 yr) = PO: 25 mg/24 hr, to be given in single dose 1 hr before bedtime; if response unsatisfactory, dose may be increased to 50 mg in children between 25–40 kg, and to 75 mg in adolescents

After a 1 mo trial without result, the drug should be discontinued as ineffective under existing circumstances. After a favorable response for a continued treatment period of 3 mo, drug should be skipped on alternate days and finally discontinued.

†, TOFRANIL; tabl

Iron preparations

℞ Daily maintenance iron requirement: elemental iron: PO: 0.5–1 mg/kg/24 hr, in single dose or divided

℞ In iron deficiency anemia, as elemental iron: PO: 6 mg/kg/24 hr, div, with meals

Note: Iron supply at this dosage level ought to be continued for 2–3 mo to compensate for the deficits in erythrocytes and iron stores. Only iron in the ferrous form (Fe^{++}) is absorbed from the gastrointestinal tract. The content of elemental iron in different preparations varies. The percentage of dry weight as elemental iron of ferrous choline citrate is 20; ferrous fumarate, 33; ferrous gluconate, 12; ferrous lactate, 19; ferrous sulfate, 20; and iron-dextran complex (ferric hydroxide), 2.

℞ Dose calculation for parenteral iron administration: elemental Fe deficit = 2.5 mg/kg × deficit of hemoglobin concentration (in grams/dl) in blood. (The deficit of the hemoglobin concentration is obtained as the difference between the measured and the desirable value, expressed in g/dl.) When iron has to be supplied by the parenteral route, deep IM injection is preferable to IV administration. In either case, a test dose of approximately 25 mg elemental Fe in the form of the dextran complex should precede the administration of the total dose. If the total dose is large, it should be divided in separate daily doses of which none should exceed 5 mg/kg/24 hr of elemental iron.

Note: An additional 20–30% of the calculated deficit is needed to restore the tissue iron reserves.

Caution: Acute overdose may lead to shock, CNS depression, death (Sec 28.10).

Isoniazid, INH, isonicotinic acid hydrazide; tuberculostatic agent

℞ in the treatment of active tuberculosis, in combination with other antituberculous drugs: IN, CH = PO, IM: 10–20 mg/kg/24 hr, div, every 8–12 hr; maximum daily dose: 500 mg/24 hr. AD-PO, IM: 5–10 mg/kg/24 hr, div, every 8–12 hr; maximum daily dose: 300 mg/24 hr

℞ for prophylaxis of complications in recent conversion to positive tuberculin reaction (primary tuberculosis), or after suspected ex-

posure: IN, CH = PO: 5–10 mg/kg/24 hr, as single dose, or div, every 12 hr; maximum daily dose: 300 mg/24 hr

Note: "Slow" acetylators (homozygous) need only about 0.20–0.50 of this dose to reach therapeutically effective plasma concentrations achieved by "rapid" acetylators (homozygous and heterozygous). Higher than necessary plasma concentrations of unmetabolized isoniazid seem not to be associated with risk of isoniazid hepatotoxicity.

†, INH; tabl, syrup, inj

Caution: Formation of toxic metabolite in some patients may lead to hepatic necrosis with usual doses (rare under 20 yr of age).

Isoproterenol hydrochloride; β-adrenergic agent

℞ to overcome atrioventricular block: IV infusion: Example: to prepare a solution containing 0.004 mg/ml, mix 1 mg isoproterenol in 250 ml 5% D/W or appropriate electrolyte solution and infuse at rate adjusted to response in patient (beginning with approximately 0.0001–0.0002 mg/kg/min)

†, ISUPREL; inj

Kanamycin sulfate; antimicrobial aminoglycoside

NB = IM, IV (over 20–30 min):

≤ 2000 g and ≤ 7 days old: 15 mg/kg/24 hr, div, every 12 hr
≤ 2000 g and > 7 days old: 20 mg/kg/24 hr, div, every 12 hr
> 2000 g and ≤ 7 days old: 20 mg/kg/24 hr, div, every 12 hr
> 2000 g and > 7 days old: 30 mg/kg/24 hr, div, every 8 hr

IN, CH = IM, IV (over 20–30 min): 6–15 mg/kg/24 hr, div, every 8–12 hr. Usual duration of therapy: 7–10 days; not indicated in long-term therapy because of ototoxic hazard. **Caution:** Ototoxic, nephrotoxic.

KANTREX; inj

Lidocaine hydrochloride; anesthetic agent used systemically for its antiarrhythmic effects; delayed slow diastolic depolarization, diminished automaticity. Does not affect normal conduction but seemingly improves conduction velocity in damaged areas of myocardium. In therapeutic doses does not depress myocardial contractility or atrioventricular conduction.

℞ against ventricular tachyarrhythmia: IN, CH = IV (slowly, as 20 mg/ml sol): 1 mg/kg/dose, to be repeated prn after 20 min, or continuous IV infusion as 1 mg/ml sol: 0.020–0.050 mg/kg/min, to a maximum total dose of 5 mg/kg/24 hr

XYLOCAINE hydrochloride IV; inj

Caution: Excessive depression of cardiac conductivity may occur; ECG monitoring indicated during treatment.

Lincomycin hydrochloride; antimicrobial macrolide

CH = PO: 30–60 mg/kg/24 hr, div, every 8 hr. IM, IV (over 1–4 hr, as 10 mg/ml sol): 10–20 mg/kg/24 hr, div, every 8–12 hr

LINCOCIN; caps, syrup, inj

"Lytic cocktail," mixture of narcotic analgesic, antihistamine, and phenothiazine

℞ for temporary heavy sedation: IM (deep, after mixing the 3 components in 1 syringe): meperidine (DEMEROL), 2 mg/kg/dose, plus promethazine (PHENERGAN), 1 mg/kg/dose, plus chlorpromazine (THORAZINE), 1 mg/kg/dose (maximum single dose not to exceed meperidine, 50 mg, promethazine, 25 mg, and chlorpromazine, 25 mg)

Magnesium hydroxide, $Mg(OH)_2$

℞ as cathartic: PO: 40 mg/kg/dose

milk of magnesia, susp, "8%" containing $Mg(OH)_2$ 80 mg/ml

Magnesium sulfate, $MgSO_4 \cdot 7H_2O$, Epsom salt; 1 g of the salt is equivalent to 98.6 mg elemental Mg or to 8.11 mEq Mg^{++}

℞ as cathartic: PO: ($MgSO_4 \cdot 7H_2O$): 250 mg/kg/dose

℞ in hypomagnesemia: IM (in solution containing $MgSO_4 \cdot 7H_2O$ 500 mg/ml, equivalent to Mg^{++} 4 mEq/ml, also labeled "50%"): $MgSO_4 \cdot 7H_2O$ 100 mg/kg/dose, equivalent to Mg^{++} 0.8 mEq/kg/dose, repeat every 4–6 hr

IV (in solution containing $MgSO_4 \cdot 7H_2O$ 100 mg/ml, equivalent to Mg^{++} 0.08 mEq/ml, also labeled "10%"): Infuse slowly $MgSO_4 \cdot 7H_2O$ up to 100 mg/kg/dose, equivalent to Mg^{++} 0.08 mEq/kg/dose

†; crystalline salt, sterile sol for inj available as 50%, 25%, and 10%

See KEY to abbreviations, p. 1814; for further information about drugs, see package insert.

Table 29–1B DRUG DOSES (Continued)

Mannitol; osmotic diuretic
  ℞ test dose for oliguria: CH = IV: 0.2 g/kg/dose, injected within 3–5 min
  ℞ in cerebral edema: CH = IV: 1–2.5 g/kg/dose, injected as 15–25% sol over 30–60 min
  †, OSMITROL, ‡; IV inj

Mebendazole; anthelmintic agent which blocks glucose uptake by the susceptible parasites and interferes with their survival
  ℞ against pinworms (*Enterobius vermicularis*; cure rate 90–100%): CH = PO: 100 mg/dose, as single dose, against whipworms (*Trichuris trichiura*; cure rate 61–75%), roundworms (*Ascaris lumbricoides*; cure rate 91–100%) and hookworms (*Ancylostoma duodenale, Necator americanus*; cure rate 96%). Alternative method = PO: 200 mg/24 hr, div, every 12 hr, for 3 consecutive days. If patient is not free of parasites 3 wk after treatment a 2nd course is indicated
  Note: Not extensively studied in children under 2 yr of age.
  VERMOX; chewable tabl

Meperidine hydrochloride; synthetic narcotic analgesic agent; addictive
  ℞ against severe pain: CH = PO, SC, IM: 6 mg/kg/24 hr, div, prn every 4–6 hr (maximum single dose; 100 mg)
  †, DEMEROL hydrochloride, ‡; tabl, elixir, inj
  Caution: May produce respiratory depression, seizures, coma in some sensitive patients. Test dose advisable. Naloxone is antidote.

Mercaptomerin sodium; mercurial diuretic
  Outmoded regimen for reducing edema in congestive heart failure, in patients with normal kidney function: CH = SC, IM: 0.035 ml "mercaptomerin sol"/kg/dose, equivalent to approximately 1.4 mg mercury/kg/dose. Dose and frequency of administration to be adjusted to the situation of the patient (once daily to once/wk). 125 mg mercaptomerin sodium is equivalent to 40 mg mercury
  THIOMERIN; inj

Metaproterenol sulfate; analogue of catecholamine; selective β_2 adrenergic agent
  ℞ bronchodilator: dosage in children not yet firmly established. PO: 1–1.5 mg/kg/24 hr, div, every 6 hr
  ALUPENT, METAPREL; syrup, tabl, inhalation

Methacycline; see Tetracyclines

Methenamine mandelate; urinary antibacterial agent effective in a nonspecific manner against microorganisms by liberating formaldehyde on decomposing in urine at pH below 5.5
  ℞ for prevention of bacterial growth in urine, provided pH is sufficiently low: CH = PO: initially 100 mg/kg/24 hr, div, every 6 hr, followed by 50 mg/kg/24 hr, div, every 6 hr
  Note: Should not be used (and is useless) when urine acidification is contraindicated or not attainable (as in infections with urea-splitting bacteria). If situation permits, acidification of urine below pH 5.5 might be implemented by adjusting acid load of intake.
  †, MANDELAMINE, tabl, oral susp ● methenamine hippurate, HIPREX; tabl

Methicillin sodium; semisynthetic penicillinase-resistant penicillin
  NB = IM, IV (over 15–30 min): according to the following criteria:
  ≤ 2000 g and < 14 days old: 50 mg/kg/24 hr, div, every 12 hr
  ≤ 2000 g and 15–30 days old: 75 mg/kg/24 hr, div, every 8 hr
  > 2000 g and ≤ 14 days old: 75 mg/kg/24 hr, div, every 8 hr
  > 2000 g and 15–30 days old: 100 mg/kg/24 hr, div, every 6 hr
  IN, CH = IV (over 15–30 min), IM: 200–400 mg/kg/24 hr, div, every 4 hr (IV) or every 6 hr (IM)
  CELBENIN, STAPHCILLIN; inj

Methyldopa; antihypertensive agent, inhibitor of aromatic amino acid decarboxylase, and precursor of α-methylnorepinephrine. Probably lowers arterial blood pressure by stimulation of central inhibitory α-adrenergic receptors, false neurotransmission, and/or reduction of plasma renin activity
  ℞ as antihypertensive in long-term treatment: CH = PO: initially 10 mg/kg/24 hr, div, every 6–12 hr; decrease or increase the dose progressively at intervals of 2 days until adequate response achieved; maximum daily dosage: 65 mg/kg/24 hr
  Caution: Positive direct Coombs test develops in 10–20% of patients on prolonged treatment, usually between 6–12 mo of continued administration. Positive indirect Coombs test, fever, and liver dysfunction occur less frequently. If evidence of hemolysis or liver dysfunction present, methyldopa should be discontinued and not reinstituted.
  ALDOMET; tabl

Methylphenidate hydrochloride; piperidine derivative structurally related to amphetamine; CNS stimulant with more prominent effects on mental than on motor activities
  ℞ in minimal brain dysfunction (MBD): drug treatment of MBD not recommended below the age of 3 yr or in nonstructured therapeutic situation. CH (over 3 yr) = PO: initiate treatment with 5 mg dose given at the onset of daytime activities and again 4–6 hr later; if needed, increase the dose at weekly intervals by increments of 5 mg/dose and adjust the size of the respective doses (early morning and mid-day) according to the response in the patient; daily dose usually should not exceed 2 mg/kg/24 hr. To avoid insomnia do not administer closer than 6 hr before bedtime
  Caution: Reduction of growth rate and weight gain might accompany prolonged use. Chronic abuse can lead to tolerance.
  ℞ in narcolepsy: PO: proceed for dosage adjustment as in MBD, with correction of the abnormal symptomatology as the end point.
  RITALIN; tabl

Miconazole; synthetic antifungal imidazole derivative effective against systemic infections with *Coccidioides immitis, Candida albicans, Cryptococcus neoformans, Paracoccidioides brasiliensis*. IV infusion alone is inadequate in the treatment of fungal meningitis and urinary bladder infection; intrathecal administration and bladder instillation must also be carried out.
  ℞ for treatment of proven coccidioidomycosis, candidiasis, cryptococcosis, or paracoccidioidomycosis: CH = IV (after dilution with isotonic saline or 5% D/W and over 30–60 min): 20–40 mg/kg/24 hr, div, every 8 hr, until clinical and laboratory tests no longer indicate activity of fungal infection. Dose may vary with type of fungus involved.
  MONISTAT IV; ampoules for IV inj

Mineral oil; indigestible liquid hydrocarbon with limited absorbability; lubricant
  ℞ mild laxative: PO: 0.5 ml/kg/dose
  †, liquid petrolatum; plain liquid or emulsion

Minocycline; see Tetracyclines

Minoxidil; direct-acting peripheral vasodilator
  ℞ in severely hypertensive patients who do not adequately respond to maximum therapeutic doses of a diuretic and 2 other antihypertensive agents. Usually a beta-adrenergic blocking agent has to be given concomitantly to prevent tachycardia and increased myocardial workload, as well as a diuretic such as hydrochlorothiazide, chlorthalidone, or furosemide to prevent serious fluid retention. CH = PO: initial dosage 0.2 mg/kg/24 hr as single dose; thereafter dosage may be increased stepwise to 0.25–1.0 mg/kg/24 hr under careful titration of the size and frequency of administration of the doses according to the individual needs of the patient.
  LONITEN; tabl

Morphine sulfate; narcotic analgesic agent; addictive
  ℞ against severe pain: CH = SC: 0.6–1.2 mg/kg/24 hr, div, prn every 4 hr, equivalent to 0.1–0.2 mg/kg/dose, to be repeated prn every 4 hr
  †; inj
  Caution: Overdose produces severe respiratory depression, hypothermia, coma. Naloxone antidotal.

Nafcillin sodium; semisynthetic penicillinase-resistant penicillin
  NB = IM, IV (over 15–30 min): ≤ 7 days old: 40 mg/kg/24 hr, div,

DRUGS

every 12 hr; > 7 days old: 60 mg/kg/24 hr, div, every 8 hr. IN, CH = PO: 50–100 mg/kg/24 hr, div, every 6 hr; IM, IV (over 15–30 min): 100–200 mg/kg/24 hr, div, every 6 hr (IM) or every 4 hr (IV)
UNIPEN; caps, tabl, oral susp, inj

Nalidixic aciu, antimicrobial agent effective against a selected group of gram-negative bacteria, apparently by inhibiting DNA synthesis
℞ for treatment of selected cases of urinary tract infection, when infective organisms can be shown to be sensitive: IN (>3 mo), CH = PO: 55 mg/kg/24 hr, div, every 6 hr, for 10–14 days
Note: If prolonged treatment is indicated, daily dose should be reduced to 33 mg/kg/24 hr, div, every 6 hr, and periodic evaluation for adverse side effects should be made. Resistance of initially sensitive microorganisms develops in about 25% of infections, and can occur within 48 hr. If resistance suspected, a therapeutic alternative must be chosen. Action of nalidixic acid is antagonized by nitrofurantoin.
NEGGRAM; oral susp, caplets
Caution: Even therapeutic doses may cause increased intracranial pressure, toxic psychosis, seizures in some patients.

Naloxone hydrochloride; opioid antagonist; nonaddictive
℞ in respiratory depression due to opioids: NB, IN, CH = IV, IM, SC: 0.01 mg/kg/dose, to be repeated prn after 2–3 min up to 3 times. After satisfactory response the dose must be repeated every 1–2 hr, as long as opioid depression persists
NARCAN, NARCAN neonatal; inj

Neomycin sulfate; antimicrobial aminoglycoside
℞ inhibition of gastrointestinal flora; justified only in selected cases (danger of hyperammonemia, enterocolitis with pathogenic *E. coli*): IN, CH = PO: 50–100 mg/kg/24 hr, div, every 6–8 hr
Caution: Against overgrowth of abnormal organisms.
†, MYCIFRADIN sulfate, ‡; oral susp, tabl

Niclosamide; anthelmintic agent useful particularly against cestodes, which under the effect of the drug become susceptible to the proteolytic action of intestinal secretions
℞ against *Diphyllobothrium latum* (fish tapeworm) and *Taenia saginata* (beef tapeworm): CH = PO: 1000 mg, as single dose; Adult = PO: 1500 mg, as single dose
℞ against *Taenia solium* (pork tapeworm): same dose as for fish and beef tapeworms. Since viability of ova contained in the segments is not affected by the drug and there is risk of cysticercosis with *Taenia solium* if ova spill out of digested segments, it is **mandatory** to give an adequate purge 1 hr after niclosamide, to clear the bowel of all dead segments before they can be digested
℞ against *Hymenolepis nana* (dwarf tapeworm): CH = PO: 1000 mg/24 hr, as single daily dose, for 5 consecutive days. Adult = PO: 1500 mg/24 hr, as single daily dose, for 5 consecutive days
Note: Niclosamide tablets must be thoroughly chewed before swallowing or finely ground and mixed with some liquid before ingested to be fully effective. Niclosamide is available in the U.S.A. from the Parasitic Disease Drug Service, Bureau of Epidemiology, Centers for Disease Control, Atlanta, GA 30333.
YOMESAN; tabl

Nitrofurantoin; nitrofuran-substituted hydantoin; antimicrobial agent effective against selected organisms, by interfering with enzyme systems of the microorganisms
℞ in the treatment of urinary tract infections, when infecting organisms are shown to be sensitive or likely to respond by clinical experience: IN (>3 mo), CH = PO: 5–7 mg/kg/24 hr, div, every 6 hr (with meals to minimize gastric upset), for 10–14 days. Repeated treatment courses with nitrofurantoin should be separated by "rest" periods. For long-term suppressive therapy dosage should be reduced, possibly to as low as 2 mg/kg/24 hr, div, every 6 hr.
Note: Because of rapid elimination by the kidneys, bacteriostatic concentrations are achieved only in urine. Better antibacterial activity is obtained in acid urine.
Caution: hemolysis occurs in G-6-PD–deficient individuals and in newborns because of insufficient detoxification capabilities. Nitro-

furantoin should not be given to pregnant women at term or to women who breast feed.
†, FURADANTIN, MICRODANTIN, ‡; oral susp, tabl, caps

Nitroprusside; sodium nitrosylpentacyanoferrate, $Na_2Fe(CN)_5 \cdot NO \cdot 2H_2O$; vasodilator by direct action on smooth muscles of blood vessels; effect appears almost immediately and ends promptly, 1–10 min after stopping of administration of nitroprusside
℞ for emergency reduction of hypertension: IV infusion: Example: to prepare a solution of nitroprusside containing 0.1 mg/ml, dissolve 50 mg nitroprusside first in 2–3 ml 5% dextrose in water, and transfer this amount to 500 ml 5% dextrose water,* and start continuous infusion using a microdrip regulator or an infusion pump that allows precise measurement of flow; begin with infusion rate of 0.003 mg/kg/min (equivalent to 0.03 ml/kg/min of solution containing 0.1 mg/ml nitroprusside), and decrease or increase dosage according to response, for which there exists a wide dosage range (0.0005–0.008 mg/kg/min)
*Only 5% dextrose in water solution should be used to prepare nitroprusside solution, and no other drug should be added. To prevent decomposition of nitroprusside by exposure to light, protect infusion bottle and possibly tubing from light; for instance, by wrapping in aluminum foil.
Caution: Fall in arterial blood pressure is dose-dependent, with risk of hypotensive circulatory failure on overdosage if careful monitoring of blood pressure does not lead to prompt adjustment of infusion rate.
Note: In patients receiving concomitant antihypertensive medications, a smaller dosage of nitroprusside is required for comparable reduction of hypertension.
NIPRIDE; powder for preparation of solution prior to inj

Nystatin; antifungal agent; 1 mg = 2000 units; seems to be active by altering permeability of cell membrane of yeasts
℞ for topical treatment of candidiasis of the buccal cavity (thrush) and the gastrointestinal tract. Very poorly absorbed. In oral candidiasis, spread nystatin suspension into recesses of mouth: NB (<2000 g) = PO: 200,000–400,000 units/24 hr, div, every 4–6 hr. NB (>2000 g), IN = PO: 400,000–800,000 units/24 hr, div, every 4–6 hr. CH = PO: 800,000–2,000,000 units/24 hr, div, every 4–6 hr
†, MYCOSTATIN, NILSTAT; oral susp, tabl

Oxacillin sodium; semisynthetic penicillinase-resistant penicillin
NB = IV (over 15–30 min), IM: for dosage same criteria apply as for methicillin in newborns; see Methicillin sodium. IN, CH = PO: 50–100 mg/kg/24 hr, div, every 6 hr; IV (over 15–30 min), IM: 100–200 mg/kg/24 hr, div, every 4 hr (IV) or every 6 hr (IM)
BACTOCILL, PROSTAPHLIN; caps, oral susp, inj

Paraldehyde; cyclic ether compound which decomposes to acetaldehyde on exposure to light and air; rapidly acting hypnotic agent
℞ in status epilepticus: CH = IM (injection remote from nerves because of risk of damage): 0.15 g/kg/dose, corresponding to 0.15 ml/kg/dose of paraldehyde solution containing 1 g/ml; occasionally 1 additional dose may be given after 30 min, prn
Note: Use glass syringe, since paraldehyde reacts with plastic equipment. When given IV, injection should be slow and paraldehyde solution should be diluted with isotonic sodium chloride solution to lessen risk of thrombophlebitis. IV use is not recommended.
℞ to calm agitation: CH = PO, IM (PR, diluted in equal amount of olive oil): 0.15 ml/kg/dose, to be repeated prn after 4–6 hr
Caution: Before use, make sure that drug is not decomposed (acetaldehyde, acetic acid).
†, PARAL; liquid for inj, oral use (risk of gastric irritation), and rectal use

Pemoline, an oxazolidone; structurally different from amphetamine and methylphenidate; CNS stimulant with minimal sympathomimetic effects
℞ in minimal brain dysfunction: drug treatment of MBD not recommended below the age of 3 yr or in nonstructured therapeutic situation: CH (so far insufficient data have been accumulated in

See KEY to abbreviations, p. 1814; for further information about drugs, see package insert.

DRUGS

Table 29–1B DRUG DOSES *(Continued)*

children below the age of 6 yr to assess efficacy and safety in this age group) = PO: initiate treatment with approximately 1 mg/kg/24 hr, as single dose each morning. If needed, increase dosage at weekly intervals by increments of 0.5 mg/kg/24 hr. On this schedule of titration of dose therapeutic response may not become evident until 4th wk of continued administration. Daily dose should not exceed 3 mg/kg/24 hr

Note: Insomnia, anorexia, and weight loss have been observed. The degree of reduced growth pattern on continued treatment is not yet established. Drug treatment of MBD should be discontinued at appropriate intervals to observe behavior of the patient and assess indication for further treatment.

CYLERT: tabl

Penicillin G benzathine, for injection: combination of 1 mole of dibenzylethylenediamine with 2 moles of penicillin G; 1 mg = 1211 units

℞ for prophylaxis of rheumatic fever: CH = IM: 600,000–1,200,000 units, equivalent to 500–1000 mg penicillin G, once a month

†, BICILLIN L-A, PERMAPEN, ‡; susp for inj

Penicillin G, benzylpenicillin; potassium penicillin G (1 mg = 1595 units); sodium penicillin G (1 mg = 1667 units). One million units of these salts of penicillin contains either 1.68 mEq K+ or Na+; in other terms, 1 g contains either 2.7 mEq K+ or 2.8 mEq Na+.

NB = IV (over 15–30 min), IM:

≤ 7 days old: 50,000 units/kg/24 hr, equivalent to 31 mg/kg/24 hr, div, every 12 hr

℞ for meningitis: 100,000–150,000 units/kg/24 hr, div, every 4 hr

> 7 days old: 75,000 units/kg/24 hr, equivalent to 47 mg/kg/24 hr, div, every 8 hr

℞ for meningitis: 150,000–250,000 units/kg/24 hr, div, every 4 hr

(The higher doses should be chosen for meningitis caused by group B streptococci.)

IN, CH = PO, IM, IV (over 15–30 min): 25,000–50,000 units/kg/24 hr, equivalent to 15.5–31 mg/kg/24 hr, div, every 4–6 hr; if given PO, administer penicillin G 0.5 hr before or 2 hr after the meal.

℞ in severe infections: IV: 200,000–400,000 units/kg/24 hr, equivalent to 125–250 mg/kg/24 hr, as continuous drip infusion or div, every 2–4 hr

℞ for prophylaxis of rheumatic fever: PO: 200,000 units/dose, equivalent to 125 mg/dose, twice daily, spaced from meals (see Sec 9.81)

†, PENTIDS, PFIZERPEN G, ‡; tabl, caps, oral susp, inj (IV)

Penicillin G procaine, for injection; combination of penicillin G with procaine, mole for mole (1 mg = 1009 units)

NB = IM: 50,000 units/kg/24 hr, equivalent to 50 mg/kg/24 hr, in single daily dose. IN, CH = IM: 25,000–50,000 units/kg/24 hr, equivalent to 25–50 mg/kg/24 hr, in single daily dose

†, CRYSTICILLIN, DURACILLIN A.S., ‡; susp for IM inj

Penicillin V, phenoxymethyl penicillin; acid-resistant penicillin; 1 mg = 1695 units

IN, CH = PO: 25,000–50,000 units/kg/24 hr, equivalent to 15–30 mg/kg/24 hr, div, every 6–8 hr. *Note:* 400,000 units = 250 mg (approx).

†, PEN-VEE K, VEETIDS, ‡; tabl, oral susp, drops

Pentazocine hydrochloride; narcotic analgesic of the benzomorphan type; addictive

℞ against severe pain: Clinical experience in children under 12 yr of age is limited. Adult = PO: 50 mg/dose, to be repeated prn after 3–4 hr; IM, SC (pentazocine lactate); 30 mg/dose, to be repeated prn after 4 hr

FORTRAL, TALWIN; tabl (hydrochloride); inj (lactate)

Caution: As for *morphine,* above.

Pentobarbital, central nervous system depressant with short duration of action; tolerance to hypnotic effect may develop on continued use; initially, hypnotic effect of 3–5 hr

℞ for sedation: IN, CH = PO, IM: 1–2 mg/kg/24 hr, div, every 6 hr

℞ for sleep: IN, CH = PO, IM: 2–3 mg/kg/dose, repeat prn after 12–24 hr

†, NEMBUTAL elixir ● pentobarbital sodium, †, NEMBUTAL sodium; inj, caps, suppos

Phenobarbital, central nervous system depressant with long duration of action; initially, hypnotic effect of 8–12 hr; tolerance to hypnotic effect may develop on continued use

℞ for sedation: IN, CH = PO, IM: 2–3 mg/kg/24 hr, div, every 8–12 hr

℞ for sleep: IN, CH = PO, IM: 2–3 mg/kg/dose, repeat prn after 12–24 hr

℞ as anticonvulsant for long-term therapy: IN, CH = PO: start with 1.5 mg/kg/24 hr, div, every 12 hr; increase according to tolerance and therapeutic effect to 4–6 mg/kg/24 hr, div, every 12 hr, or as single daily dose, preferably at bedtime in order to minimize daytime drowsiness from hypnotic effect (see also Table 20–3)

℞ as adjunct in treatment of status epilepticus: CH = IV: 5–7.5 mg/kg/1st dose, by slow IV injection; followed prn after interval of 5 min by 2.5–3 mg/kg/dose, to be repeated once prn. If status epilepticus has been interrupted by drugs not including a barbiturate, phenobarbital can be given IM: 5–10 mg/kg/dose, followed by PO anticonvulsant regimen

†, LUMINAL; elixir, tabl ● phenobarbital sodium, †, LUMINAL sodium; inj

Phenolphthalein; laxative acting primarily on the colon

CH = PO: 1 mg/kg/dose

†, tabl, oral susp; component of several preparations

Phenylephrine hydrochloride; catecholamine with exclusively α-adrenergic action; peripheral vasoconstrictor

℞ to increase blood pressure in orthostatic hypotension, or

℞ to trigger vagal reflex in response to blood pressure increase, in the treatment of atrial tachyarrhythmia: PO: 1 mg/kg/24 hr, div, every 4 hr; SC, IM: 0.1 mg/kg/dose, repeat prn by monitoring response

Caution: With regard to hypertensive state and peripheral ischemia.

†, NEO-SYNEPHRINE hydrochloride; inj, elixir; also available as nose drops for local decongestant effect

Phenytoin, diphenylhydantoin; anticonvulsant agent; effective also in certain types of cardiac arrhythmias; antiarrhythmic effects similar to those of lidocaine: delayed slow diastolic depolarization, diminished automaticity; may facilitate conduction in damaged myocardial areas; does not depress myocardial activity

℞ as anticonvulsant for long-term therapy: IN, CH = PO: 3–8 mg/kg/24 hr, div, every 12 hr

℞ as adjunct in the treatment of status epilepticus: CH = IV (slow infusion under monitoring of heart rate): 10–15 mg/kg/dose (see also Table 20–3)

℞ as adjunct in the treatment of ventricular tachyarrhythmia: CH = IV (over 5 min): 2–3 mg/kg/dose, to be repeated prn after 20 min

†, DILANTIN; oral susp ● phenytoin sodium, †, DILANTIN sodium; caps, inj

Primaquine, 8-aminoquinoline antimalarial agent, used for prophylaxis against *P. vivax, P. ovale,* and *P. malariae* and for "radical" cure for *P. vivax* and *P. ovale*

IN, CH = PO: 0.55 mg/kg/24 hr (equivalent to 0.3 mg/kg/24 hr of base), as single daily dose, for 14 days

Note: Degree of intravascular hemolysis in individuals with G-6-PD deficiency is related to dosage and particular variant of the deficiency.

Primaquine diphosphate; tabl

Primidone; a deoxybarbiturate which is partially metabolized to phenobarbital; anticonvulsant agent

℞ for long-term therapy of selected types of convulsive disorder: CH = PO: 10 mg/kg/24 hr, div, every 8–12 hr (see also Table 20–3)

MYSOLINE; oral susp, tabl

Probenecid, competitive inhibitor of tubular secretion and reabsorption of organic acids

See KEY to abbreviations, p. 1814; for further information about drugs, see package insert.

Table 29–1B DRUG DOSES *(Continued)*

Ŗ for uricosuric action (acetylsalicylic acid antagonizes this effect), or

Ŗ in conjunction with penicillin G or V, or ampicillin, methicillin, oxacillin, cloxacillin, nafcillin to achieve longer persistence of therapeutic blood and tissue concentrations of the antimicrobial agent. CH = PO: initial dose of 25 mg/kg, followed by 40 mg/kg/24 hr, div, every 6 hr
BENEMID; tabl

Procainamide hydrochloride; antiarrhythmic agent with general cardio-depressant effects; diminished myocardial excitability (decreased threshold potential, prolonged refractory period), reduced conduction velocity, diminished automaticity; decreases myocardial contractility; effects similar to those of quinidine

Ŗ against ventricular tachyarrhythmia: IN, CH = IV (infused slowly, diluted in 5% dextrose in water): 2–5 mg/kg/dose; to be repeated at intervals of 20 min up to a total of 30 mg/kg in a 24 hr period. IM: 20–30 mg/24 hr, div, every 6 hr; PO: 40–60 mg/kg/24 hr, div, every 4–6 hr

†, PRONESTYL; tabl, caps, inj

Prochlorperazine; piperazine-type phenothiazine with pronounced antiemetic effect

Ŗ for sedation: CH (over 2 yr old) = PO: 0.4 mg/kg/24 hr, div, every 6–8 hr, prn. IM: 0.2 mg/kg/24 hr, div, every 8–12 hr, prn
COMPAZINE; suppos ● prochlorperazine edisylate, COMPAZINE edisylate; oral liquid, syrup, inj

Caution: May produce parkinsonian syndrome. Diphenhydramine may be antidotal.

Promethazine hydrochloride; phenothiazine with aliphatic side chain

Ŗ for sedation, prevention or treatment of motion sickness, and as antihistamine; CH = PO: 1 mg/kg/24 hr, divided into half dose at bedtime and quarter doses every 6 hr of the remaining daytime

†, PHENERGAN; syrup, tabl, suppos

Propantheline bromide, antispasmodic synthetic antimuscarinic agent as well as partial ganglionic blocking drug

Ŗ as adjunctive therapy against spasms in the gastrointestinal tract: CH = PO: 1.5 mg/kg/24 hr, div, every 6 hr, with meals, if applicable. IM: 0.8 mg/kg/24 hr, div, every 6 hr
PRO-BANTHINE; tabl, inj

Propoxyphene hydrochloride, and propoxyphene napsylate; opioid analgesic with less dependence liability than seen with codeine

Ŗ against mild to moderately severe pain: CH = PO: 2–3 mg/kg/24 hr, div, every 6 hr
propoxyphene hydrochloride, †, DARVON, ‡; caps ● propoxyphene napsylate, DARVON-N; oral susp, tabl

Propranolol hydrochloride; β-adrenergic blocking agent (β₁ and β₂); racemic mixture of D- and L-propranolol, of which only L form has adrenergic blocking activity

Ŗ against selected forms of supraventricular and ventricular tachycardia: IN, CH = IV: 0.02–0.03 mg/kg/dose, given slowly; repeat prn every 20 min. PO: 0.3–1.2 mg/kg/24 hr, div, every 6 hr

Ŗ as antihypertensive in long-term therapy: CH = PO: initially 1 mg/kg/24 hr, div, every 6 hr, and progressive increase of dosage, if needed to achieve adequate response, up to 5 mg/kg/24 hr, div, every 6 hr. Combination with diuretic and/or hydralazine indicated, since propranolol blocks physiologic compensatory mechanisms such as adrenergic inotropic and chronotropic responses, as well as renin activity. See also Table 13–16.

Ŗ for prevention of migraine attack in severe cases and

Ŗ to combat the manifestations of thyrotoxicosis: Propranolol requirements vary widely from patient to patient because of individual differences in severity of underlying disease, endogenous sympathetic neuronal activity, sensitivity of β-adrenergic receptors to blockade, degree of protein binding, hepatic blood flow. For comparable effect, oral dose 6–10 times higher than intravenous dose in spite of good absorption from the gut because of inactivation of important fraction of propranolol in liver after entrance through portal vein.

Measures in case of exaggerated response: against bradycardia, atropine; if no response, isoproterenol, *cautiously;* against cardiac

failure, digitalization and diuretics; against hypotension, epinephrine; against bronchospasm, isoproterenol, theophylline (aminophylline)
INDERAL; tabl, inj

Pseudoephedrine hydrochloride; indirectly acting sympathomimetic

Ŗ as nasal decongestant by systemic route: CH = PO: 4 mg/kg/24 hr, div, every 6 hr

†, SUDAFED, ‡; syrup, caps; contained in many combination products

Pyrantel pamoate; anthelmintic agent effective by means of neuromuscular paralysis of the parasite

Ŗ against pinworms (*Enterobius vermicularis*), *Ascaris lumbricoides*, and hookworms (*Necator americanus, Ancylostoma duodenale*): pyrantel pamoate has not been extensively studied in infants and children below 2 yr of age, hence particular attention should be given to children of this age group during treatment of parasitic infestation with pyrantel. CH = PO: 11 mg/kg/dose, as single dose and without regard to food intake or time of day; purging not necessary prior to, during, or after therapy

Note: In pinworm infestation, in which possibility of reinfection with eggs from the host exists, a 2nd treatment 2–3 wk after the 1st might be indicated.
ANTIMINTH; oral susp

Pyridostigmine bromide, cholinesterase inhibitor

Ŗ for diagnosis of myasthenia gravis: see Edrophonium chloride

Ŗ in myasthenia gravis: NB, IN, CH = IM: 0.1 mg/kg/dose, and continue with PO medication. PO: frequency of dosage and size of dose must be adjusted individually to provide optimum compensation during cycle of daily activities; average effective dose: 7 mg/kg/24 hr, div, every 4–5 hr

Ŗ for reversal of nondepolarizing muscle relaxants (tubocurarine, gallamine, pancuronium): IV (preceded by IV injection of atropine to prevent excessive secretions and bradycardia): 0.15 mg/kg/dose, and watch for recovery that ought to occur after 15–30 min; assure appropriate ventilation until complete recovery
MESTINON; tabl, syrup, inj

Caution: As for Edrophonium chloride.

Pyrimethamine, inhibitor of dihydrofolate reductase, antimalarial agent; for use in treatment of toxoplasmosis (see Sec 10.113)

Ŗ for clinical prophylaxis of malaria, especially effective against *P. falciparum*: IN, CH = PO: 0.5–0.75 mg/kg/dose, once every 7 days. Begin prophylaxis 2 wk before entering malarious area and continue for 8 wk after leaving. To eradicate *P. vivax* and *P. ovale* infections, treatment for 14 days with primaquine should be considered immediately on leaving malarious area while pyrimethamine prophylaxis is still in effect; see also Sec 10.113

Note: Hematologic abnormalities (anemia, thrombocytopenia, leukopenia) secondary to folic and folinic acid depletion can be prevented or reversed by IM administration of folinic acid (leucovorin) without affecting the efficacy of pyrimethamine.
DARAPRIM; tabl

Quinacrine hydrochloride, mepacrine hydrochloride; acridine derivative formerly used as antimalarial agent and against infestation with tapeworms, presently regarded as drug of choice against lambliasis

Ŗ against *Giardia lamblia* (*Lamblia intestinalis*): CH = PO: 6 mg/kg/24 hr, div, every 8 hr, for 5 consecutive days; maximum daily dose: 300 mg/24 hr
ATABRINE; tabl

Quinidine gluconate, quinidine sulfate, and quinidine polygalacturonate; alkaloid with general cardiodepressant effects: diminished myocardial excitability (decrease in threshold potential), reduced conduction velocity (widening of QRS complex, possibility of A-V block), increased refractory period, diminished automaticity, especially in ectopic sites; depresses myocardial contractility with risk of congestive heart failure if myocardial damage present

Ŗ against atrial tachycardia (usually after digitalization), and/or ventricular tachyarrhythmia: IN, CH = 2 mg/kg test dose PO, IM, (IV) to exclude idiosyncrasy. For treatment: PO (quinidine

Table 29-15 DRUG DOSES (Continued)

sulfate): 30 mg/kg/24 hr, div, every 4–5 hr. IV, IM (quinidine gluconate): 2–10 mg/kg/dose, prn every 3–6 hr

quinidine gluconate, QUINAGLUTE; tabl, inj ● quinidine sulfate, †, QUINIDEX, ‡; tabl quinidine polygalacturonate. CARDIOQUIN; tabl

Caution: Overdose may lead to cardiac arrest.

Quinine sulfate and quinine dihydrochloride; alkaloid with effects on such a variety of biologic systems that it has been called "general protoplasmic poison."

℞ for treatment of chloroquine-resistant strains of *Plasmodium falciparum*, quinine used either with tetracycline or with a combination of pyrimethamine and a sulfonamide (see Table 10–55)

Oral treatment: *quinine sulfate:* CH = PO: 25 mg/kg/24 hr, div, every 8 hr, for 10–14 days, and either *tetracycline:* CH = PO: 40 mg/kg/24 hr, div, every 6 hr, for 10 days or *pyrimethamine:* CH = PO: 0.75 mg/kg/24 hr, div, every 12 hr, for 3 days, and *sulfadiazine:* CH = PO: 150 mg/kg/24 hr, div, every 6 hr, for 6 days

Intravenous treatment (severe cases when PO treatment not indicated): *quinine dihydrochloride:* IN, CH = IV (use dilute solution containing 200 mg in 200 ml half-isotonic sodium chloride solution): give 10 mg/kg/dose, by slow infusion over 1–2 hr; repeat at intervals of 12 hr until clinical response is obtained. Complete course of treatment (14 days) by oral route.

In addition: either *tetracycline:* IN, CH = IV: 20 mg/kg/24 hr, div, every 12 hr, until oral administration of oral dosage (see above) becomes possible, for a course of treatment of 10 days; or *pyrimethamine:* IN, CH = PO: 0.75 mg/kg/24 hr, div, every 12 hr, for 3 days, *and sulfadiazine:* IN, CH = IV: 100 mg/kg/24 hr, div, every 6 hr, until oral administration of oral dosage (see above) becomes possible, for a total of 6 days

Note: In case quinine dihydrochloride for injection (powder to be dissolved) not available, quinidine, the D-isomer of quinine, can be substituted until quinine becomes available. Quinidine for injection comes as the gluconate. Also see *note* under Tetracyclines.

Quinine sulfate, tabl; quinine dihydrochloride, inj, available in U.S.A. from Parasitic Disease Drug Service, Bureau of Epidemiology, Centers for Disease Control, Atlanta, GA 30333

Reserpine, alkaloid which depletes stores of catecholamines and serotonin in many organs, including the brain

℞ as antihypertensive in long-term treatment: CH = PO: initially 0.02 mg/kg/24 hr, as single daily dose or div, every 12 hr; for maintenance, dose usually reduced to 0.005–0.01 mg/kg/24 hr

Note: See Table 13–16. Reserpine may induce mental depression, nasal congestion.

†, SANDRIL, SERPASIL; tabl, elixir

Rifampin; macrocyclic antimicrobial and antimycobacterial agent, interfering with RNA-polymerase of infecting organisms

℞ in treatment of tuberculosis, in conjunction with at least 1 other antituberculous agent (isoniazid), and

℞ in carriers of *Neisseria meningitidis* resistant to penicillin and sulfonamide; treatment course of 4 consecutive days (possibility of rapid emergence of resistance): IN, CH = PO: 10–20 mg/kg/24 hr, in single daily dose (1 hr before or 2 hr after meal); maximum daily dose: 600 mg (= adult dose)

RIFADIN, RIMACTANE; caps

Salicylate sodium

℞ antipyretic, analgesic, anti-inflammatory: CH, Adolescents = PO: 25–50 mg/kg/24 hr, div, every 4–6 hr, prn

℞ antirheumatic: CH, Adolescents = PO: 50–100 mg/kg/24 hr, div, every 6 hr

†, tabl

Caution: See Sec 28.6.

Scopolamine methylbromide, also methscopolamine bromide; antimuscarinic agent and quaternary ammonium compound, which essentially lacks the central nervous system actions (sedation or excitement, amnesia, euphoria, hallucinations, unexpected behavior) of scopolamine

℞ as adjunctive therapy in the treatment of spasms in the gastrointestinal and urinary tracts: CH = PO: 0.15 mg/kg/24 hr, div, every 6 hr; SC, IM: 0.01 mg/kg/dose, repeat prn every 6–8 hr

PAMINE; tabl, inj

Caution: As for Belladonna.

Secobarbital, central nervous system depressant with short duration of action; tolerance to the hypnotic effect may develop on continued use; initially, hypnotic effect of 3–5 hr

℞ for sedation: IN, CH = PO, IM: 1–2 mg/kg/24 hr, div, every 6 hr

℞ for sleep: IN, CH = PO, IM: 2–3 mg/kg/dose, repeat prn after 12–24 hr

†, SECONAL elixir ● secobarbital sodium, †, SECONAL sodium; inj, caps, suppos

Caution: See Sec 28.8.

Senna syrup; contains anthraquinones, sennosides A and B, which stimulate the intramural nerve plexuses of the colon

℞ as laxative: CH = PO: 0.15 ml/kg/dose; to be repeated only once per wk, if indicated, so as not to interfere with normal bowel motility and not to induce laxative dependence

†; syrup

Sodium sulfate, $Na_2SO_4 \cdot 10H_2O$, Glauber salt; 1 g of salt traps about 30 ml of water to make the solution isosmotic

℞ as salinic cathartic: CH = PO: 300 mg/kg/dose

†; crystalline substance to be dissolved in a liquid for PO administration

Spironolactone; aldosterone antagonist and potassium-sparing diuretic, which interferes with sodium reabsorption

℞ as diuretic in selected cases (with normal renal function), most effective in combination with a potassium-wasting diuretic: CH = PO: 1.5–3 mg/kg/24 hr, div, every 4–8 hr

Note: Monitoring of serum concentration of potassium, of potassium intake, and of renal function is indicated during treatment with spironolactone.

ALDACTONE; tabl

Streptomycin sulfate; antimicrobial aminoglycoside

Caution: Because this drug when administered in large doses and/or for long periods can damage the 8th cranial nerve in adults, children, and transplacentally in fetuses, its indications are stringently selective today.

℞ in tuberculous meningitis and progressive tuberculosis, in association with isoniazid and other anti-tuberculous medication: CH = IM: 20–40 mg/kg/24 hr, div, every 12 hr, for 2–3 mo; maximum daily dose irrespective of weight: 1 g/24 hr. See Tables 10–33 and 10–34

†; susp, inj

Sulfonamides; analogues of para-aminobenzoic acid, interfering with the synthesis of tetrahydrofolic acid in sensitive bacteria

Sulfadiazine, sulfisoxazole, and trisulfapyrimidines: IN, CH = PO: initial dose 75 mg/kg/1st dose, followed by 120–150 mg/kg/24 hr, div, every 4–6 hr. IV (over 30 min), SC: 100–110 mg/kg/24 hr, div, every 4–6 hr

Sulfadiazine, †; tabl ● sulfadiazine sodium, †, inj ● sulfisoxazole, †, GANTRISIN; tabl sulfisoxazole acetyl, GANTRISIN acetyl; oral susp, syrup ● sulfisoxazole diolamine, GANTRISIN diolamine; inj ● trisulfapyrimidines (equal parts of sulfadiazine, sulfamerazine, and sulfamethazine), †, ‡; tabl, oral susp

Sulfamethoxazole: IN, CH = PO: initial dose 50–60 mg/kg/1st dose, followed by 50–60 mg/kg/24 hr, div, every 12 hr

GANTANOL; oral susp, tabl

Trimethoprim-sulfamethoxazole (combination of 20 mg TMP and 100 mg SMX): IN (>2 mo old), CH = PO: 8 mg TMP + 40 mg SMX/kg/24 hr, div, every 12 hr

BACTRIM, SEPTRA; tabl, oral susp

Terbutaline sulfate, catecholamine; β-adrenergic receptor agonist with preferential effect on β₂-adrenergic receptors

℞ bronchodilator: Dosage in pediatric age group not firmly established. PO: 0.10–0.15 mg/kg/24 hr, div, every 8 hr. β₂-selectivity is reduced with increasing dosage or on parenteral administra-

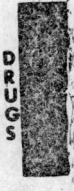

Table 29–1*B* DRUG DOSES *(Continued)*

tion. SC: 0.005 mg/kg/dose, to be repeated prn after 20 min, once only

BRETHINE, BRICANYL; tabl, inj

Tetracyclines; a group of derivatives of polycyclic naphthacenecarboxamide

Chlortetracycline hydrochloride: CH = PO: 25–50 mg/kg/24 hr, div, every 6 hr

AUREOMYCIN; caps, inj (IV)

Demeclocycline and *demeclocycline hydrochloride:* CH = PO: 7–13 mg/kg/24 hr, div, every 6–12 hr

DECLOMYCIN; pediatric drops, syrup • DECLOMYCIN hydrochloride; caps, tabl

Doxycycline monohydrate and *doxycycline hyclate:* CH = PO: 5 mg/kg/24 hr, div, every 12 hr

† , VIBRAMYCIN monohydrate; oral susp • † , VIBRAMYCIN hyclate; caps, inj (IV)

Methacycline hydrochloride: CH = PO: 7–13 mg/kg/24 hr, div, every 6–12 hr

RONDOMYCIN; caps, syrup

Minocycline hydrochloride: CH = PO, IV: initial dose 4 mg/kg, followed by 4 mg/kg/24 hr, div, every 12 hr

MINOCIN, VECTRIN; caps, syrup, inj (IV)

Oxytetracycline, oxytetracycline hydrochloride, oxytetracycline calcium: same dosage as tetracycline hydrochloride, below

TERRAMYCIN; tabl, inj (IM) • TERRAMYCIN hydrochloride; † , caps, inj (IV, IM) • TERRAMYCIN calcium; pediatric drops, syrup

Tetracycline hydrochloride: CH = PO: 25–50 mg/kg/24 hr, div, every 8 hr; IM (often very painful): 15–25 mg/kg/24 hr, div, every 8–12 hr; IV: 10–20 mg/kg/24 hr, div, every 12 hr

† , ACHROMYCIN V, PANMYCIN, ‡ ; caps, inj (IV, IM); sol for IM inj contains local anesthetic. Pediatric drops, oral susp, and syrup prepared with tetracycline base

Note: Tetracyclines have limited indications in infancy and childhood because of their accumulation in bone and teeth and their potential to interfere with growth. Their use should be avoided insofar as possible until formation of dental enamel is complete in most permanent teeth (at about 8 yr), to avoid unsightly discolored, pitted teeth. Tetracyclines may cause increased intracranial pressure in infants (pseudotumor cerebri).

Theophylline, inhibitor of phosphodiesterase, analeptic, cardiotonic, diuretic

℞ in status asthmaticus: initial loading dose IV: 7 mg/kg/dose, infused after dilution in equal volume of intravenous fluid over 20–30 min, followed by maintenance IV: 20 mg/kg/24 hr, div, every 4–6 hr, or by continuous IV drip; switch to PO maintenance as soon as possible

℞ oral maintenance: PO: 20 mg/kg/24 hr, div, every 6 hr; as conditions permit, taper to lowest effective dosage, usually around 10 mg/kg/24 hr, div, every 6 hr

Note: the content of theophylline in the following formulations: theophylline (anhydrous), 100%; aminophylline, 85%; theophylline monoethanolamine, 75%; dihydroxypropyltheophylline, 70%; oxtriphylline, choline salt, 64%; theophylline sodium glycinate, 50%; theophylline calcium salicylate, 48%.

theophylline, † , ELIXOPHYLLIN elixir, ELIXICON oral susp, SLO-PHYLLIN caps, oral susp, SOMOPHYLLIN caps, ‡ : component of many combination products • aminophylline, † , SOMOPHYLLIN oral liquid, ‡ ; inj, oral preparations

Caution: Circulatory collapse, seizures, coma may result from acute or chronic overdose.

Thioridazine hydrochloride; phenothiazine of the piperidine type

℞ for sedation and neuroleptic effect: CH = PO: 1 mg/kg/24 hr, div, every 8 hr

MELLARIL; oral liquid, tabl

Caution: Overdose may produce parkinsonian syndrome. Diphenhydramine may be antidotal.

Ticarcillin disodium; semisynthetic penicillin which is not resistant to penicillinase; low degree of toxicity permits high serum and tissue concentrations in selected severe infections; 1 g contains 5.3 mEq Na$^+$

Note: Experience with ticarcillin disodium in the pediatric age group is limited at this time and recommendations are not firmly established.

NB = IV (over 20–30 min), IM: ≤ 2000 g and ≤ 7 days old: 225 mg/kg/24 hr, div, every 8 hr; > 2000 g and ≤ 7 days old: 300 mg/kg/24 hr, div, every 6 hr; > 7 days old: 600 mg/kg/24 hr, div, every 4 hr

IN, CH = IV (over 20–30 min): 200–300 mg/kg/24 hr, div, every 4 hr

TICAR; IV and IM inj

Triamterene; potassium-sparing diuretic; inhibits the reabsorption of Na$^+$ in exchange for K$^+$ and H$^+$; its effect is potentiated by concomitant use of diuretics which act more proximally

CH = PO: initially 4 mg/kg/24 hr, div, every 12 hr (after meals).

Note: For maintenance, dosage must be adjusted to needs of individual patient; in conjunction with other diuretics dosage usually can be decreased.

Caution: Because of the risk of hyperkalemia, serum potassium concentrations and potassium intake should be watched.

DYRENIUM; caps

Trimethadione; oxazolidinedione; anticonvulsant agent

℞ as an adjunct in the treatment of convulsive disorders: CH = PO: 20 mg/kg/24 hr, div, every 8 hr; if needed, dosage can be progressively adjusted to 40 mg/kg/24 hr, div, every 8 hr

Note: The methylated metabolite of trimethadione accumulates progressively in the body and is partially responsible for anticonvulsant effect.

TRIDIONE; tabl, caps, oral susp

Trimethoprim; see Sulfonamides

Tripelennamine hydrochloride: an ethylenediamine with antihistamine, mild cholinergic, and slight sedative effects

℞ antiallergic effect: CH = PO: 5 mg/kg/24 hr, div, every 6 hr

† , PYRIBENZAMINE hydrochloride; tabl • tripelennamine citrate, PYRIBENZAMINE citrate; elixir

Valproate sodium, dipropylacetate sodium; anticonvulsant agent with singular mode of action (effective probably by increasing γ-aminobutyric acid in brain tissues)

℞ in the treatment of simple petit mal, and of complex absence seizures, either alone or in combination with other drugs (see reservation below) according to the results: CH = PO: start with 15 mg/kg/24 hr, div, every 8–12 hr; if needed, dosage increased by weekly increments of 5–10 mg/kg/24 hr up to a maximum recommended dose of 30 mg/kg/24 hr, div, every 8 hr

Caution: Concomitant use of valproate sodium and clonazepam might result in petit mal status. Blood concentrations of phenobarbital and phenytoin may be affected by addition of valproate sodium to the regimen.

DEPAKENE; caps (valproic acid), syrup (valproate sodium)

See KEY to abbreviations, p. 1814; for further information about drugs, see package insert.

SANFORD N. COHEN
LEON STREBEL

REFERENCE RANGES FOR LABORATORY TESTS

Reference ranges are valuable guidelines for the clinician, but they should not be regarded as absolute indicators of health or disease. There are several reasons for using reference ranges with caution. Most importantly, values for "healthy" individuals often overlap with values for persons afflicted with disease. In addition, laboratory values may vary due to methodological differences and mode of standardization. This is especially true for immunological tests, which utilize antibodies that may have different characteristics. As a result, laboratory values in individual institutions may differ from those listed.

For those laboratory tests where differences among the ages and sexes exist, all values are listed. Values without any age specification should be considered as those for the adult individual in the fasting state but generally apply for children as well.

In general, reference values are given as ranges. The mean values with the standard deviation (SD) or the standard error of the mean (SEM) are given in those cases in which the original author failed to give the range or detailed information regarding the distribution of values.

All laboratory values are given in conventional units, as well as in international units. In general, the international units given conform to the SI system (Systèm International d'Unités). However, in some cases the recommendations of the International Union of Pure and Applied Chemistry (IUPAC) and the Commission on World Standards of the World Association of Societies of Pathology (COWS of WASP) are used, since it is felt that these have found wider acceptance and offer certain advantages over SI units.

Throughout this appendix, we have used the prefixes for units as approved by the CGPM (Conférence Générale des Poids et Mésures), 1964, and the International Congress of Clinical Chemistry, 1966. The pertinent prefixes denoting the decimal factors are listed below.

Prefixes Denoting Decimal Factors

Prefix	Symbol	Factor
mega	M	10^6
kilo	k	10^3
hecto	h	10^2
deka	da	10^1
deci	d	10^{-1}
centi	c	10^{-2}
milli	m	10^{-3}
micro	μ	10^{-6}
nano	n	10^{-9}
pico	p	10^{-12}
femto	f	10^{-15}

To preserve space, we have used the following abbreviations commonly used in laboratory medicine.

Abbreviations

ΔA	change in absorbance
ACD	acid-citrate-dextrose
AI	angiotensin I
ALL	acute lymphocytic leukemia
AML	acute myeloid leukemia
AMML	acute myelomonocytic leukemia
AU	arbitrary unit
BMD	Boehringer Mannheim Diagnostics
cAMP	adenosine 3',5'-cyclic phosphate
cap.	capillary
CHF	congestive heart failure
CNS	central nervous system
conc.	concentration
CSF	cerebrospinal fluid
d	diem, day, days
EDTA	ethylenediaminetetraacetate; edetic acid
F	female
FDP	fibrin degradation products
G-D	General Diagnosis
h	hour, hours
Hb	hemoglobin
HbCO	carboxyhemoglobin
hpf	high power field
HPLC	high performance liquid chromatography
ICSH	International Committee for Standardization in Hematology
IFA	indirect fluorescent antibody
IRP-2-hMG	2nd International Reference Preparation of Human Menopausal Gonadotropin
IU	International Unit of hormone activity
L	liter
L→P	lactate to pyruvate reaction
M	male
MCV	mean corpuscular value
min	minute, minutes
mm³	cubic millimeter; equivalent to microliter (μL)
mo	month, months
mol	mole
M.W.	relative molecular weight
occup.	occupational
P→L	pyruvate to lactate reaction
RBC	red blood cell(s); erythrocyte(s)
RIA	radioimmunoassay
RID	radial immunodiffusion
RT	room temperature
s	second, seconds
SD	standard deviation
SE	standard error
std.	standard
therap.	therapeutic
U	International Unit of enzyme activity
V	volume
WBC	white blood cell
WHO	World Health Organization
wk	week, weeks
y	year, years

Symbols

>	greater than
≥	greater than or equal to
<	less than
≤	less than or equal to
±	plus/minus
≈	approximately equal to

Acknowledgment. We thankfully acknowledge the assistance of Nancy M. Logan, B.A., Karen D. Reeves, A.A. and Marion C. Reid, B.S., in the preparation of this material

C. CHARLTON MABRY

NORBERT W. TIETZ

Beutler E: Hemolytic Anemia in Disorders of Red Cell Metabolism. New York, Plenum, 1978.
Brown SS, Mitchell FL, Young DS (eds): Chemical Diagnosis of Disease. Amsterdam, Elsevier/North-Holland Biomedical Press, 1979.

Conn HF, Conn RB (eds): Current Diagnosis. Ed 6. Philadelphia, WB Saunders, 1980.
Gilman AG, Goodman L, Gilman A (eds): The Pharmacological Basis of Therapeutics. Ed 6. New York, Macmillan, 1980.
Henry JB (ed): Todd-Sanford-Davidsohn Clinical Diagnosis and Management by Laboratory Methods. Ed 16. Philadelphia, WB Saunders, 1979.
Miale JB: Laboratory Medicine: Hematology. Ed 5. St. Louis, CV Mosby, 1977.
Tietz NW (ed): Fundamentals of Clinical Chemistry. Ed 2. Philadelphia, WB Saunders, 1976.
Tietz NW: Reference ranges and laboratory values of clinical importance. In: Wyngaarden JB, Smith LH Jr (eds): Cecil Textbook of Medicine. Ed 16. Philadelphia, WB Saunders, 1982.
Tietz NW (ed): Clinical Guide to Laboratory Tests. Philadelphia, WB Saunders, 1983 (in press).
Tietz NW, Blackburn, RH (eds): Reference Ranges and General Information. Clinical Laboratories, A. B. Chandler Medical Center, University of Kentucky, Lexington, Ky., July, 1981.
Williams WJ, Beutler E, Erslev AJ, Rundles RW: Hematology. Ed 2. New York, McGraw-Hill, 1977.

Table 29–2   REFERENCE RANGES*

TEST	SPECIMEN	REFERENCE RANGE	FACTOR	REFERENCE RANGE INTERNATIONAL UNITS
Acetaminophen	Serum, plasma (heparin, EDTA)	Therap. conc.: 10–30 µg/mL Toxic conc.: >200	× 6.62	66–200 µmol/L >1300
Acetone *Semiquantitative*	Serum or plasma (oxalate)	Negative (<3 mg/dL)	× 0.1722	Negative (<0.5 mmol/L)
Quantitative		0.3–2.0 mg/dL		0.05–0.34 mmol/L
Semiquantitative	Urine	Negative		Negative
Activated Partial Thromboplastin Time (APTT) *Microtechnique (Miale)*	Whole blood (Na citrate) Remove plasma immediately Capillary blood (siliconized micropipets; Na citrate)	25–35 s (Differs with method) Infants: <90 s Reaches adult levels by 2–6 mo		25–35 s <90 s

Adrenocorticotropic Hormone (ACTH)	Plasma (EDTA)	*pg/mL*
		Cord: 143 ± 7.0 (1 SD)
		1–7 d postnatal: 120 ± 8.3
		Adult,
		  0800 h: 25–100
		  1800 h: <50
			× 1	*ng/L*
				143 ± 7.0 (1 SD)
				120 ± 8.3
				
				25–100
				<50

Alanine Aminotransferase (ALT, GPT)	Serum	Newborn/Infant: 5–25 U/L Thereafter: 8–20		5–25 U/L 8–20
Albumin	Serum	*g/dL* Premature: 3.0–4.2 Newborn: 3.6–5.4 Infant: 4.0–5.0 Thereafter: 3.5–5.0	× 10	*g/L* 30–42 36–54 40–50 35–50
	CSF	10–30 mg/dL		100–300 mg/L
Qualitative	Urine	<20 mg/dL		<200 mg/L
Quantitative		<80 mg/d	× 1	<80 mg/d
Aldolase	Serum	1.0–7.5 U/L (30 °C) 0.3–3.0 U/L at bed rest 1.5–12.0 U/L (37 °C) Children: 2× adults Newborn: 4× adults		1.0–7.5 U/L (30 °C) 0.3–3.0 U/L at bed rest 1.5–12.0 U/L (37 °C) Children: 2× adults Newborn: 4× adults

*The material in this appendix was partially extracted from: Clinical Guide to Laboratory Tests, NW Tietz (ed), PR Finley (asst ed); Philadelphia, WB Saunders, 1983 (in press). The main contributors are RV Blanke and RA Blouin: Drugs and Toxicology; C Hougie: Coagulation; HP Lehmann: International Units; J Leonard: Endocrinology; W Mertz and RV Blanke: Trace Metals; DA Nelson: Hematology; SE Ritzmann: Proteins; and HE Sauberlich: Vitamins. Some of the values were generated in the clinical laboratories of the University of Kentucky Medical Center, Lexington, Ky. Other sources are listed under references at the end of this section.

Table 29-2 REFERENCE RANGES (Continued)

TEST	SPECIMEN	REFERENCE RANGE	FACTOR	REFERENCE RANGE INTERNATIONAL UNITS
Aldosterone	Plasma (heparin, EDTA) or serum	ng/dL	× 0.0277	nmol/L
		Newborn: 5–60		0.14–1.7
		1 wk–1 y: 1–160		0.03–4.4
		1–3 y: 5–60		0.14–1.7
		3–5 y: <5–80		<0.14–2.2
		5–7 y: <5–50		<0.14–1.4
		7–11 y: 5–70		0.14–1.9
		11–15 y: <5–50		<0.14–1.4
		Adult, Average sodium diet		
		Supine: 3–10		0.08–0.3
		Upright, F: 5–30		0.14–0.8
		M: 6–22		0.17–0.61
		2–3× higher during pregnancy		
		Adrenal vein:		
		200–800 ng/dL		5.5–22 nmol/L
		Low sodium diet:		
		increases 2- to 5-fold:		
		Florinef suppression:		
		<4 ng/dL		<0.1 nmol/L
		ACTH or angiotensin stimulation, 1 h:		
		2- to 5-fold		

		Total Urinary Na mmol/d	Plasma Renin Activity ng AI/mL/h	Urinary Aldosterone μg/d		Urinary Aldosterone nmol/d
	Urine, 24 h	<20	5–24	>35–80	× 2.77	>97–220
		50	2–7	13–33		36–91
		100	1–5	5–24		14–66
		150	0.5–4	3–19		8–53
		200		1–16		3–44
		250		1–13		3–36

(assuming normal serum Na, K, and exracellular volume)

TEST	SPECIMEN	REFERENCE RANGE	FACTOR	REFERENCE RANGE INTERNATIONAL UNITS
Alkaline Phosphatase, Leukocyte, see Neutrophil Alkaline Phosphatase				
Alkaline Phosphatase, Serum, see Phosphatase, Alkaline				
δ-Aminolevulinic Acid (δ-ALA)	Serum	15–23 μg/dL; lower in children	× 0.076	1.1–1.8 μmol/L
	Urine, 24 h	1.3–7.0 mg/d	× 7.626	9.9–53.4 μmol/d
Ammonia Nitrogen Resin or enzymatic	Serum or plasma (Na-heparin)	μg N/dL		μmol/L
		Newborn: 90–150	× 0.714	64–107
		0–2 wk: 79–129		56–92
		>1 mo: 29–70		21–50
		Thereafter: 15–45		11–32
	Urine, 24 h	500–1200 mg/d	× 0.0714	36–86 mmol/d
Amniotic Fluid Analysis, ΔA_{450nm}	Amniotic fluid	28 wk: 0–0.048 A		0–0.048 A
		40 wk: 0–0.02 A		0–0.02 A
Amphetamine	Serum, plasma (heparin, EDTA)	Therap. conc.: 20–30 ng/mL	× 7.396	150–220 nmol/L
		Toxic conc.: >200		>1500
Amylase (Beckman; BMD)	Serum	Newborn: 5–65 U/L		5–65 U/L
		>1 y: 25–125		25–125
	Urine, timed specimen	1–17 U/h		1–17 U/h

Androstenedione	Serum	ng/dL (mean ±1 SE)				nmol/L (mean ±1 SE)	
			M	F		M	F
		Cord:	85 ± 27	93 ± 28	× 0.0349	2.9 ± 0.94	3.2 ± 1.0
		1–3 mo:	34 ± 11	19 ± 4		1.2 ± 0.4	0.66 ± 0.14
		Adult:	107 ± 25	151 ± 38		3.74 ± 0.87	5.27 ± 1.33

TEST	SPECIMEN	REFERENCE RANGE	FACTOR	REFERENCE RANGE INTERNATIONAL UNITS
Anion Gap [Na − (Cl + CO₂)]	Plasma (heparin)	7–16 mmol/L		7–16 mmol/L
Anti-Deoxyribonuclease B Titer (Anti-DNAse Titer)	Serum	≤170 units		≤170 units

Antidiuretic Hormone (hADH, Vasopressin)	Plasma (EDTA)	Plasma mOsmol/kg	Plasma ADH pg/mL		Plasma ADH ng/L
		270–280:	<1.5	× 1	<1.5
		280–285:	<2.5		<2.5
		285–290:	1–5		1–5
		290–295:	2–7		2–7
		295–300:	4–12		4–12

Table 29-2 REFERENCE RANGES *(Continued)*

TEST	SPECIMEN	REFERENCE RANGE		FACTOR	REFERENCE RANGE INTERNATIONAL UNITS
Anti-Streptolysin-O Titer (ASO Titer)	Serum	≤166 Todd Units 170–330 Todd Units in school-aged children			
α₁-Antitrypsin	Serum	Newborn: 145–270 mg/dL Thereafter: 105–200		×0.222	32.2–60.0 μmol/L 23.3–44.4
Ascorbic Acid, see *Vitamin C*					
Aspartate Aminotransferase (AST, βGOT, 30 °C)	Serum	Newborn/Infant: 15–60 U/L Thereafter: 8–20			15–60 U/L 8–20
Base Excess	Whole blood (heparin)	*mmol/L* Newborn:　(−10)–(−2) Infant:　(−7)–(−1) Child:　(−4)–(+2) Thereafter:　(−3)–(+3)			*mmol/L* (−10)–(−2) (−7)–(−1) (−4)–(+2) (−3)–(+3)
Bicarbonate	Serum	Arterial: 21–28 mmol/L Venous: 22–29			Arterial: 21–28 mmol/L Venous: 22–29
Bile Acids, Total	Serum, fasting Serum, 2 h postprandial Feces	0.3–2.3 μg/mL 1.8–3.2 μg/mL 120–225 mg/d		×1 ×1	0.3–2.3 mg/L 1.8–3.2 mg/L 120–225 mg/d
Bilirubin			*Full*		
		Premature *mg/dL*	*Term* *mg/dL*		
Total	Serum	Cord:　<2.0 0–1 d:　<8.0 1–2 d:　<12.0 2–5 d:　<16.0 Thereafter:　<2.0	<2.0 <6.0 <8.0 <12.0 0.2–1.0	×17.10	*μmol/L* <34　<34 <137　<103 <205　<137 <274　<205 <34　3.4–17.1
	Urine	Negative			Negative
	Amniotic fluid	28 wk: <0.075 mg/dL (or ΔA₄₅₀ <0.048) 40 wk: <0.025 mg/dL (or ΔA₄₅₀ <0.02)		×17.10	<1.3 μmol/L (or ΔA₄₅₀ <0.048) <0.43 μmol/L (or ΔA₄₅₀ <0.02)
Conjugated (Direct)	Serum	0–0.2 mg/dL		×17.10	0–3.4 μmol/L
Bleeding Time (BT) *Ivy*	Blood from skin puncture	Normal: 2–7 min Borderline: 7–11 min			2–7 min 7–11 min
Simplate (G-D)		2.75–8 min			2.75–8 min
Blood Volume	Whole blood (heparin)	M: 52–83 mL/kg F: 50–75 mL/kg		×0.001	M: 0.052–0.083 L/kg F: 0.050–0.075 L/kg
Brucellosis, Agglutinins	Serum	≤1:8		×1	≤1:8
C-Peptide	Serum	≤4.0 ng/mL		×1	≤4.0 μg/L
C-Reactive Protein	Serum	Cord: 10–350 ng/mL Adult: 68–8200		×1	10–350 μg/L 68–8200
CSF, see *Cerebrospinal Fluid*					
Calcitonin (hCT)	Serum or plasma (heparin or EDTA)	*pg/mL* Newborn, Term, cord:　30–240 48 h:　91–580 7 d:　77–293 Premature, cord:　30–265 48 h:　108–670 7 d:　79–570 Adult, M:　<100 F: 4 times lower (increases in pregnancy) Concentrations decrease with age		×1	*ng/L* 30–240 91–580 77–293 30–265 108–670 79–570 <100
Calcium, Ionized (ICa)	Serum, plasma, or whole blood (heparin)	*mg/dL* Cord:　5.5±0.3 Newborn, 3–24 h:　4.3–5.1 24–48 h:　4.0–4.7 Thereafter:　4.48–4.92 or　2.24–2.46 mEq/L		×0.25 ×0.5	*mmol/L* 1.37±0.07 1.07–1.27 1.00–1.17 1.12–1.23 1.12–1.23

Table 29–2 REFERENCE RANGES (Continued)

TEST	SPECIMEN	REFERENCE RANGE		FACTOR	REFERENCE RANGE INTERNATIONAL UNITS
Calcium, Total	Serum		*mg/dL*		*mmol/L*
		Cord:	9.0–11.5	× 0.25	2.25–2.88
		Newborn, 3–24 h:	9.0–10.6		2.3–2.65
		24–48 h:	7.0–12.0		1.75–3.0
		4–7 d:	9.0–10.9		2.25–2.73
		Child:	8.8–10.8		2.2–2.70
		Thereafter:	8.4–10.2		2.1–2.55
	Urine, 24 h	*Ca in Diet*	*mg/d*		*mmol/d*
		Ca Free:	5–40	× 0.025	0.13–1.0
		Low to average:	50–150		1.25–3.8
		Average			
		(20 mmol/d):	100–300		2.5–7.5
	CSF	2.1–2.7 mEq/L or		× 0.50	1.05–1.35 mmol/L
		4.2–5.4 mg/dL		× 0.25	1.05–1.35 mmol/L
	Feces	Avg.: 0.64 g/d		× 25	16 mmol/d
Carbamazepine	Serum, plasma (heparin, EDTA); collect at trough conc.	Therap. conc.: 8–12 µg/mL		× 4.233	34–51 µmol/L
		Toxic conc.: >15			>63
Carbon Dioxide, Partial Pressure (pCO₂)	Whole blood (heparin)		*mmHg*		*kPa*
		Newborn:	27–40	× 0.1333	3.6–5.3
		Infant:	27–41		3.6–5.5
		Thereafter:	35–48		4.7–6.4
			32–45		4.3–6.0
Carbon Dioxide, Total (tCO₂)	Serum or plasma (heparin)		*mmol/L*		*mmol/L*
		Cord:	14–22		14–22
		Premature:	14–27		14–27
		Newborn:	13–22		13–22
		Infant:	20–28		20–28
		Child:	20–28		20–28
		Thereafter:	23–30		23–30
Carbon Monoxide	Whole blood (EDTA)	Nonsmokers:	<2% HbCO	× 0.01	HbCO fraction: <0.02
		Smokers:	<10%		<0.10
		Lethal:	>50%		>0.5
Carboxyhemoglobin, see *Carbon Monoxide*					
β-Carotene	Serum		*µg/dL*		*µmol/L*
		Infant:	20–70	× 0.0186	0.37–1.30
		Child:	40–130		0.74–2.42
		Thereafter:	60–200		1.12–3.72
Catecholamines, Fractionated	Plasma (EDTA-sodium metabisulfite)	Norepinephrine,			
		Supine:	100–400 pg/mL	× 5.911	591–2364 pmol/L
		Standing:	300–900		1773–5320
		Epinephrine,			
		Supine:	<70 pg/mL	× 5.458	<382 pmol/L
		Standing:	<100		<546
		Dopamine:	<30 pg/mL	× 6.528	<196 pmol/L
		(no postural change)			(no postural change)
	Urine, 24 h	Norepinephrine,	*µg/d*		*nmol/d*
		0–1 y:	0–10	× 5.911	0–59
		1–2 y:	0–17		0–100
		2–4 y:	4–29		24–171
		4–7 y:	8–45		47–266
		7–10 y:	13–65		77–384
		Thereafter:	15–80		87–473
		Epinephrine,	*µg/d*		*nmol/d*
		0–1 y:	0–2.5	× 5.458	0–13.6
		1–2 y:	0–3.5		0–19.1
		2–4 y:	0–6.0		0–32.7
		4–7 y:	0.2–10		1.1–55
		7–10 y:	0.5–14		2.7–76
		Thereafter:	0.5–20		2.7–109
		Dopamine,	*µg/d*		*nmol/d*
		0–1 y:	0–85	× 6.528	0–555
		1–2 y:	10–140		65–914
		2–4 y:	40–260		261–1697
		Thereafter:	65–400		424–2611
Catecholamines, Total	Urine, 24 h	*µg/m²/d*			*µg/m²/d*
		2–3 mo:			
		12.2 ± 4 to 19.6 ± 14.5		× 5.91	12.2 ± 4 to 19.6 ± 14.5
		4–10 mo:			
		19.2 ± 18 to 29.9 ± 21.3			19.2 ± 18 to 29.9 ± 21.3
		12–18 mo:			
		19.3 ± 14.3 to 33.5 ± 14.4			19.3 ± 14.3 to 33.5 ± 14.4
		Adult: <280 µg/d			<280 µg/d

Table 29-2 REFERENCE RANGES (Continued)

TEST	SPECIMEN	REFERENCE RANGE	FACTOR	REFERENCE RANGE INTERNATIONAL UNITS
Cerebrospinal Fluid Pressure	CSF	70–180 mm water		70–188 mm water
Cerebrospinal Fluid Volume	CSF	Child: 60–100 mL Adult: 100–160	×0.001	0.006–0.10 L 0.1–0.16
Ceruloplasmin	Serum	*mg/dL* Newborn: 1–30 6 mo–1 y: 15–50 1–12 y: 30–65 Thereafter: 14–40	×0.0662	*µmol/L* 0.06–1.99 0.99–3.31 1.99–4.30 0.93–2.65
Chloral Hydrate	Serum	As Trichloroethanol: Therap. conc.: 2–12 µg/mL Toxic conc.: >20	×6.694	13–80 µmol/L >134
Chloride	Serum or plasma (heparin)	*mmol/L* Cord: 96–104 Newborn: 97–110 Thereafter: 98–106		*mmol/L* 96–104 97–110 98–106
	CSF	118–132 mmol/L		118–132 mmol/L
	Urine, 24 h	*mmol/d* Infant: 2–10 Child: 15–40 Thereafter: 110–250 (varies greatly with Cl intake)		*mmol/d* 2–10 15–40 110–250
	Sweat	*mmol/L* Normal (homozygote): 0–35 Marginal: 30–60 Cystic fibrosis: 60–200 Increases by 10 mmol/L during lifetime		*mmol/L* 0–35 30–60 60–200 Increases by 10 mmol/L during lifetime
Cholesterol, Total	Serum or plasma (EDTA)	*mg/dL* Cord: 45–100 Newborn: 53–135 Infant: 70–175 Child: 120–200 Adolescent: 120–210 Adult: 140–310 *Recommended* (desirable) range for adults: 140–250	×0.0259	*mmol/L* 1.17–2.59 1.37–3.50 1.81–4.53 3.11–5.18 3.11–5.44 3.63–8.03 3.63–6.48
Chorionic Gonadotropin, β-Subunit (β-hCG)	Serum or plasma (EDTA)	Child and M: nondetectable F, post- conception *mIU/mL* 7–10 d: >5.0 30 d: >100 40 d: >2000 10 wk: 50,000–100,000 14 wk: 10,000–20,000 Trophoblastic disease: >100,000	×1.0	*IU/L* >5.0 >100 >2000 50,000–100,000 10,000–20,000 >100,000
Clotting Time Lee-White, 37 °C	Whole blood (no anticoagulant)	Glass tubes: 5–8 min (5–15 min at RT) Silicone tubes: about 30 min prolonged		Glass tubes: 5–8 min (5–15 min at RT) Silicone tubes: about 30 min prolonged
Coagulation Factor Assays *Factor I, see Fibrinogen* Factor II	Plasma (citrate)	0.5–1.5 U/mL or 60–150% of normal	×1	0.5–1.5 kU/L 60–150 AU
Factor IV, see Calcium Factor V		0.5–2.0 U/mL or 60–150% of normal	×1	0.5–2.0 kU/L 60–150 AU
Factor VII		65–135% of normal	×1	65–135 AU
Factor VIII		60–145% of normal	×1	60–145 AU
Factor VIII antigen		50–200% of normal	×1	50–200 AU
Factor IX		60–140% of normal	×1	60–140 AU
Factor X		60–130% of normal	×1	60–130 AU
Factor XI		65–135% of normal	×1	65–135 AU
Factor XII		65–150% of normal	×1	65–150 AU
Factor XIII (Fibrin Stabilizing Factor, FSF)	Whole blood (citrate or oxalate)	Minimal hemostat U/mL or 1–2%	×1000	20–50 U/L or 1–2 AU

Table 29–2 REFERENCE RANGES (Continued)

Test	Specimen	Reference Range		Factor	Reference Range International Units
Complement Components					
Total hemolytic complement activity	Plasma (EDTA)		75–160 U/mL or >33% of plasma CH_{50}	× 1	75–160 kU/mL >0.33 of plasma CH_{50}
Total complement decay rate (functional)	Plasma (EDTA)		~10–20%	× 0.01	~0.10–0.20 (fraction of decay rate)
			Deficiency: >50%		0.50 (fraction of decay rate)
Classic pathway components					
C1q	Serum		*mg/dL*		*mg/L*
		Cord:	4.7 ± 5.1 (1 SD)	× 10	47 ± 51 (1 SD)
		1 mo:	4.2 ± 1.0		42 ± 10
		6 mo:	4.4 ± 1.6		44 ± 16
		Adult:	6.5 ± 0.7		65 ± 7
C1r	Serum		2.5–3.8 mg/dL	× 10	25–38 mg/L
C1s (C1 esterase)	Serum		2.5–3.8 mg/dL	× 10	25–38 mg/L
C2	Serum		*mg/dL*		*mg/L*
		Cord:	2.2 ± 0.3 (1 SD)	× 10	22 ± 3 (1 SD)
		1 mo:	2.9 ± 0.5		29 ± 5
		6 mo:	3.0 ± 0.3		30 ± 3
		Adult:	2.8 ± 0.6		28 ± 6
C3			*mg/dL*		*g/L*
~ *RID*	Serum	Cord:	88.4 ± 11.7 (1 SD)	× 0.01	0.884 ± 0.117 (1 SD)
		1 mo:	95.5 ± 17.4		0.995 ± 0.174
		6 mo:	111.2 ± 12.3		1.112 ± 0.123
		Adult:	141.2 ± 14.9		1.412 ± 0.149
		Maternal:	161–175		1.61 ± 1.75
		At birth, conc. is 50–75% of adult values			At birth, conc. is 50–75% of adult values
Nephelometry	Serum	Newborn:	58–120 mg/dL	× 0.01	0.58–1.20 g/L
		Adult:	80–155		0.80–1.55
C4					
RID	Serum	Newborn:	16–39 mg/dL	× 10	160–390 mg/L
		Adult:	15–45		150–450
Nephelometry	Serum	Newborn:	10–26 mg/dL	× 10	100–260 mg/L
		Adult:	13–37		130–370
C5	Serum		*mg/dL*		*mg/L*
		Cord:	4.8 ± 0.7 (1 SD)	× 10	48 ± 7 (1 SD)
		1 mo:	4.3 ± 1.0		43 ± 10
		6 mo:	4.4 ± 1.0		44 ± 10
		Adult:	6.4 ± 1.3		64 ± 13
C6	Serum		*mg/dL*		*mg/L*
		Cord:	2.6 ± 0.78 (1 SD)	× 10	26 ± 7.8 (1 SD)
		1 mo:	3.7 ± 0.75		37 ± 7.5
		6 mo:	5.4 ± 0.86		54 ± 8.6
		Adult:	5.6 ± 0.80		56 ± 8.0
C7	Serum		4.9–7.0 mg/dL	× 10	49–70 mg/L
C8	Serum		4.3–6.3 mg/dL	× 10	43–63 mg/L
C9	Serum		4.7–6.9 mg/dL	× 10	47–69 mg/L
Alternative pathway components					
C4 binding protein	Serum		18.0–32.0 mg/dL	× 10	180–320 mg/L
Factor B (C3 proactivator)					
RID	Plasma (EDTA)		*mg/dL*		*mg/L*
		Cord:	11.8 ± 2.0	× 10	118 ± 20
		1 mo:	17.4 ± 5.6		174 ± 56
		6 mo:	23.1 ± 3.1		231 ± 31
		Adult:	24.1 ± 4.7		241 ± 47
Nephelometry	Serum	Newborn:	14–33 mg/dL	× 10	140–330 mg/L
		Adult:	20–45		200–450
Properdin	Serum		*mg/dL*		*mg/L*
		Cord:	1.5 ± 0.1 (1 SD)	× 10	15 ± 1 (1 SD)
		1 mo:	1.4 ± 0.4		14 ± 4
		6 mo:	1.9 ± 0.3		19 ± 3
		Adult:	2.8 ± 0.4		28 ± 4
Regulatory proteins					
β1H-globulin (C3b inactivator accelerator)	Serum		*mg/dL*		*mg/L*
		Cord:	34.0 ± 34.1 (1 SD)	× 10	340 ± 41
		1 mo:	39.8 ± 8.1		398 ± 81
		6 mo:	46.8 ± 7.1		468 ± 71
		Adult:	56.1 ± 7.8		561 ± 78
C1 inhibitor (Esterase inhibitor)					
RID	Plasma (EDTA)		17.4–24.0 mg/dL	× 10	174–240 mg/L
Complement decay rate (functional)	Serum		<20% decay	× 0.01	<0.20 (fraction of decay rate)
			Deficiency: >50% decay		>0.50 (fraction of decay rate)

Table 29-2 REFERENCE RANGES (Continued)

TEST	SPECIMEN	REFERENCE RANGE		FACTOR	REFERENCE RANGE INTERNATIONAL UNITS
C3b inactivator (KAF)	Serum		*mg/dL*		*mg/L*
		Cord:	2.2 ± 0.2 (1 SD)	× 10	22 ± 2 (1 SD)
		1 mo:	2.7 ± 0.6		27 ± 6
		6 mo:	3.3 ± 0.5		33 ± 5
		Adult:	4.0 ± 0.7		40 ± 7
S protein	Serum	41.8–60.0 mg/dL		× 10	418–600 mg/L
Copper	Serum		*µg/dL*		*µmol/L*
		Birth–6 mo:	20–70	× 0.157	3.14–10.99
		6 y:	90–190		14.13–29.83
		12 y:	80–160		12.56–25.12
		Adult, M:	70–140		10.99–21.98
		F:	80–155		12.56–24.34
	Erythrocytes (heparin)	90–150 µg/dL		× 0.157	14.13–23.55 µmol/L
	Urine, 24 h	15–30 µg/d		× 0.0157	0.24–0.47 µmol/d
Coproporphyrin	Urine, 24 h	34–234 µg/d		× 1.5	51–351 nmol/d
	Feces, 24 h	<30 µg/g dry wt		× 1.5	<45 nmol/g dry wt
		400–1200 µg/d			600–1800 nmol/d
Corticobinding Globulin (CBG), see Transcortin					
Cortisol	Serum or plasma (heparin)		*µg/dL*		*nmol/L*
		Newborn:	1–24	× 27.59	28–662
		0800 h:	5–23		138–635
		1600 h:	3–15		82–413
		2000 h:	≤50% of 0800 h	× 0.01	Fraction of 0800 h: ≤0.50
Cortisol, Free	Urine, 24 h		*µg/d*		*nmol/d*
		Child:	2–27	× 2.759	5.5–74
		Adolescent:	5–55		14–152
		Adult:	10–100		27–276
Creatine Kinase (CK, CPK; 30 °C)					
Total	Serum		*U/L*		*U/L*
		Newborn:	68–580		68–580
		Adult, M:	12–70		12–70
		F:	10–55		10–55
		Ambulatory,			
		M:	25–90		25–90
		F:	10–70		10–70
		Higher after exercise			Higher after exercise
Isoenzymes	Serum	Fraction 2 (MB) <5% of total			Fraction of total: <0.05
Creatinine					
Jaffe, kinetic or enzymatic	Serum or plasma		*mg/dL*		*µmol/L*
		Cord:	0.6–1.2	× 88.4	53–106
		Newborn:	0.3–1.0		27–88
		Infant:	0.2–0.4		18–35
		Child:	0.3–0.7		27–62
		Adolescent:	0.5–1.0		44–88
		Adult, M:	0.6–1.2		53–106
		F:	0.5–1.1		44–97
Jaffe, manual	Serum or plasma	0.8–1.5 mg/dL		× 88.4	70–133 µmol/L
	Amniotic fluid	After 37 wk gestation:			After 37 wk gestation:
		>2.0 mg/dL		× 88.4	>180 µmol/L
	Urine, 24 h		*mg/kg/d*		*µmol/kg/d*
		Infant:	8–20	× 8.84	71–180
		Child:	8–22		71–195
		Adolescent:	8–30		71–265
		Adult:	14–26		124–230
		or:	*mg/d*		*mmol/d*
		M:	800–2000	× 0.00884	7–18
		F:	600–1800		5.3–16
Creatinine Clearance (Endogenous)	Serum or plasma and urine	Newborn: 40–65 mL/min/1.73 m² <40 y, M: 97–137 F: 88–128 Decreases ~6.5 mL/min/decade			
Cyclic AMP	Plasma (EDTA)	M: 17–33 nmol/L F: 11–27			M: 17–33 nmol/L F: 11–27
	Urine, 24 h	1000–11,500 nmol/d <6000 nmoles cAMP/g creatinine			1000–11,500 nmol/d <6000 nmoles cAMP/g creatinine

Table 29–2 REFERENCE RANGES (Continued)

TEST	SPECIMEN	REFERENCE RANGE		FACTOR	REFERENCE RANGE INTERNATIONAL UNITS
Dehydroepiandrosterone (DHEA)	Serum		*ng/mL*	×3.467	*nmol/L*
		Cord:	5.6–20.0		19.4–69.3
		Child:	1.0–3.0		3.5–10.4
		Adult, M:	1.7–4.2		5.9–14.6
		F:	2.0–5.2		6.9–18.0
		Pregnancy:	0.5–12.5		1.7–43.3
	Urine, 24 h		*mg/d*		*µmol/d*
		Child,		×3.467	
		0–1 y:	<0.1		<0.35
		10–15 y:	<0.4		<1.4
		Adult, M:	0–2.3		0–8.0
		F:	0–1.2		0–4.2
Dehydroepiandrosterone Sulfate (DHEA-SO₄)	Serum or plasma (heparin or EDTA)		*µg/mL*	×2.608	*µmol/L*
		Newborn:	<300		<780
		1–4 d:	<20		<52
		Child:	0.60–2.54		1.6–6.6
		Adult, M:	1.99–3.34		5.2–8.7
		F,			
		Premenopausal:	0.82–3.38		2.1–8.8
		Pregnancy, term:	0.23–1.17		0.6–3.0
Diazepam	Serum, plasma (heparin, EDTA); collect at trough conc.	Therap. conc.: 100–1000 ng/mL Toxic conc.: >5000		×3.512	350–3500 nmol/L >17,500
Differential Count, see *Leukocyte Differential Count*					
Digitoxin	Serum, plasma (heparin, EDTA); collect at least 6 h after dose	Therap. conc.: 20–35 ng/mL Toxic conc.: >45		×1.307	26–46 nmol/L >59
Digoxin	Serum, plasma (heparin, EDTA); collect at least 12 h after dose		*ng/mL*		*nmol/L*
		Therap. conc.,			
		CHF:	0.8–1.5	×1.281	1–1.9
		Arrhythmias:	1.5–2.0		1.9–2.6
		Toxic conc.,			
		Child:	>2.5		>3.2
		Adult:	>3.0		>3.8

TEST	SPECIMEN	REFERENCE RANGE			FACTOR	REFERENCE RANGE INTERNATIONAL UNITS	
Dihydrotestosterone (DHT)	Serum			*ng/dL*	×0.03443		*nmol/L*
		Prepubertal:		<3.5			<0.12
		Pubertal	*M*	*F*		*M*	*F*
		stage I:	<10	<10		<0.34	<0.34
		II:	<20	<15		<0.7	<0.5
		III:	<35	<25		<1.2	<0.86
		IV–V:	<75	<25		<2.6	<0.86
		Adult:	60–300	10–40		2–10.3	0.34–1.4

Diphenylhydantoin, see *Phenytoin*

TEST	SPECIMEN	REFERENCE RANGE		FACTOR	REFERENCE RANGE INTERNATIONAL UNITS
Disaccharide Absorption Test	Serum		*mg/dL*		*mmol/L*
		Change in glucose from fasting			Change in glucose from fasting value:
		value: Normal	>30	×0.055	>1.67
		Inconclusive:	20–30		1.11–1.67
		Abnormal:	<20		<1.11

Dithionite Tube Test, see *Sickle Cell Tests*

Electrophoresis, Hemoglobin, see *Hemoglobin Electrophoresis*

TEST	SPECIMEN	REFERENCE RANGE	FACTOR	REFERENCE RANGE INTERNATIONAL UNITS
Eosinophil Count	Whole blood (EDTA or heparin); capillary blood	50–350 cells/mm³ (µL)	×10⁶	50–350 × 10⁶ cells/L

Epinephrine, see *Catecholamines, Fractionated*

Table 29–2 REFERENCE RANGES (Continued)

TEST	SPECIMEN	REFERENCE RANGE		FACTOR	REFERENCE RANGE INTERNATIONAL UNITS
Erythrocyte Count (RBC Count)	Whole blood (EDTA)	*millions of cells/mm³ (μL)*			*× 10¹² cells/L*
		Cord blood:	3.9–5.5	× 1	3.9–5.5
		1–3 d (cap.):	4.0–6.6		4.0–6.6
		1 wk:	3.9–6.3		3.9–6.3
		2 wk:	3.6–6.2		3.6–6.2
		1 mo:	3.0–5.4		3.0–5.4
		2 mo:	2.7–4.9		2.7–4.9
		3–6 mo:	3.1–4.5		3.1–4.5
		0.5–2 y:	3.7–5.3		3.7–5.3
		2–6 y:	3.9–5.3		3.9–5.3
		6–12 y:	4.0–5.2		4.0–5.2
		12–18 y, M:	4.5–5.3		4.5–5.3
		F:	4.1–5.1		4.1–5.1
		18–49 y, M:	4.5–5.9		4.5–5.9
		F:	4.0–5.2		4.0–5.2
Erythrocyte Sedimentation Rate (ESR)					
Westergren, modified	Whole blood (EDTA)		*mm/h*		*mm/h*
		Child:	0–10		0–10
		Adult: M, <50 y:	0–15		0–15
		F, <50 y:	0–20		0–20
Wintrobe		Child:	0–13		0–13
		Adult, M,	0–9		0–9
		F,	0–20		0–20
ZETA		41–54%			41–54 AU
Erythropoietin					
RIA	Serum	<5–20 mU/mL		× 1	<5–20 U/L
Hemagglutination		25–125			25–125
Bioassay		5–18			5–18
Estradiol	Serum or plasma (heparin or EDTA)		*pg/mL*		*pmol/L*
		M, pubertal		× 3.671	
		stage I:	2–8		7–29
		II:	11		40
		III:	>20		>73
		Adult, M:	8–36		29–132
		F, pubertal			
		stage I:	0–23		0–84
		II:	0–66		0–242
		III:	0–105		0–385
		IV:	20–300		73–1101
		Follicular:	10–90		37–330
		Midcycle:	100–500		367–1835
		Luteal:	50–240		184–881
	Urine, 24 h		*μg/d*		*nmol/d*
		Adult, M:	0–6	× 3.671	0–22
		F,			
		Follicular:	0–3		0–11
		Ovulatory peak:	4–14		15–51
		Luteal:	4–10		15–37
Estriol (E₃), Free	Serum	*Weeks of*			
		gestation	*μg/L*		*nmol/L*
		25:	3.5–10.0	× 3.47	12.1–34.7
		28:	4.0–12.5		13.9–43.4
		30:	4.5–14.0		15.6–48.6
		32:	5.0–16.0		17.4–55.5
		34:	5.5–18.5		19.1–64.2
		36:	7.0–25.0		24.3–86.8
		37:	8.0–28.0		27.8–97.2
		38:	9.0–32.0		31.2–111.0
		39:	10.0–34.0		34.7–118.0
		40–41:	10.5–25.0		36.4–86.8
	Amniotic fluid		*ng/mL*		*nmol/L*
		Weeks	*(95% range)*		*(95% range)*
		16–20:	1.0–3.2	× 3.47	3.5–11.1
		20–24:	2.1–7.8		7.3–27.1
		24–28:	2.1–7.8		7.3–27.1
		28–32:	4.0–13.6		13.9–47.2
		32–36:	3.6–15.5		12.5–53.8
		36–38:	4.6–18.0		16.0–62.5
		38–40:	5.4–19.8		18.7–68.7

Table 29–2 REFERENCE RANGES (Continued)

Test	Specimen	Reference Range		Factor	Reference Range International Units
Estriol (E₃), Total	Serum		*ng/mL*		*nmol/L*
		Pregnancy (wk),			
		24–28:	30–170	× 3.468	104–590
		28–32:	40–220		140–760
		32–36:	60–280		208–970
		36–40:	80–350		280–1210
		Adult, M and nonpregnant F:	<2		<7
	Urine, 24 h		*mg/d*		*μmol/d*
		Pregnancy (wk),			
		30:	6–18	× 3.468	21–62
		35:	9–28		31–97
		40:	13–42		45–146
		Decrease of >40% of previous value suggests fetus at risk			Fraction of previous value of <0.60 suggests fetus at risk
Estrogens, Total	Serum		*pg/mL*		*ng/L*
		Child:	<30	× 1	<30
		M:	40–115		40–115
		F, cycle—days			
		1–10 d:	61–394		61–394
		11–20 d:	122–437		122–437
		21–30 d:	156–350		156–350
		Prepubertal:	≤40		≤40
	Urine, 24 h		*μg/d*		*μg/d*
		Child:	1.0 (mean)	× 1	1.0 (mean)
		M, Pubertal,			
		Stage I:	2.5 (mean)		2.5 (mean)
		II:	5.9 (mean)		5.9 (mean)
		III:	6.2 (mean)		6.2 (mean)
		Adult, M:	5–25		5–25
		F, Preovulation:	5–25		5–25
		Ovulation:	28–100		28–100
		Luteal peak:	22–80		22–80
		Pregnancy:	<45,000		<45,000
		Postmenopausal:	<10		<10
Ethanol	Whole blood (oxalate), serum	Toxic conc.: 50–100 mg/dL		× 0.2171	11–22 mmol/L
		Depression of CNS: >100			>22
Ethosuximide	Serum, plasma (heparin, EDTA); collect at trough conc.	Therap. conc.: 40–100 μg/mL		× 7.084	280–700 μmol/L
		Toxic conc.: >150			>1060
Fat, Fecal	Feces, 72 h		*g/d*		*g/d*
		Infant, breast-fed:	<1	× 1	<1
		0–6 y:	<2		<2
		Adult:	<7		<7
		Adult (fat-free diet):	<4		<4
		Coefficient of fat absorption (%)			*Absorbed fraction*
		Infant, breast-fed:	>93	× 0.01	>0.93
		Infant, formula-fed:	>83		>0.83
		>1 y:	≥95		≥0.95
Fatty Acids, Nonesterified (Free)	Serum or plasma (heparin)	Adults: 8–25 mg/dL		× 0.0354	0.30–0.90 mmol/L
		Children and obese adults: <31			<1.10
Ferric Chloride Test	Urine, fresh random	Negative			Negative
Ferritin	Serum		*ng/ml*		*μg/L*
		Newborn:	25–200	× 1	25–200
		1 mo:	200–600		200–600
		2–5 mo:	50–200		50–200
		6 mo–15 y:	7–140		7–140
		Adult, M:	15–200		15–200
		F:	12–150		12–150
Fetal Hemoglobin (HbF) *Alkali denaturation (White)*	Whole blood (EDTA)		*% HbF*		*Mass fraction HbF*
		1 d:	77.0 ± 7.3	× 0.01	0.77 ± 0.073
		5 d:	76.8 ± 5.8		0.768 ± 0.058
		3 wk:	70.0 ± 7.3		0.70 ± 0.073
		6–9 wk:	52.9 ± 11.0		0.529 ± 0.11
		3–4 mo:	23.2 ± 16.0		0.232 ± 0.16
		6 mo:	4.7 ± 2.2		0.047 ± 0.022
		Adult:	<2.0		<0.020

Table 29–2 REFERENCE RANGES (Continued)

TEST	SPECIMEN	REFERENCE RANGE			FACTOR	REFERENCE RANGE INTERNATIONAL UNITS	
α₁-Fetoprotein	Serum	Adult: <40 ng/mL			× 1	<40 µg/L	
		Mean: 2.6 ± 1.6 (1 SD) ng/mL				2.6 ± 1.6 (1 SD) µg/L	
		Fetal: peak of 200–400 mg/dL in first trimester			× 0.01	peak of 2–4 g/L in first trimester	
		1 y: <30 ng/mL			× 1	<30 µg/L	
	Amniotic fluid		*mg/dL* median	*±2* *log SD*		*mg/L* median	*±2* *log SD*
		weeks					
		11–12	24	10–50	× 10	240	100–500
		13–14	23	13–41		230	130–410
		15–16	18	9–35		180	90–350
		17–18	15	6–33		150	60–330
		19–20	10	5–25		100	50–250
		21–25	7	4–14		70	40–140
		26–30	6	3–10		60	30–100
		31–35	2	0.5–7		20	5–70
		36–40	1	0.2–3		10	2–30
Fibrin Degradation Products *Agglutination* *(Thrombo-Wellco test^R)*	Whole blood; special tube containing thrombin and proteolytic inhibitor	<10 µg/mL			× 1	<10 mg/L	
	Urine: 2 mL in special tube (see above)	<0.25 µg/mL			× 1	<0.25 mg/L	
Fibrinogen	Whole blood (Na citrate)	Newborn: 125–300 mg/dL			× 0.01	1.25–3.00 g/L	
		Adult: 200–400				2.00–4.00	
Folate	Serum	Newborn: 7.0–32 ng/mL			× 2.265	15.9–72.4 nmol/L	
		Thereafter: 1.8–9				4.1–20.4	
	Erythrocytes (EDTA)	150–450 ng/mL cells				340–1020 nmol/L cells	
Follicle Stimulating Hormone (hFSH)	Serum or plasma (heparin)		*mU/mL* *(IRP-2-hMG)*		× 1	*IU/L*	
		Birth–1 y, M:	<1–12			<1–12	
		F:	<1–20			<1–20	
		1–8 y, M:	<1–6			<1–6	
		F:	<1–4			<1–4	
		9–10 y, M:	<1–10			<1–10	
		F:	2–8			2–8	
		11–12 y, M:	2–12			2–12	
		F:	3–11			3–11	
		13–14 y, M:	3–15			3–15	
		F:	3–15			3–15	
			mU/mL			*IU/L*	
		Adult, M:	4–25			4–25	
		F,					
		Premenopause:	4–30			4–30	
		Midcycle peak:	10–90			10–90	
		Pregnancy: Low to undetectable				Low to undetectable	
Galactose	Serum	Newborn: 0–20 mg/dL			× 0.0555	0–1.11 mmol/L	
		Thereafter: <5				<0.28	
	Urine	Newborn: ≤60 mg/dL			× 0.0555	≤3.33 mmol/L	
		Thereafter: <14 mg/d			× 0.00555	<0.08 mmol/d	
Gastrin	Serum	<100 pg/mL			× 1	<100 ng/L	
Glucose	Serum		*mg/dL*			*mmol/L*	
		Cord:	45–96		× 0.0555	2.5–5.3	
		Premature:	20–60			1.1–3.3	
		Neonate:	30–60			1.7–3.3	
		Newborn,					
		1 d:	40–60			2.2–3.3	
		>1 d:	50–90			2.8–5.0	
		Child:	60–100			3.3–5.5	
		Adult:	70–105			3.9–5.8	
	Whole blood (heparin)	Adult:	65–95			3.6–5.3	
	CSF	Adult:	40–70			2.2–3.9	
Quantitative, enzymatic	Urine	<0.5 g/d			× 5.55	<2.8 mmol/d	
Qualitative	Urine	Negative				Negative	
Glucose, 2 h Postprandial	Serum	<120 mg/dL			× 0.0555	<6.7 mmol/L	
		Diabetes: see *Glucose Tolerance Test, Oral*					

Table 29-2   REFERENCE RANGES   (Continued)

TEST	SPECIMEN	REFERENCE RANGE	FACTOR	REFERENCE RANGE INTERNATIONAL UNITS
Glucose-6-phosphate Dehydrogenase (G-6-PD) in Erythrocytes	Whole blood (ACD, EDTA, or heparin)			
WHO and ICSH methods		Adult: 12.1 ± 2.09 U/g Hb (1 SD) 351 ± 60.6 U/10^{12} RBC 4.11 ± 0.71 U/mL RBC	$\times 0.0645$ $\times 10^{-3}$ $\times 1$	Adult: 0.78 ± 0.13 (1 SD) MU/mol Hb 0.35 ± 0.06 nU/RBC 4.11 ± 0.71 kU/L RBC
Bishop, modified		Adult: 3.4–8.0 U/g Hb 98.6–232 U/10^{12} RBC 1.16–2.72 U/mL RBC Newborn: 50% higher	$\times 0.0645$ $\times 10^{-3}$ $\times 1$	Adult: 0.22–0.52 MU/mol Hb 0.10–0.23 nU/RBC 1.16–2.72 kU/L RBC Newborn: 50% higher

Glucose Tolerance Test (GTT), Oral
Dose, Adult: 75 g
Child: 1.75 g/kg
of ideal weight up to
maximum of 75 g

Specimen: Serum

	mg/dL Normal	Diabetic	Factor	mmol/L Normal	Diabetic
Fasting:	70–105	>115	$\times 0.0555$	3.9–5.8	>6.4
60 min:	120–170	≥200		6.7–9.4	≥11
90 min:	100–140	≥200		5.6–7.8	≥11
120 min:	70–120	≥140		3.9–6.7	≥7.8

TEST	SPECIMEN	REFERENCE RANGE	FACTOR	REFERENCE RANGE INTERNATIONAL UNITS
γ-Glutamyltransferase (GGT), 37 °C	Serum	M: 9–50 U/L F: 8–40	$\times 1$	M: 9–50 U/L F: 8–40
Growth Hormone (hGH, Somatotropin) Fasting, at rest	Serum or plasma (EDTA, heparin)	ng/mL Cord: 10–50 Newborn: 10–40 Child: <5 Adult, M: <5 F: <8	$\times 1$	µg/L 10–50 10–40 <5 <5 <8
Ham's Test, see Acidified Serum Test				
Haptoglobin (Hp) RID	Serum; avoid hemolysis	30–175 mg/dL	$\times 0.155$	6.20–27.90 µmol Hb bound/L of serum = 300–1750 mg/L
Sephadex		40–180 mg Hb bound/dL of serum		
Nephelometry		Newborn: 5–48 mg/dL Thereafter: 25–175 mg/dL	$\times 10$	50–480 mg/L 250–1750 mg/L

HDL-Cholesterol (HDLC)
Specimen: Serum or plasma (EDTA)

	mg/dL M	F	Factor	mmol/L M	F
Mean:	45	55	$\times 0.0259$	1.17	1.42
Range,					
Cord blood:	5–50	5–50		0.13–1.30	0.13–1.30
0–14 y:	30–65	30–65		0.78–1.68	0.78–1.68
15–19 y:	30–65	30–70		0.78–1.68	0.78–1.81
20–29 y:	30–70	30–75		0.78–1.81	0.78–1.94
30–39 y:	30–70	30–80		0.78–1.81	0.78–2.07
40+ y:	30–70	30–85		0.78–1.81	0.78–2.20

Values for Blacks ~10 mg/dL higher

Hematocrit (HCT, Hct)
Calculated from MCV and RBC (electronic displacement or laser)

Specimen: Whole blood (EDTA)

	% of packed red cells (V red cells/V whole blood × 100)	Factor	Volume fraction (V red cells/V whole blood)
1 d (cap):	48–69	$\times 0.01$	0.48–0.69
2 d:	48–75		0.48–0.75
3 d:	44–72		0.44–0.72
2 mo:	28–42		0.28–0.42
6–12 y:	35–45		0.35–0.45
12–18 y, M:	37–49		0.37–0.49
F:	36–46		0.36–0.46
18–49 y, M:	41–53		0.41–0.53
F:	36–46		0.36–0.46

Hemoglobin (Hb)
Specimen: Whole blood (EDTA)

	g/dL	Factor	mmol/L
1–3 d (cap):	14.5–22.5	$\times 0.155$	2.25–3.49
2 mo:	9.0–14.0		1.40–2.17
6–12 y:	11.5–15.5		1.78–2.40
12–18 y, M:	13.0–16.0		2.02–2.48
F:	12.0–16.0		1.86–2.48
18–49 y, M:	13.5–17.5		2.09–2.71
F:	12.0–16.0		1.86–2.48

	Serum or plasma (heparin, ACD, EDTA)	<10 mg/dL <3 mg/dL with butterfly set-up and 18 g needle	$\times 0.1551$	<1.55 µmol/L <0.47 µmol/L with butterfly set-up and 18 g needle
	Urine, fresh random	Negative		Negative

Table 29-2 REFERENCE RANGES (Continued)

Test	Specimen	Reference Range	Factor	Reference Range International Units
Hemoglobin, glycosylated	Whole blood (heparin, EDTA, or oxalate)			Fraction of Hb
Electrophoresis		5.6–7.5% of total Hb	×0.01	0.056–0.075
Column		6–9% of total Hb		0.06–0.09
HPLC		HbA$_{1a}$ 1.6% total Hb		0.016
		HbA$_{1b}$ 0.8		0.008
		HbA$_{1c}$ 3–6		0.03–0.06
Hemoglobin A	Whole blood (EDTA, citrate, or heparin)	>95%	×0.01	Fraction of Hb: >0.95
Hemoglobin A$_2$ (HbA$_2$)	Whole blood (EDTA, oxalate)	Adult: 1.5–3.5% (2 SD) Lower in infants <1 y		Mass fraction 0.015–0.035 (2 SD)
Hemoglobin (Hb) Electrophoresis	Whole blood (EDTA, citrate, or heparin)			Mass fraction
		HbA >95%	×0.01	HbA >0.95
		HbA$_2$ 1.5–3.5%		HbA$_2$ 0.015–0.035
		HbF <2%		HbF <0.02
Hemoglobin F	Whole blood (EDTA)			
Alkali denaturation (White)		% HbF		Mass fraction HbF
		1 d: 77.0 ± 7.3		0.77 ± 0.073
		6 mo: 4.7 ± 2.2		0.047 ± 0.022
		Adult: <2.0		<0.020
Hemoglobin H (HbH) Isopropanol precipitation	Whole blood (ACD, EDTA, or heparin)	No precipitation at 40 min		No precipitation at 40 min
Homovanillic Acid (HVA)	Urine, 24 h	Child: 3–16 µg/mg creatinine	×0.621	1.9–10 mmol/mol creatinine
		Thereafter: <15 mg/d	×5.489	<82 µmol/d
17-Hydroxycorticosteroids (17-OHCS)	Urine, 24 h			µmol/d
		mg/d		
		0–1 y: 0.5–1.0	×2.76	1.4–2.8 (Conversion
		Child: 1.0–5.6		2.8–15.5 based on
		Adult, M: 3.0–10.0		8.2–27.6 hydrocortisone,
		F: 2.0–8.0		5.5–22 M.W. 362)
		or: 3–7 mg/g creatinine	×0.312	or: 0.9–2.5 mmol/mol creatinine
5-Hydroxyindole Acetic Acid (5-HIAA)				
Qualitative	Fresh random urine	Negative		Negative
Quantitative	Urine, 24 h	2–8 mg/d	×5.230	10.5–42 µmol/d
17-Hydroxyprogesterone (17-OHP)	Serum			
		ng/mL		nmol/L
		M,		
		Pubertal stage I: 0.1–0.3	×3.026	0.3–0.9
		Adult: 0.2–1.8		0.6–5.4
		F,		
		Pubertal stage I: 0.2–0.5		0.6–1.5
		Follicular: 0.2–0.8		0.6–2.4
		Luteal: 0.8–3.0		2.4–9.0
		Postmenopausal: 0.04–0.5		0.12–1.5
Immunoglobulin A (IgA)	Serum			
		mg/dL		mg/L
		Cord: 0–5	×10	0–50
		Newborn: 0–2.2		0–22
		1/2–6 mo: 3–82		30–820
		6 mo–2 y: 14–108		140–1080
		2–6 y: 23–190		230–1900
		6–12 y: 29–270		290–2700
		12–16 y: 81–232		810–2320
		Thereafter: 60–380		600–3800
Immunoglobulin D (IgD)	Serum	Newborn: None detected		None detected
		Thereafter: 0–8 mg/dL	×0.055	0–0.44 µmol/L
Immunoglobulin E (IgE)	Serum	M: 0–230 IU/mL	×1	0–230 kIU/L
		F: 0–170		0–170
Immunoglobulin G (IgG)	Serum			
		mg/dL		g/L
		Cord: 760–1700	×0.01	7.6–17
		Newborn: 700–1480		7–14.8
		1/2–6 mo: 300–1000		3–10
		6 mo–2 y: 500–1200		5–12
		2–6 y: 500–1300		5–13
		6–12 y: 700–1650		7–16.5
		12–16 y: 700–1550		7–15.5
		Adults: 600–1600		6–16
		(higher in Blacks)		(higher in Blacks)

Table 29–2 REFERENCE RANGES (Continued)

Test	Specimen	Reference Range		Factor	Reference Range International Units	
Immunoglobulin M (IgM)	Serum		mg/dL		mg/L	
		Cord:	4–24	× 10	40–240	
		Newborn:	5–30		50–300	
		1/2–6 mo:	15–109		150–1090	
		6 mo–2 y:	43–239		430–2390	
		2–6 y:	50–199		500–1990	
		6–12 y:	50–260		500–2600	
		12–16 y:	45–240		450–2400	
		Thereafter:	40–345		400–3450	
		Results vary with std. preparation				
Insulin (12 h Fasting)	Serum or plasma (no anticoagulant)	Newborn: 3–20 µU/mL		× 1.0	3–20 mU/L	
		Thereafter: 7–24			7–24	
Insulin with Oral Glucose Tolerance Test	Serum	Min	Insulin, µU/mL		mU/L	
		0:	7–24	× 1	7–24	
		30:	25–231		25–231	
		60:	18–276		18–276	
		120:	16–166		16–166	
		180:	4–38		4–38	
Iron	Serum		µg/dL		µmol/L	
		Newborn:	100–250	× 0.179	17.90–44.75	
		Infant:	40–100		7.16–17.90	
		Child:	50–120		8.95–21.48	
		Thereafter, M:	50–160		8.95–28.64	
		F:	40–150		7.16–26.85	
		Intoxicated child:	280–2550		50.12–456.5	
		Fatally poisoned child:	>1800		>322.2	
Iron-Binding Capacity, Total (TIBC)	Serum	Infant: 100–400 µg/dL		× 0.179	17.90–71.60 µmol/L	
		Thereafter: 250–400			44.75–71.60	
17-Ketogenic Steroids (17-KGS)	Urine, 24 h		mg/d		µmol/d	
		0–1 y:	<1.0	× 3.467	<3.5	(Conversion based
		1–10 y:	<5		<17	on dehydroepi-
		11–14 y:	<12		<42	androsterone,
		Thereafter, M:	5–23		17–80	M.W. 288)
		F:	3–15		10–52	
Ketone Bodies						
Qualitative	Serum	Negative			Negative	
	Urine, random	Negative			Negative	
Quantitative	Serum	0.5–3.0 mg/dL		× 10	5–30 mg/L	
17-Ketosteroids (17-KS), Total *Zimmerman rection*	Urine, 24 h		mg/d		µmol/d	
		14 d–2 y:	<1	× 3.467	<3.5	(Conversion based
		2–6 y:	<2		<7	on dehydroepi-
		6–10 y:	1–4		3.5–14	androsterone,
		10–12 y:	1–6		3.5–21	M.W. 288)
		12–14 y:	3–10		10–35	
		14–16 y:	5–12		17–42	
		Thereafter,				
		M, 18–30 y:	9–22		31–76	
		M, >30 y:	8–20		28–70	
		F:	6–15		21–52	
		Decreases with age			Decreases with age	
Chromatography	Urine, 24 h	Adult, M: 5.0–12.0		× 3.467	Adult, M: 17–42	
		F: 3.0–10.0			F: 10–35	
LDL-Cholesterol (LDLC)	Serum or plasma (EDTA)		mg/dL		mmol/L	
			M	F	M	F
		Cord blood: 10–50 / 10–50		× 0.0259	0.26–1.30	0.26–1.30
		0–19 y: 60–140 / 60–150			1.55–3.63	1.55–3.89
		20–29 y: 60–175 / 60–160			1.55–4.53	1.55–4.14
		30–39 y: 80–190 / 70–170			2.07–4.92	1.81–4.40
		40–49 y: 90–205 / 80–190			2.33–5.31	2.07–4.92
		Recommended (desirable) range for adults: 65–175 mg/dL			1.68–4.53	
Lactate	Whole blood (heparin)		mmol/L		mmol/L	
		Venous:	0.5–2.2		0.5–2.2	
		Arterial:	0.5–1.6		0.5–1.6	
		Inpatients,				
		Venous:	0.9–1.7		0.9–1.7	
		Arterial:	<1.25		<1.25	

Table 29-2   REFERENCE RANGES (Continued)

Test	Specimen	Reference Range	Factor	Reference Range International Units
Lactate Dehydrogenase (LDH), 30 °C	Serum			
Total (L→P)		*U/L*		*U/L*
		Newborn: 160–450		160–450
		Infant: 100–250		100–250
		Child: 60–170		60–170
		Thereafter: 45–90		45–90
Total (P→L)				
30 °C				
37 °C		Adult: 150–320 U/L		150–320 U/L
		Adult: 210–420		210–420
	CSF	~10% of serum value	× 0.01	~0.10 fraction of serum value
Isoenzymes	Serum			*Fraction of total*
		Fraction 1: 15–29%	× 0.01	0.15–0.29
		Fraction 2: 28–45%		0.28–0.45
		Fraction 3: 16–27%		0.16–0.27
		Fraction 4: 5–15%		0.05–0.15
		Fraction 5: 3–12%		0.03–0.12
Lead	Whole blood (heparin)			
		μg/dL		*μmol/L*
		Child: <30	× 0.0483	<1.45
		Adult: <40		<1.93
		Acceptable for industrial		
		exposure: <60		<2.90
		Toxic: ≥100		≥4.83
	Urine, 24 h	<80 μg/L	× 0.00483	<0.39 μmol/L
Lecithin/Sphingomyelin (L/S) Ratio	Amniotic fluid	2.0–5.0 indicates probable fetal lung maturity (>3.0 in diabetics)		2.0–5.0 indicates probable fetal lung maturity
Lecithin Phosphorus	Amniotic fluid	>0.10 mg/dL indicates probable adequate fetal lung maturity	× 0.3229	>0.33 mmol/L indicates probable adequate fetal lung maturity
Leukocyte Count (WBC Count)	Whole blood (EDTA)	*× 1000 cells/mm³ (μL)*		*× 10⁹ cells/L*
		Birth: 9.0–30.0	× 10⁶	9.0–30.0
		24 h: 9.4–34.0		9.4–34.0
		1 mo: 5.0–19.5		5.0–19.5
		1–3 y: 6.0–17.5		6.0–17.5
		4–7 y: 5.5–15.5		5.5–15.5
		8–13 y: 4.5–13.5		4.5–13.5
		Adult: 4.5–11.0		4.5–11.0
	CSF	*cells/μL*		*× 10⁶ cells/L*
		Premature: 0–25 mononuclear		0–25
		0–100 polymorphonuclear		0–100
		0–1000 RBC		0–1000
		Newborn: 0–20 mononuclear		0–20
		0–70 polymorphonuclear		0–70
		0–800 RBC		0–800
		Neonate: 0–5 mononuclear		0–5
		0–25 polymorphonuclear		0–25
		0–50 RBC		0–50
		Thereafter: 0–5 mononuclear		0–5
		(Numbers of cells in very young infants greater than in older individuals' CSF, without substantial implications for growth and development in most instances.)		
Leukocyte Differential Count	Whole blood (EDTA)			
Myelocytes		*%*		*Number fraction*
		0	× 0.01	0
Neutrophils—"bands"		3–5		0.03–0.05
Neutrophils—"segs"		54–62		0.54–0.62
Lymphocytes		25–33		0.25–0.33
Monocytes		3–7		0.03–0.07
Eosinophils		1–3		0.01–0.03
Basophils		0–0.75		0–0.0075
		Cells/mm³ (μL)		*× 10⁶ cells/L*
		0	× 1	0
		150–400		150–400
		3000–5800		3000–5800
		1500–3000		1500–3000
		285–500		285–500
		50–250		50–250
		15–50		15–50
Leukocyte Differential Count	CSF			
		%		*Number fraction*
Lymphocytes		62 ± 34	× 0.01	0.62 ± 0.34
Monocytes*		36 ± 20		0.36 ± 0.20
Neutrophils		2 ± 5		0.02 ± 0.05
Histocytes		rare		rare
Ependymal cells		rare		rare
Eosinophils		rare		rare
		Includes pia-arachnoid mesothelial cells.		

Table 29-2 REFERENCE RANGES *(Continued)*

TEST	SPECIMEN	REFERENCE RANGE	FACTOR	REFERENCE RANGE INTERNATIONAL UNITS
Leukocyte Peroxidase Stain	Whole blood	+ + + in AML − in ALL ± in AMML		
Lipase *Tietz method (37 °C)* *BMD (30 °C)*	Serum	0.1–1.0 U/mL ＜140 U/L	×280 ×1	28–280 U/L ＜140 U/L
Lipoprotein Electrophoresis	Serum	Distinct beta band; negligible chylomicron and pre-beta bands		
Lithium	Serum, plasma (heparin, EDTA); at least 12 h after last dose	Therap. conc.: 0.6–1.2 mmol/L Toxic conc.: ＞2		0.6–1.2 mmol/L ＞2
Long Acting Thyroid Stimulating Hormone (LATS)	Serum	Undetectable		Undetectable
Luteinizing Hormone (hLH)	Serum or plasma (heparin)	*mIU/mL* 1–3 mo, M: 22.3 ± 13.4 (1 SD) F: 17.4 ± 9.6 3–5 mo, M: 15.5 ± 11.8 F: 13.2 ± 7.6 5–7 mo, M: 17.1 ± 8.0 F: 13.4 ± 8.0 7–12 mo, M: 24.0 ± 18.3 F: 3.4 ± 1.3 Prepuberty phase I, M: 3.9 ± 2.1 F: 3.4 ± 1.3 M, 10–13 y: 4–12 12–14 y: 6–12 12–17 y: 6–16 15–18 y: 7–19 F, 8–12 y: 2.0–11.5 9–14 y: 2.0–14.0 12–18 y: 3.0–29.0 Adult, M: 6–23 F, Follicular phase: 5–30 Midcycle: 75–150 Luteal: 3–40 Postmeno- pausal: 30–200	×1	*IU/L* 22.3 ± 13.4 (1 SD) 17.4 ± 9.6 15.5 ± 11.8 13.2 ± 7.6 17.1 ± 8.0 13.4 ± 8.0 24.0 ± 18.3 3.4 ± 1.3 3.9 ± 2.1 3.4 ± 1.3 4–12 6–12 6–16 7–19 2.0–11.5 2.0–14.0 3.0–29.0 6–23 5–30 75–150 3–40 30–200
Lysergic Acid Diethylamine	Plasma (EDTA) Urine	After hallucinogenic dose: 0.005–0.009 µg/mL 0.001–0.050 µg/mL	×3089	After hallucinogenic dose: 15.5–27.8 nmol/L 3.1–155 nmol/L
Magnesium	Serum	*mEq/L* Newborn, 2–4 d: 1.2–1.8 5 mo–6 y: 1.65 ± 0.23 (2 SD) 6–12 y: 1.56 ± 0.18 12–20 y: 1.56 ± 0.21 Adult: 1.3–2.1 (Higher in females during menses)	×0.5	*mmol/L* 0.6–0.9 0.83 ± 0.12 (2 SD) 0.78 ± 0.09 0.78 ± 0.11 0.65 ± 1.05
Mean Corpuscular Hemoglobin (MCH)	Whole blood (EDTA)	*pg/cell* Birth: 31–37 1–3 d (cap.): 31–37 1 wk–1 mo: 28–40 2 mo: 26–34 3–6 mo: 25–35 0.5–2 y: 23–31 2–6 y: 24–30 6–12 y: 25–33 12–18 y: 25–35 18–49 y: 26–34	×0.0155	*fmol/cell* 0.48–0.57 0.48–0.57 0.43–0.62 0.40–0.53 0.39–0.54 0.36–0.48 0.37–0.47 0.39–0.51 0.39–0.54 0.40–0.53
Mean Corpuscular Hemoglobin Concentration (MCHC)	Whole blood (EDTA)	*%Hb/cell or g Hb/dL RBC* Birth: 30–36 1–3 d (cap.): 29–37 1–2 wk: 28–38 1–2 mo: 29–37 3 mo–2 y: 30–36 2–18 y: 31–37 ＞18 y: 31–37	×0.155	*mmol Hb/L RBC* 4.65–5.58 4.50–5.74 4.34–5.89 4.50–5.74 4.65–5.58 4.81–5.74 4.81–5.74

Table 29–2 REFERENCE RANGES (Continued)

Test	Specimen	Reference Range	Factor	Reference Range International Units
Mean Corpuscular Volume (MCV)	Whole blood (EDTA)	μm^3 1–3 d (cap): 95–121 0.5–2 y: 70–86 6–12 y: 77–95 12–18 y, M: 78–98 F: 78–102 18–49 y, M: 80–100 F: 80–100	×1	fL 95–121 70–86 77–95 78–98 78–102 80–100 80–100
Metanephrine, Total	Urine, 24 h	μg/mg creatinine <1 y: 0.001–4.60 1–2 y: 0.27–5.38 2–5 y: 0.35–2.99 5–10 y: 0.43–2.70 10–15 y: 0.001–1.87 15–18 y: 0.001–0.67 Thereafter: 0.05–1.20	×0.5735	mmol/mol creatinine 0.0006–2.64 0.15–3.08 0.20–1.71 0.25–1.55 0.0006–1.07 0.0006–0.38 0.03–0.69
Methemoglobin (MetHb)	Whole blood (EDTA, heparin, or ACD)	0.06–0.24 g/dL or 0.78 ± 0.37% of total Hb	×155 ×0.01	9.3–37.2 μmol/L 0.0078 ± 0.0037 (mass fraction)
Microsomal Antibodies, Thyroid see *Thyroid Microsomal Antibodies*				
Myoglobin	Serum Urine, random	6–85 ng/mL Negative	×1	6–85 pg/L Negative
Neutrophil Alkaline Phosphatase (Leucocyte Alkaline Phosphatase)	Finger-stick blood	Score: 13–130		
Niacin (Nicotinic Acid)	Urine, 24 h	0.3–1.5 mg/d	×8.113	2.43–12.17 μmol/d
Occult Blood	Feces, random Urine, random	Negative (<2 mL blood/d in ~100–200 g stool) Negative		Negative Negative
Osmolality	Serum Urine, random Urine, 24 h	Child, Adult: 275–295 mOsmol/kg H_2O 50–1400 mOsmol/kg H_2O, depending on fluid intake. After 12 h fluid restriction: >850 mOsmol/kg H_2O ≈300–900 mOsmol/kg H_2O		

Osmotic Fragility Test (RBC Fragility) pH 7.4, 20 °C — Whole blood (heparin)

% NaCl (g/dl)	% Hemolysis	Factor	NaCl (g/L)	Hemolyzed fraction
0.30	97–100	×10 = g/L NaCl	3.0	0.97–1.00
0.35	90–99	×0.01 = Hem. frac.	3.5	0.90–0.99
0.40	50–95		4.0	0.50–0.95
0.45	5–45		4.5	0.05–0.45
0.50	0–6		5.0	0.00–0.06
0.55	0		5.5	0.00

Sterile incubation at 37 °C

% NaCl (g/dL)	% Hemolysis	Factor	NaCl (g/L)	Hemolyzed fraction
0.20	95–100	×10 = g/L NaCl	2.0	0.95–1.00
0.30	85–100	×0.01 = Hem. frac.	3.0	0.85–1.00
0.35	75–100		3.5	0.75–1.00
0.40	65–100		4.0	0.65–1.00
0.45	55–95		4.5	0.55–0.95
0.50	40–85		5.0	0.40–0.85
0.55	15–70		5.5	0.15–0.70
0.60	0–40		6.0	0.00–0.40
0.65	0–10		6.5	0.00–0.10
0.70	0–5		7.0	0.00–0.05
0.85	0		8.5	0.00

Oxygen, Partial Pressure (pO_2) — Whole blood (heparin), arterial

	mmHg	Factor	kPa
Birth:	8–24	×0.133	1.1–3.2
5–10 min:	33–75		4.4–10.0
30 min:	31–85		4.1–11.3
>1 h:	55–80		7.3–10.6
1 d:	54–95		7.2–12.6
Thereafter:	83–108		11–14.4
(Decreases with age)			

Oxygen Saturation — Whole blood (heparin), arterial

	Reference Range	Factor	Reference Range International Units
	Newborn: 40–90% Thereafter: 95–99%	×0.01	Fraction saturated: 0.40–0.90 0.95–0.99

Table 29–2 REFERENCE RANGES (Continued)

Test	Specimen	Reference Range	Factor	Reference Range International Units
pO₂, see Oxygen, Partial Pressure				
pO_2 at half saturation (pO_2(0.5) or P_{50})	Whole blood (heparin), arterial	25–29 mmHg	×0.133	3.3–3.9 kPa
Paraldehyde	Serum, plasma (heparin, EDTA)	µg/mL		µmol/L
		Therap. conc.,		
		Sedation: 10–100	×7.567	75–750
		Anesthesia: >200		>1500
		Toxic conc.: 20–40		150–300
		Lethal conc.: >50		>375
Parathyroid Hormone (hPTH)	Serum	Vary with laboratory, e.g., Mayo Clinic, Bioscience:		
		N-terminal 230–630 pg/mL	×1	230–630 ng/L
		C-terminal 410–1760 pg/mL		410–1760 ng/L
		Nichols Institute:		
		C-terminal 40–100 µLEq/mL		40–100 mLEq/L
Partial Thromboplastin Time (PTT)	Whole blood (Na citrate)			
Nonactivated		60–85 s (Platelin)		60–85 s
Activated		25–35 s (differs with method)		25–35 s
pH	Whole blood (heparin), arterial			H⁺ concentration:
		Premature (48 h): 7.35–7.50		31–44 nmol/L
		Birth, full term: 7.11–7.36		43–77
		5–10 min: 7.09–7.30		50–81
		30 min: 7.21–7.38		41–61
		>1 h: 7.26–7.49		32–54
		1 d: 7.29–7.45		35–51
		Thereafter: 7.35–7.45		35–44
		Must be corrected for body temperature		
	Urine, random	Newborn/neonate: 5–7		0.1–10 µmol/L
		Thereafter: 4.5–8		0.01–32 µmol/L
		(average ≈6)		(average ≈1.0 µmol/L)
	Stool	7.0–7.5		31–100 nmol/L
Phenacetin	Plasma (EDTA)	Therap. conc.: 1–20 µg/mL	×5.580	5.6–110 µmol/L
		Toxic conc.: 50–250		280–1400
Phenobarbital	Serum, plasma (heparin, EDTA); collect at trough conc.	µg/mL		µmol/L
		Therap. conc.: 15–40	×4.306	65–170
		Toxic conc.,		
		Slowness, ataxia, nystagmus: 35–80		150–345
		Coma with reflexes: 65–117		280–504
		Coma without reflexes: >100		>430
Phensuximide (both parent and N-desmethyl metabolite)	Serum, plasma (heparin, EDTA)	Therap. conc.: 40–60 µg/mL	×5.71	228–343 µmol/L
Phenylalanine	Serum	mg/dL		mmol/L
		Premature: 2.0–7.5	×0.06054	0.12–0.45
		Newborn: 1.2–3.4		0.07–0.21
		Thereafter: 0.8–1.8		0.05–0.11
	Urine, 24 h	mg/d	×6.054	µmol/d
		10 d–2 wk: 1–2		6–12
		3–12 y: 4–18		24–110
		Thereafter: trace–17		trace–103
		or: 6±2 mg/g creatinine	×0.685	or: 4.1 ± 1.4 mmol/mol creatinine
Phenylpyruvic Acid, Qualitative	Urine, fresh random	Negative by FeCl₃ test		Negative by FeCl₃ test
Phenytoin	Serum, plasma (heparin, EDTA); collect at steady-state trough conc.	Therap. conc.: 10–20 µg/mL	×3.964	40–80 µmol/L
		Toxic conc.: >20		>80
Phosphatase, Acid Prostatic (RIA)	Serum	<3.0 ng/mL	×1	<3.0 µg/L
Roy, Brower, and Hayden, 37°C		0.11–0.60 U/L		0.11–0.60 U/L
Phosphatase, Alkaline (p-nitrophenyl phosphate,	Serum			
		U/L		U/L
SKI method; 30°C		Infant: 50–155		50–155
		Child: 20–150		20–150
		Adult: 20–70		20–70
Bowers and McComb, 30°C		25–90 U/L		25–90 U/L

Table 29–2 REFERENCE RANGES (Continued)

Test	Specimen	Reference Range	Factor	Reference Range International Units
Phospholipids, Total	Serum or plasma (EDTA)	*mg/dL*		*g/L*
		Newborn: 75–170	× 0.01	0.75–1.70
		Infant: 100–275		1.00–2.75
		Child: 180–295		1.80–2.95
		Adult: 125–275		1.25–2.75
Phosphorus, Inorganic	Serum	*mg/dL*		*mmol/L*
		Cord: 3.7–8.1	× 0.3229	1.2–2.6
		Premature (1 wk): 5.4–10.9		1.7–3.5
		Newborn: 4.3–9.3		1.4–3.0
		Child: 4.5–6.5		1.45–2.1
		Thereafter: 3.0–4.5		0.97–1.45
Plasma Volume	Plasma (heparin)	M: 25–43 mL/kg	× 0.001	M: 0.025–0.043 L/kg
		F: 28–45		F: 0.028–0.045
Platelet Count (Thrombocyte Count)	Whole blood (EDTA)	$\times 10^3/mm^3$ *(µL)*		$\times 10^9/L$
		Newborn: 84–478	× 10^6	84–478
		(After 1 wk, same as adult)		
		Adult: 150–400		150–400
Porphobilinogen (PBG)				
Quantitative	Urine, 24 h	0–2.0 mg/d	× 4.42	0–8.8 µmol/d
Qualitative	Urine, fresh random	Negative		Negative
Potassium	Serum	*mmol/L*		*mmol/L*
		Newborn: 3.9–5.9		3.9–5.9
		Infant: 4.1–5.3		4.1–5.3
		Child: 3.4–4.7		3.4–4.7
		Thereafter: 3.5–5.1		3.5–5.1
	Plasma (heparin)	3.5–4.5 mmol/L		3.5–4.5 mmol/L
	Urine, 24 h	2.5–125 mmol/d varies with diet		2.5–125 mmol/d varies with diet
Pregnanetriol	Urine 24, h	*mg/d*		*µmol/d*
		2 wk–2 y: 0.02–0.2	× 2.972	0.06–0.6
		2–5 y: <0.5		<1.5
		5–15 y: <1.5		<4.5
		>15 y: <2.0		<5.9
Primidone	Serum, plasma (heparin, EDTA); collect at trough conc.	Therap. conc.: 5–12 µg/mL	× 4.582	23–55 µmol/L
		Toxic conc.: >15		>69
Progesterone	Serum	*ng/mL*		*nmol/L*
		M,		
		Pubertal stage I: 0.11–0.26	× 3.18	0.35–0.83
		Adult: 0.12–0.3		0.38–1
		F,		
		Pubertal stage I: 0–0.3		0–1
		II: 0–0.46		0–1.5
		III: 0–0.6		0–2
		IV: 0.05–13.0		0.16–41
		Follicular: 0.02–0.9		0.06–2.9
		Luteal: 6.0–30.0		19–95
Prolactin (hPRL)	Serum	*ng/mL*		*µg/L*
		Adults, M: <20	× 1	<20
		F,		
		Follicular phase: <23		<23
		Luteal phase: 5–40		5–40
		Pregnancy,		
		1st trimester: <80		<80
		2nd trimester: <160		<160
		3rd trimester: <400		<400
		Newborn: >10-fold adult levels		>10-fold adult levels
Propranolol	Serum, plasma (heparin, EDTA); collect at trough conc.	Therap. conc.: 50–100 ng/mL	× 3.856	190–380 nmol/L
Protein				
Total	Serum	*g/dL*		*g/L*
		Premature: 4.3–7.6	× 10	43.0–76.0
		Newborn: 4.6–7.4		46.0–74.0
		Child: 6.2–8.0		62.0–80.0
		Adult,		
		Recumbent: 6.0–7.8		60.0–78.0
		~0.5 g higher in ambulatory patients		~5 g higher in ambulatory patients

Table 29–2 REFERENCE RANGES (Continued)

Test	Specimen	Reference Range	Factor	Reference Range International Units
Electrophoresis		*g/dL*		*g/L*
		Albumin,		
		Premature: 3.0–4.2		30–42
		Newborn: 3.6–5.4		36–54
		Infant: 4.0–5.0		40–50
		Thereafter: 3.5–5.0		35–50
		α_1-Globulin,		
		Premature: 0.1–0.5		1–5
		Newborn: 0.1–0.3		1–3
		Infant: 0.2–0.4		2–4
		Thereafter: 0.2–0.3		2–3
		α_2-Globulin,		
		Premature: 0.3–0.7		3–7
		Newborn: 0.3–0.5		3–5
		Infant: 0.5–0.8		5–8
		Thereafter: 0.4–1.0		4–10
		β-Globulin,		
		Premature: 0.3–1.2		3–12
		Newborn: 0.2–0.6		2–6
		Infant: 0.5–0.8		5–8
		Thereafter: 0.5–1.1		5–11
		γ-Globulin,		
		Premature: 0.3–1.4		3–14
		Newborn: 0.2–1.0		2–10
		Infant: 0.3–1.2		3–12
		Thereafter: 0.7–1.2		7–12
		Higher in Blacks		Higher in Blacks
Total	Urine, 24 h	1–14 mg/dL		10–140 mg/L
		50–80 mg/d (at rest)		50–80 mg/d
		<250 mg/d after intense exercise		<250 mg/d after intense exercise
Electrophoresis		*Average % of Total Protein*		*Fraction of Total*
		Albumin 37.9	×0.01	0.379
		Globulin, α_1 27.3		0.273
		α_2 19.5		0.195
		β 8.8		0.088
		γ 3.3		0.033
Total Column Turbidimetry	CSF	Lumbar: 8–32 mg/dL	×10	80–320 mg/L
		mg/dL		*mg/L*
		Lumbar,		
		Premature: 40–300		400–3000
		Newborn: 45–120		450–1200
		Child: 10–20		100–200
		Adolescent: 15–20		150–200
		Thereafter: 15–45		150–450
Electrophoresis		*% of Total*		*Fraction of Total*
		Prealbumin: 2–7	×0.01	0.02–0.07
		Albumin: 56–76		0.56–0.76
		α_1-Globulin: 2–7		0.02–0.07
		α_2-Globulin: 4–12		0.04–0.12
		β-Globulin: 8–18		0.08–0.18
		γ-Globulin: 3–12		0.03–0.12
Prothrombin Time (PT) One-stage (Quick)	Whole blood (Na citrate)	In general: 11–15 s (varies with type of thromboplastin)		11–15 s
		Newborn: prolonged by 2–3 s		Prolonged by 2–3 s
Two-stage modified (Ware and Seegers)	Whole blood (Na citrate)	18–22 s		18–22 s
Pyruvate Kinase (PK) in Erythrocytes	Whole blood (ACD, EDTA, or heparin)	Adult:		Adult:
		15.0 ± 1.99 U/g Hb (1 SD)	×0.0645	0.97 ± 0.13 MU/mol Hb (1 SD)
		435 ± 57.7 U/10^{12} RBC	×10^{-3}	0.44 ± 0.06 nU/RBC
		5.10 ± 0.68 U/mL RBC	×1	5.10 ± 0.68 kU/L RBC
		Low substrate system to detect genetic variants: 14.9 ± 3.71% of above values.		
		Low substrate + FDP: 43.5 ± 2.46% of values of full substrate system.		
Quinidine	Serum, plasma (heparin, EDTA); collect at trough conc.	Therap. conc.: 2–5 μg/mL	×3.083	6.2–15.5 μmol/L
		Toxic conc.: >6		>18.5
RBC Count, see *Erythrocyte Count*				
RBC Fragility, see *Osmotic Fragility*				

Table 29-2 REFERENCE RANGES (Continued)

Test	Specimen	Reference Range	Factor	Reference Range International Units
Red Cell Volume	Whole blood (heparin)	M: 20–36 mL/kg F: 19–31	×.001	M: 0.020–0.036 L/kg F: 0.019–0.031

Renin (Renin Activity, Plasma; PRA)	Plasma (EDTA)	*ng/mL/h*
		2–4 y: 2.37 ± 0.57 (1 SE)
		5–6 y: 1.48 ± 0.17
		7–9 y: 2.13 ± 0.44
		10–11 y: 1.96 ± 0.36
		14–15 y: 1.18 ± 0.28
		16–17 y: 1.08 ± 0.25
		Normal sodium diet:
		Supine: 1.6 ± 1.5
		Standing
		  (4 h): 4.5 ± 2.9
		Low sodium:
		Supine: 3.2 ± 1.1
		Standing
		  (4 h): 9.9 ± 4.3
			×1	*µg/L/h*
				2.37 ± 0.57 (1 SE)
				1.48 ± 0.17
				2.13 ± 0.44
				1.96 ± 0.36
				1.18 ± 0.28
				1.08 ± 0.25
				
				1.6 ± 1.5
				
				4.5 ± 2.9
				
				3.2 ± 1.1
				
				9.9 ± 4.3

Reticulocyte Count	Whole blood (EDTA, heparin, or oxalate)	Adults: 0.5–1.5% of erythrocytes or 25,000–75,000/mm³ (µL)	×0.01 ×10⁶	0.005–0.015 (number fraction) 25,000–75,000 × 10⁶/L
	Capillary	*%* 1 d: 3.2 ± 1.4 (SD) 7 d: 0.5 ± 0.4 1–4 wk: 0.6 ± 0.3 5–6 wk: 1.0 ± 0.7 7–8 wk: 1.5 ± 0.7 9–10 wk: 1.2 ± 0.7 11–12 wk: 0.7 ± 0.3	×0.01	*Number fraction* 0.032 ± 0.014 0.005 ± 0.004 0.006 ± 0.003 0.010 ± 0.007 0.015 ± 0.007 0.012 ± 0.007 0.007 ± 0.003
Reverse Triiodothyronine (rT₃)	Serum	*ng/dL* 1–5 y: 15–71 5–10 y: 17–79 10–15 y: 19–88 Adults: 30–80	×0.0154	*nmol/L* 0.23–1.1 0.26–1.2 0.29–1.36 0.46–1.23
Riboflavin (Vitamin B₂)	Urine, random, fasting	*µg/g creatinine* 1–3 y: 500–900 4–6 y: 300–600 7–9 y: 270–500 10–15 y: 200–400 Adult: 80–269	×0.3	*µmol/mol creatinine* 150–270 90–180 81–150 60–120 24–81
Salicylates	Serum, plasma (heparin, EDTA); collect at trough conc.	Therap. conc.: 15–30 mg/dL Toxic conc.: >30	×0.0724	1.1–2.2 mmol/L >2.2
Sediment *Casts*	Urine, fresh random	Hyaline: occasional (0–1) casts/hpf RBC: not seen WBC: not seen Tubular epithelial: not seen Transitional and squamous epithelial: not seen		Hyaline: occasional (0–1) casts/hpf RBC: not seen WBC: not seen Tubular epithelial: not seen Transitional and squamous epithelial: not seen
Cells		RBC: 0–2/hpf WBC, Males: 0–3/hpf Females and children: 0–5/hpf Epithelial: few; more frequent in newborn Bacteria, unspun: no organisms/oil immersion field spun: <20 organisms/hpf		RBC: 0–2/hpf WBC, Males: 0–3/hpf Females and children: 0–5/hpf Epithelial: few; more frequent in newborn Bacteria, unspun: no organisms/oil immersion field spun: <20 organisms/hpf
Sedimentation Rate, see *Erythrocyte Sedimentation Rate*				
Sickle Cell Tests *Sodium Metabisulfite*	Whole blood (EDTA, heparin, or oxalate)	Negative		
Dithionite Test	Whole blood (EDTA, heparin, or oxalate)	Negative		

Table 29–2 REFERENCE RANGES (Continued)

Test	Specimen	Reference Range	Factor	Reference Range International Units

Sodium — Serum or plasma (heparin)

	mmol/L		mmol/L
Newborn:	134–146	×1	134–146
Infant:	139–146		139–146
Child:	138–145		138–145
Thereafter:	136–146		136–146

Urine, 24 h

	40–220		40–220
	(diet dependent)		

Sweat

	10–40		10–40
Cystic fibrosis >70			>70

Somatomedin C — Plasma (EDTA)

Vary with laboratory, e.g., Nichols Institute

	U/mL			U/L	
	M	F	×1000	M	F
0–2 y:	0.10–0.72	0.10–1.7		100–720	100–1700
3–5 y:	0.12–1.5	0.15–2.3		120–1500	150–2300
6–10 y:	0.19–2.2	0.44–3.6		190–2200	440–3600
11–12 y:	0.22–3.6	1.50–6.9		220–3600	150–6900
13–14 y:	0.79–5.5	0.81–7.4		790–5500	810–7400
15–17 y:	0.76–3.3	0.59–3.1		760–3300	590–3100
18–64 y:	0.34–1.9	0.45–2.2		340–1900	450–2200

Endocrine Sciences

Cord:	0.25–0.66	250–660
0–1 y:	0.17–0.62	170–620
1–5 y:	0.14–0.94	140–940
6–12 y:	0.87–2.06	870–2060
13–17 y:	1.35–3.00	1350–3000
18–25 y:	0.92–2.06	920–2060
Thereafter:	0.70–2.04	700–2040

Specific Gravity — Urine, random

Adult: 1.002–1.030
After 12 h fluid restriction: >1.025

Adult: 1.002–1.030
After 12 h fluid restriction: >1.025

Urine, 24 h

1.015–1.025

Sucrose Hemolysis and Sugar-Water Tests for Paroxysmal Nocturnal Hemoglobinuria (PNH) — Whole blood (citrate or oxalate)

≤5% lysis	×0.01	Lysed fraction: ≤0.05
Questionable: 6–10% lysis		0.06–0.10

T₃, see Triiodothyronine

T₄, see Thyroxine

Testosterone, Free — Serum

	ng/dL (mean ± 1SE)	% of total		pmol/L (mean ± 1SD)	Fraction of total
Cord,			×34.67		
M:	1.0 ± 0.4	2.9 ± 0.6		34.6 ± 14	0.029 ± 0.006
F:	0.89 ± 0.29	3.0 ± 0.5		31 ± 10	0.03 ± 0.005
1–15 d,					
M:	0.8 ± 0.8	1.3 ± 0.2		28 ± 28	0.013 ± 0.002
F:	0.14 ± 0.06	1.2 ± 0.2		4.9 ± 2	0.012 ± 0.002
Prepubertal,					
M:	0.04 ± 0.01	0.7 ± 0.2		1.4 ± 0.35	0.007 ± 0.002
F:	0.04 ± 0.01	0.7 ± 0.1		1.4 ± 0.35	0.007 ± 0.001
Adult,					
M:	7.9 ± 2.3	1.4 ± 0.3		274 ± 80	0.014 ± 0.003
F:	0.31 ± 0.07	0.9 ± 0.2		11 ± 2	0.009 ± 0.002

Testosterone, Total — Serum

	ng/dL		nmol/L
Prepubertal,		×0.03467	
M:	6.6 ± 2.5		0.23 ± 0.09
F:	6.6 ± 2.5		0.23 ± 0.09
Adult,			
M:	572 ± 135		19.8 ± 4.7
F:	37 ± 10		1.3 ± 0.3

Theophylline — Serum, plasma (heparin, EDTA)

	μg/mL		μmol/L
Therap. conc.,			
Bronchodilator:	8–20	×5.550	44–110
Prem. apnea:	6–13		33–72
Toxic. conc.:	>20		>110

Thiamin (Vitamin B₁) — Serum

0–2.0 μg/dL	×37.68	0.0–75.4 nmol/L

Urine, acidify with HCl

	μg/g creatinine		μmol/mol
1–3 y:	176–200	×0.426	75–85
4–6 y:	121–400		52–170
7–9 y:	181–350		77–149
10–12 y:	181–300		77–128
13–15 y:	151–250		64–107
Thereafter:	66–129		28–55

Table 29–2 REFERENCE RANGES (Continued)

Test	Specimen	Reference Range	Factor	Reference Range International Units
Thrombin Time	Whole blood (Na citrate)	Control time ± 2 s when control is 9–13 s		Control time ± 2 s when control is 9–13 s
Thromboplastin Time, Activated, see *Activated Partial Thromboplastin Time (APTT)*				
Thyroglobulin (Tg)	Serum	<50 ng/mL	× 1	<50 µg/L
Thyroid Microsomal Antibodies	Serum	Nondetectable (hemagglutination) or <1:10 (IFA)		Nondetectable (hemagglutination) or <1:10 (IFA)
Thyroid Thyroglobulin Antibodies	Serum			
Tanned RBC agglutination test		Children: ≤1:4 dilution Thereafter: ≤1:10		≤1:4 dilution ≤1:10
Thyroid Stimulating Hormone (hTSH)	Serum or plasma (heparin)	*µU/L* Cord:　3–12 Newborn:　3–18 Thereafter:　2–10	× 1	*mU/L* 3–12 3–18 2–10
Thyroid Uptake of Radioactive Iodine	Activity over thyroid gland	2 h:　lt6% 6 h:　3–20% 24 h: 8–30%	× 0.01	2 h:　<0.06 6 h:　0.03–0.20 24 h: 0.08–0.30
Thyroid Uptake of ^{99m}TcO$_4^-$	Activity over thyroid gland	After 24 h: 0.4–3.0%	× 0.01	Fractional uptake: 0.004–0.03
Thyrotropin Releasing Hormone (hTRH)	Plasma	5–60 pg/mL	× 2.759	14–165 pmol/L

Thyroxine Binding Globulin (TBG)	Serum		*mg/dL*				*mg/L*	
			(Mean)	(Range)			(Mean)	(Range)
		Cord:		1.4–9.4	× 10			14–94
		1–4 wk:		1.0–9.0				10–90
		1–12 mo:		2.0–7.6				20–76
		1 y:	4.4				44	
		1–5 y:	4.2	2.9–5.4			42	29–54
		5–10 y:	3.8	2.5–5.0			38	25–50
		10–15 y:	3.3	2.1–4.6			33	21–46
		Adult:		1.5–3.4				15–34

Thyroxine, Free (FT$_4$)	Serum	0.8–2.4 ng/dL	× 12.87	10–31 pmol/L

Thyroxine, Total (T$_4$)	Serum		*µg/dL*		*nmol/L*
		Cord:	8–13	× 12.87	103–168
		Newborn:	11.5–24		148–310
		(lower in low birth weight infants)			
		Neonate:	9–18		116–232
		Infant:	7–15		90–194
		1–5 y:	7.3–15		94–194
		5–10 y:	6.4–13.3		83–172
		Thereafter:	5–12		65–155
		Newborn screen (filter paper):	6.2–22		80–284

Tourniquet Test (Capillary Fragility)		<5–10 petechiae in 2.5 cm circle on forearm (halfway between systolic and diastolic pressure for 5 min); 0–8 petechiae in 6 cm circle (50 torr for 15 min); 10–20 petechiae in 5 cm circle (80 mm Hg)		<5–10 petechiae in 2.5 cm circle on forearm (halfway between systolic and diastolic pressure for 5 min); 0–8 petechiae in 6 cm circle (50 torr for 15 min); 10–20 petechiae in 5 cm circle (80 mm Hg)

Transcortin	Serum		*mg/dL*		*mg/L*
		M:	1.5–2.0	× 10	15–20
		F, Follicular:	1.7–2.0		17–20
		Luteal:	1.6–2.1		16–21
		Postmenopausal:	1.7–2.5		17–25
		Pregnancy,			
		21–28 wk:	4.7–5.4		47–54
		33–40 wk:	5.5–7.0		55–70

Transferrin	Serum	Newborn: 130–275 mg/dL Adult:　200–400	× 0.01	1.3–2.7 g/L 2.0–4.0

Table 29–2 REFERENCE RANGES (Continued)

TEST	SPECIMEN	REFERENCE RANGE			FACTOR	REFERENCE RANGE INTERNATIONAL UNITS	
Triglycerides (TG)	Serum, after ≥12 h fast		mg/dL				g/L
			M	F	×0.01	M	F
		Cord blood:	10–98	10–98		0.10–0.98	0.10–0.98
		0–5 y:	30–86	32–99		0.30–0.86	0.32–0.99
		6–11 y:	31–108	35–114		0.31–1.08	0.35–1.14
		12–15 y:	36–138	41–138		0.36–1.38	0.41–1.38
		16–19 y:	40–163	40–128		0.40–1.63	0.40–1.28
		20–29 y:	44–185	40–128		0.44–1.85	0.40–1.28
		Recommended (desirable) levels for adults:				*Recommended* (desirable) levels for adults:	
		Male: 40–160 mg/dL				Male: 0.40–1.60 g/L	
		Female: 35–135				Female: 0.35–1.35	
Triiodothyronine, Free	Serum		*mean pg/dL*			*mean pmol/L*	
		Cord:	130 ± 10(SE)		×0.01536	2.0 ± 0.15(SE)	
		1–3 d:	410 ± 20			6.3 ± 0.3	
		6 wk:	400 ± 20			6.1 ± 0.3	
		Adults (20–50 y):	230–660 pg/dL			3.5–10 pmol/L	
Triiodothyronine Resin Uptake Test (T₃RU)	Serum					Fractional uptake:	
		Newborn: 26–36%			×0.01	0.26–0.36	
		Thereafter: 26–35%				0.26–0.35	
Triiodothyronine, Total (T₃-RIA)	Serum		*ng/dL*			*nmol/L*	
		Cord:	30–70		×0.0154	0.46–1.08	
		Newborn:	75–260			1.16–4.00	
		1–5 y:	100–260			1.54–4.00	
		5–10 y:	90–240			1.39–3.70	
		10–15 y:	80–210			1.23–3.23	
		Thereafter:	115–190			1.77–2.93	
Tyrosine	Serum		*mg/dL*			*mmol/L*	
		Premature:	7.0–24.0		×0.0552	0.39–1.32	
		Newborn:	1.6–3.7			0.088–0.20	
		Adult:	0.8–1.3			0.044–0.07	
Urea Nitrogen	Serum or plasma		*mg/dL*			*mmol urea/L*	
		Cord:	21–40		×0.357	7.5–14.3	
		Premature (1 wk):	3–25			1.1–9	
		Newborn:	3–12			1.1–4.3	
		Infant/Child:	5–18			1.8–6.4	
		Thereafter:	7–18			2.5–6.4	
Uric Acid	Serum		*mg/dL*			*μmol/L*	
Phosphotungstate		Newborn:	2.0–6.2		×59.48	119–369	
		Adult, M:	4.5–8.2			268–488	
		F:	3.0–6.5			178–387	
Uricase		Child:	2.0–5.5			119–327	
		Adults, M:	3.5–7.2			208–428	
		F:	2.6–6.0			155–357	
Urinary Sediment, see *Sediment*							
Urine Volume	Urine, 24 h		*mL/d*			*L/d*	
		Newborn:	50–300		×0.001	0.050–0.300	
		Infant:	350–550			0.350–0.500	
		Child:	500–1000			0.500–1.000	
		Adolescent:	700–1400			0.700–1.400	
		Thereafter, M:	800–1800			0.800–1.800	
		F:	600–1600			0.600–1.600	
		(varies with intake and other factors)					
Valproic Acid	Serum, plasma (heparin, EDTA); collect at trough conc.	Therap. conc.: 50–100 μg/mL			×6.934	350–700 μmol/L	
		Toxic conc.: >100				>700	
Vanillylmandelic Acid (Vanilmandelic Acid)	Urine, 24 h		*mg/d*			*μmol/d*	
		Newborn:	<1.0		×5.046	<5.0	
		Infant:	<2.0			<10.1	
		Child:	1–3			5–15	
		Adolescent:	1–5			5–25	
		Thereafter:	2–7			10–35	
		or: 1.5–7 μg/mg creatinine			×0.571	or: 0.86–4 mmol/mol creatinine	
Vitamin A	Serum		*μg/dL*			*μmol/L*	
		Newborn:	35–75		×0.0349	1.22–2.62	
		Child:	30–80			1.05–2.79	
		Thereafter:	30–65			1.05–2.27	
Vitamin B₁, see *Thiamin*							

Table 29–2 REFERENCE RANGES (Continued)

TEST	SPECIMEN	REFERENCE RANGE	FACTOR	REFERENCE RANGE INTERNATIONAL UNITS
Vitamin B$_2$, see *Riboflavin*				
Vitamin B$_6$	Plasma (EDTA)	3.6–18 ng/mL	× 4.046	14.6–72.8 nmol/L
Vitamin B$_{12}$	Serum	Newborn: 175–800 pg/ml Thereafter: 140–700	× 0.738	129–590 pmol/L 103–517
Vitamin C	Plasma (oxalate, heparin, or EDTA)	0.6–2.0 mg/dL	× 56.78	34–113 µmol/L
Vitamin D$_2$, 25-Hydroxy	Plasma (heparin)	Summer: 15–80 ng/mL Winter: 14–42	× 2.496	37–200 nmol/L 35–105
Vitamin D$_3$, 1,25-Dihydroxy (Calcitriol)	Serum	25–45 pg/mL	× 2.4	60–108 nmol/L
Vitamin E	Serum	5.0–20 µg/mL	× 2.32	11.6–46.4 µmol/L
WBC, see *Leukocyte*				
Xylose Absorption Test	Whole blood (Na-fluoride) 0.5 g/kg in H$_2$O: 25 g:	*mg/dL* Child, 1h: >20 Adult, 2h: >25	× 0.0667	*mmol/L* >1.33 >1.67
	Urine, 5 h	Child: 16–33% of ingested dose	× 0.01	Fraction ingested dose: 0.16–0.33
		Adult, *g/5 h* 5 g dose: >1.2 25 g dose: >4.0	× 6.66	*mmol/5 h* >8.00 >26.64
Zinc	Serum	70–150 µg/dL	× 0.153	10.7–22.9 µmol/L
	Hair	216 ± 87 µg/g (1 SD)	× 0.0153	3.30 ± 1.33 µmol/g (1 SD)

MILLIOSMOLAL AND MILLIOSMOLAR SOLUTIONS

The total osmotic pressure of a solution is dependent on the number of particles in the solution, regardless of their charge, size, or shape. In principle, 1 mole of an ideal substance (assumed to be a nonelectrolyte) dissolved in a kilogram of water will lower the freezing point of the solvent (water) by 1.8557°C. Such a solution would have 1 osmole *per kilogram of water.* One milliosmole is equal to one thousandth of an osmole. The osmometer used in the clinical laboratory measures the osmolality of serum, urine, or other biological fluids by comparing their freezing points with that of a carefully prepared sodium chloride solution of known osmotic pressure. The lowering of the freezing point is proportional to the mole fraction (gram-mole of solute *per kg of solvent*), and gives the millio*smolal* concentration, which is slightly different from the millio*smolar* concentration; the latter represents milliosmoles of solute *per liter of solution.* For dilute solutions these 2 values approach each other and are often used without distinction. Osmo*lality* is the preferred term, because that is what is measured by the osmometer.

In studying osmotic pressure relations in solutions containing electrolytes it is useful to express the osmotic activity in terms of ionic concentrations. The term "milliosmolar" supplements the term "millimolar" in appreciation of the additive osmotic effect of the particles formed by ionization.

For example: A millimolar solution of glucose (180 mg/l) is also a milliosmolar solution (1 milliosmole/l), because the number of osmotically active particles is not increased in solution through ionization. On the other hand, owing to the nearly complete ionization of sodium chloride in solution, a millimolar solution of sodium chloride (58.5 mg/liter) contains 1 milliequivalent of sodium ions and 1 milliequivalent of chloride ions. The milliosmolar concentration is 2 milliosmoles per liter, because 1 chemical milliequivalent of sodium or of chloride ions is equal to 1 milliosmole of sodium or of chloride ions, respectively.

A milliequivalent equals a milliosmole for all univalent ions. The chemical milliequivalence of a divalent ion is twice the milliosmolar value. In a millimolar solution of calcium chloride (CaCl$_2$), for example, there are 2 chemical milliequivalents of calcium ions, but only 1 milliosmole of calcium ions.* The millimolar solution of calcium chloride contains 2 chemical milliequivalents of chloride ions or 2 milliosmoles of chloride ions per liter. Accordingly, a millimolar solution of calcium chloride contains 3 milliosmoles per liter, because this salt ionizes into 1 calcium ion and 2 chloride ions. In blood serum containing 10 mg of calcium per dl (100 ml), there are 5 chemical milliequivalents of calcium* per liter, but only 2.5 milliosmoles of calcium per liter.

The average normal total ionic concentration of blood serum is 290 milliosmoles per *kg* H$_2$O, to which cations contribute 151 milliosmoles and anions 139. In blood plasma the milliosmoles accounted for by glucose or urea (3–6 mOsm/kg H$_2$O) or by protein (1.2–1.4 mOsm/kg H$_2$O) are small compared to the osmotic effect of the electrolytes. One milliosmole generates an osmotic pressure of about 19.3 mm Hg. The osmotic pressure of the blood serum of infants and children is comparable to that of adults.

VICTOR C. VAUGHAN III

---

*Calcium has an atomic weight of 40; a millimolar solution has 40 mg/l (4 mg/dl). (See also Table 29–3.)

CONVERSION TABLES

Table 29-3 METHOD FOR CONVERSION OF MILLIGRAMS TO MILLIEQUIVALENTS PER LITER (or to Millimoles per Liter)

mg = milligrams
gm = grams

ml = milliliter
1 ml = 1.000027 cc
dl = deciliter = 100 ml

$$mEq/l \text{ (milliequivalents per liter)} = \frac{mg \text{ per liter}}{equivalent \text{ weight}}$$

$$Equivalent \text{ weight} = \frac{atomic \text{ weight}}{valence \text{ of element}}$$

For example: A sample of blood serum contains 10 mg of Ca in 1 dl (100 ml). The valence of Ca is 2, and the atomic weight is 40. The equivalent weight of Ca is therefore 40 ÷ 2, or 20. The milliequivalents of Ca per liter are 10 (mg/dl) × 10 (dl/l) ÷ 20, or 5 milliequivalents per liter.

$$mM/l \text{ (millimoles per liter)} = \frac{mg/liter}{molecular \text{ weight}}$$

Vol. % (volumes per cent) = mM/liter × 2.24 for a gas whose properties approach that of an ideal gas, such as oxygen or nitrogen. For carbon dioxide the factor is 2.226.

Table 29-4 FACTORS FOR CONVERSION OF CONCENTRATION EXPRESSED IN MILLIEQUIVALENTS PER LITER TO MILLIGRAMS PER DECILITER (100 ml), AND VICE VERSA, FOR COMMON IONS THAT OCCUR IN PHYSIOLOGIC SOLUTIONS

ELEMENT OR RADICAL	MEQ/L	TO MG/DL	MG/DL	TO MEQ/L
Sodium	1	2.30	1	0.4348
Potassium	1	3.91	1	0.2558
Calcium	1	2.005	1	0.4988
Magnesium	1	1.215	1	0.8230
Chloride	1	3.55	1	0.2817
Bicarbonate (HCO_3)	1	6.1	1	0.1639
Phosphorus valence 1	1	3.10	1	0.3226
Phosphorus valence 1.8	1	1.72	1	0.5814
Sulfur valence 2	1	1.60	1	0.625

Example: To convert milliequivalents of magnesium per liter to milligrams per deciliter (100 ml), multiply by the factor 1.215.

To convert milligrams of potassium per deciliter (100 ml) to milliequivalents per liter, multiply by the factor 0.2558.

Table 29-5 MILLIEQUIVALENTS AND MILLIGRAMS OF CATIONS AND ANIONS PRESENT IN A MILLIMOLE OF SALTS COMMONLY USED IN PHYSIOLOGIC SOLUTIONS

SALT	mM/L	MG/L	CATION	ANION	MEQ/L	MG/L	MEQ/L	MG/L
Sodium chloride (NaCl)	1	58.5	Na^+	Cl^-	1	23.0	1	35.5
Potassium chloride (KCl)	1	74.6	K^+	Cl^-	1	39.1	1	35.5
Sodium bicarbonate ($NaHCO_3$)	1	84.0	Na^+	HCO_3^-	1	23.0	1	61.0
Sodium lactate ($CH_3CHOHCOONa$)	1	112.0	Na^+	Lactate⁻	1	23.0	1	89.0
Potassium phosphate (K_2HPO_4) dibasic	1	174.2	K^+	HPO_4^{--}	2	78.2	1	96.0
Potassium phosphate (KH_2PO_4) monobasic	1	136.1	K^+	$H_2PO_4^-$	1	39.1	1	97.0
Calcium chloride anhydrous ($CaCl_2$)		111.0	Ca^{++}	Cl^-	2	40.0	2	71.0
Calcium chloride dihydrate ($CaCl_2.2H_2O$)	1	147.0	Ca^{++}	Cl^-	2	40.0	2	71.0
Magnesium chloride anhydrous ($MgCl_2$)	1	95.2	Mg^{++}	Cl^-	2	24.3	2	71.0
Magnesium chloride hexahydrate ($MgCl_2.6H_2O$)	1	203.3	Mg^{++}	Cl^-	2	24.3	2	71.0
Ammonium chloride (NH_4Cl)	1	53.5	NH_4^+	Cl^-	1	18.0	1	35.5

Table 29-6 CONVERSION OF APOTHECARY'S MEASURES TO METRIC EQUIVALENTS

1 grain = 64 mg
60 minims = 1 fl dram = 3.7 ml
1 ml = 16.23 minims

Table 29–7 EQUIVALENT TEMPERATURE READINGS (CENTIGRADE AND FAHRENHEIT)*

°C	°F	°C	°F	°C	°F	°C	°F
0	32.0	37.2	99	39.2	102.6	41.2	106.2
20	68.0	37.4	99.3	39.4	102.9	41.4	106.5
30	86.0	37.6	99.7	39.6	103.3	41.6	106.9
31	87.8	37.8	100.1	39.8	103.7	41.8	107.2
32	89.6	38.0	100.4	40.0	104	42	107.6
33	91.4	38.2	100.8	40.2	104.4	43	109.4
34	93.2	38.4	101.2	40.4	104.7	44	111.2
35	95.0	38.6	101.5	40.6	105.1	100	212
36	96.8	38.8	101.8	40.8	105.4		
37	98.6	39.0	102.2	41.0	105.8		

*To convert centigrade readings to Fahrenheit, multiply by 1.8 and add 32. To convert Fahrenheit readings to centigrade, subtract 32 and divide by 1.8.

Table 29–8 COMPOSITION OF COMMONLY USED ORAL AND PARENTERAL SOLUTIONS

Fluid	CHO gm/dl	Prot* gm/dl	Calories per l	Na (mEq/l)	K (mEq/l)	Cl (mEq/l)	HCO3† (mEq/l)	Ca (mEq/l)	P‡ (mEq/l)	Mg (mEq/l)	Osm§ (mOsm/kgH2O)
Oral											
Apple juice¶	11.9	0.1	480	0.4	26						700
Coca-Cola¶	10.9		435	4.3	0.1		13.4	3	4.5		656
Gatorade	5.9		250	21	2.5	17					377
Ginger ale¶	9.0		360	3.5	0.1		3.6		6.8		565
Grape juice¶	16.6	0.2	672	0.4	30		32				1027
Grapefruit juice¶ (canned, sugar added)	17.8	0.6	736	0.2	35			6.5			591
Hydra-lyte	24		100	84	10	59	15	<1	<1		300
Lytren	7.0		280	30	25	25	36	4	5	4	267**
Milk	4.9	3.5	670	22	36	28	30	60	54		260**
Orange juice¶	10.4	0.7	444	0.2	49		50				654
Pedialyte	5.0		200	30	20	30	28	4		4	387
Pepsi-Cola	12.0		480	6.5	0.8		7.3				—
Pineapple juice (canned)¶	13.5	0.4	556	0.2	38						783
Prune juice¶	19	0.4	776	0.9	60			7.5	9		—
Root beer¶				3.5	3.9			7	20		588
Seven-Up¶	8.0		320	7.5	0.2			0.3			564
Tomato juice (canned, salted)¶	4.3		172	100	59	150	10	3	18		592
Parenteral											
CHO†† in H2O	5–10		200–400								
Isotonic saline	0–5		0–200	154		154					266–532
½ Isotonic saline	2.5–5		100–200	77		77					292–558
3% (M/2) saline				513		513					280–415
5% Saline				855		855					969
2.14% Ammonium chloride						400					1616
M/6 Sodium lactate				167			167				
5% Sodium bicarbonate				595			595				
Lactated Ringer solution	0–5–10		0–200–400	130	4	109	28	3			
Modified Butler 1 (a)	5		200	25	20	22	23				261–531–801
Modified Butler 2 (b)	5–10		200–400	56	25	49	26		3	3	360
Talbot (c)	5		200	40	35	40	20		12	5	423–719**
Ordway (d)	3.5		140	26	27	53			15		409
Gastric replacement (e)	5–10		200–400	63	17	150	(contains 71 mEq/l NH4+)				281**
Intestinal replacement (f)	10		390	80	36	64	60	5		3	555–812**
Protein hydrolysate 5% (g)		5	850	35	19	20		5	30	2	800**
Protein hydrolysate 10% (h)		10	1700	60	31	44		10	60	4	430**
Amino-acid preparation (i)		8.5		10		44			60		860**
									20		850**
Human plasma protein fraction (j)		5		110	2	50	50				
Blood††		3		95	4	50	40		2	1–2	
Dextran 10% (low mol. wt.) (k)	5		200								
Dextran 10% in saline (l)				154		154					
Dextran 6% (high mol. wt.) (m)	5–10		200–400								
Dextran 6% in saline (n)				154		154					
Mannitol 20%§§											

Table 29–8 COMPOSITION OF COMMONLY USED ORAL AND PARENTERAL SOLUTIONS (Continued)

AVAILABLE ADDITIVES

Glucose 50%	0.5 gm per ml
Sodium chloride	0.5, 1, 2.5 and 5 mEq per ml
Sodium lactate	4 and 5 mEq per ml
Sodium bicarbonate	5 (4.2%) and 9 (7.5%) mEq per ml
Potassium chloride	1, 2 and 3 mEq per ml
Potassium phosphate	3 mEq per ml
Potassium acetate	2 and 2.5 mEq per ml
Calcium gluconate 10%	9.0 mg (.45 mEq) calcium per ml
Calcium chloride 10%	27.2 mg (1.36 mEq) calcium per ml
Ammonium chloride	4 mEq per ml
Magnesium sulfate (Mg SO₄ · 7 H₂O) 50% (also 10%, 12.5% and 25% available)	4 mEq per ml

SELECTED U.S. COMMERCIAL PREPARATIONS
(possible slight variations in composition from values in Table)

(A, Abbott; C, Cutter; M, McGaw; P, Pharmacia; T, Travenol)

(a) Ionosol MB in D5W (A); Isolyte P with 5% Dextrose (M)
(b) Ionosol B in D5W (A); Electrolyte #2 with 10% invert sugar (C,M); 10%-Travert in Electrolyte #2 (T)
(c) Ionosol T in D5W (A); Isolyte M (M)
(d) Ordway solution with 3.5% Dextrose (C)
(e) Ionosol G in D10W (A); Isolyte G with 5% Dextrose (M)
(f) Ionosol D with 10% Invert Sugar (A); 10% Travert with Electrolyte #1 (T)
(g) Amigen 5% (T)
(h) Amigen 10% (T)
(i) Free Amine 2 (M)
(j) Plasmatein (A); Plasmanate (C)
(k)(l) LMD 10% (A); Dextran 40 (C,M); Rheomacrodex (P); Gentran 40 (T)
(m)(n) Dextran 75 (A); Macrodex (P); Gentran 75 in 10% Travert (T)

*Protein or amino acid equivalent.
†Actual or potential bicarbonate, such as acetate, lactate, citrate.
‡Calculated according to valence of 1.8.
§Osmolality except for values shown ** which are osmolarity (in mOsm/l).
¶Composition varies slightly depending on source.
**See § above.
††Glucose (dextrose, fructose or invert sugar).
‡‡Red cell contents not included in calculations.
§§Also available: mannitol 5%, 10%, 15%, and 20%.
(Sources: Church CF, Church HN: Food Values of Portions Commonly Used (Bowes and Church). Ed 11. Philadelphia, JB Lippincott, 1970; Kastrup EK, Boyd JR: Facts and Comparisons. 1978. St. Louis, Facts and Comparisons, Inc., 1978; Murray BN, Peterson LJ: Unpublished observations. Additional values in Wendland BE, Arbus GS: Canad Med Ass J 121:564, 1979.)

FOOD VALUES

Table 29–9 FOOD COMPOSITION TABLE FOR SHORT METHOD OF DIETARY ANALYSIS

Food and Approximate Measure	Weight GM	Food Energy Cal	Protein GM	Fat GM	Carbohydrate GM	Calcium MG	Iron MG	Vitamin A Value IU	Thiamine MG	Riboflavin MG	Niacin MG	Ascorbic Acid MG
Milk, cheese, cream; related products												
Cheese: blue, cheddar (1 cu in, 17 gm), cheddar process (1 oz). Swiss (1 oz)	30	105	6	9	1	165	0.2	345	0.01	0.12	Trace	0
cottage (from skim) creamed (½c)	115	120	16	5	3	105	0.4	190	0.04	0.28	0.1	0
Cream: half-and-half (cream and milk) (2 tbsp)	30	40	1	4	2	30	Trace	145	0.01	0.04	Trace	Trace
For light whipping add 1 pat butter												
Milk: whole (3.5% fat) (1 c)	245	160	9	9	12	285	0.1	350	0.08	0.42	0.1	2
fluid, nonfat (skim) and buttermilk (from skim)	245	90	9	Trace	13	300	Trace	—	0.10	0.44	0.2	2
milk beverage (1 c): cocoa, chocolate drink made with skim milk. For malted milk add 4 tbsp half-and-half (270 gm)	245	210	8	8	26	280	0.6	300	0.09	0.43	0.3	Trace
milk desserts, custard (1 c) 248 gm, ice cream (8 fl oz) 142 gm		290	8	17	29	210	0.4	785	0.07	0.34	0.1	1
cornstarch pudding (248 gm), ice milk (1 c) 187 gm		280	9	10	40	290	0.1	390	0.08	0.41	0.3	2
White sauce, med (½c)	130	215	5	16	12	150	0.2	610	0.06	0.22	0.3	Trace
Egg: 1 large	50	80	6	6	Trace	25	1.2	590	0.06	0.15	Trace	0
Meat, poultry, fish, shellfish, related products												
Beef, lamb, veal: lean and fat, cooked, inc. corned beef (3 oz) (all cuts)	85	245	22	16	0	10	2.9	25	0.06	0.19	4.2	0
lean only, cooked; dried beef (2+ oz) (all cuts)	65	140	20	5	0	10	2.4	10	0.05	0.16	3.4	0
Beef, relatively fat, such as steak and rib, cooked (3 oz)	85	350	18	30	0	10	2.4	60	0.05	0.14	3.5	0
Liver: beef, fried (2 oz)	55	130	15	6	3	5	5.0	30,280	0.15	2.37	9.4	15
Pork, lean and fat, cooked (3 oz) (all cuts)	85	325	20	24	0	10	2.6	0	0.62	0.20	4.2	0
lean only, cooked (2+ oz) (all cuts)	60	150	18	8	0	5	2.2	0	0.57	0.19	3.2	0
ham, light cure, lean and fat, roasted (3 oz)	85	245	18	19	0	10	2.2	0	0.40	0.16	3.1	0

Table 29–9   FOOD COMPOSITION TABLE FOR SHORT METHOD OF DIETARY ANALYSIS *(Continued)*

FOOD AND APPROXIMATE MEASURE	WEIGHT GM	FOOD ENERGY CAL	PROTEIN GM	FAT GM	CARBOHYDRATE GM	CALCIUM MG	IRON MG	VITAMIN A VALUE IU	THIAMINE MG	RIBOFLAVIN MG	NIACIN MG	ASCORBIC ACID MG
Luncheon meats: bologna (2 sl), pork sausage, cooked (2 oz), frankfurter (1), bacon, broiled or fried crisp (3 sl)	185		9	16	—	5	1.3	—	0.21	0.12	1.7	0
Poultry												
chicken: flesh only, broiled (3 oz)	85	115	20	3	0	10	1.4	80	0.05	0.16	7.4	0
fried (2 + oz)	75	170	24	6	1	10	1.6	85	0.05	0.23	8.3	0
turkey, light and dark, roasted (3 oz)	85	160	27	5	0	—	1.5	—	0.03	0.15	6.5	0
Fish and shellfish												
salmon (3 oz) (canned)	85	130	17	5	0	165	0.7	60	0.03	0.16	6.8	0
fish sticks, breaded, cooked (3-4)	75	130	13	7	5	10	0.3	—	0.03	0.05	1.2	0
mackerel, halibut, cooked	85	175	19	10	0	10	0.8	515	0.08	0.15	6.8	0
bluefish, haddock, herring, perch, shad, cooked (tuna canned in oil, 20 gm)	85	160	19	8	2	20	1.0	60	0.06	0.11	4.4	0
clams, canned; crab meat, canned; lobster; oyster, raw; scallop; shrimp, canned	85	75	14	1	2	65	2.5	65	0.10	0.08	1.5	0
Mature dry beans and peas, nuts, peanuts, related products												
Beans: white with pork and tomato, canned (1 c)	260	320	16	7	50	140	4.7	340	0.20	0.08	1.5	5
red (128 gm). Lima (96 gm), cowpeas (125 gm), cooked (½ c)	125		8	—	25	35	2.5	5	0.13	0.06	0.7	—
Nuts: almonds (12), cashews (8), peanuts (1 tbsp), peanut butter (1 tbsp), pecans (12), English walnuts (2 tbsp), coconut (¼ c)	15	95	3	8	4	15	0.5	5	0.05	0.04	0.9	—
Vegetables and vegetable products												
Asparagus, cooked, cut spears (⅔ c)	115	25	3	Trace	4	25	0.7	1055	0.19	0.20	1.6	30
Beans: green (¼ c) cooked 60 gm; canned 120 gm.		15	1	Trace	3	30	0.4	340	0.04	0.06	0.3	8
Lima, immature, cooked (½ c)	80	90	6	1	16	40	2.0	225	0.14	0.08	1.0	14
Broccoli spears, cooked (⅔ c)	100	25	3	Trace	4	90	0.8	2500	0.09	0.20	0.8	90
Brussels sprouts, cooked (⅔ c)	85	30	3	Trace	5	30	1.0	450	0.07	0.12	0.7	75
Cabbage (110 gm); cauliflower, cooked (80 gm); and sauerkraut, canned (150 mg) (reduced ascorbic acid value by one third for kraut) (⅔ c)		20	1	Trace	4	35	0.5	80	0.05	0.05	0.3	37
Carrots, cooked (⅔ c)	95	30	1	Trace	7	30	0.6	10,145	0.05	0.05	0.5	6
Corn, 1 ear, cooked (140 gm); canned (130 gm) (½ c)		75	2	Trace	18	5	0.4	315	0.06	0.06	1.1	6
Leafy greens: collards (125 gm), dandelions (120 gm), kale (75 gm), mustard (95 gm), spinach (120 gm), turnip (100 gm cooked, 150 gm canned) (⅔ c cooked and canned) (reduce ascorbic acid one half for canned)		30	3	Trace	5	175	1.8	8570	0.11	0.18	0.8	45
Peas, green (½ c)	80	60	4	1	10	20	1.4	430	0.22	0.09	1.8	16
Potatoes, baked, boiled (100 gm), 10 pc. French fried (55 gm) (for fried, add 1 tbsp cooking oil)		85	3	Trace	30	10	0.7	Trace	0.08	0.04	1.5	16
Pumpkin, canned (½ c)	115	40	1	1	9	30	0.5	7295	0.03	0.06	0.6	6
Squash, winter, canned (½ c)	100	65	2	1	16	30	0.8	4305	0.05	0.14	0.7	14
Sweet potato, canned (½ c)	110	120	2	—	27	25	0.8	8500	0.05	0.05	0.7	15
Tomato, 1 raw, ⅔ c canned, ⅔ c juice	150	35	2	Trace	7	14	0.8	1350	0.10	0.06	1.0	29
Tomato catsup (2 tbsp)	35	30	1	Trace	8	10	0.2	480	0.04	0.02	0.6	6
Other, cooked (beets, mushrooms, onions, turnips) (½ c)	95	25	1	—	5	20	0.5	15	0.02	0.10	0.7	7
Other commonly served raw, cabbage (½ c, 50 gm), celery (3 sm stalks, 40 gm), cucumber (¼ med, 50 gm), green pepper (½, 30 gm), radishes (5, 40 gm)		10	Trace	Trace	2	15	0.3	100	0.03	0.03	0.2	20
carrots, raw (½ carrot)	25	10	Trace	Trace	2	10	0.2	2750	0.02	0.02	0.2	2
lettuce leaves (2 lg)	50	10	1	Trace	2	34	0.7	950	0.03	0.04	0.2	9
Fruits and fruit products												
Cantaloupe (½ med)	385	60	1	Trace	14	25	0.8	6540	0.08	0.06	1.2	63
Citrus and strawberries: orange (1), grapefruit (½), juice (½ c), strawberries (½ c), lemon (1), tangerine (1)	50		1	—	13	25	0.4	165	0.08	0.03	0.3	55
Yellow, fresh: apricots (3), peach (2 med); canned fruit and juice (½ c) or dried, cooked, unsweetened: apricot, peaches (½ c)	85		—	—	22	10	1.1	1005	0.01	0.05	1.0	5
Other, dried: dates, pitted (4), figs (2), raisins (¼ c)	40	120	1	—	31	35	1.4	20	0.04	0.04	0.5	—
Other, fresh: apple (1), banana (1), figs (3), pear (#)	80		—	—	21	15	0.5	140	0.04	0.03	0.2	6
Fruit pie: to 1 serving fruit add 1 tbsp flour, 2 tbsp sugar, 1 tbsp fat												

Table 29–9 FOOD COMPOSITION TABLE FOR SHORT METHOD OF DIETARY ANALYSIS (Continued)

Food and Approximate Measure	Weight GM	Food Energy Cal	Protein GM	Fat GM	Carbohydrate GM	Calcium MG	Iron MG	Vitamin A Value IU	Thiamine MG	Riboflavin MG	Niacin MG	Ascorbic Acid MG
Grain products												
Enriched and whole grain: bread (1 sl, 23 gm), biscuit (½), cooked cereals (½ c), prepared cereals (1 oz) Graham crackers (2 lg), macaroni, noodles, spaghetti (½ c, cooked), pancake (1, 27 gm), roll (½), waffle (½, 38 gm)	65		2	1	16	20	0.6	10	0.09	0.05	0.7	—
Unenriched: bread (1 sl, 23 gm), cooked cereal (½ c), macaroni, noodles, spaghetti (½ c), popcorn (½ c), pretzel sticks, small (15), roll (½)	65		2	1	16	10	0.3	5	0.02	0.02	0.3	—
Desserts												
Cake, plain (1 pc), doughnut (1). For iced cake or doughnut add value for sugar (1 tbsp). For chocolate cake add chocolate (30 gm)	45	145	2	5	24	30	0.4	65	0.02	0.05	0.2	—
Cookies, plain (1)	25	120	1	5	18	10	0.2	20	0.01	0.01	0.1	—
Pie crust, single crust (½ shell)	20	95	1	6	8	3	0.3	0	0.04	0.03	0.3	—
Flour, white, enriched (1 tbsp)	7	25	1	Trace	5	1	0.2	0	0.03	0.02	0.2	0
Fats and oils												
Butter, margarine (1 pat, ½ tbsp)	7	50	Trace	6	Trace	1	0	230	—	—	—	—
Fats and oils, cooking (1 tbsp). French dressing (2 tbsp)	14	125	0	14	0	0	0	0	0	0	0	0
Salad dressings, mayonnaise type (1 tbsp)	15	80	Trace	9	1	2	0.1	45	Trace	Trace	Trace	0
Sugars, sweets												
Candy, plain (½ oz), jam and jelly (1 tbsp), syrup (1 tbsp), gelatin dessert, plain (½ c), beverages, carbonated (1 c)	60		0	0	14	3	0.1	Trace	Trace	Trace	Trace	Trace
Chocolate fudge (1 oz), chocolate syrup (3 tbsp)		125	1	2	30	15	0.6	10	Trace	0.02	0.1	Trace
Molasses (1 tbsp), caramel (½ oz)		40	Trace	Trace	8	20	0.3	Trace	Trace	Trace	Trace	0
Sugar (1 tbsp)	12	45	0	0	12	0	Trace	0	0	0	0	0
Miscellaneous												
Chocolate, bitter (1 oz)	30	145	3	15	8	20	1.9	20	0.01	0.07	0.4	0
Sherbet (½ c)	96	130	1	1	30	15	Trace	55	0.01	0.03	Trace	2
Soups: bean, pea (green) (1 c)		150	7	4	22	50	1.6	495	0.09	0.06	1.0	4
noodle, beef, chicken (1 c)		65	4	2	7	10	0.7	50	0.03	0.04	0.9	Trace
clam chowder, minestrone, tomato, vegetable (1 c)		90	3	2	14	25	0.9	1880	0.05	0.04	1.1	3

From Wilson ED, Fisher KH, Fuqua ME: Principles of Nutrition. Ed 2. New York, John Wiley & Sons, 1965, pp 528–33.

Table 29–10 NUTRITIVE VALUE OF BABY FOODS (PER SERVING)

FOOD	SERVING	ENERGY CALORIES	PROTEIN GM	FAT GM	CARBOHYDRATE GM	SODIUM MG	CALCIUM MG	IRON MG	VITAMIN A VALUE IU	THIAMIN MG	RIBOFLAVIN MG	NIACIN MG	ASCORBIC ACID MG
Cereals, precooked, dry and other products													
Barley, added nutrients	15 gm	50	1	0	10	5	95	7	(0)	0.2	0.3	2	0
High protein, added nutrients	15 gm	50	5	1	6	3	95	7	—	0.2	0.3	24.0	0
Mixed, added nutrients	15 gm	40	2	0	9	4	95	7	—	0.2	0.3	22.3	0
Oatmeal, added nutrients	15 gm	50	2	1	9	5	95	7	(0)	0.2	0.3	21.3	0
Rice, added nutrients	15 gm	40	1	0	9	4	95	7	(0)	0.2	0.3	19.7	0
Dinners, canned: cereal, vegetable, meat mixtures (approx. 2–4% protein)													
Beef with vegetables	128	110	7	5	9	40	10	0.7	600	0.04	0.05	2	2
Chicken with vegetables	128	130	8	7	8	35	95	0.8	2200	0.03	0.05	1.5	2
Cottage cheese with pineapple	135	150	8	2	26	200	96	0.3	0	0.05	6	0.4	3
Ham with vegetables	128	110	8	4	10	30	8	0.8	400	0.15	6	1.5	3
Turkey with vegetables	128	120	8	6	9	40	50	0.9	350	0.03	6	2	4
Veal with vegetables	128	90	8	3	9	35	8	1.0	100	0.04	7	2.5	3
Fruits and fruit products with or without thickening, canned													
Applesauce	128	50	0	0	14	2	5	0.1	40	0.01	0.02	0.1	15
Applesauce and apricots	128	80	0	1	18	5.5	5.7	0.1	288	0.01	0.04	0.2	1.5
Bananas (with tapioca or cornstarch added ascorbic acid), strained	128	80	1	0	16		13	0.1	50	0.02	0.02	0.2	15
Bananas and pineapple (with tapioca or cornstarch)	128	70	0	1	16	8.0	20	0.1	45	0.01	0.01	0.1	15
Peaches	128	70	1	1	14	5	6	0.1	300	0.01	0.02	0.7	15
Pears	128	70	1	1	15	3	7	0.1	50	0.02	0.02	0.2	15
Pears and pineapple	128	80	1	1	16	2	7	0.1	45	0.03	0.02	0.2	15
Plums with tapioca, strained	128	90	1	1	19	5	5	0.1	150	0.01	0.02	0.2	15
Prunes with tapioca	135	110	1	1	25	15	7	0.3	300	0.02	0.06	0.4	7
Meats, poultry, and eggs; canned													
Beef:													
Strained	99	90	13	4.0	0	59	7	1	91	0.01	0.16	3.5	2
Junior	99	100	14	4	1	61	6	1.6	74	0.02	0.20	3.6	2
Chicken junior, strained	99	140	14	9	0	41	8	1	52	0.02	0.16	3.5	2
Egg yolks, strained	94	180	9	16	1	57	79	3.0	542	0.12	0.22	Trace	2
Ham junior	99	120	15	6	1	43	6	1	32	0.01	0.16	2.8	2
Lamb:													
Strained	99	100	14	4	1	51	4	1	99	0.02	0.17	3.3	1
Junior	99	100	15	4	1	54	5	1.6	19	0.01	0.16	3.0	1
Liver, strained	99	90	14.1	3	2	53	4	5.6	25,000	0.05	2.00	7.6	19
Veal:													
Strained	99	0	13	4	1	55	4	1	61	0.03	0.20	4.3	3
Junior	99	100	15	4	0	55	5	1	28	0.01	0.15	4	2
Vegetables, canned													
Beans, green	128	40	2	0	7	1	40	0.7	400	0.02	0.06	0.3	6
Beets, strained	128	40	1	0	10	90	13	0.3	20	0.02	0.03	0.1	3
Carrots	128	40	1	0	8	50	25	0.5	17,000	0.02	0.03	0.4	10
Mixed vegetables, including vegetable soup	128	60	2	1	10	15	14	0.9	7000	0.05	0.04	0.6	3
Peas, strained	128	60	4	1	10	5	14	1.2	600	0.08	0.09	1.2	10
Spinach, creamed	128	70	4	2	9	65	130	1.5	7000	0.02	0.13	0.3	6
Squash	128	40	1	0	8	3	24	0.4	2000	0.02	0.04	0.3	11
Sweet potatoes	135	80	1.0	0	19	25	16	0.4	6500	0.04	0.03	0.4	11

From various manufacturers.

LIPIDS AND LIPOPROTEIN VALUES IN CHILDREN

Tables 29–11*A, B,* and *C* present data from 3 studies* which are comparable in data collection and biochemical analysis, although all age groups were not represented in each.† Both Rochester, Minnesota and Muscatine, Iowa have fewer than 1% black school-age children in

*Cardiovascular Profile of 15,000 Children of School Age in Three Communities, 1971–1975; Bogalusa, Louisiana (Louisiana State University Medical Center), Rochester, Minnesota (Mayo Clinic), Muscatine, Iowa (University of Iowa Medical Center). U.S. Department of Health, Education and Welfare, Public Health Service, National Institutes of Health, National Heart, Lung, and Blood Institute, DHEW Publication No. (NIH) 78-1472.
†Bogalusa, ages 5–14; Rochester, ages 6–18; Muscatine, ages 5–18.

their populations, hence all data are combined under white males and females. Data from Bogalusa, Louisiana for white and black children are considered separately. These tables can be used only to read "statistical normals," not to predict health or disease or to extrapolate for a single individual over time.

Although HDL cholesterol and LDL cholesterol determinations were performed by the same methods in 2 studies in which they were evaluated (Bogalusa and Rochester), the results are considerably different for unknown reasons. It was felt incorrect, therefore, to average results and they are presented separately.

Table 29–11C shows data from Bogalusa, Louisiana, only.

I. BRUCE GORDON

Table 29–11A LIPIDS AND LIPOPROTEIN BLOOD VALUES IN CHILDREN—WHITE MALES (mg/dl)

| | AGE IN YEARS | | | | | | | | | | | | | |
	5	6	7	8	9	10	11	12	13	14	15	16	17	18
Cholesterol														
mean*	152	159	157	161	164	166	165	164	159	155	156	158	156	161
no. of participants†	242	683	651	659	661	630	613	582	480	477	313	316	220	117
standard deviation‡	26–29	35–29–21	29–26–23	32–26–25	29–27–21	30–28–24	27–31–24	27–31–25	26–30–24	25–29–24	30–35	38–24	30–26	33–24
Triglycerides														
mean	64	59	60	65	68	73	73	73	78	82	85	89	86	93
no. of participants	242	683	650	658	661	629	613	582	480	477	313	316	220	117
standard deviation	27–28	32–27–27	25–29–21	31–40–26	31–44–19	34–44–95	47–44–23	34–41–38	29–48–29	32–50–30	49–28	52–31	46–42	46–31
HDL Cholesterol—Bogalusa														
mean	63	72	67	67	66	68	66	69	65	58				
no. of participants	71	91	96	102	99	123	114	134	110	93				
standard deviation	20	28	20	22	22	21	23	20	18	20				
HDL Cholesterol—Rochester														
mean		47	53	55	51	52	53	49	44	43	41	42	41	42
no. of participants		34	40	39	64	83	79	131	139	146	111	157	111	59
standard deviation		11	9	12	9	10	11	10	9	10	8	9	9	9
LDL Cholesterol—Bogalusa														
mean	91	90	88	88	94	87	89	85	82	83				
no. of participants	71	91	96	102	99	123	114	134	110	93				
standard deviation	22	24	23	26	24	24	23	22	22	21				
LDL Cholesterol—Rochester														
mean		103	105	99	103	109	104	101	99	98	99	96	100	101
no. of participants		34	40	39	64	83	79	131	139	146	111	157	111	59
standard deviation		18	20	19	23	21	21	23	21	21	31	21	22	22

*Means represent an average of studies with determinations for specific age groups.
†Sum of participants with determinations for specific age groups.
‡Since standard deviations cannot be averaged they are listed separately for each study as follows: age 5 Bogalusa–Muscatine; ages 6–14 Bogalusa–Muscatine–Rochester; ages 15–18 Muscatine–Rochester.

Table 29–11B LIPIDS AND LIPOPROTEIN BLOOD VALUES IN CHILDREN—WHITE FEMALES (mg/dl)

	5	6	7	8	9	10	11	12	13	14	15	16	17	18
							AGE IN YEARS							
Cholesterol														
mean*	153	156	161	163	167	165	166	160	164	161	166	166	166	165
no. of participants†	236	638	636	649	674	602	598	576	488	452	321	319	281	129
standard deviation‡	25–33	31–28–24	28–28–33	27–31–22	26–28–23	24–30–32	27–31–28	25–30–24	25–30–29	27–33–24	29–26	30–28	31–30	28–40
Triglycerides														
mean	63	64	68	70	76	79	83	85	87	84	78	78	78	81
no. of participants	236	637	635	647	671	601	598	576	487	453	321	320	281	129
standard deviation	24–28	30–29–13	34–36–21	31–40–21	30–46–28	42–45–26	61–44–27	35–43–26	32–49–28	31–46–25	45–24	38–27	38–29	44–38
HDL Cholesterol—Bogalusa														
mean	68	63	62	70	64	58	62	64	67	61				
no. of participants	88	77	91	96	98	105	111	122	106	82				
standard deviation	23	23	21	20	21	21	22	20	18	19				
HDL Cholesterol—Rochester														
mean		46	49	50	53	49	49	45	45	45	46	48	49	47
no. of participants		21	57	54	76	74	72	143	134	130	107	149	140	71
standard deviation		10	9	10	10	9	12	10	10	10	10	10	10	11
LDL Cholesterol—Bogalusa														
mean	84	93	92	92	95	93	93	86	86	85				
no. of participants	88	77	91	96	98	105	111	122	105	82				
standard deviation	18	21	22	23	24	23	24	19	20	21				
LDL Cholesterol—Rochester														
mean		113	115	103	110	106	107	98	100	99	102	103	106	104
no. of participants		21	57	54	76	74	72	143	134	130	107	149	140	71
standard deviation		23	42	22	20	31	26	22	26	25	23	25	27	38

*Means represent an average of studies with determinations for specific age groups.
†Sum of participants with determinations for specific age groups.
‡Since standard deviations cannot be averaged they are listed separately for each study as follows: age 5 Bogalusa–Muscatine; ages 6–14 Bogalusa–Muscatine–Rochester; ages 15–18 Muscatine–Rochester.

Table 29–11C LIPIDS AND LIPOPROTEIN BLOOD VALUES IN BLACK CHILDREN (mg/dl)

	5	6	7	8	9	10	11	12	13	14
					AGE IN YEARS					
MALES										
Cholesterol										
mean	170	172	171	165	177	169	171	173	161	167
no. of participants	30	44	49	61	80	71	70	81	68	55
standard deviation	28	40	38	30	36	29	30	31	26	25
Triglycerides										
mean	56	57	53	57	62	53	64	60	61	66
no. of participants	30	44	49	61	80	71	70	81	68	55
standard deviation	20	21	19	26	31	20	24	22	28	26
HDL Cholesterol										
mean	68	78	76	70	78	78	74	79	74	72
no. of participants	30	44	48	61	80	71	70	81	68	55
standard deviation	19	25	28	24	21	26	22	25	22	18
LDL Cholesterol										
mean	96	90	90	88	92	84	89	87	79	86
no. of participants	30	44	48	61	80	71	70	81	68	55
standard deviation	25	27	23	20	28	18	26	23	22	19
FEMALES										
Cholesterol										
mean	168	177	171	178	172	172	174	164	167	167
no. of participants	31	50	52	50	55	60	64	74	69	60
standard deviation	23	33	33	34	30	32	33	24	25	29
Triglycerides										
mean	67	61	59	63	62	67	67	62	65	63
no. of participants	31	50	52	50	55	60	64	74	69	60
standard deviation	29	22	22	20	25	38	25	17	23	20
HDL Cholesterol										
mean	67	73	75	74	74	72	69	73	77	69
no. of participants	31	50	52	50	55	60	64	74	69	60
standard deviation	19	27	22	21	21	29	23	18	18	17
LDL Cholesterol										
mean	94	98	90	96	91	92	96	84	82	89
no. of participants	31	50	52	50	55	60	64	74	69	60
standard deviation	19	22	21	28	24	26	23	18	19	23

INDEX

For DRUGS listed by indications for use, see Table 29–1A, p. 1811.   For DRUGS listed individually with dosages, see Table 29–1B, p. 1814.

For DRUGS listed by indications for use, see Table 29–1A, p. 1811. For DRUGS listed individually with dosages, see Table 29–1B, p. 1814.

For DRUGS listed by indications for use, see Table 29–1A, p. 1811. For DRUGS listed individually with dosages, see Table 29–1B, p. 1814.

For REFERENCE RANGES for laboratory tests, see pp. 1827 to 1852.

Drooling, 886
Drowning, 262, 264–266
Drug(s). See also names of specific drugs
    and names of specific classes of
    drugs, e.g., *Antibiotics.*
absorption of, 275
absorptive defects induced by, 939
abuse of, 1524–1529
additive effects of, 278
adult dosage conversions for, 1814
adverse reactions to, 278–279, 553–555.
    See also names of specific agents.
as teratogens, 316
causing displacement of other drugs,
    278
causing jaundice, 279–280
distribution of, 275–277
excretion of, 277
half-life of, 277
hemolytic anemia induced by,
    associated with glucose-6-phosphate
    dehydrogenase deficiency, 1222–1223
hepatotoxicity of, 972–973
hypoglycemia from, 1427
in human milk, 281
inhibition of metabolism by, 279
interactions of, 278, 279
interference with absorption of other
    drugs, 278
liver injury from, 972–973
metabolism of, 276
    acetylation in, 26
nephrotoxicity of, 1381–1382
neutropenia induced by, 1240–1241
poisoning by, 1786–1805. See also
    names of specific agents.
precocity from, 1449
protein binding of, 275–276
pulmonary disease from, 1009–1010
reactions to, 278–279, 553–555. See also
    names of specific agents.
side effects of, 280, 939
syndromes produced by, 280
tables of, 1811–1827
therapy with, 275–281
thrombocytopenias from, 1250
toxicity of, 278–281
Drug fever, 554
Drug-drug interactions, 278–281
Dry mouth, 886–887
Dry pleurisy, 1078–1079
D-trisomy syndrome, 299–300
Duane syndrome, 1753
Dubowitz examination, 343–344
Duchenne muscular dystrophy, 1611–1612
Ductus arteriosus, 1117–1118. See also
    Patent ductus arteriosus.
Ductus venosus, 1116
Duncan disease, 511
Duodenal web, 907
Duroziez sign, 1182
Dwarf tapeworms, 868–869
Dwarfism, 1634–1653
    due to diabetes, 1417
Dyggve-Melchior-Clausen syndrome, 1643
Dying child, 94–95, 132–134
    care of, 133
    care of parents of, 132–133
Dysautonomia, familial, 1598–1599
        ocular changes in, 1745
        tongue manifestations of, 886
Dyschondrosteosis, 1641
Dyscoria, 1750
Dysdiadochokinesis, 111–112

Dysentery, bacillary, 670
Dyserythropoietic anemia, congenital,
    1209–1210
Dysfibrinogenemias, congenital, 1247
Dysgerminomas, 1291
Dyshidrosis, 1687–1688
Dyshidrotic eczema, 1687–1688
Dyskeratosis, congenital, 1668
Dyskinetic cilia syndrome, 1043–1044
Dyslexia, 1547, 1749
Dysmenorrhea, 1520
Dysmorphology, 317–321
Dysnomia, 114
Dysorthographia, 113
Dysosteosclerosis, 1648
Dysostosis, craniofacial, 1630
Dysphagia, 888, 894
Dysplasia(s)
    acetabular, 1619
    of hip, congenital, 1617–1619
    skeletal genetic, 1634–1653
Dysplasia epiphysealis hemimelica, 1644
Dyspneic attacks, in tetralogy of Fallot,
    1123
Dystonia, 1549
Dystonia musculorum deformans, 1584–
    1585
Dystrophic epidermolysis bullosa, 1682–
    1683
Dystrophies of muscle, 1611–1612
Dysuria, 1372

Eagle-Barrett syndrome, 1391–1392
Ear, disorders of, 1022–1030
Eastern equine encephalitis, 627
EB virus, 766
Ebstein disease, 1136–1137
ECG. See Electrocardiography.
Ecchymosis, 389
Eccrine sweat glands, 1664
Echinococcosis, 869–870
Echocardiography, 1109–1112
Echoviruses
    clinical manifestations of, 796–802
    in newborn, 415–416
Ecthyma, 1712
Ecthyma gangrenosum, 675, 676
Ectodermal dysplasias, 1668–1669
Ectomorph, 22
Ectopia cordis, 1141
Ectopia lentis, 1760
Ectopic atrial tachycardia, 1173
Ectopic pancreatic tissue, 951
Ectopic pregnancy, 1520
Ectopic ureteral orifices, 1386
Ectopic ureterocele, 1387–1388
Ectrodactyly–ectodermal dysplasia, 1669
Ectropion, 1755
Eczema, 149, 1685–1689
Eczema herpeticum, 752–753
Eczema vaccinatum, 753, 763
Eczematoid dermatitis, 1025
Edema, 209, 213
    cerebral, 245, 1558
        in newborn, 358
    high altitude pulmonary, 1070
    in adult respiratory distress syndrome,
        272
    in chronic renal failure, 1365
    in near-drowning, 264–265
    in nephrotic syndrome, 1323
    in newborn, 332, 392–393

Edema (*Continued*)
    of malnutrition, 166
    pulmonary, 265, 272, 1070
        in burns, 270
        intensive care for, 258
        treatment of, 258
    scrotal, 1400
Edwards syndrome, 299
EEC syndrome, 1669
Effeminacy in boys, 92
Effusions
    pericardial, 1191–1192
    pleural, 1078–1080
    subdural, 1590
Ego, 54
Ehlers-Danlos syndrome, 1702
    type VII, 282
Eisenmenger syndrome, 1138–1139
Ejection clicks, 1103
Elastolysis, generalized, 1701–1702
Elastosis perforans serpiginosa, 1703
Elbow
    osteochondrosis of, 1629
    pulled, 1629
Electrocardiography, 1105–1108
    in anomalous origin of left coronary
        artery, 1166
    in atrial fibrillation, 1174
    in bradycardia-tachycardia syndrome,
        1176
    in complete atrioventricular block, 1175
    in paroxysmal supraventricular
        tachycardia, 1172
    in premature atrial contraction, 1171
    in premature atrial tachycardia, 1173
    in premature ventricular contractions,
        1172
    in sick-sinus syndrome, 1176
    in sinus arrhythmia with junctional
        escape, 1170
    in wandering atrial pacemaker, 1171
    in Wenckebach phenomenon, 1175
    in Wolff-Parkinson-White syndrome,
        1173
Electroencephalography, 1536–1538, 1556
Electrolytes
    in central nervous system disorders,
        239, 245
    in transcellular fluids, 213
    losses of, in disease states, 230
    maintenance requirements of, 238–239
Electromyography, 1556
Elliptocytosis, hereditary, 1219, 1220
Ellis–van Creveld syndrome, 1638
Embden-Meyerhof pathway, 1422
Embolism, 1194–1195
    pulmonary, 1070–1071
Emotional behavior, 46–99
Emotional deprivation, hypopituitarism
    and, 1437
Emotional disorders, 76–81
Emphysema, 1066–1069
    due to alpha$_1$-antitrypsin deficiency,
        1069–1070
    obstructive, 1039
Empyema, 1079–1080
    epidermal, 1590
    subdural, 1590
Encephalitic poliomyelitis, 794
Encephalitis, 626–631, 801
    behavioral sequelae of, 71
    due to herpes simplex infection, 754
    due to poliovirus, 794
    due to tetanus, 688

For DRUGS listed by indications for use, see Table 29–1A, p. 1811.   For DRUGS listed individually with dosages, see Table 29–1B, p. 1814.

Encephalitis (*Continued*)
  focal, 801
  postinfectious, 627
    due to varicella, 757
    slow virus diseases with, 627
Encephalocele, 286, 1560
Encephalomyelitis, vaccinal, 763
Encephalomyelopathy, subacute
  necrotizing, 173, 454–455, 1425, 1579,
  1745
Encephalopathy. See also *Reye syndrome.*
  acute toxic, 1591–1592
  following DPT, 189
  mental retardation in, 125
  myoclonic, 1584
Encephalotrigeminal angiomatosis, 1575
Enchondromas, 1293
Enchondromatosis, 1644–1656
Encopresis, 74, 889
Endarteritis, infective, 1151
Endocapillary proliferative
  glomerulonephritis, 1343
Endocardial cushion defects, 1148–1150
Endocardial fibroelastosis, 1185–1186
Endocardial sclerosis, 1185
Endocarditis
  bacterial acute, 648
    in tetralogy of Fallot, 1126
  due to *Campylobacter*, 702
  due to *Streptococcus viridans*, 637
  glomerulonephritis in, 1336
  infective, 1176–1179
  prevention of, 1180
Endocrine disorders of newborn, 395–399
Endocrine myopathies, 1608–1609
Endocrine system, 1432–1514
Endodermal sinus tumor, 1290
Endomorph, 22
Endophthalmitis, 652
Endoscopy, 1001, 1007
  in cystic fibrosis, 1094–1095
Endosteal hyperostosis, 1649
Endotoxemia, in burns, 271
Endotoxic shock, 271–275
Endotracheal tubes, 1007
Enophthalmos, 1767
Entamoeba histolytica, 835–837
Enteritis, necrotizing, 691–693
Enterobiasis, 858
Enterocolitis
  antibiotic-associated, 925–926
  due to meningococcal infections, 651–
    652
  due to staphylococcal infections, 648
  due to *Yersinia*, 680–681
  necrotizing, 346, 925
Enterokinase deficiency, 937
Enteroviruses, 791–804
  infection with, in newborn, 415–416
Entropion, 1755
Enucleation, for retinoblastoma, 1287
Enuresis, 59, 73, 1381, 1400
Enzyme-linked immune serum assay
  (ELISA), 599
Eosinophilia, 529, 1238
Eosinophilic fasciitis, 586
Eosinophilic gastroenteritis, 927
Eosinophilic granuloma of bone, 1273
Ependymoma, 1587
Ephelides, 1676
Epicanthal folds, 298, 1755
Epidemiology, 194–195
Epidermal inclusion cysts, 1704

Epidermal necrolysis, toxic, 1681–1682
Epidermal nevi, 1675
Epidermis, 1663
  diseases of, 1691–1696
Epidermolysis bullosa, 1682
Epidermolytic hyperkeratosis, 1698
Epididymal appendage torsion, 1395
Epididymal torsion, 1395
Epididymitis, 800, 1395, 1399
  due to mumps, 771
Epidural abscess, spinal, 1597
Epidural empyema, 1590
Epidural hemorrhage, 1595
Epigastric hernia, 988
Epiglottitis, 656–657, 1034–1035
Epilepsy, 1534–1543
  disorders simulating, 1543–1544
  psychiatric disorders with, 71
Epimembranous glomerulopathy, 1327–
  1328
Epinephrine
  for shock, 274
  in resuscitation, 259
Epinephrine tolerance test, 1429
Epiphyseal centers, 23, 24
Epiphyseal dysgenesis, 1456
Epiphyseal dysplasias, 1639–1640
Epiphyseal fractures, 1631
Epiphyseal separations, in newborn, 361
Epispadias, 1389–1390
Epistaxis, 1012
Epithelioid cell nevus, 1674
Epithelioma adenoides cysticum, 1729–
  1730
Epstein pearls, 333, 883
Epstein-Barr (EB) virus, 766
Epulis, 883, 1293
Equinovarus deformity, 1614
Erb sign, 250
Erb-Duchenne paralysis, 359
Erysipelas, 635
Erythema marginatum, 591
Erythema multiforme, 550, 609, 1680–1681
  caused by drugs, 280
  with infections, 609
Erythema multiforme exudativum, 584
Erythema nodosum, 584–585, 609
  caused by drugs, 280
  with infections, 609
Erythema toxicum, 332, 1666
Erythrasma, 1714
Erythremia, 1232
Erythredema, 1798
Erythroblastopenia of childhood,
  transient, 1209
Erythroblastosis fetalis, 383–388
  hyperinsulinism in, 1424
Erythrocytes. See *Red blood cells.*
Erythrocytosis, 1232
Erythrokeratodermia variabilis, 1698
Erythropoietic protoporphyria, 1690
Erythropoietin, 1204, 1305
Escherichia coli infections, diarrheogenic,
  661–663
Esophageal atresia, 376, 893–894
Esophageal duplication cysts, 894
Esophageal perforation, 898
Esophageal varices, 899
Esophagitis, 897–898
Esophagus, disorders, 893–899
Esophoria, 1752
Esotropia, 1752
Espundia, 852

Essential amino acids, 138
Essential fatty acids, 140
  deficiency of, 1700
Essential hypertension, 1197
Esthesioneuroblastoma, 1276
Estriol concentrations, 328
Estrogenic lesions of ovary, 1505
Estrogens, 316, 1495–1496
Ethics, 134–135
Ethosuximide, 1542
Ethrane, 256
Ethyl alcohol ingestion
  additive effects of, 278
  hypoglycemia and, 1427
E-trisomy syndrome, 299
Eunuch syndrome, 1499
Eustachian tube
  in newborn, 13
  ventilatory function of, 1023
Evans syndrome, 1230
Eventration, 362, 988–990
Ewing sarcoma, 1258, 1285–1286
Exanthem(s)
  diagnosis of, 600
  due to enteroviruses, 797
Exanthem subitum, 750–751
Exchange transfusion, 381–382, 386–387
Excretory urography, 1315
Exercise-associated hematuria, 1310
Exfoliative dermatitis, 280
Exhibitionism, 92
Exocrine pancreas, 949–953
Exocrine pancreatic insufficiency. See
  Cystic fibrosis.
Exophthalmos, 1767
Exostoses, cartilaginous, 1293
  multiple, 1644
Expiratory reserve capacity, 996–997
Expiratory reserve volume, 996–997
Expressive aphasia, 1547
Exstrophy
  of bladder, 1389, 1390
  of cloaca, 1390
External auditory canal, 1024
External otitis, 1024–1025
Extracapillary proliferative
  glomerulonephritis, 1343
Extracellular fluid, 207, 210
Extrahepatic biliary atresia, 966–967, 968
Extrahepatic portal obstruction, 984
Extramembranous gomerulopathy, 1327–
  1328
Extrapancreatic tumors, 1428
Extrapulmonary tuberculosis, 714–718
Extrapyramidal cerebral palsy, 1571
Extrasystoles, 1171
Exudates, 596, 1002
Exudative enteropathy, opportunistic
  infections in, 699
Eye(s), 1735–1769. See also names of
  specific ocular disorders and structures.
Eye strain, 1573
Eyelid(s)
  ecchymosis of, 1768
  heliotrope, 581
  swelling of, 1768
  tumors of, 1756

FAB classification of leukemias, 1262
Fabry disease, 480–481, 1672
Facial asymmetries, 875

For REFERENCE RANGES for laboratory tests, see pp. 1827 to 1852.

For DRUGS listed by indications for use, see Table 29–1A, p. 1811. For DRUGS listed individually with dosages, see Table 29–1B, p. 1814.

For **REFERENCE RANGES** for laboratory tests, see pp. 1827 to 1852.

Hydatid cysts, 869–870
Hydatid disease, 869–870
Hydranencephaly, 1565
Hydrindicuria, 431–432
Hydroa aestivale, 1690
Hydroa vacciniforme, 1690
Hydrocalycosis, 1385
Hydrocarbon pneumonia, 1056–1057
Hydrocarbon poisoning, 1793–1794
Hydrocele
    of tunica vaginalis, 1395
    transient, 335
Hydrocephalus, 33, 1566–1569
    achondroplasia in, 1636
    in acute bacterial meningitis, 620
    psychiatric disorders in, 71
Hydrogen ion
    generation of, 221
    metabolism of, 219
Hydronephrosis, 1387
Hydrophobia, 804–808
Hydrops fetalis, 384
Hydrothorax, 1082
Hydroxykynureninuria, 431
17-Hydroxylase deficiency, 1483, 1509
21-Hydroxylase deficiency, 1482–1483
Hydroxylysinase, 443–445
Hydroxylysine-deficient collagen, 443–445
Hydroxylysinemia, 445
Hydroxyproline, defects in metabolism of, 437–438
Hydroxyprolinemia, 437
Hygroma, cystic, 1294–1295
Hymen, imperforate, 1516, 1521
Hymenolepiasis, 868–869
Hymenoptera insect allergy, 556
Hyperactivity, 58, 72, 82–86, 105–119
    psychopharmacology in, 96–97
Hyperaldosteronism, 1490
Hyperammonemias, 439–441
Hyperbaric oxygen, 691
Hyperbilirubinemia, 378–381, 890
    conjugation reactions in, 955
    due to hemolytic disease of the
        newborn, 383–388
    exchange transfusion, 381–382, 386–387
    intrauterine transfusion for, 386
    with liver disease, 957
Hypercalcemia, 217
    congenital aortic stenosis with, 1161
    idiopathic, 1658
    physical signs in, 235
    renal tubular damage from, 1350
Hypercalciuria, 1376
Hypercapnia, 996, 999
Hyperchloremia, 226
Hyperdibasicaminoaciduria, 444
Hyperdynamic precordium, 1102
Hyperglycemia, 346. See also *Diabetes mellitus.*
    in cystic fibrosis, 1098
Hypergonadotropic hypogonadism, 1496–1499, 1501–1503
Hyperhemolytic crises, in sickle cell anemia, 1224
Hyperinsulinism, 396, 1423–1424
Hyperkalemia, 215, 216
    electrocardiogram of, 1108
    in acute renal failure, 1358
    signs of, 248
    treatment of, 248
Hyperkalemic periodic paralysis, 1610

Hyperlipidemia, 1200–1203
    in cholesteryl ester storage disease, 485
    in nephrotic syndrome, 1324
Hyperlucent lung, 1067
Hypermagnesemia, 218
    in newborn, 394
    signs of, 235, 249
    treatment of, 249
Hypernatremia, 213–214
    causes of, 248
    treatment of, 248
Hypernatremic dehydration, 232–233, 237–238, 240
Hyperopia, 1737–1738
Hyperosmolality, 238
Hyperosmolar coma, nonketotic, 1406–1407
Hyperostosis, 172
    endosteal, 1649
    infantile cortical, 1650
Hyperparathyroidism, 1473–1475
    muscle disease and, 1609
Hyperphosphatasemia with osteoectasia, 1649–1650
Hyperphosphatemia, 227, 1658
Hyperpigmented skin lesions, 1676–1677
Hyperpituitarism, 1441–1442
Hyperpyrexia, malignant, 257
Hyperreactivity of airways, in asthma, 539
Hypersecretion of vasopressin, 1440
Hypersensitivity, 501–502
    cell-mediated, 526
    delayed, 526
    IgE-mediated, 524–525
    immediate type, 526–529
    skin testing in, 531
    to inhaled materials, 1058
Hypersensitivity shock, 271–275
Hypersplenism, 1255
Hypertelorism, 1011, 1767
    ocular, 1631
Hypertension
    accelerated, 1197
    blood pressure ranges by age, 1101
    curable forms of, 1196
    in acute poststreptococcal
        glomerulonephritis, 1332–1334
    in acute renal failure, 1358–1359
    in chronic renal failure, 1365
    in Wilms tumor, 1278
    intracranial 258–259
    malignant, 1197
    portal, 984–985
    pulmonary, 1118–1119
        primary, 1166–1167
    pulmonary venous, 1164
    renovascular, 1379–1380
    retinopathy in, 1764–1765
    secondary, 1195–1196
    systemic, 1195–1200
Hyperthermia, in newborn, 392
Hyperthyroid myopathy, 1609
Hyperthyroidism, 395–396, 1462–1464
Hypertonic dehydration, 232–233
    deficit therapy of, 239
Hypertrichosis, 1707
Hypertrophic cardiomyopathy, 1186
Hypertrophic interstitial neuritis, 1604
Hypertrophic osteoarthropathy, in cystic fibrosis, 1095
Hyperuricemia, 469–470

Hyperventilation, 996
    as cause of tetany, 250
    fluid losses in, 231
Hyperviscosity syndrome, 1119
Hypervitaminosis A, 172
    pseudotumor cerebri in, 172
Hypervitaminosis D, 184
Hyphema, 1769
Hypoallergenic milks, 157
Hypocalcemia, 217, 250–252
    associated with hypomagnesemia, 252–253
    cow's milk–induced, 393
    due to maternal hypoparathyroidism, 1469
    electrocardiogram in, 251, 1108
    in DiGeorge syndrome, 251, 507–508
    in newborn 250, 393
    physical signs of, 235
Hypocalcemic tetany, 250–252
Hypocalcemic vitamin D–resistant rickets, 1657
Hypocapnia, 996
Hypochloremia, 226
Hypochloremic alkalosis, 905
Hypochondroplasia, 1636–1637
Hypofibrinogenemia, due to hemangioma, 1294
Hypogammaglobulinemia, 931.
Hypoglossal nerve, 1552
Hypoglycemia, 346, 1421–1431, 1570
    in infants of diabetic mothers, 396–397
    in newborn, 397–399
Hypogonadism
    hypergonadotropic, 1496–1499, 1501–1503
    hypogonadotropic, 1499–1500, 1504
Hypohidrotic ectodermal dysplasia, 1668–1669
Hypokalemia, 215
    electrocardiogram in, 1108
    in salicylate poisoning, 1790
    renal tubular damage from, 1350
    signs of, 248
    treatment of, 248
Hypomagnesemia, 218, 252–253, 939
    associated with hypocalcemia, 252–253
    in newborn, 393–394
    physical signs of, 235, 248
    primary, 939
    treatment of, 248–249
Hypomagnesemic tetany, 252–253
Hypomelanosis of Ito, 1678–1679
Hyponatremia, 213
    asymptomatic, 247
    causes of, 247
    spurious, 210
    symptomatic, 248
    treatment of, 247–248
Hyponatremic dehydration, 232–233, 237, 239–240
Hypoparathyroidism, 252, 1469–1472
    in newborn, 396
    transient, 250
Hypophosphatasia, 473, 1650, 1658
Hypophosphatemia, 227–228
    familial, 1656–1657
Hypopigmented macules, 1574
Hypopigmented skin lesions, 1678–1680
Hypopituitarism, 1434–1437, 1499, 1504
Hypoplastic left heart syndrome, 1139–1140

Hypoproteinemia
  idiopathic, 392–393
  in nephrotic syndrome, 1323
Hypoprothrombinemia, 185
Hyposensitization, 536–538
Hypospadias, 1392–1393
Hyposplenia, functional, 1255
Hypotelorism, 1767
Hypothalamic gliomas, 1588
Hypothalamus, disorders of, 1432–1451
Hypothermia, in newborn, 356
Hypothyroidism, 1453–1460
  myopathy in, 1609
  with precocious puberty, 1447–1448
Hypotonia, 1603
Hypotonic dehydration, 232–233
Hypotony of eye, 1767
Hypotrichosis, 1707
Hypouricemia, 470
Hypoventilation, due to neuromuscular
  diseases, 1084
Hypovolemia, 271–275
Hypoxemia, 996, 999
  cardiopulmonary effects of, 1120
  in drowning, 264
Hypoxia, 996
  in drowning and near-drowning, 264
  in fetus, 327–328
Hypsarrhythmia, 1536
Hysteria, 1554–1555
Hysterical fits, 1544
Hysterical gait disturbance, 1554
Hysterical neuroses, 77

I-cell disease, 486
Ichthyosis, 1696–1700
Ichthyosis linearis circumflexa, 1698
Ichthyosis syndrome, 1698–1700
Ichthyosis vulgaris, 1697
Icteric leptospirosis, 735
Id reaction, 1716
Identical twins, 341–342
IgA deficiency, 931
  selective, 506–507
IgA nephropathy, 1334–1336
IgE, 525
  in allergy, 524–525
  serum concentrations in atopic
    dermatitis, 547
  serum levels at different ages, 529
IgG subgroup deficiency, 507
IgM deficiency (selective), 507
Ileal atresia, 909
Ileal fluid, electrolytes in, 213
Ileal obstruction, 909–910
Ileostomy fluid, composition of, 231
Ileus, paralytic, 914
Imidazole aciduria, 442
Imipramine, 74, 97
Immature left colon syndrome, 917
Immotile cilia syndrome, 1043–1044
Immune complex deposition in kidney,
  1319
Immune complex determinations, 563
Immune complex disease, 526
Immune deficiency states
  malabsorption in, 931
  skeletal dysplasias with, 1635
Immune globulin, for tetanus, 688
Immune neonatal thrombocytopenia, 1251
Immune thrombocytopenic purpura, 1230

Immunization, 189–193
  adverse reactions to, 192
  against cholera, 673
  against diphtheria, 644
  against hepatitis A and B, 789
  against influenza viral infections, 192–
    193, 774–775
  against measles, 191–192, 745–746
  against mumps, 191–192, 772
  against pertussis, 660–661
  against poliomyelitis, 191–192, 803
  against pseudomonas, 676
  against rabies, 807–808
  against rubella, 191–192, 748–749
  against smallpox, 193, 761–763
  against tetanus, 688
  against tuberculosis, 712
  against typhoid fever, 669
  against varicella, 757–758
  allergic reactions to, 192
  delayed, 192
  in breast feeding, 149–150
  schedule of, 189–192
  special, 192–193
Immunodeficiency diseases, 503, 504–511.
  See also names of specific diseases.
Immunoglobulins, 500–501
  diagnostic significance of, 503
  in rheumatic diseases, 563
  levels of, 497
  serum IgE at different ages, 529
Immunology, 497–594
Immunosuppression, 511
  opportunistic infections in, 697–699
Immunotherapy, 536–538
  for insect allergy, 557
Impacted teeth, 883
Imperforate anal membrane, 918
Imperforate anus, 335
Imperforate hymen, 1516, 1521
Impetigo, 635
Impetigo contagiosa, 752, 1711–1712
Inappropriate secretion of antidiuretic
  hormone, 245, 630, 1440–1441
Inattention, 111
Inborn errors of metabolism, 313, 417–
  496. See also names of specific
  disorders.
  amino acid, 424–445
  carbohydrate, 445–467
  classification of, 418–422
  clinical patterns of, 418
  heme pigment, 488–496
  lipid, 476–487
  plasma enzyme, 473
  plasma protein, 472–473
  purine, 468–470
  pyrimidine, 470–471
  tissue protein, 473–475
Incarcerated hernia, 948–949
Incest, 92, 102–104
Incisional hernia, 988
Inclusion cysts, epidermal, 1704
Incontinentia pigmenti, 1667
Incontinentia pigmenti achromians, 1678–
  1679
Incubator care, 347–348
Indian childhood cirrhosis, 979
Indicanuria, 431
Indicator dilution curves, 1114–1115
Indicator dye test, 1114
Indolylacroylglycinuria, 432
Indomethacin, 371

Infant(s)
  anesthesia for, 255–256
  assessment of motor function in, 1553–
    1554
  breast feeding of, 149–154
  chronic subdural hematoma in, 1595–
    1596
  formula feeding of, 154–160
  growth and development of, 18–19
  maternal interaction with, 17
  mortality rates for, 186–187, 197
  neurologic examination of, 1552–1554
  newborn. See Newborn.
  of diabetic mothers, 396–397, 1424
  of low birth weight, 342–353. See also
    Low birth weight infant(s).
  reflexes of, 1552–1553
  water content of, 136
Infantile acne, 1728
Infantile autism, 93
Infantile cerebromacular degeneration,
  1577–1579
Infantile cortical hyperostosis, 1650
Infantile digital fibromatoses, 1728–1729
Infantile hemiplegia, acute, 1593
Infantile lethal agranulocytosis, 1239
Infantile microcystic disease, 1329
Infantile myoclonic seizures, 1536
  electroencephalography in, 1537
Infantile polyarteritis, 579–580
Infantile spasm, 1536
Infantile spinal muscular atrophy, 1602
Infantile tetany, 183–184
Infant-parent attachment, 55–56
Infarction, pulmonary, 1070–1071
Infection(s). See also Infectious diseases and
    names of specific diseases.
  anemia in, 1209
  congenital, with ocular changes, 1748
  cutaneous bacterial, 1711–1715
  cutaneous fungal, 1715–1721
  cutaneous viral, 1721–1722
  due to bites, 705–706
  due to substance abuse, 1525
  in acute renal failure, 1360
  in burns, 270–271
  mortality in, 3, 4
  of hip, 1619–1620
  of umbilical cord, 391
  of upper respiratory tract, 1012–1019
  of urinary tract, 1367–1373, 1396–1397
  prevention of, in prematurity, 351
  psychiatric problems in, 71
Infectious diseases, 595–873. See also
    Infection(s) and names of specific
    infectious diseases.
  anemia-associated, 1230
  arthropod-borne, 737–738
  bacterial, 632–728
  chemotherapy for, 1261
  chlamydial, 738–741
  clinical manifestations of, in newborn,
    402
  diabetes mellitus management during,
    1416
  effect of prematurity on, 400
  frequency of, in newborn, 399
  intestinal, 920–921
  isolation measures in, 631–632
  mycobacterial, 708–728
  mycoplasmal, 741–742
  mycotic, 825–834
  nosocomial, in nursery, 402–403

For DRUGS listed by indications for use, see Table 29–1A, p. 1811. For DRUGS listed individually with dosages, see Table 29–1B, p. 1814.

Junctional nevi, 1673
Junctional tachycardia, accelerated, 1173
Juvenile cerebromacular degeneration, 1578–1579
Juvenile chronic myelocytic leukemia, 1268
Juvenile colonic polyp, 946
Juvenile hypothyroidism, 1457–1458
Juvenile melanoma, 1674
Juvenile myasthenia gravis, 1607
Juvenile-onset diabetes, 1403–1404
Juvenile pernicious anemia, 938, 1213
Juvenile rheumatoid arthritis, 564–572
Juvenile xanthogranulomas, 1730
Juxtaglomerular apparatus, 1299

Kala-azar, 850–852
Kallmann syndrome, 1499
Kaolin-pectin, drug interactions of, 278
Kaposi sarcoma, acquired immune deficiency syndrome in, 701
Kaposi varicelliform eruption, 548, 752–753
Kartagener syndrome, 522, 1043–1044, 1747
Karyotypes
    abnormal, 291–293
    nomenclature for, 293
    normal, 289–291
    sex chromosome, atypical, 309–310
Karyotyping, 289
Kasabach-Merritt syndrome, 1250, 1670
Kasai operation, 966–967
Katayama fever, 865
Kawasaki disease, 580
Kayser-Fleischer rings, 978, 1584
Kearns-Sayre syndrome, 1612
Kell system, 523
Keloid, 1701
Keratitis, interstitial, 1759
Keratoconjunctivitis, due to herpes simplex infection, 754
Keratoconus, 1758–1759
Keratoderma of palms and soles, 1699
Keratolysis, pitted, 1714
Keratolytic agents, 1732
Keratoma hereditaria mutilans, 1699
Keratosis follicularis, 1694–1695
Keratosis palmaris et plantaris, 1699
Keratosis pilaris, 1693
Kernicterus, 346, 381–383, 385, 1570
Kerosene poisoning, 1793
Ketoacidosis, diabetic, 222, 1406–1407, 1408
Ketogenic diet, for epilepsy, 1543
Ketotic glycinemia, 434
Kidney(s), 1299–1385. See also *Renal.*
    acid production by, 221–222
    agenesis of, 1373–1374
    anatomy of, 1299–1303
    Ask-Upmark, 1374
    biopsy of, 1313
    calculi of, 1376–1377
    carbuncle of, 1398
    chronic insufficiency of, 222
    cystic conditions of, 1356
    developmental abnormalities of, 1373–1376
    diagnostic imaging of, 1314–1318
    disorders of. See names of specific renal disorders.
    in newborn, 390

Kidney(s) (*Continued*)
    duplication of, 1375
    electrolyte excretion by, 229–230, 1312
    hereditary disorders of, 1350–1357
    horseshoe, 1375
    in sickle cell anemia, 1355
    infections of, 1398
    physiology of, 1303–1307
    polycystic, 1356–1357
    traumatic injuries of, 1401
    tumors of, 1277–1279
Kinky hair syndrome, 473, 939, 1579
Kinsbourne syndrome, 1584
Kiss-the-knee test, 793
Klebsiella pneumonia, 1053
Kleeblattschädel, 1630, 1637
Klinefelter syndrome, 308–309, 1497–1498
    incidence of, 288
Klinefelter variation, 1498
Klippel-Feil disorder, 1627
Klippel-Trenaunay-Weber syndrome, 1671
Klumpke paralysis, 359
Knee, disorders of, 1622, 1623
Kniest dysplasia, 1640
Knock knees, 1623
Kocher-Debré-Sémélaigne syndrome, 1456
Koebner response, 1691–1692, 1695, 1696
KOH preparation, for skin examination, 1665
Kohler disease, 1617
Kohn, pores of, 944
Koplik spots, 743, 744
Korean hemorrhagic fever, 816
Krabbe disease, 483–484, 1580–1581
Kuru, 808–809
Kussmaul breathing, 221, 235
Kwashiorkor, 166–168
Kyasanur Forest disease, 816–817
Kynureninase defects, 431
Kynureninuria, 430–431
Kyphoscoliosis, 1085
Kyphosis, 1625–1626

L forms, laboratory diagnosis of, 598
Labial frenulum, 884
Labial fusion, 1484, 1485
Laboratory test tables, 1827–1852
Labyrinthine function evaluation, 1023–1024
Labyrinthine reflex, 333
Labyrinthitis, suppurative, 1029
Lactase deficiency, 938
Lactic acid, in shock, 273
Lactic acidosis, 451–455
Lactobacillus bifidus, 150
Lactoferrin, 150
Lactose intolerance, 446
Lacunar skull, 1630
Lagophthalmos, 1755
LaLeche League, 153
Lamellar ichthyosis, 1697–1698
Lancefield groupings, 633
Landau reflex, 1553
Langer-Giedion syndrome, 1644
Langer-Saldino syndrome, 1637–1638
Language
    development of, 121–123
    disorders of, 109, 119–123
    expressive, 108–110, 121–122
    receptive processing of, 108, 122
Large for gestational age (LGA), 339

Laryngitis, 1041
    acute infectious, 1035
    acute spasmodic, 1035–1036
Laron syndrome, 1436
Larsen syndrome, 1642
Laryngeal anomalies, congenital, 1031
Laryngeal atresia, 1031
Laryngeal diphtheria, 642
Laryngeal foreign body, 1038
Laryngeal stenosis, 1041
Laryngeal stridor, congenital, 1031–1032
Laryngeal trauma, 1040–1041
Laryngeal webs, 1031
Laryngomalacia, 1031–1032
Laryngoscopy, 1001
Laryngospasm, 184, 249
    in drowning, 264
Laryngotracheobronchitis, 1035
Laryngotracheoesophageal cleft, 1031
Lassa fever, 816, 817
Lateral dominance, 112
Lateral neck films, 1000
Lateral pharyngeal abscess, 1018
Lateral sinus thrombosis, 1593
Laurence-Moon-Biedl syndrome, 1500, 1744
Lavage
    in cystic fibrosis, 1094–1095
    in poisoning, 1787
Lead poisoning, 73, 1800–1803
    anemia and, 1217
    mental retardation in, 125
Learning disabilities, 105–119
Lecithin-cholesterol acyltransferase deficiency, 473
Left coronary artery anomaly, 1165
Left heart syndrome, 1139–1140
Left to right shunt or no shunt, 1142–1167
Left transposition of the great arteries, 1145
Left ventricular hypertrophy, 1107
Left ventricular–right atrial shunt, ventricular septal defect and, 1144–1145
Left-right discrimination, 106, 112
Leg, 1622–1624
Legg-Calvé-Perthes disease, 1620–1621
    recurrence risk of, 286
Legionnaires disease, 703–705
Leigh subacute necrotizing encephalomyelopathy (SNE), 173, 454–455, 1425, 1579, 1745
Leiner disease, 1688
Leiomyoma, 947
Leiomyosarcomas, 1282
Leishmaniasis, 850–853
Length
    by age, 27–32
    recumbent, 33
Lens, dislocation of, 1760
Lentigines, 1676
Lenz syndrome, 1747
Leopard syndrome, 1676
Leprechaunism, 1424
Leprosy, 726–728
Leptospirosis, 598, 734–736
Leri-Weill syndrome, 1641
Lesbianism, 91–92
Lesch-Nyhan syndrome, 468–469, 1377
Letdown reflex, 153
Lethal midline granuloma, 580–581
Letterer-Siwe disease, 1273
    with immunodeficiency, 509
Leucine, defects in metabolism of, 432–435

For REFERENCE RANGES for laboratory tests, see pp. 1827 to 1852.

For DRUGS listed by indications for use, see Table 29–1A, p. 1811.   For DRUGS listed individually with dosages, see Table 29–1B, p. 1814.

For REFERENCE RANGES for laboratory tests, see pp. 1827 to 1852.

For DRUGS listed by indications for use, see Table 29–1A, p. 1811. For DRUGS listed individually with dosages, see Table 29–1B, p. 1814.

For **REFERENCE RANGES** for laboratory tests, see pp. 1827 to 1852.

For DRUGS listed by indications for use, see Table 29–1A, p. 1811. For DRUGS listed individually with dosages, see Table 29–1B, p. 1814.

For REFERENCE RANGES for laboratory tests, see pp. 1827 to 1852.

For DRUGS listed by indications for use, see Table 29–1A, p. 1811. For DRUGS listed individually with dosages, see Table 29–1B, p. 1814.

For REFERENCE RANGES for laboratory tests, see pp. 1827 to 1852.

For DRUGS listed by indications for use, see Table 29–1A, p. 1811.   For DRUGS listed individually with dosages, see Table 29–1B, p. 1814.

For REFERENCE RANGES for laboratory tests, see pp. 1827 to 1852.

For DRUGS listed by indications for use, see Table 29–1A, p. 1811. For DRUGS listed individually with dosages, see Table 29–1B, p. 1814.

Sabin polio vaccine, 191
Saccharopinemia, 443
Sacral agenesis, 1626–1627
Sacrococcygeal teratoma, 1290
Sacrococcygeal tumor, 1290
Saddle nose, 730
Sagittal sinus thrombosis, 1593
St. Louis virus encephalitis, 627
Saldino-Noonan syndrome, 1638–1639
Salicylate. See also *Aspirin.*
   drug interactions of, 278
   effects of, on metabolism, 278
   poisoning due to, 222, 1789–1791
     treatment of, 244–245, 1791
Saliva, electrolytes in, 213
Salivary gland
   disorders of, 886–887
   tumors of, 1287–1288
Salk polio vaccine, 191
Salmon patch, 1666
Salmonella(e)
   food poisoning due to, 1783–1784
   infections due to, 612, 663–670
Salt and pepper retinitis, 412
Salt depletion, in cystic fibrosis, 1098
Salt intake, 161–162
Salt poisoning, 248
Salt-losing adrenocortical insufficiency,
   1481–1482
Salt-losing adrenogenital syndrome, 1485
Salt-losing congenital adrenal hyperplasia,
   1485
San Joaquin fever, 830–832
Sandhoff disease, 479
Sanfilippo syndromes, 1652
Sarcoidosis, 1776
Sarcoma(s), 1279–1282, 1295
   Ewing, 1258, 1285–1286
   of heart, 1295
Sarcoma botryoides, 1279, 1519
Sarcosinemia, 435
Scabies, 1723–1725
Scalded skin syndrome, 280, 410, 1713
   in graft-versus-host disease, 510
Scalp blood sampling, 327–328
Scaphocephaly, 1629
Scarlet fever, 634–635
   due to *Staphylococcus,* 647
Scheie syndrome, 1652
Scheuermann disease, 1625
Schick test, 597, 643
Schilder disease, 1581
Schilling test, 929–930
Schistosomiasis, 863–865
   bladder stones in, 1377
Schizoid child, 88
Schizophrenia, recurrence risk of, 286
Schmidt syndrome, 1461
Schönlein-Henoch syndrome, 1249, 1338–
   1340
Schönlein-Henoch vasculitis, 577–579
School, 20–21, 60–61
   dysfunction in, 105–119
School phobia, 60, 76
Schwartz-Jampel syndrome, 1640
Sciatic nerve injury, 1606
Scissoring, 1553–1554
Scleredema, 1701
Sclerema neonatorum, 1705
Scleroderma, 582–583
Sclerosing cholangitis, 979–980
Sclerosing panencephalitis, subacute, 743,
   745, 809, 1579–1580
   ocular changes in, 1745

Sclerosis
   multiple, 1581–1582
   tuberous, 1574, 1678, 1744
Sclerosteosis, 1649
Scoliosis, 1624–1625
Scombroid fish poisoning, 1785–1786
Scorbutic rosary, 177
Scorpions, 870, 1810
Screamer's nodules, 1041
Screening programs
   for hyperlipidemia, 1201
   psychological, 69
   urinary tract, 1313–1314
Scrofuloderma, 1715
Scrotal edema, idiopathic, 1400
Scrotal inflammation, 1399
Scrub typhus, 822–823
Scurvy, 176–179
Sea anemone stings, 1808
Seat belts, 261
Sebaceous glands, 1663–1664
Sebaceous hyperplasia, 1665
Seborrhea of genitalia, 1517
Seborrheic dermatitis, 548, 1025, 1688–
   1689
Seckel syndrome, 1747
Secretor substance, 314
Secretory component (SC) deficiency, 507
Secretory IgA, 506–507
Sedimentation rate, 562
Segmental hypoplasia of kidney, 1374
Segmental postural drainage, 1007
Segmental spinal reflex arc, 1601
Seip-Lawrence syndrome, 1705
Seizures, 35. See also *Epilepsy.*
   due to cerebral edema, 245
   due to hypernatremic dehydration, 237–
     238
   due to hypocalcemia, 251
   due to tetany, 250
   due to water intoxication, 246
   following DPT, 189
   from vitamin B_6 dependency, 176
   in systemic lupus erythematosus, 577
   in tetanus, 687
   of vitamin D deficiency, 184
Selenium, 143
Seminoma, 1290, 1291
Sensitivity tests for antibiotics, 597–598
Sensorineural hearing loss, 119, 1022
Sensory deprivation, 16
Sensory examination, 1549–1550
Sensory neuropathy, congenital, 1604–
   1605
Separation
   death and, 64–65
   psychosomatic illness in, 94–95
Sepsis, 600, 612–613
   due to splenectomy, 1256
   in burns, 270–271
   in neonate, 403–405
Septic arthritis, 613, 615–617
   due to *Hemophilus influenzae,* 657
   due to *Staphylococcus aureus,* 648
Septic shock, 271–275
Septicemia, 600, 612–613
Septo-optic dysplasia, 1434–1435
Sequestra of bone, 614
Sequestration crises, in sickle cell anemia,
   1224
Sequestration of lung, 1032–1033
Serine, defects in metabolism of, 436–437
Serofibrinous pleurisy, 1079
Serologic tests, 597, 600–601

Serotonin, 528
Sertoli tumors, 1291
Serum, composition of, 210
Serum hepatitis, 413–414, 785
Serum proteins, in rheumatic diseases,
   563
Serum sickness, 552–553
   caused by drugs, 280
Severe combined immunodeficiency
   (SCID), 931
Sex chromosomes, 305–310
Sex hormones, 1494–1496
Sex maturity ratings, 40–42
Sex steroids, 1494–1496
Sexual abuse, 90, 91, 92, 102–104, 1529–
   1530
Sexual behavior, 61–62
Sexual differentiation, 1506–1507
Sexual intercourse, 58, 188, 1522–1523
Sexual maturation, 21–22
Sexual precocity, 1442–1451, 1519
Sexual pseudoprecocity, 1500–1501
Sexuality, 58, 61–62
Shagreen patches, 1574, 1678
Shake lotions 1731
Shampoos, 1731
Sheep erythrocyte rosette, 499, 1263
Shellfish poisoning, 1785
Shigellosis, 670–671
Shingles, 758–759
Shipyard conjunctivitis, 754
Shock, 258, 259, 271–275
   cardiogenic, 1189–1191
   in acute renal failure, 1360
   in burns, 270
   in dengue hemorrhagic fever, 813–815
   in newborn, 363–364
   insulin, 1415
   treatment of, 236, 258, 273–275
   ventricular fibrillation in, 1174
   with poisoning, 1786
Shock lung, 265
Shoe dermatitis, 1687
Short gut syndrome, 932
Short rib–polydactyly syndromes, 1638–
   1639
Shunts
   left to right, 1142–1167
   opportunistic infection in, 696
   right to left, 1123–1142
Shwachman syndrome, 522, 951, 1240
Sialidoses, 486, 487
Sibling relationships, 59
Sibling rivalry, 59
Sick sinus syndrome, 1175–1176
Sickle cell anemia, 1223–1225
   kidney and, 1355
   pneumococcal infections in, 638–639
   complement deficiencies in, 517
Sickle cell hemoglobinopathies, 1223–1225
Sickle cell trait, 1223
Sickle cells, 1220
Sideroblastic anemias, 1216–1217
Silo filler's disease, 1058
Silver-Russell syndrome, 1437
Simian crease, 298
Singapore hemorrhagic fever, 813–815
Singer's nodules, 1041
Sinoatrial block, 1175
Sinobronchitis, 1019
Sinus(es), 13, 21, 24
   development of, 1018
   infection of, 1018–1019
   newborn, 13

For DRUGS listed by indications for use, see Table 29–1A, p. 1811. For DRUGS listed individually with dosages, see Table 29–1B, p. 1814.

For REFERENCE RANGES for laboratory tests, see pp. 1827 to 1852.

For DRUGS listed by indications for use, see Table 29–1A, p. 1811. For DRUGS listed individually with dosages, see Table 29–1B, p. 1814.

For REFERENCE RANGES for laboratory tests, see pp. 1827 to 1852.

For DRUGS listed by indications for use, see Table 29–1A, p. 1811.   For DRUGS listed individually with dosages, see Table 29–1B, p. 1814.

For REFERENCE RANGES for laboratory tests, see pp. 1827 to 1852.

For DRUGS listed by indications for use, see Table 29–1A, p. 1811. For DRUGS listed individually with dosages, see Table 29–1B, p. 1814.